his

FIFTH EDITION

INSALL & SCOTT
Surgery of the Knee

Editor

W. Norman Scott, MD, FACS

Clinical Professor
Department of Orthopaedic Surgery
Albert Einstein College of Medicine
Associate Orthopaedic Attending
Lenox Hill Hospital
Founding Director
Insall Scott Kelly Institute for
Orthopaedics and Sports Medicine
New York, New York

with 3439 illustrations

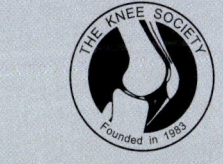

Published in association with
The Knee Society

ELSEVIER
CHURCHILL
LIVINGSTONE

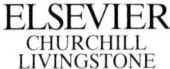

1600 John F. Kennedy Blvd.
Ste 1800
Philadelphia, PA 19103-2899

INSALL & SCOTT SURGERY OF THE KNEE ISBN: 978-1-4377-1503-3

Notices

Library of Congress Cataloging-in-Publication Data

Insall & Scott surgery of the knee / editor, W. Norman Scott.—5th ed.
    p. ; cm.
  Insall and Scott surgery of the knee
  Includes bibliographical references and index.
  ISBN 978-1-4377-1503-3 (hardcover : alk. paper)
  1. Knee–Surgery.   I. Scott, W. Norman.   II. Insall, John N.   III. Title: Insall and Scott surgery of the knee.   IV. Title: Surgery of the knee.
  [DNLM   1. Knee–surgery.   2. Arthroplasty.   3. Knee Injuries–surgery.   4. Ligaments, Articular–injuries. WE 870]
  RD561.S87 2012
  617.5'82059—dc23

                                                                    2011017158

Acquisitions Editor: Dolores Meloni
Developmental Editor: Anne Snyder
Publishing Services Manager: Catherine Jackson
Senior Project Manager: Rachel E. McMullen
Design Direction: Ellen Zanolle

Printed in the United States of America

Last digit is the print number: 9   8   7   6   5   4   3   2   1

W. Norman Scott MD, FACS
Clinical Professor
Department of Orthopaedic Surgery
Albert Einstein College of Medicine
Associate Orthopaedic Attending
Lenox Hill Hospital
Founding Director
Insall Scott Kelly Institute for Orthopaedics and
    Sports Medicine
New York, New York

Fred D. Cushner, MD
Assistant Clinical Professor
Albert Einstein School of Medicine
Bronx, New York
Director
Insall Scott Kelly Institute for Orthopaedics and
    Sports Medicine
New York, New York
Chairman, Division of Orthopedics
Southside Hospital
Bay Shore, New York

David R. Diduch, MS, MD
Alfred R. Shands Professor of Orthopaedic Surgery
Head Orthopaedic Team Physician
Fellowship Director, Sports Medicine
University of Virginia
Charlottesville, Virginia

Andrew G. Franks, Jr., MD, FACP
Clinical Professor of Dermatology & Medicine
    (Rheumatology)
Director, Skin Lupus & Autoimmune Connective Tissue
    Disease Section
New York University School of Medicine
New York, New York

George J. Haidukewych, MD
Academic Chairman of Orthopedic Surgery, Orlando
    Health;
Chief of Orthopedic Trauma;
Chief of Complex Adult Reconstructive Services;
    Residency Program;
Director, Orlando Health
Professor of Orthopedic Surgery, University of Central
    Florida
Orlando, Florida

Arlen D. Hanssen, MD
President, 2010-2011
The Knee Society,
Professor
Department of Orthopedic Surgery
Mayo Clinic
Rochester, Minnesota

Mininder S. Kocher, MD, MPH
Associate Director
Division of Sports Medicine
Children's Hospital Boston
Associate Professor of Orthopaedic Surgery
Harvard Medical School
Boston, Massachusetts

Richard D. Komistek, PhD
Fred M. Roddy Endowed Professor, Biomedical Engineering
Co-Center Director, Center for Musculoskeletal Research
University of Tennessee
Knoxville, Tennessee

Mary I. O'Connor, MD
Associate Professor, Mayo Clinic College of Medicine
Chair, Department of Orthopedic Surgery
Mayo Clinic in Florida
Jacksonville, Florida

Susan Craig Scott, MD
Clinical Assistant Professor
Orthopaedic Surgeon
New York University School of Medicine;
Surgeon, Hand Surgery
New York University Hospital for Joint Diseases
New York, New York

Giles R. Scuderi, MD
Director
Insall Scott Kelly Institute for Orthopedics and Sports
    Medicine;
Vice President
Orthopedic Service Line
North Shore/LIJ Health Care System
New York, New York

Daniel M. Walz, MD
Chief, Division of Musculoskeletal Imaging
Department of Radiology
North Shore University Hospital
Manhasset, New York;
Medical Director
North Shore-LIJ Imaging at Great South Bay
Islip, New York;
Assistant Professor of Radiology
North Shore-LIJ Hofstra University School of Medicine
Hempstead, New York

To My Wife, My Best Friend whose understated demeanor disguises her spectacular achievements, Physician, Teacher, Author, Wife, and Mother!

To our children, Eric, Will, and Kelly, Not a day goes by that we aren't so thankful to have been blessed with the three of you. All of you have worked so hard to achieve so much in such a short time and yet have maintained such a wonderful balance in your life. Your uncompromising pursuit of accomplishment will unquestionably continue to bring happiness to your lives and, of course, ours! Thank you.

CONTRIBUTORS

Aryeh M. Abeles, MD
Assistant Clinical Professor, Division of Rheumatology, Department of Medicine, University of Connecticut Health Sciences Center, Farmington, Connecticut

Paolo Aglietti, MD
Former Director of the First Orthopaedics Clinic, University of Florence, Florence, Italy

Azhar A. Ali
Computational Biomechanics Lab, University of Denver, Denver, Colorado

Annunziato Amendola, MD
Professor, Department of Orthopedic Surgery and Rehabilitation; Director and Callaghan Chair, University of Iowa Sports Medicine, University of Iowa, Iowa City, Iowa

Allen F. Anderson, MD
Tennessee Orthopaedic Alliance; Director, Lipscomb Foundation for Education and Research, Nashville, Tennessee

Christian Noel Anderson, MD
Chief Resident, Department of Orthopaedic Surgery, Vanderbilt University Medical Center, Nashville, Tennessee

Jason D. Archibald, MD
New England Orthopedic Specialists; Clinical Affiliate, Orthopaedic Surgery, Massachusetts General Hospital, Boston, Massachusetts

Elizabeth Arendt, MD
Professor and Vice Chair, University of Minnesota, Department of Orthopaedic Surgery, Minneapolis, Minnesota

Jean-Noël Argenson, MD, PhD
Professor of Orthopaedic Surgery, Chairman, Department of Orthopaedic Surgery, Aix-Marseille University, Marseille, France

Amy F. Austin, MD
Assistant Professor of Radiology, Methodist Hospital Division, Thomas Jefferson University Hospital, Philadelphia, Pennsylvania

Bernard R. Bach, Jr., MD
Claude Lambert–Helen S. Thomson Professor of Orthopedics; Director, Division of Sports Medicine; Director, RUSH Sports Medicine Fellowship; Team Physician, Chicago White Sox and Chicago Bulls, Chicago, Illinois

David Backstein, MD, MEd, FRCS
Associate Professor, University of Toronto; Head, Division of Orthopaedic Surgery, Mount Sinai Hospital; Director of Undergraduate Education, Department of Surgery, University of Toronto; Medical Lead and Chair, Mount Sinai Centre for MSK Disease, Toronto, Canada

Geoffrey S. Baer, MD, PhD
Assistant Professor, Division of Sports Medicine, Department of Orthopedics and Rehabilitation, University of Wisconsin-Madison, Madison, Wisconsin

Sarvottam Bajaj, BE
Division of Sports Medicine, Department of Orthopaedic Surgery, Rush University Medical Center, Chicago, Illinois

Andrea Baldini, MD
First Orthopaedic Clinic, University of Florence, Florence, Italy

Mark A. Baldwin
Computational Biomechanics Lab, University of Denver, Denver, Colorado

Sue Barber-Westin, BS
Director, Clinical and Applied Research, Cincinnati Sportsmedicine Research and Education Foundation, Cincinnati, Ohio

Joseph Barker
Fellow, Division of Sports Medicine, Department of Orthopedic Surgery, Rush University Medical Center, Chicago, Illinois

Christopher P. Beauchamp, MD
Associate Professor of Orthopaedic Surgery, Mayo Clinic, Phoenix/Scottsdale, Arizona

Martin Bédard, FRCS
Département de Chirurgie Orthopédique, Hôpital de l'Enfant-Jésus, Quebec, Canada

Keith R. Berend, MD
Associate, Joint Implant Surgeons; Vice-Chairman, Board of Directors, Mount Carmel New Albany Surgical Hospital; Clinical Assistant Professor, Department of Orthopaedics, Ohio State University, New Albany, Ohio

Richard A. Berger, MD
Assistance Professor of Orthopedics, Rush University, Chicago, Illinois

Thomas Bernasek, MD
Clinical Professor, University of South Florida; Orthopaedic Surgery Director, Adult Reconstruction Fellowship, Florida Orthopaedic Institute; Chief of Staff, Tampa General Hospital, Tampa, Florida

Daniel J. Berry, MD
L. Z. Gund Professor and Chairman, Department of Orthopedic Surgery, Mayo Clinic, Rochester, Minnesota

Jack M. Bert, MD
Summit Orthopedics; Adjunct Clinical Professor, University of Minnesota School of Medicine, St. Paul, Minnesota

Kevin F. Bonner, MD
Assistant Professor, Eastern Virginia Medical School, Jordan-Young Institute, Virginia Beach, Virginia

Adam C. Brekke, BA
Research Fellow, Institute of Orthopedic Research and Education, Houston, Texas

Karen K. Briggs, MBA, MPH
Department of Clinical Research, Steadman Philippon Research Institute, Vail, Colorado

Claire L. Brockett, BEng, PhD
Institute of Medical and Biological Engineering, School of Mechanical Engineering, University of Leeds, Leeds, United Kingdom

Michael K. Brooks, MD, MPH
Department of Radiology, Brigham and Women's Hospital, Boston, Massachusetts

James A. Browne, MD
Fellow in Adult Reconstruction, Department of Orthopaedic Surgery, Mayo Clinic, Rochester, Minnesota

Brandon J. Bryant, MD, MC, USN
Orthopaedic Surgeon, Sports Medicine Service, Naval Medical Center, Portsmouth, Virginia

Jarett S. Burak, MD
Division of Musculoskeletal Imaging, Department of Radiology, North Shore University Hospital; Assistant Professor of Radiology, North Shore-LIJ Hofstra University School of Medicine, Hempstead, New York

Alissa Burge, MD
North Shore University Hospital, Department of Radiology, Manhasset, New York

Charles Bush-Joseph, MD
Division of Sports Medicine, Rush University Medical Center, Chicago, Illinois

Asokumar Buvanendran, MD
Associate Professor of Anesthesiology, Division of Pain Medicine; Director of Orthopedic Anesthesia, Department of Anesthesiology, Rush University Medical Center, Chicago, Illinois

John Callaghan, MD
Professor of Orthopaedics and Rehabilitation, Dr. Lawrence and Marilyn Dorr Endowed Chair for Hip Reconstruction and Research, University of Iowa Sports Medicine, University of Iowa, Iowa City, Iowa

Tom R. Carter, MD
Orthopaedic Clinic Association, Phoenix, Arizona

Eli Chen, MD, PhD
Department of Orthopaedic Surgery, Long Island Jewish Medical Center, New Hyde Park, New York

Anikar Chhabra, MD, MS
Team Orthopaedic Surgeon, Arizona State University; Banner Good Sam Ortho Residency, Sports Medicine Director, Mayo Clinic; Adjunct Assistant Professor, Orthopaedic Clinic Association, Phoenix/Scottsdale, Arizona

Constance R. Chu, MD
Albert Ferguson Associate Professor, Vice Chair Translational Research, Department of Orthopaedic Surgery; Director, Cartilage Restoration Center, University of Pittsburgh, Pittsburgh, Pennsylvania

Randy Clark, MD
Resident, Department of Orthopedic Surgery and Rehabilitation, University of Iowa, Iowa City, Iowa

Henry D. Clarke, MD
Consultant, Department of Orthopedics, Associate Professor of Orthopedics, College of Medicine, Mayo Clinic, Phoenix/Scottsdale, Arizona

David E. Cohen
Department of Medicine, New York University School of Medicine, New York, New York

Brian J. Cole, MD, MBA
Professor, Departments of Orthopedics and Anatomy and Cell Biology, Division of Sports Medicine; Section Head, Cartilage Restoration Center, Rush University Medical Center, Chicago, Illinois

Thomas M. Coon, MD, FAAOS
Director and Founder, Coon Joint Replacement Institute, St. Helena Hospital, St. Helena, California

John H. Currier, MS
Dartmouth Biomedical Engineering Center, Thayer School of Engineering, Dartmouth College, Hanover, New Hampshire

Fred D. Cushner, MD
Director, Insall Scott Kelly Institute for Orthopaedics and Sports Medicine; Chairman, Division of Orthopedics, Southside Hospital Bay Shore; Assistant Clinical Professor, Albert Einstein School of Medicine, New York, New York

Diane L. Dahm, MD
Associate Professor of Orthopedic Surgery, Mayo Clinic College of Medicine; Mayo Clinic Sports Medicine Center, Rochester, Minnesota

Timothy A. Damron, MD, FACS
David G. Murray Professor of Orthopedic Surgery, Upstate Medical University, State University of New York, Syracuse, New York

Joseph P. DeAngelis, MD
Instructor, Harvard Medical School; Department of Orthopaedics, Beth Israel Deaconess Medical Center, Boston, Massachusetts

Bridget M. Deasy, PhD
Department of Bioengineering, Department of Orthopedic
Surgery, McGowan Institute of Regenerative Medicine;
Assistant Professor Departments of Orthopedic Surgery
and Bioengineering, University of Pittsburgh, Pittsburgh,
Pennsylvania

David DeJour, MD
Lyon-Ortho-Clinic, Lyon, France

Craig J. Della Valle, MD
Associate Professor of Orthopedic Surgery, Department of
Orthopedic Surgery, Rush University Medical Center,
Chicago, Illinois

A. Lee Dellon, MD, PhD
Professor of Plastic Surgery and Neurosurgery, Johns
Hopkins University; Dellon Institute for Peripheral
Nerve Surgery, Towson, Maryland

Guillaume Demey, MD
Hôpital de la Croix Rousse, Orthopedie Centre Albert
Trillat, University Hospital, Lyon, France

Douglas A. Dennis, MD
Adjunct Professor, Department of Bioengineering,
University of Tennessee; Adjunct Professor of
Bioengineering, University of Denver; Director, Rocky
Mountain Musculoskeletal Research Laboratory, Denver,
Colorado

Ezra Deutsch, MD, FACC, FSCAI
Director, Cardiac Catheterization Laboratory, Southside
Hospital, Bay Shore, New York; The Suffolk Heart
Group, Smithtown, New York

Ian D. Dickey, BSc, PEng (Hon), MD, FRCSC
Adjunct Professor, Department of Chemical and Biological
Engineering, University of Maine, Orono, Maine

David R. Diduch, MS, MD
Alfred R. Shands Professor of Orthopaedic Surgery; Head
Orthopaedic Team Physician, Fellowship Director, Sports
Medicine, University of Virginia, Charlottesville,
Virginia

Mark E. Easley, MD
Associated Professor of Orthopedic Surgery, Duke
University Medical Center, Durham, North Carolina

Kostas Economopoulos, MD
Banner Good Samaritan Orthopedic Surgery Residency,
Tempe, Arizona

Gerard A. Engh, MD
Anderson Orthopaedic Clinic, Alexandria, Virginia

Gregory C. Fanelli, MD
GHS Orthopaedics, Danville, Pennsylvania

Jack Farr, II, MD
Voluntary Professor of Orthopaedic Surgery, Indiana
University School of Medicine; Medical Director,
Cartilage Restoration Center of Indiana; Director,
OrthoIndy Sports Medicine; Fellowship, Indiana
Orthopaedic Hospital, Greenwood, Indiana

Christopher M. Farrell, MD
Maryland Orthopedic Specialists, Bethesda, Maryland

Thomas K. Fehring, MD
Co-Director, OrthoCarolina Hip and Knee Center; Chief
of Orthopaedics, Presbyterian-Orthopaedic Hospital,
Charlotte, North Carolina

Julian Feller, MD
Associate Professor, La Trobe University Medical Center,
Orthopaedic Surgeon, Richmond VIC Australia

Jonathan T. Finnoff, DO
Assistant Professor of Physical Medicine and
Rehabilitation, Mayo Clinic College of Medicine, Mayo
Clinic Sports Medicine Center, Rochester, Minnesota

John Fisher, PhD, DEng
Professor of Mechanical Engineering; Director, Institute of
Medical and Biological Engineering, School of
Mechanical Engineering, University of Leeds, United
Kingdom

Wolfgang Fitz, MD
Associate Orthopaedic Surgeon, Brigham and Women's and
Faulkner Hospital, Harvard Medical School, Boston,
Massachusetts

Clare K. Fitzpatrick
Computational Biomechanics Lab, University of Denver,
Denver, Colorado

John P. Fletcher, MBBS, MD, MS, FRACS, FRCS, DDU
University of Sydney and Westmead Hospital; President,
International Surgical Thrombosis Forum (ISTF);
Professor of Surgery, University of Sydney and Westmead
Hospital, Sydney, Australia

John M. Flynn, MD
Associate Chief of Orthopaedic Surgery, Children's
Hospital of Philadelphia; Associate Professor of
Orthopaedic Surgery, University of Pennsylvania School
of Medicine, Philadelphia, Pennsylvania

Andrew G. Franks, Jr., MD, FACP
Clinical Professor of Dermatology & Medicine
(Rheumatology), Director, Skin Lupus & Autoimmune
Connective Tissue Disease Section, New York University
School of Medicine, New York, New York

Richard J. Friedman, MD, FRCSC
Department of Orthopaedic Surgery, Roper Hospital,
Medical University of South Carolina; Chairman,
Department of Orthopaedic Surgery, Roper Hospital;
Clinical Professor of Orthopaedic Surgery, Medical
University of South Carolina; Medical Director,
Charleston Orthopaedic Associates, Charleston, South
Carolina

Nicole A. Friel, MS, MD
Resident, Department of Orthopaedic Surgery, University
of Pittsburgh Medical Center, Pittsburgh, Pennsylvania

Freddie H. Fu, MD, D.Sc. (Hon.), D.Ps. (Hon.)
Distinguished Service Professor, David Silver Professor, Chairman, Department of Orthopaedic Surgery, University of Pittsburgh School of Medicine; Head Team Physician, University of Pittsburgh Athletic Department, University of Pittsburgh Medical Center, Pittsburgh, Pennsylvania

John P. Fulkerson, MD
Orthopedic Associates of Hartford; Clinical Professor of Orthopedic Surgery, University of Connecticut, Farmington, Connecticut

Robert Kyle Fullick, MD
Baytown, Texas

Theodore J. Ganley, MD
Department of Orthopaedic Surgery, Children's Hospital of Philadelphia; University of Pennsylvania School of Medicine, Philadelphia, Pennsylvania

Donald S. Garbuz, MD, MHsc, FRCSC
Associate Professor and Head, Division of Lower Limb Reconstruction and Oncology, Department of Orthopaedics, University of British Columbia, Vancouver, British Columbia, Canada

Burhan Gharaibeh, PhD
Stem Cell Research Center; Department of Orthopaedic Surgery and Children's Hospital of Pittsburgh, UPMC Center for Sports Medicine, Pittsburgh, Pennsylvania

Thomas J. Gill, IV, MD
Chief, Sports Medicine Service; Associate Professor of Orthopaedic Surgery, Massachusetts General Hospital, Boston, Massachusetts

Maria S. Goddard, MD
Research Fellow, Rubin Institute of Advanced Orthopedics, Sinai Hospital, Baltimore, Maryland

Andreas Gomoll, MD
Assistant Professor of Orthopaedic Surgery, Harvard Medical School; Brigham and Women's Hospital, Cartilage Repair Center, Boston, Massachusetts

Carlos Gonzalez, MD
Cartilage Repair Center, Brigham and Women's Hospital, Boston, Massachusetts

Christopher R. Gooding, BSc, MD, FRCS
Fellow in Reconstructive Orthopaedic Surgery, Department of Orthopaedics, University of British Columbia, Vancouver, British Columbia, Canada

Robert C. Grumet, MD
Department of Orthopaedic Surgery, St. Joseph Medical Center, Orthopaedic Specialty Institute, Orange, California

F. Winston Gwathmey, Jr., MD
Resident Physician, University of Virginia, Department of Orthopaedics, Charlottesville, Virginia

Steve Haas, MD
Hospital for Special Surgery, New York, New York

Mahmoud Hafez, FRCS Ed, PhD
Professor, Head of the Orthopaedic Department, October 6 University; Arthroplasty Consultant, Al Helal (National) Orthopaedic Hospital, Cairo, Egypt

George J. Haidukewych, MD
Academic Chairman of Orthopedic Surgery, Orlando Health; Chief of Orthopedic Trauma; Chief of Complex Adult Reconstructive Services; Residency Program; Director, Orlando Health, Professor of Orthopedic Surgery, University of Central Florida, Orlando, Florida

Christopher A. Hajnik, MD
Director, STRIDE Comprehensive Joint Replacement Program, Scripps Memorial Hospital; CORE Orthopaedic Medical Center, Encinitas, California; Insall Scott Kelly Institute for Orthopaedics and Sports Medicine, New York, New York

Arlen D. Hanssen, MD
President, 2010-2011, The Knee Society; Professor, Department of Orthopaedics Surgery, Mayo Clinic, Rochester, Minnesota

Christopher D. Harner, MD
Professor, Department of Orthopaedic Surgery, University of Pittsburgh School of Medicine; UPMC Center for Sports Medicine, Pittsburgh, Pennsylvania

Joseph M. Hart, PhD, ATC
Assistant Professor, University of Virginia, Department of Orthopaedic Surgery, Department of Human Services, Charlottesville, Virginia

William L. Healy, MD
Chairman, Orthopaedic Surgery, Lahey Clinic, Burlington, Massachusetts; Professor, Orthopaedic Surgery, Boston University, Boston, Massachusetts

Peter F. Heeckt, MD, PhD
Smith & Nephew, Memphis, Tennessee

Sarah E. Henry, MD
Orthopedic Surgery Resident, University of Pittsburgh, Pittsburgh, Pennsylvania

Benton E. Heyworth, MD
Attending Orthopaedic Surgeon, Division of Sports Medicine, Department of Orthopaedic Surgery, Children's Hospital; Clinical Instructor, Harvard Medical School, Boston, Massachusetts

Richard Y. Hinton, MD, MPH
Union Memorial Orthopaedics, Baltimore, Maryland

Aaron A. Hofmann, MD
Professor, University of Utah Orthopaedic Center, Salt Lake City, Utah

Siegfried Hofmann, MD
Associate Professor Orthopedic Surgery, Vienna, Austria

Ginger E. Holt, MD, FACS
Associate Professor, Department of Orthopaedic Surgery and Rehabilitation, Vanderbilt University Medical Center, Nashville, Tennessee

Terese T. Horlocker, MD
Professor of Anesthesiology and Orthopaedics, Department of Anesthesiology, Mayo Clinic, Rochester, Minnesota

Stephen M. Howell, MD
Department of Mechanical Engineering, University of California, Davis, California

Johnny Huard, PhD
Henry J. Mankin Professor, Vice-Chair for Musculoskeletal Cellular Therapeutics, Department of Orthopaedic Surgery, Pediatrics, Microbiology, and Molecular Genetics; Director, Stem Cell Research Center, University of Pittsburgh School of Medicine; Department of Orthopaedic Surgery, Children's Hospital of Pittsburgh of UPMC, Pittsburgh, Pennsylvania

Catherine Hui, MD, FRCSC
North Sydney Orthopaedic and Sports Medicine Centre, Sydney, Australia

Christophe Hulet, MD
Orthopaedic Department, Caen University Hospital, Caen, France

Maury L. Hull, PhD
Biomedical Engineering Program, University of California, Davis, California

Marc W. Hungerford
Director of Joint Replacement and Reconstruction, Mercy Medical Center, Baltimore, Maryland

Anthony F. Infante, Jr., DO
Assistant Professor, University of South Florida, Tampa, Florida

John N. Insall, MD[†]
Formerly Clinical Professor of Orthopaedic Surgery, Albert Einstein College of Medicine, Bronx, New York; Director, Insall Scott Kelly Institute for Orthopaedics and Sports Medicine, Beth Israel Medical Center, New York, New York

David J. Jacofsky, MD
Chairman, The Core Institute, The Center for Orthopedic Research and Education, Sun City West, Arizona

James G. Jarvis, MD, FRCS(C)
Associate Professor of Surgery, University of Ottawa; Chief, Division of Pediatric Orthopaedic Surgery, Children's Hospital of Eastern Ontario, Ontario, Canada

Louise Jennings, MEng, PhD
Principal Research and Innovation Fellow, Institute of Medical and Biological Engineering, School of Mechanical Engineering, University of Leeds, Leeds, United Kingdom

Charles E. Johnston, II, MD
Assistant Chief of Staff, Texas, Scottish Rite Hospital for Children, Professor, Orthopedic Surgery, University of Texas Southwestern Medical School, Dallas, Texas

V. Karthik Jonna, MD
Resident, Maimonides Medical Center, Department of Orthopaedic Surgery, Brooklyn, New York

Thomas Keller, MD
Resident Physician, Department of Orthopaedic Surgery, University of Virginia School of Medicine, Charlottesville, Virginia

Donna R. Kesselman, MD
Attending Physician, Lenox Hill Hospital, New York, New York

Craig Kessler, MD
Professor of Medicine, Georgetown University Medical Center, Washington, DC

Saurabh Khakharia, MD, DNB
Adult Reconstruction and Sports Medicine, Department of Orthopedics, Colquitt Regional Medical Center, Moultrie, Georgia

Harpal S. Khanuja, MD
Director, Hip and Knee Replacement, Rubin Institute of Advanced Orthopedics, Sinai Hospital, Baltimore, Maryland

Raymond H. Kim, MD
Colorado Joint Replacement, Denver, Colorado

Sung Jae Kim, MD, PhD, FACS
Professor, Department of Orthopaedic Surgery, Severance Hospital, Yonsei University College of Medicine, Yonsei University Health System; Director, Yonsei University Arthroscopy and Joint Research Institute, Seoul, South Korea

Yair D. Kissin, MD
Clinical Assistant, Hackensack University Medical Center, Hackensack, New Jersey; Attending Physician, Insall Scott Kelly Institute, Lenox Hill Hospital, New York, New York

Kevin Klingele, MD
Director, Orthopaedic Education and Clinical Research; Surgical Director, Sports Medicine, Nationwide Children's Hospital; Clinical Assistant Professor, Ohio State University, Columbus, Ohio

Mininder S. Kocher, MD, MPH
Associate Director, Division of Sports Medicine, Children's Hospital Boston; Associate Professor of Orthopaedic Surgery, Harvard Medical School, Boston, Massachusetts

Richard D. Komistek, PhD
Fred M. Roddy Endowed Professor, Biomedical Engineering; Co-Center Director, Center for Musculoskeletal Research, University of Tennessee, Knoxville, Tennessee

Gabrielle P. Konin, MD
North Shore University Hospital, Department of Radiology, Manhasset, New York

Sandra L. Kopp, MD
Assistant Professor of Anesthesiology, Mayo Clinic, Rochester, Minnesota

[†]Deceased.

Nathan Kopydlowski, BA
University of Michigan Medical School, Ann Arbor,
  Michigan

Dennis Kramer, MD
Instructor, Division of Sports Medicine, Department of
  Orthopaedic Surgery, Children's Hospital Boston;
  Harvard Medical School, Boston, Massachusetts

Christopher M. Kuenze, ATC
Department of Orthopaedic Surgery, Department of Human
  Services, University of Virginia, Charlottesville, Virginia

Paul F. Lachiewicz, MD
Chapel Hill Orthopedics Surgery and Sports Medicine,
  Chapel Hill, North Carolina

Jason E. Lang, MD
Assistant Professor, Department of Orthopaedic Surgery,
  Division of Adult Reconstruction, Wake Forest School of
  Medicine, Winston-Salem, North Carolina

Joshua R. Langford, MD
Attending Orthopaedic Traumatologist, Orlando Health
  Orthopaedic Residency Program; Instructor of
  Orthopaedic Surgery, University of Central Florida
  College of Medicine; Affiliate Assistant Professor,
  University of South Florida College of Medicine,
  Orlando, Florida

Robert F. LaPrade, MD, PhD
Sports Medicine and Complex Knee Surgery, Steadman
  Clinic; Director, Biomechanics Research Department,
  Steadman Philippon Research Institute, Vail, Colorado

Peter J. Laz, PhD
Computational Biomechanics Lab, University of Denver,
  Denver, Colorado

Matthew Leidl, BA
Temple University School of Medicine, Philadelphia,
  Pennsylvania

James M. Leone, MD, FRCSC
Orthopedic Surgeon, Cambridge Memorial Hospital,
  Cambridge, Ontario, Canada

Filip Leszko, MS
Graduate Research Assistant, Mechanical, Aerospace and
  Biomedical Engineering Department, University of
  Tennessee, Knoxville, Tennessee

David Levi, MD
Radiologist, Atlantic Medical Imaging, Galloway, New
  Jersey

Gabriel Levi, MD
Joint Reconstruction and Sports Medicine Specialist,
  Orthopaedic and Rehabilitation Centers; Clinical
  Assistant Professor of Orthopaedic Surgery, University of
  Illinois, Chicago, Illinois

Randall J. Lewis
Clinical Professor, Orthopaedic Surgery, Orthopaedics and
  Sports Medicine,George Washington University Medical
  Center, Washington, DC

Martin Lind, MD
Head of Sports Trauma, Department of Orthopedics, Arhus
  University Hospital, Arhus, Denmark

Eric M. Lindvall, DO
Trauma Service, Orthopaedic Surgery Residency, University
  of California San Francisco-Fresno, Community Regional
  Medical Center-Fresno, Fresno, California

David R. Lionberger, MD
Department of Orthopedic Surgery, Methodist Hospital,
  Bellville General Hospital, Bellville, Texas

Frank A. Liporace
Associate Professor, Director of Trauma and Reconstructive
  Fellowship, University of Medicine and Dentistry, New
  Jersey/New Jersey Medical School, Newark, New Jersey

Martin Logan, MBChB, MRCS, MD, FRCS
Consultant Orthopaedic Surgeon, Windsor Knee Clinic,
  Berkshire, United Kingdom

Adolph V. Lombardi, Jr., MD, FACS
President, Joint Implant Surgeons, New Albany, Ohio;
  Clinical Assistant Professor, Department of
  Orthopaedics; Clinical Assistant Professor, Department
  of Biomedical Engineering, Ohio State University,
  Columbus, Ohio; Attending Surgeon, Mount Carmel
  Health System, New Albany, Ohio

William J. Long, MD, FRCSC
St Francis Hospital, Roslyn, New York

Jess H. Lonner, MD
Associate Professor of Orthopaedic Surgery, Thomas
  Jefferson University, Philadelphia, Pennsylvania;
  Rothman Institute, Bryn Mawr Hospital, Bryn Mawr,
  Pennsylvania

Sébastien Lustig
Hôpital de la Croix Rousse, Orthopedie Centre Albert
  Trillat, University Hospital, Lyon, France

Steven Lyons, MD
Florida Orthopaedic Institute, Tampa, Florida

Travis G. Maak, MD
Chief Resident in Orthopaedic Surgery, Hospital for
  Special Surgery, New York, New York

Jeffrey A. Macalena, MD
Department of Orthopaedic Surgery, University of
  Minnesota, Minneapolis, Minnesota

Samuel D. Madoff, MD
Department of Radiology, New England Baptist Hospital,
  Boston, Massachusetts

Shinichi Maeno, MD, PhD
North Sydney Orthopaedic and Sports Medicine Centre,
  Sydney, Australia

Robert A. Magnussen, MD
Department of Orthopaedic Surgery, Hôpital de la Croix-
  Rousse, Centre Albert Trillat, Lyon, France

Suzanne A. Maher, PhD
Hospital for Special Surgery, New York, New York

Mohamed R. Mahfouz, PhD
Chair, Career Development Professor, Program Coordinator, Biomedical Engineering; Co-Director, Center for Musculoskeletal Research, Knoxville, Tennessee

Sabine Mai, MD
Orthopedic Surgeon, Vitos Orthopaedic Center, Kassel, Germany

Patrick G. Marinello, BA
MD Candidate, Albany Medical College, Albany, New York

J. Bohannon Mason, MD
OrthoCarolina Hip and Knee Center, Charlotte North Carolina

Bassam A. Masri, MD, FRCSC
Professor and Chairman, Department of Orthopaedics, Vancouver Hospital and Health Sciences Centre, University of British Columbia, Vancouver, Canada

Henry Masur, MD
Chief, Critical Care Medicine, National Institutes of Health Clinical Center, Bethesda, Maryland

Kevin R. Math, MD
Chief of Musculoskeletal Imaging, Beth Israel Medical Center; East Manhattan Diagnostic Imaging, New York New York; Associate Professor of Clinical Radiology, Albert Einstein College of Medicine, Bronx, New York

Richard C. Mather, MD
Sports Medicine Service, Department of Orthopaedic Surgery, Duke University Medical Center, Durham, North Carolina

Kenneth B. Mathis, MD
Chairman, Center of Orthopedic Excellence, Clinical Assistant Professor, Weill-Cornell Medical College, Houston, Texas

Shuichi Matsuda, MD, PhD
Department of Orthopaedic Surgery, Kyushu University, Fukuoka, Japan

Jeremy McCandless, MD
Hofmann Arthritis Institute, Salt Lake City, Utah

Kristen E. McClure, MD
Assistant Professor of Radiology, Methodist Hospital Division, Thomas Jefferson University Hospital, Philadelphia, Pennsylvania

R. Michael Meneghini, MD
Director of Joint Replacement, Indiana University Health Saxony Hospital, Indiana University Health Physicians; Assistant Professor of Orthopaedic Surgery, Department of Orthopaedic Surgery, Indiana University School of Medicine; Indiana Clinic, Indianapolis, Indiana

Mark Miller, MD
S. Ward Casscells Professor of Orthopaedic Surgery; Head, Division of Sports Medicine; University of Virginia Team Physician, James Madison University, Charlottesville, Virginia

Douglas Mintz, MD
Department of Radiology and Imaging, Hospital for Special Surgery, New York, New York

Michael A. Mont, MD
Director, Rubin Institute of Advanced Orthopedics, Sinai Hospital, Baltimore, Maryland

Claude T. Moorman, III, MD
Sports Medicine Service, Department of Orthopaedic Surgery; Professor, Orthopaedic Surgery; Professor, Evolutionary Anthropology; Director, Duke Sports Medicine; Head Team Physician, Duke Athletics, Duke University Medical Center, Sports Medicine Center, Durham, North Carolina

Michael J. Morris, MD
Associate, Joint Implant Surgeons, New Albany, Ohio

William B. Morrison, MD
Professor of Radiology Thomas Jefferson University Hospital Philadelphia, Pennsylvania

Kenneth R. Morse, MD
Orthopaedic Surgeon, Downeast Bangor, Maine

John Kyle P. Mueller, PhD
Measurement Science and Systems Engineering Division, Oak Ridge National Laboratory, Oak Ridge, Tennessee

Thomas Muellner, MD, PhD
Sportsclinic Vienna-Tulln, Vienna, Austria

David Murray, MD
Professor of Orthopaedic Surgery, University of Oxford, Oxford, United Kingdom

Volker Musahl, MD
Assistant Professor of Orthopaedic Surgery, UPMC Center for Sports Medicine, Pittsburgh, Pennsylvania

Michael D. Neel, MD
Clinical Assistant Professor in Orthopaedics, University of Tennessee; Consultant Staff, Department of Orthopaedics, St. Jude's Children's Research Hospital, Memphis, Tennessee

Joshua Nelson, MD, PharmD
Assistant Professor, Department of Orthopaedic Surgery, Division of Sports Medicine, University of Kansas Medical Center, Kansas City, Kansas

Michael P. Nett, MD
Orthopedic Surgeon, St. Francis Hospital Roslyn, New York

Philippe Neyret, MD
Hôpital de la Croix Rousse, Orthopedie Centre Albert Trillat, University Hospital, Lyon, France

Philip C. Noble, PhD
Professor of Orthopedic Surgery, Baylor College of Medicine; John S. Dunn Professor of Orthopedic Research; Director of Research, Methodist Hospital, Houston, Texas

Frank R. Noyes, MD
Chairman and Medical Director, Cincinnati Sports
   Research and Orthopaedic Center; President, Cincinnati
   Sports Medicine Research and Education Foundation;
   Former Clinical Professor, Department of Orthopaedic
   Surgery, University of Cincinnati College of Medicine;
   Former Adjunct Professor, Noyes Tissue Engineering and
   Biomechanics Laboratory, Department of Biomedical
   Engineering, University of Cincinnati College of
   Engineering, Cincinnati, Ohio

Mary I. O'Connor
Associate Professor, Mayo Clinic College of Medicine;
   Chair, Department of Orthopedic Surgery, Mayo Clinic
   in Florida, Jacksonville, Florida

Matthew E. Oetgen, MD
Attending, Department of Orthopaedic Surgery and Sports
   Medicine, Children's National Medical Center,
   Washington, DC

Mark W. Pagnano, MD
Associate Professor of Orthopaedic Surgery, Mayo College
   of Medicine; Consultant, Division of Adult
   Reconstruction, Department of Orthopaedic Surgery,
   Mayo Clinic, Rochester, Minnesota

Christopher J. Palestro, MD
Professor of Radiology, Hofstra University School of
   Medicine, Hempstead, New York

Sebastien Parratte, MD, PhD
Center for Arthritis Surgery, Aix-Marseille University,
   Hopital Sainte-Marguerite, Marseille, France

Brian S. Parsley, MD
Associate Professor, Barnhart Department of Orthopedic
   Surgery, Baylor College of Medicine, Houston, Texas

Nilesh Patil, MD
Clinical Sports Medicine Fellow, Penn State Orthopedics,
   State College, Pennsylvania

Henrik B. Pedersen, MD
Director of Medical Multimedia, Insall Scott Kelly Institute
   for Orthopaedics and Sports Medicine, New York, New
   York

Lars Peterson, MD, PhD
Professor of Orthopaedics, Department of Orthopaedics,
   University of Gothenburg, Gothenburg, Sweden

Michael H. Pillinger, MD
Associate Professor of Medicine and Pharmacology;
   Director, Rheumatology Training, New York University
   School of Medicine; Section Chief, Rheumatology, New
   York Harbor Healthcare System, New York Campus; US
   Department of Veterans Affairs, New York, New York

Leo Pinczewski, MBBS, FRACS
Associate Professor of Orthopaedic Surgery, Notre Dame
   University, North Sydney Orthopaedic and Sports
   Medicine Centre, Sydney, Australia

William R. Post, MD
Orthopedic Surgeon, Mountaineer Orthopedic Specialists,
   Morgantown, West Virginia

Sridhar R. Rachala, MBBS
Assistant Professor Orthopedic Surgery; Consultant,
   Orthopedic Surgery, State University of New York at
   Buffalo; Buffalo General Hospital, Buffalo, New York

Craig S. Radnay, MD, MPH
Associate Orthopaedic Athending, St. Francis Hospital
   Roslyn, New York

Adam J. Rana, MD
Orthopedic Resident, Boston University, Orthopedic
   Surgery Department, Boston, Massachusetts

R. Lor Randall, MD, FACS
Department of Orthopaedics, Mayo Clinic, Jacksonville,
   Florida

Robert S. Reiffel, MD
Past President, Medical and Dental Staff, White Plains
   Hospital, White Plains, New York

Michael D. Ries, MD
Professor of Orthopaedic Surgery and Chief of Arthroplasty,
   University of California, San Francisco

Samuel P. Robinson, MD
Jordan-Young Institute, Virginia Beach, Virginia

Scott A. Rodeo, MD
Hospital for Special Surgery, New York, New York

William G. Rodkey, DVM, Diplomate ACVS
Chief Scientific Officer, Sports Medicine Fellowship,
   Deputy Director, Steadman Philippon Research Institute,
   Vail, Colorado

Jose Rodriquez, MD
Chief of Reconstruction Arthroplasty; Director,
   Arthroplasty Fellowship Program, Lenox Hill Hospital,
   New York, New York

Gregory J. Roehrig, MD
Orthopaedic Institute of Central Jersey, Spring Lake, New
   Jersey

Aaron G. Rosenberg, MD
Professor of Surgery; Director, Section of Adult
   Reconstructive Orthopedics, Rush Medical College,
   Chicago, Illinois

Pamela B. Rosenthal
Assistant Professor of Medicine, Division of Rheumatology,
   Department of Medicine, New York University School of
   Medicine, New York, New York

Paul J. Rullkoetter, PhD
Computational Biomechanics Lab, University of Denver,
   Denver, Colorado

Paulo R. F. Saggin, MD
Orthopaedic Surgeon, Instituto de Ortopedia e
   Traumatologia (IOT) de Passo Fundo, Passo Fundo,
   Brazil

Lucy Salmon, PhD
North Sydney Orthopaedic and Sports Medicine Centre, Mater Clinic, Sydney, Australia

Roy Sanders, MD
Clinical Professor of Orthopaedics, University of South Florida; Chief, Department of Orthopaedics, Tampa General Hospital; Director, Orthopaedic Trauma Services, Florida Orthopaedic Institute, Tampa, Florida

Robert C. Schenck, Jr., MD
Professor and Chair, Depertment of Orthopaedic Surgery, The University of New Mexico, Albuquerque, New Mexico

Oliver S. Schindler, MD, OFD, MFSEM, FRCSEd, FRCSE, FRCS
Consultant Orthopaedic Surgeon, Bristol, United Kingdom

Verena M. Schreiber, MD
Department of Orthopaedic Surgery, University of Pittsburgh Medical Center, Pittsburgh, Pennsylvania

Richard D. Scott, MD
Boston, Massachusetts

Susan Craig Scott, MD
Clinical Assistant Professor, Orthopaedic Surgeon, New York University School of Medicine; Surgeon, Hand Surgery, NYU Hospital for Joint Diseases, New York, New York

W. Norman Scott, MD, FACS
Clinical Professor, Department of Orthopaedic Surgery, Albert Einstein College of Medicine; Associate Orthopaedic Attending, Lenox Hill Hospital; Founding Director, Insall Scott Kelly Institute for Orthopaedics and Sports Medicine, New York, New York

Giles R. Scuderi, MD
Vice President, Orthopedic Service Line, North Shore/ LIJ Health Care System; Director, Insall Scott Kelly Institute for Orthopaedics and Sports Medicine, New York, New York

Ari D. Seidenstein, MD
Orthopaedic Surgeon, Hartzband Center for Hip and Knee Replacement; Paramus, New Jersey; Hackensack University Medical Center, Hackensack, New Jersey; Holy Name Medical Center, Teaneck, New Jersey; Hartzband Center for Hip and Knee Replacement, Paramus, New Jersey

Jon K. Sekiya, MD
Associate Professor, Sports Medicine, MedSport; Department of Orthopaedic Surgery, University of Michigan, Ann Arbor, Michigan

Elvire Servien, MD
Hôpital de la Croix Rousse, Orthopedie Centre Albert Trillat, University Hospital, Lyon, France

Erik P. Severson, MD
Adult Reconstruction Fellow, Department of Orthopaedics, Mayo Clinic, Rochester, Minnesota

Nicholas A. Sgaglione, MD
Chairman and Residency Program Director, Department of Orthopaedic Surgery; Professor of Orthopaedic Surgery, Albert Einstein College of Medicine, Hofstra North Shore-LIJ School of Medicine, North Shore Long Island Jewish Medical Center Manhasset, New York; Department of Orthopaedic Surgery, Long Island Jewish Medical Center, New Hyde Park, New York

Adrija Sharma, PhD
Research Assistant Professor, Mechanical, Aerospace and Biomedical Engineering Department, University of Tennessee, Knoxville, Tennessee

Seth L. Sherman, MD
Rush University Medical Center, Chicago, Illinois

Michael S. Shin, MD
Orthopedic Attending, St. Margaret's Hospital, Spring Valley, Illinois

Werner E. Siebert, MD
Professor of Orthopaedic Surgery, Attending Orthopaedic Surgeon, Vitos Orthopaedic Center, Kassel, Germany

Rafael J. Sierra, MD
Associate Professor, Consultant, Department of Orthopedics, Mayo Clinic, Rochester, Minnesota

C. Van Sikes, III, MD
Resident, Department of Orthopaedic Surgery, Wake Forest School of Medicine, Winston-Salem, North Carolina

David L. Skaggs, MD
Chief of Orthopaedic Surgery, Children's Hospital, Los Angeles; Professor, University of Southern California School of Medicine, Los Angeles, California

Gideon P. Smith, MD
Director of Connective Tissue Diseases, Department of Dermatology, Massachusetts General Hospital, Harvard University, Boston, Massachusetts

Gary E. Solomon, MD
Associate Director of Rheumatology, New York University Langone School of Medicine; Attending, Hospital for Joint Diseases, Orthopedic Institute; Director, Arthritis Clinic, Hospital for Joint Diseases Orthopedic Institute; Attending, Psoriasis and Psoriatic Arthritis Clinic, Tisch Hospital, New York, New York

Kurt P. Spindler, MD
Kenneth D. Schermerhorn Professor, Vice Chairman, Orthopaedics and Rehabilitation; Director, Vanderbilt Sports Medicine and Orthopaedic Patient Care Center; Head Team Physician, Vanderbilt University, Nashville, Tennessee

Andrew I. Spitzer, MD
Director, Cedars-Sinai Joint Replacement Program, Cedars-Sinai Orthopaedic Center, Los Angeles, California

Bryan D. Springer, MD
Attending Orthopaedic Surgeon, OrthoCarolina Hip and Knee Center, Charlotte North Carolina

J. Richard Steadman, MD

Kelly Stets, MD
New York, New York

Anna L. Stevens, MD, PhD
Department of Orthopaedic Surgery, University of
  Pittsburgh Medical Center, Pittsburgh, Pennsylvania

James B. Stiehl, MD
Director, Midwest Orthopaedic Biomechanical Laboratory,
  St. Mary's Hospital, Centralia, Illinois

Eric J. Strauss, MD
Assistant Professor, Division of Sports Medicine, New York
  University -Hospital For Joint Diseases, New York, New
  York; Division of Sports Medicine, Rush University
  Medical Center, Chicago, Illinois

Michael Stuart, MD
Professor and Vice-Chairman, Department of Orthopedics,
  Mayo Clinic, Rochester, Minnesota

S. David Stulberg, MD
Professor of Clinical Orthopaedic Surgery, Northwestern
  University Feinberg School of Medicine; Founder and
  Director, Joint Reconstruction and Implant Service,
  Northwestern Memorial Hospital, Chicago, Illinois

Eric Tannenbaum, BS
University of Michigan Medical School, Ann Arbor,
  Michigan

Dean C. Taylor, MD
American Board of Orthopaedic Surgery, Board Certified,
  Subspecialty Certification in Sports Medicine;
  Department of Orthopaedic Surgery, Duke University
  Medical Center; Duke Sports Medicine Center, Durham,
  North Carolina

Kimberly Templeton, MD
Professor of Orthopaedic Surgery and Health Policy and
  Management, Department of Orthopaedic Surgery,
  University of Kansas Medical Center, Kansas City,
  Kansas

Stephen R. Thompson, MD, MEd
Department of Orthopedic Surgery, University of Maryland,
  Baltimore, Maryland

Thomas Thornhill

Gehron Treme, MD
Department of Orthopaedics, University of New Mexico,
  Albuquerque, New Mexico

Alfred J. Tria Jr., MD
Chief of Orthopaedic Surgery, St. Peter's University
  Hospital; Clinical Professor of Orthopaedic Surgery,
  Robert Wood Johnson Medical School, New Brunswick,
  New Jersey

Kimberly A. Turman, MD
Division of Sports Medicine, GIKK Ortho Specialists,
  Creighton University Athletics, Omaha, Nebraska

Hans K. Uhthoff, MD, FRCSC
Professor Emeritus, University of Ottawa, Ottawa, Canada

Anthony S. Unger, MD

Thomas Parker Vail, MD
Professor and Chair, Department of Orthopaedic Surgery,
  University of California; San Francisco Orthopaedic
  Institute, San Francisco, California

Douglas W. Van Citters, PhD
Assistant Professor, Dartmouth Biomedical Engineering
  Center, Thayer School of Engineering Dartmouth
  College, Hanover, New Hampshire

Geoffrey S. Van Thiel, MD, MBA
Chief Resident, Department of Orthopedic Surgery, RUSH
  University Medical Center, Chicago, Illinois

Haris S. Vasiliadis, MD, PhD
Department of Orthopaedics, School of Medicine,
  University of Ioannina, Ioannina, Greece; Molecular
  Cell Biology and Regenerative Medicine, Sahlgrenska
  Academy, University of Gothenburg, Gothenburg,
  Sweden

Vincent J. Vigorita
Professor of Pathology and Orthopaedic Surgery, State
  University of New York Downstate Medical Center,
  Brooklyn, New York; Core Faculty, Kingsbrook Jewish
  Medical Center, Brooklyn, New York; Lenox Hill
  Hospital, New York, New York; Consultant, Department
  of Pathology, Maimonides Medical Center, Brooklyn,
  New York

Kelly G. Vince, FRCS
Orthopedic Surgeon, Northland District Health Board,
  Whangarei Hospital, Whangarei, New Zealand

Bruno Violante, MD
Adult Knee and Hip Reconstructive Surgery, Jewish
  Hospital, Rome, Italy

James E. Voos, MD
Orthopaedic and Sports Medicine Clinic of Kansas City,
  Leawood, Kansas

Shail Vyas, MD
University of Pittsburgh Sports Medicine Fellow, UPMC
  Center for Sports Medicine, Pittsburgh, Pennsylvania;
  Orange County Orthopaedic Group, Orange County,
  California

Daniel M. Walz, MD
Chief, Division of Musculoskeletal Imaging, Department of
  Radiology, North Shore University Hospital, Manhasset,
  New York; Medical Director, North Shore-LIJ Imaging at
  Great South Bay, Islip, New York; Assistant Professor of
  Radiology, North Shore-LIJ Hofstra University School of
  Medicine, Hempstead, New York

David Warwick, MD, FRCS
Consultant Hand Surgeon, Reader in Orthopaedic Surgery,
  University of Southampton, Southampton University
  Hospitals, Southampton, United Kingdom

Nicholas P. Webber, MD
David G. Murray Professor of Orthopedic Surgery, Upstate
  Medical University, State University of New York,
  Syracuse, New York

Jennifer Weiss, MD
Assisant Professor of Orthopedics, Director of the Sports Medicine Program, Children's Hospital Los Angeles, Los Angeles, California

Kurt R. Weiss, MD
Assistant Professor, Department of Orthopaedic Surgery, University of Pittsburgh Medical Center; Division of Musculoskeletal Oncology, Cancer Stem Cell Laboratory, Pittsburgh, Pennsylvania

Barbara N. Weissman, MD
Department of Radiology, Brigham and Women's Hospital, Boston, Massachusetts

Leo A. Whiteside, MD
Director, Missouri Bone and Joint Research Foundation, St. Louis, Missouri

Thomas L. Wickiewicz, MD
Professor of Clinical Orthopaedic Surgery, Weill Medical College of Cornell University; Attending Orthopaedic Surgeon, Hospital for Special Surgery, New York, New York

Bryan S. Williams, MD, MPH
Assistant Professor of Anesthesiology, Division of Pain Medicine, Department of Anesthesiology, Rush University Medical Center, Chicago, Illinois

Riley J. Williams, III, MD
Attending Orthopedic Surgeon, Associate Professor of Orthopedic Surgery, Weill Medical College of Cornell University, New York, New York

Yi-Meng Yen, MD, PhD
Clinical Instructor, Department of Orthopaedic Surgery, Division of Sports Medicine, Children's Hospital, Boston, Massachusetts

Hong Zhang
Division Chief, Professor of Orthopedics, Department of Joint Surgery and Sport Medicine, Clinic, General Hospital of CPLA, Beijing, China

Sumesh M. Zingde, MS
Graduate Research Assistant, Mechanical, Aerospace and Biomedical Engineering Department, University of Tennessee, Knoxville, Tennessee

Adam C. Zoga, MD
Associate Professor of Radiology, Thomas Jefferson University Hospital, Philadelphia, Pennsylvania

When reflecting on what has occurred in the quick six years since the fourth edition of *Insall & Scott Surgery of the Knee*, the field of knee surgery has continued to explode with the introduction of new concepts, surgical techniques, and technologies. The fifth edition once again brings the reader an updated and comprehensive reference source with an accompaniment of video and e-information for the entire scope of knee surgery. Significant updates have occurred in all areas including basic science, anatomy, surgical techniques, and prosthetic design. The fifth edition now includes 14 book sections and 153 chapters, multiple videos, quarterly updates, and a prosthesis glossary! It is not really possible to describe how comprehensive this excellent textbook has become in a short foreword.

The combination of newly described anatomical features and updates about aberrations of the knee, genetic treatment approaches, new imaging techniques, knee kinematics, articular cartilage physiology, pathophysiology of crystalline disorders, psoriatic and rheumatoid arthritis, osteonecrosis, as well as posttraumatic and osteoarthritis comprise just a short list of the new information provided. Considerable new information has also been added regarding the diagnosis and treatment of tumors, pediatric disorders, and trauma-related entities about the knee. The description, examination, imaging, and treatment options of articular cartilage disorders, ligamentous pathologies, and osseous deformities are encyclopedic and clearly represent multiple expert perspectives and philosophies. Realignment osteomety is covered in separate chapters for treatment associated with ligamentous reconstruction and for arthritic conditions.

Likewise, the chapters related to entities treated by arthroplasty are extremely thorough and encompass unicompartmental through bone–replacing megaprostheses. Excellent new additions include considerations for the "stented" patient, current recommendations for venous thrombosis prophylaxis, and treatment of complications such as postoperative bleeding. The chapter describing new multimodal preoperative pain management strategies should be read by anyone performing knee arthroplasty. The descriptions of computer navigated surgery and robotics are current yet pragmatic. Expert advice is provided for essentially every complication or untoward outcome in primary and revision surgery by description of the etiology, diagnosis, investigations required, and treatment options available.

In addition to the excellent coverage of all topics related to knee surgery, it is important that the editors of a textbook also provide the information in an organized and visually appealing manner. The fifth edition is extremely user-friendly and the liberal use of exceptional photographs, drawings, tables, and treatment algorithms categorizes this editorial effort as a first class textbook. Despite all of these attributes, a standard textbook in the current era has little chance of succeeding without a number of other nonstandard characteristics. The fifth edition of *Insall & Scott Surgery of the Knee*, both as a standard print and e-textbook, has adroitly met these needs. The accompaniment of high quality videos for many of the surgical techniques will be very popular and highly used by many readers. The use of international roundtable symposiums with multiple international experts on a variety of topics is very clever as a part of a traditional textbook and should also be well received. Finally, the organization and inclusions of the recognized global differences and perspectives provide the proper balance of information required for reader demand and desire everywhere.

It is overwhelming to think about the sheer number of topics and extent of information now encompassed within the boundaries of the field of knee surgery. Three decades have passed since the project of writing a textbook on the field of knee surgery was conceptualized by the late Dr. John Insall. It is important to note that so many of his ideas and concepts laid the essential groundwork for the eventual advances observed in knee surgery. Like most pioneers, he would likely be very surprised but highly intrigued by the current status of knee surgery and yet I suspect he would be quite amused at the retention of so many old controversies still in existence. His initial 1984 work product, the first edition of *Surgery of the Knee*, was considered to be a standard reference for knee surgery. Under the continued efforts and nurturing by his close friend and partner, Dr. W. Norman Scott, the fifth edition of *Insall & Scott Surgery of the Knee* will continue to be a highly popular textbook and remain the standard of reference for knee surgery.

Arlen D. Hanssen, MD
President, 2010-11
The Knee Society,
Professor
Department of Orthopaedic Surgery
Mayo Clinic
Rochester, Minnesota

There is nothing that "succeeds like success," and for the last five decades the treatment of knee disorders has been a major success story. From the first edition of *Surgery of the Knee* to the present fifth edition, inclusive of approximately 1000 National and International contributors, we have been fortunate to chronicle these tremendous advancements. Although history is often overlooked, we think it is important, so important in fact, that we have included the prefaces for the first four editions of Surgery of the Knee to hopefully facilitate the progressive understanding of the anatomic, physiologic, clinical, diagnostic, and therapeutic advances that allow students of the knee to "push the envelope" even further. It requires, however, an understanding of the historical failures in the scientific pursuit of helping our patients if we are to minimize the chances of repeating past mistakes and hopefully avoid future ones. The authors throughout this edition attempt to highlight these potential pitfalls.

The fifth edition of *Surgery of the Knee* contains one textbook, a complete e-version, an e-glossary of knee implants, and a video section that we believe is the most comprehensive sports and adult reconstruction video section in any knee textbook. The book has 14 sections, two more than the previous edition, and 153 chapters written by almost 200 worldwide contributors. The fifth edition will be enhanced by quarterly updates in a video journal format and updates to the glossary of knee replacement designs, past and present, as presented by all the manufacturers who chose to participate. Similar to the quarterly updates, the manufacturers will have the opportunity to update their prosthetic designs to keep the information timely.

In Section 1, Basic Science of Anatomy, Anatomic Aberrations, and Clinical Examination are updated and now include a more detailed video on the examination of the knee. Section 2, Imaging, has been rewritten by an orthopedic radiologist, Dan Walz, and presents the most current diagnostic criteria for knee imaging. Similarly, the Biomechanics section also has a new leader in Rick Komistek, who has assembled a stellar group of contributors.

The Sports Medicine section, almost a third of the book, has been spearheaded by David Diduch. It is a tremendous enhancement to the work of previous editors, and David's work in putting this section together has truly been Herculean! From articular cartilage biology and biomechanics, extensor mechanism issues, meniscal repair, resection, or replacement, isolated or combined cruciate and collateral ligament treatments, the information in the fifth edition is truly state of the art. And, of course will remain current via the aforementioned quarterly updates.

Section 7, developed by Andy Franks, pertains to the current concepts regarding the diagnosis of knee arthritis, both inflammatory and noninflammatory.

Sections 8 and 9 include updates on synovium, hemophilia, HIV, and plastic surgery as it relates to wound healing and skin coverage options about the knee.

In Section 10, George Haidukewych, once again, has done an outstanding job of organizing fractures about the knee and periprosthetic fractures, probably one of the major causes for TKR revision today.

Likewise, in Section 11, Min Kocher presents today's state of the art treatment of pediatric knee disorders, which will continue via the quarterly updates.

Section 12, Joint Replacement and Its Alternatives, includes another new feature, the International and National Roundtables Discussions. We believe that this approach really allows the reader to comprehend the international differences and similarities in understanding worldwide controversial areas. Gil Scuderi did an excellent job in organizing these discussions and the forty other chapters encompassing the totality of the treatment of the arthritic knee. Similar to the other sections, the surgical video techniques enhance the learning experience.

Section 13 includes the extremely controversial orthopedic medical issues such as DVT prophylaxes management and comprehensive pain management protocols associated with knee surgery.

In Section 14, Mary O'Connor once again has her contributors present the latest evidence on treating tumors about the knee. The mega prosthesis chapter, of course, is often apropos to the nontumor arthritic or revision TKR and is necessary reading for the TKR revision surgeon.

A new feature on the e-version, the glossary of implants, is presented in the spirit of helping the practicing physician determine the implant that he or she is evaluating whether in a primary or revision setting. We thank the companies for their cooperation and welcome their updates since the glossary is presented as an e-version which does not require the rigors of print media.

In the last five decades better understanding of the basic sciences has allowed the knee community to develop much more of a consensus in the treatment of the "sports knee" and the arthritic knee. From a surgical perspective, techniques are continuing to be refined but one has to question whether "better is now the enemy of good?" It is a fine line and the surgical techniques cannot be the sole indication for treatment. For instance, registries in joint replacement are often at odds with published series by experts. Is this an indication, surgical technique, or patient expectation problem? We must be able to address and solve these issues before the publication of the sixth edition of *Surgery of the Knee*.

In the 1980s, Dr. Insall penciled an often quoted statement that one should not perform a revision TKR, unless the etiology of the failure was thoroughly understood. If he were with us today, I am sure that he would likewise want us to ascertain the indications for procedures based on a careful analysis of resultant treatments, whether it be nonoperative or operative. Better analysis of patient demographics and expectations, design considerations, biological advances, and evidence-based results will allow us to better develop the treatment of knee disorders as a science rather than just an art. Physicians specializing in knee disorders must understand the practical consequences of all treatments to truly give our patients the best advice.

Once again, a tremendous "thanks" to all our contributors who join me in hoping that the "knee student" truly gains from studying the text, e-version, videos, and updates in the fifth edition of *Surgery of the Knee!*

W. Norman Scott, MD

In 1984, John Insall almost single-handedly wrote the first edition of *Surgery of the Knee*. There were only 24 contributors to that single volume. In 1993, the second edition had 40 contributors and four associate editors and consisted of two volumes. In 2001, we combined efforts (*The Knee*, Mosby, 1994) to enhance the third edition (159 contributors) of *Surgery of the Knee*. Thus in 17 years three editions were published, and now the fourth edition has published less than five years later. This shortened publication time reflects our interest in being current and in using the latest technology and leading experts to inform our readers. In this fourth edition of *Surgery of the Knee*, we have updated basic chapters and introduced new information utilizing text and visual aids (DVDs), and we are inaugurating a new feature, a companion online e-dition: www.scottkneesurgery.com. The e-dition website will include full text search, hyperlinks to PubMed, an image library, and monthly content updates, to minimize the customary complaint of the "perpetual lag" inherent with textbooks in general. Our goal is to create an interactive current environment for all of us students of the diagnosis and treatment of knee disorders.

The fourth edition of *Surgery of the Knee* has 12 sections, 112 chapters, and 191 international contributors. The DVD sections include (1) a classic video recorded in 1994 (Drs. Insall and Scott) detailing "Exposures, Approaches and Soft Tissue Balancing in Knee Arthroplasty"; (2) interactive anatomical and physical examination recordings, which enhance the material presented in Chapters 1, 2, 3, 5, 6, and 7; and (3) three commonly used minimally invasive surgical techniques for knee arthroplasty.

In Section I, Basic Science, Chapters 1 to 5, the core information presented in the third edition is updated. The DVD of the Anatomy Section is interactive with the imaging in Section II, so the reader can see the normal and abnormal findings side by side. Chapter 3, Clinical Examination of the Knee, now, as mentioned, has the added feature of an actual examination on the DVD to enhance the text.

Section III, Biomechanics, has been expanded under the guidance of A. Seth Greenwald, DPhil (Oxon), to include soft issue and implant considerations that are essential to executing surgical decisions.

With the plethora of Internet information available to patients today, it behooves the knee physician to be absolutely familiar with the various nonoperative and operative alternatives for the treatment of articular cartilage and meniscal disorders (Section IV). Dr. Henry Clarke has done a magnificent job in assembling the innovators in the field. The 18 chapters in this section truly capture the basic science, including the potential of gene therapy, biomechanics, and various treatment options, presented in great detail with the most current results. The section is further highlighted by Dr. Clarke's algorithm for clinical management of articular cartilage injuries.

The advances in the treatment of knee ligament injuries since 1984 are, needless to say, overwhelming. The success achieved today in the treatment of ligament injuries would have been unimaginable 25 years ago. As Section Editor of Section V, Ligament Injuries, Dr. Fred Cushner has assembled most of the people associated with these improvements. The foundations for treatments, controversies, and specific techniques are well chronicled throughout this section. Similarly, Section VI, Patellar and Extensor Mechanism Disorders, represents an updated comprehensive review by Dr. Aglietti and surgical chapters by Drs. Fulkerson and Scuderi.

Sections VII and VIII are "must reads" for all knee clinicians. In addition to discussing the normal and abnormal synovium, we have recruited distinguished authors to discuss the application of current topics of concern to both the patient and clinician, e.g., HIV and hepatitis (Chapter 59), anesthesia for knee surgery (Chapter 60), and an understanding of reflex sympathetic dystrophy (Chapter 61). The orthopaedic knee surgeon must have an absolute awareness of the potential problems inherent in the skin about the knee. In Chapter 63, Soft-Tissue Healing, Drs. Susan Scott and Robert Reiffel give us a foundation for avoiding and treating these potential problems.

Section IX focuses on fractures about the knee and has been organized by Dr. George Haidukewych. These fracture experts have covered all the fractures that occur, including the difficult periprosthetic fractures. Treatment modalities are detailed and reflect the current options with the latest equipment.

Section X, Pediatric Knee, has been reinvigorated with the help of Carl Stanitski. We decided to present the orthopaedic pediatric approach, rather than the sole view-point of the knee physician who treats pediatric injuries. The section is well organized, comprehensive, and, I believe, an improvement over the third edition of *Surgery of the Knee*.

The largest section in this two-volume edition is Section XI, Joint Replacement and Its Alternatives. Dr. Gil Scuderi has organized this section of the surgical treatment of the arthritic knee, including osteotomy, unicompartment replacement, patellofemoral arthroplasty, total knee replacement, and the more challenging revision surgery. While establishing the indications and contraindications for techniques, he has been careful to include the identification and management of difficult complications, such as infection, bone defects, extensor mechanism disruption, blood management, and thrombophlebitis. The tremendous success achieved in knee arthroplasty has paralleled the improvements in surgical instrumentation. In this section several authors have detailed the current concepts of computer and navigation surgery, a truly exciting recent development. In the aforementioned e-dition version of *Surgery of the Knee*, the first several streaming videos will focus on specific techniques. Thus, these chapters provide an excellent foundation for interpreting the subsequent e-version techniques.

Dr. Mary O'Connor has developed Section XII, Tumors about the Knee, in a concise, clinically rational framework for those physicians who do not necessarily treat many of these difficult problems. Chapters 106 to 112 are well written and are truly outstanding contributions to this text.

Surgery of the Knee is a text that includes audiovisual teaching aids and now a monthly means of communicating current information in a timely audiovisual manner. To me, it's very exciting, and I look forward to integrating the contributions of these authors into a rapidly current technology for the benefit of all our patients.

W. Norman Scott, MD

Twenty-five years ago, the adolescent with knee pain unresponsive to immobilization, with subsequent atrophy and increasing disability afterwards, underwent a totally unnecessary arthrotomy and meniscectomy, sometimes preceded by a very inaccurate athrography.

When symptoms persisted, the other meniscus was usually considered the source of discomfort, and the treatment was unsuccessfully repeated. Then, with the evolution of failed arthrotomies, the patella was believed to be the culprit. Unfortunately, there was no nonoperative or operative intervention that was universally successful. Surgically, distal and then proximal realignments were performed on almost all types of "chondromalacia" complaints. Anterior cruciate ligament injuries, if diagnosed, were treated in a spectrum from purposeful neglect to an assortment of combined intra- and extra-articular reconstructions. The recovery from these procedures was truly, in today's perspective, a tribute to the dedication of the patient and therapist and somewhat of a warning to avoid surgery!

Unfortunately, many of these patients' knee disorders led to post-traumatic arthritis unresponsive to most nonsteroidal anti-inflammatory medicines; thus, they were candidates for an osteotomy. Even though the osteotomy would probably not be indicated today, there were no other surgical options. Today, a better understanding of clinical diagnosis, imaging techniques, and rehabilitative modalities has eliminated many unnecessary surgeries. Arthroscopy has revolutionized the diagnosis and treatment of cartilage lesions and ligament disruptions. Total knee arthroplasty, on the other hand, has yielded unparalleled success in alleviating patients' discomfort while eliminating their disability.

This 25-year retrospective view is, I believe, somewhat predictive of how we will perceive the contribution of classic textbooks to continuing medical education. As we enter the digital century, if not millennium, it is increasingly difficult to accept the analog world's perpetual lag of inadequacy of the published word while attempting to enhance education and subsequently new breakthrough treatments for our patients. Thus, we have attempted in this two-volume comprehensive color text to "bridge the gap" between the analog and digital worlds. In combining our two previous textbooks, *Surgery of the Knee* and *The Knee*, we have solicited the contributions of national and international experts recognized worldwide by serious knee students.

This textbook consists of 95 chapters divided into 11 sections. In Basic Science (Section I) we have introduced an interactive CD-ROM combining the anatomical and imaging chapters. While we believe this approach, either by CD or through Internet access, is the future, practical considerations precluded us from presenting the entire book in this format at this time. The CD takes studying, browsing, and researching anatomy and imaging in a new direction. Thanks to Drs. Clarke and Pedersen, the CD contains an extensive collection of medical data pertaining to anatomy, anatomical aberrations, imaging, and surgical exposures. We believe this is truly a breakthrough in understanding comprehensive knee anatomy.

In Biomechanics (Section II), Dr. Michael Freeman has truly enhanced our understanding of the dynamics of knee motion in an extensive MRI-controlled model of knee motion. The remainder of this section reinforces basic principles of knee biomechanics and explains the relationship of the knee to normal and abnormal gait.

Healing articular cartilage defects has enticed orthopaedists since the beginning of our specialty. Today, the enthusiasm seems to be at fever pitch. Thus, we have included many, if not all, of the therapeutic approaches by the recognized international originators of the technique. From Europe to the United States, contributors lay the foundation for what will hopefully be therapeutic success in the year to come.

Although the more than 150 contributors to this edition are too numerous to focus on individually, there are some especially innovative chapters that deserve special attention. Chapter 41, "Revision ACL Surgery: How I Do It," allows the reader to see step-by-step the "pearls" of various experts on how they approach this difficult problem in the operating theater.

With increasing focus on recreational athletics, the problems with the pediatric knee are becoming more manifest. Thus, Chapters 64 to 68 give the reader the opportunity to learn from pediatric orthopaedists on normal growth and development, congenital deformities, physeal fractures, and dealing with ACL injuries in skeletally immature patients.

Almost a quarter of this text is devoted to knee replacement and surgical alternatives. The success of the former necessitates such an approach. Osteotomy, however, must not be forgotten; thanks to Drs. Hanssen and Poilvache, we get both the European and American perspective. The standard issues with knee replacement, designs, technique, thrombophlebitis, skin problems (Section VII), infection, and complications requiring revision surgery are extensively detailed. Just as with revision ACL surgery, there are six sections devoted to revision TKR surgery. The diversity of surgical approaches and "tips" is truly priceless.

It is a true honor to have collaborated with my mentor, partner, and, most importantly, friend in publishing this comprehensive text. Dr. Insall's published works on all aspects of knee surgery are unparalleled. For me to have continued my "residency" under his guidance for the past 2 years has been a gift beyond measure.

On behalf of all the authors, we hope that you, the reader, are stimulated by this text to learn, analyze your observations, challenge thoughtfully, and make a contribution that will ultimately help your patients!

W. Norman Scott, MD

This textbook is larger than before, a change made necessary by the many advances made in knee surgery since the first edition was published ten years ago. Radiology of the knee has been revolutionized by computed tomography (CT) and magnetic resonance imaging (MRI), which have added a degree of certainty to the diagnosis of meniscal and some ligament injuries. Clinical acumen and careful examination are, of course, still required, but when these state of the art investigations are available, precise diagnosis will avoid unnecessary surgery. The ligament chapters are completely new, reflecting greater understanding of the pathology of ligament injuries. The classification of these injuries was in disarray in the early 1980s without true recognition of the role of the cruciate ligaments in causing knee instability. Anteromedial and anterolateral instabilities and the tests for their diagnosis were previously discussed without mentioning the anterior cruciate ligament (ACL), and it was still widely believed that the ACL was not an important stabilizer of the knee. Lesions of the posterior cruciate ligament (PCL) were also poorly understood, and the terminology was complexed and confusing. Due to the work of the late John Marshall and his successors, ligament injuries and laxities are today logically classified. The contribution to knee stability of the ACL in particular is universally accepted. It is fitting that Russell Warren, who followed Marshall as the Director of Sports Medicine at The Hospital for Special Surgery, coauthored the chapter on acute ligament injuries.

Arthroscopy was included in the first edition only to outline general principles. Today such limited treatment is impossible because arthroscopy has become a major part of knee surgery. Norman Scott, who has himself written a text on arthroscopy, has comprehensively described the techniques and advances in this subspecialty.

The chapters on knee arthroplasty are all new. Very little has been carried over except for historical reference. Advances in knee prostheses and especially in surgical instrumentation and technique have made the operation reliable and predictable. A preeminent bioengineer, Peter Walker, has contributed the section on knee prosthesis design. Clement Sledge and C. Lowry Bames have written on PCL retention in knee arthroplasty, and Richard Scott describes the role of unicompartmental replacement. George Galante and Aaron Rosenberg make the case for cementless fixation. However, not all of these innovations have proven successful and new problems such as polyethylene wear have recently become a major clinical issue. Osteolysis caused by polyethylene debris is an even newer complication. The extent and severity of both problems will have to wait the passage of time and further evaluation.

I may have suggested in the earlier preface that I was a "complete" knee surgeon: even if this was once true, it most certainly is not today. I do not believe that one surgeon can be equally expert in all of the conditions that affect even a single joint such as the knee: for example, since 1984 over 500 articles have been published in the three major English language journals on the subject of total knee arthroplasty alone. Therefore, to prepare this edition, I have enlisted the help of four associate editors, all of whom I have trained at some stage of their careers and who have continued to work closely with me. In addition to their editorial functions, they have also contributed material of their own. Paolo Aglietti has revised his previous chapters on fractures of the knee and in this edition provides additional chapters on chronic ligament injuries and the management of the patellofemoral joint. Norman Scott, calling upon his vast experience in athletic injuries, has contributed chapters on arthroscopy and the classification of ligament injuries. Russell Windsor has written on the management of infection, arthrodesis, and soft-tissue disorders. Michael Kelly has revised the chapters on anatomy and physical examination. Between us it is hoped that we covered the material adequately.

Mrs. Martha Moore has labored on this edition as she did on the first one, again earning my profound gratitude. I also thank Ms. Virginia Ferrante and Ms. Elizabeth Roselius for the new illustrations.

John N. Insall, MD

If the 1960s saw a revolution in hip surgery, the knee had its turn during the 1970s. Much has changed and is still changing. Arthroscopic surgery has emerged as a new discipline; knee arthroplasty has become a reliable treatment for gonarthrosis; and concepts in the treatment of ligament injuries have altered radically in the last 10 years. Also, surgeons interested in the knee have separated into three groups, their major involvement being either in arthroscopy, sports medicine, or knee replacement. As one who has dabbled in all of these areas, it is my hope that this book will have some unifying benefit.

However, there is still no unanimity of opinion about how to treat all disorders of the knee joint, and for one who has the temerity to edit a textbook on the subject, there is the certain knowledge that he cannot please everyone. On the other hand, a textbook must have cohesion so that one chapter does not contradict the next. My solution to this dilemma is to present the current opinion and practice at The Hospital for Special Surgery, and, therefore, most of the contributors are past or present members of the staff. Where there are significant areas of controversy, I have also sought other viewpoints, notably on ligament surgery, the place of cruciate ligaments in knee arthroplasty, and the fixation of prosthetic components to bone. I have also reached beyond the walls of my own hospital for additional expertise, and well-known authorities have written chapters on osteochondrosis dissecans, hemophilia, surgical pathology of arthritis, and arthroscopy.

With regard to the chapter on arthroscopy, I foresee that this chapter may be considered too short in an era when arthroscopic surgery and knee surgery are becoming synonymous in the minds of many surgeons. This decision to keep this chapter short was made deliberately for two reasons: (1) Excellent textbooks devoted specifically to the techniques of arthroscopic surgery already exist, and (2) both Doctor McGinty and I felt that, because arthroscopic surgery has not been placed in full perspective, some currently popular arthroscopic techniques may become discredited with time.

I also decided not to include specific details of AO surgical techniques in the fracture chapter as these are also very well described elsewhere.

It would not have been possible to complete this book without the invaluable assistance of my secretary, Mrs. Martha Moore, who has put in as much effort as I and must now know every word and every reference by heart. I also wish to thank Ms. Joelle Pacht for her endless retyping of the manuscript, Miss Dottie Page and the Photographic Department at The Hospital for Special Surgery for their assistance in preparing the photographic material, and Mr. William Thackeray who has done most of the book's illustrations and drawings.

John N. Insall, MD

ACKNOWLEDGMENTS

To Dr. Henrik Bo Pedersen, Your knowledge, enthusiasm, and expertise make my job so easy! Thank you.

To Kathleen Lenhardt, Your involvement in the education and management of the ISK Fellows and Insall Traveling Fellows and Insall Club has afforded me an opportunity to develop and utilize a reservoir of such distinguished surgeons and authors! Thank you.

To Ruth O'Sullivan, You "just" get everything done! Thank you.

To Dina Potaris, Your first entry into the publishing world was a success and made everybody look good! Thank you.

CONTENTS

xxxi

SECTION 5

Sports Medicine: Ligament Injuries

SECTION 6

Sports Medicine: Patellar and Extensor Mechanism Disorders

SECTION 7

Knee Arthritis

SECTION 8

Miscellaneous Conditions and Treatments

SECTION 9

Plastic Surgery

SECTION 10

Fractures About the Knee

SECTION 11

Pediatric Knee

SECTION 12

Joint Replacement and Its Alternatives

SECTION 13

Medical/Surgical Consideration in Managing the Total Knee Replacement Patient

Medical Issues

Deep Vein Thrombosis

View Expertconsult.com for periodic updates.

I. GLOSSARY OF IMPLANTS

II. VIDEOS

This icon appears throughout the book to indicate chapters with accompanying video available on Expertconsult.com.

Normal Anatomy

Physical Examination of the Knee

MRI Imaging of the Knee

SECTION 1

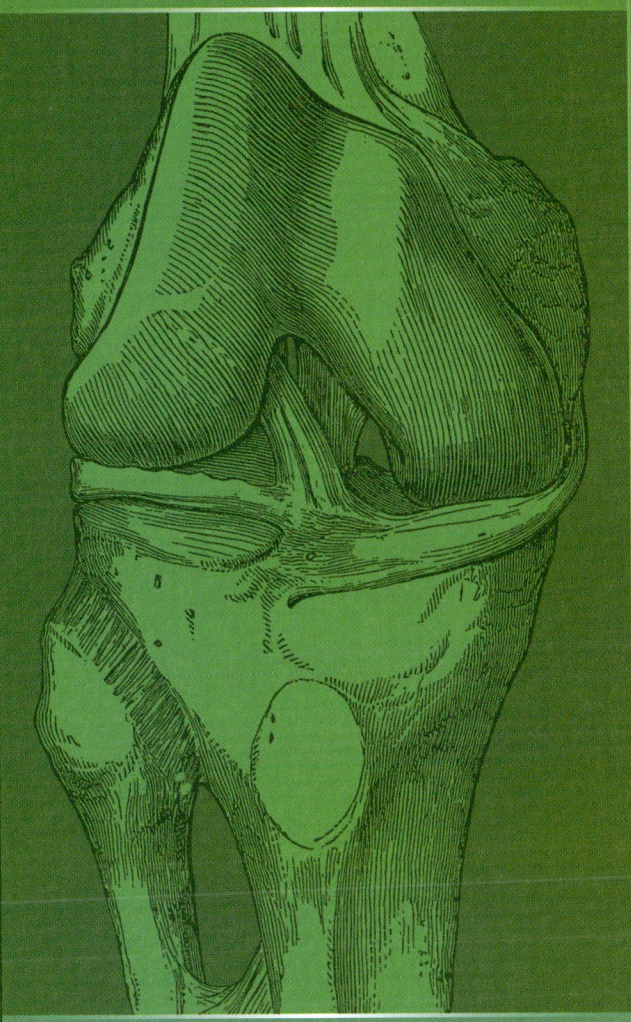

Basic Science

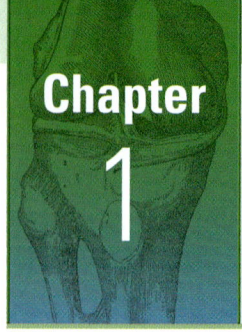

Chapter 1

Anatomy

Henry D. Clarke, W. Norman Scott, John N. Insall, Henrik B. Pedersen, Kevin R. Math, Vincent J. Vigorita, and Fred D. Cushner

The anatomy of the knee can be examined on a number of levels from microscopic to gross and with a variety of techniques, including physical examination, anatomic dissection, radiographic and cross-sectional imaging, and arthroscopic examination. Any practitioner interested in diagnosing and treating disorders of the knee must have a detailed understanding of both normal and abnormal regional anatomy. Furthermore, the ability to interpret and correlate information obtained from different sources is highly beneficial. However, it is also paramount that the clinician gain the knowledge required to be able to interpret the significance of an identifiable anatomic abnormality within the context of a patient's complaints. It is the goal of this chapter to present a thorough review of knee anatomy to help the reader successfully assimilate the material presented in subsequent chapters. To provide a comprehensive description of pertinent anatomic details, text, illustrations, arthroscopic photographs, radiographs, and pictures from cross-sectional imaging studies are used. In addition, in many situations, the same structures are presented from different perspectives. Rather than being redundant, we hope that this approach will facilitate the development of a more complete appreciation of the anatomy about the knee. The descriptions that follow are taken in part from standard anatomic texts.[3,10,73,120]

NORMAL SKELETAL STRUCTURES

Bone Physiology

Bone is composed of mineral crystals embedded in an organic matrix. Of the dry weight of bone (about 10% of the actual weight in situ), approximately 70% is due to mineral content and 30% is organic matter. The mineral consists of primarily calcium and phosphorus in a ratio of 2:1. The organic matter is composed of collagen, noncollagenized matrix, and proteins. Collagen is the major extracellular component of bone and is composed of fibrils. Collagen fibrils, which form a parallel, highly organized arrangement, are known as *intrinsic fibers*, whereas those that tend to anchor ligaments and tendons at attachment sites and often insert in a perpendicular manner are *extrinsic fibers*. The matrix is populated by mesenchymal cells, which differentiate into osteocytes, osteoblasts, and osteoclasts. These cells perform key functions in the turnover and remodeling of bone in response to both physical and metabolic stimuli. Osteoblasts are cuboid in nature and have abundant cytoplasm. The main function of osteoblasts is to produce osteoid, a collagenized protein that mineralizes at the tidemark zone as hydroxyapatite crystals are incorporated (Fig. 1-1). As the matrix becomes mineralized bone, these cells become embedded and are transformed into osteocytes. The osteocyte is in contact with the osteoblast through the cannular system. Osteoclasts are

multinucleated macrophage-like cells that perform bone resorption at mineralized bone surfaces (Fig. 1-2). Other associated tissues such as periosteum (Fig. 1-3), fatty and hematopoietic marrow elements, and tendon and ligament attachments create a complex system with mechanical, metabolic, and hematopoietic functions.

Bony Architecture

The knee joint consists of three bony structures—femur, tibia, and patella—that form three distinct and partially separated compartments: medial, lateral, and patellofemoral compartments.

Patella

The patella, the largest sesamoid bone in the body, sits in the femoral trochlea. It is an asymmetrical oval with its apex directed distally. The fibers of the quadriceps tendon envelop it anteriorly and blend with the patellar ligament distally. The articulation between the patella and the femoral trochlea forms the anterior or patellofemoral compartment (Fig. 1-4).

The posterior aspect of the patella is described as possessing seven facets. The medial and lateral facets are divided vertically into approximately equal thirds, whereas the seventh or odd facet lies along the extreme medial border of the patella. Overall, the medial facet is smaller and slightly convex; the lateral facet, which consists of roughly two thirds of the patella, has both a sagittal convexity and a coronal concavity (Fig. 1-5). Six morphologic variants of the patella have been described (Fig. 1-6). Types I and II are stable, whereas the other variants are more likely to give rise to lateral subluxation as a result of unbalanced forces.[12,119] The facets are covered by the thickest hyaline cartilage in the body, which may measure up to 6.5 mm in thickness.[119] The relationship between surface degeneration of this articular surface, or chondromalacia, seen arthroscopically in adolescents and young adults, and pain is unclear.

The femoral trochlea is separated from the medial and lateral femoral condyles by indistinct ridges; the lateral ridge is more prominent. The patella fits into the trochlea of the femur imperfectly, and the contact patch between the patella and the femur varies with position as the patella sweeps across the femoral surface. The contact patch has been investigated by dye[39] and casting techniques.[2] Both methods produce very similar results and indicate that the area of contact never exceeds about one third of the total patellar articular surface. At 10 to 20 degrees of flexion, the distal pole of the patella first contacts the trochlea in a narrow band across the medial and lateral facets (Fig. 1-7).[39,54] As flexion increases, the contact area moves proximally and laterally. The most extensive contact is made at approximately 45 degrees, where the contact area is an ellipse in continuity across the central

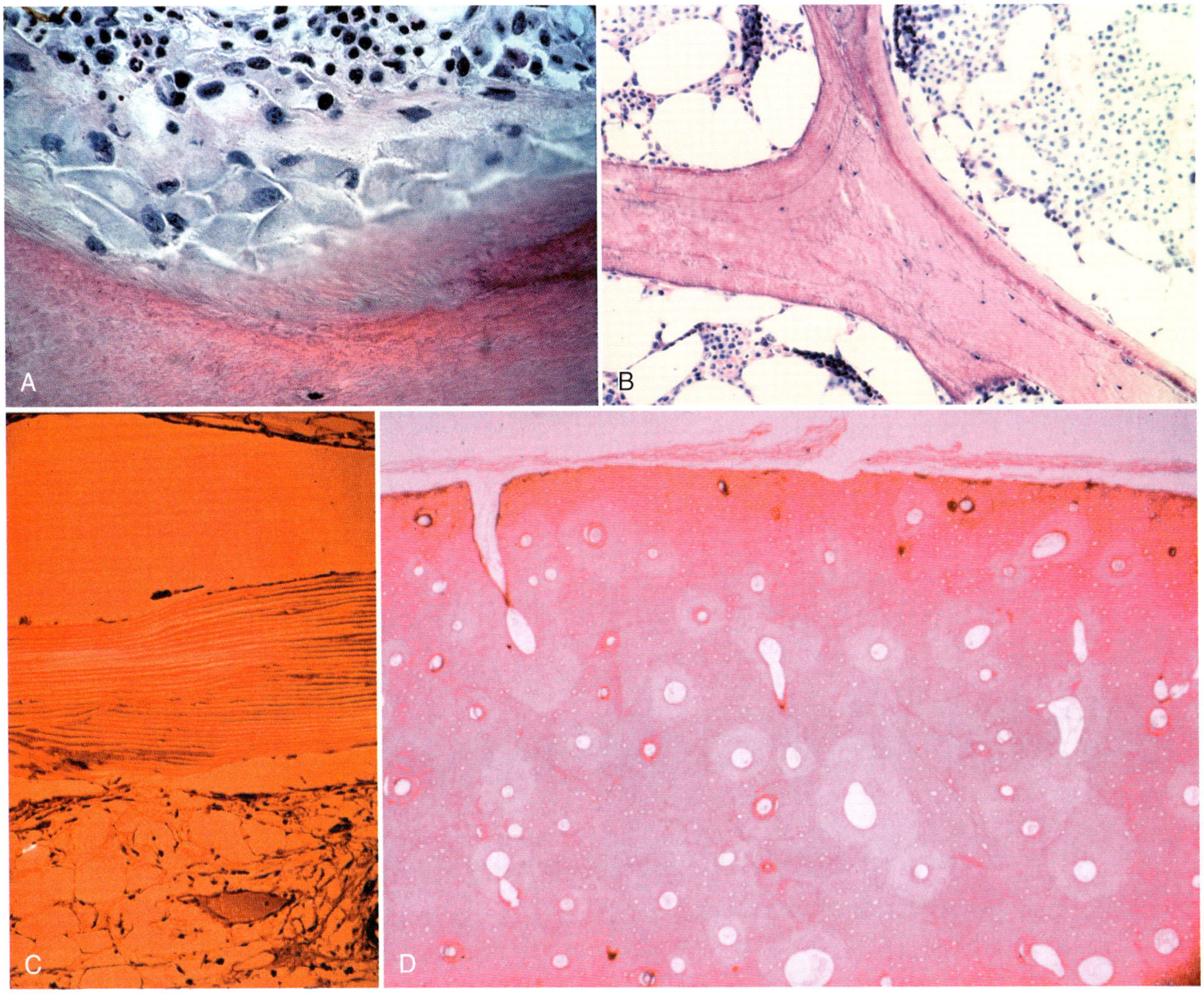

Figure 1-1. **A,** Osteoblasts. Plump, cytoplasm-rich osteoblasts actively making osteoid, the type I collagen that in the normal sequence of events becomes the fibrous matrix of mineralized bone. **B,** Normal cancellous (trabecular, spongy) bone bathed in normal hematopoietic marrow. Bone surfaces are smooth. Osteoid deposition (light pink surface) is interfaced with mature bone by the basophilic mineralization front. **C,** Normal cancellous bone. With the use of polarized light microscopy, the organized lamellar or pleated deposition of the collagen matrix of mineralized bone is appreciated. **D,** Cross-section of cortical bone showing numerous haversian systems of varying age. The cortical bone is surrounded on its surface by periosteum. The cortical bone itself is composed of haversian bone systems, which represent interwoven longitudinal, circumferential, and concentric bone-forming units (osteons) characterized by central haversian canals of various size and shape. Remodeling is ongoing throughout life; most of it occurs in an axial direction down the shaft.

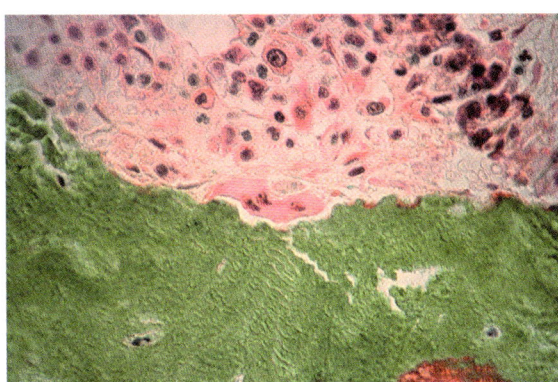

Figure 1-2. Osteoclast. A multinucleated osteoclast is resorbing bone at a crenated surface, Howship's lacuna.

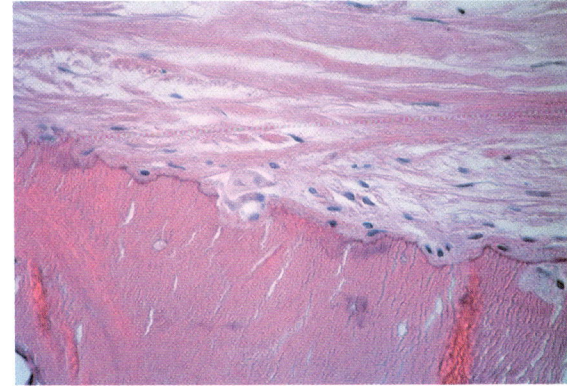

Figure 1-3. Periosteum. The often inconspicuous spindle-shaped fibroblast-like cells of the periosteum belie their remarkable capacity to become activated as bone-forming cells.

Figure 1-4. Merchant view radiograph of a normal patellofemoral joint. The tibial tubercle is superimposed over the apex of the femoral trochlea.

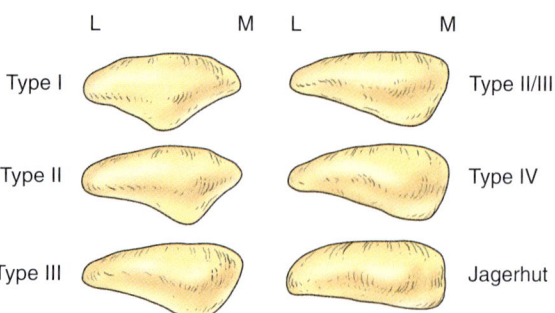

Figure 1-6. Wiberg's and Baumgartl's patella types.[12,119]

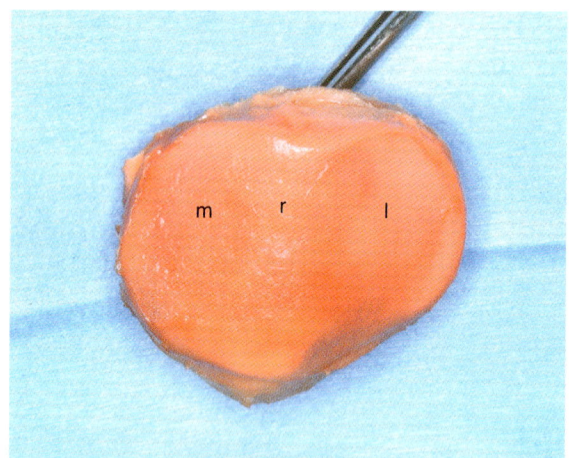

Figure 1-5. Articular surface of the patella. The median ridge (r) divides the smaller medial facet (m) from the larger lateral facet (l).

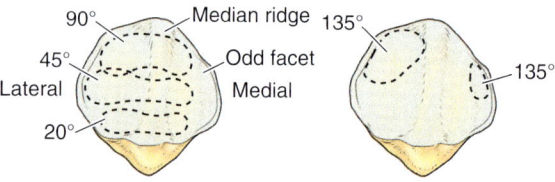

Figure 1-7. Patellofemoral contact areas at different degrees of flexion.

portion of the medial and lateral facets. By 90 degrees, the contact area has shifted to the upper part of the medial and lateral patellar facets. With further flexion, the contact area separates into distinct medial and lateral patches.[2,39,54] Because the odd facet makes contact with the femur only in extreme flexion (such as in the act of squatting), this facet is habitually a noncontact zone in humans in Western cultures—a fact that is thought to have some pathologic significance.

The main biomechanical function of the patella is to increase the moment arm of the quadriceps mechanism.[62] The load across the joint rises as flexion increases, but because the contact area also increases, the higher force is dissipated over a larger area. However, if extension against resistance is performed, the force increases while the contact area shrinks, and this may exacerbate pain from the patellofemoral region. Straight-leg raises eliminate force transmission across the patellofemoral joint because in full extension, the patella has not yet engaged the trochlea.[54]

Femur

The architecture of the distal end of the femur is complex. Furthermore, this area serves as the attachment site of numerous ligaments and tendons (Fig. 1-8). In shape and dimensions, the femoral condyles are asymmetrical; the larger medial condyle has a more symmetrical curvature. The lateral condyle viewed from the side has a sharply increasing radius of curvature posteriorly. The femoral condyles viewed from the surface, articulating with the tibia, show that the lateral condyle is slightly shorter than the medial. The long axis of the lateral condyle is slightly longer and is placed in a more sagittal plane than the long axis of the medial condyle, which is oriented at a mean angle of about 22 degrees and opened posteriorly.[61] The lateral condyle is slightly wider than the medial condyle at the center of the intercondylar notch. Anteriorly, the condyles are separated by a groove known as the femoral trochlea (Fig. 1-9). The sulcus represents the deepest point in the trochlea. Relative to the midplane between the condyles, the sulcus lies slightly laterally.[28] Reproducing this anatomic relationship is important for accurate patellofemoral mechanics after total knee replacement.

The intercondylar notch separates the two condyles distally and posteriorly. The lateral wall of the notch has a flat impression, where the proximal origin of the anterior cruciate ligament (ACL) arises. On the medial wall of the notch is a larger site, where the posterior cruciate ligament (PCL) originates. The mean width of the notch is narrowest at the distal end and widens proximally (1.8 to 2.3 cm); in contrast, the height of the notch is greatest at the midportion (2.4 cm) and decreases proximally (1.3 cm) and distally (1.8 cm).[68] The dimensions of the notch have become an important topic because of the association between narrow notch width and increased risk for ACL tear. This risk does not seem to be related to the intrinsic characteristics of the ACL because normal-size ligaments have been identified in specimens with narrow notches.[87] Therefore, the increased risk of ACL failure is probably due to impingement on the ligament.[38,70,87] Notchplasty or sculpting of the intercondylar notch to increase the dimensions has become an integral part of ACL reconstruction.

The lateral condyle has a short groove just proximal to the articular margin, in which lies the tendinous origin of the popliteus muscle. This groove separates the lateral epicondyle from the joint line. The lateral epicondyle is a small but

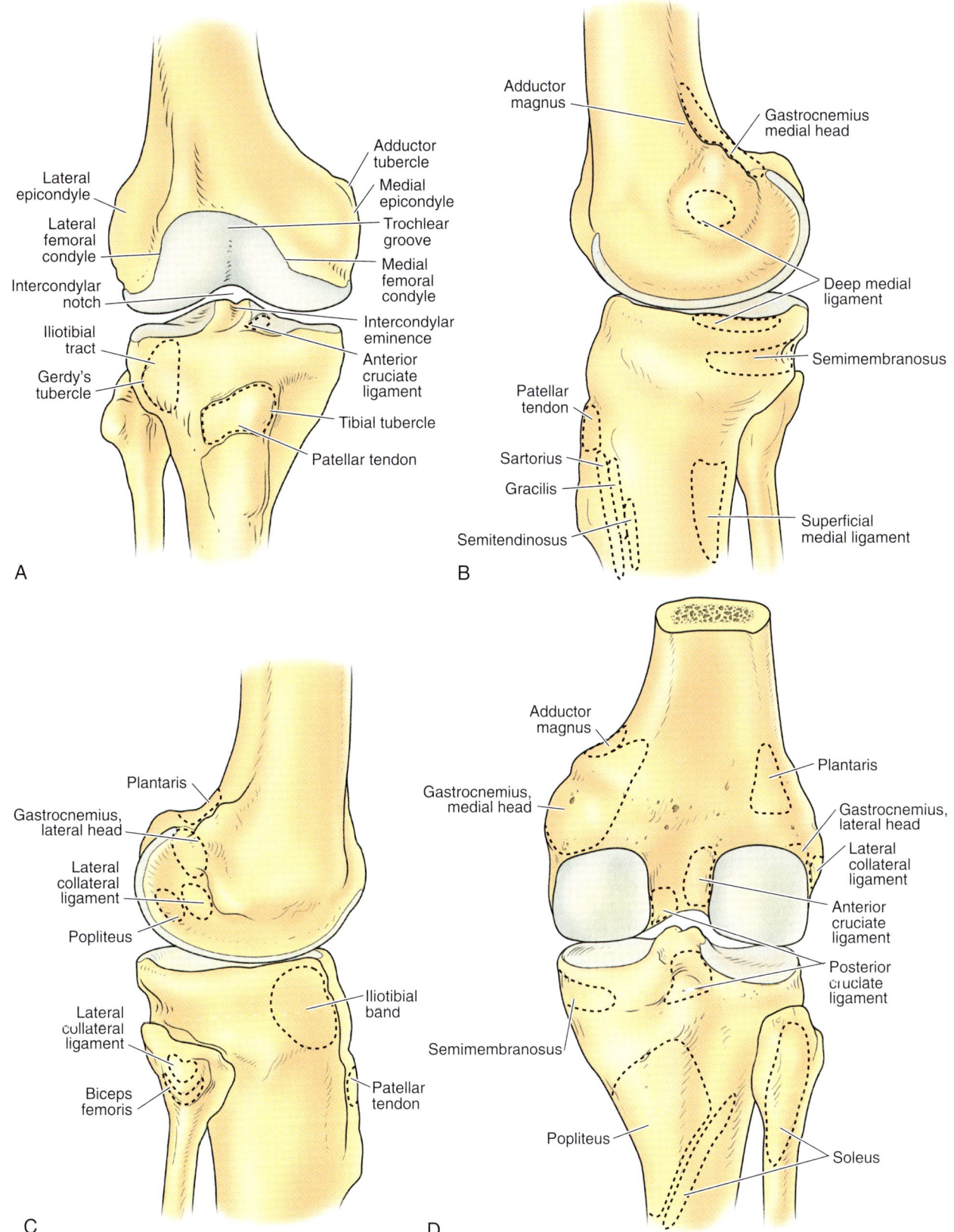

Figure 1-8. Bony landmarks with ligament and tendon attachment sites on the anterior (**A**), and medial (**B**). Medial (**C**) and posterior (**D**) aspects of the knee.

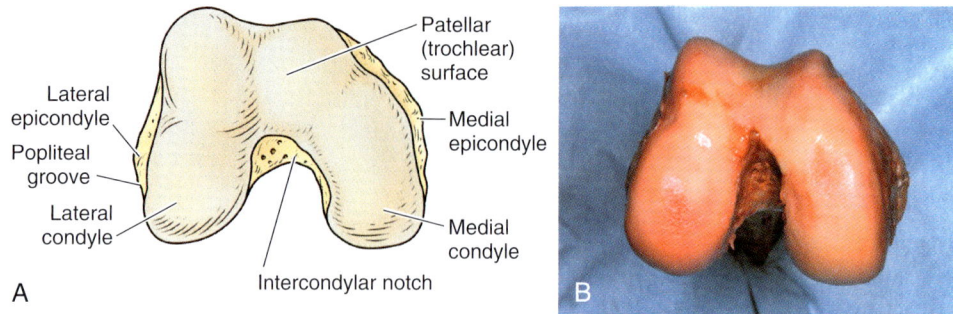

Figure 1-9. **A,** Bony architecture of the distal femur. **B,** Anatomic specimen of the distal femur. The femoral trochlea separates the lateral and medial femoral condyles. The deepest point lies slightly offset to the lateral side. The anterior aspect of the lateral condyle is more prominent than the medial side.

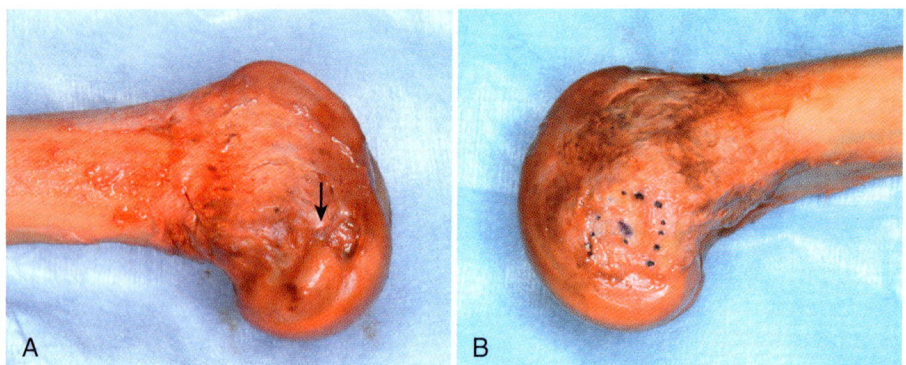

Figure 1-10. **A,** Bony landmarks of the lateral aspect of the distal femur. The characteristic groove for the popliteus tendon lies just proximal to the articular surface of the lateral condyle. The prominence of the lateral epicondyle *(arrow)* is located posterior to this groove. **B,** Bony landmarks of the medial aspect of the distal femur. The center of the sulcus of the C-shaped, ridgelike medial epicondyle *(both marked)* represents the center of attachment of the medial collateral ligament.

distinct prominence to which the lateral (fibular) collateral ligament (LCL) is attached. On the medial condyle, the prominent adductor tubercle is the insertion site of the adductor magnus. The medial epicondyle lies anterior and distal to the adductor tubercle and is a **C**-shaped ridge with a central depression or sulcus (Fig. 1-10). Rather than originating from the ridge, the medial collateral ligament (MCL) originates from the sulcus. The epicondylar axis passes through the center of the sulcus of the medial epicondyle and the prominence of the lateral epicondyle (Fig. 1-11). This line serves as an important reference line in total knee replacement. In relation to a line tangent to the posterior femoral condyles, the epicondylar axis is externally rotated about 3.5 degrees in males and 1 degree in females with normal knees.[13] In patients with osteoarthritis and valgus knee alignment, the transepicondylar axis has been shown to be externally rotated up to 10 degrees relative to the posterior condylar line.[41]

In recent years, important anatomic variations in the morphology of the distal femur have been identified in males and females and in different racial groups. Measurements of the distal femur in both Asian and Caucasian populations suggest that women have narrower femurs in the medial-lateral dimension than males, for any given anterior-posterior dimension.[14,19,21,48,77] This concept has been defined in terms of the aspect ratio of the distal femur, where the medial-lateral width is divided by the anterior-posterior dimension × 100.[19,48] In females, the aspect ratio tends to be smaller than in males in both Asian and white populations.[19,48] However, this aspect ratio is also affected by race, with Japanese females displaying a greater medial-lateral width than white females for any given anterior-posterior dimension.[110] In addition to these findings, racial differences appear to exist in the rotational anatomy of the distal femur, with more natural external rotation of the transepicondylar axis versus the posterior condylar line in Asian populations.[122] These racial differences and sexual dimorphism among humans may have significant implications for both prosthesis development and surgical technique in total knee arthroplasty.[94] This information has stimulated vigorous debate regarding whether gender-specific femoral components and knee prostheses designed for different racial groups are needed.* In particular, implants with a narrower medial-lateral geometry for a given specific anterior-posterior dimension have been advocated by some for use in females.[40,48,77] A similar prosthesis has been suggested for use in Indian populations, among which greater variability in medial-lateral width for any given anterior-posterior dimension has been noted.[112]

*References 19, 40, 77, 85, 110, and 112.

Although a gender bias has been demonstrated for some contemporary knee prostheses, it is unclear whether this bias has adversely affected the outcomes of total knee arthroplasty in females versus males.[29,48,84,85]

Tibia

In a macerated skeleton, inspection of the tibial plateau suggests that the femoral and tibial surfaces do not conform at all. The larger medial tibial plateau is nearly flat and has a squared-off posterior aspect that is distinct on a lateral radiograph.[25] In distinction, the articular surface of the narrower lateral plateau borders on convexity. Both surfaces have a

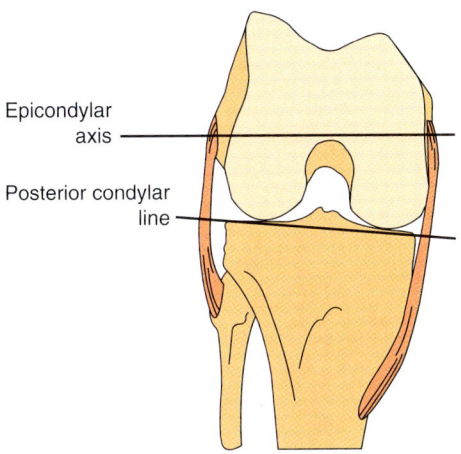

Figure 1-11. The epicondylar axis, which connects the prominence of the lateral epicondyle and the sulcus of the medial epicondyle, is externally rotated relative to the posterior condylar line.

posterior inclination of approximately 10 degrees with respect to the shaft of the tibia. However, lack of conformity between the femoral and tibial articular surfaces is more apparent than real. In an intact knee, the menisci enlarge the contact area considerably and increase the conformity of the joint surfaces. As previously noted for the femur, gender and race appear to affect the morphology of the proximal tibia.[48,69] Again, this may have implications for prosthesis design in total knee arthroplasty.[48,69] However, because flexibility in coverage and position of the tibial component is generally greater on the prepared surface of the tibial plateau in total knee arthroplasty, the implications of this variability have not been well researched at this time.

The median portion of the tibia between the plateaus is occupied by an eminence: the spine of the tibia. Anteriorly a depression is seen—the anterior intercondylar fossa—to which, from anterior to posterior, the anterior horn of the medial meniscus, the ACL, and the anterior horn of the lateral meniscus are attached. Behind this region are two elevations: the medial and lateral tubercles. They are divided by a gutter-like depression: the intertubercular sulcus. On an anteroposterior radiograph, the medial tubercle usually projects more superiorly than the lateral tubercle; on a lateral radiograph, the medial tubercle is located anterior to the lateral tubercle (Fig. 1-12). The tubercles do not function as attachment sites for the cruciate ligaments or menisci but may act as side-to-side stabilizers by projecting toward the inner sides of the femoral condyles. In concert with the menisci, the tibial spine enhances the impression of cupping seen in intact specimens. In the posterior intercondylar fossa, behind the tubercles, the lateral and then the medial menisci are attached anteriorly to posteriorly. Most posteriorly, the PCL inserts on the margin of the tibia between the condyles.

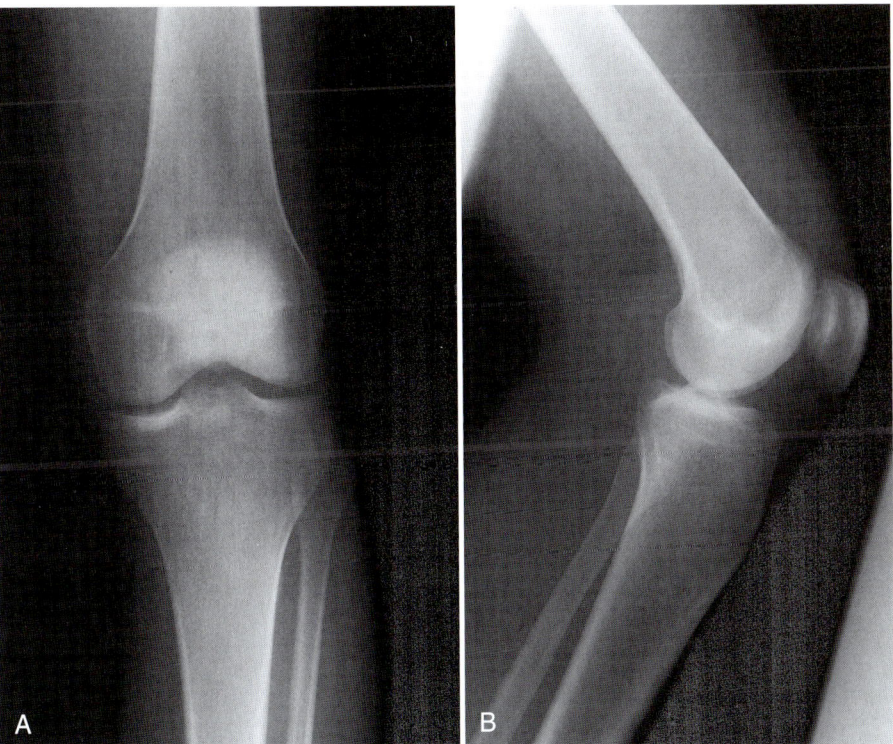

Figure 1-12. Anteroposterior (**A**) and lateral (**B**) radiographs of a normal knee.

On the anterior aspect of the tibia, the tuberosity is the most prominent feature and is the attachment site of the patellar tendon. Approximately 2 to 3 cm lateral to the tibial tubercles is Gerdy's tubercle, which is the insertion site of the iliotibial band (ITB).

Tibiofibular Joint

In an embryo, both the fibula and the tibia are in contact with the femur. However, because the tibia grows at a faster rate than the fibula does, the distance from the femorotibial articulation to the fibula increases. The portion of the capsule that initially surrounds the knee is retained by the fibula and forms the superior tibiofibular joint. The articular surface of the head of the fibula is directed superiorly and slightly anteromedially to articulate with the posterolateral portion of the tibial metaphysis. The styloid process projects superiorly from the posterolateral aspect of the fibula and is the insertion site for the LCL, biceps femoris tendon, fabellofibular ligament, and arcuate ligament.

The superior tibiofibular joint is lined with synovial membrane and possesses a capsular ligament that is strengthened by anterior and posterior ligaments. In contrast, the inferior tibiofibular joint is a syndesmosis, and the bones are joined by a strong intraosseous ligament. The intraosseous membrane originates from the intraosseous border of the fibula, and the fibers run distally and medially to attach to the intraosseous border of the tibia. A large opening that is present superiorly allows passage of the anterior tibial vessels.

The anterior aspect of the superior tibiofibular joint and the adjoining portions of the tibia and fibula give rise to the origins of the tibialis anterior, extensor digitorum longus, and peroneus longus muscles. The posterior aspect of the same region gives rise to a portion of the soleus muscle. The anterior tibial artery, the terminal branch of the popliteal artery, enters the anterior compartment of the leg through the opening in the intraosseous membrane, two fingerbreadths below the superior tibiofibular joint. A recurrent branch contributes to anastomosis around the knee. The anterior tibial nerve and a terminal branch of the common peroneal nerve also pierce the anterior intermuscular septum between the extensor digitorum longus and the fibula and come to lie at the lateral side of the artery. The superficial peroneal nerve arises from the common peroneal nerve on the lateral side of the neck of the fibula and runs distally and forward in the substance of the peroneus longus muscle.

HYALINE/ARTICULAR CARTILAGE

Articular cartilage is a specialized connective tissue composed of hydrated proteoglycans within a matrix of collagen fibrils. Proteoglycans are complex glycoproteins consisting of a central protein core to which glycosaminoglycan chains are attached. The structure of hyaline cartilage is not uniform, but rather can be divided into distinct zones based on the arrangement of the collagen fibrils and the distribution of chondrocytes. The density of chondrocytes is highest close to subchondral bone and decreases toward the articular surface (Fig. 1-13). Calcification occurs in a distinct basophilic zone at the deepest level of chondrocyte proliferation termed the *tidemark*. Beneath this region is a zone of calcified cartilage that anchors the cartilage to the subchondral plate. Cartilage is avascular, and chondrocytes in the superficial zones are believed to derive nutrition from synovial fluid. Deeper zones probably obtain nutrition from subchondral bone.

Examination of gross specimens or arthroscopic visualization reveals normal cartilage to consist of a white, smooth,

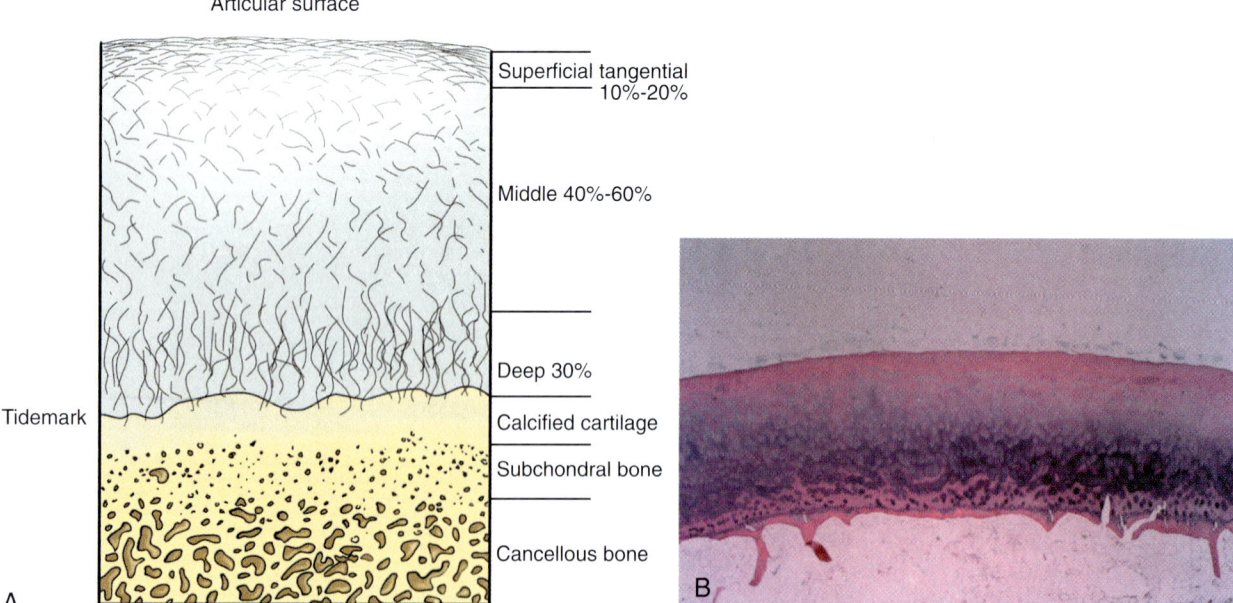

Figure 1-13. A, Diagrammatic representation of the transition from articular cartilage to bone. **B,** Normal articular (hyaline) cartilage composed of water, collagen, and proteoglycan. The sparsely cellular, smooth superficial zone becomes increasingly cellular in deeper layers. A distinct basophilic line, the mineralization front, can be seen where cartilage becomes calcified.

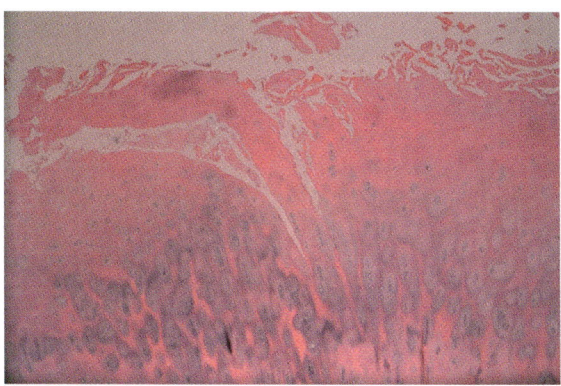

Figure 1-14. Degenerative or chondromalacic articular cartilage. Irregular thickness, surface fibrillation, longitudinal slits, increased chondrocyte cellularity, and altered matrix staining are evident.

firm material. Articular cartilage damage or degeneration, termed *chondromalacia*, can be readily identified (Fig. 1-14). These characteristic changes seen during arthroscopic examination have been classified by Outerbridge[90]: Grade 0 is normal, white-appearing cartilage; grade I is swelling or softening of an intact cartilage surface; grade II is represented by fissuring and fibrillation over a small area (<0.5 inch); grade III includes the same pathologic changes over a larger area (>0.5 inch); and grade IV changes represent erosion to subchondral bone and are indistinguishable from osteoarthritis. Chondral flap tears caused by delamination of the articular cartilage may also be encountered (Fig. 1-15). These changes in articular cartilage cannot be directly visualized on conventional radiographs but may be seen on magnetic resonance imaging (MRI) studies. However, even MRI is unreliable for detecting early stages of chondromalacia, which may appear as foci or areas of diffuse abnormal signal with a normal surface. Grade III or IV chondromalacia is visible as thinning, irregularity, and fissuring of cartilage (Fig. 1-16).

Damage to the articular cartilage and joint surface may result indirectly from pathologic changes in subchondral bone. Both osteonecrosis and osteochondritis dissecans (OCD) may lead to destruction of the articular surface. In the knee, OCD tends to occur on the intercondylar aspect of the medial femoral condyle in young people. These lesions may separate from the surface and form a loose body. The base of these lesions, if débrided, will reveal vascular subchondral bone (Fig. 1-17). Classic radiographic findings include a lucent osseous defect that may have a fragmented or corticated osseous density within the lucency (Fig. 1-18). On MRI studies, increased signal about the defect on T2-weighted images represents joint fluid surrounding the lesion; irregularity of the articular surface may also be noted (Fig. 1-19). Osteonecrosis results in a similar osteochondral fragment but tends to occur in elderly patients on the weight-bearing aspect of the medial femoral condyle (Fig. 1-20). In distinction to the lesions in OCD, fragments in osteonecrosis separate from a bed of avascular bone (Fig. 1-21). Again, radiographs may reveal a lucent defect at the involved site, but MRI is more reliable for evaluation of these defects (Fig. 1-22). A curvilinear area of low signal with variable bone edema is characteristic. Although the articular cartilage is initially normal, both processes may lead to

detachment of osteochondral loose bodies, fragmentation, and collapse of the articular surface with resultant degenerative changes.

MENISCI

The menisci are two crescentic fibrocartilage structures that serve to deepen the articular surfaces of the tibia for reception of the femoral condyles (Fig. 1-23). The most abundant components of the menisci include collagen (75%) and noncollagenized proteins (8% to 13%). Glycosaminoglycans and glycoproteins are also key constituents. Although four main types of collagen are present in the menisci, type I collagen is the predominant component and accounts for about 90% of the total collagen. Histologic examination reveals a population of fibroblasts and fibrocartilaginous cells dispersed in an organized matrix of eosinophilic collagen fibrils. The collagen bundles are arranged in a circumferential pattern that is optimal for absorption of compressive loads (Fig. 1-24). Radial fibers found at the surface and in the midsubstance parallel to the plateau may act to increase structural rigidity and help prevent longitudinal splitting.[96] Elastin fibers, which constitute approximately 0.6% of the dry weight of the meniscus, seem to help in recoil to the original shape after deformation.[113] In degenerative menisci, metaplasia of the cell population occurs with a trend toward chondroid cell appearance (Fig. 1-25).

Each meniscus covers approximately the peripheral two thirds of the corresponding articular surface of the tibia. The peripheral border of each meniscus is thick, convex, and attached to the capsule of the joint; the opposite border tapers to a thin, free edge. The proximal surfaces of the menisci are concave and in contact with the femoral condyles; the distal surfaces are flat and rest on the tibial plateau. On MRI studies, normal menisci are best seen on sagittal views and have low-signal characteristics with no or little internal signal. The posterior horn of the medial meniscus is larger than the anterior horn, whereas the anterior and posterior horns of the lateral menisci are typically of similar size (Fig. 1-26). Increased signal within the menisci may be noted and classified on a scale ranging from I to III. Patchy areas of increased signal that do not touch the inferior and superior borders of the menisci represent grade I changes. Grade II changes typically have a linear configuration, but again they do not touch the superior and inferior surfaces. These signal changes probably represent the normal aging process in the menisci. Increased signal with a linear appearance that contacts one of the articular surfaces of the menisci is classified as grade III change and represents a true meniscal tear (Fig. 1-27).[78,105] A variety of meniscal tears may be identified on MRI but are best delineated by arthroscopic examination (Fig. 1-28). Patterns include vertical and horizontal cleavage tears, radial tears, bucket handle tears (detachment of the body of the menisci at the periphery with intact anterior and posterior horn attachments), and complex degenerative tears (Fig. 1-29). The technique of arthroscopic repair and partial meniscectomy has superseded open meniscectomy; therefore, examination of intact resected specimens is rarely possible (Fig. 1-30).

Calcification may occur within the fibrocartilage of the menisci and is referred to as *chondrocalcinosis*. This

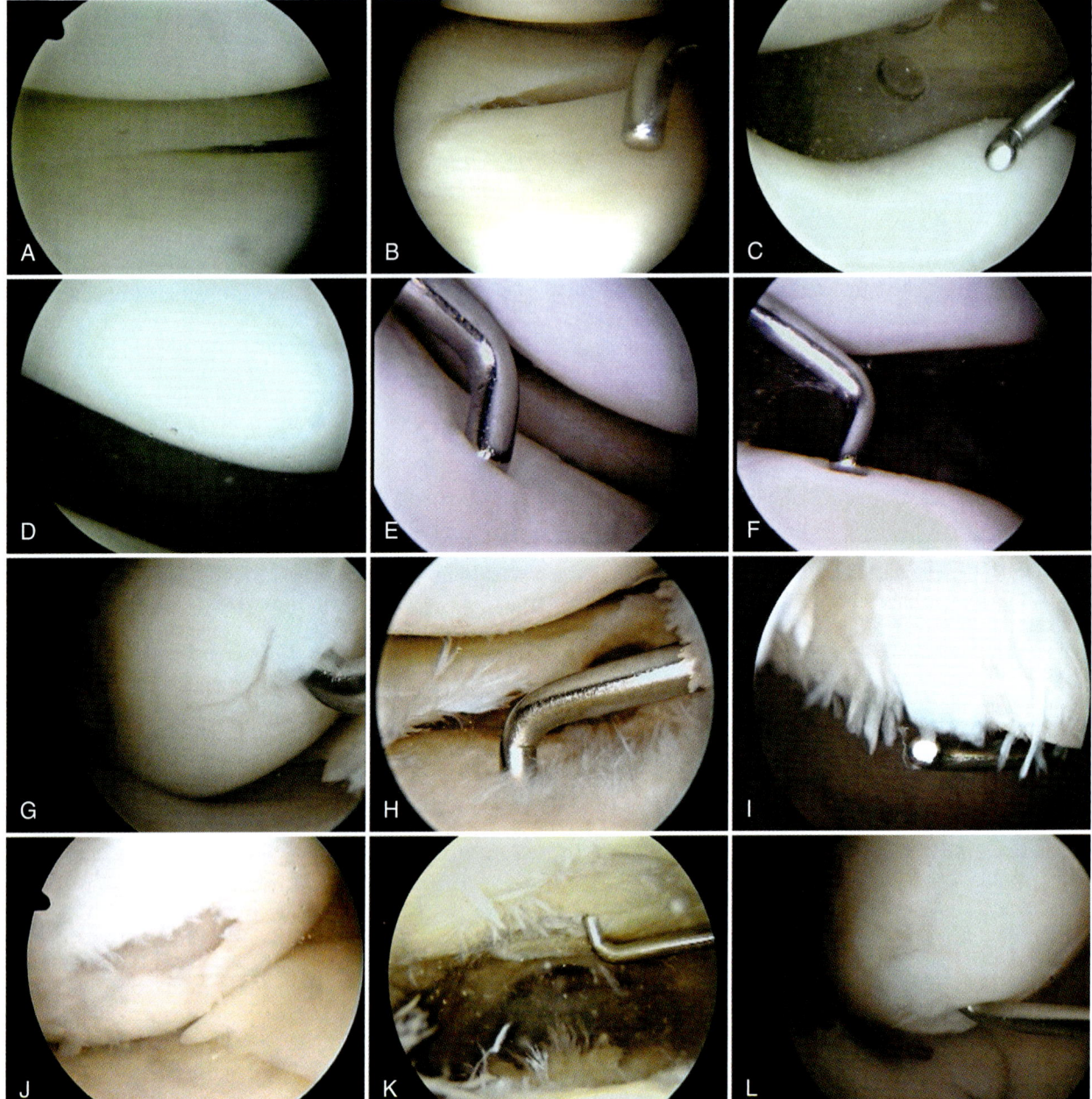

Figure 1-15. Arthroscopic views of articular cartilage. Normal white, smooth articular cartilage (Outerbridge grade 0) in the medial **(A)**, lateral **(B)**, and patellofemoral compartments **(C** and **D)**. Softening of the articular surface of the lateral tibial plateau **(E)** and the patellofemoral articulation **(F)** with indentation at the probe tip (Outerbridge grade I) is noted. **G,** A small fissure and fibrillation of the medial femoral condyle (Outerbridge grade II). Extensive fibrillation of the articular cartilage involving the tibial plateau **(H)** and the patella **(I)** (Outerbridge grade III). Erosion of articular cartilage to subchondral bone involving the medial femoral condyle **(J)** and patella **(K)** (Outerbridge grade IV). Arthroscopic view of a chondral flap tear **(L)**; the probe tip is deep to a flap of delaminated articular cartilage on the medial femoral condyle.

abnormality has classically been described in association with calcium pyrophosphate dihydrate deposition disease. However, chondrocalcinosis may be noted incidentally on radiographs or during arthroscopic examination (Fig. 1-31).

The menisci perform several important functions, including (1) load transmission across the joint, (2) enhancement of articular conformity, (3) distribution of synovial fluid across the articular surface, and (4) prevention of soft tissue impingement during joint motion. The medial meniscus also confers some stability to the joint in the presence of ACL insufficiency, in that the posterior horn acts as a wedge to help reduce anterior tibial translation.[76] However, the lateral meniscus does not perform a similar function.[75] The rapid progression of degenerative changes, first observed by Fairbank, that occur as a result of complete meniscectomy have been well documented.[30] These changes include (1) osteophyte formation on the femoral condyle projecting over the site of meniscectomy, (2) flattening of the femoral condyle, and (3) narrowing of joint space in the involved compartment.

Text continued on page 16

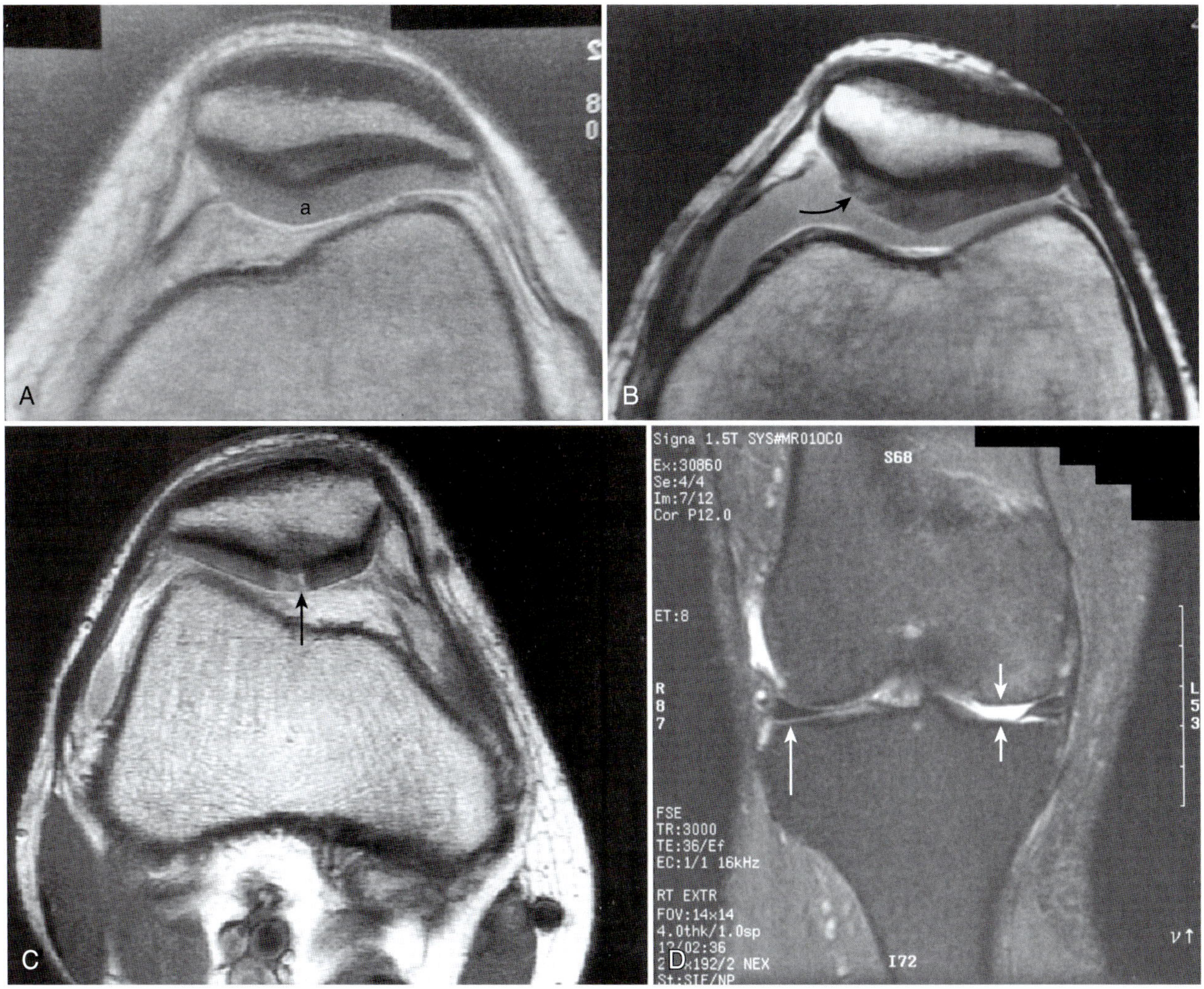

Figure 1-16. **A,** Axial magnetic resonance image (MRI) showing normal articular cartilage *(a)* on the patellar facets. The cartilage has a uniform signal thickness and appearance. **B,** Axial MRI revealing fissuring and fibrillation of articular cartilage on the medial facet of the patella *(arrow)*. **C,** Axial MRI with advanced chondromalacia of the patella. The signal irregularity extends to subchondral bone, and a deep fissure is identified *(arrow)*. **D,** Coronal MRI demonstrating complete loss of the articular cartilage of the medial compartment *(short arrows)*. For comparison, the gray band of articular cartilage on the lateral tibial plateau is also identified *(long arrow)*.

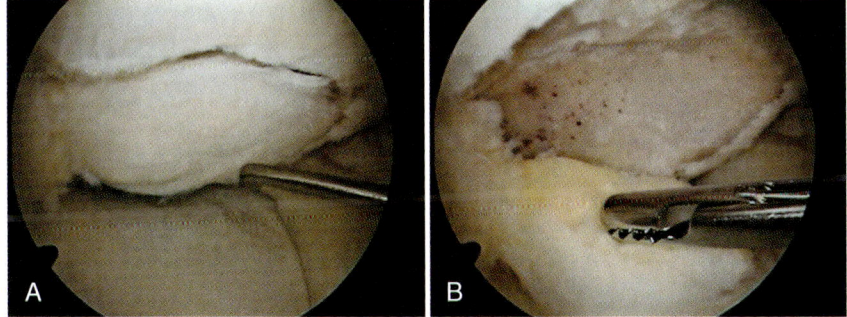

Figure 1-17. Arthroscopic view of osteochondritis of the femoral condyle. **A,** Osteochondral fragment of the articular surface of the femoral condyle. **B,** Punctate bleeding from the base of vascular subchondral bone with the osteochondral fragment mobilized.

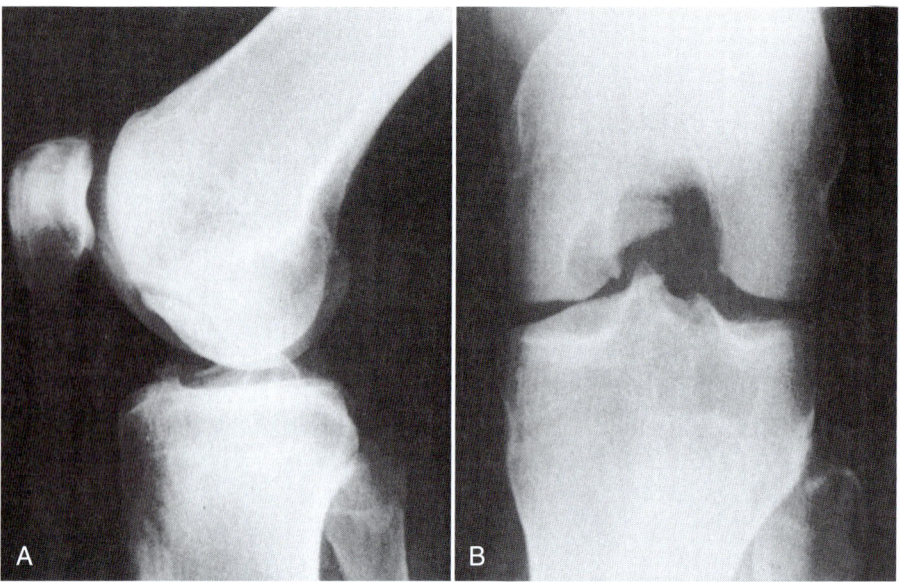

Figure 1-18. Radiographs of osteochondritis dissecans. Lateral **(A)** and tunnel **(B)** views show an osseous density within a lucent defect on the medial femoral condyle.

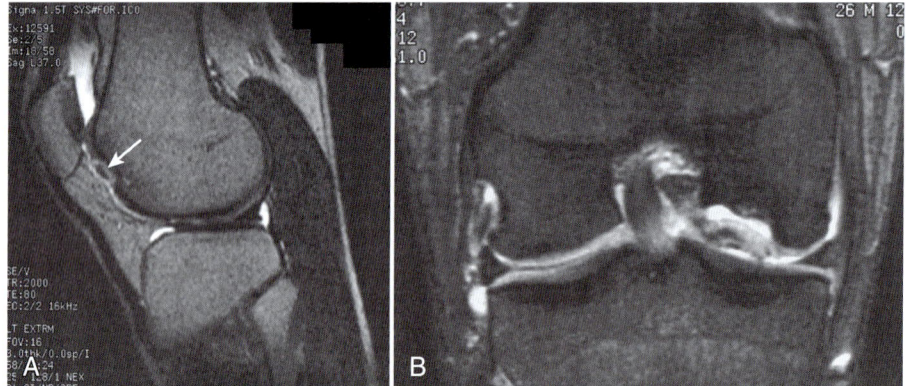

Figure 1-19. A, Sagittal magnetic resonance image (MRI) demonstrating a well-demarcated osteochondral lesion *(arrow)* in the anterior aspect of the lateral femoral condyle. **B,** Coronal MRI showing high-signal fluid about a loose osteochondral fragment of the medial femoral condyle. (Courtesy Martin Broker, MD.)

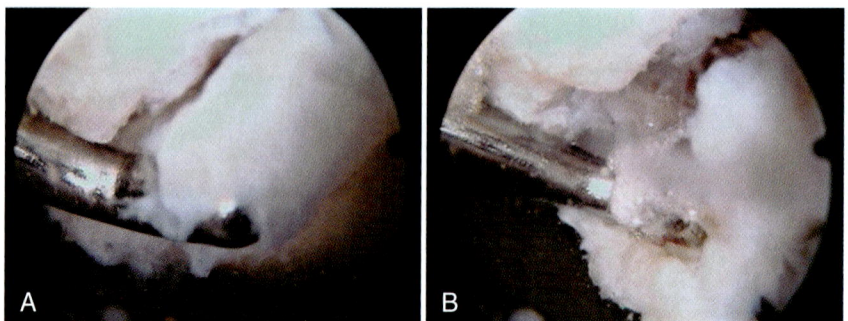

Figure 1-20. Arthroscopic views of osteonecrosis of the femoral condyle. **A,** Disruption of the articular surface by a detached osteochondral fragment. **B,** A probe elevates the loose fragment to reveal a base of almost completely avascular, dead subchondral bone.

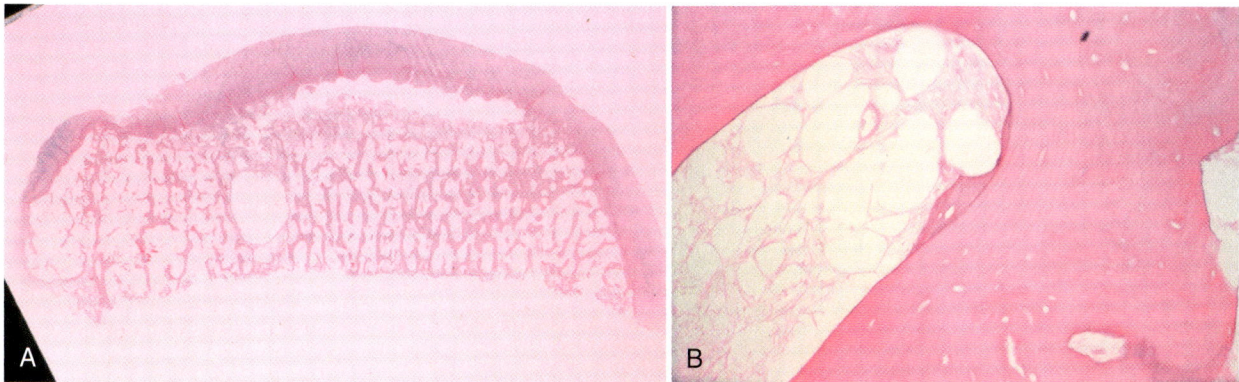

Figure 1-21. **A,** Osteonecrosis. A subchondral lucent zone is surrounded by intact articular cartilage and a thin plate of subchondral bone superficially with collapsed necrotic bone and granulation tissue inferiorly. **B,** Osteonecrosis (high power). Dead bone is characterized by marrow fat necrosis imparting a foggy, acellular appearance and bone devoid of osteocytes (empty lacunar spaces) and bone-lining cells.

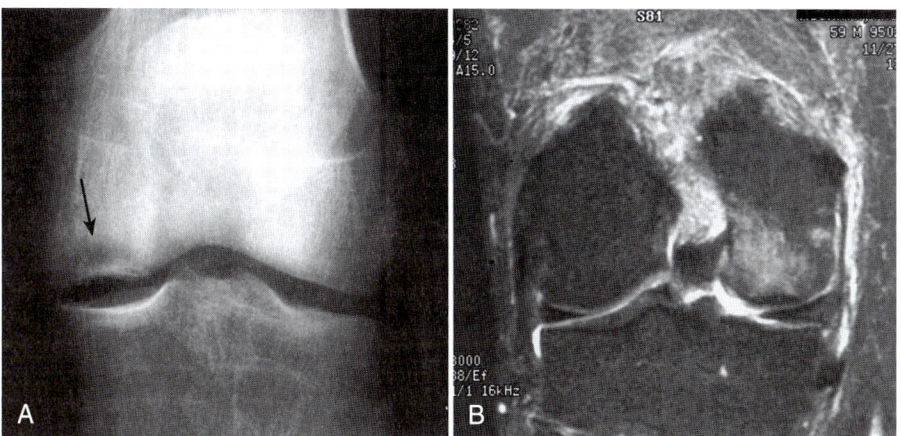

Figure 1-22. Osteonecrosis. **A,** Anteroposterior radiograph of the knee with focal lucency and flattening of the articular surface of the medial femoral condyle *(arrow).* **B,** Fat-suppressed proton density coronal magnetic resonance image with a curvilinear area of low signal in the necrotic bone and surrounding marrow edema.

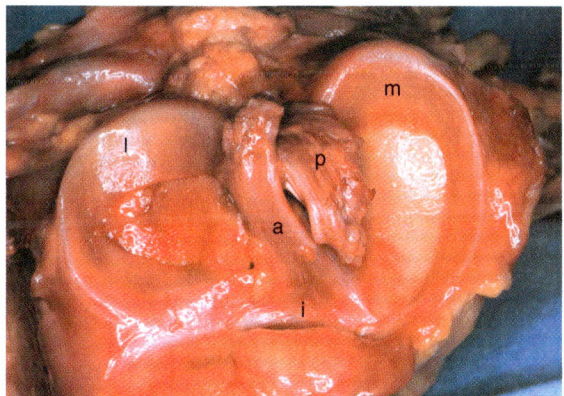

Figure 1-23. Anatomic dissection of the tibial plateau. The menisci act to increase the conformity of the articular surface of the tibial plateau. The medial meniscus *(m)* is C shaped, whereas the lateral meniscus *(l)* is more circular. Remnants of the anterior cruciate ligament *(a)* and posterior cruciate ligament *(p)* are also marked, as is the transverse intermeniscal ligament *(i).*

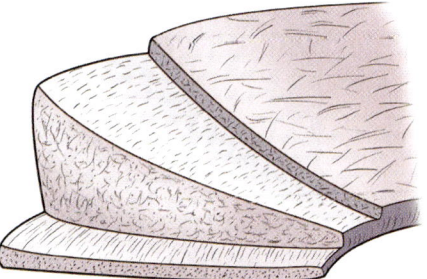

Figure 1-24. Trilaminar cross-sectional area of the meniscus.

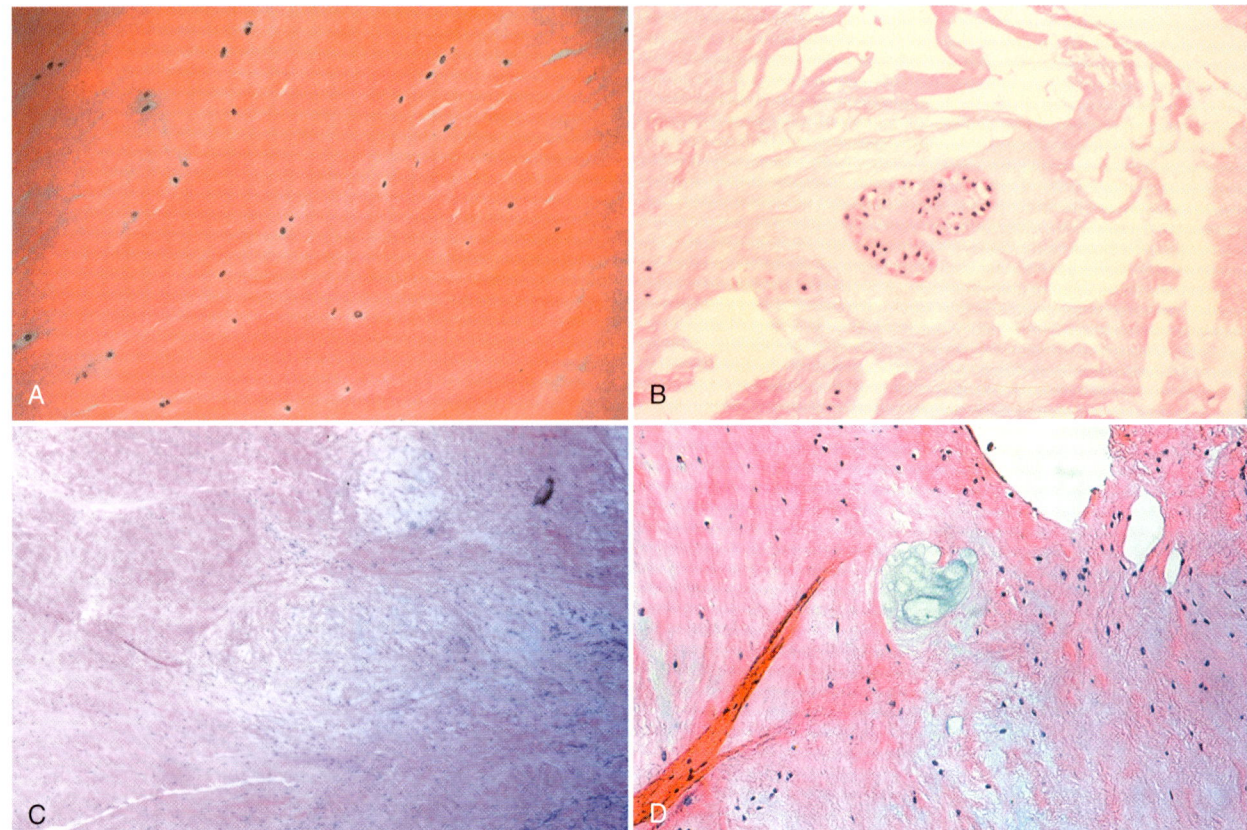

Figure 1-25. Cross-section of the medial meniscus (fibrocartilage) demonstrating the eosinophilic collagen matrix in interwoven bands, within which can be seen the nuclei of fibroblasts, here more prominent than those seen in tendons and ligaments, with occasional perinuclear spaces, often similar to immature cartilaginous cells **(A)**. With trauma or degeneration, chondroid metaplasia **(B)**, loss of matrix **(C)**, and cystic changes **(D)** take place.

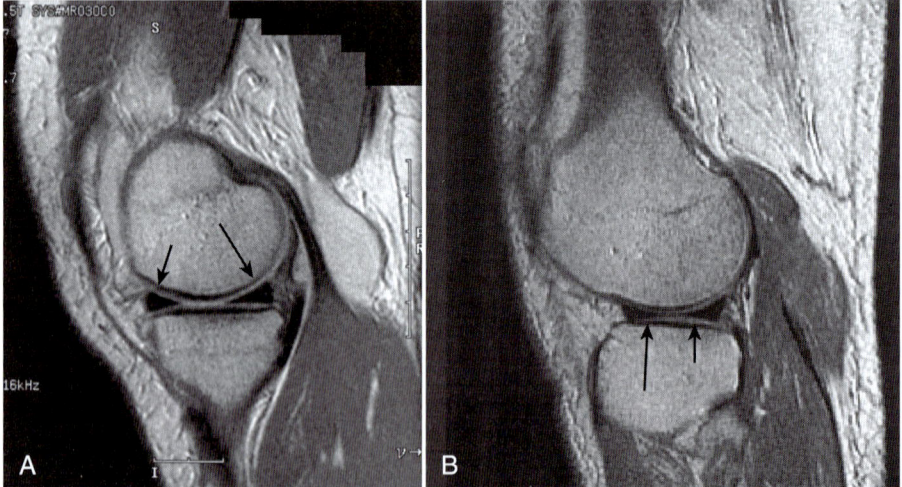

Figure 1-26. A, Sagittal magnetic resonance image (MRI) of the medial compartment with a normal medial meniscus. The posterior horn *(long arrow)* is larger than the anterior horn *(short arrow)*. **B,** Sagittal MRI of the lateral compartment of the knee. The low-signal anterior and posterior horns of the lateral meniscus *(long arrow* and *short arrow,* respectively) have a uniform appearance and a triangular shape.

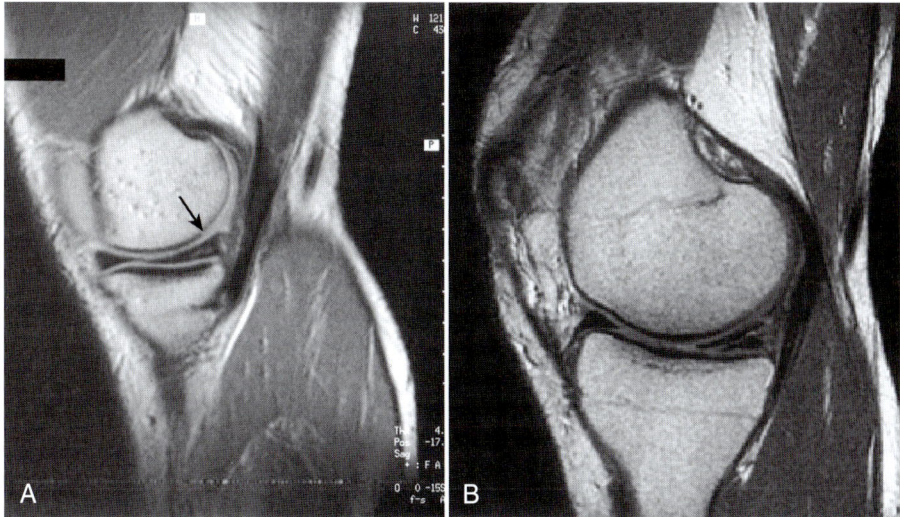

Figure 1-27. Sagittal magnetic resonance images. **A,** Linear intrameniscal signal *(arrow)* in the posterior horn that does not contact the meniscal surface (grade II). **B,** Obliquely oriented linear signal in the posterior horn of the medial meniscus. The signal abnormality touches the inferior surface and is consistent with a meniscal tear (grade III).

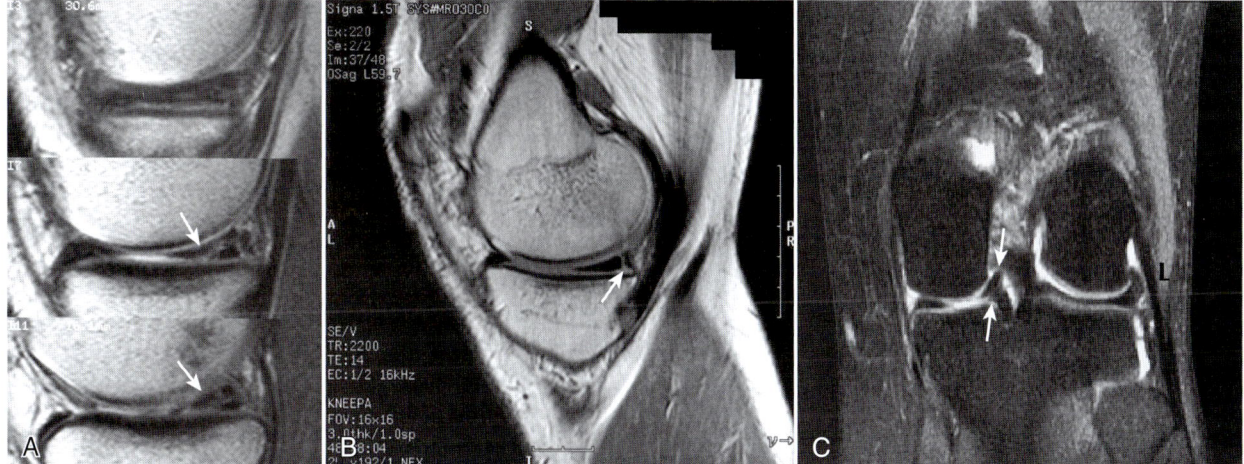

Figure 1-28. A, Three sagittal magnetic resonance imaging (MRI) views ("meniscal windows") with multiple linear intrameniscal signals that contact the superior *(arrow, lower left image)* and inferior meniscal surfaces *(arrow, middle left image)* representing a complex degenerative tear. **B,** Sagittal MRI showing a peripheral vertical cleavage tear *(arrow)* of the posterior horn of the medial meniscus. **C,** Coronal MRI demonstrating a displaced bucket handle meniscal tear with the fragment displaced into the notch *(arrows)*. The lateral collateral ligament *(L)* is also well visualized.

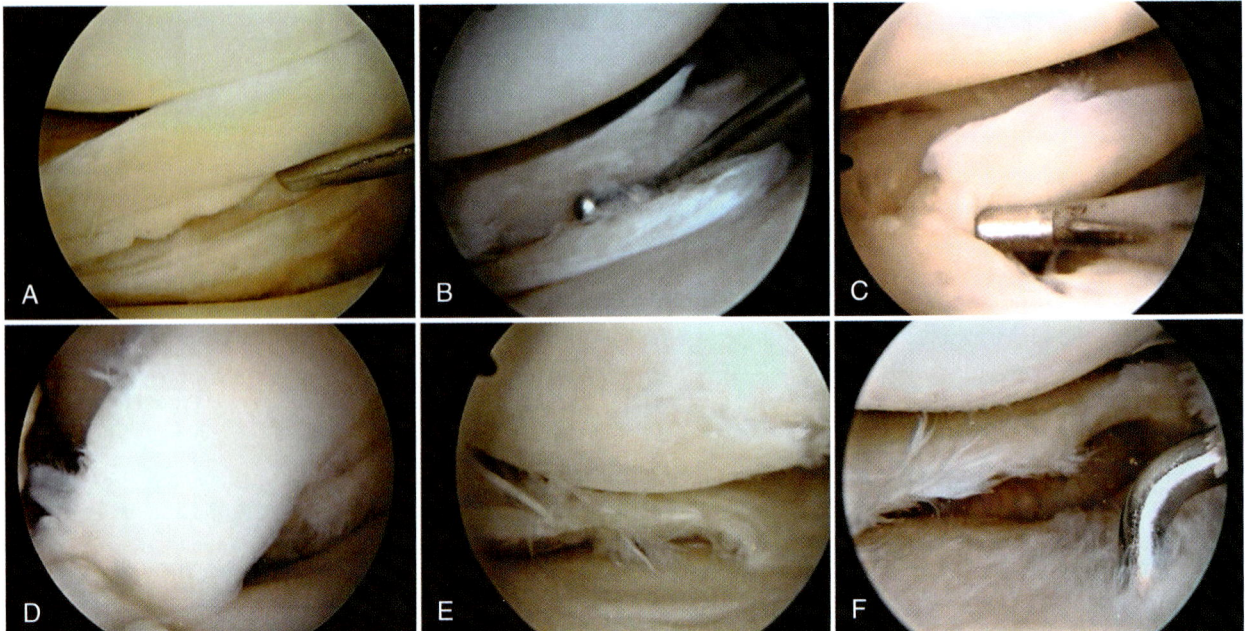

Figure 1-29. Arthroscopic views of meniscal tears. **A,** Vertical cleavage tear with separation of the meniscus from the peripheral attachment. **B,** Horizontal cleavage meniscal tear. **C,** Radial tear in the midbody of the meniscus. **D,** Detached meniscal bucket handle tear with a fragment displaced into the intercondylar notch. **E,** Complex degenerative tear of the posterior body and horn of the medial meniscus. **F,** Degenerative fraying of the meniscus without a gross tear.

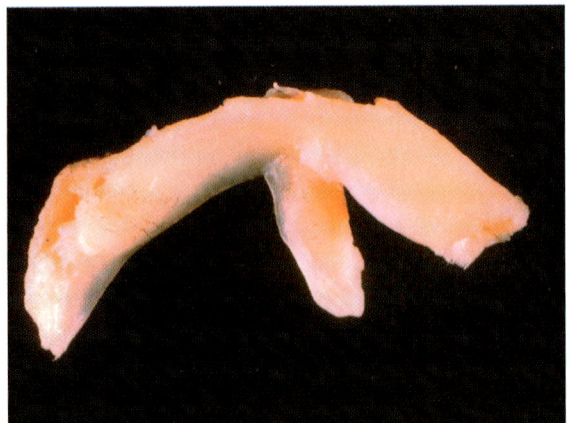

Figure 1-30. Gross anatomic specimen of a torn meniscus.

Medial Meniscus

The medial meniscus is nearly semicircular in form and measures about 3.5 cm in length. It has a triangular cross-section and is asymmetrical, with a considerably wider posterior than anterior horn. The attachment of the posterior horn, the so-called meniscal root, is firmly attached to the posterior portion of the intercondylar fossa of the tibia, directly anterior to the PCL insertion (Fig. 1-32). The functional importance of the meniscal root has become better appreciated over the past 5 years. Tears of the meniscal root destabilize the meniscus and are associated with meniscal extrusion on MRI.[74] As a result, it has been theorized that root tears appear to produce the same functional changes as total medial meniscectomy.[4,46,74,82] This is believed to be a significant risk factor in the development of early osteoarthritic changes.[4,74] In biomechanical studies, evidence to support the MRI findings has been forthcoming, with data showing increased joint contact pressures and altered knee kinematics; indeed, these changes are similar to those seen after total meniscectomy that have been associated with subsequent articular cartilage damage and osteoarthritic changes.[4,82] It is important to note that repair of a root tear appears to improve the function of the meniscus and may reduce the risk of early osteoarthritic changes.[4,46,82]

The anterior attachment of the meniscus is more variable; usually, it is firmly attached to the anterior intercondylar fossa approximately 7 mm anterior to the anterior margin of the ACL insertion, in line with the medial tibial tubercle, but this attachment can be flimsy.[56] Also, a fibrous band of variable thickness, the transverse intermeniscal ligament, connects the anterior horn of the medial meniscus with the lateral meniscus (Fig. 1-33). Peripherally, the medial meniscus is continuously attached to the capsule of the knee. The midpoint of the medial meniscus is more firmly attached to the femur via a condensation in the capsule known as the deep medial ligament (Fig. 1-34). The tibial attachment of the meniscus, sometimes known as the coronary ligament, attaches to the tibial margin a few millimeters distal to the articular surface, where it gives rise to a synovial recess. Posteromedially, according to Kaplan, the meniscus receives a portion of the insertion of the semimembranosus via the capsule.[61]

Lateral Meniscus

In contrast to the **C**-shaped medial meniscus, the lateral meniscus is nearly circular and covers a larger portion of the articular surface (see Fig. 1-32). The anterior horn is attached to the intercondylar fossa, directly anterior to the lateral tibial tubercle and adjacent to the ACL. The posterior horn

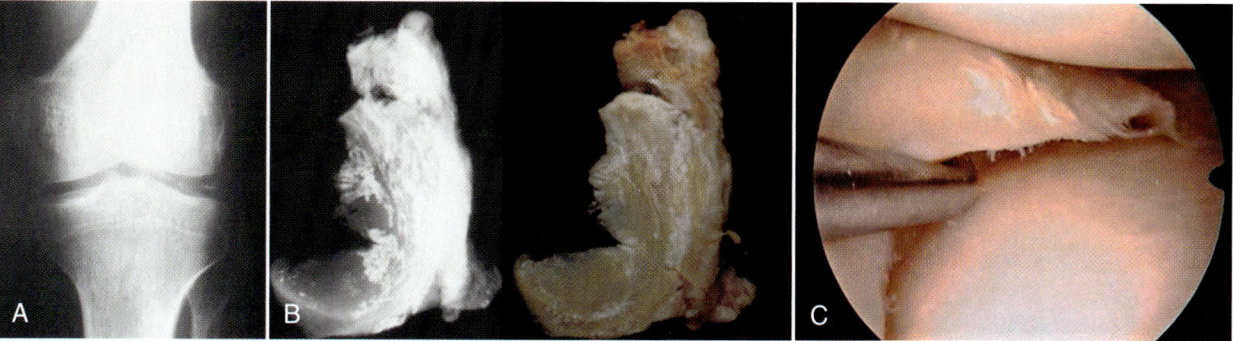

Figure 1-31. **A,** Anteroposterior radiograph of a knee with calcium pyrophosphate dihydrate deposition disease. **B,** Gross meniscus and specimen radiograph. **C,** Arthroscopic view of chondrocalcinosis of the lateral meniscus. (From Vigorita AJ: The synovium. In Orthopedic pathology, Philadelphia, 1999, Lippincott Williams & Wilkins, 1999.)

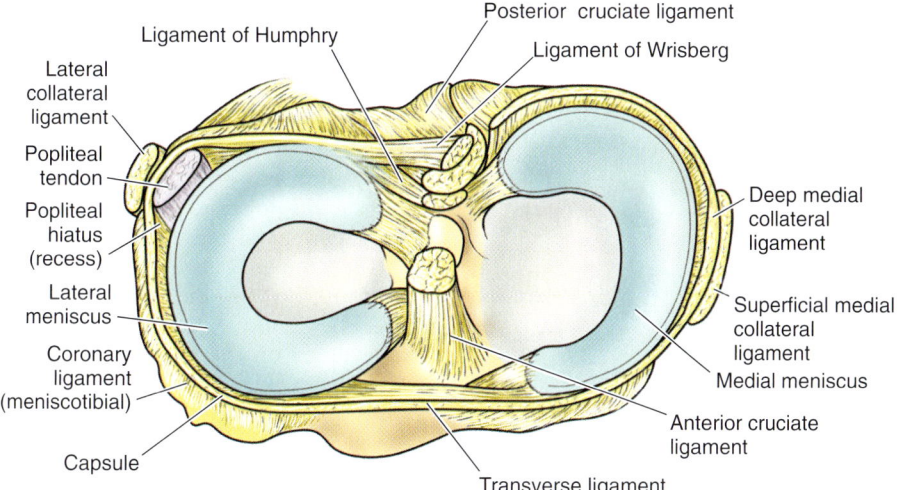

Figure 1-32. Superior aspect of the tibial plateau.

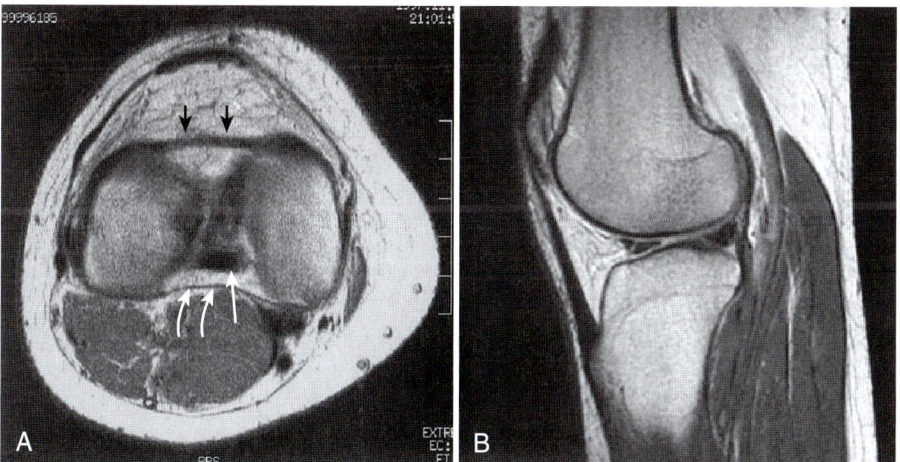

Figure 1-33. **A,** Axial magnetic resonance image (MRI) with the low-signal transverse intermeniscal ligament *(short arrows)* connecting the anterior horns of the medial and lateral menisci. The posterior capsule *(curved arrows)* and the posterior cruciate ligament *(long arrow)* are also identified. **B,** Sagittal MRI through the lateral compartment of the knee shows the interface between the transverse intermeniscal ligament and the anterior horn of the meniscus. This may be misidentified as a meniscal tear.

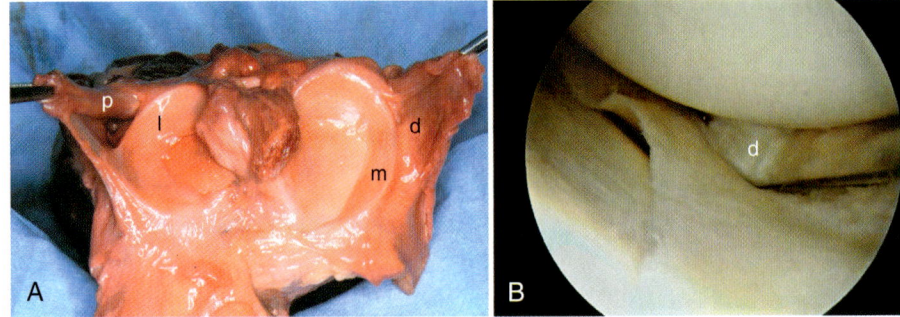

Figure 1-34. A, Tibial plateau. The C-shaped medial meniscus has a continuous attachment to the capsule. The deep medial collateral ligament (MCL) *(d,* retracted in the forceps) is directly attached to the periphery of the midbody of the medial meniscus *(m).* Laterally, the popliteus tendon *(p,* retracted in the forceps) enters the joint via the popliteal hiatus. In this location, the capsular attachment of the lateral meniscus *(l)* is interrupted. **B,** Arthroscopic view of the deep MCL. The fibers of the deep MCL *(d),* which represent a thickening in the medial capsule, can be seen at the tip of the probe.

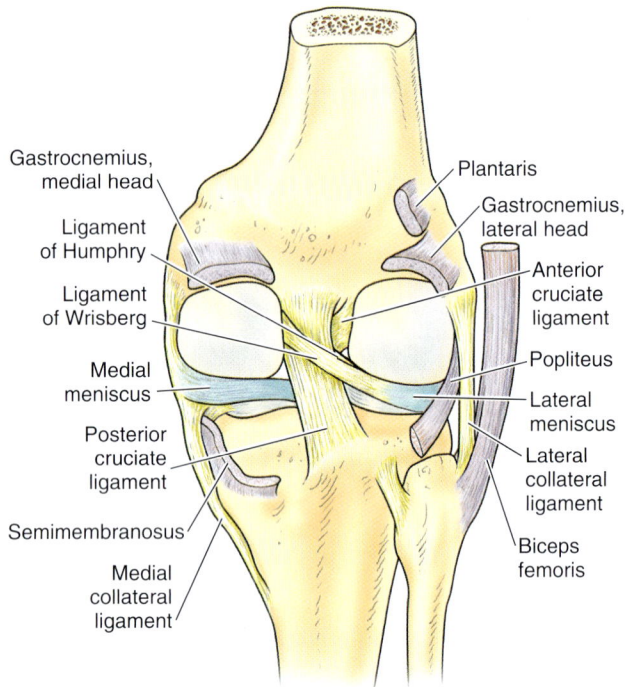

Figure 1-35. Posterior aspect of the knee. The ligaments of Humphry and Wrisberg, which attach the posterior horn of the lateral meniscus to the medial femoral condyle, embrace the posterior cruciate ligament. The popliteal tendon partially inserts into the posterolateral aspect of the lateral meniscus.

only a small percentage of specimens.[96,111,114] Meniscofemoral ligaments running from the anterior horns of the medial and lateral menisci to the intercondylar notch anterior to the ACL have also been identified. Wan and Felle[114] reported a 15% incidence of both of these structures in 60 cadaver knees, and one or the other was present in 25% of specimens. In general, the ligaments of Wrisberg and Humphry were much more robust structures than either of the meniscofemoral ligaments originating from the anterior horns.

The peripheral capsular attachment of the medial meniscus is continuous, but the attachment of the lateral meniscus is interrupted by the popliteal hiatus, through which passes the popliteal tendon (Fig. 1-37). In addition, unlike the anatomy on the medial side, the lateral meniscus does not have a direct attachment to the collateral ligament. Posterolaterally at the popliteal hiatus, the lateral meniscus is grooved by the popliteal tendon. Some fibers of the tendon insert into the periphery and superior border of the meniscus at this site.[62,63] Because the lateral meniscus is not as extensively attached to the capsule as the medial meniscus is, it is more mobile and may displace up to 1 cm. The controlled mobility of the lateral meniscus, which is guided by the popliteal tendon and meniscofemoral ligament attachments, may explain why meniscal injuries occur less frequently on the lateral side.[71,72] Although the meniscofemoral ligaments appear to perform an important function, little is known about the significance of injury to these structures.

CAPSULE

The capsule is a fibrous membrane containing areas of thickening that may be referred to as discrete ligaments. The anterior capsule is thin, and directly anteriorly it is replaced by the patellar ligament. Proximally, the capsule of the knee joint attaches to the femur approximately three to four fingerbreadths above the patella. Distally, it attaches circumferentially to the tibial margin, except where the popliteal tendon enters the joint through the hiatus. Posteriorly, the capsule consists of vertical fibers that arise from the condyles and walls of the intercondylar fossa of the femur. In this region, the capsule is augmented by fibers of the oblique popliteal ligament, which is derived from the semimembranosus tendon. This broad, flat band is attached proximally to

is attached to the intercondylar fossa directly posterior to the lateral tibial tubercle and adjacent and anterior to the posterior horn of the medial meniscus.[56] Somewhat variable fibrous bands, the meniscofemoral ligaments, connect the posterior horn of the lateral meniscus to the intercondylar wall of the medial femoral condyle. These meniscofemoral ligaments, which embrace the PCL, are also known by the eponyms Humphry and Wrisberg (Fig. 1-35). The ligament of Humphry passes anterior to the PCL, whereas the ligament of Wrisberg passes posterior to the PCL (Fig. 1-36). One or the other of these meniscofemoral ligaments has been identified in 71% to 100% of cadaver knees; the ligament of Wrisberg is a more constant finding, and both ligaments together are found in

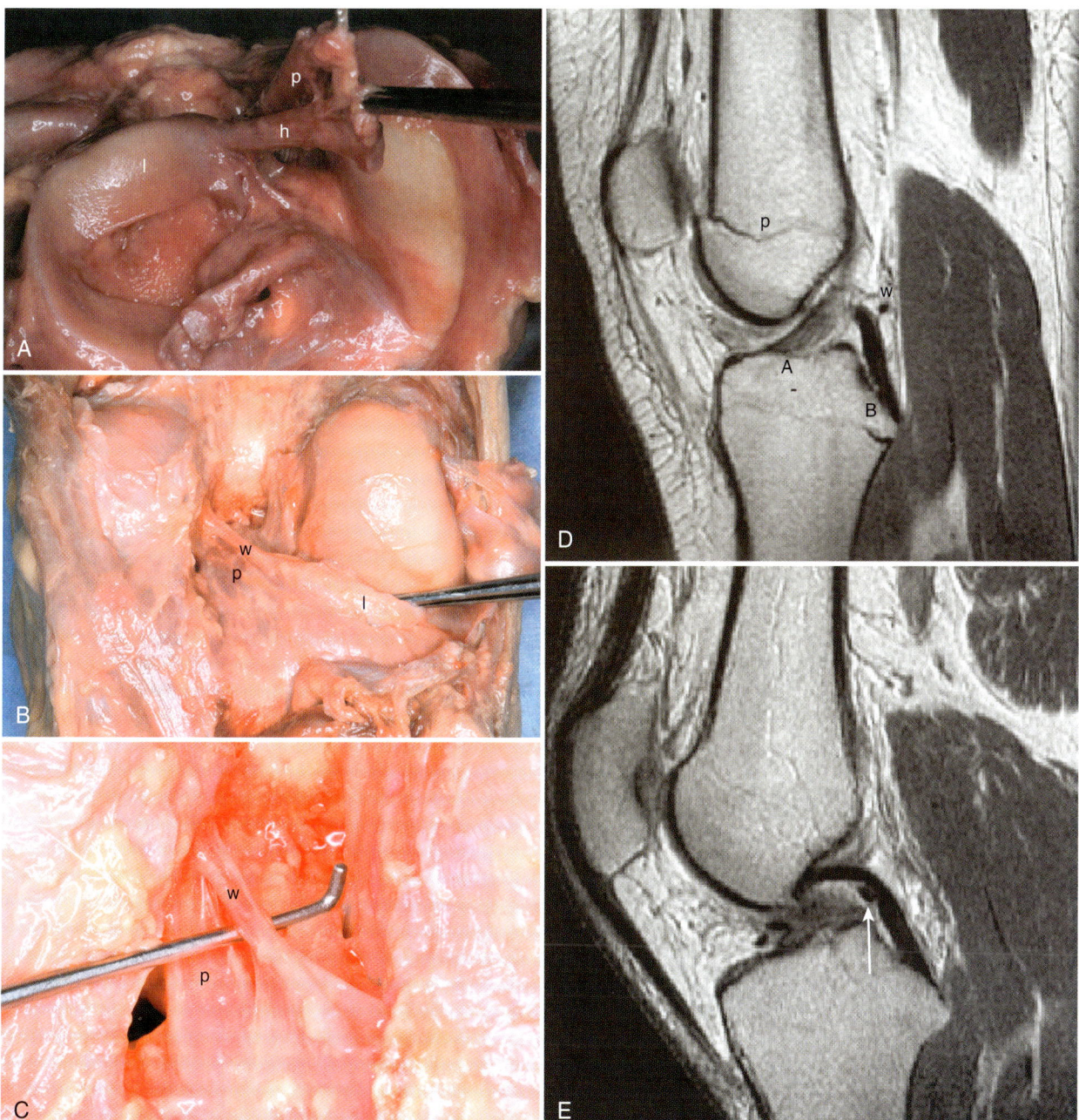

Figure 1-36. Meniscofemoral ligaments. **A,** The ligament of Humphry (*h,* retracted in the forceps) arises from the posterior horn of the lateral meniscus *(l)* and passes anterior to the posterior cruciate ligament (PCL) *(p).* **B,** Posterior view of the knee with the capsule removed laterally, revealing the ligament of Wrisberg *(w),* which originates from the lateral meniscus (*l,* tip of the forceps) and then passes posterior to the PCL *(p).* **C,** Close-up view of an anatomic dissection of the posterior aspect of the knee, with the capsule removed from the intercondylar notch. The ligament of Wrisberg *(w)* lies posterior to the PCL fibers *(p).* **D,** Sagittal magnetic resonance image (MRI) showing the ligament of Wrisberg *(w)* posterior to the PCL **(B).** Also identified are the anterior cruciate ligament *(A)* and the physeal scar *(P).* **E,** Sagittal MRI with the small oval ligament of Humphry identified anterior to the PCL *(arrow).*

the margin of the intercondylar fossa and posterior surface of the femur close to the articular margins of the condyles. The fascicles are separated by apertures for the passage of vessels and nerves. The oblique popliteal ligament forms part of the floor of the popliteal fossa, and the popliteal artery rests on it. At the site of the popliteal hiatus, the capsule is displaced inferiorly toward the fibula head, forming the arcuate ligament between the lateral meniscus and the fibular styloid.

SYNOVIAL CAVITY

Synovium is normally a smooth, translucent pink tissue. Histologically, a thin layer of synovial cells, or synoviocytes, is found at the surface (Fig. 1-38). The synoviocytes consist of two cell populations, broadly classified into those that have macrophage-type function and those with a synthetic function. Type 1 cells contain numerous mitochondria, lysosomes, phagosomes, and surface undulations indicative of their

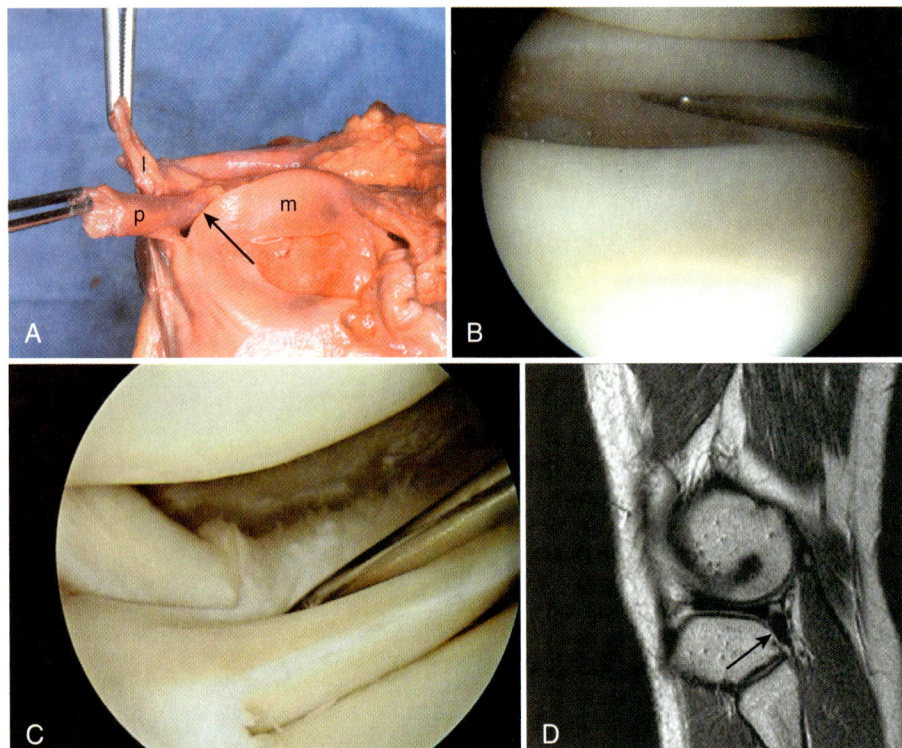

Figure 1-37. Popliteal hiatus. **A,** Anatomic dissection revealing incomplete capsular attachment of the lateral meniscus *(m)*. The popliteal tendon (*p,* anterior forceps) passes deep to the lateral collateral ligament (*l,* posterior forceps) through the hiatus *(arrow)*. **B,** Arthroscopic view of the popliteal hiatus with the lateral meniscus elevated superiorly. **C,** Arthroscopic view of the popliteal tendon passing between the periphery of the lateral meniscus and the capsule. **D,** Sagittal magnetic resonance image with the popliteus tendon *(arrow)* traversing the popliteal hiatus posterior to the lateral meniscus.

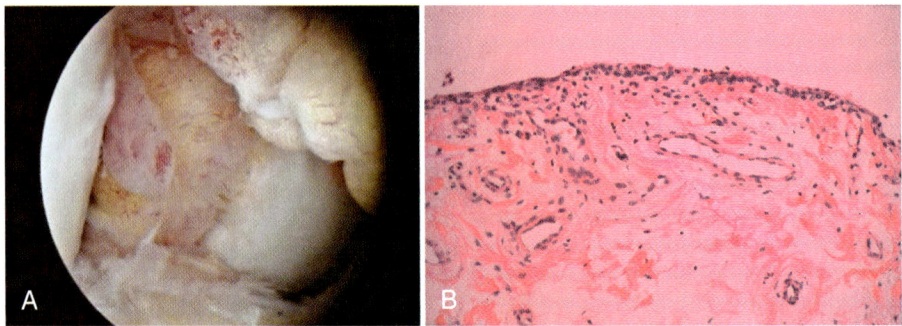

Figure 1-38. **A,** Arthroscopic view of normal synovium. Normal synovium is a fine pink layer that covers the intra-articular surfaces of the knee. **B,** Section of essentially normal synovium demonstrating the synovial intimal layer consisting of synoviocytes, one to two cells thick, beneath which rests the highly vascular subintimal layer, usually sparsely cellular, but containing fibroblasts, histiocytes, fat cells, and occasional mast cells.

macrophage function. Type 2 cells have rough endoplasmic reticulum and free ribosomes characteristic of secretory cells. This layer of cells, the intimal layer, lies above a fibrovascular zone, the subintimal layer, which contains arterioles, fat, and a variety of connective tissue cells, including fibroblasts and histiocytes. The fibrovascular zone gradually becomes more fibrous at capsular insertions. In specific disease processes, including rheumatoid arthritis, the synovium becomes hypertrophic and inflamed and contributes to intra-articular destruction (Fig. 1-39).

Synovium invests the interior of the knee joint and extends proximally into the suprapatellar pouch above the patella. The suprapatellar pouch is separated from the anterior surface of the femur by a layer of fat (Fig. 1-40). The uppermost limit of the pouch is attached to a small muscle, the articularis genus, which originates from the anterior surface of the femoral shaft. The articularis genus serves to prevent invagination of the suprapatellar pouch beneath the patella.

Intra-articularly, the synovium invests the cruciate ligaments and the popliteal tendon. A synovial recess or sleeve extends around the popliteal tendon for a variable distance beyond the posterolateral capsule. The synovium also lines the coronal recesses beneath the menisci and anteriorly invests the fat pad, which lies posterior to the patellar ligament and capsule. Although the synovium approximates the capsule, it is much more redundant. Synovial folds occur frequently, particularly in the suprapatellar pouch. Plicae

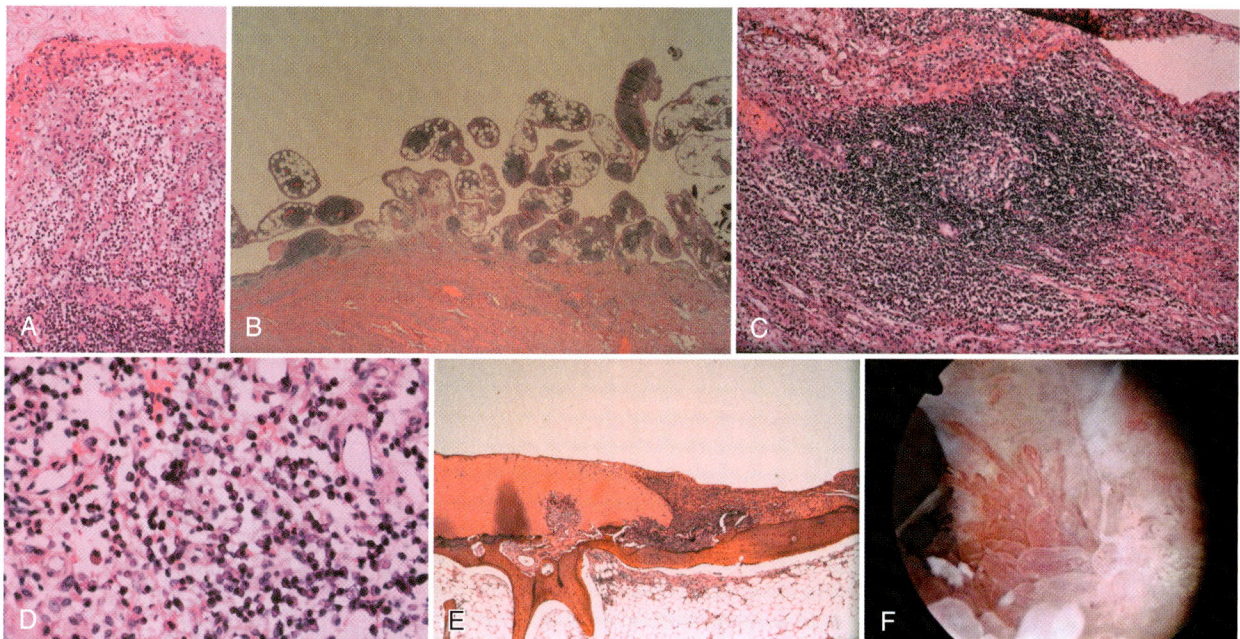

Figure 1-39. Rheumatoid synovium. In rheumatoid arthritis, the synovium becomes thickened, edematous, fibrinous, and inflamed (**A**). Marked lymphocytosis is seen (**B**, low power), along with germinal center formation (**C**) and plasma cell proliferation (**D**). The inflamed synovium or pannus (**E**) causes chondrolysis and invades the cartilage and bone. **F**, Arthroscopic view of inflamed synovium with hypertrophic, red villi.

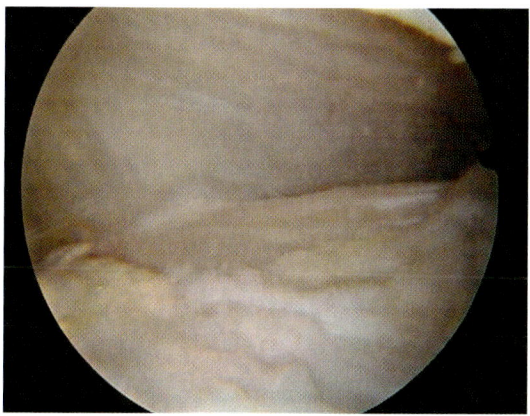

Figure 1-40. Arthroscopic view of the suprapatellar pouch. A thin layer of translucent synovium covers the interior surfaces.

probably represent remnants of synovial septa normally absorbed during embryonic development. The infrapatellar (ligamentum mucosum), suprapatellar, and medial patellar plicae are the three most common plicae (Fig. 1-41). Visualization of plicae on MRI studies can be difficult without an associated intra-articular effusion. In most cases, sagittal and axial images provide the best detail (Fig. 1-42). Rarely, plicae, especially medial patellar plicae, can become inflamed and painful; in these circumstances, arthroscopic resection may be considered.

The posterior synovial cavity communicates with a popliteal bursa that is found between the semimembranosus tendon and the medial head of the gastrocnemius in about 50% of people (Fig. 1-43).[121] This bursa may be distended when dye is injected into the knee; the bursa can also become enlarged by an intra-articular effusion, resulting in a popliteal or Baker's cyst. With this exception, the synovial cavity does

not normally communicate with any of the other bursae around the knee.

BURSAE

Of numerous bursae about the knee, those with the greatest clinical significance include the prepatellar, infrapatellar, and anserine bursae (Fig. 1-44). The prepatellar bursa is large and lies subcutaneously anterior to the patella. The infrapatellar bursa lies posterior to the patellar ligament and separates the ligament from the tibia and the lower portion of the fat pad. The pes anserinus bursa lies between the sartorius, gracilis, and semitendinosus tendons and the tibia; another bursa separates the superficial medial ligament from the pes tendons. These bursae may become inflamed as a result of trauma or overuse. The significance of the semimembranosus bursa has already been discussed.

CRUCIATE LIGAMENTS

The cruciate ligaments consist of a highly organized collagen matrix, which accounts for approximately three fourths of their dry weight. Most of the collagen is type I (90%), and the remainder is type III (10%).[27] In the ACL, collagen is organized into multiple fiber bundles 20 μm wide that are grouped into fascicles 20 to 400 μm in diameter.[23] Occasional fibroblasts and other substances, such as elastin (<5%) and proteoglycans (1%), make up the remainder of the dry weight.[27] Water constitutes 60% of the net weight under physiologic conditions. At the microscopic level, ligament and tendon insertions into bone have a characteristic structure consisting of collagen fibrils directly continuous with fibrils within the bone. A calcified front, similar to that seen between osteoid and mineralized bone, can be distinguished (Fig. 1-45).

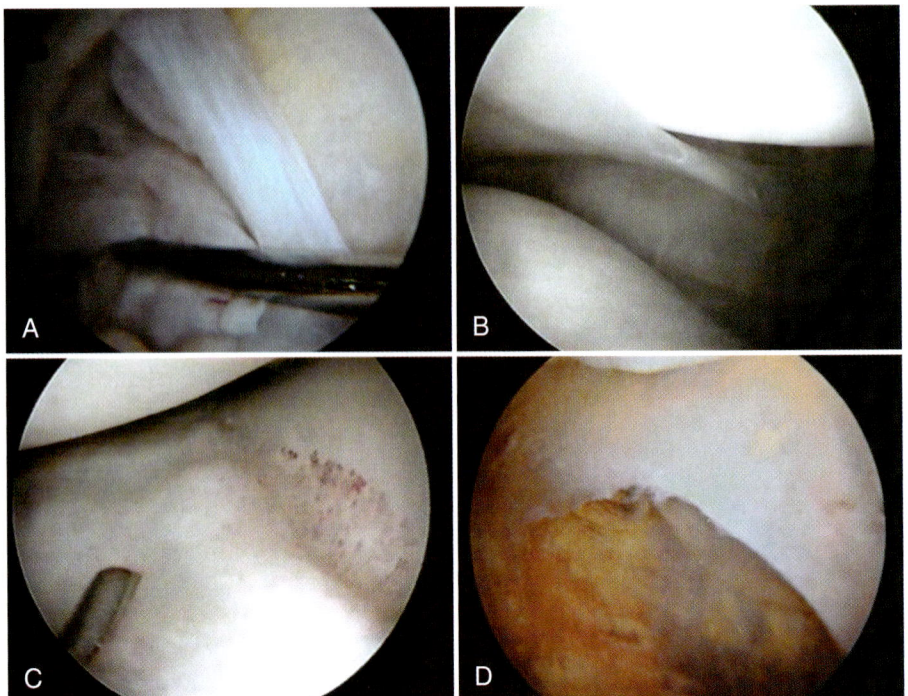

Figure 1-41. Arthroscopic views of intra-articular plicae. **A,** The infrapatellar plica (ligamentum mucosum) passes between the intercondylar notch and the anterior fat pad. **B,** A large medial patellar plica is seen interposed between the anterior surface of the medial femoral condyle and the patella. **C,** Thickening along the margin of a large medial patellar plica caused by irritation and abrasion on the femoral condyle. **D,** A suprapatellar plica may occlude the opening to the suprapatellar pouch. In some cases, this plica may be continuous with a medial patellar plica.

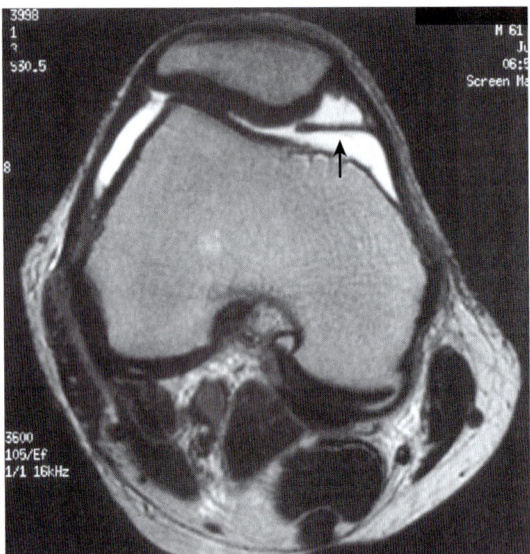

Figure 1-42. Axial magnetic resonance image with a low-signal, thick medial plica *(arrow)* that is highlighted by the large effusion.

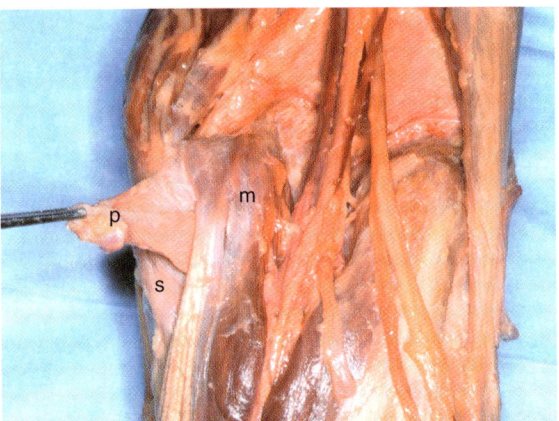

Figure 1-43. Popliteal bursa. Anatomic dissection of the popliteal fossa with a popliteal bursa *(p, forceps)* originating between the medial head of the gastrocnemius *(m)* and the semimembranosus tendon *(s)*.

The cruciate ligaments are named for their attachments on the tibia and are essential to function of the knee joint.[47,66,71,118] The cruciate ligaments act to stabilize the knee joint and prevent anteroposterior displacement of the tibia on the femur. The presence of numerous sensory endings also implies a proprioceptive function. These ligaments are intra-articular but, because they are covered by synovium, are considered extrasynovial. They receive their blood supply from branches of the middle genicular and both inferior genicular arteries. The anatomy of the cruciate ligaments has been studied by Girgis et al[36] (Fig. 1-46).

Anterior Cruciate Ligament

The ACL originates from the medial surface of the lateral femoral condyle posteriorly in the intercondylar notch in the form of a segment of a circle (Fig. 1-47). The anterior side of

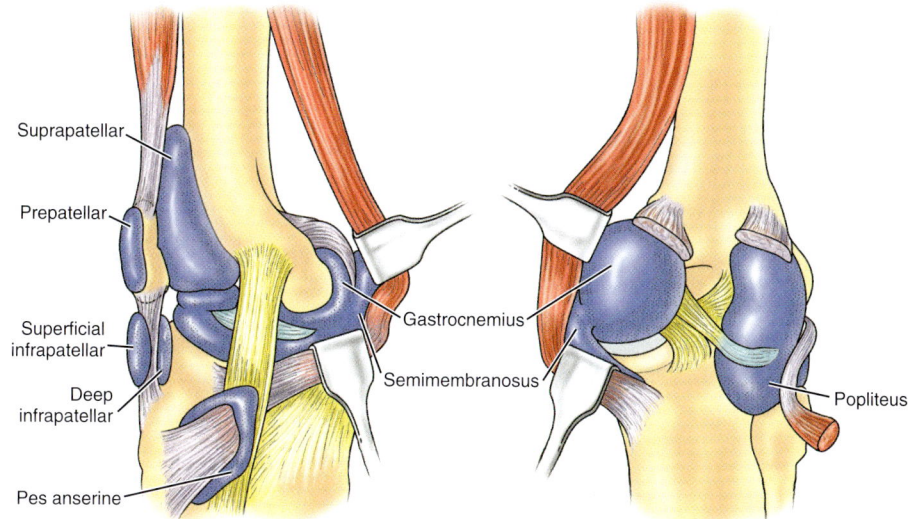

Figure 1-44. Bursae around the knee.

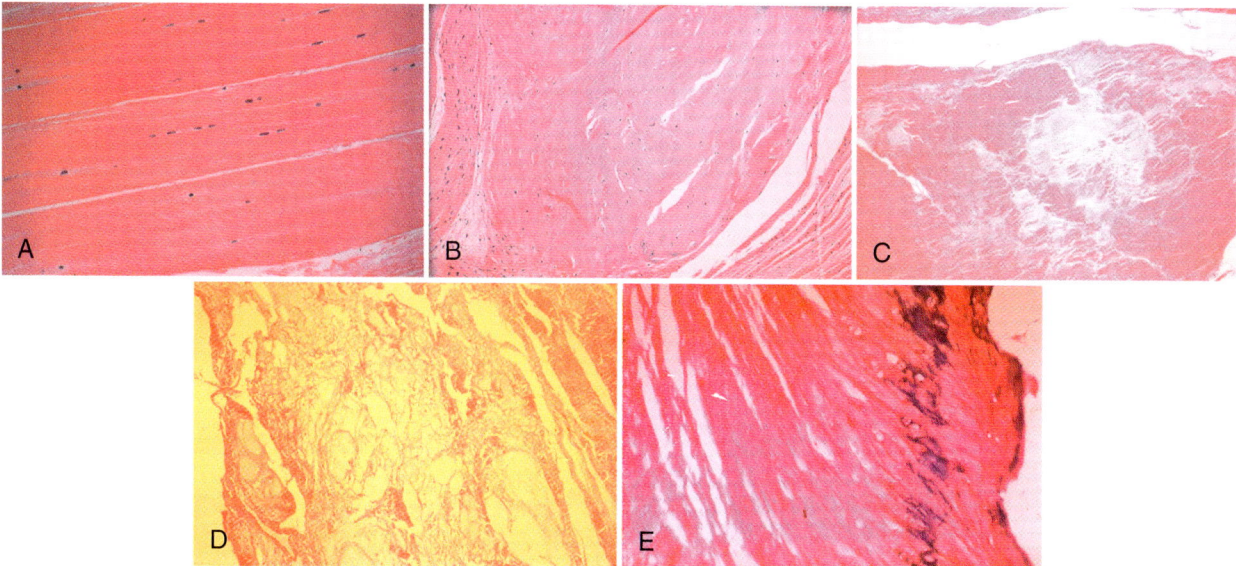

Figure 1-45. Tendon and ligament. **A,** A longitudinal segment of a ligament showing the sparsely cellular, highly eosinophilic collagenized matrix. The nuclei of the fibroblasts are relatively indistinct, dark, ovoid shapes, sometimes in columns enveloped by the collagen matrix. Chondroid metaplasia **(B),** loss of matrix **(C),** and cystic changes **(D)** occur with injury or degeneration. **E,** The fibrils of tendon and ligaments as they insert into bone provide a contiguous flow of fibrils through the calcifying zone (basophilic area) with direct continuity into the subchondral plate.

the attachment is almost straight and the posterior side convex. The ligament courses anteriorly, distally, and medially toward the tibia (Fig. 1-48). Over the length of its course, the fibers of the ligament undergo slight external rotation. The average length of the ligament is 38 mm and the average width 11 mm.[36] About 10 mm below the femoral attachment, the ligament stands out as it proceeds distally to the tibial attachment, which is a wide, depressed area anterior and lateral to the medial tibial tubercle in the intercondylar fossa (Fig. 1-49). The tibial attachment is oriented in an oblique direction and is more robust than the femoral attachment. A slip to the anterior horn of the lateral meniscus is well marked.[36]

Over the past decade, increasing importance has been placed on identification of discrete bundles within this ligament. Although the anatomic basis of this division has been debated for decades, with evidence to support a single anatomic structure, two discrete bundles, or even three bundles, the concept of two functional bundles is now well established.* The two bundles are defined by their respective tibial insertion with an anteromedial (AM) bundle and a posterolateral (PL) bundle.[5,20,93,120] The AM bundle originates in the proximal part of the femoral origin and inserts in the anteromedial portion of the tibial insertion; in distinction, the PL bundle originates distally in the femoral origin and inserts in the posterolateral aspect of the tibial insertion.[5,20,93,123] In the coronal plane, the AM bundle originates

---

*References 5, 36, 67, 89, 102, 123.

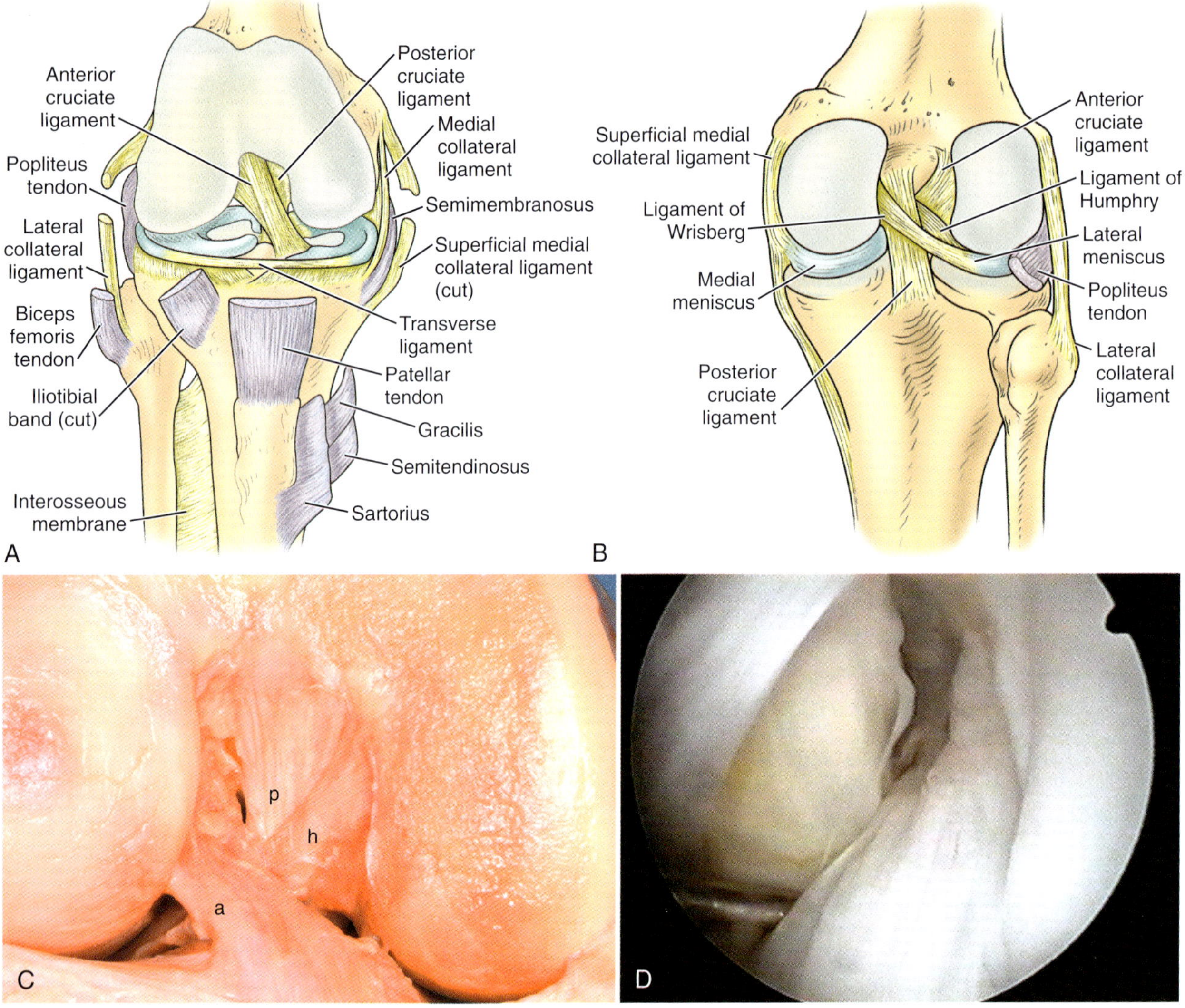

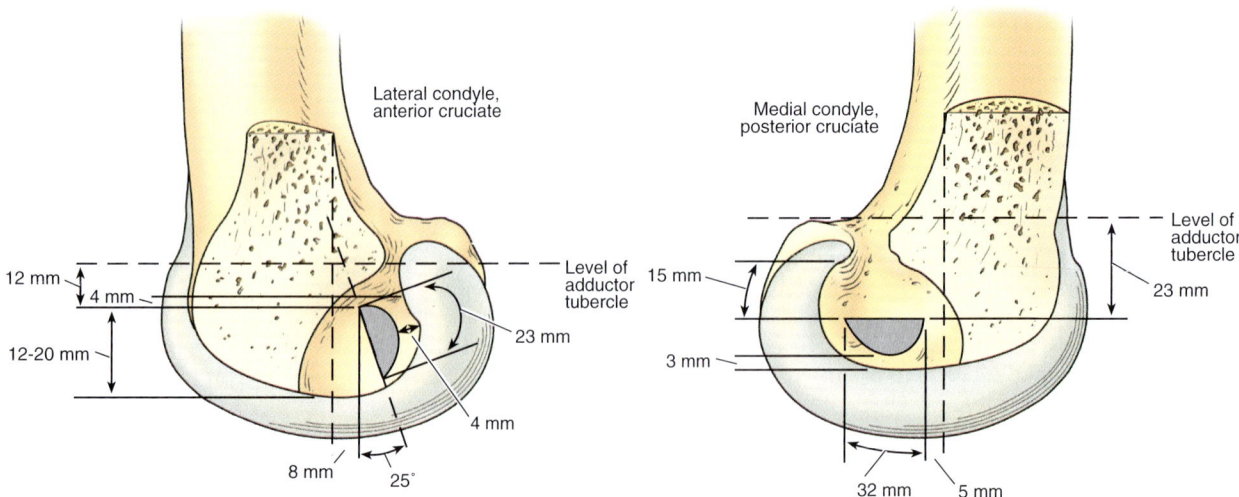

Figure 1-46. A, Anterior cruciate ligament (ACL) and **(B)** posterior cruciate ligament (PCL). **C,** Close-up of an anatomic specimen seen from the anterior aspect, demonstrating the relationship of the ACL *(a),* ligament of Humphry *(h),* and PCL *(p)* from anterior to posterior in the intercondylar notch. **D,** Arthroscopic view of the contents of the intercondylar notch showing, from left to right, the ligamentum mucosum, PCL, and ACL (probe posterior to the ACL).

Figure 1-47. Attachments of the anterior and posterior cruciate ligaments to the femur. (From Girgis FG, Marshall JL, Al Monajem ARS: The cruciate ligaments of the knee joint. Clin Orthop 106:216, 1975.)

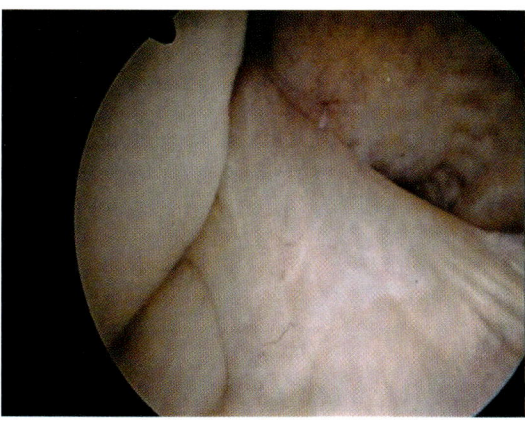

Figure 1-48. Arthroscopic view of a normal anterior cruciate ligament (ACL). The fibers of the ACL fan out distally, anteriorly, and medially to insert on the tibia. The origin of the posterior cruciate ligament can be visualized posterior to the ACL.

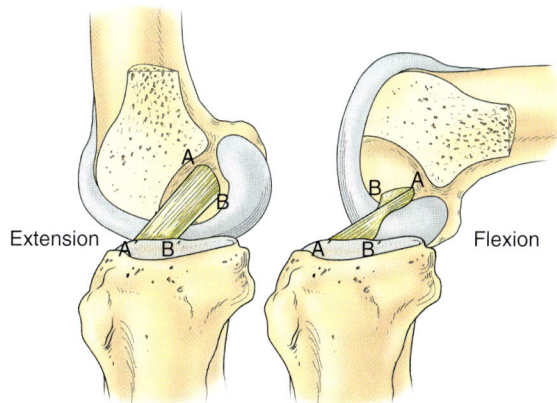

Figure 1-50. Diagram of the anterior cruciate ligament in extension and flexion. Note that in extension the posterolateral bulk is taut, whereas in flexion, the anteromedial band is tight and the posterolateral bulk is relatively relaxed. (From Girgis FG, Marshall JL, Al Monajem ARS: The cruciate ligaments of the knee joint. Clin Orthop 106:216, 1975.)

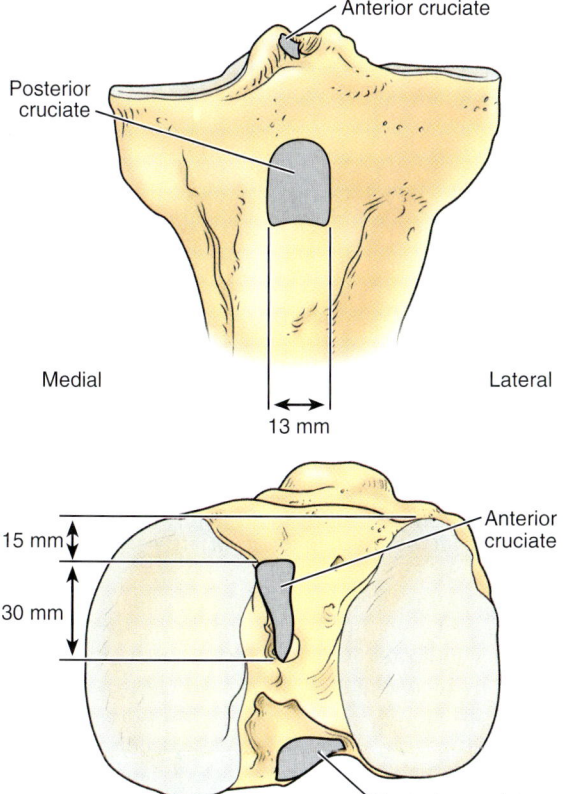

Figure 1-49. Attachments of the anterior and posterior cruciate ligaments to the tibia. (From Girgis FG, Marshall JL, Al Monajem ARS: The cruciate ligaments of the knee joint. Clin Orthop 106:216, 1975.)

at about the 10:30 clock position, and the PL bundle originates more horizontally at the 9:30 clock position.[93,123] Increased emphasis has been placed on these anatomic details during ACL reconstruction surgery, with a trend discussed in later chapters toward more anatomic ACL reconstruction with two-tunnel, double-bundle techniques, as well as through modifications to femoral tunnel placement in single-bundle techniques.[20,45,67,102]

The ACL is the prime static stabilizer against anterior translation of the tibia on the femur and accounts for up to 86% of the total force resisting anterior draw.[17,33,49,64] The bundles of the ligament are not isometric through the range of motion. Rather, at different stages of knee motion, the distinct functional bundles of the ACL have different roles in stabilizing the knee joint.[5,20,36,123] In extension, the bundles are parallel, but as the knee flexes, the femoral origin of the PL bundle moves anteriorly, and the bundles cross.[5,20,33,36,118] Functionally, the AM bundle tightens as the knee flexes and the PL bundle loosens; conversely, the PL bundle becomes tight as full extension is approached (Fig. 1-50).* Consequently, isolated rupture of the AM bundle will tend to have a greater effect on the anterior draw test (performed at 90 degrees of flexion), and failure of the PL bundle will have a greater effect on the Lachman test (performed at 30 degrees of flexion).[5,33] The PL bundle also plays an important role in resisting internal and external rotation.[5,20,123] Changes in ACL reconstruction techniques, attained through double-bundle reconstruction or by placing the femoral tunnel origin more horizontally in the notch, have been driven by the desire to better restore the functional effects of the PL bundle in resisting rotation, as well as anterior translation.[20,45,102] The current criticism of single-bundle reconstruction methods is that when these techniques are performed through a transtibial method, the resulting femoral tunnel is placed too high in the notch; consequently, only the AM bundle is effectively reconstructed. This leads to improvement in anterior tibial translation but does not accurately restore stability through the range of motion, and does not restore rotational stability.[5,45,102] In addition to the trend toward anatomic ACL reconstruction, improvements in our understanding of the anatomy and function of the ACL have stimulated the development of augmentation techniques that effectively reconstruct single functional bundles in the setting of isolated bundle tears (injuries that were previously grouped collectively under the term *partial ACL tears*).[45]

---

*References 5, 20, 33, 36, 43, 118, and 123.

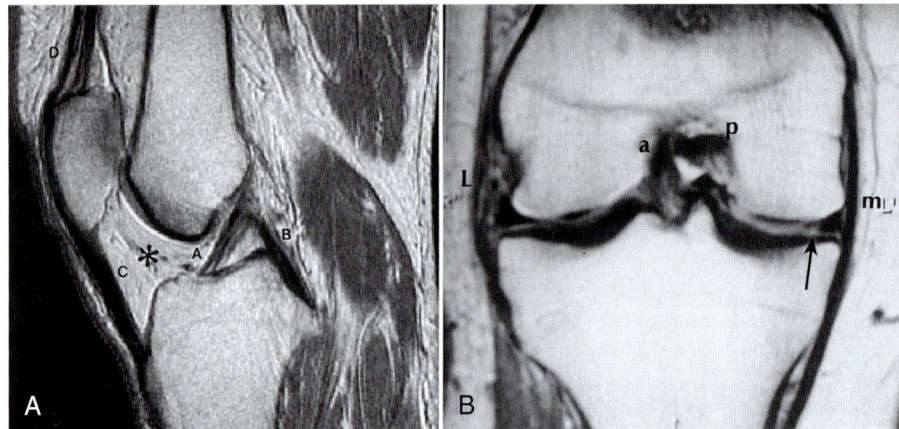

Figure 1-51. Magnetic resonance imaging of the knee. **A,** Sagittal view demonstrating a normal anterior cruciate ligament (ACL) *(A)* and posterior cruciate ligament (PCL) *(B)*. The low-signal patellar *(C)* and quadriceps *(D)* tendons and the high-signal fat pad *(asterisk)* can be identified anteriorly. **B,** Coronal view with the ACL *(a)* lateral to the PCL *(p)* in the intercondylar notch. The low-signal medial collateral ligament *(m)* runs from the femur, with the superficial fibers extending distally onto the medial aspect of the tibia. The lateral collateral ligament *(L)* and a small tear in the medial meniscus *(arrow)* can be seen.

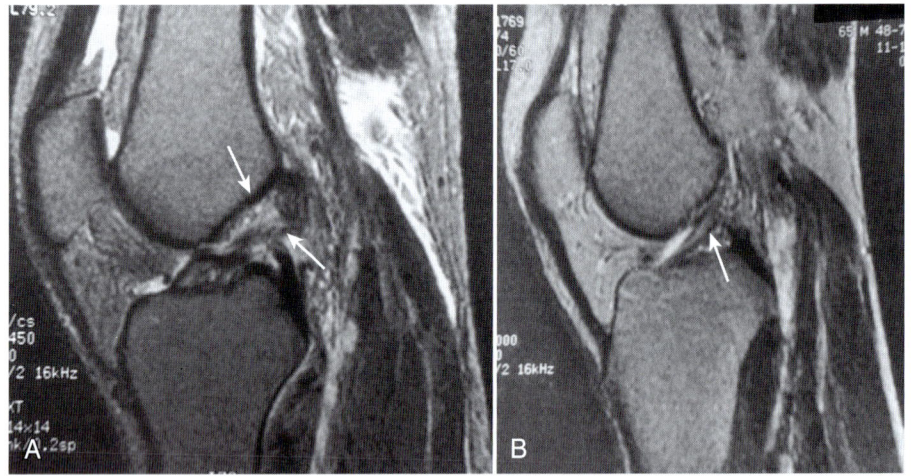

Figure 1-52. A, Sagittal magnetic resonance image (MRI) of a torn anterior cruciate ligament (ACL) with disruption at the femoral origin *(arrows)* and an abnormal wavy contour. **B,** Sagittal MRI showing hemorrhage about the ACL and intrasubstance signal *(arrow)* consistent with a partial ACL tear, later confirmed by arthroscopic examination.

The maximum tensile strength of the ACL is approximately 1725 ± 270 N, which is less than the peak force that occurs in vigorous athletic activities.[88] Stability is enhanced by dynamic stabilizers, such as the muscles that exert a force across the knee joint. For muscles to aid in protective stabilization of the knee, effective proprioceptive feedback regarding joint position is crucial. It appears that the ACL plays an important proprioceptive function because a variety of mechanoreceptors and free nerve endings have been identified.[9,27,63,99,100] In humans with ACL-deficient knees, a significantly higher threshold for detecting passive motion of the involved knee has been reported.[9] Afferent and efferent signals involving the ACL are carried by branches of the posterior tibial nerve. On MRI, the ACL is best visualized on sagittal images. Because of its oblique course, the ACL should be evaluated routinely on two or three sagittal sections. A normal ACL has a relatively low signal, but toward the distal insertion, the ACL may appear striated (Fig. 1-51). Discontinuity in the fibers or a soft tissue mass in the notch with high signal characteristics resulting from edema and

hemorrhage indicates an ACL tear. Partial ACL tears may be suggested by increased signal, thickening, or redundancy in the ligament. However, accurate diagnosis of partial injuries remains challenging (Fig. 1-52). Arthroscopic evaluation of the ACL remains the gold standard for evaluating suspected partial and complete tears (Fig. 1-53).

Posterior Cruciate Ligament

The PCL originates from the posterior part of the lateral surface of the medial femoral condyle in the intercondylar notch (see Fig. 1-47). As with the ACL, the origin is in the form of a segment of a circle and is oriented horizontally. The superior boundary of the attachment is straight and the inferior boundary is convex. The PCL has an average length of 38 mm and an average width of 13 mm.[36,111] It is narrowest in its midportion and fans out to a greater extent superiorly than it does inferiorly. The fibers are attached to the tibial insertion in a lateromedial direction, whereas in the femur they arise in an anteroposterior direction. The tibial

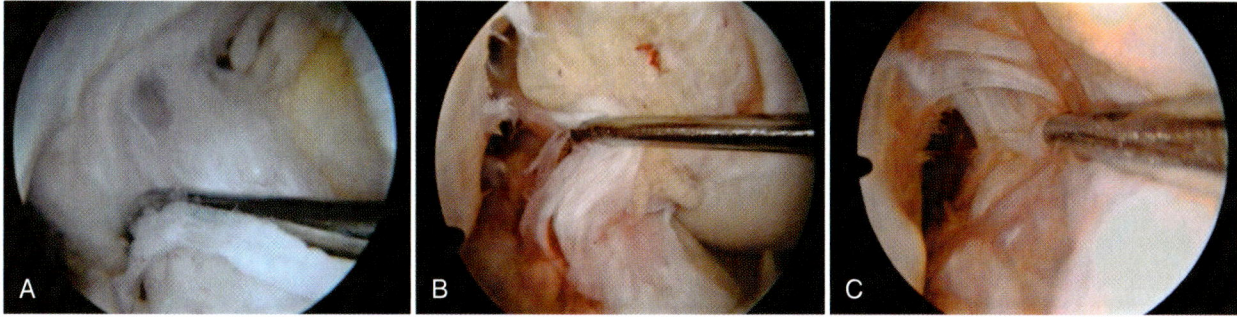

Figure 1-53. Arthroscopic views of anterior cruciate ligament (ACL) tears. **A,** A significant partial proximal ACL tear with a small number of intact fibers inferiorly. **B,** Complete ACL tear with the remaining stump of ruptured fibers at the tibial insertion retracted medially. The bare intercondylar wall (empty wall sign) of the lateral condyle is evident. **C,** Close-up view of the empty wall sign. The stump of the ACL is retracted medially to reveal that the intercondylar wall of the lateral femoral condyle is devoid of the normal ACL origin.

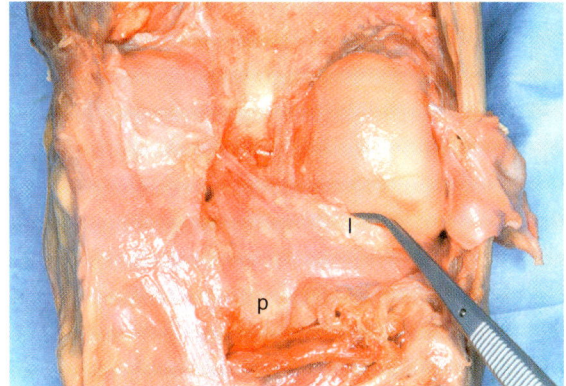

Figure 1-54. Anatomic dissection of the posterior aspect of the knee. The posterior cruciate ligament *(p)* originates on the lateral aspect of the medial femoral condyle and inserts on the posterior aspect of the tibia distal to the articular surface (*l,* probe on the superior aspect of the lateral meniscus).

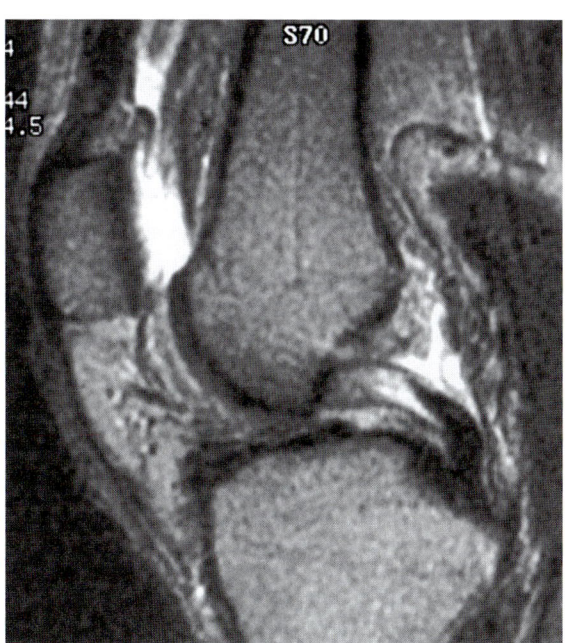

Figure 1-55. Sagittal magnetic resonance image showing increased signal within the femoral half of the posterior cruciate ligament, consistent with a partial tear.

attachment occurs in a depression posterior to the intra-articular upper surface of the tibia (see Fig. 1-49). The attachment extends up to 1 cm distally onto the adjoining posterior surface of the tibia (Fig. 1-54). Immediately proximal to the tibial attachment, the PCL sends a slip to blend with the posterior horn of the lateral meniscus.[36,111]

A normal PCL has uniformly low signal intensity on MRI studies, along with a hockey stick shape. The PCL can be well visualized in both the sagittal and coronal planes (see Fig. 1-51A and B). In addition, the meniscofemoral ligaments of Humphry and Wrisberg may be identified close to the anterior and posterior aspects of the PCL. Tears of the ligament appear as bright signal intensity within the tendon substance, indicative of discontinuity of fibers (Fig. 1-55). Chronic tears may appear as thinning or as an abnormal contour of the ligament.

The PCL is considered to be the primary stabilizer of the knee because it is located close to the central axis of rotation of the joint and is almost twice as strong as the ACL.[22,51,65,111,118] The PCL has been shown to provide approximately 95% of the total restraint to posterior translation of the tibia on the femur.[17] It is maximally taut at full flexion and becomes tighter with internal rotation (Fig. 1-56). Two inseparable components of the PCL have been identified. Anterior fibers form the bulk of the ligament and are believed to be taut in flexion and lax in extension. The opposite applies to the

thinner posterior portion. The PCL appears to function in concert with the LCL and the popliteus tendon to stabilize the knee. Cutting studies have demonstrated that posterior translation in flexion significantly increases when only the PCL is cut, but when the LCL and the popliteus are also transected, the translation is significantly greater.[37,111]

Injuries to the PCL are less common than injuries to the ACL and usually result from hyperextension or anterior blows to a flexed knee. Rarely do these injuries result in symptomatic instability, but they may be associated with chronic pain. Significant degenerative changes that involve the medial compartment in 90% of cases have been associated with chronic PCL injuries.[22]

The nature of the superior attachment of the cruciate ligaments results in twisting of the bands around their longitudinal axes on flexion. The ACL and the PCL are twisted in opposite directions because they are attached to opposing surfaces. From the front, the direction of torsion will appear to be toward the center of the joint.

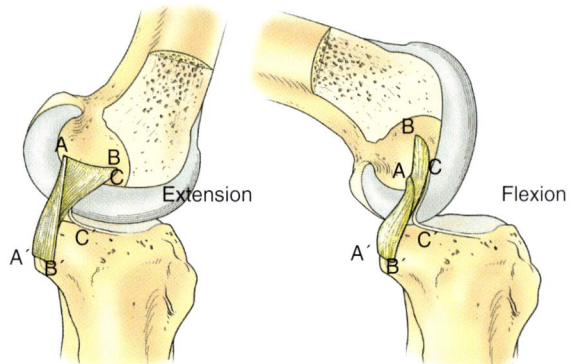

Figure 1-56. Posterior cruciate ligament. In flexion, the bulk of the ligament becomes tight, whereas in extension, it is relaxed. (From Girgis FG, Marshall JL, Al Monajem ARS: The cruciate ligaments of the knee joint. Clin Orthop 106:216, 1975.)

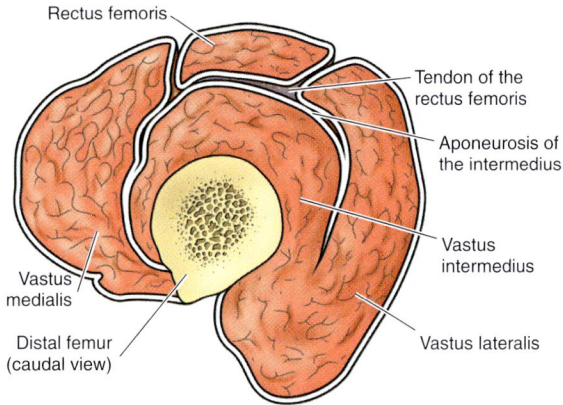

Figure 1-57. Four components of the quadriceps muscle shown through a cross-section at the junction of the middle and distal thirds of the femur. The four components then fuse to form the trilaminar tendon of the quadriceps muscle.

ANTERIOR ASPECT

The quadriceps muscle group consists of four distinct parts that share a common tendon of insertion (Fig. 1-57). The rectus femoris arises as two heads—direct and indirect—from the ilium that unite and form a muscle belly running distally in the anterior aspect of the thigh. It narrows to a tendon 5 to 8 cm proximal to the superior pole of the patella.[95] The rectus femoris accounts for about 15% of the cross-section of the quadriceps group. The vastus lateralis arises from a broad linear strip, beginning at the proximal end of the trochanteric line and extending halfway down the linea aspera. It also arises from the lateral intermuscular septum. A fibrous expansion from the distal margin of the vastus lateralis blends with the lateral patellar retinaculum, through which direct attachment to the tibia is attained. The vastus medialis originates from the distal part of the trochanteric line and follows the spiral line to the medial lip of the linea aspera. The most distal fibers of the muscle arise from the tendon of the adductor magnus and pass almost horizontally anterior to the insertion into the common tendon and the medial border of the patella. This part of the muscle is sometimes described as the vastus medialis obliquus (VMO). Like the vastus lateralis, the vastus medialis has a distal fibrous expansion that blends with

the medial patellar retinaculum. The vastus intermedius arises from the anterior and lateral aspects of the shaft of the femur; medially, it partly blends with the vastus medialis. The four muscles become confluent distally and form the quadriceps tendon, which extends anteriorly about the patella and becomes the patellar tendon (ligament) (Fig. 1-58). The fibers of the rectus femoris and vastus intermedius insert almost perpendicularly into the superior pole of the patella, whereas the fibers of the vastus medialis and lateralis insert obliquely at mean angles of approximately 55 degrees (range, 28 to 70 degrees) and 14 degrees (range, 6 to 45 degrees), respectively.[50,95]

The quadriceps tendon is often depicted as a trilaminar structure; the anterior layer is formed by the rectus femoris, the intermediate layer by the vastus medialis and lateralis, and the deep layer by the tendon of the vastus intermedius.[71,95] In reality, the organization is more complex and variable.[95] On MRI, the multilaminar nature of the tendon may produce a striated appearance on sagittal views rather than a uniformly low signal structure (see Fig. 1-51A). Discontinuity or increased signal intensity within the tendon substance and in the surrounding tissues on T2-weighted images is suggestive of quadriceps rupture (Fig. 1-59). Distally, the quadriceps tendon inserts into the patella via an expansion that passes anterior to the patella. In most cases, only fibers from the rectus femoris portion of the tendon continue in the distal expansion over the patella. However, in some cases, fibers from the vastus lateralis can also directly insert distally. In addition, extensions from the medial and lateral vasti insert into the tibia via the patellar retinaculum.

The patellar tendon runs from the lower border of the patella to the tubercle of the tibia. Because the shaft of the femur has an inclination, the quadriceps muscle does not pull in a direct line with the patellar tendon. The angle formed is always valgus, and the average angle is 14 degrees in males and 17 degrees in females.[1] This angle, the quadriceps (Q) angle, is accentuated by internal rotation of the femur (Fig. 1-60). The resulting tendency toward lateral patellar displacement is resisted by the lateral lip of the femoral trochlea, the horizontal fibers of the VMO, and the medial patellar retinaculum. Selective strengthening of the VMO has been proposed as treatment of patellofemoral pain and subluxation. Although the most visible function of the quadriceps group is to extend the knee (with a secondary function to flex the hip), the primary physiologic action is to decelerate flexion of the knee during the early stance phase of gait by contracting in an eccentric manner. The four segments of the quadriceps femoris are supplied by the femoral nerve.

The patellar tendon is a strong, flat ligamentous band about 5 cm in length. Proximally, it originates from the apex and adjoining margins of the patella and the rough depression on the posterior surface. Distally, the patellar tendon inserts into the tuberosity of the tibia; superficial fibers are continuous over the front of the patella with those of the tendon of the quadriceps femoris.[95] Medial and lateral portions of the quadriceps tendon pass down on either side of the patella and insert into the proximal end of the tibia on either side of the tuberosity. These expansions merge into the capsule and form the medial and lateral patellar retinacula. The patellar tendon normally has low signal intensity on MRI, but it is not uncommon for it to contain intermediate signal at the patella

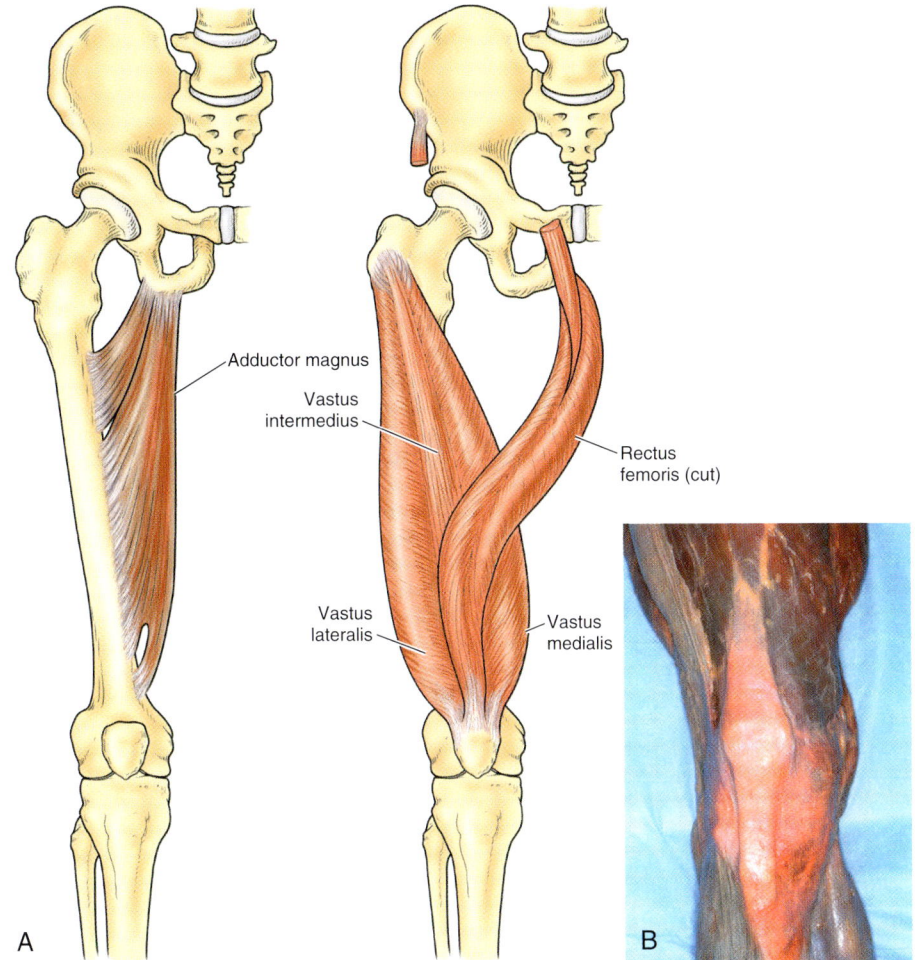

Figure 1-58. **A,** Quadriceps group. **B,** Anatomic dissection of the anterior aspect of the knee.

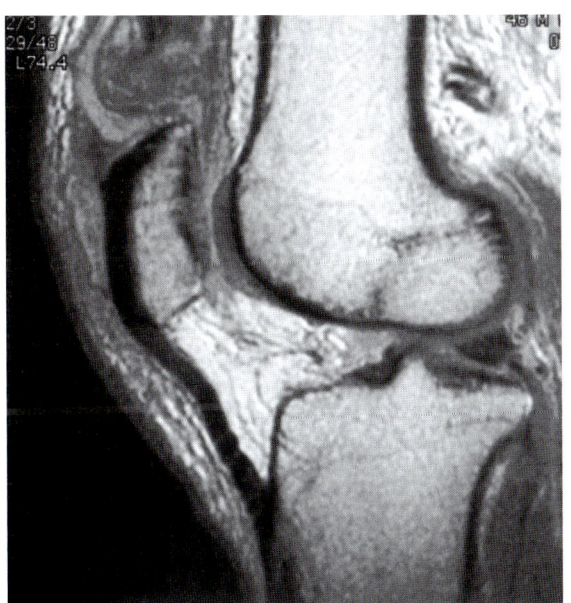

Figure 1-59. Sagittal magnetic resonance image of a complete quadriceps tendon tear with a discontinuity in the fibers at the attachment site on the superior pole of the patella.

or at tibial attachments. As elsewhere, focal discontinuity or high signal intensity in and about the tendon is indicative of a disruption or tear (Fig. 1-61).

The posterior surface of the patellar tendon is separated from the synovial membrane of the joint by a large infrapatellar pad of fat and from the tibia by a bursa. The fat pad fills the space between the femoral condyles and the patellar tendon and adjusts its shape as the size of this potential cavity varies with movement. The fat pad is pierced by numerous blood vessels derived from the genicular arteries. The patellar tendon forms an incomplete septum between the anterior intercondylar notch of the femur and the fat pad.

MEDIAL ASPECT

According to Warren and Marshall,[115] the supporting structures on the medial side of the knee can be divided into three layers. Layer 1 is the most superficial in that it is the first fascial plane encountered after a skin incision is made on the medial side of the knee. The plane is defined by the fascia that invests the sartorius muscle (Fig. 1-62). The sartorius inserts into this network of fascial fibers and does not have a distinct insertion distally on the tibia. Posteriorly, a layer of fatty tissue lies between layer 1 and the deeper structures. The gracilis and semitendinosus tendons lie in the plane between

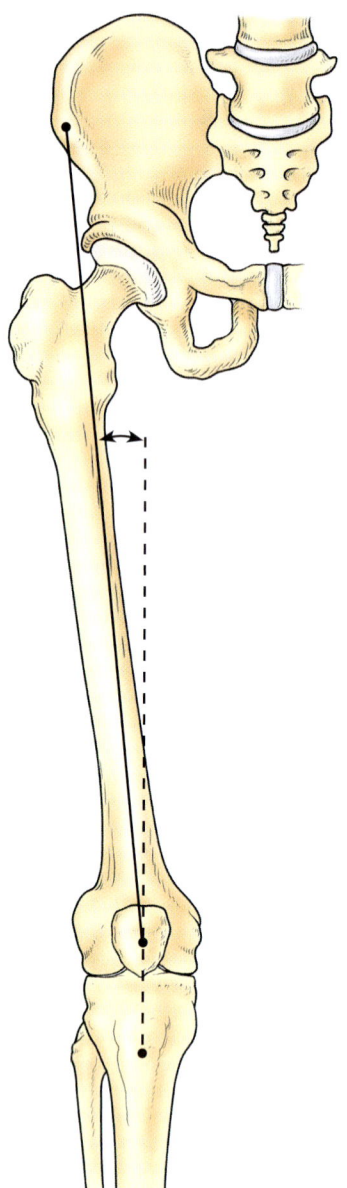

Figure 1-60. Quadriceps (Q) angle.

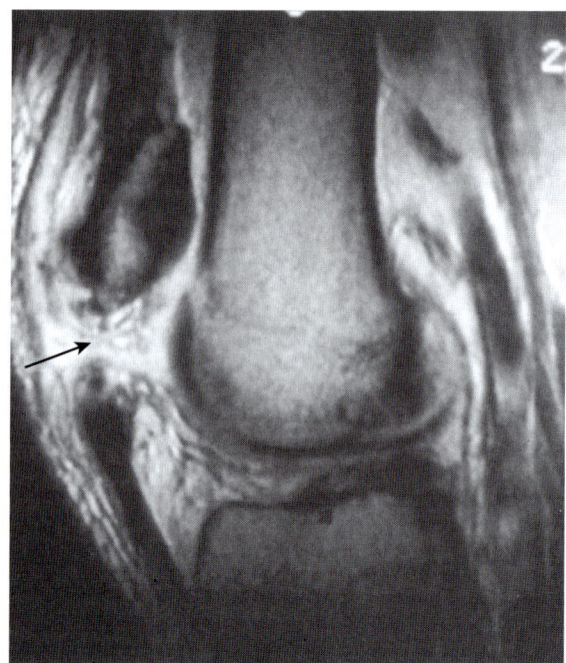

Figure 1-61. Sagittal magnetic resonance image of a patellar tendon tear at the inferior pole of the patella *(arrow)*.

distally to an insertion on the medial surface of the tibia. This insertion is on average 4.6 cm inferior to the tibial articular surface and is immediately posterior to the insertion of the pes anserinus. The posterior oblique fibers run from the medial epicondyle and blend with layer 3 to form the posteromedial joint capsule.

Anteriorly, according to Warren and Marshall,[115] layer 2 splits vertically. The fibers anterior to the split proceed cephalad to the vastus medialis and join the plane of layer 1 to form the parapatellar retinaculum. The fibers posterior to the split run cephalad to the femoral condyle, from which transverse fibers run forward in the plane of layer 2 to the patella and form the medial patellofemoral ligament. This medial patellofemoral ligament connects the patella to the medial femoral condyle and passively limits lateral patellar excursion. At the inferior border of the medial patella is the medial meniscopatellar ligament, which connects the patella to the anterior horn of the medial meniscus. The medial retinaculum can be visualized well on routine MRI. Disruptions or tears with the surrounding edema and hemorrhage that occur in association with patella dislocations can also be seen (Fig. 1-65).

Layer 3, the capsule of the knee joint, can be separated from layer 2 except toward the margin of the patella, where it becomes very thin (Fig. 1-66). Deep to the superficial MCL, layer 3 becomes thicker and forms a vertically oriented band of short fibers known as the deep MCL. The deep MCL extends from the femur to the midportion of the peripheral margin of the meniscus and tibia (Fig. 1-67). Anteriorly, the deep MCL is clearly separated from the superficial MCL, and a bursa is interposed, but posteriorly, the layers blend because the meniscofemoral portion of the deep ligament tends to merge with the overlying superficial ligament near its cephalad attachment. The meniscotibial portion of the deep MCL, however, is readily separated from the overlying superficial ligament and is referred to as the coronary ligament.

layers 1 and 2 (Fig. 1-63). Farther posteriorly, layer 1 is a fascial sheet that overlies the two heads of the gastrocnemius and the structures of the popliteal fossa. This layer serves as a support for muscle bellies and neurovascular structures in the popliteal region. Layer 1 can always be separated from the underlying parallel and oblique portions of the superficial MCL. If a vertical incision is made posterior to the parallel fibers of the ligament, the anterior portion of layer 1 can be reflected anteriorly to expose the superficial MCL. Approximately 1 cm anterior to the superficial MCL, layer 1 blends with the anterior portion of layer 2 and the medial patellar retinaculum derived from the vastus medialis. Anteriorly and distally, layer 1 joins the periosteum of the tibia.

Layer 2 is the plane of the superficial MCL. The superficial MCL, as described by Brantigan and Voshell,[16] consists of parallel and oblique portions (Fig. 1-64). Anterior or parallel fibers arise from the sulcus of the medial epicondyle of the femur and consist of heavy, vertically oriented fibers running

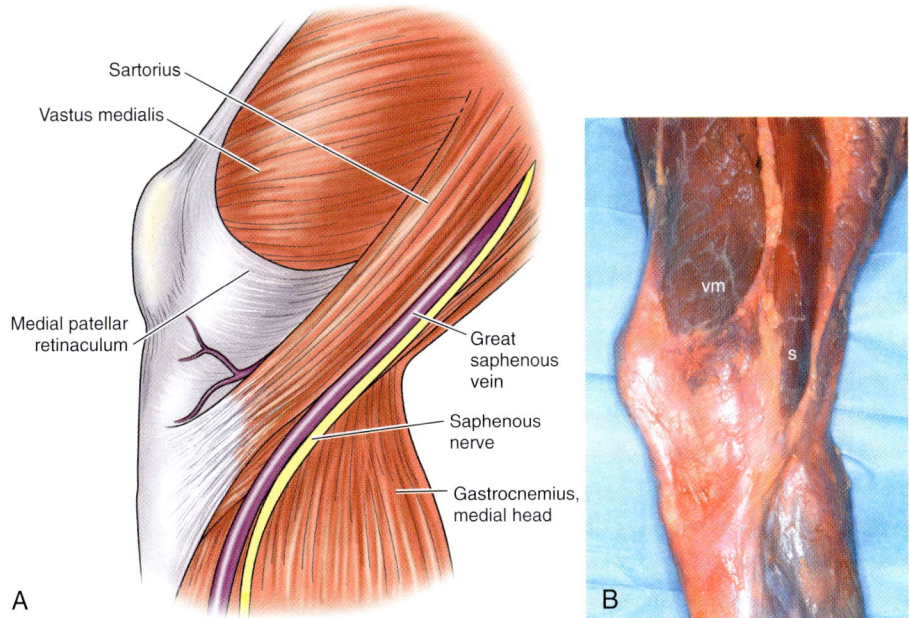

Figure 1-62. A, Medial aspect of the knee, layer 1. **B,** Anatomic dissection of the medial knee. Layer 1 on the medial aspect of the knee is defined by the fascial layer, which invests the sartorius muscle *(s)* *(vm,* vastus medialis).

Components of the MCL are well seen on MRI studies. Coronal images provide clear visualization, but axial images can provide complementary information. Normal ligament fibers have low signal intensity (see Fig. 1-51B). With partial and complete tears, the fibers become less distinct, and increased signal on T2-weighted images can be identified in the ligament as a result of edema and bleeding (Fig. 1-68).

The posteromedial region formed by the merging of layers 2 and 3 is reinforced by five insertions of the semimembranosus tendon and tendon sheath. The semimembranosus has a direct tendinous insertion on the posteromedial corner of the tibia and a second tibial insertion deep to the superficial MCL (see Fig. 1-66). A third tract blends with the oblique fibers of the superficial MCL, and a fourth doubles back to insert proximally in the capsule over the medial meniscus. The fifth tract runs proximally and laterally across the posterior capsule and forms the oblique popliteal ligament (of Winslow) (Fig. 1-69).[115]

On the medial side, the three layers are most obviously separated in the region of the superficial MCL. Anteriorly, the superficial layer and a portion of the middle layer blend and merge with the overlying retinacular expansion from the quadriceps. The other cephalad portion of the middle layer, formed where it splits anterior to the superficial medial ligament, persists as a separate layer forming the patellofemoral ligament. Anteriorly, the deep layer, although separate, becomes extremely thin and difficult to define. Posteriorly, layer 1 becomes the deep fascia, and layers 2 and 3 blend to form the joint capsule.

The superficial MCL functions as the primary restraint against valgus stress, a restraint to external rotation of the tibia, and a weak restraint to anterior tibial translation in ACL-deficient knees.[106,116] The anterior parallel fibers of the superficial MCL are under tension from full extension to 90 degrees of flexion but become maximally taut at 45 to 90 degrees of flexion.[34,86,116] During extension, the anterior fibers

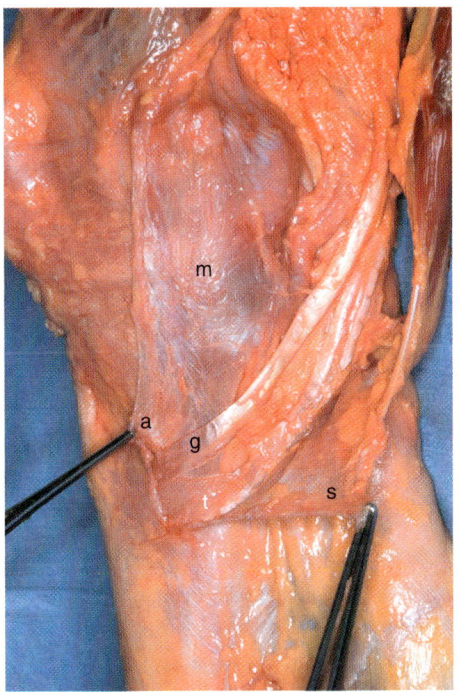

Figure 1-63. Anatomic dissection of the medial aspect of the knee. The tendons of the gracilis *(g)* and the semitendinosus *(t)* lie between layer 1 (the fascia investing the sartorius) and layer 2 *(m,* the superficial medial collateral ligament). In this specimen, layer 1 has been divided, and the sartorius insertion and fascia are retracted posteriorly *(s,* inferior forceps), and the anterior fascial margin is retracted anteriorly *(a,* superior forceps).

relax and the posterior fibers become taught.[34,86] Strain measurements in the ligament confirm that different areas of the superficial MCL experience different forces, depending on valgus load and joint position. Peak strain during valgus loading appears to occur in the fully extended position near

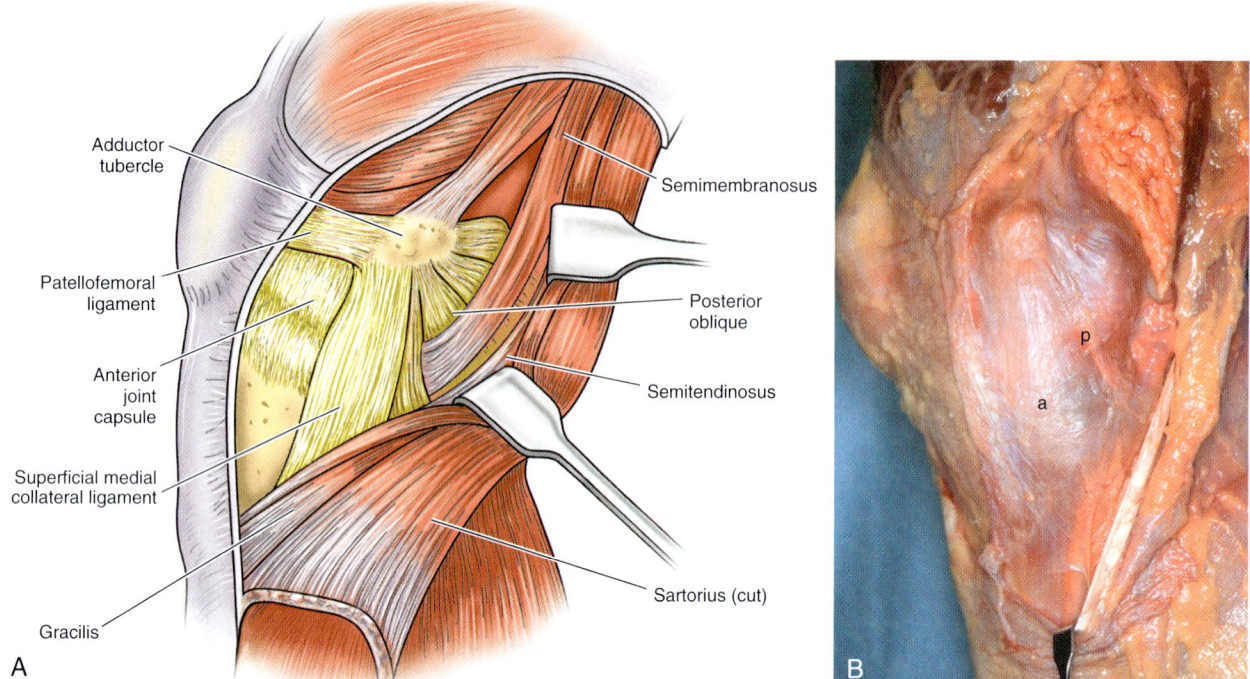

Figure 1-64. A, Medial aspect of the knee, layer 2. **B,** Anatomic dissection of the medial knee. The pes tendons are retracted distally and posteriorly to reveal the anterior parallel fibers *(a)* and the posterior oblique fibers *(p)* of the superficial medial collateral ligament (layer 2).

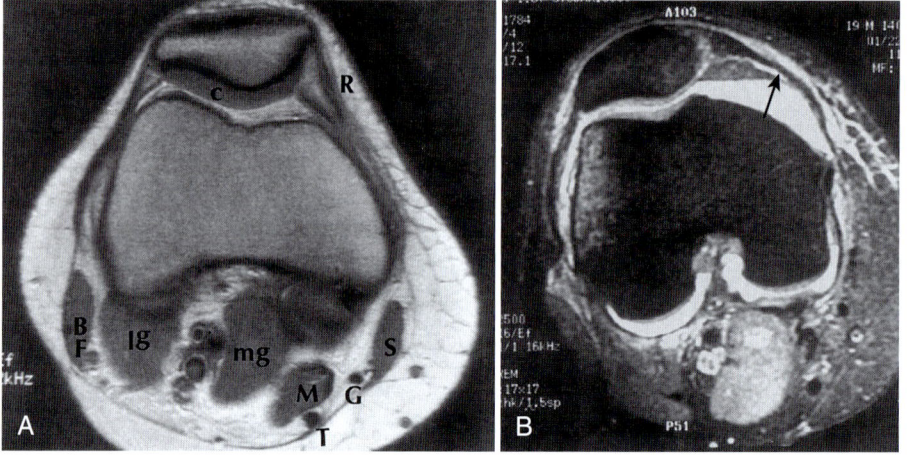

Figure 1-65. A, High-resolution axial magnetic resonance image (MRI) of the knee. The popliteal vessels and the tibial nerve can be identified between the two heads of the gastrocnemius. The other following structures are marked: patella articular cartilage *(c)*, medial patellar retinaculum *(R)*, sartorius muscle *(S)*, gracilis muscle *(G)*, semimembranosus muscle *(M)*, semitendinosus tendon *(T)*, medial head of the gastrocnemius *(mg)*, lateral head of the gastrocnemius *(lg)*, and biceps femoris *(BF)*. **B,** Axial MRI demonstrating a partial tear of the medial retinaculum *(arrow)* with increased signal on either side secondary to acute lateral patella dislocation.

the femoral insertion; this finding explains the high rate of clinical injury noted to occur in this portion of the ligament.[34] Oblique fibers seem to play a minimal role in overall function of the superficial MCL. The deep MCL performs only a weak secondary role as a stabilizer against valgus stress. Understanding of the anatomy and function of the individual portions of the MCL is important during soft tissue balancing in total knee arthroplasty, as well as during evaluation of traumatic injury.

LATERAL ASPECT

Supporting structures on the lateral side of the knee have also been described as consisting of three layers.[101] Layer 1 contains the superficial fascia (fascia lata), the iliotibial tract, and the biceps femoris with its expansion posteriorly (Fig. 1-70). Layer 2 is formed by the quadriceps retinaculum anteriorly and is incomplete posteriorly, where it consists of two patellofemoral ligaments. Layer 3 is composed of the lateral capsule

(Fig. 1-71). Posterior to the overlying iliotibial tract, the posterior capsule is divided into two laminae. The deep lamina is composed of the coronary ligament and the arcuate ligament and is newer phylogenetically. The superficial lamina represents the original capsule and consists of the LCL and the fabellofibular ligament. The inferior lateral geniculate artery passes between the two laminae (Fig. 1-72).

The ITB is a longitudinal thickening in the fascia lata that runs along the lateral side of the knee and inserts into Gerdy's tubercle on the tibia. Some of the fibers proceed across Gerdy's tubercle to the tibial tuberosity. Proximally, the fascia lata is adherent to the lateral intermuscular septum, where it is attached to the femur. Posteriorly, the fascia lata merges into the biceps fascia.[59] The biceps femoris muscle is formed from two heads; the long head arises in common with the semitendinosus from the ischial tuberosity, and the short head arises from the lateral lip of the linea aspera, the lateral supracondylar line, and the lateral intermuscular septum. The nerve supply of both heads is derived from the sciatic nerve, but from different branches; the long head is innervated by the tibial branch, and the short head by the common popliteal nerve. The two heads unite above the knee joint in a common tendon that folds around the LCL insertion on the fibular styloid and then divides into three layers.[81] The superficial layer spreads out and inserts as a wide expansion over the adjoining part of the proximal tibia. The middle layer is a thin, poorly defined layer that envelops the LCL and is separated from the ligament by a bursa. The deep layer bifurcates and inserts on the fibular styloid and on the tibia at Gerdy's tubercle. The biceps functions mainly as a knee flexor but additionally acts as a weaker hip extensor and external rotator of the tibia. The biceps is also believed to be an important static and dynamic stabilizer of the lateral aspect of the knee, especially as the knee flexes beyond 30 degrees.[87,108]

The lateral knee retinaculum has been described by Fulkerson and Gossling[32] (Fig. 1-73). The lateral patellar retinaculum is composed of two major components: the superficial oblique retinaculum and the deep transverse retinaculum. The superficial oblique retinaculum runs superficially from the ITB to the patella (Fig. 1-74). The deep transverse retinaculum is denser and consists of three major components. The epicondylopatellar band, also known as the transverse patellofemoral ligament, provides superolateral patellar support. The transverse retinaculum courses directly from the ITB to the midpatella and provides the primary support for the lateral patella. The patellotibial band, the third component, runs between the patella and the tibia inferiorly (Fig. 1-75). Overall, the lateral retinaculum provides stronger support to the patella than is provided by its medial counterpart.

In layer 3, the lateral joint capsule is a thin, fibrous layer that is circumferentially attached to the femur and tibia at the proximal and distal margins of the knee joint. The attachment at the margin of the inferior border of the lateral

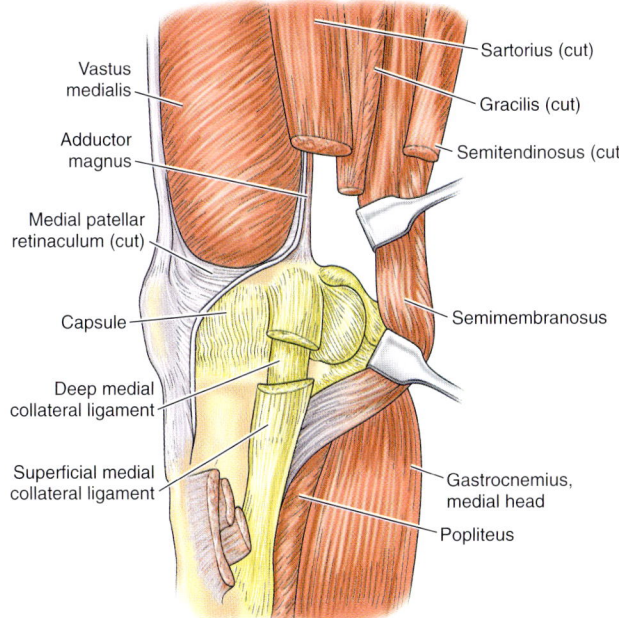

Figure 1-66. Medial aspect of the knee, layer 3.

Vastus medialis
Adductor magnus
Medial patellar retinaculum (cut)
Capsule
Deep medial collateral ligament
Superficial medial collateral ligament
Sartorius (cut)
Gracilis (cut)
Semitendinosus (cut)
Semimembranosus
Gastrocnemius, medial head
Popliteus

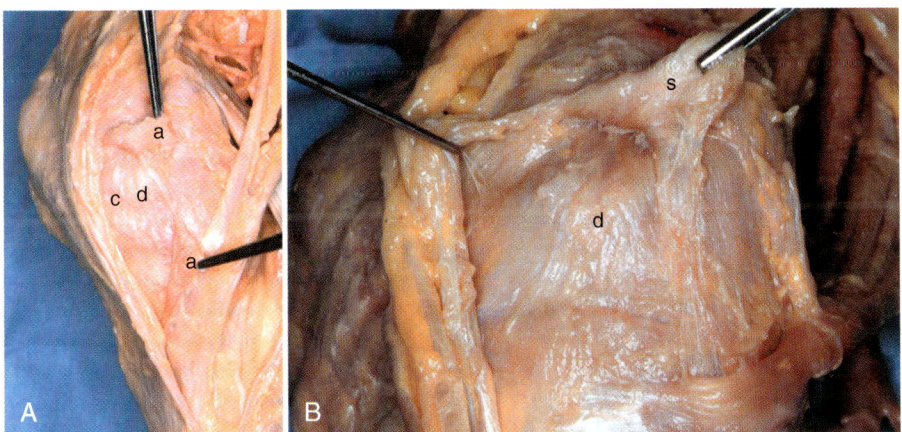

Figure 1-67. Anatomic dissections of the medial aspect of the knee. **A,** The anterior parallel fibers *(a)* of the superficial medial collateral ligament (MCL) (layer 2) have been sectioned transversely through the middle of the ligament and retracted posteriorly (both forceps) to reveal the fibers of the deep MCL *(d)* and capsule *(c,* layer 3). **B,** Close-up view of fibers of the deep MCL *(d)* from the femur to the periphery of the meniscus attachment on the tibia. The superficial MCL *(s)* has been sectioned and the proximal portion retracted proximally (forceps).

meniscus, which runs to the edge of the articular margin of the tibia, has been termed the *coronary ligament*.[72,101] The LCL originates on the lateral epicondyle of the femur anterior to the origin of the gastrocnemius. It runs beneath the lateral retinaculum to insert into the head of the fibula, where it blends with the insertion of the biceps femoris. On MRI studies, the LCL is best seen on coronal images and appears as a thin band of low signal intensity (see Fig. 1-51B). Two to three sequential images are usually required to visualize the entire structure because of the oblique course of the ligament. A tear appears as a disruption in the fibers, thickening, or increased signal on T2-weighted images in and about the ligament as a result of edema.

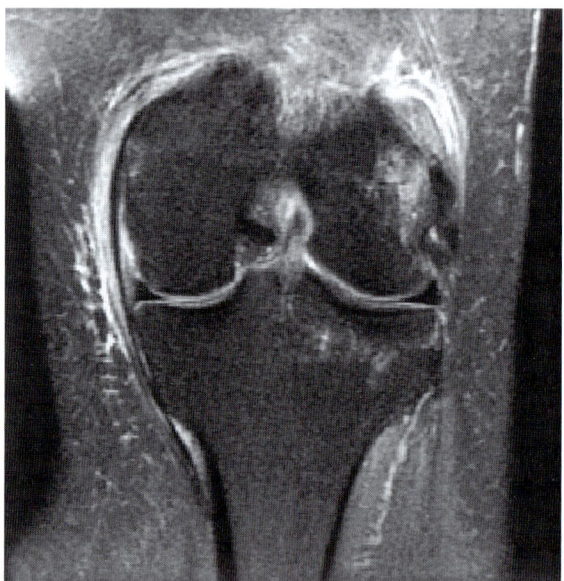

Figure 1-68. Coronal magnetic resonance image with increased fluid signal about the medial collateral ligament consistent with a sprain.

The fabellofibular ligament is a condensation of fibers lying between the LCL and arcuate ligaments that runs from the fabella, a sesamoid bone found in the lateral head of the gastrocnemius, to the fibular styloid.[60] The arcuate ligament has been variously described; according to Last, "In truth, there is at this part of the capsule such a complexity of fibers running in many directions that, by artful dissection, almost any pattern desired by the dissector could be made."[72] Some fibers extend from the lateral condyle of the femur to the posterior part of the capsule. The strongest and most consistent fibers of the arcuate ligament, however, form a triangular sheet that diverges upward from the fibular styloid. The lateral limb of this mass is dense and strong and is attached to the femur and the popliteal tendon. The weaker medial limb curves over the popliteal muscle and blends with the fibers of the oblique popliteal ligament. The free edge of this medial limb is crescentic, and the lateral or femoral part of the popliteus emerges beneath it to approach its tibial attachment. Three common variations in the fabellofibular and arcuate ligaments have been described. In most knees (67%), both the fabellofibular and arcuate ligaments are present, but in the case of a large fabella, the fabellofibular ligament dominates, and the arcuate ligament is absent (20%); however, in the absence of a fabella, only the arcuate ligament is present (13%).[101] Watanabe et al further divided these categories into a total of seven types based on the presence or absence of a fibular insertion of a portion of the popliteal tendon.[117]

The popliteal muscle arises with a strong tendon about 2.5 cm long from a depression at the anterior part of the groove on the lateral condyle of the femur. The tendon, which is invested in synovial membrane, passes beneath the medial limb of the arcuate ligament and forms a thin, flat, triangular muscle that inserts into the medial two thirds of the triangular surface, proximal to the popliteal line on the posterior surface of the tibia. A direct attachment to the fibular head has been redefined.[83,117] The tendon is also attached to the arcuate ligament, and, according to Last, up

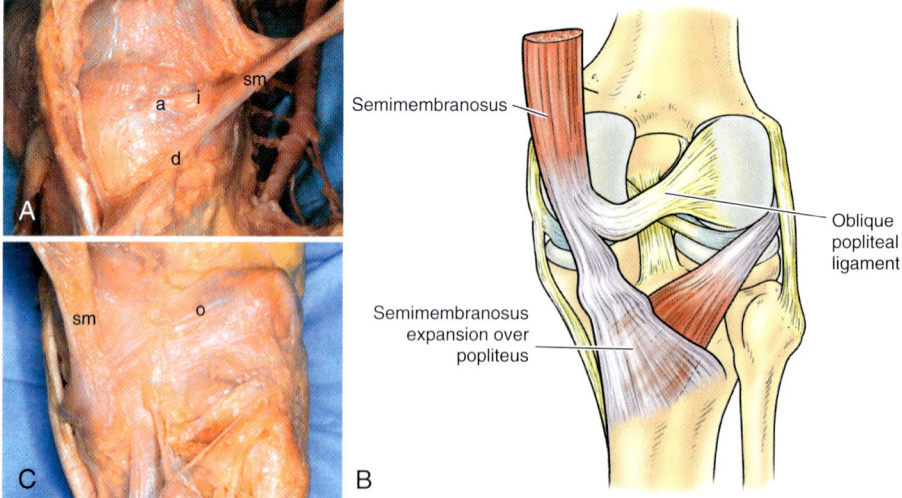

Figure 1-69. **A,** Anatomic dissection of medial aspect of the knee. The superficial medial collateral ligament (MCL) has been sectioned and retracted to reveal the direct insertion *(i)* of the semimembranosus *(sm)* on the posteromedial tibia and the anterior extension *(a)* deep to the superficial MCL. A band of fibers *(d)* also runs distally to insert into the retracted superficial MCL. **B,** Relationship of the oblique popliteal ligament *(o)* to the semimembranosus muscle. **C,** Anatomic dissection of the posterior aspect of the knee, demonstrating the oblique popliteal ligament *(o)*, which passes obliquely across the posterior capsule to insert on the lateral femoral condyle.

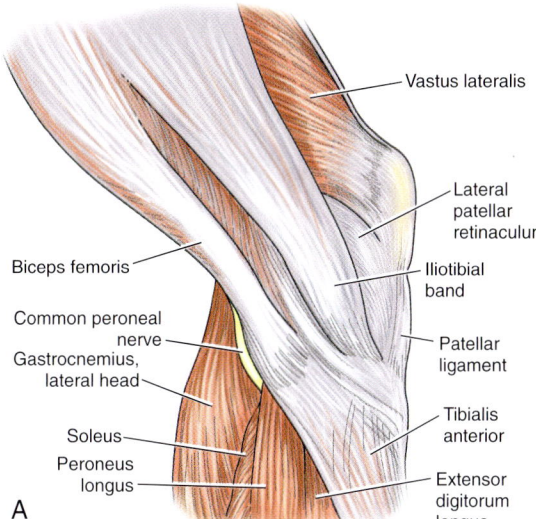

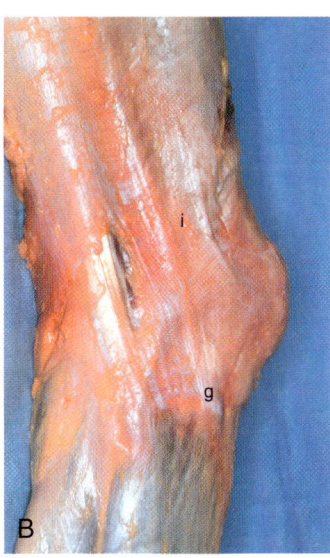

Figure 1-70. **A,** Lateral aspect of the knee, layer 1. **B,** Anatomic dissection of the lateral knee. Layer 1 on the lateral side of the knee with a prominent iliotibial band *(i)* insertion on Gerdy's tubercle *(g).*

Labels in A: Vastus lateralis, Lateral patellar retinaculum, Iliotibial band, Patellar ligament, Tibialis anterior, Extensor digitorum longus, Biceps femoris, Common peroneal nerve, Gastrocnemius, lateral head, Soleus, Peroneus longus

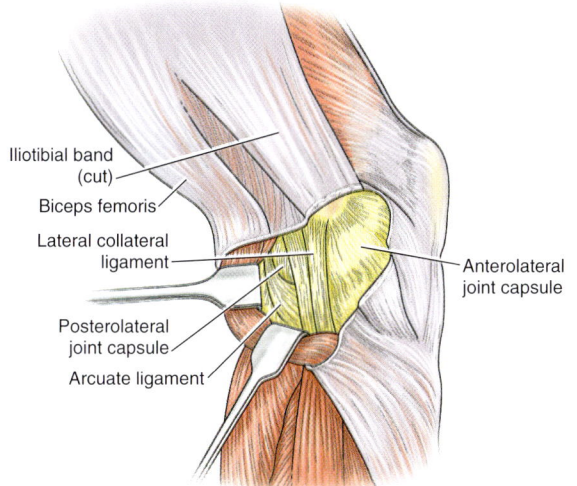

Figure 1-71. Lateral aspect of the knee, layer 3.

Labels: Iliotibial band (cut), Biceps femoris, Lateral collateral ligament, Posterolateral joint capsule, Arcuate ligament, Anterolateral joint capsule

to half of its fibers are attached to the lateral meniscus.[72] The synovial membrane below the meniscus herniates deep to the muscle as the popliteus bursa. The function of the popliteus is controversial, but it may act in conjunction with the meniscofemoral ligaments to control the motion of the meniscus as the knee flexes.[11,57,72,109] However, its primary role appears to be unlocking the knee to allow flexion by producing external rotation of the femur in the loaded position.[11,72,79] The nerve to the popliteus arises from the tibial nerve and runs distally across the popliteal vessels to reach the lower border of the muscle, where it enters the deep surface.

The LCL, PCL, and popliteal–arcuate complex act in concert to stabilize the posterolateral corner of the knee against varus stress, external tibial rotation, and posterior flexion. Damage to these structures results in posterolateral rotatory instability.[8,52,53]

POSTERIOR ASPECT

The popliteal fossa is bounded laterally by the biceps femoris and medially by the semimembranosus and tendons of the pes anserine. Distally, the space is closed by the two heads of the gastrocnemius. The roof of the fossa is formed by the deep fascia; the floor consists of the popliteal surface of the femur, the posterior capsule of the knee joint, and the popliteus muscle with its fascial covering (Fig. 1-76).

The biceps femoris lies posterior to the ITB and forms the lateral wall of the popliteal fossa; it has been described previously. The semitendinosus arises from the ischial tuberosity and runs distally and medially on the surface of the semimembranosus. The semimembranosus arises from the upper and lateral impressions on the ischial tuberosity. It passes distally and medially deep to the origin of the biceps and semitendinosus (Fig. 1-77). Its tendon forms the proximal and medial boundaries of the popliteal fossa and inserts into a groove on the posteromedial aspect of the tibia. Multiple expansions reinforce the posteromedial capsule, as previously described. Directly posteriorly, a robust expansion called the oblique popliteal ligament passes proximally and laterally and blends with the posterior capsule and arcuate ligament from the lateral side. The nerve supply to the hamstring muscles is derived from the tibial branch of the sciatic nerve. The gracilis muscle arises from the inferior pubic ramus and runs distally along the medial side of the thigh. In the lower third of the thigh, the fibers end in a long tendon that lies medial to the tendon of the semitendinosus. It is innervated by the obturator nerve. The sartorius muscle arises from the anterior superior iliac spine and runs distally and medially across the front of the thigh, where it forms the roof of the subsartorial canal. Its nerve supply is derived from the femoral nerve. Distally, the sartorius tendon is wider and less well defined than the gracilis and semitendinosus nerves. Rather than inserting directly into the tibia, the diffuse tendinous fibers blend with layer 1 of the medial aspect of the knee. Together, the tendons of the sartorius, gracilis, and semitendinosus form the pes anserinus (see Fig. 1-77). The sartorius tendon expansion lies superficially and covers the insertions of the gracilis and semitendinosus. The semitendinosus inserts into the tibia just distal to the gracilis and forms a conjoint structure with a mean width of 20 mm; the proximal-most point of the insertion begins a mean of 19 mm distal and 22.5 mm medial to the apex of the tibial tubercle.[91] The muscles, which insert at the pes, act to flex and internally rotate the knee.

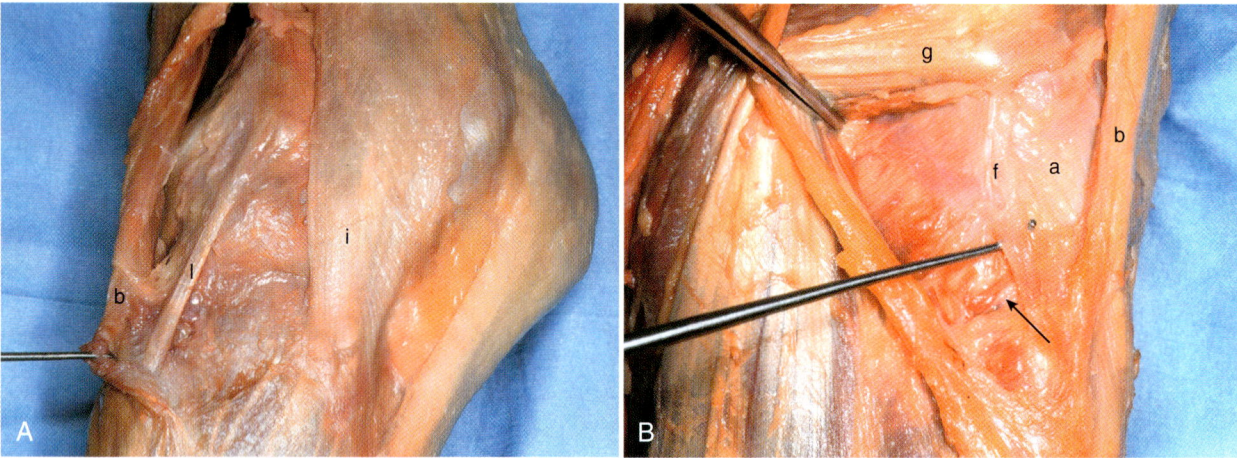

Figure 1-72. Anatomic dissections of the posterolateral aspect of the knee. **A,** The superficial layers along the posterior margin of the iliotibial band *(i)* have been incised and retracted posteriorly to reveal layer 3 of the lateral aspect of the knee. The prominent lateral collateral ligament *(l)* inserts deep to the biceps *(b,* retracted by the probe) on the fibular head. **B,** The lateral head of the gastrocnemius *(g)* has been retracted medially (forceps) to expose the fabellofibular *(f)* and arcuate ligaments *(a).* The inferior lateral geniculate artery *(arrow)* passes between the fabellofibular ligament (superficial lamina of layer 3) and the arcuate ligament (deep lamina of layer 3) just distal to the probe placed between the two laminae *(b,* biceps femoris).

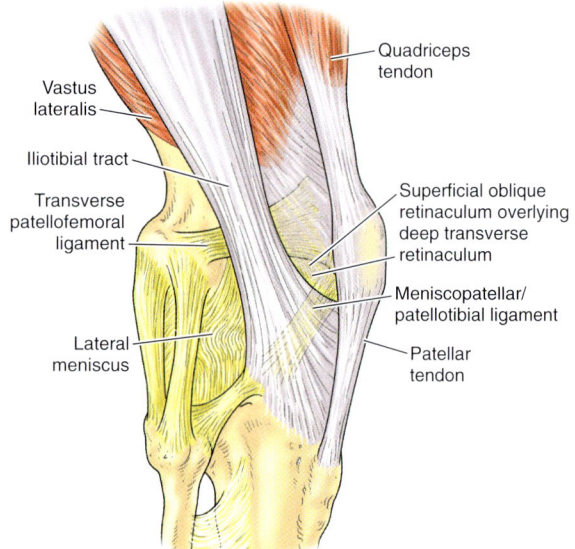

Figure 1-73. Structures of the lateral retinaculum.

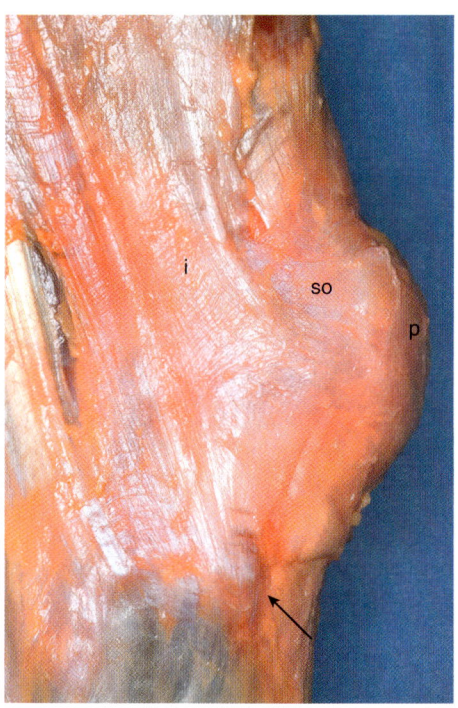

Figure 1-74. Anatomic dissection of the lateral aspect of the knee. The superficial oblique *(so)* fibers of the lateral retinaculum run between the anterior margin of the iliotibial band *(i)* and the lateral aspect of the patella *(p)* *(arrow,* Gerdy's tubercle).

When the knee is flexed, the biceps tendon can be felt subcutaneously on the lateral side. Medially, two tendons are prominent, with the gracilis lying medial to the semitendinosus.

The ischial fibers of the adductor magnus are a derivative of the hamstring group. The fibers run distally and end in a short tendon that inserts into the prominent adductor tubercle on the medial condyle of the femur. Through a gap in the insertion of this muscle, the femoral vessels enter the popliteal fossa. Similar to the hamstrings, this portion of the adductor magnus is supplied by the sciatic nerve.

The gastrocnemius muscle arises as a lateral head from the lateral aspect of the lateral femoral condyle and as a larger medial head from the popliteal surface of the femur and the medial aspect of the medial femoral condyle (Fig. 1-78). The lateral head has a largely fleshy origin, but the portion of the medial head that arises from the medial condyle

adjoining the attachment of the medial collateral ligament is tendinous. The two heads merge and form a common tendon with the soleus, which narrows distally and inserts into the tendo calcaneus.

The plantaris muscle has a small, fleshy belly that arises from the lateral supracondylar line of the femur deep to the lateral head of the gastrocnemius. It gives rise to a very long, narrow tendon that runs distally deep to the medial head of the gastrocnemius. The plantaris is absent in about 7% of individuals and is believed to represent a vestigial structure in humans.[26]

The soleus arises from multiple origins, including the upper fourth of the posterior surface of the shaft and head of the fibula, the tendinous arch crossing the posterior tibial vessels and nerve, and the soleal line of the posterior surface of the tibia. Its tendon joins the deep surface of the tendo Achilles. The gastrocnemius, plantaris, and soleus are supplied by the tibial nerve.

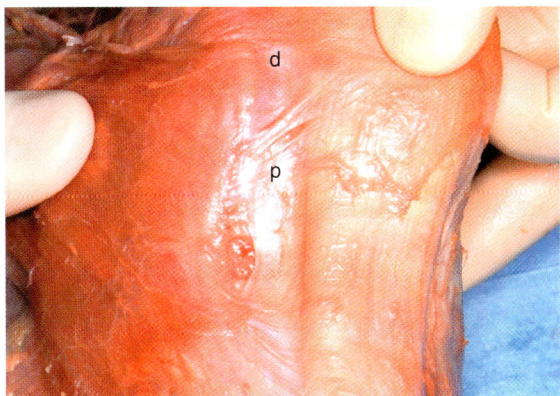

Figure 1-75. Close-up of an anatomic dissection of the lateral retinaculum. With the superficial oblique retinaculum removed, the patellotibial band *(p)* and transverse fibers *(d)* of the deep retinaculum can be identified.

NERVES

Although considerable individual variation exists, predominant patterns of innervation about the knee have been identified.[35,63] Two distinct groups of afferent nerves have been differentiated. The first, a posterior group, includes the posterior articular branch of the tibial nerve and obturator nerves. The second group is anterior and includes the articular branches of the femoral, common peroneal, and saphenous nerves.

The tibial nerve (medial or internal popliteal nerve) arises from the sciatic nerve halfway down the thigh. It runs distally through the popliteal fossa, lying at first in the fat beneath the deep fascia. More distally, it is found deeper in the interval between the two heads of the gastrocnemius. A cutaneous branch, the sural nerve, descends on the surface of the gastrocnemius (see Fig. 1-76). Muscular branches are given off to both heads of the gastrocnemius, plantaris, soleus, and popliteal muscles. In addition, several articular branches are present. The largest and most consistent branch, the posterior articular nerve, has a variable origin but often arises within the popliteal fossa. In other circumstances, it may arise from the tibial portion of the sciatic nerve in the thigh.[35] It courses laterally and wraps around the popliteal vessels before passing deep to join the popliteal plexus. Fibers from the plexus penetrate through the oblique popliteal ligament to innervate the posterior and perimeniscal capsule and the synovial covering of the cruciates. The extent of innervation of the menisci is controversial; evidence supports penetration of both nerve fibers into the outer third of the menisci and

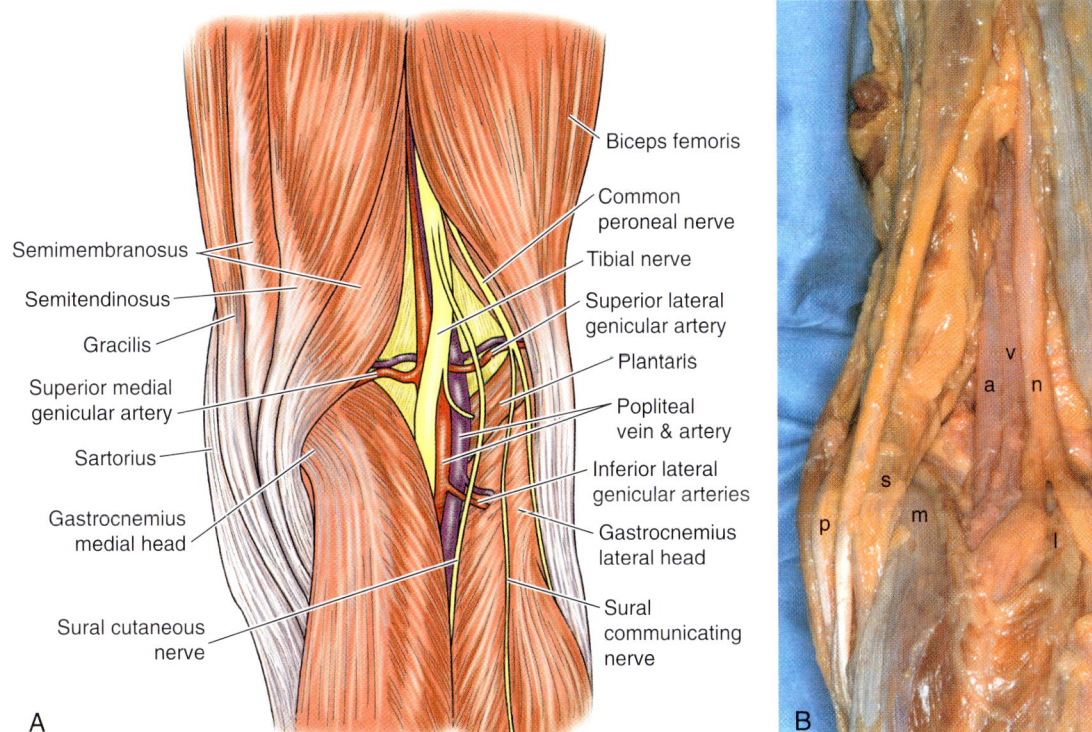

Figure 1-76. A, Posterior aspect of the knee. The tibial nerve arises from the sciatic nerve in the thigh. The popliteal artery and vein are in close proximity. **B,** Anatomic dissection of the popliteal fossa. From left to right (medial to lateral), the identified structures at the level of the joint line are the pes tendons *(p)*; semimembranosus *(s)*; medial head of the gastrocnemius *(m)*; popliteal artery *(a)*, vein *(v)*, and nerve *(n)*; lateral head of the gastrocnemius *(l)*; and biceps femoris tendon *(b)*.

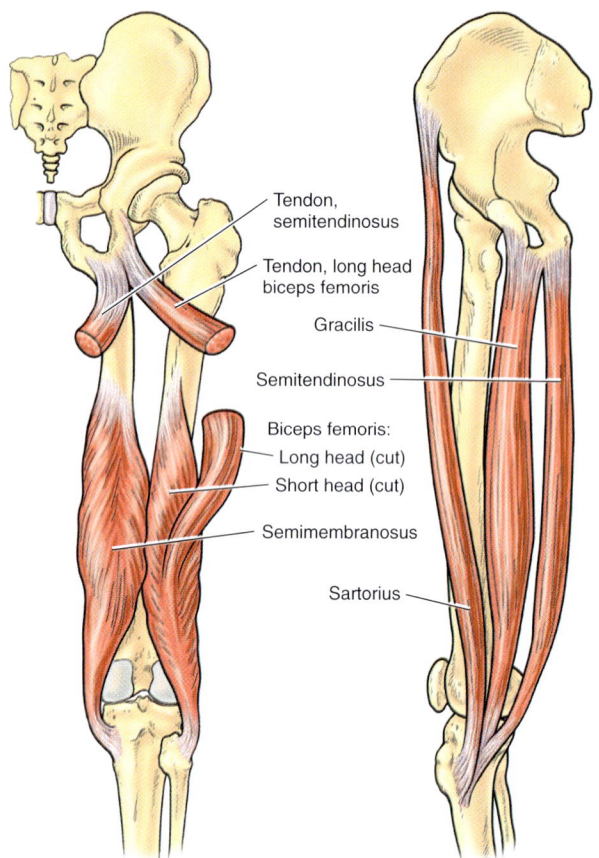

Figure 1-77. Posterior musculature.

innervation limited to the perimeniscal capsule.[63] The terminal branch of the posterior division of the obturator nerve, which follows the course of the femoral artery into the popliteal fossa, contributes to the popliteal plexus and thus to the innervation of the capsule and menisci.

The capsule and ligaments on the anteromedial and anterolateral areas of the knee are innervated by the anterior afferent group, in particular, the articular branches of the nerves, which supply the quadriceps muscles. The largest branch arises from the nerve supplying the vastus medialis and supplies a portion of the anteromedial capsule. Laterally, a branch from the nerve to the vastus lateralis innervates the superolateral capsule, and anteriorly, afferent fibers from the suprapatellar pouch join nerves to the vastus intermedius. The saphenous nerve arises from the posterior division of the femoral nerve. At the lower end of the subsartorial canal, the nerve pierces the deep fascia on the medial side of the knee between the sartorius and gracilis tendons. The infrapatellar branch traverses the sartorius muscle and joins the patellar plexus; it provides innervation to the anteromedial capsule, patellar tendon, and skin anteromedially (Fig. 1-79).[55] Distally, the sartorial branch of the saphenous nerve is joined by the long saphenous vein and runs along the medial aspect of the leg (Fig. 1-80). The patellar plexus lies in front of the patella and the patellar tendon. It is formed by numerous communications between the terminal branches of the lateral, intermediate, and medial cutaneous nerves of the thigh and the infrapatellar branch of the saphenous nerve.

The common peroneal nerve (lateral or external popliteal nerve) enters the popliteal fossa on the lateral side of the tibial nerve and runs distally along the medial side of the biceps tendon (Fig. 1-81). The common peroneal nerve

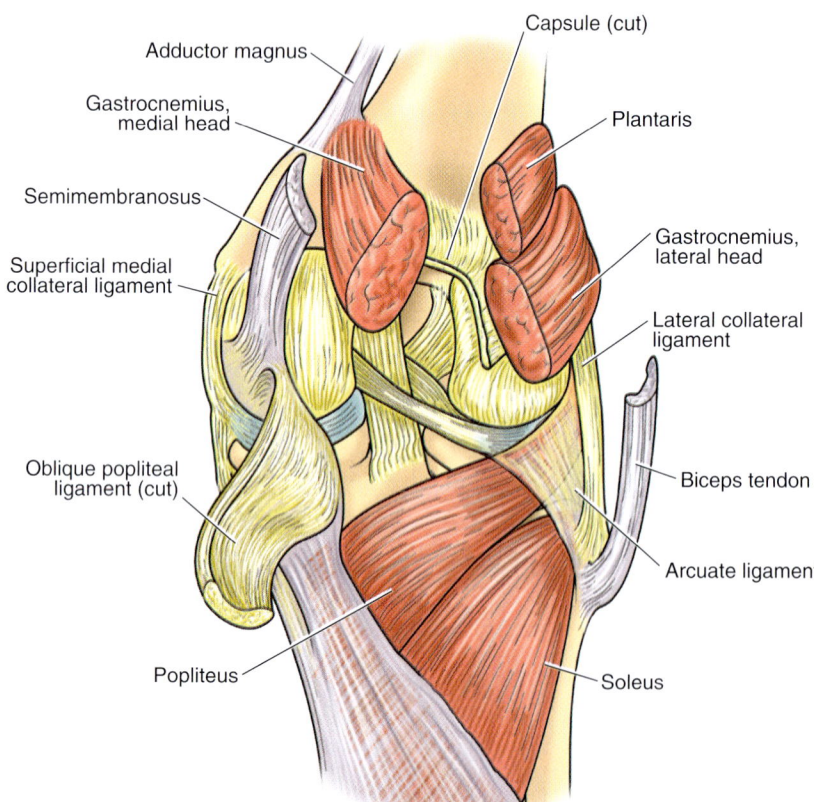

Figure 1-78. Popliteal fossa.

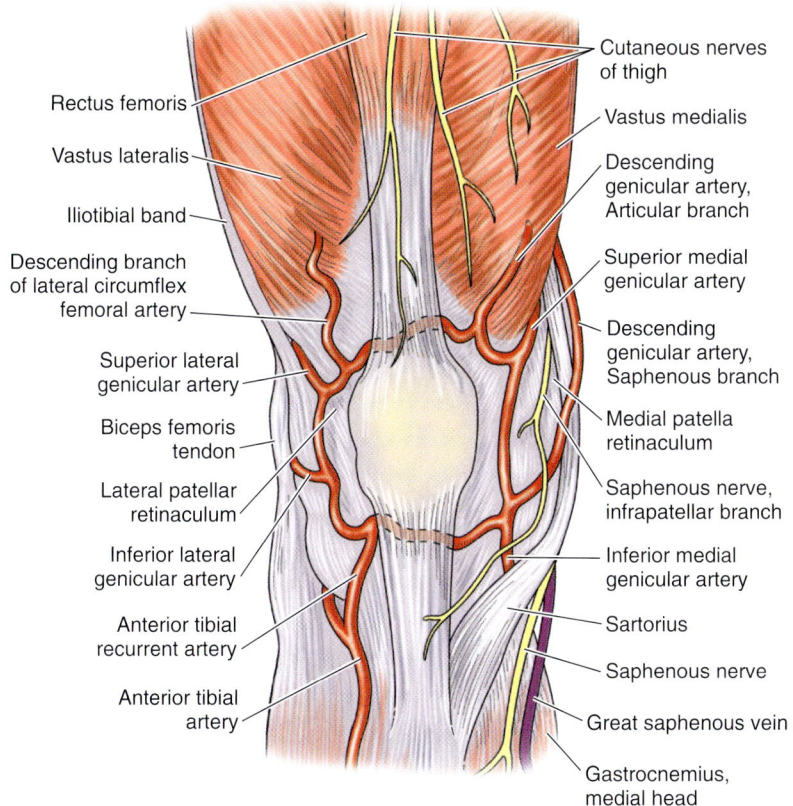

Figure 1-79. Superficial neurovascular structures of the anterior aspect of the knee.

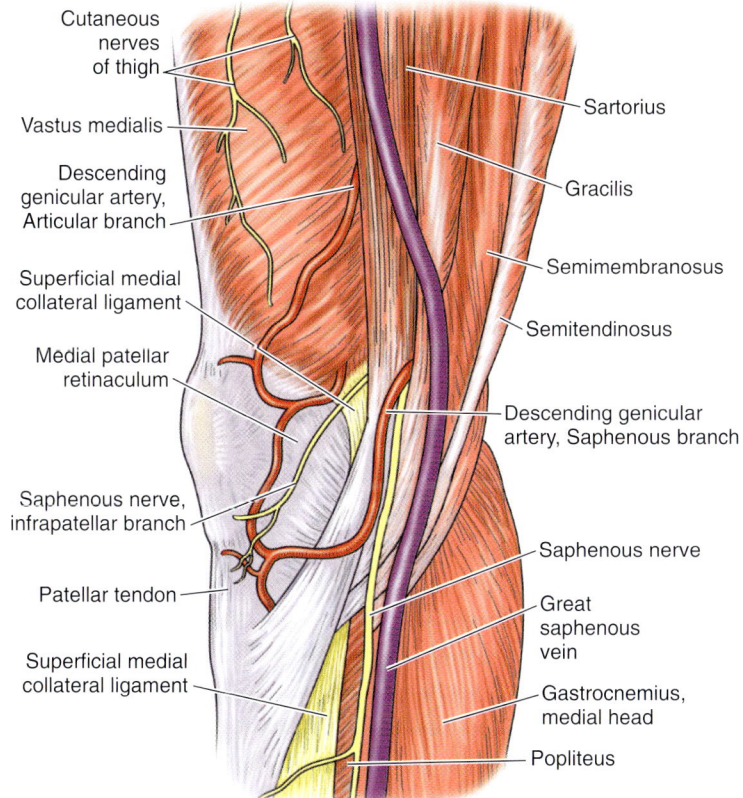

Figure 1-80. Superficial neurovascular structures of the anteromedial aspect of the knee.

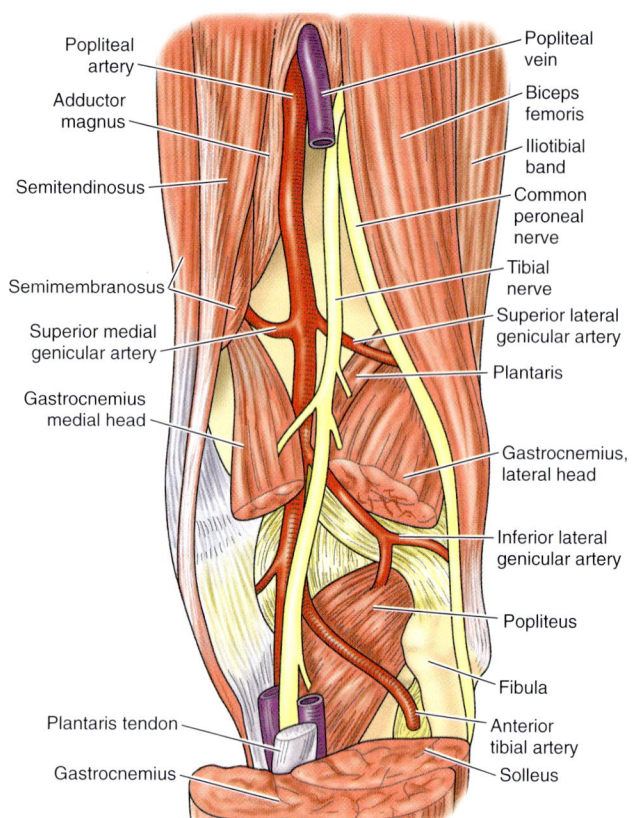

Figure 1-81. Neurovascular structures of the popliteal fossa.

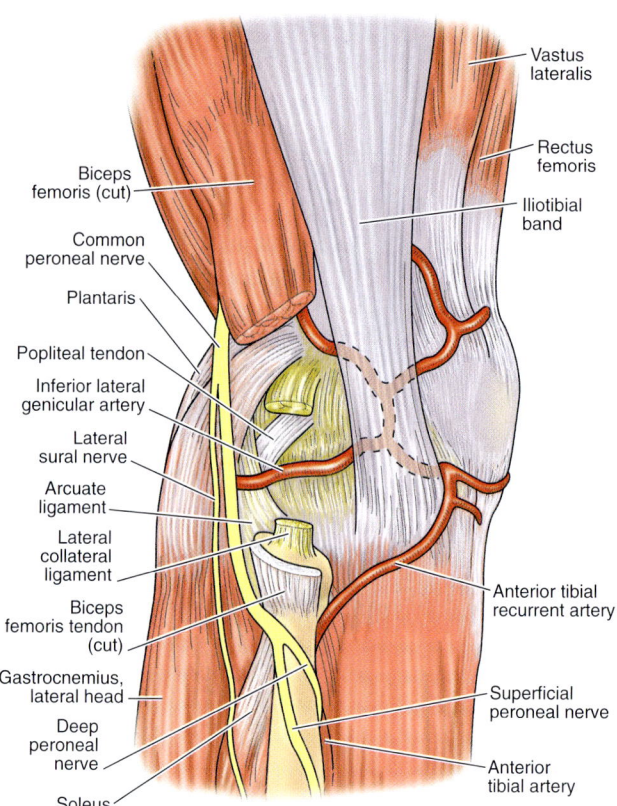

Figure 1-82. Superficial neurovascular structures of the lateral aspect of the knee.

passes between the biceps femoris tendon and the lateral head of the gastrocnemius and runs distally posterior to the fibula head (Fig. 1-82). It next winds superficially across the lateral aspect of the neck of the fibula before piercing the peroneus longus through a fibrous tunnel and dividing into the superficial peroneal (musculocutaneous) and deep peroneal (anterior tibial) nerves. The cutaneous branches are the sural communicating nerve, which joins the sural nerve, and a small branch to the skin over the upper anterolateral aspect of the leg. Two articular branches of the common peroneal nerve are the lateral articular nerve, which arises at the level of the joint line and innervates the inferior lateral capsule and LCL, and the recurrent peroneal nerve, which ascends the anterior surface of the tibia in the peroneus longus and enters the joint anterolaterally.[63]

The individual structures involved in specific functions such as pain sensation and proprioception in the knee are controversial. Kennedy et al indicated that deep fibrous structures such as the ligaments and menisci rarely contain nerve fibers, whereas both pain and specialized mechanoreceptors are found in the surrounding connective tissues of the capsule and synovium.[63] Stretching of the capsule causes pain, and effusions greater than 60 mL have been shown to cause reflex quadriceps inhibition.[63,104] Because of the numerous mechanoreceptors, the capsule also probably plays a significant role in proprioception.

BLOOD SUPPLY

Before passing through the adductor hiatus, the femoral artery gives off the descending genicular artery. This vessel,

in turn, gives off the saphenous branch, an articular branch, and the deep oblique branch. The saphenous branch travels distally with the saphenous nerve and passes the sartorius before anastomosing with the medial inferior genicular artery. The articular branch extends distally within the vastus medialis and anastomoses with the lateral superior genicular artery to contribute to the peripatellar network. The deep oblique branch courses along the medial aspect of the femur and gives off branches to the supracondylar femur, as well as collateral muscular branches. The popliteal artery exits from Hunter's canal and enters the popliteal fossa at the junction of the middle and lower thirds of the femur (Fig. 1-83). Proximally, it is separated from the femur by a thick pad of fat, but distally, in the region of the posterior joint line, it lies in direct contact with the oblique posterior ligament. Farther distally, the artery runs superficial to the popliteus fascia and ends at the lower border of the popliteus by dividing into the anterior and posterior tibial arteries.

The popliteal artery gives off numerous muscular branches and five articular branches (Fig. 1-84). The middle genicular artery arises from the anterior aspect of the popliteal artery and pierces the posterior oblique ligament to supply the posterior capsule and intracapsular structures, including the posterior horns of the menisci (Fig. 1-85).[98] Ligamentous branches of this artery traverse the synovium and form a plexus of vessels that cover both the ACL and the PCL and perforate the ligaments to anastomose with small vessels, which run parallel to the collagen fibrils.[98] The cruciates may also receive terminal branches from the inferior genicular arteries. The ACL receives essentially no blood supply from the ligament–bone insertion sites.[6] The medial and lateral

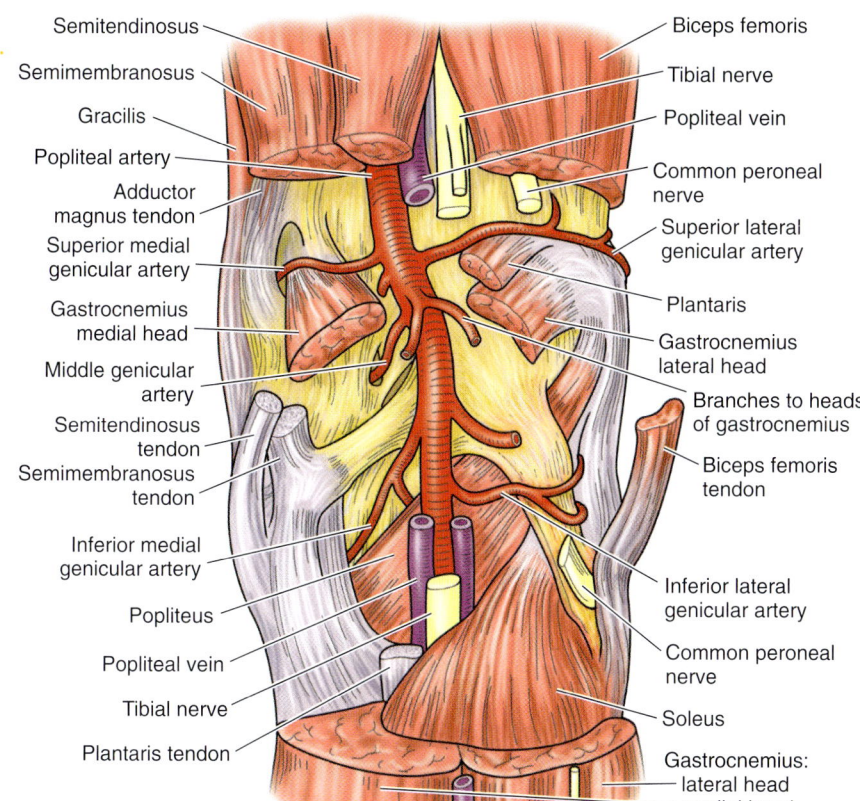

Semitendinosus
Semimembranosus
Gracilis
Popliteal artery
Adductor magnus tendon
Superior medial genicular artery
Gastrocnemius medial head
Middle genicular artery
Semitendinosus tendon
Semimembranosus tendon
Inferior medial genicular artery
Popliteus
Popliteal vein
Tibial nerve
Plantaris tendon

Biceps femoris
Tibial nerve
Popliteal vein
Common peroneal nerve
Superior lateral genicular artery
Plantaris
Gastrocnemius lateral head
Branches to heads of gastrocnemius
Biceps femoris tendon
Inferior lateral genicular artery
Common peroneal nerve
Soleus
Gastrocnemius: lateral head, medial head

Figure 1-83. Branches of the popliteal artery in the popliteal space. The artery lies on the oblique posterior ligament at the level of the joint line. More proximally, it is separated from the posterior of the femur by a layer of fat. The femoral vein is interposed between the artery and the tibial nerve.

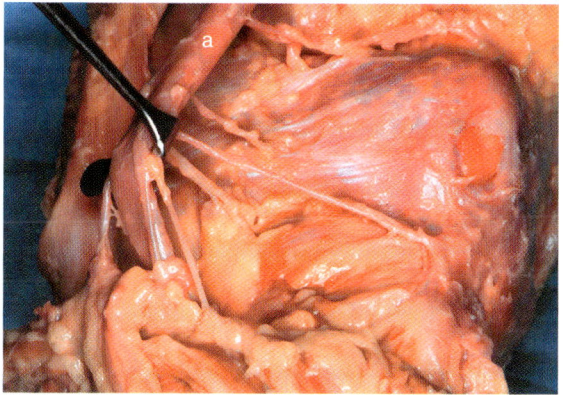

Figure 1-84. Anatomic dissection of the popliteal artery. The popliteal artery *(a)* has been elevated (probe) to reveal, from proximal to distal, the superior lateral genicular, middle genicular (passing through the posterior oblique ligament), inferior lateral and medial genicular, and two sural branches.

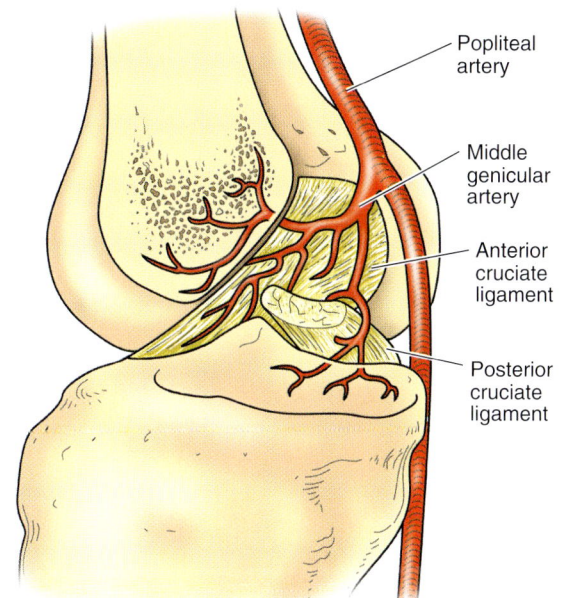

Popliteal artery
Middle genicular artery
Anterior cruciate ligament
Posterior cruciate ligament

Figure 1-85. Middle genicular artery with supply to the cruciate ligaments.

superior genicular arteries originate from the posterior aspect of the artery and then wind around the lower end of the femur immediately proximal to the condyles. The lateral superior genicular artery passes deep to the biceps femoris tendon and then anastomoses with the descending branch of the lateral femoral circumflex artery. The medial superior genicular branch courses anteriorly deep to the semimembranosus and semitendinosus and proximal to the origin of the medial head of the gastrocnemius. Arising more distally at a level below the joint line from either side of the popliteal artery are the medial and lateral inferior genicular arteries. The inferior lateral genicular artery lies immediately adjacent to the lateral joint line. It passes deep to the LCL, proximal to the fibular head, as it traverses anterolaterally to join the anterior anastomosis. The inferior medial genicular artery passes two fingerbreadths distal to the medial joint line, deep to the MCL, and also joins the anterior anastomosis.

Branches from the inferior genicular arteries form a complex capillary network in the anterior fat pad and provide abundant supply to the fat pad, synovial cavity, and patellar tendon. Terminal branches of all four medial and lateral genicular arteries also extend into the menisci, but Arnoczky and Warren[7] have shown that the predominant vascular supply comes from the superior and inferior lateral genicular

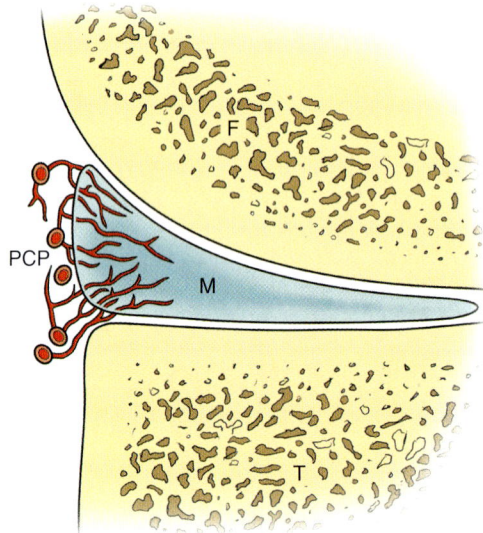

Figure 1-86. Diagrammatic representation of the peripheral blood supply to the medial meniscus *(M)*. *F,* Femur; *PCP,* perimeniscal capillary plexus; *T,* tibia.

arteries. Rather than providing a uniform supply to the entire menisci, only the peripheral 30% receive these vascular branches (Fig. 1-86). Tears that occur in this peripheral vascular zone are considered to be the best candidates for repair.

The anterior anastomosis around the knee is formed by the four inferior and superior genicular arteries, branches of the descending genicular artery, the descending branch of the lateral circumflex femoral artery, and recurrent branches of the anterior tibial artery. The anastomosis thus connects the femoral artery at the origin of its profundus branch with the popliteal and anterior tibial arteries (Fig. 1-87). Anteriorly, the anastomosis forms a vascular circle around the patella, from which, according to Scapinelli, 9 to 12 nutrient arteries arise at the lower pole of the patella and run proximally on the anterior surface of the bone in a series of furrows (Fig. 1-88).[97] These vessels penetrate the anterior surface of the patella in the middle third. Additional polar vessels penetrate the patella in the apical region. The patellar retinaculum on the medial side is supplied by the anastomosis, with the main contribution coming from the descending genicular artery. The lateral retinaculum receives almost all of its supply from the lateral anastomosis formed by the superior and inferior lateral genicular arteries.[24] The arterial supply to the patellar tendon appears to be derived from two anastomotic arches that are fed by medial and lateral pedicles.[103] The descending and inferior medial genicular arteries appear to be important contributors to the medial pedicles, whereas on the lateral side, the lateral genicular arteries and recurrent tibial anterior arteries provide the greatest contributions.[103] Perforating collateral vessels from the superior (retropatellar) and inferior (supratubercular) anastomotic arches create two distinct

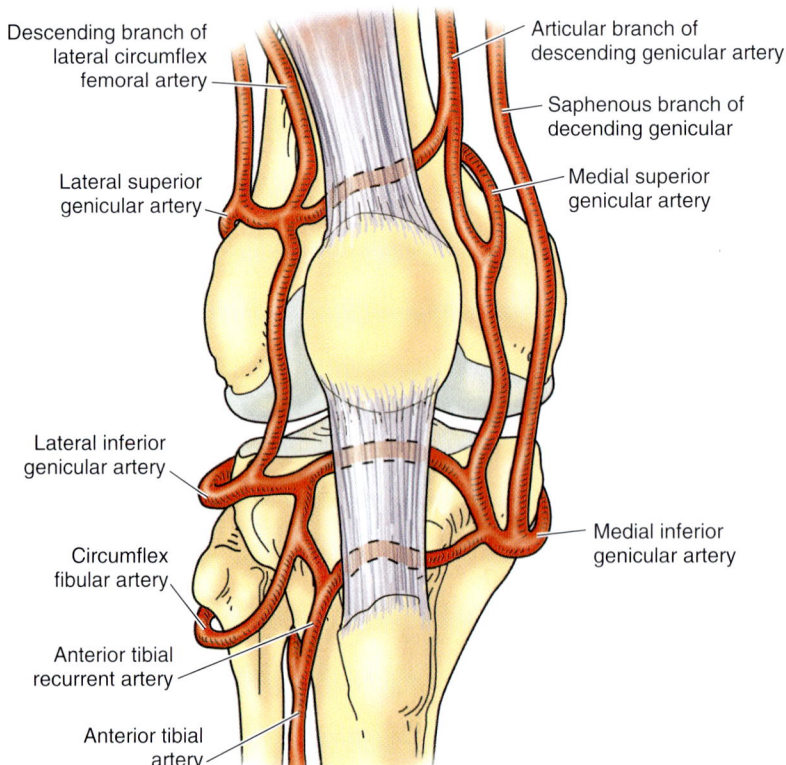

Descending branch of lateral circumflex femoral artery

Lateral superior genicular artery

Lateral inferior genicular artery

Circumflex fibular artery

Anterior tibial recurrent artery

Anterior tibial artery

Articular branch of descending genicular artery

Saphenous branch of decending genicular

Medial superior genicular artery

Medial inferior genicular artery

Figure 1-87. Genicular artery circulation and anterior artery anastomosis of the knee.

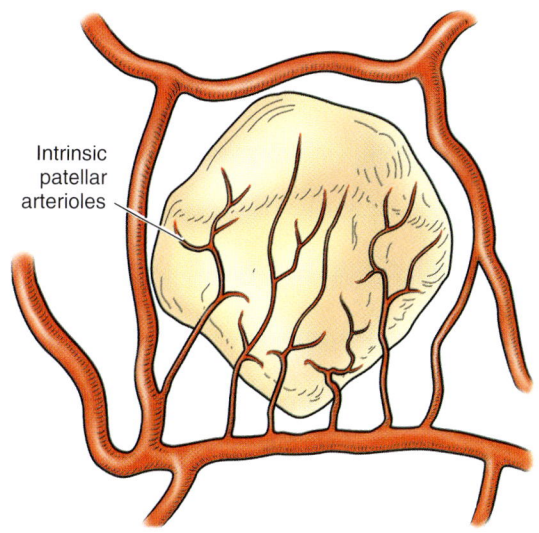

Figure 1-88. Vascular circle around the patella, which, according to Scapinelli,[97] supplies the patella via nutrient arteries that enter predominantly at the inferior pole. The genicular arteries and their branches lie in the most superficial layer of the deep fascia.

Intrinsic patellar arterioles

vascular zones that anastomose in the middle third of the tendon.[103]

The skin overlying the anterior aspect of the knee receives its blood supply via three routes: direct cutaneous, musculocutaneous, and septocutaneous (intermuscular) vessels.[18,43,44] These vessels provide arterial inflow in both random perforating and axial-type distributions. Perforating vessels include terminal branches from the anterior anastomosis, as well as additional musculocutaneous terminal branches from the rectus femoris and vastus muscle group. Once they have perforated through the deep fascia, these vessels run parallel to the skin surface for a considerable distance in the loose areolar layer that separates the deep fascia from subcutaneous fat. In this layer, these vessels form an interconnecting fascial plexus.[43,107] Branches from this fascial plexus traverse the subcutaneous tissue and anastomose with other branches to create a subdermal plexus.[42,107] Because the skin relies on the distribution from the fascial plexus just superficial to the deep fascia, the true surgical plane of the anterior knee is beneath the deep fascia; consequently, undermining of the skin in a manner that creates elevated skin and subcutaneous flaps should be minimized.[42] Furthermore, although the skin receives arterial inflow from the medial and lateral contributions to the anterior anastomosis, the principal vascular supply is provided from the medial side.[24,43] In particular, the saphenous artery, which arises in a common trunk with the descending genicular vessel from the superficial femoral artery, provides a major contribution to the fascial plexus.[24,43]

Surgical exposure of the knee interrupts flow into variable portions of this network of perforating terminal branches. In a healthy individual, a single midline anterior incision presents little problem for wound healing, but multiple previous incisions or ischemic disease can lead to wound complications or skin necrosis. In general, a previous transverse incision may be crossed perpendicularly. If multiple longitudinal incisions are present, the most lateral midline incision should be selected in the majority of circumstances to avoid creating large laterally based flaps as a result of the medially biased arterial inflow.[24]

The popliteal vein enters the popliteal fossa on the lateral side of the artery; it crosses superficial to the artery and lies on the medial side in the lower part of the fossa. Throughout the popliteal fossa, it is interposed between the artery and the tibial nerve (see Fig. 1-65A).

MOTION AND FUNCTION

The knee joint is a modified hinge that possesses limited inherent stability from the bony architecture. Lack of conformity between the bony surfaces allows 6 degrees of freedom of motion about the knee, including translation in three planes (medial-lateral, anterior-posterior, proximal-distal) and rotation in three planes (flexion-extension, internal-external, and varus-valgus). Motion and stability of the joint are controlled by additional intra-articular static stabilizers, including the menisci and cruciate ligaments, as well as extra-articular static and dynamic stabilizers, such as the collateral ligaments and muscles.[49,58,80,118] In full extension, both collateral and cruciate ligaments are taut, and the anterior aspects of both menisci are snugly held between the condyles of the tibia and the femur. At the beginning of flexion, the knee "unlocks" and external rotation of the femur on the tibia occurs, which, according to Last, is brought about by contraction of the popliteus muscle.[72] During the first 30 degrees of flexion, rollback of the femur on the tibia occurs and is more pronounced laterally. After 30 degrees, the femoral condyles spin at one point on the tibial condyles.[15,92] New evidence from dynamic MRI studies demonstrates that the medial condyle essentially remains static on the tibia as flexion occurs, with rollback basically limited to the lateral condyle.[31] The menisci, which are squeezed between the joint surfaces in extension, move posteriorly with the femur in flexion, the lateral more so than the medial. The articular surface of the medial femoral condyle is larger than that of the lateral femoral condyle; when the direction of motion is reversed, the lateral compartment reaches a position of full extension first before the medial compartment is fully extended. Terminal extension is achieved and the knee is "locked" by internal rotation of the femur on the tibia—the so-called screw home mechanism—until the medial compartment also reaches the limits of extension (Fig. 1-89).

Some portion of the superficial MCL remains taut throughout flexion, whereas the LCL is taut only in extension and relaxes as soon as the knee is flexed, thereby permitting greater excursion of the lateral tibial condyle.

The superficial MCL is the most important medial stabilizer.[116] Parallel fibers move in a posterior direction as the knee is flexed. The attachments to the femoral condyle are such that with the knee in extension, the posterior fibers are taut and the anterior fibers relax and are drawn in under the posterior part of the ligament (Fig. 1-90). With flexion of the knee, the anterior fibers move proximally and become tight and are then subjected to increasing tension as the joint is flexed (Fig. 1-91). This action, according to Palmer, is attributable to the oval shape of the femoral origin, which changes its orientation in flexion such that the attachments of the most anterior fibers are elevated.[92] As the anterior border becomes tight, the posterior fibers slacken as the knee flexes and remain relaxed throughout flexion. The posterior oblique fibers are relaxed in extension and lie partially beneath the parallel fibers. In flexion, the fibers are drawn out (Fig. 1-92);

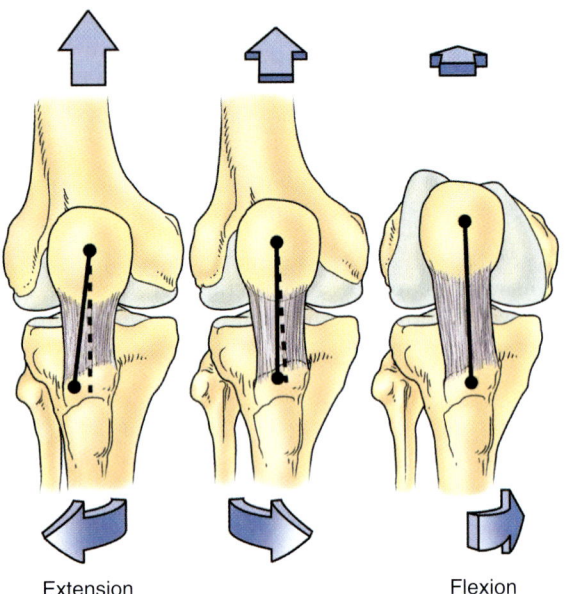

Extension   Flexion

Figure 1-89. Screw home mechanism. At full extension, the tibial tubercle lies lateral to the midpoint of the patella.

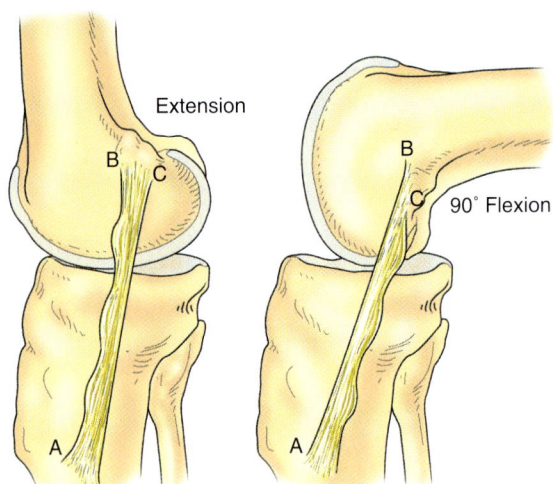

Figure 1-91. Diagram of the superficial medial ligament with flexion and extension of the knee. Because point B moves superiorly, the anterior border is tightened in flexion. Conversely, in extension, point C moves proximally and tightens the posterior margin of the ligament. (From Warren LF, Marshall JL, Girgis FG: The prime static stabilizer of the medial side of the knee. J Bone Joint Surg Am 56:665, 1974.)

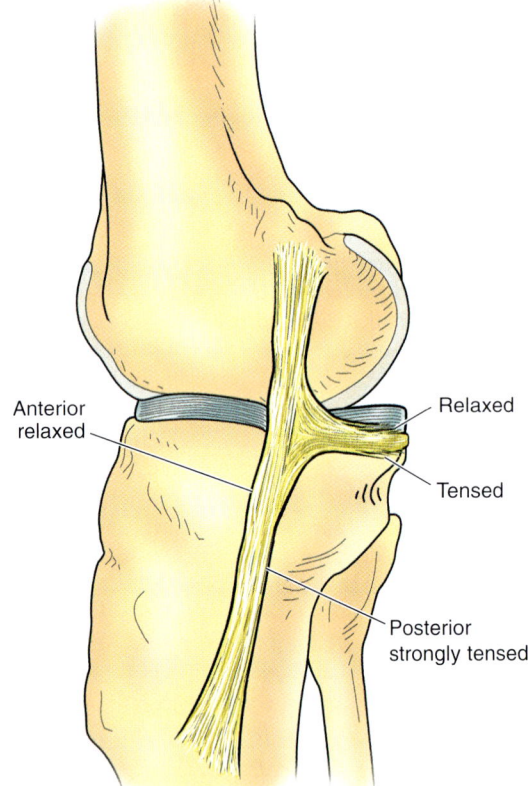

Figure 1-90. In extension, the posterior margin of the medial collateral ligament is tense and the anterior border relatively relaxed. Proximal anterior fibers are drawn underneath the posterior fibers.

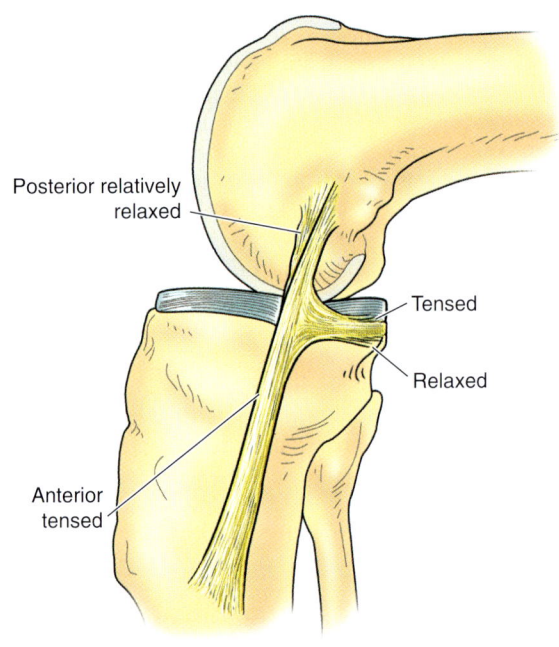

Figure 1-92. The posterior oblique fibers become more tense in flexion. (From Palmer I: On the injuries to ligaments of the knee joint: a clinical study. Acta Chir Scand 81[Suppl 53]:3, 1938.)

according to Palmer, because of their attachment to the capsule and the periphery of the medial meniscus, these fibers check the backward sliding of the meniscus that occurs in flexion. In the presence of intact parallel fibers, approximately 1 to 2 mm of medial opening to valgus stress is present.

The joint is slightly tighter in full extension, and the greatest degree of medial opening occurs at 45 degrees.[116] Parallel fibers of the superficial MCL also control rotation; sectioning these fibers not only increases the amount of medial opening to valgus stress but also causes a significant increase in external rotation. In distinction, sectioning the capsule, the deep MCL, or the oblique fibers of the superficial MCL causes little or no increase in rotation.[116]

Lateral stability is provided by several structures.[52] In extension, the fibers of the iliotibial tract are crucial, and because these fibers attach proximally to the femur and distally to the tibia, they may be regarded as a true ligament. However, Kaplan demonstrated, through electrical stimulation of the tensor fascia lata and traction on the iliotibial tract in cadavers, that contractions of the tensor fascia lata and gluteus maximus are not transmitted to the tibia; therefore, the iliotibial tract does not represent a tendon.[59] As the knee flexes, the iliotibial tract moves posteriorly and becomes somewhat relaxed; beyond approximately 30 degrees of flexion, the tendon of the biceps femoris may become an important lateral stabilizer.[81]

The lateral ligament is also taut in extension but is relaxed throughout flexion. The same is true of the arcuate ligament. Thus, in flexion, a much greater degree of rotation is possible laterally than medially. This rotation is permitted by the attachments of the lateral meniscus and by relaxation of the supporting ligaments in flexion. A greater degree of rolling of the femur on the tibia is seen, whereas medially, this motion is only slight. The attachment of the popliteal tendon to the lateral meniscus draws the meniscus posteriorly and prevents entrapment as the knee is flexed.[72]

The ACL consists of two functional bands: an anteromedial band and a stronger, thicker posterolateral part. In extension, the ligament appears as a flat band, and the posterolateral bulk of the ligament is taut (see Fig. 1-50). Almost immediately after flexion begins, the smaller anteromedial band becomes tight, and the bulk of the ligament slackens. In flexion, it is the anteromedial band that provides the primary restraint against anterior displacement of the tibia.[36]

The PCL consists of two inseparable parts. An anterior portion forms the bulk of the ligament, and a smaller posterior part runs obliquely to the back of the tibia. In extension, the bulk of the ligament is relaxed, and only the posterior band is tight. In flexion, the major portion of the ligament becomes tight, and the small posterior band is loose (see Fig. 1-56).[35,111]

The ACL is a check against both hyperextension and internal and external rotation. The PCL is a check against posterior instability in the flexed knee but not against hyperextension, provided that the anterior cruciate is intact.

According to Palmer, tightening of the anterior cruciate in extension fixes the lateral femoral condyle anteriorly; thus, continuation of movement into hyperextension is possible only when simultaneous inward rotation of the femur occurs.[92]

Rotation occurs around an axis through the center of the medial femoral condyle as a result of the tighter anchorage of this condyle by the superficial MCL. If this ligament is ruptured, the axis shifts laterally. According to Palmer, because of the medially shifted axis of rotation, external rotation of the tibia relaxes the ACL through forward travel of the lateral femoral condyle, at the same time stretching the PCL.[92] Internal rotation reverses this sequence, tensing the anterior cruciate and relaxing the posterior cruciate.

A fibrous band connects the posterior cruciate with the posterior margin of the lateral meniscus (the tibiomeniscal ligament of Kaplan). This band probably restricts the forward sliding motion of the lateral meniscus in internal rotation.

Girgis et al have shown that rotary movements of the tibia on the femur occur in all ranges of motion.[36] Their studies indicate that the anterior cruciate is a check against external rotation in flexion but does not significantly limit internal rotation. In extension, the ACL is a check against external rotation and to a lesser degree against internal rotation. Thus, the precise function of the cruciate ligaments with regard to rotation is a topic of some disagreement.

Action of the Muscles

The movements of the knee are flexion, extension, and rotation. Flexion is performed by the hamstrings and biceps femoris and, to a lesser extent, by the gastrocnemius and popliteus. Flexion is limited by the soft tissues at the back of the knee. Extension is performed by the quadriceps, and because of the shape of the articulation and the ligament attachments, the femur rotates medially on the tibia in terminal extension; this is the screw home mechanism that locks the joint. This movement is purely passive, as are other rotary movements that occur during activity, and is due to the articular geometry and static stabilizers as previously described. The exception is lateral rotation of the femur that precedes flexion by unlocking the joint. This movement is performed by the popliteus. The sartorius, gracilis, and hamstrings are weak rotators of the knee but probably do not act as such. The sartorius, gracilis, and semitendinosus medially and the iliotibial tract laterally most often act as "guy ropes" to stabilize the pelvis.

KEY REFERENCES

Agur AMR, Dalley AF: Grant's atlas of anatomy, ed 12, Philadelphia, 2009, Wolters Kluwer Health/Lippincott Williams & Wilkins.

Basmajian JV: Grant's method of anatomy, ed 10, Baltimore, 1980, Williams & Wilkins.

Brantigan OC, Voshell AF: The tibial collateral ligament: its function, its bursae, and its relation to the medial meniscus. J Bone Joint Surg 25:121, 1943.

Haertsch P: The blood supply to the skin of the leg: a post-mortem investigation. Br J Plast Surg 34:470, 1981.

Johnson DL, Swenson TM, Livesay MS, et al: Insertion site anatomy of the human menisci: gross, arthroscopic, and topographical anatomy as a basis for meniscal transplantation. Arthroscopy 11:386, 1995.

Kennedy JC, Alexander IJ, Hayes KC: Nerve supply of the knee and its functional importance. Am J Sports Med 10:329, 1982.

Last RJ: Anatomy: regional and applied, ed 6, Edinburgh, 1978, Churchill Livingstone.

Miyamoto RG, Bosco JA, Sherman OH: Treatment of medial collateral ligament injuries. J Am Acad Orthop Surg 17:152, 2009.

Petersen W, Zantop T: Anatomy of the anterior cruciate ligament with regard to two bundles. Clin Orthop 454:35, 2006.

Reider B, Marshall JL, Koslin B, et al: The anterior aspect of the knee joint: an anatomical study. J Bone Joint Surg Am 63:351, 1981.

Renstrom P, Johnson RJ: Anatomy and biomechanics of the menisci. Clin Sports Med 9:523, 1990.

Scapinelli R: Blood supply of the human patella: its relation to ischaemic necrosis after fracture. J Bone Joint Surg Br 49:563, 1967.

Seebacher JR, Inglis AE, Marshall JL, et al: The structure of the posterolateral aspect of the knee. J Bone Joint Surg Am 64:536, 1982.

Warren LF, Marshall JL: The supporting structures and layers on the medial side of the knee: an anatomical analysis. J Bone Joint Surg Am 61:56, 1979.

Williams PL, Warwick R: Gray's anatomy, ed 36, Philadelphia, 1980, WB Saunders.

Full references for this chapter can be found on www.expertconsult.com.

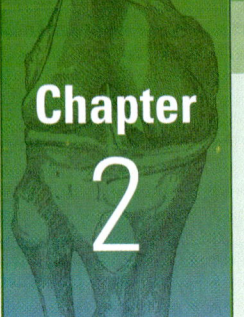

Chapter

2

Anatomic Aberrations

Henry D. Clarke, W. Norman Scott, and John N. Insall

Chapter 3

Clinical Examination of the Knee

Michael P. Nett, Henrik B. Pedersen, Gregory J. Roehrig,
Alfred J. Tria, Jr., and W. Norman Scott

HISTORY

Despite improvements in advanced imaging techniques, clinical examination of the knee remains an essential step in evaluating the knee patient. Evaluation of every patient should begin with a complete history of the symptoms and/or a full description of the mechanism of injury. Often, the history will direct the examiner to the area of knee involvement. This will sharpen the physical examination, result in a more accurate diagnosis, and allow the clinician to be more proficient.

OBSERVATION AND INSPECTION

The examination should begin with observation. Observation of the patient's gait provides critical information. The examiner should note the patient's ability to ambulate, the use of gait aids, the speed of ambulation, and the amount of discomfort present with attempted ambulation. Evaluation of the gait pattern and the stance position of the lower limb is performed while the patient ambulates. A shortened stance phase of gait (antalgic gait) will confirm the side of involvement. A short leg gait requires confirmation of limb length. This may be accompanied by a significant varus or valgus deformity at the knee or may represent an extra-articular deformity requiring further evaluation. Varus or valgus alignment should be noted, as well as any medial or lateral thrust in the stance phase of gait (Fig. 3-1). The clinical alignment of the lower part of the leg (anatomic axis) measures the femorotibial angle (Fig. 3-2) and is different from the mechanical axis of the limb (Fig. 3-3), as measured from the femoral head through the knee to the center of the ankle on a standing roentgenogram. With a goniometer applied to the anterior aspect of the thigh and the lower part of the leg and centered on the patella, the examiner can report the clinical varus or valgus alignment. This measurement should be used along with the roentgenographic measurements.

Patellar alignment must also be observed. It is influenced by femoral neck anteversion, tibial torsion, the anatomy of the individual patellar facets, and the depth and angle of the femoral sulcus (Fig. 3-4). The Q angle is drawn from the middle of the tibial tubercle to the middle of the patella and then to the anterior superior iliac spine of the pelvis. The normal angle is 10 to 20 degrees.

Clinical effusion may be apparent visually. Active range of motion should be recorded, along with any limitations to full extension or flexion. Active range of motion will be further evaluated with palpation and should be compared with passive range of motion of the knee (Fig. 3-5). It is customary that full extension should be considered 0 degrees, and flexion is recorded as an increasing number or as the distance of the heel of the foot from the buttocks. An inability to fully extend may represent lag, a locked knee, or a flexion contracture. An inability to fully flex may be due to an effusion, pain, or extension contracture.

Quadriceps atrophy is sometimes visually apparent and can help confirm the involved side. The gross appearance of quadriceps atrophy should lead to further investigation with circumferential measurement during the palpation phase of the physical examination.

PALPATION

All bony landmarks should be palpated and identified. The Q angle, Gerdy's tubercle, the fibular head, the epicondyles of the femur, the patellar margins, and the tibiofemoral joint lines can be readily palpated in most patients.

Effusions can be graded in size by compressing the suprapatellar pouch and then noting any fluid (grade 1), slight lift-off of the patella (grade 2), a ballotable patella (grade 3), or a tense effusion with no ability to compress the patella against the femoral sulcus (grade 4) (Fig. 3-6).

If muscle atrophy was noted on observation, thigh circumference should now be measured. The circumference of the thigh should be measured at a set distance (10 cm) above the patella with the knee in full extension, and then compared with the opposite side. The calf should be measured at its greatest circumference in the lower part of the leg.

Crepitation in and of itself may or may not represent evidence of a disorder. The location should be recorded for future reference. It may involve the medial or lateral patellofemoral articulation, the medial tibiofemoral articulation, or the lateral tibiofemoral articulation.

The Patellofemoral Joint

Examination of the patellofemoral joint includes both static and dynamic evaluation. Visual inspection should be performed to note any evidence of quadriceps atrophy or vastus medialis obliquus hypoplasia. Prepatellar swelling or erythema may be present, suggesting prepatellar bursitis. The Q angle should be measured with the patient supine and the hip and knee in full extension. If the knee is allowed to flex slightly, the Q angle will decrease with internal rotation of the tibia on the femur (Fig. 3-7). The average male Q angle is 14 ± 3 degrees, and the average female Q angle is 17 ± 3 degrees.[1] A Q angle greater than 20 degrees must be noted as excessive. Tracking of the patella from full extension into flexion should be recorded visually. In full extension, the patella begins with contact of the median ridge and the lateral facet with the lateral side of the sulcus. The patella moves more centrally and the facets increase their contact with the femoral condyles as flexion increases (Fig. 3-8). Excessive lateralization of the patella with full extensions will result in a pathologic "J-sign." This may be seen in patients with recurrent lateral subluxations or excessive

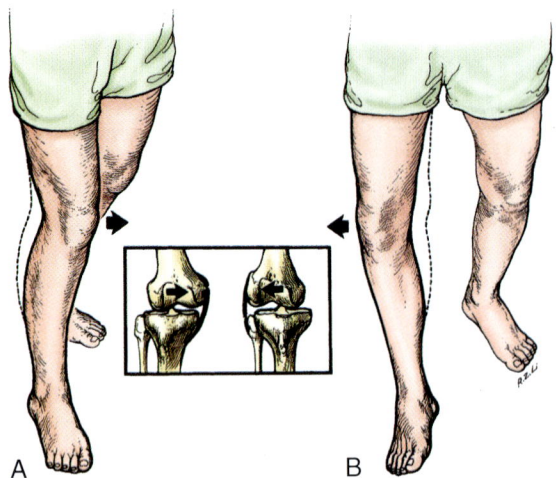

Figure 3-1. Medial thrust of the femur indicates shift of the femur medially on the tibia through the stance phase of gait in the coronal plane **(A)**. Lateral thrust indicates lateral shift of the femur in the coronal plane **(B)**. (From Tria AJ Jr, Klein KS: An illustrated guide to the knee, New York, 1992, Churchill Livingstone.)

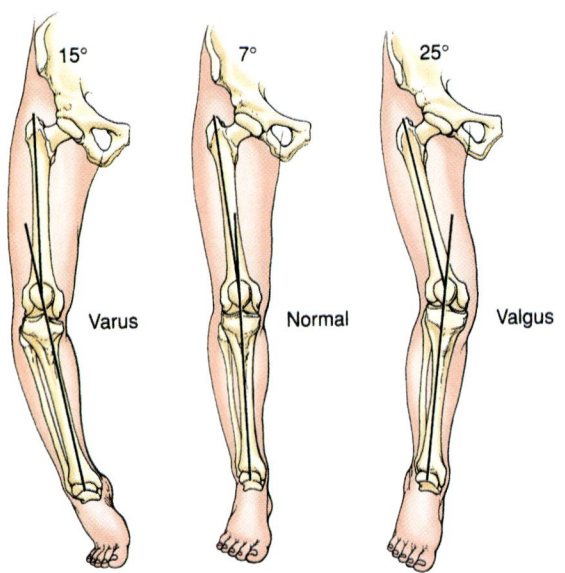

Figure 3-2. The anatomic axis is measured by drawing lines parallel to the long axis of the femur and the tibia and measuring the intercepting angle. (From Tria AJ Jr, Klein KS: An illustrated guide to the knee, New York, 1992, Churchill Livingstone.)

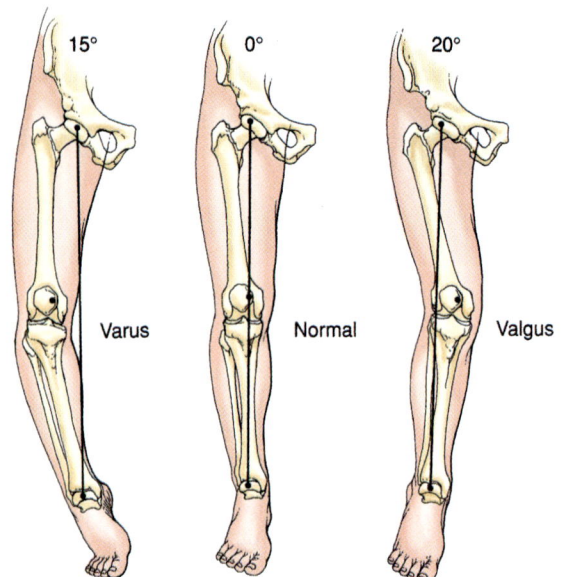

Figure 3-3. The mechanical axis of the leg is measured in the standing position with an imaginary "plumb line" dropped from the femoral head to the ground. This angular measurement gives the best functional evaluation of lower extremity alignment. (From Tria AJ Jr, Klein KS: An illustrated guide to the knee, New York, 1992, Churchill Livingstone.)

ligamentous laxity, or following a traumatic lateral patellar dislocation.

Because the patellar facets do not begin to contact the femoral sulcus until the knee is flexed 30 degrees, the medial and lateral patellofemoral articulation should be palpated at this degree of flexion. This can be accomplished by allowing the leg to bend slightly over the edge of the table or by placing a small pillow below the knee. Direct patellar compression is performed and may elicit pain over the medial or lateral facet, depending on the location of the pathology (Fig. 3-9). Direct compression can be performed at progressively increasing degrees of flexion to further isolate the location of a chondral lesion. The patellar grind test consists of quadriceps contraction while direct compression is placed on the patella. When performed in full extension, entrapped synovium can cause pain even with a normal patellofemoral joint. This is especially true in the patient with patella alta. This is an unreliable test and is not recommended. The examiner should complete the static aspect of the examination by evaluating for the presence of tenderness over the medial and lateral facets of the patella, the medial and lateral retinacula, the insertion of the quadriceps tendon, and the insertion of the patellar tendon.

Dynamic evaluation should include observation of patellar tracking with active knee flexion and extension. This is performed with the patient seated on the edge of the examination table and the knees bent over the side (Fig. 3-10). The patella can be seen engaging the trochlea at 10 to 30 degrees of flexion.[2] Any excessive lateral displacement with full extension or any maltracking should be noted. After patellar tracking is assessed, the examiner should place one hand over the anterior aspect of the patella and provide resistance to knee extension with the opposite hand. Knee extension against resistance will elicit any patellofemoral crepitus or pain from chondral pathology. The half-squat test is a different technique to load the patellofemoral joint in a similar manner. With this test, the patient is asked to hold the position of a half-squat and report the presence of anterior knee pain.

Patellar tilt, mobility, and the presence of patellar apprehension are then evaluated. The patient is placed in a supine position. In full extension, neutral or slight lateral tilt of the patella is normal. The inability to tilt the patella past neutral indicates an excessively tight lateral retinaculum (Fig. 3-11). With the knee flexed 20 to 30 degrees, patellar mobility is assessed. Both medial and lateral translation should be noted. Translation should not exceed two quadrants in either direction.[3] If less than one quadrant of medial translation is

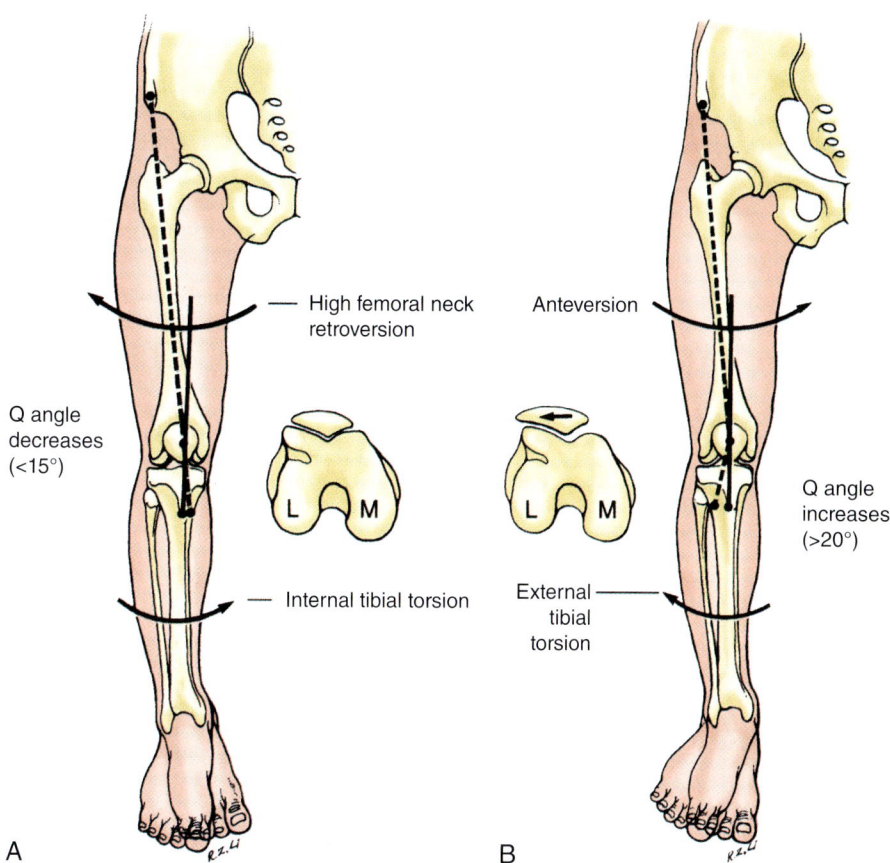

Figure 3-4. High femoral neck retroversion rotates the distal end of the femur externally. In combination with internal tibial torsion, the Q angle is decreased. Patellar tracking is improved, and patellofemoral sulcus alignment is normal. High femoral neck anteversion rotates the distal end of the femur internally. In combination with external tibial torsion, the Q angle is increased. Patellar tracking is compromised, and the patella tends to track laterally. (From Tria AJ Jr, Klein KS: An illustrated guide to the knee, New York, 1992, Churchill Livingstone.)

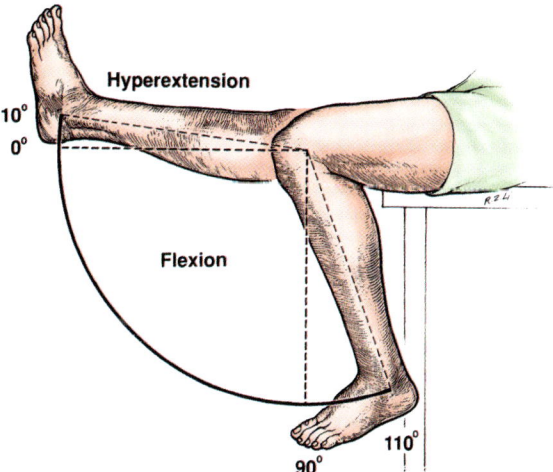

Figure 3-5. Full extension of the knee is the zero or neutral point. (From Tria AJ Jr, Klein KS: An illustrated guide to the knee, New York, 1992, Churchill Livingstone.)

present, this suggests an excessively tight lateral retinaculum. Patellar apprehension should also be assessed with the knee flexed 20 to 30 degrees (Fig. 3-12).[4] Medial apprehension may be seen but is much less frequent and often iatrogenic in nature following an excessive lateral release. Lateral apprehension is more common and may suggest recurrent subluxations, traumatic lateral patellar dislocation, or excessive ligamentous laxity.

Examination of the patellofemoral joint is not complete until the hip is examined. Passive and active range of motion of the hip should be recorded. Excessive internal rotation of the hip secondary to increased femoral anteversion will result in an increased Q angle and may be part of a "miserable malalignment" type syndrome.[5] Hip rotation and femoral anteversion should be assessed with the patient in a prone position (Fig. 3-13). Internal rotation that exceeds external rotation by greater than 30 degrees is considered pathologic and should be noted.[6] Limited range of motion or pain with hip range of motion may signify hip pathology as a source of referred pain. This suggests that further evaluation of the hip should be performed before an accurate diagnosis can be made.

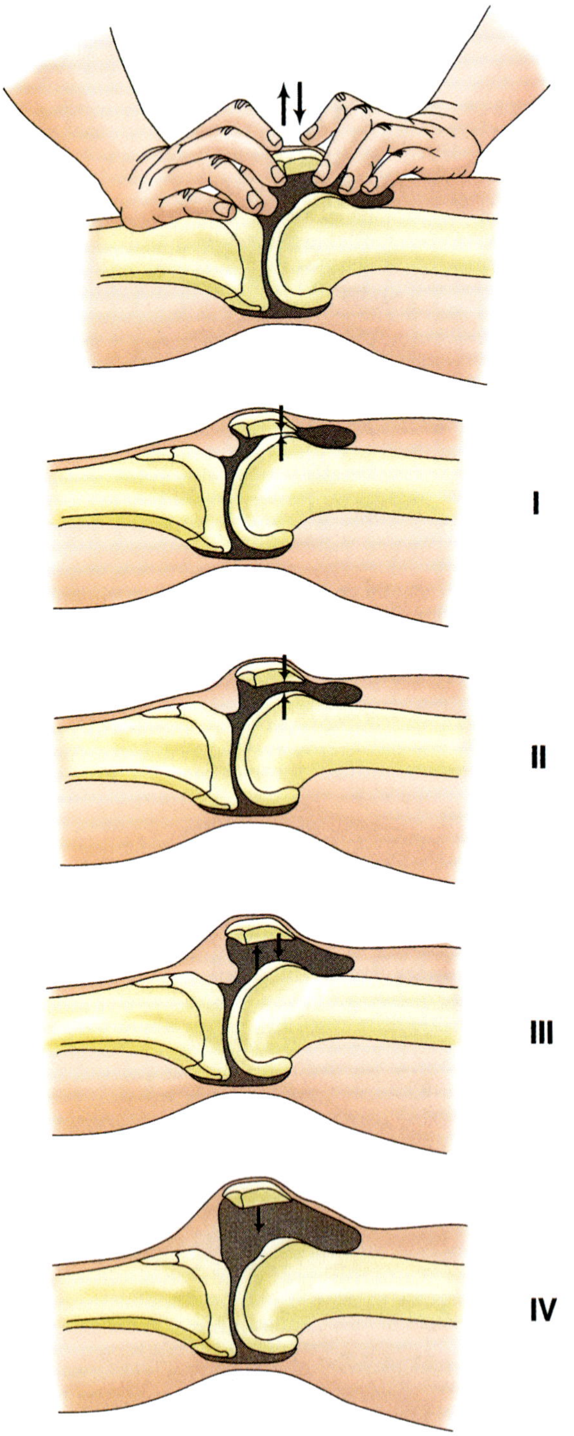

The Tibiofemoral Joint

Examination of the tibiofemoral joint should note the presence of any cystic mass (ganglion) along the joint line, localized tenderness, crepitation, snapping, or clicking.

Meniscal tears occur as a result of injury to or degeneration of fibrocartilage. Physical examination of a knee with a torn meniscus reveals joint line tenderness with a palpable click or snap and occasionally the presence of an effusion. Range of motion may be limited secondary to a displaced meniscal tear. A block to full extension may be indicative of a locked knee with a large displaced tear.

Tests for meniscal tears are divided into two groups: those that evaluate the presence of tenderness or clicks with palpation, and those that depend on symptoms of joint line pain with rotation (Table 3-1).[7]

The primary palpation tests are the Bragard, McMurray, and Steinmann second tests. The Bragard test describes that external tibial rotation and knee extension increases tenderness along the medial joint line in the presence of a medial meniscus tear. This maneuver brings the medial meniscus more anterior and closer to the examining finger, therefore eliciting more pain. Internal rotation and flexion cause less tenderness by bringing the meniscus farther from the area of palpation. In the presence of a lateral meniscus tear, internal rotation of the tibia and extension will increase tenderness along the lateral joint line, while flexion and external rotation will reduce tenderness. If an articular surface irregularity of the femur or the tibia leads to tenderness, no difference between the two positions will be noted.

Figure 3-6. Effusions of the knee are graded from 1 to 4. (From Tria AJ Jr, Klein KS: An illustrated guide to the knee, New York, 1992, Churchill Livingstone.)

Table 3-1 Meniscal Tests

Palpation	Rotation
Bragard	Apley
McMurray	Apley grind
Steinmann second	Bohler
	Duck walking
	Helfet
	Merke
	Payr
	Steinmann first

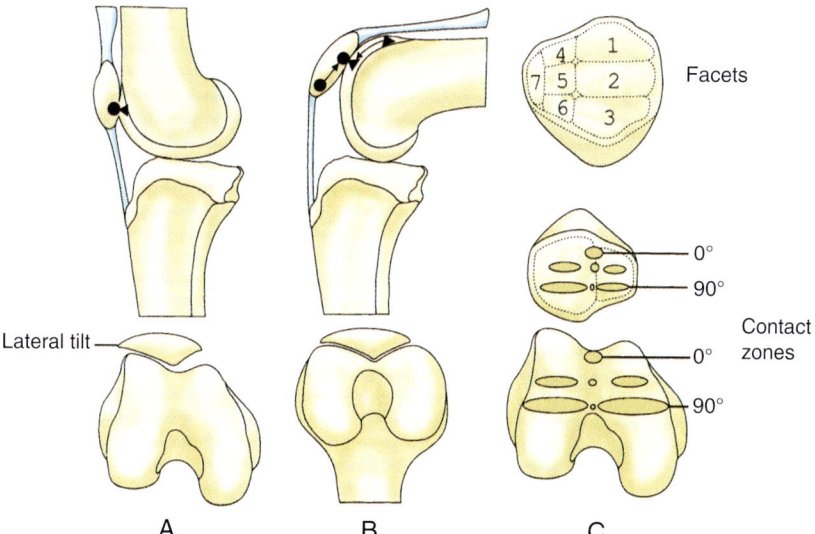

Figure 3-7. As flexion increases, the patella moves more medially, and the contact zones shift proximally and to the medial and lateral facets. (From Tria AJ Jr, Klein KS: An illustrated guide to the knee, New York, 1992, Churchill Livingstone.)

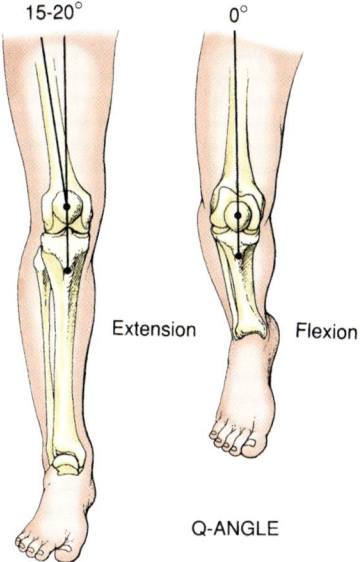

Figure 3-8. Flexion of the knee decreases the Q angle as the result of internal tibial rotation. (From Tria AJ Jr, Klein KS: An illustrated guide to the knee, New York, 1992, Churchill Livingstone.)

The McMurray test elicits a palpable click on the joint line.[21] Medially, it is demonstrated by external tibial rotation and passive motion from flexion to extension. Laterally, it is demonstrated with the tibia in internal rotation and passive motion from flexion to extension. A posterior tear may result in occurrence of the click within the initial few degrees from full flexion. If the click is palpated later as the knee is brought into greater extension, the tear is believed to be more anterior.

The Steinmann second test demonstrates joint line tenderness that moves posteriorly with knee flexion and anteriorly with knee extension. This finding is consistent with a meniscal tear that moves with range of motion of the knee. On the other hand, with a fixed joint line disorder, tenderness

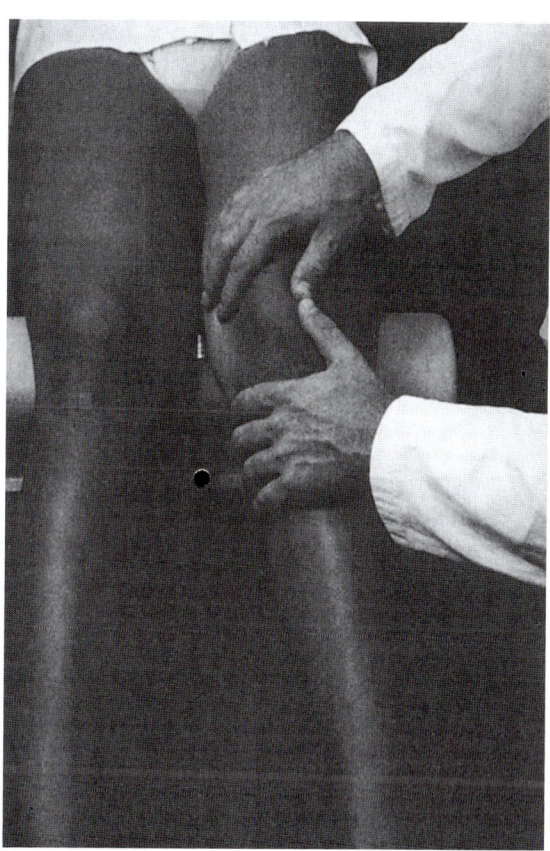

Figure 3-9. The patellar compression test. With the knee flexed slightly to engage the patella in the femoral trochlea, direct compression is applied to the patella.

should remain stationary throughout the range of motion (Fig. 3-14).

The remaining tests for meniscal pathology depend on pain with rotation. The Apley grind forces the tibiofemoral surfaces together to elicit pain. A positive finding is believed to confirm a meniscal tear. On the other hand, the Apley test is performed with the knee surfaces distracted. If Apley test (distraction) elicits less discomfort than the Apley grind (compression), the finding of a meniscal tear is favored over a fixed joint line disorder. If the distraction test and compression are equally painful, an articular surface disorder is favored (such as an irregular surface secondary to osteoarthritic erosion).

If a medial meniscus tear is expected, the Bohler test can be performed by applying a varus stress to the knee. With a medial tear, a varus stress will result in increased pain caused

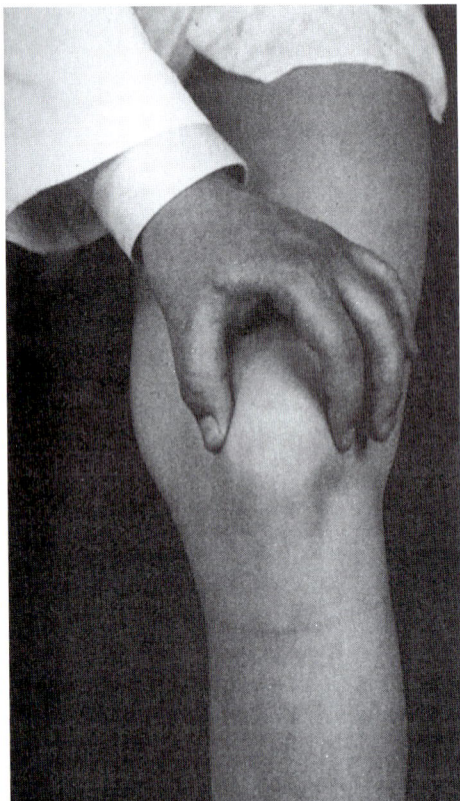

Figure 3-10. Clinical evaluation of patellar tracking is performed with the patient seated with the knee flexed to 90 degrees. During active knee extension, the examiner can detect the presence of maltracking, excessive lateral tilt, or lateral subluxation of the patella.

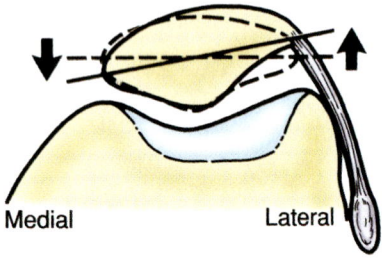

Medial   Lateral

Figure 3-11. The passive patellar tilt test. In full extension, the transverse axis of a normal patella will tilt beyond the horizontal. The inability to perform this maneuver may indicate an excessively tight lateral retinaculum.

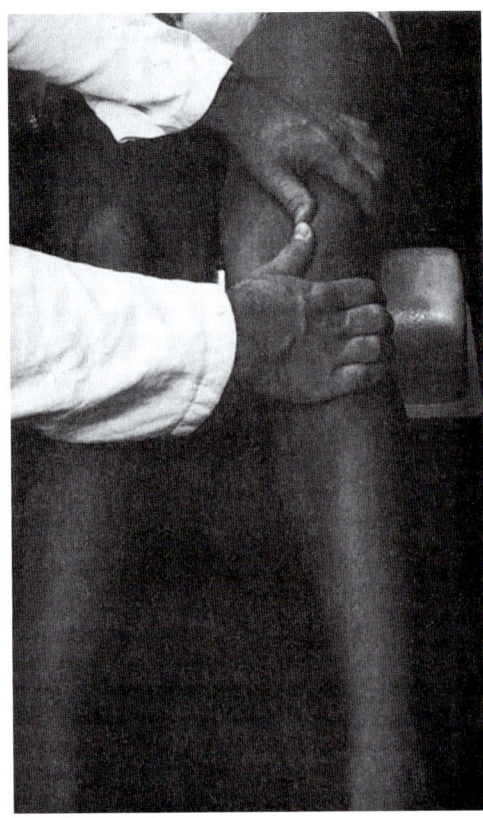

Figure 3-12. The apprehension test. With the knee flexed 20 to 30 degrees, the examiner translates the patella laterally. With a positive test, the patient experiences apprehension, contracts the quadriceps, and attempts to push the examiner's hand from the knee.

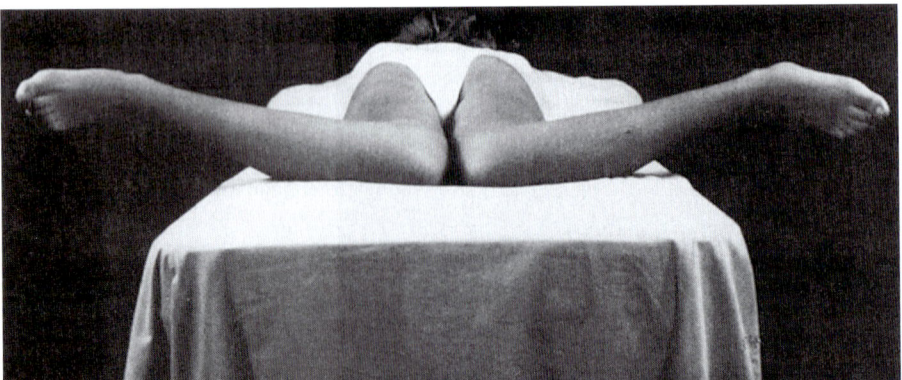

Figure 3-13. Hip rotation and femoral version. With excessive femoral anteversion, the patient will display a marked increase in hip internal rotation. This may contribute to recurrent patellar dislocations, maltracking, or lateral subluxation.

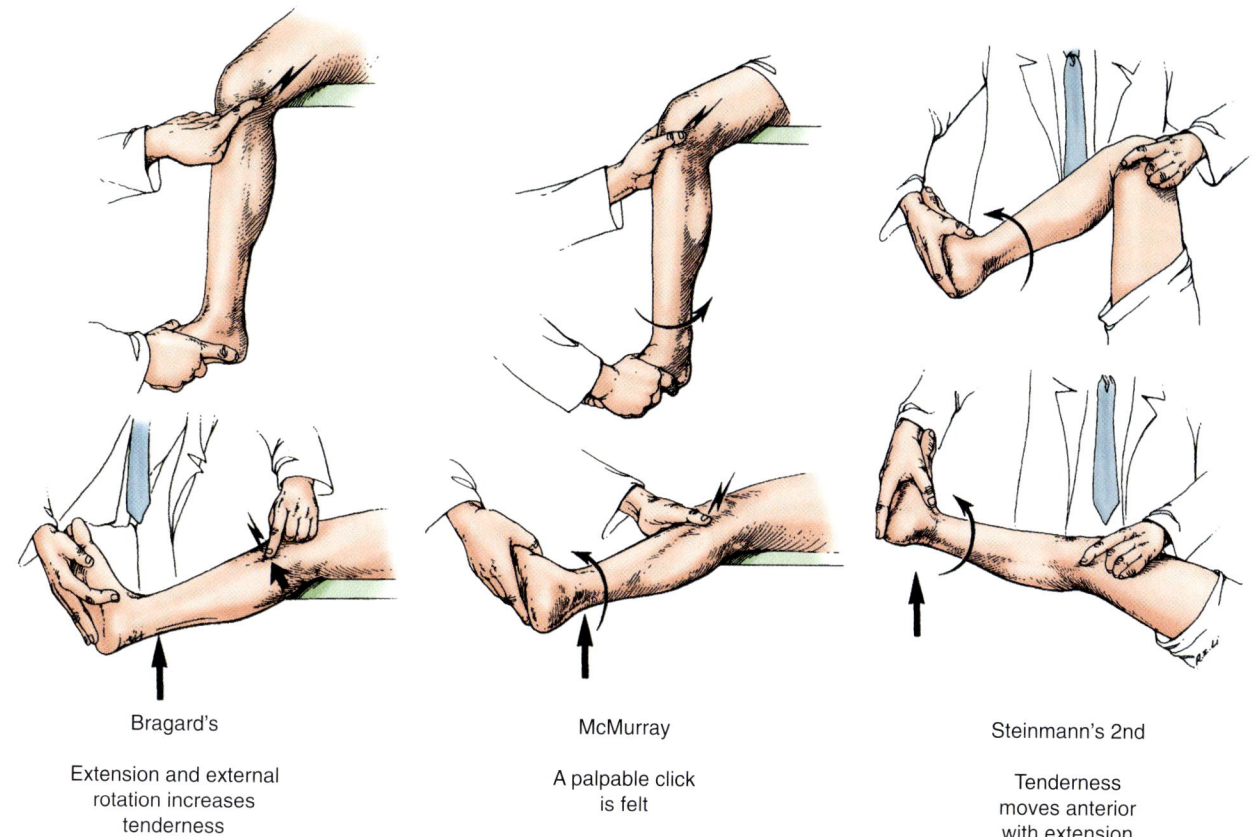

Bragard's

Extension and external
rotation increases
tenderness

McMurray

A palpable click
is felt

Steinmann's 2nd

Tenderness
moves anterior
with extension

Figure 3-14. Meniscal tests requiring palpation include the Bragard, McMurray, and Steinmann second tests. (From Tria AJ Jr, Klein KS: An illustrated guide to the knee, New York, 1992, Churchill Livingstone.)

by compression. A lateral meniscus tear can be similarly diagnosed with a valgus stress causing compression. Duck walking increases the compressive force on the posterior horns of the menisci, thus causing pain in the presence of a posterior meniscus tear.

The Helfet test is appropriate only when the knee is locked. Because a mechanical block to normal motion is present, the tibial tubercle cannot rotate externally with extension, and the Q angle cannot increase to normal with extension of the knee. Failure of the knee to externally rotate normally with extension is a positive test result.

In the Steinmann first test, the patient is seated and the knee is flexed to 90 degrees. To assess for a possible medial meniscus tear, the tibia is suddenly externally rotated by grasping the foot. A positive result produces pain along the medial joint line. Sudden internal tibial rotation is used in a similar manner to confirm a lateral meniscus tear and will result in lateral joint line pain (Fig. 3-15).

The Merke test is similar to the first Steinmann test and is performed with the patient bearing weight on the affected extremity. Internal rotation of the body over the affected limb produces external rotation of the tibia and medial joint line pain when the medial meniscus is torn. The opposite occurs with external rotation of the body over the limb when the lateral meniscus is torn.

The Payr test is performed with the patient in the "Turkish sitting position." A downward force is then applied to the knee. This results in a varus stress on the knee. A torn medial

meniscus results in medial pain from increased compression. This test can be performed only for medial joint line pathology.

EXAMINATION OF THE LIGAMENTS AND ASSOCIATED CAPSULAR STRUCTURES

Stress examination is performed to evaluate the status of the two collateral ligaments, the cruciate ligaments, and the posteromedial and posterolateral capsular structures.[14,15,20] During stress testing, the examiner should record the degree of opening and the quality of the endpoint. It can be graded from I to III or by the number of millimeters that the joint opens as determined by the examiner.[9] The authors prefer to use the grading system. Grade I corresponds to a stress examination that allows minimal to no opening with stress, but with the manipulation causing pain along the line of the collateral ligament. Grade II corresponds to a physical examination that shows some opening of the joint but with a distinct endpoint. Grade III shows no distinct endpoint to the stress evaluation.

The valgus stress test evaluates the medial collateral ligament (MCL) and the posteromedial capsule. A valgus stress applied in full extension is used to assess the MCL and the associated posteromedial capsule. In 30 degrees of flexion, the same valgus stress isolates the MCL by relaxing the capsule (Fig. 3-16). Thus, full extension evaluates the ligament and capsule; flexion evaluates the ligament alone. In similar

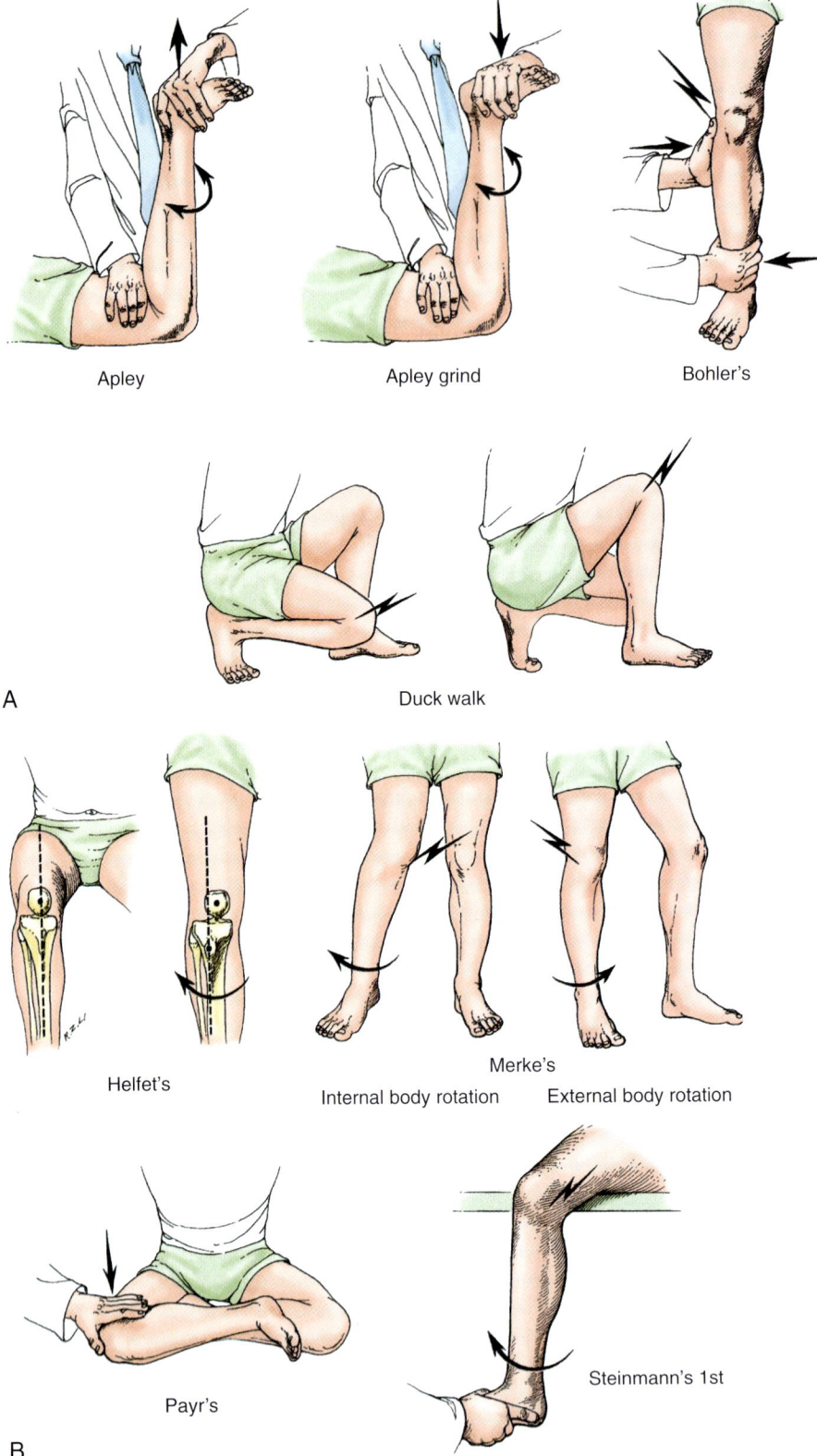

Apley

Apley grind

Bohler's

A

Duck walk

Helfet's

Merke's

Internal body rotation

External body rotation

Payr's

Steinmann's 1st

B

Figure 3-15. Meniscal tests that depend on rotation of the knee. (From Tria AJ Jr, Klein KS: *An illustrated guide to the knee,* New York, 1992, Churchill Livingstone.)

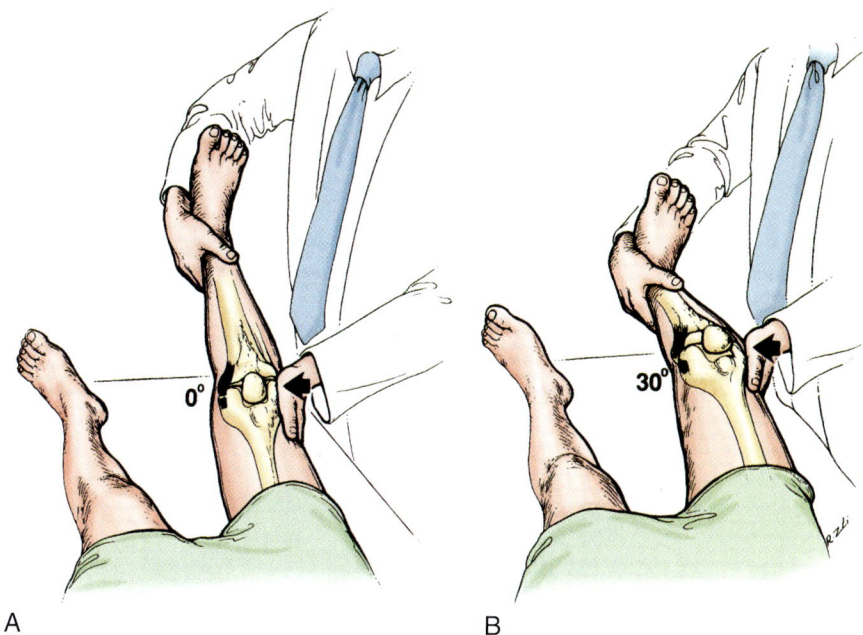

Figure 3-16. Valgus stress in extension tests the medial collateral ligament and the posteromedial capsule. Stress in 30 degrees of flexion tests only the medial collateral ligament. (From Tria AJ Jr, Klein KS: An illustrated guide to the knee, New York, 1992, Churchill Livingstone.)

A   B

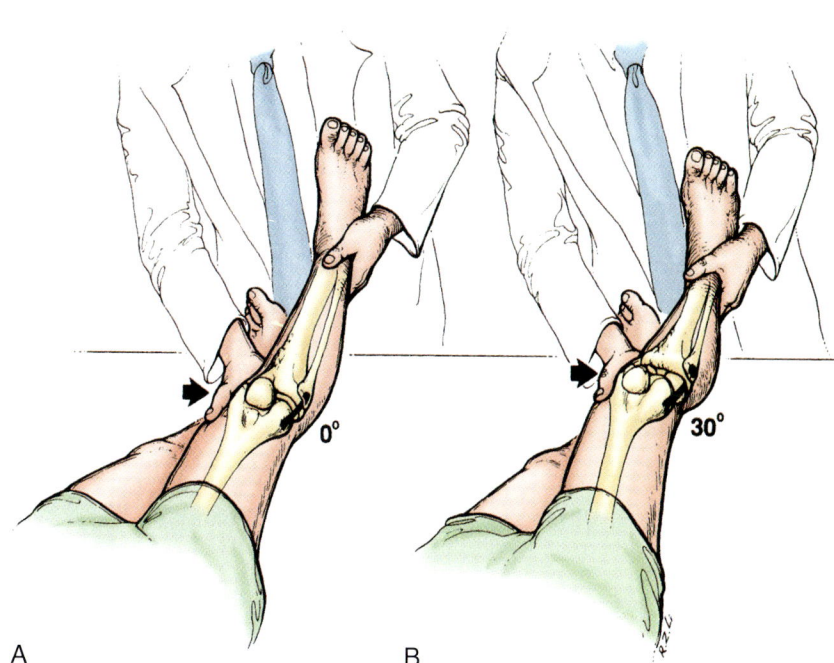

Figure 3-17. Varus stress in extension tests the lateral collateral ligament and the posterolateral capsule. Stress in 30 degrees of flexion tests only the lateral collateral ligament. (From Tria AJ Jr, Klein KS: An illustrated guide to the knee, New York, 1992, Churchill Livingstone.)

A   B

fashion, the varus stress test is performed in full extension and 30 degrees of flexion to evaluate the lateral collateral ligament and the posterolateral capsule (Fig. 3-17).

A multitude of examinations can be used to determine the integrity of the anterior cruciate ligament. The Lachman (Fig. 3-18) and anterior drawer (Fig. 3-19) tests apply anterior stress to the tibia at 30 and 90 degrees of flexion, respectively.[24] The Lachman test is thought to be more sensitive for the posterolateral bundle of the cruciate, and the anterior drawer test more sensitive for the anteromedial bundle. If the knee is held at 30 degrees of flexion and the patient is asked to contract the quadriceps muscle, an anterior cruciate–deficient knee will pull the tibia slightly forward before the

lower part of the leg begins to extend (quadriceps active test for the anterior cruciate ligament) (Fig. 3-20).[10]

The flexion rotation drawer test builds on the Lachman test and notes tibial motion and femoral rotation from 15 to 30 degrees of flexion (Fig. 3-21).[22] Anterior force is applied to the tibia, starting at 15 degrees of flexion. This maneuver leads to anterior subluxation, much as in the Lachman test. With further knee flexion, the tibia reduces beneath the femur with a noticeable "clunk" and internal rotation of the femur.

The jerk, pivot-shift, and Losee tests emphasize anterolateral motion of the tibia beneath the femur. Although the Lachman, drawer, and flexion rotation drawer tests can be

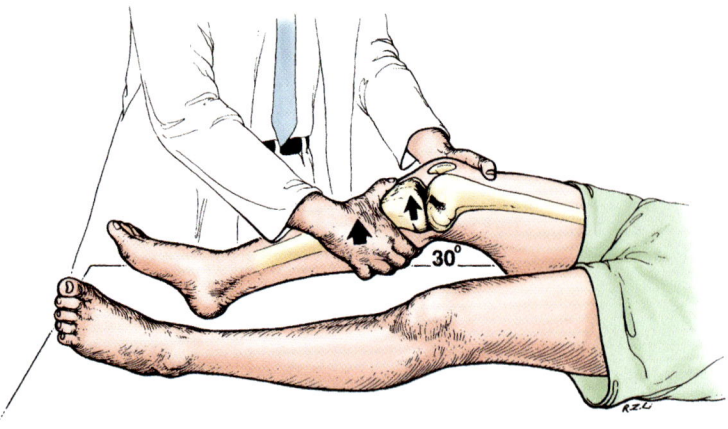

Figure 3-18. The Lachman test is performed in 30 degrees of flexion with anterior force exerted on the proximal end of the tibia. (From Tria AJ Jr, Klein KS: An illustrated guide to the knee, New York, 1992, Churchill Livingstone.)

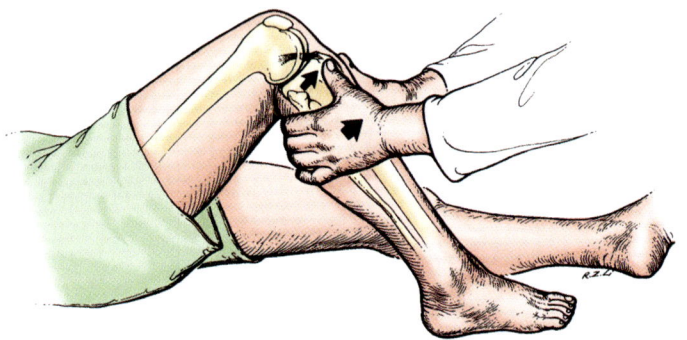

Figure 3-19. The anterior drawer test is performed with the knee flexed to 90 degrees and anterior force applied to the proximal end of the tibia. (From Tria AJ Jr, Klein KS: An illustrated guide to the knee, 1992, New York, Churchill Livingstone.)

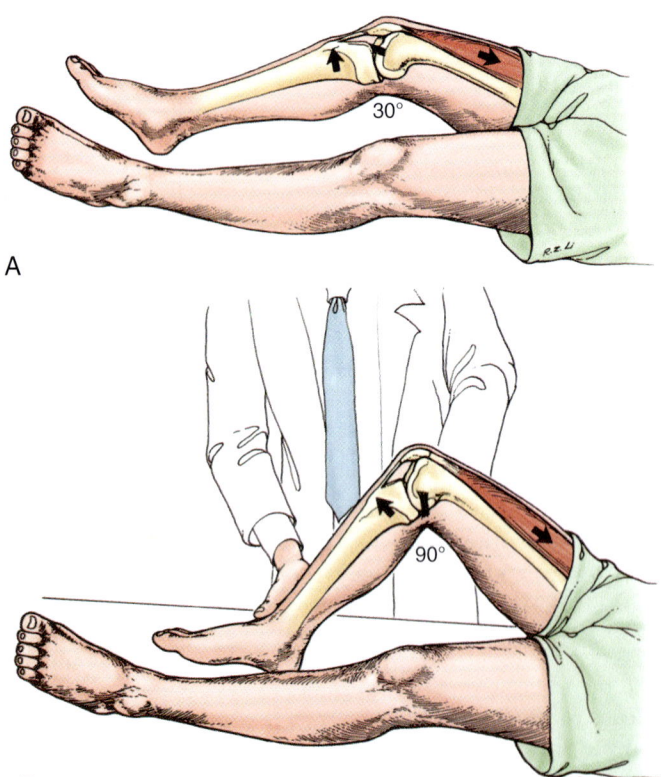

Figure 3-20. Quadriceps active test for the anterior cruciate ligament in 30 degrees of flexion (**A**) and for the posterior cruciate ligament in 90 degrees of flexion (**B**). (From Scott WN [ed]: The knee, St Louis, 1994, CV Mosby.)

performed with the patient completely awake and unmedicated, the anterolateral tests produce more discomfort for the patient and are difficult to perform on an awake patient with a knee that has been recently injured. However, in a knee with chronic instability, the anterolateral tests are easier to perform than the Lachman, drawer, and flexion rotation drawer tests. In the chronic setting, the patient will often allow the examiner to perform the test and will comment that the motion and discomfort in the knee are similar to the instability experienced when the knee is symptomatic.

The jerk test is initiated in flexion with associated internal tibial rotation, forward pressure on the fibular head, and valgus stress (Fig. 3-22). This combination subluxes the lateral tibial condyle anteriorly. As the knee is brought into extension, the tibia reduces with a palpable clunk that is sometimes visible.

The pivot-shift test begins with the knee in full extension.[11-13] Valgus stress is applied along with internal tibial rotation and forward pressure on the fibular head. As flexion is commenced, the lateral aspect of the tibia again comes forward and then reduces on further flexion with a palpable clunk (Fig. 3-23). On occasion, this test may cause medial joint line pain indicative of an associated medial meniscal tear.

The Losee test is similar to the jerk test.[17-19] It also begins with the knee in flexion and valgus stress. The tibia, however, is initially held in external rotation. As the knee is gradually extended, the tibia is rotated internally, and the clunk of the reduction is again felt as in the jerk test. The test attempts to accentuate the subluxation with external tibial rotation (Fig. 3-24).

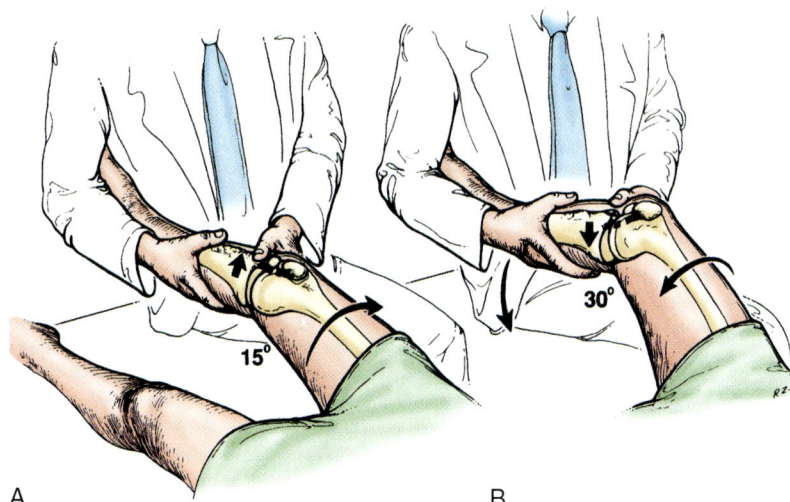

Figure 3-21. In the flexion rotation drawer test, the tibia is cradled in the examiner's hands, while the knee is flexed to demonstrate tibial reduction and internal femoral rotation. (From Tria AJ Jr, Klein KS: An illustrated guide to the knee, New York, 1992, Churchill Livingstone.)

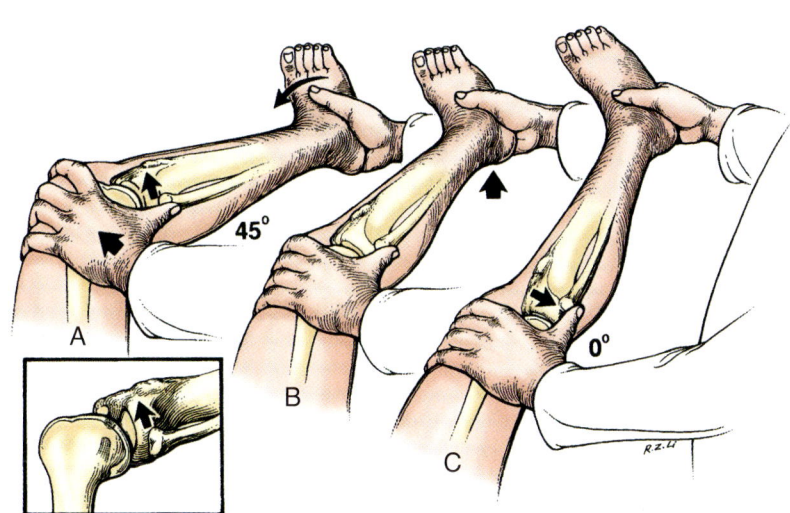

Figure 3-22. The jerk test begins with the knee in flexion, and internal rotation and valgus stress are applied to demonstrate anterolateral subluxation of the tibia. (From Tria AJ Jr, Klein KS: An illustrated guide to the knee, New York, 1992, Churchill Livingstone.)

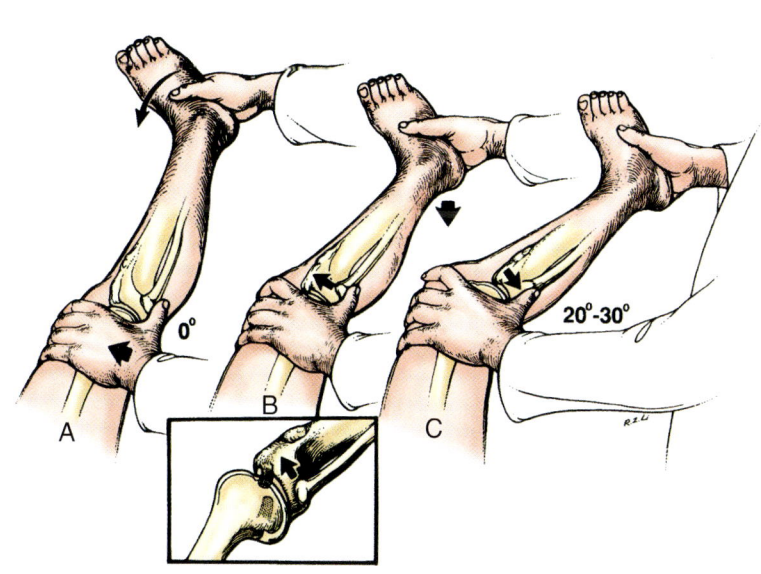

Figure 3-23. The pivot-shift test begins with the knee in full extension, and internal rotation and valgus stress are applied to demonstrate anterolateral subluxation. (From Tria AJ Jr, Klein KS: An illustrated guide to the knee, 1992, New York, Churchill Livingstone.)

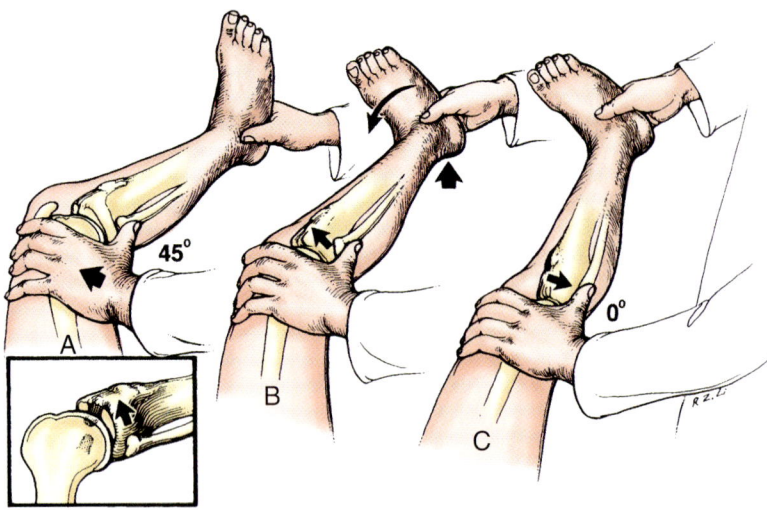

Figure 3-24. The Losee test begins with the knee in flexion, but the foot is externally rotated. Valgus stress is applied, and the tibia is internally rotated as the knee is extended. (From Tria AJ Jr, Klein KS: An illustrated guide to the knee, New York, 1992, Churchill Livingstone.)

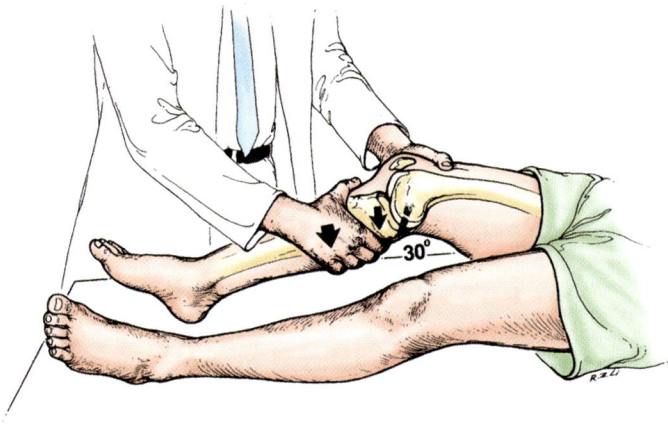

Figure 3-25. The "posterior" Lachman test applies posterior force to the proximal end of the tibia with the knee flexed 30 degrees. (From Tria AJ Jr, Klein KS: An illustrated guide to the knee, New York, 1992, Churchill Livingstone.)

The posterior cruciate ligament can be evaluated with two primary tests and one secondary test. The "posterior" Lachman test is performed in 30 degrees of flexion, and the tibia is forced posteriorly (Fig. 3-25). In the posterior drawer test (Fig. 3-26), the knee is positioned in 90 degrees of flexion, and posterior force is then applied. The varus stress examination in full extension is said to include the posterior cruciate ligament. If the lateral aspect of the knee opens with varus stress in full extension, as discussed earlier, the lateral collateral ligament and the posterolateral capsular structures are included. Some examiners believe that this opening cannot occur without posterior cruciate disruption. The authors disagree with this statement and believe that the varus stress examination can have a positive result with an intact posterior cruciate ligament. Grading of the degree of opening will sometimes help in determining the total amount of injury. A grade I or II laxity test is more likely to include a lateral collateral ligament and a posterolateral capsule tear with an intact posterior cruciate ligament, whereas grade III laxity with a completely indistinct endpoint may indeed include a posterior cruciate ligament tear.

A knee with chronic posterior cruciate ligament laxity will often have a posterior sag. If the patient attempts to contract the quadriceps muscle with the knee in 90 degrees of flexion, the tibia will come forward before the lower part of the leg begins to extend (quadriceps active test for the posterior cruciate ligament) (see Fig. 3-20).

The posteromedial capsule is evaluated with the Slocum test (anterior drawer test at 90 degrees of flexion with external rotation of the lower part of the leg).[8,23] When the tibia is rotated externally, the posteromedial capsule should tighten and allow less anterior excursion than with the drawer test in neutral rotation. When the posteromedial capsule is torn, the Slocum test demonstrates an increase in anterior motion of the tibia versus the drawer test in neutral, and the tibia tends to "roll out" (Fig. 3-27).

The posterolateral capsule is tested with the anterior drawer test at 90 degrees of flexion and internal tibial rotation of 15 degrees. If the posterolateral capsule is torn, the drawer test with internal rotation will show an increase in anterior motion versus the drawer test in neutral, and the tibia will tend to "roll in" (Fig. 3-28). The dial examination can also assess the posterior cruciate ligament and posterolateral structures. The patient is placed in the prone position. External rotation of the tibia is recorded and 30 and 90 degrees and is compared with the uninjured side. Increased external rotation with asymmetry at 90 degrees is indicative of an injury

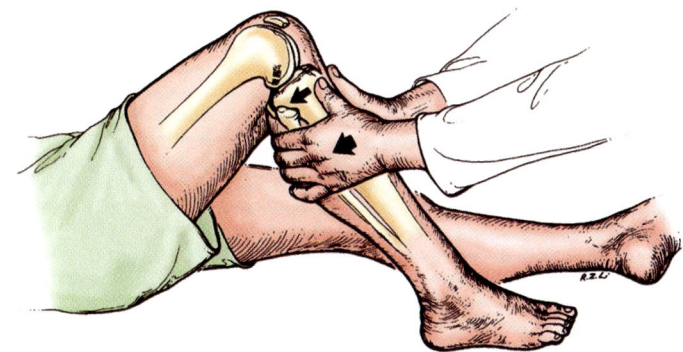

Figure 3-26. The posterior drawer test is performed in 90 degrees of flexion with posterior force on the proximal end of the tibia. (From Tria AJ Jr, Klein KS: An illustrated guide to the knee, New York, 1992, Churchill Livingstone.)

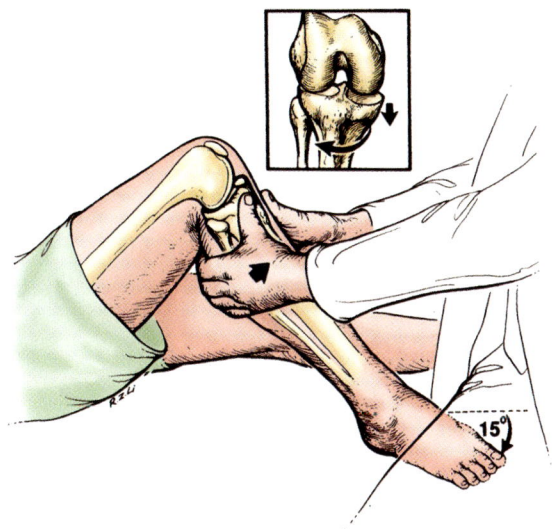

Figure 3-27. The Slocum test is performed in 90 degrees of flexion with the foot externally rotated and anterior proximal tibial force applied to test the posteromedial capsule. (From Tria AJ Jr, Klein KS: An illustrated guide to the knee, New York, 1992, Churchill Livingstone.)

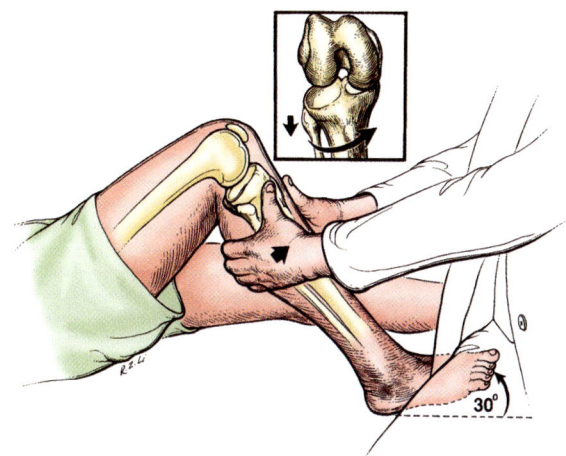

Figure 3-28. The posterolateral capsule is tested with the knee flexed to 90 degrees and anterior proximal tibial force applied with the tibia rotated internally. (From Tria AJ Jr, Klein KS: An illustrated guide to the knee, New York, 1992, Churchill Livingstone.)

Table 3-2 Stress Examination (in Order of Sensitivity)

Ligament	Test
MCL	Valgus stress (30 degrees flexion)
LCL	Varus stress (30 degrees flexion)
ACL	Lachman, flexion-rotation-drawer, anterior drawer, jerk, pivot, Losee
PCL	Posterior Lachman, posterior drawer, sag (late) (? varus laxity in full extension)
Posteromedial capsule	Valgus in full extension, Slocum
Posterolateral capsule	Varus in full extension, drawer in internal rotation, hyperextension recurvatum test

ACL, Anterior cruciate ligament; *LCL,* lateral collateral ligament; *MCL,* medial collateral ligament; *PCL,* posterior cruciate ligament.

to the PCL. Increased external rotation with asymmetry at 30 degrees is indicative of an injury to the posterolateral structures. The hyperextension recurvatum sign correlates with injury to the posterolateral capsule. If the leg is held in full extension, the knee hyperextends and the tibia rotates externally because of absence of the posterolateral capsule and its supporting structures (Fig. 3-29). The reverse pivot-shift test is performed with the tibia rotated externally and the knee flexed. When the knee flexes 20 to 30 degrees, tibial external rotation is seen with posterior subluxation of the lateral tibia. As the knee is extended, the tibia reduces with a palpable clunk, indicative of a deficient posterolateral capsule (Fig. 3-30).[16]

During examination of each ligament and capsular structure, all tests should be applied to each area as indicated. Despite sophisticated computers and measurement devices, physical examination of the knee remains the most reliable tool for diagnostic evaluation of supporting structures. On occasion, diagnostic evaluation of the knee may not be complete despite physical examination, magnetic resonance imaging, and local anesthetic infiltration. Some stress tests are more sensitive than others (Table 3-2), and the examiner may rely on that sensitivity, or it may be necessary to perform an examination under anesthesia along with arthroscopy to completely confirm the anatomy of the injury. Diagnostic accuracy is the key to appropriate therapeutic intervention.

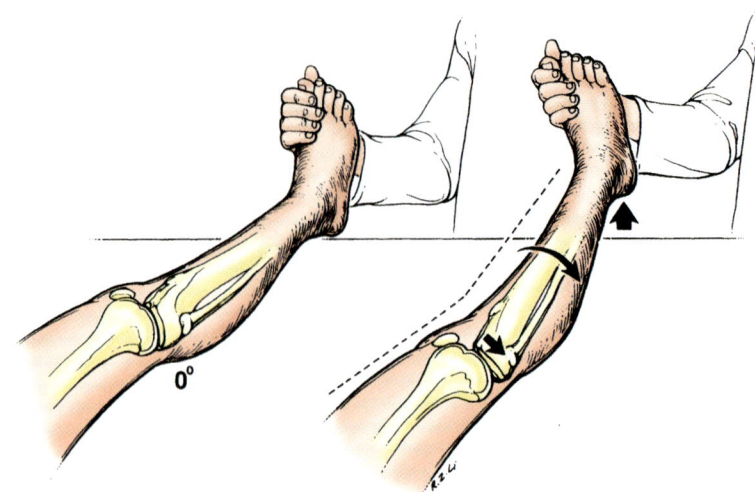

Figure 3-29. The hyperextension recurvatum test demonstrates increased extension of the knee along with external tibial rotation and drop-back. (From Tria AJ Jr, Klein KS: An illustrated guide to the knee, New York, 1992, Churchill Livingstone.)

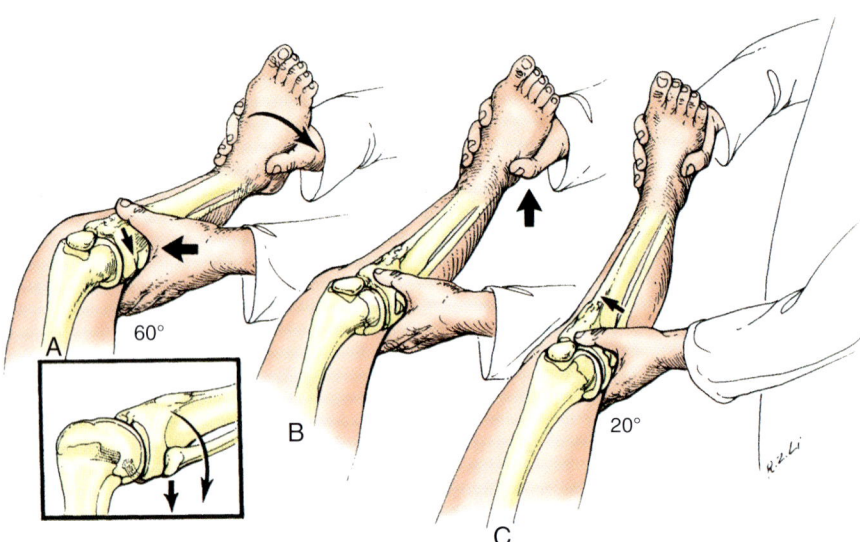

Figure 3-30. The reverse pivot-shift test begins with the knee flexed, and the tibia is externally rotated. The knee is then extended to demonstrate posterolateral capsular laxity. (From Tria AJ Jr, Klein KS: An illustrated guide to the knee, New York, 1992, Churchill Livingstone.)

KEY REFERENCES

Aglietti P, Insall JN, Cerulli G: Patellar pain and incongruence. I: Measurements of incongruence. Clin Orthop 176:217, 1983.

Apley AC: The diagnosis of meniscal injuries. J Bone Joint Surg 29:78, 1947.

Daniel DM, Stone ML, Barnett P, et al: Use of the quadriceps active test to diagnose posterior cruciate ligament disruption and measure posterior laxity of the knee. J Bone Joint Surg Am 70:386, 1988.

Fairbank HA: Internal derangement of the knee in children. Proc R Soc 3:11, 1937.

Feagin JA, Cooke TD: Prone examination for anterior cruciate ligament insufficiency. J Bone Joint Surg Br 71:863, 1989.

Fetto JF, Marshall JL: Injury to the anterior cruciate ligament producing the pivot-shift sign. J Bone Joint Surg Am 61:710, 1979.

Hughston JC, Andrews JR, Cross MJ, et al: Classification of knee ligament instabilities. Part I. The medial compartment and cruciate ligaments. J Bone Joint Surg Am 58:159, 1976.

Hughston JC, Andrews JR, Cross MJ, et al: Classification of knee ligament instabilities. Part II. The lateral compartment. J Bone Joint Surg Am 58:173, 1976.

Losee RE: Diagnosis of chronic injury to the anterior cruciate ligament. Orthop Clin North Am 16:83, 1985.

McMurray TP: The semilunar cartilages. J Bone Joint Surg 29:407, 1942.

Noyes FR, Butler D, Grood E, et al: Clinical paradoxes of anterior cruciate instability and a new test to detect its instability. Orthop Trans 2:36, 1978.

Slocum DB, Larson RL: Rotatory instability of the knee: its pathogenesis and a clinical test to demonstrate its presence. J Bone Joint Surg Am 50:211, 1968.

Full references for this chapter can be found on www.expertconsult.com.

Gene Therapy in the Treatment of Knee Disorders

Anna L. Stevens, Burhan Gharaibeh, Kurt R. Weiss, Freddie H. Fu, and Johnny Huard

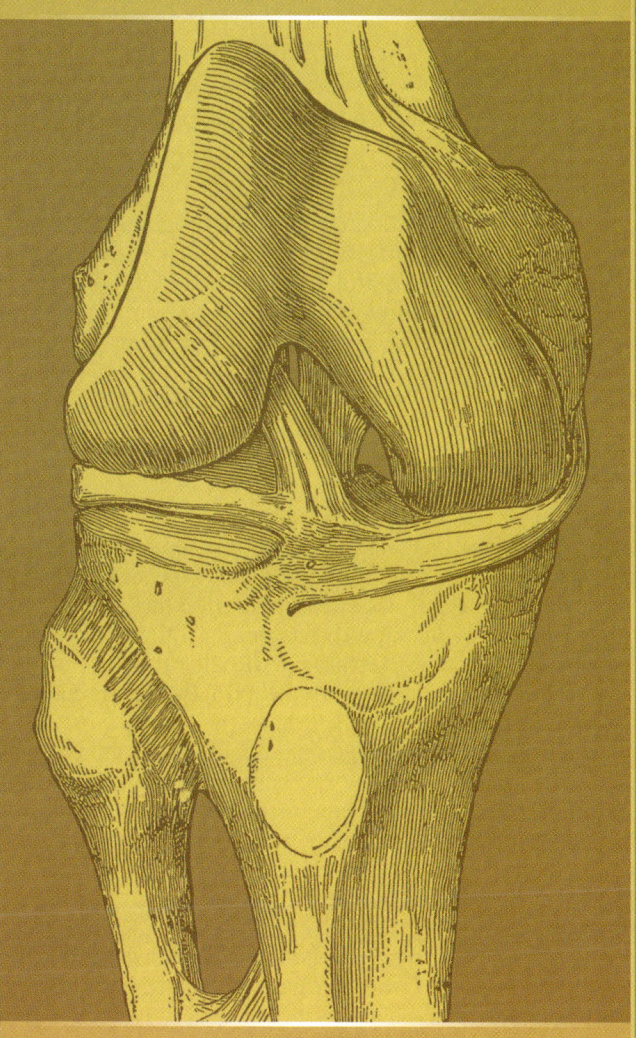

SECTION 2

Imaging of the Knee

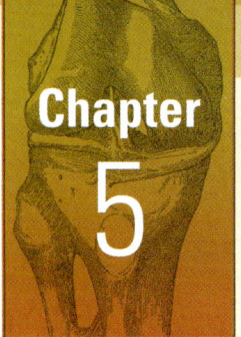

Chapter 5

Knee Imaging Techniques and Normal Anatomy

Samuel D. Madoff, Jarett S. Burak, Kevin R. Math, and Daniel M. Walz

RADIOGRAPHY

Applications

Radiographs are the workhorse of knee imaging. Nearly any symptom or sign may be initially evaluated with an x-ray. Radiographs provide useful information across the entire spectrum of knee pathology, including congenital deformities, arthritis, trauma, oncology, sports injuries, metabolic disease, and arthroplasty evaluation.[36]

Technique

A brief orientation to x-ray technology enhances an understanding of knee imaging. An x-ray tube converts electricity into a beam of high-energy photons. The x-ray beam is aimed through the knee. A cassette containing x-ray film is positioned opposite the x-ray beam on the other side of the patient. Photons that pass through the patient strike the film, exposing it. Tissue density is the primary determinant of whether a photon successfully reaches the film. A dense tissue such as bone absorbs or deflects most photons. So, few photons reach the film. Areas of unexposed film appear white, representing dense tissue. Less dense materials, such as the lung or fat, do not obstruct as many passing photons. Here the exposed film appears darker. Simplistically, a radiograph is a shadow formed by high-energy light outlining the patient's anatomy.

Traditionally, an exposed film was developed and hung for interpretation. Over the past 20 years, new cassette designs have replaced film with an imaging plate, creating computed radiography (CR). After exposure, the imaging plate is run through a CR reader and the captured image is digitized. The imaging plate is subsequently reset and can be reused thousands of times. Digital radiography (DR) represents the next evolution of filmless image capture. DR dispenses with the cassette entirely and utilizes a flat panel detector. The detail and overall image quality of DR are superior to CR.

A remaining niche for true film radiography is the standing, frontal, long-standing view radiograph of the lower extremity. This may be requested for precise knee anatomic and mechanical axis measurements.

After an image has been acquired by a CR or DR reader, it is transmitted to the picture archiving and communication system (PACS) for interpretation. The advantages of PACS are manifold, including image manipulation (windowing, zooming, etc.), transmission (electronic), and storage (online, easily accessible). The time-honored file room has given way to a well-ventilated closet housing several hard-working computers.

Radiographic Views

Standard radiographic examination of the knee consists of three views: anteroposterior (AP), lateral, and axial (sunrise or Merchant). Tunnel, posteroanterior flexion weight-bearing (Rosenberg view) and oblique views may be performed for particular indications. In the setting of knee instability and ligamentous injury, stress radiographs may be performed. If a bilateral examination has been requested, each knee should be imaged separately.

Anteroposterior Radiograph

The AP view is obtained with the knee extended, the cassette behind the knee, and the central x-ray beam perpendicular to the cassette. A standing (weight-bearing) AP radiograph more accurately assesses the joint space than one obtained with the patient supine.[1,2,31,38] For this reason, as well as to allow the estimation of valgus or varus angulation, weight-bearing images are preferable whenever possible (Fig. 5-1). Normal structures evaluated on every AP radiograph of the knee are the patella, the medial and lateral femoral condyles, the medial and lateral joint compartments, the tibial spines, the medial and lateral tibial plateaus, and the fibula. The AP view also provides a gross assessment of femoral tibial alignment (Fig. 5-2A). The lateral compartment is normally slightly wider than the medial.

Lateral Radiograph

The lateral view is obtained with the knee flexed 30 degrees and the patient lying on the affected limb. The cassette is positioned under the lateral side of the knee, and the x-ray beam is directed perpendicular to the cassette. This view depicts the quadriceps tendon, the patella, the patellar tendons, the suprapatellar bursa, the distal femur, the proximal tibia, and the proximal fibula (Fig. 5-2B).

The medial femoral condyle is slightly larger than the lateral condyle. The lateral femoral condyle can be identified by the presence of the lateral femoral sulcus at the anterior aspect of its weight-bearing portion.[34] Blumensaat's line represents the roof of the intercondylar notch. The closed physeal scar is also evident on the lateral view, and the patella should fall between it and Blumensaat's line.

The tibial plateaus slope downward as they progress posteriorly, a fact that can aid in fracture identification. The plateaus may be differentiated by several clues. The higher of the two tibial spines belongs to the medial plateau. At its posterior extent, the medial tibial plateau projects most dorsally and is squared. In contrast, the posterior aspect of the lateral tibial plateau slopes smoothly downward with a rounded contour.

The quadriceps and patellar tendons are well evaluated on a lateral view. The distal quadriceps tendon attaches to the superior pole of the patella. The patellar tendon extends from the inferior pole of the patella to the tibial tubercle. Both structures are well demarcated by a posterior fat plane. They should be straight and of uniform thickness.

In the setting of a joint effusion and suspected occult intra-articular fracture, a cross-table lateral view is useful for evaluating for lipohemarthrosis. The view is obtained with the patient supine and the knee slightly elevated. The cassette is placed

adjacent to the medial knee. This positioning, in contrast to the standard lateral view, is better tolerated by a traumatized patient. The presence of a fat fluid level indicates an intra-articular fracture (most commonly, the tibial plateau) and prompts further evaluation with computed tomography (CT) or magnetic resonance imaging (MRI) (Fig. 5-3A, B, and C).

The suprapatellar bursa is the proximal extension of the joint space. It may be identified on the standard lateral view as a slender, 1 to 2 mm, vertically oriented structure contained within the lucent area of fat formed by the anterior margin of the distal femur and the posterior margin of the quadriceps tendon.

Superoinferior positioning of the patella may be evaluated using the Insall-Salvati ratio. This is the ratio of the greatest length of the patella divided by the length of the patellar tendon. This ratio averages 1.17 and normally falls between 0.8 and 1.2 (see Fig. 5-2B). A long patellar tendon generates a ratio greater than 1.3, indicating a high patella (patella alta). Conversely, a short tendon accompanies a low patella and a ratio less than 0.8, termed patella baja.

Axial View

The axial view of choice is the Merchant view.[15,35,37] The patient is placed in the supine position on the radiography table; the knees are flexed 45 degrees (using a fixed or adjustable platform), and the cassette is placed on the proximal part of the shins. Both knees are exposed simultaneously, with the x-ray beam directed toward the feet, inclined 30 degrees from the horizontal (Fig. 5-4A). This view provides an excellent assessment of patellofemoral alignment and is ideal for

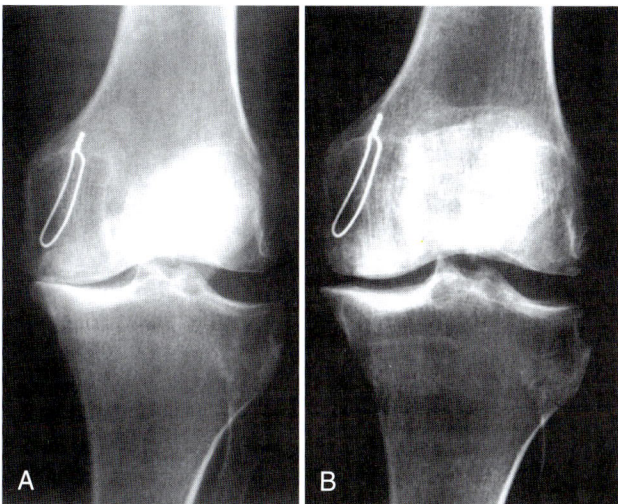

Figure 5-1. Anteroposterior supine versus weight-bearing views. Severe medial joint space narrowing is more apparent on the weight-bearing view **(A)** compared with the supine view **(B)**.

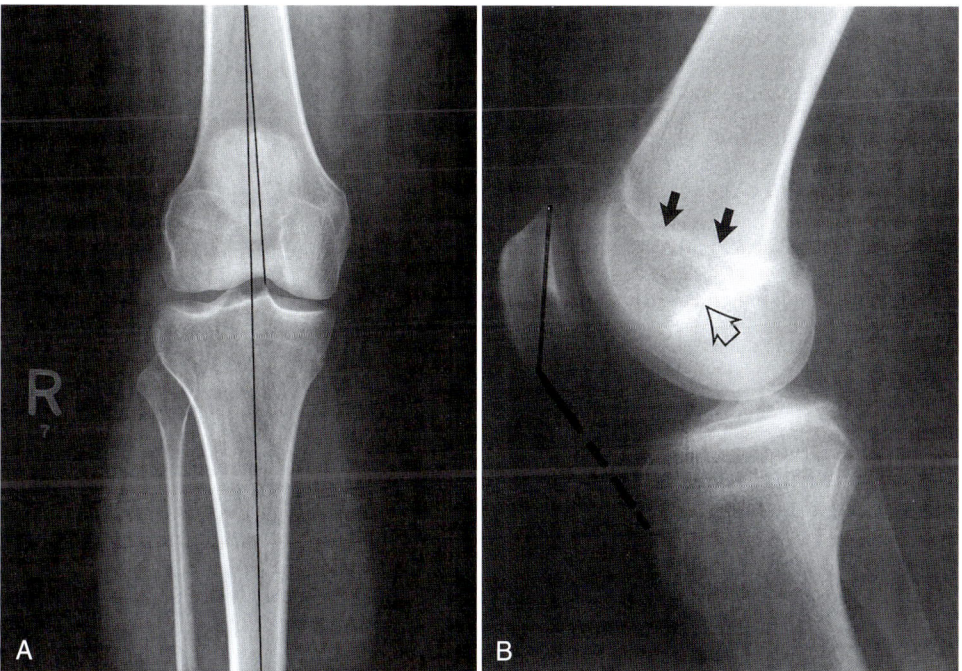

Figure 5-2. **A,** Normal anteroposterior view of the right knee. Femoral-tibial alignment is in 6 degrees of valgus angulation. The lateral compartment is normally slightly wider than the medial compartment. **B,** Lateral view of the knee. Blumensaat's line *(open arrow)* represents the roof of the intercondylar notch. The physeal scar is indicated by the *solid arrows.* The patella is commonly located between these two lines, with the lower pole approximately at the level of Blumensaat's line. The Insall-Salvati ratio is a more accurate method of assessing patellar height: the length of the patellar tendon *(dotted line)* divided by the greatest diagonal length of the patella *(solid line)* should be approximately 1 (0.8 to 1.2).

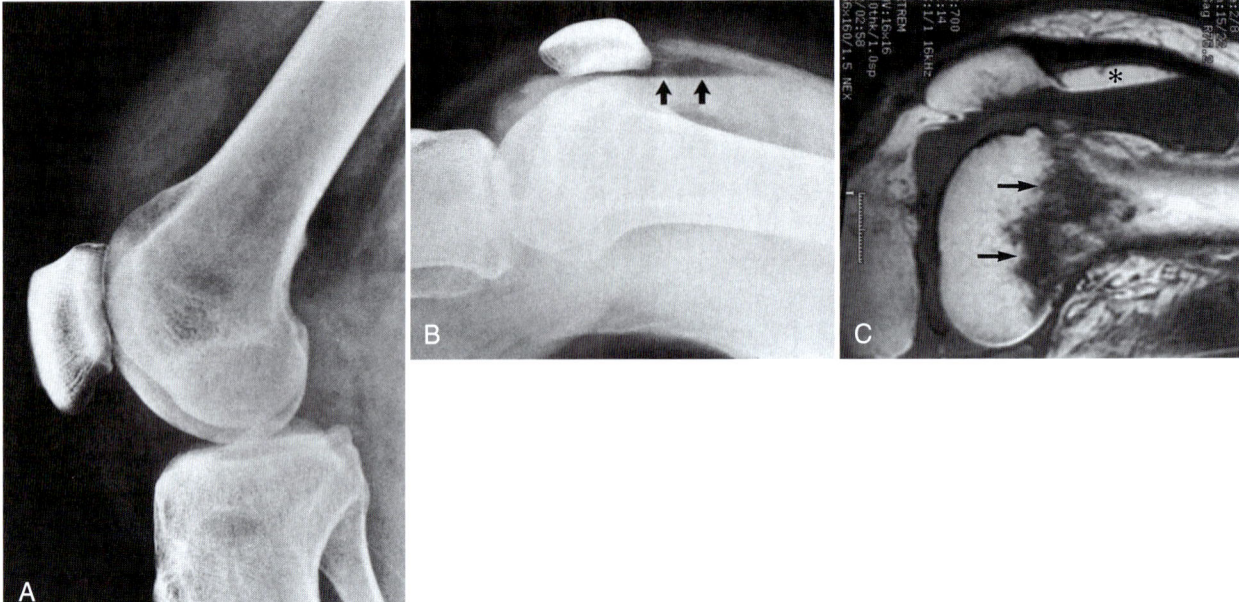

Figure 5-3. Knee joint effusion. **A,** Lateral radiograph demonstrates an oval soft tissue density representing a joint effusion within the suprapatellar pouch posterior to the quadriceps tendon. **B,** Cross-table lateral view shows a fat-fluid level *(arrows)* indicative of an intra-articular fracture with lipohemarthrosis. **C,** A sagittal T1-weighted magnetic resonance image obtained with the patient supine demonstrates high signal fat *(asterisk)* floating on top of intra-articular hemorrhage. An acute supracondylar fracture is also noted *(arrows).* (From Torg JS, Pavlov H, Morris VB: Salter-Harris type III fracture of the medial femoral condyle occurring in the adolescent athlete. J Bone Joint Surg Am 63:586, 1981.)

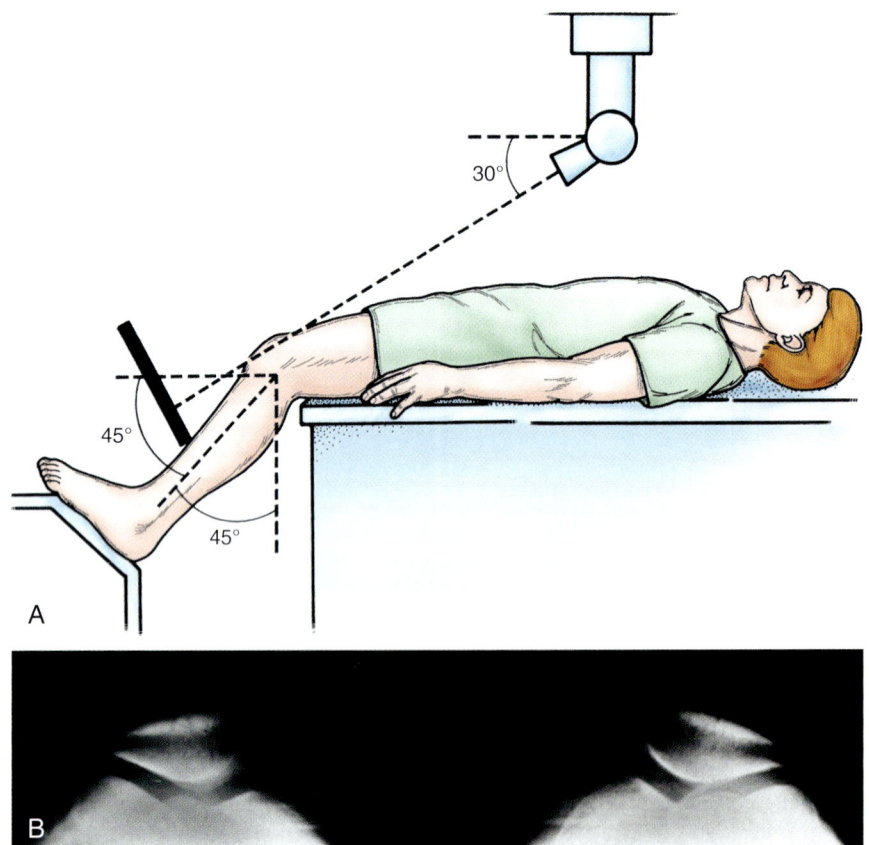

Figure 5-4. Merchant view. **A,** Technique. **B,** Normal Merchant view. Patellofemoral alignment is normal bilaterally, and the osseous structures and articular cortices are normal.

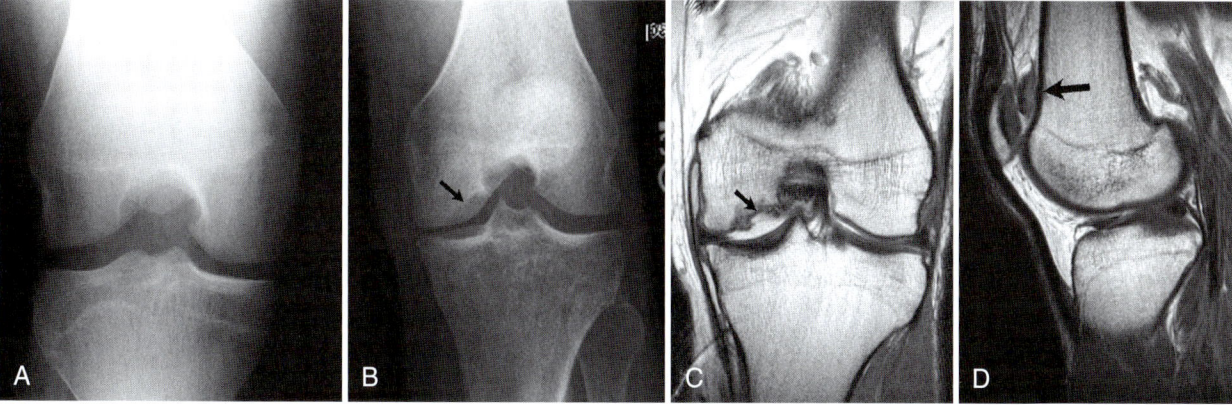

Figure 5-5. Tunnel view. **A,** Normal tunnel view demonstrates the posterior aspect of the femoral condyles, the tibial spines, the articular surfaces of the tibial plateau, and the intercondylar notch. **B,** Tunnel view from a different patient, demonstrating an ovoid area of lucency at the inner margin of the medial femoral condyle *(arrow)* suspicious for osteochondritis dessicans. **C,** Coronal and **(D)** sagittal proton density MRI confirms the large osteochondral defect *(arrow)* with a completely displaced osteochondral fragment located in the suprapatellar joint recess *(arrow).* (Case provided courtesy of the MRI Department, Hospital for Special Surgery, New York, New York.)

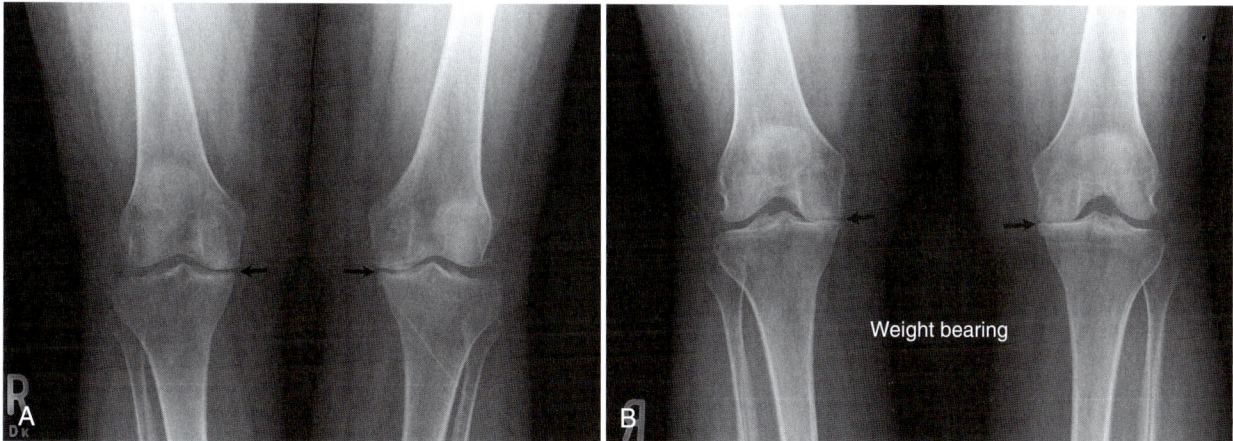

Figure 5-6. The flexed weight-bearing posteroanterior (PA) view. **A,** Routine standing anteroposterior (AP) film demonstrates moderate bilateral medial compartment joint space narrowing with proliferative changes *(arrows).* **B,** PA flexion view demonstrates the findings to be more severe with marked narrowing of bilateral medial joint compartments, complete loss of the joint space, and bone-on-bone apposition *(arrows).*

assessing the osseous patellofemoral articular surfaces (Fig. 5-4B). In contrast, a skyline (or sunrise) view is obtained with the patient prone and the knee in maximum flexion. This view demonstrates the posterior surface of the patella and the anterior surface of the femur, but the imaged femoral surface is not at the patellofemoral joint. Furthermore, accurate assessment of patellofemoral alignment is limited when the knee is flexed excessively.[7,15] Some patients have difficulty tolerating this position.

Supplemental Views

The tunnel view is a frontal view obtained with the knee flexed 60 degrees. It can be obtained AP with the patient in the supine position, or posteroanterior (PA) with the patient prone or kneeling on the cassette. The x-ray beam is directed perpendicular to the tibia. This view demonstrates the posterior aspect of the intercondylar notch, the inner posterior aspects of the medial and lateral femoral condyles, and the tibial spines and plateaus (Fig. 5-5A). It is ideal for evaluating

patients with suspected osteochondritis dissecans (OCD), which tends to occur more posteriorly in the intercondylar notch (Fig 5-5B, C, and D).

The flexed, PA weight-bearing (Rosenberg) view is a modified tunnel view. It is obtained with the patient standing and the knee flexed 45 degrees. The patellae should touch the film cassette. The x-ray beam is centered at the level of the inferior pole of the patella and is directed 10 degrees caudad. It captures the joint space at the posterior aspect of the femorotibial joint. This view is valuable for evaluating arthritis. It detects joint space narrowing due to cartilage loss that often goes unappreciated or underestimated on a conventional AP weight-bearing view (Fig. 5-6A and B).[8,9,25,47,49] Comparisons of intraoperative and radiographic findings demonstrate that the flexed PA weight-bearing view has greater accuracy, sensitivity, and specificity than the conventional extension weight-bearing radiograph.[49]

Oblique radiographs complement a routine examination. Occult fractures and tibiofibular arthritis may be more easily detected with oblique views than with routine AP

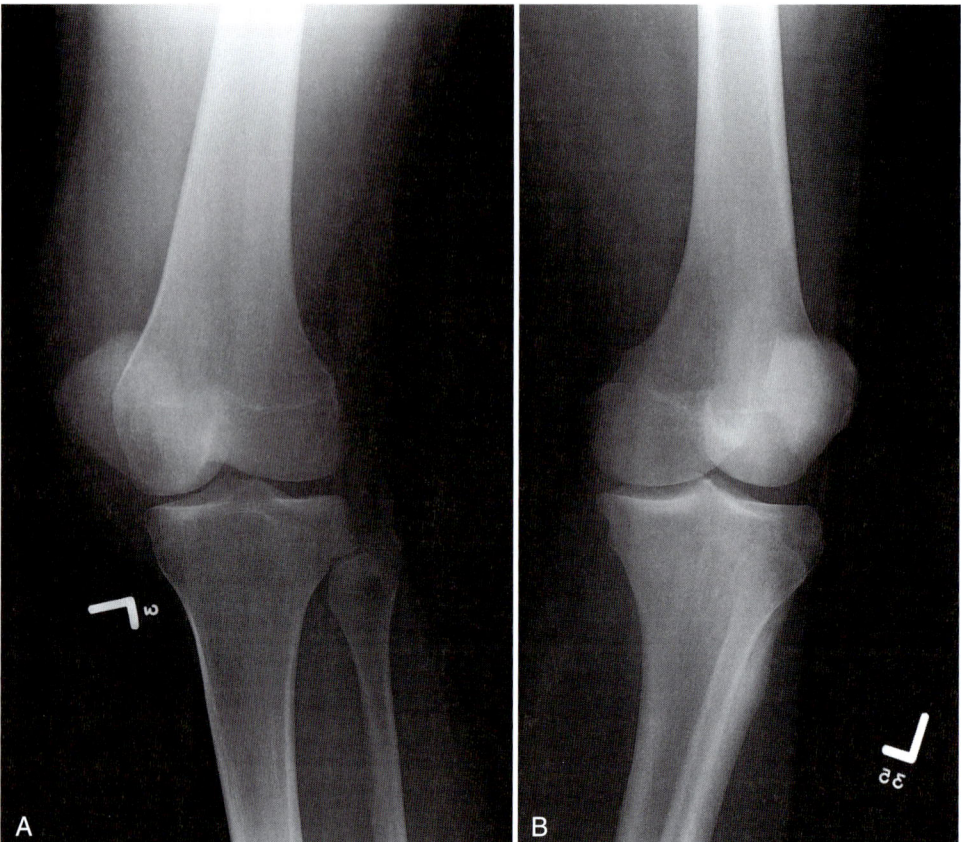

Figure 5-7. Internal **(A)** and external **(B)** rotational views of the knee in different patients. In external rotation, the tibia and fibula are superimposed on each other; with internal rotation, there should be less superimposition. A suprapatellar joint effusion is seen on the internally rotated view.

radiographs. Bilateral oblique views are obtained at 45 degrees of internal and external rotation, with the patient supine, the affected knee extended, and the cassette behind the knee. The x-ray beam should be directed 5 degrees cephalad. Views should demonstrate the patella, the femoral condyles, the tibial plateaus, and the fibula. In external rotation, the tibia and fibula are superimposed on each other. With internal rotation, there is less superimposition between the tibia and fibula (Fig. 5-7A and B).

Various stress views have been described for evaluation of instability and include *valgus and varus stress* radiographs for evaluation of the collateral ligaments, and *anterior drawer stress* radiographs for evaluation of the anterior cruciate ligament. These require use of a mechanical stress device or lead gloves worn by the x-ray technologist and manually stress the knee joint. In current clinical practice, these views are seldom ordered, as MRI is considered the gold standard for evaluation of internal derangement, and because stress views often need to be performed with local anesthesia for pain control.

Special Considerations and Anatomic Variants

Two sesamoid bones commonly identified on knee radiographs are the fabella and the cyamella. The fabella is located within the lateral head of the gastrocnemius. It overlies the lateral femoral condyle on the frontal view and sits posterior to the distal femur on the lateral view. The cyamella lives

within the popliteus tendon. On a frontal radiograph, it may be found at the insertion of the popliteus in the notch of the lateral femoral condyle (Fig. 5-8A, B, and C).

Normal variants also occur in the patella, which can have two or more osseous centers, referred to as a bipartite or multipartite patella (Fig. 5-9A and B). A bipartite patella is the more common variant, seen in 1% of the population. It is bilateral 50% of the time.[35] The smaller pieces of the patella are located superolaterally and should fit neatly together like pieces of a jigsaw puzzle. The width of a bipartite patella is usually greater than that of the contralateral patella when assessed on a tangential axial view. MRI depicts intact cartilage overlying a bipartite patella, whereas a fracture displays disrupted osteochondral integrity. These features help dismiss the suspicion of a fracture.[35] Rarely (<2% of the time), a bipartite patella can be symptomatic. MRI of the knee may demonstrate bone marrow edema on one or both sides of the synchondrosis.

A dorsal defect of the patella is another anatomic variant, usually detected incidentally. It appears as a lucent area of the superolateral patella (Fig. 5-10).[18,26] Pathologically, the lesion is composed of fibrous tissue and spicules of bone. This uncommon entity is seen in children and typically fills in with normal or sclerotic bone in adulthood.

Patellofemoral Alignment

Merchant views can evaluate patellofemoral malalignment, which can be quantified with the sulcus and congruence

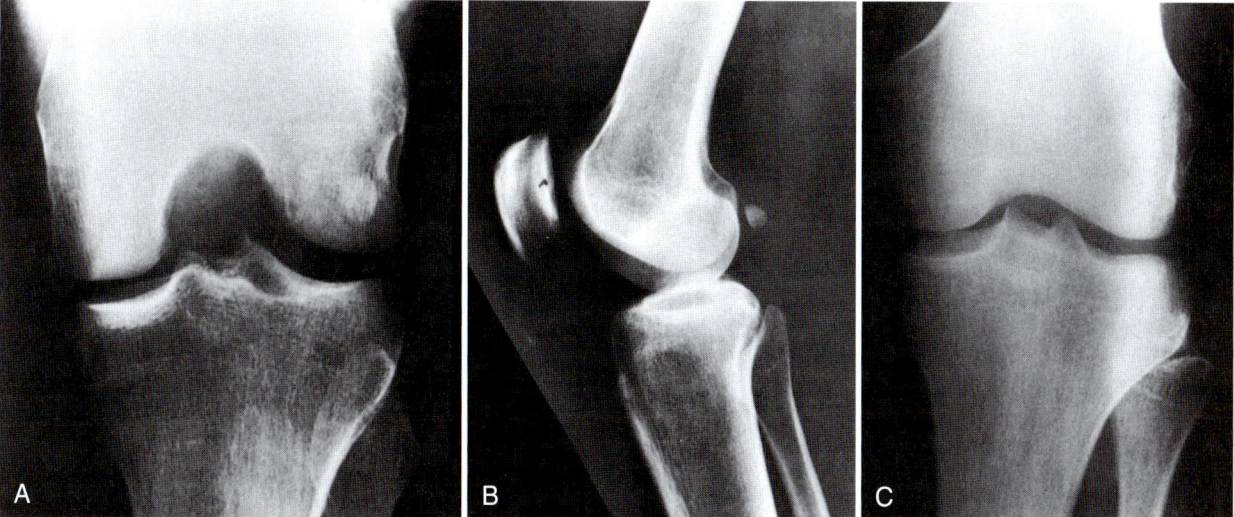

Figure 5-8. Fabella and cyamella. The fabella is a circular osseous density, a sesamoid, in the lateral head of the gastrocnemius muscle. **A,** On the anteroposterior (AP) view, it is superimposed on the lateral femoral condyle. **B,** On the lateral view, the fabella is posterior to the femoral condyles. **C,** A cyamella is a sesamoid bone in the popliteus tendon. On the AP view, the cyamella is seen within the notch at the lateral aspect of the lateral femoral condyle.

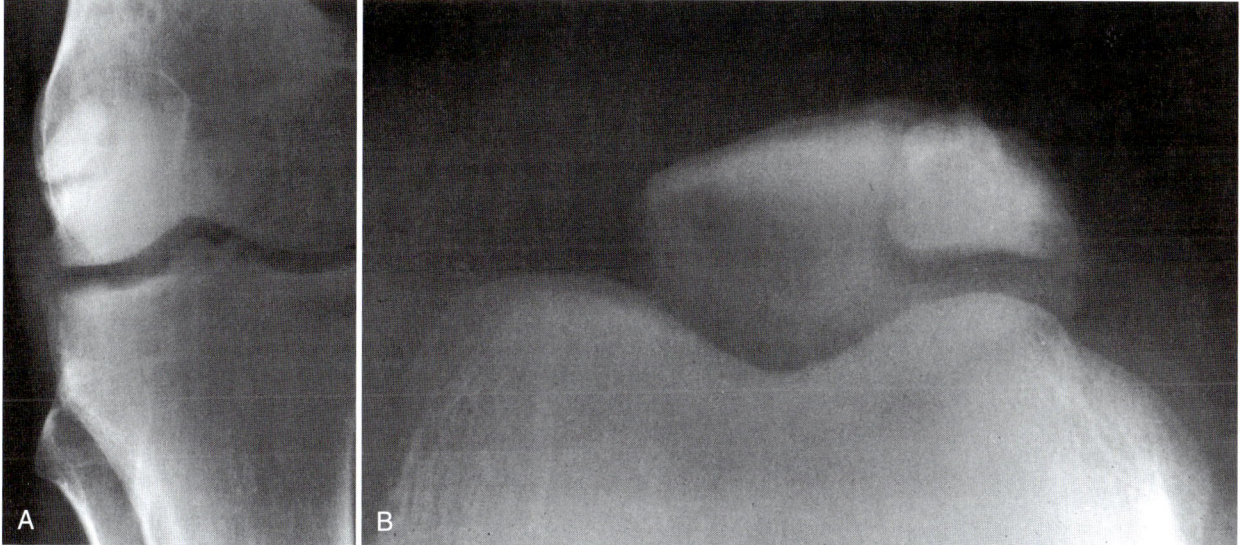

Figure 5-9. Bipartite patella. Oblique **(A)** and tangential axial **(B)** views of the patella demonstrate a crescentic radiolucency traversing the superolateral aspect of the patella. This lucency forms the interface between the two osseous centers of the bipartite patella. The superolateral location is typical of this entity.

angles. The sulcus angle is formed by drawing lines outward from the deepest portion of the trochlear sulcus to the tops of the femoral condyles. The angle normally measures 138 degrees (±6 degrees).[20] A shallow sulcus greater than 144 degrees is associated with recurrent patellar dislocation.

The congruence angle provides an index of subluxation. To measure it, the sulcus angle is bisected to create a reference line. An additional line is then drawn from the deepest portion of the trochlear sulcus to the patellar apex. The angle formed between this line and the reference line is the congruence angle. If the patellar apex falls lateral to the reference line, then the value of the congruence angle is positive. If the

apex falls medial to the reference line, then the value of the congruence angle is negative. The normal congruence angle is six degrees (±11 degrees) (Fig. 5-11).[20,37]

Patellar tilt is another measure of patellofemoral alignment. It is measured by the angle formed between a horizontal line and a line drawn between the medial and lateral corners of the patella. In the study performed by Grelsamer and colleagues, the mean tilt angle of a group of patients with signs and symptoms suggesting patellofemoral malalignment was 12 degrees (±6 degrees); in a similar group of control subjects, it was 2 degrees (±2 degrees). Tilting of 5 degrees was taken to be the limit of normal. It is noteworthy that in the Grelsamer study, the knee was held in 30 degrees of flexion, rather than 45 degrees of flexion in the normal Merchant view.[21] Other imaging techniques (CT scans performed at various degrees of flexion) are sometimes necessary to detect patients with subtle or transient lateral patellar subluxation (Fig. 5-12A and B).

Short- versus Long-standing Views

Short-standing frontal views (weight-bearing AP or Rosenberg) are typically sufficient for measuring the anatomic axis of the knee joint. The normal anatomic axis is 6 to 7 degrees of valgus angulation. If the exact quantitative measurement of the mechanical axis is required, then a

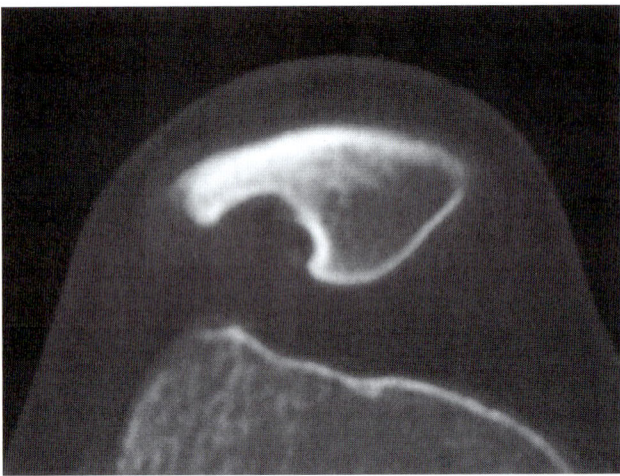

Figure 5-10. Dorsal defect of the patella. Axial computed tomography image demonstrates a large lucent dorsal defect involving the majority of the lateral facet of the patella. The patient had a smaller, similar lesion in the contralateral patella. This finding is bilateral in approximately one third of individuals.

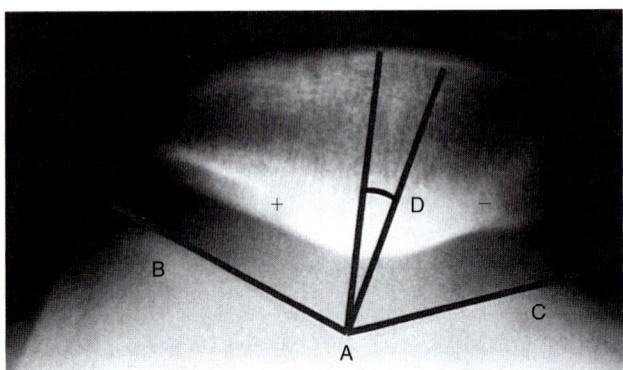

Figure 5-11. Merchant view; measurement of the sulcus and congruence angles. The sulcus angle (BAC) is bisected by the reference line. A second line (AD) is then drawn from the sulcus to the patellar ridge. If the patellar apex is lateral to the reference line, the value of the angle is positive; if it is medial, the value of the angle is negative.

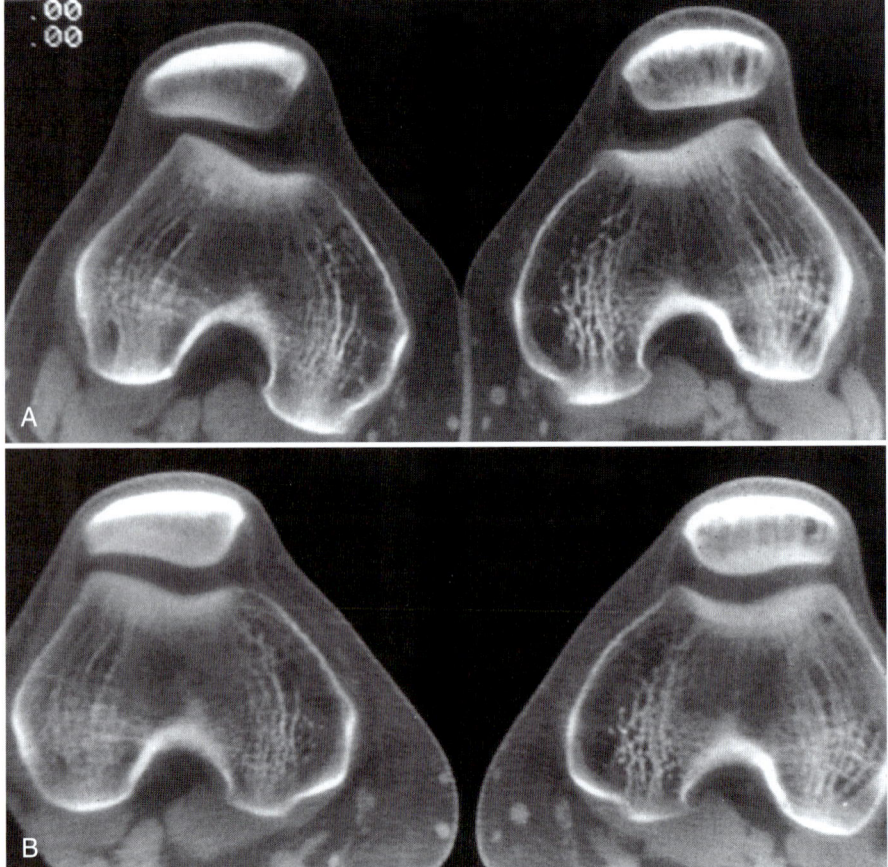

Figure 5-12. Computed tomography (CT) assessment of patellar tracking. Axial CT images obtained at 30 degrees **(A)** and 45 degrees **(B)** of flexion demonstrate transient bilateral lateral patellar subluxation. The patellar subluxation present at 30 degrees reduces at 45 degrees of flexion, thus explaining the normal Merchant view in this symptomatic patient.

long-standing frontal view of the lower extremity may be performed. The mechanical axis (weight-bearing axis) of the lower extremity is defined by a line drawn from the center of the femoral head to the center of the tibial plafond. In the normal setting, this line should pass through the inner aspect of the medial compartment of the knee joint. If genu valgus is excessive, then the mechanical axis will shift laterally. A medially shifted mechanical axis indicates genu varus. Knowledge of the mechanical axis and how it relates to the anatomic axis is important in evaluating patients who are about to undergo or have undergone total knee arthroplasty and/or revision arthroplasty. It is also helpful in evaluating patients with posttraumatic deformities, malalignment, or limb length discrepancies.

Obtaining long-standing radiographs requires a long cassette. If a long cassette is not available, a CT scanogram can be obtained. CT scanning to obtain the mechanical axis is not advocated by the authors because it is not weight bearing, does not provide functional information, and may fail to take account of ligamentous laxity. Also, CT scanograms entail higher radiation dosage exposure compared with conventional radiographs (Fig. 5-13).

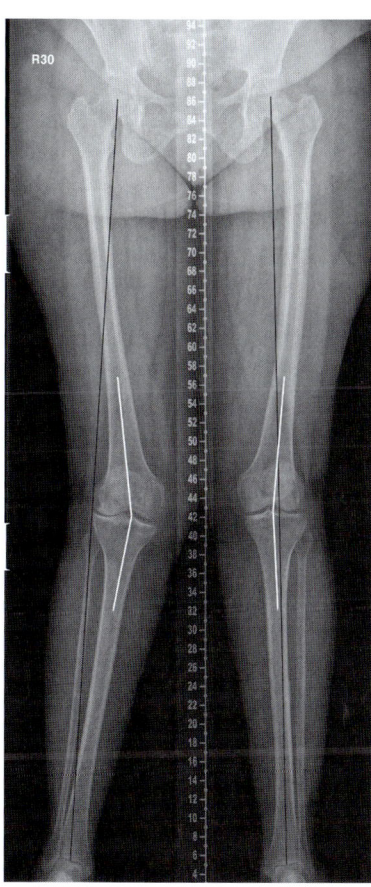

Figure 5-13. Long-standing views of bilateral lower extremities. Mechanical axis *(long black lines),* anatomic axis *(shorter white lines).* On the left, the anatomic axis is normal (6 degrees of valgus), and the mechanical axis (the line drawn from the center of the femoral head to the center of the tibial plafond) passes through the inner aspect of the medial compartment of the femorotibial joint. On the right, genu valgus angulation is excessive, and the mechanical axis is shifted laterally. Ruler included for limb length validation.

Arthrography

Radiographic arthrography entails intra-articular injection of x-ray dye, typically an iodine-based product. Arthrography has many uses, including confirming placement before joint aspiration. Commonly, once radiographs confirm dye placement within the joint space, a CT or MRI is performed to better evaluate meniscal or articular cartilage pathology and/or component loosening (Fig. 5-14).

Safety

Radiography necessitates exposing the patient to ionizing radiation. The associated risk is low, particularly in the extremities. Special consideration should be given to children and young adults to minimize their exposure.

COMPUTED TOMOGRAPHY

Applications

Computed tomography (CT) provides detailed information about osseous structures and generally functions as a problem-solving modality once the limits of radiography have been reached. Specialized knee applications include evaluation of complex trauma such as tibial plateau fractures, fracture healing, and joint loose bodies. CT is utilized with increasing frequency for preoperative joint replacement planning, arthroplasty complications, and revision arthroplasty preparation.[10,29,33,46] Extensor mechanism and patellofemoral joint evaluation in the setting of knee pain has also been reported.[22,27,28,32]

CT arthrography may be requested to evaluate menisci and/or articular cartilage when a patient is unable to undergo an MRI. This situation is commonly encountered in patients with claustrophobia or MRI-contraindicated metallic devices such as pacemakers.[41,58]

Technique

CT scanning is a radical extension of radiography. A radiograph is obtained in a single projection, but a tomogram is the fusion of multiple projections to form an image. The notion is similar to looking at an object, say a car, only from the front versus walking around the car to appreciate it from multiple perspectives. The computed element of CT involves having a computer generate an image as the x-ray beam strikes multiple detectors from multiple locations.

Similar to radiographs, CT scanners measure a single parameter, tissue density. Hounsfield units (HU) are the standard for measuring density. Water is zero HU. Less dense materials such as fat (−120 HU) and air (−1000) appear darker. Denser materials such as muscle (40 HU) and bone (400 HU) appear brighter. Thus, a CT image can be thought of as a density map plotted along a gray scale. Contrast is provided by the different densities of adjacent tissues.

CT technology has evolved quickly over the past several decades. Early on, a scanner moved stepwise through the anatomy of interest, acquiring a single slice at a time. Studies required several minutes to complete. Nowadays, scanners move helically, acquiring multiple slices in fractions of a

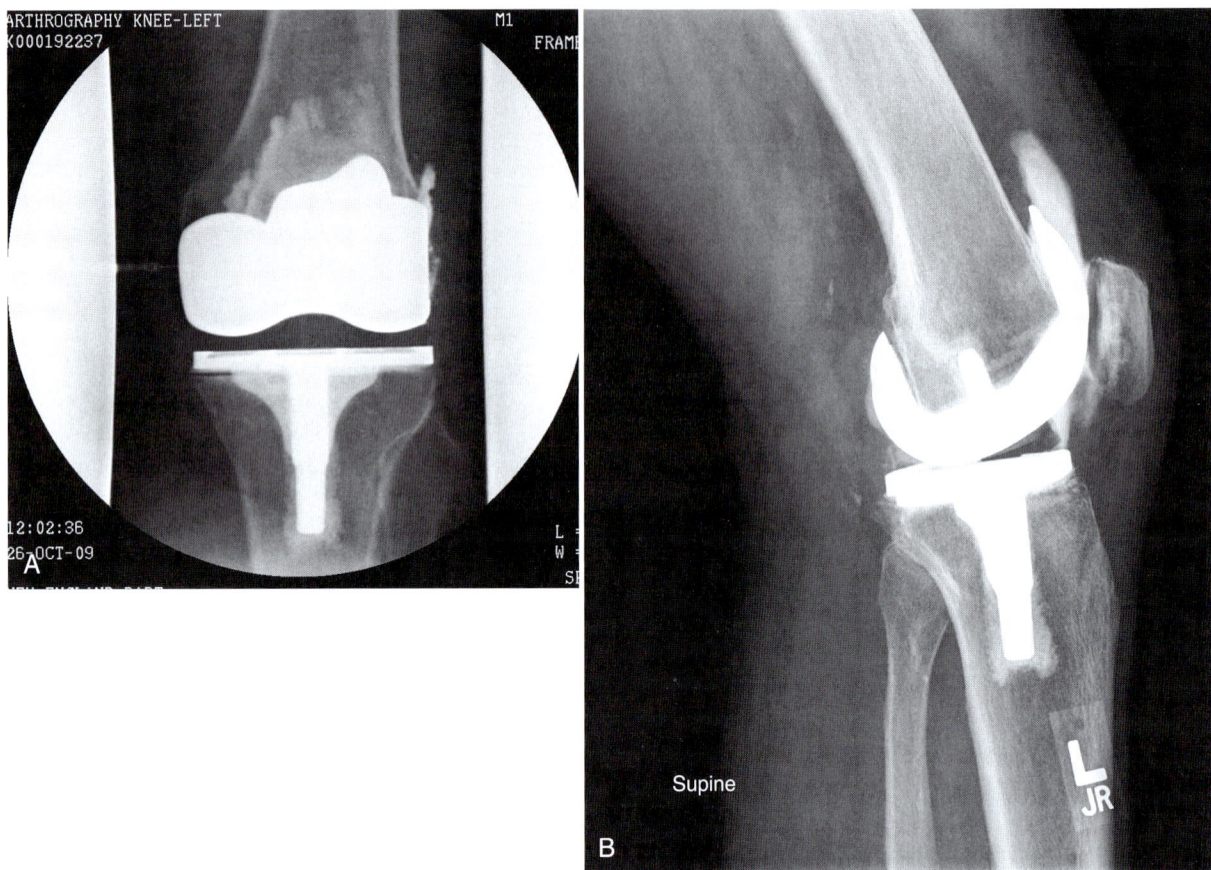

Figure 5-14. Normal knee arthrogram in a patient with a total knee arthroplasty. Anteroposterior (AP) **(A)** and lateral views **(B)** of the knee after intra-articular injection of radiopaque contrast material. Needle noted on the AP view.

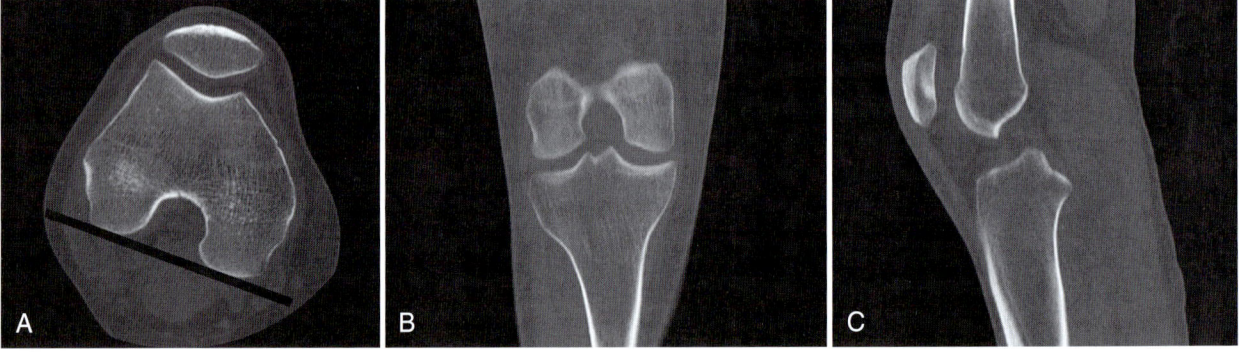

Figure 5-15. Normal axial **(A)**, coronal **(B)**, and sagittal **(C)** computed tomography (CT) images of the knee. A line drawn along the posterior aspect of the femoral condyles **(A)** on axial images demonstrates the correct plane selection for coronal reconstruction.

second. Entire examinations are routinely finished in a few seconds.

Additionally, modern technology allows the acquisition of isotropic voxels. Voxels are the three-dimensional analogues of pixels. They are the building blocks of an image. Each voxel represents a discrete density (HU) at a discrete location. A voxel is isotropic if it is equal in each of its three dimensions (i.e., cubic). This permits multiplanar reformatting. So, data acquired in a standard axial fashion with isotropic voxels can be reworked into sagittal and coronal planes, or any other plane desired. One pass of the

scanner allows you to look at the knee from any perspective you want!

Practically, the knee is imaged axially with thin sections (1.25 or 0.625 mm). The coronal reformats are prescribed via a line connecting the posterior aspects of the femoral condyles. The sagittal plane is generated along a line perpendicular to the coronal plane (Fig. 5-15A, B, and C).

Slice thickness is user dependent. Thicker slices, say 2.5 or 5 mm, reduce the number of overall images, making the dataset more manageable. It is easier and more efficient to scroll through 50 images rather than 200. In contrast, thin slices may provide finer detail that is effectively averaged out on thicker reformats. A balance is usually sought in slice thickness to provide a digestible number of images with adequate diagnostic information. Datasets are malleable, and additional reformats may be requested as necessary.

Several techniques are available for reducing metal-related artifact. First off, patient positioning is important. When possible, the goal is to position the patient so the beam penetrates the smallest cross-sectional area of metal. The high density of metal is challenging for a CT scanner because it prohibits the passage of photons. This may be partially overcome by increasing the peak kilovoltage (kVp) and milliampere seconds (mAs). kVp is the maximum voltage applied across an x-ray tube. A higher voltage results in higher energy photons, which possess greater penetrating power. mAs is the quantity of photons produced by the x-ray tube. Raising the mAs means that more photons are available to penetrate

the metal and contribute to the image. The pitch may be decreased, typically to less than one, to increase the overlap of slices (think of a tight spiral). This effectively increases the number of image-generating photons. The tradeoff in increasing each of these parameters is increased radiation exposure to the patient. During postprocessing, choosing thicker sections reduces image noise, combating metal-related artifact. Also, because bone algorithms worsen artifact, utilizing a standard reconstruction filter is preferable (Fig. 5-16).

Image Interpretation

A knee CT scan is read in any of three standard imaging planes: axial, sagittal, or coronal. An advantage of a PACS environment is that images can be instantaneously adjusted to focus on a specific range of densities to best show the tissue(s) of interest. A center density is identified, termed the level. The second setting, the window, is the range of densities around the level. For example, to evaluate fine bony detail, a level of 500 HU and a window of 2000 HU might be elected. In contrast, to assess soft tissue structures such as the menisci or cruciate ligaments, a level of 40 HU and a window of 400 may be chosen. These different bone and soft tissue settings are often programmed into the PACS and can be quickly selected at the touch of a button (Fig. 5-17A, B, and C).

In addition, three-dimensional volume and surface-rendered reconstructions can be created at an independent workstation. These are useful in the setting of complex osseous trauma, as well as in obtaining a more global view of implanted hardware (Fig. 5-18A and B).

CT Arthrography

CT arthrography is a two-step process. First, under fluoroscopic control, at least 15 mL of iodinated contrast is instilled into the knee joint. To provide double contrast, some physicians choose to instill several milliliters of air as well. The amount of air and contrast varies significantly among radiologists, but the point is to coat the joint surfaces with contrast so as to make abnormal extension of contrast into tears

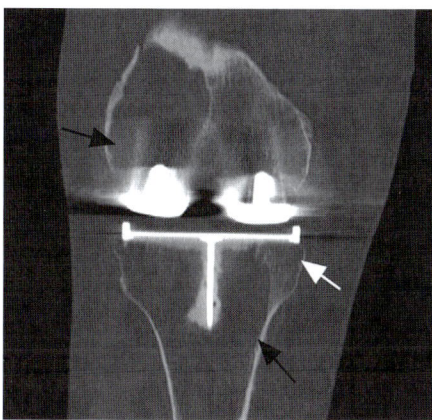

Figure 5-16. Coronal reconstructed computed tomography (CT) image of the knee using metal artifact reduction techniques clearly demonstrates large areas of osteolysis *(black arrows)* surrounding both the femoral and tibial components of a total knee arthroplasty, including a region immediately subjacent to the tibial plate *(white arrow).*

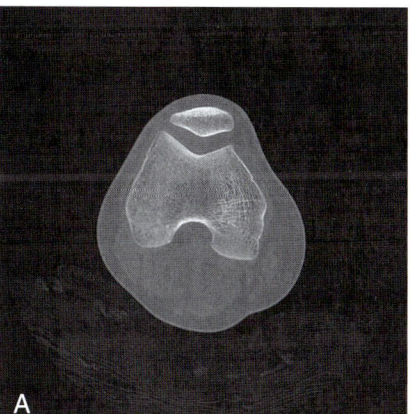
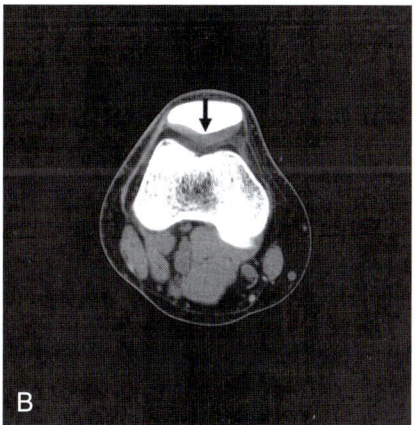
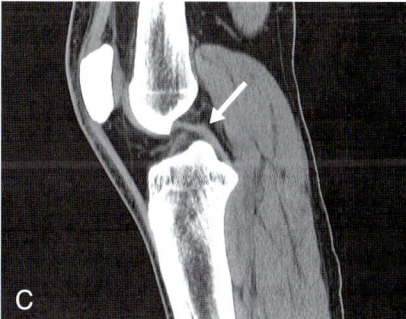

Figure 5-17. Bone and soft tissue windows. Axial computed tomography (CT) image of the knee at the level of the patellofemoral joint, using a bone reconstruction filter **(A)** is useful for demonstrating fine osseous detail. An image obtained at the same level using a soft tissue window **(B)** can evaluate soft tissue structures such as patellar cartilage *(arrow).* Sagittal image of the knee using a soft tissue window **(C)** demonstrates ligamentous structures such as the posterior cruciate ligament (PCL) *(arrow).*

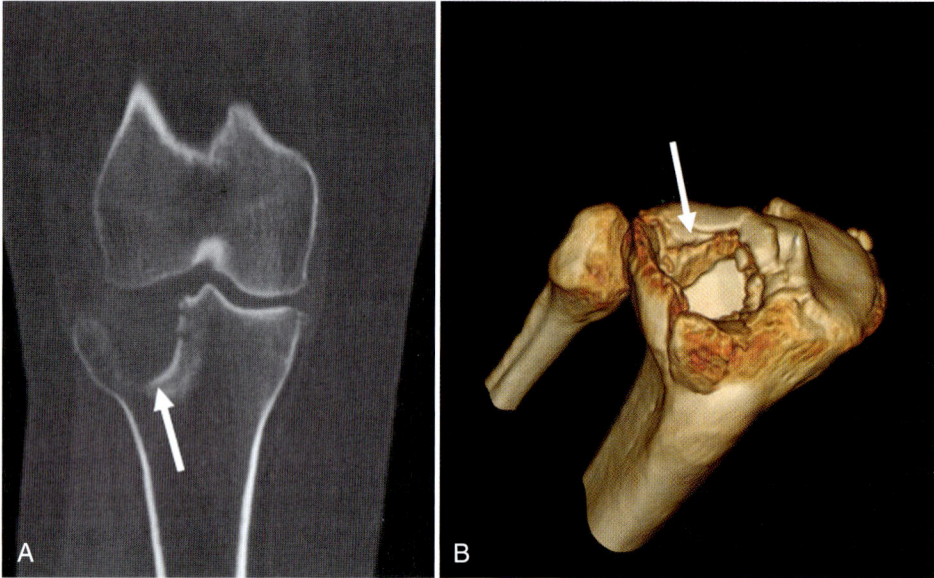

Figure 5-18. Three-dimensional (3D) reconstruction. A coronal reformatted image of the knee **(A)** demonstrating a markedly depressed fracture of the lateral tibial plateau *(white arrow)*. Postprocessed 3D volume rendered reconstruction with the soft tissues and femur cut away **(B)** shows the depressed fracture from a cranial oblique vantage point *(white arrow)* and may be useful for preoperative planning.

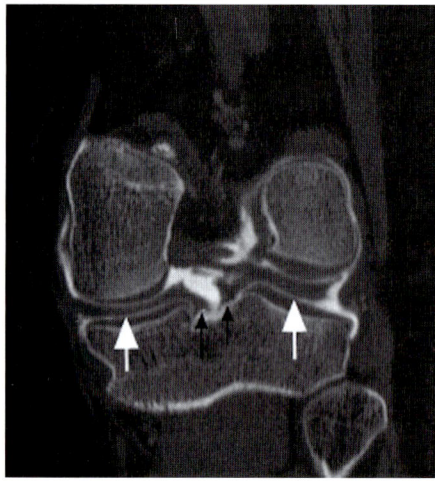

Figure 5-19. Computed tomography (CT) arthrogram. Coronal reconstructed CT arthrographic image of the knee demonstrates normal appearing medial and lateral menisci *(white arrows)*, including normal posterior root attachments *(black arrows)*. No imbibition of contrast material into the menisci occurs to indicate a meniscal tear.

visible. The patient then is transported to the CT suite and scanned. Contrast fills cartilage defects and meniscal tears. Loose bodies are outlined by contrast, appearing as filling defects (Fig. 5-19).

Artifacts/Special Considerations

Today, CT artifacts are notably few in orthopedic applications. Modern scanners have nearly eliminated several traditionally nagging artifacts. Motion artifact from patient movement renders an image blurry with indistinct margins. This now is rarely an issue because scanning a knee takes only a few seconds (or less). Partial volume effects come about when the scanner has difficulty processing adjacent tissues of markedly different density, bone and fat, for example. The scanner resolves this discrepancy by generating an average density that represents neither tissue. Sharp edges become blurred. The ability to obtain thin slices (i.e., less than 1 mm) has greatly diminished partial volume effects.

Beam hardening occurs when the x-ray beam encounters a dense material such as contrast or metal. The outcome is one of two distortions: cupping or streaks/dark bands. Cupping, as the name implies, is the appearance of a curved contour to an object when none actually exists. Streak artifact manifests as dark bands that radiate from a dense material, obscuring nearby anatomy. In the past, this artifact rendered the evaluation of metallic implants challenging. Current sophisticated software and filtration algorithms are able to minimize these artifacts (see Fig. 5-16).

It is important to keep in mind that the cost of reducing an artifact may be increased radiation to the patient. Although it is less of an issue when imaging an extremity of an adult patient, radiation exposure remains an issue at the forefront of protocol planning and patient safety, especially in the pediatric population.

Safety

Similar to radiography, CT utilizes ionizing radiation to generate an image. The difference lies in the amount of exposure. The effective dose of a CT scan is an order of magnitude greater than that of a radiograph. By virtue of comparison, a chest x-ray results in a 10 millirem effective dose, whereas a chest CT requires 600 millirem. When a CT scan is performed, determining and considering the radiation exposure is warranted, particularly in younger patients.

MAGNETIC RESONANCE IMAGING

Applications

Magnetic resonance imaging (MRI) is an extremely powerful tool that has supplanted other imaging modalities as the most versatile and effective technique for evaluating patients with internal derangement and cartilage disorders.[4,6,42] MRI is also invaluable for evaluating other pathologic processes such as tumor, infection, and metabolic bone disease. When used appropriately, after careful physical examination, MRI can be a useful tool in the surgical decision-making process and for preoperative planning.[3,40,57]

Technique

The MRI scanner is a large, powerful magnet. A 1.5 Tesla machine is 30,000 times stronger than the earth's magnetic field. This mighty device exposes a patient to strong magnetic forces and measures the resulting tiny, very fast movements of atoms.

Clinical imaging centers upon hydrogen atoms (protons), which are ubiquitous throughout the body. Inherent qualities of each tissue dictate how its protons will respond in the MRI environment. In contrast to a CT scanner that measures density, the MRI scanner is capable of measuring multiple tissue properties: T1, T2, proton density, and so forth. MRI scanners are calibrated to measure a specific property by prescribing values for several variables—altogether termed a sequence. Two of these variables are time to echo (TE) and time to repetition (TR). In general, a T2-weighted sequence necessitates a long TR on the order of several thousand milliseconds and a TE near a hundred milliseconds or so. A T1-weighted sequence uses a relatively short TR (hundreds of milliseconds) and a short TE (less than 50 milliseconds). Sequences vary considerably across manufacturers and field strengths.

Bearing this in mind, different tissues in the body behave in a reproducible manner on specific pulse sequences, and knowledge of these characteristics is helpful for detection of pathologic processes. For example, adipose tissue and acute hemorrhage are hyperintense (bright) on T1-weighted sequences; hematopoietic bone marrow is lower in signal intensity on T1- and T2-weighted images than fatty marrow because of its lower fat content (Fig. 5-20A and B). Water is bright on T2-weighted images and dark on T1-weighted images. Because pathologic processes (tumor, infection, contusion, ligament and tendon injury) are typically associated with increased water content, abnormalities usually appear hyperintense to adjacent tissues on fluid-sensitive sequences and lower in signal intensity on T1-weighted images. Increased signal intensity or bone marrow edema pattern becomes more conspicuous when fat suppression is applied. Fat suppression can be accomplished by preferentially saturating the fat protons (chemical saturation) or by a technique known as short tau inversion recovery imaging (STIR). The former technique is more commonly used in the knee. Fat suppression serves to make the presence and extent of pathologic processes more conspicuous on T2-weighted and proton density sequences.

Metal reduction techniques have been developed to permit MRI examination in areas of implanted hardware.

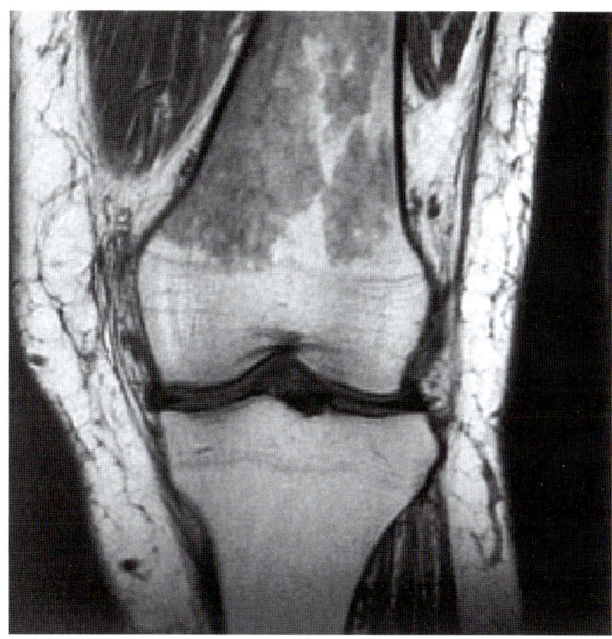

Figure 5-20. Magnetic resonance imaging (MRI) of marrow signal. A coronal T1-weighted image shows bright marrow signal in the tibia and at the distal end of the femur, which represents fatty (yellow) marrow. The dark signal in the metaphysis and distal shaft of the femur represents hematopoietic (red) marrow hyperplasia. Note that the red marrow almost never crosses the growth plate scar.

Several sequence variables are adjusted, for example, bandwidth and matrix. When hardware is present, STIR is preferred over chemical fat suppression, because it is less prone to magnetic susceptibility artifact caused by metallic prosthetic components.

As the scanner executes the sequence, protons in a patient's tissues generate signal. A receiver coil, a device analogous to a highly engineered antenna, then collects signal and transmits it back to the scanner, which then produces an image. The coil is an important determinant of image quality. The more signal that is accurately captured, the better is the image. Optimal coils are designed for a specific body part. For example, a wrist coil is used for the wrist and a knee coil is used for the knee. Using a coil not designed for the body part of interest may result in images of lower quality.

Recent advances in MRI along with decreases in cost have further placed it at the forefront in evaluation of the knee. Among these advances includes 3.0 Tesla strength magnet systems, improved cartilage imaging, three-dimensional imaging, and multichannel (8 or 16) dedicated knee receiver coils. Although these improvements have helped to create fast and sophisticated imaging protocols, one must remember that tremendous variation and quality are seen among clinically available MRI systems. The spectrum of clinically available systems ranges in strength from open 0.2 Tesla without dedicated coils to 3.0 Tesla magnets with 16 channel receiver coils. The deficiencies of these lower field strength systems are exposed most conspicuously when subtle meniscal and hyaline cartilage injuries are imaged. Therefore, the accuracy of knee MRI is variable, depending on the equipment used and the experience and subspecialty expertise of the interpreting radiologist.[15]

Plane and Protocol Selection

MRI of the knee is performed in axial, sagittal, and coronal planes. The axial plane is a true anatomic transverse plane through the knee. The coronal plane is typically prescribed from the axial plane based on a line drawn along the posterior aspect of the femoral condyles (Fig. 5-21). The sagittal plane is then chosen perpendicular to the coronal plane. Most knee structures may be evaluated in three planes, although each plane has particular advantages. For example, axial images best display the patellar cartilage and subchondral bone. In contrast, the trochlear sulcus cartilage is seen to best advantage in the sagittal plane. The sagittal and coronal planes best demonstrate meniscal and femorotibial cartilage anatomy and pathology. Although the sagittal plane is most often used for preliminary evaluation of the anterior cruciate ligament (ACL) and posterior cruciate ligament (PCL), it is essential to use the coronal and axial planes to follow the entire course of each ligament to the level of the osseous attachments.

Wide variation in protocol planning and sequence selection has been noted. Proton density (PD) sequences with or without fat suppression are commonly employed to evaluate ligaments, tendons, and articular cartilage. Fat-suppressed PD or T2-weighted sequences are useful for imaging osseous contusion and/or the bone marrow edema pattern, as well as muscle, tendon, and ligament tears and strains. T1-weighted images (with and without fat suppression and both before and after intravenous gadolinium contrast administration) are often obtained to evaluate the marrow cavity in cases of suspected tumor or osteomyelitis. Fat-saturated T1-weighted imaging is used when MR arthrography is performed after intra-articular administration of dilute gadolinium. Three example protocols are presented here. These protocols are based on the use of a 3.0 Tesla MRI (General Electric, Milwaukee, Wis) with an eight-channel dedicated knee coil (Table 5-1). MRI of knee arthroplasties can be performed to minimize metallic artifact using bandwidth and matrix manipulation and STIR sequences.[52] Although this approach is often effective in evaluating complications of and pathology surrounding total joints, it has yet to fully permeate clinical practices owing to the difficulty involved in obtaining consistently high-quality images.

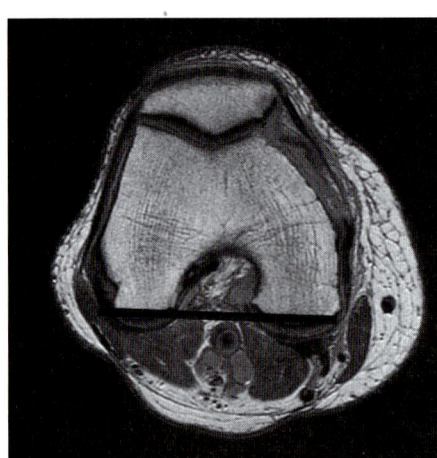

Figure 5-21. Axial proton density (PD) fast spin echo (FSE) image of the knee with a black line connecting the posterior aspects of the femoral condyles. This line is the correct plane choice for coronal imaging.

Normal Anatomy

Ligaments

The ACL functions primarily to restrain anterior tibial translation. It courses from the inner or medial aspect of the lateral femoral condyle, traveling inferiorly and obliquely, parallel to Blumensaat's line, to insert on the anteromedial tibia adjacent to the medial tibial spine. The ligament is composed of anteromedial and posterolateral bundles. In the sagittal plane, the ACL is typically visualized over several images because of its oblique course. The ACL is also well evaluated

Table 5-1 MRI Knee Protocols

Sequence	TR	TE	ETL	BW	NEX	Matrix	ST, mm	IG, mm
ROUTINE KNEE FOR INTERNAL DERANGEMENT								
Sag PD FSE	3000	42	6	50	2	384 × 224	3	1
Sag FS PD FSE	3000	42	6	50	2	384 × 224	3	1
Cor T2 FS FSE	2500	68	11	31.25	2	320 × 224	3	1
Cor PD FSE	3017	30	6	50	2	384 × 224	3	1
Ax FS PD FSE	3017	30	6	50	2	382 × 224	3	1
KNEE ARTHROGRAM (COR T2 FS FSE, SAG PD FSE, AND THE FOLLOWING SEQUENCES)								
Sag T1 FS FSE	1300	Min	2	31.25	2	320 × 224	3	0.5
Cor T1 FS FSE	1300	Min	2	31.25	2	320 × 224	3	0.5
Ax PD FS FSE	3567	45	2	50	2	384 × 224	3	1
KNEE FOR TUMOR AND INFECTION (COR T2 FS FSE, SAG FS PD FSE, SAG AND COR T1 FSE, AND THE FOLLOWING SEQUENCES)								
Ax T1 FSE	1300	Min	2	31.25	2	320 × 224	3	0.5
Sag T1 FS + Gad	1300	Min	2	31.25	2	320 × 224	3	0.5
Ax T1 FS + Gad	1300	Min	2	31.25	2	320 × 224	3	0.5

BW, Bandwidth; *ETL,* echo train length; *IG,* interslice gap; *NEX,* number of excitations; *ST,* slice thickness; *TE,* echo time; *TR,* repetition time.

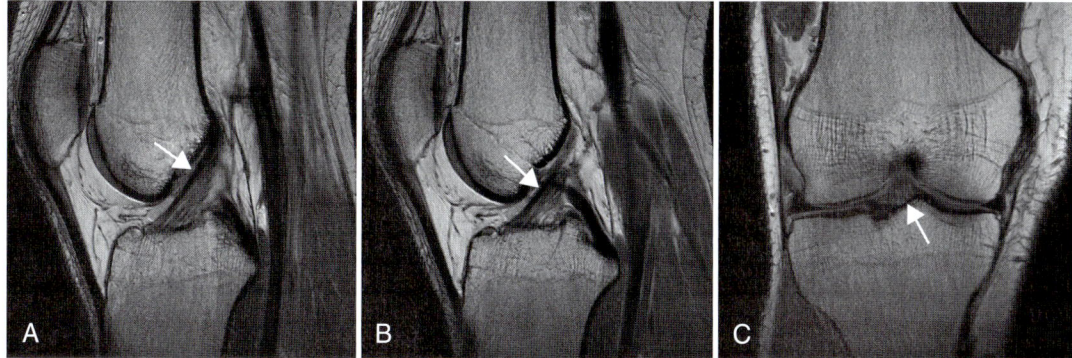

Figure 5-22. Consecutive sagittal proton density (PD) fast spin echo (FSE) images of the knee (**A** and **B**) demonstrate a normal appearing anterior cruciate ligament (ACL) *(arrow)*. Coronal PD FSE image **(C)** shows a normal tibial insertion of the ACL *(arrow)*. Intermediate to bright signal is seen interposed between the ligament fibers, consistent with fat and synovium.

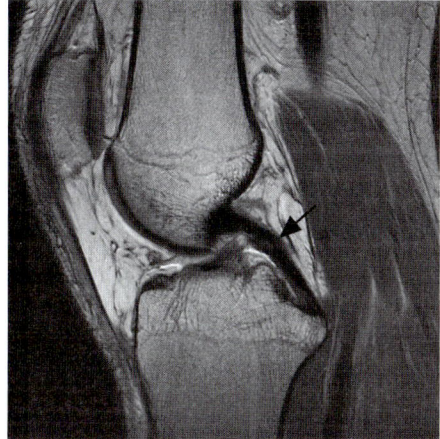

Figure 5-23. Sagittal proton density (PD) fast spine echo (FSE) image of the knee demonstrates a normal appearing posterior cruciate ligament (PCL) *(arrow)*.

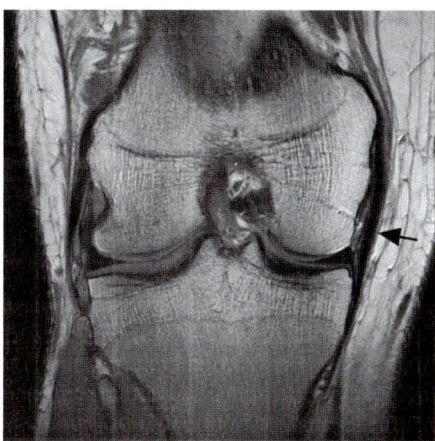

Figure 5-24. Coronal proton density (PD) fast spin echo (FSE) image of the knee demonstrates a normal appearing medial collateral ligament (MCL) *(arrow)*.

on standard images obtained in the coronal and axial planes. Dedicated imaging can be performed in an oblique sagittal plane to produce images within the same plane as the ligament. However, this is not believed to be necessary because of the accuracy of imaging ACL injuries using standard imaging planes.[30] The normal appearance of the ACL is that of a low signal band on all imaging sequences with an intrasubstance linear intermediate to bright signal from normal interposed fat and synovium (Fig. 5-22A, B, and C).

The PCL limits posterior tibial translation and is larger and stronger than the ACL. The PCL originates at the inner aspect of the medial femoral condyle and inserts on the posterior tibia. The cross-sectional area of the PCL is largest at its femoral origin and decreases toward the tibial insertion. The PCL tibial attachment extends over the dorsal rim of the posterior tibial shelf.[48] Similar to the ACL, the PCL can be divided into two functional units: anterolateral and posteromedial bundles. The normal MRI appearance of the PCL is that of a low signal band on all imaging sequences; it is typically visualized on one or two consecutive images on sagittal pulse sequences. The PCL is taut in flexion and tends to become more lax with extension—the typical position in which the knee is placed during MRI. It should have a gently curved configuration when viewed in the sagittal plane (Fig. 5-23).[48]

The medial collateral ligament (MCL) provides support to the medial aspect of the knee. Its primary functions are to stabilize the femorotibial joint when valgus stresses are applied, and to stabilize against lateral subluxation/dislocation of the patella. Although the MCL has been described as a simple bandlike structure, it is rather a ligamentous complex composed of three layers. It blends imperceptibly with the surrounding joint capsule and other medial supporting structures.[5] The MCL consists of deep and superficial components. The superficial fibers of the MCL reside in layer 2 of the medial supporting structures and take their origin at the medial femoral condyle (layer 1 primarily consists of crural fascia).[54] Superficial MCL fibers run slightly anteromedially to insert on the tibia, approximately 5 cm from the joint line, just posterior to the pes anserinus tendons.[55] The deep fibers or capsular layer includes the meniscofemoral and meniscotibial (coronary) ligaments. The deep and superficial fibers are separated by the medial collateral bursa, which in the normal setting should be collapsed and imperceptible on MRI. The MCL should appear with uniformly low signal on all pulse sequences. It is best appreciated on coronal and axial sequences (Fig. 5-24). MCL injuries range from sprains, in which the ligament will be normal in appearance with surrounding fluid signal, to partial- and full-thickness tears with disruption of the superficial and/or deep fibers.

The lateral collateral ligament (LCL) functions to resist varus stress and provide posterolateral stability. This complex is composed of three layers. The superficial layer (layer 1) includes the iliotibial band anteriorly and the superficial portion of the biceps femoris posterolaterally.[54] The iliotibial band inserts at the far anterior aspect of the lateral tibia at Gerdy's tubercle. The biceps femoris inserts on the fibular styloid. The middle layer (layer 2) includes the lateral retinaculum anteriorly and two discrete areas of ligamentous thickening that originate from the lateral patella.[54] The deep layer (layer 3) forms a portion of the lateral joint capsule. It is composed of the LCL proper (fibulocollateral ligament), the arcuate complex, and several posterolateral corner structures.[54] The fibulocollateral ligament originates from the lateral femoral condyle and courses posterolaterally to insert upon the fibular head, combining with the deep fibers of the biceps femoris tendon to form the conjoined tendon.[54] The contents of the posterolateral corner include the popliteus tendon, the LCL proper, the lateral head of the gastrocnemius muscle, and the arcuate, popliteofibular, and fabellofibular ligaments.

The components of the LCL complex and the posterolateral corner are normally of homogeneously low signal. Coronal images display them optimally (Fig. 5-25A through G), although axial images are also illustrative. Tears of any portion of the LCL complex manifest themselves as signal hyperintensity and discontinuity of ligament/tendon fibers. Tears of the LCL proper are closely associated with posterolateral corner injuries, which can lead to posterolateral instability.[5]

Menisci

The menisci are wedge-shaped, semilunar fibrocartilaginous structures that lie between the femoral condyles and the tibia.

The primary function of the menisci is to increase surface area and distribute the load evenly across the femoral condyles. The menisci also act as shock absorbers and play a role in chondrocyte nutrition and joint lubrication. In the ACL-deficient knee, the menisci act as anteroposterior stabilizers. The absence of a normal meniscus can lead to irreversible and accelerated degenerative changes.[16]

Each meniscus is arbitrarily divided into anterior horn, body, and posterior horn. The periphery of each meniscus is thick, and the inner aspect is thin. Thus the menisci appear triangular in cross-section, except at the body, where the menisci maintain a "bow-tie" appearance on sagittal images. The central edge of the meniscus is termed the free edge or apex. It should appear as a sharp point. The superior surfaces of the menisci are concave and serve to deepen the contact area with the femoral condyles; the inferior aspects are flat and rest on the tibial plateau. The menisci are almost entirely avascular structures. The posterior and peripheral aspects of the menisci have a vascular supply and therefore are termed the red zone. It has been proposed that tears in this region have a greater tendency to heal.[23,39,56]

The menisci cover 50% of the medial and 70% of the lateral surface of the tibial plateau.[16] The medial meniscus is C-shaped, and the posterior horn is approximately two times larger than the anterior horn (Fig. 5-26). The medial meniscus is attached to the joint capsule throughout its course peripherally, limiting its mobility and making it more prone to injury than the lateral meniscus. The anterior horn has a root attachment centrally, just anterior to the ACL attachment on the tibia. The posterior horn attachment is to the posterior aspect of the tibia within the intercondylar fossa.

The lateral meniscus is semicircular, and its two horns are symmetrical. The lateral meniscus is more mobile than the

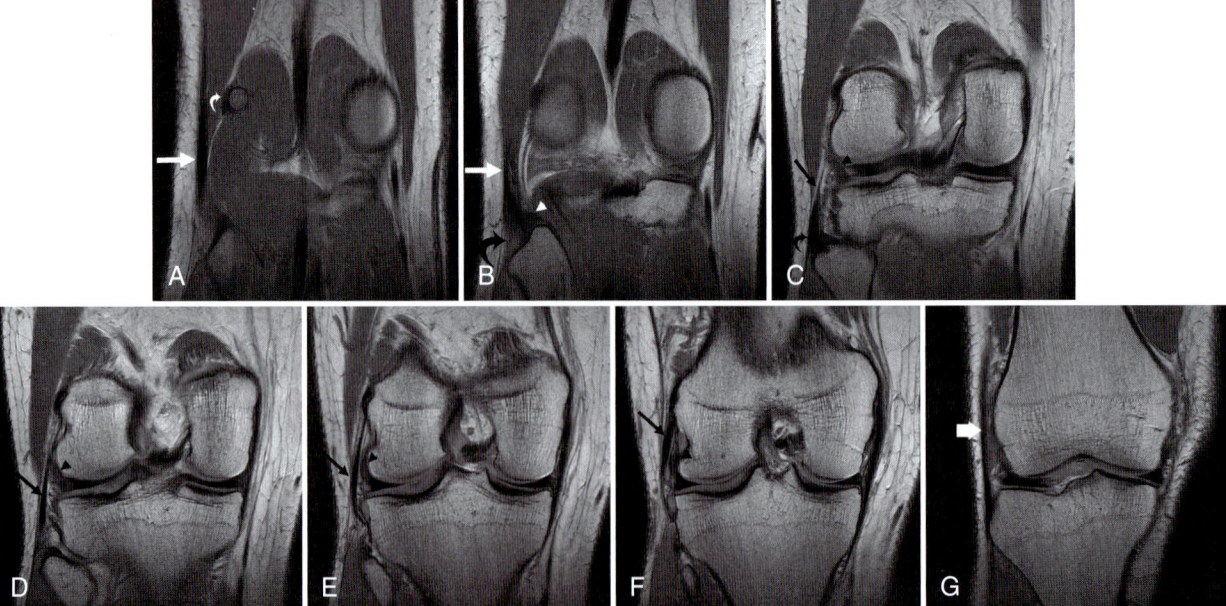

Figure 5-25. The lateral collateral ligament complex and selected structures of the posterolateral corner. Multiple coronal proton density (PD) images starting at the far posterior aspect of the knee and progressing anteriorly (**A** through **G**) demonstrate the normal appearing fabella and fabellofibular ligament *(curved white arrow)*, the biceps femoris tendon *(straight white arrow)*, the conjoined tendon inserting on the fibula *(curved black arrow)*, the poplitiofibular ligament *(white arrowhead)*, the fibulocollateral ligament *(straight black arrow)*, the popliteus tendon *(black arrowhead)*, and the iliotibial band *(wide white arrow on image **G**)*. Images **A** through **F** are consecutive, and image **G** is located more anteriorly.

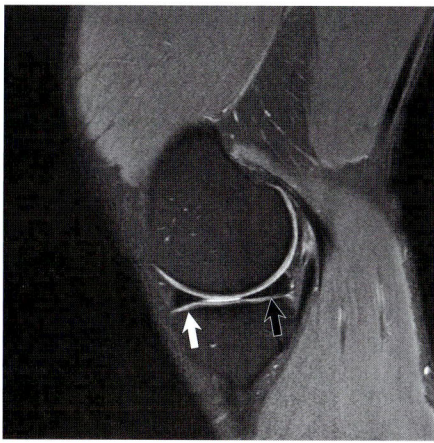

Figure 5-26. Normal medial meniscus. Sagittal fat suppressed proton density (PD) image demonstrates both the anterior and posterior horns to be normal in signal (diffusely low) and morphology (appear as triangles with a sharp free edge), with the posterior horn *(black arrow)* approximately 50% larger than the anterior horn *(white arrow)*.

medial meniscus. It attaches only to the anterior and far posterior aspects of the joint capsule. Its capsular attachment is interrupted at the body and much of the posterior horn to accommodate the popliteus tendon coursing through the popliteal hiatus (Fig. 5-27). Small fascicles attach the popliteus to the lateral meniscus, allowing the meniscus to be pulled posteriorly during knee flexion (Fig. 5-28).

The meniscofemoral ligaments of Humphrey and Wrisberg extend from the posterior horn of the lateral meniscus to the inner aspect of the medial femoral condyle. They cross anterior and posterior to the PCL, respectively (Fig. 5-29A and B). Meniscofemoral ligaments are inconsistently and variably present (i.e., patients may have one, both, or neither and may be considered normal).

The menisci are homogeneous low signal structures that should be evaluated on both sagittal and coronal images. On sagittal images, normal menisci should appear as black signal triangles with sharp central edges. The body segment, the portion between the anterior and posterior horns, appears as a low signal "bow-tie"–shaped structure at the peripheral aspect of the sagittal images. Coronal images through the

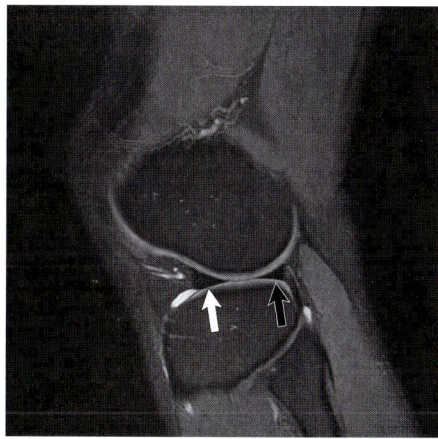

Figure 5-27. Normal lateral meniscus. Sagittal fat-suppressed proton density (PD) image demonstrates both the anterior and posterior horns to be normal in signal (diffusely low) and morphology (appear as triangles with a sharp free edge), with the posterior horn *(black arrow)* approximately the same size as the anterior horn *(white arrow)*.

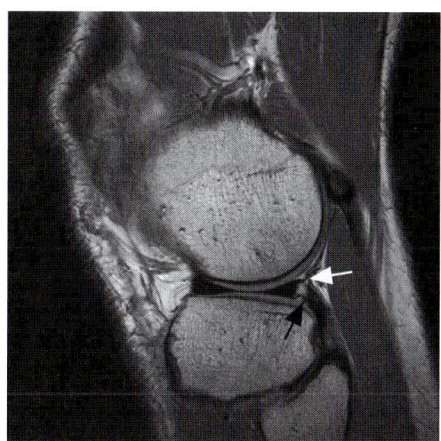

Figure 5-28. Sagittal proton density (PD) fast spin echo (FSE) image of the knee demonstrates a normal appearing posterior horn of the lateral meniscus with intact superior *(white arrow)* and inferior *(black arrow)* fascicular attachments *(arrows)* to the popliteus tendon.

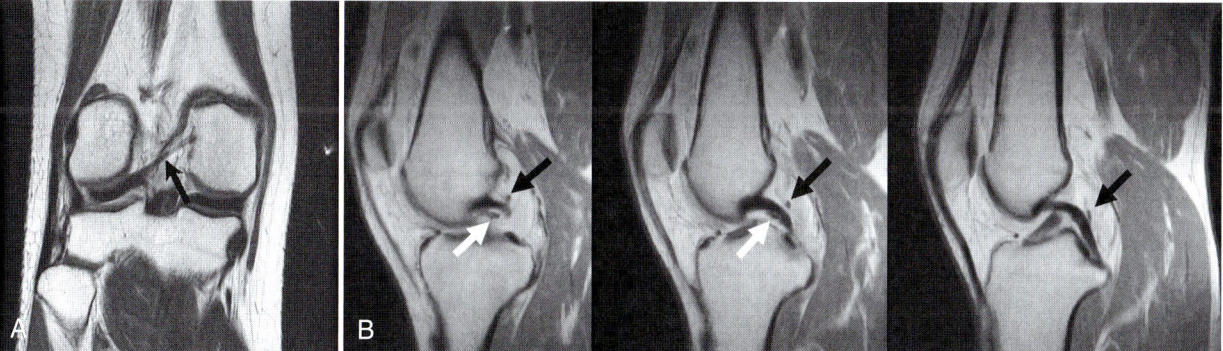

Figure 5-29. Meniscofemoral ligaments. Coronal proton density (PD) image of the knee **(A)** demonstrates the normal course of the meniscofemoral ligament *(arrow)* extending from the posterior horn of the lateral meniscus to the inner aspect of the posterior medial femoral condyle. Three consecutive sagittal PD images of the knee **(B)** in a different patient, with the meniscofemoral ligaments of Humphrey *(white arrow)* and Wrisberg *(black arrow)* noted anteriorly and posteriorly to the posterior cruciate ligament (PCL), respectively.

menisci allow evaluation of the root attachments and cross-sectional evaluation of the meniscal bodies.

Tears of the menisci manifest as linear bright signal abnormalities on fluid-sensitive sequences that reach an articular surface, or as alterations in normal meniscal morphology.[13,45,53]

Meniscal variants include the discoid meniscus and the transverse meniscal ligament. A discoid meniscus, instead of having a semicircular or **C** shape, is shaped like a disk. Discoid menisci are much more common on the lateral side and have a reported incidence of 0.4% to 16.6%. Three types of discoid menisci have been described: complete, incomplete, and Wrisberg variants. Visualization of a continuous band of meniscus on more than three contiguous peripheral sagittal images (5 mm or less in thickness) indicates a discoid meniscus (Fig. 5-30).[51] A meniscal body on coronal images greater than 15 mm wide or extending into the intercondylar notch also suggests the diagnosis. Discoid menisci have an increased incidence of tears and degeneration.[16]

The transverse or anterior intermeniscal ligament connects the anterior horns of the medial and lateral meniscus. It is present in 44% to 58% of patients.[16] On sagittal images, the interface of this structure with the anterior horn of the lateral meniscus often simulates a tear (Fig. 5-31).[14,24] Following this "pseudotear" on sequential images helps identify this normal structure.

Tendons

The extensor mechanism of the knee consists of the quadriceps and patellar tendons. The quadriceps is composed of the rectus femoris tendon anteriorly, the vastus medialis and lateralis tendons centrally, and the vastus intermedius posteriorly. The normal quadriceps tendon is low signal on all pulse sequences, with internal striations of brighter signal representing the divisions of the previously described tendons. The quadriceps inserts on the superior pole of the patella. The patellar tendon is composed primarily of fibers from the rectus femoris, which continue below the patella to insert on the tibial tubercle. Its normal appearance is homogeneously low

signal. The extensor mechanism is best visualized in the sagittal plane (Fig. 5-32). The axial plane provides ideal visualization of the medial and lateral retinaculi, which originate from the patella to insert on the medial and lateral femoral condyles, respectively (Fig. 5-33).

The semimembranosus and pes anserinus tendons course along the posteromedial aspect of the knee. They are low signal structures. The semimembranosus has multiple slips that insert on both the medial tibia and the joint capsule.

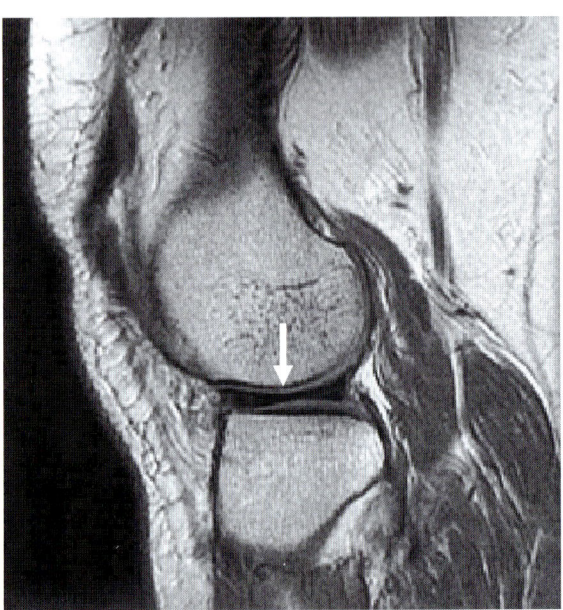

Figure 5-30. Discoid lateral meniscus. Sagittal proton density (PD) image demonstrates a blocklike continuous band of meniscus *(white arrow)*; the lateral meniscus had this configuration on nearly all sagittal images. A normal meniscus has this appearance only on the more peripheral images and assumes the appearance of two separate triangles (anterior and posterior horns) centrally in the region of the intercondylar notch.

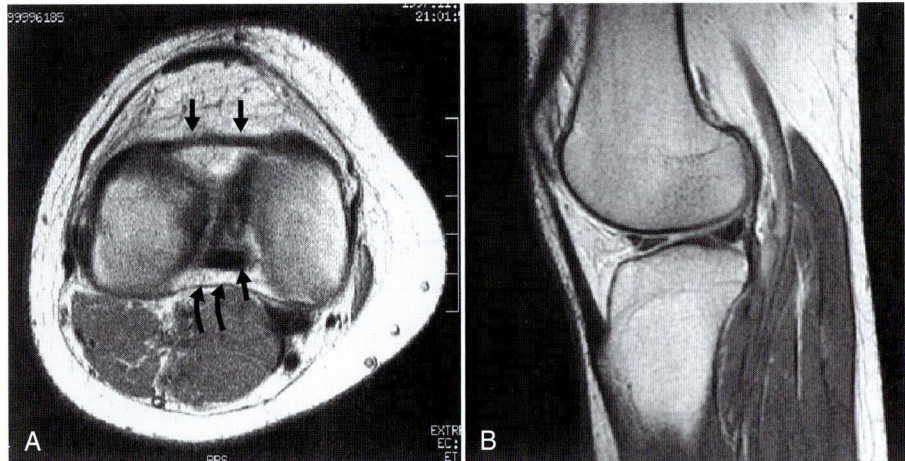

Figure 5-31. Transverse meniscal ligament. **A,** Axial proton density (PD) image shows the low signal transverse meniscal ligament (TML) *(short arrows)* connecting the anterior horns of the lateral and medial menisci. Also seen on this image are the posterior cruciate ligament *(long arrow)* and the posterior joint capsule *(curved arrows)*. **B,** Sagittal PD image through the lateral meniscus shows a linear interface between the anterior margin of the anterior horn of the lateral meniscus and the TML. The TML can be mistaken for a portion of the lateral meniscus; the interface can therefore simulate a tear.

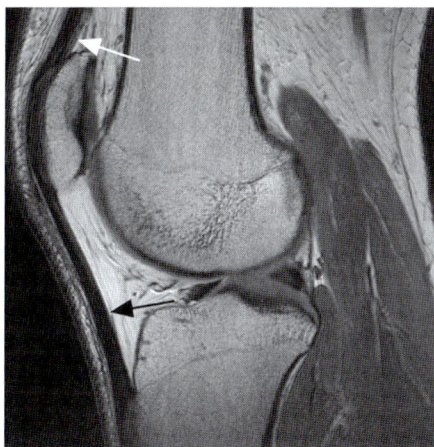

Figure 5-32. Extensor mechanism. Sagittal proton density (PD) fast spin echo (FSE) image of the knee demonstrates normal homogeneously low signal patellar *(white arrow)* and quadriceps *(black arrow)* tendons.

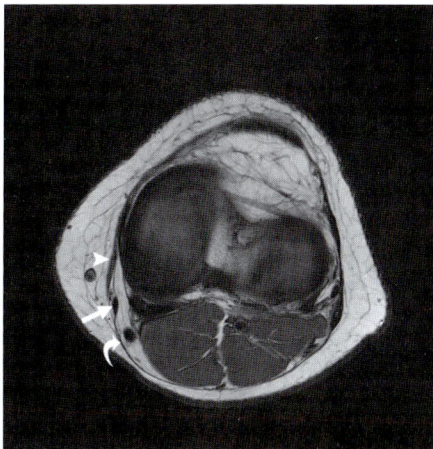

Figure 5-34. The pes anserinus. Axial proton density (PD) image demonstrates the normal appearing low signal sartorius *(white arrowhead)*, gracilis *(straight white arrow)*, and semitendinosus *(curved white arrow)* tendons coursing anteriorly and inferiorly along the medial aspect of the knee at the level of the knee joint toward their insertion on the anteromedial aspect of the tibia.

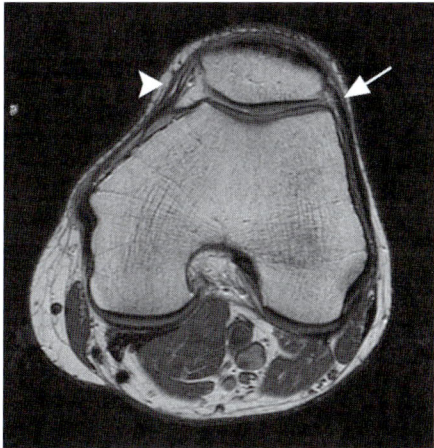

Figure 5-33. Axial proton density (PD) fast spin echo (FSE) image of the knee demonstrates intact medial *(white arrowhead)* and lateral *(white arrow)* patellar retinaculi.

The pes anserinus is made up of three tendons: gracilis, sartorius, and semitendinosus. The three tendons insert on the medial aspect of the tibia anterior to the MCL insertion. They are well demonstrated on axial images (Fig. 5-34).

The popliteus tendon originates at the lateral aspect of the lateral femoral condyle and courses posteroinferiorly to join the muscle belly, which inserts on the proximal posteromedial aspect of the tibia. Superior and inferior popliteomeniscal fascicles serve as attachments between the lateral meniscus, popliteus tendon, and capsule to form the roof and floor of the popliteal hiatus. At least one fascicle is visualized in 97% of patients with an intact lateral meniscus. The fascicles control the motion of the lateral meniscus in flexion and extension and appear as thin low signal structures that extend from the posterolateral aspect of the lateral meniscus to the joint capsule (see Fig. 5-28). Disruption of one or more of the fascicles allows increased motion of the meniscus and can result in pain and/or locking.[16]

Cartilage

Various techniques are used to evaluate cartilage within the knee joint. Fat-suppressed proton density weighted images provide increased conspicuity of lesions, given their high resolution and clear differentiation between fluid and cartilage. Properly obtained non–fat-suppressed fast spin echo (FSE) proton density images can also provide exquisite cartilage detail. Some authors believe this sequence is inferior to fat-suppressed sequences in evaluating for commonly associated subchondral bone abnormalities.[55] Other advanced but less frequently clinically used techniques include T2 mapping, T1RHO, and delayed gadolinium-enhanced MRI of cartilage. T1 fat saturation sequences can also be used after placement of intra-articular gadolinium to provide images analogous to nonarthrographic fat-saturation PD FSE. Although the optimal pulse sequence is controversial, the Articular Cartilage Imaging Committee, a subcommittee of the International Cartilage Repair Society (ICRS), recommends using FSE imaging with PD weighted imaging with or without fat saturation, T2-weighted imaging with or without fat saturation, or T1-weighted gradient echo imaging for the evaluation of both native and repaired cartilage.[50]

The articular cartilage of the femorotibial joint covers the entirety of the femoral condyles and the tibial plateau. The femoral cartilage anterior to the anterior horns is termed the trochlear cartilage. This cartilage articulates with the patella. Posteriorly on the femoral condyles is cartilage that is not in contact with the tibia during routine MRI. During flexion, this surface contacts the tibial surface. It is important not to overlook cartilaginous defects in this region. The cartilage of the patellofemoral joint is evaluated in both the axial and sagittal planes. Patellar cartilage represents the thickest cartilage in the body. Axial PD FSE sequences, either with or without fat saturation, display it nicely. The patellar cartilage comprises medial and lateral facets, as well as a median ridge (patellar apex). The medial facet sometimes contains an extra flat surface termed the odd facet. The trochlear cartilage is better evaluated in the sagittal plane owing to its obliquity within the axial plane (Fig. 5-35A through *D*).

On non–fat-suppressed FSE images performed with an intermediate TE, the zonal architecture of the articular cartilage will be apparent. The deep zone will appear

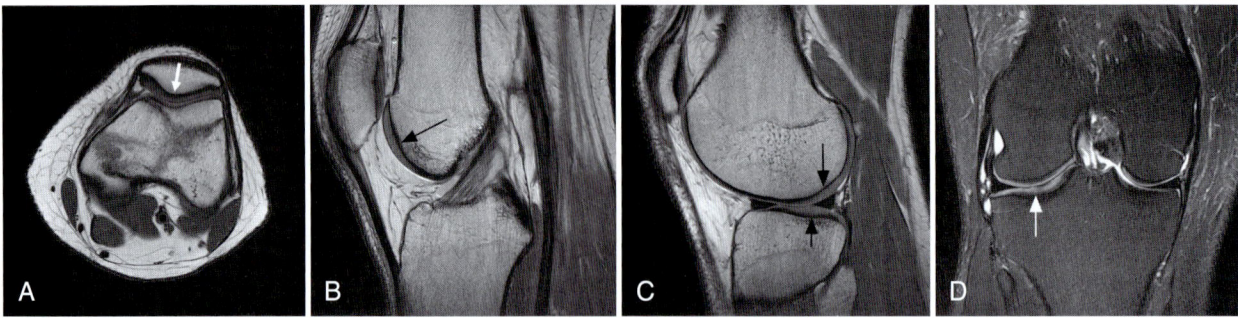

Figure 5-35. Articular cartilage. Axial and sagittal proton density (PD) images (**A, B,** and **C**) and coronal fat-suppressed PD image (**D**) demonstrating normal patellar (**A**), trochlear (**B**), and femorotibial articular cartilage (**C** and **D**). Note the higher signal in the middle and superficial zones compared with the deep zone and subchondral bone. This is normal and is referred to as gray scale stratification.

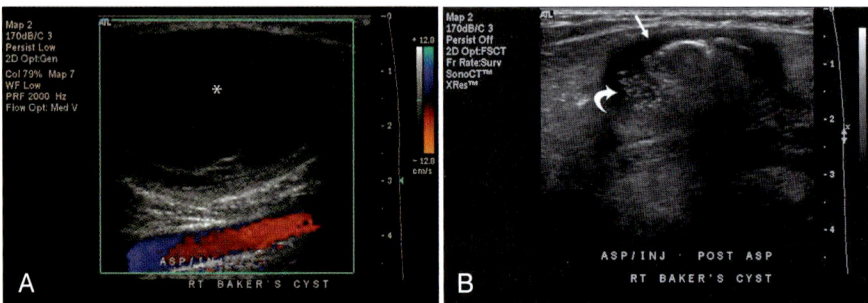

Figure 5-36. Ultrasound images performed before (**A**) and after (**B**) ultrasound-guided aspiration and injection of a Baker's cyst *(asterisk).* Postprocedure image (**B**) demonstrates the collapsed cyst *(straight arrow)* with small dependent echogenic foci *(curved arrow)* reflecting injected steroid and anesthetic.

hypointense because of the closely aligned collagen fibers of the radial zone, which are highly ordered and markedly restrict water mobility. Water is less restricted in the middle and superficial zones, which have more randomly ordered collagen fibers. Thus, these areas have a higher signal compared with the deep zone and subchondral bone. This subtly increasing signal is referred to as gray-scale stratification.[50] The most superficial layer of cartilage, the so-called lamina splendins, is extremely thin and is not visible at clinically relevant field strengths.

ULTRASOUND

Applications

Ultrasound of the knee excels in evaluation of the popliteal fossa. Vascular structures, such as popliteal artery aneurysms, can be fully depicted, and their flow characteristics analyzed. Popliteal cysts can also be imaged, often with the goal of ultrasound-guided aspiration (Fig. 5-36). Another application of ultrasound is evaluation of the extensor mechanism. A range of maladies such as patellar tendon tears and prepatellar bursitis may be identified. Ultrasound also may be used to evaluate patients with meniscal and parameniscal symptoms. The availability of high-frequency high-resolution linear transducers permits diagnosis and treatment of symptomatic parameniscal cysts.[11,12,44]

Technique

Ultrasound, as the name implies, aims high frequency sound waves through tissue to form an image. The transducer acts as both the emitter and the receiver of the signal. The image

represents a map of how much sound is reflected to the transducer from each location in an imaging plane (i.e., depth). Bright (echogenic) objects, such as calcifications, strongly reflect the ultrasound beam. Substances such as water allow the sound waves to pass through easily and reflect little signal. As a result, simple fluid appears dark (hypoechoic). The contrast in the images represents how much (or little) of the sound wave is reflected back to the transducer by any two adjacent tissues. The ultrasound machine uses high level math and the speed of sound to map the signals it receives, thereby forming a two-dimensional image.

Image Interpretation

Ultrasound is heavily operator dependent. Therefore, views are labeled according to their location and plane of imaging to orient those interpreting the images. Ultrasound affords great freedom in scanning. A handheld probe is used to investigate a structure in real time at virtually any angle, allowing appreciation of its relationship to other nearby anatomy. Cine clips are short movies saved during an examination that allow valuable segments of the real-time examination to be reviewed on the PACS.

Artifacts/Special Considerations

Ultrasound artifacts may be broadly separated into technical and tissue factors. If recognized, technical artifacts may be addressed while scanning (and hopefully eliminated). As for artifacts intrinsic to the tissue, strong reflectors such as bone, calcium, and metal distort the sound wave, thereby altering its return course to the transducer. This results in a variety of appearances, such as reverberation artifact. Interfaces between two very different tissues also disrupt ultrasound transmission. This may create a mirror image artifact.

Safety

Concerns regarding ultrasound safety are minimal, particularly in the extremities. It is notable that high-intensity exposure may cause tissue heating, but this is rarely, if ever, a factor when imaging the knee.

NUCLEAR MEDICINE

Applications

Nuclear medicine has myriad applications. Examinations of the knee are requested for occult fractures, stress injuries, infection, arthroplasty complications, arthritis, metabolic bone disease, and tumor workup. Bone scanning is also frequently used to image the entire skeleton to determine the presence and distribution of osseous metastatic disease.

Nuclear medicine scans of the knee are complementary to anatomic studies such as radiographs, CT scans, or MRI. It is useful to have correlative examinations available while interpreting a bone scan, as this helps to localize abnormal radiotracer activity. Bone scans may also elucidate pathology not visible on other modalities, such as osteomyelitis and occult fracture.

Technique

In contrast to anatomic imaging, nuclear medicine stands out in its ability to capture and characterize physiologic processes such as increased blood flow, abnormal lung ventilation, or altered renal function. Rather than pass an x-ray beam through a patient, nuclear scintigraphy relies on injecting a radiopharmaceutical and measuring the resulting gamma ray emissions coming from within the patient. A radiopharmaceutical is a combination of a tracer and a radioisotope. A tracer is a substance whose uptake, distribution, and metabolism are predictable. For example, a phosphate analogue such as methylene-diphosphate (MDP) is preferentially taken up by bone. A tracer may consist of the patient's own cells. For example, labeled white blood cells may be utilized to seek out inflammation or infection.

Radioisotopes are usually byproducts of nuclear power plants. These radioactive molecules emit gamma rays as they decay, providing measurable emissions to create an image. Examples include technetium-99m (Tc-99m) and Indium-111 (In-111). Each radioisotope is characterized by a distinctive half-life and gamma ray energy (measured in keV). Half-life is important because it guides imaging time and helps determine radiation exposure to the patient. A short half-life, 6 hours in cases of Tc-99m, necessitates imaging within a few hours. The later imaging is attempted, the fewer gamma rays will be available for detection. Conversely, a longer half-life, such as 2.8 days for In-111, allows imaging over several days. Radiation exposure is directly related to half-life (physical *and* biologic). A relatively short half-life means that the radioisotope exposes the patient to less radiation. In general, if the half-life is longer, radiation exposure is higher.

Images are acquired with cameras sensitive to the gamma rays emitted by the radioisotopes. This is known as scintigraphy. In brief, a gamma camera performs three complementary functions. It converts a gamma ray into light, assigns a location to this emission, and counts the number of emissions from a particular location over time. As the number of counts increases for a given position, the image reflects more activity at this location. The number of counts a gamma camera receives is related to the amount of pharmaceutical administered and the length of time the patient spends under the camera. It may take 30 minutes or longer to acquire sufficient counts to generate a diagnostic image. The anatomy of interest should be as close to the camera as possible to get the maximum counts within the shortest time. If pathology of the patella is suspected, the camera should be positioned anterior to the knee. If a popliteal process is being investigated, the camera is positioned posterior to the knee. Some gamma cameras simultaneously obtain images in anterior and posterior projections.

A majority of nuclear medicine images are planar (i.e., two-dimensional) frontal or oblique projections. The spatial resolution of nuclear medicine images is inherently restricted by a number of factors beyond discussion in this review. Small or closely positioned structures may not be readily identified or delineated.

Single photon emission computed tomography (SPECT) is a technique used to acquire a dataset in multiple planes, similar to a CT scan. A special camera that rotates around the patient is required. Additional imaging time is necessary, as compared with standard, static planar images. Once complete, the area of interest can be manipulated on the viewing station so that abnormalities can be more precisely localized. This is particularly helpful around hardware and in the spine.

Multiple examinations may be performed to further heighten diagnostic specificity. For example, a Tc-99m sulfur colloid performed in tandem with an In-111 white blood cell scan increases the specificity of the white blood cell scan when evaluating a joint prosthesis for infection.

Technetium 99m-Methylene Diphosphonate (Tc-MDP) Scan

The Tc-MDP bone scan is the most commonly performed nuclear medicine examination for orthopedic purposes. Imaging may be done in one or three phases. For a single-phase scan, delayed planar images are acquired 2 or 3 hours after administration of the radiotracer. This type of examination is commonly requested for metastatic disease, primary bone tumors, and metabolic disease. A three-phase scan involves acquiring images immediately and within several minutes of radioisotope dispensation. These first two phases, blood flow and blood pool, respectively, yield information about perfusion to bones and joints, as well as periosseous and periarticular soft tissues. Standard delayed whole body and spot images are obtained 2 or 3 hours later, similar to the single-phase examination, and reflect bone metabolic activity. The three-phase examination is helpful when osteomyelitis, septic arthritis, aseptic synovitis, or fractures are diagnostic considerations.

Timed images, such as the blood flow and blood pool phases, rely upon the appearance (or cessation) of activity within an appropriate time window. A normal blood flow phase reveals expected arterial activity without focal activity in the bone. A normal blood pool phase has no increased

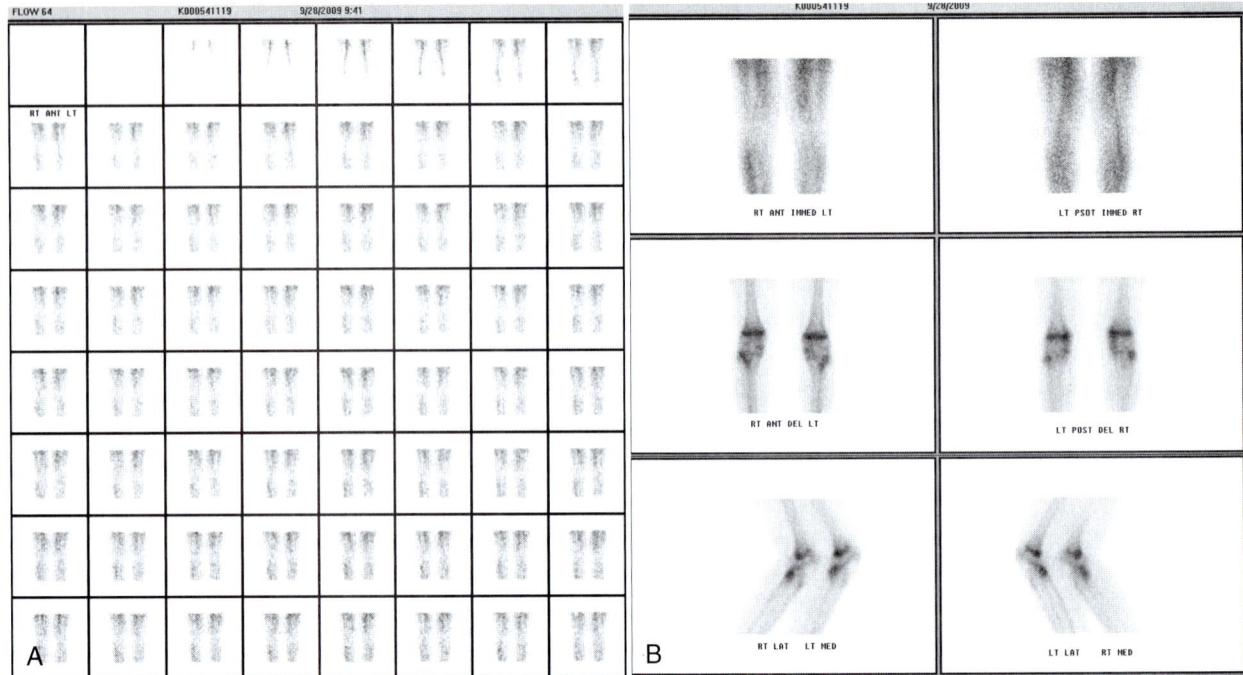

Figure 5-37. Normal triple-phase technetium-99m methylene diphosphonate (Tc-MDP) bone scan of the knees, demonstrating normal blood flow **(A)**, normal blood pool (top two images of **B**), and delayed skeletal uptake of radiotracer (bottom four images of **B**). Symmetrical areas of increased uptake in the physeal regions bilaterally reflect ossification at the growth plates in this skeletally immature patient.

bone or soft tissue activity. A normal delayed phase reveals symmetrical osseous distribution of radioisotope.

The mechanism of action of Tc-MDP is chemisorption. Tc-MDP is taken up by cortical bone and is bound to the hydroxyapatite crystal. The degree of delayed skeletal uptake is largely determined by ongoing bone formation and blood flow.[19] Areas of abnormally increased bone turnover (whether secondary to fracture, infection, inflammation, arthritis, metabolic bone disease or neoplasm, etc.) will have increased uptake relative to the remainder of the surrounding skeleton.

In all phases of imaging, it is critical to compare for symmetry. This includes comparing the right and left knees, as well as analogous structures within a single knee such as the medial and lateral femoral condyles. Skeletally immature patients have normally increased activity at the physes (Fig. 5-37A and B). Notably, implants appear as photopenic defects.

Labeled White Blood Cell Scan

Labeled white blood cell (WBC) scans augment the workup of suspected infection, whether it be osteomyelitis, septic arthritis, or soft tissue abscess. The specificity and sensitivity of this examination are superior to gallium-67 citrate. White blood cells are isolated from a sample of the patient's blood, labeled in vitro with In-111 (or Tc-99m) and reinjected into the patient. Images may be obtained 3 or 4 hours later. Some departments image at 24 hours. A normal scan demonstrates no focal area of increased uptake. Abnormal radioisotope deposition indicates inflammation or infection with sensitivity and specificity approaching 90%. Most labeled cells are

neutrophils and therefore have a strong predilection for sites of bacterial infection.

In the presence of infection, blood work for C-reactive protein and erythrocyte sedimentation rate is often elevated. For the exclusion of septic arthritis, knee aspiration is preferred, as it has the highest specificity and sensitivity. Aspirate is sent for cell count with differential, gram stain, and culture and sensitivity. In equivocal cases, nuclear medicine scanning can be useful.

Labeled leukocyte imaging is the radionuclide procedure of choice for diagnosing so-called complicating osteomyelitis. It often must be performed in conjunction with bone marrow (Tc-sulfur colloid) scanning to maximize specificity and accuracy.[43] Normal labeled leukocyte scans have a high negative predictive value for infection.

Although the sensitivity and negative predictive value of indium-WBC scans are very high, approaching 95% and 100%, respectively, a positive indium scan, in and of itself, is of limited value.[36] This dilemma is addressed by performing the labeled white cell scan in conjunction with a Tc-99m sulfur colloid scan.

Technetium-99m Sulfur Colloid Scan

A Tc-99m sulfur colloid (SC) scan is employed as a problem-solving tool. It complements the In-111 WBC scan, increasing specificity and accuracy for diagnosing infection after total knee arthroplasty.[43] Imaging occurs within a few hours of injection. Tc-99m SC localizes to the reticuloendothelial system: bone marrow, liver, and spleen.

The rationale behind Tc-99m SC examination is that accumulation of In-111 WBCs may occur in infection or

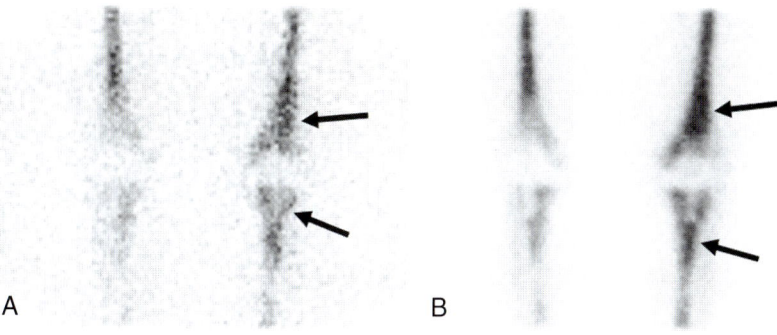

Figure 5-38. A 71-year-old male with bilateral total knee arthroplasties, left side in 2000 and right side in 2002, with pain on the left side. Apparent asymmetrical and increased uptake on the indium-111–labeled white blood cell scan in the distal left femur and proximal tibia **(A)** *(arrows)* is related to marrow expansion, and *not* infection, as demonstrated by matching (congruent) areas of uptake on the technetium (Tc)-sulfur colloid scan **(B)** *(arrows)*.

hyperplastic marrow. Hyperplastic marrow is a relatively common finding after arthroplasty implantation. Tc-99m SC differentiates these two entities, as it will localize to reactive marrow but not to a site of infection. Thus, if results are congruous on both In-111 WBC and Tc-99m SC scans, infection is unlikely (Fig. 5-38A and B). On the contrary, increased activity on the In-111 WBC scan, as compared with Tc-99m SC images, indicates a high likelihood of infection (>90%).[36]

Gallium-67 Citrate Scan

Gallium-67 citrate scans have largely been replaced by labeled leukocyte scans and are less commonly performed. Images are acquired 48 and 72 hours after injection. This radioisotope acts as both a calcium and iron analogue, resulting in its incorporation into bone and bone marrow. It localizes to sites of infection or inflammation, in part because it binds the iron-carrying proteins transferrin and lactoferrin. Gallium was traditionally used in the evaluation of infection, particularly chronic osteomyelitis and septic arthritis. In the setting of a normal white blood cell count, labeled leukocyte scans are preferred because they have higher sensitivity and specificity. In the immunocompromised patient (WBC <2000) or for spinal infection, gallium scanning may be favored.[43]

Safety

Nuclear medicine employs ionizing radiation. The patient is exposed from the time the radiotracer is administered until it has decayed sufficiently to become a negligible source of radiation, at least four half-lives. For Tc-99m, the half-life of 6 hours renders radiation exposure negligible after 24 hours for a standard 20 mCi dose. In-111 has a longer half-life of 2.8 days, resulting in greater radiation exposure.

Specific organs may receive disproportionate radiation exposure. For example, Tc-99m MDP is primarily eliminated via the kidneys and collects in the bladder. Therefore bladder exposure may be significantly higher than in most other organs.

Careful consideration should be given to pregnant women and children before requesting nuclear medicine scans. The dose to the fetus may be particularly high if the radiopharmaceutical is excreted via the genitourinary tract, given the bladder's proximity to the uterus. Consultation with a radiologist or nuclear medicine physician is recommended.

KEY REFERENCES

Beall D, Googe J, Moss J, et al: Magnetic resonance imaging of the collateral ligaments and the anatomic quadrants of the knee. Radiol Clin North Am 45:983–1002, 2007.

De Maeseneer M, Vanderdood K, Marcelis S, Shabana W: Sonography of the medial and lateral tendons and ligaments of the knee: the use of bony landmarks as an easy method for identification. Am J Roentgenol 178:1437–1444, 2002.

DeSmet AA, Norris MA, Yandow DR, et al: MR diagnosis of meniscal tears of the knee: importance of high signal in the meniscus that extends to the surface. AJR Am J Roentgenol 161:101, 1993.

Fox M: MR Imaging of the meniscus: review, current trends, and clinical implications. Radiol Clin North Am 45:1033–1053, 2007.

Greenspan A: Orthopedic imaging, a practical approach, ed 4, Philadelphia, 2004, Lippincott Williams & Wilkins.

Manester BJ, Roberts CC, Andrews CL, et al: Diagnostic and surgical imaging anatomy: musculoskeletal, ed 1, Philadelphia, 2006, Lippincott Williams & Wilkins.

Math KR, Zaidi SF, Petchprapa C, Harwin SF: Imaging of total knee arthroplasty. Semin Musculoskel Radiol 10:47–63, 2006.

Merchant AC, Mercer RL, Jacobsoen RH, et al: Roentgenographic analysis of patellofemoral congruence. J Bone Joint Surg Am 56:1391, 1974.

Palestro CJ, Love C: Radionuclide imaging of musculoskeletal infection, conventional agents. Semin Musc Radiol 11:336–339, 2007.

Parker L, Nazarian NL, Carino JA, et al: AIUM practice guidelines: musculoskeletal ultrasound, 2007. (http://www.aium.org/publications/guidelines/musculoskeletal.pdf).

Roberts CC, Towers JD, Spangehl MJ, et al: Advanced MR imaging of the cruciate ligaments. Radiol Clin North Am 45:1003–1016, 2007.

Rosenberg TD, Paulos LE, Parker RD, et al: The forty-five degree posterior anterior flexion weightbearing radiograph of the knee. J Bone Joint Surg Am 70:1479, 1988.

Shindle MK, Foo LF, Kelly BT, et al. Magnetic resonance imaging of cartilage in the athlete: current techniques and spectrum of disease. J Bone Joint Surg Am 88(suppl 4):27–46, 2006.

Stoller DW, Li AE, Anderson LJ, Cannon WD: The knee. In Stoller DW, editor: Magnetic resonance imaging in orthopedics and sports medicine, ed 3, Philadelphia, 2007, Lippincott, Williams & Wilkins.

Full references for this chapter can be found on www.expertconsult.com.

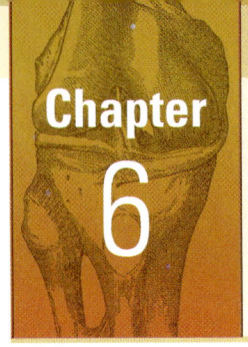

Chapter 6

Imaging of Osseous Knee Trauma

Alissa Burge and Daniel M. Walz

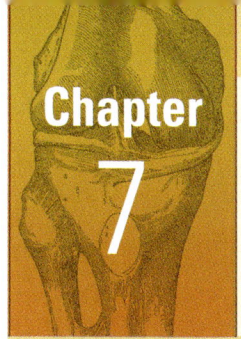

Internal Derangements: Ligaments and Tendons

Amy F. Austin and Adam C. Zoga

Noncontrast magnetic resonance imaging (MRI) is standard of care imaging in the posttraumatic knee with clinical findings suggestive of ligamentous injury. MRI findings of partial and complete, and acute and chronic ligament tears throughout the knee are well described. MRI review should be systematic, with every effort made to identify the injury mechanism, and thus should focus on osseous, ligamentous, and cartilaginous structures at risk for acute trauma, while identifying chronic and degenerative lesions that might not be related to the recent injury.

BURSAE

Bursae about the knee are not typically identified on MRI unless they are inflamed and/or fluid-filled. Bursitis fluid most commonly appears simple on MRI, demonstrating increased T2 signal and decreased T1 signal, but it may be somewhat complex, containing debris or blood products. The bursal wall is generally thin with neat borders, and postcontrast sequences show only minimal contrast enhancement. However, in an inflammatory or primary synovial process, such as rheumatoid arthritis, wall thickening and mild central enhancement can be seen.

The medial gastrocnemius-semimembranosus bursa (Baker's cyst) is commonly fluid-filled and is best demonstrated on an axial fluid-sensitive sequence, where it is seen as a comma-shaped structure between these two tendons (Fig. 7-1). It is the only knee bursa that consistently shows continuity with the joint space, and it has been associated with internal derangements such as meniscal tear, joint effusion, and degenerative joint disease. Rupture of a Baker's cyst, a cause of acute knee pain and a mimic of deep venous thrombosis, is manifest by fluid signal tracking along the adjacent fascial planes, often into the midcalf (Fig. 7-2). Baker's cysts can be a cause of refractory or recurrent posterior knee or calf pain, and they tend to recur after percutaneous aspiration. The semimembranosus–tibial collateral ligament bursa can be distinguished from a Baker's cyst by its location medial to the semimembranosus tendon. The tibial collateral ligament bursa, or Voshell's bursa, is located between its deep and superficial layers and can mimic medial meniscocapsular separation (Fig. 7-3).[15] Pes anserinus bursitis manifests as fluid tracking along the pes anserinus tendons anteromedially at the knee joint line in an oblique plane (Fig. 7-4). The pes anserinus bursa is often contiguous with the tibial collateral bursa, and both can be contiguous with a Baker's cyst. It is important to distinguish a primary bursitis in any of these locations from a parameniscal cyst, where fluid extends from a meniscal tear into one or more of these bursae.

Anteriorly, the prepatellar and infrapatellar bursae are best evaluated on sagittal sequences. Prepatellar bursitis, or housemaid's knee, may be related to repetitive trauma such as kneeling (Fig. 7-5). As the name implies, it is located superficial to the mid extensor mechanism. Infrapatellar bursitis may involve the superficial or deep infrapatellar bursae. The superficial bursa is located between the skin and the tibial tuberosity and has been referred to as clergyman's knee (Fig. 7-6). The deep infrapatellar bursa (Fig. 7-7), between the distal patellar tendon and the tibial tuberosity, may contain fluid in the setting of patellofemoral tracking syndromes or active Osgood-Schlatter disease.

Laterally, the iliotibial band bursa is located between the tibia and the distal iliotibial band. Iliotibial band bursitis can manifest as anterolateral knee pain caused by overuse, often seen in runners. The fibular collateral ligament–biceps femoris bursa (Fig. 7-8) is lateral to the distal fibular collateral ligament, extending around the anterior and anteromedial aspects of the ligament. It extends proximally to where the biceps femoris crosses the fibular collateral ligament, and distally to the insertion of the fibular collateral ligament on the fibula.[2]

A posttraumatic Morel-Lavallee lesion may be mistaken as a bursitis on MRI (Fig. 7-9A and B). This closed degloving injury results from sudden severe trauma, often caused by motor vehicle accidents, that causes a shearing injury between the skin and subcutaneous fat and the underlying fascia. The perforating vessels and lymphatic channels are severed, resulting in a complex hematoma containing varying amounts of lymph and necrotic fat. On MRI, the lesion may show layering fluid levels related to layering blood products. A capsule may surround the mass and may be indicative of a lesion requiring surgical intervention; conservative treatments such as compression may be refractory.[6]

BONE MARROW CONTUSION PATTERNS

Careful observation and assessment of osseous contusions about the knee should serve as a guide for interrogation regarding suspect soft tissue structures likely to be injured based on specific mechanisms. Osseous contusion patterns often elucidate the mechanism of injury and guide the evaluation for subsequent pathology. Five dominant osseous contusion patterns described by Sanders and associates play a key role in diagnostic MRI interpretation of knee ligament trauma.[18] These include pivot shift injury, dashboard injury, hyperextension injury, clip injury, and lateral patellar dislocation. MRI evaluation for osseous contusion is facilitated by the use of T2 fat-saturated sequences. Contusions appear as subcortical or subchondral regions of increased T2 signal and decreased T1 signal, often with a flame-shaped configuration, without a discrete fracture line.

Following a pivot shift injury, osseous contusions most commonly involve the posterolateral tibial plateau and the lateral femoral condyle (Fig. 7-10). The presence of this contusion pattern indicates acute or chronic anterior cruciate

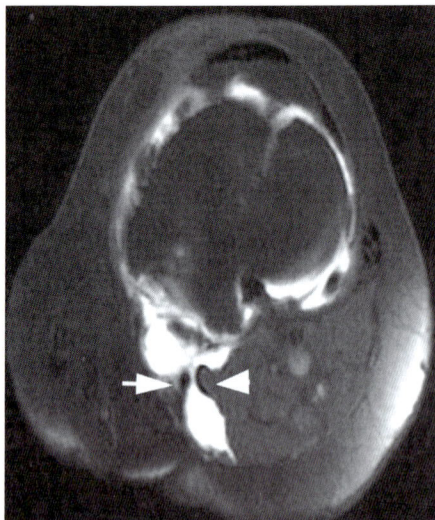

Figure 7-1. Axial T2 fat-saturated image demonstrates a Baker's cyst between the semimembranosus *(arrow)* and the medial head of the gastrocnemius *(arrowhead)* tendon.

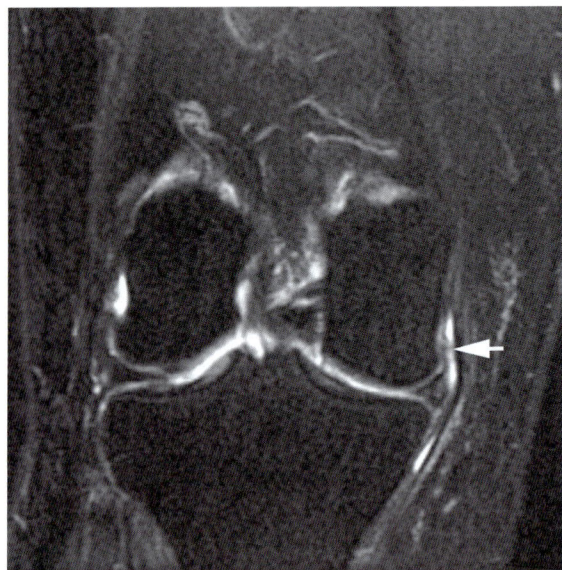

Figure 7-3. Coronal T2 fat-saturated image demonstrates tibial collateral bursitis with fluid dissecting between the deep and superficial layers of the medial collateral ligament *(arrow)*.

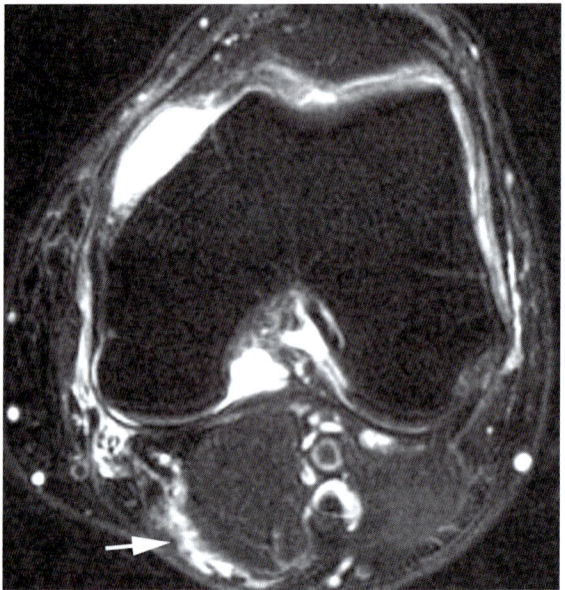

Figure 7-2. Axial T2 fat-saturated image demonstrates a ruptured Baker's cyst with fluid dissecting along the subcutaneous tissues *(arrow)*.

ligament (ACL) disruption, as it is failure of this ligament that leads to tibial subluxation and impaction. Other associated pathology includes posterolateral corner injury and subsequent instability. Osseous contusion of the medial tibial plateau has also been described with a pivot shift mechanism of injury, present in approximately 20% of cases and associated with posteromedial peripheral tears of the medial meniscus.

The dashboard injury is related to a direct blow to the knee, often during an automobile accident. This mechanism manifests as contusions involving the anterior tibia and posterior, subchondral patella. Concomitant soft tissue injury with a dashboard contusion pattern often includes posterior

cruciate ligament (PCL) and posterior capsule disruption. Hyperextension injury results in impaction of the anterior tibia and anterior femoral condyle, and subsequent osseous contusions (Fig. 7-11). Associated ligamentous pathology with this mechanism can include ACL or PCL injury.

A clip injury is related to valgus stress to the knee and results in a dominant contusion within the lateral femoral condyle from direct impaction, along with a smaller focus of bone marrow edema within the medial femoral condyle related to avulsive force at the origin of the medial collateral ligament. Injury to the medial collateral ligament is common with this mechanism, ranging from low-grade sprains to frank disruption. In addition, ACL injury and medial mensical injury have been described with clip injuries. Osseous contusions following lateral patellar dislocation involve the lateral, nonarticular portion of the lateral femoral condyle, as well as the medial patellar facet (Fig. 7-12). Associated soft tissue injuries include medial patellar retinaculum and medial patellofemoral ligament sprain or disruption. Cartilaginous injury has also been reported with transient lateral patellar dislocations, with delamination of cartilage at the medial patellar facet or at the anterolateral margin of the lateral femoral condyle, sometimes leading to intra-articular cartilaginous bodies.

ANTERIOR CRUCIATE LIGAMENT

On MRI, the ACL is low in signal relative to muscle on all sequences and parallels the intercondylar roof on sagittal images (Blumensaat's line). The normal ligament may appear striated on sagittal images, presumably related to interposition of fat and synovium between the bundles, more commonly identified close to the tibial attachment.[24] All three planes should be utilized for the most accurate assessment of the ACL. The sagittal sequence (Fig. 7-13) is most useful and can be performed in an oblique sagittal plane parallel to the

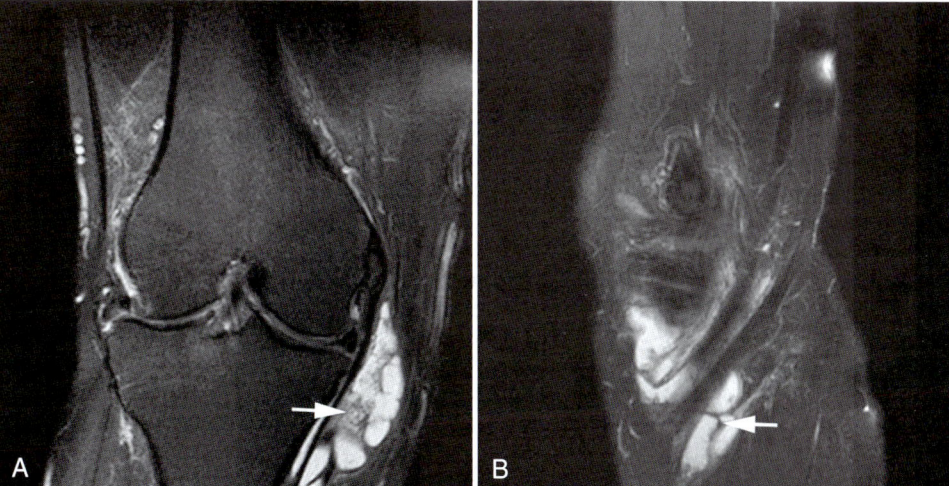

Figure 7-4. Coronal **(A)** and sagittal **(B)** T2 fat-saturated image demonstrates pes anserine bursitis *(arrows)* along the distal pes anserine tendons.

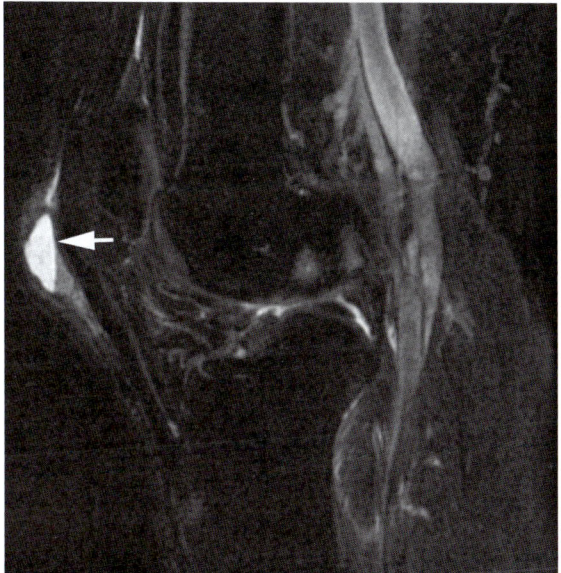

Figure 7-5. Sagittal T2 fat-saturated image demonstrates complex fluid superficial to the patella *(arrow)* with layering blood products.

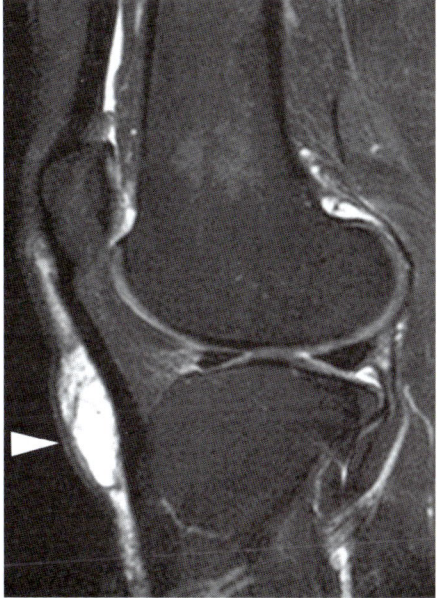

Figure 7-6. Sagittal T2 fat-saturated image shows superficial infrapatellar bursitis (pretibial bursitis) with fluid superficial to the inferior patellar tendon *(arrowhead)*.

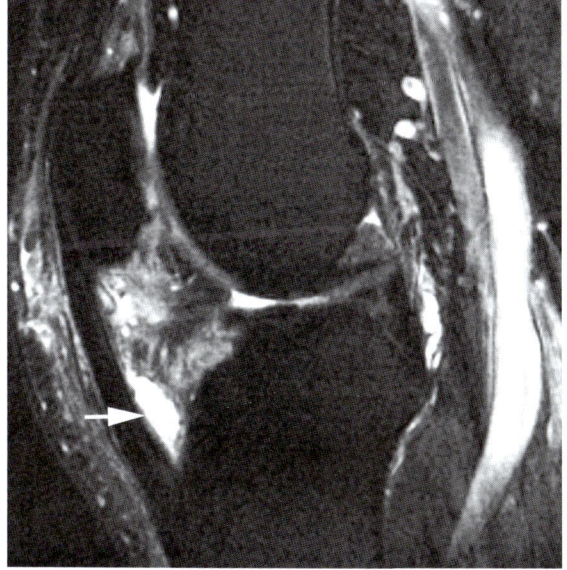

Figure 7-7. Sagittal T2 fat-saturated image shows deep infrapatellar bursitis with fluid deep to the patellar tendon *(arrow)*.

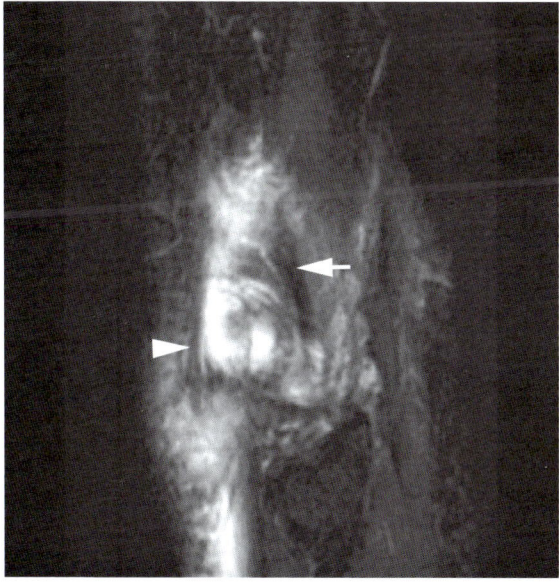

Figure 7-8. Sagittal T2 fat-saturated image shows fibular collateral ligament *(arrowhead)* with biceps femoris *(arrow)* bursitis.

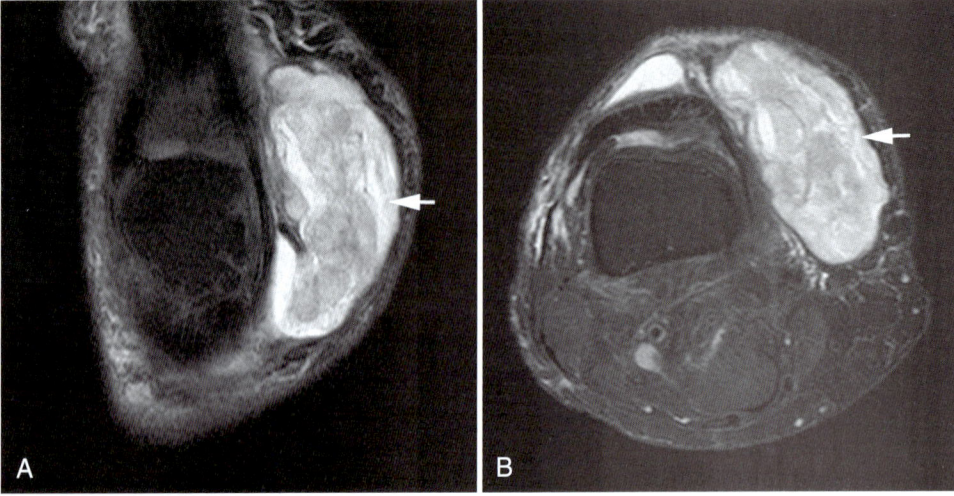

Figure 7-9. Coronal **(A)** and axial **(B)** T2 fat-saturated images demonstrate a complex subcutaneous fluid collection following motor vehicle accident, representing a closed degloving injury or Morel-Lavallee lesion *(arrows)*.

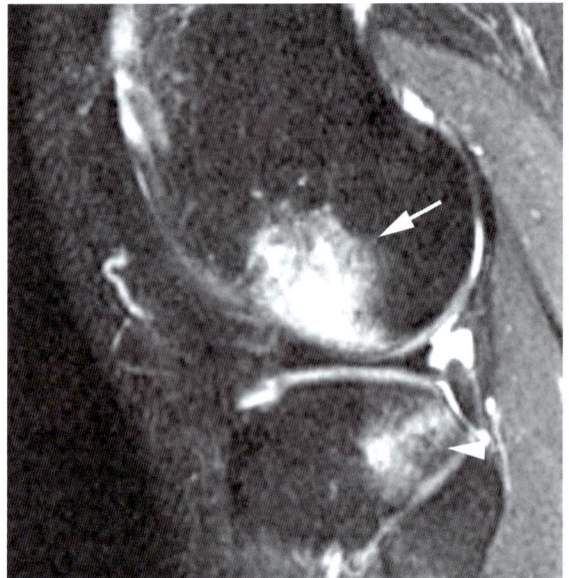

Figure 7-10. Sagittal T2 fat-saturated image demonstrates bone marrow edema, with the lateral femoral condyle *(arrow)* and the posterolateral tibia *(arrowhead)* representing osseous contusions secondary to a pivot shift injury during a fall while skiing.

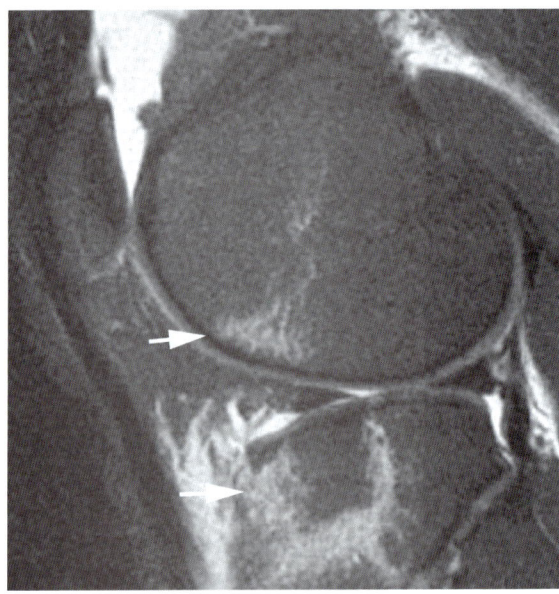

Figure 7-11. Sagittal T2 fat-saturated image shows bone marrow edema in the anterior tibia and femoral condyle compatible with osseous contusions *(arrows)* related to hyperextension injury in a 20-year-old soccer player.

orientation of the ACL as prescribed from an axial localizer image with 3 to 4 mm image thickness to decrease volume averaging. The axial and coronal images (Fig. 7-14) are useful in evaluating the ligamentous attachments and confirming abnormalities seen on the sagittal sequence. Axial images are particularly helpful for assessing the integrity of individual ACL bundles in the setting of sprain or partial tear.

Both primary and secondary signs of ACL rupture have been seen on MRI. Primary signs of rupture include a discontinuous ligament or an abnormal course of the ligament, no longer paralleling Blumensaat's line.[24] With a discontinuous ligament, the fibers may appear wavy or horizontal in orientation (Fig. 7-15A). Often the ligament is replaced with amorphous increased signal related to edema and hemorrhage

when tears are subacute; fibers appear as if they have been cut with scissors in more acute injuries (Fig. 7-15B). Secondary signs of ACL tear include buckling of the PCL, anterior translation of the tibia, uncovering of the posterior horn of the lateral meniscus, and characteristic osseous contusion patterns. Buckling of the PCL, uncovering of the posterior horn of the lateral meniscus, and anterior translation of the tibia are all related to anterior subluxation of the tibia relative to the femur secondary to ACL incompetence. Anterior translation of the tibia, referred to as the MRI equivalent of an anterior drawer sign, is assessed using the sagittal imaging plane (Fig. 7-16). The distance between the posterior tibia and the femoral condyle is measured using lines parallel to the long axis of the image. With this method, Vahey and

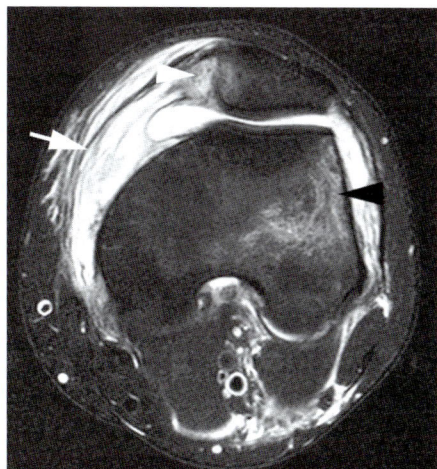

Figure 7-12. Axial T2 fat-saturated image shows bone marrow edema in the medial patella and lateral femoral condyle *(arrowheads)* representing osseous contusions secondary to prior lateral patellar dislocation in a 15-year-old field hockey player. Edema surrounds the medial patellar retinaculum *(arrow)*.

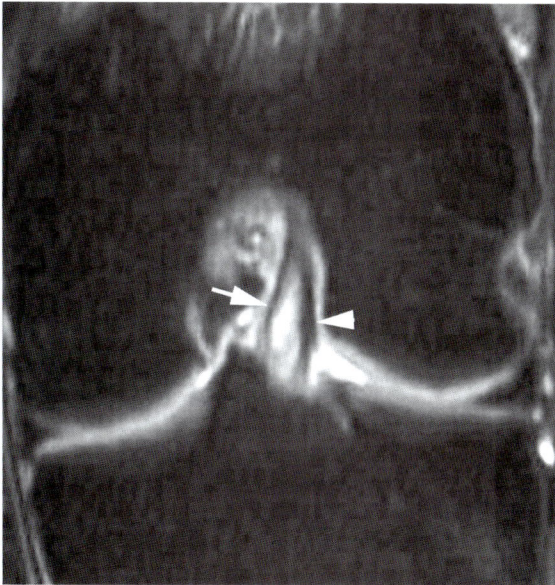

Figure 7-14. Coronal T2 fat-saturated image showing a normal anterior cruciate ligament with intact anteromedial *(arrow)* and posterolateral *(arrowhead)* bundles.

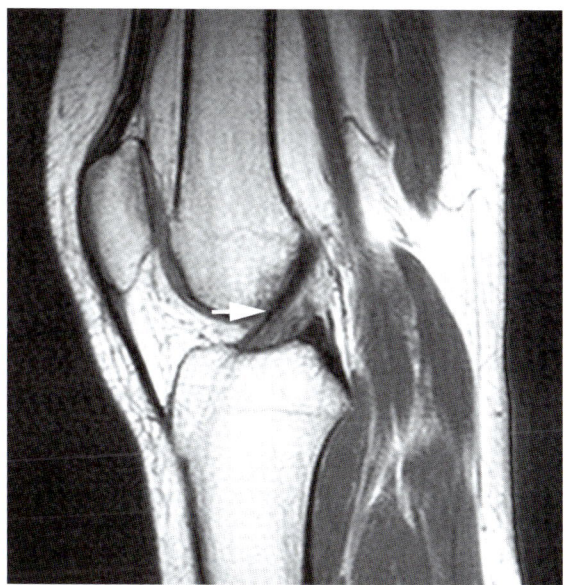

Figure 7-13. Sagittal proton density image showing a normal anterior cruciate ligament *(arrow)*.

colleagues demonstrated high specificity (93%) and positive predictive value (95%) of subluxation of 5 mm or more for ACL disruption. A 7 mm or greater subluxation had 100% specificity and positive predictive value.[25] The characteristic osseous contusion pattern for ACL disruption involves the posterolateral tibial plateau and the lateral femoral condyle. Contusion may also be seen at the posteromedial tibial plateau. Complete rupture of the ACL is often accompanied by joint effusion and hemarthrosis. A fluid-fluid level representing layering blood products may be identified in the suprapatellar recess as related to patient positioning during the examination. In skeletally immature patients, ACL injury commonly manifests as an avulsion fracture at its insertion onto the tibia. MRI will demonstrate an intact ligament with

an associated displaced osseous fragment at the medial tibial spine or the intercondylar tibial eminence (Fig. 7-17). Subchondral bone marrow edema may be seen within the proximal tibial epiphysis related to the fracture. With this injury, the immature epiphyseal bone is weaker than the mature ligament. Identification of the avulsed tibial fragment on radiography or MRI is essential, as treatment options differ considerably from those used with a traditional ACL rupture.

Partial tears of the ACL are more difficult to detect with MRI and are defined as abnormal intrasubstance signal within an otherwise intact ligament, or as discontinuity of some of the ligamentous fibers not involving the full width (Fig. 7-18). Commonly, the most proximal portion of the anterolateral bundle of the ACL is disrupted with an intact posteromedial bundle. Although this type of injury can be confidently called a partial ACL tear on MRI, ligamentous integrity is not easily established without a dedicated and properly performed physical examination. MRI is not a sensitive tool for determining the integrity of a partially torn ACL, although secondary signs such as pivot shift osseous contusions or an MRI anterior drawer can be helpful in suggesting ligamentous incompetence. In general, abnormal T2 hyperintense signal about or within a partially or completely intact ACL with a recent trauma history should be described as a partial tear of the ACL or low-grade ACL injury by MRI. This should be followed by a thorough description of the findings, the presence or lack of pivot shift contusions, and other findings that might suggest ligament incompetence.

ACL tears are often accompanied by other injuries of the ipsilateral knee. Medial collateral ligament sprain and meniscal tear are the most commonly associated injuries, with a particular prevalence of peripheral vertical tears in the posterior horn of either meniscus. Peripheral meniscus tears just above points of osseous contusion on the posterolateral or posteromedial tibial plateau are also commonly seen. Injuries to the posterolateral corner have been described

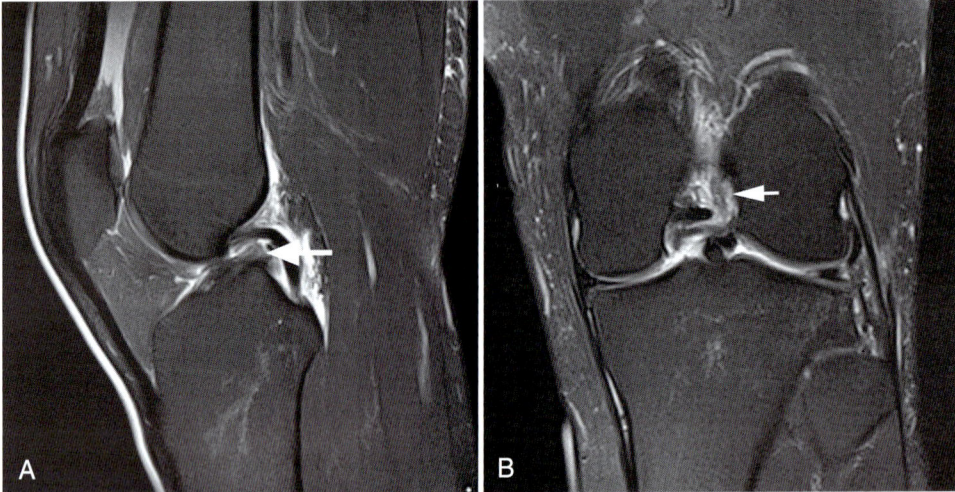

Figure 7-15. Sagittal **(A)** and coronal **(B)** T2 fat-saturated images show a complete anterior cruciate ligament tear. On the sagittal image **(A)**, the fibers are horizontally oriented *(arrow)*. On the coronal image **(B)**, hematoma replaces the expected location of the ligament *(arrow)*.

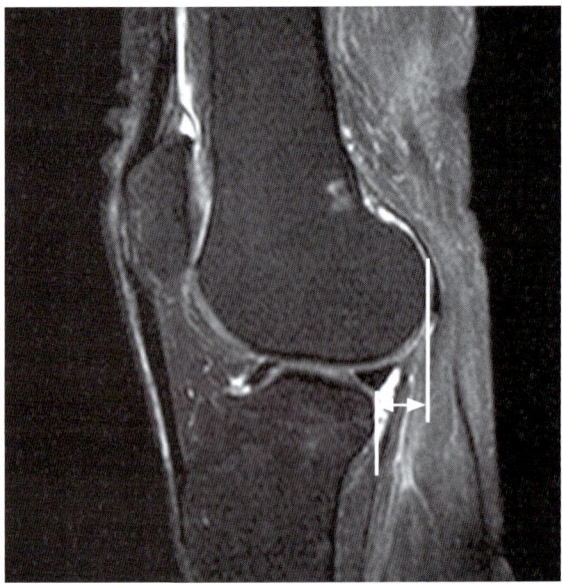

Figure 7-16. Sagittal T2 fat-saturated image shows anterior subluxation of the tibia with respect to the femur, and demonstrates the measurement used to assess anterior drawer.

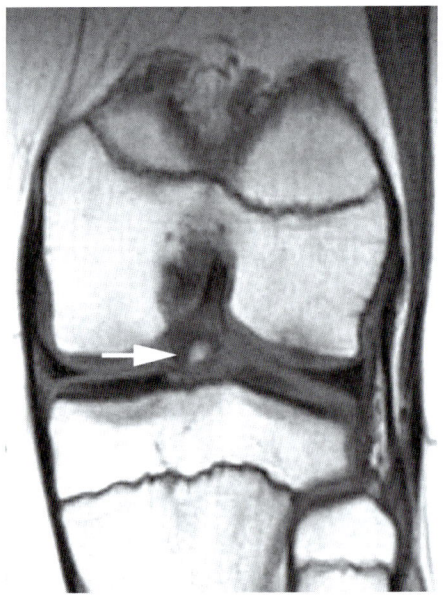

Figure 7-17. Coronal T1 image shows an avulsion fracture *(arrow)* of the intercondylar tibial eminence at the anterior cruciate ligament insertion in a skeletally immature 12-year-old football player.

in association with ACL disruption as well. The Segond fracture, an avulsion fracture from the lateral tibia at the lateral capsular ligament insertion, is an indicator of ACL disruption that can be seen on MRI, as well as on plain radiographs (Fig. 7-19).

Nonvisualization of the ACL is the most common MRI presentation of a chronic tear. On axial images, fluid in the lateral intercondylar notch, where the normal ACL is found, described as the empty notch sign, can be seen in chronic ACL tears (Fig. 7-20). The ligament may be attenuated or residual fibers may have a horizontal orientation. The chronically torn ACL may scar and adhere to the PCL, and clinically may present with an endpoint on anterior drawer examination.[24] Pivot shift contusions suggest ACL

incompetence, but not necessarily an acute tear. A patient with a chronic and long-standing ACL tear can acutely pivot shift, leading to new contusions and a hemarthrosis, as well as injury to other ligamentous and cartilaginous structures. Therefore, pivot shift contusions and no visible ACL fibers at MRI should be interpreted as an age-indeterminate ACL tear, with a recent pivot shift injury. In contrast, mucoid degeneration of the ACL manifests as increased T2 signal, enlargement, and ill definition of an otherwise intact ligament. This pattern of ACL abnormality at MRI should not show a pivot shift contusion pattern and does not suggest the presence of acute ACL trauma, but more likely, chronic and repetitive abnormal ACL biomechanics related to meniscal tear or osteoarthritis. Mucoid degeneration of the ACL or

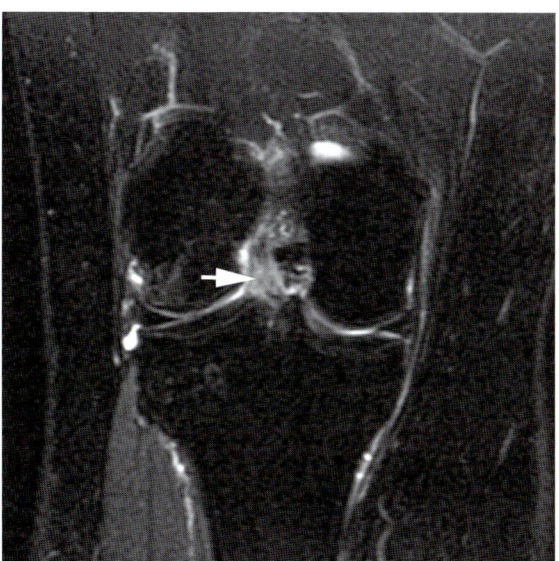

Figure 7-18. Coronal T2 fat-saturated image shows abnormal intrasubstance signal within intact anterior cruciate ligament (ACL) fibers *(arrow)* compatible with partial tear in a 35-year-old snowboarder.

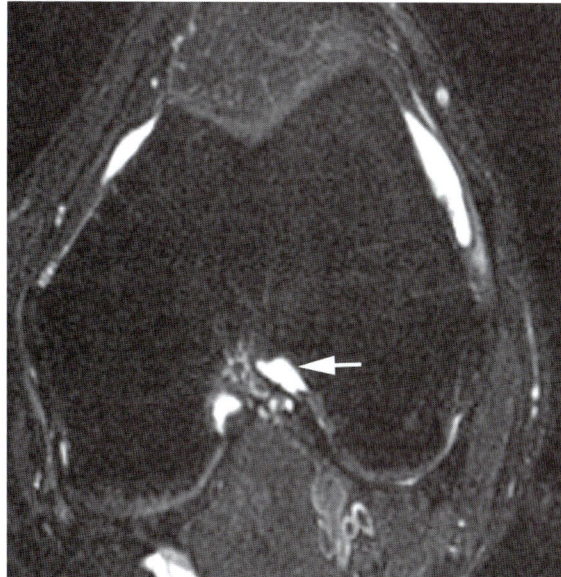

Figure 7-20. Axial T2 fat-saturated image shows absence of fibers at the lateral intercondylar notch *(arrow)* representing a chronic anterior cruciate ligament tear after a basketball injury.

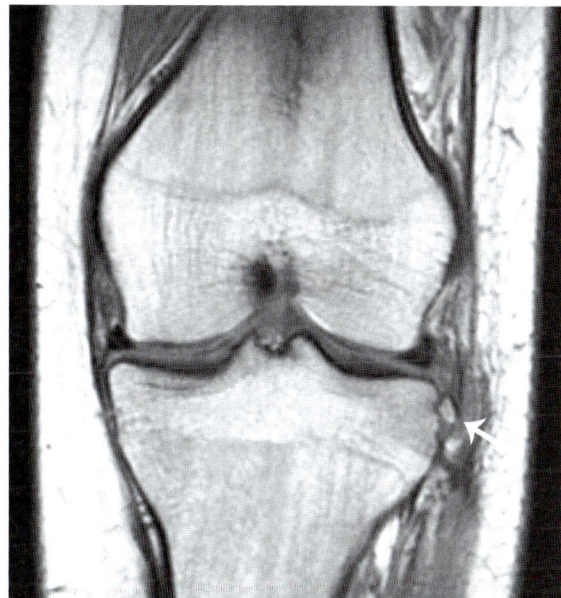

Figure 7-19. Coronal T1 image shows an avulsion fracture at the proximal tibia *(arrow)*, a Segond fracture, at the site of lateral capsular ligament insertion.

PCL can be associated with osseous cystic formation at the cruciate attachments, distal more common than proximal. These intraosseous cruciate cysts are likely a variant of cruciate ganglion cysts, which show homogeneous increased T2 signal similar to that of fluid, insinuating between intact ligament bundles. They are loculated cysts often with lobulation and generally extending along the length of the ligament (Fig. 7-21).[16]

Interpretation of postoperative imaging of ACL grafts can be difficult, especially in the first 18 months to 2 years during graft neovascularization. Through this period, the graft can

show increased T2 signal and may simulate acute ACL pathology, thereby decreasing MRI sensitivity for graft tear.[23] Further, ACL reconstruction graft tears tend to manifest on MRI as focal signal heterogeneity or attenuation as opposed to the visible discontinuity seen with a native ACL tear. MRI evidence for a recent pivot shift mechanism or hemarthrosis is a useful tool in supporting the diagnosis of an ACL graft rupture or ACL graft incompetence. MRI in the postoperative setting is also appropriately used to evaluate graft impingement, tunnel placement, anterior arthrofibrosis, tunnel widening, and graft failure. With graft impingement related to an abnormally anteriorly placed tibial tunnel, the graft will show increased signal in the distal two thirds with visible deflection or angulation at the intercondylar roof on sagittal sequences acquired in near full knee extension (Fig. 7-22).[8,24] Side wall impingement, related to a femoral tunnel low in the intercondylar notch, is best appreciated on coronal sequences. The graft will indent where it bends around the medial aspect of the lateral femoral condyle.[24] Anterior arthrofibrosis, or cyclops lesion, can be a cause of limited knee extension and is easily identified on MRI. Tissue anterior to an ACL graft at the level of the joint line on sagittal imaging should follow the signal of fat on all sequences. A nodular mass of fibrous tissue anterior to the graft at the joint line and proximal to the tibial tunnel with intermediate to low in signal on T1- and T2-weighted images is typical for postoperative arthrofibrosis (Fig. 7-23).[3,17] ACL graft tunnel widening or loosening will show as fluid signal surrounding the graft within the tunnel, tibial greater than femoral. MRI findings of graft tunnel widening are often present in conjunction with abnormal signal within the graft itself, indicating degeneration related to abnormal biomechanics. A bioabsorbable interference screw produces less susceptibility artifact than that seen with metal, so traditional noncontrast knee MRI protocols are generally diagnostic after ACL reconstruction. Intravenous contrast protocols can be useful for suspected postoperative synovitis or infection, but rarely provide much

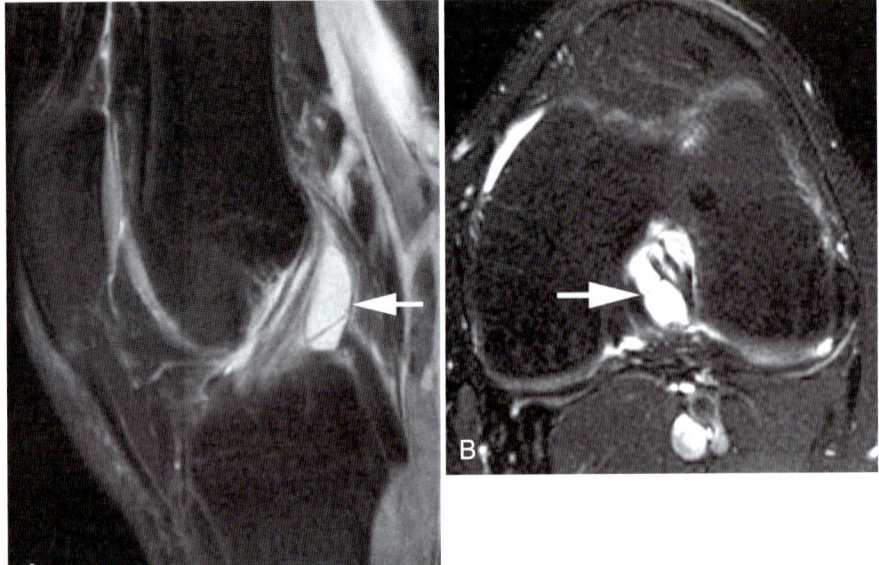

Figure 7-21. Sagittal **(A)** and axial **(B)** T2 fat-saturated images demonstrate loculated fluid extending along the length of the anterior cruciate ligament *(arrows)* representing an anterior cruciate ligament ganglion.

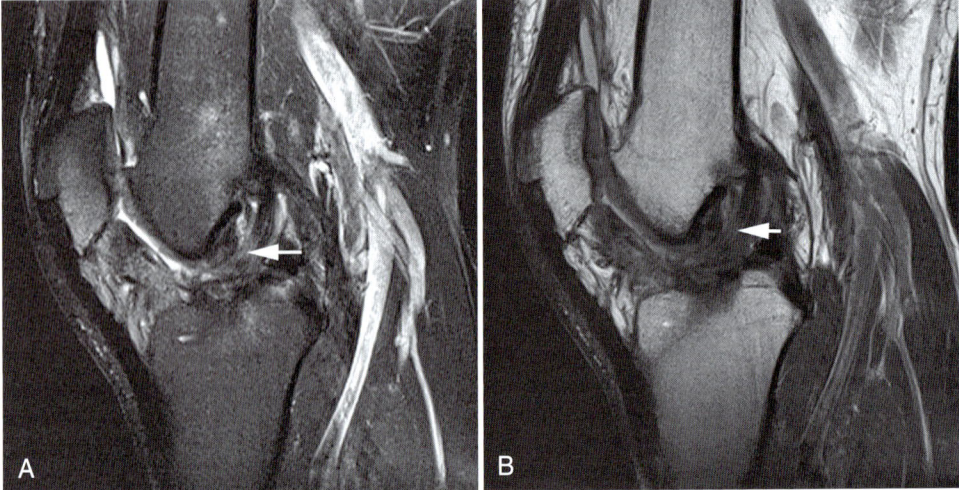

Figure 7-22. Sagittal T2 fat-saturated **(A)** and sagittal proton density **(B)** images demonstrate abnormal signal within the anterior cruciate ligament (ACL) graft *(arrows)* related to impingement by osseous proliferation at the distal femur in an NFL player 11 months after ACL reconstruction.

additional information in assessment of the graft itself. Lactide-glycolide screws may produce reactive edema, which is not seen with polylactic acid screws.[26]

POSTERIOR CRUCIATE LIGAMENT

The PCL is best evaluated on sagittal MRI sequences, where it generally exhibits homogeneously low signal with a slightly curved morphology (Fig. 7-24). Any abnormal signal on the T1 sequence should be confirmed on T2-weighted or proton density–weighted sequences, as signal alteration on T1 may be artifactual and related to magic angle phenomena.[15] Both axial and coronal images can help confirm findings on sagittal sequences and are useful for vertical and horizontal segments of the PCL, respectively.[22]

PCL injury is less frequently encountered on MRI than ACL lesions, commensurate with published ligament injury rates.[24] MRI signs of complete tear of the PCL include non-visualization of the ligament with or without hematoma in its expected location or focal, discrete disruption (Fig. 7-25).[22] Partial or intrasubstance PCL tearing, defined as abnormal MRI signal within the ligament, or fiber discontinuity, is more frequently encountered. Partial tears of the PCL more commonly involve its anterolateral bundle on MRI, and there is often focal ill definition and enlargement of the ligament at its middle third.[15] There is no pathognomonic osseous contusion pattern to confirm a PCL tear, but high-grade PCL injuries can be seen with both dashboard and hyperextension contusion patterns. Osseous avulsion injury is uncommon but most frequent at the tibial attachment, with irregularity of

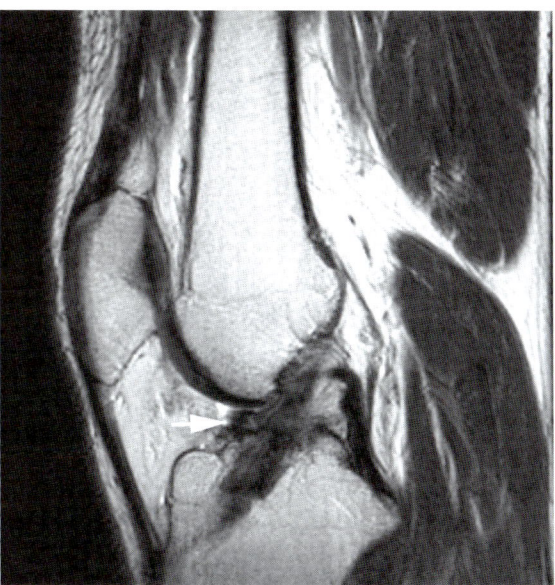

Figure 7-23. Sagittal proton density image shows a hypointense nodular mass of fibrous tissue *(arrow)* anterior to the anterior cruciate graft compatible with arthrofibrosis in a patient with limited knee extension.

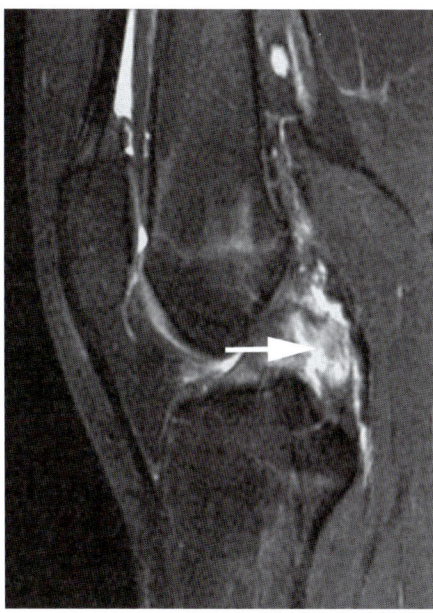

Figure 7-25. Sagittal T2 fat-saturated image shows disruption of the posterior cruciate ligament *(arrow)* compatible with complete tear after a motor vehicle accident and dashboard injury.

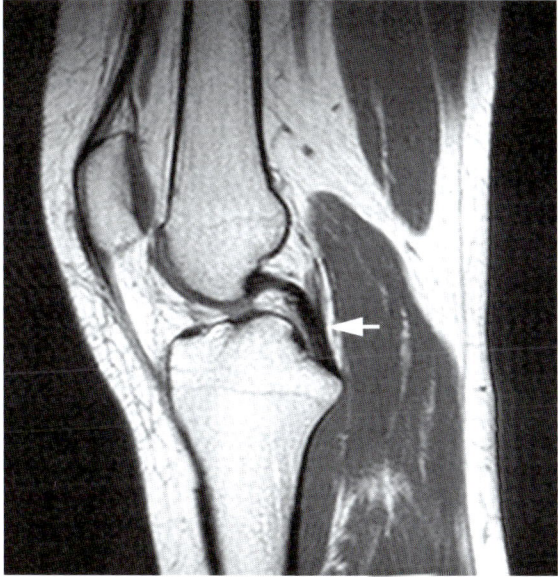

Figure 7-24. Sagittal proton density image demonstrating a normal posterior cruciate ligament *(arrow)*.

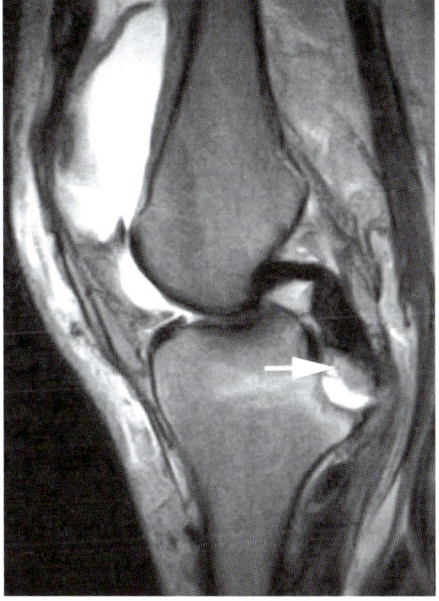

Figure 7-26. Sagittal image shows avulsion fracture of the tibia at the posterior cruciate ligament insertion *(arrow)* in a football player with knee hyperextension.

the tibial cortex and an osseous fragment attached to the free end of the otherwise intact ligament (Fig. 7-26).[22] Subchondral bone marrow edema and hemorrhage may be present between the fragment and the tibia.[24] A grading system has been described for PCL evaluation on MRI: grade 0 is normal, grade 1 is abnormal intrasubstance signal (intrasubstance tear), grade 2 injury is partial interruption of the anterior or posterior border (partial tear), and grade 3 injury is complete disruption, but correlating MRI findings with physical examination and surgery using this system can be difficult, and a descriptive MRI report may be of greater use to treating orthopedists. Osseous avulsion at the anteromedial aspect of

the medial tibial plateau has been termed a reverse Segond fracture or an anteromedial impingement fracture. This injury represents an avulsion of the deep portion of the medial collateral ligament and is an insensitive but highly specific finding for PCL tear. In fact, if an osseous fragment is identified on radiographs in this location, and there is a history of trauma, knee MRI is indicated to assess the PCL.[5]

PCL injuries are an isolated finding on MRI in only about 25% of PCL sprains or tears. Concomitant injuries include meniscal tears, medial slightly more common than lateral, and ligamentous injury, most commonly involving the ACL.

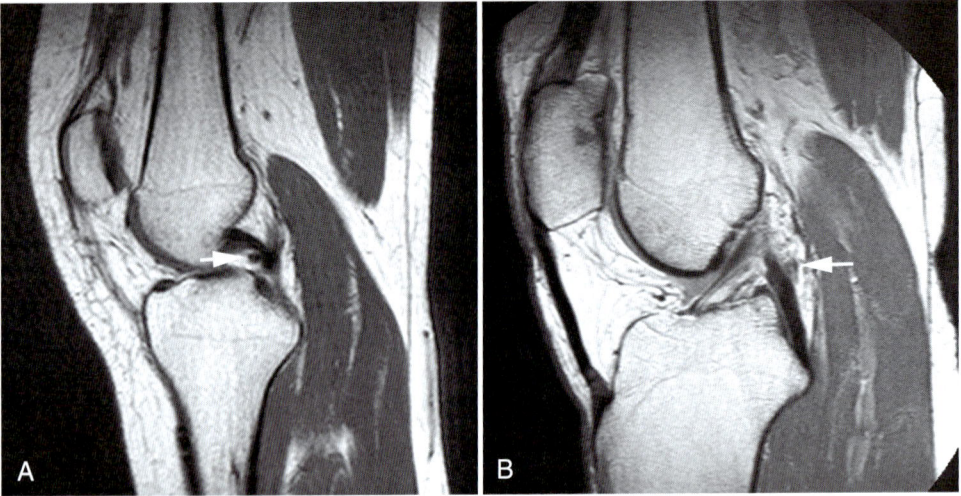

Figure 7-27. Sagittal proton density images show the meniscofemoral ligaments of Humphrey (*arrow* in **A**) and Wrisberg (*arrow* in **B**), anterior and posterior to the posterior cruciate ligament, respectively.

Posterolateral corner injury and avulsion fractures of the fibular head are also associated with PCL disruption. This fracture has been described as the arcuate sign, related to avulsion at the insertion of the arcuate complex, consisting of the fabellofibular, popliteal-fibular, and arcuate ligaments. In one small series, all patients with an avulsion at the fibular head had concomitant PCL injury.[9] In contrast to the torn ACL, at imaging follow-up, the PCL can have a normal appearance, even with complete disruption on initial MRI. Therefore, MRI appearances of a PCL tear do not correlate as well with long-term PCL dysfunction as those indicating ACL tear do with ACL dysfunction. Chronic tears may also present with abnormal morphology such as a hyperbuckled or **U**-shaped appearance,[1] or they may have intermediate intrasubstance signal.[24]

The function of the meniscofemoral ligaments is somewhat controversial. They are often identified by MRI, best in the sagittal plane, with the meniscofemoral ligament of Humphrey anterior to the PCL and the ligament of Wrisberg posterior to the PCL (Fig. 7-27). Some authors propose a mechanical role of the mensicofemoral ligaments in supplementing the PCL.[7] At imaging, the meniscofemoral ligament can mimic a tear of the posterior horn of the lateral meniscus. Following the ligament medially on subsequent sagittal images to its femoral attachment aids in interpretation. A prominent meniscofemoral ligament of Humphrey on sagittal T2-weighted images with surrounding soft tissue edema should tip the interpreter off to the possibility of a primary PCL sprain.

MEDIAL COLLATERAL LIGAMENT

The medial collateral ligament (MCL) is injured with valgus stress to a flexed knee (Fig. 7-28). On MRI, it is evaluated primarily on the coronal fat–saturated T2 or short tau inversion recovery (STIR) sequences. Axial fat–saturated fluid-sensitive sequences supplement and confirm those findings on the coronal sequence. Injury to the MCL, as with other ligaments, is graded 1 to 3 by MRI. Findings of a grade 1 injury include an intact ligament, normal in signal, with surrounding edema and/or hemorrhage (Fig. 7-29). Edema

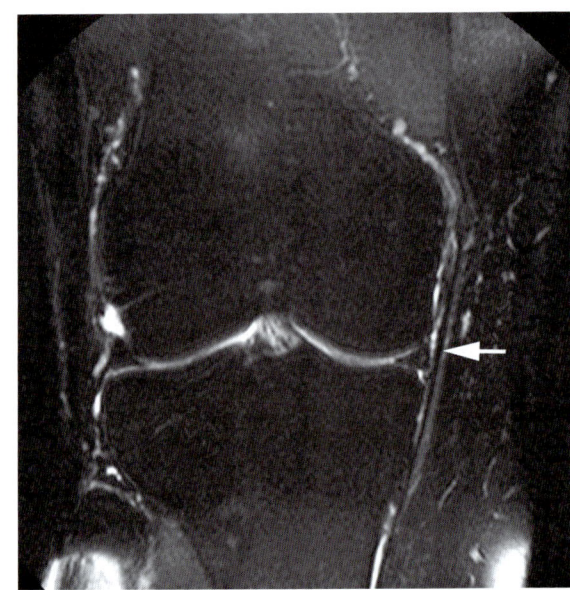

Figure 7-28. Coronal T2 fat-saturated image shows a normal medial collateral ligament *(arrow).*

surrounding the MCL should be evaluated in context with the overall knee pathology. Mimickers of grade 1 MCL injury include a ruptured Baker's cyst, medial compartment pathology such as osteoarthritis or meniscal tear, and lateral patellar dislocation. All of these injuries can present with edema insinuating around the MCL. A grade 2 injury, or partial rupture, manifests as abnormal signal within the ligament itself and/or fluid surrounding the ligament in the MCL bursa (Fig. 7-30).[19] A grade 3 injury, or complete rupture, is characterized by frank disruption and discontinuity of the ligament (Figs. 7-31 and 7-32). Osseous contusions of the medial femoral condyle or lateral tibial plateau may accompany grade 2 or 3 sprains. Injury to the MCL should prompt close evaluation of the other structures of the knee, as it is associated with tears of the ACL and medial meniscus.[19] Osseous avulsion is most common at the femoral attachment, with

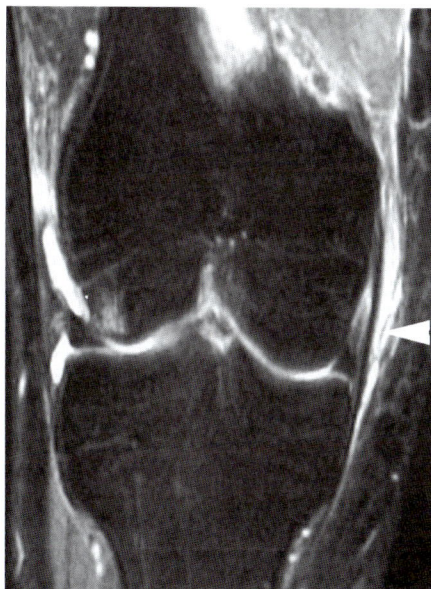

Figure 7-29. Coronal T2 fat-saturated image demonstrates edema signal *(arrowhead)* surrounding an intact medial collateral ligament representing a grade 1 sprain.

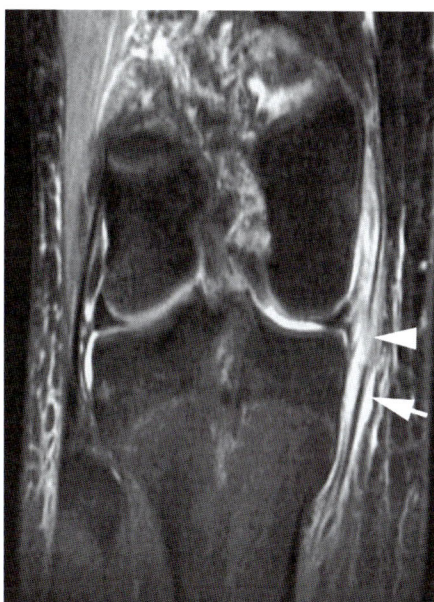

Figure 7-31. Coronal T2 fat-saturated image shows complete disruption of the midsubstance of the medial collateral ligament *(arrowhead)* and surrounding edema *(arrow)* representing a grade 3 sprain (full-thickness tear) sustained in a football injury with a blow to the lateral knee.

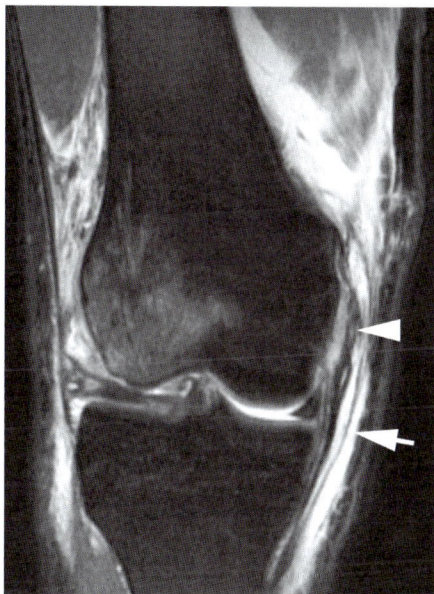

Figure 7-30. Coronal T2 fat-saturated image shows abnormal intrasubstance signal *(arrowhead)* and edema surrounding *(arrow)* the medial collateral ligament compatible with a grade 2 sprain in a soccer player.

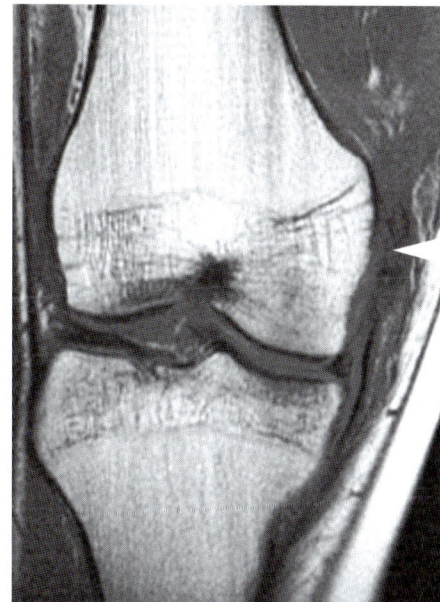

Figure 7-32. Coronal T1 image demonstrates disruption of the proximal medial collateral ligament *(arrowhead)* representing a grade 3 sprain in a skier after a valgus injury.

the osseous fragment best appreciated on T1 non–fat saturated images.[15]

Because MCL injuries often present clinically with medial joint line tenderness, the medial meniscus and meniscocapsular attachments should be carefully interrogated on MRI in the setting of a valgus trauma or MCL sprain. Additionally, especially with contact sports injuries, the lateral knee structures should be evaluated thoroughly for osseous and soft tissue contusions and for fibular head fractures that may be occult to radiographs. A peroneal neuropathy paired with an

MCL sprain is a common scenario identified on MRI, as the common peroneal nerve can be contused or impinged at the site of lateral impaction that led to the valgus stress. Chronic injury to the MCL may result in ligamentous thickening or the radiographic finding of calcification or ossification along the medial knee, also known as a Pellegrini-Steida lesion. On MRI, the chronically sprained MCL is often hypointense on all sequences and larger and more irregular than the normal MCL.

LATERAL COLLATERAL LIGAMENT AND POSTEROLATERAL CORNER

Injury to the static and dynamic stabilizers of the posterolateral corner of the knee, including the fibular collateral ligament, popliteus and biceps femoris muscles and tendons, popliteal-fibular ligament, arcuate ligament, and fabellofibular ligaments, can be evaluated with MRI. Coronal and axial T2 fat-saturated sequences are most frequently employed in examination of the posterolateral corner. Isolated injury is uncommon and therefore should prompt close inspection of the other structures of the knee. Cruciate ligament pathology is often encountered with posterolateral corner injury, as well as MCL, meniscal, and peroneal nerve pathology. Posterolateral corner injury and instability can be somewhat occult clinically, especially in the setting of a recent pivot shift mechanism, so interrogation of these structures at MRI is essential. In one series by Miller and associates, 3 of 30 posterolateral corner injuries were detected by physical examination. Posterolateral instability has been cited as a cause of ACL graft failure and persistent instability following PCL repair. Therefore preoperative assessment of these structures can be of clinical import for surgical planning.

Fibular collateral ligament (lateral collateral ligament proper, FCL) injury is less common than MCL injury (Fig. 7-33). In a prospective study by La Prade and colleagues,[10] MRI detected fibular collateral ligament injury with 94% sensitivity and 100% specificity. Most commonly, FCL injury manifests as complete midsubstance disruption with surrounding soft tissue edema. Injury to the lateral collateral ligament complex can be graded on MRI, with a similar system used for other ligamentous structures about the knee. Edema surrounding an intact ligament is defined as a grade 1 sprain. Intrasubstance ligamentous signal, possibly with ligamentous thickening or thinning and surrounding edema, is considered a grade 2 sprain. Frank disruption and discontinuous fibers represent a grade 3 injury (Fig. 7-34). Osseous

avulsion fractures at the ligamentous attachments, most commonly involving the fibular head, can also be seen at MRI (Fig. 7-35), although radiographs are more sensitive for small avulsed bony fragments. Biceps femoris tendon injury is usually related to chronic repetitive trauma. On MRI, the tendon will appear thickened just proximal to its insertion and may demonstrate abnormal signal. Acute injury may manifest as abnormal intrasubstance signal with surrounding edema or an avulsion fracture at its insertion with the FCL on the fibular head.

With its oblique course, the popliteus muscle and tendon are best evaluated with both sagittal and coronal MRI sequences (Fig. 7-36). They are most commonly injured at the musculotendinous junction (Fig. 7-37).[15] Increased T2 signal extends along the distal muscle fibers to the tendon, giving a feathery or herringbone appearance. Injury to the popliteus tendon manifests as increased intrasubstance signal, or complete disruption. Subjacent bone marrow edema within the lateral femoral condyle has also been described (Fig. 7-38). A strain at the proximal myotendinous junction of the popliteus, a dynamic posterolateral stabilizer, should raise concern for traumatic injury to the static posterolateral corner stabilizers. In fact, in the setting of a traumatic knee injury and subsequent MRI, the popliteus can be considered the "window to the posterolateral corner." Smaller static posterolateral stabilizers include the arcuate ligament, the popliteal-fibular ligament, and the fabellofibular ligament. These are variable in size and, in the case of the fabellofibular ligament, may or may not be present in the normal knee. The arcuate ligament is a multidirectional condensation of ligamentous and capsular fibers, often out of plane and difficult to identify on standard MRI sequences. Therefore, nonvisualization of these structures in isolation cannot be interpreted as disruption. Yu and colleagues[27] proposed using an oblique coronal plane, paralleling the course of the popliteus tendon for better visualization of these structures; however, this has not become a part of the routine evaluation of the knee at most institutions. Injury to the popliteal-fibular ligament was detected at MRI with a reported sensitivity of 69% and specificity of 68% in one series.[10] However, a systematic approach using standard T2-weighted fat-suppressed coronal imaging

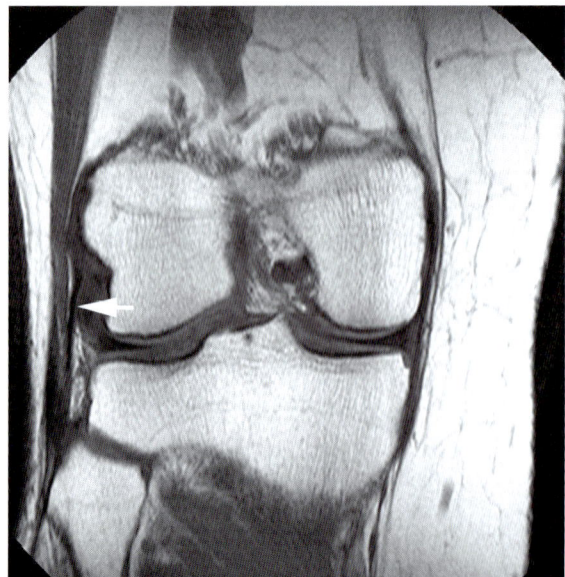

Figure 7-33. Coronal T1 image shows a normal fibular collateral ligament *(arrow)* extending from the femoral condyle to the fibula.

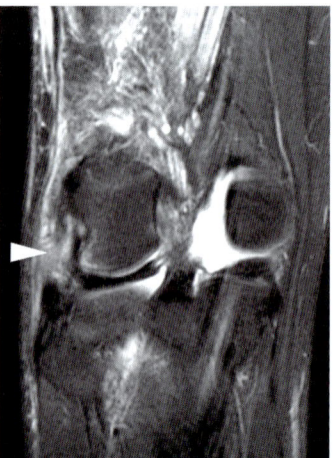

Figure 7-34. Coronal T2 fat-saturated image shows disruption of the fibular collateral ligament *(arrowhead)* representing a grade 3 sprain after a basketball injury.

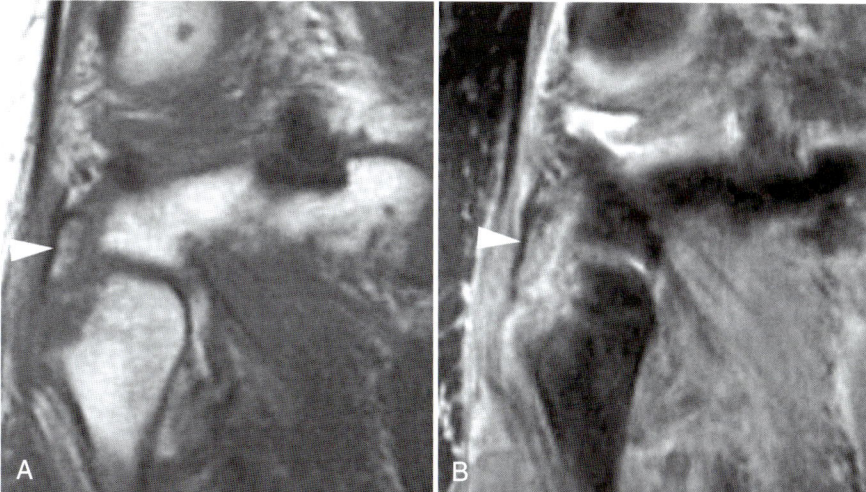

Figure 7-35. Coronal T1 **(A)** and coronal T2 fat-saturated **(B)** images show an avulsion fracture of the proximal fibula at the insertion of the fibular collateral ligament *(arrowhead)*.

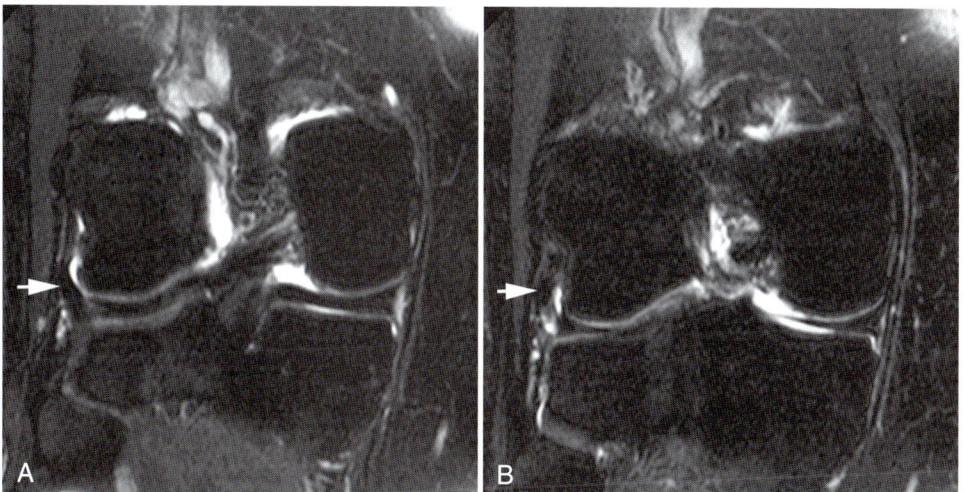

Figure 7-36. Consecutive coronal T2 fat-saturated images **(A** and **B)** demonstrate a normal popliteus tendon *(arrows).*

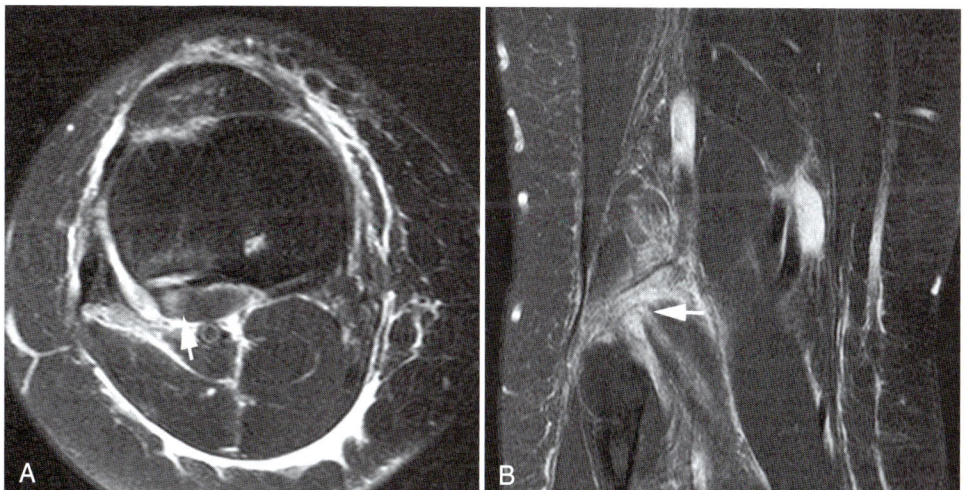

Figure 7-37. Axial **(A)** and coronal **(B)** T2 fat-saturated images demonstrate increased signal at the musculotendinous portion of the popliteus muscle indicative of a strain *(arrows)* without injury to the posterolateral corner stabilizers in a football player.

should increase this sensitivity. If a traumatic strain is evident at the proximal myotendinous junction of the popliteus, as well as edema about the posterolateral soft tissues, an irregular or ill-defined and injured popliteal-fibular ligament can often be identified as a dark structure bridging the popliteus to the fibula amidst the bright edema. With this constellation of findings, especially in the presence of pivot shift contusions, concern for posterolateral corner stabilizer injury should be reported (Fig. 7-39).[27]

POSTEROMEDIAL CORNER

Components of the posteromedial corner of the knee include the posterior oblique ligament, the semimembranosus expansions, the meniscotibial ligaments, the oblique popliteal ligament, and the posterior horn of the medial meniscus. Although physical examination is the most reliable diagnostic tool for posteromedial corner injuries,[20] MRI can aid in evaluation. The intimate relationship of the meniscus, posterior oblique ligament, and capsule is demonstrated on MRI.

Injury can manifest as increased signal within the semimembranosus tendon on a fluid-sensitive fat-saturated sequence, or as meniscocapsular disruption. Evaluation of the posteromedial corner is best on sagittal and coronal imaging sequences. On MRI, posteromedial corner injuries are frequently associated with peripheral (red zone) meniscus tears. Occasionally, patients with focal medial joint line tenderness without evidence of internal derangement will have abnormal signal within the distal semimembranosus insertion, representing an underlying tendinopathy.

EXTENSOR MECHANISM

The extensor mechanism is composed of the quadriceps muscle and tendon, the patella and patellar tendon, and the retinacula. Injuries to the extensor mechanism can be characterized by MRI. The quadriceps tendon routinely exhibits a trilaminar appearance on MRI, where it converges on the superior pole of the patella (Fig. 7-40). The most anterior component consists of fibers of the rectus femoris, middle component fibers from the vastus medialis and vastus lateralis, and posterior component fibers from the vastus intermedius. Quadriceps tendon tears most often occur in the occasional athlete or weekend warrior, and have been associated with systemic conditions such as chronic renal failure, rheumatoid arthritis, diabetes, and long-term steroid therapy.[15] The quadriceps tendon can be evaluated on MRI on the sagittal fluid-sensitive sequences. Partial tears appear as abnormal increased signal within the tendon, with intact fibers coursing around or through the tear.[21] With a complete tear, T2 or fluid-sensitive signal is increased at the site of the tear, and no intact fibers can be identified (Fig. 7-41). The proximal tendon edge may be wavy or balled up owing to quadriceps muscular contraction. The patella may be tilted anteriorly and displaced inferiorly.[21] An assessment of the cranial-caudal gap or retraction should be made on sagittal MRI in the setting of quadriceps rupture.

Patellar tendon injury is more commonly attributed to overuse and repetitive microtrauma. Patellar tendinitis, or jumper's knee, is seen in adolescent and young adult basketball players, volleyball players, and other athletes as the result of repetitive quadriceps muscle contraction. Although this condition may be asymptomatic, patients can present with focal infrapatellar pain. Therefore, it is important to identify

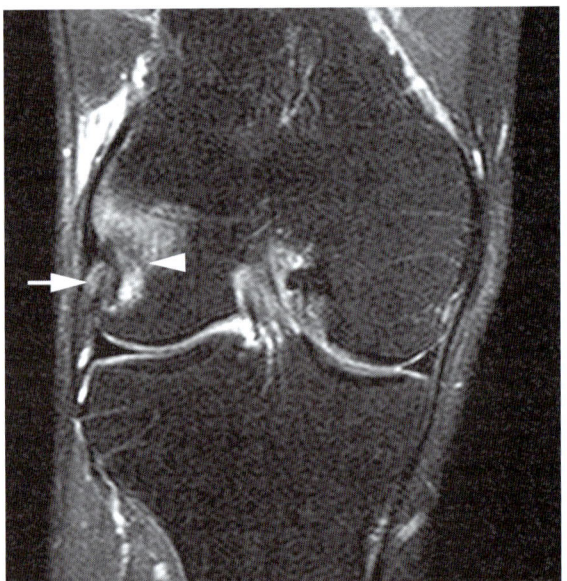

Figure 7-38. Coronal T2 fat-saturated image shows popliteus tendinopathy (arrow) and subjacent bone marrow edema within the lateral femoral condyle (arrowhead).

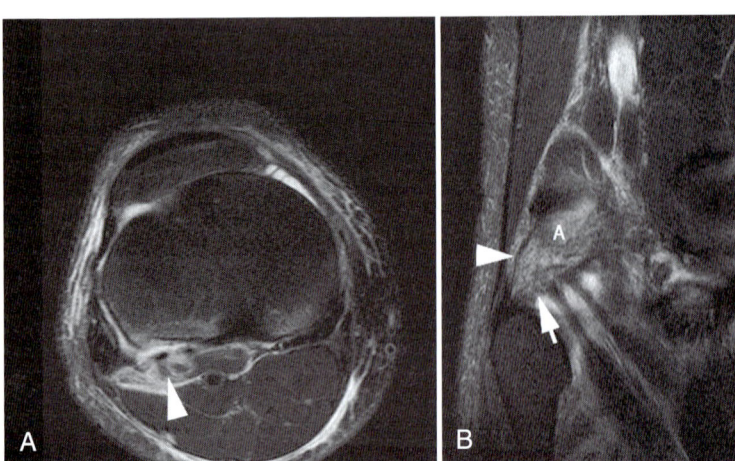

Figure 7-39. Axial (A) and coronal (B) T2 fat-saturated images show a severe posterolateral corner injury following a skiing accident. Along with a complete anterior cruciate ligament tear (not shown), images reveal a strain of the popliteus muscle, sprain of the fabellofibular ligament (arrowhead in B), soft tissue edema (arrow in B), and a sprain of the popliteofibular ligament (arrow in A). Arcuate fibers are denoted by A in part B.

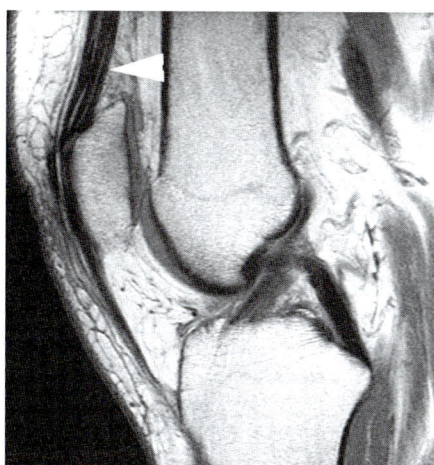

Figure 7-40. Sagittal proton density image demonstrates a normal quadriceps tendon with a trilaminar appearance *(arrowhead).*

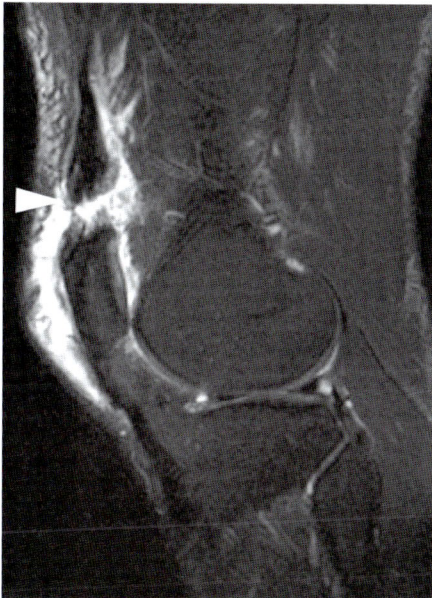

Figure 7-41. Sagittal T2 fat-saturated image shows a complete tear of the quadriceps tendon with fluid signal at the site of disruption *(arrowhead)* in a middle-aged recreational basketball player.

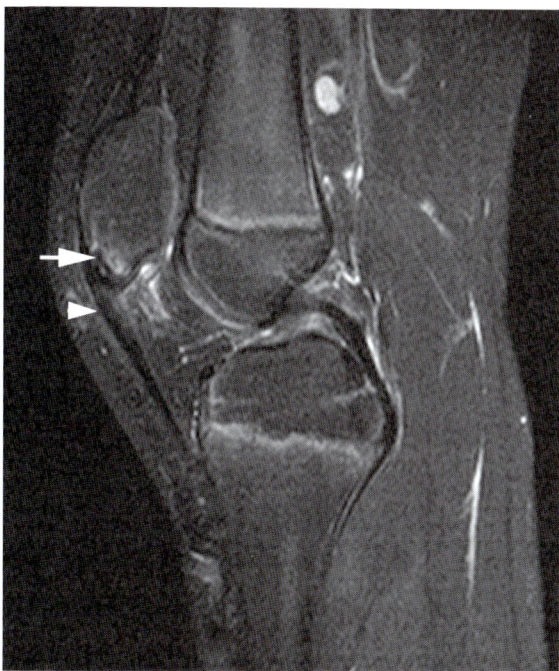

Figure 7-42. Sagittal T2 fat-saturated image shows abnormal signal within the proximal patellar tendon *(arrowhead)* and bone marrow edema within the inferior patella *(arrow)* in this skeletally immature patient (note femoral and tibial physes). Findings represent patellar tendinitis or jumper's knee.

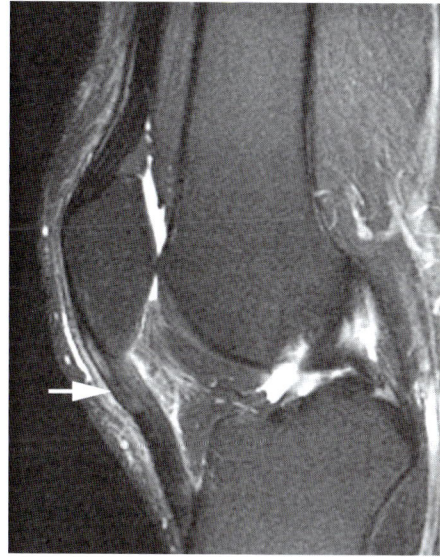

Figure 7-43. Sagittal T2 fat-saturated image demonstrates thickening and abnormal signal within the proximal patellar tendon *(arrow),* suggesting a chronic patellar tendinosis.

early signs of patellar tendon disease with imaging. On MRI, the proximal patellar tendon will appear thick with foci of increased T2 signal (Fig. 7-42).[15] Chronic patellar tendon degeneration, a disease of adulthood, can be seen anywhere along the length of the tendon. Imaging reveals areas of intermediate T1 and T2 foci within the tendon, with or without tendon thickening (Fig. 7-43). Foci of increased fluid-sensitive signal may be related to mucinous degeneration and interstitial cyst formation. Using the quadriceps tendon as a reference is often helpful, as a patellar tendon that is equal in thickness to the quadriceps tendon is abnormal.[21] Rupture of the patellar tendon may be related to chronic degeneration, most commonly at the proximal aspect, or to acute forced flexion against a contracted quadriceps muscle, most commonly at its midportion.[15] The patellar tendon will be discontinuous on sagittal imaging sequences, with superior displacement of the patella (Fig. 7-44).

Acute and chronic avulsion injuries of the patellar tendon affect adolescents and include patellar sleeve avulsion, Osgood-Schlatter disease, and Sinding-Larsen-Johansson syndrome. Patellar sleeve avulsion occurs secondary to an acute forceful contraction of the quadriceps muscle and results in a tear of the proximal patellar tendon with an avulsed osteochondral fragment from the patella. On MRI, the fracture line through the patella will be seen on fluid-sensitive sequences with the retracted patellar tendon and its bony fragment distally (Fig. 7-45). Osgood-Schlatter disease and Sinding-Larsen-Johansson syndrome are similar in pathology and mechanism, affecting the distal and proximal patellar tendon, respectively. Both are related to chronic microavulsion of the patellar tendon. In Osgood-Schlatter disease, MRI will demonstrate enlargement of the tendon with foci of ossification (Fig. 7-46). Although there is normal variant anatomy of the tibial eminence ossification centers, the presence of surrounding edema and fluid in the deep infrapatellar bursa supports a diagnosis of Osgood-Schlatter disease. Sinding-Larsen-Johansson syndrome has similar MRI characteristics at the proximal patellar tendon with tendon

thickening, abnormal intrasubstance signal, and areas of ossification.[21]

Lateral patellar dislocation is often transient, and patients as well as clinicians may not realize that it has occurred. MRI plays an important role with this lesion, as it has been reported that between 45% and 73% of lateral patellar dislocations are clinically unsuspected. Characteristic MRI findings in lateral patellar dislocation include joint effusion and hemarthrosis, medial retinacular injury, and osteochondral injury to the anterolateral lateral femoral condyle and medial patella. Osseous contusions secondary to patellar dislocation and subsequent relocation will be seen as foci of increased signal at the nonarticular, subcortical lateral femoral condyle, and at the medial patellar facet on bone marrow edema–sensitive images (Fig. 7-47). The medial retinaculum is invariably injured and may be thickened or disrupted. However, injury to the medial patellofemoral ligament (MPFL) may hold greater clinical importance and should be recognized at MRI. With disruption of the MPFL, fluid signal dissects under the distal, oblique fibers of the vastus medialis, which has been disrupted from its adductor tubercle attachment. Often, a torn MPFL can be identified as a wavy hypointense structure amid this soft tissue edema.[4] Injury can also be seen within the infrapatellar fat pad, manifested by increased fluid-sensitive signal, or even shear injury, as fluid-filled clefts within the fat pad.[15]

Patellar malalignment and abnormal tracking are related to incongruence between the patella and the femur that results in patellofemoral joint instability. The patellofemoral compartment is best evaluated in the axial plane. Excessive lateral pressure syndrome manifests on MRI with lateral patellar tilt (Fig. 7-48), cartilage abnormality along the lateral patellar facet, and/or edema within the lateral patella (Fig. 7-49).[15] Dynamic assessment of patellar tracking with varying degrees of flexion and quadriceps contraction have been described with MRI using gradient echo sequences. The Insall-Salvati ratio has also been used with MRI. The longest patellar measurement and the length of the patellar tendon at its mid portion are used. If the ratio of patellar tendon length to patellar length is 1.3 or greater, then patella alta is

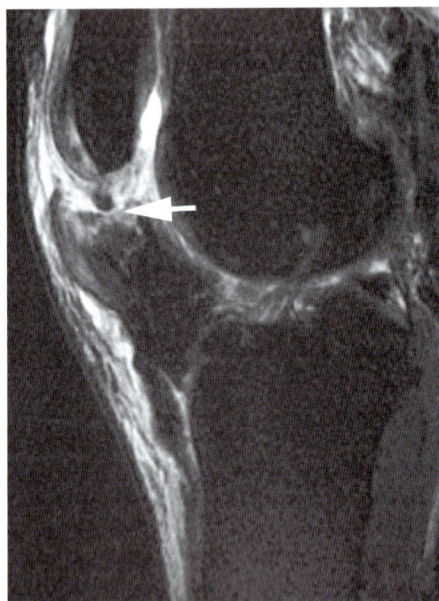

Figure 7-44. Sagittal T2 fat-saturated image shows a complete tear of the patellar tendon with fluid signal at the site of the tear and retraction of tendon fibers *(arrow)* in a middle-aged soccer player.

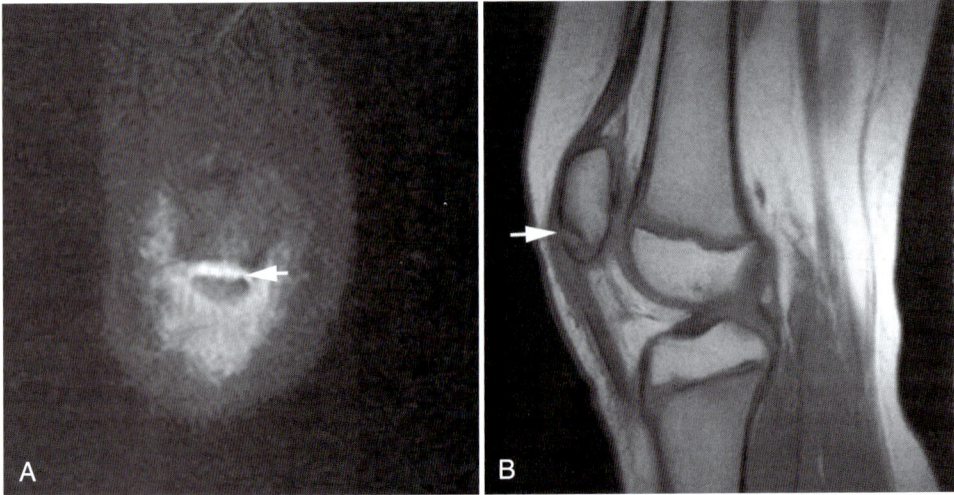

Figure 7-45. Coronal T2 fat-saturated **(A)** and sagittal proton density **(B)** images show a patellar sleeve avulsion in a 15-year-old basketball player with abnormal signal in the patellar tendon and a transverse fracture through the inferior patella *(arrow* in **A)** with mild inferior displacement of the osteochondral fragment *(arrow* in **B)**.

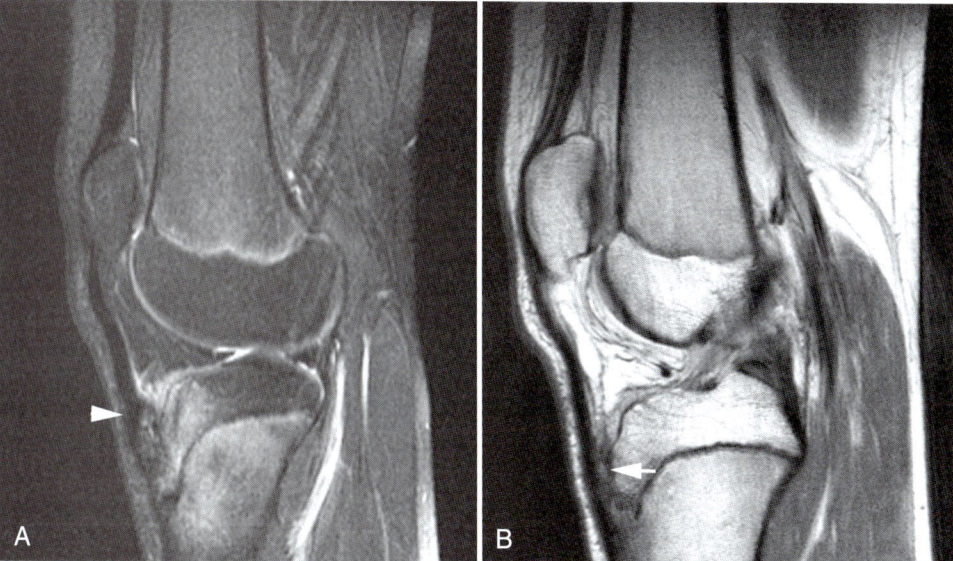

Figure 7-46. Sagittal T2 fat-saturated (**A**) and sagittal proton density (**B**) images demonstrate bone marrow edema at the tibial tuberosity and abnormal signal within the distal patellar tendon (*arrowhead* in **A**). Osseous fragmentation is evident at the tibial tuberosity (*arrow* in **B**). Findings represent Osgood-Schlatter disease.

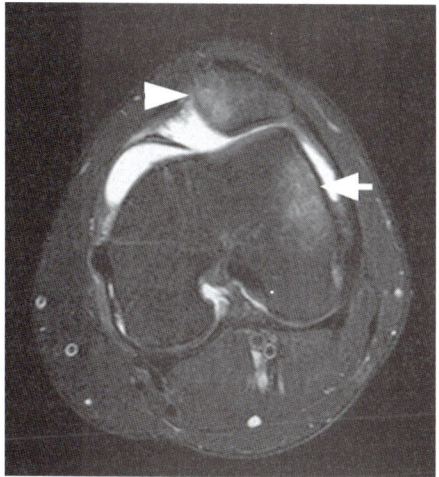

Figure 7-47. Axial T2 fat-saturated image shows bone marrow edema and osseous contusions within the medial patella (*arrowhead*) and lateral femoral condyle (*arrow*) compatible with recent transient lateral patellar dislocation in this 16-year-old lacrosse player.

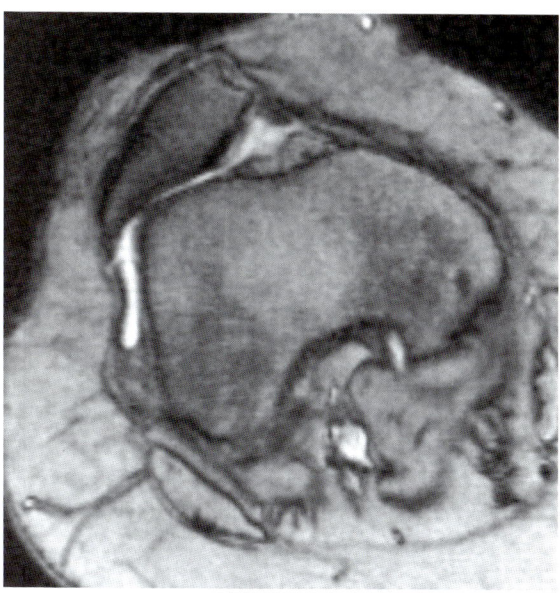

Figure 7-48. Axial gradient echo image shows lateral patellar tilt in a female with a long-standing lateral patellofemoral tracking syndrome.

present. Patella infera or patella baja occurs with a ratio of 0.8 or less.

ILIOTIBIAL BAND

The iliotibial band (ITB) is an aponeurosis formed from the more proximal tensor fascia lata, gluteus maximus muscle, and gluteus medius muscle. It inserts onto the lateral femoral condyle and more distally onto the anterolateral tibia at Gerdy's tubercle. Iliotibial band friction syndrome is a condition most often seen in runners and cyclists, and is related to repetitive flexion and extension, causing compression of vascularized and innervated fat between the ITB and the lateral femoral condyle.[15] Fluid-sensitive fat-saturated coronal and

axial images are most sensitive, demonstrating increased signal or soft tissue edema deep to the iliotibial band adjacent to the lateral femoral condyle (Fig. 7-50). Increased signal may extend into and even superficial to the ITB, and focal fluid collections have been described.[13,14] The iliotibial band itself may be normal in signal and morphology or mildly enlarged with this overuse syndrome, and reciprocal bone marrow edema is occasionally present in the nonarticular lateral femoral condyle (Fig. 7-51).

MULTILIGAMENT KNEE INJURIES

Although this term is more prevalent in the orthopedics and sports medicine literature than in radiology journals, it is

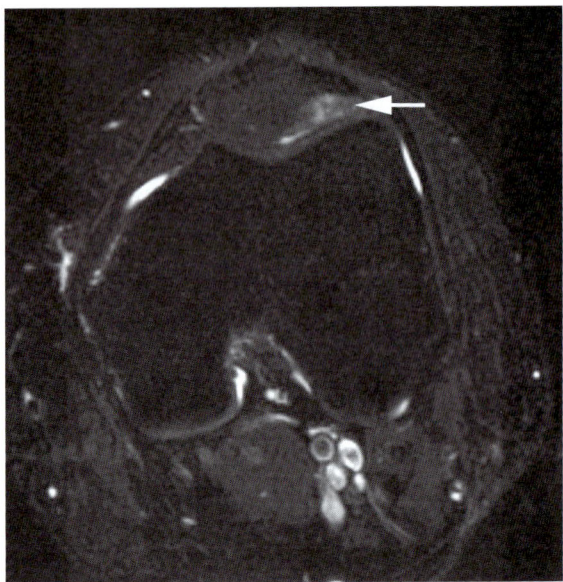

Figure 7-49. Axial T2 fat-saturated image shows edema within the lateral patella *(arrow)* and within the lateral aspect of Hoffa's fat typical for abnormal patellofemoral tracking.

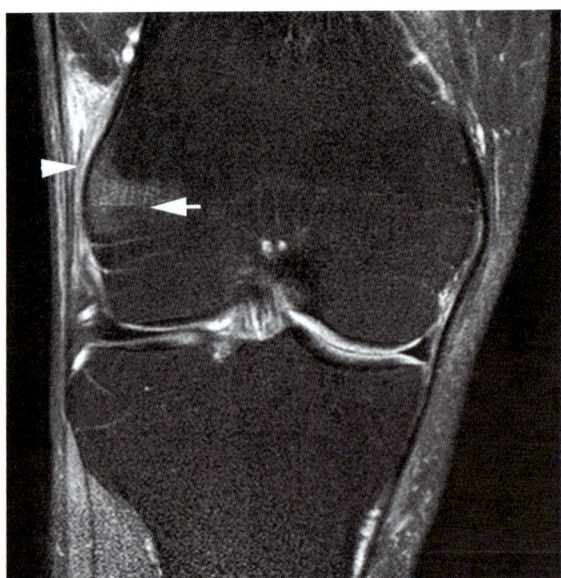

Figure 7-51. Sagittal T2 fat-saturated image demonstrates a more advanced case of iliotibial band friction syndrome with edema deep to the iliotibial band *(arrowhead)* and bone marrow edema within the lateral femoral condyle *(arrow)*.

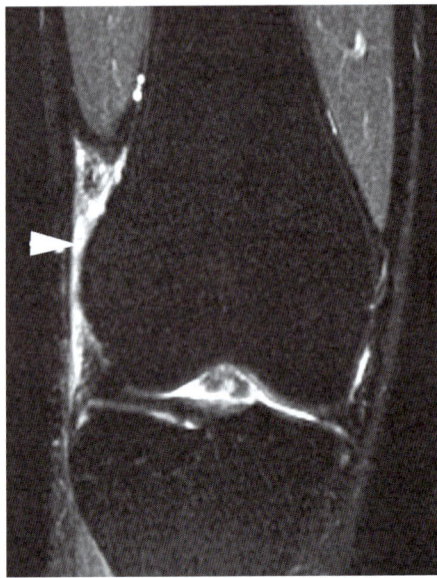

Figure 7-50. Sagittal T2 fat-saturated image demonstrates extensive soft tissue edema deep to the iliotibial band (ITB) *(arrowhead)* compatible with ITB friction syndrome in a 33-year-old distance runner.

important for imagers to accept and even expect associated soft tissue injuries in the knee, once an injury mechanism or ligamentous lesion has been identified. Injuries previously labeled as knee dislocations are now often more appropriately categorized under the term multiligament knee injury, indicating that at least two of the knee-stabilizing structures discussed in this chapter have been injured during a traumatic episode. Rather than review each MRI with a checklist, investigating each tendon and ligament individually, a more effective mechanism for interpretation of the traumatized knee is to identify the mechanism and primary ligamentous

injury, and then interrogate the other structures likely to be secondarily involved. Often, imaging findings can raise concern for a ligament sprain or tendon strain, but the actual integrity and stability of the secondarily injured structure must be confirmed at physical examination, or sometimes at surgery. Common multiligament knee injury patterns include ACL tear with posterolateral corner injury with or without an MCL sprain, PCL tear and FCL sprain with or without posterolateral corner injury, and tears of both cruciate ligaments with FCL and posterolateral corner injury—a pattern more appropriately labeled as a knee dislocation (Figs. 7-52 and 7-53).[11,12]

Often articular cartilage defects, lesions, and meniscal tears in specific locations are associated with ligament injuries and mechanisms; these associations should drive the imager to take a second look at structures in jeopardy. A transient lateral patellar dislocation is associated not only with medial patellofemoral ligament injury, but also with a shear-type, delaminating articular cartilage lesion at the anterolateral margin of the lateral femoral condyle. In this regard, effective MRI interpretations often log specific lesions under an umbrella mechanism such as "constellation of MRI findings" consistent with a recent pivot shift injury at the right knee including an acute, midsubstance, complete tear of the ACL, a grade 2 sprain of the popliteal-fibular ligament, a vertical tear at the posteromedial periphery of the medial meniscus, and a 4 mm × 3 mm focal grade 4 articular cartilage lesion at the terminal sulcus of the lateral femoral condyle.

CONCLUSION

The posttraumatic knee MRI review should be injury mechanism based, including a second look or careful evaluation of soft tissue and osseous structures likely to be injured based on the biomechanics of the injury. Recognition of reproducible injury patterns will lead to a thorough and useful imaging interpretation that can effectively guide therapeutic options.

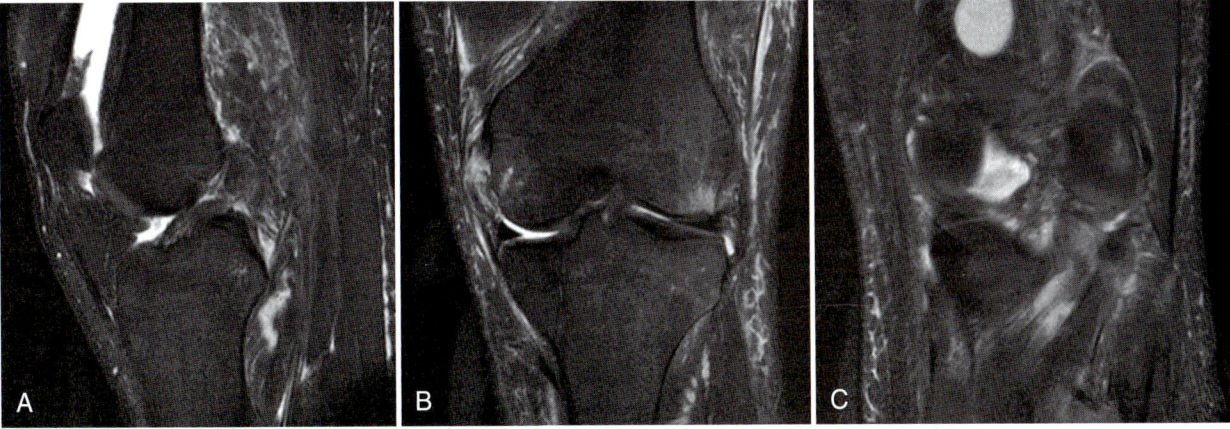

Figure 7-52. Sagittal **(A)** and coronal **(B** and **C)** T2 fat-saturated image shows tears of the anterior cruciate, posterior cruciate, and medial collateral ligaments with associated posterolateral corner injury **(C)**.

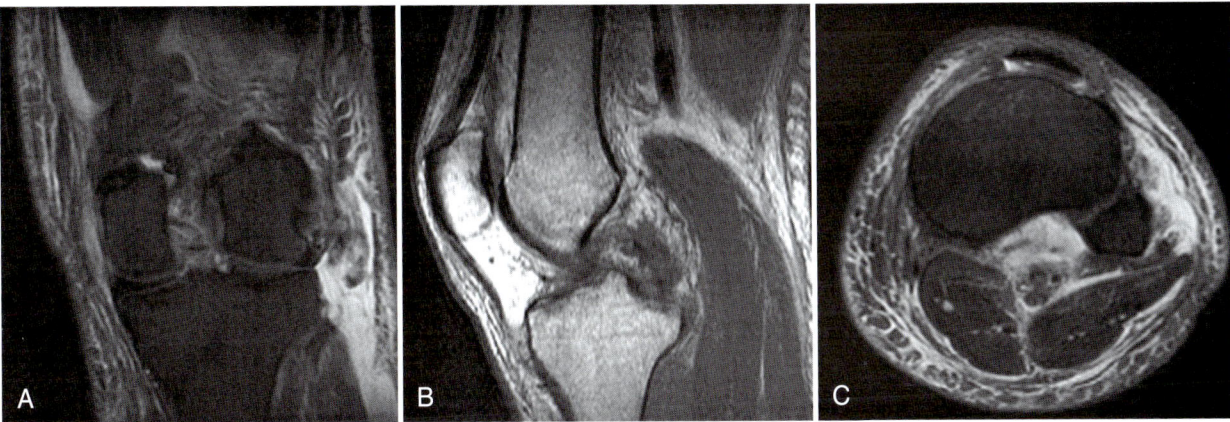

Figure 7-53. Coronal **(A)** T2 fat-saturated, sagittal proton density **(B)**, and axial T2 fat-saturated **(C)** images show tears of the anterior cruciate, posterior cruciate, and lateral collateral ligaments.

KEY REFERENCES

Beaman FD, Peterson JJ: MR imaging of cysts, ganglia, and bursae about the knee. Radiol Clin North Am 45:969–982, 2007.

Elias DA, White LM: Imaging of patellofemoral disorders. Clin Radiol 59:543–557, 2004.

Huang GS, Yu JS, Munshi M, et al: Avulsion fracture of the head of the fibula (the "arcuate" sign): MR imaging findings predictive of injuries to the posterolateral ligaments and posterior cruciate ligament. Am J Roentgenol 180:381–387, 2003.

LaPrade RF, Gilbert TJ, Bollom TS, et al: The magnetic resonance imaging appearance of individual structures of the posterolateral knee: a prospective study of normal knees and knees with surgically verified grade III injuries. Am J Sports Med 28:191–199, 2000.

Sanders TG, Medynski MA, Feller JF, et al: Bone contusion patterns of the knee at MR imaging: footprint of the mechanism of injury. Radiographics 20:S135–S151, 2000.

Sims WF, Jacobson KE: The posteromedial corner of the knee. Am J Sports Med 32:337, 2004.

Full references for this chapter can be found on www.expertconsult.com.

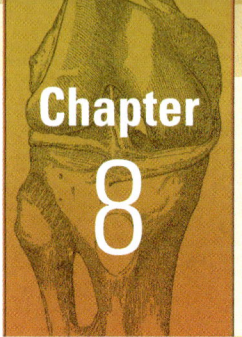

Chapter 8

Internal Derangements: Menisci and Cartilage

Kristen E. McClure and William B. Morrison

MENISCUS

Anatomy

The medial and lateral menisci of the knee are fibrocartilaginous semicircular structures that act as shock absorbers and transmit forces between the femur and the tibia. The menisci are composed of longitudinal collagen bundles, circumferentially oriented in a C-shaped configuration, as well as transversely oriented collagen fibers that radiate from the free edge of the meniscus to the peripheral margin. Together, these longitudinal and radial collagen fibers act to provide hoop tensile strength, resist axial loading extrusive forces, and prevent separation of the menisci in a radial direction.

Both menisci are thicker in craniocaudad dimension along the periphery and taper to a thinner margin along the free edge. Although the medial and lateral menisci serve the same purpose in the medial and lateral compartments of the knee, they are not symmetrical in size or shape. The medial meniscus is a larger C-shaped structure, and the lateral meniscus is a tighter, near complete circle (Fig. 8-1). Because of these morphologic differences, the medial meniscus covers approximately one half of the tibial plateau contact surface, and the lateral meniscus covers approximately three quarters of the tibial plateau contact surface.

The medial meniscus can be differentiated from the lateral meniscus by position and size, and also by its distinct morphologic characteristics and regional attachments. The posterior horn of the medial meniscus is wider in an anteroposterior dimension than the anterior horn. This can be demonstrated on sagittal imaging of the knee when the posterior horn appears two to three times larger than the anterior horn (Fig. 8-2). The posterior horn of the medial meniscus attaches to the tibia at the posterior intercondylar fossa, anterior to the posterior cruciate ligament insertion, but behind the posterior horn of the lateral meniscus. The anterior horn of the medical meniscus attaches to the tibia at the anterior intercondylar fossa, in front of both the anterior horn of the lateral meniscus and the insertion of the anterior cruciate ligament. The periphery of the medial meniscus is attached to the joint capsule along its entire length via meniscotibial and coronary ligaments.[12]

In comparison, the lateral meniscus is symmetrical from front to back (Fig. 8-3). Therefore, on sagittal imaging of the knee, the posterior horn and the anterior horn are similar in size. The posterior horn of the lateral meniscus attaches to the tibia behind the intercondylar eminence, anterior to both the posterior cruciate ligament insertion and the posterior horn of the medial meniscus. The anterior horn of the lateral meniscus attaches to the tibia in front of the intercondylar eminence, behind both the anterior horn of the medial meniscus and the anterior cruciate ligament insertion. The fibers of the anterior cruciate ligament partially blend with the lateral meniscus at its tibial attachment. The periphery of the lateral meniscus cannot attach directly to the joint capsule because of the intra-articular course of the popliteus tendon between the lateral meniscus and the joint capsule. The lateral meniscus actually attaches to the joint capsule through small fascicles or struts.

Meniscal nutrition is supplied by two routes. The vascular supply is confined to the outer one third of the meniscus, also known as the red zone. The vessels arise from the medial and lateral genicular arteries, forming a perimeniscal synovial capillary plexus that bathes the periphery of the menisci. The central portion of the meniscus receives nutrients from the synovial fluid, which diffuses into or is forced through the joint with activity. This avascular portion of the meniscus is known as the white zone. The presence or absence of vascular supply at the location of a meniscal tear can determine whether the tear has a possibility of healing without intervention. A peripheral meniscal tear with adequate vascular supply is capable of healing and may not require surgical intervention.

Function

The menisci have many biomechanical functions. They act to increase contact area and joint congruity, transmit load and absorb shock, prevent radial extrusive forces during axial loading, and aid in joint lubrication. Because fibrocartilage is less stiff than hyaline cartilage, the menisci intrinsically have a higher shock-absorbing capacity. Functional meniscal studies have found that 50% to 85% of the load placed across the joint is transmitted by the meniscus. Following total meniscectomy, the contact area between the femur and the tibia decreases by approximately 75%; thus contact stresses between the femur and the tibia increase by more than 200%. Studies have demonstrated that contact stresses at the knee joint proportionately increase in relation to the amount of meniscus removed.[12]

Discoveries such as these have altered the surgical management of meniscal tears. Preservation and conservation of meniscal tissue are now the ultimate goals to maximize the function of the residual meniscus and prevent progression to osteoarthritis.

Magnetic Resonance Imaging of the Meniscus

The normal meniscus demonstrates homogeneous low signal intensity on all imaging sequences because of its short T2 relaxation. Increased signal intensity within the meniscus is abnormal and represents a meniscal tear or degeneration. A short time to echo (TE) imaging sequence is necessary to evaluate the meniscus on magnetic resonance imaging (MRI).

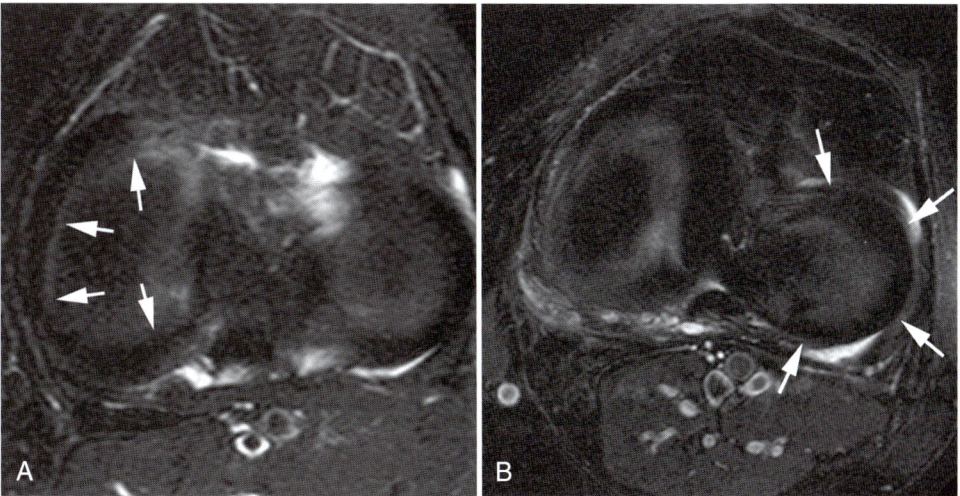

Figure 8-1. A and **B,** Normal meniscal anatomy. Axial T2-weighted fat-suppressed images at the level of the menisci demonstrate the larger C-shaped medial meniscus (*arrows* in **A**) and the smaller near complete circle lateral meniscus (*arrows* in **B**).

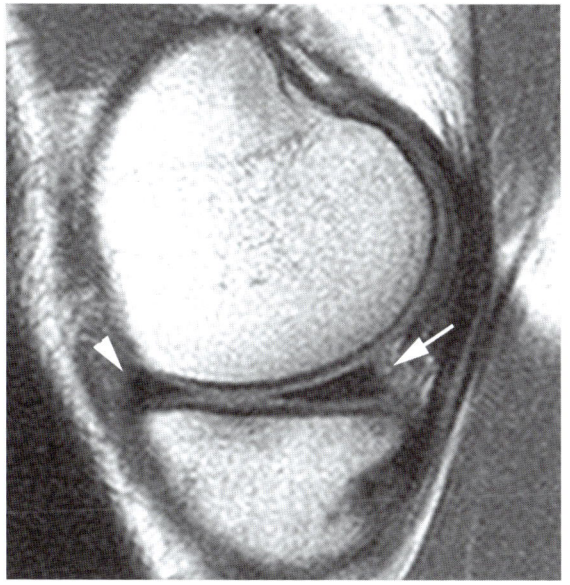

Figure 8-2. Normal meniscal anatomy. Sagittal proton density image through the medial compartment shows that the posterior horn of the medial meniscus (*arrow*) typically appears two to three times larger than the anterior horn (*arrowhead*).

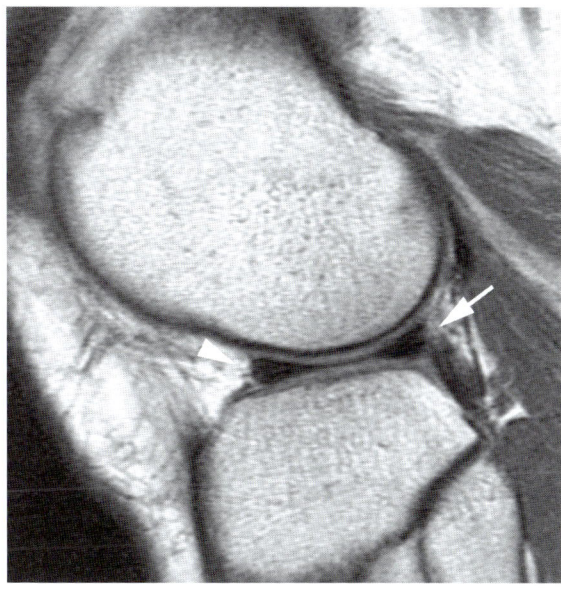

Figure 8-3. Normal meniscal anatomy. Sagittal proton density image through the lateral compartment shows that the lateral meniscus is symmetrical from back (*arrow*) to front (*arrowhead*).

This can be accomplished with proton density, gradient echo, or traditional spin echo T1-weighted imaging sequences. The utility of fast spin echo has been debated in the literature, with some describing blur artifact limitations, and others reporting similar sensitivities and specificities as conventional spin echo.

T1-weighted images (i.e., low TE images) are the most sensitive for detecting signal alteration within the meniscus; however, they are the least specific for meniscal tear. Meniscal vascularity and degeneration, as well as tear, are bright on low TE images. As TE increases, fluid in true meniscal tears becomes relatively more prominent. However, not all tears contain fluid. Therefore, T2-weighted images (i.e., high-TE images) are specific but not sensitive for tear and are more useful for confirmation, as fluid signal may be present at the

site of the tear. The best imaging sequence to evaluate for meniscal tear is a proton density–weighted imaging sequence that achieves a balance between sensitivity and specificity. Sagittal proton density images are typically more valuable in diagnosing a tear of the anterior or posterior horns. However, meniscal root tears and flipped fragments may be better seen on coronal imaging, and correlation with two imaging planes has been encouraged in the interpretation of meniscal pathology.[25] Slice thickness can affect sensitivity as well. It has been recommended that slice thickness be no greater than 4 mm, and that minimal gap exist between each slice.

At our institution, we routinely acquire fast spin echo sequences, including sagittal proton density images, coronal T2-weighted images with fat suppression, and sagittal T2-weighted images with fat suppression. We also acquire coronal T1-weighted spin echo images, without fat suppression. We use a slice thickness of 3 mm with 0.5-mm gaps between slices. Protocols will vary depending on vendor, field strength, and user preference.

MRI Criteria for Meniscal Injuries

A meniscal tear can be diagnosed by identifying abnormal intrameniscal signal, abnormal morphology, or a displaced meniscal fragment. MRI criteria for diagnosing meniscal tear were first investigated just over 20 years ago. Abnormal MRI signal (hyperintensity) within the meniscus in symptomatic patients was evaluated and subjectively classified prior to surgery. Intrameniscal signal abnormality was graded according to its confluence and extension to the articular surface on sagittal imaging. Histologic grading of the same menisci was performed following surgery, thereby differentiating degeneration from meniscal tear. This histologic grading was correlated with MRI signal grade, as classified below:

Grade 1: punctuate or amorphous signal abnormality without extension to the articular surface.

Grade 2: linear signal abnormality without extension to the articular surface.

Grade 3: signal abnormality extending to at least one articular surface.

In this study, 100% correspondence was noted between MRI grade signal alteration and histologic grade. MRI grade 1 and 2 signal alterations corresponded with meniscal degeneration. MRI grade 3 signal alteration corresponded with meniscal tear.[20]

Later it was described that as the number of sequential images with abnormal surfacing meniscal signal increased, the accuracy of diagnosing a meniscal tear also increased. In two separate studies conducted in 1993 and 2005, the positive predictive value for diagnosing meniscal tears increased when two or more images with surfacing signal abnormality were required compared with only a single abnormal image.[8] This concept was presented as the two-slice-touch rule and is used by many radiologists today in diagnosing meniscal tear.

These basic MRI criteria were created in the early days of MRI. Today, with higher-field-strength MRI and dedicated extremity coils and imaging systems, the original MRI diagnostic criteria for meniscal tear may not be entirely applicable. No recent studies have been performed on MRI at different field strengths to evaluate the difference in diagnostic accuracy between two sequential images with surfacing signal abnormality and only a single image with surfacing signal abnormality. With higher signal-to-noise ratio and improved imaging techniques, the two-slice-touch rule may not be necessary for accurate diagnosis of meniscal tears. Although the original MRI criteria are still used as guidelines at our institution, they are not always strictly adhered to. Furthermore, secondary signs of meniscal tear have become more important in our interpretations.

Secondary signs of meniscal tear can enhance confidence in diagnosis, particularly in cases where the signal abnormality within the meniscus is equivocal, or when the study is degraded by artifact. Indirect evidence of meniscal pathology includes adjacent cartilage loss, parameniscal cyst (also referred to as meniscal cyst), meniscal extrusion, parameniscal soft tissue edema, bowing of the ipsilateral collateral ligament, joint effusion, perivascular bone marrow edema, and subchondral bone marrow edema (Table 8-1).[1]

The presence of a parameniscal cyst has a 100% positive predictive value for an associated meniscal tear in some studies. Parameniscal cysts are believed to result from extruded joint fluid through an adjacent meniscal tear.[2] Parameniscal cysts are seen in 7% of meniscal tears (Fig. 8-4). They have the same incidence for medial and lateral meniscal tears but are seen more commonly medially owing to higher prevalence of medial tears. Medial meniscal cysts are most frequently located posteriorly, and lateral meniscal cysts are most frequently located anteriorly.[2]

Adjacent collateral ligament edema and linear subchondral bone marrow edema have been shown to have high specificity and positive predictive values in the diagnosis of meniscal tear.[1] Collateral ligament edema can be seen in the setting of primary ligamentous injury and osteoarthritis. However in the setting of meniscal tear, collateral ligament edema likely reflects inflammatory hyperemia, reactive synovitis, and increased fluid formation related to the tear (Fig. 8-5). The sensitivity of this sign is greater for medial meniscal tears, indicating the closer apposition of the medial collateral ligament to the periphery of the medial meniscus as compared

Table 8-1 Positive Predictive Value (PPV), Sensitivity, and Specificity of Indirect Signs for Meniscal Tears at Arthroscopy

Indirect Signs	PPV	MEDIAL Sensitivity	MENISCUS Specificity	PPV	LATERAL Sensitivity	MENISCUS Specificity
Cartilage loss near tear	0.94	0.54	0.88	0.68	0.23	0.91
Meniscal extrusion	0.78	0.57	0.94	0.49	0.09	0.93
Collateral ligament bowing	0.96	0.58	0.91	1.00	0.11	1.00
Collateral ligament edema	0.98	0.70	0.94	0.95	0.23	0.99
Parameniscal cyst	1.00	0.09	1.00	1.00	0.23	0.61
Parameniscal soft tissue edema	0.97	0.44	0.91	0.59	0.23	0.58
Perivascular bone marrow edema	0.95	0.22	0.97	0.99	0.09	0.95
Effusion	0.77	0.95	0.21	0.37	0.80	0.08
Linear subchondral edema	0.99	0.67	0.97	0.95	0.89	0.99

Adapted from Bergin D, Hochberg H, Zoga AC, et al: Indirect soft-tissue and osseous signs on knee MRI of surgically proven meniscal tears. AJR Am J Roentgenol 191:86–92, 2008. Statistics provided are an average of Reader 1 and Reader 2 values.

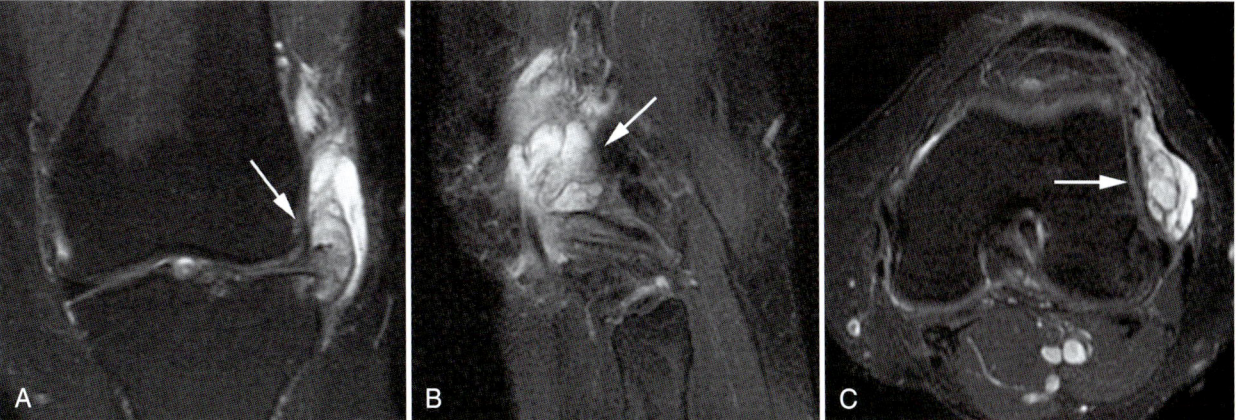

Figure 8-4. **A** through **C,** Secondary signs of meniscal tear: parameniscal cyst. Coronal **(A)**, sagittal **(B)**, and axial **(C)** fluid-sensitive sequences depict a large parameniscal cyst *(arrows)* emanating from an underlying lateral meniscal tear.

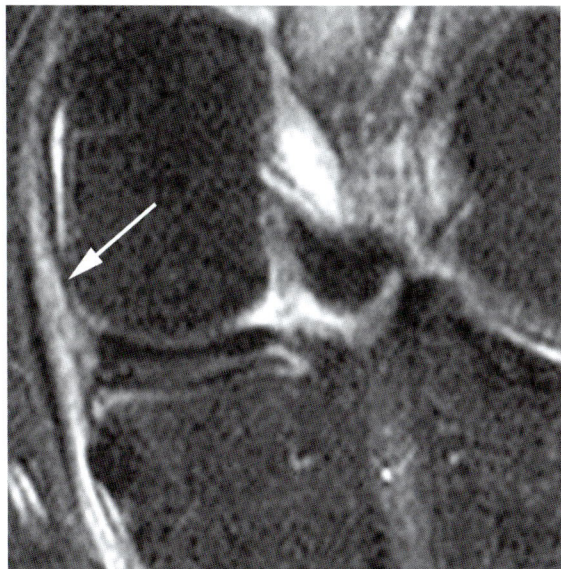

Figure 8-5. Secondary signs of meniscal tear: collateral ligament edema. Coronal T2-weighted fat-suppressed image shows medial collateral ligament bowing and edema *(arrow)* related to underlying medial meniscal tear.

with the lateral collateral ligament and the lateral meniscus. Periarticular bone marrow edema can be seen with trauma and osteoarthritis. However, in the setting of meniscal tear, linear subchondral bone marrow edema is located directly adjacent to the meniscus and probably represents hyperemia at the junction of the bony cortex, cartilage, and meniscus (Fig. 8-6). These secondary signs can help guide attention to the meniscus on MRI and can increase confidence when primary diagnostic criteria are equivocal.[1]

Meniscal extrusion can also be used as a secondary sign of meniscal tear. It is defined as extension of the peripheral meniscus past the tibial margin, and it results from a tear that destabilizes the circumferential collagen fibers of the meniscus and allows it to expand in a radial direction (Fig. 8-7). Major meniscal extrusion (>3 mm) is more highly associated with extensive tears, advanced meniscal degeneration, complex tears, and large radial tears. Tears that extend into the meniscal root are also more likely to result in substantial meniscal extrusion. Identifying meniscal extrusion is important, not only in the detection of meniscal tear, but also because it is strongly associated with the development of osteoarthritis.[3,13]

Errors in Interpretation

Some normal variants may cause confusion in the diagnosis of meniscal tears. For instance, the anterior horn of the lateral meniscus can have a speckled appearance with foci of increased signal. This may be related to blending of the fibers of the anterior cruciate ligament with the anterior horn, or splaying of the fibers of the meniscus at its attachment.[11] This abnormal signal should not be mistaken for a tear or degeneration (Fig. 8-8).

Meniscal flounce is a rare normal variant of the medial meniscus in which there is an undulating appearance of the inner margin, possibly related to ligamentous laxity (Fig. 8-9). This buckling along the free edge may be confused for a meniscal tear, but is not said to increase the risk of tearing. Its prevalence is approximately 0.2%.[11]

The meniscofemoral ligaments of Wrisberg and Humphrey connect the posterior horn of the lateral meniscus to the lateral aspect of the medial femoral condyle. The ligament can divide and course anterior to the posterior cruciate ligament named the ligament of Humphrey, or posterior to the posterior cruciate ligament named the ligament of Wrisberg (Fig. 8-10). The ligaments of Humphrey and Wrisberg are noted in approximately one third of cases. If soft tissue or fluid is interposed between the origin of the meniscofemoral ligament and the posterior horn of the lateral meniscus, this interface can be misinterpreted as a meniscal tear. Care must be taken to follow the ligament over several successive images while avoiding this pitfall.[15]

The transverse intermeniscal ligament courses horizontally between the anterior horns of the medial and lateral menisci, in front of the anterior cruciate ligament. The interface between the ligament and the anterior meniscal horns can also be confused for a tear.[15]

The popliteus tendon travels superiorly from its muscle belly in an oblique, intra-articular course, separating the lateral meniscus from the joint capsule, to insert on the

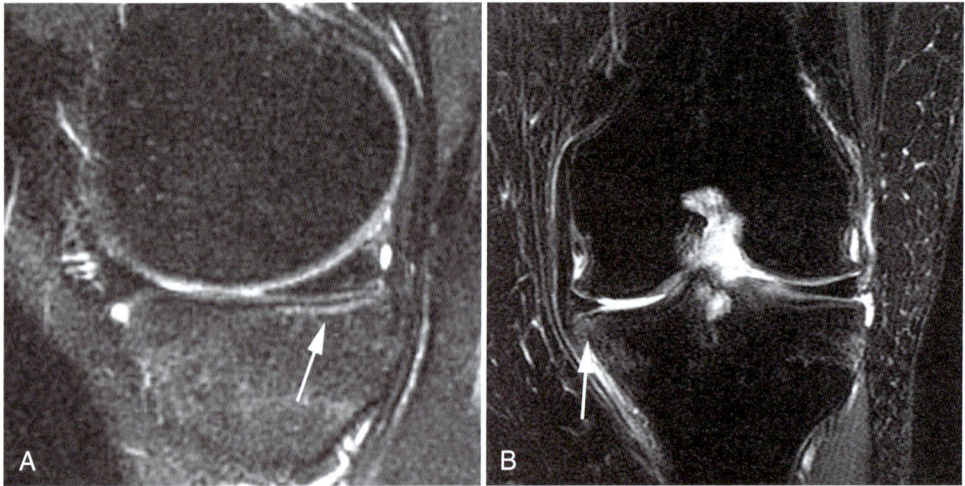

Figure 8-6. **A** through **B,** Secondary signs of meniscal tear: subchondral edema. Sagittal T2-weighted fat-suppressed image **(A)** demonstrates linear subchondral bone marrow edema *(arrow)* adjacent to the posterior horn of the medial meniscus, which contains surfacing signal consistent with tear. Coronal T2-weighted fat-suppressed image in a different patient **(B)** demonstrates cartilage loss in the medial compartment with underlying bone marrow edema *(arrow),* findings commonly seen in association with a meniscal tear.

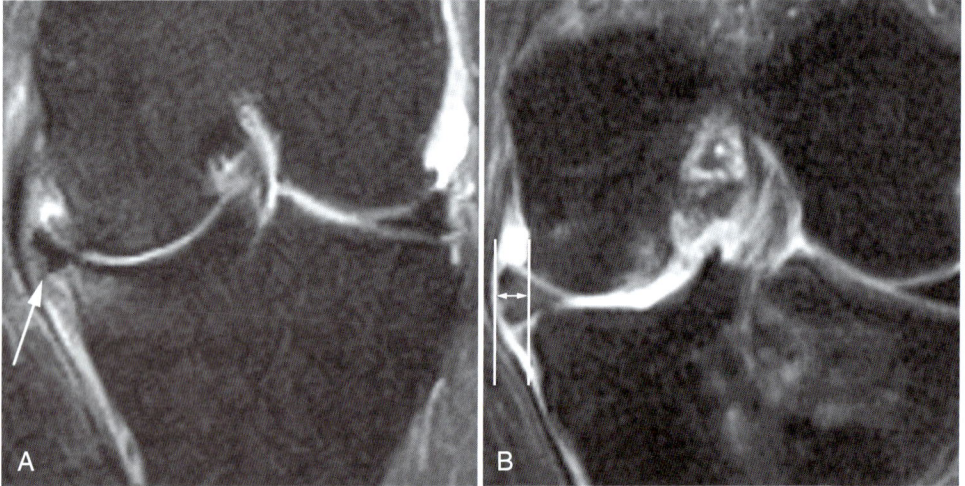

Figure 8-7. **A** and **B,** Secondary signs of meniscal tear: meniscal extrusion. Coronal T2-weighted fat-suppressed images depict extrusion of the periphery of the medial meniscus *(arrow* in **A**) beyond the periphery of the tibial margin. Major meniscal extrusion, demarcated by lines in **(B),** is classified as >3 mm; this finding has a high association with complex, radial, or root tear of the associated meniscus.

popliteal groove along the lateral aspect of the lateral femoral condyle. The popliteal bursa is the opening created by the fascicles of the lateral meniscus, which allow the popliteal tendon to course from its muscle belly into its intra-articular location, and finally to insert on the femur. The medial margin of the popliteal hiatus is the body of the lateral meniscus (Fig. 8-11). Fluid within the popliteus tendon sheath or the popliteal hiatus may be mistaken for a meniscal tear.[7,23]

A meniscal contusion occurs during an acute traumatic event, typically described with an acute anterior cruciate ligament disruption. The meniscus is compressed between the femur and the tibia, becomes contused, and demonstrates altered signal on MRI. The increased signal within the con-tused meniscus is more likely to be amorphous in shape, will

not extend to the articular surface, and may be accompanied by a bone bruise. This may simulate a meniscal tear and result in a false-positive MRI interpretation.[11]

Magic angle phenomenon describes the artifact that occurs when collagen fibers are oriented at 55 degrees relative to the main magnetic field on short TE images. This artifact causes falsely increased signal intensity and can imitate a meniscal tear. This is particularly a dilemma in the posterior horn of the lateral meniscus as it angles upward from its root to the insertion on the tibia behind the intercondylar eminence.[6]

Chondrocalcinosis within the fibrocartilage of the menis-cus can cause a false-positive interpretation for tear. Chon-drocalcinosis results in increased signal on proton density and T1-weighted images, which can be confused with a meniscal

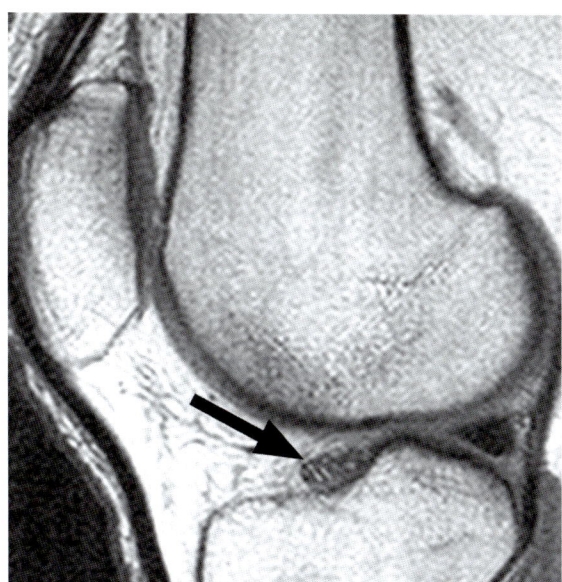

Figure 8-8. Pitfall for meniscal tear: normal intrameniscal signal. Sagittal proton density image shows fibers of the anterior horn of the lateral meniscus spreading apart at the root attachment *(arrow)*. This creates a normal speckled pattern and should not be confused for a meniscal tear.

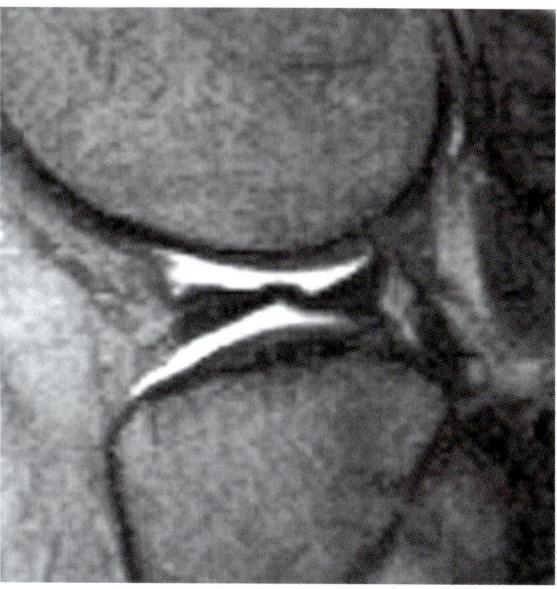

Figure 8-9. Pitfall for meniscal tear: meniscal flounce. Sagittal fluid-sensitive sequence demonstrates buckling of the meniscal body (lateral meniscus pictured), referred to as a meniscal flounce, a normal finding.

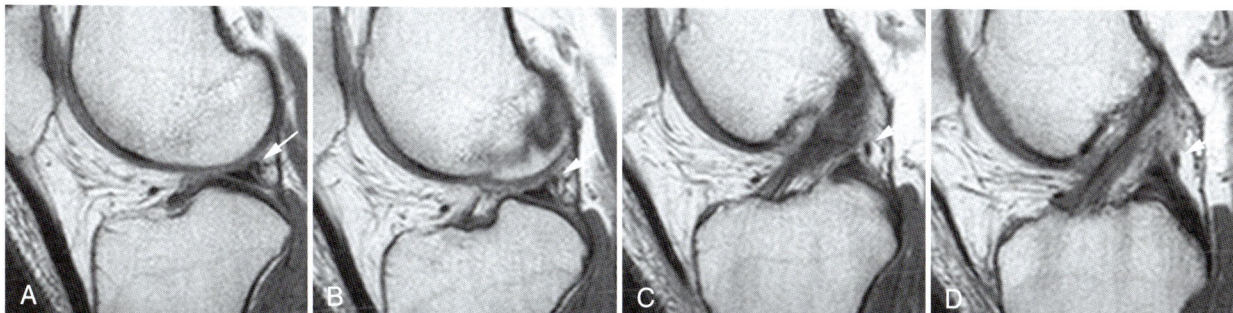

Figure 8-10. **A** through **D,** Pitfall for meniscal tear: meniscofemoral ligament. Consecutive sagittal proton density images show the ligament of Wrisberg *(arrows)* coursing from the posterior horn of the lateral meniscus, posterior to the posterior cruciate ligament (PCL), inserting onto the lateral aspect of the medial femoral condyle; the ligament is seen on magnetic resonance imaging (MRI) in approximately one third of individuals. A similar structure, the ligament of Humphrey, is also seen in about one third of individuals and courses anterior to the PCL. The point of attachment on the meniscus can simulate a tear on MRI.

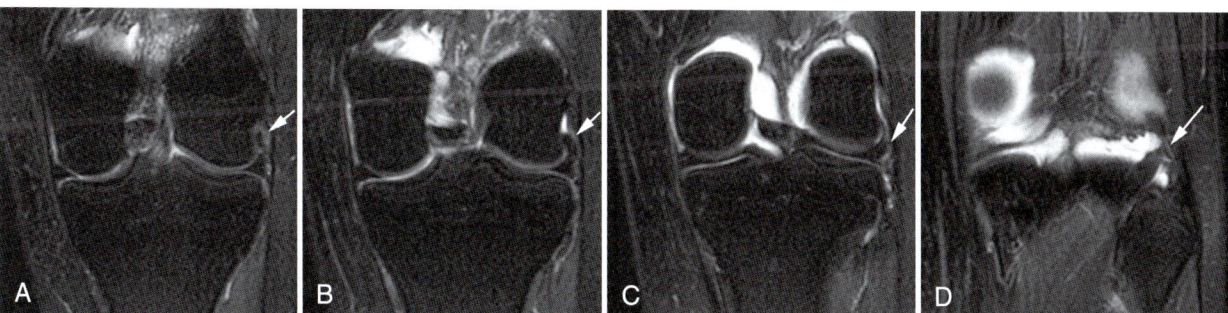

Figure 8-11. **A** through **D,** Pitfall for meniscal tear: popliteus tendon. Consecutive coronal T2-weighted fat-suppressed images show the popliteus tendon *(arrows)* as it originates from the lateral femoral condyle and courses posterolaterally through the popliteal hiatus and inferiorly past the tibial plateau. As the tendon passes by the lateral meniscus, the intervening fluid can be misinterpreted for meniscal tear.

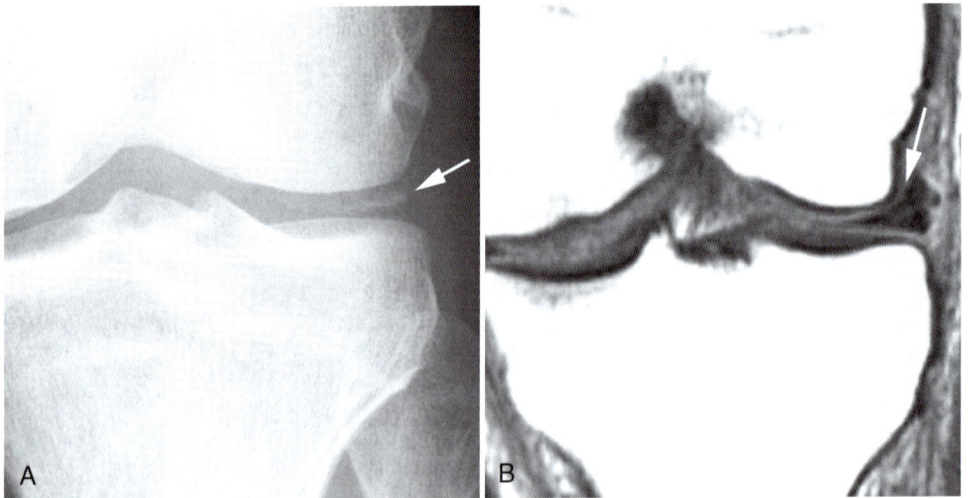

Figure 8-12. **A** and **B,** Pitfall for meniscal tear: chondrocalcinosis. Frontal radiograph **(A)** shows lateral meniscal calcification *(arrow)* representing calcium pyrophosphate crystal deposition. Coronal T1-weighted image **(B)** shows increased lateral meniscal signal corresponding to chondrocalcinosis seen on radiographs. This can simulate a meniscal tear.

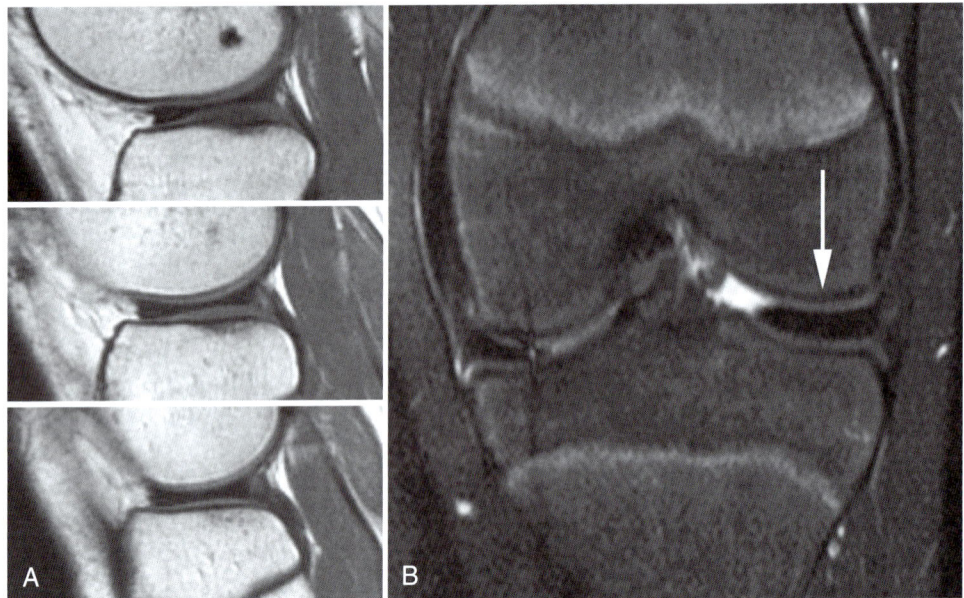

Figure 8-13. **A** and **B,** Discoid meniscus. Three consecutive sagittal proton density images **(A)** suggest discoid morphology of the lateral meniscus, with continuity of the anterior and posterior horns on three consecutive sagittal images. Coronal T2-weighted fat-suppressed image **(B)** through the midpoint of the knee shows a large, pancake-like lateral meniscus extending centrally, consistent with discoid morphology.

tear.[11] Correlation with radiographs may help to detect and confirm the presence of chondrocalcinosis within the meniscus (Fig. 8-12).

Some authors propose that a delay between MRI diagnosis of meniscal tear and arthroscopy may allow for spontaneous healing.[17] When the tear is not identified at surgery, it is documented as a false positive. Others report that healed or surgically repaired meniscal tears may have persistent signal that extends to the articular surface and can be mistaken for a new meniscal tear or retear. Some meniscal tears are more difficult to visualize at arthroscopy, particularly along the inferior surface of the medial meniscus.[7] If these tears are not documented by arthroscopy, which is the gold standard, then they are also reported as false positive.

Other Meniscal Disorders

Discoid meniscus occurs almost exclusively in the lateral meniscus with an incidence of approximately 1% in the general population. Discoid morphology is defined by continuity of the anterior and posterior horns on three or more consecutive sagittal images. It also can be diagnosed on coronal images, if the inner margin of the meniscus courses under or extends past the apex of the femoral condyle (Fig. 8-13). Some propose that a transverse measurement greater than 15 mm, or more than 20% of the tibial width on axial images, can be used to diagnose discoid meniscus. Discoid meniscus can be categorized into three types according to its peripheral attachments. The type that is most commonly symptomatic is the Wrisberg type, which lacks posterior

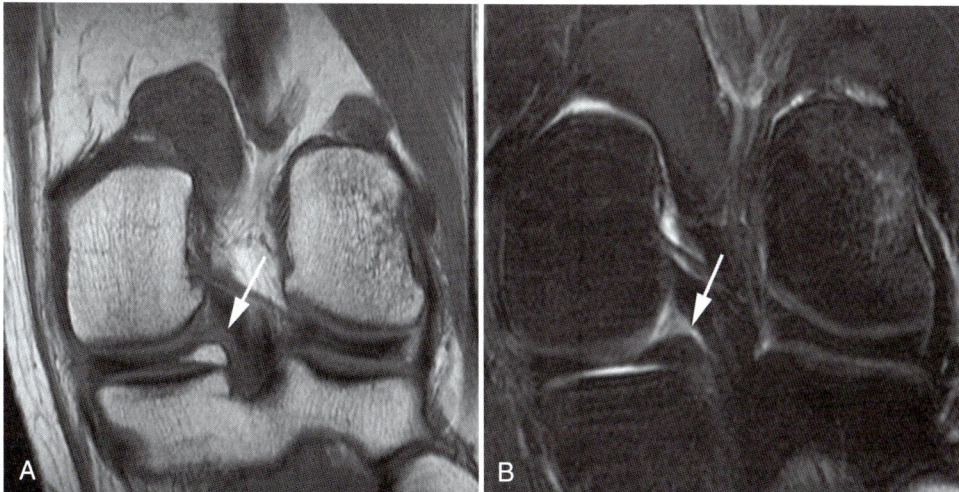

Figure 8-14. **A** and **B,** Meniscal ossicle. Coronal T1- **(A)** and T2-weighted fat-suppressed **(B)** images show ossification *(arrows)* of the posterior root of the medial meniscus, following the signal characteristics of bone marrow on all imaging sequences.

capsular attachments. Discoid menisci are believed to be at increased risk for tear owing to increased mechanical stresses and hypermobility. Medial discoid menisci have been reported, but are rare. The incidence of bilateral lateral discoid menisci has been reported as high as 20%.[12]

Meniscal ossicles are rare and are most commonly seen in young men, with a reported prevalence of 0.15%. The origin of the meniscal ossicle is unknown and is hypothesized to be developmental or related to previous trauma, representing a form of heterotopic ossification. Meniscal ossicles are most commonly found in the posterior horn of the medial meniscus near the root attachment, following the signal characteristics of bone marrow on all imaging sequences (Fig. 8-14). Meniscal ossicles may be asymptomatic or may present with functional impairment and pain. Therapy is guided by the patient's symptoms. Care must be taken not to mistake a meniscal ossicle for an intra-articular body, an avulsion fracture, or even chondrocalcinosis. The diagnosis can be made radiographically, with computed tomography (CT), or on MRI.[14]

Types of Meniscal Tears

Meniscal tears are described according to morphology, location, orientation, and extent. Location and extent are described in reference to the anterior horn, body, and posterior horn. Orientation is described as longitudinal (i.e., along the circumference of the meniscus, paralleling the central meniscal fibers) or radial (i.e., perpendicular to the circumference, crossing through the central fibers). Longitudinal tears can be horizontal (separating the meniscus into top and bottom portions), oblique, or vertical. Vertical longitudinal tears commonly lead to fragment displacement and bucket-handle configuration. Radial tears can be straight or curved (parrot-beak configuration); parrot-beak tears can result in displaced flaps. Tears with variegated type are referred to as complex tears. Tears should also be described as mainly involving the central avascular portion or the peripheral vascularized portion. Small tears of the inner margin or free edge are also described; these tears may not be mechanically significant. Some types of tears are more mechanically

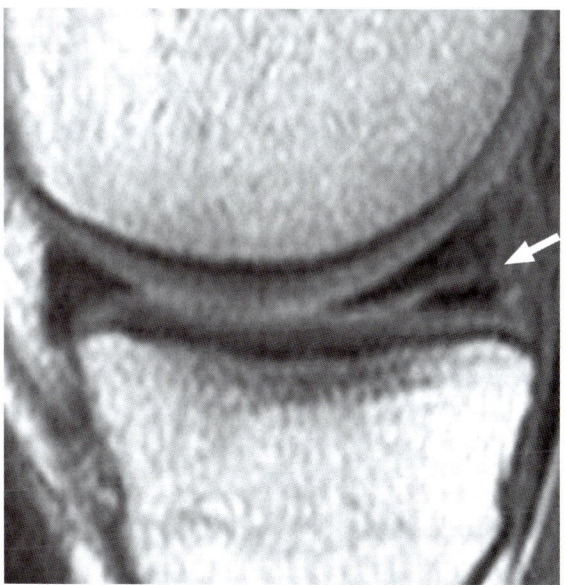

Figure 8-15. Meniscal tear. Sagittal proton density image depicts a longitudinal oblique tear, with surfacing signal to the inferior margin of the posterior horn of the medial meniscus *(arrow).*

significant, including tears involving the root attachments, radial tears, complex tears, and tears with displaced flaps. Tears with meniscal extrusion greater than 3 mm from the tibial margin are associated with more rapid compartmental cartilage loss and can predispose susceptible patients (i.e., those with osteopenia and lack of buttressing from underlying osteoarthritis) to subchondral insufficiency fracture.

Oblique or horizontal tears are most commonly degenerative, often extend to the inferior articular surface, and divide the meniscus into superior and inferior fragments (Fig. 8-15). These tears are typically stable, although an oblique tear extending to the undersurface can lead to development of a flap tear extending from the posterior horn, with the fragment displaced inferior to the meniscal body, in the meniscotibial recess. Frequently, this morphologic pattern of tearing occurs in the posterior horn of the medial meniscus.

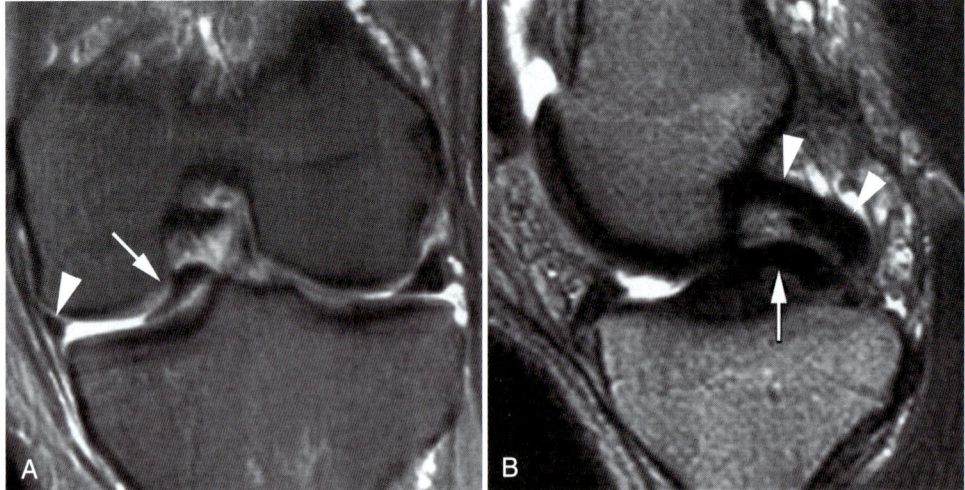

Figure 8-16. A and **B**, Bucket-handle type of meniscal tear. Coronal and sagittal T2-weighted fat-suppressed images show typical findings. The coronal image **(A)** demonstrates truncation of the body of the medial meniscus *(arrowhead)*; the flipped fragment *(arrow)* is displaced centrally. The sagittal image **(B)** shows the double PCL sign, with the flipped meniscal fragment *(arrow)* located beneath the posterior cruciate ligament *(arrowheads)*.

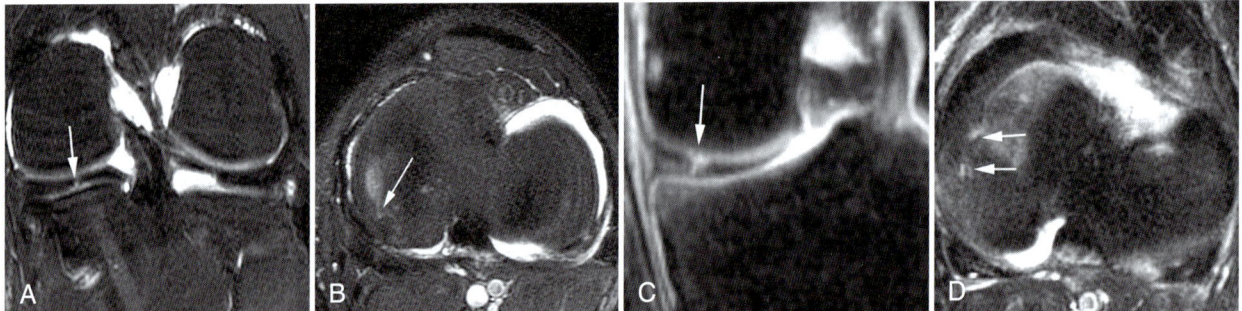

Figure 8-17. A through **D**, Radial tear and parrot-beak meniscal tears. Coronal **(A)** and axial **(B)** T2-weighted fat-suppressed images show a notch in the inner margin of the posterior horn medial meniscus representing a small radial tear, extending vertically perpendicular to the meniscal circumference. Coronal **(C)** and axial **(D)** T2-weighted fat-suppressed images of a different patient show an obliquely oriented radial tear with a shape resembling a parrot's beak *(arrows)*.

If a vertical longitudinal tear extends to involve the anterior horn, body, and posterior horn, the inner fragment may displace centrally into the intercondylar notch, creating a bucket-handle–type tear (Fig. 8-16). On sagittal imaging, the displaced fragment may be seen below the posterior cruciate ligament, creating the double PCL sign (this occurs only in medial bucket-handle tears; lateral fragments are blocked by the intact anterior cruciate ligament). Approximately 95% of bucket-handle tears involve the medial meniscus and are detected by noting an abnormal meniscal size or meniscal truncation. A bucket-handle tear can be mimicked by a torn anterior cruciate ligament or an intra-articular body. Care should be taken not to confuse postsurgical truncation related to débridement from a meniscal tear with displaced fragment.

A radial tear is a type of vertical tear that occurs along the inner margin of the meniscus, perpendicular to the circumference of the meniscus (Fig. 8-17). On sagittal and coronal images, these tears result in a blunted appearance of the normal triangular morphology of the meniscus. Radial tears may be seen only on one slice—a noted exception to the two-slice rule. A parrot-beak tear has a radial tear component, which then extends along the longitudinal axis of the meniscus (curved radial tear). When scrolling through adjacent images, this type of tear will look as though it migrates through the meniscal substance.

A peripheral tear occurs in the outer one third of the meniscus, the area known as the red zone, in reference to its vascular supply (Fig. 8-18). A peripheral tear is amenable to meniscal repair because of the increased vascularity. Alternatively, some surgeons may wait to repair the meniscus, given the possibility that the tear may heal on its own. Care should be taken not to miss these types of tears, which can be difficult to detect, as they tend to blend with the hyperintense perimeniscal tissues and/or joint recesses.

Meniscal root attachments prevent meniscal displacement in a radial direction and act as primary resistance to hoop strain during axial load bearing. Meniscal root tears are often missed and can lead to accelerated osteoarthritis. A root tear should be suspected if, while looking at sagittal images, it appears that the posterior horn has disappeared; these tears are typically radial tears. Meniscal root tears occur medially more often than laterally and are often associated with extrusion and the development of degenerative joint disease (Fig. 8-19).

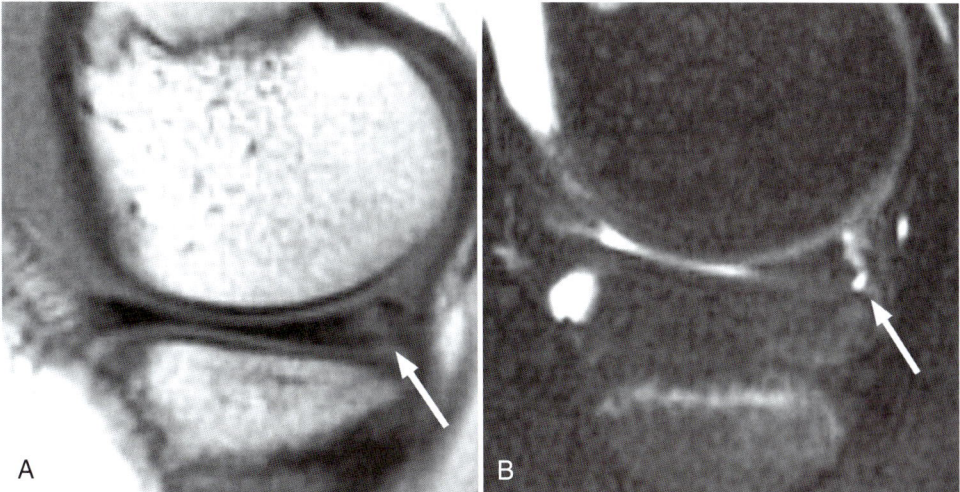

Figure 8-18. A and **B**, Peripheral meniscal tear. Sagittal proton density **(A)** and T2-weighted fat-suppressed images **(B)** show vertical signal extending through the outer margin of the posterior horn medial meniscus *(arrows)*.

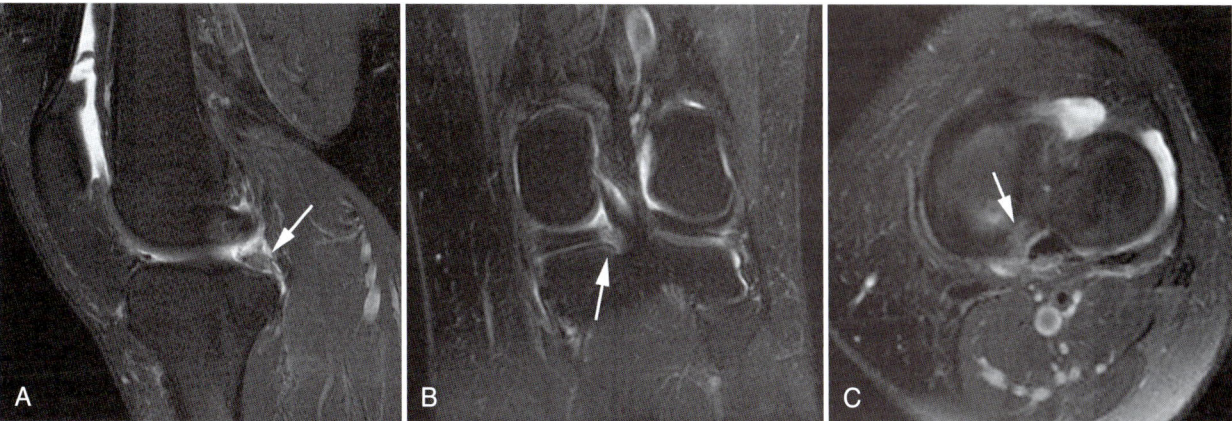

Figure 8-19. A through **C**, Meniscal root tear. Sagittal **(A)**, coronal **(B)**, and axial **(C)** T2-weighted fat-suppressed images show fluid signal extending through the posterior root attachment of the medial meniscus *(arrows)*. Root tears are often radial type, as seen in this example; resultant meniscal destabilization causes extrusion and is strongly associated with subsequent cartilage loss.

A complex tear is a meniscal tear with more than one cleavage plane. Frequently, the tear extends to both the superior and inferior articular surfaces. These tears are more likely to be unstable, lead to meniscal extrusion, and progress to osteoarthritis.

A flap tear is a meniscal tear that results in an isolated fragment, which becomes displaced (Fig. 8-20); flaps commonly become displaced into the meniscotibial or meniscofemoral recess. If the meniscus appears diminutive and there has been no history of meniscectomy, care must be taken to evaluate for a flap tear with a displaced meniscal fragment. Meniscal fragments can also flip anteriorly, creating an enlarged appearance of the anterior horn, or the entire meniscal horn can flip centrally, often posterior to the posterior cruciate ligament (Fig. 8-21).

Meniscal Tear Stability

An unstable meniscal tear is defined as a tear in which a fragment of the meniscus can be displaced by a probe into the femorotibial joint at the time of arthroscopy. Unstable tears lead to meniscal extrusion and accelerated osteoarthritis. Therefore, predicting the stability of a meniscal lesion on MRI helps guide management of the tear, pointing toward spontaneous healing, repair, or resection. The following MRI criteria have been used to evaluate unstable meniscal lesions and have been compared with findings at arthroscopy:

1. A displaced meniscal fragment is visible on MRI.
2. A lesion is visible on more than two 4-mm-thick sagittal and on three 3-mm-thick coronal images.
3. More than one lesion pattern or more than one cleavage plane is present within the meniscus.
4. Fluid signal is present within the meniscus on T2-weighted images.

These MRI criteria for unstable meniscal lesions were found to have high specificity and positive predictive value when compared with findings at arthroscopy. This was important because it meant that unstable meniscal tears could be identified by MRI, and therefore patients who would benefit from arthroscopy could be delineated.[21]

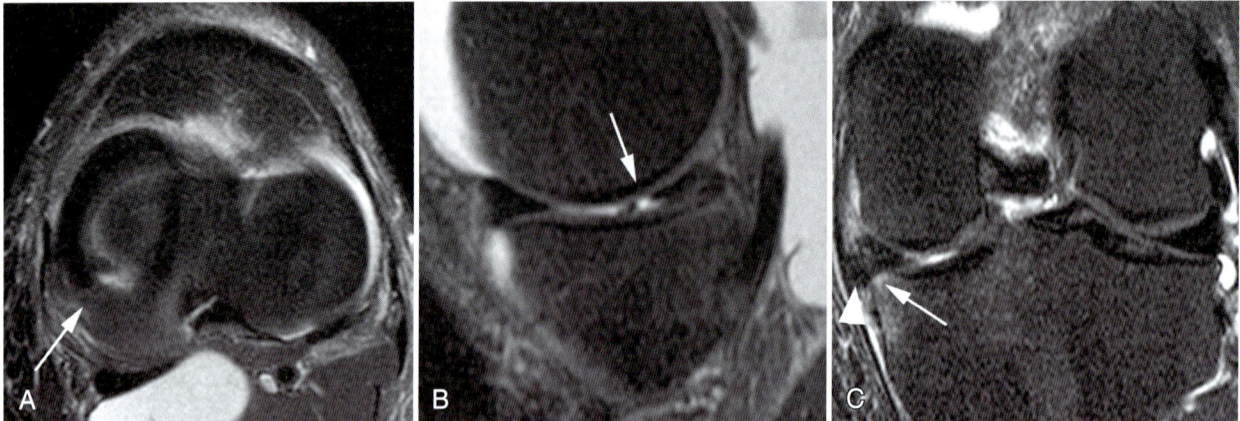

Figure 8-20. A through **C,** Meniscal flap tears. Axial **(A)** and sagittal **(B)** T2-weighted fat-suppressed images show a parrot-beak–type tear at the junction of the body and the posterior horn of the medial meniscus *(arrows)* with displacement of the inner margin fragment. Coronal T2-weighted fat-suppressed image **(C)** of a different patient shows a meniscal fragment *(arrowhead)* flipped under the body of the medial meniscus, into the meniscotibial recess. Note underlying reactive bone marrow edema in the medial tibial plateau *(arrow).*

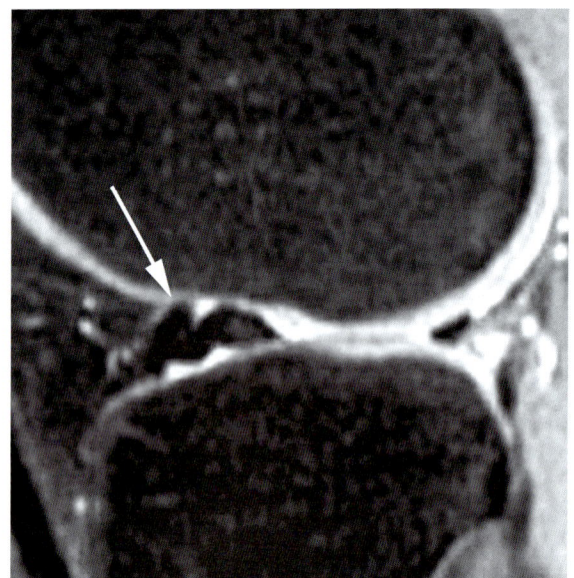

Figure 8-21. Anteriorly flipped meniscal fragment. Sagittal T2-weighted fat-suppressed image though the lateral compartment shows that a large meniscal fragment *(arrow)* originating from the posterior horn has flipped anteriorly and is positioned next to the native anterior horn. This can block full range of motion on extension.

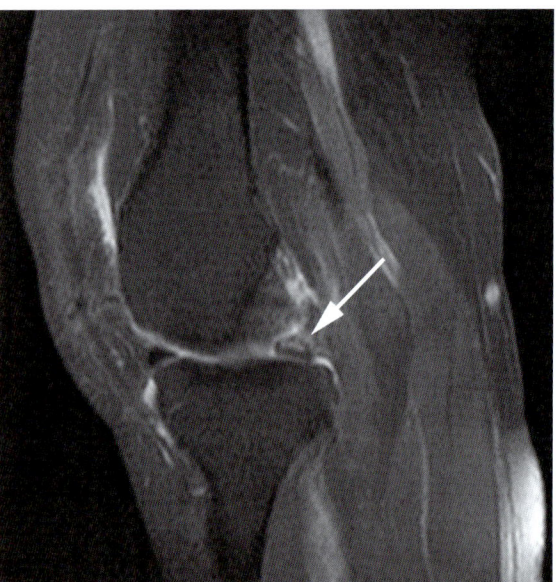

Figure 8-22. Sagittal T1-weighted fat-suppressed image from an indirect magnetic resonance arthrogram (delayed imaging following an intravenous dose of gadolinium contrast) demonstrates contrast within the posterior horn of the medial meniscus *(arrow)* at the site of prior débridement, consistent with recurrent tear.

Postoperative Meniscus

After meniscal repair or meniscal healing, MRI findings of surfacing signal abnormality may persist and may appear no different from the tear initially noted on preoperative imaging. For this reason, standard MRI diagnostic criteria for meniscal tears cannot be applied to the postoperative or healed meniscus. This creates a diagnostic dilemma in the postoperative patient with recurrent or residual symptoms.

Magnetic resonance (MR) arthrography has been promoted for assessment of the postoperative meniscus. With direct MR arthrography, dilute gadolinium contrast is placed directly into the joint under fluoroscopic guidance. The joint is distended by the contrast. Theoretically, intra-articular

contrast will dissect into a residual or recurrent meniscal tear in the postoperative patient, highlighting the abnormality. With indirect MR arthrography, gadolinium contrast is administered intravenously. After an appropriate delay, the knee joint is imaged. A residual or recurrent meniscal tear should enhance beyond adjacent meniscal tissue, accentuating the abnormality (Fig. 8-22). Unfortunately, granulation tissue in a healed meniscus can also enhance, confounding the importance of the finding. Studies comparing diagnostic accuracy between direct and indirect arthrography found no significant difference. CT arthrography has also been suggested as useful for evaluation of the postoperative meniscus (Fig. 8-23). CT is insensitive to the internal degenerative signal that causes confusion on MRI in the postoperative meniscus, and contrast entering the meniscus is specific for retear.[4]

Noncontrast MRI can also evaluate for a retear in the postoperative meniscus. In a symptomatic patient with clinical suspicion for meniscal retear, the fluid-sensitive sequence is most specific for diagnosis. Fluid signal within the meniscus tracking to the articular surface is highly predictive of retear. This represents free fluid tracking through the meniscal tear and simulates the arthrographic effects of contrast insinuating into the tear.[4] Secondary signs of meniscal tear, including associated subchondral bone marrow edema, parameniscal

cyst, and adjacent collateral ligament edema, may also prove to be important.

Spontaneous Osteonecrosis of the Knee (SONK)

Spontaneous osteonecrosis of the knee, also referred to as SONK, is an outdated term that describes subchondral insufficiency fractures typically found along the weight-bearing aspect of the medial femoral condyle in middle-aged to elderly patients, more commonly females. The entity can also involve the lateral femoral condyle or the tibial plateau and is believed to be related to altered biomechanics and weight bearing following a meniscal tear or meniscal surgery. On MRI, the subchondral fracture line is hypointense on T1- and T2-weighted images with extensive adjacent bone marrow edema. Bone marrow edema may even extend to the femoral notch (Fig. 8-24). Following intravenous gadolinium administration, the subchondral fracture line will not enhance.

Subchondral insufficiency fractures are usually treated conservatively. However, if treatment is not effective or is delayed, the insufficiency fracture can progress to osteonecrosis and articular collapse, requiring surgery. In later stages, the subchondral fracture line becomes less visible, bone marrow edema decreases, and findings of osteonecrosis and osteoarthritis dominate.

CARTILAGE

Cartilage and Osteochondral Injuries

Hyaline cartilage covers the articular surface of the knee joint and is composed of chondrocytes surrounded by a medium of collagen, proteoglycans, and electrolytes. Hyaline cartilage acts to aid in resistance against compressive and shearing forces, predominantly by dissipating the forces to the menisci and subchondral bone.[19] Because of the prevalence of degenerative osteoarthritis, imaging of hyaline cartilage has become an important focus of diagnostic radiology research.

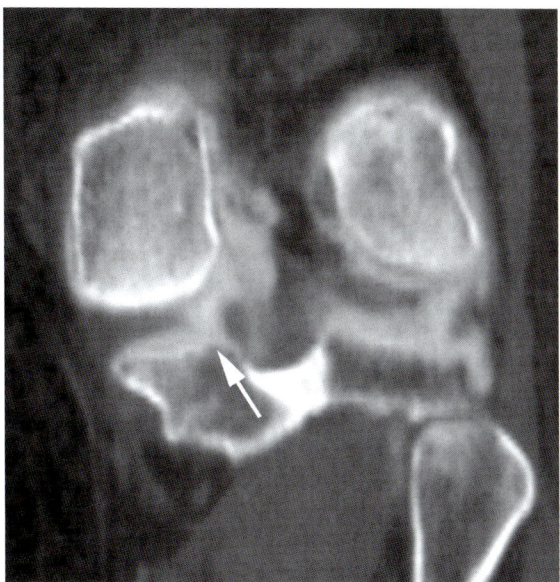

Figure 8-23. Meniscal tear on computed tomography (CT) arthrogram. Coronal reconstruction CT image through the posterior aspect of the knee following intra-articular injection of contrast in a patient with prior meniscal surgery and recurrent knee pain shows contrast dissecting through a large radial tear in the posterior horn of the medial meniscus *(arrow),* near its posterior root attachment.

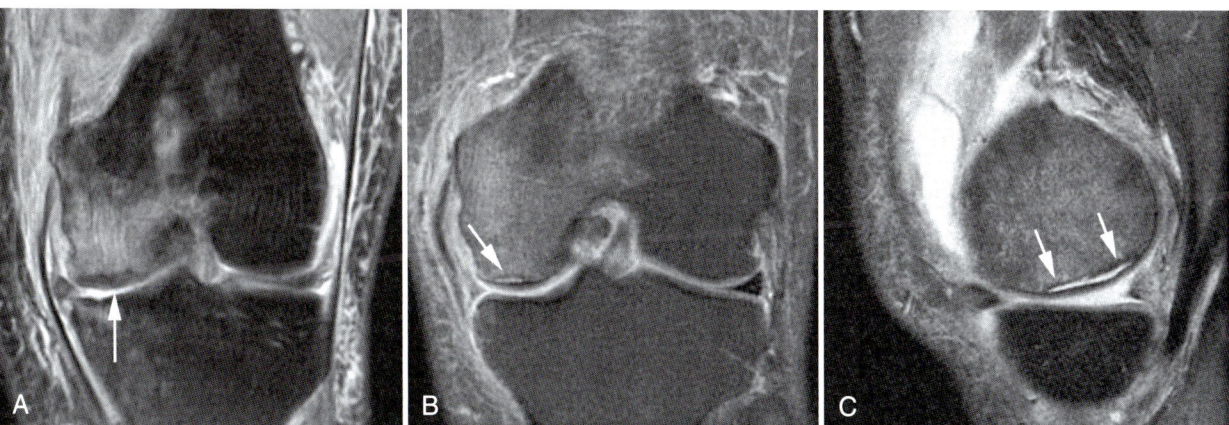

Figure 8-24. A through **C,** Spontaneous osteonecrosis of the knee (SONK), also known as a subchondral insufficiency fracture (SIFK). Coronal T2-weighted fat-suppressed image **(A)** shows the classic magnetic resonance features, with diffuse bone marrow edema in the medial femoral condyle and a low signal crescent in the subchondral bone *(arrow)* representing the fracture line. Note associated meniscal extrusion that is often seen with this phenomenon. Surrounding soft tissue edema related to hyperemia is also commonly seen. The fracture can progress to osteonecrosis. Coronal **(B)** and sagittal **(C)** T2-weighted fat-suppressed images of a different patient demonstrate articular collapse at the site of subchondral fracture *(arrows),* with delamination of the overlying hyaline cartilage.

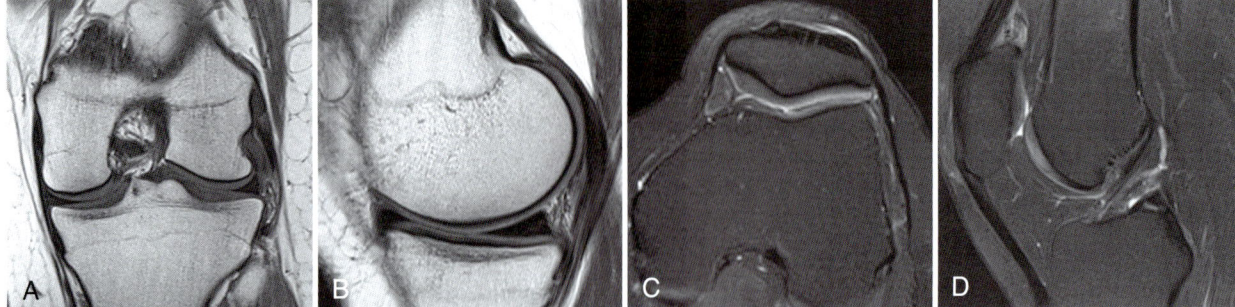

Figure 8-25. A through **D,** Normal articular cartilage. Normal cartilage is demonstrated on coronal T1 **(A),** sagittal proton density **(B),** axial T2-weighted fat-suppressed **(C),** and sagittal T2-weighted fat-suppressed **(D)** images. Articular cartilage has intermediate signal on T1- and T2-weighted images; on most sequences, fat suppression results in higher relative cartilage signal. Achieving high resolution and a pronounced difference in brightness of cartilage and joint fluid is essential for imaging cartilage abnormalities. Note poor contrast between cartilage and joint fluid on the T1-weighted image **(A).**

MRI of Hyaline Cartilage

To adequately image hyaline cartilage in the knee, adequate differences in signal intensity (contrast) must be evident between joint fluid, hyaline cartilage, and subchondral bone. Additionally, spatial resolution must be optimized, allowing for differentiation between cartilage thinning, fissuring, and partial-thickness and full-thickness defects.

No universal MRI sequence has been dedicated for hyaline cartilage imaging. Proton density and T2-weighted fast spin echo sequences with fat suppression provide sufficient contrast between higher signal joint fluid and intermediate signal cartilage to detect chondral abnormalities. Both proton density and T2-weighted fast spin echo sequences produce high signal-to-noise ratio images with relatively short acquisition times. Short T1 inversion recovery (STIR) images may also provide sufficient contrast resolution to evaluate for chondral abnormalities, but intrinsically have lower signal-to-noise ratio and spatial resolution. Two- or three-dimensional (2D or 3D) gradient imaging sequences can improve resolution and can more accurately evaluate the superficial surface of the cartilage; however, these sequences generally require a longer acquisition time, are limited for use in evaluation of deeper cartilage layers, and are more susceptible to imaging artifacts.[19] MRI diagnostic capabilities in low-grade cartilage lesions are limited by contrast and spatial resolution, partial volume averaging, and artifact.

Normal articular cartilage has a homogeneous or laminar appearance with a smooth surface contour. Articular cartilage has intermediate signal on both T1- and T2-weighted images (Fig. 8-25). Fat-suppression techniques can be used on any sequence and have the advantage of increasing apparent signal of the hyaline cartilage relative to other tissues (i.e., cartilage appears bright on fat-suppressed images, regardless of the sequence used).

Chondral abnormalities are diagnosed on MRI by recognizing a contour defect within the cartilage, focal thinning compared with the thickness of the adjacent cartilage, and/or signal alteration within the cartilage (Figs. 8-26 through 8-30). A secondary sign of cartilage defect includes underlying bone marrow edema, as manifested by increased signal in the subchondral bone on fat-suppressed proton density and T2-weighted images. Subchondral bone marrow edema is a nonspecific finding that may be seen with acute injury (bone contusion or bruise, fracture), mechanical disturbance such

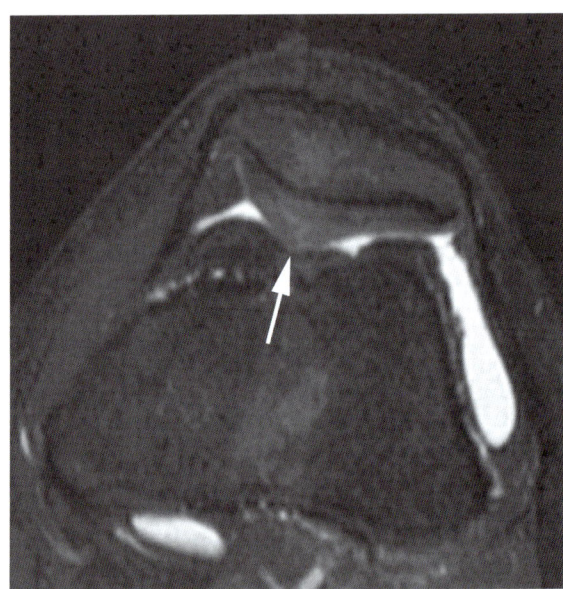

Figure 8-26. Low-grade chondromalacia. Axial T2-weighted fat-suppressed image shows swollen, T2 hyperintense cartilage *(arrow)* along the median ridge of the patella.

as stress response or overlying meniscal tear, and many other conditions, including metabolic and neoplastic lesions. However, a flame-shaped or rounded focus of marrow edema in the subchondral bone should initiate a search for overlying hyaline cartilage abnormality.

Cartilage damage can be related to acute trauma, prolonged and repetitive stress, and degeneration. Numerous classifications have been proposed to grade cartilage lesions based largely on arthroscopic findings, and less so on MRI findings. These classification systems describe articular cartilage damage ranging from swelling and signal heterogeneity to fissuring, ulceration, partial-thickness defects, and full-thickness defects with exposure of the subchondral bone.

The Outerbridge scale classifies cartilage abnormalities based on arthroscopic findings. Grade I includes softening or swelling of the articular cartilage, Grade II describes cartilage fragmentation and fissuring less than 1.5 cm in diameter, Grade III describes cartilage fragmentation and fissuring greater than 1.5 cm in diameter, and Grade IV involves cartilage erosion to bone.[18] The International Cartilage Repair Society has adopted the classification system described by Yulish and associates. Grade 0 represents normal cartilage, Grade 1 describes increased T2 signal within the cartilage, Grade 2 refers to a partial-thickness defect less than 50% of normal cartilage thickness, Grade 3 represents a partial-thickness defect greater than 50% of normal cartilage thickness, and Grade 4 describes a full-thickness defect.[16] In the Noyes system, Grade 1 depicts an intact cartilage surface, Grade 2A reflects cartilage damage with less than 50% cartilage thickness involved, Grade 2B cartilage defects involve greater than half of the cartilage thickness, and Grade 3 represents full-thickness cartilage defects with exposed subchondral bone (3A cortical surface is intact, 3B cortical surface shows cavitation) (Table 8-2).

Aside from grading cartilage loss, assessing the location, size, and morphology of the cartilage defect is also important. Chondral injuries in weight-bearing areas have a worse prognosis and different treatment implications than those in non–weight-bearing areas. Traumatic chondral injuries are usually focal and may have acute margins with adjacent shoulders. They may be partial thickness or full thickness and can shear off from the cortex, resulting in an intra-articular body.[22]

In osteoarthritis, the cartilage thins particularly along weight-bearing aspects and degenerates with fraying, fissuring, ulceration, and sometimes delaminating defects. Accompanying osteophyte formation, subchondral cystic change,

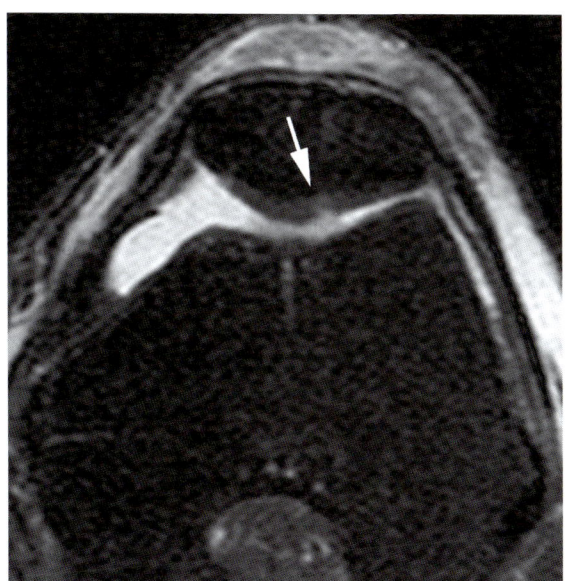

Figure 8-27. Partial-thickness cartilage defect. Axial T2-weighted fat-suppressed image demonstrates diffuse patellar cartilage thinning with focal partial-thickness cartilage loss at the lateral facet *(arrow)*, accounting for <50% of the normal cartilage thickness.

Table 8-2 Chondral Injury Classifications

Outerbridge	ICRS	Noyes
Grade I: softening and swelling of cartilage	Grade 0: normal cartilage	Grade 1: intact cartilage surface
Grade II: cartilage fragmentation and fissuring <1.5 cm diameter	Grade 1: increased T2 signal in the cartilage	Grade 2A: cartilage surface damaged with <50% thickness involved
Grade III: fragmentation and fissuring >1.5 cm diameter	Grade 2: partial-thickness defect <50% of normal cartilage thickness	Grade 2B: cartilage defects involve >50% cartilage thickness
Grade IV: cartilage erosion to bone	Grade 3: partial-thickness defect >50% of normal cartilage thickness	Grade 3: bone exposed (3A cortical surface intact, 3B cortical surface cavitation)
	Grade 4: full-thickness defect	

ICRS, International Cartilage Repair Society.

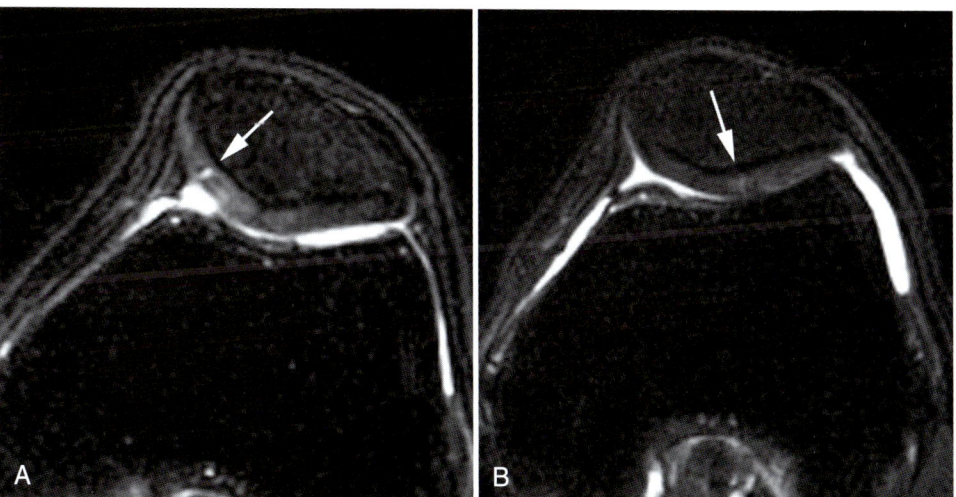

Figure 8-28. **A** and **B,** Full-thickness cartilage fissuring. Axial T2-weighted fat-suppressed image **(A)** depicts a small fissure at the medial patellar facet *(arrow)*. Axial T2-weighted fat-suppressed image of a different patient **(B)** shows a broader area of cartilage surface irregularity at the lateral facet with a full-thickness fissure *(arrow)*.

bone marrow edema, and sclerosis may occur. Several studies have demonstrated that meniscal root tears, large radial meniscal tears, and severe meniscal degeneration are strongly associated with major meniscal extrusion and may precede or even accelerate the development of osteoarthritis with cartilage loss.[22]

Inflammatory arthritides result in diffuse, uniform cartilage thinning throughout the joint, with uniform joint space narrowing. Focal cartilage defects are not typical. However, in areas of inflammatory pannus, focal cartilage and bony erosions may be found. Significant osteophyte formation should not occur.[22]

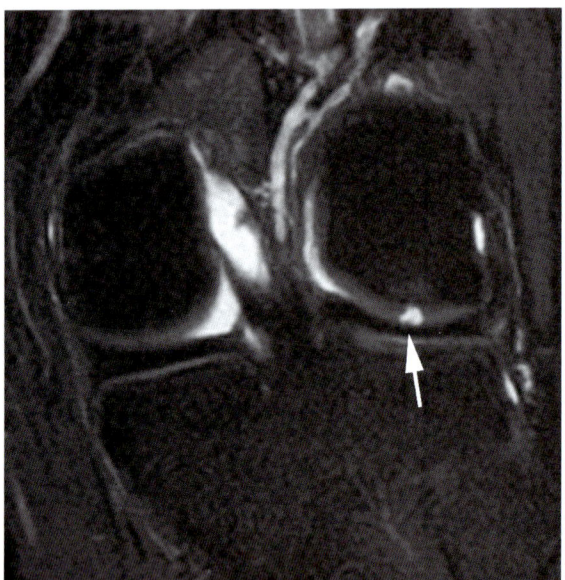

Figure 8-29. Focal full-thickness defect. Coronal T2-weighted fat-suppressed image shows a focal full-thickness cartilage defect *(arrow)* along the lateral femoral condyle. Reactive underlying subchondral bone marrow edema is evident.

Osteochondral Lesions

The term osteochondral lesion is used to describe a spectrum of disease from traumatic osteochondral injury to chronic osteochondritis dissecans. Lesions may arise from forces applied to the chondral surface in a single traumatic event or over time as the result of repeated minor injury. Damage to the underlying subchondral bone ensues. The bone may become necrotic and collapse. If the cartilage surface is damaged, fluid can extend from the joint into the bone and the fragment can separate, eventually detaching and forming a loose body. Alternatively, especially if the overlying cartilage remains intact, the underlying bone can heal. Overlying cartilage can itself delaminate and become displaced as an intra-articular body, or it may degenerate and become thinned and fissured. Most commonly, osteochondral lesions are encountered in the talus, femoral condyles, and elbow.

Traumatic Osteochondral Lesions

A traumatic osteochondral lesion occurs when shearing, compressive, or rotational forces are transmitted between two articular surfaces, resulting in a chondral or subchondral fracture (Fig. 8-31). A cartilage flap or an osteochondral fragment may form, depending on the depth of the fracture line. This injury is typically associated with tenderness, a joint effusion, and sometimes even hemarthrosis. Elevated intra-articular pressure is thought to force synovial fluid into the cartilage flap or beneath the osteochondral fragment, resulting in resorption of the subchondral bone and cystic change. Sometimes the cartilage flap or osteochondral fragment dissociates from the underlying bone, resulting in an intra-articular body.[16]

Osteochondritis Dissecans

Osteochondritis dissecans (OCD) is a somewhat outdated term, although it is still in common use; a better term is *osteochondral lesion.* Nevertheless, the term OCD typically refers to an osteochondral lesion that is discovered

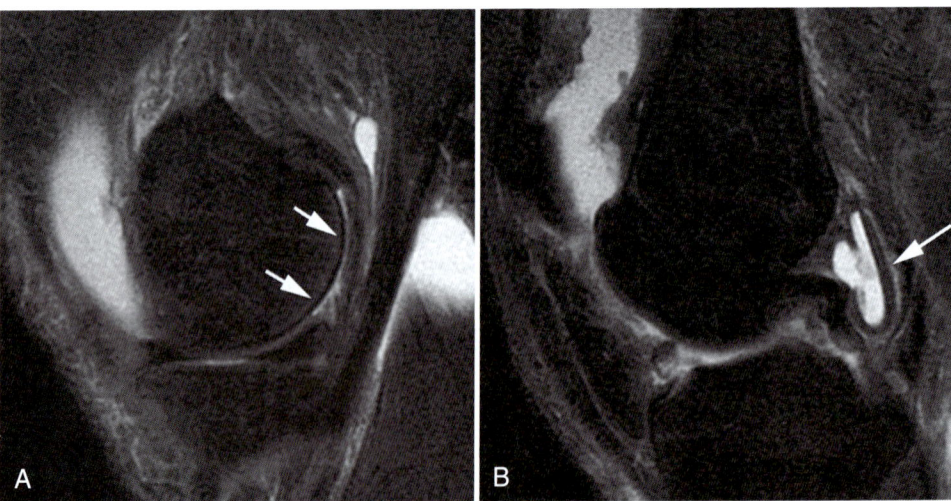

Figure 8-30. **A** and **B,** Cartilage delamination. Sagittal T2-weighted fat-suppressed images demonstrate a broad area of full-thickness cartilage loss from the posterior aspect of the medial femoral condyle *(arrows* in **A**). The cartilage has delaminated from the femoral condyle and is seen displaced into the posterior joint space *(arrow* in **B**).

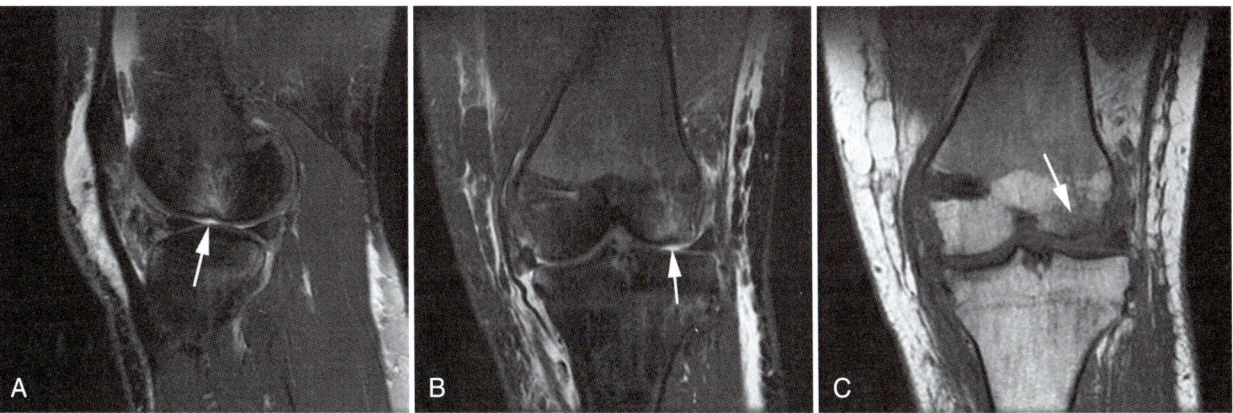

Figure 8-31. **A** through **C,** Osteochondral impaction injury. Sagittal T2-weighted fat-suppressed **(A),** coronal T2-weighted fat-suppressed **(B),** and coronal T1-weighted **(C)** images show an osteochondral impaction injury along the lateral femoral condyle *(arrows)* consistent with a pivot shift mechanism of injury.

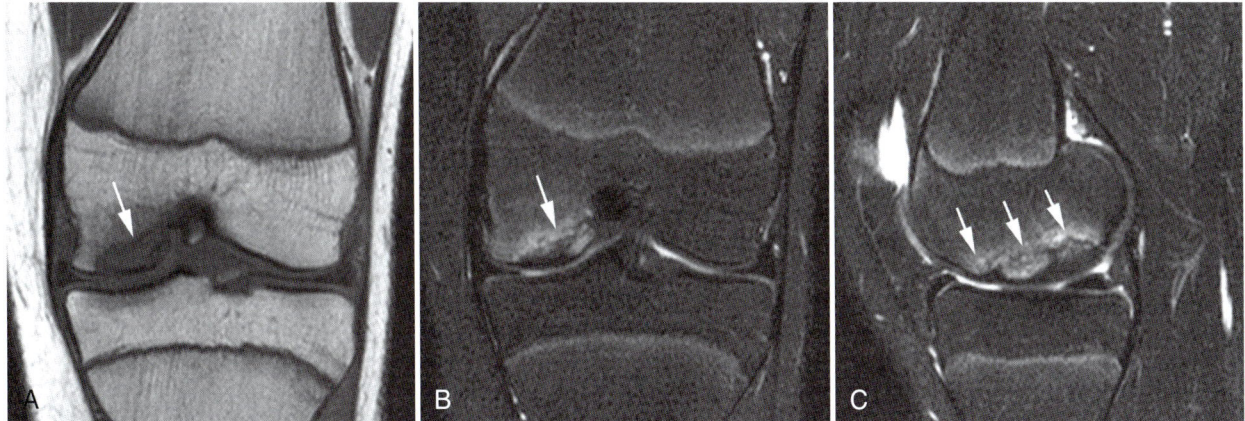

Figure 8-32. **A** through **C,** Osteochondral lesion. Coronal T1-weighted **(A),** coronal T2-weighted fat-suppressed **(B),** and sagittal T2-weighted fat-suppressed **(C)** images show a chronic osteochondral lesion *(arrows)* along the lateral aspect of the medial femoral condyle. This is also referred to as osteochondritis dissecans. Underlying cystic change seen in **(B)** suggests instability; black signal in **(A)** in the subchondral bone suggests underlying necrosis.

incidentally and is presumed to represent a chronic injury. Classic OCD is most commonly seen in young patients between 10 and 20 years of age. The idiopathic variety of OCD often occurs in the lateral aspect of the medial femoral condyle, along the non–weight-bearing aspect near the intercondylar notch, possibly related to microtrauma between the tibial spine and the medial femoral condyle during internal rotation of the tibia. Repetitive microinjuries are thought to disrupt blood supply to the subchondral bone, sometimes resulting in osteonecrosis and progressing to an osteochondral lesion. The natural progression of stable OCD (i.e., with intact overlying cartilage) is spontaneous healing. However, if the lesion is painful and unstable, surgery is usually indicated.

MRI should be performed to accurately characterize OCD, to evaluate size and location, and to determine the stability of the lesion (Fig. 8-32). The osteonecrotic fragment has low signal intensity on T1- and T2-weighted images. Measurement is generally performed using T1-weighted images. Surrounding bone marrow edema is variable and may represent healing response or irritation from lesion instability, so this finding is nonspecific; however, it is often the case that the

more bone marrow edema is present, the more painful the lesion is. An unstable lesion is identified by one or more of the following findings on T2-weighted fat-suppressed images or STIR images: (1) linear high signal intensity surrounding the osteochondral fragment, (2) cystic change interposed between the osteochondral fragment and normal bone, or (3) overlying cartilage defect or fissuring.[5] Intra-articular gadolinium may dissect beneath the osteochondral fragment, also indicating lesion instability.

OCD was initially graded by Berndt and Harty into four stages, with the first two stages indicating lesion stability, and the last two stages signifying instability. Stage 1 demonstrates no discontinuity between the osteochondral lesion and surrounding bone, Stage 2 describes a partially detached but stable osteochondral lesion, Stage 3 refers to a completely detached osteochondral lesion that is not dislocated, and Stage 4 represents a completely detached and displaced osteochondral fragment. The Anderson MRI classification of OCD is more widely used; it was initially created to describe osteochondral lesions of the talus (OLT), but can be applied to the knee and other areas. Stage I refers to the presence of bone marrow edema, Stage IIa describes underlying

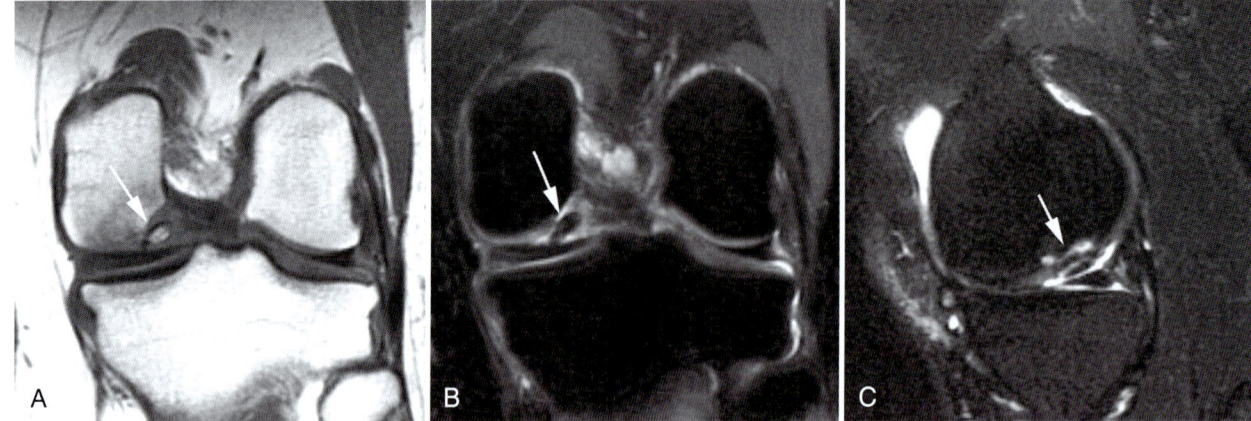

Figure 8-33. A through **C,** Osteochondral lesion. Coronal T1-weighted **(A),** coronal T2-weighted fat-suppressed **(B),** and sagittal T2-weighted fat-suppressed **(C)** images demonstrate an unstable osteochondral lesion along the lateral aspect of the medial femoral condyle. Fluid is interposed between the osteochondral lesion and the normal femoral condyle. The fragment is partially detached. This corresponds to Anderson stage IV.

subchondral cystic change, Stage IIb refers to a partially detached osteochondral lesion with bone marrow edema, Stage III lesions have fluid undermining a nondisplaced and completely detached osteochondral lesion, and Stage IV describes a completely detached and displaced osteochondral fragment (Fig. 8-33). One criticism of this classification is that bone marrow edema may be present at any stage and appears to be a nonspecific finding.[9,16]

A healed osteochondral lesion will not demonstrate fluid bright signal between the osteochondral fragment and the host bone. Normal bone marrow fat signal will return to the osteochondral fragment once it heals. The overlying articular cartilage may be intact, without contour irregularities, or may exhibit degeneration, thinning, or fraying.

Recent Advances in MRI of Cartilage

Current MRI of articular cartilage utilizes 2D multislice acquisitions with small gaps between slices. Three-dimensional imaging, typically spoiled gradient recalled echo with fat suppression, allows for volumetric image acquisition, producing high contrast between the signal of cartilage and adjacent joint fluid. Three-dimensional spoiled gradient recalled (SPGR) sequence is the standard for evaluating cartilage volume and thickness, but is limited for use in evaluating internal cartilage abnormalities (e.g., degeneration, delamination) and other joint pathology.

Driven equilibrium Fourier transform (DEFT) imaging uses a 90-degree pulse to return magnetization to the z-axis, and increases signal from tissues with long T1 relaxation time. This results in high signal synovial fluid and improved contrast between cartilage and fluid at a short time to repetition (TR). The contrast between cartilage and synovial fluid with DEFT imaging is superior to that with SPGR, proton density fast spin echo, and T2-weighted fast spin echo images.[10]

Balanced steady-state free precession (SSFP) is also known as trueFISP (true fast imaging with steady-state precession, Siemens Healthcare, Malvern, Pa), FIESTA (fast imaging employing steady-state acquisition, GE Healthcare, Buckinghamshire, UK), or BFFE (balanced fast-field echo imaging,

Philips Healthcare, Andover, Mass), depending on the MRI scanner manufacturer. Images are 3D volumetric acquisitions, synovial fluid is hyperintense, and tissue contrast is sufficient for evaluation of cartilage and for imaging internal derangement.[10]

T2 relaxation time mapping is based on the knowledge that T1 and T2 relaxation times are constant for a given tissue at specific MRI field strengths. Alteration of relaxation time within a given tissue may be related to pathology or introduction of a contrast agent. T2 relaxation time mapping detects the water content within cartilage, with altered water content correlating with cartilage damage. A color or gray scale map depicting the T2 relaxation time is created, illustrating areas of cartilage damage.[10]

Delayed gadolinium-enhanced MRI of cartilage (dGEMRIC) refers to the use of Magnevist, or gadopentetate dimeglumine, in the evaluation of cartilage damage. Magnevist carries a negative ionic charge, which facilitates its diffusion into cartilage and concentration in areas of decreased glycosaminoglycan (GAG) content. A T1 map is created, demonstrating glycosaminoglycan content. Areas of decreased GAG correspond to damaged cartilage.[10]

KEY REFERENCES

Bergin D, Hochberg H, Zoga AC, et al: Indirect soft-tissue and osseous signs on knee MRI of surgically proven meniscal tears. AJR Am J Roentgenol 191:86–92, 2008.

Campbell SE, Sanders TG, Morrison WB: MR imaging of meniscal cysts: incidence, location, and clinical significance. AJR Am J Roentgenol 177:409–413, 2001.

Costa CR, Morrison WB, Carrino JA: Medial meniscus extrusion on knee MRI: is extent associated with severity of degeneration or type of tear? AJR Am J Roentgenol 183:17–23, 2004.

DeSmet AA, Norris MA, Yandow DR, et al: MR diagnosis of meniscal tears of the knee: importance of high signal in the meniscus that extends to the surface. AJR Am J Roentgenol 161:101–107, 1993.

DeSmet AA, Tuite MJ: Use of the "two-slice-touch" rule for the MRI diagnosis of meniscal tears. AJR Am J Roentgenol 187:911–914, 2006.

Elias I, Jung JW, Raikin SM, et al: Osteochondral lesions of the talus: change in MRI findings over time in talar lesions without operative intervention and implications for staging systems. Foot Ankle Int 27:157–166, 2006.

Gold GE, Chen CA, Koo S, Hargreaves BA, Bangerter NK: Recent advances in MRI of articular cartilage. AJR Am J Roentgenol 193:628–638, 2009.

Helms CA: The meniscus: recent advances in MR imaging of the knee. AJR Am J Roentgenol 179:1115–1122, 2002.

Kocher MS, Klingele K, Rassman SO: Meniscal disorders: normal, discoid, and cysts. Orthop Clin North Am 34:329–340, 2003.

Lerer DB, Umans HR, Hu MX, Jones MH: The role of meniscal root pathology and radial meniscal tear in medial meniscal extrusion. Skeletal Radiol 33:569–574, 2004.

Pope TL, Bloem HL, Beltran J, Morrison WB, Wilson DJ: Imaging of the musculoskeletal system, ed 1, Philadelphia, 2008, Saunders Elsevier, pp 567–596, 665–689.

Rodríguez-Merchán EC, Gómez-Cardero PG: The Outerbridge classification predicts the need for patellar resurfacing in TKA. Clin Orthop Relat Res 468:1254–1257, 2010.

Sonin AH, Pensy RA, Mulligan ME, Hatem S: Grading articular cartilage of the knee using fast spin-echo proton density weighted MR imaging without fat suppression. AJR Am J Roentgenol 179:1159–1166, 2002.

Vande Berg BC, Poilvache P, Duchateau F, et al: Lesions of the menisci of the knee: value of MR imaging criteria for recognition of unstable lesions. AJR Am J Roentgenol 176:771–776, 2001.

Verstraete KL, Almqvist F, Verdonk P, et al: Magnetic resonance imaging of cartilage and cartilage repair. Clin Radiol 59:674–689, 2004.

Full references for this chapter can be found on www.expertconsult.com.

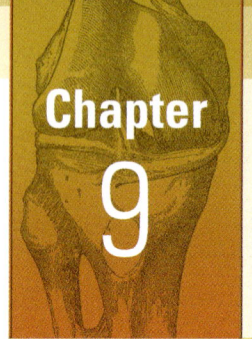

Chapter 9

Arthropathies, Osteonecrosis, and Bursitis

Gabrielle P. Konin and Daniel M. Walz

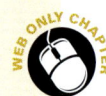

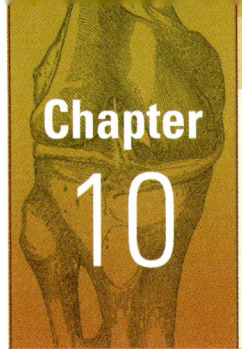

Imaging of Total Knee Arthroplasty

Michael K. Brooks, Christopher J. Palestro, and Barbara N. Weissman

Total knee arthroplasty results in improvement in overall quality of life in more than 90% of patients.[79] This remarkable success and factors such as an aging population have led to a dramatic increase in the number of procedures performed and to corresponding increases in the number of imaging studies obtained for assessment (http://www.cdc.gov/nchs/data/nhsr/nhsr005.pdf). In addition to radiography, computed tomography (CT), magnetic resonance imaging (MRI), ultrasonography (US), arthrography, and a number of nuclear medicine studies are now available for evaluation of knee arthroplasty. It is the responsibility of both imagers and clinicians to provide the most efficacious and cost-effective examinations in a particular clinical situation. This chapter reviews some available imaging techniques, expected findings in uncomplicated and complicated cases, and the efficacy of various techniques in assessing complications.

IMAGING

Radiographs

Preoperative Radiographs

Preoperative radiographs often include supine anteroposterior (AP) and lateral and tangential patellar views of the affected knee, as well as standing AP and flexed PA views of both knees and an AP standing radiograph of both legs.[68] At the Brigham and Women's Hospital, lateral radiographs are usually obtained cross-table lateral with the knee in maximal extension. When digital radiographs are used, a standard-sized reference object is placed alongside the knee to allow assessment of magnification.

The standing view of both legs allows the mechanical axis (a line drawn from the center of the femoral head to the center of the tibial plafond) and the femoral (along the femoral shaft) and tibial anatomic axes to be defined. Normally, the mechanical axis passes through the center of the knee, and the angle between the anatomic and mechanical axes measures 5 to 8 degrees.[73] Standing radiographs of the legs are used to plan the femoral resection, so as to re-create normal mechanical alignment. McGrory and associates, however, found that this examination did not significantly aid in obtaining a neutral mechanical axis as compared with performing a standard femoral cut of 5 degrees.[68] Huang and colleagues found measurement of the mechanical axis to have a variability of 1 to 3 degrees.[45]

Postoperative Radiographs

At the Brigham and Women's Hospital, in most cases, imaging is not performed immediately after surgery but is done at the first postoperative visit. Usually, both supine radiographs (AP, lateral, and tangential patellar views) and standing radiographic[100] views are obtained.

Normal Postoperative Radiographic Appearances

Alignment

Because coronal malalignment can lead to decreased implant survival[22] and accelerated wear, careful analysis of component position and leg alignment is warranted. Radiographs are an effective means of evaluating component position in sagittal and coronal planes.

AP and Lateral Knee Radiographs. Component position on AP and lateral knee radiographs can be assessed as in Figure 10-1. Tibial resection is generally perpendicular to the anatomic axis of the tibia.[9] Femoral resection is more complex owing to the desire to resect the femur perpendicular to its mechanical axis. Approximately 5 to 8 degrees of valgus is present between the femoral condyles and the anatomic axis of the femur.[73] The posterior/inferior tilt of the tibial component can be assessed on the lateral radiograph. Increased downsloping of the tibial component (with posterior cruciate ligament [PCL] retaining components) can increase maximum flexion, but excessive tibial downslope can lead to anterior tibial subluxation, posterior polyethylene wear, and lack of extension.[12]

Standing Radiographs

Axial Alignment. Angulation of the knee in the coronal plane can be measured on standing radiographs of the legs. The angle between the mechanical axis of the femur (drawn from the center of the femoral head to the center of the intercondylar notch) and a line from the middle of the intercondylar eminence to the center of the talus demonstrates the angulation of the knee. Conventional radiographs or digital radiographs can be utilized for this assessment.[102]

The Mechanical Axis. The mechanical axis (a line drawn from the center of the femoral head to the center of the tibial plateau) should intersect the center of the knee[73] (Fig. 10-2). The femoral and tibial components should be perpendicular to this line,[73] and the joint space should be parallel to the ground.[115] Deviations from this alignment should be minimal (within 3 degrees of the normal mechanical axis).[121] Some authors consider axial malalignment as mechanical alignment outside the range of 1 degree varus to 2 degrees valgus.[14]

The Joint Line. In 1986, Figgie and associates noted that restoration of the tibial patellofemoral relationships had an impact on function in patients receiving posterior stabilized condylar knee prostheses.[32] Change of 8 mm or less in the height of the joint line (measured as the perpendicular distance from the weight-bearing surface of the tibial plateau to the tibial tubercle) resulted in better functional knee scores, improved range of motion, and absence of patellofemoral pain or mechanical symptoms (Fig. 10-3).

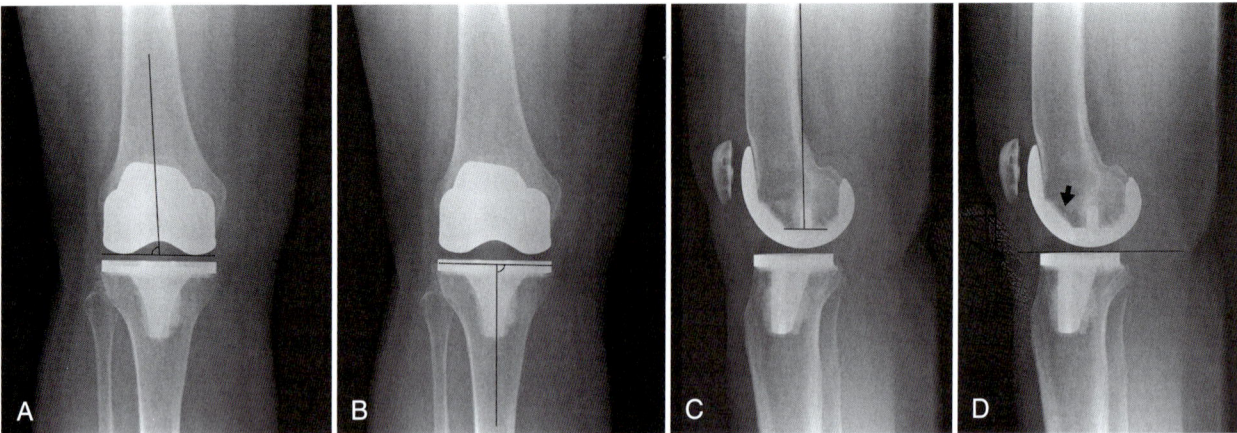

Figure 10-1. Normal component positioning on standing knee radiographs. **A,** Anteroposterior (AP) view of the knee demonstrates the method of measuring femoral component alignment. **B,** The tibial tray should be 90 degrees to the long axis of the tibial shaft. **C,** Lateral radiographs show the femoral component parallel to the femoral shaft. **D,** The tibial tray is at approximately 90 degrees to the tibial shaft. Osteopenia *(arrow)* is seen about the femoral component, consistent with stress shielding.

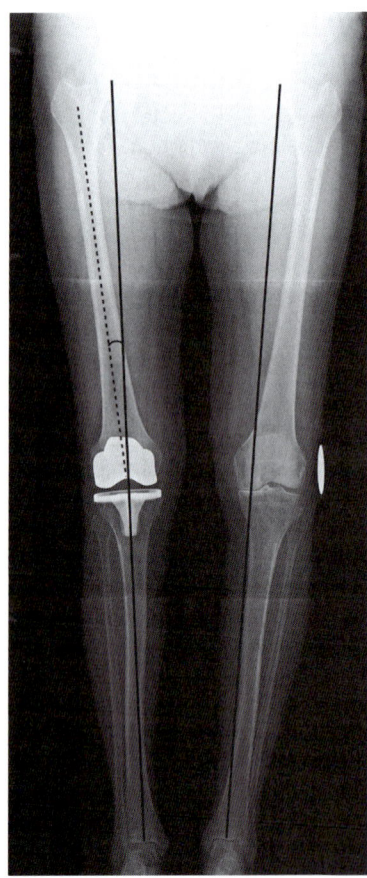

Figure 10-2. The mechanical axis. Ideally, the mechanical axis (drawn from the center of the femoral head to the center of the tibial plafond) falls through the center of the knee. Standing anteroposterior radiograph of both legs shows that the mechanical axis on the right *(solid line)* falls through the center of the knee arthroplasty, while the anatomic femoral axis *(dashed line)* is 6 degrees valgus to the mechanical axis. On the left, the mechanical axis passes through the medial tibial plateau indicating varus alignment, in this case due to osteoarthritis with medial joint space narrowing.

Hofmann and colleagues used measurements from the adductor tubercle to the joint line of the distal femur (in comparison with the normal side or the preoperative radiograph) to assess "proximalization" or "distalization" of the joint line[42] (Fig. 10-4). Restoration of the joint line (to within 4 mm of the preoperative or contralateral side) is said to avoid problems such as patella baja, patella alta, extensor mechanism maltracking, lack of motion, and midflexion instability.[42]

Radiolucent Lines. Development of thin radiolucent lines at the bone/cement or bone/prosthesis interface of less than 2 mm within the first 6 months in a cemented implant or during the first 1 to 2 years in noncemented implants without evidence of progression is considered normal (Fig. 10-5). Evaluation of low contact stress total knee arthroscopy (TKA) with meniscal bearings showed that 99% of radiolucent lines were nonprogressive, but even progressive radiolucent lines did not appear to affect fixation.[2] A scoring system for monitoring loosening developed by The Knee Society delineates specific areas to be assessed[27] (see Fig. 10-5). This method is complex, and a simplified system has been proposed.[7]

Stress Shielding. Areas of decreased stress around femoral or tibial components show a diffuse decrease in bone density. These usually can be distinguished from radiolucent lines by absence of the thin delimiting sclerotic line in areas of stress shielding (see Fig. 10-1).

Patellofemoral Joint. The patellofemoral articulation can be an important cause of postoperative knee pain and prosthetic failure.[120] However, the relationship between patellar abnormalities on radiographs and knee symptoms is imperfect.[8]

Imaging Techniques. Both lateral and tangential patellar views are important for assessing the patellar component and alignment. Numerous methods can be used for obtaining tangential patellar views in preoperative or postoperative individuals. Radiographic positioning alterations such as degree of flexion and weight bearing may significantly alter imaging findings.[120] Baldini and associates evaluated weight-bearing tangential patellar radiographs obtained with patients standing and semisquatting with the knees in 45 degrees of flexion.[8] Correlation was made between anterior knee symptoms and signs and imaging findings.[8] Persistence of patellar

tilt of >5 degrees on the patellar dome on the weight-bearing study correlated positively with anterior knee pain.[8] None of the measurements made on non–weight-bearing radiographs correlated with pain and clinical scores.[8]

Radiographic evaluation of the patellofemoral joint includes assessment of patellar tilt, patellar dislocation or subluxation, asymmetry in patellar component positioning,[8] "overstuffing," patellar height, and patellar fracture.[32,35] Often postoperative measurements are compared with preoperative ones.

Patellar Height. Figgie and colleagues proposed measuring patellar height as the perpendicular distance from the inferior

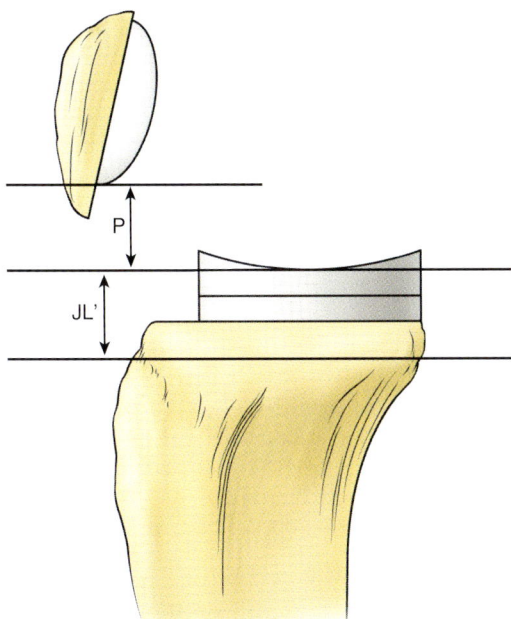

Figure 10-3. Assessing joint line and patellar height. Diagram of a method for measuring joint line (JL) and patellar (P) height. (From Figgie HE, Goldberg VM, Heiple KG, et al: The influence of tibial-patellofemoral location on function of the knee in patients with the posterior stabilized condylar knee prosthesis. J Bone Joint Surg Am 68:1035–1040, 1986.)

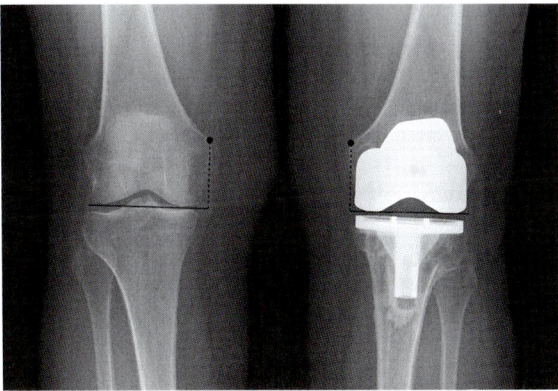

Figure 10-4. Anteroposterior method of measuring the joint line according to Hofmann and associates. The distance from the adductor tubercle to the joint line on the operated side is comparable with that on the nonoperated side (38.3 mm vs. 40.1 mm on the operated side).

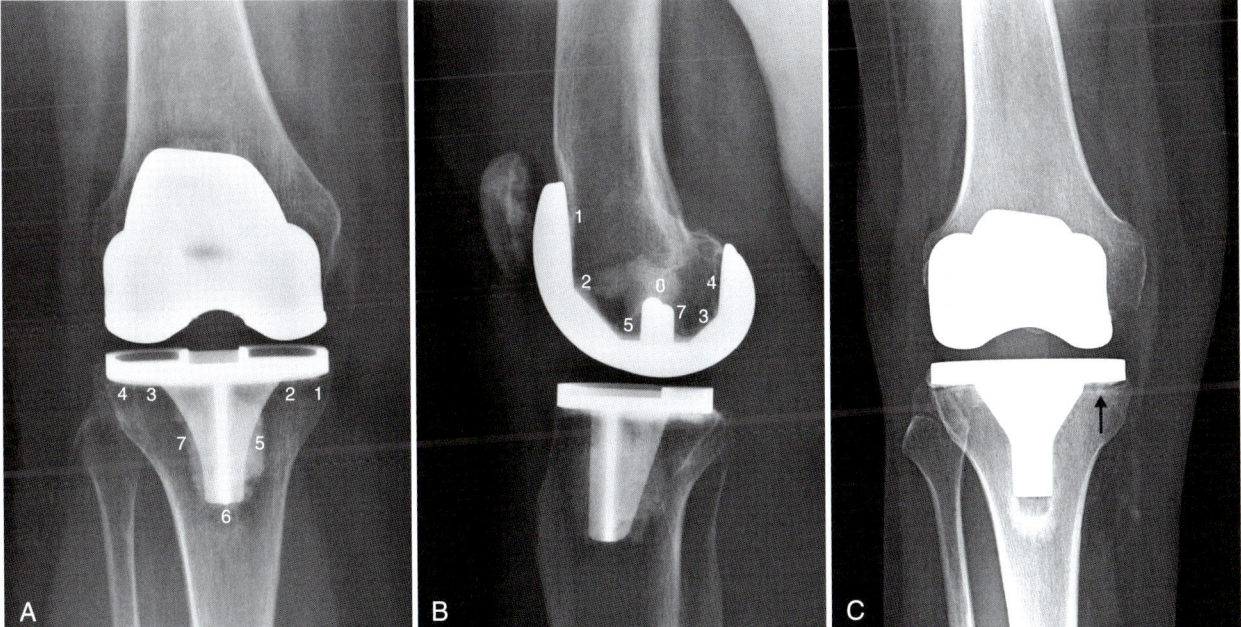

Figure 10-5. Nomenclature for localization of periprosthetic lucent lines proposed by Ewald and colleagues. **A,** Anteroposterior and **(B)** lateral views demonstrating the seven zones of the tibial and femoral components, respectively. Patellar zones can be viewed on tangential projections. A modification of this system has been proposed by Bach and coworkers. **C,** A less than 2 mm lucent line is present under the medial and lateral tibial baseplate with an adjacent thin sclerotic line *(arrow)*. Such lucencies are seen in asymptomatic patients.

pole of the patellar implant to the joint line of the prosthesis (see Fig. 10-3). Measurements of between 10 and 30 mm were associated with the best clinical results.[32]

Patellar Tilt. Patellar tilt is measured as the angle formed between a line drawn along the anterior femoral condyles and a line along the prosthesis/bone interface.[53]

Patellar tilt is not uncommon (Fig. 10-6). For example, Bindelglass and associates found patellar tilt in 31.2% of 234 primary total knee prostheses.[17] Patellar tilting in relation to the femoral component changes the contact area and permits the thinner peripheral portion of the patellar component to be subjected to maximum forces.[53] Polyethylene deformation, particle shedding, and early failure may occur. Laughlin and coworkers found that patellar tilt may change during the course of postoperative follow-up examinations.[53]

Articulation (impingement) between the patellar bone and the femoral component may occur. When this is extensive and is associated with sclerosis of the patella on a weight-bearing tangential patellar view, a positive correlation with pain has been found.[8]

Asymmetry of Patellar Component Placement. Asymmetrical resection greater than 4 mm in the mediolateral dimension or asymmetry of component position in the superior/inferior position as demonstrated on lateral views has been shown to correlate with anterior knee pain.[8] Lateral placement may cause retinacular tightness that may be avoided by medial positioning of the patellar component.[73]

Overstuffing. The postoperatively resurfaced patella should have a thickness equal to or thinner than that of the native patella.[53] A too large femoral component may produce stress on the lateral retinaculum, resulting in lateral patellar subluxation.[73]

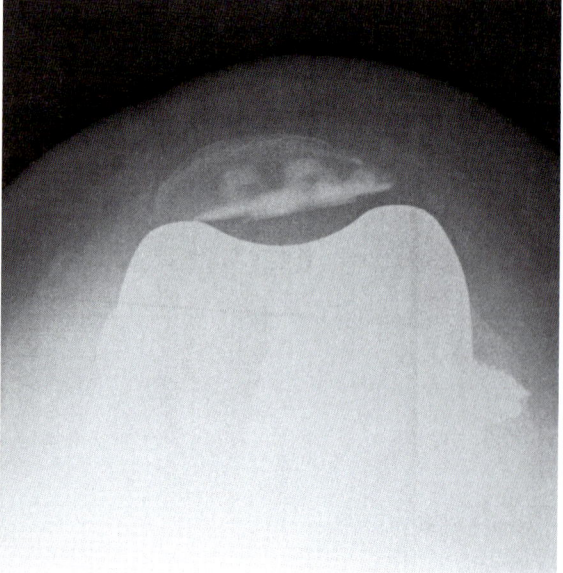

Figure 10-6. Patellar tilt. Tangential patellar view demonstrates patellar tilt with articulation between the medial patella and the femoral component.

Computed Tomography

Scout View

A relatively low-dose scout view obtained supine has been shown to allow accurate determination of the mechanical and anatomic axes of the femur for surgical planning.[115]

Improvement in CT techniques has made this modality considerably useful in evaluating complications of TKA. Multidetector helical CT with a higher applied kilovolt peak (140 kVp) improves x-ray penetration and produces superior image quality (although it also increases effective dose).[61,92,97] Use of soft tissue reconstruction filters in the setting of metallic prostheses and of wide window settings (width, 3000 to 4000 Hounsfield units [HU]; level, 800 HU) allows evaluation of bone near a prosthesis and is useful in the detection of focal areas of osteolysis.[19,108,122] Reformatted images may be helpful in minimizing artifact and demonstrating granuloma extent. Three-dimensional volume-rendered images minimize artifacts usually seen on conventional multiplanar reformatted images.[28]

Chauhan and associates described CT assessment of component position with relation to the mechanical axis as determined by CT scanning from the acetabular roof to the talar dome.[20,56] One potential limitation of this technique is the absence of weight bearing during the examination.

Rotational Alignment of Components

Several methods have been utilized surgically to align the femoral component, such as the Whiteside line (the AP axis of the distal femur),[123] the posterior femoral condylar axis, and the transepicondylar axis. The surgical transepicondylar axis connects the point of the lateral epicondyle to the medial sulcus of the medial epicondyle.[16] The femoral component should be parallel to this line or slightly externally rotated. Errors in femoral component rotation are common and may lead to patellofemoral complications and anterior knee pain.[109] Berger and colleagues found that patellofemoral complications were associated with combined (tibial and femoral) internal rotation, and the greater the rotational abnormality, the worse were the symptoms.[14]

CT scanning can be used to measure the rotation of tibial and femoral components. Berger and coworkers used the transepicondylar axis as a reference to evaluate femoral component rotation and the tibial tubercle as the reference to assess tibial component rotation on CT scans[14] (Fig. 10-7). They noted that normal rotation of the femoral condyles is 0.3 ± 1.2 degrees of internal rotation for females and 3.5 ± 1.2 degrees of internal rotation for males in comparison with the surgical epicondylar axis. On the tibial side, the native tibial articular surface (and the correctly positioned tibial component) is in 18 degrees ± 2.6 degrees of internal rotation relative to the tibial tubercle.[14] The AP tibial component axis is drawn perpendicular to the posterior edge of the tibial component.[16] When the femoral component is parallel to the transepicondylar axis and the tibial component is aligned in 18 degrees of internal rotation in relation to the tibial tubercle, normal patellar tracking results.[16] The degree of excessive combined internal rotation of the components was shown to be directly proportional to the severity of patellofemoral complications.[16]

This method has been difficult to use because the sulcus in the medial epicondyle is frequently difficult to identify.

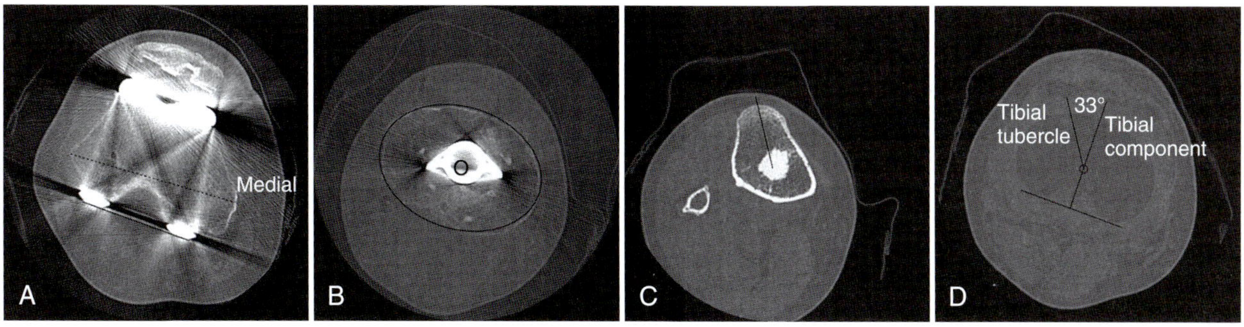

Figure 10-7. Analysis of component rotation on computed tomography (CT) according to Berger and associates. **A,** Femoral component rotation. The CT slice that passes through the femoral epicondyles is used to assess femoral component rotation. The transepicondylar axis is constructed by connecting the prominence of the lateral epicondyle with the trough in the medial epicondyle *(dashed line)*. The posterior condylar line is drawn along the posterior aspects of the medial and lateral posterior condylar surfaces *(solid line)*. Ideally, the femoral component is parallel to this line or in external rotation. The angle between these lines is measured. If the angle opens medially, the component is internally rotated. Because women normally have a posterior condylar angle of 3.1 (±1.2) degrees of internal rotation, this angle may be subtracted from any measured internal rotation to determine the degree of "excessive internal rotation." **B,** Tibial component rotation. Axial CT image obtained below the tibial baseplate. This image allows the center of the tibia to be located, establishing a reference point. **C,** The center reference point in **B** is transposed onto the image showing the most prominent portion of the tibial tubercle, and the axis is drawn between these two points. **D,** On the image through the articular polyethylene, a line is drawn along the posterior surface of the polyethylene liner, and a perpendicular line is drawn to that. The tibial tubercle axis from **C** is superimposed on the image, and the angle is measured. A total of 18 degrees is subtracted from the measured internal rotation to determine the excessive internal rotation. (This case demonstrates excessive internal rotation of 15 degrees.)

When the prominences of both epicondyles (instead of the medial sulcus) are used, the clinical transepicondylar axis produces a baseline that is more anteriorly and externally rotated (by about 6 degrees).[73] The angle between the epicondylar prominences and the posterior condyles is termed the twist angle.[3,114]

Mismatch between femoral and tibial component rotation may also be problematic.[114]

MRI

Despite the presence of metal components, MRI has become a viable (and valuable) technique for investigating complications of knee arthroplasty, particularly wear (Fig. 10-8). As summarized by Malchau and Potter and the Implant Wear Group, modifications in pulse sequence parameters and optimized protocols allow soft tissues and areas of osteolysis around the knee and hip prostheses to be evaluated.[61] MRI metal suppression techniques include increasing the bandwidth, which diminishes the frequency shift caused by metallic components, and increasing the signal-to-noise ratio by increasing the number of acquisitions and by using fast spin-echo techniques with longer echo-train lengths.[61,118] The interested reader is referred to the reference by Malchau and Potter for specific protocol information.[61]

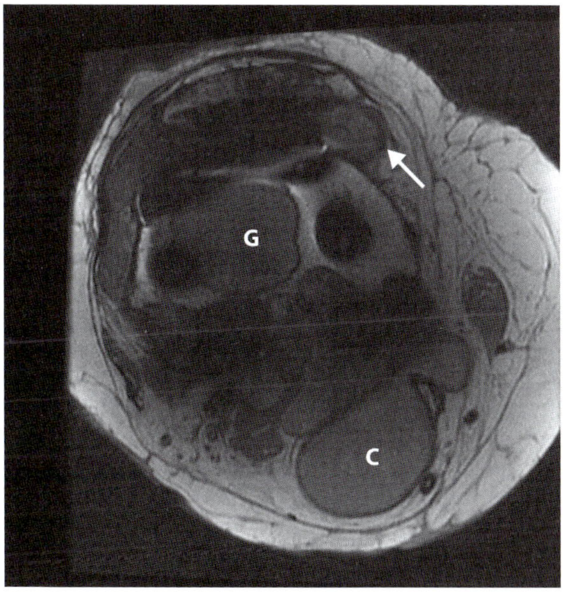

COMPLICATIONS

The most commonly cited reasons for failed total knee replacement include aseptic loosening, instability, infection, hardware failure, and malalignment, with more than 50% of revisions occurring within the first 2 years following primary surgery.[105] The most common causes of early failure (within 2 years) were infection and instability; long-term complications included polyethylene wear and aseptic loosening.[31,105]

Figure 10-8. Magnetic resonance imaging demonstrating bone and soft tissue changes in granulomatous disease. Axial fast spin-echo image shows intermediate signal intensity synovitis *(arrow)*, as well as an intermediate signal lesion (granuloma *[G]*) adjacent to the fixation plug. A popliteal cyst *(C)* is also noted.

Disorders of the Patella and Extensor Mechanism

A retrospective review of 1272 consecutive total or partial knee arthroplasties by Melloni and associates disclosed patellar complications in 3.6%.[70] Complications included instability/dislocation, fracture, osteonecrosis, infection, erosion, impingement, patellar or quadriceps tear, and

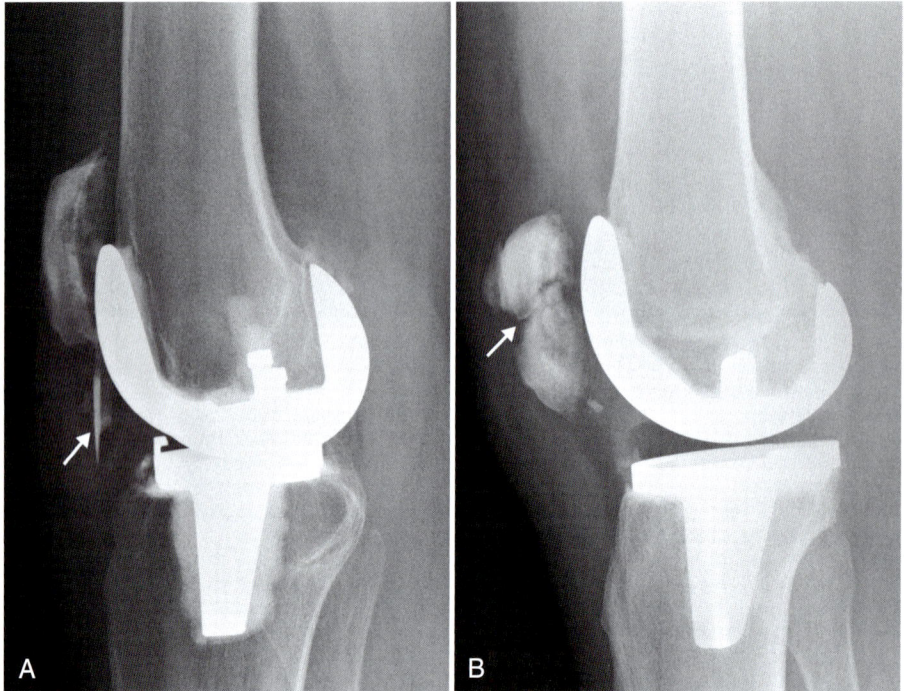

Figure 10-9. Patellar complications. **A,** Lateral radiograph shows the displaced polyethylene component *(arrow)* to lie caudal to the patella. **B,** Lateral radiograph in another patient shows a patellar fracture *(arrow).* Increased density of the fragments suggests osteonecrosis.

loosening of the patellar component (Fig. 10-9). The most common complication is patellar instability related to maltracking, often due to internal rotation of the tibial or femoral component.[70] Many patellar complications can be detected on radiography, but any underlying rotatory malalignment of components is best assessed on CT.

Patellar fragmentation and sclerosis have been attributed by Melloni and colleagues to osteonecrosis (see Fig. 10-9). Patellar fractures may be difficult to identify on radiography and may be asymptomatic.[70] Over-resection of the patella may predispose to fracture.[73] Evaluation of any accompanying patellar component loosening and of remaining bone stock of the patella helps classify fractures for treatment planning.[73] Quadriceps or patellar tendon disruption may be confirmed on ultrasound examination.[70]

Polyethylene Liner Wear

Multiple factors influence tibial component polyethylene liner wear, including weight and activity level of the patient, polyethylene thickness, alignment, relationship between the polyethylene component and the metal surface of the femoral and tibial components, and physical properties of the polyethylene.[34,37,40,73] The thickness of the polyethylene liner depends on the tensile forces needed to balance the knee ligaments, but it should measure at least 8 mm initially.[37,40]

In TKA, polyethylene wear may be evaluated on standing AP and lateral views with the x-ray beam parallel to the tibial baseplate (Fig. 10-10). The distance from the femoral condyles to the tibial baseplate can then be measured. Large amounts of polyethylene wear will be detected as moderate to severe narrowing of the distance between the femoral

component and the metal backing (baseplate); early or mild joint space narrowing may be more subtle and may be appreciated only if comparison is made between serial examinations.[73] Eventually, wear may progress to allow metal-to-metal contact, erosion of the tibial metal backing, and metal synovitis (Fig. 10-11). Development of a popliteal cyst in patients with a TKA may be an indirect sign of prosthetic wear or loosening.[77,83] Ultrasonography has been shown to accurately evaluate polyethylene thickness.[107,126]

Loosening, Particle Disease, and Osteolysis

Particle shedding, especially that caused by polyethylene wear, is the primary reason for long-term failure of TKA.[13,30,80,81,105] The natural response to particulate debris begins with the release of inflammatory cytokines, which stimulate osteoclasts and inhibit osteoblasts. The biologic cascade of polyethylene wear–related osteolysis is dependent on several factors, including the number of wear particles, the size and surface morphology of the wear particles, and the rate at which particles accumulate in periprosthetic tissues.[43] Particles migrate along the "effective joint space"[103] and produce changes in the joint, along the bone cement or prosthesis bone interfaces, and sometimes in adjacent soft tissues and lymph nodes.

Loosening

The tibial component loosens more frequently than the femoral component. Radiographic indicators that are suggestive of loosening include the development of focal radiolucencies greater than 2 mm, interval increases in the width

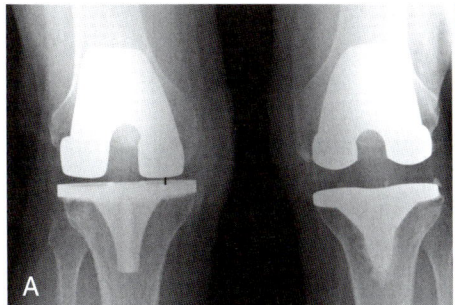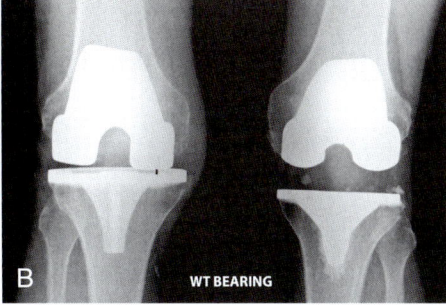

Figure 10-10. Polyethylene wear. **A,** Standing flexed posteroanterior (PA) view of both knees and **(B)** a similar view 3 years later show that the distance between the medial femoral condyle (*vertical line* in **A** and **B**) and the tibial baseplate has decreased, indicating wear of the polyethylene liner. Ideally, positioning should be identical to make this assessment. A mobile bearing left total knee prosthesis is shown in the opposite knee with the solid appearing metallic tibial component.

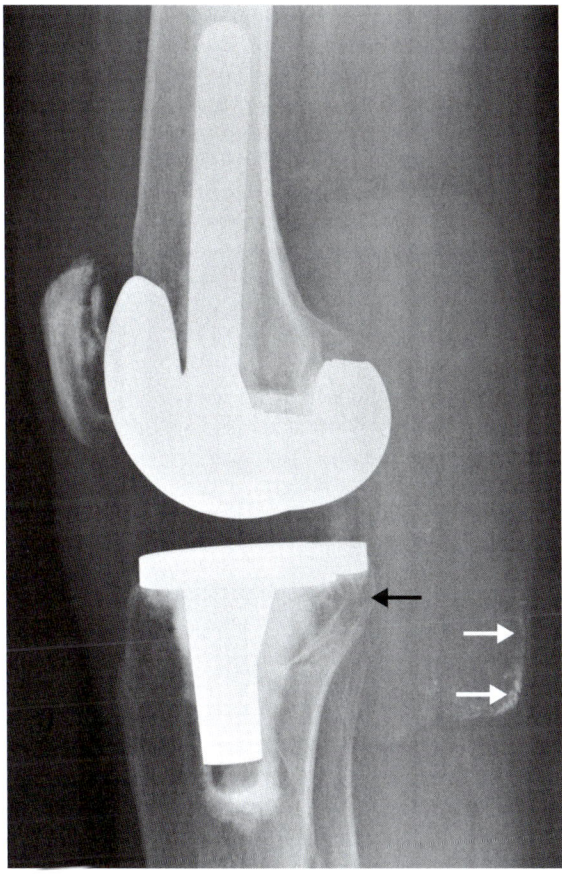

Figure 10-11. Metal synovitis. Lateral radiograph following revision of a total knee arthroplasty demonstrates a dense line outlining a distended popliteal cyst (metal line sign, *white arrows*), which is diagnostic of metal synovitis. Osteolysis is also seen at the posterior tibial baseplate *(black arrow)*, along with loosening of the patellar component.

of an existing radiolucency, cement fracture, and changes in component position.[73] Radiolucent zones in both noncemented and cemented implants are often bordered by a thin layer of lamellar bone, which is produced by remodeling (Fig. 10-12). Wide lucent lines around the stem are more likely to be indicators of loosening than are peripheral lucent zones. Detection of radiolucent lines requires that they be seen in

tangent, and this is facilitated by fluoroscopy or by special views (such as an oblique posterior condylar view).[29,66,74,75,81] The tibial component tends to shift into a varus position with subsidence into the medial plateau and collapse of the cancellous bone,[62,66] while a loose femoral component tends to shift into flexion (see Fig. 10-12).

Disappearance of the bordering line of sclerosis may suggest infection. However, in most cases, loosening due to infection and loosening due to mechanical factors or histiocytic response cannot be distinguished on radiographs.[73]

Granulomas

Focal areas of bone destruction due to particle disease produce well-defined areas of osteolysis (Fig. 10-13). Usually these are located adjacent to the components, although marked extension of the process may occur and large soft tissue masses may result. Osteolysis can occur at the interfaces of a loose component. With well-fixed components, osteolysis occurs in the posterior aspects of the femoral condyles and condylar attachments of collateral ligaments, near the edges of the tibial baseplate, along the stem or screw holes, and along the patellar component interface or margins.[73]

Most patients with evidence of loosening present with pain; however, patients with osteolysis may be asymptomatic. Radiographs can underestimate the extent of bone involvement.[28,90,108] CT examination can be helpful, as it can demonstrate synovitis, detect more granulomas than are visible on the radiograph, and allow assessment of component rotation on the same study (see Fig. 10-13).

Because of its direct multiplanar capabilities and superior soft tissue contrast (and with the added benefit of the absence of ionizing radiation), tailored MRI can evaluate both periprosthetic osteolysis[93,119] and synovitis (that may precede bone loss)[61,93] (see Fig. 10-13). Metallic implants created from oxidized zirconium alloy have demonstrated less susceptibility artifact when compared with conventional cobalt-chromium alloy because of the diminished magnetic moment of zirconium.[98] Modifications in pulse sequences have also improved imaging by reducing artifact even when cobalt chrome components are present. MRI may demonstrate radiographically occult osteolytic lesions and may offer more accurate extent and localization of osteolysis prior to revision surgery. MRI with metal suppression may be indicated in specific cases in which osteolysis is suspected clinically but is

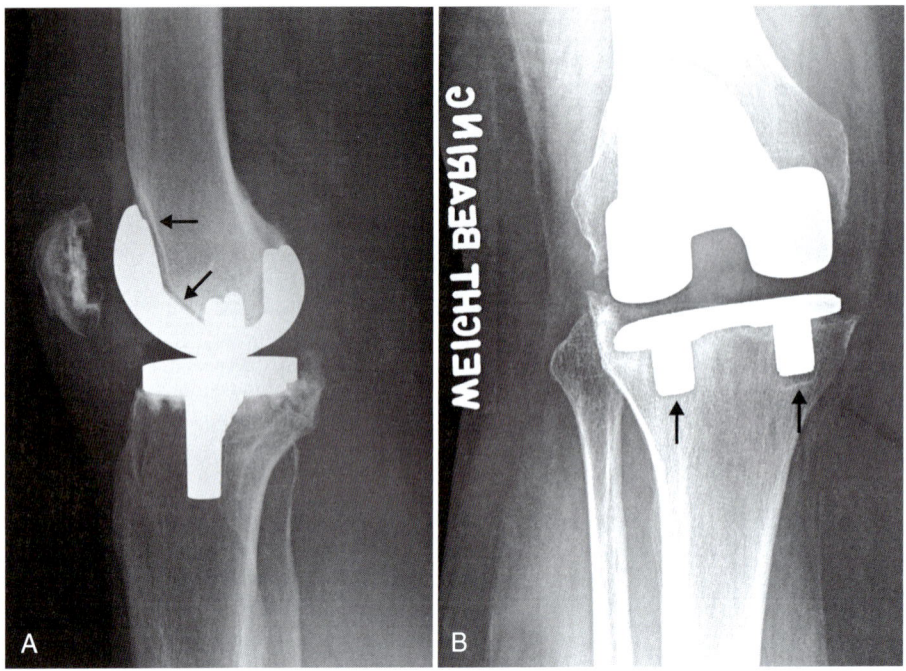

Figure 10-12. Loosening. **A,** Lateral radiograph shows radiolucent lines *(arrows)* along the femoral component (Ewald zones 1, 2, and 5). This component was proven to be loose at the time of revision surgery. **B,** Weight-bearing view in another patient demonstrates radiolucent lines greater than 2 mm along the tibial baseplate *(arrows)* and subsidence of the tibial component, indicating loosening.

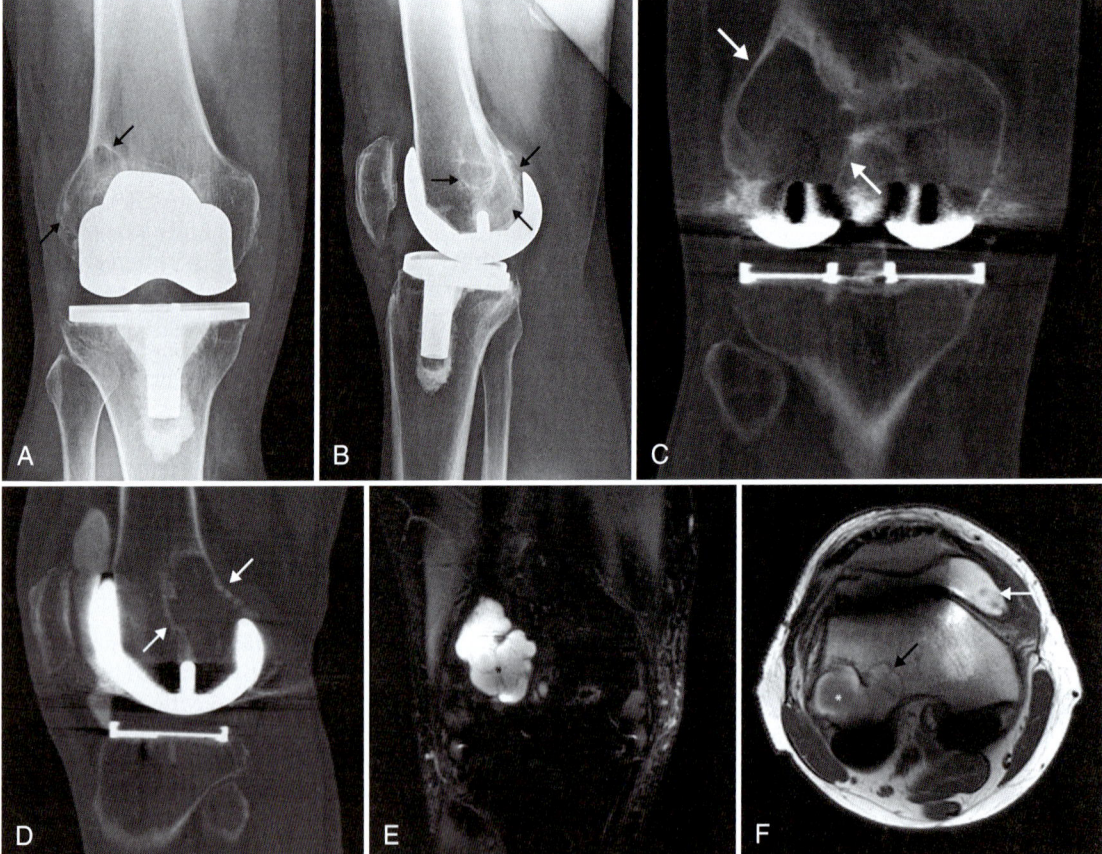

Figure 10-13. Granulomatous disease. This 47-year-old man presented with a painful right total knee replacement, as well as a deep venous thrombosis (DVT) and effusion 5 years after initial surgery. Pathologic examination revealed synovium with mononuclear histiocytic proliferation and foreign body giant cell reaction. **A,** Anteroposterior and **(B)** lateral radiographs demonstrate an eccentric lytic lesion with thin sclerotic margins in the lateral femoral condyle *(arrows* in **A** and **B**). **C,** Coronal and **(D)** sagittal images from a computed tomography (CT) arthrogram clearly demonstrate the large lytic lesion *(arrows)* with sclerotic margins in the posterolateral femoral condyle with disruption of the cortex posteriorly. **E,** Coronal short tau inversion recovery (STIR) and **(F)** axial T1-weighted postcontrast images demonstrate the multilobulated lesion (*) in the posterior aspect of the lateral femoral condyle with a hypointense rim and peripheral enhancement consistent with a large granuloma. Joint distention *(arrow)* is present.

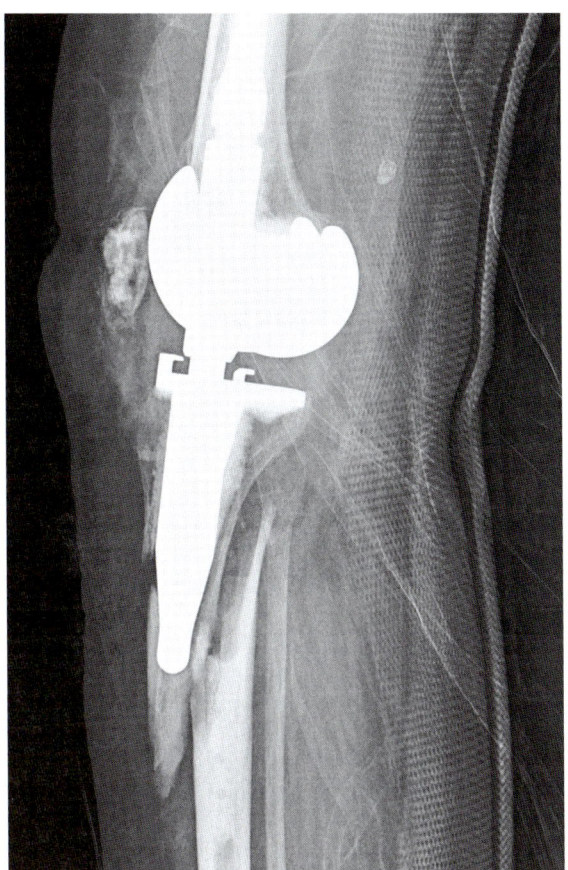

Figure 10-14. Periprosthetic fracture. Constrained total knee arthroplasty (TKA) with a periprosthetic fracture at the distal tibial stem.

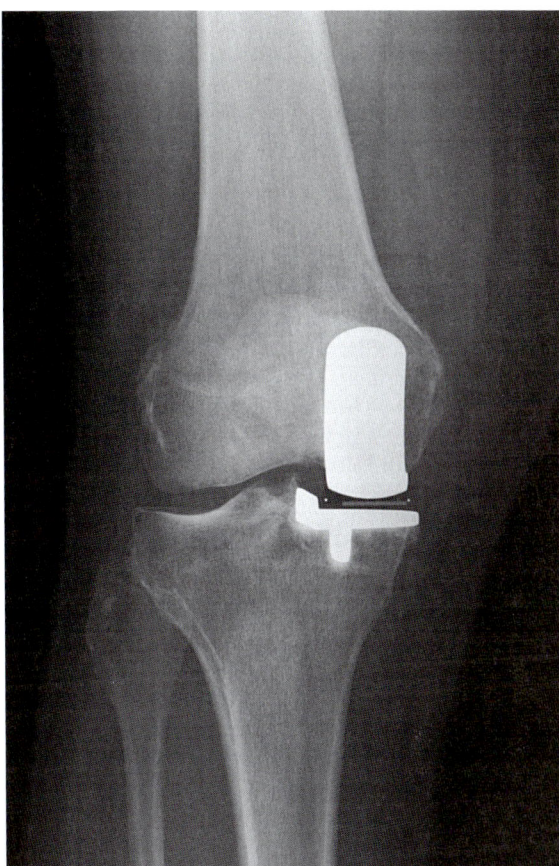

Figure 10-15. Normal unicompartmental arthroplasty of the medial compartment (Oxford Bearing). The metallic markers in the bearing allow assessment of its position.

not visible radiographically, as well as in instances in which the extent or volume of osteolysis needs to be determined preoperatively.[34,61,118]

Metal Synovitis

Metal-induced chronic synovitis is the result of metal wear debris caused by abrasion of metal components that occurs after failure of the interposed polyethylene-bearing surfaces.[21] A dense line outlining a distended knee capsule or an articular surface on radiographs, also known as the metal-line sign, is diagnostic of metal synovitis[120] (see Fig. 10-11). Erosion of the tibial metal backing may reveal the site of wear. On MRI, thickened synovium in cases of metal synovitis shows low signal intensity on all pulse sequences.

Periprosthetic and Component Fractures

The overall incidence of periprosthetic fracture is very low, with supracondylar femoral fractures reportedly in the range between 0.3% and 2.5%.[39] Risk factors for postoperative supracondylar fracture include osteopenia, femoral notching, and poor flexion,[113] as well as focal osteolysis and component loosening.[73] A decrease in the torsional strength of the femur has been reported when a 3-mm notch is present in the anterior femoral cortex,[106] with others reporting that nearly 50% of periprosthetic femur fractures have associated

anterior femoral notching.[1] The significance of femoral notching is controversial, however. Periprosthetic fractures of the proximal tibia have been reported less often than supracondylar and patellar fractures, with only a few cases reported (Fig. 10-14). Fractures may also occur following medial or lateral[18,52,117,125] unicompartmental knee arthroplasty.

Fracture of the femoral or tibial component is uncommon, with a rate of 0.2%.[44] Malalignment, uneven cement fixation, severe polyethylene wear, and undersizing of the tibial tray have been described as causes of tibial component failure.[4,41,65] Femoral component fracture is due to metal defects or cracks.[110,123] The polyethylene stabilizing post in posterior stabilized total knee replacement may also fracture, resulting clinically in an extension clunk.[67]

Unicompartmental Complications

Utilization of the unicompartmental knee arthroplasty (UKA) has grown in acceptance and has seen a resurgence over the past several years, primarily because of the introduction of minimally invasive techniques (Fig. 10-15). The aim of UKA is to resurface the medial or lateral tibiofemoral compartment in patients with uncontrolled symptoms due to arthritis predominantly confined to a single compartment. Unicondylar implants with a freely mobile meniscal bearing are now available, distributing forces over a larger surface area, theoretically decreasing contact stresses and polyethylene wear. An intact anterior cruciate ligament is required to maintain near-normal joint kinematics and mechanics.[24,26] Although some studies have shown comparable survival rates for total and unicompartmental knee arthroplasties,[6,15,82,94,111] a direct comparative study of UKA and TKA revealed a lower 5-year survivorship for UKA (85%) versus TKA (98%).[5] In patients younger than 50 years old, a recent study demonstrated 12-year survivorship of 80% in patients who underwent UKA, concluding that polyethylene wear remains a concern affecting the survival of unicompartmental knee replacements in younger patients.[89]

Complications of UKA include infection, polyethylene wear, osteolysis, subsidence and loosening, development of degenerative arthritis in the opposite compartment, and stress fractures below the tibial component.[16,18,47,73] Radiolucent lines are commonly observed under the tibial component of Oxford unicompartmental knee implants, and although the cause remains unknown, they are not thought to lead to loosening.[38,99] Polyethylene wear and axial malalignment can be evaluated by standing AP radiographs,[50] and radiographs in flexion and extension have been described for evaluation of femoral component loosening.[76]

Infection

Infection complicates 0.8% to 1.9% of knee arthroplasties.[23] Predisposing causes are categorized as those related to the patient (such as prior revision arthroplasty, prior infection of a prosthesis in the same joint, rheumatoid arthritis, and diabetes) and those related to the surgery and the postoperative period (such as simultaneous bilateral arthroplasty, long operating time, allogenic blood transfusion, wound complications, and urinary tract infection).[23]

Infection often is not obvious prior to revision surgery. Low-grade or chronic infections are particularly difficult to identify.

More than half of cases are due to staphylococci. Organisms may be introduced at the time of surgery (usually skin bacteria) or through hematogenous spread or direct contamination from compromised adjacent tissues.[23] Microorganisms adhere to the prosthesis, residing in a biofilm that limits the effects of antimicrobial agents.[23]

The primary symptom of infection is pain, typically night pain or pain at rest.[54] If other signs of infection (erythema, sinus tract) are not present, differentiation from other causes of pain, particularly aseptic loosening, can be problematic. The American Academy of Orthopaedic Surgeons (AAOS) proposes that testing strategies be planned according to the probability of infection. (AAOS, American Academy of Orthopaedic Surgeons, The diagnosis of periprosthetic joint infections of the hip and knee. Adopted by the American Academy of Orthopaedic Surgeons Board of Directors June 18, 2010) Higher probability is suggested when one or more symptoms are present and at least one or more risk factors (such as prior knee infection, superficial surgical site infection, operative time >2.5 hours, or immunosuppression) or physical exam finding or early implant loosening/osteolysis on radiographs is present.

Nonimaging techniques such as C-reactive protein (CRP) may be helpful. DelPozo and Patel noted that CRP levels return to normal within 2 months, and a normal CRP level generally excludes infection.[23] A CRP of 13.5 mg or more per liter is 73% to 91% sensitive and 81% to 86% specific for the diagnosis of infected TKA.[23] The AAOS recommends joint aspiration of patients being assessed for periprosthetic infection who have an abnormal erythrocyte sedimentation rate and/or C-reactive protein results. (AAOS, American Academy of Orthopaedic Surgeons, The diagnosis of periprosthetic joint infections of the hip and knee. Adopted by the American Academy of Orthopaedic Surgeons Board of Director June 18, 2010.)

Joint aspiration is the most valuable test for infection.[23] A cell count of >1.7 × 10^3 per cubic millimeter or >65% neutrophils is consistent with knee joint infection.[23] Barrack and colleagues noted that in contrast to aspiration of total hip replacement, where false-positive results are more common, aspirations of knee joints are more likely falsely negative.[10] This was thought to result most often from antibiotic treatment.[10] At least 2 weeks off antibiotics is recommended before the aspiration is performed (with careful clinical monitoring for sepsis), but as long as 1 month may be necessary for cultures of aspirated fluid to become positive. In questionable cases, aspiration should be repeated.

Radiographs

Generally, radiographs are insensitive for diagnosing prosthetic infection (Fig. 10-16). Radiographs may not be helpful because loosening, periostitis, focal osteolysis, and radiolucent lines have been seen in infected and uninfected knees. Also, infection may be present with a "normal" radiographic appearance.

Increasing soft tissue swelling with blurring of fat lines and joint effusion, periosteal reaction, and loosening (especially with loss of the thin sclerotic demarcation lines) should suggest infection. Arthrography may show sinus tracts.

CT and MRI

In the absence of a prosthesis, CT and MRI are well-recognized tools for evaluating infection. MRI can be used to evaluate soft tissues for edema, fistulas, sinus tracts, abscesses, and fluid collections. Abscess cavities can often be differentiated from bland postoperative fluid collections, as abscesses have thick, irregular, diffusely enhancing walls, and fluid collections are bounded by thin, minimally enhancing walls. CT has less soft tissue contrast and suffers image degradation by metallic components. In spite of these limitations, considerable information can be gleaned with the use of these modalities (see Fig. 10-16).

Radionuclide Imaging

Bone Scintigraphy

Bone scintigraphy, performed with technetium-99m (Tc-99m)-labeled diphosphonates, is highly sensitive for detecting complications of lower extremity prosthetic joint surgery. Although sensitive for identifying failed joint replacement, this test cannot determine the cause of failure. Evaluation of knee replacements is especially problematic because, even in the absence of complications, increased periprosthetic activity can persist for some time after implantation.[57] Rosenthall and colleagues[101] observed persistent periprosthetic activity around more than 60% of the femoral components and nearly 90% of the tibial components of asymptomatic knee replacements more than 1 year after implantation. Hofmann and associates[42] studied asymptomatic knee replacements with

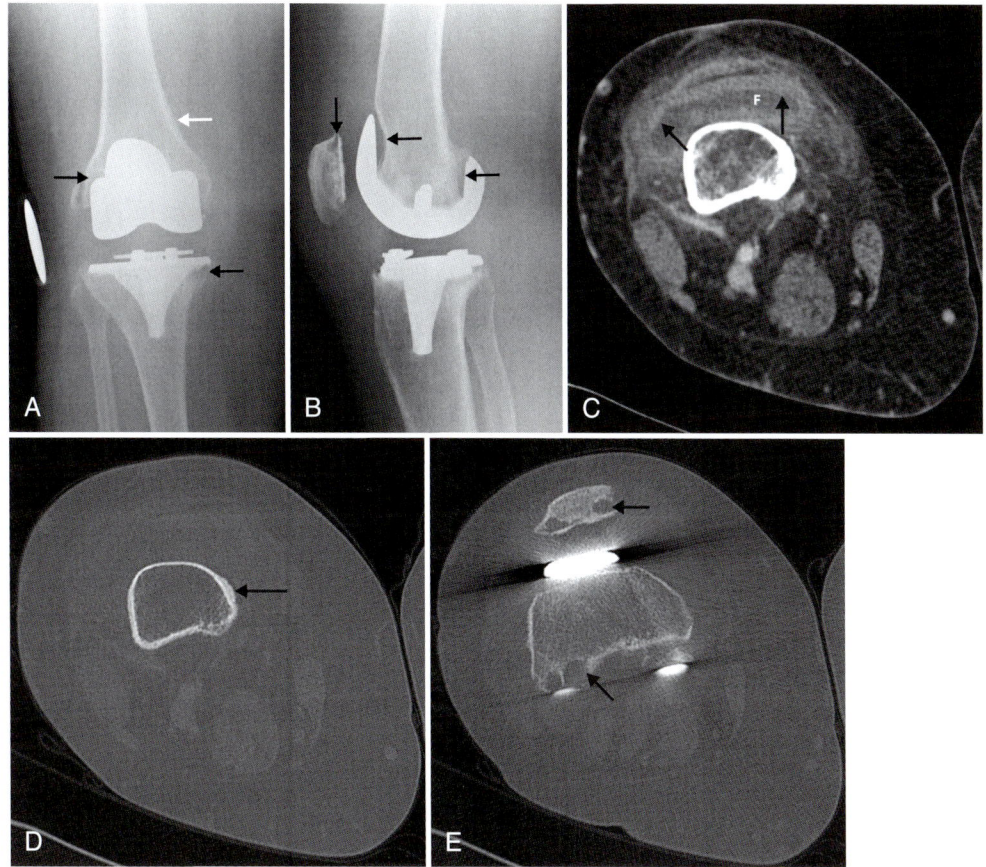

Figure 10-16. Infected total knee arthroplasty. This 55-year-old woman presented with a history of painful right total knee replacement 1½ years following arthroplasty. C-reactive protein (CRP) (33.1) and sedimentation rate (67 mm per hour) were both elevated. Aspiration showed a white count of 28,000 mm³ with 86% polymorphonuclear leukocytes. The *Abiotrophia* species was cultured. **A,** Anteroposterior and **(B)** lateral radiographs show extensive soft tissue swelling, bone resorption along the femoral and patellar interfaces *(black arrows),* and periosteal reaction *(white arrow* in **A**). A magnification marker of known size is placed alongside the knee. **C,** Axial computed tomography (CT) image with soft tissue algorithm shows marked thickening of the suprapatellar pouch *(arrows),* which is distended with low attenuation fluid *(F).* **D,** Axial CT images using a bone algorithm at the same level as **C. E,** Axial image at the level of the patella shows periosteal reaction *(black arrow* in **D**), as well as confirmation of bone loss adjacent to the femoral and patellar components *(arrows* in **E**). These lytic areas are not specific and may be seen with granulomatous disease. Pathologic examination showed fibrin and granulation tissue with acute inflammation.

serial bone scans over a 2-year period and found that although periprosthetic activity usually decreased over time after implantation, considerable patient-to-patient variation was evident. They concluded that a single study cannot reliably detect prosthetic failure, and that sequential scans are needed. Palestro and coworkers[88] reported that bone scintigraphy was not specific for infection (Fig. 10-17).

Performing the bone scan as a three-phase study does not improve the accuracy of the test (Fig. 10-18). Magnuson and associates[60] reviewed 49 painful lower extremity joint replacements and found that although three-phase bone scintigraphy was 100% sensitive, it was only 18% specific for diagnosing infection. Levitsky and colleagues[55] in an investigation of 72 lower extremity joint replacements reported a sensitivity of 30% and a specificity of 86%. Palestro and coworkers[88] reported that the three-phase bone scan was neither sensitive (67%) nor specific (76%) for diagnosing the infected knee replacement.

Although the overall accuracy of bone scintigraphy in evaluation of the painful prosthetic joint is about 50% to 70%, this study does have a high negative predictive value,

and it can be used as an initial screening test or in conjunction with other diagnostic tests.[86]

Sequential Bone/Gallium Imaging

In an effort to improve the accuracy of the radionuclide diagnosis of prosthetic joint infection, gallium imaging often is performed along with a bone scan and the two studies are interpreted together.[57] Although Tehranzadeh and associates[112] reported 95% accuracy for the combined study, most other investigators have reported less satisfactory results. Merkel and colleagues[72] found that the sensitivity, specificity, and accuracy of sequential bone/gallium imaging for diagnosing joint replacement infection in an animal model were 61%, 71%, and 67%, respectively. In 130 patients with painful orthopedic prostheses, these investigators reported that the test was 66% sensitive, 81% specific, and 77% accurate for diagnosing infection.[71] Gomez-Luzuriaga and associates[36] reported sensitivity, specificity, and accuracy of 70%, 90%, and 80%, respectively. Kraemer and colleagues[51] reported a sensitivity of 38%, a specificity of 100%, and an accuracy of 81% for diagnosing prosthetic hip infection.

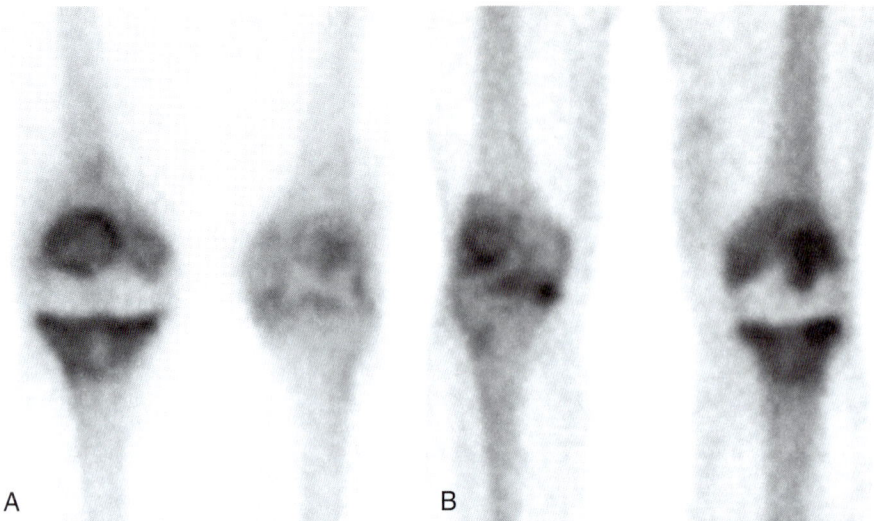

Figure 10-17. **A,** Infected 1-year-old right total knee replacement. Periprosthetic activity is increased, especially around the tibial component, on the bone scan. **B,** Aseptically loosened 2-year-old left total knee replacement. Increased periprosthetic activity around this knee prosthesis is virtually indistinguishable from that in **A.**

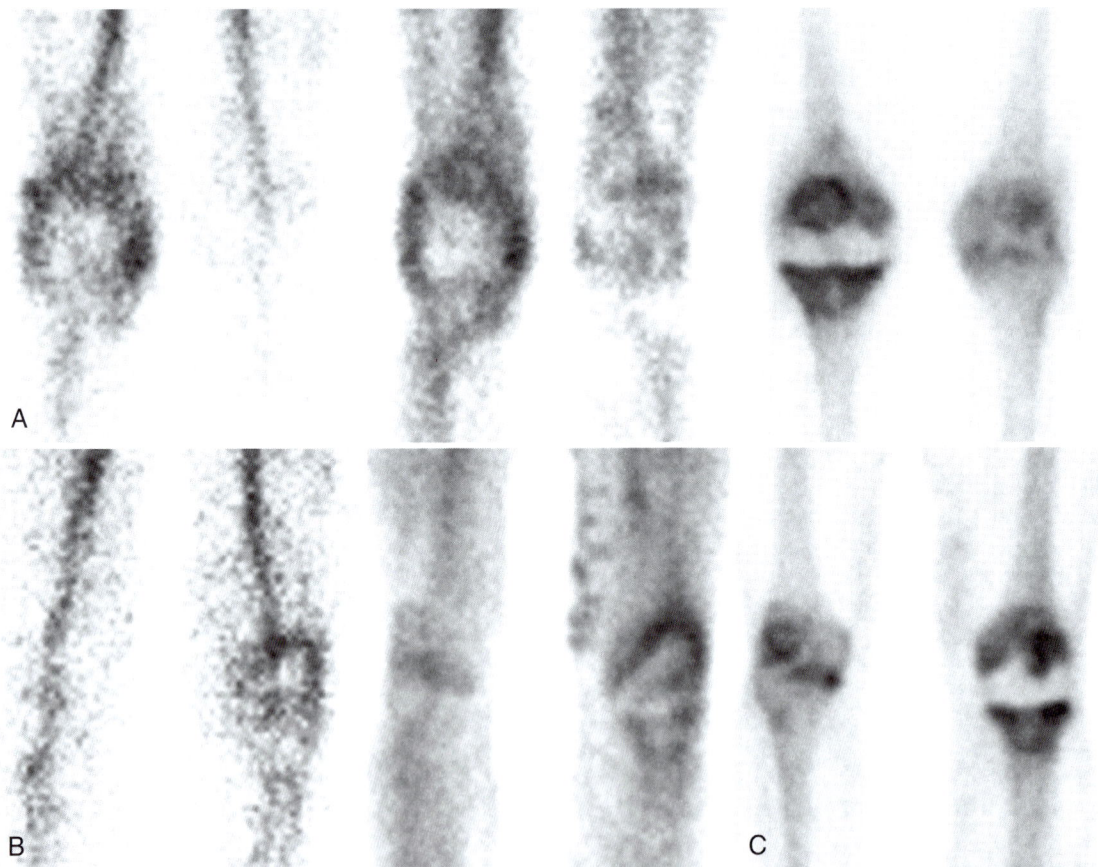

Figure 10-18. **A,** Infected 1-year-old right total knee replacement (same patient illustrated in Fig. 10-17*A*). Hyperperfusion and hyperemia are seen around the right knee on the flow *(left)* and blood pool *(center)* images, with increased periprosthetic activity on the delayed image *(right)* of the three-phase bone scan. **B,** Aseptically loosened 2-year-old left total knee replacement (same patient illustrated in Figure 17*B*). Hyperperfusion and hyperemia are evident around the left knee on the flow *(left)* and blood pool *(center)* phases, with increased periprosthetic activity on the delayed image *(right)* of the three-phase bone scan. Although bone scintigraphy is sensitive, it is not specific, even when performed as a three-phase study, and it cannot be used to differentiate aseptic loosening from infection.

Sequential bone/gallium imaging, with an accuracy ranging from 65% to 80%, offers only a modest improvement over bone scintigraphy alone and is of limited value in differentiating prosthetic joint infection from other causes of prosthetic failure (Fig. 10-19).[57]

Labeled Leukocyte Imaging

Although labeled leukocyte (white blood cell [WBC]) imaging is the radionuclide procedure of choice for diagnosing prosthetic infection, early results were inconsistent, with some investigators reporting that the test was sensitive but not specific, and others reporting that the test was specific but not sensitive.* Low sensitivity was attributed to the chronic nature of prosthetic joint infection, and poor specificity was ascribed to nonspecific inflammation. Although chronicity and nonspecific inflammation may be part of the explanation for the inconsistent results reported, a more fundamental problem with WBC imaging is related to interpretation of the images themselves. Standard practice for interpreting WBC images is to compare activity in the region of interest with activity in some normal reference point.

_____

*References 48, 60, 69, 85, 88, 95, 96, and 124.

Thus, WBC studies are interpreted as positive for osteomyelitis when uptake in the region of interest exceeds uptake in the predetermined reference point, or when activity outside the normal distribution of the radiotracer is observed. Unfortunately, both the intensity of uptake in prosthetic knee infection and the normal distribution of labeled WBCs are variable[57] (Fig. 10-20).

Efforts to improve the accuracy of the test for diagnosing prosthetic joint infection have focused on the use of two combined modalities: WBC/bone and WBC/marrow imaging. Wukich and coworkers[124] reported that the specificity improved from 45% for WBC alone to 85% for WBC/bone imaging. Sensitivity decreased, however, from 100% to 85%. Johnson and associates[48] in an assessment of hip arthroplasties observed that the combined technique was more specific (95% vs. 50%) but less sensitive than WBC imaging alone (88% vs. 100%). Results reported by other investigators, however, have been less satisfactory. Palestro and colleagues[88] investigated 25 painful knee replacements and reported that the sensitivity (67%) and specificity (78%) of WBC/bone imaging were not better than those of WBC imaging alone (89% sensitivity and 75% specificity). Oswald and coworkers[84] observed incongruent WBC/bone images in 15% of asymptomatic patients with porous-coated hip

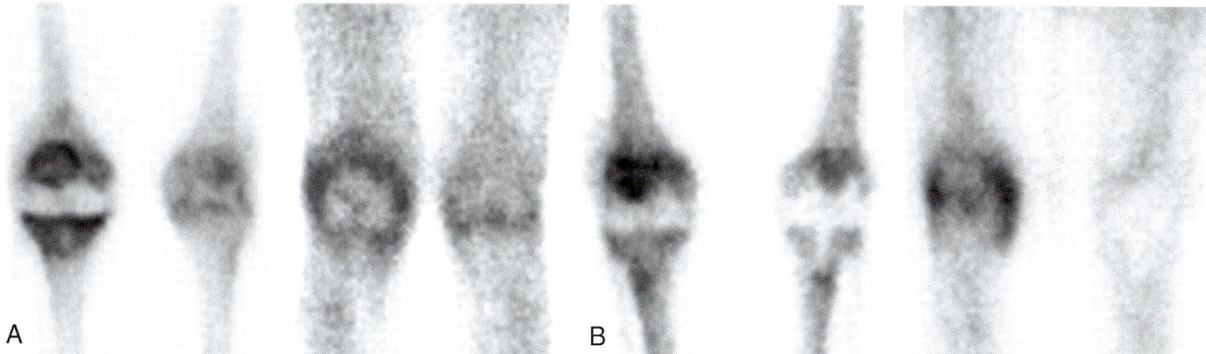

Figure 10-19. **A,** Infected 1-year-old right total knee replacement (same patient illustrated in Fig. 10-17*A*). Abnormal activity on the bone scan *(left)* is located primarily around the tibial component, and abnormal activity on the gallium scan *(right)* is located primarily around the femoral component. When the distribution of the two tracers is spatially incongruent, as in this case, the combined study is positive for infection. **B,** Aseptically loosened 2-year-old right total knee replacement. Abnormal activity on the bone scan *(left)* is located primarily around the femoral component, and abnormal activity on the gallium scan *(right)* is located primarily along the lateral and medial margins of the knee joint itself. In this case, the combined study is false-positive for infection.

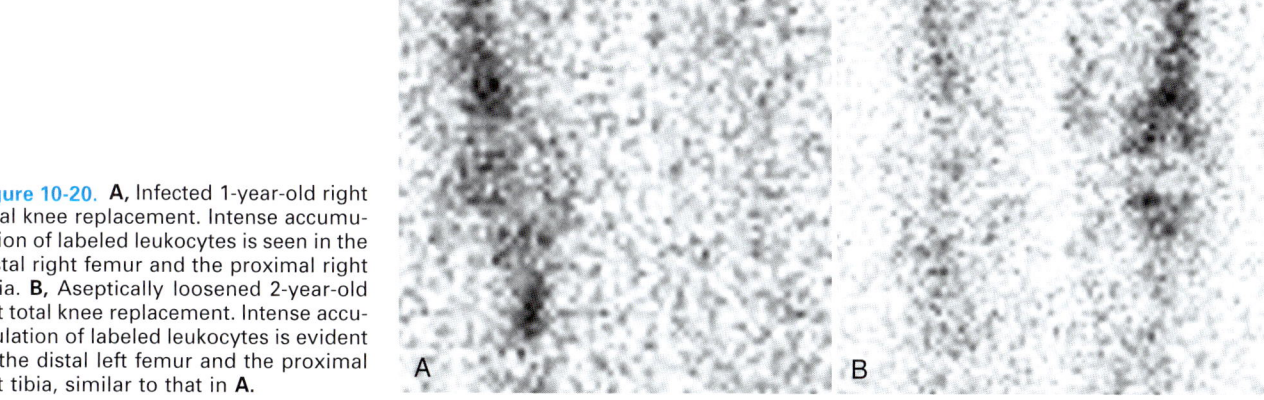

Figure 10-20. **A,** Infected 1-year-old right total knee replacement. Intense accumulation of labeled leukocytes is seen in the distal right femur and the proximal right tibia. **B,** Aseptically loosened 2-year-old left total knee replacement. Intense accumulation of labeled leukocytes is evident in the distal left femur and the proximal left tibia, similar to that in **A.**

arthroplasties and concluded that, in patients with this type of hip replacement, incongruence of activity at the prosthetic tip is of little clinical utility.

Although some investigators have focused on WBC/bone imaging, others have studied the combination of WBC with Tc-99m sulfur colloid bone marrow imaging.* The principle of combined WBC/marrow imaging is based on the fact that WBC and marrow images both reflect radiotracer accumulation in the reticuloendothelial cells, or fixed macrophages, of the marrow. The distribution of marrow activity is similar, or spatially congruent, on WBC and marrow images in normal individuals and in those with underlying marrow abnormalities. The exception is osteomyelitis, including prosthetic joint infection, which stimulates uptake of leukocytes but suppresses uptake of sulfur colloid, resulting in spatially incongruent images (Fig. 10-21).[87]

Over the years, the results of WBC/marrow imaging have been remarkably consistent, with reported accuracies ranging from 88% to 98%.[57] Palestro and associates[88] reported that WBC/marrow imaging was 89% sensitive and 100% specific for diagnosing prosthetic knee infection and was superior to bone (including three-phase) alone, WBC alone, and WBC/bone. Love and colleagues[58] reported that in 19 patients with surgically, histopathologically, and microbiologically confirmed diagnoses, the test was 100% accurate for diagnosing prosthetic knee infection. El Espera and associates[25] compared WBC/bone versus WBC/marrow imaging for diagnosing prosthetic joint infection and reported that far fewer equivocal results and much better interobserver agreement were noted for WBC/marrow than for WBC/bone imaging.

¹⁸F-Fluorodeoxyglucose Positron Emission Tomography

Despite its utility, significant disadvantages are associated with WBC/marrow scintigraphy, and investigators continue to search for suitable alternatives. One radionuclide procedure that has generated considerable interest for diagnosing prosthetic joint infection is ¹⁸F-fluorodeoxyglucose positron emission tomography (FDG-PET). FDG is transported into cells via glucose transporters, but unlike glucose, it is not metabolized and remains trapped within the cell. Increased FDG uptake in inflammation presumably is due, at least in part, to increased expression of glucose transporters in inflammatory cells and increased affinity of these glucose transporters for deoxyglucose.[59]

FDG-PET has several potential advantages over conventional nuclear medicine tests. Degenerative bone changes usually show only faintly increased FDG uptake compared with infection. Normal bone marrow has only a low glucose metabolism under physiologic conditions, which could facilitate the differentiation of inflammatory cellular infiltrates from hematopoietic marrow and obviate the need for bone marrow imaging. The small FDG molecule enters poorly perfused areas quickly, and the procedure is completed within 2 hours after tracer injection. Images have higher spatial resolution than those obtained with single photon emitting tracers. Semiquantitative analysis by means of standardized uptake values (SUVs), which is readily available with PET but less feasible with conventional nuclear techniques, could be useful for differentiating infectious from noninfectious conditions, and for monitoring response to therapy.[57]

Manthey and associates[63] studied 14 painful knee prostheses and reported that FDG-PET correctly identified the 1 infected device and was true negative in 13 uninfected devices (100% accuracy). However, results of most other investigations have been less satisfactory. Zhuang and colleagues[127] evaluated FDG-PET in knee replacements and reported sensitivity, specificity, and accuracy of 92%, 72%, and 78%, respectively, for diagnosing infection. VanAcke and coworkers[116] evaluated FDG-PET in 21 patients with suspected prosthetic knee infection and reported that the test was 100% sensitive but only 73% specific for diagnosing infection. When FDG-PET was interpreted together with bone scintigraphy, specificity improved to 80%. Love and associates[58] compared coincidence detection FDG-PET versus WBC/marrow imaging for diagnosing prosthetic knee infection in 19 patients, and reported an accuracy of 58% for FDG-PET compared with an accuracy of 100% for

---

*References 25, 49, 58, 78, 85, 88, and 91.

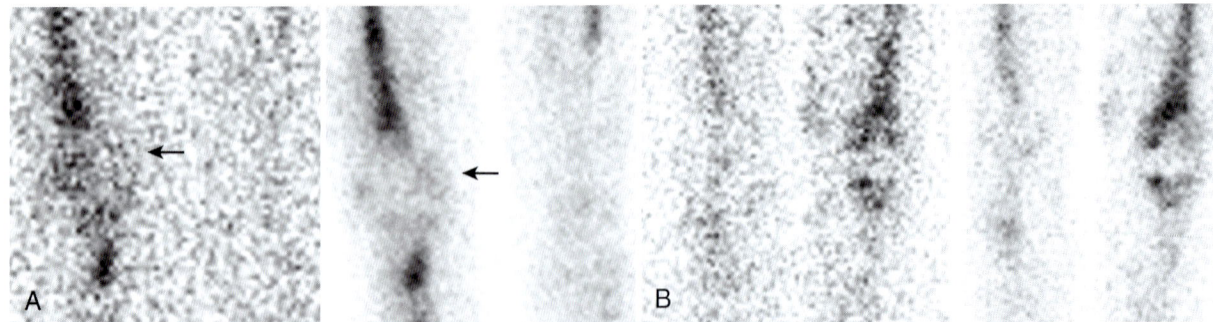

Figure 10-21. **A,** Infected 1-year-old right total knee replacement (same patient illustrated in Fig. 10-20*A*). Distribution of activity on the labeled leukocyte *(left)* and bone marrow *(right)* images is the same, except in the knee joint region *(arrows)*, where there is accumulation of labeled leukocytes, but not sulfur colloid. The images are incongruent, and the combined study is positive for infection. Areas of most intense activity on the labeled leukocyte image correspond to areas of activity on the bone marrow image and reflect marrow activity, not infection. Abnormal labeled leukocyte activity, which is seen in the joint region, is much less intense. **B,** Aseptically loosened 2-year-old left total knee replacement (same patient illustrated in Fig. 10-20*B*). Distribution of activity on the labeled leukocyte *(left)* and bone marrow *(right)* images is virtually identical, and the combined study is negative for infection. Neither intensity nor distribution of labeled leukocyte activity around a joint prosthesis is a reliable criterion for diagnosing infection.

WBC/marrow imaging. In a recent meta-analysis, overall sensitivity and specificity of FDG-PET imaging for diagnosing prosthetic knee infection were reported as 87% and 75%, respectively. Based on these results, there appears to be no role for FDG-PET in evaluation of the painful knee prosthesis.

SUMMARY

The principal role of nuclear medicine in evaluation of the painful knee replacement is to diagnose infection. Nonspecific indicators of inflammation, such as gallium and FDG, are of limited value because of the frequency with which inflammation accompanies aseptic loosening. Bone scintigraphy is useful for screening purposes, but combined WBC/marrow scintigraphy is the radionuclide procedure of choice for diagnosing infection.

KEY REFERENCES

Berger RA, Rubash HE: Rotational instability and malrotation after total knee arthroplasty. Clin Orthop Relat Res 32:639–647, 2001.

Del Pozo J, Patel R: Infection associated with prosthetic joints. N Engl J Med 361:787–793, 2009.

Fayad LM, Patra A, Fishman EK: Value of 3D CT in defining skeletal complications of orthopedic hardware in the postoperative patient. AJR Am J Roentgenol 193:1155–1163, 2009.

Figgie HE, Goldberg VM, Heiple KG, et al: The influence of tibial-patellofemoral location on function of the knee in patients with the posterior stabilized condylar knee prosthesis. J Bone Joint Surg Am 68:1035–1040, 1986.

Frick MA, Collins MS, Adkins MC: Postoperative imaging of the knee. Radiol Clin North Am 44:367–389, 2006.

Love C, Marwin SE, Palestro CJ: Nuclear medicine and the infected joint replacement. Semin Nucl Med 39:66–78, 2009.

Malchau H, Potter HG: Implant Wear Symposium clinical work: how are wear-related problems diagnosed and what forms of surveillance are necessary? J Am Acad Orthop Surg 16(Suppl 1):S14–S19, 2008.

McGrory JE, Trousdale RT, Pagnano MW, et al: Preoperative hip to ankle radiographs in total knee arthroplasty. Clin Orthop Relat Res 404:196–202, 2002.

Melloni P, Valls R, Veintemillas M: Imaging patellar complications after knee arthroplasty. Eur J Radiol 65:478–482, 2008.

Miller TT: Imaging of knee arthroplasty. Eur J Radiol 54:164–177, 2005.

Naudie DD, Ammeen DJ, Engh GA, et al: Wear and osteolysis around total knee arthroplasty. J Am Acad Orthop Surg 15:53–64, 2007.

Palestro CJ, Love C: Radionuclide imaging of musculoskeletal infection: conventional agents. Semin Musculoskelet Radiol 11:335–352, 2007.

Palestro CJ, Love C, Tronco GG, et al: Combined labeled leukocyte and technetium 99m sulfur colloid bone marrow imaging for diagnosing musculoskeletal infection. Radiographics 26:859–870, 2006.

Sofka CM, Adler RS, Laskin R: Sonography of polyethylene liners used in total knee arthroplasty. AJR Am J Roentgenol 180:1437–1441, 2003.

Sofka CM, Potter HG, Adler RS, et al: Musculoskeletal imaging update: current applications of advanced imaging techniques to evaluate the early and long-term complications of patients with orthopedic implants. HSS J 2:73–77, 2006.

Vessely MB, Frick MA, Oakes D, et al: Magnetic resonance imaging with metal suppression for evaluation of periprosthetic osteolysis after total knee arthroplasty. J Arthroplasty 21:826–831, 2006.

Weissman BN, Scott RD, Brick GW, et al: Radiographic detection of metal-induced synovitis as a complication of arthroplasty of the knee. J Bone Joint Surg Am 73:1002–1007, 1991.

Full references for this chapter can be found on www.expertconsult.com.

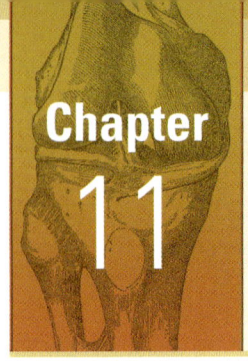

Chapter 11

Tumor and Tumor-like Conditions

David Levi and Daniel M. Walz

WEB ONLY CHAPTER

SECTION 3

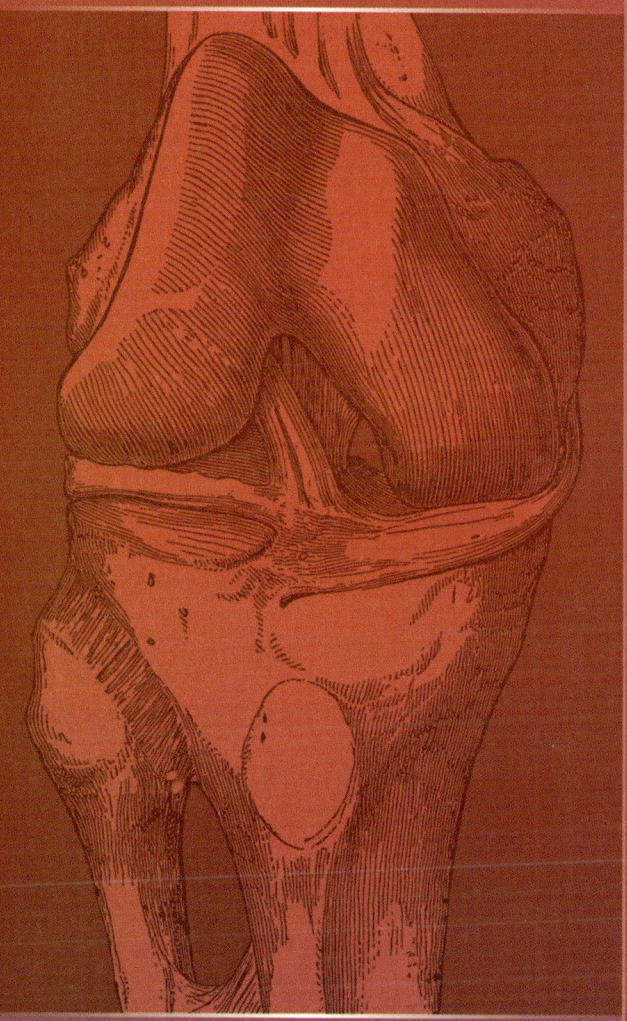

Biomechanics

Chapter 12

Three-Dimensional Morphology of the Knee

Mohamed R. Mahfouz

Chapter 13

Fluoroscopic Analysis of Total Knee Replacement

John Kyle P. Mueller, Richard D. Komistek, Mohamed R. Mahfouz, and Douglas A. Dennis

Chapter 14

Biomechanics and Vibroarthrography of the Patellofemoral Joint

Filip Leszko

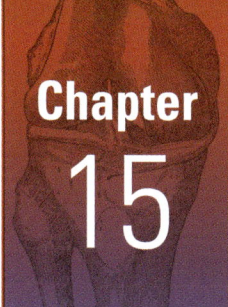

Chapter 15

Contact Mechanics of the Human Knee

Adrija Sharma and Richard D. Komistek

Chapter 16

In Vivo Mechanics and Vibration of the Knee Joint

Sumesh M. Zingde

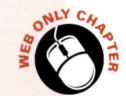

Chapter 17

Does Strain in the Patella Change After TKA? A Finite Element Investigation of Natural and Implanted Patellae

Clare K. Fitzpatrick, Mark A. Baldwin, Azhar A. Ali, Peter J. Laz, and Paul J. Rullkoetter

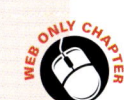

Chapter 18

Simulation Testing of Knee Implants

John Fisher, Louise Jennings, and Claire L. Brockett

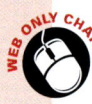

Chapter 19

Knee Wear

John H. Currier and Douglas W. Van Citters

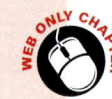

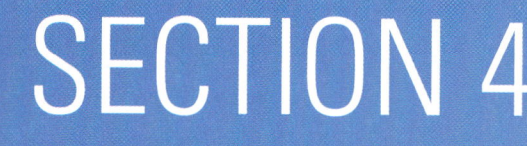

SECTION 4

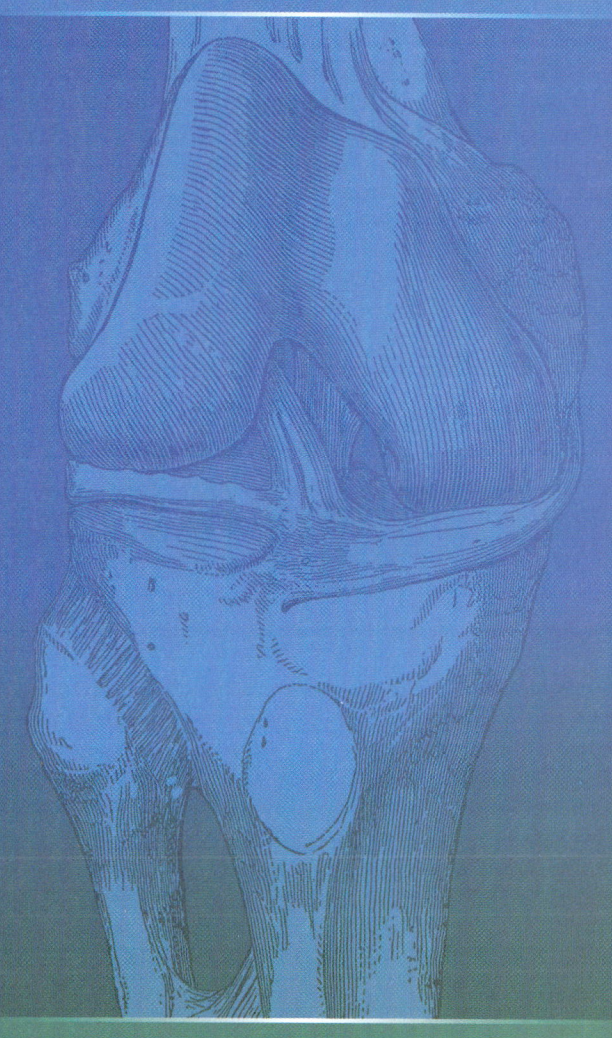

Sports Medicine: Articular Cartilage and Meniscus

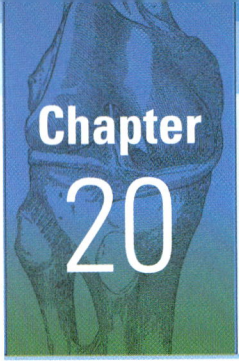

Chapter 20

Articular Cartilage: Biology, Biomechanics, and Healing Response

Sarah E. Henry, Bridget M. Deasy, and Constance R. Chu

Articular cartilage forms the load-bearing surfaces of all synovial joints. Its highly organized structure provides the biomechanical properties necessary for the tissue to withstand multiple forces created during movement.* Following injury, articular cartilage has limited healing potential because the cells have minimal mitotic activity and the matrix lacks a vascular supply[10,35,36] It is important for orthopedic surgeons to understand the basic science of articular cartilage because advances in the treatment of cartilage defects are utilizing tissue engineering repair techniques in an attempt to regenerate and develop tissue with structural and mechanical properties similar to those of normal cartilage.[19,31,37] Also, identification of biochemical biomarkers that detect early cartilage degradation may lead to the development of treatments to prevent, halt, or reverse cartilage damage before the onset of severe degeneration.[4]

BIOLOGY AND STRUCTURE

The main functions of articular cartilage in synovial joints are to provide a low-friction surface for motion and to resist tensile, shear, and compressive forces.[2,3,45] Articular cartilage varies in specific composition within the same joint and between different joints, but it consists of the same basic components and structure throughout all joints.[2] Grossly, articular cartilage appears as a smooth, homogeneous tissue approximately 2 to 5 mm thick (Fig. 20-1). When probed, healthy cartilage is firm and resists deformation. Diseased cartilage is soft, deforms when probed, and may contain visible surface disruptions.

Articular cartilage consists of a sparse population of chondrocytes embedded within a highly hydrated extracellular matrix composed of collagen and proteoglycans. The composition of articular cartilage varies with depth from the surface, and it is divided into four structural zones.[3,31] The matrix is also divided into three regions, and its composition varies with distance from the chondrocyte.[13] This precise arrangement of the tissue components provides specific mechanical properties for each zone.[45] Chondrocytes synthesize matrix components and regulate homeostasis of articular cartilage.[17]

Chondrocytes

Chondrocytes, the single cell type in articular cartilage, account for a small amount of cartilage tissue (5% of weight, <10% of volume) but perform the vital roles of extracellular matrix synthesis and regulation.[29] Chondrocytes are derived from pluripotential mesenchymal stem cells (MSCs) and differentiate into chondroblasts and mature chondrocytes.[42]

Articular cartilage is avascular, thus chondrocytes must derive nutrition and oxygen from the synovial fluid by diffusion and must meet energy requirements through glycolysis.[17] Each chondrocyte is surrounded by extracellular matrix and forms few cell-cell contacts[2] (Fig. 20-2A). Despite this isolated arrangement, chondrocytes are able to respond to a variety of mechanical and biochemical factors.[42]

Chondrocytes differ in size, shape, and metabolic activity in the different structural zones, but all cells contain endoplasmic reticulum and Golgi apparatus for matrix synthesis.[17,46] Chondrocytes synthesize the two major articular cartilage macromolecules—type II collagen and aggrecan—and organize the structure of the matrix.[2] Specific interactions between chondrocytes and the extracellular matrix are unknown, but detection of a variety of mechanical and biochemical factors by the chondrocyte is vital for matrix synthesis and homeostasis. A few mechanisms have been discovered, including the presence of binding proteins (integrins) and osmotically sensitive ion channels on the cell surface of chondrocytes.[29,42]

Development and maintenance of the chondrocyte phenotype is an important research topic because current and future treatments for articular cartilage damage include implantation of stem cells and chondrocytes into defects.[19,25,39] In vitro study of chondrocytes has shown that proliferation and expansion of chondrocytes in monolayer results in loss of cell phenotype and subsequent synthesis of type I collagen. However, culture conditions that include high cell density, cell-cell contact, and a three-dimensional environment appear to maintain the chondrocyte phenotype and the production of type II collagen.[37,47] Growth factors such as transforming growth factor-β (TGF-β), fibroblast growth factor (FGF), and insulin-like growth factor-1 (IGF-1) also appear important for maintenance of the chondrocyte phenotype, with identification of receptors on chondrocytes.[42] A range of other molecules such as oxygen and common injectable anesthetics have been shown to have an impact on chondrocytes. In a recent study, sustained hypoxia in vitro increased type II collagen gene expression and proteoglycan synthesis.[6] Also, a one-time dose of 0.25% to 0.5% bupivacaine has been reported to be toxic to human chondrocytes in vitro in a dose- and time-dependent manner.[5] Further research is required to understand the complex interactions of numerous biochemical factors with chondrocytes.

Extracellular Matrix

Most of the articular cartilage (90%) is composed of the extracellular matrix. The matrix consists of tissue fluid and macromolecules.[2] The composition of the zonal structure of the matrix determines its interaction with tissue fluid and thus is responsible for determining the mechanical properties of the cartilage.[31] The main functions of the matrix are to

---

*References 3, 18, 31, 38, 44, and 45.

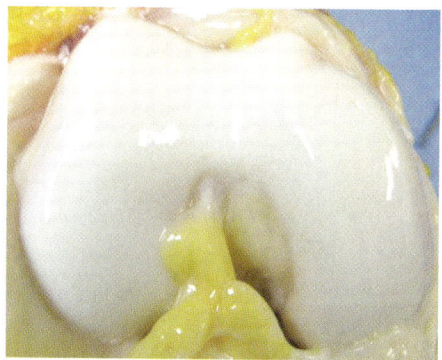

Figure 20-1. Gross image of articular cartilage on the femoral condyle of a healthy 20-year-old female. This image displays the smooth, homogeneous surface appearance of normal articular cartilage.

resist tensile and shear forces through the arrangement of collagen fibrils, and to resist compressive forces through alteration in hydrostatic pressure.[9,18,24]

Tissue Fluid

Water is the major component of the extracellular matrix (75% weight) and tissue fluid.[2] Tissue fluid also consists of high concentrations of cations, gases, and small proteins. The volume of water present in the cartilage tissue depends on the concentration and organization of the macromolecules, specifically, proteoglycans. The concentration of proteoglycans varies between cartilage zones, contributing to differences in water concentration, porosity, and permeability of the tissue.[29,31] Throughout joint movement, water continually moves into and out of the cartilage to aid in distribution of compressive forces and lubrication of the cartilage surface.[18]

Macromolecules

The macromolecules of the extracellular matrix include collagens (20% of the matrix), proteoglycans (5%), and noncollagenous proteins and glycoproteins (1%).[2] Type II collagen fibrils provide structural integrity and tensile and shear strength to the articular cartilage.[44] Proteoglycans, mainly aggrecan, attract water, providing resistance to compression.[45] The noncollagenous proteins and glycoproteins help to bind chondrocytes to the matrix, stabilize matrix macromolecules, and assist in regulation of matrix homeostasis.[29]

Collagens

Articular cartilage contains multiple types of collagen, including II, VI, IX, X, and XI.[29] Type II collagen accounts for 90% of the collagen in articular cartilage.[2] Type II collagen is composed of three alpha chains, which intertwine into a triple helix. These helices covalently cross-link in a lateral array to form collagen fibrils.[34] This network of fibrils contributes to maintenance of the volume, shape, and tensile and shear strength of the cartilage. Levels of type II collagen are highest in the superficial zone and decrease in concentration with increasing depth from the surface[33] (see Fig. 20-2A and B). The collagen fibril network restrains the proteoglycans in the matrix and prevents swelling of the cartilage to greater than 450 mOsm when water flows into the tissue.[33] This allows creation of high tissue pressure, which is vital for resistance of compressive forces.

Under physiologic conditions, type II collagen metabolism is slow and fibrils have a half-life of years. In early stages of cartilage degeneration, degradation of collagen fibrils is observed.[26] Enzymes called matrix metalloproteinases (MMPs) are thought to contribute to this degradation, specifically collagenases and aggrecanases. Collagenases mediate cleavage of type II collagen and produce two main fragments.[26] Antibodies to specific neoepitopes on these fragments can be detected by synovial fluid, serum, or urine assays and are being studied for use as potential biomarkers of early cartilage degradation.[1,4,26]

Other collagen types are less prevalent but perform important functions, including stabilization and regulation of type II collagen fibrils. Type IX collagen forms cross-links along the surface of type II collagen fibrils and interconnects the fibrils with proteoglycan aggregates.[29] Type XI collagen binds to the interior structure of type II collagen fibrils and regulates the diameter of the fibrils. Type X collagen is localized near the calcified cartilage zone and the hypertrophic zone of the growth plate and is thought to contribute to cartilage mineralization.[29] Type VI collagen is located in the pericellular matrix and aids in the attachment of chondrocytes to the extracellular matrix.[13]

Proteoglycans

Proteoglycans (PGs) consist of a protein core with glycosaminoglycan (GAG) side chains.[29] GAGs consist of long unbranched polysaccharide chains containing repeating disaccharides of amino sugars with negatively charged carboxylate or sulfate groups.[28] Specific GAGs include hyaluronic acid (HA), chondroitin sulfate (CS), keratan sulfate (KS), and dermatan sulfate (DS). The major proteoglycan (90% of mass) in articular cartilage is aggrecan.[8] Aggrecan has many CS and KS side chains and noncovalently associates with an HA backbone to form aggregates (see Fig. 20-2A). HA is a long-chain nonsulfated GAG capable of binding a large number of aggrecan molecules. Link protein, a glycoprotein, stabilizes the association between HA and each aggrecan molecule.[29]

Aggrecans play a key role in generating hydrostatic pressure. The negatively charged aggrecans attract cations, increasing the osmolality of the tissue. Water is then attracted into the tissue, decreasing the osmolality.[45] Hydrostatic pressure created by the interaction of collagen, PGs, and water provides stiffness to the cartilage to absorb compressive mechanical loads without damage to the matrix. Displacement of water from PGs during compression of the superficial zone of matrix lubricates the joint.[45]

Under physiologic conditions, aggrecan turnover occurs over a period of years.[26] Similar to collagen, degradation of aggrecan is observed in early cartilage degeneration, and aggrecanases are thought to contribute.[1] Aggrecan synthesis and degradation can also be measured by antibodies to specific neoepitopes on fragments by synovial fluid or serum assays. Inhibitors of aggrecanases are being investigated for potential treatments for cartilage degeneration.[11]

Smaller PGs include decorin, fibromodulin, and biglycan.[29] The function of each PG is related to the specific core protein and GAG chains that it contains. Decorin contains DS side chains and is located at the surface of type II collagen fibrils. It is thought to inhibit the lateral growth of fibrils and contributes to organization and stabilization of the fibrils.

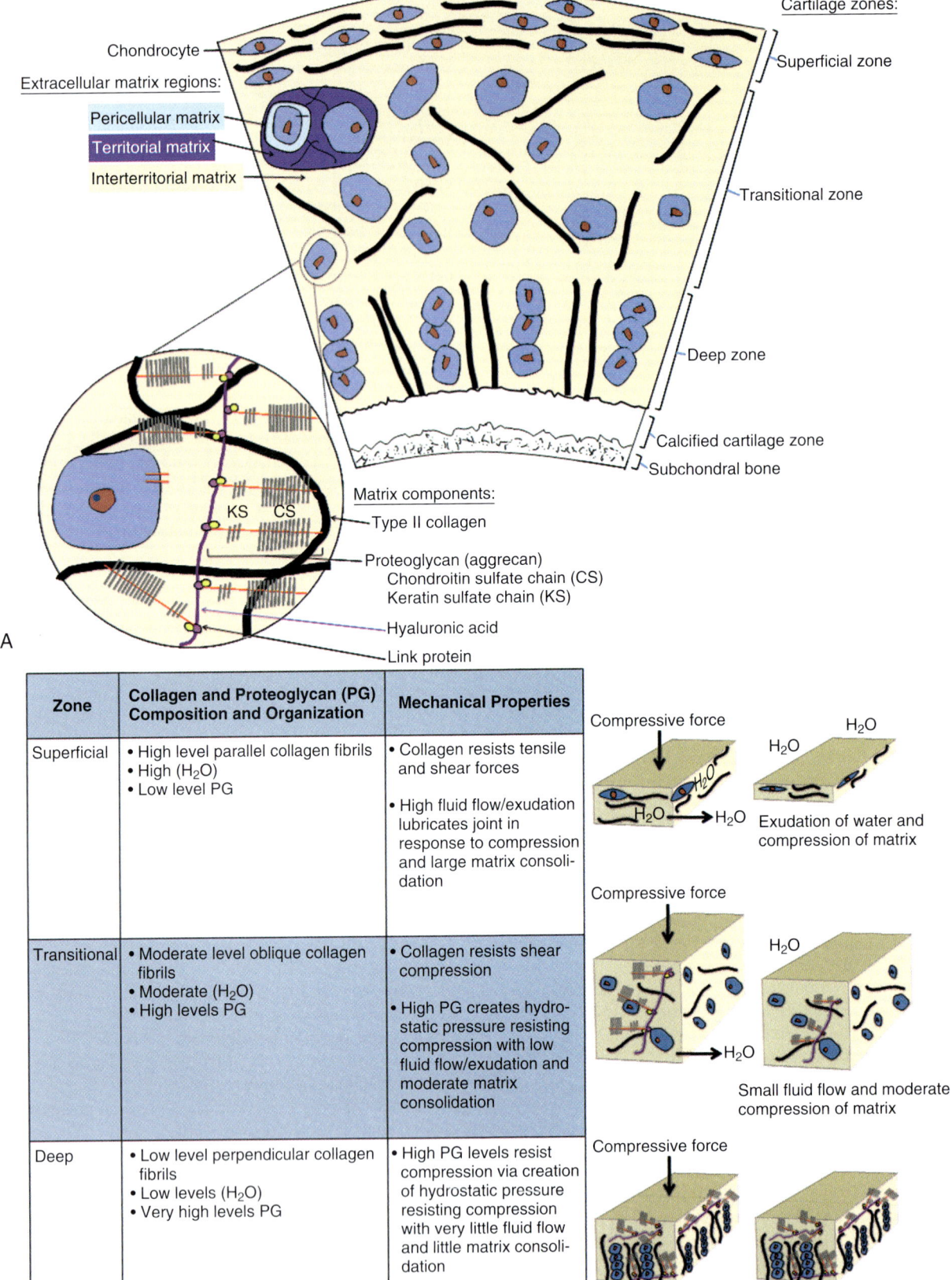

Figure 20-2. A, Schematic of articular cartilage matrix regions and structural zones. The three matrix regions depicted with increasing distance from the chondrocyte are, respectively, pericellular, territorial, and interterritorial. The matrix regions are present in all zones but are depicted in only one area in the schematic. As described, chondrocyte morphology and organization vary between zones. Collagen fibril concentration and organization also vary between zones. Superficial zone: high collagen content, parallel organization; transitional zone: moderate collagen content, oblique orientation; deep zone: low collagen content, vertical orientation. *Inset,* A chondrocyte is surrounded by the type II collagen fibril network and proteoglycans. (Aggrecan molecules are shown with keratin and chondroitin sulfate glycosaminoglycan chains on a hyaluronic acid backbone. The aggrecan molecules are bound to collagen by link protein.) **B,** Table and schematic of composition, organization, and mechanical properties of articular cartilage zonal layers.

Fibromodulin has KS side chains and binds type II collagen fibrils, providing stabilization. Biglycan contains DS side chains, binds TGF-β, and interacts with type VI collagen in the pericellular matrix.[29] Expression of smaller PG changes within zones and with mechanical stress likely contributes to cell stabilization and signaling through interaction with other proteins.[29]

Noncollagenous Proteins and Glycoproteins

The matrix contains many additional proteins that represent a small volume but a large molarity of the tissue.[2] Cartilage oligomeric matrix protein (COMP), anchorin, and fibronectin function to bind chondrocytes to the matrix. COMP binds to chondrocytes in the territorial matrix.[7] Anchorin binds to chondrocyte surface protein, anchoring chondrocytes to collagen fibrils. Fibronectin is an adhesion molecule expressed on the surface of chondrocytes.[7] Ongoing research is investigating the roles of these proteins, but most appear to aid in organization and stabilization of the chondrocytes and matrix.[29]

Other proteins include growth factors and cytokines, which bind to chondrocyte receptors, altering rates of matrix synthesis and degradation. Effects of these proteins depend on their concentration, cofactors, type of target cell, and number of cell receptors. TGF-β, IGF-1, FGF, bone morphogenetic protein (BMP), and platelet-derived growth factors (PDGFs) stimulate matrix synthesis and proliferation.[42] TGF-β, FGF, and PDGFs also promote proliferation and chondrogenic differentiation of mesenchymal stem cells in combination with many other factors. Matrix degradation is stimulated by interleukin-1 (IL-1), tumor necrosis factor-alpha (TNF-α), and MMPs.[42]

Regions Surrounding the Chondrocyte

Matrix composition and organization vary with distance from the chondrocyte. Three regions have been identified: pericellular matrix, territorial matrix, and interterritorial matrix[2] (see Fig. 20-2A). The pericellular matrix directly surrounds the chondrocyte; the territorial matrix surrounds the pericellular matrix and assists in binding the chondrocyte cell membranes to the matrix. The pericellular and territorial regions also transmit mechanical signals to the chondrocytes when the matrix deforms.[13] Most of the matrix is contained in the interterritorial region, which consists of collagen fibrils and PG aggregates and provides the mechanical properties of the cartilage.[3]

Pericellular Matrix

In all cartilage zones, the individual chondrocyte is directly surrounded by the pericellular matrix. Chondrocyte cell membranes attach to the rim of the pericellular matrix covering the cell surface. This region contains many PGs and proteins, including type VI collagen, decorin, anchorin, and fibronectin.[13] This region contains little to no fibrillar collagen. The function of this region is not fully understood, but it serves to regulate the microenvironment of the chondrocyte. The presence of type VI collagen defines this region and anchors the chondrocyte cell membrane to the matrix.[13]

Territorial Matrix

The territorial matrix surrounds the pericellular matrix, forming clusters of chondrocytes. In the deep zone, the territorial matrix surrounds each column of chondrocytes. In this region, thin collagen fibrils adhere to the pericellular matrix and form fibrillar baskets around the cells.[26] This region protects the chondrocytes from damage during joint loading.[3]

Interterritorial Matrix

Most of the matrix is contained in the interterritorial region. Compared with the other two regions, the interterritorial region possesses the largest-diameter collagen fibrils and is responsible for the mechanical properties of the cartilage.[3] The orientation of the collagen fibers in this region changes with depth from the surface, as described in the section on the zonal structure of articular cartilage.[45]

Many advances have been made in the knowledge of articular cartilage biology, but many more questions remain, including questions related to the factors involved in regulation of matrix homeostasis and formation of the zonal structure of articular cartilage.

Zones

In addition to specific matrix regions, articular cartilage has a precise zonal structure, with the composition, organization, and mechanical properties of the tissue varying with depth from the surface.[31] Four zones have been identified from the surface to the subchondral bone, respectively: superficial zone, transitional zone, deep zone, and calcified cartilage[21] (see Fig. 20-2A and B). Each zone has unique chondrocyte morphology, arrangement of type II collagen fibers, and levels of proteoglycans and water. This structure creates different mechanical properties for each specific zone.[31,45,46]

Signals that regulate the development and maintenance of the zonal structure of articular cartilage remain unknown but are the topic of current research.[31] A recent study isolated bovine articular chondrocytes from each zone, seeded the cells in a fibrin hydrogel, and subjected the cells to oscillatory tensile loading.[40] Tensile loading was found to stimulate PG synthesis in superficial zone chondrocytes, and deep zone chondrocytes were found to secrete matrix, exhibiting properties similar to the superficial zone.[40] This suggests that synthesis and organization of the matrix by chondrocytes are partially dependent on the mechanical environment.[40] An understanding of zonal structure is important for the development of artificial cartilage constructs or for induction of a cartilage reparative response for future treatment of chondral injuries.

Superficial Zone

The superficial zone, the thinnest zone (10% to 20% of the matrix, ≈0.2 to 0.5 mm), consists of two layers.[2] The top layer is a clear film called the lamina splendens, which contains no cells, little polysaccharide, and few collagen fibrils. The main layer consists of flattened ellipsoid, densely packed, and horizontally arranged chondrocytes that synthesize a matrix with high collagen and low PG content.[2,45,46] The thick collagen fibrils are arranged parallel to the surface (see Fig. 20-2A). The abundance and parallel organization of collagen to the joint surface permits the superficial zone to provide strength to resist tensile and shear forces.[24] The high concentration of water also provides lubrication and resistance to compression.[18] Removal of this layer, as observed in early cartilage degeneration, results in increased permeability and decreased resistance to tensile forces. This leads to softening of the cartilage and increased loading of the remainder of the matrix.[45]

Transitional Zone

The transitional zone, the largest zone (40% to 60% of the matrix, ≈1 to 1.75 mm), functions to resist shear and compressive forces.[3,24] The chondrocytes are spheroidal and synthesize matrix with larger-diameter collagen fibrils oriented obliquely to the surface into rotational arches[46] (see Fig. 20-2A). This arrangement allows the fibers to resist shear forces.[18] The higher PG and the lower water content of the matrix compared with the superficial zone permit increased compressibility and thus shock absorption and load distribution.[45]

Deep (Radial) Zone

The deep zone is of intermediate thickness (30% of the matrix, ≈0.6 to 1 mm) and functions to resist compressive forces.[45] The chondrocytes are spheroidal, are arranged in vertical columns perpendicular to the surface, and synthesize matrix with the greatest amount of PG[33,46] (see Fig. 20-2A). The collagen fibrils are the largest in diameter and are arranged vertically to resist compression, provide stiffness, and anchor the cartilage to the subchondral bone.[18] Removal of the deep vertical fibrils increases the tensile strain in the superficial fibrils and the junction with subchondral bone.[3]

Calcified Cartilage Zone

The thin calcified cartilage zone between the deep zone and subchondral bone anchors the cartilage to the bone via type X collagen. The tidemark is located in this zone and is the boundary between calcified and uncalcified cartilage.[2]

BIOMECHANICS

The composition and structure of the articular cartilage extracellular matrix formed by chondrocytes create a low-friction surface capable of sustaining a wide range of static and dynamic mechanical loads. The coefficient of friction estimated at 0.002 in synovial joints allows the tissue to withstand millions of cycles of loading each year without degeneration.[45] The precise zonal structure of cartilage gives the tissue its biomechanical properties: The superficial zone consisting of parallel collagen fibrils and high collagen levels resists tensile and shear forces; the transitional zone consisting of oblique collagen fibrils and high PG levels resists shear and compressive forces; the deep zone consisting of perpendicular collagen fibrils and high PG levels resists compressive forces* (see Fig. 20-2B). Normal movement results in peak static stresses reaching 3.5 MPa, occurring over a long duration (5 to 30+ minutes), and resulting in compressive strains of 35% to 45%. Peak dynamic stresses reach as high as 20 MPa (3000 lb per square inch), occur during very short durations (<1 second), and lead to compressive strains of 1% to 3%.[3,18,45] Resistance to compressive loading is a function of the level of PGs and interaction with the collagen fibril network. In response to compression, cartilage exhibits biphasic viscoelastic properties: The solid matrix deforms, increasing the contact area and decreasing stress; the tissue fluid is exuded and redistributed, lubricating the surface and decreasing friction.[38,44] Fluid pressurization provides the main strength of cartilage to resist compressive loads.[9,38] PGs have a large

negative charge owing to the carboxylate and sulfate groups of GAGs. This high fixed negative charge density attracts mobile cations, generating increased osmolality.[9,28] Water is attracted to the tissue, decreasing osmolality and generating high fluid pressure. The collagen fibril network restrains the PG, preventing swelling and maintaining high fluid pressure.[9,45] The deep zone provides the majority of resistance to compressive load via deformation of its solid matrix. The high PG content and low permeability of the deep zone trap water, creating a high fluid pressure.[38] Increased permeability of the superficial zone also provides resistance to compression via extrusion of fluid into the joint space.[9,44] After the load is removed, the cartilage matrix reabsorbs the fluid and returns to its hydrated status.[45] Distribution of compressive loads minimizes stress on subchondral bone, chondrocytes, and other matrix zones.

In addition to different types of stresses (tensile, shear, compressive), physiologic movement creates mechanical stresses of different magnitudes, durations, rates, and frequencies. A critical yet unknown level and pattern of mechanical stress are required to maintain the normal balance of matrix homeostasis beyond which leads to degeneration.[23,27,32] Simplifying these complex interactions, static compression suppresses matrix synthesis, while dynamic loading stimulates matrix synthesis.[32]

Static compression even within the physiologic range inhibits matrix synthesis, downregulating gene expression and synthesis of type II collagen and aggrecan and increasing expression of MMPs.[32] Similarly, both immobilization and excessive loading (high magnitude or long duration) result in decreased matrix synthesis.[45] Decreased levels of PG decrease the ability of the tissue to resist compressive forces, increasing the susceptibility of tissue to microdamage. Loss of PG caused by immobilization appears to be reversible on remobilization of the joint, but excessive loading often results in irreversible chondrocyte death and surface disruptions.[41]

On the contrary, dynamic loading increases synthesis of collagen type II and aggrecan and increases expression of tissue inhibitors of metalloproteinases (TIMPs), enzymes that counteract MMPs.[27] Moderate exercise is reported to increase PG synthesis and cartilage stiffness, but the specific type, intensity, duration, and frequency necessary to produce these beneficial changes are difficult to define.[27,45] The effects of these different variables on matrix homeostasis and details of the mechanosignaling processes are not well understood and require further research.

HEALING RESPONSE

Articular cartilage has a limited capacity for natural healing owing to lack of blood supply, absence of chondrogenic progenitor cells, and decreased mitotic activity.[2] Cartilage injuries occur through a variety of mechanisms, including a single load of great magnitude or repetitive joint overloading of lesser magnitude.[35,36] Cartilage lesions are common in patients sustaining knee injuries, with lesions present in approximately 60% at arthroscopy.[43] Cartilage injuries have been divided into three categories based on depth of injury: (1) cell and matrix damage without visible surface changes; (2) cartilage disruption with visible fibrillations, fissures, flaps, or defects; and (3) visible cartilage and subchondral bone disruption. Each injury type has a different healing response

---

*References 3, 9, 24, 31, 38, and 44.

dependent mainly on viability of the chondrocytes and penetration of the damage into the subchondral bone.[2] Both the initial impact and subsequent altered mechanics contribute to cartilage degeneration.[35,36] Current surgical treatments for cartilage damage include arthroscopic débridement, microfracture, autologous chondrocyte implantation, and osteochondral transplantation.[19] Joint arthroplasty is the last option in young patients because multiple revisions are often necessary. Although some patients receive symptomatic relief with these treatments, none is capable of restoring articular cartilage with the same volume, zonal structure, and biomechanical properties as healthy cartilage.* Therefore, research is ongoing to develop novel techniques to reconstruct or repair damage to the articular cartilage surface.

Cell and Matrix Damage

Almost every joint injury includes damage to chondrocytes and the matrix through impact.[35,36] Following impact injury, studies report increased expression of proteins involved in cartilage degradation (TNF-α, IL-1, and MMPs).[35] Further investigation is needed to determine the biochemical changes that occur with an impact injury and to identify factors that differentiate a reversible injury from an irreversible injury. One important variable in determining the severity of cartilage damage is the survival of chondrocytes. Damage that results in injury only to the matrix components and spares chondrocytes has the potential for restoration of the matrix by chondrocyte matrix synthesis.[2] If the damage involves chondrocyte death, spontaneous repair to damaged tissue is limited and results in matrix with altered structure. If chondrocytes are not able to synthesize new matrix, the damaged matrix loses PG and has a decreased ability to resist mechanical forces.[15] Development of techniques such as biomarkers to detect this early damage to chondrocytes and the matrix is important to understand the natural history of this "invisible" injury and to further advance early treatment options.[4]

Cartilage Disruption

Because of lack of access to the vascular system, visible damage to the cartilage surface that does not extend into the subchondral bone does not initiate a reparative response.[2] Transient proliferation of chondrocytes near the edges of the defect has been observed, but the cells do not proliferate into the defect or produce a significant amount of matrix.[15,30] The cells briefly increase synthesis of type II collagen and PG, but injury results in chondrocyte apoptosis and cessation of matrix synthesis.[30] Damage to the superficial zone disrupts the collagen network and increases the permeability of the matrix, thereby decreasing the ability of the matrix to resist tensile and compressive loads. This results in increased stress in the matrix and subchondral bone with eventual progression to osteoarthritis.[20]

One treatment option for partial-thickness cartilage lesions is arthroscopic lavage and débridement. This involves lavage of the joint with saline and removal of fibrillated or chondral flaps of cartilage with a mechanical shaver to create a smooth surface. Débridement results in improvement of symptoms in some patients but is not clearly superior to placebo.[22] Because full-thickness cartilage defects left untreated rarely heal spontaneously, surgical treatments include microfracture, autologous chondrocyte implantation (ACI), and oteochondral autografts or allografts.* Microfracture is a treatment option for full-thickness cartilage defects measuring less than 2 cm² on a weight-bearing region of a limb with normal alignment. Through penetration of the subchondral bone with an awl, microfracture results in formation of fibrocartilage (predominately type I cartilage) at the defect site.[12,16] When compared with microfracture in a recent 2-year follow-up report, patients undergoing ACI were reported to have similar clinical outcomes but structurally superior repair tissue more similar to normal cartilage.[39] ACI has been used for treatment of symptomatic full-thickness cartilage disruption in patients with lesions measuring greater than 2 cm².[2,25,39] ACI involves obtaining chondrocytes from a cartilage biopsy of the patient and culturing the cells in vitro. Then, following chondrocyte expansion, the cells are injected beneath a periosteal/collagen flap or membrane covering the cartilage defect, which is sealed with fibrin glue.[25,39] Advances in this technique continue to be developed, including use of three-dimensional natural and synthetic scaffolds, addition of bone marrow mesenchymal stem cells, and addition of growth factors.[37] Osteochondral auto/allograft transplantation can also be performed for full-thickness cartilage disruption. Osteochondral autograft transfer (OATS) involves harvesting osteochondral plugs from a limited weight-bearing area of the joint and inserting the plugs into a full-thickness or osteochondral defect measuring greater than 2 cm².[12,14] ACI and osteochondral grafting result in formation of cartilage with structure and mechanical properties intermediate between fibrocartilage and normal cartilage.[12,14,25,39] Additional long-term outcome studies are needed to further evaluate the success of current treatment methods of cartilage disruption.

Cartilage and Subchondral Bone Disruption

Cartilage injuries penetrating the subchondral bone gain access to the vascular system and elicit a reparative response.[2] This response includes formation of a hematoma, a fibrin clot, an inflammatory response, and migration of mesenchymal stem cells from the bone marrow.[12,19,20,26,30] Platelets release vasoactive mediators, growth factors, and cytokines, including TGF-β and PDGF. Although the force required to produce a fracture of the subchondral bone is severe and also causes chondrocyte death and matrix damage, the reparative response does reliably result in formation of fibrocartilage within 6 to 8 weeks.[10,26] Fibrocartilage cells appear similar to fibroblasts, the matrix consists mainly of type I collagen, and the matrix is different in composition and structure compared with normal cartilage.[10,30]

Although some patients with intra-articular fracture have good function following surgical restoration and stabilization of the joint surface, the chondral repair tissue formed following most osteochondral injuries begins to degenerate, with the presence of fibrillations, within the first year.[10]

---

*References 12, 14, 16, 20, 25, and 39.

*References 12, 14, 16, 25, 30, and 39.

Penetration of the subchondral bone induces a reparative response, but the synthesized cartilage does not have the same composition, structure, and mechanical properties as normal cartilage.[19,20,26,30] Many patients develop posttraumatic arthritis following intra-articular fracture. This is due to a combination of the initial impact injury and alterations in joint contact forces resulting in chondrocyte death and disruption of matrix integrity.[10] Treatment options for posttraumatic arthritis include osteochondral auto/allograft transplantation for focal defects and joint arthroplasty for more diffuse osteoarthritis.[12,14]

FUTURE DIRECTIONS

Major challenges to the development of treatments for damage to articular cartilage include maintenance of cells with chondrocyte phenotypes, restoration of the zonal structure of cartilage, and integration of repair tissue with the surrounding matrix.[31,42] Current research is also investigating potential chondroprotective agents to stimulate repair, such as matrix metalloproteinase inhibitors, growth factors, and cytokines.[11,37] The goal is development of a treatment aimed at the early stages of cartilage degeneration with restoration of normal articular cartilage structure and function. Research is ongoing to investigate the mechanical and biochemical factors necessary to develop tissue-engineered cartilage repair techniques and to stimulate a reparative response.

KEY REFERENCES

Chu CR, Izzo NJ, Coyle CH, et al: The in vitro effects of bupivacaine on articular chondrocytes. J Bone Joint Surg Br 90:814–820, 2008.
Furman BD, Olson SA, Guilak F: The development of posttraumatic arthritis after articular fracture. J Orthop Trauma 20:719–725, 2006.

Glasson SS, Askew R, Sheppard B, et al: Deletion of active ADAMTS5 prevents cartilage degradation in a murine model of osteoarthritis. Nature 434:644–648, 2005.
Gudas R, Kalesinskas RJ, Kimtys V, et al: A prospective randomized clinical study of mosaic osteochondral autologous transplant versus microfracture for the treatment of osteochondral defects in the knee joint in young athletes. Arthroscopy 21:1066–1075, 2005.
Hangody L, Vasarhelyi G, Hangody LR, et al: Autologous osteochondral grafting: technique and long-term results. Injury 39(Suppl 1):S32–S39, 2008.
Hunziker EB, Kapfinger E: Repair of partial-thickness defects in articular cartilage: cell recruitment from the synovial membrane. J Bone Joint Surg Am 78:721–733, 1996.
Lee KB, Bai LB, Yoon TR, et al: Second-look arthroscopic findings and clinical outcomes after microfracture for osteochondral lesions of the talus. Am J Sports Med 37(Suppl 1):63S–70S, 2009.
Magnussen RA, Dunn WR, Carey JL, Spindler KP: Treatment of focal articular cartilage defects in the knee. Clin Orthop Relat Res 466:952–962, 2008.
Szczodry M, Coyle CH, Kramer SJ, et al: Progressive chondrocyte death after impact injury indicates a need for chondroprotective therapy. Am J Sports Med 37:2318–2322, 2009.
Thomas GC, Asanbaeva A, Vena P, et al: A nonlinear constituent based viscoelastic model for articular cartilage and analysis of tissue remodeling due to altered glycosaminoglycan-collagen interactions. J Biomech Eng 131:101–112, 2009.
Van Assche D, Staes F, Van Caspel D, et al: Autologous chondrocyte implantation versus microfracture for knee cartilage injury: a prospective randomized trial, with 2-year follow-up. Knee Surg Sports Traumatol Arthrosc 18:486–495, 2010.
Wescoe KE, Schugar RC, Chu CR, Deasy BM: The role of the biochemical and biophysical environment in chondrogenic stem cell differentiation assays and cartilage tissue engineering. Cell Biochem Biophys 52:85–102, 2008.
Wong M, Carter DR: Articular cartilage functional histomorphology and mechanobiology: a research perspective. Bone 33:1–13, 2003.
Youn I, Choi JB, Cao L, et al: Zonal variations in the three-dimensional morphology of the chondron measured in situ using confocal microscopy. Osteoarthritis Cartilage 14:889–897, 2006.

Full references for this chapter can be found on www.expertconsult.com.

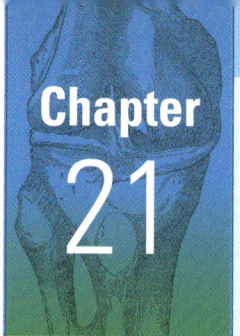

Chapter 21

Articular Cartilage Injury and Adult OCD: Treatment Options and Decision Making

Nicole A. Friel, Sarvottam Bajaj, and Brian J. Cole

Osteochondritis dissecans (OCD) is a pathologic process in which the subchondral bone and the overlying articular cartilage detach from the underlying bony surface.[10,40,55] The disease results in subchondral bone loss and destabilization of the overlying articular cartilage, leading to separation and increased susceptibility to stress and shear.[43] Fragmentation of both cartilage and bone leads to early degenerative changes and loss of function in the affected compartment. The true cause is unknown but is likely related to repetitive microtrauma, an acute traumatic incident, ischemia, an ossification abnormality, or endocrine or genetic predisposition.[2,39,53]

The prevalence of OCD is estimated at 15 to 30 cases per 100,000, most frequently occurring in the knee, with medial femoral condyle involvement in 80% of cases, lateral femoral condyle in 15%, and patellofemoral in 5%.[27,36] The lateral aspect of the medial femoral condyle is the classic site of the OCD lesion. In addition to the knee, OCD has the propensity of occurring in the elbow, wrist, and ankle.[2,10,55]

Osteochondritis dissecans is divided into juvenile (JOCD) and adult (AOCD) forms.[9] The distinction between JOCD (open growth plates) and AOCD (closed growth plates) may be important in treatment and prognosis. JOCD often resolves with nonoperative management and has a much better prognosis compared with adult OCD, which, once symptomatic, can follow a progressive, unremitting course.

Nonoperative treatments for symptomatic AOCD are rarely an option because of the inherent poor regenerative capacity of articular cartilage. Thus, cases of AOCD usually require surgical intervention, such as loose body removal, drilling, internal fixation, marrow stimulation, autologous chondrocyte implantation, or osteochondral autograft/allograft transplantation, to replace the damaged cartilage. In advanced cases, joint replacement may be the only feasible solution.

PRESENTATION

A patient with an OCD lesion complains primarily of pain and swelling of the affected joint, which can be triggered by physical activity. In the presence of a loose body, mechanical symptoms such as clicking, popping, and locking may accompany the primary complaints.

On physical examination, patients present with tenderness overlying the OCD region. Patients often present with an antalgic gait. If the OCD lesion is present in the classic location, the lateral aspect of the medial femoral condyle, the patient will ambulate with the affected leg in relative external rotation (Wilson sign) to decrease contact of the lesion with the medial tibial eminence. Joint effusion, decreased range of motion, and quadriceps atrophy are also variably present, depending on the severity and duration of the lesion.[20,42]

Patellar OCD most often presents with patellofemoral pain, followed by swelling. Feelings of a loose body, locking, or giving way, or episodes of patellar subluxation may also be noted. On examination, patients have retropatellar crepitus or pain and effusion.

IMAGING

Unfortunately, none of the physical findings observed during the examination can be used specifically to diagnose OCD; therefore confirmatory x-ray, magnetic resonance imaging (MRI), or computed tomography (CT) scans are required. Plain x-ray films should include standard anteroposterior, flexion weight-bearing anteroposterior (tunnel view), lateral, and Merchant views (Fig. 21-1). Flexion weight-bearing anteroposterior in addition to standard anteroposterior allows better visualization of lesions along the posterolateral aspect of the medial femoral condyle.[26] Radiographic images of patients with adult OCD show a lesion that typically appears as an area of osteosclerotic bone, with a high-intensity line between defect and epiphysis.

MRI is the mainstay in the diagnosis of OCD lesions and is the most informative imaging modality in the preoperative workup of OCD. Specifically, the quality of bone edema, subchondral separation, and cartilage condition are evaluated before treatment.[1] MRI can reliably indicate lesion size, location, and depth, providing insight into a patient's knee condition (Fig. 21-2). MRI images are assessed according to the criteria presented below; meeting one of the four criteria offers up to 97% sensitivity and 100% specificity in predicting lesion stability.[15,16,20,43]

- Thin, ill-defined or well-demarcated line of high signal intensity, measuring 5 mm or more in length at the interface between the OCD lesion and underlying subchondral bone
- Discrete rounded area of homogeneous high signal intensity, 5 mm or more in diameter beneath the lesion
- Focal defect with an articular surface of the lesion with a width of 5 mm or more
- High signal intensity line traversing the articular cartilage and subchondral bone plate into the lesion

Furthermore, OCD lesions can be classified by MRI findings according to whether the lesion is attached, partially attached, or completely detached from the parent bone[37,43,49] (Table 21-1).

Other imaging modalities such as CT scans are also used, as they can be greatly beneficial in revealing the exact location and extent of the lesion.

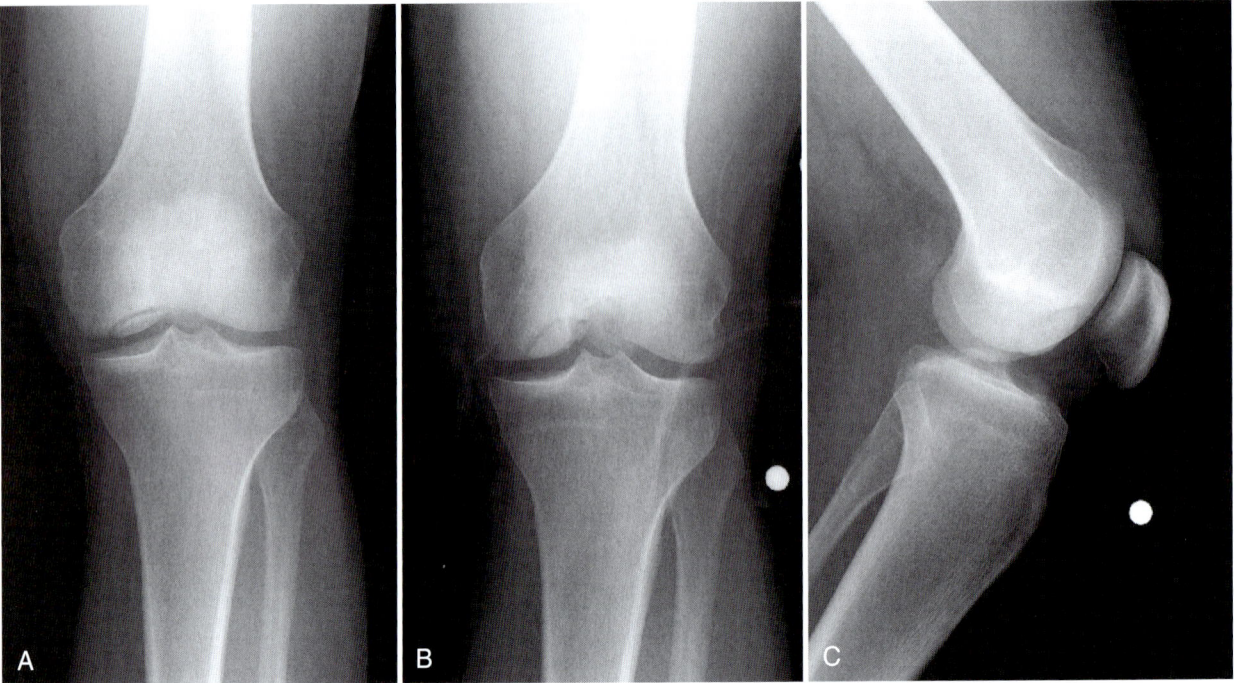

Figure 21-1. Radiograph of an osteochondritis dissecans (OCD) lesion in the classic location of the lateral aspect of the medial femoral condyle. **A**, Standard anteroposterior. **B**, Flexion weight-bearing anteroposterior. **C**, Lateral.

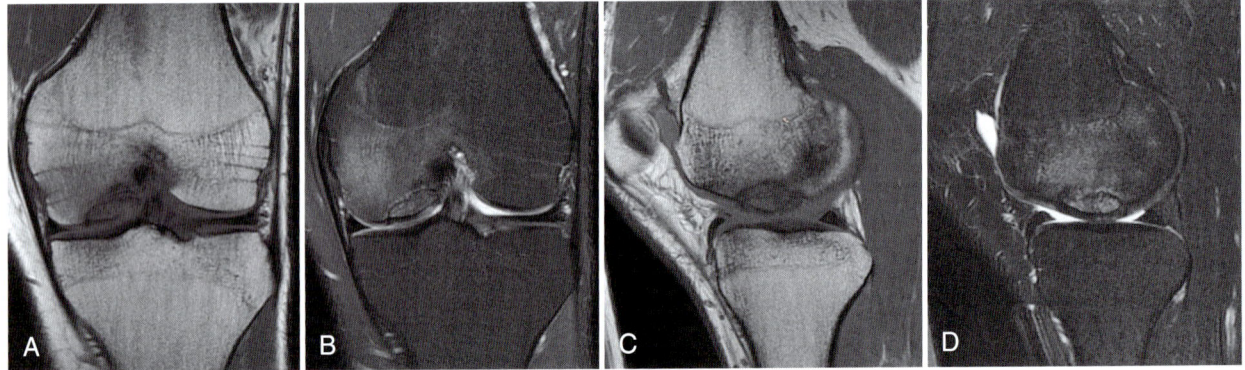

Figure 21-2. Magnetic resonance imaging (MRI) of an osteochondritis dissecans (OCD) lesion at the lateral aspect of the medial femoral condyle. Anteroposterior T1-weighted **(A)** and T2-weighted **(B)** views. Sagittal T1-weighted **(C)** and T2-weighted **(D)** views.

Table 21-1 MRI Staging for Evaluation of Osteochondral Fracture[27,33,38]

Stage	MRI Findings
0	Normal
I	Signal changes consistent with articular cartilage injury, without disruption, and with normal subchondral bone
II	High-grade signal intensity; breach of the articular cartilage with a stable subchondral fragment
III	Partial chondral detachment with a thin high-signal rim (on T2-weighted images) behind the osteochondral fragment, representing synovial fluid
IV	Loose body in the center of the osteochondral fragment or free in the joint space

ETIOLOGY, NATURAL HISTORY, AND PROGNOSIS

The definitive cause of OCD has yet to be established. A number of factors may contribute, such as repetitive micro-trauma, acute stress and injury, restricted blood supply, endocrine abnormalities, and genetic predisposition.[2,39,53] Physical trauma is thought to be one of the major contributory factors in the development of OCD. Repetitive trauma to the joint leads to redundant healing and fibrosis, interrupting the blood supply to subchondral bone and possibly leading to avascular necrosis.[13] In adults, high-impact sports such as soccer, basketball, football, and weightlifting may put a participant at higher risk of developing OCD. Endocrine abnormalities affecting calcium and phosphorous homeostasis or anomalies of bone formation can compromise the blood supply to subchondral bone and progress to avascular necrosis. Recent reports have suggested a genetic predisposition to OCD.[39]

Most adult OCD cases arise from established but untreated or asymptomatic juvenile OCD. However, many patients with adult OCD present with a history of knee pain that began when they had open physes. These cases probably represent juvenile OCD that did not heal and evolved to adult OCD. An exception to this progression is juvenile OCD that heals spontaneously; however, such lesions usually are not present in the classic location (lateral aspect of the medial femoral condyle).[13,55] Adult OCD may also arise de novo.[9,21]

The natural history of untreated OCD is poorly defined. Neither the literature nor our experience allows us to definitively determine whether untreated OCD has a higher likelihood of progressing to symptomatic degenerative joint disease (DJD) in the future. Linden performed a long-term retrospective follow-up study on patients with OCD of the femoral condyles with an average follow-up of 33 years after initial diagnosis.[35] The author concluded that OCD occurring prior to closure of the physes (JOCD) does not lead to additional complications later in life, but patients who manifest OCD after closure of the physes (AOCD) develop osteoarthritis 10 years earlier than the normal population. In contrast, Twyman and associates evaluated 22 knees with juvenile OCD and found that 50% had some radiographic signs of osteoarthritis at an average follow-up of 34 years.[56] The likelihood of developing osteoarthritis was also found to be proportional to the size of the area involved. The authors believe that lateral femoral condyle OCD has a poorer prognosis, but not all of these cases will become symptomatic over time despite radiographic changes.

NONOPERAIVE TREATMENT

The ideal goal of conservative treatment is to attain lesion healing, which occurs more often before physeal closure.

Stable OCD lesions in young patients have a favorable prognosis when treated initially with nonoperative treatment. Nonoperative treatment options include modified activity with decreased weight-bearing, anti-inflammatory medications, and management of patient symptoms. Traditional nonoperative treatment consists of an initial phase of knee immobilization with partial weight-bearing to prevent repeated microtrauma lesions. Once the patient is pain free, weight-bearing as tolerated is permitted and a rehabilitation program emphasizing knee range of motion and low-impact strengthening exercises ensues. The goal is to promote healing in the subchondral bone and prevent chondral separation. X-rays are usually taken 3 months after the start of nonsurgical therapy to assess the status of the lesion and the condition of the subchondral bone. If the lesion reveals adequate healing, patients are allowed to gradually return to activities; if no change is observed, x-ray assessment is repeated in 3 months.

SURGICAL TREATMENT

Surgical options are considered more often than not for adult OCD, as articular cartilage presents with an inherent poor ability to repair itself. Surgical options include loose body removal, drilling of the subchondral bone, internal fixation of the fragment, microfracture, osteochondral autografting and allografting, and autologous chondrocyte implantation.[9,19,21,43] The overall goal of such intervention is to enhance the healing potential of the subchondral bone, fix the unstable fragment, and replace damaged bone and cartilage with implantable tissue.

The type and extent of surgery necessary for OCD depend on the patient's age, characteristics of the lesion (quality of articular cartilage; size of associated subchondral bone; and shape, thickness, and location of the lesion), diagnostic information provided by MRI and arthroscopy, and preference of the operating surgeon. The author's preferred algorithm for treatment of OCD lesions is shown in Figure 21-3.

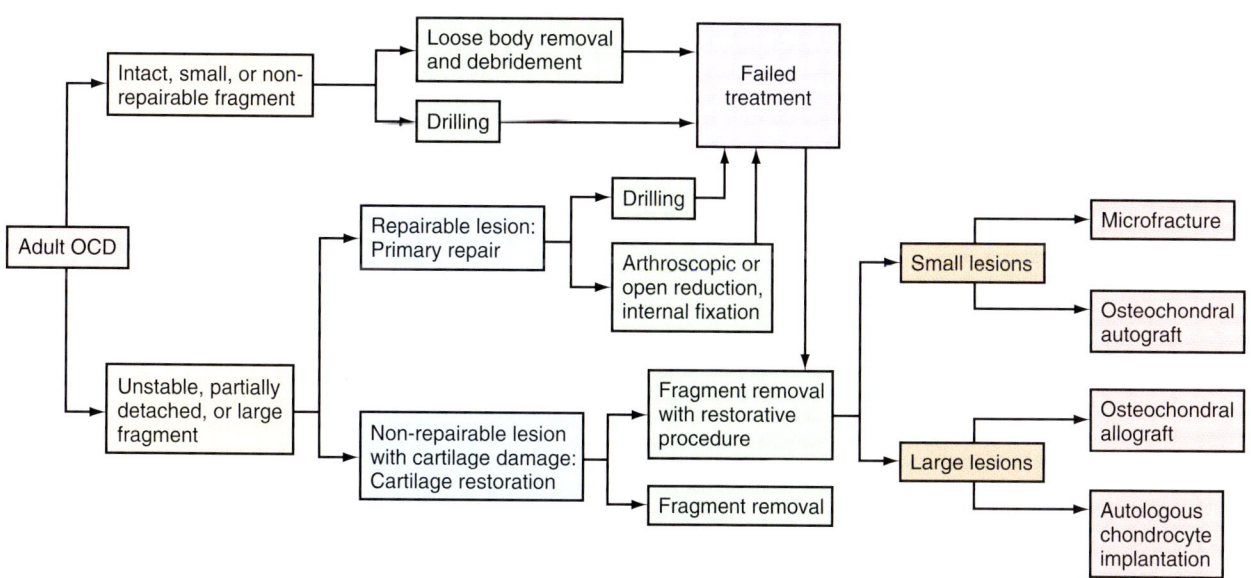

Figure 21-3. Algorithm for surgical treatment of adult osteochondritis dissecans (OCD).

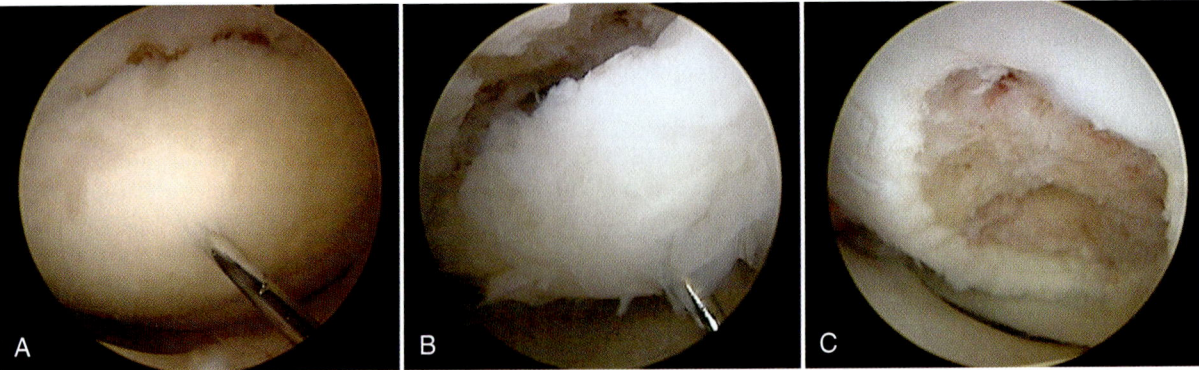

Figure 21-4. Unstable osteochondritis dissecans (OCD) fragment. **A,** OCD lesion palpable at arthroscopy. **B,** Palpation reveals unstable lesion. **C,** Subchondral bone following removal of the OCD lesion.

Table 21-2 Guhl's Classification[18]

Stage	Arthroscopic Findings
I	Normal
II	Fragmentation in situ
III	Partial detachment
IV	Complete detachment, loose body present

Positioning, Examination Under Anesthesia, and Diagnostic Arthroscopy

All patients are placed supine, with the leg supported by a standard thigh holder and the knee flexed at 90 degrees. The affected extremity is prepared and draped to the proximal thigh to ensure easy access to the knee. Examination under anesthesia assesses range of motion and ligamentous integrity. Lesions on the surfaces of the femoral condyle can usually be accessed using an arthroscopic approach. Standard portals are used and accessory portals are added when needed to improve visibility. More challenging locations, such as the patella and tibial plateau, may require an arthrotomy for better visualization and treatment.

A complete diagnostic arthroscopic evaluation of the structures in each compartment is performed. When the lesions are identified, a probe is used to determine the stability of the fragment (Fig. 21-4). Guhl's intraoperative classification is defined by cartilage integrity and fragment stability[25] (Table 21-2).

Loose Body Removal

In a small number of cases, when the fragment is comminuted, avascular, deformed, or otherwise irreparable, fragment removal is an isolated treatment option.[3] In cases involving chronic symptomatic lesions, fibrous tissue may impede anatomic reduction and adequate healing. In addition, the fragment may be associated with only small amounts of subchondral bone with limited ability to heal.

Although OCD lesions should be reduced, stabilized, bone grafted, or restored when possible, patients with small or non–weight-bearing lesions may have good outcomes with isolated loose body removal. Ewing and Voto showed 72% satisfactory results in patients treated with fragment excision with or without drilling or abrasion.[19] A recent study showed successful outcomes in 8 of 9 patients treated with loose body removal alone for small (<2 cm^2) AOCD lesions.[50] These results, however, are controversial and may pertain only to short-term outcomes. Anderson and Pagnani excised OCD fragments in 11 patients with JOCD and 9 patients with AOCD. At an average of 9 years postoperatively, five failures and six poor outcomes were reported, and equally disappointing outcomes were seen with JOCD and AOCD.[4] Similarly, Wright and coworkers had 65% fair or poor results at an average 8.9 years postoperatively in 17 patients treated with fragment excision, and suggested the use of aggressive cartilage preservation techniques and avoidance of fragment excision.[58]

REPARATIVE PROCEDURES

The goal of reparative procedures is to restore the integrity of the native subchondral interface and preserve the overlying articular cartilage.[42]

Drilling

As mentioned previously, disruption of the blood supply to the subchondral bone is thought to be an important factor in the development of OCD.[5] Thus, treatment incorporates creation of vascular channels to the affected region. Arthroscopic drilling can be used to generate such channels and is usually performed in young patients.[1]

This technique is performed using an antegrade or a retrograde approach. Antegrade drilling is performed from the joint space, through the articular cartilage, and into the subchondral bone. Lesions of the medial femoral condyle can be drilled through an anterolateral or anteromedial portal, and lesions of the lateral femoral condyle are usually accessible through the anterolateral portal. If the lesion is not accessible via standard portals, accessory portals are created to obtain an orthogonal drilling angle.[5] Multiple holes are drilled using a K-wire, making certain to uniformly cover the lesion. Return of blood and fat droplets from the drilled region is used to confirm the depth of the penetration.

Antegrade drilling has the undesirable consequence of violating the articular cartilage surface causing the violation to fill with fibrocartilage. Retrograde drilling, although more difficult, avoids damage to the articular cartilage. The drill enters behind the lesion and penetrates the bony fragment without violating the cartilage or entering the joint. C-arm visualization or the use of an anterior cruciate ligament (ACL) guide is necessary to avoid joint penetration or dislodgement of the OCD fragment.[32]

Overall, outcomes of OCD drilling are generally favorable, and patient age is the best prognostic factor. Younger patients who have undergone this procedure demonstrate higher levels of radiographic healing and favorable relief of symptoms.[5,8,18,31] Louisia and associates compared outcomes of JOCD versus AOCD, reporting radiographic healing in 71% of JOCD cases, and only 25% in adult AOCD cases.[38]

It is our opinion that drilling should be utilized when the defect is stable to palpation despite MRI evidence of fluid behind the fragment, indicating biologic instability. When possible, drilling is performed through the intercondylar notch (i.e., adjacent to the posterior cruciate ligament [PCL] femoral origin for OCD of the medial femoral condyle [MFC]) or along the lateral nonarticulating border of the distal femur using a 0.45-mm K-wire. When no gross ballotable instability is noted, we often place one or two bioabsorbable compression screws that are buried deep to the level of the subchondral plate (BioCompression Screw, Arthrex, Inc., Naples, Fla). With any evidence of instability, we make every effort to "hinge" the lesion open to expose the base, which is often covered in fibrovascular scar tissue.

Arthroscopic or Open Reduction and Internal Fixation

Adult OCD lesions that have become detached from the subchondral bone may present with articular cartilage flaps or loose bodies that require fixation.[43] Fixation is advised for symptomatic unstable lesions, provided that the lesion has sufficient subchondral bone to provide support for the fixation system. A cartilage flap, sometimes referred to as a hinged lesion, can be fixed using pins and screws. Unstable "trap door" lesions, which are partially elevated off the subchondral bone, require bed fixation, which can be achieved using microfracture awls to restore/improve blood supply, followed by fixation.[47]

Internal fixation can be achieved using a variety of fixation devices, as well as bone pegs and osteochondral grafts.[11,22] Internal fixation devices include cannulated screws, metal pins/K-wires, and bioabsorbable pins. The method of fixation is based largely on surgeon preference.

Constant thread pitch (AO) and variable thread pitch (Herbert, Accutrak) cannulated screws allow for compression across the lesion. AO screws, available in varying sizes, must

be placed below the articular surface to avoid damage to the opposing articular surface. Variable pitch Herbert (partially threaded) and Accutrak (fully threaded) screws have a headless design that allows excellent compression of the fragment into the defect bed. Some surgeons bury the head of these screws, so as to allow early range of motion and prevent subsequent damage to the opposing tibial surface. However, it is the author's preference to utilize variable pitch metal screws and remove them at 8 weeks postoperatively to assess for healing and to avoid the consequences of fragment collapse, which can lead to prominent hardware. Bioabsorbable screws have been recommended by some to avoid removal, but questions remain as to the degree of compression they provide and the fact that they remain in situ for a prolonged time before enzymatic breakdown occurs.[28]

Before screw placement, unstable lesions are opened to expose the sclerotic bed. If necessary, lesions on the lateral aspect of the medial femoral condyle may require superficial release of PCL fibers to expose the lateral margin of the lesion.[22] Cartilage at the lesion site is hinged open, the undersurface is débrided and curetted, and microfracture awls are used to stimulate bleeding from the subchondral bone. To place a screw, a guide wire is drilled through the fragment into the femoral condyle. The guide wire is then overdrilled and the screw is placed, compressing the fragment into the bed (Figs. 21-5 and 21-6). Another option is retrograde fixation, which most often is used for OCD lesions of the patella. Screws are placed from behind the lesion through the subchondral bone and into the bony portion of the fragment. Accurate screw placement is crucial for the success of this procedure and often involves the use of intraoperative fluoroscopy. Following any OCD procedure with internal fixation, the knee should be ranged to ensure that the screw head does not abrade the opposing surface.

K-wires and metal pins are advantageous because of their ease of insertion and availability in the operating room. However, K-wire use is limited because K-wires do not provide compression, may break or bend, and can migrate from the osteochondral fragment.

Bioabsorbable pins, both smooth and barbed, offer adequate fixation when a smaller device is used without the need for removal. Pins are placed by an anterograde method, and the small-head or headless pin can be impacted beneath the surface. Bioabsorbable pins have the disadvantages of implant fracture and foreign body reaction, resulting in aseptic synovitis. In addition, they provide minimal compression across the defect junction.

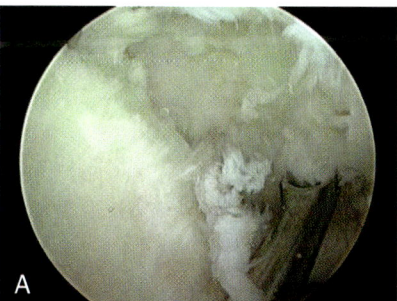 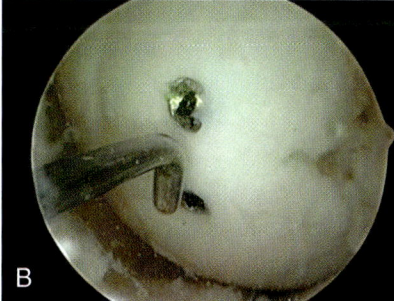 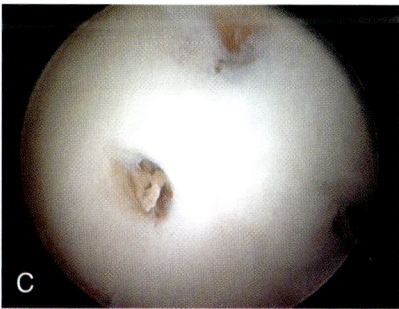

Figure 21-5. Arthroscopic reduction, internal fixation of the osteochondritis dissecans (OCD) fragment. **A,** Unstable fragment with curettage of the underlying subchondral bone. **B,** Fragment fixation with two metallic compression screws. **C,** Hardware removal at second-look arthroscopy 8 weeks postoperatively.

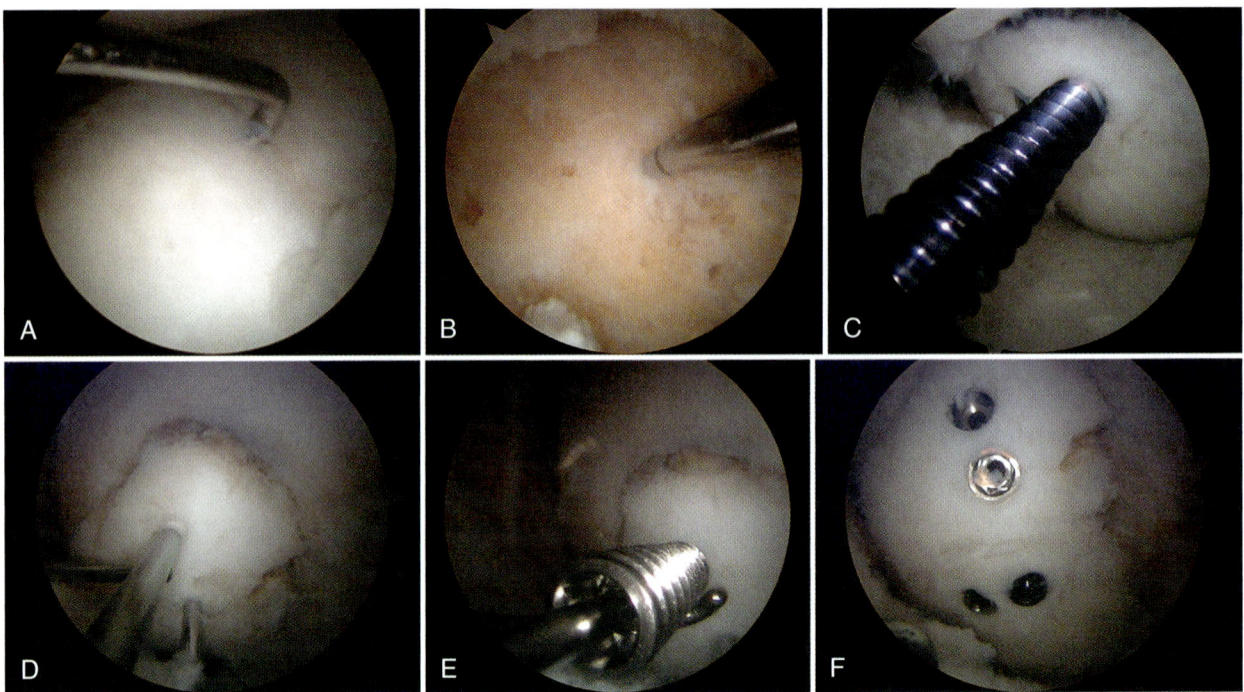

Figure 21-6. A, Unstable osteochondritis dissecans (OCD) fragment palpable at arthroscopy. **B,** Débridement and microfracture of the subchondral bone. **C,** Screw placement for fixation. **D,** Evaluation of reduced fragment. **E,** Placement of additional screws to provide further compression and rotational stability. **F,** Final fixation of two large fragments, each with two screws.

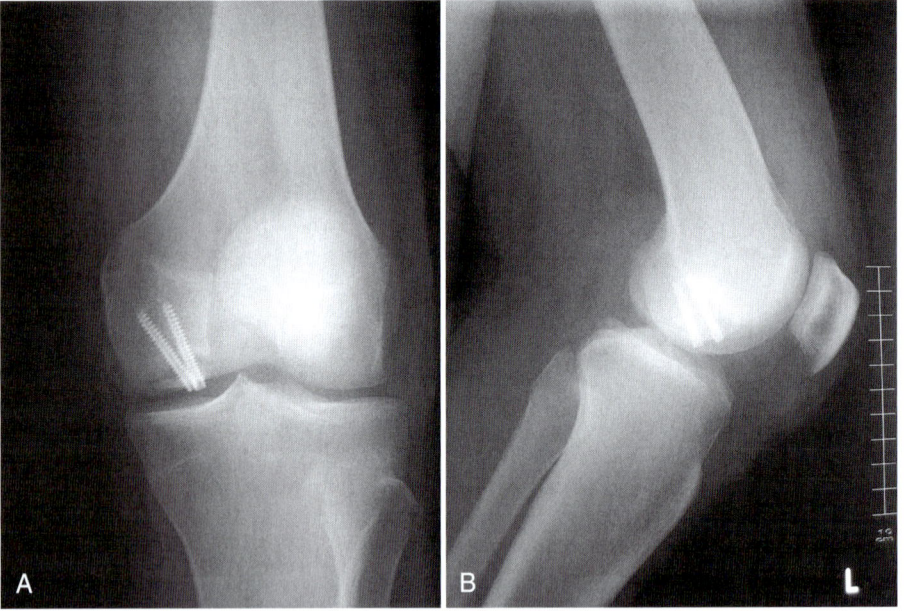

Figure 21-7. Anteroposterior **(A)** and lateral **(B)** views of an osteochondritis dissecans (OCD) lesion after screw fixation. Note that the screws are placed in the center of the lesion and are recessed below the cartilage surface.

In general, unless the lesion is very small, at least two fixation points are utilized to ensure compression and rotational stability. Screws are tightened until the fragment is compressed, but overtightening should be avoided to prevent fracture of the osteochondral fragment. All devices with a prominent head should be recessed beneath the cartilage surface to avoid further injury to the juxtaposing cartilage (Fig. 21-7). As mentioned before, nonabsorbable screws often require a second procedure for hardware removal; this affords the opportunity for a second look at the lesion site to verify healing.[43]

Large, displaced fragments should be augmented with bone grafting. After the base of the lesion has been examined, and débridement and penetration of the lesion bed have been performed with microfracture awls, the fragment still may not sit congruently within the defect site. Cancellous autograft can be harvested from Gerdy's tubercle on the ipsilateral limb. The bone graft is impacted into the defect site, and reduction of the fragment is reassessed until adequate reduction is achieved. Alternatively, small dowels of bone can be harvested arthroscopically using small-diameter instrumentation from the osteochondral autograft transfer systems. Once adequate reduction is achieved, the fragment is held in place with provisional K-wires until appropriate final fixation is achieved, as described earlier. Osteochondral plugs help to provide fixation and bone grafting across the lesion.

Postoperatively, all patients who have undergone arthroscopic or open reduction and internal fixation may heel-touch weight-bear and, when available, may utilize continuous passive motion machines for 4 to 6 hours per day.

Favorable outcomes have been reported after internal fixation of OCD fragments using absorbable and nonabsorbable screws. A study of Herbert compression screw fixation yielded 13 of 15 normal knees based on International Knee Documentation Committee (IKDC) clinical scoring, including 6 of 8 in skeletally mature patients.[41] Kouzelis and colleagues treated patients with grade III and IV osteochondral lesions using reverse drilling and Herbert screw fixation and reported 90% normal or nearly normal results using IKDC scoring.[32] Magnussen reported healing in 92% of patients undergoing open reduction and internal fixation (ORIF) of grade IV OCD lesions, including healing in all seven skeletally mature patients.[40] Similarly, Pascual-Garrido and coworkers reported satisfaction in 13 of 15 adult OCD cases treated with arthroscopic reduction internal fixation.[50]

Similar outcome scores have been reported with the use of bioabsorbable screw, nail, and pin fixation. Nagawana and associates used fixation with bioabsorbable poly-L-lactide (PLLA) pins and showed 100% union and a clinical score of good (4/8) or excellent (4/8) in all patients.[48] Good and excellent clinical results were also achieved in all eight patients undergoing fixation with PLLA nails for OCD.[17] Weckstrom and colleagues compared bioabsorbable nails and pins in 30 patients with AOCD and showed significantly better fixation with nails (73% good to excellent) versus pins (35% good to excellent), suggesting that the barbs and the head of the nail allow for increased compression and rigid fixation.[57]

Summary of Author's Preferred Reparative Treatment Method

The method of fixation is based largely on the surgeon's preference because no specific treatment has produced far superior outcomes. We prefer two to three partially threaded cannulated screws with a second-look arthroscopy to remove the hardware and verify defect healing at 6 to 8 weeks. Bioabsorbable screws are also an option, especially when only one screw is needed for adequate stabilization of a macroscopically stable lesion, as is often seen with the early diagnosis and treatment of JOCD.

RESTORATIVE PROCEDURES

Restorative procedures attempt to replace damaged articular cartilage with hyaline or hyaline-like tissue.[34] These techniques should be considered as the next option if the patient has failed reparative treatments and presents with recurrent joint effusion, pain, and reduced range of motion. Multiple restorative techniques can be used for the treatment of OCD; however, the treatment algorithm should start with the least invasive options and progress to the more invasive options.

Marrow Stimulation (Microfracture)

Microfracture involves production of tiny fractures in the subchondral bone, allowing an influx of pluripotent stem cells from the marrow into the defect site and forming a superclot. The presence of pluripotent cells allows differentiation and results in the production of fibrocartilage.[54] Microfracture is indicated in patients with a small, localized cartilage defect, typically measuring less than 4 cm² (Fig. 21-8). Postoperatively, rehabilitation requires 6 weeks of non–weight bearing with use of continuous passive motion (CPM) for 6 hours a day.

Gudas and colleagues randomized patients with posttraumatic, symptomatic full-thickness cartilage lesions (56%) and OCD lesions (44%) to treatment with microfracture or osteochondral autograft transplantation (OAT). Clinical outcomes were significantly worse for the microfracture group, and the authors noted that whether treated with microfracture or OAT, patients with OCD had worse outcomes than those with full-thickness cartilage defects.[24] Another similarly conducted study by Knutsen and coworkers randomized femoral condyle (28% with OCD lesions) cartilage defects to treatment with microfracture or autologous chondrocyte implantation. Both groups demonstrated satisfactory results in 77% of patients at 5 years, with younger patients having better results in both groups. Overall, microfracture should be considered as a first-line treatment, especially in the setting of fragment removal with shallow defects

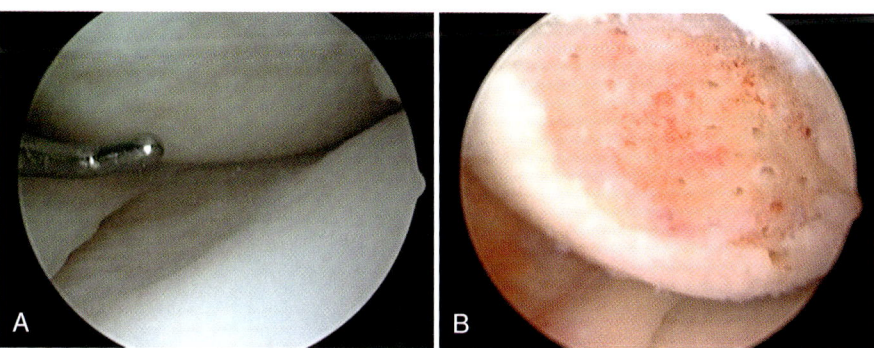

Figure 21-8. A, Osteochondritis dissecans (OCD) lesion of the femoral condyle. **B,** Treatment with microfracture.

that are relatively small. Whether fragment removal and microfracture fare better than fragment removal alone is not known, and we know little about which OCD lesions are optimal for initial microfracture treatment.[30]

Osteochondral Autograft Transplantation

In situations where the underlying subchondral bone integrity cannot support microfracture, osteochondral autograft transplantation (OAT) can be considered. The OAT procedure involves transplantation of osteochondral tissue from a low–weight-bearing region, such as the area just above the intercondylar notch or the lateral edge of the trochlea, with insertion of the plug into the defect.[52] A single autograft plug is preferred for defects smaller than 1 cm[2]; however, some authors perform mosaicplasty with multiple smaller plugs for larger defects.

Good clinical results have been reported with osteochondral autografts. Miniaci and associates have reported normal postoperative knee scores at 18 months for all 20 OCD patients (11 immature and 9 mature) treated with OAT used as a biologic splint placed through the unstable fragment into the defect bed. In addition, radiographic evidence obtained 6 months postoperatively demonstrated adequate healing.[46] Outerbridge used osteochondral plugs taken from the ipsilateral lateral patella to treat patients with large osteochondral defects. The authors noted that all patients had increased function, and 81% returned to a high level of function. However, use of OAT is limited to small lesions because of limited supplies and donor site morbidity.

Autologous Chondrocyte Implantation

With limited supplies and donor site morbidity associated with the OAT procedure, treatment for larger lesions requires a different technique. Autologous chondrocyte implantation (ACI) is ideal for large, isolated osteochondral defects measuring up to 10 cm[2]. This two-step procedure involves an initially healthy chondrocyte biopsy, performed arthroscopically with tissue extracted from the non–weight-bearing intercondylar notch region. Extracted cells are expanded in vitro over 4 to 6 weeks and then are reimplanted at the lesion site. At the time of implantation, defect preparation involves débridement of the calcified cartilage base and creation of vertical walls of healthy cartilage. A patch, periosteal, or synthetic collagen membrane is attached to the perimeter using absorbable sutures. The edges are sealed using fibrin glue, and in vitro cultured cells are injected beneath the patch[14,45] (Fig. 21-9). As with microfracture, 6 weeks of non–weight bearing postoperatively and CPM are indicated for both OAT and ACI.

Peterson and colleagues evaluated 58 patients (60% JOCD and 40% AOCD) who underwent an ACI procedure. At 2- to 10-year follow-up, the authors reported the presence of repair tissue at the lesion site with good to excellent clinical outcomes in 91% of patients.[51] As noted previously, Knutsen and coworkers reported 77% satisfactory results in patients with femoral condyle lesions treated with ACI.[30] In a large population of patients undergoing ACI, including 24% with OCD lesions, Bentley and associates reported 88% good to excellent outcomes based on clinical assessment.[7] Krishnan and colleagues performed ACI using a collagen membrane to treat 37 OCD patients (27 JOCD and 9 AOCD).[33] Among patients with juvenile-onset OCD, 91% good to excellent outcomes were achieved in patients treated before skeletal maturity compared with 77% in those treated after skeletal maturity, suggesting that early treatment is optimal. Furthermore, adult-onset OCD patients had 44% good to excellent outcomes, and better clinical outcomes were seen in those with smaller (<6 cm[2]) lesions.

Defects deeper than 8 to 10 mm can still be treated with ACI, but concomitant or staged bone grafting is recommended. Prior to bone grafting, drilling through the bed following débridement allows appropriate blood flow into the defect, ensuring subsequent bone graft incorporation. When

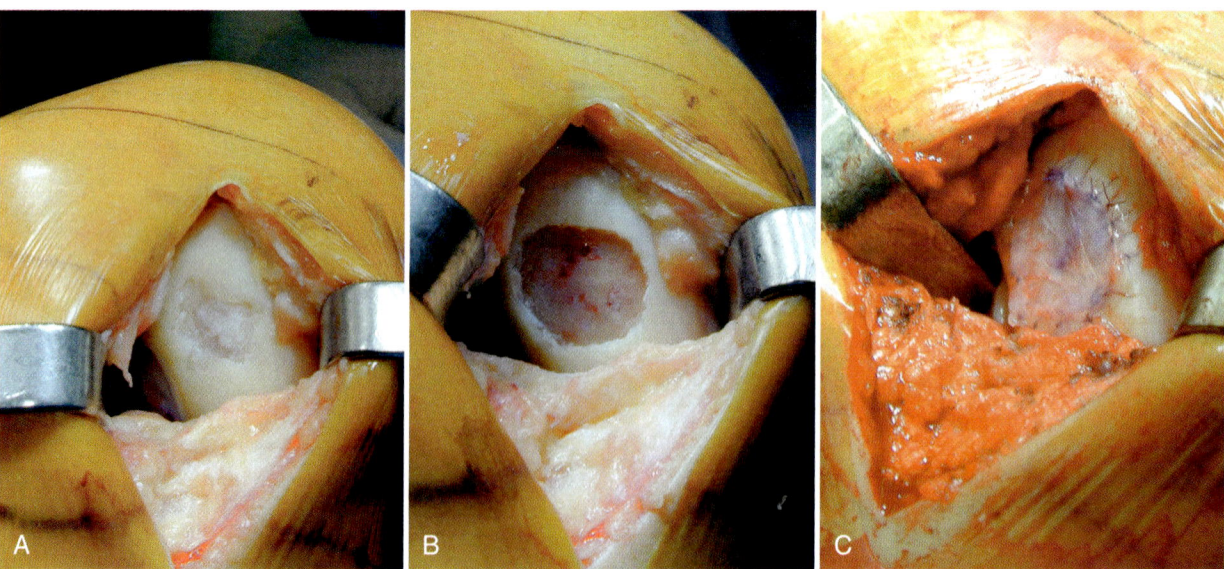

Figure 21-9. A, Lesion at the lateral aspect of the medial femoral condyle. **B,** Lesion prepared for autologous chondrocyte implantation (ACI). **C,** Completed ACI.

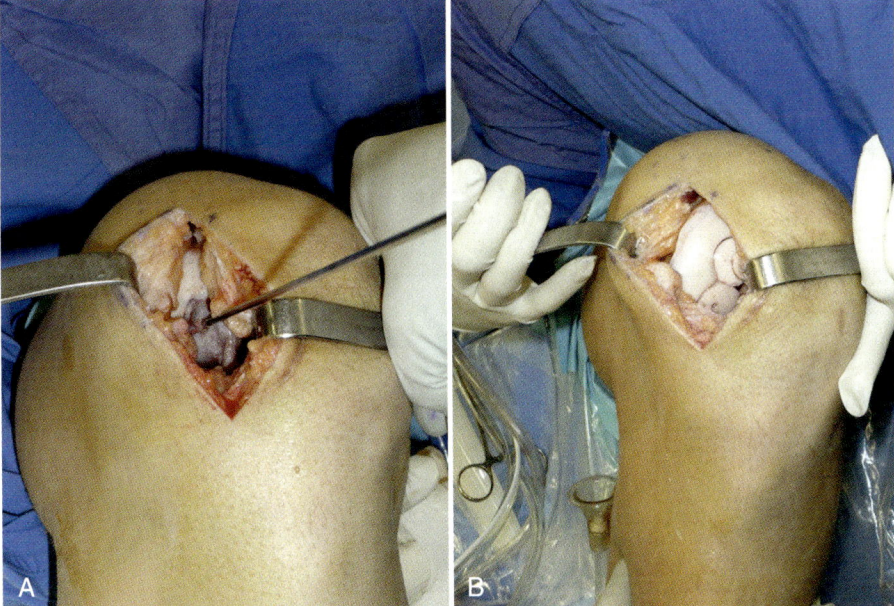

Figure 21-10. A, Large osteochondritis dissecans (OCD) lesion of the femoral condyle. **B,** Treatment with two osteochondral allograft plugs.

bone grafting is performed as a primary procedure in an effort to stage definitive treatment with ACI, most surgeons wait a minimum of 6 months to allow bone graft incorporation. Alternatively, a bilayer collagen membrane (periosteal "sandwich" technique) can be employed without the need to stage the ACI.[6,12] A layer of periosteum or collagen membrane is used to seal the bone graft, and it is fixed with 6-0 Vicryl suture. A second layer is placed on top of the first and is similarly sewn; this is followed by injection of cultured cells between the two layers. Limited experience with this technique has been documented. Bartlett and associates reported three excellent results, one good, and one fair in five patients treated using ACI with a bilayer collagen membrane with bone graft.[6]

Osteochondral Allograft

Large OCD lesions may also be treated with osteochondral allograft (OA) transplantation.[23] The OA graft provides the ability to resurface larger and deeper defects with mature hyaline cartilage and addresses the underlying subchondral bone deficiency, which is a hallmark of OCD. The donor tissue is generally fashioned in a cylindrical plug matching the diameter of the initial lesion (Fig. 21-10). To ensure proper fixation, bioabsorbable compression screws or headless variable pitch titanium screws can be used. Postoperative rehabilitation is similar to that utilized following OAT or ACI.

It has been reported that fresh OA graft transplantation provides good to excellent clinical outcomes with long-term follow-up. Garrett presented a series of AOCD lesions of the femoral condyle, reporting 94% clinical success at a mean follow-up of 3 years.[21] McCulloch and associates, in 25 patients with full-thickness defects including 6 OCD lesions, presented an 84% success rate.[44] In a large study of 66 OCD lesions in 64 patients, treatment with a fresh OA yielded good to excellent results in 72% of patients. Overall, treatment of OCD with an OA graft can result in subjective

improvement in 75% to 85% of patients, as supported by long-term follow-up.[29]

CONCLUSIONS

Adult OCD of the knee is a challenging problem that results in poor outcomes without surgical intervention once patients present with symptoms. Timely diagnosis can prevent compromise of the articular cartilage and can maximize the successful outcome of restorative procedures. Several surgical treatments have been used to treat OCD lesions. Reestablishment of the joint surface by improving blood supply via drilling or internal fixation is the primary goal of osteochondral fragment preservation. When the symptomatic fragment is not suitable for preservation, cartilage restoration techniques should be considered as an option. The overall goal for the treatment of adult OCD lesions is to relieve pain, restore function, and prevent development of secondary osteoarthritis.

KEY REFERENCES

Adachi N, Deie M, Nakamae A, et al: Functional and radiographic outcome of stable juvenile osteochondritis dissecans of the knee treated with retroarticular drilling without bone grafting. Arthroscopy 25:145–152, 2009.

Alford JW, Cole BJ: Cartilage restoration, part 2: techniques, outcomes, and future directions. Am J Sports Med 33:443–460, 2005.

Bartlett W, Gooding CR, Carrington RW, et al: Autologous chondrocyte implantation at the knee using a bilayer collagen membrane with bone graft: a preliminary report. J Bone Joint Surg Br 87:330–332, 2005.

Day JB, Gillogly SD: Autologous chondrocyte implantation in the knee. In Cole BJ, Sekiya JK, editors: Surgical techniques of the shoulder, elbow, and knee in sports medicine, Philadelphia, 2008, Saunders Elsevier, pp 559–566.

Gomoll AH, Flik KR, Hayden JK, et al: Internal fixation of unstable Cahill Type-2C osteochondritis dissecans lesions of the knee in adolescent patients. Orthopedics 30:487–490, 2007.

Gudas R, Stankevicius E, Monastyreckiene E, et al: Osteochondral autologous transplantation versus microfracture for the treatment of articular cartilage defects in the knee joint in athletes. Knee Surg Sports Traumatol Arthrosc 14:834–842, 2006.

Kang RW, Gomoll AH, Cole BJ: Osteochondral allografting in the knee. In Cole BJ, Sekiya JK, editors: Surgical techniques of the shoulder, elbow, and knee in sports medicine, Philadelphia, 2008, Saunders Elsevier, pp 549–557.

Kouzelis A, Plessas S, Papadopoulos AX, et al: Herbert screw fixation and reverse guided drillings, for treatment of types III and IV osteochondritis dissecans. Knee Surg Sports Traumatol Arthrosc 14:70–75, 2006.

Lewis PB, McCarty LP 3rd, Kang RW, et al: Basic science and treatment options for articular cartilage injuries. J Orthop Sports Phys Ther 36:717–727, 2006.

McCarty LP III: Primary repair of osteochondritis dissecans in the knee. In Cole BJ, Sekiya JK, editors: Surgical techniques of the shoulder, elbow, and knee in sports medicine, Philadelphia, 2008, Saunders Elsevier, pp 517–526.

McCulloch PC, Kang RW, Sobhy MH, et al: Prospective evaluation of prolonged fresh osteochondral allograft transplantation of the femoral condyle: minimum 2-year follow-up. Am J Sports Med 35:411–420, 2007.

Pascual-Garrido C, Friel NA, Kirk SS, et al: Midterm results of surgical treatment for adult osteochondritis dissecans of the knee. Am J Sports Med 37(Suppl 1):125S–130S, 2009.

Peterson L, Minas T, Brittberg M, et al: Treatment of osteochondritis dissecans of the knee with autologous chondrocyte transplantation: results at two to ten years. J Bone Joint Surg Am 85(Suppl 2):17–24, 2003.

Rabalais RD, Swan KG Jr, McCarty E: Osteochondral autograft for cartilage lesions of the knee. In Cole BJ, Sekiya J, editors: Surgical techniques of the shoulder, elbow, and knee in sports medicine, Philadelphia, 2008, Saunders Elsevier, pp 539–548.

Steadman JR, Rodkey WG, Briggs KK: Microfracture technique in the knee. In Cole BJ, Sekiya JK, editors: Surgical techniques of the shoulder, elbow, and knee in sports medicine, Philadelphia, 2008, Saunders Elsevier, pp 509–515.

Full references for this chapter can be found on www.expertconsult.com.

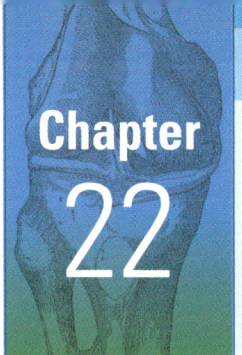
International Experience With Autologous Chondrocyte Implantation With Periosteum (Autologous Chondrocyte Implantation), Including Scaffold Guided Techniques and Tissue Engineered Matrix Support

Lars Peterson and Haris S. Vasiliadis

Articular cartilage is a unique tissue with no vascular, nerve, or lymphatic supply. Lack of vascular and lymphatic circulation may be one of the reasons why articular cartilage has such a poor intrinsic capacity to heal. No inflammatory response to tissue damage occurs unless subchondral bone in the damaged area shows involvement. Subsequently, there will be no macrophage invasion to phagocytose and remove damaged and devitalized tissue; furthermore, no cells with repair capacity will migrate into the damaged area. The chondrocyte itself, encapsulated in its own matrix, is incapable of migrating and repopulating the damaged area.

Chondral injuries that penetrate down to subchondral bone will not heal but may progress to osteoarthritis over time by enzymatic degradation and mechanical wear. Osteochondral injuries that penetrate subchondral bone into trabecular bone with bleeding will result in inflammatory repair tissue filling the lesion with fibrocartilage produced by mesenchymal stem cells or fibroblasts. Unfortunately, fibrocartilage repair tissue has been shown to be unable to withstand mechanical wear over time; fibrocartilage may degenerate and the lesion may progress to osteoarthritis.[6,18]

Good results can be achieved with treatment of severe osteoarthritis of the knee by total joint replacement in elderly patients. However, this treatment exposes patients to increasing risk of potentially serious complications, and it has a limited duration of life, finally demanding a revision surgery. Total knee arthroplasty burns the bridges to any other treatment options and is considered the last treatment option, indicated only for severe cases in older patients. In young and middle-aged patients, however, no optimal treatment is available for chondral injuries. The spectrum of treatment alternatives for articular cartilage defects in young and middle-aged patients can range from simple lavage and débridement, drilling, microfracturing, and abrasion to osteochondral grafting and autologous chondrocyte implantation (ACI).[36]

Optimal healing of an articular cartilage injury should consist of regeneration with tissue identical to hyaline cartilage; however, repair of chondral injury involves filling with tissue not identical to hyaline cartilage (i.e., fibrocartilage). The repair tissue should be able to fill and seal off the defective area with good adhesion to subchondral bone and complete integration to surrounding cartilage. It should be able to withstand mechanical wear over time and should gradually be included in the natural turnover of normal cartilage, thus providing longer symptom relief.[6]

The functional unit of articular cartilage includes not only the different layers of cartilage, but also subchondral and trabecular bone. Any treatment technique that interferes with subchondral and trabecular bone may not be able to restore the functional unit of cartilage, especially its shock-absorbing function.

Techniques that affect the subchondral bone plate include abrasion arthroplasty, multiple drilling, and microfracture. All these techniques may result in stiffening of subchondral and trabecular bone, leading to osteophyte formation underneath the repair tissue.[20,35] Osteochondral grafting may affect subchondral and trabecular bone function because the osseous part of the plug has to undergo resorption, revascularization, remodeling, and healing to the surrounding bone. Periosteal and perichondrial grafting also affects subchondral bone by drilling and abrading the subchondral bone plate.

Chondrocyte implantation does not violate subchondral or trabecular bone. On the contrary, for success with this technique, bleeding from subchondral bone should be avoided so that fibroblasts or stem cells are not introduced, resulting in fibroblastic repair tissue.[5]

HISTORICAL BACKGROUND OF AUTOLOGOUS CHONDROCYTE IMPLANTATION (TRANSPLANTATION)

In 1965, Smith was successful in isolating and growing chondrocytes in culture for the first time.[11] Epiphyseal chondrocytes grown in culture were injected into tibial articular defects in the rabbit knee but did not show any significant repair.

In 1982, experimental work was begun at the Hospital for Joint Diseases–Orthopedic Institute in New York to design an experimental rabbit model using articular chondrocytes isolated and grown in culture for implantation into a defect made in the patella and covered with a periosteal flap. The idea was to use articular chondrocytes because they are the only cells committed to form hyaline cartilage.

Initial results of ACI in this rabbit model were presented in 1984 and showed hyaline-like cartilage filling 80% of the patellar defect. No significant filling was seen in the control side, where the defect was treated with periosteal cover but no cells.

Since 1984, extensive animal studies have been ongoing at the University of Göteborg, Sweden. The results from New York have been confirmed and improved.

In 1985, work started on transferring the cell-culturing technique to human chondrocytes, and in 1987 the first ACI (or *transplantation*, as first named) was performed in the human knee at the Department of Orthopaedics, University of Göteborg, after approval by the Ethical Committee of the Medical Faculty of the University of Göteborg (Fig. 22-1).

A pilot study of 23 patients with 39 months' follow-up reported in the *New England Journal of Medicine* in October 1994 showed that of 16 patients who underwent femoral condyle procedures, 14 had a good or excellent result. Eleven of 15 biopsy specimens showed hyaline-like cartilage. Among seven patients who underwent ACI of the patella, however,

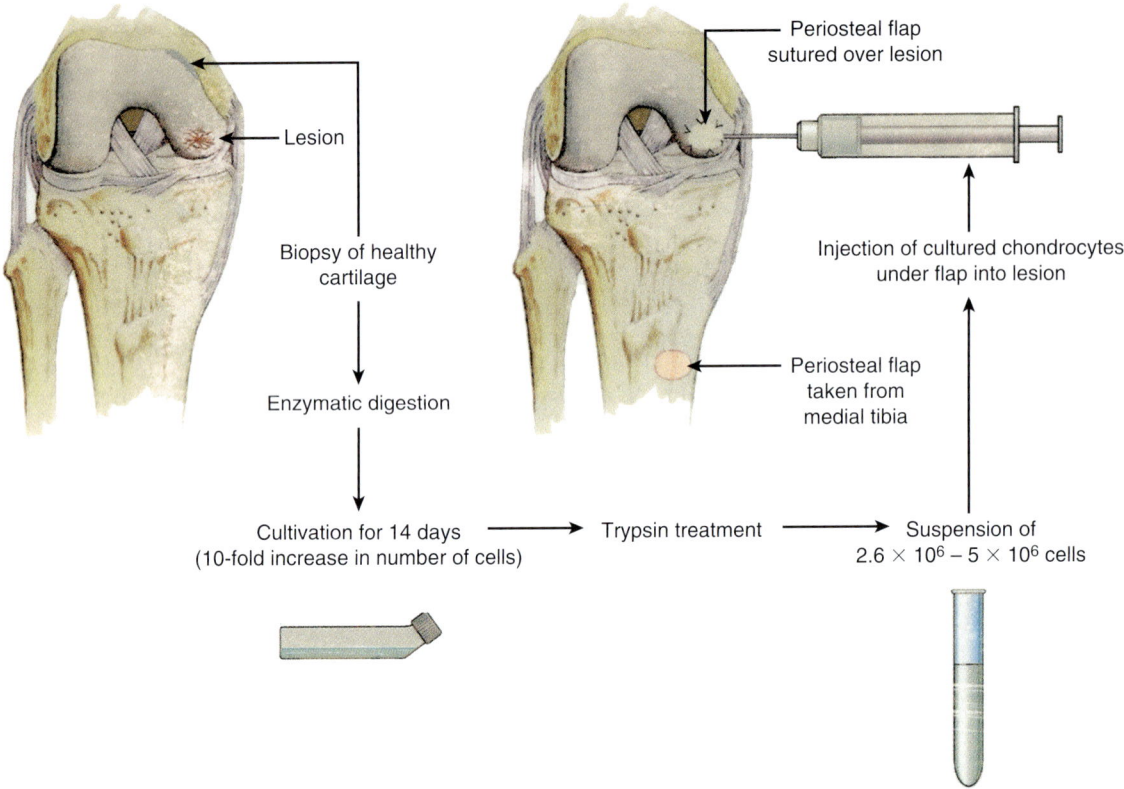

Figure 22-1. Diagram of the autologous chondrocyte implantation procedure.

only two good or excellent results were achieved, and one biopsy specimen showed hyaline-like cartilage.[5]

Since 1987, more than 1800 patients have been operated on in Göteborg, Sweden, and since 1995, more than 400 surgeons have performed ACI on more than 30,000 patients outside Sweden.

Clinical results from Sweden were reported at the American Academy of Orthopaedic Surgeons in 1996, 1997, 1998, 2000, 2001, 2002, 2003, and 2004, and long-term results obtained 10 to 20 years after the ACI were first presented at the International Cartilage Research Society meeting in 2009.[29,34]

INDICATIONS FOR AUTOLOGOUS CHONDROCYTE IMPLANTATION

Autologous chondrocyte implantation is indicated in patients between 15 and 55 years old with symptomatic, full-thickness Outerbridge or International Cartilage Repair Society (ICRS) grade III to IV cartilage injuries of the knee with a diameter larger than 10 mm up to an area of 10 to 16 cm[2] (Fig. 22-2). The defect should be located on the femoral or patellar articular surface and should be accessible for implantation via open arthrotomy. Only grade I to II Outerbridge or ICRS classification changes on the reciprocal articular surface should be included.

Osteochondritis dissecans of the medial or lateral femoral condyles with an unstable fragment, a separated but attached flap, or an empty bed is another indication for ACI (Fig. 22-3).

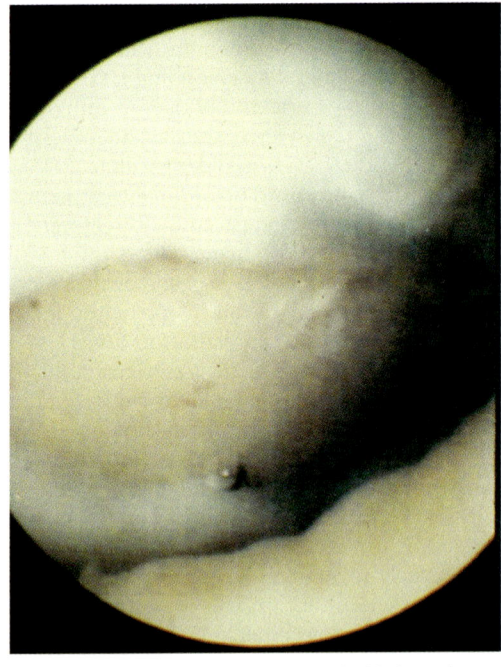

Figure 22-2. Arthroscopic view of a chondral injury down to bone on the medial femoral condyle, an indication for autologous chondrocyte implantation.

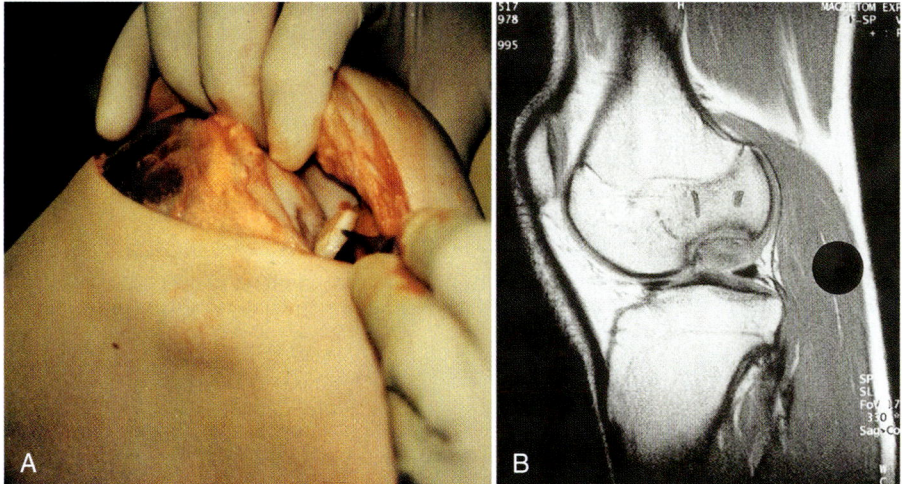

Figure 22-3. **A,** Arthrotomy of a right knee with osteochondritis dissecans of the lateral femoral condyle and an avulsed but attached flap, an indication for autologous chondrocyte implantation. **B,** Magnetic resonance image showing a deep osseous defect on the lateral femoral condyle.

Bipolar chondral injuries (i.e., osteoarthritis) are undergoing investigational study and at present could be considered as requiring a salvage procedure or as a relative indication. A recent long-term follow-up study described very good results 10 to 20 years after implantation, even for large bipolar lesions, for which ACI had been performed as a salvage procedure.[29,34] Evidence supports that ACI is indicated even for large bipolar lesions, delaying total knee arthroplasty. A definite decision regarding the indication is made during arthroscopic evaluation.

CLINICAL EVALUATION

A thorough history of symptoms, trauma, or repetitive loading is important, as is a careful record of previous surgeries. Clinical examination, including assessment of signs of local tenderness, swelling, range of motion, and crepitation, is performed.

Varus and valgus deformities are assessed, and patellar malalignment, maltracking, or instability is evaluated. Ligament instability is clinically tested.

BACKGROUND FACTORS TO CONSIDER

An understanding of the optimal environment for survival of repair tissue in the short or long term is of utmost importance. Varus or valgus malalignment should be evaluated on standing x-ray films of the knee in the extended position and in 45 degrees of knee flexion. Additional information could be gathered by examining the hip, knee, and ankle axis on long, standing x-ray films. Varus or valgus deformity should be corrected. Magnetic resonance imaging (MRI) could be helpful in evaluating articular cartilage injury and the condition of the subchondral bone in greater detail, as well as the status of the menisci. Previous meniscal surgery should be assessed, and after total or subtotal meniscectomy, meniscal transplantation should be considered.

Instability should be evaluated clinically, and any instability noted should be corrected. Osseous defects deeper than 8 to 10 mm should be considered for autologous bone grafting and chondrocyte implantation. MRI could be a helpful tool in evaluating bone pathology.

ARTHROSCOPIC EVALUATION— CARTILAGE RETRIEVAL

Under general or spinal anesthesia, complete stability testing of the knee is performed, and results are compared with those on the healthy side. Complete examination of the knee joint should be performed, including visualization and probing of articular cartilage surfaces, synovial lining, menisci, and cruciate ligaments, and the presence of any fragment or loose body should be identified. Undiagnosed pathology may be critical to the outcome of surgery. The cartilage injury is visualized, probed, and assessed for depth, size, and location. The opposing articular surface should be assessed and should be normal or should have only fibrillation or superficial fissuring, Outerbridge or ICRS grade I to grade II. The defect should be evaluated regarding containment and shouldering. An uncontained lesion extends into the synovial lining of the joint. It may be unilateral or bilateral, for example, extending from the synovial lining of the articular surface of the medial femoral condyle into the synovial lining of the intercondylar notch (Fig. 22-4).

A shouldered defect is a defect surrounded by normal cartilage in which the bone in the center of the defect is not in contact with the opposing articular surface. An unshouldered defect is so large that in a weight-bearing position, the subchondral bone in the center of the defect is in contact with the opposing articular surface (Fig. 22-5). During arthroscopy, the proposed implantation is evaluated regarding different possibilities for the surgical approach, the intended amount of débridement, the extent of shouldering, containment of the defect, and so forth.

Meniscal lesions should be treated at this time, but only after cartilage has been harvested for cell culture. Cartilage fragments and loose bodies should be removed before the cartilage is harvested.

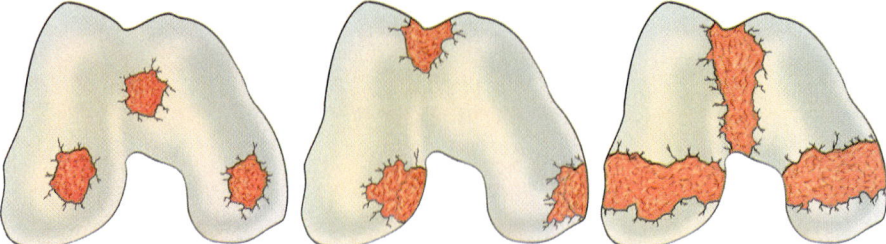

Figure 22-4. Schematic drawing showing containment of defects. The *left* drawing shows contained defects; the *middle* drawing, unilateral uncontained defects extending to the synovial lining; and the *right* drawing, bilateral uncontained defects.

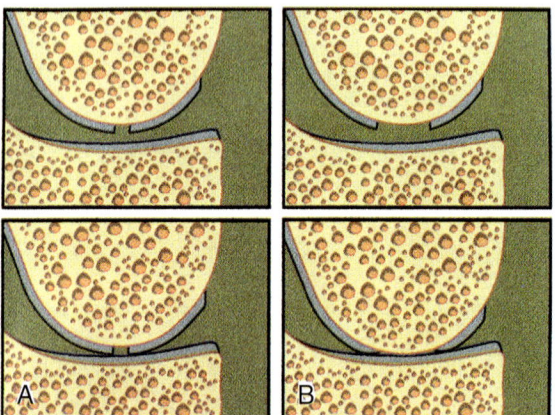

Figure 22-5. A, Shouldered defects are usually smaller than 10 mm and are contained. **B,** Unshouldered defects are larger. During weight bearing, the center of the defect is in contact with the opposing articular surface.

Only gentle or no débridement of the injury should be performed at this time. When the specifics of the indication have been fulfilled, cartilage is harvested from the upper medial or upper lateral femoral condyle on minor weight-bearing areas (Fig. 22-6). It can also be harvested from the intercondylar notch. In 98% of our cases, cartilage is harvested from the upper medial femoral condyle. With a curette, three to four slices of cartilage 3 to 4 mm wide by 10 mm long should be taken down to subchondral bone on the upper medial femoral condyle.[6] Approximately 200 to 300 mg of articular cartilage is required for enzymatic digestion and cell culturing. The harvesting area should extend to the synovial lining to allow fibrous and synovial ingrowth to cover the harvest area. In more than 1600 patients who have had cartilage removed for cell culturing, no complications or late symptoms from the donor site have occurred. Optimal harvesting of cartilage is of greatest importance for the success of cell culturing, and optimal cell quality is necessary for the best possible result of this procedure.

CELL CULTURING

The retrieved cartilage is transferred to the cell culture laboratory in a sterile tube containing 0.9% NaCl. Upon arrival, the cartilage is mechanically minced into smaller pieces (1 mm of diameter) and washed in medium supplemented with antibiotics (gentamicin sulfate, amphotericin B, L-ascorbic acid, and glutamine). Then it is subjected to overnight collagenase digestion, allowing isolation of the chondrocytes. The chondrocytes are then cultured in DMEM/F12

with 10% autologous serum supplement and antibiotics. Primary cultures are performed in 25-cm^2 flasks incubated in 7% CO_2 in air at 37° C. After 1 week, the cells are trypsinized and passed into bigger culture flasks (75 cm^2), where they are cultured for an additional week. Two weeks after the culture begins, the cells are trypsinized again, washed, counted, and resuspended in 0.3 to 0.4 mL of implantation medium, in a tuberculin syringe, to a treatment density of 30 million cells/mL. A second surgery is performed for implantation of cells into the cartilage defect area.

SURGICAL PROCEDURE—CHONDROCYTE IMPLANTATION

Chondral Lesions

The patient is placed under general or spinal anesthesia. With a tourniquet-controlled bloodless field, a minor parapatellar incision is made. The joint is opened and the injury assessed. For good surgical technique, it is important to obtain good access to the defect, and the arthrotomy might need to be adjusted accordingly (Fig. 22-7). The patella may have to be dislocated in the case of implantation to multiple femoral or patellar lesions.

Clinical and radiologic assessment has to be performed before surgery is undertaken, revealing a potential indication for a realignment procedure. A realignment procedure is then scheduled in patients with patellar lesions and patellofemoral malalignment or instability. Tibial or femoral osteotomies are performed when needed, in cases of excessive varus or valgus deformity, for protection of the implanted area. Corrective operations (osteotomy, reconstruction of extensor mechanism, ACL reconstruction) are performed before the cells are implanted. In tibial osteotomy, medial transfer of the tibial tuberosity, or ACL reconstruction, fixation is performed at the end of the procedure before the cells are implanted.

Excision and Débridement of the Lesion

The cartilage lesion area is assessed, incised, and débrided with a curette down to the subchondral bone and until healthy cartilage is reached in the periphery of the defect. Radical excision is the key to success. Resulting lesions should be as circular or as oval as possible. If the lesion is not contained by healthy cartilage, it is better to leave a 3- to 4-mm rim of acceptable cartilage than to have the lesion border bone or synovium. Gentle débridement of the excised area is performed down to subchondral bone without causing any bleeding. If bleeding occurs, an epinephrine sponge or a drop of fibrin glue can stop it. The excised defect is then measured in its longest diameter and longest perpendicular diameter.

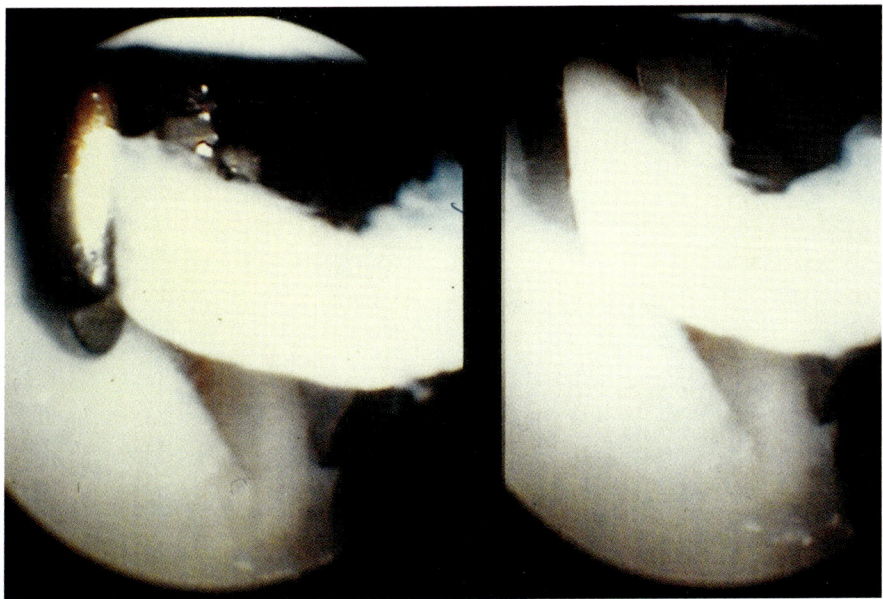

Figure 22-6. Arthroscopic views show harvesting of articular cartilage from the upper medial femoral condyle with a grasper (*left picture*) and a ring curette (*right* picture).

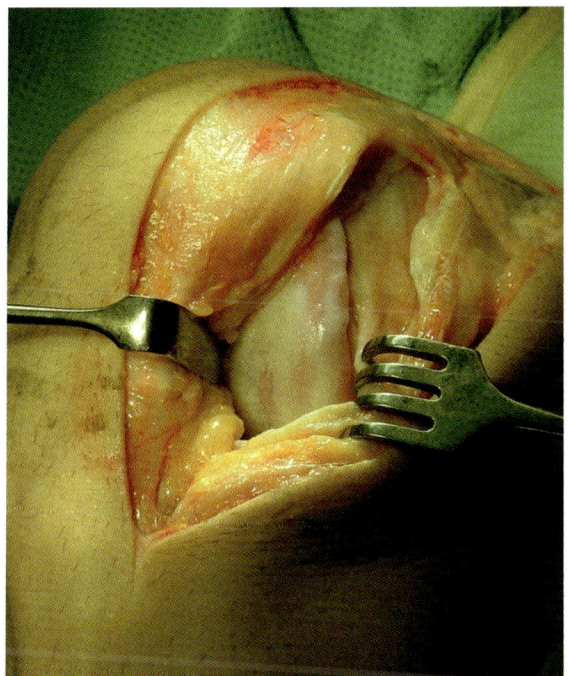

Figure 22-7. The arthrotomy is adjusted for good exposure of the defect.

The defect should be shaped as geometrically as possible. A template of sterile aluminum foil or paper is used to model the exact size of the defect (Fig. 22-8).

Harvesting of the Periosteal Flap

Through a separate incision on the upper medial aspect of the tibia, the periosteum is dissected free of fascia, fat, and fibrous tissue. Even passing vessels should be dissected off the flap. Measure the intended periosteal flap, or use the template to create the exact size and form. Oversize the periosteal flap by adding 1 to 2 mm to the periphery of the intended flap.

Incise the periosteum and use a sharp elevator to remove the periosteal flap. Use small movements to avoid rifts in the periosteum (Fig. 22-9). Mark the side of the periosteum to allow identification of the cambium layer. Saline is used to keep the periosteal flap moist. The periosteal flap should be as thin as possible and transparent to achieve more volume in the defect and to allow the cells to spread and expand. The thinner the periosteal flap, the less is the risk for hypertrophy, fibrillation, or other complications.

Suturing of the Periosteal Flap

Anchor the periosteal flap in four corners with the cambium layer facing the inside of the bone of the defect. Then adapt the periosteum to the surrounding cartilage by placing 6-0 resorbable suture at 4- to 6-mm intervals. Insert the suture to a depth of at least 5 to 6 mm to avoid cutting through the cartilage. Intervals between sutures are sealed with fibrin glue. An opening in the upper part of the defect is left for injection of the cells.

Before injecting the cells, check that there is no leakage by introducing a soft catheter with a syringe into the defect. Inject saline slowly into the defect and check for any leakage. Then aspirate the saline and inject the cells into the defect, starting distally and withdrawing the syringe proximally as the cells are injected. Close the injection site with suture and fibrin glue (Fig. 22-10).

Osteochondral Lesions (Osteochondritis Dissecans)

When osteochondritis dissecans is treated by ACI, attention must be paid to the depth of the defect. If the bony defect is shallower than 6 to 8 mm, the lesion is treated the same way as a chondral lesion. Gently débride the sclerotic bottom of the defect, but be careful to not cause bleeding. The cartilage is incised and débrided to vertical edges of healthy cartilage. Cover the defect with a periosteal flap, seal, and check for leakage. Then implant the chondrocytes and close the last opening.

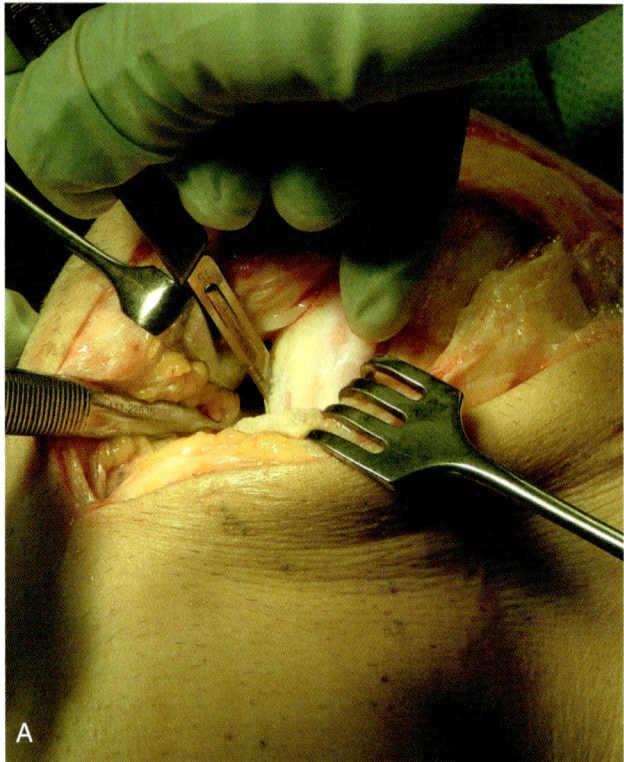

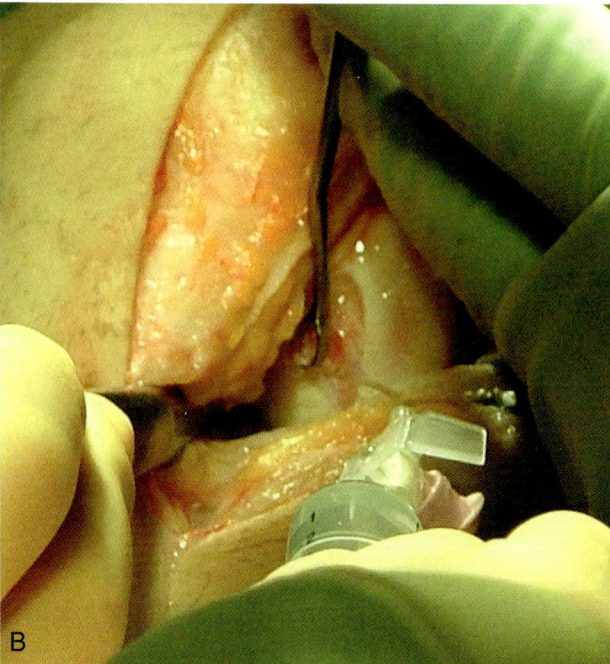

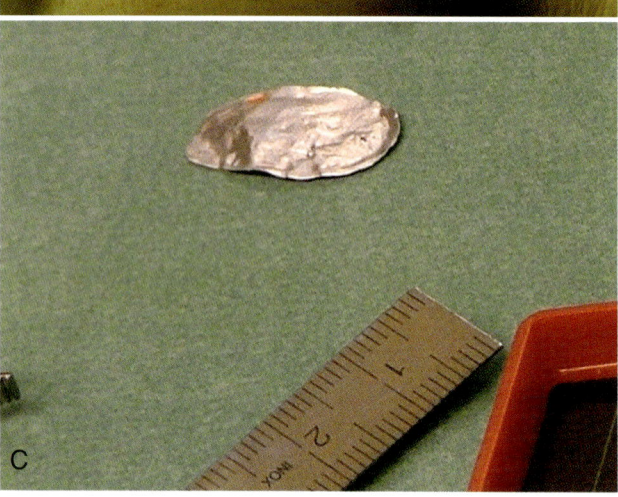

Figure 22-8. All damaged or undermined cartilage is excised (**A**) and carefully débrided (**B**). A template of the defect is made from sterile aluminum foil (**C**).

If the bony defect is deeper than 6 to 8 mm, ACI is not enough, and concomitant autologous bone grafting is needed ("sandwich technique"). Start by abrading the sclerotic bottom of the defect to spongy bone and undercut the subchondral bone plate. Use a 2-mm bur and drill multiple holes into the spongy bone. The cartilage is débrided to healthy cartilage with vertical edges. Then harvest cancellous bone for grafting of the bony defect. If the bony defect is small, use bone from the tibial or femoral condyle, but if the defect is larger, bone has to be harvested from the iliac crest. Pack the bone from the bottom up and try to shape the bone graft to the contour of the condyle.

Harvest a periosteal flap to cover the bone graft at the level of subchondral bone, with the cambium layer facing the joint. Anchor it with horizontal or mattress sutures placed into the cartilage or through small drill holes in the subchondral bone plate, and use fibrin glue under the flap for fixation to the bone graft. This technique will avoid bleeding into the cartilage defect. Another periosteal flap is harvested and sutured to the cartilage edges, with the cambium layer facing the defect. Use fibrin glue to seal the intervals between sutures. Test for a watertight seal with a gentle saline injection. If no leakage is present, aspirate the saline and inject the chondrocytes. Close the last opening and seal with fibrin glue (Fig. 22-11).

THE CONCEPT OF OPTIMAL ENVIRONMENTAL CONDITIONS FOR THE SHORT- AND LONG-TERM SURVIVAL OF REPAIR TISSUE

Over the years, it has become obvious that for ACI and concomitant procedures, it is mandatory to create optimal

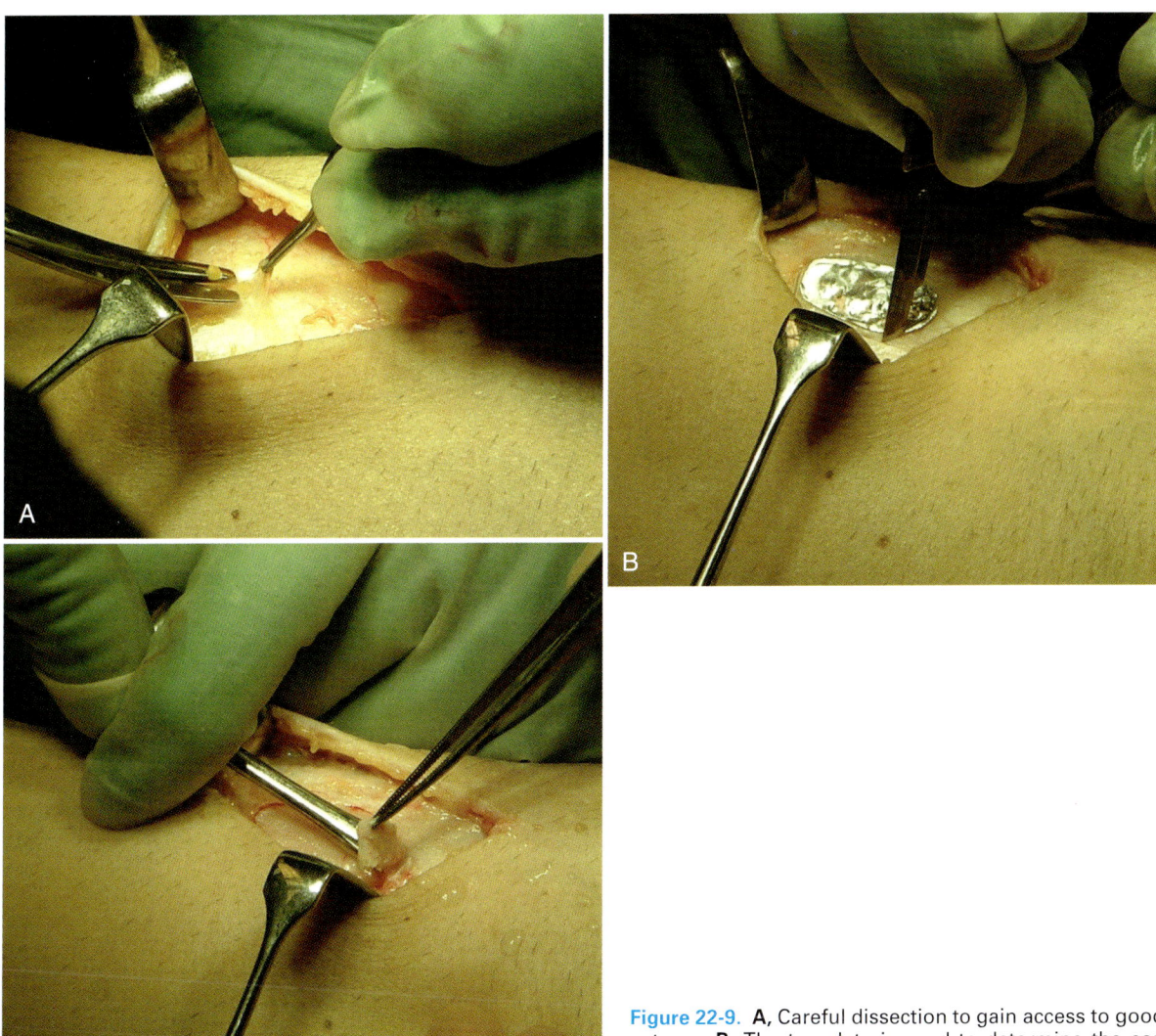

Figure 22-9. **A,** Careful dissection to gain access to good-quality periosteum. **B,** The template is used to determine the correct size and form of the periosteal flap. **C,** With careful technique, the flap is removed.

local environmental conditions for the short- and long-term survival of the repair. Malalignment and instability will need corrective surgery for a good result. Procedures such as anterior cruciate ligament (ACL) reconstruction or high tibial osteotomy may be performed at the same time that the biopsy specimen is harvested. Otherwise, they could be done concomitant with the implantation. Pathologic mechanics in the joint reduces the chance of successful repair. Patellar lesions are often related to a maltracking or unstable patella; the patella must thus be realigned or stabilized for good healing. Stabilizing procedures may include anteromedialization of the tibial tuberosity, lateral release, proximal medial soft tissue shortening, and trochlear grooveplasty (if it is dysplastic). In patients with trochlear and patellar lesions, especially large and uncontained ones, unloading with ventralization of the tibial tuberosity should be considered. A torn ACL is reconstructed after the cartilage lesion is débrided and covered with periosteum, but before the chondrocytes are injected. To unload the transplanted area when a varus or valgus deformity is present, a high tibial or distal femoral osteotomy is performed. When these corrective surgeries are performed, a brace-limiting range of motion of 0 to 60 degrees

is used postoperatively for 3 weeks, and for the following 3 weeks, range of motion is limited to 0 to 90 to 120 degrees. In patients with previous total or subtotal meniscectomy, meniscus allograft implantation should be considered.

POSTOPERATIVE TREATMENT

The patient is given antibiotic and thrombotic prophylaxis for 48 hours. Six to 8 hours after surgery, a continuous passive motion machine is used with a range of motion of 0 to 40 degrees. Range of motion, as well as isometric quadriceps training, is allowed on the day after surgery. Weight bearing is limited during the first weeks. Depending on the size, location, and containment of the lesion and concomitant procedures, weight bearing consists of loading to the pain threshold for 6 weeks, loading with 30 to 40 lb to 8 weeks, and then gradually increased weight bearing for another 6 weeks. Cycling on a stationary bike with low resistance could be started when the patient has reached 90 to 100 degrees of knee flexion. When full weight bearing is achieved, long-distance walking with increasing distances is encouraged. Swimming is allowed, as well as wet vest training, when the

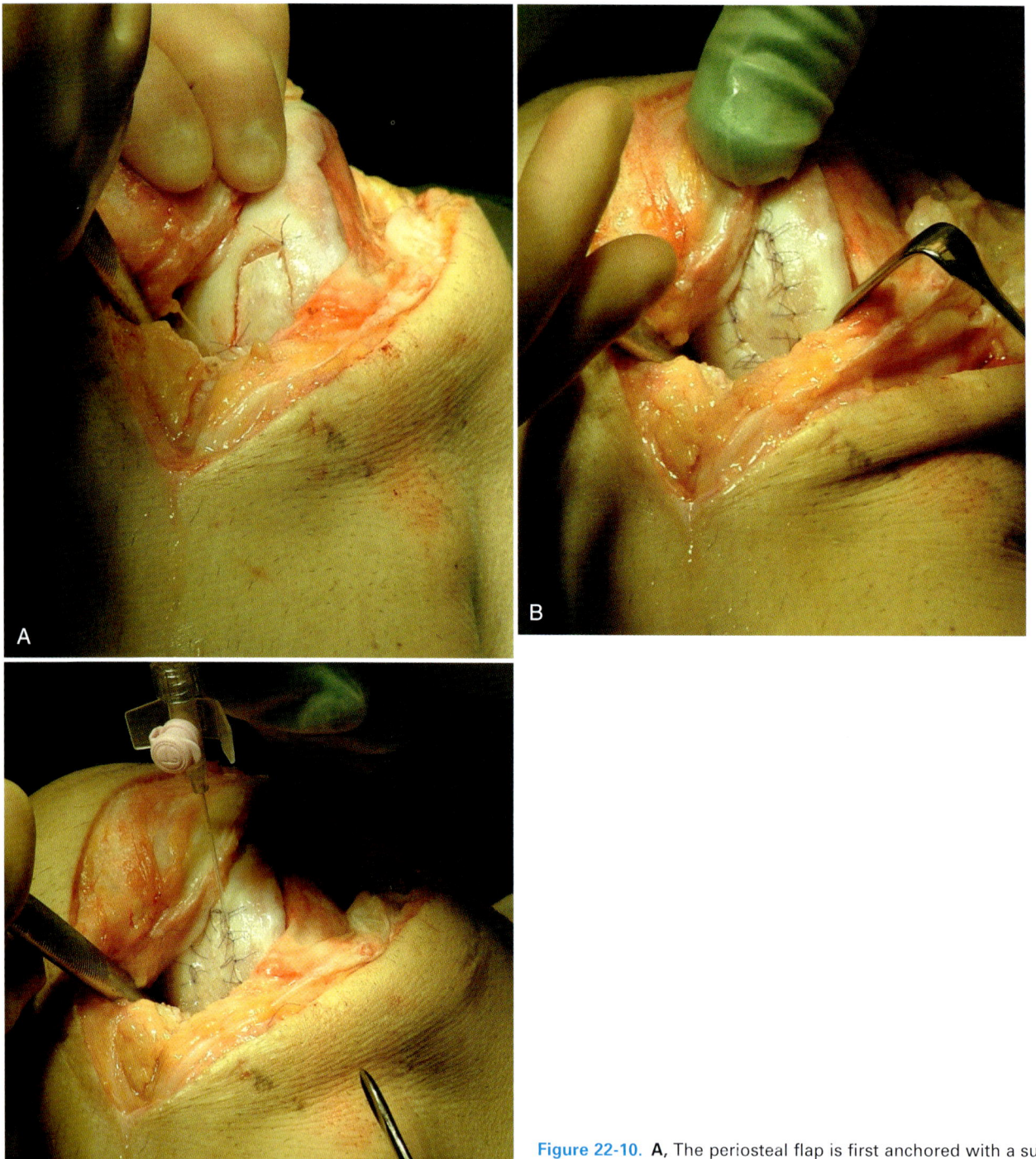

Figure 22-10. A, The periosteal flap is first anchored with a suture in each corner. **B,** The flap is then sutured to the cartilage rim. **C,** The integrity of the chamber under the flap is tested with an injection of saline.

wounds are healed. Cross-country skiing, in-line skating, or outdoor skating, if the patient is used to these activities, can be allowed when full weight bearing has been achieved. Running is not allowed until 9 months.

Return to professional sports is permitted after individual assessment, including overall clinical and functional tests and arthroscopic evaluation with the indentation test and probing, to determine the hardness and condition of the repair tissue.

It is very important to inform the patient about the healing process, starting with cells in a suspension changing to cotton-like tissue in the first 2 to 3 months and gradually maturing to a rubber-like tissue within 6 months. Continuous maturation with hardening is an ongoing process that is stimulated by gradually increased weight bearing, as well as by motion. Such maturation will continue for 12 months or longer. The return of proteoglycans to the repair area and to the cartilage in general can be assessed by MRI enhanced

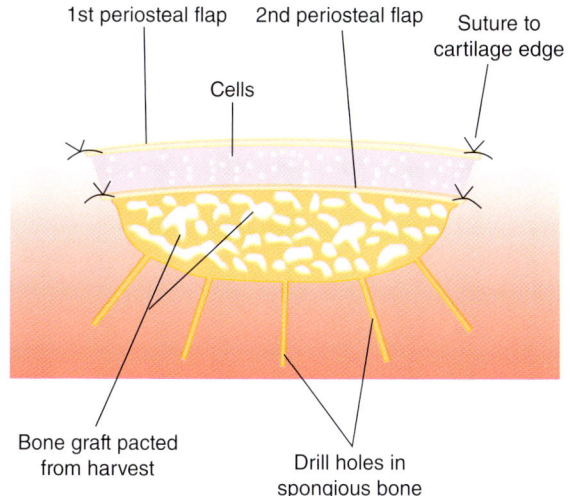

Figure 22-11. Schematic drawing of the sandwich procedure with layers of transplanted bone, periosteal flap, chondrocytes, and periosteal flap.

with gadolinium (dGEMRIC) showing normalization of proteoglycan concentrations at 9 to 12 to 15 months postoperatively.[9]

RESULTS OF AUTOLOGOUS CHONDROCYTE IMPLANTATION: LONG-TERM SWEDISH EXPERIENCE

Since October of 1987, more than 1800 patients have undergone ACI in Göteborg, Sweden. Several follow-up studies have been published.[27,28] In our latest study, conducted in 2009, we presented 224 patients evaluated 10 to 20 years after the ACI.[29] Follow-up evaluation was performed 12.8 years from the time of implantation (range, 10 to 20 years). Average patient age was 33.3 years (range, 14 to 62 years) at the time of the ACI.

Seventy-four percent of patients had isolated cartilage lesions, and 26% had multiple lesions. Forty patients had two lesions, 12 patients had three lesions, and 4 patients had more than three lesions. The locations of the lesion varied; 52% had an isolated lesion on a femoral condyle, 22% had an isolated patellar or trochlear lesion, 10% had kissing lesions, and 16% had multiple but not kissing lesions. The mean size of lesions per patient was 7 cm² (range, 1 to 27 cm²), and the mean size per lesion was 5.2 cm² (range, 1 to 16 cm²).

Concomitant procedures were performed with ACI mainly because of ligamentous insufficiency. Forty-six patients had an ACL reconstruction; 42 of them had it at the same time as the ACI, and 4 had it before the ACI. Twenty-one patients underwent a high tibial osteotomy before or during the ACI, five had reconstruction of a collateral ligament, and two had a posterior cruciate ligament (PCL) reconstruction. One in three patients (37%) had undergone a previous operation before ACI that involved shaving or drilling of the subchondral bone of the lesion area. Thirty-four percent (76/224 patients) had a history of a meniscal lesion and partial or total meniscectomy before or during the ACI. Sixty-six percent (148/224 patients) did not have meniscal involvement at least until the time of implantation.

Patients were evaluated with the use of multiple functional scales and activity scores. Reported results mainly relate to the injury locations considered an indication for ACI.[29,34] Indentation tests were also performed in previous studies to measure the stiffness of the repair tissue, and biopsy tissue was harvested for analysis of microscopic appearance and biochemistry.[25] Indirect measurement of glycosaminoglycans (GAGs) of the repair tissue has been performed using the dGEMRIC technique.[9,35]

Isolated Injury to the Femoral Condyle

A total of 52 patients with isolated femoral lesions were evaluated. Forty-one lesions were located on the medial condyle and 11 on the lateral; the size per lesion varied between 0.6 and 14 cm² (average, 4.9 cm²). Average patient age at the time of surgery was 35.5 years (range, 17 to 62 years).

Forty-seven patients (90%) responded that they had benefited from the treatment and would undergo the operation again. Thirty-six patients (69%) thought that they were the same or had improved in comparison with previous years.

Average Tegner-Wallgren score was 8 (range, 2 to 14), and 37 patients (84%) had a score of 6 or greater. The average Lysholm score was 60.1 (range, 46 to 81) before surgery and 72.6 (range, 25 to 96) 10 to 20 years postoperatively. The overall Brittberg-Peterson score was 65.9 preoperatively (range, 31 to 107) and 38.4 postoperatively (range, 3 to 102.8), thus suggesting overall improvement in quality of life and knee function. Noyes score was 5.4 (range, 1 to 9); Knee injury and Osteoarthritis Outcome Scores (KOOS) were 77.3 for pain, 65 for symptoms, 83.1 for activities of daily living (ADL), 45.1 for sports, and 51 for quality of life.

Femoral Condyle Lesions With ACL Reconstruction

Forty-six patients had a femoral condyle lesion and underwent ACL reconstruction. In 42 cases, ACL reconstruction was performed at the time of implantation; 4 patients had been reconstructed earlier. Thirty-seven patients had a lesion on the medial femoral condyle and 13 on the lateral. Thirty-seven had an isolated femoral condyle lesion, and the remaining nine had between two and four lesions (six with two lesions, two with three, and one with four lesions).

The average size of medial femoral condyle lesions was 4.5 cm² (range, 1.2 to 10 cm²) and of lateral femoral condyle lesions 4.6 cm² (range, 2.4 to 10.5 cm²). Average age at the time of implantation was 31.1 years (range, 17.5 to 50.5 years).

Thirty-four patients evaluated their current status as better or the same compared with previous years; 41 of them (91.1%) would undergo the operation again.

The Tegner-Wallgren score was 8.1 (range, 3 to 15), and the Lysholm 69.2 (range, 34 to 100). Total Brittberg-Peterson was 41.1 (range, 2 to 103.4), and Noyes was 5.2 (range, 1 to 9). KOOS was 72.8 for pain, 67.5 for symptoms, 81.3 for ADL, 41.1 for sports, and 48.2 for quality of life. Preoperative values for Tegner-Wallgren and Lysholm were 7.2 and 59.1, respectively; for Brittberg-Peterson (total), the value was 56.3.

Osteochondritis Dissecans of the Femoral Condyle

Twenty-six patients with osteochondritis dissecans were evaluated in the study of 2009. All lesions were isolated. Fifteen lesions were located on the medial femoral condyle, nine on the lateral, and two on the patella. Average size was 6.2 cm^2 (range, 1 to 12 cm^2). Average patient age at the time of implantation was 26.8 years (range, 15.7 to 52.4 years).

Twenty-one patients (81%) replied that they were better or the same compared with previous years. Twenty-five (96.2%) would undergo the operation again.

The Tegner-Wallgren score was 8.6 in the latest follow-up (range, 5 to 13). Twenty-four patients had a Tegner-Wallgren score equal to or greater than 6. The mean Lysholm score was 67.4 (range, 31 to 95). Preoperatively, Tegner-Wallgren was 6.4 (range, 1 to 9) and Lysholm was 56.2 (range, 13 to 85). Total Brittberg-Peterson score was 38.6 (range, 2.7 to 99) and 51.8 preoperatively (range, 9.4 to 104). Noyes score was 5.7 (range, 3 to 9), and KOOS was 78 for pain, 65.2 for symptoms, 85.6 for ADL, 46.9 for sports, and 54.3 for quality of life.

Arthroscopic Assessment and Biopsies

In our previous follow-up study, arthroscopic assessment was performed in 46 patients. Macroscopic evaluation of the defect area showed a maximal defect score of 12 points. Isolated femoral condyle injuries in 20 patients showed an average of 10.3 points. Isolated femoral condyle lesions plus ACL reconstruction had an average score of 10.9 points and, with osteochondritis dissecans, an average score of 10.5 out of 12 maximum, which is complete filling of the defect until total integration to the surrounding cartilage and a normal surface. Biopsy samples were harvested and judged by unbiased scientists; 80% showed hyaline-like cartilage (Fig. 22-12).[25]

Indentation Test of Repair Tissue

In the study of 2002, the indentation test with an arthroscopic probe showed no significant difference in stiffness between normal articular cartilage and hyaline-like repair tissue in the transplanted area. Patients with fibrous tissue in the repair area had a significant decrease in stiffness when compared with normal cartilage and the repair tissue of hyaline-like cartilage.[25]

Immunohistochemical Analysis

Twenty-two biopsy specimens were taken from both repair tissue ($n = 19$) and healthy cartilage ($n = 3$). Analysis was done in blinded fashion and involved the content of type I and II collagen, cartilage oligomeric matrix protein, and aggrecan. Hyaline-like repair tissue had characteristics very similar to those of normal articular cartilage, whereas fibrous repair tissue differed in all analyzed parameters (Table 22-1).

Complications

No serious complications, no infections, no chronic synovitis, and no thrombosis were reported. The reoperation rate was 5%. The main complications included periosteal hypertrophy with a clicking or crepitating sensation, sometimes with swelling early in the postoperative period. Most of these symptoms disappeared with time and continued rehabilitation. If symptoms remained, patients were treated arthroscopically by débridement of the hypertrophic periosteum or fibrillation (Fig. 22-13). This complication had no impact on the long-term result. A few patients sustained partial delamination of the grafted area, with or without a new trauma episode. These patients were treated by reimplantation of autologous chondrocytes and achieved good and excellent results.

Evaluation With dGEMRIC

Thirty-six knees in 31 patients were assessed 9 to 18 years after treatment with ACI.[35] All patients had isolated lesions: 27 on a femoral condyle, 1 on the trochlea, and 8 on the patella. Knees were evaluated with the dGEMRIC technique. Measurement of the concentrations of gadolinium compounds on MRI T1 sequences (T1 mapping) provides information regarding the concentrations of GAGs in normal cartilage or repair tissue at the cartilage lesion area.

The quantity of proteoglycans in the repair tissue was found to be equal to that in surrounding cartilage. This indicates equal quality of the transplant and surrounding cartilage, thus successful coverage of the defect area. This study shows that 9 to 18 years after the ACI, the cartilage defect area is restored in most cases.

Long-Term Durability

Fifty of 61 patients with femoral condyle injuries had good or excellent results at 2 years' follow-up. Fifty-one patients had a good or excellent result 5 to 10 years postoperatively,

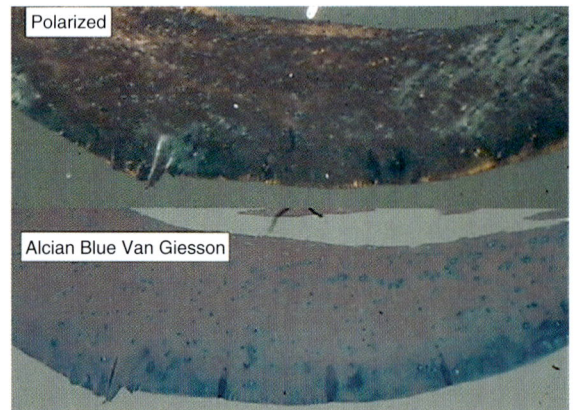

Figure 22-12. Biopsy specimen from repair tissue 9 years after autologous chondrocyte implantation.

Table 22-1 Immunohistochemical Analysis Comparing Normal Cartilage With Hyaline and Fibrous Repair Tissue

	Normal Cartilage	Hyaline Repair	Fibrous Repair
Collagen type I	$- \rightarrow +$	$- \rightarrow +$	$++ \rightarrow +++$
Collagen type II	$+++$	$++ \rightarrow +++$	$-$
Cartilage oligomeric protein	$+++$	$++ \rightarrow +++$	$+ \rightarrow ++$
Aggrecan	$+++$	$++ \rightarrow +++$	$+ \rightarrow ++$

+, Normal finding; −, not present.

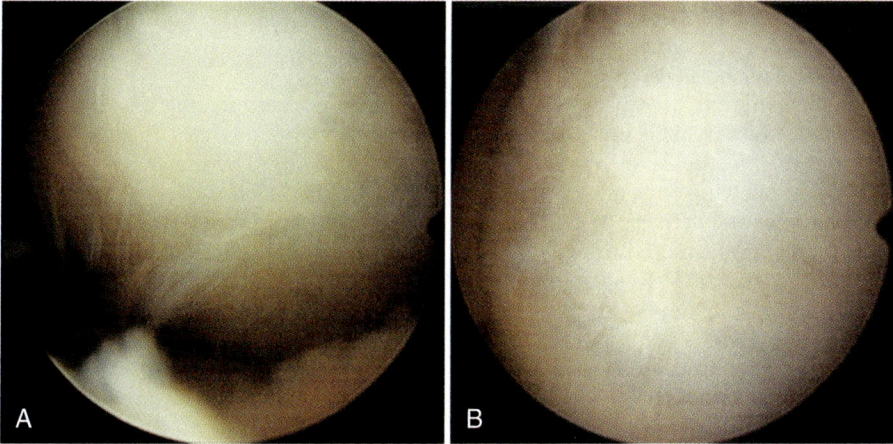

Figure 22-13. **A,** Complication consisting of fibrillation of the periosteal flap 1 year after autologous chondrocyte implantation of the medial femoral condyle and **(B)** after débridement of the superficial fibrillation of the periosteal flap. The fibrillation had no impact on the long-term results.

with an average follow-up of 7.4 years. Ten to 20 years after implantation, 74% of patients replied that they were better or the same compared with previous years. Ninety-two percent were satisfied and would undergo the ACI again. Lysholm, Tegner-Wallgren, and Brittberg-Peterson scores were improved compared with preoperative values. These outcomes indicate high durability of the repair tissue after ACI. This is also indicated by the evaluation of repair tissue performed with biopsies or the dGEMRIC technique.

According to findings at 10 to 20 years' follow-up, patient improvement was similar regardless of the number or size of lesions, and regardless of whether patients had a previous history of ACL reconstruction. Moreover, average final values of Lysholm, Tegner-Wallgren, and Brittberg-Peterson scores were statistically not different between patients with single or multiple lesions, and between patients with or without previous or concomitant meniscal or ACL reconstruction surgery.

Shaving or drilling of cartilage lesions before the ACI did not seem to affect clinical improvement in the medium term (3 years) or at final (10 to 20 years') follow-up. However, patients who had undergone previous bone surgeries (shaving or drilling) showed deterioration ($P = .06$) of Lysholm scores between medium- and long-term follow-up. Long-term evaluation with dGEMRIC revealed that lesions that had been treated previously with bone marrow–stimulating surgeries (microfractures, drilling) had a higher incidence of intralesional osteophytes.

This evidence suggests that previous bone marrow–stimulating surgeries may affect the long-term durability of ACI repair tissue.

CARTILAGE REGISTRY REPORT

All patients treated by ACI in the United States and Europe are monitored in a registry outcome study. In a cohort of patients with single ($n = 28$) and multiple lesions ($n = 11$) on the medial and lateral condyles and the trochlea with 72 months' follow-up, the modified Cincinnati Knee Rating Scale went from 3.15 preoperatively to 6.93 at 72 months. Eighty-two percent of patients had functional improvement.

A cohort of 15 patients with multiple lesions and a minimum of 60 months' follow-up were evaluated with the modified Cincinnati Knee Rating Scale for overall patient evaluation, pain, and swelling. All parameters increased. The overall patient evaluation category increased from 2.73 to 7.53, pain from 2.80 to 7.33, and swelling from 3.73 to 7.47, and the overall condition was improved in 93% of patients.

Complications

No infections have been reported since the start of the study in 1995. Adverse events or complications were reported by 5.8% after implantation, and 2.9% had a complication considered to be at least possibly related to the autologous cultured chondrocytes. The most frequently reported adverse events included hypertrophic tissue at the repair site, intraarticular adhesions, superficial wound infection, hypertrophic synovitis, and postoperative hematoma.

Both clinical results and complications were on a level with the Swedish results.

TISSUE ENGINEERED MATRIX SUPPORT (TEMS) USING MEMBRANES, CARRIERS, SCAFFOLDS, AND GELS IN AUTOLOGOUS CHONDROCYTE IMPLANTATION

Tissue Engineered Matrix Support (TEMS)

First-generation ACI with the use of periosteum has been performed since 1987 with good to excellent results for most treated patients.

However, the procedure is technically demanding, requiring suturing of the periosteum on healthy cartilage to achieve a water-sealed environment for the injected suspension of chondrocytes. It also requires an open arthrotomy for the implantation with an additional incision for harvesting of the periosteum. Besides this, it has been reported that an increased number of periosteal hypertrophies required a second arthroscopy.

Interest is increasing in the development of new materials and techniques of ACI that could overcome the limitations and difficulties of first-generation ACI and further improve and perfect the regeneration of hyaline articular cartilage. Remarkable progress has been made in the development of supportive materials (e.g., scaffolds, membranes) for initial support of repair tissue, allowing to some extent the use of arthroscopic techniques for the delivery of cells.

At present, resorbable membranes are used to replace the periosteum and to carry cells seeded onto the membrane for delivery into the defect. Different techniques for fixation of the membranes are under development. Membranes made of collagen type I/III of porcine origin are used, as well as synthetic materials (polyglycolic–polylactic acids) with resorption times of about 6 to 12 weeks. Cells are also cultured in collagen membranes and in tridimensional scaffolds of esterified hyaluronic acid with a resorption time of about 4 months. Chondrocytes are grown for 3 weeks in the scaffold and can be delivered arthroscopically and fixed by press-fit technique into smaller defects.

Membranes and scaffolds provide a bed for the seeding and culturing of cells in two- or three-dimensional cultures. The aim is to reduce intraoperative time and postoperative morbidity, while avoiding the harvesting and use of periosteum. Scaffold-guided ACI is still a two-stage operation; however, it may be faster and easier and may result in fewer complications for the patient. The mechanical and functional properties of scaffolds could contribute to the viability, redifferentiation, and matrix production of cells. However, the mechanical properties (e.g., the friction coefficient of the surface facing the joint, stiffness in comparison with normal surrounding cartilage) are not specified or regulated. Longer resorption times may be required for mechanical support of the tissue during rehabilitation for earlier return to work and sports.

What Is the Optimal Scaffold?

The ideal scaffold has to fulfill several requirements in terms of safety, material features, and regenerative properties.

First of all, it has to be safe for the patient, that is, noncarcinogenic and biocompatible, without causing any inflammatory or immune reaction. It has to have the ability to be effectively sterilized without losing its biomechanical properties. The scaffold when implanted has to be free of live tissue (except from the autologous chondrocytes) or heterologous biologic material.

It should not be cytotoxic for seeded cells or for surrounding tissues. It must be capable of supporting and holding the cells. Those cells have to stay viable and must be effectively attached to the scaffold and mechanically supported so they do not spread into the joint cavity after implantation; however, at the same time, the scaffold has to be permeable to allow diffusion of factors that promote cellular production of extracellular matrix.

The mechanical support should be applied until cells start to produce extracellular matrix. Then, the ideal scaffold has to start being gradually reabsorbed and substituted for by the hyaline-(like) matrix produced by the cells.

The structure of the scaffold has to be effectively reproducible. Finally, it must be easily transferred and handled by the surgeon so as to be effectively applied to the defect area. The possibility of a less invasive but still effective fixation technique allows for transarthroscopic implantation, limiting the postoperative morbidity caused by an open incision.

Matrix-Induced Autologous Chondrocyte Implantation (MACI)

Autologous periosteum has been used as coverage for implanted chondrocytes (first-generation ACI with periosteum [ACI-P]). The use of porcine type I/III collagen membranes in medicine led to the development of matrix-induced ACI (MACI, Verigen AG, Leverkusen, Germany). Chondrocytes are seeded on the MACI type I/III collagen membrane before implantation. The membrane is fixed to the cartilage defect area with fibrin glue, resorbable pins, or additional sutures. This approach seeks to provide and stabilize cells in the cartilage defect area, seeded on the bilaminate collagen membrane. Thus, the membrane is used as a carrier for delivery of cells into the cartilage lesion. At present, the cells are seeded to the membrane and cultured for 48 hours before they are implanted in smaller lesions using arthroscopic technique and fixation with fibrin glue or resorbable pins. More than 7000 patients have been treated with MACI since 1998. However, the method has not been validated with long-term clinical studies. Only a few cohort studies have been performed with promising results.

In one cohort study, MACI showed clinical efficacy 3 years (range, 2 to 5 years) after implantation, but the number of participants was low.[3] Gigante and associates reported significant improvement in all measured clinical scores 3 years after treatment of patellofemoral lesions with distal realignment of the patella and MACI.[8] However, it was not clear from this study whether improvement was the result of patellofemoral realignment or treatment of the cartilage lesion. Another recent study has demonstrated the ability to generate hyaline-like cartilage as early as 6 months after MACI.[37] Two randomized controlled trials with MACI have been published. Basad and colleagues reported significantly better outcomes compared with microfracture, and the study of Bartlett and coworkers showed no differences compared with autologous chondrocyte implantation—collagen covered (ACI-C) 12 months after surgery.[1,2] A comparative study between ACI-C and MACI showed no great differences in clinical results, histology or hypertrophy of the graft, or reoperation rate, revealing an incidence of graft hypertrophy of 9% in each group.[1]

Limited literature supports the efficacy of MACI and its superiority over other treatment options for large, full-thickness cartilage defects. Additional studies of better quality and with longer follow-up are needed.

The term *MACI* has been used improperly in the literature to represent any scaffold (i.e., matrix)-induced ACI technique. However, MACI is an established brand name, and any other use of this term can easily lead to misunderstanding. Therefore, we support the use of tissue engineered matrix support (TEMS) for methods that use three-dimensional matrices as scaffolds for the culturing and seeding of cells.

Collagen-Covered Autologous Chondrocyte Implantation (CACI) (Chondro-Gide, Restore, Maci)

Collagen type I/III membranes of porcine origin have been used instead of the periosteal patch to cover the cartilage lesion area (Chondro-Gide, Geistlich, Wolhausen, Switzerland; Restore, DePuy, Warsaw, Ind; Maci, Genzyme,

Cambridge, Mass).[13,32] Chondro-Gide is a porcine-derived bilayer collagen type I/III. It consists of a porous layer of collagen fibers in a loose open-weave arrangement that favors cell invasion and attachment, and a compact membrane layer with a smooth surface, which is cell occlusive. The aim of using CACI is to reduce operative time and the need for a second incision for the periosteal harvest. CACI may also reduce the periosteal hypertrophy that has been reported in about 26% to about 5% of cases.[12,13,32] Chondro-Gide can be seeded with cells and fixed by fibrin glue, but the procedure needs to be done via an arthrotomy.[31] Only short-term results have been reported.

Three-Dimensional Scaffolds for Autologous Chondrocyte Implantation

With third-generation techniques, chondrocytes are cultured in three-dimensional matrices (scaffolds) such as hyaluronic acid (Hyalograft C, Fidia Advanced Biopolymers, Abano Terme, Italy) before implantation in the cartilage defect area.[17,19]

Hyaluronic Acid Scaffolds (Hyalograft C)

Evidence shows that hyaluronic acid is an ideal molecule for use in tissue engineering in cartilage repair, given its multifunctional involvement in cartilage homeostasis.

Hyalograft C is a three-dimensional hyaluronan-based scaffold made of HYAFF 11, a benzyl ester of hyaluronic acid with 20-μm fibers. Autologous chondrocytes harvested from the patient are expanded in vitro and are seeded in a three-dimensional culture onto the scaffold. They are cultured in the scaffold for 3 additional weeks before arthroscopic implantation into small, contained cartilage defects using a press-fix technique (Fig. 22-14). Hyalograft C was introduced in 1999 for the treatment of full-thickness cartilage defects.[10,21]

Hyalograft C constructs can be implanted in the lesion without the need for periosteal collagen membrane coverings, while avoiding suturing to the surrounding cartilage, thus limiting operative time and simplifying the whole procedure. The features of the scaffold also permit the development of an arthroscopic implantation, without the need for an open arthrotomy, contributing to decreases in postoperative morbidity. However, this is possible only for small and contained lesions.

Several studies have provided the first medium-term clinical results, which are promising for the treatment of cartilage lesions. A prospective study of Kon and coworkers presented significant improvement 2 to 5 years postoperatively. Although microfracture provided comparable results at 2 years, significant deterioration was noted at 5 years' follow-up, revealing the superiority of repair tissue after Hyalograft C, in terms of quality and tolerance.[17] Marcacci and associates reported improvement in 91.5% of treated patients 2 to 5 years postoperatively; Nehrer and colleagues showed significant improvement even 7 years after treatment.[19,22] Gobbi and coworkers found significant improvement in objective and subjective International Knee Documentation Committee (IKDC) scores 24 months after treatment with Hyalograft C for cartilage defects of the patellofemoral joint.[11]

Evidence derived from histologic evaluation of repair tissue is limited. Among 22 cases, Marcacci and associates reported 12 cases with hyaline, 6 with mixed fibrohyaline, and 4 with fibrocartilage at 10 to 30 months postoperatively.[19] Gobbi and associates biopsied six specimens, four of which were hyaline-like and two of which were fibrohyaline.[11] Indirect evaluation of repair tissue using dGEMRIC shows an increase in GAGs. Although the content of GAG is significantly higher compared with microfracture, it is still lower than that of normal articular cartilage.[33]

The complication rate reported after Hyalograft C is relatively low. Complications such as repair tissue hypertrophy occur rarely; this fact, along with reduced postoperative morbidity, is considered an advantage over first-generation ACI.

However, additional studies with greater numbers of participants and longer follow-up times are needed to confirm currently available results and determine the long-term efficacy of the technique.

Suggested Classification of ACI Techniques

Following the introduction of new materials and techniques, different classifications of ACI techniques have been developed and used in the literature. Usually, ACI techniques are separated into two or three generations. However, there is no commonly accepted classification, especially regarding the clarification of second and third generations.

Therefore, we suggest the use of the following classification and terminology.

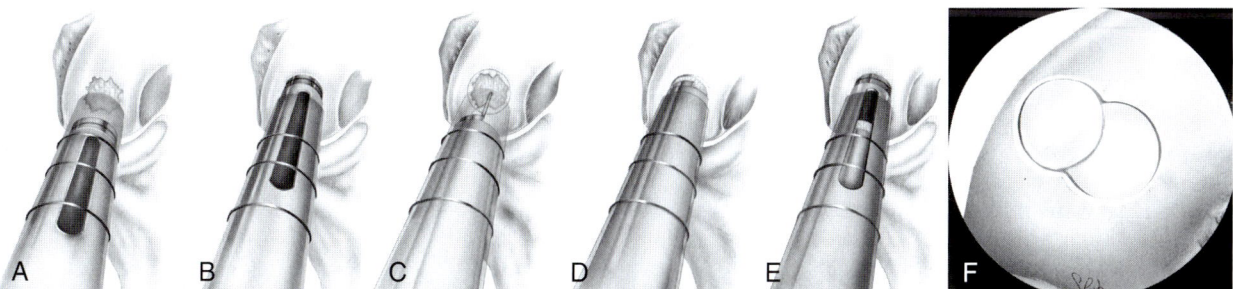

Figure 22-14.   A and **B,** A delivery device of variable diameter (6.5 to 8.5 mm) with a sharp edge is used to evaluate the size of the defect. **C,** A circular area with regular margins for graft implantation is prepared with a specially designed cannulated low-profile drill. **D** and **E,** The delivery device is then filled with a hyaluronic acid patch, which is transported and positioned in the prepared area. **E** and **F,** The graft is pushed out of the delivery device and is precisely positioned within the defect, where it remains tightly adhered to the subchondral bone. Because of the physical adhesive characteristics of the graft, no fibrin glue or sutures are used to fix the implant. (Courtesy Stefano Zaffagnini, Elizaveta Kon, and Maurilio Marcacci, Istituti Ortopedici Rizzoli, Bologna, Italy.)

First-generation ACI: ACI as first described in 1994, with the use of autologous periosteal membrane as a patch for the covering of chondrocytes in suspension.[5]

Second-generation ACI: ACI with tissue engineered matrix support (TEMS) of animal tissue origin (bovine or porcine collagen or others) or chemically synthesized matrix support (polyglycolic–polylactic acids, or others) used as membranes (e.g., Chondrogide) or as cell carriers (e.g., MACI).

Third-generation ACI: ACI with three-dimensional TEMS of animal or chemical origin used as scaffolds for growing and delivering chondrocytes into the joint (e.g., Hyalograft C).

INTERNATIONAL EXPERIENCE WITH AUTOLOGOUS CHONDROCYTE IMPLANTATION

Ochi and coworkers have done interesting research with autologous chondrocytes evenly distributed and transplanted in a collagen gel. Twenty-eight knees in 26 patients treated with chondrocytes in collagen gel (covered with a periosteal patch sutured to the defect) were monitored for at least 25 months. Treatment resulted in significant improvement in the Lysholm score. Pain and swelling were reduced in all patients, and locking was not present in any patient postoperatively. Arthroscopic assessment indicated that 26 knees had a good or excellent outcome.[23]

From Australia, Hart and Henderson have confirmed the Swedish results in medium-term follow-up.[14] From different centers in Europe, short- to medium-term results of ACI have been reported.[7] Pavesio and Marcacci published promising short-term results on arthroscopic ACI with the use of Hyalograft, a hyaluronic acid derivative.[24] Guillen and colleagues reported good to excellent short-term results with type I collagen membranes. Nehrer and coworkers have shown promising results with matrix-assisted chondrocyte implantation.[21]

Prospective randomized studies with short- and medium-term results have been published by Knutsen and associates,[15,16] with comparison between ACI and microfracture, as well as by Bentley and colleagues,[4] who randomized between ACI and mosaicplasty. Promising clinical results are presented, but the follow-up is too short to allow any conclusions regarding which technique is better suited for the lesions treated.[30]

FUTURE INDICATIONS

In young patients with multiple lesions (two or more in one joint) or bipolar lesions (i.e., bone-to-bone articulation), it is possible to try ACI. In treating this patient group, it is of utmost importance to address background factors such as ligament instability, varus/valgus deformity, total/subtotal meniscectomy, bony defects in osteochondritis dissecans or after fracture, and patellar malalignment or instability.

It is very important that the surgeon have optimal access to the defects, especially in the posterior part of the femur and the tibia. To attain this, the surgeon may need to detach the anterior insertion of the meniscus and its capsular insertion to the tibia. If this is not enough to reach the posterior

part of the defect, the second step is to incise behind the collateral ligament. If this is not acceptable, do not hesitate to take down the collateral ligament from the femoral epicondyle with a bone block measuring 2 × 2 cm; then open the joint to achieve excellent access to the posterior part of the tibia and femur.

Postoperative rehabilitation is longer in young, early osteoarthritic patients (bipolar lesions), especially those who undergo concomitant procedures. Usually, we recommend partial weight bearing with 20 kg for 8 weeks, then progressively increased weight bearing up to full weight bearing at 4 months.

Patients with multiple lesions and a minimum of 3 years' follow-up had 84% good or excellent results. Those with bipolar tibial-femoral lesions had 75% good or excellent results, and patients with bipolar patellofemoral lesions had 75% good or excellent results.

OTHER JOINTS

Autologous chondrocyte implantation has been used in the ankle joint with osteochondritis dissecans, as well as for cartilage lesions in the shoulder, elbow, and wrist. In principle, this technique can be used in any joint with a localized articular cartilage lesion or osteochondritis dissecans.

The longest follow-up in the talus is now over 8 years, and the results are good in 80%. The approach to medial or lateral localized injuries in the talus usually mandates a medial or sometimes a lateral osteotomy for optimal surgical access to the defect.[26]

The hip has been operated on in six young patients with osteochondritis dissecans or chondral lesions on the caput femoris. The shoulder has been operated on in three cases, two of which had lesions of both the glenoid and the head of the humerus. Results seem promising in other joints, but we need more patients and longer follow-up to establish these indications.

Further data collection and long-term results are needed before indications for these joints can be approved.

SUMMARY

At present, clinical experience with ACI is now longer than 22 years. Isolated articular cartilage injuries on the femoral condyles show good to excellent results in 90% of cases. Treatment of osteochondritis dissecans produces good to excellent results in 89% of cases. No serious complications have occurred, and a low number of adverse reactions have been reported. Biopsy specimens have shown hyaline-like cartilage in 80%, and indentation tests have indicated no significant difference between the indentation stiffness of hyaline-like repair tissue and of normal surrounding cartilage.

Results from the Swedish study have been confirmed by Cartilage Repair Registry data, with longest follow-up being 6 years, and by data from surgeons in Boston and Atlanta, with longest follow-up being 14 years. In the United States, more than 15,000 operations have been performed since 1995 (worldwide, more than 25,000).

Promising results are emerging with several new techniques using scaffolds and membranes as carriers, or growing the cells in before implantation with arthroscopic techniques.

Research continues regarding different cell types and how to safely use growth factors. We are moving forward to simplify and to optimize the regeneration of articular cartilage.

KEY REFERENCES

Bartlett W, Skinner JA, Gooding CR, et al: Autologous chondrocyte implantation versus matrix-induced autologous chondrocyte implantation for osteochondral defects of the knee: a prospective, randomised study. J Bone Joint Surg Br 87:640–645, 2005.

Bentley G, Biant LC, Carrington RW, et al: A prospective, randomised comparison of autologous chondrocyte implantation versus mosaicplasty for osteochondral defects in the knee. J Bone Joint Surg Br 85:223–230, 2003.

Brittberg M, Lindahl A, Nilsson A, et al: Treatment of deep cartilage defects in the knee with autologous chondrocyte transplantation. N Engl J Med 331:889–895, 1994.

Gobbi A, Kon E, Berruto M, et al: Patellofemoral full-thickness chondral defects treated with second-generation autologous chondrocyte implantation: results at 5 years' follow-up. Am J Sports Med 37:1083–1092, 2009.

Gooding CR, Bartlett W, Bentley G, et al: A prospective, randomised study comparing two techniques of autologous chondrocyte implantation for osteochondral defects in the knee: periosteum covered versus type I/III collagen covered. Knee 13:203–210, 2006.

Henderson IJ, Tuy B, Connell D, et al: Prospective clinical study of autologous chondrocyte implantation and correlation with MRI at three and 12 months. J Bone Joint Surg Br 85:1060–1066, 2003.

Kon E, Gobbi A, Filardo G, et al: Arthroscopic second-generation autologous chondrocyte implantation compared with microfracture for chondral lesions of the knee: prospective nonrandomized study at 5 years. Am J Sports Med 37:33–41, 2009.

Minas T, Gomoll AH, Rosenberger R, et al: Increased failure rate of autologous chondrocyte implantation after previous treatment with marrow stimulation techniques. Am J Sports Med 37:902–908, 2009.

Peterson L, Brittberg M, Kiviranta I, et al: Autologous chondrocyte transplantation: biomechanics and long-term durability. Am J Sports Med 30:2–12, 2002.

Peterson L, Minas T, Brittberg M, Lindahl A: Treatment of osteochondritis dissecans of the knee with autologous chondrocyte transplantation: results at two to ten years. J Bone Joint Surg Am 85(Suppl 2):17–24, 2003.

Peterson L, Minas T, Brittberg M, et al: Two- to 9-year outcome after autologous chondrocyte transplantation of the knee. Clin Orthop Relat Res 374:212–234, 2000.

Peterson L, Vasiliadis HS, Brittberg M, Lindahl A: Autologous chondrocyte implantation: a long-term follow-up. Am J Sports Med 38:1117–1124, 2010.

Vasiliadis HS, Concaro S, Brittberg M, et al: Autologous chondrocyte implantation: 10-20 years follow up. Paper presented at the 8th World Congress of the International Cartilage Repair Society, Miami, Fla, May 23–26, 2009.

Vasiliadis HS, Danielson B, Ljungberg M, et al: Autologous chondrocyte implantation in cartilage lesions of the knee: long-term evaluation with magnetic resonance imaging and delayed gadolinium-enhanced magnetic resonance imaging technique. Am J Sports Med 38:943–949, 2010.

Vasiliadis HS, Wasiak J, Salanti G: Autologous chondrocyte implantation for the treatment of cartilage lesions of the knee: a systematic review of randomized studies. Knee Surg Sports Traumatol Arthrosc 18(12):1645–1655, 2010.

Full references for this chapter can be found on www.expertconsult.com.

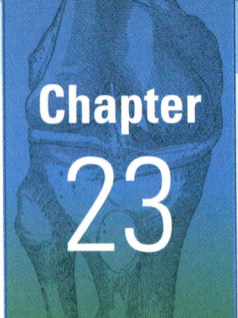

Chapter 23

Osteochondral Autograft Plug Transfer

Eli Chen and Nicholas A. Sgaglione

The treatment of symptomatic focal articular cartilage defects continues to present a clinical dilemma for many orthopedists. Surgical approaches to this problem can be categorized into those that attempt to resurface focal defects through tissue repair or regeneration and those that reconstitute articular cartilage surfaces through transplantation of intact osteochondral grafts. The former group includes repair strategies such as marrow stimulation and cell-based therapies such as implantation of chondrocytes expanded ex vivo. The results of these resurfacing procedures have been associated with tissue repair predominated by fibrocartilage, which has been shown to have inferior wear characteristics compared with hyaline tissue.[61] Osteochondral autograft plug transfer (OAT) involves the direct transplantation of osteochondral segments from less loaded regions of cartilage to areas with symptomatic focal defects. Despite concerns of donor site morbidity and limited availability, this method has been demonstrated to reliably restore native hyaline cartilage architecture and the underlying subchondral bone.

Early work on autologous hyaline cartilage transplantation to the femoral or tibial condyles involved direct transfer of patellar osteochondral grafts. The procedure was first described using a pedunculated patellar graft by d'Aubigné in 1945; in more recent times, Campanacci et al reported on a case series of 19 patients who underwent similar transfer of a free patellar graft.[13] Indications included primarily giant cell tumors and involved resection of almost the entire osteochondral segment of the patella and screw fixation to the tibial or femoral condyle. Attempts to restore native articular cartilage contour were made through careful orientation of the patellar graft, but with obvious donor–recipient mismatches. Patients were noted to have overall success, with the main complication being loss of range of motion.

Later reports described the transfer of autogenous osteochondral fragments for treatment of osteochondritis dissecans of the knee. Yamashita et al in 1985 described two patients who underwent graft harvest from the superomedial femoral trochlea in a region which "in extension was in contact with neither patella nor meniscus."[90] Donor sites were filled with iliac crest bone graft, and all segments were fixed using orthogonal mini-cancellous screws. Second-look arthrotomy for screw removal revealed macroscopically intact hyaline cartilage with mild irregularities at the interface between graft and native tissue. Slight surface contour irregularities were noted at both donor and graft sites, but with negligible clinical sequelae. Outerbridge et al in 1995 described the transfer of an osteochondral graft from the lateral facet of the patella to repair a large osteochondral defect in the ipsilateral femoral condyle in 10 patients.[68] A manual press-fit technique was used for graft fixation. Preoperative and postoperative function was assessed using the Cincinnati Knee Score; an average improvement from 43 points (range, 24 to 64) to 93 points (range, 79 to 100) was reported. All patients were satisfied with the procedure, and 70% were able to resume full, unrestricted activity. Success was offset by increased patellofemoral pain and progression of degeneration of the medial facet of the patella. Second-look arthroscopy revealed solid graft fixation and intact surface hyaline cartilage.

Current OAT procedures benefit from improvements in technique and instrumentation. Although the principle of restoration of hyaline cartilage by direct transfer from articular cartilage of less significant loading remains unchanged, the use of smaller grafts decreases donor site morbidity and allows for more limited exposure. Improvements in surgical technique have resulted in more predictable success rates and fewer complications, with greater attention toward restoring native articular cartilage topography. Indications for resurfacing have also expanded, reflecting more defined pathoetiology and a more precise approach with regard to site, size, and geometry of pathologic sites. In this chapter, we review the current approach to OAT, including indications, technical considerations, pearls and pitfalls, postoperative regimens, and clinical results.

INDICATIONS

Numerous treatment algorithms have been proposed for the management of articular cartilage lesions.[15,77,82] Smaller lesions (<10 mm) are typically managed with simple débridement, citing the limited increase in biomechanical loading and rim stresses around the edges of the defect.[25] Primary treatment options typically include marrow stimulation techniques such as microfracture, which has been demonstrated to provide good symptomatic relief and restoration of function in defects with intact edges and good containment.[62,84] However, more recent studies have raised concerns about the durability of fibrous/fibrocartilaginous repair tissue.[61] Larger lesions (surface area >200 mm²) and those with defects extending into subchondral bone represent a more complex scenario.

OAT is indicated for the management of focal articular cartilage lesions of the medial or lateral femoral condyles, the trochlear groove, and the patella. Reports of retrograde methods to address tibial plateau lesions have been discussed but are not clinically common. Indications as far as size considerations are concerned have traditionally been described as ranging from 10- to 25-mm-diameter lesions to 150- to 250-mm²-area lesions.[14,55] Overall, the optimal lesion size indicated for treatment includes symptomatic lesions that measure from 50 to 250 mm². Smaller osteochondritis dissecan (OCD) lesions and osteochondral fractures represent a good indication for OAT in that restoration of both the surface hyaline and the underlying subchondral bone can be successfully addressed. A variation on the typical OAT procedure has been described for the treatment of unstable OCD lesions. Rather than conventional hardware fixation, single or multiple osteochondral plugs may be used as biologic pegs to secure OCD lesions following débridement and backfill of underlying fibrous tissue.[60,63] Age is a consideration; patients younger than 50 years of age with an absence of degenerative pathology are indicated for OAT, depending on the quality and availability of donor tissue. Other patient factors include compliance with postoperative weight-bearing restrictions.

TECHNICAL CONSIDERATIONS

In 1982, Osterman and colleagues reported on a series of animal model experiments in rats, in which different strategies were taken toward reconstituting medial femoral condyle defects.[51] Fixation of a loose osteochondral fragment with a bone peg or with tissue adhesive was studied along with comparison of fresh-frozen allografts versus autogenous grafts harvested from the lateral femoral condyle. The authors concluded that precise reconstruction of the articular surface was essential because failures were seen in cases where restoration of joint surface congruity was inadequate. Subsequent studies have expanded on our understanding of the factors influencing outcomes from OAT. These include topography, contact pressures, fill pattern, depth of insertion, graft harvest, and graft insertion. Although advances in instrumentation and surgical techniques are essential and important, challenges remain, and several technique-related resurfacing factors must be addressed.

TOPOGRAPHY

In 1991, Ateshian et al described an analytic stereophotogrammetry technique through which the articular surface topography and the cartilage thickness of the knee joint were mapped (Fig. 23-1).[3] In a later study, Bartz et al described a method to be used for computerized matching of the topography of donor and recipient sites for OAT, allowing analysis of which commonly used donor site is best matched to a specific defect.[7] They concluded that cartilage defects in the weight-bearing regions of the medial and lateral femoral condyles are best treated with grafts taken from the most inferior parts of the superomedial and superolateral borders of the trochlea (Fig. 23-2). Similarly, lesions in the saddle-shaped trochlea may be addressed with grafts from the intercondylar notch.[1]

It has been proposed that matching of cartilage thickness between donor and recipient sites is important, and avoiding underlying subchondral step-off may result in a better loading response.[87] Although no biomechanical or animal studies have proven this to be the case, the structural composition of cartilage and the means by which contact pressures are distributed support this theory. Hydrostatic pressures within cartilage and the rate of increase with joint loading can be expected to vary with different cartilage thicknesses. Studies have shown that cartilage thickness is correlated with local joint load, with central condylar thickness up to 3.65 mm compared with sulcus terminalis thickness of as little as 0.22 mm.[85] Typical graft sites measure 1.2 to 1.6 mm in cartilage thickness compared with condylar thicknesses in the 1.6- to 2.0-mm range.

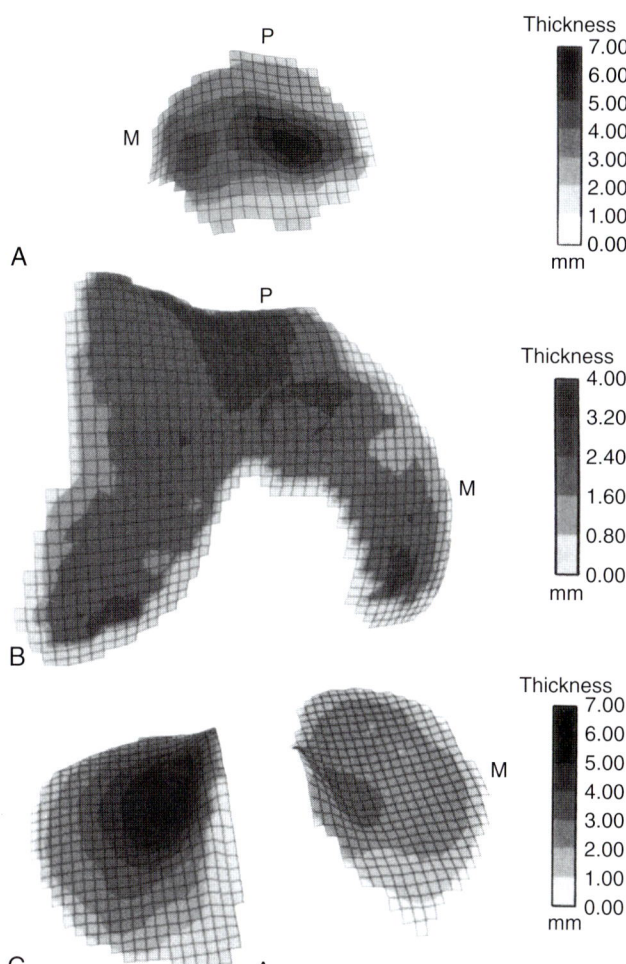

Figure 23-1. Grayscale of cartilage thickness superimposed on the topographic map of **(A)** patellar, **(B)** femoral, and **(C)** tibial articular surfaces. *A,* Anterior; *M,* medial; *P,* proximal. (From Ateshian GA, Soslowsky LJ, Mow VC: Quantitation of articular surface topography and cartilage thickness in knee joints using stereophotogrammetry. J Biomech 24:766–768 [Figure 6], 1991.)

The concept of split line orientation of surface cartilage may also merit consideration during osteochondral autografting. In 1898, Hultkrantz demonstrated a distinct orientation to collagen fibers along the articular cartilage surface, postulating that this was related to directional variation in stiffness and strength. Benninghoff in 1925 further described the microarchitecture of articular cartilage to include collagen fibers oriented perpendicular to the joint surface in the deep layer, with parallel orientation superficially. Below et al mapped the split line pattern of articular cartilage at the distal femur, demonstrating a characteristic pattern of collagen fiber orientation (Fig. 23-3).[8] Although this may have no significant clinical effect, it is a theoretical concern that deserves consideration.

CONTACT PRESSURES

Contact pressures of the patellofemoral articulation have been examined by several investigators.[1,21,83] Simonian et al[83] reported that commonly used donor sites along the periphery of the femur at the patellofemoral joint and within the

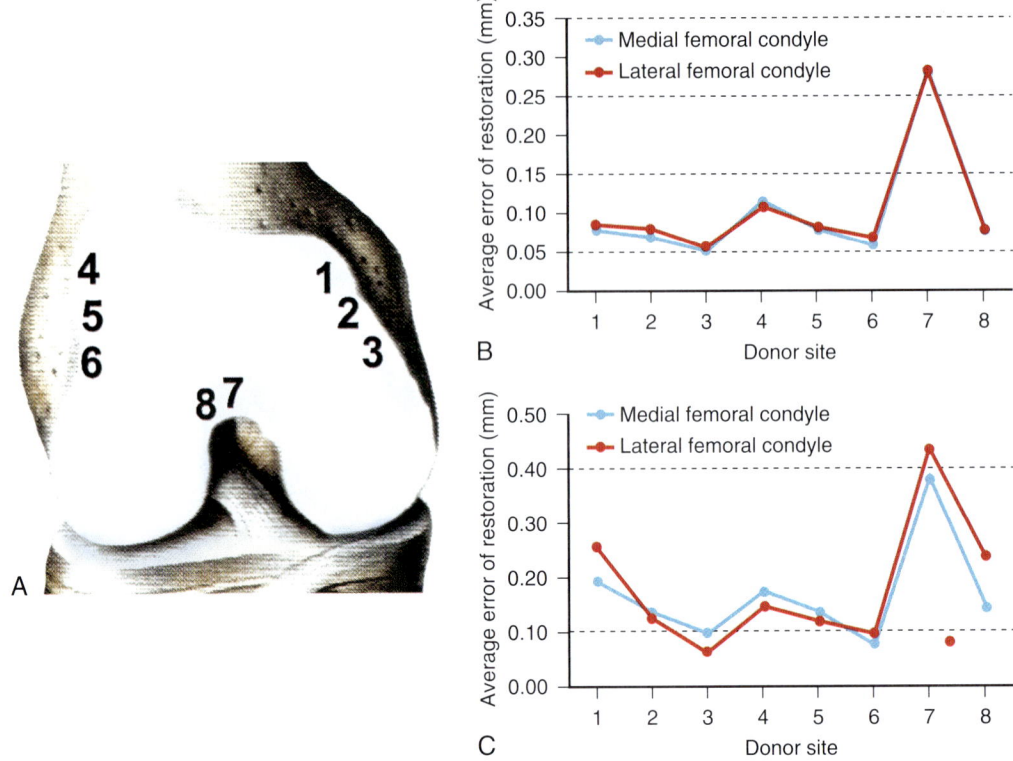

Figure 23-2. A, Surface topography measurements and calculations of topographic mismatches to a central weight-bearing defect in the medial femoral condyle for the eight most common OAT donor sites. **B,** Average errors of restoration of surface topography for a 6-mm defect with osteochondral autograft plugs from each of the regions in **(A)**. **C,** Average errors of restoration of surface topography for an 8-mm defect. (From Bartz RL, Kamaric E, Noble PC, et al: Topographic matching of selected donor and recipient sites for osteochondral autografting of the articular surface of the femoral condyles. Am J Sports Med 29:209–210 [Figures 4, 6, 7], 2001.)

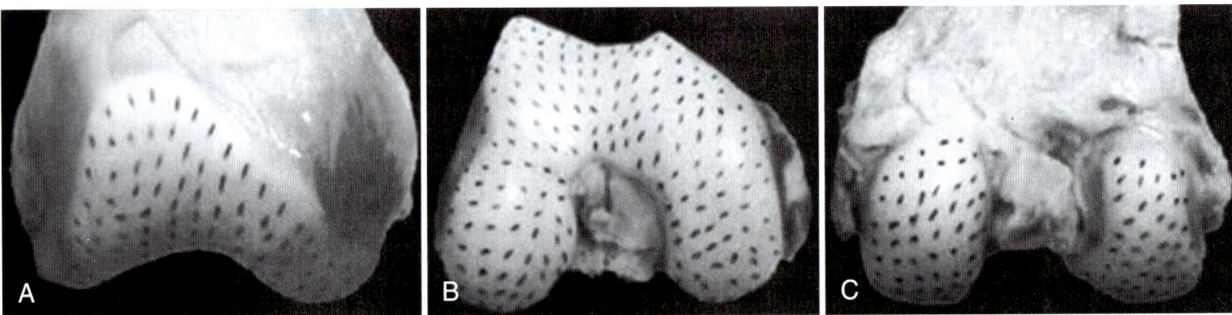

Figure 23-3. Split line pattern of the distal femur. Photographs of the cartilage surface show split lines created with a dissecting needle dipped in India ink. **A,** Anterior view; **C,** distal view; **C,** posterior view. (From Below S, Arnoczky SP, Dodds J, et al: The split-line pattern of the distal femur: a consideration in the orientation of autologous cartilage grafts. Arthroscopy18:615 [Figure 3], 2002.)

intercondylar notch were not completely free of joint loading forces. Ahmad et al[1] quantified a patellofemoral contact map exhibiting the differences in contact pressures at various sites along the distal femur, showing lowest contact forces at the superomedial border of the femur, as well as along the most inferior part of the intercondylar notch (Fig. 23-4). Garretson et al[21] measured contact pressures under two different loads through the entire range of knee flexion. Contact pressures were noted to be lower along the medial condyle; however, no significant differences were noted along the far medial or far lateral edges of the distal femur. The authors concluded that harvesting of grafts from the medial femoral flare may have less impact on patellofemoral biomechanics, but is limited by the fact that the medial condyle is narrower and more sloped than the lateral condyle. They recommend that grafts 5 mm in diameter or smaller should be harvested from the medial femoral flare, and that larger grafts be harvested from the lateral femoral flare. The consensus from these studies is that although all articular surfaces bear some load, the edges of both medial and lateral flares bear the least force during patellofemoral articulation and may represent optimal surface match contours for condyle lesions. Depending on the size of the recipient site and the number and size of donor plugs needed, individualized strategies for harvesting may be devised, with the goal of minimizing alterations in patellofemoral biomechanics.

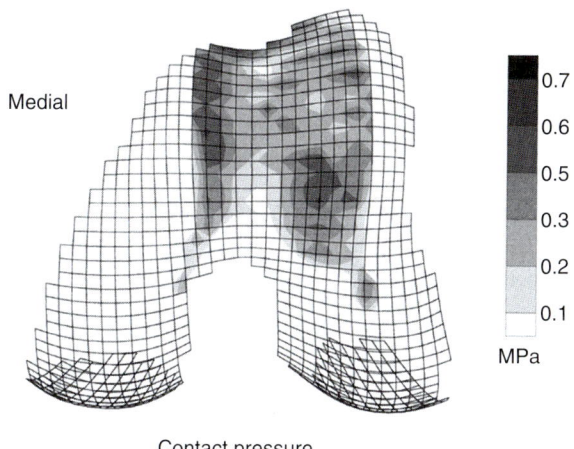

Medial

Contact pressure

Figure 23-4. Grayscale of typical patellofemoral contact pressures superimposed on the topographic map of the distal femur. (From Ahmad CS, Cohen ZA, Levine WN, et al: Biomechanical and topographic considerations for autologous osteochondral grafting in the knee. Am J Sports Med 29:203 [Figure 2], 2001.)

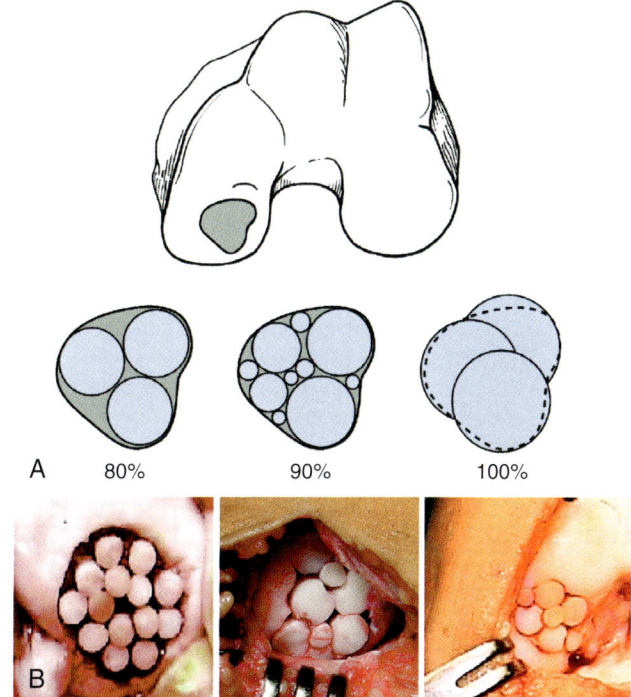

A   80%   90%   100%

B

Figure 23-5. Filling pattern for a complex lesion. **A,** Arrangement of osteochondral autograft plugs within a defect to achieve 80%, 90%, and 100% coverage. Note the different sizes of plugs used, as well as the trimming of plugs to achieve greater coverage. **B,** Representatative photos demonstrating mosaic filling of large, complex lesions. (From Hangody L, Ráthonyi GK, Duska Z, et al: Autologous osteochondral mosaicplasty: surgical technique. J Bone Joint Surg Am 86[Suppl 1]:68 [Figure 5], 2004.)

FILL PATTERN

Depending on the size and pattern of the lesion, different technical strategies for coverage may be used. Smaller lesions can be covered with a single donor graft, depending upon condyle size and topography. Larger lesions may require multiple grafts. Biomechanical studies of osteochondral defects in cadaveric knees have demonstrated increased rim stress concentration in defects measuring 10 mm or greater in diameter.[25] Smaller defects did not demonstrate significant load redistribution. The implication for OAT is that complete fill is not required for adequate reconstitution of lesions. Hangody et al illustrated how multiple osteochondral plugs may be arranged to fill a large defect (Fig. 23-5).[32] Given the limited nature of donor plugs, as well as the biomechanical considerations outlined previously, defects are typically tiled with multiple plugs of different sizes with fibrous fill in the intervening gaps. It has been proposed that the gaps between these osteochondral plugs may be filled with hyaline-like tissue, but no evidence indicates that this additional measure results in appreciably improved outcomes.[34]

Burks et al in 2006 demonstrated that incomplete fill of a larger lesion better preserved the contour of a femoral condyle than of untreated or bone-grafted defects.[12] In an ovine model, a 6-mm plug was placed in the center of a 10-mm defect. While surrounded by fibrous tissue, this method better preserved the articular surface and contour compared with unfilled defects. Hyaline cartilage was noted in the central plug, and composite cartilage scores on histologic evaluation were significantly higher in incompletely filled defects than in unfilled defects.

DEPTH OF INSERTION

Early concerns over subsidence of osteochondral plugs led to recommendations that osteochondral autograft plugs be placed slightly proud. In 2001, Pearce et al performed a study on sheep comparing grafts placed flush with the joint surface and those placed 2 mm proud.[73] Contrary to the authors' hypothesis, grafts placed proud showed poor bony

incorporation evidenced by surrounding fibroplasia and chondroplasia consistent with hypertrophic nonunion attributed to micromotion or shear of the grafts. Grafts placed flush with surrounding cartilage revealed good alignment and continuity, with interstices filled by well-attached repair tissue. In a subsequent series of biomechanical studies, Koh et al studied contact pressures in elevated and countersunk osteochondral plugs placed in porcine knees, as well as grafts inserted at an angle with surface asymmetry.[44,45] Contact pressures were markedly elevated (roughly 50% increase in peak pressure) in grafts placed as little as 0.5 or 1 mm above the surface. Countersunk grafts exhibited approximately 10% increases in peak pressures over those placed flush, although still less than defects left unfilled (20% increase). Similarly, angled grafts placed with any part of the graft protruding above the surrounding cartilage resulted in significant increases in peak contact pressures, whereas those placed partially countersunk were similar to plugs placed orthogonally and flush. These results were corroborated in a case series by Nakagawa et al.[65] Clinical outcomes and second-look arthroscopy were compared in five patients following OAT; two had proud grafts and three had countersunk grafts. Patients with proud grafts complained of catching sensation about 4 months postoperatively, as well as occasional knee sensations. Second-look arthroscopy showed fibrillation and fissuring around the grafts. Patients with countersunk grafts reported no clinical symptoms and exhibited fibrocartilaginous tissue overlying the grafts with a smooth joint surface. These data clearly demonstrate that although the ideal osteochondral plug placement is flush with surrounding cartilage, there is far greater tolerance for plugs placed slightly countersunk as opposed to elevated. Any prominence of the transferred tissue results in significant elevation of contact pressures and may lead to toggling, clefting, and perimeter breakdown of the graft with degradation of the transplanted cartilage.

GRAFT INSERTION

Fixation of osteochondral autograft plugs is achieved through a press-fit technique. This method allows all-arthroscopic delivery of grafts, as well as arrangement of several grafts within a single defect bed. Several investigators have studied the effects of different parameters on graft stability. Kock et al compared push-in forces for different lengths of plugs, as well as the effects of matching donor to recipient plug depth.[41] They found that longer plugs (>12 mm) were more stable when unmatched to recipient site depth, owing to higher frictional forces along the edge of the graft. In contrast, donor plugs that matched recipient site depth (e.g., those that contacted the base of the prepared defect) were more stable when shorter lengths were used. Kordas et al found that grafts with larger diameters withstood greater push-in forces, but that multiple grafts regardless of arrangement (row vs. circle) were less stable than individual plugs.[47] Similarly, overlap of multiple plugs with breach of interplug native bone (socket wall) was found to decrease stability.[27] It is hypothesized that this decreased stability may be related to less adjacent native articular cartilage and bone available to buttress the graft. Dilatation of the recipient bed has been described as a means of obtaining an optimal press-fit. Shorter dilatation lengths allow for more of a tapered fit between donor plug and recipient site. Similarly, slight oversizing of donor plugs relative to recipient sites increased stability by compensating for extraction blade width. In a rabbit model, Makino et al demonstrated increased stability and better preservation of cartilage thickness when grafts oversized by 1 mm relative to the recipient site were used.[54]

One disadvantage of the press-fit technique is the force required for graft impaction. Several studies have documented a decrease in chondrocyte viability following impaction, although the clinical relevance of this has yet to be determined.[6,10,26,89] Lower forces used to gently seat plugs into well-matched recipient sites may be benign, whereas the markedly increased forces required to compress a graft that would otherwise be left proud may adversely affect chondrocyte viability.[71]

GRAFT HARVEST

Harvesting of osteochondral autografts has been a focus of several studies, with emphasis on cell viability. Evans et al reported superiority of manual punches over power trephines, with inadvertent skidding, ragged cartilage edges, and separation of cartilage from subchondral bone seen in the latter.[19] Chondrocyte viability was also decreased when power trephines were used for graft harvest. Duchow et al, in a study of pull-out strengths with porcine osteochondral autografts harvested using a manual punch, noted that plugs extracted by levering of the plug were less stable than those extracted by turning of the punch.[18] They also noted that failure loads

were significantly less frequent in 10-mm-long plugs compared with those 15 mm or 20 mm long. Moreover, repeated insertion and extraction led to decreased stability. The cutting profile of manual punches also had an effect on chondrocyte survival, with subtle compression of the articular cartilage resulting in a marginal zone of death.[35,36]

A critical concept in graft harvest is perpendicularity.[16] Although this may be achieved through an open or an arthroscopic approach, it is critical that grafts that are orthogonal to the articular surface are harvested.[39] This allows for improved articular congruity, in addition to more precise restoration of the condylar bevel and radius of curvature, which is of particular importance in defects requiring multiple plugs.

Donor site morbidity remains a technical concern when OAT is considered. Early reports used iliac crest cortical bone grafts to fill lesions following graft harvest. Similar fill using the bone remaining from recipient site preparation with a trephine cutting technique has been documented.[64] In a canine model, Feczkó et al in 2003 compared several biodegradable materials for donor site filling, including hydroxyapatite, carbon fiber, polyglyconate-B, compressed collagen, and polycaprolactone.[20] They found on second-look arthroscopy and histologic evaluation that compressed collagen yielded the best fibrocartilage coverage of harvest site defects. Several composite bone graft substitute polymer plugs are now commercially available and have been used to fill donor site defects (TruFit, Smith & Nephew, Andover, Mass; OsseoFit, Kensey Nash Corp., Exton, Pa).[80]

PEARLS AND PITFALLS

Many of the complications associated with OAT can be directly attributable to technical details. Hemarthrosis has been reported, and filling of the donor site, as well as placement of a postoperative drain, may reduce this problem.[29] Donor site collapse has been reported and may be avoided by maintaining a 1- to 2-mm spread between harvest sites and from the edge of the condyle, as well as by taking into account the natural convergence of the bases of individual grafts caused by the curvature of the condylar surface. Graft failure may occur for a number of reasons. Impaction forces may be minimized by careful matching of recipient site and donor plug depth. Although this has already been incorporated into several commercial systems, optimization of the difference between plug diameter and recipient bed diameter to allow good press-fit without excessive force is important. Careful removal of donor plugs limits collateral damage to surrounding cartilage. Likewise, meticulous handling of the donor plug from the osseous side minimizes microtrauma to the graft cartilage surface, which can affect chondrocyte viability; OCD lesions and other bony defects extending into subchondral bone may require longer grafts. In cases where multiple grafts are used, minimizing the step-off between grafts and relative to the surrounding cartilage will decrease surface fibrillation and edge-loading of grafts.

POSTOPERATIVE REGIMEN

The standard postoperative regimen involves initial protection from weight bearing, followed by gradual transition to weight bearing. Early range of motion is instituted, but with limited joint loading. Non–weight bearing generally lasts 3 weeks and is followed by gradual advancement. Postoperative stiffness (particularly in the setting of hemarthrosis) may be prevented by early range of motion, and continuous passive motion machines may be useful. Active physical therapy includes patellar mobilization, stretching, and progressive strengthening beginning with isometrics. Subsequent proprioceptive neuromuscular reeducation occurs with conditioning, including swimming, leg press, and closed chain kinetic exercises. Normal daily activity can be achieved at 8 to 10 weeks, but progression to high-demand sports may be delayed for as long as 6 months.

RESULTS

Several case series have been reported, all with generally positive results from the procedure. Outcome measures include validated outcome scores such as the Knee Injury and Osteoarthritis Outcome Score (KOOS), the International Cartilage Repair Society (ICRS) cartilage repair assessment score, the International Knee Documentation Committee (IKDC) score, Lysholm scores, subjective activity level assessments using Tegner scores, and radiologic measures such as magnetic resonance observation of cartilage repair tissue (MOCART). Second-look arthroscopy and histologic analysis of biopsy samples also provide objective evidence of structural articular cartilage resurfacing. Table 23-1 summarizes results obtained from several level 4 case series. In the most extensive longitudinal study, Hangody et al documented long-term data from his own case series, including 967 mosaicplasties, 789 involving the femoral condyles, 147 the patellofemoral joint, 31 the tibial plateau, and the remainder other joints (talar dome, femoral head, and humeral head).[30] Good to excellent results were achieved in 92% of femoral condyle lesions, 87% of tibial plateau lesions, and 74% of patellofemoral lesions. This trend among sites within the knee has been reported by other groups as well, with greatest success uniformly achieved in treating femoral condyle lesions. Another prognostic factor was age, with patients older than 45 years faring less well than younger patients.

Several prospective randomized controlled studies have compared OAT to microfracture and autologous chondrocyte implantation (ACI) (Table 23-2). Bentley et al in 2003 in a level 1 therapeutic study reported on 100 patients (mean age, 31.3 years; range, 16 to 49 years) who were randomized to ACI versus OAT.[9] Most lesions were posttraumatic, with a mean defect size of 4.66 cm². Cincinnati scores were good to excellent in 88% of ACI versus 69% of OAT patients, and second-look arthroscopy at 1 year showed good to excellent articular cartilage resurfacing in 82% of ACI versus 34% of OAT patients. However, a major limitation of this study was a technical one: the authors reported placing the osteochondral autograft plugs slightly prominently to allow contact during normal movement and to "ensure that nutrition was maintained by loading and by the passage of fluid through the articular cartilage." Subsequent work has shown that plugs placed prominently fare worse, with micromotion resulting in possible nonunion, and differential loading of the articular surface resulting in fibrillation and early degeneration of the graft.

Gudas et al in 2005 in a level 1 therapeutic study compared 60 patients (mean age, 24.3 years; range, 15 to 40 years) who were competitive athletes at the regional or national level and were randomized to microfracture or OAT.[23] Clinical improvement was seen in both groups, but good to excellent results were achieved in 96% of patients who had undergone OAT versus 52% who had undergone microfracture. Hospital for Special Surgery (HSS) and ICRS scores were significantly better in patients treated with OAT compared with those treated with microfracture at 12, 24, and 36 months after surgery. It was reported that 93% of OAT patients and 52% of microfracture patients returned to sports activities at the preinjury level at an average of 6.5 months (range, 4 to 8 months). Magnetic resonance imaging (MRI) findings revealed similar success, with joint surface congruity achieved in 94% of patients following OAT versus 49% following microfracture. Repair tissue thickness appeared the same as surrounding cartilage in 68% of the OAT group compared with 18% of the microfracture group. Of note, only all-arthroscopic procedures were included in this study.

Horas et al in 2003 in a level 2 therapeutic study compared 40 patients (mean age, 33.4 years; range, 18 to 44 years) who underwent ACI or OAT.[34] Lesions ranged from 3.2 to 5.6 cm² in area (mean, 3.75 cm²). Postoperative Lysholm scores were higher in patients treated with OAT compared with those treated with ACI at 6, 12, and 24 months. However, Meyers and Tegner activity scores were equivalent 2 years after treatment. Biopsy at 2 years showed consistent fibrocartilage with localized areas of hyaline-like regenerative cartilage near the bone following ACI compared with intact hyaline cartilage that could not be differentiated from surrounding native cartilage following OAT. One weakness of this study was failure to achieve >80% follow-up of the patient study group.

In general, patients do well following OAT procedures, with significant improvement in knee function and satisfaction. Complications include hemarthrosis, loosening of plugs, fibrous overgrowth, graft subsidence, and donor site morbidity. Careful attention to technique is critical, as many of the complications can be directly attributed to user error. It is difficult to isolate morbidity from graft harvest in the setting of baseline knee pathology. Several studies in which OAT was performed in other joints, including talar dome, capitellum, and femoral head, document significant morbidity to the knee following graft harvest.[2,76] In multiple cases, knees that were asymptomatic prior to graft harvest developed some degree of impairment postoperatively. This morbidity may be independent of patient age or the size and number of grafts.[72] Although this may be an important consideration in OAT harvest for other joints, the morbidity associated with graft harvest in the same knee is usually offset by improvements achieved through the OAT procedure.

GROSS MORPHOLOGY AND HISTOLOGY

Examination of articular surfaces following OAT during second-look arthroscopy has generally revealed good incorporation of the graft. Articular surfaces consistently show good restoration of surface congruity with fibrous fill at the periphery of grafts (Fig. 23-6). Probing of grafts on occasion demonstrates some fibrillation or fraying of cartilage edges (Fig. 23-7), but more often grade I chondromalacia or better appearance of the articular cartilage surface.

Text continued on page 190

Table 23-1 Level 4 Case Series Reports of OAT Procedures

Authors	Number	Age, Yr	Follow-up	Scoring System	Subjective	Supplemental	Complications	Location	Size
Atik Bull HJD 2005	12 (6M, 6F)	20-63 (38)	2-8 yr (4)	Lysholm 56 >86	85% pain free	2nd look in 5, used screw removal set	Slight joint effusion	9 MFC, 1 LFC, 1 patella	Up to 5 plugs, 3.5 × 10 mm
Barber Arthroscopy 2006	36 (20M, 16F)	17-69 (43)	24-89 mo (48)	Lysholm 44 >84 Tegner 5 at flu		2nd look in 14, good incorporation, donor sites with fibrocartilage		27 MFC, 9 LFC	1-5 plugs (1.9), 6 mm
Braun Arthritis Res Ther 2008	33 (23M, 10F)	15-59 (34.3)	46-98 mo (66.4)	Lysholm 12-79 (49) >40-100 (86)	27/33 return to sports 31/33 satisfied, would redo	X-ray: remodeling of posterior condyle concurrent HTO in 15		27 MFC, 6 LFC	MegaOATS: 2-10.5 cm² (6.2)
Chow Arthroscopy 2004	30 (13M, 17F)	19-66 (44.6)	24-63 mo (45.1)	Lysholm 18-61 (43.6) >57-100 (87.5) IKDC 63.3% D, 36.7% C >26.7% A, 60% B, 6.7% C, 6.7% D	83.3% excellent/good	2nd look in 9 (6-15 mo, mean 8.8); 7/9 complete healing; 2/9: fibrillation; donor sites all fibrocartilaginous; 2 concurrent ACL, 5 partial meniscectomy, 8 removal of loose body	Hematoma	28 MFC, 2 LFC	1-4 plugs (2.2)
Duany Arch Orthop Trauma Surg 2009	9 (5M, 4F)	18-74 (43.4)	11-120 mo (42.1)	KSS 39-75 (57.9) >43-100 (80.2)	88.9% survivorship (1 conversion to TKA)	Patients with SONK who failed nonop treatment		6 MFC, 3 LFC	
Gaweda Int Orthop 2006	19	Mean, 25.5 (vs. 21.7)	24 mo	Marshall 36.3 ± 2.1 >46.2 ± 1.8 (vs. 40.7 ± 3.7 >47.1 ± 1.6)		Patients undergoing patellar realignment, comparison of procedure alone/with OAT	Joint effusion decr ROM	19 patella	
Hangody KSSTA 1997	44 (26M, 18F)	17-45 (30)	12-54 mo (25.1)	HSS 62.2 >67-100 (94.2) (vs. abrasion arthroplasty 21 pts 59.6 >78.2)	Aborted dual-arm study mosaicplasty vs. abrasion arthroplasty due to HSS score diff	2.7, 3.5, 4.5 × 15 mm plugs, 25 mm for osteochondral defects, 10 control arthroscopies—good result	3 hematomas (aspiration)	25 MFC, 15 LFC, 4 both	
Hangody Orthopedics 1998	57 (26M, 31F)	17-45 (31.4)	36-56 mo (48.7)	HSS 64-100 (90.7)	54 return to normal activity	2nd look in 19 (12 wk to 5 yr): 16 smooth, 3 grade II changes	2 hematomas	25 MFC, 22 LFC, 8 patella	1-8.5 cm² 3-17 plugs (8): 2.7, 3.5, 4.5 mm
Hangody J Sports Traumatol 1998	55 (32M, 23F)	16-41 (23.1)	12-62 mo (29.5)	HSS 67-100 (89)	51 return to normal activity	2nd look in 17: 2 grade II chondromalacia, 1 grade III	4 hematomas	24 MFC, 27 LFC, 4 patella	1-9 cm² (5.1) 3-19 plugs (7): 3.5, 4.5 mm
Hangody CORR 2001	578			HSS, Cincinnati, Lysholm, ICRS	Femoral 92% excellent/good, tibial 88% excellent/good, troch/patella 81% excellent/good	86% concomitant procedures (ACL, realignment, meniscus surgery). 2nd look in 68 pts: 85.3% good, 14.7% with degenerative changes; Bandi scores: 3% donor site disturbances; Artscan in 22: 80% with similar stiffness as surrounding cartilage	4 deep infections, 34 painful hemarthroses, 2 thromboembolic	461 femoral condyles, 93 patellofemoral joints, 24 tibial condyles	2.7, 3.5, 4.5, 6.5, 8.5 mm plugs 80%-90% coverage

Study	N (sex)	Age range (mean)	Follow-up range (mean)	Outcome measures	Results	Comments	Complications	Location	Plug size/coverage
Hangody JBJS 2003, Szerb Bull HJD 2005	740			HSS, Cincinnati, Lysholm, ICRS	Femoral 92% excellent/good, tibial 87% excellent/good, troch/patella 79% excellent/good	85% concomitant procedures (ACL, realignment, meniscus surgery), 2nd look in 83 pts: 83.1% good, 16.9% with degenerative changes; Bandi scores: 3% donor site disturbances	4 deep infections, 36 painful hemarthroses, 2 thromboembolic	597 femoral condyles, 118 patellofemoral joints, 25 tibial condyles	2.7, 3.5, 4.5, 6.5, 8.5 mm plugs 80%-90% coverage
Hangody Injury 2008	967			HSS, Cincinnati, Lysholm, ICRS	Femoral 92% excellent/good, tibial 87% excellent/good, troch/patella 74% excellent/good	81% concomitant procedures (ACL, realignment, meniscus surgery), 2nd look in 98: 82.7% good, 17.3% with degenerative changes; Artscan in 25: 80% with similar stiffness as surrounding cartilage; Bandi scores: 3% donor site disturbances	4 deep infections, 56 hemarthroses, 4 thromboembolic	789 femoral condyles, 147 patellofemoral joints, 31 tibial condyles	2.7, 3.5, 4.5, 6.5, 8.5 mm plugs 80%-90% coverage
Jakob CORR 2002	52 (34M, 18F)	14-66 (33)	24-56 mo (37)	Improvement in ICRS Grading vs. preop	93% no/slight limitations, 52% incr sports activity, 88% satisfaction/ would, redo	Concurrent ACL, realignment, meniscectomy, HTO 2nd look in 10	Catching/locking, 4 graft failure (reop)		1.5-16 cm² (4.9) 1-16 plugs (6), mostly 6.3 mm plugs, 70%-85% coverage 7 contralateral donor site
Karataglis Knee 2005	36 (23M, 13F)	18-48 (31.9)	18-73 (36.5)	Tegner 1-8 (3.76) ADLKOOS 18-98 (72.3)	86.5% improvement, 18 return to sports			18 MFC, 8 LFC, 7 trochlea, 4 patella	0.8-12 cm² (2.73) 1-8 plugs, 6-10 mm diam >90% coverage
Klinger KSSTA 2003	21 (15M, 6F)	22-44 (29)	32-62 mo (38)	IKDC 43% C, 57% 0 >24% A, 57% B, 19% C Lysholm 29-90 (62) >46-100 (90), Tegner 1-5 (3.9) >3-8 (6.1)	VAS 4-9 (6), preop to >6 (2), postop all but 2 returned to full activities	Concurrent ACL reconstructions	2 hematomas (aspirated)	21 MFC	2.0-5.0 cm² (3.5)
Kotani J Orthop Surg 2003	16 (2M, 14F)	58-74 (64.9)	28-111 mo (67)	JOA preop 60-75 (68.1) >80-100 (88.8)		Indications: osteonecrosis follow-up arthroscopy at 18-21 mo			
Koulalis KSSTA 2004	18 (12M, 6F)	24-53 (36)	24-42 mo (27.2)	ICRS 16.7% C, 83.3% D >66.7% A, 33.3% B	MRI at 12 mo: osseous integration between 3 and 6 mo postop. 2nd look in 4: color and firmness similar to native surrounding cartilage		Effusion in 7 pts (persisted 3-8 mo), patellar chondropathy in 4 pts	11 MFC, 2 LFC, 3 patella, 1 MFC + LFC, 1 trochlea	1.0-7.0 cm² (2.5) 1-7 (2.9) plugs

Continued

Table 23-1 Level 4 Case Series Reports of OAT Procedures—cont'd

Authors	Number	Age, Yr	Follow-up	Scoring System	Subjective	Supplemental	Complications	Location	Size
Lahav J Knee Surg 2006	16 knees (15 patients)		40 mo	KOOS pain 56-94 (80.6), symptoms 25-71 (53.6), ADL 79-100 (93.4), sports 20-100 (65.3), QOL 6-88 (51.0), IKDC 68.2	Would redo: 86%				
Laprell Arch Orthop Trauma Surg 2001	35 (17M, 22F)	Avg 26	6-12 yr (8.1)	CSE/ICRS 12-1, 14-11, 3-111	Subjective increases in activity levels	27 OCD at MFC near PCL insertion; 2 lateral patellar facet MRI: Kellgren/Lawrence progression of OA in 12 (17 no change), cystic changes at donor sites	Hemarthrosis (asp): 13, numbness (16), infrapatellar injury		1.1-2.4 cm² large grafts (e.g., megaOATS) from posterior MFC/LFC: 11-23 mm diam (15.6), 10-21 mm depth
Lonner J Arthroplasty 2007	4 (1M, 3F)	28-48 (39.5)	2-4 yr (2.7)	KSS clinical 40-60 (46.8) >94-95 (94.5); functional 30-70 (48.8) >90-100 (92.5)		Concurrent patellofemoral arthroplasty with plugs from ipsilateral femoral trochlea		3 MFC, 1 LFC	1-3 grafts (1.5)
Ma Injury 2004	18 (12M, 6F)	16-51 (29)	24-64 mo (42)	Lyshclm 35-60 (47.5) >79-100 (92.4), Tegner 1-4 (2.22) >4-8 (6.11)	11 excellent, 5 good, 2 fair (89% excellent/good)	10 concomitant procedures (5 ACL, 3 menisc, 2 ROH), 9 MRI, 8 2nd look (3-36 mo), 2 biopsy	Fibrillation in tib plat OAT	11 MFC, 5 LFC, 2 LTP	2.25-6 cm² (4.1)
Marcacci AJSM 2007	30 (22M, 8F)	17-46 (29.3)	7 yr	IKDC 7A, 16B, 4C, 3D at 7 yr; 11A, 12B, 4C, 3D at 2 yr; IKDC subjective 34.8 >71.7	2 yr: 22 return to sports same level, 4 return to sports lower level; 7 yr: 7 same level, 14 lower level	19 associated procedures (13 menisc, 9 ACL, 1 MCL repair), MRI for 24/27: complete integration cartilage: 75%, bone: 96%	3 failures treated with ACI (2 with 3 plugs, 1 with 4)	17 MFC, 13 LFC	1.1-2.5 cm² (1.9) 8:1,12:2,7:3,3:4 plugs (6.5, 8.5 mm)
Marcacci Arthroscopy 2005	37 (27M, 10F)	Avg 29.5	24-48 mo	IKDC 78.3% excellent/good 14A, 15B, 5C, 3D	27 return to sports at same level, 5 lower level	23 associated procedures (12 ACL, 19 menisc, 1 MCL repair)	2 failures (insufficient graft integration)	23 MFC, 14 LFC	1.8-2.5 cm² (2.1) 8:1,20:2,5:3,4:4 plugs (4.5, 6.5, 8.5 mm)
Marcacci Orthopedics 1999	13 (7M, 6F)	16-52 (31)	13-141 mo (61.5)	Cincinnati 3 excellent/8 good, Swedish 4 excellent/8 good, Lysholm 8 excellent/4 good, IKDC 4 excellent/8 good		4 press-fit, 9 screw fixation 2nd look at screw removal: good survival in all	1 flexion deformity/stiffness	11 MFC, 1 LFC, 1 LFC + LTP	1.5-3 cm diam
Miniaci Arthroscopy 2007	20	12-27 (14.3)	2-6 yr (3.4)	Preop IKDC 0A, 5B, 8C, 7D; postop 19A, 1B at 24 mo		Fixation of OCD with OAT 2nd look in 2 pts (ACL recon): congruent articular surface		19 MFC, 1 LFC	3-7 plugs (4.1) 4.5 mm diam

Study	N (sex)	Age (mean)	Follow-up (mean)	Outcome scores	Results	Methods / Concomitant procedures	Complications	Location	Lesion size / plugs
Nho AJSM 2008	22 (12M, 10F)	15-57 (30)	17.7-57.8 mo (28.7)	IKDC 21-71 (47.2) >52-87 (74.4), ADL 24-94 (60.1) >65-94 (84.7), SF-36 39-86 (64.0) >44-92 (79.4)		Concomitant procedures (realignment): MRI in 14 cases: 67%-100% fill; cartilage thickness mismatch in all; proud in 28.6%	1 reoperation for chondromalacia of plugs	22 patella	0.72-5 cm² (1.66 ± 1.28) 1-7 plugs (1.8 ± 1.4), 6-11 mm (9.7 ± 1.1) diam
Outerbridge CORR 2000	16 (13M, 3F)	17-50 (27)	2-14.6 yr (7.6)	Cincinnati 8-64 (35) >19-100 (85)	100% improved function, 81% high level of functioning	Use of patella for autograft	5 reoperations due to pain: detached in 1, meniscus tear in 1,3 normal (all resolved)	10 MFC, 8 LFC	1.5-10.8 cm² (4.5) 21%-46% patella used as graft (36%)
Ozturk Int Orthop 2006	19 (13M, 6F)	20-46 (33.1)	24-84 mo (32.4)	Lysholm 21-60 (45.8) >74-100 (87.5)	85% excellent/good	MRI: congruency restored in 84.2%			10-23 mm diam (15) 1-3 plugs (2.3)
Rose Arch Orthop Trauma Surg 2005	27 (21M, 6F)	22-43 (32)	5-28 mo (13.5)	Lysholm postop 45-98 (80)		13 concomitant procedures (ACL, menisc) 2nd look in 8: biopsy taken; MRI: osseous integration in all; protuberance in 15 cases up to 2 mm	Hemarthrosis in 3 (revision), broken plugs in 2	13 MFC	1.0-3.0 cm² (1.2) 1-3 plugs (1.5); 8 and 11 mm diam
Rue AJSM 2008	15 (13M, 2F)	19-47 (36.8)	1.9-5.0 yr (2.9)	Lysholm 42.0 ± 14.5 >68.2 ± 21.3, Tegner 4.4 ± 3.7 >6.2 ± 2.9, IKDC 31.4 ± 12.8 >57.1 ± 17.8		Combined meniscal allograft + ACI/OAT concurrent procedures: 1 HTO, 2 ROH		13 MFC, 2 LFC	2.3-9.5 cm² (5.5)
Sharpe JBJS-B 2005	13 (8M, 5F)	24-48 (42)		KSS 63.9 ± 18.9 >84.6 ± 12.3/6 mo, 90.2 ± 8.3/1 yr, 88 ± 14.1/3 yr		ACI + OAT		7 MFC, 5 LFC, 1 patella	2.2-15.3 cm² (4.8)
Tanaka Knee 2009	6 (5M, 1F)	50-57 (54.2)	23-45 mo (27.7)	Lysholm 47-70 (54.7) >85-100 (92.3)		Patients with SONK who failed nonop treatment		6 MFC	Lesion size 39.4%-58.9% (50.5) plugs 6.4, 7.45 mm diam
Tetta Eur J Radiol 2009	24 (17M, 7F)	29.9 ± 8.7	96-125 mo (113)	IKDC 31 >82; CSE/ICRS 15C, 9D >7A, 12B, 4C, 1D; Tegner 3 >6	25% return to sports at same preinjury level, 54.2% lower level, 20.8% no sports	MRI evaluation at follow-up: 62.5% complete fill, integration in 75%; intact repair surface in 62.5%, <50% damage in 20.8%, >50% damage in 16.7%	Adhesions in 12.5%, effusion in 41.6%	13 MFC, 10 LFC, 1 mixed	1.9 ± 0.5 cm² 1-3 plugs (1.9 ± 0.7); 6.1 ± 1.2 mm diam
Unnithan Knee 2008	5 (2M, 3F)	36-65 (48.2)	18-84 mo (45.6)	Oxford 28-48 (42) >15-46 (25.5)	1 converted to TKA, 1 awaiting stage II revision to TKA	Concurrent patellofemoral arthroplasty with plugs from ipsilateral femoral trochlea	1 deep infection	MFC 1, both MFC + LFC 1 (1 pt: bilateral lesions)	

ACI, Autologous chondrocyte transplantation; *ACL*, anterior cruciate ligament; *ADL*, activities of daily living; *CSE*, cartilage standard evaluation form; *HSS*, Hospital for Special Surgery scoring system; *HTO*, high tibial osteotomy; *ICRS*, International Cartilage Repair Society; *IKDC*, International Knee Documentation Committee; *JOA*, Japanese Orthopaedic Association; *KOOS*, Knee Injury and Osteoarthritis Outcome Score; *KSS*, Knee Society for pain and mobility score; *LFC*, lateral femoral condyle; *LTP*, lateral tibial plateau; *MCL*, medial collateral ligament; *menisc*, meniscectomy; *MFC*, medial femoral condyle; *MRI*, magnetic resonance imaging; *OA*, osteoarthritis; *OAT*, osteochondral allograft plug transfer; *OCD*, osteochondritis dissecans; *PCL*, posterior collateral ligament; *QOL*, quality of life; *ROH*, removal of hardware; *SONK*, spontaneous osteonecrosis of the knee; *ROM*, range of motion; *TKA*, total knee arthroplasty; *VAS*, visual analog scale.

Table 23-2 Controlled Trials Comparing OAT With Alternate Techniques

Authors	Study Arm	Number	Age	Follow-up	Scoring System	Secondary Scoring System	Supplemental	Complications	Location	Size
Bentley JBJS-B 2003 Level Ia—Therapeutic	ACI	58	30.9 (16-49)	19 months (12-26)	Cincinnati	>80 (excellent): 40% 55-79 (good): 48% 30-55 (fair): 12% <30 (poor):0%	ICRS (2nd look arthroscopy)	16% excellent 66% good 16% fair 2% poor		24 MFC 13 LFC 20 patella 1 trochlea	4.66 cm² (1-12.2)
	OAT	42	31.6 (20-48)			>80 (excellent): 21% 55-79 (good): 48% 30-55 (fair): 14% <30 (poor): 17%	0% excellent 34% good 44% fair 22% poor	plugs placed proud to increase nutrition, passage of fluid		29 MFC 5 LFC 5 patella 2 trochlea 1 LTP	
Dozin Clin J Sport Med 2005 Level II—Therapeutic (poor follow-up and compliance to treatment)	ACI	22 (17M, 5F) (12 proceeded to surgery)	29.6 ± 7.3	291 days (0-1339)	Lysholm	<60 (failure):1 60-90 (partial success): 5 90-100 (complete success): 10 lost to f/u: 6		poor follow-up, low percentage of surgery after randomization		14 MFC 2 LFC 6 patella	2.0 ± 0.4
	OAT	22 (10M, 12F) (11 proceeded to surgery)	27.9 ± 8.1	300 days (0-994)		<60 (failure):0 60-90 (partial success): 2 90-100 (complete success): 15 lost to f/u: 5				12 MFC 3 LFC 7 patella	1.9 ± 0.5
Gudas Arthroscopy 2005, KSSTA 2006 Level Ia—Therapeutic	MFx	29	24.3 (15-40)	37.1 months (36-38)	HSS	77 preop 83 at 12 months 82 at 24 months 81 at 36 months	ICRS (2nd look arthroscopy)	15% excellent 30% good 30% fair 25% poor	MRI: repair tissue thickness: 18% relative to adjacent cartilage Joint surface congruity restored in 52%	9 reoperation (conversion to OAT)	23 MFC 6 LFC	2.8 ± 0.68
	OAT	28				78 preop 88 at 12 months 91 at 24 months 91 at 36 months	50% excellent 29% good 21% fair	MRI: repair tissue thickness: 68% relative to adjacent cartilage Joint surface congruity restored in 96%	2 superficial infection, 1 reoperation (single plug revision)	25 MFC 3 LFC	2.8 ± 0.65

Study	Treatment	n	Age	Follow-up	Lysholm	Tegner		Complications	Location	Size
Horas JBJS 2003 Level II – Therapeutic (<80% follow-up)	ACI	20 (8M, 12F)	31.4 (18-42)	24 mos	24.9 preop 27.55 at 3 months 45.75 at 6 months 57.50 at 12 months 66.75 at 24 months	1.60 preop 1.55 at 3 months 2.95 at 6 months 4.25 at 12 months 5.10 at 24 months	scanning electron microscopy—regenerated tissue tightly united with original cartilage		17 MFC 3 LFC	3.86 cm²
	OAT	20 (15M, 5F)	35.4 (21-44)		28.45 preop 27.95 at 3 months 53.45 at 6 months 68.25 at 12 months 72.70 at 24 months	1.60 preop 1.55 at 3 months 3.55 at 6 months 5.00 at 12 months 5.20 at 24 months	scanning electron microscopy—gap at the cartilage level; osseous integration	mild pain while squatting (posterior femoral condyle donor site)	16 MFC 4 LFC	3.63 cm²

ACI, Autologous chondrocyte implantation; ICRS, International Cartilage Repair Society; LFC, lateral femoral condyle; LTP, lateral tibial plateau; MFC, medial femoral condyle; MFx, microfracture; MRI, magnetic resonance imaging; OAT, osteochondral autograft plug transfer.

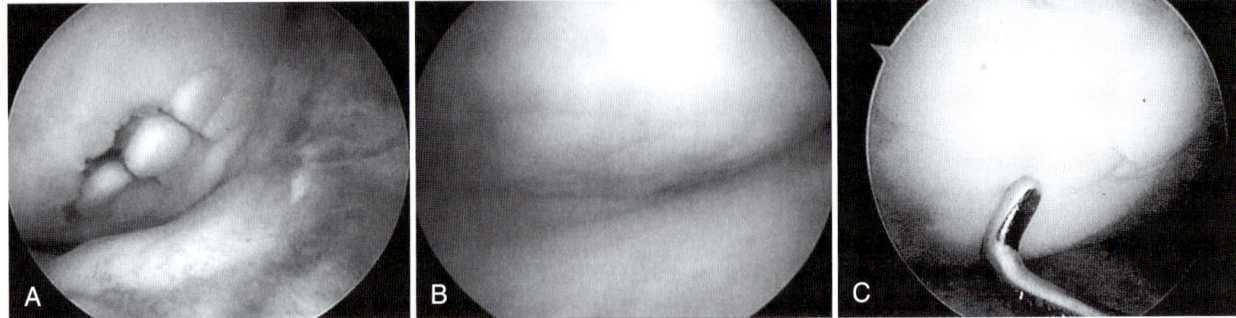

Figure 23-6. Arthroscopic views of defect repair using osteochondral autograft plug transfer (OAT). **A,** Arrangement of multiple 5.5-mm-diameter osteochondral autograft plugs to restore a 3.5-cm² osteochondritis dissecans lesion of the lateral femoral condyle. **B,** Second look at 3 years shows complete restoration of joint surface congruence with no evidence of fibrillation or degeneration. **C,** Second-look arthroscopy 1 year after OAT of a medial femoral condyle defect. Probing of the repair tissue shows good alignment with surrounding healthy articular cartilage and similar firmness. (From Gudas R, Stankevicius E, Monastyreckiene E, et al: Osteochondral autologous transplantation versus microfracture for the treatment of articular cartilage defects in the knee joint in athletes. Knee Surg Sports Traumatol Arthrosc 14:837 [Figure 2], 2006; Hangody L, Füles P: Autologous osteochondral mosaicplasty for the treatment of full-thickness defects of weight-bearing joints: ten years of experimental and clinical experience. J Bone Joint Surg Am 85[Suppl 2]:31 [Figure 10], 2003.)

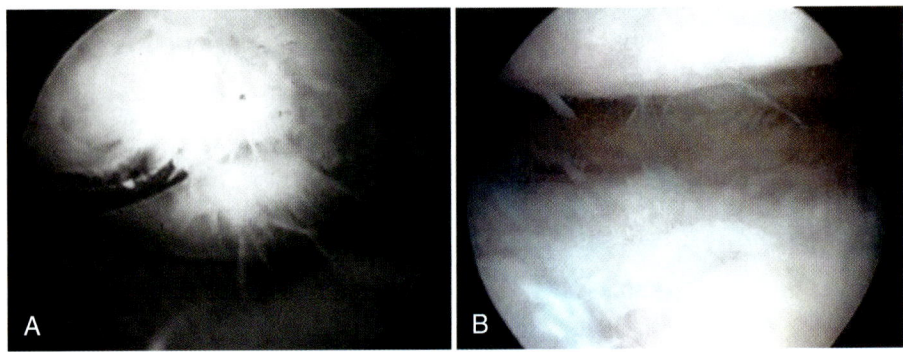

Figure 23-7. Arthroscopic views of defect repair using osteochondral autograft plug transfer (OAT). **A,** Second-look arthroscopy at 2 years following mosaicplasty of the medial femoral condyle shows fibrillation of the osteochondral plugs and incomplete filling of the spaces between them. **B,** Second-look arthroscopic view of lateral tibial surface after 26 months shows an uneven surface and degenerative changes with fibrillation. (From Bentley G, Biant LC, Carrington RW, et al: A prospective, randomised comparison of autologous chondrocyte implantation versus mosaicplasty for osteochondral defects in the knee. J Bone Joint Surg Br 85:226 [Figure 6], 2003; Ma HL, Hung SC, Huang ST, et al: Osteochondral autografts transfer for post-traumatic osteochondral defect of the knee—2 to 5 years follow-up. Injury 35:1290 [Figure 3], 2004.)

Several detailed reports have described postoperative histologic analysis of OAT resurfacing. These include biopsies taken at second-look arthroscopy, as well as entire joint surfaces resected during total knee arthroplasty.[34,42] In all cases, a persistent cleft is seen in the cartilage layer between transplanted osteochondral segments and neighboring tissue (Fig. 23-8A). However, good integration at the osseous level is seen, with reconstitution of articular cartilage topography (see Fig. 23-8B through *D*).

IMAGING

MRI has emerged as the gold standard used for noninvasive monitoring and evaluation of structural outcomes of cartilage resurfacing procedures. This is true in part because of its superior soft tissue contrast, direct multiplanar capabilities, and lack of ionizing radiation.[74] An added advantage is that MRI can reveal concomitant pathology such as meniscal lesions or ligament tears that may affect joint biomechanics. Several techniques have been developed for cartilage-specific imaging. Potter and Foo reported on several studies in which diagnostic MRI was compared with arthroscopic visualization of articular surfaces.[74] The authors concluded that fat-suppressed fast spin echo (FSE) imaging results in the least interobserver variability, as well as the highest sensitivity and specificity. This technique allows for differential contrast between fluid, subchondral bone, and meniscus. Moreover, based on different levels of water sequestration, one can differentiate between articular cartilage, fibrocartilage, and synovial fluid. This can provide valuable information about structural restoration and repair, including viability of the repair site, tissue fill volume, surface congruence, status of underlying subchondral bone, and perimeter integration (Fig. 23-9). Additional cartilage-specific sequences have been reported, including T1 rho-weighted fast spin echo, T1 three-dimensional gadolinium-enhanced MRI of cartilage (dGEMRIC), gradient refocused acquisition in the steady state and iterative decomposition of water and fat with echo asymmetry and least-squares estimation (GRASS-IDEAL), isotopic three-dimensional steady-state free procession (SSFP), and driven equilibrium Fourier transform. These imaging methods, which can assess the physiologic status of the tissue, are promising but await further validation in advance of clinical application.

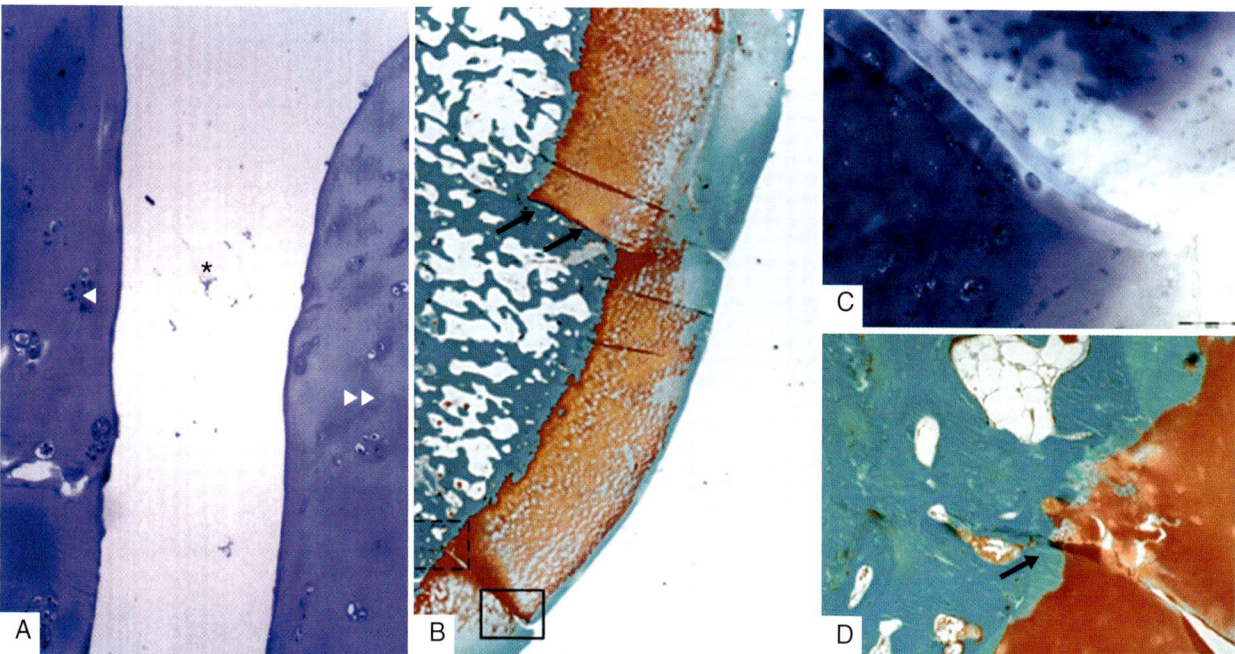

Figure 23-8. A, Histologic appearance of a biopsy specimen taken 22 months after osteochondral transplantation. A cleft (*) remains between the native cartilage *(single arrowhead)* and the osteochondral transplant *(double arrowhead)* in the cartilage layer (toluidine blue, original magnification ×200). **B,** Histologic appearance of three adjacent plugs at the recipient site. Note adequate restoration of the joint surface with hyaline cartilage and the relative deep placement of one plug (Masson's trichrome, ×12.5). **C,** Enlargement of boxed area in **(B).** Note cluster formation of chondrocytes at the boundary of each plug and less staining, indicating loss of proteoglycans (toluidine blue, ×100; bar = 200 μm). **D,** Enlargement of dotted boxed area in **(B).** Note reconstruction of the tidemark *(arrow)* at the transition zone, a clearly visible fissure between the two cartilage plugs, and full incorporation of the plugs in the subchondral bone (Masson's trichrome, ×100; bar = 200 μm). (From Horas U, Pelinkovic D, Herr G, et al: Autologous chondrocyte implantation and osteochondral cylinder transplantation in cartilage repair of the knee joint: a prospective, comparative trial. J Bone Joint Surg Am 85:190 [Figure 6], 2003; Kock N, Van Susante J, Wymenga A, Buma P: Histological evaluation of a mosaicplasty of the femoral condyle–retrieval specimens obtained after total knee arthroplasty—a case report. Acta Orthop Scand 75:507 [Figure 2], 2004.)

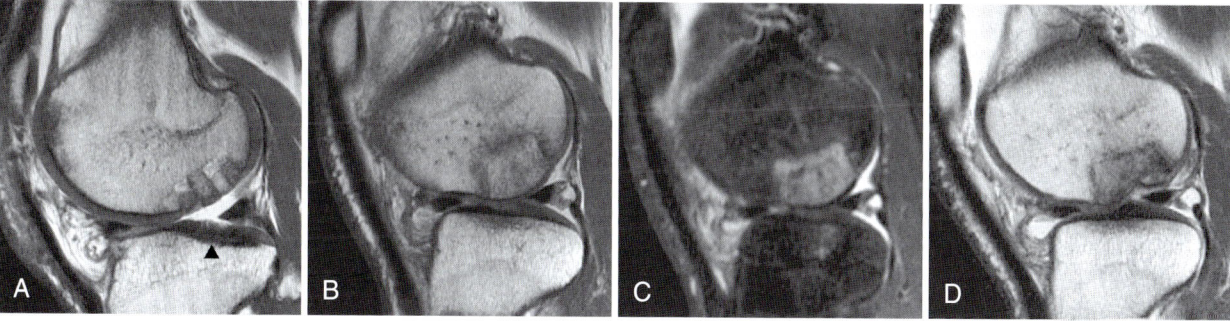

Figure 23-9. A, Sagittal cartilage-sensitive magnetic resonance image of the knee in a 21-year-old man treated with mosaicplasty for a large osteochondral defect of the lateral femoral condyle. Restoration of the radius of curvature using multiple plugs is seen. Note the thinning of cartilage over the more posterior plugs and the fibrillation of cartilage over the tibial plateau *(arrowhead).* **B,** Sagittal cartilage-sensitive magnetic resonance image of the knee in a 17-year-old boy 7 months after mosaicplasty for osteochondritis dissecans using a fresh osteochondral allograft. Intact cartilage is evident over a graft that is slightly proud. **C,** A corresponding fat-suppressed magnetic resonance image demonstrates an intense bone marrow edema pattern in the graft. **D,** A sagittal magnetic resonance image obtained 6 months later shows interval collapse and fragmentation of the allograft, with debris in the posterior recess of the joint. (Modified from Potter HG, Foo LF: Magnetic resonance imaging of articular cartilage: trauma, degeneration, and repair. Am J Sports Med 34:670–671 [Figures 16, 17], 2006.)

Collagen organization within the extracellular matrix can be assessed to obtain information about the ultrastructural composition of cartilage. T2 relaxation time mapping has been shown to correlate with specific regions of cartilage.[67] Collagen is highly organized in the deep (radial) zone of cartilage, with fibers oriented perpendicular to the articular surface, resulting in low T2 values. In the transitional zone, collagen fibers have a more random orientation and

correspondingly increased T2 values. The superficial zone, which consists of fibers oriented in a more ordered fashion parallel to the joint surface, has shorter T2 values. This detailed information allows identification of cartilage defects, as well as monitoring of the postoperative integrity of cartilage resurfacing (Fig. 23-10).[43,67]

Several investigators have reported on the correlation between postoperative MRI and clinical measures. The

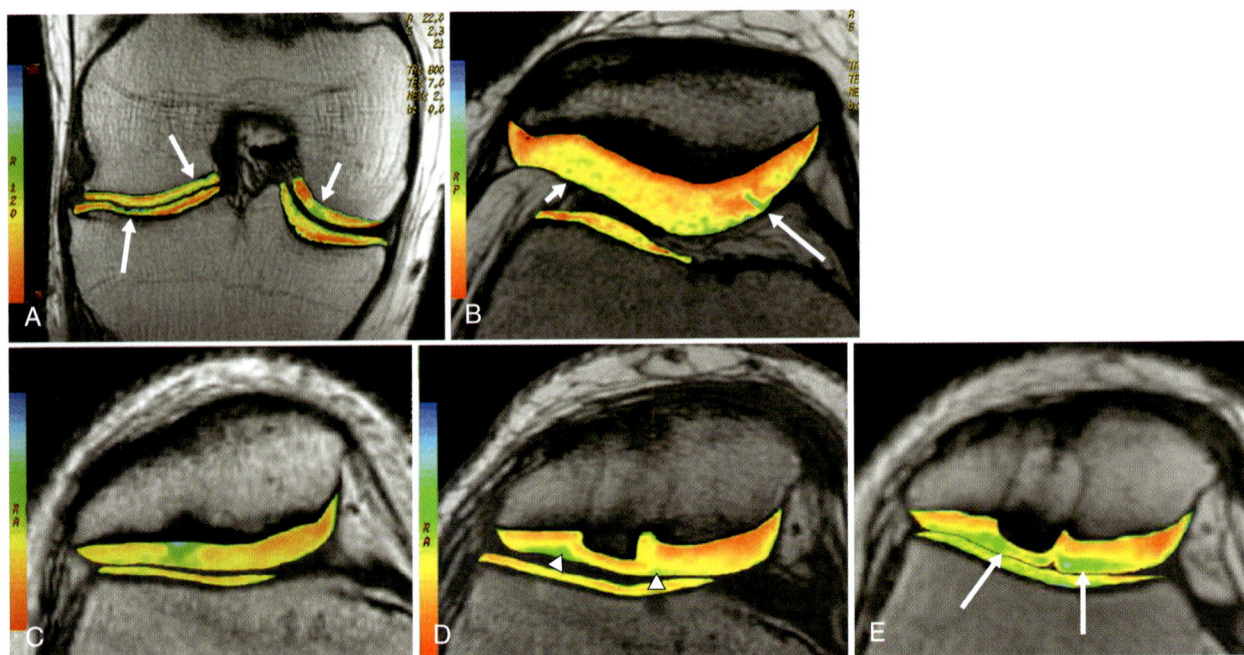

Figure 23-10. A, Quantitative T2 map demonstrates prolongation over the central portion of the lateral tibial plateau, as well as over the inner margin medial and lateral femoral condyles *(arrows)*. **B,** Quantitative magnetic resonance imaging in a 25-year-old woman with patellofemoral pain and normal radiographs. Axial quantitative T2 map, color coded according to relaxation times stratified from 10 *(red)* to 90 *(blue)* milliseconds, demonstrates a discrete fissure, yielding prolonged T2 values in the central portion of the medial facet *(long arrow)*. Also of note is global prolongation of T2 values without the superficial 75% of the lateral patella facet *(short arrow)*, consistent with lateral facet overload. **C** through **E,** Corresponding axial T2 relaxation time maps in an 18-year-old patient with a patellar autologous osteochondral plug. The color maps are coded to capture T2 values ranging from 10 to 90 milliseconds, with orange/red reflecting shorter values and green/blue reflecting longer T2 values. Before surgery **(C),** expected focal T2 prolongation is seen at the site of the full-thickness cartilage defect. Adjacent cartilage demonstrates normal color stratification. Four months after surgery **(D),** the repair cartilage maintains color stratification of normal cartilage. The repair/native interface and adjacent cartilage, however, demonstrate T2 prolongation *(white arrowheads)*. Sixteen months after surgery **(E),** marked and more diffuse T2 prolongation is demonstrated over the repair and adjacent cartilage *(white arrows)*. The opposite cartilage also demonstrates similar prolongation of T2 values, compared with before. (Modified from Koff MF, Potter HG: Noncontrast MR techniques and imaging of cartilage. Radiol Clin North Am 47:498–499 [Figures 5, 6], 2009; Nho SJ, Foo LF, Green DM, et al: Magnetic resonance imaging and clinical evaluation of patellar resurfacing with press-fit osteochondral autograft plugs. Am J Sports Med 36:1107 [Figure 4], 2008.)

MOCART grading system has been described (Box 23-1), but reports have shown mixed correlation with clinical outcomes.[46,86] In particular, the significance of bone marrow edema following OAT is unclear, as several studies have noted persistence of edema as long as 3 years postoperatively.[52,66] This edema does not correlate with knee pain and may represent normal remodeling following graft transfer. Similarly, MRI findings consistent with osteonecrosis do not necessarily bear clinical relevance. Ex vivo MRI with contrast of articular cartilage following OAT in a patient who subsequently underwent total knee arthroplasty showed direct correlation between histology and MRI. The prognostic significance of such findings is unknown; however, MRI was able to identify differences in cartilage thickness and in the level of integration of subchondral bone. It remains to be seen whether specific examination of plugs for signs of common complications will have greater clinical relevance.

FUTURE DIRECTIONS

Clinical use of OAT has been described, and the procedure has been available for longer than 15 years. Despite its reported success in restoring focal articular cartilage defects,

it remains a narrowly defined surgical option. Several factors are responsible for this, most notably, concerns about donor site morbidity, technical challenges, and learning curves. As more sophisticated biomaterials are developed and validated in clinical trials, donor site morbidity may be minimized. Adjuvant therapy, such as catabolic inhibitors or joint cytoprotective agents, may improve the environment in which chondrocytes subjected to transplantation and impaction loads are able to recover. Computer-assisted navigation may improve the precision of graft harvesting and implantation and may aid restoration of native articular surface contours. Future studies should examine the effects of mismatches between cartilage thicknesses, which are most notably seen in OAT of patellar defects.

SUMMARY

Osteochondral autograft plug transfer has been demonstrated to be a successful method of repairing symptomatic focal articular cartilage defects in the knee. Best results have been seen in isolated lesions of the femoral condyles, with trochlear, patellar, and tibial lesions showing less predictable success. Traditional size constraints have indicated OAT for

---

Box 23-1   Cartilage Repair Tissue Assessment: Grading and Point Scale

Variables

I. Degree of defect repair and filling of the defect
- Complete (on a level with adjacent cartilage)
- Hypertrophy (over the level of adjacent cartilage)
- Incomplete (under the level of adjacent cartilage: underfilling)
  - >50% of adjacent cartilage
  - <50% of adjacent cartilage
  - Subchondral bone exposed (complete delamination or dislocation and/or loose body)
2. Integration to border zone
- Complete (complete integration with adjacent cartilage)
- Incomplete (incomplete integration with adjacent cartilage)
  - Demarcating border visible (split-like)
  - Defect visible
    - <50% of length of repair tissue
    - >50% of length of repair tissue
3. Surface of repair tissue
- Surface intact (lamina splendens intact)
- Surface-damaged fibrillations, fissures, and ulcerations
  - <50% of repair tissue depth
  - >50% of repair tissue depth or total degeneration
4. Structure of repair tissue
- Homogenous
- Inhomogenous or cleft formation
5. Signal intensity of repair tissue
- Dual T2-FSE
  - Isointense
  - Moderately hyperintense
  - Markedly hypointense
6. Subchondral lamina
- Intact
- Not intact
7. Subchondral bone
- Intact
- Edema
- Granulation tissue, cysts, sclerosis
8. Adhesions
- No
- Yes
9. Synovitis
- No synovitis
- Synovitis

From Marlovits S, Striessnig G, Resinger CT, et al: Definition of pertinent parameters for the evaluation of articular cartilage repair tissue with high-resolution magnetic resonance imaging. Eur J Radiol 52:313 (Table 2), 2004.

lesions that measure 50 to 250 mm², but individual factors such as patient age, condyle size, concomitant knee pathology including malalignment, and patient expectations and goals may influence the decision-making process. As long-term studies reveal more about the durability of fibrocartilage, OAT may prove to be a more appropriate management strategy for symptomatic focal osteochondral defects in younger or high-demand patients. Meticulous attention to technique is essential; careful review of the literature reveals higher failure rates when recipient site plug positioning is suboptimal. Histologic evaluation of OAT resurfacing sites reveals incorporation of grafts at the subchondral level, but no integration at the articular cartilage level. Although the literature favors second-look arthroscopy, advances in articular cartilage–specific MRI techniques may allow more accurate, noninvasive monitoring of surgical structural outcomes, which have been shown to correlate with clinical outcomes.

A continued limitation of OAT is the availability of donor tissue. Although certain regions of the knee experience higher relative demand than others, studies have shown that no areas are free of contact. As the indications and the demand for treating complex lesions expand, donor site availability will become the rate-limiting factor. Improved strategies for filling of donor sites may limit the morbidity associated with harvest. Hybridization methods and carrying out OAT with other procedures, such as microfracture, or with newer bone graft substitutes, scaffolds, and other biologics may play a role in maximizing the utilization of donor plugs. In comparison with several other strategies aimed at reconstituting articular cartilage defects, it remains to be seen whether the long-term benefit of restoring native hyaline cartilage can outweigh donor site morbidity. However, current evidence suggests that with stringent indications, meticulous techniques, and comprehensive attention to donor harvest sites, OAT can result in successful outcomes in active patients with symptomatic focal articular cartilage defects of the knee.

KEY REFERENCES

Ahmad CS, Cohen ZA, Levine WN, et al: Biomechanical and topographic considerations for autologous osteochondral grafting in the knee. Am J Sports Med 29:201–206, 2001.

Bartz RL, Kamaric E, Noble PC, et al: Topographic matching of selected donor and recipient sites for osteochondral autografting of the articular surface of the femoral condyles. Am J Sports Med 29:207–212, 2001.

Bentley G, Biant LC, Carrington RW, et al: A prospective, randomised comparison of autologous chondrocyte implantation versus mosaicplasty for osteochondral defects in the knee. J Bone Joint Surg Br 85:223–230, 2003.

Duchow J, Hess T, Kohn D: Primary stability of press-fit-implanted osteochondral grafts: influence of graft size, repeated insertion, and harvesting technique. Am J Sports Med 28:24–27, 2000.

Garretson RB, 3rd, Katolik LI, Verma N, et al: Contact pressure at osteochondral donor sites in the patellofemoral joint. Am J Sports Med 32:967–974, 2004.

Gudas R, Kalesinskas RJ, Kimtys V, et al: A prospective randomized clinical study of mosaic osteochondral autologous transplantation versus microfracture for the treatment of osteochondral defects in the knee joint in young athletes. Arthroscopy 21:1066–1075, 2005.

Guettler JH, Demetropoulos CK, Yang KH, Jurist KA: Osteochondral defects in the human knee: influence of defect size on cartilage rim stress and load redistribution to surrounding cartilage. Am J Sports Med 32:1451–1458, 2004.

Hangody L, Ráthonyi GK, Duska Z, et al: Autologous osteochondral mosaicplasty: surgical technique. J Bone Joint Surg Am 86(Suppl 1):65–72, 2004.

Horas U, Pelinkovic D, Herr G, et al: Autologous chondrocyte implantation and osteochondral cylinder transplantation in cartilage repair of the knee joint: a prospective, comparative trial. J Bone Joint Surg Am 85:185–192, 2003.

Huntley JS, Bush PB, McBirnie JM, et al: Chondrocyte death associated with human femoral osteochondral harvest as performed for mosaicplasty. J Bone Joint Surg Am 87:351–360, 2005.

Koh JL, Wirsing K, Lautenschlager E, Zhang LO: The effect of graft height mismatch on contact pressure following osteochondral grafting: a biomechanical study. Am J Sports Med 32:317–320, 2004.

Marcacci M, Kon E, Delcogliano M, et al: Arthroscopic autologous osteochondral grafting for cartilage defects of the knee: prospective study results at a minimum 7-year follow-up. Am J Sports Med 35:2014–2021, 2007.

Nho SJ, Foo LF, Green DM, et al: Magnetic resonance imaging and clinical evaluation of patellar resurfacing with press-fit osteochondral autograft plugs. Am J Sports Med 36:1101–1109, 2008.

Pearce SG, Hurtig MB, Clarnette R, et al: An investigation of 2 techniques for optimizing joint surface congruency using multiple cylindrical osteochondral autografts. Arthroscopy 17:50–55, 2001.

Thaunat M, Couchon S, Lunn J, et al: Cartilage thickness matching of selected donor and recipient sites for osteochondral autografting of the medial femoral condyle. Knee Surg Sports Traumatol Arthrosc 15:381–386, 2007.

Full references for this chapter can be found on www.expertconsult.com.

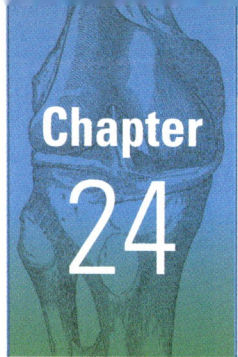

Chapter 24

Osteochondral Allograft Transplantation

Samuel P. Robinson and Kevin F. Bonner

Articular cartilage defects present a challenging clinical problem for orthopedic surgeons. The limited healing capacity of cartilage has led to the development of various treatment options for symptomatic defects. Currently available techniques with at least midterm published outcome reports include marrow-stimulating techniques (subchondral drilling, microfracture), autologous osteochondral transfer system (OATS; mosaicplasty), autologous chondrocyte implantation, and osteochondral allograft transplantation. Each of these techniques has potential benefits and limitations. Resulting repair tissue and clinical outcomes may be variable with some of these techniques; as a consequence, the optimal treatment of many defects is controversial. Treatment algorithms have been proposed that take into account both patient and lesion factors, but minimal level 1 evidence exists to validate these algorithms.[9,21,45,53]

The use of fresh osteochondral allografts has a fairly extensive clinical history, extending over three decades.* Allograft transplantation is currently gaining in popularity owing to increasing appreciation that it reliably restores viable hyaline cartilage when compared with alternative treatment options for larger defects.[7] Although logistic issues are associated with obtaining allografts, including waiting for an appropriate graft, the procedure itself is not very technically demanding in most cases. Fresh allografts are most useful in treating large chondral or osteochondral lesions (>2 cm), such as those seen with osteochondritis dissecans, trauma, osteonecrosis, and selected cases of degenerative arthrosis. Allografts can also be used as a salvage procedure after other cartilage resurfacing procedures are performed in young patients in whom arthroplasty options are undesirable.

Both patients and physicians have an interest in biologic resurfacing solutions for damaged cartilage in an effort to postpone or prevent arthroplasty procedures. Because most biologic resurfacing procedures are performed in younger individuals, most resurfacing options should realistically be considered a bridging procedure to improve pain and function until the patient is a more appropriate arthroplasty candidate.

BASIC SCIENCE

The long-term success of osteochondral allografts is dependent on preservation of the hyaline cartilage surface, healing of the osseous base to the host bone, and maintenance of structural integrity during the remodeling process.[66] Investigators have shown that chondrocyte viability is paramount in maintaining the normal extracellular architecture of hyaline cartilage and in preventing the development of degenerative joint disease, but the acceptable degree of

chondrocyte viability required is unknown at this time.[34,64] Although nonviable cartilage will appear grossly normal for a peroid of time, it will not maintain its histologic, biochemical, or biomechanical properties. As a result, the cartilage will fibrillate, develop clefts, and erode over time.[34,64]

Freezing of articular cartilage, although attractive in terms of decreasing immunogenicity and allowing storage, causes chondrocyte cell death to a variable degree with current preservation methods.[63,70] Although up to 90% of isolated chondrocytes are able to survive the freezing process, freezing of chondrocytes embedded within their matrix has not been nearly as successful.[62,63,70] This discrepancy is thought to result from poor penetration of cryopreservative, unequal rate of cooling, and high water content within the extracellular matrix.[63,70] Because cryopreservation techniques have not been shown to preserve an acceptable degree of cartilage viability, fresh allografts are considered the mainstay for allograft transplantation of articular cartilage.[22,27,61] However, whether or not the transplantation of fresh viable osteochondral grafts avoids a degenerative course superior to that of frozen grafts is a topic of ongoing controversy.[34,71] It is important to note that current "fresh" allografts are actually refrigerated (not frozen) for a time prior to implantation, in contrast to historical fresh allografts, which were transplanted much closer to the time of procurement.[41]

Immune compatibility testing and postoperative immunosuppression are not required with osteochondral allograft transplantation despite the fact that both chondrocytes and subchondral bone have been shown to have immunogenic potential.[38-40,59] Chondrocytes are surrounded by a matrix that isolates them from the host immune cells and makes them relatively "immunologically privileged."[13,31] Although donor cells within the osseous component are immunogenic, their immunogenicity is muted and probably is not clinically significant in most patients because the cells are nonviable.[15,23] When an osteochondral allograft is implanted into a host bed, a local inflammatory response is stimulated by both surgical trauma and the graft itself.[67] This response is thought to peak between the second and third weeks and is primarily directed against the bone constituent of the graft that contains the marrow elements and other immunogenic elements.[65] Therefore, pulse lavage of the bone just before implantation is recommended in an attempt to cleanse the graft and remove unbound antigenic elements. After the initial response, the inflammatory reaction may burn out or may persist for up to 18 months.[17,67]

In general, the osseous component of osteochondral allografts retains its structural integrity and is replaced with host bone via creeping substitution over a period of years.[16,29,51,54] If the nonviable bony trabeculae cannot withstand mechanical stresses during the remodeling process, subchondral microfracture, collapse, and fragmentation may occur. Based on our understanding of the remodeling process

---

*References 4, 8, 14, 15, 31, and 42.

and the stresses placed on grafts before completion of this process, it is somewhat surprising how relatively infrequently this occurs clinically. One potential benefit of minimizing the donor graft depth is a theoretical decrease in remodeling time.

Although cartilage matrix, glycosaminoglycan content, and biomechanical properties are not initially altered, percent chondrocyte viability, viable cell density, and metabolic activity have been found to progressively decrease over time following procurement.* Fresh osteochondral allografts harvested within 24 hours of donor death and preserved at 4° C have been shown to maintain up to 100% chondrocyte viability at 4 days.[18,25,62] Contemporary allograft storage techniques preserve reasonably high chondrocyte viability with a significant decline in survival after 15 to 20 days.* By 44 days, chondrocyte viability falls to approximately 67%.[57] Malinin et al showed in a primate model that osteoarticular allografts transplanted after 21 days of storage underwent more severe degenerative changes than allografts that had been stored for less than 21 days.[44] Although increased cell viability is certainly optimal, acceptable chondrocyte viability appropriate for clinical implantation is controversial. This is due to reports of successful clinical outcomes and favorable histologic biopsy analysis of grafts implanted 4 to 6 weeks following procurement.[24] Because of concerns related to infections, fresh osteoarticular allografts are currently stored hypothermically for a minimum of 14 days to allow serologic and microbiologic testing. After this time, grafts theoretically should be transplanted as soon as possible to optimize chondrocyte viability. Research continues regarding the optimal media composition for maximal preservation of chondrocyte viability while in cold storage.[58,68]

Long-term chondrocyte viability following osteochondral allograft transplantation has been shown in multiple biopsy and retrieval reports.† Researchers have biopsied transplants at various time intervals following the index procedure. Williams et al found 82% chondrocyte viability at 4-year follow-up with no significant immune reaction to the cartilage or the bone within the allograft.[76] Davidson et al reported no significant detectable differences in graft versus native cartilage cell density or viability.[24] Grafts were stored for 4 to 6 weeks before transplantation and were biopsied at a mean of 40 months postoperatively. Jamali et al confirmed that actual implanted donor chondrocytes were the source of cell viability by showing that female chondrocytes were still viable 29 years following transplantation into a male recipient.[36] This potential for long-term survival supports the use of osteochondral allografts in an attempt to maintain extracellular matrix and thus prevent long-term articular degeneration within the graft.

INDICATIONS

At this time, it is unknown why some chondral or osteochondral lesions are asymptomatic, while others cause significant morbidity.[73] Because we do not understand the natural history of most chondral lesions, surgery generally is indicated only for the treatment of symptomatic lesions. Debate continues regarding the treatment of asymptomatic full-thickness

*References 1, 5, 44, 55, 57, 74, and 77.
†References 28, 33, 36, 49, 52, and 76.

defects found at the time of surgery performed for other primary procedures (e.g., anterior cruciate ligament [ACL] reconstruction), but that discussion is beyond the scope of this chapter. The objectives of any biologic resurfacing procedure, including fresh allograft transplantation, are pain relief and functional improvement. Although our goal is the prevention of progressive joint deterioration and subsequent need for arthroplasty, most biologic resurfacing is performed in younger individuals with long life expectancies. Realistically, these biologic procedures should be considered a bridging procedure to improve pain and function until the patient is a more appropriate arthroplasty candidate.

Fresh osteochondral allografts are most useful in treating large chondral or osteochondral lesions (>2 cm), such as those seen with osteochondritis dissecans, trauma, osteonecrosis, and selected cases of degenerative arthrosis in young patients in whom arthroplasty options are undesirable. Allografts can also be used in a salvage procedure following failed cartilage resurfacing procedures. Patients with localized, unipolar, traumatic, nondegenerative, chondral lesions, osteochondritis dissecans, or osteonecrosis are believed to be optimal candidates for fresh osteochondral allografting and have obtained the best results.[7,13,31] Relatively focal nonacute chondral lesions, which tend to be degenerative in nature, may also benefit from allografting procedures in the appropriate setting. However, results are often dependent on the status of the surrounding articular surface, and whether or not the underlying mechanical and physiologic factors that contributed to the initial chondral loss continue. Patients with associated pathology are more likely to benefit from a concomitant procedure, such as an unloading osteotomy or a meniscus transplant, in an effort to delay the progression of degeneration.

Primary treatment with an osteochondral allograft is often the optimal treatment when there is significant subchondral bone involvement of greater than 5 to 10 mm.[13,21,53] The authors tend to favor osteochondral autograft or allograft for any lesion with subchondral bone involvement. Fresh osteochondral allografts are well suited for these types of lesions because they can restore the subchondral plate, in addition to hyaline cartilage.

Absolute contraindications to osteochondral allograft transplant include active infection and patients who are of appropriate age and activity level for prosthetic replacement. Associated grade III or IV kissing lesions of the tibiofemoral or patellofemoral articulation are generally considered a relative contraindication, unless both lesions are addressed at the time of the procedure.[7] Malalignment, ligamentous instability, and meniscal insufficiency must be addressed before or at the time of the resurfacing procedure.[31] Patients with inflammatory arthropathy, crystal-induced arthropathy, and synovitis are also relative contraindications. The effects of altered bone metabolism due to long-term steroid use or smoking have not been studied, although we generally consider this a contraindication.

PROCUREMENT, SCREENING, AND STORAGE

Allograft tissue should be obtained from an accredited tissue bank that adheres to the guidelines established by the American Association of Tissue Banks (AATB) and the U.S.

Federal Drug Administration (FDA).[2,72] Graft procurement should be carried out within 24 hours of death under strict aseptic conditions.[4,6,32] Donors are screened for risk of disease transmission, including detailed medical and social history for risk factors of exposure to human immunodeficiency virus (HIV), hepatitis B, and hepatitis C.[3,72] The FDA had previously mandated titers for HIV-1 and HIV-2 antibody, hepatitis B surface antigen, hepatitis core antibody, hepatitis C antibody, human T-lymphocyte virus 1 antibody, HIV p24 antigen, and the rapid plasma reagin test for syphilis. Beginning in 2005, all AATB-accredited tissue banks were required to perform nucleic acid testing (NAT) for both HIV-1 and the hepatitis C virus to further reduce the window period associated with conventional (enzyme immunoassay [EIA] method) donor screening antibody or antigen tests.[10]

One of the issues of greatest concern surrounding the use of fresh allograft material is the risk of infectious organism transmission, including viral and bacterial disease. Current tissue bank processing and donor screening reduce the risk of disease transmission to very low levels, although the exact risk estimate is unknown for fresh osteochondral allografts.[3,10-12,69] Not all cases are detected, and surveillance systems have not been designed to define the true incidence of these infections. In 1995, based on reports in the literature, the incidence of infection was estimated to be 0.02% from approximately 20,000 organ transplants per year, and 0.0004% from approximately 900,000 allografts per year.[19] In 2007, AATB-accredited tissue banks distributed just over 1.1 million musculoskeletal allografts. Most of these were processed grafts, which went through proprietary washing and sterilization. Only approximately 2200 of the distributed grafts were classified as osteochondral allografts.[10] Heightened awareness among clinicians and improved diagnostic tests have enhanced the detection of tissue-associated infection.

The risk of bacterial transmission from contaminated fresh allograft tissue is of greater concern compared with processed nonviable grafts because cytotoxic cleansing treatments cannot be utilized. One case report describes a fatal bacterial infection following implantation of a fresh osteochondral allograft contaminated with *Clostridium*.[37] A subsequent

investigation by the Centers for Disease Control and Prevention identified 26 potential patients with allograft-associated infection: 13 with *Clostridium* species and 14 associated with a single processing agency.[37] Malinin et al found that 64 of 795 consecutive donors of musculoskeletal tissue (8.1%) had *Clostridium* contamination.[43] They also found that the risk of *Clostridium* contamination increased with the length of time between donor death and allograft harvest. In addition to a review of the medical records, cultures of tissue, donor blood, and donor blood marrow are used as screening tools to limit the risk of transmitted bacterial infection.[46,47] Episodes of allograft-associated infection in the past decade have improved awareness, enhanced our understanding of the problem, and may decrease this risk in the future.

Harvested tissues are typically stored in antimicrobial solutions at temperatures just above freezing. Screening tests (except final fungal cultures) typically are not completed for approximately 14 days from the time of procurement; thus grafts are not released until at least that time. Although debate is ongoing regarding reasonable cell viability and graft expiration to optimize graft utilization, most tissue banks currently consider fresh, hypothermically stored osteoarticular grafts expired at a maximum of 42 days from procurement.

PREOPERATIVE PLANNING

Confirming that the patient is an appropriate candidate for a fresh allograft is important before tissue is ordered. This often can be accomplished with high-quality magnetic resonance imaging (MRI), in addition to weight-bearing radiography (Fig. 24-1A and B). When concern arises about whether a patient is a candidate for an allograft, we typically perform a diagnostic arthroscopy to evaluate the lesion of interest, as well as the remainder of the knee. If the patient had a recent arthroscopy performed elsewhere, arthroscopic pictures, operative reports, and radiographic studies are often sufficient. Long-alignment films are required to determine whether associated malalignment necessitates a concurrent unloading osteotomy.

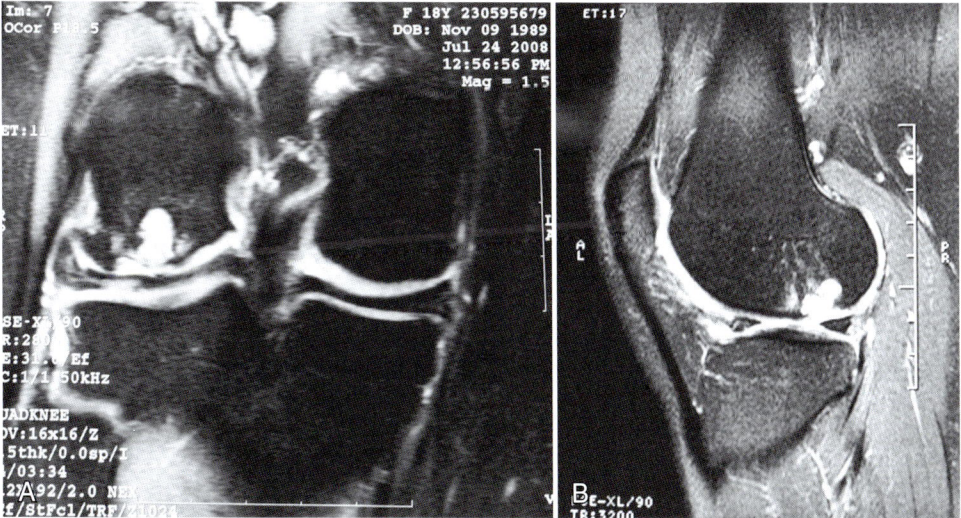

Figure 24-1. **A** and **B,** Coronal and sagittal T2-weighted magnetic resonance imaging (MRI) shows an osteochondral lesion of the distal lateral femoral condyle.

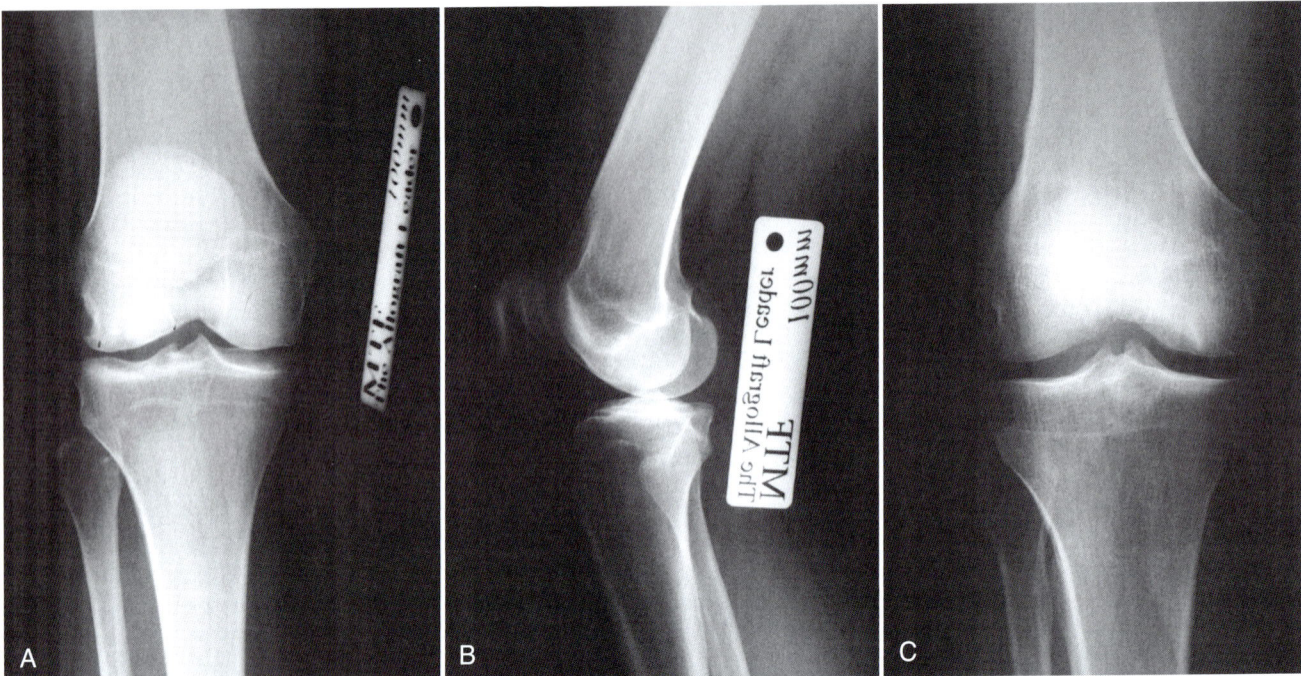

Figure 24-2. Anteroposterior (AP) and lateral radiographs of the knee with evidence of osteochondral pathology. Magnification markers are present. **A** and **B**, AP and lateral radiographs of an osteochondral lesion of the lateral femoral condyle. **C**, AP radiograph of an osteochondral lesion of the medial femoral condyle.

Obtaining an acceptable donor graft from an AATB-accredited tissue bank is a key component of the procedure. Size matching from an appropriately screened donor is the main criterion for obtaining an acceptable osteochondral graft. Graft size is measured radiographically. Anteroposterior and lateral radiographs with magnification markers placed at the patient's joint can be used to calculate dimensions (Fig. 24-2A through C). Care must be taken to allow for appropriate correction of magnification error. A match is considered acceptable at ±2 mm; however, significant variability in anatomic morphology may be noted. Differences between men and women may be particularly apparent. Larger defects typically require more precise graft matches to optimize articular congruity. However, when an osteoarticular plug or dowel technique (mega-OATS [osteochondral autograft transfer system]) is used, a same-size or larger donor surface is often acceptable. Accepting a smaller donor for a large graft is not recommended. Wait times for an acceptable graft vary and can be both lengthy and frustrating for patients. It is common to send measurements to several trusted AATB-certified tissue banks in an effort to increase the odds for procuring a compatible graft within a reasonable time frame.

SURGICAL TECHNIQUE

Before anesthesia is administered, the osteochondral allograft should be examined to confirm the adequacy of the size match and the quality of the tissue. Allograft tissue is soaked in a normal saline/antibiotic solution and is kept safe on a back table, which is set up with the allograft workstation. The patient is positioned supine on the operative table with a tourniquet on the proximal thigh. A leg holder is valuable for accessing the lesion by positioning the leg at between 70 and 100 degrees of knee flexion. Alternatively, a sandbag may

be taped on the table to help keep the knee flexed to an optimal position. In most cases, we perform a diagnostic arthroscopy before making the arthrotomy, to assess the remainder of the joint and confirm that the patient is a good candidate for the procedure.

This procedure is performed through a medial or lateral arthrotomy. The extent of exposure varies depending on the position and magnitude of the lesion. Exposure for a typical osteochondritis dissecans lesion on the lateral side of the medial femoral condyle is more extensile in that the patella will be retracted farther laterally to allow access to the lesion. Eversion of the patella typically is not necessary. More central or peripheral lesions often can be treated through a more limited approach. Because high degrees of knee flexion are required to access very posterior lesions, the patella can compromise access to these areas of the articular surface. A more extensile proximal parapatellar, midvastus, or subvastus approach often is helpful in mobilizing the patella. If needed, a tibial tubercle osteotomy can be performed to enhance exposure.

Great care is taken when entering the joint to avoid injuring the articular cartilage or the anterior horn of the meniscus. In cases where the lesion is posterior or very large, the meniscus may need to be taken down at the meniscocapsular junction and may be repaired as part of the closure. Larger bulk allografts may require more extensive exposure. For a typical condylar lesion, retractors are placed medially and laterally, including one in the notch, to retract the patella and gain exposure to the joint (Fig. 24-3). The knee is then flexed or extended until the lesion is exposed through the arthrotomy site. Once visualization is achieved, the lesion is inspected and palpated to determine its depth, size, and margins.

The two most commonly used techniques for the preparation and implantation of osteochondral allografts are the

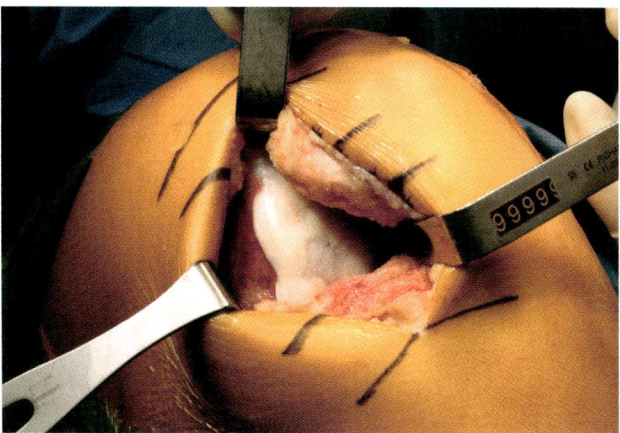

Figure 24-3. Exposure of osteochondral lesion of the lateral femoral condyle through lateral parapatellar arthrotomy.

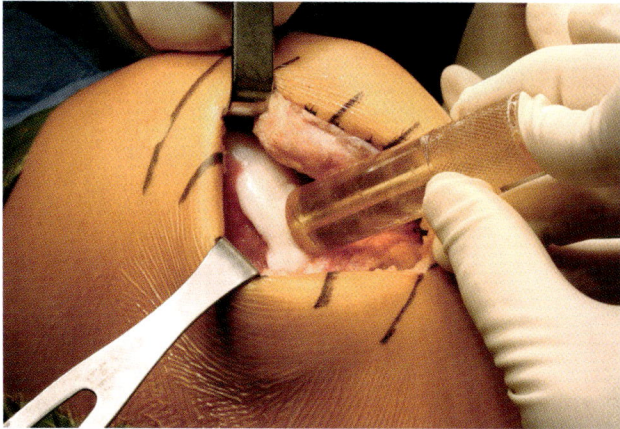

Figure 24-4. Sizing of the lesion for proposed dowel graft.

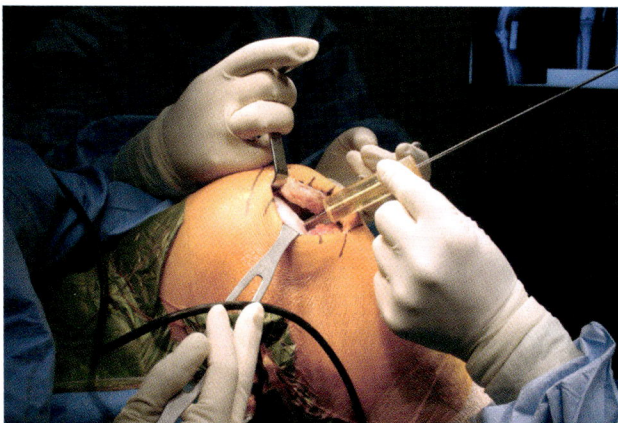

Figure 24-5. Using a commercially available sizing guide, a guide wire is placed in the center of the osteochondral lesion. The guide wire is placed perpendicular to the articular surface.

press-fit plug technique and the shell graft technique. Each technique has advantages and disadvantages. The press-fit plug technique is similar in principle to OATS and is optimal for contained condylar lesions between 15 and 35 mm in diameter. This technique is certainly the most commonly used in practice. In most cases, a stable press fit is achieved, and additional fixation is not required. One disadvantage of this technique is the sacrifice of adjacent areas of normal cartilage and bone to convert the lesion into a circular recipient defect. In addition, limitations on where the circular coring system can be used have been identified; specifically, tibial and far posterior condylar lesions are not conducive to this technique. The large plug transplant technique may occasionally be used for patellar and trochlear lesions, but these areas can be technically challenging. Shell grafts, on the other hand, have the advantages of minimizing normal cartilage and bone sacrifice and accommodating cartilage lesions of the tibia and patella and many trochlear lesions. Disadvantages of shell grafts include technical difficulty and less inherent graft stability, thus typically requiring the need for fixation.

Press-Fit Plug Allograft Technique

Several proprietary instrumentation systems are currently available for the preparation and implantation of press-fit plug allografts between 15 and 35 mm in diameter. Although we describe only one of the instrumentation systems in our technique, most systems are similar. The size of the proposed graft is determined by using a sizing dowel to cover as much of the defect as possible while limiting the sacrifice of normal tissue (Fig. 24-4). Sometimes a lesion is more amenable to the use of two overlapping cylindrical plugs (termed "snowman" or "mastercard" configuration). Once the sizing dowel is in the appropriate position, a guide wire is driven several centimeters into the center of the lesion (Fig. 24-5). It is important that the guide wire be drilled perpendicular to the curvature of the articular surface.

An appropriately sized cannulated scoring reamer is used initially over the guide pin to cut through just the articular cartilage and create a sharp circumferential edge (Fig. 24-6A). A cannulated coring drill is used to ream the subchondral bone and create the recipient site (see Fig. 24-6B and C). Debate continues regarding optimal reaming depth. Proper

preparation of the lesion will result in a healthy, bleeding bone recipient site; therefore, the depth of the preparation will depend on the quality of the subchondral bone. Without bone involvement, the recipient site should be in the range of 6 to 10 mm deep, which typically translates into 3 to 8 mm of bone preparation. A trend toward reaming less and having only 3 to 6 mm of bone on the donor plug has been noted. The benefits of creating a more shallow defect include less bone sacrifice, potentially increased bone density, and less bone volume to be incorporated over time. Potential negatives include the theoretical loss of stability from the circumferential press fit and increased reliance on an exact depth match, which may be more technically difficult. The effects of these issues on short- and long-term outcomes are currently unknown. In cases of bone loss, reaming needs to advance slowly until a healthy recipient bone bed is achieved.

Before the guide pin is removed, debris is removed from the recipient site, and the cannulated dilator is placed into the defect. The dilator not only makes delivery of the graft easier but allows preliminary recipient site measurements. The guide pin is removed, and precise depth measurements are made in all four quadrants of the recipient site. The corresponding anatomic location of the recipient site is identified and marked with a surgical marker on the graft (Fig. 24-7), which is secured onto the commercially available

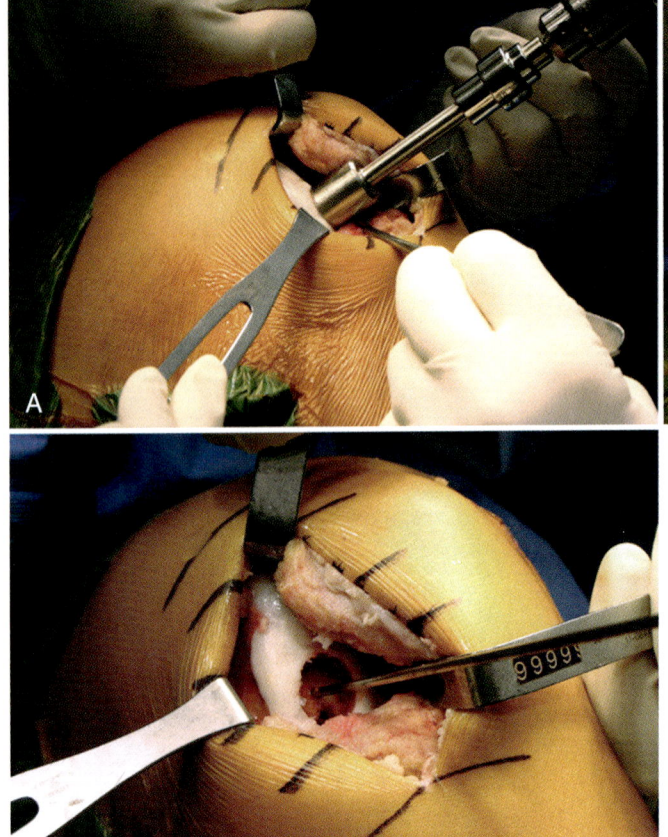

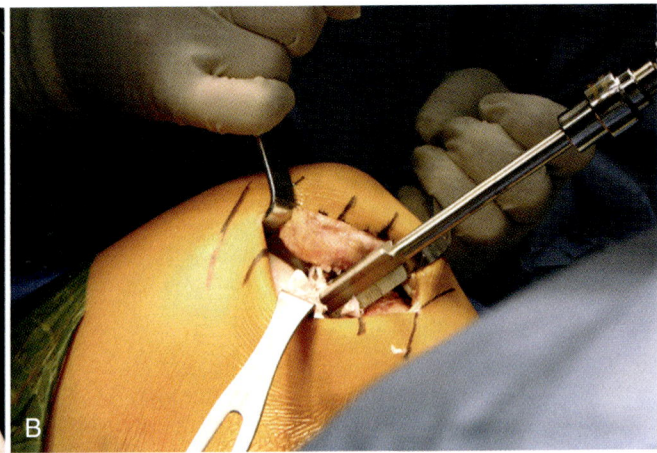

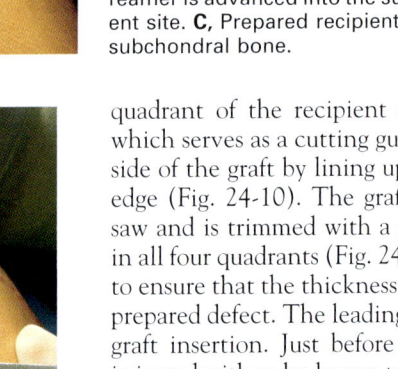

Figure 24-6. Reaming the recipient site over the guide wire. **A,** Initially, a scoring reamer is used to create a sharp edge on the adjacent articular cartilage. **B,** Next, the appropriately sized reamer is advanced into the subchondral bone to create the recipient site. **C,** Prepared recipient site bordered by healthy, bleeding subchondral bone.

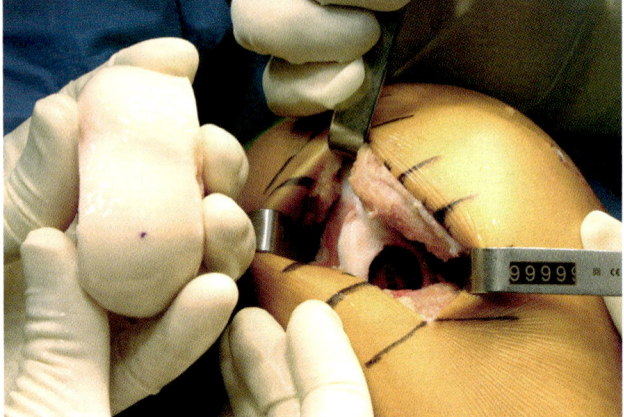

Figure 24-7. The corresponding anatomic location of the recipient site is identified on the graft.

workstation (Fig. 24-8). The 12 o'clock position on the future donor plug is marked to ensure proper orientation once removed. The workstation contains a mobile coring reamer guide, which needs to be secured in such a way that the coring reamer will harvest the graft from the appropriate anatomic location (see Fig. 24-8A through C). Placing the original sizing dowel down the guide and letting it rest perpendicular on the articular cartilage will greatly assist in properly securing the mobile guide. The appropriately sized coring reamer can then be used to core out the graft (Fig. 24-9). Once the graft has been removed, depth measurements from each

quadrant of the recipient site are marked. A graft clamp, which serves as a cutting guide, is used to secure the articular side of the graft by lining up the depth marks with the guide edge (Fig. 24-10). The graft is then cut with an oscillating saw and is trimmed with a rasp to the appropriate thickness in all four quadrants (Fig. 24-11A and B). Care must be taken to ensure that the thickness of the graft precisely matches the prepared defect. The leading edges are chamfered to facilitate graft insertion. Just before insertion, the graft is copiously irrigated with pulse lavage to remove donor marrow elements. The dilator is again inserted into the recipient site to ease the insertion of the graft and prevent excessive impact loading on the articular surface (Fig. 24-12).

The graft is inserted by hand in the appropriate orientation and is gently tamped into place until it is flush with the surrounding cartilage (Fig. 24-13A through C). Care is taken to minimize impact loading of the allograft during insertion, as this has been shown to cause chondrocyte death.[56] The articular congruity is matched as perfectly as possible, and the graft is not left proud. Small edge mismatches can be débrided with a No. 15 blade if needed. Countersinking and surface mismatches greater than 1 mm from the surrounding joint surface are not accepted. If the graft does not fit properly, the recipient site or the graft itself is refashioned carefully. When necessary, a threaded pin can be placed centrally to remove the graft. Once the graft is seated, a determination is made whether additional fixation with bioabsorbable polydioxanone pins is required. Rarely do press-fit dowel plugs require additional fixation. If the graft is large and uncontained, fixation may be necessary. The knee is brought through a

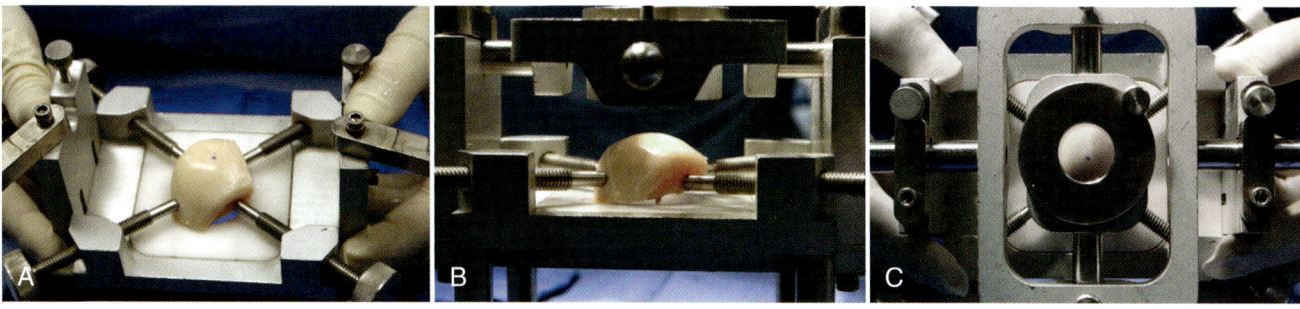

Figure 24-8. A commercially available allograft workstation is used to secure the graft (Arthrex, Naples, Fla).

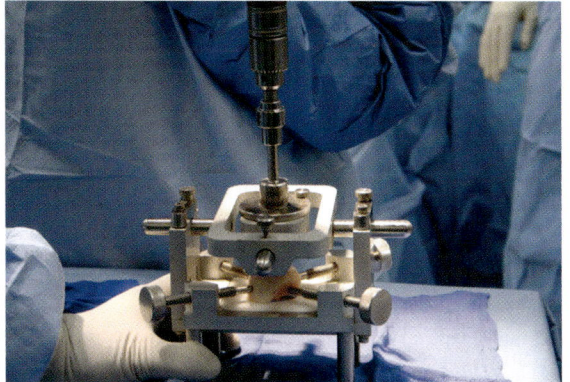

Figure 24-9. The osteochondral graft is harvested with a coring reamer.

complete range of motion to confirm that the graft is stable. The wound is copiously irrigated, and a routine closure is performed.

Shell Allograft Technique

The cartilage defect is identified through the previously described arthrotomy, and the circumference of the lesion is marked with a surgical pen. An attempt is made to create a geometric shape that will be amenable to hand crafting of the graft and minimizing the sacrifice of normal cartilage. A No. 15 blade is used to cut around the lesion, and sharp ring curettes are used to remove all tissue inside this border. With a motorized 4.0-mm burr and sharp curettes, the defect is débrided to a depth of 4 to 5 mm. A foil template can be used to achieve a precisely sized graft. A large piece of foil from suture packs can be manually fashioned over the articular cartilage of the involved compartment. The foil is manually pressed into the defect while the foil mold of the surrounding bone is maintained. The mold of the defect is then cut out of the foil and is confirmed to be a precise match with the lesion. The foil template is placed over the matched allograft and is used to outline the corresponding area on the donor graft. This demarcated cartilage is used as a guide for meticulous preparation of a shell of osteochondral allograft, with 4 to 5 mm of subchondral bone remaining.

We recommend slightly oversizing the graft initially and carefully removing bone and cartilage as necessary to provide appropriate fitting. This takes multiple trials and an abundance of patience. If deeper bone loss is seen within the defect, more bone can be left on the graft and/or the defect can be grafted with cancellous bone before graft insertion.

The graft is meticulously modified until it is flush with the articular surface (Fig. 24-14). Once the graft has been seated, graft stability can be determined. Typically, graft fixation is required.

An alternative shell graft technique, which may be technically easier than the procedure just described, utilizes a saw blade to make a cut similar to those made in unicompartmental or total knee arthroplasty. The depth of the resection is measured, and a graft is fashioned from the matching donor site. Sites that typically benefit from this method include the tibial plateau, the patella, and the trochlea. These types of shell grafts require fixation with compression screws or bioabsorbable devices.

POSTOPERATIVE MANAGEMENT

Intravenous antibiotics are discontinued after the first 24 hours postoperatively. We advocate the avoidance of nonsteroidal anti-inflammatory drugs (NSAIDs) for the first 6 to 8 weeks to optimize bone-to-bone healing. Deep venous thrombosis (DVT) prophylaxis ranges from mechanical methods and aspirin to low-molecular-weight heparin injections. Postoperative radiographs are performed routinely after the procedure to assess graft–host integration. Postoperative MRI is not performed routinely. Persistent high T2 signal abnormalities within and adjacent to the graft site are very common, and the clinical significance of such phenomena is unknown.

Postoperative rehabilitation is based on the size, location, stability, and containment of the graft, as well as concomitant procedures. Early postoperative management focuses on controlling pain and swelling while working on range of motion. This includes the use of a continuous passive motion (CPM) machine, starting in the immediate postoperative period. Extended CPM use is desirable but is not required. Alternatively, a low-resistance stationary bike can be used. Patients are generally allowed full range of motion, unless prohibited by concurrent reconstructive procedures such as meniscal repair or transplantation. Patellofemoral grafts or shell grafts with less inherent stability may require limitations in range of motion.

Weight bearing is assessed on the basis of size and stability of the graft. Smaller and inherently more stable grafts may start toe-touch weight bearing immediately for the first 6 weeks and then may progress to weight bearing as tolerated beyond that point. When concern arises regarding the stability of a plug graft, and in all cases of nonpatellofemoral shell graft, we are conservative with the use of a non–weight-bearing regimen for the first 6 to 8 weeks. Isolated

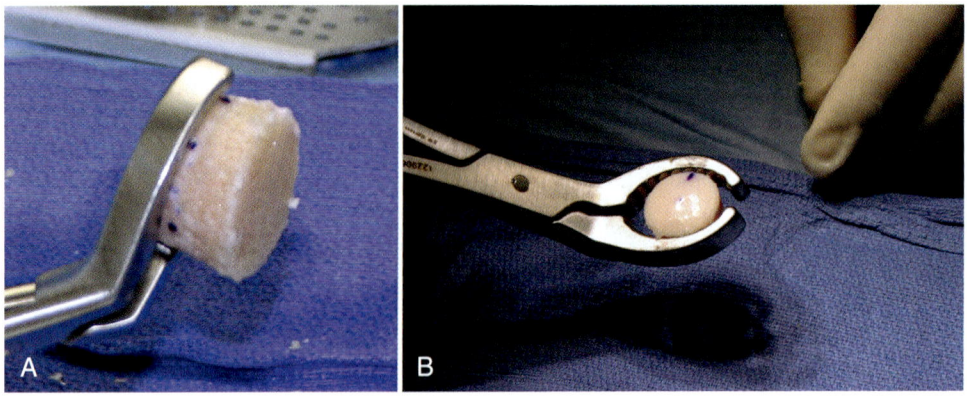

Figure 24-10. Preparation of the allograft with quadrant depth measurements **(A)** and orientation marks on the cartilage **(B)**.

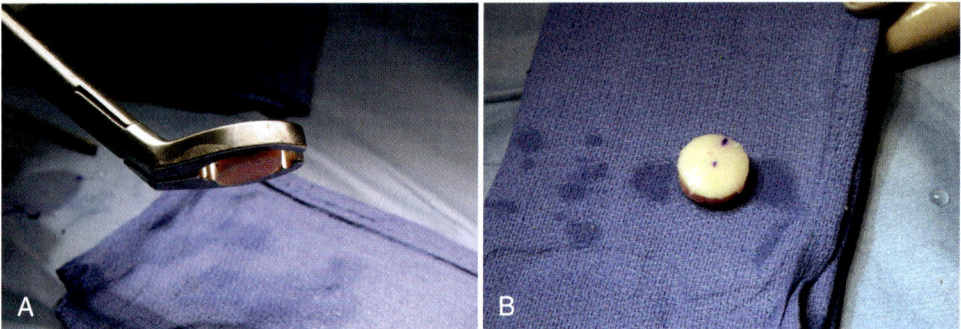

Figure 24-11. A, The graft is cut with an oscillating saw at the appropriate depth. **B,** The final graft is ready for implantation.

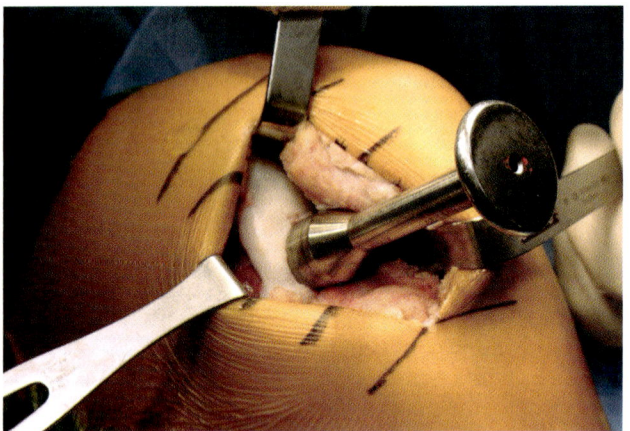

Figure 24-12. The recipient site is dilated to ease insertion of the graft and prevent excessive impact loading on the articular surface.

patellofemoral grafts can often weight-bear as tolerated with a brace locked in extension. In these patients, weight bearing is progressed slowly at 6 to 8 weeks as tolerated over a 4- to 6-week period.

For most press-fit dowel grafts, braces may be utilized to help protect the extremity until quadriceps strength returns. When grafting involves the patellofemoral joint, braces are locked in extension for the first 6 weeks. In patients undergoing large shell or bipolar tibial-femoral grafting, an unloader brace may be used to prevent excessive stress on the grafted surfaces.

The postoperative strengthening and rehabilitation program is dictated on the basis of graft stability, current understanding of allograft healing, symptoms, and evidence of radiographic incorporation. Typically, patients are started on a quadriceps strengthening program. At 4 weeks, patients are allowed closed-chain exercises such as cycling. Strengthening of the lower extremity continues with a focus on hamstring and quadriceps, using an isometric program and avoidance of open-chain exercises. When it is believed that functional rehabilitation has been completed appropriately, patients are able to return to recreation and sports 6 to 12 months after surgery. Patients generally are cautioned about excessive impact loading of the allograft, particularly for larger grafts.

RESULTS

Similar to other cartilage resurfacing procedures, the results of fresh or prolonged refrigerated osteoarticular allografts are variable, depending on defect location, origin of the lesion, status of the surrounding articular cartilage and meniscus, degree of bipolar disease, patient age, and alignment. In general, focal, posttraumatic, well-shouldered femoral condylar defects and osteochondritis dissecans of the medial femoral condyle tend to have the best outcomes in clinical practice and in the literature (Fig. 24-15). Certainly, other lesions can also do well in this often challenging patient population. Although the results are far from optimal, outcomes with osteoarticular grafts compare favorably with those of other biologic resurfacing options in the treatment of larger defects.

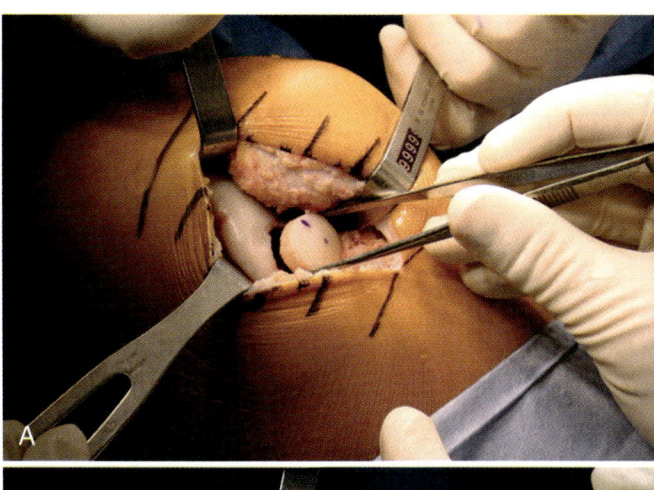

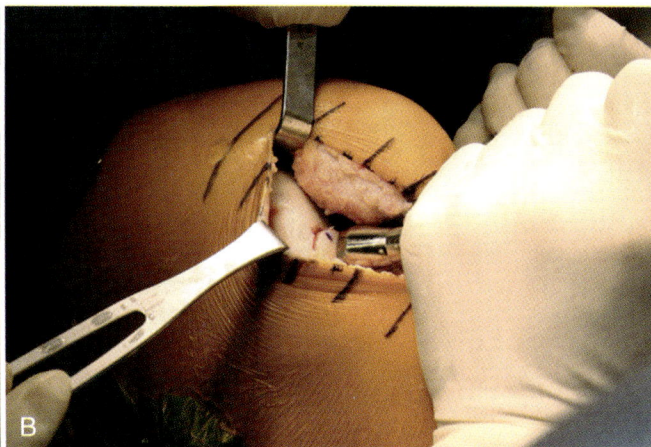

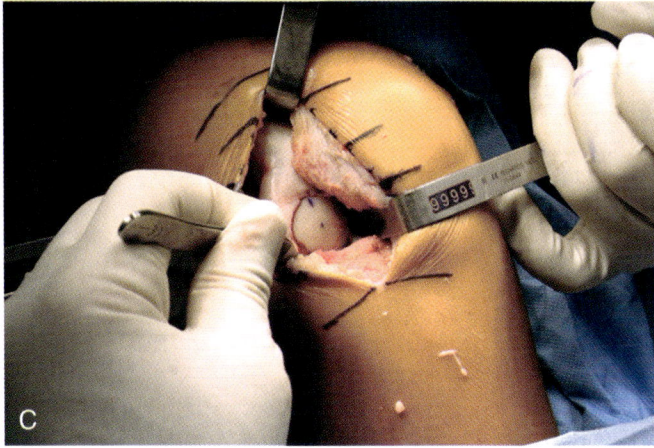

Figure 24-13. A, The graft is inserted by hand in the appropriate rotation and **(B)** is gently tamped into place. **C,** The osteochondral allograft in final position (press-fit plug technique).

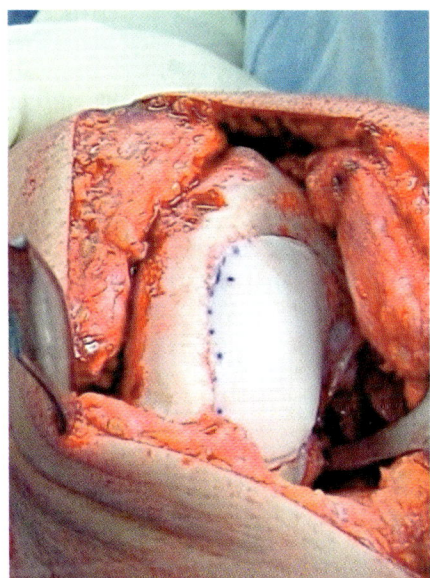

Figure 24-14. Photograph of shell allograft after implantation for a medial lesion.

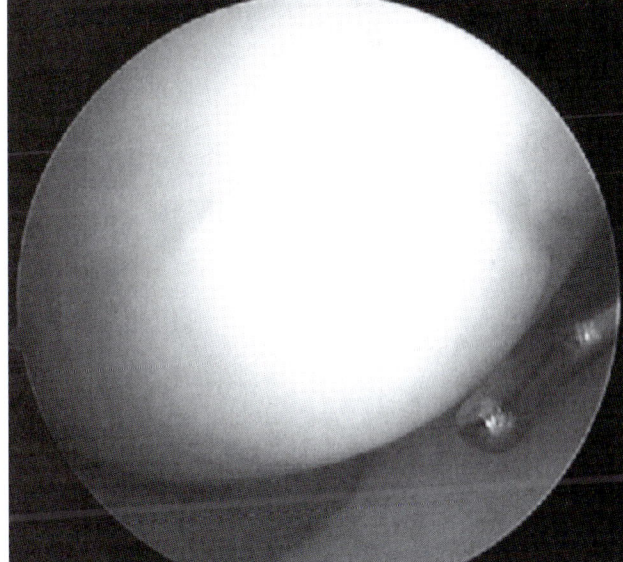

Figure 24-15. Arthroscopy photograph of fresh, refrigerated, osteochondral allograft plug of the medial femoral condyle 7 years postoperatively. The graft is well incorporated with maintenance of the hyaline cartilage.

Following is a summary of work by authors who have reported from large centers with vast allograft experience.

Emmerson et al reported a series of individuals with osteochondritis dissecans of the femoral condyle treated with fresh osteochondral allografts.[26] This series included 66 knees in 64 patients with average follow-up of 7.7 years (range, 2 to 22 years). In this series, the size of the lesions varied, and average size was 7.5 cm². Of 65 knees available for follow-up, 47 (72%) were rated good or excellent; 7 (11%) were rated fair; and 1 (2%) was rated poor. Ten patients (15%) underwent reoperation. The average clinical score improved from 13.0 preoperatively to 16.4 postoperatively on an 18-point scale ($P < .01$). Subjective knee function improved from a mean of 3.4 to 8.4 on a 10-point scale ($P < .01$).

Chu et al reported on 55 consecutive knees undergoing osteochondral allografting.[20] This study evaluated patients with a variety of diagnoses, including traumatic chondral injury, avascular necrosis, osteochondritis dissecans, and patellofemoral disease. Of 55 procedures, 43 were unipolar replacements, and 12 were bipolar resurfacing replacements. Among these knees, 42 of 55 (76%) were rated good to excellent, and 3 of 55 (5%) were rated fair. It is important to note that 84% of knees that underwent unipolar femoral grafting were rated good to excellent, and only 50% of knees with bipolar grafts achieved good or excellent status. No realignment osteotomies were reported in this series. Many patients who underwent unipolar replacement were allowed to return to recreational and competitive sports. McDermott et al reported on fresh osteochondral allografts implanted within 24 hours of harvest.[51] In this study, patients with a unifocal traumatic defect of the tibial plateau or femoral condyle had a 75% success rate after an average follow-up of 3.8 years. Patients with osteoarthritis and osteonecrosis fared worse, with failure rates of 58% and 79%, respectively.

Ghazavi et al reported on 126 knees in 123 patients with posttraumatic lesions of the distal femur at an average follow-up of 7.5 years.[32] Eighty-five percent of patients were rated as successful, while the remaining procedures failed. Factors related to failure included age over 50 years, bipolar defects, malalignment, and workers' compensation cases. Aubin et al later reported on the long-term results of these same allografts.[4] Kaplan-Meier survivorship analysis showed 85% graft survival at 10 years and 74% survival at 15 years. Patients with surviving grafts had HSS (Hospital for Special Surgery) scores of 83 points at 10-year follow-up. Radiographic analysis revealed that 52% of knees had moderate to severe arthritis at latest follow-up.

Garrett reported on his experience with the use of fresh osteochondral allografts with both press-fit and large shell techniques in the treatment of osteochondritis dissecans.[30,31] Six patients had undergone concomitant correctional osteotomy for angular malalignment of 5 degrees or greater. Patients were counseled to refrain from running and jumping sports postoperatively. Of 113 patients with follow-up ranging from 1 to 18 years, 103 (91%) reported that they were free of pain, stiffness, and swelling.[30] All 10 failures were due to fragmentation of the graft. McCulloch et al found 84% patient satisfaction in 25 consecutive patients who had undergone fresh, refrigerated, osteochondral allografting for the treatment of localized osteochondral defects of the femur. At an average of 3 years of follow-up, 79% of knees were functioning at the same level as unaffected knees.[50] Radiographically, 88% of the grafts had incorporated with the host bone surrounding the defect. Average IKDC (International Knee Documentation Committee) scores in this population improved from 29 preoperatively to 58 at follow-up.

Williams et al reported on 19 patients with an average age of 34 years who were treated with fresh stored allografts implanted an average of 30 days following procurement (range, 17 to 42 days).[75] Mean lesion size was 602 mm², and average follow-up was 48 months. MRI was used to assess the grafts at an average of 25 months following implantation.

Activities of daily living scale score increased from a baseline of 56 to 70 at the time of final follow-up. The mean Short Form-36 score increased from a baseline of 51 to 66 at the time of final follow-up. Normal articular cartilage thickness was preserved in 18 implanted grafts. Allograft cartilage signal properties were isointense relative to normal articular cartilage in 8 of the 18 grafts. Osseous trabecular incorporation of the allograft was complete or partial in 14 patients and poor in 4 patients. Complete or partial trabecular incorporation positively correlated with Short Form-36 scores at the time of follow-up.

LaPrade et al studied 23 consecutive patients who underwent osteoarticular grafting of focal articular cartilage defects of the femoral condyle using refrigerated grafts that were implanted an average of 20.3 days (range, 15 to 28 days) following procurement.[41] At an average follow-up of 3 years, investigators found an increase in mean IKDC score from 52 points to 68.5 points with good osseous incorporation into host bone. No graft failures were noted in this group. Davidson et al reported on 67 patients treated with massive osteoarticular allografts of the distal femur.[24] Grafts were stored in a cell culture medium at 4° C for 4 to 6 weeks before transplantation. Mean IKDC scores improved from 27 preoperatively to 79 postoperatively ($P = .002$). Ten knees underwent second-look arthroscopic evaluation and biopsy at a mean of 40 months (range, 23 to 60 months) after implantation. Mean graft and native cartilage cellular density and viability were not statistically different.

Jamali et al described the outcomes of 20 knees in 18 patients who were treated with fresh osteochondral allografting of the patellofemoral joint.[35] Bipolar grafting of the trochlea and the patella was performed in 12 patients, and isolated patellar lesions were treated in 8 patients. Five failures occurred, but the remaining knees showed improvement from 11.7 to 16.3 on an 18-point scale after surgery. Radiographically, four patients had no evidence of patellofemoral arthritis, and six patients had only mild arthrosis.

COMPLICATIONS

The most common complications after any knee arthrotomy include quadriceps inhibition, DVT, arthrofibrosis, synovitis, persistent knee pain, and superficial or deep surgical wound infection. Allograft-related complications include graft-related infection transmission, delayed graft union or nonunion, graft fragmentation and collapse, graft subsidence, and inflammatory-mediated pain. When present, most of these complications are treated in keeping with general practice guidelines. Some complications that are specific to allograft transplantation warrant specific discussion.

Local infection following the implantation of a fresh osteochondral allograft is rare, but its consequences can be devastating. It is critical to differentiate deep infection from superficial infection with the use of physical examination findings and joint aspiration. Although deep infection following allograft implantation is more likely related to the surgical procedure than to graft transmission, management of the infection, once recognized, is the same.[19] Deep infections involving the allograft need to be addressed immediately and aggressively. Death in the immediate postoperative period has resulted from implantation of a contaminated fresh osteochondral graft.[60] We recommend removal of the allograft in the setting of a deep infection because the tissue may be the source of infection, or the donor bone may serve as a nidus for a deep surgical infection. Patients considering fresh osteochondral allograft transplant need to be informed of the infection risk preoperatively and counseled to look for signs of infection before the time of discharge from the hospital.

Although delayed union and nonunion are always possible, problems with donor–host bone healing are actually rare. This complication is more common in larger bulk allografts or in the setting of compromised bone at the recipient site. Complete healing occasionally may take a more extended period of time and may alter the postoperative activity level. MRI or computed tomography (CT) may assist in diagnosis in the setting of clinical suspicion, but these are not necessarily performed as part of routine follow-up after surgery.[75]

Graft fragmentation or collapse is a complication that may occur months to years after surgery.[30] Fragmentation and collapse of nonvascularized allograft bone is a much more common cause of graft failure than problems with the cartilage component of the allograft. In fact, cartilage-related complications of the allograft are rare in short- to medium-term follow-up. Patients with graft fragmentation or collapse typically present with new-onset pain or mechanical symptoms. Radiographs may show graft fragmentation or collapse, joint space narrowing, cyst formation, or mixed sclerotic regions. MRI typically shows areas of graft collapse and edema. However, care must be taken in interpreting postoperative allograft MRI images because even asymptomatic, well-functioning osteochondral allografts may demonstrate significant signal abnormalities.

Allograft subsidence can be a unique problem after this procedure. According to some reports, many grafts subside by 1 to 3 mm, but up to 30% may subside up to 4 to 5 mm.[48] Other authors have not regarded subsidence as a significant problem.[75] As long as frank collapse does not occur, most of these patients are relatively asymptomatic and can be observed.[48] Whether from subsidence, fragmentation, or collapse, individual patient and specific graft considerations must be taken into account when treatment options for a failed osteochondral allograft are evaluated. In some cases, it is not unreasonable to expect a successful result from repeat fresh allograft transplantation. When degenerative arthritic changes prohibit revision allograft transplant, and when symptoms warrant intervention, unicompartmental or total knee arthroplasty is often the best salvage option.

Persistent pain following graft implantation may be multifactorial; therefore, it may be difficult to elucidate the specific cause. Some patients with pain beyond what is considered "normal" have a low-grade inflammatory reaction related to the transplanted graft. An immune response to fresh osteochondral allografts has been observed in some individuals, as shown by the development of anti–human leukocyte antigen (HLA) antibodies.[65] The clinical consequences of this finding, however, are unclear. Histologic evaluation of failed fresh allografts has not revealed evidence of immune-mediated rejection.[54] Although immunosuppression is not required, a subset of patients may produce a more significant inflammatory reaction, which may be an underlying cause of low-grade discomfort and pain. At this time, however, this hypothesis is without scientific evidence, and additional study is required.

CONCLUSIONS AND RECOMMENDATIONS

Cartilage and osteochondral injuries in young active individuals who are not candidates for arthroplasty procedures present a challenge to orthopedic surgeons. Symptomatic smaller lesions can often be treated successfully with alternative approaches such as débridement, microfracture, and autograft transfer procedures. However, when clinical failure occurs in this setting, revision with a fresh allograft can often lead to a successful outcome. We have found this to be especially true following marrow-stimulating techniques in high-activity individuals. Larger chondral or osteochondral defects (>2 cm^2) often benefit from osteochondral allograft transplantation as the primary treatment. Although autologous chondrocyte implantation (ACI) may also be a reasonable option in some patients, we have found fresh allografts to yield more reliable results on the femoral condyle and tibia. As a result, we currently consider the use of ACI only for the patellofemoral compartment.

Significant advantages and disadvantages are associated with the use of allograft tissue. Advantages when compared with alternative treatment options include lack of donor site morbidity, the ability to treat large defects including associated subchondral bone deficiency or pathology, and the ability to reliably restore viable hyaline cartilage. Disadvantages include supply issues and costs and the logistics of delivering an aseptic, size-matched graft with a high percentage of viable chondrocytes. Many clinical and basic scientific studies support the theoretical foundation and efficacy of osteochondral allografting. The surgical technique for most femoral condyle lesions is fairly straightforward with large dowel instrumentation systems. Other techniques are more demanding but can still be used with success. Enhanced understanding and advances in graft procurement and storage, refinement of indications, and progress made in surgical techniques should continue to improve clinical outcomes in this challenging patient population.

KEY REFERENCES

Aubin PP, Cheah HK, Davis AM, Gross AE: Long-term follow up of fresh femoral osteochondral allografts for posttraumatic knee defects. Clin Orthop 391S:S318–S327, 2001.

Bugbee WD: Fresh osteochondral allografting. Oper Tech Sports Med 8:58–162, 2000.

Chu CR, Convery FR, Akeson WH, et al: Articular cartilage transplantation—clinical results in the knee. Clin Orthop Relat Res 360:159–168, 1999.

Cole BJ, Farr J: Putting it all together. Oper Tech Orthop 11:151–154, 2001.

Davidson PA, Rivenburgh DW, Dawson PE, Rozin R: Clinical, histologic, and radiographic outcomes of distal femoral resurfacing with hypothermically stored osteoarticular allografts. Am J Sports Med 35:1082–1090, 2007.

Garrett J, Wyman J: The operative technique of fresh osteochondral allografting of the knee. Oper Tech Orthop 11:132–137, 2001.

Gross AE, Kim W, Las Heras F, et al: Fresh osteochondral allografts for posttraumatic knee defects: long-term followup. Clin Orthop Relat Res 466:1863–1870, 2008.

Jamali AA, Emmerson BC, Chung C, et al: Fresh osteochondral allografts: results in the patellofemoral joint. Clin Orthop Relat Res 437:176–185, 2005.

LaPrade RF, Botker J, Herzog M, Agel J: Refrigerated osteoarticular allografts to treat articular cartilage defects of the femoral condyles: a prospective outcomes study. J Bone Joint Surg Am 91:805–811, 2009.

Malinin T, Temple HT, Buck BE: Transplantation of osteochondral allografts after cold storage. J Bone Joint Surg Am 88:762–770, 2006.

McCulloch PC, Kang RW, Sobhy MH, et al: Prospective evaluation of prolonged fresh osteochondral allograft transplantation of the femoral condyle: minimum 2-year follow-up. Am J Sports Med 35:411–420, 2007.

McDermott AG, Langer F, Pritzker PH, Gross AE: Fresh small-fragment osteochondral allografts: long term follow-up study on first one hundred cases. Clin Orthop 197:96–102, 1985.

Pearsall AW, 4th, Tucker JA, Hester RB, Heitman RJ: Chondrocyte viability in refrigerated osteochondral allografts used for transplantation within the knee. Am J Sports Med 32:125–131, 2004.

Williams RJ, 3rd, Ranawat AS, Potter HG, et al: Fresh stored allografts for the treatment of osteochondral defects of the knee. J Bone Joint Surg Am 89:718–726, 2007.

Williams SK, Amiel D, Ball ST, et al: Analysis of cartilage tissue on a cellular level in fresh osteochondral allograft retrievals. Am J Sports Med 35:2022–2032, 2007.

Full references for this chapter can be found on www.expertconsult.com.

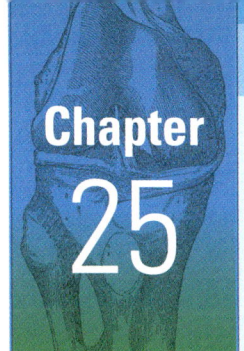

Débridement and Microfracture for Full-Thickness Articular Cartilage Defects

J. Richard Steadman, William G. Rodkey, and Karen K. Briggs

BACKGROUND

Full-thickness articular cartilage defects in the knee are common, and the lesions may present in a variety of clinical settings and at different ages.[11] A single event, the shearing forces of the femur on the tibia, may result in trauma to the articular cartilage, causing the cartilage to fracture, lacerate, and separate from the underlying subchondral bone or to separate with a piece of the subchondral bone. Alternatively, chronic repetitive loading in excess of normal physiologic levels may result in the fatigue and failure of the articular surface, especially in the presence of meniscus deficiency or axial malalignment. The single events are usually found in younger groups, whereas chronic degenerative lesions are seen in the middle-aged and older groups. It has been shown that repetitive impacts can cause cartilage swelling, an increase in collagen fiber diameter, and an alteration in the relationship between collagen and proteoglycans. Thus, acute events may not result in full-thickness cartilage loss but rather start a degenerative cascade that can lead to chronic full-thickness loss. The degenerative cascade typically includes early softening and fibrillation (grade I), fissures and cracks in the surface of the cartilage (grade II), severe fissures and cracks with a "crab meat" appearance (grade III) and, finally, exposure of the subchondral bone (grade IV).

Articular cartilage defects that extend full thickness to subchondral bone rarely heal without intervention.[13-18,21] Some patients may not develop clinically significant problems from acute full-thickness chondral defects, but most eventually suffer from degenerative changes that can be debilitating. Techniques used to treat chondral defects include marrow stimulation, osteochondral autografts, osteochondral allografts, and autologous cell transplantation. The senior author (JRS) developed the microfracture technique to enhance chondral resurfacing by providing a suitable environment for new tissue formation and taking advantage of the body's own healing potential. The senior author's clinical experience now includes more than 3500 patients in whom microfracture has been done.

We have found that arthroscopic débridement accompanied by microfracture of subchondral bone is a reliable and repeatable procedure to stimulate biologic repair of cartilage defects of the knee in patients in whom nonoperative treatment has failed or in whom acute lesions were encountered during arthroscopy. Thus, more invasive procedures, such as osteotomy, cartilage grafting, or unicompartmental arthroplasty, might be avoided or at least delayed for several years. Specifically, the goals of this procedure are to alleviate the pain and attendant disabilities that result from the chondral lesions and also to prevent late degenerative changes in the joint by restoring the joint surface.[13,15]

Indications for Microfracture

Microfracture was developed initially for patients with post-traumatic articular cartilage lesions of the knee that had progressed to full-thickness chondral defects. The microfracture technique still is most commonly indicated for full-thickness loss of articular cartilage in either a weight-bearing area between the femur and tibia or in an area of contact between the patella and trochlear groove.[13-18] Unstable cartilage that overlies the subchondral bone is also an indication for microfracture. If a partial-thickness lesion is probed and the cartilage simply scrapes off down to bone, we consider this to be a full-thickness lesion. Degenerative joint disease in a knee that has proper axial alignment is another common indication for microfracture. These lesions all involve loss of articular cartilage at the bone-cartilage interface.

Patients with acute chondral injuries are treated as soon as practical after the diagnosis is made, especially if the knee is being treated concurrently for meniscus or anterior cruciate ligament pathology. Patients with chronic or degenerative chondral lesions often are treated nonoperatively (conservatively) for at least 12 weeks after a suspected chondral lesion is diagnosed clinically. This treatment regimen includes activity modification, physical therapy, nonsteroidal anti-inflammatory drugs, joint injections, and perhaps dietary supplements that may have cartilage-stimulating properties. If nonoperative treatment is not successful, surgical treatment is considered.[13-18]

No limitations are placed on how large an acute lesion can be and still be considered suitable for microfracture.[15,18] We have observed that even very large acute lesions respond well to microfracture.[13] We have noted empirically that traumatic lesions, acute or chronic, smaller than 400 mm^2 tend to respond better to microfracture than those lesions larger than 400 mm^2, but we have not observed this difference to be statistically significant.[12] Treatment of chronic degenerative lesions is not specifically limited by size, but more emphasis is placed on proper axial alignment and the presence of global degenerative changes throughout the knee.

General considerations for the use of the microfracture procedure include patient age, acceptable biomechanical alignment of the knee, patient's activity level, and patient's expectations.[12-17] If all these criteria define a patient who could benefit from chondral resurfacing, then microfracture is considered.

Contraindications for Microfracture

Specific contraindications for microfracture include axial malalignment (see later), patients unwilling or unable to follow the required strict and rigorous rehabilitation protocol, partial-thickness defects, and inability to use the opposite leg for weight bearing during the minimal or non–weight-bearing time.[15,16] Other specific contraindications include any systemic immune-mediated disease, disease-induced arthritis, or cartilage disease. A relative contraindication is for patients older than 65 years because we have observed that some patients older than 65 years experience difficulty with crutch walking and the required rigorous rehabilitation. Other contraindications to microfracture include global degenerative osteoarthrosis or the cartilage surrounding the lesion is too thin to establish a perpendicular rim to hold the marrow clot.[12] In these advanced degenerative cases, axial malalignment often is also a confounding factor.

Two methods for radiographic measurement of the biomechanical alignment of the weight-bearing axis of the knee are used in our facility: (1) the angle made between the femur and tibia on anteroposterior (AP) views obtained with the patient standing; and (2) the weight-bearing mechanical axis drawn from the center of the femoral head to the center of the tibiotarsal joint on long standing (~51 inch [130 cm]) radiographs. If the angle drawn between the tibia and femur is greater than 5 degrees of varus or valgus compared with the normal knee, this amount of axial malalignment would be a relative contraindication for microfracture. Preferably, the mechanical axis weight-bearing line should be in the central 25% of the tibial plateau of the medial or lateral compartment. If the mechanical axis weight-bearing line falls outside the centralmost 25% of the plateaus, medial or lateral, this weight-bearing shift also would be a relative contraindication if left uncorrected. In such cases, a realignment procedure should be included as part of the overall treatment regimen.[12,13]

PREOPERATIVE PLANNING

Patients who present with knee joint pain undergo a thorough physical and orthopedic examination. The chondral lesions can be on the joint surfaces of the femur, tibia, and/or patella. At times, the physical diagnosis can be difficult and elusive, especially if only an isolated chondral defect is present. Identification of point tenderness over a femoral condyle or tibial plateau is a useful finding, but is not in itself diagnostic. If compression of the patella elicits pain, this finding might be indicative of a patellar or trochlear lesion.

For diagnostic imaging, we use long standing radiographs, as described earlier, to observe for angular deformity and for joint space narrowing, which is often indicative of loss of articular cartilage. We also obtain standard AP and lateral radiographs of both knees as well as weight-bearing views with the knees flexed 30 to 45 degrees. Axial patellar views are also useful to evaluate the patellofemoral joint. Magnetic resonance imaging (MRI) that uses newer diagnostic sequences specific for articular cartilage has become a mainstay of our diagnostic workup of patients with suspected chondral lesions. A 3-T MRI scanner adds to the diagnostic accuracy.

SURGICAL TECHNIQUE

Three portals are routinely made about the knee for use of the inflow cannula, the arthroscope, and the working instruments. We typically do not use a tourniquet during the microfracture procedure; rather, we vary the arthroscopic fluid

pump pressure to control bleeding. An initial, thorough, diagnostic examination of the knee should be done. We carefully inspect all geographic areas of the knee, including the suprapatellar pouch, the medial and lateral gutters, the patellofemoral joint, the intercondylar notch and its contents, the anterior interval between the patellar tendon and tibia, and the medial and lateral compartments, including the posterior horns of both menisci. We do all other intra-articular procedures before doing the microfracture. This technique helps prevent loss of visualization when the fat droplets and blood enter the knee from the microfracture holes, and the marrow clot is less likely to be dislodged. Importantly, we pay particular attention to soft tissues such as plicae and the lateral retinaculum, which potentially could produce increased compression between cartilage surfaces.[13-18]

After carefully assessing the full thickness articular cartilage lesion, we débride the exposed bone of all remaining unstable cartilage. We use a hand-held curved curette and a full-radius resector to débride the cartilage. It is critical to débride all loose or marginally attached cartilage from the surrounding rim of the lesion. The calcified cartilage layer that remains as a cap to many lesions must be removed, preferably by using a curette. Thorough and complete removal of the calcified cartilage layer is extremely important based on animal studies we have completed.[2,3] Care should be taken to maintain the integrity of the subchondral plate by not débriding too deeply. This prepared lesion, with a stable perpendicular edge of healthy, well-attached, viable cartilage surrounding the defect, provides a pool that helps hold the marrow clot (or *superclot*, as we have termed it) as it forms (Fig. 25-1).[15]

After preparation of the lesion, we use an arthroscopic awl to make multiple holes, or microfractures, in the exposed subchondral bone plate. We use an awl with an angle that permits the tip to be perpendicular to the bone as it is advanced, typically 30 or 45 degrees. There also is a 90-degree awl that typically is used only on the patella or other soft

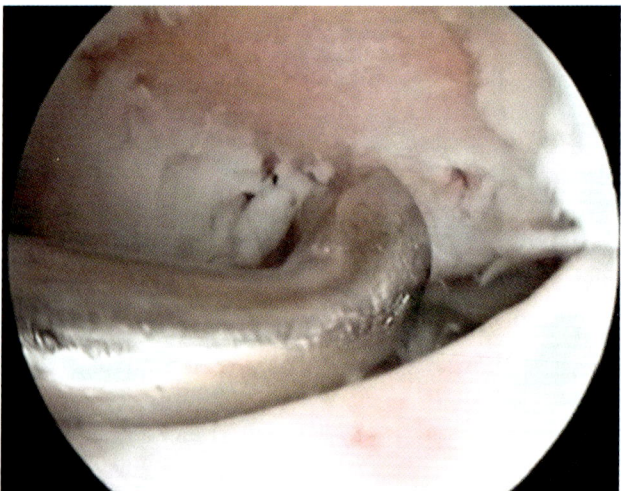

Figure 25-1. A curette is used to remove the calcified cartilage layer of a full-thickness chondral defect. Damaged cartilage has been débrided to form a stable perpendicular edge of healthy cartilage. (From Steadman JR, Rodkey WG, Briggs KK: Microfracture chondroplasty: indications, techniques, and outcomes. Sports Med Arthrosc Rev 11:236–244, 2003.)

bone. The 90-degree awl should only be advanced manually, not with a mallet. The holes are made as close together as possible, but not so close that one breaks into another, thus damaging the subchondral plate between them. This technique usually results in microfracture holes that are approximately 3 to 4 mm apart. When fat droplets can be seen coming from the marrow cavity, the appropriate depth ($\approx$2 to 4 mm) has been reached. The arthroscopic awls likely produce essentially no thermal necrosis of the bone compared with hand-driven or motorized drills. We make microfracture holes around the periphery of the defect first, immediately adjacent to the healthy stable cartilage rim (Fig. 25-2). Then we complete the process by making the microfracture holes toward the center of the defect (Fig. 25-3). We assess the treated lesion at the conclusion of the microfracture to ensure that a sufficient number of holes have been made before we reduce the arthroscopic irrigation fluid flow (Fig. 25-4). After the arthroscopic irrigation fluid pump pressure is reduced, we are able to observe under direct visualization the release of marrow fat droplets and blood from the microfracture holes into the subchondral bone. We judge the quantity of marrow contents flowing into the joint to be adequate when we observe marrow emanating from all microfracture holes (Fig. 25-5). We then remove all instruments from the knee and evacuate the joint of fluid.[15,16] Intra-articular drains should not be used because the goal is for the surgically induced marrow clot, rich in marrow elements, to form and stabilize while covering the lesion.[2,3]

Chronic degenerative chondral lesions commonly have extensive eburnated bone and bony sclerosis, with thickening of the subchondral plate,[6,12] thus making it difficult to carry out an adequate microfracture procedure. In these cases, and when the axial alignment and other indications for microfracture have been met, we first make a few microfracture holes with the awls in various locations of the lesion to assess

the thickness of the subchondral plate. We often use a motorized burr to remove the sclerotic bone until punctate bleeding is seen. After the bleeding appears uniformly over the surface of the lesion, a microfracture procedure can be performed as previously described.[12,15] We have observed noticeably improved results for these patients with chronic chondral lesions since we began using this technique. However, if the surrounding cartilage is too thin to establish a perpendicular rim to hold the marrow clot, we likely would not do a

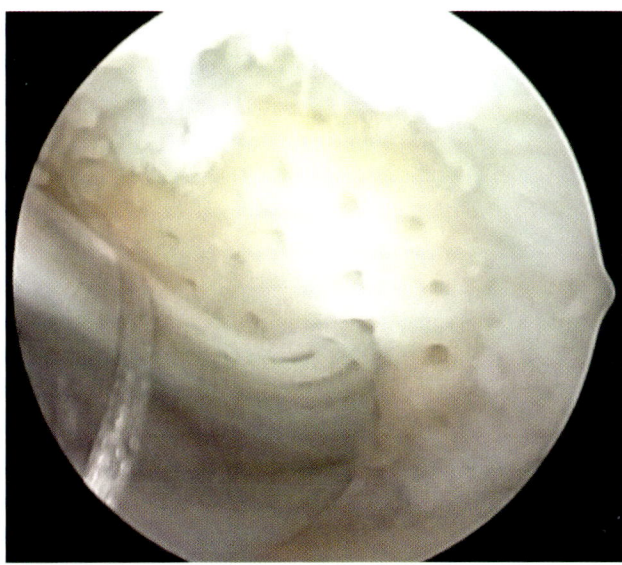

Figure 25-3. Microfracture holes are continued into the central portion of the defect. The microfracture awl is penetrating the subchondral bone approximately 2 to 4 mm in depth. (From Steadman JR, Rodkey WG, Briggs KK: Microfracture chondroplasty: indications, techniques, and outcomes. Sports Med Arthrosc Rev 11:236–244, 2003.)

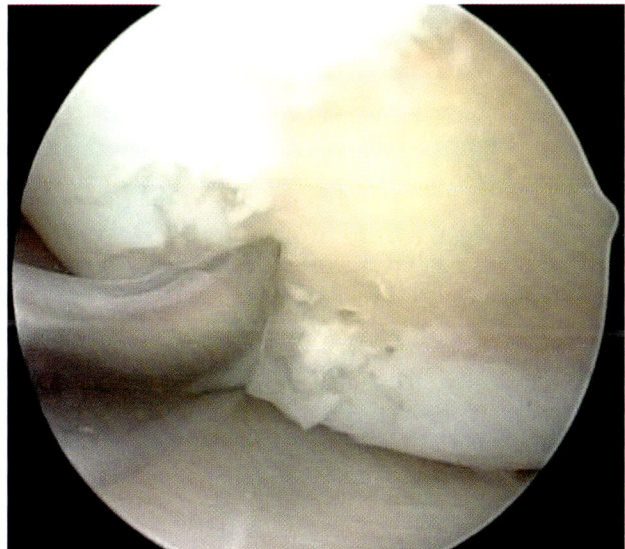

Figure 25-2. A chondral defect has been débrided and is being microfractured. The microfracture holes are started at the periphery of the defect adjacent to the stable cartilage. (From Steadman JR, Rodkey WG, Briggs KK: Microfracture chondroplasty: indications, techniques, and outcomes. Sports Med Arthrosc Rev 11:236–244, 2003.)

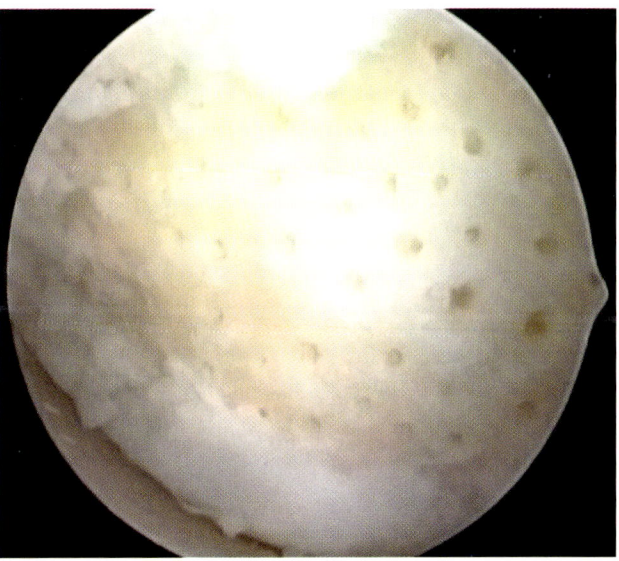

Figure 25-4. The microfracture procedure has been completed. Note the proximity of the microfracture holes, usually no more than 3 to 4 mm apart. (From Steadman JR, Rodkey WG, Briggs KK: Microfracture chondroplasty: indications, techniques, and outcomes. Sports Med Arthrosc Rev 11:236–244, 2003.)

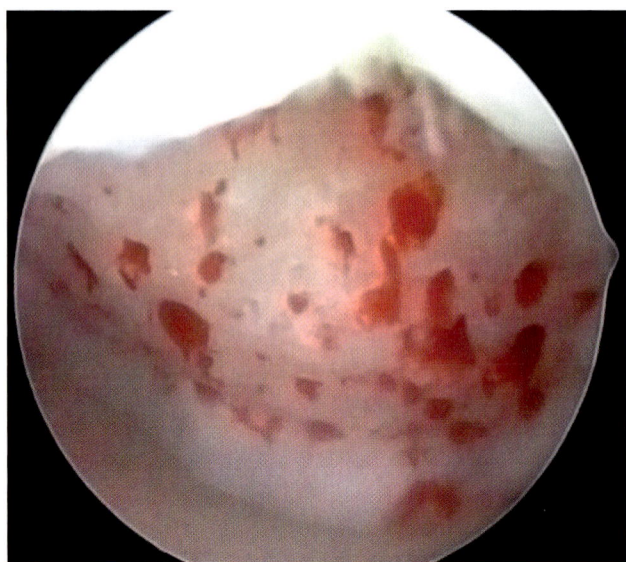

Figure 25-5. Marrow elements, including blood and fat droplets, accessed by the subchondral bone microfracture can be seen coming from essentially all the microfracture holes after the arthroscopic irrigation fluid pressure has been reduced. (From Steadman JR, Rodkey WG, Briggs KK: Microfracture chondroplasty: indications, techniques, and outcomes. Sports Med Arthrosc Rev 11:236–244, 2003.)

microfracture procedure in patients with such advanced degenerative lesions.

The microfracture awl produces a rough surface in the subchondral bone to which the marrow clot can adhere more easily, yet the integrity of the subchondral plate is maintained for joint surface shape. The microfracture procedure almost eliminates thermal necrosis and provides a roughened surface for blood clot adherence, and the different angles of arthroscopic awls available provide easier access to difficult to reach areas of the knee. The awls not only provide perpendicular holes but also improved control of depth penetration compared with drilling. We believe that the key to the entire procedure is to establish the marrow clot to provide the optimal environment for the body's own pluripotential marrow cells (mesenchymal stem cells or progenitor cells) to differentiate into stable tissue within the lesion.[2,3]

POSTOPERATIVE MANAGEMENT

We have designed the postoperative program to promote the ideal physical environment in which the newly recruited mesenchymal stem cells from the marrow can differentiate into the appropriate articular cartilage-like cell lines.[4,13-17] These differentiation and maturation processes must occur slowly but consistently.[5] Our animal studies have confirmed that cellular and molecular changes are an essential part of the development of a durable repair tissue.[2,3]

Our patients are counseled carefully so they understand that they likely will not start to experience improvement in their knees for at least 6 months after microfracture. Our experience and clinical research data indicate that improvement can be expected to occur slowly and steadily for at least 2 years.[13,15,17] During this protracted period, the repair tissue matures, pain and swelling resolve, and the patients regain confidence and comfort in their knees during increased levels of activity.[13]

REHABILITATION

The rehabilitation program after microfracture for treatment of chondral defects in the knee should be followed closely and is crucial to optimize the results of the surgery.[13] The rehabilitation protocol promotes the optimal physical environment for the mesenchymal stem cells to differentiate and produce new extracellular matrix that eventually matures into a durable repair tissue. The surgically induced marrow clot provides the basis for the most ideal chemical environment to complement the physical environment.[2,3] This newly proliferated repair cartilage then fills the original defect.

The postoperative rehabilitation program after microfracture necessitates consideration of several factors. The specific protocol recommended depends on the anatomic location and size of the defect. These factors are critical to determine the ideal postoperative plan. For example, if other intra-articular procedures are done concurrently with microfracture, such as anterior cruciate ligament reconstruction, we do not hesitate to alter the rehabilitation program as necessary. All the possible variations of the rehabilitation program are not within the scope of this chapter, but in the following paragraphs we describe two different protocols.

Rehabilitation Protocol for Patients With Lesions on the Femoral Condyle or Tibial Plateau

After microfracture of lesions on the weight-bearing surfaces of the femoral condyles or tibial plateaus, we commence immediately with a continuous passive motion (CPM) machine in the recovery room. The initial range of motion (ROM) typically is 30 to 70 degrees, which is increased as tolerated by 10 to 20 degrees until full passive ROM is achieved. The rate of the machine is usually one cycle/min, but the rate can be varied based on patient preference and comfort. Many patients tolerate use of the CPM machine at night. For those who do not, we have observed that intermittent use during the day likely is as beneficial. Regardless of when the CPM machine is used, the goal is to have the patient in the CPM machine for 6 to 8 hours every 24 hours. If the patient is unable to use the CPM machine, then instructions are given for passive flexion and extension of the knee, with 500 repetitions three times daily. We encourage patients to gain full passive ROM of the injured knee as soon as possible after surgery.

We also prescribe cold therapy for all patients postoperatively. Our experience and observations indicate that the cold helps control pain and inflammation, and most patients state that the cold provides overall postoperative discomfort relief. Cold therapy is generally used for 1 to 7 days postoperatively.

We prescribe crutch-assisted, touch-down, weight-bearing ambulation for 6 to 8 weeks, depending on the size of the lesion. For most patients, 6 to 8 weeks seems an adequate time to limit weight bearing. However, for patients with small lesions (<1 cm diameter), weight bearing may be hastened by a few weeks. Patients with lesions on the femoral condyles or tibial plateaus rarely use a brace during the initial postoperative period. However, we now prescribe an unloading-type brace when the patient becomes more active and the postoperative swelling has resolved.

We begin mobilization immediately after surgery with an emphasis on knee ROM and patella and patellar tendon mobility. Patients are touch-down weight bearing, with 10% of their body weight on their injured leg during weight bearing. They begin stationary biking without resistance and a deep water exercise program at 1 to 2 weeks after microfracture. The deep water exercises include use of a flotation vest for deep water running. It is critical and imperative that the foot of the injured leg does not touch the bottom of the pool during this exercise. Patients progress to full weight bearing after approximately 8 weeks and begin more vigorous biking with increasing resistance. They also begin knee flexion exercises at approximately 8 weeks after microfracture. An elastic resistance cord is added to the exercise regimen at about 12 weeks. A detailed description of use of the cord and the exercises has been published.[4] Our observations indicate that the ability to achieve predetermined maximum levels for sets and repetitions of elastic resistance cord exercises is an excellent indicator for progressing to weight training. We permit free or machine weights when the patient has achieved the early goals of the rehabilitation program, but not before 16 weeks after microfracture. We strongly emphasize the importance of proper technique when beginning a weight program. Depending on the clinical examination, size of the patient, sport, and size of the lesion, we usually recommend that patients do not return to sports that involve pivoting, cutting, and jumping until at least 4 to 9 months after microfracture.

Rehabilitation Protocol for Patients with Patellofemoral Lesions

All patients treated by microfracture for patellofemoral lesions must use a brace set at 0 to 20 degrees for at least 8 weeks. The brace limits compression of the regenerating surfaces of the trochlea or patella, or both. We allow passive motion with the brace removed, but otherwise the brace must be worn at all times. Patients with patellofemoral lesions are placed into a continuous CPM machine immediately postoperatively. We also use cold therapy, as described earlier. With this regimen, patients typically obtain a pain-free and full passive ROM soon after surgery.

For patients with patellofemoral joint lesions, we carefully observe joint angles at the time of arthroscopy to determine where the defect comes into contact with the patellar facet or the trochlear groove. We make certain to avoid these areas during strength training for approximately 4 months. This avoidance allows for training in the 0- to 20-degree range immediately postoperatively because there is minimal compression of these chondral surfaces with such limited motion.

Patients with lesions of the patellofemoral joint treated by microfracture are allowed weight bearing as tolerated in their brace 2 weeks after surgery. It is essential for patients to use a brace that prevents placing excessive shear force on the maturing marrow clot in the early postoperative period. We routinely lock the brace between 0 and 20 degrees ROM to prevent flexion past the point where the median ridge of the patella engages the trochlear groove. After 8 weeks, we open

the knee brace gradually before it is discontinued. When the brace is discontinued, patients are allowed to advance their training progressively. Stationary biking is allowed 2 weeks postoperatively, and increased resistance is added at 8 weeks after microfracture. Starting 12 weeks after microfracture, the exercise program is the same as that used for femorotibial lesions.

POTENTIAL COMPLICATIONS FROM MICROFRACTURE

In our experience, most patients progress through the postoperative period with little or no difficulty.[13-18] However, some patients present with mild transient pain, most frequently after microfracture in the patellofemoral joint. Small changes in the articular surface of the patellofemoral joint may be detected by a grating or gritty sensation of the joint, especially when a patient discontinues use of the knee brace and begins normal weight bearing through a full ROM. Patients rarely complain of pain at this time, and this grating sensation usually resolves spontaneously in a few days or weeks.

Similarly, if a steep perpendicular rim was made in the trochlear groove, patients may notice catching or locking as the apex of the patella rides over this lesion during joint motion. Some patients may even perceive these symptoms while in the CPM machine. These symptoms usually dissipate within 3 months. If this perceived locking is painful, the patient is advised to limit weight bearing and avoid the symptomatic joint angle for an additional period.

Swelling and joint effusion typically resolve within 8 weeks after microfracture. Occasionally, a recurrent effusion develops between 6 and 8 weeks after microfracture, usually when a patient begins to bear weight on the injured leg after microfracture of a defect on the femoral condyle. Although this effusion may mimic the preoperative or immediate postoperative effusion, it is usually painless. We treat this type of painless effusion conservatively. It generally resolves within several weeks after onset. A second arthroscopy has rarely been required for recurring effusions.

PATIENT OUTCOMES

Database Management

The Steadman Philippon Research Institute clinical research database currently has data on over 17,000 knee operative procedures. Of these surgical procedures, 3500 knees underwent microfracture by the senior author (JRS; Table 25-1). Information in this database includes preoperative physician and patient subjective assessment, findings at arthroscopy and treatments, and postoperative physician and patient subjective assessments. At the time of first examination, patients are asked to complete a self-administered questionnaire. They are then sent the questionnaire annually for evaluation of symptoms, function, return to sports, activities of daily living, and satisfaction. All patient information is stored anonymously in a relationship database. Database files are linked and queried to obtain the desired data. Data analysis is performed using an SPSS statistical software package (SPSS, Chicago). All statistics are reviewed by an independent statistician.

Table 25-1 Distribution of Locations of Grade IV Chondral Lesions Treated With Microfracture*

Area	Patients (%)
MFC	17
LFC	8
MTP	4
LTP	4
TG	15
PAT	6
MFC and MTP	16
LFC and LTP	12
TG and PAT	4
Other	14

LFC, Lateral femoral condyle; *LTP*, lateral tibial plateau; *MFC*, medial femoral condyle; *MTP*, medial tibial plateau; *PAT*, patella; *TG*, trochlear groove.

*Steadman Hawkins clinical research database, *N* > 3600.

Outcome Measures

Lysholm Score

Knee function in our database is measured using the Lysholm score. The scale of Lysholm and Gillquist is a condition-specific score that consists of eight domains related to function of the knee—walking with a limp, support, locking, instability, pain, swelling, stair climbing, and squatting.[10] Pain and instability receive the highest point allocation followed by locking, swelling, and stair climbing. A total score of 95 to 100 points is associated with normal function, 84 to 94 points indicates symptoms related to vigorous activity, and less than 84 points suggests symptoms related to activities of daily living. The Lysholm score has been widely used for various disorders of the knee, and our group has validated it for use with chondral disorders of the knee.[9]

Kocher and colleagues have determined the reliability, validity, and responsiveness of the Lysholm score.[9] These psychometric properties were analyzed in a group of 1657 patients with chondral disorders of the knee. Test-retest, which entailed the same patient completing the questionnaire twice within 4 weeks, determined the reproducibility of the score between patients, or the reliability. Validity of the score, which included content validity, criterion validity, and construct validity, was also measured. To determine whether the score can assess change, the responsiveness was determined. This study showed that the overall Lysholm score performs acceptably for the assessment of outcomes following treatment of chondral disorders. Some individual domains of the score, however, did not perform as well.

Tegner Activity Scale

Activity level in our database is measured with the use of the Tegner activity scale.[20] With the Tegner scale, a numeric value, 0 to 10, is assigned to specific activities. An activity level of 10 corresponds to competitive sports, including soccer, football, and rugby at the elite level, an activity level of 6 corresponds to recreational sports, and a level of 0 corresponds to a person on sick leave or disability pension because of knee problems. Activity levels of 5 to 10 can be achieved only if the patient participates in recreational or competitive sports. The Tegner activity scale is easy to use; however, not all sports are represented in the categories.

Western Ontario and McMaster University Osteoarthritis Index

In studies documenting the outcomes of patients with osteoarthritis of the knee, we use the WOMAC score in addition to other scores. The Western Ontario and McMaster University Osteoarthritis Index (WOMAC) is a general musculoskeletal instrument for patients who have osteoarthritis of the hip or knee.[1] It has been validated in randomized clinical trials and has been shown to be a responsive tool in measuring outcomes following treatments for osteoarthritis of the knee. The WOMAC has three domains: pain (five items), stiffness (two items), and physical functioning (17 items). The questions are ranked on a five-point Likert scale: 0 = none, 1 = slight, 2 = moderate, 3 = severe, and 4 = extreme. The score is reported as the sum of the scores for each domain.

Patient Satisfaction

As health care becomes more patient-driven, assessing patient satisfaction is a major objective of our data collection. Our objectives are to evaluate patient satisfaction with outcomes of treatment and to identify parameters that are related to such satisfaction. With determinants of patient satisfaction from these studies, we can identify the elements that are most important to the patients following surgery. We determine satisfaction with outcomes of treatment on a scale of 1 to 10, with 10 being very satisfied and 1 being very dissatisfied.

Results of Microfracture

In 2003, the first long-term outcomes paper was published on the microfracture technique.[13] This study followed 72 patients an average of 11 years following microfracture, with the longest follow-up being 17 years. This study only included knees with no joint space narrowing, no degenerative arthritis, and no ligament or meniscus pathology which required treatment. All patients were younger than 45 years. The microfracture technique used on these patients did not include recent improvements to the technique (see earlier). With a 95% follow-up rate, the results showed improvement in symptoms and function. Patient reported pain and swelling decreased at postoperative year 1 and continued to decrease at year 2, and the clinical improvements were maintained over the study period. The study identified age as the only independent predictor of Lysholm improvement. Patients older than 35 years improved less than patient younger than 35; however, both groups showed improvement.

One study has compared the outcomes of autologous chondrocyte implantation (ACI) with microfracture treatment in a randomized trial.[8] Forty patients were treated in each group. At 2 years, both groups showed significant improvement in Lysholm scores and pain, with no difference between the groups. However, the microfracture group had more improvement in the Short Form (36) Health Survey (SF-36) physical component score. A high physical functioning score corresponds to a person who performs all types of physical activities, including the most vigorous ones, without limitations because of health. The authors theorized that this difference may be to the result of the fact that microfracture is one arthroscopic procedure compared with ACI that requires one arthroscopic and one open procedure. This study also found age to be a predictor of improvement with microfracture. It also identified activity level and lesion size as predictors of better clinical results. Histologic evaluations showed no differences between the groups. The same patients were reevaluated at 5 years, and there was significant improvement for both groups, but the microfracture group continued to have better SF-36 physical component outcomes.[7] Both groups had 23% failures, but the ACI failures occurred earlier than the microfracture failures. Based on these results, with both techniques resulting in similar outcomes, we believe that microfracture should be the recommended treatment for isolated chondral defects.

Cartilage injuries are common in high-impact sports. We documented the outcomes of microfracture in patients who played professional football in the United States.[14] Between 1986 and 1997, 25 active National Football League players were treated with microfracture. The study found that 76% of players returned to play the next football season. Following return to play, those same players played an average of 4.6 additional seasons. All players showed decreased symptoms and improvement in function. Of those players who did not return to play, most had preexisting degenerative changes of the knee.

Arthroscopic treatment of the degenerative knee is controversial. However, we documented the outcomes at 2 years in patients with degenerative chondral lesions treated with microfracture.[12] The goals of this procedure are to alleviate pain, maximize function, and prevent further degenerative changes. With strict patient selection, proper surgical technique, and compliance with a well-defined rehabilitation program, patients showed improvement in function and had decreased symptoms. Pain and swelling significantly decreased, with most patients reporting only mild symptoms. Patients were highly satisfied with their results. Factors that were associated with less Lysholm score improvement included bipolar lesions, lesions larger than 400 mm^2, and knees with absent menisci. Repeat arthroscopy was reported in 15.5% of these patients. Failures, as defined by revision microfracture or total knee replacement, were documented in 6% of patients. These results confirm excellent short-term outcomes; however, further studies will be needed to determine how long the results last.

A contraindication to microfracture in the degenerative knee is malalignment of the joint. Medial opening wedge high tibial osteotomy (HTO) has gained popularity as a means of correcting malalignment in patients with medial compartment arthrosis and varus malalignment who wish to stay active. We have reported on 39 patients who underwent an opening wedge osteotomy on the medial side of the proximal tibia in conjunction with the microfracture procedure in their degenerative varus knee.[19] Patients showed improvement in function and activity level, as well as decreased symptoms. Most patients had a more than 20-point increase in their Lysholm scores. This study also showed that patients with no prior surgeries had more improvement. Two patients went on to total knee replacement at 3 and 5 years following the HTO. The study concluded that at a minimum of 2 years following surgery, patients with varus alignment and chondral surface lesions of the knee can be treated effectively with HTO and microfracture. These patients returned to an active lifestyle, as demonstrated by their high Tegner scores in Table 25-2.

Table 25-2 Average Functional Scores of All Patients

Parameter	Patient Age Range (Yr)	Score	
		Lysholm	Tegner
Traumatic lesions[13]	13-45	89	6
Traumatic lesions[8]	18-45	76	4
National Football League players[14]	22-36	90	9
Degenerative knees[12]	40-70	83	4.5
HTO and microfracture[19]	34-79	78	5

SUMMARY

Based on our extensive experience, we conclude that arthroscopic débridement with microfracture of subchondral bone is safe and effective to treat full-thickness chondral defects of the knee in clinical patients, both acute and chronic. Microfracture significantly improves functional outcomes and decreases pain in most patients treated. This repair tissue appears tough and durable, yet is smooth enough to function similarly to normal articular cartilage in clinical patients. We believe that microfracture should be considered as the initial treatment of choice for full-thickness articular cartilage defects of the knee.

KEY REFERENCES

Bellamy N, Buchanan WW, Goldsmith CH, et al: Validation study of WOMAC: a health status instrument for measuring clinically important patient relevant outcomes to antirheumatic drug therapy in patients with osteoarthritis of the hip or knee. Rheumatology 15:1833–1840, 1988.

Frisbie DD, Morisset S, Ho CP, et al: Effects of calcified cartilage on healing of chondral defects treated with microfracture in horses. Am J Sports Med 34:1824–1831, 2006.

Frisbie DD, Oxford JT, Southwood L, et al: Early events in cartilage repair after subchondral bone microfracture. Clin Orthop Relat Res 407:215–227, 2003.

Knutsen G, Drogset JO, Engebretsen L, et al: A randomized trial comparing autologous chondrocyte implantation with microfracture. Findings at five years. J Bone Joint Surg Am 89:2105–2112, 2007.

Knutsen G, Engebretsen L, Ludvigsen TC, et al: Autologous chondrocyte implantation compared with microfracture in the knee. J Bone Joint Surg Am 86:455–464, 2004.

Kocher MS, Steadman JR, Briggs KK, et al: Reliability, validity, and responsiveness of the Lysholm knee scale for various chondral disorders of the knee. J Bone Joint Surg Am 86:1139–1145, 2004.

Lysholm J, Gillquist J: Evaluation of knee ligament surgery with special emphasis on use of a scoring scale. Am J Sports Med 10:150–154, 1982.

Miller BS, Steadman JR, Briggs KK, et al: Patient satisfaction and outcome after microfracture of the degenerative knee. J Knee Surg 17:13–17, 2004.

Steadman JR, Briggs KK, Rodrigo JJ, et al: Outcomes of microfracture for traumatic chondral defects of the knee: average 11-year follow-up. Arthroscopy 19:477–484, 2003.

Steadman JR, Karas SG, Miller BS, et al: The microfracture technique in the treatment of full-thickness chondral lesions of the knee in National Football League players. J Knee Surg 16:83–86, 2003.

Steadman JR, Rodkey WG, Briggs KK: Microfracture to treat full-thickness chondral defects. J Knee Surg 15:170–176, 2002.

Steadman JR, Rodkey WG, Briggs KK: Microfracture chondroplasty: indications, techniques, and outcomes. Sports Med Arthrosc Rev 11:236–244, 2003.

Steadman JR, Rodkey WG, Rodrigo JJ: "Microfracture": Surgical technique and rehabilitation to treat chondral defects. Clin Orthop Relat Res 391S:S362–S369, 2001.

Tegner Y, Lysholm J: Rating systems in the evaluation of knee ligament injuries. Clin Orthop Relat Res 198:43–49, 1985.

Full references for this chapter can be found on www.expertconsult.com.

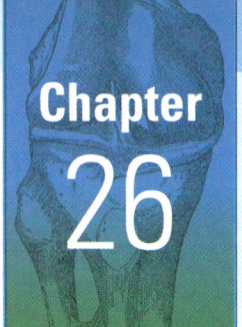

Articular Cartilage Repair With Bioscaffolds

Jack Farr, II and Andreas Gomoll

The goal of articular cartilage restoration is to recreate normal hyaline cartilage at the site of a cartilage defect. Currently, this has only been achieved through osteochondral transfer, noting that limitations of autograft and allograft implants preclude widespread use. Although hyaline-like tissue properties may be demonstrated using cell therapy alone, the tissue lacks the natural stratification of normal hyaline cartilage. As with most bodily tissues, the natural structure serves a distinct purpose—efficiency of resources and energy, function (low coefficient of friction, dispersal of loads to underlying bone both spatially and temporally), and durability. If the goal is to restore these articular cartilage attributes, all aspects of normal hyaline cartilage must be addressed: basilar integration with bone and calcified cartilage, marginal integration, filling of the defect level to the surrounding normal cartilage walls, and natural stratification duplicating the variability of the morphology and density of chondrocytes, as well as the regional differences in the extracellular matrix. To achieve these goals, one approach uses a scaffold to influence the cells. There are many variations on this theme, ranging from the most basic scaffold, the fibrin clot that occurs with any marrow stimulation procedure, to three-dimensional multiphasic (osteochondral promoting) scaffolds, with chondrocytes seeded and cultured in a stratified manner.[5,18,29,41]

Scaffolds used in cartilage defect repair techniques are often categorized by their structure (e.g., monophasic, biphasic, multiphasic) and whether they are with or without cells. As an alternative terminology, the term *scaffolds without cells* may replace the term *cell-free scaffolds*. The basis for this is to highlight that although the scaffolds are cell-free at the time of implantation, they are thought to function by providing a structural guidance for endogenous pluripotential cells. Therefore, these techniques may be better categorized as scaffolds populated with migrated host cells or scaffolds populated with exogenous cells; these exogenous cells may range from acutely harvested minced autograft cartilage, stored particulated allograft, or cultured chondrocytes seeded at surgery or grown on the scaffold. Part I of this chapter is a review of the basic scientific aspects of the scaffolds used to restore articular cartilage—that is, in theory, what is the best scaffold? Part II outlines the currently available scaffolds, those in clinical use and those in preclinical development.

PART I: SCIENTIFIC BASIS FOR DESIGN CONSIDERATIONS OF BIOSCAFFOLDS

Cartilage, like most other tissues, is comprised of two components, the extracellular matrix (ECM), composed of various macromolecules and water, and the cells contained within the ECM, which produce and maintain the former. Cartilage repair requires restoration of both components to produce a tissue that is biomechanically and biochemically able to withstand the demands of repetitive joint loading without early

degeneration and failure. In addition, as an organ, the joint is composed of and depends on the integration and interplay of various building block materials. Without transgressing into a discussion of the interaction of the menisci, ligaments, capsule, synovium, and cartilage, it is necessary to couple cartilage with the underlying bone. Without complete basilar integration through the calcified cartilage layer, a supposedly perfect cartilage construct will fail through delamination. Classic cell-based approaches, such as microfracture (marrow stimulation) and autologous chondrocyte implantation (ACI), rely on a cellular component to produce ECM, thus filling the lesion and achieving basilar and marginal integration. These procedures require activity restrictions to protect the immature tissue and are associated with long recovery times and complex postoperative rehabilitation, mainly because of the slow production and maturation of the ECM component by the cells. Many current and future approaches have the objective of modifying the classic cell-based techniques through the addition of bioscaffolds, with the goal of simplifying the surgical technique, decreasing postoperative restrictions on the patient, speeding up recovery and return to full activity, and improving outcomes. This exciting area is fluid and in constant change, so this section can only provide a snapshot of current scientific knowledge, with an attempt to delineate the characteristics of an ideal scaffold for cartilage repair.

Scaffold Requirements

Scaffold function can generally be divided into two roles, cell delivery and structural support for cell migration or stratification with composite maturation. The former uses the scaffold as a carrier substrate to help deliver cells into the defect and maintain them in situ until the new cartilage construct can achieve marginal and basilar integration. Theoretically, after the scaffold has fulfilled its purpose, it could be removed or, more realistically, resorb on its own. This function is comparatively simple, with the demands in terms of mechanical properties minimal, and therefore a number of materials have been found to be suitable for this, including the fibrin clot from microfracture, fibrin glue, alginate or agarose, collagen, hyaluronic acid, and artificial polymers, such a polylactic acid (PLA) and polyglycolic acid (PGA) and their modifications.

The second role, to act as a support structure during cell and ECM maturation, is far more complex and may require more advanced engineering to produce a scaffold that optimizes the physical and biochemical structure of the ECM while providing adequate porosity to allow cell invasion and growth (Table 26-1).[27] The ideal scaffold should allow early or even immediate weight bearing; thus, it would require mechanical properties strong enough to protect the cells while at the same time not being so stiff as to completely

Table 26-1 Desirable Attributes for Bioscaffolds Used in Cartilage Repair

Structure and Chemistry	Mechanical Properties, Strength, and Integrity	Clinical Application
Biocompatible synthetic versus naturally derived	Mechanical properties comparable to hyaline cartilage	Preformed intraoperatively versus custom shape or contour versus injectable
Porosity-permeability—optimal porosity with three-dimensional architecture	High porosity (does not apply to gel-type scaffolds)	Ease of intraoperative handling and fixation
Optimized geometry to regenerate native matrix (ECM) orientation	Composite structure with varying properties throughout its thickness	Delivery attributes—arthroscopic (air or liquid) versus miniopen versus formal open
Resorption without local or systemic adverse effect versus benign particulate breakdown scavenging	Biocompatible	Chondral versus osteochondral defects
Resorption temporal profile follows new cartilage deposition	No toxic degradation products	Reproducibility
Surface chemistry (protein absorption-deposition, enabling cell adhesion, migration, and outgrowth)	Assists in cell and tissue differentiation Resorbable	Regulatory approval pathway and final indications Cost, value

shield the cells from all stresses, which are important signals for tissue maturation. The scaffold should provide secure fixation and enhance basilar integration with the subchondral bone and circumferential integration with the surrounding cartilage. To allow cell growth, the scaffold must consist of a system of interconnected pores; the material should be hydrophilic to ease cell seeding, penetration, and adhesion. Furthermore, certain modifications can improve cell adhesion to a scaffold, such as binding of adhesion ligands to the scaffold material. It should slowly resorb with time, at a pace that allows gradual replacement through host tissue, and this process should not generate degradation products that are toxic or inflammatory.

Basic Science

The following section will review basic aspects and concepts, including the physical and biologic characteristics of bioscaffolds for cartilage repair. More specific information on individual membranes currently in clinical practice or under development will be provided in the second part of this chapter.

Physical Characteristics

Mechanical Strength

Mechanical characteristics of hyaline cartilage vary with the joint in question, as well as the specific location within the respective joint. A bioscaffold allowing early or even immediate weight bearing is desirable and should closely mirror the mechanical properties of hyaline cartilage until it has been replaced by mature repair tissue. The scaffold functions to protect the growing tissue while ensuring an appropriate level of physiologic loading to enhance the reparative process,[47] an effect first described by Pauwels,[48] who recognized the influence of physical stimuli on cell differentiation pathways of mesenchymal stem cells.

Elasticity (Young's modulus) of human hyaline cartilage has been reported as between 1 and 20 Mpa, depending on the layer and location, several orders of magnitude lower than that of immature (1000 MPa) or cortical (17,000 MPa) bone.[34] It appears from computer modeling

that an inhomogeneous three-dimensional scaffold with higher stiffness in the superficial layer, which gradually decreases toward the base of the defect, might be best suited to encourage cartilage, rather than fibrous tissue, regeneration. This theory has been substantiated by findings of a tensile modulus 6 to 20 times higher in the superficial regions than in the deeper regions, whereas permeability demonstrated a reverse distribution, increasing with increasing depth. The higher stiffness at the surface better protects the immature tissue from the high shear forces experienced at this level and the lower stiffness at the base allows sufficient strain rates to encourage chondrogenic differentiation.

Structure

Studies have investigated effects of the overall three-dimensional structure of scaffolds on cells and tissue production. Although chondrocytes attach and grow even on flat nonphysiologic surfaces (two-dimensional growth, such as in a Petri dish), they gradually dedifferentiate into a more fibroblastic phenotype with increased type I collagen production. Conversely, chondrocytes maintain their spherical appearance when grown in three-dimensional culture, such as open-pored scaffolds or alginate beads, and matrix production is improved quantitatively and qualitatively with increased type II collagen.[41] Cartilage ECM consists of a mesh of collagen fibers 10 to 140 nm in diameter[53] and studies have demonstrated improved cell adherence to fibers of submicron size.[65] Many studies have therefore investigated the use of spun or woven nanofibers of various materials for use in bioscaffolds.[76]

A system of interconnected open pores facilitates cell seeding of bioscaffolds to produce a three-dimensional structure. The normal pore area of hyaline cartilage has been reported as 5 to 33 nm,[52] but this is not directly comparable to the requirements of a bioscaffold. The former reflects the size of a lacuna, but pores in a bioscaffold have to be large enough to allow cell seeding, penetration, and proliferation, followed by production of ECM. However, increased pore size beyond a threshold value has been demonstrated to decrease attachment for a variety of cells, whereas increased specific surface area (a measure of overall porosity) was found to have a positive effect.[45] In general terms, a material porosity of 80% to 90% has been found to be beneficial in terms of quantity and quality of regenerated tissue.[28] In addition to the pore size, which allows cell migration, the nanostructure of the material must allow cell adherence during migration.

Biologic Characteristics

Biocompatibility

More commonly an issue with synthetic bioscaffolds, biocompatibility refers to tissue reactivity toward the implanted material. Biocompatibility can be improved by surface modification of the material to improve cell adhesion—for example, the wettability of hydrophobic polymers, such as the polyesters PGA and PLA, can be improved by gas plasma treatment to polymerize specific monomers to the scaffold surface.[46] Biomolecules can also be attached, such as arginine-glycine-aspartic acid (RGD), which interact with integrin receptors to anchor the cell cytoskeleton to the ECM.[57] However, even within the group of biologic scaffold materials, such as collagen and hyaluronic acid, subtle variations exist that influence cell adhesion. In a review of several collagen membranes, type II collagen appeared to be better suited to enhance cell attachment than type I collagen membranes.[23,36]

Degradation

Generally a concern with artificial scaffold materials, degradation products seen during absorption can lead to foreign body reactions and inflammatory responses. For example, both PGA and PLA degradation through hydrolytic cleavage of ester bonds can result in acidic byproducts[62] that have been implicated in foreign body and other inflammatory reactions. Buffer substances can be added to influence the rate of resorption as well as the acidity of degradation products.

Bioactivity

Ideally, a bioscaffold will provide not only mechanical support but guide the cells contained within to produce a better repair tissue. Attaching growth factors to the scaffold material has been investigated by several authors, who reported a shift to a more hyaline-like appearance of regenerated cartilage after the addition of various factors, including the bone morphogenic protein (BMP), insulin-like growth factor (IGF), and transforming growth factor (TGF) families.[2]

Summary of Desired Scaffold Attributes

An ideal bioscaffold should provide a mechanically stable environment for cells, either delivered with the membrane or absorbed from the local environment—for example, after microfracture. The scaffold should be strong enough to allow early weight bearing while conducting sufficient stress to the cells to encourage differentiation and production of a hyaline cartilage–like ECM. The scaffold should resorb over time without residual degradation products and the resorption time should be timed to coincide with tissue maturation. Bioactive substances such as ligand factors to improve cell attachment, and growth factors that aid in cell differentiation, may be bound to the scaffold material to produce a better or more rapid repair tissue. At this time, various types of bioscaffolds are being actively explored, but no approach has been demonstrated to be clearly superior to others, and

significant changes will evolve as these are brought into clinical practice.

PART II: SCAFFOLDS IN DEVELOPMENT

Part I of this chapter established the scientific basis for the use of scaffolds in the repair of articular cartilage defects of the knee. However, at the time of this writing, none are clinically available in the United States. Although the list of desirable attributes for an articular cartilage repair scaffold represents realistic goals, attempting to achieve all the attributes in one scaffold remains elusive.[59] As with all aspects of medicine, if there were a true best method or best scaffold, then all physicians would adopt that single technique. However, in this relatively new field, the reality is that many approaches remain under evaluation,[11] because none has provided the stated end goal: to produce a true stratified hyaline cartilage, with full basilar and marginal integration implanted, using a minimally invasive technique with minimal inconvenience to the patient and cost to society. Nevertheless, from the view point of demand matching, the laudable but possibly unobtainable stated goal may not be necessary for many knee lesions. Consider that many first-generation cartilage repair techniques appear to work satisfactorily in up to 70% of patients. Therefore, the goal may need to be restated from a patient function and pain perspective, and not from a histologic perspective. That is, the cartilage repair goal may be the most cost-effective and acceptably durable treatment for a specific patient and specific cartilage lesion, rather than a fully integrated hyaline cartilage. This on the ground clinical approach should not deter basic science research, but illustrates the difference between preclinical results and clinical applications. It is important to keep the patient's knee in mind while exploring the newer scaffold cartilage repair options.[43]

The first clinical application of a scaffold for knee cartilage repair was reported in 1998 by Behrens.[8] The two-stage technique was an extension of the original ACI. After an autologous biopsy was cultured, the chondrocytes were seeded onto a porcine collagen I-III scaffold (Chondro-Gide, Geistlich Biomaterials, Wolhusen, Switzerland) and allowed to grow on the scaffold before implantation. It was termed *matrix-associated autologous chondrocyte implantation* (MACI; Genzyme, Cambridge, Mass). Shortly thereafter, in 1999, Hyalograft C was introduced. The scaffold was a benzylic ester of hyaluronic acid (HYAFF 11, Fidia Advanced Biopolymers Laboratories, Padova, Italy).[69] Like the two-stage MACI, the autologous cartilage was harvested from the patient, followed by expansion and seeding onto the scaffold, where they are allowed to grow. Both of these three-dimensional scaffolds have been shown to improve the maintenance of a chondrocyte-differentiated phenotype when compared with two-dimensional culturing. These initial biodegradable polymers remain in active clinical use in Europe, with many reports of efficacy over time, and have been joined by several other seeded, cultured scaffold applications. In addition, these scaffolds allowed arthroscopic implantation in certain regions of the knee, typically the femoral condyles and trochlea, which was not possible with first-generation ACI. Because this is a rapidly changing field, our goal here is to show current scaffold applications in a general sense, with the understanding that the initiated reader will review current literature and conference presentations before making any clinical decisions. In addition, it is necessary for the reader to fully understand the regulatory process in his or her respective country because allowed clinical use may vary over time.

As an overview, it is important to reemphasize that not all cutting edge cartilage techniques use scaffolds. This is well documented elsewhere in this text. In fact, there is a certain degree of overlap of topics. For example, in the subset of cell therapies, scaffolds are obviously a further subset. Understanding the importance of marrow stimulation, osteochondral autograft, and allograft as stand-alone techniques, the subset of cell therapies may be classified by the following: (1) cells alone; (2) scaffolds without cells at time of implantation (host cell source); (3) scaffolds with seeded cells; and (4) scaffolds with seeded and cultured cells. This section will focus only on those applications using scaffolds.

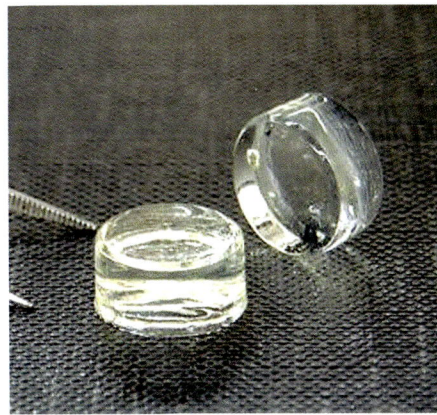

Figure 26-1. In situ implant, Gelrin*C*. (Courtesy Regentis Biomaterials, Or-Akiva, Israel.)

Scaffolds Without Cells at Time of Implantation (Host Cell Source)

Autologous Matrix-Induced Chondrogenesis

Autologous matrix-induced chondrogenesis (AMIC) is a porcine collagen I-III matrix (Chondro-Gide) that is applied over the defect immediately following microfracture. This scaffold is thicker than the original one used in MACI to allow potential filling of a full bottom to top defect. The goal is to provide a matrix that allows host cells to migrate into the scaffold and have an environment that improves the chondrogenesis from that of marrow stimulation alone.[22,31]

Matrix-Modulated Marrow Stimulation

This system uses BST-CarGel (Piramal, Mubai, India) which is a mixture of chitosan (structural component of crustacean shells) liquid and autologous blood (1:3 ratio) to form a viscous material (in situ polymerized hydrogel) implanted into marrow stimulation prepared defects (microfracture or drilling).[25,39] It has intrinsic cytocompatibility and is completely biodegradable. The construct allows both reinforcement of the clot and impedance of clot retraction.[9] The cationic charge of the chitosan increases the adhesiveness of the mixture to cartilage lesions, potentially allowing longer clot residency. This maintenance of critical blood components above the marrow access holes common to these subgroups of scaffolds may allow a more optimal tissue repair process, noting that in this case, the chitosan has some intrinsic ability to stimulate wound repair.[55]

Matrix-Modulated Marrow Stimulation

GelrinC

GelrinC (Regentis Biomaterials, Or-Akiva, Israel) is an in situ biodegradable photopolymerized hydrogel made from polyethylene glycol diacrylate (PEG-DA) covalently conjugated to a structural backbone of separated, denatured, disulfide-reduced fibrinogen chains. The scaffold (Fig. 26-1) is for use in conjunction with marrow stimulation techniques for the local repair of damaged cartilage and bone. It fills discontinuities across a focal cartilage defect and may include bone. The degradation of this implant is controlled and mediated by protease activity on the fibrinogen moieties and

by hydrolysis of the PEG. This allows a longer time frame (when compared with degradation of blood clot alone) for formation of tissue at the repair site, with implications that this altered temporal sequence will allow for more mature repair tissue—in the case of cartilage, more hyaline-like than fibrocartilage. This may allow functional tissue to fill the space occupied previously by the implant. The scaffold completely degrades within 6 to 12 months. The major degradation products are PEGylated peptides, amino acids, and PEG, and have been shown to be nontoxic to chondrocytes, bone, and the body.[49,50]

Polyglycolic Acid Scaffolds with Hyaluronan and Autologous Serum

Autologous serum and hyaluronan, combined with PGA scaffolds, are implanted into full-thickness articular cartilage defects pretreated with microfracture. Human serum is used as a chemoattractant and efficiently recruits mesenchymal progenitors. Chondrogenic differentiation of progenitor cells on stimulation with hyaluronan was demonstrated by Erggelet and associates[15] and Wakitani and coworkers.[64]

Biologic Adhesive and Photopolymerized Hydrogel With Microfracture

ChonDux (Biomet, Warsaw, Ind) combines a biologic adhesive and photopolymerized hydrogel with microfracture.[52] The biologic adhesive is a processed chondroitin sulfate that bonds with defect cartilage and defect base to aid in bonding the hydrogel in the defect. The hydrogel is a combination of PEG and hyaluronic acid; it aids in the retention of the marrow stimulation elements, is conducive to chondrogenesis, and potentially reduces fibrosis tissue production.[7,10]

Multiphase Scaffold to Fill Osteochondral Defect

There are many experimental models using a multiphase scaffold to address the bone and cartilage component of an osteochondral defect as detailed by Lynn and colleagues.[42]

TRUFIT BGS Plug

One commercially available biphasic scaffold plug option is the TRUFIT BGS plug (Smith & Nephew Endoscopy, Andover, Mass; Fig. 26-2). This is entirely synthetic and is

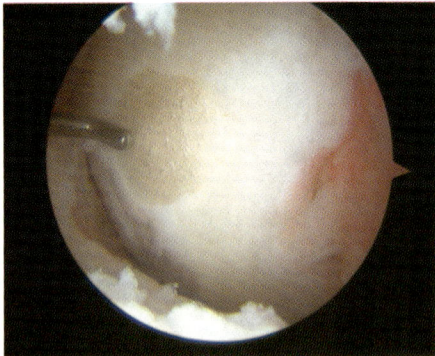

Figure 26-2. TRUFIT BGS plug after arthroscopic placement. (From Cole BJ, Gomoll AG: Biologic joint reconstruction: alternatives to arthroplasty. Thorofare, NJ, 2009, Slack.)

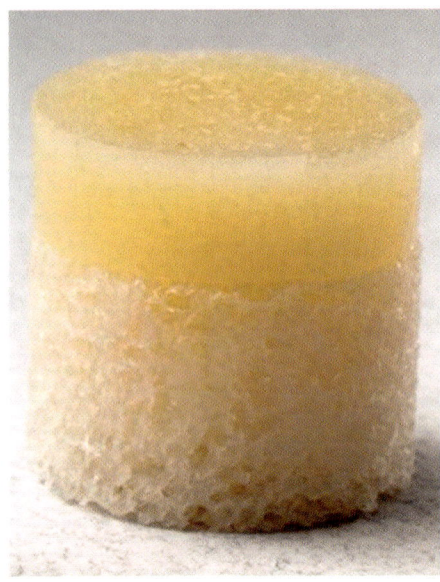

Figure 26-3. CR Plug. This sterile allograft bone plug consists of cancellous bone and demineralized cortical human bone. (Courtesy RTI Biologics, Alachua, Fla.)

designed to mimic the physical and mechanical properties of cartilage and bone. It is composed of POLYGRAFT (Smith & Nephew Endoscopy), a porous hydrophilic material comprised of an 85:15 poly(D,L-lactide–coglycolide) copolymer (PLDG), PGA fibers, calcium sulfate (bone phase only), and a trace amount of surfactant. PGA reinforcement fibers improve the early structural integrity of the scaffold and provide a mechanically stable environment for possible cell migration and tissue repair.[54] The superficial phase is malleable to allow contouring with the adjacent articular surface after implantation. Calcium sulfate in the bone phase resorbs in the first several months, releasing calcium ions, which may enhance osteoconductivity.[19] The material of the scaffold degrades in approximately 6 to 9 months[56] by hydrolysis of ester linkages into lactic and glycolic acids, which are metabolites of the Krebs cycle and have very minimal toxicity.

MaioRegen

MaioRegen is an osteochondral biomimetic scaffold (Fin-Ceramica Faenza, Faenza, Italy), which has a porous, three-dimensional, composite trilayered structure, mimicking the osteochondral unit.[61] Each layer is separately synthesized using an atelocollagen aqueous solution (1%) in acetic acid, isolated from equine tendon.[17] The layer that promote cartilaginous tissue consists of type I collagen and has a smooth surface. The intermediate layer (tide mark–like) consists of a combination of type I collagen (60%) and hyaluronic acid (HA; 40%), whereas the bone-specific layer consists of a mineralized blend of type I collagen (30%) and HA (70%).

Chondromimetic

Chondromimetic (OrthoMimetics, Cambridge, England) is a biphasic, porous, resorbable implant that contains the biocompatible and resorpable materials collagen and glycosaminoglycan, with calcium phosphate added to the bone layer phase of the dual-layer porous implant.[42] The scaffold is rehydrated with sterile fluids and autologous blood products in an effort to optimize its biologic effectiveness through cell infiltration and tissue regeneration.

Other scaffold plug options that are currently only for osseous fill include Osseofit Kensey (Kensey Nash, Exton, Pa[35]) and OsteoSponge and OsteoSponge filler (Bacterin International, Belgrade, Mont[3]).

Composite Bone Allograft Plug

CR-Plug

The CR-Plug (RTI Biologics, Alachua, Fla; Fig. 26-3) is a composite bone allograft plug that consists of cancellous bone covered with a thinner layer of demineralized bone. Although demineralized bone has been shown to allow for the formation of hyaline-like cartilage in animal models,[20,67,68] this allograft implant is being promoted by the manufacturer as a bone void filler. Demineralized bone provides a scaffold for cell migration, and the growth factors inherent to bone are retained even after demineralization. At the time of implantation, the firmness of the demineralized bone is similar to hose cartilage. It is currently undergoing clinical evaluation and is not available for use outside of this evaluation.

Polymer Scaffold

Aseed Scaffold

The Aseed scaffold[12] (Coloplast A/S, Humlebaek, Denmark) is composed of a methoxypolyethyleneglycol-poly(l,d[lactide]-co-glycolide, (MPEG-PGLA) polymer. The scaffold has a thickness comparable to that of human cartilage. The scaffold is cut to fit the defect and secured by fibrin glue. Its canal-like design allows for host cells to integrate into the scaffold fully with the goal of augmenting the outcome of marrow stimulation alone.

Scaffolds With Seeded Cells (Single-Stage)

Autologous Chondrocyte Transplant, Collagen Patch–Seeded

An autologous chondrocyte transplant (ACT), collagen patch–seeded, is a standard ACI cell suspension seeded onto a collagen patch immediately before implantation. After several minutes, the cells have adhered sufficiently for implantation. The advantage over conventional cultured chondrocytes on scaffolds is that no cells are discarded, as noted by Steinwachs.[58]

Cartilage Autograft Implant System

In a cartilage autograft implant system (CAIS; DePuy Mitek, Raynham, Mass), autologous cartilage is minced arthoscopically by a custom harvester into 1- to 2-mm pieces. These pieces are uniformly dispersed by a custom device onto a synthetic scaffold (35% polycaprolate [PCL], 65% PGA and polydiaxanone [PDS] mesh) where they are fixed on the scaffold with fibrin glue. The minced cartilage scaffold construct is implanted and fixed with bioabsorble staples during the same surgery through a miniarthrotomy.[16,21]

Cell Replacement Technology

Instruct Products

Cell Replacement Technology (CRT) Instruct products (Cell-CoTec; Bilthoven, The Netherlands) consist of a cell processor, a mechanically functional scaffold, and reusable surgical instrumentation.[67] In the operating room, autologous cartilage is harvested and bone marrow is aspirated. Chondrocytes are then isolated and mixed with the bone marrow aspirate and seeded onto a rehydrated scaffold. This is performed during a single, minimally invasive surgical procedure. Advantages may include a comparatively short rehabilitation time because of the use of a mechanically functional scaffold.[44]

Scaffolds With Cells Cultured on or Within a Scaffold (Two-Stage)

Seeded With Autologous Chondrocytes

Matrix-Associated Autologous Chondrocyte Implantation: MACI

Matrix-associated ACI (MACI; Genzyme; Fig. 26-4) is an autologous chondrocyte that is expanded, seeded onto a type I-III collagen membrane, and cultured. It is then implanted with suture or fibrin glue. A number of clinical reports from studies done outside the United States have reported similar efficacy to ACI, with a lower complication rate.[4,30,69]

CartiGro on Chondro-Gide

CartiGro ACT[60] (Stryker, Montreux, Switzerland) is similar to MACI, but is currently using a different (thicker) scaffold (Chondro-Gide; Geistlich Biomaterials, Switzerland) porcine I/III) onto which cells (CartiGro ACT) are cultured (Fig. 26-5). Since 2000, CartiGro has been implanted in more than 800 patients.[11]

NeoCart

NeoCart (Histogenics, Waltham, Mass; Fig. 26-6) is a three-dimensional bovine collagen scaffold seeded with expanded autologous chondrocytes, which are then grown on the scaffold in hydrostatic bioreactor and implanted with proprietary bioadhesive (greater adherence than fibrin glue).[13,66]

CaRes and CartiPlug

CaRes and CartiPlug (ArthroKinetics, Boston) are autologous chondrocytes seeded onto three-dimensional collagen type I gel. The diameter and thickness of the transplant can be chosen individually, depending on the nature of the defect. The cells are isolated from the patient's biopsy, mixed with the collagen gel and, after the complete gelling and 2 weeks of culture in the patient's serum cultivation medium, the chondrocyte-loaded gel is available for transplantation. The

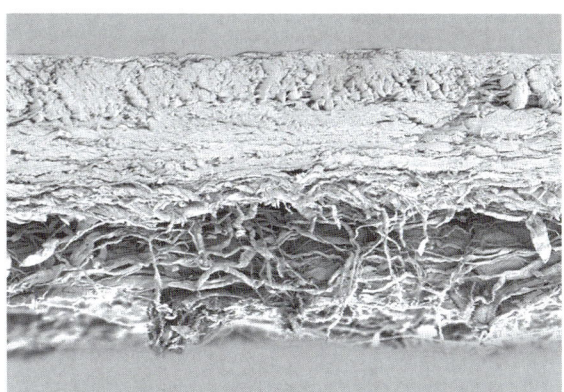

Figure 26-5. Chondro-Gide collagen type I-III matrix with unique bilayer structure. (Courtesy Geistlich, Wolhusen, Switzerland.)

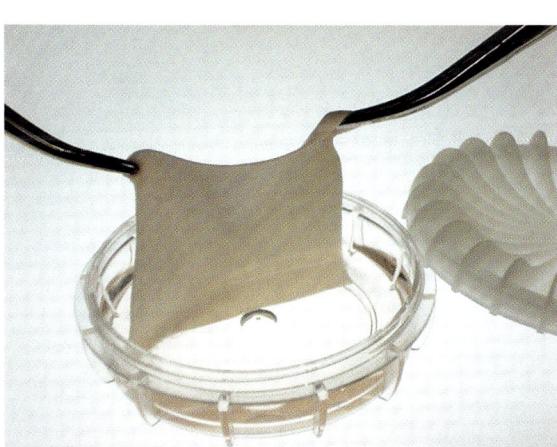

Figure 26-4. MACI membrane. (Courtesy Genzyme, Cambridge, Mass.)

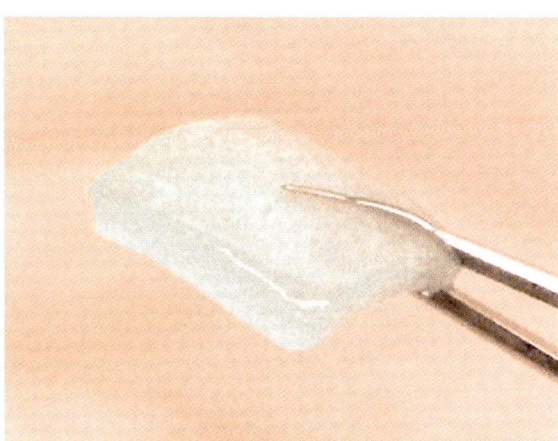

Figure 26-6. NeoCart. This autologous hyaline neocartilage implant is ready for transplantation. (Courtesy Histogenics, Waltham, Mass.)

transplantation is performed by a miniopen technique using a thin layer of fibrin glue.

Hyalograft C

Hyalograft C (Fidia Advanced Biopolymers, Abano Terme, Italy) is a hyaluronan-based biodegradable polymer (Hyaff-11) scaffold with a nonwoven three-dimensional structure. It is 20 μm thick and is seeded with expanded autologous chondrocytes, which are grown on the scaffold for 2 weeks. The construct is implanted by miniarthrotomy or arthroscopically. Intermediate-term use in studies done outside the United States have been well documented in the peer-reviewed literature.[24,38]

Bioseed C

Bioseed C (BioTissue Technologies, Freiburg, Germany) is a polyglactin poly-p-dioxanon fleece with a standard size of 2×3 cm or 2×1 cm. Autologous chondrocytes are expanded ex vivo and then loaded on a 2-mm thick porous scaffold using a fibrin glue to distribute the cells, providing a three-dimensional environment and securing the bioengineered tissue.[14,32,33]

Cartipatch

Cartipatch (TBF Tissue Engineering, Bron, France) consists of autologous chondrocytes that are implanted on a hydrogel composed of agarose and alginate. This hydrogel is of vegetal origin (ultrapurified agarose-alginate suspension [GelForCel; TBF Tissue Engineering]). It is mixed with an isolated autologous cell suspension and can be modulated at 37° C into complex shape implants, which solidify at approximately 25° C. Matrix elasticity improves handling.[1,37,51]

Novocart 3D

Novocart 3D (TETEC Tissue Engineering Technologies, Reutlingen, Germany) is an autologous chondrocyte implanted onto a collagen-based biphasic scaffold. A specific, protective, dense layer was developed to cover the collagen sponge to prevent synovial cells from invasion and improve the mechanical properties of the scaffold. The transplantation is performed by a miniopen technique using a dedicated instrumentation. For the fixation of the graft, resorbable minipins can be used.[37]

BioCart Cartilage Regeneration System Implant

The BioCart Cartilage Regeneration System implant (ProChon, Ness Ziona, Israel; Fig. 26-7) uses a fibrin scaffold, which is a natural homologous biopolymer (it constitutes part of the normal scaffold of wound healing) and is copolymerized with hyaluronan to produce a matrix that serves as a three-dimensional scaffold for chondrocyte transplantation. Pore sizes range from 10 to 15 μm. The scaffold degrades almost completely in 3 to 4 weeks. The degradation products of fibrin are fragments of polypeptides produced when the protein is broken down by the enzyme plasmin. Hyaluronan is degraded by a family of enzymes called hyaluronidases. The degradation products of hyaluronan are oligosaccharides and very low-molecular-weight hyaluronan, which are known to exhibit proangiogenic properties. The scaffold is seeded and cultured with chondroctyes that have been in the presence of the fibroblast growth factor FGF2v, which allows a more robust chondrocytic phenotype and matrix production, with a lower number of passages.[63]

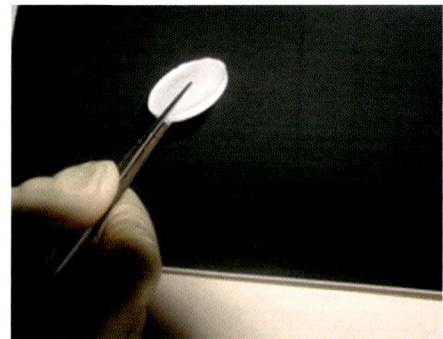

Figure 26-7. BioCart—dry, lyophilized, fibrin–hyaluronic acid three-dimensional bioscaffolds with interconnection pores ranging from 10 to 50 μm. (Courtesy ProChon Biotech, Ness Ziona, Israel.)

Cartilink-3

Cartilink-3 (Interface Biotech A/S, Hørsholm, Denmark) is an ACI based on scaffold technology (Aseed). It was developed in collaboration with Coloplast A/S. The Aseed scaffold is a fully synthetic and resorbable scaffold. The thickness is similar to that of articular cartilage and it is fixed by fibirin glue. Chondrocytes are already integrated into the Aseed scaffold, with a concentration of more than 1 million viable cells/cm^2.[12] While the Cartilink = 3 product may still be a viable option in the future, at time of printing Interface Biotech was not an active company.[6]

KEY REFERENCES

Ait T, Selmi S, Neyret P: Autologous chondrocyte transplantation in combination with an alginate-agarose based hydrogel (Cartipatch). Tech Knee Surg 6:253–258, 2007.

Buschmann M, Hoemann C, Hurtig M, et al: Cartilage repair with chitosan-glycerol phosphate-stabilized blood clots. In Williams R, editor: Cartilage repair strategies, Totowa, NJ, 2007, Humana Press, pp 85–105.

Chan BP, Leong KW: Scaffolding in tissue engineering: general approaches and tissue-specific considerations. Eur Spine J 17:467–479, 2008.

Endres M, Neumann K, Schroder SE, et al: Human polymer-based cartilage grafts for the regeneration of articular cartilage defects. Tissue Cell 39:293–301, 2007.

Garrido C, L'Heureux D, Cole B: Recommendations and treatment outcomes for patellofemoral articular cartilage defects with autogolous chondrocyte implantation (ACI): prospective evaluation at average 4-year follow-up. Paper presented at the American Orthopaedic Society for Sports Medicine Annual Meeting, Keystone, Colo, August 2009.

Gobbi A, Kon E, Berruto M, et al: Patellofemoral full-thickness chondral defects treated with second-generation autologous chondrocyte implantation: results at 5 years follow-up. Am J Sports Med 37;1083–1092, 2009.

Kon E, Delcogliano M, Filardo G, et al: Second-generation issues in cartilage repair. Sports Med Arthrosc 16:221–229, 2008.

Lynn AK, Best SM, Cameron RE, et al: Design of a multiphase osteochondral scaffold. I. Control of chemical composition. J Biomed Mater Res A 92:1057–1065, 2010.

Pauwels F: A new theory on the influence of mechanical stimuli on the differentiation of supporting tissue. The tenth contribution to the functional anatomy and causal morphology of the supporting structure. Z Anat Entwicklungsgesch 121:478–515, 1960.

Seliktar D, Peled E, Livnat M, et al: Articular cartilage repair using in situ polymerizable hydrogel implant in osteochondral defects. Paper presented at the International Cartilage Repair Society 7th World Congress, Warsaw, Poland, September 2007.

Wakitani S, Nawata M, Tensho K, et al: Repair of articular cartilage defects in the patello-femoral joint with autologous bone marrow mesenchymal cell transplantation: three case reports involving nine defects in five knees. J Tissue Eng Regen Med 11:74–79, 2009.

Full references for this chapter can be found on www.expertconsult.com.

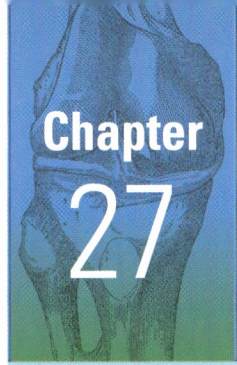

Chapter 27

Failed Cartilage Repair

Robert C. Grumet, Sarvottam Bajaj, and Brian J. Cole

The management of traumatic and degenerative cartilage lesions is a known challenge given the limited vascularity and lack of pluripotent cells that contribute to the tissue's inherently poor regenerative capacity. Many surgical techniques have been described in an effort to palliate symptoms, promote substitute tissue growth, and/or restore normal hyaline cartilage. Surgical failure of these techniques, however, may occur when the patient experiences incomplete or recurrent symptoms, or an inability to return to his or her desired activity level. Unfortunately, when all techniques are considered in aggregate, there remains a clinical failure rate that approaches 25% in most series. Technical error, graft dislodgment, graft resorption, and the failure to recognize concomitant injury leading to premature graft destruction are common causes for surgical failure. Successful revision of articular cartilage repair requires a thorough evaluation of comorbid conditions such as ligament instability, malalignment, and meniscal deficiency. These complications, left untreated, can have a detrimental effect on the cartilage repair procedure because of abnormal shear stress, increased contact pressure, and decreased contact area.

CLINICAL EVALUATION

History

Articular cartilage injuries may be caused by a direct trauma associated with impact or an indirect injury usually involving a twisting or shearing movement associated with an axial load. Patients with a history of a previous cartilage repair procedure may not describe their additional symptoms as a new injury to the knee. However, a thorough discussion about the patient's additional symptoms such as mechanical clicking, locking, or instability may help discern whether an associated pathology may have contributed to cartilage failure.

Similar to patients with a primary focal cartilage defect, pain is most often the patient's chief complaint, which is aggravated by certain positions or activities. Pain at the ipsilateral joint line is often associated with a condylar injury and can be aggravated by weight-bearing activities. Joint line pain caused by meniscal deficiency may be difficult to discern from a focal cartilage defect. However, a previous history of meniscectomy may heighten the surgeon's awareness to the possibility of meniscal deficiency causing or contributing to continued symptoms. Patients presenting with pain in the anterior compartment of the knee may be suffering from a trochlear or patellar lesion, which can be aggravated by activities that increase patellofemoral contact pressure, such as stair climbing or squatting. In addition to pain, patients may also report activity-related effusions in the knee.

Prior attempts at treatment should be reviewed with the patient. If prior surgeries have been performed, the timing and type of surgery, type of rehabilitation that followed, and whether the patient experienced a period of symptomatic relief postoperatively should be thoroughly discussed preoperatively. In addition, nonsurgical management such as oral medications, injections, bracing, physical therapy, and lifestyle modification should also be discussed as an important part of the patient's prior treatment.

Physical Examination

The physical examination of a patient with a symptomatic cartilage lesion begins with observation of the patient's gait and body habitus. Gait evaluation may reveal any antalgia caused by pain or weakness, malalignment or a varus or valgus thrust associated with ligament insufficiency or clinical malalignment. The physician should also observe and measure any associated quadriceps atrophy and effusions, and determine the location of any previous surgical incisions.

Palpation of bony and soft tissue structures about the knee may provide some insight into the location of the patient's symptoms, associated conditions such as meniscal deficiency, or presence of a subtle effusion. Patients with chondral injuries of the condyle typically present with ipsilateral joint line tenderness. Meniscal injury or deficiency may also present similarly to condylar pain with joint line tenderness; however, the pain is usually appreciated more posteriorly. Patellofemoral lesions may have pain and crepitus in the anterior compartment. Patellar tilt and glide should be evaluated for tightness of the lateral retinaculum and potential patellar instability. Finally, range of motion should be assessed in both knees, noting limitation in range and/or flexion contractures.

Identification of associated pathology is critical to the successful outcome of revision and complex articular cartilage restoration. As noted, persistent instability, malalignment, or meniscal deficiency is often a cause of premature failure of articular cartilage repairs and poor outcomes. Stability of the anterior cruciate ligament (ACL), posterior cruciate ligament (PCL), medial collateral ligament (MCL), as well as the lateral collateral ligament (LCL) and posterolateral complex, should be a routine part of any knee examination.

Imaging

Standard radiographs for cartilage injury should include bilateral knees in at least three views: anteroposterior (AP) weight-bearing view; non–weight-bearing, 45-degree flexion lateral view; and axial (Merchant) view of the patellofemoral joint. Additional views include a 45-degree flexion posteroanterior (PA) view, which may be useful to identify subtle joint space narrowing. A full-length alignment view of the affected and unaffected limb may help evaluate the mechanical axis and associated varus or valgus malalignment (Fig. 27-1). A computed tomography (CT) scan may be useful to

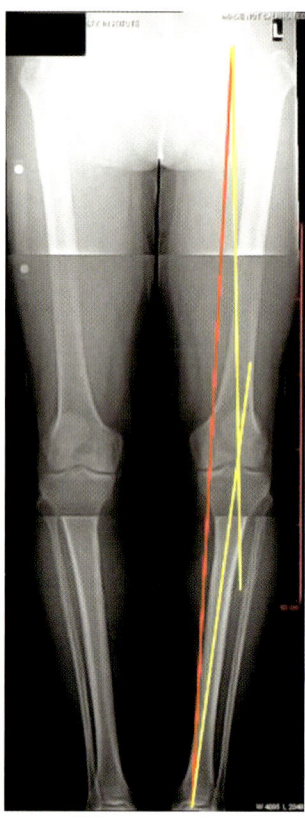

Figure 27-1. Standing long-leg alignment x-rays. The mechanical axis of the extremity is represented by the red line from the center of the femoral head to the center of the talus. This patient has an obvious varus deformity to the lower extremity. The desired correction for this patient is just beyond neutral. This angle is calculated by a line drawn from the center of the femoral head to the desired correction level at the joint line and a second line from the center of the talus to the same correction point at the joint line *(yellow).*

assess the patellofemoral joint and the associated tibial tubercle–trochlear groove (TT-TG) distance.[1,13] This measurement is particularly useful in patients with patellar instability when associated with chondrosis. Magnetic resonance imaging (MRI) scans are often used in the preoperative assessment of previously failed cartilage repair procedure. They provide a detailed assessment of lesion size, depth, quality of subchondral bone, and presence or absence of bony fractures. MRI may also confirm the presence of associated ligamentous, meniscal, or other soft tissue pathology.

TREATMENT

The appropriate treatment of a specific cartilage lesion is individualized to each patient and special considerations should be given to their postoperative goals and expectations. The overall goal of surgical intervention is to improve joint congruency, eliminate instability, and protect the repaired cartilage.

Nonoperative Treatment

Nonoperative therapies play a role for patients with previous cartilage repair surgery. Patients with unreasonable expectations or goals, failed multiple procedures, advanced

physiologic age with low demand, or unwilling to have further surgery may be amenable to these conservative modalities. These therapies include oral medications, physical therapy, weight loss, and injections (cortisone and hyaluronic acid derivatives). Oral medications such as nonsteroidal anti-inflammatory drugs and oral chondroprotective agents (e.g., glucosamine, chondroitin sulfate) are commonly used in symptomatic patients. Although the precise mechanism of action of these medications has not been elucidated, it has been hypothesized that glucosamine stimulates chondrocytes and synoviocytes to increase production of extracellular matrix, whereas chondroitin manages to inhibit fibrin clot formation and degradative enzymes.[2]

Cortisone injections are commonly used in practice for short-term pain relief because of the anti-inflammatory action of the steroids. Similarly, intra-articular injections containing hyaluronic acid provides viscosupplementation, resulting in significant pain reduction and improved function.[5,7,12,14]

Operative Treatment

Surgical managements of articular cartilage lesions can be grouped into three categories:

1. Palliative procedures, which include arthroscopic débridement and lavage to provide symptomatic relief to patients with little potential for cartilage regeneration
2. Reparative procedures, which include marrow stimulation techniques that create a pluripotent fibrin clot, ultimately resulting in fibrocartilage replacement
3. Restorative procedures, which attempt to restore the natural hyaline surface of articular cartilage using cultured chondrocytes or an osteochondral graft

The appropriate treatment for any given cartilage lesion is patient- and defect-specific. Lesion-specific variables include lesion size, location, depth, geometry, and bone quality; patient-specific variables include the patient's physiologic age, activity level, goals and expectations, and previous surgeries. Consideration of these variables and the associated comorbid conditions allow the management of cartilage lesions to be considered as part of an algorithm from the least invasive to the most invasive intervention (Fig. 27-2). The overall goal is to restore the patient's function and ameliorate symptoms using the least invasive technique. In the setting of a revision procedure, the least invasive procedure can often be exhausted, with undesirable outcomes requiring the surgeon to consider more invasive techniques for cartilage restoration while also addressing the reasons for primary failure, as noted earlier.

Palliative Procedures

Arthroscopic débridement and lavage are usually performed as a first-line treatment and considered for patients suffering from an acute injury causing pain and incongruency caused by a dislodged piece of cartilage (<2 cm²). Simple irrigation to remove debris, inflammatory cytokines, and proteases may help alleviate the patient's symptoms. In a revision setting, an arthroscopic débridement may temporarily alleviate the patient's symptoms and may also be used as a diagnostic tool to assess cartilage abnormalities and concomitant pathology. This may be especially true in the setting of previous autologous chondrocyte implantation (ACI) with resultant graft

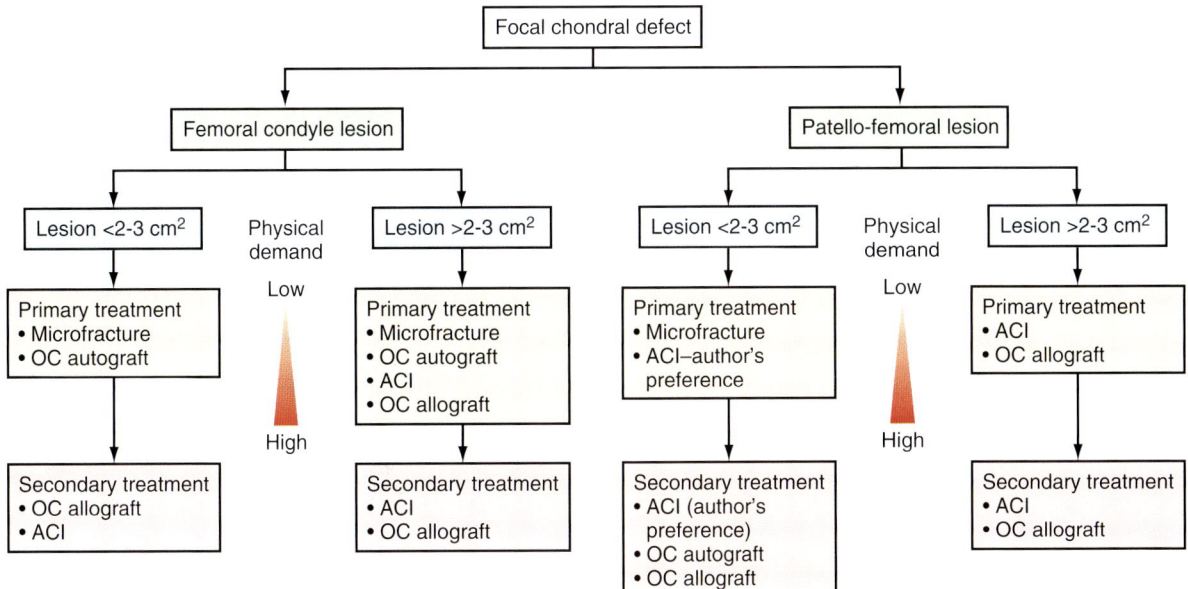

Figure 27-2. Algorithm used to guide decision making for primary and revision articular cartilage repair.

hypertrophy,[4] graft resorption with loose bodies, or advanced joint degeneration.

Reparative Procedure

Small- to medium-sized (2 to 3 cm^2), full-thickness chondral defects can be managed using marrow stimulation techniques, such as microfracture, subchondral drilling, and abrasion arthroplasty. Microfracture involves the use of a surgical awl on the subchondral bone to allow migration of marrow elements (mesenchymal cells). This migration results in the formation of a surgically induced fibrin clot at the defect site and the production of fibrocartilage. The newly formed repair tissue possesses a preponderance of types I and II collagen,[11] rendering it biologically and mechanically inferior to hyaline cartilage. This is especially helpful when prior procedures have been only partially successful in creating a complete defect repair (Fig. 27-3).

Restorative Procedures

Larger lesions and/or previously failed reparative procedures are often managed with restorative procedures. Restorative procedures include autologous chondrocyte implantation (ACI), osteoarticular autograft transplantation (OAT), and osteochondral allograft (OA) transplantation.

ACI is a two-stage procedure, with the first involving an arthroscopic biopsy of normal articular cartilage from a non–weight-bearing area. The biopsy tissue is used for in vitro dedifferentiation and culture of chondrocytes. The second step involves the implantation of the cultured cells with the off-label use of a synthetic collagen membrane patch to hold the cells in place.[4] The senior author soaks the membrane with a vial of cells prior to suturing rather than using saline. These cultured dedifferentiated cells produce a hyaline-like cartilage with superior biomechanical properties when compared with fibrocartilage. ACI is indicated for large defects measuring 2 to 10 cm^2, with limited bone loss, and may be used as a revision procedure for a previous palliative or reparative procedure. However, some concerns regarding the use

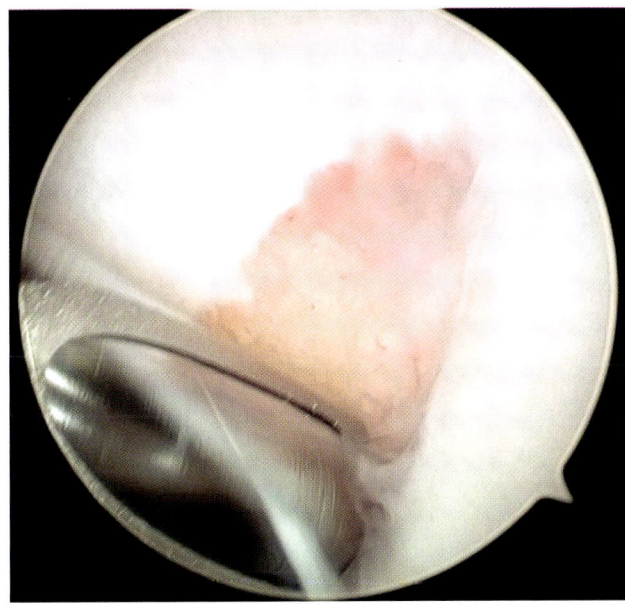

Figure 27-3. Second-look arthroscopy of a trochlear defect previously treated by ACI, with partial delamination of the repair site being prepared for microfracture.

of ACI as a revision procedure following microfracture have recently been raised, especially when the subchondral bone is highly involved, as seen by MRI.[9]

Lesions that present with subchondral bone loss are more commonly treated using osteochondral grafting. The source of the cylindric plug can be from the host (autograft) or from a cadaveric donor (allograft).

OAT is advantageous by virtue of using the patient's own tissue, eliminating immunologic concerns. Harvested tissue from non–weight-bearing regions are transplanted to the areas of defect, resulting in the replacement of the damaged articular cartilage. The OAT procedure is indicated for symptomatic patients presenting with full-thickness defects and can be used as first-line treatment for a high-demand patient or as a revision to a previously performed microfracture or even ACI, assuming that the defect is small enough. This technique is indicated for smaller defects (<2 cm²) because of limited supply of donor tissue as well as donor site morbidity.

Larger defects require the use of an OA graft in many cases. An OA graft involves transplantation of cadaveric mature hyaline cartilage with living chondrocytes and subchondral bone matrix to enhance osteointegration. In general, an OA graft is used as a secondary revision procedure and is considered the last biologic procedure before a total knee replacement.

Revision Procedures

Patients in the setting of revision articular cartilage surgery who have previously undergone and failed a simpler palliative or reparative procedure require the operating surgeon to consider more aggressive management techniques to achieve the goals.

As noted, a firm understanding of the reason(s) for failure is crucial before a revision procedure is performed to ensure prevention of further complications. Often, a comorbid condition, such as malalignment, instability, or meniscal deficiency, can lead to a premature degradation of the surgically induced replacement tissue. A diagnostic arthroscopy is often required to evaluate the extent of these comorbid conditions as well as to determine the integrity of the cartilage lesion and subchondral bone. In addition, not uncommonly, cartilage deterioration might have continued locally, adjacent to the initially treated cartilage defect, or might have developed in new locations or on opposing surfaces.

Cartilage or Meniscus Deficiency With Malalignment

A focal cartilage defect in association with meniscal deficiency and/or with varus or valgus alignment can be managed simultaneously or in stages. Focal cartilage defects previously treated with a reparative technique can be followed by a restorative technique, such as with ACI, OAT, or OA grafting, depending on the location of defect. In the presence of varus or valgus alignment, a high tibial osteotomy (Fig. 27-4) or a distal femoral osteotomy (Fig. 27-5) can be performed simultaneously with the revision articular cartilage procedure, especially in young and active patients. Older, less active patients with lower physical demands may benefit from a staged procedure. An osteotomy is performed first in an effort to offload the symptomatic compartment, followed by a period of observation. If patients present with satisfactory symptomatic relief, an additional restorative cartilage procedure may not be warranted. In the case of cartilage preservation, an osteotomy should be performed to correct the mechanical axis to neutral; however, in the setting of pain and arthrosis, the osteotomy should be corrected slightly beyond neutral. Patellofemoral lesions are most often treated with a distal realignment procedure of the tibial tubercle to decrease the contact pressure of the patellofemoral joint with the cartilage procedure. The degree of anteriorization versus medialization can be titrated based on the patient's history of instability, maltracking (TT-TG distance), or arthrosis (Fig. 27-6).

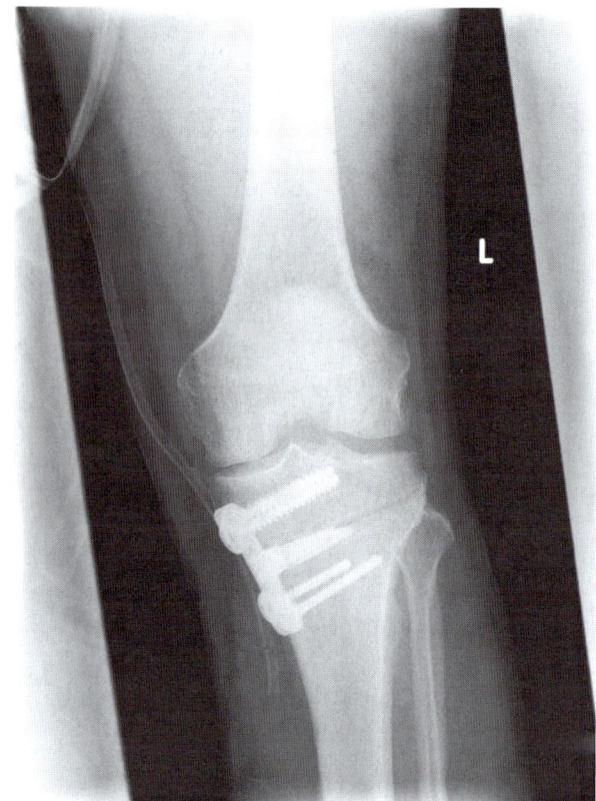

Figure 27-4. A high tibial osteotomy has been performed to correct the mechanical axis in this patient with medial knee pain and varus deformity.

Cartilage or Meniscus Deficiency With Ligament Deficiency

Cartilage lesions or meniscal deficiency with instability caused by ACL deficiency (Fig. 27-7) can be managed with an ACL reconstruction and a concomitant cartilage restoration or meniscal transplantation procedure, with an overall goal of restoring joint kinematics. Previously failed ACL reconstruction with bony tunnel expansion is often managed with a staged bone-grafting procedure. After successful grafting, an ACL reconstruction can follow simultaneously with the appropriate cartilage restorative procedure. Allografts are most commonly used for the ACL reconstruction in this setting.

Cartilage or Meniscus Deficiency With Malalignment and Ligament Deficiency

The most difficult clinical challenge is the patient who presents with focal cartilage lesions, compartment malalignment, and instability caused by ligament deficiency. Joint restorative efforts in such patients often require multiple procedures; with an ideal sequence of procedure considered on a case by case basis after a thorough assessment of the patient's symptoms and postoperative goals and expectations. Patients with pain as their primary symptom may be managed with a corrective osteotomy to unload the affected compartment. However, if instability is described as the chief complaint, a ligament reconstruction should be considered as first-line surgery. In rare cases, patients present with both pain and instability, and these should be managed in a staged

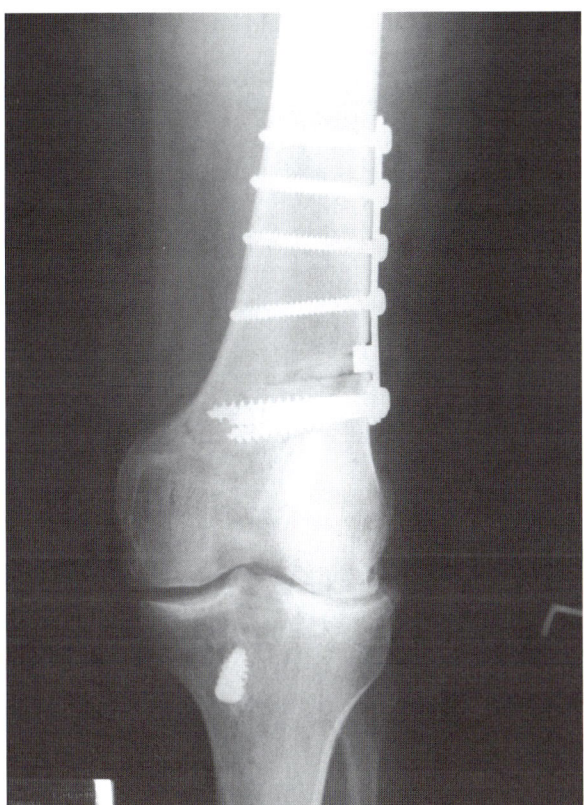

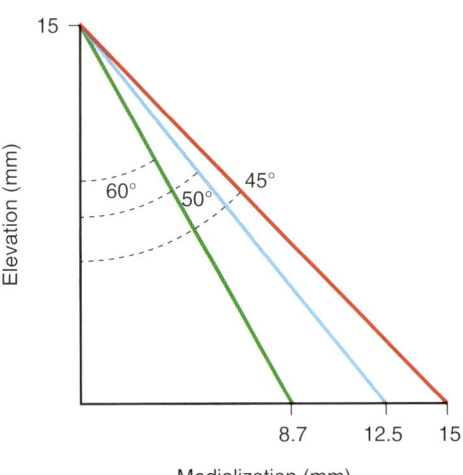

Figure 27-6. The amount of medialization may be adjusted by the angle of the osteotomy and degree of elevation. For a standard elevation of approximately 15 mm, the degree of medialization increases from 8.7 mm for a 60-degree cut relative to the anterior tibia to 15 mm for a 45-degree cut, as shown here. The amount of medialization may be titrated based on factors such as the patient's history of instability versus arthrosis.

Figure 27-5. Distal femoral osteotomy in this patient with obvious lateral compartment arthrosis and valgus malalignment is performed in an effort to offload the affected lateral compartment and relieve the patient's symptoms.

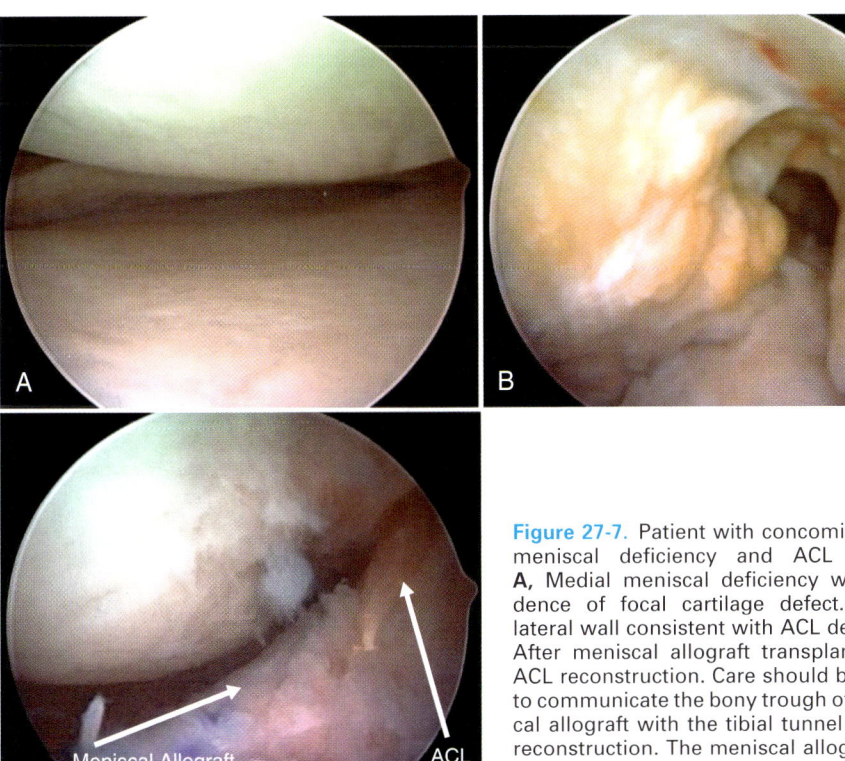

Figure 27-7. Patient with concomitant medial meniscal deficiency and ACL deficiency. **A,** Medial meniscal deficiency with no evidence of focal cartilage defect. **B,** Empty lateral wall consistent with ACL deficiency. **C,** After meniscal allograft transplantation and ACL reconstruction. Care should be taken not to communicate the bony trough of the meniscal allograft with the tibial tunnel of the ACL reconstruction. The meniscal allograft should be placed and secured before passage and fixation of an ACL graft.

algorithm, with ACL reconstruction first followed by restoration of alignment and cartilage resurfacing.

Additional Situations

Patients with a known ACL deficiency and malalignment may be managed with an ACL reconstruction alone, osteotomy alone, or as a combined procedure. The decision is again guided by the patient's symptoms, goals, and postoperative expectations. If a high tibial osteotomy is to be performed in isolation, the surgeon may consider a biplanar osteotomy whereby the varus alignment is addressed with an opening wedge medially; however, the ACL deficiency may be managed by simultaneously decreasing the tibial slope with the osteotomy cut. Alternatively, patients who are PCL-deficient with concomitant malalignment may have their tibial slope increased with an anterior-based opening wedge osteotomy to aid in reduced posterior tibial translation.

Finally, perhaps the most common scenario is the patient with a known focal cartilage defect and a history of previous meniscectomy who now has persistent joint line pain. As discussed earlier, it can often be difficult to discern whether the source of pain is the cartilage lesion or the loss of meniscal tissue. These patients are then managed with a concomitant meniscal transplantation and cartilage restorative procedure. They have generally been treated with a previous primary cartilage procedure, such as marrow stimulation or débridement, and are often revised with an osteochondral allograft in addition to the meniscal transplantation as a salvage procedure (Fig. 27-8).

Preferred Treatment

Revision procedures isolated to the femoral condyle, with no additional copathology (e.g., malalignment, instability, meniscal deficiency), are generally treated with an OA graft after a failed marrow stimulation technique or débridement. Alternatively, a failed microfracture procedure for smaller lesions can be managed with an OAT procedure. Cartilage lesions on the patella or trochlea are treated with ACI and a simultaneous anteromedialization of the tibial tubercle after a failed primary treatment. In the presence of a concomitant pathology, surgical procedures are addressed in a staged

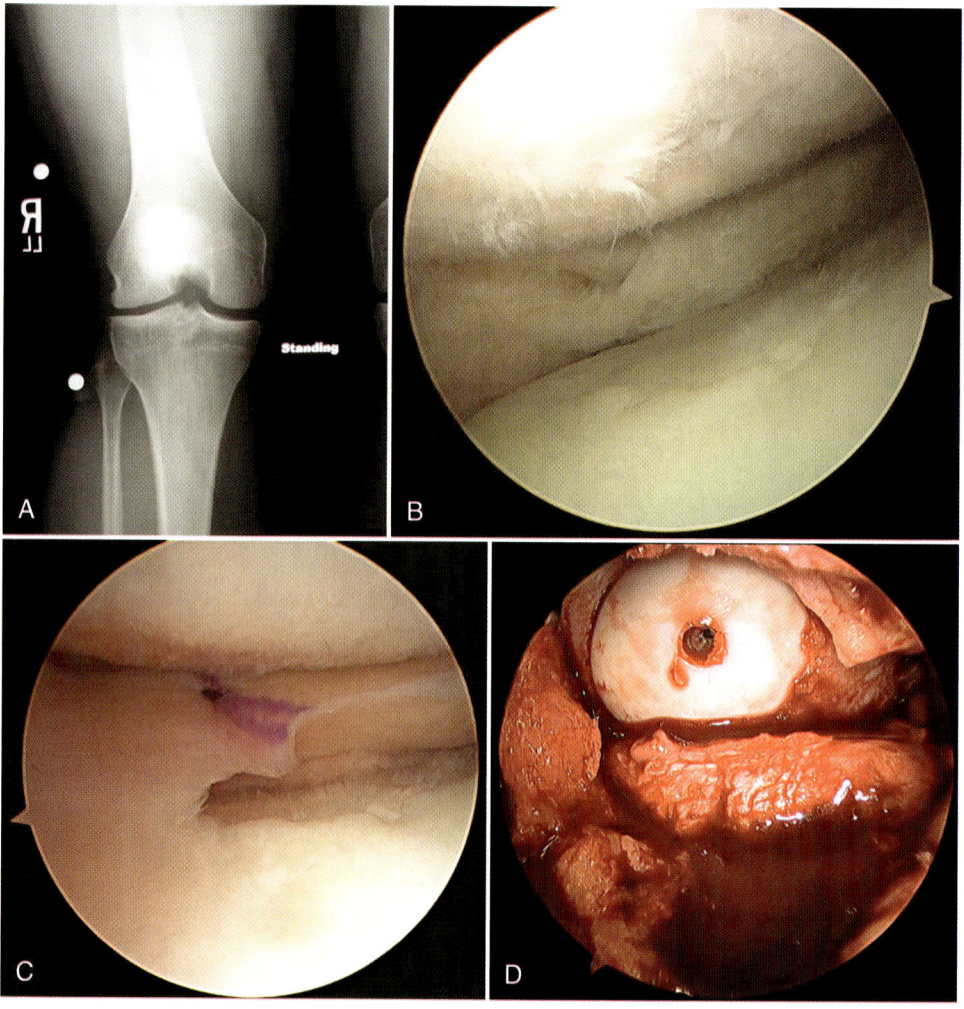

Figure 27-8. Patient with a combined meniscal deficiency and focal cartilage defect on the lateral side. **A,** Preoperative standing radiograph showing minimal evidence of joint space narrowing. **B,** Arthroscopic image of lateral compartment showing evidence of loss of meniscal tissue of the lateral compartment and a focal cartilage defect of the lateral femoral condyle. **C,** Arthroscopic image after placement of lateral meniscal allograft. **D,** Osteochondral allograft placed through a lateral parapatellar arthrotomy to restore articular cartilage architecture and surface congruence.

fashion or in combination with a revision cartilage procedure, as outlined earlier. Failed ACI of the patellofemoral (PF) joint are also revised with an OA graft.

REHABILITATION

Rehabilitation protocols vary according to the procedure(s) performed. In general, patients are placed in a hinged knee brace postoperatively and advised to use a continuous passive motion machine for 4 to 6 weeks for up to 6 hours/day. Patients who have a revision procedure on the femoral condyle or required an osteotomy with their revision procedure are protected with partial weight bearing and often use a postoperative hinged unloader brace (TROM Adjuster, DonJoy, Carlsbad, Calif). Rehabilitation of a revision procedure performed on the PF compartment allows for weight-bearing as tolerated, with a knee brace locked in extension, as long as the tibial tuberosity is not performed at that time, which would also require a period of protected weight-bearing. The goals of early rehabilitation are increased range of motion, patellar mobilization, quadriceps sets, isometrics, and proximal core strengthening. Six to 12 weeks postoperatively, patients begin to focus on a functional strengthening program. At about 3 months postoperatively, patients are advanced to muscular endurance with progressive running activities, advanced closed-chain strengthening, and plyometrics.

CONCLUSIONS

The variable algorithm and concomitant procedures often performed in revision cartilage restoration result in less predictable patient outcomes when compared with primary procedures. Minas and colleagues,[9] in a cohort study, evaluated outcomes of 321 patients (325 joints) who underwent an ACI. Of the 325 joints, 214 joints had no prior treatment affecting the subchondral bone whereas 111 joints had undergone a marrow stimulation procedure penetrating subchondral bone. Of the 214 joints with no prior treatment, 17 joints (8%) failed their restorative procedures. Revision procedures on the remaining 111 joints reported failure of 29 joints (26%), a rate three times that of the nontreated defects. Another group, in a prospective multicenter cohort study, evaluated 154 patients undergoing ACI as a revision after a failed previous marrow stimulation or débridement. Zaslav and associates[15] reported a success rate of 76% in these patients, with no statistical difference in outcome between patient groups at an average postoperative time of 48 months. There was a high reoperation rate noted at 49%; of this, 40% was related to the ACI procedure, including graft hypertrophy caused by periosteal patch use. Graft hypertrophy is believed to be less of an issue with the use of newer synthetic patches.[4]

Osteochondral allografting performed as a revision because of a failed primary or revision procedure has been described. McCulloch and coworkers[8] evaluated outcomes of 25 patients who underwent fresh OA of the femoral condyle. Of these patients, 25 had undergone at least one previous surgical treatment, including débridement and lavage, microfracture, or ACI. Thirteen patients underwent a concomitant procedure for malalignment (osteotomy), instability (ligament reconstruction), or meniscal transplantation. Patients overall reported an 84% satisfaction with their surgical procedure,

with no significant outcome difference between an isolated and combination OA grafting procedure. A similarly study conducted by LaPrade and associates[6] evaluated a group of 23 patients, of whom 20 had undergone a prior surgery and reported significant improvement in the International Knee Documentation Committee (IKDC) and Cincinnati outcomes.

Rue and coworkers,[10] in a prospective study, evaluated a group of 30 patients who underwent 31 combined meniscal transplantation and cartilage restoration procedures. Of these 31 procedures, 16 were an ACI and 15 were an OA graft; the patients were followed up for a minimum of 2 years. Of these, 28 patients reported an overall satisfaction of 76%, and 48% scored as normal or near-normal for functional outcome using IKDC at 2 years of follow-up. On rare occasions, a patient will present with articular lesions, meniscal deficiency, and malalignment. Gomoll and colleagues[3] evaluated seven patients at an average of 2 years. They reported that six of seven patients were able to return to their previous level of activity and demonstrated statistically significant improvement in outcome measures, with the exception of knee injury and osteoarthritis outcome score (KOOS) for pain ($P = .053$), KOOS symptoms ($P = .225$), and Short Form Health Survey SF-12 score ($P = .462$).

Revision articular restoration procedures remain a challenge for the operating surgeon. The goals of these procedures are to preserve joint function, improve congruity, and alleviate symptoms, thereby allowing patients to return to their desired level of activity. Treatment is guided by a thorough history and examination, discussion of the desired postoperative expectations, and consideration of the reason(s) for the failure of the primary cartilage procedure to avoid recurrence. Previous literature reports serve as a guide for expected outcomes; however, extreme caution should be taken when counseling this patient group because there are many confounding variables that may positively or negatively affect outcomes following revision procedures.

KEY REFERENCES

Biedert RM: Pathogenesis of patellofemoral pain. In Biedert RM, editor: Patellofemoral disorders: diagnosis and treatment, West Sussex, England, 2004, John Wiley & Sons, pp 55–68.

Black C, Clar C, Henderson R, et al: The clinical effectiveness of glucosamine and chondroitin supplements in slowing or arresting progression of osteoarthritis of the knee: a systematic review and economic evaluation. Health Technol Assess 13:1–148, 2009.

Gomoll AH, Kang RW, Chen AL, Cole BJ: Triad of cartilage restoration for unicompartmental arthritis treatment in young patients: meniscus allograft transplantation, cartilage repair and osteotomy. J Knee Surg 22:137–141, 2009.

Gomoll AH, Probst C, Farr J, et al: Use of a type I/III bilayer collagen membrane decreases reoperation rates for symptomatic hypertrophy after autologous chondrocyte implantation. Am J Sports Med 37: S20–S23, 2009.

Hepper CT, Halvorson JJ, Duncan ST, et al: The efficacy and duration of intra-articular corticosteroid injection for knee osteoarthritis: a systematic review of level I studies. J Am Acad Orthop Surg 17:638–646, 2009.

LaPrade RF, Botker J, Herzog M, Agel J: Refrigerated osteoarticular allografts to treat articular cartilage defects of the femoral condyles. A prospective outcomes study. J Bone Joint Surg Am 91:805–811, 2009.

Latterman C, Kang R, Cole B: Sports medicine update: What is new in treatment of focal chondral defect of the knee? Orthopedics 29:898–905, 2006.

McCulloch PC, Kang RW, Sobhy MH, et al: Prospective evaluation of prolonged fresh osteochondral allograft transplantation of the femoral condyle: minimum 2-year follow-up. Am J Sports Med 35:411–420, 2007.

Minas T, Gomoll A, Rosenberger R, et al: Increased failure rate of autologous chondrocyte implantation after previous treatment with marrow stimulation technique. Am J Sports Med 37:902–908, 2009.

Rue JP, Yanke AB, Busam ML, et al: Prospective evaluation of concurrent meniscus transplantation and articular cartilage repair: minimum 2-year follow-up. Am J Sports Med 36:1770–1778, 2008.

Steadman J, Rodkey W, Singleton S, et al: Microfracture technique for full-thickness condral defects: technique and clinical results. Oper Tech Orthop 7:300–304, 1997.

Strauss EJ, Hart JA, Miller MD, et al: Hyaluronic acid viscosupplementation and osteoarthritis: current uses and future directions. Am J Sports Med 37:1636–1644, 2009.

Teitge RA: Plain patellofemoral radiographs. Oper Tech Sports Med 9:134–151, 2001.

Watterson JR, Esdaile JM: Viscosupplementation: therapeutic mechanisms and clinical potential in osteoarthritis of the knee. J Am Acad Orthop Surg 8:277–284, 2000.

Zaslav K, Cole B, Brewster R, et al: A prospective study of autologous chondrocyte implantation in patients with failed prior treatment for articular cartilage defect of the knee: results of the Study of the Treatment of Articular Repair (STAR) clinical trial. Am J Sports Med 37:42–55, 2009.

Full references for this chapter can be found on www.expertconsult.com.

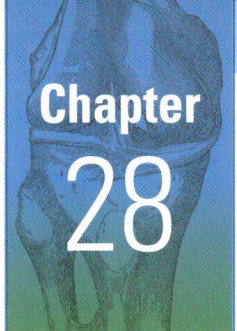

Chapter 28

Arthroscopic Treatment of Degenerative Arthritis of the Knee

Jack M. Bert

Significant controversy exists regarding the arthroscopic treatment of osteoarthritis (OA) of the knee. The indications for arthroscopic treatment of OA of the knee alone and in conjunction with other arthroscopic procedures will be reviewed.

HISTORICAL PERSPECTIVE

Arthroscopic débridement for OA of the knee was initially reported by Burman and colleagues[20] in 1934. They reviewed the first 30 cases in which knee arthroscopy was used to diagnose a "possible meniscal injury, arthritis in the knee, or suspected tumor."[19,20,28] In the group of arthritic cases, they had "the pleasant surprise of seeing a marked improvement in the joint following arthroscopy." They noted that "arthroscopy involves only minimal risk, and in some cases has actually had a beneficial therapeutic effect, probably due to the thorough flushing and distention of the joint which it necessitated." In 1941, Magnuson introduced the term *joint débridement* to describe an operation of the knee in which "all the accessible synovial membrane, osteophytes, diseased cartilage, and normal soft tissues were removed in an effort to relieve the symptoms of osteoarthritis"; this was performed as an open procedure in which "complete recovery of symptoms" occurred in 60 of 62 patients.[51]

During and after World War II, arthroscopy waned, and the open Magnuson procedure consisting of total synovectomy, osteophyte resection, cruciate ligament excision (if torn), as well as patellectomy was performed in most cases, with reported symptomatic improvement in 66% of patients. This procedure became widely accepted as the treatment of choice for OA of the knee as reported by Haggart[33] in 1947 and Isserlin[41] in 1950. These open débridement procedures, therefore, became the treatment of choice for arthritis of the knee until the resurgence of arthroscopy in the early 1970s.

CARTILAGE REPAIR

In 1743, William Hunter stated that "from Hippocrates to the present age, it is universally allowed that ulcerated cartilage is a troublesome thing and that once destroyed it is not repaired."[39] In 1849, Leidy confirmed this principle, stating that "a rupture of cartilage fragments is never united and that articular cartilage lacks regenerative power and fracture gaps extending into the joint become filled with tough fibrous tissue"[42,48]

Redfern, in 1851, described the histology of induced wounds of the articular cartilage of dog joints and stated that the wound "healed perfectly by the ingrowth of fibrous tissue,"[71] which he believed arose from the intercellular substance of the chondrocytes of the articular cartilage. However, as Mankin concluded in 1952, superficial lacerations of cartilage "neither heal nor progress to more serious disorders if they are small lesions."[52] On the basis of multiple animal studies, these superficial lacerations, therefore, are generally limited in progression and do not lead to clinical osteoarthritis. It was further noted that deep lacerations may be clearly visible years after injury.[53-55] When the subchondral bone is thus disrupted, intraosseous blood vessels expose bone matrix growth factors, causing fibrin clot formation. Inflammation introduces new cells into the cartilage defect and these cells proliferate and begin matrix repair.[16]

The native matrix of articular cartilage has extraordinary biochemical characteristics. It is a hyperhydrated tissue, with estimates of water content ranging as high as 80%. Connective tissue contains type I collagen, consisting of two alpha and one alpha-2 chains. The type II collagen of articular cartilage contains three alpha-1 chains. Furthermore, the alpha-1 chains of type II collagen have a different structure from those of type I. It is this type I collagen that is formed when fibrous tissue regenerates in attempts to repair injured articular cartilage.* Furthermore, mature fibrocartilage repair tissue has a relatively low proteoglycan concentration, and the proteoglycans do not resemble the large elaborate molecules found in native articular cartilage. Therefore, the healing response does not produce tissue with the unique composition, structure, and biochemical properties of normal articular cartilage.[16,62]

After cartilage injury or during the progression of osteoarthritis, some chondrocytes do proliferate but do not migrate through the matrix to enter the site of tissue injury. Any repair tissue matrix is formed by undifferentiated cells arising from the bone marrow and contains primarily type I collagen; thus, the normal articular cartilage properties cannot be restored. These reparative cells fail to organize the molecules they produce to create a strong cohesive structure similar to that of articular cartilage, and they produce other types of molecules that may interfere with the assembly of the cartilage matrix. This abnormal matrix, with its different composition and structure, therefore, adversely alters the material properties of the tissue.[26,69,72] These alterations compromise the ability of cartilage to survive and function in the highly stressed mechanical environment found in load-bearing joints and may lead to further cartilage degeneration and osteoarthritis. Disruption of collagen cross-linking causes cartilage to lose its intrinsic tensile stiffness, strength, and shear stiffness; the loss of proteoglycans and increased water content compromise its compressive and permeability properties.[4,56,80]

A number of treatments have been attempted to stimulate repair or reformation of the articular surface of the knee joint. Arthroscopically, these treatments include marrow stimulation procedures, débridement and shaving of fibrillated cartilage, and joint lavage. Other biologic articular cartilage

---

*References 13-15, 17, 18, 52-55, 63, and 67.

229

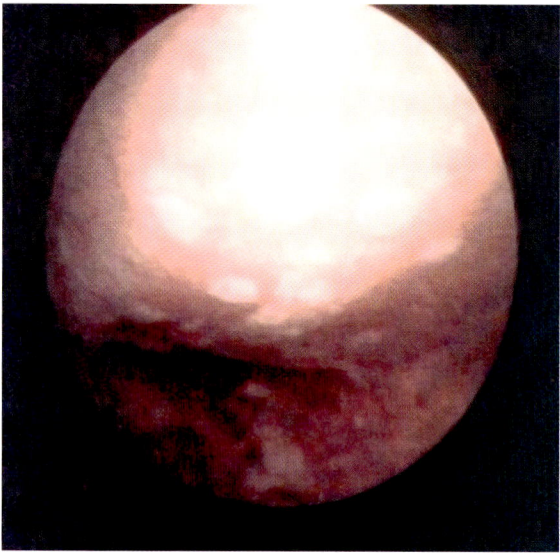

Figure 28-1. Pridie procedure illustrating fibrocartilage formation in medial femoral condylar drill holes.

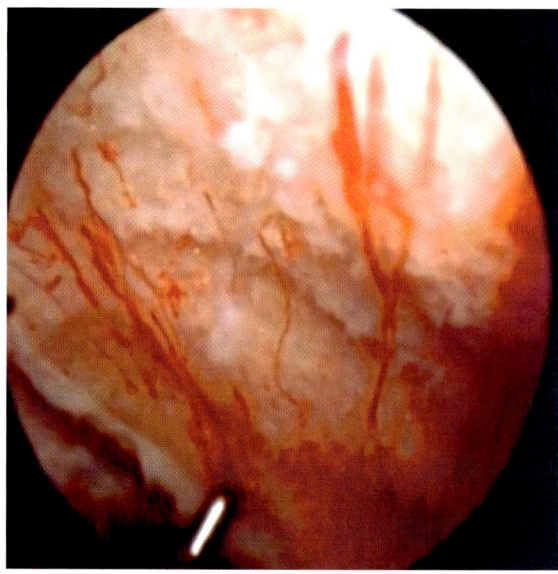

Figure 28-2. Abrasion arthroplasty. This figure depicts bleeding bone.

treatment options, including osteochondral autografting or allografting, will be described in other chapters of this text.

Marrow Stimulation Procedures

The concept of drilling through eburnated bone to stimulate reparative cartilage formation was originally described by Pridie in 1959 (Fig. 28-1); of 62 patients, 74% (46) believed that their operation was a success and stated that they would "have the operation again under similar circumstances."[68] To reconfirm these findings, Akeson surgically removed the articular cartilage of the femoral heads of dogs and drilled the subchondral bone. It was noted that after 1 year, at the time of retrieval, "excessive loading destroyed the initial repair tissue or prevented formation of repair tissue."[2] The results also indicated that 1 year after surgery, the concentration of proteoglycans in the reparative cartilage was less than half of that found in normal cartilage. Mitchell and Shepard[58,59] found that multiple small drill holes made in the subchondral bone of rabbit knee joints stimulates repair from large areas of the articular surface. They determined that repair tissue grows from the drill holes and spreads over the exposed bone. However, large areas of repair tissue that initially had the appearance of hyaline cartilage begin to fibrillate and deteriorate within 1 year. These experiments were the first to show that abrasion or perforation of subchondral bone could stimulate repair of large areas of joint surface with fibrocartilaginous tissue, but the retrieved repair tissue lacked the proteoglycan concentration found in previous studies of normal hyaline cartilage.

Abrasion arthroplasty of grade IV eburnated chondral lesions using motorized instrumentation was introduced by Johnson in 1981. This procedure is essentially an extension of the Pridie procedure except that in abrasion arthroplasty, a superficial layer of subchondral bone, approximately 1 to 3 mm thick, is removed to expose interosseous vessels (Fig. 28-2). Theoretically, the resulting hemorrhagic exudate forms a fibrin clot and allows for the formation of fibrous repair tissue over the eburnated bone (Fig. 28-3). In some

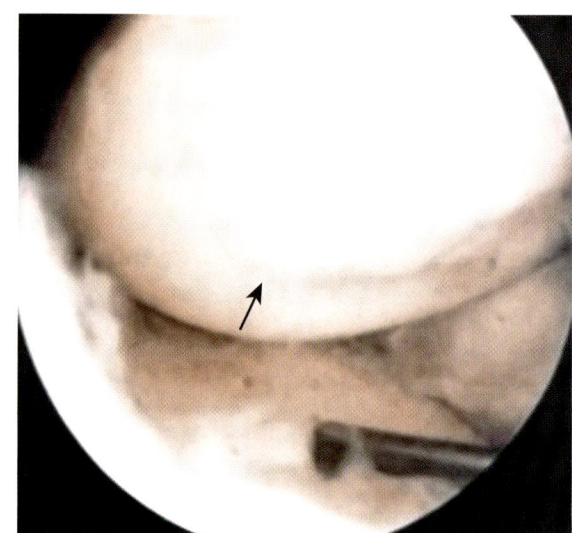

Figure 28-3. Arthroscopic view of patient 4 years after abrasion arthroplasty showing resurfacing with fibrocartilage.

patients, this fibrocartilaginous tissue lasted up to 4 years but in Johnson's series, only one of eight biopsy specimens showed any type II collagen typical of hyaline cartilage at the time of arthroscopic review and biopsy, and the rest had types I and III collagen.[9,45] In a series of patients at our institution who had abrasion arthroplasty, at 5-year follow-up examinations, 15 had been converted to total knee replacement (TKA) and biopsies were obtained at the time of TKA. All patients had fibrocartilage and type I collagen in their biopsy specimens (Fig. 28-4).

In our series of 126 patients who had treatment of unicompartmental gonarthrosis with abrasion arthroplasty or arthroscopic débridement alone, at 5-year follow-up examinations, 51% had good to excellent results with abrasion arthroplasty; 66% had good to excellent results with arthroscopic débridement alone.[9] However, all these patients had complete obliteration of the medial joint space

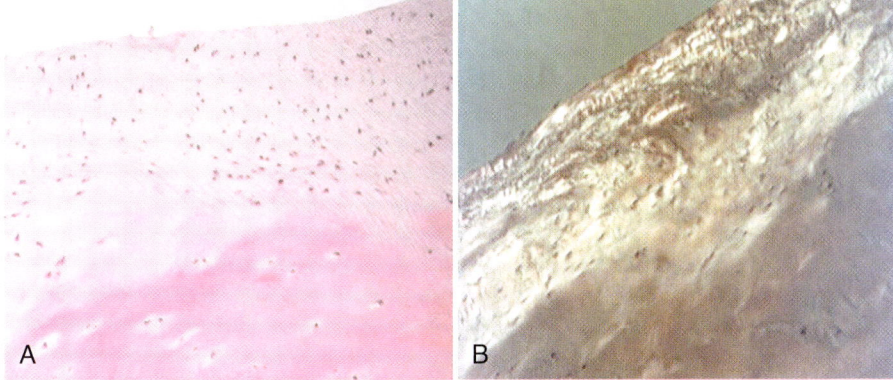

Figure 28-4. High power, hematoxylin-eosin stained, microscopic view of regenerated fibrocartilage **(A)** compared with polarized light view **(B)** of same section showing the disorganized surface fibrocartilage compared with the hyaline cartilage cells beneath. (Courtesy Dr. Steven Arnoczky, Laboroatory for Comparative Orthopedic Research, Michigan State University, East Lansing, Mich.)

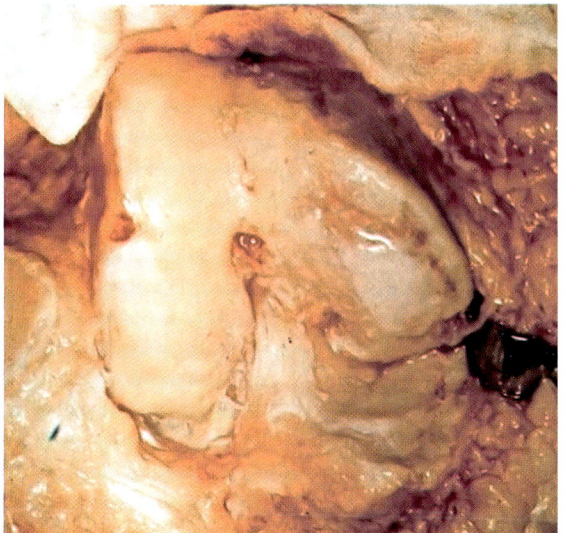

Figure 28-5. Patient after valgus upper tibial osteotomy showing formation of fibrocartilage on medial femoral condyle. (Courtesy Dr. Mark Coventry, Department of Orthopedics, Mayo Clinic, Rochester, Minn.)

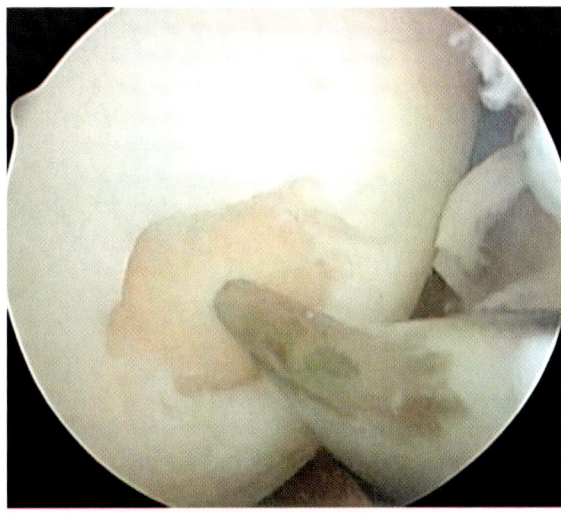

Figure 28-6. Intraoperative photograph of femoral condyle using awl to begin microfracture technique.

preoperatively. The results in our series were unrelated to age, presence of previous surgery, weight, extent of unicompartmental disease, presence or absence of joint space widening after surgery, and extent of residual varus or valgus deformity. Coventry and Bowman[23] noted that formation of hyaline-like cartilage occurred in the unloaded medial compartment of several patients after valgus upper tibial osteotomy (Fig. 28-5). This finding was confirmed arthroscopically by Fujisawa and associates[30] 12 to 18 months after upper tibial osteotomies, which implies that regeneration of reparative cartilage can occur secondary to unloading of bone alone, without additional surgery.

Microfracture

Blevens and coworkers[12] have recommended a microfracture technique in which they use an arthroscopic awl to create multiple perforations into the subchondral bone arthroscopically. They reported on 266 patients between 1985 and 1990, with a 3.7-year follow-up using a similar grading system to

the Outerbridge classification.[66,73] The indications for the microfracture technique include a full-thickness, well-circumscribed cartilage defect on a weight-bearing surface of the knee, with exposed subchondral bone (i.e., grade IV lesions). After chondral surface débridement, the bone is perforated to a depth of 3 to 4 mm using an awl, with the holes placed approximately 4 to 5 mm apart (Fig. 28-6). Blood should be seen emanating from the microfracture holes after perforation is complete. A postoperative rehabilitation program was used to provide motion without applying high load stress to the treated chondral defect. Repeat arthroscopies were performed in 80 patients. In most chondral defects, subchondral bone was covered with cartilage of varying quality and the term *hyaline-like* was introduced to describe the fibrocartilage surface. There was no evidence that hyaline cartilage was present at the second-look arthroscopy, and the authors confirmed that the only type of tissue that was seen to regenerate over these surfaces was fibrocartilaginous repair tissue. Furthermore, they stated that they were unable to determine the biochemical composition and durability of the presumed fibrocartilage repair tissue. Clearly, there is no evidence that hyaline cartilage is regenerated by marrow stimulation.

Arthroscopic Débridement

Arthroscopic débridement as a treatment option for OA was initially reported by Sprague in 1981, who arthroscopically débrided 330 knees diagnosed as having "degenerative arthritis … in two or more compartments of the knee."[76] Meniscectomy, chondroplasty of all surfaces, and loose body and debris removal were performed. At 1-year follow-up, 74% of these patients stated that the "knee was improved and more functional" than before surgery. The extent of arthritis, however, was not correlated clinically or roentgenographically with success rates. In the early to mid-1980s, others also reported that the results of arthroscopic débridement were not correlated with age or the extent of arthritis, either roentgenographically or arthroscopically, with up to 11-year follow-up.[44,75] However, Gross[32] and Ogilvie-Harris and Fitsialos[65] concluded in 1991 that OA severity was the best predictor of success after arthroscopic débridement and that normally aligned knees with mild arthritis had the best results with 8-year follow-up.

It is certainly not clear, however, that shaving damaged articular cartilage relieves pain. O'Donoghue[64] reported that chondroplasty in rabbit knees did not stimulate cartilage repair nor did it result in joint deterioration. Bentley[7,8] reported that chondroplasty during arthrotomy produced unpredictable results, and only 25% of patients treated with patellar chondroplasty had satisfactory results beyond 1 year. Timoney and colleagues[78] retrospectively reviewed 109 patients who had arthroscopic débridement for degenerative arthritis of the knee, with 4.2-year follow-up. Only 45% reported good results; 21% of patients experienced worsened symptoms and subsequently underwent TKA.

In 1996, Moseley[60] was one of the first to suggest that arthroscopic débridement for OA of the knee was no better than placebo. In that study, 10 patients with OA of the knee were randomized into a placebo group, an arthroscopic lavage group, and an arthroscopic débridement group. All patients at 6 months reported improvement in their pain scores and satisfaction with their surgery with the exception of one placebo patient. This study was repeated in 2002[61] with a larger patient group at a Veterans Administration hospital; 70% of these patients had moderate to severe OA. No significant differences were found among the three groups who had arthroscopy with débridement, arthroscopy with lavage, and placebo knee surgery. Those patients who had positive magnetic resonance imaging (MRI) scans with meniscal tears were excluded from the study. It was concluded that there is no clear role for arthroscopy in knees with OA.

Steadman and associates[77] recently reported a 71% success rate at 2 years for arthroscopic débridement of OA using the Western Ontario and McMaster Index (WOMAC) and Lysholm scoring systems. Wai and coworkers[79] and Hawker and colleagues[37] reported that up to 9.2% of patients had a TKA after 1 year and 18.4% had a TKA after 3 years subsequent to arthroscopic débridement, indicating the transient nature of improvement in some patients undergoing this procedure. A number of studies have claimed that arthroscopic débridement and shaving help relieve the symptoms of OA

of the knee, but it is unclear why these patients improve and why they remain improved for as long as 5 years postoperatively.*

Alignment and Arthroscopic Débridement

Correlation of preoperative angular deformity with the results of arthroscopically debrided knees was originally reported by Salisbury and associates[74] in 1985. In patients with residual varus deformity, 32% noted improvement in pain at 1 year. Normal knee alignment was considered as 1 to 7 degrees of femorotibial valgus alignment preoperatively. Harwin[35] and Baumgartner and coworkers[6] concluded that abnormal varus or valgus angulation was a statistically significant factor in predicting a failed result after arthroscopic débridement, Similar findings were reported by Ogilvie-Harris and Fitsialos.[65] Those patients who have varus or significant valgus knee deformities with medial or lateral compartment disease, respectively, will have worse results than those with postoperative neutral or mild valgus alignment.

Arthroscopy, Radiography, and Degenerative Joint Disease

The correlation between degenerative joint disease viewed on x-ray films and at arthroscopy was reported by Lysholm and colleagues[50] in 1987. Chondral damage was graded arthroscopically according to Outerbridge,[66] and radiographic examination was evaluated according to the Ahlback classification.[1] In one group of patients, there were Outerbridge grade II changes involving both the tibia and the femur, with space narrowing consistent with Ahlback grade I changes on x-ray. In a second group with Outerbridge grades III and IV changes, complete joint space obliteration occurred, consistent with Ahlback grade II changes. Involvement of the lateral compartment as assessed on arthroscopy was significantly more common in patients with medial compartment Outerbridge grades II and III changes as well as Ahlback grades II and III changes on x-ray.[50]

Arthroscopy and Lavage

In 1978, Bird and Ring[11] reported on a series of 14 patients who had arthroscopic lavage of the knee. Of these patients, 13 (93%) improved by 1 week, but by 4 weeks only 7 (50%) had noted mild to moderate improvement. In 1988, Jackson and associates[43] reported on more than 207 patients with "femoral tibial arthritic disease in either the medial or lateral compartment" who had lavage versus arthroscopic débridement, with 2-year follow-up. They found that débridement of chondral and meniscal tissue produced 68% improvement, and lavage alone resulted in 45% symptomatic improvement. In 1991, Livesley and coworkers[49] compared 37 knees with OA treated by arthroscopic lavage and physiotherapy with a control group of 24 knees treated by physiotherapy alone. Those treated by joint lavage improved to a greater degree than the control group and the improvement lasted longer.

---

*References 35, 36, 49, 57, 70, and 81.

The physiotherapy group initially experienced an improvement, but by the end of the study they had returned to their pretreatment state.

In 1992, Ike and colleagues[40] compared a group of patients treated with standard medical treatment (nonsteroidal antiinflammatory drugs [NSAIDs], steroid injections, physical therapy, analgesics) with those receiving tidal lavage in the office using local anesthesia. In this study, 1000 mL of saline was injected into the joint in multiple stages and aspirated, and the patient was sent home. At the conclusion of this prospective 12-week study, 62% of the tidal irrigation group of patients and 36% of the medically managed patients were improved functionally and symptomatically. In 1993, Chang[22] reported on two groups of patients, one that had undergone arthroscopic surgery and débridement, and another receiving needle joint lavage. At 1 year, 44% of patients who underwent arthroscopic surgery reported improvement and 58% of patients who underwent joint lavage noted improvement. Patients with tears of the medial or lateral meniscus had a higher probability of improvement after arthroscopic surgery as opposed to closed-needle lavage. Only two of the 27 measures of outcome showed statistically significant differences between the arthroscopy and lavage groups. It was concluded that the removal of soft tissue abnormalities via arthroscopic surgery does not generally improve pain and knee dysfunction associated with non–end-stage osteoarthritis any more than simple joint lavage, unless a meniscal tear was present. Many explanations for symptomatic relief secondary to arthroscopic lavage have been postulated, such as removal of cartilage debris, crystals, and inflammatory factors. Temporary improvement in signs of inflammation may support the hypothesis that lavage removes inflammatory agents, but the nature of these inflammatory agents remains undetermined.[21,25,31,34]

CONCLUSIONS

Arthroscopic débridement of the degenerative knee has been described as a worthwhile procedure in young patients and in older patients who desire symptomatic improvement and do not wish to risk the morbidity of a total knee replacement. Success rates for arthroscopic débridement vary between 50% and 67%, depending on many factors, including patient age, degree of arthritis, activity level, and extent of follow-up. Arthroscopic lavage success rates vary between 45% and 51% and do not appear to have the same longevity of success as arthroscopic débridement.[5] Furthermore, from at least two studies comparing arthroscopic débridement alone with abrasion arthroplasty in conjunction with arthroscopic débridement, it is apparent that abrasion arthroplasty and the Pridie procedure do not appear to offer any greater benefit in the treatment of degenerative arthritis of the knee than débridement alone.[9,70] There appears to be no advantage in performing arthroscopy in conjunction with upper tibial osteotomy compared with upper tibial osteotomy alone. The results are similar.

Furthermore, the results of upper tibial osteotomy in conjunction with abrasion arthroplasty were identical to those in a similar series of patients who had upper tibial osteotomy alone.[27] Arthroscopic procedures, therefore, in conjunction with upper tibial osteotomy, seem to be of limited value. Furthermore, the prognostic value of the arthroscope in determining whether or not to proceed with upper tibial osteotomy is minimally helpful, as noted by Fujisawa and associates[30] and Keene and Dyravy.[46] They concluded that there is no correlation in terms of prognosis and arthroscopic evaluation prior to tibial osteotomy compared with the clinical results subsequent to osteotomy.

Since Moseley and colleagues' study,[61] published in 2002, the Center for Medicare and Medicaid Services has disallowed the arthroscopic code for débridement in a patient on Medicare. This is because of the study's conclusion that success rates for arthroscopic débridement are no greater than other sham operations for OA in older patients. This opinion was reaffirmed by Kirkley and associates[47] in 2008, when they published a similar study. In their study, at 2 years, they compared 86 patients who had arthroscopic lavage for grades II to IV changes with a larger group that had physical therapy, NSAIDs, steroid injections, and viscosupplementation. They excluded patients with meniscal lesions or mechanical symptoms and, using WOMAC and Short Form Health Survey (SF-36) scoring systems, concluded that there is no role for arthroscopic débridement in OA of the knee. Recently, Bin and coworkers[10] reported on 68 patients (mean age, 63 years), with grade IV medial compartment OA. In this group, 90% improved after surgery using visual analogue scale (VAS) and Lysholm scoring systems. However, 5% required TKA at 4 years postoperatively and 25% required further surgery at a mean of 6.3 years.

The three clinical variables associated with improvement after arthroscopic débridement are preoperative medial joint line tenderness, a positive Steinman test indicative of a torn medial meniscus, and the presence of unstable meniscal tissue at the time of arthroscopy.[24] The reported predictors of improved outcomes from arthroscopic débridement are preoperative mechanical symptoms resulting from loose bodies, displaced articular chondral lesions, and meniscal tears.[29] In contrast, the reported predictors for poor outcomes after arthroscopic débridement for OA of the knee are marked malalignment, restricted range of motion, prior surgery, and severe OA in most published articles.[38] The American Academy of Orthopaedic Surgeons (AAOS) guideline on treatment of OA of the knee[3] stated that in joints with mechanical symptoms, including locking, catching, or giving way, arthroscopic removal of loose bodies, chondral flaps, and/or unstable meniscal tissue with débridement in the arthritic joint improves symptoms and clearly is indicated.

In conclusion, the arthroscope is useful in the treatment of degenerative arthritis of the arthritic knee when a patient has preoperative symptoms indicating a mechanical abnormality. Arthroscopy has an extremely low morbidity. However, based on the series reviewed in the literature, arthroscopic débridement has minimal value in association with upper tibial osteotomy or marrow stimulation procedures.

KEY REFERENCES

American Academy of Orthopaedic Surgeons: Clinical practice guideline on the treatment of osteoarthritis of the knee (non-arthroplasty), Rosemont, Ill, 2008, American Academy of Orthopaedic Surgeons (AAOS).

Bert JM: Arthroscopic treatment of degenerative arthritis of the knee. In Insall JN, Scott WN, editors: Surgery of the knee, ed 3, New York, 2001, Churchill Livingstone, p 381.

Bert JM, Maschka K: The arthroscopic treatment of unicompartmental gonarthrosis: a five-year follow-up study of abrasion arthroplasty plus arthroscopic débridement and arthroscopic débridement alone. Arthroscopy 5:25–34, 1989.

Buckwalter JA, Rosenberg LC, Hunziker EB: Articular cartilage: Composition, structure, response to injury and methods of facilitating repair. In Ewing JW, editor: Articular cartilage and knee joint function: basic science in arthroscopy, New York, 1990, Raven Press, p 19.

Coventry MB, Bowman PW: Long-term results of upper tibial osteotomy for degenerative arthritis of the knee. Acta Orthop Belg 48:139–156, 1982.

Dervin G, Stiell I, Rody K, Grabowski J: Effect of arthroscopic débridement for osteoarthritis of the knee on health related quality of life. J Bone Joint Surg Am 85:10–17, 2008.

Harwin SF, Stein A, Stern R, et al: Arthroscopic débridement of the osteoarthritic knee: a step toward patient selection. Arthroscopy 1:7–15, 1991.

Hunt S, Jazrawi L, Sherman O: Arthroscopic management of osteoarthritis of the knee. J Am Acad Orthop Surg 10:356–363, 2002.

Mow VC, Rosenwasser MP: Articular cartilage: biomechanics. In Woo SL, Buckwalter JA, editors: Injury and repair of the musculoskeletal soft tissues, Park Ridge, Ill, 1988, American Academy of Orthopaedic Surgeons, p 427.

Ogilvie-Harris DJ, Fitsialos DP: Arthroscopic management of the degenerative knee. J Arthroscopy 7:151–159, 1991.

Steadman R, Ramappa A, Maxwell B, Briggs K: An arthroscopic treatment regimen for osteoarthritis of the knee. Arthroscopy 23:948–955, 2007.

Wai E, Kreder J, Williams J: Arthroscopic débridement of the knee for osteoarthritis in patients fifty years of age or older: utilization and outcomes in the Province of Ontario. J Bone Joint Surg Am 84:17–22, 2002.

Full references for this chapter can be found on www.expertconsult.com.

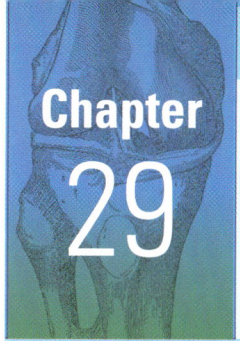

Treatment of Juvenile Osteochondritis Dissecans of the Knee

Matthew Leidl and Jon K. Sekiya

Juvenile osteochondritis dissecans (JOCD) is a condition in which a portion of subchondral bone and its overlying cartilage become damaged; it usually affects the knee.* This results in a spectrum of pathology beginning with a lesion to the bone only, followed by eventual cartilage separation, bone separation, and loose body formation.

JOCD may result in myriad nonspecific clinical symptoms, ranging from mild pain to joint effusion to locking,[13,31,38,55] which can complicate the diagnosis. Furthermore, the cause of and most effective treatment for osteochondritis dissecans (OCD) and JOCD still remain largely unclear today because of conflicting reports, studies that combine lesion types, small study population sizes, and short follow-up periods.[7,9,23,78] Regardless, treatment should seek to prevent early-onset osteoarthritis, which is associated with unhealed lesions and may show favorable results in up to 77.7% of cases.[1]

HISTORY

Osteochondritis dissecans exists in both juvenile and adult forms, distinguished as originating before or after closure of the distal femoral epiphysis, respectively.[12,73] Cahill and Ahten[10] have proposed a further subdivision of quiescent JOCD (QJOCD) as an asymptomatic form of JOCD, which will become symptomatic if left untreated.

Paget first described OCD in 1870 as resulting from a "quiet necrosis" of the bone.[65] It was König, however, who named the condition osteochondritis dissecans in 1887, under the false impression that the lesion arose from an inflammatory process.[47] König later rejected this hypothesis, but the misnomer remained.[4]

EPIDEMIOLOGY

It is difficult to determine the true prevalence of JOCD largely because papers tend to report OCD and JOCD cases as single populations.[9,12,23] The lesion may also be confused with normal variants in ossification, which could lead to over- or underreporting of its true incidence.[30] Finally, patients with JOCD often wait several months before seeking treatment, leading some to speculate that many lesions may heal spontaneously and hence will never be diagnosed. Most authors agree, however, that the condition is relatively uncommon.[13]

Historically, more boys present with JOCD than girls; the ratio of boys to girls affected ranges from 2:1 to 3:2, although this seems to be decreasing.[3,9,23,38,39] The average age of children afflicted with JOCD is reported as between 11.3 and 12.9 years.[13,69,83] This, too, seems to be changing; some have noted that the average patient age has gone down in recent years.

Right and left knees are affected in approximately equal proportions, although some report a slight preponderance for right knee involvement.[38,61] Bilateral lesions have been reported in 21.1% to 47% of affected children.[11] Lesions tend to be located in the medial femoral condyle, with most being in the lateral aspect of the medial femoral condyle.[3,13] Lesions in the central and medial aspects of the medial femoral condyle are somewhat less common. The lateral femoral condyle has been reported as the lesion site in 15% to 16.5% of cases. The patella tends to be involved less often, with reports ranging from 4.8% to 6.5% involvement. Lesions have also been reported in the tibial plateau, the entirety of the femoral trochlea,[72] and both the lateral and medial condyles of a single femur,[35] although these are not common findings.

CAUSE

There is a great deal of uncertainty regarding the cause of JOCD, and many theories have attempted to explain the condition.[9] König initially described OCD as stemming from inflammation, but even König himself has rejected this theory since its first proposal[4,47] because no evidence of inflammation had been noted.[25]

It has also been suggested that aseptic necrosis is responsible because of a proposed poor blood supply to the medial femoral condyle.[31,70] Another report, however, found no evidence of necrosis in excised OCD lesions, challenging this idea.[14]

Some studies have postulated that there is a familial form of OCD, with an autosomal dominant inheritance pattern.[34,60,64,68,75] Petrie,[67] however, conducted a study of 86 first-degree relatives in 34 patients with OCD lesions and found only one relative who also had the disease. Additionally, Hefti and colleagues[38] have found that only 4.2% of their 452 patients with OCD reported having family members with the condition. It is possible that conditions such as multiple epiphyseal dysplasia, which has both autosomal dominant and recessive inheritance patterns, may be mistaken for familial OCD.[15] Various other theories for the cause of JOCD have been proposed, including links to embolism,[25] ossification abnormalities,[71,73] patient height, endocrine dysfunction, and Osgood-Schlatter disease, but these hypotheses have not been well supported.[61,67]

The remaining proposals largely center on some type of trauma as the cause of JOCD. Fairbank[25] has suggested that the lesion results from internal tibial torsion, which drives the tibial spine into the femoral condyle thereby causing a fracture, leading to OCD. A more recent study by Bramer and associates[6] have shown that individuals with OCD have a significantly greater degree of external tibial torsion as compared with unaffected individuals.

These theories have been questioned, however, because several studies have observed large percentages of lesions in

---

*References 5, 11, 12, 22, 29, 33, 39, 40, 46, 66, and 83.

areas that could not have been from such an injury.[41,61] Additionally, direct trauma is reported in only 21.2% to 46% of patients with OCD or JOCD and in less than 10% of patients with JOCD.[3,10,38,83]

The currently prevailing theory relates JOCD to repetitive trauma. Several reports have supported the idea that repeated microtraumatic events lead to stress fractures in the subchondral bone, compromising vascular supply to the area and causing lesion formation.[3,9,10,12,40,48] This is supported by the observation of joint deformities in several patients, which may increase joint stress and the location of many lesions in weight-bearing areas of the knee. The theory is further strengthened by the fact that many JOCD sufferers are active athletes,[23,25,38,41,83] although it is questionable whether they are significantly more active than their unaffected peers.[61]

Finally, there may be a link between JOCD of the lateral femoral condyle and discoid meniscus, with speculation that the altered meniscus has a decreased capacity to absorb loads.[19,37,74] This lends further support to the microtrauma theory.

PROGNOSTIC INDICATORS

JOCD lesions tend to show greater healing rates than OCD lesions.[7,38,42,69] Additionally, younger children may show an increased propensity for healing than older children, although this has been challenged.[78] It is generally accepted that smaller JOCD lesions have a greater ability to heal than larger lesions[12,62] and that unstable lesions have a poorer prognosis than stable lesions. Despite these generalities, each theory has been questioned.[45,79] Although many have speculated that lesion location may be related to prognosis, reports vary[38,45,62,69,83]; thus, it seems best to disregard location when determining a patient's outlook.

CLINICAL PRESENTATION AND DIAGNOSIS

Early JOCD lesions tend to show nonspecific symptoms, such as pain, swelling, and quadriceps atrophy.[13,38,55] Later lesions may show more severe symptoms, including limping, effusion, decreased range of motion, and locking, especially if loose bodies are present. Even with such varied symptoms, Green and Banks[31] have observed no clinical abnormalities in half of their 27 patients. Similarly, physical examinations for JOCD tend to yield few definitive results. Palpation may elicit tenderness, although this has been reported in from 36.2% to 74.6% of patients.

Wilson[80] has indicated that children with JOCD may walk with their ipsilateral foot laterally rotated to relieve pain from contact between the ACL, tibial spinous process, and lesion and described a technique for using this finding to diagnose JOCD. The patient lies supine and the knee is flexed by the examiner to 90 degrees; the tibia is medially rotated and the knee is extended, which should elicit pain that is relieved with lateral rotation or successful treatment. Unfortunately, a more recent study found the test to be positive in only 25% of 32 cases of known OCD.[16]

Therefore, imaging studies may be the best means of diagnosing JOCD. Anteroposterior, lateral, skyline, tunnel, and notch radiographs are always indicated to detect the presence of a bony lesion[11,31,36] (Fig. 29-1).

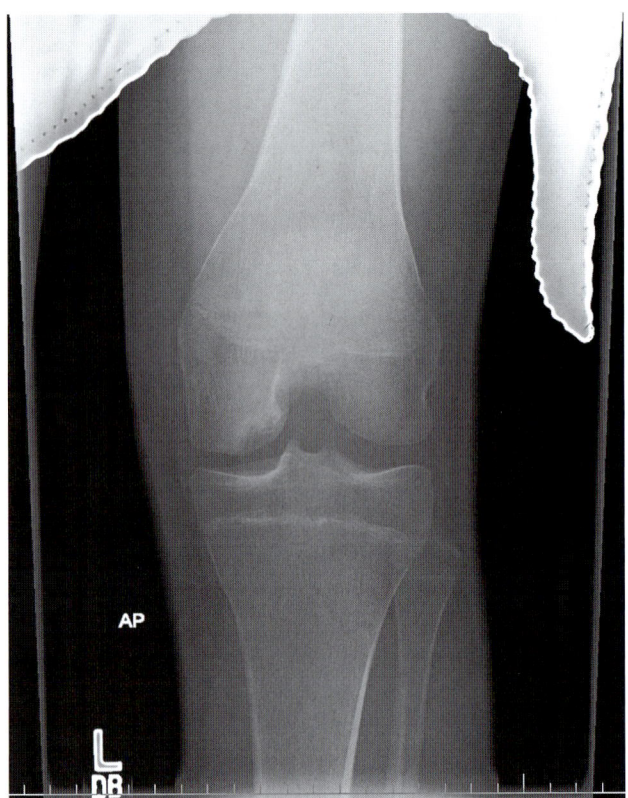

Figure 29-1. Notch posteroanterior (PA) radiograph of an unstable OCD lesion.

Many have advocated the use of magnetic resonance imaging (MRI) to visualize the cartilaginous aspects of the lesion to determine its size.* MRI may also be useful in ascertaining lesion stability and prognosis, because lesions surrounded by a high T2 signal intensity line may be unstable, particularly if the line has the same intensity as the joint fluid around it, is surrounded by a second low T2 intensity line, is present along with breaks in the subchondral bone plate as seen on T2-weighted MRI, or is surrounded by cysts.[83] Dipaola and coworkers[22] noted a better correlation between MRI and arthroscopic staging than between radiographic and arthroscopic staging, suggesting that MRI is a superior technique. Gadolinium-enhanced MRI may further aid in diagnosis[49] (Fig. 29-2).

Cahill and colleagues[9,11,12] have recommended the use of technetium scans to determine the healing status of the lesion and rule out normal ossification variants as potential JOCD lesions, but not to ascertain lesion prognosis. Cepero and associates[13] have also suggested that computed tomography (CT) scans are helpful for discerning the extent and location of JOCD lesions, especially in younger patients who might have difficulty staying still for an MRI. Regardless of the study, normal ossification variants common in the femoral condyles of children may resemble JOCD lesions.[8,30] Thus, care must be taken when interpreting images to ensure an accurate diagnosis.

To further assist with assessing OCD lesion prognosis, several classification systems have been developed; these are summarized in Table 29-1.

---

*References 17, 18, 21, 38, 42, and 69.

TREATMENT

Untreated JOCD lesions have been shown to lead to early-onset osteoarthritis; treatment is aimed its prevention.[1,7] Although many treatment options exist for JOCD, they are difficult to evaluate because authors often mix OCD and JOCD and stable and unstable lesions into the same study populations.[9,78]

Initial Management

In spite of the mixed study population, there is a general consensus that stable JOCD lesions should initially be managed nonsurgically.[38] Whether this management should include immobilization or continuous motion is uncertain. Healing has been reported in up to 50% of JOCD lesions at an average of 10 months after management by restricting activities, but not mobility or weight bearing.[9,10,12] Others have also found good results with similar activity modifications and quadriceps exercises to avoid quadriceps atrophy, stiffness, and potential cartilage degeneration that may be associated with immobilization,[3,16,83] as noted by Hughston and coworkers.[41]

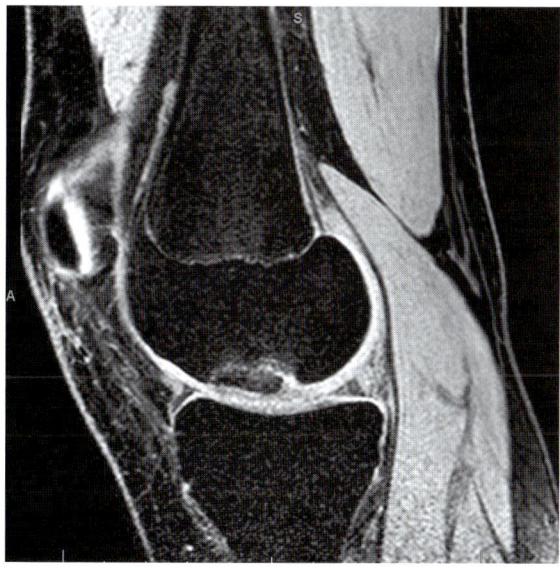

Figure 29-2. Saggital MRI scan of an unstable OCD.

In contrast, several studies have recommended that conservative treatment include some form of immobilization. Green and Banks[31] reported excellent results in 17 of 25 knees that were kept in braces or casts. Others have also found favorable results following treatment with a cast[69] or cast followed by a brace.[78] In spite of these differing theories, Hefti and colleagues[38] were able to find no statistically significant difference between a number of conservative treatment methods used for 154 patients in their study, which included the use of casts and braces, no treatment, or physical therapy.

It is important to note that noncompliance may be a significant hindrance to successful conservative treatment, especially among the active population typically affected by JOCD. This has prompted some to recommend a shortened period of conservative treatment followed by surgery, which has shown positive results in this group.[10,23,38] Similarly, Cepero and associates[13] have reported that 89.5% of their 67 patients required surgical intervention and that compared with conservative management, arthroscopic treatment decreased clinical healing time by an average of 4.8 months and radiographic healing by an average of 3.4 months.

Surgical Treatment

Although nonsurgical treatment may show favorable results in many patients with JOCD, it is not always successful. For unstable lesions, lesions in patients approaching epiphyseal closure, and stable lesions that have failed to heal following conservative management, surgery is recommended.[9,10,12,38] The goal of surgical treatment should be to ensure stable fixation of the lesion and to encourage healing of cartilage and restoration of the blood supply.[56] Most recommend the use of arthroscopic procedures whenever possible to reduce healing time.[13] If a lesion cannot be fully visualized or realigned arthroscopically, however, an open procedure is indicated.

Surgical methods tend to vary depending on the stage of the lesion. Kocher and coworkers[45] have recommended that stage II lesions undergo chondroplasty followed by fixation, stage III lesions be débrided and fixed, and stage IV lesions be treated by débridement of avascular bone and fibrous tissue, with autogenous bone grafting to fill large lesion craters. Success rates for surgical procedures vary widely based on procedure type, with reports ranging from 35% to 75%,

Table 29-1 Staging Classifications for Osteochondritis Dissecans Lesions

Stage	Radiographic Classification[5]	Arthroscopic Classification[33]	MRI Classification[22]	Scintigraphic Classification[11]
0	None	None	None	Normal knee
I	Stable lesion	Intact lesion	Thickening of articular cartilage; signal change	Normal scintigram; radiograph suggestive of OCD
II	Partially detached lesion	Lesion with early signs of separation	Articular cartilage breached; low signal rim behind fragment indicating fibrous attachment	Focal validity at OCD lesion site
III	Completely detached fragment	Partially detached lesion	High signal changes behind fragment indicating synovial fluid between fragment and subchondral bone	Stage II appearance and increased activity in the femoral condyle containing the lesion
IV	Detached lesion that has been displaced within the joint	Loose bodies	Loose body	Stage III appearance and increased activity at the ipsilateral tibial plateau

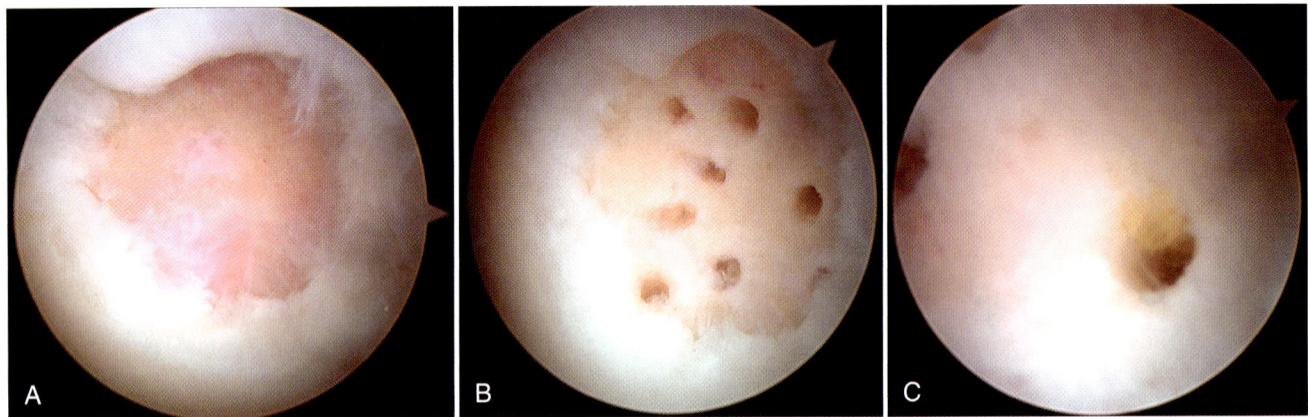

Figure 29-3. Microfracture of an unsalvageable displaced OCD lesion. **A,** Lesion outlined and prepared for microfracture. **B,** Multiple microfracture holes created. **C,** Note the marrow elements coming out of the microfracture hole when the tourniquet was released and the arthroscopic fluid pressure turned off.

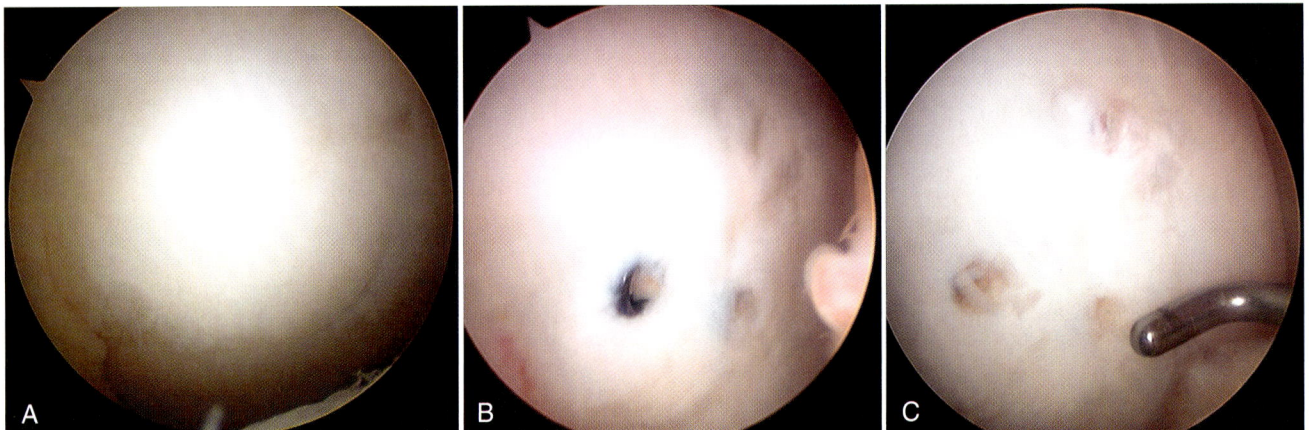

Figure 29-4. Nondisplaced but unstable OCD lesion. **A,** Arthroscopic view of the OCD lesion. **B,** Healed in situ fixation of the OCD lesion. **C,** Lesion completely stable to probing after screw removal.

up to 95%.[1,38,55] This range is likely influenced by fact that many papers report results based on mixed study populations, as noted earlier.[9,78]

Arthroscopic drilling is the primary surgical method used to treat stable JOCD.[23] The technique requires a series of holes to be drilled into the subchondral bone beneath a lesion to promote revascularization.[13,48] This can be performed transarticularly, drilling through the articular cartilage on the exposed side of the lesion, or retroarticularly, drilling through a proximal section of the femur, usually the femoral condyle, to penetrate the lesion without drilling through the articular cartilage.[1] Additionally, retroarticular drilling is often accompanied by bone grafting, in which bone plugs from the ipsilateral anterosuperior iliac spine (ASIS) may be harvested and tamped into the drill holes in the lesion to promote healing, according to a newer method proposed by Lebolt and Wall.[52]

Some authors have suggested that transarticular drilling damages the articular surface, which has a very limited ability to heal. For this reason, they recommend retroarticular drilling, although it is noted that this process is more challenging to carry out. Despite this, each procedure has demonstrated positive outcomes[1,13,23] and Bruns and colleagues[7] have observed no significant difference in knee function based on drilling method, but retroarticular drilling may result in a slower onset of osteoarthritis. In spite of these positive results, Hefti and associates[38] have reported no significant difference in the healing rate between conservative treatment or drilling alone used to treat patients with OCD and JOCD lesions that demonstrated moderate or marked sclerosis, highlighting a possible limitation to the procedure.

Lesions that are unstable are typically treated with some form of internal fixation.[9] To accomplish this, most recommend that the fragment fit as closely as possible into the crater; fragments that are too large should be débrided and craters that are too large should be packed with autogenous bone to approximate the lesion size.[45,63]

Additionally, some suggest that the lesion bed be curetted or drilled to the point of bleeding to promote healing before the fragment is fixed.[53,54] Alternatively, microfracture may be performed, in which unstable cartilage is removed from the lesion crater and an awl is used to bore holes in the subchondral bone to stimulate bleeding and healing[32,57] (Fig. 29-3). When the lesion fits properly into the crater, it is set in place using one of a variety of devices.

Herbert screws[48,54] and metal cortex screws[53] have each shown positive results when used to reattach or stabilize in situ OCD and JOCD lesions. An oft-cited drawback to the use of metal screws for fixation is the likely need for future hardware removal[21] (Figs. 29-4 and 29-5).

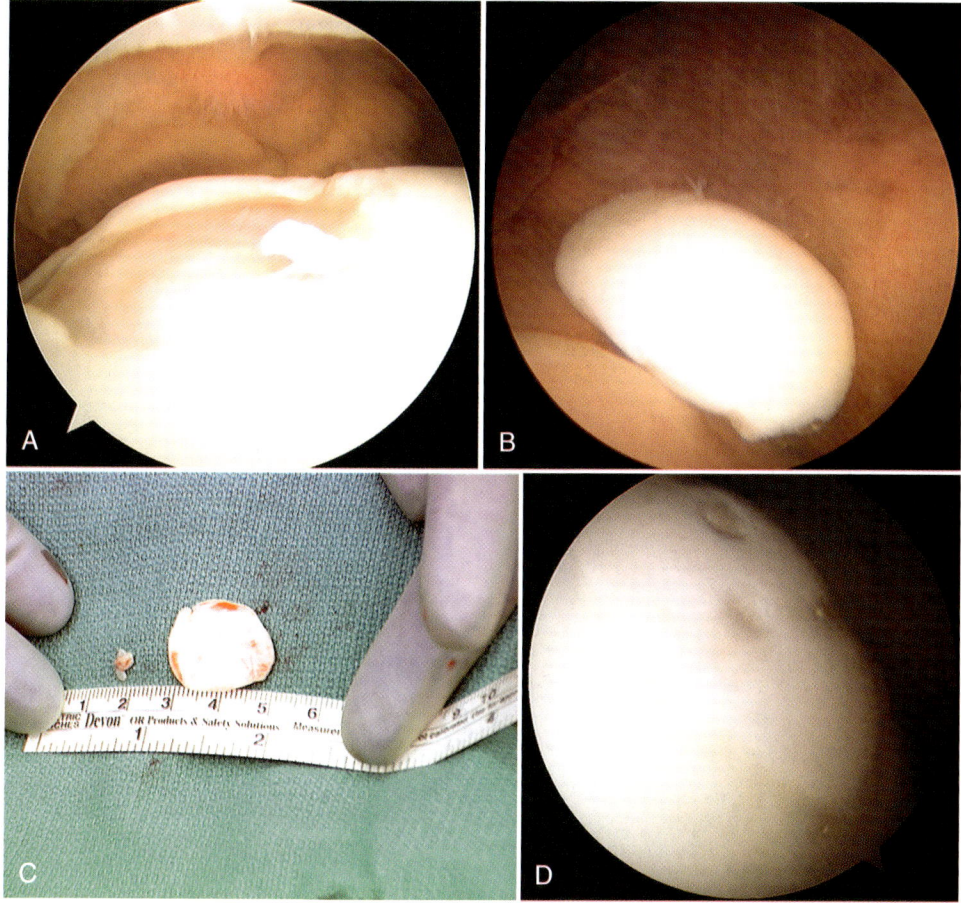

Figure 29-5. Displaced trochlear OCD lesion in a 12-year-old patient. **A,** OCD lesion missing the osteoarticular fragment. **B,** Fragment loose in the lateral gutter. **C,** 2- × 1.5-cm osteoarticular lesion. **D,** Healed OCD lesion after screw removal.

If salvage and repair are not possible, autologous osteochondral plugs have also been used to fix lesions. In this procedure, plugs are harvested from the medial and/or lateral femoral trochlea, the lesion is drilled through and into the healthy bone beneath it, and a bone plug is inserted into the drill hole. Plugs are then inserted until rigid fixation is achieved. This technique has shown favorable results in several studies and has an apparent advantage over the use of screws in that no articular defects are created, so more plugs than screws can be inserted.[44,56,58] Potential drawbacks to the procedure include limited graft size because of the risk of donor site morbidity and the added step of harvesting the osteoarticular bone.[21]

Moreover, several surgeons have written about the use of various bioabsorbable devices to fix JOCD and OCD lesions. Bioabsorbable pins have shown favorable clinical results in a number of trials,[2,20,63] as have bioabsorbable nails,[21] although Weckström and coworkers[79] have shown that bioabsorbable nails obtained significantly better results than pins in their study. They speculated that the barbs on the nails allow for more rigid fixation and better compression than the smooth pins. Drawbacks to the use of bioabsorbable devices include the risk for development of synovitis and the potential for hardware breakage and presentation as loose bodies within the joint space.[13,28]

Staples have also been used to fix fragments, although they were noted to be prone to breakage.[43] Finally, meniscus arrows

have shown potentially promising results in a biomechanical study, although the repetitive stresses on the knee inherent in locomotion could not be accounted for.[81]

In spite of these varying outcomes, Kocher and colleagues[45] have compared the results of four different devices for fixation of JOCD lesions—cannulated variable pitch screws, partially threaded cannulated screws, bioabsorbable tacks, and bioabsorbable pins. They found no significant difference among the devices with regard to healing rate.

If a lesion cannot be fixed, excision of the fragment is sometimes performed, although this procedure has widely been associated with a poor prognosis and early evidence of osteoarthritis.[38,41,45,62,82] Some, however, have suggested that removal of the fragment may yield good results.[3,77] Cahill[9] has further suggested that fragment removal may show positive results if the lesion is located in a non–weight-bearing region of the knee. Patient satisfaction may not always correlate with positive radiographic outcomes, however, which may explain the high number of initially favorable results. If the fragment must be excised, crater resurfacing or grafting techniques are available and recommended.

Autologous chondrocyte implantation (ACI) is a relatively new two-stage technique that may be performed as an open procedure or arthroscopically, and has shown promising results in a number of studies. In the first stage, a specimen of healthy articular cartilage is removed from the patient and the chondrocytes enzymatically released and cultured for 2 to

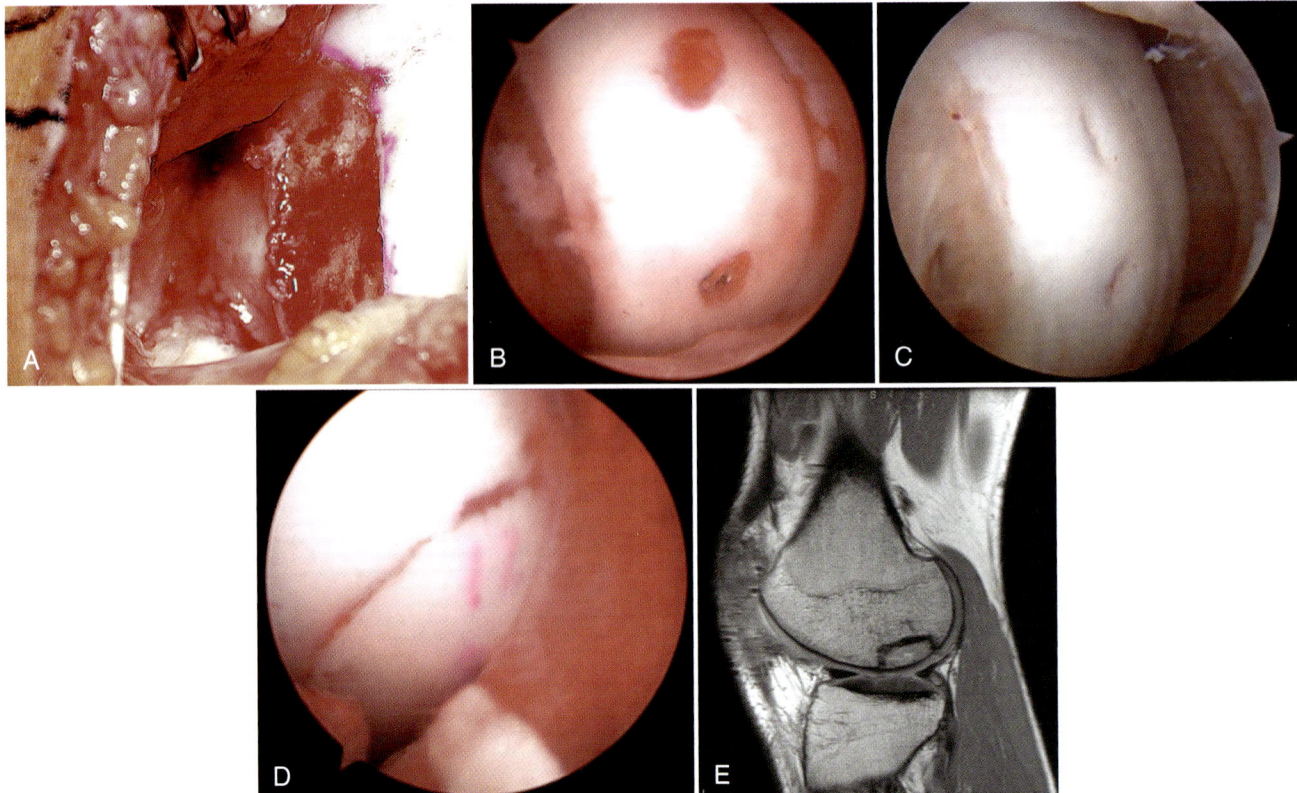

Figure 29-6. Osteoarticular allograft (OA) reconstruction of unsalvageable OCD lesions. **A,** The OCD lesion area was prepared for reconstruction using the OA on the lateral aspect of the medial femoral condyle. **B,** OA reconstruction. **C,** Healed and stable OA reconstruction following screw removal. **D,** OA reconstruction using a circular bone plug. **E,** Saggital MRI scan showing a healed OA allograft. Note the continuity of the articular cartilage.

3 weeks. At the time of implantation with the open technique, the lesion is débrided, a periosteal flap from the patient's tibia is secured over the lesion with one corner left open, and the cultured chondrocytes are inserted beneath the flap, which is then sealed.[26,66] In the arthroscopic procedure, chondrocytes are harvested and cultured in a three-dimensional hyaluronic acid scaffold. At the time of implantation, the lesion is débrided, after which the chondrocyte scaffold is cut and packed into the crater until the defect is filled.

Although the arthroscopic technique is an emerging procedure of unclear benefit at present, some have shown positive results for the open ACI technique.[50,66] Additionally, Steinhagen and associates[76] have demonstrated good to excellent results in 18 of 21 patients treated for OCD lesions with a new technique involving autologous bone grafts coupled with ACI.

Regardless of these favorable clinical results, several studies have noted that biopsies of such ACI grafts often demonstrate the presence of inferior fibrocartilage or a mixture of hyaline-like and fibrocartilage in many patients.[50,59] In further contrast to these positive results, LaPrade and coworkers[51] have reported six failures in a study of nine patients with OCD lesions treated by ACI. Graft biopsies showed fibrous tissue or fibrocartilage, with no evidence of integration into the surrounding tissue. The authors also noted that the term *hyaline-like cartilage* in other papers is misleading, because it is subjectively determined and inconsistently defined.

A final option for treatment is osteochondral allografting. In this procedure, fresh donor osteochondral tissue is acquired, which may be shaped to fit the OCD lesion and inserted. Alternatively, the lesion may be reshaped and the donor tissue then modified to fit, after which the graft can be placed. This technique has been correlated with positive clinical results and is recommended because the graft can be as large as needed, without fear for donor site morbidity (Fig. 29-6).[24,27]

SUMMARY

Juvenile osteochondritis dissecans presents myriad difficulties for the clinician. With an unclear cause and epidemiology, it can be troublesome to decide on an appropriate course of treatment, a situation further complicated by small study populations involving a combination of lesion types.

It seems clear, however, that small, stable JOCD lesions treated conservatively will generally show a favorable outcome. Surgery is indicated in the event of lesion detachment, failure to heal in response to nonsurgical management, or impending skeletal maturity. The method of surgical treatment should be determined by the stage of the lesion, with every attempt made to avoid excising the lesion fragment. If preservation is impossible, surgeons should consider following one of several options for crater resurfacing. When properly managed, JOCD lesions show a high propensity for healing, allowing these young patients to return to their normal active lives.

KEY REFERENCES

Cahill BR, Ahten SM: The three critical components in the conservative treatment of juvenile osteochondritis dissecans (JOCD). Physician, parent, and child. Clin Sports Med 20:287–298, 2001.

Cahill BR, Phillips MR, Navarro R: The results of conservative management of juvenile osteochondritis dissecans using joint scintigraphy. Am J Sports Med 17:601–606, 1989.

Cahill BR: Osteochondritis dissecans of the knee: treatment of juvenile and adult forms. J Am Acad Orthop Surg 3:237–247, 1995.

Green WT, Banks HH: Osteochondritis dissecans in children. J Bone Joint Surg Am 35:26–64, 1953.

Kocher MS, Czarnecki JJ, Andersen JS, Micheli LJ: Internal fixation of juvenile osteochondritis dissecans lesions of the knee. Am J Sports Med 35:712–718, 2007.

Mubarak SJ, Carroll NC: Juvenile osteochondritis dissecans of the knee: Cause. Clin Orthop Relat Res (157):200–211, 1981.

Murray JRD, Chitnavis J, Dixon P, et al: Osteochondritis dissecans of the knee; long-term clinical outcome following arthroscopic debridement. Knee 14:94–98, 2007.

Peterson L, Minas T, Brittberg M, Lindahl A: Treatment of osteochondritis dissecans of the knee with autologous chondrocyte transplantation: Results at two to ten years. J Bone Joint Surg Am 85:17–24, 2003.

Pill SG, Ganley TJ, Milam RA, et al: Role of magnetic resonance imaging and clinical criteria in predicting successful nonoperative treatment of osteochondritis dissecans in children. J Pediatr Orthop 23:102–108, 2003.

Wall EJ, Vourazeris J, Myer GD, et al: The healing potential of stable juvenile osteochondritis dissecans knee lesions. J Bone Joint Surg Am 90:2655–2664, 2008.

Yoshida S, Ikata T, Takai H, et al: Osteochondritis dissecans of the femoral condyle in the growth stage. Clin Orthop Relat Res (346):162–170, 1998.

Full references for this chapter can be found on www.expertconsult.com.

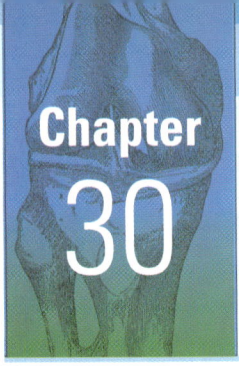

Chapter 30

Secondary, Spontaneous, and Postarthroscopy Osteonecrosis of the Knee: Diagnosis and Management

Eric J Strauss, Charles Bush-Joseph, and Bernard R. Bach, Jr.

Defined as the in situ death of a segment of bone, osteonecrosis occurs secondary to a compromise in osseous blood supply. Although more commonly seen affecting the femoral head, osteonecrosis of the knee has the potential to progress to irreversible changes, causing significant symptomatology, which may eventually require operative intervention. In addition to the secondary osteonecrosis (also termed *avascular necrosis* [AVN]) associated with corticosteroid exposure, alcohol consumption, sickle cell disease, and other common predisposing factors, two other types of osteonecrosis of the knee have been described, spontaneous osteonecrosis of the knee (SPONK) and osteonecrosis in the postoperative knee (ONPK).

First described in 1968 by Ahlback and colleagues,[3] spontaneous osteonecrosis of the knee has been recognized as a distinct clinical entity, with the potential to cause significant morbidity.[39,63] In contrast to cases of secondary osteonecrosis, spontaneous osteonecrosis of the knee tends to affect a different patient population with a different pattern of bony involvement. More recently, osteonecrosis of the knee following arthroscopic surgery has been described, most commonly following arthroscopic meniscectomy. Initially reported by Brahme and associates[14] in 1991, postarthroscopic osteonecrosis has also been noted to occur subsequent to anterior cruciate ligament reconstruction and chondroplasty procedures.[10,24,58]

This chapter will review the current knowledge of these entities, describing their clinical and radiographic presentation, hypothesized cause, and strategies for management.

SPONTANEOUS OSTEONECROSIS OF THE KNEE

SPONK is a disorder of uncertain cause, classically described as a focal lesion occurring in the medial femoral condyle of a patient in the fifth or sixth decade of life, with women affected almost three to five times as commonly as men.[3,8,34,39,63,70] Typically, patients present with the sudden onset of severe pain, localizing to the medial aspect of the knee just proximal to the joint line. Although a traumatic cause has been implicated in SPONK, only a minority of patients recall a specific injury that precipitated their symptoms. In the acute phase of the disease, patients will often report pain with weight-bearing activities and an increase in the severity of their pain at night. Depending on the stage of the lesion and its size, this acute-phase pain will either gradually resolve or become chronically debilitating.

Clinical Evaluation

Examination of the affected knee in the acute phase of SPONK, typically the first 6 to 8 weeks following symptom onset, will demonstrate a small to moderate effusion with limitation of range of motion secondary to pain and associated muscle spasm. Palpation will often elicit a localized area of tenderness over the medial femoral condyle, just proximal to the joint line in the flexed knee. Although the medial femoral condyle is most commonly affected in spontaneous osteonecrosis of the knee, lesions involving the medial tibial plateau, the lateral femoral condyle and, rarely, the patella have also been reported in the orthopedic literature.* Identifying the area of maximal tenderness to palpation can serve as a guide to localizing the involved area. Ligamentous examination of the affected knee is typically normal in cases of SPONK.

Causes

Similar to the proposed mechanisms associated with osteonecrosis of the femoral head, two main causes have been suggested in the pathogenesis of SPONK, traumatic and vascular. With most affected patients being older women with osteoporotic bone, some believe that SPONK develops as a consequence of microfractures occurring in weak subchondral bone secondary to minor trauma.[40] It has been suggested that following an episode of trauma to the knee, fluid enters the intercondylar region, filling the potential space created by the subchondral microfractures in the femoral condyle.[9,33,70] This fluid increases the intraosseous pressure in the area, leading to focal osseous ischemia and eventual necrosis. Researchers have questioned this theory as the mechanism of SPONK. Mears[43] performed histopathologic evaluation of specimens taken from 24 patients diagnosed with SPONK and found that only 1 patient had evidence of bone necrosis. Of the specimens in this study, 75% had demonstrable osteoporosis, implying that osteonecrosis is more of a secondary phenomenon following insufficiency fracture, rather than the primary mechanism of the disease. Others have supported the insufficiency stress fracture theory as the cause of SPONK, believing that when bony necrosis develops, it occurs as a consequence of physiologic resorption and remodeling following fracture.[34,55,67]

Where a vascular cause continues to be the dominant theory for osteonecrosis of the femoral head, with up to 75% of affected patients showing evidence of an underlying thrombophilia or coagulopathy, these predisposing factors have yet to be consistently demonstrated in patients with SPONK.[32,39] In the hip, many believe that the presence of a coagulation disorder, including resistance of activated protein C, low tissue plasminogen activator activity, and hypofibrinolysis, causes intraosseous venous occlusion that culminates in the hypoxic death of bone. Evaluation of the coagulation profiles of patients affected with SPONK is necessary to determine whether this mechanism is present in the pathogenesis of the disease.

---

*References 8, 21, 22, 34, 40, 41, 57, 63, and 70.

The presence of a medial meniscal tear has been proposed as a potential third cause behind the development of SPONK.[52,56] Case series have identified medial meniscal tears in 50% to 78% of patients of patients with SPONK, with a recent series by Robertson and colleagues[65] noting that tears, specifically in the area of the meniscal root, coexisted with spontaneous osteonecrosis in 24 of their 30 patients (80%). They theorized that in older patients with osteoporotic bone, discontinuity of the medial meniscus results in loss of hoop stress distribution in the medial compartment, increasing the load experienced in the femoral condyle and potentially predisposing patients to the development of subchondral insufficiency fracture.

Radiographic Evaluation and Staging

Cases of suspected SPONK should be initially evaluated with a plain, weight-bearing x-ray series of the knee, including an anteroposterior, 45-degree flexion posteroanterior, lateral, and skyline or Merchant views. Early in the disease process, plain x-rays may fail to identify any abnormalities, despite the presence of significant symptomatology. As the condition progresses, plain film findings may include a radiolucent lesion with a surrounding sclerotic halo in addition to subtle flattening of the involved femoral condyle (Fig. 30-1). In advanced cases, with significant subchondral collapse, secondary degenerative changes may be evident with loss of joint space, sclerosis in the medial tibial plateau, and osteophyte formation (Fig. 30-2).

Several staging systems have been described for SPONK based on plain x-ray appearance.[2,39,63,70] In the four-tiered system described by Koshino,[36] stage I disease is defined as incipient, with patients reporting pain with activity; however, plain x-rays are negative for pathology. In stage II SPONK, or the avascular stage, a round to oval subchondral lucency in the weight-bearing area is present with associated increased density in the surrounding femoral condyle. Subchondral collapse heralds stage III SPONK. During the collapse or developed stage of disease (stage III), x-rays demonstrate a sclerotic halo bordering the radiolucent lesion. Further subchondral

collapse with associated development of arthritic changes in the affected compartment define stage IV disease.

Aglietti and coworkers[2] have modified the Koshino staging system to include five stages of disease. In stage I, the x-rays are normal in appearance.[39] Subtle flattening of the affected femoral condyle characterizes stage II SPONK, which indicates the potential for subsequent collapse. Stage III describes the characteristic radiolucent lesion with a circumferential sclerotic border, and stage IV disease is heralded by an increase in the size of the sclerotic halo as the subchondral bone begins to collapse. Stage V SPONK includes continued subchondral collapse, with the development of associated secondary degenerative changes.

Prognostic implications can be made based on the plain x-ray appearance of the lesion, primarily based on its size. The width of the lesion can be measured on the anteroposterior view, with those measuring less than 1 cm classified as small and those more than 1 cm classified as large.[3,50,70] In many of the early studies of SPONK, the area of the lesion within the condyle was used to predict which cases would progress to severe degenerative arthritis.[40,51] Cases in which the lesion was less than 2.5 cm^2 were unlikely to progress, whereas those with an area more than 5 cm^2 were considered to have a poor prognosis. Another useful plain x-ray measure is the ratio of the width of the lesion compared with the overall width of the femoral condyle on the anteroposterior view.[2,7] This measure is not affected by differences in magnification of the view and has been shown to correlate with prognosis. Studies have demonstrated that good outcomes were common in lesions with a size ratio less than 0.45 whereas those with a ratio more than 0.5 typically progress to severe degenerative arthritis.[39]

In both the hip and knee, magnetic resonance imaging (MRI) has become the standard imaging modality for the detection of osteonecrosis. MRI is both sensitive and specific for the evaluation of SPONK, often demonstrating more extensive involvement than was evident on plain radiography.* T1-weighted imaging in cases of spontaneous osteonecrosis of the knee shows a discrete low-signal area, often surrounded by an area of intermediate signal intensity. A serpiginous low signal line is often present at the margin of the lesion, delineating the necrotic area from the adjacent area of bone marrow edema. T2-weighted images will typically show a high signal intensity at lesion edge, in the region of the bone marrow edema. Some have suggested using gadolinium-enhanced MRI for the evaluation of cases of SPONK. The addition of gadolinium is believed to provide information on the extent of osseous activity and turnover at the edges of the lesion, with enhanced adjacent activity believed to be a positive prognostic sign indicative of healing potential.

Clinical Course

The course and prognosis of patients with spontaneous osteonecrosis of the knee are dependent on the size and stage of the lesion. Most patients present with a similar history and physical examination. Pain is often severe at symptom onset, and is present with weight bearing, with a typical increase in

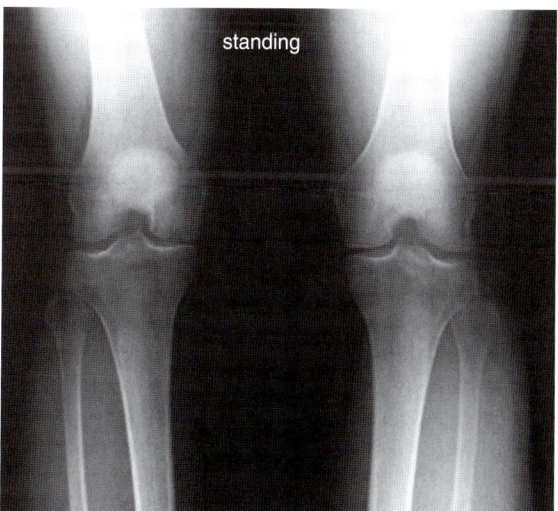

Figure 30-1. Anteroposterior x-rays of early-stage SPONK affecting the right medial femoral condyle developing in a 67-year-old man.

---

*References 12, 14, 39, 61, 69, and 70.

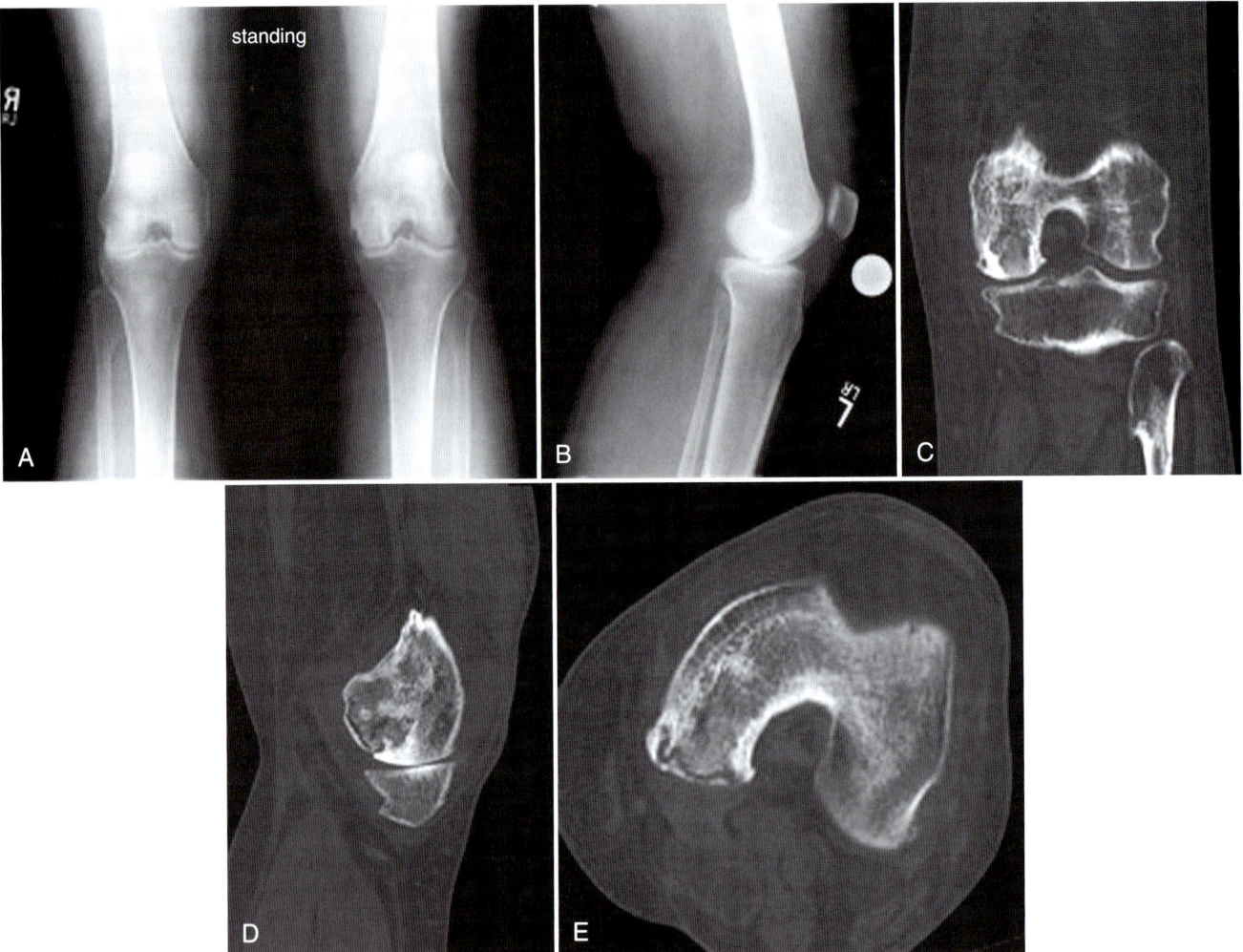

Figure 30-2. Anteroposterior and lateral x-rays and CT scan cuts depicting late-stage SPONK with collapse and associated degenerative changes in a 71-year-old male patient who went on to require total knee arthroplasty.

severity at night, and has a significant impact on the patient's daily activities. The intense pain associated with the acute phase of SPONK may last up to 6 weeks, at which point the extent of the patient's symptoms divides them into two main groups.[39] Those who will have with a satisfactory outcome will typically report improvement in their pain and intermittent swelling after the 6-week time point, although mild symptoms with activity may continue for up to 12 to 18 months. These patients most commonly have smaller lesions evident on imaging studies, with lesions usually less than 40% of the width of the involved femoral condyle. Despite significant improvement in their symptoms and the ability to resume normal daily activities, the vast majority of patients with SPONK will eventually develop osteoarthritic changes in the involved compartment. Insall[29] has reported that at 2-year follow-up, almost all patients with osteonecrosis of the knee have evidence of at least grade I osteoarthritis, with joint space narrowing. Patients whose symptoms fail to improve after 6 weeks tend to follow a more relentless and progressive disease course. They are more typically those with large lesions encompassing more than 50% of the width of their femoral condyle. These patients, in the poor prognosis group, often never report improvement in their knee function or extent of pain. Serial imaging will often demonstrate a rapid progression with collapse and the subsequent development of degenerative changes in the affected compartment.

POSTARTHROSCOPY OSTEONECROSIS OF THE KNEE

First reported by Brahme and associates[14] in a series of seven patients who developed radiographic evidence of osteonecrosis following the arthroscopic treatment of meniscal pathology, ONPK has been recognized as a rare potential complication of arthroscopic surgery.[58,70] Many early case reports describing this entity found it subsequent to arthroscopic meniscectomy, leading it to be referred to as postmeniscectomy osteonecrosis of the knee. However, more recently, osteonecrosis lesions have been noted to occur following other arthroscopic procedures, including chondroplasty and anterior cruciate ligament reconstruction.[10,24,31]

Considering the large number of arthroscopic procedures performed annually and the relatively few reports of cases of postarthroscopy osteonecrosis, the prevalence of ONPK is very low.[31] At present, ONPK following arthroscopic meniscectomy has been described in nine clinical studies, including a total of 47 patients.[58] In all 47 cases, postoperative MRI demonstrated evidence of osteonecrosis that was not present

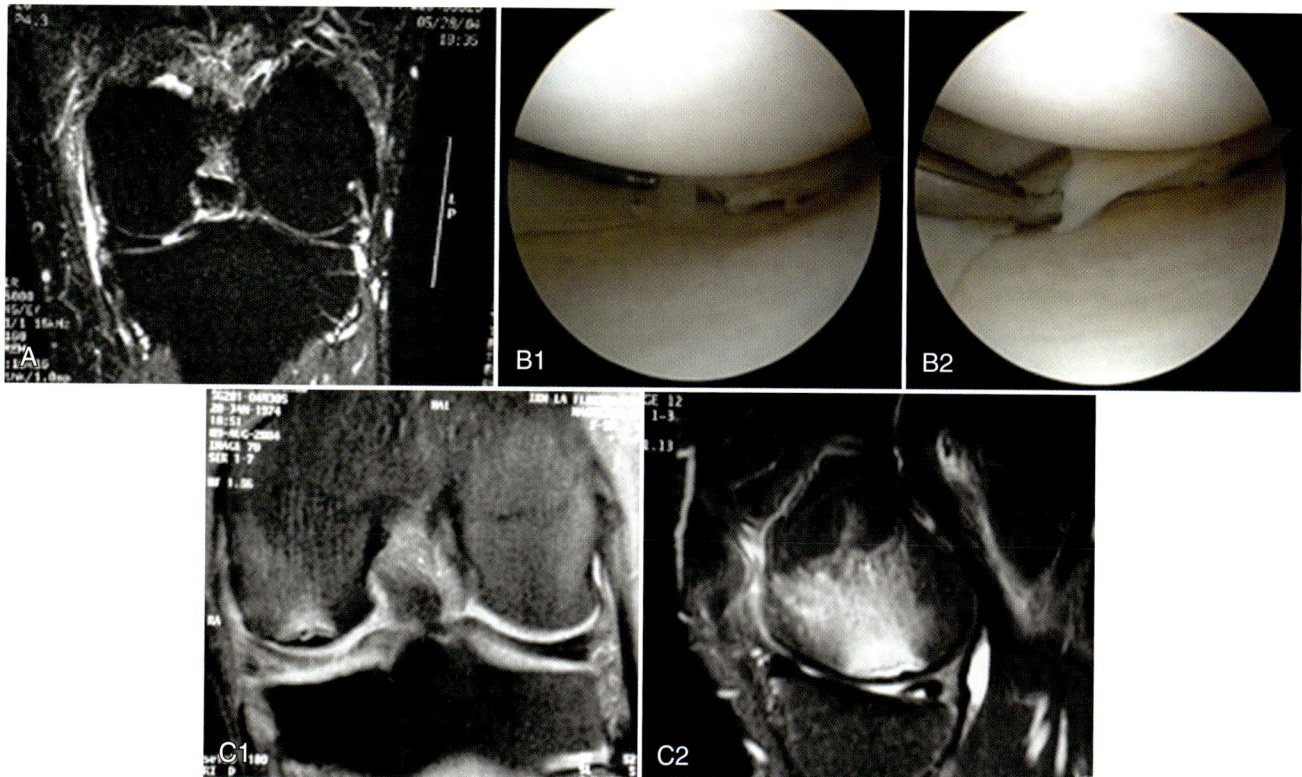

Figure 30-3. **A,** Preoperative MRI scan demonstrating medial meniscal tear with no evidence of pathology affecting the medial femoral condyle. **B,** Intraoperative arthroscopic images demonstrating radial tear of the posterior horn of the medial meniscus. **C,** Postoperative MRI scan demonstrating changes within the medial femoral condyle indicative of ONPK.

in preoperative imaging studies. In contrast to the patient population typically affected by SPONK, ONPK tends to affect slightly younger patients (mean, 58 years; range, 21 to 82 years), with an equal gender distribution (23 women and 24 men).[70]

In these 47 patients, lesions of ONPK predominantly affects the medial femoral condyle (39 [82%]), followed by the lateral femoral condyle (4), lateral tibial plateau (2), and medial tibial plateau (1). In each of the reported cases, osteonecrosis developed in the geographic location of the patient's pathology and arthroscopic procedure, with none arising in the contralateral compartment postoperatively (Fig. 30-3). Concomitant chondral lesions in the region of the meniscal tear were reported to exist in 65% of patients who went on to ONPK, with chondromalacia of the medial compartment noted to exist in 33 of these 47 published cases.

In patients who develop osteonecrosis of the knee following arthroscopic surgery, symptoms of pain, swelling, and limited range of motion may persist or even worsen postoperatively, despite the fact that an adequate resection of their meniscal tear was performed.[24,31,53,58] Cases of persistent or worsening symptoms after knee arthroscopy need to be considered for the possibility of an evolving osteonecrosis lesion, a diagnosis that needs to be distinguished from SPONK, bone marrow edema syndrome, and recurrent meniscal tear.

Clinical Evaluation

Patients with ONPK typically report continued or increased pain in the medial aspect of their knee postoperatively.

Examination of the affected knee will often demonstrate a small to moderate effusion with limitation of range of motion secondary to pain and associated muscle spasm, similar to what was seen preoperatively. Palpation will elicit localized tenderness over the medial joint line and medial femoral condyle. The ligamentous examination will often be normal.

Cause

At present, the exact cause of ONPK has yet to be fully elucidated. Similar to the previously described correlation of meniscal tears with the development of spontaneous osteonecrosis of the knee, some believe that altered knee biomechanics following meniscectomy is responsible for the pathogenesis of the disease.[53,58,68] Previous studies have shown that approximately 50% of joint compressive forces are transmitted through the meniscus in extension and up to 85% of the load in 90 degrees of knee flexion.[4] Partial meniscectomy increases tibiofemoral contact pressures in the treated compartment, potentially leading to subchondral insufficiency fractures from altered load transmission. Histopathologic evaluation of specimens from cases of ONPK have supported this theory, demonstrating evidence of subchondral insufficiency fractures, with bony necrosis present distal to the fracture site.[67] A corollary to the insufficiency fracture theory of ONPK is the possibility that overly aggressive postoperative rehabilitation contributes to the development of this condition. In an attempt to restore function, rapid resumption of weight-bearing activities and exercise are often started within days of the operative procedure. It is possible that if aggressive therapy is resumed prior to bony remodeling in response to the altered load distribution that occurs post-meniscectomy, insufficiency fractures may develop.

Others have hypothesized that the pathologic articular cartilage in the affected compartment has increased permeability to arthroscopic fluid.[58,62] This increase in fluid permeability may also occur following the instrumentation of the articular surface, during shaving chondroplasty, or with inadvertent contact of arthroscopic instruments with the femoral condyle during meniscectomy. Influx of arthroscopy fluid may cause subchondral edema and subsequent osteonecrosis from increased intraosseous pressure. Localized osteoarticular injury from the use of a laser or radiofrequency probe during the arthroscopic procedure has been described as a third potential cause of ONPK.[23,27,37,70] It has been proposed that direct thermal injury or injury from photoacoustic shock from these instruments induces an inflammatory response, leading to bony edema, increased local intraosseous pressure, and eventual osteonecrosis.

Radiographic Evaluation and Staging

In the early stages of osteonecrosis in the postoperative knee, because the disease is primarily one of the bone marrow, plain x-rays are of limited value in the initial workup. Although the bone scan will often be positive in cases of ONPK, with a high level of sensitivity for changes in local osseous vascularity, its specificity and spatial resolution are poor. The diagnosis of osteonecrosis in the postoperative knee is dependent on an MRI of the affected joint, with two specific criteria that need to be filled, the absence of osteonecrosis on preoperative MRI performed 4 to 6 weeks after the onset of symptoms and a time association between the arthroscopic procedure and the development of a suspicious bone marrow edema pattern on postoperative MRI scans.[31,52,58,59]

To distinguish cases of ONPK from those of SPONK, the preoperative MRI must be normal with respect to the condition of the bone and bone marrow of the femoral condyle and tibial plateau. However, it is important to acknowledge that in the very early stages of spontaneous osteonecrosis of the knee, MRI of the affected knee may be devoid of findings; this is described as the window period of SPONK, between symptom onset and MRI evidence of signal changes. Most authors have reported using a period of 4 to 6 weeks following the development of symptoms as sufficient time for radiographic evidence of SPONK to be present.[31,58] This is largely based on an animal study by Nakamura and coworkers[54] in which MRI changes developed in all specimens by 4 weeks following surgically induced femoral head osteonecrosis. Distinction between SPONK and ONPK may not be possible with imaging studies performed prior to this 4- to 6-week time point.

A temporal association between the arthroscopic procedure and postoperative MRI signal changes must be present for the diagnosis of ONPK to be made. In the nine clinical studies reporting cases of osteonecrosis in the postoperative knee, the mean time between arthroscopy and MRI establishing the diagnosis of ONPK was 18 weeks (range, 3 to 176 weeks).[58] This criterion is more difficult to assess and qualify, because bone marrow edema commonly occurs following arthroscopic knee procedures. In a study of 93 patients with a mean age of 36.6 years undergoing arthroscopic

meniscectomy, Kobayashi and colleagues[35] found that 34% had MRI evidence of bone marrow edema in the operative compartment within 8 months of their procedure. Although it may be related to the age of the patients in this study, none progressed to ONPK.

MRI performed in the early stages of ONPK will demonstrate a nonspecific large area of bone marrow edema in the femoral condyle, ipsilateral to the prior meniscectomy, with heterogenous signal present on T2 imaging. By 3 months postoperatively, the extent of edema typically decreases and MRI findings in cases of ONPK are similar to those seen in cases of SPONK, with T1 imaging showing a discrete low-signal area surrounded by an area of intermediate signal intensity. A line of low signal is often present at the margin of the lesion, delineating the necrotic area from the adjacent area of bone marrow edema. T2 images will typically show a high signal intensity at the lesion edge, in the region of the bone marrow edema. As the lesion progresses to its final stages, bone sequestration may be present, with a surrounding high signal rim, along with condylar flattening and the possibility of loose body development.[6,58]

Clinical Course

Review of the 47 reported cases of ONPK shows that 93.6% (44 of 47) had permanent lesions evident on MRI or progressed to irreversible stages of disease. Of these cases, 17 required additional operative intervention, with 9 undergoing total knee arthroplasty, 6 having repeat arthroscopy, and 2 treated with high tibial osteotomy.

In contrast to the correlation of clinical course and prognosis with the size of the lesion in SPONK, this correlation has been less reliable in cases of ONPK. Rapid progression of disease occurred in five of seven cases of ONPK, with a mean lesion size of 40% of the width of the femoral condyle in a series by Johnson and associates,[31] but a similar series by Muscolo and coworkers[53] found a mean lesion size of 24%. From the available data, it appears that in susceptible patients, even small areas of postoperative bone marrow signal changes have the potential to progress to osteonecrosis. Further study of cases of osteonecrosis in the postoperative knee is required in an effort to identify useful factors for predicting prognosis.

COMPARISON OF SPONTANEOUS OSTEONECROSIS OF THE KNEE, OSTEONECROSIS IN THE POSTOPERATIVE KNEE, AND SECONDARY OSTEONECROSIS OF THE KNEE

During the evaluation of patients with suspected SPONK or ONPK, the treating orthopedic surgeon must also consider other potential causes of osteonecrosis affecting the knee. In contrast to cases of SPONK or ONPK, in which patients tend to be older, have isolated, unilateral joint involvement, and no identifiable risk factors for disease, secondary osteonecrosis or AVN occurs in a younger patient population ($\leq$45 years), tends to affect multiple condyles simultaneously, and is bilateral in approximately 80% of affected patients. Additionally, patients with secondary osteonecrosis of the knee have involvement of other sites, including the femoral head (in 90% or more of cases) and proximal humerus[22] (Table 30-1).

In the early stages, patients with secondary osteonecrosis often present with the gradual onset of atraumatic, mild, bilateral knee pain.[70] The location of the pain may vary depending on the number, size, and distribution of the necrotic foci, with most patients reporting symptoms on both the medial and lateral aspects of their knees. In addition to coincident symptoms in their hips and shoulders, most patients with secondary osteonecrosis have identifiable risk factors for disease, including corticosteroid exposure, alcohol consumption, sickle cell disease, and systemic lupus erythematosus (Box 30-1). Compared with the small focal disease seen in cases of SPONK and ONPK, the radiographic workup of patients with secondary osteonecrosis of the knee will typically identify large lesions involving multiple sites within the femoral condyles and tibial plateaus (Fig. 30-4). Secondary osteonecrosis lesions within the knee are pathologically similar to those in SPONK and ONPK and tend to progress to collapse, eventually requiring operative intervention.

TREATMENT OPTIONS

Various treatment options are available for the management of cases of secondary osteonecrosis, spontaneous osteonecrosis of the knee, and osteonecrosis in the postoperative knee. These range from nonoperative and pharmacologic treatment to joint-preserving operative procedures and joint arthroplasty. Because these diseases are relatively rare, a validated treatment algorithm has yet to be developed, and management is taken on a case-individualized basis.

Table 30-1 Comparison of Spontaneous Osteonecrosis and Osteonecrosis in the Postoperative Knee With Secondary Osteonecrosis

Parameter	Secondary Osteonecrosis of the Knee (AVN)	SPONK, ONPK
Affected patient population, age (yr)	≤45	≥55-60
Onset of symptoms	Gradual	Acute
Bilateral disease	>80%	<5%
Number of lesions	Multiple foci present	One focus
Lesion size	Large	Small
Location of lesion	Multiple sites within femoral condyles and tibial plateaus	Typically, medial femoral condyle
Other sites of disease	Femoral head (>90%) and proximal humerus	Rare
Identifiable risk factors	Present	Absent

Adapted from Mont MA, Ragland PS: Osteonecrosis of the knee. In Scott WN (ed): Insall & Scott surgery of the knee, ed 4, Philadelphia, 2006, Churchill Livingstone, pp 460–480.

Box 30-1	**Risk Factors for Secondary Osteonecrosis**

Alcoholism
Coagulopathies
Caisson's disease
Chemotherapy
Corticosteroids
Cushing's syndrome
Diabetes
Familial thrombophilia
Gaucher's disease
Gout
Hyperlipidemia
Inflammatory bowel disease
Liver disease
Organ transplantation
Pancreatitis
Pregnancy
Radiation
Renal disease
Sickle cell disease (and other hemoglobinopathies)
Smoking
Systemic lupus erythematosus (and other connective tissue disorders)
Tumors

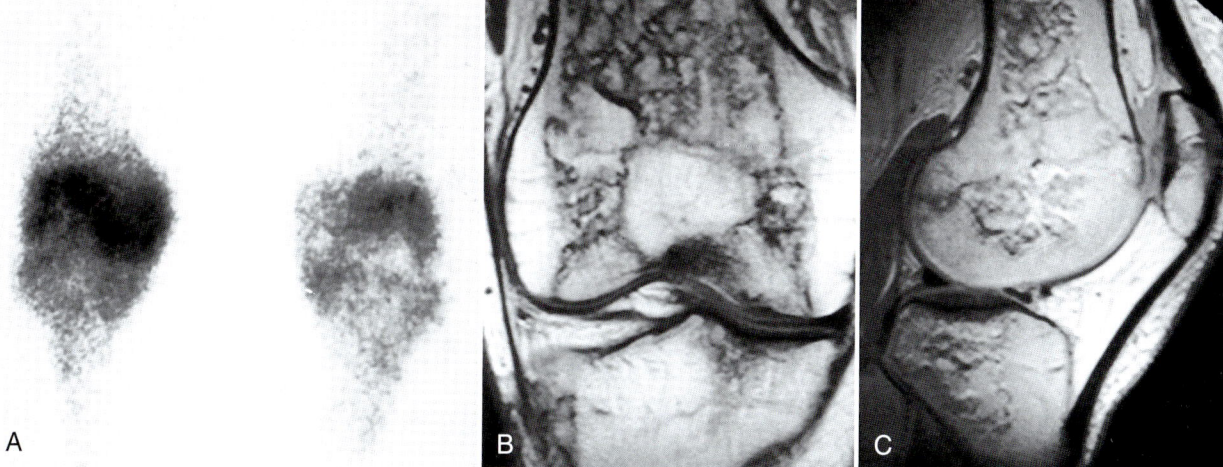

Figure 30-4. Bone scan (**A**) and coronal and sagittal MRI cuts (**B**) demonstrating a case of secondary osteonecrosis affecting the distal femur and tibial plateau in a 33-year-old man with a history of corticosteroid exposure. (From Mont MA, Ragland PS: Osteonecrosis of the knee. In Scott WN (ed): Insall & Scott surgery of the knee, ed 4, Philadelphia, 2006, Churchill Livingstone, pp 460–480.)

Nonoperative Treatment and Pharmacologic Therapy

Nonoperative Management

Once a lesion is identified, an attempt at nonoperative management is often undertaken. Protected weight bearing with crutches, coupled with analgesics and anti-inflammatory medication, is the mainstay of nonoperative treatment. Typically, the restrictions on weight bearing are maintained for a 4- to 8-week period. As the patient's symptoms improve, a resumption of normal activities of daily living, as well as the use of physical therapy for quadriceps and hamstring strengthening, is allowed.

Secondary to their large size and occurrence in a young, active patient population, nonoperative management of cases of secondary osteonecrosis tends to fair poorly. In a series of 248 knees in 136 patients with secondary osteonecrosis of the knee, Mont and colleagues[46] have reported successful outcomes (Knee Society score ≥80 and no surgical intervention) in only 20% of the 41 knees treated, with protected weight bearing and analgesic medication at a mean of 8 years of follow-up.

In contrast to Mont and associates' experience with secondary osteonecrosis, good to excellent results have been reported for cases of SPONK following nonoperative management if the lesion size is small (less than 40% of the width of the femoral condyle).[8,39,50] In a series of 79 cases of medial femoral condyle SPONK, Lotke and coworkers[40] reported that 32 of 36 patients (88.9%) with stage I disease had resolution of their symptoms after a period of protected weight bearing and analgesic treatment. In this series, only 1 patient with stage I disease went on to require total knee arthroplasty. Similar good results of nonoperative treatment were reported by Yates and colleagues[69] in their series of 20 cases of stage I SPONK. Resolution of the lesion was evident on follow-up MRI in 19 of 20 patients at a mean of 8 months (range, 3 to 18 months). As the lesion size and stage increases, the success of nonoperative treatment for cases of SPONK becomes less reliable, with most authors reporting a slow relentless progression to degenerative arthritis. Based on the available data, it appears that the nonoperative treatment of cases of ONPK is less successful in improving patient symptoms, functional outcome, and lesion resolution. Of the 47 reported cases in the orthopedic surgery literature, 3 patients (6.4%) had improvement in the MRI appearance of their lesion following 6 weeks of protected weight bearing.[58]

In an effort to reduce the weight-bearing forces experienced at the site of an osteonecrotic lesion and protect the weakened subchondral bone from collapse, an unloader brace may be used as part of a nonoperative management approach. Although there are little data in the orthopedic surgery literature to support their use in cases of secondary osteonecrosis, SPONK, or ONPK, unloader braces have been shown to be useful for patients with symptomatic varus gonarthrosis. In an evaluation of 11 patients with medial compartment osteoarthritis, Lindenfeld and associates[38] have found that a valgus-producing unloader brace reduces the adduction moment experienced at the knee during gait, leading to a 48% reduction in pain scores and a 79% increase in function during activities of daily living. Similar benefits to unloading the medial compartment with a valgus-producing brace were

reported by Draganich and coworkers[19] in their study of 10 patients with varus gonarthrosis. They found that both off-the-shelf and custom unloader braces significantly reduce knee pain and stiffness while improving functional scores compared with an unbraced state. Specific study is required for patients with osteonecrosis but, by reducing the adduction moment at the knee and the joint forces experienced in the medial compartment, unloader braces may protect lesions of the medial femoral condyle, potentially improving symptoms and allowing for successful healing.

Pharmacologic Treatment

Little has been published on the pharmacologic treatment of osteonecrosis of the knee, with most of the data extrapolated from the literature on femoral head osteonecrosis. Available medical treatment options include bisphosphonates, vasodilators, statins, and anticoagulants. As stable analogues of pyrophosphate, bisphosphonates function to promote bone formation via a reduction of osteoclast activity.[26,60] Alendronate has shown efficacy in relieving pain and reducing the incidence of collapse in cases of femoral head osteonecrosis.[1,15] Whether this early success translates to cases of secondary osteonecrosis, SPONK, or ONPK has yet to be demonstrated. In a recent report in the rheumatology literature, Corrado and colleagues[16] have described a case of SPONK affecting the medial femoral condyle of a 59-year-old woman, which was successfully treated with the intramuscular bisphosphonate neridronate (administered monthly) combined with calcitriol and analgesics. The authors reported that significant symptom improvement occurred within 2 months of treatment and evidence of lesion improvement was present on follow-up MRI performed 4 months after the initiation of neridronate. Attention has also been given to vasodilators such as iloprost[5,18,44] and anticoagulants such as enoxaparin[28] as potential disease-modifying agents in early-stage, precollapse osteonecrosis. Further study is required to determine whether these medical interventions will effectively alter the clinical course in cases of secondary osteonecrosis, SPONK, and ONPK.

Surgical Management

Arthroscopic Débridement

The use of arthroscopic débridement in the management of secondary osteonecrosis, SPONK, and ONPK has limited applications. Because the primary pathology is intraosseous, arthroscopic débridement has little likelihood of altering the course of the disease process; however, it may lead to symptomatic improvement in patients in whom mechanical symptoms are present secondary to unstable chondral fragments or loose bodies. In a series of five cases of SPONK treated with arthroscopic débridement and chondroplasty, Miller and associates[45] have reported good postoperative outcomes in four of five patients at a mean follow-up of 31 months, with Hospital for Special Surgery (HSS) knee scores improving from 52 to 82. However the natural history and progression of the osteonecrosis lesions in these patients was not altered by the arthroscopic procedure.

Some authors have reported performing arthroscopic retrograde drilling (through the articular cartilage layer to reach the lesion site) for cases of SPONK or ONPK.[17] Although retrograde drilling may stimulate revascularization within the lesion, the potential for damage to the intact articular surface and the difficulty associated with localizing the focus of the lesion accurately in the precollapse stage makes antegrade drilling (toward the articular surface without violating the cartilage layer) and core decompression more attractive treatment options.

Core Decompression

Relief of elevated intraosseous pressure via extra-articular drilling has been used frequently in early-stage, precollapse cases of osteonecrosis of the femoral head with variable results. Core decompression as a treatment for osteonecrosis of the knee was first described in 1989 by Jacobs and

coworkers[30] in their series of 28 patients. They reported good results in their stage I and II cases (7 patients) and in 52% of their stage III cases. Mont and colleagues[49] reviewed their experience with core decompression in 47 knees in patients with secondary osteonecrosis and reported good to excellent results in 72% at a mean follow-up of 11 years. More recently, in a series of 16 patients with a mean age of 64 years, Forst and associates[25] found that core decompression provided symptom relief and successful healing (normalization of bone marrow signal on MRI) in 15 stage I cases and 1 stage II case of SPONK at 3-year follow-up.[39] Based on their findings, they recommended core decompression as a useful treatment option for early-stage osteonecrosis of the knee (Fig. 30-5). However, it is important to note that these studies lacked

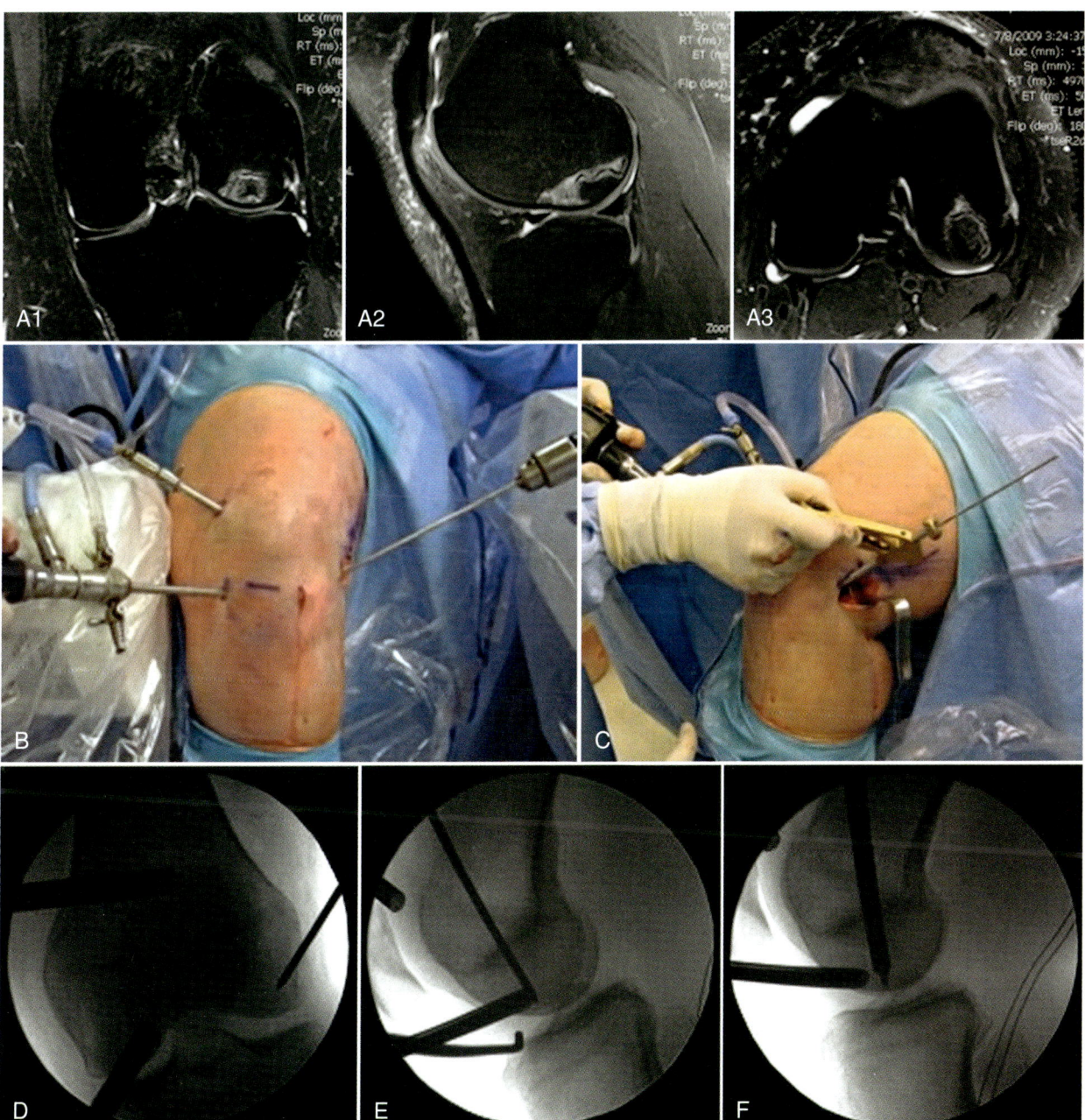

Figure 30-5. A, Preoperative coronal, sagittal, and axial MRI cuts of SPONK affecting the lateral femoral condyle. **B-F,** Arthroscopy-assisted, fluoroscopic-guided core decompression of the lateral femoral condyle.

control groups, with the possibility that these cases of early-stage disease might have improved without intervention.

High Tibial Osteotomy

Appropriately selected patients with SPONK or ONPK may be managed with a high tibial osteotomy as a joint-preserving treatment option.[20,39,63] Typically reserved for younger active patients, high tibial osteotomy can function to offload the affected femoral condyle by shifting the weight-bearing axis laterally. In their series of 105 cases of SPONK diagnosed and treated over a 20-year period, Soucacos and coworkers[66] reported using high tibial osteotomy as an effective treatment for patients with stage III disease. Although no details regarding the technique or patient outcome were described, better results were reported for patients younger than 65 years and for lesions less than 50% of the width of the femoral condyle in size. Koshino,[36] in a study of 37 cases of SPONK managed with high tibial osteotomy, with or without a concomitant drilling–bone grafting procedure, have found that the outcomes are best when the combined procedures were performed and the mechanical axis was corrected to at least 10 degrees of valgus alignment. Follow-up radiographic evaluation in this series demonstrated that the lesion improved in 17 patients and resolved completely in 13 patients. In a study including 10 patients with SPONK managed with high tibial osteotomy (6 patients) or nonoperative treatment (4 patients), Marti and associates[42] found that patients treated with high tibial osteotomy had a higher incidence of improvement in the appearance of their lesion on follow-up MRI (83% vs. 25%) and a higher incidence of symptom improvement (100% vs. 50%). Johnson and coworkers[31] reported 2 cases of ONPK treated with high tibial osteotomy, one performed 8 months and the other 10 months after the index arthroscopic medial meniscectomy; however, clinical outcome and follow-up were not described.

The use of high tibial osteotomy for cases of secondary osteonecrosis of the knee is typically not recommended secondary to the multifocal nature of this variant of disease, with most patients having bicondylar femoral involvement and coincident lesions present within the tibial plateau.

Knee Arthroplasty

For patients in whom joint-preserving treatments fail to provide symptomatic improvement and in those with large or advanced lesions, knee arthroplasty is the treatment of choice. Depending on patient factors, lesion characteristics, and condition of the remainder of the joint, unicompartmental knee arthroplasty (UKA) or standard total knee arthroplasty (TKA) may be used.[39,63] Unicompartmental arthroplasty is an effective treatment method for those with disease isolated to a single femoral condyle or tibial plateau, with the benefit of preserving the patient's bone stock and functioning cruciate ligaments. For cases of secondary osteonecrosis and extensive cases of SPONK or ONPK in patients with evidence of degenerative change in the contralateral compartment or patellofemoral joint, tricompartmental replacement is a better treatment option.

In a series of 31 patients with a mean age of 36 years whose secondary osteonecrosis was treated with total knee arthroplasty, Mont and Hungerford[47] reported good to excellent results in 55% of their cases at a mean follow-up of 8.2 years.

Of patients in this study, 37% required revision for aseptic loosening and 10% developed deep infection. Bonutti and colleagues[13] have reported the outcome of arthroplasty in 19 patients with osteonecrosis in the postoperative knee, with 4 patients undergoing UKA and 15 undergoing TKA. At a mean follow-up of 62 months, 18 patients had a good or excellent outcome based on Knee Society score (mean, 92; range, 60 to 100). Data on TKA for cases of osteonecrosis of the knee have demonstrated good outcomes, but in the long term they do not appear to function as well as TKA performed for cases of osteoarthritis. In a series of 32 knees with SPONK of the medial femoral condyle, Ritter and associates[64] have reported results inferior to those seen in a comparison group treated for osteoarthritis. Patients treated for SPONK had worse pain relief (82% vs. 90%) and a higher incidence of revision surgery (17% vs. 0%) compared with the osteoarthritis patients. Similar results were reported by Bergman and Rand[11] in their series of 36 cases of osteonecrosis of the knee managed with TKA. Good to excellent results were reported to occur in 87% of the study patients at a mean of 4 years of follow-up. Whereas implant survivorship at 5 years was predicted to be 85%, with revision surgery defined as the endpoint, survivorship was predicted to be 68% when moderate or severe pain was used as the endpoint. It was theorized that if foci of osteonecrosis exist in the supporting subchondral or metaphyseal bone, persistent pain may complicate the outcome of total knee arthroplasty. Other studies have shown better outcomes of TKA for cases of SPONK. In a series of 32 total knee arthroplasties performed in 30 patients, of which 8 were done as treatment of SPONK, Mont and coworkers reported excellent results with a Knee Society score of 98 at a mean of 108 months postoperatively.[48]

SUMMARY AND CONCLUSIONS

Secondary osteonecrosis, spontaneous osteonecrosis of the knee, and osteonecrosis in the postoperative knee are clinical entities that have the potential to cause significant morbidity in affected patients. In addition to the knowledge about the patient population at risk, classic presentation, and imaging characteristics, the treating orthopedic surgeon needs to maintain a high index of suspicion for these disorders, because early diagnosis and treatment may allow for an improved clinical outcome. Continued study of patients with SPONK and ONPK is needed in an effort to identify specific risk factors that predispose certain patients to their development. In the future, it is possible that pharmacologic intervention and alterations in postarthroscopy rehabilitation protocols in susceptible patients may alter the course of disease for those who develop SPONK and ONPK.

KEY REFERENCES

DeFalco RA, Ricci AR, Balduini FC: Osteonecrosis of the knee after arthroscopic meniscectomy and chondroplasty: A case report and literature review. Am J Sports Med 31:1013–1016, 2003.

Duany NG, Zywiel MG, McGrath MS, et al: Joint-preserving surgical treatment of spontaneous osteonecrosis of the knee. Arch Orthop Trauma Surg 130(1):11–16, 2010.

Ecker ML: Spontaneous osteonecrosis of the distal femur. Instr Course Lect 50:495–498, 2001.

Ecker ML, Lotke PA: Spontaneous osteonecrosis of the knee. J Am Acad Orthop Surg 2:173–178, 1994.

Faletti C, Robba T, de Petro P: Postmeniscectomy osteonecrosis. Arthroscopy 18:91–94, 2002.

Johnson TC, Evans JA, Gilley JA, DeLee JC: Osteonecrosis of the knee after arthroscopic surgery for meniscal tears and chondral lesions. Arthroscopy 16:254–261, 2000.

Kattapuram TM, Kattapuram SV: Spontaneous osteonecrosis of the knee. Eur J Radiol 67:42–48, 2008.

Marti CB, Rodriguez M, Zanetti M, Romero J: Spontaneous osteonecrosis of the medial compartment of the knee: a MRI follow-up after conservative and operative treatment, preliminary results. Knee Surg Sports Traumatol Arthrosc 8:83–88, 2000.

Mont MA, Baumgarten KM, Rifai A, et al: Atraumatic osteonecrosis of the knee. J Bone Joint Surg Am 82:1279–1290, 2000.

Mont MA, Tomek IM, Hungerford DS: Core decompression for avascular necrosis of the distal femur: long term followup. Clin Orthop Relat Res 334:124–130, 1997.

Muscolo DL, Costa-Paz M, Ayerza M, Makino A: Medial meniscal tears and spontaneous osteonecrosis of the knee. Arthroscopy 22:457–460, 2006.

Pape D, Seil R, Anagnostakos K, Kohn D: Postarthroscopic osteonecrosis of the knee. Arthroscopy 23:428–438, 2007.

Robertson DD, Armfield DR, Towers JD, et al: Meniscal root injury and spontaneous osteonecrosis of the knee: an observation. J Bone Joint Surg Br 91:190–195, 2009.

Yamamoto T, Bullough PG: Spontaneous osteonecrosis of the knee: The result of subchondral insufficiency fracture. J Bone Joint Surg Am 82:858–866, 2000.

Zywiel MG, McGrath MS, Seyler TM, et al: Osteonecrosis of the knee: a review of three disorders. Orthop Clin North Am 40:193–211, 2009.

Full references for this chapter can be found on www.expertconsult.com.

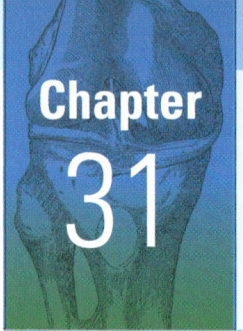

Chapter 31

Healing of Knee Ligaments and Menisci

Seth L. Sherman and Scott A. Rodeo

Muscle, ligaments, and menisci complement the bony architecture of the knee and allow for normal kinematics throughout the range of motion. Ligaments are critical to the static stability of the knee joint. The menisci serve to guide the femoral condyles in their articulation with the tibial plateau, distribute the weight more evenly, and act as shock absorbers. Structural damage to the ligaments or menisci can result in altered joint kinematics and joint forces, ultimately leading to degenerative changes in the knee. Therefore, it is imperative to restore homeostatic balance within the knee through preservation of the meniscus and through ligament healing, repair, or reconstruction.

It is the purpose of this chapter to review the basic science aspects of ligament and meniscal healing, as well as the biology of current repair and reconstructive strategies, to provide a fundamental basis for the care and treatment of these injuries.

LIGAMENTS

Structure and Function

Anatomy and Biochemistry

Ligaments are fibrous bands that span two or more bones and are critical to the static stability of the knee joint.[53] All ligaments are composed of densely organized, fibrous connective tissue consisting of mainly water and type I collagen (approximately 70% to 90% of dry weight).[65] Water is attracted into the extracellular matrix of the ligament by negatively charged proteoglycans, including decorin sulfate, chondroitin sulfate, and keratin sulfate (less than 1% of dry weight). This accounts for the ligament's rate-dependent response to mechanical load, or viscoelasticity.

Collagen is responsible for the ligaments characteristic form and tensile strength. Collagen molecules orient along the long axis of the ligament to form fibrils.[65] Ligaments contain a bimodal distribution of collagen fibril diameters. There is a group of fibrils between 40 and 75 µm in diameter and a second group between 100 and 150 µm in diameter.[44,53] The fibrils are grouped into fibers that range from 1 to 20 µm in diameter, which are then grouped into fascicles from 360 to 1500 µm in diameter. The collagen in ligaments contain stable and unstable collagen cross links and has a characteristic crimp pattern.

Other components of the extracellular matrix of ligaments include types III, IV, V, and VI collagen (3% to 90% of dry weight), elastic fibers, including elastin, fibrillin, and microfibrillar-associated glycoprotein (usually less than 5%), and a small percentage of noncollagenous proteins, including fibronectin, laminin, thrombospondin, and tenascin.[53]

Fibroblasts are the dominant cell type in ligaments, responsible for forming and maintaining the extracellular matrix. Other cell types present include endothelial cells, peripheral nerve cells, and tissue mast cells.[53] Compared with tendons, ligaments are more metabolically active.[45] Intrinsic ligament fibroblasts possess plump nuclei and have a higher DNA content compared with tenoblasts. The higher metabolic activity in ligaments may be to the result of a functional need for more rapid adaptation.

The normal ligament insertion site into bone is a highly specialized tissue that functions to transmit complex mechanical loads from soft tissue to bone.[65] Ligaments, in general, have two distinct types of insertion sites: direct and indirect.[110] The femoral insertion of the anterior cruciate ligament is an example of a direct insertion site. At a direct insertion site, the ligament often enters the bone directly at a right angle to the bony surface. This transition contains four distinct zones—ligament, unmineralized fibrocartilage, mineralized fibrocartilage, and bone (Fig. 31-1). Cartilage-specific collagens including types II, IX, X, and XI are found in the fibrocartilage of the insertion site, with collagen X playing a fundamental role in maintaining the interface between mineralized and unmineralized fibrocartilage.[57,102] Proteoglycans are also abundant in the fibrocartilaginous region of the insertion site, probably functioning to decrease stress concentration at the insertion.

An example of an indirect insertion is the tibial insertion of the medial collateral ligament. At this insertion site, collagen fibers blend with the periosteum, which are then anchored to bone via Sharpey's fibers. These Sharpey's fibers are obliquely oriented to the long axis of the bone, securely anchoring the ligament into bone and conferring mechanical strength (Fig. 31-2).[65]

Biomechanics and Function

The biomechanical characterization of a healing ligament is based on two elements, functional testing and tensile testing. Functional testing determines the contribution of the ligament to knee kinematics as well as the in situ forces of the ligament in response to external loading conditions. Tensile testing assesses the structural properties of the bone-ligament-bone complex and the material properties of the ligament substance.[147,149]

There are four basic aspects of ligament mechanical functional testing. These include laxity, stiffness, strength, and viscoelasticity.[53] Failure or overload of these functions may result in ligamentous injury and loss of critical joint-stabilizing properties of the ligament (Fig. 31-3). Healing of a ligament may be assessed using these parameters as outcome measures for success.

Laxity refers to the displacement of bones to which a ligament is attached from an anatomic position to a position in which the ligament takes up load. It is a function of both joint position and direction of load.[53] Structurally, the laxity of a ligament is partly a function of number of fibers recruited

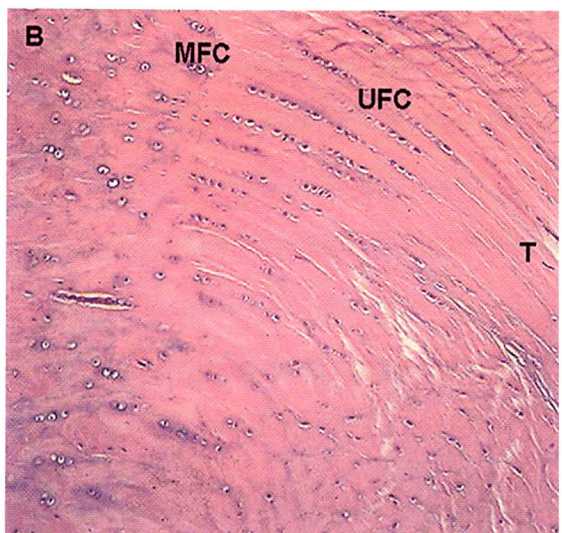

Figure 31-1. Normal tendon to bone direct insertion site of the rabbit ACL. Note the four zones—tendon *(T)*, unmineralized fibrocartilage *(UFC)*, mineralized fibrocartilage *(MFC)*, and bone *(B)*. (From Gulotta LV, Rodeo SA: Biology of autograft and allograft anterior cruciate ligament reconstruction. Clin Sports Med 26:509–524, 2007.)

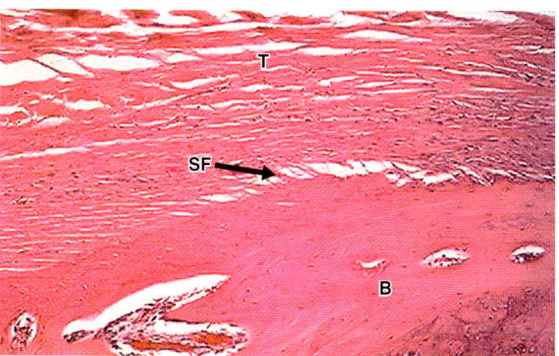

Figure 31-2. Normal tendon to bone indirect insertion site of the rabbit MCL with Sharpey's fibers. *B,* Bone, *SF,* Sharpey's fibers, *T,* tendon. (From Gulotta LV, Rodeo SA: Biology of autograft and allograft anterior cruciate ligament reconstruction. Clin Sports Med 26:509–524, 2007.)

by a specific movement and the orientation of these fibers to resist displacement.

Stiffness is the amount of load required to displace the bones to which a ligament is attached. The more load required, the stiffer the ligament-joint complex. Stiffness is also a function of fiber recruitment, with stiffer ligament having more fiber recruitment. In injured or damaged ligaments, either fibers are not recruited or those recruited are not as stiff as normal ligament fibers.[54]

Strength refers to the maximum tensile load that a bone-ligament-bone complex can withstand before it fails. Failure load is a function of both the number of fibers that tighten within a ligament, and the quality of those fibers. The direction of applied force during ligament testing also influences the structural and mechanical properties. Applying the force in the direction of the ligament will recruit a greater proportion of fiber bundles and thus result in higher forces.[27] Therefore, load direction is a critical determinant of ligament strength.

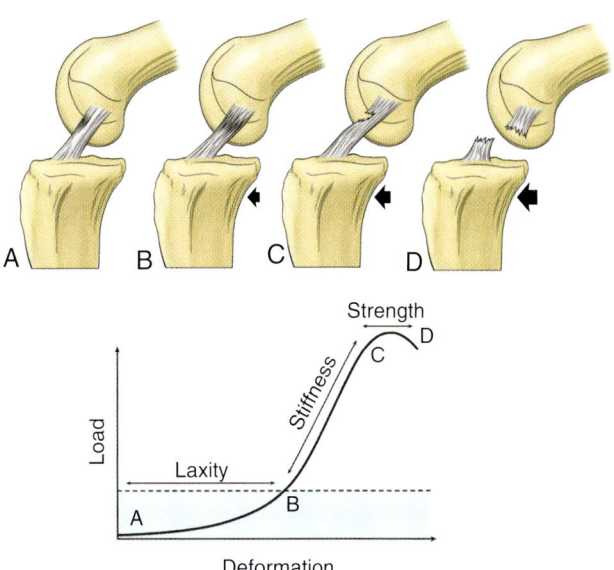

Figure 31-3. Schematic and graphic descriptions of laxity, stiffness, and strength. (From Frank CB: Ligament healing: current knowledge and clinical applications. J Am Acad Orthop Surg 4:74–83, 1996.)

Viscoelasticity refers to the ability of tissues to respond to repeat loading by altering length or load over time. Variations can account for as much as 10% changes in ligament length and up to 60% to 70% of changes in ligament loads under physiologic conditions. Creep is a viscoelastic property in which there is an increase in ligament length that occurs over time when the ligament is subjected to a constant load (Fig. 31-4). Another property, load or stress relaxation, occurs when less load is required over time to hold a ligament at a specific deformation.

Tensile testing provides information on the strength and quality of healing tissue and allows comparisons with intact ligaments. Two sets of information can be obtained from uniaxial tensile testing. The load-elongation curve demonstrates the structural properties of the bone-ligament-bone complex, and the stress-strain curve demonstrates the material properties of the ligament substance[148] (Figs. 31-5 and 31-6). Both curves demonstrate characteristic toe, linear, and failure regions. In the initial low-stiffness toe region, elongation of a ligament occurs because of straightening of the crimp pattern.[27] With further load, there is increasing recruitment of ligament fiber bundles. The slope of the linear region reflects the stiffness of the ligament or ligament complex. Structural properties that are evaluated with the load-elongation curve include linear stiffness, ultimate load, and energy absorbed at failure. The stress-strain curve provides information on modulus of elasticity, tensile strength, ultimate strain, and strain energy density.

Biology of Ligament Injury and Healing

Ligament healing involves the restoration of the structural integrity of the tissue following an injury. The ability of an injured ligament to heal is affected by a number of variables, including the site and severity of the injury, presence of multiligamentous injury, various intrinsic factors (e.g., age,

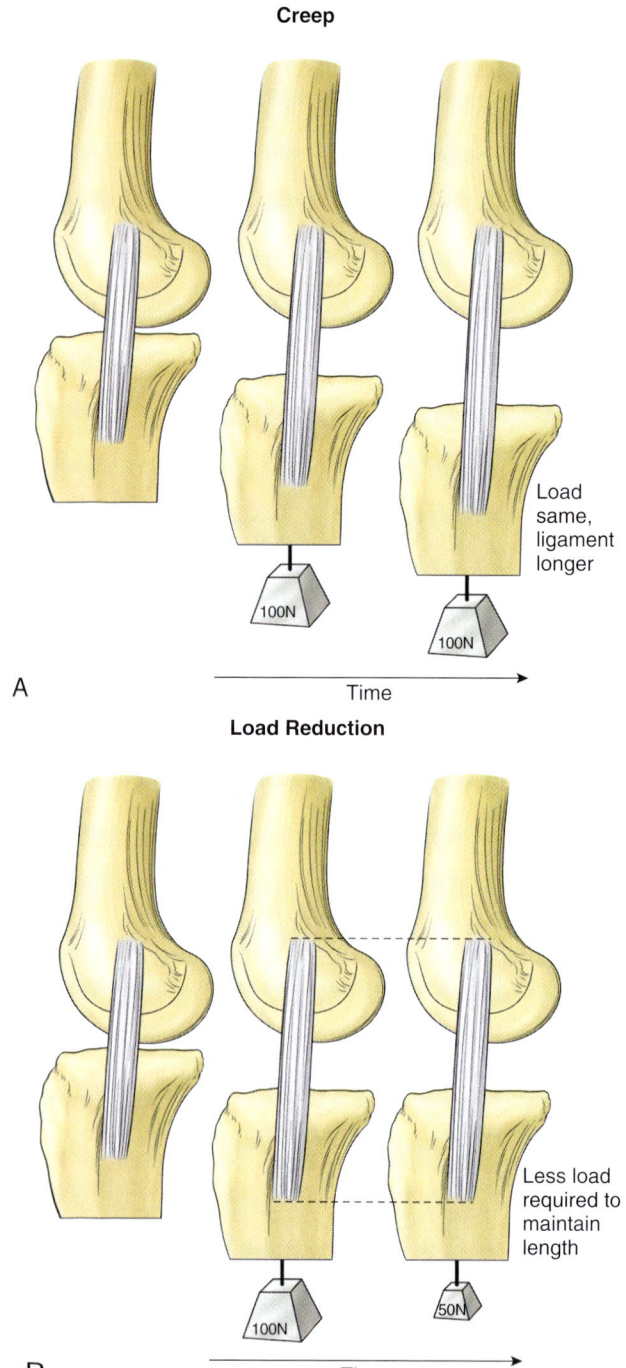

Figure 31-4. The viscoelastic properties of ligaments. **A,** Creep is the increase in the length of a ligament that occurs over time when a ligament is subjected to a constant load. **B,** Load relaxation is the decrease in load that a ligament experiences over time when it is held at a specific deformation. (From Frank CB: Ligament healing: Current knowledge and clinical applications. J Am Acad Orthop Surg 4:74–83, 1996.)

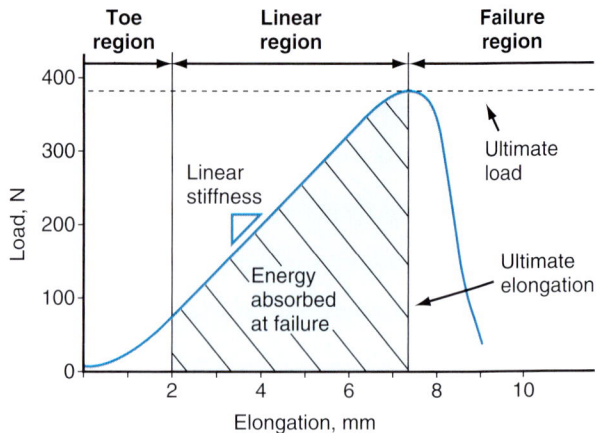

Figure 31-5. Typical load-elongation curve of the bone-MCL-bone complex. (From Woo SL, Vogrin TM, Abramowitch SD: Healing and repair of ligament injuries in the knee. J Am Acad Orthop Surg 8:364–372, 2000.)

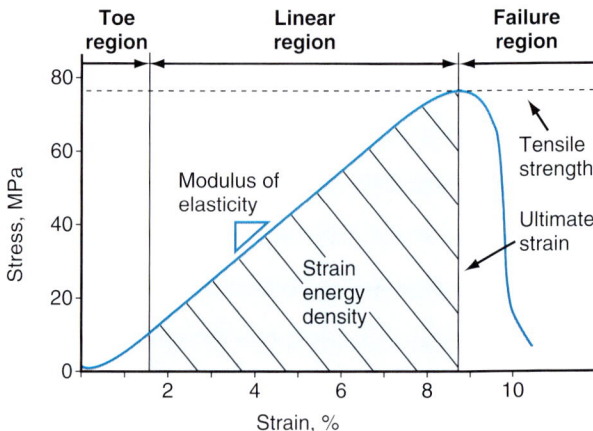

Figure 31-6. Typical stress-strain curve describing the mechanical properties of the MCL midsubstance. (From Woo SL, Vogrin TM, Abramowitch SD: Healing and repair of ligament injuries in the knee. J Am Acad Orthop Surg 8:364–372, 2000.)

Age-Related Changes in Ligament and Ligament Degeneration

The structural and mechanical properties of ligaments change with skeletal maturation.[6,122] In the setting of open physes, ligaments often fail by bone avulsion, whereas ligaments fail in the midsubstance in the skeletally mature. Structural and mechanical properties of ligaments are also positively correlated with age; specimens from younger donors demonstrate superior properties compared with specimens from older donors.[138] Water content, as well as rate of collagen synthesis, decreases with age in both the medial collateral ligament (MCL) and anterior collateral ligament (ACL) in a rabbit model.

The gross and microscopic changes of ligament degeneration can occur in acute and chronic settings. Following acute, full-thickness ligament disruption, an initial inflammatory response occurs whether the ligament is intra-articular or extra-articular. As an example, the torn ends of an acutely ruptured ACL rapidly involute. These changes are related to an increase in collagenase activity, apparently in response to

circulation status), type of treatment initiated, and degree of immobilization and rehabilitation after injury.[148] Knowledge of the basic science of ligament injury and healing is instrumental in making informed treatment decisions in a clinical setting.

local cell damage.[4] Chronic degeneration of a ligament is uncommon, but when it occurs several histologic changes are involved, including collagen fragmentation and mucoid degeneration.[120]

Healing of Extra-articular Ligaments

Extra-articular healing proceeds in three phases: (1) inflammation; (2) cellular and matrix proliferation; and (3) remodeling.[48,146] During phase I, a fibrin clot forms at the injury site. Potent vasodilators are released, including histamine and serotonin. There is infiltration of inflammatory cells and phagocytosis of necrotic debris by macrophages, followed by proliferation of capillary endothelial buds and fibroblast proliferation near the end of phase I. These fibroblasts begin early matrix synthesis. This early matrix is disorganized.[83]

Matrix and cellular proliferation are characterized by a proliferation and migration of fibroblasts to the site of injury.[83] Proliferating cells are derived from intrinsic and extrinsic populations. Collagen and glycosaminoglycan (GAG) synthesis is upregulated. Type III collagen, formed in the initial healing period, is removed and replaced by type I collagen. The mechanical strength of the repair tissue begins to increase as new matrix is deposited.

There is a relative decrease in cellularity and vascularity during the remodeling phase of healing. There is an increase in collagen density and a gradual decrease in the content of collagen type III. Collagen fibrils gradually become organized along the axis of the ligament. Collagen cross linking and post-translational modifications occur during this phase and result in an increased tensile strength. Collagen fibril diameters and collagen cross links remain abnormal for at least 1 year after ligamentous injury.[84,98] Alpha smooth muscle actin containing fibroblasts, or myofibroblasts, may be responsible for tensioning the ligament during the remodeling phase of healing.[48]

There is increased matrix synthesis and cellularity seen throughout the entire ligament (not just at the injury site) during the healing phase. Near the end of the remodeling phase, the uninjured ligament returns to normal cellularity and matrix organization, whereas scar tissue persists at the injury site.[67,87] A few early studies optimistically noted apparent ligament regeneration, but subsequent studies have shown that although normal ligament strength may recover in some instances, this is not because of formation of true ligament tissue.[54,147] Although the strength and stiffness of the collateral ligaments have been restored to 40% to 90% of normal values in animal studies, only about 30% to 70% of the material strength has returned. This scar tissue has inferior material properties compared with normal ligament matrix. It is weaker and creeps more than normal ligament and is also associated with an increased concentration of minor collagens (types III, V, and VI), decreased collagen cross links, and an increased amount of glycosaminoglycans (Table 31-1).[74]

Anterior Collateral Ligament Injury and Healing Response

In adults, most ACL ruptures occur in the midsubstance of the ligament. Murray and co-workers found that following rupture, the human anterior cruciate ligament undergoes four histological phases: inflammation, epiligamentous regeneration, proliferation, and remodeling.[96] Postinjury, the initial hemarthrosis results in inflammation that creates a hostile

Table 31-1 Differences Between Normal Ligaments and Scars

Normal (Uninjured) Ligaments	Ligament Scars
Collagen aligned	Collagen disorganized
Collagen densely packed	Defects between collagen fibers
Large collagen fibrils	Small collagen fibrils
Mature fiber cross links	Immature cross links
Primarily collagen type I (<10% type III)	More collagen type III
Small proteoglycans	Some large proteoglycans
Other components minor	Excesses of other components
Low cell density	Increased cell density
Low vascularity	Increased vascularity

From Frank CB: Ligament healing: current knowledge and clinical applications. J Am Acad Orthop Surg 4:74–83, 1996.

environment for ligament healing. The torn ends of the ACL do not touch, and there is no fibrin clot that forms between the ruptured ends in order to act as a scaffold for subsequent repair.[97] Matrix metalloproteinases (MMPs) and other degradative enzymes, including fibrinolysates that degrade fibrin clot, are normally present in the synovial fluid but are upregulated following injury. These molecules degrade the remnants of the ACL and make healing even more difficult. They also observed the formation of an alpha-smooth muscle actin-expressing synovial cell layer on the surface of the ruptured ends of the ligament and postulate that it is this layer that may inhibit a healing response following anterior cruciate ligament injury and direct repair. For these reasons, the ACL rarely heals following rupture. Therefore, ACL reconstruction is the preferred surgery for patients with symptomatic knee instability.

Biologic Differences Between Anterior Collateral Ligament and Medial Collateral Ligament Healing

In direct contrast to the findings in ACL injuries, both clinical experience and animal studies of MCL injuries have indicated a relatively good, but seldom perfect, healing response.[54,78,79] Numerous studies have examined the mechanisms accounting for the different healing potentials of the ACL and MCL.[5] Multiple factors account for the differences, including ligament ultrastructure, local environment, and cellular properties. There are differences in fibril diameter, fibril diameter distributions, and subfascicular area fractions. Medial collateral ligament fibril diameters are larger and the subfascicular area fraction is higher in the MCL, indicating more densely packed fibrils.[6] Cellular metabolism may also play a role in healing potential. MCL fibroblasts proliferate more rapidly than ACL fibroblasts in vitro and they have differential response to growth factors. There are also differences in cellular response to various chemotactic agents, such as cytokines. ACL and MCL cells demonstrate differential mitogenic, chemotactic, and matrix synthetic responses to mechanical load. There is increased expression of specific integrins on the cell surface of MCL fibroblasts in the healing MCL as compared with minimal integrin expression in the healing ACL cells. Messenger RNA for procollagen expression is also higher in the healing MCL compared with the healing ACL.

Biomechanical factors may also play a role in the ability to heal. The ACL contributes to knee stability in multiple directions whereas the MCL primarily restrains valgus rotation. Therefore, a ruptured MCL receives some protection from other structures, such as the ACL and capsule, and may not be subjected to the same forces that could impede ACL healing.[148] The ACL may not be able to accommodate the multidirectional demands so as to allow healing.[149] Knowledge of the in vivo ligamentous loads would help determine the optimal load and amount of strain to optimize ligament healing.

Combined Ligamentous Injuries

The prognosis for combined ACL-MCL injuries is generally worse than for single-ligament injury, regardless of selected treatment modality.[56,76,148] Although the clinical treatment of these combined injuries remains controversial, evidence from recent animal models may assist in clinical decision making with regard to optimization of ligament healing potential.

Rabbit and canine models have studied the effects of ACL deficiency on the healing of the injured MCL. In these models, knees with untreated combined injury demonstrated increased valgus laxity and significant reduction in the tissue quality of the healed MCL.[149] In contrast, another rabbit study demonstrated that reconstruction of the ACL combined with nonoperative full weight bearing and mobilization of the MCL leads to successful MCL healing.[150] Studies of ACL reconstruction combined with MCL repair have demonstrated improved structural properties and functional testing of the MCL in the short term, with no biochemical or biomechanical difference versus nonoperative MCL treatment after 52 weeks.

Intrinsic Factors

The healing response of ligaments is affected by a variety of endocrine or metabolic abnormalities, systemically or locally. Systemic factors include diabetes mellitus and its effect on the circulatory system, insulin deficiency, and alteration of collagen synthesis and cross linking, and the effect of various changes in the endocrine system on ultimate load of the repaired ligament, and the rates of collagen and glycosaminoglycan synthesis or degradation.[135] Local factors, such as poor circulation or infection, impede the proliferation of cells and prolong the inflammatory phase of healing.[148]

Treatment of Ligamentous Injuries

Immobilization versus Controlled Motion and Exercise

Rehabilitation of an injured ligament often depends on whether there is joint instability associated with the injury. Stable joints may be treated with immobilization for varying time periods, followed by exercise protocols to gain motion and strength. Unstable joints may additionally be treated with specific bracing techniques or surgical intervention. The effects of proper techniques in rehabilitation on patient outcome have been studied in several areas. Injured ligaments have abnormal proprioception and training regimens may improve this. Supervised rehabilitation of postural and balance training may reduce the number of re-injuries in the ankle and play a role in injury prevention.[77] Joint position sense (JPS) in ACL-deficient knees has been described as

impaired. Although knee stability can improve with exercise therapy, there may be no improvement in JPS.[31] The role of JPS in the stability of ACL-deficient knees remains unclear.[62]

Postoperative rehabilitation contributes greatly to the success of ACL reconstruction. Early joint motion is beneficial for reducing pain, improving articular cartilage nutrition, and minimizing scar formation that limits joint motion. Functional sports agility programs during the early rehabilitation period after ACL reconstruction are well tolerated and beneficial to overall outcome.[124]

Aggressive rehabilitation programs that involve contraction of the dominant quadriceps muscles have now become popular. Closed kinetic chain exercises (foot fixed against a resistance) are the mainstay of rehabilitation of ACL-insufficient or ACL-reconstructed knees. Some authors have suggested that open- and closed-chain exercises can be modified to minimize the risk of applying excessive strain on the ACL graft and of excessive patellofemoral joint stress.[44,51] However, open kinetic chain exercises (foot not fixed against a resistance) may result in increased anterior-posterior knee laxity compared with the normal knee.[89] The relationship between rehabilitation exercises and the healing response of an ACL graft is still not completely understood.

Bracing

Functional knee braces provide a protective strain-shielding effect on the normal ACL when anterior shear loads and internal rotation torques are applied to the knee in non–weight-bearing and weight-bearing conditions.[19] However, this protective effect is at loads that are less than those seen in normal walking. Future studies should strive to determine the actual loads transmitted across the knee and ACL graft strain during various rehabilitation exercises and relate these to the healing response of the knee and graft.[18]

Electrical Stimulation

Electrical stimulation has been shown to enhance the repair of biologic tissues such as bone and tendon. The use of direct current yielded improvements in maximum rupture force, energy absorbed, stiffness, and laxity in the rat MCL.[87]

Intra-articular Ligament Reconstruction

Tendon Graft Biology

When surgical intervention is indicated for the treatment of a damaged ligament, a tendon graft is often used for the reconstruction. The tendon is placed in a new biologic and mechanical role. There is a gradual biologic transformation of tissues that are transplanted to an intra-articular environment, such as in ACL reconstruction. This process has been termed *ligamentization*[5] (Fig. 31-7). This gradual biologic transformation of the transplant begins with graft avascular necrosis. The intrinsic graft cells do not survive transplantation to the new environment. Cell necrosis occurs over the first 3 weeks. This is followed by cellular repopulation, which occurs prior to revascularization of the ligament. Repopulating cells appear to be derived from synovium and obtain their nutrition by synovial diffusion. Other possible sources of repopulating cells include mesenchymal stem cells, marrow cells, blood cells, and cells from the residual ACL stump.[4,96] It is also possible that there is a surviving subset of cells in the graft, although this is much less likely. The eventual

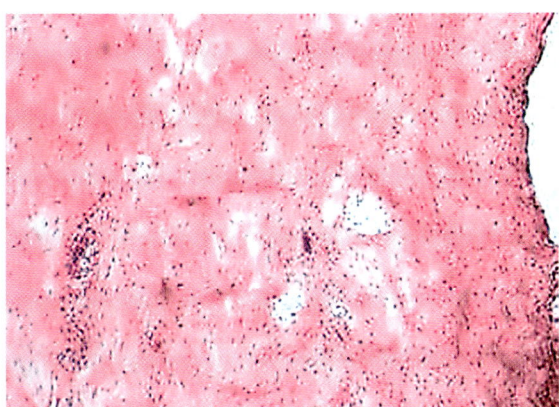

Figure 31-7. Histology of intra-articular graft ligamentization in a rabbit ACL reconstruction. The graft has been repopulated by the host cells. (Courtesy Dr. David Amiel, University of California, San Diego.)

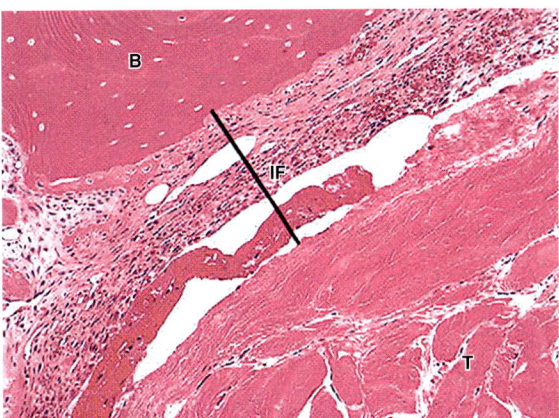

Figure 31-8. Tendon to bone interface after ACL reconstruction with a tendon graft in a rabbit at 1 week. Note the fibrovascular interface (scar) tissue between the tendon and the bone. *B,* Bone; *IF,* interface tissue; *T,* tendon. (From Gulotta LV, Rodeo SA: Biology of autograft and allograft anterior cruciate ligament reconstruction. Clin Sports Med 26:509–524, 2007.)

phenotype of the repopulating cells is not known. It is not known whether these cells assume the phenotype of normal ACL cells. These cells remain metabolically active for a prolonged period of time during the healing process of intra-articular ligament grafts.

The revascularization phase begins 6 to 8 weeks following graft transplantation.[5] Vascular synovial tissue forms around the graft. New blood supply to the graft is derived from the fat pad, tibial remnant, and posterior synovial tissues. Growing capillary buds are seen histologically. Revascularization progresses from the periphery of the graft to the central portion of the graft.

Matrix synthesis occurs in the ligament graft following cellular repopulation and revascularization.[5] Over time, the collagen and glycosaminoglycan content of the graft becomes similar to a normal ligament.[23] Similarly, the collagen crimp pattern and reducible cross link profile becomes more like that of a normal intra-articular ligament as compared with the extra-articular tendon graft. However, there is a persistent abnormal unimodal distribution of small diameter collagen fibrils in the graft. There is variable return of the pyridinoline collagen cross links. Type III collagen also has been found to remain elevated for a variable period of time following graft transplantation. These persistent abnormalities in collagen cross links, collagen type, and collagen fibril diameter probably contribute to the inferior biomechanical properties of the graft.

The last phase in the graft incorporation process is the remodeling phase.[5] There is a gradual decrease in cellularity and vascularity and an increase in matrix organization. This process occurs for a minimum of 1 year following graft transplantation.

Graft Attachment Site Biology

Surgical reconstruction of a ligament relies on the grafted tendon to attach to the bones previously connected by the torn ligament. Tendon to bone healing occurs by the formation of a fibrovascular interface tissue between the tendon and bone. In this way, the tendon becomes anchored to the bone. There is gradual reestablishment of collagen fiber continuity between the tendon and bone. Some animal studies have demonstrated direct collagen fiber continuity between the tendon and bone (Sharpey's fibers), whereas other studies

have demonstrated formation of a fibrocartilage interface between tendon and bone.[110,111] The concomitant bone formation is generally an intramembranous process. The attachment strength gradually increases as collagen fiber continuity improves.

Bone plug healing, such as seen in bone-tendon-bone ACL reconstructions, involves incorporation of the bone plug into the bone tunnel over a 12-week period.[5] The original insertion site of the patellar tendon may remain histologically normal. The comparative strength of the healed tendon to bone attachment versus the healed bone plug attachment is unknown.

Healing of a tendon graft in a bone tunnel, as is required in ACL reconstruction using semitendinosus tendon, begins with the formation of a fibrovascular interface tissue between the tendon and bone.[110] There is progressive bone ingrowth into this interface tissue, with gradual reestablishment of an indirect type of insertion by intramembranous bone formation. The increase in strength of the healing tendon to bone attachment correlates well with the progressive bone ingrowth and maturation of the interface (Figs. 31-8 and 31-9).

Healing of tendon to the surface of bone also occurs by bone ingrowth into the fibrous interface tissue that forms between the tendon and bone.[116] In a larger animal model (goats), an indirect insertion forms, whereas studies in lower animals have demonstrated formation of a direct insertion. Further study is required to determine the basic cellular mechanism of tendon to bone healing. Studies have demonstrated that bone morphogenetic protein-2, a potent osteoinductive agent, can augment tendon healing in a bone tunnel.[111]

Future Directions in Ligament Healing

Researchers are actively exploring methods to improve the quality of healing ligament tissue and to find novel ways to accelerate the healing process. Advances in the fields of molecular biology and biochemistry may have applications in the ligament healing process.[148] These approaches include innovative biologic and bioengineering techniques of using

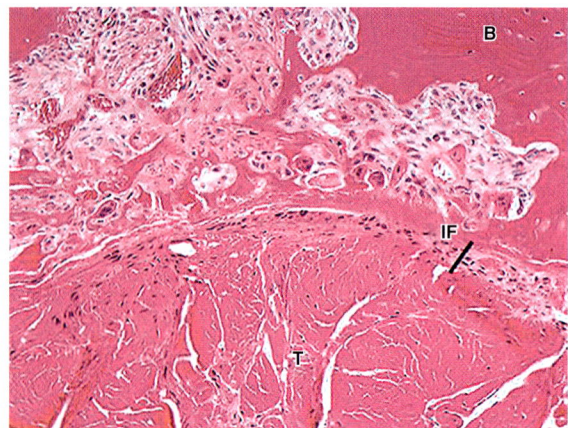

Figure 31-9. Tendon to bone interface at 2 weeks. Note the decrease in interface tissue at 2 weeks. *B,* Bone; *IF,* interface tissue; *T,* tendon. (From Gulotta LV, Rodeo SA: Biology of autograft and allograft anterior cruciate ligament reconstruction. Clin Sports Med 26:509–524, 2007.)

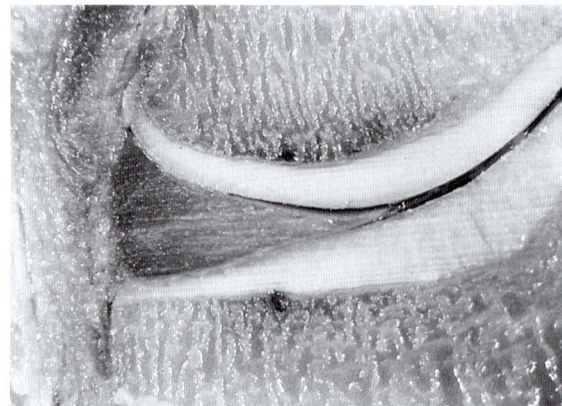

Figure 31-10. Frontal section of the medial compartment of a human knee illustrating the articulation of the menisci with the condyles of the femur and tibia. (From Warren R, Arnoczky SP, Wickiewicz TL: Anatomy of the knee. In Nicholas JA, Hershman EB [eds]: The lower extremity and spine in sports medicine, St Louis, 1986, CV Mosby, p 657.)

growth factors, gene transfer therapy, cell therapy, scaffolding materials, and mechanical stimuli.[22]

Growth Factors

Growth factors such as epidermal growth factor (EGF), basic fibroblast growth factor (bFGF), acidic fibroblast growth factor (aFGF), platelet-derived growth factor BB (PDGF-BB), and transforming growth factor beta (TGF-β) are currently being evaluated for their effects on fibroblast proliferation, matrix synthesis, and cell migration. Animal models have shown that TGF-β is a good promoter of matrix synthesis, whereas PDGF-BB, EGF, and bFGF are positive mitogens on fibroblasts of the ACL and MCL.[118,148] Investigators have demonstrated the possibility that growth factors can enhance the in vivo healing of injured ligaments.[84,145] In one rabbit model, high doses of PDGF delivered with a fibrin sealant led to significant increases in the structural properties of the femur-MCL-tibia complex.[75]

Gene Transfer

Gene transfer technology has been developed to design and enhance delivery vehicles for growth factors. Controlling and regulating the expression of proteins within a host cell will enable researchers to administer treatments over a prolonged period of time.[148] Although the technology for treating ligamentous injuries is still somewhat novel, preliminary studies have shown positive effects on collagen fibril diameter and distribution, as well as significant increases in mechanical properties.[100]

Cell Therapy

The concept of cell therapy is that implantation of genetically manipulated cells can enhance the repair of ligaments as those cells become constituents of the healing tissue.[148] Both in vivo and in vitro studies have already demonstrated that mesenchymal stem cells are capable of differentiating into many cell types involved in ligamentous healing. A study by Watanabe and colleagues[141] has demonstrated the ability of nucleated donor bone marrow cells to migrate to the area of MCL injury after transplantation. Cell therapy

may lead to new methods of treatment for ligament injuries in the future.

Biologic Scaffolds

Biologic scaffolds offer the potential to accelerate ligament and tendon healing and regeneration. Particular interest has been on the porcine small intestine submucosa. Research has shown that this submucosa can be modified in vitro by seeding marrow stromal cells on the scaffold and by applying cyclic stretching to increase cell alignment. When applied in vivo, the tissue-engineered scaffold could potentially accelerate the healing process.[22] Further research is needed in this area before these scaffolds gain widespread clinical applications.

MENISCI

Structure and Function

The menisci of the knee are **C**-shaped wedges of fibrocartilage interposed between the condyles of the femur and tibia. They are actually extensions of the tibia that serve to deepen the articular surfaces of the tibial plateau to accommodate the condyles of the femur better. The peripheral border of each meniscus is thick and convex and attached to the joint capsule, whereas the inner border tapers to a thin, free edge.[140] The proximal surfaces of the menisci are concave and in contact with the condyles of the femur; their distal surfaces are flat and rest on the tibial plateau (Fig. 31-10).

The medial meniscus is somewhat semicircular in form, approximately 3.5 cm in length and considerably wider posteriorly than anteriorly. The anterior horn of the medial meniscus is attached to the tibial plateau in the area of the anterior intercondylar fossa, anterior to the ACL (Fig. 31-11). The posterior fibers of the anterior horn merge with the transverse ligament, which connects the anterior horns of the medial and lateral menisci.[140] The posterior horn of the medial meniscus is firmly attached to the posterior intercondylar fossa of the tibia between the attachments of the lateral meniscus and posterior cruciate ligament. The periphery of the medial meniscus is attached to the joint capsule

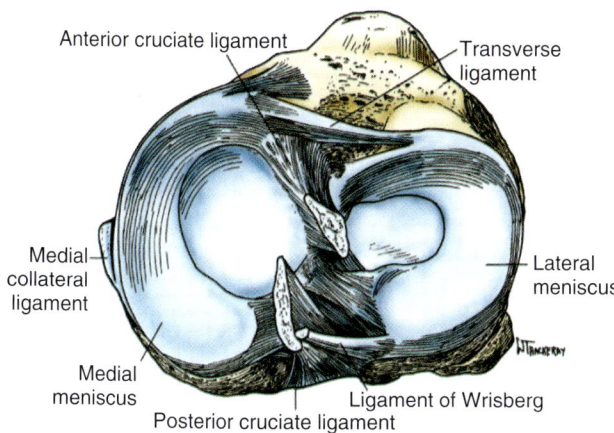

Figure 31-11. Human tibial plateau showing the relative size and attachments of the medial and lateral menisci. (From Warren R, Arnoczky SP, Wickiewicz TL: Anatomy of the knee. In Nicholas JA, Hershman EB [eds]: The lower extremity and spine in sports medicine, St Louis, 1986, CV Mosby, p 657.)

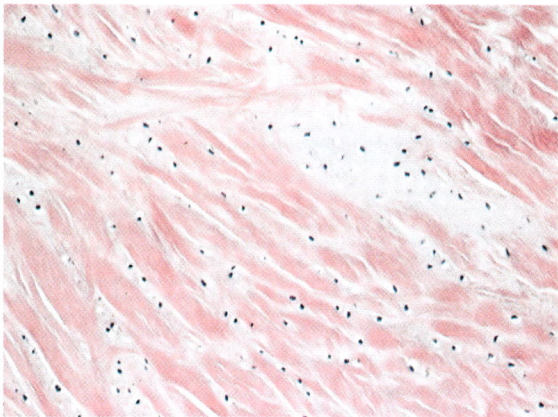

Figure 31-12. Photomicrograph of a longitudinal section of human meniscus showing the histologic appearance of meniscal fibrocartilage (hematoxylin-eosin, ×100).

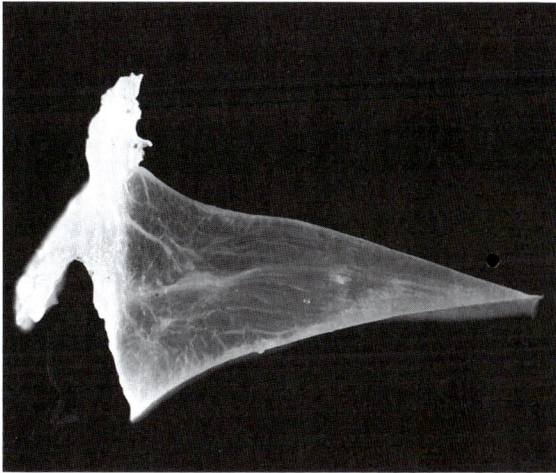

Figure 31-13. Cross-section of a lateral meniscus showing the radial orientation of fibrous ties within the substance of the meniscus. (From Arnoczky SP, Torzilli PA: The biology of cartilage. In Hunter LY, Funk FJ Jr [eds]: Rehabilitation of the injured knee, St Louis, 1984, CV Mosby, p 148.)

throughout its length. The tibial portion of the capsular attachment is referred to as the coronary ligament. At its midpoint, the medial meniscus is more firmly attached to the femur and tibia through a condensation in the joint capsule known as the deep medial collateral ligament.

The lateral meniscus is more circular in shape and covers a larger percentage of the articular surface of the tibial plateau than the medial meniscus does. The anterior and posterior horns are approximately the same width (see Fig. 31-11). The anterior horn of the lateral meniscus is attached to the tibia anterior to the intercondylar eminence and posterior to the attachment of the ACL, with which it partially blends.[140] The posterior horn of the lateral meniscus is attached posterior to the intercondylar eminence of the tibia, anterior to the posterior horn of the medial meniscus. In addition to this posterior attachment to the tibia, two ligaments may run from the posterior horn of the lateral meniscus to the medial femoral condyle, passing in front of or behind the origin of the posterior cruciate ligament. These attachments are known as the anterior meniscofemoral ligament (ligament of Humphrey) and the posterior meniscofemoral ligament (ligament of Wrisberg). Although there is no attachment of the lateral meniscus to the lateral collateral ligament, it has a loose peripheral attachment to the joint capsule.

Histologically, the meniscus is a fibrocartilaginous tissue composed primarily of an interlacing network of collagen fibers interposed with cells (Fig. 31-12).[11] The predominant type of collagen in the meniscus is type I, but types II, III, and V are present as well.[94] Although other components, such as proteoglycans, glycoproteins, and water, also contribute to the makeup of the extracellular matrix of the meniscus, it is the specific orientation of the collagen fibers that appears to be most directly related to the function of the meniscus. Even though the principal orientation of the collagen fibers is circumferential, a few small, radially disposed fibers appear on both the femoral and tibial surfaces of the menisci, as well as within the substance of the tissue. It is theorized that these radial fibers act as ties to provide structural rigidity and help resist longitudinal splitting of the menisci as a result of overcompression (Fig. 31-13).[25] Tissackt and associates[137] have measured the tensile modulus in the radial and

circumferential directions in the human meniscus. Their study showed that the meniscus is much stronger and stiffer in the circumferential direction than the radial direction, and the low circumferential shear strength is thought to be at least partly responsible for the occurrence of longitudinal tears.[7,155]

Subsequent light and electron microscopic examination of the menisci have revealed three different collagen framework layers—a superficial layer composed of a network of fine fibrils woven into a meshlike matrix, a surface layer just beneath the superficial layer composed, in part, of irregularly aligned collagen bundles, and a middle layer in which the collagen fibers are larger, coarser, and oriented in a parallel, circumferential direction (Fig. 31-14).[25,151] It is this middle layer that allows the meniscus to resist tensile forces and function as a transmitter of load across the knee joint. When an axial load is applied to the knee joint, the meniscus is compressed, but because of its wedge-shaped structure and firm anterior and posterior attachments to the tibia, it is displaced away from the joint center, resulting in tensile stress (hoop stress) in the circumferential collagen fibers.[132] There are significant

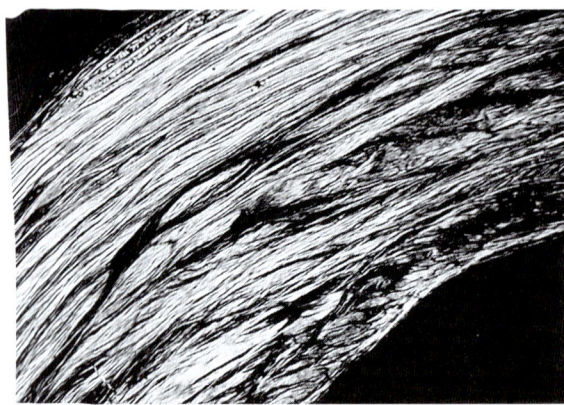

Figure 31-14. Photomicrograph of a longitudinal section of a meniscus under polarized light demonstrating the orientation of the coarse, deep, circumferentially oriented collagen fibers.

regional variations in the circumferential tensile strength and stiffness, with lower values in the posterior two thirds of the medial meniscus than in the anterior or the lateral meniscus.[50] These variations are probably because of differences in collagen fiber ultrastructure, because the variations in material properties are not correlated with differences in biochemical composition.[137]

The function of the menisci may be clinically inferred by the degenerative changes that accompany their removal. Fairbank[47] has described radiographic changes after meniscectomy that included narrowing of the joint space, flattening of the femoral condyle, and formation of osteophytes. These changes were attributed to loss of the weight-bearing function of the meniscus. Biomechanical studies have shown that the medial meniscus transmits 50% of the joint load in the medial compartment whereas the lateral meniscus transmits 70% of the joint load in the lateral compartment.[34] At least 50% of the compressive load of the knee joint is transmitted through the meniscus in extension, which increases to approximately 85% of load transmission in 90 degrees of flexion. In a meniscectomized knee, the contact area is reduced by approximately 50%.[2,58] This reduction significantly increases the load per unit area and results in articular damage and degeneration. Partial meniscectomy has also been shown to increase contact pressure significantly.[16] In an experimental study, resection of as little as 15% to 34% of the meniscus increased contact pressure by more than 350%.[121] Thus, even partial meniscectomy does not appear to be a benign procedure.*

Another proposed function of the meniscus is that of shock absorption. The meniscus can be viewed as a biphasic medium comprised of a fluid phase (the interstitial water) and solid phase (collagen, GAGs, and the other matrix proteins).[127] The collagen network and GAGs form a porous, permeable solid matrix. Interstitial fluid flow and solid matrix deformation during loading cause the meniscus to act as a viscoelastic material. By examining the compressive load deformation response of normal and meniscectomized knees, it has been suggested that the viscoelastic menisci may function to attenuate the intermittent shock waves generated by impulse loading of the knee during gait. Studies have shown that a normal knee has a shock-absorbing capacity about 20% higher than that of knees that have undergone meniscectomy.[139] Because the inability of a joint system to absorb shock has been implicated in the development of osteoarthritis, the shock absorption mechanism would appear to play a role in maintaining the health of the knee joint.[108]

In addition to the role of the meniscus in load transmission and shock absorption, the menisci are thought to contribute to knee joint stability and overall joint conformity.[86,90] The menisci serve to increase congruity between the condyles of the femur and tibia. The superior concave and inferior flat surface of the meniscus conforms to the femoral and tibial condyles, and the wedge shape of the meniscus contributes to its function in joint stabilization. Medial meniscectomy in the ACL-intact knee has little effect on anteroposterior motion; however, in the ACL-deficient knee, medial meniscectomy results in an increase in anterior tibial translation of up to 58% at 90 degrees of flexion.[3,85,105] These findings support the concept that medial meniscal transplantation should be considered at the time of reconstruction of the ACL in the medial meniscus–deficient knee.

The joint conformity provided by the menisci may promote the viscous hydrodynamic action required for fluid-film lubrication. This function assists in the overall lubrication of the articular surfaces of the knee joint. Water may be extruded into the joint space during compressive loading, aiding in joint lubrication.[12,107] The meniscus may also aid in articular cartilage nutrition by helping maintain a synovial fluid film over the articular surface and by compressing synovial fluid into articular cartilage.[50] However, the exact contribution of the meniscus to joint lubrication has yet to be fully elucidated.

Finally, the menisci may provide proprioceptive feedback for joint position sense. Neural elements are most abundant in the outer portion of the meniscus, particularly types I and II nerve fibers. The anterior and posterior horns of the meniscus are innervated with mechanoreceptors that may play a role in proprioceptive feedback during extremes of motion.[43,80] These neural elements are thought to be part of a proprioceptive reflex arc that may contribute to the functional stability of the knee.[12]

In summary, the proposed functions of the menisci include load bearing, shock absorption, joint stability, lubrication, and proprioception. Loss of the meniscus, partially or totally, significantly alters these functions and predisposes the joint to degenerative changes. Because acute traumatic tears of the meniscus usually occur in young (13- to 40-year-old) and active individuals, the need to preserve the meniscus, and thus minimize these degenerative changes, is of paramount importance.[11] The development of techniques to save the meniscus has all but replaced traditional total meniscectomy in the treatment of many meniscal lesions. Although partial meniscectomy may be the only option for some central avascular tears, research into new techniques of meniscal repair may eliminate even partial meniscectomy and the undesirable consequences of loss of this important structure.

Biology of Meniscal Injury and Healing

Thomas Annandale was credited with the first surgical repair of a torn meniscus in 1883.[9] It was not until 1936, when King published his classic experiment on meniscus healing in dogs,

---

*References 8, 33, 38, 49, 82, and 117.

that the actual biologic limitations of meniscus healing were set forth. King[81] demonstrated that for meniscus lesions to heal, they must communicate with the peripheral blood supply. Enhancing vascularity at or near the site of meniscal injury has remained a major focus in the techniques of surgical repair. In addition, advances in cellular and molecular biology now allow researchers to investigate the role of specific growth factors and cytokines in the cellular response to injury. Further application of these findings will continue to provide for means of enhancing meniscal repair.

Vascular Anatomy of the Meniscus

The vascular supply to the medial and lateral menisci of the knee originates predominantly from the medial and lateral genicular arteries (inferior and superior branches).[13] Branches from these vessels give rise to a perimeniscal capillary plexus within the synovial and capsular tissues of the knee joint. The plexus is an arborizing network of vessels that supply the peripheral border of the meniscus about its attachment to the joint capsule (Figs. 31-15 and 31-16). These perimeniscal vessels are oriented in a predominantly circumferential pattern, with radial branches being directed toward the center of the joint (Fig. 31-17). Anatomic studies have shown that the degree of peripheral vascular penetration is 10% to 30% of the width of the medial meniscus and 10% to 25% of the width of the lateral meniscus.[39] The middle genicular artery, along with a few terminal branches of the medial and lateral genicular vessels, also supplies vessels to the menisci through the vascular synovial covering of the anterior and posterior horn attachments. These synovial vessels penetrate the horn attachments and give rise to smaller vessels that enter the meniscal horns for a short distance and end in terminal capillary loops.

A small reflection of the vascular synovial tissue is also present throughout the peripheral attachment of the medial and lateral menisci on the femoral and tibial articular surfaces.[13] This synovial fringe extends for a short distance over the peripheral surfaces of the meniscus and contains small, terminally looped vessels. Although the synovial fringe is adherent to the articular surfaces of the menisci, it does not contribute vessels to the meniscus per se. The clinical significance of these fringe vessels lies in their potential contribution to the reparative response of the meniscus, as seen in synovial abrasion techniques.

Vascular Response to Injury

The vascular supply of the meniscus is the essential element in determining its potential for repair. This blood supply must have the ability to support the inflammatory response characteristic of wound repair. Clinical and experimental observations have demonstrated that the peripheral meniscal blood supply is capable of producing a reparative response similar to that in other connective tissue.[14,70]

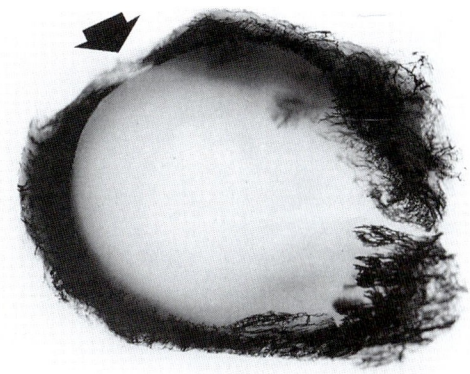

Figure 31-16. Superior aspect of a lateral meniscus after vascular perfusion with India ink and tissue clearing with a modified Spalteholz technique. Note the absence of vascularity at the posterior lateral aspect of the meniscus *(arrow)*. This is adjacent to the popliteal hiatus. (From Arnoczky SP, Warren RF: Microvasculature of the human meniscus. Am J Sports Med 10:90–95, 1982.)

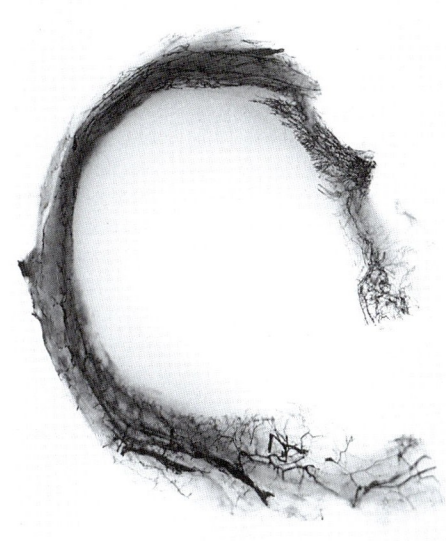

Figure 31-15. Superior aspect of a medial meniscus after vascular perfusion with India ink and tissue clearing with a modified Spalteholz technique. Note the vascularity at the periphery of the meniscus, as well as at the anterior and posterior horn attachments. (From Arnoczky SP, Warren RF: Microvasculature of the human meniscus. Am J Sports Med 10:90–95, 1982.)

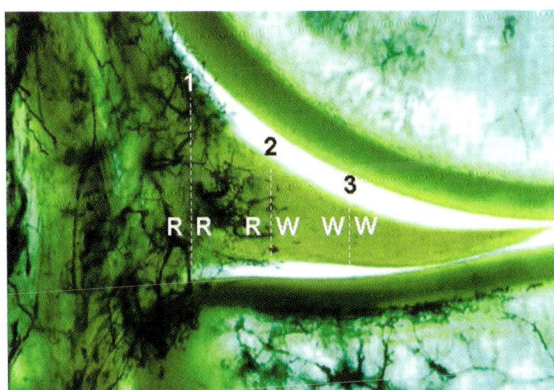

Figure 31-17. A 5-mm-thick frontal section of the medial compartment of a human knee (Spalteholz preparation). Branching radial vessels from the perimeniscal capillary plexus penetrate the peripheral border of the medial meniscus. *RR*, Red-red zone; *RW*, red-white zone; *WW*, white-white zone. (From Arnoczky SP, Warren RF: Microvasculature of the human meniscus. Am J Sports Med 10:90–95, 1982.)

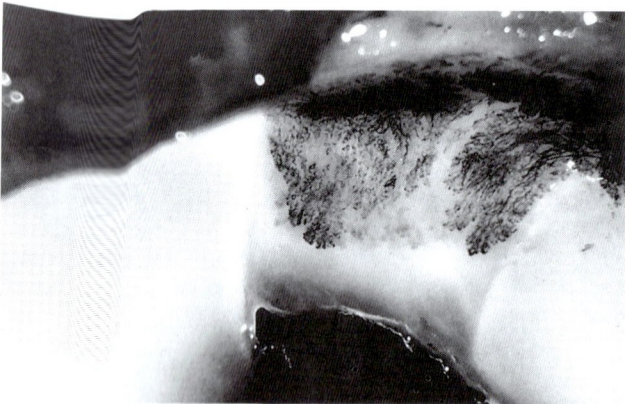

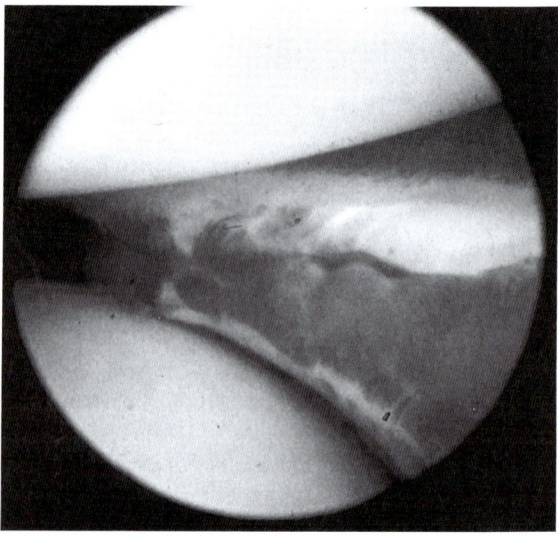

Figure 31-18. A meniscus 6 weeks after the creation of a radial lesion. Fibrovascular scar tissue has filled the defect, and vascular proliferation from the synovial fringe can be seen. (From Arnoczky SP, Warren RF: The microvasculature of the meniscus and its response to injury: An experimental study in the dog. Am J Sports Med 11:131–141, 1983.)

Figure 31-20. Arthroscopic view of a peripheral tear in a human meniscus. Note the vascular granulation tissue present at the margin of the lesion. This is classified as a red-white tear. Also note the proliferation of the synovial fringe over the femoral surface of the meniscus. (From Arnoczky SP, Torzilli PA: The biology of cartilage. In Hunter LY, Funk FJ Jr [eds]: Rehabilitation of the injured knee, St Louis, 1984, CV Mosby, p 148.)

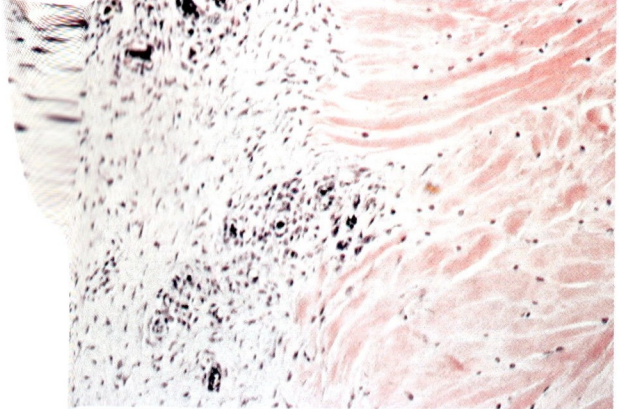

Figure 31-19. Photomicrograph of the junction of the meniscus and fibrovascular repair tissue at 10 weeks (hematoxylin-eosin, ×100). (From Arnoczky SP, Warren RF: The microvasculature of the meniscus and its response to injury: An experimental study in the dog. Am J Sports Med 11:131–141, 1983.)

After injury within the peripheral vascular zone, a fibrin clot forms that is rich in inflammatory cells. Vessels from the perimeniscal capillary plexus proliferate through this fibrin scaffold, accompanied by the proliferation of undifferentiated mesenchymal cells.[14] Eventually, the lesion is filled with a cellular fibrovascular granulation tissue that glues the wound edges together and appears to be continuous with the adjacent normal meniscal fibrocartilage.[28] Increased collagen synthesis within the granulation tissue slowly results in a fibrous scar (Fig. 31-18). The exact phenotype of the cells that initiate and regulate the healing process is unknown. Like other connective tissues, the lesion heals with scar tissue that likely has inferior material properties. For example, the tensile strength of the healed lesion did not reach the strength of normal meniscus even by 12 to 16 weeks in one animal study.[12] Furthermore, the long-term histologic and biomechanical characteristics of the reparative tissue are unknown.

Experimental studies have shown that radial lesions of the meniscus that extend to the synovium are completely healed with fibrovascular scar tissue by 10 weeks (Fig. 31-19).[14,28] Modulation of this scar into normal-appearing fibrocartilage,

however, requires several months. Further study is required to delineate the biomechanical properties at each stage of this repair process.

The ability of meniscal lesions to heal has provided the rationale for the repair of peripheral meniscal injuries, and a number of reports have demonstrated excellent results after primary repair of peripheral meniscal injuries.[32,40,41,93,113] Follow-up examination of these peripheral repairs has revealed a process of repair similar to that noted in experimental models.

When examining injured menisci for potential repair, lesions are often classified by the location of the tear relative to the blood supply of the meniscus and the vascular appearance of the peripheral and central surfaces of the tear (see Fig. 31-17).[10] The so-called red-red tear (peripheral capsular detachment) has a functional blood supply to the capsular and meniscal side of the lesion and obviously has the best prognosis for healing. Red-white tears (meniscus tears through the peripheral vascular zone) have an active peripheral blood supply; however, the central (inner) surface of the lesion is devoid of functioning vessels (Fig. 31-20). These lesions have sufficient vascularity to heal by the aforementioned fibrovascular proliferation. White-white tears (meniscus lesions completely in the avascular zone) are without blood supply and theoretically cannot heal. However, as discussed later, specific meniscal repair enhancement techniques have been developed to address tears in the white-white zone.

Cellular Response to Injury

The ability of fibrochondrocytes within a meniscus to mount a reparative response is dependent in part on its cellular activity. Cytokines and growth factors present during the inflammatory response to injury may promote meniscal healing through enhancement of cell migration, cell division, and production of extracellular matrix. Although no specific growth factor has been shown to enhance meniscus healing, researchers are beginning to identify how the meniscal fibrochondrocyte responds to various growth factors.* Meniscal repair augmentation methods such as fibrin clot and platelet-rich plasma (PRP) are based on the concept that growth factors have a positive impact on meniscal healing. Understanding which growth factors positively affect the healing potential of the meniscal fibrochondrocyte matrix will undoubtedly provide future strategies for treating meniscal injuries.

Meniscal Pathology

Intrinsic meniscal degeneration begins around 30 years of age, progresses with age, occurs in men and women, and occurs in active and inactive subjects.[101] Histologic analysis demonstrates mucinous degeneration, hypocellularity, and loss of normal collagen fiber organization.[143] The cause of such changes is unknown, but may reflect recurrent chronic microtrauma to the meniscus. Studies in animals have demonstrated that following ACL transection, the menisci undergo alterations in their extracellular matrices, including an increase in water content.[1,94] An initial decrease in the concentration of GAGs has also been observed following ACL transection. However, in joints with chronic ACL insufficiency, the concentration of GAGs was found to increase substantially. This reflects a remarkable ability of meniscal fibrochondrocytes to replenish the lost GAGs.

Degenerative meniscal tissue is believed to have a poorer potential for healing.[12] Careful attention should be paid to the appearance and consistency of the meniscus at the time of surgery. Although preservation of the meniscus may be more important in a knee with axial malalignment, the rate of healing may be lower because of concomitant degenerative changes.[66]

Meniscal Repair

Indications

Based on the established important functions of the meniscus and the clinical results of meniscectomy, most clinicians try to preserve the meniscus via repair whenever possible. Although the treatment of meniscal tears should be individualized, the most commonly accepted criteria for meniscal repair include the following: (1) a complete vertical longitudinal tear more than 10 mm in length; (2) a tear within the peripheral 10% to 30% of the meniscus or within 3 or 4 mm of the meniscocapsular junction; (3) a peripheral tear that can be displaced toward the center of the plateau by probing, thus demonstrating instability; (4) the absence of secondary degeneration or deformity; (5) a tear in an active patient; and (6) a tear associated with concurrent ligament stabilization.

Although it is most critical to perform meniscal repair on young patients in an attempt to decrease the eventual articular cartilage wear of a meniscectomized knee, meniscal repair can also be successful in older patients.[29] Well-vascularized longitudinal red-red tears and red-white tears are ideal for repair and also have the highest rate of healing. Stable longitudinal tears (<1 cm in length) and partial-thickness tears often remain asymptomatic or heal without suturing.[123] Even

though degenerative tears and radial tears can also be repaired, the function of a repaired meniscus has yet to be proved.

The onset of degenerative change has been linked to the amount of meniscus removed.[8] Large bucket handle tears as seen in young active patients would require a large portion of the meniscus to be removed if not repaired. In these younger patients, meniscal repair is often extended into the white-white (avascular) zone by using the vascular enhancement techniques discussed later. A poorer prognosis in a meniscectomized knee has also been associated with varus alignment and ACL deficiency, so meniscal repair should likewise be considered in these situations, when possible.[26,49] In addition, decreased healing rates are seen in ACL-deficient knees, so any instability of the knee should also be addressed.[95,134]

Enhancement of Meniscal Repair

The desire to preserve meniscal tissue has led to efforts to extend the region of viable meniscal repair to the central, avascular portion of the meniscus (white-white tears).[10] Experimental and clinical observations have shown that these lesions are incapable of healing under usual circumstances and have provided the rationale for partial meniscectomy.[13,81] In an effort to extend the level of repair into these avascular areas, techniques have been developed to provide vascularity to these white-white tears, as well as enhance the repair of red-white tears. Such techniques include débridement, creation of vascular access channels, trephination, use of synovial pedicles, and synovial abrasion. Also discussed will be the use and delivery of growth factors to promote meniscal healing and the role of mechanical load on healing of meniscal repairs. Finally, innovations in gene therapy and tissue engineered menisci will be explored.

Vascular Access Channels and Trephination

The creation of vascular access channels (VACs) was one of the early techniques used to extend the vascular response into the avascular zone of the meniscus.[13,70] The premise of this technique is to create full-thickness channels connecting the avascular lesion to the peripheral vasculature of the meniscus. Experimental studies in animals have demonstrated that lesions in the avascular portion of the meniscus, when connected to the peripheral vasculature by means of a full-thickness VAC, heal through the proliferation of fibrovascular scar tissue from the VAC into the tear (Fig. 31-21). VACs can allow for an extensive influx of vessels into a white-white tear, but they also cut across the predominantly circumferential orientation of the collagen fibers of the meniscus. This disruption in collagen architecture may adversely affect the function of the meniscus, especially if the VAC is carried out through the peripheral rim of the meniscus. Consequently, the original VAC technique has not been used extensively in the clinical situation.

The technique of trephination was introduced as a means of creating a pathway for vascular migration without imparting significant damage to the collagen architecture of the meniscus.[112] In this procedure, a series of horizontally oriented trephinations are made with a hypodermic needle (18-gauge needle or larger) through the peripheral aspect of the meniscal rim to produce a series of bleeding puncture sites, which provide an avenue for vascular ingrowth. This modification of the VAC technique minimizes the damage done

---

*References 20, 35, 68, 99, 128, 129, 131, 133, and 142.

to the collagen architecture of the meniscus but still allows for the influx of a vascular response. Initially developed in an animal model, clinical application of this technique has been described with and without the use of sutures.[153,154] In the first clinical report of trephination, this technique was used to treat incomplete lesions in the peripheral and middle third of the meniscus.[52] Although a 90% success rate was reported in this series, there was no control group with which to compare the specific efficacy of the technique. More recently, controlled studies have found trephination alone to be successful in treating stable meniscal lesions, as well as a means of augmenting traditional suture repair.[125,152]

Synovial Pedicles (Flaps) and Abrasion

An additional approach to extend the vascular supply to an avascular meniscal tear involves the use of a synovial pedicle or flap. In this technique, a pedicle of the highly vascular

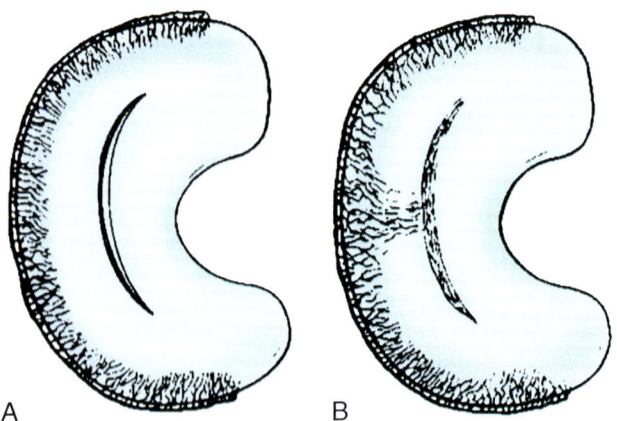

Figure 31-21. Schematic drawing showing the concept of connecting a lesion in the avascular portion of the meniscus with the peripheral blood supply through the use of a vascular access channel. **A,** Tear in an avascular zone. **B,** Vascular proliferation through an access channel. (From Arnoczky SP, Warren RF: The microvasculature of the meniscus and its response to injury: an experimental study in the dog. Am J Sports Med 11:131–141, 1983.)

synovial tissue immediately adjacent to the peripheral attachment of the meniscus is rotated into the avascular lesion and sutured in place. Although animal experiments using this technique suggest excellent potential for augmenting repairs in the white-white zone of the human meniscus, there is a paucity of clinical research in this area, possibly because of the technical difficulties in adapting synovial pedicle use to an arthroscopic approach.[59,61]

Synovial abrasion is a technique in which the synovial fringe of the femoral and tibial surfaces of the meniscus is abraded with a rasp to stimulate a proliferative response (Fig. 31-22). During the normal repair process of peripheral lesions, a vascular pannus develops from the synovial fringe and extends over the femoral and tibial surfaces of the meniscus (see Fig. 31-18). The combination of this vascular response with the peripheral meniscal blood supply provides support for the repair process. Because the vascular pannus observed in the repair process is often extensive, it was theorized that stimulation of the synovial fringe could accentuate this response and help extend it into avascular or marginally vascularized areas.[11,70] The ability of synovial abrasion to enhance the healing potential of tears in avascular areas of the meniscus has been demonstrated in several animal models.[104,109] Clinical application of synovial abrasion alone, as well as in conjunction with other enhancement techniques (including trephination and fibrin clot), has been shown to be effective in treating stable or partial-thickness meniscal tears.[70,125] Additionally, the efficacy of synovial abrasion and the simplicity of the surgical technique have led to recommendations for its use in augmenting suture repairs.[17,69,119]

Marrow-Stimulating Techniques

Cannon and Vittori[30] have found that meniscal healing rates improve from 53% to 93% when the repair is performed in conjunction with ACL reconstruction. Shelbourne and Heinrich's long-term follow-up[124] of lateral meniscal tears left in situ at the time of ACL reconstruction has demonstrated 96% normal or near-normal results. These clinical findings suggest that blood and marrow elements may produce a milieu bathing the healing meniscus, thus providing essential

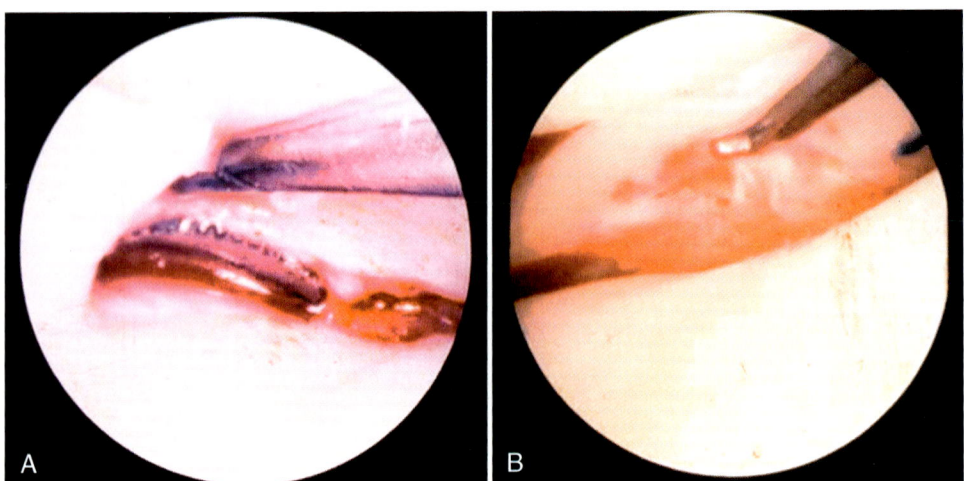

Figure 31-22. A, Arthroscopic photograph demonstrating abrasion of the synovial fringe on the surface of the meniscus with a rasp. **B,** Arthroscopic photograph taken 8 weeks after synovial abrasion demonstrating a vascular pannus extending into a white-white tear. (Courtesy Dr. Charles Henning.)

mitogenic and chemotactic elements. Assuming that the cytokines and growth factors in the blood and marrow elements introduced into the knee after notchplasty and tunnel drilling in ACL reconstruction are responsible for the improved repair rates, there would be a theoretical advantage to reproducing the presence of blood and marrow elements during meniscal repair in an ACL-intact knee. Microfracture of the intercondylar notch has been proposed as a means of re-creating the hemarthrosis present after ACL reconstruction in the hope of improving meniscal repair outcomes.[55] However, the clinical results of microfracture as a stimulus to enhance meniscal repair have not been documented.

Growth Factors

Recent emphasis has been directed toward applications of cell and molecular biology to promote meniscal healing and regeneration. Numerous growth factors have been identified as signaling molecules that control mitogenic behavior and differentiation of cells. These growth factors have been used on meniscal cells to test their effects on the healing of tears or defects, as well as their effects on extracellular matrix synthesis in tissue and cell culture (Table 31-2). Cells from the peripheral part of the meniscus have an increased ability to synthesize collagen in cell culture compared with cells derived from the inner part of the meniscus.[129] There are other differences in cellular physiology between the cells in the inner and outer regions of the meniscus, including the responsiveness to growth factors and cytokines. Webber and colleagues[142] have tested the effect of fibroblastic growth factor (FGF) and human platelet lysate (PL), both of which were found to stimulate proliferation of meniscal cells. TGF-β increased proteoglycan synthesis of fibrochondrocytes from all different regions of the meniscus in a dose-dependent manner.[35,133] Spindler and associates[128,129] have demonstrated that the cells in the inner, central region of the tissue are much less responsive to platelet-derived growth factor-AB (PDGF-AB) than the cells in the peripheral portion of the tissue. Conversely, Bhargava and coworkers[20] have demonstrated that at optimal concentrations, PDGF-AB, hepatocyte growth factor (HGF), and bone morphogenetic protein-2 (BMP-2) are equally effective in stimulating DNA synthesis in cells isolated from different zones of the meniscus. BMP-2 and insulin-like growth factor-1 (IGF-1) stimulated the migration of fibrochondrocytes from the middle zone by 40% to 50%. This study also reported that interleukin-1 (IL-1) and EGF stimulated migration of meniscal cells. Other studies have reported that hyaluronan and hyaluronic acid increased healing in a cylindric meniscal defect and stimulated collagen remodeling in the peripheral zone.[126,131] Endothelial growth factor (ECGF) was reported to accelerate healing of an allograft to the joint capsule.[99] Hashimoto and colleagues[68] have tested the effect of ECGF on a cylindric defect in the canine meniscus and found that defects that contained both the fibrin sealant and ECGF have the best healing.

The major challenge for growth factor application at this time is delivery of the selected factor into the target tissue. Because of rapid dilution and short half-lives, single doses of growth factors may not provide adequate local concentrations to induce significant biologic effects. Thus, it is evident that a carrier vehicle, such as an absorbable material, will be required to localize the growth factor at the repair site in a biologically relevant concentration. Alternatively, gene therapy techniques may be used to induce local production of the desired protein.

Research has focused on the use of a fibrin clot to induce and support a healing response in the avascular portion of the meniscus. An in vitro study has shown that when meniscal fibrochondrocytes are exposed to growth factors normally found in a blood clot, the cells demonstrate a marked increase in proliferation and matrix synthesis.[142] An in vivo study in animals has demonstrated that when a defect in the avascular portion of the meniscus is filled with a fibrin clot, the defect is able to heal with connective tissue similar to that seen in normal meniscal repair.[15] A fibrin clot is formed by gently stirring whole blood in a glass container. Approximately 50 to 60 mL of whole blood is obtained from the patient and placed in a sterile glass beaker. Then, with the sintered glass barrel from a 20-mL glass syringe, the blood is stirred gently until a fibrin clot is precipitated on the surface of the barrel (Fig. 31-23). This process usually takes between 3 and 5 minutes. The consistency of the clot formed in this manner is similar to that of wet chewing gum and is capable of holding sutures placed through its substance. Although use

Table 31-2 Effects of Various Growth Factors on Meniscal Tissue

Type	In Vitro or In Vivo (Animal)	Cell Source	Result
FGF[6]	In vitro	Rabbit	Stimulates proliferation
Human PL[6]	In vitro	Rabbit	Stimulates proliferation
ECGF[53]	Dog	No	Improves healing in cylindrical defect
ECGF[52]	Dog	No	Increases short-term healing in tears
PDGF-AB[48]	In vitro	Ovine	Affects mitogenic response from outer third of meniscus
TGF-β[47]	In vitro	Ovine	Increases proteoglycan synthesis
Hyaluronic acid[51]	Rabbit	No	Increases rate of healing in a cylindrical defect
TGF-β[46]	In vitro	Human	Increases proteoglycan synthesis
PDGF-AB[49]	In vitro	Bovine	Stimulates cell migration, increased DNA synthesis
HGF[49]	In vitro	Bovine	Stimulates cell migration, increased DNA synthesis
BMP-2[49]	In vitro	Bovine	Some cell migration, increased DNA synthesis
IGF-1[49]	In vitro	Bovine	Some cell migration
IL-1[49]	In vitro	Bovine	Some cell migration
EGF[49]	In vitro	Bovine	Some cell migration
Hyaluronan[50]	Rabbit	No	Stimulate collagen remodeling in peripheral zone

From Sweigart MA, Athanasiou KA: Toward tissue engineering of the knee meniscus. Tissue Eng 7:111–129, 2001.
HGF, Human growth factor.

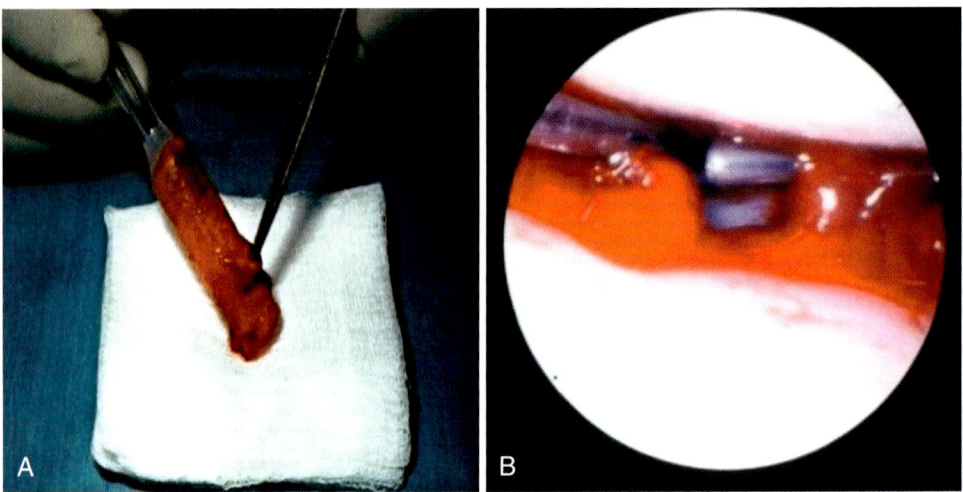

Figure 31-23. A, Fibrin clot precipitated onto the surface of a glass syringe barrel. **B,** Arthroscopic photograph of a fibrin clot being sutured into a meniscal tear. (From McAndrews PT, Arnoczky SP: Meniscal repair enhancement techniques. Clin Sports Med 15:499–510, 1996.)

of the fibrin clot technique in white-white tears has been limited, clinical studies have suggested improved healing rates in red-white meniscal tears in which a fibrin clot was used.[71,72]

The use of PRP is another potential way to provide growth factors to the area of an avascular meniscal lesion, but in greater concentrations than possible in a normal fibrin clot. PRP is defined as a platelet concentration of at least 1,000,000 platelets/μL in 5 mL of plasma.[92] This represents a threefold to fivefold increase in concentration over normal circulating platelet numbers. PRP contains increased concentrations (above normal circulating plasma levels) of several growth factors, including PDGF, TGF-β, EGF, and IGF-I.[115,144,146] Although numerous clinical studies have shown improved healing in bone and soft tissue, the use of PRP in meniscal repair has not been reported.[136]

A corollary to the use of a fibrin clot or PRP is the proposed use of a synthetic fibrin glue. The fibrin adhesive, which is formed by combining various factors in the normal clotting cascade (fibrinogen, thrombin, $CaCl_2$, and factor XIII) with an antifibrinolysate (aprotinin), has been used in other surgical applications to hold biologic tissues in approximation. Although the adhesive property of fibrin glue is superior to that of a natural fibrin clot, the synthetic material lacks the biologically active growth factors normally found in the clot. Thus, even though it may be able to hold wound edges in apposition more securely than a natural fibrin clot can, it has not been shown to play an active role in stimulating the repair process.[24]

Mechanical Load

There is very little information available about the effect of mechanical load and knee range of motion on meniscal healing. One study using a dog model has found that cast immobilization of repaired meniscal lesions in the vascular zone of canine menisci result in a decrease in collagen formation after 10 weeks of immobilization compared with nonimmobilized controls.[42] An experimental study in rabbits has found that immobilization of the normal meniscus results in diminished matrix permeability and degenerative changes in

the deep layers of the meniscus.[103] The adverse effect of such immobilization was associated with a significant reduction in blood flow compared with the nonimmobilized joint.[71] In clinical situations, a period of joint immobilization may be necessary for initial postoperative protection of articular tissues, but normal mobility of the joint should be restored as soon as possible to promote long-term joint homeostasis. Further studies are required to determine the optimal type, magnitude, and duration of loading for meniscal healing.

Future Techniques for Meniscal Healing: Gene Therapy and Tissue-Engineered Meniscus

Research is currently ongoing into methods to enhance meniscus healing and to regenerate meniscus tissue (see Fig. 31-5). Recent studies have demonstrated the ability to transfect meniscal fibrochondrocytes with novel genes using gene therapy techniques, suggesting that bioactive factors could be delivered to the meniscus by transferring growth factor genes to meniscal cells.[46,63,64,73,91] Tissue engineering techniques using absorbable polymer scaffolds seeded with cells and growth factors are also being explored as a means to heal meniscus lesions, as well as potentially to regenerate meniscus tissue.*

Creating a tissue-engineered meniscus requires that specific biologic considerations such as cell type, matrix scaffold, bioreactor design, and environmental conditions be addressed. Meniscal cells, fibroblasts, chondrocytes, and mesenchymal stem cells have been proposed as potential cell sources and have been grown (both in vivo and in vitro) on various scaffolds, including collagen-based scaffolds, chondrocyte-seeded cartilaginous scaffolds, biodegradable polymers, and small intestine submucosa (SIS).† Gastel and associates[60] have

---

*References 36, 37, 60, 88, 106, and 130.
†References 36, 37, 88, 106, 114, and 130.

shown that SIS grafts are capable of supporting the complete healing of meniscal defects in rabbits. Cook and coworkers have found that the use of SIS grafts in dogs with large (>50%), completely avascular meniscal defects resulted in superior clinical function, greater and more representative replacement tissue, and increased cartilage protection when compared with ungrafted controls.[36] Although the mechanism of tissue regeneration using SIS grafts remains unclear, the presence of collagen types I, III, IV, and VI, GAGs, fibroblast growth factor, and TGF-β in SIS may contribute to structural, chemotactic, mitogenic, and stimulatory effects on cells and matrix.

Recent emphasis in meniscal research has been directed toward applications of molecular biology to promote meniscal regeneration. Gene transfer has emerged as a new approach for growth factor delivery.[46] Several investigators have demonstrated the ability to transfer specific genes into meniscal chondrocytes using retroviral and adenoviral vectors.[64,73,91] Goto and colleagues[63] have implanted an adenoviral suspension with a fibrin clot into experimentally created canine and lapine meniscal lesions. They demonstrated successful delivery with gene expression lasting for the 3-week duration of the experiment. In the same study, they observed successful transgene expression 6 weeks after transplantation of retrovirally transduced cells into meniscal defects.

The future ability of gene therapy to treat meniscal injuries depends on precise identification of appropriate growth factors and finding the most effective means for gene delivery. Understanding the appropriate length of time for gene expression and finding a means to control levels of gene expression are important.[64] Future research in gene therapy will also focus on methods to accelerate meniscal allograft healing and enhance bioengineered meniscal tissue.

Acknowledgments. We acknowledge the contributions of Matthew J. Crawford, Julie A. Dodds, and Steven P. Arnoczky from the previous edition of the chapter.

KEY REFERENCES

Allen CR, Wong EK, Livesay GA, et al: Importance of the medial meniscus in the anterior cruciate ligament-deficient knee. J Orthop Res 18:109–115, 2000.

Andersson-Molina H, Karlsson H, Rockborn P: Arthroscopic partial and total meniscectomy: A long-term follow-up study with matched controls. Arthroscopy 18:183–189, 2002.

Arnoczky SP MC: The meniscus: structure, function, repair, and replacement. In Buckwalter JA, Einhorn TA, Simon SR, editors: Orthopaedic basic science, Rosemont, Ill, 2000, American Academy of Orthopaedic Surgeons, pp 531–545.

Chatain F, Adeleine P, Chambat P, et al: A comparative study of medial versus lateral arthroscopic partial meniscectomy on stable knees: 10-year minimum follow-up. Arthroscopy 19:842–849, 2003.

Cole BJ, Carter TR, Rodeo SA: Allograft meniscal transplantation. Background, techniques, and results. J Bone Joint Surg Am 84:1236–1250, 2002.

Freedman KB, Nho SJ, Cole BJ: Marrow stimulating technique to augment meniscus repair. Arthroscopy 19:794–798, 2003.

Gulotta L, Rodeo SA: Basic science aspects of ACL: graft healing, vascularity, microscopic anatomy. In Bach BR, Jr, editor: ACL surgery: How to get it right the first time and what to do if it fails, Thorofare, NJ, 2010, Slack.

McCarty EC, Marx RG, DeHaven KE: Meniscus repair: considerations in treatment and update of clinical results. Clin Orthop Relat Res 402:122–134, 2002.

Murray MM, Martin SD, Martin TL, et al: Histological changes in the human anterior cruciate ligament after rupture. J Bone Joint Surg Am 82:1387–1397, 2000.

Papageorgiou CD, Gil JE, Kanamori A, et al: The biomechanical interdependence between the anterior cruciate ligament replacement graft and the medial meniscus. Am J Sports Med 29:226–231, 2001.

Peretti GM, Caruso EM, Randolph MA, et al: Meniscal repair using engineered tissue. J Orthop Res 19:278–285, 2001.

Scheller G, Sobau C, Bulow JU: Arthroscopic partial lateral meniscectomy in an otherwise normal knee: clinical, functional, and radiographic results of a long-term follow-up study. Arthroscopy 17:946–952, 2001.

Shelbourne KD, Heinrich J: The long-term evaluation of lateral meniscus tears left in situ at the time of anterior cruciate ligament reconstruction. Arthroscopy 20:346–351, 2004.

Shelbourne KD, Rask BP: The sequelae of salvaged nondegenerative peripheral vertical medial meniscus tears with anterior cruciate ligament reconstruction. Arthroscopy 17:270–274, 2001.

Woo SL, Vogrin TM, Abramowitch SD: Healing and repair of ligament injuries in the knee. J Am Acad Orthop Surg 8:364–372, 2000.

Full references for this chapter can be found on www.expertconsult.com.

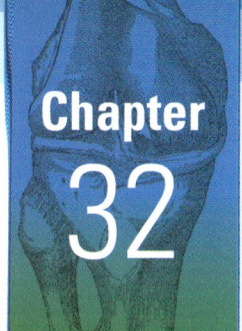

Arthroscopic Meniscal Resection

Yair D. Kissin, W. Norman Scott, and Fred D. Cushner

The medial and lateral menisci are two semilunar fibrocartilaginous structures that were once thought of as nonessential. Now it is known that they provide several important functions in the knee, including lubrication, joint stability, nutrition, shock absorption, and weight distribution. Damage to the menisci is common, resulting in disruption of the equilibrium of the knee, and can lead to early degenerative changes. Once nonoperative treatment modalities fail, operative intervention generally involves resection, repair, or transplantation. The purpose of this chapter is to review the indications, technique, and implications of arthroscopic meniscal resection.

The menisci act to cushion the loads that cross the knee joint by mediating these forces through both longitudinal and radial fibers within its core structure. These fibers distribute hoop stresses as well as shear stresses across the entire meniscus. Maintenance of as much meniscal tissue as possible is therefore essential in decreasing overall contact stresses across the knee joint. However, the menisci are mostly avascular structures, as illustrated in landmark work done by Arnoczky and Warren, which has helped our understanding of the limited healing potential of torn meniscus.[1]

The perimeniscal capillary plexus arises from the medial and lateral superior and inferior geniculate arteries and supplies approximately the peripheral third of the menisci. The lateral meniscus has even less perfusion than the medial meniscus, given the lack of capsular attachment at the popliteal hiatus. The zones of the menisci are commonly described in relation to this limited blood supply as red-red in the well-perfused periphery, red-white in the middle, and white-white in the avascular center. Generally speaking, if a tear is more than 5 mm from the meniscosynovial junction, it is considered avascular.[1] This imperfect matchup of poor perfusion to an essential structure within our knee leaves scarce amount of tissue that is amenable to healing and repair. It is for this reason that most meniscal tears that are approached surgically undergo resection rather than repair (Fig. 32-1).

According to the American Board of Orthopaedic Surgeons, arthroscopic meniscal resection, code 29881, heads the list of the Current Procedural Terminology (CPT) codes in the candidate case submissions for Part II of the orthopedic certification examination. Medial meniscal tears, code 836.0, and lateral meniscal tears, code 836.1, are in the top three ICD-9 codes submitted for the examination as well.[8]

It is important to distinguish arthroscopy for meniscal tears from arthroscopic débridement for degenerative joint disease, which has received much negative press recently as providing no benefit when compared with nonoperative treatment.[9] Meniscal tears can be described by zone, as noted, or by type of tear. The first classification deals with healing potential, whereas the more commonly used categorization is by type, which describes the orientation of the tear pattern. Tears can be vertical, both longitudinal or radial, as well as horizontal, or they can be complex. Displaceable tears consist of parrot beak, flap, horizontal cleavage, and bucket handle types.[11]

In addition to vascularity and type, chronicity of the tear and associated injuries also play an important role in classifying meniscal tears. Acute tears, less than 2 to 3 weeks old, are more amenable to repair, whereas more chronic tears become ragged and frayed, making the tissue less likely to be repaired successfully. Associated injuries, such as anterior cruciate ligament (ACL) tears, also affect meniscal tears. Meniscal tears are seen in over 50% of knees with associated ACL tears. It has been shown that ACL-deficient knees fare worse with partial meniscectomy than stable knees.[2] Some believe that a short (<1-cm) stable tear may be left untreated at the time of ACL reconstruction with no meniscal complications noted in follow-up.[12] The degree of degenerative change in the compartment with the diagnosed meniscal tear must also be assessed, because the more advanced the arthritis, the less chance a patient will likely benefit from arthroscopic meniscal resection.

Several patient-related factors to consider in the categorization of meniscal tears are age, activity level, ability to comply with physical therapy, and body mass index. Young athletes have a higher success rate than older, more sedentary patients as far as meniscal repairs are concerned. Partial meniscectomy requires less cooperation with physical therapy from the patient than meniscal repair, which may require an extended period of limited weight bearing and range of motion. An inability to participate in a more stringent rehabilitation protocol may make resection a better choice than repair. Finally, significant associations have been shown between an increase in a patient's body mass index (BMI) and the number of meniscal surgeries in both genders, including obese and overweight adults, especially in those with a BMI higher than 40.[6]

CLINICAL ASSESSMENT

Meniscal tears are common. Many studies have found that even in asymptomatic knees, the rate of meniscal tears detected on magnetic resonance imaging (MRI) is very high. One recent study has shown that in patients with radiographic signs of osteoarthritis, more than 60% of patients were found to have meniscal tears on MRI scans, regardless of the presence or lack of symptoms. In knees without radiographic evidence of osteoarthritis, meniscus tears were seen in 23% of asymptomatic knees.[3,7,14]

MRI is a useful tool for assessing meniscal tears, but should be used to confirm the clinical suspicion of a tear, rather than to screen for tears (Fig. 32-2). Another important application is to use the images, especially in multiple planes, to help anticipate arthroscopic findings (Fig. 32-3).

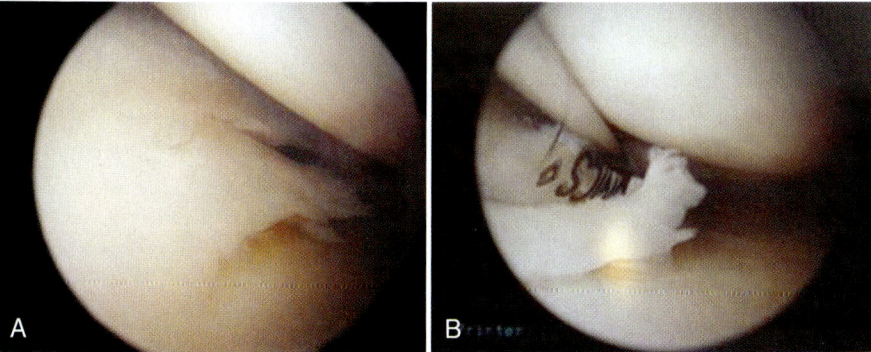

Figure 32-1. **A,** Flap tear of the medial meniscus in the avascular zone. **B,** Resection of the tear with a mechanical shaver.

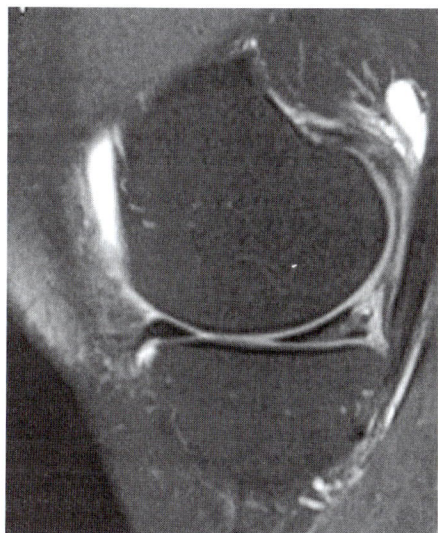

Figure 32-2. Sagittal MRI image of a posterior horn medial meniscus tear.

MRI findings alone should never be used to dictate treatment of patients with meniscal tears. Many patients present to the orthopedic surgeon with positive MRI scans, never having undergone radiographs of the knee or even an appropriate physical examination. Occasionally, a weight-bearing radiograph is sufficient to diagnose and determine a treatment plan for a patient and obviates the need for MRI, because it would add no further information that would change management. Radiographic findings always need to be properly correlated to the patient's complaints and the surgeon's physical examination findings. An acute injury with subsequent mechanical symptoms rather than a vague spontaneous onset of symptoms, along with findings of joint line tenderness and rotatory pain, with provocative tests such as the McMurray and Apley grind tests, are likely to correlate with symptomatic meniscal tears.[11]

Once a symptomatic meniscal tear has been diagnosed, proper guidance by the surgeon is essential to reach an appropriate treatment decision. Not all meniscal tears require surgical intervention. Many tears become asymptomatic with a course of activity modification, physical therapy, and

nonimpact strengthening. Those that fail nonoperative measures are indicated for surgery, which usually involves arthroscopic excision versus repair, and occasionally transplantation. Although this chapter will deal mainly with excision, the final choice between repair and resection is made at the time of surgery, on careful assessment of the tear.

Preoperative counseling is crucial for patients to be made aware of the associated risks, because surgery should never be portrayed as a benign procedure. The surgeon must endeavor to gauge a patient's expectations of the surgery, and align those expectations with the anticipated outcome of the procedure. The postoperative course should be discussed in great detail, and the unlikely possibility that symptoms may not resolve or even worsen should also be mentioned. Pain management should be discussed as well, because many patients may be led to believe that arthroscopy is a painless procedure, when occasionally, this is not the case.

Once the decision has been made to proceed with arthroscopic surgery, the procedure should not be postponed for long to avoid articular cartilage damage resulting from unstable meniscal flaps (Fig. 32-4). Rarely, a delay of several weeks is necessary to allow for a decrease in swelling and to regain a functional range of motion of the knee.

TECHNIQUE

The operative setup is that of standard arthroscopy and can be done on an outpatient basis under general or regional, and in certain circumstances, local anaesthesia. A pneumatic tourniquet can be used but is not mandatory, and flow can be obtained with a pump or gravity. The patient is positioned supine on the operating room table with a lateral post to aid in obtaining valgus stress during the procedure or with the leg placed in a circumferential leg holder. An experienced assistant can be helpful in positioning the limb in appropriate degrees of flexion and extension and varus or valgus to aid in the surgeon's visualization, but iatrogenic injury to the collateral ligaments can occur with overly aggressive force and must be avoided.

Most meniscal work can be done using a standard 30-degree arthroscope, but some surgeons also use a 70-degree arthroscope for visualization of the posterior corners of the knee. A standardized, systematic evaluation of the knee should be performed at each procedure to avoid missing pathology that may need to be addressed, as well as to identify normal intact structures in a reproducible fashion (Fig. 32-5). Portal

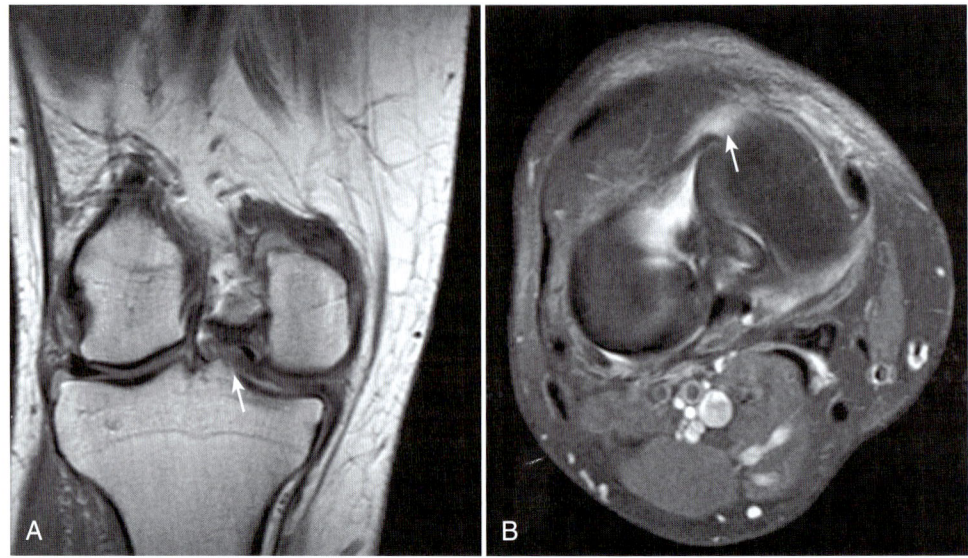

Figure 32-3. **A,** Coronal MRI image of a bucket handle medial meniscus tear with meniscal fragment seen in the intercondylar notch *(arrow).* **B,** Axial MRI image of a flipped bucket handle medial meniscus tear *(arrow).*

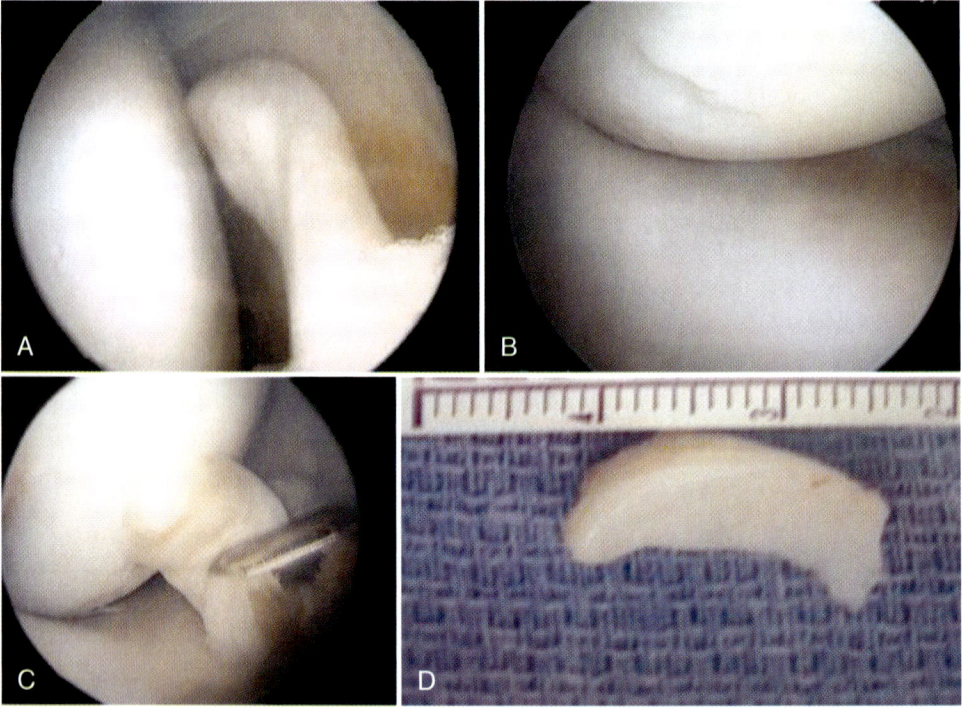

Figure 32-4. Unstable chronic lateral meniscus tear with fragment causing articular indentation of lateral femoral condyle. **A,** Unstable, flipped meniscal fragment. **B,** Aticular indentation from entrapment. **C,** Removal of the meniscal fragment. **D,** Meniscal tear after removal.

placement is essential; although most meniscal work is done through the anteromedial portal and is visualized through the anterolateral portal, anterior portions of the medial meniscus may be approached by switching portals.

By not violating the vastus medialis obliquus, the two-portal technique for standard arthroscopy appears to afford an earlier return of quadriceps strength and function and faster return to work and activities compared with the three-portal technique.[13] The menisci should be probed on the superior and inferior surfaces to assess the presence and extent of damage, and displaceable tears can be brought into the field of view to plan resection (Fig. 32-6). It is also critical to run the articular rim beneath the menisci with the probe, because this may reveal hidden flaps of meniscus that would not otherwise be seen (Fig. 32-7). Visualization of the posterior medial corner of the knee, which lies between the posterior collateral ligament (PCL) and medial femoral condyle, commonly referred to as the Gillquist view (Fig. 32-8), is essential to assess the meniscocapsular attachment of the posterior horn or the medial meniscus. This is also where a flipped segment of meniscus can be missed and mistakenly left untreated if not detected (Fig. 32-9).

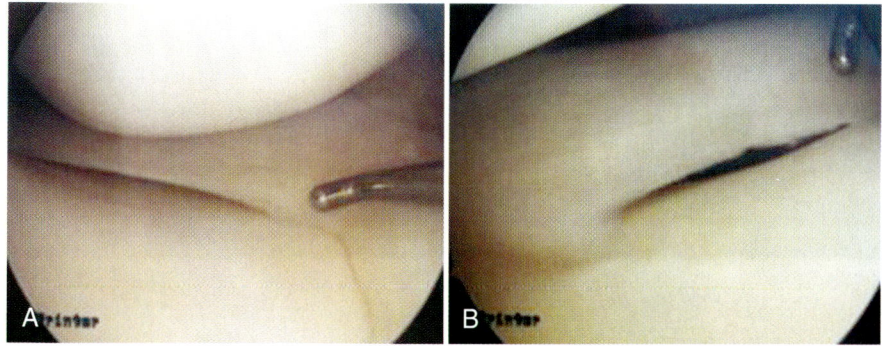

Figure 32-5. **A**, Normal medial meniscus. **B**, Normal lateral meniscus.

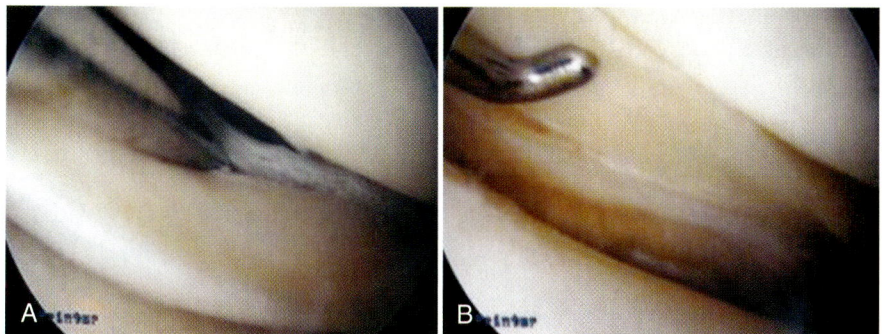

Figure 32-6. The arthroscopic probe demonstrates a tear in the lateral meniscus. Superior surface **(A)** and inferior surface **(B)** of the meniscus.

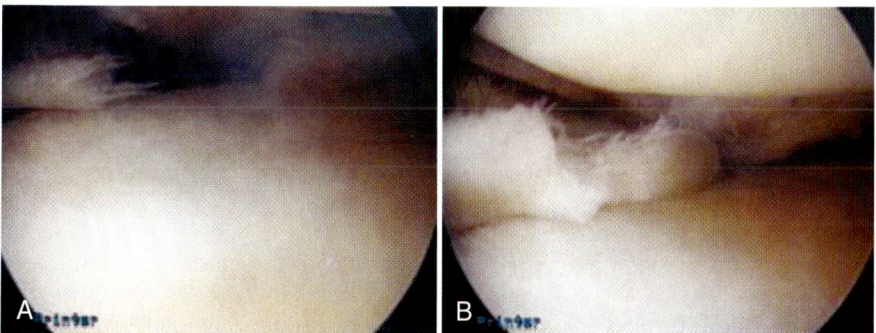

Figure 32-7. **A**, A hidden flap tear of the medial meniscus trapped around the corner of the medial tibial plateau. **B**, The unstable flap of the meniscus is reduced into the joint by running the articular rim with the arthroscopic probe.

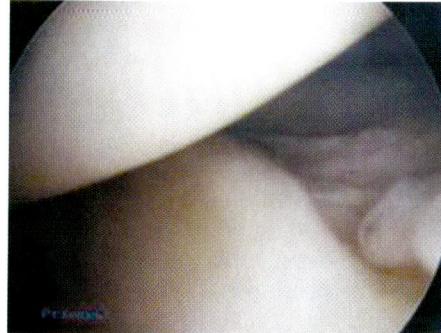

Figure 32-8. Visualization of the posterior medial corner of the knee, which lies between the PCL and medial femoral condyle. This is commonly referred to as the Gillquist view.

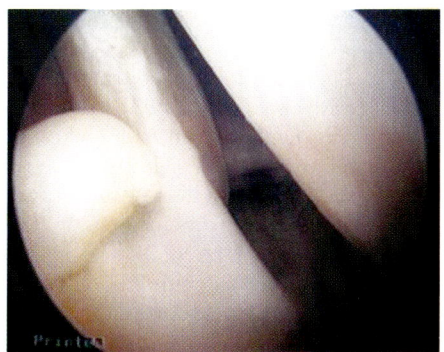

Figure 32-9. Gillquist view with flipped posterior horn medial meniscal fragment.

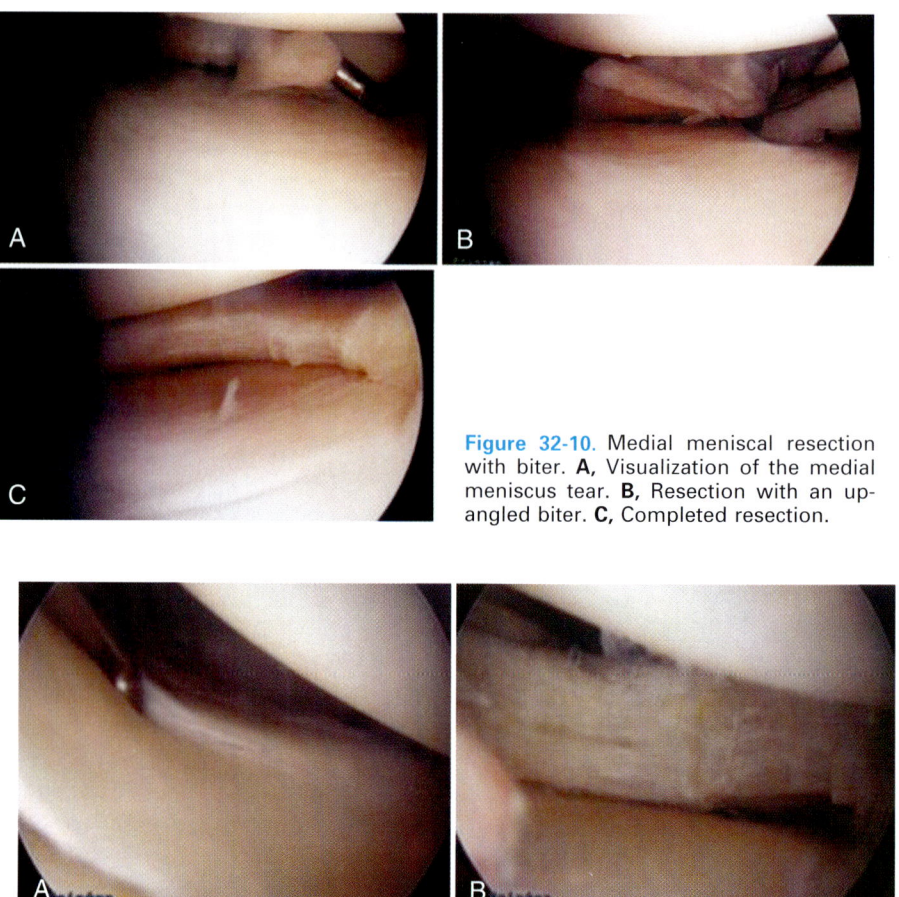

Figure 32-10. Medial meniscal resection with biter. **A**, Visualization of the medial meniscus tear. **B**, Resection with an up-angled biter. **C**, Completed resection.

Figure 32-11. **A**, Complete vertical tear of the lateral meniscus in the avascular region of the popliteal hiatus. **B**, Post-resection of the tear.

Most medial meniscal resection is carried out with an upbiter and lateral meniscal resection with a straight biter (Fig. 32-10). Curved and 90-degree biters may also be useful for contouring certain tears. The mechanical shaver is then used to smooth the resected edges of the tear and rid the knee of debris.

Certain tears that may be difficult to access are those involving the posterior horns of both menisci, especially in patients with tight collateral ligaments and those with an associated ACL or bucket handle tear (Fig. 32-11). The biter may need to be inverted when resecting the posterior horn of the lateral meniscus, because the instrument may commonly be blocked by the tibial spines. If performing a simultaneous ACL reconstruction, performing a notchplasty prior to meniscectomy may allow easier access to this region of the lateral meniscus. The posterior horn of the medial meniscus may be accessed best by placing the knee in slight flexion and external rotation. However, with an ACL-deficient knee, the knee may shift and thereby close down the posteromedial corner. A skilled assistant's help may be necessary to provide a posterior drawer force on the knee to obtain access in this situation.

Bucket handle tears are commonly encountered and require careful assessment. Tears that can be reduced must be assessed for stability and reparability. If the reduced tear subluxes each time the knee is brought through a range of motion, it will likely fail repair. Similarly, if the tear is chronic,

it is likely better off being resected. One efficient method of resecting a bucket handle tear begins by using an arthroscopic scissor to detach the posterior limb of the tear; the low profile of the scissor allows easy access to a tight area without damaging surrounding articular cartilage. The next step involves near-complete detachment of the anterior limb of the tear using a scissor or biter. The final step is grasping the torn segment of meniscus and completing the detachment by applying a twisting motion to pull the remnant out of the knee in its entirety. The portal may need to be enlarged, depending on the size of the resected segment. Alternatively, a spinal needle can be introduced into the knee to stabilize the torn segment in the intercondylar notch as the limbs are detached. An arthroscopic shaver is then used to smooth down the areas where the tear was attached (Fig. 32-12).

The overall principle of meniscal resection is to remove only the torn meniscal tissue while maintaining as much intact meniscus as possible, especially peripherally, and avoiding iatrogenic injury to the surrounding intact meniscus and articular cartilage (Fig. 32-13). Repeated passes of hand and motorized instruments can be unforgiving to the articular cartilage, and small-diameter and curved instruments may be useful for avoiding such injury. Maintenance of a stable rim of intact meniscus, free of edges from where a new tear could theoretically propagate, is the final objective of meniscal resection (Fig. 32-14). Incomplete tears need to be identified and can be left unresected if they are truly incomplete.

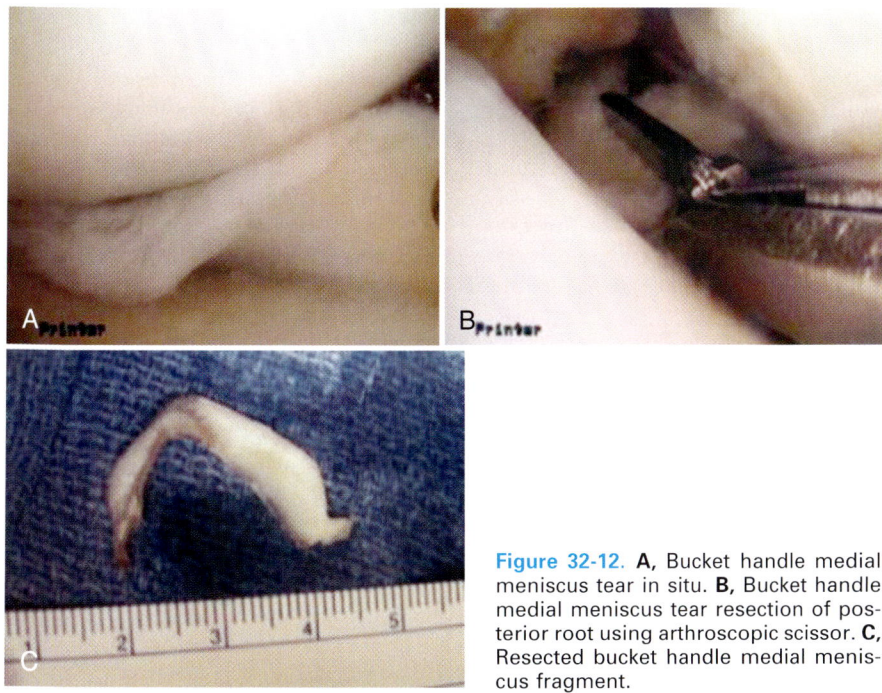

Figure 32-12. A, Bucket handle medial meniscus tear in situ. **B,** Bucket handle medial meniscus tear resection of posterior root using arthroscopic scissor. **C,** Resected bucket handle medial meniscus fragment.

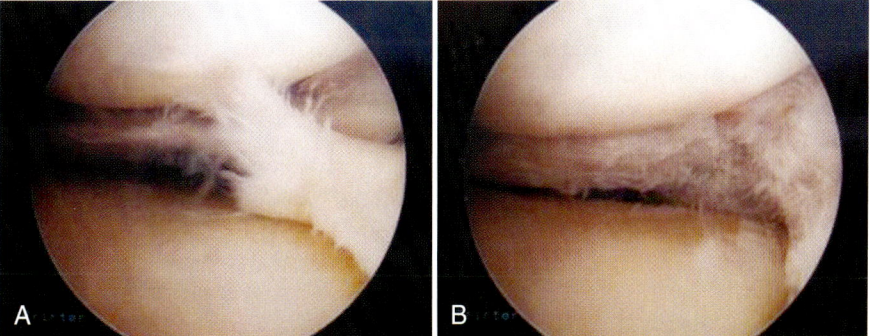

Figure 32-13. A, Medial meniscus complex degenerative tear. **B,** After resecting the torn meniscus to achieve a stable rim.

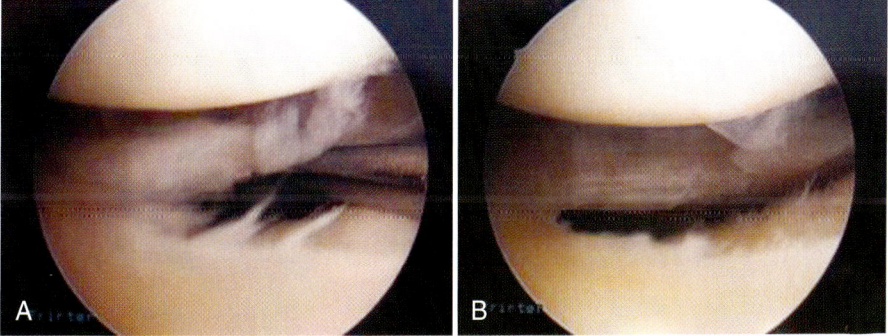

Figure 32-14. A, Lateral meniscus tear with central or free-edge fraying. **B,** After resection of the torn portion of the meniscus.

As patients become more sophisticated and informed of their medical conditions, recording clear pictures or videotaping the procedure becomes more important to share the experience with the patient in the postoperative period. Explanations of the arthroscopic findings in terms of meniscal pathology versus the extent of articular cartilage damage can help correlate with a patient's expectations for recovery.

POSTOPERATIVE COURSE AND COMPLICATIONS

Physical therapy is largely unnecessary following arthroscopic meniscectomy, because a home exercise program emphasizing range of motion and nonimpact strengthening is usually sufficient to regain function. Patients can expect to return to sedentary work in several days to 1 week, and full recovery after 3 to 6 months. There are essentially no restrictions following meniscal resection other than those mediated by pain and swelling, which can differ tremendously among patients. Return to sports occurs once range of motion, strength, and perceived confidence in the knee have returned to normal.

Complications such as deep vein thrombosis, infection, compartment syndrome, and bleeding are extremely rare, but vigilance must be used to avoid missing a potential problem.[11]

IMPLICATIONS AND OUTCOMES OF MENISCAL RESECTION

Given that the meniscus is as a crucial load-bearing structure, optimizing contact area and minimizing contact stress, the procedure of meniscal resection alters these factors and is not without consequence. Loss of meniscal fibers resisting hoop stresses as a result of partial meniscectomy can be equivalent to total meniscectomy as far as load-bearing forces are concerned. The peripheral portion of the medial meniscus has been shown to provide a greater contribution to increasing contact areas and decreasing mean contact stresses than does the central portion. In a recent study of meniscal resection, peak contact stresses increased proportionally to the amount of meniscus removed cadaveric.[10] Posterior meniscal resection, even when segmental rather than total, appeared to result in considerable negative effects on the articular surface.[10]

Clinically, these results have been correlated with faster progression of osteoarthritis, especially following posterior meniscal resection. In a recent meta-analysis, age, gender, and medial versus lateral meniscectomy did not seem to affect outcome.[4] The amount of meniscal tissue removed and degrees of osteoarthritis at the time of meniscectomy were directly related to outcome. Patients with resected bucket handle tears returned to work and sports significantly faster than those with flap tears, and repeat arthroscopy was significantly more common with flap tears, possibly reflecting the difficulty in removing the torn meniscal tissue completely.

In a Danish study,[5] 44% of patients were found to have function-related pain following arthroscopic meniscal resection. Furthermore, the combination of varus alignment and medial meniscectomy or valgus alignment and lateral meniscectomy resulted in significantly greater osteoarthritis than resection in knees with normal alignment.

CONCLUSION

Treatment for meniscal tears is still controversial. Various treatment options are difficult to randomize in an optimal way for a definitive level I study, and our ability to measure outcomes well is not ideal when comparing the different treatments. What we sometimes promote as a minor procedure may have serious implications, such as significant disruption of homeostasis of the knee, and can lead to more changes than previously thought. This rather recent recognition of the importance of maintaining an intact meniscus, especially peripherally, has led to more conservative resection compared with open meniscectomies of the past, but better understanding has not fully explained the problems associated with the procedure. To optimize outcome, proper patient selection and communication, along with skilled planning and execution of the surgical procedure, play an important role.

KEY REFERENCES

Arnoczky SP, Warren RF: Microvasculature of the human meniscus. Am J Sports Med 10:90–95, 1982.

Burks RT, Metcalf MH, Metcalf RW: Fifteen-year follow-up of arthroscopic partial meniscectomy. Arthroscopy 13:673–679, 1997.

Englund M, Guermazi A, Gale D, et al: Incidental meniscal findings on knee MRI in middle-aged and elderly persons. N Engl J Med 359:1108–1115, 2008.

Fabricant PD, Jokl P: Surgical outcomes after arthroscopic partial meniscectomy. J Am Acad Orthop Surg 15:647–653, 2007.

Fauno P, Nielson AB: Consequences of arthroscopic meniscal resection. Ugeskr Laeger 155:3388–3390, 1993.

Ford GM, Hegmann KB, White GL, Jr, Holmes ET: Associations of body mass index with meniscal tears. Am J Prev Med 28:364–368, 2005.

Fritz RC: MR imaging of meniscal and cruciate ligament injuries. Magn Reson Imaging Clin N Am 11:283–293, 2003.

Garrett WE, Jr, Swiontkowski MF, Weinstein JN, et al: American Board of Orthopaedic Surgery Practice of the Orthopaedic Surgeon: Part-II, certification examination case mix. J Bone Joint Surg Am 88:660–667, 2006.

Kirkley A, Birmingham TB, et al: A randomized trial of arthroscopic surgery for osteoarthritis of the knee. N Engl J Med 359:1097–1107, 2008.

Lee SJ, Aadalen KJ, Malaviya P, et al: Tibiofemoral contact mechanics after serial meniscectomies in the human knee. Am J Sports Med 34:1334–1344, 2006.

Scott WN, editor: Insall & Scott surgery of the knee, ed 4, New York, 2006, Churchill Livingstone.

Shelbourne KD, Heinrich J: The long-term evaluation of lateral meniscus tears left in situ at the time of anterior cruciate ligament reconstruction. Arthroscopy 20:346–351, 2004.

Stetson WB, Templin K: Two- versus three-portal technique for routine knee arthroscopy. Am J Sports Med J 30:108–1111, 2002.

Zanetti M, Pfirrmann CW, Schmid MR, et al: Patients with suspected meniscal tears: Prevalence of abnormalities seen on MRI of 100 symptomatic and 100 contralateral asymptomatic knees. AJR Am J Roentgenol 181:635–641, 2003.

Full references for this chapter can be found on www.expertconsult.com.

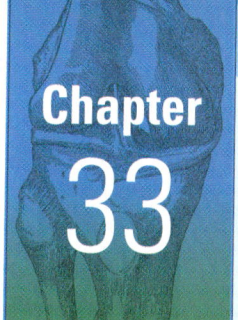

Chapter 33

Arthroscopy-Assisted Inside-Out and Outside-In Meniscus Repair

Robert A. Magnussen, Richard C. Mather, Dean C. Taylor, and Claude T. Moorman, III

Meniscal tears are an extremely common cause of knee disability. Symptoms can range from persistent low-grade pain to a locked knee. Patients in the former group with mild symptoms may be treated with a regimen of rest, anti-inflammatory medications, and various other modalities, but surgical intervention is common. We are unaware of any published prospective data describing the percentage of patients with magnetic resonance imaging (MRI)—confirmed meniscus tears that eventually require surgical intervention.[25]

Surgical treatment options for meniscal tears include excision, repair, and replacement. Partial meniscectomy has been associated with increased risk of osteoarthritis at 10- to 20-year follow-up compared with normal controls in some series.[16,21] However, lower rates of osteoarthritis have been noted in patients in whom smaller portions of meniscus were removed.[9,20] It is thus desirable to pursue treatment options that preserve or restore functional meniscal tissue. Although it has not been shown that meniscal repair results in the restoration of functional meniscal tissue, some long-term studies have shown less joint space narrowing following meniscal repair than following partial meniscectomy.[32] Meniscal repair should be attempted when possible.

INDICATIONS

Indications for meniscal repair are constantly evolving. Treatment decisions should take into account tear location and orientation, ligamentous stability, and articular cartilage status. Because only the peripheral 10% to 30% of the meniscus is vascularized, tears in this region have significantly higher healing rates than more central tears.[2] In retrospective studies using second-look arthroscopy, Buseck and Noyes[11] (98% peripheral and 79% central) and Scott and associates[31] (80% peripheral and 73% central) have noted significant differences in healing rates based on tear location. Similarly, Tenuta and coworkers[39] noted that all repaired menisci with a peripheral rim greater than 4 mm failed to heal completely in their series.

Tear orientation is also important, because current reconstruction techniques generally only allow for reconstructions of tears with a significant component in the vertical plane parallel to the circumferential meniscal fibers, such as vertical longitudinal tears, bucket handle tears, and certain large flap tears. Radial tears that disrupt circumferential fibers and complex degenerative tears are more difficult to repair and generally heal less reliably.[19]

Knee stability and concurrent procedures also significantly influence outcomes. Tenuta and Arciero,[39] Cannon and Vittori,[13] and Barber and Click[4] have all demonstrated a better prognosis for repairs performed in conjunction with anterior collateral ligament (ACL) reconstruction. They reported healing rates between 90% and 92% for repairs

concomitant with ACL reconstruction and healing rates between 57% and 67% for isolated meniscus repair in stable knees. Similarly, repairs in ACL-deficient knees have been characterized as faring poorly. Steenbrugge and associates[38] and Morgan and coworkers[27] have found 96% to 100% healing in those with intact or reconstructed ACLs but only 76% to 77% healing in those with ACL deficiency. Open meniscal repairs have demonstrated similar effects of knee stability on healing.[14]

Finally, patient factors play a large role in determining whether meniscal repair should be performed, because outcomes are generally poorer in older patients and those with articular cartilage degeneration. One must also consider the significantly increased healing time required after meniscal repair when compared with partial meniscectomy and the willingness and ability of the patient to comply with required postoperative restrictions.

TECHNIQUES FOR MENISCAL REPAIR

A number of techniques are available for meniscal repair. All generally include preparation of the tear with synovial abrasion, which induces peripheral bleeding in an attempt to promote migration of undifferentiated mesenchymal cells, or meniscal trephination, which attempts to create vascular channels through the induction of holes in the avascular portions of the meniscus. Available arthroscopic repair options include outside-in, inside-out, and all-inside techniques. This chapter will address outside-in and inside-out techniques. All-inside techniques are discussed elsewhere (see Chapter 34).

Inside-Out Technique

Inside-out techniques remain the standard for meniscal repair yielding reproducible, solid fixation of tears in the posterior and middle thirds of the meniscus.[12,34,40] The procedure begins with arthroscopic inspection of the joint, identification of meniscal tears, and determination of whether repair is appropriate. If an appropriate tear is identified, an accessory incision is made depending on the location of the tear.

Medial Meniscal Tear

An accessory posteromedial incision is used for repair of medial meniscus tears. A longitudinal incision just posterior to the medial collateral ligament is created and centered, with two thirds of its length below the joint line (Fig. 33-1). The pes anserine fascia is identified and split, retracting the medial hamstring tendons posteriorly (Fig. 33-2). This allows visualization of the medial head of the gastrocnemius muscle and protects the vulnerable saphenous nerve posteriorly (Fig. 33-3). The medial head of the gastrocnemius is dissected free

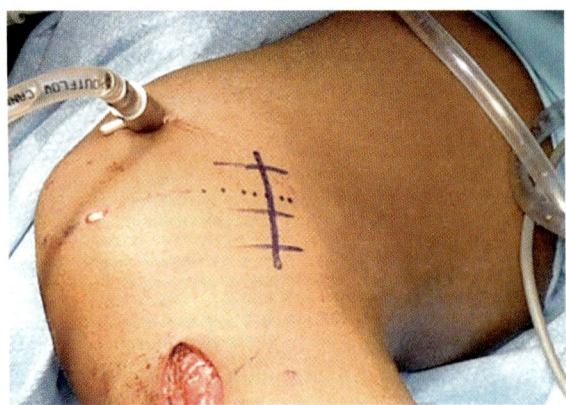

Figure 33-1. The posteromedial accessory incision for meniscal repair has been marked, posterior to the superficial medial collateral ligament extending one third above and two thirds below the joint line (dashed line).

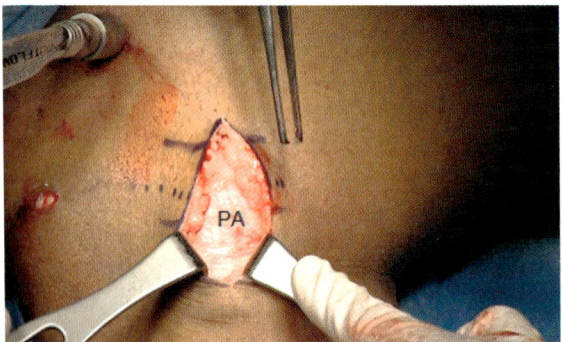

Figure 33-2. The incision has been taken through skin and subcutaneous fat to the pes anserine fascia (PA).

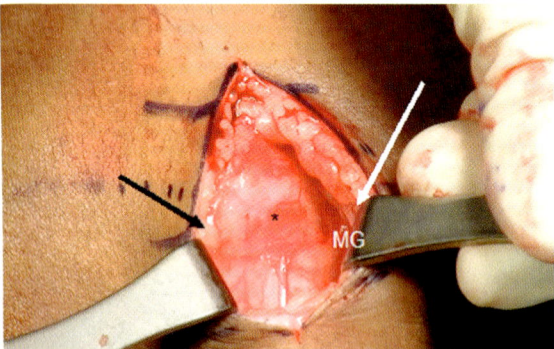

Figure 33-3. The pes fascia has been incised longitudinally and the anterior portion (black arrow) has been retracted forward. The posterior portion along with the medial hamstring tendons (white arrow) have been retracted posteriorly. The medial head of the gastrocnemius (MG) is also being retracted posteriorly, revealing the underlying posteromedial joint capsule (*).

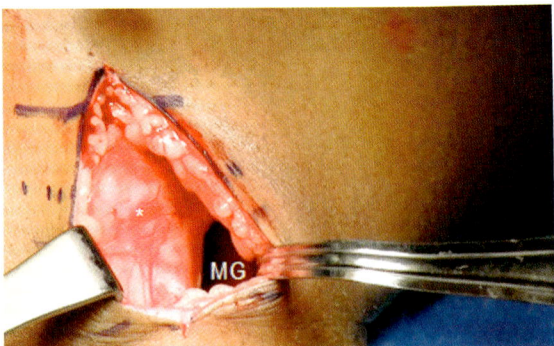

Figure 33-4. The gastronemius muscle (MG) has been retracted posteriorly behind the spoon, isolating the joint capsule (*).

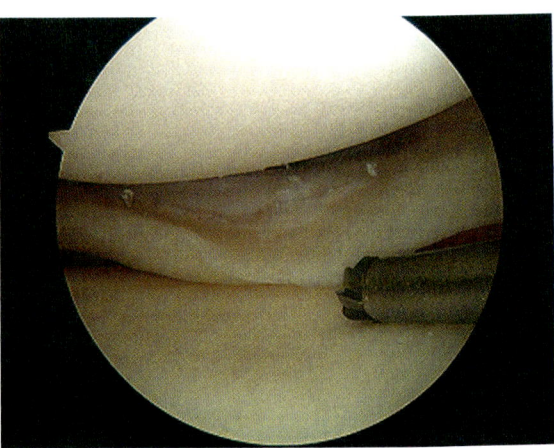

Figure 33-5. An arthroscopic rasp to be used to roughen the edges of the tear prior to repair to facilitate healing.

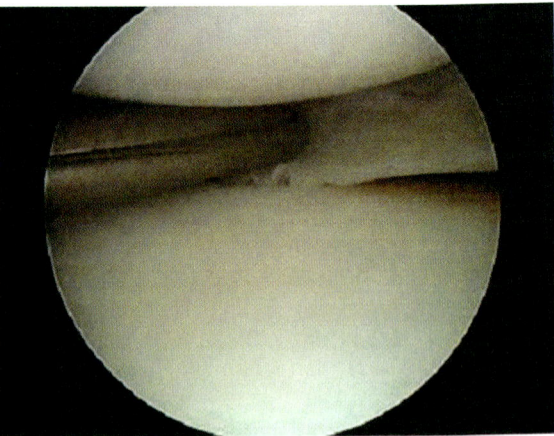

Figure 33-6. A long flexible needle is directed through a cannula, through the meniscus tear and out through the posteromedial capsule.

from the posteromedial joint capsule and retracted posteriorly with a spoon or popliteal retractor (Fig. 33-4).

The tear is visualized through the arthroscope and an arthroscopic rasp is used to roughen the edges of the tear (Fig. 33-5). With the arthroscope in the anterolateral portal, a cannula is passed into the anteromedial portal and directed toward the tear for needle passage. Alternatively, the arthroscope can be placed in the anteromedial portal and the anterolateral portal can be used for needle passage. Cannuli

of different curvatures are available to facilitate access to any portion of the posterior and middle thirds of the meniscus. A long flexible needle with attached nonabsorbable suture is passed through the cannula, across the meniscus tear, and out through the posteromedial capsule (Fig. 33-6). An assistant ensures capture of the needle by the spoon and guides the needle out of the accessory incision. The procedure is repeated with a second needle attached to the other end of the suture, completing a vertical mattress suture (Fig. 33-7). If more than one suture is required, they are generally placed in an alternating manner on the femoral and tibial surfaces of the meniscus to reduce the meniscus appropriately. After passing all sutures, they are tied in a posterior to anterior direction (Fig. 33-8). It is important to tie the sutures with the knee near full extension because tying them in 90 degrees of flexion

could tether the posteromedial capsule and limit knee extension.[6]

Lateral Meniscal Tears

An accessory longitudinal incision is made on the posterolateral knee just posterior to the fibular collateral ligament centered over the joint line (Fig. 33-9). Flexion of the knee helps displace the neurovascular structures further posteriorly to reduce the risk of injury. The interval between the iliotibial band and biceps femoris tendon is developed (Fig. 33-10) until the lateral border of the lateral head of the gastrocnemius is visualized (Fig. 33-11). The lateral gastrocnemius is dissected off the posterolateral capsule and a spoon or popliteal retractor is placed anterior to the tendon, effectively protecting the neurovascular structures located posteriorly and medially (Fig. 33-12).

With the arthroscope in the anterolateral portal, zone-specific cannuli can then be used as described to place vertical mattress sutures in the torn lateral meniscus. Repair of tears in certain locations may be facilitated by switching the camera to the anteromedial portal and while working through the anterolateral portal. After passing all sutures, they are again tied in a posterior to anterior direction.[6]

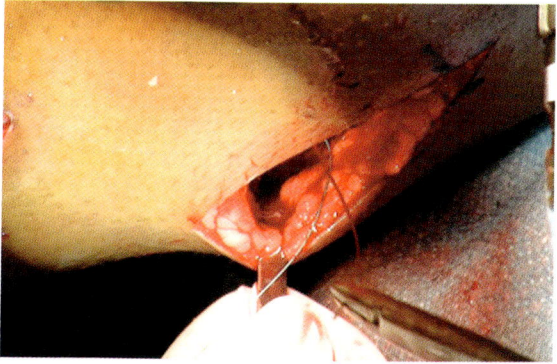

Figure 33-7. A second needle is passed through the meniscus and pulled out of the posteromedial incision in the same manner. The suture connecting the two needles forms a vertical mattress suture and reduces the meniscus tear.

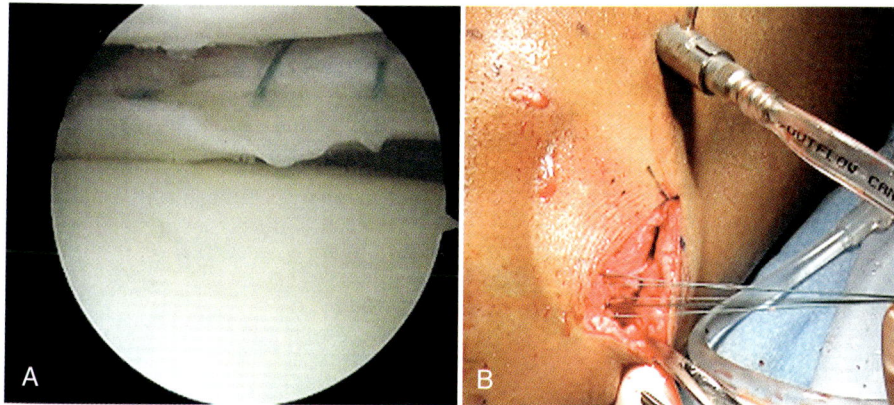

Figure 33-8. A, Additional sutures are placed in the same manner, reducing the tear. **B,** After all are placed, they are tied sequentially from posterior to anterior, with the knee in approximately 20 degrees of flexion.

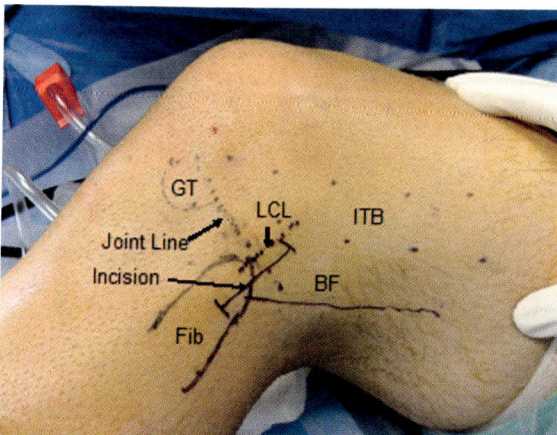

Figure 33-9. The posterolateral accessory incision has been marked, posterior to the lateral collateral ligament *(LCL)* and spanning the joint line. Gerdy's tubercle *(GT)*, the iliotibial band *(ITB)*, and biceps femoris *(BF)* have been labeled.

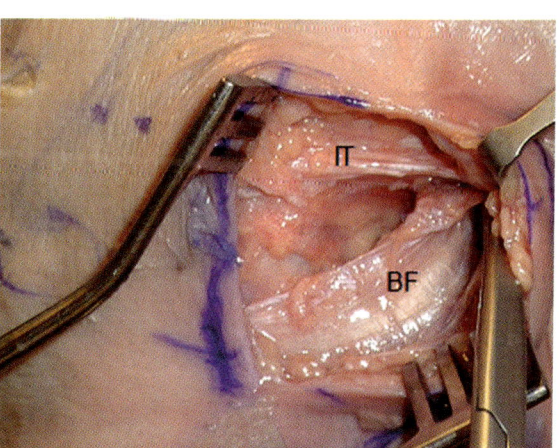

Figure 33-10. The incision has been taken down through skin and subcutaneous tissue. The interval between the iliotibial band *(IT)* anteriorly and the biceps femoris *(BF)* posteriorly has been separated. The common peroneal nerve lies posterior to the biceps femoris.

Outside-In Technique

Outside-in techniques allow repair of tears of the anterior and middle thirds of the meniscus. After arthroscopic identification and preparation of the tear, the arthroscope is used to transilluminate the skin and localize the tear (Fig. 33-13). A spinal needle is introduced through the skin and across the meniscus tear (Fig. 33-14). A wire suture shuttle is then advanced through the needle and into the joint, where it is retrieved out of an anterior portal (Fig. 33-15). The suture to be used in the repair is passed through the loop in the wire and pulled out through the meniscus (Fig. 33-16). A second

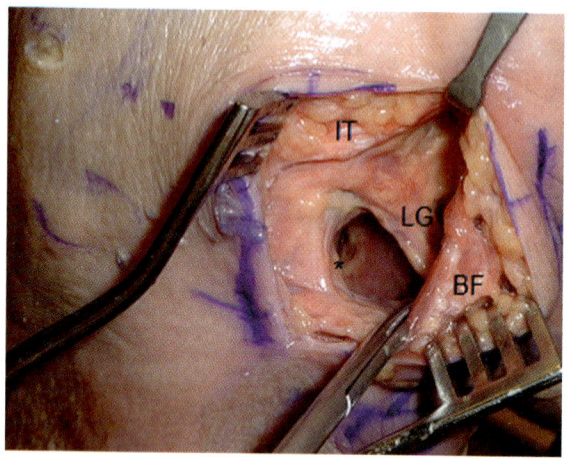

Figure 33-11. Spreading the iliotibial band *(IT)* and biceps femoris *(BF)* allows visualization of the lateral head of the gastrocnemius *(LG)* inserting into the distal femur. The posterolateral joint capsule *(*)* is visible.

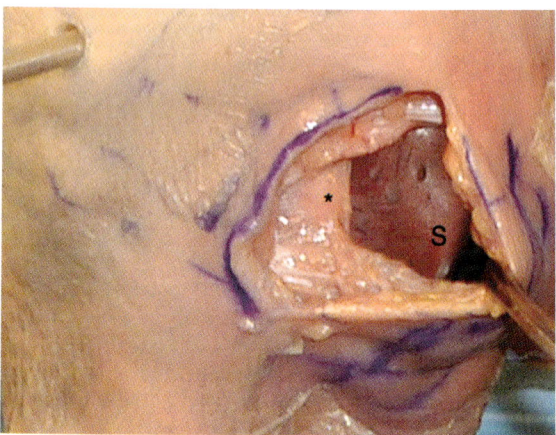

Figure 33-12. The lateral head of the gastrocnemius has been elevated off the joint capsule and a spoon *(S)* has been placed in the incision, retracting the gastrocnemius and biceps posteriorly, protecting the common peroneal nerve. The joint capsule *(*)* is now easily visualized.

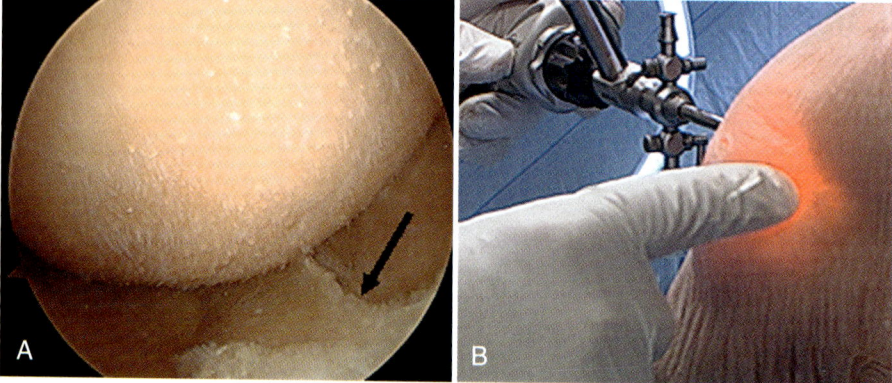

Figure 33-13. **A,** A meniscus tear is visualized arthroscopically. **B,** Light from the arthroscope is used to mark the approximate location of the tear on the outside of the knee.

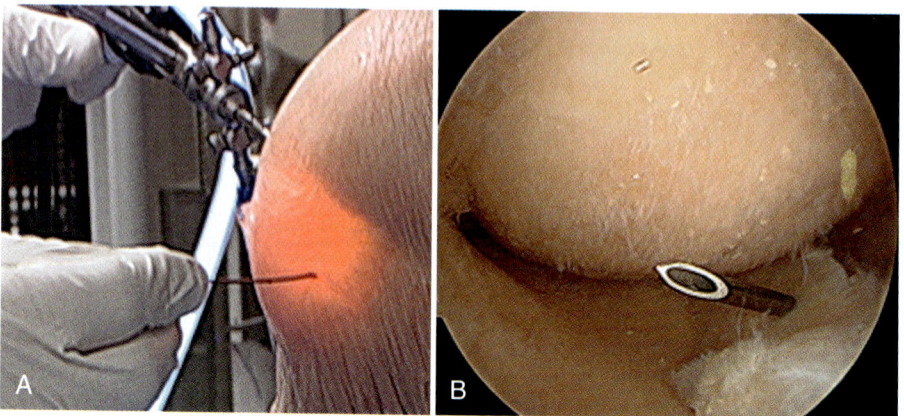

Figure 33-14. **A,** A spinal needle is passed through the skin and into the joint. **B,** Arthroscopically, the needle is seen crossing the meniscus tear.

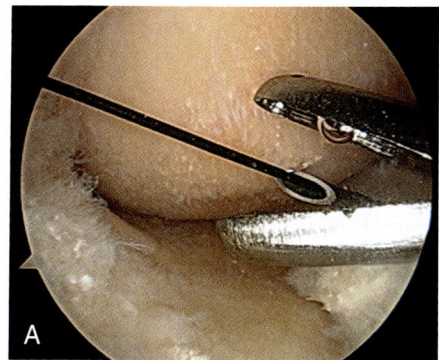

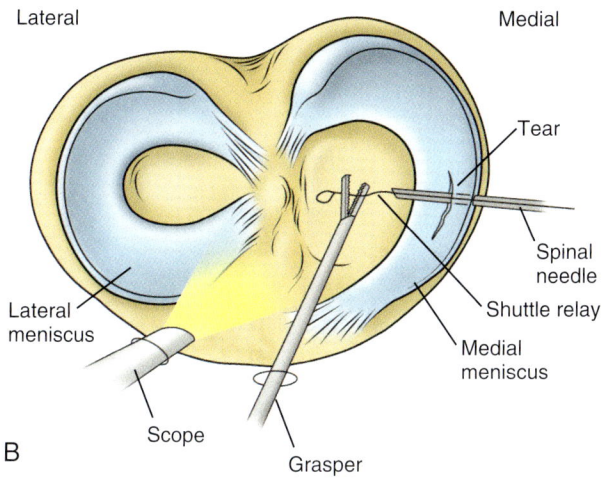

Figure 33-15. **A,** A wire is passed through the needle and retrieved into an anterior portal. **B,** Line drawing from superior perspective demonstrating wire loop retrieval.

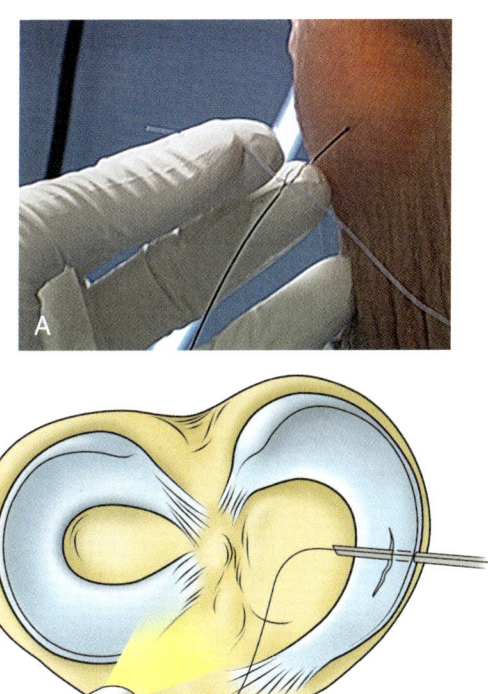

Figure 33-16. **A,** Suture to be used in the repair is threaded through a loop in the wire and pulled into the joint and through the meniscus tear as the needle is removed. **B,** Line drawing from superior perspective demonstrating suture passed through the wire loop.

needle is placed relative to the first needle in such a manner as to make a vertical mattress stitch, and a wire is pulled through this needle and out an anterior portal in the same manner (Fig. 33-17). The other end of the suture is passed through the wire (Fig. 33-18). Pulling this suture out through the meniscus completes the repair (Fig. 33-19).

After the sutures are secured inside the knee, a small incision is made between the two sutures' exit sites and the sutures are tied together over the capsule, reducing the tear. Alternatively, a second spinal needle can be used and the incision made between the needles to reduce the risk of inadvertently cutting the suture. If additional sutures are required, they can generally be placed through the same incision.

Numerous alternative methods have been described, allowing placement of sutures in a standard vertical mattress configuration. In one method, two sutures are passed into the joint through two spinal needles and retrieved through an anterior portal. They are tied together with a square knot. The knot is then pulled back through the meniscus and out of the skin by traction on either suture, resulting in a standard vertical mattress suture. Passage of the knot through the meniscus can be difficult and is facilitated by tying a smaller dilator knot in one suture prior to tying the square knot and pulling this knot through the meniscus first.[33]

Alternatively, specific devices have been developed to facilitate this repair method, including a shuttle relay that can be passed through the second needle instead of suture.

Suture from the first needle is then passed through the shuttle relay, which is withdrawn along with the second needle. This technique obviates the need to pull a knot through the meniscus and avoids extracting suture from anterior portals, where soft tissue could become entrapped.[33] The same technique can be used with a wire loop stylet that is passed through the spinal needle to retrieve the second suture.

Another technique involves passing suture through one needle and retrieving it anteriorly as above, tying a three- or four-throw mulberry knot, and then pulling the suture back into the joint against the meniscus, reducing the tear.[26,40] If this method is used, the second needle should be directed to the opposite surface of the meniscus from the first to reduce and secure the repair appropriately. However, this technique does not result in the creation of true vertical mattress sutures and may have inferior strength; also, there may be concerns for chondral abrasion.

As noted, the outside-in technique is frequently used to repair tears in the anterior and middle thirds of the meniscus. We have found this technique to be particularly useful when used in association with an all-inside technique on large meniscal tears extending anteriorly from the posterior third of the meniscus. One can use an all-inside technique to address the posterior extent of the tear and then repair the anterior portion with an outside-in technique (Fig. 33-20). This hybrid technique can be used to stabilize even the largest tears rapidly.

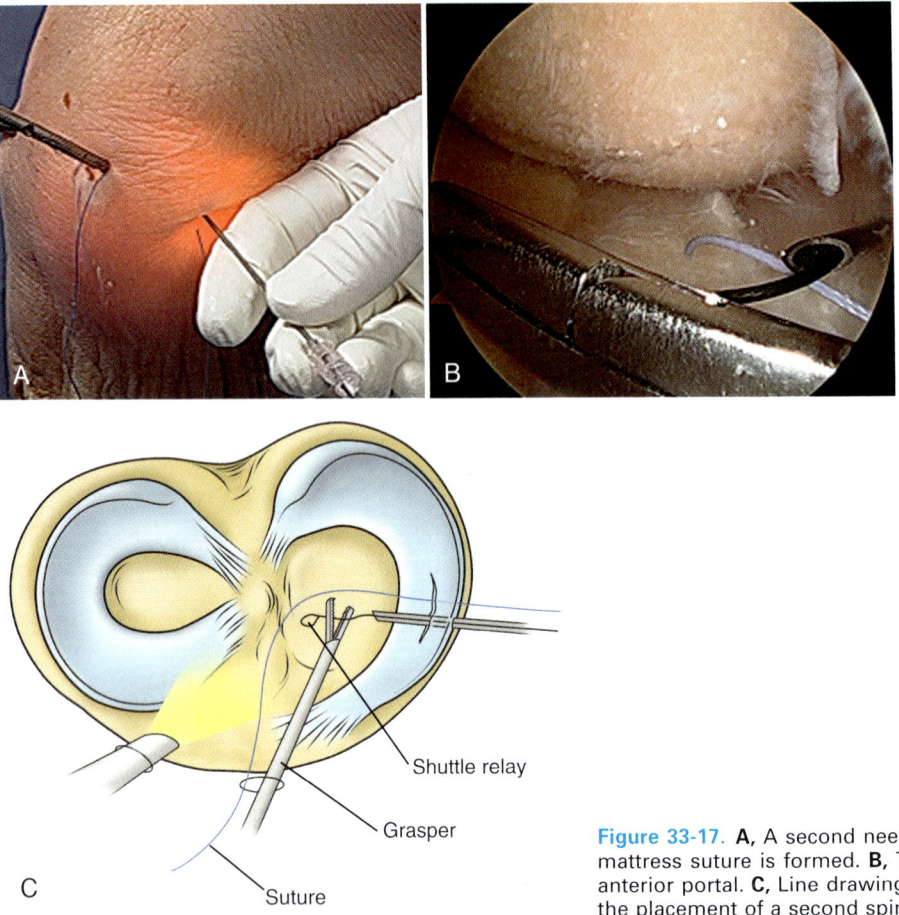

C   Shuttle relay

Grasper

Suture

Figure 33-17. A, A second needle is passed in such a way that a vertical mattress suture is formed. **B,** The wire is again retrieved via an anterior anterior portal. **C,** Line drawing from superior perspective demonstrating the placement of a second spinal needle and wire for suture retrieval.

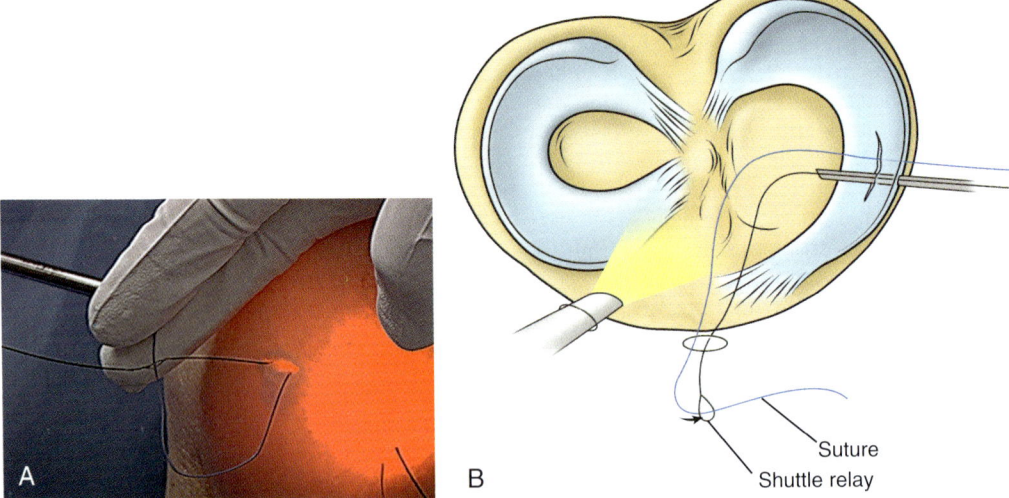

Suture
Shuttle relay

Figure 33-18. A, The other end of the suture is passed through a loop in the suture. **B,** Line drawing from superior perspective demonstrating the other end of the suture passing through the wire loop.

SELECTION OF REPAIR TECHNIQUE

With multiple repair techniques available, the surgeon must consider numerous factors in formulating a treatment plan. In addition to surgeon expertise and comfort level with a given technique, one should consider tear location, as well as biomechanical and clinical outcome data associated with

each technique. The relative advantages and disadvantages of each technique are summarized in Table 33-1.

Tear Location

Inside-out meniscal repair techniques are generally indicated for tears located in the posterior and middle thirds of the

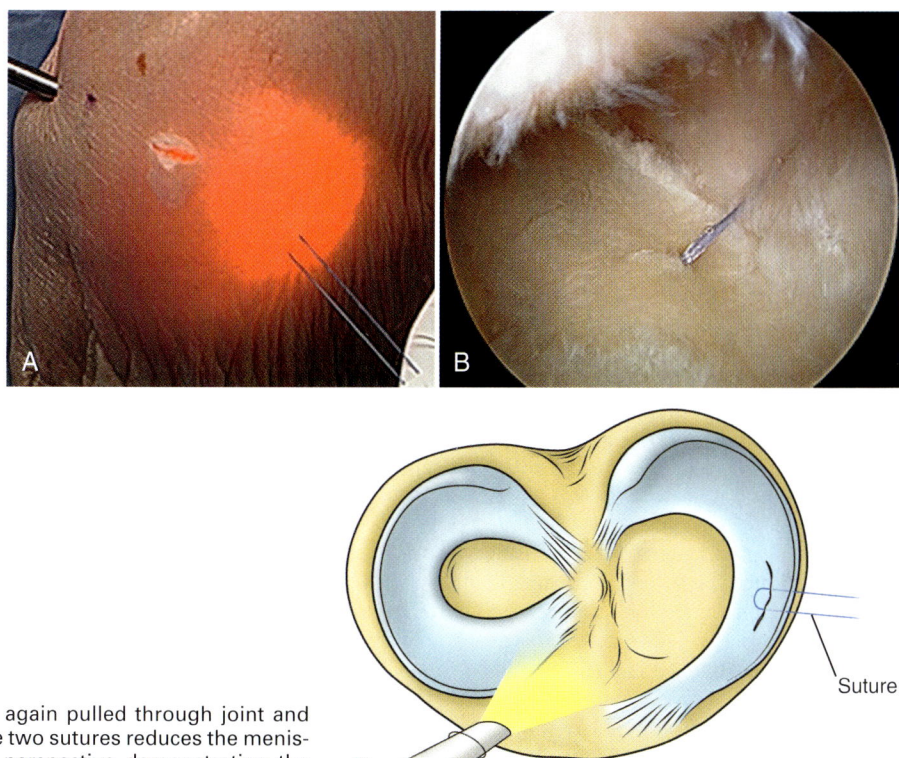

Figure 33-19. A, The wire and suture are again pulled through joint and through the meniscal tear. **B,** Pulling on the two sutures reduces the meniscus tear. **C,** Line drawing from superior perspective demonstrating the completed repair.

Table 33-1 Advantages and Disadvantages of Repair Techniques

INSIDE-OUT TECHNIQUE		OUTSIDE-IN TECHNIQUE	
Advantages	**Disadvantages**	**Advantages**	**Disadvantages**
Quickly pass many sutures with preloaded needles	Requires a significant accessory incision	Relatively rapid	Facilitated by the use of a shuttle relay (increased cost)
Easy passage of braided sutures without a shuttle relay	Increased time in surgery	Easy access to anterior two thirds of meniscus	Not useful for tears of the posterior third of the meniscus
Protection of neurovascular structures for posterior horn tears	Requires capable assistance	Can easily place sutures in any desired orientation	Difficult to pass braided suture without a shuttle relay

meniscus, whereas outside-in techniques are generally used for tears in the anterior and middle portions of the meniscus.

Biomechanical Testing

A number of studies have evaluated the pullout strength and stiffness under cyclic loading of sutures placed in vertical mattress or horizontal mattress configurations. It has been well demonstrated that a vertical mattress suture configuration is stronger than a horizontal configuration.[17,23,28,31] Any technique whereby a surgeon can place vertical mattress sutures precisely (inside-out or outside-in) can thus be considered the ideal meniscal repair technique from a biomechanical standpoint.

Numerous studies have compared the in vitro strength of a variety of all-inside repair devices with vertical mattress sutures, with similar results. Rigid devices as well as all-inside suture techniques generally had significantly lower strength than vertical mattress sutures, often similar to or significantly less than horizontal sutures.[5,8,15,17,29]

Clinical Outcome Data

Hantes and colleagues[18] have compared the three methods described in a randomized controlled trial, using Rapidloc (DePuy Mitek, Raynham, Mass) for their all-inside repairs. They noted no difference in success rates between the inside-out (100%) and outside-in (95%) techniques, but a significantly lower success rate (65%) in the Rapidloc group.

Multiple studies have compared the outcomes of all-inside techniques with inside-out suture techniques. Two randomized controlled trials[1,10] and a prospective cohort study[36] have compared meniscal arrows (Biofix) with inside-out suture techniques. None of the studies demonstrated a difference in short-term failure rates of repairs of peripheral tears.

REHABILITATION AFTER MENISCAL REPAIR

During the postoperative period following meniscal repair, importance should be placed on protecting the integrity of the repair, avoiding disuse changes in bone and soft tissue,

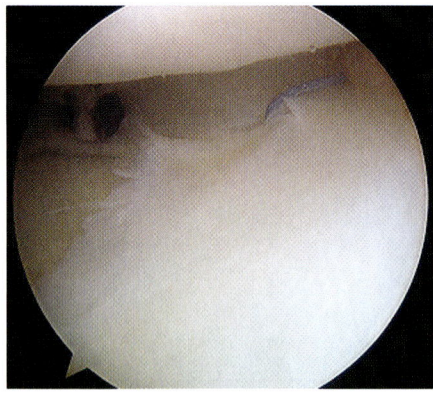

Figure 33-20. Hybrid meniscal repair technique. All-inside fixation is used for the posterior portion of the meniscal tear and an outside-in technique is used for the anterior extent of the tear.

and restoring and preserving knee range of motion. Biomechanical studies have suggested that loading of the knee in extension helps reduce longitudinal tears, whereas loading in flexion and tibial torsion produce stresses on the meniscus likely to be detrimental to healing.[7,22,30,37]

Significant research has focused on the safety of accelerated rehabilitation protocols. Shelbourne and associates[35] and Barber[3] have compared patients placed in accelerated rehabilitation protocols that included immediate, full weight bearing with patients placed in conservative rehabilitation protocols that restricted range of motion and weight-bearing status for 6 weeks after inside-out suture repair. No statistically significant differences in failure rates were noted in either study, with failure rates ranging from 9% to 19%. Both studies noted a more rapid return to full range of motion with the accelerated protocols, but no differences in final range of motion were noted. Similar results have been reported when allowing patients undergoing concurrent ACL and meniscal repair to progress with standard ACL rehabilitation protocols.[24]

CONCLUSION

Meniscal tears are commonly encountered and should be repaired whenever possible to maximize meniscal function. Repair is more frequently successful in acute, peripheral tears in younger patients. Concurrent ACL repair enhances meniscal healing but ligamentous instability is detrimental. Vertical mattress sutures placed using an inside-out technique remain the standard. Care must be taken to protect vulnerable vascular structures when using these techniques. Tears that extend more anteriorly in the meniscus are amenable to repair with an outside-in technique, particularly augmenting an inside-out or all-inside technique used posteriorly. Recent studies have demonstrated the effectiveness and safety of accelerated rehabilitation protocols.

KEY REFERENCES

Albrecht-Olsen P, Kristensen G, Burgaard P, et al: The arrow versus horizontal suture in arthroscopic meniscus repair. A prospective randomized study with arthroscopic evaluation. Knee Surg Sports Traumatol Arthrosc 7:268–273, 1999.

Arnoczky SP, Warren RF: Microvasculature of the human meniscus. Am J Sports Med 10:90–95, 1982.

Barber FA: Accelerated rehabilitation for meniscus repairs. Arthroscopy 10:206–210, 1994.

Bryant D, Dill J, Litchfield R, et al: Effectiveness of bioabsorbable arrows compared with inside-out suturing for vertical, reparable meniscal lesions: a randomized clinical trial. Am J Sports Med 35:889–896, 2007.

Cannon WD, Jr, Morgan CD: Meniscal repair: arthroscopic repair techniques. Instr Course Lect 43:77–96, 1994.

Cannon WD, Jr, Vittori JM: The incidence of healing in arthroscopic meniscal repairs in anterior cruciate ligament-reconstructed knees versus stable knees. Am J Sports Med. 20:176–181, Mar-Apr 1992.

Hantes ME, Zachos VC, Varitimidis SE, et al: Arthroscopic meniscal repair: a comparative study between three different surgical techniques. Knee Surg Sports Traumatol Arthrosc 14:1232–1237, 2006.

McCarty EC, Marx RG, Wickiewicz TL: Meniscal tears in the athlete. Operative and nonoperative management. Phys Med Rehabil Clin N Am. 11:867–880, Nov 2000.

Morgan CD, Wojtys EM, Casscells CD, Casscells SW: Arthroscopic meniscal repair evaluated by second-look arthroscopy. Am J Sports Med 19:632–637, 1991.

Rockborn P, Messner K: Long-term results of meniscus repair and meniscectomy: a 13-year functional and radiographic follow-up study. Knee Surg Sports Traumatol Arthrosc 8:2–10, 2000.

Rodeo SA: Arthroscopic meniscal repair with use of the outside-in technique. Instr Course Lect 49:195–206, 2000.

Scott GA, Jolly BL, Henning CE: Combined posterior incision and arthroscopic intra-articular repair of the meniscus. An examination of factors affecting healing. J Bone Joint Surg Am 68:847–861, 1986.

Spindler KP, McCarty EC, Warren TA, et al: Prospective comparison of arthroscopic medial meniscal repair technique: inside-out suture versus entirely arthroscopic arrows. Am J Sports Med 31:929–934, 2003.

Tenuta JJ, Arciero RA: Arthroscopic evaluation of meniscal repairs. Factors that effect healing. Am J Sports Med 22:797–802, 1994.

Warren RF: Arthroscopic meniscus repair. Arthroscopy 1:170–172, 1985.

Full references for this chapter can be found on www.expertconsult.com.

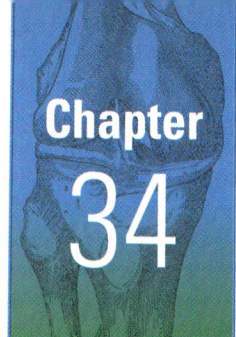

Chapter 34

All-Inside Arthroscopic Meniscal Repair

Kimberly A. Turman, F. Winston Gwathmey, Jr., and David R. Diduch

The concept of meniscal repair was first described by Annandale in 1885.[5] It is well established that the meniscus contributes several key functions to the knee, including joint stability,[38] shock absorption and load transmission,[17] proprioception,[20] and articular cartilage nutrition.[24] Furthermore, the long-term consequences of total meniscectomy include the predictable development of degenerative joint changes.[2,3,18,23] Meniscal repair is therefore preferred to meniscectomy whenever feasible.

Techniques of meniscal repair have evolved over time and include open, outside-in, inside-out, and all-inside repairs. Numerous devices to achieve the all-inside techniques have also evolved over recent years. These all-inside techniques have been developed in efforts to decrease surgical time, technical difficulty, and risk to neurovascular structures. Although inside-out vertical mattress suture repairs remain the gold standard, the use of all-inside techniques continues to expand.

INDICATIONS FOR ALL-INSIDE MENISCAL REPAIR

The basic prerequisites for inside-out meniscal repairs also apply to all-inside repairs. Not all meniscal tears are amenable to repair and several factors must be considered to determine repair suitability and healing potential. Although magnetic resonance imaging (MRI) may aid in predicting repair versus meniscectomy, the final determination of repair suitability is often made during arthroscopy. Meniscal tissue is relatively avascular. Only the peripheral 10% to 30% of the meniscus is vascularized, supplied by the medial and lateral genicular arteries[6] (Fig. 34-1). The remaining meniscus receives its nutrition through synovial fluid diffusion. The popliteal hiatus also creates a relatively hypovascular area in the posterior lateral meniscus. DeHaven[19] classified tears in the peripheral 3 mm as vascular (also referred to as the red-red zone), those more than 5 mm from the meniscocapsular junction as avascular (white-white zone), and those in between as variable (red-white zone). Based on the blood supply pattern, tears in the vascular periphery of the meniscus have the best ability to heal, whereas tears in the central white-white zone demonstrate poorer healing rates and are less amenable to repair[31] (Fig. 34-2).

In addition to location, meniscal tear orientation and complexity must also be considered. Longitudinal vertical tears, bucket handle tears, and meniscocapsular separations are most amenable to repair (Fig. 34-3). Although radial tears were previously a contraindication to repair, some of these tears may also be repaired successfully, but this remains somewhat controversial. Conversely, tears with increasing complexity may be better managed with partial meniscectomy. These include degenerative tears and tears with horizontal cleavage planes or multiple flaps.[48] Oblique undersurface tears can also be problematic because they often extend from the vascular to avascular zone.

Patient factors also play a substantial role in determining appropriate indications for meniscal repair. It is well known that meniscal repair is more successful in the setting of concurrent anterior cruciate ligament (ACL) reconstruction. All-inside techniques may be particularly indicated in this setting, as opposed to isolated repairs. Furthermore, meniscal healing rates are typically lower in an ACL-deficient knee,[29] and repair may be contraindicated if the ACL is not also reconstructed. Patient age and tear chronicity are other important variables. Older patients with chronic degenerative tears are better served with partial meniscectomy. Finally, meniscal repair requires a patient willing to comply with a prolonged rehabilitation course as opposed to resection.

TECHNIQUES

All-inside repairs were first introduced in 1991 and have subsequently been developed in successive generations of improvements in device and technique.[53] With each of these devices, an intact meniscal rim is required to anchor the repair device. Therefore, meniscocapsular separations are preferentially repaired with an alternate technique (Fig. 34-4). Anterior horn tears are also a relative contraindication because of difficulty in accessing the tear with these techniques.

First-Generation All-Inside Repairs

The first generation of all-inside repairs was described by Morgan[43] in 1991 and used curved suture hooks through accessory posterior portals to pass sutures across the tear. Sutures were then retrieved and tied arthroscopically (Fig. 34-5). The technique was technically demanding and continued to place the neurovascular structures at risk. It was subsequently abandoned with the development of second-generation repairs.

Second-Generation All-Inside Repairs

The second generation of all-inside meniscal repairs introduced the concept of technique-specific devices placed across the tear and anchored peripherally. The prototype of this generation was the T-Fix (Smith & Nephew, Andover, Mass; Fig. 34-6). The T-Fix consisted of a polyethylene bar with attached no. 2-0 braided polyester suture that was deployed through a sharp needle or cannula to capture the peripheral meniscus or capsule. Adjacent sutures were then secured with arthroscopic knots pushed onto the meniscal surface. This generation was a significant advance because meniscal repair was now achievable through standard anterior arthroscopic portals without the need for accessory incisions and with minimal risk to neurovascular structures when performed

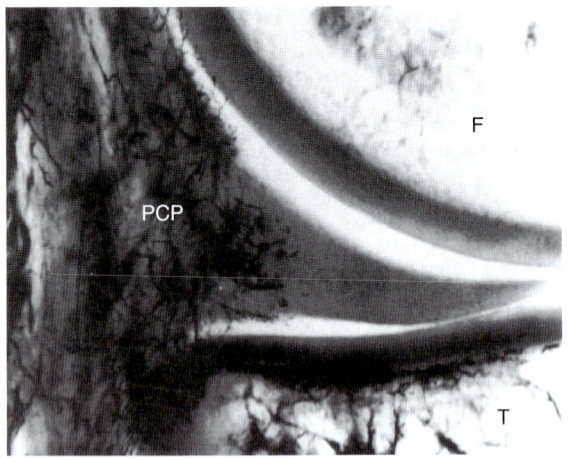

Figure 34-1. Microvasculature of the meniscus. A perimeniscal capillary plexus supplied by the medial and lateral genicular arteries perfuses the periphery of the meniscus. The remaining central portion of the meniscus is essentially avascular and has limited healing potential. *F,* Femur; *PCP,* perimeniscal capillary plexus; *T,* tibia. (From Arnoczky SP, Warren RF: The microvasculature of the human meniscus. Am J Sports Med 10:90–95, 1982.)

properly. The device confirmed that it was possible and safe to repair the meniscus by deploying an anchor across the tear and into the periphery of the meniscus and capsule. However, the need for arthroscopic knots, with potential chondral abrasion and the inability to tension the knots after placement, were technical drawbacks of the device. Early results were encouraging, with short-term success rates of 80% to 90%.[11,22] Despite the early results, the desire for a simpler device with improved compression across the meniscal repair led to the development of third-generation devices.

Third-Generation All-Inside Repairs

The third generation consisted of the development of bioabsorbable meniscal repair devices including arrows, screws, darts, and staples (Fig. 34-7). Most of these devices are composed of the rigid poly-L-lactic-acid (PLLA), which retains its strength for up to 12 months and requires 2 to 3 years or longer to resorb completely. The most commonly used device was the Meniscal Arrow (ConMed Linvatec, Largo, Fla) because of its ease of insertion and early success rates.

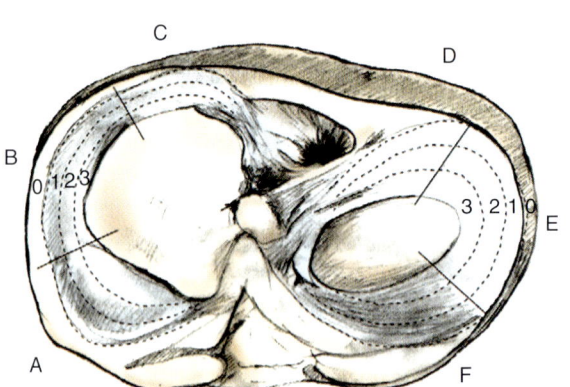

Figure 34-2. Circumferential and radial Cooper's zones of the meniscus. Tears in zones 0 and 1 are considered peripheral and have a higher healing capacity. (From Stärke C, Kopf S, Petersen W, Becker R: Meniscal repair. Arthroscopy 25:1033–1044, 2009.)

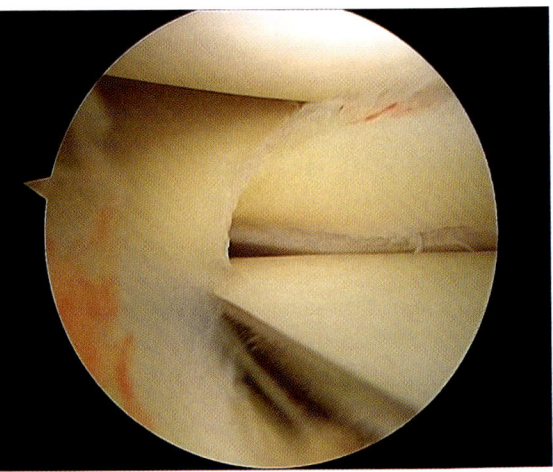

Figure 34-3. A vertical tear in the peripheral lateral meniscus is demonstrated during arthroscopy. Because of its vertical configuration, peripheral location, and size of approximately 2 cm, this tear is amenable to repair.

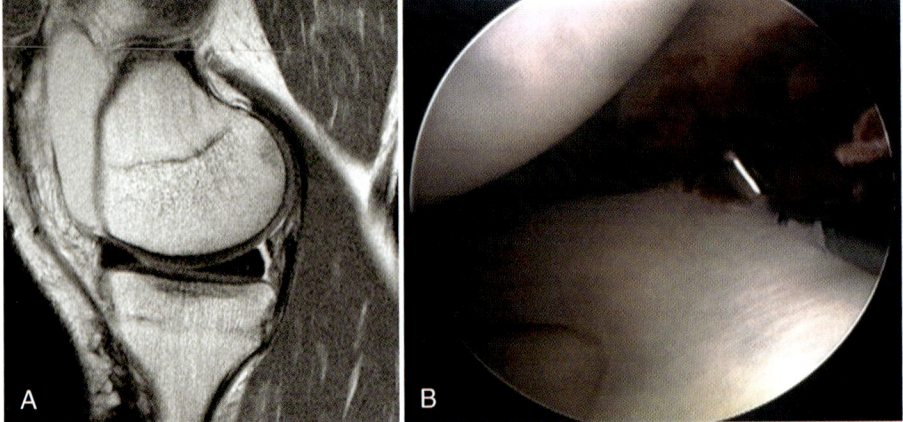

Figure 34-4. A meniscocapsular separation is demonstrated on MRI (**A**) and during arthroscopy (**B**). This tear cannot be repaired by an all-inside technique because an intact meniscal rim is required. (**A** from Choi NH, Kim TH, Victoroff BN: Comparison of arthroscopic medial meniscal suture repair techniques: Inside-out versus all-inside repair. Am J Sports Med 37:2144–2150, 2009.)

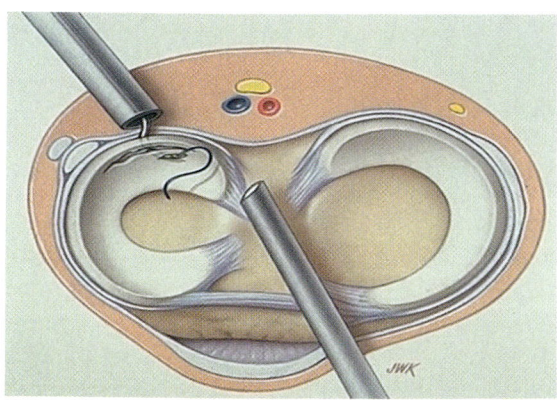

Figure 34-5. First-generation all-inside meniscal repair techniques used curved suture hooks inserted through accessory posterior portals. (From Miller MD: Atlas of meniscal repair. Oper Tech Orthop 5:70–71, 1995.)

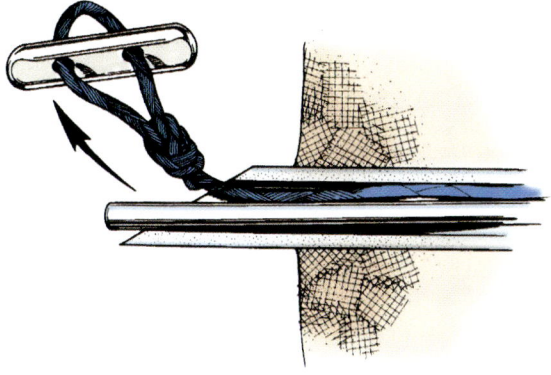

Figure 34-6. The T-Fix implant is composed of a braided suture attached to a polyethylene anchor that is deployed though a delivery needle to capture the peripheral meniscus or capsule. This device requires arthroscopic suture tying to connect adjacent anchors securing the tear. (From Smith & Nephew: Endoscopic meniscal repair using the T-Fix. Smith & Nephew Endoscopy, Andover, Mass, 1997.)

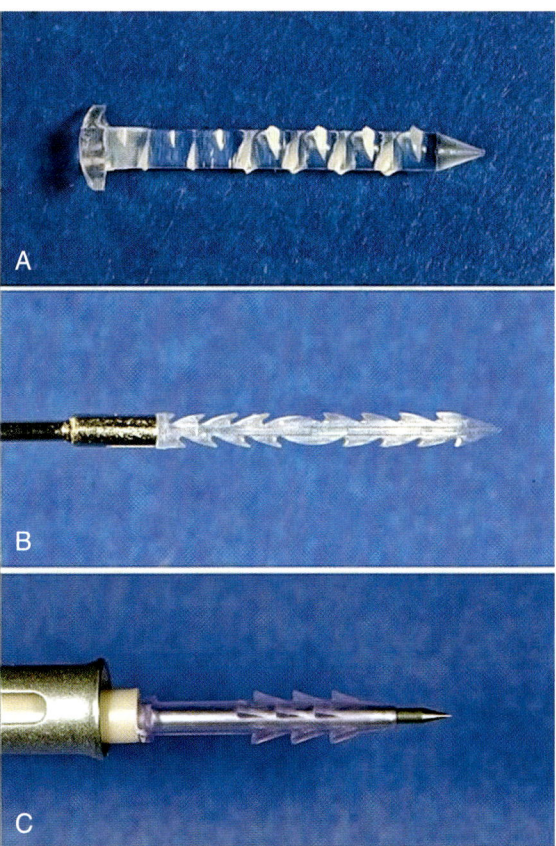

Figure 34-7. Third-generation bioabsorbable all-inside meniscal repair devices. **A,** Meniscus Arrow (ConMed Linvatec). **B,** Meniscal Dart (Arthrex). **C,** BioStinger (ConMed Linvatec). (From Stärke C, Kopf S, Petersen W, Becker R: Meniscal repair: arthroscopy 25:1033–1044, 2009.)

The current version of the meniscal arrow (Contour Meniscus Arrow and ConMed Linvatec, Largo, Fla) has a low-profile head and is barbed along the entire length of the implant shaft to improve fixation strength. It is composed of a faster resorbing self-reinforced copolymer, 80L/20D,L PLA, which retains its strength for up to 24 weeks and then gradually resorbs. When seating the arrow across the meniscal tear, it is important to indent the head of the arrow into the meniscus to reduce the risk of chondral damage. One prospective, randomized study used second-look arthroscopy to assess healing rates of 91% with the arrow versus 75% with horizontal mattress suture repairs.[1] Unfortunately, these results did not prove durable. Another study with the Meniscus Arrow revealed a 90.6% success rate at 2 years in patients undergoing concurrent ACL reconstruction.[27] However, these results deteriorated significantly at longer term follow-up, with a success rate of only 71.4% at 6 years in the same group of patients.[37] Other studies have documented similar deterioration of results.[21,49] Kurzweil and colleagues[36] reported an overall failure rate of 28% with the Meniscus Arrow at average follow-up of 54 months. Furthermore, in isolated meniscal repairs without concurrent ACL

reconstruction, the failure rate was a striking 42%. Yet another study reported a failure rate of 41% at 4.7 years.[26]

Numerous device-specific complications have also been reported with the Meniscus Arrow, including transient synovitis, inflammatory reaction, cyst formation, device failure, device migration, and chondral damage (Fig. 34-8).*

Chondral damage is a potential complication with any of the rigid third-generation devices (Fig. 34-9). If these devices are placed too proudly or loosen or migrate prior to dissolving, significant chondral damage can result, which often consists of grooving of the adjacent femoral condyle.[36] Because of the deterioration of results and numerous complications, the rigid third-generation devices have generally fallen out of favor.

Fourth-Generation All-Inside Repairs

The concerns discussed earlier, combined with the lack of adjustable tensioning, led to the development of the fourth and current generation of all-inside meniscal repair devices. These devices are flexible, suture-based, and of lower profile and allow for variable compression and retensioning across the meniscal tear. The two prototypical devices include the FasT-Fix (Smith & Nephew, Andover, Mass) and the Rapid-Loc (DePuy Mitek, Raynham, Mass).

---

*References 4, 14, 30, 33, 40, 44, 45, 47, 50, and 51.

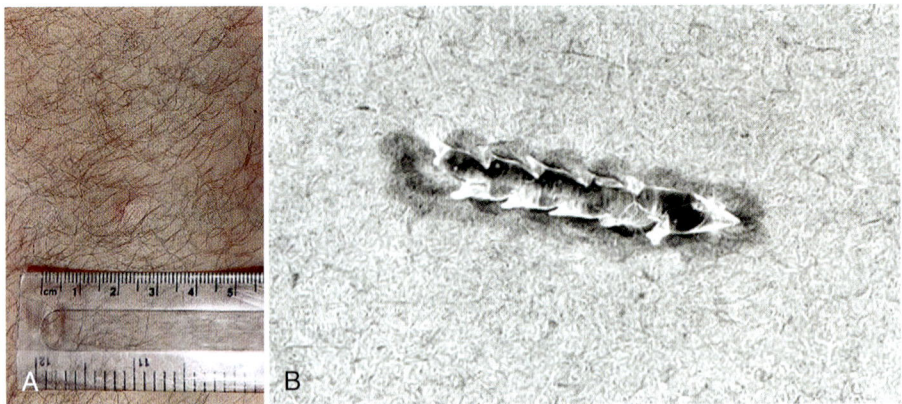

Figure 34-8. Device migration has been reported with rigid all-inside meniscal repair devices. **A,** This patient complained of a painful nodule that developed at his knee joint line after meniscal repair. **B,** Exploration of the nodule revealed a broken meniscal arrow that was excised. (From Bonshahi AY, Hopgood P, Shepard GJ: Migration of a broken meniscal arrow: a case report and review of the literature. Knee Surg Sports Traumatol Arthrosc 12:40–51, 2004.)

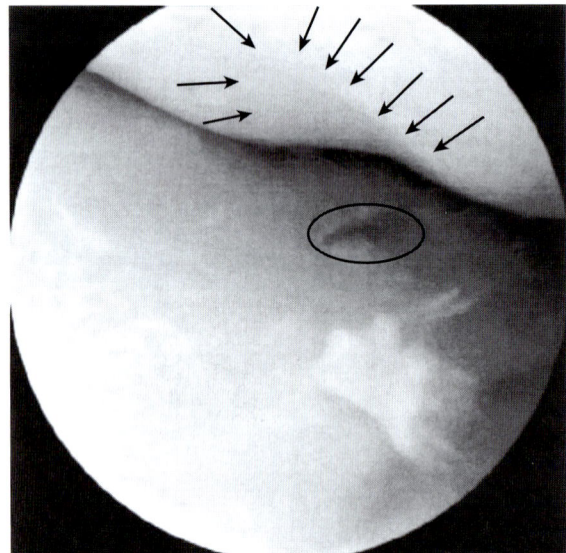

Figure 34-9. Rigid all-inside meniscal repair devices have been associated with chondral damage. Chondral grooving *(arrows)* is demonstrated in this second-look arthroscopy 6 weeks after implantation of a Meniscus Arrow *(visible within circle)*. (From Ménétrey J, Seil R, Rupp S, Fritschy D: Chondral damage after meniscal repair with the use of a bioabsorbable implant. Am J Sports Med 30:896–899, 2002.)

The FasT-Fix, first introduced in 2001, is composed of two 5-mm suture anchors connected by a no. 0 nonabsorbable polyester suture with a pretied slip knot (Fig. 34-10). A newer version of the FasT-Fix (Ultra FasT-Fix) consists of polyetheretherketone (PEEK) anchors with ultra–high-molecular-weight polyethylene (UHMWPE) sutures (Ultrabraid) to improve strength and ease of use. It is also available with absorbable PLLA anchors. A depth-limiting sleeve on the inserter may be precut to any desired length, with 12 to 13 mm generally considered a sufficient length that is also safe to the neurovascular structures.[42] The curved or straight inserter, with both anchors loaded, is introduced into the joint and advanced across the tear. After deploying the first anchor, the needle inserter is withdrawn from the meniscus, but maintained in the joint. The second anchor is advanced to the tip of the inserter, which is then advanced across the

meniscus a second time and deployed. The anchors and resultant suture bridge may be placed in a vertical or horizontal mattress configuration, simulating inside-out suture repairs. The pretied slip knot is advanced with a push-pull technique to apply variable compression across the tear. The suture is then cut or, alternatively, may be left in place until all devices are placed to allow for retensioning. One of the primary advantages of the FasT-Fix is the ability to place a suture-based device in a vertical mattress configuration (Fig. 34-11). Unfortunately, the device can be difficult to place posteriorly and misfires, device breakage, anchor pull-out, and tangled sutures are not uncommon (Fig. 34-12).

The RapidLoc provides even greater ease of insertion and is composed of a smaller absorbable backstop anchor connected to a top hat by a no. 2-0 absorbable or nonabsorbable suture (Fig. 34-13). The top hat was originally composed of PLLA, but is also available in polydioxanone (PDS) in efforts to reduce the risk of chondral damage further because it resorbs more rapidly (3 to 6 months versus 2 years or longer with PLLA). The device is available with a 0-, 12-, or 27-degree curved inserter that is introduced into the joint and across the meniscal tear in a single pass. A silicone hub on the inserter limits the insertion depth to 13 mm. The anchor is deployed and the inserter removed. The pretied slip knot and top hat are advanced into position with a knot pusher to provide variable compression against the backstop anchor (Fig. 34-14). The top hat should dimple the meniscal surface (Fig. 34-15). Again, sutures may be cut at the time of placement or after all devices have been placed to allow for retensioning if desired. Although the RapidLoc is more expedient and less technically demanding than the FasT-Fix, it does not currently allow for vertical mattress–based repair. However, a newer version, Omnispan, has recently been developed, which will allow for this technology[9] (Fig. 34-16). It is composed of two PEEK backstop anchors with a UHMWPE suture that would allow for mattress configurations. Because the slip knot is on the periphery at one of the backstops, no knot rests on the surface of the meniscus.

Other fourth-generation devices now currently available include the MaxFire meniscal repair device (Biomet, Warsaw, Ind), the Meniscal Cinch (Arthrex, Naples, Fla), and the CrossFix (Cayenne Medical, Scottsdale, Ariz) (Fig. 34-17). The Meniscal Cinch consists of two PEEK implants or

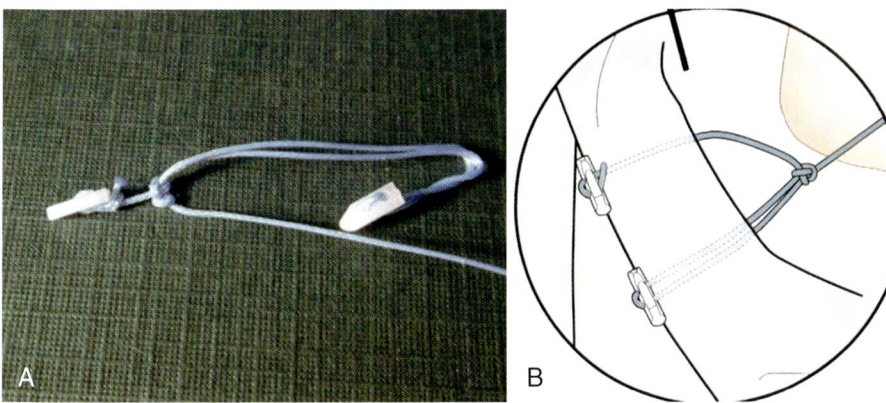

Figure 34-10. The FasT-Fix all-inside meniscal repair device is composed of two suture anchors connected by a pretied slip knot. (**A** from Barber FA, Schroeder FA, Oro FB, et al: FasT-Fix meniscal repair: mid-term results. Arthroscopy 24:1342–1348, 2008; **B** from Smith & Nephew: Meniscal repair with FasT-fix suture system. Smith & Nephew Endoscopy, Andover, Mass, 2008.)

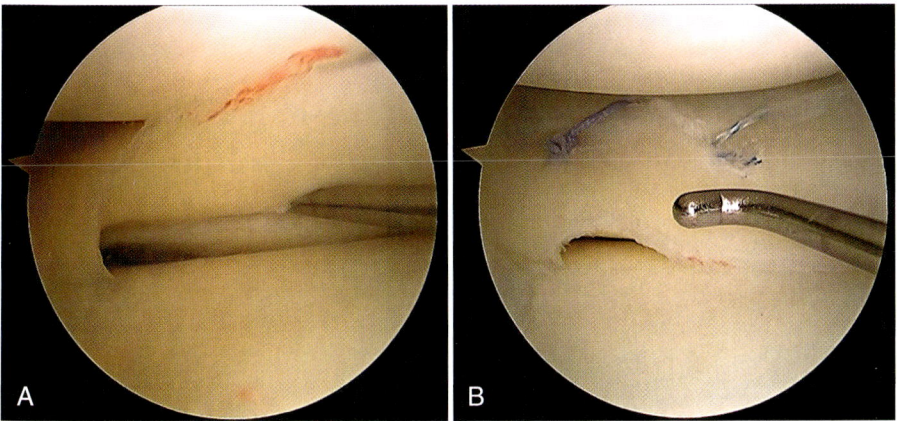

Figure 34-11. A, This lateral meniscal tear was repaired with two FasT-Fix all-inside devices inserted with oblique mattress technique (**B**).

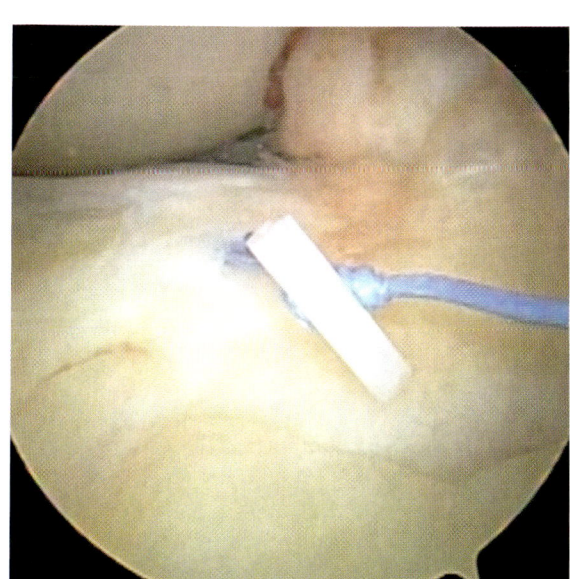

Figure 34-12. Deployment errors, tangled sutures, and anchor pullout, as shown in this figure, are potential pitfalls of the FasT-Fix. (From Barber FA, Schroeder FA, Oro FB, Beavis RC: FasT-Fix meniscal repair: mid-term results. Arthroscopy.24:1340–1348, 2008.)

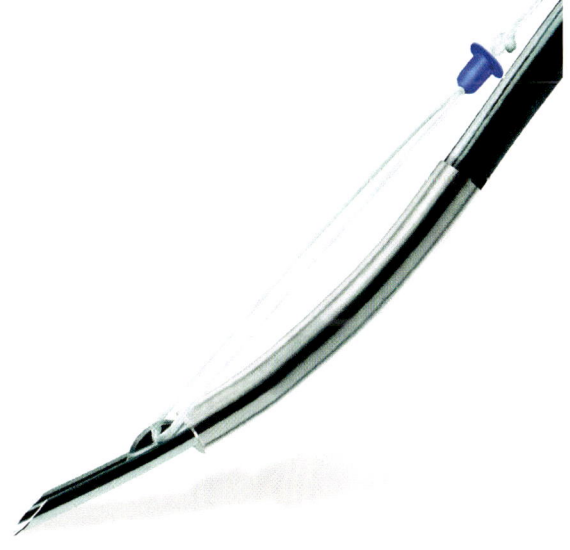

Figure 34-13. The RapidLoc all-inside meniscal repair device consists of a backstop anchor connected by a slip knot to an absorbable top hat, which secures the tear once tensioned. Straight, 12-degree, and 27-degree delivery needles are available for insertion. A silicone hub limits insertion depth to 13 mm. (From Quinby JS, Golish SR, Hart JA, et al: All-inside meniscal repair using a new flexible, tensionable device. Am J Sports Med.34:1281–1286, 2006.)

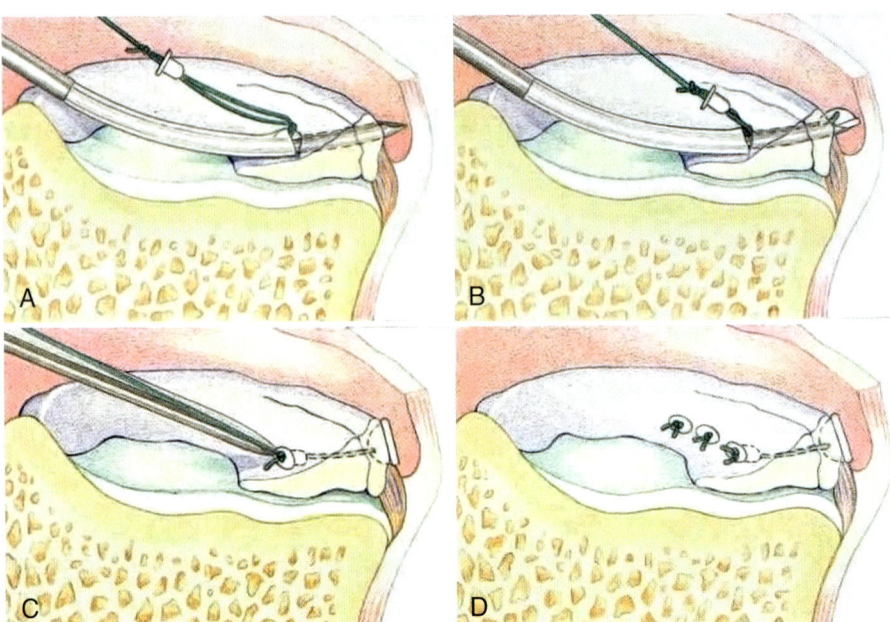

Figure 34-14. RapidLoc all-inside meniscus repair technique. **A,** The delivery needle is inserted into the meniscus and across the tear. A depth limiter prevents overpenetration. **B,** The backstop anchor is deployed behind the meniscus by firing the trigger on the device handle. **C,** The knot pusher is used to advance the top hat on the slip knot, which reduces and secures the tear. **D,** Multiple devices may be inserted with this technique to secure the entirety of the meniscal tear. (From Miller MD, Blessey PB, Chhabra A, et al: Meniscal repair with the Rapid Loc device: a cadaveric study. J Knee Surg 16:79–82, 2003.)

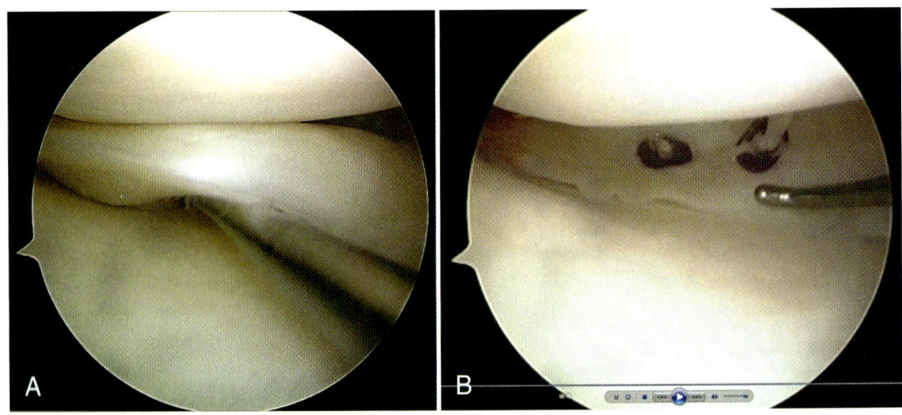

Figure 34-15. A, This medial meniscal tear has been repaired using two RapidLoc all-inside repair devices **(B).**

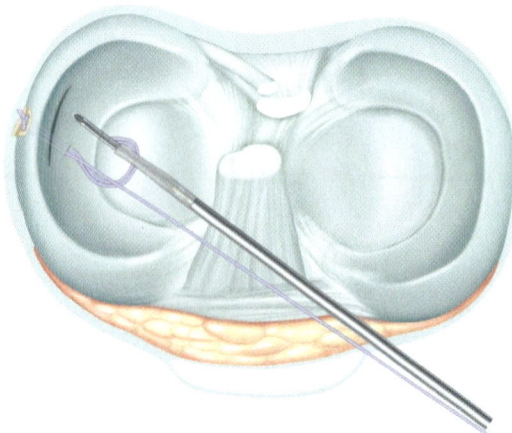

Figure 34-16. The recently developed Omnispan (Depuy Mitek, Raynham, Mass) allows mattress configuration with a sliding knot located on the periphery. (From Omnispan Meniscal Repair System Surgical Technique Manual, Figure 10. DePuy Mitek, Inc. 2010.)

anchors connected by a no. 2-0 FiberWire with a pretied slip knot. Similar to the FasT-Fix, it may be placed in horizontal or vertical mattress configuration. The MaxFire uses two all-suture anchors connected to each other with ZipLoop technology, allowing mattress placement without the need for a pretied sliding knot. The concern is that the all-suture anchors may pull out if the device is tensioned too aggressively. The CrossFix is also an all-suture device that deploys a preset 3-mm mattress stitch with a pretied sliding knot.

Biomechanical studies have demonstrated favorable results with both the FasT-Fix and RapidLoc. Strength and load to failure characteristics for each were reported to be comparable to mattress suture constructs and significantly better than earlier generation devices.[8,13] A more recent study has demonstrated improved strength in load to failure with vertical FasT-Fix constructs (125 N) as compared with horizontal FasT-Fix constructs (90 N) and the RapidLoc (87 N).[35] The vertical FasT-Fix also displayed less displacement with cyclic

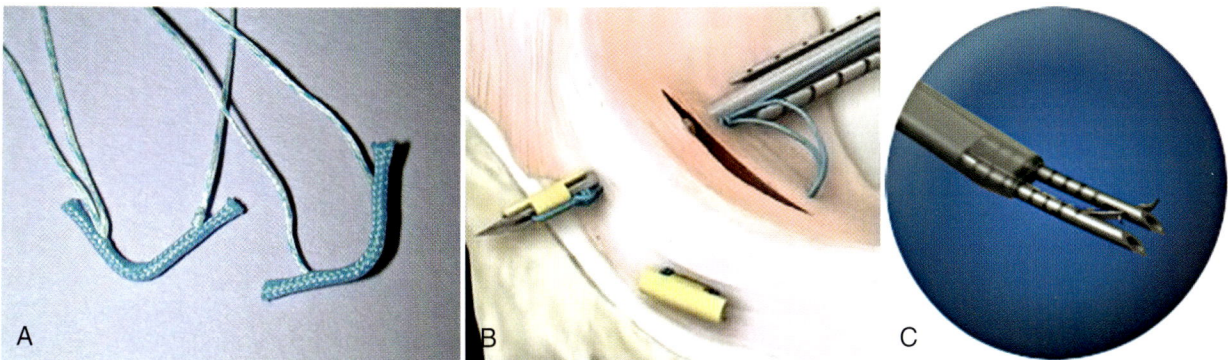

Figure 34-17. Other fourth-generation all-inside devices. **A,** Biomet MaxFire. **B,** Arthrex Meniscal Cinch. **C,** Cayenne CrossFix. (**A** from Barber FA, Herbert MA, Schroeder FA, et al: Biomechanical testing of new meniscal repair techniques containing ultra high-molecular weight polyethylene suture. Arthroscopy 25:959–967, 2009; **B** from Arthrex: Arthroscopic meniscal repair using the meniscal cinch, surgical technique (https://www.arthrex.com/myarthrex/surgicaltechniques/loader.cfm?url=/commonspot/security/getfile.cfm&pageid=56929); **C** from Cayenne Medical: CrossFix meniscal repair system, surgical technique guide, 2009 [http://www.cayennemedical.com/products/crossfix]).

loading (3.2 mm versus 4.4 and 4.6 mm, respectively). Because some displacement or loosening is expected with all these devices, it is recommended to overtighten the construct slightly at the time of insertion.

CLINICAL RESULTS

The clinical results of all-inside meniscal repairs must be compared with those for inside-out suture repairs. Success rates with inside-out techniques average 60% to 80% for isolated meniscal repairs and 90% in the setting of concurrent ACL reconstruction, because of the enhanced healing environment.[15,55] Fourth-generation all-inside techniques are showing comparable early results.

A prospective study of 42 meniscal tears repaired with the FasT-Fix with 2-year follow-up revealed success rates of 91% and 80% in patients with and without concurrent ACL reconstruction, respectively.[28] No complications were reported. At the time of the second-look arthroscopy in eight knees, the sutures were noted to be almost or completely incorporated into the meniscal tissue and no chondral damage was documented.

A similar clinical study of the PLLA RapidLoc reviewed 54 meniscal repairs in the setting of concurrent ACL reconstruction, with mean follow-up of 3 years. Results displayed a 90.7% success rate, similar to the equivalent group in the FasT-Fix study, as well as inside-out suture repairs.[46] Second-look arthroscopies in this group also revealed healing and incorporation of the top hat into the meniscal tissue with lack of chondral abrasion (Fig. 34-18). Predictors for failure included bucket handle tears, tears more than 2 cm in length, multiplanar morphology, and chronic tears longer than 3 months from injury. A subsequent study with the more rapidly absorbing PDS RapidLoc revealed similar clinical success rates of 86.8% in the setting of concurrent ACL reconstruction.[12] Again, no chondral damage was evident in patients undergoing repeat arthroscopy.

Another recent study of meniscal repair in the setting of concurrent ACL reconstruction with 2-year follow-up documented 92.4% success rates with the FasT-Fix and 86.5% with the RapidLoc.[34] A 2-year follow-up study of the MOON cohort revealed a 96% overall success rate for meniscal repair with concurrent ACL reconstruction.[52] All-inside techniques

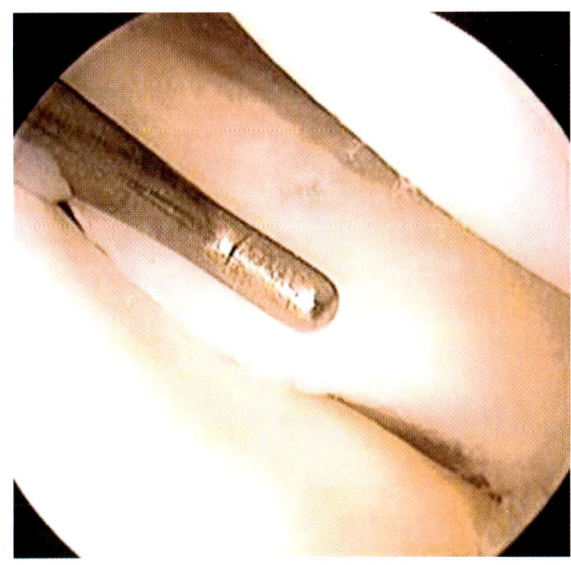

Figure 34-18. Second-look arthroscopy 14 months after meniscal repair using the RapidLoc device reveals healing of the tear and incorporation of the device into the healed meniscus. (From Quinby JS, Golish SR, Hart JA, et al: All-inside meniscal repair using a new flexible, tensionable device. Am J Sports Med 34:1281–1286, 2006.)

accounted for 80% of the repairs. All failures in this cohort were in the medial meniscus. Other authors have also shown poorer healing rates in the medial meniscus.[15,34,39]

Further studies are now becoming available evaluating the results of isolated all-inside meniscal repairs. One study of the FasT-Fix reviewed 41 meniscal repairs, 12 of which were isolated repairs.[10] The clinical success rate at an average 30-month follow-up was 83%. Of particular interest, there was no difference in success rates between patients with and without concurrent ACL reconstruction. All patients in this study underwent an accelerated rehabilitation protocol with no postoperative bracing and full immediate weight bearing, which may have contributed to the overall lower success rate. Another study of isolated meniscal repairs reviewed results of 22 all-inside, 14 inside-out, 13 hybrid, and 3 outside-in repairs at an average 38-month follow-up.[16] The overall healing rate

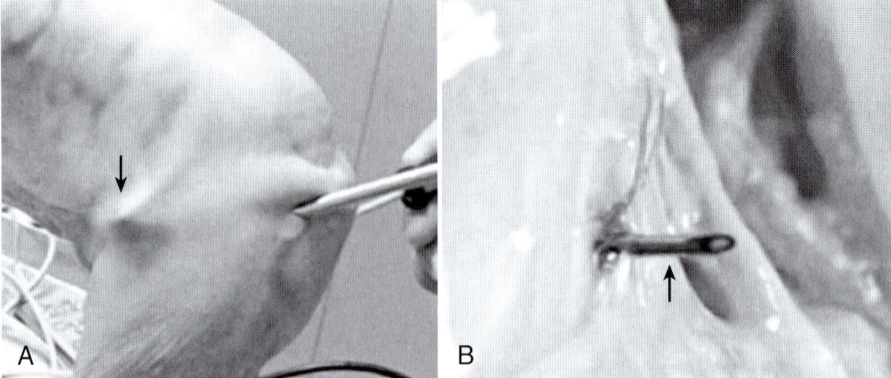

Figure 34-19. A FasT-Fix cadaveric study demonstrated penetration of the skin **(A)**, collateral ligaments **(B)**, and iliotibial tract with the preset inserter length of 22 mm. (From Miller MD, Kline AJ, Gonzales J, et al: Pitfalls associated with FasT-Fix meniscal repair. Arthroscopy 18:939–943, 2002.)

was 88.5%, with similar rates of healing and return to function among all groups. Hybrid repairs, however, showed the highest functional scores.

Although these early results are encouraging, longer term studies are necessary because we know from results with the Meniscal Arrow that successful outcomes may deteriorate over time. It should also be remembered that a repaired meniscus is not a normal meniscus and long-term studies of knee function and development of degenerative changes are also warranted following meniscal repair.

COMPLICATIONS

Despite the advances of these fourth-generation devices, they are not without complications. Device misfires and breakage are possible, as noted. Chondral damage as a result of a prominent device (top hat or suture knot) may still occur, although it is much less likely than with the rigid meniscal arrow. Iatrogenic chondral damage is also a potential complication at the time of insertion if precise technique is not used. Soft tissue penetration or entrapments are also possible, but are less common with the use of the appropriate depth-limiting devices. Finally, neurovascular complications are significantly less common with these devices than inside-out repairs, which is one of the factors that led to their development. When repairing the posterior horn of the lateral meniscus, however, it is recommended to use the contralateral portal for device placement to aim away from, and thereby reduce potential injury to, the neurovascular structures, which are located just lateral to midline.

Cadaveric studies have been performed to study the potential complications associated with insertion of these devices. In a study of the FasT-Fix, only 27 of 45 experimentally placed anchors were determined to be ideally positioned.[42] The preset inserter length of 22 mm resulted in penetration of the collateral ligaments, iliotibial tract, and skin (Fig. 34-19). Based on these results, it was recommended to trim the optional depth limiter to no longer than 15 mm to avoid potential entrapments and neurovascular injury.

A similar cadaveric study of the RapidLoc evaluated the placement of 48 devices.[41] More than 80% of devices were correctly positioned and no cartilage or vascular injuries were documented. Entrapment of the popliteus tendon and superficial medial collateral ligament (MCL) by the backstop

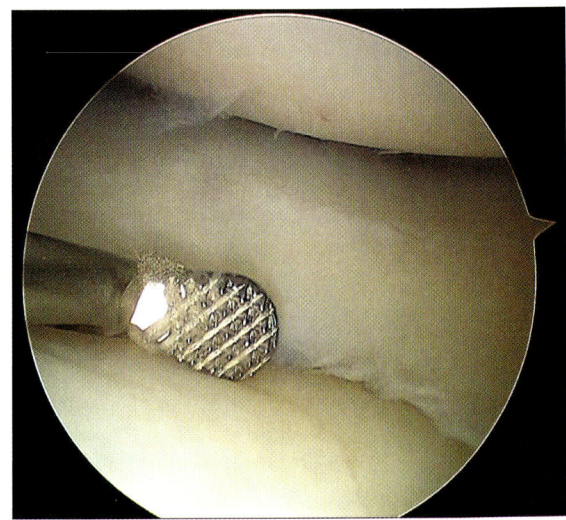

Figure 34-20. Rasping of the tear and adjacent meniscus augments the healing response.

anchors were the only potential complications encountered. These findings are also common with suture techniques and are of doubtful clinical significance.

ADJUNCTS TO MENISCAL REPAIR

Regardless of the meniscal repair technique chosen, several adjuncts may be used to enhance meniscal healing. First, meniscal or synovial rasping is routinely used to stimulate enhanced blood supply and generate a healing response (Fig. 34-20). Less commonly, trephination may be used to improve short-term vascular access to the red-white zone of the meniscus.[25] Finally, exogenous fibrin clot may be useful in the setting of isolated meniscal repair.[7,48] Fibrin clot enhances the local healing environment by placing factors found in the peripheral blood, such as growth factors, fibrin, and platelets, at the site of repair. This produces a healing milieu similar to the setting of concurrent ACL reconstruction. One study, in particular, documented a 41% failure rate in isolated meniscal repairs without the addition of exogenous fibrin clot versus 8% failure rate with its use.[32]

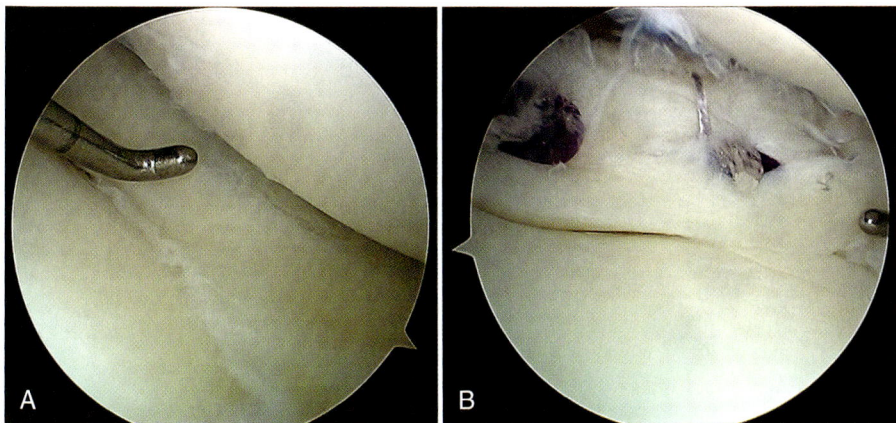

Figure 34-21. Some larger or more complex tears may require hybrid repairs. **A,** This lateral meniscal tear was 3.5 cm long and extended into the lateral body. **B,** It was repaired using a combination of RapidLoc all-inside devices and an inside-out suture technique.

REHABILITATION

The postoperative protocol must take into consideration restrictions in range of motion, weight bearing, and return to activity. In patients undergoing concurrent ACL reconstruction, a standard postoperative ACL protocol is appropriate, with a few modifications.[54] It has been shown that the menisci transmit 50% of the joint load when the knee is fully extended and 85% to 90% of the joint load when the knee is in flexion.[17] A hinged brace limiting motion during weight bearing to 0 to 90 degrees for the initial 4 to 5 weeks is typically recommended. Active, non–weight-bearing range of motion is gradually advanced, but extremes of flexion or hyperextension should be avoided. Deep squatting should be avoided for 4 to 5 months. In addition, restricted weight bearing with crutches for the initial 6 weeks following meniscal repair is also recommended to protect the repair site. Return to athletics is primarily determined by the ACL protocol, which includes a full release to activity by 6 months. Isolated meniscal repairs proceed with similar restrictions, with an expected return to athletics at 4 to 5 months.

A more accelerated postoperative protocol is advocated by some, with no restrictions on weight bearing or range of motion. However, as noted earlier, this may be a contributing factor to decreased success rates. In another study, an aggressive postoperative protocol was initially used with immediate unrestricted weight bearing and unlimited braceless range of motion.[32] Half of these patients had failure of the meniscal repair and the authors subsequently modified their protocol to include restricted weight bearing with crutches for 4 weeks and no squatting for 4 months. These modifications reduced their failure rate to 24% in the remaining patients. Postoperative restrictions in weight bearing and motion may be particularly important for all-inside meniscal repairs as opposed to suture-based repairs. Further study is warranted comparing conservative with aggressive rehabilitation protocols and results based on repair technique.

SUMMARY

The preservation of meniscal tissue is ideal and meniscal repair techniques continue to evolve. It is critically important, however, to assess meniscal tears for repair suitability because not all tears can or should be repaired. Characteristics of both the meniscal tear and patient must be considered. The final determination of partial meniscectomy versus repair and method of repair is frequently made at the time of arthroscopy. The surgeon must therefore be prepared for several options.

All-inside techniques were previously reserved for cases with an optimal healing environment, such as in the setting of concurrent ACL reconstruction. Whereas a few early studies documented similar results to inside-out sutures for isolated repairs as well, this remains a reasonable approach until further studies with the fourth-generation devices are available that demonstrate long-term success. Hybrid meniscal repairs, with all-inside devices used in the far posterior aspect of the tear, where neurovascular risk is increased, and inside-out sutures used for the body of the tear, are another potential indication (Fig. 34-21). Hybrid techniques may also be an effective fixation strategy for meniscal transplantation. Potential contraindications to all-inside repairs are meniscocapsular separations (lack intact meniscal rim to anchor the device) and anterior horn tears (difficult to access).

Although all the fourth-generation devices have in common a suture-based design and the ability to adjust tension for enhanced compression, each device is unique, with its own inherent limitations. Therefore, one must be careful not to extrapolate the results with one device to all devices to justify the use of the latest available device without supporting research. Long-term studies of the fourth-generation all-inside devices and further direct, comparative studies in the setting of isolated meniscal repairs are needed.

KEY REFERENCES

Albrecht-Olsen P, Kristensen G, Burgaard P, et al: The arrow versus horizontal suture in arthroscopic meniscus repair: a prospective randomized study with arthroscopic evaluation. Knee Surg Sports Traumatol Arthrosc 7:268–273, 1999.

Barber FA, Herbert MA, Richards DP: Load to failure testing of new meniscal repair devices. Arthroscopy 20:45–50, 2004.

Barber FA, Herbert MA, Schroeder A, et al: Biomechanical testing of new meniscal repair techniques containing ultra high-molecular weight polyethylene suture. Arthroscopy 25:959–967, 2009.

Barber FA, Schroeder FA, Oro FB, Beavis RC: FasT-Fix meniscal repair: mid-term results. Arthroscopy 24:1342–1348, 2008.

Billante MJ, Diduch DR, Lunardini DJ, et al: Meniscal repair using an all-inside, rapidly absorbing, tensionable device. Arthroscopy 24:779–785, 2008.

Cohen SB, Khurana S, Corraine C, et al: The result of isolated meniscal repairs: evaluation of return to function and incidence of re-tear. Arthroscopy 25:e19–e20, 2009

Kalliakmanis A, Zourntos S, Bousgas D, Nilolaou P: Comparison of arthroscopic meniscal repair results using 3 different meniscal repair devices in anterior cruciate ligament reconstruction patients. Arthroscopy 24:810–816, 2008.

Kocabey Y, Chang HC, Brand JC, et al: A biomechanical comparison of the FasT-Fix meniscal repair suture system and the RapidLoc device in cadaver meniscus. Arthroscopy 22:406–413, 2006.

Lee GP, Diduch DR: Deteriorating outcomes after meniscal repair using the Meniscus Arrow in knees undergoing concurrent anterior cruciate ligament reconstruction: increased failure rate with long-term follow-up. Am J Sports Med 33:1138–1141, 2005.

Logan M, Watts M, Owen J, Myers P: Meniscal repair in the elite athlete: results of 45 repairs with a minimum 5-year follow-up. Am J Sports Med 37:1131–1134, 2009.

Miller MD, Kline AJ, Gonzales J, Beach WR: Pitfalls associated with FasT-Fix meniscal repair. Arthroscopy 18:939–943, 2002.

Quinby JS, Golish SR, Hart JA, Diduch DR: All-inside meniscal repair using a new flexible, tensionable device. Am J Sports Med 34:1281–1286, 2006.

Toman CV, Dunn WR, Spindler KP, et al: Success of meniscal repair at anterior cruciate ligament reconstruction. Am J Sports Med 37:1111–1115, 2009.

Turman KA, Diduch DR: Meniscal repair: indications and techniques. J Knee Surg 21:154–162, 2008.

Turman KA, Diduch DR, Miller MD: All-inside meniscal repair. Sports Health 1:438–444, 2009.

Full references for this chapter can be found on www.expertconsult.com.

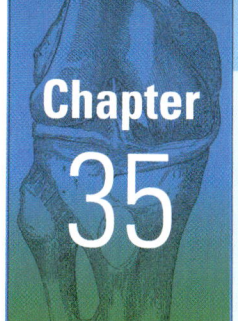

Chapter 35

Meniscal Allograft Transplantation

Kostas Economopoulos, Tom R. Carter, and Anikar Chhabra

Our understanding of the function of the meniscus has evolved over the past half- century. Historically, the meniscus was considered a vestigial remnant of leg muscle that could be removed without any harmful effect.[66] Our views of the meniscus changed when Fairbanks[23] reported the importance of the meniscus in the protection of articular cartilage of the knee and described the radiologic changes that occur following meniscectomy. Currently, every attempt at preserving the meniscus is made; however, meniscal repair or a partial meniscectomy is not always possible, and total meniscectomy may be the only available option. Meniscal allograft transplantation has become a viable option for patients who develop pain following total or near total meniscectomy. The first meniscal allograft was associated with complete knee transplantation over a century ago.[43] In 1984, Milachowski and colleagues[45] performed the first modern meniscal allograft transplantation in humans. Since the first meniscal transplantations, our techniques have improved and transitioned from open procedures to arthroscopy-assisted procedures. As of 2002, almost 4000 transplants have been performed worldwide and almost 800 procedures are performed annually.[62] The number of meniscal transplants performed each year continues to increase, making it important for the orthopedic surgeon to understand the indications, complications, multiple techniques, and results of this procedure.

MENISCAL ANATOMY AND FUNCTION

Anatomy

Menisci are fibrocartilaginous biphasic structures containing solid and fluid phases. Water makes up roughly 75% of the meniscus and collagen fibers and a small amount of proteoglycans and cells make up the other 20% to 25%. Collagen makes up between 60% to 95% of the dry weight of the meniscus, with type I collagen constituting 90% of the collagen and types II, III, V, and VI contributing a small amount to the dry weight of the meniscus. The solid phase also contains proteoglycans, which are covalently attached to negatively charged glycosaminoglycans. The charged extracellular matrix allows water to bind, leading to a slower flow of water through the meniscus. The biochemical makeup of the meniscus allow it to serve several functions.

The structural orientation of the collagen fibers is related to its function. Collagen fibers are primarily oriented in a circumferential manner. Radially oriented fibers function as ties for the circumferentially oriented fibers and resist longitudinal splitting of the meniscus. During axial loading, the femoral condylar surfaces displace the menisci radially because of their concave wedge shape. The menisci convert axial load into tensile strain. Because menisci are anchored anteriorly and posteriorly, this displacement generates circumferential hoop stress that resists extrusion of the menisci from between the femoral condyle and tibial plateau. Biomechanical studies have shown that the meniscus is 100 times stronger and stiffer in the circumferential direction compared with the radial direction. The low circumferential shear strength is believed to be in part responsible for the occurrence of longitudinal tears.[56]

The menisci are relatively avascular, especially in the inner third of their body. The limited peripheral blood supply mainly comes from the lateral and medial genicular arteries. A perimeniscal capillary plexus within the synovial and capsular tissues of the knee joint arises from these feeding vessels. In the adult, vascular penetration is 10% to 30% of the width of the medial meniscus and 10% to 25% of the width of the lateral meniscus.[6] Because the menisci are predominantly avascular, nutrition to the meniscus must be derived through diffusion or mechanical pumping.

Knowledge of the meniscal anatomy, in particular bony attachment sites, is imperative when performing meniscal transplantation. The menisci form a semilunar wedge-shaped structure that fills the void created by the incongruous femoral condyle and tibial plateau. The medial meniscus is an oval-shaped fibrocartilaginous structure covering almost 30% of the medial tibial plateau. The anterior and posterior horns of the medial meniscus are further apart than the anterior and posterior horns of the lateral meniscus. The anterior horn of the medial meniscus is a flat fan-shaped structure that inserts in line with the medial tibial eminence 6 to 8 mm anterior to the anterior cruciate ligament (ACL) tibial insertion. The insertion site is under the patellar fat pad at the junction of the medial tibial plateau and anterior tibia, and often requires anterior fat pad débridement for good visualization. Landmarks demarcating the bony insertion of the anterior horn of the medial meniscus include the anterior border of the ACL tibial insertion, articular margin of the anteromedial tibial plateau, and anterior intercondylar fossa.[36] The anterior horn of the medial meniscus is often also secured by the intrameniscal ligament, which connects to the anterior horn of the lateral meniscus. The posterior horn of the medial meniscus inserts directly anterior to the tibial insertion of the posterior cruciate ligament (PCL), on the downslope of the posterior intercondylar fossa, behind the posterior horn insertion of the lateral meniscus. The PCL, medial tibial spine, and articular margin of the posteromedial tibial plateau serve as arthroscopic landmarks for the insertion of the posterior horn of the medial meniscus.

The lateral meniscus covers approximately 50% of the lateral plateau and has a more circular shape compared with the medial meniscus. The insertion site of the anterior horn of the lateral meniscus is directly anterior to the lateral tibial spine and adjacent to the tibial insertion of the ACL. Arthroscopic landmarks include the anterior half of the ACL tibial insertion, lateral tibial spine, and articular margin of the anterolateral tibial plateau. The posterior horn of the lateral meniscus inserts directly posterior to the lateral tibial spine, adjacent and anterior to the insertion of the posterior horn of the medial meniscus. Arthroscopic landmarks identifying the insertion of the posterior horn of the lateral meniscus include the posterior border of the ACL tibial insertion, lateral tibial spine, and articular margin of the posterolateral tibial plateau.[36]

Compared with the lateral meniscus, the medial meniscus is firmly attached to the peripheral structures and has less anteroposterior mobility. In flexion, the medial meniscus has only up to 5 mm of translation compared with the 11 mm of the lateral meniscus. The medial meniscus has several peripheral attachments, including the coronary ligaments anteriorly, joint capsule and medial collateral ligament centrally, and joint capsule posteriorly. The popliteus interrupts the posterior capsular attachments of the lateral meniscus, and there are no attachments to the lateral collateral ligament.

Function

The meniscus serves several important functions in the knee, including load bearing, shock absorption, joint stability, and joint lubrication. During weight bearing, the meniscus experiences several stresses including tensile, compressive, and shear stresses. The medial meniscus transmits 50% of the joint load of the medial compartment whereas the lateral meniscus transmits 70% of the joint load of the lateral compartment. This increases to 85% of the joint load when the knee is flexed to 90 degrees.[2] Radin and colleagues[54] have demonstrated that these loads are well distributed when the menisci are intact. Total medial meniscectomy leads to 50% to 70% decreased contact area and an increase in contact stress of 100%.[27,37] Because the lateral meniscus carries a higher proportion of the joint load because of the surface area, a lateral meniscectomy leads to a significantly higher increase in contact force compared with a medial meniscectomy. Total lateral meniscectomy leads to a 40% to 50% decrease in contact area and an increase in contact force of 200% to 300% compared with the intact meniscus.[7]

The biphasic nature of the meniscus allows it to function as shock absorber. Interstitial fluid flow and solid matrix deformation during loading cause the meniscus to act as a viscoelastic material, leading to creep and stress relaxation. Knees with an intact meniscus have a 20% higher shock absorption capacity compared with knees that do not have intact menisci.[73] In addition to their other functions, the menisci also play an important role in enhancing joint stability.[41] Medial meniscectomy in the ACL-intact knee has little effect on anteroposterior motion, but in the ACL-deficient knee, it results in an increase in translation of almost 60% at 90 degrees of flexion. Force on the medial meniscus increases by 52% in extension and 197% at 60 degrees of flexion in the ACL-deficient knee.[3] The conformity created by the meniscus promotes the viscous hydrodynamic action required for fluid film lubrication. This lubrication assists in the overall lubrication of the articular surfaces of the knee joint.[56] The multiple functions of the meniscus depend on their microstructure and macrostructure, both of which can be addressed by meniscal transplantation.

NATURAL HISTORY OF THE MENISCUS-DEFICIENT KNEE

In 1948, Fairbanks[23] described the changes that occur in the knee following meniscectomy, including ridge formation, narrowing of the joint space, and flattening of the femoral condyles. These changes lead to alterations in the biomechanics of the knee joint. Cox and associates[19] have studied the effects of partial and total meniscectomy in dogs. Partial meniscectomy led to less severe degenerative changes, with the degree of degeneration directly related to the amount of meniscus resected. In the dogs with total meniscectomy, the degree of degenerative change was directly related to the amount of missing fibrocartilage. It was concluded that the knee menisci function to protect the articular cartilage from degenerative damages. McGinty and coworkers[44] have compared the outcomes of patients undergoing total and partial meniscectomy. Using the Fairbank criteria, they found that patients with partial meniscectomy have less narrowing of the joint line compared with patients with a total meniscectomy. They identified early radiographic degenerative changes in 62% of 89 patients treated with total meniscectomy compared with 36% of 39 treated with partial meniscectomy. Because the lateral meniscus carries a higher percentage of the load force of the knee, degenerative changes generally progress more rapidly in the lateral compartment following lateral meniscectomy.[35,78]

BIOLOGY OF THE TRANSPLANTED MENISCAL ALLOGRAFT

Several characteristics of the meniscus make it optimal tissue to transplant. First, meniscal tissue elicits a minimal immune response. Immune reactions have been described in 1.3% of transplants reported in the literature.[64] Ochi and colleagues[48] placed fresh meniscal allograft in the subcutaneous tissue of mice and evaluated their immune response. They detected no specific antibodies in the serum throughout the 24-week period after grafting. They concluded that in mice, fresh meniscus was not immunogenic. Although the normal meniscus consists of relatively few chondrocytes embedded in an extracellular matrix, it also contains class II and ABH-positive endothelial cells and class II–positive synovial cells.[40] These antigens are present at the moment of transplantation and could evoke an immune response in the host that would modulate the results of meniscal allografting. Rodeo and associates[57] have performed an immunologic study that identified class I and II human leukocyte antigens (HLAs) on frozen meniscal allografts. Twenty-eight deep frozen and nonirradiated samples were evaluated. Overall, 9 of 12 specimens contained immunoreactive cells, including B lymphocytes or cytotoxic T cells in the meniscus or synovial tissue. No frank immunologic rejection was identified. The immune response to the meniscal allograft does not seem to affect the clinical outcome of the transplantation.

The primary functions of the meniscus can be accomplished, even if the structure is devoid of live cells. The meniscus is for the most part acellular, and most of its function is derived from its structure. The fate of the meniscal cells that accompany the meniscal allograft is unknown. Arnoczky and coworkers[4] have studied the cellular repopulation of deep-frozen meniscal allografts. The menisci appeared to be repopulated with cells that originated from the adjacent synovium; however, the central core of the meniscus remained acellular. There was also loss of collagen orientation in the superficial layer of the meniscus. The structural remodeling associated with the cellular repopulation of deep-frozen meniscal allografts may make the transplanted meniscus more susceptible to injury. Jackson and colleagues[33] have used DNA probes to determine the fate of donor fibrocytes following meniscal transplantation. The results of this study demonstrated that host cells rapidly repopulate the transplanted meniscus. There is no evidence that these new cells will maintain the extracellular matrix of the meniscus on a long-term basis. Similarly, DeBeer and associates[20] have shown that human cryopreserved meniscal allograft donor cells are 95% replaced by host cells 1 year after transplantation. Wada and coworkers[76] have noted that frozen meniscal allografts show collagen remodeling coincident with revascularization and cellular repopulation. Types I and III procollagen mRNA levels were elevated, representing active remodeling. These data indicate the adaptation of the repopulating cells from the host to the frozen allograft at 26 weeks after transplantation. In the goat model, Jackson and colleagues[34] have shown the proteoglycan concentration to be decreased in the meniscal allograft. They also noted that transplanted menisci undergo gradual, incomplete revascularization, with new capillaries derived from the capsular and synovial attachments. Our understanding of meniscal biology following transplantation has improved, but further research is necessary to answer several unanswered questions.

GRAFT PREPARATION AND DISEASE TRANSMISSION

Prevention of disease transmission with meniscal transplantation begins with careful donor screening. Transmission of HIV with frozen connective tissue allografts is estimated to be 1 in 8 million.[10] Blood and tissue from the donor are sampled at the time of graft harvest and remain in quarantine while being tested for hepatitis B and C, syphilis, and human immunodeficiency virus (HIV). Tissue is procured within 12 hours of death for fresh grafts or within 24 hours if the body is stored at 4° C. Grafts are processed by débridement, pulsatile ultrasonic washing, and use of ethanol to denature proteins. Beginning in early 2005, HIV and hepatitis C screening were performed using direct nucleic acid testing by the polymerase chain reaction (PCR) assay. This method decreases the window that these viral infections can be missed, from 4 to 6 weeks down to 10 days.[11] Harvesting is done in a sterile

fashion or a clean nonsterile environment and secondarily sterilized. Secondary sterilization methods include the use of ethylene oxide, gamma radiation, or chemical means. Negative effects to the meniscal allograft have been reported with secondary sterilization. Gamma radiation at the level required to eliminate viral DNA may adversely affect the material properties of the meniscus.[68] Yahia and Zukor[75] have shown that exposure to more than 2.5 mrad of gamma radiation negatively affects the mechanical properties of collagen-containing tissues. Because 3 mrad of gamma radiation are recommended to eliminate HIV DNA, gamma radiation is not recommended. Ethylene oxide has been discontinued because of reports of graft failure and synovitis. Ethylene chlorohydrin, a byproduct of ethylene oxide, has been found to induce synovitis in musculoskeletal allografts.[34]

The optimal method for meniscal graft preservation has yet to be determined. Currently, there are four primary preservation methods, including fresh, cryopreserved, fresh-frozen (deep-frozen), and freeze-dried (lyophilization; Table 35-1).

Fresh graft preservation leads to logistic issues for transplantation. The short period of time to size and perform serologic testing properly makes finding a suitable recipient difficult. Because of these issues, fresh grafts have limited use in clinical practice today. The question still remains whether fresh graft is superior to grafts preserved using the three other methods. Good results have been reported in patients transplanted with fresh grafts. Verdonk[70] has found intact grafts of all 40 transplanted meniscal allografts using follow-up magnetic resonance imaging (MRI). One of the benefits of using a fresh graft includes viable cells present in the graft, which may be important in cartilage transplantation. However, Jackson and associates[33] have shown that donor DNA in the transplanted meniscus was entirely replaced by host DNA at 4-week follow-up. The importance of viable cells in the meniscal transplant remains to be determined.

Cryopreservation has provided a useful alternative to fresh grafts in terms of safety and function. The graft is thawed in the operating room just prior to surgery. Arnoczky and associates[5] have shown that the material properties of transplanted cryopreserved allografts in dogs are similar to those of normal menisci after 6 months. Cell viability ranging between 5% and 54% has been described in the literature. Gelber and coworkers[29] have shown that meniscal cryopreservation does not alter the meniscal ultrastructure or the biomechanical properties. Fabbriciani and colleagues[22] reported no difference in appearance or healing between meniscal allografts that were cryopreserved and deep-frozen. The expense and difficulty of this process, along with the uncertainty of donor

Table 35-1 Graft Preservation Techniques

Parameter	PRESERVATION TECHNIQUE			
	Fresh	Cryopreserved	Fresh-Frozen	Freeze-Dried (Lyophilization)
Viable cells	Yes	Yes	Acellular	Acellular
Method of maintenance	Lactated Ringer's solution at 4° C	Controlled freezing process	Stored at −80° C	Vacuum freezing
Duration of maintenance	7 days	10 yr	Up to 5 yr	Indefinite
Advantages	Donor cell preservation and minimal disruption of meniscal integrity	Main collagen framework maintained	Low cost	Low cost

cell viability, have decreased the popularity of this preservation process.

Fresh-frozen meniscal preservation is a simpler and less expensive method than cryopreservation. Deep freezing has been shown to destroy viable cells of connective tissue and to denature histocompatibility antigens, making frozen allografts less likely to provoke an immune response.[9] Milachowski and colleagues[45] have reported shrinkage in one of five deep-frozen grafts by MRI. At 48 weeks, deep-frozen grafts showed little revascularization or remodeling, but good preservation.

Lyophilization has been shown to destroy viable cells of connective tissue and to denature histocompatibility antigens.[9] Milachowski and associates[45] have reported shrinkage in 9 of 10 lyophilized and gamma-sterilized allografts. All lyophilized allografts were remodeled and completely revascularized at 48 weeks. The same group of patients was reviewed 14 years postoperatively.[77] Second-look arthroscopy and MRI showed shrinkage of the lyophilized grafts. Gelber and associates[29] have evaluated the collagen meniscal architecture of excised meniscal transplants at the time of total knee replacement. They found the fibrils in frozen meniscal allografts to be of smaller diameter and in more disarray compared with nonfrozen controls. These findings may explain the shrinking associated with this type of preservation.

INDICATIONS AND CONTRAINDICATIONS FOR MENISCAL TRANSPLANTATION

The indications for meniscal transplantation continue to evolve as long-term clinical results become available. Currently, meniscal transplantation is a salvage procedure for patients with meniscus-deficient knees. The goal of meniscal transplantation is to reduce pain and prevent progression of arthritis. Consideration of meniscal transplantation should only be entertained when nonsurgical measures to control pain have been exhausted, including activity modification, anti-inflammatories, injections, and unloading bracing. With concurrent ACL reconstruction, earlier meniscal transplantation may improve clinical outcomes.[30,41,61] Veltri and coworkers[69] have defined the ideal meniscal transplantation candidate to be skeletally mature, younger than 50 years, post-total or subtotal meniscectomy, with a ligamentously stable knee or planned stabilization, with no evidence of malalignment, and with minimal arthrosis. Although they used 50 years old as the upper age limit in patients with minimal arthritis, this is controversial because physiologic age is more accurate than absolute age.[49]

Outerbridge published a classification of cartilage lesions associated with chondromalacia patellae in 1961 (Table 35-2).[49] This classification system has been modified to describe articular cartilage lesions seen at the time of arthroscopy. It can be used to classify the patient's arthrosis to determine whether he or she is a candidate for meniscal transplantation. Garret,[28] Noyes and coworkers,[46] and Cole and colleagues[16] have demonstrated improved results in meniscal transplantation in patients whose degenerative changes are Outerbridge grade I or II. Patients with Outerbridge grade III or IV degeneration levels had less predictable outcomes. No studies were able to define whether the poor

Table 35-2 Outerbridge Classification

Grade	Features
Original Description*	
I	Softening and swelling of the cartilage
II	Fragmentation and fissuring $<\frac{1}{2}$ inch in diameter
III	Fragmentation and fissuring $>\frac{1}{2}$ inch in diameter
IV	Erosion of cartilage down to bone
Currently Accepted Description	
I	Softening
II	Partial-thickness fissures
III	Full-thickness fissures
IV	Exposed subchondral bone

*Initial description was based on macroscopic changes of the patella. This system was modified to describe arthroscopic changes in the articular cartilage.

results found in patients with advanced degenerative changes was caused by the degenerative disease itself or associated knee malalignment.

Another critical factor in determining a successful candidate is the mechanical alignment of the knee. Malalignment is defined as valgus or varus asymmetry between 2 and 4 degrees compared with the contralateral knee, or the mechanical axis falling into the affected meniscus-deficient compartment on weight-bearing films. Meniscal transplantation in a malaligned knee causes abnormal pressure on the meniscal allograft, resulting in impaired vascularization, degeneration, and failure of the graft.[55] In cases of malalignment, meniscal transplantation is contraindicated until a concurrent corrective osteotomy is performed. Cameron and Saha[12] have reported 85% good results in patients undergoing meniscal transplantation and corrective osteotomy. It remains to be determined whether the osteotomy or the meniscal transplantation led to the clinical improvement.

Meniscal transplantation can be considered for patients with concomitant ACL instability. Garret[28] has reported significantly improved KT-1000 arthrometer results for ACL reconstruction when performed in combination with medial meniscal allograft transplantation compared with a group of patients who underwent ACL reconstruction only, with persistent medial meniscal deficiency.

The primary absolute contraindication to meniscal transplantation is advanced arthrosis of the meniscus-deficient knee. Other contraindications to meniscal transplantation include previous infection and inflammatory arthritis. Obesity is a relative contraindication to surgery because of the increased force across the joint, leading to an increased failure rate. The indications and contraindications for meniscal transplantation will continue to evolve as long-term results become available. A summary of indications and contraindications is listed in Table 35-3.

PREOPERATIVE CONSIDERATIONS

Evaluation

The key to successful meniscal transplantation includes patient selection and appropriate preoperative evaluation. The operative report of all previous surgeries should be

Table 35-3 Contraindications
to Meniscal Transplantation

Contraindication	Features
Absolute	Advanced arthritis Joint space narrowing Femoral flattening Osteophytes Outerbridge grades III and IV changes Joint incongruity
Relative	Malalignment Focal chondral defects Ligament instability Obesity Rheumatoid arthritis Gout Immune compromise Metabolic disease Infection Lack of commitment to postoperative restrictions

reviewed. In addition, any available intraoperative photographs can be used to determine the extent of articular damage and degeneration, along with the status of the remaining meniscus. If previous arthroscopic pictures are not available, and appropriateness for meniscal transplant is unknown, diagnostic arthroscopy is indicated to determine the degree of meniscus loss and arthrosis.

The preoperative physical examination should include gait inspection, stance, and the ability for the patient to get in the squatting position. Prior incisions should be evaluated. Palpation of the joint line, McMurray's test, knee range of motion, presence of effusion, and muscle strength and wasting should all be evaluated. The examination must include a thorough ligamentous evaluation and definition of axial alignment of the limb. Patient compliance should be gauged throughout the evaluation.

Radiograph studies should include weight-bearing, 45-degree flexion posteroanterior, Merchant, and weight-bearing lateral views using magnification markers for sizing. Long-leg alignment radiographs are imperative to evaluate lower limb mechanical alignment. MRI is important for determining the status of the hyaline cartilage, subchondral bone, and menisci.

Graft Sizing

Good clinical outcomes following meniscal transplantation rely on selection of an appropriately sized meniscal allograft. The tolerance of size mismatch in knees undergoing meniscal transplantation is not known. Although too small a meniscal allograft does lead to uneven contact forces, more meniscus is not always better. The meniscus must be properly sized for optimum reduction of contact pressures. Dienst and associates[21] have shown that oversized lateral meniscal allografts lead to greater forces across the articular cartilage, whereas undersized allografts result in normal forces across the articular cartilage but greater forces across the meniscus. They concluded that grafts within 10% of the native meniscus were able to reproduce contact mechanics close to the intact state. Huang and coworkers[32] have found increased contact pressures when allografts did not match the native menisci. The

greatest predictor of differences in contact pressure was the difference in the width of the menisci. It was concluded that protocols used to select allografts should focus on cross-sectional parameters to match the native meniscus.

Sizing of allografts is done using plain radiography, computed tomography (CT), or MRI or by making direct measurements. The use of the contralateral knee in patients with prior meniscectomy has been described to help sizing. However, Johnson and colleagues[38] have shown that there is variability in meniscal size between opposite knees. The most commonly used method for sizing today is plain radiographs. Pollard and associates[52] have found that the meniscal width equals the distance (coronal) from the peak of the tibial eminence to the periphery of the tibial metaphysis on anteroposterior films. Medial meniscal length is 80% and lateral meniscal length is 70% of the measured sagittal length of the tibial plateau on the lateral radiograph. Measurement error averaged 7.8% by these parameters. Axial CT scans can size the meniscus without concern for rotation or magnification. However, the patient must endure a much larger load of radiation. Shaffer and coworkers[63] have compared the accuracy of plain x-rays and MRI for preoperative sizing of meniscal allografts. Overall, MRI was slightly more accurate than plain radiography; however, only 35% of the menisci measured with MRI were within 2 mm of the actual meniscal size. Carpenter and colleagues[13] have compared the accuracy of MRI with both plain radiograph and CT in estimating the size of the meniscal allograft. MRI was found to be the most accurate for meniscal height but consistently underestimated the anteroposterior and mediolateral sizes. Prodromos and associates[53] have compared MRI with plain radiography in estimating the appropriately sized meniscal allograft. They concluded that human knee menisci are bilaterally symmetric in size, and direct MRI measurement of the contralateral intact meniscus predicts actual meniscal size better than estimation of size indirectly from measurement of the tibial plateau on which it is located. They proposed contralateral MRI meniscal measurement as a new gold standard to size menisci before transplantation. Although plain radiographs are currently the gold standard, it appears that MRI techniques are improving and will eventually be the study of choice for determining meniscal allograft size.

SURGICAL TECHNIQUES

Several techniques have been described for meniscal allograft transplantation. The main differences between the techniques include open versus arthroscopically assisted, soft tissue fixation versus bony fixation, and bone plug versus bone-bridge.[64] Initial studies discussing meniscal transplantation described open techniques; however, arthroscopy-assisted techniques have become more popular. Both techniques have shown equivalent outcomes, but the arthroscopic approach decreases surgical morbidity, avoids collateral ligament injury, and promotes early rehabilitation.[12,14,27,45,67] Regardless of the technique used, the most important factor in successful meniscal transplantation is appropriate sizing and anatomic placement of the transplanted meniscus.[16] Although it is technically easier to anchor the meniscus with soft tissue alone, bone promotes improved load transmission and provides more normal biomechanics of the transplanted meniscus.[1,15,51] There remains debate whether bone plugs or bone-bridge is the optimal method for meniscal transplantation. The bone plug method is primarily used in the medial meniscus, where the anterior and posterior horns of the meniscus are separated by greater than 1 cm. Bone plugs allow for minor modifications in the final position of the meniscal horn position, which is useful because of some variation in meniscal horn anatomy.[8,39] Because the distance between the meniscal horns in the lateral compartment is 1 cm or less, use of bone plugs presents the risk of tunnel communication, which may compromise fixation.[36] Lateral meniscal transplantation is typically performed using a bone-bridge technique, in which the two horns of the meniscus are maintained on the same bone block. Proponents of the bone-bridge technique cite ease of insertion and maintenance of the anatomic relationship of the anterior and posterior horns.[18,24] Regardless of the technique used, care must be taken to size the allograft properly and securely fix it to its anatomic anterior and posterior horn footprints along with the capsule peripherally.

Patient Positioning and Initial Evaluation

Once general anesthesia is induced, appropriate prophylactic antibiotics are given. A thorough examination under anesthesia is performed on all patients to determine the stability and range of motion of the knee. A tourniquet should be placed as high as possible on the thigh, but not inflated. Depending on surgeon preference, the operative leg may be placed in a cushioned leg holder or unsupported in the supine position. Visualization of the posteromedial or posterolateral corner is important for medial or lateral allograft transplantation, respectively, facilitating inside-out repair. The contralateral leg should have thromboembolic deterrent (TED) hose and sequential compression devices (SCDs) placed to prevent deep venous thrombosis (DVT). Once the patient is prepped and draped, a diagnostic arthroscopy should be performed to confirm meniscal deficiency and evaluate the status of the articular cartilage and ligaments. The remaining body of the involved meniscus is débrided to a 1- to 2-mm synovial rim, which leaves a vascular source to help graft healing. The anterior and posterior horn attachments are initially preserved to serve as guide points for drilling the tibial tunnels if the bone plug technique is planned. In the lateral compartment, the meniscal rim anterior to the popliteus tendon can often be saved.

Bone Plug Technique

Graft Preparation

The appropriate graft size and side should be confirmed before preparing the meniscal allograft. If the size or side of the meniscal allograft is incorrect, the procedure should be abandoned until the appropriate allograft is available. The allograft will be delivered as a meniscus on a hemi tibial plateau or a complete tibial plateau. The allograft is thawed in warm saline. Once thawed, the first step in preparing the allograft is to remove all ligament tissue from the graft periphery. The anterior and posterior horn insertion sites should be isolated. Preparation of the posterior bone plug begins by placing a guide pin in the center of the attachment site of the posterior horn at roughly a 60-degree angle. A collared pin is then

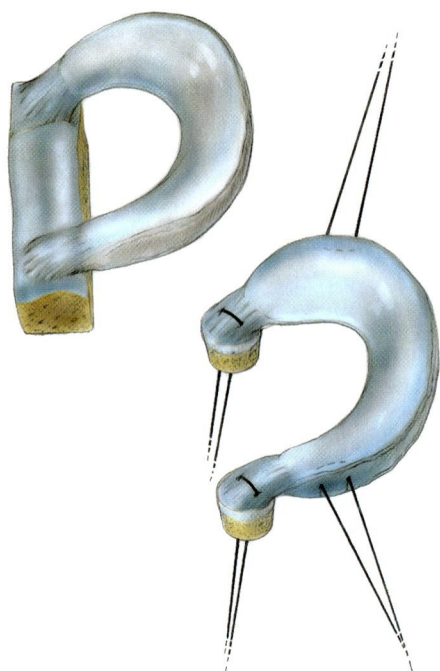

Figure 35-1. Nonabsorbable sutures are placed retrograde through the bone plugs. Guide sutures are preinserted into the posteromedial and anterior portions of the allograft.

placed through the hole in the center of the posterior horn insertion. A coring reamer is placed over the collared pin, creating a bone plug measuring 6 to 7 mm. The posterior bone plug should be beveled to make insertion easier. The top of the posterior horn of the meniscus is marked with a marking pen for orientation. Preparation of the anterior bone plug is performed in the same manner. A guide pin is placed through the anterior horn of the meniscus. Compared with preparation of the posterior bone plug, the guide wire is placed more antegrade for the anterior bone plug. A collared pin is placed over the guide wire in the center of the anterior horn insertion site and a 9- to 10-mm reamer is used to create the bone plug. Two 2-0 nonabsorbable Ethibond sutures are passed retrograde through each bone plug, creating sutures that can be passed through the tibial tunnel for proper allograft placement (Fig. 35-1). A traction suture to facilitate the introduction of the meniscus is created by placing a 0 polydiaxonone suture (PDS) at the junction of the posterior and middle thirds of the meniscus (Fig. 35-2). The anterior aspect of the posterior bone plug is marked with a sterile ink marking pen to assist in orientation.

Preparation of the Recipient Bed

Starting just adjacent to the tibial tubercle, the posterior tibial tunnel is made by placing a guide pin into the anatomic posterior horn attachment of the old meniscus. A tibial tunnel is drilled over the guide wire to a diameter of 9 mm (Fig. 35-3). If ACL reconstruction is to be done, this posterior tunnel is brought out through the lateral side of the tibia so that it will diverge from the ACL tibial tunnel. The rim of this tunnel is smoothed and any remaining posterior horn meniscal tissue is removed. A limited notchplasty of the medial femoral condyle is performed, if necessary. At least

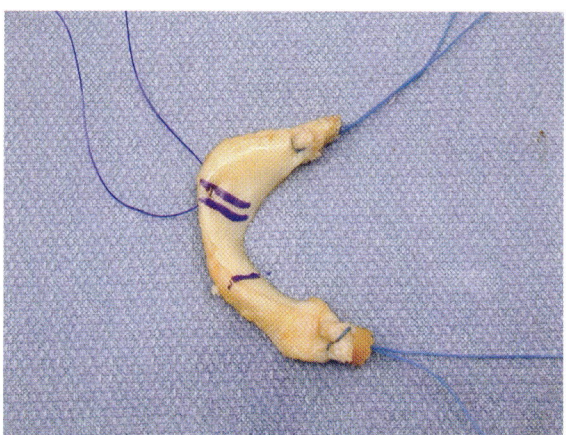

Figure 35-2. A traction suture is placed at the junction of the posterior and middle thirds of the allograft to facilitate the introduction of the meniscus.

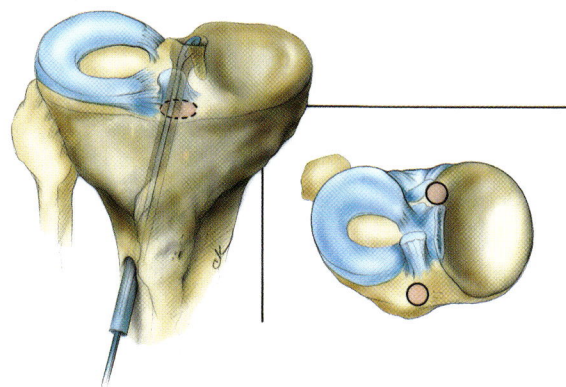

Figure 35-3. The posterior tibial tunnel is created by drilling over a guide pin that has been placed through the footprint of the native posterior horn attachment.

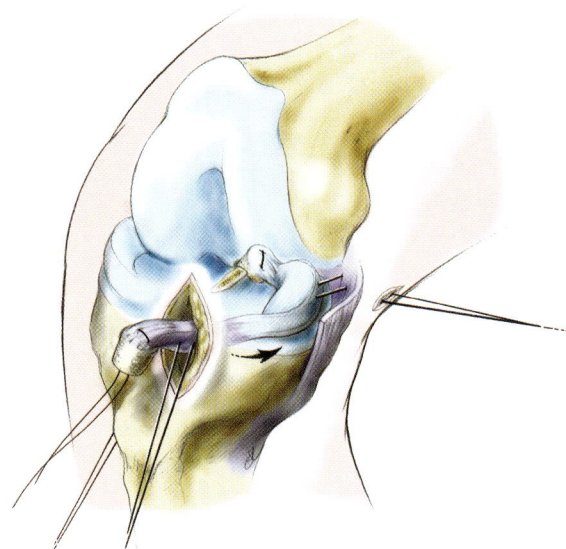

Figure 35-4. The posterior bone plug is passed through the anteromedial arthrotomy with the assistance of the secondary meniscal body suture.

8 mm of opening adjacent to the posterior cruciate ligament in the femoral notch is needed to pass the posterior osseous portion of the graft.[47]

Meniscus Implantation

The tourniquet is inflated for the first portion of implantation. A 3-cm vertical posteromedial incision is made just posterior to the superficial medial collateral ligament. The fascia anterior to the sartorius is incised and the pes anserinus muscles are retracted posteriorly. The plane between the semimembranosus tendon and capsule is established. Blunt dissection is used to separate the medial aspect of the gastrocnemius tendon and posteromedial aspect of the capsule. A 3-cm anteromedial incision is created just medial to the patellar tendon. The posterior bone plug with attached meniscus is passed through the anteromedial arthrotomy, along with the secondary meniscal body suture (Fig. 35-4). The secondary meniscal body suture is passed out through the posteromedial approach. The knee is then flexed to 90 degrees for best visualization. The posterior attachment guide wire is retrieved and the sutures attached to the posterior bone are passed. To assist in passage of the posterior bone portion of the graft, the knee is flexed to 20 degrees and a maximum

valgus load placed on the knee. Pulling on the posteromedial suture and using a blunt instrument helps reduce the meniscus into its proper anatomic location. The knee can be flexed and extended to assess meniscal fit and displacement.

A guide pin is then passed through the insertion site of the anterior horn footprint. A 9-mm tunnel is reamed over the guide pin. A Houston suture passer is passed up the anterior tunnel and the sutures on the anterior bone plug are captured and brought down the anterior tunnel. The bone plug is press-fit into the anterior tunnel using a tamp. The sutures attached to the anterior and posterior bone plugs are tied to each other over an anterior bone bridge or button.

The anterior arthrotomy is closed and peripheral attachment of the meniscus is performed by passing sutures arthroscopically. An inside-out technique is used to attach the periphery of the meniscus to the capsule. Eight to 10 vertically placed 2-0 nonabsorbable mattress sutures are placed from posterior to anterior using standard inside-out technique. The sutures should be placed superiorly and inferiorly, with constant tensioning of the meniscus from posterior to anterior. After final inspection with the knee in flexion and extension, the remaining wounds are closed in typical fashion.

Bone-Bridge Technique

Graft Preparation

Following thawing and inspection of the meniscal allograft block, the attachment sites of the anterior and posterior horn are identified on the bone block (Fig. 35-5). Using an oscillating saw, the bone-bridge is cut to a width of 7 mm, a height of 1 cm, and a length of 35 mm. Care must be taken not to detach the anterior or posterior horn from their bony attachment. A rasp that is used to create the slot in the tibia can be used to template the bone-bridge. A meniscal bridge sizing jig is used to establish the definitive width of the box at 7 to 8 mm. The bone-bridge should loosely fit though the sizing

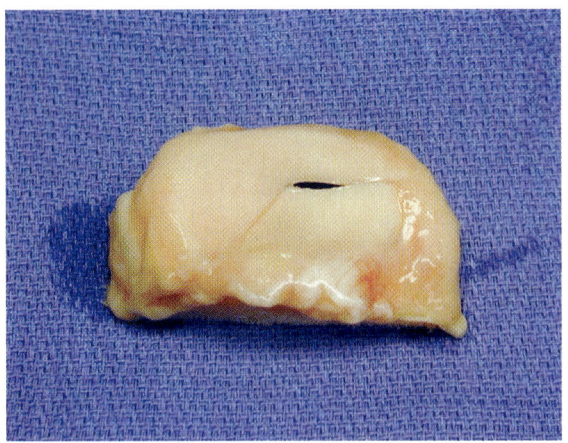

Figure 35-5. The meniscal allograft block is thawed and inspected. The anterior and posterior horns are then identified and marked.

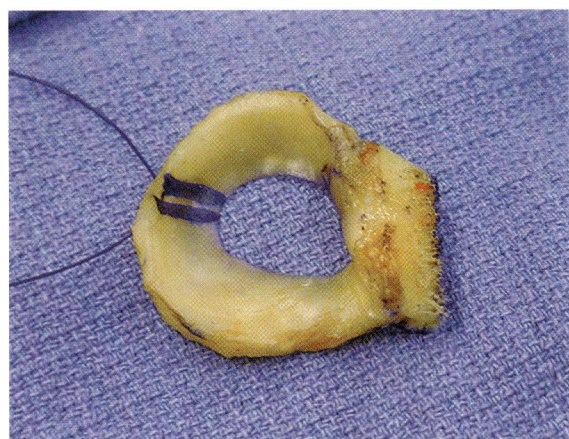

Figure 35-7. A nonabsorbable suture is placed at the junction of the posterior and middle thirds of the allograft meniscus. The suture will assist in meniscal placement.

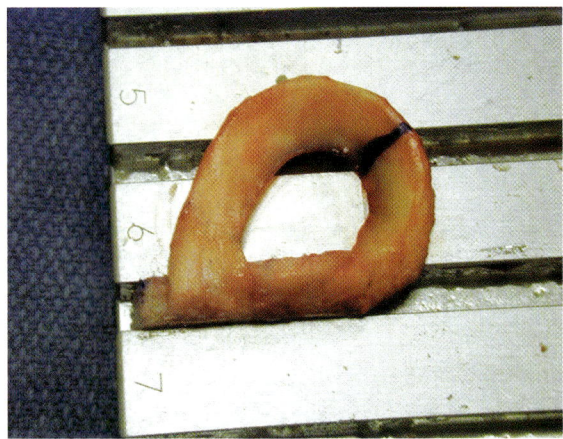

Figure 35-6. A sizing jig is used to confirm that the bone-bridge will loosely pass through the created slot.

jig (Fig. 35-6). A no. 0 PDS is placed at the junction of the posterior and middle thirds of the meniscus to function as a reduction suture, which will be used for meniscal placement (Fig. 35-7).

Tibial Preparation

The remaining meniscus is trimmed down to a 1- to 2-mm rim until punctuate bleeding occurs. The remnants of the anterior and posterior horns are left to act as footprints and assist in graft placement. A 3-cm anterolateral arthrotomy is made adjacent to the patellar tendon. A spinal needle may be used to create a reference line with the anterior and posterior horns. Electrocauterization is used to mark the correct center of the anterior and posterior horn attachment sites. A superficial reference line is created between the two horns, initially using an arthroscopic shaver and then a 4-mm burr. The reference slot should bury the 4-mm burr and be parallel to the saggital slope of the tibial plateau. A depth gauge is used to determine whether the slot is level by placing the hook of the depth gauge over the posterior cortex. An insertion pin is placed through a drill guide parallel to the tibial plateau in the saggital plane. The pin should not penetrate the posterior cortex to protect the neurovascular bundle. The

drill guide is removed and a cannulated 7- or 8-mm reamer is used to drill over the guide pin. The reamer can be followed arthroscopically as it passes through the provisional slot. A 7- or 8-mm box cutter is gently impacted into the provisional slot to the level of the posterior cortex. The slot is smoothed out using a 7- or 8-mm bone rasp.

Allograft Implantation

A 3-cm posterolateral accessory incision is made, centered behind the lateral collateral ligament. The interval between the biceps tendon insertion and iliotibial band is identified and incised. Dissection is performed anterior to the biceps femoris to prevent injury to the peroneal nerve. Sharp dissection allows the lateral head of the gastrocnemius to be freed from the posterior capsule at the joint line. Care must be taken not to extend the dissection too far proximally to avoid entering the joint. A capsular repair will be necessary if this does occur. Blunt dissection is used to enlarge the space between the posterolateral capsule and lateral head of the gastrocnemius. A popliteal retractor is then placed behind the lateral meniscal bed. A single-barrel zone-specific cannula for an inside-out suture technique is placed through the medial portal and is used to advance a long, flexible, nitinol suture-passing pin through the knee capsule site at the junction of the posterior and middle thirds of the meniscus. The pin should exit out through the accessory posterolateral incision (Fig. 35-8). The proximal end of the nitinol pin is then withdrawn through the arthrotomy site. The traction suture is placed through the loop of the nitinol pin and the sutures are withdrawn through the accessory incision. The meniscus is inserted through the anterolateral arthrotomy. The bone-bridge is aligned with the recipient slot by gently pulling on the reduction suture. The meniscus is properly captured by the tibiofemoral articulation by cycling the knee. Final fixation of the bone-bridge in the slot is performed by placing an interference screw on the far side of the bone block (Fig. 35-9).

The periphery of the meniscus is fixed to the capsule using 8 to 10 vertically placed 2-0 nonabsorbable mattress sutures. The sutures are placed from posterior to anterior using standard inside-out technique. Sutures are placed both on the dorsal surface and undersurface of the meniscus for more

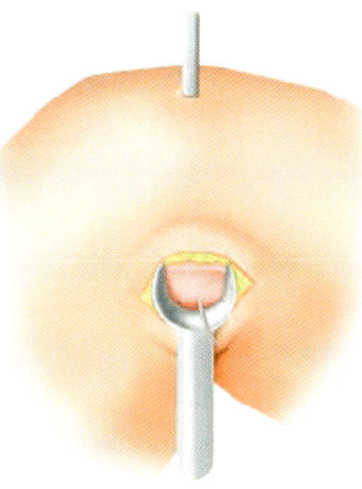

Figure 35-8. The meniscus is peripherally attached to the postero-lateral capsule using long, flexible, nitinol needles passed through the accessory posterolateral incision.

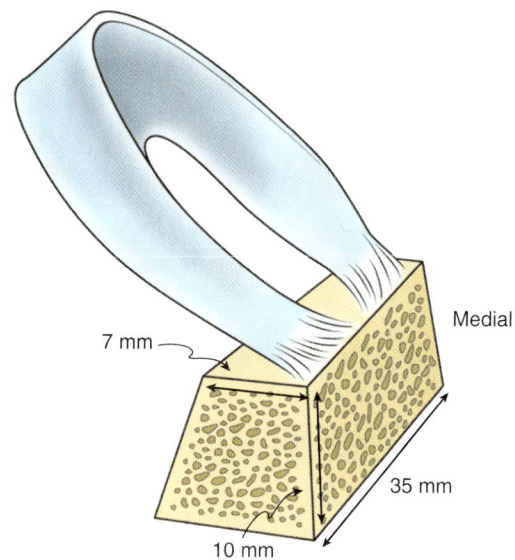

Figure 35-10. The dovetail bone block is prepared into a trapezoidal shape measuring 7 × 10 × 35 mm.

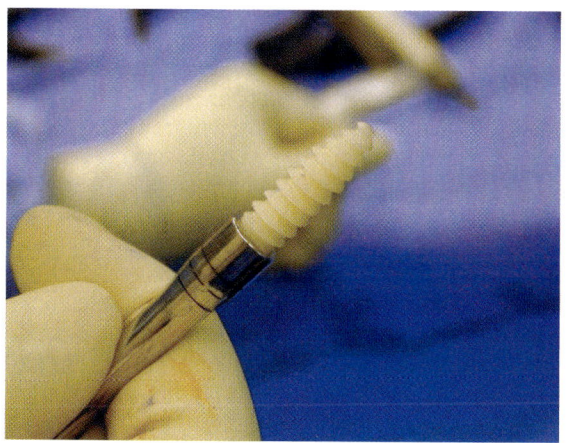

Figure 35-9. An interference screw is used for final fixation of the bone-bridge in its slot.

anatomic attachment. The sutures are tied with the knee in full extension. Arthroscopic visualization of the meniscus is helpful for confirming appropriate placement of the meniscus while the sutures are tied.

The bone-bridge technique is a technically demanding procedure, with several pitfalls. One of the technical problems is caused by the anatomy of the anterior horn insertion site on the tibia. The meniscal insertion site is 8 to 9 mm whereas the bone-bridge is typically only 7 mm wide. To deal with this problem, the anterior portion of the bone-bridge is cut slightly wider than the rest of the bridge to accommodate for the widened insertion site. Another situation that may be encountered while performing the bone-bridge technique is avulsion of the insertion site of the meniscus. If this occurs, a no. 2 Ethibond suture can be placed through the substance of the meniscus and then passed through the bone-bridge using a Kirschner wire (K wire) or free needle. The meniscus is anchored down to the bone by tying the two ends of the Ethibond together. If bone fracture occurs, a K wire can be

used as an internal splint during introduction of the meniscus. The interference screw can be used to fix the fracture once in its final position and the K wire removed. If the fracture is not amenable to repair, the bone-bridge can also be converted to a double bone plug allograft.

Dovetail Technique

The dovetail technique attempts to simplify graft preparation with a time-saving series of cuts preparing the bone component of the graft to sit securely in a semitrapezoidal recipient slot created in the tibia. A matching semitrapezoid-shaped recipient slot created in the tibia with a series of step drills, rasps, and dilators matches the bone block preparation.

Allograft preparation begins with trimming off excess soft tissue so that the anterior and posterior horns can be easily identified. The allograft tibial plateau is cut to the desired anteroposterior length. Using the trapezoidal rasp for tibial slot preparation, an outline of the dovetail bone block is drawn on the end of the bone plug. Using an oscillating saw, the bone plug is fashioned into a trapezoid-shaped bone-bridge, with the vertical wall being on the medial side and the angled wall on the lateral side (Fig. 35-10).

The tibial slot is created by initially burring a shallow trough between the anterior and posterior horns of the meniscus. To determine the AP depth of the tibial plateau, an osteotome is advanced to the posterior cortex following the path of the previously created trough. Using drill guides, drills are used to create an initial slot (Fig. 35-11). Trapezoidal rasps and dilators are used to create a trapezoidal slot in which the trapezoidal bone bridge is placed (Fig. 35-12). A tamp may be used to position the bone block into the slot. The knee is brought into a figure-of-four position to open the lateral compartment, making the passage of the trapezoidal bone bridge easier. The posterior horn must clear the femoral condyle before the bone plug will seat fully against the posterior cortex.

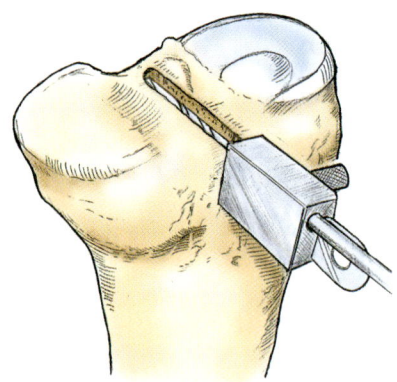

Figure 35-11. A drill guide and drill are used to create an initial bone slot that will eventually be formed into a trapezoid-shaped bone slot.

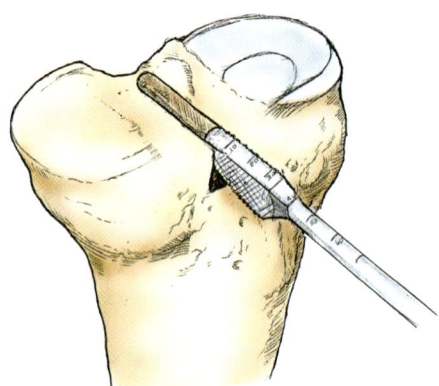

Figure 35-12. A trapezoid-shaped rasp is used to smooth out the bone-bridge slot.

Soft Tissue Technique

An alternative technique to bony fixation procedures is a soft tissue–only technique. The graft is prepared similar to the bone plug method; however, the bone plugs are removed from the allograft. Transosseous tunnels are drilled and the graft is passed in a similar manner to the bone plug method with conventional ACL guides. No. 2 braided nonabsorbable sutures secure the graft after it is passed through the transosseous tunnels to their anatomic insertion sites. Fixation is performed over a bone bridge or over a button. The remaining meniscal allograft is then secured with the use of arthroscopic inside-out suture techniques.

COMBINED TECHNIQUES

Meniscal Transplantation With Anterior Cruciate Ligament Reconstruction

Meniscal transplantation with ACL reconstruction can be performed together in combined injuries, particularly in cases of failed ACL surgery secondary to total or subtotal medial meniscectomy. Standard femoral and tibial tunnels are drilled and prepared before meniscal allograft insertion. Autograft or allograft tissue can be used for ACL reconstruction, depending on patient and surgeon preference, but allograft tissue use

in this situation is increasing in an attempt to decrease donor site morbidity. The tibial tunnel often encroaches on the bone used for the trough for the meniscus, so care must be taken while drilling the tunnel.[60] When using the medial double-plug technique, the soft tissue and osseous portions of the transplantation are performed first.[16] The tibial tunnel for the ACL reconstruction is drilled slightly more medially than usual to avoid communication between it and the tunnel for the posterior horn of the meniscus. Caution must be taken when using a trough technique for a medial meniscal allograft in combination with ACL reconstruction because the anterior and posterior horns of the native medial meniscus are often in line with the ACL, which can lead to ACL damage or encourage potential medialization of the horn attachments. When performing a bone-bridge technique for lateral meniscal transplantation, the tibial trough is created and the meniscal graft placed before the tibial tunnel for the ACL is drilled. To avoid the lateral slot, the tibial tunnel for the ACL is drilled slightly distally and medially.

Meniscal Transplantation With High Tibial Osteotomy

High tibial osteotomy should be performed in combination with meniscal transplantation in patients with axial malalignment. Similar to high tibial osteotomy performed for isolated medial compartment arthritis, the high tibial osteotomy in combination with meniscal transplantation should correct the knee to just past neutral to unload the affected limb. Most authors recommend using an opening medial osteotomy to create a valgus correction rather than a closing lateral osteotomy. All soft tissue and osseous portions of the meniscal transplantation are completed before proceeding with the tibial osteotomy. Fixation of the graft is performed once the osteotomy is completed. The osteotomy should be performed as distally as possible to avoid interference with the meniscal transplant tunnel or trough. Fluoroscopy is appropriate when placing the proximal screw to avoid the previously placed tunnels or trough. Rigid fixation of the osteotomy is recommended because the tibia is under great stresses to place the meniscal graft.

Articular Cartilage Repair With Meniscal Transplantation

Preoperative planning is important when considering performing a combined meniscal transplantation with articular cartilage repair in the same compartment. Typically, all the steps of the meniscal transplant are performed first, followed by the chondrocyte transplantation. This sequence helps avoid inadvertent damage to the transplanted chondrocytes.

RESULTS

Results of meniscal allograft transplantation reported in the literature are difficult to interpret because of the small number of patients in the studies, the heterogeneous population of patients studied, lack of outcome measure evaluation of the allografts, and validity of methods used. Few studies are available describing the outcome of an isolated medial or lateral meniscus transplantation. Multiple studies with concurrent procedures of ACL reconstruction, tibial osteotomy, and chondral resurfacing have been performed. However, lack of unified outcome measures for meniscal transplantation makes interpretation of the current literature difficult. Current studies use several knee outcome measures to evaluate meniscal transplantation, including the Lysholm, modified Hospital for Special Surgery (HSS), IKDC, Tegner, and Cincinnati scores, Western Ontario and McMaster Universities Osteoarthritis Index (WOMAC), and Knee Injury and Osteoarthritis Outcome Score (KOOS).[50] Long-term results are now available, allowing us to evaluate better the efficacy of meniscal transplantation in decreasing pain, improving patient function, and preventing the progression of arthritis.

Short-term studies of meniscal transplant uniformly show good results over the initial 2- to 3-year period. Milachowski and colleagues[45] have reported their early results on 22 patients with at least 14 months of follow-up. All patients underwent simultaneous ACL reconstruction in addition to meniscal transplantation. Second-look follow-up at 3 years showed meniscal shrinkage, which was thought to be secondary to freeze-drying the graft. In the entire series of 22 patients, there were only three failures that required removal (one fresh-frozen graft and two freeze-dried grafts). Generally, the fresh-frozen grafts were found to have a more normal gross appearance than the freeze-dried grafts. Noyes and associates[47] have reported their results of 40 meniscal transplantations in 38 knees. Concomitant procedures such as osteochondral autograft and ACL reconstruction did not increase the rate of complications. It was concluded that meniscal transplantation is encouraging in reducing pain and increasing function in the short term. Short-term results (2 to 3 years) are summarized in Table 35-4.

Medium-term follow-up appears to maintain the improvement in pain and function following meniscal allograft transplantation. Cole and coworkers[17] have reported on 44 meniscal transplants in 39 patients with a minimum of 2-year follow-up. They found that patients demonstrated statistically significant improvements in standardized outcome surveys and Visual Analogue Scale (VAS) pain and satisfaction scores. They concluded that meniscal transplantation alone or in combination with other reconstructive procedures shows reliable improvements in knee pain and function over the first 2 years. Van Arkel and de Boer[67] reported their results of 23 isolated meniscal transplantations with a follow-up of 2 to 5 years. The three unsuccessful results were caused by detachment of the graft from the capsule, leading to graft failure. Second-look arthroscopy was performed on 12 of the transplants at different time periods following transplantation. Five of the 12 menisci showed detachment from the capsule. The study concluded that lack of revascularization caused by malalignment of the knee led to the graft failures. Verdonk[71] has reported that the cumulative survival rates at 10 years were 74.2% for the medial meniscus and 69.8% for the lateral meniscus following transplantation.

Sekiya and colleagues[61] have also reported intermediate results of isolated lateral meniscal transplantation. There was no significant difference in joint space narrowing between the transplanted lateral meniscus and contralateral lateral compartment. Stollsteimer and associates[65] have shown that clinical results continue to be favorable at an average of 40 months post–meniscal transplantation. On average, the allograft was 63% the size of the native meniscus. Although the patients reported good results following the procedure, the allograft shrinkage was a concern. Kim and coworkers[38] have reviewed 14 meniscal allografts performed in patients with a total or near-total meniscectomy for torn discoid lateral menisci. All patients showed improvement in their symptoms, and Lysholm scores increased from 71.4 preoperatively to 91.4. Secure peripheral integration into the capsule was seen in all patients on MRI scans. It was determined that meniscal allograft transplantation after total meniscectomy for torn discoid lateral menisci could be a reasonable option for symptomatic patients. Results of medium-term follow-up (3 to 10 years) are summarized in Table 35-5.

The results of meniscal allograft transplantation after 10 years are less conclusive. Von Lewinski and colleagues[74] have reported on Milachowski's original cohort of patients at 20-year follow-up. The radiologic results revealed clear degenerative changes with long-term follow-up after the meniscal transplantation, even though some patients were doing well regarding the subjective and clinical results at the 20-year follow-up examination. Using MRI, Hommen and associates[31] have reported a 25% failure rate of medial meniscal transplantation and 50% failure of lateral transplantation at an average of 141 months. Of 15 patients in the study with postoperative radiographs, 10 showed narrowing of the involved tibiofemoral compartment. Although meniscal transplantation improved knee pain and function, the average knee function was fair at long-term follow-up. Long-term follow-up studies (>10 years) are summarized in Table 35-6.

The results of combined ACL and meniscal transplantation show good short- and intermediate-term results. Graf and coworkers[30] reported on eight patients undergoing concomitant ACL reconstruction and medial meniscal transplantation, with an average follow-up of 9.7 years. Of the eight patients, six were extremely pleased with their knee function and were active in recreational sports. They concluded that the addition of the knee-stabilizing procedure improved the outcomes of the eight patients. Rueff and colleagues[59] compared the 5-year outcomes of

Table 35-4 Summary of Short-Term Results*

Study (Year)	Follow-Up (mo)	Allografts	Combined Procedures	Results
Milachowski et al (1989)[46]	14	22	All combined with ACL reconstruction	Three failures by second-look arthroscopy
Noyes et al (1995)[48]	30	96		56 of 96 (58%) failed
Cameron and Saha (1997)[13]	31	67	21 isolated, 5 ACL, 34 HTO, 7 HTO + ACL	58 successful (92%)

*Up to 3 years.

Table 35-5 Summary of Intermediate Results*

Study (Year)	Follow-Up	No. of Allografts	Combined Procedures	Results
Cole et al (2006)[18]	36 mo	31	16 ACI, 15 osteochondral allograft	48% (60% ACI , 36% OCA normal or almost normal by IKDC score)
Garrett (1993)[28]	2-7 yr	43	7 isolated, 24 ACL, 13 HTO	35 of 43 (81%) successful
Van Arkel and de Boer (1995)[67]	2-5 yr	23		Three failures
Carter (1999)[15]	48 mo (mean)	51		45 of 51 (88%) successful
Sekiya et al (2006)[61]	3.3 yr (mean)	32		96% of patients thought their overall function improved following surgery.
Stollsteimer et al (1994)[65]	40 mo (mean)	23		13 of 23 normal or almost normal IKDC scores
Kim (2006)[†]	58 mo (mean)	14		Modified Lysholm score increased from 71.4 preoperatively to 91.4 postoperatively
Verdonk et al (2005)[71]	7.2 yr (mean)	100	13 HTO	Modified HSS scores improved from 60.1 to 88.6.
Noyes et al (2004)[48]	40 mo	38		89% successful

ACI, Autologus chondrocyte implantation; *OCA*, osteochondral allograft.
*3-10 years.
†From Kim JM, Bin S: Meniscal allograft transplantation after total meniscectomy of torn discoid lateral meniscus. Arthroscopy 22: 1344–1350, 2006.

Table 35-6 Summary of Long-Term Results*

Study (Year)	Follow-Up	No. of Allografts	Combined Procedures	Results
Hommen et al (2007)[32]	141 mo (mean)	22	—	35% failure rate
Von Lewinski et al (2007)[74]	20 yr	5	5 ACL	Two normal IKDC scores, two abnormal, one severely abnormal

*Longer than 10 years.

patients undergoing primary ACL reconstruction and either meniscal transplantation or meniscal repair–partial meniscectomy. At 5 years, the pain levels of the meniscal allograft group were similar to the meniscal repair–partial meniscectomy group.

Short- and intermediate-term results are also available for combined meniscal transplantation with articular cartilage repair. Farr and coworkers[25] have studied 36 patients undergoing combined meniscal allograft transplantation and femoral condyle autologous chondrocyte implantation (ACI), with a minimum of 2-year follow-up. Statistically significant improvements in the standardized outcomes surveys, VAS score, and satisfaction were reported. It was noted that the improvements were less than the literature-reported outcomes of either procedure performed in isolation; however, the results are promising for the combined pathology. Of the 36 patients, 8 patients had kissing chondral defects secondary to previous meniscectomy; significant improvement was seen in 6 of these 8 patients at 1 year. Each patient was able to lead an active lifestyle and five maintained the improvement at a mean follow-up of more than 3 years. Rue and colleagues[58] have reported on 16 patients undergoing combined meniscal allograft transplantation with ACI and 15 patients undergoing combined meniscal transplantation with osteochondral allograft (OA). These studies showed good initial results of combined meniscal transplantation with chondral allograft.

The importance of correct axial alignment has been well described in the literature. Cameron and Saha[12] described 63

meniscal transplantations with 34 of these performed in combination with a valgus high tibial osteotomy (HTO), varus high tibial osteotomy, or varus distal femoral osteotomy to correct for preoperative malalignment. Of the patients undergoing combined osteotomy and meniscal transplant, 29 (85.3%) attained good to excellent results. Verdonk and associates[72] presented the clinical, radiologic, and MRI outcomes of the menisci and articular cartilage of 42 meniscal transplantations at a minimum 10-year follow-up. Patients undergoing HTO and medial meniscal transplantation showed better modified HSS scores than patients undergoing medial meniscal transplantation alone at the final follow-up. Fairbanks' changes remained stable in 9 of 32 knees (28%). These results show encouraging trends in pain relief and function following meniscal transplantation combined with osteotomy.

The short- and intermediate-term results of meniscal transplantation indicate decreased pain and improved function in the treated knee. Scrutiny of these studies shows considerable variability in indications, type of graft, surgical technique, presence of concomitant surgery, duration of follow-up, and outcome evaluation. The long-term results begin to show degenerative changes and shrinkage of the allograft; however, most patients continue to have decreased pain and improved function. Current studies show a mutually beneficial effect of combined meniscal transplantation with other procedures such as ACL reconstruction, HTO, or cartilage restoration. It is evident that these procedures work synergistically and do not increase the complication rate when performed together. Long-term studies are necessary to determine the durability of the grafts and status of arthritis in these patients.

COMPLICATIONS

Complication rates associated with meniscal transplantation range from 10% to 50% in the literature. Graft tearing is the most common complication encountered with meniscal transplantation. Tears of meniscal allograft are approached the same way as tears in the native meniscus are treated, including meniscal repair if possible or partial meniscectomy. Matava[43] performed a systematic review of meniscal transplantation and identified 45 tears in 547 patients, for a tear rate of 8.2%. Allograft tears led to reoperation in 25% of Graf and associates'[30] patients and 26% of Stollsteimer and coworkers'[65] subjects. Infection and immune reactions are uncommon complications following meniscal transplantation. Cameron and Saha[12] have reported wound infections in 2 of 67 transplanted knees. Both were treated by antibiotics and resolved. Stollsteimer and colleagues[65] have described 1 of 22 patients who developed a pyogenic infection requiring removal of the meniscal allograft. Matava[43] reported only three studies specifically describing a postoperative immune response. No reports of HIV transmission have been described in the literature from the use of allografts. Other complications that may occur with meniscal transplantation include loss of graft fixation, hemarthrosis, synovitis, and arthrofibrosis. Complications associated with meniscal transplantation are summarized in Box 35-1.

POSTOPERATIVE REHABILITATION

Postoperative rehabilitation following meniscal allograft transplantation is similar to the protocols followed after meniscal repair (Box 35-2). Rehabilitation following meniscal transplantation consists of five phases. Phase I consists of the first 6 weeks following surgery and includes bracing and 50% weight bearing. Pain control, quadriceps strengthening, and full extension are the primary goals of this phase. Phase II consists of full weight bearing, with encouragement of full range of motion. Pivoting, twisting, hopping, jumping, and running are not allowed. Months 3 to 4 make up phase III. Progress to open- and closed-chain resistance exercises take place during this phase, including isokinetic exercises. Phase IV occurs during months 4 to 6; the patient continues to progress with strengthening and flexibility along with single-leg squats and light jogging. Sport-specific drills and plyometrics occur during phase V, 6 months postoperatively. There is no consensus regarding the timing of return to athletic activities.

CONCLUSION

Meniscal allograft transplantation is an increasingly popular treatment for young symptomatic patients with meniscus-deficient knees. The ideal candidate for the procedure is a patient who is physiologically young, has a stable, well-aligned knee, with minimal arthritis, and is complaining of focal pain on the meniscal deficient side of the knee. Meniscal allograft transplantation should be considered as a salvage operation for these patients, and only used once other conservative measures have been exhausted. Many techniques have been described for performing the transplantation and much debate continues about which technique is superior. The important guidelines for successful meniscal replacement include bony fixation and anatomic replacement of the anterior and posterior horns. Typically, the bone plug technique is used for medial meniscal replacement because the anterior horns are separated by a larger distance compared with the lateral meniscal horns. Because the lateral meniscal horns are

---

Box 35-1   Complications

Graft tearing
Infection and immune reaction
HIV transmission
Loss of graft fixation
Hemarthrosis
Synovitis
Arthrofibrosis

Box 35-2   Rehabilitation Protocol

Phase I: 0-6 Weeks
- Brace 0-90 degrees for 4 weeks postoperatively
- 50% weight bearing for 4 weeks postoperatively
- Wean off crutches beginning 4 weeks postoperatively
- Limit flexion to 90 degrees until 4 weeks postoperatively
- Pain, edema control, patellar mobilizations
- Quadriceps sets, hamstring cocontractions at multiple angles
- Straight leg raise in brace at 0 degree until quadriceps can maintain knee locked
- Heel slides in brace
- Obtain full extension

Phase II: 6-12 Weeks
- Stationary bike with seat high, lower as tolerated
- Leg press with 50% body weight (BW) maximum
- Leg extensions with range of motion (ROM) restrictions, high volume, light weight
- Leg curls with ROM restrictions, high volume, light weight
- Full weight bearing
- No pivoting, twisting, hopping, jumping, running
- Encourage full ROM
- Normalize gait mechanics

Phase III: 3-4 Months
- Progress open-, closed-chain resistance exercises
- Isokinetic exercises
- Treadmill forward and retro walking
- Single-leg stance for proprioception
- Cardiovascular fitness
- Slide board—initially short distance, increase as tolerated
- Manage patellofemoral signs and symptoms

Phase IV: 4-6 Months
- Continue and progress strengthening and flexibility
- Single leg squats
- Plyometrics – (4 months)
- Light jogging on treadmill (4 months)

Phase V: 6+ Months
- Sport-specific drills
- Plyometrics

separated by 1 cm or less on average, a bone-bridge technique is recommended. Clinical trials have shown favorable outcomes for cryopreserved or fresh-frozen allografts. Negligible rates of disease transmission because of careful procurement and sterilization protocols have been reported in the literature. Mid- and long-term reports have demonstrated predictable improvements in pain, swelling, and knee function following meniscal allograft transplantation. Despite these results, there is minimal evidence that meniscal transplantation restores meniscal function. Further long-term studies are necessary to determine the efficacy of meniscal transplantation in slowing down the degenerative process that occurs with meniscal deficiency.

KEY REFERENCES

Bhosale AM, Myint P, Roberts S, et al: Combined autologous chondrocyte implantation and allogenic meniscus transplantation: a biological knee replacement. Knee 14:361–368, 2007.

Cole BJ, Cater TR, Rodeo SA: Allograft meniscal transplantation. J Bone Joint Surg Am 84:1236–1250, 2002.

Dienst M, Greis PE, Ellis BJ, et al: Effect of lateral meniscal allograft sizing on contact mechanics of the lateral tibial plateau: an experimental study in human cadaveric knee joints. Am J Sports Med 35:34–42, 2007.

Farr J, Rawal A, Marberry KM: Concomitant meniscal allograft transplantation and autologous chondrocyte implantation: minimum 2-year follow-up. Am J Sports Med 35:1459–1166, 2007.

Graf KW, Jr, Sekiya JK, Wojtys EM: Long-term results after combined medial meniscal allograft transplantation and anterior cruciate ligament reconstruction: minimum 8.5-year follow-up study. Arthroscopy 20:129–140, 2004.

Hommen JP, Applegate GR, Del Pizzo W: Meniscus allograft transplantation: ten-year results of cryopreserved allografts. Arthroscopy 23:388–393, 2007.

Matava MJ: Meniscal allograft transplantation. A systematic review. Clin Orthop Relat Res (455):142–157, 2007.

Packer JD, Rodeo SA: Meniscal allograft transplantation. Clin Sports Med 29:259–283, 2009.

Rodeo SA, Seneviratne A, Suzuki K, et al: Histological analysis of human meniscal allografts. A preliminary report. J Bone Joint Surg Am 82:1071–1082, 2000.

Sekiya JK, Elkousy HA, Harner CD: Meniscal transplant combined with anterior cruciate ligament reconstruction. Oper Tech Sports Med 10:157–164, 2002.

Sohn DH, Toth AP: Meniscus transplantation. Current concepts. J Knee Surg 21:163–172, 2008.

Verdonk PC, Demurie A, Almqvist KF, et al: Transplantation of viable meniscal allograft. Survivorship analysis and clinical outcome of one hundred cases. J Bone Joint Surg Am 87:715–724, 2005.

Verdonk PC, Verstraete KL, Almqvist KF, et al: Meniscal allograft transplantation: long-term clinical results with radiological and magnetic resonance imaging correlations. Knee Surg Spots Traumatol Arthrosc 14:694–706, 2006.

Von Lewinski G, Milachowski KA, Weismeier K et al: Twenty-year results of combined meniscal allograft transplantation, anterior cruciate ligament reconstruction and advancement of the medial collateral ligament. Knee Surg Sports Traumatol Arthrosc 15:1072–1082, 2007.

Wirth CJ, Peters G, Milachowski KA, et al: Long-term results of meniscal allograft transplantation. Am J Sports Med 30:174–181, 2002.

Full references for this chapter can be found on www.expertconsult.com.

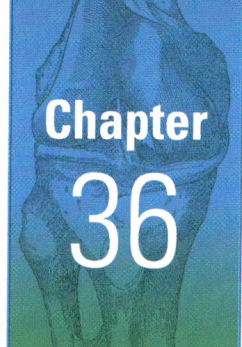

Chapter 36

Synthetic Meniscal Substitutes and Collagen Meniscal Implantation

Patrick G. Marinello, Suzanne A. Maher, and Scott A. Rodeo

The structure and composition of the **C**-shaped fibrocartilaginous menisci enable the functional performance of the knee joint during activities of daily living. Wedged between the incongruent surfaces of the tibia and femur, the menisci help distribute loads across the articulating surfaces and, in doing so, help protect adjacent articular cartilage. The tissue contains an inhomogeneous anisotropic arrangement of collagen type I fibers combined with proteoglycans, glycoproteins, and elastin.[4] The circumferentially oriented collagen fiber bundles are contiguous with the anterior and posterior horns that anchor the meniscus to the tibial plateau. These anchor sites help the tissue resist extrusive forces and allow the menisci to contribute to joint stability.[24]

Sometimes, the meniscus cannot withstand the mechanical burdens placed on it. Traumatic tears are most commonly observed in young, athletically active individuals, whereas degenerative meniscal tears tend to occur in patients older than 40 years. If damage occurs in a vascularized zone, the tissue can heal with a cellular fibrovascular scar similar to that which occurs in other soft tissues. However, healing is slow, with months or even years required for the scar tissue to mature to normal fibrocartilage. The mechanical function and strength of the repair tissue are unknown, so even when healing is complete, the residual strength and thus the function of the meniscus may be compromised. When meniscal injuries occur in the avascular region of the meniscus, common for degenerative tears, no reparative response is possible. Surgeries to treat damaged menisci number 850,000 per year in the United States but despite the prevalence of meniscal injuries, surprisingly few treatment options exist.[28]

TREATMENT OPTIONS

The ultimate goal of any surgical intervention is to relieve pain while restoring the function of the meniscus so that it can contribute to knee stability and protect surrounding musculoskeletal tissues from degeneration. There are four options to treat a damaged meniscus: (1) removal; (2) repair; (3) substitution (allograft or synthetic implant); and (4) scaffold implantation. The treatment used depends on the location and extent of the damage, age and activity level of the patient, and presence of concomitant injuries, such as rupture of the anterior cruciate ligament, which places increased mechanical demands on the healing tissue.[14]

Removal of Meniscal Tissue

The deleterious effects of total meniscectomy include pain, recurrent swelling, limited mobility and ultimately osteoarthritic degeneration.[1,11,13,19] The subsequent deterioration of the joint leads to disability, the need for multiple surgeries

and, often, total knee joint replacement. Although complete meniscectomy has fallen from favor, removal of a portion of the meniscus remains a commonly performed procedure. A recent cadaveric study reported a direct relationship between the amount of the posterior medial meniscus removed and the increase in articular cartilage contact stress.[23] However, the minimum amount of meniscal tissue that can be removed without negatively impacting the functional performance of the joint remains unclear.

Meniscal Repair

The ability to repair a torn meniscus is dependent on the location and type of tear. Whereas tears in the vascular periphery of the meniscus have the ability to heal, most of the inner meniscal tissue is avascular and therefore has poor healing potential. There is much interest in developing methods to augment healing by using cytokines and other bioactive moieties.[16,37]

Early work by Arnoczky and colleagues,[5] for example, evaluated the use of a fibrin clot in meniscus healing. Full-thickness lesions in the avascular portion of the medial meniscus of 12 adult dogs were filled with an exogenous fibrin clot. The defects filled with a fibrin clot healed through a proliferation of fibrous connective tissue that eventually modulated into fibrocartilaginous tissue. It was concluded that the fibrin clot acts as a chemotactic and mitogenic stimulus for reparative cells and provides a scaffold for the reparative process. Scotti and associates[31] have suggested augmenting repair sites with a chondrocyte-rich solution encapsulated within an acellular fibrin glue. Harvested swine menisci were used to create a trilayered construct consisting of a layer of chondrocyte-fibrinogen solution glue sandwiched between two layers of harvested swine menisci and wrapped in acellular fibrin glue. After 4 weeks of implantation into the subcutaneous tissue of nude mice, the acellular fibrin glue exterior had been replaced with a neovascular capsule, which allowed for tissue growth between the two sections of the meniscus. Hypercellular fibrocartilaginous tissue, active remodeling of the meniscal tissue, and bonding across the interface were evident.

The effect of insulin-like growth factor-1 (IGF-1) on meniscus healing was recently assessed in a goat model.[41] Full-thickness meniscal defects were created in the avascular region of the meniscus in 48 goats and bone marrow stromal cells transfected with the hIGF-1 gene were delivered to the healing meniscus using a calcium alginate gel delivery vehicle. At 16 weeks, the repaired meniscal defects were filled with white tissue similar to that in normal meniscal fibrocartilage. The repair tissue was composed of cells embedded within matrix that filled the interfibrillar spaces. Notably, the proteoglycan content in the gene-enhanced group was higher than that in the control groups.

Meniscal Substitution

Despite limitations, which include incomplete graft incorporation, difficulty in sizing, availability, immunologic rejection, disease transmission, and tissue integrity, meniscal substitution in the form of an allograft has been indicated for patients who have had a complete meniscectomy.[27] Short-term studies have demonstrated improvements in symptoms (pain and swelling) following meniscus transplantation; however, the ability of a meniscus allograft transplant to provide long-term chondroprotection is unproven.

Replacing the entire meniscus with a synthetic nondegradable implant that can carry and distribute load without damaging the articular surfaces of the joint has been a longstanding goal in the field of musculoskeletal soft tissue research. However, finding the optimal combination of synthetic materials to allow for a wear-resistant functional substitute has been difficult, with the result that no synthetic implant is clinically available as yet. Nondegradable hydrogels, such as polyvinyl alcohol (PVA), have been suggested as suitable meniscal substitute materials because of their high water content, low coefficient of friction, and stability when implanted. In small animal models, PVA-based total meniscal replacements demonstrated an ability to protect cartilage and remain intact for periods of up to 12 months.[22] PVA-based implants were also followed for up to 12 months in an ovine model and, at 2 months postoperatively, the implants demonstrated an ability to protect the knee joint from degeneration as compared with the meniscectomized knee.[21] At 4 months, however, the tibial plateau was significantly more degenerated when compared with that of the allograft implanted group, with degenerative changes particularly evident on the peripheral region of the tibial plateau. By 12 months, radial tears in the posterior aspect of the implant were evident. These studies highlight the challenges of designing a substitute that can withstand the rigorous mechanical environment of the knee.

Scaffold Implantation

Synthetic scaffolds are currently available for the repair or partial replacement of the meniscus. These acellular scaffolds are intended to be populated with matrix-generating cells after implantation. Two such scaffolds are clinically available for implantation at this time, a collagen meniscal implant, known more recently by its trade name Menaflex in the United States and Europe, and a polyurethane-based scaffold known by its trade name Actifit in Europe. In the remainder of this chapter, we review the basic science that led to the development of the current implants, indications for use, method of implantation, and clinical follow-up data. The challenge in assessing the long-term efficacy of these new devices is also reviewed.

Collagen Meniscal Implant

In December 2008, the U.S. Food and Drug Administration (FDA) approved the first collagen-based meniscal implant for commercial use in the United States, known as Menaflex (ReGen Biologics, Franklin Lakes, NJ).[25] Note that through its development, this was referred to as a collagen meniscal implant (CMI). When ReGen Biologics received FDA approval to market the device for sale in the United States, Menaflex became its preferred (trade) name. We will use the term *collagen meniscal implant* (CMI) in this chapter to refer to the Menaflex product.

CMI is manufactured from type I collagen harvested from bovine Achilles tendon (Fig. 36-1). The harvested tendon is washed, the collagen fibers are isolated and purified using sequential chemical treatments and organic solvents, and the purified collagen fibers are swollen in the presence of equal quantities of hyaluronic acid and chondroitin sulfate. Glycosaminoglycans are added and the resulting compound is coprecipitated by the addition of ammonium hydroxide. The collagen fibers and associated extracellular components are then dehydrated and manually oriented in a mold. The resulting structure is lyophilized and sterilized by gamma irradiation. The end product is an acellular scaffold intended to support cell migration and de novo tissue growth from existing meniscal tissue, the synovium, and synovial fluid.[34] The collagen meniscal implant can be trimmed to match the specific dimensions of a patient's meniscal defect. The resulting implant has the tensile strength to support attachment of the implant to a rim of the native meniscus with sutures and immediately withstand the sheer and compression forces within the knee joint, while maintaining a porous matrix to allow tissue regeneration. The collagen meniscal implant has been studied in humans to replace partial meniscal defects of the medial and lateral meniscus. In Europe, both medial and lateral implants are available for surgical implantation,

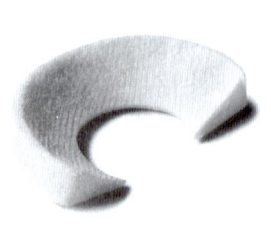
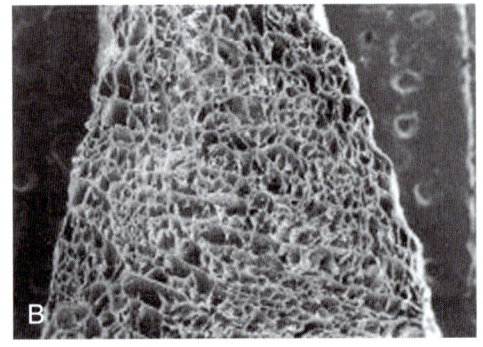

Figure 36-1. A, Collagen meniscal implant, Menaflex (RenGen Biologics). **B,** Scanning electron micrograph of a cross-section of the collagen meniscal implant, Menaflex. (From Stone KR, Steadman JR, Rodkey WG, Li ST: Regeneration of meniscal cartilage with use of a collagen scaffold. Analysis of preliminary data. J Bone Joint Surg Am 79:1770–1777, 1997.)

whereas in the United States, only the medial implant is currently available for use.

Pathway to Clinical Use

Although CMI has only been recently approved for use in the United States, it has been available in Europe for several years. CMI developed involved almost 2 decades of research and consequently its performance in vitro and in vivo has been studied extensively.[29,30,32-34] The construct has been shown to support cellular ingrowth and encourage tissue regeneration in many small and large animal models. Stone and associates,[33] for example, have evaluated CMI in a canine model. An 80% subtotal resection of the medial meniscus was created and the defect was then treated with the collagen-based scaffold. The investigators found that the implant was compatible with meniscal fibrochondrocyte ingrowth and concluded that it could induce regeneration of the meniscus in the mature dog.

Clinical Indications

CMI is indicated for use in individuals who have acute or chronic medial meniscal damage that is irreparable via suturing. A peripheral portion of the native meniscus must be intact to allow for secure attachment of the scaffold and to allow for cell ingrowth. Significant chondral damage, knee malalignment, and instability are contraindications. Concomitant ACL reconstruction or an osteotomy to correct malalignment may be done with scaffold implantation. The clinical trials that have been completed thus far have been primarily conducted on men, but gender is not an inclusion or exclusion criterion.[30]

Surgical Technique, Postoperative Care, and Rehabilitation

CMI is intended to be implanted arthroscopically. The medial meniscus is débrided to the vascular zone and, using a customized measuring device, an implant is chosen for the specific defect. A standard inside-out suturing technique is used to secure the implant. A posteromedial incision is used for placement of a posterior retractor. Before the implant is inserted (Fig. 36-2), a temporary suture is placed in the

midlesion and oriented to capture the collagen meniscal implant once introduced. The implant is introduced via the ipsilateral working portal using a specially designed delivery mechanism and subsequently guided by the initial suture, which serves to lasso and temporarily secure the meniscal implant. Vertical mattress sutures are placed to secure the implant to the rim of the existing meniscus. The implant is secured to the anterior and posterior horn of the existing meniscus via horizontal mattress sutures (Figs. 36-3 and 36-4). Use of 2-0 nonabsorbable sutures is recommended. After the implant is properly secured to the existing meniscal tissue, the initial temporary suture is removed and the newly placed meniscal implant is checked for fixation integrity (Fig. 36-5).[30]

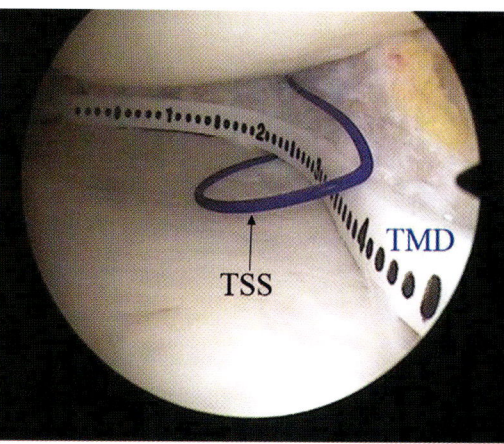

Figure 36-3. Following the partial meniscectomy, the size of the meniscal defect was measured using specific instrumentation. The numbers on the Teflon measuring device (TMD) represent centimeters, and the hash marks represent millimeters. The temporary stay suture (TSS; *arrow*) can be used to guide the TMD and stabilize the collagen meniscus implant during suture fixation. The temporary stay suture is removed after the collagen meniscus implant has been sutured to the meniscus rim. (From Rodkey WG, DeHaven KE, Montgomery WH 3rd, et al: Comparison of the collagen meniscus implant with partial meniscectomy. A prospective randomized trial. J Bone Joint Surg Am 90:1413–1426, 2008.)

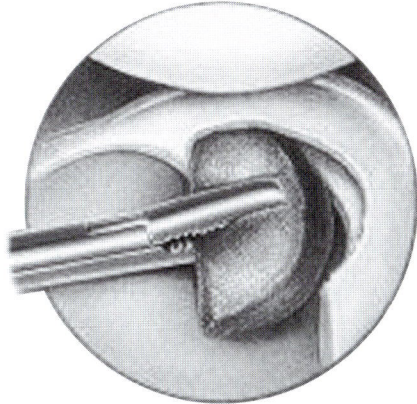

Figure 36-2. Illustration depicting insertion of the collagen meniscal implant. (From Stone KR, Steadman JR, Rodkey WG, Li ST: Regeneration of meniscal cartilage with use of a collagen scaffold. Analysis of preliminary data. J Bone Joint Surg Am 79:1770–1777, 1997.)

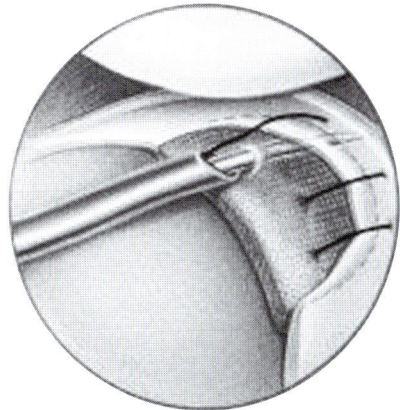

Figure 36-4. Illustration depicting suturing of the collagen meniscal implant. (From Stone KR, Steadman JR, Rodkey WG, Li ST: Regeneration of meniscal cartilage with use of a collagen scaffold. Analysis of preliminary data. J Bone Joint Surg Am 79:1770–1777, 1997.)

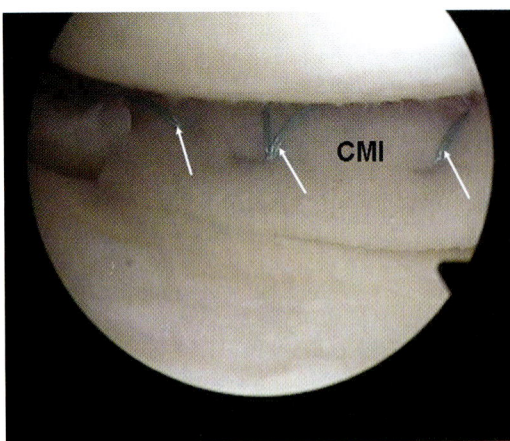

Figure 36-5. After the CMI was delivered into the joint, it was sutured to the host meniscus remnant with nonabsorbable sutures *(white arrows)* and an inside-out technique. (From Rodkey WG, DeHaven KE, Montgomery WH 3rd, et al: Comparison of the collagen meniscus implant with partial meniscectomy. A prospective randomized trial. J Bone Joint Surg Am 90:1413–1426, 2008.)

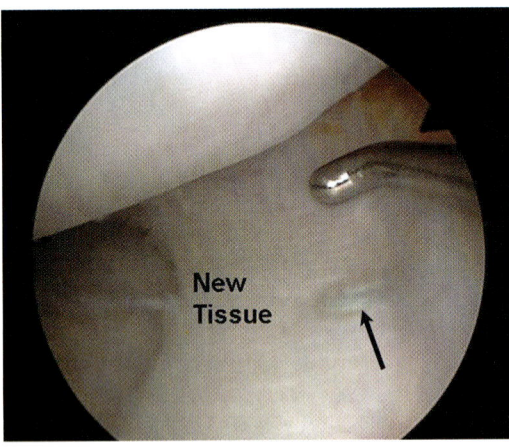

Figure 36-6. One-year second-look arthroscopy showed that the collagen meniscus implant had been replaced by new tissue. One of the sutures can still be seen *(arrow)*, although it is covered by synovial tissue. The probe demonstrates the approximate interface between the new tissue generated by the collagen meniscus implant and the host meniscus rim. (From Rodkey WG, DeHaven KE, Montgomery WH 3rd, et al: Comparison of the collagen meniscus implant with partial meniscectomy. A prospective randomized trial. J Bone Joint Surg Am 90:1413–1426, 2008.)

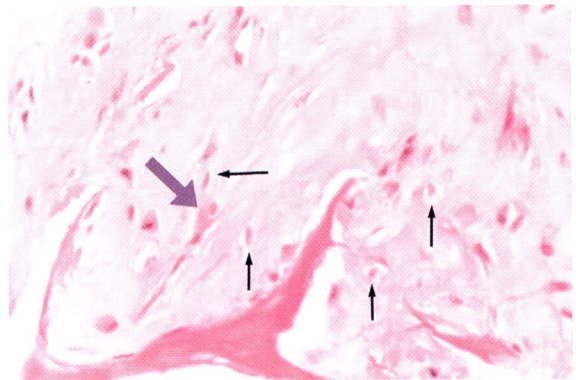

Figure 36-7. In this biopsy specimen, obtained at 1 year, the CMI appears to provide a scaffold for meniscus-like fibrochondrocytic matrix production by the host. The collagen meniscus implant was integrated into this tissue as it was assimilated and/or resorbed *(large purple arrow)*. Cells that appear to be meniscal fibrochondrocytes *(small black arrows)* are noted to be surrounded by lacunae, suggesting that they are viable and active cells (hematoxylin and eosin, ×100). (From Rodkey WG, DeHaven KE, Montgomery WH 3rd, et al: Comparison of the collagen meniscus implant with partial meniscectomy. A prospective randomized trial. J Bone Joint Surg Am 90:1413–1426, 2008.)

The postoperative rehabilitation protocol is designed to limit excessive loads on the implant prior to tissue ingrowth. Immediately following implantation, the knee is placed in a knee brace locked in full extension and kept non–weight bearing for 6 weeks. Knee motion is started immediately postoperatively with flexion limited to 60 degrees for the first 4 weeks and 90 degrees for the following 2 weeks. After 6 weeks, the brace is unlocked, the patient is allowed to be fully weight bearing, and physical therapy starts and continues until 6 months postoperatively, at which point the patient resumes normal activities.[30]

Clinical Outcomes

Most of the clinical trials have been completed by the developers of the device, starting with an initial study focused on the feasibility of implantation.[34] A subsequent study was used to assess its short-term clinical effectiveness.[30] These two studies corresponded with the phase I and II clinical trials as required by the FDA, which led to a multicenter, multisurgeon prospective randomized trial[29] in which 311 patients from 16 centers and 26 surgeons were divided into two cohorts, acute and chronic injury, to determine the effectiveness of the CMI. Patients were randomized to receive a CMI implant or to undergo a partial meniscectomy (considered the standard of care). Inclusion criteria were age (18 to 60 years), presence of an acute irreparable medial meniscus tear (acute group), or failed previous meniscectomy (chronic group). Patients were excluded if they had posterior cruciate ligament (PCL) insufficiency, an abnormal mechanical axis, and/or a significant chondral lesion. Of these 311 patients, 157 were allocated to the acute study arm (75 CMI treatment, 82 controls) and 154 were allocated to the chronic study arm (85 CMI treatment, 69 controls). No patients were lost in the acute arm follow-up and 3 patients were lost in the chronic study, allowing for final analysis of 308 patients.

The defect size for the CMI implanted patients was recorded at the time of surgery and was reassessed via arthroscopy at 1 year after the index surgery (Fig. 36-6). A significant increase in the amount of meniscus tissue in the experimental group was found in the acute and chronic groups. This suggested that the meniscal implant provided a significant contribution of new tissue surface area when compared with the control, which was assumed to have no new growth.[2,7,23] A needle biopsy taken of the scaffold showed fibrochondrocyte-like cells residing within lacunae, which is suggestive of matrix generation (Figs. 36-7 and 36-8). Remnants of the scaffold (10% to 25% of the initial area) were seen in the biopsy specimens but most of the scaffold had been reabsorbed and replaced with meniscus-like tissue. At the junction between the matrix and the native meniscal rim, there was evidence of vascular infiltration into the site of scaffold implantation. There were no obvious inflammatory infiltrates or evidence of adverse immune response.

Clinical outcome scales included the visual analogue pain score, the Lysholm score, and the patient self-assessment score; all scores increased in the treatment and control groups in both the chronic and acute arms of the study as a function

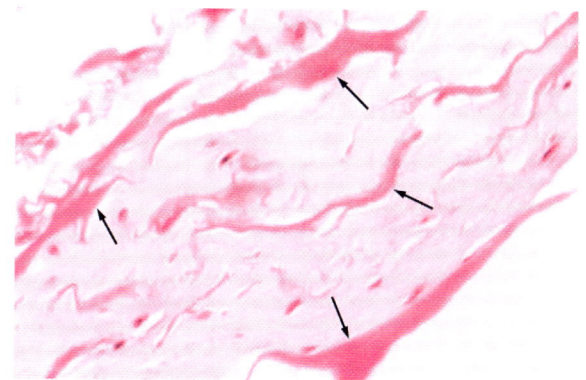

Figure 36-8. In this biopsy specimen, obtained at 1 year, it can be seen that most of the collagen meniscus implant has been resorbed or assimilated into the new matrix. The *arrows* point to darker staining structures that are remnants of the collagen meniscus implant (hematoxylin and eosin, ×100). (From Rodkey WG, DeHaven KE, Montgomery WH 3rd, et al: Comparison of the collagen meniscus implant with partial meniscectomy. A prospective randomized trial. J Bone Joint Surg Am 90:1413–1426, 2008.)

of time. Patients in the chronic group who were treated with the CMI were able to regain more of their preinjury activity when compared with the control (partial meniscectomy) cohort as measured by the Tegner index, which was considered a primary benefit of the CMI implant.

This study has several weaknesses, including a relatively short follow-up time of 5 years, the unblinded nature of the index procedure, and reliance on subjective patient satisfaction scores.[29] In addition, radiologic outcomes of the implanted collagen matrix were not provided. Overall, this longitudinal, randomized, prospective, controlled study supported the previous findings and demonstrated de novo tissue formation at the site of scaffold implantation. However, the function of the newly formed tissue and its ability to protect the adjacent cartilage from degeneration over the long term remains unknown.

Genovese and coworkers[15] have examined the radiologic outcomes (magnetic resonance imaging [MRI] and MR arthrography) of CMI in 40 patients at 6, 12, and 24 months postoperatively (Figs. 36-9 to 36-11). The implant position, signal intensity, and incorporation into the host tissue was assessed. A progressive reduction in the signal intensity of the regenerating tissue was found, indicating gradual tissue incorporation and maturation. There was a strong hyperintense signal in 80% of the implants at 6 months whereas only 35% of the implants imaged at 12 months had a hyperintense signal. None of the implants showed normal meniscus signal intensity at 6 or 12 months; however, at 24 months,

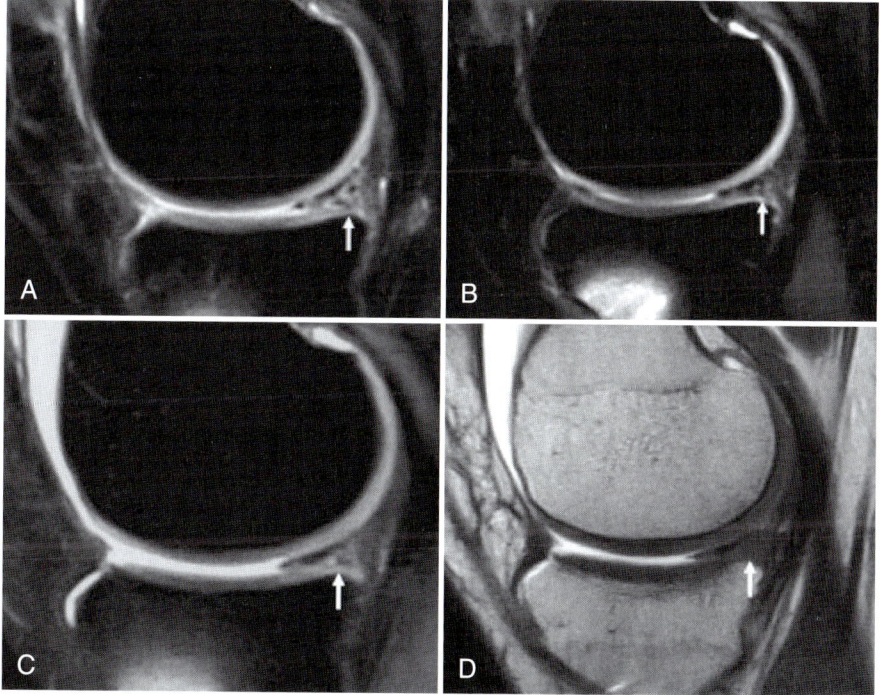

Figure 36-9. A, Examination at 6 months. CMI size is identical to that of the normal meniscus, type 3 *(arrow)*. The sagittal images obtained with fat-suppressed T2/DP show an inhomogeneous and marked increase in signal intensity, type 1 *(arrow)*. **B,** Same patient as in **A;** follow-up at 12 months. On the T2/DP-weighted sagittal images with fat suppression, scaffold size is type 3 *(arrow)*, but signal intensity is reduced compared with the previous examination; signal characteristics are type 2 *(arrow)*. **C,** Same patient, follow-up at 24 months. Scaffold size is still type 3 *(arrow)*, but signal intensity is reduced with respect to the examination at 12 months; signal characteristics are type 3 *(arrow)*. **D,** Same patient, follow-up at 24 months. On the spin-echo (SE) T1-weighted sagittal images obtained after intra-articular injection of contrast material, CMI size is type 3 *(arrow)*. The implant has integrated, and there is no infiltration of contrast agent. (From Genovese E, Angeretti MG, Ronga M, et al: Follow-up of collagen meniscus implants by MRI. Radiol Med 112:1036–1048, 2007.)

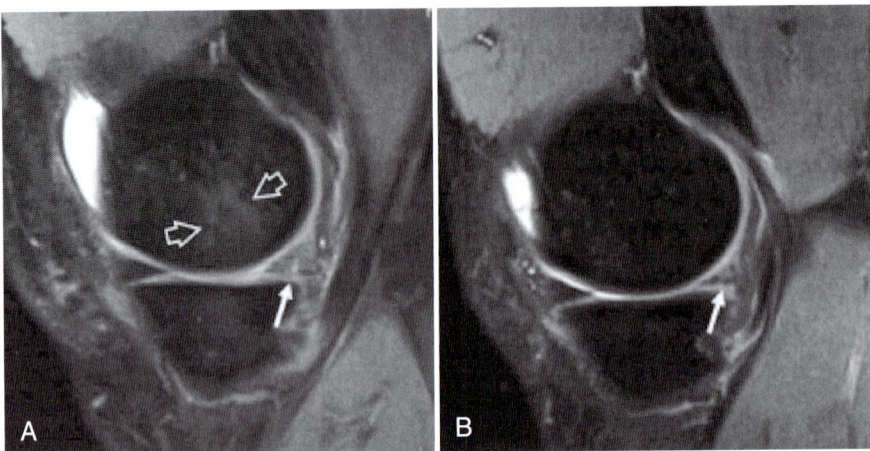

Figure 36-10. **A,** Examination at 6 months. In the T2/DP sagittal images with fat suppression, CMI size is type 3, and the signal intensity has inhomogeneously increased, reaching type 1 *(white arrow)*. The femoral condyle bone marrow shows an area with edema and interstitial hemorrhage identified by its high signal *(empty white arrows)*. **B,** Same patient, follow-up at 12 months. The complex size has decreased to type 2 *(white arrow)*, but the CMI size has decreased to type 2 *(white arrow)*. CMI signal intensity is reduced compared with the previous examination and is now type 2 *(white arrow)*. In comparison with the examination at 6 months, the bone marrow edema and interstitial hemorrhage have completely resolved. (From Genovese E, Angeretti MG, Ronga M, et al: Follow-up of collagen meniscus implants by MRI. Radiol Med 112:1036–1048, 2007.)

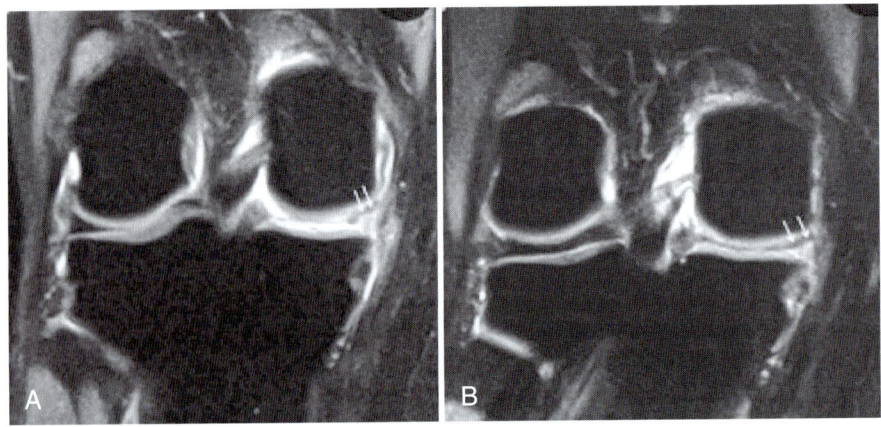

Figure 36-11. On the T2/DP-weighted and fat-suppressed coronal images, the interface between the prosthetic meniscus and native meniscus is indicated by a sharp hyperintense line at both 6 *(white arrows* in **A)** and 12 *(white arrows* in **B)** months. (From Genovese E, Angeretti MG, Ronga M, et al: Follow-up of collagen meniscus implants by MRI. Radiol Med 112:1036–1048, 2007.)

approximately 27% of the patients showed characteristics similar to those of the normal meniscus. A limitation of the study was the inability to determine chondral damage.

Bulgheroni and colleagues[9] followed 34 patients who underwent placement of a CMI to repair medial meniscal injuries for up to 5 years. Evaluation included Lysholm II and Tegner activity scores, as well as plain films, traditional MRI, and MR arthrography. The Lysholm and Tegner scores were found to be significantly improved when compared with preoperative status. Radiologic analysis of the CMIs showed that the chondral surfaces of the medial compartment, corresponding to the location of implant placement, did not show any further progression of chondral degeneration when compared with the patient's preoperative status. The MRI signal generated by the CMI gradually decreased over the 5-year follow-up period, suggesting progressive tissue maturation. Contracture of the meniscal implant was also observed but this did not seem to be detrimental to clinical outcomes.

Of note, two smaller studies, with eight and four patients enrolled, respectively were conducted by two separate groups in Italy. The results were similar to those already reported in the larger, more comprehensive studies.[26,40] Overall, the CMI scaffold reduced pain and allowed patients to return to their preoperative activity levels, in addition to providing protection from continued chondral degeneration.

Long-term longitudinal studies are needed to highlight the clinical usefulness of CMI better and its ability to offer protection against articular cartilage damage. Currently, the implant appears to work well in the short term for the indicated patient population and, as such, is a viable option for treating a medial meniscal injury. There is a need for further studies to determine the efficacy of the CMI clearly.

Porous Synthetic Scaffolds

Actifit (Orteq Sports Medicine, London) is a porous, biodegradable, aliphatic polyurethane with a porosity of 80% and pores ranging in size from 150 to 355 μm (Fig. 36-12).[17] Approved for use in Europe, it is currently being assessed by the FDA. A considerable body of work has been published on the development, characterization, and in vivo performance of the porous scaffold. Tienen and associates[35,36] and Welsing and coworkers[39] have followed the performance of the scaffold as a total meniscal replacement in a dog model. Up to 24 months postoperatively, the scaffold was fully integrated with newly formed tissue and did not elicit an adverse foreign body reaction. However, the scaffold did not prevent degeneration of the articular cartilage of the tibial plateau. This may, in part, have been caused by the method used to attach the implant to the tibia, which involved drilling holes through the tibial plateau. More recently, its use as a partial meniscal replacement scaffold has been explored, with indications that the scaffold can carry loads after implantation.[8]

The clinical indications for the use of the Actifit implant are similar to those of CMI although, unlike CMI, Actifit has been used for lateral meniscus repair. A prospective, nonrandomized, single-arm, multicenter clinical study was undertaken to determine the clinical efficacy, safety, and performance of the implant. At 3 months postoperatively, Verdonk and colleagues[18,38] observed tissue growth into the scaffold in 36 of 42 subjects using dynamic contrast-enhanced MRI (DCE-MRI). At 12 months, tissue ingrowth was evident in all subjects and, in 10 of 33 subjects, the meniscal lesion was completely filled (Figs. 36-13 and 36-14). Importantly, no evidence of articular cartilage damage related to the presence of the implant was found. Although long-term comprehensive clinical outcomes are warranted, these preliminary results are promising and encourage continued investigation.

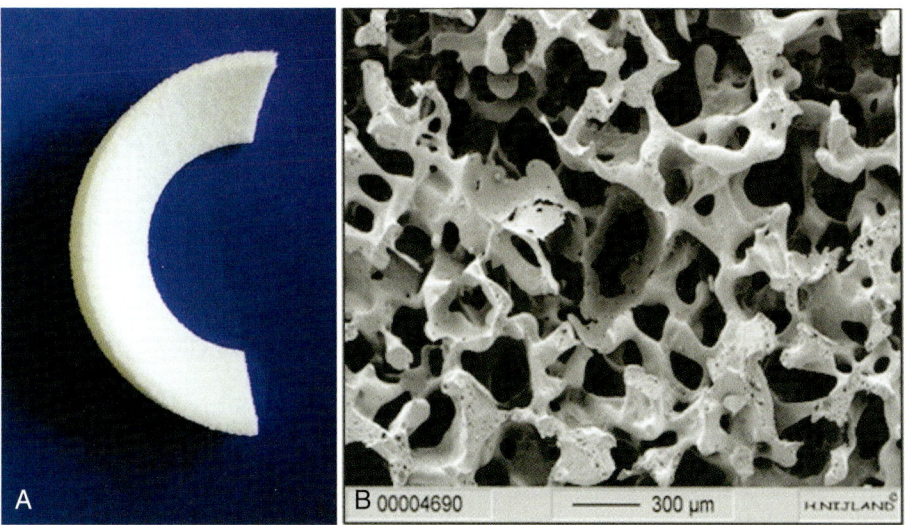

Figure 36-12. **A,** The Actifit implant. **B,** Microscopic view demonstrating the porosity of the polyurethane material. The average porosity is 80%, with pores ranging in size from 150 to 355 μm.

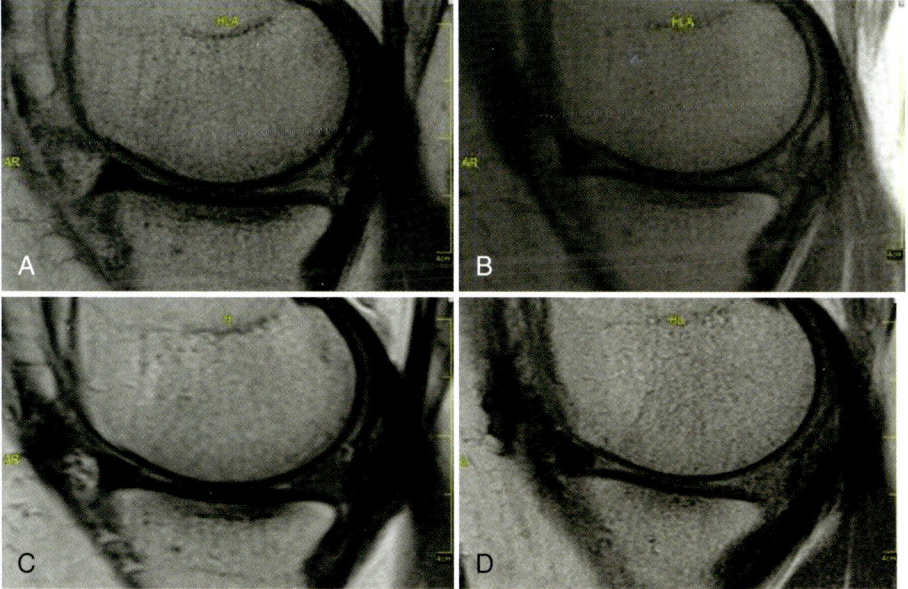

Figure 36-13. MR images of Actifit implant. **A,** 1 week postimplantation. **B,** 3 months postimplantation. **C,** 12 months postimplantation. **D,** 24 months postimplantation. (Courtesy Dr. Rene Verdonk.)

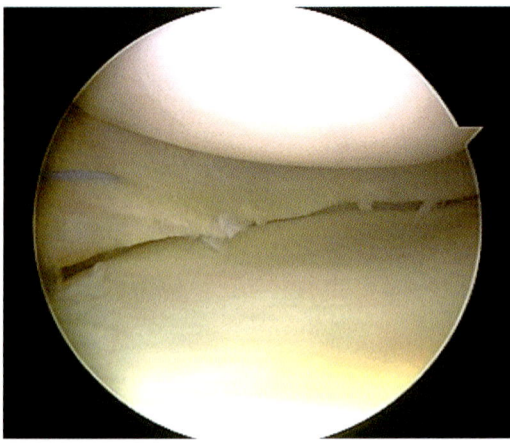

Figure 36-14. Arthroscopic appearance at 12 months postimplantation. (Courtesy Professor Johan Bellemans, Leuven, Belgium.)

Hyaluronic Acid–Based Scaffolds

Although not yet used clinically, resorbable hyaluronic acid–based scaffolds combined with polycaprolactone were designed by Chiari and colleagues,[11] with pores ranging in size from 200 to 300 μm. Two types of meniscal implants were designed, one indicated for total meniscal replacement and one for partial meniscal replacement. The total meniscal implant was augmented with circumferential polylactic acid fibers that protruded from the anterior and posterior horns of the implant to facilitate attachment to the tibial plateau. The partial meniscal implant was augmented with a polyethylene terephtalate net, which provided attachment sites for the sutures used to secure the implant to the remaining native meniscal tissue. On the basis of 6-week follow-up data, it was found that for both total and partial meniscal replacement, the implants incorporated well into the native synovium and did not cause any adverse reactions. Gross and histologic inspection confirmed the presence of new tissue growth in the total meniscal replacement implant and adhesion to the native meniscus in the partial meniscal replacement. Extrusion of the implant, primarily in the posterior area of the joint capsule, was reported, leading to some concern about the mechanical strength of the attachment sites.

REGENERATIVE MEDICINE AND THE STEM CELL FRONTIER

Advances in tissue engineering have also affected the field of meniscal repair. Aufderheide and associates[6] have explored the use of a scaffold-free method for growing self-assembled meniscus-shaped constructs. It was determined that the biochemical and biomechanical properties of the construct could be altered, depending on the relative concentrations of meniscal fibrochondrocytes and articular chondrocytes. This suggests the ability to tailor the self-assembling construct to mimic the native tissue most efficaciously. Kang and coworkers[20] have developed a meniscal scaffold consisting of polyglycolic acid (PGA) fiber meshes cross linked with poly(lactic-co-glycolic acid). The scaffold was seeded with allogenic rabbit meniscal cells, cultured in vitro for 1 week and then transplanted in the rabbits following medial meniscectomy. At 10 weeks, neovascular tissue formation and tissue growth were observed, demonstrating the feasibility of using allogenic cells to form a transplantable seeded scaffold into the knee.

Stem cells undoubtedly hold powerful regenerative potential that will affect our ability to enhance the repair of the damaged musculoskeletal system. However, no stem cell–based therapy is currently used clinically for the purposes of meniscal repair. Angele and colleagues[3] implanted a hyaluronan–bovine collagen composite scaffold seeded with marrow-derived mesenchymal stem cells into a rabbit model and found increased tissue ingrowth in cell-seeded scaffolds when compared with the acellular controls. Cristino and associates[12] seeded mesenchymal stem cells (MSCs) onto a hyaluronic acid–based scaffold (HYAFF 11, Fidia Advanced Biopolymers, Abano Terme, Italy). MSC growth and development were dependent on the density of cells and the expression of the CD 44 receptor. Advances in characterizing the differentiation process of an MSC population are needed to help advance their use for meniscal tissue regeneration. The clinical usefulness of stem cells will be advanced by further information about the signals (i.e., chemical and mechanical signals) necessary for differentiation of stem cells into meniscal fibrochondrocytes.

SUMMARY

The clinical use and development of meniscal implants is in its infancy. Our ability to transition the rich array of novel materials and therapies that are being explored for the repair or replacement of damaged menisci from the bench to clinical use successfully will ultimately rely on the ability to assess their functional performance preclinically. Questions about the ability of a construct to withstand physiologic loads, aid with knee joint stability, and ultimately help avoid knee joint degeneration should and will become a crucial part of the product design process. The use of appropriate load-bearing animal models,[10] combined with experimental models capable of measuring the functional performance of constructs,[8] can at least start to address these issues. In conclusion, replicating the complex structure and function of the meniscus in scaffolds or substitutes will prove challenging. However, already in the United States, a novel scaffold, CMI, is available for the treatment of partial medial meniscal injuries. Further clinical trials are needed to understand the long-term functional performance of the construct, but its clinical benefit thus far is most convincing in patients who suffer from chronic meniscal injuries.

KEY REFERENCES

Arnoczky S, McDevitt C: The meniscus: structure, function, repair, and replacement. In Buckwalter J, Einhorn T, Simon S, editors: Orthopaedic basic science: biology and biomechanics of the musculoskeletal system, Rosemont, Ill, 2000, American Academy of Orthopaedic Surgeons, pp 532–545.

Genovese E, Angeretti MG, Ronga M, et al: Follow-up of collagen meniscus implants by MRI. Radiol Med 112:1036–1048, 2007.

Kelly BT, Robertson W, Potter HG, et al: Hydrogel meniscal replacement in the sheep knee: preliminary evaluation of chondroprotective effects. Am J Sports Med 35:43–52, 2007.

Mow V, Flatow E, Ateshian G: Biomechanics. In Buckwalter J, Einhorn T, Simon S, editors: Orthopaedic basic science: biology and biomechanics of the musculoskeletal system, Rosemont, Ill, 2000, American Academy of Orthopaedic Surgeons, pp 135–180.

Reguzzoni M, Manelli A, Ronga M, et al: Histology and ultrastructure of a tissue-engineered collagen meniscus before and after implantation. J Biomed Mater Res B Appl Biomater 74:808–816, 2005.

Rodkey WG, DeHaven KE, Montgomery WH, 3rd, et al: Comparison of the collagen meniscus implant with partial meniscectomy. A prospective randomized trial. J Bone Joint Surg Am 90:1413–1526, 2008.

Rodkey WG, Steadman JR, Li ST: A clinical study of collagen meniscus implants to restore the injured meniscus. Clin Orthop Relat Res (367):S281–S292, 1999.

Scotti C, Pozzi A, Mangiavini L, et al: Healing of meniscal tissue by cellular fibrin glue: an in vivo study. Knee Surg Sports Traumatol Arthrosc 17: 645–651, 2009.

Steadman JR, Rodkey WG: Tissue-engineered collagen meniscus implants: 5- to 6-year feasibility study results. Arthroscopy 21:515–525, 2005.

Stone KR, Rodkey WG, Webber R, et al: Meniscal regeneration with copolymeric collagen scaffolds. In vitro and in vivo studies evaluated clinically, histologically, and biochemically. Am J Sports Med 20:104–111, 1992.

Stone KR, Steadman JR, Rodkey WG, Li ST: Regeneration of meniscal cartilage with use of a collagen scaffold. Analysis of preliminary data. J Bone Joint Surg Am 79:1770–1777, 1997.

Full references for this chapter can be found on www.expertconsult.com.

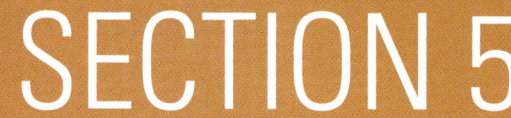

SECTION 5

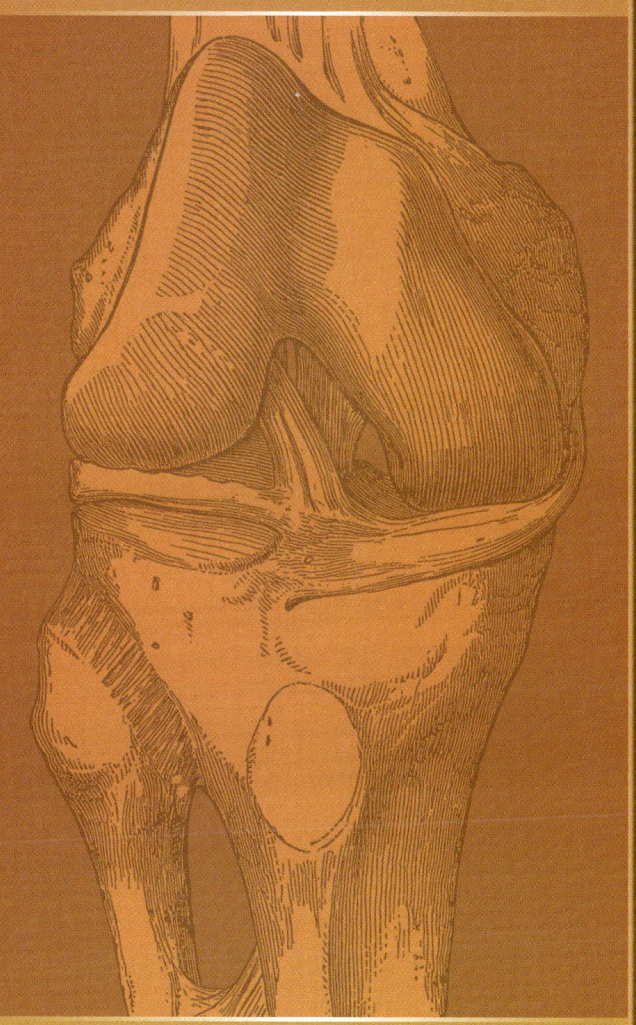

Sports Medicine: Ligament Injuries

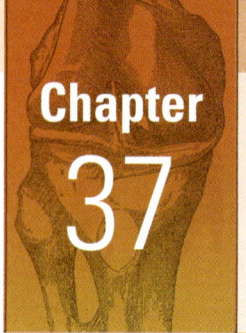

Classification of Knee Ligament Injuries

Christopher A. Hajnik, Craig S. Radnay, Giles R. Scuderi, and W. Norman Scott

Given the extensive investigation of ligamentous injuries of the knee, it is essential that a standardized, valid, reproducible, and universally accepted classification system be adopted. Effective systems of classification necessitate agreement on both the meaning and appropriate use of terms to describe abnormal knee kinematics such that there is no ambiguity. Furthermore, clinical examination findings, operative findings, and anatomic studies must be correlated in an attempt to clarify the classification of these injuries. By reviewing the current and classic literature, this chapter discusses the relationship of knee anatomy and kinematics, defines terms, and attempts to classify knee ligament injuries in an understandable fashion.

RELATIONSHIP OF CAPSULAR AND LIGAMENTOUS STRUCTURES

Critical to defining stability of the knee is understanding the relationship of the surrounding capsular and ligamentous structures.

Medial Structures

Hughston and colleagues[36] Warren and Marshall,[92] and LaPrade and colleagues[50] have clearly described the supporting structures on the medial side of the knee (Fig. 37-1). The medial collateral ligament (MCL) and the posteromedial capsular ligament, termed the *posterior oblique ligament*, are augmented by the dynamic stabilizing effect of the capsular arm of the semimembranosus tendon and its aponeurosis, the oblique popliteal ligament. The medial head of the gastrocnemius provides dynamic support to the medial compartment. Brantigan and Voshell[10] have described the MCL as having vertical and oblique portions that behave differently as the knee flexes. The parallel anterior fibers of the superficial medial ligament are arranged around the axis of flexion so that tension remains constant throughout the arc of motion. Posteriorly, the oblique fibers of the superficial ligament blend with the deeper layer within the posteromedial corner to form the posterior oblique ligament, which relaxes in flexion (Fig. 37-2).

Hughston and associates[35,36,41] have indicated that the posterior oblique ligament is the primary medial support against valgus stress to the knee. Although somewhat lax as the knee goes into flexion, the posterior oblique ligament is dynamized by the muscular attachment to the semimembranosus tendon, and it has a significant influence on stability throughout the first 60 degrees of flexion (Fig. 37-3). Muller[61] has also stated that the posterior oblique ligament is paramount in abolishing any valgus laxity in the extended knee. Even though the posterior oblique ligament and tibial collateral ligament are functionally independent, they are both dynamized, the former by the semimembranosus tendon and the latter by the

vastus medialis. This study also claims that the MCL has some function in preventing external rotation of the tibia on the femur with the knee flexed. However, the main deterrent to external rotation is the posterior oblique ligament.

In contrast to Hughston and Muller, Warren and coworkers[92] have noted that most fibers of the MCL are the prime static stabilizers on the medial side of the knee. The anterior 5 mm of the MCL remains tight in flexion and thus resists valgus stress in external rotation in this position (Fig. 37-4). According to their study, the posterior two thirds of the superficial MCL is slightly lax with the knee in flexion and therefore serves as a backup restraint against valgus and external rotatory forces. In their reports, Hughston and colleagues[35,36,41] have labeled the oblique fibers of the posterior aspect of the superficial MCL as the posterior oblique ligament. This is a thickening of the posteromedial capsule of the knee and it is firmly attached to and contiguous with the medial meniscus in this location.

Still another viewpoint, presented by Kennedy and Fowler,[47] has identified the deep medial capsular ligament as a primary restraint against external rotatory instability. They concluded that external rotatory instability is caused by a tear in the medial capsular ligament, with or without a partial or a complete tear of the MCL. Grood and associates,[33] in a biomechanical study of cadaveric knees, have concluded that the long parallel-oriented fibers of the tibial collateral ligament are the prime medial static stabilizers of the knee that resist medial opening to valgus stress. Although this ligament contributes to medial support with the knee close to full extension, as the knee flexes, the importance of this ligament increases from providing 57% of the restraining force to providing 78% of the restraining force. This increase is caused by the relaxation or laxity that develops with flexion in the other contributing structures, mainly the posteromedial capsule. The deep medial capsular ligament, although important in that it provides a firm attachment site for the medial meniscus, does not serve as a primary restraint against straight medial opening.[42]

Although these previous qualitative assessments are useful in developing an understanding of medial-sided knee injuries, LaPrade and coworkers[50] have made a quantitative assessment of the medial structures of the knee. Claiming that the layered approach is not helpful for surgical exposure, because it often leads to an oversimplification of structures with frequent inaccuracies regarding ligamentous attachment sites, they sought to verify the relationships of medial knee structures to pertinent osseous anatomy through cadaveric dissection. They confirmed that the medial epicondyle lies anterior and distal to the adductor tubercle. They also consistently recognized a third, previously undescribed osseous prominence, which lies distal and posterior to the adductor tubercle, near the attachment depression of the medial gastrocnemius tendon. They labeled this new structure the

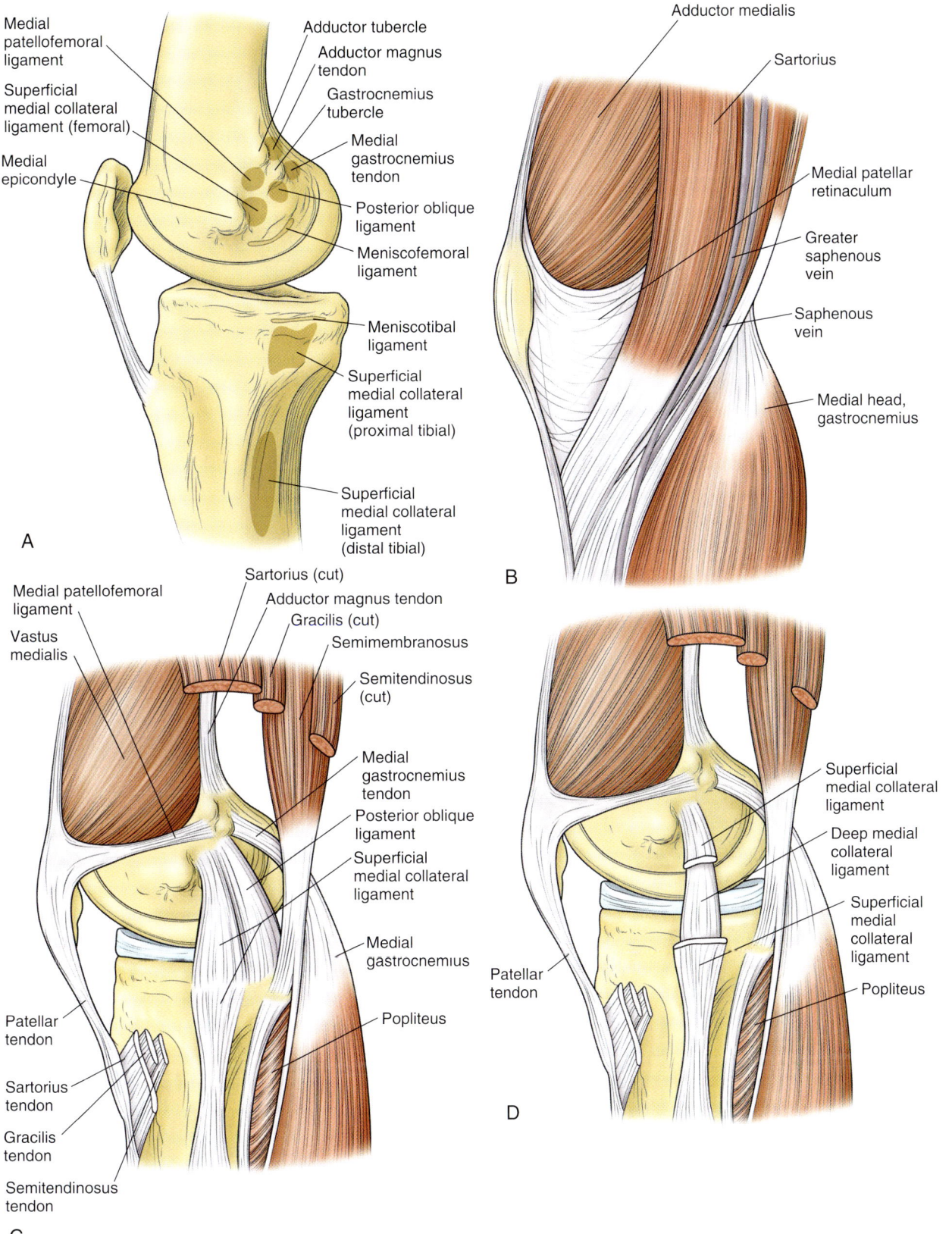

Figure 37-1. **A,** Medial knee bony anatomy. **B,** Layer 1, medial side of the knee. **C,** Layer 2, medial side of the knee with the medial collateral ligament and posterior oblique ligament. **D,** Layer 3, medial side of the knee. (**A** redrawn from LaPrade, RF, Engebretsen AH, Ly TV, et al: The anatomy of the medial part of the knee. J Bone Joint Surg Am 89:2000, 2007.)

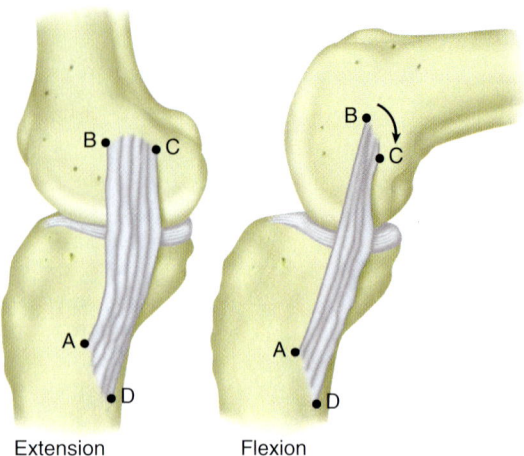

Figure 37-2. Medial collateral ligament in flexion and extension. (From Scott WN [ed]: The knee, St Louis, 1994, CV Mosby.)

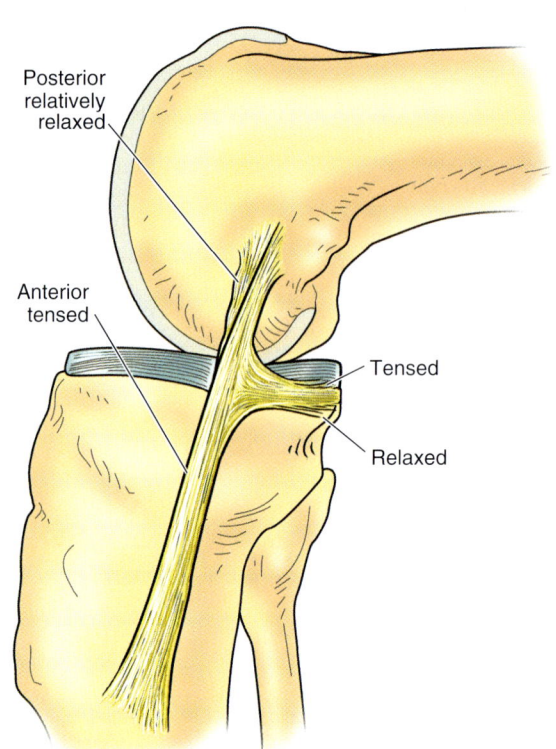

Figure 37-3. The posterior oblique fibers become more tense in flexion. (From Palmer I: On the injuries to ligaments of the knee joint. A clinical study. Acta Chir Scand 81[Suppl 53]:3, 1938.)

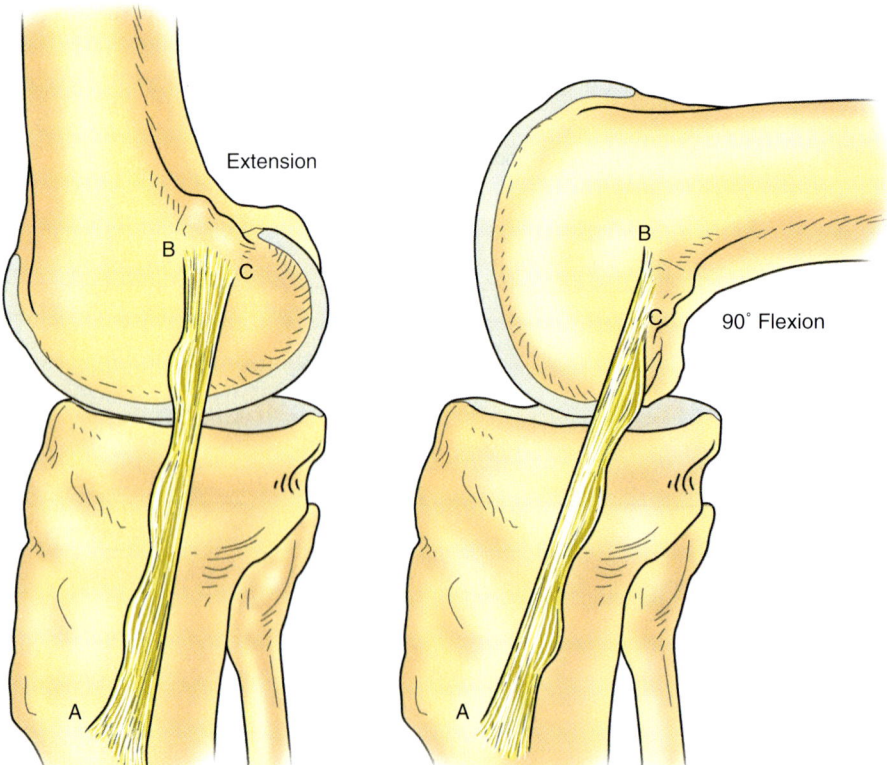

Figure 37-4. Diagram of the superficial medial ligament with flexion and extension of the knee. Because point B moves superiorly, the anterior border is tightened in flexion. Conversely, in extension, point C moves proximally, and the posterior margin of the ligament is tightened. (From Warren RF, Marshall JL, Girgis F: The prime static stabilizer of the medial side of the knee. J Bone Joint Surg Am 56:665, 1974.)

gastrocnemius tubercle and noted that the posterior oblique ligament attachment was actually closer to this structure than to the adductor tubercle.

The superficial MCL is the largest medial knee structure, measuring between 10 and 12 cm in length, but it does not attach directly to the medial epicondyle, as previously described.[10,41,91] Its femoral attachment lies slightly proximal and posterior.[50] There are two distinct tibial attachments. Proximally, it attaches to the soft tissues directly over the anterior arm of the semimembranosus. Distally, it attaches to bone approximately 6 cm from the joint line.

The superficial, central, and capsular arms of the posterior oblique ligament are readily identifiable, with the central arm forming the largest component of this structure. The central arm contributes most fibers for femoral attachment and adheres to the medial meniscus as it merges distally with the posteromedial capsule.[50]

A subsequent study by Wijdicks and colleagues[94] has concluded that the attachments of medial ligamentous structures could be correlated to the location of osseous landmarks seen on plain radiographs. This may aid in pre- and intraoperative assessment of surgical repairs and reconstructions of these structures.

Lateral Structures

The lateral supporting structures have been described by Hughston and associates[37] and Seebacher and coworkers[74] (Fig. 37-5). The lateral collateral ligament (LCL) is the major static support to varus stress, whereas the iliotibial tract provides both dynamic and static support. Terry and colleagues[85] have investigated the role of the iliotibial tract, iliopatellar band, and iliotibial band as dynamic and static stabilizers of the lateral side of the knee.

The posterolateral corner is composed of the LCL, popliteus aponeurosis, popliteofibular ligament (PFL), and posterolateral capsule. Although these individual static structures have often been grouped together as the arcuate ligament complex, other studies have highlighted their individual importance. Together, their function is augmented by the dynamic effects of the biceps femoris, popliteus, and lateral head of the gastrocnemius.[5]

On the femoral side, the LCL attaches to a small depression between the lateral epicondyle and supracondylar process, and it attaches distally to the posterior aspect of the fibular head.[12,51] The popliteus originates from the posteromedial aspect of the proximal tibia, courses intra-articularly, and inserts anterior and distal to the LCL attachment. Its function in providing dynamic stability to the lateral meniscus is controversial—countering views on its role in retraction and protection of the meniscus have been espoused.[78,88,89] The PFL arises from the myotendinous junction of the popliteus and inserts on the fibular styloid process.

Anterior Cruciate Ligament

The anterior cruciate ligament (ACL; Fig. 37-6) is the primary structure that controls anterior displacement in the unloaded knee. The anatomic and functional aspects of the ACL have undergone extensive investigation.[57-59,84] For reconstruction purposes, the focus has often centered on the relationship of the ligament to osseous landmarks. On the femoral side, the anterior border of the ACL is a bony ridge on the medial wall of the lateral femoral condyle, commonly referred to as resident's ridge.[71] On the tibial side, the ACL posterior border lies at a ridge between the medial and lateral intercondylar tubercles at the base of the tibial eminence.

The ACL has been described as a single ligament, with different portions taut throughout the range of motion (ROM).[6] In investigating the functional anatomy of the ACL, Odensten and Gillquist[67] found no anatomic separation of the ligament into different bundles. However, they did confirm that the ligament is twisted through 90 degrees, and that both the length[49,86,89,90] and tension[27] of different fibers in the ligament change as knee flexion occurs. Therefore, they believe that there are different functional portions of the ACL.[93] Based on this concept of different functional portions of the ACL, Girgis and associates[29] have divided the ACL into anteromedial and posterolateral bands. Norwood and Cross[62] further divided the ACL into three functional bundles and described their different actions in resisting rotatory instability. Amis and Dawkins[3,4] have supported this multifascicular structure of the ACL; although not necessarily separate entities, the bundles interact as three functional bundles. They found that the fiber bundles were not isometric; the anteromedial bundle lengthens and the posterolateral bundle shortens during flexion (Fig. 37-7). These changes in fiber length correlate with their changing participation in total ACL action as the knee is flexed.

Tibial rotation is better resisted by a combination of capsular structures, collateral ligaments, the joint surface, and meniscal geometry, whereas the cruciates play only a secondary role.[3,4,65] However, recent evidence suggests a larger role for the ACL in rotational stability if both bundles remain functionally intact.[14] Despite this, the MCL is anatomically better suited than the ACL and has the mechanical advantage to control torsion or laxity because its attachments are further removed from the axis of tibial rotation.[77] The MCL will provide significant resistance to the anterior drawer test only after the ACL is gone and when both ligaments are lost. In this scenario, the knee will exhibit large tibial excursions and response to anterior force if it is unchecked by muscle action. Injuries to the medial structures further compromise anterior stability when they accompany ACL injuries.[81]

Posterior Cruciate Ligament

The posterior cruciate ligament (PCL; Fig. 37-8) is believed to be the most important of the knee ligaments because of its cross-sectional area, tensile strength, and location in the central axis of the knee joint.* Its position provides 95% of the total resistance to posterior displacement of the tibia. Both James and associates[44] and Kennedy and coworkers[48] have shown that the tensile strength of the PCL is almost twice that of the ACL. Hughston and colleagues[36] have described the PCL as the fundamental stabilizer of the knee because it is located in the center of the knee joint and functions as the axis about which the knee moves in flexion and extension, as well as in rotation.

The PCL prevents posterior translation at all angles of flexion.[13,26,34] Patients who have an isolated injury of the PCL

---

*References 13, 15, 17, 18, 39, and 40.

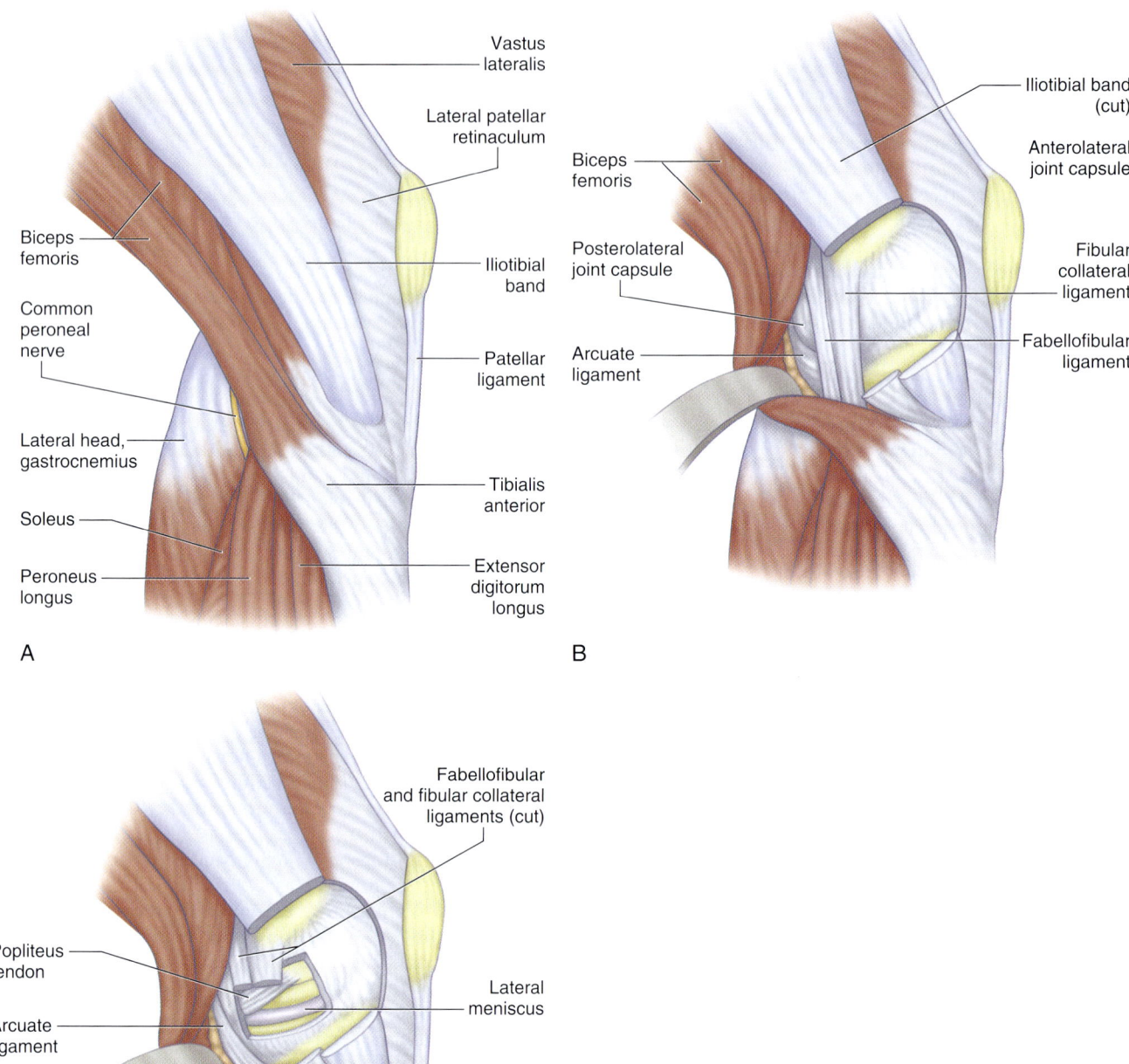

A

- Vastus lateralis
- Lateral patellar retinaculum
- Biceps femoris
- Common peroneal nerve
- Lateral head, gastrocnemius
- Soleus
- Peroneus longus
- Iliotibial band
- Patellar ligament
- Tibialis anterior
- Extensor digitorum longus

B

- Biceps femoris
- Posterolateral joint capsule
- Arcuate ligament
- Iliotibial band (cut)
- Anterolateral joint capsule
- Fibular collateral ligament
- Fabellofibular ligament

C

- Popliteus tendon
- Arcuate ligament
- Fabellofibular and fibular collateral ligaments (cut)
- Lateral meniscus

Figure 37-5. **A**, Layer 1, lateral side of the knee. **B**, Layer 2, lateral side of the knee with the lateral collateral ligament. **C**, Layer 3, lateral side of the knee with the arcuate complex. (From Scott WN: Ligament and extensor mechanism injuries of the knee: diagnosis and treatment, St Louis, 1991, Mosby–Year Book.)

may maintain fairly good function of the knee.[25] Gollehon and associates[30] have found that isolated sectioning of the PCL produces increased posterior translation of the tibia at all degrees of flexion of the knee, with the greatest increase occurring from 75 to 90 degrees. Absence of the PCL has no effect on primary varus or external rotation of the tibia as long as the LCL and capsular structures are intact.

Like the ACL, the PCL is a continuum of fascicles, with different portions being taut throughout ROM. The anterior portion, which forms the bulk of the ligament, tightens in flexion, whereas the smaller posterior portion tightens in extension (Fig. 37-9).[6] The PCL originates from the posterior part of the lateral aspect of the medial femoral condyle and inserts on the posterior surface of the tibia. The femoral footprint consists of a medial intercondylar ridge at its proximal border and a medial bifurcate ridge that occasionally divides the two functional bundles.[24] The insertion reaches approximately 1 cm below the articular surface in a

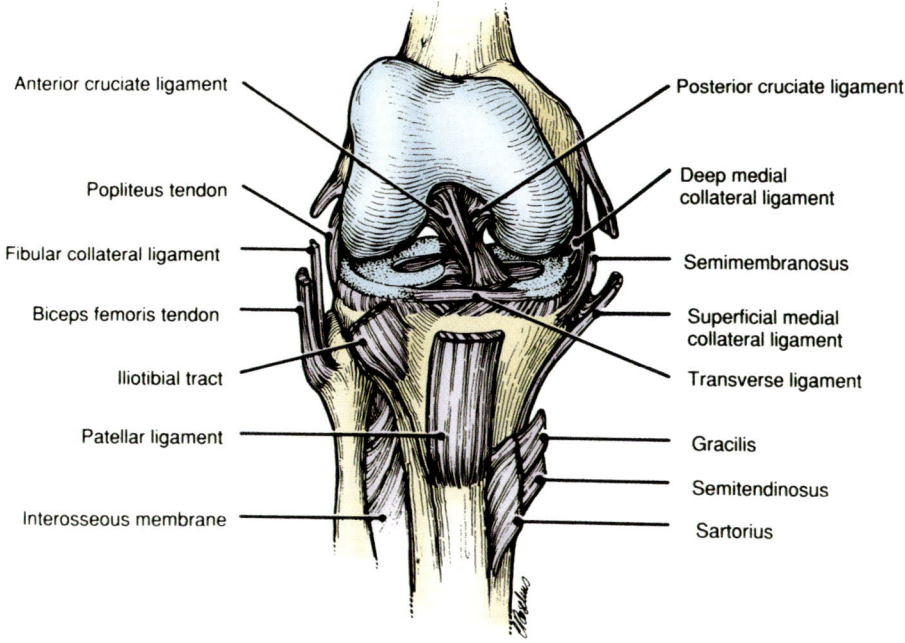

Figure 37-6. The anterior cruciate ligament has been described as a single ligament with different portions taut throughout the range of motion. (From Scott WN: Ligament and extensor mechanism injuries of the knee: diagnosis and treatment, St Louis, 1991, Mosby–Year Book.)

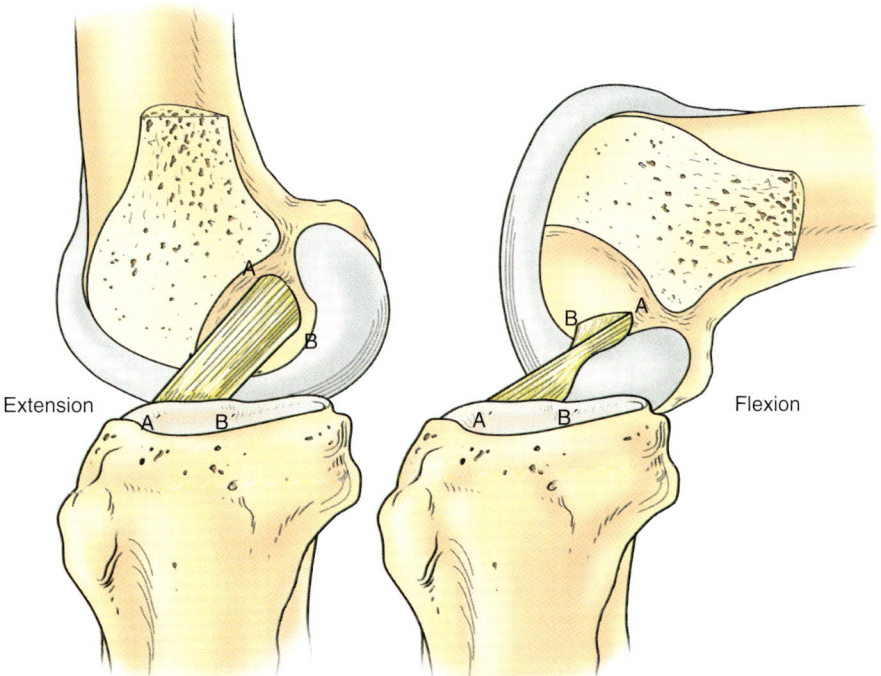

Figure 37-7. Diagram of the anterior cruciate ligament in extension and flexion. Note that in extension the posterolateral bulk is taut, whereas in flexion the anteromedial band is tight and the posterolateral bulk is relatively relaxed. (From Girgis FG, Marshall JL, Al Monajem ARS: The cruciate ligaments of the knee joint: anatomical, functional and experimental analysis. Clin Orthop 106:216, 1975.)

nonarticular area that Jacobsen[43] has termed the *area intercondylaris posterior*. Tajima and coworkers[82] have further investigated the tibial insertion site and noted that the insertions of its two bundles are located in different planes, with a change in slope beween them. Lying anterior to the PCL and connecting the posterior horn of the lateral meniscus to the medial femoral condyle is the ligament of Humphry (Fig.

37-10). The ligament of Wrisberg passes posterior to the PCL to attach on the PCL. The ligaments of Humphrey and Wrisberg (Fig. 37-11) are so intimately related that early authors described them as separate portions of a single ligament.[55] Clancy and colleagues[15] have noted that the meniscofemoral ligament may serve as a secondary stabilizer in a posterior cruciate-deficient knee. The presence of these structures may

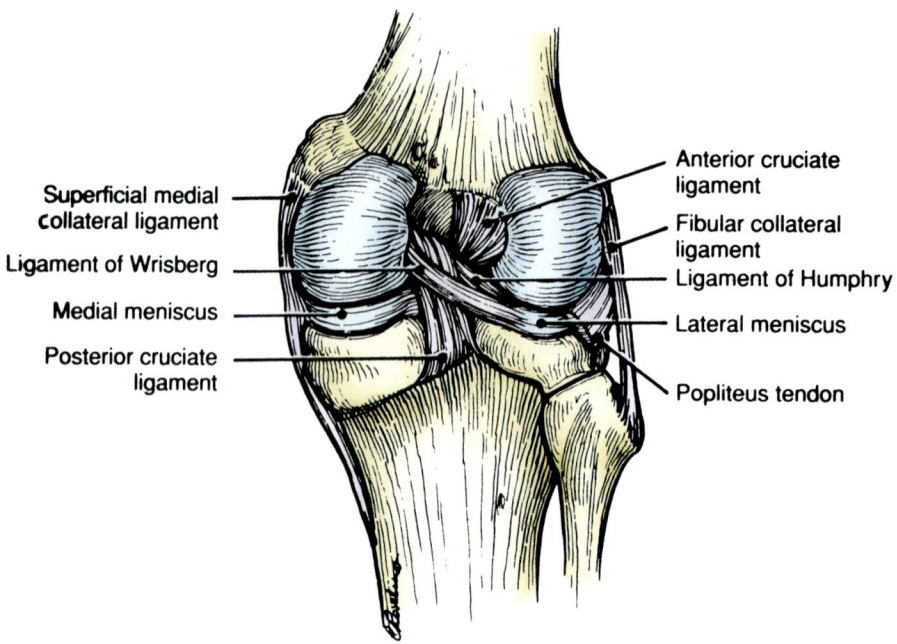

Figure 37-8. The posterior cruciate ligament is an important ligament because of its cross-sectional area, tensile strength, and location in the central axis of the knee joint. (From Scott WN: Ligament and extensor mechanism injuries of the knee: diagnosis and treatment, St Louis, 1991, Mosby–Year Book.)

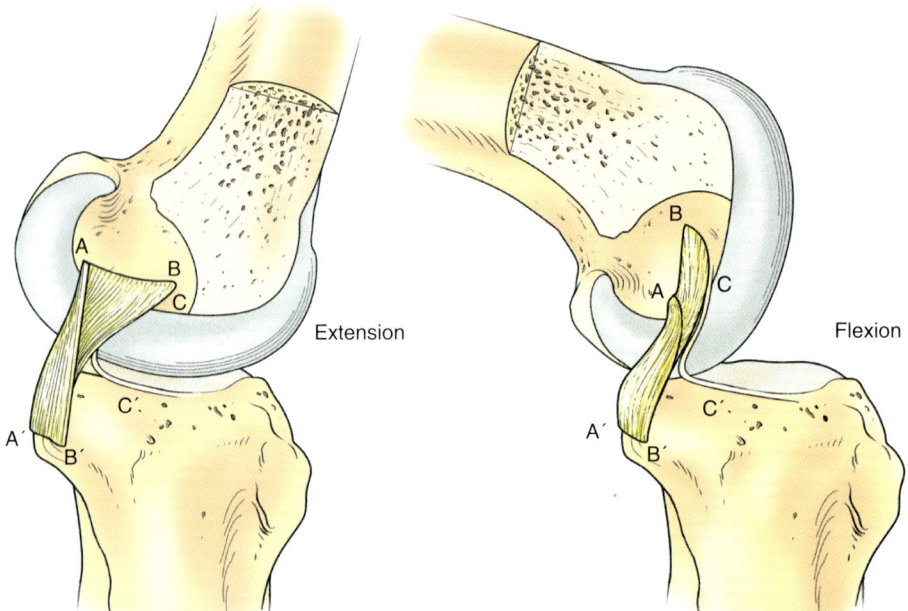

Figure 37-9. Posterior cruciate ligament. In flexion, the bulk of the ligament becomes tight, whereas in extension it is relaxed. (From Girgis FG, Marshall JL, Al Monajem ARS: The cruciate ligaments of the knee joint: anatomical, functional and experimental analysis. Clin Orthop 106:216, 1975.)

account for the absence of posterior drawer in isolated PCL tears.

KINEMATICS

In classifying knee ligamentous instabilities, it is important that the terms be clearly understood and used in a lucid and universally accepted manner. The terms in the literature should be specific to define positions of the knee, motions of the knee, and ligamentous injury. Noyes and associates[66] have taken the time to review the literature and define terms that are in common orthopedic usage.

Position

Position refers to the orientation of the tibia with respect to the femur and determines the tension in each of the ligaments and supporting structures. Dislocation is a term indicating a complete noncontact position of both the tibia and femur or the patellofemoral joint. Dislocations of the knee are classified by the final tibial position-anterior, posterior, medial, lateral, or rotary.[52] Subluxation is defined as an incomplete partial dislocation and does not have limits. It can be described in an anteroposterior, medial lateral, or rotary position.

Motion

Motion is the process of changing position and describes the displacement between the starting and ending points. Displacement is the change in position and is described according to 6 degrees of freedom, a combination of three translations and three rotations. Translation is the parallel displacement of a rigid body or, in the case of the knee joint, the tibia with respect to the femur. Translation of the tibia is composed of

three independent components or translational degrees of freedom—medial lateral translation, anteroposterior translation, and proximal distal translation. Rotation describes motion or displacement about an axis and, in the knee, has 3 degrees of freedom—flexion-extension, internal-external rotation, and abduction-adduction. Range of motion is defined as the displacement that occurs between the two limits of movement for each degree of freedom. There is a ROM for each of the translational and rotational degrees of freedom. For motions other than flexion-extension, ROM generally depends on the angle of knee flexion. The limits of motion are defined as the extreme positions of movement that are possible in each of the 6 degrees of freedom. Injury to the ligamentous and osseous structures about the knee alters the limits of motion. By convention, the limits of flexion and extension are described relative to the neutral position or extension of 0 degrees, with flexion described in positive terms and hyperextension in negative terms. Coupled displacement concerns motion in 1 or more degrees of freedom that is caused by a load applied in another degree of freedom. The amount of coupled rotation depends on where the force is applied to the tibia or on whether the center of rotation is constrained or allowed to move freely. An example is the internal rotation that results when an anterior load is applied to the tibia.[26] When assessing ligamentous stability, motion of the knee joint may occur freely or be constrained, based on the integrity of the ligamentous structures. The ligaments determine the constraint of the knee joint. Elongation or stretching of the ligament limits joint motion and is also supported by compressive joint contact forces that act in an opposite direction. Two ligaments are required to limit translation and rotation, one for each direction. A single ligament alone is unable to resist rotation. If the motion is unconstrained, the tibia displaces into its maximum position. Most clinical tests performed on the knee, however, are constrained.

The force that displaces the knee has three properties, an orientation or line of action, a sense (forward or backward) along its line of action, and a magnitude. The effect of a force

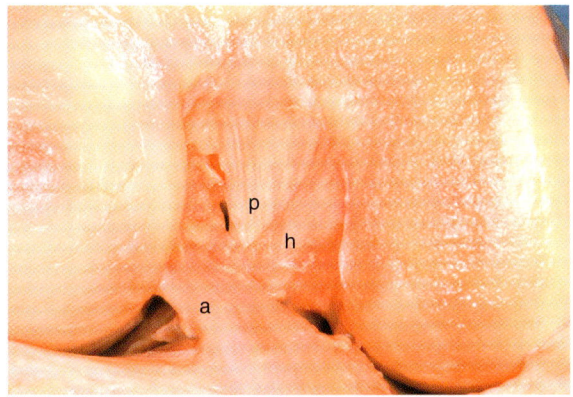

Figure 37-10. Close-up of an anatomic specimen seen from the anterior aspect demonstrating the relationship of the ACL *(a)*, ligament of Humphry *(h)*, and PCL *(p)* from anterior to posterior in the intercondylar notch.

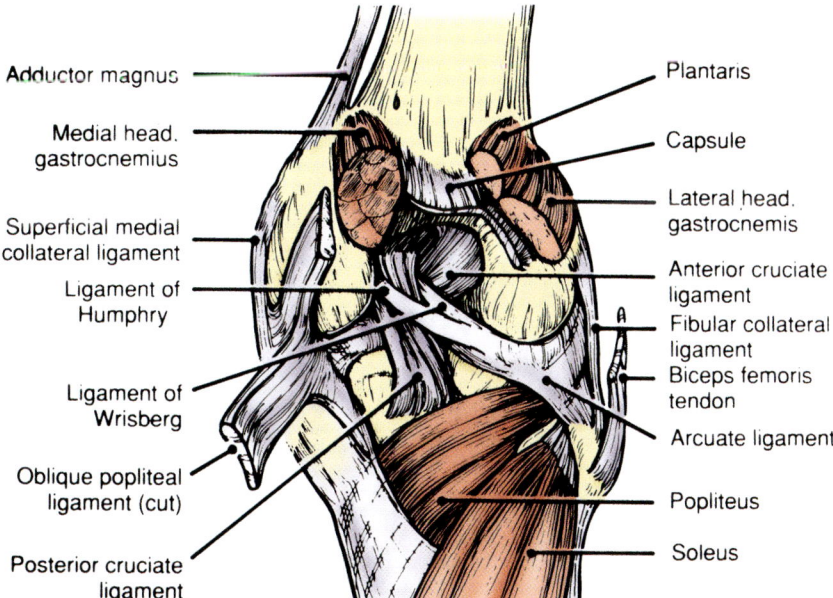

Figure 37-11. The ligaments of Humphry and Wrisberg are so intimately related that early authors described them as separate portions of a single ligament. (From Scott WN: Ligament and extensor mechanism injuries of the knee: diagnosis and treatment, St Louis, 1991, Mosby–Year Book.)

depends on all three of its properties and its point of application. The moment causes an angular or rotational acceleration and has three properties, an orientation or line of action, a sense (clockwise or counterclockwise) about its line of action, and a magnitude. When indicating the moment of the knee joint, it is essential that the axis of rotation be defined.

Laxity

Laxity is a term used to describe the looseness of the joint, which can be normal or abnormal. To avoid confusion, it is better to measure the amount of displacement in millimeters of translation and rotation. The differences between the involved and uninvolved knee should also be reported clearly. Instability is characterized by increased or excessive displacement of the tibia caused by a traumatic injury.

CLASSIFICATION OF LIGAMENT INJURIES

Several terms have been used to describe an injury to a ligament.

Sprain

A sprain is an injury to a joint ligament that stretches or tears ligamentous fibers but does not completely disrupt the ligament. In the handbook *Standard Nomenclature of Athletic Injuries*,[1] sprains were characterized on the basis of indirect evidence of ligament injury, including the history, symptoms, and physical examination (Fig. 37-12). A first-degree sprain is a tear involving a minimal number of fibers of a ligament, with localized tenderness and no instability. A second-degree sprain tears more ligamentous fibers, with slight to moderate abnormal motion. In a third-degree sprain, there is a complete tear of the ligament, with disruption of fibers and demonstrable instability. Third-degree sprains are further

subdivided as follows: grade I, less than a 0.5-cm opening of the joint surfaces; grade II, a 0.5- to 1-cm opening of the joint surfaces; and grade III, a rupture larger than a 1-cm opening. Rupture of a ligament implies complete tearing of the ligament, with concomitant loss of function. Because a ligament may undergo a complete tear but still retain continuity between displaced fibers, it is the loss of function (resistance to displacement) that defines a tear, not the property of continuity.[66] Deficiency of a ligament implies that the ligament is absent or that there is loss of function, such as when the ligament still exists but is stretched and nonfunctional.[60]

Instability

The most elaborate classification system of knee ligament instability was developed by Hughston and colleagues[36,37] and the American Orthopaedic Society of Sports Medicine Research and Education Committee in 1976.[2] This classification system attempts to describe the instability by the direction of tibial displacement and, when possible, by structural deficits. The classification of knee ligament instability is based on rotation of the knee about the central axis of the PCL. All rotatory instabilities indicate subluxation about the intact PCL. Once the PCL is damaged, the instability is designated as straight instability, which indicates subluxation or translation without rotation around a central axis. The subluxation hinges on the intact MCL or LCL.

Rotatory Instability

Rotatory instability includes anteromedial, anterolateral, posterolateral, posteromedial, and combined (Fig. 37-13).[72] Combined instability is not as clearly defined as rotatory or straight instability.

Anteromedial Rotatory Instability

External tibial rotation plus anterior translation is manifested as anteromedial rotatory instability, which causes the medial

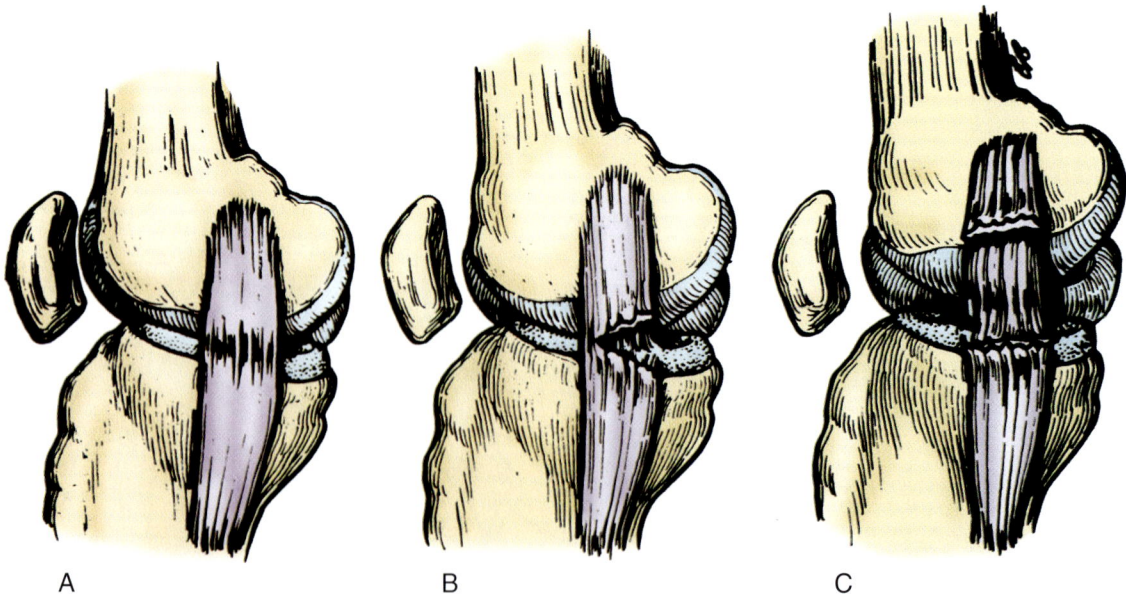

A   B   C

Figure 37-12. Sprains have been characterized on the basis of ligament injury: first-degree **(A)**, second-degree **(B)**, and third-degree **(C)** sprains. (From Scott WN: Ligament and extensor mechanism injuries of the knee: diagnosis and treatment. St Louis, 1991, Mosby–Year Book.)

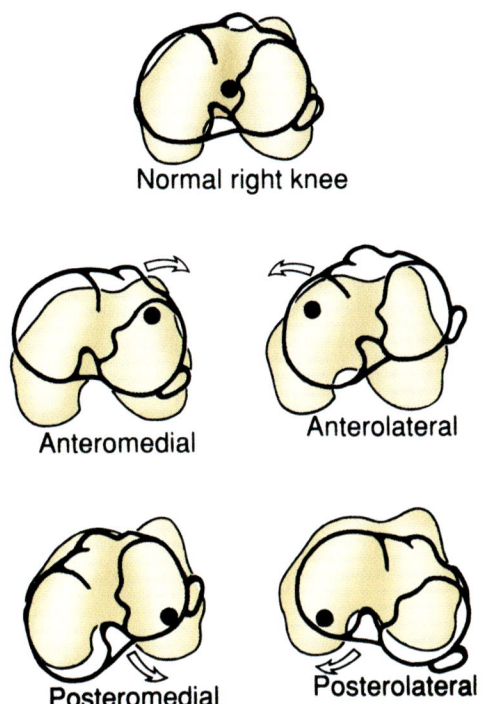

Figure 37-13. Rotatory instability includes anteromedial, anterolateral, posteromedial, and posterolateral instability, which are described in terms of abnormal tibial rotation. (From Scott WN: Ligament and extensor mechanism injuries of the knee: diagnosis and treatment, St Louis, 1991, Mosby–Year Book.)

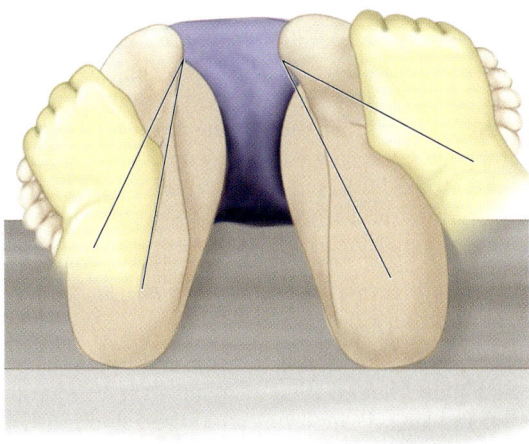

Figure 37-14. The prone external rotation test, which is performed at both 30 and 90 degrees of knee flexion. Forceful external rotation is exerted by the examiner, and the amount of external rotation is measured by comparison of the axis of the medial border of the foot with the femur. (From Veltri DM, Warren RF: Isolated and combined posterior cruciate ligament injuries. J Am Acad Orthop Surg 1:70, 1993.)

tibial plateau to subluxate anteromedially on the medial femoral condyle.[38] This motion implies disruption of the medial capsular ligament, MCL, posterior oblique ligament, and ACL.[41,46,47,80] The medial meniscus is considered an important stabilizing structure and may also be injured.[70] On clinical examination, the abduction stress test result is positive, with abnormal excess opening of the medial joint space at 30 degrees, along with positive anterior drawer and Lachman test results.

Anterolateral Rotatory Instability

This instability results in excessive internal tibial rotation and anterior subluxation, which implies disruption of the lateral capsular ligament, the arcuate complex, and the ACL. The iliotibial band may be damaged to a varying degree, with most of the injury occurring to the deep fibers, which are attached to the posterior cortex of the lateral femoral condyle. Clinical examination reveals positive results for an adduction test at 30 degrees of flexion and for the anterior drawer, Lachman, and pivot-shift tests. The anterior drawer test result with the tibia rotated externally will be negative because the tibia will not be able to rotate internally. The radiographic presence of a Segond fracture implies an avulsion fracture of the attachment of the anterior oblique band of the lateral capsule from the tibia. This finding, associated with a tear of the ACL, is pathognomonic for anterolateral rotatory instability.[73]

Posterolateral Rotatory Instability

This instability is apparent when the lateral tibial plateau rotates posterior to the lateral femoral condyle.[9,16,37] The pathologic condition involves tears of the PFL, popliteus

tendon, and LCL, with possible injury to the biceps tendon. The PCL is not torn and is the axis on which the knee rotates. The anterior drawer, Lachman, and pivot-shift test results will be negative. The patient may be observed walking with a lateral thrust.

On examination, numerous specific tests to help diagnose injuries of the posterolateral corner of the knee have been described; most should be performed with any posterior subluxation of the knee reduced.[17] The posterior drawer test should be performed at 30 and 90 degrees of flexion. If posterior translation, varus rotation, and external rotation are increased at 90 degrees but are normal at 30 degrees, a tear of the PCL should be suspected. With posterior translation, increased at 30 degrees but normal at 90 degrees, posterolateral injury should be assumed. Combined injury should be suspected if posterior translation, varus rotation, and external rotation are increased at all degrees of flexion. The Dial test (tibial external rotation test) is best done with the patient prone at both 30 and 90 degrees of flexion (Fig. 37-14). Increased external rotation at 30 but not 90 degrees is characteristic of injury to the posterolateral corner; increased external rotation at both angles suggests injury to both the PCL and the posterolateral corner. The posterolateral external rotation test is performed with the knee flexed 30 and 90 degrees, with components of posterior and external force applied to the proximal end of the tibia while palpating for posterolateral tibial subluxation. Again, subluxation at 90 degrees implies injury only to the PCL; subluxation at both 30 and 90 degrees suggests injury to both the PCL and posterolateral corner. Veltri and Warren[89] have reported that the most useful tests for the diagnosis of posterolateral knee injury are the Dial test at 30 and 90 degrees of flexion and the varus stress test at 0 and 30 degrees of flexion.

Posteromedial Rotatory Instability

This instability is manifested by posterior rotation of the medial tibial plateau on the medial femoral condyle. It implies disruption of the MCL, the medial capsular ligament, the posterior oblique ligament, the ACL, and the posteromedial capsule. There may be stretching or major injury to the semimembranosus tendon. The PCL is intact. Hughston and associates[36] do not believe that posteromedial rotatory instability occurs if the PCL is intact because the tightening of the PCL that accompanies internal rotation would prevent this type of instability. If the PCL is disrupted, there would be no fixed axis of rotation, and the instability would be straight posterior.

Combined Anteromedial and Anterolateral Rotatory Instability

This instability results in simultaneous anterior subluxation of the medial and lateral tibial plateaus. It implies injury to the medial and lateral supporting structures, along with a tear of the ACL. Medially, the injury involves the middle third of the medial capsular ligament, the posterior oblique ligament, and the MCL. Laterally, there is a tear of the middle third of the lateral capsular ligament, the iliotibial band, and the short head of the biceps. Clinically, the knee demonstrates positive results for the anterior drawer, Lachman, pivot-shift, and abduction stress tests at 30 degrees of flexion; the results of the adduction stress test at 30 degrees are equivocal.

Combined Anterolateral and Posterolateral Rotatory Instability

This instability is the result of disruption of all of the lateral capsular ligaments, with or without a tear of the iliotibial band. Although the ACL is torn, the PCL remains intact. There is a high incidence of lateral meniscal tears. On clinical examination, results of the adduction stress test are markedly positive, along with positive results for the Lachman and anterior drawer tests.

Combined Anteromedial and Posteromedial Rotatory Instability

This instability occurs when all the medial and posteromedial structures, including the semimembranosus complex, are torn along with an injury to the ACL. The PCL is intact.

Straight Instability

The four types of straight instability are medial, lateral, posterior, and anterior.

Straight Medial Instability

This instability is caused by disruption of the medial supporting structures, including the MCL, middle third of the medial capsular ligament, and the posterior oblique ligament. Although the ACL is usually torn, Hughston[36] has noted that the PCL must be torn for straight medial instability to exist. This opinion is not held by all clinicians; some investigators believe that the PCL may not be disrupted. Because the axis of rotation is the LCL, the clinical examination will demonstrate medial joint space opening with an abduction stress test at 30 and 0 degrees. If the ACL is torn, the anterior drawer result will be positive in all three rotational positions. With a torn PCL, the posterior drawer result is positive.

Straight Lateral Instability

This instability is the result of a tear of the lateral supporting structures and the PCL, with an axis hinging on the MCL. It is manifested by lateral opening with an adduction stress test in the fully extended position. The injury involves disruption of the lateral capsular ligament, the LCL, the arcuate complex, and the PCL. Clinically, the adduction stress test result is positive at 30 and 0 degrees, but the degree of opening depends on the level of injury to the iliotibial band. The posterior drawer result is positive in the neutral position and will show increased translation with the knee rotated externally. If there is an ACL tear, the anterior drawer and Lachman test results will be positive. The pivot-shift result may not be positive if there is an injury to the iliotibial band.

Straight Posterior Instability

This instability occurs in patients with isolated injury to the PCL. Although there might be injury to the arcuate ligament and the posterior oblique ligament, the MCL, LCL, and ACL are intact. On examination, the knee demonstrates a posterior drop-back of the tibia without evidence of rotation. Whereas the posterior drawer test result is markedly positive, medial, lateral, and anterior test results are negative.

Straight Anterior Instability

This instability is the result of disruption of the ACL and is demonstrated by a positive result of the anterior drawer test in neutral rotation with an equal amount of medial and lateral subluxation. There is no evidence of rotational displacement. In contrast, Hughston and colleagues defined straight instability as an injury to the PCL and related supporting structures, with loss of the central axis of rotation. Therefore, they did not regard straight anterior instability as an injury to the ACL, but rather as an injury to the PCL. With this in mind, Hughston and coworkers[36,37] claimed not to have encountered any anterior displacement great enough to rupture the PCL without also rupturing the MCL and LCL.

Noyes and Grood Rotatory Instability Model

Noyes and Grood[32,64,65] have maintained that the terms for rotatory instability, as discussed earlier, are imprecise and do not represent a specific definable motion or set of motions. An almost infinite number of combinations of joint motion actually exist and can occur, depending on the abnormalities in any of 1, 2, or 3 of the degrees of freedom. Accurate diagnosis requires knowledge of the precise abnormalities and biomechanical data as to which ligaments limit the use of motion. As a result of such information, they developed the bumper model of the knee. They found this model to be useful in understanding how the ligaments and capsular structures limit anterior and posterior translation and internal and external rotation.

Noyes and Grood developed a knee ligament evaluation form (Fig. 37-15). The clinician examines and tests the knee for integrity of the primary and secondary ligament restraints. It is important to select a laxity test to diagnose a specific ligament injury. The extent of damage to each structure is reported as follows: I, partial damage, still functional; II, partial damage, compromised function; and X, complete damage, nonfunctional. The assessment of the functional capacity of the injured ligaments and capsule is only an approximation. Ultimately, it is necessary to quantitate the damaged structures. In the bumper model, the bumpers do not represent exact ligament structures; instead, they

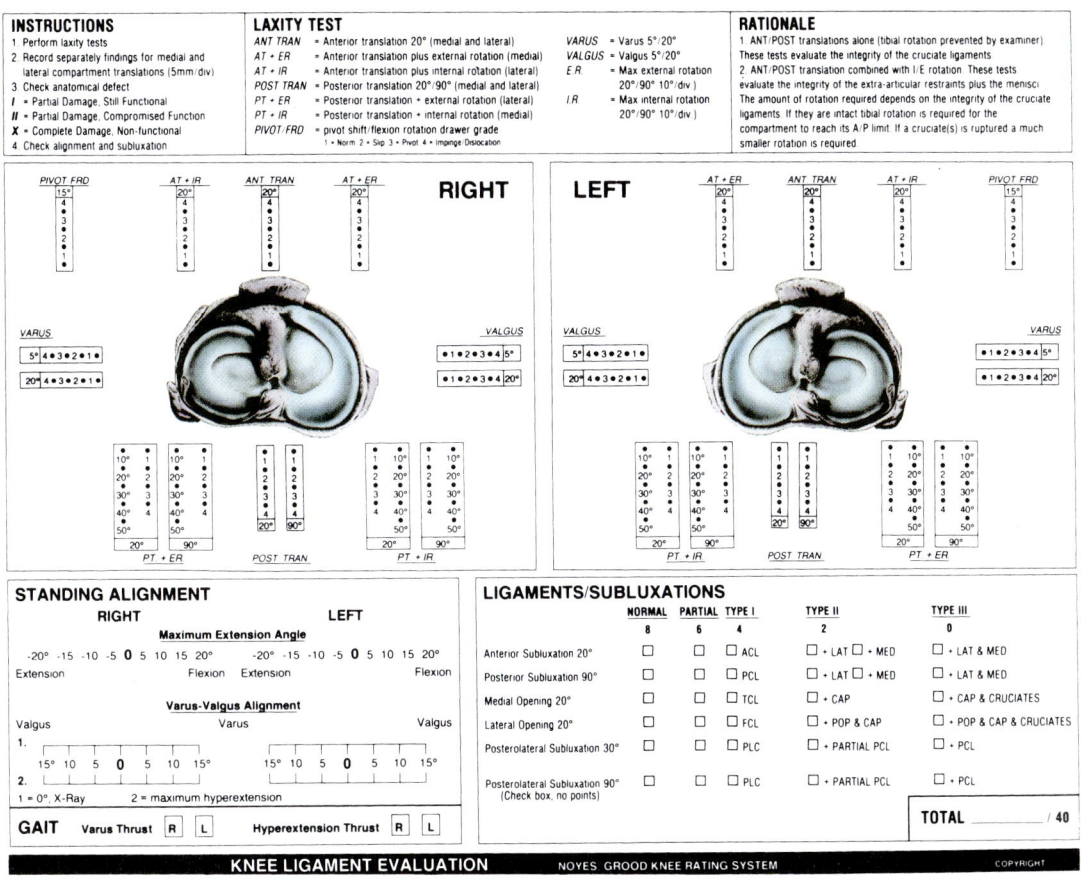

Figure 37-15. The knee ligament evaluation form used in the Noyes-Grood rating system. (From Noyes FR, Grood ES: Classification of ligament injuries: why an anterolateral laxity or anteromedial laxity is not a diagnostic entity. Instr Course Lect 36:185, 1987.)

represent the final restraints to tibial motion, with summation of the effect of the ligament, menisci, and capsular structures.

Type I motion is described as normal, and there are three clinically identifiable types of anterior knee subluxation that can occur after a rupture of the ACL. Noyes and Grood[32,64,65] have recommended performing the anterior drawer and Lachman tests in a neutral position without rotation for initial evaluation of the ACL. The anterior drawer test is then repeated with internal and external rotation to determine the maximum excursion of the lateral and medial tibiofemoral compartments to provide information on the laxity of the extra-articular ligamentous restraints. The results of the laxity tests are indicated on the evaluation form by recording first, the amount of central subluxation and, second, the amount of translation of the medial and lateral compartments when tibial rotation is added. The clinical significance of identifying these three types of anterior subluxation rests in their different natural histories and treatment programs. Type II subluxation is characterized by tight extra-articular structures; the amount of anterior and lateral tibial translation is only slightly increased. Type III subluxation consists of anterior subluxation with increased translation of the medial and lateral tibial compartments. The translation of the lateral tibial compartment will be greater because of associated increases in the internal rotation units. Type IV anterior subluxation indicates gross subluxation with increased

translation of the medial and lateral compartments. As the degree of subluxation increases, the axis of rotation is shifted medially outside the joint.

The final diagnosis of a ligament defect must be made in precise anatomic terms; in cases of partial disruption or after healing occurs, the clinician must analyze the remaining functional capacity of the ligaments. It has been suggested that identifying these types of anterior subluxation has clinical significance because each carries a different prognosis. Type II subluxation, characterized by tight extra-articular structures, has a better prognosis than that of types III and IV subluxation; ACL reconstruction is recommended.[64] With type IV subluxation, it is important to restore the associated damaged ligamentous structures, especially the lateral extra-articular structures.

DETERMINATION OF KNEE LIGAMENT INSTABILITY

The joint motion assessed on clinical examination determines the classification of knee ligament instability. It is important that the objective findings on the clinical examination correlate with the pathologic knee motion and allow standardized classification of knee ligament instability. Clinical findings have been substantiated by biomechanical studies.

Ligament Injury Tests

Valgus Stress Test

This test should be performed first on the normal extremity for later comparison. The involved knee is flexed to 30 degrees, and a gentle valgus stress is applied to the knee, with one hand placed on the lateral aspect of the thigh and the other hand grasping the foot and ankle (Fig. 37-16). Placing the hip in relative extension helps relax the hamstring musculature. The valgus stress test must also be performed with the knee in full extension or in the amount of recurvatum present in the opposite uninvolved limb. The degree of opening of the medial side of the knee should be quantified, graded, and recorded.

Varus Stress Test

This test is similar to the valgus stress test. The varus stress test is carried out with the knee in full extension and in 30 degrees of flexion. The degree of lateral opening should be quantified, graded, and recorded (Fig. 37-17).

Anterior Drawer Test

The hip is flexed to 45 degrees, with the knee flexed to 80 to 90 degrees (Fig. 37-18). The examiner sits on the table and, using the buttocks, stabilizes the patient's foot. The examiner places his or her hands about the upper part of the tibia and palpates the hamstrings to make sure that they are relaxed. The examiner then gently pulls and pushes the proximal

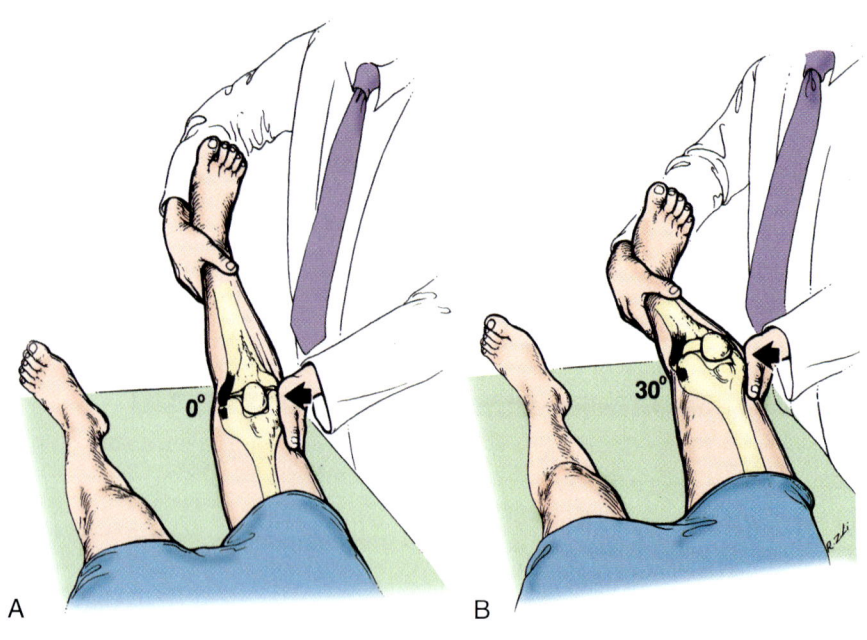

Figure 37-16. **A,** Valgus stress in extension tests the medial collateral ligament and the posteromedial capsule. **B,** Stress in 30 degrees of flexion tests only the medial collateral ligament. (From Tria AJ Jr, Klein KS: An illustrated guide to the knee, New York, 1992, Churchill Livingstone.)

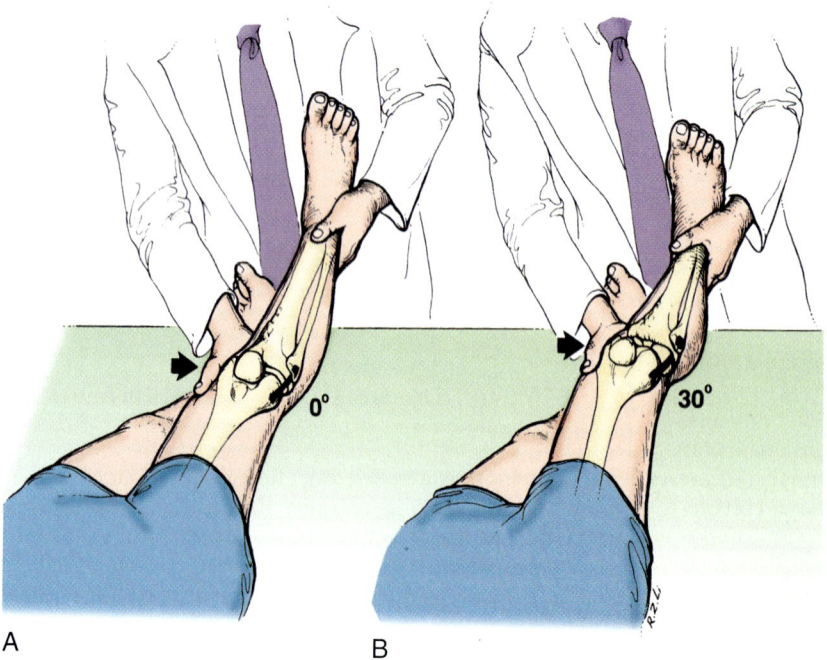

Figure 37-17. **A,** Varus stress in extension tests the lateral collateral ligament and the posterolateral capsule. **B,** Stress in 30 degrees of flexion tests only the lateral collateral ligament. (From Tria AJ Jr, Klein KS: An illustrated guide to the knee, New York, 1992, Churchill Livingstone.)

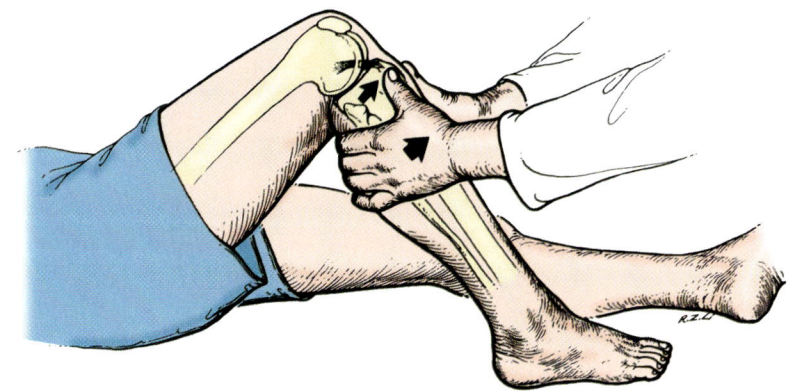

Figure 37-18. The anterior drawer test is performed with the knee flexed to 90 degrees and with anterior force applied to the proximal end of the tibia. (From Tria AJ Jr, Klein KS: An illustrated guide to the knee, New York, 1992, Churchill Livingstone.)

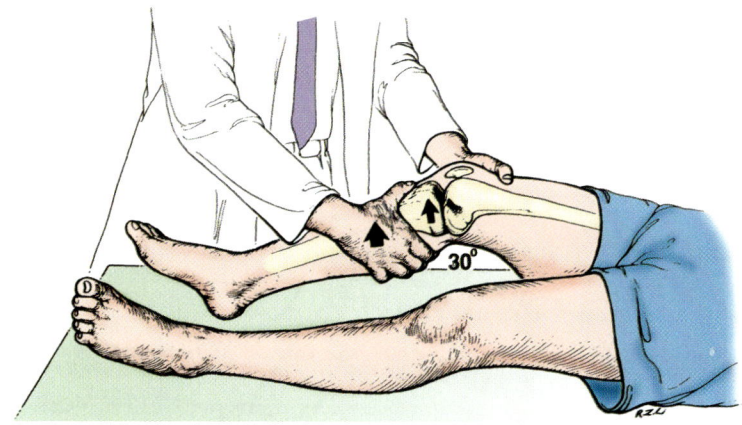

Figure 37-19. The Lachman test is performed in 30 degrees of flexion with anterior force exerted on the proximal end of the tibia. (From Tria AJ Jr, Klein KS: An illustrated guide to the knee, New York, 1992, Churchill Livingstone.)

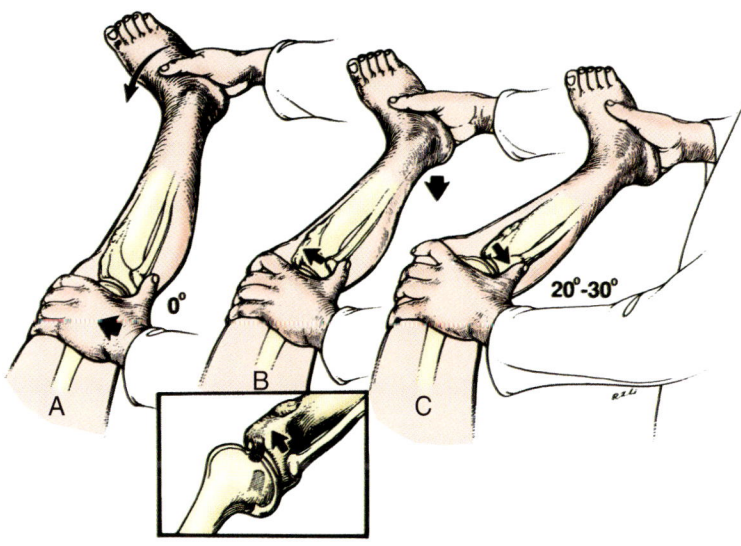

Figure 37-20. The pivot-shift test begins with the knee in full extension **(A)** and applies internal rotation **(B)** and valgus stress **(C)** to demonstrate anterolateral subluxation. (From Tria AJ Jr, Klein KS: An illustrated guide to the knee, New York, 1992, Churchill Livingstone.)

portion of the tibia in a to-and-fro manner. The test is performed in neutral, internal, and external rotated postures of the foot. The degree and type of anterior drawer should be reported.

Lachman Test

This test has been the standard examination for evaluating the integrity of the ACL and is used to assess anterior knee laxity and stiffness, with the knee in about 20 degrees of flexion (Fig. 37-19). In this position, an anterior drawer is applied to the proximal part of the calf, at which time the examiner perceives displacement of the tibia and assesses the end point stiffness.[45] The slightest increase in anterior displacement of the tibia would be considered a positive test result when compared with the contralateral knee. End point stiffness should be clearly documented.

Pivot-Shift Test

The pivot-shift test[28] (Fig. 37-20) and the Losee test[53] (Fig. 37-21) demonstrate anterior subluxation and reduction of the

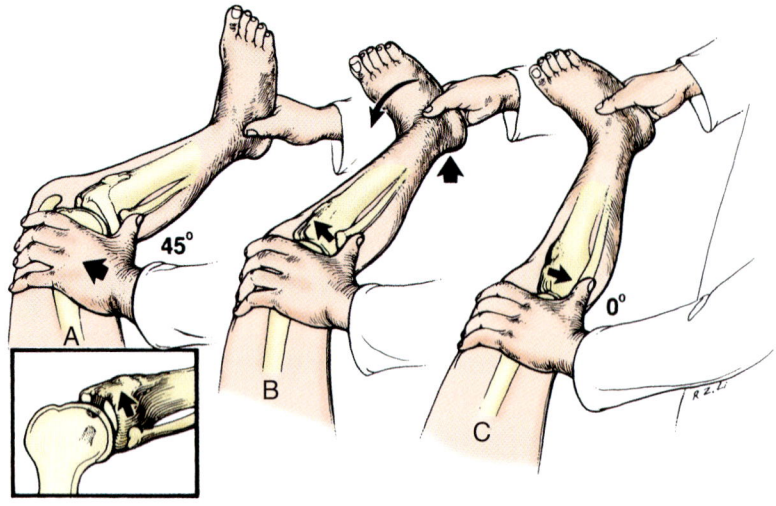

Figure 37-21. **A,** The Losee test begins with the knee in flexion but externally rotates the foot. Valgus stress is applied **(B)**, and the tibia is internally rotated as the knee is extended **(C)**. (From Tria AJ Jr, Klein KS: An illustrated guide to the knee, New York, 1992, Churchill Livingstone.)

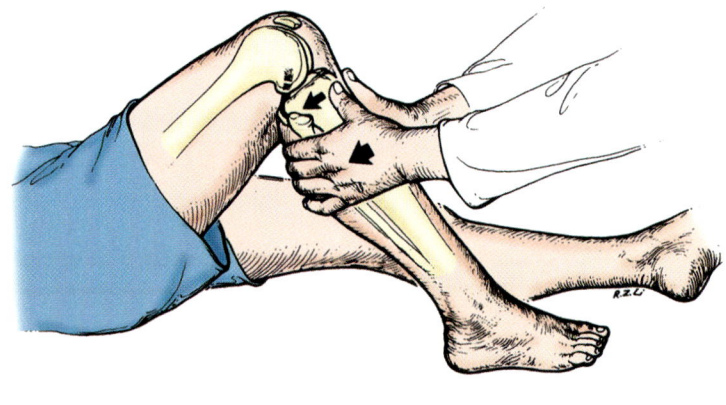

Figure 37-22. The posterior drawer test is performed in 90 degrees of flexion with posterior force applied to the proximal end of the tibia. (From Tria AJ Jr, Klein KS: An illustrated guide to the knee, New York, 1992, Churchill Livingstone.)

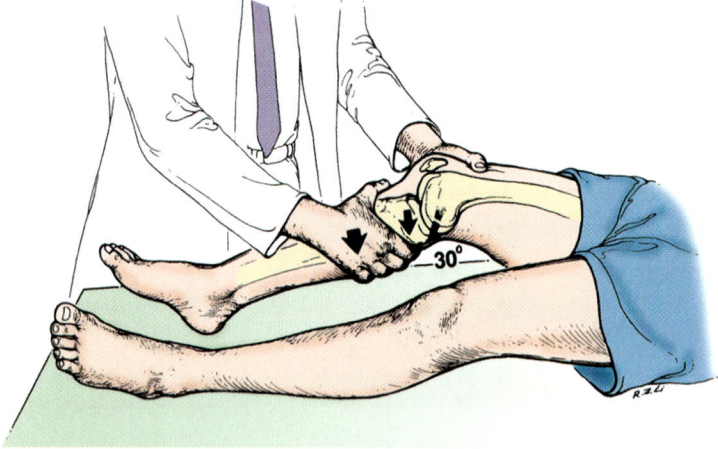

Figure 37-23. The posterior Lachman test applies posterior force to the proximal end of the tibia with the knee flexed 30 degrees. (From Tria AJ Jr, Klein KS: An illustrated guide to the knee, New York, 1992, Churchill Livingstone.)

tibia, with the knee in flexion-extension from 10 to 40 degrees as a result of ACL disruption. Patients with an MCL disruption or previous iliotibial tract surgery may have less dramatic findings on physical examination.[20]

Posterior Drawer Test

The standard test to assess the PCL has been the posterior drawer test. The knee is flexed to 90 degrees and posterior force is exerted on the tibia in an attempt to sublux it posteriorly in relation to the femur (Fig. 37-22). Before initiating the test, to avoid a potential false-negative examination finding, it is important to ensure that the tibia rests at its normal anatomic position approximately 1 cm anterior to the femoral condyles. A grade III posterior drawer in addition to more than 10 mm of posterior tibial translation on stress radiographs has been shown to represent a combined PCL and posterolateral corner injury.[75] A posterior Lachman test result has also been described for acute PCL injuries (Fig. 37-23). The knee is held in 30 degrees of flexion and the tibia is forced posteriorly. Any motion in this direction correlates with a tear of the PCL.[87]

Quadriceps Active Test

A knee with chronic PCL deficiency may demonstrate posterior sag when the knee and hip are flexed to 90 degrees. To perform the 90-degree quadriceps active test, the clinician sits beside the examining table, with the patient's knee flexed to 90 degrees at eye level (Fig. 37-24). The foot is stabilized by the clinician, and the patient is asked to slide her or his foot gently down the table. The clinician's hand prevents the foot from moving forward, thereby allowing anterior translation of the tibia, which occurs when the tibia is posteriorly subluxated secondary to PCL disruption.

Reverse Pivot-Shift Test

This test is used to diagnose injuries to the posterolateral ligament complex. The clinician supports the patient's limb with a hand under the heel, with the knee in full extension and neutral rotation (Fig. 37-25). A valgus stress is applied and the knee is flexed. In a positive test, at about 20 to 30 degrees of flexion the tibia will rotate externally, and the lateral tibial plateau will subluxate posteriorly and remain in this position during further flexion. When the knee is then extended, the tibia reduces. In the standard pivot-shift test, the tibia is subluxated anteriorly in early flexion and reduces between 20 and 40 degrees of flexion. In the reverse pivot-shift test, the tibia

is initially reduced and then the lateral tibial plateau posteriorly subluxates at 20 to 30 degrees of flexion. In a patient with a combined ACL and posterolateral ligament complex injury, one may observe the tibia go from anterior subluxation to a reduced position and then to a posterior subluxated position.[20] A knee with a posterolateral injury should be tested at 0 to 30 degrees of flexion for maximum primary posterior translation and at 75 to 90 degrees of external rotation for minimum translation. A knee in which an isolated PCL injury is suspected should be tested at 75 to 90 degrees of flexion for maximum primary posterior translation and at 0 to 30 degrees for minimum translation. In an isolated PCL injury, no change should be expected in primary external rotation. If both the posterolateral structures and PCL are ruptured, there will be a substantial increase in primary posterior translation, external rotation, and varus rotation at all angles of flexion of the knee as compared with an intact knee or one in which either structure has been injured in isolation.[30]

Ligament Testing Devices Used in Classification

It is important that the classification of ligament injuries be precise and that the clinician understand the remaining functional capacity of the ligaments. Difficulties still remain in the evaluation of these injuries, and it is anticipated that newer diagnostic devices will provide detailed information to

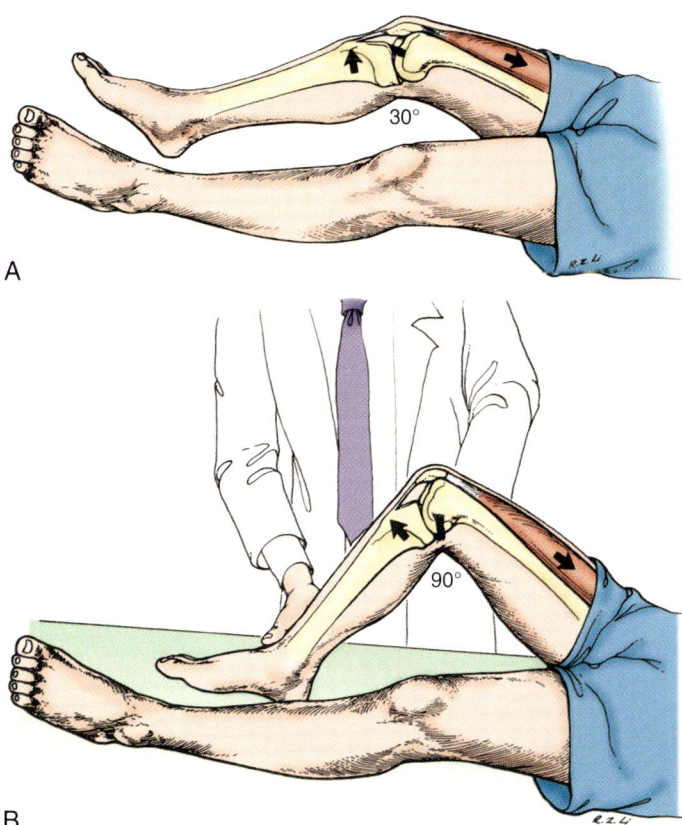

Figure 37-24. Quadriceps active test for the anterior cruciate ligament in 30 degrees of flexion **(A)** and for the posterior cruciate ligament in 90 degrees of flexion **(B).** (From Scott WN [ed]: The knee, St Louis, 1994, CV Mosby.)

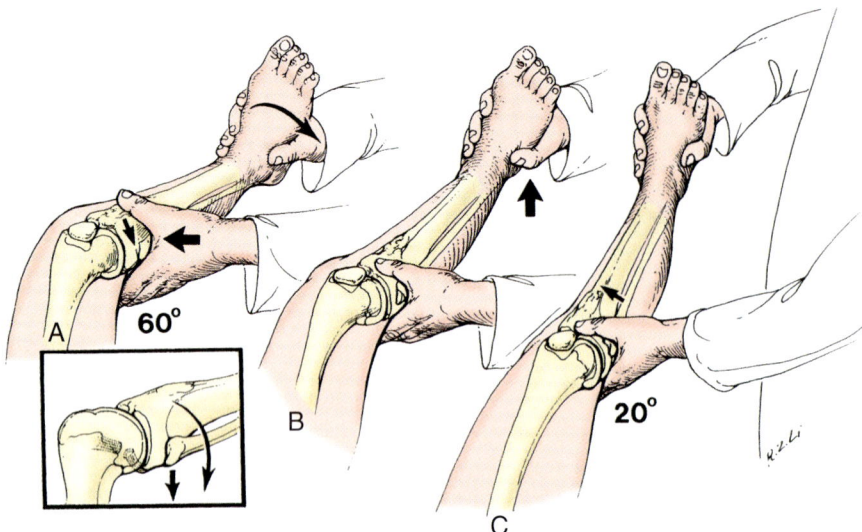

Figure 37-25. **A,** The reverse pivot-shift test begins with the knee flexed and the tibia externally rotated. **B, C,** The knee is then extended and posterolateral capsular laxity demonstrated. (From Tria AJ Jr, Klein KS: An illustrated guide to the knee, New York, 1992, Churchill Livingstone.)

enable the clinician to determine the different types of instability under defined loading conditions.

In the 1980s, several ligament testing devices were developed in an attempt to quantitate anteroposterior displacement of the knee joint objectively.* The variability in subjective clinical grades given to many testing maneuvers makes it difficult to compare injuries and clinical results. Objective quantitative ligament testing devices provide the opportunity to more accurately compare populations of patients. The pathologic anteroposterior motion of cruciate ligament injuries can be diagnosed with the KT-1000 arthrometer (MEDmetric, San Diego, Calif). Daniel and colleagues[23] have reported that 97% of 120 normal subjects tested with the KT-1000 arthrometer demonstrated less than a 3-mm right-left difference, whereas the right-left difference was 3 mm or greater in 90% of 33 patients with an acute ACL injury with the manual maximum test. Miyasaka and associates[59] have found that use of the KT-1000 arthrometer and quadriceps active tests helped them diagnose a PCL injury with high accuracy. In another study, 40 of 41 patients with documented PCL rupture were found to have pathological laxity by this method.[21] Objective quantification of knee laxity in ACL and PCL injury with instrumented testing is useful. Daniel and coworkers[22] have shown that 96% of patients with an arthroscopically confirmed tear of the ACL had a maximum manual KT-1000 test result with a more than 3-mm side to side difference. It has been suggested that further quantitative reporting should include 89 N, maximum manual, compliance index, and side-to-side difference because variations in testing parameters have been noted.[7] There are pitfalls and limitations with the use of current instrumented testing devices. Bach and colleagues[8] found that the KT-1000 is useful only for anteroposterior translation because it does not allow assessment of rotational or varus-valgus instability. The clinical applicability of the Genucom computerized system appears to be limited by variability in measurements of knee laxity.[31] The problem is that this device assumes that the change in stiffness of the soft tissues can be accurately predicted from one angle of flexion of the knee to another. However, major variations in the effect of the position of the knee are expected between subjects and even between repeated examinations of the same individual.

Objective quantitation of knee laxity in ligamentous injuries is an important diagnostic adjunct. Testing devices that objectively measure laxity permit the clinician to evaluate the injured or postsurgical knee and predict the functional outcome. In a prospective study, Daniel and associates[22] have shown that the early KT grade is a predictor of the late KT grade.

KNEE LIGAMENT RATING SYSTEMS

In the course of developing knee ligament rating systems, investigators have attempted to correlate function and clinical findings. Although universal acceptance has not been achieved, several rating systems have been popularized. The Lysholm scale[54] (Table 37-1) is based solely on the patient's subjective evaluation of function, with no weight given to objective findings. In an effort to rate a patient's level of function, Tegner and Lysholm[83] have developed a knee activity assessment that questions patients about their participation in sports and work (Table 37-2). Twenty-five years after their introduction, the Lysholm score and Tegner activity scale have demonstrated acceptable responsiveness and psychometric parameters as patient-administered scores.[11]

Because it is important to include objective clinical findings with the level of activity, Noyes and colleagues[63] designed a knee rating system that uses subjective and objective criteria (Table 37-3). The subjective criteria include a system rating scale, assessment of function, and sports rating scale. Objective testing includes ROM, the presence of crepitus, KT-1000 testing, and a radiographic review. The scale includes a scheme for a final rating of excellent, good, fair, or poor. Although these rating systems have gained regional or institutional acceptance, the American Orthopaedic Society of Sports Medicine and its European equivalent, under the auspices of the International Knee Documentation Committee, have published a knee ligament injury evaluation form (Fig. 37-26).

---

*References 19, 23, 24, 56, 68, 69, and 76.

Table 37-1 Lysholm Scale

Parameter	Finding	Score	Parameter	Finding	Score
Limp	None	5	Pain	None	25
	Slight or periodic	3		Inconstant and slight during strenuous activities	20
	Severe and constant	0			
Support	None	5		Marked during or after walking >2 km	10
	Stick or crutch needed	2		Marked during or after walking <2 km	5
	Weight bearing impossible	0		Constant	0
Locking	None	15	Swelling	None	10
	None, but catching sensation present	10		After strenuous activities	6
	Occasional	6		After ordinary activities	3
	Frequent	2		Constant	0
	At examination	0	Squatting	No problem	5
Stairs	No problem	10		Slight problem	4
	Slight problem	6		Not beyond 90 degrees of knee flexion	2
	One step at a time	3		Impossible	0
	Impossible	0			
Instability	Never	25			
	Rarely during athletic activities	20			
	Frequently during athletic activities	15			
	Occasionally during daily activities	10			
	Often during daily activities	5			
	Every step	0			

Adapted from Lysholm J, Gillquist J: Evaluation of knee ligament surgery results with special emphasis on using a scoring scale. J Sports Med 10:150, 1982.

Table 37-2 Tegner and Lysholm Activity Scales

Level	Type of Sport or Activity	Example(s)
10	Competitive sports	Soccer—national or international level
9	Competitive sports	Soccer—lower divisions Ice hockey Wrestling Gymnastics
8	Competitive sports	Bandy Squash or badminton Athletics (e.g., jumping) Downhill skiing
7	Competitive sports	Tennis Athletics (e.g., running) Motocross or speedway Handball or basketball
	Recreational sports	Soccer Bandy or ice hockey Squash Athletics (e.g., jumping) Cross-country track finding (orienteering), both recreational and competitive
6	Recreational sports	Tennis or badminton Handball or basketball Downhill skiing Jogging at least five times weekly
5	Work Competitive sports Recreational sports	Heavy labor (e.g., construction, forestry) Cycling Cross-country skiing Jogging on uneven ground at least twice weekly
4	Work Recreational sports	Moderately heavy work (e.g., truck driving, scrubbing floors) Cycling Cross-country skiing Jogging on uneven ground at least weekly
3	Work Competitive and recreational sports	Light work (e.g., nursing) Walking on rough forest terrain
2	Work	Light work Walking on uneven ground
1	Work	Sedentary work Walking on uneven ground
0	Sick leave or disability pension because of knee problems	

Adapted from Tegner Y, Lysholm J: Rating systems in evaluation of knee ligament injuries. Clin Orthop 198:43, 1985.

THE SEVEN GROUPS	THE FOUR GRADES				GROUP GRADE (see footnotes)			
	A: normal	B: nearly normal	C: abnormal	D: sev. abnorm.	A	B	C	D
1 Patient subjective assessment On a scale of 0 to 3 how did you rate your pre-injury activity level?	☐ 0	☐ 1	☐ 2	☐ 3				
On a scale of 0 to 3 how did you rate your current activity level?	☐ 0	☐ 1	☐ 2	☐ 3				
If your normal knee performs 100%, what percentage does your operated knee perform?	_____ %				☐	☐	☐	☐

2 Symptoms	(Grade at highest activity level known by patient)							
	I Strenuous activities	II Moderate activities	III ADL/Light activities	IV ADL problems				
Pain	☐	☐	☐	☐				
Swelling	☐	☐	☐	☐				
Partial giving way	☐	☐	☐	☐				
Full giving way	☐	☐	☐	☐	☐	☐	☐	☐

3 Range of motion	Flex/Ext: Index side: __ /__ /__ Opposite side: __ /__ /__							
Lack of extension (from zero degrees)	☐ <3°	☐ 3–5°	☐ 6–10°	☐ >10°				
Δ Lack of flexion	☐ 0–5°	☐ 6–15°	☐ 16–25°	☐ >25°	☐	☐	☐	☐

4 Ligament examination								
Δ Lachman (25° flex)	☐ 1 to 2 mm	☐ 3 to 5 mm	☐ 6 to 10 mm	☐ >10 mm				
(manual, instrumented, x-ray) Endpoint: ☐ firm ☐ soft	☐ firm		☐ soft					
Δ Total a.p. transl. (70° flex)	☐ 0 to 2 mm	☐ 3 to 5 mm	☐ 6 to 10 mm	☐ >10 mm				
Δ Post. sag in 70° flex	☐ 0 to 2 mm	☐ 3 to 5 mm	☐ 6 to 10 mm	☐ >10 mm				
Δ Med. joint opening (valgus rotation)	☐ 0 to 2 mm	☐ 3 to 5 mm	☐ 6 to 10 mm	☐ >10 mm				
Δ Lat. joint opening (varus rotation)	☐ 0 to 2 mm	☐ 3 to 5 mm	☐ 6 to 10 mm	☐ >10 mm				
Pivot shift	☐ neg.	☐ + (glide)	☐ ++ (clunk)	☐ +++ (gross)				
Reversed pivot shift	☐ equal	☐ glide	☐ marked	☐ gross	☐	☐	☐	☐

5 Compartmental findings								
Crepitus patellofemoral	☐ none		☐ moderate	☐ severe				
Crepitus medial compartment	☐ none		☐ moderate	☐ severe				
Crepitus lateral compartment	☐ none		☐ moderate	☐ severe (palpable & audible)	☐	☐	☐	☐

6 X-ray findings								
Med. joint space narrowing	☐ none		☐ <50%	☐ >50%				
Lat. joint space narrowing	☐ none		☐ <50%	☐ >50%				
Patellofemoral joint space narrowing	☐ none		☐ <50%	☐ >50%	☐	☐	☐	☐

7 Functional test								
Δ One leg hop (% of opposite side)	☐ 100–90%	☐ 90–76%	☐ 75–50%	☐ <50%	☐	☐	☐	☐
Final evaluation					☐	☐	☐	☐

Footnotes:
- Group grade: The lowest grade within a group determines the group grade.
- Final evaluation: The worst group determines the final evaluation.
- In a final evaluation all 7 groups are to be evaluated; for a quick knee profile the evaluation of groups 1–4 are sufficient.

Figure 37-26. International Knee Documentation Committee knee rating system. (From the International Knee Documentation Committee: knee ligament injury and reconstruction evaluation. In Aichroth PM, Dilworth Cannon WD Jr [eds]: Knee surgery: Current practice, New York, 1992, Martin Dunitz/Raven Press, p 760.)

Table 37-3 Cincinnati Knee Rating System

Activity	Function	Points
A. Assessment of Function		
Activities of Daily Living		
Walking	Normal, unlimited	40
	Some limitations	30
	No more than 3-4 blocks possible	20
	Less than 1 block with cane or crutch	0
Stair climbing	Normal, unlimited	40
	Some limitations	30
	No more than 11-30 steps possible	20
	No more than 1-10 steps possible	0
Squatting, kneeling	Normal, unlimited	40
	Some limitations	30
	No more than 6-10 possible	20
	No more than 0-5 possible	0
Sports Activities		
Straight running	Fully competitive	100
	Some limitations, guarding	80
	Run half-speed, definite limitations	60
	Not able to do so	40
Jumping, landing on affected leg	Fully competitive	100
	Some limitations, guarding	80
	Definite limitations, half-speed	60
	Not able to do so	40
Hard twisting, cutting, pivoting	Fully competitive	100
	Some limitations, guarding	80
	Definite limitations, half-speed	60
	Not able to do so	40

B. Symptom Rating Scale

Symptoms	Activities	Points
None	Able to do strenuous work, sports with jumping and hard pivoting	10
With strenuous work, sports	Able to do moderate work, sports with running, turning, and twisting	8
With moderate work, sports	Able to do light work, sports with no running, twisting, or jumping	6
With light work, sports	Able to perform activities of daily living alone	4
Frequent and limiting	Activities of daily living produce moderate symptoms	2
Constant and not relieved	Activities of daily living produce severe symptoms	0

C. Sports Activities Rating Scale

Level	Participation	Motion	Sport	Points
I	4-7 days/wk	Jumping, hard pivoting, cutting	Basketball, volleyball, football, gymnastics, soccer	100
		Running, twisting, turning	Tennis, racquetball, handball, baseball, ice hockey, field hockey, skiing, wrestling	95
		No running, twisting, jumping	Cycling, swimming	90
II	1-3 days/wk	Jumping, hard pivoting, cutting	Basketball, volleyball, football, gymnastics, soccer	85
		Running, twisting, turning	Tennis, racquetball, handball, baseball, ice hockey, field hockey, skiing, wrestling	80
		No running, twisting, jumping	Cycling, swimming	75
III	1-3 times/mo	Jumping, hard pivoting, cutting	Basketball, volleyball, football, gymnastics, soccer	65
		Running, twisting, turning	Tennis, racquetball, handball, baseball, ice hockey, field hockey, skiing, wrestling	60
		No running, twisting, jumping	Cycling, swimming	55
IV	None	No problems with activities of daily living	40	
		Moderate problems with activities of daily living	20	
		Severe problems with activities of daily living (uses crutches, full disability)	0	

Continued

Table 37-3 Cincinnati Knee Rating System—cont'd

D. Scheme for Final Rating

Signs	Excellent	Good	Fair	Poor
Pain	10	8	6-4	2-0
Swelling	10	8	6-4	2-0
Partial giving way	10	8	6-4	2-0
Full giving way	10	8	6-4	2-0
Walking	40	30	20	0
Stairs or squatting (choose lower score)	40	30	20	0
Running	100	80	60	40
Jumping	100	80	60	40
Hard twists, cuts, pivots	100	80	60	40
Effusion (mL)	Normal	<25	26–60	>60
Lack of flexion (degrees)	0-5	6-15	16-30	>30
Lack of extension (degrees)	0-3	4-5	6-10	>10
Tibiofemoral crepitus*	Normal	—	Moderate	Severe
Patellofemoral crepitus*	Normal	—	Moderate	Severe
Anterior displacement (KT-1000; mm)	<3	3–5	6	>6
Pivot-shift test, joint space narrowing	Negative	Slip	Definite	Severe
Medial tibiofemoral (radiographs)[†]	Normal	Mild	Moderate	Severe
Lateral tibiofemoral (radiographs)[†]	Normal	Mild	Moderate	Severe
Patellofemoral (radiographs)[†]	Normal	Mild	Moderate	Severe
Functional testing (limb symmetry, %)[‡]	85-100	75-84	65-74	<65

Adapted from Noyes FR, Barber SD, Mangine RE: Bone-patellar ligament-bone and fascia lata allografts for reconstruction of the anterior cruciate ligament. J Bone Joint Surg Am 72:1125, 1990.

*Moderate indicates definite fibrillation and cartilage abnormality of 25 to 50 degrees; severe, cartilage abnormality of more than 50 degrees.

[†]Moderate indicates narrowing of less than half the joint space; severe, more than half the joint space.

[‡]Use an average of at least three one-legged hop-type tests.

KEY REFERENCES

Amis AA: Anterior cruciate ligament replacement: knee stability of the effect of implants. J Bone Joint Surg Br 71:819, 1989.

Amis AA, Dawkins GPC: Functional anatomy of the anterior cruciate ligament. J Bone Joint Surg Br 73:260, 1991.

Andrews JR, Baker CL, Curl WW, et al: Surgical repair of acute and chronic lesions of the lateral capsular ligamentous complex of the knee. In Feagin JA, Jr, editor: The crucial ligaments, New York, 1987, Churchill Livingstone, p 425.

Arnoczky SP, Warren RF: Anatomy of the cruciate ligaments. In Feagin JA, Jr, editor: the crucial ligaments, New York, 1987, Churchill Livingstone, p 179.

Daniel DM, Stone ML, Dobson BE, et al: Fate of the ACL-injured patient: a prospective outcome study. Am J Sports Med 22:632, 1994.

Daniel DM, Stone ML, Sachs R, et al: The measurement of anterior knee laxity in patients with acute anterior cruciate ligament disruption. Am J Sports Med 13:401, 1985.

Girgis FG, Marshall JL, Al Monajem ARS: The cruciate ligaments of the knee joint: anatomical, functional and experimental analysis. Clin Orthop 106:216, 1975.

Grood ES, Noyes FR: Diagnosis and classifications of knee ligament injuries: biomechanical precepts. In Feagin JA, Jr, editor: The crucial ligaments, New York, 1987, Churchill Livingstone, p 245.

Hughston JC, Andrews JR, Cross MJ, et al: Classification of knee ligament instabilities: the medial compartment and cruciate ligaments. J Bone Joint Surg Am 58:159, 1976.

Hughston JC, Andrews JR, Cross MJ, et al: Classification of knee ligament instabilities: the lateral compartment. J Bone Joint Surg Am 58:173, 1976.

LaPrade, RF, Engebretsen AH, Ly TV, et al: The anatomy of the medial part of the knee. J Bone Joint Surg Am 89:2000–2010, 2007.

LaPrade RF, Ly TV, Wentorf FA, Engebretsen L: The posterolateral attachments of the knee. Am J Sports Med 31:854, 2003.

Larson RL, Jones DC: Dislocation and ligamentous injuries of the knee. In Rockwood CA, Jr, Green DP, editors: Fractures in adults, vol 2, ed 2, Philadelphia, 1984, JB Lippincott, pp 1, 480, 591.

Norwood LA, Cross MJ: Anterior cruciate ligament: functional anatomy of its bundles in rotatory instabilities. Am J Sports Med 7:23, 1979.

Noyes FR, Grood ES: Classification of ligament injuries: why an anterolateral laxity or anteromedial laxity is not a diagnostic entity. Instr Course Lect 36:185, 1987.

Noyes FR, Grood ES: Diagnosis of knee ligament injuries: clinical concepts. In Feagin JA, Jr, editor: The crucial ligaments, New York, 1987, Churchill Livingstone, p 261.

Noyes FR, Grood ES, Torzilli PA: Current concepts review: the definition of terms for motion and position of the knee and injuries of the ligaments. J Bone Joint Surg Am 71:465, 1989.

Seebacher JR, Linglis AE, Marshall JL, et al: The structure of the posterolateral aspect of the knee. J Bone Joint Surg Am 64:536, 1982.

Tegner Y, Lysholm J: Rating systems in evaluation of knee ligament injuries. Clin Orthop 198:43, 1985.

Warren RF, Marshall JL, Girgis F: The prime static stabilizer of the medial side of the knee. J Bone Joint Surg Am 56:665, 1974.

Full references for this chapter can be found on www.expertconsult.com.

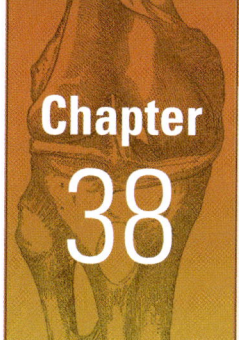

Chapter 38

Sports Knee Rating Systems and Related Statistics

Joseph M. Hart and Christopher M. Kuenze

Outcomes following orthopedic injury are typically determined by the physical examination or other objective or physician or evaluator assessment. Patient Reported Outcomes (PRO) instruments in the form of survey-style questionnaires are important in the orthopedic literature to determine outcomes following injury and/or surgery. These instruments are designed to ask a series of pertinent questions and quantify the values on a scale that can be compared across the entire population and over time. The challenge is selecting the most appropriate PRO instrument. Instruments can be used in single or multisite prospective databases. They can be used, for example, to compare outcomes over short or long periods of time or before and after surgery, or to determine the natural history of injuries or disease processes. These instruments can also be used to compare factors such as patient groups, treatments, surgical techniques, and other medical therapies. Subjective instruments may be designed to evaluate general quality of life or can be region-specific or injury-specific. For example, an instrument to evaluate outcomes following shoulder function may ask questions about overhead activities, grooming, or dressing whereas an outcomes instrument to evaluate outcomes following knee or ankle injury may ask questions about lower extremity function such as pain with stair climbing, walking, or running.

Patient-reported outcomes remain paramount in determining the success or failure of treatment following orthopedic injury; however, they can be considered one of many tools in the armamentarium of medical research used to understand outcomes and guide treatment decision making. In this chapter, several PRO instruments commonly used for persons with knee injuries will be identified and discussed. In addition, a review of basic statistical concepts will help clarify how these instruments can be used to test hypotheses relevant to the practice of orthopaedic surgery.

SELECTING THE MOST APPROPRIATE SELF-REPORT OUTCOME INSTRUMENT

Familiarity with outcomes instruments is important when making decisions about which one is most appropriate. Outcomes scales selected for evaluating patient outcomes need to be reproducible, accurately represent the patients' condition, and detect changes in a self-reported condition caused by changes in disease or injury state. A great deal of time and thought are required to develop a series of questions that will be provocative enough to represent the patient's condition accurately, be sensitive to subtle changes, and be reliable with repeated measurements and when administered by different health care professionals in different settings. The reliability and validity of outcomes instruments are typically reported in the literature. Relevant instruments that are found to be highly valid and reliable through well-designed research studies should be considered first.

GENERAL OUTCOME AND QUALITY OF LIFE SCALES

Medical Outcomes 36-Item Short Form Health Survey

The medical outcomes 36-item Short Form Health Survey (SF-36) is a common general health questionnaire used in health science research that includes 36 questions about general health status. This generic general health scale is not specific to a disease or pathology and therefore allows for wide-ranging comparisons across patient populations.[44] It is also available in a shorter 12-item form, known as the SF-12, which shares all 12 of its items with the SF-36. Both the SF-12 and SF-36 have been shown to be reliable and valid when administered in several languages both in person and via telephone, and are easily compared with previously established normative values.[22,45] Research[14] has shown that these scales are most reliable when administered in subjects between the ages of 18 and 75 years, and the SF-12 may be more appropriate when used in studies with large sample sizes. Currently, these scales have been used widely in research involving knee and hip osteoarthritis, anterior cruciate ligament (ACL) reconstruction, patellofemoral pain syndrome, and other sports injury populations.[19,23,39,40]

The SF-36 and SF-12 scales consist of eight subscales (physical function, role-physical, bodily pain, general health, vitality, social functioning, role-emotional, and mental health), which allow for individual scoring as well as calculation of a physical and mental composite score.[44,45] Composite and subscale scoring are based on a 0 (worst health) to 100 (most healthy) scale. The SF-36 has shown better specificity (Table 38-1) and is less likely to experience floor and ceiling effects in injured populations whereas the SF-12 offers easier scoring and a shorter amount of time to administer.[48] Most commonly, this scale is used in combination with a more region-specific or injury-specific scale to allow for a more global assessment of patients' general health status in conjunction with region-specific function through the use of another outcome instrument.

Global Rating of Change

The global rating of change (GROC) scale is a PRO instrument that allows for simple tracking of patient outcomes by determining how much better or worse the patient is feeling after an injury, treatment, surgery, and so on. The GROC scale can have multiple forms. One commonly used GROC form consists of the rating of change consists of a 15-point scale, ranging from patients reporting they feel "a great deal worse" (positive values, maximum +7) to great decrement (negative values, minimum −7). A score of 0 means that the patient has perceived no change in his or her condition.[12,35]

Table 38-1 Summary of Research Studies Reporting Minimal Clinically Important Differences for Specific Injury Populations[*]

Scale	Population	Follow-up	Scale Range (Total Score)	MCID (Units)
SF-36	Severe knee OA[2]	3 mo	0-100 points	7.8
	Total knee arthroplasty[9]			10.0
Tegner activity rating	ACL injury[5]	6, 9, 12, 24 mo	0-10 levels	1.0
VAS	Knee OA[43]		0-100 mm	19.9 mm
	Anterior knee pain[7]			20.0 mm
IKDC	Knee injury[17]		0-100 points	11.5
	Articular cartilage surgery[17]	7 wk		12.7
Cincinnati Knee Scale	Articular cartilage surgery[26]	5 day	0-100 points	27.5
KOOS	Knee injury[32]		0-100 points	10.0
WOMAC	Knee OA		0-100 points	18.0
	Total knee replacement[9]	1 yr		15.0
	Severe knee OA[2]	3 mo		13.3
Kujala scale (AKPS)	Anterior knee pain[41]		0-100 points	7.0
	Anterior knee pain[20]			10.0
	Anterior knee pain[46]			14.0
Lysholm scale	Articular cartilage surgery[21]	5 day	0-100 points	11.6
	Articular cartilage surgery[26]	4 wk		15.8

This table presents the population and follow up duration for which each instrument was validated. The MCID value indicates the magnitude of the difference (whether the difference is an improvement or deterioration in outcome) that is necessary to be interpreted as a clinically important change. For example, a difference of 11.5 points (based on a 100-point scale).

Scoring of the global rating of change varies throughout the literature and can be manipulated to fit the research question at hand best. In many cases, a value of −7 is assigned to the descriptor of greatest decrement whereas a value of +7 is assigned to the descriptor of greatest improvement.[12,35] This scoring system allows for easy comparison of patient-reported changes over time with regard to function, symptoms, and affective outcome measures. Its use can be modified based on the question asked. For example, a patient can provide a global rating of change score when asked, "How would you rate your outcome following your shoulder surgery?" Clearly, the scale can be used for various conditions and patient groups at various time points following injury or surgery to provide an overall (global) understanding of how a patient perceives the outcome following their injury, condition, or procedure.

Currently, this rating scale is most commonly used in research involving surgical interventions, knee osteoarthritis, and patellofemoral pain.[7,34] Although this scale allows for a easy comparison over time, it is generally combined with a region- or pathology-specific scale, such as the SF-36 and SF-12, to provide a more comprehensive review of patient outcome. No minimal clinically important differences have yet been established for this scale in patients with knee pathology because of the wide scope of populations and injury severities represented.

Visual Analogue Scale

The Visual Analogue Scale (VAS) is possibly the most easily understood and widely used pain rating scale in clinical research. Although there are many iterations of this scale, the concept remains consistent throughout. In general, patients are asked to place a mark intersecting a 100-mm line with two polar descriptors—for example "no pain" on one end and "worst imaginable pain" on the other. Patients make a mark along the line at the point between the two polar descriptors

that represents their current level of pain or discomfort. The distance (in millimeters) from one end of the scale (the zero point, or the point representing no pain) is then measured to represent the subjective level of pain perceived by the patient. Other VAS scales will ask to identify a number from 0 to 10 that represents their current level of perceived pain at a specific time or during an activity.[10] In many cases, more than one VAS can be used to characterize better the pain experienced by the patient. These scales include such questions as current pain, worst pain in the previous 24 hours, worst pain during work-related activity, average pain over the previous 24 hours, and least pain in the previous 24 hours. Although these are representative of some commonly used scales, the questions used can easily be altered to attain a better fit of the patient population and pathology being studied.

The VAS has been shown to be valid and reliable in many forms throughout the literature and often is used as a gold standard when attempting to validate a new assessment instrument.[*] Sensitivity is highly variable, depending on the scale used and the population in which the measurement is taken. This flexibility is a strength of the VAS but results in difficulty when attempting to show clear cutoff points for patient improvement. Currently, minimal clinically important differences have been shown in patients with knee osteoarthritis, hip osteoarthritis, and anterior knee pain, reported as 19.9, 15.3, and 20.0 mm, respectively (Table 38-1).

The VAS has been used as a framework for knee-specific outcomes scales. For example, the Knee Disorders Subjective History[10] has been used to characterize function following knee joint injury or surgery. This scale involves 28 questions about knee joint function during specific activities. It is a series of visual analogue scales with different polar descriptors that enable patients to rate their function from best to worst for each specific question. For example, the question, "Do you

---

[*]References 7, 10, 24, 31, 33, 34, 37, and 43.

feel grinding when your knee moves?" is rated on a 10-point scale ranging from none to severe; the question, "Is your knee stiff?" is rated on a 10-point scale ranging from none to "I can barely move my knee due to stiffness." Questions can be reviewed individually or assigned a specific score (from 1 to 10) for each of the 28 questions and then combined for a total score, normalized to 100%, which represents highest possible function.

Another VAS-based knee-specific outcome score was proposed as a general quality of life outcomes score specific to patients with ACL deficiency. The ACL deficiency quality of life (ACL-QOL) measure[27] incorporates scores from a series of visual analogue scales (100-mm lines with polar descriptors) for 31 total questions. Scores for each question are combined to form a single score on a 100% scale in which 100% indicates highest function or quality of life in ACL-deficient patients. The scale is divided into subsections that ask specific questions about symptoms and physical complaints (four questions), work-related concerns (four questions), recreational activities and sports participation or competition (12 questions), lifestyle (six questions) and social and emotional (five questions). ACL-deficient patients who scored low on this scale were more likely to go on to have reconstruction surgery compared with patients who scored high.

Tegner Activity Scale

The Tegner activity scale was developed in 1985 as a patient-reported score describing typical daily activities. This scale offers patients the choice of 10 distinct levels. The patient provides a rating (values are from 0 to 10, with 10 indicating the highest level of activity) for current level of activity and level of activity prior to injury.[42] The available ratings are broken into four distinct regions, with a rating of 0 corresponding to disability caused by knee problems, 1 to 5 representing levels of work-related activity and recreational sport, 6 to 9 representing competitive and higher levels of recreational and organized or competitive sports, and 10 representing the highest and most elite international or professional level competitive sport. These levels, depending on the population of interest, may not adequately represent the spectrum of daily function and activity and therefore may not allow for clear comparisons among patients. In practice, this scale is commonly associated with the Lysholm score and can allow for a reasonable characterization of patient activity levels, especially when measured in a preinjury, physically active population. Currently, this scale has been shown to be valid and reliable in patients with meniscal injury, patellar instability, and ACL injury.[4,5,33] In patients with ACL injury, a minimal clinically important change of 1.0 has been established. This suggests that a change in activity rating following ACL injury of at least 1 point needs to be met for the change to be considered clinically important. When the scale is used for young patients involved in high levels of activity, it is important to note that transitions from the higher ratings (competitive or elite sports) to lower levels (work and recreational activity) may reflect the natural course of time as an athlete graduates from competitive sports and begins to pursue other professional or life interests. Whether this change is the result of injury or other noninjury-related factors is a potential limitation to the interpretation of this score.

KNEE-SPECIFIC OUTCOMES SCALES

International Knee Documentation Committee Subjective Knee Form

The International Knee Documentation Committee Subjective Knee Form (IKDC) was developed as a standardized assessment tool for knee injury and treatment. It was first published as a patient-reported outcome measure in 1993 and revised to its current form in 1997. This scale is knee-specific but allows for measurement of subjective outcomes of various pathologies. Currently, the IKDC includes 18 total items, those regarding symptoms (7 items), general function (2 items), and sport activities (9 items).[16] Patients are encouraged to complete all of included items; however, scoring is possible as long as 16 of 18 items are completed. Following completion, the scores are converted to a 100-point scale with 100 representing the best possible score and highest knee function. The strength of this rating scale lies in the diversity of items regarding patient-reported knee joint symptoms and function during activities that specifically involve the knee joint (e.g., walking, jogging, stair climbing), which allows for a better representation of the limitations or improvements that may be expected in different populations and pathologies.

The IKDC has been shown to be reliable and valid for a number of pathologies, including ACL injury, meniscal injury, articular cartilage injury, patellofemoral pain syndrome, and knee osteoarthritis.[1,15,17] Normative values have been established to allow for easy comparison of healthy and pathologic populations. A minimally important difference of 11.5 has been suggested but has not been validated in all pathologic populations (see Table 38-1). This form is available in several languages and can be completed in less than 10 minutes. The IKDC represents a clear and concise assessment tool for knee-related research that can be applied across pathologies and population characteristics.

Western Ontario and McMaster Universities Osteoarthritis Index

The Western Ontario and McMaster Universities Osteoarthritis Index (WOMAC) was developed to assess symptoms and function in patients with lower extremity osteoarthritis. This scale is composed of 24 items divided among three subscales—pain (5 items), stiffness (2 items), and function (17 items). Each item asks the patient to provide a Likert rating (none, mild, moderate, severe, or extreme) in response to each item. Each item is scored and combined in total or within each subscale and normalized to a 100-point scale, in which a score of 100 represents no symptoms and a score of 0 represents the worst symptoms.[38,48] The WOMAC is most commonly used for assessing changes in patient reported outcomes related to post-traumatic osteoarthritis in older populations but has been used more broadly to measure changes in symptoms and subjective outcomes in a spectrum of knee injuries.[3]

The WOMAC has become the most widely reported subjective outcome measure for patients with lower extremity osteoarthritis and has been shown to be valid, reliable, and sensitive to change over time.[3] Minimal clinically important difference has been established as 9.1 in the knee osteoarthritis (OA) population, indicating that the total WOMAC score must change by a minimum of 9.1 points for the change to be clinically important. This difference has also been calculated when the WOMAC is compared with the SF-36 in a rehabilitation population, with 12% at baseline and a 6% difference at maximum score considered to be important.[2] This value has not been validated in other populations but may act as a benchmark for comparison within the population of OA patients. The WOMAC is currently available in several languages and several methods of administration and has been shown to take an average of 10 to 15 minutes to complete.[48,49] Although the WOMAC has several strengths and weaknesses, its widespread use in the knee and hip OA literature makes it an important consideration when assessing PRO in patients with OA.

Knee Injury and Osteoarthritis Outcome Score

The Knee Injury and Osteoarthritis Outcome Score (KOOS) was first published in 1998 and was developed as a patient-reported instrument to assess subjective opinion regarding knee injury. As the name implies, this scale is used in patients with knee osteoarthritis. Aptly, the KOOS includes the pain, stiffness, and function sections of the WOMAC scale, which allows for easy comparison of KOOS and WOMAC scores. This scale is directed toward knee injury that can result in post-traumatic OA and allows for prospective assessment of subjective functional and sport-specific outcomes.[36,38] The KOOS consists of 42 items divided into five subscales; pain (9 items), symptoms (7 items), function in daily living (17 items), knee-related quality of life (4 items), and function in sport and recreation; these are scored on a 5-point Likert scale. After completion, each subscale is normalized to a 100-point scale, in which a score of 100 represents no symptoms and a score of 0 represents the worst possible symptoms. The KOOS generally requires 10 to 15 minutes to complete and is available in several languages.

Validity and reliability of the KOOS have been established in patients following ACL reconstruction, partial meniscectomy, and tibial osteotomy, and OA.[8,36-38,47] It has been reported that a change of 8 to 10 points on a transformed subscale score may represent the minimal clinically important difference. The KOOS has been shown to be most sensitive to change in young active populations, with greatest responsiveness on the function in sport and recreation and knee-related quality of life subscales. Despite this fact, the KOOS has been used in the literature in wide range of ages (18 to 78 years) and levels of physical activity. Reference values for the healthy population stratified by age and gender are available and allow for easy comparison between healthy and pathologic populations.[36]

Kujala Anterior Knee Pain Scale

The Kujala scale, or anterior knee pain scale (AKPS), is a patient-reported, knee-specific scale that was developed in 1993 for patients with anterior knee pain. This 13-item scale contains questions related to symptoms reported by patients both at rest and during specific functional tasks, including walking, running, jumping, squatting, sitting for long periods of time, and stair climbing. Each item in the AKPS includes specific responses from which the patient can choose; each is assigned a point value to allow for easy scoring. The AKPS is based on a 100-point scale, with a score of 100 representing pain-free function and a score of 0 representing the maximum presence of pain, and therefore worst function.[24]

The AKPS has been shown to be valid and reliable in differentiating the difference in severity of anterior knee pain as well as the effect of treatment on anterior knee pain. Sensitivity has shown to be good to excellent in most cases, with the exclusion of differentiating among patients with repetitive patellar dislocation and those with one-time dislocations.[33] This may be because of the lack of questions relating to the progression of the patient's condition, with exhaustive focus instead on the effects of the condition on daily symptoms and function. Minimal clinically important differences have been established in three different studies at a value of 7, 10, and 14 points, respectively[20,41,46] (see Table 38-1). In all cases, these differences were reported as improvements over time or following treatment. The AKPS is a widely used scale, both clinically and in clinical research, for monitoring longitudinal changes in patient-reported symptoms and function, and should be considered when attempting research regarding anterior knee or patellofemoral pain.

Other Common Scales

There are several other commonly used scales for various assessments of knee symptoms and functions. The Cincinnati knee rating scale[28-30] assesses knee symptoms as well as functional activity to allow for assessment of six subscales scores as well as a 100-point composite score. The scale is a clinician- and patient-reported score most commonly used for the assessment of ACL injury. Although it is considered to be comprehensive, it has only been partially validated.

Similar to the Cincinnati knee rating scale, the Lysholm knee scale[4,5,21] is widely used for the assessment of knee ligament injury and surgical outcomes. It consists of eight items (limp, support, stair climbing, squatting, instability, locking, catching, pain, and swelling) that are weighted and scored on a 100-point scale. The Lysholm scale has been validated for several knee pathologies and is commonly combined with activity scales in an effort to achieve a comprehensive assessment of knee function.

Similarly, the ACL quality of life scale[27] (ACL-QOL) is a 32-item scale specifically designed as an outcome measure for chronic ACL deficiency. The 32 items are divided among five subscales (symptoms and physical complaints, work-related concerns, recreational activities and sport competition, lifestyle, and social and emotional function) and transformed to a 100-point scale. This scale has been shown to be valid and reliable, and may have some value in predicting which patients may eventually require surgical intervention. However, it has not been specifically developed for a particular knee pathology.

Finally, the Hospital of Special Surgery knee score[11] (HSS) was developed as an assessment for total knee replacement outcomes. It is based on a 100-point scale divided into seven categories. This scale uses both patient- and clinician-reported outcomes and has been shown to be valid and reliable when assessing patients with knee replacements.

Table 38-2 Common Epidemiologic Measures and Their Interpretation

Measure	Calculation	Interpretation
Prevalence	$\dfrac{\text{\# existing instances of outcome}}{\text{Total Population at Risk}}$	Proportion of individuals within a population who exhibit an outcome of interest
Incidence	$\dfrac{\text{\# new instances of outcome}}{\text{Total Population at Risk}}$	Proportion of new cases of outcome of interest within a specific time interval
Absolute risk	$\dfrac{\text{\# new outcomes}}{\text{Total Population at Risk}}$	Proportion of population of interest at risk for developing outcome of interest
Relative risk	$\dfrac{\text{Incidence in an Exposed Group}}{\text{Incidence in an UNexposed Group}}$	1.0: Risk of outcome identical between groups >1.0: Risk of outcome greater in exposed vs. unexposed group
Odds ratio	$\dfrac{\text{Probability of outcome in an Exposed Group}}{\text{Probability of an outcome in an UNexposed Group}}$	<1.0: Odds of outcome less in exposed vs. unexposed group
Specificity	$\dfrac{\text{True negatives}}{\text{Total patients without disease}}$	Of all patients who *do not* have the disease or outcome of interest, the proportion who tested negative; specific clinical tests have high true-negative and low false-positive rates.
Sensitivity	$\dfrac{\text{True positives}}{\text{Total patients with disease}}$	Of all patients who have the disease or outcome of interest, the proportion who tested positive. Sensitive clinical tests have high true positive and low false negative rates.
Positive predictive value	$\dfrac{\text{True positives}}{\text{Total patients with positive test result}}$	Proportion of patients with positive test result who were correctly diagnosed
Negative predictive value	$\dfrac{\text{True negatives}}{\text{Total patients with negative test result}}$	Proportion of patients with negative test result who were correctly diagnosed
Positive likelihood ratio	Sensitivity/(1 − specificity)	Example: (+) LR = 5—a positive test indicates that the patient is five times more likely to have the outcome of interest than patient with negative result
Negative likelihood ratio	(1 − Sensitivity)/specificity	Example: (−) LR = 0.2—a negative test will be present in only 2 of every 10 patients who actually have the outcome of interest

COMMON STATISTICAL CONCEPTS IN OUTCOMES RESEARCH

Outcomes scores can be used to describe the distribution and determinants of disease and response to treatment and to test specific hypotheses related to outcomes research. Epidemiology is the study of the distribution, frequencies and determinants of injury and/or disease. Common measures of frequency include prevalence and incidence; common measures of association include relative risks and odds ratios (Table 38-2).

Prevalence and Incidence

Prevalence is calculated as the proportion of individuals in a population who have an outcome of interest now, or at a particular point in time. Prevalence values are calculated as the number of existing cases of disease of injury divided by the total population who are identified to be at risk. Incidence is the proportion of new cases of an outcome or disease within a specific time interval. Therefore, to calculate incidence, a follow-up period or time interval is required. Incidence is calculated as the number of new cases of disease of injury divided by the total population at risk. It is interpreted as the occurrence of new cases over a period of time. Absolute risk is an incidence in which the number of new occurrences of disease or injury over a period of time is divided by the total number of patients at risk. For example, if 6 of 100

patients undergoing ACL reconstruction report poor subjective outcome at a 6-month follow-up evaluation, the absolute risk for poor outcome is 6% (6/100).

Relative Risk and Odds Ratio

Relative risk (RR) is used to compare the incidence of injury/disease between two cohorts of patients. RR is calculated as the incidence of injury or disease in one group divided by the incidence of injury or disease in another group. Groups can be defined as a cohort of patients who were exposed to risk or an intervention. RR values range from 0 to ∞ and are interpreted relative to a value of 1.0. An RR value equal to 1.0 indicates that the incidence of the outcome of interest is identical in the exposed and unexposed groups. An RR value less than 1 indicates an inverse relationship, or decreased risk in the exposed group, and an RR value greater than 1 indicates increased risk among patients in the exposed group (group presented in the numerator of the RR calculation). When comparing a treatment (exposed) with a control group for a particular outcome of interest, an RR value of 0.5 indicates that treated patients have half the risk for developing the outcome of interest, whereas an RR value of 2.5 indicates a 2.5 times increased risk of developing the outcome of interest when in the treatment group. Because RR values are calculated from incidence rates (requiring a follow-up period), they are most appropriate for prospective cohort studies or clinical trials.

Odds ratios (ORs) can be calculated as the proportion of patients with an injury, disease, or outcome of interest divided by the proportion of patients who do not have the injury, disease, or outcome of interest. An OR compares odds in a group of patients who have been exposed to a particular risk factor or treated in an intervention study with a cohort of patients who were not exposed to risk or treated. ORs are more commonly used in retrospective studies. The interpretation of an OR value is similar to the interpretation of an RR value.

Reliability, Validity, Accuracy, and Precision

Reliability is concerned with the reproducibility of a measure, whereas validity describes the ability of a measure, test, or instrument to represent truth and reality effectively. Accuracy describes the ability of a test or measure to differentiate between positive (+) and negative (−) diagnoses. Therefore, the accuracy of a particular diagnostic test or outcome instrument can be calculated by dividing the number of times the test correctly diagnosed the disease of interest with a positive result (true positives) added to the number of times the test correctly determined the absence of a disease with a negative result (true negatives) divided by the total number of patients in a given study. Precision describes the repeatability of a test result with multiple testing; that is, is the test yielding similar scores or results when the same specimen or patient is tested on multiple occasions?

Sensitivity, Specificity, and Likelihood Ratios

Sensitivity, specificity, and positive and negative predictive values can be calculated from a contingency table (Table 38-3). Sensitivity describes the ability to detect true positive test results whereas specificity describes the ability to detect true negative test results. When a highly sensitive (Sn) test

Table 38-3 Sensitivity, Specificity,[3,4] and Positive and Negative Predictive Values[1,2]: Calculated from a Contingency Table*

	Disease Present (+)	Disease Absent (−)	
Diagnostic Test (+)	True positives	False positives	1
Diagnostic Test (−)	False negatives	True negatives	2
	3	4	

[1]Positive predictive value = true positives/total patients with positive test result.
[2]Negative predictive value = true negatives/total patients with negative test result.
[3]Sensitivity = true positives/total patients with disease.
[4]Specificity = true negatives/total patients without disease.
*The effectiveness of diagnostic tools can be measured by constructing a 2 × 2 contingency table that compares the outcome of a specific diagnostic test with a gold standard. In a person who has the disease or outcome of interest, a positive diagnostic test will indicate a true positive, whereas a negative diagnostic test will indicate a false negative. Similarly, in a person who does not have the disease or outcome of interest, a positive test result will indicate a "false positive" whereas a negative diagnostic test will indicate a "true negative".

is negative (N), it is good for ruling OUT an injury because high sensitivity indicates few false negatives (mnemonic: SnNOUT). When a highly specific (Sp) test is positive (P), the test is good for ruling IN an injury or disease because high specificity indicate few false positives (mnemonic: SpPIN).

A likelihood ratio (LR) is calculated from sensitivity and specificity. A positive likelihood ratio describes the impact of a positive examination finding (clinical test) on the probability that a disease exists:

$$(+)\, LR = sensitivity/(1 - specificity)$$

A negative likelihood ratio describes the impact of a negative clinical test on the probability that the disease is present:

$$(-)\, LR = (1 - sensitivity)/specificity$$

Receiver operating characteristic (ROC) curves are graphic representations of the relationships between sensitivity and specificity, in which the sensitivity value is plotted on the vertical axis and specificity is plotted on the y axis. The area under the ROC curve is an estimate of the overall diagnostic value of a given test. When the area under the ROC curve equals 1.0, the test has perfect diagnostic value. An area of 0.5 indicates that the diagnostic value of a particular test is no better than random guessing.

Hypothesis Testing Using Outcomes Data

Outcomes data collected during a research study can be subjective (provided by the research participant) or objective (measured by an instrument or other device). Dependent variables are measured subjectively or objectively. The data can be summarized with descriptive statistics. The mean (arithmetic average), median (value dividing the data set into equal halves), and mode (most commonly occurring data value) are descriptive statistics commonly used to describe the basic features of a data set. Data distributions are presented as histograms to visualize these descriptive statistic concepts. When the items in a data set are normally distributed, the mean, median, and mode are the same value (Fig. 38-1).

Data collected from a patient, subject, or specimen, for example, can be classified as continuous or categorical. Continuous data such as height, weight, time, or age have an infinite number of possible values. In contrast, categorical or discrete data can be binary (e.g., yes or no, failure or success, satisfactory or unsatisfactory, gender), ordered (e.g., severity—mild, moderate, severe; outcome—excellent, good, fair, poor), or unordered (race). Categorical data have a discrete number of possible values.

A confidence interval (CI) quantifies the precision of a mean or another statistic such as an odds ratio or relative risk. A 95% confidence interval describes a range of data values around a sample statistic (mean, OR, RR) in which it is 95% certain that the actual value representative of the entire population lies somewhere within the calculated upper and lower limits of the CI. CIs can provide an estimate of the variability of sample data; hence, they can estimate the precision of the measure. Furthermore, CIs present accuracy of the test statistic to represent reality. Large CIs have poorer

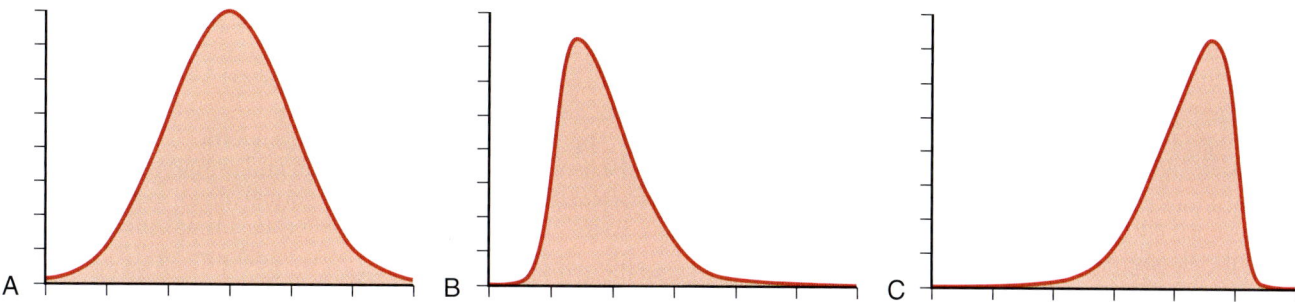

Figure 38-1. A, Histogram showing graphic depiction of tabulated data frequencies. The data are normally distributed; therefore, the mean, median, and mode are the same value. Examples of non-normally distributed data are skewed to the right (positive skew; **B**) and skewed to the left (negative skew; **C**).

Table 38-4 Basic Decision Making for Statistical Tests

Parameter	STATISTICS* Parametric	STATISTICS* Nonparametric
Descriptive statistic	Mean and standard deviations	Median, ranks, range
Two groups†		
Paired	Dependent (paired) samples t-test	Wilcoxon signed rank test
Unpaired	Independent samples t-test§	Mann-Whitney U test
Three groups or more‡		
One dependent variable	Analysis of variance (ANOVA)	Kruskal-Wallis test
Multiple dependent variables	MANOVA	
Analysis including a covariate	ANCOVA	
Repeated observation in same patient	Repeated measures ANOVA	
Relationship or association	Pearson product-moment correlation coefficient	Spearman rank correlation coefficient
Prediction		
From one predictor variable	Simple regression	Logistic regression
From >one predictor variables	Multiple regression	
Categorical data		
Two or more variables	Chi-square test	Chi-square test
Better for low sample size	Fisher's exact test	Fisher's exact test

*Parametric statistics are good for continuous data that are normally distributed. If the assumption of normal distributed data (among others) is violated, the use of a parametric statistic is unreliable and a nonparametric equivalent should be used. Nonparametric tests are also good for categorical data, where appropriate.
†The threshold for defining "statistical significance" can be made more conservative if multiple dependent variables are being simultaneously compared. The Bonferroni correction is peiformed by dividing the typical P-value threshold ($P = 0.05$) by the number of comparisons being made. If 3 comparisons are being made, then the test is only statistically significant if the P-value is less than 0.05/3 or 0.017. There is some debate about whether or not this correction is appropriate for reducing type I error.
‡If measurements are recorded in the same subjects or patients on multiple occasions, a repeated measures ANOVA is appropriate. If there are multiple, related dependent variables being analyzed in three groups or more, a multivariate analysis of variance is appropriate (MANOVA). If there is a need to correct for a covariate or other confounding factor, an analysis of covariance (ANCOVA) is appropriate.
§Because these tests are appropriate for categorical data, they may be considered parametric or nonparametric.

precision and are less likely to be accurate. Small CIs are more precise and more likely to be accurate.

Parametric and Nonparametric Inferential Statistics

Inferential statistics attempt to generalize findings from a representative sample to the entire population. Inferential statistics can be divided into parametric and nonparametric statistics. Parametric tests use the mean and standard deviations when comparing groups or identifying associations and are best suited for normally distributed continuous data. Nonparametric statistical tests use medians and ranks and are therefore more powerful alternatives when data are not normally distributed, because they are less sensitive to outliers (more robust) or when sample sizes are low. The goal of

inferential statistics is to estimate parameters (descriptors of the entire population) and therefore statistical tests should be parametric, if possible (Table 38-4)

Statistical Tests for Comparing Two Groups

If a research study proposes to compare two groups of data, whether they are paired or independent, the t-test is appropriate. There are two basic types of t-tests. Paired t-tests are used to compare data from paired samples or data collected from the same person. The independent samples t-test is used to compare continuous data between two independent groups. The nonparametric equivalent to the paired samples t-test is the Wilcoxon signed rank test and the nonparametric equivalent to the independent samples t-test is the Mann-Whitney U test.

Statistical Tests for Comparing More Than Two Groups

If a research study proposes to compare three or more groups, an analysis of variance (ANOVA) is the appropriate inferential statistical test. The ANOVA can be used to compare three or more independent groups of data. For example, an ANOVA would be used when comparing patient reported outcomes among patients treated with treatment A, treatment B, and treatment C. When comparing data collected from the same subjects (e.g., at multiple time points), the repeated measures ANOVA is used. When a confounding factor exists and influences the outcome of a study, an analysis of covariance (ANCOVA) is appropriate. An ANCOVA is a more sophisticated ANOVA model that will take into account the confounding factor when comparing groups. The nonparametric equivalent for the ANOVA is the Kruskal-Wallis test; Friedman's test is a nonparametric test similar to the repeated measures ANOVA.

Post Hoc Tests

Specific between-group comparisons are necessary after a statistically significant (e.g., $P \leq .05$) ANOVA or F-test to determine the exact location of the group differences. The P value associated with the ANOVA test only indicates that a difference exists somewhere between the groups compared. In the hypothetical example given earlier, post hoc tests would be used to compare outcomes between the following: (1) treatment groups A and B; (2) treatment groups A and C; and (3) treatment groups B and C. Each of these post hoc tests would have an associated P value indicating the presence of a statistically significant difference (i.e., $P \leq 0.05$). Examples of common post hoc tests include the Tukey, Sidak, Dunnet, and Scheffe tests.

Statistical Tests for Categorical Data

The chi-square test and Fisher exact test are appropriate when data are categorical. For example, when comparing patient outcomes (good, fair, poor) between treatment A and treatment B, these tests would be appropriate. In the example given earlier, a statistically significant test is interpreted to mean that a relationship exists between outcome and treatment. Constructing a contingency table to evaluate frequencies would aid in interpreting the relationship. The Fisher exact test may be used when sample sizes are low or when the number of occurrences in one of the categories is very small (e.g., only one person with treatment B had a poor outcome).

Statistical Tests for Describing Relationships

Correlations describe the strength of a relationship between two variables. A Pearson product moment correlation coefficient (r) is used to correlate two arrays of continuous, normally distributed data. The value of a correlation coefficient can range from −1 to 0 to +1. Values closer to + or −1 indicate stronger relationships. Values closer to 0 indicate weaker relationships. Positive correlation coefficients represent direct relationships and indicate a relationship in which patients who score high on one scale tend to also score high on the other scale. Correlation coefficients that are negative indicate indirect relationships in which patients who score high on one scale tend to score low on another scale. Although several interpretations of the magnitude of a correlation coefficients have been proposed, a common method describes the strength of a correlation coefficient that is less than 0.33 to be weak, between 0.33 and 0.66 as moderate, and more than 0.66 as strong.

Spearman rho is the nonparametric equivalent to the Pearson correlation coefficient and is appropriate for non-normally distributed or categorical data. Both correlation coefficients have associated P values that describe whether the coefficient represents a true relationship ($P \leq .05$) or is caused by chance ($P > .05$).

Probability Values and Statistical Error

Test statistics are typically reported with an associated probability value (P value) that helps interpret the test statistics as being statistically significant or statistically nonsignificant. This decision is made based on an arbitrary decision regarding an acceptable rate of committing a type I error. In statistics, a type I error is the probability of being wrong when concluding that a relationship among test variables exists—that is, observing differences when there actually are none. As a matter of tradition, we typically accept this type of error 5% of the time or less. Therefore, if $P \leq .05$, we conclude that a statistically significant relationship exists. The correct interpretation of $P \leq .05$ is that the observed relationship or difference is most likely not caused by chance. Conversely, a $P > .05$ indicates that observed differences or relationships are likely caused by chance alone and not by hypothesized differences or relationships. The P value is influenced by the variability of the data, the number of subjects from which data was collected, and the magnitude of the differences between groups. Statistically, it is most difficult to observe significant differences if data variability is high, if the number of subjects is low, and/or if the magnitude of difference is minimal.

Minimal Clinically Important Difference

Descriptive and inferential statistics tools in the researchers' toolbox that describe study data and highlight group differences and/or relationships. Typically, P associated with a particular statistical test used to determine whether a statistical difference or relationship is statistically significant (i.e., likely not caused by chance when $P \leq .05$). When interpreting study data, it is important not only to consider statistical test findings and P values that describe statistically significant relationships, but also to determine the clinical importance or meaningfulness of the observed differences or relationships. The concept of a minimal clinically important difference (MCID) has been described as a difference in outcome score in a clinical research study that a patient perceives as beneficial or that would necessitate a change in treatment.[6,13,18] For example, very small differences or changes that are observed in a clinical research study (or clinical trial) that are statistically significant may or may not be large enough to result in a benefit to patients. Therefore, both statistical significance and/or clinical importance should be considered when drawing conclusions from study data.

MCID values can be calculated using a distribution approach, anchor approach, and expert opinion approach.[25] In the distribution approach, confidence intervals are calculated and compared between groups. If there is no overlap among the ranges of the confidence intervals from two independent groups, then the difference is said to have achieved clinical importance. Another way to interpret study differences is to calculate an effect size. Effect sizes measure the magnitude of a treatment effect. These statistics not only describe the mean difference between treatment groups, but also account for data variability. To calculate an effect size, the difference between treatment groups is divided by the standard deviation; therefore, if data are highly variable, then the estimated effect size will weaken. Effect sizes range in value from 0 to ∞; values closer to 0 indicate no treatment effect. Effect sizes are interpreted as being stronger or larger as values increase. Although there are different ways to interpret the magnitude of effect sizes, one common method is to consider an effect size <0.2 as small, <0.5 as medium, and 0.8 and higher as large.

The anchor method for determining the MCID is to compare the changes detected with a particular outcomes instrument with an existing, validated gold standard. This will allow development of a 2 × 2 contingency table and calculation of specificity, sensitivity, and other statistics described earlier in this chapter. Finally, the expert opinion method of determining MCID takes into consideration input from patients or expert health care professionals.

In summary, the MCID value describes the minimum difference that needs to be observed following a treatment for the change to be considered clinically meaningful or important. Table 38-1 contains MCID values from several self-report outcomes instruments used in outcomes research about knee joint injuries. The MCID values can be used to determine the minimum necessary reduction or improvement in patient reported outcome score to be considered clinically important.

KEY REFERENCES

Kocher MS, Zurakowski D: Clinical epidemiology and biostatistics: a primer for orthopaedic surgeons. J Bone Joint Surg Am 86:607–620, 2004.

Make B: How can we assess outcomes of clinical trials: the MCID approach. COPD 4:191–194, 2007.

Marx RG: Patient-reported measure of knee function. J Bone Joint Surg Am 82:1199–1202, 2000.

McKeon PO, Medina JM, Hertel J: Hierachy of research design in evidence-based sports medicine. Athletic Ther Today 11:42–45, 2006.

Medina JM, McKeon PO, Hertel J: Rating the levels of evidence in sports medicine research. Athletic Ther Today 11:38–41, 2006.

Redelmeier DA, Guyatt GH, Goldstein RS: Assessing the minimal important difference in symptoms: a comparison of two techniques. J Clin Epidemiol 49:1215–1219, 1996.

Wang D, Bakhai A, Maffulli N: A primer for statistical analysis of clinical trials. Arthroscopy 19:874–881, 2003.

Wright RW: Knee injury outcomes measures. J Am Acad Orthop Surg 17:31–39, 2009.

Wright RW: Knee sports injury outcome measures. J Knee Surg 18:69–72, 2005.

Full references for this chapter can be found on www.expertconsult.com.

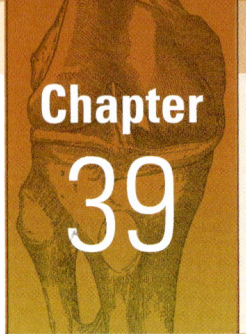

Chapter 39

Medial Ligamentous Injuries of the Knee: Acute and Chronic

Gehron Treme and Robert C. Schenck, Jr.

INTRODUCTION

Injuries to the medial collateral ligament (MCL) are commonly encountered by orthopedic surgeons. Knowledge of anatomy, biomechanics, treatment rationales, and potential associated injuries allows physicians to develop treatment plans that lead to good outcomes for their patients. Most MCL injuries can be treated without surgery with an expectation of good functional results at completion of rehabilitation. Less commonly, some injuries to the medial side of the knee require surgical reconstruction to give the patient the best chance of an acceptable outcome.

ANATOMY AND BIOMECHANICS

Sound treatment rationales and reproducible reconstruction results require a working knowledge of the structures of the medial side of the knee. Several studies have made useful contributions to the current understanding of the anatomy and biomechanics of these structures.

The anatomic study by Warren and Marshall provides the basis for knowledge of the medial side of the knee.[43] In their classic paper, these authors described medial knee anatomy using a spatial concept of three distinct layers (Fig. 39-1). Layer 1 consists of the crural fascia of the knee and is present from the patella anteriorly to the popliteal fossa posteriorly. The sartorius fascia is found in this layer and blends with the crural fascia anteriorly as it attaches to the tibia. The gracilis and semitendinosus tendons are found between layers 1 and 2.

Layer 2 is the superficial medial collateral ligament (sMCL), which, in the absence of scarring, can be easily identified deep to the gracilis and semitendinosus tendons once the crural fascia is incised. In a quantitative study, LaPrade found that the sMCL was attached to the femur an average of 3.2 mm proximal and 4.8 mm posterior to the medial epicondyle[25] (Fig. 39-2). The tibial attachment of the sMCL has two divisions, with the proximal division attaching to soft tissue and the distal division attaching directly to the posteromedial tibia. Vertically oriented fibers of the sMCL anteriorly blend with more obliquely oriented fibers in the posterior portion of the knee capsule and semimembranosus insertion at the posteromedial corner (Fig. 39-3). This blending of tissue planes forms the posteromedial capsular pouch enveloping the medial femoral condyle.

The third and final layer of the knee consists of the knee joint capsule. This capsule thickens from anterior to posterior, and a distinct component of the capsule deep to the sMCL represents the deep medial collateral ligament (dMCL), which has meniscofemoral and meniscotibial attachments but no attachment to the overlying sMCL.[25] The nomenclature describing the structures of the posteromedial corner has become better defined in the orthopedic literature.[20,25,35] The posterior oblique ligament (POL) has been identified as a thickening of the posterior medial capsule (PMC) in this region, and its importance in medial stability has become increasingly recognized. The POL attaches proximally and posteriorly to the attachment site of the sMCL on the femur. The previously described oblique portion of the sMCL is now recognized as the POL. The POL has superficial, central, and capsular arms; the central arm is the most robust of the three and is the primary portion of the POL that should be repaired or reconstructed upon medial injury (Fig. 39-4). The posteromedial capsule is further reinforced by contributions from the semimembranosus and its sheath through multiple attachments.

In contrast to the anatomic nomenclature, little debate exists regarding the biomechanical role of the medial knee structures. Robinson found that the anterior aspect of the sMCL remained taut throughout motion, while the PMC consistently loosened in flexion and tightened in full extension and internal rotation.[35] Griffith et al demonstrated that both divisions of the sMCL serve as primary restraints to valgus load and external rotation, and that the degree of knee flexion affects the load response.[15] Additionally, the POL serves as a restraint to internal rotation and valgus at and approaching full extension, and exhibits a flexion-dependent reciprocal role in resistance to internal rotation with the sMCL. In a second biomechanical study, Griffith et al further defined the primary static stabilizers of the knee.[14] These authors found that the proximal division of the sMCL serves as the primary stabilizer to valgus stress, the distal division of the sMCL serves as the primary stabilizer to external rotation at 30 degrees of flexion, and, when viewed as a single functional unit, the sMCL serves as a primary restraint to valgus and internal rotation at all flexion angles and to external rotation at 30 degrees of flexion. The primary restraints to internal rotation were the POL and the distal sMCL division at all flexion angles. Additionally, investigators found that the dMCL made an important contribution to flexion-dependent internal rotation stability. Wijdicks et al reported that these relationships and load values changed with sequential cutting of structures, demonstrating the intricate load-sharing properties of the medial knee structures.[45]

DIAGNOSIS

As with any injured extremity, examination of the knee with a suspected medial side injury should follow a standard stepwise process. A thorough history can frequently lead the examiner to suspect an MCL injury. Asking the patient to describe the injury as might be viewed by an observer can be a useful way to extract valuable information. Isolated MCL injuries occur with a valgus moment across a flexed knee and may occur in a contact or noncontact situation. Rotational

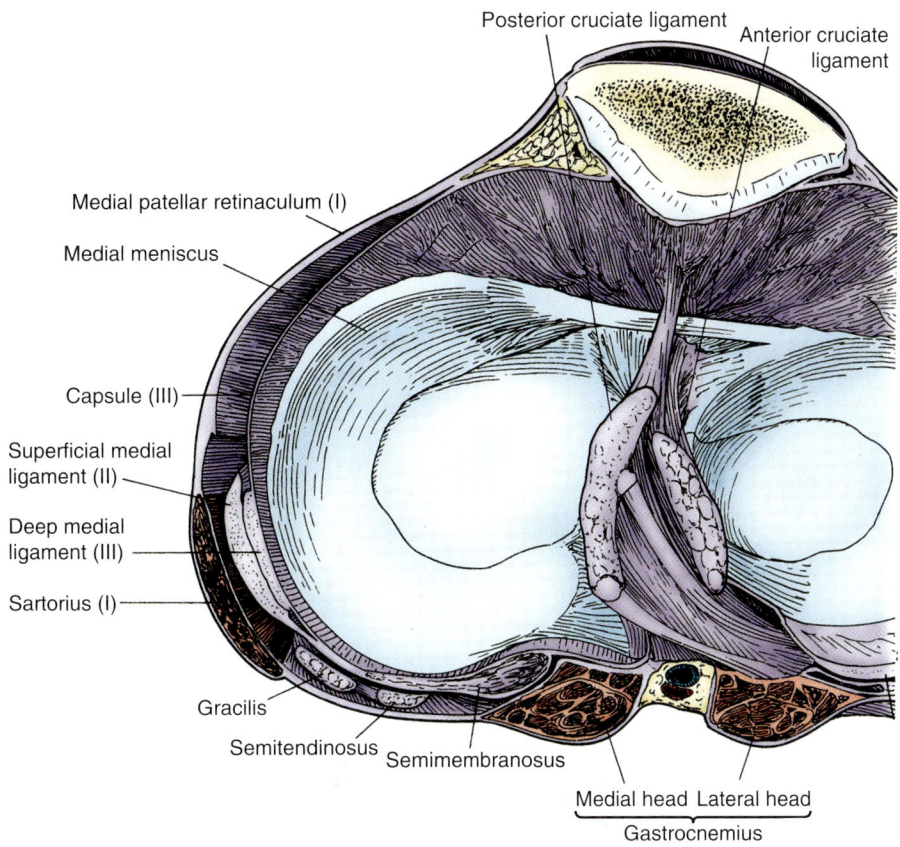

Figure 39-1. Cross-section of the knee demonstrating the layering concept as described by Warren and Marshall. Note the sartorius fascia, superficial medial collateral ligament (sMCL), and deep medial collateral ligament (dMCL), with the pes tendons between layers 1 and 2. (From Radnay CS, Silver SG: Medial ligament injuries of the knee. In Scott WN [ed]: Insall and Scott surgery of the knee, ed 4, Philadelphia, 2006, Churchill Livingstone.)

mechanisms associated with a direct blow more commonly result in multiple ligament damage.

Inspection of knee alignment and the soft tissue envelope can give clues to the severity of the injury. A hemarthrosis raises suspicion of intra-articular involvement, as opposed to localized swelling usually seen with isolated MCL injury. Depending on the acuity, bruising can be seen along the medial side of the knee as well. The patient's neurovascular status should be evaluated and documented, particularly in the case of suspected multiligamentous injury. Patients with an MCL injury typically will have pain along the expanse of the ligament with a point of focal maximal tenderness depending on the point of rupture. Although frequently challenging secondary to patient discomfort, a standard cruciate examination and evaluation of the lateral structures should always be completed. In the acute situation, resting the flexed knee on a pillow improves patient tolerance to the ligamentous examination and enhances the quality of information obtained.

The amount of joint line opening with valgus stress at 0 and 30 degrees determines the grade of the MCL injury. Comparison is made with the uninjured knee, with <5 mm of increased opening indicating a grade I injury, 5 to 10 mm indicating a grade II, and >10 mm termed grade III. Placing a finger along the joint line and comparing with the uninjured knee helps to quantify the amount of joint line opening. The quality of the endpoint should also be recorded. Increased

laxity in full extension is indicative of injury to the POL and often indicates a combined ligament injury, most commonly an ACL tear. Fetto found an 80% incidence of combined ligament injury with grade III MCL tears.[9] Attention should be paid to rotational instability as well. The posteromedial corner complex limits internal rotation (IR) of the knee, and increased rotational motion should raise suspicion of injury to this structure. Increased external rotation (ER) has been primarily attributed to lateral side and posterior cruciate ligament (PCL) injury. However, Griffith demonstrated that the sMCL serves as a primary restraint to ER, and this should be considered during that portion of the examination.[14] Visual inspection of the tibia during ER will help determine whether the increased ER is related to medial or lateral injury. Injury to the medial structures will result in rotation of the anteromedial tibia anteriorly; in contrast, the posterolateral tibia will effectively fall away when increased ER results from a lateral injury. Often, with multiligamentous injuries, an examination under anesthesia is needed to determine the degree of functional integrity of collateral ligaments.

IMAGING

Initial imaging examination should begin with standard radiographs. With acute or subacute injury, standard anterior-to-posterior, lateral, and sunrise patellar views are obtained, with special attention given to the potential for fracture and

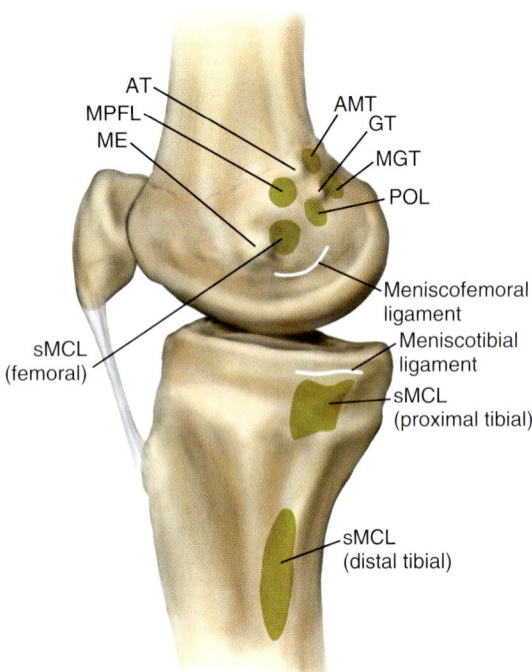

Figure 39-2. Illustration of the femoral osseous landmarks and attachment sites of the main medial knee structures. *AMT,* Adductor magnus tendon; *AT,* adductor tubercle; *GT,* gastrocnemius tubercle; *ME,* medial epicondyle; *MGT,* medial gastrocnemius tendon; *MPFL,* medial patellofemoral ligament; *POL,* posterior oblique ligament; *sMCL,* superficial medial collateral ligament. (Reprinted with permission from LaPrade RF, Engebretsen AH, Ly TV, et al: The anatomy of the medial side of the knee. J Bone Joint Surg Am 89:2000, 2007.)

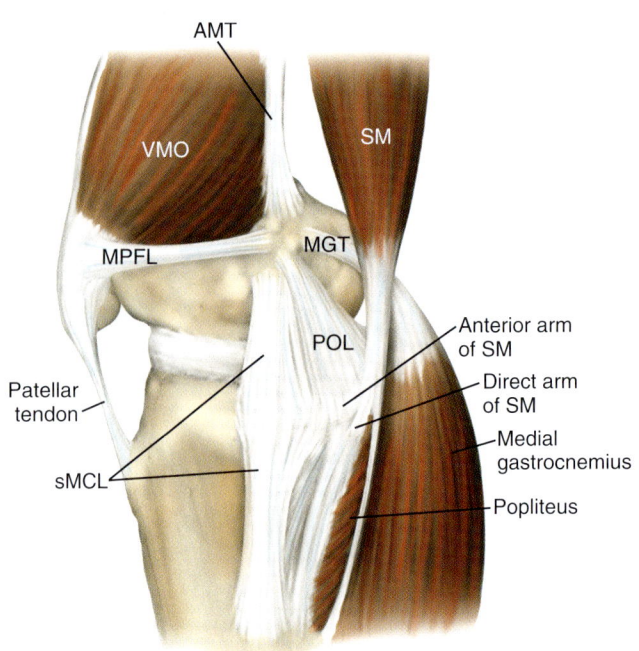

Figure 39-3. Illustration of the main medial knee structures (right knee). *AMT,* Adductor magnus tendon; *MGT,* medial gastrocnemius tendon; *MPFL,* medial patellofemoral ligament; *POL,* posterior oblique ligament; *SM,* semimembranosus muscle; *sMCL,* superficial medial collateral ligament; *VMO,* vastus medialis obliquus muscle. (Reprinted with permission from LaPrade RF, Engebretsen AH, Ly TV, et al: The anatomy of the medial side of the knee. J Bone Joint Surg Am 89:2000, 2007.)

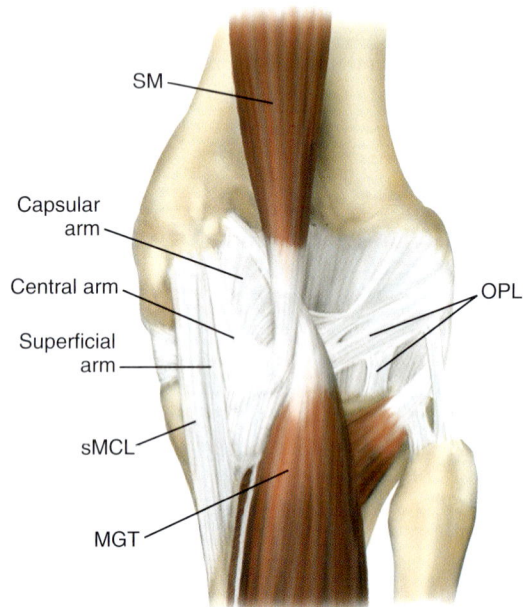

Figure 39-4. Illustration of the three arms of the posterior oblique ligament (posteromedial aspect, right knee). *MGT,* Medial gastrocnemius tendon; *OPL,* oblique popliteal ligament; *SM,* semimembranosus muscle; *sMCL,* superficial medial collateral ligament. (Reprinted with permission from LaPrade RF, Engebretsen AH, Ly TV, et al: The anatomy of the medial side of the knee. J Bone Joint Surg Am 89:2000, 2007.)

to joint malalignment indicating multiligament injury. Widening of the joint space on non–weight-bearing films is frequently seen in the multiligament-injured knee. The chronically injured knee should have a full complement of weight-bearing radiographs, with the addition of a Rosenberg view to assess the amount of joint wear resulting from the chronic injury.

Magnetic resonance imaging (MRI) has become an invaluable tool in assessment of the medial ligamentous structures; it can define the location and quality of the MCL injury (Figs. 39-5 and 39-6). In addition, MRI allows evaluation of the knee for meniscal lesions, osteochondral injury, and damage to other ligaments. Distal avulsion of the MCL with displacement superficial to the pes tendons, similar to a Stener lesion in the thumb, may indicate the need for operative repair. Rubin compared MRI findings versus findings at the time of surgery and noted diagnostic sensitivity and specificity of 94% and 99%, respectively, for ligament and meniscal damage with an isolated injury.[36] These values decreased to 88% and 84%, respectively, when two or more structures were damaged. Additionally, Rasenberg et al noted a high degree of agreement between instrumented grading of MCL injury and grading by MRI.[33] Miller et al noted that trabecular microfractures or "bone bruises" occurred in 45% of patients with isolated MCL tears, and that all of these injuries resolved in 2 to 4 months on follow-up imaging.[28] The information obtained on MRI should be correlated with the history and physical examination findings to determine the extent of injury and develop an appropriate plan of care for the patient.

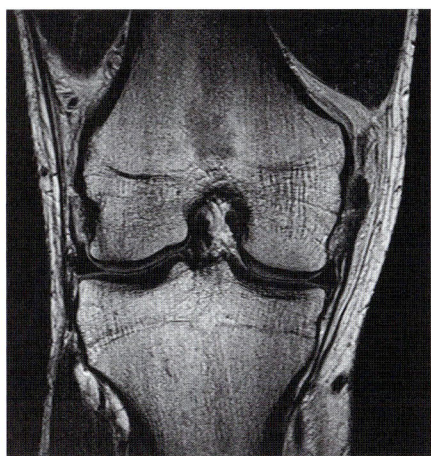

Figure 39-5. Coronal magnetic resonance imaging (MRI) of a proximal medial collateral ligament (MCL) rupture.

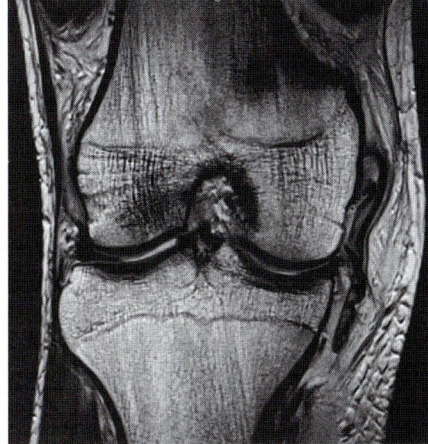

Figure 39-6. Coronal magnetic resonance imaging (MRI) of a distal medial collateral ligament (MCL) rupture.

TREATMENT

Brace Wear

Prevention of MCL injuries has been studied extensively. Prophylactic knee braces (PKBs) are commonly used in collegiate down linemen football players to protect the medial knee structures. Several studies have shown that PKBs decrease strain on the MCL.[5,10,11] Surrogate modeling in vitro testing demonstrates that bracing decreases forces across the MCL by 20% to 30%, and that custom bracing provides improved protection over off-the-shelf versions.[5] Although these models have been validated, obvious limitations are seen when a surrogate knee model loaded in an in vitro setting is compared with an athlete's knee injured during competition.

Similar to laboratory testing, clinical studies have demonstrated some limited protective benefit of PKBs in certain sporting populations.[1,2,40] Sitler analyzed the effects of prophylactic knee bracing on knee injury in West Point cadets playing full contact American football.[40] The incidence of MCL injury was decreased in braced defensive players compared with unbraced controls. However, the severity of injury was not affected by brace wear. Additionally, in a study sponsored by the Big Ten football conference, Albright et al

showed that linemen, linebackers, and tight ends were at highest risk for MCL injury, and that bracing consistently decreased injury rates both at practice and in games.[2] The linebacker and tight end groups were less likely to wear PKBs, citing concern for performance limitations with the brace.

Performance effects of prophylactic knee bracing have been well documented. Styf et al showed that intramuscular pressures increased with brace wear and raised the potential for early muscle fatigue as a result.[41] Greene demonstrated that some braces worn to protect against knee injury might cause decreased speed and agility.[13] With the trade-off of protection for performance, a decision must be made as to which athletes benefit most from prophylactic bracing.[29] The most common practice consists of PKB use in offensive and defensive down linemen, with skill position players opting to perform without braces.

ISOLATED MCL INJURY

Injury to the MCL results in a robust healing response because of its blood supply, relatively wide surface area, association with other secondary stabilizers, and extra-articular location. These factors contribute to the well-documented ability of the MCL to heal without the need for surgical repair or reconstruction. In the absence of injury to secondary stabilizers, particularly the ACL, acute MCL injuries will heal with rare exception. In a rabbit model, Frank showed that MCL injuries at the proximal or distal insertion sites were slower to heal than those seen with midsubstance disruption.[12]

The mainstay of treatment for isolated MCL injury has long been nonoperative with an expectation of good outcomes.* Lundberg et al reported that patients treated nonoperatively with grade I or II MCL injury can expect good return of function, normal to near normal stability, and no increased risk of osteoarthritis at 10-year follow-up.[27] The authors believed that exclusion of additional ligament injury, namely, anterior cruciate ligament (ACL) injury, was imperative for successful treatment of these injuries. Indelicato et al followed 21 athletes for a mean of 46 months with isolated grade III MCL injuries treated nonoperatively and demonstrated 95% good and excellent results.[21] Average return to full contact sport occurred 9.2 weeks after injury for the group, and all athletes with remaining college eligibility returned to play football. Holden et al treated 51 football players with grade I and II MCL injuries nonoperatively, and 80% of the players returned to sport in an average of 21 days.[19] The 20% of players who failed to complete rehabilitation were found to have previously unrecognized injury associated with the ACL and/or the medial meniscus. The authors stressed that truly isolated injury to the MCL could be treated nonoperatively with an expectation of good functional results, and that vigilance is required to detect other potential injuries, because their presence consistently compromised the results of rehabilitation. Jones et al reported on 24 high school football players with isolated grade III MCL injury treated nonoperatively.[22] Twenty-two of the 24 athletes returned to football in an average of 34 days.

Although no standardized rehabilitation protocol for isolated MCL injury exists, several basic tenets of treatment are

---

*References 6, 19, 21, 22, 27, 34, and 42.

typically employed. First, the knee is stabilized in a brace to protect against a second valgus insult. Bracing may also improve pain control and may allow the injured athlete to participate more actively in the rehabilitation program. Second, early motion and weight bearing are encouraged and improve the rate and quality of the healing response.[42] Third, quadriceps and hamstring strengthening is started early in the process to prevent deconditioning and to optimize the function of the knee's dynamic stabilizers. The decision to allow athletes to return to play is dictated by their pain level, functional improvement, and stability on examination. In a prospective study of athletes with grade III MCL injury, Reider instituted a functional rehabilitation program that adhered to these principles.[34] At 5-year follow-up, the mean Hospital for Special Surgery (HSS) knee score was 45.9, and the authors believed that the functional, nonoperative treatment of these injuries with functional rehabilitation produced results as good as those attained with surgical treatment or immobilization, without the treatment-related morbidity noted with those two approaches.

COMBINED INJURIES

ACL/MCL

Although recommendations for the treatment of isolated MCL injuries have been well established, appropriate treatment for patients with combined ACL and MCL injuries continues to evolve. The ACL acts as a secondary stabilizer to valgus stress in the knee, and as such contributes to the innate healing potential of the MCL when intact. Similarly, an intact MCL improves healing of a reconstructed ACL. Loss of a functional ACL has been shown to diminish the capacity of the MCL to heal with nonoperative treatment.[46]

Some concerns have been raised regarding residual laxity in valgus after ACL reconstruction and the effects this may have on the reconstructed knee. Zaffagnini et al compared the immediate postoperative stability of combined ACL/MCL injuries treated with reconstruction of both ligaments or reconstruction of the ACL only.[48] The authors found that addressing the ACL alone led to greater immediate postoperative laxity than did reconstruction of both ligaments. These findings raised concerns regarding abnormal stresses across the ACL graft that might compromise outcomes in knees treated with ACL reconstruction and nonoperative treatment of the MCL injury. Despite these findings, the outcomes literature has not consistently shown residual valgus laxity if the ACL is successfully reconstructed in the acute phase once motion is regained.[16-18,31,37,39]

In a prospective randomized trial evaluating knee range of motion and quadriceps power, Halinen et al compared two treatment groups of knees with combined ACL/MCL injuries.[16] In group 1, patients were treated with early ACL reconstruction and MCL repair, while group 2 knees underwent ACL reconstruction only. Both groups regained acceptable knee motion and quadriceps strength, but the knees in group 2 saw both variables return more quickly. In a second portion of this study, the authors followed these patients for a mean of 27 months and evaluated both subjective and objective outcomes measures.[17] No differences were noted in motion, power, instrumented stability, or Lysholm or International Knee Documentation Committee (IKDC) scores. Once

postinjury motion was regained, the authors recommended nonoperative treatment of combined injuries when the ACL was reconstructed acutely.

Noyes and Barber-Westin demonstrated that operative treatment of the medial structures in ACL/MCL injuries resulted in an increased rate of flexion loss and patellofemoral pain.[32] They recommended nonoperative treatment of the MCL with early reconstruction of the ACL. Shelbourne and Porter reported similar results with acute ACL reconstruction and nonoperative MCL treatment.[39] They stated that residual laxity at the MCL tended to be asymptomatic, and that outcomes for ACL reconstruction alone with this combined injury pattern were similar to those for ACL reconstruction for an isolated ACL tear. Finally, Hillard-Simbell recommended that patients with combined ACL/MCL injuries could be treated with ACL reconstruction only.[18] Additionally, the authors compared patients with combined ACL/MCL injuries treated with ACL reconstruction only versus a group of patients treated with ACL reconstruction for an isolated ACL tear, and found no differences between groups with respect to laxity, return to sport, functional limitation, strength, or one-legged hop testing for distance.

Less has been written on combined ACL/MCL injuries in the pediatric patient. Sankar et al reported on 12 patients with this injury pattern and described similar results to those seen in the adult literature.[37] Patients had similar outcomes and return to sport with ACL reconstruction alone compared with ACL reconstruction in patients with isolated ACL injury. Again, the authors recommended nonoperative treatment of MCL injury if the ACL injury is reconstructed acutely.

ACL/PCL/MCL

The existing orthopedic literature is much less clear regarding the most effective treatment of those knees with medial-sided injury in association with multiligament disruption. The combination of the relative rarity of the injury, the heterogeneity of injury patterns, the treatment approach and technique, and associated medical and trauma issues makes clarification of this condition difficult and elusive. A recent review of the literature by Kovechevich found no consensus with regard to reconstruction or repair of the medial structures, although patients had good results with both approaches.[24] No direct comparison has been made of nonoperative treatment versus operative reconstruction, and most of the information available on this condition has been gleaned from reports on treatment of knee dislocation, with multiple patterns and frequently multiple techniques.

Treatment protocols vary among surgeons. Some surgeons prefer early reconstruction/repair of all injured ligaments, some prefer to brace for 4 to 6 weeks to regain motion and reconstruct the cruciates alone if valgus stability is restored, and others prefer to address the MCL and PCL acutely and reconstruct the ACL if needed later; still others reconstruct or repair the collaterals and address the cruciates in a delayed fashion. Although final results seem to be similar with all approaches, note should be made that risk of arthrofibrosis is associated with early reconstruction or repair of all structures.[31,38,44]

In a study of multiligamentous knee injury with 2- to 10-year follow-up, Fanelli reported on outcomes of operative and nonoperative treatment of combined ligament injuries with MCL involvement with reconstruction of the cruciates.[7] Fifteen patients in the study had injury to the MCL; 7 were treated with surgical reconstruction, and 8 were treated with a brace. All patients treated operatively and 7 of 8 patients treated nonoperatively had normal valgus testing at 30 degrees of flexion.

RECONSTRUCTION TECHNIQUES

Although some authors advocate repair of the medial stabilizing structures, many surgical techniques for medial collateral reconstruction are available; most are variations on the technique originally described by Bosworth.[4] Bosworth described transplantation of the semitendinosus (ST) beneath a fascial, periosteal, and cortical flap at the femoral attachment of the MCL. The tendon is left attached both proximally and distally. The Bosworth technique has been modified to detach the tendon proximally and secure it to the femur at the MCL origin, with the remaining portion of the graft secured to the tibia distally. Similar single- and double-bundle techniques have been described with the use of free tendon grafts.[3,8] In a cadaver study, Feeley et al tested four reconstruction options, including single-bundle reconstruction, the Bosworth technique, a double-bundle technique, and the modified Bosworth reconstruction.[8] The authors found that the modified Bosworth and anatomic double-bundle techniques provided better stability to valgus stress and ER at 30 and 0 degrees of flexion. As the anatomy of the posteromedial corner has become better defined, attention has been turned to reconstructing its functional components, namely, the POL. Because of this, some discussion is ongoing as to the best site of attachment for the posterior limb of the reconstruction. Support exists for routing the posterior limb beneath the direct head of the semimembranosus, through a posterior tibial tunnel, or directly onto the proximal sMCL tibial attachment.[23,26,47] All techniques have yielded similar clinical results.

AUTHORS' PREFERRED TREATMENT

We treat isolated MCL injury nonoperatively with full-time brace wear and a functional rehabilitation program. Immediate weight bearing is encouraged, with active and passive range of motion started as soon as the patient can tolerate it. A full-length brace is used if needed initially for swelling, until a short-hinged knee brace can be applied. Bracing continues full time for 4 to 6 weeks and daytime for another 4 to 6 weeks, or through completion of the current season, if applicable. Athletes are allowed to return to sport once they demonstrate restoration of valgus stability at 0 and 30 degrees of flexion, full range of motion, and successful completion of sport-specific functional rehabilitation. Time to return to play depends on the degree of injury, the athlete's recovery, and the sport/position involved, with typical return times of between 2 and 6 weeks after injury. Exceptions to the nonoperative treatment of isolated MCL injury include large bony avulsions identified on radiographs, Stener-type lesions of the distal MCL, and patients with persistent functional valgus instability after nonoperative treatment.

Regardless of MCL injury grade, most acute ACL/MCL combination injuries are treated with ACL reconstruction once range of motion has been reestablished. Standard post–ACL reconstruction rehabilitation is followed, with the

exception of continued brace wear similar to that for an isolated MCL injury, for a total of 3 months. For chronic ACL tears with residual valgus instability, we recommend simultaneous reconstruction of the ACL and MCL. We prefer to address ACL/PCL/MCL injuries with reconstruction of all injured ligaments once range of motion has been regained. The cruciate ligaments are reconstructed initially, and the functional integrity of the MCL is then assessed.

Surgical Technique

The patient is placed in a supine position, and the knee is examined to determine the extent of ligamentous injury present. Arthroscopic evaluation of the joint line opening aids in determining the amount of laxity present from the collateral injury. Greater than 10 mm of joint space opening indicates injury to the sMCL and POL.[30] Standard, arthroscopically assisted reconstruction of the ACL and PCL is performed as indicated, and any lateral-sided injury is addressed before the MCL is assessed. If valgus instability or abnormal joint line opening remains, the MCL is reconstructed using a modified Bosworth technique. A long curvilinear incision is made over the medial side of the knee with exposure of the crural fascia (Fig. 39-7). The fascia is split longitudinally, with care taken to preserve the gracilis and ST. The ST is identified, isolated, and harvested using an open-ended tendon stripper, leaving its distal attachment in place (Figs. 39-8 and

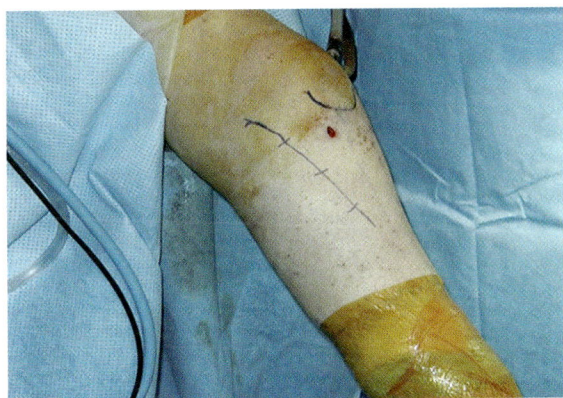

Figure 39-7. A curvilinear incision is made over the medial side of the knee for reconstruction of the medial collateral ligament (MCL).

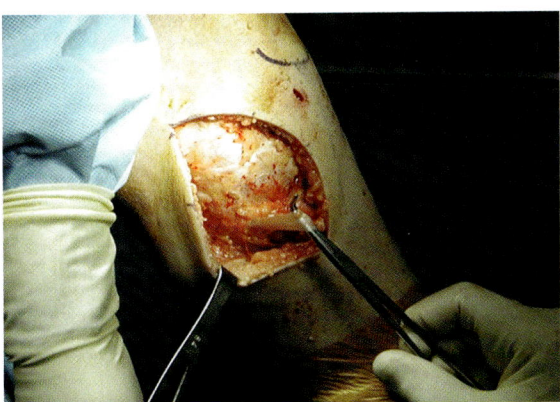

Figure 39-8. The distal extent of the ST is identified, with care taken to protect the distal insertion of the tendon.

39-9). A whipstitch is placed into the free end of the tendon to improve control of the graft (Fig. 39-10). The femoral insertion point for the sMCL is identified proximal and posterior to the medial epicondyle. A 6.5-mm screw with a spiked washer is inserted, with the graft looped around the screw (Fig. 39-11). Alternatively, a shallow trough can be prepared and the graft secured to the femur with a staple. The tendon is then tensioned at 30 degrees of flexion with an axial load and varus stress across the knee (Fig. 39-12). The

remaining portion of the graft is then routed distally beneath the gracilis tendon and is secured to the tibia with a staple at the level of the tibial sMCL insertion (Figs. 39-13 and 39-14). Remaining medial structures can be incorporated into the reconstruction during closure to effect a repair of the POL. Caution should be exercised to avoid overtensioning the posteromedial corner structures, as this can lead to a flexion contracture. The patient is started on a rehabilitation program that involves early motion and progressive weight

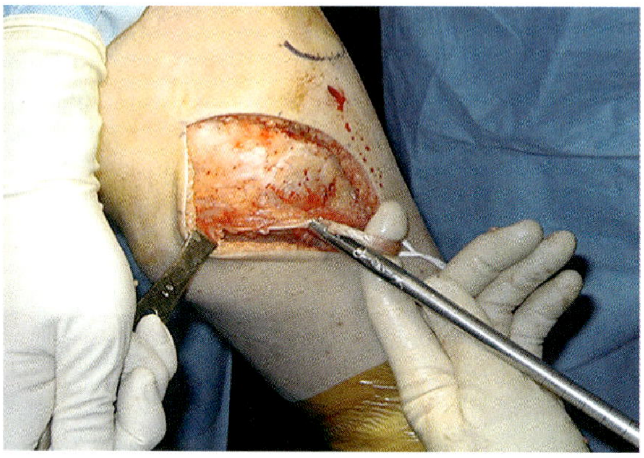

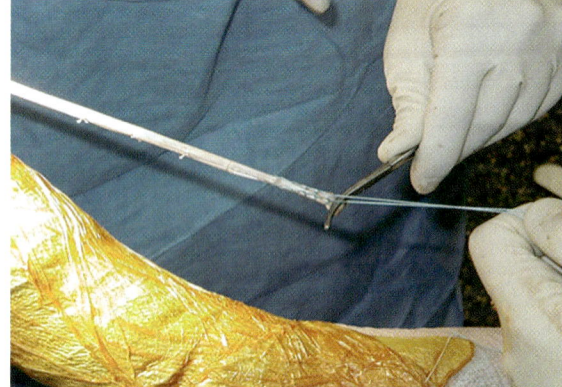

Figure 39-9. The ST is isolated and harvested with an open-ended tendon stripper.

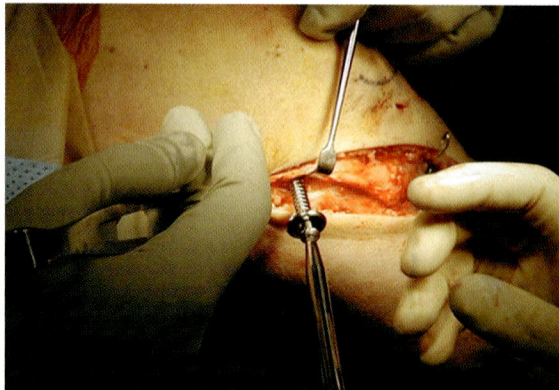

Figure 39-10. A locking running suture is placed into the proximal end of the harvested ST tendon.

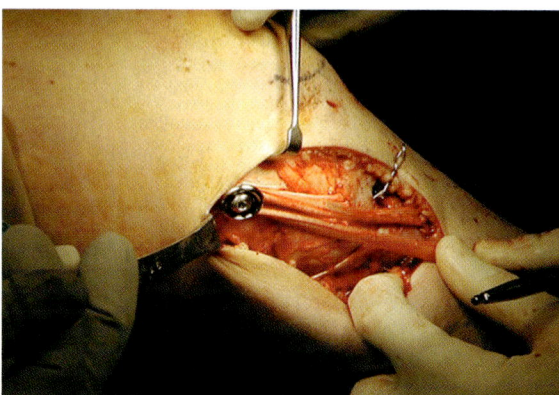

Figure 39-12. The proximal stitched end of the graft is looped around the screw and secured to the femur beneath the spiked washer. The graft is tensioned with the knee in 30 degrees of flexion and a varus stress placed across the knee.

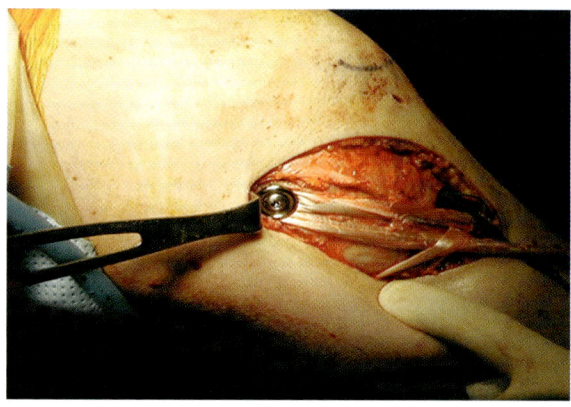

Figure 39-13. The remainder of the graft is then passed beneath the gracilis tendon distally.

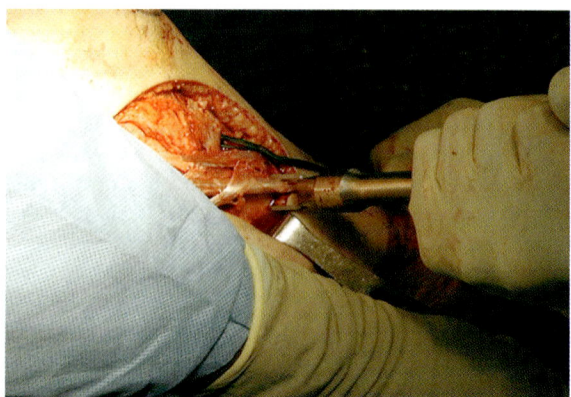

Figure 39-14. The graft is secured to the tibia with a single staple, and the reconstruction is complete.

Figure 39-11. Layer 1 has been incised, and the injured superficial medial collateral ligament (sMCL) is identified as layer 2. The femoral insertion for the sMCL is identified, and a 6.5-mm screw and spiked washer are placed to secure the graft.

bearing in a long, hinged knee brace. The brace is continued for a total of 3 months to give added stability to the collateral repair.

KEY REFERENCES

Albright JP, Powell JW, Smith W, et al: Medial collateral ligament knee sprains in college football: effectiveness of preventive braces. Am J Sports Med 22:12, 1994.

Bosworth DM: Transplantation of the semitendinosus for repair of lacerations of the medial collateral ligament of the knee. J Bone Joint Surg Am 34:196, 1952.

Feeley BT, Muller MS, Allen AA, et al: Biomechanical comparison of medial collateral ligament reconstructions using computer-assisted navigation. Am J Sports Med 37:1123, 2009.

Griffith CJ, LaPrade RF, Johansen S, et al: Medial knee injury: Part 1, Static function of the individual components of the main medial knee structures. Am J Sports Med 37:1762, 2009.

Griffith CJ, Wijdicks CA, LaPrade RF, et al: Force measurements on the posterior oblique ligament and superficial medial collateral ligament proximal and distal divisions to applied loads. Am J Sports Med 37:140, 2009.

Halinen J, Lindahl J, Hirvensalo E, Santavirta S: Operative and non-operative treatments of medial collateral ligament rupture with early anterior cruciate ligament reconstruction: a prospective randomized study. Am J Sports Med 34:1134, 2006.

Holden DL, Eggert AW, Butler JE: The nonoperative treatment of grade 1 and 2 medial collateral ligament injuries to the knee. Am J Sports Med 11:340, 1983.

Indelicato PA, Hermansdorfer J, Huegel M: Nonoperative management of complete tears of the medial collateral ligament of the knee in intercollegiate football players. Clin Orthop Relat Res 256:174, 1990.

Kovachevich R, Shah JP, Arens AM, et al: Operative management of the medial collateral ligament in the multi-ligament injured knee: an evidence based systematic review. Knee Surg Sports Traumatol Arthrosc 17:823, 2009.

LaPrade RF, Engebretsen AH, Ly TV, et al: The anatomy of the medial side of the knee. J Bone Joint Surg Am 89:2000, 2007.

Lundberg M, Messner K: Ten-year prognosis of isolated and combined medial collateral ligament ruptures: a matched comparison in 40 patients using clinical and radiographic evaluations. Am J Sports Med 25:2, 1997.

Reider B, Sathy MR, Talkington J, et al: Treatment of isolated medial collateral ligament injuries in athletes with early functional rehabilitation: a five-year follow-up study. Am J Sports Med 22:470, 1994.

Rubin DA, Kettering JM, Towers JD, et al: MR imaging of knees having isolated and combined ligament injuries. AJR Am J Roentgenol 170:1207, 1998.

Sitler M, Ryan J, Hopkinson W, et al: The efficacy of a prophylactic knee brace to reduce knee injuries in football: a prospective randomized study at West Point. Am J Sports Med 18:310, 1990.

Warren LF, Marshall JL: The supporting structures and layers on the medial side of the knee: an anatomical analysis. J Bone Joint Surg Am 61:56, 1979.

Wijdicks CA, Griffith CJ, LaPrade RF: Medial knee injury: Part 2, Load sharing between the posterior oblique ligament and superficial medial collateral ligament. Am J Sports Med 37:1771, 2009.

Full references for this chapter can be found on www.expertconsult.com.

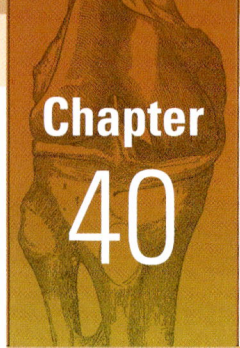

Chapter 40

Fibular Collateral Ligament and the Posterolateral Corner

Robert F. LaPrade and Jeffrey A. Macalena

Although less commonly injured than the cruciate ligaments or the medial knee ligament complex, injuries to the fibular collateral ligament and posterolateral corner comprise a significant portion of knee ligament injuries.[25] Associated posterolateral corner injuries provide a potential source of residual instability following anterior cruciate ligament and posterior cruciate ligament reconstruction and can lead to reconstruction graft failure.[10,21,22] A high index of suspicion is necessary when initially evaluating the injured knee to detect these sometimes occult injuries. Furthermore, a diligent physical examination and comprehensive review of radiographic studies is necessary to identify these injuries. We will provide a review of the anatomy and clinically relevant biomechanics of the fibular collateral ligament and posterolateral corner. We will then present nonoperative and operative treatment options, as well as the postoperative rehabilitative protocol and potential complications.

ANATOMY

An understanding of the complex anatomy of the lateral aspect of the knee is required prior to performing a physical examination, reviewing the radiographic images, or embarking on a complex reconstruction. We will review the major components of the lateral knee ligament complex, as well as their insertions and actions (Fig. 40-1).

Fibular Collateral Ligament

The fibular collateral ligament is the primary stabilizer to varus stress of the knee.[7,8,24] The femoral attachment of the fibular collateral ligament (FCL) is in a small bony depression 1.4 mm proximal and 3.1 mm posterior to the lateral epicondyle.[19] At its femoral origin, the cross-section of the FCL is 0.48 cm^2. As the FCL travels distally to its attachment on the fibular head, the cross-sectional area decreases slightly to 0.43 cm^2. The FCL fibular attachment site is 8.2 mm posterior to the anterior margin of the fibular head and 28.4 mm distal to the tip of the fibular styloid. The FCL occupies 38% of the width of the fibular head at its attachment; the average length of the FCL is 69.6 mm.

Popliteus Tendon

The popliteus muscle courses proximally and laterally from its distal insertion on the posteromedial tibia. It becomes tendinous in the lateral third of the popliteal fossa and becomes intra-articular as it courses deep to the FCL. The cross-section of the popliteus tendon at its femoral insertion is 0.59 cm^2.[19] Its proximal insertion is along the proximal half of the popliteal sulcus and is always anterior (18.5 mm) to the insertion of the FCL femoral attachment (Fig. 40-2). The

tendinous portion of the popliteus is approximately 55 mm in length.

Popliteofibular Ligament

The popliteofibular ligament originates from the musculotendinous junction of the popliteus muscle and inserts onto the fibular styloid. It has two divisions (Fig. 40-3), anterior and posterior; the posterior division is larger at its fibular attachment site (3 vs. 6 mm, respectively).[19] The popliteofibular ligament provides an important restraint to external rotation.[24]

Lateral Gastrocnemius Tendon and Fabellofibular Ligament

The lateral gastrocnemius tendon originates along the supracondylar process of the distal femur (see Fig. 40-1). This attachment averages 13.8 mm posterior to the femoral attachment site of the FCL.[19] Because it is less frequently injured than the other structures of the posterolateral knee, it can be an important landmark during surgical reconstruction. As the lateral gastrocnemius tendon courses distally, it becomes inseparable from the lateral capsule, just proximal to the fabella. The fabella (Latin for "little bean") is a sesamoid bone that is found within the lateral gastrocnemius tendon in 30% of individuals.[11] If not fully ossified, a cartilaginous analogue is frequently found up to 66% of the time. The fabellofibular ligament is a thickening of collagen that extends in a vertical orientation from the fibular styloid to the fabella. It is the distal edge of the capsular arm of the short head of the biceps femoris. It courses between the biceps tendon and gastrocnemius tendon.

Biceps Femoris Tendon: Long and Short Heads

The two heads of the biceps tendon also provide important stabilization of the lateral knee complex. The main tendon of the long head of the biceps femoris divides approximately 1 cm proximal to the fibular head into direct and anterior arms.[19] The direct arm inserts onto the posterolateral fibular head and is the more important of the two. The anterior arm has a small insertion site on the more distal and anterior fibular head before most of the tendon continues on as a broad fascial aponeurosis over the anterior compartment of the leg. The anterior arm forms a bursa as it passes superficial to the fibular collateral ligament and the interval between the direct arm and the anterior arm, which provides a crucial access point to the FCL during reconstruction. The long head of the biceps tendon is also an important anatomic landmark for identification of the peroneal nerve, which lies just to its posterior (Fig. 40-4).

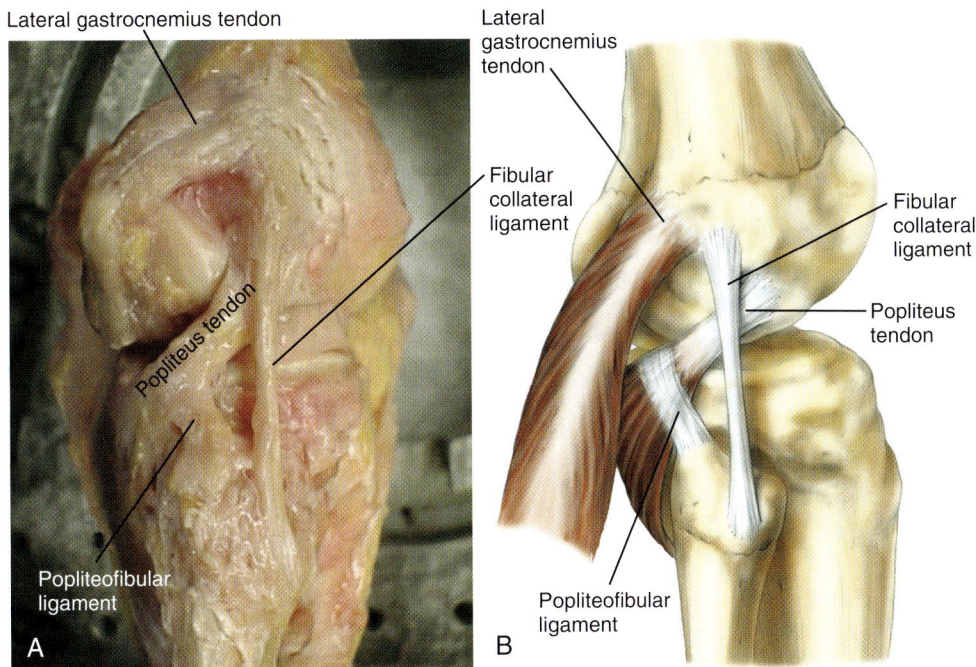

Figure 40-1. **A,** Lateral knee dissection showing the fibular collateral ligament, popliteofibular ligament, popliteus tendon, and lateral gastrocnemius tendon. **B,** Drawing of lateral knee dissection. (From LaPrade RF, Ly TV, Wentorf FA, et al: The posterolateral attachments of the knee. A qualitative and quantitative morphologic analysis of the fibular collateral ligament, popliteus tendon, popliteofibular ligament, and lateral gastrocnemius tendon. Am J Sports Med 31:854–860, 2003.)

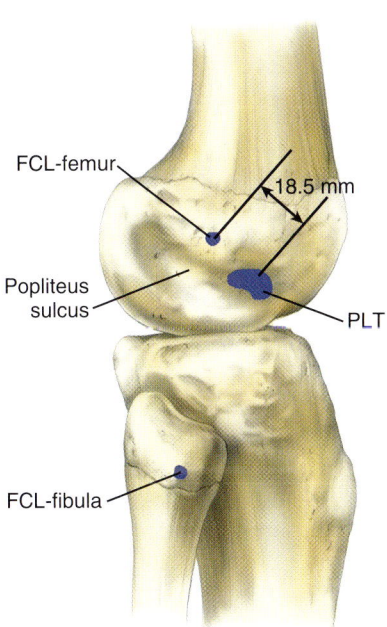

Figure 40-2. Drawing of the attachments sites of the insertions of the popliteus tendon and fibular collateral ligament. The popliteus tendon inserts on average 18.5 mm anterior to the fibular collateral ligament on the femur. (From LaPrade RF, Ly TV, Wentorf FA, et al: The posterolateral attachments of the knee. A qualitative and quantitative morphologic analysis of the fibular collateral ligament, popliteus tendon, popliteofibular ligament, and lateral gastrocnemius tendon. Am J Sports Med 31:854–860, 2003.)

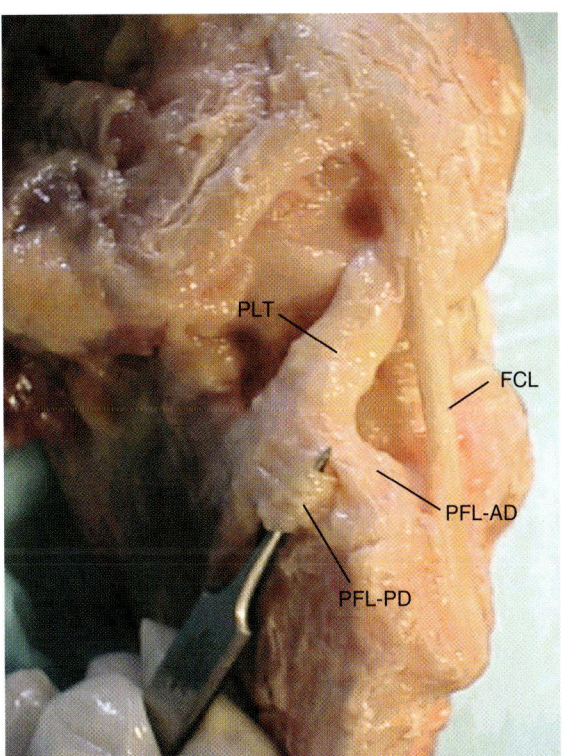

Figure 40-3. Photograph of a cadaveric dissection of the popliteus tendon (PLT), FCL, and anterior division (AD) and posterior division (PD) of the PFL. (From LaPrade RF, Ly TV, Wentorf FA, et al: The posterolateral attachments of the knee. A qualitative and quantitative morphologic analysis of the fibular collateral ligament, popliteus tendon, popliteofibular ligament, and lateral gastrocnemius tendon. Am J Sports Med 31:854–860, 2003.)

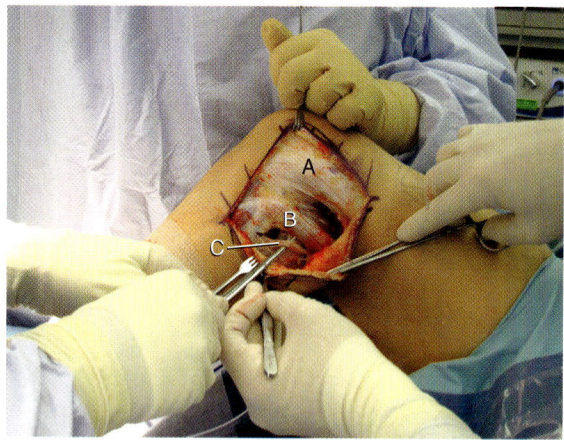

Figure 40-4. Intraoperative photograph of a lateral knee dissection showing the iliotibial band (**A**), long head of the biceps femoris tendon (**B**), and peroneal nerve (**C**). A neurolysis has been performed.

The short head of the biceps tendon also has arms that attach along the posterolateral aspect of the knee. This insertion is medial to the direct arm attachment of the long head, along the lateral aspect of the fibular styloid. The anterior arm of the short head of the biceps tendon passes deep to the FCL and inserts on the tibia just posterior to Gerdy's tubercle. At this point, the anterior arm of the short head of the biceps tendon blends with the meniscotibial ligament, a thickening of the lateral capsule that attaches the capsule to the meniscus and tibia. This capsular arm of the short head of the biceps tendon courses proximally until it blends with the lateral gastrocnemius tendon and posterolateral capsule.

Iliotibial Band

The iliotibial band is the most superficial of the layers of the lateral aspect of the knee. Its broad superficial layer is the first structure encountered deep to the subcutaneous tissues and covers a significant portion of the lateral knee (see Fig. 40-4). Its insertion is at Gerdy's tubercle, along the anterolateral aspect of the tibia. The other components of the iliotibial band include an anterior expansion known as the iliopatellar band, a deep layer that blends with the lateral intermuscular septum, and a capsulo-osseous layer that attaches to the tibia just posterior and proximal to the main attachment at Gerdy's tubercle.[33]

Lateral Capsular Thickenings

The meniscofemoral and meniscotibial ligaments are capsular connections of the meniscus to the femur and tibia, respectively. A Segond injury is an avulsion of the meniscotibial ligament from the tibia. The coronary ligament is an attachment of the lateral meniscus to the joint capsule. This helps anchor the lateral meniscal root posteriorly.

CLINICALLY RELEVANT BIOMECHANICS OF THE POSTEROLATERAL KNEE

The structures of the lateral knee and posterolateral corner provide the primary restraint to varus stress of the knee,[7,8] as well as posterolateral rotation of the tibia in relationship to the femur.[24] These structures are also important secondary stabilizers to anterior and posterior tibial translation when the cruciate ligaments are torn.[13] We will next review these static and dynamic stabilizers in regard to the stresses experienced by the knee.

Varus Stress

The fibular collateral ligament is the primary restraint to varus stress across the knee. Cutting studies have demonstrated that selective sectioning of the FCL results in an increase in varus opening.[7,8] In cutting series in which the FCL remains intact, varus stability has been preserved. The popliteus, popliteofibular ligament (PFL), iliotibial band, lateral gastrocnemius tendon, and short and long heads of the biceps tendon, as well as the cruciate ligaments, are secondary restraints to varus force; their contribution has been noted after sectioning of the FCL.[13]

External Tibial Rotation

The FCL and popliteus complex are the primary restraints to tibial external rotation.[24] With sectioning of the FCL, popliteofibular ligament, and popliteus tendon, an increase in tibial external rotation has been shown in a number of studies; it is most prevalent at approximately 30 to 40 degrees of knee flexion.[30]

Just as the FCL and popliteus complex act as a secondary restraint to the posterior cruciate ligament (PCL) in resisting posterior tibial translation, the PCL acts as a secondary restraint to prevent external rotation of the tibia on the femur.[13] Because of this relationship, combined posterior cruciate ligament and posterolateral corner injuries are particularly unstable to external rotation forces.

Internal Tibial Rotation

The fibular collateral ligament and posterolateral corner structures are secondary restraints to internal rotation. Their contribution becomes better appreciated in the anterior cruciate ligament (ACL)–deficient knee.

Anterior Tibial Translation

The ACL is the primary restraint to anterior tibial translation.[34] In knees with an intact ACL, the lateral ligament complex does not provide significant restraint to anterior tibial translation. However, in an ACL-deficient knee, the structures of the posterolateral corner provide an important secondary anterior translation stabilization role.[22] This is particularly true during the first 40 degrees of knee flexion.

Posterior Tibial Translation

The PCL is the primary restraint to posterior tibial translation, but the structures of the posterolateral corner (PLC) also play a primary role in preventing posterior translation of the tibia on the femur.[7] This contribution is noted most in full extension and at lower degrees of flexion.[8,34] The contribution of the PLC increases in the PCL-deficient knee, in which the popliteus tendon appears to contribute the most to secondary stability of the structures of the PLC.[9]

INJURIES TO THE FIBULAR COLLATERAL LIGAMENT AND POSTEROLATERAL CORNER

Mechanism of Injury

A direct blow to the medial (particularly the anteromedial) knee is a common mechanism of injury to the FCL and PLC, although noncontact hyperextension and noncontact varus stress injuries have also been well described.[23] Only 40% of PLC injuries are sports-related.[30] Motor vehicle accidents, falls, and other high-energy trauma comprise a significant portion of these injuries. Usually, injuries to the PLC are associated with ACL or PCL tears because only approximately 25% of PLC injuries are isolated knee ligament tears.[15,25]

History and Physical Examination

Patients usually highlight a discrete event in regard to the onset of their knee injury. However, in chronic settings, previous surgeries and a prolonged time since the injury may make the details of the actual injury less clear.

Common symptoms include pain, subjective side to side instability (near extension), difficulty with stairs, difficulty on uneven ground, swelling, and ecchymoses. A varus thrust gait can be noted by the patient and physician. Patients may also report parasthesias in the peroneal nerve distribution, as well as a footdrop. It has been reported that common peroneal nerve injury can be seen in up to one third of posterolateral corner injuries.[23,34]

A complete history, including details of the accident, subsequent injuries, previous surgeries, and other associated injuries should be ascertained. Furthermore, a review of the patient's past medical history (including problems with bleeding, clotting, or anesthesia), medications, tobacco use, and goals regarding return to sports and activities should be obtained.

A detailed physical examination is an important and required component of a patient's evaluation. A patient's gait should be examined to assess for evidence of a varus thrust with the initiation of the stance phase.[6] The alignment of the limbs should be evaluated and the skin examined for any evidence of penetrating trauma, open wounds, or ecchymoses. A detailed neurovascular examination with diligent recording of distal pulses, as well as muscle grading of ankle dorsiflexion, plantar flexion, inversion, and eversion strength, is also completed. Sensory examination of the distal extremity is performed with attention to the dorsum of the foot, which is supplied by the superficial peroneal nerve, and to the first web space, which is supplied by the deep peroneal nerve.

A detailed examination of the knee is then performed with active and passive range of motion measurements. Stability examination of the ACL using a Lachman and pivot shift examination and of the PCL using the posterior draw test is also completed. The patella is evaluated for evidence of chronic or acute subluxation or dislocation. Palpation is performed along the deep infrapatellar bursa, Gerdy's tubercle, pes anserine bursa, and patellar tendon attachment on the inferior pole of the patella. The structures of the PLC are then palpated, with specific attention to any tenderness along

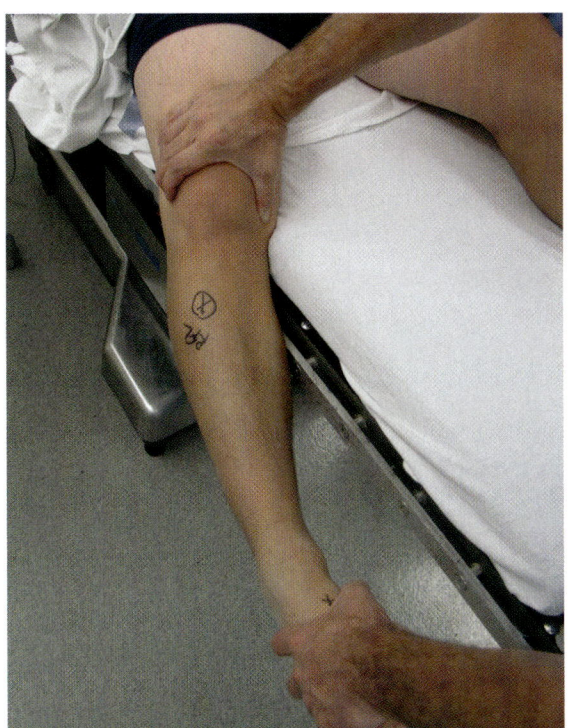

Figure 40-5. A varus stress test is performed by stabilizing the femur with the examiner's right hand and palpating the lateral joint line. The other hand provides a varus stress to the ankle. The test is performed at 0 and 30 degrees.

the femoral attachment of the FCL and popliteus tendon and to tenderness at the fibular head. Tibiofemoral joint stability is then assessed. Specific tests to assess for PLC injuries will be presented in the following sections.

Varus Stress Test

With the knee in full extension and at 30 degrees of flexion, the femur is stabilized to the examination table with the examiner's hand (Fig. 40-5). A varus force is applied through the patient's foot or ankle. The lateral knee joint line is palpated by the examiner's finger (from the hand that is stabilizing the knee) and the amount of lateral compartment gapping is assessed. All stability examinations should be graded on amount of opening (as compared with the contralateral side) and firmness of the end point. Opening of the lateral compartment with the knee flexed to 30 degrees requires an injury to the FCL and possibly the secondary stabilizers of the PLC. The knee is then brought up to full extension; if the stability is restored, an isolated injury to the FCL and PLC is presumed. If the varus instability persists in full extension, a combined FCL and PLC and cruciate ligament injury is presumed.

Dial Test

The dial test measures external rotation of the tibia in regard to the femur. The test is performed in the prone or supine position. The femur is fixed with one hand while the ankle and foot are externally rotated (Fig. 40-6). This is done with the knee flexed to 30 degrees. An increase of more than 10 degrees of external rotation compared with the uninvolved

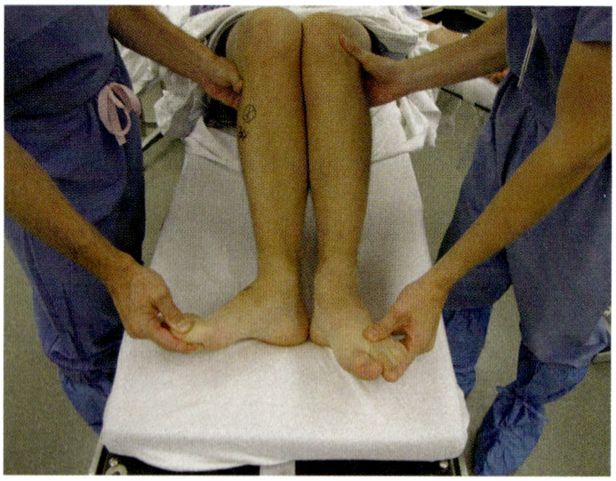

Figure 40-6. The dial test evaluates for external rotation of the tibia on the femur. It is performed at 30 and 90 degrees. Here, a positive dial test at 90 degrees is shown on the patient's right side. This suggests a combined posterolateral corner and posterior cruciate ligament injury.

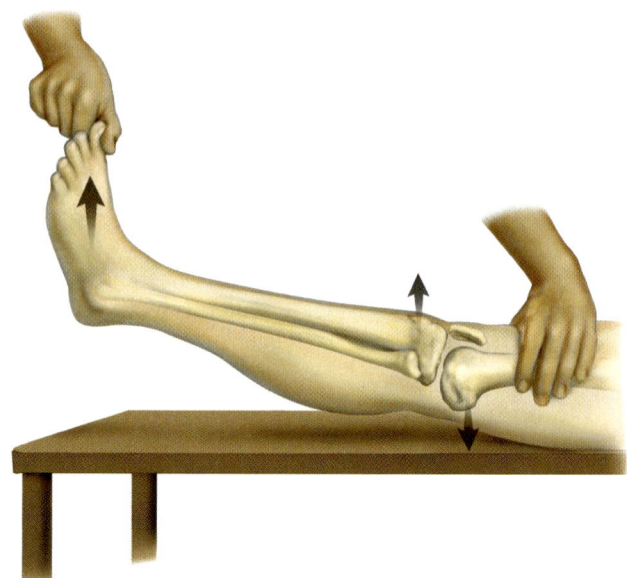

Figure 40-7. Drawing of the external rotation recurvatum test. The femur is fixed to the examination table and the patient's leg is lifted by the great toe. Increase in recurvatum through the knee as compared with the uninjured side is considered a positive test. (From LaPrade RF, Ly TV, Griffith C: The external rotation recurvatum test revisited. Am J Sports Med 36:709–771, 2008.)

side suggests an injury to the PLC.[8] The knee is then flexed to 90 degrees. Because of its role as an important secondary stabilizer, a knee with an intact PCL will see a decrease in external rotation. If, at 90 degrees, there is an increase in external rotation, as compared with 30 degrees, a combined PLC and PCL injury is presumed. A sequential sectioning study by Bae and coworkers[2] have demonstrated increased external rotation following sectioning of at least three ligaments of the PCL and PLC. It was cautioned that the dial test may not be sufficiently sensitive to identify one- or two-ligament injuries.

External Rotation Recurvatum Test

In the external rotation recurvatum test, the patient is placed supine, with the knees and hips extended. The great toe is grasped and the leg lifted from the table with gentle pressure applied to the proximal knee (Fig. 40-7). The height of the heel in centimeters or degrees of hyperextension of the knee is recorded and compared with the contralateral side. A wide variation of the sensitivity of this test has been reported. Recently, LaPrade and colleagues[18] evaluated this test and found it to identify less than 10% of a series of 134 patients with posterolateral corner injuries. However, in their study, a positive external rotation recurvatum test predicted a combined anterior cruciate ligament and posterolateral corner injury.

Posterolateral Drawer Test

The posterolateral drawer test is performed in the same position as the conventional drawer test, with the patient supine and the knee flexed to 90 degrees and with the foot stabilized by the examiner. With the examiner's fingers grasping the femoral condyles, a posteriorly directed force is applied with the tibia in external rotation. An increase in translation with external rotation as compared with the contralateral normal knee suggests an injury to the posterolateral corner.

Reverse Pivot Shift

The reverse pivot shift is performed by positioning the patient supine with the knee flexed to almost 90 degrees. A valgus load is applied across the knees and an external rotation force applied to the tibia. The knee is then slowly extended. Reduction of the previously subluxated lateral tibial plateau at approximately 35 to 40 degrees of flexion is a positive result. A positive reverse pivot shift and injuries to the PLC have been correlated.[30] It is important to compare the results with the contralateral knee because the test has been reported to be positive in 35% of normal knees.[5]

Imaging

Plain Radiographs

Standing anteroposterior (AP) and lateral radiographs of the knee should be obtained, as well as a bent knee patellofemoral view. Radiographs are frequently normal in acute injuries. The presence of Segond fractures[15] (Fig. 40-8), tibial spine avulsions, or fibular head fractures or avulsions (arcuate sign[27]; Fig. 40-9) may be visualized. A standing long-leg anterior-posterior alignment radiograph is a requirement for chronic posterolateral corner injuries because malalignment needs to be recognized and corrected prior to or at the time of surgical reconstruction (Fig. 40-10). Varus and posterior stress radiographs are also an important component of the radiographic workup of a patient with a suspected FCL or PLC injury (Fig. 40-11). Contralateral knee stress films are obtained for comparison. Varus stress radiographs have been shown in cadaveric sectioning studies to be sensitive and reproducible. LaPrade and associates[16] have demonstrated that sectioning of the FCL results in 2.7 mm of increased lateral gapping with varus stress and that sectioning of the entire PLC allows 4.0 mm of increased lateral gapping. Combined injuries to the posterolateral corner and posterior cruciate ligament should be suspected when posterior drawer

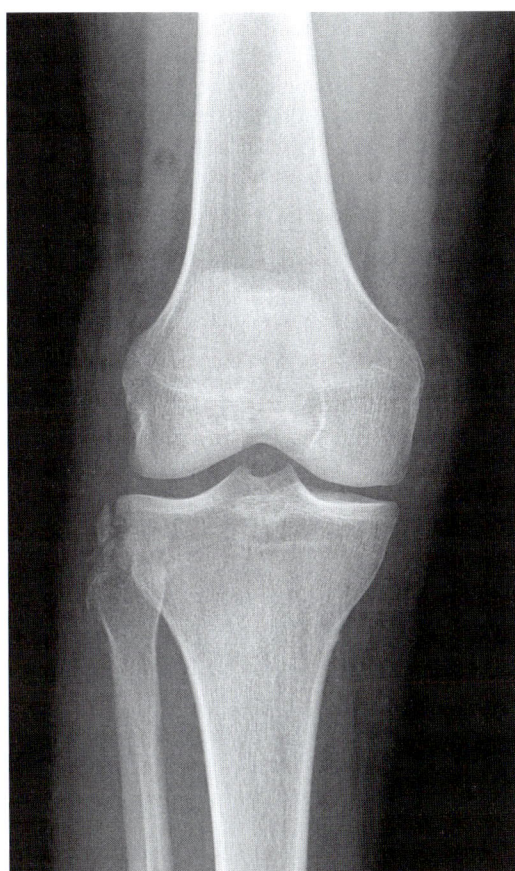

Figure 40-8. AP radiograph of the knee demonstrating a Segond fracture of the lateral tibial plateau.

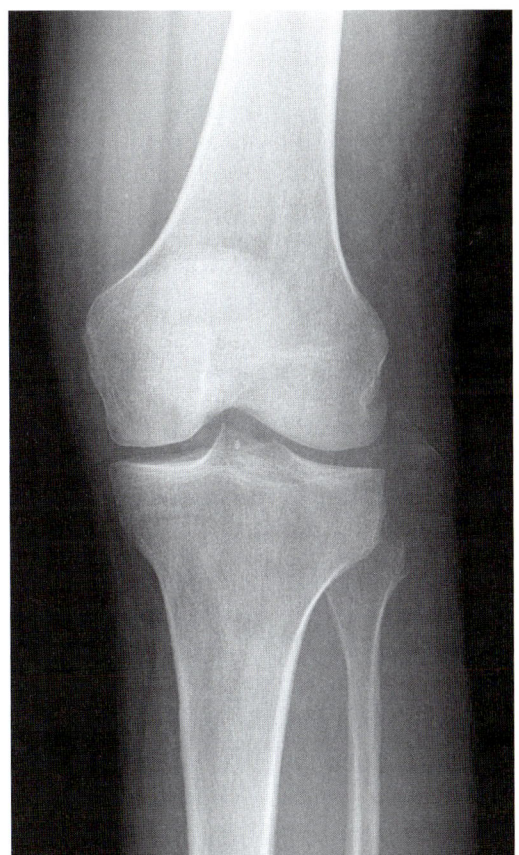

Figure 40-9. AP radiograph of the knee demonstrating a fracture of the fibular head (arcuate sign).

testing demonstrates more than 12 mm of posterior translation of the tibia.

Magnetic Resonance Imaging

Magnetic resonance imaging (MRI) is an important diagnostic tool for evaluating the structures of the posterolateral corner, especially in acute injuries. Both T1- and T2-weighted MRI series have provided important information regarding the structures involved and extent of injury. Coronal and saggital series should be obtained. The sensitivity and specificity for identifying injuries to specific components of the posterolateral corner are high, more than 90% for identifying injuries to the superficial layer of the iliotibial band, anterior arm of the biceps femoris tendon, midthird capsular ligaments, and FCL (Fig. 40-12).[12] The popliteofemoral origin and fabellofibular ligaments had sensitivities in the 80% to 90% range. Only the popliteofibular ligament had sensitivity and specificity less than 80% (68.8% and 66.7%, respectively).[15] The cartilage, menisci, and cruciate ligaments should also be evaluated for associated injuries.

Diagnostic Arthroscopy

The intra-articular structures of the posterolateral corner can be visualized with arthroscopy. These include the popliteal tendon's origin (Fig. 40-13), meniscofemoral ligament, coronary ligament of the lateral meniscus, and meniscotibial

ligaments. LaPrade[12] has evaluated these structures arthroscopically and noted injuries to them in 33%, 37%, 73%, and 80% of knees with grade III posterolateral corner injuries. This study also indicated that concomitant injuries are frequently observed as well, because 63% of knees had ACL tears, 23% had PCL tears, and 22% had lateral meniscus tears. Chondromalacia was noted 23% of the time. A drive-through sign (increased laxity of the lateral compartment) is an indirect indicator of a FCL and possibly a PLC injury.

TREATMENT

Grades I and II injuries to the fibular collateral ligament can be usually treated nonoperatively.[30] Knee bracing with a knee immobilizer or hinged knee brace locked in full extension for 3 to 6 weeks is usually sufficient. Full weight bearing is usually allowed and passive and active prone knee flexion are performed to prevent stiffness. In more involved injuries, a course of protected weight bearing is sometimes prescribed. Stress radiographs can be used at the time of injury and prior to return to play to compare side to side differences. After 3 to 6 weeks, sports-specific therapy is initiated and a return to play can be considered once pain is absent and full range of motion, strength equal to the contralateral side, and clinical stability to varus stress testing are attained. Bracing can be continued after return to play, depending on the type of sport and the severity of the injury. Injuries to the anterior cruciate ligament and posterior cruciate ligament should be treated with reconstruction and grades I and II injuries of the PLC treated nonoperatively.

Grade III injuries to the posterolateral corner are best treated with surgery because the risk for continued symptomatic instability is significant.[30] In combined PLC and ACL or PCL-injured knees, concurrent repair or reconstruction of the PLC is recommended because the PLC-deficient knee places significant stress on the newly placed ACL or PCL graft, increasing the risk of graft failure.[10,21,22] We will review the available treatments, including repair and reconstruction.

Repair

Intrasubstance repairs of the fibular collateral ligament and popliteus have not fared well and therefore should not be performed. However, other structures of the PLC are amenable to intrasubstance repair. These include the coronary ligament of the lateral meniscus, meniscofemoral and meniscotibial ligaments, and fibers of the popliteomeniscal

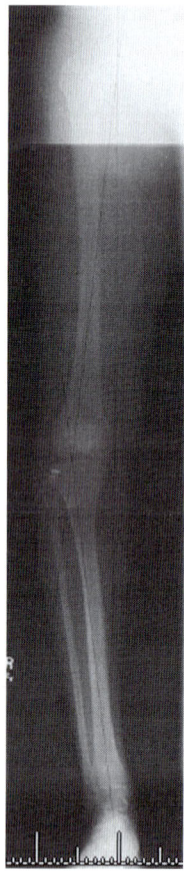

Figure 40-10. Long-leg standing AP radiograph demonstrating varus malalignment. The pencil mark outlining the mechanical axis of the limb is visualized medial to the knee joint.

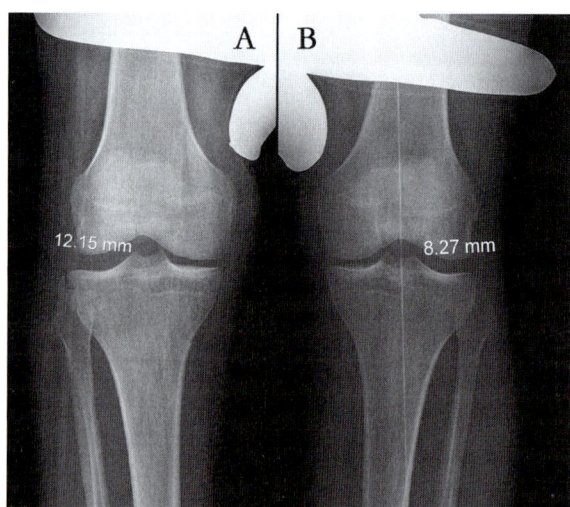

Figure 40-11. A, Stress radiographs of the injured knee demonstrate 12.15 mm of lateral compartment opening of the injured knee. **B,** Stress films of the patient's contralateral uninjured knee demonstrate an 8.27-mm opening.

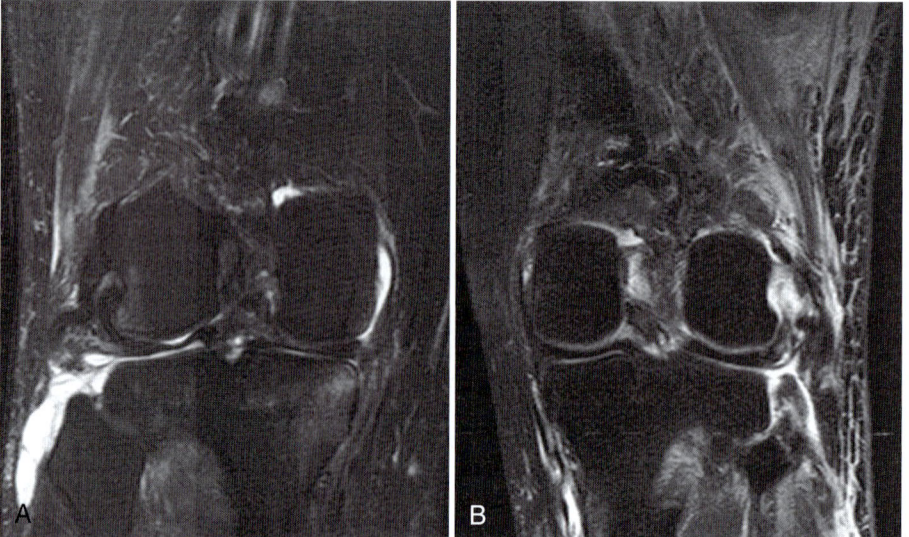

Figure 40-12. A, Coronal T2-weighted MRI image of a right knee demonstrating an avulsion of the fibular collateral ligament from its fibular attachment site. The popliteus tendon is visualized deep to the ruptured fibular collateral ligament. **B,** Coronal T2-weighted MRI image of a left knee demonstrates avulsion of the femoral attachment of the popliteus tendon.

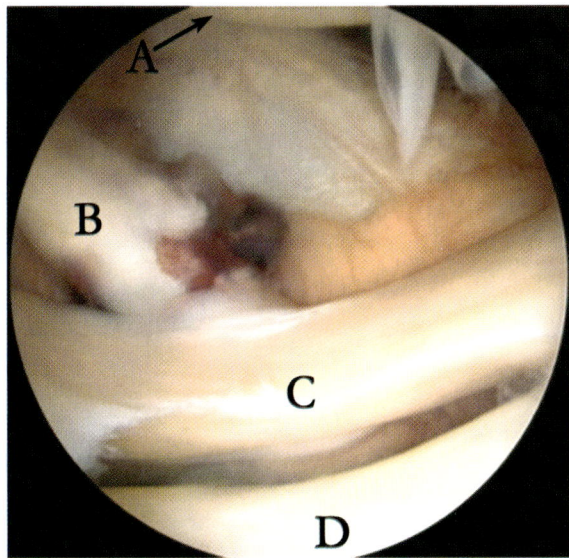

Figure 40-13. Arthroscopic image of the lateral compartment of the knee. The femoral and tibial articular surfaces are seen at the *top* and *bottom* of this figure. The lateral meniscus is seen traveling across the *center portion*. The popliteus tendon has been avulsed from its femoral insertion. Hematoma is seen along its course. A drive-through sign is shown by the increased lateral compartment gapping.

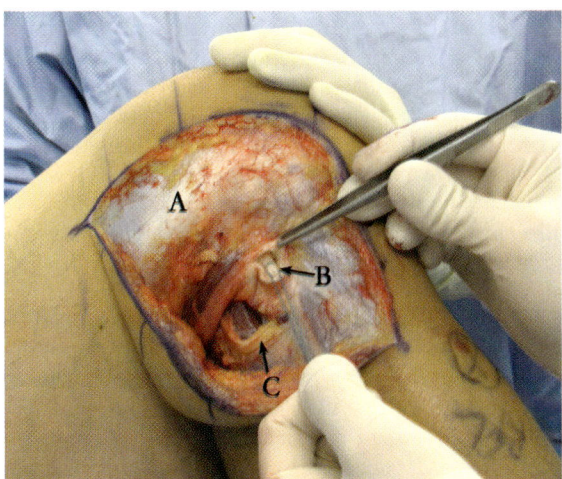

Figure 40-14. Lateral knee dissection. The iliotibial band **(A)**, fibular collateral ligament **(B)**, with a stay suture at its fibular attachment, and peroneal nerve **(C)** are visualized following neurolysis.

ligaments. Horizontal or vertical sutures are placed through these structures after adequate visualization has been achieved. We recommend using of 0-0 braided, nonabsorbable suture for this. These sutures should be tensioned with the knee in full extension. Early range of motion up to 90 degrees is immediately allowed.

Techniques have been described in which the avulsed ends of the popliteus and/or the fibular collateral ligament have been placed within a bone tunnel or tied down with suture anchors at the femoral origin. This recession technique uses an eyelet-passing pin for passage of sutures across the distal femur.[13,26] Prior to passage of the sutures, a 5-mm reamer is used to create a bone tunnel. The sutured ends of the FCL or popliteus are then placed into the Beath pin, which is advanced medially. The tendon is seen to pass into the freshly drilled tunnel and the passing suture is tied down medially over a button. The location of the starting point for the tunnel is at the anatomic origin of the involved structure.

A prospective review by Stannard and coworkers[32] has compared repair with reconstruction. In their review, repair was inferior to reconstruction in the management of acute posterolateral corner injuries. They compared a suture anchor and repair of damaged structures with a modified two-tailed reconstruction (see later). The reconstruction group fared better and had fewer failures (9% vs. 37%) than the repair group.

Reconstruction

Numerous posterolateral knee reconstructive techniques have also been described. These include nonanatomic and anatomic techniques. Nonanatomic techniques such as the biceps tendon tenodesis, initially described and popularized by Clancy,[3] redirect the biceps tendon, or a slip of the biceps tendon, from its distal attachment on the fibular head to a

site along the distal lateral femur approximately 1 cm anterior to the origination of the FCL, theoretically to reconstruct the FCL.[31] This technique requires harvesting 6 to 8 cm of biceps tendon and looping it over a screw and spiked washer.

The Stannard reconstruction technique is a nonanatomic reconstruction of the fibular collateral ligament, popliteofibular ligament, and popliteus tendon.[32] A tibialis anterior or tibialis posterior allograft is used. After exposure of the lateral knee, a bone tunnel is drilled along the posterior tibia in an anterior to posterior direction. This tunnel will be the anchor point of one end of the allograft and approximates the tibial position of the popliteus tendon. The allograft is then advanced proximally over a previously placed screw at the reported isometric point of the lateral femoral condyle to re-create the popliteus. The allograft is then brought back inferiorly toward the fibular head and passed through a tunnel drilled in the fibular head. This arm of the allograft reportedly reconstructs the popliteofibular ligament. The allograft is passed in a posterior to anterior direction through the fibula and returned to the screw in the distal femur. This final arm re-creates the fibular collateral ligament. The screw and spiked washer are advanced and the graft tensioned at 40 to 60 degrees of knee flexion.

Preferred Techniques

Fibular Collateral Ligament Reconstruction

For isolated fibular collateral ligament injuries, we recommend reconstruction using a semitendinosus autograft. After harvesting the semitendinosus via a standard technique, attention is turned to the open reconstruction of the FCL.[4] An incision is made along the lateral knee over the lateral epicondyle, along the posterior border of the iliotibial band. This is extended proximally and distally for approximately 10 cm. The common peroneal nerve is identified posterior to the biceps tendon and protected. A neurolysis is performed. The iliotibial band is opened in line with its fibers along its posterior third (Fig. 40-14). A horizontal incision into the biceps bursa generally identifies the fibular collateral ligament. Injuries to the FCL usually leave the midsubstance of the ligament intact although functionally incompetent because of elongation. A stay suture is placed into the FCL remnant just proximal to the fibular head and gentle tension applied (Fig. 40-15). The femoral attachment site can then be identified. Sharp dissection with a knife is used to lift the FCL femoral attachment site subperiosteally, which is slightly proximal and posterior to the femoral epicondyle. An eyelet-passing pin is placed through the center of the FCL femoral attachment site and directed proximomedially across the distal femur. We ream a 6-mm tunnel to a depth of 25 mm and tap with a 7-mm tap (Fig. 40-16). The previously tubularized graft is recessed into the femoral tunnel by pulling on the passing sutures and a 7- × 23-mm bioabsorbable screw is placed (Fig. 40-17). The distal attachment of the fibular collateral ligament is then identified along the lateral aspect of the fibular head. A guide pin is placed through this depression with an ACL-targeting guide. The exit point of the guide pin is along the posteromedial fibular head, distal to the insertion of the popliteofibular ligament (Fig. 40-18). A 6-mm reamer is used to create a tunnel. A tract is made deep to the superficial layer of the iliotibial band and passing sutures are used to place the graft into the fibular tunnel (Fig. 40-19). A 7- × 23-mm bioabsorbable interference is screw-placed with

tension applied to the graft and a valgus force applied to the knee to prevent any lateral compartment gapping, with the knee flexed to 20 degrees (Fig. 40-20). After the screw is placed, the free end of the graft is continued posteriorly around the fibular head, between a split in the anterior arm of the biceps femoris and sutured to itself using a nonabsorbable suture (Fig. 40-21).

Posterolateral Corner Reconstruction

When a posterolateral corner injury is present in addition to a fibular collateral ligament injury, we recommend an anatomic reconstruction of both the PLC and FCL. Described by LaPrade and colleagues in 2004,[17] this technique anatomically reconstructs the FCL, popliteus tendon, and popliteofibular ligament. Following a lateral approach and peroneal nerve neurolysis, the attachment sites of the fibular collateral ligament on the lateral fibular head and the popliteofibular ligament on the posteromedial fibular head are identified. An ACL-cannulated guide is then used to drill a guide pin from the FCL attachment on the lateral aspect of the fibular head posteromedially to the popliteofibular ligament attachment site (Fig. 40-22). This is overreamed with a 7-mm reamer. The posterior tibial popliteal sulcus is then identified with

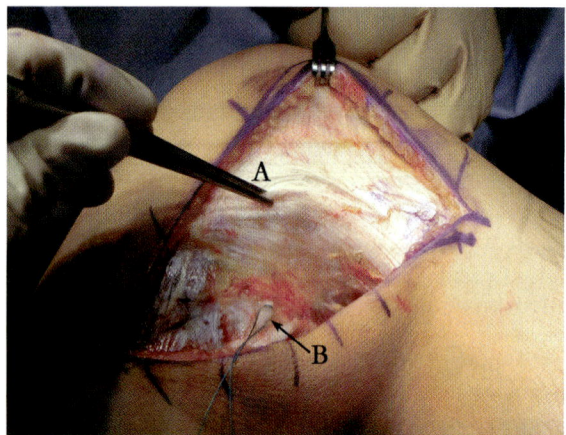

Figure 40-15. **A,** The iliotibial band is split in line with its fibers and reflected, demonstrating the femoral insertion of the fibular collateral ligament **(B)**. The stay suture is again visualized at the fibular insertion of the FCL.

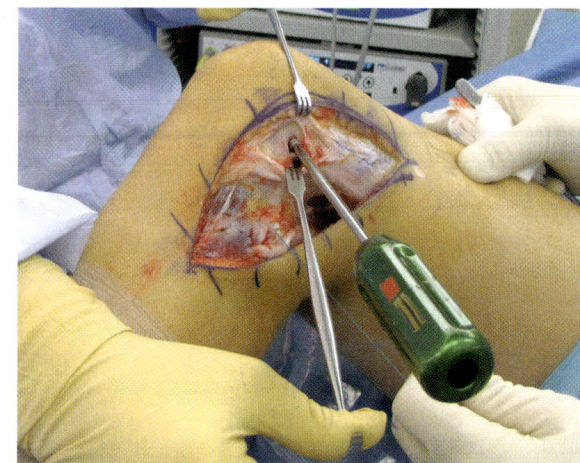

Figure 40-16. The femoral tunnel is tapped in preparation for placement of the graft and interference screw.

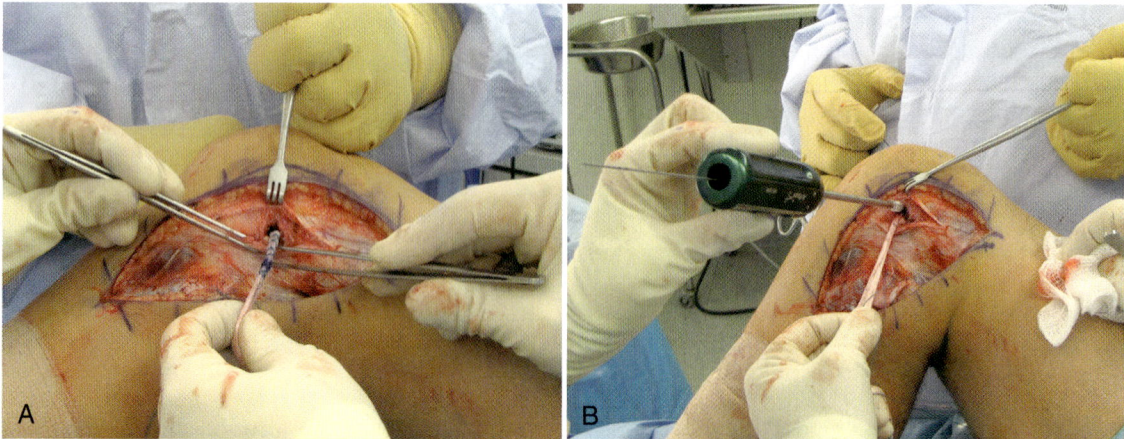

Figure 40-17. **A,** The graft is placed within the femoral tunnel. **B,** A bioabsorbable interference screw is placed to secure the graft.

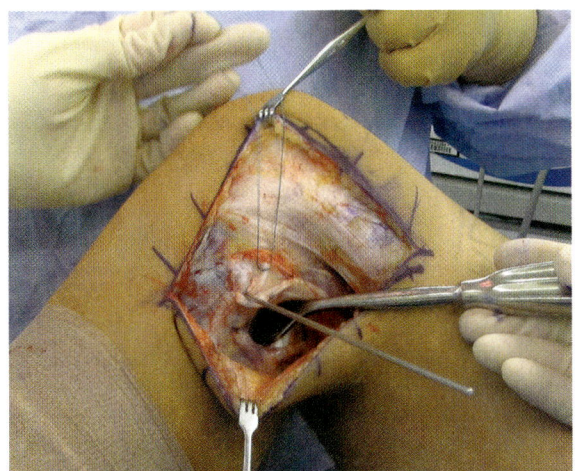

Figure 40-18. A guide pin is placed across the fibular tunnel. The pin is started at the anatomic insertion of the fibular collateral ligament.

direct palpation in the interval between the lateral gastrocnemius and soleus muscles. This marks the musculotendinous junction of the popliteus. With a retractor protecting the neurovascular structures, an ACL-cannulated guide is used to place a guide pin from anterior to posterior (Fig. 40-23). The pin is overreamed with a 9-mm reamer. The femoral attachment of the popliteus and the fibular collateral ligament are then identified. Eyelet pins are placed at their anatomic attachments sites and advanced anteromedially (Fig. 40-24). The distance between these two pins is measured and should be approximately 18.5 mm.[19] The lateral cortex is reamed to a depth of 25 mm for both of these pins.

An Achilles allograft is split lengthwise and the tendons tubularized. Two 9- × 20-mm bone blocks are fashioned. Passing sutures in the bone block are used to reduce the bone blocks into the femoral tunnel and 7-mm metal interference screws are placed (Fig. 40-25). The FCL graft is routed deep

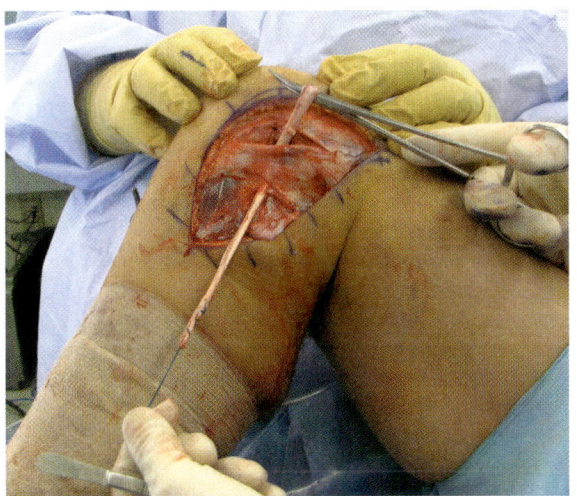

Figure 40-19. The graft is routed deep to the iliotibial band.

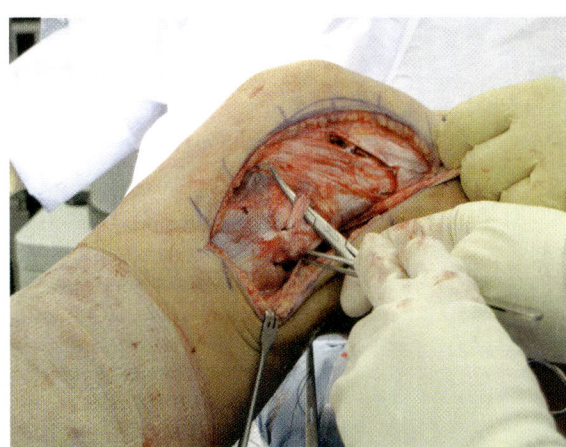

Figure 40-20. The fibular collateral ligament graft in place is seen deep to the hemostat. A valgus force is applied across the knee, the graft tensioned, and an interference screw placed within the fibular head.

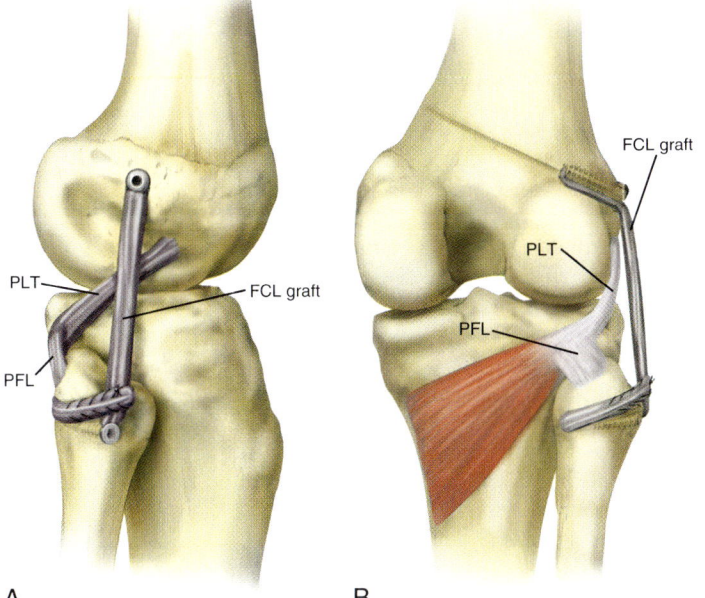

A   B

Figure 40-21. Drawing of lateral (**A**) and posterior (**B**) views of the anatomically reconstructed fibular collateral ligament (FCL graft). The free tail of the graft is brought around the posterior aspect of the fibular head and sutured to itself to provide an extra point of fixation. The popliteus tendon (PLT) and PFL are shown as well. (From Coobs BR, LaPrade RF, Griffith CJ, Nelson BJ. Biomechanical analysis of an isolated fibular [lateral] collateral ligament reconstruction using an autogenous semitendinosus graft. Am J Sports Med 35:1521–1527, 2007.)

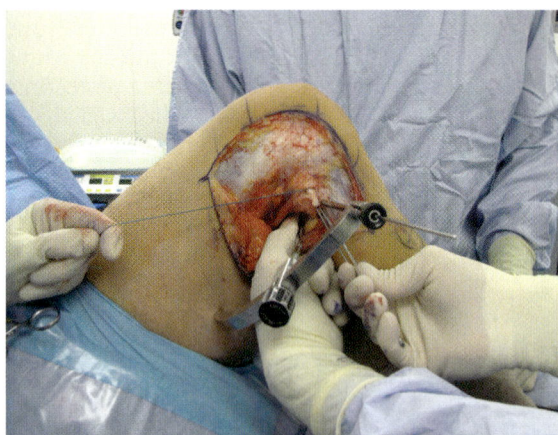

Figure 40-22. An ACL cannulated guide is used to place a guide pin for the fibular tunnel for the posterolateral corner reconstruction. The anatomic insertion of the fibula collateral ligament is the starting point. The guide pin should exit at the insertion of the popliteofibular ligament on the fibular styloid.

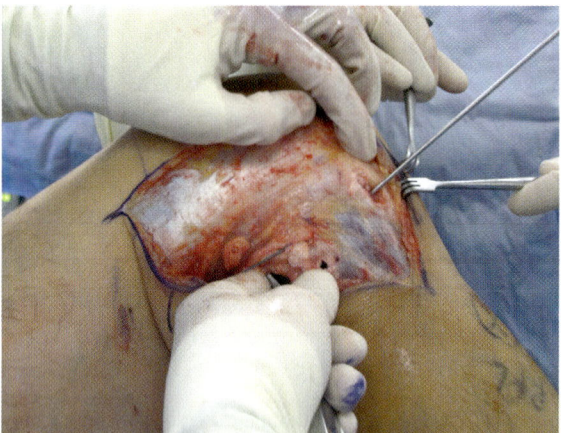

Figure 40-23. The guide pin is placed for the popliteus tunnel. This is drilled anterior to posterior, with the exit point at the popliteal sulcus on the posterior tibia. Retractors are placed to protect the neurovascular structures.

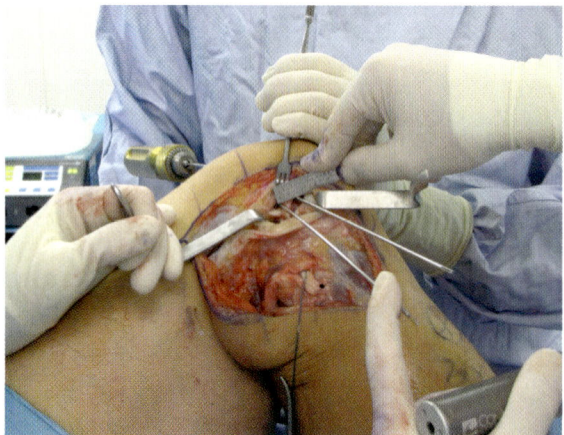

Figure 40-24. Guide pins are placed for the femoral insertion of the fibular collateral ligament and popliteus tendon reconstruction. The popliteus tendon inserts on average 18.5 mm anterior to the fibular collateral ligament. This figure shows both guide pins in place and a ruler confirming the appropriate relationship.

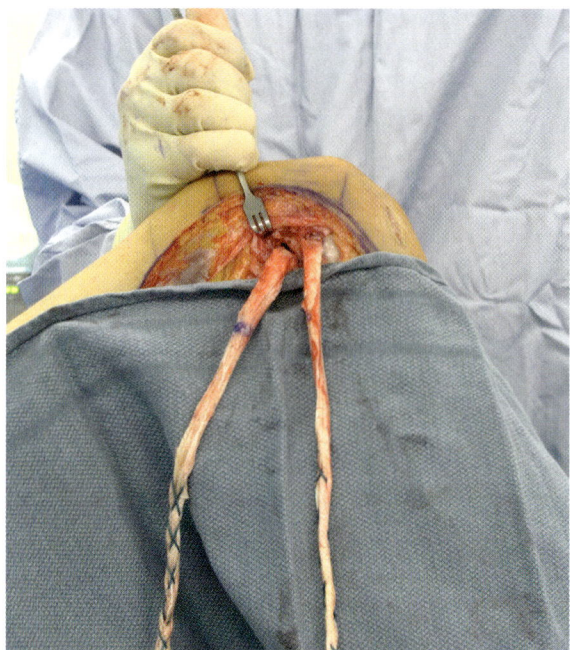

Figure 40-25. The grafts reconstructing the popliteus *(right)* and fibular collateral ligament *(left)* are shown after being placed within the femoral tunnel. These are held in place with interference screws.

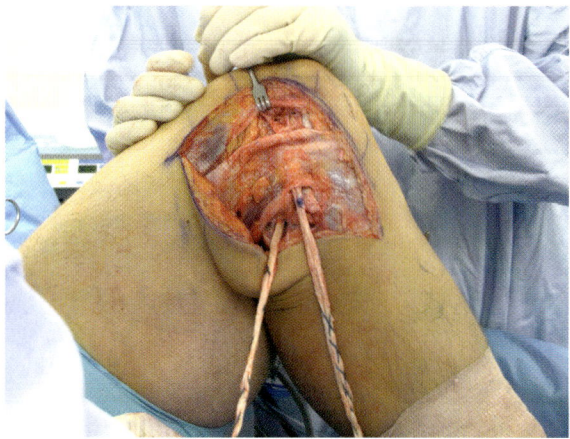

Figure 40-26. The grafts are routed into position. The fibular collateral ligament graft has been routed deep to the iliotibial band and is now seen on the *right*. The popliteus graft is routed deep to the fibular collateral ligament graft and is now on the *left*.

to the iliotibial band (Fig. 40-26) and through the tunnel in the fibular head. A 7-mm biointerference screw is placed with the knee in 20 degrees of flexion, with a valgus force across the knee to reconstruct the fibular collateral ligament. The tail of the just placed FCL graft is continued to the posterior aperture of the popliteus tunnel, re-creating the popliteofibular ligament (Fig. 40-27). Both the popliteofibular graft (the continued free tail of the FCL graft) and popliteus tendon graft are combined and routed through the tibial tunnel posteriorly to anteriorly and held in place with a 9-mm interference screw (Fig. 40-28). The knee is flexed to 60 degrees and an anterior force is placed across the tibia as the screw is advanced to complete the reconstruction (Fig. 40-29). An examination under anesthesia is then performed

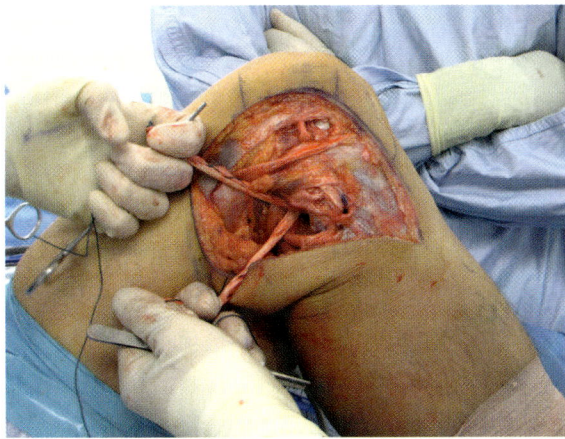

Figure 40-27. The fibular collateral ligament graft has been routed through the fibular tunnel. Valgus stress is applied to the knee, the graft tensioned, and an interference screw placed within the fibular head. The free tail is then continued to the posterior aspect of the tibia and combined with the popliteus graft, reconstructing the popliteofibular ligament.

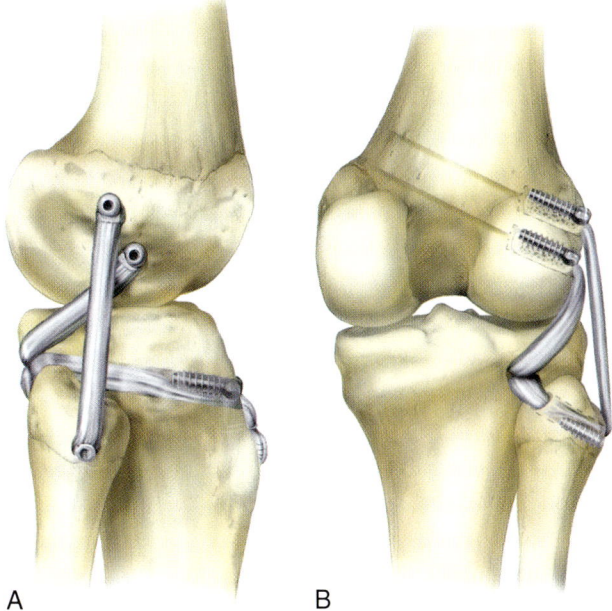

A   B

Figure 40-29. Drawings of the lateral **(A)** and posterior **(B)** knee demonstrating the fibular collateral ligament and posterior lateral corner reconstruction. (From LaPrade RF, Johansen S, Wentorf FA, et al:An analysis of an anatomical posterolateral knee reconstruction: An in vitro biomechanical study and development of a surgical technique. Am J Sports Med 32:1405–1414, 2004.)

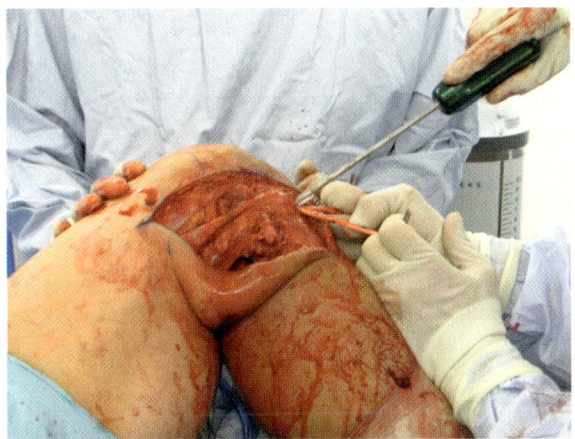

Figure 40-28. The grafts are combined and passed from posterior to anterior through the tunnel drilled in the proximal tibia. An interference screw is placed from anterior to posterior to fixate the grafts.

to verify graft stability. The remainder of the graft tails are cut and the wounds are closed in layers.

As part of any open management of posterolateral corner reconstruction, we recommend initial identification of the common peroneal nerve on the posterior border of the biceps femoris tendon. This allows for protection of the nerve during the surgical procedure and provides an opportunity for in situ neurolysis and decompression. We recommend particular attention to the peroneal nerve, distal to the biceps tendon, to ensure that it is decompressed as it crosses the fascial bands of the lateral compartment.

Postoperative Management

Postoperatively, a knee immobilizer is worn for 6 weeks following surgery. Weight bearing is limited for 6 weeks. Quadriceps sets and straight leg raises are initiated immediately postoperatively in the knee immobilizer only. At the 1- to 2-week mark, range of motion exercises are initiated. Closed-chain strengthening exercises are not initiated until

6 weeks. This focuses on quadriceps strength. Hamstring strengthening is limited so as not to stress the repair or reconstruction until at least 4 months postoperatively. Weight bearing is slowly progressed, starting at 6 weeks. An exercise bike is added when enough knee flexion is present to allow for rotation of the pedals. Sport-specific training is initiated at 4 months, with a return to sports or activity allowed when normal knee range of motion, and normal strength and stability comparable to the contralateral side, have been achieved (frequently at 6 to 9 months, although it may be 12 months). Finally, the athlete should have completed sport-specific therapy prior to returning to competitive athletics.

Results

Levy and associates[28] have completed a systematic literature review and found that operative management provides improved outcomes compared with nonoperative management. They also reported that surgical management completed early (within 3 weeks) improves outcomes as compared with procedures performed after 3 weeks, and that reconstruction provides better outcomes than repair of posterolateral corner injuries. No recommendations were given with regard to the type of reconstruction (anatomic vs. nonanatomic). Yoon and coworkers[35] have compared a sling technique with an anatomic reconstruction. They demonstrated improved Lysholm scores, less varus laxity, and less external rotation laxity in the anatomic reconstruction group. Concerns for the anatomic technique include its technically demanding nature and the concern regarding potential overconstraint of the knee.[29] High-quality studies with long-term follow-up are needed to gain a better understanding of the outcomes of posterolateral corner reconstruction.

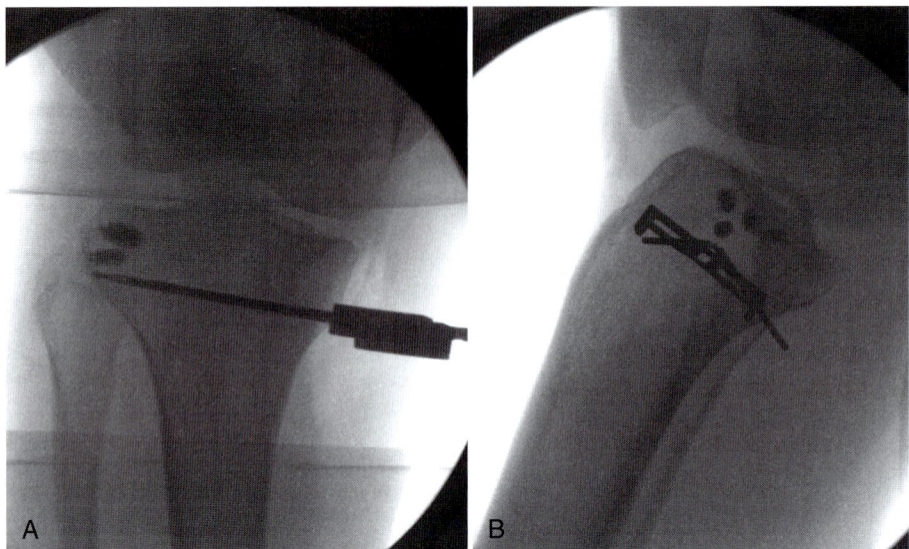

Figure 40-30. A, AP intraoperative image of the guide pins for a proximal medial opening wedge osteotomy. There are suture anchors in place in the lateral proximal tibia from a prior failed lateral ligament reconstruction. **B,** Lateral intraoperative radiograph of the knee showing guide pins in place for a proximal tibial opening wedge osteotomy. The final desired slope is approximated by the slope of the guide pins. Previously placed suture anchors are seen.

Chronic Posterolateral Corner Injuries

Posterolateral corner injuries of longer than 3 months' duration are classified as chronic injuries. These injuries present specific challenges that are not always present in the management of acute injuries. When evaluating a chronic PLC injury, standing long-leg AP alignment radiographs are mandatory to evaluate the patient's alignment. The reconstructed FCL, popliteus, and popliteofibular ligament will not tolerate any varus malalignment.[10,14,21,22] Varus malalignment is defined as being present when a line from the center of the femoral head to the center of the ankle joint (the mechanical axis) falls medial to the tip of the medial tibial spine on a long-leg alignment radiograph.[1] When varus malalignment occurs, a corrective osteotomy needs to be performed prior to reconstruction. We recommend a proximal tibial medial opening wedge osteotomy. As compared with a lateral tibial closing wedge osteotomy, the medial opening wedge osteotomy has the theoretical benefit of tightening the posterior capsule[20] and decreasing external rotation and varus motion.[34] Furthermore, an opening wedge osteotomy allows for the opportunity for a biplanar osteotomy in the setting of a cruciate-deficient knee or in a knee with recurvatum or a flexion contracture. In a knee with a deficient ACL, the tibial slope should be decreased; in a knee with a deficient PCL, the tibial slope should be increased. Genu recurvatum can be addressed by increasing the tibial slope and a flexion contracture at the knee can be addressed by decreasing the tibial slope.

Preferred Technique: Medial Tibial Opening Wedge Osteotomy for Chronic Posterolateral Corner Injury With Varus Malalignment

The patient is positioned supine on a radiolucent table with a tourniquet. A bump can be placed under the contralateral hip to improve exposure to the proximal medial tibia. A standard vertical incision is made midway between the tibial tubercle and posterior medial border of the tibia at the distal

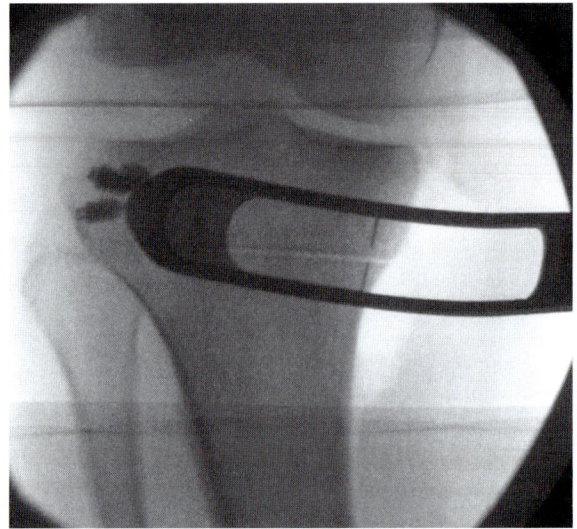

Figure 40-31. A radiolucent retractor is used to facilitate the osteotomy. An oscillating saw is used to perform the osteotomy. Note that the lateral cortex was not violated by the osteotomy.

aspect of the tibial tubercle. The dissection is carried straight to bone to avoid devascularization of the skin flaps. The distal aspect of the patellar tendon and superficial medial collateral ligaments are identified and protected. The dissection is continued posteriorly and a radiolucent retractor is placed to protect the neurovascular bundle. A retractor is placed deep to the patellar tendon. Two guide pins are placed parallel to the joint line (in the AP plane), just distal to the metaphyseal flare. In the lateral plane, the guide pins approximate the desired tibial slope (Fig. 40-30). An oscillating saw is used to osteotomize the medial cortex (Fig. 40-31). This is followed by osteotomes anteriorly and posteriorly. A hinge of bone (approximately 1 cm in width) is maintained along the

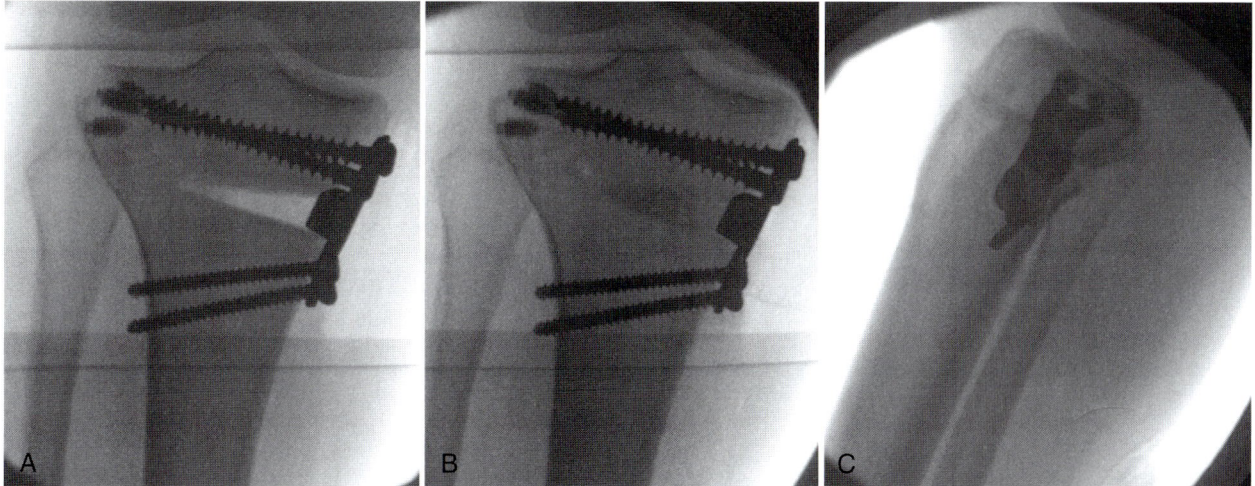

Figure 40-32. **A,** A plate is placed across the osteotomy site and screws are placed proximally and distally to the osteotomy. The lateral cortex remains intact. **B,** Bone graft or bone graft substitute is packed into the osteotomy site. **C,** Lateral intraoperative radiograph demonstrating the bone graft as well as the medial plate and screw construct.

proximal lateral tibia. A spreader is used to distract the medial cortex until the desired correction is obtained. A staple is placed laterally if propagation of the osteotomy occurs through the lateral cortex. A plate is placed along the medial cortex, with two screws above and below the osteotomy (Fig. 40-32). A wide variety of osteotomy plates are commercially available. Autologous or allograft bone is placed into the osteotomy site. The wound is closed in layers and a knee immobilizer is placed.

Postoperative Management

A patient with a proximal tibial osteotomy is continued in a knee immobilizer for 8 weeks. Quadriceps sets and straight leg raises are initiated immediately. Prone flexion and extension are initiated four times daily. Progressive weight bearing is initiated at 8 weeks, with a goal of full weight bearing at 3 months. Enteric-coated aspirin, 325 mg orally daily, or other anti-coagulant agent, as indicated, is initiated for deep venous thrombosis prophylaxis. Standing radiographs are obtained at 3 months and the alignment is reviewed. Complete healing is ensured prior to proceeding with PLC reconstruction (Fig. 40-33). We do not recommend this type of osteotomy for patients who use tobacco given the risk of soft tissue healing and delayed or nonunion. Gradual return to activities is then allowed. If instability persists, a staged reconstruction can be performed at the 6- to 9-month mark.

Results

Arthur and coworkers[1] have reviewed their results of valgus osteotomy for chronic PLC injuries. They found that 8 of 21 patients (38%) had sufficient improvement of knee function that subsequent posterolateral corner reconstruction was not necessary. High-velocity injuries and patients with concomitant cruciate injuries were more likely to proceed to a second-stage reconstruction compared with patients with low-velocity injuries and isolated PLC injuries.

Complications

Routine surgical complications such as infection and wound breakdown can be encountered. Preoperative evaluation of the skin and soft tissues should be performed to minimize this

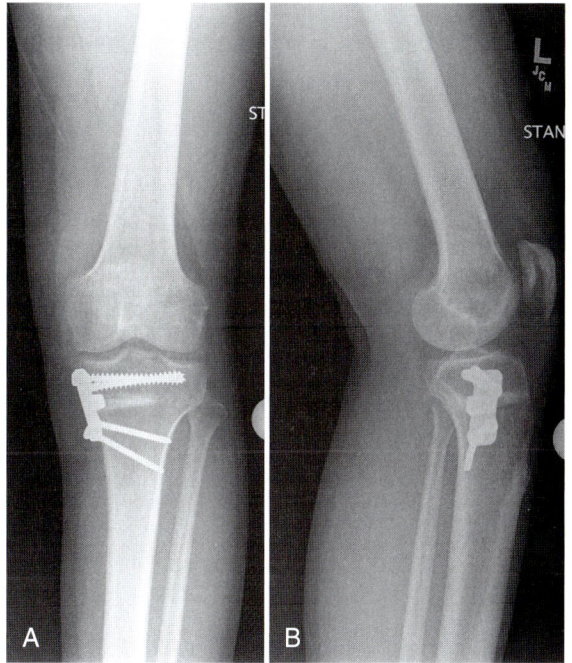

Figure 40-33. **A,** Final AP radiograph of a healed proximal tibial opening wedge osteotomy. **B,** Lateral radiograph of a healed proximal tibial opening wedge osteotomy.

risk. Up to 30% of patients with a PLC injury demonstrate a peroneal nerve injury[23,34] and there is also an iatrogenic risk of peroneal nerve injury at the time of surgery. Careful dissection is paramount to avoid injury to the peroneal nerve. Deep venous thrombosis is a risk following this procedure, and consideration for venous thromboembolism prophylaxis should be entertained. No data exist about the incidence of deep venous thrombosis following PLC reconstruction, although patients with a positive family history, smokers, or those on oral contraceptives warrant particular consideration of chemical prophylaxis. We routinely use enteric-coated aspirin, 325 mg orally daily, for 6 weeks. Graft failure or recurrent varus laxity is also reported. This complication is hopefully minimized by attention to graft choice, anatomic tunnel placement, and correction of existing malalignment and associated cruciate injury.

KEY REFERENCES

Cooper DE: Tests for posterolateral instability of the knee in normal subjects. Results of examination under anesthesia. J Bone Joint Surg Am 73:30–36, 1991.

Gollehon DL, Torsilli PA, Warren RF: The role of the posterolateral and cruciate ligament in the stability of the human knee. A biomechanical study. J Bone Joint Surg Am 69:233–242, 1987.

Grood ES, Stowers SF, Noyes FR: Limits of movements in the human knee. Effect of sectioning the posterior cruciate ligament and posterolateral structures. J Bone Joint Surg Am 70:88–97, 1988.

LaPrade RF: Arthroscopic evaluation of the lateral compartment of the knees with posterolateral complex grade 3 complex knee injuries. Am J Sports Med 25:596–602, 1997.

LaPrade RF: Posterolateral knee injuries: anatomy, evaluation, and treatment, New York, 2006, Thieme.

LaPrade RF, Gilbert TJ, Bollom TS, et al: The magnetic resonance imaging appearance of individual structures of the posterolateral knee: a prospective study of normal knees and knees with surgically verified grade III injuries. Am J Sports Med 28:191–199, 2000.

LaPrade RF, Terry GC: Injuries to the posterolateral aspect of the knee: association of anatomic injury patterns with clinical instability. Am J Sports Med 25:433–438, 1997.

LaPrade RF, Ly TV, Wentorf FA, et al. The posterolateral attachments of the knee. A qualitative and quantitative morphologic analysis of the fibular collateral ligament, popliteus tendon, popliteofibular ligament, and lateral gastrocnemius tendon. Am J Sports Med 31:854–860, 2003.

Veltri DM, Deng XH, Torzilli PA, et al: The role of the cruciate and posterolateral ligaments in stability of the knee. Am J Sports Med 23:436–443, 1995.

Full references for this chapter can be found on www.expertconsult.com.

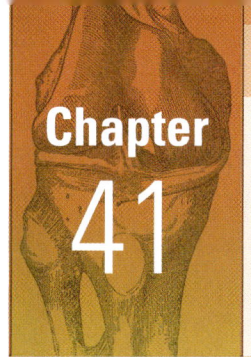

Chapter 41

Anterior Cruciate Ligament Injuries and Reconstruction: Indications, Principles, and Outcomes

William J. Long and W. Norman Scott

Injury to the anterior cruciate ligament (ACL) is the most common ligament injury in the knee and results in between 50,000 and 105,000 reconstructions/year in the United States.[51,82] Greater participation in sporting and recreational activities by the general population continues to expose more individuals to the risk of ACL rupture. As the experience of orthopedic surgeons with ACL injuries has expanded, so have the science and technique of ACL reconstruction. Numerous methods for reconstructing the ligament exist, including the use of patellar tendon autograft, hamstring tendons, and allograft material. The most extensive research has been performed on the use of patellar tendon autograft, and this technique remains the gold standard for ACL reconstruction.[66] Since the last edition of this text, there have been a significant number of meta-analyses and systematic reviews of the literature in this area in an attempt to combine studies and achieve greater success. We have revised this chapter to include these important additions to the literature.

HISTORY OF ANTERIOR CRUCIATE LIGAMENT RECONSTRUCTION

Use of the central third of the patellar tendon for reconstructing a torn ACL was first described by Jones[71] in an effort to provide a more physiologic procedure than those previously described. His technique involved transferring the patellar tendon with a patellar bone block to the intercondylar region of the femur while maintaining the distal attachment of the tendon to the tibial tubercle. Other authors subsequently modified Jones' technique by using the medial third of the patellar tendon.[5,47] Marshall and colleagues[84] have described using the central third of the patellar tendon along with the prepatellar fascia and central portion of the quadriceps tendon. These modifications of Jones' technique also involved creating a more anatomic placement of the reconstructed ligament by passing it through a tibial tunnel, from the anterior aspect of the tibia to the normal tibial ACL insertion site, and leaving the distal attachment of the patellar tendon in place on the tubercle. The femoral side of the graft was passed either through bone tunnels in the femur or over the top of the lateral femoral condyle and secured with sutures or staples. Clancy and associates,[39] in an effort to obtain bony union at the femoral fixation site, first described harvesting a block of patellar bone along with the proximal portion of the patellar tendon. They also described detaching the tibial origin of the graft along with a block of bone when the graft was found to be too short. The bone-patellar tendon-bone graft (BPTB) is now the gold standard in ACL reconstruction. Advantages of this type of autograft include its increased stiffness and energy to failure, as well as its ability to revascularize.[11] It has been shown that a 14- to 15-mm-wide BPTB graft has a mean strength that is approximately 168% that of a normal ACL.[98] Current graft widths are closer to 10 mm,

but continue to possess greater tensile strength than a native ACL.[140] In addition, the BPTB autograft has a superior ability to achieve stable initial fixation as a result of the bone plugs providing bone to bone healing.

PREDISPOSING FACTORS AND ASSOCIATED INJURIES

Several studies have attempted to identify factors predisposing to ACL injury and have found an association between such injury and intercondylar notch stenosis.[79,133] Souryal and Freeman[132] prospectively examined 902 high school athletes and noted that athletes who sustained ACL tears had statistically significant stenosis of the intercondylar notch when compared with those who did not have such injuries. Harner and coworkers[63] compared 31 patients with noncontact, bilateral ACL injuries with 23 controls who had no history of knee injury. Computed tomography (CT) analysis of the lower extremities revealed that the width of the lateral femoral condyle was significantly larger in the injured knee group and was the predominant contributor to intercondylar notch stenosis. A study comparing notch width measurements in men and women with and without ACL tears revealed a narrower intercondylar notch width in women than in men, as well as a narrower width in patients with ACL tears than in controls.[120] These results may enable identification of individuals at increased risk for unilateral and, in particular, bilateral ACL tears, which have an overall incidence of approximately 4%. In addition, this may be one factor responsible in part for the increased incidence of ACL tears in female athletes.

Much attention has been focused on the cause of ACL tears in women. Studies investigating injury rates noted that women sustain four to eight times the number of ACL injuries as men in the same sports.[10,24] Possible reasons for this discrepancy include extrinsic factors, such as muscle strength, and intrinsic factors, such as joint laxity, notch dimensions, and lower stiffness to applied load.[116] Little objective evidence is currently available, however, to support a single hypothesis. The association between female athletes' menstrual cycle and ACL injuries has been examined.[20,103] More injuries than expected were noted during the preovulatory and ovulatory[142] phases of the cycle, when a surge in estrogen production occurs. This finding suggests that noncontact ACL tears in female athletes may be related in part to hormonal fluctuations. The hormones responsible for this observed association and the effect of the mechanism of action on the mechanical properties of the ACL have yet to be determined. A recent meta-analysis has concluded that neuromuscular training and strengthening can reduce the risk of ACL injury in female athletes, particularly those less than 18 years of age.[144]

Associated injuries at the time of ACL tear affect surgical management and outcomes. Jumping versus nonjumping ACL injuries were reviewed in 263 patients. Those associated with a jumping mechanism were associated with a significantly higher rate of meniscal tears.[8,107] Postulating that anthropomorphic characteristics were associated with intra-articular injury at the time of ACL tear, Bowers and colleagues[26] reviewed their ACL database, for height, weight, and body mass index (BMI). Increases in all three variables were associated with higher rates of associated specific intra-articular pathologies at the time of ACL reconstruction. It was thus hypothesized that by reducing weight and BMI, patients could reduce associated injuries and improve outcomes following ACL reconstruction.

INDICATIONS FOR RECONSTRUCTION

Identification of patients with an ACL injury can usually be made on the basis of the history and physical examination. Patients commonly describe a history of a deceleration injury, with or without contact, during such maneuvers as cutting and pivoting. Patients with this injury mechanism associated with an audible pop, severe pain, and significant swelling of the knee can be assumed to have a torn ACL. Physical examination confirms the diagnosis by demonstrating a positive pivot shift, Lachman,[138] or anterior drawer test in the injured knee as opposed to a contralateral normal knee (Fig. 41-1).

After the acute phase of knee pain and swelling subsides, symptomatic patients complain of persistent instability and giving way of the knee, which can be associated with intermittent episodes of swelling. Once a torn ACL is diagnosed, one must decide whether to recommend nonoperative or operative treatment. Satisfactory results from conservative treatment of ACL tears have been reported.[52] McDaniel and Dameron[89] have noted that 70% of patients with complete ACL tears treated conservatively return to strenuous sports. Similarly, Giove and associates[55] reported a 59% rate of return to sports activities after a program emphasizing hamstring strengthening. However, sports requiring sudden stopping and pivoting had the lowest rate of return to participation. Buss and coworkers[32] evaluated the results of conservative treatment of acute, complete ACL injuries in older, lower demand patients. They noted that 70% of patients were able to continue with moderate-demand sports at an average follow-up of 46 months. They concluded that conservative treatment in this group of patients can be successful, despite a modest amount of residual instability.

Numerous other studies, however, have reported less successful outcomes of non-operative treatment.[8,49,98,99,129] Noyes and colleagues[100] have studied 103 athletically active patients an average of 5.5 years after ACL injury. Despite an initial return to sports activity by 82% of the participants,

Fifty-five percent sustained a significant reinjury within 1 year of the original injury and only 35% were participating in strenuous sports at the most recent follow-up. Hawkins and associates[65] reported on 40 patients treated nonoperatively with an average follow-up of 4 years and noted 87.5% fair or poor results; only 14% of patients were able to return fully to unlimited athletic activity. Similarly, Barrack and coworkers[17] reported 69% fair or poor results after nonoperative treatment in an active naval midshipmen population. Daniel and colleagues[43] have determined that the best predictor for later meniscal or ligament reconstruction surgery is total hours per year of levels I and II sports participation before injury. This observation highlights the fact that individuals who engage in demanding recreational or vocational activities do not respond well to nonoperative treatment of ACL injuries.

The decision to reconstruct an ACL tear should be based not only on the presence of symptomatic instability, but also on the lifestyle and activity level of the patient. In a prospective nonrandomized trial of an ACL reconstruction algorithm by Fithian and associates,[50] patients were categorized as low, medium, or high activity level and had reconstructions if they fell into the medium or high level group. At an average 6.6-year follow-up, early reconstruction was associated with a reduced rate of knee laxity, symptomatic instability, late meniscal tears, and further surgery.

We do not use guidelines based on age in our practice because the more important factor is the overall level of activity. It is generally agreed that younger individuals have higher levels of activity and, therefore, place greater demands on their knees. However, many older individuals are participating in higher levels of recreational sports and are doing so for longer periods. Consequently, age itself should not be a

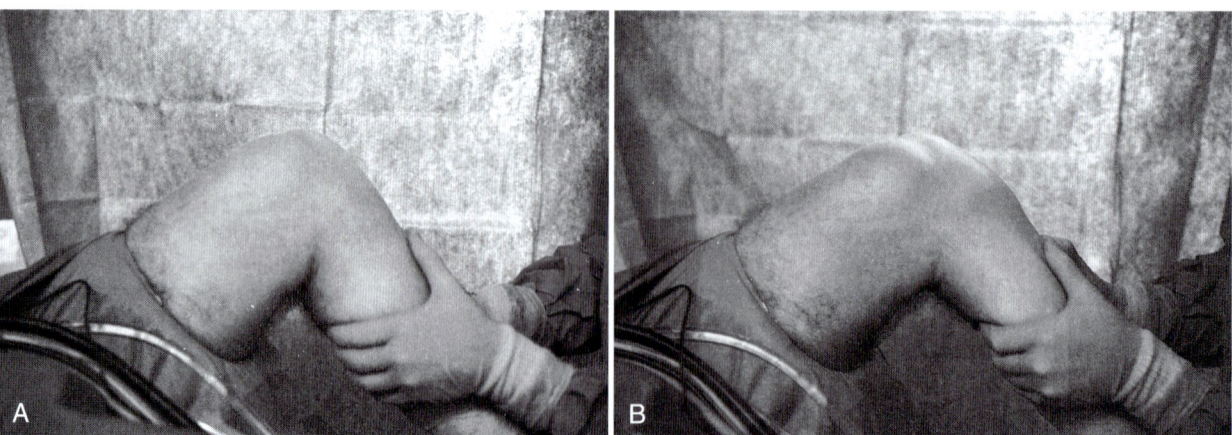

Figure 41-1. Demonstration of the anterior drawer sign. **A,** Knee in neutral position. **B,** Increased anterior translation of the knee secondary to anterior cruciate ligament rupture.

contraindication to ACL reconstruction. Plancher and coworkers[109] have reported 97% good or excellent results after ACL reconstruction in patients older than 40 years at a mean follow-up of 55 months. All patients were satisfied with the procedure, and most were able to return fully to their sports activities, including tennis and skiing.

Symptomatic patients with a more sedentary lifestyle and those who are willing to modify their level of activity can be considered for nonoperative treatment, consisting of a supervised rehabilitation program. One option is initially to treat all patients with an ACL rupture nonoperatively and perform reconstruction on those for whom this form of treatment fails. This approach can involve several months of rehabilitation, followed by several more months if reconstruction is ultimately performed. In our experience, we have found that most patients are unwilling to accept this amount of time away from their recreational activities; therefore, we recommend early reconstruction for symptomatic patients with greater lifestyle demands. The goal of early reconstruction in this patient population is to provide stability, which allows a return to previous activity levels without further damage to the knee, such as meniscal tears and arthrosis. The significant reinjury rates in nonreconstructed knees[50,99] emphasizes the potential sequelae of continued high levels of activity in patients with ACL injury.

In a review of 3475 patients in the Norwegian National Knee Ligament Registry undergoing ACL reconstruction between 2004 and 2006,[59] timing of reconstruction was examined for its relationship to meniscal tears and cartilage lesions. The odds of cartilage lesion increased by almost 1% for each month elapsed between injury and reconstruction.

TIMING OF SURGERY

The timing of ACL reconstruction has been debated; however, no consensus has yet been reached regarding the ideal timing. Initial concern existed over reconstruction of the ACL during the early postinjury period because of the increased risk for arthrofibrosis and difficulty gaining full motion of the knee postoperatively. Shelbourne and colleagues[128] have demonstrated a higher rate of arthrofibrosis in patients undergoing ACL reconstruction within the first week after injury than in those who underwent reconstruction 21 days or longer after injury. The same authors noted, however, that when an accelerated rehabilitation protocol was followed postoperatively, the rates of arthrofibrosis in the two groups were comparable. Noyes and Barber-Westin[97] reported that 69% of knees with chronic rupture scored in the normal or very good range after reconstruction as compared with 100% of knees with an acute rupture. Other studies have also found earlier return to sporting activities as well as better clinical and laxity testing results in knees undergoing early reconstruction.[83] Hunter and associates[69] have shown that the use of modern arthroscopic surgical techniques and an aggressive rehabilitation protocol can yield results that are independent of the timing of surgery. We agree that the specific number of days after injury when the reconstruction should be performed is not as important as the preoperative condition of the knee. Criteria for successful results of ACL reconstruction are minimal or no swelling, good leg control, and full range of motion, including full hyperextension.[125]

SURGICAL TECHNIQUE

Arthroscopic reconstruction of a torn ACL with a BPTB autograft is our procedure of choice and is the technique described here. Steps of the reconstructive procedure include diagnostic arthroscopy, harvesting the graft, preparing the graft, performing the notchplasty, drilling of the tibial and femoral tunnels, passing the graft, and femoral and tibial fixation of the graft. Before beginning the reconstructive procedure, however, the knee is examined under anesthesia. A positive Lachman test and pivot shift sign are sought on the injured knee as clinical evidence of a torn ACL. These maneuvers are repeated on the uninjured contralateral knee for comparison and to determine the degree of normal laxity in the knee for the individual patient. A positive pivot shift under anesthesia is the most sensitive clinical test of the functional status of the ACL because it demonstrates a loss of rotational stability imparted by an intact ligament.[15,81] The injured extremity is then prepared and draped in the usual sterile fashion after the application of a thigh tourniquet well above the operative site.

Diagnostic Arthroscopy

After inflation of the thigh tourniquet, the arthroscope is inserted into the knee through a standard lateral portal, and the ACL is visualized to confirm the injury. The ACL is most commonly torn from its proximal attachment on the femur, which results in a stump of tissue that is usually easily visualized through the arthroscope. At times, however, the appearance of the ACL can be deceiving. A torn ACL can become scarred to the surface of the posterior cruciate ligament (PCL) and give the erroneous impression of an intact ligament. Visualization of the ACL with the leg in the figure-of-four position enables adequate assessment of its proximal attachment site in these cases. This view clearly demonstrates absence of the ACL attachment to the femur in ACL-deficient knees. In cases in which poor visualization is obtained, a large persistent vertical septum is present, or synovitis obscures the ligament, we do not hesitate to make a second medial working port, insert the full-radius resector, and remove this tissue.

Meniscal resection or repair can also be performed at the diagnostic examination or can be addressed during preparation of the graft. A second medial working portal is established if the menisci are addressed at this stage. Otherwise, the arthroscope is removed and attention turned to the graft.

Graft Harvesting

The patellar and tibial tubercle landmarks are drawn on the skin and a vertical incision is made from the inferior pole of the patella to 1 cm medial to the tibial tubercle. Skin flaps are developed to identify the full width of the tendon and the paratenon is incised in line with the skin incision and reflected. A 9- or 10-mm catamaran blade is used to make the incision in the tendon from the patella to the tibial tubercle, with care taken to remain parallel to the tendon fibers. In general, no more than one third of the patellar tendon is used. The incision is carried proximally over the patella for a distance of 25 mm from the tendon insertion, as well as distally over the tibial tubercle, also 25 mm from the attachment site of the tendon. A small oscillating saw is used to cut bone plugs to a depth of approximately 8 mm. We apply a Steri-Strip at a 10-mm depth along the blade as a simple reference when performing these cuts. The bone plugs are then carefully removed with a curved osteotome.

We have examined the effect of graft diameter on postoperative knee stability by testing ACL-reconstructed knees with the KT arthrometer after the use of a 9- or 10-mm-diameter graft.[56] The average time from surgery to KT arthrometer testing was 6.6 months, and at the time of testing the average side to side difference for the 9-mm group was 1.02 mm. The average side to side difference for the group receiving 10-mm grafts was 1.14 mm. No significant differences between the two groups could be identified with regard to knee stability.

Graft Preparation

Excess soft tissue is first removed from the graft, and the diameter of the bone plugs is trimmed with a rongeur to the appropriate width (9 or 10 mm). The plug from the tibial tubercle is prepared for placement in the femoral tunnel, where its anatomy and less curved geometry provide maximum bone fill. The edges of the plugs are rounded to permit smooth passage of the graft and the diameters are checked by passing the graft through a tunnel template of the correct size. Three drill holes are then made in the patellar bone plug and one in the tibial tubercle bone plug, followed by passage of no. 5 nonabsorbable suture through these holes (Fig. 41-2). The suture facilitates passage and tensioning of the graft. Finally, the total length of the graft is measured. In general, if the total length is between 92 and 97 mm, fixation with interference screws can be achieved. Fixation with a screw and washer on the tibial side is usually required for grafts measuring outside this range.

Notchplasty

A second arthroscopic portal is made medial to the patellar tendon, if not done previously, as well as a superomedial inflow portal to improve visualization. The remnants of the ACL are then removed with an intra-articular punch and full-radius resector. The lateral wall of the intercondylar notch is cleared of soft tissue attachments while taking care not to injure the adjacent PCL. The motorized bur is then inserted into the medial portal and the notchplasty is begun. The amount of bone to be removed remains controversial and ultimately depends on intra-operative assessment by the surgeon.

Several studies have attempted to establish guidelines for assessing the adequacy of the notchplasty.[57,137] Odensten and Gillquist[102] have noted an average maximum distance of 21 mm between the inner surfaces of the medial and lateral femoral condyles in 20 normal cadaver knees. As a result, they suggested that the notchplasty should restore the notch width to this diameter. Berg[18] has defined an adequate notchplasty on the basis of the notch width index[133] and stated that this index, which is the ratio of the intercondylar width to the total femoral condylar width at the level of the popliteal groove, should be at least 0.250 to prevent impingement of the graft. Howell and associates[68] have described the relationship between the placement of the tibial tunnel and the required size of the notchplasty. A more anteriorly placed tibial tunnel requires up to 6 mm of bone removal from the intercondylar roof as compared with only minimal removal of bone for tunnels placed 2 to 3 mm posterior to the ACL tibial insertion site. Berns and Howell[19] have further defined the requirements for notchplasty by determining the flexion angle at which the graft contacts the roof through the use of a force transducer in cadaver knees. The angle at which contact occurs averages 12.8 degrees for knees with an eccentrically placed tibial tunnel and requires 4.6 mm of bone removal to achieve zero impingement. This angle of contact decreases to 4.1 degrees when the tibial tunnel is placed 4 to 5 mm posterior to the slope of the intercondylar roof and requires only 1.3 mm of bone removal to prevent impingement. We prefer a generous notchplasty, in which up to 6 mm of bone is removed from the anterior edge of the lateral wall of the notch to prevent any possible impingement on the graft (Fig. 41-3).

The effect of the extent of the notchplasty on the patellofemoral articulation has been investigated. Morgan and coworkers[93] have measured patellofemoral contact area and pressure after increasing degrees of notchplasty (3, 6, and 9 mm) and found no statistical differences among the groups. They concluded that routine notchplasty, including up to

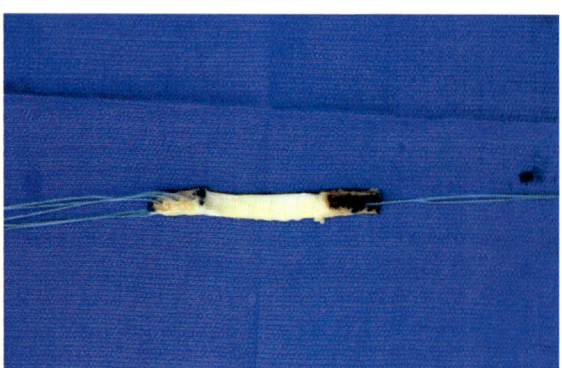

Figure 41-2. Completed preparation of a bone-patellar tendon-bone graft. Methylene blue ink is placed on the cancellous surfaces of the plugs to facilitate their orientation during graft passage.

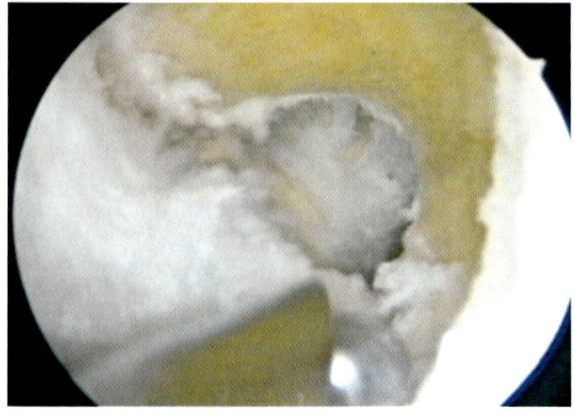

Figure 41-3. Arthroscopic view of a completed femoral notchplasty. The posterior edge of the notch roof must be visualized for correct femoral tunnel position.

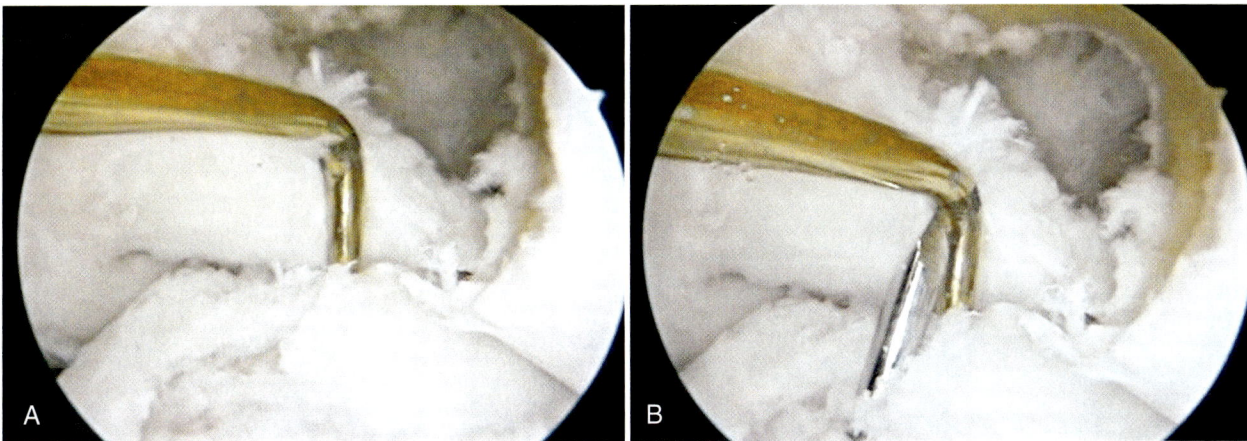

Figure 41-4. Optimal position of the tibial guide. **A,** Proper positioning of the tibial pin guide adjacent to the posterior cruciate ligament. **B,** The tip of the guide pin should be at the level of the posterior edge of the anterior horn of the lateral meniscus such that the graft will drape over the posterior cruciate ligament.

9 mm, does not affect the patellofemoral articulation. Patellofemoral complications related to the size of the notchplasty have similarly not been a problem in our experience.

The notchplasty is continued posteriorly to the posterior edge of the lateral wall. It is important to identify and remove the resident's ridge to prevent inadvertent anterior placement of the femoral tunnel. This ridge is located at the level of the anterior border of the PCL. Therefore, care must be taken to extend the notchplasty posterior to this border. A hooked probe is useful in ensuring that the over the top position and posterior edge of the lateral wall have been reached. The surface of the lateral wall should be smooth, with no rough edges, which could impinge on and abrade the graft.

Tunnel Placement

The choice of location for the tibial and femoral tunnels can have a significant effect on the outcome of ACL reconstructive surgery. Several studies have examined the effect of tunnel site on graft impingement,[67,143] range of motion,[111] and overall clinical results.[73] It is recognized that anterior placement of the femoral tunnel is to be avoided to prevent excessive tightness of the graft and thus limit full knee flexion. Similarly, excessive anterior placement of the tibial tunnel may result in graft impingement and early failure. In an attempt to identify definitive landmarks for reproducible tibial tunnel placement, Morgan and colleagues[93] have determined that the ACL central insertion point on the intercondylar floor averages 7 mm anterior to the anterior border of the PCL with the knee flexed to 90 degrees; therefore, this is the ideal location for the tibial tunnel.

We routinely set the tibial drill guide at 55 degrees. The guide tip is placed through the medial portal and positioned with the use of several landmarks, including the anterior border of the PCL, posterior border of the anterior horn of the lateral meniscus, and interspinous area of the tibial plateau. The tunnel is positioned to enable the graft to drape the PCL (Fig. 41-4). The starting point for the guide pin on the proximal end of the tibia is approximately one fingerbreadth medial to the tibial tubercle and two fingerbreadths distal to the medial joint line. After insertion of the guide pin, the tunnel is drilled with a reamer, and the intra-articular

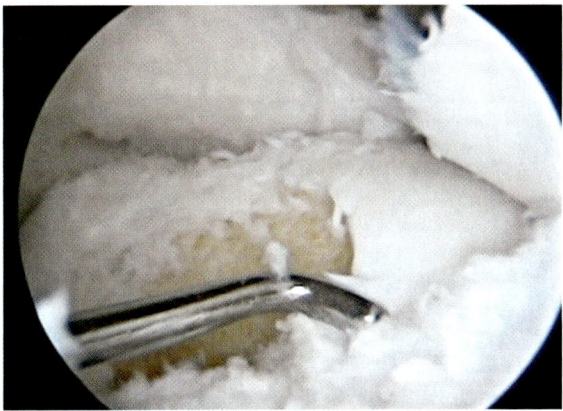

Figure 41-5. Arthroscopic view of the intra-articular rim of the tibial tunnel showing the relationship to the posterior edge of the anterior horn of the lateral meniscus (located at the tip of the probe).

edges of the tunnel are smoothed with a rasp to prevent abrasion of the graft (Fig. 41-5). Attempts have been made to produce the correct tibial tunnel length consistently to prevent graft extrusion with tunnels that are too short, as well as prevent difficult distal fixation and femoral tunnel placement with tunnels that are too long.[92] We have found, however, that this is not always accurate and may be altered by small variations in operative technique.[105]

Attention is then turned to the femoral tunnel. We use a transtibial technique for placement of this tunnel. The guide pin, which represents the center of the tunnel, is placed in the 1:30- to 2-o'clock position for the left knee or the 10- to 10:30-o'clock position for the right knee and 6 or 7 mm anterior to the over the top position, depending on whether a 9- or 10-mm graft, respectively, is used (Fig. 41-6). It is inserted to a depth of 35 mm, or 1.5 inches, to ensure that there is room for the tunnel without violating the posterior cortex (Fig. 41-7). An indentation, or footprint in the bone is then made with the reamer by hand over the guide pin to confirm the correct position in relation to the posterior cortex. This also ensures that the posterior cortex is intact (Fig. 41-8). The tunnel is then reamed to 30 mm with the

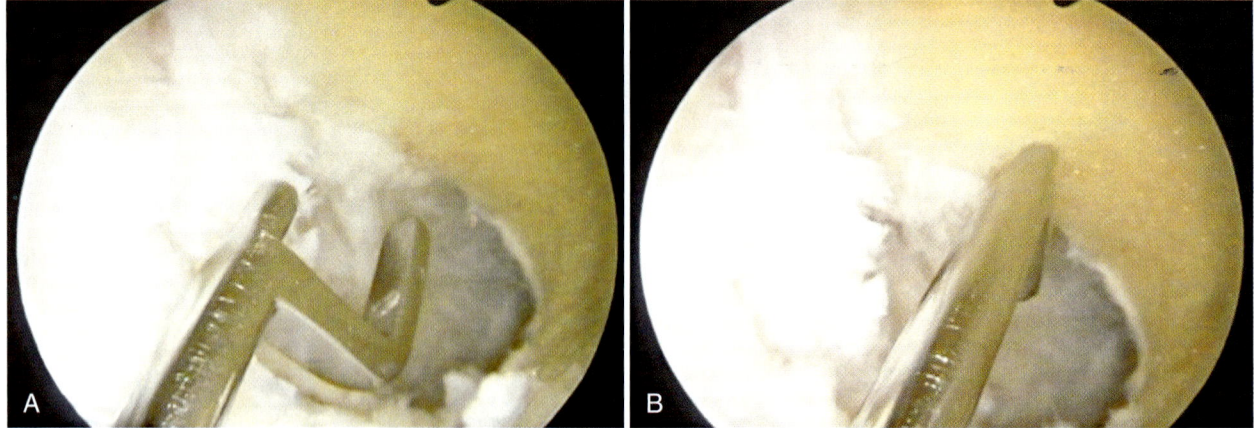

Figure 41-6. **A,** Femoral guide with a 6-mm offset. **B,** Positioning of the femoral guide in the 11-o'clock position for a right knee. The guide is placed in the 1-o'clock position for a left knee. Note that the posterior tip of the guide is in the over-the-top position on the femur.

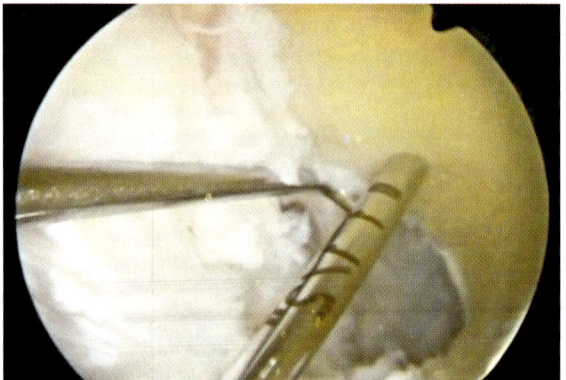

Figure 41-7. Femoral pin inserted to a depth of 1.5 inches.

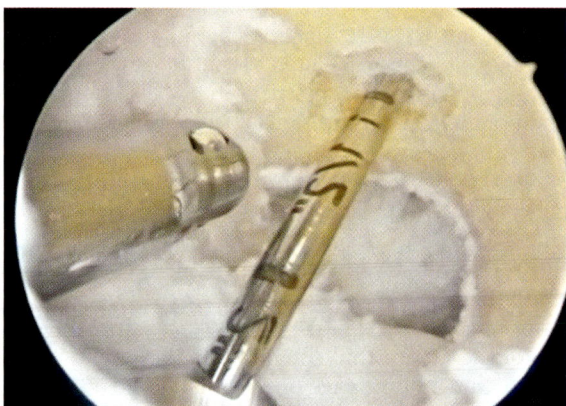

Figure 41-8. Initial reaming over the guide pin to create a femoral footprint. This allows visual inspection of the posterior rim to verify adequate wall thickness before completion of the reaming.

knee in a flexed position. The reamer is removed, and the arthroscope is placed in the medial port, to assess the integrity of the posterior cortex by visualizing the tunnel directly before passage of the graft (Fig. 41-9).

Testing for isometry can be performed at this point or just before committing to the femoral tunnel. Isometer readings are obtained to determine the position of the graft that will result in equal length and tension throughout a full range of motion. However, it has been shown that these readings may vary widely from the final graft isometry because of eccentric placement of the graft within the bone tunnels.[40] Additionally, because the normal ACL is nonisometric, intra-articular testing for isometry is not required if anatomic zones are maintained.[141]

GRAFT PASSAGE

A Beath pin is drilled through the femoral tunnel while maintaining the hip and knee in a hyperflexed position. This position allows the tip of the needle to be pushed through the soft tissues and exit the skin on the anterolateral aspect of the distal part of the thigh. The Beath pin is used to pull the suture in the femoral bone plug through the femoral tunnel. The graft is passed through the tunnels by grasping the sutures on either end of the bone plugs and pulling the graft into the joint. The graft is inserted so that the

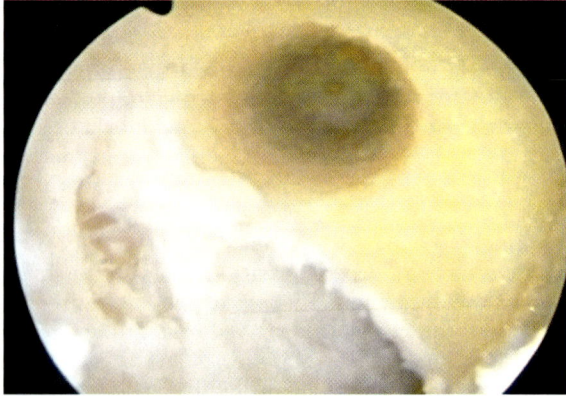

Figure 41-9. Arthroscopic view of a reamed femoral tunnel to confirm the integrity of the posterior wall. The distance between the posterior rim of the tunnel and the posterior edge of the notch roof should be approximately 2 mm.

cancellous bone of the femoral plug is facing anterolaterally in the femoral tunnel (Fig. 41-10). This allows interference screw placement against the cancellous surface of the graft, because insertion of a fixation screw on the cortical surface of the plug may lead to disruption of the ligamentous

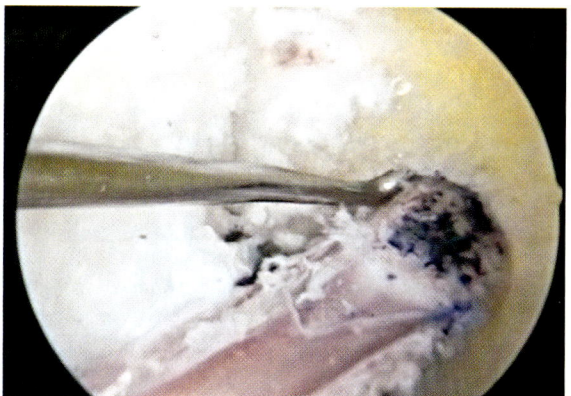

Figure 41-10. Passage of the femoral bone plug into the femoral tunnel, with the cancellous surface oriented superolaterally in the tunnel.

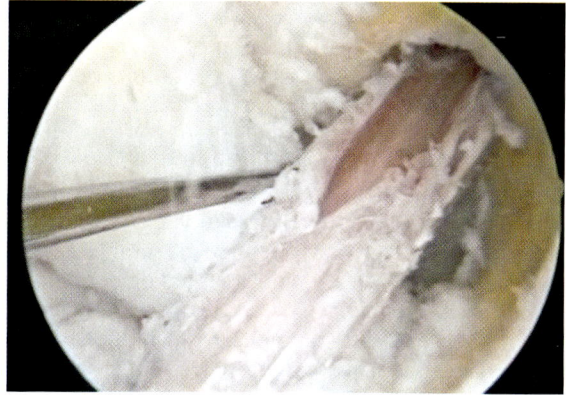

Figure 41-11. Appearance of the graft under manual tension before fixation.

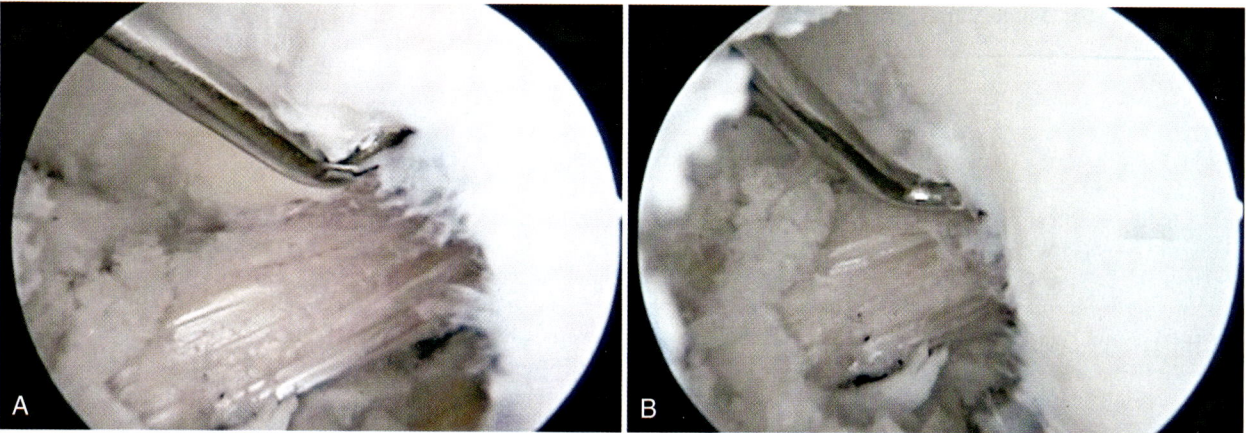

Figure 41-12. An arthroscopic probe is used to assess graft clearance from the roof of the notch with the knee in 30 degrees of flexion (**A**) and in the fully extended position (**B**). No impingement should occur in either position.

attachment. Tension is applied to the graft through manual pull on the bone plug sutures and the orientation of the graft is assessed (Fig. 41-11). The arthroscope is used to visualize the intra-articular side of the tibial tunnel to verify that the tibial bone plug does not enter into the joint. Assessment of graft clearance from the notch roof is performed both at 15 degrees of flexion and in full knee extension (Fig. 41-12).

Graft Fixation

Kurosaka and associates[77] introduced the self-tapping interference screw, which demonstrated improved mechanical properties when compared with buttons or staples. Regardless of technique, failure occurred at the fixation site. Interference screw fixation demonstrated an increase in ultimate failure load. Paschal and coworkers[106] have compared fixation strengths between 9-mm interference screws and sutures tied over a cancellous screw and washer (post fixation) in porcine knees. Higher ultimate failure loads and less displacement of the bone graft were noted with interference screw fixation. Matthews and colleagues[87] found no difference in the force to failure of patellar tendon-bone grafts in cadaveric knees when comparing interference screw fixation with post fixation. They did note, however, that post fixation strength is dependent on the type of suture used; no. 5 nonabsorbable

suture material provided optimal strength. Despite the conflicting biomechanical results, no studies to date have demonstrated any differences in clinical outcome when comparing interference screw fixation with post fixation.

Absorbable interference screws have been introduced, and several studies have examined the biomechanical properties and clinical results of these screws versus standard metal interference screws.[70] Pena and associates[108] investigated the insertional torque and failure load for metallic and absorbable interference screws in young and middle-aged cadaveric knees. They noted a higher mean insertional torque for the metal screws as well as a greater mean failure load. Other laboratory studies, however, did not demonstrate any differences between the two types of screws.[35,70] Caborn and coworkers[36] have compared the maximum load to failure of titanium alloy interference screws with that of absorbable screws in a human cadaveric model with the approximate physiologic strain rate of in vivo BPTB graft loading. No statistical differences were noted between the two groups in the failure mode or the maximum load to failure. Similarly, clinical studies did not demonstrate significant differences in use of the screw types.[85] Barber and colleagues[16] performed a randomized, prospective, multicenter comparison of bioabsorbable and metallic interference screws in 110 patients undergoing arthroscopic ACL reconstruction with patellar tendon autografts. At a minimum 12-month follow-up, postoperative Tegner and Lysholm scores and KT arthrometer maximum side to side differences were not statistically different between the two groups. It was concluded that the absorbable screw is a reasonable alternative to the metal interference screw for bone plug fixation.

Potential problems with the use of interference screws include length mismatch in the tunnel, graft, and screw, divergence of the screw, graft fracture, and suture laceration.[12] Screw divergence has been implicated in failure of graft fixation[87]; however, others have observed that screw divergence less than 30 degrees does not appear to lead to early failure provided that intraoperative stability is noted.[46] Similarly, we examined the effect of divergence between the femoral interference screw and femoral bone plug.[117] Radiographs and KT-2000 values from 100 consecutive endoscopic autologous BPTB ACL reconstructions were reviewed at a minimum follow-up of 1 year. The mean anteroposterior divergence angle was 6.6 degrees (range, 0 to 32 degrees), and no association was found between the divergence angle and KT-2000 measurements.

The guide pin for the femoral interference screw should be inserted between the edge of the femoral tunnel and the cancellous surface of the bone plug in a direction parallel to the orientation of the graft. The interference screw is passed over the guide pin and advanced into the femoral tunnel. The screw should engage at least 75%, if not 100%, of the bone block (Fig. 41-13). A 7-mm interference screw is recommended if the bone plug-tunnel gap is 2 mm or less. A gap greater than 2 mm requires the use of a 9-mm screw.

Several studies have examined the effect of twisting the graft 90 to 180 degrees before fixation of the tibial plug in an attempt to reproduce the normal helicoid orientation of the ACL fibers. In vitro studies noted enhanced isometry of the graft fibers,[45] improved graft strength,[41] and restoration of normal tibial rotation in relation to the femur[114] as a result of graft twisting. The clinical significance of these findings, however, remains unclear. Diduch and associates[44] have performed a prospective randomized study examining the clinical and arthrometric results of patients undergoing ACL reconstruction with and without pretwisting of the graft. They reported no clinical failures in either group and no statistically significant differences clinically or by arthrometry between the two groups. The study concluded that pretwisting of the graft has no short-term effect on knee laxity.

The precise amount of initial tension applied to the graft before fixation has not been determined. This will have a direct effect on the stability of the knee because inadequate tension will lead to persistent instability, whereas excessive tensioning may lead to elongation of the graft or early fixation failure. Previous studies investigating graft tension concluded that excessive tightness may result in abrasion on the edges of the bone tunnels or the intercondylar roof; in addition, revascularization of these overly tight grafts may be impaired.[29,145]

Burks and Leland[30] have noted that the tension applied to an ACL graft to obtain normal anteroposterior translation is dependent on the graft tissue; less stiff grafts require more tension. They determined that 3.6 lb of tension applied to the knee at 20 to 25 degrees of flexion is required for patellar tendon grafts.

In addition to the amount of tension, the position of the knee during application of the tension has also been investigated. Bylski-Austrow and coworkers[34] reconstructed cadaveric knees with a flexible cable and examined the effect of varying degrees of tension and knee position during tensioning. They noted that knees tensioned in 30 degrees of flexion are overconstrained and that this is independent of the initial tension used. Similarly, Melby and colleagues[90] also reported overconstraint of reconstructed cadaveric knees when tensioned at 30 degrees of flexion. In addition, greater quadriceps force was necessary to achieve full extension as the graft tension increased, particularly when tensioned in 30 degrees of flexion. Nabors and associates[95] evaluated 57 patients after ACL reconstruction with a patellar tendon autograft in which the graft was tensioned by a maximal sustained one-handed pull on the tibial end, with the knee in full passive extension. At a minimum 2-year follow-up, the Lysholm score improved from 65 preoperatively to 90 postoperatively, the mean side to side difference on instrumented laxity testing was reduced from 7.6 to 0.8 mm, and only one patient had a postoperative contracture. It was concluded that tensioning of the graft in full extension ensures that the knee will come to full extension without compromising the stability of the knee. We use a similar technique of graft tensioning, in which a manual pull is exerted on the sutures in the tibial end of the graft so that there is no laxity in the suture strands. Fixation of the graft is then performed with the knee in full extension.

Fixation of the tibial plug is dependent on the length of the plug with respect to the extra-articular edge of the tibial tunnel. Interference screw fixation is used when the end of the plug is within 5 mm of the extra-articular edge of the tibial tunnel. The bone plug can be visualized in the tibial tunnel with the arthroscope to ensure that the interference screw is placed on the cancellous side of the bone plug. If the tibial plug is positioned more than 5 mm from the extra-articular tunnel edge (long or short), fixation is achieved by tying the sutures over a tibial post. We use a burr to create a trough in the anterior tibia distal to the tunnel. This allows the graft to sit flush against the tibia. The post screw is then placed at least 1 cm distal to the trough and a 6.5-mm partially threaded screw with a washer is placed in a unicortical fashion, for the post.

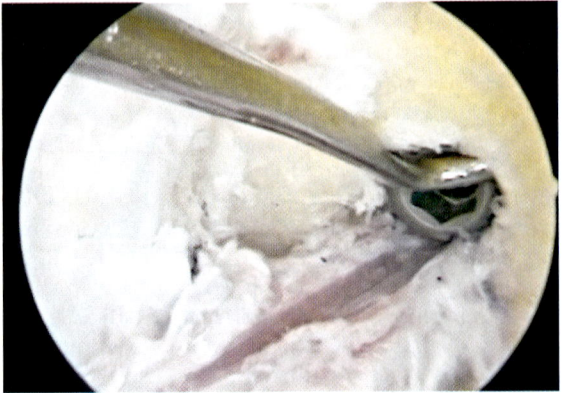

Figure 41-13. Fixation of the femoral bone plug with an interference screw. The screw should be fully seated with no protrusion from the rim of the tunnel into the joint.

The functional adequacy of the graft is then tested by performing a manual Lachman test, directly visualizing the graft with the arthroscope, and probing the graft to verify proper tension throughout a range of motion. A bone graft is placed in the patella defect, followed by closure of the paratenon and skin in successive layers.

POSTOPERATIVE MANAGEMENT

Radiographs can be obtained in the recovery room to assess placement of the bone tunnels, if not done intraoperatively (Fig. 41-14). At the completion of the procedure, a femoral nerve block is placed by the anesthesiologist prior to returning to the recovery room. The knee is placed in a hinged knee brace. All patients are dismissed home on the day of surgery. Because of the nerve block, patients are instructed to use the brace and crutches until the block has resolved, usually within 24 hours. They are then permitted to mobilize without the crutches and discontinue the brace as they feel comfortable.

A continuous passive motion (CPM) machine is delivered to the home. Patients begin with 4 hours/day on the CPM, which may be split into two 2-hour sessions. Range of motion on the CPM machine starts at 0 to 60 degrees and is increased daily, as tolerated. The CPM machine is discontinued when full motion is obtained or when they are comfortable shifting to a stationary bike for active motion activities.

All patients undergo a standardized, supervised, postoperative rehabilitation protocol that focuses on immediate weight bearing and obtaining full range of motion, including early full extension. Rehabilitation of the knee is considered complete when equal quadriceps strength is achieved, which is defined as being within 10% of the strength of the contralateral uninjured leg by isokinetic testing. When this goal has been attained, the patient may return to full activities, including return to sports.

COMPLICATIONS

Complications associated with ACL reconstruction can be classified as intraoperative and postoperative. Intraoperative complications include patellar fracture, incorrect tunnel placement, violation of the posterior cortex of the femur, graft fracture, and suture laceration. Postoperative complications include patella fractures, quadriceps or patellar tendon avulsion, loss of motion, graft stretching and failure, patellofemoral symptoms, and quadriceps weakness.

Intra-Operative Complications

Correct placement of the tunnels is crucial to the outcome of ACL reconstruction. Careful evaluation of the position of the guide pins before reaming can prevent erroneous tunnel placement. It is much easier to reposition the guide pin than to correct the position of a tunnel that has already been reamed. If, however, a reamed tunnel is noted to be slightly malpositioned, the orientation of the graft plug and interference screw may compensate. For example, if the tibial tunnel is noted to be slightly anterior, placing the graft posteriorly and the screw anteriorly in the tunnel will effectively move the insertion site of the graft posterior to the center of the hole.[12] When there is gross malpositioning of the reamed tunnel, rereaming of the tunnel in the correct position should be performed, followed by the use of a larger diameter interference screw and bone graft, if necessary, to achieve adequate fixation.

Violation of the posterior cortex of the femur can occur from inadvertently reaming too far into the femoral tunnel and not maintaining the femur in a flexed position during the reaming. When this complication occurs, fixation with an interference screw is no longer possible because the graft will be pushed out of the posterior aspect of the femur by the screw. Fixation with a screw and post on the lateral aspect of

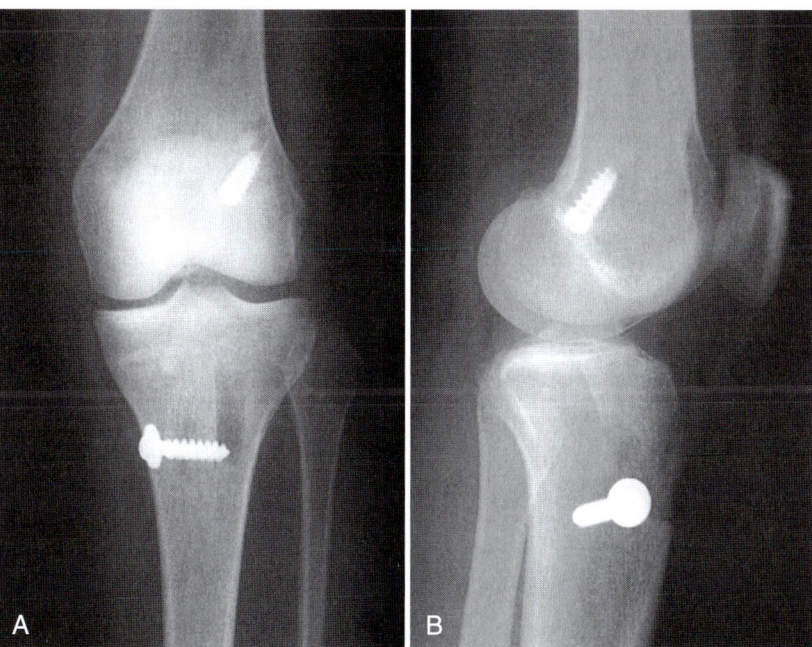

Figure 41-14. Postoperative anteroposterior **(A)** and lateral **(B)** radiographs after anterior cruciate ligament reconstruction showing correct placement of the bone tunnels. In this case, fixation of the femoral plug was achieved with an interference screw and the tibial plug was secured by tying sutures over a screw and washer.

the distal end of the femur through a separate incision is necessary, or the traditional two-incision technique with a more anteriorly placed tunnel can be used.[31] This problem can be avoided by maintaining clear visualization during advancement of the reamer into the femoral tunnel and not exceeding 30 mm in the depth of insertion.

Both graft fracture and suture laceration can be caused by inadequate space for the plug and screw in the tunnel. In this situation, as the screw is inserted, the graft becomes overly compressed and can fracture. A tight fit can also predispose to the screw engaging the sutures and causing laceration and loss of tension on the graft. Overreaming of the tunnels by 1 mm can prevent an overly tight fit of the interference screw. In addition, we routinely place a single suture in the end of the femoral bone plug and use an interference screw that is shorter than the length of the plug. This prevents the screw from reaching the suture and possibly causing laceration. On the tibial side, the screw should be inserted under direct visualization to avoid entangling the sutures. If laceration occurs at this end, the tibial plug can be passed into the joint and pulled through the patellar tendon defect and new holes can be drilled. The plug is then passed back into the joint and pulled through the tibial tunnel from inside-out. In the event of bone plug fracture, sutures can be placed in the end of the tendon with a Krackow-type stitch and tied over a screw and post.

Patella fracture after ACL reconstruction is infrequent, and the literature on this complication consists mostly of case reports.[38,88] Both direct force and indirect force have been implicated in the cause of this fracture. Simonian and coworkers[131] have suggested that an indirect force can result in different patellar fracture patterns, depending on the time elapsed from harvesting. They determined that stellate fractures can occur without direct injury in the early postoperative period (within 5 weeks). After this period, the fracture pattern is more likely to be transverse. Fracture of the patella during graft harvesting can be avoided by not deepening the cuts more than 8 mm and by maintaining a 45-degree orientation of the sagittal saw blade to the perpendicular surface of the patella. The cuts should also not extend beyond the limits of the fragment to avoid a possible stress riser. In the event of an intraoperative patellar fracture, the patellar fragments should be rigidly fixed to facilitate early range of motion postoperatively.

Postoperative Complications

Despite initially good results after ACL reconstructive surgery, postoperative complications may occur that are detrimental to the long-term outcome. Fortunately, patellar and tibial avulsions are rare, but they are devastating when they do occur. Several case reports have documented this complication, with some occurring up to 6 years after the reconstructive surgery.[25,86] Nixon and colleagues[96] noted that the patellar tendon donor site, left open at the time of surgery, was histologically identical to normal tendon at 2 years. Others have shown that the ultrasound signal of the tendon returns to normal by 1 year.[1] This time frame may explain why most of these avulsions occur within the first 10 months after surgery.

Much attention has been focused on postoperative loss of motion after ACL reconstruction. This complication may result from preoperative, intraoperative, or postoperative

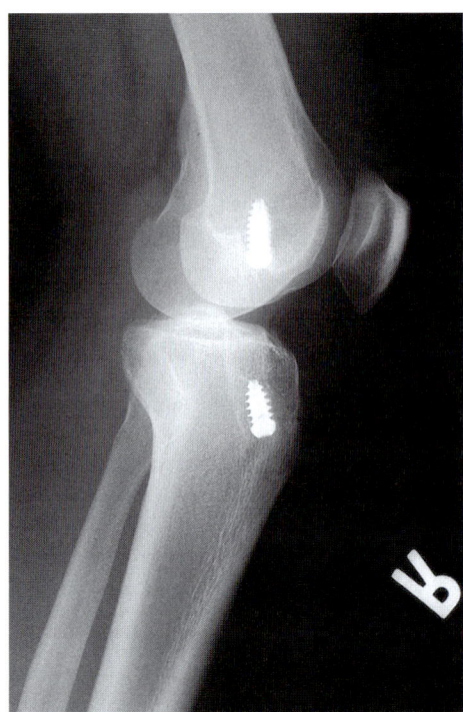

Figure 41-15. Lateral radiograph after anterior cruciate ligament reconstruction showing anterior femoral placement of the graft and interference screw.

factors. The presence of an effusion, limited range of motion, and concomitant ligamentous injuries of the knee preoperatively are factors that predispose to poor postoperative motion.[61,125] Intraoperative factors include erroneous tunnel placement and inadequate notchplasty. Anterior placement of the femoral tunnel results in overtightening of the graft and loss of full flexion (Fig. 41-15). Placement of the tibial tunnel too far anteriorly can result in impingement of the graft and lead to loss of full extension. Similarly, an inadequate notchplasty can also lead to extension loss secondary to impingement. Finally, postoperative immobilization and the rehabilitation protocol can have a significant effect on ultimate range of motion. Previous methods of cast immobilization after reconstruction and therapy emphasizing limited knee extension resulted in significant rates of postoperative arthrofibrosis. The trend toward limited or no immobilization and more aggressive rehabilitation has decreased these rates.[42,58,124] The concern over possible stretching and failure of the graft as a result of aggressive rehabilitation has not been realized. Histologic analysis of the patellar tendon autografts used for ACL reconstruction has revealed that the grafts undergo ligamentization over a period of months to years,[6,48] but that a necrotic stage may not occur and the grafts may be viable as early as 3 weeks postoperatively.[112]

The incidence of arthrofibrosis after ACL reconstructive surgery has decreased as postoperative rehabilitative protocols emphasizing early motion have been instituted. The cause of the arthrofibrosis may be poor patient motivation or compliance with the therapy regimen or other factors, such as incorrect bone tunnel placement or the development of reflex sympathetic dystrophy. Treatment of postoperative arthrofibrosis begins with recognition of the problem. Initial treatment with physical therapy should focus on stretching exercises and may also involve the use of static or dynamic braces to regain motion, particularly extension. Manipulation under anesthesia may be necessary if no significant improvement is noted with physical therapy alone. Manipulation is most effective if performed within the first 6 weeks after reconstructive surgery, and aggressive physical therapy must follow the manipulation to prevent recurrence. Adequate anesthesia with an indwelling epidural catheter can facilitate this early rehabilitation. If the manipulation is unsuccessful or it is longer than 6 weeks after surgery, arthroscopic or possibly open release of the adhesions will be required. Revision of the notchplasty may be needed at this time if scar tissue has developed in this area. Once again, aggressive physical therapy must follow any release to prevent recurrence. If the limited range of motion is to the result of improper tunnel placement, revision of the tunnels will need to be performed to prevent recurrence.

Stretching of the graft results in recurrence of instability symptoms and a positive Lachman test on examination. This may occur acutely or gradually over time and may be the result of improper tunnel placement, inadequate tension at the time of the reconstruction, or loss of fixation. Treatment of this complication must start with determining the reason for the failure. Graft incompetence immediately postoperatively is most likely caused by inadequate tensioning at surgery. Tunnel-graft mismatch may result in incarceration of the plug in the tunnel and lead to fixation of the plug with laxity in the graft. Proper tunnel sizing and evaluation of graft tension after fixation is achieved should prevent this unnecessary complication. Early (within 6 weeks) acute failure indicates a loss of fixation of one of the plugs because this is the weak link in the construct until bony union occurs. Removal of the interference screw and insertion of a larger diameter screw or fixation with the screw and post technique are required. Improper tunnel placement can result in loss of motion, as noted, or stretching and failure of the graft. In the latter case, treatment consists of graft revision with correct tunnel placement.

The most common and persistent complication of ACL reconstruction may be postoperative patellofemoral pain. The exact cause of this problem has not been determined, but several studies have suggested that a relationship exists among persistent flexion contracture, patellofemoral pain, and quadriceps weakness. Sachs and colleagues[113] have reported on 126 patients undergoing ACL reconstruction and noted a 19% rate of patellofemoral pain, which correlated positively with the presence of a flexion contracture. Similarly, Aglietti and associates[3] noted a 5% incidence of patellofemoral pain and a 20% incidence of patellofemoral crepitus without pain in 226 patients after ACL reconstruction. A positive correlation was found between patellofemoral symptoms and flexion and extension losses. Although some studies have suggested that the morbidity of the donor site in autologous patellar tendon reconstructions may contribute to patellofemoral pain,[139] Shelbourne and Trumper[126] have shown that the incidence of anterior knee pain is related more to failure to obtain full knee hyperextension. In their study, 602 patients who underwent ACL reconstruction, followed by a rehabilitation protocol emphasizing full knee hyperextension, were compared with 122 control patients with no history of knee injury. No differences in patellofemoral symptoms were found between the two groups. It was concluded

that anterior knee pain can be prevented through a program of early motion and full knee hyperextension. No detrimental effects on stability of the knee from the hyperextension protocol have been noted, provided that precise location of the graft is achieved.

OUTCOMES

Early results of open reconstruction of the ACL were encouraging in terms of restoration of knee stability.[47,78,115] Marshall and coworkers[84] have reported on 40 patients with an average follow-up of 22 months. Four patients were considered failures because of recurrent giving way in two, inability to return to sports in one, and persistent synovitis in one. Clancy and colleagues[39] have reported good or excellent results in 94% of 50 patients at an average 33-month follow-up. None of the patients had any postoperative episodes of instability, and all but six were able to return to full sports activity. O'Brien and associates[101] have reviewed 79 patients undergoing intra-articular ACL reconstruction with use of a free, non-vascularized autologous graft from the central third of the patellar tendon. Augmentation with an extra-articular lateral sling of iliotibial band was performed in 60% of the reconstructions. Episodes of giving way were eliminated in 95% of patients; however, nine were unable to return to previous activity levels, and 40% of those who did maintain previous levels of activity continued to wear a brace. Addition of a lateral sling had no effect on the outcome.

Despite these early results, persistent problems associated with ACL reconstruction became evident; these included flexion contracture, patellofemoral pain, limited range of motion, and quadriceps muscle atrophy, in addition to a prolonged rehabilitation period. Technologic advances in orthopedic surgery have resulted in the emergence of arthroscopically assisted ACL reconstruction. This reduces the surgical morbidity associated with open reconstruction and facilitates rehabilitation and return to activity. Several studies have shown that when compared with open reconstruction, the arthroscopically assisted technique results in a decreased incidence of patellar symptoms, knee stiffness, and need for manipulation, with no difference in knee stability.[2,14,33] Current techniques of ACL reconstruction have evolved further and now involve the use of a single-incision arthroscopic approach that reduces the surgical morbidity further and has been shown to yield consistently good results.[13,104,127] Despite concern with this newer technique regarding potential divergence of interference screw fixation, graft breakage, and posterior cortical violation, comparison studies between the single-incision and two-incision techniques have shown similar results in terms of outcome and complications.[9,62,118]

Harner and coworkers[62] have prospectively compared patients undergoing the two-incision rear entry technique for ACL reconstruction with another group undergoing the single-incision arthroscopic reconstruction technique. At an average follow-up of 35 months, no significant functional or radiographic differences were noted between the two groups. It was concluded that the single-incision technique yields reliable results, provided that tunnel placement and graft fixation were accurately performed, and that this technique is less invasive and more cosmetic. They also noted that less postoperative pain and therefore a faster rehabilitation period are other potential benefits of this technique. Reat and Lintner[110] prospectively studied 30 patients with chronic ACL injuries. The patients were randomly assigned to undergo reconstruction with the one- or two-incision technique. At a mean follow-up of 17 months, no statistically significant differences were found between the two groups, including early postoperative pain and range of motion. It was concluded that the two techniques are interchangeable and that both should be familiar to surgeons, because the two-incision technique allows for salvage of intraoperative loss of arthroscopic fixation of the femoral bone plug.

Sgaglione and Schwartz[118] have retrospectively reviewed 90 patients who underwent ACL reconstruction with the endoscopic single-incision or arthroscopically assisted two-incision technique. Similar outcomes were noted in subjective, functional, and objective data for the two groups. Four cases of posterior cortical violation occurred in the endoscopic group; however, all of them occurred early in the series. A 33% rate of screw divergence in the endoscopic group versus 14% in the two-incision group was also noted, but no clinical differences in these patients and those with parallel screw placement were found.

George and colleagues[54] have performed a systematic review of four prospective randomized controlled trials comparing two-incision (rear entry) with one-incision (all-endoscopic) techniques. There was no significant difference in objective test scores and outcomes.

Several studies have reported on the longer term follow-up of ACL reconstruction with autologous patellar tendon graft. Bach and associates[14] have retrospectively reviewed the results of 97 patients 5 to 9 years after arthroscopically assisted ACL reconstruction with patellar tendon autograft. A manual maximum side to side difference of 3 mm or less was noted in 70% of the patients, and 82% had excellent or good results according to the modified Hospital for Special Surgery scoring system. In addition, all patients had a pivot shift result of 1+ or less, and no patient demonstrated clinical findings of chronic patella tendinitis. It was concluded that this technique of ACL reconstruction yields reliable stability and a high level of patient satisfaction. Shelbourne and Gray[121] reported on the 2- to 9-year follow-up of ACL reconstruction performed through a medial miniarthrotomy, followed by accelerated rehabilitation. A total of 1057 patients were prospectively monitored and objective data were available for 806 of these patients. The mean manual maximum KT-1000 knee arthrometer score was 2.0 mm; quadriceps muscle strength testing revealed 94% strength after acute reconstruction and 91% strength after chronic reconstruction. Patients were able to return to sports-specific activities at a mean of 6.2 weeks postoperatively and to athletic competition at full capacity at 6.2 months postoperatively. Otto and coworkers[104] have retrospectively reviewed the 5-year results of 68 patients who underwent single-incision ACL reconstruction with patellar tendon autograft. Three patients experienced rerupture of their ACL grafts before the 5-year evaluation; of the remaining patients, 98% exhibited 5 mm or less of laxity on the Lachman test, and 77% were participating in level I or II activities according to the International Knee Documentation Committee (IKDC) score. Extension loss of more than 3 degrees was seen in 5% of the patients; however, the postoperative therapy regimen consisted of the use of a brace, which did not allow full extension for the first 4 weeks after

reconstruction. It was concluded that this technique results in excellent stability of the knee and allows return to a high level of function, and that even better results are anticipated with newer postoperative therapy regimens.

When comparing surgical results, one must consider the postoperative rehabilitation protocol. Previous ACL reconstruction rehabilitation was characterized by periods of immobilization and non–weight bearing in casts. More recent protocols now emphasize early range of motion and full weight bearing, as tolerated, with or without brace support. These aggressive programs have been shown to restore range of motion, reduce patellofemoral complications, and hasten return to activities without compromising knee stability.[121,124] As a result, overall outcomes of ACL reconstruction have improved.

Gender differences have not only been noted with respect to predisposing factors to ACL injury, but outcome studies have also demonstrated a poorer outcome in women postreconstruction. A meta-analysis by Biau and colleagues[22] has demonstrated persistent laxity following reconstruction, with increased rates of postoperative pivot shift in females. Shelbourne and Gray[122] have reported the rates of reinjury in 1415 patients at 5 years postreconstruction. They noted a similar rate of rerupture in the operative knee, but a significantly higher rate of rupture in the contralateral knee in women (7.8%) than in men (3.7%). The incidence of injury to either knee was associated with a younger age and higher level of activity.

A medium-term follow-up study by Spindler and coworkers[135] has reviewed patients at an average 5.4 years following reconstruction. Only 69% of patients (217 of 314) were available for follow-up. Predictors of poor outcome on multiple scales included the patient's recollection of hearing or feeling a pop at the time of the injury, a weight gain of more than 15 lb (6.8 kg), and no change in educational level since the surgery. Of note, there was a lack of association between the outcome and either the occurrence or form of treatment of a meniscal tear or chondromalacia of the articular cartilage.

Anterior Cruciate Ligament Reconstruction and Development of Arthrosis

One concern that has existed since the advent of surgical reconstruction is whether stabilizing the knee reduces the risk of developing arthritis. There is still a lack of definitive evidence, but in a study by Louboutin and colleagues,[80] reconstruction of the ligament reduced the rate of developing osteoarthritis (OA) from 60% to 100% with untreated knees down to 14% to 26% with a normal medial meniscus, and 37% with a meniscectomy at 20 years following ACL reconstruction. A systematic review demonstrated low rates of OA at more than 10 years following reconstruction. When isolated ligament reconstruction was required, the rate of arthritis was 0% to 13%, but when a meniscectomy was performed, it rose to 21% to 48%. They pointed out the nonuniform manner in which OA was determined in these studies.[103] Hart and associates[64] used single-photon emission computed tomography (SPECT) to determine the rates of arthritis at an average of 10 years following reconstruction in 31 patients, using the contralateral knee as a control. They found that 31% of patients had uptake; 13% of those were symptomatic and had a meniscectomy at about the time of reconstruction, but only 7% (one patient) was symptomatic in the nonmeniscectomized knees. In a review of 502 patients at a mean of 14.1 years postoperatively, another factor noted to be associated with more arthritis and pain was the loss of full extension following surgery.[122]

Fifty-five patients with established medial knee arthritis and a chronic ACL tear underwent reconstruction and were followed up at an average of 10 years by Shelbourne and Benner.[119] They concluded that reconstruction provides long-term pain relief and improves function. Two patients underwent osteotomy or total knee arthroplasty (TKA), and the importance of obtaining full motion postoperatively was noted. Plancher and coworkers[109] also demonstrated excellent outcomes (97% good to excellent at 5.5 yrs) following ACL reconstruction in patients older than age of 40 years, many of whom had preexisting arthritis.

At the other end of the age spectrum, adolescent athletes also sustain ACL injuries to the knee. Concern exists regarding ACL reconstruction because of the possibility of growth and angular deformities following standard tunnel placement across an open physis. Traditionally, options included avoiding twisting or pivoting sports versus physical therapy, rehabilitation, and return to sport with or without a brace. Because of the increased demands in this age group, and unwillingness to modify activities to such an extent, surgical reconstruction has been proposed. Reconstruction has been addressed in one of two ways—traditional tunnel positioning[7,75,123] or a modified physeal-sparing technique.[74] Both techniques demonstrate low complication rates without significant growth disturbance, indicating that successful reconstruction can be obtained in the adolescent athlete with open growth plates.

Graft Choice

Graft selection has remained a topic of discussion. In a prospective, randomized controlled trial (RCT) of a BPTB versus a two-strand hamstring graft at 3-year follow-up, the objective results of ACL replacement with a BPTB autograft were superior to those of replacement with a two-strand semitendinosus-gracilis graft with regard to knee laxity, pivot shift grade, and strength of knee flexor muscles. However, comparable results were noted in patient satisfaction, activity level, and knee function. Differing fixation techniques, and the fact that only two strands were used in the hamstring reconstructions, likely contributed to the poorer outcomes in this group.[21]

There have been a number of meta-analyses performed on graft selection and outcomes. The first combined nine RCTs and found the only differences to be a slight increase in arthrometer testing laxity with hamstrings, and more pain with kneeling in patents with patellar tendon grafts. It was concluded that graft type may not be the primary determinant in outcomes following ACL reconstruction.[134] A second meta-analysis was performed to explore outcome differences between the two graft sources, combining 14 studies with 1263 patients. This review demonstrated no significant difference in IKDC score and return to preinjury activity level. Of note, at latest follow-up, only 41% and 33% of patients, respectively, had patellar and hamstring grafts reconstructed reported as normal based on their IKDC score.[23] A more recent meta-analysis of randomized clinical trials comparing

BPTB with hamstring autograft included six combined studies, with a total of 423 patients. Results demonstrated decreased instability on postoperative pivot shift testing with the use of BPTB reconstructions.[22]

Two review articles combined the results of smaller studies examining the results of autograft versus allograft for ACL reconstruction. The meta-analysis by Krych and coworkers[76] focused only on patellar tendon grafts, whereas the systematic review by Carey and colleagues[37] incorporated one study with hamstring grafts. When one specific study with a sterilization method that compromised the graft was excluded, there were no differences in outcome scores, laxity, clinical failure rates, and return to sports. The authors did point out a significant limitation in these studies, because none of the studies included were randomized.

Rates of ACL reconstruction were examined in a review of the state database for New York over a 10-year period from 1997 to 2006. These rates were used to extrapolate a national rate of approximately 105,000 ACL reconstructions in 2006. Observed trends included increasing rates (22%) over the 10-year time period and a 6.5% rate of surgery on either knee within 1 year following ACL reconstruction. Predictors of further surgery include female gender, other interventions in the knee at the time of ligament reconstruction, and treatment by a lower volume surgeon.[82]

Following up on their success with national joint registries, Scandinavian countries have instituted ACL registries. Begun in 2004 in Norway, and a year later in Sweden and Denmark, these will have collected information regarding epidemiology, associated injuries, techniques, perioperative and postoperative protocols, and outcomes.[60]

New Directions

Proponents of double-bundle reconstruction of the ACL have noted that it better re-creates the two-bundle anteromedial and posterolateral anatomy of the native ligament. Three recent RCTs have compared single-bundle (SB) to double-bundle (DB) hamstring reconstructions. The first study randomized 68 patients into two equal arms. Results at a mean of 25 months indicated that DB ACL reconstruction via a four-strand semitendinosus tendon is superior to the SB technique with regard to anterior and rotational stability.[94] The second study of 70 patients at an average 18-month follow-up demonstrated a significant advantage in anterior and rotational stability as well as objective IKDC scores for four-tunnel DB ACL reconstruction compared with SB ACL reconstruction.[130] A third prospective RCT also examined 70 patients receiving an SB or DB hamstring graft for ACL reconstruction. At a minimum 2-year follow-up, DB ACL reconstructions showed better visual analogue scale (VAS) scores, less anterior knee laxity, and improved final objective IKDC scores than SB.[4]

Other investigators have found no significant differences. This includes a meta-analysis by Meredick and associates,[91] which combined the results of four RCTs and demonstrated no clinically significant differences in KT-1000 arthrometer or pivot shift testing. Another recent RCT of 50 male athletes reconstructed with an SB or DB technique was designed to investigate results in this high-demand subset of patients at a minimum 2-year follow-up. The SB group was reconstructed with a graft placed at a more horizontal position (10 or 2 o'clock) and it was thought that this may have contributed to the comparable results in the SB group, because there were no differences in laxity, rotational stability, or outcome scores.[136]

Conversion to a DB technique also has implications for operative time and cost to the health care system. Brophy and coworkers[27] have performed a cost-benefit analysis on this technique modification. They concluded that the DB technique has the potential to introduce considerable new expense into the procedure, and thus does not appear to be cost-effective at this time. These results have been criticized by proponents of the technique because of the limited scope of the comparisons and the short duration of clinical outcomes used for comparison in this review.[53]

A recent all-inside arthroscopic technique for ACL reconstruction has been described. This modification avoids the cortical disruption associated with standard tibial techniques. Outcomes and clinical results have not yet been published.[28]

It has long been known that the ACL provides more than simple mechanical restraint to the knee. A recent study comparing functional brain magnetic resonance imaging (MRI) scans noted central nervous system reorganization in several motor-related areas in patients with chronic ACL-deficient knees, when compared with controls.[72] This may lead to further studies, and modifications to rehabilitation protocols, in an effort to address this nonmusculoskeletal aspect of ACL injuries.

CONCLUSION

The goal of ACL reconstruction is to restore stability of the knee without loss of motion and thereby allow patients to return to their preinjury level of function. The patellar tendon autograft has proved to be a reliable substitute for the native ligament and has yielded good long-term results. Refinements in surgical technique and postoperative therapy regimens have reduced complication rates and decreased recovery times after the procedure. Future challenges for ACL reconstruction are to decrease rates of injuries in athletes, improve surgical techniques, and further optimize rehabilitation protocols. Newly developed registries, similar to those in the arthroplasty literature, will provide increased objective outcome data that can be used to advance techniques.

Acknowledgment. We thank Dr. Henrik Bo Pedersen for his valuable assistance in preparation of the illustrations in this chapter.

KEY REFERENCES

Alm A, Gillquist J: Reconstruction of the anterior cruciate ligament by using the medial third of the patellar ligament. Acta Chir Scand 140:289, 1974.

George MS, Huston LJ, Spindler KP: Endoscopic versus rear-entry ACL reconstruction: a systematic review. Clin Orthop Relat Res (455):158, 2007.

Gotlin R, Cushner FD, Scott WN: Influence of graft diameter on knee stability: KT arthrometry study (unpublished data).

Granan LP, Bahr R, Lie SA, Engebretsen L: Timing of anterior cruciate ligament reconstructive surgery and risk of cartilage lesions and meniscal tears: a cohort study based on the Norwegian National Knee Ligament Registry. Am J Sports Med 37:955, 2009.

Granan LP, Forssblad M, Lind M, Engebretsen L: The Scandinavian ACL registries 2004-2007: baseline epidemiology. Acta Orthop 80:563, 2009.

Hospodar SJ, Miller MD: Controversies in ACL reconstruction: bone-patellar tendon-bone anterior cruciate ligament reconstruction remains the gold standard. Sports Med Arthrosc 17:242, 2009.

Krych AJ, Jackson JD, Hoskin TL, Dahm DL: A meta-analysis of patellar tendon autograft versus patellar tendon allograft in anterior cruciate ligament reconstruction. Arthroscopy 24:292, 2008.

Louboutin H, Debarge R, Richou J, et al: Osteoarthritis in patients with anterior cruciate ligament rupture: a review of risk factors. Knee 16:2394, 2009.

Lyman S, Koulouvaris P, Sherman S, et al: Epidemiology of anterior cruciate ligament reconstruction: trends, readmissions, and subsequent knee surgery. J Bone Joint Surg Am 91:2321, 2009.

Morgan CD, Kalman VR, Grawl DM: Definitive landmarks for reproducible tibial tunnel placement in anterior cruciate ligament reconstruction. Arthroscopy 11:275, 1995.

Nabors ED, Richmond JC, Vannah WM, et al: Anterior cruciate ligament graft tensioning in full extension. Am J Sports Med 23:488, 1995.

Noyes FR, Mooar PA, Matthews DS, et al: The symptomatic anterior cruciate-deficient knee: Part I. The long-term functional disability in athletically active individuals. J Bone Joint Surg Am 65:154, 1983.

Plancher KD, Steadman JR, Briggs KK, et al: Reconstruction of the anterior cruciate ligament in patients who are at least forty years old. A long-term follow-up and outcome study. J Bone Joint Surg Am 80:184, 1998.

Shelbourne KD, Gray T: Anterior cruciate ligament reconstruction with autogenous patellar tendon graft followed by accelerated rehabilitation: a two- to nine-year follow-up. Am J Sports Med 25:786, 1997.

Shelbourne KD, Gray T, Wiley BV: Results of transphyseal anterior cruciate ligament reconstruction using patellar tendon autograft in tanner stage 3 or 4 adolescents with clearly open growth plates. Am J Sports Med 32:1218, 2004.

Shelbourne KD, Nitz P: Accelerated rehabilitation after anterior cruciate ligament reconstruction. Am J Sports Med 18:292, 1990.

Shelbourne KD, Trumper RV: Preventing anterior knee pain after anterior cruciate ligament reconstruction. Am J Sports Med 25:41, 1997.

Full references for this chapter can be found on www.expertconsult.com.

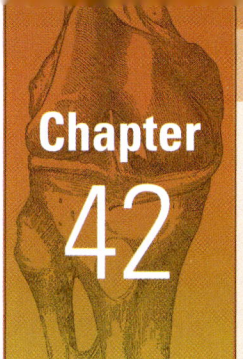

Bone-Patellar Tendon-Bone Autograft Anterior Cruciate Ligament Reconstruction

Robert A. Magnussen, Joseph P. DeAngelis, and Kurt P. Spindler

ADVANTAGES OF AND CONTRAINDICATIONS TO BONE-PATELLAR TENDON-BONE AUTOGRAFT PROCEDURES

Although general indications for anterior cruciate ligament (ACL) reconstruction are discussed elsewhere in this text, it is important to review advantages and disadvantages of patellar tendon autograft reconstruction. Numerous systematic reviews published since 2000 have shown that both bone-patellar tendon-bone (BTB) autograft and three- or four-strand hamstring grafts (HGs) produce reliable ACL reconstruction results with few clinical outcome differences between the two.* A recent systematic review of the one-versus two-incision BTB autograft technique has shown no reproducible difference in pain medication requirement, rehabilitation time, laxity, or other outcome measure.[11]

Advantages

- Interference screw fixation provides immediate strength to allow aggressive early rehabilitation.
- Bone to bone graft healing leads to improved strength compared with tendon to bone healing in the early (less than 6 weeks) postoperative period.[25]
- It avoids injury to the hamstring musculature, whose the function is critical for certain explosive athletes (sprinters) and protective to the ACL.

Contraindications

- Patients requiring repetitive kneeling for recreational, occupational, or religious reasons: More anterior knee discomfort and pain with kneeling have been noted following patellar tendon graft harvest.[14,17,20,21,30]
- History of extensor mechanism rupture: The potential risk of patellar fracture, patellar tendon rupture or avulsion has been described.[5,7]
- Small patellar tendon width (<25 mm), significant patellar tendinosis, or presence of a large Osgood-Schlatter ossicle: All may compromise graft strength.[4]

SURGICAL TECHNIQUE

Patient Positioning

The patient is positioned supine with a proximal thigh tourniquet in place, taking care to leave adequate room for an anterolateral incision on the femur, if needed. The foot of the table is flexed beyond 90 degrees or removed, allowing the knee to bend to 90 degrees. The patient should be positioned so that the thigh extends 3 to 4 inches beyond the edge of the table to avoid displacement of neurovascular structures anteriorly, decreasing the risk of injury. The contralateral leg should be padded to protect the common peroneal nerve and bony prominences from intraoperative compression. Much of the procedure, including notch preparation, tunnel drilling, and graft passage, is performed with the thigh resting on the operative table and the knee flexed to approximately 90 degrees. A padded bolster under the distal thigh can assist in maintaining this position.

Diagnostic Arthroscopy

The procedure begins with a systematic diagnostic arthroscopy. Each articular surface in the knee (patella, trochlea, medial and lateral tibial plateaus, and femoral condyles) should be inspected and graded. Treatment of unstable articular cartilage flaps, removal of loose bodies, and marrow stimulation techniques such as microfracture or abrasion should be performed prior to ACL reconstruction. Similarly, both menisci should be inspected and probed for tears. In general, small stable or partial tears should be left alone, with the decision to repair or excise the tear dependent on its location and orientation. Following documentation and treatment of any articular cartilage and meniscal injuries, ACL reconstruction proceeds.

Graft Procurement

There are many techniques for harvesting the BTB graft from the extensor mechanism. General principles include atraumatic harvest, maintenance of a solid bone-tendon attachment on either end of the graft, and careful preservation of remaining patellar tendon attachment sites on the tibia and patella. Careful harvest is critical for minimizing damage to articular surfaces of the patella and trochlea as well as the risk of patella fracture, patellar tendon rupture, and graft disruption.

The harvest can be approached through a single longitudinal incision or two smaller transverse incisions. Because it provides easy visualization of the entire length of graft, a longitudinal incision is recommended. Using the anteromedial portal and tibial tubercle as landmarks, an incision is made from 1 cm proximal to the anteromedial portal to the tibial tubercle distally, incorporating the anteromedial portal. Ensuring that the incision extends distally to the inferior aspect of the tibial tubercle allows graft harvest and tibial tunnel drilling with a single incision. A scalpel is used through the skin, dermis, and subcutaneous tissues until the transverse prepatellar fascia is encountered. Skin flaps are developed in the plane just superficial to this fascia, more laterally than

---

*References 3, 9, 10, 12, 19, 24, 27, and 29.

medially. Use of an Army-Navy retractor should allow visualization of the entire patella proximally and 2.5 cm of the tibial tubercle distally.

The transverse fascia (peritenon) is divided longitudinally in the center of the patellar tendon from the superior pole of the patella distal to the tibial tubercle. Based on surgeon preference, this layer may or may not be closed after harvest. Dissection should be carried medially and laterally to expose the central portion of the patellar tendon (15 to 20 mm). If peritenon closure in not planned, it is important to avoid dissecting too far medially or laterally, which could cause fat pad herniation. The width of the tendon is measured with the knee flexed 90 degrees. The maximum width of BTB graft is one third of the entire width of the patellar tendon. A 10-mm graft is standard in our practice because a typical patellar tendon measures 30 mm in width. For a 27-mm tendon, most would harvest a 9-mm graft and adjust tunnel size accordingly. Some authors have recommended avoidance of patellar tendon harvest in patients with a tendon width of less than 25 mm[4]; however, as little as 14 mm of patellar tendon following harvest has been left, without subsequent patellar tendon rupture.[23]

Following determination of tendon width and desired graft size, harvest begins. The tendinous portion of the graft is divided first. A scalpel is used with the knee flexed to 90 degrees to put tension on the patellar tendon. Once the tendon is divided, the surgeon can mark the size of the anticipated rectangular bone blocks with electrocautery (Fig. 42-1). Bone plugs are generally between 20 and 25 mm in length and the same width as the graft. However, the length of the patellar block is adjusted to preserve a minimum of 1 cm of intact proximal patellar bone to avoid patellar fracture.

Harvesting the patellar block should proceed with careful attention to detail to avoid iatrogenic compression injury of patellar or trochlear articular cartilage, because the knee is in flexion during harvest. This goal is accomplished through the use of an oscillating saw with a narrow blade. Cuts should begin distally, extending just through the anterior cortex of the patella to avoid injury to the deep surface. As the cuts are extended proximally, they should not exceed a depth of 6 to 7 mm. The cuts should be angled toward the center of the patella so that the resulting bone block is trapezoidal. Thickness of the cortex varies by patient age and size and should be anticipated by the surgeon. Next, the proximal horizontal cut is completed, with care taken not to extend the cut more medially or laterally than the respective vertical limbs. Failure to make the cuts square ("T-ing" the cuts) leads to stress risers and potential postoperative fracture (Fig. 42-2).

After the saw cuts are completed, a ¼-inch osteotome is gently tapped into the horizontal cut and two-finger pressure is used to elevate the block (Fig. 42-3). If only two-finger pressure is used, the bone block will not fracture. Work with osteochondral autografts has demonstrated that the vigorous tapping to insert plugs can generate chondrocyte death.[28] These data suggest avoidance of vigorous tapping on the patella during graft harvest.

The tibial cut can be completed with an oscillating saw or osteotome because there is no articular cartilage to injure with compression. Our preferred technique is to use ½-inch osteotomes for the vertical cuts and ¼-inch osteotomes for the distal horizontal cut (Fig. 42-4). When harvesting the tibial bone block, care must be taken to ensure that the

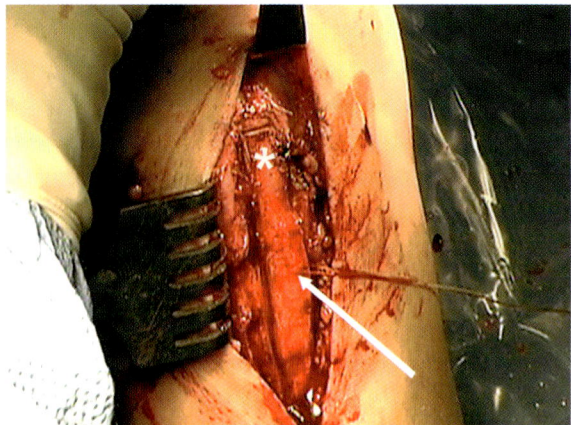

Figure 42-1. The patellar tendon has been divided sharply and the desired size of the patellar bone block (*) has been marked with electrocautery. Note the stitch securing the graft to the drape *(arrow)* to avoid accidently dropping it during harvest.

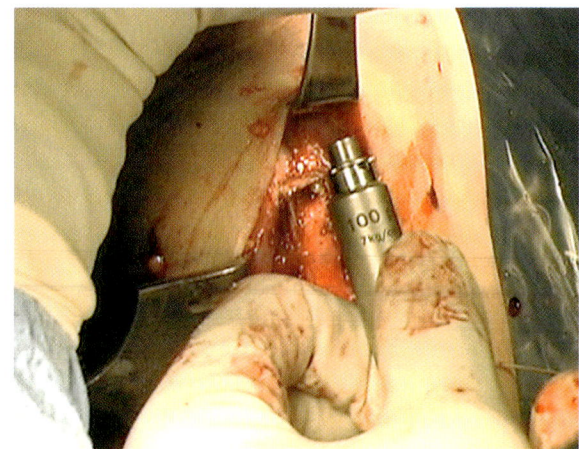

Figure 42-2. A small oscillating saw is used to cut the cortical bone of the patella, outlining the bone block. Care is taken not to "T" the cuts.

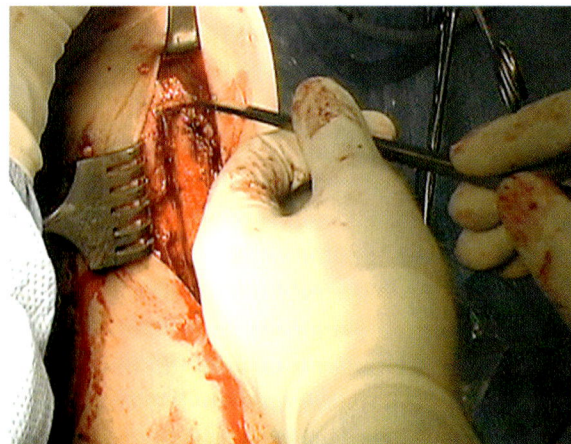

Figure 42-3. A ¼-inch osteotome is used in the transverse cut to free the bone block from its bed. Only two-finger pressure should be used to avoid bone block fracture.

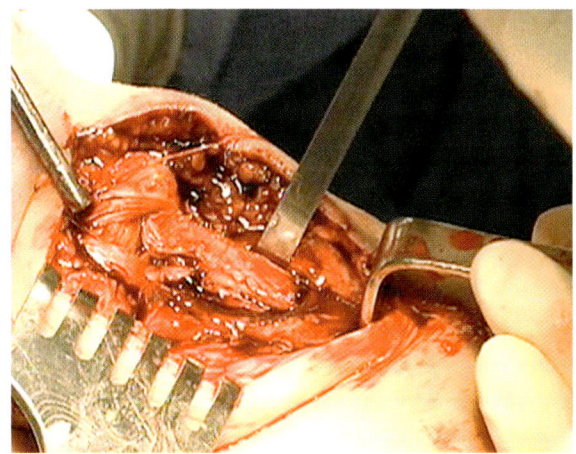

Figure 42-4. The tibial bone block is harvested with osteotomes.

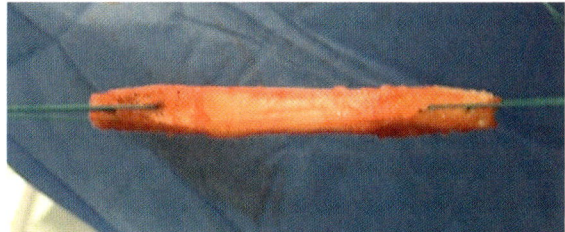

Figure 42-5. Prepared patellar tendon graft demonstrating placement of passing sutures through the shaped bone blocks.

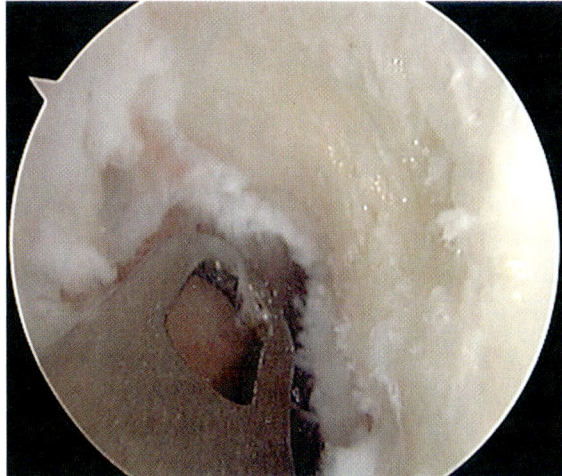

Figure 42-6. Prepared notch demonstrating clear visualization of the lateral wall and the posterior extent of the notch.

proximal end is at the insertion of the patellar tendon into bone, not the proximal end of the tibia. If the surgeon does not carefully visualize this point, a shorter than desired bone block can inadvertently be harvested. Again, two-finger pressure is used with an osteotome to lever the block out, avoiding bone block fracture. The shape of this bone block is generally more triangular than the patellar block to avoid damage to remaining tibial attachments.

To avoid inadvertent dropping of the graft on the floor, we recommend putting a stitch in the middle and securing it to the drapes during harvest. The patellar tendon defect is closed with interrupted figure-of-eight heavy absorbable suture, with the knee flexed 90 degrees. Bone graft resulting from graft preparation is used to fill the patellar defect, with any remaining bone used for the tibial defect.

Graft Preparation

The graft is prepared on the back table. Extreme caution must be used to avoid damage to the tendon or bone blocks and avoid inadvertently dropping the graft on the floor and contaminating it. One way to prevent the tendon from falling on the floor is to leave the stitch that was in the tendon in place and secure it to the back table drape with a hemostat. In general, the goal during bone block preparation is to size the blocks to fit comfortably and snugly within the tunnels. The bone blocks are usually brought down to size to fit easily within their respective sizing sleeves with rongeurs. If a graft passer is to be used to pass the graft up into the femur, the bone block going into the femur should be downsized by 1 mm. Thus, if you plan to have a 10-mm tunnel and use a graft passer, you should size the femoral block to fit easily into a 9-mm sleeve. This will allow you to place the graft into the graft passer and slide it up through the tunnel with relative ease. For the tibial tunnel, the graft is sized to fit comfortably within a sleeve that is the same size as the tibia tunnel.

To pass the graft, the surgeon will need to place holes in the patellar and tibial bone block for sutures. If one is using a suture that could be cut by metallic screws or the metal taps required for bioabsorbable screws, one should consider placing the suture tunnels perpendicular to one another so that one will remain intact, even if the other is cut. The use of the newer, high-strength polyethylene sutures, which are not easily cut with any of the taps, allows placement of both tunnels in the

same direction, usually straight through the cortex. The size of the hole in the bone should be just large enough to pass the metal needle of the suture through it and no larger to minimize stress risers in the graft. Once the graft is appropriately sized and the surgeon's suture of choice is placed into the two bone blocks, the graft is rinsed with saline and placed in a moist saline-soaked sponge until needed (Fig. 42-5).

Notch Preparation and Consideration of Notchplasty

Significant disagreement exists among surgeons regarding the need to débride ACL remnant from the lateral wall of the notch, the need for and degree of notchplasty, and the amount of Hoffa's fat pad that should be excised. Sufficient ACL tissue and fat pad should be débrided for the surgeon to visualize appropriate entry points for the femoral and tibial tunnels accurately (Fig. 42-6). Some surgeons prefer to preserve residual ACL stump to aid in graft placement, whereas others débride all ACL tissue and rely on other landmarks. One must then ensure that the notch is wide enough to avoid graft impingement at any point of knee motion. A good rule of thumb is to be certain that one can easily place a 5.5-mm burr between the lateral wall of the notch and posterior cruciate ligament (PCL), with a few millimeters on either side. If the notch is too narrow for this maneuver to be performed, notchplasty should be considered. Notchplasty is generally performed anteriorly to posteriorly using a burr. The need for further notchplasty should be rechecked later in the procedure, after the graft passer is placed through the tunnels. One should ensure that the graft passer slides easily without impingement through the full normal range of knee motion. Any impingement should be adjusted by further notchplasty.

Tunnel Preparation

Tibial Tunnel

The goal in tibial tunnel placement is to position the tunnel within the ACL footprint so that the graft will neither impinge anteriorly or laterally on the intercondylar notch in extension nor wrap around the PCL in full flexion. Numerous anatomic landmarks have been described as references to aid in tunnel placement, including the posterior edge of the anterior horn of the medial or lateral meniscus or the anterior aspect of the PCL. Various commercial guides are available to reference off these structures. Placement can be checked prior to reaming by bringing the knee into full extension following guide pin placement. Some surgeons prefer to leave behind a sufficient stump of the ACL to seal the tunnel once the graft is placed through, whereas others prefer to remove all residual ACL tissue to facilitate visualization. It is currently unknown which technique is most beneficial.

Our standard technique is to set the tibial targeting guide at an angle of 50 to 55 degrees, placed at the posterior edge of the anterior lateral meniscus centered halfway between the PCL and lateral wall of the notch (Fig. 42-7). Care should be taken when drilling this guide pin to make sure that the starting point is sufficiently distal on the tibia to leave a sufficient anterior bone bridge. The tunnel is generally placed at about the level of the tibial tubercle. Placing the starting point too far medially will result in damage to the pes anserine tendons or medial collateral ligament, whereas starting too far laterally could damage the patellar tendon insertion.

Once the guide pin is placed, the knee is brought into full extension to check the position, as noted earlier. If the location is not acceptable, the pin can be moved with either a Gatling gun type of drill guide or 3- to 5-mm offset guides to the correct position. Once the pin is appropriately placed, the tunnel is drilled to the appropriate size. A curette should be placed over the intra-articular end of the guide pin during drilling to avoid inadvertent pin migration during overdrilling. Care should be taken to avoid plunging with the drill because the PCL, the lateral wall of the notch, or the lateral femoral condyle could be damaged. The intra-articular mouth of the tunnel is then smoothed with rasps to avoid graft laceration on a sharp bony lip.

Femoral Tunnel

Femoral tunnel location has been the source of renewed interest in recent years. There is considerable debate about how far down the lateral wall the center of tunnel should be. Using the clock face method, recommendations range from 11 to 9 o'clock (right knee) or 1 to 3 o'clock (left knee). Classic teaching is to place the graft at the 10 o'clock (right knee) or 2 o'clock (left knee) position. Recently, increased focus on anatomic placement has led numerous authors to recommend placement farther down the lateral wall of the notch.[6,8] It is believed that a more horizontal graft can better restore rotational stability than a vertical graft.[16,18,22] Anteroposterior position of the femoral tunnel has been shown to influence graft isometry more significantly than a medial-lateral position in the notch.[13] Therefore, excellent visualization is required to ensure that the graft is not placed too anteriorly in the notch. The recommended position is 7 mm anterior to the over the top position at the back of the femoral notch when drilling a 10-mm tunnel (Fig. 42-8). There are three basic techniques frequently used to drill the femoral tunnel—transtibial, two-incision, and accessory medial portal.

Transtibial Technique

A frequently used technique for drilling the femoral tunnel involves drilling it through the tibial tunnel. A guide pin is placed through the tibial tunnel in a retrograde manner and centered on the desired femoral tunnel location. Care must be taken to avoid the vertical graft placement that can commonly occur using this technique. After the guide pin has been placed, one must check to ensure that adequate posterior bone is present to avoid posterior wall blowout while drilling the tunnel. After the guide pin is appropriately placed, the femoral tunnel is overdrilled with the appropriately sized cannulated drill. The tunnel should be deeper than the bone block's length (usual tunnel depth is about 35 mm),

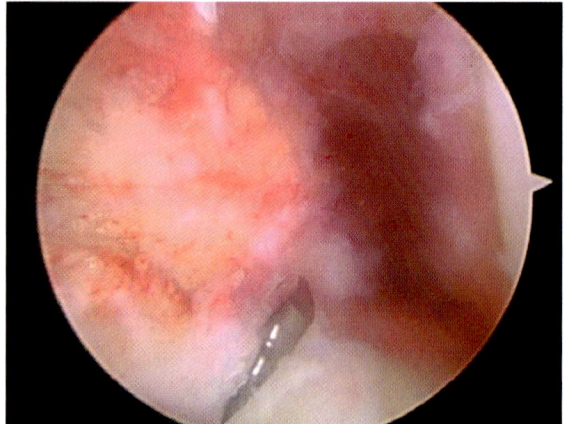

Figure 42-7. Appropriate placement of the tibial tunnel guide wire just posterior to the anterior horn of the lateral meniscus, centered between the PCL and the lateral wall of the notch.

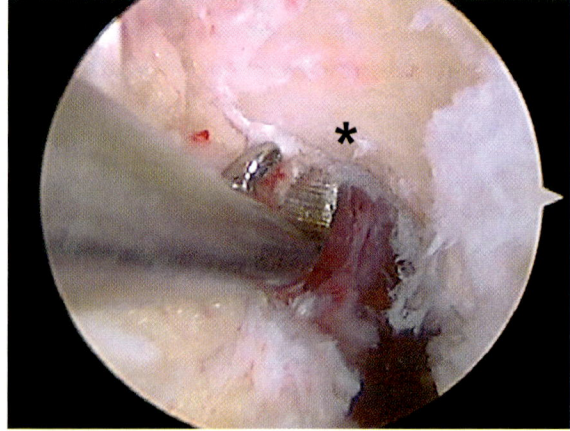

Figure 42-8. 7-mm offset guide demonstrating an appropriate entry point for the femoral tunnel into the notch (*).

but it is not necessary to penetrate the lateral cortex of the femur. After drilling, the drill and guide pin are removed and a rasp is used to smooth the sharp edges of the tunnel to avoid graft laceration. Advantages of this technique include its relative ease and efficiency as well as the avoidance of an incision on the anterolateral femur.

Accessory Medial Portal Technique

The accessory medial portal technique for femoral tunnel placement was developed to solve the problem of vertical graft placement noted to occur frequently with a transtibial technique. After desired femoral tunnel position has been identified, the location of the accessory medial portal is determined by spinal needle localization. The portal should be placed so that the spinal needle can easily touch the desired location of the tunnel in the notch without touching the medial femoral condyle. Hyperflexion of the knee is generally required to reach the desired tunnel entry point. A portal is created in the desired location and the guide pin is drilled into the desired tunnel entry point via the portal. The pin site is then inspected to ensure that adequate posterior bone is present to avoid posterior wall blowout during drilling.

The appropriately sized cannulated drill is then advanced over the guide pin and into the notch. Extreme caution must be used to avoid damage to the articular cartilage of the medial femoral condyle when advancing the drill toward the notch. The tunnel is then overdrilled to a depth exceeding the length of the bone block. The hyperflexed knee position and more horizontal graft position obtained with this technique generally lead to a shorter femoral tunnel than the transtibial technique, and it may be necessary to drill through the lateral cortex to obtain adequate tunnel length. The drill and guide pin are then carefully removed, again taking care to avoid damage to the articular surface of the medial femoral condyle.

Two-Incision Technique

The two-incision technique allows a wide range of femoral tunnel positions without constraints imposed by tibial tunnel or portal drilling. Ex vivo data have shown a better ability to reproduce the native femoral insertion of the ACL with an independent drilling technique than a transtibial technique.[1,15]

Numerous guide systems exist to facilitate drilling of the femoral tunnel in an outside-in manner. Our preferred guide system includes a stylus that enters the notch from the front via the anteromedial portal, with an adjustable aimer that extends anteriorly to the anterolateral thigh. With the arthroscope in the anterolateral portal, the hooked stylus of the guide is inserted through the anteromedial portal and centered over the desired intra-articular entry point of the tunnel (Fig. 42-9). The other end of the guide is positioned over the anterolateral thigh and the drill sleeve is inserted to mark the entry point into the skin (Fig. 42-10).

The sleeve is removed and a 2-cm incision is made parallel to the long axis of the femur, one third proximal and two thirds distal to the skin mark. The incision is carried down sharply to the iliotibial band and tissue overlying the iliotibial band is cleared with a Cobb elevator. The iliotibial band is then incised anterior to the lateral intermuscular septum and parallel to its fibers. The vastus lateralis muscle is swept anteriorly off the septum and lateral border of the femur. A Z knee retractor is placed along the anterior femur and used to pull

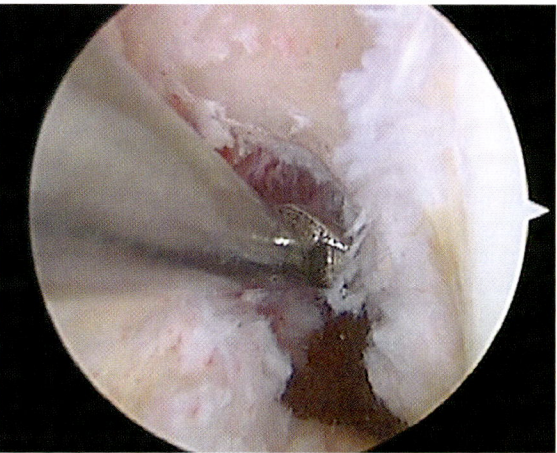

Figure 42-9. Femoral drill guide positioned in the notch and centered on the position marked with the 7-mm offset guide.

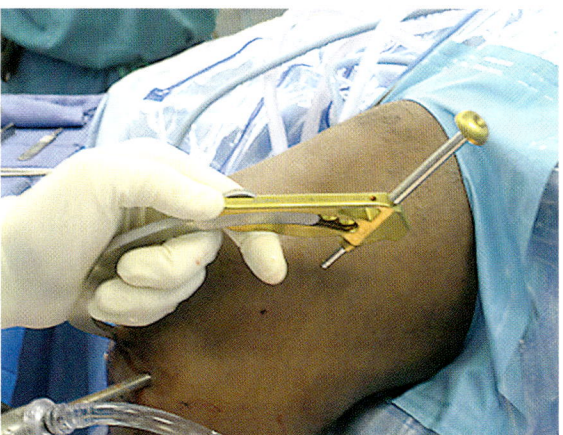

Figure 42-10. The opposite end of the femoral guide is centered over the anterolateral thigh to localize placement of the accessory anterolateral incision.

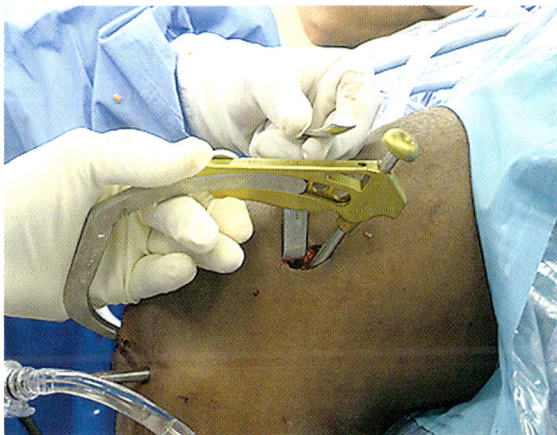

Figure 42-11. The anterolateral incision has been created and the drill guide advanced to bone on the anterolateral femoral metaphysis.

the vastus lateralis anteriorly. The drill sleeve is again placed through the femoral drill guide and advanced to bone (Fig. 42-11). An entry position on the lateral femur is chosen, taking care that sufficient bone remains posteriorly to maintain the posterior wall of the femoral tunnel.

After ensuring that the intra-articular portion of the guide remains in the desired position, a 2-mm drill is drilled through the sleeve in an antegrade manner and advanced into the joint under arthroscopic visualization. The femoral drill guide and sleeve are then removed, leaving the 2-mm drill in place. The lateral femoral cortex is again palpated to ensure that sufficient posterior bone remains. A cannulated drill is then used to overdrill the femoral tunnel in an antegrade manner, again under direct visualization (Fig. 42-12). Careful attention should be paid not to plunge. Once the drills are removed, a curved rasp is used to clean out the intra-articular portions so that there are no rough edges to abrade the graft. One should clean the lateral cortex to ensure that there are no impinging soft tissues that could interfere with graft passage or with screw placement.

Graft Passage

Regardless of drilling technique, grafts are general passed from distal to proximal. The first step is to pull the sutures attached to the graft through the tunnels. With a transtibial or accessory medial portal technique, this is generally accomplished by drilling a Beath pin through the femoral tunnel (either via the tibial tunnel or accessory medial portal) and out through the anterolateral thigh. If an accessory medial portal technique is used, one must then advance the Beath pin into the knee joint and retrieve it through the tibial tunnel using a grasper. The leading sutures for the graft are then placed through the Beath pin and pulled through both tunnels (Fig. 42-13). With a two-incision technique, a commercially available graft passer can be passed through the femoral tunnel in a retrograde manner, pulled through the tibial tunnel using a grasper, and used to pull the graft's sutures through the tunnels. Alternatively, a free suture can be passed through the femoral tunnel, retrieved through the tibial tunnel, and used to pull the graft's sutures through the tunnels. Use of a suture passage device may facilitate passage of the suture through the femoral tunnel.

The graft is then passed through the tibial tunnel, into the knee joint, and up into the femoral tunnel. Passage should be performed under arthroscopic visualization. The most common cause of difficult passage is difficulty passing the proximal bone block into the femoral tunnel. Guiding the graft into the tunnel with a probe via the anteromedial portal may be helpful. Another sticking point may be entry of the distal bone block into the tibial tunnel. This location should be checked if passage is difficult. If a graft passer is used, the femoral block of the graft (which has been downsized by 1 mm) is placed into the graft passer and brought up approximately 1 to 2 cm. This leaves the tibial block out of the graft passer because it is the same size as the tibial tunnel and would have difficulty fitting through the tunnel inside the graft passer. At this point, the surgeon pulls the graft and graft passer up through the tibial tunnel and into the femur. Once the leading bone block has engaged the femoral tunnel, the plastic graft passer is completely removed and passage continues until the bone block is completely within the femur.

Graft Fixation

Fixation of patellar tendon autografts is most commonly performed with interference screws. Alternatively, buttons can be used proximally and sutures can be tied over a post, either proximally or distally. Interference screws (metal or bioabsorbable) are the most popular choice for fixation for several reasons. First, interference fixation is more rigid than button or post fixation because it is more apical and effectively shortens the graft. Second, tying over a post, at least on the tibia, has been associated with more postoperative hardware-related pain. Thus, the technique presented here focuses exclusively on interference screws.

Regardless of the specific type of screw used, there are several principles that guide screw selection and placement. First, the screw should not be longer than the bone block to avoid damage the graft as it moves during knee range of motion. Second, the screw should be inserted until it is flush with the cortex of the femur or tibia so that it is secured in the most rigid bone and is not prominent. Third, the width of the chosen screw should be based on the size difference between the bone block and the tunnel. If the size difference is 1 mm, a 7-mm screw is used. If the gap is 2 mm, an 8-mm screw is used. If the gap is 3 to 4 mm, a 9-mm screw is used. Screw size can be modified based on the relative softness of bone, with a larger screw used for the same gap size in softer bone. Finally, some bioabsorbable screws require tapping but

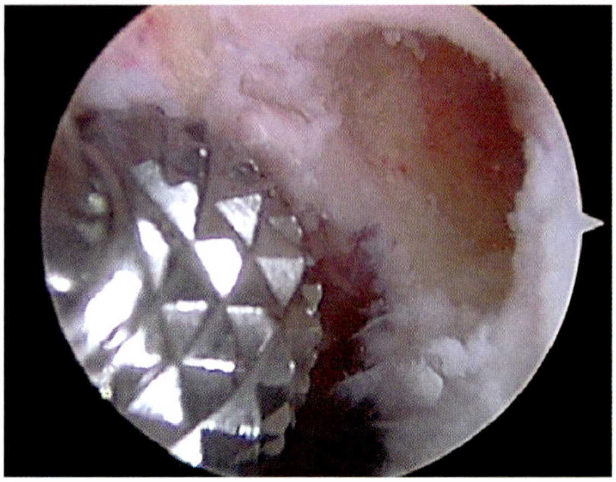

Figure 42-12. Completed femoral tunnel in the 2 o'clock position in the notch.

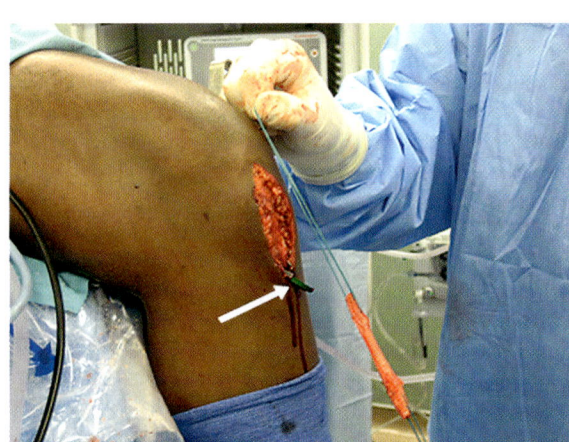

Figure 42-13. The bone-patellar tendon-bone graft ready for passage. The graft passer can be visualized protruding from the distal end of the tibial tunnel *(arrow).*

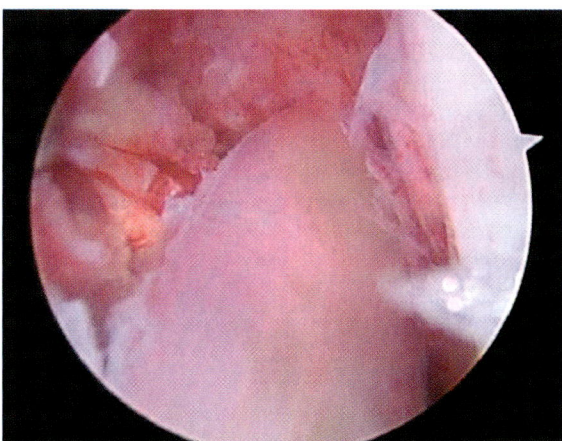

Figure 42-14. Completed ACL graft visualized in the notch.

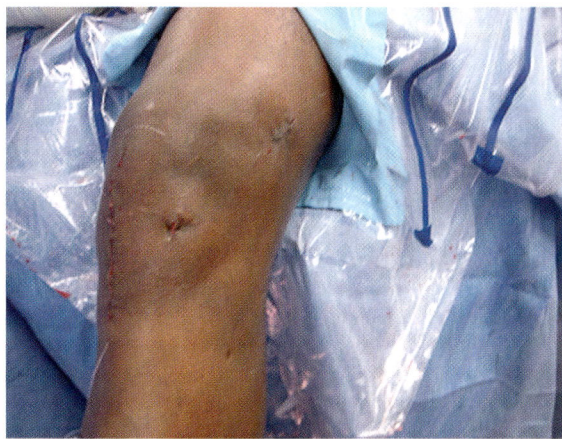

Figure 42-15. Closed incisions. The subcuticular closure allows for excellent cosmetic appearance of all incisions.

others do not. This requirement depends on the specific type of screw and its mechanical properties. If a screw requiring tapping is to be used, it is wise to ensure that the sutures in the bone blocks are in such a position that they will not lacerate when tapping.

The femoral interference screw is generally placed first, with the technique dependent on the technique used in drilling the femoral tunnel. If a transtibial or accessory medial portal technique has been used, the femoral interference screw is placed from within the joint in a retrograde manner. First, a small awl is used through a medial portal to create a starting point for the screw between the graft and the edge of the tunnel. A guide wire is then placed via the medial or accessory medial portal into the tunnel next to the graft. A tap is used if needed, followed by insertion of the screw. The distal sutures on the graft should be held to ensure that the graft does not migrate proximally with screw insertion.

In a two-incision ACL reconstruction, the femoral interference screw is inserted from outside to inside in an antegrade manner. This technique eliminates the possibility that the tap or interference screw could cut the graft, as has been reported with retrograde interference screw placement.[2] A tap is used if needed, followed by insertion of the screw. It is critical to provide tension on the proximal sutures to avoid distal migration of the graft during screw placement.

After femoral fixation is achieved, the tibial screw can be secured under tension. The ideal tension is unknown at present. Some surgeons prefer to cycle the knee a few times prior to fixation; others do not. Graft fixation can be performed in full extension or in 20 degrees of flexion. When fixing the tibial side, the tibia should be translated maximally posteriorly against the PCL. The tibial screw is then inserted with or without a guide wire. Care is again taken not to push the graft proximally into the tunnel because this error could result in a lax graft. Once the graft is fixed, the knee should be ranged from hyperextension to 100 degrees, a Lachman test performed on the table, and the position and tension of the graft checked arthroscopically to ensure that no impingement occurs at any degree of flexion (Fig. 42-14).

Closure

After graft placement and fixation are satisfactory, the knee is rinsed and drained and all open incisions are irrigated.

Bone graft is then placed in the patellar harvest defect and any remaining graft is placed in the tibial defect. The patellar tendon is closed with interrupted, figure-of-eight heavy absorbable sutures, with the knee bent at 90 degrees. The transverse fascia over the patellar tendon may be left open or closed; however, if one elects not to close the patellar tendon defect, it is recommended that this fascia be closed. The iliotibial band can be closed with interrupted absorbable sutures or left open according to surgeon preference. The skin is closed with inverted, absorbable, deep dermal sutures and a subcuticular running suture (Fig. 42-15). Drains are not routinely used during this procedure and efforts should be taken to maintain good hemostasis, except for unavoidable bone bleeding.

Pearls and Pitfalls

Pearls

1. The key to obtaining a reproducible ACL reconstruction is to have adequate visualization of the notch and native femoral and tibial ACL attachments for placement of the femoral and tibial tunnels.
2. Excellent visualization of the patellar tendon is the key to an atraumatic harvest of the patellar tendon bone blocks. Care must be taken to avoid compression injury to the articular surfaces of the patella and trochlea and to avoid damage to the remaining tibial attachment of the patellar tendon on the tibia.
3. There are many commercially available guide systems and templates. The surgeon should be familiar with the nuances, strengths, and weaknesses of the guide system they choose so that they can confirm a reproducible, anatomic tunnel position.
4. It is recommended that the patellar bone block be more trapezoidal in profile, which would reduce the depth of the harvested bone and potentially minimize any possibility of intra-articular violation or extra stress at the donor site. At the tibial site, the graft should be more triangular, which maximizes the remaining bone deep to the medial and lateral portions of the remaining tendon so as to maintain a sturdy attachment.
5. Adequate confirmation of each step is required so that the optimal position and fixation is maintained:

- For example, one should confirm the accurate position of guide pins for the femur and tibia.
- Second, one should confirm that there is adequate lateral and posterior bone for the femoral tunnel.
- Third, one should confirm after drilling these tunnels that the intra-articular openings are chamfered and that the graft passer passes through the notch without impingement throughout range of motion.
- Fourth, once the graft is passed and fixed in the femur, isometry is checked.
- Fifth, after tibial fixation, stability is checked by a manual Lachman test as well as arthroscopic inspection for impingement and tension.

6. When placing metal or bioabsorbable interference screws, the specific gap sizes of the tunnel, screw width and length, and fixation of the graft without twisting or pushing it into the tunnel are critical.
7. Finally, when harvesting the patellar bone block, at least 1 cm of proximal patella should be preserved and bone graft should be placed at the patella defect to provide complete healing of the patella and decrease the risk of iatrogenic patellar fracture.

Pitfalls

1. Adequate confirmation of the guide pins should be visualized arthroscopically as well as through the incisions to ensure that the proper position is achieved and maintained. If not, these pins should be moved by various methods (Gatling gun or fixed parallel pin guides).
2. Notchplasty should be performed first when needed for visualization and later to avoid impingement.
3. Avoidance of intra-operative fracture of the patella or damage to the patellar block or patellar tendon requires meticulous attention to detail, the use of an oscillating saw, and gentle harvesting of the graft from the bone, as noted.
4. Graft fixation is achieved when the sutures are held, gap sizes are understood, and properly sized screws are inserted without pushing the bone block into the tunnel or rotating the block.
5. Prior to incision closure, consideration should be given to thorough irrigation of the open wounds to minimize potential for infection.

POSTOPERATIVE MANAGEMENT AND REHABILITATION

The goals after reconstructing the ACL are to manage pain, decrease swelling, restore range of motion, gain quadriceps control and strength, participate in neuromuscular education, and engage in sport-specific retraining. Our practice is to allow immediate weight bearing as tolerated on the operative extremity with crutches used until the patient is able to walk without a limp. We do not currently use a brace following surgery, although bracing should be considered if patients have undergone regional anesthesia that could lead to postoperative quadriceps weakness. Factors that modify the typical ACL reconstruction protocol include concurrent performance of meniscus repair or articular cartilage stimulating procedures, such as microfracture. The rehabilitation protocol should be adjusted and be in sync with the surgeon's operative technique, rehabilitation specialist's skill, and patient factors, including age, compliance, and level of activity to which the patient plans to return. Randomized trials have demonstrated the safety and efficacy of accelerated rehabilitation protocols following patellar tendon autograft ACL reconstruction.[26]

KEY REFERENCES

Abebe ES, Moorman CT, 3rd, Dziedzic TS, et al: Femoral tunnel placement during anterior cruciate ligament reconstruction: an in vivo imaging analysis comparing transtibial and 2-incision tibial tunnel-independent techniques. Am J Sports Med 37:1904–1911, 2009.

Biau DJ, Tournoux C, Katsahian S, et al: Bone-patellar tendon-bone autografts versus hamstring autografts for reconstruction of anterior cruciate ligament: meta-analysis. BMJ 332:995–1001, 2006.

Busam ML, Provencher MT, Bach BR, Jr: Complications of anterior cruciate ligament reconstruction with bone-patellar tendon-bone constructs: care and prevention. Am J Sports Med 36:379–394, 2008.

DuMontier TA, Metcalf MH, Simonian PT, Larson RV: Patella fracture after anterior cruciate ligament reconstruction with the patellar tendon: a comparison between different shaped bone block excisions. Am J Knee Surg 14:9–15, 2001.

George MS, Huston LJ, Spindler KP: Endoscopic versus rear-entry ACL reconstruction: a systematic review. Clin Orthop Relat Res 455:158–161, 2007.

Hame SL, Markolf KL, Hunter DM, et al: Effects of notchplasty and femoral tunnel position on excursion patterns of an anterior cruciate ligament graft. Arthroscopy 19:340–345, 2003.

Ibrahim SA, Al-Kussary IM, Al-Misfer AR, et al: Clinical evaluation of arthroscopically assisted anterior cruciate ligament reconstruction: patellar tendon versus gracilis and semitendinosus autograft. Arthroscopy 21:412–417, 2005.

Kaseta MK, DeFrate LE, Charnock BL, et al: Reconstruction technique affects femoral tunnel placement in ACL reconstruction. Clin Orthop Relat Res 466:1467–1474, 2008.

Lee MC, Seong SC, Lee S, et al: Vertical femoral tunnel placement results in rotational knee laxity after anterior cruciate ligament reconstruction. Arthroscopy 23:771–778, 2007.

Liden M, Ejerhed L, Sernert N, et al: Patellar tendon or semitendinosus tendon autografts for anterior cruciate ligament reconstruction: a prospective, randomized study with a 7-year follow-up. Am J Sports Med 35:740–748, 2007.

Loh JC, Fukuda Y, Tsuda E, et al: Knee stability and graft function following anterior cruciate ligament reconstruction: comparison between 11 o'clock and 10 o'clock femoral tunnel placement. 2002 Richard O'Connor Award paper. Arthroscopy 19:297–304, 2003.

Roe J, Pinczewski LA, Russell VJ, et al: A 7-year follow-up of patellar tendon and hamstring tendon grafts for arthroscopic anterior cruciate ligament reconstruction: differences and similarities. Am J Sports Med 33:1337–1345, 2005.

Sajovic M, Vengust V, Komadina R, et al: A prospective, randomized comparison of semitendinosus and gracilis tendon versus patellar tendon autografts for anterior cruciate ligament reconstruction: five-year follow-up. Am J Sports Med 34:1933–1940, 2006.

Scopp JM, Jasper LE, Belkoff SM, Moorman CT, 3rd. The effect of oblique femoral tunnel placement on rotational constraint of the knee reconstructed using patellar tendon autografts. Arthroscopy 20:294–299, 2004.

Thompson J, Harris M, Grana WA: Patellofemoral pain and functional outcome after anterior cruciate ligament reconstruction: an analysis of the literature. Am J Orthop 34:396–399, 2005.

Van Grinsven S, van Cingel RE, Holla CJ, van Loon CJ: Evidence-based rehabilitation following anterior cruciate ligament reconstruction. Knee Surg Sports Traumatol Arthrosc 18:1128–1144, 2010.

Zaffagnini S, Marcacci M, Lo Presti M, et al: Prospective and randomized evaluation of ACL reconstruction with three techniques: a clinical and radiographic evaluation at 5 years follow-up. Knee Surg Sports Traumatol Arthrosc 14:1060–1069, 2006.

Full references for this chapter can be found on www.expertconsult.com.

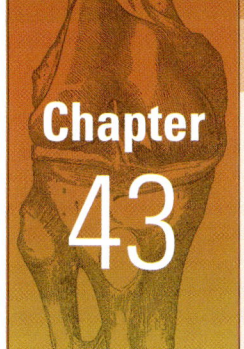

Chapter 43

Anterior Cruciate Ligament Reconstruction With Hamstring Tendons

Leo Pinczewski, Lucy Salmon, Shinichi Maeno, and Catherine Hui

The evolution of anterior cruciate ligament (ACL) reconstructive surgery has been from open surgery to arthroscopy-assisted to current all-arthroscopic techniques. There are many options in the armamentarium of the surgeon treating these injuries regarding graft choice, fixation, and surgical technique.

Graft options include hamstring tendon autograft, patellar tendon autograft, and allograft. The ideal graft should be easy to harvest with minimal donor site morbidity, have the strength of the native ACL, incorporate quickly, and allow rigid fixation to enable early mobilization and rehabilitation. Most surgeons prefer autograft because of ready availability, decreased cost, and faster graft incorporation and because of the risk of disease transmission associated with the use of allograft.[17,20,36] Historically, patellar tendon autograft is the gold standard; however, because of the associated complications related to donor site morbidity,[88,90,95] many surgeons are now using hamstring tendon autografts.

Biomechanical advantages of hamstring tendon grafts include increased strength, stiffness, and larger cross-sectional area for vascular ingrowth and ligamentization (Table 43-1).[37,79,80,108]

An understanding of the process of graft healing is required to manage the reconstructed ACL safely through the rehabilitation process. Over time, the graft undergoes a process of remodeling and revascularization, referred to as ligamentization.[5] Most studies on graft healing have been conducted using various animal models.[35,87] Few studies have examined the process of ligamentization in humans and the true process is not completely understood. Several authors have found, using core biopsy of traumatically failed hamstring autografts, that complete graft integration with the surrounding bone occurs, with the presence of Sharpey-like fibers as early as 12 weeks with interference screw fixation.[78,82] Other biopsies have shown the graft to be enveloped with a layer of granulation tissue and that macroscopically and histologically, no direct connection between the tendon graft and the bone could be found. There are no neural elements in the reconstructed ACL[9] and some have suggested that a normal ligament never forms after ACL reconstruction.[32,68]

There have been several well-conducted prospective studies and meta-analyses comparing the results of hamstring and patellar tendon autografts. The results of these studies suggest that a functionally stable knee is achieved in more than 95% of patients with hamstring tendon or patellar tendon autograft ACL reconstructions.[30] The most consistent difference between the two graft options in these studies is increased kneeling and anterior knee pain* and greater loss of postoperative extension† with patellar tendon reconstructions. Over the short term, the hamstring tendon graft has been associated with tendon discomfort for up to 6 to 8 weeks after surgery, weakness with high knee flexion, and greater laxity.[6,22,28] The issue of increased laxity seemed to be related to inadequate fixation, which has subsequently been resolved with alternate fixation devices. Over the long term, the patellar tendon graft may be associated with higher rates of radiographic degenerative change. In studies in which fixation, surgical technique, and rehabilitation are standardized, the incidence of ACL graft rupture is equivalent with hamstring and patellar tendon autograft.[92,103] It is generally well accepted that reconstruction of the ACL with hamstring tendon autograft is effective for restoring anteroposterior laxity to the knee, has good subjective outcomes, and allows a high proportion of patients to return to their desired activity level.

For immediate postoperative mobilization, the ACL graft-fixation construct should be strong enough to withstand the everyday forces required for walking and activities of daily living, which has been estimated to be up to 450 N.[40,44,74,79] Currently, there are a multitude of fixation options for hamstring tendon autografts. These are classified into aperture versus suspensory fixation and metal versus bioabsorbable materials. There are several considerations when selecting a fixation device. First, the process of graft healing and maturation is poorly understood, as is the effect of rehabilitation protocols on these processes. Second, most studies on fixation devices and their biomechanical properties have been conducted on animal or cadaver models and in vivo results may differ. Commonly used fixation devices and their biomechanical properties are summarized in Table 43-2.

Aperture fixation with interference screws is commonly used in ACL surgery. Soft tissue interference screws with blunt threads were designed for hamstring tendon grafts to enable compression of the graft against the tunnel wall without graft damage. Improved initial soft tissue graft fixation strength can be achieved with the use of a longer[13] and larger diameter screw.[113] Proper graft-tunnel fit with the tunnel sized 0.5 mm larger than the graft diameter also improves fixation strength.[104] Nurmi and colleagues[81] have found that there is no difference in initial fixation strength between compaction and extraction drilling using a porcine model. However, extraction drilling often leaves sharp bony edges within the tunnel that can damage the graft on insertion, and compaction drilling may still be beneficial to avoid graft damage. Concentric or eccentric screw placement does not influence initial fixation properties.[97,99]

Suspensory fixation has been reported to result in an increased incidence of tunnel widening compared with aperture fixation.[11,43] The exact mechanism of this is unknown, but proposed reasons include a greater distance between the fixation point and tunnel aperture, leading to micromotion between the graft and bone. Clinical studies have shown, however, that there is no difference between aperture and suspensory fixation methods with respect to physical examination, instrumented

---

*References 8, 25, 26, 29, 62, 85, 88, 95, and 117.
†References 1, 26, 27, 34, 48, and 83.

Table 43-1 Biomechanical Characteristics of Various Anterior Cruciate Ligament Graft Types

Graft Type	Ultimate Tensile Load (N)	Stiffness (N/mm)	Cross-Sectional Area (mm²)
Native ACL[116]	2160	242	50
10-mm patellar tendon autograft[115]	1784	210	45
Four-strand gracilis and semitendinosus hamstring tendon autograft[37]	4090	776	53

Table 43-2 Commonly Used Fixation Options in Hamstring Tendon Anterior Cruciate Ligament Reconstruction

Implant	Manufacturer*	Type of Fixation (A or S)	Material	Ultimate Strength (N)	Stiffness (N/m)	Slippage Under Cyclic Load
Metal interference screw (BPTB)	—	A	—	559[60]	74[60]	—
Femoral Devices						
RCI screw	Smith & Nephew	A	Ti	546[57]	68[57]	3.9 mm after 1500 cycles of 200 N[57]
BioScrew	ConMed Linvatec	A	PLLA	589[59]	66[59]	4.0 mm after 1500 cycles of 200 N[59]
Endopearl + BioScrew	ConMed Linvatec	A	PLLA	659[114]	42	
Endobutton CL	Smith & Nephew	S	Ti	864[2] 1086[59]	79	1.75 mm after 100 sec of 250 N cyclic loading[2]; 3.9 mm after 1500 cycles of 200 N[59]
Cross pin	DePuy Mitek	S	Ti	35 mm: 1003 70 mm: 1604[21]	—	—
RigidFix (bioabsorbable cross pin)	DePuy Mitek	S	PLLA	639[118] 868[59]	226[118] 77[59]	6.02 mm after 100 sec of 250 N cyclic loading[2]; 3.7 mm after 1500 cycles of 200 N[59]
TransFix	Arthrex	S	Ti	1470	207	2.8 mm after 1000 cycles of 150 N[70]
Bio-TransFix	Arthrex	S	PLLA	746[2] 1492[70]	210[70]	1.4 mm after 100 sec of 250 N cyclic loading[2]; 2.6 mm after 1000 cycles of 150 N[70]
Bone mulch screw	Biomet	S	Ti	1112[59]	115[59]	2.2 mm after 1500 cycles of 200 N[59]
Sutures tied over a 6.5-mm screw post	—	S		573[107]	18[107]	
Tibial Devices						
Intrafix	Mitek	A	Ti	1332[58]	223[58]	1.5 mm after 1500 cycles of 200 N[58]
WasherLoc	Biomet	S	Ti	975[58] 905[67]	87[58] 200[67]	3.2 mm after 1500 cycles of 200 N[58]; 0.6 mm at 250 N; 2.0 mm at 500 N[67]
AO washer-screw + sutures around screw post	Synthes	S	—	442[67]	60[67]	4.9 mm at 500 N
RCI screw	Smith & Nephew	A	Ti	350[67]	226[67]	1.8 mm at 150 N; 3.7 mm at 500 N[67]
BioScrew	Arthrex	A	PLLA	647[16] 612[58]	65[16] 91[58]	4.1 mm after 1500 cycles of 200 N
Double soft tissue staple	—	S	—	785[67]	118[67]	3.3 mm at 500 N[67]

A, Aperture; *BPBT*, bone-patellar tendon-bone; *PLLA*, poly-L-lactic acid; *S*, suspensory; *Ti*, titanium.
*Arthrex, Naples, Fla; Biomet, Warsaw, Ind; DePuy Mitek, Raynham, Mass; Synthes, West Chester, Pa.

testing, Lysholm, Tegner, and International Knee Documentation Committee (IKDC) scores.[11,65,100]

Graft fixation is also affected by bone mineral density.[13,18,40] The bone mineral density of the proximal tibia is lower than that of the distal femur. Hill and associates[42] have found that females undergoing ACL reconstruction with hamstring tendon autograft and 7- × 25-mm interference screw fixation may develop increased postoperative laxity compared with their male counterparts; they recommended supplemental

tibial fixation with a staple, which successfully restored normal laxity at the expense of increased kneeling pain at 2-year follow-up. Older patients are another subgroup of patients with decreased bone mineral density for whom supplemental tibial fixation may need to be considered.

There has been a recent trend toward using bioabsorbable fixation devices. Possible advantages of bioabsorbable devices include easier revision surgery, minimal interference with future imaging such as magnetic resonance imaging (MRI),[40,76] and decreased risk of graft laceration during insertion of bioabsorbable interference screws.[14,119] Ultimately, the benefit of bioabsorbable screws is resorption of the device, with subsequent bony replacement of the device in the tunnel. Unfortunately, this has not consistently been the case in vivo. Studies have found no evidence of screw resorption up to 4 years postoperatively and no evidence of new bone formation in the tunnels.[10,86,111] Other disadvantages of bioabsorbable devices include synovitis[12,31] and device breakage, leading to loss of fixation, a potentially catastrophic complication.[19] With current software and imaging techniques, the metal artifacts from titanium screws can largely be eliminated. If revision is required, a small, screw-shaped femoral defect is superior to a larger fibrous defect or a partly resorbed bioscrew with remnant material adhering to the tunnel wall. Thus, our preferred technique is to use metallic interference screw fixation of hamstring tendon autografts, which have had excellent clinical success for over 15 years.

When assessing the outcome of ACL reconstruction, it is imperative to acknowledge that variations in the surgical technique and selection of patients have a direct effect on outcomes. The surgical technique described in this chapter, using the anteromedial portal and a four-strand hamstring tendon autograft, has been used in an ongoing prospective study of 200 patients with an isolated ACL injury since 1994. A summary of the 7-year outcome of 200 patients and the 10-year outcome of a subgroup of 90 patients from this group is shown in Table 43-3.[83,94] Ongoing longitudinal assessment is continuing, and we are currently collecting the 15-year outcomes.

Successful ACL reconstruction relies on anatomic placement of the graft. The ACL is intricately involved in knee kinematics and proper graft placement is needed to ensure knee function and stability. Recreating a functional ACL graft requires both the graft within the tunnel and the tunnel itself to be in an anatomic position.

Corry and coworkers[22] have found a left- to right-sided difference in knee laxity measurement. It was hypothesized that this difference is related to graft rotation during femoral screw insertion. With a standard screw, clockwise graft rotation occurs, leading to a posterior final graft position in left knees but a relatively anterior final graft position in right knees. This was improved with the use of a reverse thread screw for right-sided ACL reconstructions.[75]

Improper tunnel placement is one of the most common, yet avoidable, reasons for early graft failure.* Single-incision arthroscopic ACL reconstruction was introduced and popularized using transtibial femoral tunnel drilling.[73] When constrained by the tibial tunnel, proper placement of the femoral tunnel can be more difficult to achieve reproducibly and often results in vertical graft placement, leading to residual anterolateral rotatory instability.[7,41,54] Subsequent research has confirmed that lower, more anatomic, tunnel placement in the lateral femoral condyle results in increased rotational stability of the knee, with elimination of the pivot shift phenomenon.[38,50,53,64]

The low anteromedial portal technique was first described by the senior author (LP) and has been used since 1989. It has recently gained popularity because of recognition of the importance of femoral tunnel placement and the advent of double-bundle ACL reconstruction techniques.[106,120] The principle of the low anteromedial portal technique is drilling of the femoral tunnel independent of, and before, drilling the tibial tunnel, allowing the tunnels to be placed within their respective ACL footprints.[54] Another advantage of this technique is improved visualization. In the transtibial technique, once the tibial tunnel is drilled, the irrigation solution escapes through this tunnel, decreasing the intra-articular pressure and obscuring visualization required for femoral tunnel placement.

The key to successful femoral drilling via the anteromedial portal requires that the knee be flexed to 120 degrees at the time of drilling and screw insertion (see Fig. 43-5). This helps prevent posterior wall blowout.[39] A low central anteromedial portal, 1 cm proximal to the medial joint line, helps prevent injury to the medial femoral condyle during femoral tunnel drilling and screw insertion[105] and allows an anterior orientation to the femoral tunnel direction.

Tunnel placement, assessed postoperatively with routine radiographs, is one of the greatest advances in ACL reconstructive surgery. The intended tunnel position is determined arthroscopically from intraoperative landmarks. The information that can be obtained from routine anteroposterior (AP) and lateral radiographs of the knee allows the surgeon to correlate perceived intraoperative tunnel placement to an objective measure and to learn the subtle variations in intraoperative anatomy between patients. Without this feedback, improvement in surgical technique is difficult.

Successful results 7 years after surgery are strongly associated with the radiologic position of the tunnels. The center of the femoral tunnel should be located 86% posteriorly along Blumensaat's line and, on the AP view, it should be at a distance of 43% lateral to the lateral femoral epicondyle. Anterior placement of the femoral tunnel is associated with adverse clinical outcomes as a result of excessive constraint, leading to loss of movement or elongation of the graft with cyclic loading. The tibial tunnel should be centered 48%

Table 43-3 7- and 10-year Outcomes of Isolated Anterior Cruciate Ligament Reconstruction*

Parameter	OUTCOME	
	7-year	10-year
No. of patients reviewed	165/200	86/90
ACL graft rupture (%)	11	13
Contralateral ACL rupture (%)	6	10
Mean KT-1000 (mm)	1.6	1.6
Lachman grade 0 (%)	75	79
Grade 0 pivot (%)	85	86
Normal or nearly normal IKDC range of motion grade (%)	99	98
Lysholm median	95	89
Patients able to hop >90% of contralateral limb (%)	79	80
No knee-related decrease in activity (%)	89	89
Overall IKDC grade A or B (%)	83	83
Grade A radiograph (%)	83	81

*Using four-strand hamstring tendon graft, interference screw fixation, and anteromedial portal.

*References 3, 15, 23, 39, 49, 55, 71, and 101.

posteriorly along the tibial plateau on the lateral radiograph. Placement of the tibial tunnel center 50% or more posteriorly is associated with loss of knee flexion and increased incidence of graft rupture. More anterior placement is associated with graft impingement and decreased range of motion. In the coronal plane, the tibial tunnel should be centered 47% across the width of the tibial plateau from the medial cortex. More lateral placement is associated with impingement of the graft, whereas medial placement will result in loss of flexion. The graft inclination angle should be measured from a 30-degree weight-bearing posteroanterior radiograph. This angle is subtended by a line connecting the medial wall of the femoral tunnel and the medial wall of the tibial tunnel and a line perpendicular to the tibial plateau[84] (see Fig. 43-8).

SURGICAL TECHNIQUE

Management of ACL injury involves preoperative, operative, and postoperative considerations. The surgical technique and its rationale described in this chapter has been used by the senior author (LP) in over 7500 hamstring tendon ACL reconstructions.

Timing of Surgery

It is now well accepted that ACL reconstruction should not be performed until the knee has recovered from the acute injury—after the effusion has resolved and almost full pain-free range of motion has been achieved. Early intervention should only be considered in the acutely locked knee caused by a displaced bucket handle meniscal tear; however, most patients with fixed flexion deformity have a medial ligament strain preventing terminal extension, rather than a bucket handle tear of the meniscus, which is extremely rare in an acute, first-time cruciate ligament injury.[51]

Preoperative Considerations

The evolution of ACL reconstructive surgery, advent of day surgery, and anesthetic technique have resulted in this operation being an elective outpatient procedure. All patients receive antibiotic prophylaxis. The most common bacteria causing infection are coagulase-negative staphylococci and *Staphylococcus aureus.*[52,110] Coagulase-negative staphylococci are often resistant to first-generation cephalosporins but are susceptible to vancomycin. Accordingly, patients receive 1 g vancomycin and 2 g of a cephalosporin IV 1 hour prior to induction of anesthesia for prophylaxis against these common bacteria. We understand that this antibiotic regimen is controversial; however, using this antibiotic regimen, our infection rate has dropped to less than 0.2%. Vancomycin resistance has never been reported using the antibiotic in this manner.

Positioning and Examination

Following induction of anesthesia, the patient is positioned supine on the operating table lying close to the edge of the table on the operative side. A tourniquet is placed high on the thigh and inflated after the limb is exsanguinated and a straight leg raise is performed to stretch the hamstrings. The knee is positioned at 70 degrees of flexion using a foot rest and a lateral thigh post (Fig. 43-1). The foot rest is placed at

the end of the operating table, which allows the surgeon to stand at the foot of the table to harvest the graft, rather than leaning over the limb toward the center of the table.

The knee is examined for range of motion and ligamentous stability with the Lachman, pivot shift, and anterior and posterior drawer tests and varus and valgus stability at 0 and 30 degrees of flexion; tests for posterolateral rotary instability as required.

Hamstring Tendon Harvest and Graft Preparation

A sound knowledge of the surface anatomy around the knee is imperative for successful graft harvest. The hamstring tendons insert at the pes anserine, 1 cm medial to the tibial tubercle and 1 to 3 cm distal to the tubercle. The gracilis and semitendinosus tendons are harvested through a 2-cm oblique incision centered over the pes anserine to decrease the incidence of injury to the infrapatellar branch of the saphenous nerve (Fig. 43-2). However, until a level of surgical comfort is achieved in harvesting the tendons, a vertical incision, which is extensile, should be used. Although this places the infrapatellar branch of the saphenous nerve at greater risk, it is preferable to an insufficient graft. A vertical skin incision is also recommended for patients in whom palpation of the tendons is difficult or for whom prior trauma or surgery may have created scar tissue about the pes anserine, making a difficult harvest. If palpation of the tendons is difficult, centering the incision three fingerbreadths below the joint line approximates the correct position.

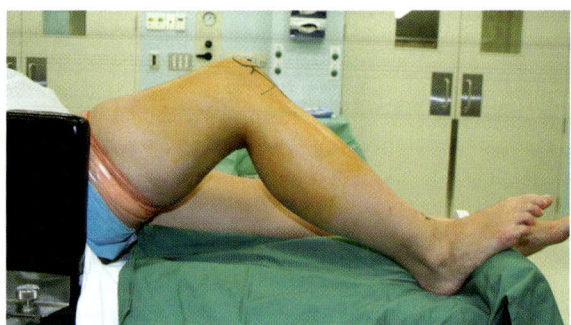

Figure 43-1. Positioning of limb for surgery.

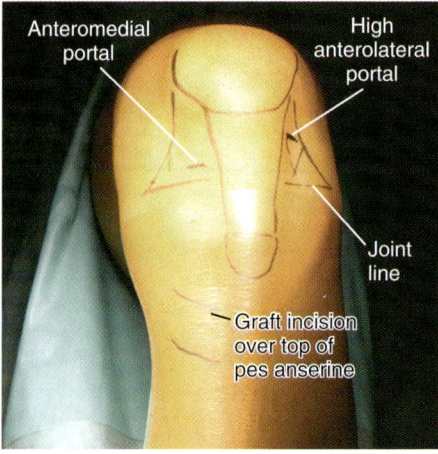

Figure 43-2. Incisions and surface anatomy.

Following incision of the skin and subcutaneous fat, a gauze is used to dissect the fat bluntly from the sartorial fascia. The tendons are palpated and a 1-cm incision is made in the fascia along the superior margin of the sartorius tendon and Metzenbaum scissors are used to enlarge this fascial incision bluntly along the line of the tendon to expose the gracilis and semitendinosus tendons. Until both tendons are clearly and separately identified, neither tendon should be harvested to ensure that the semitendinosus tendon is not mistaken for the gracilis tendon and that there is no inadequate harvest because of lack of attention to the vinculi. The gracilis tendon, being more proximal, can be hooked out of the subsartorial space with a right-angled forceps and is harvested first. It rarely has any significant vinculi. The tendon stripper applied to the tendon should be passed beyond the proximal tibia and then aimed at the muscle origin on the pubic symphysis. A tendon stripper that may be mechanically closed around an attached tendon is used (ConMed Linvatec, Largo, Fla). It is advanced to 22 cm and, by rotating the handle, the graft is amputated from its muscular attachment at this length. With the harvest of the gracilis tendon, the semitendinosus tendon is thus exposed and extreme care must be taken to identify all of its vinculi to prevent partial harvest of the tendon. These pass distally and medially from the body of the tendon toward the medial gastrocnemius fascia.

Using a right-angled forceps to hook around the tendon, providing distal traction, an arthroscopy probe is used to palpate its inferior and medial surface for vinculi. There are usually two vinculi along the semitendinosus tendon, one distally near its insertion and one more proximally.[109] Because the proximal vincula is not usually found more than 12 cm from the distal insertion into the tibia, it can be hooked and pulled out of the wound or divided close to the tendon, depending on its mobility. Once the vinculi have been divided, the tendon stripper is applied and 22 cm of tendon is harvested, with the instrument aimed at the ischial tuberosity. Prior to amputating the tendons, 50 mL of local anesthetic solution (40 mL of 0.5% bupivacaine with adrenaline diluted in 100 mL of normal saline, corrected for weight) is administered along the track of the tendon stripper through multiple percutaneous punctures using a 19-gauge spinal needle (Fig. 43-3). This provides significant postoperative pain relief from the graft harvesting.

The tendons are left attached distally at the pes anserine while the graft is prepared (Fig. 43-4). Muscle tissue is meticulously removed from the tendons, as is the mesotendon tissue near its tibial insertion, which can cause ganglion formation if transplanted into the tibial tunnel. The free ends of the tendons are clipped together at a 22-cm length, folded over two no. 5 nonabsorbable leading sutures back to their tibial insertion, and then whipstitched using a no. 2 Vicryl absorbable suture over a length of 40 mm to form a four-stranded bundle. No. 1 dyed Vicryl is then used to suture 25 mm of tendon on the looped femoral end, which is then sized for diameter. A surgical pen is used to place a mark 30 mm from the end of the graft. The graft is left attached at its distal insertion until it is passed through the joint. This eliminates the risk of losing the graft from the sterile field. Preconditioning of the graft is not performed.

Arthroscopy and Notch Preparation

Proper portal placement is crucial. A high anterolateral portal is made toward the top of the lateral triangle soft spot, adjacent to the lateral border of the patellar tendon. A low anteromedial portal is made 1 cm above the medial joint line (see Fig. 43-2), which allows anterior orientation to the drilling of the femoral tunnel. The position of this portal can be checked with a small-gauge needle to ensure that the anterior horn of the medial meniscus is avoided. Diagnostic arthroscopy is then performed and any meniscal or chondral injuries are addressed prior to starting the reconstruction.

ACL reconstruction begins with the establishment of a field of view by dividing the ligamentum mucosum to allow the fat pad to retract anteriorly. The ACL stump is then débrided as close to the tibia as possible and the lateral wall of the notch is exposed. Notchplasty is not performed except in rare cases of chronic ACL deficiency with osteophytes overgrown in the notch. Notchplasty was popularized in the 1980s and 1990s to improve visualization and to avoid

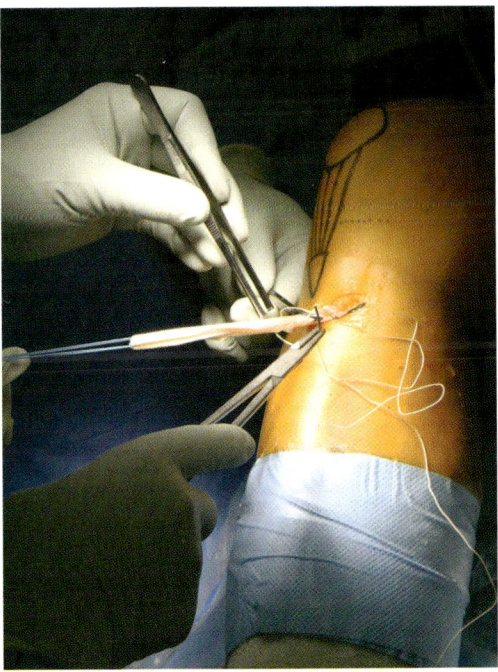

Figure 43-4. Graft preparation.

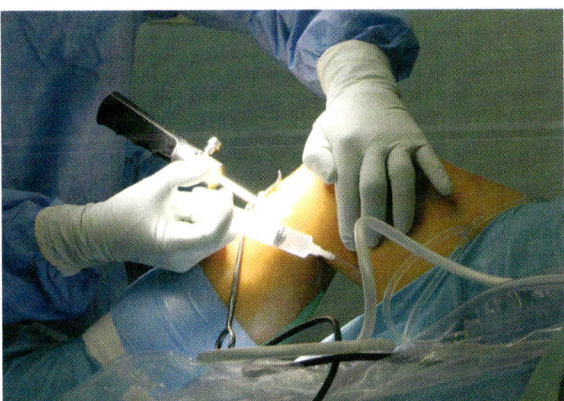

Figure 43-3. Local anesthetic injection along hamstring tendon track.

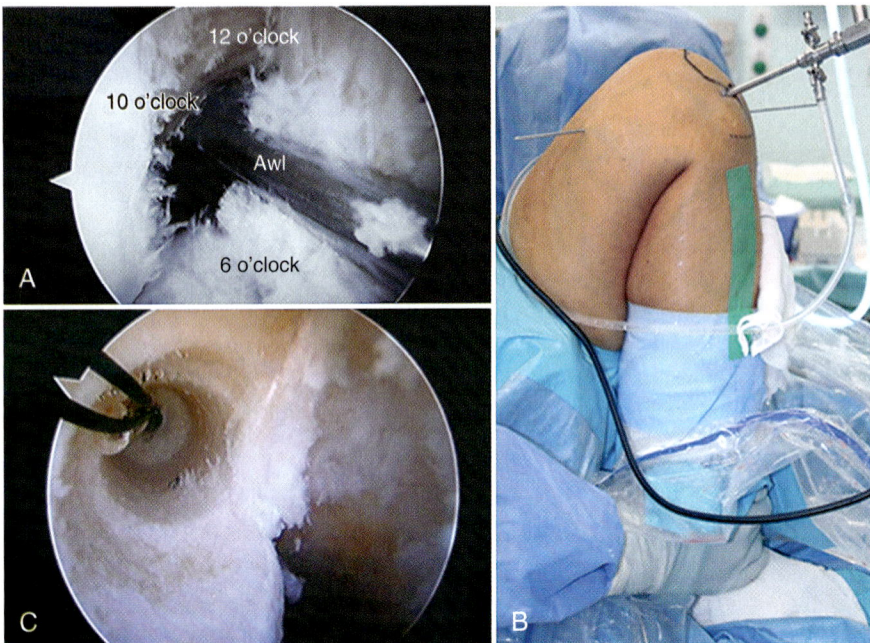

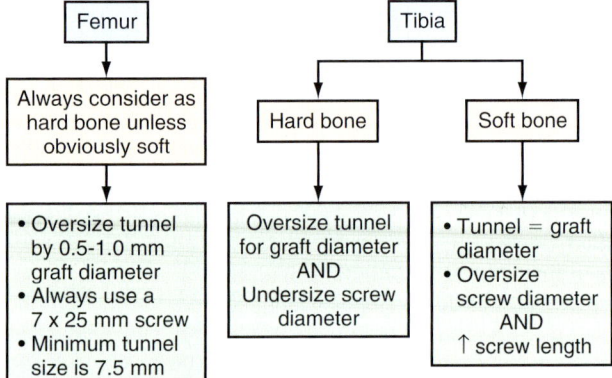

Figure 43-5. **A,** Awl confirmation of femoral tunnel placement on lateral wall of intercondylar notch. **B,** Beath pin inserted through the anteromedial portal, through the femoral tunnel, and exiting the lateral thigh with the knee in full flexion. **C,** Femoral tunnel placement with reference to the posterior cortex of the lateral femoral condyle.

impingement.[56,90] However, with a high anterolateral viewing portal, the femoral ACL footprint can be seen without difficulty and anatomic placement of the graft will prevent impingement.

Exposure of the lateral wall begins at the most inferior, anterior aspect of the notch adjacent to the articular surface of the lateral femoral condyle. A curette is used in a curved, upward sweeping motion to remove the fibrous tissue along the lateral wall to expose the femoral attachment of the ACL. The posterior border of the lateral intercondylar notch is confirmed visually and with an arthroscopic probe. It is critical to avoid mistakenly identifying resident's ridge as the posterior border leading to anterior tunnel placement.

Tunnel Placement

Femoral Tunnel

The femoral tunnel for hamstring tendons should be centered 5 mm anterior to the posterior capsular insertion on the lateral femoral condyle. This should be checked arthroscopically to be at the 10 o'clock position on the clock face in the right knee (2 o'clock in the left knee). A bone awl, inserted through the anteromedial portal into the center of the femoral tunnel site, provides an indication of the position of the proposed tunnel. The arthroscope is then withdrawn to view the lateral wall of the intercondylar notch, which should be aligned vertically along the 6 to 12 o'clock line. The position of the femoral tunnel, as indicated by the awl, can now be confirmed with reference to the roof of the intercondylar notch (Fig. 43-5).

Once the position of the femoral tunnel has been confirmed, the knee is fully flexed and a bicortical femoral tunnel is drilled using a 4.5-mm drill. A 2.4-mm Beath pin is introduced through the anteromedial portal, into the femoral tunnel and out the anterolateral thigh (see Fig. 43-5). The femoral tunnel is then reamed to a 30-mm depth using a cannulated RCI femoral stepped reamer (Smith & Nephew,

Andover, Mass), with a 10-mm aperture to accommodate the head of the screw and graft. The minimum tunnel diameter with a 6.5-mm graft is 7.5 mm with the use of a 7-mm screw. Otherwise, the tunnel should be reamed at a diameter 0.5 to 1 mm greater than the diameter of the graft, depending on the hardness of bone (Fig. 43-6). Care must be taken to avoid damage to the PCL and the femoral articular surfaces with the reamer during this part of the procedure. With the knee still fully flexed, a doubled nylon suture is pulled through the anteromedial portal and out the lateral thigh using the Beath pin. It is then folded on itself and held taut using a hemostat on the anterolateral thigh. This will subsequently be used to pull the leading sutures of the graft.

Tibial Tunnel

The knee is brought out to its resting position at 70 degrees of flexion. The tibial aperture entering the joint should be centered at 5 mm (or half a tunnel diameter) medially along a line that joins the apex of the medial tibial spine to the posterior margin of the anterior horn of the lateral meniscus at its attachment to the tibia. This places the tibial aperture

Figure 43-6. Algorithm for selection of interference screw size.

Femur	Tibia	
Always consider as hard bone unless obviously soft	Hard bone	Soft bone
• Oversize tunnel by 0.5-1.0 mm graft diameter • Always use a 7 × 25 mm screw • Minimum tunnel size is 7.5 mm	Oversize tunnel for graft diameter AND Undersize screw diameter	• Tunnel = graft diameter • Oversize screw diameter AND ↑ screw length

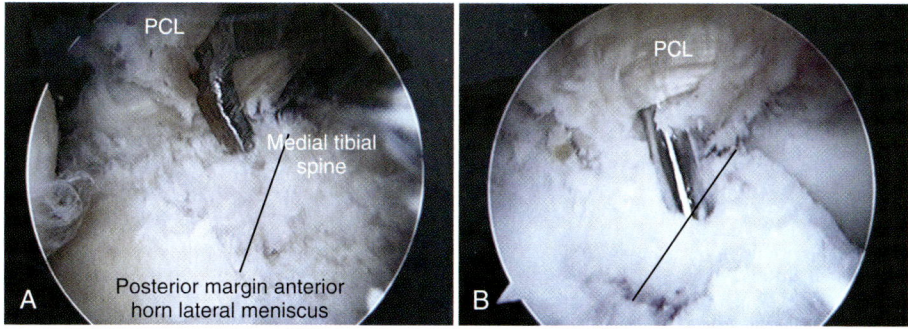

Figure 43-7. Tibial tunnel. **A,** Elbow-aiming tibial guide placement. **B,** Beath pin piercing PCL.

both medial and posterior in the native ACL footprint. It has been shown that placing the graft in the center of the tibial ACL footprint leads to graft impingement.[45] Furthermore, this medial tibial placement and lateral femoral placement creates an obliquity in the coronal plane that has been documented to control rotary stability better.[84] An elbow-aiming ACL tibial guide (Acufex, Smith & Nephew) is placed through the anteromedial portal. A 4.5-mm drill, centered in the graft incision, is used first. A Beath pin is then introduced into the joint and held in place by piercing the PCL with the tip of the pin (Fig. 43-7). A 45-mm tibial tunnel is then drilled using the RCI tibial stepped reamer. The tibial tunnel is drilled at the same diameter as the graft diameter.

Passage of the Graft

With the knee flexed at 70 degrees, the hemostat on the lateral thigh securing the nylon suture is released and a grasping forcep is inserted through the tibial tunnel to bring the looped end of the nylon suture out the tibial tunnel. This nylon loop has now been passed through both tunnels and is used to pass the no. 5 lead sutures from the graft construct, first through the tibial tunnel and then into the femoral tunnel. The tendons are carefully released from the pes anserine and the graft is drawn into the femoral hole until the 30-mm mark on the graft is at the entrance of the femoral tunnel.

Femoral Fixation

A 2.0-mm titanium RCI screw guide wire is introduced through the anteromedial portal. The tip of the guide wire is placed at the femoral tunnel entrance between the anterior edge of the tunnel and the graft, and the knee is then fully flexed to advance the guide wire to its 25-mm mark. A 7- × 25-mm titanium RCI screw is used for all fixations, with a reverse threaded screw used for right-sided femoral tunnels. The screw should be advanced 5 to 10 mm deep into the tunnel aperture such that the head of the screw is not visible once the screwdriver is removed. The knee is then put through a range of motion and the graft is checked to ensure that it does not impinge on the notch. Our algorithm for screw size selection is shown in Figure 43-6.

Graft Tensioning and Tibial Fixation

The graft is tensioned following femoral fixation. With the knee in its resting position at 70 degrees of flexion, tension is applied to the four-stranded graft and its sutures at the external tibial aperture using a hemostat to wind up the sutures and graft exiting the tibial tunnel. The 2.0-mm RCI screw guide wire is then inserted between the graft and the posterior aspect of the distal tibial tunnel. While maintaining tension on the graft with the hemostat, an RCI screw is advanced until the screw captures the graft lightly. The knee is then slowly extended to full hyperextension, allowing any slippage of the bundles to occur, which equalizes bundle tension. With the knee in full hyperextension, the screw is advanced up the tibial tunnel until the head is 5 to 10 mm up the tunnel. The tibial graft is then divided 5 mm longer than the tunnel, allowing a plug of tendon tissue to fill the external tibial aperture, covering the screw head.

The knee is put through a full range of motion and restoration of stability is confirmed with the Lachman, pivot shift, and anterior drawer tests. The joint is irrigated and suctioned of any remaining debris and the proximal lead sutures are removed from the lateral thigh puncture.

Closure

Skin closure is achieved using a subcuticular resorbable suture so that removal is not required. Local anesthetic, 50 mL (40 mL of 0.5% bupivacaine with adrenaline diluted in 100 mL of normal saline, corrected for weight) is infiltrated into the wounds, the surrounding soft tissues, and the vastus medialis muscle prior to closure using a 19-gauge spinal needle. With recent studies confirming the toxicity of local anesthetics to chondrocytes, intra-articular injections are not recommended.[63] Furthermore, clinical experience is that capsular infiltration is far more effective than intra-articular injection for pain relief. A compression dressing is then applied.

POSTOPERATIVE MANAGEMENT

Immediate, full weight-bearing and joint motion are encouraged. An accelerated rehabilitation program, as detailed in Table 43-4, is routinely used. Although initially described for use with patellar tendon autografts, equal success has been shown with this program in four-strand hamstring tendon autografts with rigid fixation.[46,66] The rehabilitation protocol is provided to the patient and treating physical therapist. Patients are recommended to attend physiotherapy starting on postoperative day 1. A wound check is performed at 7 to 10 days following surgery and patients should be walking normally without support at this time. Routine follow-up is

Table 43-4 Rehabilitation Protocol Following Anterior Cruciate Ligament Injury and Hamstring Tendon Reconstruction

Stage	Aims	Goals	Treatment Guidelines
Prehabilitation	Prepare patient for surgery	Full range of motion Pain-free mobile joint Teach simple postoperative exercises	Operating on pain-free mobile joints minimizes complications. May take many months Do not be pressured by patient into early surgery. Preprogramming postoperative rehabilitation is beneficial.
I: Acute recovery (day 1 to 10-14)	Postoperative pain relief and management of soft tissue trauma Wean off crutches and progress to normal gait.	Wound healing Manage graft donor-site morbidity. ↓ swelling Restore full extension (including hyperextension). Establish muscle control.	↓ swelling and pain with ice, elevation, and cocontractions Aim for full range of motion using active and passive techniques. Patella mobilizations Gait retraining with full extension at heel strike Return of coordinated muscle function encouraged with biofeedback Begin quadriceps strengthening as static cocontraction with hamstrings, emphasizing VMO control at various angles of knee flexion. Gentle hamstring stretching to minimize adhesions Active hamstring strengthening begins with static weight-bearing cocontractions and progresses to active free hamstring contractions by day 14. Resisted hamstring strengthening should be avoided for at least 6 wk.
II: Hamstring and quadriceps control (2-6 wk)	Return patient to normal function. Prepare patient for stage III.	Develop good muscle control and early proprioceptive skills. If not done sooner, restore normal gait. Reduce any persistent or recurrent effusion.	Progress cocontractions for muscle control by ↑ repetitions, length of contraction, and more dynamic positions, Gradually introduce gym equipment (e.g., stepper, leg press, minitramp). Hamstring strengthening progresses with ↑ complexity and repetitions; open-chain hamstring exercises are commenced. Watch for hamstring strains. Low-resistance, high-repetition weights aim to ↑ hamstring endurance. Continue with intensive stretching exercises. Eccentric hamstring strengthening is progressed as pain allows at wk 6.
III: Proprioception (6-12 wk)	Improve neuromuscular control and proprioception.	Continue to improve total leg strength. Improve endurance capacity of muscles. Improve confidence.	Progress cocontractions to more dynamic movements (e.g., step lunges, half-squats). Proprioceptive work more dynamic (e.g., lateral stepping, slide board) Can begin jogging in straight lines on the flat Progress resistance on gym equipment (e.g., leg press, hamstring curls). Solo sports (e.g., cycling, jogging, swimming) are usually permitted with little or no restrictions. Open-chain exercises commence (if no patellofemoral symptoms) 40 to 90 degrees, progressing to 10 to 90 degrees by 12 wk.
IV: Sport-specific (12 wk-5 mo)	Prepare to return to sport	Incorporate more sport-specific activities. Introduce agility and reaction time into proprioceptive work. Increase total leg strength. Develop patient confidence.	Progress strength work. Proprioceptive work should include hopping and jumping activities and emphasize good landing technique; incorporate lateral movements. Agility work may include shuttle runs, ball skills, sideways running, skipping. Sport-specific activities (e.g., tennis—lateral step lunges, forward and backward running drills; volleyball, basketball—vertical jumps)
V: Return to sport (5-6 mo)		Return to sport safely and with confidence.	Continue progression of plyometrics and sport specific drills. Return to training and participating in skill exercises. Continue to improve power and endurance. Add PEP* program[33] to warmup to reduce further ACL injury. Complete PEP program for 30 consecutive days prior to return to sport.

*PEP, Prevent injury, enhance performance.

at 6 weeks and 6 months postoperatively. Patients report an inability to detect a difference in their knee joints and have regained full confidence during athletic activities by 18 months.

Routine radiographs are obtained at the first postoperative visit. Tunnel and screw position are scrutinized. Recommended radiologic positions of the tunnels in the coronal and sagittal views are shown in Figure 43-8.[84]

Gilchrist and colleagues[33] have shown that ACL injury may be decreased with the implementation of a specific motor-retraining rehabilitation program.[77] Patients who suffer one ACL injury have a 30% incidence of rupturing their contralateral ACL or the graft.[93] The reported incidence of ACL rupture in a normal athletic population is 1.5% to 1.7%/year.[61,102] If only one in three patients will sustain a

further ACL injury following reconstruction, the addition of these programs to the rehabilitation of ACL-reconstructed patients to reduce this risk is a worthwhile consideration.

COMMON COMPLICATIONS AND THEIR TREATMENT

The common complications of ACL reconstruction using ipsilateral hamstring tendon autograft, treatment options, and strategies for prevention are shown in Table 43-5.

Summary

This technique of endoscopic ACL reconstruction through a low anteromedial portal using a four-strand ipsilateral

Table 43-5 Potential Common Complications of Anterior Cruciate Ligament Reconstruction

Intraoperative Complications	Reported Incidence (%)	Treatment Options	Preventive Strategies
Femoral tunnel blowout	1.2[4]	Suspensory fixation Outside-in femoral screw insertion	Deep knee flexion during femoral tunnel placement
Graft contamination (dropped graft)	1.0[4]	4% chlorhexidine gluconate soak[72]	Leave graft attached to proximal tibia until graft passage.
Graft amputation	6.0[4]	Alternate graft Three-strand graft Suspensory fixation	Careful identification of all vinculi prior to graft amputation Harvest the gracilis tendon first to improve visualization of the semitendinosus.
Screw tunnel divergence	0.6[4]		Use the anteromedial portal.
Bioabsorbable screw breakage	0.9[4]	Alternate fixation device	Use a titanium screw unless contraindicated.
Significant graft rotation around screw during insertion	—	Remove screw and reinsert.	Tension the proximal and distal ends of the graft during screw insertion.
Early Postoperative Complications			
Infection	0.14 to 1.7[110]	Varies according to severity and cultures	Use of antiseptic soap for 2 wk prior to surgery. Antibiotic prophylaxis, including vancomycin. Larger medial portal to allow easy instrument passage
Loss of motion/stiffness (≥5 degrees at 4 wk)	25[69]	Aggressive physiotherapy; MUA if required	Appropriate surgical timing Anatomic graft placement Tension the graft in full hyperextension under axial compression. Accelerate rehabilitation.
Deep vein thrombosis	1.5[24]	Anticoagulant therapy	Immediate weight bearing and early mobilization
Pulmonary embolus	0.2[47]	Anticoagulant therapy	Immediate weight bearing and early mobilization
Late Postoperative Complications			
Tunnel widening	36 to 94,[98,112] depending on fixation	No known clinical implications	Aperture fixation
Cyclops lesion	2 to 3.6[69,83]	Arthroscopic excision of lesion	Anatomic graft placement Look for ACL stump remnant after graft placement.
Traumatic graft failure	1.0/yr[92]	Revision ACL reconstruction	Neuromuscular training program during rehabilitation
Contralateral ACL rupture	1.0/yr[92]	ACL reconstruction	Neuromuscular training program during rehabilitation
Pretibial subcutaneous cyst	2[83]	Removal of tibial screw and ganglion	Filling of tibial aperture with remnant graft material

MUA, Manipulation under anesthesia.

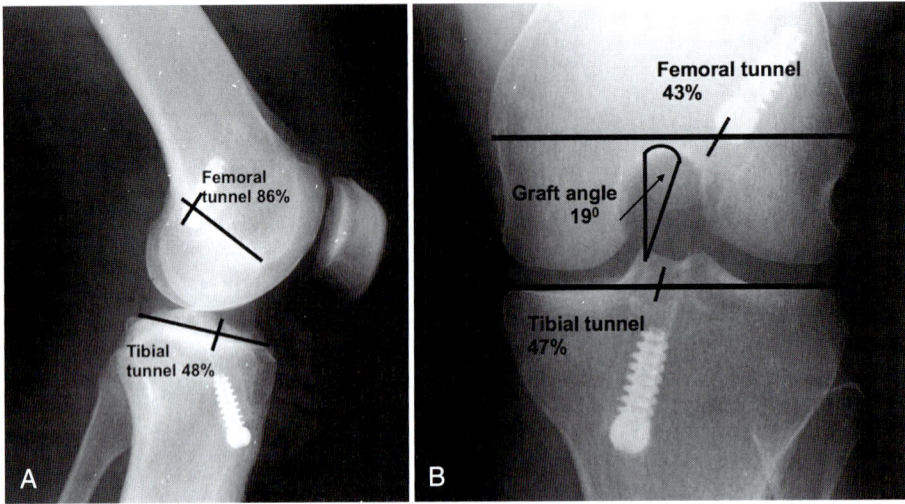

Figure 43-8. Recommended radiologic tunnel positions after ACL reconstruction. **A,** Sagittal view. **B,** Coronal view.

hamstring tendon autograft and aperture fixation allows the femoral and tibial tunnels to be made independently. It is advantageous with respect to allowing more anatomic placement of the graft within the native ACL footprints compared with transtibial procedures. It reliably reestablishes a stable joint and enables immediate weight bearing and accelerated rehabilitation. Although controversy still remains regarding the ideal graft and method of graft fixation, the goals remain as follows: in the short term, to ensure secure, anatomic graft placement, allowing immediate rehabilitation and a stable knee that permits return to sports; and in the long term, prevention of further intra-articular injury and osteoarthritis. Accurate placement of the ACL graft is crucial in obtaining a successful outcome after reconstruction.

KEY REFERENCES

Almazan A, Miguel A, Odor A, et al: Intraoperative incidents and complications in primary arthroscopic anterior cruciate ligament reconstruction. Arthroscopy 22:1211–1217, 2006.

Crawford C, Nyland J, Landes S, et al: Anatomic double bundle ACL reconstruction: a literature review. Knee Surg Sports Traumatol Arthros 15:946–964, 2007.

Freedman KB, D'Amato MJ, Nedeff DD, et al: Arthroscopic anterior cruciate ligament reconstruction: a meta-analysis comparing patellar tendon and hamstring tendon autografts. Am J Sports Med 31:2–11, 2003.

Gilchrist J, Mandelbaum BR, Melancon H, et al: A randomized controlled trial to prevent noncontact anterior cruciate ligament injury in female collegiate soccer players. Am J Sports Med 36:1476–1483, 2008.

Harvey A, Thomas NP, Amis AA: Fixation of the graft in reconstruction of the anterior cruciate ligament. J Bone Joint Surg Br 87:593–603, 2005.

Heming JF, Rand J, Steiner ME: Anatomical limitations of transtibial drilling in anterior cruciate ligament reconstruction. Am J Sports Med 35:1708–1715, 2007.

Kousa P, Järvinen TL, Vihavainen M, et al: The fixation strength of six hamstring tendon graft fixation devices in anterior cruciate ligament reconstruction. Part I: Femoral site. Am J Sports Med 31:174–181, 2003.

Kousa P, Järvinen TLN, Vihavainen M, et al: The fixation strength of six hamstring tendon graft fixation devices in anterior cruciate ligament reconstruction. Part II: Tibial site. Am J Sports Med 31:182–188, 2003.

Lo IKY, Sciore P, Chung M, et al: Local anesthetics induce chondrocyte death in bovine articular cartilage disks in a dose- and duration-dependent manner. Arthroscopy 25:707–715, 2009.

Myers P, Logan M, Stokes A, et al: Bioabsorbable versus titanium interference screws with hamstring autograft in anterior cruciate ligament reconstruction: a prospective randomized trial with 2-year follow-up. Arthroscopy 24:817–823, 2008.

Pinczewski LA, Lyman J, Salmon LJ, et al: A ten-year comparison of hamstring tendon and bone-patellar tendon-bone anterior cruciate ligament reconstructions. A controlled, prospective trial. Am J Sports Med 35:564–574, 2007.

Pinczewski LA, Salmon LJ, Jackson WFM, et al: Radiological landmarks for placement of the tunnels in single-bundle reconstruction of the anterior cruciate ligament. J Bone Joint Surg Br 90:172–179, 2008.

Rue J-PH, Lewis PB, Parameswaran AD, et al: Single-bundle anterior cruciate ligament reconstruction: technique overview and comprehensive review of results. J Bone Joint Surg Am 90(Suppl 4):67–74, 2008.

Salmon LJ, Refshauge KM, Russell VJ, et al: Gender differences in outcome after anterior cruciate ligament reconstruction with hamstring tendon autograft. Am J Sports Med 34:621–629, 2006.

Steiner ME: Independent drilling of tibial and femoral tunnels in anterior cruciate ligament reconstruction. J Knee Surg 22:171–176, 2009.

Full references for this chapter can be found on www.expertconsult.com.

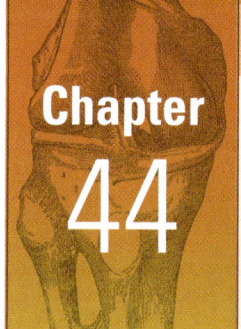

Chapter 44

Anterior Cruciate Ligament Reconstruction With Central Quadriceps Free Tendon Graft

John P. Fulkerson

Since the introduction of the central quadriceps free tendon (CQFT) graft as an alternative for ACL reconstruction,[1] long-term results of this procedure have been reviewed by DeAngelis[2] and Geib.[3] Results were comparable to both hamstring and bone tendon bone anterior cruciate ligament (ACL) reconstruction and to reconstructions with central quadriceps using bone from the patella. The primary benefit of central quadriceps free tendon is that no bone is harvested from the patella, thereby minimizing the risk of fracture. Rehabilitation is rapid,[4] pain medication requirements are less than for other autograft alternatives, and postoperative problems, particularly anterior knee pain, are less common. Central quadriceps as a free tendon graft therefore is a desirable, readily available, low-morbidity autograft alternative for ACL reconstruction.

TECHNIQUE

After establishing that ACL reconstruction is necessary, the CQFT graft is harvested through a short longitudinal incision immediately above the center of the patella. The central quadriceps tendon is about 9 mm thick, almost twice as thick as the patellar tendon, so a graft measuring 7 mm in depth by 9 to 10 mm wide by 7 cm long is consistently possible to be used. After defining the entire quadriceps tendon above the patella, a 9- to 10-mm-wide graft is delineated centrally, leaning somewhat toward the medial side of the quadriceps tendon where the quad tendon is thickest. Using a no. 10 scalpel blade, medial and lateral borders of the graft are defined, cutting to a 7-mm depth (the depth of a no. 10 scalpel blade). A hemostat is then used to define the posterior border of the graft, leaving about 1 mm of quadriceps tendon posteriorly as a border in front of the suprapatellar pouch. The graft then has portions of both rectus and intermedius components of the quadriceps tendon. The hemostat is spread to define the posterior border of the graft and the free tendon autograft is released from the proximal pole of the patella. Using a uterine T clamp to hold the distal end of the tendon graft, it is dissected sharply and bluntly from distal to proximal, preserving all fibers of the quadriceps tendon. At any point during this procedure, whipstitches may be placed in the end of the graft to hold it better. I use two no. 5 sutures at each end. The graft is dissected bluntly and sharply to a distance 7 cm from the proximal patella (Fig. 44-1) and then released at a 7-cm length after which no. 5 whipstitches are placed at the proximal end. At this point, there are two sets of no. 5 sutures (four strands) coming off each end of the graft, and the graft is marked at the levels desired so that at least 2 cm of CQFT graft will be in each socket (Fig. 44-2).

At this point, the notchplasty is completed and both the tibial tunnel and femoral socket are drilled at the appropriate locations. The 8- or 9-mm femoral socket (depending on the graft diameter) is drilled to a depth of 30 mm, after which an EndoButton drill (Smith & Nephew, Andover, Mass) is used to complete a drill hole through the femoral socket, up through the lateral femoral metaphysis, for passage of the EndoButton fixation.

After measuring the depth of the femoral socket and EndoButton tunnel, the sutures at the end of the quadriceps free tendon graft are placed through one of the EndoButton central holes; these are brought back through the other central hole so that they may be tied to the other whipstitch sutures immediately adjacent to the tendon graft. Thus, the knot itself is almost incorporated into the end of the free tendon graft. The length of the sutures to the EndoButton is determined by the total length necessary to allow 2 cm of the CQFT graft to be locked into the femoral socket. If the total tunnel length on the femoral side is 40 mm and the goal is to have 20 mm of tendon graft in the socket, then the length of the sutures would be 20 mm, so that 20 mm of graft would constitute the remaining total of 40 mm in the femoral socket. Using a guide pin, the EndoButton and trailing grafts are delivered into the femoral socket. The lead sutures on the EndoButton are pulled through the lateral cortex of the femur, and the EndoButton is deployed by flipping it using the trailing sutures on the EndoButton. The CQFT graft is thereby fixed securely into the femoral socket that has been appropriately rasped and prepared for the graft.

On the tibial side, I prefer a biointerference screw placed on the anterior aspect of the graft. After cycling the graft thoroughly, the screw is placed over a guide pin and recessed back from the knee joint by about 5 mm, depending on the graft length (Fig. 44-3). I recommend using a biointerference screw that is the same diameter as the tunnel diameter. In most cases, both the femoral and tibial tunnels measure 8 or 9 mm in diameter, just enough to accommodate the graft snugly. For softer bone, the sutures can be tied over a ligament button as back-up fixation at the tunnel aperture.

DOUBLE-BUNDLE RECONSTRUCTION USING QUADRICEPS FREE TENDON

If a surgeon wants to use quadriceps free tendon for double-bundle ACL reconstruction, it is well suited because the quadriceps tendon graft has two components—the rectus femoris and the vastus intermedius. My approach to this has been to drill the two femoral sockets (Fig. 44-4) but use one tibial tunnel. Figure 44-5 shows the graft preparation for this construct. In my opinion, the safest and easiest way to use a CQFT graft for a double-bundle ACL reconstruction is to pass the two separate components (rectus and intermedius) of the CQFT graft into the respective sockets for anteromedial and posterolateral bundles and then tie the sutures together on the lateral femur. This allows for balanced tension in the two bands on flexion and extension of the knee. I have

403

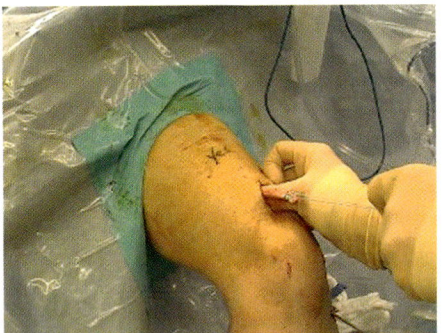

Figure 44-1. Short anterior incision to allow harvest of the central quadriceps free tendon graft (without bone).

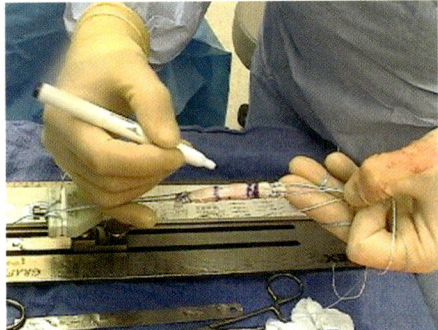

Figure 44-2. Preparation of a roughly 7-cm-long graft with whip-stitches at both ends and reference lines marked.

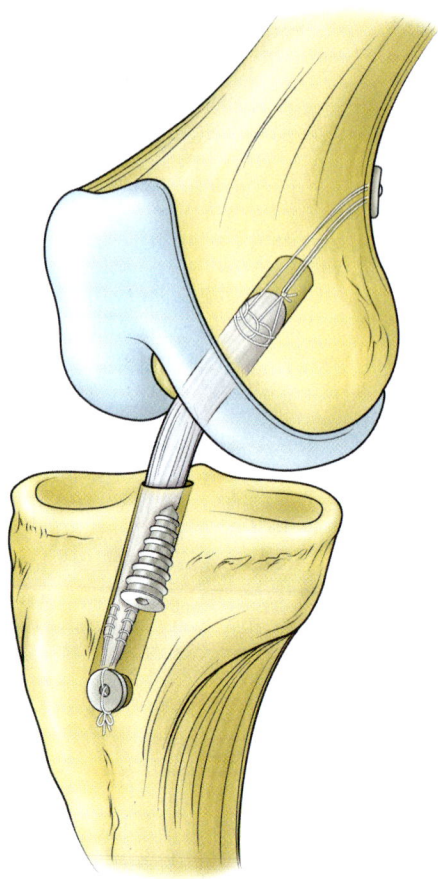

Figure 44-3. Final construct with EndoButton fixation on the femur and biointerference screw plus optional button for tibial fixation.

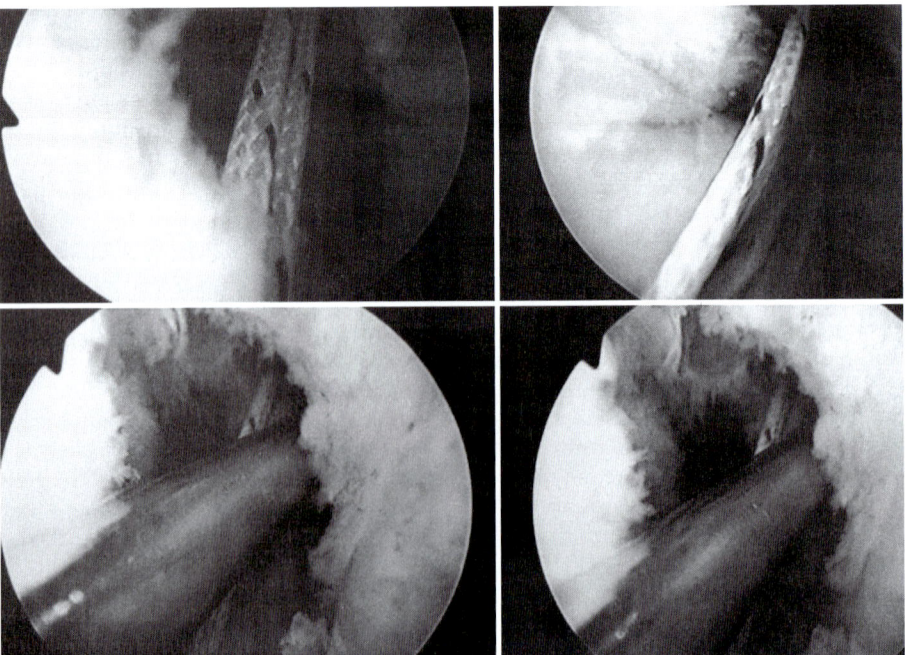

Figure 44-4. Arthroscopic image of dual femoral tunnels prior to graft passage.

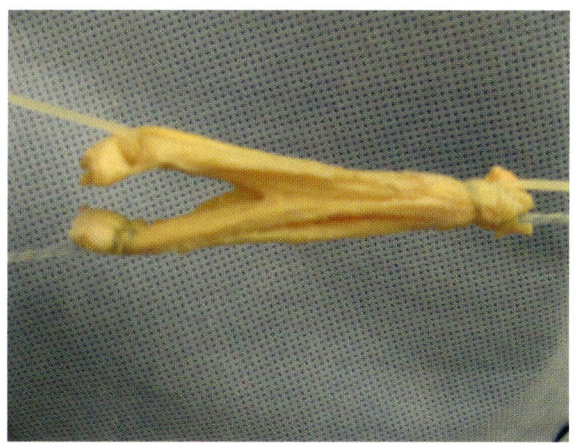

Figure 44-5. Double femoral bundle graft construct from central quadriceps free tendon, split into its respective portions from the rectus and intermedius.

no experience with separate tunnels on the tibial side using quadriceps tendon and recommend a biointerference screw on the tibial side, as in the single-bundle reconstruction. Using a button for fixation on the tibial side would allow for controlled rotation of the graft within the socket as necessary to produce orientation of the anteromedial and posterolateral bundles appropriately.

REHABILITATION

Immediate range of motion and full extension are achieved as soon as possible following CQFT ACL reconstruction. Partial weight bearing is initiated with crutches and a home exercise program. At 2 weeks, physical therapy begins for further motion, weight bearing, and closed-chain strengthening. Open-chain exercises begin at 8 weeks postoperatively. Effort should be made to control hemarthrosis and effusion vigorously. Many patients will start straight-ahead running 3 to 4 months after quadriceps free tendon ACL reconstruction. At least 6 months should be allowed for secure healing before returning to sports.

KEY REFERENCES

1. Fulkerson J: Central quadriceps free tendon for anterior cruciate ligament reconstruction. Oper Tech Sports Med 7:195–200, 1999.
2. DeAngelis J, Fulkerson J: Central quadriceps tendon for ACL reconstruction. Clin Sports Med 26:587–596, 2007.
3. Geib T, Shelton W, Phelps R, Clark L: ACL reconstruction using quadriceps tendon autograft. Arthroscopy 25(12):1408–1414, 2009.
4. Joseph M, Fulkerson J, Nissen C, et al: Short-term recovery after anterior cruciate ligament reconstruction: a prospective comparison of three autografts. Orthopedics 29:243–248, 2006.

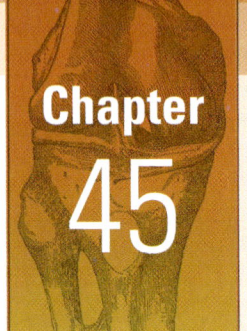

Allograft Anterior Cruciate Ligament Reconstruction

Shail Vyas and Christopher D. Harner

Allograft usage in orthopedic operations has increased significantly over the last 2 decades.[19] Approximately 20% of the estimated 300,000 anterior cruciate ligament (ACL) reconstructions done annually are performed with an allograft.[63] Because of certain drawbacks of autogenous graft ACL reconstruction, allograft usage has gained popularity. There are a variety of allograft options available to the orthopedic surgeon for ligamentous reconstruction operations. Allografts have their own unique risks and disadvantages that the surgeon and patient must consider as part of the informed consent.

ALLOGRAFT CONSIDERATIONS

Graft Options

ACL reconstruction using autograft patellar tendon was first described by Jones in 1963.[40] Now, patellar tendon autograft is considered the gold standard for ACL reconstruction.[77] Patellar tendon autograft offers high initial strength, earlier bone-to bone healing, and proven success by a multitude of outcome studies.[1,6,16,20,53] However, despite being the gold standard graft choice, there are several disadvantages to autogenous patellar tendon harvest. These include anterior knee pain, patellar shortening, decreased range of motion, longer surgical time, infrapatellar fat pad fibrosis, patellar fracture, and patellar chondrosis.* Dynamic disadvantages of autograft patellar tendon harvest include decreased quadriceps strength, quadriceps inhibition, altered patellar alignment, and decreased active range of motion.[36,44,51]

Quadrupled hamstring autografts (semitendinosus and gracilis tendon autograft) have been shown to have the highest tensile strength and excellent clinical results. However, disadvantages include decreased knee flexion and hip extension strength, which can be detrimental to athletes who rely on knee flexion strength beyond 90 degrees of flexion (e.g., sprinters, wrestlers, gymnasts, martial arts practitioners).[36,74,79] Furthermore, hamstring strength has been shown to be protective of ACL reconstruction by way of the ACL-hamstring reflex arc. Taking the semitendinosus and gracilis tendons results in disruption of this arc and a decrease in the protective effect of the hamstrings on the ACL graft.[9]

Quadriceps tendon autograft is also being used in some centers for ACL reconstruction. Limited outcome data are available but early studies have suggested equivalent results between quadriceps tendon (with patellar bone plug) autograft and patellar tendon autograft. After a 2-year follow-up, a recent study has found that kneeling pain is significantly less than with a bone-patellar tendon-bone (BPTB) autograft but anterior knee pain in the two groups is similar.[45]

Because of the potential drawbacks of autograft ACL reconstruction with patellar tendon, hamstring, or quadriceps tendon, allograft ACL reconstruction is increasing in the United States.[5,77] Advantages of an allograft include elimination of donor site morbidity, decreased surgical time, smaller incisions, lower incidence of arthrofibrosis, decreased postoperative pain, no loss of donor graft function, faster subjective recovery time, and predictable graft sizes.[19,27,41] Allograft options include patellar tendon, hamstring, anterior tibialis, posterior tibialis, Achilles, and fascia lata. However, allograft drawbacks also exist, such as disease transmission, slower incorporation, possible immunologic reaction, finite supply, tunnel expansion, inferior biomechanical strength, possibly increased failure rate, and cost.[31,33,65,71,73]

Graft Procurement and Sterilization

There are over 150 individual tissue banks that provide allograft for surgical use. Most of these tissue banks are members of the American Association of Tissue Banks (AATB). Beginning in May 2005, federal legislation was passed mandating that all United States tissue banks be subject to the U.S. Food and Drug Association (FDA) "Good Tissue Practice" guidelines. These guidelines specify a minimum standard for tissue procurement, as well as testing and processing, require periodic inspections of tissue bank facilities, and necessitate reporting adverse events to the FDA.[19,77]

Graft procurement begins with donor screening to eliminate donors who are at high risk for transmitting communicable diseases. This involves screening prior to death and evaluating cause of death. High-risk donors are eliminated; these include those who have a known communicable disease, show active signs of infection despite not having a diagnosis, or whose lifestyle places them at high risk for infection. Physical examination is the next step to assess the potential donor for high-risk behavior (e.g., needle marks, skin findings). Third, blood tests and tissue cultures are taken from the potential donor to rule out an otherwise undetermined communicable disease. Required serologic tests include human immunodeficiency virus (HIV) types 1 and 2, hepatitis B, hepatitis C, and syphilis. The AATB-affiliated tissue banks also test donors for human T-lymphotropic virus (HTLV) types 1 and 2. Certain tissue banks may accept positive bacterial cultures, relying on the sterilization process to eliminate the infection. Tissue banks that are part of the AATB require destruction of all tissue that demonstrates positive cultures for Clostridia or group A streptococcus.[19] Once these criteria are met and passed, the graft is suitable for procurement in the standard sterile surgical fashion. Each tissue bank has a specific time window for acceptable retrieval of graft tissue. Once obtained, the graft is placed in an antimicrobial solution and taken to the sterilization plant.

---

*References 5, 10, 17, 23, 56, 57, 66, 67, and 74.

Sterilization is performed via two techniques, tissue irradiation and chemical processing. It has been found that high levels of irradiation (>25 kGy) can reliably inactivate HIV and spores. However, these same high levels of irradiation can be detrimental to the biomechanical properties of the graft itself.[43,71,77] Thus, most tissue banks use lower dose irradiation, which inactivates most organisms but does not alter the strength of the graft. Low-dose radiation may not inactivate viruses such as HIV.[76] Various tissue banks will use different radiation dosages and some banks have abandoned irradiating as a sterilization technique because of adverse effects on graft biomechanics. Chemical processing involves a succession of cleansing, disinfection, and rinsing of the tissue to remove viable cells, lipids, and microorganisms. Penetration into the deepest parts of the tissue is the primary challenge in chemical sterilization. Various tissue banks have their proprietary chemical cleansing solutions. Tissue "sterility" (sterility assurance level) is defined by the tissue banking industry as $P < .000001$ that a viable microbe is present in tissue after having undergone the sterilization process. Once the sterilization process is complete, the graft is then frozen at $-70°$ C to $-80°$ C until surgery. Deep freezing has been shown to decrease the risk of graft rejection by causing cell necrosis and loss of immunogenicity.[27] Freezing of allograft tissue has led to variable results in biomechanical properties, with some studies suggesting no difference, whereas others demonstrating that freezing is detrimental to graft strength.[54,60] Deep freezing does not destroy HIV or the hepatitis C virus. Tissue irradiation, chemical processing, and deep freezing have been found in some studies to result in decreased graft biomechanical strength. Because the procurement and sterilization protocols of tissue banks can vary, the surgeon and hospital should be well aware of the quality and techniques of tissue processing of the company that they choose to use as their source of graft tissue.

Infection

The risk of disease transmission is an important factor when weighing the options of allograft versus autograft ACL reconstruction. Possible infectious agents include HIV, hepatitis B, hepatitis C, HTLV, syphilis, aerobic bacteria, and anaerobic bacteria. With tissue banks adopting varying procedures on graft sterilization, the risk of disease transmission is also variable. The risk of HIV infection has ranged in the literature from 1 to 400,000 to 8,000,000, with a commonly quoted figure of 1 to 1,600,000.[5,11,12,19] The risk of hepatitis B and C virus infection has consistently been shown to be higher than that of HIV transmission. Bacterial infection is also a concern with regard to disease transmission with *Clostridium* spp. (a spore-forming anaerobe) being a common pathogen. In a Centers for Disease Control and Prevention (CDC) study performed in 2002, 26 cases (18 used for ACL reconstruction) of allograft-associated bacterial infections were identified in approximately 1 million transplanted allografts. Half of these were found to be caused by *Clostridium* spp., with one death.[13] In another CDC study,[42] published in 2004, 70 cases of allograft-associated infection were reported; it was found that since 1995, 6 were caused by hepatitis C and none by HIV. Of these patients, 14 were found to have *Clostridium* infections.

Routine culture of allografts prior to implantation has yielded 4.8% to 9.7% positive cultures for bacterial organisms, but no clinical infection was correlated with these positive culture results.[14,30] Thus far, routine preimplantation cultures have not been recommended. Because tissue banks differ in their methods of sterilization, the surgeon should be familiar and comfortable with the tissue processing of the bank selected and be able to discuss possible infection transmission risks with patients as part of the informed consent.

Graft Biology

Allograft incorporation and healing is critical to the success of ACL reconstruction. One commonly cited disadvantage of allograft usage for ACL reconstruction is slower and less extensive incorporation compared with autograft ACL reconstruction.[24] Allograft versus autograft ACL reconstruction has been compared from histologic, biomechanical, and radiographic perspectives. A recent sheep study[72] comparing native ACL, reconstructed soft tissue autograft ACL, and reconstructed soft tissue allograft ACL has suggested that allograft demonstrated delayed remodeling histologically at 6 and 12 weeks postoperatively. However, at 52 weeks, the differences were less apparent. Biomechanically, allografts at 52 weeks demonstrated statistically significant anteroposterior laxity compared with autografts; this was not present at 6 and 12 weeks. Allograft healing was improved in a rabbit histologic study when the fresh-frozen Achilles allografts were coated with mesenchymal stem cells compared with controls (Achilles allograft only).[75] Radiographically, BPTB allografts were found to have less revascularization by contrast-enhanced magnetic resonance imaging (MRI) at 1, 4, 6, and 12 months after surgery, but were found to equalize at 18 months postoperatively. The authors suggested that revascularization is slower in BPTB allografts compared with BPTB autografts.[58] However, computed tomography (CT) imaging of BPTB bone plugs at 1 week, 2 months, and 5 months did not show a significant difference in bony incorporation of BPTB allograft versus BPTB autograft.[50]

For allograft ACL reconstruction to be successful, the graft must heal adequately in the bone tunnel. The intra-articular portion of the allograft must undergo the process of ligamentization in which the graft remodels to resemble the histology of a native ligament more closely.[31]

Soft tissue allografts must undergo tendon to bone tunnel healing. The native ACL insertion site is an example of direct insertion from tendon to bone. Four distinct histologically appreciable zones comprise this insertion site—tendon, unmineralized fibrocartilage, mineralized fibrocartilage, and finally bone. With soft tissue ACL reconstruction, this direct insertion site is not replicated. Rather, indirect insertion is relied on for soft tissue graft healing within the bone tunnel. Indirect insertion is naturally exemplified by other ligaments, such as the medial collateral ligament (MCL), which broadly inserts along the surface of the bone through fibers that travel obliquely from the long axis of the ligament to the long axis of the bone. These fibers, known as Sharpey's fibers, are also seen histologically in ACL reconstruction with tendon grafts and correlate with the biomechanical properties of the graft insertion site.[28,31,70]

A number of strategies have been used to improve the strength and healing of the soft tissue graft within the bone tunnel. Creating a longer tunnel has been shown to increase the strength of the graft-tunnel interface, presumably by increasing the amount of contact between the graft and the bone.[81] Impregnating the graft with mesenchymal stem cells, as suggested earlier, has shown superior healing as well as more normal tendon to bone insertion histology.[49,62,75] The application of bone morphogenic proteins to the graft has also been shown to increase bone formation around the graft as well as graft pull-out strength.[55] Inhibition of osteoclast activity has been investigated with the use of osteoprotegerin (OPG). OPG-treated grafts in rabbits demonstrated greater bone formation and smaller sized bone tunnels around the graft.[25] Inhibiting degrading matrix metalloproteinases (MMPs) in rabbit allograft ACL reconstruction has shown more Sharpey's fibers and a stronger load to failure.[21] The primary healing response after graft implantation involves the arrival of inflammatory cells facilitated by cyclooxygenase-2 (COX-2). Studies have shown that avoiding anti-inflammatory medications such as COX-2 inhibitors allows the primary healing phase to proceed without chemical interruption. Some have cautioned against the use of nonsteroidal anti-inflammatory drugs (NSAIDs) to prevent inhibition of the primary healing response.[18,31,61]

Compared with soft tissue grafts, which require soft tissue to bone healing within the osseous tunnel, BPTB grafts require bone to bone healing. This bone to bone healing is widely accepted as the strongest form of healing for ACL reconstruction. Histologic studies have demonstrated that the implanted bone plug demonstrates initial osteonecrosis and hypocellularity followed by revascularization, fibroblast invasion, and collagen synthesis, with subsequent rapid incorporation of the plug by surrounding bone.[22,39,64,80] These changes have been found to be similar in autograft versus allograft BPTB healing. Within 3 weeks, histologic incorporation is visible, but still fragile. At 3 weeks after implantation, the weakest point of a BPTB autograft remains the graft-tunnel interface. However, at 6 weeks, this interface has healed so that the site of graft failure is at the patellar tendon insertion into the bone plug.[31] Although some studies evaluating timing of incorporation have suggested no significant difference between autograft and allograft bone plugs, others have shown that allograft bone plugs require a longer time to incorporate and central portions of the plug may not incorporate at long-term evaluation.[37,38,52] Healing of the bone plug likely occurs from the end of the tunnel furthest from the influences of degradative enzymes in the synovial fluid.[8]

Ligamentization of the graft is the phase of graft incorporation in which the intra-articular portion of the graft undergoes changes that more closely resemble the histologic properties of a native ligament. Whether autograft or allograft, this process takes several months and undergoes a series of steps.[31,38] Similar to the initial events of bone plug incorporation, the ligamentous portion also undergoes an initial phase of avascular necrosis and acellularity. Despite being devoid of cells, the graft maintains its collagenous structure, which serves as a scaffold for subsequent steps—cellular repopulation, revascularization, and ligament maturation.[3,4] The timing of these steps, outlined in a rabbit model, has demonstrated that at 2 weeks, necrosis of the graft begins. At 4

weeks, the graft is completely devoid of cellularity but the collagen scaffold remains intact. At 12 weeks, vascular proliferation and cellular repopulation are appreciated. At 6 months, the cellularity of the graft is similar to that of a native ligament. Finally, at 9 months, the graft is mature and histologically similar to a native ACL.[61] In humans, surface blood flow studies have suggested that after an initial period of increased flow, ACL allografts demonstrate normal surface blood flow at 18 months, implying the end of graft remodeling.[71]

RESULTS OF ALLOGRAFT ANTERIOR CRUCIATE LIGAMENT RECONSTRUCTION

Autograft ACL reconstruction has generally been accepted as the gold standard for ACL graft choice, providing optimal graft strength and healing. Nonetheless, the use of allograft ACL reconstruction is increasing because of disadvantages specific to autogenous graft harvest. There have been several studies comparing subjective and objective outcomes of allograft versus autograft ACL reconstruction, with the best of these being prospective cohort studies. Randomization of graft is difficult because the patient must be informed of graft type and the inherent and specific advantages and drawbacks. Recent relevant studies are briefly reviewed in this section.

One randomized study in the literature by Sun and colleagues[76] have compared three groups: BPTB autograft, irradiated (2.5 Mrad) BPTB allograft, and nonirradiated BPTB allograft. In ths study, 99 patients were randomized to one of these three groups on the day of surgery with almost evenly sized comparison groups (34, 33, and 32 patients). At 31 months postoperatively, these patients were evaluated subjectively and objectively. No statistically significant difference was found among the three groups with regard to International Knee Documentation Committee (IKDC) functional and subjective evaluations, but a trend toward inferior outcome scores was noted in the irradiated group. However, statistically significant differences were found for stability testing in the irradiated allograft group compared with the other two groups. KT-2000 testing found that only 31.3% of irradiated patients had less than a 3-mm side to side difference compared with 87.8% in the autograft group and 85.3% in the nonirradiated allograft group. Furthermore, graft failure in the irradiated group occurred in 34.4% of patients compared with 6.1% in the autograft group and 8.8% in the nonirradiated allograft group. The authors concluded that they do not recommend the use of irradiated allograft tissue, but nonirradiated allograft BPTB provides similar results to autogenous BPTB graft. The same group published another prospective randomized study comparing autograft BPTB with nonirradiated allograft BPTB and evaluated 5.6-year follow-up data.[78] No statistically significant difference was found except shorter surgical time and longer postoperative fever for the allograft group (80 patients, average age 32.8 years) compared with the autograft group (76 patients, average age 31.7 years). It was concluded that nonirradiated allograft is a reasonable alternative to autograft use for ACL reconstruction.

In contrast, Rihn and associates[69] have prospectively compared 39 irradiated (2.5 Mrad) BPTB allograft ACL reconstructions with 63 BPTB autograft ACL reconstructions, with an average follow-up of 50.4 months. It was found that both cohorts have similar clinical outcomes, as measured by IKDC scores and KT-1000 translation. It was concluded that irradiated BPTB allograft has results similar to those of BPTB autograft ACL reconstruction. Two other prospective BPTB allograft versus autograft prospective cohort studies have found equivalent functional outcomes, one at 25.6-month and another at 47.1-month follow-up.[7,47]

Believing that the prospective trials in the literature comparing BPTB autograft with BPTB allograft ACL reconstruction were underpowered, Krych and coworkers[46] performed a meta-analysis of six prospective trials to compare the two groups. They compiled a group of 256 patients who underwent BPTB autograft ACL reconstruction and 278 who underwent BPTB allograft ACL reconstruction. Their analysis demonstrated that those in the allograft group were more likely to rerupture in comparison with those in the autograft group (odds ratio [OR], 5.03; $P = 0.01$) and more likely to have a hop test less than 90% of the contralateral nonoperated limb (OR, 5.66; $P < .01$). However, when irradiated and chemically processed grafts were excluded, there was no difference between the allograft and autograft groups with regard to graft rerupture, rate of reoperation, IKDC normal and near-normal scores, Lachman, pivot shift, and hop tests, patellar crepitus, or return to sport.

One recent study has prospectively evaluated autograft quadrupled hamstring tendon versus allograft quadrupled hamstring tendon without complete randomization.[26] A cohort of 37 autograft hamstring ACL reconstructions was compared with 47 allograft BPTB patients. No difference was found in Tegner, Lysholm, KT-1000, or IKDC scores at follow-up periods of 52 months (autograft cohort) and 48 months (allograft cohort).

Soft tissue graft irradiation was compared in a study evaluating irradiated (2 to 2.5 Mrad) versus nonirradiated Achilles allograft in regard to early failure.[68] With at least 6-month follow-up, the nonirradiated group had a 1/42 (2.4%) graft failure rate compared with 11/33 (33%) failure rate in the irradiated Achilles allograft group ($P < .01$). This significantly higher failure rate led the authors to cease using irradiated allografts for ACL reconstruction.

A noncomparative long-term outcome study evaluated 61 patients with a mean age of 20.9 years who underwent free tendon allograft ACL reconstruction.[59] Mean long-term follow-up of 11.5 years was compared with 2-year postoperative data in the same group of patients; of these, 87% of patients maintained a negative Lachman test result whereas 85% of patients maintained a negative pivot shift test result. Mean KT-2000 laxity measurements were a 1.6-mm side to side difference at long-term follow-up and no more than 3 mm in 92% of patients. All patients except one assessed their knee as normal or near-normal by IKDC score. It was concluded that free tendon allograft ACL reconstruction affords knee stability for the long term. Another long-term follow-up study also found good clinical results (IKDC, Lysholm, Tegner, one-leg hop test) in 55 patients followed for a mean of 10 years after having undergone free tendon allograft ACL reconstruction.[2] Harreld and colleagues[34] have described self-reported patient outcomes at short-term (mean, 2.8 years) and long-term (mean, 7.8 years) follow-up after ACL allograft (mix of BPTB and free tendon allograft)

reconstruction. No differences were found in the short-term group compared with the long-term group with regard to IKDC subjective evaluation or Knee Outcome Survey Activities of Daily Living Scale (KOS-ADLS) scores. However, there was a statistically significant decrease in the KOS-ADLS score in the long-term cohort, suggesting that over the long term, patients have a decreased perception of sporting activity knee function.

OPERATIVE CONSIDERATIONS

Choice of Surgical Technique

The senior author (CH) prefers to perform an anatomic ACL reconstruction, regardless of graft choice. It is believed that this is best done through femoral tunnel placement from the medial portal rather than the transtibial position. It is preferable to avoid interference screws to allow circumferential healing of the graft within the tunnel. Graft fixation of choice is the EndoButton (Smith & Nephew, Andover, Mass) for the femoral side and the graft tied over a post for the tibial side.

Patient Evaluation

Selecting the appropriate patient for ACL reconstruction begins with a thorough history and physical examination. This includes a full assessment of mechanism of injury, activity level, comorbidities, and expectations. Physical examination should include evaluation for other injuries about the knee, including meniscal, medial collateral ligament, and posterolateral corner injuries. With regard to imaging, flexion weight-bearing plain radiographs are routinely used to evaluate for acute fractures, bony avulsions, status of the growth plate, and presence of arthritis. MRI scans are also obtained to confirm an ACL-deficient knee, but more to evaluate for other injuries about the knee associated with the ACL tear, such as menisci, collateral structures, and articular cartilage. History, physical examination findings, and imaging studies are correlated to establish the complete diagnosis for each injured knee. Indications for ACL reconstruction include an active patient with episodic knee pain and subjective instability that correlates with an ACL-deficient knee on physical examination and MRI.

Prior to ACL reconstruction, the patient undergoes knee rehabilitation with the goal of full active range of motion, symmetric quadriceps strength, and a normal heel to toe gait. We prefer to familiarize our patients with the physical therapy protocol prior to surgery. On occasion, if a large knee effusion is hindering preoperative rehabilitation, an aspiration will be performed in the office. This rehabilitation process generally requires 3 to 6 weeks.

Approximately 5% to 10% of our patients will present with an ACL tear with an associated ligamentous injury. If an acute (<3 weeks) posterior lateral corner injury is present, we will repair the posterior lateral corner and stage the ACL reconstruction. If the patient presents with a concomitant MCL injury, we may delay surgery for 4 to 6 weeks, allowing the MCL to heal.

A thorough discussion regarding the nature of the surgery as well as the attendant risks, benefits, and alternatives, should take place with the patient. We think that this should only be performed by the surgeon ultimately responsible for the care of the patient. Only after the patient has a thorough understanding of all these considerations is he or she asked to sign the consent form.

Graft Selection

Graft choice for ACL reconstruction is influenced by patient age, activity level, gender, associated injuries, degree of laxity, and planned concomitant operations. As a general guideline, autografts are recommended for patients younger than 35 years because it is presumed that these patients are more active. Those older than 35 years are counseled to use allograft tissue. We recommend BPTB autografts to all high-level athletes involved in cutting sports (e.g., football, basketball, rugby), patients with a history of hamstring injury, and larger patients. With bone to bone healing, a more aggressive rehabilitation course may be taken. Hamstring autografts are recommended to most women because of better donor site cosmesis, unless their activity level dictates otherwise, and for augmentation in the young athlete. Allografts tend to be reserved for older athletes and most multiligamentous injury reconstructions. Allograft BPTB is preferred for older athletes but, occasionally, we will use tibialis anterior allograft in older women. In the setting of ACL augmentation, soft tissue allograft (e.g., tibialis anterior) is more amenable to graft passage and requires smaller diameter bone tunnels while allowing preservation of the remaining native bundle. In revision ACL surgery, a variety of grafts are used. BPTB and occasionally hamstring autografts are preferred. If these are unavailable, then BPTB is the allograft of choice in most cases.

Anesthesia

Our preferred anesthesia for an ACL reconstruction involves a combined femoral and sciatic nerve block administered in the preoperative holding area. Intraoperatively, a general anesthetic with an laryngeal mask airway (LMA) can be used. Postoperatively, our patients are discharged with a 72-hour indwelling femoral nerve catheter. Ultimately, anesthesia should be individualized taking into account the patient's comorbidities and preferences, and surgical team needs.

Examination Under Anesthesia

A thorough bilateral knee examination under anesthesia is performed after the general anesthetic is administered. For the ACL, we use the Lachman, anterior drawer, and pivot shift test and compare side to side differences. Discrepancies among these test results may signify an isolated bundle rupture amenable to augmentation. The results are considered along with previously collected data (i.e., history, prior examination, and imaging studies) to confirm the diagnosis of an ACL tear.

Positioning and Setup

The patient is positioned supine on the operating table with the heels at the end of the table (Fig. 45-1A). The surgical site is shaved appropriately with an electric razor, taking into consideration other procedures that may be necessary during the operation (e.g., meniscal repairs). No tourniquet or leg holders are used. The operative leg is brought into neutral rotation by placing an appropriate sized bump under the ipsilateral buttock. A 10-pound sandbag is affixed to the table in a location that holds the leg flexed at 90 degrees of flexion. A side post is placed at the midthigh level to support the leg without assistance when the leg is flexed to 90 degrees. Bony prominences of the nonoperative leg are well padded to prevent pressure sores and peroneal nerve palsies. With the knee flexed to 90 degrees, anatomic landmarks are marked. Standard anterolateral and anteromedial portals are marked (see Fig. 45-1B). A 3-cm tibial tunnel incision is drawn on the anteromedial tibial surface. Proposed incisions for possible medial and/or lateral meniscal inside-out repairs are also marked. With the leg in extension, a standard anterolateral outflow portal is marked. All incisions are then infiltrated with 0.25% bupivacaine hydrochloride with 1:200,000 epinephrine. The surgical team then scrubs, allowing time for the local anesthetic and, more importantly, hemostatic agents to take effect. The limb is then prepped with alcohol and povidone-iodine (Betadine) and draped in a standard sterile fashion. The inflow is connected to a pump while the outflow drains to gravity.

Arthroscopic Evaluation

Prior to thawing the allograft, a diagnostic arthroscopy is usually performed. If a repairable meniscal tear is encountered, we prefer to repair it using an inside-out suture technique. If a meniscal root tear is encountered, we prefer to repair these as well through bone tunnels, as described by Harner and associates.[32] With all meniscal repairs, we tie the

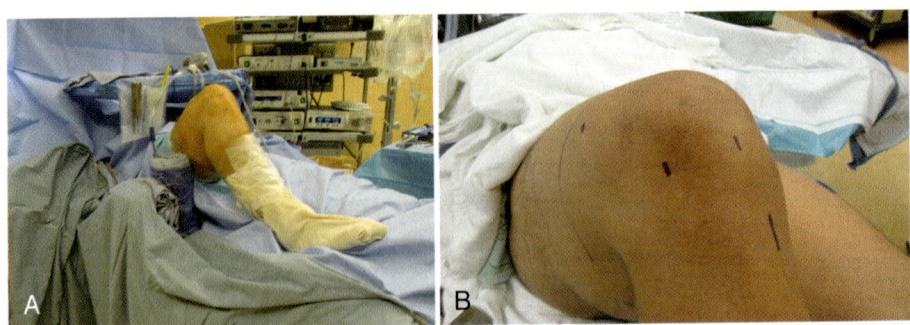

Figure 45-1. A, Patient setup. The patient is positioned supine with a lateral leg rest and a bump holding the right knee at 90 degrees of flexion. **B,** Incision. A tibial tunnel incision as well as standard anterolateral, anteromedial, and superlateral portals are shown on this right knee.

suture after the graft is secured. Focal full-thickness articular injuries are initially managed at the time of ACL reconstruction with microfracture.

PROCEDURE

Graft Preparation

Once the graft has thawed, it is ready for preparation. With BPTB allograft preparation, the bone on either side of the tendon is trimmed to 20 mm in length by 10 mm in diameter (Fig. 45-2). The plug dimensions are verified by graft sizing tubes. The tendinous portion is trimmed to a 10- to 11-mm width. The leading bone plug is tapered to facilitate graft passage. Two 1.5-mm holes are drilled into the tibial bone plug, from cancellous to cortical, at approximately 5 and 15 mm from the end. A no. 5 braided polyester nonabsorbable suture (Ethibond Excel, Ethicon, Somerville, NJ) is then threaded through each hole. An EndoButton CL BPTB (Smith & Nephew) is attached to the femoral bone plug. The appropriate loop size is determined for full bone plug length to reside within the femoral tunnel. A mark is placed at the soft tissue to bone interface of the leading bone plug. The graft is then wrapped in a moist sponge to protect the graft from desiccation until the time of implantation.

For soft tissue allograft, anterior tibialis is our graft of choice. The graft is doubled over an EndoButton CL (Smith & Nephew). We generally use the shortest loop available (15 mm) to maximize the amount of graft material in the tunnel because this has been shown to maximize pull-out strength.[29] The free ends of the graft are individually whipstitched and the graft is tensioned on a graft board. The graft is then wrapped in a moist sponge to protect the graft from desiccation until the time of implantation.

Notch Preparation

While the graft is being prepared, attention is turned to the femoral notch. The ACL tear pattern is evaluated. Partial tears in which a functionally intact bundle (anteromedial or posterolateral) may be treated differently are assessed, which may also explain physical examination irregularities. When possible, we prefer to attempt augmentation of an intact bundle with our graft. The torn portion of the ACL is removed with a shaver. With a complete tear, the femoral stump is totally removed to permit observation as far posteriorly in the notch as possible. We prefer to leave as much tibial stump as we can, removing only that which impairs visualization and graft passage. It a has been shown that maximal preservation of the tibial remnant enhances proprioceptive and vascular properties.[48] We do not think that a notchplasty is routinely necessary. If needed for visualization, a minimal (1- to 2-mm) notchplasty is performed for better visualization and/or to relieve graft impingement. The fat pad is left intact to prevent scarring, pain and potential patella baja.

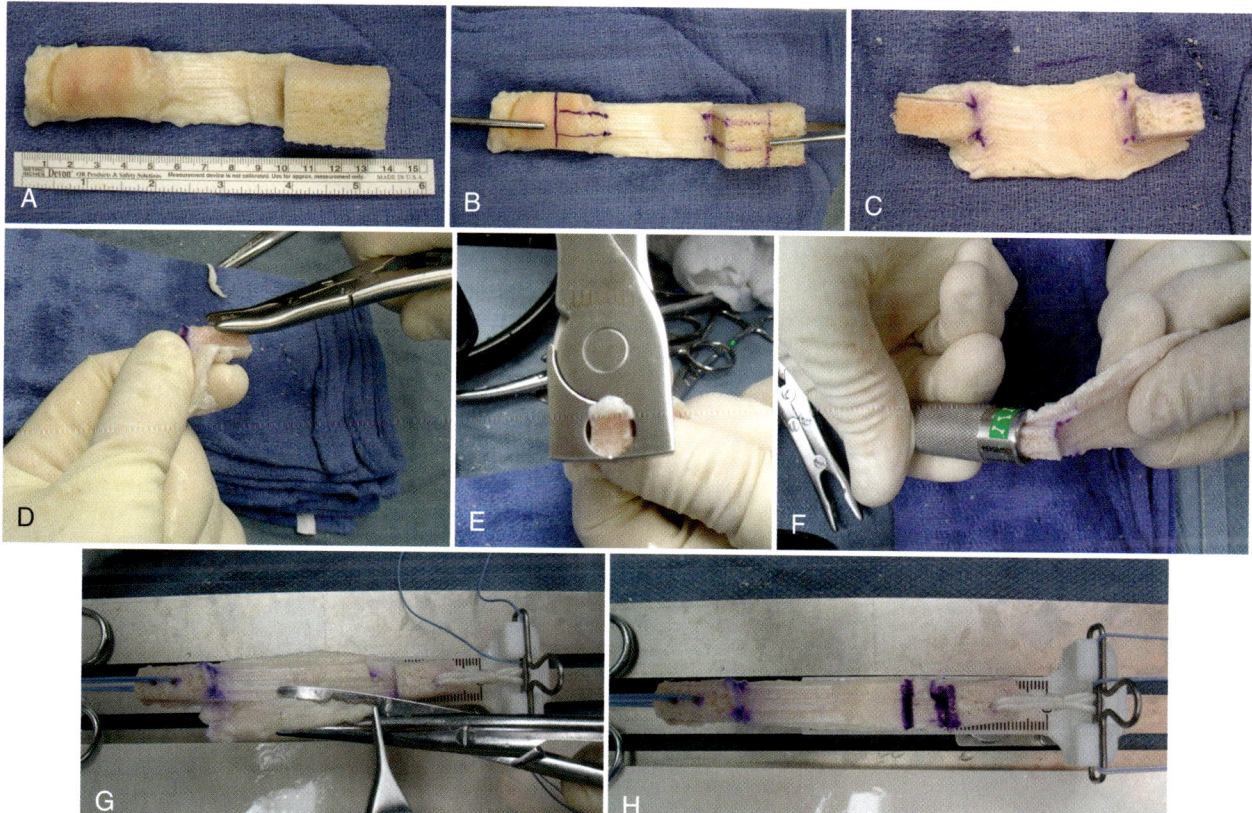

Figure 45-2. A, Thawed BPTB allograft. **B,** Projected bone plug markings (20- × 10-mm plugs). **C,** Bone plugs cut with oscillating saw. **D,** Rongeur used to size and taper plug. **E,** Compaction pliers used to finalize plug dimensions. **F,** Sizing tube to confirm plug size. **G,** Graft placed in tension to cut excess fibers that do not exhibit tension. **H,** Final graft construct.

Tunnel Site Selection

Our goal is to make femoral and tibial tunnels in their anatomic positions. We believe that an anatomic femoral tunnel position is best achieved through the anteromedial portal because it allows us to place the femoral tunnel independently of the confines of the tibial tunnel. This technique may be used regardless of graft type, instrumentation, or fixation method. Medial portal femoral tunnel preparation also allows for flexibility of tunnel creation, whether a single-bundle, double-bundle, or revision situation exists. Medial portal femoral tunnel preparation has been shown to decrease tunnel widening and minimize interference screw divergence.[15]

After the notch is prepared, the next step is to identify the femoral tunnel starting point. The center of the femoral footprint of the ACL is identified. This is typically 4 to 6 mm anterior to the posterior wall of the notch in the 10 o'clock (right knee) or 2 o'clock (left knee) position. Note that this is an approximation and that this footprint can vary based on ACL size and bony anatomy. A 30-degree awl is used to first identify the over the top position at the 10 o'clock or 2 o'clock location. The awl is then impacted into the bone approximately 6 mm anterior to this position (Fig. 45-3A). If the femoral footprint of the ACL is visible, the starting point should also acknowledge the position of the native ACL. Intraoperative fluoroscopy is used to confirm the starting position with the awl in place with the goal of the starting point to be in the superoposterior quadrant of the lateral femoral condyle, with adequate distance between the awl and the back wall (see Fig. 45-3B).

Tibial Tunnel

Once the femoral starting point is marked with the awl, anatomic tibial tunnel placement is accomplished with arthroscopic landmarks and fluoroscopic imaging. An elbow ACL tibial guide (Acufex, Smith & Nephew) is preferred (Fig. 45-4A). The point of the guide is placed at the intersection of the line made by the free edge of the anterior horn of the lateral meniscus (in the coronal plane) and the mid–medial half of the distance between the medial and lateral tibial spines (in the saggital plane). This point should also be in the mid to posterior half of the existing tibial stump, if

available for confirmation (see Fig. 45-4B). The tip of the guide is held in place while the base of the guide is adjusted so that the bullet portion of the guide will contact the tibia midway between the anterior and medial crests of the tibia. The bullet of the guide is advanced, scoring the skin. A 2-cm skin incision is then made centered around the skin marking. The skin and subcutaneous tissues are sharply dissected until the tibial periosteum is encountered. A ³⁄₃₂-inch Kirschner wire (K wire) is advanced through the bullet into the knee joint until it reaches the elbow portion of the guide. The guide is then disassembled and removed. The pin position is confirmed with respect to the above mentioned landmarks (see Fig. 45-4C). The knee is brought to full extension to confirm that the graft will not impinge in extension. The pin position is evaluated on lateral and anteroposterior (AP) fluoroscopic imaging (Fig. 45-5). On the lateral view (with the knee fully extended), the pin should enter the tibial plateau at approximately the junction of the anterior and middle thirds of the plateau. Also, it should be in line with the radiographic shadow indicating the roof of the notch (Blumensaat's line) with the knee flexed 90 degrees for BPTB allografts and 2 to 4 mm more posteriorly if a soft tissue graft is used. On the AP view, the pin should emerge into the joint on the downslope of the medial tibial spine. If fluoroscopy demonstrates a slightly misplaced pin, a 3- or 5-mm tibial pin offset guide is used to fine-tune the pin placement. The tibial tunnel is then created with a cannulated compacting reamer 0.5 to 1.0 mm smaller than the graft size. Tunnel dilators are then used to dilate the tibial tunnel sequentially to the size of the soft tissue graft or 0.5 mm larger than the graft if using a BPTB allograft (see Fig. 45-4D). The final dilator is left in place and, again, the knee is brought to extension to check for impingement of the dilator with the notch. If the graft impinges, an appropriate notchplasty is performed.

Femoral Tunnel

Attention is then returned to the femoral insertion site. Through the anteromedial portal, a ³⁄₃₂-inch K wire is introduced to the hole previously made by the awl. Once engaged in this hole, the knee is flexed to 120 degrees to improve visualization of the insertion site, prevent breaching the posterior cortex, increase tunnel length, and avoid risk to posterior neurovascular structures. The K wire is then impacted

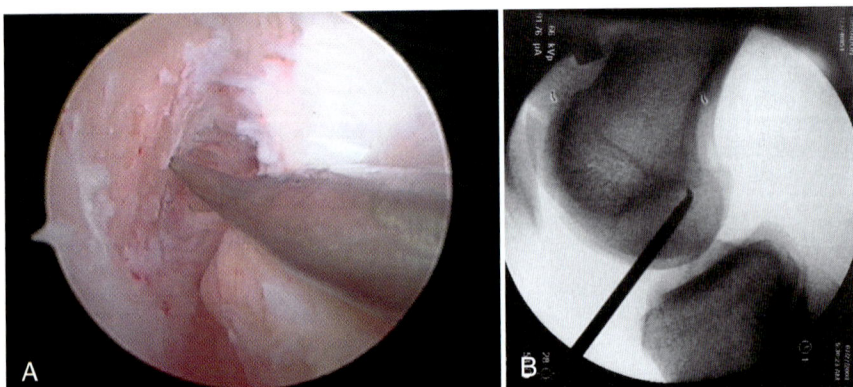

Figure 45-3. A, Femoral starting point is marked with a pointed awl. Note the approximate 10 o'clock position for this right knee. **B,** Femoral starting point confirmed on lateral fluoroscopy. Note the posterior and midcondylar position on the lateral femoral condyle as well as the approximate 5-mm distance from the over the top position.

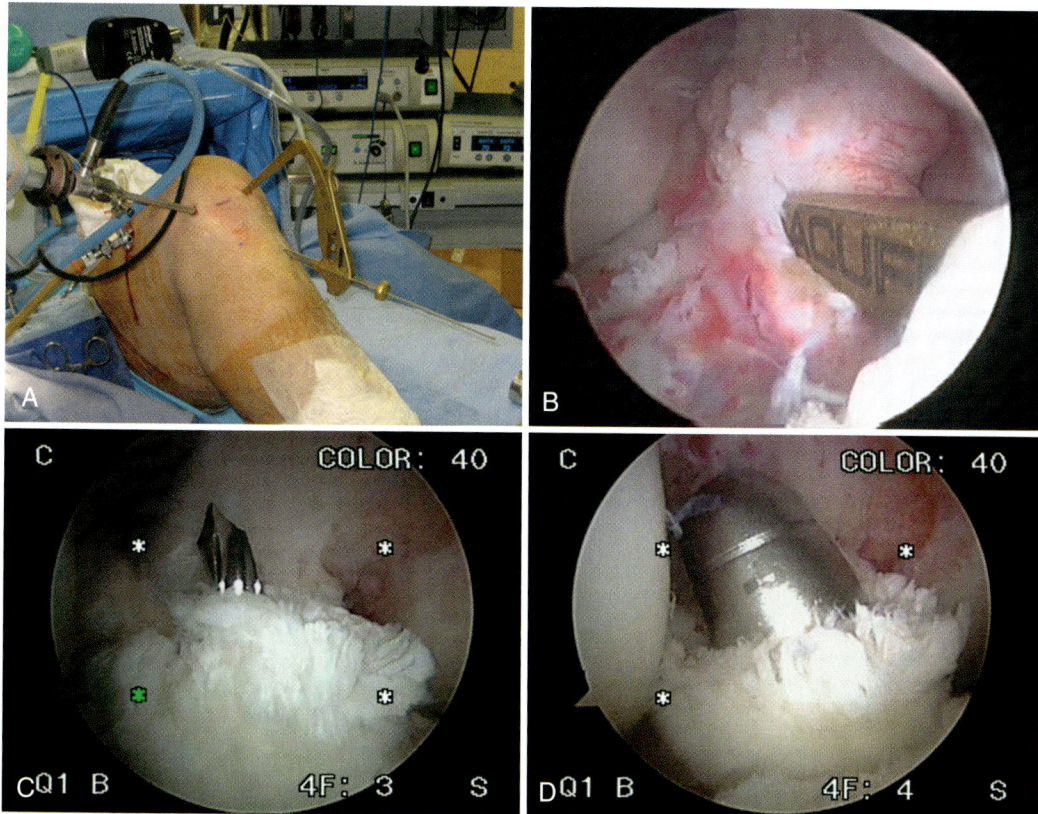

Figure 45-4. **A,** External view of tibial elbow guide in right knee. The guide pin is passed with the knee in 90 degrees of flexion. **B,** Tibial elbow guide placed in center of native ACL tibial insertion site for this right knee. **C,** Arthroscopic view of tibial guide pin in right knee. Note the preservation of the ACL stump. **D,** Arthroscopic view of tibial tunnel dilator after tibial tunnel underdrilled by 0.5 to 1.0 mm in right knee. Again, note preservation of the tibial stump.

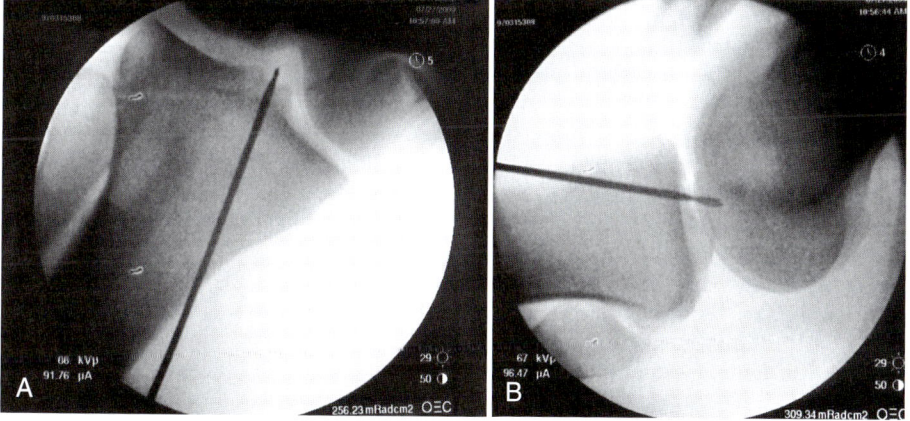

Figure 45-5. **A,** Fluoroscopic AP view of tibial guide pin. Note that the guide pin emerges into the knee at the downslope of the medial tibial eminence. **B,** Lateral fluoroscopic view of the tibial guide pin, taken with the knee in extension. Note that the pin is in line or slightly posterior to Blumensaat's line, entering the knee in the anterior third of the tibial plateau.

into the insertion site with the knee flexed to 120 degrees (Fig. 45-6A). A 1.0-mm undersized acorn reamer is advanced over the wire taking care not to abrade the medial condyle or patella. If this proves to be difficult, a half-round reamer can be used with the smooth portion facing the at-risk cartilaginous surface until it is seated against the lateral condyle. The position of the drill is checked to confirm adequate distance from the back wall and desired trajectory. The drill is then advanced by hand to begin the footprint of the insertion site, reevaluated, and drilled by power to the depth mandated by the fixation technique. A shaver is introduced in the tunnel to remove the bone and soft tissue debris (see Fig. 45-6B). Dilators are next introduced through the antero-medial portal to dilate the tunnel to the size of the soft tissue graft (or 0.5 mm larger than the graft if using a BPTB allograft). Our fixation of choice is the EndoButton (Smith & Nephew). A 3.2-mm EndoButton drill is used to breach the lateral femoral cortex. A Beath pin with an affixed a no. 5 Ethibond looped suture is then advanced through the drilled femoral tunnel, through the EndoButton drill track,

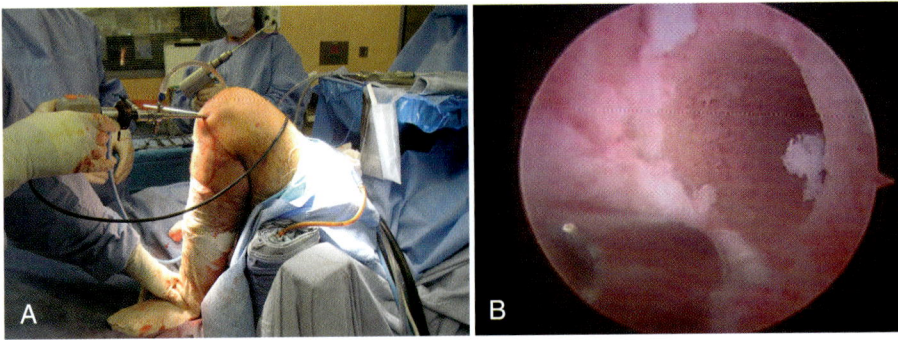

Figure 45-6. A, The femoral tunnel is drilled through the anteromedial portal with the knee in deep flexion in this left knee. **B,** Arthroscopic view of femoral tunnel in deep flexion in left knee.

and through the lateral thigh soft tissue. This looped Ethibond suture is then retrieved intra-articularly from the tibial tunnel. The Beath pin is left in place. The knee is now ready for graft passage.

Graft Passage

The knee is now flexed to 90 degrees. Passing sutures that are threaded through the two eyes of the EndoButton on the femoral side of the graft are placed around the Ethibond loop, which is now exiting the tibial tunnel. The Beath pin is then pulled from the lateral thigh and the passing sutures are delivered through the femoral tunnel and out the lateral thigh. One set of passing sutures is pulled (allowing the Endo-Button to slant through the drilled tunnel) while the other set of passing sutures is intermittently pulled, only relieving their slack. If a BPTB allograft is used, the cancellous portion of the bone plug is anterior, allowing the graft to reside posteriorly in the tunnel. To facilitate graft passage, a right angle clamp can be used that acts as an intra-articular pulley to help get an appropriate angle into the femoral tunnel. Also, with BPTB allografts, the bone plug can be gently impacted to encourage passage through the tunnel. Finally, the knee can be further flexed to help ease passage of the graft. Once the EndoButton has exited the cortex (determined by appropriate graft markings and confirmed by fluoroscopy), the EndoButton is flipped by applying tension to the lagging strand of the femoral passing sutures. Tension is placed on the tibial side of the graft to seat the EndoButton flush with the femoral cortex. Appropriate seating is also confirmed by fluoroscopy. With tension on the tibia-sided lead sutures, the graft is cycled to reduce creep within the graft. Graft isometry is also evaluated, as is impingement in extension.

Graft Fixation

We prefer tibial post fixation, regardless of graft type. A standard 4.5-mm large-fragment cortex screw with a washer is placed bicortically, approximately 5 to 10 mm distal to the tibial tunnel. When the far cortex is engaged but prior to final seating of the screw and washer, the two pairs of tibial lead sutures are individually tied around the post with the knee in 15 to 30 degrees of flexion. The screw is then fully seated. The graft is arthroscopically evaluated for tension and impingement (Fig. 45-7). Postoperative Lachman and pivot shift tests are repeated to confirm reversal of preoperative

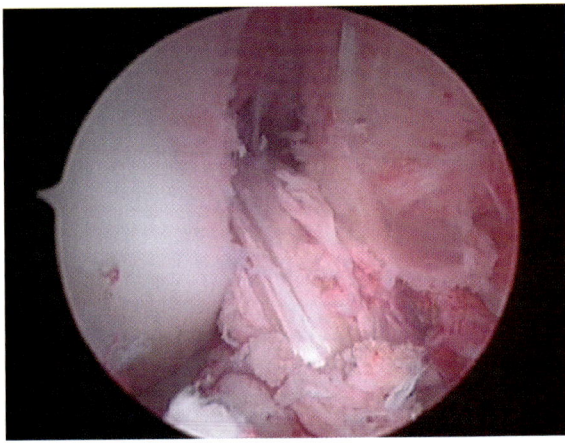

Figure 45-7. Final view of reconstructed ACL with BPTB allograft in right knee.

findings. Final radiographs are taken to verify hardware placement and tunnel position (Fig. 45-8). The wounds are irrigated and closed in layers. A sterile dressing is applied. A cold therapy sleeve is placed over the dressing. A hinged knee brace is then centered over the joint line, locking the knee in full extension.

POSTOPERATIVE MANAGEMENT

The patient is discharged the same day after the nerve catheters are redosed. Deep venous thrombosis prophylaxis is individualized, depending on specific risk factors. Smokers, patients on oral contraceptives, patients with a family history of clotting disorders, and those with a previous DVT all receive prophylaxis. Rehabilitation follows a standard protocol in which full return to activity is expected by 6 to 12 months, depending on graft choice and patient-specific factors. We allow a longer time for allografts to incorporate.

In the first week after surgery, patients are allowed to bear weight with crutches, with the brace locked in full extension. A recent study has shown that brace wear does not affect pain or range of motion within the first 2 weeks atfter surgery, but we think that it protects the newly reconstructed graft and gives patients a feeling of safety.[35] Basic home exercises, including quadriceps sets, straight leg raises, and heel slides, are permitted out of the brace with the goal of achieving full

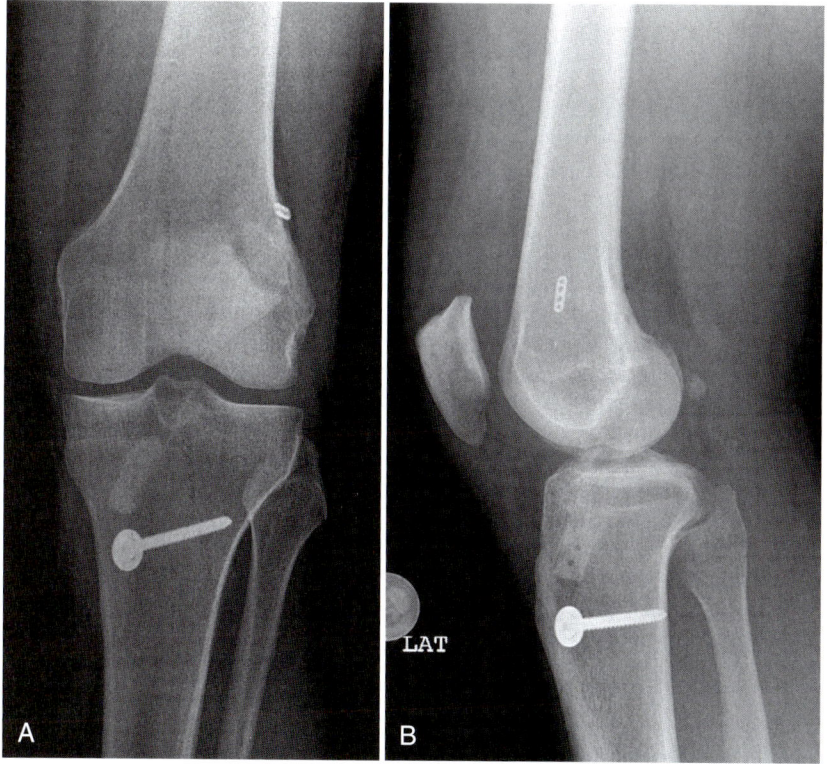

Figure 45-8. Postoperative AP **(A)** and lateral **(B)** x-ray demonstrating a well-positioned femoral EndoButton and tibial post in this left knee.

extension and full flexion, and initializing return of quadriceps strength. The patient is seen in 1 week and sutures are removed. Patients are sent to formal physical therapy after this visit. The added focus at this time is to begin gait training with the brace unlocked to practice a heel to toe gait. The goal at 1 month is full range of motion and a normal heel to toe gait. The brace is discontinued when this is confirmed at the second appointment, 1 month after surgery. Strengthening of the lower extremity is the subsequent focus, with gradually increasing light resistance training (e.g., exercise bicycle, closed-chain low-resistance weights). At the third postoperative visit (at 3 months after surgery), the patient should exhibit significant return of quadriceps and hamstring strength. More aggressive strengthening exercises are permitted, taking care to avoid open-chain knee extensions. The delicate decision is made at this time as to when the patient can begin in-line exercises, generally between 3 and 6 months. At 6 to 12 months from surgery, full return to sport is gradually permitted.

KEY REFERENCES

Almqvist KF, Willaert P, De Brabandere S, et al: A long-term study of anterior cruciate ligament allograft reconstruction. Knee Surg Sports Traumatol Arthrosc 17:818–822, 2009.

Baer GS, Harner CD: Clinical outcomes of allograft versus autograft in anterior cruciate ligament reconstruction. Clin Sports Med 26:661–681, 2007.

Cohen SB, Sekiya JK: Allograft safety in anterior cruciate ligament reconstruction. Clin Sports Med 26:597–605, 2007.

Edgar CM, Zimmer S, Kakar S, et al: Prospective comparison of auto and allograft hamstring tendon constructs for ACL reconstruction. Clin Orthop Relat Res 466:2238–2246, 2008.

Gulotta LV, Rodeo SA: Biology of autograft and allograft healing in anterior cruciate ligament reconstruction. Clin Sports Med 26:509–524, 2007.

Harreld K, Nyland J, Cottrell B, Caborn DN: Self-reported patient outcomes after ACL reconstruction with allograft tissue. Med Sci Sports Exerc 38:2058–2067, 2006.

Krych AJ, Jackson JD, Hoskin TL, Dahm DL: A meta-analysis of patellar tendon autograft versus patellar tendon allograft in anterior cruciate ligament reconstruction. Arthroscopy 24:292–298, 2008.

Kustos T, Bálint L, Than P, Bárdos T: Comparative study of autograft or allograft in primary anterior cruciate ligament reconstruction. Int Orthop 28:290–293, 2004.

Marrale J, Morrissey M, Haddad F: A literature review of autograft and allograft anterior cruciate ligament reconstruction. Knee Surg Sports Traumatol Arthrosc 15:690–704, 2007.

Nakata K, Shino K, Horibe S, et al: Arthroscopic anterior cruciate ligament reconstruction using fresh-frozen bone plug-free allogeneic tendons: 10-year follow-up. Arthroscopy 24:285–291, 2008.

Penn D, Willet TL, Glazebrook M, et al: Is there significant variation in the material properties of four different allografts implanted for ACL reconstruction? Knee Surg Sports Traumatol Arthrosc 17:260–265, 2009.

Rihn JA, Irrgang JJ, Chhabra A, et al: Does irradiation affect the clinical outcome of patellar tendon allograft ACL reconstruction? Knee Surg Sports Traumatol Arthrosc 14:885–896, 2006.

Scheffler SU, Schmidt T, Gangéy I, et al: Fresh-frozen free-tendon allografts versus autografts in anterior cruciate ligament reconstruction: delayed remodeling and inferior mechanical function during long-term healing in sheep. Arthroscopy 24:448–458, 2008.

Sun K, Tian S, Zhang J, et al: Anterior cruciate ligament reconstruction with BPTB autograft, irradiated versus non-irradiated allograft: a prospective randomized clinical study. Knee Surg Sports Traumatol Arthrosc 17:464–474, 2009.

Sun K, Tian SQ, Zhang JH, et al: Anterior cruciate ligament reconstruction with bone-patellar tendon-bone autograft versus allograft. Arthroscopy 25:750–759, 2009.

Full references for this chapter can be found on www.expertconsult.com.

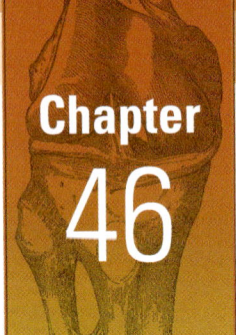

Double-Bundle Anterior Cruciate Ligament Reconstruction

Kenneth R. Morse, Verena M. Schreiber and Freddie H. Fu

Single-bundle anterior cruciate ligament (ACL) reconstruction has largely been a successful surgery over the last several decades, with satisfactory subjective patient outcomes in the short term.[5] However, more recent long-term studies have found significant sequelae of ACL injury and its reconstruction with the development of early arthritic changes in a large percentage of patients. Pinczewski and colleagues[19] have reported arthritic changes in 39% of patients who underwent patellar tendon autograft ACL reconstruction at 10 years postoperatively. Additionally, others have reported a subset of patients, between 30% and 40%, who have persistent instability or are unable to return to their previous level of activity.[2] Although these results compare favorably with the nonoperative treatment of ACL injuries, potential areas for improvement obviously remain.

In an attempt to improve these clinical results, surgeons have revisited a technique that once received little interest, the double-bundle ACL reconstruction. With the primary goals of recreating the two functional bundles of the ACL and individualizing each surgical procedure, the double-bundle reconstruction was first described in the 1980s. Over the last decade, the technique has gained in popularity as a better understanding of the normal anatomy and biomechanics of the ACL has been achieved.

This chapter will explore the native anatomy and biomechanics of the anterior cruciate ligament and the double-bundle reconstruction technique.

ANATOMY AND BIOMECHANICS

The anatomy of the ACL has been studied for many years, with the assumption that a better understanding of the anatomy would lead to a better reconstructive procedure. In general terms, the ACL originates on the medial aspect of the lateral femoral condyle and runs obliquely to its insertion at the medial tibial eminence. It is narrowest in the midsubstance, with an average cross-sectional area of 36 mm^2 in females and 44 mm^2 in males.[1] It then fans out to a broad insertion at both ends.[18] The length of the ACL is depends on which fibers are measured; it can range from 22 to 41 mm.[17]

It is widely accepted that the ACL is composed of two functional bundles. This was first described in the 1930s and has since been confirmed by others.[27] These two bundles, anteromedial (AM) and posterolateral (PL), are named for their tibial insertion and have distinct functional properties (Fig. 46-1). Recent literature has shown that in response to an anteriorly directed tibial load, the in situ force in the PL bundle is highest at full extension and decreases with flexion, whereas the AM bundle is lower in full extension and increases to maximum at 60 degrees of flexion.[7] Additionally, the PL bundle also resists anterior translation when the knee is subjected to a combined rotatory load (simulated pivot shift) when near full extension.[18]

Although researchers continue to investigate the anatomy and function of the ligament itself, others have revisited the insertional anatomy of the ACL. The last several years have provided a much greater detailed understanding of both the femoral and tibial insertions. On the femoral side, the overall shape is that of a segment of circle, with its anterior border straight and its posterior border convex. Ferretti and associates[4] have studied the area of the femoral insertion site and found it to average 196.8 mm^2. Individually, the AM bundle averaged 120 mm^2 and the PL bundle averaged 76.8 mm^2; however, there may be some ethnic variation. To help identify each bundle, there are distinct bony landmarks that signify the anatomic extents of each bundle as well as the ACL as a whole. The lateral intercondylar ridge (resident's ridge) is the anterior border of the ACL. This bony landmark runs from proximal to distal with the knee straight, and no cruciate fibers insert anterior to this point. The lateral bifurcate ridge, which is subtle but often present, separates the anterior portion of the AM bundle from the PL bundle. Of importance is the understanding that these two insertion sites are vertical with the knee extended and horizontal with the knee in flexion. Therefore, the two bundles are parallel with the knee in extension but crossed with flexion.[10] This explains the biomechanical features of the two bundles and aides in reconstruction.

On the tibial side, the insertion varies in shape in size.[13,24] Medially, the ACL inserts up to a bony ridge that is an anterior extension of the medial intercondylar tubercle.[22] Posteriorly, no fibers extend beyond a ridge of bone at the anterior aspect of the tibial spine between the medial and lateral tibial intercondylar tubercles. The portion of the ACL, the PL bundle, lies just anterior to the insertion of the posterior horn of the lateral meniscus. The anterior and lateral borders are less well defined and consist of diffuse expansions. Similarly, there is no bony landmark that separates the two bundles on the tibial side.

Understanding the biomechanical function and insertional anatomy of the ACL highlights the importance of each bundle. This is critical to the correct application of the double-bundle technique.

PREOPERATIVE CONSIDERATIONS

Patient Evaluation

Patient evaluation progresses in a similar fashion despite whether a single- or double-bundle reconstruction is preferred by the surgeon. A thorough history and careful physical examination are critical to the identification of an ACL tear and to the development of a treatment plan. In the history, the mechanism of injury should be explored and can help determine whether other ligamentous injuries may be present.

Symptoms such as locking or catching may suggest meniscal injuries.

A complete physical examination is performed on both lower extremities for comparison. Visual inspection for overall limb alignment, ecchymosis, joint effusion, and muscular atrophy is performed. A complete range of motion followed by palpation of the parapatellar area, joint line, and bony prominences aids in the diagnosis of the ACL tear and any concomitant pathology. Special tests, including the anterior drawer, posterior drawer, Lachman, pivot shift, reverse pivot shift, McMurry, dial, and varus-valgus tests, may be difficult to perform in the acute setting but are crucial to a complete evaluation. The degree of anterior laxity can be better quantified with the KT2000 arthrometer (MEDmetric, San Diego, Calif); a 3-mm or greater side to side difference is suggestive of an ACL injury.

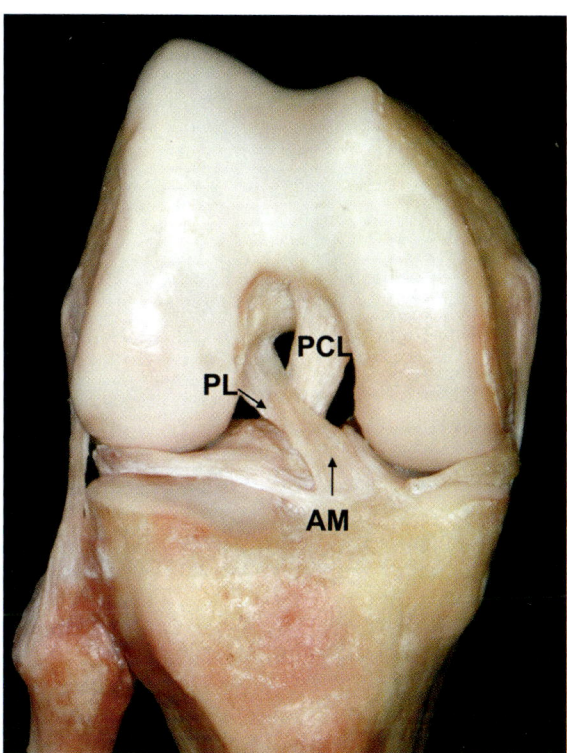

Figure 46-1. Cadaveric specimen showing the AM and PL bundles of the ACL.

Imaging

Plain radiographs are first obtained and consist of weight-bearing extension and 45-degree flexion posteroanterior views. Non–weight-bearing 45-degree lateral and axial (Merchant) views are also obtained. Standard magnetic resonance imaging (MRI) sequences are helpful for diagnosing the ACL tear as well as any additional injuries. Oblique coronal views, taken in the plane of the ACL, are helpful for visualizing the two bundles of the ACL (Fig. 46-2). For cases involving revision ACL reconstruction, computed tomography (CT) with three-dimensional reconstructions provide better bone detail than MRI and are used to evaluate prior tunnel placement and the degree of bone lysis (Fig. 46-3).

Indications and Contraindications

Double-bundle reconstruction is indicated for patients with ACL tears or for patients with persistent instability after single-bundle reconstruction. This typically includes high-level athletes in cutting sports or patients with demanding employment or activities. Those with a sedentary lifestyle or with lower demand activities can possibly be treated nonoperatively.

Contraindications to reconstruction in general include advanced degenerative changes, infection, and patient noncompliance. In patients with open growth plates or multiligament injuries, consideration should be made to performing a single-bundle reconstruction. However, each individual case requires an in-depth conversation between the treating surgeon and patient to develop an appropriate plan acceptable to both.

TECHNIQUE

As noted, the goal of double-bundle ACL reconstruction is to re-create the patient's native anatomy. This requires attention to the detail of the ligament insertion sites, which can be more time-consuming than a single-bundle reconstruction but is necessary to optimize clinical outcomes.

Setup

As with all surgical procedures, the patient and appropriate extremity are identified and marked in the preoperative area.

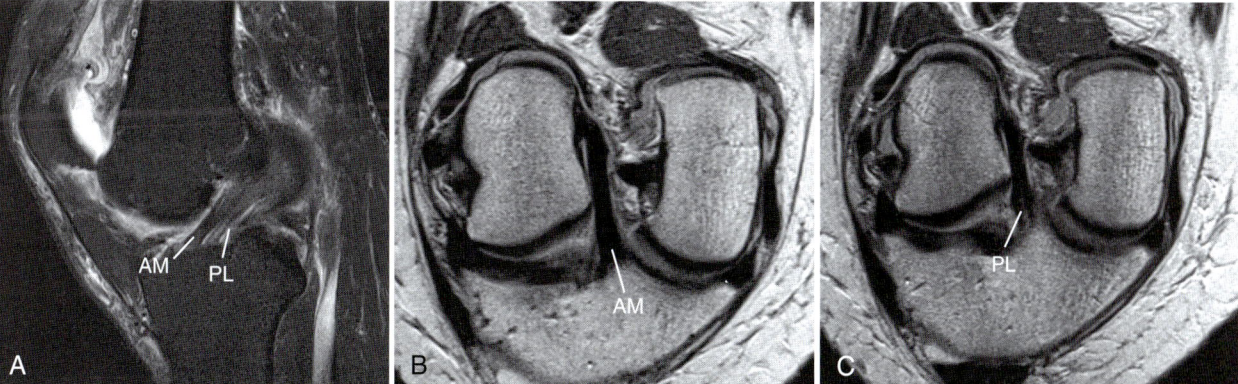

Figure 46-2. MRI of the ACL. **A,** T2-weighted sagittal ACL with AM and PL bundle. **B,** Coronal oblique cut shows the AM bundle. **C,** Coronal oblique cut shows the PL bundle.

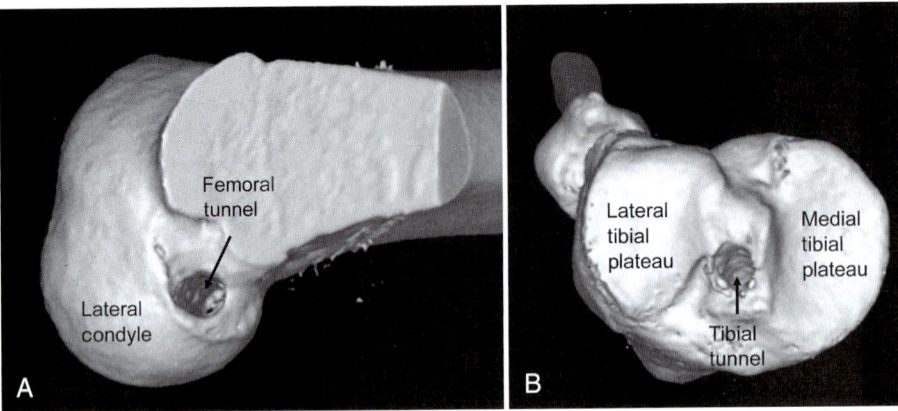

Figure 46-3. Three-dimensional CT scan of the right femur and tibia. **A,** Femur after single-bundle reconstruction. **B,** Tibia after single-bundle reconstruction.

The patient is brought to the operating room where the anesthetic of choice is administered. While under anesthesia, a thorough examination is performed. Careful attention is paid to rotational instability.

The nonoperative extremity is placed in a well-leg holder, which is padded to protect the peroneal nerve. A pneumatic tourniquet is placed on the thigh of the operative extremity and is insufflated to 350 mm Hg after elevation of the extremity for 3 minutes. The leg is then placed in an arthroscopic leg holder with the foot of the table dropped. Range of motion is verified to allow full extension and flexion beyond 120 degrees. Alternatively, the reconstruction can be performed without the leg holder as long as hyperflexion is possible. The leg is then prepped and draped in a sterile fashion.

Additional setup considerations include the presence of a portable fluoroscopy device that can be used to verify guidewire position, if necessary.

Graft Selection and Preparation

Both autograft and allograft options exist for the double-bundle reconstruction and one must consider the patient's age, anatomy, prior surgical history, activities, and occupation when discussing this with the patient. Although allograft tissue eliminates donor site morbidity, one must counsel the patient regarding possible disease transmission and potentially higher failure rate.[24] If allograft is chosen, tibialis anterior tendons are preferable because of the large diameter and length. Two grafts are chosen, each at least 24 cm in length. After the graft diameters are determined (see later), each graft is trimmed so that its doubled-over diameter will be the desired size. Each end is stitched with a strong nonabsorbable suture to facilitate graft passage and fixation.

For autograft, options include hamstring and quadriceps tendon grafts. Hamstring grafts are harvested and prepared in standard fashion. However, because the diameters of the harvested hamstring tendons may be smaller than those required for the double bundle reconstruction, the surgeon can hybridize the reconstruction with the addition of an allograft tendon to supplement the autograft or perform the reconstruction with smaller bundles.

With the use of quadriceps tendon, an 11-mm-wide, full-thickness quadriceps graft is obtained. This is detached as proximally as possible to maximize graft length, and distally

a 20-mm-long bone plug is harvested from the patella. This soft tissue portion of the graft can be split and trimmed to provide the two bundles for reconstruction. However, with the bone plug, only one femoral tunnel is used, as will be described.

Portal Establishment

A three-portal technique is used to visualize the ACL footprints properly. The anterolateral (AL) portal is established first in a slightly higher position to avoid the infrapatellar fat pad.[20] The AM and accessory anteromedial (AAM) portals are established with the aid of a spinal needle. The AM portal is established along the medial border of the inferior patellar tendon. The spinal needle should project along the path of the native ACL without injuring the intermeniscal ligament. Following the establishment of the anteromedial portal, the shaver is introduced and some of the fat pad is removed to facilitate visualization. The AAM portal is established at the level of the joint line, approximately 1.5 cm medial to the AM portal. The spinal needle should pass safely by the medial meniscus and reach the center of the femoral ACL footprint. With the needle in the center of the footprint, one needs to ensure that there is room between it and the medial femoral condyle to allow safe passage of instruments without damaging the articular cartilage (Fig. 46-4).

Defining the Rupture Pattern and Anterior Cruciate Ligament Footprints

The ACL tear is carefully studied to identify each bundle and tear pattern (Fig. 46-5). The tibial and femoral footprints are then established with the use of a thermal device on a very low setting. The bony anatomy of the lateral femoral condyle, as noted, is helpful in locating the boundaries of each bundle (Fig. 46-6). Once the footprints are identified, several measurements are made to tailor each reconstruction to the individual patient. The length and width of the AM and PL bundle insertion sites on the tibia and femur are measured with an arthroscopic ruler (Fig. 46-7). The smaller insertion size for each bundle determines the graft size and the grafts are prepared accordingly. Additionally, the entire ACL footprint is measured on the tibial and femoral side to determine the feasibility of a double-bundle reconstruction. In our

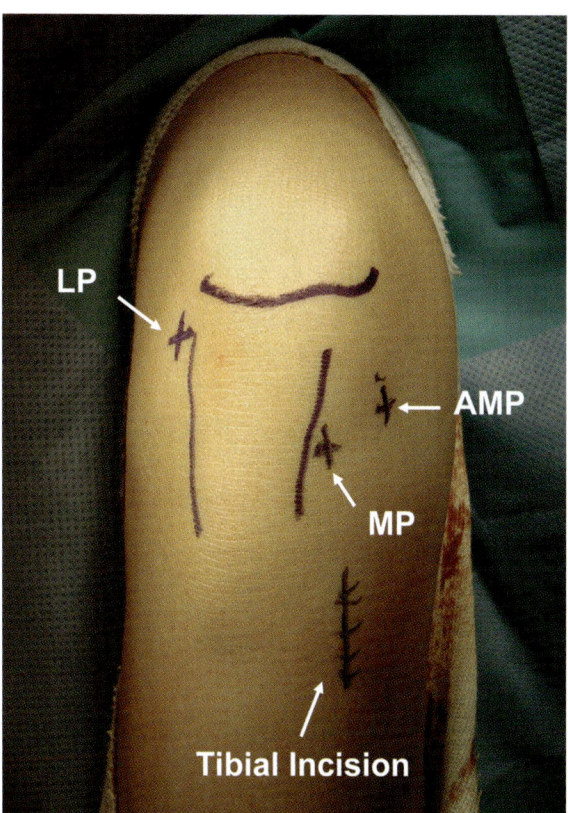

Figure 46-4. Portal establishment using the three-portal-technique—anterolateral portal *(LP)*, anteromedial portal *(AM)*, and accessory anteromedial portal *(AMP)*.

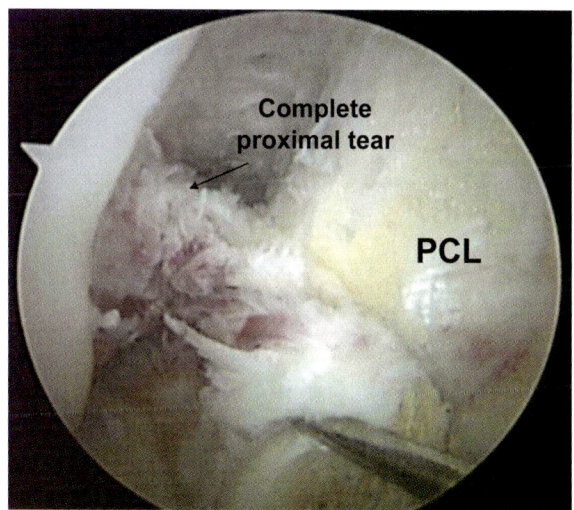

Figure 46-5. Complete proximal tear of AM and PL bundle.

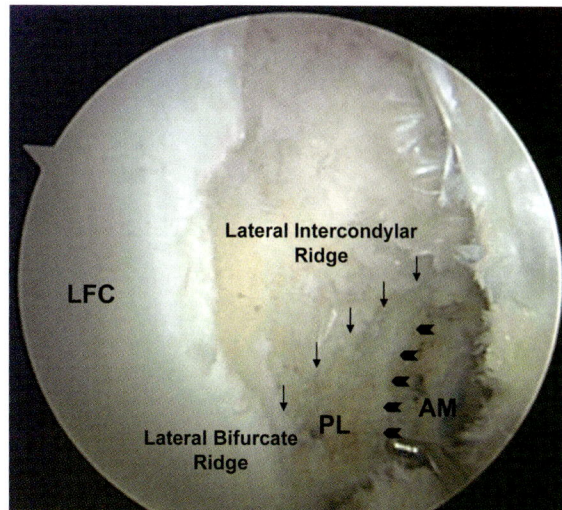

Figure 46-6. Marking of the femoral insertion sites (AM and PL bundles) with a thermal device. *Long arrows* depict the lateral intercondylar ridge (resident's ridge); *arrowheads* depict the lateral bifurcate ridge.

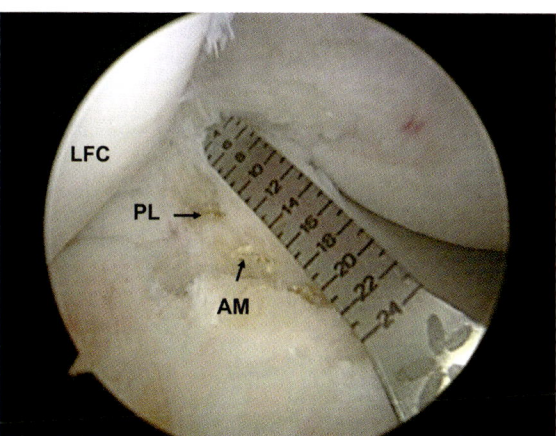

Figure 46-7. Measurement of the tibial insertion site of the ACL after marking with a thermal device. The insertion site measures 20 mm.

Tunnel Placement

The PL femoral tunnel is prepared first through the AAM portal. An awl is used to mark the center of the PL bundle femoral insertion. A 3.2-mm guide wire is placed through the AAM portal to the marked center of the PL insertion and is malleted in place as the knee is brought to full flexion. Next, an acorn drill bit 1 mm smaller in diameter than the previously determined PL bundle size is used to drill the PL femoral tunnel to a depth of approximately 20 mm. A drill bit is used to pierce the lateral cortex and the tunnel length is measured. If the tunnel is more than 30 mm, our preference is to use a button as a suspensory method of fixation. If a short tunnel is encountered (less than 30 mm), a number of fixation techniques can be used, including a polyethylene button or screw and washer. The final tunnel length is determined by accounting for the clearance necessary to flip the button; it is prepared with the correct acorn drill size by hand. In cases in which a quadriceps tendon graft is used, one central

experience, the AM bundle typically measures 6 to 8 mm in diameter and the PL bundle typically measures 5 to 7 mm. Therefore, to accommodate the two bundles and a bony bridge, an ACL footprint of at least 14 mm is required. If these conditions are not met, it is best to proceed with an anatomic single-bundle reconstruction. Similarly, the inter-condylar notch is measured and should be no less than 14 mm to ensure that there will not be any graft impingement with the posterior cruciate ligament (Fig. 46-8).

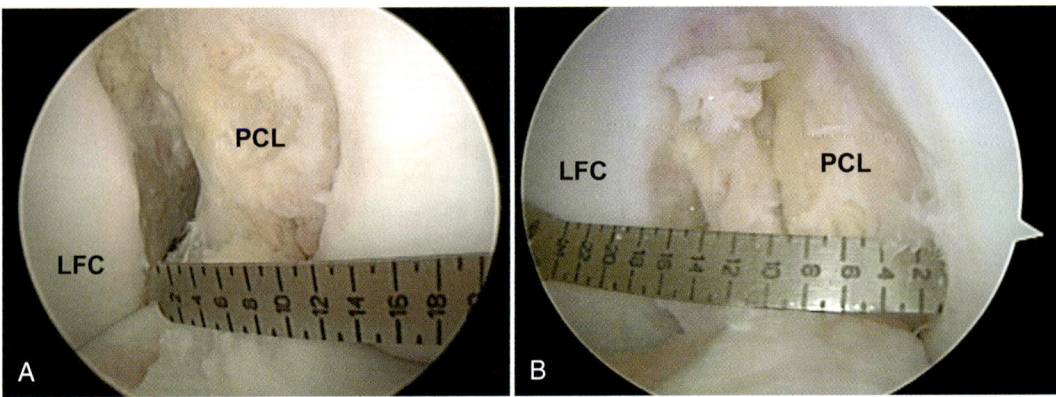

Figure 46-8. Measurement of the intercondylar notch. **A,** Narrow notch measuring 12 mm. **B,** Wide notch measuring 20 mm.

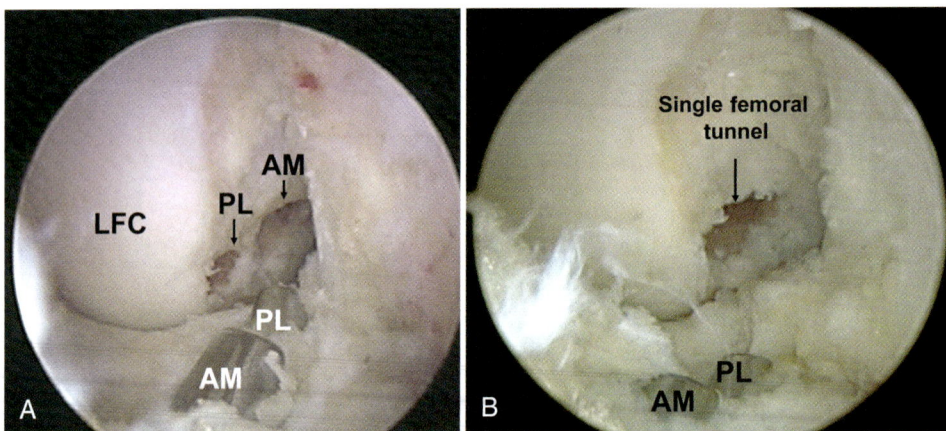

Figure 46-9. Views of femoral and tibial tunnels. **A,** Four tunnels in double-bundle reconstruction with soft tissue graft. **B,** Single femoral and two tibial tunnels in double-bundle reconstruction with quadriceps tendon autograft and femoral bone plug.

tunnel is created in the center of the entire ACL femoral insertion.

Next, the tibial tunnels are prepared. A 5-cm incision is created over the anteromedial tibia distal to the level of the tibial tubercle. The PL tibial tunnel is drilled first with the ACL tip guide set at 45 degrees. The tip is placed in the center of the tibial PL bundle insertion site, with care taken to avoid any damage to the insertion of the lateral meniscus. A 3.2-mm guide wire is drilled from the tibial cortex, just anterior to the superficial fibers of the medial collateral ligament, to the tip of the guide. Similarly, the tibial AM tunnel is drilled with the guide set at 55 degrees and the tunnel located midway between the PL tunnel and tibial tubercle. There should be adequate distance between the two pins to allow for at least a 2-mm bone bridge between the two tunnels at the ACL footprint. The tunnels are then drilled over the guide wires and expanded to the appropriate size with dilators.

Finally, in cases in which two soft tissue grafts are used, the femoral AM tunnel is established. Often, the femoral AM tunnel can be approached through the tibial PL tunnel. If a guide wire can be placed through the PL tunnel into the center of the femoral AM insertion, it is used and drilled with a half-round half-fluted drill so as not to expand the tibial PL tunnel. In cases in which this cannot be performed, the AAM

portal is used in the same fashion as for the PL tunnel (Fig. 46-9).

Graft Passage and Fixation

A Beath pin with a looped suture is placed through the AAM portal into the femoral PL tunnel and brought out through the anterolateral thigh. A suture-grasping device is placed through the tibial PL tunnel and the suture is retrieved. A second Beath pin is used for the AM bundle. The PL bundle is passed first and the button device is flipped on the lateral femoral cortex, followed by the AM bundle. When using the quadriceps tendon graft, a Beath pin with looped suture is used to bring the bone plug in through the AAM portal and it is seated into the femoral tunnel. Again, the bone plug button device is flipped on the lateral cortex. The sutures from each limb are retrieved and brought out through their respective tunnel. Arthroscopy is used to visualize the position of the two bundles and the knee is cycled approximately 25 times. The PL bundle is fixed first with an interference screw in full extension. The AM bundle is fixed in 45 degrees of flexion. Arthroscopy is again performed to verify graft position and the knee is brought through a full range of motion (Fig. 46-10).

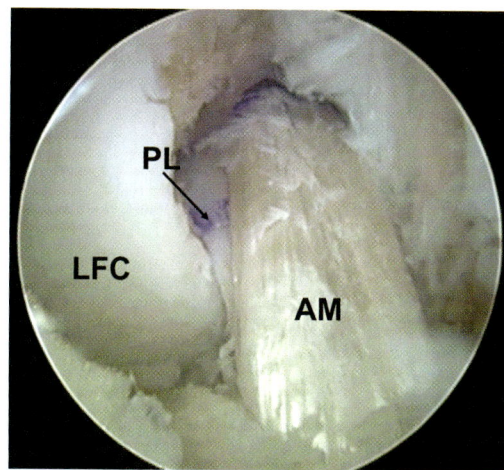

Figure 46-10. Anatomic double-bundle ACL reconstruction. Both grafts (AM and PL bundles) can be visualized.

POSTOPERATIVE REHABILITATION

Standard postoperative rehabilitation programs are used, with particular attention paid to minimizing inflammation, gaining full range of motion, and brace use. A continuous passive motion machine is used initially until the patient achieves 120 degrees of flexion and formal physical therapy is begun at 1 week. Particular milestones include discontinuation of the brace and crutches when full extension without a lag has been achieved (typically, 6 weeks), jogging when quadriceps strength is near-normal (typically, 4 months), and return to cutting activities with normal strength, motion, and stability (typically, 9 months). A functional ACL brace is used initially if the patient desires to return to a cutting activity.

POTENTIAL PITFALLS AND RECOMMENDATIONS

The potential pitfalls of double-bundle reconstruction are the same as for the single-bundle technique. However, concern has been expressed regarding the potential injury to the lateral and posterolateral structures, including the peroneal nerve, with drilling of the femoral PL tunnel. Several recent cadaveric studies have shown that this risk is minimal if the femoral tunnels are drilled in at least 120 degrees of flexion, as has been recommended.[8,16]

There are several points that must be made to optimize surgical outcome and avoid potential mistakes, the most important of which is to visualize the femoral and tibial ACL insertions properly. As noted, this is accomplished by viewing through multiple arthroscopy portals. By properly identifying the insertions, the anatomic location of the reconstruction can be identified and mismatching of the tibial and femoral tunnels can be avoided. Similarly, one should avoid referring to the reconstruction in the "o'clock" terminology. The femoral notch is a three-dimensional structure and to describe it using a two-dimensional process leads to nonanatomic placement of the reconstruction. Finally, one must properly restore the tension pattern in the two bundles of the ACL, as described. Nonphysiologic tensioning may lead to over- or undertensioning at certain flexion angles, which could result in graft failure.[3]

RESULTS

The biomechanical results of the double-bundle reconstruction have been studied extensively in the cadaveric and in vivo settings. Woo and coworkers[25] have evaluated the single-bundle reconstruction in response to an anterior tibial and combined rotatory load in cadavers. Although the reconstruction was successful at limiting anterior translation, it was ineffective at providing stability to the combined load. A similar study evaluated both the single- and double-bundle reconstruction with better biomechanical stability, particularly in rotatory testing, found in the double-bundle anatomic approach.[26] One possible benefit to better normalization of stability is an improvement in contact areas and stresses within the knee. Morimoto and colleagues[14] have evaluated the contact area and pressure in a normal knee; after single- and double-bundle reconstruction, they found that the single-bundle reconstruction resulted in a smaller contact area and higher contact pressures, but the double-bundle reconstruction approached that of the normal knee.

Clinical results have also been promising for the double-bundle technique. Jarvela and associates[9] have reported on the 2-year follow-up of a randomized, controlled clinical trial comparing double-bundle and single-bundle reconstructions. Rotational stability was best in the double-bundle group, with no significant difference in anterior stability. Additionally, Fu and coworkers[6] conducted a 2-year prospective study and found that the double-bundle reconstruction results in good restoration of joint stability with a normal or near-normal Lachman examination in 98% of patients and a normal pivot shift test in 94% of patients. Patient-reported measures were also promising, with scores similar to those reported for the single-bundle approach. The results of these two studies are similar to other reports in the literature.[11,12,15,21,23] However, despite objective evidence of improved rotational stability after double-bundle reconstruction, these studies fail to show significant differences in subjective measures. The reason for this remains perplexing, but possibly relates to lack of knowledge regarding how these small differences affect the patient's interpretation of the outcome and the outcome measure's ability to detect these subtleties. Nevertheless, future long-term studies are required to determine the true benefits of the double-bundle reconstruction.

CONCLUSION

The last several decades have seen significant advances in the understanding of the anatomy and biomechanics of the ACL. Using this information, surgical techniques have been developed in an attempt to replicate better what is seen in dissection and in the laboratory. The double-bundle reconstruction is one such technique because it more accurately reproduces the native anatomy of the ACL. It is a complex procedure that should be performed only by those with an understanding of the anatomic approach and with advanced training. Although initial biomechanical and clinical reports appear promising, better evaluation tools and longer term studies are required.

KEY REFERENCES

Biau DJ, Tournoux C, Katsahian S, et al: ACL reconstruction: a meta-analysis of functional scores. Clin Orthop Relat Res 458:180–187, 2007.

Colvin AC, Shen W, Musahl V, Fu FH: Avoiding pitfalls in anatomic ACL reconstruction. Knee Surg Sports Traumatol Arthrosc 17:956–963, 2009.

Ferretti M, Ekdahl M, Shen W, Fu FH: Osseous landmarks of the femoral attachment of the anterior cruciate ligament: an anatomic study. Arthroscopy 23:1218–1225, 2007.

Fu FH, Shen W, Starman JS, et al: Primary anatomic double-bundle anterior cruciate ligament reconstruction: a preliminary 2-year prospective study. Am J Sports Med 36:1263–1274, 2008.

Gabriel MT, Wong EK, Woo SL, et al: Distribution of in situ forces in the anterior cruciate ligament in response to rotatory loads. J Orthop Res 22:85–89, 2004.

Jordan SS, DeFrate LE, Nha KW, et al: In vivo kinematics of the anteromedial and posterolateral bundles of the anterior cruciate ligament during weight-bearing knee flexion. Am J Sports Med 35:547–554, 2007.

Kopf S, Musahl V, Tashman S, et al: A systematic review of the femoral origin and tibial insertion morphology of the ACL. Knee Surg Sports Traumatol Arthrosc 17:213–219, 2009.

Morimoto Y, Ferretti M, Ekdahl M, et al: Tibiofemoral joint contact area and pressure after single- and double-bundle anterior cruciate ligament reconstruction. Arthroscopy 25:62–69, 2009.

Muneta T, Koga H, Mochizuki T, et al: A prospective randomized study of 4-strand semitendinosus tendon anterior cruciate ligament reconstruction comparing single-bundle and double-bundle techniques. Arthroscopy 23:618–628, 2007.

Petersen W, Zantop T: Anatomy of the anterior cruciate ligament with regard to its two bundles. Clin Orthop Relat Res 454:35–47, 2007.

Pombo MW, Shen W, Fu FH: Anatomic double-bundle anterior cruciate ligament reconstruction: where are we today? Arthroscopy 24:1168–1177, 2008.

Prodromos CC, Joyce BT, Shi K, et al: A meta-analysis of stability of autografts compared to allografts after anterior cruciate ligament reconstruction. Knee Surg Sports Traumatol Arthrosc 15:851–856, 2007.

Purnell ML, Larson AI, Clancy W: Anterior cruciate ligament insertions of the tibia and femur and their relationships to critical bony landmarks using high-resolution volume-rendering computed tomography. Am J Sports Med 36:2083–2090, 2008.

Siebold R, Dehler C, Ellert T: Prospective randomized comparison of double-bundle versus single-bundle anterior cruciate ligament reconstruction. Arthroscopy 24:137–145, 2008.

Zelle BA, Vidal AF, Brucker PU, Fu FH: Double-bundle reconstruction of the anterior cruciate ligament: anatomic and biomechanical rationale. J Am Acad Orthop Surg 15:87–96, 2007.

Full references for this chapter can be found on www.expertconsult.com.

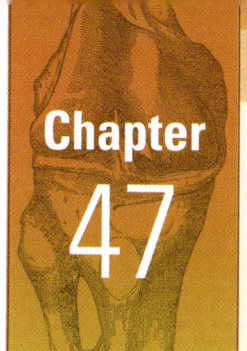

Chapter 47

Anterior Cruciate Ligament Reconstruction via the Anteromedial Portal and Single-Tunnel, Double-Bundle Techniques

Benton E. Heyworth and Thomas J. Gill, IV

ANTERIOR CRUCIATE LIGAMENT RECONSTRUCTION VIA THE ANTEROMEDIAL PORTAL

Use of the anteromedial portal (AMP) for establishment of the femoral tunnel in anterior cruciate ligament reconstruction (ACLR) surgery is an area of growing clinical and research interest. Traditionally, femoral tunnel creation has been performed by placing instruments through the previously reamed tibial tunnel. Several studies[3-6,8,14,15,26] have suggested that use of the AMP eliminates the constraint in instrumentation positioning imposed by the transtibial technique, which can lead to the creation of a more vertical femoral tunnel or one with a nonanatomic aperture. The AMP is meant to allow for more anatomic, lower placement of the femoral tunnel and better re-creation of the native origins of the anteromedial and posterolateral bundles on the femoral condyle. However, some reports[3,19,20] have underscored the technical challenges and steep learning curve associated with application of the AMP technique. Complications that have been described include lateral femoral condyle back wall blowout, iatrogenic damage to the anterolateral cartilage of the medial femoral condyle (MFC), bending or breakage of the guide pin or Beath pin, and difficulty with graft passage.

Additionally, technical considerations related to graft-length mismatch, shortening of femoral tunnel length, and inadequate femoral tunnel fixation can arise with use of the AMP technique. Because the femoral tunnel angle is typically smaller, or less steep, than that used with the transtibial technique, and because the tunnel is directed toward the lateral cortex, rather than the anterior cortex, of the distal femur, the length of the femoral tunnel is generally shorter. With the use of bone-patellar tendon-bone (BPTB) grafts, either autograft or allograft, shorter femoral tunnel length can cause the graft to be longer than the overall distance from the proximal extent of the femoral tunnel to the distal extent of the tibial tunnel on the anterior cortex of the tibia—that is, graft-length mismatch. Although this situation is rarely seen with the technique to be described, detailed preoperative planning can avoid this pitfall[13] and several approaches can be used to address it when it occurs. Shortening of the bone plug lengths, seating the distal end of the femoral bone plug several millimeters deep to the aperture of the femoral tunnel, use of a free tibial bone block, and rotation of the tibial bone plug within the tibial tunnel are all acceptable, well-described techniques for addressing length issues and should be familiar to surgeons performing ACLR.[34,35]

When using soft tissue grafts, there are a number of options for femoral fixation. The growing popularity of the AMP technique and its shorter femoral tunnel has increased the demand for soft tissue fixation constructs with flexibility in length. For example, because the commonly used EndoButton CL (Smith & Nephew, Andover, Mass) uses suspensory cortical fixation and the construct contains a continuous loop of suture, with a minimum length of 15 mm, shorter femoral tunnels may leave a relatively short or unsatisfactory amount of graft contained within the tunnel. The newer EndoButton Direct (Smith & Nephew) device allows direct fixation of the graft onto the button, which maximizes the amount of graft in the femoral tunnel and may therefore be better suited for AMP techniques. The ACL Tightrope (Arthrex, Naples, Fla) is another suspensory fixation option for soft tissue grafts and allows the doubled-over end of the graft to be advanced to the most proximal aspect of the femoral tunnel. The Femoral Intrafix (DePuy Mitek, Raynham, Mass) uses aperture fixation via a sheath and screw construct. Because it allows for separation of different portions of the graft, thereby replicating the two bundles,[10] it represents the senior author's current implant of choice when using the AMP technique with soft tissue grafts. The AperFix femoral implant (Cayenne Medical, Scottsdale, Ariz) can also offer aperture fixation. However, AMP technique with this device requires a slightly larger portal, because both the implant and all graft limbs must be passed through the portal, and the smallest length of the implant is 29 mm, requiring a femoral tunnel length of at least 30 to 35 mm.

Here we describe our approach for creation of the AMP for ACLR with a BPTB graft and offer technical tips related to avoidance of common complications.

Technique

Creation of an appropriately located anteromedial portal is the most essential, primary step in ACLR surgery that uses the AMP technique (Fig. 47-1). Although some favor the use of an accessory AMP, we prefer instead to use a single AMP that is slightly more inferior than the standard portal in ACLR. The only exception to this approach is the need to perform a concomitant procedure that requires standard portal placement, such as meniscal repair, in which case two AMP portal incisions may be made. In this scenario, the first portal is established 1 to 2 mm inferior to the inferomedial pole of the patella and the second, femoral tunnel–creating AMP is 1 to 2 mm superior to the superior rim of the tibial plateau. Arthroscopic visualization of AMP creation from a standard anterolateral portal (ALP) is advised to avoid damage to the anterior horn of the medial meniscus, given the relatively inferior position of the AMP. In addition, some surgeons have recommended a more medial position of the portal compared with the AMP placement typically used in ACLR. However, we have found that damage to the cartilage of the medial femoral condyle can be a significant complication that is best avoided with AMP placement 2 to 3 mm medial to the medial edge of the patellar tendon.

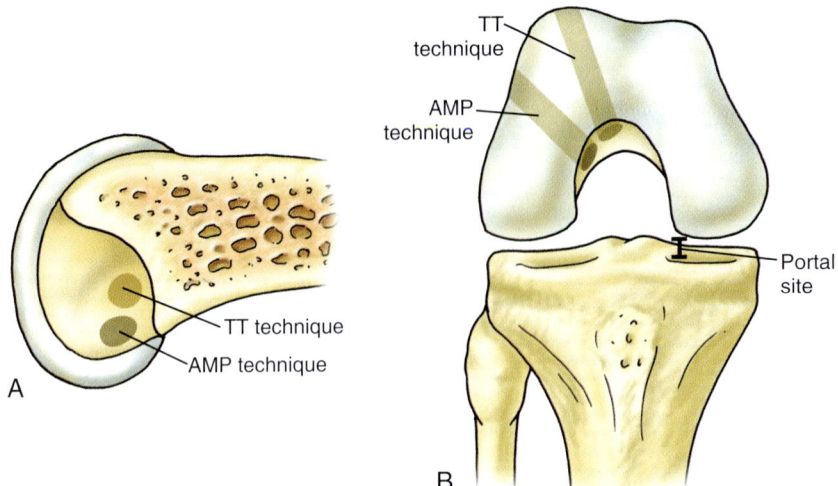

Figure 47-1. A, In some knees, where the anatomic footprint for the femoral tunnel cannot be reached using transtibial (TT) technique, or in certain revision cases, use of the AMP for guide wire and reamer advancement may allow for optimal tunnel position. **B,** An anterior view of the knee demonstrates the angle of the femoral tunnel when the AMP is used to establish the tunnel, relative to the TT technique.

Following standard diagnostic arthroscopy and débridement of the torn ACL, a notchplasty may be performed, but we have found this necessary only in the minority of cases with abnormally narrow notches, less than 15 mm in width. Given the relatively inferior position of graft placement on the femoral condyle, compared with traditional transtibial technique, graft impingement is rarely encountered. The posterior aspect of the soft tissue at the ACL footprint on the tibial surface is used as a landmark for tibial tunnel creation, in conjunction with the posterior aspect of the anterior horn of the lateral meniscus. We prefer to completely débride the soft tissues and mark the center of the footprint with the electrocautery device or a small curette prior to insertion of a standard ACL guide. Following standard tibial tunnel reaming and use of the motorized shaver to eliminate bony debris, a reverse chamfer drill is used to smooth the posterior intra-articular edge of the tibial tunnel to prevent bony abrasion of the graft during cyclic knee flexion.

A similar approach as described for the tibial footprint is used to identify and mark the center of the femoral ACL footprint. The soft tissues are then completely débrided from the lateral wall of the intercondylar notch while preserving the mark for the center of the footprint. An arthroscopic probe is used to identify the back wall of the femoral condyle definitively to avoid back wall blowout. The AMP is used to introduce the offset femoral guide and the guide wire as a unit past the medial femoral condyle, just as Cain and colleagues[8] initially described introduction of the guide wire and reamer as a unit. The knee must be hyperflexed 110 to 120 degrees to allow the trajectory of the guide wire directly into the center of the femoral footprint. Alternatively, flexible guide pins and reamers have been introduced in an effort to avoid the need for hyperflexion, minimize articular cartilage damage on the medial femoral condyle, and allow the length of the femoral tunnel to be maximized via a more proximally directed orientation. The guide wire is advanced to the level of the anterolateral femoral cortex and the offset guide is removed. A second guide wire is introduced through the AMP to the femoral footprint, just adjacent and parallel to

the first, to allow for measurement of the approximate length from footprint to cortex to ensure adequate tunnel length. If insufficient tunnel length is anticipated, the angle of the guide wire can be altered to increase tunnel length or other techniques to address mismatch can be planned, such as slight shortening of one or both bone plugs, depending on the estimated length. The second guide wire is removed and the reamer is then introduced into the notch under arthroscopic visualization, taking care to avoid damage to the MFC cartilage by the edges of the reamer.

Provided the angle of knee flexion is not changed and the trajectory of the guide wire maintained, we have found the risk of damage to the cartilage or bending of the guide wire to be minimal. In addition, the 30-degree arthroscope may be replaced with a 70-degree arthroscope if adequate visualization of the femoral footprint cannot be achieved with instrumentation in the notch, although this is not necessary in most cases. The reamer is advanced 5 to 10 mm into the femoral ACL footprint and withdrawn slightly to allow for reassessment of the adequacy of the back wall, with a goal of 1 to 2 mm of intact posterior bone. The reamer is then advanced to the appropriate depth, which varies according to graft type and graft length. The guide wire–reamer unit is removed. A Beath pin with a looped passing suture is introduced through the AMP into the notch, and the knee is again hyperflexed, with direct assessment of avoidance of contact between the Beath pin and MFC before advancement into the femoral tunnel. The pin is passed through the skin of the anterolateral thigh. The loop of the passing suture is left in the notch, an arthroscopic grasper is introduced through the tibial tunnel, and the passing is suture brought out of the tibial tunnel.

Graft passage is performed in standard fashion, with free sutures on the femoral side of the graft having been fed through the looped passing suture. An arthroscopic probe or grasper is used to orient the femoral bone block of the graft in the proper trajectory for smooth advancement into the femoral tunnel. Graft fixation is performed in standard fashion, with a femoral interference screw passed through the

AMP over a nitinol wire. Care must be taken to advance the screw into the tunnel with the knee in the same degree of hyperflexion that was used during femoral reaming. This avoids the complication of graft-screw divergence that has been reported for the AMP technique. Standard cycling of the graft and tibial interference screw fixation, with the knee in full extension and maximal manual traction on the graft, is then performed. A routine approach to wound closure is used.

Discussion

Use of the anteromedial portal in ACL reconstruction has the advantage of allowing for placement of a femoral tunnel in a more anatomic location than that seen with classic transtibial techniques. It can be particularly useful in revision surgery, in which the primary surgery may have involved placement of a more vertical femoral tunnel (e.g., at 11:00 or 1:00 o'clock, if not higher). Not only can a vertical primary position be responsible for graft failure through retear or persistent rotational instability, but the more anatomic placement may be performed without significant primary graft or tunnel débridement, interference screw removal, or bone grafting. In addition, use of the AMP has gained interest because of the growing popularity in double-bundle surgery, in which a more complex tibial tunnel configuration may warrant great flexibility in femoral tunnel placement, as is afforded by the AMP technique.

Despite its advantages in revision or double-bundle procedures, use of the AMP may have its greatest role as a new standard technique in primary ACL reconstruction, given the increasingly recognized importance of femoral tunnel position on restoration of native knee kinematics.[10,39,40] Despite the technical challenges associated with its use, complications can be avoided by a thorough understanding of the potential pitfalls and technical principles. Critical to success with AMP techniques are an understanding of native footprint anatomy, appropriate inferior AMP placement, introduction and advancement of instruments into the joint and notch under arthroscopic visualization, meticulous measurements of graft and tunnel length, and experience with appropriate flexion and hyperflexion angles of the knee for the different portions of the procedure. Although more clinical outcomes studies related to use of this technique are warranted, early, lower level evidence, cadaveric studies, and descriptions of its technique have been favorable.[4,5,12,14,19]

It remains unclear how widespread AMP use will be in the future, but we believe that it should become a technique familiar to all surgeons performing ACLR, especially in the revision setting. One approach favored by many surgeons for primary ACLR is creation of the tibial tunnel and assessment of potential femoral tunnel positioning through the transtibial tunnel. Because even minute variations in knee anatomy and tibial tunnel position can influence the ability to achieve anatomic placement of the femoral tunnel, this step allows for use of the AMP technique at this time if the transtibial approach does not allow for optimal graft placement. In the senior author's experience, an optimal femoral tunnel can often be achieved transtibially, and the transtibial approach can be used for the single-tunnel, single-bundle technique and the single-tunnel, double-bundle technique, as will be described.

ANTERIOR CRUCIATE LIGAMENT RECONSTRUCTION VIA SINGLE-TUNNEL, DOUBLE-BUNDLE TECHNIQUE

Although a number of clinical outcomes studies have demonstrated good results using single-bundle ACLR,[2,23,29] several long-term studies have shown unsatisfactory rates of osteoarthritis and knee pain following this technique.* Therefore, double-bundle ACLR has gained increasing interest based on clinical and biomechanical evidence suggesting that re-establishment of the separate anteromedial (AM) and posterolateral (PL) bundles may more closely restore native knee joint stability and kinematics.[9-11,21,22,31,36-38] However, double-bundle reconstruction techniques involving the creation of two tibial tunnels, and either one or two femoral tunnels, are more technically challenging, with longer operative times and more bone loss, thereby potentially increasing complication rates and making revision surgery more difficult. In addition, clinical and biomechanical studies have been performed that fail to demonstrate improved outcomes.[28,32]

Here we describe a technique of single-tunnel, double-bundle (STDB) ACLR that was developed in our laboratory. It takes advantage of the potential biomechanical advantage of separate AM and PL bundles while avoiding the technical challenges and pitfalls associated with the creation of two bony tunnels.

Technique

Knee arthroscopy is performed through standard anteromedial and anterolateral portals to confirm the ACL tear, and the ACL remnant is débrided with a motorized shaver. A notchplasty is performed only if necessary. The lower extremity is then exsanguinated and a thigh tourniquet inflated to 280 mm Hg. The semitendinosus and gracilis tendons are harvested in standard fashion through a 2- to 3-cm incision in the skin overlying the pes anserinus insertion on the anteromedial surface of the proximal tibia. The harvested grafts are pretensioned on a graft preparation board (DePuy Mitek) with 20 lb of force while the tibial and femoral tunnels are prepared in standard fashion. If optimal anatomic positioning of the femoral tunnel cannot be achieved through a transtibial technique, an anteromedial portal technique is used to centralize the tunnel on the femoral ACL footprint, as described earlier.

Two different femoral fixation devices, with slightly different techniques, may be used to achieve a STDB soft tissue graft construct, depending on surgeon preference. The first STDB technique involves use of the Femoral Intrafix (DePuy Mitek) device. This has the dual advantage of aperture fixation using a femoral sheath and interference screw construct, while maximizing biologic healing, via compression of the graft against cancellous bone throughout the length of the tunnel. The semitendinosus and gracilis tendons are looped over a single strand of suture and only the AM bundle is colored on the proximal end of the graft to identify the bundle easily. To achieve the desired anatomic position for the AM and PL bundles, a graft-positioning tool from the Intrafix set is used. The graft is placed in the fork of the

---

*References 1, 16, 17, 24, 25, and 27.

positioning tool with one bundle on either side of the fork. When the passing suture is used to pull the graft into the tunnel, the graft positioning tool is advanced through the tibial tunnel until it reaches the aperture of the femoral tunnel, at which time the AM and PL bundles are rotated by rotating the positioning tool. When the desired positions of the two bundles are achieved, the construct is then fully advanced into the femoral tunnel. The keel of a sheath trial is then placed between the strands to maintain the separation of the two bundles within the single tunnel. The femoral Intrafix sheath is then inserted into the tunnel, taking care not to alter the position of the two bundles. The graft is secured by the Intrafix screw into the sheath. Tibial tunnel fixation involves placement of the tibial Intrafix sheath with the AM and PL bundles placed in two opposite quadrants of the sheath at their anatomic insertion sites on the tibial plateau. A 40-N graft tension is applied to the graft while the tibial Intrafix screw is advanced with the leg in full extension.

An alternative STDB construct that may be used, provided that femoral tunnel length is adequate (>30 to 35 mm), is the AperFix (Cayenne Medical, Scottsdale, Ariz) femoral implant. In this technique, the semitendinosus and gracilis tendons are passed through the device and looped to form four strands (Fig. 47-2B). Because the device allows for isolation of the separate tendons of the hamstrings, the two strands of the semitendinosus tendon are used to represent the AM bundle and the two gracilis tendon strands represent the PL bundle (Fig. 47-3A). The implant is passed through the tibial tunnel into the femoral tunnel. Before deployment, the two bundles are positioned inside the femoral tunnel in the native ACL bundle positions. The semitendinosus limbs of the graft construct are placed in a slightly deeper and higher position on the femoral condyle, with the knee in the flexed position, and the gracilis limbs of the graft construct are placed in an anteroinferior position on the femoral condyle. The implant is then deployed in standard fashion, with the deployment knob expanding the teeth of the implant

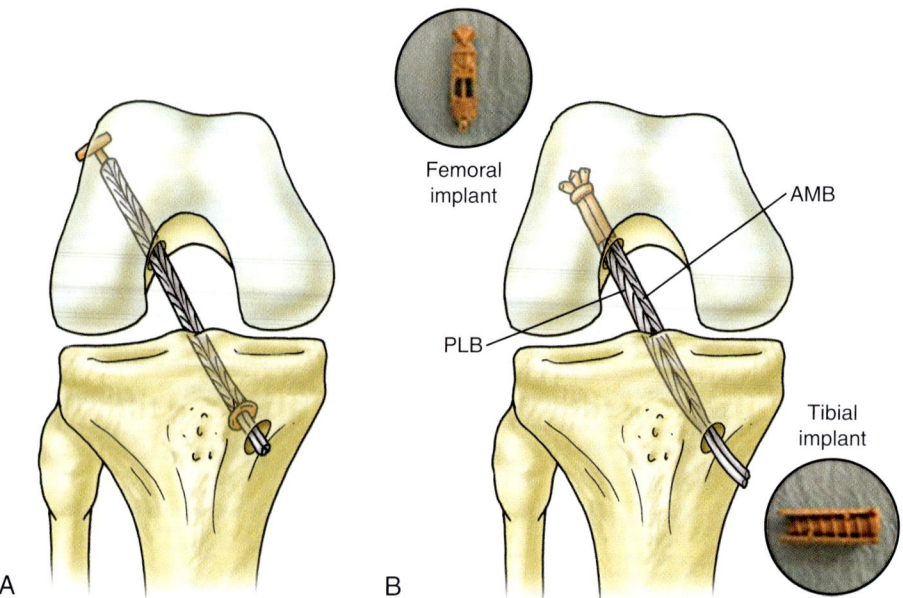

Figure 47-2. Schematic representation of single-bundle **(A)** and STDB **(B)** ACL reconstruction. *AMB*, Antermedial bundle; *PLB*, posterolateral bundle. (From Gadikota HR, Seon JK, Kozanek M, et al: Biomechanical comparison of single-tunnel-double-bundle and single-bundle anterior cruciate ligament reconstructions. Am J Sports Med 37:962–969, 2009.)

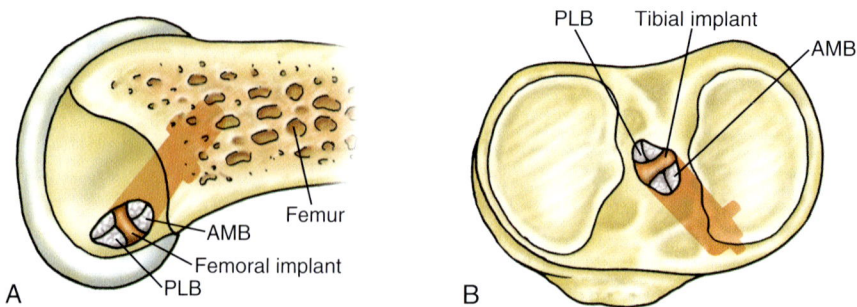

Figure 47-3. Schematic illustration of the femoral implant and separation of the two bundles in the femoral tunnel **(A)** and the tibial implant and separation of the two bundles in the tibial tunnel **(B)**. *AMB*, Anteromedial bundle; *PLB*, posterolateral bundle. (From Gadikota HR, Seon JK, Kozanek M, et al: Biomechanical comparison of single-tunnel-double-bundle and single-bundle anterior cruciate ligament reconstructions. Am J Sports Med 37:962–969, 2009.)

into the femoral cancellous bone. With the graft now secured at the femoral end, the distal end of the graft is rotated by 90 degrees in a clockwise direction for the left knee (counterclockwise for the right knee), giving rise to the native anatomic relationship of the AM and PL bundles as they pass into the tibial tunnel in the location of the ACL footprint (see Fig. 47-3B). This degree of rotation is based on the in vivo biomechanical study performed by Jordan and associates[18] that demonstrates approximately 80 degrees of ACL rotation as the knee flexes from 0 to 120 degrees. After cycling the knee five times, the graft is tensioned under maximal manual axial graft tension, with the knee in full extension, using the AperFix tensioning device. The graft is secured on the tibial side using the AperFix sheath and interference screw.

In either technique, the skin incisions at the two portal sites are repaired using 4-0 monofilament sutures, and the incision at the tibial footprint is approximated at the deep dermal layer by 2-0 braided suture and then by a running subcuticular monofilament suture. The postoperative rehabilitation protocol involves 50% partial weight bearing with the use of crutches for the first 6 weeks. An unlocked hinged knee brace is used for weight bearing, but removed for therapy, which includes the use of a continuous passive motion machine. Strength and stretching exercises are advanced according to standard post-ACL reconstruction principles.

Discussion

Although interest in double bundle ACL reconstruction continues to grow, there is also increasing evidence that its purported advantages may not be replicated in clinical outcomes or patient satisfaction. Interestingly, a cadaveric study by Rue and coworkers[26] has demonstrated that a well-oriented, laterally angled tibial tunnel in single-bundle, single-tunnel surgery allows for re-creation of the femoral footprints of both the AM and PL bundles, bringing into question the need for double tunnels at all. A separate clinical study with 2-year follow-up[32] failed to show any difference in the functional outcomes of two cohorts of 19 patients undergoing single-bundle, single-tunnel versus double-tunnel, double-bundle reconstructions, respectively.

To date, few clinical studies have been published regarding the use of a STDB construct for ACL reconstruction. Caborn and Chang[7] have described their technique, in which a tibialis anterior allograft is folded over to replicate the AM and PL bundles, which are separated in single femoral and tibial tunnels and secured with interference screws. However, their technique does not involve rotation of the graft limbs prior to tibial fixation, as described for our technique (see earlier). Shino and associates[30] have described several alterations in the reaming for and positioning of a BPTB autograft, which therefore causes different portions of the graft to mimic the two bundles of the native ACL, but the authors do not support this interpretation with biomechanical or clinical data. Takeuchi and coworkers[33] have reported on a technique

involving a bone-hamstring-bone composite graft, in which a bone block is removed from the tibia at the pes insertion, divided in two, and sutured to the ends of a standard hamstring autograft. This composite graft allows for separation of the limbs of the semitendinosus and gracilis autograft, similar to our technique. They reported ultimate fixation strength in their composite graft superior to that of a standard BPTB autograft.

Two biomechanical cadaveric studies from our institution have investigated the AperFix and Intrafix STDB techniques described earlier. In 2009, Gadikota and colleagues[11] showed that the STDB approach with the AperFix reduces anterior tibial translation at all flexion angles, compared with the ACL-deficient state. Interestingly, when compared with ACL-intact specimens, knees with STDB reconstructions showed comparable anterior tibial translation at low flexion angles, but decreased translation at 60 and 90 degrees, suggesting slight overconstraint. However, the maximum difference was less than 3 mm in all cases. A second 2010 study investigating femoral interference screw fixation with soft tissue grafts demonstrated that the STDB technique restores anterior knee stability better when compared with a conventional single-bundle reconstruction.[10] The advantage of both techniques is that they represent technically simple methods of re-creating double-bundle anatomy without introducing many of the technical challenges and risk of complications inherent in the technique.

KEY REFERENCES

Bedi A, Altchek DW: The "footprint" anterior cruciate ligament technique: an anatomic approach to anterior cruciate ligament reconstruction. Arthroscopy 25:128–138, 2009.

Gadikota HR, Seon JK, Kozanek M, Oh LS, Gill TJ, Montgomery KD, et al: Biomechanical comparison of single-tunnel-double-bundle and single-bundle anterior cruciate ligament reconstructions. Am J Sports Med 37:62–69, 2009.

Gadikota HR, Wu JL, Seon JK, Sutton K, Gill TJ, Li G, et al: Single-tunnel double-bundle anterior cruciate ligament reconstruction with anatomical placement of hamstring tendon graft: can it restore normal knee joint kinematics? Am J Sports Med 38:13–20, 2010.

Gavriilidis I, Motsis EK, Pakos EE, et al: Georgoulis AD, Mitsionis G, Xenakis TA. Transtibial versus anteromedial portal of the femoral tunnel in ACL reconstruction: a cadaveric study. Knee 15:64–67, 2008.

Harner CD, Honkamp NJ, Ranawat AS: Anteromedial portal technique for creating the anterior cruciate ligament femoral tunnel. Arthroscopy 24:13–15, 2008.

Lubowitz JH: Anteromedial portal technique for the anterior cruciate ligament femoral socket: pitfalls and solutions. Arthroscopy 25:95–101, 2009.

Rue JP, Ghodadra N, Bach BR, Jr: Femoral tunnel placement in single-bundle anterior cruciate ligament reconstruction: a cadaveric study relating transtibial lateralized femoral tunnel position to the anteromedial and posterolateral bundle femoral origins of the anterior cruciate ligament. Am J Sports Med 36:3–9, 2008.

Zantop T, Diermann N, Schumacher T, et al: Anatomical and nonanatomical double-bundle anterior cruciate ligament reconstruction: importance of femoral tunnel location on knee kinematics. Am J Sports Med 36:78–85, 2008.

Zantop T, Herbort M, Raschke MJ, et al: The role of the anteromedial and posterolateral bundles of the anterior cruciate ligament in anterior tibial translation and internal rotation. Am J Sports Med 35:23–27, 2007.

Full references for this chapter can be found on www.expertconsult.com.

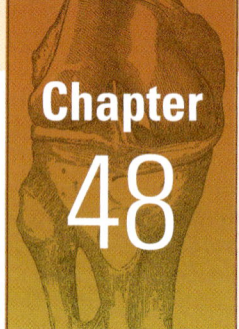

Chapter 48

Complications of Anterior Cruciate Ligament Reconstruction

Jason D. Archibald and Geoffrey S. Baer

Rupture of the anterior cruciate ligament (ACL) is one of the most common ligament injuries to the knee. More than 100,000 ACL reconstructions are performed each year in the United States. The goal of these procedures is to re-create a stable and functional knee joint that allows return to the level of activity prior to injury. Current arthroscopic techniques have success rates reported between 75% to 95%. However, as many as 5% to 10% of ACL reconstructions are revisions.[20] As with all surgical procedures, there are inherent risks to the reconstruction of the ACL. Complications from ACL reconstruction can be viewed as intraoperative or postoperative. Intraoperative complications include malpositioned tunnels, improper tensioning, and failure of graft fixation. Postoperative failures include infection, arthrofibrosis, graft failure, and osteoarthritis. The choice of graft also precludes an inherent set of complications, whether it is autologous bone-patellar tendon-bone, autologous hamstring, or allograft.

INTRAOPERATIVE COMPLICATIONS

Tunnel Placement

Intraoperative complications often result from technical errors. Wetzler and colleagues[83] have found that 77% of ACL revision cases are the result of technical shortcomings, including nonanatomic tunnel placement, graft impingement, improper tensioning, and inadequate graft fixation. Proper positioning of the femoral and tibial tunnels is essential to successful reconstruction of the ACL. Among these intraoperative complications, improper tunnel placement is the most common, specifically an anteriorly located femoral tunnel,[38] which leads to excessive strain during flexion and restricted range of motion. A femoral tunnel that is too vertically oriented (the 12-o'clock position) may control anterior-posterior forces on the knee joint but will lack the rotational control of the native ACL.[61] A femoral tunnel located too posteriorly in the notch risks blowing out the posterior wall of the tunnel, which may compromise fixation of the graft. If this occurs, one may move from interference to suspensory fixation, or another option is to redrill the femoral tunnel using an outside-in technique. Jepsen and coworkers[36] randomized 60 patients undergoing ACL reconstruction to low or high femoral tunnel positions and found no difference in laxity at 25 and 70 degrees, but a significant increase was found in subjective knee stability in the group with low (2-o'clock) femoral tunnels. While drilling the femoral tunnel, one should attempt to recreate the anatomic attachment of the native ACL, whether it is through a transtibial, anteromedial, or retrodrill technique.[1]

The tibial tunnel is more forgiving than the femoral tunnel but malpositioning can also lead to complications. The tunnel should be located posterior to Blumensaat's line when viewed on a lateral x-ray. When the tibial tunnel is drilled too anterior of the native footprint, the graft will impinge and likely fail. When too posterior, the graft becomes too vertical and loses rotational stability in the same fashion as the anteriorly drilled femoral tunnel.[49] Medial or lateral malpositioning of the tibial tunnel can lead to impingement, increased laxity, or chronic synovitis.[49,55]

Some complications regarding tunnel placement are inherent to the technique used for reconstruction. During ACL reconstructions using a double-bundle technique, one must avoid convergence of the two tunnels in the femur and tibia. This can be accomplished by measuring the footprint to ensure appropriate size, careful pin placement, avoiding tunnels over 9 mm in diameter, and potentially drilling tunnels using an outside-in technique. Recently, several systems have been developed to help prevent tunnel convergence. An anteromedial portal may be used to drill the femoral tunnels. Anteromedial drilling allows anatomic placement of the femoral tunnels that is independent of the tibial tunnels. If an anteromedial portal is used, care must be taken to avoid damage to the medial femoral condyle as the guide pin or reamer pass closely by the articular surface. We recommend careful visualization during creation of the anteromedial portal and the use of half-fluted reamers to help avoid cartilage damage (Fig. 48-1). Additionally, an anteromedial drilling technique may lead to shorter femoral tunnels than typically encountered with a transtibial technique. Fixation strategies should be adjusted to ensure an adequate amount of graft within the femoral tunnel to allow graft integration.

Impingement of the graft is often caused by nonanatomic tunnel placement but can also result from oversized grafts and inadequate notchplasty. Impinging ACL grafts will deform with strain and will likely become lax or fail.[24] Abrasion of the graft on the lateral femoral condyle or intercondylar roof can cause chronic synovitis, ligament attenuation, and failure.[74] However, aggressive notchplasty may damage articular cartilage. A dog model demonstrated histopathologic changes at 6 months similar to those of early degenerative arthritis in groups undergoing aggressive notchplasty.[45] Others have noted that although notchplasty may assist in visualization during arthroscopy, there does not appear to be a clinical difference in patients who did or did not receive a notchplasty during their ACL reconstruction.[58] Minimizing the notchplasty may reduce postoperative pain, bleeding, swelling, and potential notch regrowth.[21,60]

Graft Tension

Another complication of ACL reconstructions arises from improper tensioning of the graft. Inadequate tensioning creates a loose graft that will not re-create joint stability and kinematics. Overtensioning of the graft can lead to loss of

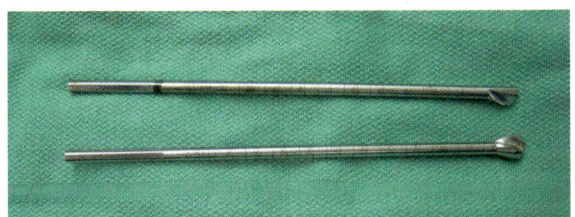

Figure 48-1. Half-fluted reamers may be used during femoral tunnel drilling from an anteromedial portal technique to prevent damage to the articular cartilage during drilling.

motion, graft stretching, excessive stress on the articular cartilage, poor vascularity, and subsequent graft degeneration.[33,85] Failure to precondition a graft cyclically can decrease forces within the graft by 30% soon after fixation.[29] A review of the randomized controlled trials evaluating graft tension in ACL reconstructions using bone-patellar tendon-bone (BPTB) autograft and hamstring autografts found no statistically or clinically relevant differences in various graft tensions.[5] The amount of tension that should be applied to optimize outcome is unknown at this time.

Graft Contamination

Graft contamination caused by the graft being dropped onto the floor of the operating room is a rare but dangerous intraoperative complication which can lead to early septic arthritis. Cooper and associates[15] investigated the incidence of positive cultures in dropped grafts in an operating room environment. Six of 10 grafts (60%) that were dropped on the floor for 3 minutes had a positive culture at 10 days. Three of 10 grafts (30%) that were dropped on the floor for 3 minutes and then soaked in sterile saline containing bacitracin and polymyxin B for 15 minutes also had positive cultures at 10 days. Similarly, Molina and coworkers[54] harvested native ACLs during total knee arthroplasties, dropped them onto the operating room floor for 15 seconds, and then cultured them. In this study, 29 of 50 specimens (58%) were found to have positive cultures. Grafts soaked in solutions exhibited drops in the positive culture rate—12 of 50 (24%) in the povidone-iodine solution group, 3 of 50 (6%) in the antibiotic solution group, and 1 of 50 (2%, in broth only) in the chlorhexidine gluconate group. Although data regarding dropped grafts are limited, a survey of surgeons found that many recommend cleansing the graft and proceeding with the ACL reconstruction rather than harvesting a different autograft or switching to allograft.[33] A combination of chlorhexidine gluconate and triple antibiotic solution in sterile saline appears to be the most effective for preventing positive cultures.[28] The most effective way to prevent graft contamination caused by a dropped graft is clearly prevention. We recommend minimizing hand-offs during the reconstruction, clear communication between staff when the graft is being moved, and clamping the graft on the field.

Graft Fixation and Maturation

Until a graft has incorporated into the host bone tunnels, it is dependent on adequate fixation strength for stability. Current rehabilitation protocols emphasize early range of motion and strengthening, underscoring the need for stable fixation. One study has found no difference in clinical outcome among interference screws, whether they were metallic, titanium, or bioabsorbable.[21] Furthermore, good results have been found with soft tissue grafts when using EndoButton, femoral transfix, soft tissue screws, or a tibial-sided screw and washer. BPTB grafts begin to incorporate between 6 and 12 weeks. At 16 to 24 weeks, a normal bone-ligament junction forms. However, caution must be exercised in patients with low bone mineral density, because interference screw fixation has low stiffness in osteopenic cancellous bone. This may necessitate switching to fixation based on cortical rather than cancellous bone. Cortical bone may also be used as backup fixation (e.g., tie sutures around a screw and washer or a staple).

A graft goes through morphologic changes over time and becomes similar to a native ACL, a process termed *ligamentization*. This process consists of several steps, including necrosis (0 to 4 weeks), revascularization and cellular proliferation (4 to 12 weeks), and remodeling (3 to 6 months).[67] Arthroscopically collected samples of patellar tendon and hamstring ACL grafts taken at 6 and 12 months after ACL reconstruction have demonstrated the amount of collagen cross-linking in the ACL graft returns to the level of native ACLs within 1 year of reconstruction.[51] Ligamentization takes a longer period of time in allografts and hamstring autografts. Animal studies have shown a delay of revascularization and proliferation in allograft compared with autograft at 6 and 12 weeks of healing whereas at 52 weeks the differences are less distinct.[33,66] Although labeled as ligamentization, the incorporated graft does not have the same physical properties of the native ACL. The collagen fibers of the graft are uniform in length and diameter, unlike the various fibers of the native ACL, which are able to distribute loads throughout the range of motion. Furthermore, there are different proportions of glycosaminoglycans and collagen-reducible cross-links. These can contribute to biologic failure of the graft.[24] The processes of graft incorporation and ligamentization should be taken into account when determining advances in rehabilitation, as well as return to sporting activities, to prevent an early failure of the graft.

POSTOPERATIVE COMPLICATIONS

Infection

Infection is a rare but devastating complication following ACL reconstruction. It can lead to the loss of articular cartilage and increase the risk of arthrofibrosis. Once identified, infection should be treated with prompt arthroscopic irrigation and débridement. Broad-spectrum antibiotics should be initiated until a more culture-specific regimen can be identified. If still functional, the graft can often be maintained. Risk factors for infection include previous arthroscopic or open knee surgery and tibial ACL graft fixation with a post and washer.[39] In a retrospective review of 3126 ACL reconstructions, Barker and colleagues[9] have identified 18 infections (0.58%). Infections occurred in 6 of 1349 allografts (0.44%), 7 of 1430 BPTB autografts (0.49%), and 5 of 347 hamstring autografts (1.44%). The most common organism was *Staphylococcus aureus*. The increased rate of infection in hamstring grafts was statistically significant. A higher risk of infection or need for graft removal was not seen with allografts. Another review in China demonstrated a similar rate of infection (0.52%) among 4068 patients over a 10-year period. Of these 21 infections, 20 were autologous hamstring grafts and 1 was a patellar tendon allograft.[82] Katz and associates[41] have reviewed 801 reconstructions and found an infection rate of 0.75% (6 patients). Their analysis showed that autograft (2 of 170) had twice the risk of infection compared with allograft (4 of 628) but this difference was not statistically significant ($p = 0.77$).

Stiffness

Loss of motion is the most common complication after ACL reconstruction, occurring in 4% to 35% of cases.[23] The causes are often multifactorial and the aforementioned complications can all contribute to joint stiffness. Other factors include prolonged immobilization, poor patient compliance, intercondylar notch scarring, capsulitis, cyclops lesion, and reflex sympathetic dystrophy.[12] Harner and coworkers[31] have retrospectively reviewed 244 ACL reconstructions for postoperative stiffness and found an incidence of 11.1%. Factors associated with loss of motion included acute reconstruction less than 1 month from injury, male gender, and concomitant medial collateral ligament (MCL) repair. Shelbourne and coworkers' retrospective review[70] of 169 ACL reconstructions found that acute reconstructions are not associated with increased risk of arthrofibrosis (4%) when an accelerated postoperative rehabilitation program is followed. Loss of both extension and flexion is more common, with loss of extension thought to be more detrimental to function. A knee flexion contracture greater than 10 degrees prevents a normal gait and increases loads across the patellar femoral joint. Loss of flexion past 125 degrees interferes with activities of daily living, including sitting, stair climbing, and running. Historically, ACL reconstructions were initially immobilized and motion was slowly advanced. This led to increased rates of arthrofibrosis. Current physical therapy protocols have emphasized early range of motion, which has decreased rates of stiffness without adversely affecting clinical outcomes.

Treatment of arthrofibrosis includes physical therapy and dynamic braces. A manipulation under anesthesia may aid in the recovery of motion, especially when performed within the first 6 weeks of the postoperative course. Arthroscopic lysis of adhesions or resection of a cyclops lesion may be necessary. Loss of motion resulting from technical errors (e.g., misplaced tunnels) during the initial surgery may require revision ACL reconstruction. Administration of a tapered course of oral steroids in the early postoperative period for patients with decreased range of motion has also been described as a method to improve flexion by reducing inflammation and intra-articular scar formation.[62]

Extensor mechanism dysfunction is uncommon after ACL reconstruction but can play a role in the development of arthrofibrosis. Early postoperative rehabilitative protocols emphasize quadriceps strengthening. Deficits in quadriceps strength can often be found in up to 20% of patients at 6 months post–ACL reconstruction.[59] Although the magnitude and incidence of quadriceps weakness decrease with time, its role in maintaining knee joint stability underscores the importance of early aggressive strengthening of this muscle group.

Graft Failure

Biologic graft failure may occur in the early postoperative course (first 6 months) before full incorporation and ligamentization. As noted, this is usually a result of an intraoperative technical error. Other causes of early graft failure include premature return to sports, infection, and graft insufficiency. Late graft failures occur in 5% to 10% of individuals who have returned to their preinjury level of activity.[30,37] Spindler and colleagues[73] have reviewed nine randomized controlled trials comparing patellar tendon and hamstring autografts. There was no significant difference in failure between the two choices of graft with an overall incidence of 3.6% and a minimum of 2 years of follow-up. Salmon and associates[64] followed 760 ACL reconstructions over a 5-year period. They reported a 6% risk of ACL graft rupture as well as a 6% risk of contralateral native ACL injury, which was not affected by choice of patellar tendon or hamstring autograft. In the first year, there was an increased risk of graft failure on the operative knee, but by 12 months there is an equal chance of rupturing the unaffected ACL or reconstructed ACL graft. This is significantly higher than the 1.5% to 1.7% risk of primary ACL injury in a young athletic population.[43] Similarly, Wright and coworkers[85] have reported on data collected in the MOON (Multicenter Orthopaedic Outcomes Network) cohort study. In their report, 235 patients who underwent ACL reconstructions were followed for 2 years. There were 14 ACL injuries, 7 in the contralateral knee (3%) and 7 in the reconstructed knee (3%). Although females are 2 to 8 times more likely to tear their native ACL than their male counterparts, there does not appear to be any differences in failure rates of ACL reconstructions between males and females.[64] Recent data have suggested that allograft reconstructions may suffer from a higher failure rate compared to autograft.[32]

Arthritis

Osteoarthritis (OA) is a common postoperative disease complicating ACL reconstructions. The risk of OA has been reported to be 50% after an ACL injury and as high as 70% when associated with a meniscal injury.[26] Keays and colleagues[42] followed 56 ACL reconstructions for 6 years after surgery and noted that meniscectomy and chondral damage are associated with a higher risk of tibiofemoral and patellofemoral arthritis. Øiestad and associates[57] have reviewed 7 prospective and 24 retrospective studies on the development of knee OA following ACL reconstruction. At 10 years follow-up, the prevalence of radiographic OA in isolated ACL injuries was 0% to 13% and higher with combined injuries (21% to 48%). They concluded that previous data overestimated the prevalence of osteoarthritis after ACL reconstruction. No differences were seen in patients who were treated nonoperatively versus those who underwent ACL reconstruction, regardless of graft selection.

GRAFT-SPECIFIC COMPLICATIONS

The choice of ACL graft carries an inherent set of complications, whether the surgeon uses patellar tendon autograft, hamstring autograft, or allograft.

Bone-Patellar Tendon-Bone Autograft

The BPTB autograft is considered the gold standard and is often the graft of choice in high-demand athletes. It is thought that the bone plug to bone tunnel healing occurs more quickly than soft tissue grafts.[33] Anterior knee pain is the most frequently noted complication associated with patellar tendon autograft. Sachs and coworkers[63] have studied 126 patients who had undergone BPTB autograft ACL reconstructions and found patellofemoral pain in 19% of patients, which correlated positively with a flexion contracture. Aglietti and colleagues[3] reviewed their series of 226 patellar tendon ACL reconstructions and reported a 5% incidence of painful patellofemoral crepitus with pain and 20% with crepitus and no pain. In a review of nine randomized trials, Spindler found a range of anterior knee pain between 13% and 43%, with no significant differences between hamstring (HS) and BPTB autografts.[73] However, all four studies that evaluated kneeling pain found significantly more pain in the patellar tendon groups (36% to 67% of patients).

Graft tunnel mismatch is an intraoperative complication that may occur when the BPTB graft is too long and less than 20 mm of the bone plug remains within the tibial tunnel, preventing effective use of interference screw fixation. This is more likely to occur when the patellar tendon is more than 50 mm.[69] Strategies to remedy this problem include recession of the graft further into the femoral tunnel, insertion of a bone plug into the tibial tunnel, and fixation at the tibia with a post and screw. Furthermore, the graft may be rotated to decrease the amount of mismatch. Rotation of 540 degrees will decrease length by 10%[81] and 630 degrees by 25%,[6] without any statistical difference in ultimate failure strength (Fig. 48-2). Furthermore, Barber[8] reported on 50 patients who underwent flipping of the bone plug 180 degrees onto the tendon to shorten the length of tendon between bone plugs. No significant complications were found at a mean follow-up of 28 months.

Patellar fractures following patellar tendon harvest are rare but have been reported in the literature. Tay and colleagues[77]

have reviewed five case reports and eight series reports and found an incidence rate of 0.55%. These fractures may be direct, the intraoperative result of a technical error during the harvest, or indirect, occurring on average 11 weeks after the ACL reconstruction. They are usually stellate or transverse-shaped. Many authors recommend primary bone grafting of the harvest sites intraoperatively to reduce the risk of fracture.[15] Lee and associates[46] have reviewed 1725 consecutive patients who underwent primary ACL reconstruction using a BPTB autograft and reported three complications related to harvest of the patellar tendon graft—one intraoperative fracture, one postoperative fracture, and one patellar tendon rupture. With a 0.2% acute complication rate, they concluded that the patellar tendon is a safe and viable choice of graft for ACL reconstruction.

The shape of the patellar tendon bone plugs affects the risk of fracture. Using a porcine model, Moholkar and associates[53] have shown that the shape of the bone plug affects the risk of fracture. The impact energy required to create a 1% probability of complete fracture was 7 J for a sharp-cornered defect, 17 J for a trapezoidal plug, 22 J for a sharp-cornered defect with a drill hole at the corner, 40 J for a round-cornered defect, and 49 J for a normal patella. They concluded that the use of a round-cornered patellar defect would reduce the risk of patellar fracture intraoperatively and postoperatively. DuMontier and coworkers[16] used a cadaveric model to demonstrate that the mean ultimate tensile strength of the patellar tendon after harvesting is not altered (2500 to 3000 N) whether the defect left in the patellar is circular, rectangular, or triangular. To avoid patellar fractures, it is recommended to avoid the primary use of osteotomes during harvest of the tendon. The graft should be located in the central portion of the patellar tendon. The bone plugs should be 25 mm or less in length and 10 mm or less in width. Two thirds of the patellar depth should be preserved and the bone plugs should be cut in a triangular or trapezoidal shape with the saw. Cross-hatching at the corners should be avoided. We use an oscillating saw with a Steri-Strip around the blade to mark 1 cm of depth and fill in the patellar defect with autologous bone graft in an attempt to reduce fracture risk and anterior knee pain (Fig. 48-3).

Hamstring Autograft

Hamstring autograft reconstructions have become more prevalent in the past decade. Initial concerns of inadequate

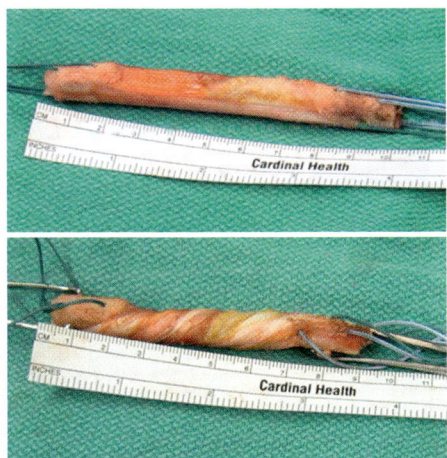

Figure 48-2. Graft tunnel mismatch can be a concern in patients with patella alta or a long patellar tendon. Twisting of the graft by 540 degrees can shorten the graft by 10% without weakening the reconstruction. **A,** Patellar tendon graft prior to twisting. **B,** Patellar tendon graft twisted 540 degrees, shortening the graft by over 1 cm to help correct for graft tunnel mismatch.

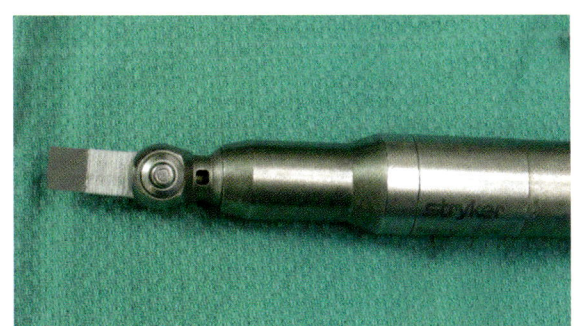

Figure 48-3. A Steri-Strip may be used to mark the saw blade at 1 cm to prevent overpenetration of the blade, reducing the risk for patellar fracture or cartilage damage.

strength of single- or double-stranded grafts have been addressed with the use of four-stranded semitendinosus and gracilis autografts. Current literature reveals few clinical differences in range of motion, isokinetic strength, laxity, or long-term results between hamstring and BPTB autografts.[73] A common complication seen in HS ACL reconstructions is intraoperative premature amputation of the gracilis or semitendinosus tendons, usually caused by an incomplete release of the tendon from the fascial bands. Solman and Pagnani[72] have documented up to five accessory bands or insertions of the semitendinosus alone that must be mobilized prior to harvest. There is a consistent band to the medial head of the gastrocnemius approximately 5.5 cm proximal to the pes anserinus. Tuncay and colleagues[79] have studied the anatomy of the fascial band between the semitendinosus and gastrocnemius in 23 cadaveric knees. The mean width of the band was 2.6 cm and the mean distance from the semitendinosus insertion to the fascial band was 7 cm. The size of the harvested hamstring tendons can be difficult to predict. If there is insufficient hamstring length, the surgeon may need to select an alternate graft. When the tendons have a small caliber but a long length, the grafts may be tripled to provide a graft of greater caliber (Fig. 48-4).

Another complication associated with hamstring tendon harvesting for ACL reconstruction is injury to the saphenous nerve, which is located between layers I and II and is at risk for injury when the tendon stripper is moved proximally. Sanders and associates[65] have reviewed the results of 164 patients who had undergone ACL reconstruction using hamstring autograft over a 4-year period. Of the patients surveyed, 74% reported postoperative sensory disturbance. Injury to the sartorial branch of the saphenous nerve (SBSN) and infrapatellar branch of the saphenous nerve (IPBSN) occurred in 32%, and isolated injury to the SBSN occurred in 23% and to the IPBSN in 19%. This was followed by an examination of the saphenous nerve anatomy in 11 cadavers. They found that the saphenous nerve is intimately associated with the gracilis over a span of 4.6 cm, between 7.2 and 11.8 cm proximal to its insertion. Placing the knee in a figure-of-four position or knee flexion to 90 degrees will relax the saphenous nerve as it passes over the medial hamstrings and may reduce the risk of injury to the saphenous nerve.[58]

Another complication of hamstring tendon harvest for ACL reconstruction is hamstring weakness. Initial studies by Lipscomb and coworkers[48] have demonstrated the mean strength of the hamstrings to be 99% of the contralateral leg after HS ACL reconstruction, a finding confirmed by others.[4,13] Later data have raised questions regarding hamstring function after harvesting. Nakajima and colleagues[56] have found decreased hamstring strength in deep flexion after ACL reconstruction. More recently, Tashiro and associates[76] randomly assigned 90 patients to gracilis and semitendinosus or semitendinosus alone ACL reconstructions. They found significant decreases in hamstring muscle strength at 70 degrees or more of flexion in both groups, but less so in the semitendinosus only group. Similarly, Gobbi and coworkers[27] prospectively followed a group of 97 patients who were also randomized to gracilis and semitendinosus hamstring or semitendinosus alone. They found no differences in clinical results and flexion and extension strength, but found a significant deficit in internal rotation. It has been suggested by Adachi and associates[2] that although peak flexion torque and total work are not significantly altered by hamstring harvesting, the more hamstring tendons are harvested, the more peak torque angle is shifted to a shallower angle, which may explain weakness in deep flexion. Regrowth of the harvested hamstring tendons has been observed,[25] and magnetic resonance imaging (MRI) studies have correlated the extent of tendon regrowth with the amount of strength regained after hamstring harvest for ACL reconstruction.[75]

Both femoral and tibial tunnels widen in hamstring ACL reconstructions postoperatively.[47,68,84] Clatworthy and coworkers[14] have evaluated the incidence and degree of tunnel widening in a prospective series of 73 patients receiving a hamstring or patellar tendon autograft. Tunnel widening was evaluated with anteroposterior and lateral radiographs after validation with MRI. At a minimum 1-year follow-up, the tunnel area for HS grafts was increased 100.4% in the femur and 73.9% in the tibia, whereas the tunnel area for BPTB grafts decreased 25% in the femur and 2.1% in the tibia. Despite these observations, no clinical significance has been correlated with tunnel widening in long-term studies. However, tunnel widening may pose a difficult problem in revision ACL reconstruction, requiring a two-stage reconstruction initially to treat the bone defects prior to proceeding with ACL reconstruction (Fig. 48-5).

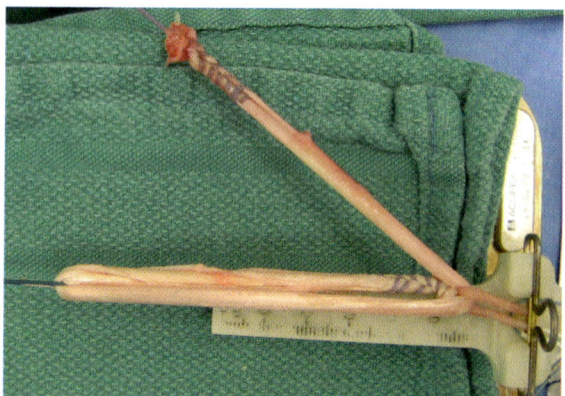

Figure 48-4. Tripling of a hamstring tendon graft of adequate length allows the creation of a graft with greater caliber than simply doubling over each graft. In this case, by tripling the semitendinosus tendon and doubling the gracilis tendon, the graft size was increased from 6.5 to 8.5 mm.

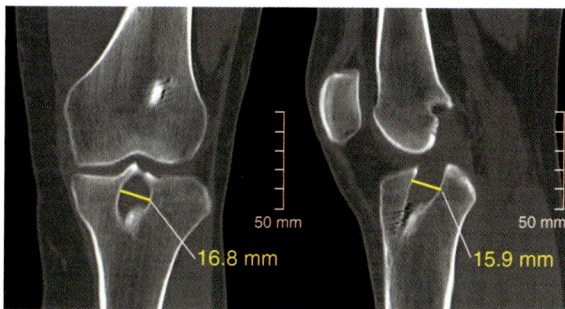

Figure 48-5. Tunnel dilation can pose a significant problem when approaching revision ACL reconstruction. In this case, a two-stage reconstruction was undertaken to allow treatment of the significant bone defects prior to revision of the ACL reconstruction.

Allograft Tissue

Allograft tissue has been advocated as an alternative to autograft tendons in ACL reconstructions secondary to shortened surgical times, less postoperative pain, and lack of donor site morbidity.[7,32] Complications associated with allograft ACL reconstructions include disease transmission and slower incorporation of the graft.

Viral transmission of human immunodeficiency virus (HIV) and hepatitis are among the most concerning diseases that may be transmitted through allograft use. Since a blood test for HIV has been available, there has been one transmission of HIV in 1985 through the surgical use of allograft tissue.[78] Since then, more than several million grafts have been implanted in the United States without a documented transmission of HIV.[71] With current serologic tests to screen donors and tissue processing and storage, the estimated risk of HIV transmission with connective tissue allografts is 1:8,000,000.[6] Two cases of hepatitis C transmission were reported in 1991, one of which occurred before a specific blood test for hepatitis C was available. A third case of hepatitis C transmission was reported by the Centers for Disease Control and Prevention (CDC) in 2002 in a patient receiving a patellar tendon allograft.[80] Freeze-dried grafts appear to have lower risk of viral transmission than fresh-frozen or frozen allograft tissue; however, freeze drying, ethylene oxide sterilization, and irradiation higher than 2.5 Mrad have been shown to decrease the biomechanical properties of the allograft.[33,52]

Bacterial infection is another complication that may occur following allograft ACL reconstruction. In 2002, the CDC reported on 26 cases of allograft-associated bacterial infections. Of these, 14 grafts had been processed by a single facility and 18 of the infections followed anterior cruciate reconstruction.[80] Between 1998 and 2003, 14 patients were infected with *Clostridium septicum* following musculoskeletal allograft implantation. This resulted in one death. The others were treated with hospitalization, intravenous antibiotics, and joint irrigation and débridement; 10 patients required removal of their allografts.[40] Other isolated bacterial species include gram-negative bacilli and *Streptococcus pyogenes*. The CDC has made specific recommendations regarding tissue processing to decrease the risk of microbial contamination. We recommend using an accredited tissue bank and reviewing their processing techniques.

There has been concern that allograft ACL reconstructions may have a higher failure rate than autograft reconstructions. Both autografts and allografts go through a similar process of ligamentization, as discussed earlier. The remodeling of allografts has been demonstrated to occur at a slower rate than in autografts.[34] Consequently, many surgeons will delay a patient's return to activity after allograft ACL reconstruction to allow the graft time to mature fully. Consistent with longer incorporation times, failure rates do appear to be higher in allograft reconstructions. Carey and colleagues[11] have performed a systematic review of nine studies comparing autograft and allograft anterior cruciate reconstructions. The short-term clinical outcomes between both grafts did not differ significantly. Another systematic review by Foster and associates[19] analyzed the results from 31 prospective studies comparing autograft and allograft ACL reconstructions. Their meta-analysis found few statistical differences between the two graft choices. The graft failure rate was $4.7/100 \pm 0.5/100$ for autograft and $8.2/100 \pm 2.1/100$ for allograft. Although not statistically significant, this could represent a concerning trend. They concluded that the choice of graft had minimal effect on the clinical outcome for the patients. However, the authors in both of these reviews noted that the results are not stratified to control for patient age or activity level.

Edgar and coworkers[17] have prospectively compared identical quadrupled hamstring autografts with allograft constructs in 84 patients. The two cohorts were similar in age, acute or chronic nature of their ACL injury, and incidence of concomitant meniscal injuries. At a mean follow-up of 50 months, there were no differences in subjective or objective outcomes. Laxity did not appear to be increased in the allograft group. An additional review of prospective studies comparing autograft BPTB and allograft BPTB grafts was presented by Krych and colleagues.[43] Six studies met their inclusion criteria comprised of 256 autograft and 278 allograft patients. Allograft patients were more likely to rupture their graft than autograft patients (odds ratio, 5.03; $P = .01$). However, when irradiated and chemically processed grafts were excluded, no significant difference between the two groups was seen. More recent data presented from the Multicenter Orthopaedic Outcomes Network (MOON) study at the American Orthopaedic Society for Sports Medicine (AOSSM) 2008 meeting in Orlando, Florida, showed an odds ratio of failure of 6.77 in allograft ACL reconstructions in 10- to 19-year-old patients when compared with autografts.[32]

MEDICAL COMPLICATIONS

Deep venous thrombosis (DVT) is a potentially life-threatening complication of ACL reconstruction that may lead to pulmonary embolism (PE). The American College of Chest Physicians has recommended that patients undergoing knee arthroscopy who do not have additional thromboembolic risk factors should use early mobilization alone as thromboprophylaxis.[22] The risk of DVT for routine arthroscopy is reported to be between 0.6% and 17.9%, depending on the diagnostic technique.[10] However, ACL reconstruction is often associated with longer operative times and has a theoretically higher risk. Marlovits and associates[50] prospectively followed 175 patients following ACL reconstruction who were randomized to enoxaparin or placebo for 20 days postoperatively. Of the enoxaparin group, 2.8% developed DVT as confirmed by magnetic resonance venography compared with 41.2% of the placebo group. Risk factors for DVT were age older than 30 years and immobilization before surgery. No cases of PE were diagnosed in either group.

KEY REFERENCES

Abebe ES, Moorman CT, 3rd, Dziedzic TS, et al: Femoral tunnel placement during anterior cruciate ligament reconstruction: an in vivo imaging analysis comparing transtibial and 2-incision tibial tunnel-independent techniques. Am J Sports Med 37:1904–1911, 2009.

Arneja S, McConkey MO, Mulpuri K, et al: Graft tensioning in anterior cruciate ligament reconstruction: a systematic review of randomized controlled trials. Arthroscopy 25:200–207, 2009.

Baer GS, Harner CD: Clinical outcomes of allograft versus autograft in anterior cruciate ligament reconstruction. Clin Sports Med 26:661–681, 2007.

Barker JU, Drakos MC, Maak TG, et al: Effect of graft selection on the incidence of postoperative infection in anterior cruciate ligament reconstruction. Am J Sports Med 38:281–286, 2010.

Carey JL, Dunn WR, Dahm DL, et al: A systematic review of anterior cruciate ligament reconstruction with autograft compared with allograft. J Bone Joint Surg Am 91:2242–2250, 2009.

Foster TE, Wolfe BL, Ryan S, et al: Does the graft source really matter in the outcome of patients undergoing anterior cruciate ligament reconstruction? An evaluation of autograft versus allograft reconstruction results: a systematic review. Am J Sports Med 38:189–199, 2010.

Fu FH, Bennett CH, Ma CB, et al: Current trends in anterior cruciate ligament reconstruction. Part II. Operative procedures and clinical correlations. Am J Sports Med 28:124–130, 2000.

Harner CD, Lo MY: Future of allografts in sports medicine. Clin Sports Med 28:327–340, 2009.

Jepsen CF, Lundberg-Jenson AK, Faunoe P: Does the position of the femoral tunnel affect the laxity or clinical outcome of the anterior cruciate ligament–reconstructed knee? A clinical prospective, randomized, double-bind study. Arthroscopy 23:1326–1333, 2007.

Krych AJ, Jackson JD, Hoskin TL, Dahm DL: A meta-analysis of patellar tendon autograft versus patellar tendon allograft in anterior cruciate ligament reconstruction. Arthroscopy 24:292–298, 2008.

Marumo K, Saito M, Yamagishi T, Fujii K: The "ligamentization" process in human anterior cruciate ligament reconstruction with autogenous patellar and hamstring tendons: a biochemical study. Am J Sports Med 33:1166–1173, 2005

Øiestad BE, Engebretsen L, Storheim K, Risberg MA: Knee osteoarthritis after anterior cruciate ligament injury: a systematic review. Am J Sports Med 37:1434–1443, 2009.

Salmon L, Russell V, Musgrove T, et al: Incidence and risk factors for graft rupture and contralateral rupture after anterior cruciate ligament reconstruction. Arthroscopy 21:948–957, 2005.

Spindler KP, Kuhn J, Freedman KB, et al: Anterior cruciate ligament reconstruction autograft choice: bone-tendon-bone versus hamstring. Does it really matter? A systematic review. Am J Sports Med 32:1986–1995, 2004.

Wright RW, Dunn WR, Amendola A, et al: Risk of tearing the intact anterior cruciate ligament in the contralateral knee and rupturing the anterior cruciate ligament graft during the first 2 years after anterior cruciate ligament reconstruction: a prospective MOON cohort study. Am J Sports Med 35:1131–1134, 2007.

Full references for this chapter can be found on www.expertconsult.com.

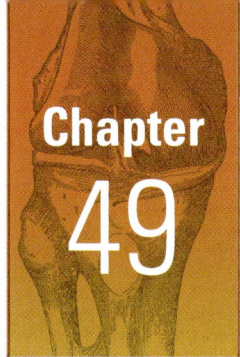

Chapter 49

Revision Anterior Cruciate Ligament Reconstruction

James E. Voos, Travis G. Maak, Riley J. Williams, III, and Thomas L. Wickiewicz

Although primary anterior cruciate ligament (ACL) reconstruction is commonly a successful procedure, failure rates of 3% to 15% have been reported.[3,26] Revision ACL reconstruction presents a significant challenge for the orthopedic surgeon, and the success of revision surgery relies on determining the cause of failure for the primary operation. Recurrent trauma, technical errors, concomitant injuries, loss of motion, and failure of graft incorporation can all contribute to a poor outcome.* The results of revision ACL reconstruction have been inferior to primary reconstructions. Increasing knowledge of ACL anatomy, kinematics, and surgical technique may allow patients undergoing revision ACL reconstruction to return to a high level of function.

CAUSATIVE FACTORS

For revision ACL reconstruction to be successful, it is paramount to determine the underlying factors leading to failure of the index reconstruction. The goal of revision ACL surgery is to provide knee stability to maximize patient function and protect articular cartilage and the meniscus from further injury.[2] The cause of failure may be related to loss of motion or recurrent trauma but often is the result of surgical technique and failure to recognize concomitant pathology.[11,15,17,22] At the time of revision surgery, the causative factors must be addressed to provide an optimal clinical result.

Loss of Motion

Motion loss is one of the most common and potentially debilitating complications following ACL reconstruction.[19] Specifically, extension loss is encountered more frequently and is less tolerated than flexion loss.[28] The cause of motion loss may be attributed to a number of causes, such as time from injury to ACL reconstruction, tunnel position on the tibia and femur, excessive graft tension, extensor mechanism and patellar tendon scarring, arthrofibrosis, multiple ligament injury, and prolonged immobilization.[23]

The cause of motion loss must be addressed prior to proceeding with revision ACL reconstruction. Although prevention is the best strategy, early recognition of developing stiffness allows for the appropriate conservative or surgical intervention to provide the best outcome. Importance is placed on maximizing knee range of motion, decreasing inflammation, and improving muscle strength prior to revision ACL reconstruction.

Assessment of tunnel placement, graft impingement, and fibrosis location can be ascertained by physical examination, diagnostic imaging, and surgical visualization. A systematic evaluation of the knee, as described by Millet and colleagues,[30] allows for careful débridement of fibrotic structures through arthroscopic or open procedures. When motion loss is significant, a staged revision procedure may be indicated.

Persistent Pain

Persistent pain after ACL reconstruction is often multifactorial. Articular cartilage loss, meniscal pathology, prominent hardware, neuromas, graft site morbidity, prolonged inflammatory response, painful scars, and infection have all been implicated as confounding variables. Often, the exact source of pain is difficult to ascertain. However, selection of an optimal treatment plan relies on accurately determining the cause.

Recurrent Instability

Instability after ACL reconstruction can be divided into three categories: traumatic failure, atraumatic failure, and failure caused by graft malposition or fixation loss. Analysis of these categories relies on careful history, physical examination, imaging, and review of prior operative reports.

Patients with traumatic failure report a single traumatic event in a previously well-functioning stable knee. The mechanism is often the same as that occurring in a native rupture of the ACL. Instability that occurs in the early postoperative course may be the result of trauma to the ACL before full graft incorporation.[23] Other studies have shown that returning to athletics prior to full return of neuromuscular coordination and strength may increase the risk of recurrent injury.[15,17] In most of these cases, it can be assumed that the primary reconstruction was appropriately performed, and thus the same tunnels may be reused for the revision. It is crucial, however, to consider the primary reconstruction graft type and ensure appropriate graft selection for the revision procedure. Controversy exists regarding the ideal graft type for revision surgery.[32]

Atraumatic failure of ACL reconstructions can occur for a number of reasons. Although the primary reconstruction may have been technically acceptable, the progressive return of instability in the absence of trauma may still occur. Causes for this failure include failure of graft biologic integration, improper graft tension, failure of bone healing, or missed associated instabilities, such as persistent medial laxity or posterolateral corner deficiency.* Determining the type of graft tissue used in the primary operation is important to avoid similar problems in the revision setting. For example, Singhal and associates[38] have reported unacceptably high reoperation rates with the use of allograft tibialis anterior tissue in patients younger than 25 years. Studies have also shown high levels of gamma irradiation (4 Mrad) in some

---

*References 1, 5, 13, 31, 42, and 45.

*References 15, 17, 22, 29, 31, and 42.

allograft tissue may weaken the graft structural properties leaving it prone to failure.[35] Tunnel widening may also be present as a result of mechanical and biologic factors related to graft motion within the tunnel and release of inflammatory cytokines.[44] A thorough physical examination to assess for other instability patterns that can predispose an ACL reconstruction to early failure should be performed. Secondary causes of instability should be addressed at the time of revision to provide the best chance for an optimal outcome.

With no evidence of concomitant pathology, the location of the tibial and femoral tunnels should be assessed with preoperative imaging. In many cases, the tunnel position is optimal and the same tunnels may be used for the revision procedure. If tunnel widening is present, a decision should be made as to whether the widening can be addressed at the time of revision with techniques that will be outlined later in the chapter or whether a two-stage procedure is required.

The third cause of recurrent instability is a malpositioned graft or loss of graft fixation (Table 49-1). Errors in surgical technique related to placement of tunnels and graft fixation are the most common cause of failure in ACL reconstruction.[15,17] Graft malposition can occur on both the tibial and femoral sides, although anterior femoral tunnel placement is the most common error. Anterior femoral tunnel placement leads to flexion deficits and early graft failure as a result of excessive tension and impingement in extension. This failure can occur when using an endoscopic technique secondary to difficulty visualizing the over the top position. Revision surgery may require placement of a new tunnel posterior to the original anterior tunnel. If preexisting hardware is not impeding proper tunnel placement, the prior hardware should be left in place to avoid creating a larger defect. When a posterior femoral tunnel position with femoral cortical compromise is identified as the primary problem, revision using a two-incision, outside-in technique to create divergent tunnels is recommended. If this technique is not possible, a two-stage revision should be considered. Central femoral tunnel positioning may produce a vertical graft that provides anteroposterior stability without rotational control.[9,27] This

problem can manifest on physical examination with a negative Lachman examination and a persistent pivot shift. If adequate bone stock remains, a proper femoral tunnel can be created with an endoscopic or two-incision technique. Recent discussion regarding anatomic ACL reconstruction has identified femoral tunnel placement lower on the intracondylar notch as a potential solution to this issue.[7,10] The use of an accessory anteromedial portal has also been described as a means of drilling a more anatomic femoral tunnel site.[18] Independent drilling of femoral and tibial tunnels has recently been shown to outperform conventional transtibial drilling in a cadaver model.[39] However, Rue and coworkers[34] have demonstrated that it is technically possible to create an obliquely oriented single-bundle femoral tunnel down the femoral wall through a tibial tunnel angled approximately 60 degrees from the proximal tibial joint surface. This correlates with a femoral tunnel approximately midway between the anteromedial and posterolateral bundle origins of the ACL.

Errors in tibial tunnel placement can also lead to graft failure. A tibial tunnel placed too anteriorly will result in graft impingement on the intracondylar notch in extension and early graft failure.[20,21] A posterior position will result in a vertical graft and loss of rotational control.[8] Posterior tibial tunnel placement can also lead to excessive laxity in flexion and impingement on the posterior cruciate ligament. Specifically, when using an endoscopic technique, it is important to consider the affect of coronal plane obliquity of the tibial tunnel on femoral tunnel position. In cases of tibial tunnel malposition, an attempt can be made to drill a properly oriented tibial tunnel if adequate bone stock is present.[41] Kopf and colleagues[24] have reported in a meta-analysis that there is wide variability in the location of the footprint of the ACL and stressed the importance of using anatomic landmarks when creating tunnels.

Loss of graft fixation may occur secondary to poor bone quality, screw breakage, screw divergence, or graft damage during screw insertion. Poor bone quality may require other revision techniques, including compaction drilling or bone grafting. Additional fixation may be warranted such as the use of a suspensory device such as the EndoButton (Smith & Nephew, Andover, Mass) on the femoral side. A lateral screw post or ligament button may be placed through a separate incision. This technique may also be used on the tibia. Nevertheless, aperture fixation should be used whenever possible because interference screws have been shown to be stronger than staples, suture fixation around a post, or a soft tissue washer with screw fixation.[15,40] However, interference screws can be complicated by poor fixation in osteopenic bone, disruption of the bone plug, and transection of the graft. If graft damage occurs during femoral screw placement, the graft can be reversed so that the tibial bone block is placed on the femoral side and soft tissue fixation techniques are used on the tibial side.

PATIENT EVALUATION

A thorough history is important to obtain complete information related to the patient's current symptoms and prior treatment course. A description of the index event that resulted in the initial ACL injury is extremely important during this process because clues to other concomitant injuries that may have occurred are closely related. The length of time from injury to ACL reconstruction is also important when

Table 49-1 Common Technical Errors and Results

Error	Result
Femoral tunnel malposition	
Anterior	Graft impingement and/or loss of extension
	Excessive graft length changes (tension in flexion)
Vertical	Rotational instability
Tibial tunnel malposition	
Anterior	Graft impingement and/or loss of extension
Posterior	Excessive graft length changes (tension in flexion)
	Excessive graft length changes (tension in extension)
Inadequate notchplasty	Graft impingement and/or loss of extension
Inadequate graft tensioning	Translational and/or rotational instability
Unrecognized ligament injury	Translational and/or rotational instability
Unrecognized chondral or meniscal injury	Persistent pain and/or mechanical symptoms
Poor fixation	Translational and/or rotational instability

discussing issues of motion loss or arthrofibrosis. When possible, a review of the operative report is useful to record the type of graft used, fixation methods, concomitant procedures, and status of the articular cartilage and meniscus. The patient's postoperative course should be evaluated regarding rehabilitation, recurrent feelings of instability, signs of infection, and traumatic episodes that may have resulted in graft failure.

Physical examination begins with assessment of the patient's gait and overall limb alignment. Range of motion should also be evaluated, with particular attention to loss of extension. Comparison of contralateral quadriceps strength and circumference is similarly important. The knee is then evaluated for presence of an effusion, painful hardware, and joint line tenderness. Signs of patellar tendinitis and mobility in the medial-lateral and superior-inferior planes are crucial to document after prior bone-patellar tendon-bone (BPTB) reconstructions. A stability examination is performed, including anterior-posterior drawer, Lachman, and pivot shift tests. Finally, the collateral ligaments and posterolateral corner structures are assessed, because these structures have been reported as a cause of early failure of ACL reconstruction.

Imaging begins with standard weight-bearing anteroposterior (AP), lateral, Merchant, and 45-degree flexion views. The presence and location of hardware are noted. The femoral and tibial tunnels can be assessed for position and presence of tunnel widening. Several radiographic methods of quantifying tunnel widening have been described.[12,25] The femoral tunnel is typically easier to assess on the AP view, and the lateral view better delineates the position of the tibial tunnel by using Blumensaat's line as a reference.[21] The 45-degree flexion view allows for assessment of early loss of joint space.[33] If limb alignment is in question, standing full length views are helpful.

Magnetic resonance imaging (MRI) provides detailed information regarding the integrity of the graft, incorporation of bone plugs or bioabsorbable screws into the native bone, articular cartilage, meniscus, and surrounding ligaments. The presence of an effusion and bone marrow edema patterns can provide clues about the acuity of the trauma and degree of injury. Cartilage sensitive sequences have been developed to quantify articular cartilage injury.[36] MRI has also been used to calculate the cross-sectional area (CSA) of the femoral and tibial tunnels for tunnel widening.[14,37]

SURGICAL TECHNIQUE

Preoperative Planning

Once the preoperative patient evaluation is complete and the cause of failure of the primary ACL reconstruction has been ascertained, revision ACL reconstruction can be performed. Proper preoperative planning is critical to anticipate challenges during the revision procedure. Many important factors should be considered when planning for revision procedures (Table 49-2). A methodical approach is necessary to account for each technical aspect of the case. Reviewing prior operative reports and imaging studies provides valuable information about surgical approach, hardware used, type of graft, and coexisting pathology at the time of the primary procedure.

The first step is to select the graft type to be used for the revision procedure. There are a number of graft tissue options available for the revising surgeon (Box 49-1). If allograft

Table 49-2 Technical Considerations in Planning Revision ACL Reconstruction

Parameter	Technical Consideration
Motion loss	Rehabilitation pre- and postoperatively; arthroscopic or open débridement
Limb malalignment	Prior osteotomy; concurrent high tibial osteotomy
Tunnel osteolysis	Débridement; bone grafting
Graft removal	Intact vertical graft; malpositioned incompetent graft; synthetic graft
Hardware removal	Location and need for removal based on location
Revision graft selection	Determine original graft used; autologous tissue options; allograft tissue options
Revision tunnel placement	Location and quality of bone
Graft fixation	Aperture versus suspensory fixation
Associated injuries	Meniscus, articular cartilage, collateral ligaments, posterolateral corner, capsule

Box 49-1   Graft Sources

Autogenous
(Ipsilateral, contralateral)
Bone-patellar tendon-bone
Hamstring (semitendinosus and gracilis)
Quadriceps tendon-bone

Allograft
Bone-patellar tendon-bone
Hamstring
Achilles tendon-bone
Tibialis anterior

tissue was used for the primary procedure, use of ipsilateral autograft tissue is recommended because of the possibility of a previous rejection of the allograft and presence of tunnel widening. Although some studies have shown improved outcomes of revision surgery with the use of autograft tissue, recent reports have found no difference in outcomes of revision surgery with autograft versus allograft.[1,5,16] Allograft tissue is commonly selected as the graft of choice for revision procedures. The primary advantages of allograft tissue are the absence of donor site morbidity and decreased operative time. Second, the large bone blocks of Achilles tendon and BPTB allografts provide versatility in shaping bone blocks to fill preexisting bone tunnels. It is important to note that allograft tissue runs the risk of disease transmission, increases cost, and recellularizes more slowly and less completely than autograft tissue.[32]

The next step is to identify potential problems related to existing tunnel placement, tunnel widening, and hardware placement. Review of previous operative reports and radiographs allows for identification of the manufacturer and size of implants used in the primary reconstruction. Tibial hardware can often be removed directly through the old anterior tibial incision. Removal of femoral hardware can present a more difficult challenge. In many cases, femoral screws may not need to be removed. If a two-incision or accessory anteromedial portal technique is planned, the divergent nature of the new femoral tunnel often avoids the existing femoral screw. In cases in which the femoral tunnel is placed too anteriorly, there is often room to drill the new femoral tunnel in the proper posterior position without obstruction from the existing hardware. Regardless of hardware position, it is important to have the appropriate screwdrivers, staple extractors, and broken hardware removal sets available in case they are needed. When tunnel widening is present, the surgeon must plan the technique and potential instrumentation or bone graft needed to address the defect ahead of time. If a previous double-bundle reconstruction has been performed, the two tunnels may have eroded into one another and a larger bone defect may be present.

Anesthesia and Setup

The patient is placed on the operating table in the supine position. Regional anesthesia should be used whenever possible. Frequently, a combined spinal-epidural anesthetic with or without a femoral nerve block for postoperative pain management is administered. The leg is then placed in a cradle leg holder or a lateral post. Care should be taken to position the patient so that the knees fall below the distal break in the table. This position enables the bottom of the table to be dropped during surgery, allowing knee flexion. The ability to flex the knee more than 90 degrees is of particular importance when using an anteromedial portal technique. The routine use of antibiotic prophylaxis is recommended. Prior to sterile preparation of the extremity, an examination under anesthesia is performed and compared with the contralateral knee. Passive range of motion is measured with care to document any flexion or extension deficits. The medial and lateral collateral ligament integrity are assessed in full extension and 30 degrees of flexion. The posterolateral corner is assessed with the external rotation spin at 30 degrees of knee flexion. It is important to recognize and address persistent varus, valgus, or posterolateral instability because they are known causes of early ACL graft failure. The posterior cruciate ligament is assessed with the posterior drawer test, posterior sag, and external rotation spin at 90 degrees of knee flexion. Finally, the integrity of the ACL is determined with the pivot shift and Lachman tests. The Lachman maneuver provides feedback for graft function in the AP plane. A graft that is intact but placed in a vertical position may have a negative Lachman test result. Therefore, the pivot shift test is used to measure rotational instability. The leg is then prepped in a sterile fashion and prior skin incisions are marked to protect skin integrity. A portable fluoroscopic image intensifier may also be used during the procedure to assess tunnel placement.

Operative Procedure

At the initiation of the procedure, a diagnostic arthroscopy is performed. The meniscus is visualized and probed from posterior to anterior to assess the integrity. The articular cartilage surfaces are then evaluated, taking care to flex and extend the knee in each compartment to visualize the entire condyle completely. If there is concern for medial or lateral ligament instability, valgus or varus stress can be applied to

the compartment with a 3-mm probe in place to measure the degree of opening. Concomitant pathology is then addressed accordingly.

The graft is then assessed in the intracondylar notch. In addition to direct visualization of the graft, a probe is used to assess graft tension. An arthroscopic Lachman examination can be performed. The attachment of the graft on the femur and tibia should be carefully scrutinized.

When the decision is made to proceed with revision reconstruction, the existing graft is removed with a combination of arthroscopic biters, motorized shaver, and electrocautery device. On the femoral side, the over the top position and integrity of the back wall are visualized. If the patient has a narrow notch or visualization of the back wall is impeded, a revision notchplasty is performed. The notchplasty also ensures that the revision graft does not impinge on the roof of the notch with the knee in extension. Next, the existing femoral tunnel and hardware are identified and a decision made as to whether the existing hardware needs to be removed. If a new tunnel can be correctly positioned without interference with the existing hardware, then the prior hardware should be retained to avoid creating a larger defect in the bone. However, if the hardware conflicts with proper femoral tunnel positioning, it should be removed.

On the tibial footprint of the ACL, the existing graft material is removed. The anatomic landmarks for a proper tibial tunnel position are visualized, including the anterior edge of the posterior cruciate ligament, tibial spines, and posterior border of the anterior horn of the lateral meniscus. The tibial tunnel is evaluated in a similar fashion as the femoral tunnel to determine whether the original tunnel can be used and whether previously placed hardware may interfere with tunnel placement. Next, the tibial tunnel entrance site is generally exposed through the prior tibial incision. Subperiosteal dissection is carried out and existing hardware removed, if necessary. A guide wire can be placed through an endoscopic technique as well as accessory anteromedial portal technique to determine which position provides the best tunnel position prior to drilling (Fig. 49-1).

At this point in the procedure, there are four revision options available to the surgeon. The first option is to proceed with single-stage revision using the previously well-placed

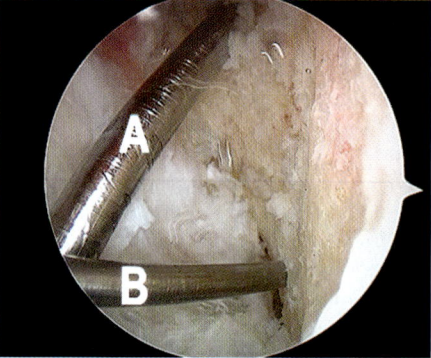

Figure 49-1. A guide wire is initially placed through the original tibial and femoral tunnels (transtibial technique). This wire placement is followed by a new guide wire placed through an accessory anteromedial portal for the femoral tunnel. Optimal position is then determined and this placement is selected for drilling.

tunnels if bone stock is sufficient. If this option is selected, the tunnels should be rereamed to remove sclerotic bone or fibrous tissue to allow biologic graft incorporation. The procedure is then continued in a fashion similar to that for primary ACL reconstruction. The second option is the divergent tunnel or funnel technique in the setting of a previous anatomic tunnel with moderate bone loss and adequate bone quality (Fig. 49-2). This technique creates a new tunnel by using the original intra-articular footprint of the primary reconstruction while creating a bone tunnel with a new extra-articular orientation. The new orientation of this tunnel establishes a bone bridge for adequate fixation. If aperture fixation was used in the primary reconstruction, this can remain or can be removed and bone-grafted. Once the tunnels have been placed, the graft is passed using standard techniques. Fixation on the femoral side is usually secured with

an interference screw. Secondary fixation can be provided using a lateral incision on the femur. When femoral fixation is complete, the graft is tensioned and the knee is cycled to remove creep. The graft is visualized arthroscopically with the knee in full extension to confirm that no impingement on the femoral notch exists. Fixation on the tibial side is carried out using an interference screw. Secondary fixation can be provided using a soft tissue button or staple. The Lachman and pivot tests should be performed when fixation is complete to ensure that they are negative.

The second option may be selected when previous tunnels were placed in a nonanatomic fashion and there is absence of significant tunnel widening. New tunnels can be easily drilled bypassing the previous tunnels and hardware. As noted earlier, a number of options are available to provide anatomic tunnel placement, including transtibial, two-incision, and anteromedial portal.

When tunnel widening is present, a third option is available. Tunnel widening is a challenging problem during revision ACL reconstruction and familiarization with several techniques allows the surgeon to address the bone loss effectively and provide a stable graft construct. Options available in this setting include the divergent tunnel–funnel technique, stacked interference screws, matchstick bone grafting, large bone plug–graft constructs, allograft dowels (Fig. 49-3), and structural bone void fillers.[3,4,6,43] In the senior author's experience, aperture fixation with metal interference screws should be used whenever possible, given the association of bioabsorbable screws and suspensory fixation with tunnel widening. However, suspensory fixation may be added as supplemental fixation, especially in the setting of posterior cortical compromise.

The final option is primary bone grafting of the tibial or femoral tunnels if widening is greater than 100% of the original tunnel or approximately 16 to 20 mm in any dimension on preoperative imaging (Fig. 49-4). In addition, if placing an isometric anatomic graft is not possible using the aforementioned techniques, primary bone grafting and staged reconstruction should strongly be considered. The widened tunnels require meticulous preparation, with a focus on adequate débridement of the sclerotic tunnel rim and fibrous material within the tunnels. Primary bone grafting requires removal of all previous hardware prior to placing either morsellized autograft iliac crest or allograft bone chips in the

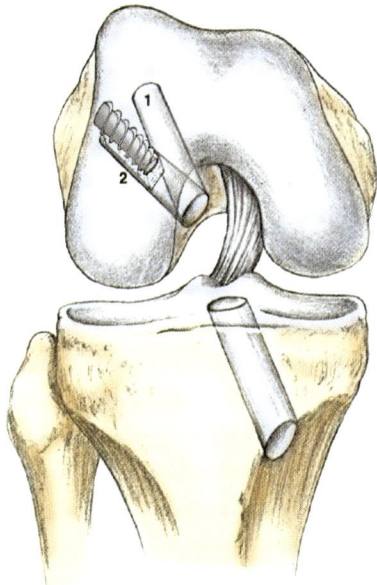

Figure 49-2. The funnel technique. This technique is used for a widened but anatomically placed tunnel in which the aperture of the new tunnel remains unchanged but the angle and direction of the tunnel are new, thereby creating an anatomic tunnel in new bone stock. (From Bach, BR Jr: Revision anterior cruciate ligament surgery. Arthroscopy 19[Suppl 1]:14–29, 2003.)

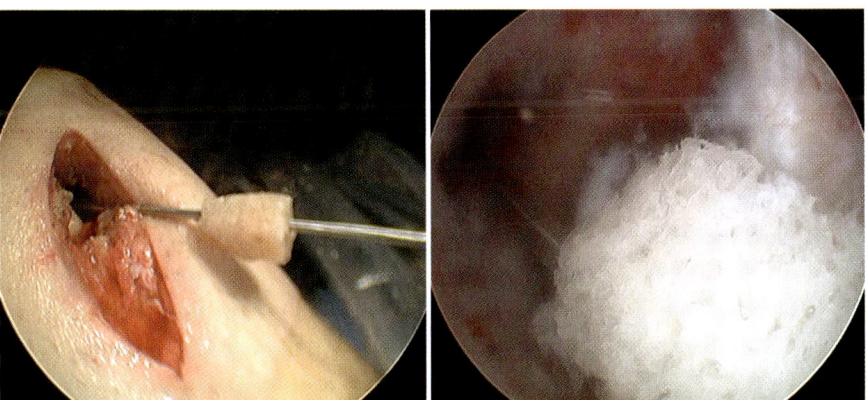

Figure 49-3. Guided bone plug placement over a guide wire. This method can be used for grafting of the tibial (*left, open view*) and femoral tunnels (*right, arthroscopic view*). A new guide wire is placed prior to drilling of the new tunnel.

femoral and tibial tunnels. A large allograft bone dowel may also be fashioned to fill the defect. Other injectable bone substitutes such as demineralized bone matrix and calcium phosphate have also been used with some success in this setting. Although these injectable forms offer the advantage of ease of arthroscopic placement, little data exist regarding their efficacy. Revision reconstruction should be staged at 3 to 4 months following bone grafting when sufficient consolidation has occurred (Fig. 49-5).

REHABILITATION

Although the goal of most patients is to return to full athletic activity, the first priority is to return to functional activities of daily living. The postoperative protocol for revision ACL reconstruction is similar to that used for primary reconstruction, but it should be amended depending on the quality of fixation achieved at revision surgery and concomitant procedures performed.

For isolated revision ACL reconstruction with allograft tissue, our immediate postoperative protocol consists of partial weight bearing with the knee locked in extension. Early range of motion with an emphasis on extension is started immediately. At 6 weeks postoperatively, when the patient has a normal gait and quadriceps strength, the brace is discontinued and the patient is allowed to bear weight as tolerated. Straight-ahead jogging is allowed at 4 months, followed by sport-specific rehabilitation. Return to athletics is allowed at 6 months if the knee is stable on examination and quadriceps strength is at least 80% of the opposite side.

CONCLUSION

As more ACL reconstructions are being performed, the demand for revision ACL reconstruction is increasing. Although recent studies have shown good outcomes with revision surgery, the results do not match those of primary ACL reconstruction. Revision ACL surgery is a technically demanding procedure and meticulous preoperative planning and determining the cause of failure are necessary for a successful result. Associated disorders must be diagnosed and treated. To optimize outcome, graft selection, tunnel placement, addressing tunnel widening, and graft fixation must be carefully planned. Revising surgeons should be familiar with a variety of techniques and instruments at their disposal for performing each of these steps.

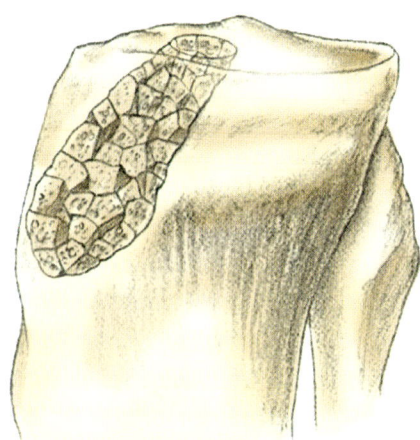

Figure 49-4. Tunnel widening greater than 100% (16 to 20 mm) or such that anatomic graft placement is not possible should be reconstructed in a staged fashion. Removal of all implants and débridement of old graft and fibrotic material within the tunnels should be followed by primary bone grafting of both tunnels. (From Bach BR Jr: Revision anterior cruciate ligament surgery. Arthroscopy 19[Suppl 1]: 14–29, 2003.)

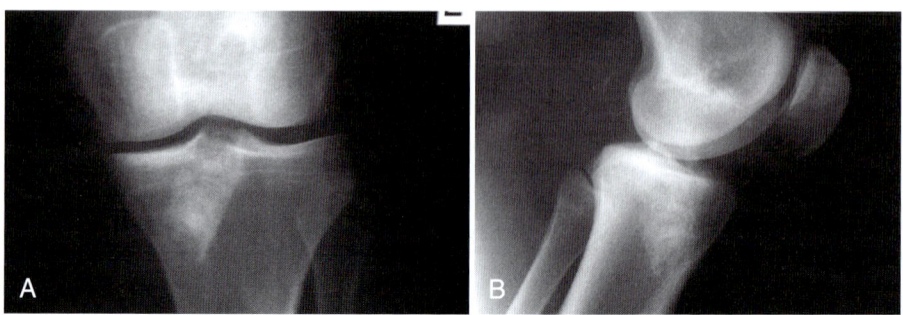

Figure 49-5. Anteroposterior **(A)** and lateral **(B)** projections following staged bone grafting of a widened tibial tunnel.

KEY REFERENCES

Ahn JH, Lee YS, Ha HC: Comparison of revision surgery with primary anterior cruciate ligament reconstruction and outcome of revision surgery between different graft materials. Am J Sports Med 36:1889–1895, 2008.

Bach BR, Jr: Revision anterior cruciate ligament surgery. Arthroscopy 19(Suppl 1):14–29, 2003.

Battaglia MJ, 2nd, Cordasco FA, Hannafin JA, et al: Results of revision anterior cruciate ligament surgery. Am J Sports Med 35:2057–2066, 2007.

Battaglia TC, Miller MD: Management of bony deficiency in revision anterior cruciate ligament reconstruction using allograft bone dowels: surgical technique. Arthroscopy 21:767, 2005.

George MS, Dunn WR, Spindler KP: Current concepts review: revision anterior cruciate ligament reconstruction. Am J Sports Med 34:2026–2037, 2006.

Harner CD, Giffin JR, Dunteman RC, et al: Evaluation and treatment of recurrent instability after anterior cruciate ligament reconstruction. Instr Course Lect 50:463–474, 2001.

Harner CD, Honkamp NJ, Ranawat AS: Anteromedial portal technique for creating the anterior cruciate ligament femoral tunnel. Arthroscopy 24:113–115, 2008.

Harner CD, Irrgang JJ, Paul J, et al: Loss of motion after anterior cruciate ligament reconstruction. Am J Sports Med 20:499–506, 1992.

Howell SM, Barad SJ: Knee extension and its relationship to the slope of the intercondylar roof. Implications for positioning the tibial tunnel in anterior cruciate ligament reconstructions. Am J Sports Med 23:288–294, 1995.

Loh JC, Fukuda Y, Tsuda E, et al: Knee stability and graft function following anterior cruciate ligament reconstruction: comparison between 11 o'clock and 10 o'clock femoral tunnel placement. 2002 Richard O'Connor Award paper. Arthroscopy 19:297–304, 2003.

Millett PJ, Wickiewicz TL, Warren RF: Motion loss after ligament injuries to the knee. Part II: prevention and treatment. Am J Sports Med 29:822–828, 2001.

Noyes FR, Barber-Westin SD: Revision anterior cruciate ligament reconstruction using a 2-stage technique with bone grafting of the tibial tunnel. Am J Sports Med 34:678–679, 2006.

Rue JP, Ghodadra N, Lewis PB, Bach BR, Jr: Femoral and tibial tunnel position using a transtibial drilled anterior cruciate ligament reconstruction technique. J Knee Surg 21:246–249, 2008.

Singhal MC, Gardiner JR, Johnson DL: Failure of primary anterior cruciate ligament surgery using anterior tibialis allograft. Arthroscopy 23:469–475, 2007.

Steiner ME, Murray MM, Rodeo SA: Strategies to improve anterior cruciate ligament healing and graft placement. Am J Sports Med 36:176–189, 2008.

Full references for this chapter can be found on www.expertconsult.com.

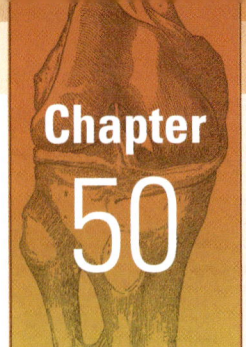

Chapter 50

Revision Anterior Cruciate Ligament Surgery: One-Stage versus Two-Stage Technique

John M. Minnich, Mark S. Haro, Mark Miller, and David R. Diduch

As the need for anterior cruciate ligament (ACL) revisions increases, it will be imperative for surgeons to identify the causes of failure of the primary procedure accurately and address them in a systematic fashion. Pitfalls must be recognized and avoided to optimize the success of the revision procedure. The accurate placement of femoral and tibial tunnels should not be compromised by the index tunnel placement.[9] Depending on the type and location of the fixation, the location and size of the existing tunnels, and the quality of the bone, the surgeon must be prepared to use a number of different techniques.

The revision surgery can be performed all at once (one-stage) or as two separate procedures (two-stage), if necessary. The two-stage surgery ensures adequate healing of bone tunnels, which will then provide a good bed for fixation of the ACL graft without compromising the location of the bone tunnels.[23] However, this technique exposes the patient to the inherent risks of two surgeries and the hazards of an unstable knee while waiting for the graft to incorporate, causing meniscal injury or cartilage damage. An obvious advantage of the one-stage surgery is to avoid the need for a second surgery. For the technique to be successful, it requires good bone quality with acceptable tunnel size and location or the ability to bypass existing tunnels or fill bone defects with adequate density and strength.[3,5,13,17,25] This chapter presents a treatment algorithm based on different scenarios and describes the surgical techniques for both procedures.

Approximately 100,000 to 175,000 ACL reconstructions are performed in the United States annually.[6,16,22] With respect to pain relief, stability, and return to function, the reported long-term results after primary ACL reconstruction are 75% to 95% good to excellent.[10,27]

With an increasing number of ACL reconstructions being performed each year,[16] however, there will inevitably be an increasing need for revision procedures. The Danish registry recently published a report indicating that 3% of all ACL reconstructions were revised within the first 2 years.[15] Historically, the failure rate of primary ACL reconstructions caused by instability has been reported to be as low as 0.7% and as high as 8% in the United States.[8,10,27] Based on our calculations, there are potentially 700 to 14,000 revision ACL procedures to be performed annually in the United States alone.

Chapter 49 addressed the causes of ACL failure and the planning and decision making for revision surgery. One of the most challenging aspects of ACL revision surgery is how to deal with the previous technical errors, methods of fixation, and tunnel widening. Old tunnels may be poorly positioned and interfere with new tunnel location, hardware may block the path of the new tunnel or fixation device, and an enlarged tunnel or large bone defect may jeopardize graft security and incorporation.

PREOPERATIVE WORKUP

Determining the cause of failure is crucial to achieving a successful outcome and avoiding a repeat failure. The most common cause of failure of the primary ACL reconstruction is related to errors in surgical technique.[11,14,18,24] A vast majority of the time (70% to 80%), this is caused by nonanatomic tunnel placement.[1,20,27] Other technical errors include improper graft tensioning, inadequate fixation, graft impingement, and failure to address unrecognized pathology.

Poor tunnel location results in excessive changes in graft length, plastic deformation, and ultimately failure. It can occur on the femoral and tibial sides (one or both) and in the saggital (too anterior or too posterior) and coronal planes (too vertical or too horizontal). Usually, the femoral tunnel is nonanatomic. Specifically, it is usually placed too far anterior because the posterior femoral cortex is not adequately visualized (Fig. 50-1).[9,12]

Careful preoperative planning should be undertaken to evaluate the cause of failure of the primary ACL reconstruction. A thorough history and physical examination should be obtained and a meticulous review of operative notes with details about previous hardware and location should be performed. Specific attention should be paid to the previous surgical technique, the type of graft used, and the type of fixation. Each of these factors may affect the revision procedure.

Posteroanterior (PA), lateral, sunrise, and lateral hyperextension radiographic views should be obtained to determine previous tunnel and hardware position, whether tunnel expansion has occurred, and whether any degenerative changes are present (Fig. 50-2). Consider standing views on a long cassette to determine the mechanical axis. If significant bony defects are present on the radiographs, a computed tomography (CT) scan is often beneficial in planning new tunnel placement and to help determine whether bone graft or void fillers will be needed (Fig. 50-3).

The hospital or surgery center must have the necessary equipment and implants for the revision surgery (Fig. 50-4). Custom-sized allograft materials should be ordered in advance, if needed. Consider having soft tissue allografts in stock as a backup for unexpected occurrences. A variety of sizes and types of bone graft should be readily accessible (Fig. 50-5). Specific instrumentation (if possible) or a universal screw removal set (Fig. 50-6) should be available to remove the previous hardware. It is also often useful to use fluoroscopic guidance to facilitate removing retained hardware or assist in tunnel placement, especially if one is attempting to bypass the previously placed hardware.

The patient must be appropriately counseled preoperatively about the surgery and expected outcomes. The patient should have realistic goals and understand that the results of revision surgery are less predictable and generally less favorable.[4,6,24,27] Occasionally, it is not possible to determine preoperatively whether a one- or two-stage procedure will be performed, and the patient should consent to the possibility of additional surgery if necessary.

TREATMENT OPTIONS

In general, one-stage surgery can be performed in the setting of adequate bone quality and tunnel placement, when the hardware is not in the way. In the ideal scenario, the alignment of the initial tunnels is so malpositioned that the normal landmarks and bone stock will be preserved (see Fig. 50-1). If this is the case, the previous tunnels and hardware can simply be bypassed with new anatomically placed tunnels.[17] Frequently, however, it is not this simple.

If small or moderately sized bony defects are present, either caused by tunnel widening or from the removal of previous hardware, these must be addressed intraoperatively. The defect can be filled with autograft plugs[7,19] or allograft dowels.[3,5] Other techniques use structural grafts, including bioabsorbable interference screws[2,13] or calcium phosphate cement,[25] to fill the void. These rigid bone void fillers allow new tunnels to be drilled anatomically (without compromising location) and the graft to be securely fixed in one procedure.

Paessler[19] has described a technique in which iliac crest corticocancellous autograft bone plugs can be used during a one-stage procedure. The iliac crest graft is harvested through a 2- to 3-cm incision using a specialized harvesting tube. The trajectory for the tube harvester is marked with a Kirschner wire (K wire) passed into the iliac crest. A harvesting tube is used that matches the diameter required for the corticocancellous plug and the plug is removed with a removal device. The harvested plugs can then be inserted into the tunnel defects in an arthroscopic or open fashion.

Battaglia and Miller[5] have recommended using cylindric bone allografts, or Cloward dowels, to fill bone voids (Fig. 50-7). The previous tunnel is aggressively débrided and reamed and the corresponding sized dowel is inserted. The most common sizes are 12 mm in diameter by 25 to 35 mm in length, although up to 18-mm diameter dowels have been used successfully. A variety of different sized dowels must be available. This study noted that even with meticulous preoperative planning, the exact size of the defect is often difficult to predict.

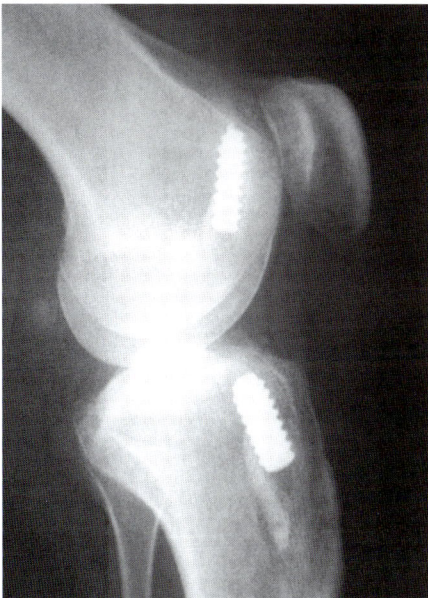

Figure 50-1. Lateral knee x-ray with excessive anterior femoral tunnel location.

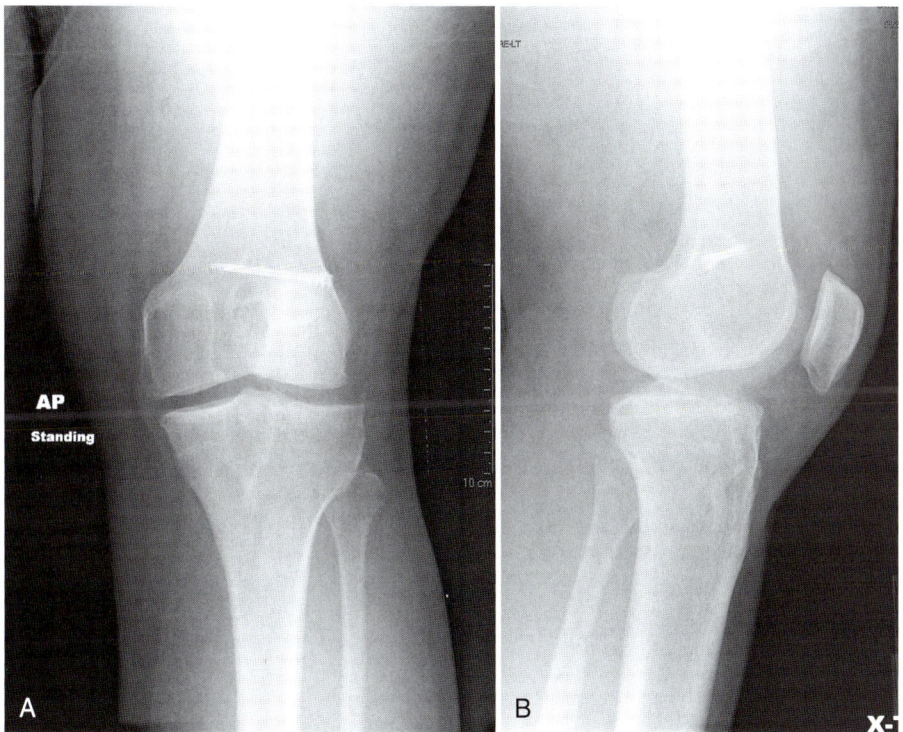

Figure 50-2. PA **(A)** and lateral **(B)** x-rays of the knee showing tunnel lysis and early degenerative changes.

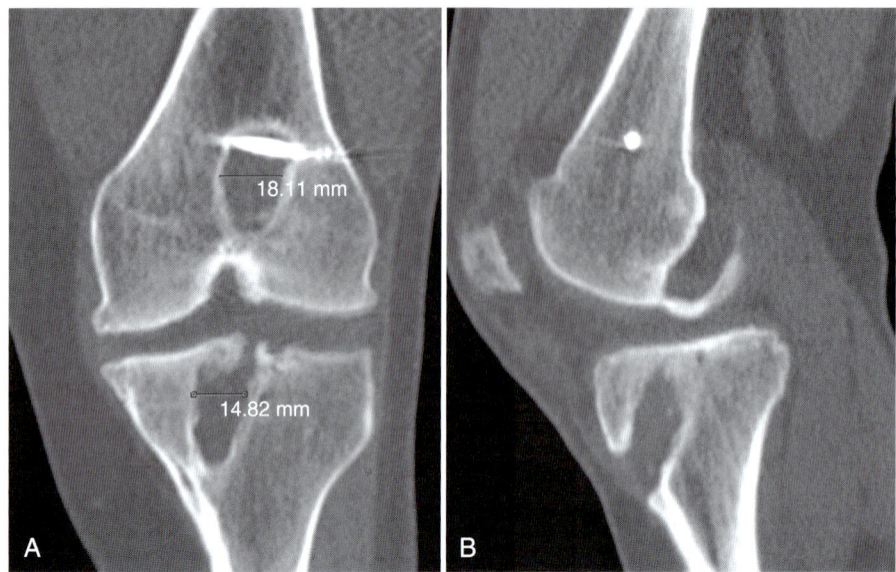

Figure 50-3. Coronal **(A)** and saggital **(B)** CT images showing femoral tunnel widening >18 mm and tibial tunnel widening >14 mm.

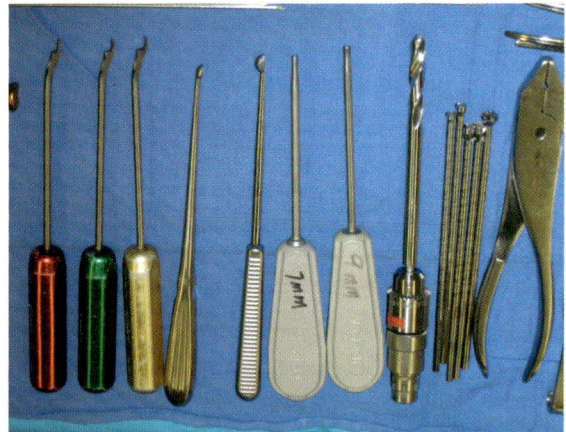

Figure 50-4. Revision ACL instrumentation set.

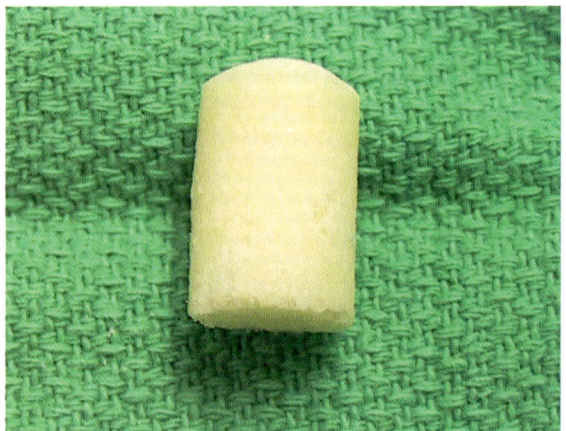

Figure 50-5. Cloward dowel cylindric bone allograft measuring 12 × 16 mm.

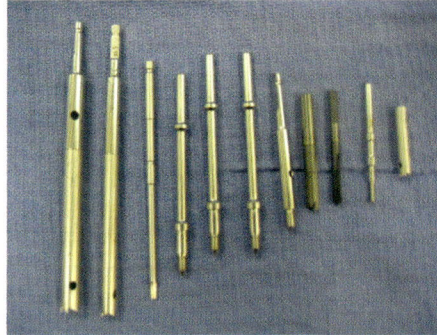

Figure 50-6. Universal screw removal set.

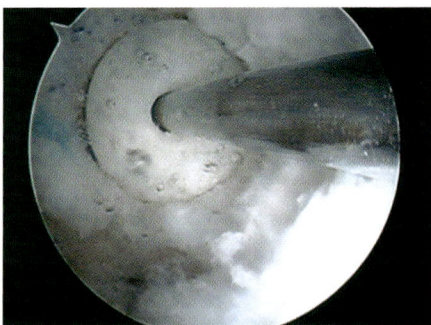

Figure 50-7. Bone allograft dowel insertion in bone defect.

A similar technique involves replacing an existing metal interference screw in the femoral tunnel with a bioabsorbable screw.[13] If the existing tunnel is partially overlapped by the new tunnel, the reamer can drill through the corner of the absorbable screw; the remaining screw fills the void and provides structural support. The stacked interference screw concept specifically refers to inserting a second interference screw, adjacent to the one providing structural support, to reinforce fixation.[2]

In a recent study by Vaughn and colleagues,[25] the authors performed a cadaveric study to determine the load to failure of a bone-patellar tendon-bone graft (BPTB) placed after filling bone defects with calcium phosphate cement. They found that using standard fixation techniques and anatomically drilled tunnels, the load to failure of the reconstruction using the bone cement was not significantly different from that of the control group, a primary ACL reconstruction with standard interference screw fixation. However, although it has been shown that calcium phosphate bone cement is stronger than cancellous bone, this biomechanical study on cadavers did not necessarily correlate to in vivo results. A significant question that remains is whether the cement would inhibit incorporation of the graft into bone.

Two-stage surgery should be considered for significant widening of the tunnels when tunnels are close but not ideal (causing an hourglass shape or tunnel confluence) and when an excessive amount of bone is removed during the hardware extraction process. Many authors suggest bone grafting and staged revision if the amount of cystic widening (or osteolysis) is greater than 15 mm.[1,12] The initial procedure involves removing the existing hardware and filling the bony defects with bone graft. Typically, the bone graft is incorporated over a period of several months. Then, during the second stage, new tunnels can be drilled and the ACL revision procedure can be performed.

A two-stage technique should also be considered in the setting of decreased range of motion (arthrofibrosis) following index ACL surgery. If there is a flexion contracture more than 5 degrees or a flexion loss more than 20 degrees, a manipulation under anesthesia, lysis of adhesions, and aggressive physical therapy should be performed to improve motion prior to revision.[12] In addition, a staged revision must be performed in the setting of an underlying infection. Obviously, the definitive reconstruction should be delayed until the infection is eradicated.

Thomas and associates[23] have advocated a two-stage procedure if the tibial tunnel from the index procedure would overlap the correctly placed new tibial tunnel either partially or fully. After débriding the old tunnel, bone was harvested from the iliac crest in the form of dowels and impacted in the tunnel. The femoral tunnel was not grafted because it was later drilled in virgin bone via a different technique (outside-in). A CT scan was obtained 4 months later to confirm adequate healing of the bone graft. A revision ACL procedure was then performed similar to a primary procedure.

The decision to perform one-stage or two-stage revision ACL surgery is complex and multifactorial. It must take into consideration technical factors from the previous surgery, such as tunnel location and previous graft type, and patient-dependent factors, such as activity level and bone quality. The following scenarios provide a treatment algorithm to facilitate the decision making process in a stepwise manner. The decision tree starts by first identifying whether the tunnels are in an acceptable location.

Acceptable Femoral and Tibial Tunnel Locations

Remove fixation?
- Yes
  - Easily performed without large defect
  - Difficult; metal cross pins may require overdrilling with a hollow drill, causing a large defect (see Fig. 50-2)
- No
  - Retain screw and drill through portion of screw to avoid complications of screw removal.[17]

Assess for large bone defect secondary to cystic widening or implant removal.
- Small to moderate (<15 mm; Fig. 50-8)
  - One-stage bone grafting with autograft or allograft
  - Structural graft
  - Bioabsorbable interference screws
  - Bone cement
  - Use Achilles or BPTB allograft with larger bone plug (rotate plug to fill defect).
- Large (>15 mm; Fig. 50-9): Bone grafting and staged revision

Drill tunnel.
- Endoscopic transtibial
- Two-incision outside-in technique
- Accessory medial port—divergent

Graft fixation. Consider dual fixation if there is any question of bone quality (Fig. 50-10)
- Femoral side: Interference screw and lateral cortex (over the top) fixation (EndoButton, Smith & Nephew, Andover, Mass)
- Tibial side: Interference screw plus post and washer or staple

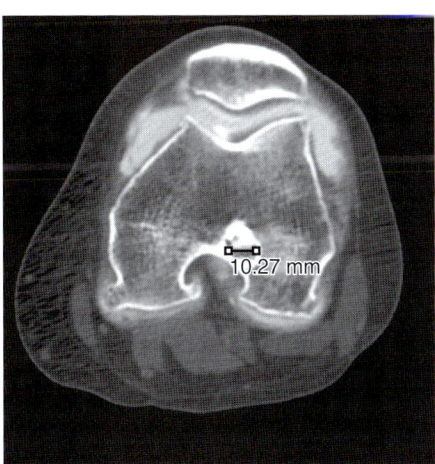

Figure 50-8. Axial CT image showing moderately sized femoral tunnel measuring approximately 10 mm.

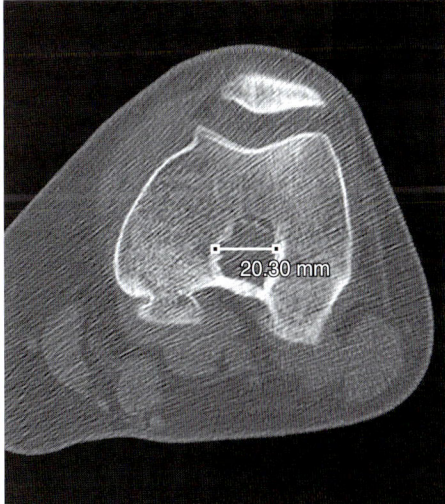

Figure 50-9. Axial CT image showing large femoral tunnel >20 mm.

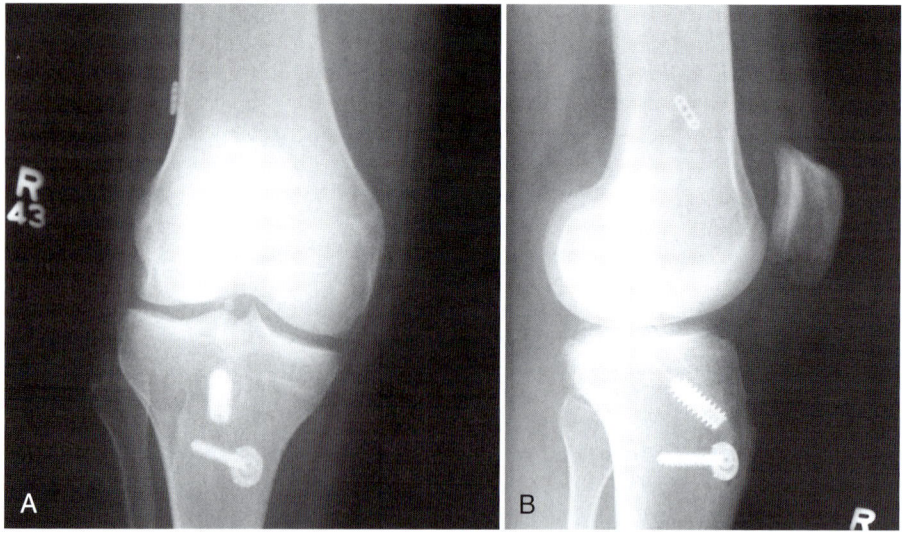

Figure 50-10. Postoperative anteroposterior (AP; **A**) and lateral **(B)** x-rays with dual fixation of the femoral and tibial tunnels.

Unacceptable Femoral Tunnel Location

Is hardware blocking new tunnel path?
- Yes; remove hardware.
- No; leave hardware in place.

Femoral tunnel
- Cystic widening?
  - <15 mm; consider one-stage bone grafting.
  - >15 mm; consider two-stage revision with bone grafting.
- Consider surgical approach used at index procedure.
  - Transtibial? Consider accessory medial port drilling.
  - Two-incision? Use endoscopic technique to change trajectory and avoid hardware.
- Evaluate tunnel location.
  - Too anterior? (most common)

More than one tunnel diameter?
- Bypass old tunnel and redrill new tunnel endoscopically.

Less than one diameter? (hourglass shape or tunnel confluence)
- Hamstring graft with small diameter. Drill small tunnel posteriorly that fits without overlap.
- Simultaneous bone grafting
  - Autograft bone plug
  - Allograft bone dowel
  - Bioabsorbable interference screws
  - Bone cement
- Use Achilles or BTPB allograft with larger bone plug (rotate plug to fill defect).
- Bone grafting and staged revision
  - Too posterior? (usually with deficient posterior wall; Fig. 50-11)
  - Drill anatomic tunnel using two-incision or accessory medial portal technique.
  - Too vertical? (Fig. 50-12)
  - Drill tunnel from same starting point but at a different angle or orientation to create a new intact femoral tunnel (funnel or tunnel diversion concept[2]; Fig. 50-13)

Graft fixation: Consider dual fixation.

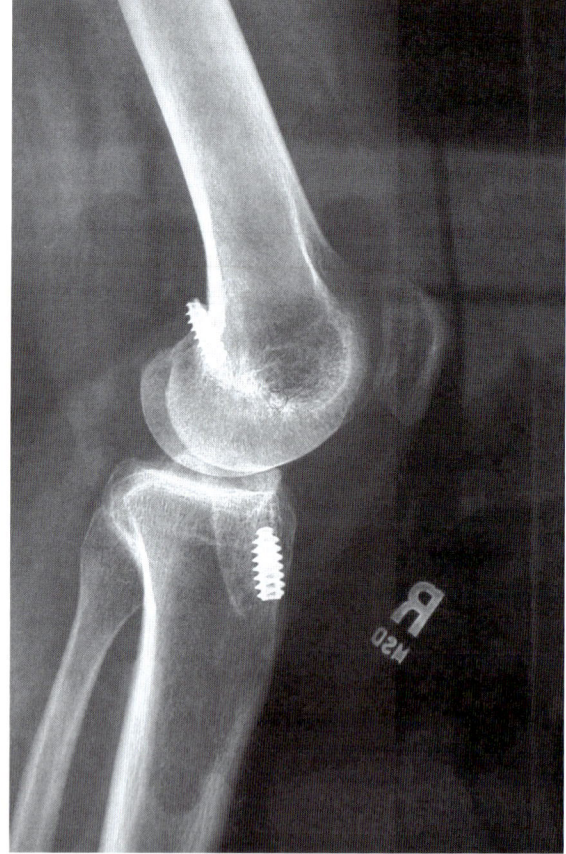

Figure 50-11. Lateral x-ray with penetration through the posterior femoral cortex with the interference screw.

Unacceptable Tibial Tunnel Location

Is hardware blocking new tunnel path?
- Yes; remove hardware.
- No; leave hardware in place.

Tibial tunnel
- Cystic widening?
  - <15 mm; consider one-stage bone grafting.

- >15 mm; consider two-stage revision with bone grafting.
- Evaluate tunnel location (similar principles to femoral side).

Too anterior?

- More than one diameter?
  - Drill new tunnel posterior to the original tunnel without removing fixation.

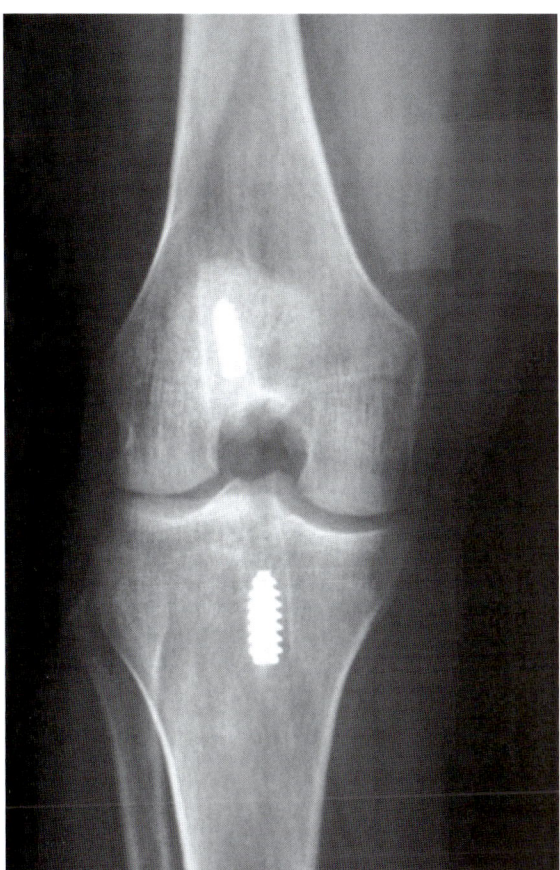

Figure 50-12. AP x-ray with vertically oriented femoral and tibial tunnels.

- Less than one diameter?
  - Expand existing tunnel until center is optimal position. Fill the void between the anterior wall and new graft with allograft bone, core reamings, structural graft, or BPTB allograft with large bone plug.
  - Create new tibial tunnel with new extra-articular starting point that ends at the optimal intra-articular position.[6]

Too posterior?

- More than one diameter?
  - Drill new tunnel anteriorly to the original tunnel without removing fixation.
- Less than one diameter?
  - Expand existing tunnel until center is optimal position. Fill the void between the posterior wall and new graft with allograft bone, core reamings, and structural graft or BPTB allograft with large bone plug.
  - Potential for tunnel overlap causing the graft to fall posteriorly into the old tunnel: Recommend bone grafting and staged revision.[6]

Graft fixation: Consider dual fixation.

SURGICAL PROCEDURES

One-Stage Technique

Perform examination under anesthesia and diagnostic arthroscopy.

Débride the previous ACL graft.

- Once the available landmarks are visible, a complete evaluation of the tunnel location is possible.

Remove tibial interference screw (if necessary).

- The remaining tibial defect can be filled by packing it with bone graft from the drilling of the revised tunnel or allograft croutons.
- Consider replacing a metal interference screw with a bioabsorbable screw and drill through a portion of the screw.

Insert guide pins for new femoral tunnel prior to hardware removal.

- If the previous interference screws can be bypassed with the new tunnels, simply drill the tunnel in standard fashion.[17]

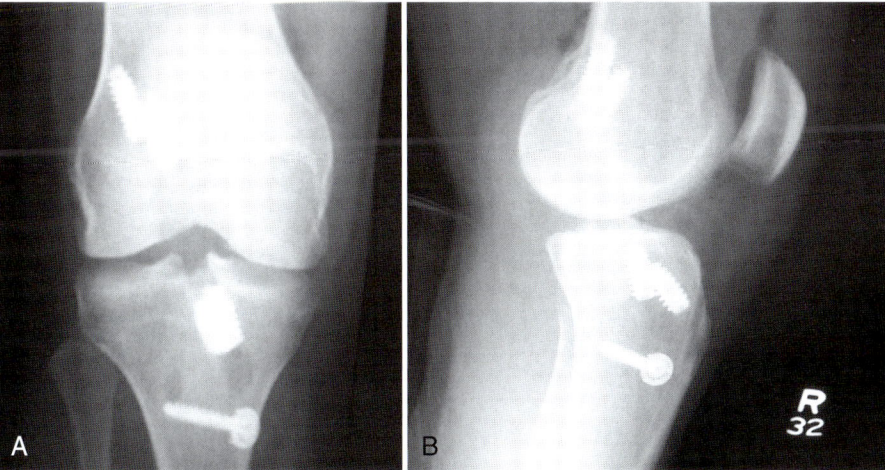

Figure 50-13. Postoperative ACL revision AP **(A)** and lateral **(B)** x-rays showing divergently placed femoral and tibial tunnels.

- If the guide pin placement is satisfactory, with the retained hardware partially interfering with new tunnel placement, and it appears that adequate fixation can be obtained with the hardware in place, then drill through a portion of the retained hardware.[17]
  - Bioabsorbable interference screws are easily drilled through.
  - Metal screws and implants are typically made from softer alloys, making it possible to drill through a small portion thereof.
- If the retained hardware blocks guide pin placement or completely interferes with drilling the new tunnel, or if there is excessive tunnel widening that would prevent adequate fixation, the hardware should be removed and bone void filler should be used (multiple options; see earlier).

Use of allograft bone dowels[3,5] (Fig. 50-14).
- First, débride the previous tunnel.
- Insert the Beath pin into the center of the tunnel (confirm fluoroscopically).
- Sequential reaming of the tunnel is performed.
  - Start with a 8-mm diameter reamer and continue until a satisfactory tunnel is created for the allograft bone dowel, with fresh bone margins.
- Select correct size of dowel and insert arthroscopically (Fig. 50-15).
- Use an over the top guide to insert the guide pin in an acceptable position.

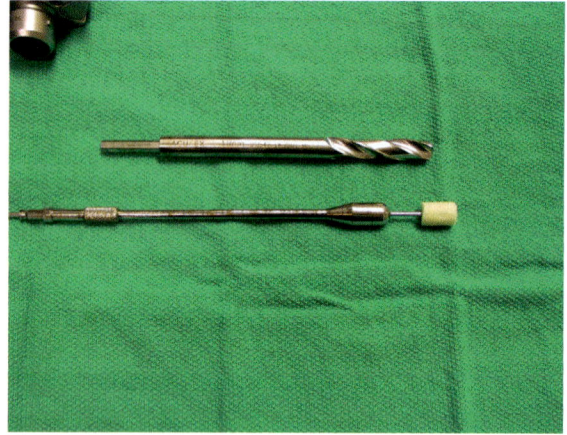

Figure 50-14. Allograft bone dowel and instrumentation for insertion.

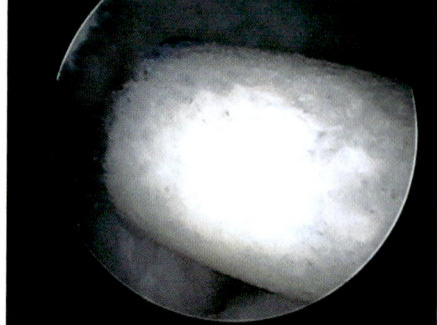

Figure 50-15. Intraoperative photo of dowel being inserted arthroscopically.

- Drill the tunnel over the guide pin.
- Allograft bone dowel provides sufficient support to allow redrilling of the new tunnels immediately adjacent to the old tunnels (Fig. 50-16).

Alternatively, replace metal interference screw with bioabsorbable screw of same size.
- Drill the tunnel in standard fashion.
- Insert an ACL graft through the tunnels.
- Use dual fixation (see Fig. 50-10).

Carry out accelerated rehabilitation protocol postoperatively.

Two-Stage Technique

First Stage

Plan skin incisions carefully to avoid skin sloughing and infection.
- Use previous incision when possible.

Perform examination under anesthesia.
- Assess medial collateral ligament (MCL) and posteromedial and posterolateral corners.

Perform diagnostic arthroscopy.
- Address meniscal and chondral lesions.

Send cultures and biopsy tissue (if infection is suspected).

Remove hardware (if necessary).
- Universal screw removal sets (see Fig. 50-6) should be available.
- Use adequate soft tissue débridement for proper seating of screw and proper angle of screwdriver to avoid stripping.
  - Metal cross pins (Mitek Slingshot, DePuy Mitek, Raynham, Mass; see Fig. 50-2) may be especially challenging. The bone grows into the hex head, so there is usually a need to overdrill and pull out as a plug, leaving a larger defect than anticipated.
- Bioabsorbable screws may soften or fragment on removal.
  - May still be present several years after implantation, depending on the type of polymer

Remove previous tendon graft,
- Autograft or allograft should be débrided completely.
- Prosthetic graft should be removed en bloc.[21]
  - Create synthetic fiber particles that incite inflammatory response.
  - May cause more synovitis and scarring[23]

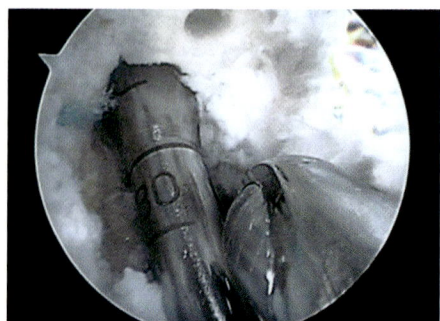

Figure 50-16. New tunnel being drilled adjacent to old tunnel. Note that the allograft bone is partially overdrilled.

Perform revision notchplasty as needed,
- Notch overgrowth and osteophyte formation are common after primary procedure.
- Resect bone from roof and lateral wall of notch similar to primary procedure.

Bone graft tunnel
- Identify previous tunnels.
- Débride sclerotic walls of tunnel.
  - A reamer is most effective (Fig. 50-17).
  - A drill, curette, or rasp may also be used.
  - Preserve as much bone as possible.
- Autograft versus allograft bone is patient- and cost-dependent.
  - Harvest bone in form of dowel grafts from the iliac crest.
  - Allograft croutons (dried morsellized bone) or freeze-dried cylindrical bone graft
- Pack graft into tunnel.
  - On the femoral side, use a bone tamp or screwdriver to ensure that graft is well packed (Fig. 50-18).
  - On the tibial side, be careful not to breach the joint.

Confirm arthroscopically that the graft is not within the joint.

Interim

Repeat imaging (x-ray or CT scan) 12 to 16 weeks later to assess healing of the bone graft (Fig. 50-19).

Second Stage

Examination under anesthesia, diagnostic arthroscopy
- Assess previous tunnel sites that were bone-grafted during the first stage.

Graft harvest
- Choice of graft is dependent on its availability and individualized to the patient.

Revision ACL technique is similar to the primary procedure.
- Drill tunnels anatomically.
  - Landmarks may be less distinct; consider intraoperative imaging.
- Consider dual fixation.

Carry out accelerated rehabilitation protocol postoperatively.

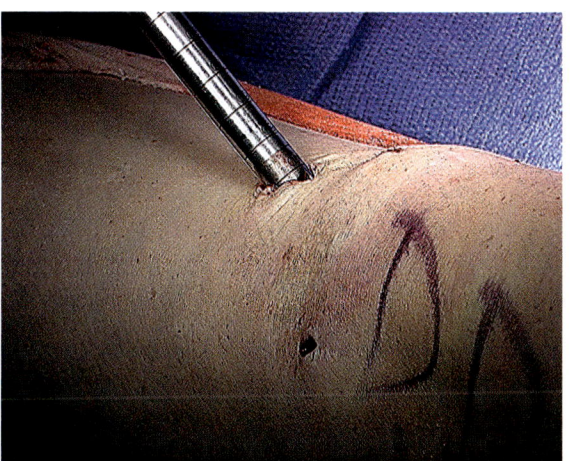

Figure 50-17. Débriding sclerotic bone of old tibial tunnel with reamer.

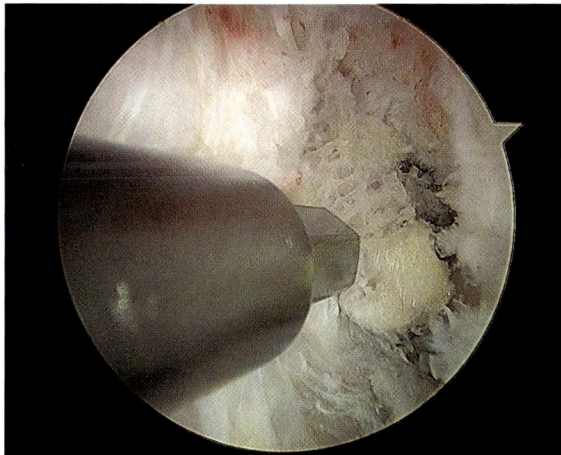

Figure 50-18. Packing allograft cancellous bone chips in femoral tunnel with screwdriver.

CASE EXAMPLES

Case 1

(See video on website.)

A 23-year-old female soccer player with a history of a left knee ACL reconstruction with a hamstring allograft 5 years ago presented complaining of left knee pain and instability after a noncontact injury 1 week prior to presentation. She had an uneventful postoperative course, participated in aggressive rehabilitation, and returned to full activity without difficulty until the most recent injury. Her physical examination revealed a trace effusion, a 3+ Lachman test with no end point, and a 3+ pivot shift test. Her x-rays (Fig. 50-20) and magnetic resonance imaging (MRI) scans (Fig. 50-21) confirmed a complete tear of the ACL graft and showed adequate tibial and femoral tunnel location with a metal cross pin fixation device on the femur. The patient was consented for a two-stage revision ACL reconstruction because of the expected challenges in removing the metal cross pin device and potential for creating a large transverse bone defect after removal.

During the first procedure, the screw was removed through the previous lateral incision and the resulting defect was packed with cancellous allograft chips. Next, a diagnostic arthroscopy was performed and a small area of chondromalacia was addressed with a shaving chondroplasty. The intercondylar notch was débrided and the previous tunnel was identified (Fig. 50-22). The tibial and femoral tunnels were reamed to remove sclerotic bone. The articular surface of the tibial tunnel was preserved so that the bone graft did not enter the joint. The femoral and tibial tunnels were then packed tightly with cancellous chips using a bone tamp.

Consolidation of the bone graft was confirmed 4 months postoperatively radiographically (Fig. 50-23). Subsequently, the patient underwent the second-stage procedure. Once again, the notch was débrided and a revision notchplasty was performed. The lateral wall of the femoral condyle was

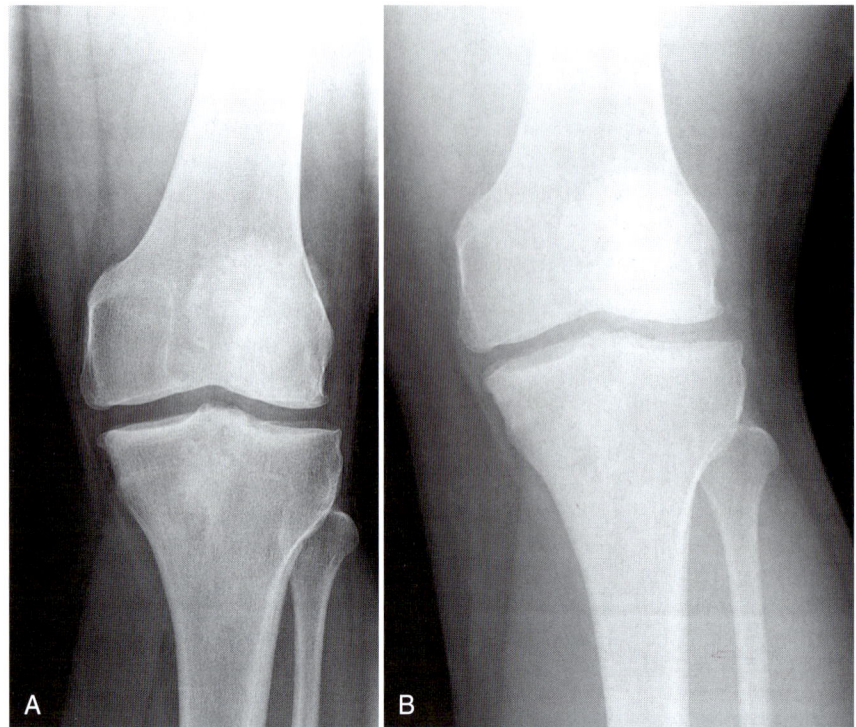

Figure 50-19. **A,** AP x-ray at 6 weeks postoperatively showing bone graft in tunnels. **B,** AP x-ray at 16 weeks postoperatively showing consolidated and healed bone graft.

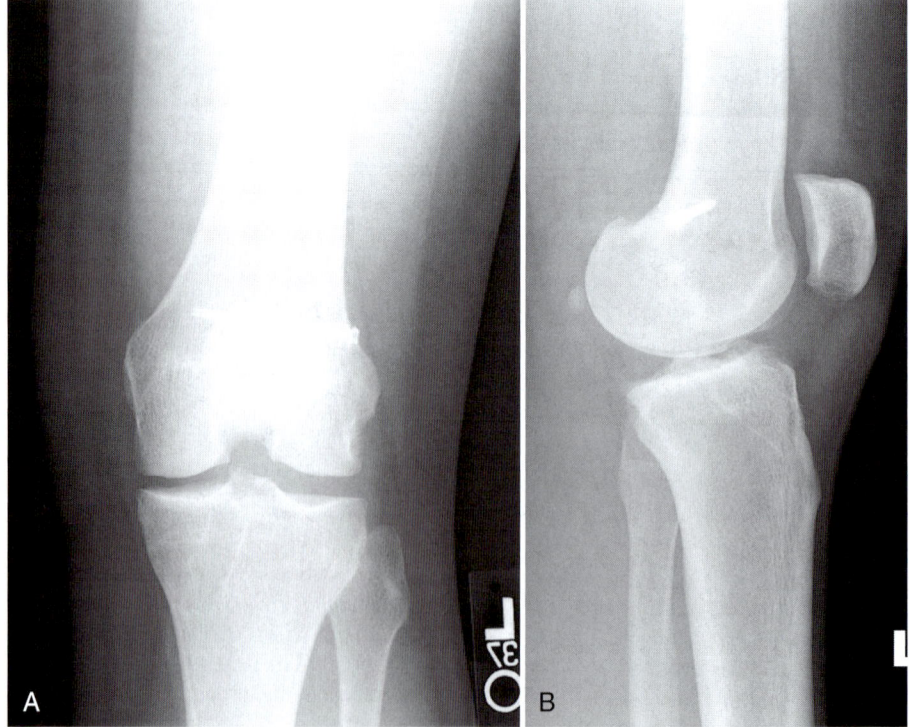

Figure 50-20. AP **(A)** and lateral **(B)** x-rays showing metal cross pin fixation in the femur.

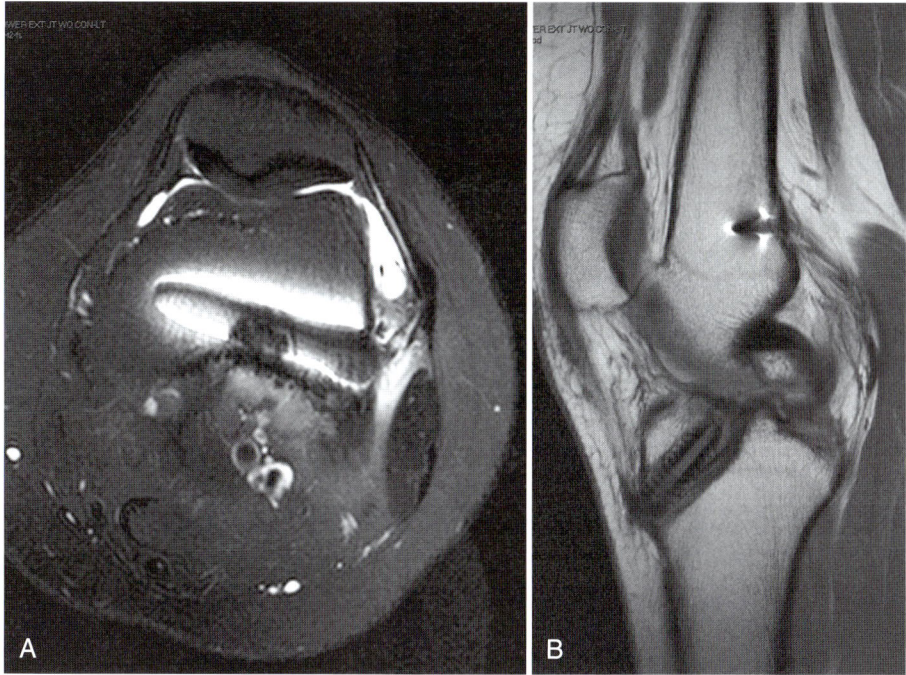

Figure 50-21. Axial **(A)** and saggital **(B)** MRI images confirming adequate tunnel location and minimal osteolysis.

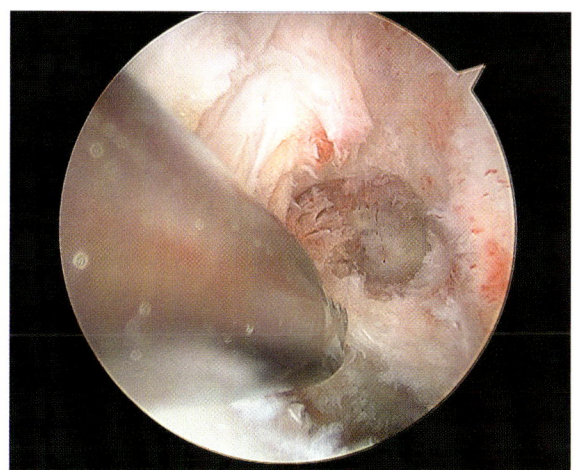

Figure 50-22. Débridement of notch and identification of old femoral tunnel.

carefully assessed and there was no evidence of a previous tunnel (Fig. 50-24). The new tibial and femoral tunnels were drilled in standard fashion (Fig. 50-25).

Case 2

(See video on website.)

A 17-year-old male with a history of a right knee ACL reconstruction with a BPTB autograft and a partial lateral meniscectomy 1 year ago presented complaining of right knee pain and swelling after being kicked in his knee playing soccer. He had returned to full activity without difficulty. In the clinic, he was noted to have a positive Lachman test and an effusion. Radiographs demonstrated acceptable but not ideal tunnel positioning, without evidence of significant widening and metal interference screws (Fig. 50-26). The femoral

tunnel appeared slightly anterior. An MRI was obtained, which confirmed the diagnosis of an ACL tear and further defined tunnel location. Based on the preoperative workup, the surgical plan was to keep the existing hardware in place, attempt to bypass the old tunnels, and drill new tunnels in more anatomic alignment. If the tunnels could not be bypassed, an attempt would be made to drill through a portion of the screw or remove the screw and fill it with bone void filler (bioabsorbable screw or allograft bone dowel).

At surgery, the diagnostic arthroscopy demonstrated a complete tear of his ACL graft. A hamstring tendon autograft (semitendinosus and gracilus [ST and G]) was harvested from the ipsilateral side. The ACL stump on the tibial and femoral surfaces was débrided and the previous tunnel locations were identified. The femoral tunnel was noted to be slightly vertical and anterior (Fig. 50-27). Next, an attempt was made to drill the tibial tunnel. A guide wire was passed into the tibial tunnel in a satisfactory position; however, the previous metal interference screw blocked the drill (Fig. 50-28). The old interference screw was then removed (Fig. 50-29A) and a matching bioabsorbable interference screw was inserted and used as a bone void filler (see Fig. 50-29B). The tibial tunnel was then drilled partly through the edge of the new bioabsorbable screw. Next, an over the top guide was used to insert the femoral guide pin in a more horizontal and posterior location to bypass the previous hardware completely. The femoral tunnel was drilled without interference and the posterior cortex remained intact (Fig. 50-30). The graft was then passed (Fig. 50-31) and satisfactory fixation was obtained. The patient was discharged home and participated in an accelerated ACL rehabilitation without complications.

Case 3

A 29-year-old man who had previously had an ACL reconstruction with an allograft 2 years earlier presented to our

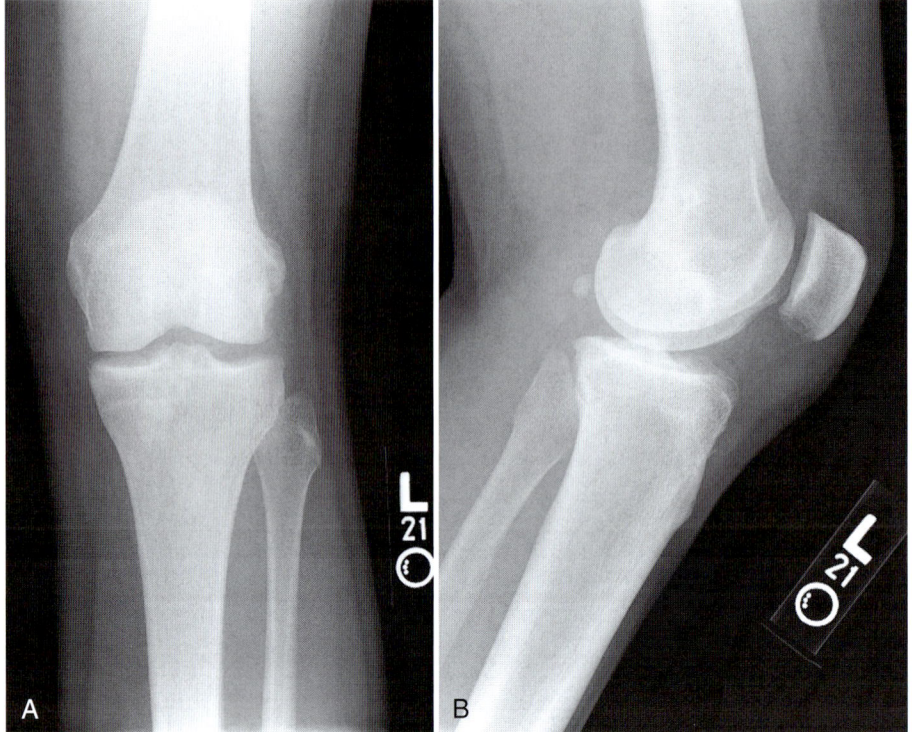

Figure 50-23. AP **(A)** and lateral **(B)** x-rays at 4 months postoperatively confirming healing of bone graft in tunnels.

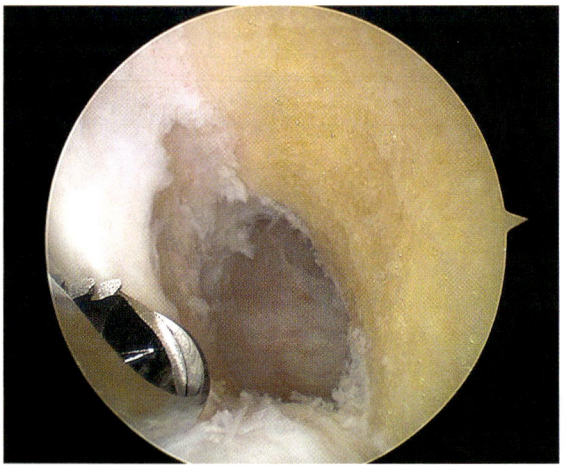

Figure 50-24. Revision notchplasty with no evidence of previous femoral tunnel.

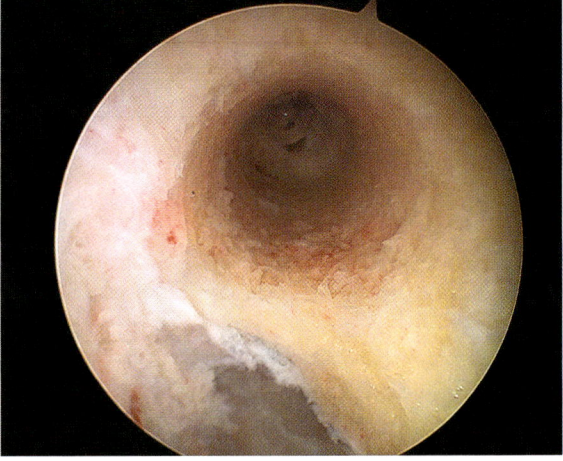

Figure 50-25. New femoral tunnel drilled in anatomic location with intact posterior wall.

clinic complaining of left knee pain and swelling after a twist-ing injury while playing softball. On examination, he had positive Lachman and pivot shift tests.

Radiographs revealed a metal interference screw in the femur and a screw and washer construct on the tibia. There was significant tunnel osteolysis and a malpositioned femoral tunnel (vertical and anterior; Fig. 50-32). An MRI was sub-sequently performed, which confirmed the diagnosis of an ACL graft tear (Fig. 50-33A), and again demonstrated sig-nificant tunnel osteolysis (see Fig. 50-33B). The patient was consented to undergo a single-stage ACL revision using a hamstring autograft. Although it was felt that this could be

done in one procedure with the use of a cylindric allograft dowel, the patient was informed that if adequate fixation could not be obtained intraoperatively, the surgery might have to be staged.

The patient was subsequently taken to the operating room and a diagnostic arthroscopy confirmed a complete tear of the ACL graft (Fig. 50-34). The graft was débrided, previous hardware was removed, and the tunnels were débrided with a 12-mm reamer (Fig. 50-35). A 12- × 18-mm cylindrical allograft dowel was then inserted into the prepared femoral tunnel, completely filling the bone void. A guide pin was inserted in the standard fashion and the tunnel was drilled

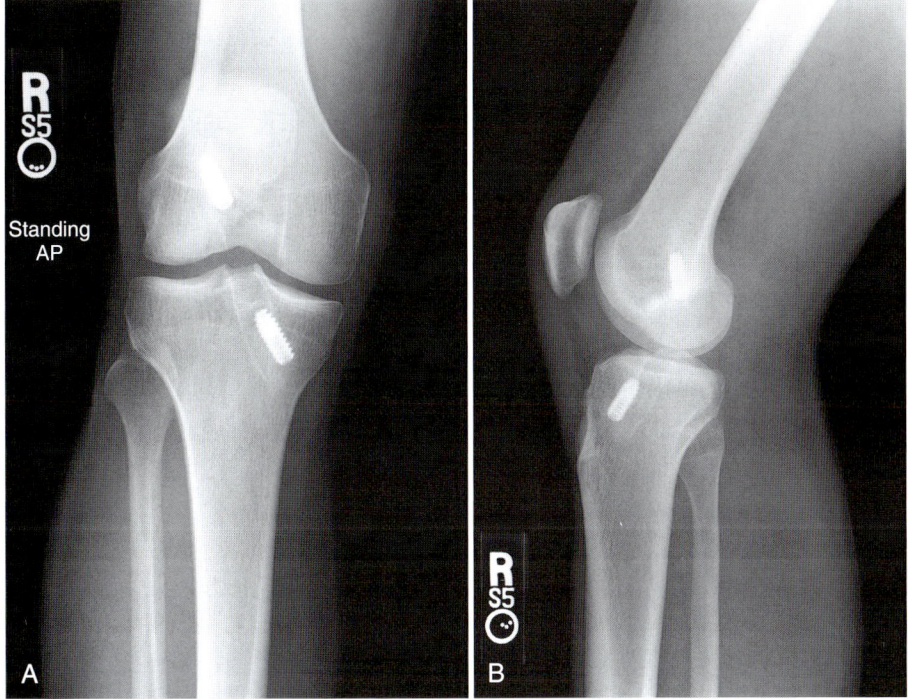

Figure 50-26. AP **(A)** and lateral **(B)** x-rays showing acceptable but not ideal tunnel position without significant tunnel widening.

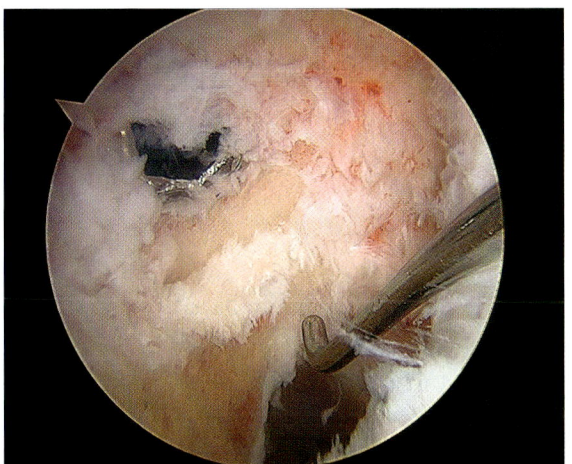

Figure 50-27. Previous tunnel with metal interference screw in a slightly anterior location.

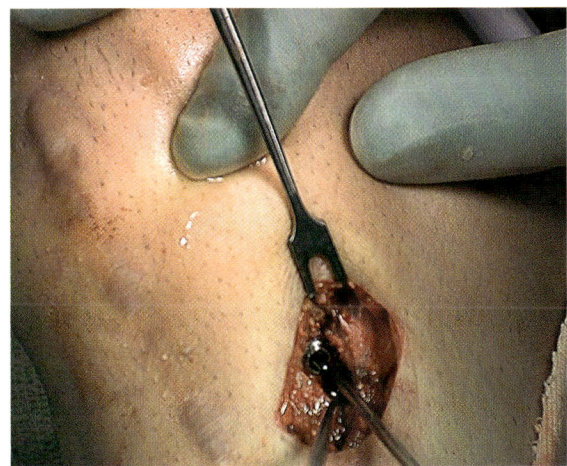

Figure 50-28. Guide wire placed for new tibial tunnel. Metal interference screw blocks drilling of tunnel.

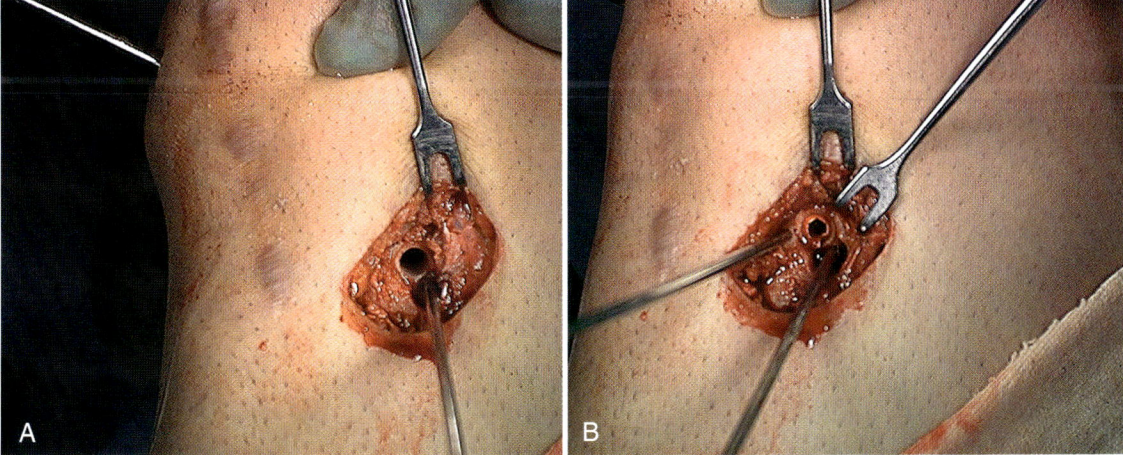

Figure 50-29. **A, B,** Metal interference screw removed and replaced by bioabsorbable screw.

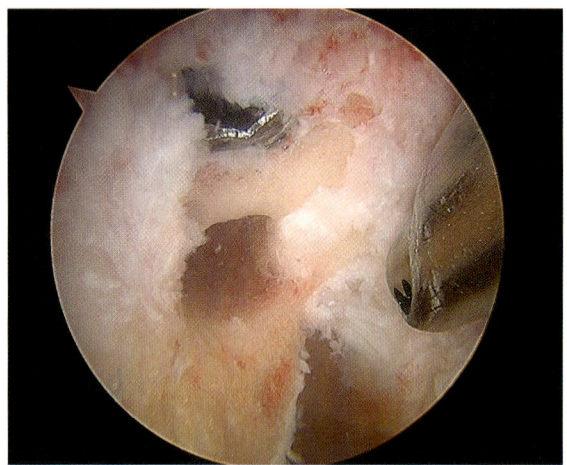

Figure 50-30. New femoral tunnel drilled without interference from previous tunnel.

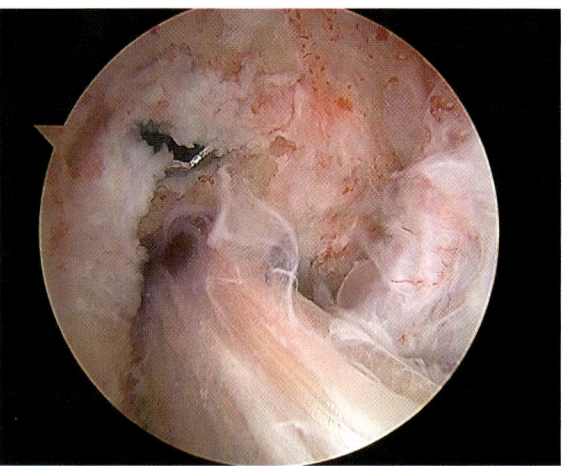

Figure 50-31. Graft inserted and fixed.

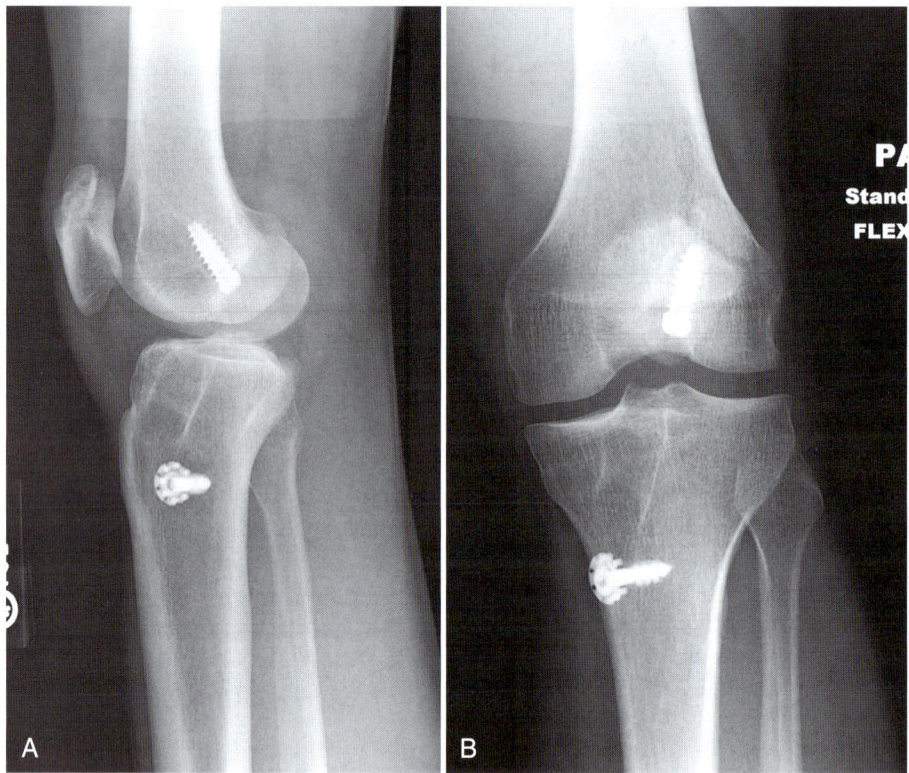

Figure 50-32. Lateral **(A)** and AP **(B)** x-rays showing a vertical and anterior femoral tunnel and moderate tunnel widening.

through a portion of the allograft (Fig. 50-36). The graft was passed into position and two methods of fixation were used to secure it into position.

OUTCOMES

Currently, no study has directly evaluated the outcomes of one-stage versus two-stage revision ACL reconstructions. However, there have been a few studies that have evaluated one-stage and two-stage revisions versus primary ACL reconstructions. Weiler and coworkers[26] have evaluated the outcomes of single-stage revision ACL reconstructions versus primary ACL reconstructions with autologous hamstring grafts. In their prospective study, 62 patients met the inclusion criteria and were compared with a matched control group. The postoperative results demonstrated no statistical significance in the objective International Knee Documentation Committee (IKDC) rating between the primary and single-stage revisions. Despite no objective differences, there were differences in the subjective Lysholm scores and functional testing in which the primary reconstruction group fared considerably better. The authors concluded that factors other than objective measures were responsible for the inferior results in the revision group.

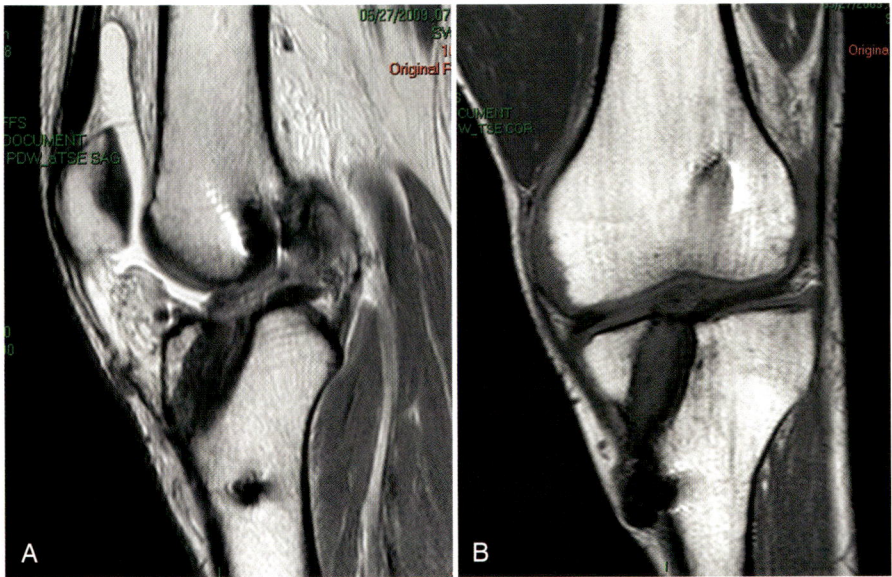

Figure 50-33. Coronal **(A)** and saggital **(B)** MRI images confirming tear of ACL graft and moderate tunnel widening.

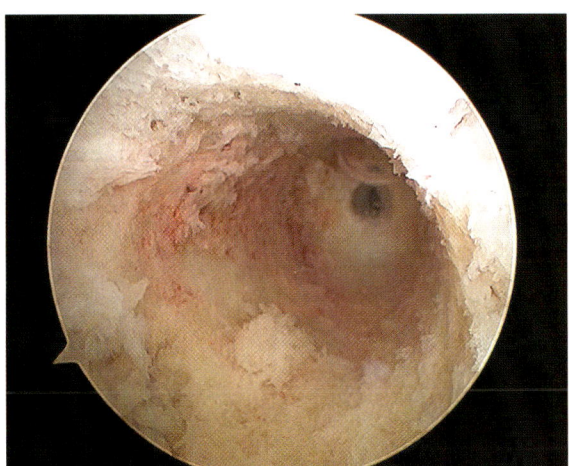

Figure 50-34. Sclerotic wall of old femoral tunnel débrided.

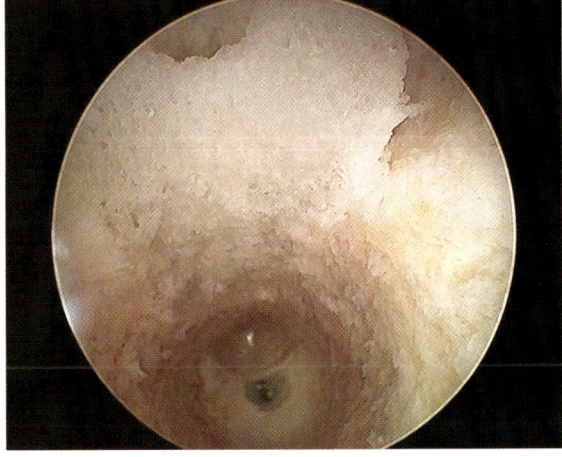

Figure 50-36. New tunnel drilled through portion of allograft dowel.

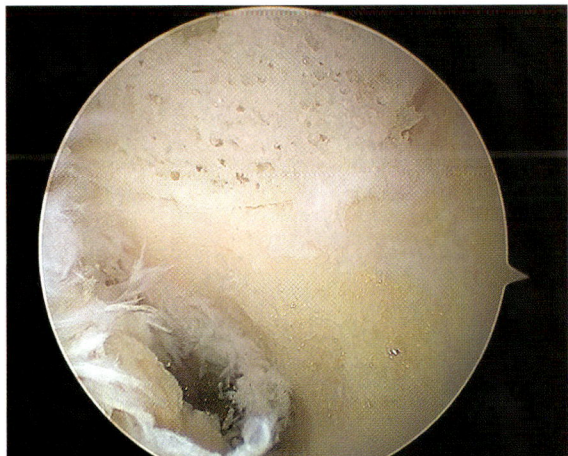

Figure 50-35. Allograft bone dowel inserted in prepared femoral tunnel.

In another study by Thomas and colleagues,[23] a prospective study comparing the results of a two-stage revision versus a primary ACL reconstruction was performed. They looked at 49 consecutive two-stage revisions and compared the results to that of a matched group that underwent a primary ACL reconstruction. Unlike in the study by Weiler and associates,[26] a significant difference between the objective IKDC scores was found in those who underwent primary and two-stage revisions. Overall, the patients who underwent a two-stage ACL revision had a greater degree of passive range of motion deficits as well as crepitus. Subjectively, the IKDC subjective score was 61.2 in the revision ACL group whereas it was 72.8 in the primary group. They also found that although objective scores were often similar, there were statistically significant worse subjective outcomes in patients who underwent a two-stage ACL revision compared with those who underwent a primary ACL reconstruction.

CONCLUSION

As the need for ACL revisions increases, it will be imperative for surgeons to identify the causes of failure of the primary procedure accurately and address them in a systematic fashion (Figs. 50-37 to 50-39). Pitfalls must be recognized and avoided to optimize the success of the revision procedure. The accurate placement of femoral and tibial tunnels should not be compromised by the index tunnel placement.[9] Depending on the type and location of the fixation, the location and size of

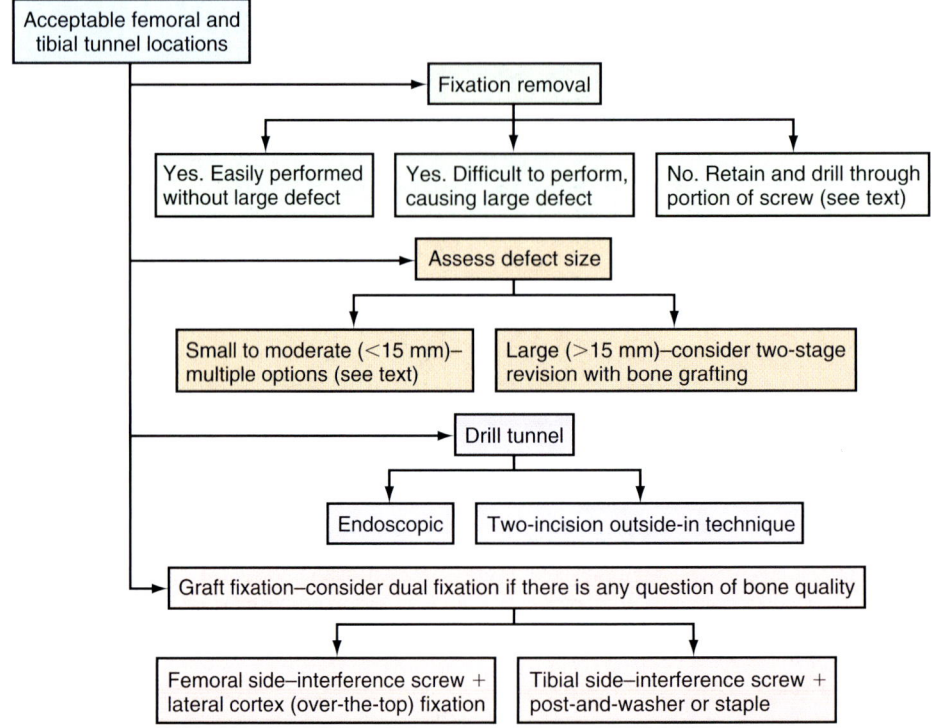

Figure 50-37. Acceptable femoral and tunnel locations.

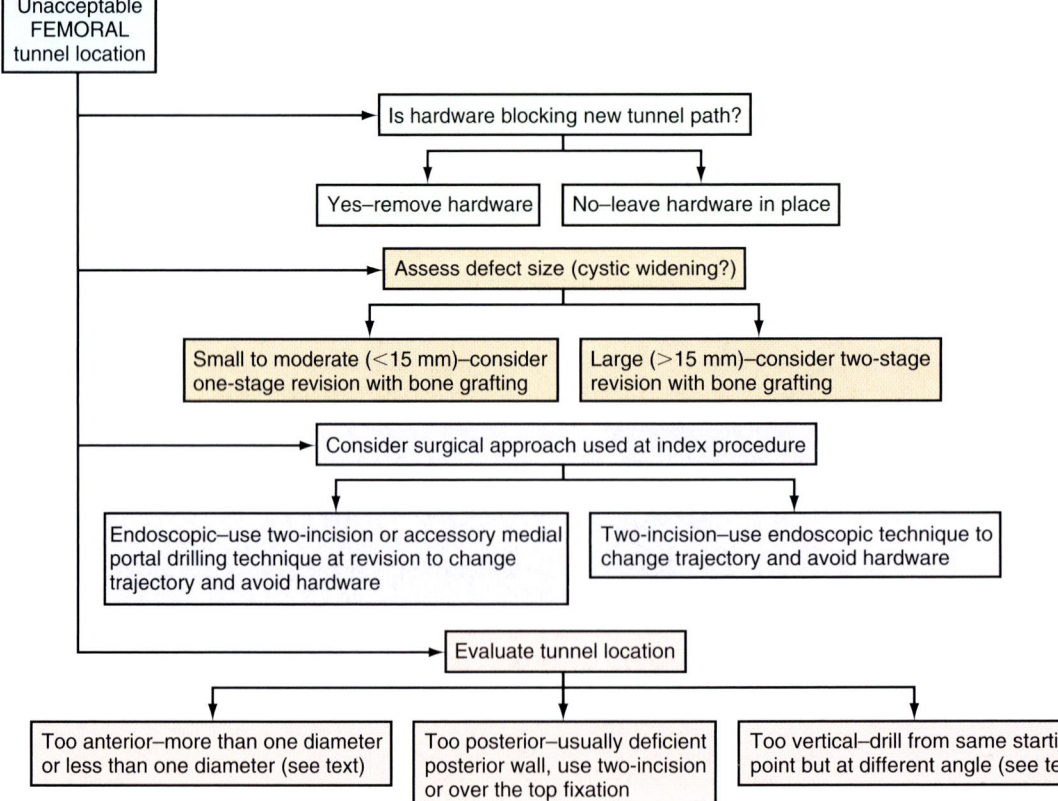

Figure 50-38. Unacceptable femoral tunnel location.

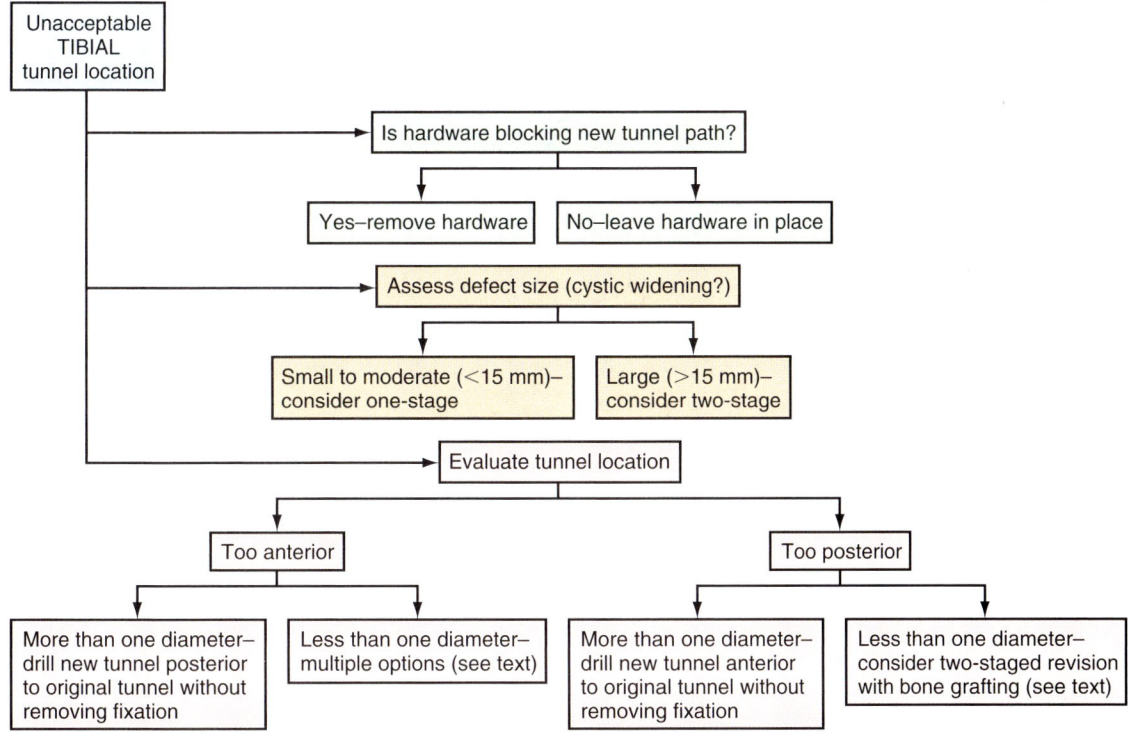

Figure 50-39. Unacceptable tibial tunnel location.

the existing tunnels, and the quality of the bone, the surgeon must be prepared to use a number of different techniques. Regardless of whether a one-stage or a two-stage procedure is performed, the goal must be to choose an appropriate graft and fix it in anatomic position in good quality bone, similar to a primary procedure.[23] Both surgical techniques have advantages and disadvantages and should be carefully considered to meet the needs of the individual patient.

KEY REFERENCES

Bach BR, Jr: Revision ACL Reconstruction: indication and technique. In Miller MD, Cole BJ, editors: Textbook of arthroscopy, Philadelphia, 2004, WB Saunders, pp 675–686.

Battaglia TC, Miller MD: Management of bony deficiency in revision anterior cruciate ligament reconstruction using allograft bone dowels: Surgical technique. Arthroscopy 21:767, 2005.

Brown CH, Jr, Carson EW: Revision anterior cruciate ligament surgery. Clin Sports Med 18:109–171, 1999.

Diamantopoulos AP, Lorbach O, Paessler HH: Anterior cruciate ligament revision reconstruction: results in 107 patients. Am J Sports Med 36:851–860, 2008.

George MS, Dunn WR, Spindler KP: Current concepts review: revision anterior cruciate ligament reconstruction. Am J Sports Med 34:2026–2037, 2006.

Harner CD, Giffin JR, Dunteman RC, et al: Evaluation and treatment of recurrent instability after anterior cruciate ligament reconstruction. J Bone Joint Surg Am 82:1652–1664, 2000.

Lind M, Menhert F, Pedersen AB: The first results from the Danish ACL reconstruction registry: epidemiological and 2-year follow-up results from 5,818 knee ligament reconstructions. Knee Surg Sports Traumatol Arthrosc 17:117–124, 2009.

Miller MD: Revision cruciate ligament surgery with retention of femoral interference screw. Arthroscopy 14:111–114, 1998.

Thomas NP, Kankate R, Wandless F, Pandit H: Revision anterior cruciate ligament reconstruction using a 2-stage technique with bone grafting of the tibial tunnel. Am J Sports Med 33:1701–1709, 2005.

Weiler A, Schmeling A, Stohr I, et al: Primary versus single-stage revision anterior cruciate ligament reconstruction using autologous hamstring tendon grafts: a prospective matched-group analysis. Am J Sports Med 35:1643–1652, 2007.

Full references for this chapter can be found on www.expertconsult.com.

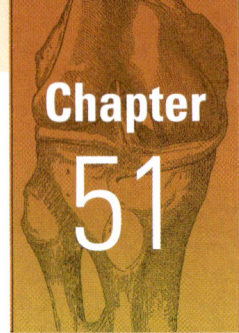
Osteotomy and the Cruciate-Deficient Knee

Randy Clark and Annunziato Amendola

Estimates report 100,000 new anterior cruciate ligament (ACL) injuries each year in the United States, with an overall incidence of 1/300,000 people.[15] ACL injuries are frequently associated with dysfunction and impairment caused by knee joint instability, loss of proprioception, chondral and meniscal injuries, reduced quadriceps strength, and changes in the biomechanics of knee, with the risk of subsequent post-traumatic arthritis. Risk factors associated with ACL injury and implicated in the development of post-traumatic knee arthritis are meniscal injury, osteochondral pathology, malalignment, high levels of activity, genetic predisposition, obesity, age, and participating in high-level sports activities involving cutting, pivoting, and twisting.[9,26] No previous studies have demonstrated that ACL reconstruction prevents the development of post-traumatic arthritis.[11,25]

CRUCIATE INJURY AND ARTHROSIS

In general, instability of the knee is not well tolerated and eventually post-traumatic arthritis develops. There is a significant amount of literature regarding ACL deficiency and post-traumatic arthritis. Some authors have reported the development of knee osteoarthritis (OA) after ACL injury in 50% of patients on average.[9,25] Others have reported the development of OA in up to 70% of patients with combined ACL and meniscal injuries at 15 to 20 years after injury.[20] Øiestad and colleagues,[32] in a recent systematic review, indicated that the most accurate report of knee OA after isolated injury could be as low as 0% to 13%, and a prevalence of knee OA in combined ACL and meniscal injuries as high as 21% to 48%.

Patients with ACL and/or posterior cruciate ligament (PCL) deficiency, concomitant chondral and meniscal injuries, and preexisting malalignment of the knee are at increased risk of post-traumatic joint arthritis. In the case of ACL deficiency and underlying malalignment, with the loss of neuromuscular control, the knee is more likely to go into increased varus and overload the medial compartment. The varus knee with radiographic separation of the lateral tibiofemoral compartment and increased external rotation and hyperextension with an abnormal varus recurvatum position is referred to as a triple-varus knee.[6,31] Medial joint pain, instability, and early degenerative joint disease may result in patients with this clinical scenario.

The medial compartment tends to have a posterior medial tibial plateau wear pattern in triple-varus knees (Fig. 51-1). This is thought to be caused by a chronic anterior subluxation of the tibia with respect to the femur.[5] This pattern is further exacerbated by medial meniscal insufficiency. As the degenerative process progresses and the arthritic changes occur, the knee becomes less unstable. The patient begins to have arthritis-type complaints rather than instability complaints.

It is important to differentiate the cause of the patient's complaints. The surgeon must determine whether he or she is suffering from underlying instability or if the complaints are caused by degenerative joint disease. The surgeon can differentiate between the two by determining which activities cause symptoms. It is important to distinguish whether the patient is complaining of pain with aggressive activities and pivoting types of movement, indicating instability, or of pain with activities of daily living, indicating arthrosis.

PCL-deficient knees are susceptible to posterior tibial subluxation and posterior instability.[27] Mavrodontidis and associates[30] have discussed two cases of rapid development of post-traumatic arthritis after failed PCL reconstruction. Instability of the knee joint leads to progressive knee arthritis. Much attention is devoted to soft tissue reconstruction, but surgeons may choose to ignore correctable risk factors for reconstruction failure such as joint malalignment. Frequently, joint malalignment contributes to the ligamentous injury prior to the discussion of reconstruction ever occurring. Geissler and Whipple[16] found a 49% incidence of chondral defects and 36% incidence of meniscal tears in patients with chronic PCL instability. Keller and colleagues[22] reviewed 40 PCL-deficient patients treated nonoperatively and found that 90% complained of knee pain with activity at 4 years from the time of injury, and only 12% of patients had normal-appearing radiographs. Clancy and associates[8] found that 48% of patients with chronic PCL injuries had moderate to severe articular injury to the medial femoral condyle at the time of surgical reconstruction.

Posterior tibial slope and its relationship to instability in cruciate deficiency is also something to consider, particularly when considering osteotomy in these patients. Bonin and colleagues[5] have described the relationship of pathologic tibial slope and incidence of ACL injury. The greater the slope, the greater the incidence of ACL instability. Giffin and associates,[18,19] Agneskirchner and coworkers,[1] and Dejour and Bonin[12] have shown that increasing tibial slope alters tibial translation, and this is augmented in the cruciate-deficient knee (Fig. 51-2).

INDICATIONS FOR OSTEOTOMY

Osteotomies have been used for localized medial and lateral compartment gonarthrosis with varus and valgus malalignment. The principle supporting the use of tibial osteotomy is redistribution of the mechanical force across the joint. Coventry[10] initially described the indications for high tibial osteotomy to include stable knees with no subluxation or thrust, range of motion (ROM) of at least 15 to 100 degrees, localized medial compartment OA, minimal or no patellofemoral symptoms, and age younger than 65 years. Indications for high tibial osteotomies have since expanded for cases of posterior instability, ACL deficiency, and correcting

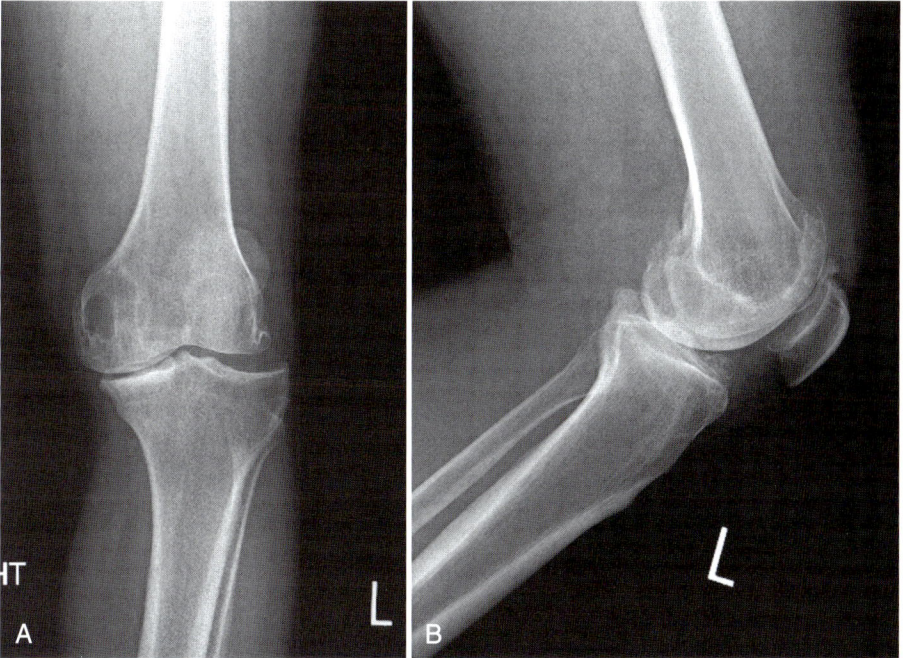

Figure 51-1. AP **(A)** and lateral **(B)** views of a 50-year-old male chronic ACL-deficient patient with medial compartment OA, varus align-ment, and no previous surgery. Note the medial wear on the AP view, and the posterior wear pattern on the lateral view caused by chronic anterior subluxation.

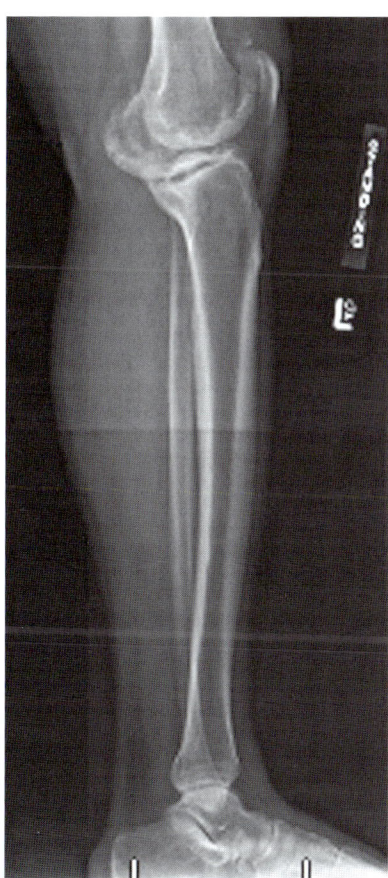

Figure 51-2. Long lateral view of the tibia in a chronic ACL-deficient patient. Note the increased posterior slope and anterior subluxation of the proximal tibia.

> **Box 51-1** Indications for Osteotomy Based on Clinical Signs Of Instability
>
> 1. Posterolateral or lateral laxity and varus malalignment ± thrust
> 2. Cruciate deficiency and varus alignment ± thrust
> 3. Combined ligamentous laxity and varus alignment ± thrust
> 4. Repeat failures of cruciate reconstruction
>
> Adapted from Phisitkul P, Wolf BR, Amendola A: Role of high tibial and distal femoral osteotomies in the treatment of lateral-posterolateral and medial instabilities of the knee. Sports Med Arthrosc 14:96–104, 2006.

tibial slope in sagittal instability.[13,31] The senior author's indi-cations for osteotomy in the setting of instability are found in Box 51-1.

In the setting of ACL insufficiency with symptomatic instability and pathologic sagittal tibial slope, one should consider correction of the underlying malalignment issue in addition to ligamentous reconstruction. Previous observa-tions of an increased incidence of ACL tears with increased tibial slope and biomechanical studies demonstrating increased anterior tibial translation with increasing tibial slope have suggested that decreasing the tibial slope would provide a more stable biomechanical environment.[12,18,19] The PCL-deficient knee presents a contrary situation in which decreasing tibial slope causes an increase in posterior tibial translation and symptoms of instability (Fig. 51-3).

TREATMENT OF CRUCIATE DEFICIENCY AND ARTHROSIS

If the patient is diagnosed with chronic ACL deficiency with early medial compartment arthritis and varus malalignment with overload, the physician should optimize conservative

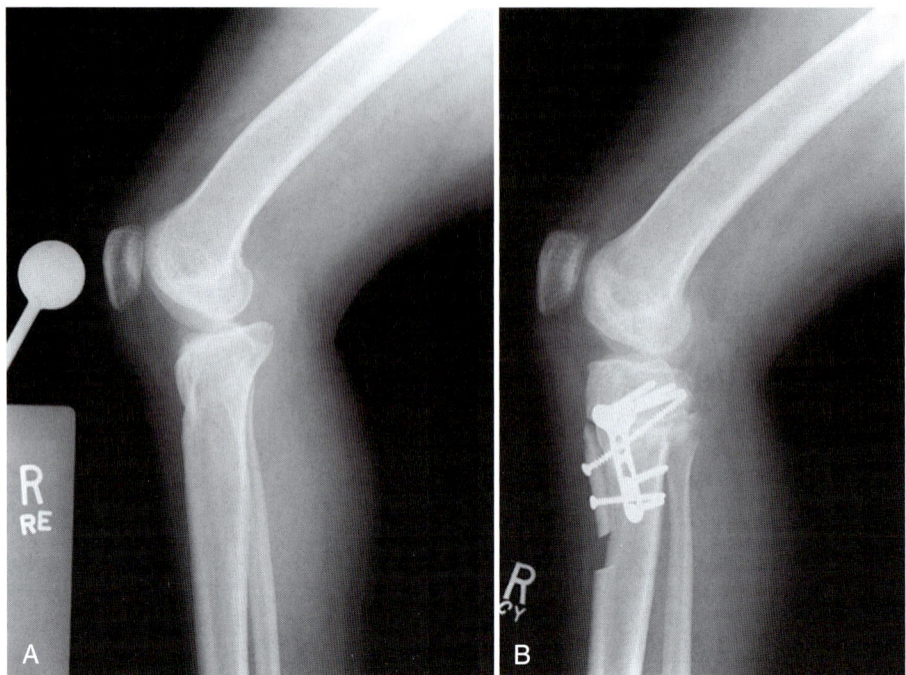

Figure 51-3. **A,** Lateral view of the knee. Posterior instability of the knee and decreased posterior tibial slope accentuates posterior subluxation and hyperextension. **B,** Same patient treated with proximal tibial osteotomy to increase the slope and prevent hyperextension and posterior instability. Note the improved slope and decreased posterior subluxation. The tibial tubercle osteotomy was performed to move the tubercle proximally to prevent patella baja.

care, including unloader bracing, physical therapy, and activity modification. Patients who are experiencing arthritis-type symptoms related to previous meniscectomy, mechanical axis deviation into the medial compartment, and early medial compartment degenerative changes may benefit from a high tibial osteotomy (HTO). The painful symptoms from degenerative joint disease secondary to underlying instability and previous injury are termed *pseudoinstability*. In the setting of previously failed soft tissue reconstruction, one must consider malalignment as a contributing factor.

In the setting of a younger patient who is experiencing symptoms of instability with underlying malalignment and other meniscal or chondral pathology, the surgeon could consider ACL reconstruction in addition to an osteotomy. Surgeons are currently pushing the envelope for ACL reconstruction in older yet active patients with complaints of instability.

To determine whether an ACL reconstruction is indicated in addition to HTO, the physician must consider the patient's complaints at the time of initial presentation. If an older or less active patient is suffering from mechanical overload and pain, they will likely respond to the osteotomy alone. It is important to assess the entire clinical picture and differentiate pseudoinstability from true instability. If the patient continues to complain of instability after HTO, ACL reconstruction can be considered as a secondary procedure. However, ACL reconstruction alone in the face of malalignment is doomed for continuing symptoms of compartment overload and early failure of the ACL surgery.

PREOPERATIVE EVALUATION

Factors considered in the preoperative evaluation and prior to indication for osteotomy include the following: (1) pure

valgus or varus malalignment; (2) loss of neuromuscular control associated with ligament injury and loss of proprioceptive feedback (thrust during stance); (3) abnormal sagittal slope in the setting of ACL or PCL insufficiency; (4) triple-varus knee; and (5) unicompartmental degeneration (usually a postmeniscectomy knee).

The preoperative examination should include a detailed history, clinical examination, and imaging studies. Physical examination findings supportive of an osteotomy include joint line tenderness, abnormal gait patterns, with special attention to lateral thrust, and limb alignment in stance. Attention is directed toward instability tests including Lachman, pivot shift, anterior and posterior drawer, reverse pivot shift, and external rotation tests. The examiner should note the double- or triple-varus knee associated with ACL, PCL, or posterolateral corner deficiency.

Radiographic evaluation begins with assessment of the extent of knee arthrosis and lower extremity alignment with bilateral standard weight-bearing long-leg (hip to ankle) anteroposterior views, standard anteroposterior views in full extension, bilateral weight-bearing posteroanterior tunnel views in 30 degrees of flexion, and lateral and Merchant patellar views. Dugdale and coworkers[14] have described the technique used to calculate the HTO correction. The mechanical axis and weight-bearing axis are determined and the correction to be made is calculated just lateral to the lateral tibial spine (Fig. 51-4).

MRI evaluation is helpful for preoperative planning. The astute clinician can determine ACL or PCL insufficiency from the examination, but advanced imaging provides additional information that is often useful in determining soft tissue repair and reconstruction in addition to the osteotomy, which is determined from plain films and the clinical

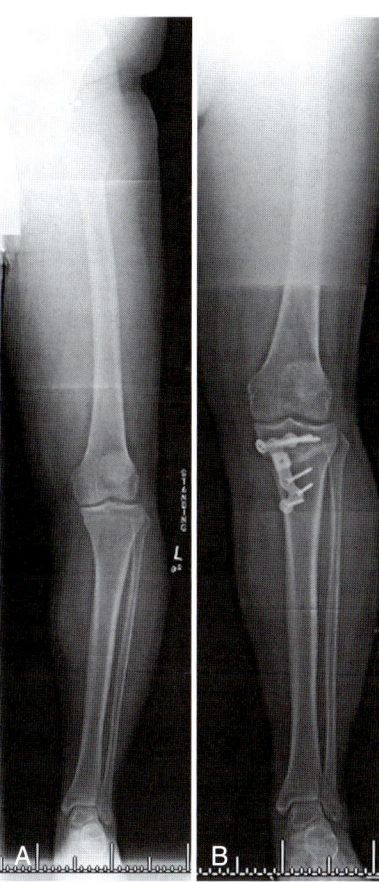

Figure 51-4. **A,** Hip to ankle x-ray (the patient is standing with equal weight on both legs) to measure preoperative varus deformity. **B,** Postoperative correction of varus deformity with medial opening wedge osteotomy.

examination. The senior author uses MRI imaging to evaluate chondral, meniscal, and soft tissue injury in addition to subtle osseous findings that plain film radiographs are often not sensitive enough to demonstrate.

In active patients who hope to return to a high activity level, we plan the osteotomy so that it will place the weight-bearing line—as measured from the center of the femoral head to the center of the tibiotalar joint—through the center of the knee joint. This is described as just lateral to the tibial spine (or 62% of the width of the joint surface referenced from medial joint line). Some authors have recommended overcorrection in the setting of medial compartment arthritis. We do not perform significant overcorrection in younger patients; rather, our goal is to re-create neutral alignment and unload the previously overloaded medial compartment in the varus knee. In the setting of an arthritic knee with ACL or PCL insufficiency, the goal of the osteotomy is to achieve the desired posterior tibial slope in the sagittal plane and thus obtain enhanced stability of the knee.[1,13,18,19,33]

The surgeon must exercise caution in the setting of severe deformity, because the accuracy of correction may be more difficult to determine (Fig. 51-5). Patients with osteoporosis present challenges in obtaining suitable fixation and can require prolonged periods for healing. Other considerations must be given to risk factors for failure, including smokers, prolonged dependency of corticosteroids, immunosuppressants, and chronic illness.

SURGICAL PROCEDURE

Authors' Preferred Technique

We prefer the medial opening wedge osteotomy to the lateral closing wedge osteotomy because, in our experience, precise correction is more likely and overcorrection is less likely. Although this approach increases the stability of a malaligned knee, it also avoids osteotomy of the proximal fibula, thereby avoiding potential instability through the tibiofibular joint and posterolateral corner structures and injury to the peroneal nerve.[7,23,38] The medial opening wedge incision also provides access to the hamstring autograft in the setting of ACL reconstruction. This approach also allows for correction in the coronal and sagittal planes. We use an opening wedge plating system from Arthrex (Naples, Fla). Another advantage of the medial opening wedge tibial osteotomy is that the risk of inadvertently altering the normal tibia slope is decreased. Amendola and colleagues[2] have shown that by avoiding osteotomy of the proximal fibula, as with a lateral closing wedge technique, the tibial slope will be forced to decrease because of hinging at the proximal tibiofibular joint.

Operative Procedure With Anterior Cruciate Ligament Reconstruction

The patient is administered prophylactic intravenous antibiotics preoperatively. The patient is then positioned supine and the involved limb is prepared and draped in standard fashion. Arthroscopy using low pressures and frequent compartment checks is performed to evaluate the condition of the articular cartilage and menisci. Once the arthroscopy has been completed, the extremity is elevated and exsanguinated and the tourniquet is used for the remainder of the osteotomy procedure.

The senior author does not perform any articular cartilage resurfacing procedures such as autologous chondrocyte implantation (ACI) or meniscal transplantation at the time of this surgery. If they are required, surgery is staged; the osteotomy is performed first, followed by soft tissue reconstruction once the patient has recovered from the osteotomy.

To close the osteotomy wedge anteriorly, a bump is placed underneath the leg to hyperextend the knee. This decreases the tibial slope and thus decreases anterior tibial translation in the ACL-deficient knee.

A vertical incision is made over the pes anserinus insertion halfway between the medial border of the patellar ligament and the posterior margin of the tibia. This is followed by exposure and incision of the sartorial fascia and finally by subperiosteal elevation of the medial collateral ligament (MCL). Blunt retractors are then placed anteriorly to protect the patellar ligament and posteriorly to protect the hamstring tendons and superficial MCL.

Under fluoroscopic control, a guide wire is drilled across the proximal tibia from medial to lateral. The guide is positioned at the level of the superior aspect of the tibial tubercle and oriented obliquely to end at least 1 cm below the joint line at the lateral tibial cortex. By aiming approximately 1 cm below the lateral joint line, we can stay proximal to the patellar tendon insertion and still be sufficiently inferior to the articular surface to prevent intra-articular fracture during the cut. The osteotomy maximizes the metaphyseal location and

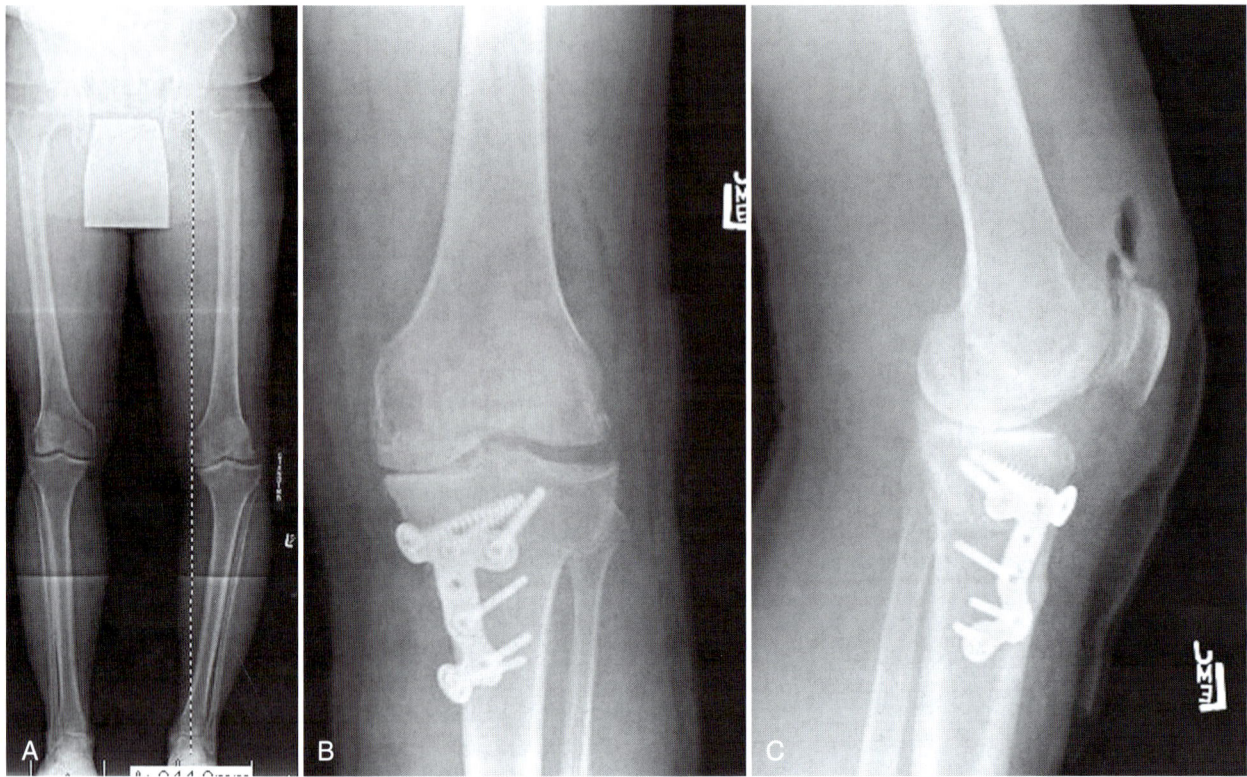

Figure 51-5. **A,** Preoperative long-leg standing view from hips to ankles in a chronic ACL-deficient patient with severe deformity. **B,** Postoperative AP view after dome osteotomy, which was performed rather than opening wedge for a large deformity. **C,** Postoperative lateral view with decreased slope following a dome osteotomy to help the ACL instability.

likelihood of healing. If the osteotomy cut is too distal, it becomes extracapsular, thereby reducing the stability of the osteotomy site. The osteotomy is performed with an oscillating saw below the guide pin to prevent superior migration and decrease risk of an intra-articular fracture. The osteotomy is deepened with flexible and rigid osteotomes using fluoroscopic confirmation.

Once the osteotomy has been completed, the medial opening is created with an osteotomy wedge to the predetermined depth. Intraoperative femorotibial alignment is verified by fluoroscopy and an extramedullary alignment guide is used to ensure that the weight-bearing axis is passing through the center of the knee joint. Sabharwal and Zhao[34] have recently cautioned that for obese patients or those with substantial malalignment, supine fluoroscopy alignment measurements without loading of the knee joint does not reflect the axis as accurately as preoperative standing films. In such cases, we believe careful scrutinizing of the preoperative weight-bearing films and the intraoperative fluoroscopic images can still lead to favorable results.

The posterior tibial slope is also assessed intraoperatively and can be changed by distracting the osteotomy more anteriorly or posteriorly if the patient has any symptomatic cruciate deficiency or excessive anteroposterior translation preoperatively. If the opening is more than 1 cm anteriorly, a tibial tubercle osteotomy is performed to advance the tubercle the same height of the osteotomy. When the desired opening has been achieved, the osteotomy is secured with a plate and bone graft (corticocancellous wedges cut from a femoral head allograft).

The plate is fixed proximally with 6.5-mm cancellous screws and distally with 4.5-mm cortical screws. Placement of fixation is confirmed with fluoroscopic imaging. The tourniquet is released and hemostasis controlled. The wound is closed in layers over a drain placed in the subcutaneous space.

The osteotomy is performed prior to drilling the tunnels for ACL reconstruction to prevent the creation of a possible stress riser through the ACL tunnel. Arthroscopically assisted ACL reconstruction is done using standard technique with the following considerations. We drill the tibial tunnel anterior and superior to the osteotomy site. A retro drill (Arthrex) technique is useful to avoid the osteotomy site.

A femoral tunnel is drilled in the usual technique. The ACL graft is passed through the tibial tunnel and out the femoral tunnel. The senior author's preference is to use extracortical button fixation. A tibial side interference screw is placed for primary fixation proximal to the osteotomy site. Secondary fixation can be placed below the osteotomy site, if desired. Bone grafting of the osteotomy site is performed at this point (Fig. 51-6).

POSTOPERATIVE PROTOCOL

Following surgery, the patient is allowed toe-touch weight bearing with ROM performed within a 0- to 90-degree arc for 6 weeks. It is important to begin early postoperative range of motion to prevent stiffness in the knee joint. Radiographs are obtained at the 6-week postoperative appointment. If there is evidence of consolidation, the brace is discontinued and full weight bearing is initiated with a strengthening

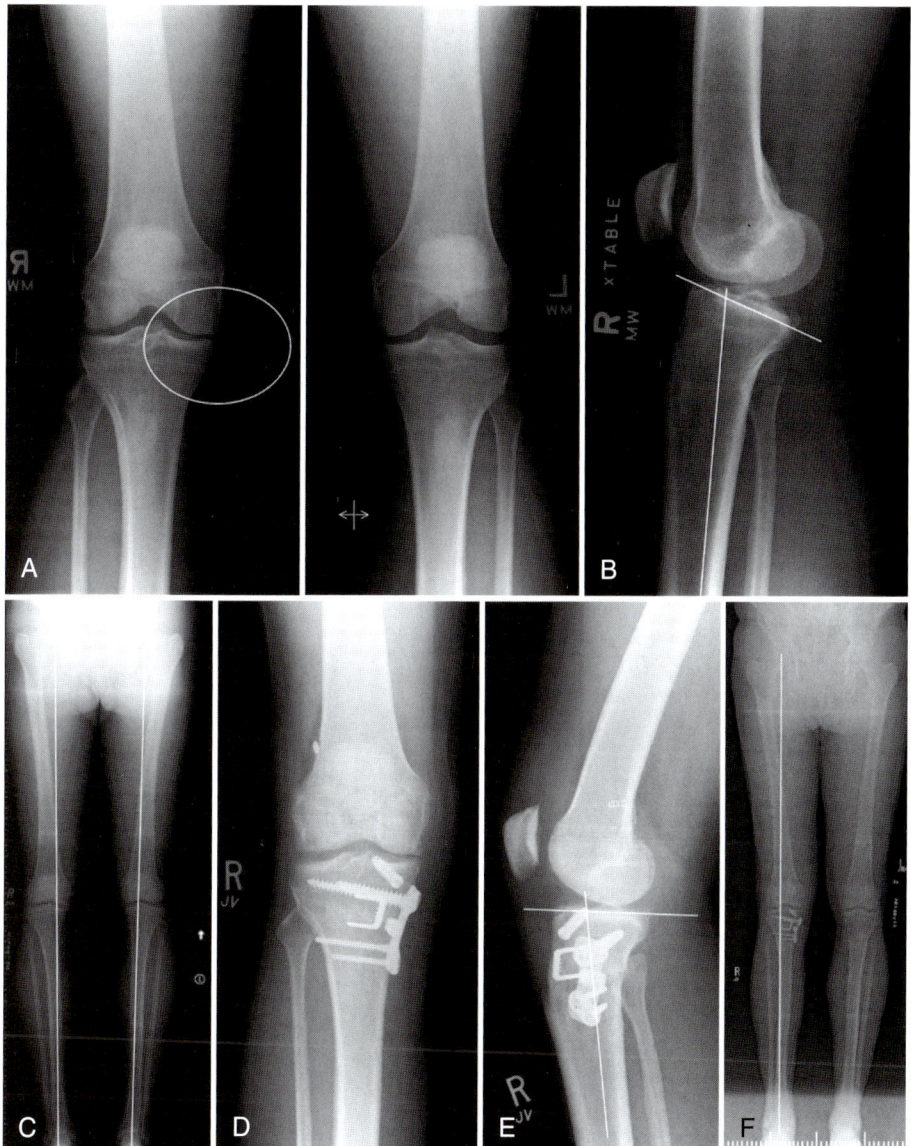

Figure 51-6. **A,** Preoperative standing tunnel view in a 30-year-old ACL-deficient patient with no previous surgery. **B,** Preoperative lateral view with increased lateral slope, ACL deficiency. **C,** Preoperative long-leg hip to ankle radiograph demonstrating medial axis deviation, used for operative planning on the amount of correction. **D,** Postoperative AP view with opening wedge osteotomy plus ACL reconstruction using allograft and interference screw fixation on the tibia and EndoButton fixation on the femur. **E,** Postoperative lateral view demonstrating decrease in tibial slope to help the ACL deficiency. Often, fixation can be augmented anteriorly to close the wedge and thereby decrease the slope. **F,** Postoperative long-leg standing x-ray demonstrating correction of the weight-bearing axis to the lateral tibial spine, avoiding overcorrection.

program. At the 10-week postoperative appointment, radiography is repeated. If osseous consolidation has been achieved, sport-specific rehabilitation is initiated.

OUTCOMES

High tibial osteotomy in addition to ACL reconstruction in patients with early medial compartment arthrosis has been shown to reduce symptoms and possibly reduce the progression of arthritis.[5] The older patient with ACL deficiency who is suffering from symptoms consistent with advanced arthritis rather than instability would benefit most from joint realignment and unloading of the diseased medial compartment. Lattermann and Jakob[24] have shown that many patients older

than 40 years do well with the osteotomy alone and do not require later ACL reconstruction. In patients with ACL deficiency that would be indicated for an HTO alone, it is important to consider reduction of the tibial slope to reduce the tendency of the tibia to translate anterior to the femur, as is expected with chronic ACL insufficiency.

There is some discussion as to whether the young patient who is experiencing ACL-related instability in addition to medial compartment degeneration and malalignment should undergo a one-step or staged ACL reconstruction with HTO. We prefer to perform one definitive procedure with modern techniques and minimal morbidity. If the surgeon feels inclined to perform a two-stage reconstruction, the senior author recommends performing the HTO first because this is likely to improve symptoms of the degenerative medial compartment in addition to improving symptoms of instability. Performing an ACL reconstruction alone will lead to inferior results, with a propensity to failure and progression of arthritic symptoms.

COMPLICATIONS

Complications associated with HTO include nonunion, fracture, hardware failure, symptomatic hardware, infection, peroneal nerve palsy, and compartment syndrome. Matthews and associates[29] and Hernigou and colleagues[21] have noted intra-articular fractures to occur in 11% of cases in medial opening HTO and in 10% to 20% in lateral closing HTO. To avoid this complication, we stay inferior to a guide pin during the osteotomy. The guide pin is aimed 1 cm below the joint line on the lateral side to help reduce the risk of intra-articular fracture. In the setting of an intra-articular fracture, the priority becomes congruity of the tibial plateau with stable fixation. Nonunion is a more common complication in opening wedge techniques, with risks reported from 0.7% to 4.4%.[3,36,37] Bone autograft and allograft, bone substitutes, and growth factors have been used to fill the void in opening HTO and decrease nonunion. We routinely use a femoral head allograft.

Recent research supports use of a locking plate design to enhance fixation and allow earlier weight-bearing to help decrease risk of nonunion.[39,40] The Contour Lock System (Arthrex) offers polyaxial locked fixation and less often is symptomatic than larger traditional locking plates. In our experience, the Arthrex plate usually does not require a second surgery for hardware removal and has not been associated with hardware failure or nonunion. Infection risk with ORIF has been reported to be 4%.[4] The senior author has not encountered the complication of compartment syndrome; the exact incidence of compartment syndrome in HTO is unknown.[21] Nonetheless, concomitant arthroscopic procedures should increase concern and suspicion for compartment syndrome during HTO.[28] When arthroscopy is necessary, we use lower pressures and perform frequent compartment checks during the operation. Reports of the incidence of peroneal nerve palsy associated with closing wedge HTO range from 2% to 16%.[17,35]

KEY REFERENCES

Agneskirchner JD, Hurschler C, Stukenborg-Colsman C, et al: Effect of high tibial flexion osteotomy on cartilage pressure and joint kinematics: a biomechanical study in human cadaveric knees. Winner of the AGA-DonJoy Award 2004. Arch Orthop Trauma Surg 124:575–584, 2004.

Amendola A, Rorabeck CH, Bourne RB, et al: Total knee arthroplasty following high tibial osteotomy for osteoarthritis. J Arthroplasty 4(Suppl):S11–S17, 1989.

Bonin N, Ait Si Selmi T, Donell ST, et al: Anterior cruciate reconstruction combined with valgus upper tibial osteotomy: 12 years follow-up. Knee 11:431–437, 2004.

Brinkman JM, Lobenhoffer P, Agneskirchner JD, et al: Osteotomies around the knee: Patient selection, stability of fixation and bone healing in high tibial osteotomies. J Bone Joint Surg Br 90:1548–1557, 2008.

Clatworthy M, Amendola A: The anterior cruciate ligament and arthritis. Clin Sports Med 18:173–198, 1999.

Daniel DM, Stone ML, Dobson BE, et al: Fate of the ACL-injured patient. A prospective outcome study. Am J Sports Med 22:632–644, 1994.

Dugdale TW, Noyes FR, Styer D: Preoperative planning for high tibial osteotomy. The effect of lateral tibiofemoral separation and tibiofemoral length. Clin Orthop Relat Res 274:248–264, 1992.

Giffin JR, Vogrin TM, Zantop T, et al: Effects of increasing tibial slope on the biomechanics of the knee. Am J Sports Med 32:376–382, 2004.

Hernigou P, Medevielle D, Debeyre J, et al: Proximal tibial osteotomy for osteoarthritis with varus deformity. A ten- to thirteen-year follow-up study. J Bone Joint Surg Am 69:332–354, 1987.

LaPrade RF, Engebretsen L, Johansen S, et al: The effect of a proximal tibial medial opening wedge osteotomy on posterolateral knee instability: a biomechanical study. Am J Sports Med 36:956–960, 2008.

Lattermann C, Jakob RP: High tibial osteotomy alone or combined with ligament reconstruction in anterior cruciate ligament–deficient knees. Knee Surg Sports Traumatol Arthrosc 4:32–38, 1996.

MacDonald P, Miniaci A, Fowler P, et al: A biomechanical analysis of joint contact forces in the posterior cruciate deficient knee. Knee Surg Sports Traumatol Arthrosc 3:252–255, 1996.

Phisitkul P, Wolf BR, Amendola A: Role of high tibial and distal femoral osteotomies in the treatment of lateral-posterolateral and medial instabilities of the knee. Sports Med Arthrosc 14:96–104, 2006.

Full references for this chapter can be found on www.expertconsult.com.

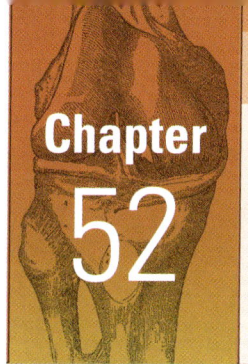

Chapter 52

Unicompartmental Knee Arthroplasty in Anterior Cruciate Ligament–Deficient Knees

Carlos Gonzalez, Andreas H. Gomoll, and Wolfgang Fitz

Management of unicompartmental osteoarthrosis of the knee continues to generate controversy. The 1970s and 1980s cast doubt on the benefit of a unicompartmental knee arthroplasty (UKA) as a surgical option for knee arthritis. However, more recent studies support the increased use of UKA based on lower morbidity, cost efficiency, longevity, and efficacy of unicompartmental arthroplasty.[11,17] Symptomatic unicompartmental gonarthrosis in young and active patients with preexisting anterior cruciate ligament (ACL) deficiency has been a challenging problem that is being encountered on a more frequent basis with younger patients presenting for surgical intervention. The goal of surgical management remains the same—to offer the patient an intervention that will provide lasting symptom relief of both instability and osteoarthritic symptoms. With the advancements in implant designs and surgical techniques, various options exist for the treatment of unicompartmental knee gonarthrosis. Surgical options such as arthroscopic débridement, cartilage replacement techniques, with or without realignment osteotomy, and concomitant ACL reconstruction have their limitations, because ACL reconstruction addresses the instability but not the degenerative process. Realignment osteotomy with or without ACL reconstruction may improve the patient's symptoms but does not completely relieve pain, and progression of contralateral compartment gonarthrosis remains an issue.[14] In ACL-deficient knees, previous studies have demonstrated disappointing results when UKA alone, without ACL reconstruction, was performed to address unilateral gonarthrosis.[7,9]

INDICATIONS AND CONTRAINDICATIONS

Scott and colleagues[13] have provided a framework for describing recommended indications and contraindications for unicompartmental knee arthroplasty. Their initial inclusion criteria include a diagnosis of unicompartmental gonarthrosis, age older than 60 years, low activity demand, weight less than 82 kg, minimal pain at rest, arc of motion more than 90 degrees, less than 5 degrees flexion contracture, and an angular deformity less than 15 degrees that is passively correctable to neutral. Initial contraindications to UKA were inflammatory arthritis, patient age younger than 60 years, high activity level, patellofemoral or pain in the contralateral compartment, and ACL-deficient knees.[3,13] However, recent studies have reported good or excellent results in patients who underwent UKA despite not falling within the traditional indications. A retrospective series of patients with UKA aged 60 years or younger (range, 35 to 60 years) demonstrated an excellent survivorship of 92% at 11 years.[15,16] Moreover, a series published by Tabor and associates[20] has demonstrated comparable survival and clinical outcomes of UKA in obese patients with a body mass index (BMI) more than 30 at up to 20 years compared with nonobese patients.

In general, there are reports of fixed-bearing UKA designs, such as the Miller-Galante (Zimmer, Warsaw, Ind) and Marmor UKAs (Smith & Nephew, Memphis, Tenn) reporting no higher failure rates in heavier patients.[19] Therefore, increased weight and activity are not considered an absolute contraindication of fixed- or mobile-bearing UKAs. Failures in these types of patients may in part also be attributed to certain implant designs and/or surgical technique.[1]

Preoperative weight-bearing anteroposterior (AP) standing, flexed posteroanterior (PA) or Rosenberg standing, and lateral standing radiographic views are necessary and helpful. A lateral standing x-ray is useful for identifying wear pattern and predicting whether the ACL is intact.[12] Preoperative films clearly demonstrate a more posterior wear pattern on the lateral standing x-ray, suggesting ACL insufficiency (Fig. 52-1). Preservation of the lateral tibiofemoral and patellofemoral compartment may provide further support for considering a combined UKA and ACL reconstruction. Obtaining a preoperative magnetic resonance imaging (MRI) scan may also be useful in identifying other unforeseen soft tissue abnormalities and evaluating the integrity of the articular surface and meniscus in the contralateral compartment.

UNICOMPARTMENTAL KNEE ARTHROPLASTY IN THE ANTERIOR CRUCIATE LIGAMENT–DEFICIENT KNEE

The debate continues as to whether a functional ACL is necessary for successful implantation of a unicompartmental knee arthroplasty. Most adult reconstruction surgeons agree that an intact and functional ACL is necessary to have a successful outcome with a UKA.[8] However, two large series with a minimum of a 9- to 10-year follow up demonstrated good to excellent results with UKA, even in ACL-deficient knees.[4,5] A 10-year follow up of 60 Marmor UKAs included 10 knees with ACL deficiency at the time of surgery, none of which required revision arthroplasty surgery; 7 of 10 were asymptomatic, 2 knees demonstrated mild instability, and 1 knee required a revision ACL reconstruction. It remains unclear whether these patients were young and active or older and less active. Cartier and coworkers[4] have suggested that these osteoarthritic ACL deficient knees were stable because there was no other soft tissue disruption and additional stability was provided by the formation of osteophytes. However, removal of these osteophytes during implantation of a UKA, especially meniscus-bearing designs, could accentuate instability and potentially lead to changes in wear pattern or even dislocation of the meniscal component. Hernigou and colleagues[10] have also demonstrated that the degree of posterior slope is associated with the outcome of a UKA. In their series, 81 of 99 knees had an intact ACL at the time of unconstrained UKA implantation. Of the 18

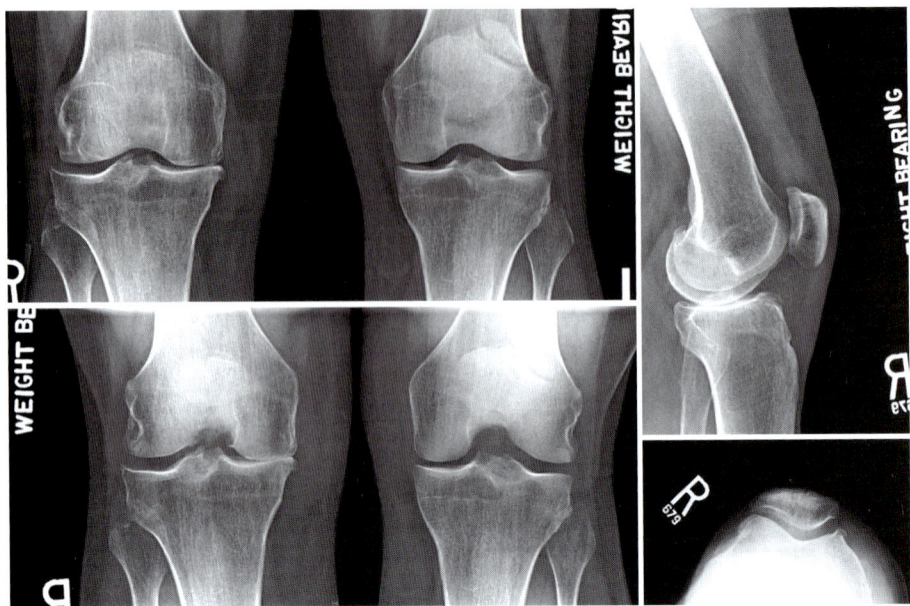

Figure 52-1. Preoperative standing AP, Rosenberg, lateral standing and skyline views demonstrate isolated medial TF osteoarthritis and a central to posterior wear pattern on the lateral standing view.

knees in which the ACL was absent at the time of implantation, 11 still had the implant in situ at a mean follow-up of 17 years. In these 11 knees, the posterior slope was less than 5 degrees. Of the 7 ACL-deficient knees that required revision, mean slope was greater than 8 degrees and anterior tibial translation was greater than 10 mm, as observed on a single-stance lateral radiograph. Previous studies have also demonstrated that every 10-degree increase in posterior tibial slope is associated with a 6-mm increase in anterior tibial translation in monopodal stance.[6]

Furthermore, increased anterior tibial translation ultimately leads to an increased sliding motion or tibiofemoral subluxation that may result in accelerated wear and failure of the polyethylene (PE) component or dislocation in mobile-bearing designs. Fixed-bearing designs may have an advantage over mobile-bearing designs by eliminating the possibility of a meniscus-bearing dislocation; however; at this time; no data exist to support this. Argenson and associates[2] used videofluoroscopy to evaluate the tibiofemoral contact areas in 20 subjects implanted with a UKA. Normal axial rotation was observed in 12 of 17 patients after medial UKA and 2 of 3 patients after lateral UKA. Abnormal axial rotation seen in the other subjects may have been caused by the inability of the ACL to pull the femur anteriorly in full extension. The authors suggested that the ACL plays a significant role in knee kinematics and may ultimately contribute to UKA longevity. Suggs and coworkers[18] have performed an in vitro robotic study to determine the role of the ACL in the anterior-posterior stability of the knee after UKA. After UKA, the knee exhibited tibial translation and forces in the ACL similar to those of the native knee. The ACL-deficient knee after UKA, however, demonstrated significantly greater anterior tibial translation than both the native knee and the knee after UKA with an intact ACL. Their data suggest that medial UKA does not alter the anterior stability in the knee with an intact ACL, but that a functional ACL is necessary to ensure normal mechanics after UKA.

AUTHOR'S PREFERRED TECHNIQUE

The procedure is performed under general or spinal anesthesia. The patient is placed in the supine position and the extremity is prepped and draped in a sterile fashion. A foot bump is positioned on the bed distally to allow for 90 degrees of constant knee flexion during various portions of the surgical procedure. A midline incision extending from the medial third of the patella to the medial aspect of the tibial tubercle is performed. Access to the knee joint is accomplished through a short medial parapatellar approach. The knee is inspected to verify the deficient ACL and the preservation of the lateral tibiofemoral and patellofemoral joint. The posterior wear pattern is confirmed. Using an extramedullary alignment guide, the tibia is resected and 3 to 4 mm are taken off the deepest tibial point. Using a 7- or 8-mm spacer block, the flexion gap is confirmed and attention drawn to the femur. The intramedullary canal is opened and great care is taken to place a fluted rod. The femoral sizer is placed on a spacer block or on the 3-mm metal shim for femoral condyle sizing. The posterior cutting block is placed to perform a posterior condylar cut. The distal femur is prepared using a 0 spigot. After balancing flexion and extension gaps, trial implants are placed and attention given to the ACL reconstruction.

A limited notchplasty may be performed if necessary. The deficient ACL is débrided. The knee is hyperflexed, and a guide pin is drilled into the center of the ACL tibial origin slightly more lateral than normal to avoid interference with the tibial base plate and overreamed with an appropriately sized acorn reamer. Soft tissue is stripped off the wall of the femoral tunnel. The femoral tunnel is drilled with an appropriate offset drill guide and reamer (Fig. 52-2). If a cortical button-type fixation device is used, the tunnel is overdrilled to the cortex with a 4.5-mm drill. A tibialis allograft is whipstitched on both ends. Using an EndoButton system (Smith & Nephew, Andover, Mass), the graft is pulled through the tibial tunnel into the femur. Toggling of the EndoButton is confirmed or alternative femoral fixation performed. After sufficient femoral fixation of the graft is achieved with the prosthetic trial components in place, the knee is taken through a range of motion to exclude notch impingement in full extension. Final gap balancing is performed and trial UKA components are removed to allow for pulse lavage of the joint surfaces. The tibia is cemented first, followed by the femoral component. After cement polymerization (Fig. 52-3), the final meniscus-bearing polyethylene component is inserted in flexion (Fig. 52-4). Attention is then given to tibial fixation of the ACL graft. After taking the graft through flexion and extension, the ACL graft is finally tensioned and fixed on the tibial side with an interference fit screw or alternative device (Fig. 52-5). Fixation may be augmented with the use of one or two staples. Again, the knee is taken through a range of motion to evaluate for notch impingement in full extension (Fig. 52-6). The stability of the graft is verified by performing a Lachman test. Wounds are closed in the usual fashion. Drains may be placed at the surgeon's discretion.

Postoperative radiography (Fig. 52-7) demonstrates correction of the varus deformity and satisfactory graft placement. The slope of the tibial component is decreased to reduce anteroposterior translation and strain on the ACL.

Postoperative rehabilitation is crucial to the success of this combined procedure. Most patients experience increased knee swelling. A 2-week period of partial weight bearing on crutches following surgery with unrestricted range of motion has been helpful and is our preferred protocol.

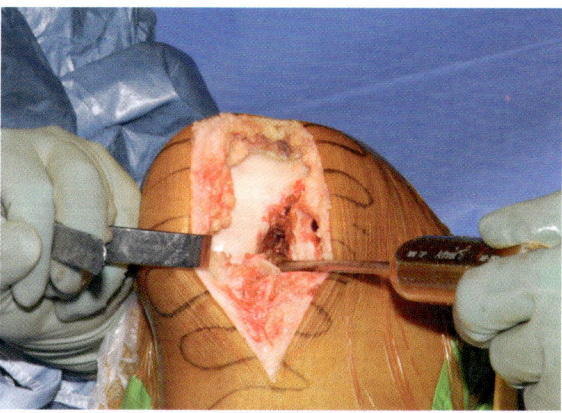

Figure 52-2. The approach for a UKA provides good visualization of the placement of the femoral tunnel using the offset drill guide.

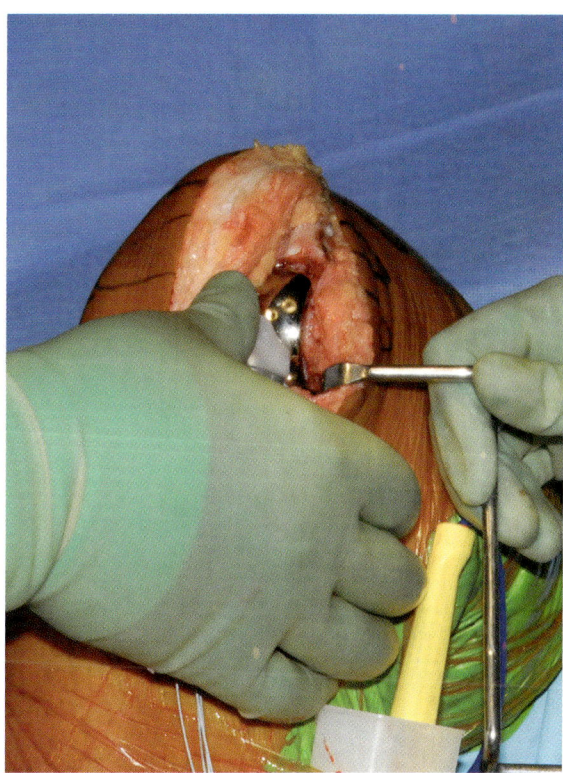

Figure 52-4. The meniscal bearing is inserted in flexion before the graft is secured on the tibial side.

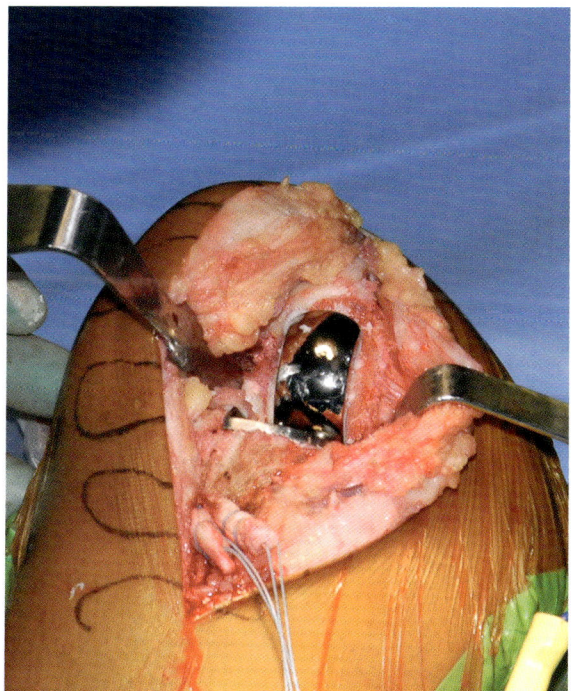

Figure 52-3. Cementation of tibial and femoral components.

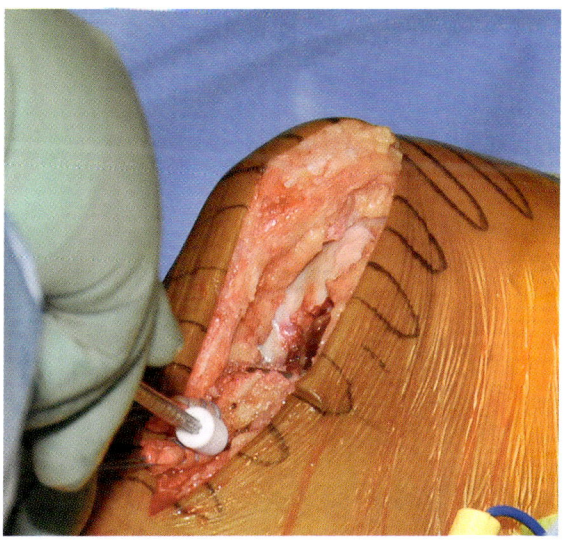

Figure 52-5. Tibial graft fixation.

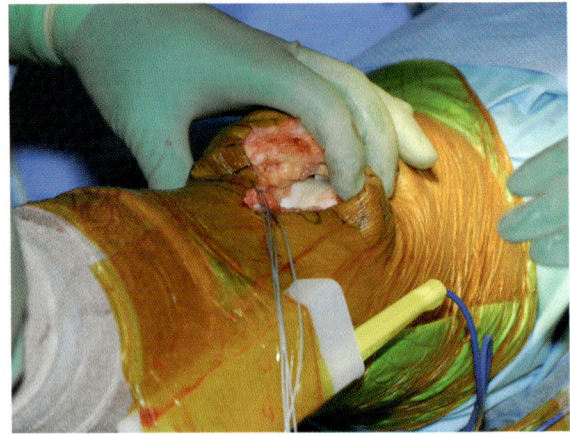

Figure 52-6. Notch impingement is excluded in extension.

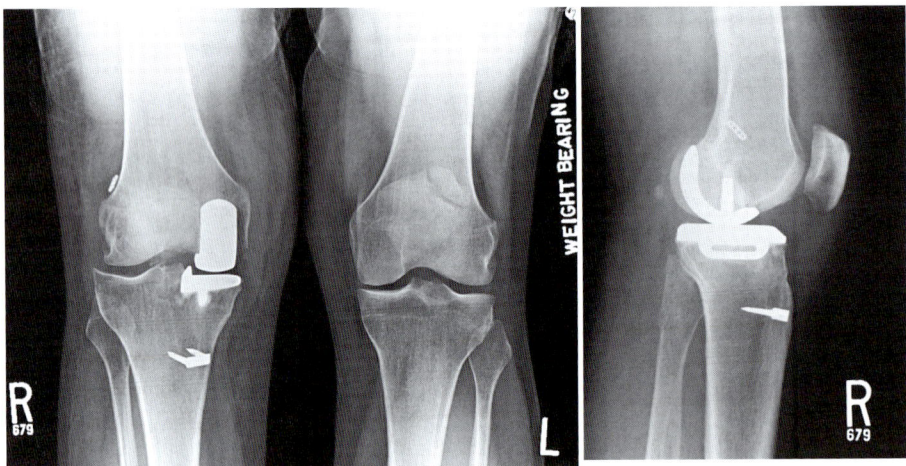

Figure 52-7. Postoperative AP standing and lateral x-rays.

Controversy and debate over performing unicompartmental knee arthroplasty in patients with anterior cruciate ligament insufficiency will continue. Establishing an algorithm to identify patients who are candidates for this type of combined procedure remains difficult.

Preoperative imaging studies or arthroscopy may be helpful in deciding whether an ACL reconstruction and concomitant UKA are indicated. Patients must be made aware of the controversy, concerns, and limited long-term data regarding this procedure. Therefore, the experienced knee surgeon must continue to individualize selection criteria to ensure the most successful outcome.

KEY REFERENCES

Cartier P, Sanouiller JL, Grelsamer RP: Unicompartmental knee arthroplasty surgery. 10-year minimum follow up period. J Arthroplasty 11:782–788, 1996.

Engh GA, Ammeen D: Is an intact anterior cruciate ligament needed in order to have a well-functioning unicondylar knee replacement? Clin Orthop Relat Res 428:170–173, 2004.

Hernigou P, Deschamps G: Posterior slope of the tibial implant and the outcome of unicompartmental knee arthroplasty. J Bone Joint Surg Am 86:506–511, 2004.

Kozinn SC, Scott R: Unicondylar knee arthroplasty. J Bone Joint Surg Am 71:145–150, 1989.

Pennington DW, Swienckowski JJ, Lutes WB, Drake GN: Unicompartmental knee arthroplasty in patients sixty years of age or younger. J Bone Joint Surg Am 85:1968–1973, 2003.

Price AJ, Dodd CA, Svard UG, Murray DW: Oxford medial unicompartmental knee arthroplasty in patients younger and older than 60 years of age. J Bone Joint Surg Br 87:1488–1492, 2005.

Suggs JF, Li G, Park SE, Steffensmeier S, et al: Function of the anterior cruciate ligament after unicompartmental knee arthroplasty. J Arthroplasty 19:224–229, 2004.

Swienckowski JJ, Pennington DW: Unicompartmental arthroplasty in patients sixty years of age or younger: surgical technique. J Bone Joint Surg Am 86(Suppl 1):131–142, 2004.

Full references for this chapter can be found on www.expertconsult.com.

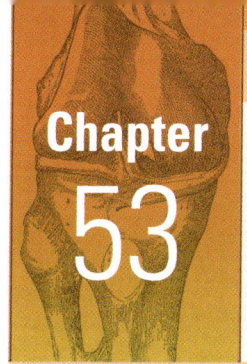

Chapter 53

Rehabilitation of the Surgically Reconstructed and Nonsurgically Treated Anterior Cruciate Ligament

Jonathan T. Finnoff and Diane L. Dahm

The anterior cruciate ligament (ACL) serves a number of roles within the knee. The ACL is the primary restraint to anterior tibial translation relative to the femur. It also assists in varus and valgus knee stability, provides proprioceptive feedback, guides the screw-home mechanism that occurs during knee extension, and prevents knee hyperextension.[43] Consequently, ACL injuries may result in significant functional deficits. Recurrent episodes of joint instability have been associated with meniscal injury and damage to the articular cartilage. Furthermore, ACL injuries, whether treated surgically or nonsurgically, predispose to the development of knee osteoarthritis.[24,26,78] Whether a patient chooses surgical or nonsurgical management, rehabilitation is an integral part of the treatment program. Rehabilitation techniques have evolved substantially over the past 25 years. The goals of nonoperative and postoperative ACL rehabilitation programs include return of neuromuscular control, strength, power, and functional symmetry.[77] This chapter will discuss current recommendations for nonoperative and postoperative rehabilitation of ACL injuries.

NONOPERATIVE REHABILITATION OF ANTERIOR CRUCIATE LIGAMENT INJURIES

Traditionally, nonoperative management of ACL injuries has been offered primarily to those participating in International Knee Documentation Committee (IKDC) level III or IV activities (Table 53-1).[62] A number of studies have reported poor outcomes and limited success in returning to IKDC level I and II sports with nonoperative treatment of ACL injuries.* Furthermore, other studies have demonstrated that the incidence of medial meniscal tears increases over time in ACL-deficient knees, which may predispose to early-onset knee osteoarthritis.† A study by Levy and Meier[66] found the incidence of meniscal tears in chronically ACL-deficient patients to be 40% at 1 year, 60% at 5 years, and 80% by 10 years postinjury. The ACL has been referred to as "the guardian of the meniscus."[87] Ultimately, the goal of treatment following ACL injury is to provide the patient with the best functional outcome and to minimize the risk of future injury and/or development of knee osteoarthritis.

For individuals with an isolated ACL injury who lead a sedentary lifestyle, do not experience instability during activities of daily living (ADLs), and have no concomitant injury requiring surgical intervention, nonoperative treatment is an appropriate option. However, in patients who participate in IKDC level I or II activities, correct identification of individuals who can dynamically stabilize their knee (copers) is

imperative to meet the goals of optimizing functional outcome and minimizing the risk of future knee injuries and knee osteoarthritis. There is evidence that individuals who meet specific post-ACL injury screening criteria and successfully complete a rehabilitation program involving perturbation training and a sport-specific functional progression can return to cutting, pivoting, and jumping types of sports 63% to 79% of the time without subsequent episodes of instability, injury, or reduced functional status.[27,35,56,57]

Dynamic knee stability can be defined as the ability to stabilize the knee during the rapidly changing loads created by activity.[57] Dynamic knee stability is dependent on neuromuscular control when static restraints (e.g., the ACL) are absent. Also affecting the ability to regain dynamic knee stability are the proprioceptive deficits that occur in the knee following an ACL injury.[6,7,10,112] Correction of proprioceptive deficits has become a focus of modern nonoperative and postoperative rehabilitation programs following ACL injury.[17,23,77] This is achieved through controlled stimulation of joint mechanoreceptors and muscle spindles using proprioceptive and balance exercises to increase the sensitivity of mechanoreceptors and muscle spindles and improve the readiness of muscles to respond to destabilizing forces.

There are a number of stabilization strategies used by those who sustain an ACL injury. Patients who tend to experience instability episodes and poor functional outcomes (noncopers) following ACL injury attempt to stabilize their knees through excessive cocontraction of thigh musculature, reduced knee flexion during the load acceptance phase of gait, and a greater posterior tibial displacement when compared with copers and uninjured controls.[18,19,94,95] By restricting knee flexion during load acceptance, noncopers maintain a relatively extended position of the knee, which may predispose to future subluxation episodes.[53] Noncopers also preferentially recruit their quadriceps during unilateral stance postural perturbations, which may further destabilize the ACL deficient knee.[26] Thus, noncopers stabilize the knee through abnormal muscular recruitment patterns and by limiting knee movement whereas copers attempt to normalize knee movement and recruitment patterns.

Based on the earlier work of Eastlack and colleagues,[27] Fitzgerald and associates[35] have developed a screening examination whereby potential copers and noncopers could be distinguished. This screening examination has been used successfully by other investigators.[57,58] According to these criteria, patients were not considered candidates for the screening examination and were referred to an orthopedic surgeon for ACL reconstruction surgery if they had any of the following: a fracture, reparable meniscal tear, multiligament knee injury, or full-thickness articular cartilage lesion. They also could not have experienced more than one instability episode since sustaining the ACL injury. Prior to the screening test, patients participated in a rehabilitation program to resolve their knee

---

*References 2, 3, 5, 29, 32, 47, 63, and 104.
†References 16, 20, 21, 32, 82, 110, and 120.

469

Table 53-1 International Knee Documentation Committee Activity Levels

Level	Sports Activity	Occupational Activity
I	Jumping, cutting, pivoting	Jumping, cutting, pivoting
II	Lateral movements, but less pivoting than level I sports	Heavy manual labor on uneven surfaces
III	Linear activities with no jumping or pivoting	Light manual work
IV	Sedentary activities	Activities of daily living

Adapted from Haggmark T, Eriksson E: Cylinder or mobile cast brace after knee ligament surgery: a clinical analysis and morphological and enzymatic study of changes in quadriceps muscle. Am J Sports Med 7:48–56, 1979.

effusion, restore full knee range of motion (ROM), strengthen their quadriceps muscle to 70% or more of the isometric strength of their contralateral extremity, and improve their weight-bearing status to the point at which they could hop on the injured leg without pain. Patients who did not meet these criteria after 1 month of rehabilitation were not considered candidates for the screening examination and were referred for ACL reconstruction surgery.

The screening examination included a timed 6-m single-leg hop test, global rating of knee function, and knee outcome survey–ADL rating. Potential copers were identified by hop test scores 80% or more of their contralateral limb, global rating of knee function of 60% or more, and a knee outcome survey–ADL score of 80% or more. Patients who met these criteria were enrolled in a physical therapy program that involved exercises for strength, endurance, agility, balance, and proprioception. A sport-specific functional progression was also included in the physical therapy program. Approximately two thirds of individuals identified as copers were able to return to IKDC level I or II sports without subsequent episodes of instability, injury, or reduced functional status after completing the physical therapy program.[27,35,56,57]

Using the screening test of Fitzgerald and coworkers,[35] Hurd and colleagues[56,57] were able to identify several additional characteristics that assist in differentiating ACL deficient copers from noncopers. A timed single-leg hop test demonstrating less than 10% difference between the injured and uninjured sides was the greatest predictor of a high level of self-assessed global function postinjury. In addition, noncopers were more likely to be female, to have sustained an ACL injury via a noncontact mechanism, and to have less quadriceps strength than copers. Furthermore, noncopers participated in fewer hours of IKDC level I or II sports preinjury.

For patients with isolated ACL injuries who have not experienced a postinjury subluxation episode and who only participate in IKDC level III or IV activities, we suggest a trial of nonoperative management. We recommend ACL reconstruction surgery for the following individuals: patients who participate in IKDC level I or II activities or who have experienced at least one postinjury subluxation episode, have sustained a multiligament knee injury, or have a concomitant repairable meniscal and/or significant chondral injury. If a patient who participates in IKDC level I or II activities sustains an isolated ACL injury and requests a trial of nonoperative treatment, we recommend performing the screening

Table 53-2 Nonoperative ACL Rehabilitation Summary

Examination Phase	Goals
Prescreening	Decrease pain and effusion. Reestablish ROM. Normalize gait pattern. Maintain cardiovascular fitness. Strengthen trunk, hip girdle, and thigh musculature.
Postscreening	Restore full dynamic stability. Prepare for return to sports.

examination outlined by Fitzgerald and associates.[35] If the patient does not pass the screening examination, we recommend ACL reconstructive surgery. If the screening examination is passed, the patient is enrolled in a nonoperative ACL injury rehabilitation program. The following is a description of this nonoperative ACL injury rehabilitation program (Table 53-2).

Prescreening Examination Rehabilitation Phase

The goals of the prescreening examination rehabilitation phase are to reduce the patient's pain and effusion, reestablish full knee ROM, normalize the gait pattern, maintain cardiovascular fitness, and strengthen the trunk, hip girdle, and thigh musculature. The patient is given crutches and instructed in progressive weight bearing as tolerated as pain, knee ROM, and ability to stabilize the knee dynamically improves. Crutches are discontinued when the patient is able to ambulate without a limp.

Pain can be reduced through local physical modalities such as cryotherapy and electrical stimulation and the judicious use of analgesic medications.[112] Resolution of any knee effusion facilitates knee ROM, improves the patient's ability to ambulate, and reduces reflex quadriceps inhibition.[25,60,107] Active contraction of the calf musculature with active ankle ROM exercises also facilitates edema reduction and may prevent complications of venous stasis. Knee ROM exercises include heel slides, active knee ROM, active assisted knee flexion with the arms or uninvolved leg, stationary bicycle–assisted knee flexion, towel stretches, overpressure knee extension with 2.5 to 10 pounds of weight, prone hangs, and passive knee extension while propping the heel up on a towel.

Isometric quadriceps-strengthening exercises can be initiated immediately following the injury and include quadriceps setting and straight leg raises. If the patient is unable to contract their quadriceps muscle actively either because of reflex inhibition from a large knee joint effusion or significant pain, high-intensity neuromuscular electrical stimulation can be applied to the quadriceps musculature to facilitate quadriceps contraction.[105] Closed kinetic chain (CKC) exercises can also be safely used during the prescreening phase of rehabilitation and will produce minimal anterior tibial displacement forces across the knee.[11,49,80,81,116] CKC exercises promote normal muscle activation patterns, enhance joint stability through muscular cocontraction, provide proprioceptive input through joint compressive forces and mechanoreceptor stimulation, mimic normal functional movements, and assist in strengthening the quadriceps muscles and ACL antagonist muscles (e.g., gastrocnemius and hamstrings).[42] Open kinetic chain (OKC) exercises for the quadriceps can also be used during the prescreening examination phase of rehabilitation, but should be limited to the ROM within 90 to 45 degrees of knee flexion because of the increased anterior displacement of the tibia at lower knee flexion angles.[12,76] OKC hamstring exercises can be performed through the entire knee ROM.

Proprioceptive exercises begin in this phase of rehabilitation. Early proprioceptive exercises can be accomplished with a combination of joint repositioning drills and with CKC exercises, such as weight shifts and joint repositioning exercises.[114] A compressive sleeve used for edema control may also improve knee proprioception and should be worn during rehabilitation exercises.[65] Minisquats can be progressed to be done on an unstable surface, such as a foam pad, based on the patient's functional improvements. Functional activities, such as three-way lunges, step-ups, and cone step-over drills can also be incorporated into the rehabilitation program. As the patient's ability to bear full weight and sense of knee stability improve, progression to single-leg balance exercises while standing on a stable surface can be attempted. Initially, single-leg balance exercises can be performed between parallel bars so that the subject can use the arms for support, if needed. Eventually, the patient can begin moving the non–stance leg in adduction-abduction and flexion-extension directions, and the upper extremities in flexion, extension, abduction, adduction, and diagonal patterns with or without weight, while maintaining knee stability.[112] The amount of extremity excursion, rate of movement, and amount of resistance can be manipulated to alter the level of challenge posed by the exercise. The patient can eventually progress to standing on an unstable surface such as a foam pad (Fig. 53-1).

To complete the screening examination, the patient will need to be able to perform various single-leg jump tasks. Therefore, this phase of rehabilitation should prepare the patient for single-leg jumping. Initially, jumping should be performed with two legs in a submaximal vertical direction and only involve a single jump. Correct landing mechanics should be emphasized, which include avoidance of excessive lower extremity coronal and transverse plane motions, good balance, and adequate ankle, knee, and hip flexion for shock absorption. When the patient displays good technique during a submaximal double-leg vertical jump, he or she can progress to a maximal double-leg vertical jump. Next, a single, forward, double-leg jump can be introduced, in which the patient lands softly, with proper technique, and holds the knee in a flexed position for 5 to 10 seconds after landing. This can progress to a double-leg triple jump. When forward jumping can be performed successfully, backward and side to side double-leg jumping can be introduced. Eventually, double-leg jumping while rotating clockwise or counterclockwise can be performed. Single-leg jumps should be introduced after the double-leg jump progression has been successfully completed, but the single-leg jumps should not progress beyond the forward direction until the screening examination has been completed.

Finally, during the prescreening examination rehabilitation phase, the patient should maintain cardiovascular fitness through low-impact aerobic conditioning, progressing from a stationary bike to an elliptical machine. Running should not occur during this phase. The patient should also incorporate trunk and hip girdle strengthening exercises. In particular, the hip extensors, external rotators, abductors, and flexors should be strengthened to provide concentric (hip extensors, external rotators, and abductors) and eccentric (hip flexors) control of femoral adduction and internal rotation motions, which have been implicated as potential contributing factors to ACL injuries.[52]

While participating in the rehabilitation program, the patient should be monitored for an escalation in pain, increased knee effusion, and/or sensation of knee instability during or following activity. If any of these signs and/or symptoms should occur, the patient should be instructed to rest, ice, compress, and elevate the lower extremity until they resolve, at which time the rehabilitation program should be reinstituted at a lower level and progressed more slowly. If the patient experiences a subluxation episode, she or he should be encouraged to discontinue the nonoperative rehabilitation program and meet with a surgeon for consideration of ACL reconstructive surgery.

Postscreening Examination Rehabilitation Phase

After the patient has passed the screening examination, he or she will enter the second phase of the rehabilitation program. The goal of the postscreening examination phase of the rehabilitation program is to restore full dynamic stability to the knee and prepare the patient to return to sports. The patient's primary sport should be identified, and the program tailored accordingly.

A key component to this phase of the patient's rehabilitation program is the addition of perturbation training. Perturbation training has been shown to improve the functional outcomes in ACL-deficient patients when compared with rehabilitation without perturbation training.[38] Perturbation training may be performed on a roller board and a tilt board (Fig. 53-2), and should occur two or three times/week. The

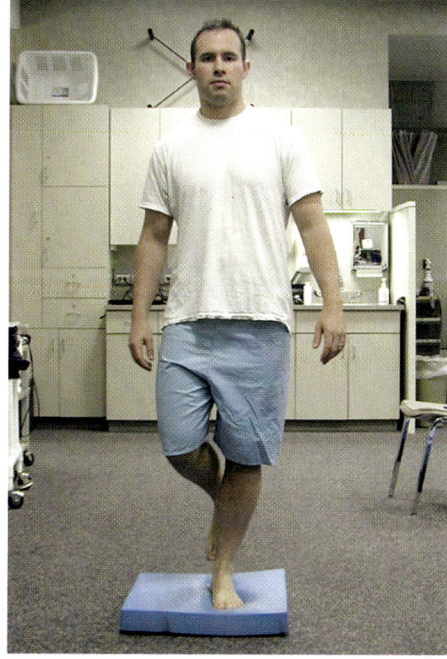

Figure 53-1. Single-leg balance exercises on a foam pad.

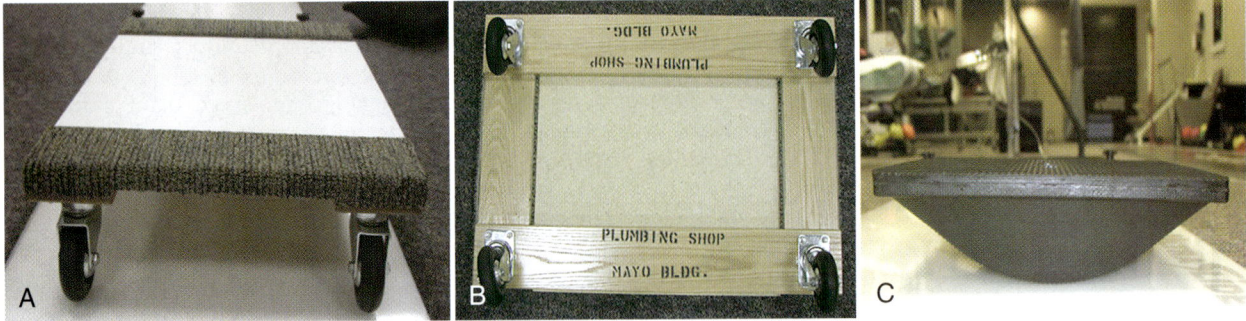

Figure 53-2. Top **(A)** and bottom **(B)** views of a roller board. The roller board casters rotate freely allowing multiple planes of movement during perturbation training. **C,** Side view of a tilt board.

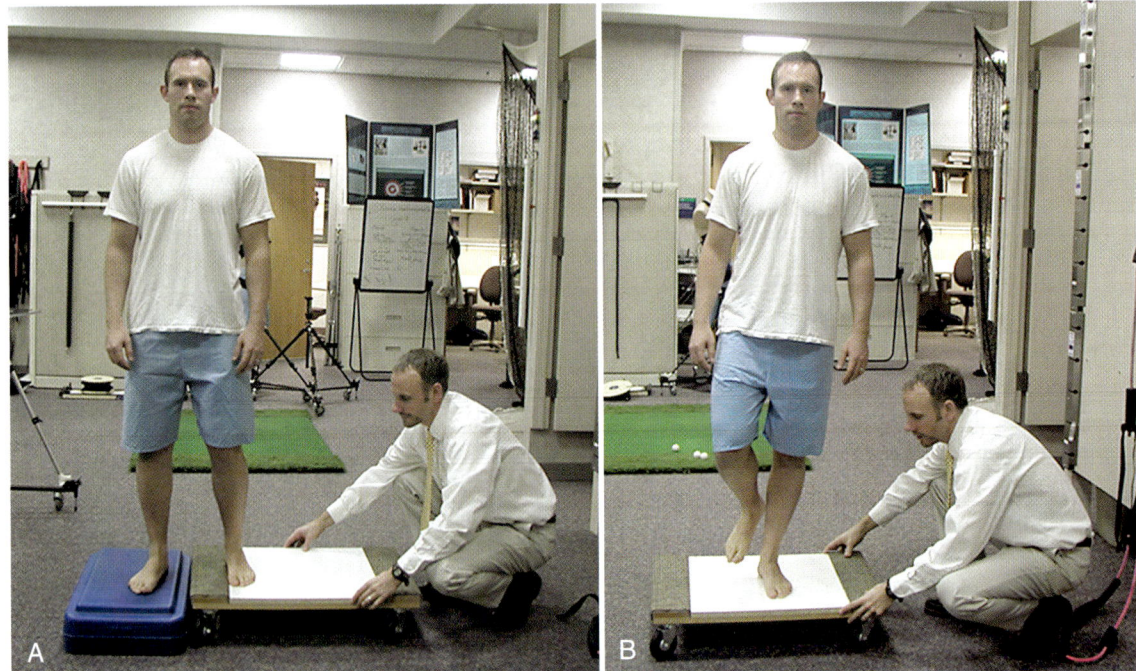

Figure 53-3. **A,** During the initial phase of perturbation training, the roller board is placed next to a stable platform so that the patient can place one foot on the roller board and the other foot on the stable platform while a perturbation force is applied to the roller board. A walker or parallel bars can be used initially for safety (not shown). **B,** Eventually, the patient is advanced to balancing on a single leg on the roller board while perturbation forces are applied to the roller board.

speed, direction, and amplitude of perturbations should be varied by the therapist and applied in a random order as the patient becomes more proficient with the exercises. When the patient is able to perform all perturbation exercises in a single-limb position on the tilt board and roller board, with minimal disturbance in balance, sport-specific and functional tasks should be added to the program with the goal of creating learned compensatory responses to sport-specific and functional activities (Figs. 53-3 and 53-4). By performing perturbation training during sport-specific and functional tasks, improved carryover to real life situations may occur, thereby minimizing the chance of a subluxation episode or recurrent knee injury.

The patient should continue strengthening exercises focusing on the quadriceps, hamstring, gastrocnemius-soleus complex, hip girdle, and trunk. The principles of progressive resistance exercises and periodization are applied during this phase of rehabilitation. A periodized resistance training program may be divided into three phases.[109]

The first phase is the hypertrophy and endurance phase, which involves low to moderate weight (50% to 75% of the patient's one repetition maximum) and moderate to high repetitions (10 to 20) and sets (three to six). The goals of the hypertrophy and endurance phase are to develop good technique during resistance exercises, increase lean body mass, and provide a base of strength in preparation for the later phases of resistance training.

During the second, or basic strength, phase of resistance training, muscle strength is increased by progressively increasing the intensity (weight = 80% to 90% of one repetition maximum) and decreasing the volume (three to five sets of four to eight repetitions). Emphasis should be placed on technique, slow movement, and strengthening the muscles required for the patient's particular sport.

The final resistance training phase, the strength and power phase, involves sport-specific exercises performed at or near competition pace, at a high intensity (85% to 95% of one repetition maximum) and low volume (three to five sets of

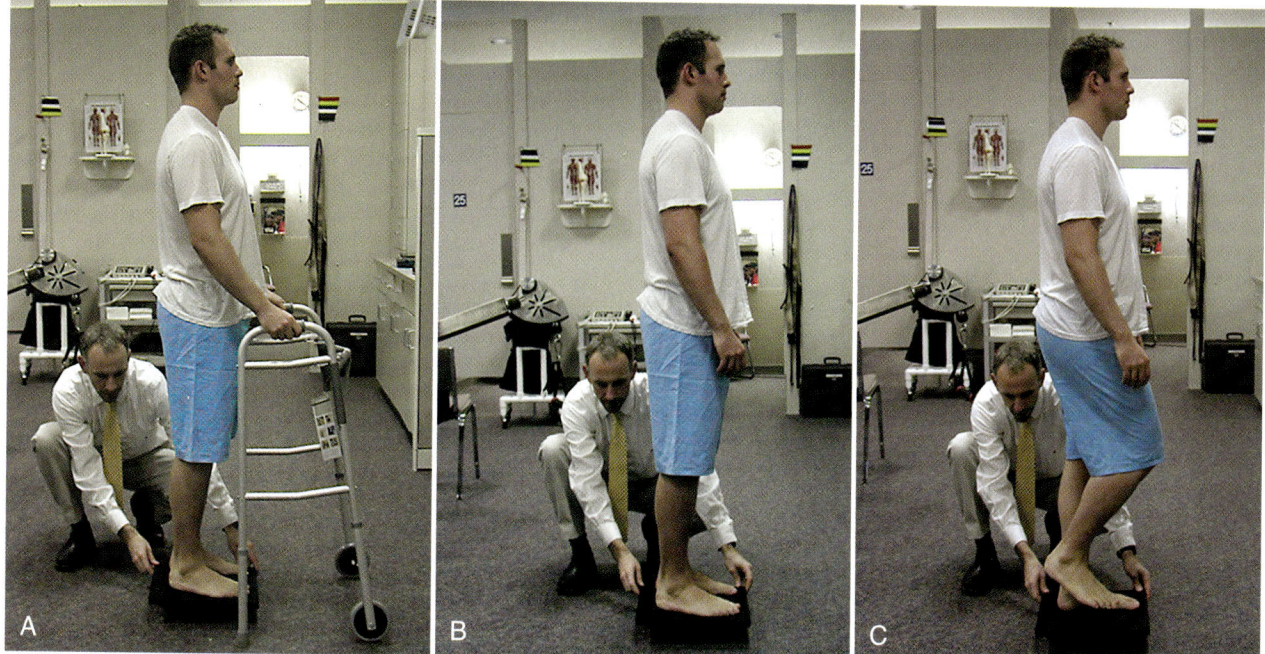

Figure 53-4. A, The patient begins perturbation training by standing with both feet on the tilt board while a perturbation force is applied to the tilt board. Parallel bars or a walker can be used initially for patient safety. The patient is progressed to double-leg perturbation exercises on the tilt board without parallel bars or a walker **(B)**, and finally to single-leg perturbation exercises on the tilt board **(C)**.

two to five repetitions). Throughout the periodized resistance training program, the patient's one repetition maximum for the primary exercises should be determined every 2 to 4 weeks and the amount of resistance applied during the exercises adjusted accordingly.

A combination of CKC and OKC exercises can be used during this phase, with an emphasis on functional movement patterns and strengthening muscles involved in the patient's primary sport. OKC quadriceps strengthening exercises should continue to be limited to knee flexion angles between 45 and to 90 degrees for the first 4 weeks after the injury to minimize anterior tibial displacement forces, but can be performed through the entire knee ROM after this time. Other strengthening exercises may include leg curls, squats, calf raises, three-way lunges, lunges with trunk rotation, front and lateral step-ups, front step-downs, four-way hip resistance exercises (hip adduction, abduction, extension, and flexion), and hip external rotation resistance exercises. Trunk stability exercises may include prone, supine, and side-lying stability ball bridges, bird dog exercises, stability ball straight and oblique crunches, and stability ball partial crunches with medicine ball trunk rotations. Single-leg and/or single-arm bridges can add difficulty to the trunk exercise. As the patient's program progresses, the exercises should become more sport-specific, not only strengthening the muscles that will be required for their sport, but also improving the neuromuscular movement patterns required for participation in their sport.

Plyometric training should begin in this phase of the rehabilitation program. The therapist should continually reinforce appropriate landing technique, which includes landing softly on the toes with the knees slightly flexed and absorbing the ground reaction forces associated with landing through

adequate hip, knee, and ankle flexion. Plyometric exercises should include double-leg and single-leg tasks.

If the patient participates in running sports, running should be introduced during this phase of the rehabilitation program. The running program should begin on a treadmill at a slow speed on a level surface. A running analysis should be performed to detect gross abnormalities in running gait, including asymmetries in stride length and stance time and lower extremity joint angles during the load acceptance phase of gait. After the patient's running gait has been normalized and no gross asymmetries are present, the speed and incline of the treadmill workouts can gradually be increased and the patient may transition to running off the treadmill, if desired. The patient should begin running on a level surface. Hills can be introduced when the patient can run 20 to 30 minutes on a level surface without experiencing symptoms. Finally, the patient can begin performing sprint drills. When the patient can successfully perform sprint drills, she or he can begin drills that involve deceleration and direction change. Finally, sport-specific drills should be incorporated into the patient's rehabilitation program in preparation of the return to sports. Sport-specific training should simulate the functional movement patterns of the patient's sport while incorporating peripheral afferent stimulation (e.g., proprioceptive challenges) to facilitate neuromuscular reeducation and train dynamic knee stability during functional sport-specific tasks. For sports that involve running, cutting, and jumping, such as football or soccer, sport-specific drills may include cone drills, side shuffling, carioca, sudden starts and stops, cutting drills, jumping drills, and ball handling drills. For skating sports, sport-specific drills may include sudden starts and stops, direction changes, figure-of-eights, and forward-backward skating.

After the athlete has successfully performed this rehabilitation program, he or she may return to unrestricted sports with the use of a functional derotational brace, as needed. If the patient has pain, recurrent effusions, or a sensation of knee instability despite completing the rehabilitation program or experiences a subluxation episode during the rehabilitation program, she or he is referred to a surgeon for consideration of ACL reconstructive surgery.

REHABILITATION AFTER ANTERIOR CRUCIATE LIGAMENT RECONSTRUCTIVE SURGERY

Surgical Considerations

Graft healing following ACL reconstruction is a complex biologic process influenced by a number of surgical and postoperative variables.[28] These include graft type, graft position, graft tensioning and fixation, and individual patient factors. In general, the graft healing process following ACL reconstruction occurs in several phases. An initial inflammatory response occurs almost immediately.[64] Graft revascularization occurs over the next several months and originates primarily from the infrapatellar fat pad, posterior synovial tissue, and endosteal vessels within the femoral and tibial tunnels.[4] Over the ensuing months to years, remodeling or ligamentization of the intra-articular portion of the graft occurs, which is characterized by cellular repopulation, collagen remodeling, and ligament maturation.[71]

In general, options for graft type in ACL reconstruction include bone-patellar tendon-bone (BPTB) autograft, quadruple hamstring autograft, quadriceps tendon bone autograft, BPTB allograft, Achilles tendon bone allograft, and tibialis anterior allograft. The rates and characteristics of the graft healing process among these grafts clearly differ, and the specifics of these differences are not well understood. Several animal models have shown slower bone tunnel incorporation with soft tissue autograft and allograft compared with BPTB autograft.[28,92] Although complete incorporation at the bone-tunnel interface has been shown to occur at 6 to 8 weeks with the use of patellar tendon autograft,[83] the incorporation of soft tissue graft has been shown to be considerably longer, at 12 weeks.[41,92] Although allograft tissue appears to heal in a similar manner to autograft tissue, this occurs at a much slower rate.[44] In addition, compared with autograft tissue, allografts lose more of their time zero strength during remodeling. ACL reconstruction with allograft tissue has not been definitively shown to be associated with a poorer prognosis.[52] Nonetheless, these differences should be taken into account when designing a rehabilitation program. Although a prospective randomized trial[14] has shown that an accelerated rehabilitation program produces no difference in knee laxity, functional performance, synovial fluid biomarkers, or articular cartilage metabolism in patients reconstructed with a BPTB autograft, insufficient evidence exists regarding the safety of an accelerated rehabilitation program for patients undergoing ACL reconstruction with allograft tissue.

Secure mechanical fixation is required in the early postoperative period. A number of different fixation devices are available and include metallic and bioabsorbable interference screws for femoral and tibial fixation, suspensory and transfixion devices for femoral fixation, and combinations of aperture and augmentation devices for tibial fixation. A large number of studies have examined differences in biomechanical properties between various fixation devices at time zero; however, few studies have explored differences in biologic incorporation of grafts relative to individual fixation methods.[28] Graft fixation is influenced by various physical properties, including graft material, bone density, fixation device, and fixation site.[46] Although most fixation techniques have been demonstrated to perform well in clinical studies, it is important that the surgeon be familiar with the biomechanical properties of the individual system being used because the rehabilitation program may need to be adjusted accordingly.

Anatomic tunnel placement has recently been emphasized to achieve physiologic graft loading, promote bone graft healing, and restore knee stability.[28] In particular, a more anatomic femoral graft placement has been shown to offer significant biomechanical advantages.[119] With respect to graft tension, both excessively low tension and excessively high tension have been postulated to reduce the biomechanical properties of the graft. Further study is required to determine the optimal tension that should be applied relative to each graft type and fixation method. Delayed graft healing and tunnel enlargement have been postulated to occur secondary to excessive graft tunnel motion.[54] Motion between the graft and bone tunnel has been correlated with the type of fixation used and the postoperative rehabilitation program. Although early knee ROM and weight bearing are considered to be beneficial, an early aggressive rehabilitation protocol may increase graft tunnel motion, thus affecting healing of the graft to bone. This phenomenon may be more likely to occur in the setting of nonanatomic femoral tunnel placement. Further study is required to determine the optimal load and optimal timing of the loads required for successful graft healing after ACL reconstruction.

Timing of Surgery and General Rehabilitation Considerations

Prior to undergoing surgery, the patient should demonstrate minimal knee effusion, and full symmetrical extension to minimize the postoperative complications of arthrofibrosis.[73,102] The patient is allowed sufficient time to cope with the injury psychologically and prepare for the surgery and postoperative rehabilitation process, which requires significant commitment from the patient to optimize surgical outcome. Postoperatively, it has been reported by Shelbourne and Klotz[103] that reestablishment of symmetrical knee ROM is a critical factor related to patient satisfaction. Thus, reestablishment of full symmetrical knee ROM should be a primary focus of the early postoperative rehabilitation program.

Cryotherapy

Several studies have demonstrated that cryotherapy reduces pain, edema, and inflammation in the postoperative setting.[95,109] In an experimental knee swelling model, cryotherapy was found to be effective in reducing arthrogenic muscle inhibition induced by swelling.[88] In a meta-analysis of cryotherapy following ACL reconstruction, it was found that cryotherapy has a statistically significant benefit in postoperative pain control.[86] The study concluded that because cryotherapy is fairly inexpensive, easy to use, has a high level of patient satisfaction, and is rarely associated with adverse events, its use is justified.

ROM and Weight Bearing

Immediate postoperative motion has been shown to reduce complications associated with joint immobilization, including detrimental effects to knee ligaments, cartilage, bone, and musculature.[13] Five prospective, randomized controlled trials have demonstrated the benefits of immediate versus delayed knee motion following ACL reconstructive surgery.[45,51,79,85,93] These studies have noted improved ACL graft healing and capsular mobility, as well as decreased postoperative pain, scar formation, and adverse articular cartilage changes.

There have been six prospective, randomized controlled trials investigating the use of continuous passive motion (CPM) machines post-ACL reconstructive surgery.* Four of the studies demonstrated no significant benefit when CPM was added to the postoperative rehabilitation regimen.[89,93] However, a study by Yates and colleagues[117] has reported decreased hemarthrosis, narcotic use, and swelling in patients who received CPM 16 hours/day for the first 3 postoperative days, followed by 6 hours/day for 11 days, when compared with patients who did not receive CPM. In addition, McCarthy and associates[69] have demonstrated decreased narcotic pain medication use in patients who received CPM for the first 3 postoperative days when compared with patients who did not receive CPM. Therefore, it appears that CPM may have a limited role in the early reduction of pain and edema following ACL reconstructive surgery.

There appears to be no benefit to delaying weight bearing post-ACL reconstructive surgery. In a randomized trial comparing immediate versus delayed weightbearing for 2 weeks, Tyler and coworkers[108] found a decreased incidence of anterior knee pain in the weight-bearing group. This was thought to be secondary to earlier recruitment of the vastus medialis obliquus in the weight-bearing group.

Bracing

The use of rehabilitation braces during the early postoperative phase of ACL reconstructive surgery appears to reduce effusion, wound drainage, prevalence of hemarthrosis, and pain but does not appear to affect the long-term clinical outcome.[13] Wright and Fetzer[114] have published a systematic review of 11 studies of postoperative rehabilitative bracing. None showed an increase in adverse effects when bracing was not used. Specifically, there was no evidence found for increased pain, decreased ROM, or increased knee laxity in the control groups that were not braced following surgery. Furthermore, functional derotational braces after ACL reconstructive surgery do not appear to affect long-term functional outcomes and should therefore be reserved for special circumstances.[70,91]

Electrical Stimulation

Several studies have demonstrated that the use of neuromuscular electrical stimulation of the quadriceps during volitional exercises results in more quadriceps strength and a better gait pattern when compared with volitional exercises alone.[105,106] Fitzgerald and associates[37] have evaluated neuromuscular

electrical stimulation in a prospective randomized study of 48 patients who underwent ACL reconstruction. The electrical stimulation group was found to demonstrate improved quadriceps strength at 12 weeks. ADL scores and the time to begin agility training were improved in the electrical stimulation group versus controls. Based on these studies, neuromuscular electrical stimulation appears to have a beneficial effect; however, for it to be successful, it must be applied in the early postoperative setting and at a high intensity. This requires that the treatment be administered by a physical therapist in a supervised setting. Insufficient data exist regarding the beneficial effect of home-based electrical stimulation units.[115]

Supervised versus Home-Based Rehabilitation

There have been several randomized controlled trials comparing the efficacy of predominantly home-based rehabilitation programs that require intermittent supervision by a physical therapist, with supervised clinic-based rehabilitation programs following ACL reconstructive surgery.[8,34,96] None of the studies demonstrated a higher level of subjective and/or objective outcome measures between the two rehabilitation conditions. These findings suggest that intermittent supervision by a physical therapist to monitor the patient's progress and direct the home-based rehabilitation program may be as effective as a supervised, clinic-based rehabilitation program, assuming that patient compliance and ability to follow the protocols is not a problem.

Proprioceptive Training

A number of studies have demonstrated proprioceptive deficits in knees following ACL injury, regardless of whether the injury was treated with or without surgery.[6,7,10,113] It has been suggested that exercises designed to stimulate joint mechanoreceptors and muscle spindles (e.g., proprioceptive and balance exercises) may increase their sensitivity, thereby improving the muscle's ability to stabilize the joint in response to destabilizing joint forces.[61] Thus, prospective, randomized controlled studies have been performed to evaluate the effectiveness of proprioceptive and balance exercises on post-ACL reconstructive surgery rehabilitation programs.* All the studies but one[22] demonstrated better subjective and/or objective outcome measures following post-ACL reconstructive surgery rehabilitation with proprioceptive and balance exercises rather than standard post-ACL reconstructive surgery rehabilitation without proprioceptive and balance exercises. Therefore, it appears that the addition of proprioceptive and balance exercises to post-ACL reconstructive surgery rehabilitation programs is warranted.

Closed Kinetic Chain versus Open Kinetic Chain Exercises

The addition of OKC exercises to a post-ACL reconstructive surgery rehabilitation program may provide additional quadriceps strength when compared with CKC exercises alone,[73] and does not appear to be detrimental as long as the OKC exercises are limited to 40 to 90 degrees of knee flexion.[15,55,75,76] For patients treated with a BPTB graft, it appears that OKC exercises between 0 and 40 degrees of knee flexion can be safely introduced 4 weeks postoperatively; however, the exact

---

*References 30, 68, 69, 89, 93, and 117.

*References 1, 9, 22, 67, 89, and 118.

timing of introducing these exercises when using other graft materials, such as the four-strand hamstring graft, has not been well defined.[115] Furthermore, it has been suggested that early use of OKC quadriceps exercises after hamstring ACL reconstruction may result in significantly increased anterior knee laxity in comparison with both late start and early and late start after BPTB ACL reconstruction.[50]

Accelerated Rehabilitation

Finally, there have been limited studies determining the optimal duration of the post-ACL reconstruction rehabilitation program. Shelbourne and associates[97-99] were some of the first researchers to report that early postoperative weight bearing and early return to sports was safe and effective. This form of rehabilitation has frequently been referred to as accelerated rehabilitation. Two prospective randomized, controlled trials have confirmed that accelerated rehabilitation protocols produce similar results in a shorter duration of time when compared with traditional (i.e., delayed) rehabilitation programs.[14,59] One study also suggested that 2.5 hours of rehabilitation performed three to five times/week produced better knee joint position sense, higher Lysholm scores, and returned people to work earlier than a rehabilitation program that involved 30 minutes of rehabilitation performed two to three times weekly.[38] Further research is required to determine the optimal duration and intensity required for an accelerated post-ACL reconstructive surgery rehabilitation program, particularly in the setting of hamstring and allograft reconstruction.[28,39] Based on the currently available research, and considering the goals of returning patients safely and expeditiously to their preinjury level of function, we propose the following postoperative rehabilitation program shown in Table 53-3.

Table 53-3 Postoperative Rehabilitation Summary

Week(s)	Goals
1	Pain control Decreased swelling and edema Improved quadriceps activation Achieving full passive knee extension
2-4	Maintaining full passive knee extension Improving knee flexion Reestablishing patellar mobility Resolving effusion Strengthening thigh and hip girdle and trunk musculature Improving aerobic fitness—nonimpact or low impact Improving joint proprioception
5-12	Maintaining full active and passive knee extension Achieving normal patellar mobility Reestablishing full knee flexion Advancing thigh, hip girdle, and trunk strengthening Introducing more advanced proprioceptive and functional exercises Improving aerobic fitness—low or medium impact
13-24	Reestablishing symmetric lower extremity strength Introducing plyometrics Progressing to higher impact aerobic conditioning as tolerated Enhancing proprioception and neuromuscular control Beginning a functional progression of sport-specific drills

Preoperative Rehabilitation

The rehabilitation program for patients who undergo ACL reconstructive surgery begins at the initial postinjury visit, prior to surgery. The indications for ACL reconstructive surgery, risks and benefits of the surgery, postoperative rehabilitation process, and expected return to sports date are discussed with the patient during the initial appointment with the physician. Following this, ideally the patient meets with a sports psychologist as well as a physical therapist. The sports psychologist suggests coping strategies, teaches the patient relaxation and pain management techniques that assist in the rehabilitation process, and discusses ways to enhance performance during rehabilitation and return to sports. The physical therapist instructs the patient on the appropriate use of crutches, which the patient uses until he or she can ambulate without a limp and has regained adequate dynamic stability of the knee. The patient is instructed on edema control measures, including compression, which is achieved through the use of a compressive sleeve, elevation, ankle pumps, and cryotherapy. Cryocompression devices are occasionally used to assist with resolution of the effusion. The patient is taught knee ROM exercises, including wall heel slides, heel props, and towel stretches. A stationary bicycle can be used to assist with the reestablishment of knee ROM. Strengthening exercises during the preoperative phase include quadriceps sets and straight-leg raises progressing to CKC exercises such as minisquats, lunges, and step-ups. OKC knee extension exercises can be performed within the knee flexion ranges of 45 and 90 degrees, whereas knee flexion exercises can be performed throughout the entire knee ROM. Neuromuscular electrical stimulation can be used to facilitate quadriceps contraction if the patient is unable to contract the quadriceps adequately volitionally. The patient should also perform trunk stability exercises (e.g., prone, side-lying, supine bridges) and hip girdle strengthening exercises (e.g., hip flexion, abduction, extension, adduction, external rotation against resistance). The patient should be educated about appropriate forms of low-impact aerobic conditioning exercises, such as a stationary bicycle, elliptical machine, or rowing machine, which can be performed to maintain cardiovascular fitness. The therapist also assists the patient in the reestablishment of a normal gait pattern.

Postoperative Rehabilitation

Week 1

During the first week, our emphasis is on pain control, decreasing swelling and edema, and improving quadriceps activation. Knee ROM exercises include heel slides, active knee ROM, active assisted knee flexion using the upper extremities or the uninvolved leg, stationary bicycle assisted knee flexion, towel stretches, sustained overpressure knee extension, prone hangs, and passive knee extension while propping the heel up on a towel. Full knee extension should be achieved within the first 2 to 5 postoperative days.

Cryotherapy is used regularly. A compressive wrap or sleeve is applied to the knee and the knee is elevated in full extension whenever the patient is not performing rehabilitation exercises. Cryocompression devices may be used to assist with effusion resolution. Active ankle ROM exercises help reduce postoperative edema and venostasis. The patient is provided with a knee-immobilizing brace, which is used only until the patient has regained the ability to activate the quadriceps to prevent risk of falls caused by quadriceps inhibition. This is typically done for up to 1 week following surgery as a safety precaution. A proper crutch gait is reviewed and the patient is allowed to bear weight as tolerated.

Strengthening exercises are begun immediately following the surgery. Early strengthening exercises should include multiangle isometric thigh-strengthening exercises (between 60 and 90 degrees of knee flexion), quadriceps sets with the knee in full extension, three-direction straight-leg raises (hip flexion, abduction, extension), weight shifts, and minisquats. Early quadriceps neuromuscular electrical stimulation is frequently used during volitional exercises to enhance quadriceps muscle recruitment and strengthening. Standing hamstring curls without resistance may begin within the first few days, but should be performed with the patient using parallel bars for stability.

In addition to strengthening exercises, the patient should also participate in proprioceptive training, trunk strengthening and stability exercises, and aerobic conditioning exercises. Early proprioceptive training can include knee repositioning exercises, weight shifts, and CKC exercises such as minisquats. Aerobic conditioning can be maintained initially by using an upper extremity ergometer. Early trunk stability exercises can include transversus abdominus muscle isometrics, straight and oblique abdominal crunches on a stable surface, and lightweight and low-speed medicine ball trunk rotations while sitting on a stable surface.

One potential complication following ACL reconstructive surgery is patellar hypomobility, which can lead to pain, decreased ROM, and inability to recruit the quadriceps muscle adequately.[112] Therefore, the patient should be instructed on the performance of medial-lateral and superior-inferior patellar mobilization exercises. If the patient's ACL was reconstructed using a BPTB autograft, particular attention should be paid to superior-inferior patellar mobilization exercises to prevent excessive infrapatellar scaring, often referred to as infrapatellar contracture syndrome.[84]

Weeks 2 to 4

By the beginning of the second postoperative week, the patient should have achieved full passive knee extension, at least 90 degrees of knee flexion, and satisfactory patellar mobility and quadriceps control, and any knee effusion should be almost resolved. The goals of this rehabilitation phase are to maintain full passive knee extension, improve knee flexion, reestablish normal patellar mobility, resolve the knee effusion, strengthen the thigh, hip girdle, and trunk musculature, and improve aerobic fitness and knee joint proprioception. The patient may discontinue crutches whenever he or she is able to ambulate comfortably without a limp (typically by postoperative days 10 to 14). Edema control measures, including cryotherapy, elevation, and compression, should continue until the knee effusion has fully resolved. The patient should continue to work on reestablishing full passive knee ROM during this rehabilitation phase, with the goal of achieving full knee flexion by postoperative week 4.

In addition to the strengthening exercises for the hip girdle and thigh musculature that were initiated in the first postoperative week, various exercises can be gradually incorporated into the strengthening program during this

rehabilitation phase. The patient may begin the following CKC exercises as tolerated: leg press, squats from 0 to 50 degrees of knee flexion, three-way lunges, front and lateral step-ups, and forward and lateral cone step-overs. OKC quadriceps strengthening exercises between 40 and 90 degrees of knee flexion can begin. Quadriceps contraction during CKC and OKC exercises can be facilitated with neuromuscular electrical stimulation. OKC hamstring curls with resistance may also be introduced during this phase of rehabilitation unless the patient's ACL was reconstructed with a hamstring graft, in which case hamstring resistance exercises are delayed until 6 weeks after ACL reconstructive surgery to avoid irritation of the graft harvest site.[112]

Early proprioceptive exercises should be emphasized during this rehabilitation phase. These should include the proprioceptive exercises performed during the first postoperative week (e.g., CKC strengthening exercises, weight shifts, joint repositioning exercises). The compressive sleeve used for edema control may also improve knee proprioception and should be worn during rehabilitation exercises.[65] Minisquats can be progressed to an unstable surface, such as a foam pad, based on the patient's functional improvements. When able, the patient should begin single-leg balance exercises on a stable surface between parallel bars so that she or he can use the arms for support, if needed. The proprioceptive challenge can be increased by moving the nonstance limbs while standing on one leg.[112] The amount of extremity excursion, rate of movement, and amount of weight can be manipulated to alter the level of challenge posed by the exercise. The patient can eventually be progressed to standing on an unstable surface, such as a foam pad (see Fig. 53-1).

As the patient's knee ROM improves, the aerobic conditioning program can switch from an upper extremity ergometer to a stationary bicycle, which has the advantage of promoting knee ROM and lower extremity strengthening while developing cardiovascular fitness. Furthermore, when the patient's incision site has completely healed, the patient can be allowed to begin aerobic conditioning in the pool with activities such as pool walking. Hip girdle strengthening exercises can be advanced to include standing four-way hip (abduction, adduction, extension, flexion) isotonic strengthening exercises performed on a stable surface. Trunk strengthening and stability exercises should be incorporated into the routine, including medicine ball trunk rotations performed at different speeds and at different trunk inclination angles while sitting on a stability ball. Double-leg prone, supine, and side bridges on a stable surface can be added during this phase of rehabilitation and progressed to single-leg bridges as tolerated. The patient can also begin straight and side abdominal crunches and back extension exercises while on a stable surface.

Weeks 5 to 12

By the beginning of postoperative week 5, the patient should have achieved almost full knee flexion and have minimal or no knee effusion. The patient's quadriceps strength should be at least 60% of the contralateral side if isometric and/or isotonic strength testing is performed at this time. The goals of this rehabilitation phase are to maintain full passive knee extension and normal patellar mobility, reestablish full knee flexion, continue to advance thigh, hip girdle, and trunk strengthening exercises, introduce more advanced proprioceptive and functional exercises, and improve aerobic fitness.

The patient should continue the knee flexion and extension ROM exercises and patellar mobility exercises described earlier. The patient's strengthening exercise program should continue using isometric and CKC and OKC isotonic exercises, but the principles of progressive resistance exercises and periodization, as described for the nonoperative ACL injury rehabilitation program, can now be emphasized. During this rehabilitation phase, the patient is in the hypertrophy-endurance phase of a periodized strength training program, which involves low to moderate weight and moderate to high repetitions and sets with an emphasis on developing good technique during resistance exercises, increasing lean body mass, and providing a base of strength in preparation for the later phases of resistance training. Isometric exercises can include multiangle quadriceps strengthening from 0 to 90 degrees of knee flexion. Isotonic exercises for the hip girdle and thigh can include four-way (abduction, adduction, flexion, extension) standing hip exercises, front and side step-ups, three-way lunges, squats, and hamstring curls. A functional CKC hip external rotator strengthening exercise involves step-ups while the therapist exerts a medially directed force on the patient's knee with resistance tubing (Fig. 53-5). For patients treated with a BPTB autograft, OKC knee extension exercises between 0 and 40 degrees of knee flexion are typically introduced at postoperative weeks 6 to 8; however, patients who have undergone ACL reconstruction using a hamstring graft or allograft typically do not perform OKC knee extension exercises in this range of knee flexion until approximately 12 weeks after hamstring graft ACL reconstructive surgery.[50]

Single-leg CKC and OKC exercises should be added to the patient's resistance training program during this rehabilitation phase to improve strength, balance, and coordination. When able, the patient should begin performing single-leg squats focusing on correct technique, including avoidance of contralateral hip drop (e.g., Trendelenburg), and adduction and internal rotation of the femur, which commonly presents as dynamic knee valgus or corkscrewing. As noted, this abnormal movement pattern may lead to traumatic and atraumatic knee injuries and should be corrected. Initially, single-leg squats can be performed to between 20 and 30 degrees of knee flexion. As the patient's ability to perform this exercise improves, the knee should be flexed to 60 degrees. Weight and speed can gradually be added to the single-leg squat exercises, as tolerated.

Proprioceptive training, which appears to be one of the keys to successful post-ACL reconstructive surgery rehabilitation, should continue to progress during this rehabilitation phase. In addition to the CKC exercises on stable surfaces (see earlier), these exercises can also be performed on unstable surfaces such as foam or air pads. Single-leg squatting exercises are also proprioceptively demanding and assist in reestablishing normal neuromuscular patterns required for a variety of activities. Additional proprioceptive exercises can include single-leg balance on an unstable surface, with or without extremity movements. The patient can be given a medicine ball or weights to hold and then perform functional movements while standing on one leg. A ball can also be thrown to the patient who is standing on one leg to increase the challenge and sport specificity of this proprioceptive exercise.

Finally, the patient should continue trunk strength and stability exercises and aerobic conditioning exercises. The patient should continue to use the exercises introduced in the previous rehabilitation phase with the addition of one- and two-legged prone, side-lying, and supine bridges on an

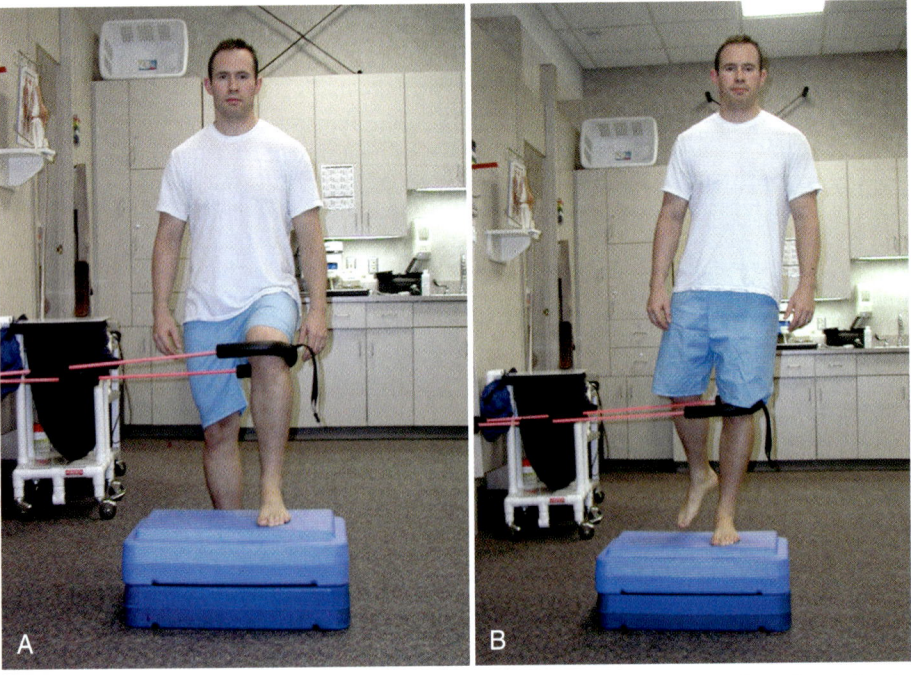

Figure 53-5. A, B, Patient performing a step-up exercise while a medially directed force is placed on the patient's left knee using resistance tubing.

unstable surface, forward and side crunches on an unstable surface, back extensions on an unstable surface, and four-way hip strengthening exercises while standing on an unstable surface. Aerobic conditioning may continue on the stationary bicycle, but the patient can progress to using an elliptical machine if she or he would like to return eventually to activities that involve running or a slide board to return to activities that involve skating. We do not typically encourage athletes to begin running or plyometric activities during this rehabilitation phase, regardless of the type of graft used to reconstruct the ACL.

Weeks 13 to 24

By postoperative week 12, the patient should have achieved full knee ROM, resolution of the knee effusion, and isokinetic and/or isometric strength quadriceps strength of at least 75% of the uninjured limb if strength testing is performed at this time. The goals of this phase of rehabilitation are to reestablish symmetric lower extremity strength, introduce plyometrics, enhance proprioception and neuromuscular control, and complete a functional progression of sport-specific drills prior to releasing the patient to sports.

All the previously described exercises should continue during this phase of rehabilitation, with the following additions. The patient should begin the second or basic strength phase of the periodized resistance training program, which increases the weight and decreases the volume of their resistance exercises. Proper technique, slow controlled movements, and strengthening of the muscles required for the patient's particular sport should be emphasized. Toward the end of this rehabilitation phase, the patient should transition into the strength and power phase of the periodized strength training program, which involves the performance of high-intensity, low-volume, sport-specific exercises at or near competition pace.

Perturbation training should be incorporated into the proprioceptive exercise regimen of this rehabilitation phase. It should follow the same roller board and tilt board progression as described for the nonoperative ACL injury postscreening examination rehabilitation program. After completing the standard perturbation training progression, sport-specific perturbation training exercises can be added; these may include swinging a bat, club, or stick, or catching a ball or hitting a puck while standing on a roller board or tilt board.

The patient should complete the plyometric double-leg jumping progression and progress to the single-leg jumping progression. After finishing the single-leg jumping progression, sport-specific plyometric drills should be incorporated into the patient's rehabilitation program such as catching a weighted or unweighted ball thrown by the physical therapist to the patient while performing a jumping drill or performing a continuous jumping drill that incorporates unforeseen direction and leg changes as directed by the physical therapist (e.g., double-leg straight, right single-leg forward, left single leg 180 degrees left rotation).

The patient should begin running or skating at the beginning of this rehabilitation phase, and may follow the same functional progression outlined in the nonoperative ACL injury postscreening rehabilitation program. Sport-specific agility drills, as described for the nonoperative ACL injury postscreening examination rehabilitation program,

should be introduced after having completed the running or skating functional progression. Particular attention should be paid to proper technique and neuromuscular control during deceleration, cutting, and jumping activities to prevent future knee injury.

Return to Sports Criteria

After successful completion of the rehabilitation program, the patient is prepared to begin reintegration into his or her respective sport. Objective tests include single-leg hop for distance, single-leg hop for height, single-leg triple hop for distance, single-leg triple cross-over hop for distance, 6-m single-leg hop test for speed, technique during single-leg squat to 60 degrees of knee flexion, double-leg jumping technique, and concentric quadriceps and hamstring isokinetic strength testing at 60 and 180 degrees/second. To be clear to resume practice activities and gradually return to unrestricted sports participation, the performance on the injured leg single-leg hop tests should be at least 90% of the uninjured leg. Also, the patient should exhibit satisfactory neuromuscular control and correct movement patterns during a single-leg squat to 60 degrees of knee flexion and double-leg jumping, and isokinetic strength should be at least 80% of the uninjured leg. Athletes who attain symmetry with respect to sports performance in both limbs prior to sports reintegration after ACL reconstruction may significantly reduce their potential for recurrent ACL injury.[77]

Rehabilitation Variations Based on Concomitant Procedures

ACL injuries frequently are associated with injuries to other ligaments, the menisci, or articular cartilage. Treatment of these injuries, whether surgical or nonsurgical, frequently leads to changes in the rehabilitation program. Common associated injuries and their effect on the rehabilitation process will be discussed in this section.

The incidence of medial collateral ligament (MCL) injuries associated with acute ACL injuries is approximately 13%.[112] If the MCL injury is treated nonoperatively, ACL reconstruction may be delayed to allow for MCL healing, reduction of the patient's effusion, and reestablishment of knee ROM.[100] If an MCL repair or reconstruction is also performed at the time of ACL reconstruction, a postoperative brace to prevent valgus stress is typically used for the first 6 weeks postoperatively. Patients with combined ACL and MCL injuries frequently have more pain, effusion, and difficulty achieving full passive knee ROM after ACL reconstructive surgery. Therefore, the physical therapist should pay close attention to effusion control and reestablishment of knee ROM, with an emphasis on achieving full passive knee extension.

Combined ACL–posterior cruciate ligament (PCL) injuries appear to have improved short- and long-term functional outcomes with ligament reconstructive surgery versus nonoperative treatment.[72] The primary differences between the standard post-ACL reconstruction rehabilitation program and the combined ACL-PCL reconstruction rehabilitation program are a slower progression in weight bearing, reestablishment of knee flexion, and introduction of strengthening exercises.[31,112] In general, these patients undergo protected weight bearing for a total of 6 weeks. A gradual progressive knee ROM program is emphasized, with early establishment of full knee extension and 90 degrees of flexion by the beginning of postoperative week 7. A PCL brace can be used during the first 8 to 12 postoperative weeks to reduce posterior tibial sagging. CKC exercises and bicycling can begin during postoperative weeks 8 to 12. Open kinetic chain quadriceps exercises performed in the 0 to 45 degree ROM can also begin during this period. Aerobic conditioning with low-impact activities such as walking and use of an elliptical trainer may begin at 3 to 4 months postoperatively. Light jogging may begin at 5 to 6 months postoperatively. Open kinetic chain resisted knee flexion should not occur until at least 6 months postoperatively. More aggressive agility drills should be delayed until 6 to 9 months postoperatively. Return to sports and heavy labor occurs thereafter once sufficient ROM, strength, and proprioceptive skills have returned.

Of all ACL injuries, 64% to 77% are accompanied by traumatic meniscal injuries.[111,112] If a partial meniscectomy is performed, the post-ACL reconstructive surgery rehabilitation program will remain essentially unchanged, although it may take longer to reintroduce running and jumping activities. However, if the meniscal injury is treated with surgical repair, the patient will use crutches with partial weight bearing to be performed with a brace locked in extension for the first 3 to 4 postoperative weeks. During this time, patients are allowed to perform non–weight-bearing ROM exercises as tolerated, with limits of flexion anywhere from 90 to 120 degrees, depending on the complexity of the repair. Rehabilitation then progresses similarly to that of the previously mentioned post-ACL reconstructive surgery rehabilitation program; however, the patient is instructed to avoid deep knee flexion with weight bearing for at least 4 to 6 postoperative months, again depending on the complexity of the repair.

If the patient requires surgical microfracture treatment of an articular cartilage lesion sustained at the time of the ACL injury, activities that increase articular cartilage shear stress need to be delayed.[112] Although passive ROM exercises should be encouraged because of the nutritional benefits of joint movement on articular cartilage, the postoperative weight-bearing progression should be postponed considerably. The actual postoperative weight-bearing status depends on the location of the chondral lesion within the knee.[40] Lesions of the patella and trochlea may bear weight as tolerated in a hinged brace with a 30-degree flexion stop; however, if the location of the chondral lesion is in the medial or lateral compartment, the patient is kept strictly touch weight bearing for 6 weeks. A continuous passive motion machine is used for 6 to 8 hours/day during the first 6 weeks postoperatively. After 6 weeks, the patient begins gradually progressive weight bearing with progression to full weight bearing by 12 weeks, or as tolerated. Return to sports that require cutting, pivoting, or jumping are restricted for 4 to 6 months postoperatively.

SUMMARY

An optimal rehabilitation program is essential for full functional return to sports and other activities for patients who have suffered an ACL tear, whether these patients have chosen operative or nonoperative management. It is essential that patients progress through the varying stages of the ACL rehabilitation protocol and that they are able to demonstrate adequate return of neuromuscular control, strength, power, lower extremity symmetry, and proficiency in their sport or activity prior to return. For the postoperative patient, it is critical that the surgeon have an understanding of the biomechanical and biologic properties of the specific ACL graft and fixation construct used and the potential implications for the rehabilitation process. Finally, various aspects of these protocols can be modified based on the individual patient's goals, resources, and response to treatment.

KEY REFERENCES

Beynnon B, Fleming BC, Johnson RJ, et al: Anterior cruciate ligament strain behavior during rehabilitation exercises in vivo. Am J Sports Med 23:24–34, 1995.

Chmielewski T, Hurd WJ, Rudolph KS, et al: Perturbation training improves knee kinematics and reduces muscle co-contraction after complete unilateral anterior cruciate ligament rupture. Phys Ther 85:740–754, 2005.

Church S, Keating JF: Reconstruction of the anterior cruciate ligament: timing of surgery and the incidence of meniscal tears and degenerative change. J Bone Joint Surg Br 87:1639–1642, 2005.

Cooper R, Taylor NF, Feller JA: A systematic review of the effect of proprioceptive and balance exercises on people with an injured or reconstructed anterior cruciate ligament. Res Sports Med 13:163–178, 2005.

Fitzgerald G, Axe MJ, Snyder-Mackler L: A decision-making scheme for returning patients to a high-level activity with nonoperative treatment after anterior cruciate ligament rupture. Knee Surg Sports Traumatol Arthrosc 8:76–82, 2000.

Gulotta LV, Rodeo SA: Biology of autograft and allograft healing in anterior cruciate ligament reconstruction. Clin Sports Med 26:509–524, 2007.

Hurd W, Axe MJ, Snyder-Mackler L: A 10-year prospective trial of a patient management algorithm and screening examination for highly active individuals with anterior cruciate ligament injury. Part 1, Outcomes. Am J Sports Med 36:40–47, 2008.

Hurd W, Axe MJ, Snyder-Mackler L: A 10-year prospective trial of a patient management algorithm and screening examination for highly active individuals with anterior cruciate ligament injury. Part 2, Determinants of dynamic knee stability. Am J Sports Med 36:48–56, 2008.

Morrissey M, Hudson ZL, Drechsler WI, et al: Effects of open versus closed kinetic chain training on knee laxity in the early period after anterior cruciate ligament reconstruction. Knee Surg Sports Traumatol Arthrosc 8:343–348, 2000.

Shelbourne K, Nitz P: Accelerated rehabilitation after ACL reconstruction. Am J Sports Med 18:292–299, 1990.

Shelton W, Barrett GR, Dukes A: Early season anterior cruciate ligament tears: a treatment dilemma. Am J Sports Med 25:656–658, 1997.

Wilk K, Reinold MM, Hooks TR: Recent advances in the rehabilitation of isolated and combined anterior cruciate ligament injuries. Orthop Clin North Am 34:107–137, 2003.

Wojtys E, Huston LJ: Neuromuscular performance in normal and anterior cruciate ligament–deficient lower extremities. Am J Sports Med 22:89–104, 1994.

Full references for this chapter can be found on www.expertconsult.com.

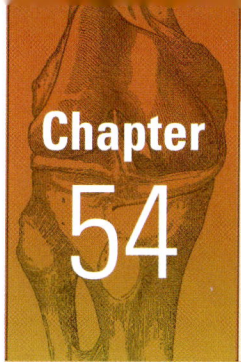

Chapter 54

Knee Bracing for Athletic Injuries

Geoffrey S. Van Thiel, Joseph Barker, and Bernard R. Bach, Jr.

Knee injuries represent the most common problem facing the sports medicine community. As sports participation continues to increase, so does the likelihood of sustaining a debilitating knee impairment. Thus, prevention, treatment, and rehabilitation of these injuries are important to both the athlete and the treating physician. Surgery is often a viable option; however, most of these injuries are treated conservatively with rest, therapy, and bracing.

The use of braces in sports medicine has long been surrounded by debate. Does the benefit of a brace justify the potential discomfort and cost? This question must be evaluated in the context of brace use and the desired purpose. Different braces serve different functions. The American Academy of Orthopaedic Surgeons (AAOS) has defined three categories of knee braces[24]:

1. Rehabilitative braces—postoperative braces designed to allow protected range of motion
2. Functional braces—provide stability to the unstable knee and improve function
3. Prophylactic braces—prevent injury to a normal knee

In addition to the three proposed categories, unloader and patellofemoral braces have become popular in contemporary orthopedics. Unloader (knee osteoarthritis) braces are designed to improve the function in patients with unicompartmental arthritis and supplement other conservative management. This chapter will evaluate the current literature available for braces in each of these categories and clarify their purpose, function, and usefulness.

REHABILITATIVE BRACES

Rehabilitative braces are designed to provide two functions, to protect a reconstructed/repaired ligament and allow early motion. However, the effectiveness of attaining and the clinical need for both of these purposes has been called into question by the contemporary literature. These braces can be off-the-shelf types with thigh and calf enclosures, hinges, hinge-brace arms, and straps that encircle the brace components (Fig. 54-1). The hinges can be unlocked to allow restricted range of motion and the braces are typically long to improve the lever arm and stability. Custom braces are available at an added cost. Rehabilitation braces are most prevalent in the context of anterior cruciate ligament (ACL) reconstruction and postoperative protocols.

Post–Anterior Cruciate Ligament Reconstruction Bracing

There are two main reasons to brace after ACL reconstruction—to protect the repair and avoid loss of extension. Various authors and surgeons have different opinions and protocols regarding bracing; some are based on experience and some based on the literature. This was clearly illustrated in a survey conducted by Marx and colleagues[45] of 397 AAOS members with regard to ACL surgery. When surgeons were asked whether they braced patients postoperatively for 6 weeks, 40% responded "no" and 60% "yes." Then, when asked if they recommended braces postoperatively for sports participation, 38% responded "no" and 62% "yes." Despite the disparity in clinical opinion, there have been many prospective randomized clinical trials that evaluated the effect of a postoperative rehabilitation brace and a multitude of systematic reviews (Table 54-1).

Harilainen and associates[28,29] completed a randomized controlled study with a braced and an unbraced group. The braced group used a rehabilitation brace for 12 weeks postoperatively with a gradual increase in weight bearing, whereas the unbraced group was allowed immediate range of motion with the use of crutches for 2 weeks. The 1-, 2- and 5-year follow-up examinations revealed no differences in Tegner activity level, Lysholm knee score, laxity, or isokinetic thigh muscle strength.

Brandsson and coworkers[12] also completed a prospective randomized clinical trial on the usefulness of postoperative rehabilitation braces in 50 patients. ACL reconstruction was completed with a bone-patellar tendon-bone (BPTB) autograft and patients were randomized to undergo rehabilitation for 3 weeks with or without a brace. Patients were followed for 2 years and, at the early follow-up visits rehabilitation with a brace resulted in fewer problems with swelling, a lower prevalence of hemarthrosis and wound drainage, and less pain throughout the early recovery period compared with rehabilitation without a brace. The 2-year follow-up revealed no differences between groups with regard to Tegner activity level, International Knee Documentation Committee (IKDC) rating, one-legged hop and isokinetic strength, or KT-1000 knee laxity.

Another randomized prospective clinical trial was completed by Moller and colleagues.[50] They randomized 62 patients to 6 weeks of rehabilitation with or without a brace followed by a specific program for up to 6 months. In the early follow-up period, the braced group had slightly higher Tegner scores. At the 2-year follow-up, there were no differences in Lysholm, visual analogue scale (VAS) scores, range of motion, isokinetic strength, or laxity. The authors concluded that a postoperative knee brace provides no additional benefit. Risberg and associates,[65] in a prospective randomized study, compared an unbraced population with a braced population that included the use of a postoperative rehabilitative knee brace for 2 weeks and then a functional brace for an additional 10 weeks. There were no differences between the groups except at the 3-month point. Despite greater thigh atrophy, the braced group showed an improved Cincinnati knee score. Otherwise, KT-1000 laxity, Cincinnati knee score, goniometry-measured range of motion testing, computed tomography (CT), thigh atrophy measurement, Cybex

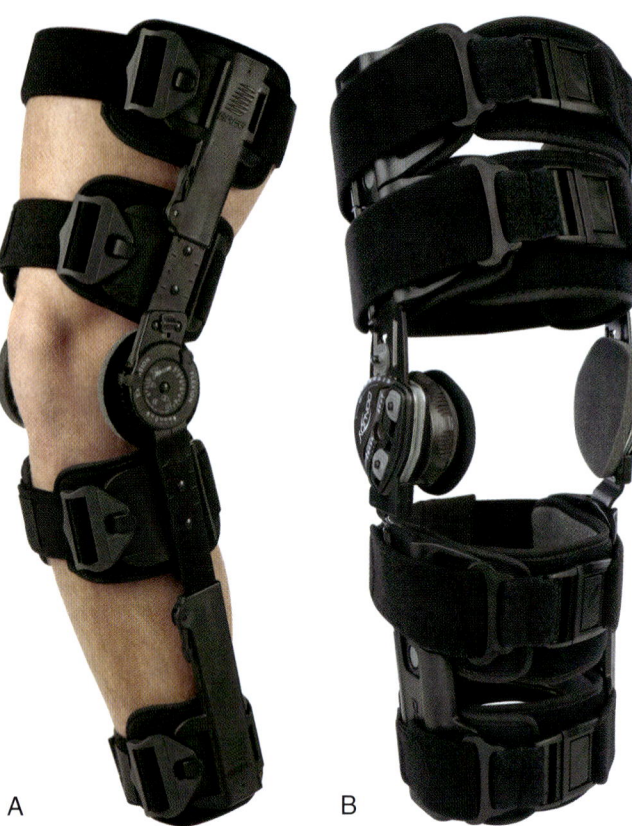
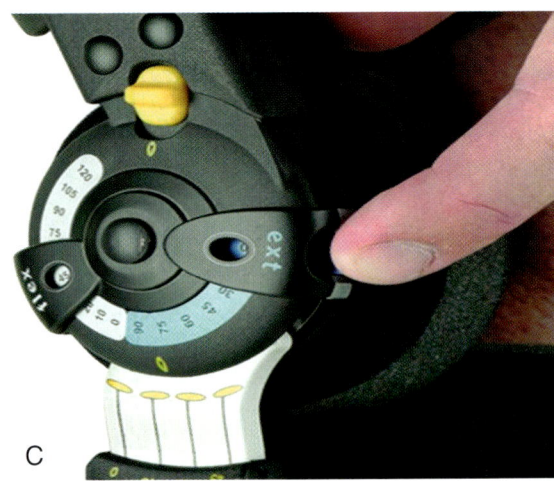

A   B

Figure 54-1. ACL rehabilitation braces. **A,** Breg T-Scope; postoperative ACL brace. **B,** Donjoy TROM adjuster; postoperative brace. **C,** Össur Innovator DLX; dial for the postoperative brace.

Table 54-1 Summary of Literature: Bracing After Anterior Cruciate Ligament Reconstruction

Study (Year)	Type	No. of Patients	Groups	Graft	Follow-Up	Results
Harilainen and Sandelin (2006)[28]	RCT	60	Brace, 12 wk No brace, crutches, 2 wk	BPTB	1, 2, 5 yr	No difference: Tegner, Lysholm scores; laxity, muscle strength
Brandsson et al (2001)[12]	RCT	50	Brace, 3 wk; no brace	BPTB	2 yr	Early: Brace had less swelling, drainage, pain 2 yr: No differences in Tegner, IKDC scores, strength, laxity
Moller et al (2201)[50]	RCT	62	Brace, 6 wk; no brace	BPTB	2 yr	No differences in Lysholm, VAS, range of motion, strength, laxity
Risberg et al (1999)[65]	RCT	60	Rehabilitation brace, 2 wk; functional brace,10 wk; no brace	Various	2 yr	No differences in laxity, range of motion, strength, functional tests, pain
McDevitt et al (2004)[46]	RCT	95	Functional brace, 1 yr; no brace	BPTB	2 yr	No differences in stability, functional testing, IKDC, Lysholm scores, range of motion, strength
Hiemstra et al (2009)[32]	RCT	88	Brace—knee immobilizer, 2 wk; no brace	Hamstring	2 wk	No differences in VAS scores, pain medication, range of motion
Melegati et al (2003)[47]	Clinical trial	36	Brace locked in extension, 1 wk; brace not locked in extension	BPTB	8 wk, 4 mo	Significant differences at 8 wk: Extension greater in extension lock group No differences in KT-1000
Mikkelsen et al (2003)[48]	RCT	44	Brace set at –5 degrees for 3 mo; brace set at 0 degree for 3 mo	BPTB	3 mo	Significant differences in 0-degree group; loss of full extension No differences in flexion, laxity, pain

RCT, Randomized controlled trial.

testing, functional knee tests, and VAS scores all were equal at 6 weeks, 3 and 6 months, and 1 and 2 years. It should also be noted that 24% of subjects in the brace group discontinued use prior to the 3-month time period.

A complete analysis of bracing after ACL reconstruction was done by McDevitt and coworkers.[46] The authors prospectively randomized 95 patients over three institutions to brace wear for 1 year post–ACL reconstruction or no brace. All patients had a BPTB autograft and were held in extension for 3 weeks postoperatively and then followed up at 2 years. No significant differences were found between the groups in knee stability, functional testing with the single-leg hop test, IKDC scores, Lysholm scores, knee range of motion, or isokinetic strength testing. Two braced subjects had reinjuries and three nonbraced subjects had reinjuries.

The referenced studies are, for the most part, high-quality prospective randomized clinical trials that showed no quantifiable long-term benefit to postoperative bracing following ACL reconstruction with regard to activity level, subjective outcome, or knee laxity. However, some surgeons believe that a brace in the immediate postoperative period can provide the patient additional comfort. Hiemstra and colleagues[32] looked at patients braced for the first 2 days, with a follow-up of 14 days. They found that bracing did not provide any additional pain relief in the acute period above and beyond that for nonimmobilized patients.

Bracing has also been proposed as a way to reduce any potential flexion contracture. Petsche and Hutchinson[56] have identified loss of knee extension as the biggest problem after ACL reconstruction. Potential causes include surgical technique, graft placement, and postoperative contracture. Melegati and coworkers[47] have evaluated the effect of bracing BPTB ACL reconstructions in extension for the first week. In this study, 36 subjects were allocated to an extension bracing group or a brace group with 0 to 90 degrees of motion for the first week. All patients were then allowed unrestricted motion after the first week. They found that at the 4- and 8-week postoperative points, there was a significant difference with regard to the two groups; the extension brace group had extension closer to that of the normal knee.

Mikkelsen and coworkers[48] have evaluated the concept that the 0-degree setting on a brace does not represent true anatomic 0 degree and that this discrepancy affects the postoperative knee extension in patients who have undergone ACL reconstruction. Five subjects were placed in postoperative dressings and extension braces. Radiographs were taken to determine alignment. With the brace set at 0 degree, no subject had an anatomically straight leg (mean, +2.8 degrees) when compared with the −5-degree (mean, −2.5 degrees) and −10-degree (mean, −4.1 degrees) settings. Then, in a prospective study of ACL-reconstructed knees, they compared the differences between a hyperextension brace (−5 degrees) and an extension brace (0 degree) postoperatively. No significant differences were found between the groups in terms of knee flexion, sagittal knee laxity, or postoperative pain. However, only 2 of 22 patients in the hyperextension brace group had an extension loss more than 2 degrees, whereas 12 of 22 in the extension brace group had a loss more than 2 degrees.

In summary, knee bracing in the postoperative period continues to be used by many practicing surgeons for a variety of reasons. However, the evidence that a brace confers additional stability, improves range of motion, protects the graft, reduces pain, or improves subjective outcomes is limited. Most prospective randomized clinical trials have shown no difference between braced and unbraced subjects at long-term follow-up. To the contrary, if the brace is used to maintain extension, there is a moderate amount of literature that supports bracing in the acute postoperative period to prevent flexion contractures.

PROPHYLACTIC KNEE BRACES

Many athletes at all levels of competition have experienced the agony and devastation of significant knee injuries. Thus, prevention and prophylactic knee bracing have received considerable attention over the last 50 years. This is perhaps most evident in football, in which there is a high percentage of knee injuries; 20% of professional football players never return from ACL reconstruction and those that do often do not reach their preinjury level of play.[15] Anderson and colleagues[4] were the first to report a prophylactic brace that was predominantly used to protect the MCL of professional football players; however, they also speculated that the brace provided increased anterior and posterior stability. They noted that there was no adverse impact on performance for the braced athlete. No controlled studies were completed at that time, yet bracing in professional and collegiate football experienced a rapid increase. In this section, we will review studies regarding the benefits and drawbacks of prophylactic bracing (Fig. 54-2; Table 54-2).

The reports by Anderson and associates[4] led to a significant increase in brace use and studies to evaluate their efficacy in the early and mid-1980s. These early studies failed to demonstrate an appreciable benefit to brace wear, and some documented increased injuries and performance impairments, In 1985, the American Academy of Orthopaedic Surgeons stated that "Efforts need to be made to eliminate the unsubstantiated claims of currently available prophylactic braces and to curtail the inevitable misuse, unnecessary costs, and medical legal problems."[24] The American Orthopaedic Society of Sports Medicine and the *Journal of Bone and Joint Surgery* took a similar position.[19] The American Academy of Pediatrics went a step further and recommended that prophylactic lateral knee bracing not be considered standard equipment for football players because of lack of efficacy and the potential for causing harm.[44]

There are two basic types of prophylactic knee braces designed to prevent or reduce the severity of knee injuries. One type includes lateral bars with a single axis, dual axis, or polycentric hinges. The second type uses a plastic shell that encircles the thigh and calf and has polycentric hinges. The effect on performance and degree of protection provided must be evaluated on an individual basis. There have been a few large studies regarding brace usefulness and functional effects (see later).

Advantages and Disadvantages

No Benefit to Prophylactic Bracing

Teitz and coworkers[79] used the members of Division I in the National Collegiate Athletic Association as its study population. They reviewed statistics from 71 colleges in 1984 and

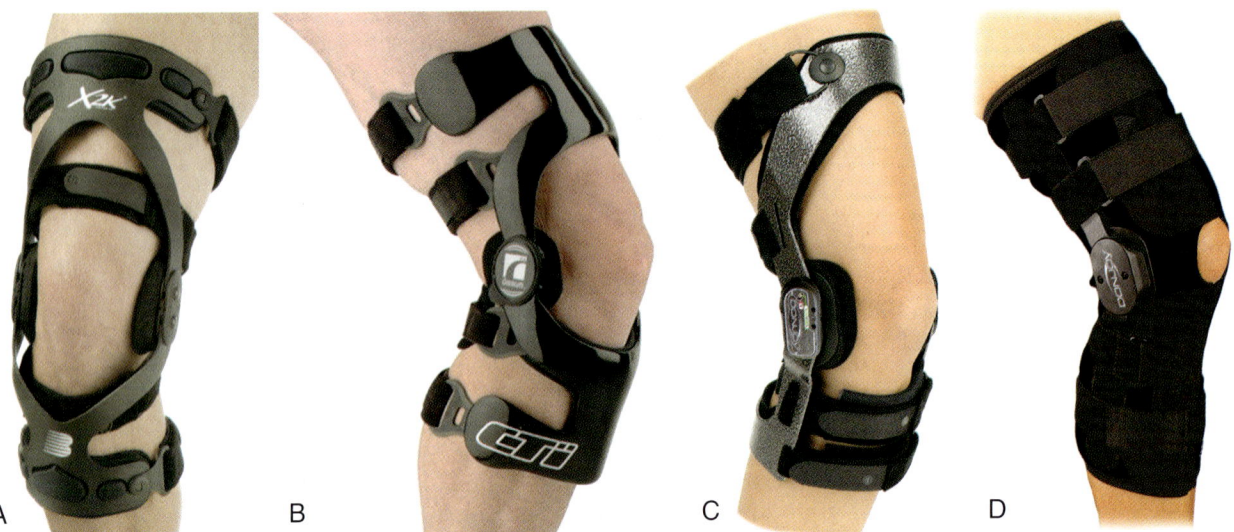

Figure 54-2. Prophylactic and functional knee braces. **A,** Breg X2K High Performance; indicated for ACL, PCL, MCL, and lateral collateral ligament (LCL) instabilities. **B,** Össur CTi Custom; custom-made brace; indicated for ACL, MCL, LCL, PCL, rotary, and combined instabilities. **C,** DonJoy AirArmor; moderate to severe ACL, PCL, MCL, and LCL instabilities. **D,** DonJoy Playmaker; neoprene with hinges, for mild to moderate ligament instabilities.

Table 54-2 Summary of Literature: Prophylactic Knee Braces

Study (Year)	Type	Subjects	Groups	Follow-Up	Results and Comments
Teitz et al (1987)[79]	Retro case	11,752 players	Brace; no brace	One season	Players who wore braces had higher injury rates and more meniscal injuries; no controls and four braces used; college football players
Hewson et al (1986)[31]	Case control	57,484 exposures	Anderson Knee Stabler; brace; no brace	8 yr	No differences in injury rates or severity of injury; college football players
Rovere et al (1987)[66]	Case control	742 player seasons	Anderson Knee Stabler; brace; no brace	One season	No differences in injury rate; cramping and financial expenditure larger in brace group; college football players
Grace et al (1988)[26]	Prospective clinical trial	580	Single-hinged brace (247); double-hinged brace (83); no brace (250)	2 yr	High school football players; significantly greater injury rate in single hinge; significantly greater foot and ankle injuries in brace group
Sitler et al (1990)[70]	RCT	1396 players	Double-hinged brace; biaxial brace; no brace	2 yr	Football—military cadets; shoe-, compliance-, and brace-controlled; significantly greater injury rate in unbraced group
Albright et al (1994)[2,3]	Prospective clinical trial	987	Brace; no brace		Analyzed injury patterns for college football MCL; trend toward decreased injury rates with brace wear, especially for linemen and linebackers

61 colleges in 1985; 6307 players in 1984 and 5445 players in 1985 were analyzed. The player's position, incidence of injury, type, mechanism, and severity of injury, playing surface, level of skill, and prior knee injury were considered contributing factors. The results showed that in 1984 and 1985, players who wore braces had a significantly higher injury rate than players who did not wear braces. Four different types of prophylactic knee braces were worn, and no attempt was made to differentiate between them with data analysis. The severity of injuries did not differ between the two groups. Player position, playing surface, mechanism of injury, or type of brace did not affect the rates of injury. Injuries were more common during contact and at every skill level in players who used braces. The incidence of ACL injury was similar in both groups, but braced players had more

meniscal injuries. The severity of injury was assessed by measuring playing time lost and the need for surgery. Surgical rates were similar for both groups. Although the average playing time lost was less for players who used braces, the increased incidence of injury produced an overall time lost that was greater in players using braces. They concluded that prophylactic bracing would not prevent injuries and might actually be harmful.

Hewson and colleagues[31] also completed a study of braced and unbraced football populations over an 8-year period (1977 to 1985). The nonbraced period was reviewed from 1977 to 1981. Following this, the Anderson Knee Stabler (Omni Life Science, Vista, Calif) was mandatory for all practices and games for players at greatest risk, including linemen, linebackers, and tight ends. In the mandatory brace group,

28,191 exposures occurred and, in the nonbraced group, 29,293 exposures. Information was analyzed by type of injury, severity of injury, player's position, days lost from practice or games, and rate of knee injury/season/100 players at risk. Results showed that the number of knee injuries was similar for the braced and nonbraced groups and the type and severity of injury were similar in all categories. Rovere and associates[66] also performed a 2-year study that included all players on the Wake Forest football team using the Anderson Knee Stabler prophylactically during practice and games. A 2-year nonbrace group control period was evaluated and compared with a subsequent braced group. The time and mechanism of injury, diagnosis, and treatment were noted. Brace use did not significantly alter the relative frequency of injuries by player or position, and it was noted that brace wearing was associated with cramping and added financial expenditures.

Grace and coworkers[26] evaluated 580 high school football players over a 2-year period; 250 nonbraced athletes were matched according to size, weight, and position with 247 athletes wearing single-hinged braces and 83 athletes wearing double-hinged braces. The athletes who wore the prophylactic single-hinged braces had a significantly higher knee injury rate ($P < .001$), and the athletes wearing double-hinged braces had a greater number of injuries (no statistical significance). Foot and ankle injuries occurred three times more frequently in the braced group ($P < 0.01$). Different playing surfaces were used, and no documentation of prophylactic ankle taping was noted. The study results not only questioned the efficacy of prophylactic knee braces, but also called attention to the potential adverse effects on adjacent joints.

Potential Benefit to Prophylactic Bracing

The previous studies suggested no benefit and potential detrimental effects to prophylactic bracing. However, there have also been well-designed studies that purported a benefit for specific football positions. Initially, Garrick and Requa[25] completed a review of available studies and noted two studies that suggested a benefit to bracing, those by Schriner[67] and Taft and Funderburk.[76] However, these studies were only presented at a conference and were never published. Furthermore, there were significant methodologic concerns with the study designs. Garrick and associates were unable to develop a conclusion with regard to brace use secondary to the lack of well-designed clinical trials.

Then, in 1990, Sitler and colleagues[70] reported the results of a prospective, well-controlled research study regarding the effectiveness of a single, upright biaxial brace in a 2-year study of 1396 U.S. Military Academy cadets playing intramural tackle football as their mandatory competitive sport. The military population afforded control of the athletic shoe, athlete exposure, brace assignment and compliance, playing surface, and knee injury history. The study was completed over 2 years and at the beginning of each year the subject was assigned to a braced or unbraced group. The brace selected was the DonJoy Protective Knee Guard (DonJoy Braces, Coconut Creek, Fla) a double-hinged, single, upright, off-the-shelf brace applied to the leg with a brace-constrained, no-slip strap and neoprene thigh and calf straps. Individuals with ACL deficiencies, reconstructions, or repairs were excluded from the study. Knee injuries were defined as those that were severe enough to cause a missed practice or game. Nonsurgical evaluation was confirmed by at least two of the three orthopedic surgeons, and the injury was classified accordingly. There were 71 injuries and the overall knee injury rate was 2.46/1000 athlete exposures. The unbraced group had a significantly higher rate of injury than the braced group (3.40/1000 versus 1.50/1000 athlete exposures, respectively). There was also a trend noted toward decreased severity of injury in the braced group. This was a well-designed study with significant control, and the authors concluded that in this study population there is a benefit to prophylactic brace use.

Another well-done study was completed by the Big Ten Sports Medicine Committee. They conducted a 3-year prospective, multi-institutional analysis of medial collateral ligament (MCL) sprains in college football players.[2,3] In their study, 987 previously uninjured participants were classified according to their frequency of wearing preventive knee braces. These subjects were then studied and the brace use patterns from 100 injuries were analyzed. The investigators evaluated the following factors:

- Patterns of MCL sprains that occurred in unbraced knees
- Daily brace wear records of the study group
- Importance of the relationship between unbraced knee injury patterns and brace wear tendencies in study group participants

Confirmation that a reportable MCL sprain had occurred was the combined responsibility of the team athletic trainer and the team physician; this was based on clinical determination and examination. The total number of injuries was recorded. With regard to brace use, 50.7% of the 55,722 knee exposures were with braces. The pattern of where, when, and how often an individual participant chose to wear braces most closely paralleled those of his peers playing the same position and their string. The line players tended to wear braces almost 75% of the time in both games and practices. The linebackers and tight ends wore braces 50% of the time in practices and 40% during games. Finally, players in the skill positions wore braces only 26% of the time in practices and 10% during games. The effectiveness of preventive braces was examined by comparing only those injury rates for players with and without braces who were in the same position groups playing during the same sessions. For players in practice, all position groups displayed lower injury rates with brace use. During games, the same trend held true for the linemen and linebacker–tight end group but not for the skill position players. Although none of these numbers were statistically significant, a consistent trend in favor of the braces did emerge. For those in the two position groups (linemen and linebackers–tight ends) who were at greatest risk of such injury, the injury rates were lower for those players wearing braces. The protective tendency of the braces to reduce risk of injury was greatest in the linebacker–tight end positions. However, this group did not wear braces as often as expected because they were allegedly torn between protecting their knees and keeping up with the speed of their competition.

Performance Impairments With Bracing

There does appear to be a potential role for prophylactic brace use in specific situations with specific athletes. However, this preventative benefit must be weighed against any potential performance impairments that the brace could cause.

These impairments may be a direct effect of increased intramuscular pressures, muscle performance, knee joint kinematics, and associated energy costs. The following studies must be reviewed in the context of the time during which they were conducted. Many braces now in use have improved on the initial concepts and shortcomings of the braces historically used and reported in the studies reviewed here.

Styf and associates[73] have studied the intramuscular pressures associated with functional braces. The intramuscular pressures of eight healthy athletes were recorded at rest and during and after exercise in the supine, sitting, and standing positions. There were three braces used in this study, a catheter was connected to an electromagnetic transducer, and intramuscular pressures were measured by an infusion technique. Pressures at rest increased significantly, in all positions, in braced study participants. Muscle relaxation pressure during exercise also increased significantly. Muscle relaxation pressures decreased to prebracing levels after removal of the brace or the distal straps. The results of this study suggested that external compression from a knee brace on leg muscles may induce premature muscle fatigue by reducing perfusion of the working muscle. More recently, Lundin and Styf[43] have demonstrated that there is a direct correlation between thigh and tibial strap tensions and intramuscular values. There is also an inverse relationship with local blood perfusion.

Houston and Goemans[35] evaluated the performance of braced and unbraced knees. Seven athletes with knee instability underwent four tests. Maximal torque output was measured during knee extension. Isometric torque was measured at a knee angle of 90 degrees at increasing velocities (30, 90, 180, and 300 degrees/second). Maximal unloaded angular velocity was measured during leg extension. Vertical velocity and power were determined using a short stair run. In addition, blood lactate concentration was measured 1 minute after a 15-minute ride on a bicycle ergometer. Maximal torque during isokinetic knee extension without braces was found to be significantly higher, and the differences between braced and unbraced study participants increased as velocity increased. Maximal unloaded knee extension velocity was 20% faster for unbraced individuals during the stair run. In addition to reporting impaired performance for braced study participants, an increased energy expenditure was observed; the blood lactate level increased 41% for braced participants.

This finding of ncreased energy expenditure was also supported by Zetterlund and associates[84] who showed increased energy cost during treadmill running at a slow rate in 10 players. They found that oxygen consumption and heart rate significantly increase for braced athletes. However, energy consumption is not the only adverse effect reported with bracing. In the context of proprioception, Osternig and Robertson[53] noted significant changes in joint position sense and electromyographic activity in six healthy volunteers when a brace was worn compared with when it was not worn.

Furthermore, Sforzo and colleagues[68] showed that wearing a dual-hinged brace did not affect the performance of 25 male football players but did inhibit 10 women's collegiate lacrosse team members. The testing protocol involved the use of a Cybex II lower extremity isokinetic dynamometer to measure peak quadriceps torque, rise time, and time to fatigue. A Monark cycle ergometer (HealthCare International, Langley,

Wash) fitted with a Lafayette impulse counter (Lafayette Instrument Company, Lafayette, Ind) was then used to perform a 30-second maximal effort Wingate test of anaerobic power. Serum lactate accumulation was determined as the difference between postexercise and resting lactate levels. Although the overall performance score was significantly different, the differences were not significant for any one of the parameters.

On the other hand, Veldhuizen and associates[81] did not support the theory that bracing weakens the knee. There was no significant difference between braced and unbraced healthy study participants performing testing for isokinetic muscle strength, a 60-m dash, a vertical jump height test, and treadmill running. Knutzen and coworkers[37-39] have studied the knee joint kinematics of six braced individuals who ran a 12- to 13-km/hour pace. Knee stability and function were studied during maximum knee flexion in the swing phase, maximum knee flexion during the support phase, maximum external tibial rotation, and maximum internal tibial rotation. It was concluded in this and other reports that rotation and abduction-adduction decrease for braced individuals but does not affect performance.[78]

Greene and colleagues[27] have demonstrated the effects of bracing on speed and agility, as well as the tendency of the brace to migrate, in 30 college football players. Players in full gear ran a 40-yard dash and performed a four-cone agility drill either wearing braces on both knees or wearing no brace, serving as matched controls. Brace migration and subjective measures were recorded after each trial. In the 40-yard dash, times did not significantly differ when using the AirArmor 1 (AirArmor Sports, Scottsdale, Ariz) and OMNI (OMNI Life Science, East Taunton, Mass) braces compared with nonbraced control times. Times with other braces were significantly slower, with the Breg (Breg, Vista, Calif) having the slowest time, followed by DonJoy, McDavid (McDavid USA, Woodridge, Ill) and AirArmor. The AirArmor 1 and McDavid braces showed significantly less superior-inferior migration in the 40-yard dash than the other braces. These findings indicate that specific braces have differential effects on the athlete and that fit is an important factor if migration is prevented.

In summary, prophylactic knee bracing remains controversial. These braces have not consistently been shown to prevent or reduce the severity of injuries to the ACL or menisci. Several studies have shown a trend toward a reduced incidence of serious MCL injuries, but other studies have shown no change in the incidence of these injuries. There is evidence suggesting that brace use for specific positions and athletes is beneficial (e.g., for football lineman). However, this recommendation must be weighed against the fact that other studies have shown decreased performance and increased muscle fatigue in braced subjects. Many of the studies reviewed used older braces that are no longer on the market, and the possibility that newer braces have improved on previous shortcomings is acknowledged. Further brace and sport-specific studies need to be completed before any definitive conclusions can be drawn.

FUNCTIONAL KNEE BRACES

Functional knee braces (see Fig. 54-2) have shown limited clinical usefulness in various studies, but many studies

Table 54-3 Summary of Clinical Studies: Functional Knee Bracing

Study (Year)	Type	Subjects	Groups	Follow-Up	Results/Information
McDevitt et al (2004)[46]	RCT	95	Functional brace, 1 yr; no brace	2 yr	No differences in stability, functional testing, IKDC, Lysholm score, range of motion, strength
Risberg et al (1999)[65]	RCT	60	Postoperative rehabilitation brace, 2 wk; functional brace, 10 wk; no brace	2 yr	No differences in laxity, range of motion, strength, functional tests, pain, patient satisfaction
Birmingham et al (2008)[10]	RCT	150	Brace at 6 wk postoperative ACL recon; neoprene sleeve at 6 wk postoperative	2 yr	No differences in questionnaire, KT-1000, Tegner score
Sterett et al (2006)[71]	Prospective clinical trial	820	Brace—Post– ACL reconstruction; no brace	One season	Skiers: Brace group significantly less knee injuries
Swirtun et al (2005)[75]	RCT	42	Brace for ACL deficiency; no brace	6 mo	Management of acute ACL tears; no differences in functional knee scores; significantly lower subjective instability in brace group

reported improved subjective knee stability with brace use (Table 54-3). Although the scientific evidence supporting the clinical efficacy of functional knee braces is limited, they continue to have widespread use. In 1995, a survey of practice patterns for functional bracing revealed that most sports medicine orthopedic surgeons surveyed prescribed braces for ACL-deficient and ACL-reconstructed patients.[20] Only 1% reported never bracing ACL-deficient patients and 7% reported never bracing ACL-reconstructed patients. In a follow-up study in 2003, 13% of physicians reported never bracing ACL-reconstructed patients, whereas only 3% never braced ACL-deficient patients. Half of the respondents reported bracing less frequently than 5 years ago.

The theory behind functional bracing is that normal gait patterns at a low cadence rate generally do not pose any difficulty to these patients, but instability and risk of further injury are possible if above-normal cadence or sudden deceleration movements are encountered. Instability is primarily caused by knee subluxation and tibial rotation during the terminal aspect of knee extension. The contributing factor for such instability seems to be the increased angular velocity of the knee during fast cadence rates when anatomic deficiencies allow increased impact energy at extension, resulting in anterior displacement and rotation of the tibia relative to the femur.[1] Functional braces attempt to control these abnormal moments.

McDevitt and associates[46] have completed a prospective randomized clinical trial comparing rehabilitation using functional bracing for 1 year with rehabilitation without bracing after ACL reconstruction in 100 patients. Both groups were treated for the first 3 weeks after surgery with a rehabilitation brace locked in extension. Then, in the functional brace group, the knee was mobilized gradually from 3 to 6 weeks, with the rehabilitation brace used intermittently. The patient was then fitted for a functional brace at 6 weeks and allowed full range of motion. The brace was worn full time for the following 6 months and thereafter during all rigorous activities until 1 year after surgery. In the nonbraced group, bracing was discontinued after 3 weeks. At the 2-year follow-up, there were no differences between the groups with regard to anterior-posterior knee laxity, one-legged hop distance, IKDC

and Lysholm scores, range of motion, and isokinetic strength. Two braced subjects and three nonbraced subjects sustained reinjuries to their ACL graft. It was concluded that there are no significant differences between braced and nonbraced treatment groups.

In a second prospective randomized clinical trial, Risberg and coworkers[65] compared rehabilitation with functional bracing to rehabilitation without bracing after ACL reconstruction in 60 patients. The braced group was protected by a rehabilitation brace for 2 weeks, and a functional brace was used almost full time for the following 10 weeks. Thereafter, the functional brace was used as needed for sports. The nonbraced group had no brace at any time postoperatively. The authors found no evidence that bracing has an effect on knee joint laxity, range of motion, strength, functional knee tests, patient satisfaction, or pain at the final 2-year follow-up. Birmingham and colleagues[10] have also completed a randomized prospective study of bracing versus a neoprene sleeve for functional use post-ACL reconstruction. In this study, 150 patients were given a brace or neoprene sleeve at the 6-week postoperative follow-up and then followed for 2 years. There were no significant differences in any objective score or adverse events.

However, Sterett and associates[71] prospectively evaluated skiers who had an ACL reconstruction and used or did not use functional bracing; 257 subjects used functional knee bracing and 563 did not. Despite the fact that the braced skiers had a significantly higher percentage of grade II Lachman tests, there was a significantly decreased rate of subsequent knee injuries; 8.9 injuries/100 knees/ski season in the nonbraced group and 4.0 injuries/100 knees/ski season in the braced subset.

Swirtun and coworkers[75] have prospectively evaluated functional knee braces in the nonoperative management of acute (<5 weeks) ACL tears. In this study, 95 patients were randomized to a brace group for 12 weeks or to a no-brace group, with 42 patients completing the study. There were no differences in functional knee scores at the 6-month follow-up; however, the brace group had significantly lower subjective instability ratings.

Studies of the Lenox Hill brace (Lenox Hill Brace Shop, New York, NY) by Colville and colleagues[17] have shown that the absolute laxity of the deficient knee is unchanged by the brace, but that the relative resistance to displacement is increased. Branch and associates[11] have evaluated the contribution of functional bracing to muscle-firing amplitude, duration, and timing, which may result in improved dynamic stability. Ten ACL-deficient subjects and five normal controls were evaluated using foot switches and dynamic electromyography. Bracing did not alter the relative electromyography activity and did not change firing patterns compared with the unbraced situation. All muscles showed a similar reduction in activity, suggesting that functional braces do not have a proprioceptive influence.

Cook and coworkers[18] performed a dynamic analysis of functional knee braces for ACL-deficient athletes. Foot switch, high-speed photography, and force plate data were recorded with and without the custom-fitted CTi braces (Össur, Foothill Ranch, Calif). Cutting angle, approach time to cut, and time on the force plate showed no significant differences during brace wear. Athletes who did not achieve 80% of the isokinetic quadriceps torque of the normal limb generated significantly more forces during cutting maneuvers while wearing their braces. Athletes also reported better subjective results while snow skiing and waterskiing compared with playing basketball and racket sports. They noted subjectively fewer subluxation episodes and better performance with the brace. Improvements were even more significant in the quadriceps-deficient patients, suggesting that athletes who rehabilitate incompletely may obtain increased benefit from functional knee bracing.

Rink and colleagues[64] compared the CTi, OTI (DJ Orthopedics, Vista, Calif), and TS7 (Omni Scientific, Springfield, Utah) knee braces in 14 patients with arthroscopically shown ACL-deficient knees. The subjects evaluated the braces and underwent testing with physical examination, KT-1000 arthrometry, and timed running events. All braces reduced subjective symptoms of knee instability, and a reduction in anterior tibial displacement was seen with all braces at low loads. This reduction decreased, however, as forces increased. A timed figure-eight running event did not show any functional advantage, and five subluxation events occurred in four subjects while braced.

Mishra and associates[45] have evaluated four functional knee braces and their effect on anterior knee laxity. All braces reduced giving-way episodes and the grade of pivot shift testing. Brace use decreased anterior displacement on KT-1000 measurements at 89-N, high-load passive anterior displacement and with quadriceps contraction active displacement. There was no significant effect on functional test results. Patients with the most functional limitations improved the most, whereas patients minimally affected had diminished performance.

Several studies have evaluated metabolic costs of knee brace wear. Highgenboten and coworkers[33] have studied four braces in 14 normal subjects undergoing horizontal treadmill running. The braces caused increases in oxygen consumption, heart rate, and ventilation of 3% to 8% compared with running without the brace. Subjective exertion also was increased 9% to 13%. They concluded that these braces cause a consistent increase in metabolic cost, which was related to their weight. These results are consistent with past research on prophylactic braces showing increased energy costs and intramuscular pressures.[35,72,73,84]

In summary, definitive studies supporting or refuting functional brace use have not been done. Thus, the treating physician must make an educated, patient-specific decision with regard to recommendations. In the post–ACL reconstruction patient, there does not appear to be a clear benefit (objective or subjective) to brace use. However, in the setting of ACL deficiency or instability, there is a subjective and biomechanical advantage to brace use. Although this benefit has not translated into a significant functional improvement, brace use should still be considered in this patient subset. Further studies are needed to clarify the usefulness and benefit of functional knee bracing.

BIOMECHANICAL FINDINGS

Clinical studies may provide the highest usefulness and practice application; however, it is notoriously difficult to control all extraneous variables. Thus, biomechanical corollaries provide important information and can direct good clinical research and decision making. The studies reviewed here provide a solid foundation for future clinical research.

Beynnon and colleagues[8] have critically evaluated nine ACL-deficient subjects to determine the effect of functional ACL bracing on chronic ACL-deficient knees in non–weight bearing and weight bearing, and the transition between the two states. They used the Vermont Knee Laxity Device (DJ Orthopedics) and recorded tibial translation relative to the femur in simulated conditions. Bracing resulted in a significant reduction of anterior translation values, to a level within normal limits in the non–weight-bearing and weight-bearing states. However, as the knees transitioned from non–weight bearing to weight bearing, the brace group had translation 3.5 times greater than the normal knees. They concluded that this is why patients gain partial control of their pathologic laxity, but may continue to experience subluxation episodes during activity. Hinterwimmer and associates[34] also have shown a decrease in tension in the collateral ligaments in an ACL-deficient cadaver model with brace use.

Furthermore, Theoret and Lamontagne[80] used electromyographic and three-dimensional kinematic data to evaluate functional bracing in ACL-deficient knees during running, with 11 patients participating in the study. Few differences were found in the kinematic analysis and no significant differences were reported in the electromyographic findings; however, based on the data, it was concluded that bracing the ACL-deficient knee during running has the effect of placing the injured limb in a safer kinematic position, particularly in preparation for and during weight bearing. Bracing also has the effect of increasing the efficiency of the stride by increasing stride length.

Beck and colleagues[7] tested seven functional knee braces on three ACL-deficient knees with KT-1000 and Stryker knee laxity testers. They found that the hinge, post, and shell types of braces performed consistently better in controlling anterior tibial displacement at low loads. The effectiveness of the functional knee braces in controlling anterior tibial displacement decreased as forces increased. Liu and associates[41] evaluated 10 functional knee braces on a knee model and found the bilateral hinge–shell models provide the greatest resistance to anterior displacement, whereas the unilateral hinge–shell models provided the least resistance. None of these braces were capable of controlling displacement at high loads. Baker and coworkers[6] evaluated commercially available athletic braces for their effect on abduction forces applied to a cadaveric knee with no instability and with medial instability. Under computer control, abduction forces were applied while simultaneously data were obtained from an electrogoniometer and transducers applied to the ACL and superficial MCL at 0, 15, and 30 degrees of flexion. Results showed a reduction in abduction angle using functional braces, whereas prophylactic braces showed little or no protective effect.

Beynnon and colleagues,[9] in 1992, used strain transducers applied to the ACL to test scientifically the protective effect of bracing in vivo when different loads were applied to the knee. They found a protective effect of bracing when low anterior shear loads were applied to the knee. However, these low loads were lower than those during activities of daily living.

Cawley and associates[16] have performed a biomechanical comparison of eight commonly used rehabilitative knee braces using a mechanical limb. Most of the braces significantly reduced translations and rotations compared with the unbraced limb under static test conditions. Factors believed to be important in brace design included overall brace stiffness, the use of nonelastic straps, which adapt to leg contour better, and hinge design, including the presence or absence of joint line contact.

Paulos and coworkers,[54,55] in a biomechanical study using fresh-frozen cadaveric knees, measured ligament tension and joint displacement at static nondestructive valgus forces and at low-rated destructive forces. After nonbraced controls were examined, knees were braced with two different laterally applied preventive braces, the McDavid Knee Guard and the Anderson Knee Stabler. The effects of lateral bracing were analyzed according to valgus force, joint line opening, and ligament tension. Valgus applied forces, with or without braces, consistently produced MCL disruption at ligament tension surprisingly higher than the ACL and higher than or equal to the posterior cruciate ligament (PCL). In the first part of their study, no significant protection could be documented with the two preventive braces used. Also, four potentially adverse effects were noted—MCL preloading, center axis shift, premature joint line contact, and brace slippage. In the second part of their study, brace-induced MCL preload in vivo was negated by joint compressive forces. They concluded that most prophylactic knee braces presently available are biomechanically inadequate. They noted that before prophylactic knee braces can be categorically recommended, more biomechanical and clinical studies should be initiated.

In 1991, Paulos and colleagues[54] also evaluated the effects of six different prophylactic knee braces on ACL ligament strain under valgus loads using a mechanical surrogate limb. The results indicated that these braces have a beneficial effect in protecting the knee against direct lateral blows, greater for the ACL than for the MCL. Brace hinge contact with the lateral joint line of the knee reduced the effectiveness. These results should be confirmed clinically and there is a definite need for improved designs.

Patellofemoral Braces

Patellofemoral pain is a common clinical problem presenting to the sports medicine physician. A retrospective chart review by Taunton and associates[77] found that patellofemoral pain is the primary complaint in patients presenting to a sports medicine clinic. Anterior knee pain has a predilection toward the young female athlete and patients often present with a history of nontraumatic peripatellar or retropatellar knee pain of gradual onset. The pain is usually worse after exercise activity or after prolonged inactivity, particularly when sitting with the knee in a flexed position. It can be aggravated with ascending and descending stairs. These symptoms are often attributed to the patella and are manifestations of a lateral subluxation force. This can be evident radiographically as a lateral tilt or on examination with lateral laxity. Regardless, initial treatment consists of activity modifications, nonsteroidal anti-inflammatory drugs, and physical therapy. The role of bracing in these patients has yet to be clearly delineated (Fig. 54-3).

The primary goal of bracing is to centralize the patella within the trochlear groove, thus improving alignment and tracking. Several studies have demonstrated decreases in pain with bracing; however, the mechanism whereby braces reduce symptoms has not been elucidated. Although it is assumed that bracing improves patellar kinematics, imaging studies have reported that bracing has little or no effect on patellar alignment or tracking. Apart from changing patellar kinematics, it has been suggested that bracing may have a more subtle effect on patellofemoral joint mechanics. For example, the compressive force applied to the patellofemoral joint as a result of bracing could seat the patella more firmly within the trochlear groove, thereby increasing contact area.

In a randomized prospective study, Lun and coworkers[42] evaluated 186 knees with patellofemoral pain in four distinct treatment groups at 3-, 6-, and 12-week follow-up. The treatment groups included patellofemoral brace only, home exercise, home exercise with patellofemoral brace, and home exercise with knee sleeve. All groups showed a reduction in pain and an improvement in function, but there were no differences between the treatment groups. These findings were also supported by Miller and colleagues[49] in their study of 59 military cadets during basic training. Subjects presented with anterior knee pain were randomized to therapy only, therapy plus brace type A, and therapy plus brace type B. At the completion of basic training (6 to 8 weeks), there were no differences between the groups with regard to pain.

Warden and associates[83] have completed a systematic review of studies that evaluated patellar bracing and taping. The results of 10 moderate-quality studies demonstrated that on a 100-mm scale, medially directed patellar tape reduces chronic knee pain by 16 mm compared with no tape. This effect was not dependent on the time course of tape application; pain reductions were observed immediately following tape application and after repeated applications over the short term (3 to 12 weeks), with reductions in pain of 17 and 14 mm, respectively. Similarly, the reduction in pain with tape use was independent of diagnosis; medially directed tape reduced pain associated with anterior knee pain and knee osteoarthritis (OA) by 15 and 20 mm, respectively. In contrast to the evidence for the benefits of patellar tape, there was disputable evidence for the benefits of patellar bracing. Braces reduced anterior knee pain by 15 mm on a 100-mm scale compared with no brace. This outcome was attributable to the immediate effects in one study,[58] with no differences

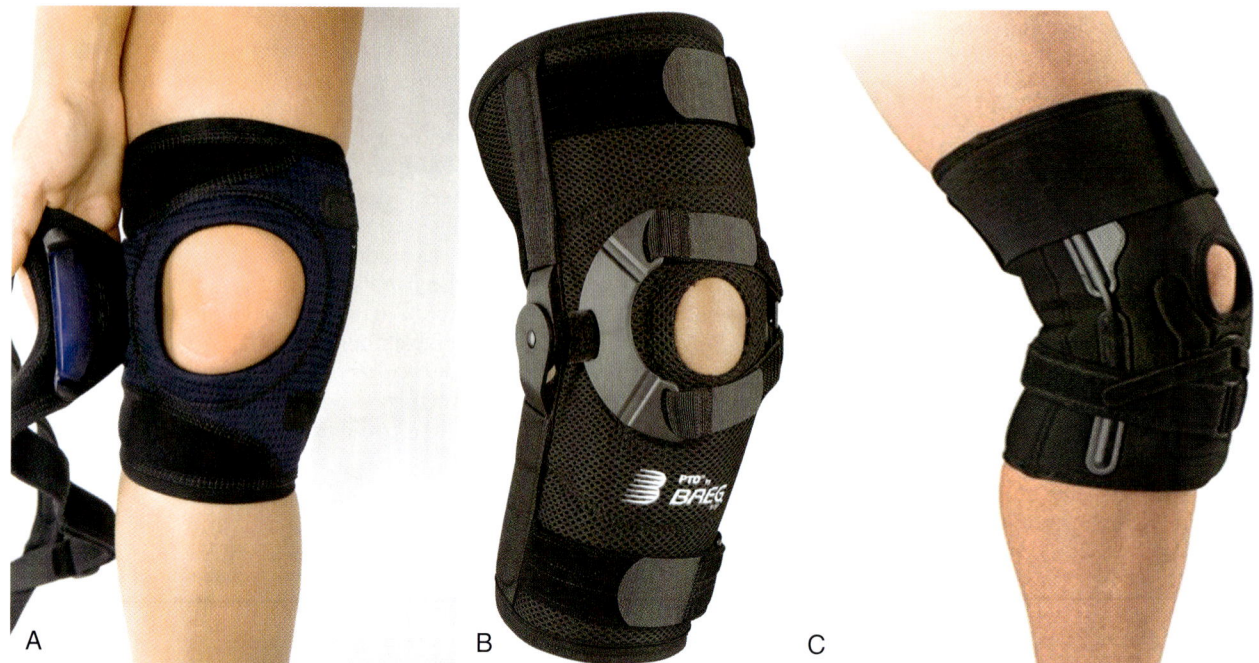

Figure 54-3. Patellofemoral braces. **A,** DonJoy Tru-Pull Lite. **B,** Breg PTO. **C,** Össur patella-stabilizing brace.

being found in two studies on the short-term effects of medially-directed bracing.[42,49]

Another option is to use an infrapatellar strap. The evidence is limited, but Villar[82] looked at the infrapatellar strap in military recruits. The brace was effective in only 24% of recruits in the short term and in 22% at 1 year. However, despite these less than ideal results, the strap seems to help some individuals and have relatively few drawbacks.

The question of whether patellofemoral braces improve knee kinematics has also been evaluated from a biomechanical standpoint. Draper and colleagues[23] used magnetic resonance imaging (MRI) to evaluate patellar mechanics with and without a patellofemoral brace and sleeve. They found an improvement in lateral translation and patellar tilt with the patellofemoral braces. Furthermore, Powers and associates[59] evaluated patellar mechanics and contact pressures in 15 subjects with both MRI and gait analysis for walking and fast walking. They found a significant decrease in peak patellofemoral contact pressures and an increase in patellofemoral contact area in the brace group, with an average 56% decrease in pain perception, thus suggesting that a possible cause for clinically decreased pain with bracing may be the result of increased contact area between the patella and trochlea. However, in a corollary study, they found no significant decrease in peak patellar contact pressure between a braced and nonbraced state for stair climbing. There was an increase in patella contact area, but the corresponding increase in extensor moment negated any decrease in overall peak contact pressure.[60]

Previously, Shellock and coworkers[69] studied 21 patellofemoral joints with the brace in place. There was restraint to lateral displacement of the patella in 16 knees. They concluded that the other four knees did not have a change because these subjects had patella alta. Muhle and colleagues[51] also used MRI data to evaluate the usefulness of a brace in altering patella kinematics. They looked at 24 knees

and found no significant improvement in patellar tilt angle, bisect offset, or lateral patellar displacement before or after wearing the patellar brace.

Conclusion

Bracing for patellofemoral pain has not reliably shown clinical efficacy. However, given the dearth of functional evidence, according to Arroll and associates,[5] patients continue to have subjective improvement. There also exists a moderate amount of evidence showing that taping may provide short-term relief. Regardless, patellar bracing cannot be recommended or denied at this point. More controlled studies must be completed with defined patient populations. The clinical data are inconclusive, but there are biomechanical data that may suggest improvement in knee kinematics.

Unloader Braces

As patients remain active longer into their lives and physiologic age becomes more important than chronologic age, unicompartmental arthritis can pose a significant treatment paradox. Excellent pain relief can be achieved with operative techniques, but the risk of postoperative limitations is significant. Thus, a brace that relieves pain can be an attractive option for patients with mild to moderate disease (Fig. 54-4). The question then becomes whether braces work for these patients.

Once a patient begins having medial unicompartmental disease, the adduction moment of the knee can change. Various compensatory mechanisms are then put into play: the redistribution of condylar loads; contraction of antagonist muscle groups; increased tension in the lateral convex soft tissues and cruciate ligaments; increased body sway in the lateral direction; decreased stride length; and decreased inversion moment at the ankle accomplished by out-toeing. Once the degeneration overcomes these protective

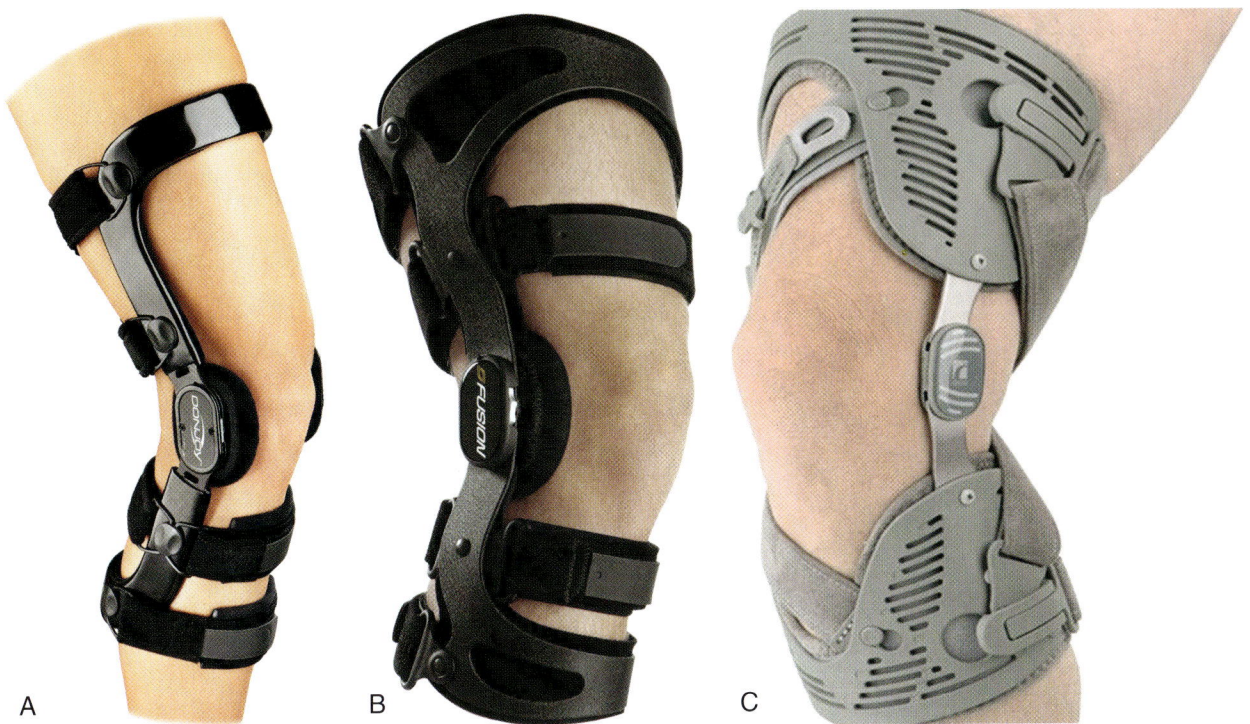

Figure 54-4. Osteoarthritis and unloader braces. **A,** DonJoy OA Defiance. **B,** Breg Fusion OA. **C,** Össur Unloader One; custom knee brace.

mechanisms, the load becomes excessive and the result is medial knee pain.

The AAOS has published a consensus statement that does not recommend for or against the use of valgus or varus unloading braces[63] and the Osteoarthritis Research Society International has given bracing for unicompartmental OA an 76% SOR (strength of recommendation).[85] These conclusions were based largely on the results of one systematic review[13] and two randomized clinical trials[14,36] in the valgus-directing brace group and zero clinical trials in the varus-directing brace group. Kirkley and coworkers[36] were the first to evaluate brace treatment in varus gonarthrosis with a randomized controlled study. In their study, 119 patients with varus gonarthrosis were randomized to a control group of medical treatment alone, a combined group of medical treatment and a neoprene sleeve, and a combined group of medical treatment and an unloader brace. At the 6-month evaluation, there was a significant improvement in the quality of life and function of the neoprene sleeve group and the unloader brace group. The unloader brace group had significant improvement over the neoprene sleeve group with regard to pain after a 6-minute walking test and a 30-second stair-climbing test. The combination of an unloader brace and medical treatment was the best treatment regimen for varus gonarthrosis.

Furthermore, Brouwer and colleagues[14] completed a multicenter randomized controlled trial comparing brace treatment with standard conservative management. In this study, 117 patients were enrolled and allocated to a brace with conservative treatment arm (60 patients) or conservative management alone (57 patients). Follow-up was completed at 3-, 6-, and 12-month intervals with VAS, Hospital for Special Surgery (HSS), and walking distance scores recorded.

The only significant improvement was noted in walking distance, with VAS and HSS scores trending toward a decrease in the brace group. Of note, 25 of the patients in the brace group and 14 in the nonbrace group discontinued treatment. Of the patients who stopped brace treatment, 13 switched to conservative management only and cited "no effect" as the reason. This study led the authors to conclude that brace treatment has a small effect on unicompartmental arthritis, but it also suggests that some patients will not maintain this treatment regimen for an extended period.

The previous studies suggest a benefit of the valgus-unloading braces for a varus knee. However, the question of whether the unloading brace or a simple knee brace provides variable levels of relief was evaluated by Richards and associates.[62] In this study, 12 patients were randomly divided into a hinged and unloader group and, at 6 months, the unloader group displayed significantly lower VAS and higher HSS knee scores. Although the number of patients was low, this study suggests an added benefit with a valgus unloader brace. Along these same lines, Draganich and coworkers[22] compared the use of an off-the-shelf with a custom valgus-directing brace in patients with medial compartment disease; 10 patients participated in a crossover study and served as their own controls. It was concluded that the custom brace is more effective than the off-the-shelf brace in improving the results for pain, stiffness, and function, and in reducing the varus angle of alignment of the knee and the peak external adduction moments about the knee during gait and stair stepping.

Hewett and colleagues[30] have prospectively evaluated 18 patients with symptomatic medial compartment arthritis and fitted them with a valgus-producing brace. All subjects were evaluated after 9 weeks of brace use, and 13 subjects were evaluated at 1 year. At the 9-week evaluation, pain with activities of daily living decreased from 78% to 39% and walking tolerance improved from 51 to 138 minutes. At the 1-year evaluation, pain with activities decreased to 31% and walking tolerance was 107 minutes. A gait analysis also was performed for this study, but no differences were found in dynamic gait parameters.

Nonetheless, the effectiveness of valgus-unloading braces and the cause of pain relief remain controversial. The leading theory—that these valgus-producing braces unload the medial compartment of a varus malaligned knee—has been challenged by some. Ramsey and associates[61] have suggested that bracing reduces pain and improves function by stabilizing the knee and decreasing antagonistic muscle cocontraction. In their study, 16 subjects were evaluated with no brace and a custom unloader brace in neutral and in 4 degrees of valgus. Pain and function were improved in the brace group, but not significantly different between the neutral and 4 degrees of valgus brace groups. Thus it was concluded that there may be another mechanism for patient improvement in the brace group other than unloading.

Pollo and coworkers[57] have studied 11 patients with medial compartment arthritis. The subjects were custom-fitted with a valgus brace. Pain and activity level improved in all patients. Using gait analysis, the varus moment about the knee was decreased and the medial compartment load decreased in the 4-degree calibrated brace setting. Lindenfeld and colleagues[40] also confirmed these findings with the use of an automated gait analysis to study the adductor moment of a valgus-producing brace. Eleven patients with confined medial arthritis were custom-fitted with a valgus-producing brace and compared with 11 healthy controls. The mean adduction moment with the use of the brace decreased 10%, approaching the normal controls. The VAS pain score decreased 48% and the Cincinnati Knee Rating System increased 79%. This study showed that pain, function, and biomechanics of the knee are improved with the use of an appropriately fitted unloader brace.

Dennis and coworkers[21] and Naudad and associates[52] have published results of a three-dimensional imaging study on the effect of valgus unloading braces and found a small benefit to these with the most significant improvement at heel-strike and the smallest effect at mid-stance. They also noted that obese patients experienced less benefit both clinically and radiographically. They also found a wide variability between different manufacturers.

Conclusions

As with the other brace categories, additional randomized controlled studies need to be completed before solid conclusions can be made regarding unloader braces. However, there are currently studies that do suggest a benefit from clinical and biomechanical standpoints. The cause of this pain relief remains under debate. Given the mild adverse effects of bracing (cost and inconvenience), it can be considered for the nonobese active patient with mild to moderate unicompartmental arthritis.

SUMMARY

Knee bracing for the prevention and treatment of athletic injuries is controversial and prevalent. With a relatively small downside, bracing gives physicians a tool that can potentially avoid more extensive treatment protocols associated with greater risks. However, the literature fails to support some of these regimens fully. Given the increased complexity and improvements in current knee braces, further studies are needed to define the role of each specific brace for specific patient subsets.

In the post-ACL reconstruction period, the evidence that a brace confers additional stability, improves range of motion, protects the graft, reduces pain, and/or improves subjective outcomes is limited. However, there are data that support brace use to maintain extension and prevent flexion contractures. Prophylactic knee braces have not consistently been shown to prevent or reduce the severity of injuries to the ACL, MCL, or menisci in the general population. However, there is evidence suggesting that brace use for specific athletic positions and athletes is beneficial (e.g., for a football lineman).

Studies that definitively support or refute functional brace use have not been carried out. Thus, the treating physician must make an educated, patient-specific decision with regard to recommendations. In the setting of ACL deficiency or instability, there is a subjective and biomechanical advantage to brace use. Although this benefit has not translated into a significant functional improvement, brace use should still be considered for this patient subset.

Bracing for patellofemoral pain has not reliably shown clinical or functional efficacy; nevertheless, some patients continue to have subjective improvements. Biomechanically, an increased patellar contact area has been described in the laboratory, but more clinical studies are needed to determine the potential patient benefit.

Lastly, unloader braces have been shown to have a biomechanical and clinical advantage in limited studies. However, the cost of the brace must be weighted against the potential improvements in pain and function. These braces have been shown to be more effective in the non-obese active patient with mild disease. Overall, prescribing patterns for knee braces should follow explicit guidelines, with a distinct goal for each patient's treatment.

KEY REFERENCES

Beaudreuil J, Bendaya S, Faucher M, et al: Clinical practice guidelines for rest orthosis, knee sleeves, and unloading knee braces in knee osteoarthritis. Joint Bone Spine 76:629–636, 2009.

Beynnon BD, Fleming BC, Churchill DL, Brown D: The effect of anterior cruciate ligament deficiency and functional bracing on translation of the tibia relative to the femur during nonweightbearing and weightbearing. Am J Sports Med 31:99–105, 2003.

Birmingham TB, Bryant DM, Giffin JR, et al: A randomized controlled trial comparing the effectiveness of functional knee brace and neoprene sleeve use after anterior cruciate ligament reconstruction. Am J Sports Med 36:648–655, 2008.

Draganich L, Reider B, Rimington T, et al: The effectiveness of self-adjustable custom and off-the-shelf bracing in the treatment of varus gonarthrosis. J Bone Joint Surg Am 88:2645–2652, 2006.

Draper CE, Besier TF, Santos JM, et al: Using real-time MRI to quantify altered joint kinematics in subjects with patellofemoral pain and to evaluate the effects of a patellar brace or sleeve on joint motion. J Orthop Res 27:571–577, 2009.

Harilainen A, Sandelin J: Postoperative use of knee brace in bone-tendon-bone patellar tendon anterior cruciate ligament reconstruction: 5-year follow-up results of a randomized prospective study. Scand J Med Sci Sports 16:14–18, 2006.

Hiemstra LA, Heard SM, Sasyniuk TM, et al: Knee immobilization for pain control after a hamstring tendon anterior cruciate ligament reconstruction: a randomized clinical trial. Am J Sports Med 37:56–64, 2009.

McDevitt ER, Taylor DC, Miller MD, et al: Functional bracing after anterior cruciate ligament reconstruction: a prospective, randomized, multicenter study. Am J Sports Med 32:1887–1892, 2004.

Mikkelsen C, Cerulli G, Lorenzini M, et al: Can a postoperative brace in slight hyperextension prevent extension deficit after anterior cruciate ligament reconstruction? A prospective randomised study. Knee Surg Sports Traumatol Arthrosc 11:318–321, 2003.

Najibi S, Albright JP: The use of knee braces, part 1: prophylactic knee braces in contact sports. Am J Sports Med 33:602–611, 2005.

Sterett WI, Briggs KK, Farley T, Steadman JR: Effect of functional bracing on knee injury in skiers with anterior cruciate ligament reconstruction: a prospective cohort study. Am J Sports Med 34:1581–1585, 2006.

Van Tiggelen D, Witvrouw E, Roget P, et al: Effect of bracing on the prevention of anterior knee pain—a prospective randomized study. Knee Surg Sports Traumatol Arthrosc 12:434–439, 2004.

Warden SJ, Hinman RS, Watson MA, Jr, et al: Patellar taping and bracing for the treatment of chronic knee pain: a systematic review and meta-analysis. Arthritis Rheum 59:73–83, 2008.

Wright RW, Fetzer GB: Bracing after ACL reconstruction: a systematic review. Clin Orthop Relat Res (455):162–168, 2007.

Wright RW, Preston E, Fleming BC, et al: A systematic review of anterior cruciate ligament reconstruction rehabilitation: Part I: continuous passive motion, early weight bearing, postoperative bracing, and home-based rehabilitation. J Knee Surg 21:217–224, 2008.

Full references for this chapter can be found on www.expertconsult.com.

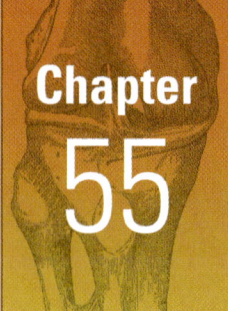

Chapter 55

Decision Making and Surgical Treatment of Posterior Cruciate Ligament Ruptures

Frank R. Noyes and Sue Barber-Westin

The proper management of injuries to the posterior cruciate ligament (PCL) and other ligaments of the knee involves a series of decisions based on knowledge of diagnosis, reconstruction options and techniques, and rehabilitation concepts.[70,76] The clinician must be able to diagnose and treat a spectrum of knee injuries, from an isolated PCL rupture to a combined injury involving other knee ligaments (Box 55-1). This chapter will review the current knowledge of the function of the PCL—both alone and in concert with other ligament systems—that form the basis for the diagnosis of abnormal translations and rotations that result in different types of knee subluxations requiring surgical restoration (Box 55-2). Legitimate controversy exists about the treatment of complete PCL ruptures because of the absence of a true natural history study, short-term clinical results of PCL reconstructions, and lack of randomized controlled trials of sufficient numbers of patients to form conclusions.

The steps to diagnose and treat associated problems in knees with PCL ruptures must be systematically accomplished; they are reviewed in this chapter. These include varus malalignment, deficiency of the posterolateral structure (PLS) abnormal gait mechanics including knee hyperextension, and severe muscle atrophy. The detection and treatment of these problems are critical, because failure to correct associated conditions properly may result in an undesirable outcome. Many of these problems are found in patients with chronic knee instabilities who may also have lost one or both menisci and demonstrate advanced articular cartilage damage. In these knees, the goal is to restore knee function for daily activities. Surgical advances in treating acute PCL ruptures hopefully will prevent the chronically unstable knee and resultant arthritis that often occur in younger athletes.

This chapter will also review advances from our center in PCL graft selection and surgical techniques designed to reduce the morbidity of the procedure. There are different surgical approaches available for acute knee injuries, dislocated knees with multiple ligament ruptures, chronic knees, and revision knees. Important decisions must be made regarding the placement of single- and two-strand graft constructs. In addition, differences exist in the postoperative rehabilitation program, depending on the surgical procedure(s) performed.[82] A detailed analysis and surgical treatment of other knee disorders that accompany PCL ruptures has been previously published; this chapter represents a synopsis of this work.[76]

POSTERIOR CRUCIATE LIGAMENT ANATOMY

The PCL arises from a depression posterior to the intra-articular upper surface of the tibia and courses anteromedially behind the ACL to the lateral surface of the medial femoral condyle (Fig. 55-1).[122] The PCL has an average length of 38 mm and width of 13 mm.[36,131] The cross-sectional area of the PCL varies and increases from tibial to femoral insertions.[42] The PCL is approximately 50% larger than the ACL at its femoral origin and 20% larger at its tibial insertion. The anterior meniscofemoral ligament (ligament of Humphry) courses anterior to the PCL, and the posterior meniscofemoral ligament (ligament of Wrisberg) runs obliquely behind the PCL. At least one meniscofemoral ligament is present in 91% of knees, and both ligaments may be found in 50% of knees in young individuals (Box 55-3).[41,42,65]

Free nerve endings and mechanoreceptors that are believed to have a proprioceptive function in the knee[49] have been identified in the femoral and tibial attachment sites and on the surface of the PCL.[47,106]

The traditional division of the PCL into separate anterolateral and posteromedial bundles oversimplifies PCL fiber function. The PCL is a complex anatomic structure comprised of a continuum of fibers of different lengths and attachment characteristics. The length-tension behaviors of the fibers that resist posterior tibial translation (with knee flexion) are controlled primarily by femoral attachment regions.* The distal fibers lengthen with increasing knee flexion and the proximal fibers shorten with knee flexion.[65,105]

Variation exists among knees in the shape of the PCL femoral attachment, from the common elliptical shape to a more rounded and thicker shape (Fig. 55-2).[65] The most accurate measurement system that describes the femoral attachment site uses a clock reference position, with one set of measurement lines perpendicular to the articular cartilage edge and the other set parallel to the femoral shaft.

In general, the PCL attachment extends from high in the notch (11:30 to 5 o'clock on a right knee) along the medial femoral condyle. The anterior portion of the PCL attachment follows the articular cartilage within 2 to 3 mm of its edge and gradually recedes deeper with the notch until, at the 5 o'clock position, the posterior third is 5 mm from the articular margin. Therefore, the distal boundary of the PCL femoral attachment is furthest away from the cartilage margin posteriorly.

The distance of the distal edge of the attachment to the articular cartilage margin is 3.2 ± 0.8 mm at the roof, 5.8 ± 2.2 mm at its midportion, and 7.9 ± 2.2 mm at its "lowest" extent.[105] The proximal edge of the PCL is usually straight or partially oval, with the attachment tapered in width along its posterior portion.

A clear understanding of the anatomy of the native PCL is critical in determining what portion of the ligament will be reconstructed. The terms *high, low, shallow,* and *deep* are only general descriptors. Because there may be confusion regarding femoral graft tunnel placement during PCL reconstruction, the PCL femoral attachment is described using the rule of thirds (Fig. 55-3A, B) to define the proximal-middle-distal

---

*References 1, 17, 31, 40, 56, 57, 105, 110, and 115.

Box 55-1   Spectrum of Posterior Cruciate Ligament Injuries

Posterior Cruciate Ligament Rupture, Isolated

A. Partial
B. Complete
   1. Bone avulsion
   2. Ligament insertion peel-off
   3. Ligament substance

Posterior Cruciate Ligament Rupture Combined With Other Knee Joint Abnormality

Lateral, posterolateral structures
Medial, posteromedial structures
Anterior cruciate ligament
Meniscus tears, partial or complex, medial or lateral
Joint arthrosis, articular cartilage damage*
   1. Medial tibiofemoral
   2. Lateral tibiofemoral
   3. Patellofemoral
Extensor mechanism malalignment, subluxation

Posterior Cruciate Ligament Rupture Combined With Other System Abnormality

Lower limb malalignment
Neuromuscular system
Peripheral vascular system
Cutaneous, skin

*Classified according to the system described in Noyes FR, Stabler CL: A system for grading articular cartilage lesions at arthroscopy. Am J Sports Med 17:505–513, 1989.

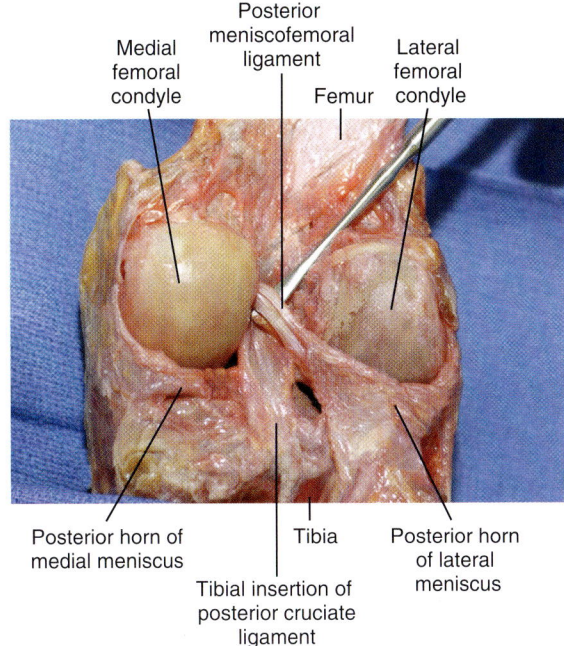

Figure 55-1. The PCL femoral and tibial attachments. Note the prominent posterior meniscofemoral ligament and broad posterior tibial attachment. (From Noyes FR, Barber-Westin SD: Posterior cruciate ligament: diagnosis, operative techniques, and clinical outcomes. In Noyes FR [ed]: Noyes' knee disorders: surgery, rehabilitation, clinical outcomes, Philadelphia, 2009, Saunders, pp 503–576.)

Box 55-2   Clinical Effects of Posterior Tibial Subluxation of the Posterior Cruciate Ligament–Deficient Knee

- PCL forces up to 50% body weight occur during level walking
- Higher PCL forces occur during stair climbing, ascending and descending stairs
- Posterior tibial subluxation occurs in PCL-deficient knees during activities of daily living in high knee flexion positions, but not at low flexion positions, when medial-lateral ligaments are intact and smaller posterior shear forces are present
- Patients with chronic PCL deficiency frequently note an anterior shifting of the tibia as the tibial moves forward from its subluxated position when they attempt to stand from a seated position.
- Significantly increased contact pressures in medial tibiofemoral and patellofemoral compartments in PCL-deficient knees
- Loss of medial meniscus function because of posterior tibial subluxation

From Noyes FR, Barber-Westin SD: Posterior cruciate ligament: diagnosis, operative techniques, and clinical outcomes. In Noyes FR (ed): Noyes' knee disorders: surgery, rehabilitation, clinical outcomes, Philadelphia, 2009, Saunders, pp 503–576.

Box 55-3   Meniscofemoral Ligaments

- Most knees have at least one meniscofemoral ligament (MFL).
- One third of knees have both meniscofemoral ligaments.
- There are insufficient data to support a functional role of these structures.
- Identify anterior MFL and posterior MFL (when present) to determine true PCL anatomic footprint for graft placement.
- In some knees with isolated PCL ruptures, secondary ligament restraints, including the MFL structures, resist posterior tibial subluxation, particularly at low knee flexion angles.
- The best position to test for maximum posterior translation is 90 degrees of knee flexion, neutral tibial rotation.
- The amount of posterior translation after PCL rupture is determined by secondary restraints and will vary depending on physiologic laxity.

From Noyes FR, Barber-Westin SD: Posterior cruciate ligament: diagnosis, operative techniques, and clinical outcomes. In Noyes FR (ed): Noyes' knee disorders: Surgery, rehabilitation, clinical outcomes, Philadelphia, 2009, Saunders, pp 503–576.

Vascular Anatomy and Variations

The PCL is covered with a well-vascularized synovial sleeve that contributes to its blood supply. The distal portion also receives some vascular supply from capsular vessels originating from the inferior and middle genicular arteries and the popliteal artery.

Detailed knowledge of posteromedial knee anatomy, especially the vascular structures, is required to avoid

thirds (deep to shallow in the femoral notch), and anterior-middle-posterior thirds (high to low), with a small posterior oblique portion in the sagittal plane.[65,67] This provides a grid for the identification of the tunnel locations for the graft strands and is preferred over the historical division of an anterolateral or posteromedial bundle (see Fig. 55-3C).

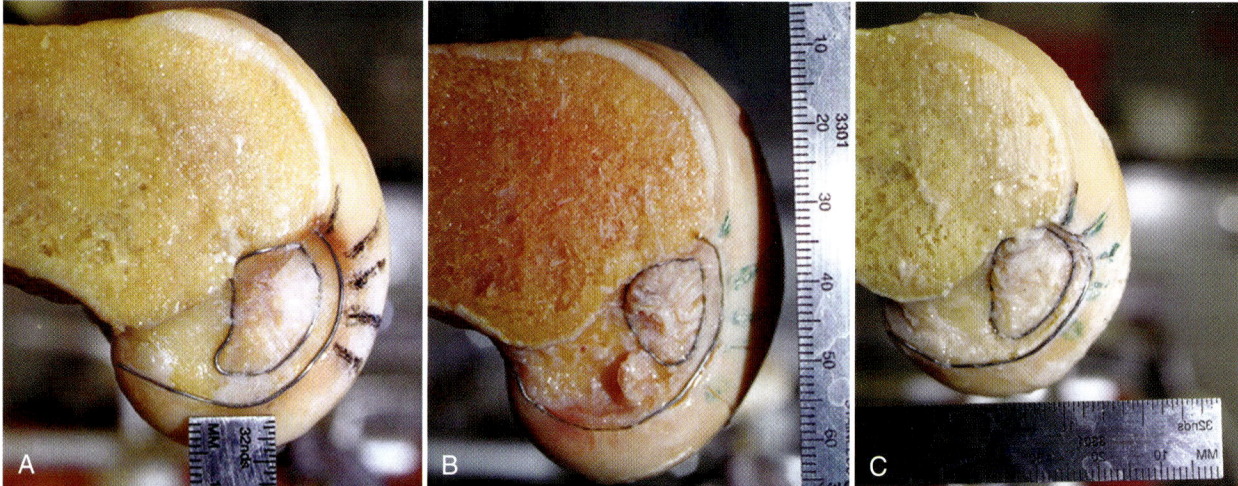

Figure 55-2. Composite of the shapes of different PCL insertion sites as seen on lateral views. Variability is noted between specimens from an oval to an elliptical PCL footprint configuration. Note the differences in the anterior to posterior and proximal to distal dimensions in the PCL footprint. The most common shape of the PCL footprint is elliptical. **A,** Fibers insert proximally to the intercondylar roof. The PCL footprint is smaller in its anteroposterior dimension. **B,** Prominent posterior meniscofemoral ligaments. **C,** More oval PCL attachment, with greater proximal to distal width. (From Mejia EA, Noyes FR, Grood ES: Posterior cruciate ligament femoral insertion site characteristics. Importance for reconstructive procedures. Am J Sports Med 30: 643–651, 2002.)

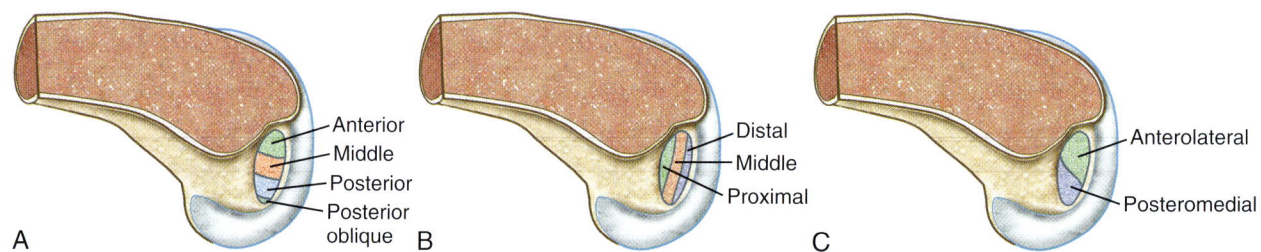

Figure 55-3. A, Rule of thirds. The PCL footprint is divided into anterior, middle, and posterior thirds. The anterior third extends past the midline (12:30 o'clock, left knee) and the posterior region extends to 5 o'clock. The smaller posterior oblique portion of the PCL footprint is also represented. The PCL footprint is elliptical in most knees, but variations exist. **B,** Rule of thirds. The PCL footprint is further divided into distal, middle, and proximal thirds. This allows for more exact referencing of graft strand placement during PCL reconstruction. The PCL fibers in the distal two thirds lengthen with knee flexion whereas the proximal fibers shorten. The reverse occurs with knee extension. **C,** Typical division of anterolateral and posteromedial bundles provides an incorrect description of PCL fiber length change, because it describes anterior PCL fibers that lengthen (AL) and posterior fibers (PL) that shorten with knee flexion. (From Noyes FR, Barber-Westin SD: Posterior cruciate ligament: diagnosis, operative techniques, and clinical outcomes. In Noyes FR [ed]: Noyes' knee disorders: surgery, rehabilitation, clinical outcomes, Philadelphia, 2009, Saunders, pp 503–576.)

complications when using a posteromedial approach for a tibial inlay PCL reconstruction. The popliteal artery originates at the adductor hiatus and passes through the popliteal fossa. Before passing deep to the fibrous arch over the soleus muscle, it divides into the anterior and posterior tibial arteries at the distal aspect of the popliteus muscle.

At the level of the knee joint, four major arteries are distributed—the medial and lateral sural arteries, a cutaneous branch that travels with the small saphenous vein to supply superficial tissues, and the middle genicular artery. The medial and lateral inferior genicular arteries are given off just distal to the knee joint.

Two branches deserve particular attention. The medial inferior genicular artery arises from the medial aspect of the distal portion of the popliteal artery and runs medially, deep to the medial head of the gastrocnemius, and approximately 2 to 3 mm from the superior surface of the popliteus muscle. It continues around the medial aspect of the proximal tibia,

deep to the superficial MCL (SMCL). The middle genicular artery arises at the level of the femoral condyles proximal to the joint line and passes anteriorly to pierce the oblique popliteal ligament and posterior joint capsule and supply the cruciate ligaments.

This normal vascular pattern has been reported to occur in approximately 88% of knees.[20,63] In approximately 5% to 7%, the popliteal artery will divide at least 1 inch or more proximal to the distal border of the popliteus muscle.[14] In slightly less than half of these knees, with a high division of the popliteal artery, the anterior tibial artery passes anteriorly, not posteriorly, to the popliteus muscle belly.[129] A number of variations of the anterior tibial artery were described by Mauro and colleagues.[63] Therefore, with a tibial inlay approach, the dissection is always performed proximal to the popliteus muscle using a meticulous technique, because the anterior tibial artery is at risk for transection in approximately 3% to 4% of knees.

An unusual variation in the vascular pattern involves the popliteal artery passing medially and then beneath the medial head of the gastrocnemius. Various subtypes of this abnormal pattern have been described. An abnormal vascular pattern may manifest clinically as the popliteal artery entrapment syndrome, which is characterized by vascular claudication symptoms.[52,102,118] Arterial insufficiency occurs most commonly with entrapment of the artery deep to the medial gastrocnemius muscle, but may also occur when the artery is entrapped deep to the popliteus muscle (persistence of ventral component of artery), or entrapped deep to an abnormal accessory head of the gastrocnemius. A history of pain in the lower extremity with activity but none at rest, particularly in a young patient, should alert the surgeon to the possibility that an abnormal vascular pattern may exist. Further evaluation with magnetic resonance imaging (MRI) or angiography may be warranted.[30,55]

POSTERIOR CRUCIATE LIGAMENT FIBER FUNCTION

The femoral attachment location of a PCL graft strongly influences graft tension and the ability of the reconstruction to restore posterior stability.* Investigations by Grood and

---

*References 1, 3, 32, 93, 105, 110, and 130.

associates[38] and Sidles and coworkers[115] have demonstrated that the femoral attachment location, and not the tibial attachment location, determines the graft tibiofemoral separation distance with knee flexion-extension.

On the femur, the proximal-distal location of a graft has a greater effect on the attachment separation distance than the anterior-posterior location (Figs. 55-4 and 55-5), which forms the basis for the rule of thirds. A graft placed in the distal and middle thirds lengthens with knee flexion, whereas a graft placed in the proximal third lengthens with knee extension.

In an investigation at our laboratory,[105] the changes in tibiofemoral length for seven peripheral attachment sites at the proximal and distal origins located around the circumference of the PCL femoral attachment were studied. The data confirm that proximal PCL fibers lengthen with knee extension and distal fibers lengthen with knee flexion (Fig. 55-6). In Figure 55-7, the flexion angles in which the fiber length elongations were the least (within 5% of the maximum length and, therefore, the functional zone) are graphed for each attachment point. The data as a whole show a progressive loading of fibers from distal to proximal within the PCL attachment with increasing knee flexion. There is a smaller effect proceeding from anterior to posterior. These data contradict the description of PCL fiber function that divides the PCL into an anterolateral bundle (which lengthen with knee flexion) and posteromedial bundle (which shorten with knee flexion).

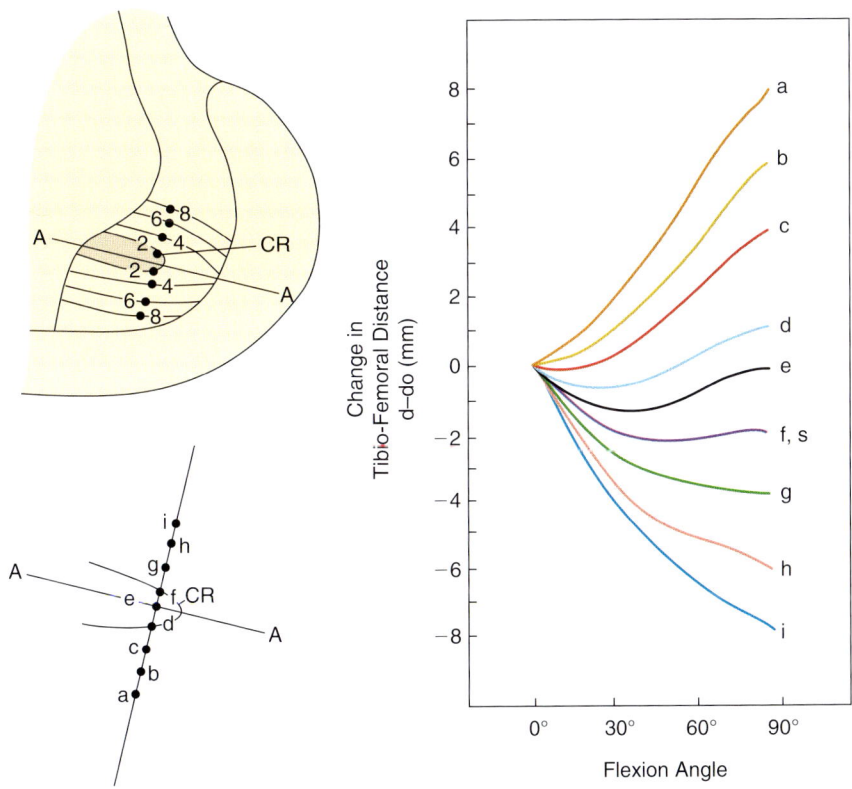

Figure 55-4. Contour map for a typical knee. The number on each contour line indicates the magnitude of the maximum length change. Line A-A represents the most isometric line and runs almost in the AP direction. Point CR indicates the intersection of the best-fit flexion axis with the lateral surface of the medial femoral condyle. Note that line A-A passes near point CR. The curves at the *right* show the changes in the tibiofemoral separation distances that occurred for selected femoral attachments. Attachments proximal to the isometric line were shorter at 90 degrees than at full extension. Attachments distal to the line were longer at 90 degrees. Attachments along line A-A had a length at 90 degrees that was almost identical to its length at 0 degrees. (From Grood ES, Hefzy MS, Lindenfeld TN: Factors affecting the region of most isometric femoral attachments. Part I: The posterior cruciate ligament. Am J Sports Med 17:197–207, 1989.)

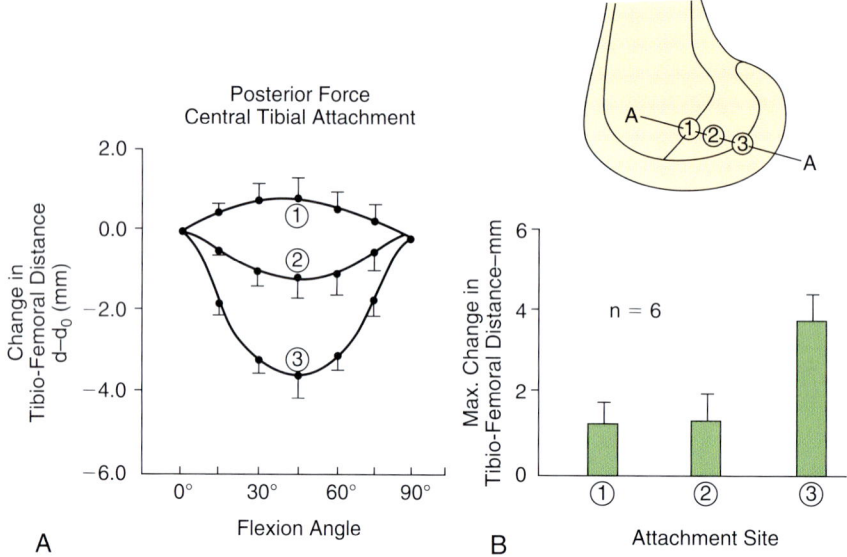

Figure 55-5. *Left,* The curves show the average tibiofemoral separation distance versus knee flexion for three femoral attachment sites located along the most isometric line. *Right,* The bar chart shows the average and standard deviation of the difference between the maximum and minimum tibiofemoral separation distance for each of the three femoral attachment sites. (From Grood ES, Hefzy MS, Lindenfeld TN: Factors affecting the region of most isometric femoral attachments. Part I: The posterior cruciate ligament. Am J Sports Med 17:197–207, 1989.)

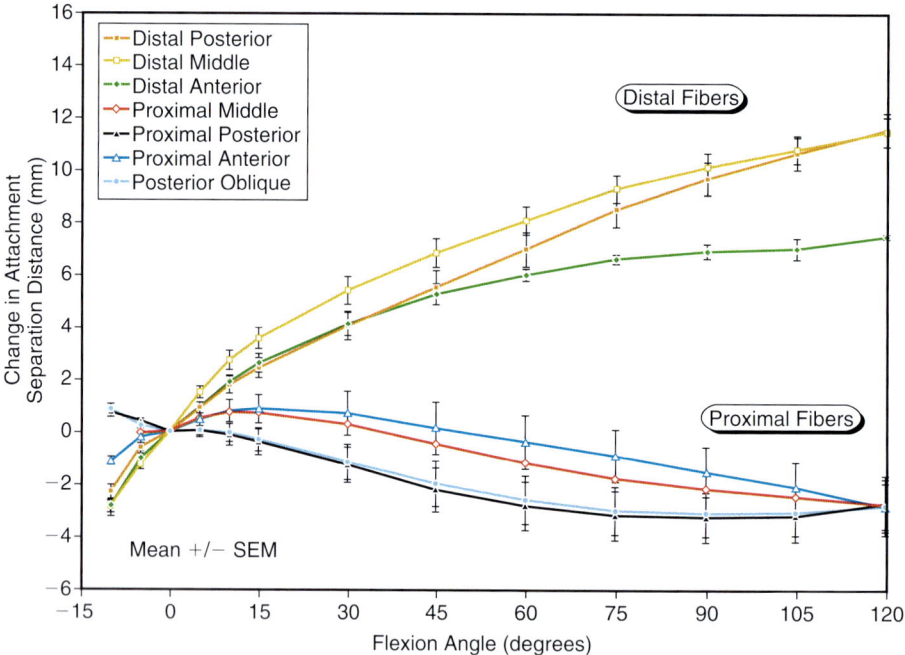

Figure 55-6. Changes in attachment separation distance (in mm) are measured with progressive knee flexion under a 100-N posterior load. Distal fibers lengthen with knee flexion; proximal fibers shorten with knee flexion. (From Saddler SC, Noyes FR, Grood ES, et al: Posterior cruciate ligament anatomy and length-tension behavior of PCL surface fibers. Am J Knee Surg 9:194–199, 1996.)

The surgeon has the option of placing a PCL graft strand into different regions of the PCL femoral attachment site that determine the functional range of the graft with knee flexion and the knee flexion position to tension the graft. In a study from our laboratory,[57] one- and two-stand PCL reconstructions were attached in three different locations within the PCL femoral footprint. A 50-N posterior force was applied to the tibia for the single-stand construct and a 100-N force was applied to the two-strand PCL reconstruction. The tension in the graft stands was adjusted to restore posterior translation to within ±1 mm of the intact knee. The complex behavior of a two-strand PCL reconstruction is shown in Figure 55-8, in which the two strands were placed into the more distal locations and tensioned at 90 degrees. Both strands shared the applied load as shown. In contrast, a two-strand construct, in which one strand was placed anterior and the

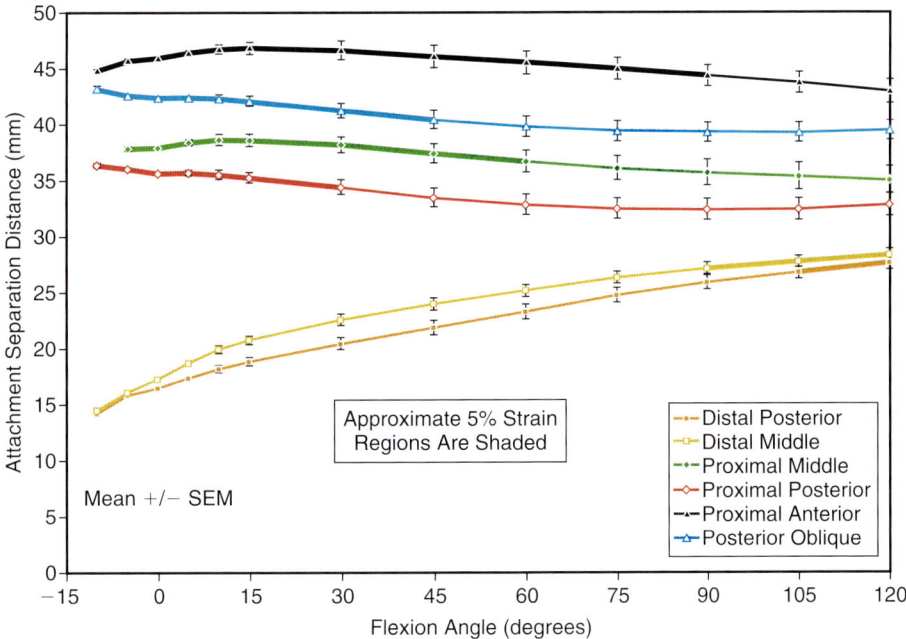

Figure 55-7. The change in attachment separation distance curves have been shifted to begin at the measured absolute length of each fiber. The darker area for each curve represents the 5% strain for each fiber. This in theory represents the functional range of knee flexion for each fiber. Note that this model predicts that the proximal-anterior fiber will function over the longest functional range. (From Saddler SC, Noyes FR, Grood ES, et al: Posterior cruciate ligament anatomy and length-tension behavior of PCL surface fibers. Am J Knee Surg 9:194–199, 1996.)

second strand was placed more proximally, resulted in a reciprocal loading relationship between strands (Fig. 55-9). In both situations, posterior translation limits were restored to normal.

Another investigation at our laboratory[110] confirmed that a proximal to distal change in the femoral position of the second bundle of a two-bundle construct markedly affects bundle tension and function. A middle placement of the second bundle produced load sharing, which is more ideal in terms of graft function in the long term for preventing posterior tibial subluxation with increasing knee flexion. These concepts are used to select PCL graft attachment locations and tensioning, described in the operative techniques section (see later). The surgeon should select graft attachment locations that have the least amount of change in tibiofemoral length, and tension the graft at the knee flexion position at which the graft length is the longest (and therefore functional). If a graft is tensioned at a knee flexion angle at which the tibiofemoral fiber length is at its shortest, the graft will initially constrain knee flexion or extension and fail as the graft (tibiofemoral distance) lengthens with further knee flexion or extension.

DIAGNOSIS OF POSTERIOR CRUCIATE LIGAMENT FUNCTION AND KNEE JOINT SUBLUXATIONS

Posterior Translation

The normal anterior and posterior translation knee limits are shown in Figure 55-10A.[40] The increase in these limits when the PCL is cut is shown in Figure 55-10B and the further

increase in these limits when the PLS is also sectioned is shown in Figure 55-10C.

The PCL is a primary restraint to posterior tibial translation throughout knee flexion, with the exception of a small increase in posterior translation at full extension when the PLS is cut. A knee that demonstrates increased posterior translation at 30 to 45 degrees of knee flexion, similar to the posterior translation limit at 90 degrees, indicates associated injury to the PLS and the medial structures. In a knee with a combined deficiency of the PCL and PLS, the abnormal posterior tibial translation is at least four to five times the normal limit throughout knee flexion.

The PLS represents one of the most important secondary restraints and has a major effect on lateral tibiofemoral compartment translation. There are marked differences in the amount of posterior tibial translation between isolated and combined PCL injuries. Although the amount of posterior translation may vary among knees,[40] it is generally appreciated clinically that a 10-mm or greater abnormal displacement at 90 degrees flexion indicates some deficiency of the secondary restraints in addition to the PCL. Furthermore, the posterior tibial displacement progressively increases at low flexion angles with injury or stretching of the secondary ligament restraints. The abnormal forces placed on the patellofemoral and tibiofemoral compartments are expected to increase as greater posterior tibial displacements occur.[116] Clinically, it is advantageous to reconstruct the PCL before the loss of these secondary restraints. Otherwise, the PCL graft is placed under greater forces because the secondary restraints are not able to share a portion of the load in resisting posterior tibial subluxation. In chronic cases, in which the secondary restraints are deficient, we recommend surgical

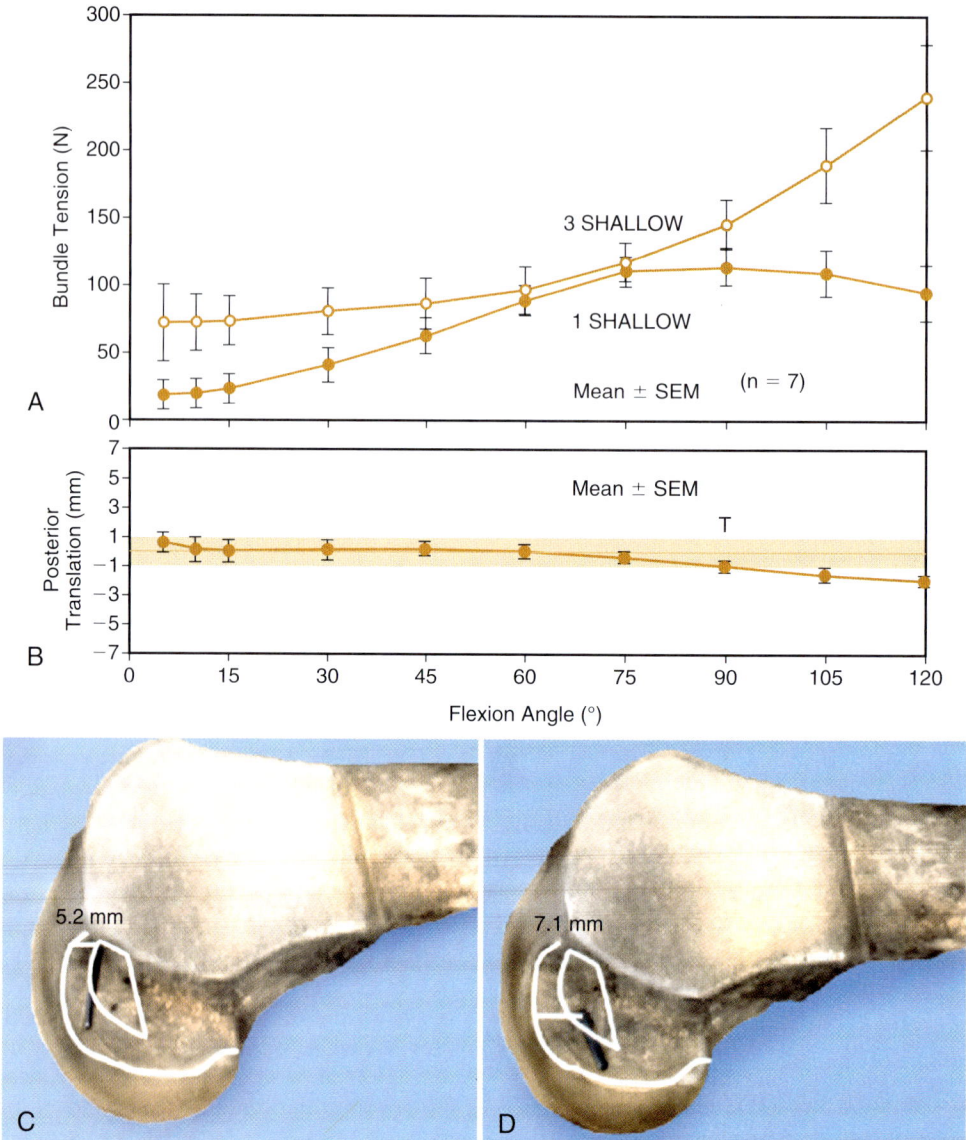

Figure 55-8. The graph shows the strand tension **(A)** and change in posterior translation from intact **(B)** for the one shallow and two shallow two-strand reconstruction with a 100-N posterior force. The T indicates the flexion angle at which the strands were tensioned. The shaded area for posterior translation represents the translation for the intact knee ±1 mm. The photographs show the **(A)** one shallow and **(B)** three shallow femoral tunnel placements. (From Mannor DA, Shearn JT, Grood ES, et al: Two-bundle posterior cruciate ligament reconstruction. An in vitro analysis of graft placement and tension. Am J Sports Med 28: 833–845, 2000.)

reconstruction of these structures during the PCL reconstruction to allow load sharing and protection of the PCL graft during the healing process. The individual function of each of the posterolateral structures has been previously published.[71]

Varus and Valgus Rotations

Injury to the fibular collateral ligament (FCL) and posterolateral structures (popliteus muscle–tendon–ligament unit [PMTL], popliteofibular ligament [PFL], and posterolateral capsule) results in increases in lateral joint opening under varus loads and increases in posterior subluxation of the lateral tibial plateau with external tibial rotation. With these ligament injuries, the PCL is placed under higher than normal loading conditions. Figures 55-11 and 55-12 show the

relationship of the primary ligamentous restraints to medial and lateral joint opening and the PCL.[39] Normally, a small force is present in the PCL to both varus and valgus loads.[61] With injury to medial or lateral structures, the PCL and anterior cruciate ligament (ACL) may be placed in the role of a primary restraint that is not ideal, because their mechanical advantage in the center of the knee joint is not suited to resist medial and lateral joint openings. These biomechanical findings indicate the importance of determining an abnormal medial or lateral joint opening (subluxation) that requires surgical reconstruction. The failure to correct such associated subluxations places the PCL graft reconstruction under high in vivo forces postoperatively and risks graft failure.

Careful examination of the knee preoperatively and under anesthesia is required to determine whether abnormal motions and other ligament injuries are present that require

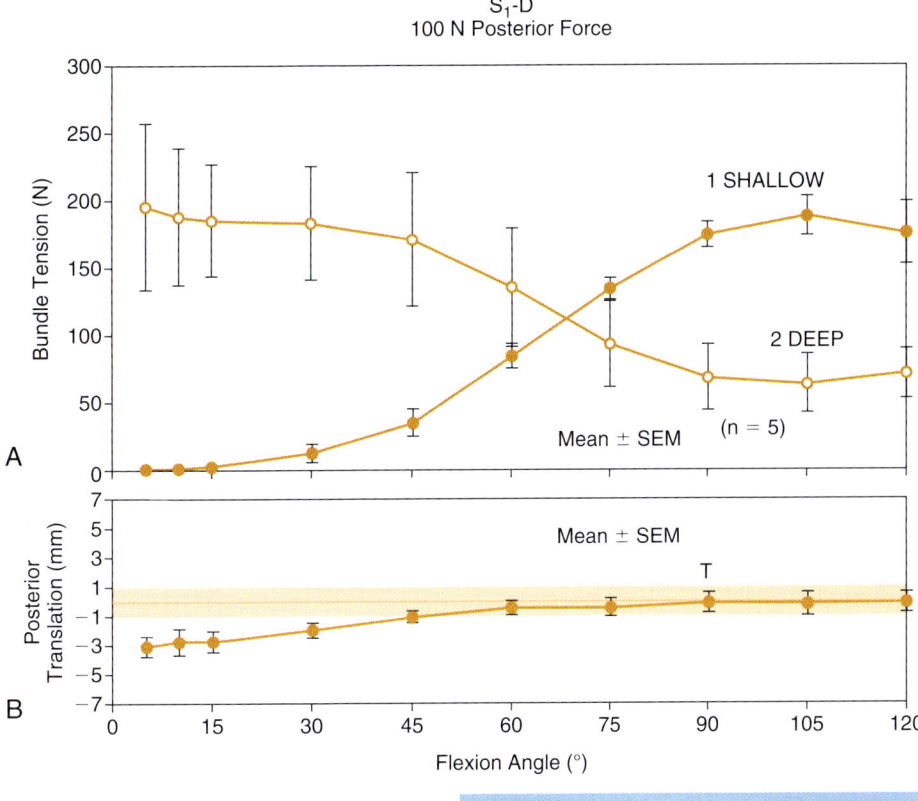

Figure 55-9. The graph shows the strand tension **(A)** and change in posterior translation from intact **(B)** for the one shallow and two-deep two-strand reconstruction with a 100-N posterior force. The T indicates the flexion angle where the strands were tensioned. The shaded area for posterior translation represents the translation for the intact knee ±1 mm. **C,** Photograph shows the two-deep femoral tunnel placement. (From Mannor DA, Shearn JT, Grood ES, et al: Two-bundle posterior cruciate ligament reconstruction. An in vitro analysis of graft placement and tension. Am J Sports Med 28: 833–845, 2000.)

reconstruction at the same time as the PCL. During the arthroscopic examination, the gap test confirms that excessive medial or lateral joint opening is not present, which would place abnormal loads on a PCL graft (Fig. 55-13). The goal is to restore function of any insufficient ligamentous structure in one surgical setting. Both the ACL and PCL function in combination with the medial and lateral ligamentous structures in a complex system of primary and secondary restraints that establish the limits to rotations and translations that normally occur in the knee joint. Any insufficiency of two ligamentous structures results in a combination of subluxations involving the medial and lateral tibiofemoral compartments (see later).

Tibiofemoral Rotational Subluxations

Injury to the FCL and PLS produces an increase in external tibial rotation and a posterior subluxation of the lateral tibial plateau. There are two primary restraints to external tibial rotation, the PLS at low flexion angles and both the PLS and PCL at high flexion angles (Fig. 55-14). Careful examination of knees with suspected injury to these structures may show a marked increase in external tibial rotation and posterior translation of the lateral tibial plateau or only a slight increase in these abnormal knee motions.[91] The clinician's first goal is to diagnose all the possible knee subluxations and define the extent of injury to the PLS. In 1989, we first reported on a modification of existing rotation tests to diagnose tibial rotatory subluxations of the medial and lateral tibiofemoral compartments more accurately (dial or spin rotation test).[88] We then studied the amount of increased posterior subluxation of the medial and lateral tibial plateaus that result from injury to the PCL and PLS.[91] We found that sectioning of the PLS results in a significant mean increase in posterior translation of the lateral tibial plateau of 8.0 mm at 30 degrees of flexion over the intact state ($P < .01$). No significant increase of the

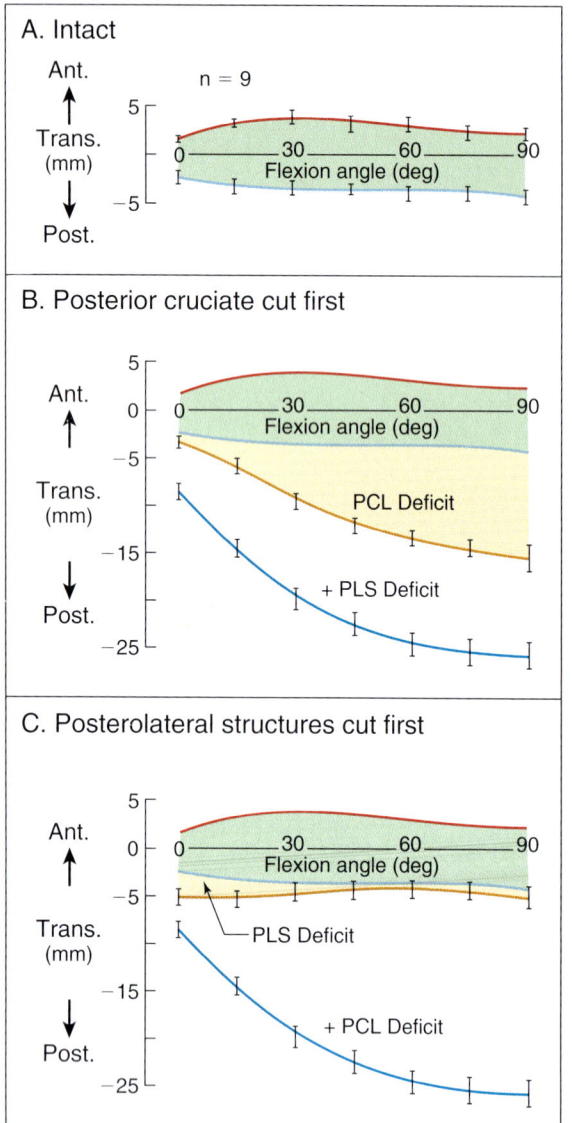

Figure 55-10. The curves show the limits of anterior and posterior translation *(vertical axis)* when a 100-N AP force was applied. **A,** Intact knees. The curves show the average limits of motion and the standard deviation for nine knees. The range of total AP translation of the intact knee is shown shaded green in **A-C. B,** Posterior cruciate ligament (PCL) cut first. The increase in posterior translation after cutting the PCL is shown in the blue shaded area (PCL deficit). The limit of posterior translation, and therefore the amount of increase, is controlled by the remaining intact structures. The unshaded portion (+ PLS deficit) shows the added increase when the posterolateral structures (FCL, capsule, PMTL) were cut after the PCL had first been removed. A concurrent external rotation took place with this cut. **C,** Posterolateral structures cut first. There was only a small increase (PLS deficit) in the posterior limit near full extension when the posterolateral structural elements were cut first. A concurrent external rotation was also present. (Adapted from Noyes FR, Barber-Westin SD: Function of the posterior cruciate ligament and posterolateral ligament structures. In Noyes FR [ed]: Noyes' knee disorders: surgery, rehabilitation, clinical outcomes, Philadelphia, 2009, Saunders, pp 467–502.)

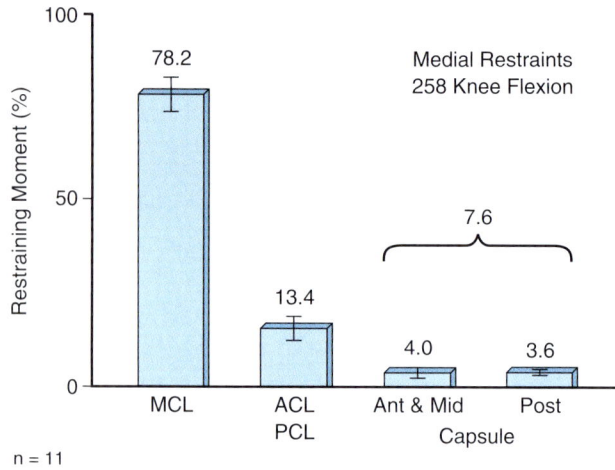

n = 11
5 mm Joint Opening

Figure 55-11. The percentage contributions to the medial restraints by the ligaments and capsule at 5 mm of medial joint opening and 25 degrees of flexion. The error bars represent ± one standard error of the mean. (Adapted from Noyes FR, Grood ES: The scientific basis for examination and classification of knee ligament injuries. In Noyes FR [ed]: Noyes' knee disorders: surgery, rehabilitation, clinical outcomes, Philadelphia, 2009, Saunders, pp 47–88.)

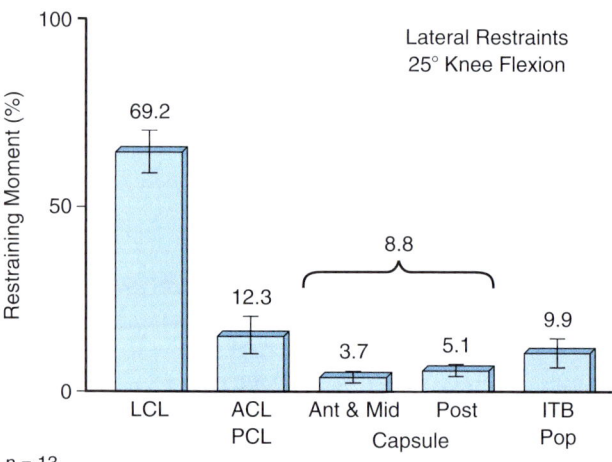

n = 13
5 mm Joint Opening

Figure 55-12. The percentage contributions to the lateral restraints by the ligaments and capsule at 5 mm of lateral joint opening and 25 degrees of flexion. The error bars represent ± one standard error of the mean. (Adapted from Noyes FR, Grood ES: The scientific basis for examination and classification of knee ligament injuries. In Noyes FR [ed]: Noyes' knee disorders: surgery, rehabilitation, clinical outcomes, Philadelphia, 2009, Saunders, pp 47–88.)

lateral tibial plateau occurred at 90 degrees of flexion. There was no significant increase in posterior translation of the medial tibial plateau at either flexion angle. After sectioning both the PCL and PLS, significant increases in posterior translation of the medial and lateral tibial plateaus occurred at 30 and 90 degrees of flexion ($P < .01$). The increase in posterior translation of the lateral tibial plateau averaged 17.8 and 23.5 mm at 30 and 90 degrees of flexion, respectively, and the increase in posterior translation of the medial tibial plateau averaged 7.6 and 12.3 mm at 30 and 90 degrees, respectively.

From the results of this study, we concluded that the diagnosis of injury to the PLS should be made based on the final

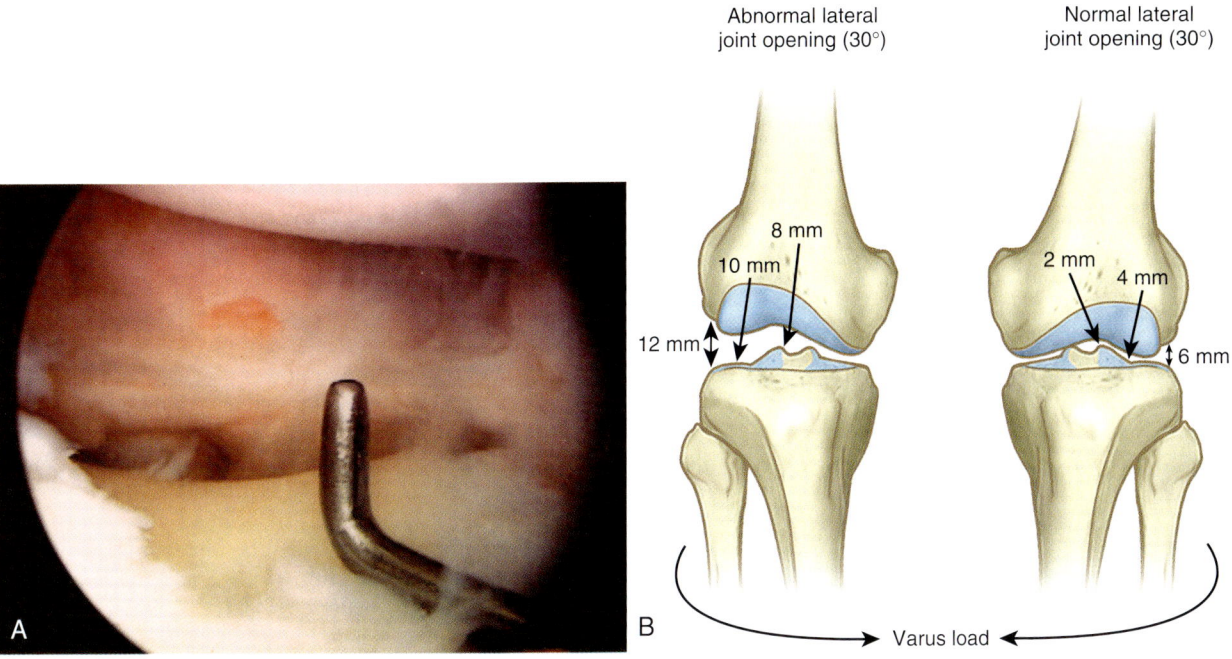

Figure 55-13. **A,** Arthroscopic demonstration of the lateral joint opening—gap test. The amount of lateral joint opening is measured with the knee at 25 degrees flexion. **B,** Knees with insufficiency of the posterolateral structures will demonstrate 12 mm of joint opening at the periphery of the lateral tibiofemoral compartment, 10 mm of opening at the midportion of the compartment, and 8 mm at the inner most medial edge. (From Noyes FR, Barber-Westin SD: Primary, double, and triple varus knee syndromes: diagnosis, osteotomy techniques, and clinical outcomes. In Noyes FR [ed]: Noyes' knee disorders: surgery, rehabilitation, clinical outcomes, Philadelphia, 2009, Saunders, pp 821–895.)

position of the lateral tibial plateau and not on the amount of increased external tibial rotation alone. An increase in external tibial rotation can occur with anterior subluxation of the medial tibial plateau, posterior subluxation of the lateral tibial plateau, or a combination of both subluxations. In a prior investigation,[86] we found that clinicians often misdiagnose injuries to the PLS because of misinterpretation of the increase in external tibial rotation as a posterior subluxation of the lateral tibial plateau, when in fact there was a subluxation of the medial tibial plateau caused by injury to the medial collateral ligament (MCL) alone or in combination with the ACL.

We have recommended that during the rotation tests to determine rotatory subluxations of the tibial plateaus, the examiner carefully palpate the position of each tibial plateau to determine qualitatively whether an anterior or posterior subluxation is present. We and others[15,16] have reported that it is not possible to determine the actual millimeters of translation of the medial and lateral tibial plateaus in reference to the femoral condyle. Thus, a qualitative determination of whether the reference tibial plateau is anteriorly or posteriorly subluxated is recommended. The inability to measure tibiofemoral compartment translations precisely, and to quantify the amount of posterolateral subluxation, creates problems in deciding whether surgical correction is warranted.

A classification system of rotatory subluxations was previously described based on two concepts—determining the final position of the medial and lateral tibial plateaus under defined loading conditions (e.g., with either internal or external tibial rotation at a defined knee flexion angle) and classifying the position of each plateau.[91] There are three possible positions for each plateau: anterior subluxation, normal

position, or posterior subluxation. For each of these positions of the lateral tibial plateau, there are three corresponding positions for the medial tibial plateau (Fig. 55-15).

When a posterior subluxation of the lateral tibial plateau is positively identified by the described tibiofemoral rotation test, the examiner performs additional tests to determine whether ruptures exist to other ligamentous structures. The amount of lateral joint opening at 0 and 20 degrees of knee flexion should be determined (and quantified by stress radiography when possible) to determine the integrity of the FCL and PLS.[40] The presence of a varus recurvatum in both the supine and standing positions must be carefully assessed. The difference in results of these tests between the injured and contralateral normal knee is compared because of inherent physiologic looseness that is present in some individuals. The different type of subluxations after posterolateral injuries depends on whether there is a concomitant rupture to the ACL or PCL.

CLINICAL EVALUATION

Physical Examination

A comprehensive examination of the knee joint is required to detect all abnormalities (Fig. 55-16). This includes assessment of the following: (1) patellofemoral joint and extensor mechanism malalignment; (2) patellofemoral and tibiofemoral crepitus, indicative of articular cartilage damage; (3) gait abnormalities (excessive hyperextension or varus thrust) during walking and jogging[87]; and (4) abnormal knee motion limits and subluxations compared with the contralateral knee.[88]

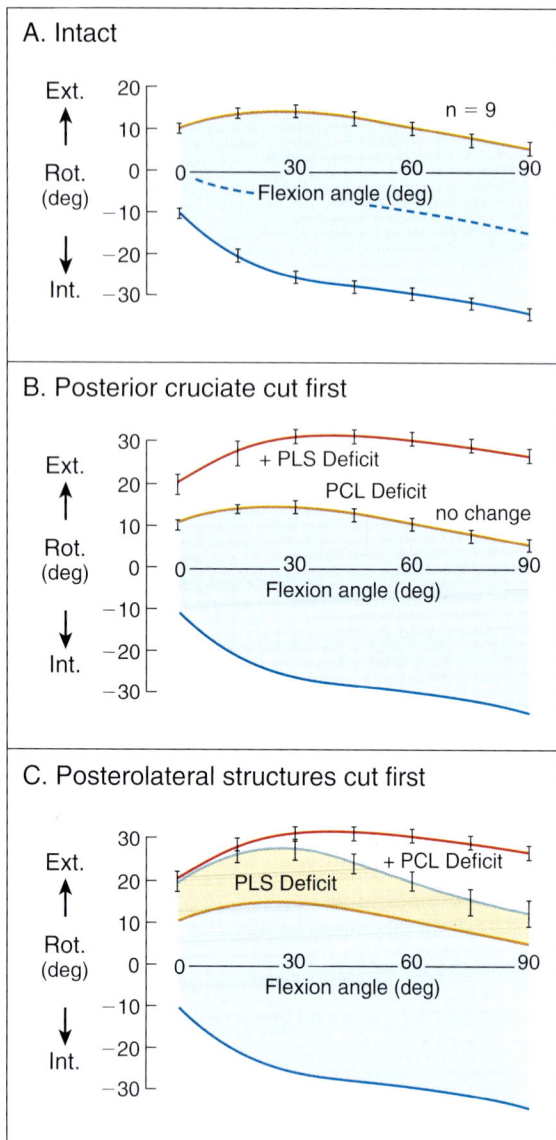

Figure 55-14. The limits of internal and external rotation of the tibia when a 5-N torque was applied. The fully extended position, measured in the intact knee, was used as the zero rotation reference. **A,** Intact knees. The upper curve shows the limit of external rotation. The *dashed line* shows the average position of the knee during passive flexion with the tibia hanging freely. The range of tibial rotation in the intact knee is shaded in **A-C. B,** Posterior cruciate ligament cut first. No change was found in external tibial rotation. **C,** Posterolateral structures (FCL, capsule, PMTL) cut first. Increases in external tibial rotation occurred at low flexion angles. With added PCL sectioning, the increase in external tibial rotation occurred at high flexion angles. (Adapted from Noyes FR, Barber-Westin SD: Function of the posterior cruciate ligament and posterolateral ligament structures. In Noyes FR [ed]: Noyes' knee disorders: surgery, rehabilitation, clinical outcomes, Philadelphia, 2009, Saunders, pp 467–502.)

Experienced clinicians are aware that patients with chronic deficiency of the PCL and PLS may develop an abnormal gait pattern, which is characterized by excessive knee hyperextension during the stance phase.[87] Subjective complaints of knee instability and giving way during routine daily activities, along with severe quadriceps atrophy, often accompany this gait abnormality. Gait analysis and retraining

are required in patients who demonstrate abnormal knee hyperextension patterns before proceeding with any ligament reconstruction. The failure to do so may lead to failure of reconstructed ligaments if the abnormal gait pattern is resumed postoperatively.

Diagnostic Clinical Tests

The medial posterior tibiofemoral step-off on the posterior drawer test is performed at 90 degrees of flexion. The amount of posterior tibial translation will vary among knees with isolated PCL ruptures because of physiologic laxity or injury to the secondary posterolateral or medial soft tissue restraints. Posterior tibial translation progressively increases with injury to the secondary restraints.

The exact determination of the extent of a PCL tear (partial versus complete) can be difficult, but is essential from a therapeutic standpoint. The clinical posterior drawer test can be highly subjective, with the forces applied too variable to allow accurate determination of the status of the PCL. MRI is not always accurate for diagnosing partial PCL tears. Frequently, this test may indicate that the ligament is completely ruptured; however, ligament continuity may still exist, with some portions functioning to limit posterior tibial subluxation to only a few millimeters.[96]

The quantitative measurement of posterior tibial subluxation in knees with PCL ruptures or reconstruction is therefore important.[43] The knee arthrometer is the most frequently used device to measure posterior tibial translation following PCL injury and reconstruction. However, this device underestimates the true amount of posterior translation in PCL-deficient and reconstructed knees, often by several millimeters.[58,121] Stress radiography is the most accurate and reproducible technique currently available.[25,28,98,107] We recommend that PCL clinical investigations incorporate stress radiography to provide a more valid measure of posterior tibial translation (Figs. 55-17 and 55-18).

The integrity of the ACL is determined by Lachman and pivot shift tests. The result of the pivot shift test is recorded on a scale of 0 to 3, with a grade of 0 indicating no pivot shift; grade 1, a slip or glide; grade 2, a jerk with gross subluxation or clunk; and grade 3, gross subluxation, with impingement of the posterior aspect of the lateral side of the tibial plateau against the femoral condyle. Knee arthrometer testing may be done at 20 degrees of flexion (134-N force) to quantify total anteroposterior (AP) displacement.

Medial and lateral ligament insufficiency are determined by varus and valgus stress testing at 0 and 30 degrees of knee flexion. The surgeon estimates the amount of joint opening (in millimeters) between the initial closed contact position of each tibiofemoral compartment, performed in a constrained manner to avoid internal or external tibial rotation, to the maximal opened position. The result is recorded according to the increase in the tibiofemoral compartment of the affected knee compared with that of the opposite normal knee.

The tibiofemoral rotation dial test at 30 and 90 degrees is done to determine whether increases in external tibial rotation exist with posterior subluxation of the lateral tibial plateau (see earlier).[88]

The presence of a varus recurvatum in both the supine and standing positions is carefully assessed.

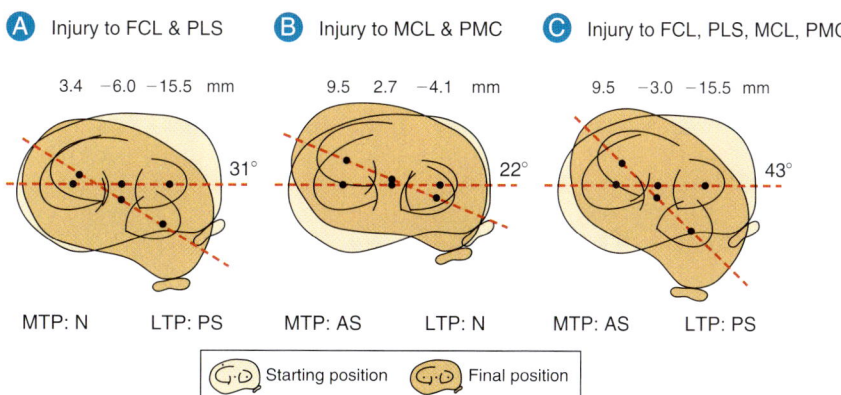

A Injury to FCL & PLS
B Injury to MCL & PMC
C Injury to FCL, PLS, MCL, PMC
3.4 −6.0 −15.5 mm
9.5 2.7 −4.1 mm
9.5 −3.0 −15.5 mm
31°
22°
43°
MTP: N LTP: PS
MTP: AS LTP: N
MTP: AS LTP: PS
Starting position
Final position

Figure 55-15. Three types of tibiofemoral situations observed with increased external tibial rotation. **A,** Abnormal posterior translation of the lateral tibial plateau (at 30 degrees of knee flexion under the loading conditions described in the study). **B,** Abnormal anterior translation of the medial tibial plateau under loading conditions of 5 Nm at 30 degrees of knee flexion. **C,** Abnormal posterior translation of the lateral tibial plateau plus abnormal anterior translation of the medial tibial plateau after sectioning both the medial and lateral ligament structures. *AS,* Anterior subluxation; *FCL,* lateral collateral ligament; *LTP,* lateral tibial plateau; *MCL,* medial collateral ligament; *MTP,* medial tibial plateau; *N,* normal position; *PLS,* posterolateral structures (FCL, PMTL); *PMC,* posterior medial capsule; *PS,* posterior subluxation. (From Noyes FR, Stowers SF, Grood ES, et al: Posterior subluxations of the medial and lateral tibiofemoral compartments. An in vitro ligament sectioning study in cadaveric knees. Am J Sports Med 21:407–414, 1993.)

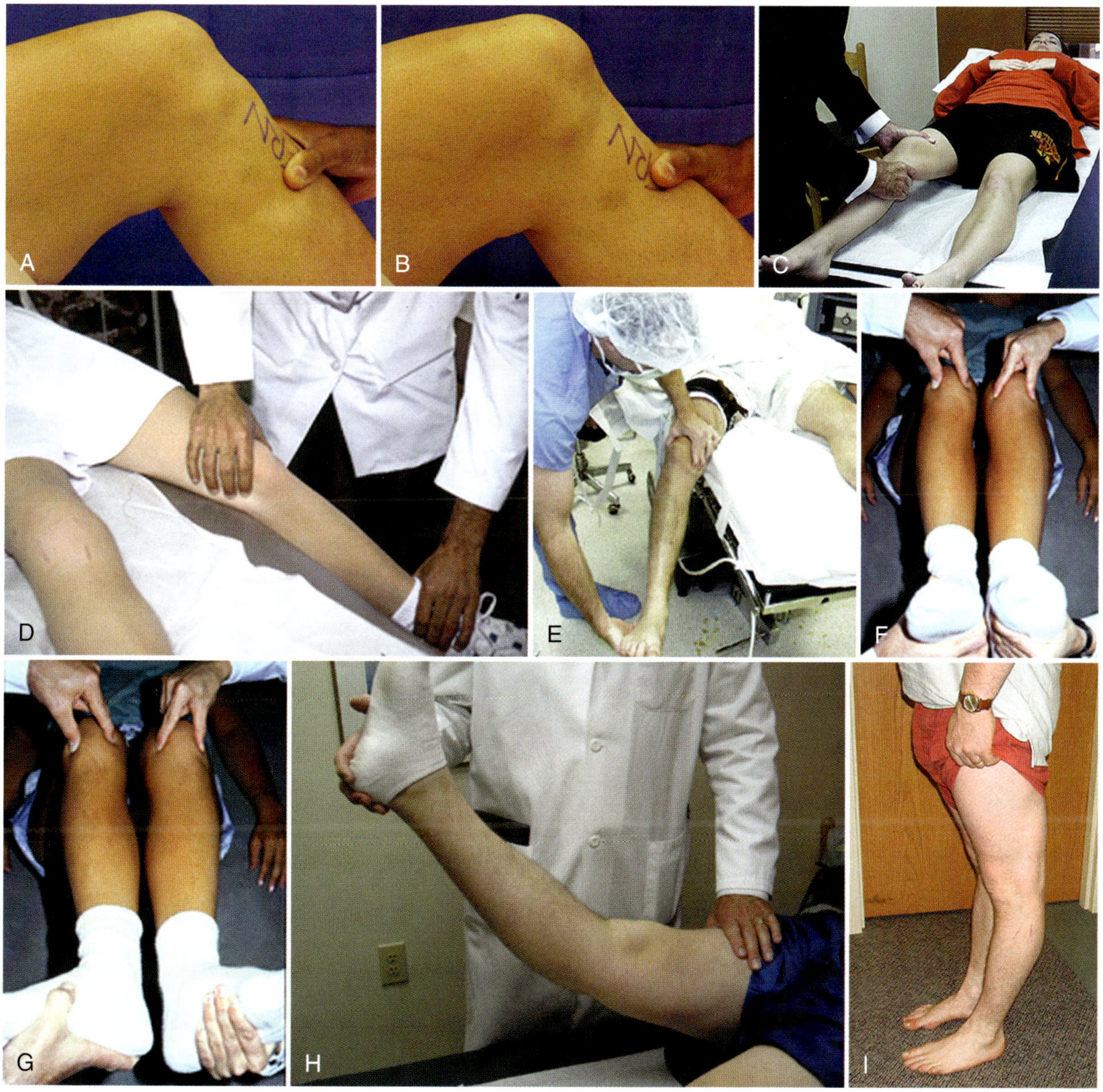

Figure 55-16. Manual knee tests. **A** and **B,** Posterior drawer test at 90 degrees knee flexion. **C,** Lachman test. **D,** Valgus manual test for medial joint opening. **E,** Valrus manual test for lateral joint opening. **F,** Dial test at 90 degrees of knee flexion in neutral tibial rotation and maximum external tibial rotation **(G)**. Varus recurvatum in the supine **(H)** and standing **(I)** positions. (From Noyes FR, Barber-Westin SD: Primary, double, and triple varus knee syndromes: diagnosis, osteotomy techniques, and clinical outcomes. In Noyes FR [ed]: Noyes' knee disorders: surgery, rehabilitation, clinical outcomes, Philadelphia, 2009, Saunders, pp 821–895.)

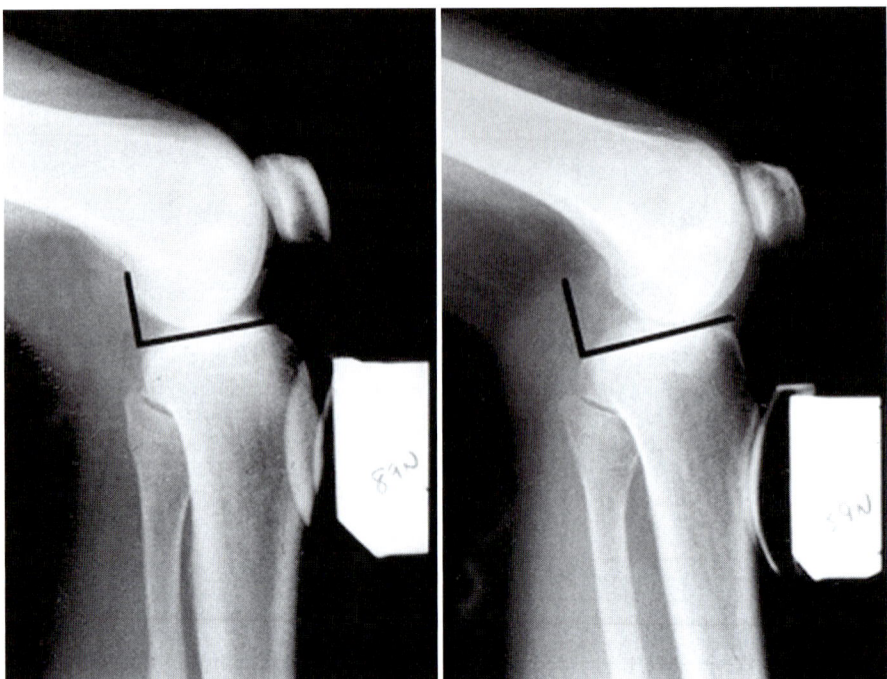

Figure 55-17. Lateral stress radiograph of a PCL-deficient knee demonstrating a 19-mm posterior drop-back (involved-noninvolved knee, 70 degrees knee flexion, 89 N). (From Noyes FR, Barber-Westin SD: Treatment of complex injuries involving the posterior cruciate and posterolateral ligaments of the knee. Am J Knee Surg 9: 200–214, 1996.)

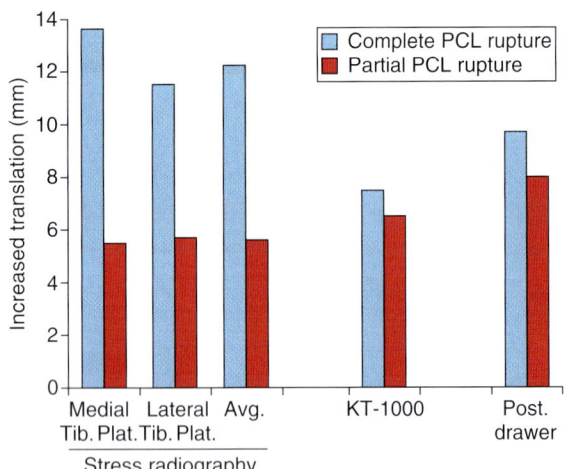

Figure 55-18. Results of lateral stress radiography on 20 patients with PCL deficiency (9 complete ruptures and 11 partial ruptures). The differences in the measurements between complete and partial PCL ruptures for the medial tibial plateau, lateral tibial plateau, and average of both plateaus were statistically significant ($P < .01$). Differences in the KT-1000 and posterior drawer measurements between complete and partial PCL ruptures were not significant. The KT measurements at 70 degrees flexion underestimated the magnitude of posterior tibial subluxation for complete PCL ruptures. (From Hewett TE, Noyes FR, Lee MD: Diagnosis of complete and partial posterior cruciate ligament ruptures. Stress radiography compared with KT-1000 arthrometer and posterior drawer testing. Am J Sports Med 25: 648–655, 1997.)

Imaging Studies

Radiographs taken during the initial examination include AP, lateral at 30 degrees of knee flexion, weight-bearing posteroanterior (PA) at 45 degrees of knee flexion, and patellofemoral axial views.

Posterior stress radiographs are done with an 89-N force applied to the proximal tibia (see Figs. 55-17 and 55-18).[43] A lateral radiograph is taken of each knee at 90 degrees of flexion. The limb is placed in neutral rotation with the tibia unconstrained and the quadriceps relaxed. The difference in posterior tibial displacement between the injured knee and contralateral knee is recorded. More than 8 mm of increase in posterior tibial translation on stress testing indicates a complete PCL rupture.[107]

Medial or lateral stress radiographs may be required of both knees. The patient is seated (0 degree of knee extension) in neutral tibial rotation with the tibia unconstrained. Approximately 89 N of varus or valgus force is applied and comparison made of the medial or lateral tibiofemoral compartment opening between knees (in millimeters).

Full standing radiographs of both lower extremities, from the femoral heads to the ankle joints, are done in knees in which varus lower extremity alignment is detected on clinical examination. The mechanical axis and weight-bearing line are measured to determine whether a high tibial osteotomy (HTO) is indicated before PCL reconstruction.[24,85] If the varus malalignment is not corrected, there is a risk that a PCL or ACL graft may fail because of the varus thrusting forces and concurrent increased lateral joint opening, producing high graft tension loads.[74]

MANAGEMENT CONSIDERATIONS

Posterior Cruciate Ligament Natural History

The treatment of complete isolated PCL ruptures remains controversial because of the unknown natural history of this injury in regard to long-term symptoms, functional limitations, and risk of joint arthritis. Although some studies that included patients with partial PCL deficiency have reported that patients do well when treated conservatively,* others[6,19,23,48] have described noteworthy symptoms and functional limitations years after the injury, which can be disabling. A high percentage of knees with complete PCL ruptures develop articular cartilage deterioration over time; this usually occurs on the medial femoral condyle and patellofemoral surfaces because of increased joint pressures.[6,34,35,123] Posterior tibial subluxation after PCL rupture has a deleterious effect to the knee, similar to that of a medial meniscectomy, because there is loss of medial meniscus function and increased joint contact stress. Posterior tibial subluxation results in a loss of normal joint kinematics (see Box 55-2) and in coupled external tibial rotation with joint loading.

*References 18, 29, 95, 111-113, 124, and 125.

Accordingly, a PCL rupture has a more deleterious effect in a varus-angulated knee with associated loss of the medial meniscus and, in particular, larger athletes desiring a return to strenuous athletics. All these factors result in substantial medial tibiofemoral loads and risk of joint deterioration.

Treatment of Acute Posterior Cruciate Ligament Ruptures

Controversy exists in regard to the treatment of midsubstance complete PCL ruptures, primarily because of the lack of a scientifically proven operative procedure that can restore posterior stability and PCL function predictably. In comparison, surgical procedures to reattach the native PCL in cases of bony avulsion injuries or peel-off injuries directly at the PCL attachment site have more predictable healing rates.[5,54,127,128] Even in cases of PCL rupture directly at the attachment site, there is usually sufficient ligament substance for a direct repair.

Augmentation of partial PCL tears is controversial.[2,46,132] Graft reconstruction of the so-called posteromedial portion of the PCL has been described in which the anterolateral bundle is still intact and functional. The senior author (FN) has not performed augmentation procedures to date.

The treatment rationale for patients with acute PCL ruptures is shown in Figure 55-19.[76] The algorithm is divided into

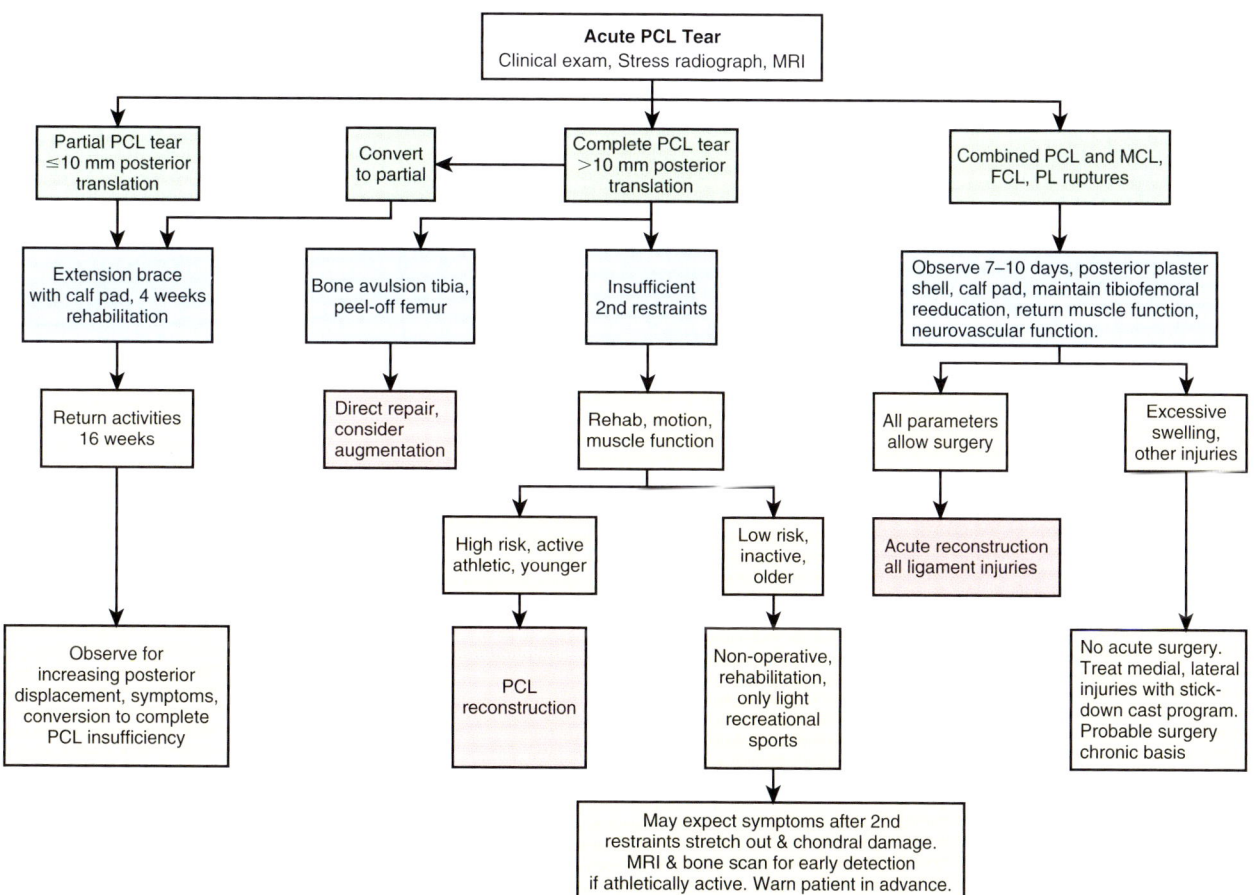

Figure 55-19. Treatment algorithm for acute PCL ruptures. (From Noyes FR, Barber-Westin SD: Posterior cruciate ligament: diagnosis, operative techniques, and clinical outcomes. In Noyes FR [ed]: Noyes' knee disorders: surgery, rehabilitation, clinical outcomes, Philadelphia, 2009, Saunders, pp 503–576.)

three major sections based on the PCL tear (partial, complete, or combined with other ligament ruptures). The 10-mm division is somewhat arbitrary.

The rules to treat partial or acute isolated PCL tears are shown in Box 55-4. In our experience, 4 weeks of protection to allow initial healing of a complete PCL rupture will frequently restore partial PCL function, with less than 10-mm residual posterior tibial subluxation. The initial PCL healing process involves low tensile strength and an additional 4 to 6 weeks of protection is recommended, including avoiding athletics, running, walking on downhill grades, walking down stairs, or other high knee flexion activities that load the PCL. Even in knees with a complete PCL tear and more than 10 mm of increased posterior tibial displacement, healing of the disrupted PCL fibers may still occur, although a residual posterior tibial subluxation of a few millimeters (with a hard end point) will remain. Knees in which partial PCL function has been restored should be routinely followed, with repeat stress radiographs obtained at 6 months and over the next few years to determine PCL function. These partial PCL tears seldom require reconstruction. A repeat MRI with fast spin-echo cartilage sequences[101] helps determine the integrity of the articular cartilage and provides important information for counseling the patient on athletic activities to decrease the risk of future joint arthritis.

In cases of complete isolated midsubstance PCL ruptures that have more than 10 mm of increased posterior tibial displacement, and the patient is seen late after the injury and the above program cannot be instituted, one treatment approach in athletes and strenuous occupations is PCL graft reconstruction before the secondary restraints stretch out, with subsequent reinjuries. We believe that in athletic individuals, PCL reconstructive procedures have advanced to the point where more predictable results can be expected to restore sufficient PCL function to prevent gross posterior tibial subluxation. Studies have demonstrated, at least in the short term, that most patients with acute PCL ruptures treated with reconstruction are able to return to various levels

of sports activities.[73] Additional factors to be weighed in the decision to perform early surgery on an isolated PCL rupture (with >10 mm posterior displacement at 90 degrees flexion) include athletic goals, body weight, medial meniscus or tibiofemoral joint damage, patellofemoral joint damage, and varus malalignment, because these factors add to the effects of the residual posterior subluxation in increasing knee joint loads and subsequent joint deterioration. Sedentary patients with a complete PCL rupture and more than 10 mm of posterior translation (90 degrees flexion) are not considered surgical candidates; however, they are followed as described earlier.

Patients with a PCL disruption and other ligament injuries have an obvious posterior tibial drop back without a firm end point on posterior drawer testing, and 10 mm or more of posterior tibial subluxation. In almost all these knees, some increase in medial or lateral joint opening or external tibial rotation can be detected, although the findings may be subtle. There may be physiologic laxity of other ligament structures without a true injury that allow for the gross posterior tibial subluxation.

In knees that have associated posterolateral ruptures, acute anatomic repair is required within 14 days before scarring occurs and the ability to restore these structures anatomically is lost. A similar situation exists for the medial ligament structures; however, these tissues are easier to reconstruct later if surgery cannot be performed during the ideal time period for anatomic repair. There may exist a displaced meniscus tear requiring early treatment. As a word of caution, a displaced meniscus should be reduced into the tibiofemoral joint by 3 weeks to prevent meniscus shortening and scarring, which compromise a future repair and result in loss of meniscus function. Even in knees that have marked soft tissue swelling and edema, and in which major ligament reconstruction is contraindicated, a meniscus repair procedure using all-inside techniques can be performed to reduce the meniscus to a normal tibiofemoral position. The mistake is to wait until 6 weeks or later, expecting that the meniscus repair can be performed at that time.

Too frequently, major ligament surgery in dislocated knees performed under acute conditions results in joint arthrofibrosis, compromising the result. Patients should be carefully selected for acute multiligament repairs, realizing that there are proven techniques for reconstruction of the ruptured ligaments performed later under more ideal conditions. When surgery is performed on acute combined PCL and posterolateral ruptures, the procedure includes the use of appropriate grafts to restore lateral stability and allow an early protected range of knee motion program.[77] Most acute knee dislocations should be treated in a staged approach, first by treating the acute injury and then determining whether a ligament reconstruction should be performed within the 10- to 14-day envelope or delayed. When early surgery is not advisable, the knee is protected for the first 4 weeks to prevent posterior tibial subluxation, as described earlier for acute isolated PCL ruptures. A lateral radiograph is obtained with the knee placed in a posterior plaster shell and a soft bolster positioned beneath the calf to prevent posterior tibial subluxation. The capsular tissues heal in 7 to 10 days to provide enough stability to prevent recurrence of dislocation.

There is a select group of morbidly obese patients who sustain serious knee dislocations with minimal trauma. The lack of protective muscle function and extreme body weight place abnormal tensile loads on ligament reconstructions, and a high rate of failure of a PCL reconstruction is expected. The preferred treatment for these patients is short-term plaster immobilization (and occasionally external fixation) to allow healing of soft tissues, followed by rehabilitation to return muscle function and knee motion. Only in exceptional circumstances would operative repair (acute or chronic) be warranted in these patients, although consideration for surgical reconstruction is warranted after appropriate weight reduction.

If a nonoperative approach is selected with associated MCL and posteromedial capsular disruptions, the same program is followed, with the lower limb placed in a cylinder cast to allow "stick-down" of the medial soft tissues. Plaster immobilization is required because a soft hinged brace, even

if maintained at 0 degree of extension, does not provide sufficient protection to maintain medial joint line closure to allow the disrupted medial tissues to heal. At 7 to 10 days, the cylinder cast is split into an anterior and posterior shell and the therapist assists the patient with range of motion from 0 to 90 degrees in a figure-of-four position, with the hip joint externally rotated to protect the healing medial tissues.

Treatment of Chronic Posterior Cruciate Ligament Ruptures

The algorithm for the treatment of chronic PCL ruptures is shown in Figure 55-20. The symptoms and clinical examination determine the functional limitations, particularly the component of symptoms caused by medial tibiofemoral or patellofemoral arthritis, because these problems are likely to

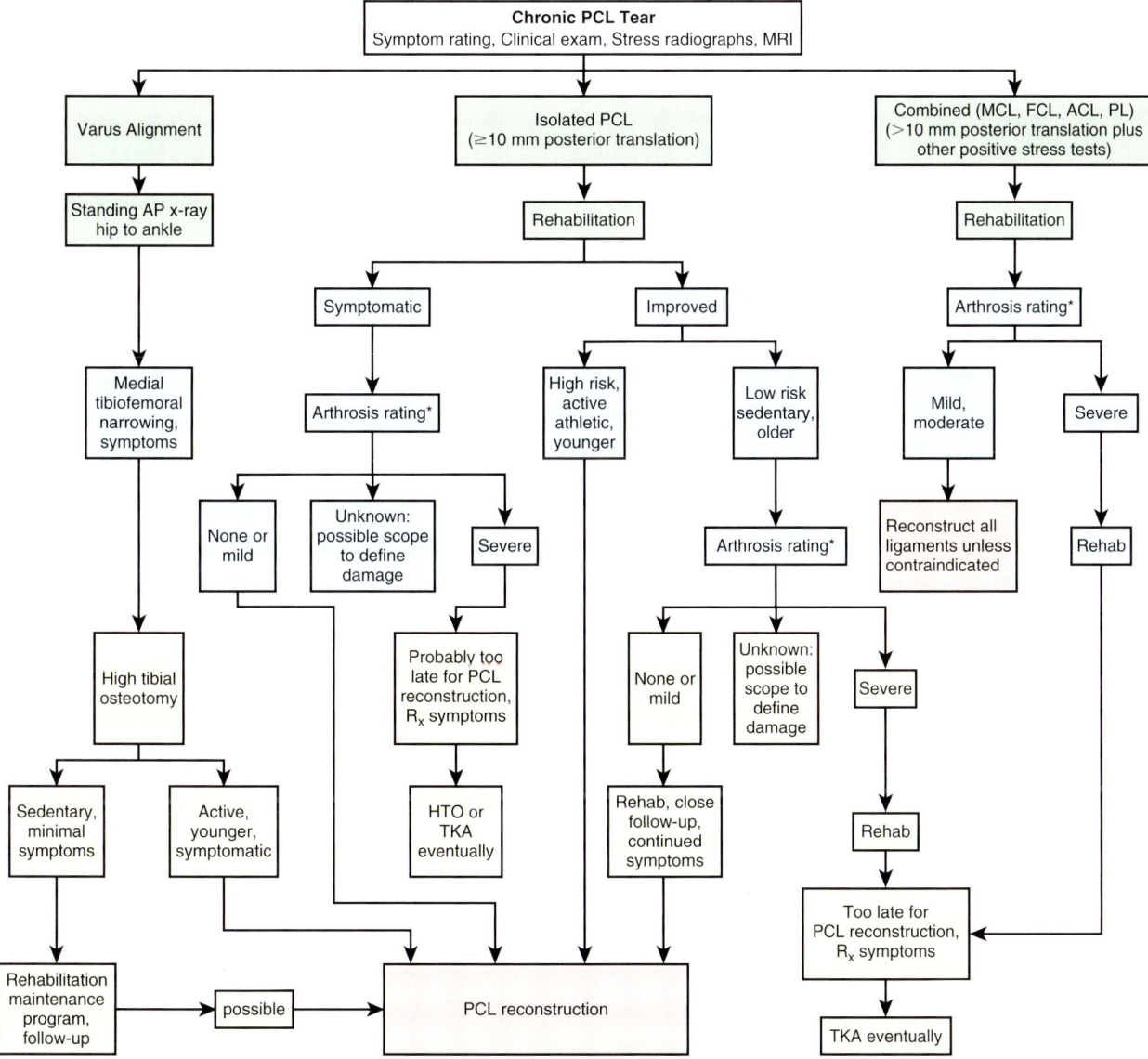

Figure 55-20. Treatment algorithm for chronic PCL ruptures. (From Noyes FR, Barber-Westin SD: Posterior cruciate ligament: diagnosis, operative techniques, and clinical outcomes. In Noyes FR [ed]: Noyes' knee disorders: surgery, rehabilitation, clinical outcomes, Philadelphia, 2009, Saunders, pp 503–576.)

persist after surgical stabilization. Knees with chronic PCL ruptures are arbitrarily divided into three categories—those with varus osseous malalignment (and, rarely, valgus malalignment) in which an osteotomy must be considered, those with an isolated PCL rupture in which reconstruction may or may not be necessary, and those with significant combined ligament injuries that require reconstruction.

Patients are entered into a formal rehabilitation program to correct muscular weakness and gait-related problems (hyperextension) when required. The amount of joint arthritis must be determined with accuracy. Radiographs (Merchant view, standing PA at 45 degrees) and MRI articular cartilage fast spin-echo sequences provide valuable information.

In knees with no or only mild articular cartilage damage, an assessment of the patient's goals and athletic desires may indicate the need to proceed with PCL reconstruction. The indications for surgical reconstruction in these knees are pain and instability with athletics or other activities, swelling, and 10 mm or more of increased posterior tibial translation at 90 degrees flexion.

Patients with chronic PCL deficiency who have severe muscle atrophy, loss of knee motion, or hyperextension gait abnormalities require extensive rehabilitation and gait retraining before reconstruction.[87]

Combined ligament ruptures that produce complex instability patterns require careful clinical assessment to detect all the joint subluxations and ligament deficiencies present. PCL reconstruction is most frequently performed in dislocated knees with gross instability caused by other ligament injuries to the ACL, MCL, or PLS.

The results of PCL reconstruction in knees with chronic ruptures are not as favorable as those that undergo reconstruction for acute injuries. This is because patients present with pain and swelling caused by joint deterioration, which often persists, even though some benefit may be gained from improved knee stability obtained from the operative procedure.[73] In these knees, areas of exposed bone are frequently encountered in the medial tibiofemoral compartment, along with diffuse cartilage fragmentation in the patellofemoral joint. In these individuals, even mildly strenuous exercises aggravate the joint arthritis symptoms and cannot be performed. The patient's initial experience with rehabilitation, and the inability to perform the required rehabilitation exercises, provides important information regarding the amount of joint arthritis that is present and joint symptoms, which are likely permanent.

If a nonoperative approach is elected, the clinician should warn the patient that the return to athletic activities may carry an uncertain prognosis and that although sports may be resumed in the short term, some form of joint arthritis will eventually ensue. It is therefore important to follow the patient at regular intervals. A bone scan may be used to provide some indication of abnormal blood flow dynamics; however, it is our experience that the onset of pain and swelling usually indicates more advanced joint damage and a poor prognosis after PCL reconstruction. An MRI scan with fast spin-echo[101] sequences provides a baseline for repeated studies at 1- to 2-year intervals. The nonoperative treatment protocol of chronic PCL injuries involves educating the patient to avoid activities such as lunges and other high knee flexion activities that increase posterior tibial subluxation.

OPERATIVE TECHNIQUES: CURRENT CONCEPTS

PCL operative techniques continue to evolve and clinical outcome studies remain limited to allow precise decision making. The senior author's (FN) recommended surgical approaches and relative advantages and disadvantages of each procedure are shown in Box 55-5.

First, the surgical approach of the all-inside or tibial inlay technique is chosen. The all-inside approach simulates the tibial inlay approach by placing the bone portion of the PCL graft directly at the posterior tibial attachment. In our experience, soft tissue grafts placed through a large tibial tunnel have an increased risk of failure because of delayed graft incorporation. When a soft tissue graft is placed at the tibia, the use of two tibial tunnels is preferred to allow better graft tunnel healing, although sometimes this is not possible in smaller knees. Others have described the historical technique that places the bone plug at the femoral site (inside-out or outside-in tunnel) and the collagenous portion through a single tibial tunnel. The most frequently used graft for this technique is the Achilles tendon-bone (AT-B) allograft. This technique is perhaps the easiest to master and is useful when surgical time is an issue, because it can be more difficult to pass the bone portion of the graft through the tibial tunnel.

Box 55-5   Recommended Surgical Approaches

All-Inside

Single tibial tunnel approach
- Bone plug in tunnel at posterior PCL attachment (same as inlay except tunnel)
- Avoids posterior dissection, operative time
- Projected results similar to tibial inlay

Two-tunnel femoral approach
- Provides better anatomic positioning along oval PCL attachment
- Advantage of graft incorporation over single large diameter graft
- Outside-in tunnel, graft interference screw with suture post
- Second option: single femoral tunnel for multi-ligament reconstruction where time, operative complexity warrants single tunnel, outside-in, screw and suture post

Tibial Inlay

Reserved for revision knees to bypass misplaced tibial tunnel (staged bone graft may be required)

Graft Selection

Isolated PCL rupture
1. Quadriceps tendon-patellar bone autograft, ipsilateral (rarely contralateral)
2. Bone-patellar tendon-bone allograft
3. Achilles tendon-bone allograft

PCL combined with other ligament rupture
- Use allograft listed above.
- Avoid large-diameter soft tissue allograft through tibial tunnel.
- Place bone plug at posterior tibia tunnel.
- No autograft should be harvested from the same knee.

Adapted from Noyes FR, Barber-Westin SD: Posterior cruciate ligament: diagnosis, operative techniques, and clinical outcomes. In Noyes FR (ed): Noyes' knee disorders: surgery, rehabilitation, clinical outcomes, Philadelphia, 2009, Saunders, pp 503–576.

Second, a large graft must be used that fills most of the PCL anatomic femoral and tibial footprints. At the femoral attachment, either a two-tunnel or a single rectangular bone plug placement will fulfill this requirement. A single large-diameter femoral tunnel may also be used; however, from a theoretical standpoint, this is considered less ideal, because portions of the graft may be outside the femoral footprint.

Third, the use of a bone-tendon-bone or bone-tendon graft offers the advantage of more secure fixation and superior healing of a bone plug compared with a soft tissue graft without bone plugs. It is important that high-strength graft fixation methods be used to withstand the large forces expected postoperatively.

The fourth principle is to use an autogenous graft in isolated PCL surgical procedures, when possible, because of higher success rates and healing compared with allografts.[72,73] In multiligament knee injuries, allograft tissues are usually required, although an autogenous graft may be harvested from the contralateral side in select knees. In combined ligament reconstructions, a quadriceps tendon–patellar bone (QT-PT) autograft is not removed from the same knee, because this adds to the morbidity of the operative procedure.

Surgical Options

Tibial Attachment Techniques: Arthroscopic All-Inside versus Open Tibial Inlay Approach

The arthroscopic all-inside technique is the senior author's (FN) preferred procedure because it avoids the added operative time and complexity of the posteromedial tibial inlay approach. The surgeon must have extensive arthroscopic experience to perform this procedure safely to identify the PCL posterior tibial attachment site, avoid penetration into the posterior capsule and subsequent damage to the neurovascular structures, and place the tibial tunnel into the anatomic PCL tibial footprint. Specially designed instruments, drill guides with safety stops for guide pins, and drills are available to lessen the serious risk of inadvertent penetration of instruments posteriorly and damage to neurovascular structures.

The all-inside arthroscopic technique is particularly advantageous in knees with multiple ligament ruptures. High-strength grafts are used to reconstruct the PCL and ACL, which are appropriately tensioned and fixed to reduce the tibiofemoral joint to its normal anteroposterior position. Medial or lateral operative approaches are used for concurrent medial and posterolateral ligament and soft tissue repairs or reconstructions. A combined ACL-PCL-MCL injury requires an all-arthroscopic approach for the ACL and PCL, followed by a limited medial dissection for repair of the medial tissues and meniscus attachments.

Exceptions include a PCL avulsion fracture from the tibial attachment and a PCL revision knee in which a prior tibial tunnel was used; a tibial inlay graft is required to bypass this tunnel. In these cases, loss of the normal bony architecture about the posterior tibial PCL attachment may be encountered and a tibial inlay bone graft is therefore required. In other PCL revision cases that have enlarged tibial tunnels, a staged bone graft procedure may be indicated, with the preference to use autogenous bone, supplemented with allograft bone when required. The bone grafting of the enlarged or misplaced tibial tunnel is first done from an anterior approach.

After the tunnel has healed, a tibial tunnel or tibial inlay PCL reconstruction may be performed, as indicated.

The open posteromedial tibial inlay technique places a tibial inlay graft securely into the posterior PCL tibial attachment site. This approach may be selected when only the PCL requires reconstruction. The tibial inlay graft provides ideal graft fixation and early healing. A two-strand autogenous QT-PB graft with two femoral tunnels has been described.[68,69]

The all-inside technique has the theoretical disadvantage of the collagenous portion of the graft abrading against the angulated posterior tibial tunnel. There are operative techniques designed to reduce this problem. These include creating a more oblique tibial tunnel drilled through the anterolateral tibia and carefully chamfering the tunnel exit. Collagen grafts with a large cross-sectional area and diameter are favored over those with a smaller area and diameter, in which any abrasion compromises graft strength. To decrease soft tissue graft abrasion at the tibial tunnel, the bone portion of the graft is placed in a tibial tunnel directly adjacent to the tunnel exit. The intent is to match the beneficial effect of the tibial inlay procedure and allow prompt osseous healing.

Biomechanical studies of PCL reconstructions have also shown the potential for graft abrasion and failure at the femoral attachment.[109] Operative techniques to protect against graft failure and abrasion are therefore required at both tibial and femoral attachment sites.

Posterior Cruciate Ligament Femoral Attachment Technique: Two-Tunnel versus Single-Tunnel Options

It is not difficult from a technical standpoint to use two well-placed femoral tunnels within the PCL femoral footprint from outside-in and, in our opinion is the most ideal technique to master. When the tibia inlay or tibial tunnel bone plug two-strand graft procedure is selected, two femoral tunnels are created, using the outside-in technique with a limited anteromedial subvastus approach. This allows graft tensioning, a long femoral tunnel for graft incorporation, and graft fixation with a suture post. This is our preferred technique with an autograft or allograft.

The 4 o'clock posterior PCL graft strand is shorter by at least 15 mm compared with the 1 o'clock anterior graft strand. The outside-in tunnel approach allows accurate tensioning, fixation, and visualization of the graft length change during knee flexion. This allows the surgeon to determine the ideal knee flexion position for graft fixation.

In the alternative technique described, in which the bone portion of the graft is placed at the femoral site, a rectangular femoral slot technique is preferred. The bone plug is fixed with an inside-out arthroscopic technique. The rectangular slot technique places the bone within the PCL femoral footprint, which is more ideal than a single large diameter tunnel, although either technique may be used. One or two tibial tunnels are used for the collagenous portion of the graft. In a PCL revision procedure, there may be a misplaced femoral tunnel, in which the bone portion of the graft is preferred over one or two soft tissue femoral graft tunnels.

A single femoral tunnel drilled from an inside-out anterolateral portal is more difficult because of the narrow intercondylar notch, proximity of the lateral femoral condyle, placement of the tunnel within the PCL footprint, and need to avoid too proximal (deep) placement of the tunnel with portions of the graft outside the PCL footprint. For these reasons, the outside-in drilling approach for a single large-diameter femoral graft tunnel is recommended.

There are techniques for inside-out drilling of tunnels and fixation of soft tissue grafts at the femoral attachment site using interference screws, similar to those performed in ACL reconstructions.[44] However, these techniques result in lower attachment strength. The outside-in approach allows graft sutures and a suture post to be incorporated. PCL reconstructions are under high in vivo loads and it is advantageous to select graft fixation methods that provide for maximum tensile strength of the graft construct.[8,60,117]

Single-Strand versus Two-Strand Posterior Cruciate Ligament Graft Constructs

The advantages and disadvantages of one- and two-strand PCL graft techniques are summarized in Table 55-1. The goal of adding a second strand is to place additional collagenous tissue within the PCL footprint to increase the cross-sectional area of the graft and replicate the native PCL attachment more closely. This theoretical advantage is sometimes referred to as the mass action effect of adding additional collagen within the PCL footprint. The improved stability and clinical success of a two-strand graft construct compared with a single-strand graft have not been demonstrated clinically. However, some studies have shown that a single graft strand obtains results similar to a two-strand procedure.[10,22,26]

The incorporation of a second graft strand has the theoretical advantage of providing additional collagen tissue for load sharing, which decreases stress in the collagen fibers, increases graft strength, and reduces cyclic fatigue of the graft construct.[109,133] The two graft strands are tensioned at surgery to share loads that decrease the loads compared with those of a single PCL graft construct.

Studies have shown that a single graft will restore posterior translation limits to normal after PCL sectioning,[4,57,110] but often at the expense of high graft tensile forces. Therefore, the theoretical advantage of the second graft strand is to lower the high graft forces placed on a single graft strand and decrease graft failure from cyclic loading.

A justification to add a second PCL graft strand is the frequent notation in clinical studies that at high knee flexion angles, there is a residual posterior tibial drop-back in most

Table 55-1 Basis for the Selection of One- Versus Two-Strand Posterior Cruciate Ligament Reconstruction

Parameter	Single Strand	Two-Strand
Greater area	−	+
Load sharing (decreased tensile forces in each graft strand)	−	+
Operative complexity	+	−
Cyclic fatigue	−	+
Clinical results (residual posterior tibial translation)*	Unknown	Unknown

From Noyes FR, Barber-Westin SD: Posterior cruciate ligament: diagnosis, operative techniques, and clinical outcomes. In Noyes FR (ed): Noyes' knee disorders: surgery, rehabilitation, clinical outcomes, Philadelphia, 2009, Saunders, pp 503-576.

+, Relative advantage; −, relative disadvantage.

*Proven by objective measurements, including stress radiography at 90 degrees of knee flexion.

PCL reconstructions.[73] There is no question that current PCL surgical procedures are not uniformly accomplishing a functional restoration of normal joint kinematics and stability postoperatively. The concern is that residual posterior tibial displacement decreases the ability of the medial meniscus, and perhaps the lateral meniscus as well, to function,[97] thereby increasing tibiofemoral contact pressures.[53,116] Increases in patellofemoral contact pressures have also been reported.[35]

There are two types of two-strand PCL graft constructs. The first is a QT-PB graft with the bone plug placed at the femoral or tibial attachment and the tendon split into two strands, which are tensioned separately and ideally placed in two separate tunnels. The second option is use of two separate grafts that are placed into two separate femoral and tibial tunnels. It is not known for purposes of load sharing between graft strands with knee flexion whether there is any difference between a single and two separate bone attachments. In our opinion, there is no functional difference between these two graft constructs that can be measured.

Another technique passes two bone plugs through a single tibial tunnel; one bone plug is sutured to the tendon just proximal to the other bone plug, placing the two bone plugs in series. Sutures are inserted into each bone plug and an interference screw is added in the tibial tunnel. It is difficult to pass the double graft construct into the tibial bone tunnel, which is drilled 1 to 2 mm larger in diameter. This technique is not recommended; we prefer instead to use a larger diameter single tibial tunnel with an appropriately sized single bone plug and two graft strands and tunnels at the femoral attachment.

When an AT-B allograft is selected, it is important that the graft be inspected and discarded if it has a narrow tendon section just adjacent to the bone attachment. A QT-PB allograft is a more suitable PCL substitute because of the larger cross-sectional area of the tendon; however, this graft is more difficult to obtain from tissue banks.

Multicenter randomized controlled trials of one- and two-strand PCL reconstructions are required in the future to provide a more scientific basis for selection of one type of graft procedure over another. The surgeon is currently faced with small clinical trials with level 4 evidence (see later). Thus, more than one PCL technique is described, with recommendations made regarding the technical issues to maximize the clinical result. Our preferred PCL graft procedures are provided, along with the justification and rationale for these selections. In addition, it is necessary to use a case by case basis for selecting the appropriate surgical procedure in multiligament knee injuries.

In summary, it appears that there are sound theoretical reasons to warrant a two-strand PCL reconstruction when clinically feasible. These conditions include isolated PCL reconstructions when the added time required to perform a two-strand PCL graft does not represent a contraindication in terms of operative time and complexity. In multiligament reconstructions, the primary goal is to repair and reconstruct all ruptured ligaments. Adding a second femoral tunnel, and tensioning and securing two graft strands, may be time-consuming in an already complex surgical reconstruction. Therefore, the surgeon should be prepared, based on the operative findings, to modify the preoperative plan when required. In certain multiligament injured knees, a single-strand PCL graft construct may offer a reasonable opportunity to restore functional stability.[59] Given the complex PCL fiber microgeometry, a single- or two-strand graft construct still represents an imperfect substitution, providing only a check rein effect for controlling joint motions and subluxations.

Posterior Cruciate Ligament Grafts for Tibial Inlay and All-Inside Techniques

The goal of PCL surgery is to select a graft that matches the structural properties of the PCL as closely as possible. The problem is that the PCL is a highly complex ligament, composed of fibers of different lengths that are brought into the loading configuration based on knee flexion and tibial rotation positions. The data show initial graft mechanical properties that are expected to decline after graft implantation and in vivo remodeling. It is thus not possible to match the complex PCL microgeometry with any tendon substitute. The principles for the selection of all-inside grafts are summarized in Table 55-2.

INTRAOPERATIVE EVALUATION

The patient is instructed to use a chlorhexidine soap scrub of the operative limb (toes to groin) the evening before and

Table 55-2 All-Inside PCL Graft Options

Two-Strand Grafts	Single Strand Grafts
Preferred	**Preferred**
QT-PB autograft 1. Single tibial tunnel bone plug at posterior tunnel exit 2. Femur—two strand, two tunnels	QT-PB autograft 1. Tibial tunnel—bone plug at posterior tunnel exit 2. Femoral tunnel—one strand outside-in tunnel, interference screw plus suture post
Alternatives	**Alternatives**

Femoral attachment, two tunnels
  BPTB allograft
  QT-PB allograft
  AT-B allograft
	BPTB allograft
	QT-PB allograft
	AT-B allograft

Principles	**Principles**
• Allografts have lower success rate, delayed healing • Bone graft plug provides secure fixation, faster healing, increased graft construct tensile strength compared with soft tissue grafts • Rehabilitation, return to activity delayed with allografts • Avoid single small-diameter BPTB autograft; second graft required to achieve native PCL width • Graft selection rules still empirical until randomized controlled clinical trials performed	• Allograft provides acceptable results in multiligament reconstructions, dislocated knees with operative complexity, when time warrants single-tunnel procedure • Preference for bone plug at posterior tibial tunnel to avoid large-diameter soft tissue graft through tibia with delayed graft incorporation

From Noyes FR, Barber-Westin SD: Posterior cruciate ligament: diagnosis, operative techniques, and clinical outcomes. In Noyes FR (ed): Noyes' knee disorders: surgery, rehabilitation, clinical outcomes, Philadelphia, 2009, Saunders, pp 503–576.

morning of surgery. Lower extremity hair is removed by clippers and not a shaver. Antibiotic infusion is begun 1 hour prior to surgery. In complex multiligament surgery, the antibiotic is repeated at 4 hours and continued for 24 hours. Both the patient and surgeon initialize the knee skin area before entering the operating room, with a nurse observing the procedure. The identification process is repeated with all operative personnel, with a time out before surgery to verify the knee undergoing surgery, procedure, allergies, antibiotic infusion, and special precautions that apply.

All knee ligament subluxation tests are performed after the induction of anesthesia in both the injured and contralateral limbs. The amount of increased anterior tibial translation, posterior tibial translation, lateral joint opening, and external tibial rotation is documented. In acute knee injuries, arthroscopic pressure is maintained at a low setting, with adequate outflow at all times to prevent fluid extravasation. A thorough arthroscopic examination should be conducted, documenting articular cartilage surface abnormalities[90] and the condition of the menisci.

The medial and lateral tibiofemoral gap test is done during the arthroscopic examination.[83] The knee is flexed 30 degrees and a varus and valgus load of approximately 89 N is applied. A calibrated nerve hook is used to measure the amount of lateral and medial tibiofemoral compartment opening. Twelve mm or more of joint opening at the periphery of the compartment indicates the need for a combined lateral or medial ligament reconstructive procedure to protect and unload the PCL reconstruction.

Appropriate arthroscopic procedures are performed as indicated, including meniscal repairs or partial excision, débridement, and articular cartilage procedures.

Posterior Cruciate Ligament Graft Harvest Options

Quadriceps Tendon–Patellar Bone Autograft

A tourniquet is inflated to 275 mm of pressure.[76] This is usually the only time that the tourniquet is used in the reconstructive procedure, except when the open tibial inlay approach is selected. An incision is made just medial to the superior pole of the patella and extended proximally 5 to 6 cm (Fig. 55-21). The incision also allows access to the anteromedial aspect of the medial femoral condyle and vastus medialis oblique (VMO) for subvastus placement of the femoral tunnels. A cosmetic approach is used, with subcutaneous dissection performed circumferentially about the incision to allow the skin to be mobilized superiorly and inferiorly for the graft harvest. With this technique, there is no incision required over the patella.

The graft length and thickness are marked on the tendon and the proximal musculotendinous junction is avoided, which would weaken the extensor mechanism. The quadriceps tendon appears more narrow proximally and it is important not to remove more than one third of the tendon. In some patients, there is a shortened quadriceps tendon that is not suitable for harvest; the patient is advised preoperatively and provides consent for an autograft or allograft approach. The quadriceps tendon graft should ideally be 70 mm in length, not counting the patellar bone plug. The full-thickness quadriceps tendon graft is taken from the central tendon and

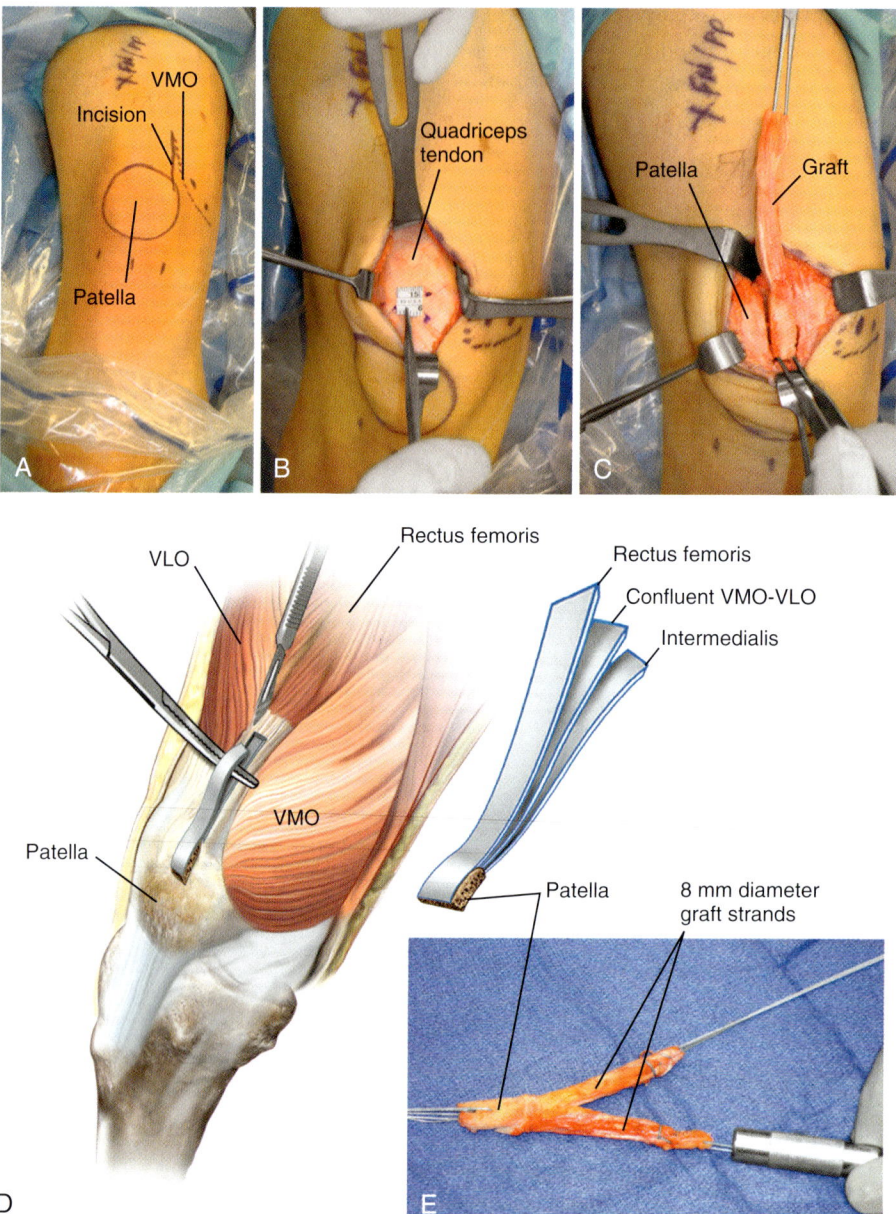

Figure 55-21. QT-PB autograft harvest. **A,** Medial incision. **B,** The quadriceps tendon is carefully marked to only remove 30% of its width and not extend to the musculotendinous junction. **C,** A central 10- to 11-mm wide full-thickness quadriceps tendon graft is harvested. The defect is later closed to maintain arthroscopic joint distention. **D,** Graft harvest. **E,** Two-strand 8-mm tendon graft with patellar bone is prepared. (From Noyes FR, Barber-Westin SD: Posterior cruciate ligament: diagnosis, operative techniques, and clinical outcomes. In Noyes FR [ed]: Noyes' knee disorders: surgery, rehabilitation, clinical outcomes, Philadelphia, 2009, Saunders, pp 503–576.)

is 10 to 11 mm in width and thickness. The quadriceps tendon consists of three layers—rectus tendon, VMO–vastus lateralis oblique (VLO) combined tendon, and vastus intermedius tendon. A meticulous technique is followed to incise all three layers in a perpendicular fashion with a new blade. There is a tendency not to harvest the deep layer or to allow the blade to assume an oblique plane rather than a perpendicular plane. A curved instrument is placed behind the three tendon layers at the proximal aspect of the tendon harvest site to protect the underlying joint synovium. If the synovium is entered, it is closed along with the remaining quadriceps tendon closure to maintain joint distention for the arthroscopic procedure.

An Ellis clamp is placed about the three ends of the tendon to maintain tension. Care is taken at the quadriceps tendon attachment to the patella, because the tendon attachment is located at the proximal and anterior third of the proximal patella. There is a plane established at this point just behind the quadriceps tendon attachment to preserve the posterior underlying synovial attachment and adjacent soft tissues. These tissues provide a superior buttress for the bone grafting of the patella to close the defect and secure the bone graft.

The patella bone block matches the quadriceps width, which is usually 10 to 11 mm wide. The bone block length is 22 to 24 mm and the depth is 8 to 10 mm. A thin powered saw blade is marked with a Steri-Strip to a depth of 10 mm to prevent overly deep penetration. The saw is kept perpendicular to the patella for all cuts. After the anterior bone cuts are made, the quadriceps tendon is lifted superiorly at its attachment site. The inferior portion of the bone block is cut with the saw blade in a perpendicular manner beneath the quadriceps tendon attachment to a depth of 8 to 10 mm. This allows the bone block to be removed gently for graft preparation. The tourniquet is deflated and hemostasis obtained.

The graft is prepared based on whether the one-strand or two-strand technique is selected. With two femoral tunnels (our preference), the tendon is split in a longitudinal manner and two graft strands are fashioned. The two tendon graft strands are sutured in a meticulous manner using three nonabsorbable 2-0 sutures with two or three whipstitches beginning and exiting at the end of the graft strand. With one graft strand and a single femoral tunnel, all three tendon layers are sutured together. The graft diameter is sized for the appropriate tunnel to be drilled. A blood-soaked sponge from the wound site is wrapped around the graft to provide protection, keep the tissues moist, and potentially maintain cell viability.

The quadriceps tendon and synovium are closed to provide a fluid-tight closure, allowing joint distention. The quadriceps tendon defect is closed with nonabsorbable 0 sutures. The tendon is closed in a Z-plasty manner, in which portions of the quadriceps tendon layers are brought together to avoid the use of circumferential tight sutures placed through all three tendon layers to decrease medial to lateral tension in the extensor mechanism.

The patellar bone defect is later bone-grafted in a meticulous manner with bone obtained with a coring reamer during preparation of the femoral graft tunnels. It is important to obtain a bone graft that completely fills the defect, because bone shavings from the tunnel preparations are insufficient. Postoperatively, a bone defect that is meticulously grafted heals without a palpable patellar defect and decreases the incidence of graft harvest site pain.

Achilles Tendon-Bone Allograft

The preparation of an AT-B allograft is performed in a similar manner to that of QT-PB described earlier. The only difference is that it is necessary to tube each portion of the single- or double-strand graft because the tendon has a wide proximal fan shape. Care is taken when performing the incision of the tendon into two strands close to the bone attachment because the tendon narrows in this area. For these reasons, the AT-B graft is generally used for single tibial and femoral tunnel applications, with the bone plug placed in a posterior tibial tunnel location.

SURGICAL PROCEDURES

Anteromedial Approach and Outside-In Femoral Tunnels

This approach is selected when two femoral tunnels are used and is less traumatic than a muscle-splitting approach, because it is necessary to split the VMO for 5 to 6 cm for proper visualization, which is traumatic to the muscle tissue. In addition, this approach allows for good visualization of the graft and suture post fixation. When a single femoral tunnel

is selected, this approach is not used but, instead, a skin incision is placed directly over the drill guide and a limited muscle splitting approach is performed.

A vertical skin incision of 3 to 4 cm is made over the anteromedial vastus medialis proximal to the knee joint and just medial to the quadriceps tendon. When an ipsilateral QT-PB is harvested, the same skin incision is used.

The key to the anteromedial approach is to identify the VMO anterior attachment to the medial retinaculum and medial patellofemoral ligament and dissect in this plane to achieve a subvastus elevation of the VMO. Only a 1-cm incision is made into the VMO attachment to the patella and the medial patellofemoral ligament is not incised. The synovium beneath the VMO is protected and not entered. The VMO nerve innervation proximally is not disturbed. A branch of the superior genicular artery that traverses the inferior border of the VMO is protected.

The outside location of the 1 o'clock femoral tunnel entrance is identified with the drill guide. The guide pin is placed 12 mm proximal to the articular cartilage of the medial femoral condyle and an equal distance medially from the medial trochlear border that is easily palpated without entering the joint. The tunnel should be in line with the obliquity of the PCL graft, but not located too far distally adjacent to the articular cartilage; this would risk breakout of the tunnel into the distal femoral condyle. To maintain an adequate bone bridge at both the entrance and exit of both tunnels, the location of the 4 o'clock femoral tunnel is also 12 mm from the medial articular cartilage margin and just anterior to the femoral epicondyle.

At the time of graft fixation, the surgeon uses a headlight to view the graft in the tunnels. The graft length is observed as the knee is flexed, which determines the knee flexion angle at which the greatest graft length is produced; this is usually 70 to 90 degrees flexion. In addition, the headlight provides for adequate visualization for the placement of the interference screw and additional graft fixation over a suture post. Routine closure is performed with absorbable sutures used for the VMO retinaculum attachment and subcutaneous tissues.

Posterior Cruciate Ligament All-Inside Technique: One- and Two-Strand Graft Reconstructions

Our graft preference for an all-inside technique is a QT-PB autograft for isolated PCL reconstruction (see Table 55-2). The preference for multiligament reconstructions is a bone-patellar tendon-bone (BPTB) allograft for the PCL procedure, using two femoral tunnels and a single tibial tunnel. The bone plug is placed and fixated in a posterior tibial tunnel or socket directly at the posterior entrance under fluoroscopic control. The goal is to match the results of the tibial inlay procedure, with the bone plug placed directly at the posterior PCL attachment using an oblique tunnel instead of a tibial inlay, which requires an open posteromedial approach. The operative steps for these techniques are described in the following sections.

Patient Positioning and Setup

An examination under anesthesia is performed to confirm the diagnosis and carefully compare the injured knee to the

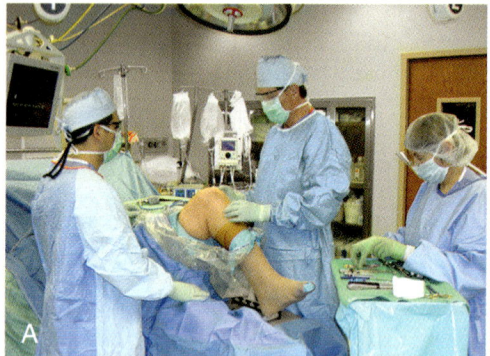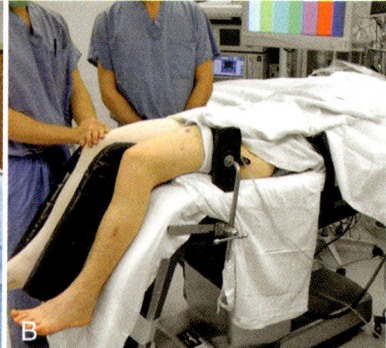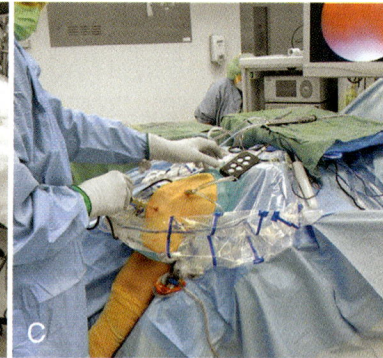

Figure 55-22. A, Patient position used in multiligament surgery with foot in leg holder and knee flexed to 70 degrees. **B** and **C,** Patient position with the knee flexed to 70 degrees as an alternative position. Note that the bed is flexed to maintain hip flexion. There is no pressure against the posterior popliteal space. The opposite leg is well padded. (From Noyes FR, Barber-Westin SD: Posterior cruciate ligament: diagnosis, operative techniques, and clinical outcomes. In Noyes FR [ed]: Noyes' knee disorders: surgery, rehabilitation, clinical outcomes, Philadelphia, 2009, Saunders, pp 503–576.)

opposite normal knee, as described earlier. It is important to palpate the medial tibiofemoral step-off at 90 degrees of flexion in both knees. At surgery, the PCL grafts will be tensioned at 70 to 90 degrees of knee flexion and the medial tibiofemoral step-off used as verification that the abnormal posterior translation has been corrected. In multiligament operative procedures, the patient is in a supine position with appropriate padding under all extremities with an Alverado foot and leg holder or similar device used to flex the knee joint to 60 to 70 degrees (Fig. 55-22). This allows the lower limb to be secured and positioned throughout the operative procedures. After appropriate cruciate ligament surgery, any associated medial or lateral ligament procedure is performed, with the knee flexion angle adjusted as necessary.

An alternative approach is used with isolated PCL surgery. The patient is placed supine on the operating table with appropriate padding. The operating table is placed in a 15-degree reflexed position to prevent hyperextension of the spine and produce mild flexion of the hip to relieve undue tension on the right and left femoral nerves. The knee portion of the bed is flexed to 60 degrees. A thigh tourniquet is placed over cast padding. The opposite limb is positioned in a foam leg holder, with the hip slightly flexed. A thigh-high compression hose is placed on the opposite extremity. After appropriate draping, a 4-inch flat padded bolster is placed underneath the operative thigh to protect the tissues and allow for knee flexion during the operative procedure. The operative procedure is performed with the knee flexed from 60 to 90 degrees; however, further knee flexion is possible by adjusting the operative table or using an additional thigh bolster. It is important that no undue pressure be placed against the posterior thigh and sciatic nerve during the operative procedure. For this reason, an arthroscopic thigh holder is not used. In prolonged surgical procedures, there may exist abnormal pressures on the posterior thigh that compromise the neurovascular structures. As a result, posterior thigh muscle ischemia and peroneal tibial nerve damage, although rare, may occur.

When a meniscal repair is required, an arthroscopic thigh holder is initially used to allow for adequate joint opening for an inside-out meniscus repair using the patient and limb positioning described. The knee position of the bed is flexed as required. After the meniscal repair is performed, the thigh holder is removed and appropriate posterior thigh padding placed as necessary.

Arthroscopy of the knee begins with a pressure-regulated pump that is adjusted to provide mild joint distention and prevent fluid extravasation. The pump is required to maintain joint distention, particularly during the drilling of the tibial tunnel, so that the fluid expands the posterior capsule out of the operative field. Modern pressure- and volume-regulated pumps allow for a controlled inflow and outflow that maintains a safe pressure. In addition, sufficient fluid inflow is maintained so that a tourniquet is not required during the operative procedure.

Routine arthroscopic anteromedial, anterolateral, and superolateral portals are created. During the PCL reconstruction, a transpatellar central portal is required. The posteromedial portal to débride the PCL tibial fibers is not required and avoids inadvertent fluid extravasation into the popliteal fossa; this would limit posterior capsule distention and posterior joint arthroscopic visualization.

A standard arthroscopic examination is performed. The gap test is used to assess lateral and medial joint opening at 30 degrees knee flexion with a varus and valgus stress (see earlier). Any meniscal repairs or partial resections, débridement, or other arthroscopic procedures are performed. The PCL graft harvest procedure on the operative or contralateral limb is carried out as required.

Tibial Tunnel Preparation

The most difficult part of the operative procedure is to prepare the tibial tunnel, located in the distal PCL attachment position, without injuring the popliteal neurovascular structures. To maintain joint distention and allow full visualization, a pressure-regulated arthroscopic pump is used and the femoral tunnels are placed after the tibial tunnel has been prepared.

The knee is positioned at 60 degrees of flexion to prevent pressure against the popliteal structures posteriorly. This allows the posterior neurovascular structures to drop away from the posterior aspect of the knee. Matava and colleagues[62] have reported that the mean distance of the PCL from the popliteal artery from 0 to 100 degrees of flexion is 7.6 mm in the axial plane and 7.2 mm in the sagittal plane; however, there may be individual variation between knees. During the operative procedure, the surgeon is constantly aware of the joint pressure, fluid inflow and outflow, increased thigh tension, and any lack of joint distention. Intermittent palpation of the popliteal and calf regions is performed during the operative procedure to detect fluid extravasation by an inadvertent puncture of the posterior capsule.[89] An accessory posteromedial portal and arthroscopic approach (described by others to remove the PCL or visualize the PCL attachment) is not recommended because posterior fluid extravasation may occur. With the operative steps described, the PCL attachment may be viewed through the anteromedial portal.

The preparation of the tibial tunnel is more difficult when the ACL is intact. It is first necessary to identify residual PCL fibers adjacent to the ACL, which are removed through the anteromedial portal with the arthroscope in the anterolateral portal. The middle genicular artery enters into the proximal aspect of the PCL and requires electrocoagulation. Some PCL fibers are left on the femoral attachment for later identification and placement of the graft tunnels. The anterior meniscofemoral ligament (aMFL) and posterior meniscofemoral (pMFL) ligament are identified and, if present, are preserved. It is usually possible to preserve the pMFL, but is more difficult to preserve the aMFL, especially when both

meniscofemoral ligaments are present. When these ligaments are present, additional care is required in preparation of the tibial tunnels because the instruments are passed adjacent to these structures and the passage of grafts posteriorly may be temporarily blocked. If these structures impede visualization, they may be removed as long as the lateral meniscus has a confirmed posterior horn attachment to the posterior tibia and is not an anatomic variant, in which the posterior horn is attached by a meniscofemoral attachment.

The 30-degree arthroscope is next placed into the anteromedial portal and positioned high in the notch adjacent to the PCL femoral attachment. This allows the posterior capsular recess and remaining PCL stump at the tibial attachment to be viewed and instruments to be passed medially to the ACL.

A critical step is the passage of a curved Cobb elevator or commercially available Acufex (Smith & Nephew Endoscopy, Andover, Mass) PCL Elevator (Fig. 55-23), which has a 90-degree curve and is used to free up the space gently in front of and behind the remaining PCL fibers. In some knees, the posterior capsule becomes adherent to the PCL fibers. The PCL Elevator is used to tease the capsule gently off the

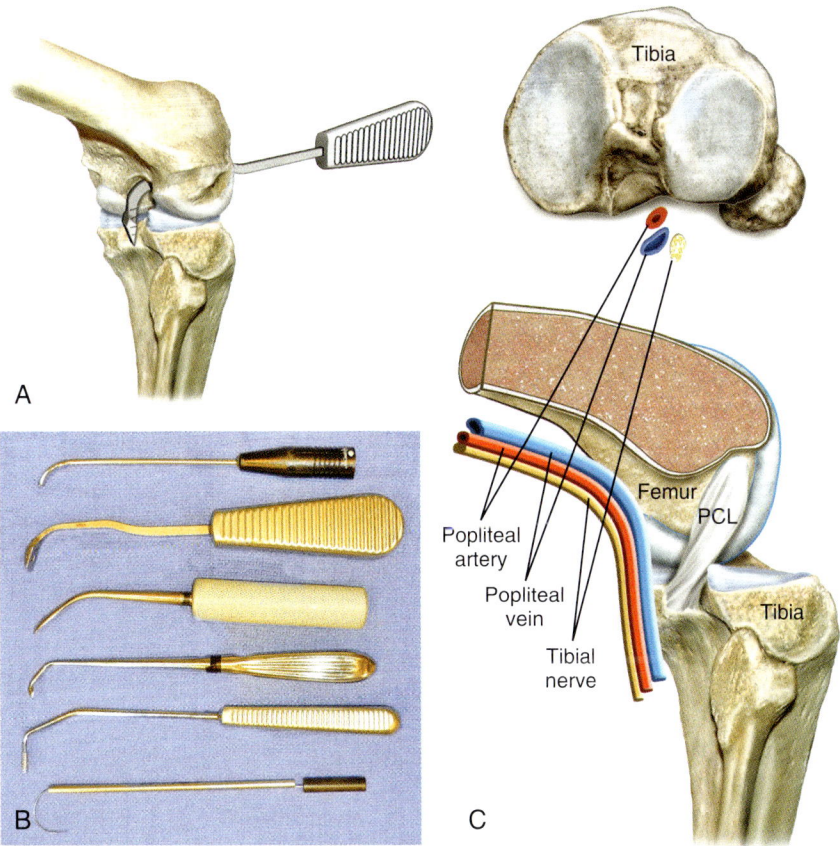

Figure 55-23. **A** and **B,** Tibial preparation. A 30-degree arthroscope is placed through the anteromedial portal. The arthroscope is placed high in the notch adjacent to the medial condyle to view the posterior region of the joint. Instruments are placed through a central portal, medial to the ACL, carefully protecting the ligament. **A,** Acufex PCL Elevator is inserted through the notch to free the posterior capsule carefully and re-create the normal capsular recess behind the PCL, because the capsule may be adherent to the ruptured PCL fibers. This step allows the capsule to displace posteriorly, with fluid distention protecting the neurovascular structures. **B,** The tibial PCL stump is removed under direct visualization using curved shavers, baskets, Cobb elevators, and radiofrequency instruments. The posterior medial and lateral meniscus attachments are protected at all times. **C,** Anatomic illustration shows the close proximity of popliteal neurovascular structures. (From Noyes FR, Barber-Westin SD: Posterior cruciate ligament: diagnosis, operative techniques, and clinical outcomes. In Noyes FR [ed]: Noyes' knee disorders: surgery, rehabilitation, clinical outcomes, Philadelphia, 2009, Saunders, pp 503–576.)

PCL fibers and avoid rupture of the posterior capsule. This step requires a gentle approach to push the posterior capsule distally to the level of the distal PCL and capsule attachments, which are at the level of the posterior tibial step-off.

If the posterior capsule is violated, a decrease in pump pressure is required and a large anterior fluid outflow portal is established. Close monitoring of any fluid extravasation into the popliteal space and calf is done. It is usually safe to proceed under low-pressure conditions; however, if there is any question of visualization and popliteal space distention, the operative procedure is postponed to allow for capsule healing.

The medial and lateral meniscal posterior tibial attachments adjacent to the PCL tibial fossa are viewed and protected at all times during the preparation of the tibial tunnels. These meniscal attachments are located within a few millimeters of the PCL attachment and may be easily damaged during drilling of one or two tunnels.

The PCL stump is removed with arthroscopic instruments of the surgeon's preference. There are a variety of curved instruments, including baskets, suction cutting blades, and curettes that are helpful. Particularly valuable are electrocoagulation instruments that are manually bent to an appropriate curve to facilitate removal of the PCL fibers in the posterior tibial fossa. At the conclusion of these steps, the entire posterior PCL tibial fossa (to the level of the posterior capsule attachment) is viewed for identification of the correct placement of the tibial tunnel.

Drilling of the Tibial Tunnel

A medial skin incision 3 to 4 cm is made 1 cm medially to the tibial tubercle. The tunnel entrance is medial or lateral to the tibial tubercle (Fig. 55-24). There may be a theoretical advantage for the tunnel to be started just lateral to the tibial tubercle to produce less posterior tunnel graft angulation. However, either tunnel location is acceptable. The senior author (FN) usually prefers an entrance medial to the tibial tubercle. When an ACL reconstruction is also performed with a medial tunnel, the PCL graft is placed through a tunnel lateral to the tibial tubercle.

The arthroscope is placed in the anteromedial portal and positioned high in the notch to view the posterior aspect of the tibial PCL attachment to the capsular attachment. In most cases, the 30-degree arthroscope provides an excellent view. On occasion, a 70-degree arthroscope is required.

The drilling of the tibial tunnel is shown in Figure 55-25. The drill guide is placed through the transpatellar portal. The tip of the guide is placed at the desired position of the tunnel as far distally as possible, which is to the level of the posterior capsule insertion on the tibia just before the posterior tibial step-off. The distal placement of the guide pin is a critical step for success; an error is to place the guide pin too proximally in the PCL fossa, which produces a near-vertical PCL graft with limited ability to resist posterior tibial subluxation. The tip of the guide rests on the distal posterior capsule attachment, with the guide pin target just 5 mm proximal to

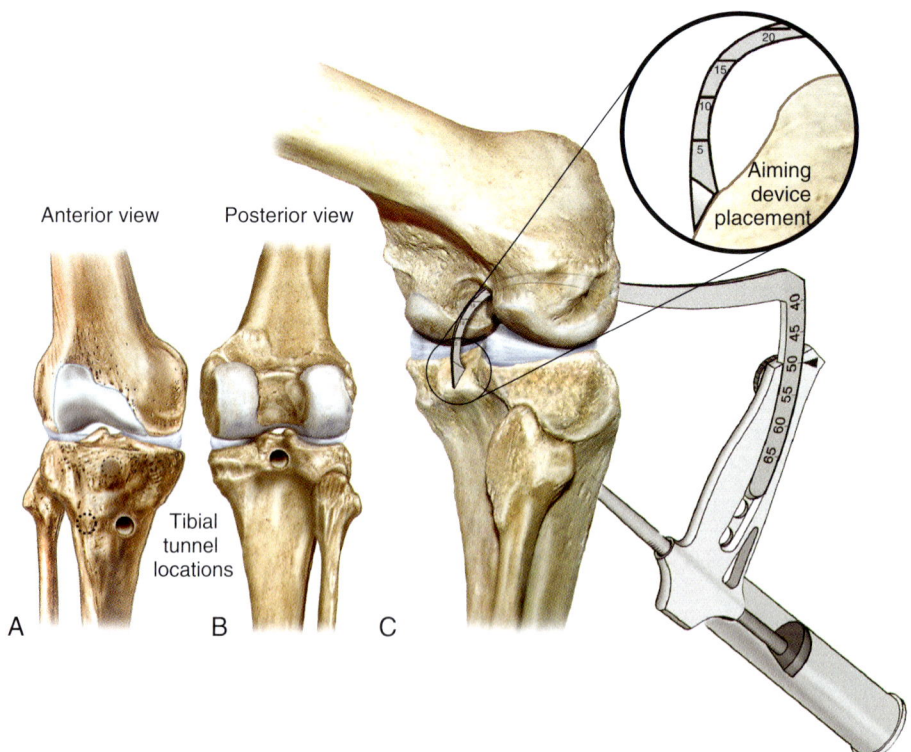

Figure 55-24. Location of the tibial tunnel. **A,** Tunnel position may be medial or lateral *(dotted circle)* to the tibial tubercle 3 to 4 cm distal to the joint line. The tunnel position is at a 50-degree angle or more to decrease the acute angulation at the posterior tibia. **B,** Posterior tibial tunnel at distal PCL attachment site. **C,** Acufex Director PCL Tibial Aimer is placed through the central portal with the tip of the guide resting on the posterior capsule insertion, with the target 5 mm proximal to the distal aspect of the PCL footprint. This allows sufficient tibial bone proximal to the tunnel to prevent anterior graft migration. (From Noyes FR, Barber-Westin SD: Posterior cruciate ligament: diagnosis, operative techniques, and clinical outcomes. In Noyes FR [ed]: Noyes' knee disorders: surgery, rehabilitation, clinical outcomes, Philadelphia, 2009, Saunders, pp 503–576.)

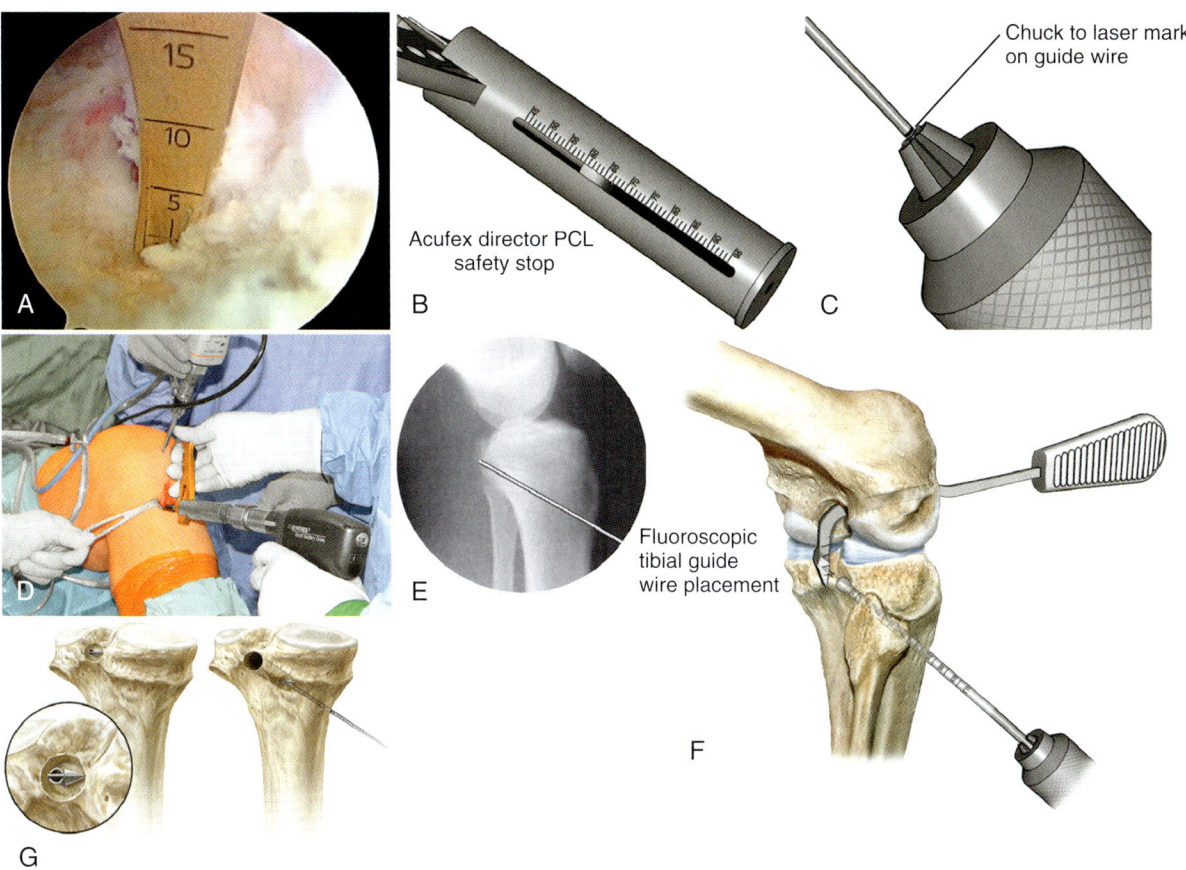

Figure 55-25. Drilling of the tibial tunnel. **A,** Drill guide at distal PCL attachment adjacent to posterior capsule insertion. **B,** Acufex guide pin safety stop is attached to the drill guide. **C,** The guide wire is chucked on the power drill to the laser mark, which is the maximum length from the safety stop to the drill guide tip. This prevents the guide wire from being advanced beyond the drill guide after passing through the posterior cortex. **D,** Placement of guide pin using drill guide system at surgery. **E,** Fluoroscopy verifies guide wire placement. **F,** Tibial tunnel drilling with PCL Elevator–Wire Catcher (Acufex) to protect posterior neurovascular structures. **G,** Alternative technique using a flip-drill to make a posterior tibial socket for the PCL graft bone plug. Four FiberWire sutures (Arthrex) placed through the plug are passed to the anterior tibia for graft fixation. (From Noyes FR, Barber-Westin SD: Posterior cruciate ligament: diagnosis, operative techniques, and clinical outcomes. In Noyes FR [ed]: Noyes' knee disorders: surgery, rehabilitation, clinical outcomes, Philadelphia, 2009, Saunders, pp 503–576.)

the tip. This prevents the drill from proceeding too far distally beyond the posterior tibial step-off where the drill tip would not be visualized and could penetrate neurovascular structures. The goal is to place the guide pin in the distal central portion of the PCL fossa, 20 to 25 mm from the proximal entrance of the PCL fossa. This leaves 15 mm of the posterior fossa to retain the posterior graft position and prevent a vertical PCL graft. This is a key step of the procedure. The drill guide is angled 50 to 55 degrees to produce an oblique tibial tunnel, which will decrease graft angulation effects.

The next step involves use of the drill guide safety stop system (Acufex). The guide pin is chucked to a fixed distance with the safety stop mounted on the drill guide. The safety stop controls the depth of guide pin penetration into the tibia, irrespective of the angle or position of the PCL tibial aimer, and prevents the guide pin from passing beyond the guide tip and damaging neurovascular structures.

The guide pin is drilled into the selected tibial tunnel location. The depth of the guide pin is measured and used during the drilling process to determine the depth of drill penetration. The final position of the guide pin(s) is viewed and again it is confirmed that the guide pin is distal in the

PCL fossa. Fluoroscopic confirmation of the guide pin position is recommended.

The tibial tunnel is drilled to the desired diameter using safety procedures to be described. A commercially available PCL guide pin protector (Acufex) has a wide shape, with a central recess 5 mm from its tip to engage the tibial guide pin before and during the drilling procedure. The tip of the pin is viewed at all times during the drilling process. The instrument prevents posterior migration of the pin and drill bit. The drilling process involves use of a drill with a drill tip and not a drill twist extending the length of the drill. The drill tip only extends 10 mm with a smooth shank. The drill is advanced in a slow manner. The depth of drill penetration is measured by the calibrated drill and prior drill guide pin measurements. As the drill tip reaches the posterior cortex, there is a noticeable resistance. At this point, the drill is slowly advanced without sudden penetration. A second option is to remove the power and place a hand chuck over the drill bit to complete the tunnel through the posterior tibial cortex.

When the flip-drill technique (FlipCutter, Arthrex, Naples, Fla) is selected, a 4-mm drill is initially used to establish the tibial tunnel. The flip-drill is then advanced under arthroscopic visualization to exit the posterior tibial tunnel. The drill is flipped and held against the posterior tibial cortex and the tunnel is carefully drilled in a retrograde manner to the desired depth that is determined by the measured length of the flip-drill. The PCL dilator remains in place posteriorly at all times to displace the posterior capsule away from the drilling procedure and prevent inadvertent capsule penetration.

To summarize, there are specific safety procedures built into this technique to protect the neurovascular structures.

1. Identification of the entire PCL attachment and PCL tibia fossa
2. Drill guide system with the safety stop and controlled depth of guide pin penetration, with the guide pin placed 5 mm proximal to the distal posterior capsule insertion, verified by fluoroscopy
3. Placement of the PCL guide pin protector and slow drill penetration with direct viewing of the guide pin
4. Final drill penetration of the posterior tibial cortex with complete protection posteriorly by the PCL Elevator to prevent inadvertent deep drill penetration

The proximal edge of the tibial tunnel is carefully chamfered with a rasp to limit graft abrasion effects (Fig. 55-26). Any remaining PCL fibers are removed so that the tibial tunnel entrance does not have soft tissue that would limit graft passage and to ensure that the graft will lie flat against the PCL tibial fossa. Again, it is necessary to have 15 mm of the posterior tibial fossa proximal to the tunnel to maintain the normal angulation of the PCL tibial attachment to prevent a vertical PCL graft and decrease graft tunnel enlargement (windshield wiper effect). The most common technical

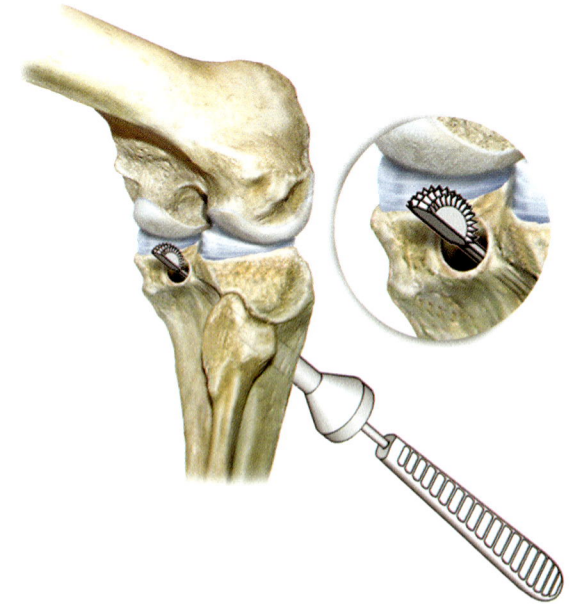

Figure 55-26. Chamfering of the tibial tunnel with a rasp to decrease graft abrasion effects. It is necessary to have 15 mm of bone retained in the posterior tibial fossa above the PCL footprint to prevent the graft from migrating through the tibia. (From Noyes FR, Barber-Westin SD: Posterior cruciate ligament: diagnosis, operative techniques, and clinical outcomes. In Noyes FR [ed]: Noyes' knee disorders: surgery, rehabilitation, clinical outcomes, Philadelphia, 2009, Saunders, pp 503–576.)

mistake is to place the tibial tunnel at the proximal entrance of the PCL fossa, which is proximal to the native PCL tibial attachment.

Posterior Cruciate Ligament Femoral Graft Technique

As described earlier, the PCL attachment is elliptical in shape, extending from high in the notch over the lateral aspect of the distal medial condyle, from an approximate 11:30 to 5 o'clock position (left knee). The PCL footprint follows the articular cartilage, with the anterior portion within 2 to 3 mm of its edge, depending on the reference system used (see earlier).[65] At the 4 o'clock position, the PCL attachment is approximately 4 mm from the articular cartilage edge.[105] However, if the aMFL is present, the footprint will appear to be 1 to 2 mm from the cartilage edge. There is anatomic variability in the normal proximal to distal width of the PCL, and in some knees a more oval appearance exists because of an increased width of the middle third of the PCL attachment. Because of anatomic variability in the PCL femoral attachment, it is necessary to map out the attachment using remaining PCL fibers to locate the desired graft position. The reference system axis used to describe the PCL attachment is distal to proximal and anterior to posterior with the knee in full extension (see Fig. 55-3). However, the surgeon views the PCL with the knee flexed and it is also helpful to communicate a graft position as deep or shallow and high or low in the femoral notch on the medial femoral condyle.

There are two main techniques used for PCL graft femoral placement and fixation. The first technique (our preference) incorporates two separate femoral tunnels with two separate graft strands. The second technique involves a single femoral tunnel when operative time and complexity of the surgery is a factor.

Femoral Placement of Two Tunnels and Graft Passage

The technique for femoral placement of two tunnels and graft passage is shown in Figure 55-27. The PCL footprint is mapped with a calibrated probe and electrocoagulation. The 12, 1, and 4 o'clock position marks on the medial femoral condyle are made. The goal is to create two separate femoral tunnels in the distal two thirds of the native PCL attachment. This places a graft with an approximate area of 100 mm² in cross section, occupying up to 75% of the PCL attachment.

If the PCL graft is placed too distal or shallow in the notch, it will be subject to high tensile forces with knee flexion, resulting in constraining flexion and probable graft failure. If the graft is placed too proximal or deep in the notch, the graft will slacken with knee flexion and allow posterior tibial subluxation. The correct placement of two guide pin marks within the PCL footprint is shown in Figure 55-27, in which the graft replaces the distal two thirds of the PCL that functions in resisting posterior tibial subluxation with knee flexion.

The PCL guide is used for two separate femoral tunnels to prevent overlap of the tunnels. The anterior tunnel is centered at the 1 o'clock position, 6 mm deep to the articular cartilage. The posterior tunnel is centered at the 4 o'clock position, 8 mm proximal (deep) to the articular cartilage

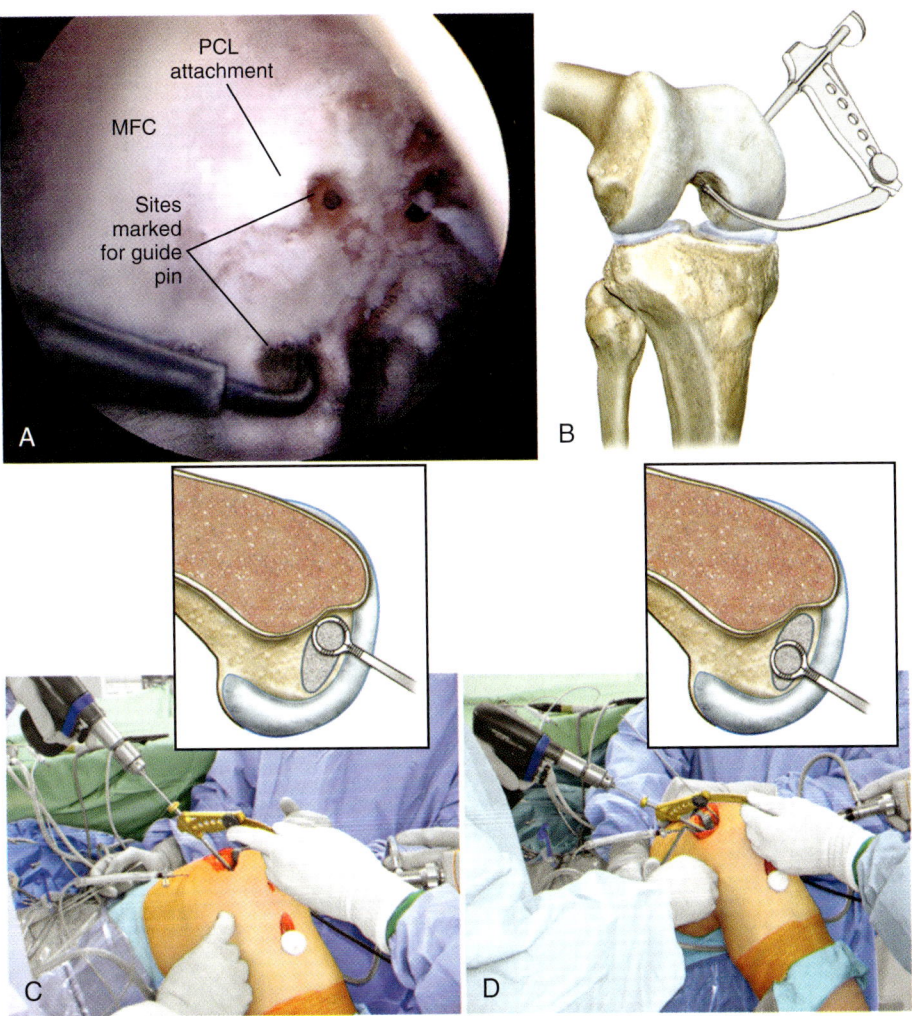

Figure 55-27. Placement of two femoral tunnels. **A,** Arthroscopic view of two PCL attachment shows 1 and 4 o'clock guide pin marks, 6 and 8 mm from the articular cartilage. **B,** PCL guide 15 mm proximal to the outside articular cartilage border. **C,** Placement of 1 o'clock tunnel. **D,** Placement of 4 o'clock tunnel. (From Noyes FR, Barber-Westin SD: Posterior cruciate ligament: diagnosis, operative techniques, and clinical outcomes. In Noyes FR [ed]: Noyes' knee disorders: surgery, rehabilitation, clinical outcomes, Philadelphia, 2009, Saunders, pp 503–576.)

edge. A mark is made at the center position of each tunnel with cautery, and then defined with a curette or sharp awl passed from the anterolateral portal. The bone beneath the PCL attachment is dense and requires making a well-defined small entrance hole for the two drill guide pins. Following this technique, the first tunnel is located in the anterior third of the PCL attachment and in the distal two thirds in the proximal to distal direction. The second tunnel is located in the posterior third of the PCL attachment and also in the distal two thirds. The tunnels are carefully placed in the anterior to posterior direction to allow for a 2- to 3-mm bone bridge between tunnels. This placement of the two tunnels ensures that both graft strands will resist posterior tibial translation with knee flexion, sharing the load and not being placed too deeply in the notch.

The two femoral tunnels are drilled using the outside-in (VMO-sparing approach) subvastus technique. As noted, the entrance of the 1 o'clock tunnel is 12 mm proximal to the femoral articular cartilage border and medial to the trochlea. The 4 o'clock tunnel entrance is also 12 mm proximal to the articular cartilage border and anterior to the femoral

epicondyle. A core reamer is used for the 1 o'clock tunnel to obtain a bone graft for the patellar defect (QT-PB graft; Fig. 55-28). Careful chamfering of the tunnel edges is performed to decrease graft abrasion. A flexible ruler is passed through the tibial and femoral tunnels to measure the intra-articular length of the two graft strands.

The passage of the graft is performed in a stepwise fashion (Fig. 55-29). A 20-gauge wire is passed through the tibial tunnel and brought out the anterolateral portal, which is enlarged sufficiently to accept the PCL graft. A 22-gauge wire is passed through each of the two femoral tunnels and a grasper or nerve hook is used to bring the two wires out the same anterolateral portal. The 1 and 4 o'clock wires are marked.

The tibial bone is first passed into the knee joint with the arthroscope placed in the anteromedial portal. A nerve hook facilitates passage adjacent and medial to the ACL and into the tibial tunnel. It is important that all soft tissues have been removed about the tibial tunnel, which is 1 mm larger than the graft to facilitate passage. The nerve hook is used to angle the bone to facilitate the initial entrance into the tibial

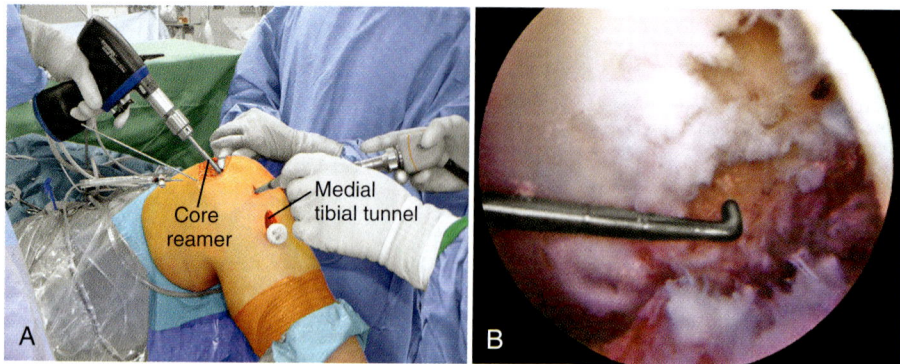

Figure 55-28. A, Use of core reamer to obtain bone graft for patellar bone defect. **B,** Arthroscopic view shows final appearance of two femoral graft tunnels. (From Noyes FR, Barber-Westin SD: Posterior cruciate ligament: diagnosis, operative techniques, and clinical outcomes. In Noyes FR [ed]: Noyes' knee disorders: surgery, rehabilitation, clinical outcomes, Philadelphia, 2009, Saunders, pp 503–576.)

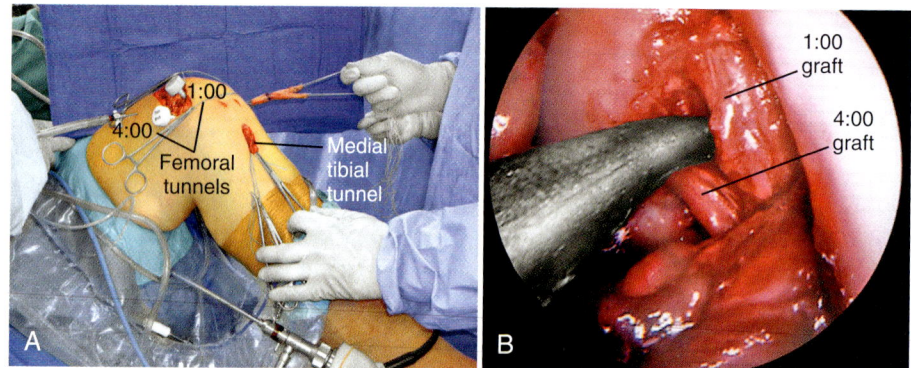

Figure 55-29. A, Passage of the quadriceps-bone two-strand graft through enlarged anterolateral portal. **B,** Final appearance of two-strand graft within femoral tunnels. (From Noyes FR, Barber-Westin SD: Posterior cruciate ligament: diagnosis, operative techniques, and clinical outcomes. In Noyes FR [ed]: Noyes' knee disorders: surgery, rehabilitation, clinical outcomes, Philadelphia, 2009, Saunders, pp 503–576.)

tunnel. The two femoral graft strands are then passed through the enlarged anterolateral portal and viewed through the anteromedial portal to have the correct orientation in the 1 and 4 o'clock tunnels. It is preferable to first pass the 4 o'clock and then the 1 o'clock graft.

Fluoroscopy is used to confirm final placement of the bone plug in the tibial tunnel. The graft is marked at the collagenous fiber-bone junction and is viewed arthroscopically to confirm that the bone plug is entirely within the tibial tunnel and placed directly at the posterior tibial tunnel entrance. The patellar bone plug sutures are tied over a tibial suture post, maintaining its position at the posterior tibial tunnel entrance. An absorbable interference screw (1 mm smaller than the diameter of the tunnel) is used for bone plug fixation at the tibial tunnel, verified by fluoroscopy. The final tensioning of the graft at the femoral site is performed next. In the alternative flip-drill technique of drilling a posterior tibial socket, four high-strength sutures placed in the bone plug are tied over a suture post.

Graft Tensioning and Fixation for All-Inside Grafts

The graft tensioning and fixation steps are the same for all grafts. For grafts with the bone block in the tibial tunnel, initial fixation is performed at the tibia (as described) and final tensioning and fixation are performed at the femoral site. (For alternative techniques in which the bone block is

placed and fixed at the femoral site and the final tensioning and fixation are performed at the tibial site, follow the same procedure described next.)

After the initial fixation of the bone plug at the tibial site, the knee is taken through a full range of motion, with an assistant displacing the tibia forward to correct for the weight of the leg and maintain joint reduction.

The knee flexion position for graft fixation is checked by determining the flexion angle at which the graft strand is the longest (functional zone) to ensure that the graft is not tensioned in its shortest position, which would overconstrain the joint and produce graft failure. A nonserrated hemostat is placed on each set of graft strand sutures exiting from the femoral tunnel(s) and circumferentially wound onto the clamp. The clamp is used to apply a 10-lb (44-N) load to each graft strand. The graft strands are conditioned by taking the knee joint through 0 to 120 degrees of flexion. The knee is placed at 90 degrees flexion and a normal medial tibiofemoral step-off is palpated and confirmed. This is done with the assistant placing approximately 10 lb (44 N) of pressure against the calf to apply an anterior tibial force (assuming that the ACL is intact). The knee is again taken through a full range of motion and the change in length of both graft strands noted. With increasing knee flexion, there will be increased tension and a pulling of the sutures and clamp into the tunnel of only 0 to 2 mm as the 90-degree position is reached.

The graft is longest at high knee flexion angles, which is the position selected for graft fixation. In most knees, the 70-degree flexion angle has the same graft length behavior as 90 degrees and this position is selected. There are commercially available graft-tensioning devices[27] (as used in ACL reconstructions) that provide measurable length-tension data and may be used for the measurement of graft-tensioning loads. The sutures for each graft stand are tied over a femoral post, maintaining the 10 lb of graft load and 10 lb of anterior tibial load.

The final position of the medial tibiofemoral joint is again verified. An absorbable interference screw is added to the fixation. The arthroscope is placed and, with a nerve hook, the tension in the PCL graft strand is confirmed. The knee is taken through 0 to 110 degrees flexion.

It should be noted that if one femoral tunnel is too proximal (deep in the notch), the graft strand length decreases with knee flexion (allowing posterior subluxation), because the graft strand is longest closer to full extension. In this situation, the final graft fixation is done at a low flexion position. The proximal graft strand will function in a reciprocal manner with the other graft strand and the desired load sharing between grafts will not be achieved.

Alternatively, if the graft is progressively pulled into the femoral tunnel starting at 45 to 60 degrees, then the femoral tunnels are too distal (shallow). This is not an acceptable position and the femoral tunnel is reconfigured, removing 5 mm of the proximal aspect of the tunnel to allow the graft to assume a deeper and more ideal position. The interference femoral screws are placed distal in the femoral tunnels to secure the grafts in a more proximal (deep) position. With the technique described for the placement of the femoral tunnels, it would be unusual for this graft tunnel adjustment to be performed.

In knees that undergo ACL reconstruction, it is important to determine the neutral anteroposterior position of the medial and lateral tibiofemoral joints as accurately as possible, without added internal or external tibial rotation. There is a tendency to displace the tibia into an abnormal anterior position by overtensioning the PCL graft. When the ACL is intact, the graft forces displace the tibial anteriorly, loading the ACL under low loads. When the ACL is insufficient, to prevent anterior tibial subluxation, the following steps are performed:

1. Place the knee at full extension with a 10-lb (44-N) force on each graft (or 20 lb for a single graft) and 10 lb anterior force on the calf to overcome the gravity weight effects of the leg. This achieves a reduced tibiofemoral joint position when one or both of the medial or fibular collateral ligaments are present.
2. Flex the knee to 90 degrees, maintaining the same approximate graft load and anteriorly directed load on the calf. An anteriorly subluxated tibia at 90 degrees (compared with 0 degrees) will have abnormally increased tibiofemoral attachment site distances and the graft can be observed to piston into the tibial tunnel. In essence, the graft tension and length should be similar at both 0 and 90 degrees of flexion.
3. Palpate for a normal tibiofemoral step-off and arthroscopically visualize a normal anterior relationship of the anterior portion of the medial and lateral meniscus in relationship to the respective femoral

condyles. If there is any question, a lateral fluoroscopic or radiograph may be obtained intraoperatively. This is especially helpful in large limbs in which the neutral anteroposterior position is difficult to determine with accuracy.

Femoral Placement of a Single Tunnel: Outside-In Technique

The drill guide is introduced into the anteromedial portal and the desired femoral tunnel position is located. The arthroscope is placed in the anterolateral portal. The goal is to place the tunnel into the anterior half of the PCL attachment, avoiding too proximal a placement. The entrance of the guide pin is at the 2 o'clock position, approximately 7 to 8 mm from the articular cartilage edge. This should produce a tunnel that is 2 to 3 mm from the articular cartilage edge. A note of caution is that there is a tendency to place the drill tunnel too proximal (deep in the femoral notch) and out of the PCL femoral footprint, producing a graft that only functions at low flexion angles. The ability to determine the native PCL footprint in the patient's knee carefully is important for correct tunnel placement. The preference is for a tunnel of 10 mm in most knees, and 11 mm in larger knees. If the drill diameter is larger, portions of the graft will be too deep in the notch and outside of the normal PCL footprint.

The entrance position of the guide pin in the outside-in technique is midway between the femoral epicondyle and trochlea, at least 12 mm proximal to the articular cartilage edge. A more proximally placed guide pin would increase the tunnel angulation entering the joint and potentially increase graft abrasion effects.

A subvastus VMO approach is used, as already described for fixation of the tendon portion of the QT-PB or AT-B graft to gain exposure for the interference screw and suture post.

A small skin incision and VMO muscle-splitting incision is used with an alternative graft with a bone plug because the bone plug fixation is done with an interference screw without a suture post. The guide pin is reamed or a coring reamer may be used to harvest a bone graft. The tunnel entrance into the knee joint is chamfered to limit graft abrasion effects. A modification of this technique is possible with a BPTB allograft, in which a flip-drill is placed from outside-in instead of the guide pin and the femoral socket drilled from inside-out.

At the time of graft passage, an inside-out passage (preferred; enlarged anterolateral portal used for graft passage into the knee) or an outside-in passage (retrograde guide wire from tibial tunnel out through femoral tunnel) is used. The final graft conditioning, tensioning, and fixation are the same as described earlier. All grafts at the tibia have double fixation with a cancellous interference screw and suture post.

There are reports that have described the all-inside drilling of a large single tunnel at the femoral attachment. However, the outside-in approach is preferred for a large-diameter tunnel. From a technical standpoint, the drilling of a large-diameter tunnel is difficult because of the proximity of the lateral condylar articular cartilage and the ACL, and the tendency exists to have a tunnel entrance that is markedly angled distally. In the senior author's (FN) experience, a more precise and less angulated tunnel is obtained with the outside-in approach. The single femoral tunnel technique is used when operative time must be limited because this approach is the least technically demanding of all approaches used for PCL femoral graft fixation.

Alternative Posterior Cruciate Ligament All-Inside Techniques

Femoral Placement of Rectangular (Oval) Tunnel for Bone Plug

An all-inside technique using the QT-PB autograft or BPTB or AT-B allograft is described in which the bone plug is placed at the femoral site and the soft tissue graft is placed through a tibial tunnel. This procedure has the advantage of easy passage of the soft tissue graft through the tibial tunnel. It is used in select knees in which operative time is a factor. In addition, in revision knees, there may be displaced femoral tunnels in which the bone plug provides a more stable fixation at the femoral site. As noted, the senior author (FN) prefers to reverse the graft with the bone plug at the posterior tibial tunnel. It is unknown from a clinical standpoint which procedure provides the best outcome related to return of joint stability.

The patient positioning and initial surgical approach are similar to the all-inside technique described. The posterior PCL stump is removed and PCL tibial attachment is prepared for one or two tibial tunnels.

When a two-strand PCL reconstruction is selected, with the collagen graft strands placed in a tibial tunnel, there is an advantage of using two tibial tunnels because of the smaller diameter tunnel required. This avoids creating a large-diameter single tunnel in which both graft strands are passed. Two smaller diameter tunnels provide for better healing potential and ingrowth into the graft in comparison to a single large-diameter tunnel (see earlier). However, the procedure is more technically demanding and

time-consuming. Thus, two tibial tunnels are only used with an isolated PCL reconstruction. The two tibial tunnels are placed on the medial and lateral aspects of the tibial tubercle. Two tunnels are difficult to drill in small knees in which the width of the PCL attachment is narrow and a single tunnel is required. In multiligament reconstructions when operative time is a factor, a single tibial tunnel is selected. The single tibial tunnel (or double tunnels) is drilled with the technique previously described.

The technique for the femoral PCL graft attachment of the bone portion of the graft involves using a rectangular femoral slot or femoral tunnel. The all-inside technique for the rectangular slot is preferred to place a greater portion of the graft within the PCL femoral footprint, in which approximately 75% of the footprint is occupied by the graft. A single circular tunnel of 10 to 11 mm (outside-in approach described earlier) replicates only the anterior and middle portions of the PCL attachment and remains an option, but is less ideal from a theoretical standpoint.

The goal is to create an 8- × 12-mm rectangular slot that extends from 1 to 4 o'clock in the distal two thirds of the PCL footprint. The 12 and 4 o'clock marks are made on the medial femoral condyle. Again, the guide pin mark is 6 and 8 mm from the articular cartilage of the medial femoral condyle for the anterior and posterior tunnels (Fig. 55-30), verified by observing the PCL footprint and determining that the two tunnels are in the distal two thirds of the footprint. A small curette or awl is used to penetrate and define the pilot hole for each tunnel. A 2.4-mm guide pin is placed through the anterolateral portal into the anterior tunnel location, the knee is flexed to 90 degrees, and the guide pin is advanced through the medial femoral condyle approximately 25 mm deep, based on the patellar bone length.

The second guide pin is placed into the second marked position. The guide pins are overreamed with an endoscopic

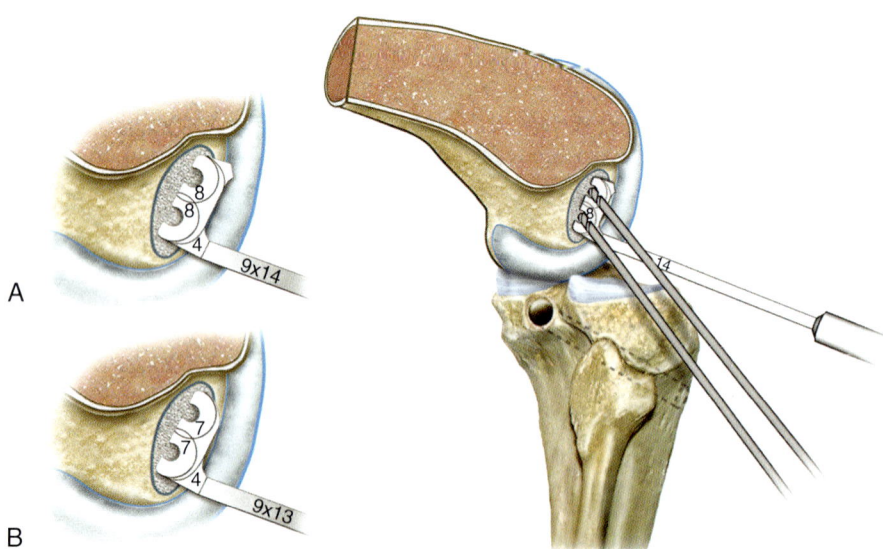

Figure 55-30. **A** and **B,** All-inside femoral tunnel. The PCL femoral template is placed through the anteromedial portal with the arthroscope in the central portal. This defines the position of two overlapping 7- or 8-mm tunnels. The top edge of the template is placed 2 mm from the articular margin and the bottom edge is 4 mm from the articular margin. This places the center of the anterior tunnel 6 mm from the articular cartilage margin and the center of the posterior tunnel 8 mm from the articular cartilage margin. (From Noyes FR, Barber-Westin SD: Posterior cruciate ligament: diagnosis, operative techniques, and clinical outcomes. In Noyes FR [ed]: Noyes' knee disorders: surgery, rehabilitation, clinical outcomes, Philadelphia, 2009, Saunders, pp 503–576.)

drill (Fig. 55-31) to form an oblong tunnel entrance to a depth that corresponds to the graft bone. Care is taken to avoid the lateral femoral condyle articular cartilage as the drill is introduced into the knee joint. The remaining central bone bridge is removed with a curette or burr.

The PCL Dilator (Fig. 55-32) dilates the attachment into an oval 9- × 13-mm shape that is approximately 1 mm larger than the bone portion of the graft. Care is taken at this point to use low forces in dilating the rectangular slot to avoid fracture of the femoral condyle. In our experience, this has not been reported; however, it is worth a cautionary note. The PCL Dilator has a graft sizing slot on the handle for a 9- × 13-mm bone block that is used for preparation of the graft.

The distal aspect of the femoral oval opening is chamfered and rasped to create a gentle slope to limit graft abrasion.

The femoral tunnel has an oval appearance and approximates two thirds or more of the PCL attachment site. The bone portion of the graft is initially rectangular and the graft corners are contoured to a more oval shape for easier passage into the femoral tunnel.

The passage of the graft begins with the passage of a 22-gauge wire through the tibial tunnel that is grasped with a nerve hook and brought out through the anterolateral portal (Fig. 55-33). The tendon graft strands are passed through the enlarged anterolateral portal that is increased 2 to 3 cm in length to prevent soft tissues from impeding graft passage. When a two-tunnel tibial technique is used, two wires are passed and the graft strands marked for the 1 o'clock graft to the lateral tunnel and the second 4 o'clock graft to the medial tibial tunnel. A towel clip or suture is used to close the anterolateral portal after graft passage to maintain joint distention.

The graft strands are viewed through the anterolateral portal adjacent to the ACL (when present), and a nerve hook through the central portal is used to assist gently and angulate the graft to enter into the respective tibial tunnel. It is easier first to pass the medial graft strand and then the lateral graft strand, maintaining the orientation of the bone portion of the graft so that the lateral tibial strand corresponds to the 1 o'clock femoral position and the medial tibial strand corresponds to the 4 o'clock femoral position.

A guide pin (with an end to carry the sutures) is passed through the anterolateral portal into the rectangular femoral slot to exit anterior and proximal to the medial femoral epicondyle. The bone block with sutures is passed into the knee joint. The arthroscope views the bone block and the orientation is controlled with the cancellous surface oriented proximally (deep) in the rectangular slot. The bone block is positioned flush (not recessed) at the femoral attachment. Fixation is performed with an interference screw passed through the anterolateral portal with the knee flexed to 110 degrees (Fig. 55-34). The interference screw is placed anterior to the bone block and snugly secures the graft.

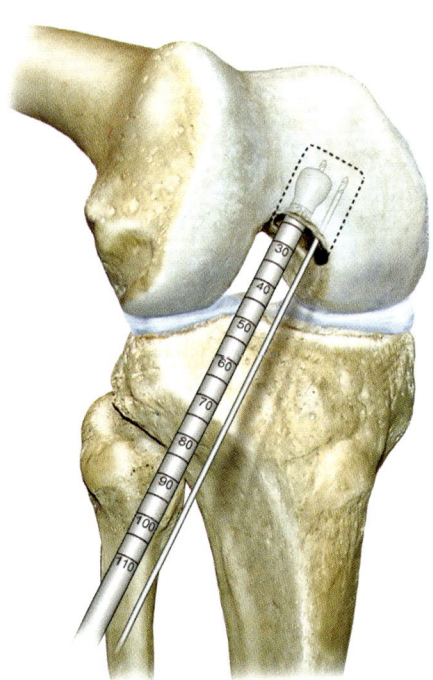

Figure 55-31. The guide pins are placed and then overreamed with an endoscopic drill to a depth of 25 mm, avoiding passage of the drill through the femoral cortex. The central bone bridge is removed with a curette and burr. (From Noyes FR, Barber-Westin SD: Posterior cruciate ligament: diagnosis, operative techniques, and clinical outcomes. In Noyes FR [ed]: Noyes' knee disorders: surgery, rehabilitation, clinical outcomes, Philadelphia, 2009, Saunders, pp 503–576.)

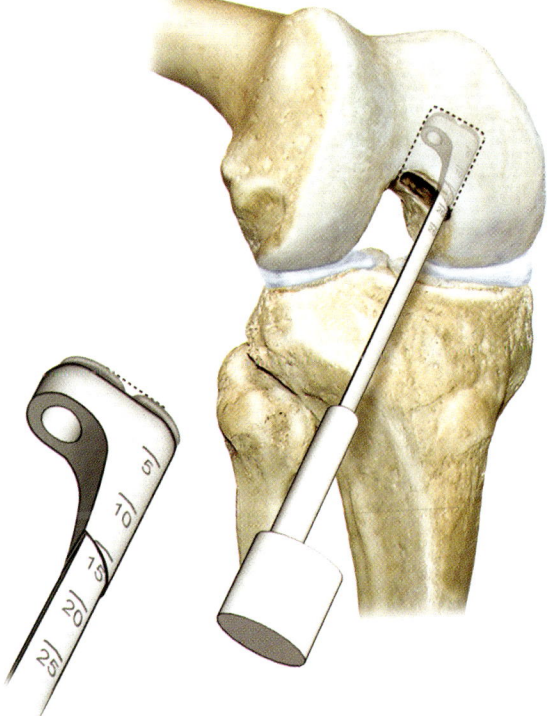

Figure 55-32. The PCL Dilator is used to gently conform the femoral oval footprint to 9 × 13 mm and to an appropriate depth. There is a matching oval opening in the PCL Dilator handle of 9 × 13 mm to size the bone block. (From Noyes FR, Barber-Westin SD: Posterior cruciate ligament: diagnosis, operative techniques, and clinical outcomes. In Noyes FR [ed]: Noyes' knee disorders: surgery, rehabilitation, clinical outcomes, Philadelphia, 2009, Saunders, pp 503–576.)

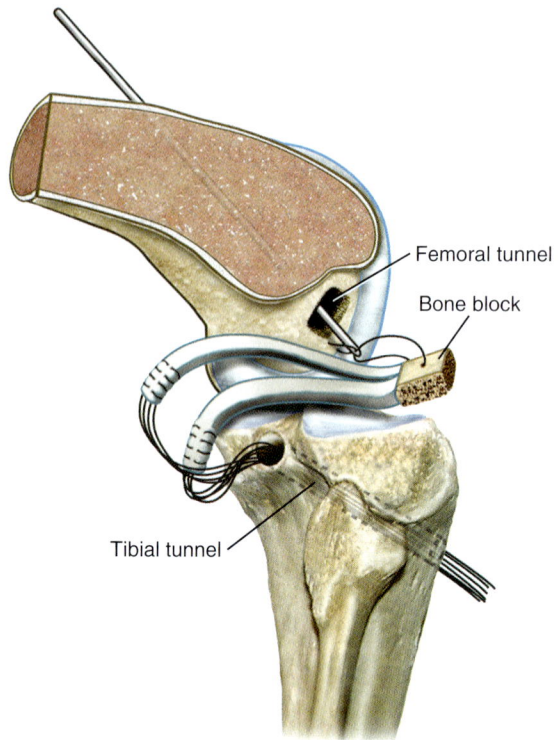

Figure 55-33. All-inside graft passage. A 20-gauge wire is passed through the tibial tunnel and grasped anteriorly through the anterolateral arthrotomy. The tibial portion of the graft is passed through the single tibial tunnel. The pin is then passed through the anterolateral portal into the femoral tunnel. The bone block is passed through the enlarged anterolateral portal and carefully oriented into the correct position, with the cancellous bone surface oriented deep in the oval opening. (From Noyes FR, Barber-Westin SD: Posterior cruciate ligament: diagnosis, operative techniques, and clinical outcomes. In Noyes FR [ed]: Noyes' knee disorders: surgery, rehabilitation, clinical outcomes, Philadelphia, 2009, Saunders, pp 503–576.)

The conditioning and graft tensioning are the same as described for the all-inside technique, except that the final fixation is performed at the tibial site with an interference screw and suture post.

Two Separate Femoral and Tibial Tunnels and Two Separate Grafts

This technique uses two separate BPTB grafts, one autograft and one allograft. The tibial and femoral outside-in tunnels are placed and drilled as described. The passage of the two bone grafts is technically more demanding when the ACL is present and requires patience. Two tibial tunnel guide wires are passed and brought out the anterolateral portal. The medial tibial (4 o'clock) femoral graft is passed first, with the tibial portion gently eased into the tibial tunnel. The femoral bone plug with a 4-cm loop lead suture is advanced through the anterolateral portal into the knee joint. A suture retrieval instrument is used at the posterior 4 o'clock femoral tunnel to grasp the suture and gently lift the bone block into the tunnel, assisted with a nerve hook. The arthroscope is placed in the central or anterolateral portal to view correct placement of the femoral bone plug. The procedure is repeated for the lateral tibial 1 o'clock femoral graft. It is important in the

preparation of the femoral tunnel that all soft tissues in the posterior aspect of the notch behind the PCL femoral attachment be removed to allow for the graft to pass and to provide sufficient visualization.

Through the anteromedial approach for the VMO, the outside aspect of the femoral tunnels is visualized. Through the arthroscope, the bone block is placed flush with the femoral tunnel opening within the joint. Each bone block is fixed with an absorbable interference screw. The visualization of the bone block deep in the tunnel is facilitated by use of the surgeon's headlight and graft position is verified by arthroscopy. In revision knees or if obvious femoral bone osteopenia is present and the fixation compromised, a suture post is used for added fixation, with the sutures placed in each bone block.

In the all-inside placement of the two femoral tunnels for two separate bone plugs when a BPTB graft is used, the graft passage is in the same order, except that the femoral portion of the graft is advanced through the anterolateral portal by a guide wire–suture carrier placed through the respective femoral tunnel. Interference screw fixation is performed through the anterolateral portal for each graft strand with the knee flexed to 110 degrees. The final placement of the bone block in the femoral tunnel is more ideal (less graft angulation) when the cancellous side of the bone block is posterior (deep) and the bone block is advanced flush with the femoral tunnel. Graft conditioning, tensioning, and fixation are performed as already described. The femoral interference screw is placed anterior to the 1 o'clock graft strand and distal (shallow) to the 4 o'clock graft strand; after appropriate tensioning, the final fixation is performed at the tibial site with an interference screw and suture post.

The senior author (FN) has used this technique and publications occasionally reference this procedure using a variety of grafts. The recommendation provided in this chapter is to use a single tibial tunnel with a bone plug without the added complexity of two tibial and two femoral tunnels.

Posterior Cruciate Ligament Arthroscope-Assisted Open Tibial Inlay Technique

We have described in detail all the operative steps required for the open tibial inlay and arthroscope-assisted femoral tunnel PCL reconstruction (Fig. 55-35).[76] The current recommended approach is to use the all-inside technique described here, in which the bone plug is positioned at the posterior tibial tunnel entrance, simulating the tibial inlay approach. The goal is to avoid the added time and potential morbidity of the open posteromedial approach. However, with added experience, it should be noted that the open posteromedial approach and tibial inlay procedure remain suitable techniques to use in select cases.

Posterior Cruciate Ligament Avulsion Fractures

Avulsion fractures of the PCL occasionally occur, particularly in younger patients. Treatment options are based on the type and size of the fracture, displacement, comminution, and orientation of the fragment.[37,66] These injuries usually occur at the tibial attachment and may involve a small area at the posterior region of the attachment or a large area that extends anteriorly and outside the PCL attachment. The avulsion

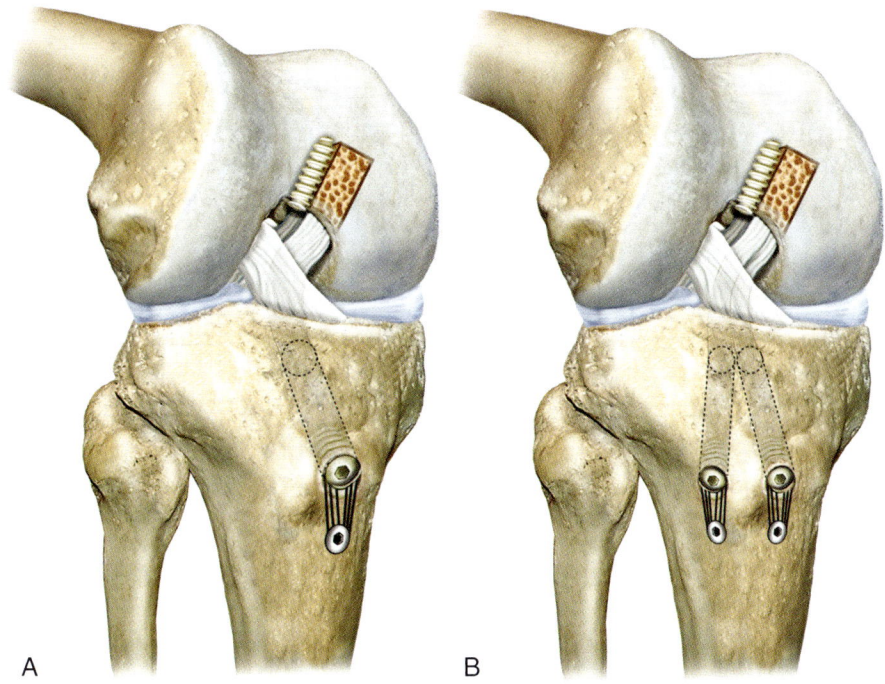

A   B

Figure 55-34. Final configuration of the single **(A)** or alternative two-tunnel **(B)** technique. (From Noyes FR, Barber-Westin SD: Posterior cruciate ligament: diagnosis, operative techniques, and clinical outcomes. In Noyes FR [ed]: Noyes' knee disorders: surgery, rehabilitation, clinical outcomes, Philadelphia, 2009, Saunders, pp 503–576.)

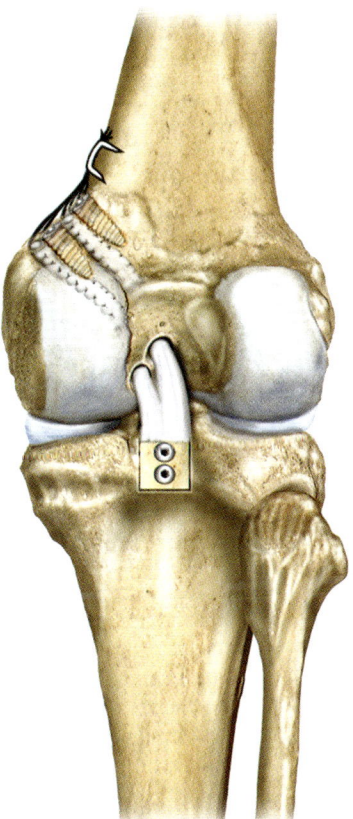

Figure 55-35. Final tibial and femoral fixation of the QT-PB two-strand graft. (From Noyes FR, Barber-Westin SD: Posterior cruciate ligament: diagnosis, operative techniques, and clinical outcomes. In Noyes FR [ed]: Noyes' knee disorders: surgery, rehabilitation, clinical outcomes, Philadelphia, 2009, Saunders, pp 503–576.)

fracture is obvious on routine radiographs but, on occasion, a computed tomography (CT) scan is required to define the extent of the facture pattern in major avulsion fractures extending into the joint.[7,37]

Patients who have small, partial PCL avulsion fractures, with a negative posterior translation test at 90 degrees knee flexion, are kept in a brace locked in full extension and remain partial weight bearing for 4 weeks to allow healing. The brace is removed for gentle range of motion (avoiding posterior tibial translation) and quadriceps exercises. Overall, the prognosis for healing and PCL function is good to excellent, although there may be a subtle increase in posterior tibial translation.[134]

Complete avulsion of the PCL attachment at the tibia, and less frequently, at the femoral attachment[100,104] (peel-off avulsion) with posterior tibial subluxation, is an indication for surgical repair. Numerous authors have reported good results with the open reduction and internal fixation of PCL avulsion fractures at the tibial insertion site.[45,66,126] Along with the tibial avulsion, an abnormal MRI signal intensity may be observed within the PCL fibers, indicating partial tearing; this is responsible for a residual posterior tibial translation after healing of the bone avulsion.

Arthroscopic techniques have been reported for fixation of PCL tibial avulsion injuries.[7,21,114] Kim and and coworkers[51] have reported on 14 knees that had an avulsion fracture of the PCL at the tibial attachment. The arthroscope was placed through the posteromedial portal and a plastic sheath with a waterproof diaphragm passed through the posterolateral portal. Large bone fragments were fixed using one or two transtibial cannulated screws placed from the anterior tibia. Small bony fragments were fixed with multiple sutures through one or two tibial tunnels. All avulsion fractures healed with only a small amount of residual posterior tibial translation. However, postoperative arthrofibrosis developed in 3 of 14 knees, which compromised the final result. It was speculated that an early range of motion program might be beneficial to prevent arthrofibrosis.

Shino and colleagues[114] have reported on six knees that had arthroscopic fixation of a PCL tibial bone avulsion. Fixation was achieved with a single cannulated screw or by suture fixation with comminuted injuries. A pullout button was introduced through the posteromedial portal and the sutures passed through two tibial drill holes and tied at the anterior aspect of the tibia.

The surgeon should select an arthroscopic or open technique for tibial avulsion fractures based on experience. In general, it is relatively straightforward to use an arthroscopic approach for cannulated screw fixation for large and medium-sized avulsion fractures. For PCL tibial avulsions with small bony fragments that require a combination of sutures and bone fixation, an open posterior tibial approach is favored by the senior author (FN) because it provides good exposure and allows for secure fixation. The therapist should begin protected knee motion within the first postoperative week, applying an anteriorly directed load to protect the relatively weak suture fixation. The use of a posterior calf pad and careful positioning in the brace are required for the first 4 postoperative weeks, until suitable healing has occurred. Knees with suture or pin fixation have relatively low tensile strength repairs and require expert postoperative rehabilitation.

A peel-off type of PCL rupture from the femoral attachment has been described as a hyperextension knee injury[64] or in patients suffering from trauma from a motor vehicle accident.[13,94] This type of PCL rupture directly at the femoral attachment may occur at the fibrocartilaginous junction with minor associated damage to most PCL fibers. The PCL attachment may be repaired with sutures passed through small drill holes, avoiding the proximal physeal growth plate.

Ross and colleagues[104] have described an arthroscopic approach for repair of acute femoral peel-off tears. Three no. 2 nonabsorbable sutures are passed through the PCL substance, through a femoral tunnel at the PCL footprint, and tied over the medial cortex. Park and Kim[94] have reported an arthroscopic technique that uses two transfemoral tunnels for the anterior strand and two posterior tunnels for suture repair of the posterior strand. They noted that femoral avulsion injuries were exceedingly rare.

The senior author's (FN) preferred technique for femoral peel-off or proximal PCL repairs is to use an arthroscope-assisted approach in which two or three guide pin tunnels are placed at the anterior and posterior aspects of the PCL footprint, distal to the physis, to fan out the PCL fiber attachment. A VMO-sparing approach is used and suture passers are brought into the knee joint. Through a limited medial arthrotomy and under direct visualization using a headlight, multiple nonabsorbable baseball looped sutures are placed at appropriate sites in the PCL fibers to approximate the broad elliptical femoral PCL attachment. Secure fixation is achieved along with anatomic placement of disrupted PCL fibers.

The decision is made at this point as to whether a tendon augmentation of the repair through separate femoral and tibial drill holes is required. In such cases, the arthroscopically assisted tendon augmentation drill holes are first placed in the respective tibial and femoral sites, the graft is passed, and the tibiofemoral joint reduced. A nonirradiated tendon allograft is the senior author's (FN) first choice for skeletally immature patients and the second choice is a doubled semitendinosus autograft.

The sutures in the proximal PCL stump are placed and brought out through anteriorly and posteriorly placed femoral drill holes. In children, the physis is not crossed at the tibial or femoral site and the augmentation tunnel is 4 to 5 mm in diameter. In most cases of a peel-off fracture, a tendon augmentation is not necessary because the bulk of the PCL fibers can be brought back to the PCL femoral attachment.

In PCL injuries that extend away from the femoral attachment and involve the proximal third of the PCL fibers, an augmentation is favored. The postoperative protocol for a direct suture repair should take into account the low repair tensile strength, requiring maximum protection. The knee is maintained in full extension and the therapist assists in gentle range of knee motion for the first 4 weeks postoperatively. Only toe-touch weight bearing is permitted during this time period. Then, the patient may progress to 50% weight bearing with the brace locked at full extension. At 6 weeks postoperatively, weight bearing is progressed in the brace. Knee motion is advanced to 0 to 90 degrees. The brace is removed at 8 weeks.

POSTOPERATIVE REHABILITATION

Our rehabilitation program is summarized in Table 55-3.[82] The protocol consists of a careful incorporation of exercise concepts supported by scientific data and clinical experience. The protocol was developed for a two-strand PCL graft reconstruction (QT-PB, BPTB). The goal is to progress a patient at a rate that takes into account athletic and occupational goals, condition of the articular surfaces and menisci, return of muscle function and lower limb control, and postoperative graft healing. Modifications to the program may be required if articular cartilage deterioration is found during surgery.

The supervised rehabilitation program is supplemented with home exercises that are performed daily. Therapeutic procedures and modalities and routine examinations are used as required for successful rehabilitation. Patients are warned to avoid any exercises or activities that place high posterior shear forces on the tibia, such as walking down inclines or squatting, for the first 6 postoperative months. In addition, patients are cautioned that an early return to strenuous activities postoperatively carries a risk of a repeat injury or the potential of compounding the original injury.

Passive knee motion from 0 to 120 degrees is begun the first day postoperatively, along with patellar mobilization. Although patients are encouraged to regain full extension as soon as possible, knee flexion is limited for the first 7 to 8 postoperative weeks to avoid high posterior shear forces. The total number of daily knee motion cycles is limited to 60 (20 cycles, three times daily) for the first 4 weeks to lessen abrasion effects on the graft.

A long-leg hinged postoperative brace with a posterior calf pad is worn for the first 6 weeks postoperatively, 24 hours a day. A functional PCL brace is indicated when patients return to a higher level of occupational or sports activities. In patients who undergo a combined PCL-posterolateral procedure, a bivalved cast is used for 4 weeks postoperatively to limit lateral joint opening during ambulation and daily

Table 55-3 Rehabilitation Protocol Following Posterior Cruciate Ligament Reconstruction

Parameter	POSTOPERATIVE WEEKS					POSTOPERATIVE MONTHS			
	1-2	3-4	5-6	7-8	9-12	4	5	6	7-12
Hinged long-leg postoperative brace	X	X	X						
Patellar knee sleeve				X	X	X	X		
Functional brace								X	X
Range of motion, minimum goals (degrees)									
0-90	X								
0-110		X							
0-120			X						
0-135					X				
Weight bearing									
25% body weight	X								
50% body weight		X							
Full				X					
Patella mobilization	X	X	X	X					
Modalities									
Electrical muscle stimulation (EMS)	X	X	X	X	X				
Pain, edema management (cryotherapy)	X	X	X	X	X	X	X	X	X
Stretching									
Hamstring, gastroc-soleus, iliotibial band, quadriceps	X	X	X	X	X	X	X	X	X
Strengthening									
Quad isometrics, straight leg raises, active knee extension	X	X	X	X	X				
Closed-chain—gait retraining, toe raises, wall sits, minisquats				X	X	X	X	X	
Knee flexion hamstring curls (90-0 degrees)					X	X	X	X	X
Knee extension quads (90-30 degrees)		X	X	X	X	X	X	X	X
Hip abduction-adduction, multihip		X	X	X	X	X	X	X	X
Leg press (70-10 degrees)			X	X	X	X	X	X	X
Balance, proprioceptive training									
Weight shifting, cup walking, BBS			X	X					
BBS, BAPS, perturbation training, balance board, minitrampoline					X	X	X	X	X
Conditioning									
UBC	X	X	X	X	X				
Bike (stationary)				X	X	X	X	X	X
Aquatic program					X	X	X	X	X
Swimming (kicking)					X	X	X	X	X
Walking					X	X	X	X	X
Stair climbing machine					X	X	X	X	X
Ski machine					X	X	X	X	X
Running, straight								X	
Cutting–lateral carioca, figure eights									X
Plyometric training									X
Full sports									X

From Noyes FR, Barber-Westin SD, Heckmann T: Rehabilitation of posterior cruciate ligament and posterolateral reconstructive procedures. In Noyes FR (ed): Noyes' knee disorders: surgery, rehabilitation, clinical outcomes, Philadelphia, 2009, Saunders, pp 631– 657.

BAPS, Biomechanical Ankle Platform System (Camp, Jackson, Mich); *BBS,* Biodex Balance System (Biodex Medical Systems, Shirley, NY); *UBC,* Upper Body Cycle (Biodex).

activities. The cast is removed four times daily and active range of knee motion is performed in a seated position. The cast is then carefully reapplied to protect the knee joint during walking activities. After the first 4 postoperative weeks, sufficient healing of the posterolateral ligamentous reconstructive procedure should occur and the patient is placed in a long-leg hinged brace.

Patients are allowed to bear 25% of their body weight during the first 1 to 2 postoperative weeks. Weight bearing is then slowly progressed and crutches are usually discontinued at postoperative week 6. The entire program is described in detail elsewhere.[82]

CLINICAL STUDIES

All of our clinical studies involved a prospective, consecutive patient enrollment, using the validated Cincinnati Knee Rating System for the analysis of function and symptoms.

The minimum follow-up duration of each study described here was 24 months; the results were evaluated by a senior clinical research associate and not the surgeon.

Posterior Cruciate Ligament Two-Strand Procedures

Quadriceps Tendon-Patellar Bone Autograft, Tibial Inlay

Nineteen knees with chronic PCL ruptures treated with a two-strand PCL QT-PB autograft reconstruction (tibial inlay approach) were followed for a mean of 35 months (range, 24 to 84 months) postoperatively.[69] The PCL reconstructions were done at a mean of 43 months (range, 4 to 216 months) after the original knee injury. In nine knees, prior PCL procedures had been done elsewhere and failed. Associated procedures included posterolateral procedures in five knees, ACL reconstruction in two knees, MCL semitendinosus-gracilis reconstruction in two knees, and meniscus transplantation[84] in one knee.

The mean increase in posterior tibial translation (compared with the contralateral knee) on stress radiography improved from 11.6 ± 2.9 mm preoperatively to 5.0 ± 2.6 mm at follow-up ($P < .0001$). Preoperatively, all knees were graded C or D (International Knee Documentation Committee [IKDC] rating) according to stress radiographic data. At follow-up, 2 knees (10%) were graded A, 12 knees (63%) as B, 3 knees (16%) as C, and 2 knees (10%) as D. All the associated knee ligament procedures were rated A or B at follow-up. There were no infections, permanent limitations of knee motion, donor site problems, or patellar fractures.

All patients except 1 rated their knee condition as improved. Before surgery, 11 patients (58%) had pain with daily activities, but only 1 (5%) had such pain at follow-up. Significant improvements were noted for symptoms and limitations with daily and sports activities. Eleven patients (58%) were participating in low-impact sports and two were participating in more strenuous sports without problems.

The results affirmed the recommendation for early operative treatment for PCL ruptures, because by the time surgical reconstruction is necessary for problems with daily activities, the reconstruction may not be effective because of arthritic joint damage. The posterior stability obtained in this study was superior to that previously reported in our single-strand PCL allograft investigation.[73] Stress radiographs revealed that 68% of the knees had no more than 5 mm increase in posterior tibial displacement, compared with 37% of the knees in the allograft population. Still, in acute injury situations, or in dislocated knees that require multiligament reconstructive procedures, allografts may be more suitable.

Quadriceps Tendon-Patellar Bone Autograft, Tibial Tunnel

Twenty-nine knees that received a two-strand PCL QT-PB autograft reconstruction (all-inside tibial tunnel) were followed for a mean of 43 months (range, 24 to 84 months) postoperatively.[81] Eighteen patients had the PCL reconstruction for chronic ruptures and 11, for acute injuries. Fifteen knees had an associated ligament reconstruction, including ACL reconstruction in nine knees, MCL repair or reconstruction in six, posterolateral procedures in five, and meniscus transplantation in one.

The mean increase in posterior tibial translation measured with stress radiography improved from 10.5 ± 2.9 mm preoperatively to 6.5 ± 4.3 mm at follow-up ($P = .06$). Preoperatively, all knees were rated C or D (IKDC) according the stress radiographic data. At follow-up, 3 knees (10%) were rated A, 7 knees (24%) as B, 17 knees (59%) as C, and 2 knees (7%) as D. Eight of the associated ACL reconstructions were rated A or B and 1 was rated C. All the MCL and posterolateral procedures were rated as A or B. There were no infections or patellar fractures. Two patients reported residual pain at the patellar donor site.

Of these patients, 94% rated their knee condition as improved. Before surgery, 87% of patients with chronic PCL ruptures had pain with daily activities compared with 11% at follow-up. Significant improvements were noted for pain, swelling, giving way, walking, stairs, running, jumping, and twisting or turning ($P < .01$). For all 29 patients, 15 (52%) returned to low-impact sports and 7 (24%) were participating in strenuous sports without problems.

Revision Quadriceps Tendon-Patellar Bone Autograft Reconstruction

PCL revision reconstructions with a two-strand QT-PB autograft were performed in 15 knees that were followed for a mean of 44 months (range, 23 to 84) postoperatively.[75] A mean of 46 months (range, 4 to 187 months) had elapsed between the failed PCL procedures and the revision. Before the PCL revision reconstruction, a staged HTO was required in three knees and an autogenous bone grafting of prior graft tunnels was done in one knee.

The tibial inlay technique was used in nine knees and the tibial tunnel technique was done in six knees. Six knees had one or more concomitant ligament reconstructive procedures with the PCL revision. Four knees had a ACL allograft reconstruction,[70] one had an MCL autograft reconstruction,[80] and four had a posterolateral reconstruction.

Stress radiograph posterior tibial translation values improved from 11.7 ± 3.0 mm preoperatively to 5.1 ± 2.4 mm at follow-up ($P < .001$). Before the revision, all knees were rated as C or D according to stress radiographic data. At follow-up, one knee was rated A, nine knees as B, four knees as C, and one knee as D. Associated knee ligament reconstructive procedures restored anterior, medial, and posterolateral stability.

Significant improvements occurred in pain, function, and patient perception scores, and 87% thought that their overall knee condition was better postoperatively. However, the subjective and functional results were inferior to those reported after primary acute PCL reconstruction. Only 53% returned to light sports without problems.

The QT-PB two-strand revision provided reasonable results in this group of complex knees; however, this is a small series of PCL revision cases, and definitive conclusions cannot be reached. In this study, 13 of 15 knees (87%) had compounding problems of articular cartilage damage, prior meniscectomy, need for associated ligament procedures, or varus malalignment with medial tibiofemoral compartment damage. The results were inferior to those obtainable from primary PCL reconstructions, because most patients were in a salvage knee situation.

Results of Posterior Cruciate Ligament Two-Strand Reconstructions from Other Investigators

Whereas many reports have described two-strand PCL reconstruction,* only a few investigators outside our center have reported on the outcome of two-strand PCL reconstruction using objective measuring instruments. Most of these used the KT-2000 to quantify the results of the operations, and not stress radiography,[92,120] which unfortunately underestimates the true amount of posterior tibial translation in PCL-deficient and reconstructed knees at 70 degrees of knee flexion. To date, only three investigations[33,69,81] have used stress radiography to ascertain the results of two-strand PCL reconstruction. The range of patients with 5 mm or less of increased posterior tibial translation in these studies was 34% to 73%. The number of patients in each study was too small to perform valid comparisons. Therefore, to date, there remain too few evidence-based studies to determine the indications for a two-strand versus a single-strand technique, the most advantageous graft to select for different circumstances, and the failure rate for autografts and allografts.

Stannard and associates[120] have reported on 29 patients who sustained acute traumatic multiligament injuries and received a two-strand AT-B PCL allograft and were followed from 15 to 39 months postoperatively. The technique used two femoral tunnels and a tibial inlay approach. The anterolateral strand was tensioned at 70 degrees of knee flexion and the posteromedial strand was tensioned at 20 degrees of flexion. Both strands were secured with absorbable interference screws. The report noted that 20% of the patients had a 1+ posterior laxity and 80% had no increased posterior laxity at follow-up. However, 40% of the patients developed some degree of arthrofibrosis and required a manipulation or arthroscopic lysis of adhesions. The KT-2000 data showed that 50% of the operated knees had less posterior tibial displacement at 70 degrees of flexion than the contralateral knees. Stress radiographs were not performed. Fifty-five percent returned to their pre-injury level of activities, 41% returned to a lower level, and 3% did not return to sports.

Nyland and coworkers[92] have reported on the short-term (27 ± 2 months) clinical results of a two-strand anterior tibialis allograft reconstruction in 19 knees with chronic PCL injuries. The technique used two femoral tunnels and a single tibial tunnel. One femoral tunnel was located at the 3 o'clock position, 12 mm posterior to the anterior articular edge, and the second tunnel was placed at 1 o'clock, 5 mm posterior to the anterior cartilage edge. Both femoral strands were secured with the knee flexion to 80 to 90 degrees of knee flexion with interference screws. Postoperatively, KT-1000 testing revealed a mean of 2.4 ± 2 mm posterior displacement. Posterior drawer testing showed normal (11 knees) or near-normal (8 knees) test results. Seventeen patients were graded as normal or near-normal in the overall IKDC score, one was graded as abnormal, and one as severely abnormal.

Garofalo and colleagues[33] used two autografts to reconstruct chronic PCL ruptures in 15 patients. A B-PT-B graft was used to replace the posteromedial strand and a semitendinosus graft was used for the anterolateral strand. A single

transtibial tunnel and two femoral tunnels were used, one of which was placed at the 11 o'clock position, 8 mm proximal from the cartilage edge, and the other at the 9 o'clock position (left knee). The anterolateral strand was tensioned and fixed at 70 degrees of flexion and the posteromedial strand was fixed at 30 degrees of flexion. At follow-up, 2 to 5 years postoperatively, 40% of the patients had 6 mm or more of increased posterior tibial translation on stress radiographs. It was concluded that the procedure offers no advantage over that of single-strand constructs in terms of restoration of normal posterior translation.

POSTEROLATERAL SURGICAL TECHNIQUE OPTIONS

Fibular Collateral Ligament Anatomic Reconstruction

Perhaps the most common injury associated with PCL ruptures is posterolateral ligament ruptures. We have described in detail the surgical options for correcting lateral and posterolateral ligamentous deficiency.[77] These options are based on the quality and integrity of these tissues determined at the time of surgery and the anatomic structures that are disrupted. Indications for reconstruction of the posterolateral structures include abnormal lateral joint opening, increased external tibial rotation, and a varus recurvatum position with hyperextension of the knee.

In cases of acute ligamentous disruptions, primary repair of the FCL is only indicated for bony avulsions that are amenable to internal fixation. Otherwise, graft reconstruction is recommended. We prefer to perform acute posterolateral reconstruction procedures within the first 10 days of injury. Because posterolateral ruptures are usually accompanied by injuries to one or both cruciates and may represent a knee dislocation, we observe these patients for 1 week to evaluate the neurovascular structures and skin condition. This short delay also allows appropriate planning of the surgical procedure and, most importantly, the institution of rehabilitation to initiate supervised range of motion and muscle exercises prior to surgery.

Our preferred technique for acute posterolateral injuries not amenable to primary repair or chronic ruptures is an anatomic FCL reconstruction with a B-PT-B graft. A 10- to 12-cm skin incision is made in a straight line centered over the joint line and 1 cm posterior to the iliotibial band (ITB) attachment at the tibia (Fig. 55-36). The skin flaps are mobilized beneath the subcutaneous tissue and fascia to protect the vascular and neural supply. The peroneal nerve is identified and protected throughout the procedure and usually is not dissected from its anatomic position.

The ITB is incised at the posterior edge and anterior to the biceps tendon. The ITB attachments are excised to the short head of the biceps femoris muscle and the ITB is gently lifted anteriorly to expose the entire lateral aspect of lateral femoral condyle and attachments of the popliteus, FCL, and lateral gastrocnemius muscle tendon attachment.

The interval anterior to the lateral gastrocnemius tendon at the joint line, and directly at the top of the fibula, is entered, avoiding the inferior geniculate artery. The approach is similar to that described for meniscal repairs.[72] This allows exposure of the PMTL junction, posterolateral capsule, and

---

*References 9, 11, 12, 50, 99, 103, 108, and 119.

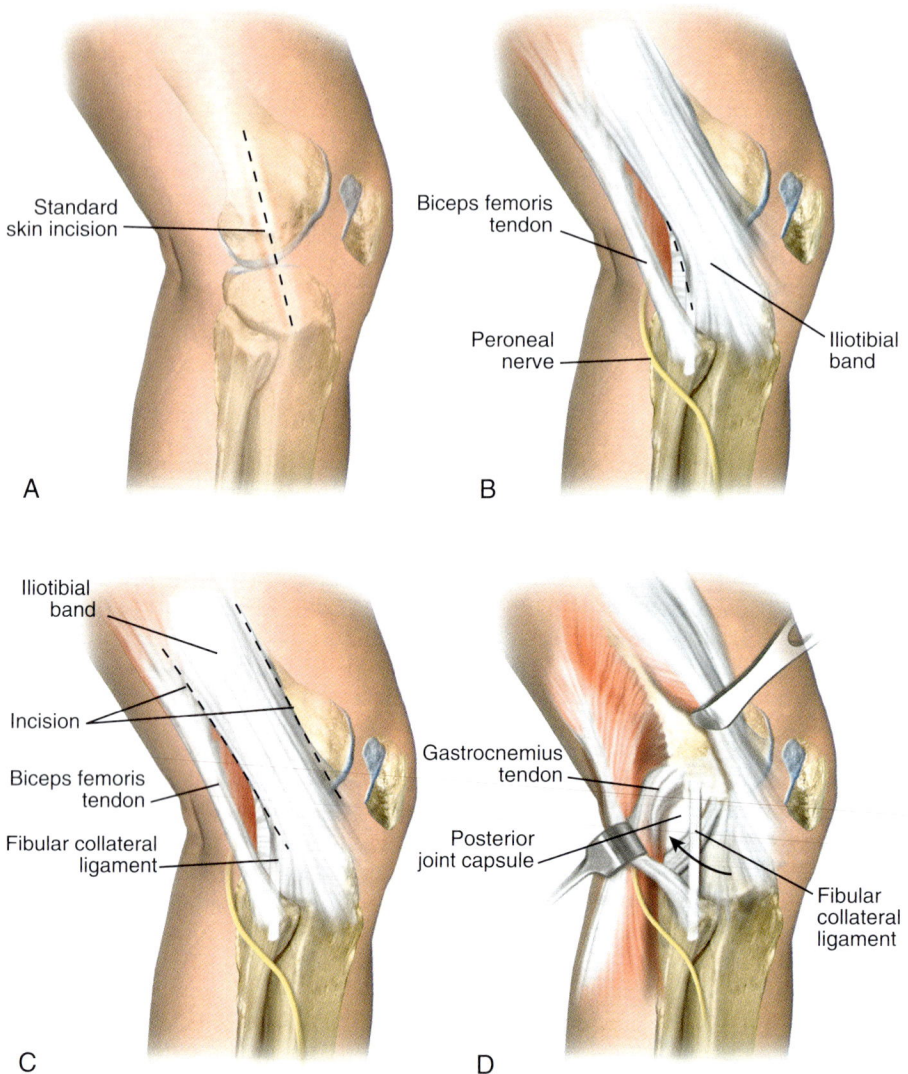

Figure 55-36. Posterolateral surgical technique. **A,** Site for the skin incision. **B,** Incision site in the interval between the posterior edge of the iliotibial band (ITB) and the anterior edge of the biceps tendon. **C,** In chronic cases with severe scarring, it may be necessary to add an anterior incision and displace the ITB posteriorly during the reconstructive procedure to allow better exposure. **D,** With the ITB retracted anteriorly, the interval between the lateral head of the gastrocnemius and the posterolateral aspect of the capsule is opened bluntly, just proximal to the fibular head, without entering the joint capsule proximally. (From Noyes FR, Barber-Westin SD: Posterolateral ligament injuries: diagnosis, operative techniques, and clinical outcomes. In Noyes FR [ed]: Noyes´ knee disorders: surgery, rehabilitation, clinical outcomes, Philadelphia, 2009, Saunders, pp 577–630.)

PFL. A second anterior ITB incision may be required when there is extensive scar involving all of the posterolateral structures. The VLO is lifted gently in an anterior direction and an S retractor is placed beneath the muscle fibers. A vertical incision approximately 2 cm in length is made into the capsule, just anterior to the popliteus tendon attachment. The joint is entered and the lateral meniscus attachments are inspected and later repaired if torn about the popliteal hiatus.

The normal anatomic attachment sites of the FCL to the lateral femur and anterolateral aspect of the fibular head are identified and a suture is placed between the two attachment sites; the length is measured to determine the required graft size. The bone portion of each end of the graft is 22 to 25 mm in length. The fibular graft attachment is performed using a

tunnel at the anatomic attachment site. The femoral graft is attached by placing a femoral tunnel at the anatomic attachment site. A second option is a femoral inlay of the proximal bone portion of the graft; this is useful if there is a 5- to 8-mm discrepancy of graft length, which would not allow full coverage of the bone in a femoral tunnel. The patellar tendon graft must normally be 50 mm or longer to be suitable for an anatomic FCL reconstruction. In some patients, the autogenous patellar tendon is too small and therefore an allograft of the desired size is required. We ensure that sufficient allograft tissue is available during surgery.

The bone portion of the graft is gently taped into the fibular tunnel so that the bone is entirely seated into the tunnel and level with the proximal fibular head to preserve

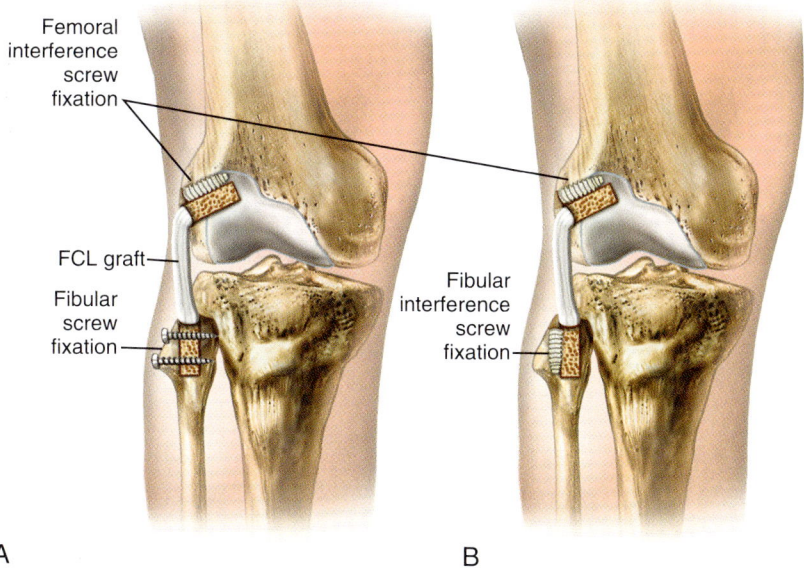

Figure 55-37. Anatomic substitution of the FCL with a B-PT-B autograft or allograft showing two methods for fibular graft fixation. **A,** Two small fragment screws are used to fix the bone into a tunnel created in the proximal fibula (our preference). Interference screw fixation is used at the femoral anatomic site of the FCL. **B,** A fibular tunnel is made, the graft is seated, and an interference screw is used for fixation. (From Noyes FR, Barber-Westin SD: Posterolateral ligament injuries: diagnosis, operative techniques, and clinical outcomes. In Noyes FR [ed]: Noyes' knee disorders: surgery, rehabilitation, clinical outcomes, Philadelphia, 2009, Saunders, pp 577–630.)

graft length. The ideal graft fixation is with two small fragment cortical screws placed from anterior to posterior, engaging both fibular cortices, in the proximal and distal thirds of the bone portion of the graft (Fig. 55-37). The proximal bone of the graft is advanced into the femoral tunnel. The graft is conditioned by cycling the knee 20 to 30 times. The graft is fixed with a soft tissue interference screw at 30 degrees of knee flexion, in neutral tibial rotation, under an approximate 5-lb tensile load (22 N) on the sutures, which have been advanced by the Beath needle to the medial aspect of the knee. The graft is purposely not overtensioned to avoid over-constraining the lateral tibiofemoral joint.

Popliteus Muscle–Tendon–Ligament Procedures

In acute cases in which partial PMTL function exists and the joint external tibial rotation (PL subluxation) is deemed only moderate (10 degrees increased tibial rotation at 30 degrees of knee flexion), a surgical repair of disrupted tissues is performed. The FCL graft reconstruction protects the PMTL repair and provides the necessary resistance against abnormal lateral joint opening and external tibial rotation. In acute cases, in which the popliteus is avulsed at its femoral site, a direct repair may be performed. In most cases, the tear is at the distal muscle-tendon junction or fiber attachment.

In chronic cases in which no PMTL function is found, a graft replacement is required (Fig. 55-38). The senior author (FN) prefers to use an AT-B allograft. The bone portion of the graft is placed at the anatomic femoral insertion site and the collagenous portion of the graft is passed in the tibial tunnel. Alternative grafts to consider are a B-PT-B allograft (which is more difficult to pass through the tibial tunnel) or a semitendinosus and gracilis (STG) two-strand autograft (which is less ideal because there is no bone attachment on the femur). An incision is made just beneath Gerdy's tubercle,

extending from the bare area of the anterior fibula to the tibial tubercle, and then 3 cm distally along the anterolateral tibia. A retractor is placed anterior to the lateral gastrocnemius muscle and tendon to expose the popliteus muscle. The final tibial 8-mm tunnel is at the most lateral aspect of the tibial margin and 15 mm distal to the joint line, passing through the popliteus muscle attachment and just medial to the tibiofibular joint. The total length of the graft is determined from the femoral to tibial insertion, including added length for the tibial suture fixation distal to the anterior tibial tunnel.

The graft is passed through the femoral tunnel, through the tibial tunnel, and fixed at the femoral site by an interference screw. The graft is conditioned by repetitive knee flexion and extension, and fixation is performed with an absorbable interference screw in the tibial tunnel with the leg at 30 degrees of knee flexion, neutral tibial rotation, and approximately 5 lb (22 N) of tension placed on the graft. A backup suture fixation post with a screw is used on the anterolateral aspect of the tibia. A final assessment of the graft is done to determine that it is under adequate tension and is blocking abnormal external tibial rotation and knee hyperextension. A direct suture of the PMT graft to the FCL graft at the level of the fibular head is done (see Fig. 55-38F, G). A plication procedure of the posterolateral structures is performed at 10 degrees of flexion, avoiding overtension, which would limit normal extension (see Fig. 55-38H, I). For knees which have severe hyperextension (>15 degrees), advancement of the posterolateral capsule will note be sufficient to block the hyperextension postoperatively. We have described elsewhere a posterlateral capsule reconstruction using an AT allograft.[77]

Femoral-Fibular Reconstruction

Another operative option that we have described for posterolateral instability is a nonanatomic femoral-fibular

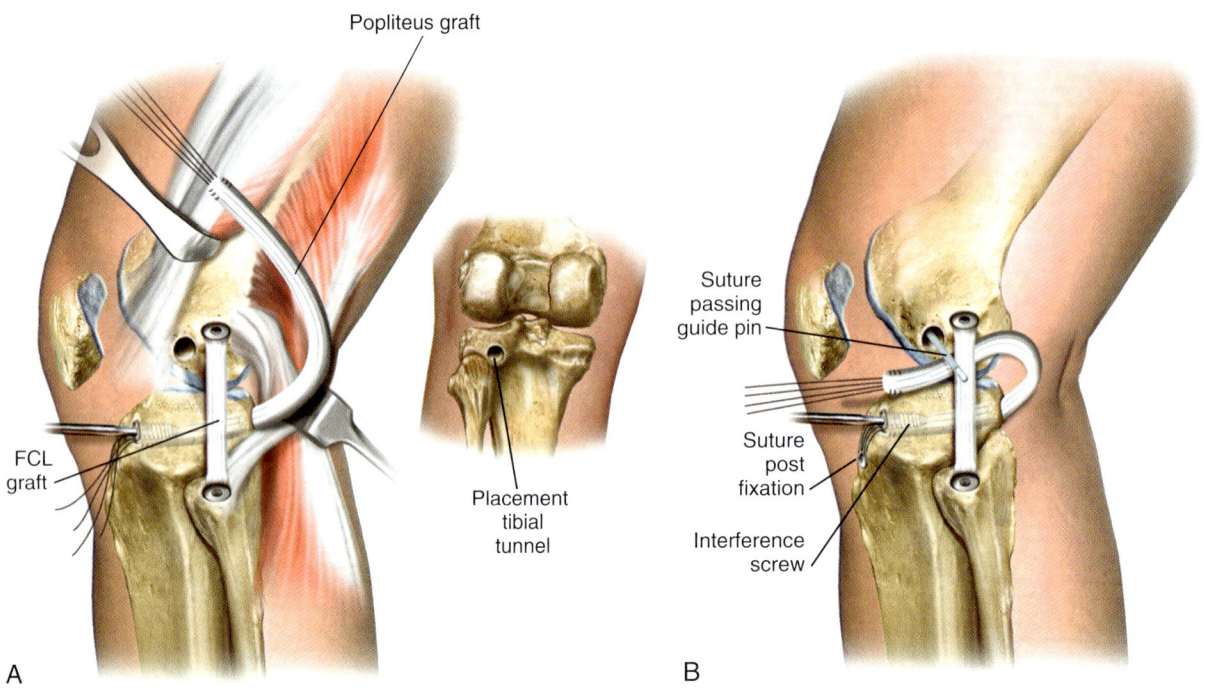

A

B

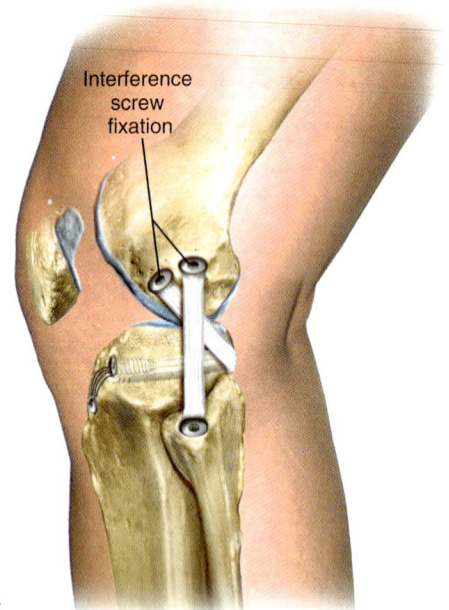

C

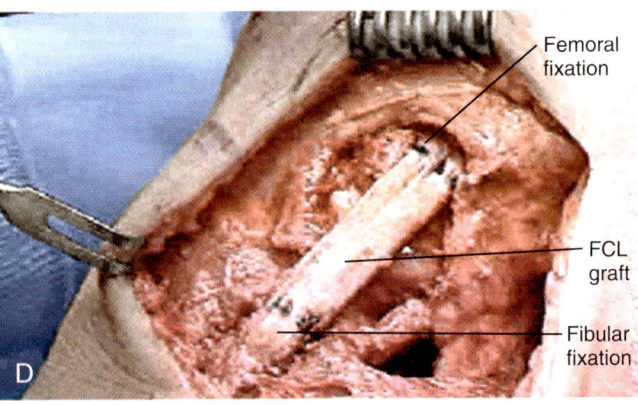

Figure 55-38. Anatomic PMTL reconstruction and FCL reconstruction with B-PT-B autograft or allograft. **A,** Location of posterolateral tibial tunnel and graft passage. A soft tissue interference screw and suture post are used for tibial fixation of the popliteus graft. **B,** Passage of popliteus graft beneath the FCL B-PT-B graft. **C** and **D,** Final fixation of the popliteus and FCL graft reconstructions.

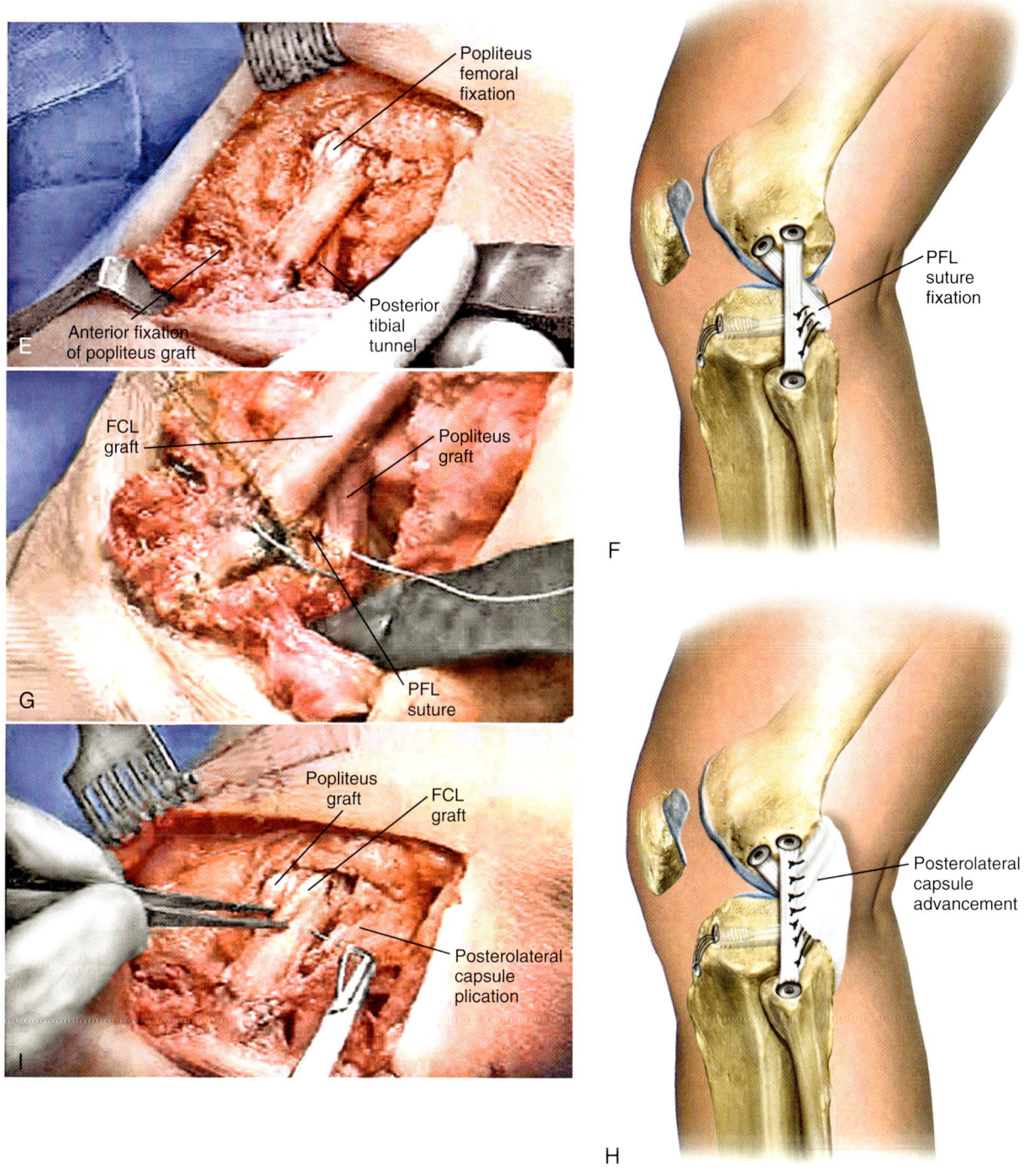

Figure 55-38, cont'd. E, Final fixation of the popliteus and FCL graft reconstructions. **F, G,** Suture of popliteus graft to posterior margin of the FCL graft at the fibular attachment site to restore the popliteofibular ligament. **H** and **I,** Suture plication of posterolateral capsule to posterior margin of the FCL graft. (From Noyes FR, Barber-Westin SD: Posterolateral ligament injuries: diagnosis, operative techniques, and clinical outcomes. In Noyes FR [ed]: Noyes' knee disorders: surgery, rehabilitation, clinical outcomes, Philadelphia, 2009, Saunders, pp 577–630.)

graft reconstruction.[78] This procedure is indicated when the FCL is intact but deficient and the PMTL does not require graft substitution. In addition, the procedure is advantageous when operative time needs to be considered in dislocated knees and a relatively easy stabilizing procedure can be performed.

The femoral-fibular reconstruction provides a large graft reconstruction of the FCL and a posterior graft arm to augment the posterolateral structures (Fig. 55-39). The posterolateral capsule reconstruction is performed by a plication procedure. The popliteus tendon is plicated to the fibular FCL reconstruction to restore the PFL. The procedure is considered a nonanatomic reconstruction because the femoral-fibular graft is placed adjacent but not directly at the FCL femoral and fibular anatomic attachment sites.

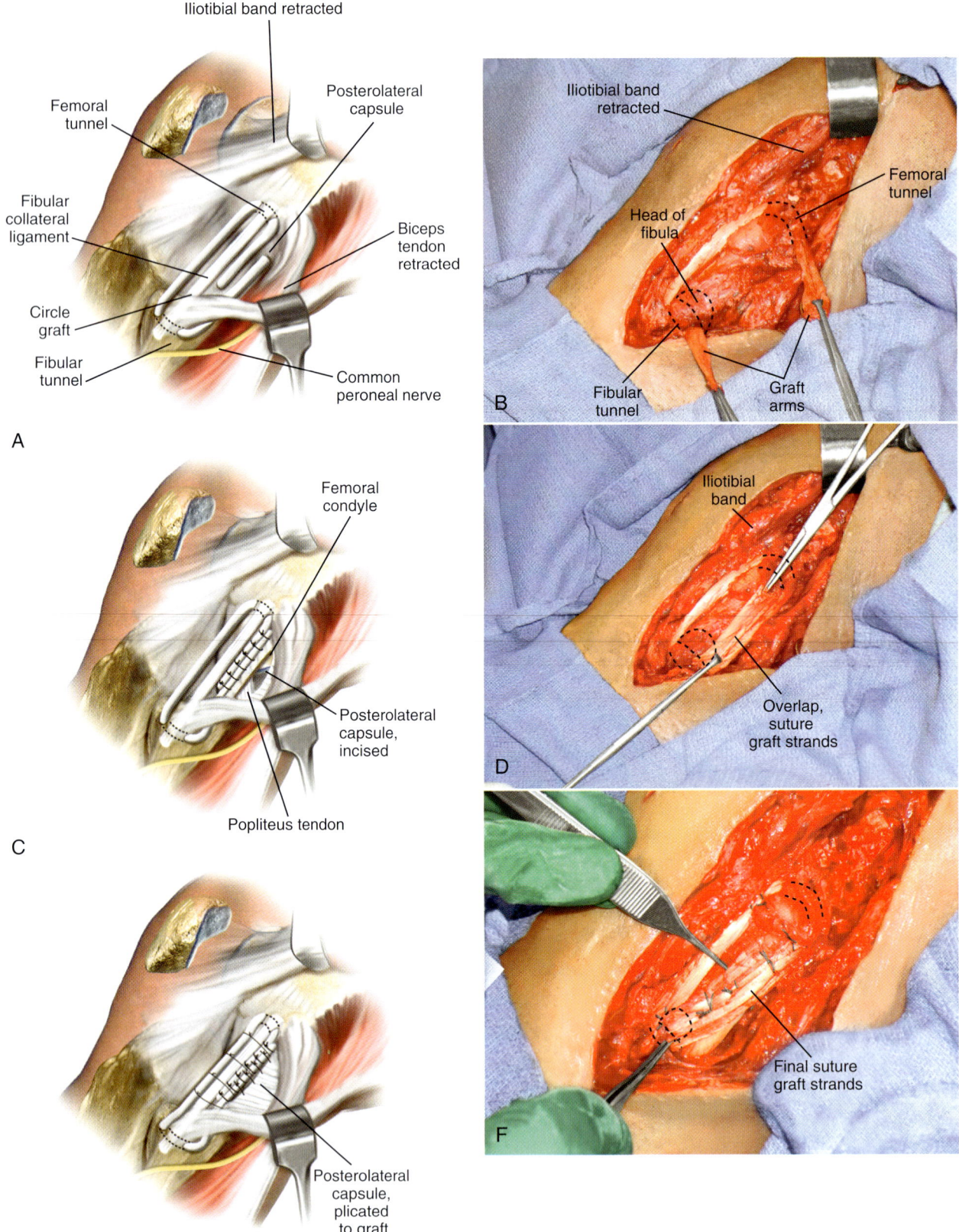

Figure 55-39. Femoral-fibular reconstruction. **A, B,** Placement of femoral and fibular tunnels and FCL graft. **C, D,** Suturing and tensioning of graft arms. **E, F,** Multiple sutures used through both arms of the graft and the slack FCL. Plication of the posterolateral capsule is performed to the graft. (From Noyes FR, Barber-Westin SD: Posterolateral ligament injuries: diagnosis, operative techniques, and clinical outcomes. In Noyes FR [ed]: Noyes' knee disorders: surgery, rehabilitation, clinical outcomes, Philadelphia, 2009, Saunders, pp 577–630.)

Proximal Advancement
of the Posterolateral Structures

A third operative approach may be considered in knees in which chronic insufficiency of the posterolateral structures results from a minor injury (without a traumatic disruption) or from varus osseous malalignment and a varus recurvatum thrust on walking. The posterolateral insufficiency is caused by interstitial tearing; a definitive FCL of normal width and integrity (although lax) can be identified and the

PMTL appears functionally intact, even though elongated. A graft reconstruction is not indicated for these knees. Instead, the posterolateral tissues are proximally advanced in a more simplified manner, which avoids the added operative complexity and morbidity that may occur with major graft reconstructive procedures (Fig. 55-40).[79] Importantly, the FCL must be at least 5 to 7 mm in width and the posterolateral structures must be at least 3 to 4 mm thick to be functional when the residual slackness is removed by the advancement procedure. The goal is to advance the FCL in a proximal

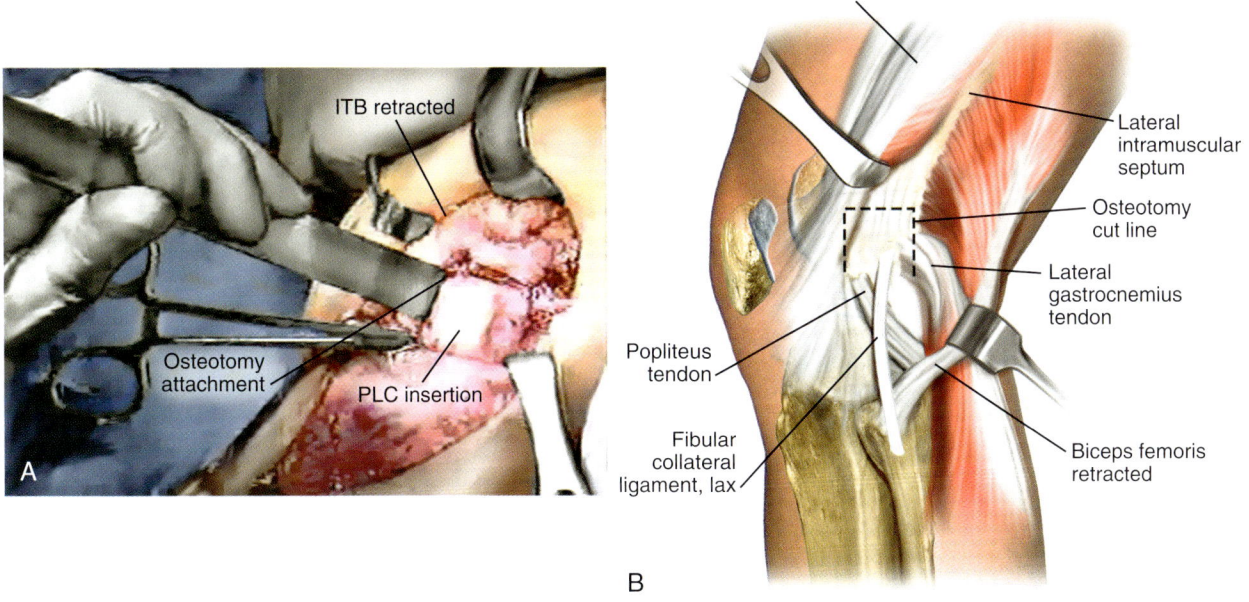

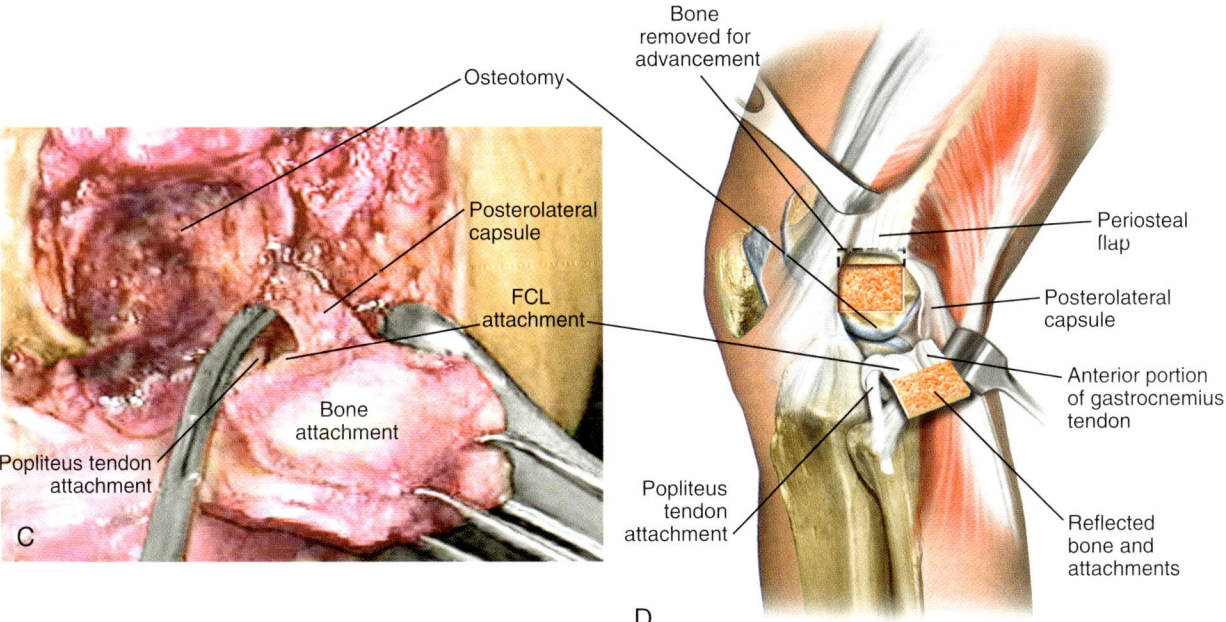

Figure 55-40. Proximal advancement of intact but lax posterolateral structures. **A** and **B,** Posterolateral structures are identified and have a normal appearance, although lax. The line for the osteotomy of the femoral attachment of the FCL, PMT, and anterior portion of the gastrocnemius tendon is shown. **C** and **D,** The osteotomy is 8 mm deep to provide sufficient bone to maintain the attachments of the FCL, popliteus tendon, anterior gastrocnemius tendon, and posterolateral capsule. The posterolateral capsule is incised 15 mm in length.

Continued

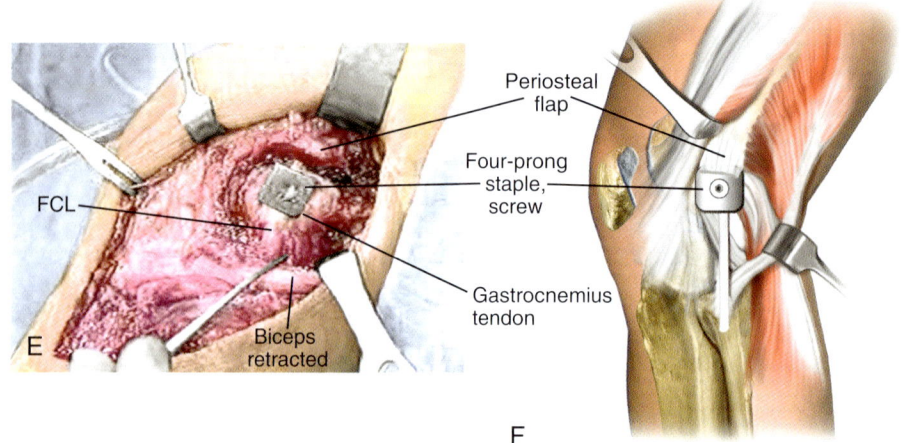

Figure 55-40, cont'd. E and **F,** The bone attachment of the posterolateral structures is advanced proximally in line with the FCL, with the knee in neutral tibial rotation and 30 degrees flexion. Reattachment of the bone is achieved with a four-pronged staple and screw. (From Noyes FR, Barber-Westin SD: Posterolateral ligament injuries: diagnosis, operative techniques, and clinical outcomes. In Noyes FR [ed]: Noyes' knee disorders: surgery, rehabilitation, clinical outcomes, Philadelphia, 2009, Saunders, pp 577–630.)

direction to remove excessive slack and to use staple fixation at the normal anatomic site. This procedure will not be effective if the posterolateral structures consist of scar tissue or if the distal attachment site has been disrupted.

KEY REFERENCES

Galloway MT, Grood ES, Mehalik JN, et al: Posterior cruciate ligament reconstruction. An in vitro study of femoral and tibial graft placement. Am J Sports Med 24:437–445, 1996.

Mannor DA, Shearn JT, Grood ES, et al: Two-bundle posterior cruciate ligament reconstruction. An in vitro analysis of graft placement and tension. Am J Sports Med 28:833–845, 2000.

Markolf KL, Feeley BT, Jackson SR, McAllister DR: Biomechanical studies of double-bundle posterior cruciate ligament reconstructions. J Bone Joint Surg Am 88:1788–1794, 2006.

Mejia EA, Noyes FR, Grood ES: Posterior cruciate ligament femoral insertion site characteristics: importance for reconstructive procedures. Am J Sports Med 30:643–651, 2002.

Noyes FR, Barber-Westin S: Posterior cruciate ligament replacement with a two-strand quadriceps tendon-patellar bone autograft and a tibial inlay technique. J Bone Joint Surg Am 87:1241–1252, 2005.

Noyes FR, Barber-Westin SD: Posterior cruciate ligament revision reconstruction, part 1: causes of surgical failure in 52 consecutive operations. Am J Sports Med 33:646–654, 2005.

Noyes FR, Barber-Westin SD: Posterior cruciate ligament revision reconstruction, part 2: results of revision using a 2-strand quadriceps tendon-patellar bone autograft. Am J Sports Med 33:655–665, 2005.

Noyes FR, Barber-Westin SD: Function of the posterior cruciate ligament and posterolateral ligament structures. In Noyes FR, editor: Noyes' knee disorders: surgery, rehabilitation, clinical outcomes, Philadelphia, 2009, Saunders, pp 467–502.

Noyes FR, Barber-Westin SD: Posterior cruciate ligament: diagnosis, operative techniques, and clinical outcomes. In Noyes FR, editor: Noyes' knee disorders: surgery, rehabilitation, clinical outcomes, Philadelphia, 2009, Saunders, pp 503–576.

Noyes FR, Barber-Westin SD: Posterolateral ligament injuries: diagnosis, operative techniques, and clinical outcomes. In Noyes FR, editor: Noyes' knee disorders: surgery, rehabilitation, clinical outcomes, Philadelphia, 2009, Saunders, pp 577–630.

Noyes FR, Barber-Westin SD, Heckmann TP: Rehabilitation of posterior cruciate ligament and posterolateral reconstructive procedures. In Noyes FR, editor: Noyes' knee disorders: surgery, rehabilitation, clinical outcomes, Philadelphia, 2009, Saunders, pp 631–657.

Shearn JT, Grood ES, Noyes FR, Levy MS: One- and two-strand posterior cruciate ligament reconstructions: cyclic fatigue testing. J Orthop Res 23:958–963, 2005.

Shearn JT, Grood ES, Noyes FR, Levy MS: Two-bundle posterior cruciate ligament reconstruction: how bundle tension depends on femoral placement. J Bone Joint Surg Am 86:1262–1270, 2004.

Sidles JA, Larson RV, Garbini JL, et al: Ligament length relationship in the moving knee. Journal of Orthopaedic Research 6:593–610, 1988.

Strickland JP, Fester EW, Noyes FR: Lateral, posterior, and cruciate knee anatomy. In Noyes FR, editor: Noyes' knee disorders: surgery, rehabilitation, clinical outcomes, Philadelphia, 2009, Saunders, pp 20–43.

Full references for this chapter can be found on www.expertconsult.com.

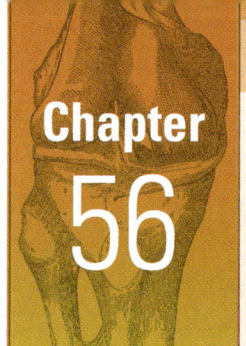

Chapter 56

Posterior Cruciate Ligament Reconstruction: Posterior Inlay Technique

Thomas Keller and Mark Miller

Injuries to the posterior cruciate ligament (PCL) occur much less frequently than injuries to the anterior cruciate ligament (ACL). PCL injuries are present in up to 3% of knee injuries in the general population and as many as 37% of knee injuries in trauma patients with acute hemarthrosis.[9,28] Isolated injuries of the PCL can lead to progressive instability and degenerative joint disease when left untreated. Although PCL reconstruction has become more common with improved diagnostic and surgical techniques, operative management of PCL injuries remains a controversial subject. There is a considerable amount of debate regarding the preferred technique of tibial graft fixation. The tibial inlay technique is advantageous in that it avoids the "killer turn," which is thought to be a major drawback of the transtibial tunnel technique.[1] Additionally, proponents have argued that the tibial inlay technique facilitates less anteroposterior (AP) laxity, greater biomechanical strength, and less risk to neurovascular structures.[2,19,23] This chapter describes the traditional tibial inlay technique for PCL reconstruction using a single-bundle autograft.

ANATOMY

The PCL is approximately 32 to 38 mm long, measuring 11 mm^2 in cross section at its midpoint.[11] The ligament originates from the anterolateral aspect of the medial femoral condyle approximately 1 cm proximal to the articular surface. The PCL inserts in a central sulcus on the posterior aspect of the tibia approximately 1 to 1.5 cm distal to the posterior edge of the tibial plateau. Despite being present within the joint capsule of the knee, the PCL is considered extra-articular because it is enclosed within a synovial sheath.

The ligament is functionally divided into an anterolateral (AL) bundle and a posteromedial (PM) bundle, referencing the location of the division's femoral origin (anterior or posterior) to its tibial insertion (lateral or medial). The thicker and stronger AL bundle is taut with knee flexion, whereas the smaller PM bundle is taut with knee extension.[8,14,16] Although the AL bundle provides the greatest resistance to posterior tibial translation,[18] research has verified the importance of the PM bundle as well as the meniscofemoral ligaments.

The meniscofemoral ligaments (ligaments of Humphrey and Wrisberg) commonly remain intact following PCL rupture. These ligaments may provide additional knee stability following PCL injury. The meniscofemoral ligaments contribute as much as 28% of the resistive forces to posterior tibial displacement in intact knees.[13]

HISTORY AND PHYSICAL EXAMINATION

PCL injury typically results following an excessive posteriorly directed force on the tibia with the knee in 90 degrees of flexion. Foot positioning at the time of impact may be predictive of the resultant injury. A posteriorly directed force on the tibia with the foot in dorsiflexion often leads to patellofemoral injury, whereas the same force directed on the tibia with the foot in plantar flexion is more likely to result in PCL injury. Unlike ACL injuries, PCL injuries often occur without a definitive pop or subjective feeling of instability. Athletes will often continue to play on a PCL-injured knee, delaying medical consultation until pain develops days later. Patients with chronic PCL injuries may complain of generalized aching in the knee, pain while walking down stairs, or subjective instability with ambulation.

When a PCL injury is suspected, the possibility of additional knee pathology must be considered prior to conducting a physical examination. Although injury to the ACL and collateral ligaments can occur in conjunction with PCL injury, combined PCL and posterolateral corner (PLC) injuries are more common. The physical examination is an important tool in the diagnosis of these injuries. The gold standard examination for the diagnosis of PCL injury is the posterior drawer test[22] (Fig. 56-1). When performing this test, the examiner must consider the concept of the starting point to assess PCL and ACL integrity properly. ACL pseudolaxity, occurring during posterior tibial sagging, can be deceptive to the examiner, resulting in a false-positive anterior drawer test and subsequently misdiagnosed ACL injury (Fig. 56-2). PCL tears can be classified by measuring the amount of posterior tibial displacement in comparison to the uninjured contralateral knee (grade I, 1 to 5 mm; grade II, 6 to 10 mm; grade III, >10 mm).[27] Because grade III injuries rarely represent isolated PCL tears, additional ligamentous injuries must be considered. Injury to the PLC is frequently associated with grade III PCL laxity. An external rotation asymmetry of more than 15 degrees at 30 and 90 degrees of knee flexion supports the diagnosis of combined PCL and PLC injury.

Plain films, stress views, and magnetic resonance imaging (MRI) scans have all been used to confirm clinical suspicion of PCL injury. Plain films may reveal subtle posterior tibial subluxation, bony avulsions, or fibular head fractures suggestive of PLC injury (Fig. 56-3). Stress views, used to quantify the degree of posterior tibial subluxation, are taken with the knee in 90 degrees of flexion (Fig. 56-4). The sensitivity of MRI in diagnosing acute PCL tears is approximately 100%[4] (Fig. 56-5). Although MRI better facilitates the visualization of associated soft tissue injuries, PLC injuries may be overdiagnosed as a result of substantial local edema.

Low-grade isolated PCL injuries are typically treated nonoperatively with an emphasis on reducing inflammation, reestablishing knee motion, and strengthening the quadriceps to counteract the tendency toward posterior tibial subluxation. Return to activity within 3 to 6 weeks is dependent on the goals of the patient as well as the severity of the injury.[26,27] Operative indications following PCL injury include multiligamentous injuries, symptomatic chronic grade II or III

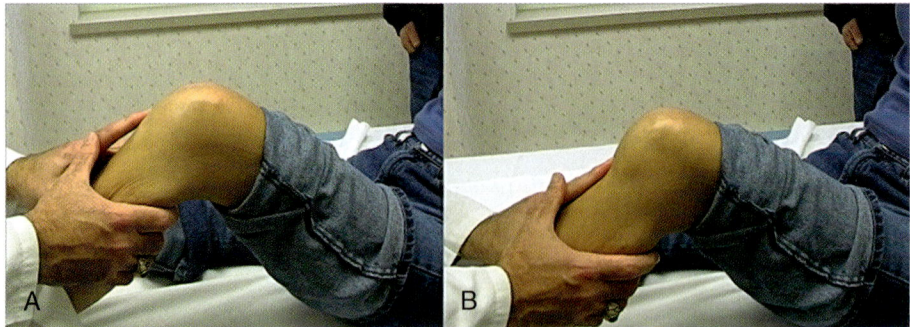

Figure 56-1. Posterior drawer test demonstrating proper starting point **(A)** with obvious posterior laxity **(B)** suggestive of PCL pathology.

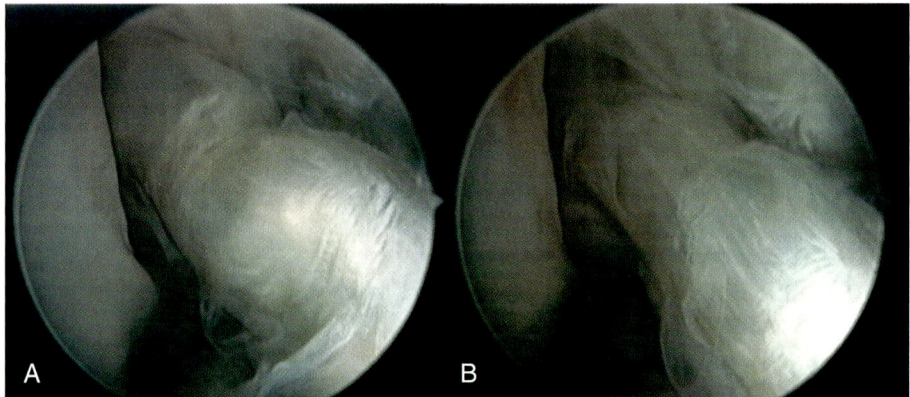

Figure 56-2. A, Arthroscopic view demonstrating ACL pseudolaxity. **B,** ACL tension is subsequently restored following anterior drawer.

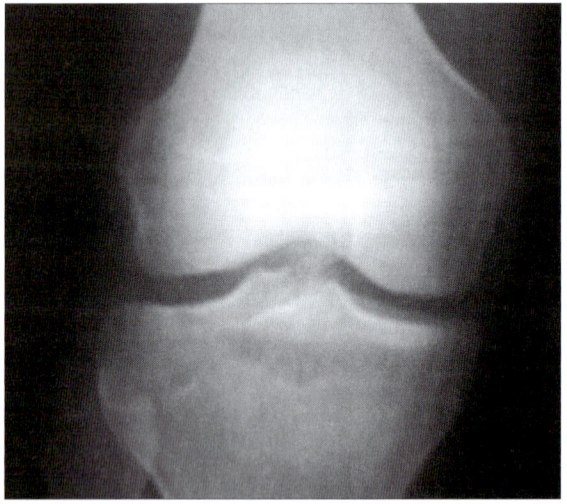

Figure 56-3. Plain film demonstrating PCL avulsion injury.

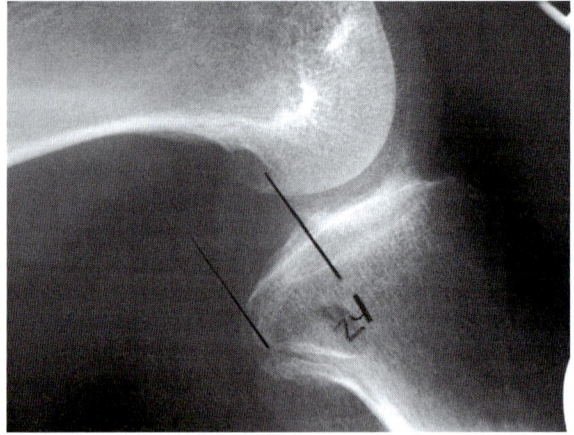

Figure 56-4. PCL stress radiograph demonstrating posterior tibial translation suggestive of PCL injury.

injuries that fail rehabilitation, PCL avulsions, and PCL injuries in active patients who are unwilling to change their lifestyle to comply with conservative treatment options.

Posterior tibial avulsion injuries involving the PCL insertion are repaired anatomically with lag screws or suture fixation. Midsubstance tears of the PCL require ligamentous reconstruction. Proponents prefer the tibial inlay technique for PCL reconstruction because it reproduces the most anatomic PCL reconstruction while avoiding the killer turn associated with tibial tunneling. Patients with tibial osteopenia or a history of prior osteotomies or fractures may require the tibial inlay procedure instead of the transtibial tunneling procedure to prevent proximal graft migration.[25] Contraindications to PCL reconstruction using the tibial inlay technique include a history of vascular repair or bypass grafting procedures.

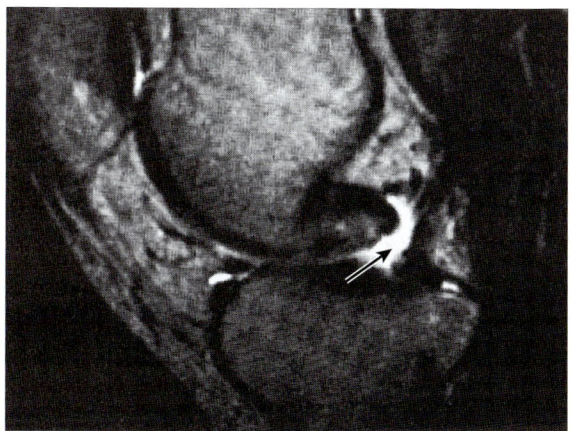

Figure 56-5. PCL tear *(black arrow)* as seen on MRI scan.

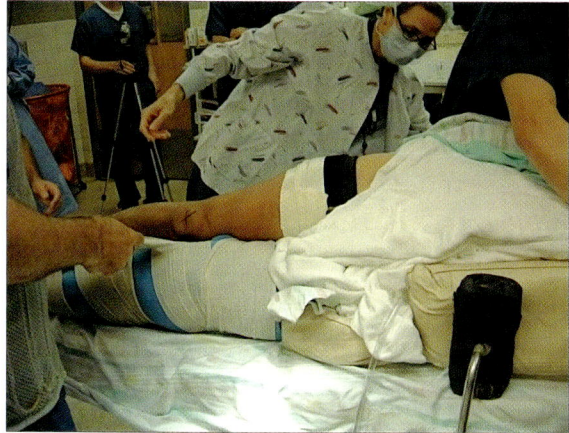

Figure 56-6. The patient is placed in the lateral decubitus position in preparation for PCL reconstruction. The nonoperative extremity is generously padded. A tourniquet is applied to the proximal operative thigh.

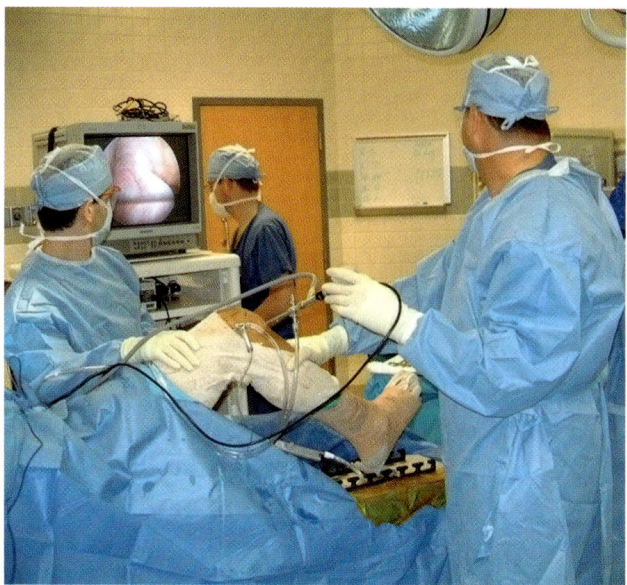

Figure 56-7. Diagnostic arthroscopy and graft harvest are performed with the operative hip placed in abduction and external rotation while the knee is secured in flexion using a leg holder. Standard arthroscopic portals are used during diagnostic arthroscopy.

TIBIAL INLAY TECHNIQUE

Examination Under Anesthesia, Patient Positioning, and Diagnostic Arthroscopy

A general anesthetic is preferred to facilitate patient positioning and an examination under anesthesia. Prior to beginning the procedure, the patient is examined under anesthesia to confirm PCL injury and rule out any additional unrecognized ligamentous injuries. The patient is then placed in the lateral decubitus position with the uninjured leg against the table in extension. The uninjured leg is padded in its entirety, paying special attention to the bony prominences. The fibular head is padded to prevent peroneal nerve injury. The foot and ankle of the operative extremity are placed in a commercially available leg holder, with plenty of padding. A tourniquet is applied to the proximal operative thigh and the patient is prepped and draped in typical sterile fashion (Fig. 56-6).

The leg is then positioned for graft harvest and arthroscopy by abducting and externally rotating the hip, flexing the knee, and locking the operative extremity in place using the leg holder. Diagnostic arthroscopy is performed using standard arthroscopic portals (Fig. 56-7). Bony avulsions, degenerative changes, and complete versus partial PCL tears can

be visualized during arthroscopy. The joint is visually inspected, addressing any meniscal or cartilage pathology prior to PCL reconstruction. The presence of a torn PCL is confirmed before proceeding on to graft harvest (Fig. 56-8). Indicators of PCL injury include hemorrhage and ACL pseudolaxity. After identifying the torn PCL, the stump is débrided using a combination of biting rongeurs, suction shaver, and thermal ablation. Residual PCL fibers remaining in continuity should be maintained. The anterior edge of the PCL footprint may be preserved to serve as a reference point for the inlay.[5]

Patellar Graft Harvest

The patellar autograft is harvested from the ipsilateral knee with the operative extremity placed in abduction and external rotation. A longitudinal anterior knee incision is made medial to the midline of the patella tendon at the inferior pole of the patella and carried approximately 2 cm distal to the tibial tubercle. Skin flaps are raised as the dissection is carried down to the paratenon. A sharp blade is then used to demarcate the central third (approximately an 11- to 12-mm width) of the patellar tendon from the patella to the tibial tubercle. An oscillating saw is used to remove bone plugs from both the tibial tubercle and patella. Bone plug length is typically 20 to 25 mm.

Graft Preparation

Patellar tendon autograft preparation is performed on a side table while the knee is being prepared for graft incorporation. The patellar portion of the graft is contoured into a cylinder with a rounded tip, mimicking the shape of a bullet. The contoured patellar bone plug is sized to fit through a 10- to 12-mm wide femoral tunnel and should be at least 18 mm long. Two perpendicular drill holes are placed approximately

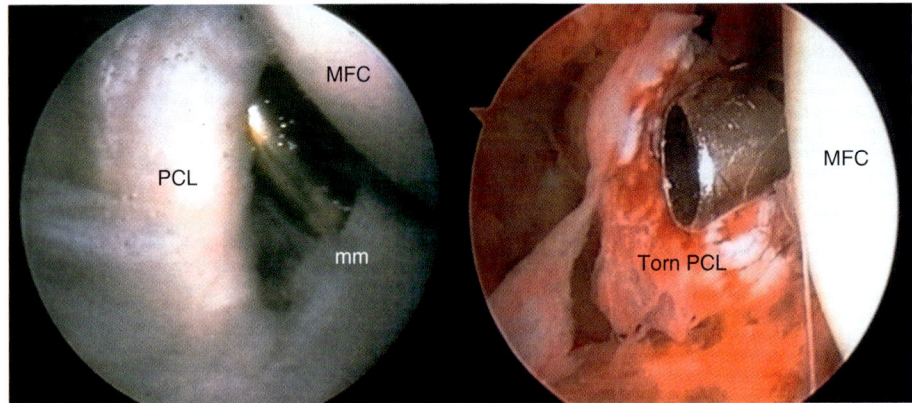

Figure 56-8. Arthroscopic view of an intact PCL *(left)* and a torn PCL with hemorrhage *(right)*.

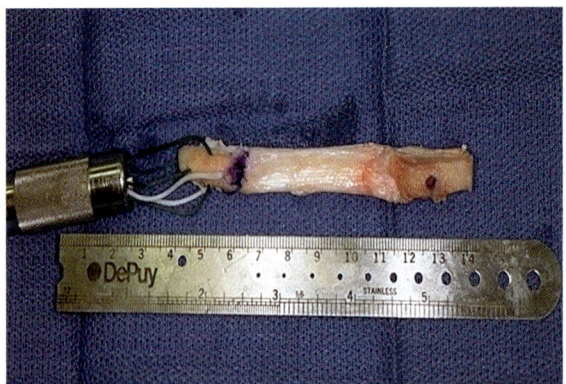

Figure 56-9. Harvested bone-patellar tendon-bone autograft. Pre-drilled rectangular tibial bone block *(right)* with tapered bone plug and perpendicular sutures for femoral fixation *(left)*.

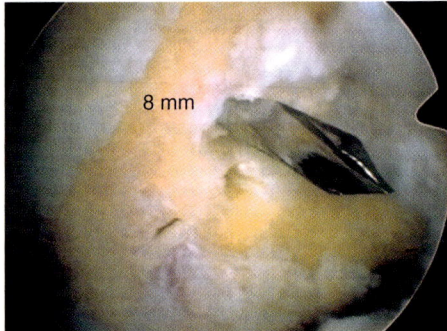

Figure 56-10. Arthroscopic view during femoral guide pin placement. Guide pin entry occurs 8 mm from the articular surface of the medial femoral condyle *(top left)*.

5 and 10 mm from the tip of the patellar bone plug. Two no. 5 sutures are passed through the drill holes to assist in graft placement. Additionally, a no. 2 Ethicon or Ticron suture may be placed at the junction of the tendon and patellar bone plug to facilitate easier entry into the femoral tunnel. The tibial bone block is shaped into a trapezoid, creating a flat surface on the side that will lay directly on the tibia (Fig. 56-9).

Femoral Tunnel Placement

Prior to femoral tunnel placement, the lateral aspect of the medial femoral condyle, in addition to any remaining soft tissue in the notch, is débrided arthroscopically. A standard PCL femoral guide is introduced into the knee through the anteromedial portal. The PCL femoral guide is placed approximately 8 mm from the articular surface of the anteromedial portion of the intercondylar notch at the 1 o'clock position for the right knee, and the 11 o'clock position for the left knee. An adequate bone bridge separating the articular cartilage of the femur from the bone tunnel will minimize the risk of avascular necrosis of the medial femoral condyle. A 2-cm incision is made along Langer's lines over the medial portion of the knee at the medial femoral condyle. The incision is carried down through the subcutaneous tissue and along the inferior border of the vastus medialis muscle to the level of the condyle. An external tunnel guide is then placed

on the cortical surface of the condyle, away from the articular surface of the femur. A guide pin is drilled from outside in and pin placement within the femoral footprint is verified arthroscopically (Fig. 56-10). Using a cannulated drill bit reamer appropriately sized for the harvested graft, the guide pin is overdrilled from outside in, creating the femoral tunnel. The margins of the tunnel are then rasped to reduce graft abrasion. After the femoral tunnel is fully prepared, a looped, smooth, 18-gauge wire, or commercially available graft passer, is placed into the tunnel from outside to inside. The guide wire is passed into the posterior aspect of the knee joint to facilitate graft passage at a later stage. The arthroscopic equipment is then removed from the knee to begin the tibial inlay portion of the case.

Posterior Approach and Inlay

In preparation for the tibial inlay portion of the procedure, the leg is placed in full extension and neutral rotation on a padded Mayo stand (Fig. 56-11). A horizontal incision made in the flexion crease superficial to the popliteal fossa provides excellent exposure and preserves cosmesis (Fig. 56-12). The underlying fascia is separated in a hockey stick fashion, incising the fascia perpendicular to the skin incision laterally and curving distally between the medial head of the gastrocnemius and semimembranosus muscles. Using blunt dissection, the interval between the gastrocnemius and

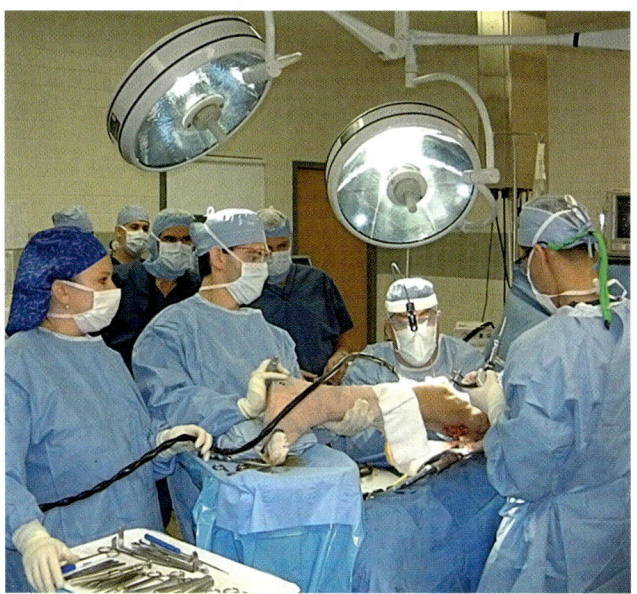

Figure 56-11. The operative extremity is placed in full extension and neutral rotation during the inlay portion of the procedure to facilitate access to the popliteal fossa.

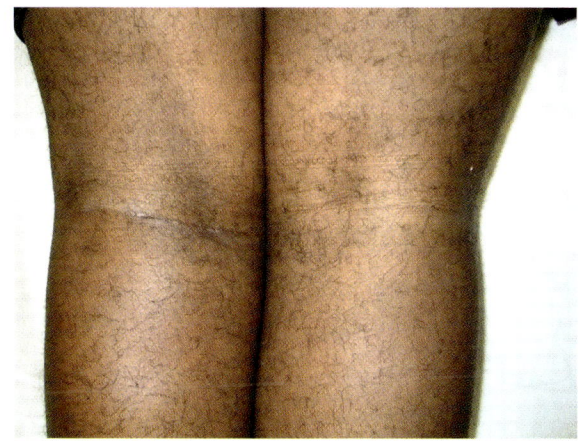

Figure 56-12. Healed surgical scar in the flexion crease of the left knee demonstrating excellent cosmetic results.

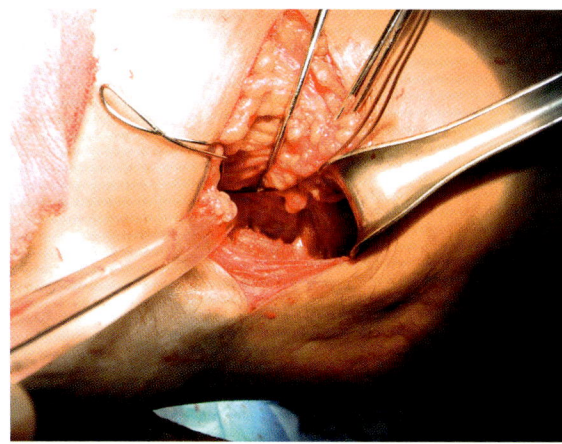

Figure 56-13. Smooth Steinman pins placed in the posterior tibia allow for static retraction of the medial head of the gastrocnemius, facilitating exposure of the posterior capsule.

semimembranosus is developed, minding the proximity of the medial sural cutaneous nerve as well as the middle and inferior medial genicular arteries. The medial head of the gastrocnemius is retracted laterally after mobilization and separation from the semimembranosus. Slight knee flexion will improve exposure of the posterior knee capsule by allowing for increased lateral retraction of the medial head of the gastrocnemius. Smooth Steinman pins may be inserted into the posterior tibia and bent laterally to hold lateral retraction on the gastrocnemius (Fig. 56-13). In addition to allowing excellent exposure of the posterior knee capsule, lateral retraction of the medial head of the gastrocnemius provides innate protection of the neurovascular structures of the popliteal fossa.

The tibial footprint of the PCL is then identified by palpating the sulcus between the medial and lateral prominences of the posterior tibia. The PCL sulcus is palpated through the fibers of the popliteus muscle, using the relatively larger and more easily identifiable medial prominence as a guide. Electrocauterization and an elevator are used to clear the soft tissues away from the sulcus, exposing the posterior cortex of the tibia. Using an osteotome, high-speed burr, and bone tamp, a unicortical window is created in the naked PCL sulcus to match the dimensions of the tibial bone block portion of the graft. Next, a vertical posterior arthrotomy is performed, extending distally to the PCL sulcus to facilitate graft passage. The PCL graft is retrieved from the preparation table and fitted into the unicortical window that was created in the PCL sulcus. Care is taken to ensure that the bone plug of the graft lays flush and snug on the posterior surface of the tibia.

After verifying an adequate fit of the tibial bone plug, the graft is returned to the preparation table where one or two guide pins are placed provisionally through the anterior cortex of the tibial bone block. These guide pins will allow for provisional graft fixation and assessment of screw length for definitive fixation. Next, the graft is retrieved from the preparation table and prepared for fixation. The guide wire placed during the femoral tunneling step is identified and retrieved through the posterior capsular incision. Using this guide wire, the no. 5 sutures previously placed through the drill holes in the patellar portion of the graft are used to pull the graft into the joint and femoral tunnel. If a no. 2 suture has been placed at the junction of the tendon and patellar interface of the graft to facilitate toggling during femoral tunnel fixation, an additional looped wire guide may be used to pull the no. 2 suture through the anteromedial arthroscopic portal. Once the tibial component of the graft is positioned and the rest of the graft is passed into the knee joint, the tibial bone block is secured to the tibia. Preliminary fixation is achieved by driving the guide pins through to the anterior tibial cortex. The guide pins are adjusted to achieve proper bicortical purchase and measurements are taken to determine screw length. A cannulated drill bit is used to overdrill the guide pins and 4.5-mm bicortical screws and flat washers are placed to lag the tibial bone block to the tibia. The guide pins are then removed, leaving the graft well secured to the posterior tibia (Figs. 56-14 and 56-15).

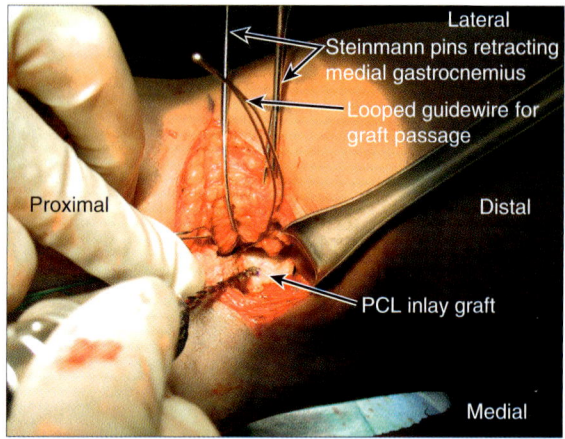

Figure 56-14. Preparing the tibial bone block for definitive fixation.

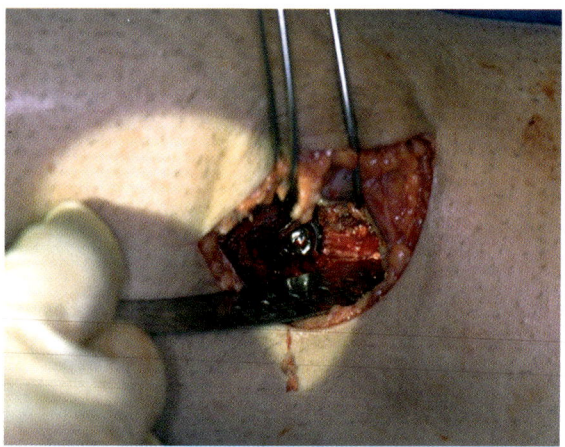

Figure 56-15. Posterior view of the knee following graft passage and tibial bone block fixation.

Graft Passage and Fixation

After the tibial bone block has been secured to the PCL sulcus, the patellar end of the graft is passed through the joint and into the previously prepared femoral tunnel using the guide wire (Fig. 56-16). The knee should be cycled through a full range of motion at this point to ensure that the tibial bone block is secure and the graft is free from impingement at the site of the posterior capsulotomy. The leg is then repositioned in the initial position used for arthroscopy. The no. 5 sutures are passed through the femoral tunnel and tensioned to bring the patellar bone plug–tendon interface of the graft flush with the articular margin of the femoral tunnel. The no. 2 suture, passed through the anteromedial portal, may be used here to help toggle the patellar bone plug into position. Failure to position the patellar bone plug properly can result in early graft failure caused by excessive shear stress on the graft. Once the graft is correctly positioned in the femoral tunnel, a moderate amount of tension is applied to the no. 5 sutures. The knee is again cycled through a full range of motion to remove any residual kinking in the graft and reconfirm a lack of impedance at the site of the posterior capsulotomy. A 9- × 20-mm interference screw is then seated into the femoral tunnel while an anterior drawer force is applied with the knee in 70 to 90 degrees of flexion. This secures the graft under tension. Care should be taken during this step to ensure that the patellar tendon-bone junction remains at the desired intra-articular position. Additional fixation is achieved by tying the no. 5 nonabsorbable suture to a plastic button over the cortex at the femoral tunnel entrance. The graft is then visualized arthroscopically to ensure proper bone plug fixation. Restoration of PCL stability is confirmed by posterior drawer testing.

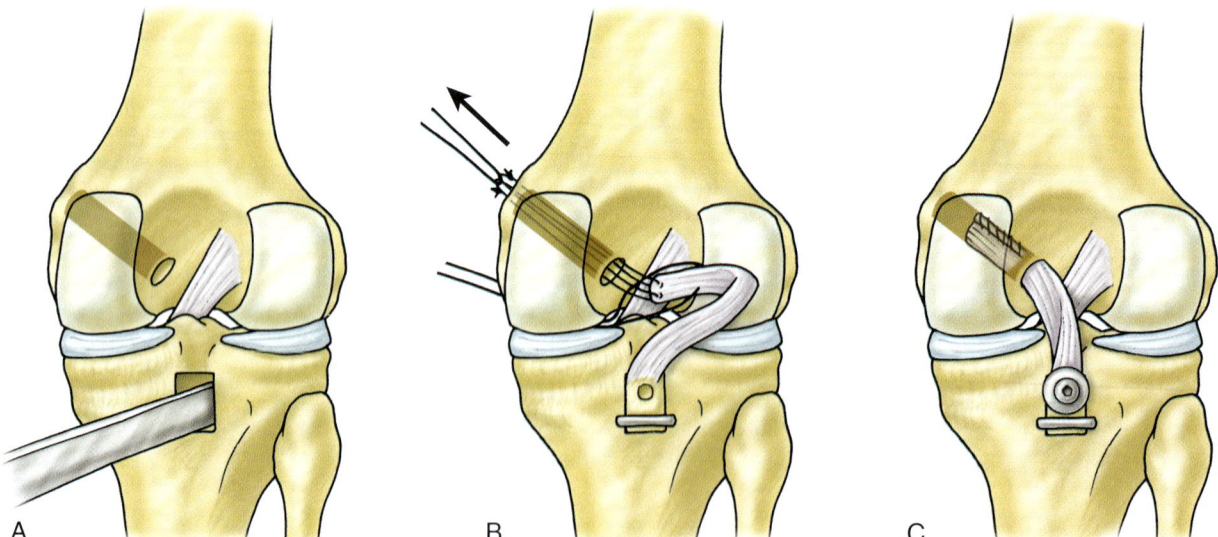

Figure 56-16. Overview of tibial inlay technique. **A,** The tibial footprint of the PCL is placed in the sulcus between the medial and lateral prominences of the posterior tibia. **B,** Prior to fixation, the graft is pulled through the posterior arthrotomy and into the femoral tunnel using the looped guide wire. **C,** After verifying appropriate bone block fitting and graft clearance, the graft is tensioned and definitively secured. (Redrawn from Miller MD, Gordon WR: Posterior cruciate ligament reconstruction: tibial inlay technique. Oper Tech Orthop 9:289–297, 1999.)

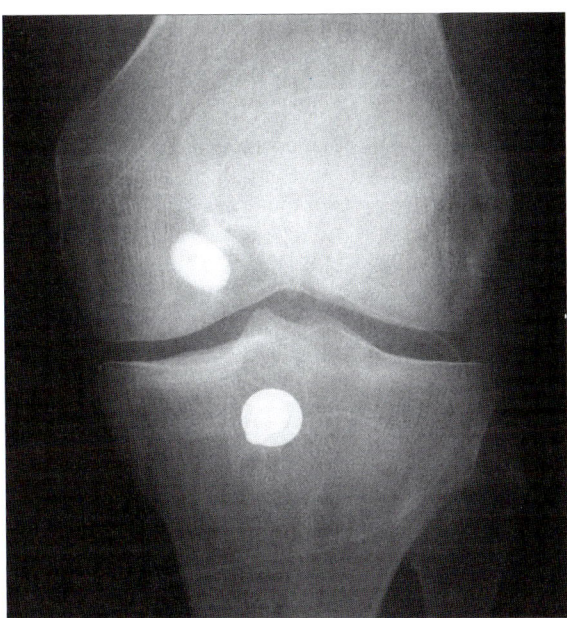

Figure 56-17. Postoperative AP radiograph.

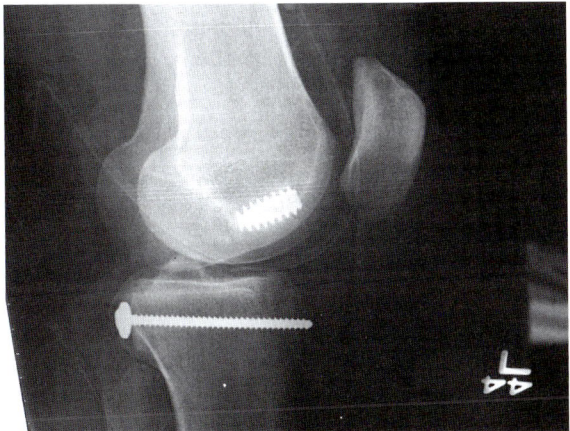

Figure 56-18. Lateral radiograph.

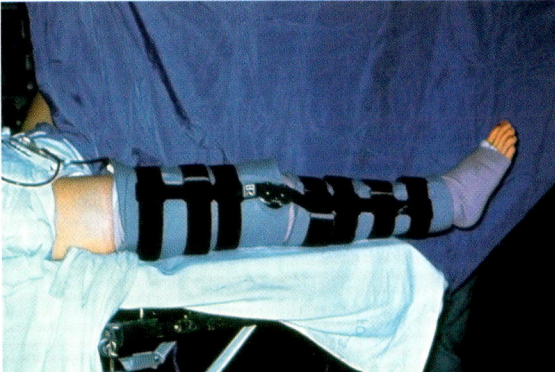

Figure 56-19. Postoperative hinged knee brace with knee locked in extension.

Closure

Bone graft set aside following femoral tunneling and graft preparation is used to pack the remaining defects at the patellar and tibial tubercle graft harvest sites. The anterior knee is closed in standard fashion and sterile dressing is applied. Posteriorly, the capsule is repaired and a Hemovac drain is placed deep to the medial head of the gastrocnemius to reduce the risk of postoperative hematoma formation. The posterior wound is then closed in standard fashion and sterile dressings are applied. AP and lateral radiographs of the knee are taken following the procedure to ensure appropriate graft and hardware placement (Figs. 56-17 and 56-18). The knee is braced in extension to support the posterior tibia and prevent posterior translation.

POSTOPERATIVE REHABILITATION PROGRAM

Postoperative rehabilitation following PCL reconstruction is often more difficult than rehabilitation following ACL reconstruction. Full recovery may take up to 1 year. Rehabilitative efforts should be focused on regaining full knee range of motion, reducing pain and edema, and strengthening the quadriceps while preventing posterior tibial translation. Excessive graft stress must be avoided until adequate healing has occurred. Open-chain hamstring exercises place excessive posterior force on the tibia and should be avoided for approximately 3 months following PCL reconstruction.

Immediately following the procedure, the knee is placed in a hinged knee brace that is locked in extension to support the tibia and prevent posterior translation (Fig. 56-19). Continuous passive motion, isometric quadriceps training, and straight leg raises should be initiated as soon as the patient can tolerate such exercises. Weight bearing with the knee brace strictly locked at 0 degrees is permitted on the first postoperative day, using crutches to assist with ambulation. The brace is to remain locked in extension at all times, except during supervised passive range of motion activities, for the first 2 weeks. Range of motion exercises are typically performed with the patient in the prone position to prevent posterior tibial translation. After 1 month, the hinged knee brace is transitioned to the unlocked position and the patient is allowed to ambulate and perform activities under therapist supervision. Between the 1- and 2-month time points, the crutches are discontinued and the brace is removed. The stationary bicycle, slide boards, VersaClimber, elliptical trainers, and Nordic track are introduced after 2 months. Jogging on a treadmill is typically permitted after 3 months. Between 3 and 9 months, the patient is allowed to progress within her or his own level of function and symptoms. Assuming a return of knee stability, quadriceps strength, and range of motion, the patient may resume normal activities 9 to 12 months after PCL reconstruction.

COMPLICATIONS

The most common complication following PCL reconstruction is residual posterior laxity.[21,24] PCL laxity following surgical reconstruction can be attributed to inappropriate tensioning during graft placement, failure to diagnose and treat other associated ligamentous injuries, poor graft fixation, and overly aggressive rehabilitation. Intraoperatively, the surgeon should ensure that the graft is not loose, kinked, or impinging on the posterior arthrotomy site by palpating the inlay site and visualizing the PCL under arthroscopy while the knee is passively ranged. Additionally, care should be taken to ensure that the tendon–patellar bone junction of the graft rests at the intra-articular margin of the femoral tunnel. Failure to do so can result in graft fraying and residual laxity. Cadaveric studies have shown that PCL reconstruction using the tibial inlay technique achieves significantly less residual posterior laxity than knees reconstructed using the transtibial tunneling technique.[2,19] Although double-bundle reconstruction using the tibial inlay technique arguably decreases residual posterior laxity by more closely restoring the biomechanics of the intact knee, double-bundle reconstruction may result in overconstraint of the knee at certain angles of flexion.[7,29]

The most feared complication during PCL reconstruction is injury to the neurovascular structures in the popliteal fossa (Fig. 56-20). Fully mobilizing and retracting the medial heel of the gastrocnemius functions to protect these structures. Steinman pins placed in the posterior tibia can be used to retract the gastrocnemius continually, avoiding further risk of injury associated with repetitive repositioning of retractors. Revision surgeries place the popliteal neurovascular structures in jeopardy because residual scarring can distort normal anatomic planes.

Avascular necrosis of the medial femoral condyle has been reported as well. Symptoms present months to years after PCL reconstruction and typically include medial knee pain exacerbated by palpation of the medial femoral condyle. This complication is thought to be caused by femoral drilling in close proximity to the articular surface of the knee, resulting in trauma to the subchondral blood supply. To avoid this potential problem, the femoral tunnel should be started approximately 10 mm posterior to the articular margin.

Other complications include infection, wound breakdown, anterior knee pain, and heterotopic ossification.[15] Metallic screws used in inlay fixation may pose a problem for patients requiring future revision surgery, osteotomies, or knee arthroplasty. Alternatives to traditional metallic screws for tibial bone plug fixation have been proposed, including sutures and bioabsorbable screws. Studies have shown no difference in acute fixation strength among metallic screws, bioabsorbable screws, and sutures.[6,12]

SUMMARY

Indications to perform PCL reconstruction include multiligamentous injuries, symptomatic chronic grade II or grade III injuries that fail rehabilitation, PCL avulsions, and PCL injuries in active patients who are unwilling to change their lifestyle to comply with conservative treatment options. Chronic PCL insufficiency leads to an increased incidence of knee pain, effusion and chondrosis.[3,10] Following reconstruction of the PCL, the patient can expect to return to grade I laxity or better. Although residual posterior laxity is one of the most common complications following PCL reconstruction, patients rarely complain of functional instability and are often subjectively unaware of any laxity present on physical examination.

Tibial fixation, graft options, and surgical techniques for PCL reconstruction continue to evolve.[20] In comparison to the transtibial tunneling technique, the tibial inlay technique more closely replicates the anatomy of the PCL while avoiding the killer turn thought to be responsible for residual laxity seen following reconstruction with a transtibial tunnel. Double-bundle PCL reconstruction using the tibial inlay technique has gained interest as a method to replicate more closely the biomechanics of the native PCL, which is composed of two main fiber bundles. Double-bundle reconstruction of the PCL may offer increased stability to rotation and posterior translation, especially in cases of combined PCL and posterolateral corner injury. In cases of isolated PCL injury, however, double-bundle PCL reconstruction may result in excessive constraint to motion at certain angles of flexion.[29] The all-arthroscopic tibial inlay techniques, although technically challenging, do not require an extensive surgical dissection in the popliteal space and eliminate the need for patient repositioning in the middle of the procedure.[5,17] Long-term studies examining the theoretical improvements offered by double-bundle reconstruction and all-arthroscopic techniques are unavailable to date. Improvements in graft options, methods of graft fixation, surgical techniques, and surgical instrumentation, in conjunction with long-term results, will guide the evolution of PCL reconstruction in the future.

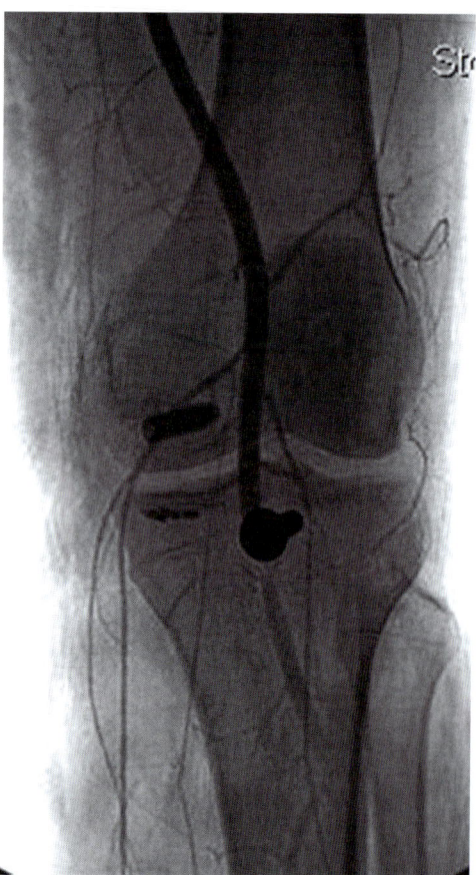

Figure 56-20. Postoperative angiogram demonstrating occlusion of the popliteal artery.

KEY REFERENCES

Ahn JH, Yang HS, Jeong WK, Koh KH: Arthroscopic transtibial posterior cruciate ligament reconstruction with preservation of posterior cruciate ligament fibers. Am J Sports Med 34:194–204, 2006.
Bergfeld JA, McAllister DR, Parker RD, et al: A biomechanical comparison of posterior cruciate ligament techniques. Am J Sports Med 29:129–136, 2001.

Campbell RB, Jordan SS, Seikya JK: Arthroscopic tibial inlay for posterior cruciate ligament reconstruction. Arthroscopy 23:1356.e1–1356.e4, 2007.

Campbell RB, Torrie A, Hecker A, Sekiya JK: Comparison of tibial graft fixation between simulated arthroscopic and open inlay techniques for posterior cruciate ligament reconstruction. Am J Sports Med 35:1731–1738, 2007.

Carson EW, Deng XH, Allen A, et al: Evaluation of in situ graft forces of a 2-bundle tibial inlay posterior cruciate ligament reconstruction at various flexion angles. Arthroscopy 23:488–495, 2007.

Edwards A, Bull AM, Amis AA: The attachments of the fiber bundles of the posterior cruciate ligament: an anatomic study. Arthroscopy 23:284–290, 2007.

Gupta A, Lattermann C, Busam M, et al: Biomechanical evaluation of bioabsorbable versus metallic screws for posterior cruciate ligament inlay graft fixation: A comparative study. Am J Sports Med 37:748–753, 2009.

Lopes OV, Jr, Ferretti M, Shen W, et al: Topography of the femoral attachment of the posterior cruciate ligament. J Bone Joint Surg Am 90:249–255, 2008.

Mariani PP, Margheritini F: Full arthroscopic inlay reconstruction of posterior cruciate ligament. Knee Surg Sports Traumatol Arthrosc 14:1038–1044, 2006.

Markolf KL, Feeley BT, Tejwani SG, et al: Changes in knee laxity and ligament force after sectioning the posteromedial bundle of the posterior cruciate ligament. Arthroscopy 22:1100–1106, 2006.

Markolf KL, Zemanovic JR, McAllister DR: Cyclic loading of posterior cruciate ligament replacments with tibial tunnel and tibial inlay methods. J Bone Joint Surg Am 84:518–524, 2001.

Noyes FR, Medvecky MJ, Bhargava M: Arthroscopically assisted quadriceps double-bundle tibial inlay posterior cruciate ligament reconstruction: an analysis of techniques and a safe operative approach to the popliteal fossa. Arthroscopy 19: 894–905, 2003.

Sekiya JK, Whiddon DR, Zehms CT, Miller MD: A clinically relevant assessment of posterior cruciate ligament and posterolateral corner injuries. Evaluation of isolated and combined deficiency. J Bone Joint Surg Am 90:1621–1627, 2008.

Whiddon DR, Zelms CT, Miller MD, et al: Double- compared with single-bundle open inlay posterior cruciate ligament reconstruction in a cadaver Model. J Bone Joint Surg Am 90:1820–1829, 2008.

Full references for this chapter can be found on www.expertconsult.com.

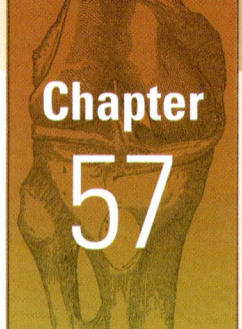

Chapter 57

Posterior Cruciate Ligament Reconstruction: Transtibial Double-Bundle Technique

Gregory C. Fanelli

Posterior cruciate ligament (PCL) surgical reconstruction may be unsuccessful because of failure to recognize and treat associated ligament instabilities (posterolateral instability and posteromedial instability), failure to treat varus osseous malalignment, and incorrect tunnel placement.[32-34] The keys to successful PCL reconstruction are to identify and treat all pathology, utilize strong graft material, accurately place tunnels in anatomic insertion sites, minimize graft bending, use a mechanical graft tensioning device, use primary and backup graft fixation, and employ the appropriate postoperative rehabilitation program. Adherence to these technical points results in successful single- and double-bundle arthroscopic transtibial tunnel (TTT) PCL reconstruction, documented by stress radiography, arthrometer, knee ligament rating scales, and patient satisfaction measurements.[7-9,11,13-16,18-25,29] The purpose of this chapter is to describe our surgical techniques for arthroscopic TTT PCL reconstruction and posterolateral reconstruction.

The incidence of PCL injury is reported to range from 1% to 40% of acute knee injuries. Incidence is dependent on the patient population reported and is approximately 3% in the general population and 38% in reports from regional trauma centers.[3,6,17] Our practice at a regional trauma center has a 38.3% incidence of PCL tears in acute knee injuries, and 56.5% of these PCL injuries occur in multiple-trauma patients. Of these PCL injuries, 45.9% are combined anterior cruciate ligament (ACL)/PCL tears, and 41.2% are PCL/posterolateral corner tears. Only 3% of acute PCL injuries seen in our trauma center are isolated.

This chapter illustrates my surgical technique for the arthroscopic, double-bundle/double–femoral tunnel TTT PCL reconstruction surgical procedure, and presents our results of PCL reconstruction using this surgical technique. Because isolated PCL reconstruction is rarely performed in my practice, this chapter has been written with PCL reconstruction viewed within the context of the multiple ligament–injured knee.

SURGICAL INDICATIONS

Double-bundle/double–femoral tunnel (DB/DFT) TTT PCL reconstruction approximates the anatomy of the PCL by reconstructing the anterolateral and posteromedial bundles of the PCL. This double-bundle reconstruction more closely approximates the broad femoral insertion of the PCL, enhancing the biomechanics of PCL reconstruction.[30] Although the DB/DFT TTT PCL reconstruction does not perfectly reproduce the normal PCL, certain components lead to success with this surgical technique:

1. Identify and treat all pathology (especially posterolateral instability).
2. Provide accurate tunnel placement.
3. Identify anatomic graft insertion sites.

4. Use strong graft material.
5. Minimize graft bending.
6. Perform final tensioning at 70 to 90 degrees of knee flexion.
7. Apply graft tensioning.
   a. Use a mechanical tensioning device.
8. Provide primary and backup fixation.
9. Choose an appropriate rehabilitation program.

Our indications for surgical treatment of acute PCL injuries include insertion site avulsions, tibial step-off decreased by 10 mm or more, and PCL tears combined with other structural injuries. Our indications for surgical treatment of chronic PCL injuries are evident when an isolated PCL tear becomes symptomatic, or when progressive functional instability develops.

Surgical Timing

Surgical timing is dependent upon vascular status, reduction stability, skin condition, systemic injuries, open versus closed knee injury, meniscus and articular surface injuries, other orthopedic injuries, and the collateral/capsular ligaments involved. Certain ACL/PCL/medial collateral ligament (MCL) injuries can be treated with brace treatment of the MCL, followed by arthroscopic combined ACL/PCL reconstruction within 4 to 6 weeks after healing of the MCL. Other cases may require repair or reconstruction of the medial structures and must be assessed on an individual basis.

Combined ACL/PCL/posterolateral injuries are addressed as early as safely possible. ACL/PCL/posterolateral repair–reconstruction performed between 2 and 3 weeks post injury allows sealing of capsular tissues to permit an arthroscopic approach, and still permits primary repair of injured posterolateral structures.

Open multiple-ligament knee injuries/dislocations may require staged procedures. The collateral/capsular structures are repaired after thorough irrigation and débridement, and the combined ACL/PCL reconstruction is performed at a later date, after wound healing has occurred. Care must be taken in all cases of delayed reconstruction to confirm that the tibiofemoral joint is reduced by serial anterior-posterior (AP) and lateral radiographs.

The surgical timing guidelines outlined previously should be considered in the context of the individual patient. Many patients with multiple-ligament injuries of the knee are severely injured multiple-trauma patients with multisystem injuries. Modifiers to the ideal timing protocols outlined earlier include the vascular status of the involved extremity, reduction stability, skin condition, open or closed injury, and other orthopedic and systemic injuries. These additional considerations may cause knee ligament surgery to be performed earlier or later than desired. We have previously reported excellent results with delayed reconstruction in the multiple ligament–injured knee.*

Graft Selection

Our preferred graft source for PCL, ACL, posteromedial, and posterolateral reconstruction is allograft tissue. The antero-lateral bundle of the PCL is reconstructed with Achilles tendon allograft, and the posteromedial bundle of the PCL is reconstructed with tibialis anterior allograft tissue. Postero-lateral reconstruction is performed with semitendinosus allograft for fibular-based reconstructions combined with a posterolateral capsular shift procedure. Fibular head- and tibia-based posterolateral reconstructions are performed with a split Achilles tendon allograft or a semitendinosus allograft for the fibular arm, and a tibialis anterior allograft for the tibial arm, also combined with a posterolateral capsular shift procedure. Anterior cruciate ligament reconstruction is per-formed with Achilles tendon allograft or tibialis anterior allograft. Posteromedial reconstruction is performed with a posteromedial capsular shift procedure combined with allograft augmentation as indicated.

Posterior Cruciate Ligament Reconstruction Surgical Technique

The patient is positioned on the operating table in the supine position, and the surgical and nonsurgical knees are examined under general or regional anesthesia. A tourniquet is applied to the operative extremity, and the surgical leg is prepped and draped in a sterile fashion. Allograft tissue is prepared before the surgical procedure is begun, and autograft tissue is harvested before the arthroscopic portion of the procedure is undertaken. Standard arthroscopic knee portals are used. The joint is thoroughly evaluated arthroscopically, and the PCL is evaluated using the three-zone arthroscopic technique.[4,25] The PCL tear is identified, and the residual stump of the PCL is débrided with hand tools and the syno-vial shaver.

An extracapsular posteromedial safety incision approxi-mately 1.5 to 2.0 cm long is created.[9,11,13-16,18-25,29] The crural fascia is incised longitudinally, with precautions taken to protect the neurovascular structures. The interval is devel-oped between the medial head of the gastrocnemius muscle and the posterior capsule of the knee joint, which is anterior. The surgeon's gloved finger is positioned so that the neuro-vascular structures are posterior to the finger, and the poste-rior aspect of the joint capsule is anterior to the surgeon's finger. This technique enables the surgeon to monitor surgical instruments such as the over-the-top PCL instruments and the PCL/ACL drill guide as they are positioned in the poste-rior aspect of the knee. The surgeon's finger in the postero-medial safety incision also confirms accurate placement of the guide wire before tibial tunnel drilling is begun in the medial-lateral and proximal-distal directions (Fig. 57-1). This is the same anatomic surgical interval that is utilized in the tibial inlay posterior approach.

Curved over-the-top PCL instruments are used to elevate the posterior knee joint capsule away from the tibial ridge on

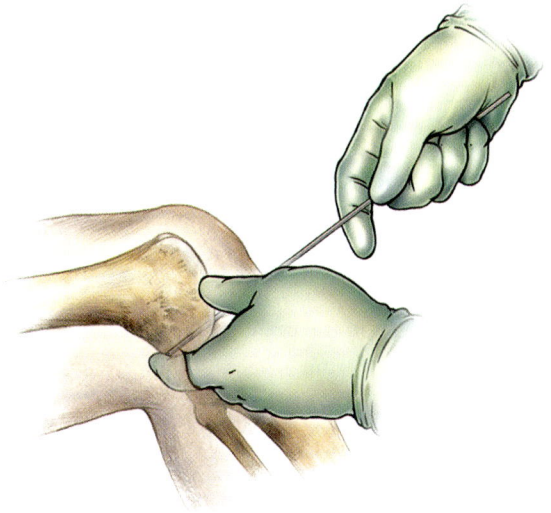

Figure 57-1. The surgeon is able to palpate the posterior aspect of the tibia through the extracapsular extra-articular pos-teromedial safety incision. This enables the surgeon to accurately position guide wires, create the tibial tunnel, and protect neuro-vascular structures. (With permission, Biomet Sports Medicine, Inc., Warsaw, Ind.)

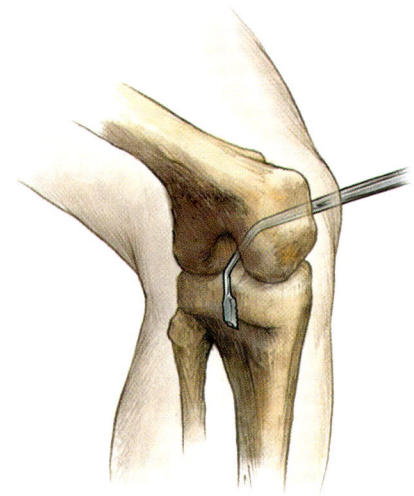

Figure 57-2. Posterior capsular elevation using Arthrotek Biomet Sports Medicine posterior cruciate ligament (PCL) instruments. (With permission, Biomet Sports Medicine, Inc., Warsaw, Ind.)

the posterior aspect of the tibia. This capsular elevation enhances correct drill guide and tibial tunnel placement (Fig. 57-2).

The arm of the Biomet Sports Medicine PCL-ACL drill guide (Biomet Sports Medicine, Warsaw, Ind) is inserted into the knee through the inferior medial patellar portal and is positioned in the PCL fossa on the posterior tibia (Fig. 57-3). The bullet portion of the drill guide contacts the anterior medial aspect of the proximal tibia approximately 1 cm below the tibial tubercle, at a point midway between the tibial crest anteriorly and the posterior medial border of the tibia. This drill guide positioning creates a tibial tunnel that is relatively vertically oriented and has its posterior exit point in the inferior and lateral aspect of the PCL tibial anatomic insertion site. This positioning creates an angle of graft orientation such that the graft will turn two very smooth 45-degree angles on the posterior aspect of the tibia (Fig. 57-4).

The tip of the guide in the posterior aspect of the tibia is confirmed with the surgeon's finger through the extracapsular posteromedial safety incision. Intraoperative AP and lateral x-rays may be used, as well as arthroscopic visualization, to confirm drill guide and guide pin placement. A blunt spade-tipped guide wire is drilled from anterior to posterior, and can be visualized with the arthroscope, in addition to being palpated with the finger in the posteromedial safety incision. We consider placement of the finger in the posteromedial safety incision the most important step for accuracy and safety.

An appropriately sized standard cannulated reamer is used to create the tibial tunnel. The closed curved PCL curette may be positioned to cup the tip of the guide wire. The arthroscope, when positioned in the posteromedial portal, may visualize the guide wire being captured by the curette, and may help in protecting neurovascular structures, in addition to the surgeon's finger in the posteromedial safety incision. The surgeon's finger in the posteromedial safety incision is monitoring the position of the guide wire. The standard cannulated drill is advanced to the posterior cortex of the

tibia. The drill chuck is then disengaged from the drill, and the tibial tunnel reaming is completed by hand. This gives an additional margin of safety for completion of the tibial tunnel. The tunnel edges are chamfered and rasped with the PCL/ACL system rasp.

The PCL femoral tunnel may be created from outside in or from inside out. When the PCL femoral tunnel is created from outside in, the PCL/ACL drill guide is positioned to create the femoral tunnel. The arm of the guide is introduced through the inferomedial patellar portal and is positioned in such a way that the guide wire will exit through the center of the stump of the anterior lateral bundle of the PCL (Fig. 57-5A and B). The spade-tipped guide wire is drilled through the guide, and just as it begins to emerge through the center of the stump of the PCL anterior lateral bundle, the drill guide is disengaged. Accuracy of placement of the wire is confirmed arthroscopically with probing and visualization. By arthroscopically examining the patellofemoral joint prior to drilling, care is taken to ensure that the patellofemoral joint has not been violated, and that the distance between the

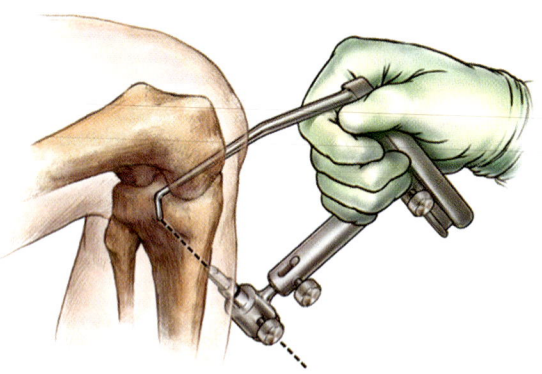

Figure 57-3. Posterior cruciate ligament (PCL)–anterior cruciate ligament (ACL) drill guide positioned to place guide wire in preparation for creation of the transtibial PCL tibial tunnel. (With permission, Biomet Sports Medicine, Inc., Warsaw, Ind.)

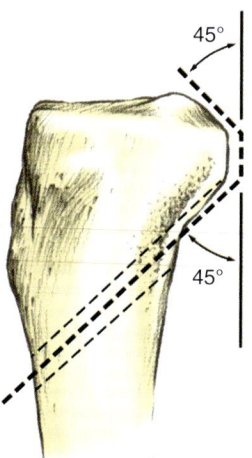

Figure 57-4. Drawing demonstrating the desired turning angles that the posterior cruciate ligament (PCL) graft will make after creation of the tibial tunnel. (With permission, Biomet Sports Medicine, Inc., Warsaw, Ind.)

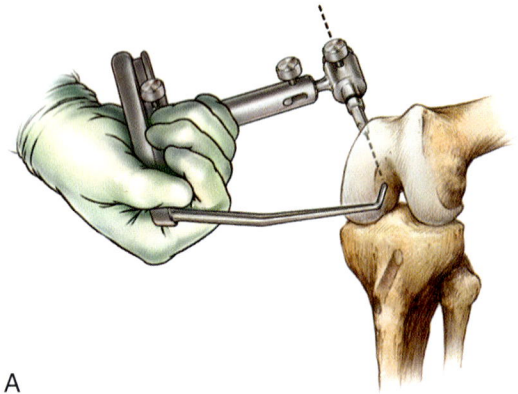

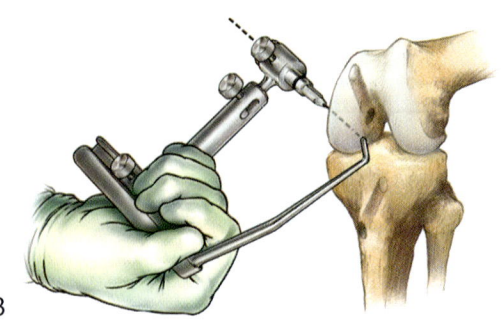

A   B

Figure 57-5. **A** and **B,** The posterior cruciate ligament (PCL)–anterior cruciate ligament (ACL) drill guide is positioned to drill the guide wire from outside in. The guide wire begins at a point halfway between the medial femoral epicondyle and the medial femoral condyle trochlea articular margin, approximately 2 to 3 cm proximal to the medial femoral condyle distal articular margin, and exits through the center of the stump of the anterolateral bundle of the PCL stump. (With permission, Biomet Sports Medicine, Inc., Warsaw, Ind.)

femoral tunnel and the medial femoral condyle articular surface is adequate. An appropriately sized standard cannulated reamer is used to create the femoral tunnel. A curette is used to cap the tip of the guide wire, so no inadvertent advancement of the guide wire occurs; this movement may damage the ACL or the articular surface. As the reamer is about to penetrate interiorly, the reamer is disengaged from the drill and the final reaming is completed by hand. This provides an additional margin of safety. The reaming debris is evacuated with a synovial shaver to minimize fat pad inflammatory response with subsequent risk of arthrofibrosis. The tunnel edges are chamfered and rasped.

The PCL/ACL drill guide is positioned to create the second femoral tunnel. The arm of the guide is introduced through the inferior medial patellar portal and is positioned in such a way that the guide wire will exit through the center of the stump of the posterior medial bundle of the PCL. The blunt spade-tipped guide wire is drilled through the guide, and just as it begins to emerge through the center of the stump of the PCL posterior medial bundle, the drill guide is disengaged. Accuracy of placement of the wire is confirmed arthroscopically with probing and visualization. Care must be taken to ensure that an adequate bone bridge (approximately 5 mm) will be present between the two femoral tunnels prior to drilling. This is accomplished using the calibrated probe and direct arthroscopic visualization. An appropriately sized standard cannulated reamer is used to create the posterior medial bundle femoral tunnel. A curette is used to cap the tip of the guide wire, so no inadvertent advancement of the guide wire occurs; this movement may damage the ACL or the articular surface. As the reamer is about to penetrate interiorly, the reamer is disengaged from the drill and the final reaming is completed by hand. This provides an additional margin of safety. The reaming debris is evacuated with a

synovial shaver to minimize fat pad inflammatory response with subsequent risk of arthrofibrosis. The tunnel edges are chamfered and rasped.

The author's preferred method is to perform a double-bundle PCL reconstruction by making the PCL femoral tunnels from inside out. PCL single-bundle or double-bundle femoral tunnels are made from inside out using the Biomet Sports Medicine double-bundle aimers. Inserting the appropriately sized double-bundle aimer through a low anterior lateral patellar arthroscopic portal creates the PCL anterior lateral bundle femoral tunnel. The double-bundle aimer is positioned directly on the footprint of the femoral anterior lateral bundle PCL insertion site. An appropriately sized guide wire is drilled through the aimer, through the bone, and out a small skin incision. Care is taken to ensure that there is no compromise of the articular surface. The double-bundle aimer is removed, and an acorn reamer is used to endoscopically drill from inside out the anterior lateral PCL femoral tunnel. The tunnel edges are chamfered and rasped. The reaming debris is evacuated with a synovial shaver to minimize fat pad inflammatory response with subsequent risk of arthrofibrosis. The same process is repeated for the posterior medial bundle of the PCL. Care must be taken to ensure that an adequate bone bridge (approximately 5 mm) will be present between the two femoral tunnels prior to drilling. This is accomplished using the calibrated probe and direct arthroscopic visualization (Fig. 57-6A and B).

The Biomet Sports Medicine Magellan suture-passing device is introduced through the tibial tunnel and into the knee joint, and is retrieved through the femoral tunnel with an arthroscopic grasping tool. The traction sutures of the graft material are attached to the loop of the suture-passing device, and the PCL graft material is pulled into position.

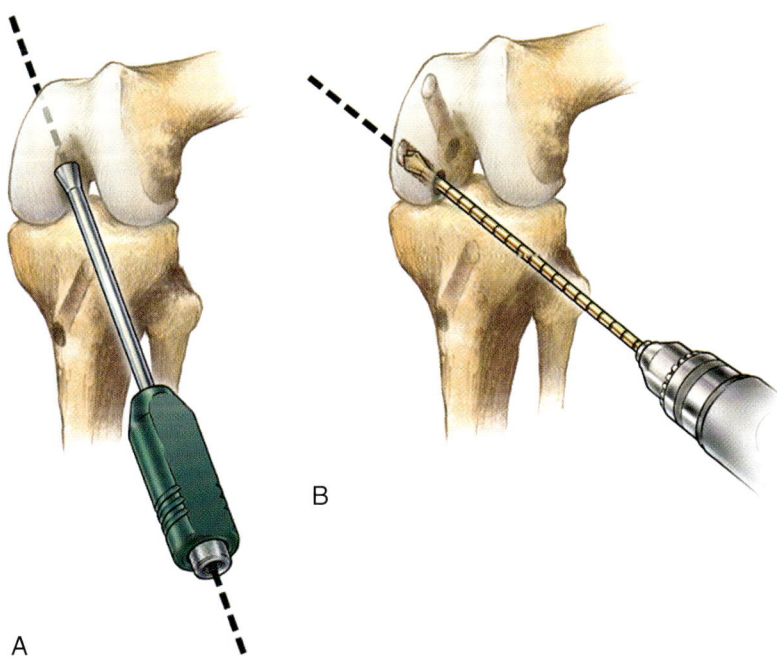

A

B

Figure 57-6. A, Biomet Sports Medicine double-bundle aimer positioned to drill a guide wire for creation of the posterior cruciate ligament (PCL) posteromedial bundle femoral tunnel through the low anterolateral portal. (With permission, Biomet Sports Medicine, Inc., Warsaw, Ind.) **B,** Endoscopic acorn reamer is used to create the posterior cruciate ligament (PCL) posteromedial bundle through the low anterolateral patellar portal. (With permission, Biomet Sports Medicine, Inc., Warsaw, Ind.)

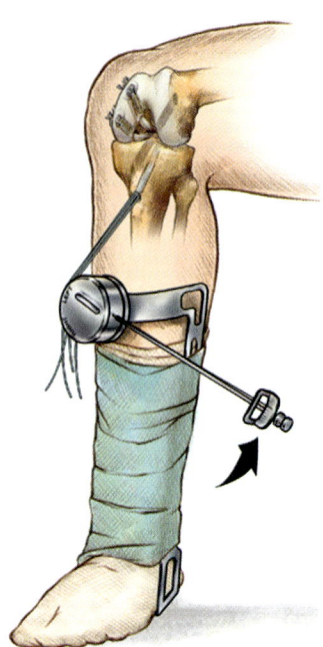

Figure 57-7. Biomet Sports Medicine knee ligament graft-tensioning boot. This mechanical tensioning device uses a ratcheted torque wrench device to assist the surgeon during graft tensioning. (With permission, Biomet Sports Medicine, Inc., Warsaw, Ind.)

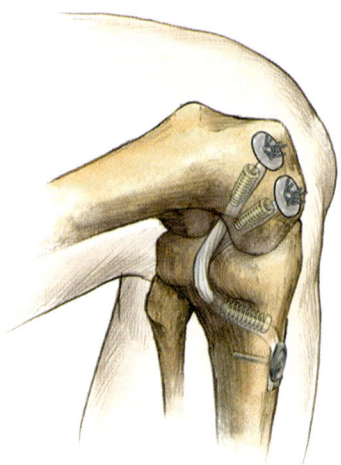

Figure 57-8. Final posterior cruciate ligament (PCL) graft fixation using primary and backup fixation. (With permission, Biomet Sports Medicine, Inc., Warsaw, Ind.)

Fixation of the PCL substitute is accomplished with primary and backup fixation on both the femoral and tibial sides. Our most commonly used graft source for PCL reconstruction is the Achilles tendon allograft alone for single-bundle reconstructions, and the Achilles tendon and tibialis anterior allografts for double-bundle reconstructions, although other allografts and autografts may be used as preferred by an individual surgeon. Femoral fixation is accomplished with cortical suspensory backup fixation using polyethylene ligament fixation buttons and aperture opening fixation with bioabsorbable interference screws. The Biomet Sports Medicine graft-tensioning boot is applied to the traction sutures of the graft material on its distal end and is tensioned to restore the anatomic tibial step-off. The knee is cycled through several sets of 25 full flexion-extension cycles for graft pretensioning and settling (Fig. 57-7). The PCL reconstruction graft is tensioned in physiologic knee flexion ranges. Graft fixation is achieved with primary aperture opening fixation using the bioabsorbable interference screw and backup fixation with a ligament fixation button, or screw and post, or screw and spiked ligament washer assembly (Fig. 57-8).

ACL Reconstruction

With the knee in approximately 90 degrees of flexion, ACL tunnels are created using the PCL/ACL drill guide single-incision endoscopic surgical technique. The arm of the Fanelli drill guide enters the knee joint through the inferior medial patellar portal. The bullet of the drill guide contacts the anterior medial proximal tibia externally at a point 1 cm proximal to the tibial tubercle, midway between the posterior medial border of the tibia and the tibial crest anteriorly. The guide wire is drilled through the guide to emerge through the

center of the stump of the ACL tibial footprint. A standard cannulated reamer is used to create the tibial tunnel. Reaming debris is evacuated, and the tunnel edges are chamfered and rasped.

With the knee in approximately 90 degrees of flexion, an over-the-top femoral aimer is introduced through the tibial tunnel and is used to position a guide wire at the 10 o'clock position (right knee) or the 2 o'clock position (left knee) on the medial wall of the lateral femoral condyle. The femoral tunnel is created to approximate the ACL anatomic insertion site, and the offset of the femoral aimer will leave a 1- to 2-mm posterior cortical wall, so interference fixation can be used. The ACL graft is positioned and fixation achieved on the femoral side using an interference screw and backup fixation with a polyethylene fixation button.

The ACL graft is tensioned on the tibial side using the graft-tensioning boot. Traction is placed on the ACL graft sutures, and tension is set at 20 pounds. The knee is then cycled through 25 full flexion and extension cycles to allow settling of the graft. This process is repeated until no further change is seen in the torque setting on the graft tensioner, indicating that all laxity is removed from the system. The knee is placed in 20 degrees of flexion; fixation is achieved on the tibial side of the ACL graft with an interference screw and backup fixation with a polyethylene ligament fixation button (Fig. 57-9).

Posterolateral Reconstruction Surgical Technique

The free graft figure-of-eight technique for posterolateral reconstruction utilizes semitendinosus autograft or allograft, Achilles tendon allograft, or other soft tissue allograft material. This technique, combined with capsular repair and/or posterolateral capsular shift procedures, mimics the function of the popliteofibular ligament and the lateral collateral ligament, tightens the posterolateral capsule, and provides a post of strong autogenous tissue to reinforce the posterolateral corner.[9,10,12,28,31] A curvilinear incision is made in the lateral aspect of the knee, extending from the lateral femoral epicondyle to the interval between Gerdy's tubercle and the fibular head. The peroneal nerve is dissected free and is protected throughout the procedure. The fibular head is exposed and a 7-mm tunnel is created in an anterior inferior–to–posterior superior direction at the area of maximal fibular diameter. The tunnel is created by passing a guide pin followed by a cannulated drill, usually 7 mm in diameter. The peroneal nerve is protected during tunnel creation and throughout the procedure. The free tendon graft is then passed through the fibular head drill hole. An incision is made in the iliotibial band in line with the fibers directly overlying the lateral femoral epicondyle. A longitudinal incision is made in the lateral capsule just posterior to the fibular collateral ligament. The graft material is passed medial to the iliotibial band and is secured to the lateral femoral epicondylar region with a screw and spiked ligament washer, with the

allograft insertion sites corresponding to the anatomic insertion sites of the fibular collateral ligament and the popliteus tendon. The posterolateral capsule that had been previously incised then is shifted and sewn into the strut of figure-of-eight graft tissue material to eliminate posterolateral capsular redundancy. The anterior and posterior limbs of the figure-of-eight graft material are sewn to each other to reinforce and tighten the construct. The final graft-tensioning position is approximately 30 to 40 degrees of knee flexion. The iliotibial band incision is closed.

When a disrupted proximal tibiofibular joint or a hyperextension external rotation recurvatum deformity occurs, two-tailed (fibular head, proximal tibia) posterior lateral reconstruction is used.[9,10,12,28,31] The semitendinosus allograft is passed through the fibular head and is secured to the lateral femoral epicondylar area, as described earlier. A tibial arm of the reconstruction is passed through a 7-mm drill hole made 2 cm below the joint line through the proximal lateral tibia. This tibial arm of the posterolateral reconstruction follows the course of the popliteus tendon, providing additional support to the posterolateral corner. The procedures described are intended to eliminate posterolateral and varus rotational instability (Fig. 57-10A through C).

Medial Posteromedial Reconstruction

Posteromedial and medial reconstructions are performed through a medial hockeystick incision (Fig. 57-11A and B). Care is taken to maintain adequate skin bridges between incisions. The superficial MCL is exposed, and a longitudinal incision is made just posterior to the posterior border of the superficial MCL. Care is taken to avoid damaging the medial meniscus during the capsular incision. The interval between the posteromedial capsule and the medial meniscus is developed. The posteromedial capsule is shifted anterosuperiorly.

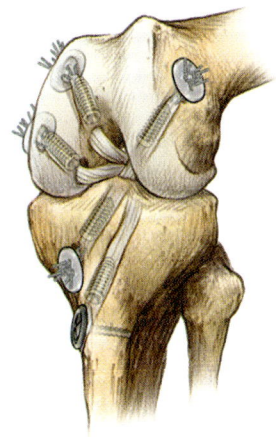

Figure 57-9. Anterior cruciate ligament (ACL) reconstruction. (With permission, Biomet Sports Medicine, Inc., Warsaw, Ind.)

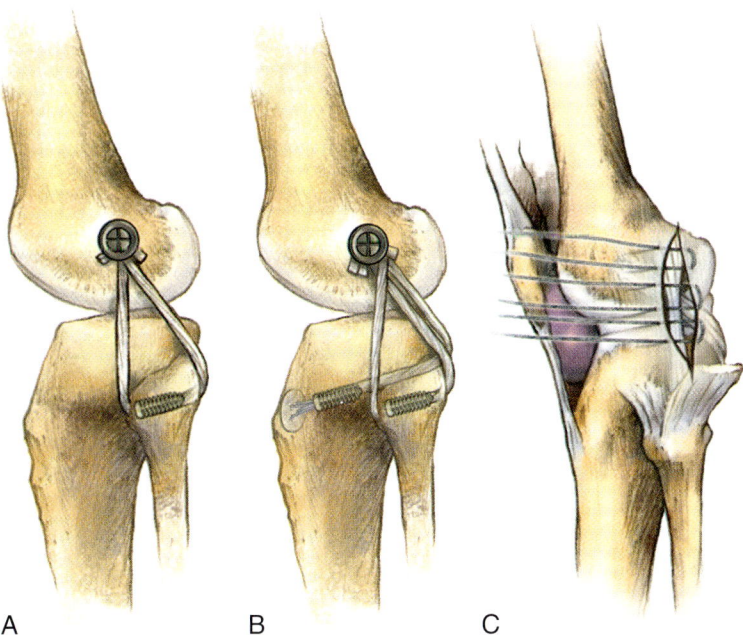

A   B   C

Figure 57-10. Posterolateral reconstruction using single- and double-tailed graft. Transfibular head figure-of-eight semitendinosus allograft mimics the force vectors of the fibular collateral ligament and the popliteofibular ligament. Transtibial tibialis anterior allograft mimics the force vectors of the popliteus tendon. Posterolateral capsular shift is also performed. (With permission, Biomet Sports Medicine, Inc., Warsaw, Ind.)

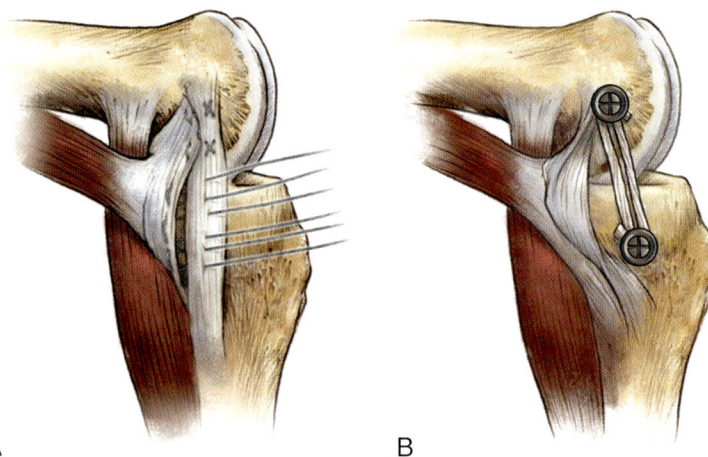

A   B

Figure 57-11. Posteromedial reconstruction using primary repair, posteromedial capsular shift, and free graft as indicated. (With permission, Biomet Sports Medicine, Inc., Warsaw, Ind.)

The medial meniscus is repaired to the new capsular position, and the shifted capsule is sewn into the MCL. When superficial MCL reconstruction is indicated, this is performed using allograft or autograft tissue. This graft material is attached at the anatomic insertion sites of the superficial MCL on the femur and tibia using a screw and spiked ligament washer, or suture anchors. The posteromedial capsular advancement is performed and is sewn into the newly reconstructed MCL. The final graft-tensioning position is approximately 30 to 40 degrees of knee flexion.[9,26,27]

Incorporation of autologous platelet-rich fibrin matrix into the grafts used in PCL and posterolateral reconstructive procedures has been found to enhance the biologic healing response and graft incorporation.[1,5] Our clinical results demonstrate earlier soft tissue graft incorporation documented radiographically, enhanced wound healing, and decreased wound inflammation and pain.

OVERVIEW OF GRAFT TENSIONING AND FIXATION

The PCL reconstruction is commonly done within the context of the multiple ligament–injured knee. When multiple ligaments need to be reconstructed, the PCL is reconstructed first, followed by the ACL, followed by the posterolateral complex and the medial ligament complex. Tension is placed on the PCL graft distally using the Biomet Sports Medicine knee ligament–tensioning device with the knee in full extension, and the tension is set at 20 pounds. This reduces the tibiofemoral joint and restores the anatomic tibial step-off. The knee is cycled through a full range of motion 25 times to allow pretensioning and settling of the graft. The knee is placed in 70 degrees of flexion, and fixation is achieved on the tibial side of the PCL graft with a bioabsorbable interference screw, and a bicortical screw and spiked ligament washer. The knee ligament–tensioning device is applied to the ACL graft and is set at 20 pounds with the knee in full extension. This reduces the tibiofemoral joint and balances PCL and ACL reconstructions. The knee is placed in 20 degrees of flexion, and final fixation of the ACL graft is achieved with a bioabsorbable interference screw and a polyethylene ligament fixation button for cortical

suspensory backup fixation. The knee is placed in 30 to 40 degrees of knee flexion, with the tibia slightly internally rotated, slight valgus force applied to the knee, and final tensioning and fixation of the posterolateral corner achieved. The MCL reconstruction is tensioned with the knee in 30 to 40 degrees of knee flexion and with the leg in a supported figure-of-four position. Full range of motion is confirmed on the operating table.

Postoperative Rehabilitation

The knee is maintained in full extension for 5 weeks of non–weight bearing. Progressive range of motion occurs during weeks 3 through 6. Progressive weight bearing occurs at the beginning of postoperative week 6, progressing at a rate of 20% bodyweight per week during postoperative weeks 6 through 10. Progressive closed kinetic chain strength training, proprioceptive training, and continued motion exercises are initiated very slowly, beginning at postoperative week 11. The long leg range of motion brace is discontinued after the 10th week, and the patient wears a PCL functional brace for all activities. Return to sports and heavy labor occurs after the ninth postoperative month, when sufficient strength, range of motion, and proprioceptive skills have returned.[8]

AUTHOR'S RESULTS OF PCL RECONSTRUCTION

Fanelli and Edson, in 2004, published 2- to 10-year (24- to 120-month) results of 41 chronic, arthroscopically assisted, combined PCL/posterolateral reconstructions evaluated preoperatively and postoperatively using Lysholm, Tegner, and Hospital for Special Surgery (HSS) knee ligament rating scales, KT 1000 arthrometer testing, stress radiography, and physical examination.[16] Posterior cruciate ligament reconstructions were performed using the arthroscopically assisted, single–femoral tunnel/single-bundle TTT PCL reconstruction technique with fresh-frozen Achilles tendon allografts in all 41 cases. In all 41 cases, posterolateral instability reconstruction was performed with combined biceps femoris tendon tenodesis and posterolateral capsular shift procedures. Postoperative physical examination revealed normal posterior drawer/tibial step-off for the overall study group in 29 of 41 (70%) knees. Normal posterior drawer and tibial step-offs were achieved in 91.7% of knees tensioned with the mechanical graft tensioner. Posterolateral stability was restored to normal in 11 of 41 (27%) knees and was tighter than the normal knee in 29 of 41 (71%) knees evaluated with the external rotation thigh foot angle test. In 40 of 41 (97%) knees, 30 degree varus stress testing was normal, and grade 1 laxity was noted in 1 of 41 (3%) knees. Postoperative KT 1000 arthrometer testing revealed that mean side-to-side difference measurements were 1.80 mm (PCL screen), 2.11 mm (corrected posterior), and 0.63 mm (corrected anterior). This is a statistically significant improvement from preoperative status for the PCL screen and corrected posterior measurements (P = .001). Postoperative stress radiographic mean side-to-side difference measurements at 90 degrees of knee flexion and with 32 lb of posterior directed force applied to the proximal tibia using the Telos device was 2.26 mm. This is a statistically significant improvement from preoperative measurements (P = .001). Postoperative Lysholm, Tegner, and HSS knee ligament rating scale mean values were 91.7, 4.92, and 88.7, respectively, demonstrating statistically significant improvement from preoperative status (P = .001). The authors concluded that chronic combined PCL/posterolateral instabilities can be successfully treated with arthroscopic PCL reconstruction using fresh-frozen Achilles tendon allograft combined with posterolateral corner reconstruction with biceps tendon tenodesis combined with a posterolateral capsular shift procedure. Statistically significant improvement is noted (P = .001) from the preoperative condition at 2- to 10-year follow-up when objective parameters of knee ligament rating scales, arthrometer testing, stress radiography, and physical examination are used.

Fanelli et al, in 2005, published the results of allograft multiple ligament–knee reconstructions using the Biomet Sports Medicine mechanical graft-tensioning device.[18] These data present 2-year follow up results of 15 arthroscopic-assisted ACL/PCL allograft reconstructions using the *Biomet Sports Medicine* graft-tensioning boot. This study group consisted of 11 chronic and 4 acute injuries. Injury patterns included 6 ACL/PCL/posterolateral corner injuries, 4/ACL/PCL/MCL injuries, and 5 ACL/PCL/posterolateral corner/MCL injuries. The tensioning boot was used during these procedures, as in the surgical technique described earlier. All knees had grade III preoperative ACL/PCL laxity and were assessed preoperatively and postoperatively using Lysholm, Tegner, and HSS knee ligament rating scales, KT 1000 arthrometer testing, stress radiography, and physical examination.

Arthroscopic-assisted combined ACL/PCL reconstructions were performed using the single-incision endoscopic ACL technique and the single–femoral tunnel/single-bundle TTT PCL technique. PCLs were reconstructed with allograft Achilles tendon in all 15 knees. ACLs were reconstructed with Achilles tendon allograft in all 15 knees. MCL injuries were treated surgically using primary repair, posteromedial capsular shift, and allograft augmentation as indicated. Posterolateral instability was treated with allograft semitendinosus free graft, with or without primary repair, and posterolateral capsular shift procedures as indicated. The graft-tensioning boot was used in this series of patients.

Postreconstruction physical examination results revealed normal posterior drawer/tibial step-off in 13 of 15 (86.6%)

knees. Normal Lackman test findings were reported in 13 of 15 (86.6%) knees, and normal pivot shift test results in 14 of 15 (93.3%) knees. Posterolateral stability was restored to normal in all knees with posterolateral instability when evaluated with the external rotation thigh foot angle test (nine knees equal to the normal knee, and two knees tighter than the normal knee). In all 11 knees with posterolateral lateral instability, 30-degree varus stress testing was restored to normal. In all nine knees with medial-side laxity, 30- and 0-degree valgus stress testing was restored to normal. On postoperative KT-1000 arthrometer testing, mean side-to-side difference measurements were 1.6 mm (range, −3 to 7 mm) for the PCL screen, 1.6 mm (range, −4.5 to 9 mm) for corrected posterior measurements, and 0.5 mm (range, −2.5 to 6 mm) for corrected anterior measurements—a significant improvement from preoperative status. Postoperative stress radiographic side-to-side difference measurements at 90 degrees of knee flexion and with 32 lb of posteriorly directed proximal force using the Telos stress radiography device were 0 to 3 mm in 10 of 15 knees (66.7%), 4 mm in 4 of 15 knees (26.7%), and 7 mm in 1 of 15 knees (6.67%). Postoperative Lysholm, Tegner, and HSS knee ligament rating scale mean values were 86.7 (range, 69 to 95), 4.5 (range, 2 to 7), and 85.3 (range, 65 to 93) respectively, demonstrating a significant improvement from preoperative status.

The authors concluded that the study group demonstrates the efficacy and success of using allograft tissue and a mechanical graft-tensioning device (*Biomet Sports Medicine* graft-tensioning boot) in single-bundle/single–femoral tunnel arthroscopic PCL reconstruction.

AUTHOR'S DOUBLE-BUNDLE COMPARED WITH SINGLE-BUNDLE PCL RECONSTRUCTION RESULTS

Multiple studies have reported good outcomes with both single-bundle and double-bundle PCL reconstruction.* We have compared the results of arthroscopic TTT single-bundle and double-bundle PCL reconstructions using allograft tissue in PCL-based multiple ligament–injured knees in a level 3 retrospective comparative study, and we provide those results in this chapter.[13,20]

Ninety consecutive PCL reconstructions were evaluated: 45 single-bundle and 45 double-bundle reconstructions. All PCL reconstructions were performed using the arthroscopically assisted TTT PCL reconstruction technique described in this chapter, using fresh-frozen allograft tissue from the same tissue bank. Achilles tendon allograft was used for the anterolateral bundle (ALB), and tibialis anterior allograft for the posteromedial bundle (PMB). The knees were evaluated postoperatively with comparison of single-bundle results to double-bundle results, and with KT 1000 arthrometer testing, three different knee ligament rating scales, and Telos stress radiography.

On postoperative KT 1000 arthrometer testing, mean side-to-side difference measurements were 1.91 mm (PCL screen, 90 degrees), 2.11 mm (corrected posterior, 70 degrees), and 1.11 mm (30 degrees) in the single-bundle group,

---

*References 2, 13, 15, 16, 18, 20, 23, and 24.

and 2.46 mm (PCL screen, 90 degrees), 2.94 mm (corrected posterior, 70 degrees), and 0.44 mm (30 degrees) in the double-bundle group (P = .289694, .231154, and .315546, respectively). Postoperative stress radiographic mean side-to-side difference measurements 90 degrees of knee flexion with 32 lb of posterior directed force applied to the proximal tibia using the Telos device were 2.56 mm in the single-bundle group and 2.36 mm in the double-bundle group (P = .895792). Postoperative Lysholm, Tegner, and HSS knee ligament rating scale mean values were 90.3, 5.0, and 86.2, respectively, in the single-bundle group, and 87.6, 4.6, and 83.3 in the double-bundle group, respectively (P = .226327, .308564, and .282588, respectively). All objective parameters demonstrated no statistically significant differences between single- and double-bundle PCL reconstructions in acute (P = .395962) and chronic (P = .416085) cases.

We were able to conclude that both single-bundle and double-bundle PCL reconstruction surgical techniques using allograft tissue provide successful results in the PCL-based multiple ligament–injured knee when evaluated with stress radiography, arthrometer measurements, and knee ligament rating scales.

Summary

Both single-bundle and double-bundle arthroscopic assisted TTT PCL reconstruction techniques are successful surgical procedures. We have documented results demonstrating statistically significant improvement from preoperative to postoperative status evaluated by physical examination, knee ligament rating scales, arthrometer measurements, and stress radiography. Factors contributing to the success of this surgical technique include identification and treatment of all pathology (especially posterolateral and posteromedial instability), accurate tunnel placement, placement of strong graft material at anatomic graft insertion sites, minimization of graft bending, performance of final graft tensioning at 70 to 90 degrees of knee flexion using the graft-tensioning boot, utilization of primary and backup fixation, and selection of the appropriate postoperative rehabilitation program.

KEY REFERENCES

Fanelli GC editor: Posterior cruciate ligament injuries: a practical guide to management. New York, 2001, Springer-Verlag.

Fanelli GC editor: The multiple ligament injured knee: a practical guide to management. New York, 2004, Springer-Verlag.

Fanelli GC: Posterior cruciate ligament rehabilitation: how slow should we go? Arthroscopy 24:234–235, 2008.

Fanelli GC: Rationale and surgical technique for PCL and multiple knee ligament reconstruction: surgical technique guide. Warsaw, Ind, 2008, Biomet Sports Medicine, Inc.

Fanelli GC, Beck JD, Edson CJ: Double bundle posterior cruciate ligament reconstruction surgical technique and results. Sports Med Arthrosc 18(4):242–248, 2010.

Fanelli GC, Edson CJ: PCL injuries in trauma patients, part II. Arthroscopy 11:526–529, 1995.

Fanelli GC, Edson CJ: Arthroscopically assisted combined ACL/PCL reconstruction: 2-10 year follow-up. Arthroscopy 18:703–714, 2002.

Fanelli GC, Edson CJ: Combined posterior cruciate ligament—posterolateral reconstruction with Achilles tendon allograft and biceps femoris tendon tenodesis: 2-10 year follow-up. Arthroscopy 20:339–345, 2005.

Fanelli GC, Edson CJ, Orcutt DR, et al: Treatment of combined ACL PCL medial lateral side injuries of the knee. J Knee Surg 28:240–248, 2005.

Fanelli GC, Edson CJ, Reinheimer KN, Beck J: Arthroscopic single bundle v double bundle posterior cruciate ligament reconstruction. Arthroscopy 24(Suppl):e26, 2008.

Fanelli GC, Giannotti BF, Edson CJ: Current concepts review: the posterior cruciate ligament: arthroscopic evaluation and treatment. Arthroscopy 10:673–688, 1994.

Fanelli GC, Giannotti BF, Edson CJ: Arthroscopically assisted combined anterior and posterior cruciate ligament reconstruction. Arthroscopy 12:5–14, 1996.

Fanelli GC, Giannotti BF, Edson CJ: Arthroscopically assisted combined posterior cruciate ligament/posterior lateral complex reconstruction. Arthroscopy 12:521–530, 1996.

Fanelli GC, Harris JD: Late MCL (medial collateral ligament) reconstruction. Technique Knee Surg 6:99–105, 2007.

Fanelli GC, Orcutt DR, Edson CJ: Current concepts: the multiple ligament injured knee. Arthroscopy 21:471–486, 2005.

Giffin JR, Haemmerie MJ, Vogrin TM, Harner CD: Single- versus double-bundle PCL reconstruction: a biomechanical analysis. J Knee Surg 15:114–120, 2002.

Noyes FR, Barber-Westin SD: Posterior cruciate ligament revision reconstruction, part 1. Am J Sports Med 33:646–654, 2005.

Robinson JR, Bull AMJ, Thomas RR, Amis AA: The role of the medial collateral ligament and posteromedial capsule in controlling knee laxity. Am J Sports Med 34:1815–1823, 2006.

Sekiya JK, Haemmerle MJ, Stabile KJ, et al: Biomechanical analysis of a combined double bundle posterior cruciate ligament and posterolateral corner reconstruction. Am J Sports Med 33:360–369, 2005.

Full references for this chapter can be found on www.expertconsult.com.

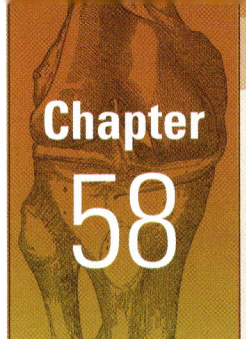

Chapter 58

Posterior Cruciate Ligament Reconstruction: Remnant-Preserving Technique Through the Posteromedial Portal

Sung-Jae Kim and Sung-Hwan Kim

The posterior cruciate ligament (PCL) is the strongest ligament in the knee and provides primary restraint to tibial posterior translation. Although the anatomy and biomechanics of the PCL have been examined in detail, controversy continues regarding the optimal treatment for PCL injuries. If surgical reconstruction is elected, the goals of surgery are to replicate the anatomy and biomechanics of the native PCL. Various surgical options are currently available for PCL reconstruction: the transtibial or inlay technique, single- or double-bundle reconstruction, and the one- or two-incision technique.[22] Surgeons observe preserved continuity of the attenuated PCL in most PCL-insufficient patients.[1,4,14] However, many surgeons have lost sight of the importance of these remaining fibers and surrounding structures. In conventional PCL reconstruction, the surgeon generally removes the residual stump of the PCL to facilitate visualization and technical performance. In fact, ligaments around the joints contain mechanoreceptors that are involved in providing the central nervous system with information about joint position and movement.[15] The cruciate ligaments have recently attracted interest and have been studied not only as mechanical and structural stabilizers, but also as sensory structures.[7,9,10,15] In addition, it has been suggested that the meniscofemoral ligaments (MFLs) contribute significantly to the cross-sectional area of the PCL complex and act as secondary restraints to tibial posterior translation.[3,24]

Accordingly, it may be of benefit to attempt to preserve the remnant tissue during PCL reconstruction. In this chapter, we describe the scientific rationale, surgical indications, and surgical technique for transtibial PCL reconstruction with remnant preservation.

SCIENTIFIC RATIONALE

Mechanoreceptors in the Posterior Cruciate Ligament

The presence of mechanoreceptors in the cruciate ligaments has led surgeons to suppose that these receptors influence the motor function of the knee joint. Several studies on anterior cruciate ligament (ACL) reconstruction revealed that success of surgery depends not only on the stability of the reconstructed ligament, but also on the quality of proprioception.[13,21,27] Unfortunately, in comparison with the ACL, very little research has been carried out exclusively on PCL receptors and proprioception. Franchi et al[8] found that the PCL possesses a neural network, and that mechanoreceptors occupy 1% of the total area of the ligament in histologic study. Afferents from these mechanoreceptors such as Ruffini endings, Ruffini corpuscles of the Golgi tendon organ-like type, and Pacinian corpuscles are thought to be involved in the control of proprioception.[5,8,31] Loss of proprioception after ligament injury leads to changes in gait pattern, muscle strength, and timing of muscle activation, which may inhibit protective reflexes and result in degenerative changes.[10]

Mechanoreceptors on the Remnant Fibers

The PCL is known to have better synovial coverage, blood circulation, and healing potential than the ACL.[29,30] Arthroscopic examination of the PCL-insufficient knee usually demonstrates well-maintained continuity of the PCL, even though it might be attenuated.[1,4,14] However, no histologic reports have indicated whether the remnant of the ruptured PCL contains mechanoreceptors. Some studies have revealed the presence of mechanoreceptors even 3 years after ACL injury,[9] and reproducible cortical somatosensory-evoked potentials induced by electrical stimulation were detected in patients with an ACL remnant bridging the femur and tibia or adherent to the PCL.[26] In this respect, the importance of the remnant of the PCL as a proprioceptive organ can be considered similar to that of the ACL.

Functions and Anatomy of the Meniscofemoral Ligaments

The MFLs are composed of the ligament of Humphrey (anterior) and the ligament of Wrisberg (posterior), which originate from the posterior horn of the lateral meniscus and insert on the lateral aspect of the medial femoral condyle. The anterior MFL passes anterior to the PCL and attaches adjacent to the femoral condylar articular cartilage, indenting the attachment of the anterolateral fibers of the PCL.[6] The posterior MFL passes posterior to the PCL and attaches proximally, close to the roof of the intercondylar notch.[2] Studies investigating the prevalence of MFLs have shown that 82% to 93% of all knees have at least one MFL, and 26% to 50% possess both.[3,24] The mean strength of the MFLs is approximately 300 N, which is mechanically equivalent to that of the posteromedial bundle of the PCL.[3] Nagasaki et al[24] reported that the cross-sectional area of MFLs accounted for 17.2% of the area of the PCL proper. Regarding a functional role in knee stability and protection, the slanting arrangement of the MFLs from the posterior horn of the meniscus up to the femoral intercondylar notch can help to withstand a tibial posterior drawer.[11] Amis et al[2] indicated that the MFLs contributed 28% of the resistance to posterior drawer in the intact knee at 90 degrees flexion; this contribution rose to 70% in the PCL-deficient knee. Moran et al[23] showed that MFLs allowed the posterior horn of the lateral meniscus to be effectively restrained relative to the femur. In some PCL-insufficient knees, where the distal attachment of the MFLs is seen at the relatively mobile lateral meniscus, it is possible for the MFLs to remain intact despite rupture of the PCL.[3]

Consequently, preservation of the MFLs may promote stabilization of knees that require PCL reconstruction.

SURGICAL INDICATIONS

Indications for PCL reconstruction are as follows: (1) pain and instability during daily activities of living, with 10 mm or more of increased posterior laxity of the affected knee compared with the intact contralateral knee on posterior stress radiographs or KT-2000 arthrometer (MedMetric Corp., San Diego, Calif) despite appropriate rehabilitation; and (2) PCL tears combined with other ligament injuries.

SURGICAL TECHNIQUE

Arthroscopic Portals

For more convenient reconstruction of the PCL, three unique portals are used: a high medial parapatellar portal, a far anterolateral portal, and a high posteromedial portal (Fig. 58-1). The high medial parapatellar portal is made first at the highest position on the medial parapatellar line, which is just off the medial edge of the patella tendon and the inferior border of the patella. This portal is more proximal than the conventional anteromedial portal and facilitates access to the attachment area of the PCL through the intercondylar notch, as well as to the posterior capsule, with a 30 degree arthroscope. The far anterolateral portal is made just above the joint line and 5 mm anterior to the lateral femoral condyle. Then, under direct visualization through the high medial parapatellar portal, the high posteromedial portal is made. A spinal needle is inserted through the posteromedial side of the knee as high as possible and just beside the medial gastrocnemius, aiming for the tibial footprint of the PCL. A scalpel is inserted alongside the entry point of the needle and is run parallel with the needle. The back of the scalpel blade

should face the femoral condyle to avoid damage to articular cartilage (Fig. 58-2). Through this portal, the tibial attachment of the PCL can be accessed directly while viewing through the intercondylar notch. Furthermore, the high posteromedial portal facilitates excellent visualization of the tibial stump and the posterior capsule as an additional viewing portal.

Tibial Tunnel Preparation

In preparing the tibial footprint of the PCL, the remnant is laterally peeled from the tibial attachment with a narrow osteotome (Fig. 58-3). To create a tibial tunnel, a PCL guide is inserted through the high medial parapatellar portal and is passed through the intercondylar notch while viewing through the high posteromedial portal. The PCL guide is located about 1.5 cm below the articular surface and just lateral to the midline on the fossa for the PCL. A 3- to 4-cm longitudinal skin incision is made just lateral to the tibial tuberosity. The tibialis anterior muscle is stripped off and retracted laterally, exposing the starting point of the tibial tunnel 2 cm posterolateral from the anterior tibial crest. Using calibrations on the PCL guide, the distance from the anterolateral cortex of the tibia to the tip of the guide in the fossa for the PCL is accurately measured. The same length as measured on the guide system is marked on the guide pin to prevent past-point drilling (Fig. 58-4). Placement of the guide pin at the ideal site of the PCL footprint is confirmed by visualization through the high posteromedial portal. To enhance visualization during the following procedures, the previously stripped PCL stump and the posterior capsule are pushed back with the arm of the PCL guide. The tibial tunnel is reamed incrementally with a 6- to 11-mm-diameter cannulated reamer. The final tibial tunnel reaming is completed manually to avoid damage to neurovascular structures (Fig. 58-5). Then, chamfering of the upper sharp edge of the

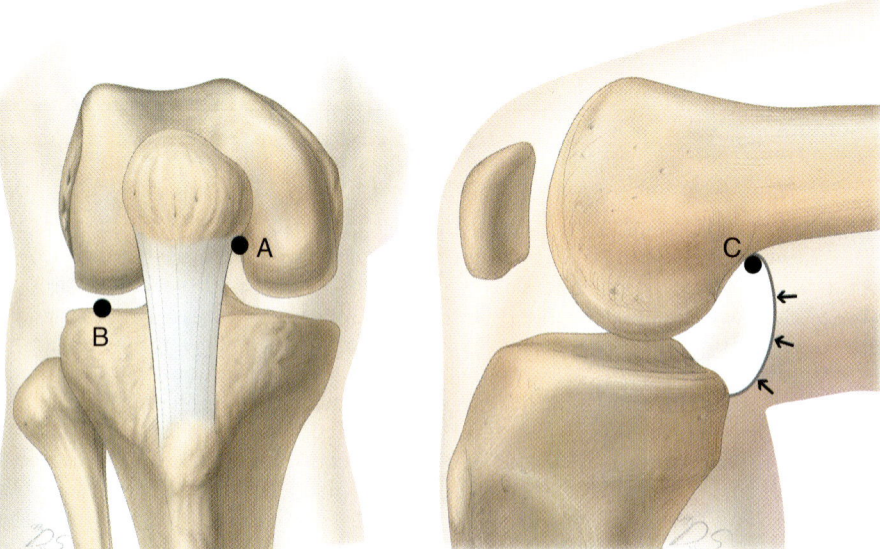

Figure 58-1. A, The high medial parapatellar portal is located at the highest position on the medial parapatellar line, which is just off the medial edge of the patella tendon and the inferior border of the patella. **B,** The far anterolateral portal is made just above the joint line and 5 mm anterior to the lateral femoral condyle. **C,** The high posteromedial portal is situated 3 to 5 cm above the joint line and in the superomedial corner of the capsule *(black arrows).*

aperture is performed using the half-round–shaped rasp to reduce abrasion of the graft.

Author's Tips

In the tibial attachment of the native PCL, the anterolateral fibers are on the anterior (deep) aspect, and the posteromedial fibers are posterior (superficial). Because of this arrangement, when a surgeon performs a single-bundle PCL reconstruction with reproduction of the anterolateral fibers, the graft should be brought up from the tibia underneath (anterior to) the remnant of the PCL.[3] In this respect, lateral

peeling of the remnant from the tibial attachment with the osteotome enables not only preservation of the remnant but also restoration of the anatomic arrangement. In addition, as described earlier, we are in favor of anterolateral tibial tunnel drilling for PCL reconstruction. Concentration of stress from the acutely angled graft at the proximal tibial tunnel margin can cause friction and stretching, followed by failure of the graft during motion against the abrasive edge, in the early postoperative incorporation period. A biomechanical laboratory study showed that the lateral approach for tibial tunnel drilling had the lowest values for maximum shear stress.[19] Moreover, in a cadaveric experiment using pressure films, the lateral tunnel showed a lower reactive force than that of the medial tunnel.[19] A recent clinical study in our institute supports the superiority of this lateral approach. When cases of

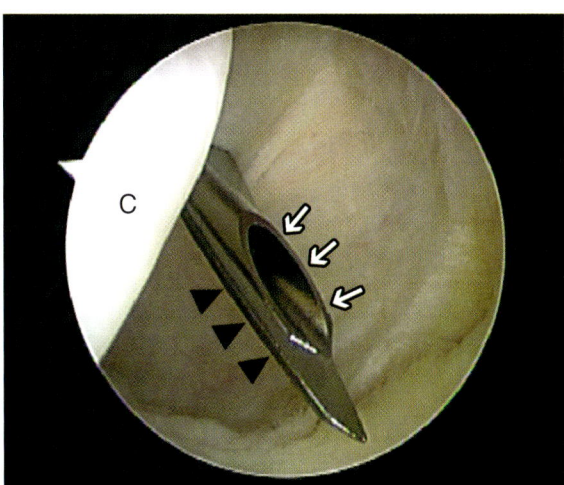

Figure 58-2. Arthroscopic view through the high medial parapatellar portal as the posteromedial portal is created. A scalpel is inserted just beside the entry point of the needle *(white arrows)* and is run parallel with the needle. The back of the scalpel blade *(black arrowheads)* should face the femoral condyle *(C)* to avoid damage to articular cartilage.

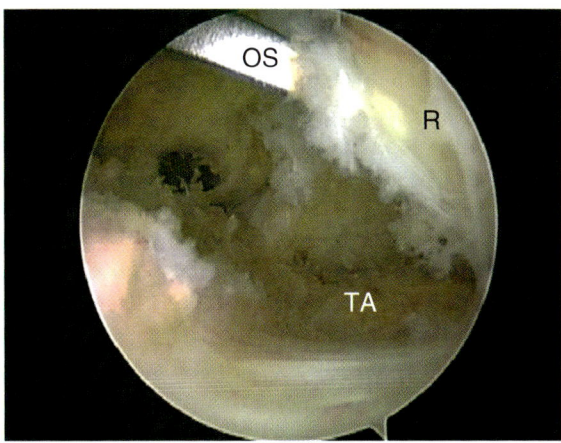

Figure 58-3. Arthroscopic view through the high medial parapatellar portal. The remnant *(R)* is laterally peeled from the tibial attachment *(TA)* with a narrow osteotome *(OS)* through the posteromedial portal.

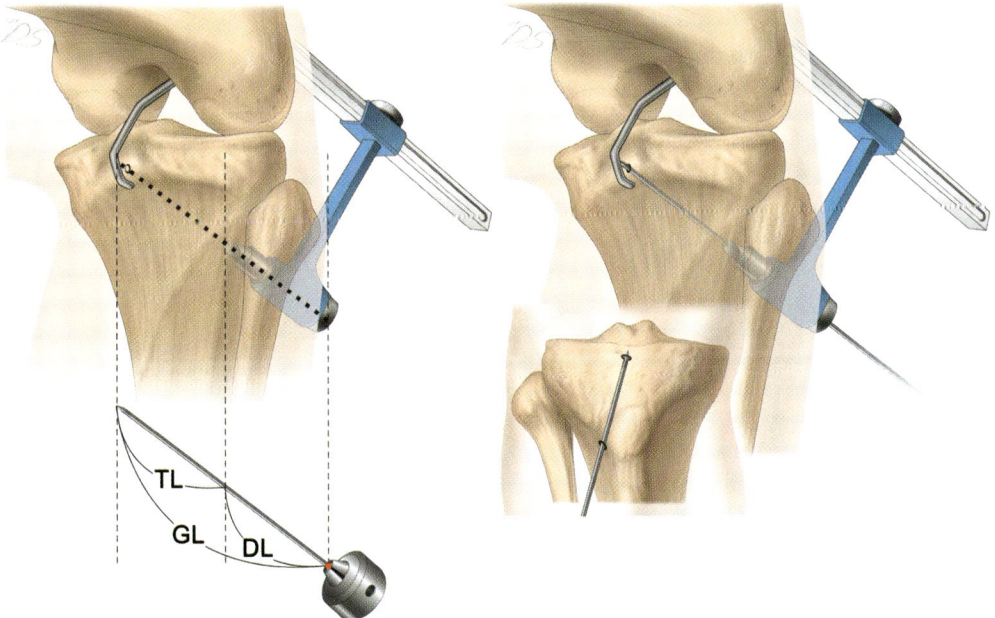

Figure 58-4. **A,** The length of the guide pin *(GL)* to prevent past-point drilling is determined as the distance from the anterolateral cortex of the tibia to the tip of the guide tunnel length *(TL)* in the fossa for the posterior cruciate ligament *(PCL)* plus the length of the device *(DL).* **B,** The ideal site of the PCL footprint is about 1.5 cm below the articular surface and just lateral to the midline in the fossa for the PCL. The entry point of the tibial tunnel is 2 cm posterolateral from the anterior tibial crest.

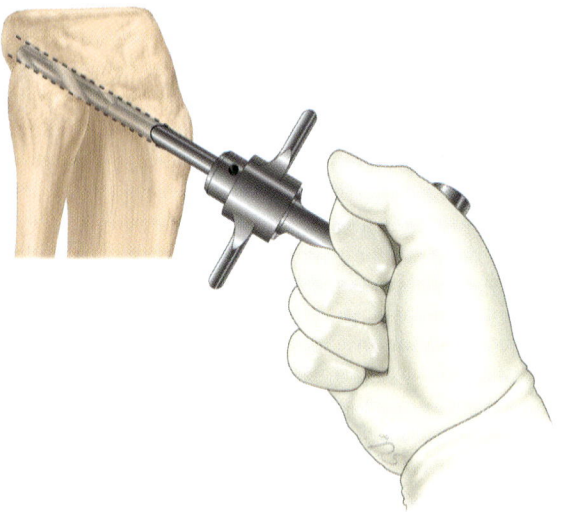

Figure 58-5. The final tibial tunnel reaming is completed manually to avoid damage to neurovascular structures.

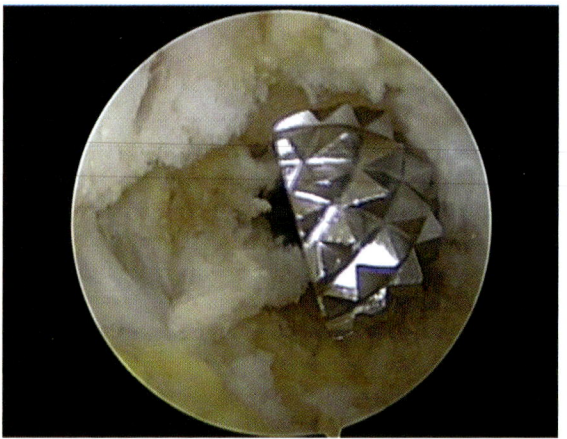

Figure 58-6. Arthroscopic view through the high posteromedial portal. With inspection of the inside of the tibial tunnel aperture, chamfering of the upper sharp edge of the tunnel is performed.

anteromedial tibial tunnel and anterolateral tibial tunnel were compared, side-to-side differences in posterior tibial translation were significantly less with the anterolateral tibial tunnel technique (2.87 ± 1.25 mm) than with the anteromedial tibial tunnel technique (3.98 ± 1.27 mm).[16] In addition to decreased stress concentration, technical advantages of the anterolateral tibial tunnel direction include easy inspection of the inside of the tibial tunnel aperture through the posteromedial portal view, making it more convenient to chamfer the abrasive edge (Fig. 58-6), and shorter tibial tunnel length with less surgical damage.

Femoral Socket Preparation

The landmark of the femoral socket is prepared in the center of the footprint of the anterolateral bundle using a blade and osteotome along the fiber direction (Fig. 58-7). This technique minimizes damage to the remnant, including adjacent MFLs. The center of the femoral socket is located 8 mm posterior from the articular junction and at the 10:30 position for the left knee and the 1:30 position for the right knee. A cannulated headed reamer with a plastic sheath is introduced through the far anterolateral portal. The plastic sheath covering the shaft of the reamer prevents damage to the articular surface of the lateral femoral condyle during reaming. To reduce graft socket divergence in the femur, the following unique tips are applied: (1) the knee is flexed more than 100 degrees; (2) the proximal tibia is pushed backward as much as possible; and (3) the cannulated headed reamer is introduced through the far anterolateral portal with a plastic sheath, which is pushed posteriorly to contact the lateral femoral condyle (Fig. 58-8). The direction of rotation of the reamer is counterclockwise to allow the socket to be made in the intended location without waggling during reaming, and to preserve as much of the PCL remnant as possible. The femoral socket is created to a 35-mm depth, and chamfering the edge of the femoral socket, especially the posterior half, is important for reducing abrasion.

Author's Tips

For creation of the femoral tunnel, one-incision (inside-out) and two-incision (outside-in) techniques have been described.

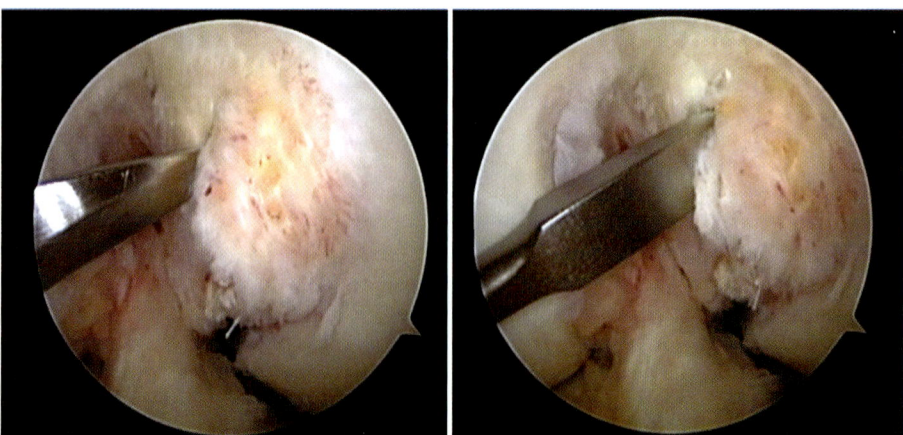

Figure 58-7. Arthroscopic view through the high medial parapatellar portal. The site of the femoral socket is prepared in the center of the footprint of the anterolateral bundle using a blade **(A)** and an osteotome **(B)** along the fiber direction.

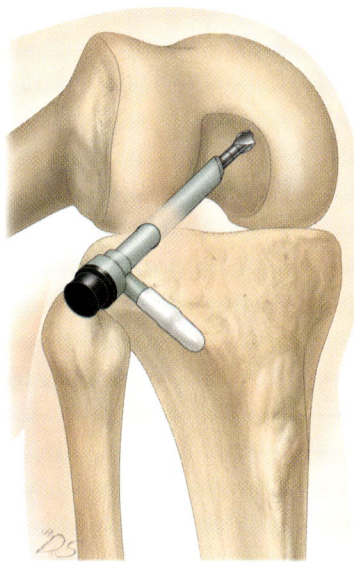

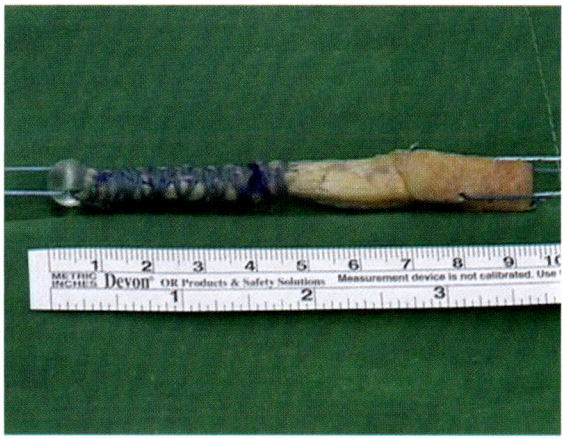

Figure 58-9. The Achilles tendon, of which the tendinous end is to be used for femoral fixation, is threaded in whipstitch fashion for up to 30 mm; then a 9-mm EndoPearl is attached.

Figure 58-8. With the knee flexed more than 100 degrees and maintaining posterior translation of the proximal tibia, the cannulated headed reamer is introduced through the far anterolateral portal with a plastic sheath to protect the lateral femoral condyle.

We prefer the one-incision technique, which avoids potential injury to the extensor mechanism, especially the vastus medialis obliquus muscle and the medial patellofemoral ligament.[20] A few authors have alleged that this technique resulted in a greater graft-socket angle, which could lead to attrition of the graft at the edge of the femoral aperture.[12,28] However, this is counteracted by using the three unique tips previously mentioned. A comparison study of one- and two-incision techniques showed no significant postoperative side-to-side differences in posterior translation between the two groups as measured by the KT-1000 or KT-2000 arthrometer (2.38 vs. 2.10 mm; $P = .26$), Lysholm scores (90.6 vs. 90.0; $P = .72$), and Tegner activity level scales (6.5 vs. 6.4; $P = .38$). Moreover, mean Hospital for Special Surgery values were significantly higher in the one-incision group than in the two-incision group (92.6 vs. 87.7; $P = .037$).[20]

Graft Preparation

An Achilles tendon–bone allograft is currently used at our institute because of its high tensile strength, lack of harvest site morbidity, rigid fixation of the osseous end, and short operation time. The bone plug for tibial fixation with the attached Achilles tendon is designed with a width of 11 mm and a length of 25 mm. The Achilles tendon is prepared to be 60 mm in length and 11 mm in width. The end of the Achilles tendon that is to be used for femoral fixation is threaded in whipstitch fashion for up to 30 mm, then a 9-mm EndoPearl (Linvatec, Largo, Fla) is attached to the tip of the tendon to enhance fixation strength (Fig. 58-9).[33]

Graft Passage

The curved portion of plastic tube (intravenous tube) connected to a passing suture is passed through the tibial tunnel and pulled out through a cannula in the far anterolateral portal using a grasper (Fig. 58-10). A Beath pin is introduced

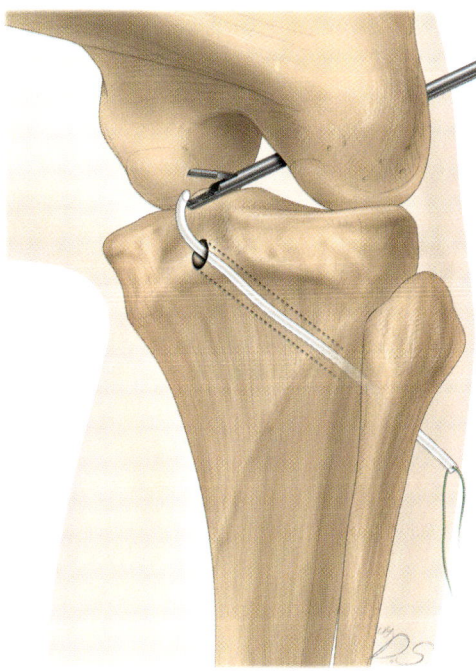

Figure 58-10. A plastic tube (intravenous tube) connected to a passing suture is passed through the tibial tunnel and pulled out using a grasper.

into the femoral socket through the cannula in the far anterolateral portal and then is drilled further through the medial femoral cortex to exit through the skin anteromedially. The passing suture is threaded into the eyelet of the Beath pin, and the pin is pulled out of the medial femoral condyle (Fig. 58-11). The leading suture of the graft is tied to the tibial end of the passing suture and is pulled out of the medial femoral condyle. Then, under arthroscopic guidance, the leading suture is pulled to pass the graft from distal to proximal, and the graft is engaged into the femoral socket.

Graft Fixation

Femoral fixation is achieved with an absorbable interference screw through the far anterolateral portal with the knee at

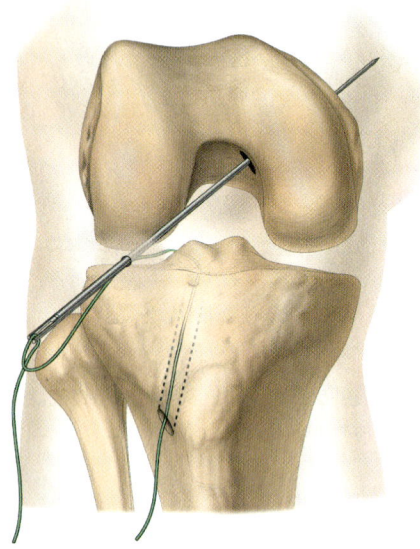

Figure 58-11. The Beath pin is pulled out of the medial femoral condyle with the passing suture.

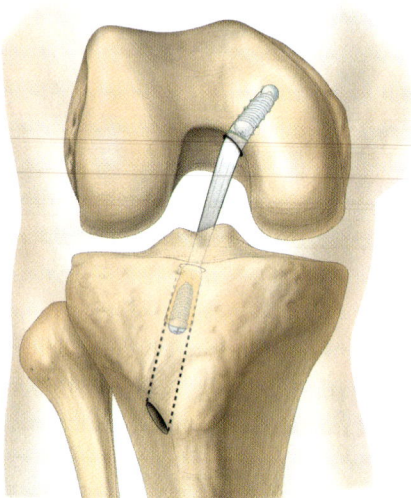

Figure 58-12. Final graft fixation is achieved with absorbable interference screws.

100 degrees of flexion. The graft is pretensioned through a range of motion 20 times. This cyclic motion helps to precondition the graft and eliminates creep.[25] The distal bone peg is secured with an absorbable interference screw with the knee in 70 degrees of flexion while an anteriorly directed force is applied to restore the normal anterior tibial step-off (Fig. 58-12).

ADDITIONAL SURGERY

Most PCL injuries are accompanied by a posterolateral corner injury or a medial injury. PCL reconstruction is performed first, followed by posterolateral or medial reconstruction. We have developed and use the following techniques.[17,18]

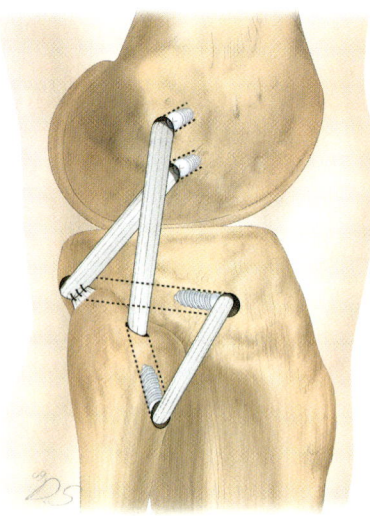

Figure 58-13. For posterolateral corner insufficiency, lateral collateral ligament and popliteus tendon reconstructions are performed with posterior tibialis tendon allograft.

For posterolateral corner insufficiency, lateral collateral ligament (LCL) and popliteus tendon (PT) reconstructions are performed with tibialis posterior tendon (TPT) allograft (Fig. 58-13). A cryopreserved TPT allograft more than 260 mm long is placed in warm saline 30 minutes before surgery for complete thawing. A skin incision is made on the lateral aspect of the knee just anterior to the fibular head and is extended proximally to the lateral femoral epicondyle in an extended position. The interval between the iliotibial tract and the biceps tendon is dissected. The lateral epicondyle of the femur, the fibular head, the posterolateral corner of the tibia, and the lateral head of the gastrocnemius muscle are exposed. Using an ACL guide, the tip is placed on the point 10 mm inferior to the posterior joint line and 5 mm medial to the posterior aspect of the tibiofibular joint, and the anterior portion is placed on Gerdy's tubercle. A guide pin is inserted under fluoroscopic guidance. The tunnel is created with a 7-mm-diameter cannulated reamer. A double-stranded looped wire is inserted into the tibial tunnel in an anterior-to-posterior direction. Then, using the ACL guide, the tip is placed at the point just posteromedial to the LCL of the fibular head, and the other end is placed at the anteroinferior aspect of the fibular head 10 mm above the peroneal nerve. The tunnel is at an angle of 70 degrees to the axial plane in an anteroinferior-to-posterosuperior direction. The direction of rotation of the reamer is counterclockwise, avoiding cortical destruction of the fibular head and peroneal nerve injury. A double-stranded looped wire is passed through the fibular tunnel in a posterior-to-anterior direction. To make the leading portion of the graft, the TPT is sutured from the tip with a whipstitch technique. A No. 2 Ethibond suture is whipstitched at the other end of the tendon for approximately 25 mm, and a 7-mm-diameter EndoPearl device is attached to the end. Using the looped wire in the tibial tunnel, the leading suture of the graft is pulled anteriorly through the tibia; then, using the same method, the graft is passed posteriorly through the fibular tunnel. The graft is fixed in the tibial and fibular tunnels using bioabsorbable interference screws through the anterior aperture, respectively.

The lateral femoral epicondyle is then exposed. The position of the patient is changed to lateral decubitus to eliminate the gravitational force of the lower leg in the supine position, and 0.045-inch Kirschner wires are provisionally inserted at tentative isometric points. A PT insertion site is placed at the superior margin of the anterior one-third portion of the popliteal sulcus, which is located about 15 mm distal to the femoral epicondyle. An LCL insertion site is placed at the anterosuperior lateral femoral epicondyle. Isometricity is confirmed by migration of less than 2 mm during flexion and extension of the knee. A femoral socket, 40 mm in depth, is created with a 7-mm-diameter cannulated reamer in the anterosuperior direction to the transverse line of the femoral shaft at an angle of 20 degrees for the PT socket and LCL socket, respectively. Using a Beath pin, the graft for the PT, which was passed underneath the LCL, is pulled through the femoral socket and then is fixed at the femur using a bioabsorbable interference screw. Distal popliteal graft is sutured to the posterosuperior ligamentous tissue of the fibular head to restore the popliteofibular ligament. The other band of graft from the fibular head is managed and fixed using the same method as for LCL reconstruction.

For medial instability, medial collateral ligament (MCL) and posterior oblique ligament (POL) reconstructions are performed using the autogenous semitendinosus tendon (ST) with preservation of its tibial attachment (Fig. 58-14). A curvilinear skin incision is made from a point 3 cm proximal to the medial femoral epicondyle to the insertion of the pes anserinus. The fascia is incised along the anterior border of the sartorius muscle in line with the muscle fibers, and the sartorius and gracilis are retracted medially. After the ST is exposed, the tendon fibers attached to the medial head of the gastrocnemius are carefully dissected to prevent premature cutting of the tendon. The ST is transected at the musculotendinous junction, and then the proximal end of the tendon is whipstitched with a No. 2 Ethibond suture for a 2-cm length. The accessory tibial insertion of the tendon is dissected for the graft to overlap with the anterior bundle of

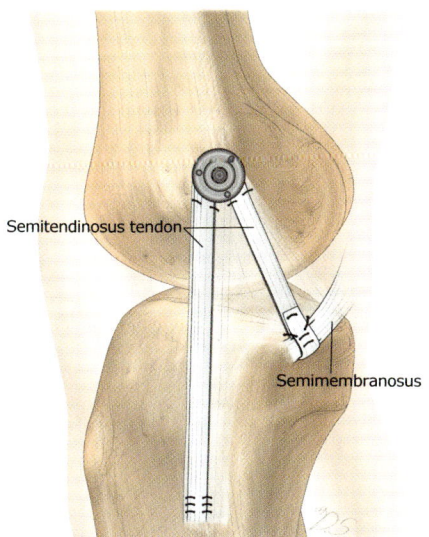

Figure 58-14. For medial instability, medial collateral ligament and posterior oblique ligament reconstructions are performed using the autogenous semitendinosus tendon with preservation of its tibial attachment.

Semitendinosus tendon

Semimembranosus

the MCL. A 0.045-inch Kirschner wire is inserted tentatively at the anterior half of the medial femoral epicondyle. After the ST is looped around the wire, isometricity is tested by pulling the suture at the tendon end during flexion and extension of the knee. After the isometric point is confirmed, a 3.2-mm hole is drilled 9 mm (the radius of a washer) proximally. After decortication under the washer, a 6.5-mm-diameter cancellous screw and an 18-mm washer are placed in the drill hole. The ST is looped around the shank of the screw to allow fixation of the tendon at the isometric point on the epicondyle. The screw is tightened with the knee in 30 degrees flexion. After dissection to find the insertion of the direct head of the semimembranosus (SM), the free end of the graft is pulled through the bisected insertion of the direct head to overlap the central arm of the POL. In 30 degrees of knee flexion, the end of the graft is fixed by No. 2 Ethibond sutures at the insertion of the direct head of the SM. Additional suture fixation using absorbable sutures is done at the femoral and tibial insertion of the MCL, and at the proximal insertion of the POL.

POSTOPERATIVE REHABILITATION

The reconstructed graft is protected by immobilization in extension with a hinge knee brace for 4 weeks with passive range-of-motion exercise allowed three times a day. Isometric quadriceps-strengthening exercise and mobilization of the patella are initiated immediately after surgery. Toe-touch weight bearing is allowed for the first 4 weeks; then patients are allowed to bear their weight and flex their knee as tolerated with progressive increase in flexion to 90 degrees. At 8 weeks, the brace is removed, and closed kinetic chain exercise is started; after 12 weeks, swimming and cycling are permitted. Return to sports involving jumping, pivoting, or side-stepping is permitted after 6 months.

CLINICAL RESULTS

A few authors have presented several techniques and clinical results for preserving remnants of the PCL.[1,14,32] Ahn et al[1] reported clinical results of 61 patients who underwent transtibial PCL reconstruction with preservation of PCL fibers. At an average follow-up of 40.8 months, mean Lysholm knee scores improved from 65.8 to 92.9, and International Knee Documentation Committee (IKDC) objective evaluation was rated as normal or nearly normal in 59 patients (97%). The mean side-to-side difference on the KT-2000 arthrometer was 2.79 mm. Jung et al[14] analyzed clinical outcomes of 49 patients who underwent tensioning of the remnant PCL and reconstruction of the anterolateral bundle of the PCL using a modified inlay technique. They found significant improvement in side-to-side differences in posterior translation on posterior stress radiography, KT-1000 arthrometer (2.2 ± 1.1 mm and 1.9 ± 1.0 mm, respectively), functional scores (the Orthopadische Arbeitsgruppe Knie score, 91 ± 7.3), and final IKDC scores (normal or nearly normal, 87.7%) at a mean follow-up of 45.7 months (range, 24 to 78 months).

AUTHOR'S EXPERIENCE

The clinical outcomes of double-bundle PCL reconstruction (DB) and transtibial single-bundle econstruction with remnant preservation (rSB) were compared. The study population consisted of 42 patients who had undergone PCL reconstruction using either technique (rSB group, 33 patients; DB group, 19 patients) combined with anatomic reconstruction of the LCL and PT for posterolateral corner insufficiency between March 2002 and July 2006. The mean follow-up period was 51.2 months (range, 24 to 70 months) in the rSB group and 44.5 months (range, 27 to 62 months) in the DB group. No significant differences were noted between rSB and DB groups in mean side-to-side differences in posterior laxity as measured with Telos stress radiographs (4.2 vs. 3.9 mm; P = .628) and KT-2000 arthrometer (2.9 vs. 1.4 mm; P = .400) at latest follow-up. Average Lysholm knee scores were 85.7 in the rSB group and 87.7 in the DB group (P = .392). No significant difference was noted between groups in IKDC knee score (P = .969). Conclusions drawn from this study were that DB PCL reconstruction combined with posterolateral corner reconstruction did not seem to offer advantages over rSB PCL reconstruction combined with posterolateral corner reconstruction with respect to clinical outcomes or posterior stability.

Conclusions

During the past two decades, arthroscopic technology has advanced and the anatomy and biomechanics of the cruciate ligaments have been elucidated. This allows surgeons to preserve the remnants of cruciate ligaments during arthroscopic ligament reconstruction. Although remnant-preserving PCL reconstruction is more demanding than the conventional technique, and consensus regarding clinical improvement has not yet been reached, preserving the remnants as much as possible deserves consideration with respect to restoring proprioceptive sensory and mechanical functions. Additional investigations are needed to clearly define the benefits of preserving remnants in PCL reconstruction.

Acknowledgments. The authors thank Dae-Young Lee, MD, for contributions with his view and comments to the manuscript.

KEY REFERENCES

Ahn JH, Nha KW, Kim YC, et al: Arthroscopic femoral tensioning and posterior cruciate ligament reconstruction in chronic posterior cruciate ligament injury. Arthroscopy 22:340–344, 2006.

Amis AA, Bull AM, Gupte CM, et al: Biomechanics of the PCL and related structures: posterolateral, posteromedial and meniscofemoral ligaments. Knee Surg Sports Traumatol Arthrosc 11:271–281, 2003.

Amis AA, Gupte CM, Bull AM, Edwards A: Anatomy of the posterior cruciate ligament and the meniscofemoral ligaments. Knee Surg Sports Traumatol Arthrosc 14:257–263, 2006.

Fontbote CA, Sell TC, Laudner KG, et al: Neuromuscular and biomechanical adaptations of patients with isolated deficiency of the posterior cruciate ligament. Am J Sports Med 33:982–989, 2005.

Georgoulis AD, Pappa L, Moebius U, et al: The presence of proprioceptive mechanoreceptors in the remnants of the ruptured ACL as a possible source of re-innervation of the ACL autograft. Knee Surg Sports Traumatol Arthrosc 9:364–368, 2001.

Grassmayr MJ, Parker DA, Coolican MR, Vanwanseele B: Posterior cruciate ligament deficiency: biomechanical and biological consequences and the outcomes of conservative treatment: a systematic review. J Sci Med Sport 11:433–443, 2008.

Gupte CM, Bull AM, Thomas RD, Amis AA: The meniscofemoral ligaments: secondary restraints to the posterior drawer. Analysis of anteroposterior and rotary laxity in the intact and posterior-cruciate-deficient knee. J Bone Joint Surg Br 85:765–773, 2003.

Jung YB, Jung HJ, Tae SK, et al: Tensioning of remnant posterior cruciate ligament and reconstruction of anterolateral bundle in chronic posterior cruciate ligament injury. Arthroscopy 22:329–338, 2006.

Katonis P, Papoutsidakis A, Aligizakis A, et al: Mechanoreceptors of the posterior cruciate ligament. J Int Med Res 36:387–393, 2008.

Kim SJ, Chang JH, Kang YH, et al: Clinical comparison of anteromedial versus anterolateral tibial tunnel direction for transtibial posterior cruciate ligament reconstruction: 2 to 8 years' follow-up. Am J Sports Med 37:693–698, 2009.

Kim SJ, Shin JW, Lee CH, et al: Biomechanical comparisons of three different tibial tunnel directions in posterior cruciate ligament reconstruction. Arthroscopy 21:286–293, 2005.

Lee BI, Min KD, Choi HS, et al: Immunohistochemical study of mechanoreceptors in the tibial remnant of the ruptured anterior cruciate ligament in human knees. Knee Surg Sports Traumatol Arthrosc 17:1095–1101, 2009.

McAllister DR, Miller MD, Sekiya JK, Wojtys EM: Posterior cruciate ligament biomechanics and options for surgical treatment. Instr Course Lect 58:377–388, 2009.

Moran CJ, Poynton AR, Moran R, Brien MO: Analysis of meniscofemoral ligament tension during knee motion. Arthroscopy 22:362–366, 2006.

Nagasaki S, Ohkoshi Y, Yamamoto K, et al: The incidence and cross-sectional area of the meniscofemoral ligament. Am J Sports Med 34:1345–1350, 2006.

Full references for this chapter can be found on www.expertconsult.com.

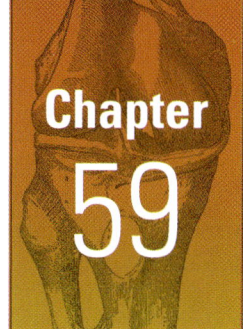
The Dislocated Knee

Brandon J. Bryant, Volker Musahl, and Christopher D. Harner

Traumatic knee dislocation represents one of the most serious and limb-threatening injuries to the lower extremity. Damage to multiple soft tissue and stabilizing structures can result in devastating complications. Dislocation of the knee is defined as complete disruption of the tibiofemoral articulation, whereas knee subluxation is defined as partial disruption of the joint with some tibiofemoral contact remaining. Associated injuries may involve neurovascular structures (i.e., popliteal artery, tibial and peroneal nerves), compartment syndrome, cruciate ligaments, collateral ligaments, medial and lateral capsular structures, medial and lateral menisci, and articular cartilage. The potential for catastrophic complications is high; these injuries therefore require timely and accurate diagnosis, stabilization, and treatment. Patients may present with a dislocated knee or, more commonly, an occult dislocation that has reduced, but the condition should be treated as a knee dislocation until ruled otherwise, even in the absence of a witnessed dislocation event. Knee dislocation results from high-energy mechanisms, such as motorcycle, motor vehicle, and car accidents versus pedestrian and sports-related injuries.[17,48,58]

In the acute setting, treatment goals include prompt reduction and stabilization of the knee joint and, if necessary, revascularization. Initial stabilization should be temporary, and assessment of the patient's neurovascular status should not be delayed. The severity of these injuries is emphasized by the fact that, despite modern vascular reconstructive techniques, 13% of knee dislocations result in amputation secondary to vascular compromise.[10] Historically, patients were largely managed nonoperatively; however, current beliefs and trends in the literature have shown that this often leads to poor results. Improvements in ligament reconstruction and repair techniques have yielded superior results.[42,48,50] Current treatment approaches include acute, staged repair/reconstruction, and chronic reconstruction strategies. Acute repair and reconstruction may yield lower subjective scores and higher rates of residual anterior instability when compared with staged treatment strategies.[32]

Because of the severity of these injuries, patients typically require an extensive preoperative workup to identify the specifics of the injury. Meticulous preoperative planning is required to ensure medical stability for surgery. The surgeon must prioritize with an evaluation and workup that include factors that may predicate early surgical intervention. Initial evaluation that reveals open dislocation, irreducible dislocation, arterial injury, or compartment syndrome requires emergent surgical intervention. In the case of arterial injury, knee-spanning external fixation is required for stabilization of the vascular repair or graft. The locations of future incision sites for ligamentous reconstruction should be discussed with the vascular surgeon. Recovery of associated soft tissue injury dictates the ability to perform later reconstruction or repair of the ligaments.

After limb-threatening injuries have been identified and treated, treatment of knee instability may be pursued. Surgical management remains controversial with respect to timing of surgery, specific surgical techniques used, which structures to repair versus reconstruct, and graft choice. Factors that influence early repair typically involve avulsion injuries, particularly of the lateral knee structures, that is, biceps femoris, lateral collateral ligament, and popliteus. Early range of motion rehabilitation combined with staged reconstruction of the cruciate ligaments can then be performed. Allograft tissue is used most commonly with the goal of reduction of patient morbidity and overall operative time during these complex cases.

INCIDENCE

Knee dislocations are thought to account for less than 0.5% of all joint dislocations.[41] The yearly incidence of knee dislocation at various institutions is reported to range from 1/10,000 to 1/100,000.[27,49] Accurate incidence data are difficult to obtain because approximately half of all knee dislocations reduce spontaneously, and the condition is often misdiagnosed at the time of injury.[31,33] Dislocation should be suspected in a knee with gross instability of two or more ligaments despite a reduced knee on clinical and radiographic examination.[48] Subsequent evaluation and treatment should be performed on the assumption that a dislocation has occurred.

MECHANISM

Knee dislocation occurs as the result of severe high-energy direct or indirect trauma to the knee. Most of these injuries are seen in cases of vehicular trauma, which is often higher in energy and more destructive to the soft tissue envelope of the knee.[11] Knee dislocation can also occur as the result of sports-related and lower-energy trauma. Shelbourne and colleagues reported that the most common at-risk sports are football (35%), wrestling (15%), and running (10%).[47,48]

Distinguishing between high-energy injuries, such as automobile accidents, and low-energy, sports-related injuries may have prognostic value because lower-velocity injuries may be less severe. Shelbourne and associates[48] reported on the incidence of associated vascular injuries (4.6%) in a series of low-velocity injuries. Green and Allen[10] reported an incidence of 32% in a series of high-velocity traumatic knee dislocations.

VASCULAR INJURY

The incidence of vascular injury associated with knee dislocation varies in the literature from 5% to 80%.[14,48] Treatment of an established or suspected arterial injury should take

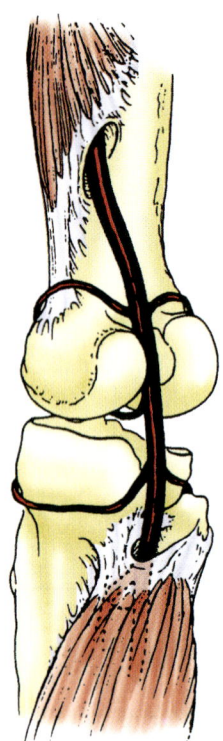

Figure 59-1. Anatomy of the popliteal artery posterior to the knee joint. (From Bloom MH: Traumatic knee dislocation. In Chapman MW [ed]: Operative orthopaedics, Philadelphia, 1988, JB Lippincott, p 1636.)

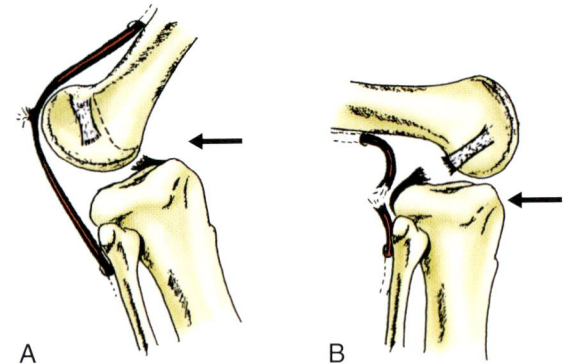

Figure 59-2. Mechanism for popliteal artery injury for anterior (**A**) and posterior (**B**) dislocations.

precedence over musculoskeletal management and should involve a qualified vascular surgeon. Timing is critical, and the presence of ischemic compromise to an extremity following reduction mandates emergent exploration by a vascular surgeon to restore arterial flow.[9,17,31,55] Amputation rates are reported to increase from 13% to 86% when revascularization is delayed more than 8 hours from the time of initial injury.[10]

The popliteal artery provides the main blood supply to the lower leg and is the primary vascular structure at risk during knee dislocation. The popliteal artery is the continuation of the superficial femoral artery as it passes through the fibrous opening in the adductor magnus and enters the popliteal fossa. It lies in the subcutaneous tissue of the popliteal fossa, tethered proximally at the adductor hiatus and distally by a fibrous arch covering the soleus (Fig. 59-1).[31] This motion restriction on the vessel and its proximity to the joint increase its susceptibility to injury during dislocation events. Within the popliteal space, the medial superior, lateral superior, medial inferior, lateral inferior, and middle geniculate arteries branch from the popliteal artery. These vessels do not provide adequate collateral flow to the lower extremity in the case of a severe popliteal artery injury.[10] Although the rate of popliteal artery injury is nearly equal with respect to anterior versus posterior knee dislocations, a higher rate of arterial transection injury has been reported with posterior dislocations.[10] Anterior dislocations more often result in traction injuries to the vessel and associated intimal tears. Kennedy[18] pointed out that anterior dislocations are more likely associated with intimal injuries because the vessel is stretched over the distal femur. In cadaveric experiments, he showed that

popliteal artery injury occurs at 50 degrees of hyperextension (Fig. 59-2A). Posterior dislocations have a higher association with artery transection, as the proximal tibia is thrust posteriorly into the vessel (Fig. 59-2B).

Intimal tears or flap tears are injuries to the endothelial lining of the arterial wall. These injuries are frequently difficult to diagnose by physical examination alone; adjunct imaging is often required for diagnosis. Arteriography has long been regarded as the gold standard for diagnosis of arterial injury. One series showed 100% correlation between magnetic resonance angiography and arteriogram following knee dislocation, although this has yet to be validated at other centers.[38] Vascular insufficiency in this setting may present acutely or in a delayed fashion, as a clot can slowly form on the injured endothelial wall, resulting in vessel occlusion hours or days after injury. Historically, many patients with intimal tears have undergone exploratory vascular surgery because it was believed that the tears would progress to complete arterial occlusion.

Multiple studies have focused on evaluation of vascular injury in knee dislocation. Many surgeons still advocate the routine use of arteriography in all suspected knee dislocations, to avoid the potentially devastating complications of a missed vascular injury.[18] Other authors have published studies questioning the need for routine arteriography in patients with a normal neurovascular examination. Mills and associates[29] published a study assessing the usefulness of the ankle-brachial index (ABI) in diagnosing arterial injury in patients with knee dislocations. Their prospective study comprised 38 patients with knee dislocation, among whom 11 had ABIs of less than 0.90 and 27 had ABIs of greater than 0.90. The authors found that all 11 patients with ABIs of less than 0.90 had vascular injuries requiring surgical treatment, whereas none of the 27 patients with ABIs of greater than 0.90 were found to have vascular injury on clinical examination or on duplex ultrasound. This study supports the current treatment algorithm of vascular assessment with ABI and observation (if >0.9) with frequent neurovascular checks.

Other studies have focused on the clinical neurovascular examination as a predictor of vascular injury. Klineberg and colleagues[20] reported a retrospective series of 57 knee dislocations, of which 32 had normal vascular examination findings compared with the contralateral side (including ABIs), and 25 knees had abnormal examination findings. None of the 32 knees with initially normal vascular examinations were found later to have vascular damage requiring surgical intervention. Therefore, the authors determined that knee dislocation might not require arteriography if the initial neurovascular examination is normal. These findings were corroborated in a study by Stannard and colleagues[51] that looked at the role of physical examination in determining the need for arteriography. Investigators used an algorithm by which all affected limbs were examined carefully for dorsalis pedis and posterior tibial pulses and were examined grossly for skin color and temperature. Patients who had an asymmetrical examination with respect to the contralateral side underwent subsequent arteriography. None of the patients with initially normal vascular examination findings went on to develop vascular complications requiring surgical intervention. Investigators subsequently recommended the selective use of arteriography in the acutely dislocated knee.

The current recommendation in the literature is to perform arteriography in those patients with abnormal clinical findings. Abnormal findings include asymmetrical pulses, skin temperature differences, skin color changes, poor Doppler waveforms, and ABIs of less than 0.90.[22] Missed arterial injury can have catastrophic consequences; as a result of this fact, and because anecdotal cases of late thrombosis have occurred following knee dislocation, we routinely use angiography at our institution.[45]

NEUROLOGIC INJURY

A thorough neurologic examination is mandatory in all patients with acute knee dislocation, as neurologic injury has been reported in 16% to 50% of patients.[27,49,59] Although it is most commonly seen with posterolateral knee dislocation, injury to the peroneal or posterior tibial nerve has been reported with all types of dislocations. The peroneal nerve is at greatest risk for injury because it is anatomically tethered around the fibular head, whereas the tibial nerve is less constrained within the popliteal space (Fig. 59-3). Injury to the peroneal nerve is caused most commonly by traction on the nerve, resulting in varying degrees of neuropraxia or axonotmesis. Treatment options for nerve dysfunction vary depending on the nature and severity of the injury. Patients with peroneal nerve injuries have been reported to regain function in only about 50% of cases.[60,62] Although the role of neurolysis remains controversial, it is occasionally performed when evidence suggests significant intraneural hematoma.

CLASSIFICATION

Two accepted classification systems have been used to describe knee dislocations: descriptive and anatomic. These classifications can aid in predicting associated injuries and in planning for surgical intervention.

Descriptive

Knee dislocations are classified according to the direction of the tibia in relation to the femur.[18] As described by Kennedy, this system was divided into five main types: anterior, posterior, medial, lateral, and rotatory (Fig. 59-4). Associated vascular and neurologic injuries have been described with every known type of dislocation.

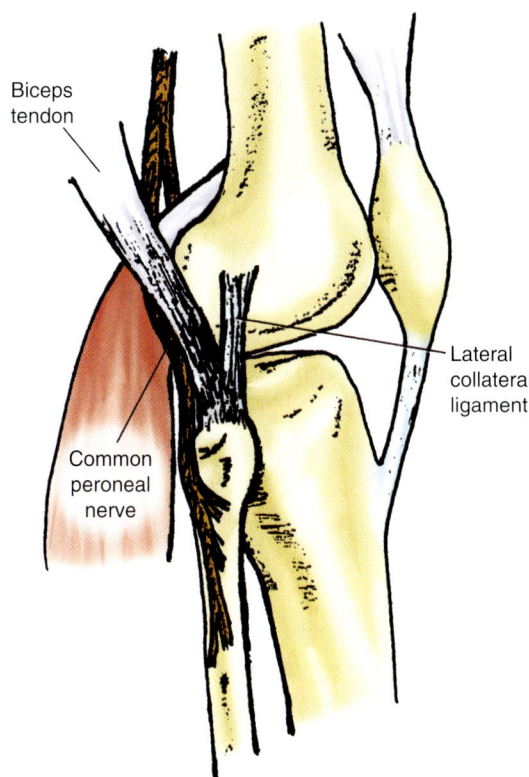

Figure 59-3. Anatomy of peroneal nerve near the knee joint.

This classification system is limited by the fact that spontaneous reductions are known to occur, and unless the patient or a witness can accurately describe the mechanism of injury, the type of dislocation remains unknown. Additionally, this classification system is not helpful in surgical planning for ligament reconstruction because the degree of individual ligament injury can vary dramatically.

Anterior Dislocation

Green and Allen[10] reported that anterior dislocations account for approximately 40% of knee dislocations. The mechanism of this injury pattern is believed to be hyperextension. Because the anterior cruciate ligament (ACL) is the primary restraint to anterior tibial translation, it is always disrupted. Biomechanical studies have shown that, with hyperextension, the posterior capsule ruptures first, followed by the ACL, and then the posterior cruciate ligament (PCL).[35] At approximately 50 degrees of hyperextension, the popliteal artery sustains injury.[18] Arterial injury in this setting typically occurs as a traction injury causing an intimal tear, which can lead to acute or delayed thrombosis.

The force required to produce an anterior dislocation may be of high or low energy. Anterior dislocations have been described to occur from a variety of different situations, ranging from vehicular trauma to stumbling after missing a step.

Posterior Dislocation

Posterior dislocation accounts for slightly fewer dislocations (33%).[18] In contrast to anterior dislocation, posterior dislocation requires a significant force. In his biomechanical study, Kennedy[18] had difficulty producing a posterior dislocation.

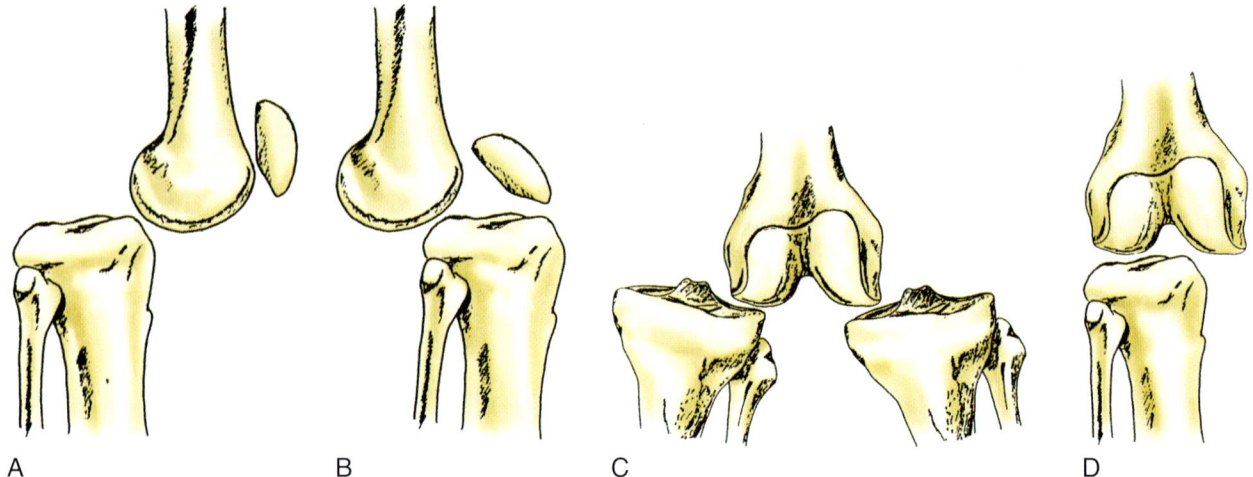

A   B   C   D

Figure 59-4. Descriptive classification system of knee joint dislocations. **A,** Posterior. **B,** Anterior. **C,** Medial or lateral. **D,** Rotatory.

These dislocations most commonly are associated with automobile accidents as "dashboard" injuries. In this setting, a seated passenger's proximal tibia is driven into the dashboard, creating a posteriorly directed force on the flexed knee.

The PCL provides the primary restraint to posterior tibial translation and by definition is disrupted in these injuries. The ACL is frequently torn, although reports have described posterior dislocation without ACL disruption.[49] Injury to the medial collateral ligament (MCL) and the lateral collateral ligament (LCL) varies. Injury to the popliteal artery in this setting traditionally has been described as a transection injury, in that the posteriorly translated tibia tears the popliteal artery. Intimal tears may be present in cases where the popliteal artery remains intact.

Medial and Lateral Dislocations

Medial and lateral dislocations are considerably less common, accounting for 18% and 4% of all dislocations, respectively.[10] It is difficult to produce pure ligamentous medial and lateral dislocation injuries experimentally. Most case reports describe high-energy varus or valgus trauma. Pure ligamentous injuries are perhaps the exception rather than the rule, as many individuals with these injuries have associated fractures on the tibial plateau or distal femur.

In contrast to anterior and posterior dislocations, with medial and lateral dislocations, both collateral ligaments are injured, along with at least one of the cruciate ligaments. Lateral dislocations can be additionally problematic because they may be irreducible as a result of entrapment of the MCL within the medial joint.

Rotatory Dislocation

Rotatory dislocation accounts for about 5% of knee dislocations and is produced by a rotational force.[10] Rotation occurs about one of the collateral ligaments, along with rupture of both cruciate ligaments and of the other collateral ligament. The most common type of rotatory dislocation is posterolateral.[13] This type of dislocation can be irreducible as the result of "buttonholing" of the medial femoral condyle through the medial capsule and invagination of the MCL. These structures become entrapped within the femoral notch, making attempts at reduction extraordinarily difficult. Physical

examination is often remarkable for subcutaneous palpation of the medial femoral condyle and a furrow or skin dimple along the medial joint line. Attempted reduction may accentuate these physical findings. Expeditious open reduction is indicated in this setting because prolonged vascular compromise to the overlying skin may result in significant skin loss.

Anatomic

An anatomic classification scheme has been developed that focuses on the ligamentous structures injured.[44] This system facilitates preoperative planning with respect to identifying those specific structures that require surgical attention. Significant differences in the healing potential have been noted between MCL and LCL.[48] The MCL heals much more readily than the LCL, and residual instability is much less of a problem with the MCL.[48] Tibial-sided MCL avulsions have a lower healing potential than avulsions from the femoral side of the ligament. Stiffness in flexion can be a problem with operative repair of the MCL. Knowing and understanding these differences and appreciating the full extent of these injuries can help with selection of the surgical approach and timing.

This classification system is limited by the difficulty involved in performing an accurate examination in the face of a severely traumatized knee. It is not unusual, despite physical examination and magnetic resonance imaging (MRI), for the clinician to not appreciate the true extent of the injury until an examination is performed with the patient under anesthesia. Nevertheless, some recognized patterns of injury have been established. Typically, the ACL and the PCL are disrupted, although this is not universally true (case reports of knee dislocations without an ACL or PCL tear have been published[3,4]). Commonly recognized patterns of injury include ACL/PCL/MCL, ACL/PCL/LCL, ACL/PCL/posterolateral corner (PLC), ACL/PCL/LCL/PLC, and ACL/PCL/LCL/PLC/MCL.[15]

This classic anatomic system has been further modified to focus additionally on injured vascular and neural structures.[7] Injuries are classified according to the number of major ligaments injured, from I to IV, with V denoting a fracture dislocation. These numbers are prefaced by KD, denoting knee dislocation. Additional designations of C and N are used to denote associated vascular and neurologic injury. A single cruciate tear would be denoted as KDI, and bicruciate tears as KDII. A dislocation resulting in disruption of the ACL, PCL, and MCL would be described as KDIIIM, with M denoting the third injured ligament as the MCL. A bicruciate and lateral collateral or posterolateral corner injury (LCL, PLC), would be described as KDIIIL. A dislocation involving all four major ligament complexes is denoted as KDIV, and KDV describes a fracture dislocation. Addition of C or N would describe associated vascular or neurologic injury. In general, higher KD numbers denote greater degrees of injury to the knee.

EVALUATION

Acute knee dislocation requires an expeditious but thorough evaluation consisting of a targeted history and physical examination, with particular attention paid to the mechanism of injury and potential associated injuries. Evaluation of patients with multiple ligamentous injuries to the knee requires a high index of suspicion to exclude the possibility of knee dislocation followed by spontaneous reduction. Two distinct categories of knee dislocation patients have been identified: those seen acutely in the emergency or trauma room, and those seen as an outpatient in the office setting. Figure 59-5 shows our algorithm for the evaluation and management of these injuries. Our institution is a level 1 trauma center, which uses an integrated multidisciplinary team approach to trauma

care. An orthopedic surgeon and a general trauma surgeon are present in the trauma room at the time of patient arrival and evaluation. This allows accurate and efficient exchange of information between treating staff and emergency medical service technicians. As the general trauma surgeon assesses the patient using an Advanced Trauma Life Support (ATLS) protocol, the orthopedic surgeon evaluates the extremities. With respect to knee dislocation injury, the orthopedist focuses on inspection of the limb, skin integrity, color, vascular assessment, and visual and tactile joint examination. If the knee is found to be acutely dislocated, a detailed neurovascular examination must be performed and documented following reduction of the joint. The extremity distal to the involved knee should be examined thoroughly for color, temperature, and capillary refill. Posterior tibial and dorsalis pedis pulses are palpated and are compared with the contralateral side. ABIs are performed to establish a baseline and for diagnostic purposes. Vascular surgery consultation is obtained immediately in the event that pulses in the affected distal extremity are absent or decreased compared with the uninvolved limb, and/or the postreduction ABI is <0.9. With regard to the peroneal nerve, sensation in the distribution of both superficial and deep peroneal nerves should be assessed and peroneal nerve motor function graded and documented.

After a detailed history and physical examination, radiographs should be obtained to determine the direction of dislocation and to assess for concomitant bony injury. Following reduction maneuvers, radiographs should be obtained again

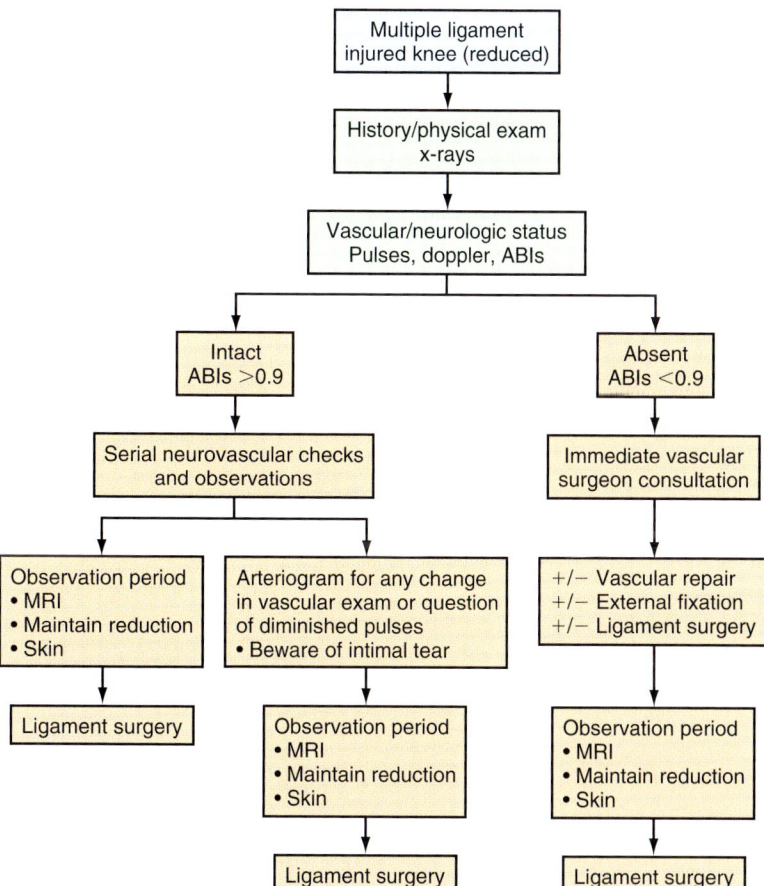

Figure 59-5. Treatment algorithm for the multiple ligament–injured knee. *ABI,* Ankle-brachial index.

to verify the reduction and to rule out any additional osseous trauma. If the knee is grossly unstable following reduction, splinting or external fixation may be required to maintain an adequate reduction.

If it has been determined that the patient requires arteriography, this should be done on an emergent basis, as the risk for amputation increases when limb ischemia exceeds 8 hours. Depending on the setting, significant delays may occur in obtaining arteriograms in the angioplasty suite versus the operating room. Performing arteriography in the operating room may preserve valuable ischemia time. Any present vascular injuries take precedence over musculoskeletal injury, and the role of the orthopedic surgeon may be limited to reducing the joint and providing temporary stabilization for the limb and the vascular repair.

When the patient is medically stable and a complete neurovascular examination has been performed, more attention can be focused on ligamentous damage to the knee. In the acute setting, it is often difficult to perform a thorough clinical ligamentous examination secondary to significant pain and edema. However, a knee that has limited motion (from 0 to 30 degrees) can be assessed for varus/valgus instability, Lachman test findings, and integrity of the extensor mechanism. The standard tests for ligamentous laxity are performed. The gold standard for testing of the ACL is the Lachman test, which is performed with the knee in 30 degrees of flexion.[6] The PCL is tested with the posterior drawer and sag tests.[25,28] Collateral ligaments are assessed with varus/valgus stress to the knee joint both in full extension and at 30 degrees of flexion.[6] PLC injuries should be evaluated by the external rotation dial test at 30 and 90 degrees.[25,28]

Radiographs should be obtained to confirm adequate reduction and to assess the presence of any associated bony injuries. MRI is obtained to evaluate these injuries after the patient has been appropriately medically stabilized. MRI allows full ligamentous, meniscal, and osteochondral evaluation and aids in preoperative planning. The actual site of cruciate and collateral ligament injury (i.e., avulsion vs. midsubstance rupture) can be defined; this may be of tremendous help in the planning of reconstruction or primary repair of structures. MRI is additionally helpful in assessing PLC injury and popliteus tendon status. This study is always obtained at our institution before operative reconstruction is begun, and we have found it to be extremely useful in planning our operative approach.

TREATMENT

The following sections analyze the early results of nonoperative management, along with the more contemporary results of different surgical techniques for stabilizing acute knee dislocations. Additionally, we address the indications for acute operative management and the approach to neurovascular injuries that frequently accompany these injuries. Finally, we describe in detail our approach to evaluating and treating knee dislocations.

Urgent Surgical Intervention

Some situations require immediate surgical intervention. As mentioned previously, any evidence of vascular injury requires immediate consultation and treatment by a qualified vascular surgeon. Patients with prolonged vascular compromise should undergo fasciotomies at the time of revascularization, as they are at significant risk for the development of compartment syndrome. Open dislocations require immediate surgical intervention, with irrigation and débridement (often multiple), intravenous antibiotics, and soft tissue coverage procedures as needed.[42] Ligament repair or reconstruction should be delayed until the soft tissue envelope has healed, especially in the face of complex soft tissue reconstruction.

Irreducible dislocations provide a unique case in which urgent surgical intervention is needed. The most common pattern of an irreducible dislocation is posterolateral, with buttonholing of the medial femoral condyle through the medial joint capsule with subsequent invagination of the capsule into the joint.[56] Multiple other causes of irreducible knee dislocation have been described; several case reports include interposition of the vastus medialis,[21] muscular buttonholing,[19] and interposed menisci.[2]

Nonoperative Management

Immediate reduction and casting was once the preferred treatment. Much of the support provided for this approach was based on the experience of Taylor and colleagues,[53] who in 1972 described 26 cases without neurovascular injury. After immediate reduction, patients were immobilized in slight flexion for approximately 6 weeks, then were given aggressive physical therapy. Eighteen of 26 patients were judged as having good results with this approach, defined as flexion of 90 degrees or more, combined with a stable, painless knee. Only two patients had a poor result by these criteria, mainly as a result of stiffness. At that time, based on this study, nonoperative treatment was thought to be the method of choice for uncomplicated knee dislocations. Subsequently, many studies have criticized the clinical outcome measurements chosen to evaluate these patients, questioning the appropriateness of the treatment method. In a meta-analysis of 132 retrospectively evaluated knee dislocations, improved motion and Lysholm scores were seen in operatively treated patients.[5] Additional studies have supported these findings, showing improvement in Lysholm scores, higher International Knee Documentation Committee (IKDC) scores, and greater return to previous activity levels with surgical treatment.[12,24,40]

Operative Management

Historically, multiple types of operative stabilization procedures have been proposed for treatment of knee dislocation, with generally good results.[1,8,27,50] It has been difficult, however, to establish a consensus regarding these injuries: reports generally contain few patients with different degrees of knee injury approached in different ways. Early reports emphasized primary ligamentous repair of collateral and cruciate ligament injuries. As described by Marshall and colleagues,[26] this recommendation was later modified for cruciate injuries in which ligament repair was performed with multiple looped sutures brought out through drill holes in the tibia and femur.[31,50] Meyers and associates[27] recognized the shortcomings of these previous studies and, in 1975, published a follow-up article to their original report on 33 patients treated with immobilization (13 patients) or early ligamentous primary repair (20 patients). Outcomes were based on patients' pain, stability, and ability to perform previous occupational tasks. Types of injuries in the two groups were thought to be equivalent and without complications. Patients who underwent early operative primary repair of all ligamentous injuries had the best results, as measured by the authors' criteria. Subsequently, other studies have supported this approach. Sisto and Warren[50] reported on 20 knee dislocations; similarly, patients treated with early primary repair had results superior to those seen following immobilization. The authors stressed generally modest clinical results in both groups, however, and clinical instability generally was not a problem. Almekinders and Logan[1] also described modest results with these injuries, regardless of the treatment method used. Although the operatively treated group seemed to exhibit superior motion and increased objective stability in the anteroposterior plane compared with nonoperatively treated patients, resultant pain, swelling, and degenerative changes by radiographic criteria were similar for the two groups.

As techniques in single-ligament surgery have advanced for isolated anterior and posterior cruciate intrasubstance ruptures, reconstruction (as opposed to primary ligamentous repair) has produced the best functional results.[37] Shapiro and Freedman[46] reported on seven patients treated with early allograft stabilization of both cruciates in combination with primary repair of medial and lateral collateral structures. Results at 4 years were graded as good to excellent in six patients; arthrofibrosis was the most common postoperative complication encountered, in four patients, all of whom required manipulation under anesthesia. Similarly, Noyes and Barber-Westin[34] reported on 11 patients with combined allograft and autograft reconstruction for bicruciate knee dislocations. At 5 years' follow-up, 8 of 11 patients (73%) were asymptomatic with daily activities, and 6 of 11 (55%) had returned to sporting activities. Reconstructive approaches to cruciate injury in knee dislocations involving only one of the two cruciate ligaments in combination with medial or lateral injuries have been reported with good results.[3,4]

More recent studies show improved outcomes for multiple ligament–injured knees with operative intervention. A retrospective study by Richter and associates[40] looked at 89 traumatic knee dislocations, 63 of which were treated surgically and 26 of which were treated nonoperatively. At greater than 8 years' average follow-up, Lysholm and Tegner scores were found to be better in the surgically treated group. Functional rehabilitation following surgical treatment was the most prognostic factor. Another study by Rios and colleagues[43] looked at results obtained after 26 traumatic dislocations. Eight of the patients (31%) were determined to have a poor result based on the Lysholm scoring system. Five of the eight with poor scores were treated nonoperatively secondary to concomitant visceral or skeletal injuries, making their surgery inadvisable. The other three poor results occurred in patients who had undergone primary repair of avulsed LCL and posterolateral structures, without addressing the cruciate ligaments. The authors advocated acute reconstruction of all injured structures to try to obtain the best postoperative result. Wong and colleagues[61] also showed superior results following knee dislocations treated surgically. The surgically treated group in their study did not show decreased range of motion when compared with the

nonoperatively treated group. The authors in this study recommended surgical treatment with repair of all ligamentous structures to achieve the most stable knee and the greatest degree of patient satisfaction. These studies validate the current trend suggesting that acute ligament repair or reconstruction is indicated in all but the most severely debilitated patients to achieve the most stable functional result.

Other reports in the literature describe a slightly different operative approach to these injuries. Several authors recommend reconstruction of the PCL with autograft or allograft tissue, in combination with primary medial or lateral ligament repair. These reports are based on Hughston's[16] experience of addressing the PCL first when both cruciates are injured. In doing so, one reestablishes the center of rotation on which all subsequent repairs can be based. This approach delays reconstruction of the ACL until a later time, if persistent instability remains a problem. If bicruciate knee dislocations are approached in this manner, the risk of postoperative arthrofibrosis may be lessened. Advocates of this theory believe that stability is much less of a problem than knee stiffness and pain.[50] Shelbourne and colleagues[48] reported on 16 low-velocity knee dislocations treated with reconstruction of both cruciate ligaments or only the PCL, in combination with anatomic medial or lateral repairs and aggressive postoperative physical therapy. Patients in this series who underwent PCL reconstruction in combination with collateral ligament repair had less postoperative stiffness compared with those undergoing simultaneous bicruciate reconstructions. Walker and colleagues[57] reported on nine patients treated in a similar manner combined with aggressive physical therapy. The average range of motion for these patients was 0 to 130 degrees at 3 years, with three patients (all with injury to the lateral structures in combination with ACL/PCL rupture) requiring manipulation at 4 weeks for flexion less than 90 degrees.

Vascular Injury

In most cases, injury to the popliteal artery requires surgical treatment. The most common method involves resection of the damaged portion of the vessel, with reverse saphenous vein interposition grafting. Four-compartment fasciotomies should be performed at the same time because the edema that ensues following revascularization can often be associated with development of compartment syndrome.[8] Injury to the popliteal vein, if noted, should be addressed. Repair of ligamentous structures at the same time as revascularization is ill advised, as the prolonged surgical time required and manipulation of the knee could potentially jeopardize the arterial repair. Reduction and stabilization of the knee joint is required, however. Often an external fixator can be placed before or after the revascularization to ensure skeletal stability, while protecting the vascular repair. Definitive ligamentous repair often can be performed within the next 10 to 14 days without significant risk to vascular structures, but this remains controversial.[31]

Neurologic Injury

Treatment of neurologic injury remains controversial, with comparably poor results regardless of the treatment strategies used. Immediate and delayed treatment of nerve injuries varies, depending on the physician and the setting. In general, nerve recovery is unpredictable, with more than half of these injuries having residual (partial to complete) nerve damage.[23,50,52] In the acute setting, repair typically is not possible because of the diffuse nature of the injury, and because of the absence of a specific lesion that would benefit from repair. Most authors approach these injuries nonoperatively for the first 3 months after injury.[60] Patients with clinical footdrop should be treated with an ankle-foot orthosis (AFO) and physical therapy (for range of motion) to prevent equinus contracture. If spontaneous resolution does not occur, reconstructive procedures, including nerve grafting, tendon transfer, and permanent bracing, are considered at that time. Results of operative decompression of the peroneal nerve reported after an initial period of observation showed improvement in 97% of patients studied.[30] Although this study suggests better results with early exploration and decompression, the findings may be misleading. Only a small subset of the patients included in this study had traumatically induced peroneal nerve injuries, and direct comparisons with previous reports should not be made.

Our approach to these injuries in the acute setting involves exploration and decompression of the peroneal nerve at the time of the initial operative procedure. Postoperatively, the foot is braced in an AFO, and recovery is closely monitored over the ensuing 3 months. If residual deficits are present at this time, tendon transfers are discussed with the patient. In our experience, nerve grafting has been less successful and has not been performed for these injuries.

Current Surgical Controversies

Although most authors agree that ligamentous instability should be addressed with surgical treatment, debate continues with respect to surgical timing, need to stage the repair/reconstruction, which ligaments to repair/reconstruct, and what types of grafts to use. It has been advocated that a staged ligamentous repair/reconstruction should be performed, including early PCL reconstruction followed by ACL reconstruction and long-term management of lateral injuries.[36] Staged repair has been associated with decreased risk of postoperative arthrofibrosis. Good results were reported at follow-up, with full range of motion and stable varus/valgus rotation. Other studies have shown that concomitant reconstruction of the ACL and the PCL, along with repair or reconstruction of the collaterals or the PLC, can be done in the acute setting (<3 weeks) without increasing the risk of late arthrofibrosis.[12,24,61] Tissue quality, injury severity, and stability dictate the ability to repair MCL, LCL, or PLC injury. If the repair is deemed inadequate, it is augmented or reconstructed. Our current preference is to acutely repair bony avulsion injuries of the lateral knee and reconstruct ruptures and midsubstance injury patterns. This single-stage procedure eliminates the morbidity of a second surgical procedure. Several studies have shown good results with acute ligament repair or reconstruction. Liow and colleagues[24] reported on a series of 22 knee dislocations. Eight patients were treated with acute ligament repair/reconstruction (<2 weeks), and 14 required reconstruction more than 6 months post injury. Investigators showed that at an average follow-up of 32 months, the mean Lysholm score was 87 in the acute group versus 75 in the delayed group. Likewise, the Tegner

activity rating was 5 in the acute group versus 4.4 in the delayed group. In addition to improved results in the acute group, the authors noted no increase in the risk of arthrofibrosis.

These results were corroborated in a study by Harner and colleagues.[12] Following knee dislocation, 31 patients were followed postoperatively for a minimum of 24 months. Of these patients, 19 underwent acute repair/reconstruction (within 3 weeks), and 12 patients underwent delayed reconstruction. Mean Lysholm scores, Knee Outcome Survey Activities of Daily Living scores, and Knee Outcome Survey Sports Activity scores all were significantly higher in the acutely treated group than in the delayed group. Overall, according to the Meyers ratings, 23 patients had an overall excellent or good score, whereas 8 had a fair or poor score. Sixteen of 19 patients (84%) with acutely treated knees and 7 of 12 (58%) with delayed reconstruction achieved an excellent or good Meyers score. All poor results were found in the delayed reconstruction group. Additionally, no difference in postoperative range of motion was noted between acute and delayed reconstruction groups. Laxity tests showed improved stability in all patients, with more predictable results seen in the acute surgical group. Overall, patients treated acutely within 3 weeks of injury showed better patient-reported subjective outcomes and objective knee laxity than patients who underwent delayed reconstruction.

AUTHORS' APPROACH

The primary goals in treating knee dislocation include anatomic reduction and restoration of knee motion and stability. It is important to counsel the patient preoperatively regarding the severity of the injury and expected outcomes. Associated injuries, patient age, and preoperative level of function influence the final result. From a technical perspective, variables such as surgical timing, operative technique, graft selection, and postoperative rehabilitation are crucial components of the overall treatment plan. A generalized treatment algorithm is presented in Figure 59-6.

Timing

Optimal timing for repair of multiligamentous injuries to the knee, including the collateral ligaments, is within 10 to 14 days from the time of injury. Within this time, the soft tissue envelope surrounding the knee has typically had sufficient time to recover and heal, and the knee's range of motion has been partially restored. Anatomic definition and repair of collateral ligament structures is often possible at this time. Following reduction and confirmation of vascular integrity, the patient is placed into a long-leg hinged knee brace and is instructed to begin range-of-motion exercises in the brace in conjunction with quadriceps strengthening exercises until definitive surgical treatment is performed. Although manipulation under anesthesia may be necessary in 50% of these injuries, rarely has further reoperation for stiffness been necessary.[23]

In the presence of collateral ligament injury requiring surgical intervention, operative treatment is delayed up to 3 weeks in the face of vascular or other associated injuries, without compromising the surgeon's ability to perform a primary repair. Beyond 3 weeks, the surgical approach

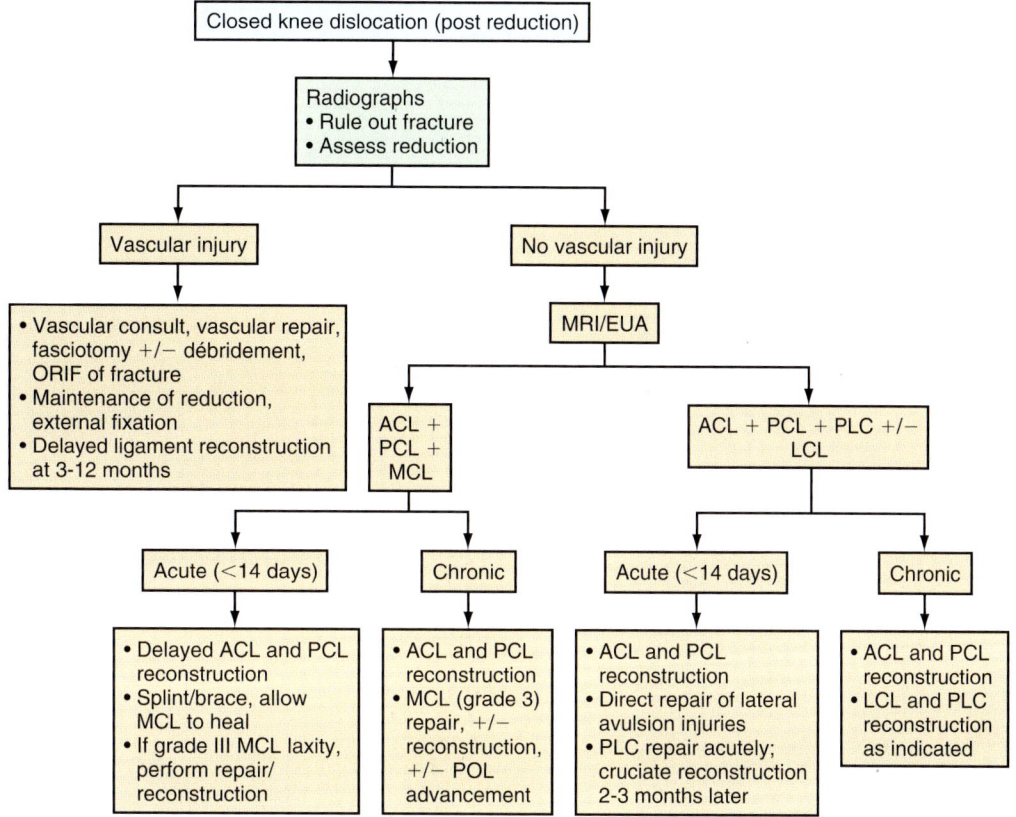

Figure 59-6. Evaluation and management of the dislocated knee. *ACL,* Anterior cruciate ligament; *EUA,* examination under anesthesia; *LCL,* lateral collateral ligament; *MCL,* medial collateral ligament; *ORIF,* open reduction internal fixation; *PLC,* posterolateral corner; *POL,* posterior oblique ligament.

becomes more difficult as the result of scar formation, making anatomic reattachment of collateral structures difficult and nonanatomic.[52] Reconstruction of the cruciate ligaments is less affected by surgical delay. In situations where the severity of the injury prohibits acute operative treatment of ligamentous injury, it is best to take a conservative approach, allowing full restoration of motion in a long-leg hinged brace before further decisions regarding surgical management are made.

In the presence of vascular injury, orthopedic management is secondary until vascular perfusion has been reestablished. The definitive repair and reconstruction of ligamentous structures is a major undertaking requiring manipulation and dissection of the extremity that potentially could threaten the vascular repair if done simultaneously. Provided that normal perfusion has been reestablished, it is typically considered safe to perform the definitive ligamentous repair and reconstruction at 10 to 14 days after revascularization.[31] A tourniquet is not routinely used in this setting because of concern over iatrogenic thrombosis. For this reason, and because of the potential duration of these cases, we no longer use a tourniquet for any of these reconstructions, although a sterile tourniquet should be available if needed.

Anesthesia, Positioning, Surface Anatomy, and Examination Under Anesthesia

The choice of anesthesia is made collaboratively by the patient, the surgeon, and the anesthesiologist. This choice often depends on patient age, other medical comorbidities, and the patient's previous anesthesia history if any. General anesthesia is our preference. At our institution, preoperative femoral or sciatic nerve block or both are routinely used as an adjunct for additional postoperative pain relief.[54] We recommend that a vascular surgeon be "on call" during the procedure because unexpected vessel injury may occur.

The site for the surgery is confirmed and marked while the patient is in the preop holding area. A thorough neurovascular examination is again performed and documented, with particular attention paid to the popliteal, dorsalis pedis, and posterior tibial pulses and the function of the tibial and peroneal nerves. Doppler ultrasound is used occasionally and vessel location marked for later ease of assessment.

The patient is brought into the operating suite and is placed in the supine position on the operating table. Our goal with positioning is to have a full free range of motion of the knee during the procedure, with the ability to have the knee statically flexed at 80 to 90 degrees without manual assistance. This is accomplished by placing a small gel pad bump under the ipsilateral hip and positioning a post on the side of the bed just distal to the greater trochanter. A 10-lb sandbag is taped to the bed during initial positioning to hold the foot stable when the knee is flexed. Additionally, a sterile bump of towels or drapes is used as a wedge between the thigh and the lateral post at various points in the procedure (Fig. 59-7).

A skin marker is used to identify surface anatomy and the incisions that will be used. Important osseous landmarks include the patella, the tibial tubercle, Gerdy's tubercle, and

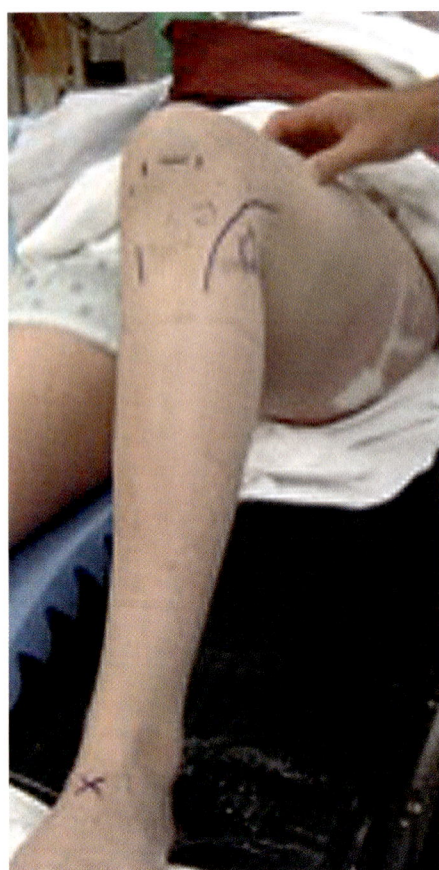

Figure 59-7. Supine operative positioning that includes a tourniquet, arthroscopic assistance, mini C-arm fluoroscopy, and intraoperative Doppler ultrasound capability, when indicated.

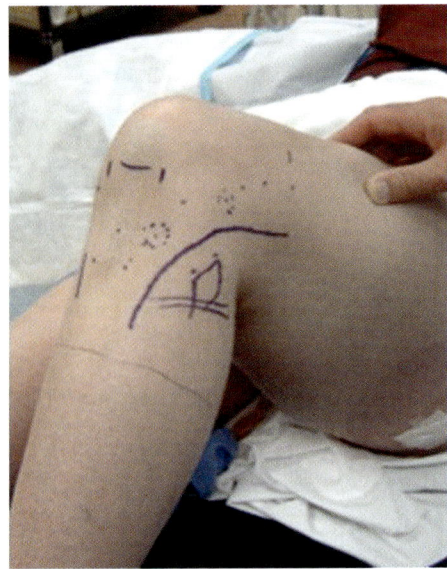

Figure 59-8. Skin incision for combined surgical exposure of a lateral-sided injury, anterior cruciate ligament, and posterior cruciate ligament.

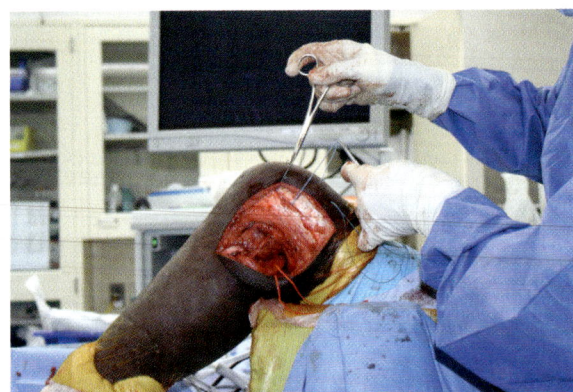

Figure 59-9. Lateral dissection, showing borders of iliotibial band and identification of peroneal nerve, protected with a red vessel loop.

the fibular head. The peroneal nerve is palpated, and its course is marked superficial to the fibular neck. The medial and lateral joint lines are identified and the course of the MCL and LCL are marked. The anterolateral arthroscopy portal is positioned adjacent to the lateral border of the patella, above the joint line, and is adjusted for patella baja if indicated. The anteromedial arthroscopy portal is positioned approximately 1 cm medial to the patellar tendon at the same level. A superolateral outflow portal is established proximal to the superior border of the patella and posterior to the quadriceps tendon. A posteromedial portal, if needed, is made under direct visualization using an outside-in technique and is not marked initially. A longitudinal 3-cm incision approximately 2 cm distal to the joint line and 2 cm medial to the tibial tubercle is drawn on the anteromedial proximal tibia for the ACL and PCL tibial tunnels. Additionally, a 2-cm incision is placed medial to the medial trochlear articular surface along the subvastus interval for the PCL femoral tunnel. If an MCL injury is present, the distal incision for the tibial tunnels is traced proximally to the medial epicondyle and is extended to the level of the vastus medialis in a curvilinear fashion. The incision for the lateral and posterolateral injuries is a curvilinear 12-cm incision that is drawn midway between Gerdy's tubercle and the fibular head and is traced proximally just inferior to the lateral epicondyle, while the knee is flexed to 90 degrees (Fig. 59-8). The proximal extent of this incision parallels the plane between the biceps femoris tendon and the iliotibial band (Fig. 59-9).

When both collateral ligaments are disrupted, we prefer the above medial and lateral incisions versus a midline incision because of potential complications of skin breakdown over the patella and limited access to the collateral ligaments.

Following successful anesthesia induction, a thorough examination is performed with the patient under anesthesia, and findings are correlated with the preoperative impression. It is crucial to examine the opposite extremity and use it as a reference. The knee range of motion is documented. The anterior drawer, Lachman test, and the pivot-shift test are used to assess the integrity of the ACL. PCL integrity is assessed by the posterior drawer and posterior sag tests, with associated step-off at 90 degrees of flexion. The MCL is examined with a valgus stress test at both 0 and 30 degrees of knee flexion. The LCL is palpated in the figure-of-four position and is tested with varus stress at both 0 and 30 degrees of knee flexion. The PLC, which consists of the LCL, the popliteus, and the popliteal-fibular ligament, is tested at 30 degrees and with external rotation of the tibia. In addition, applying an external rotation force on the proximal tibia tests the PLC and fibula while the knee is flexed 90 degrees to feel for lateral dropout. A mini C-arm fluoroscope is in the operating suite and is draped on the opposite side of the table, while a sterile Doppler is used on the surgical field before the initial incision and throughout the case to confirm the presence of the dorsalis pedis and posterior tibial pulses.

Surgical Approach

The two most common combined injury patterns with knee dislocation include the ACL/PCL/MCL and the ACL/PCL/PLC ± LCL. Less commonly, the PCL is intact or is only partially torn and does not require reconstruction. At our institution, we attempt to augment the PCL if possible. Most commonly, the anterolateral (AL) bundle is ruptured, and the meniscofemoral ligament (MFL) and the posteromedial (PM) bundle are intact. If this injury pattern is identified as present, we preserve the intact portion of the PCL and the meniscofemoral ligament and reconstruct the torn AL bundle via a single-bundle technique.

Our approach includes repair/reconstruction of all injured structures. The ACL and the PCL most commonly are intrasubstance tears that are treated with ligament reconstruction. We perform primary repair of ACL and PCL tibial avulsions, if indicated. Primary repair can be accomplished by passing large nonabsorbable sutures into the bony fragment and through bone tunnels in the tibia. Primary repair of the PCL insertion by a similar technique may be advocated in the case of a "peel-off" or a soft tissue avulsion of the PCL at its femoral insertion.

Regarding the MCL, LCL, and PLC, it is our experience that a primary repair is possible if performed within 3 weeks of injury. Chronic injuries are limited by scar formation and soft tissue contractures and often require a ligament reconstruction. The MCL can be repaired directly with intrasubstance sutures or with suture anchors if avulsed off the bone. Repair of the PLC structures and the LCL can be accomplished by direct suture repair, or by repair to bone via drill holes versus suture anchors. If direct repair is limited by poor tissue quality, the involved structures are augmented with allograft (preferred), hamstring tendons, biceps femoris, or iliotibial band. Delayed treatment involves reconstruction. In addition, concomitant injuries to the articular cartilage and the menisci are operatively addressed at the time of surgery. Arthroscopic assistance is useful but must be used with caution. Extravasation of arthroscopy fluid can lead to compartment syndrome in rare cases, secondary to capsular injury.

Graft Selection

Many different options are available for graft selection in the multiple ligament–injured knee. Graft choice is made according to the extent of injury, the timing of surgery, and the experience of the surgeon. At our institution, we recommend the use of allograft over autograft in multiple ligament–reconstruction surgery. Advantages of using allograft tissue include decreased operative time, smaller skin incisions in a knee that has been severely traumatized, and absence of donor site morbidity. We also believe that the use of allograft decreases postoperative pain and stiffness. One must be willing to assume the risks of using allograft tissue, however, which include increased cost, delayed incorporation of the graft, and minimal risk of disease transmission.[11] Autograft

tissue may be harvested from the ipsilateral or contralateral extremity and provides the advantage of improved graft incorporation and remodeling when compared with allograft tissue.

We prefer the use of bone–patellar tendon–bone allograft for reconstruction of the ACL. The bone–patellar tendon–bone allograft provides adequate biomechanical strength combined with rigid bony fixation at both the femoral and tibial attachment sites.

We use Achilles tendon allograft for reconstruction of the PCL. If a double-bundle technique is indicated (rarely in knee dislocation), an ipsilateral hamstring tendon (semitendinosus) autograft is also harvested. The allograft Achilles tendon is an attractive choice for PCL reconstruction because of its long length, significant cross-sectional area, and calcaneal bone plug, which provides rigid bony fixation in the femoral tunnel.

The LCL is reconstructed with an Achilles tendon allograft with a calcaneal bone plug. The bone plug can be fixed into the LCL insertion at the fibula through a bone tunnel. We do not tubularize the tendon because it is often reinforced to the native LCL tissue. Alternatively, the remaining bone–patellar tendon–bone allograft may be used for LCL reconstruction.

For the PCL, our graft choice for reconstructing the popliteofibular ligament (PFL) is a tibialis anterior tendon allograft or an ipsilateral hamstring (semitendinosus) autograft. These are prepared using a whipstitch on both ends with heavy nonabsorbable suture.

Intra-articular Preparation

The arthroscope is introduced through the anterolateral portal, and gravity inflow is used in combination with superolateral outflow. Care must be taken to avoid a compartment syndrome, and the posterior leg and calf region must be palpated intermittently during the procedure. Factors that influence a potential compartment syndrome include an acute reconstruction (<2 weeks from the time of injury) in which the capsular healing was insufficient to maintain joint distention, or a case in which the capsule has been breached iatrogenically during the procedure. If extravasation is noted, and a potential compartment syndrome is suspected, the arthroscopic technique is abandoned, and the remainder of the procedure is performed with an open technique.

All compartments within the knee are assessed. A PM portal is established to completely visualize the tibial insertion of the PLC. The PM portal is established under direct visualization through the Gilchrist portal. The 70-degree arthroscope is placed into the anterolateral portal and through the intercondylar notch adjacent to the posterior aspect of the medial femoral condyle. An 18-gauge spinal needle is used for placement, anterior to the saphenous nerve and vein, posterior to the MCL, and 1 cm above the joint line.

After completion of diagnostic arthroscopy, with confirmation of all intra-articular pathology, any concomitant meniscal or cartilaginous injury is addressed. Every effort is made to preserve torn meniscal tissue. Peripheral meniscal tears are repaired via an inside-out technique with zone-specific cannulas and meniscal sutures. Central or irreparable meniscal tears are débrided to a stable rim. Should the meniscus require repair, the sutures are tied down directly onto the capsule at 30 degrees of flexion at the end of the procedure after all grafts have been passed and secured.

The notch and the stumps of the torn cruciates are débrided, and any remaining intact PCL tissue is preserved, as previously described. The tibial insertion of the PCL is removed using an arthroscopic shaver, a curette, or both, via the PM portal, and the plane between the PCL and the posterior capsule is gently developed, while visualization through the anterolateral portal with the 70-degree arthroscope continues. Alternatively, the 30-degree arthroscope may be introduced through the PM portal, and a PCL curette and rasp used through the anterolateral or anteromedial portals. Every attempt is made to débride the distal-most aspect of the tibial PCL insertion, as this assists in tibial tunnel guide wire placement, later in the procedure.

Cruciate Tunnel Preparation, Graft Passage, and Proximal Fixation

We prefer to address the PCL tibial tunnel initially because of the significant risks that accompany this portion of the procedure. A PCL offset guide is used via the anteromedial portal, with the tip of the guide placed at the distal and lateral third of the insertion site of the PCL on the tibia, approximately 10 to 15 mm below the joint line. A proximal anteromedial tibial skin incision is made, and the periosteum is sharply dissected from the bone. The starting point of the guide wire is approximately 3 to 4 cm distal to the joint line. The trajectory of the tibial PCL tunnel roughly parallels the angle of the proximal tibiofibular joint. The guide wire is passed in the desired position until it just perforates the far posterior cortex of the tibia at the PCL insertion, under direct arthroscopic visualization. Caution must be taken when the guide wire is passed through the posterior tibial cortex, to avoid neurovascular structures. The PCL insertion often has a soft "cancellous" feel when the posterior tibial cortex is breached, thus lending to increased risk when the guide wire is passed. Proper guide wire location is then confirmed on a true lateral projection of the knee with a mini C-arm fluoroscopy unit. Occasionally, the wire is too proximal on the PCL insertion site, and a 3-mm or 5-mm parallel pin guide is used to obtain ideal guide wire placement. The guide wire for the PCL tibial tunnel is then left in place while attention is directed to the tibial tunnel of the ACL.

The ACL tibial tunnel guide is used via the anteromedial portal, and a guide wire is placed in the center of the ACL footprint, adjacent to the anterior horn of the lateral meniscus. The guide wire should rest posterior to Blumensaat's line on the full-extension lateral mini C-arm projection to ensure proper placement of the ACL tibial tunnel. The ACL tibial tunnel is proximal and anterior to the PCL tunnel at the proximal medial tibia.

Once acceptable placement of the ACL and PCL guide is confirmed, the PCL tunnel is reamed to the predetermined graft diameter (Fig. 59-10). A curette is placed directly on top of the guide wire posteriorly, to prevent protrusion of the wire into adjacent neurovascular structures. The PCL tunnel is expanded using dilators in 0.5-mm increments to the diameter of the graft. The ACL tibial tunnel is reamed in a similar manner. We prefer at least a 1- to 2-cm bone bridge between the ACL and PCL tibial tunnels anteriorly on the tibia (Fig. 59-11).

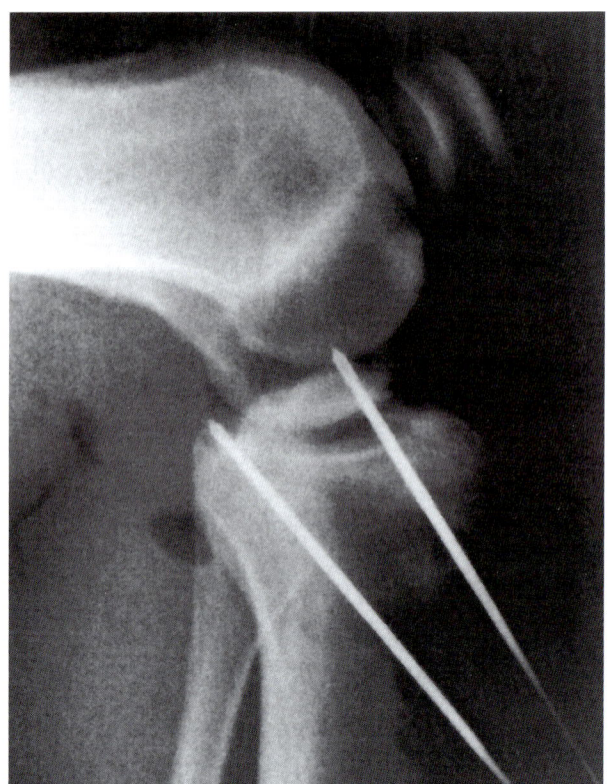

Figure 59-10. Intraoperative lateral knee radiograph confirms proper placement of anterior cruciate ligament and posterior cruciate ligament tunnels.

Attention is turned to preparation of the femoral ACL and PCL tunnels. For a single-bundle PCL reconstruction, the insertion of the PCL on the intercondylar notch is identified, and the guide wire is placed from the anterolateral portal to a point approximately 7 to 10 mm from the articular margin, within the anterior portion of the PCL femoral footprint at approximately 1 o'clock (right knee), and the knee is flexed to 100 degrees. After reaming over the guide wire, the tunnel is dilated to the size of the graft by 0.5-mm increments. If a double-bundle PCL reconstruction is chosen (in the delayed setting), the anterolateral tunnel is drilled at the 1 o'clock position, approximately 5 to 6 mm off the articular cartilage, and the posteromedial bundle is placed at the 3 to 4 o'clock position, approximately 4 mm off of the articular cartilage. These tunnels are prepared to a depth of 25 to 30 mm.

The ACL femoral tunnel is established with the knee flexed to 120 degrees. The anteromedial portal is used to introduce the guide wire into the desired position on the posterolateral femoral footprint below the lateral intercondylar ridge. The guide wire is placed in the center of the anatomic femoral ACL footprint, approximately 6 mm anterior to the back wall, or over the top position of the femur. We prefer the medial portal technique to the traditional transtibial technique because the location of the femoral tunnel is not limited by the position or angulation of the tibial tunnel (Fig. 59-12). If any question about femoral tunnel placement arises, the mini C-arm fluoroscopic machine is used for visualization.

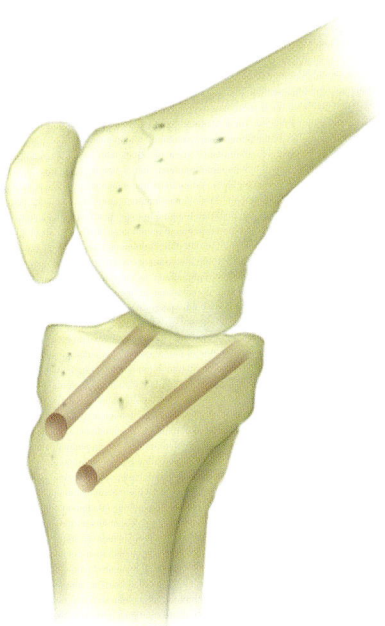

Figure 59-11. Lateral knee schematic shows anterior cruciate ligament and posterior cruciate ligament tibial tunnels.

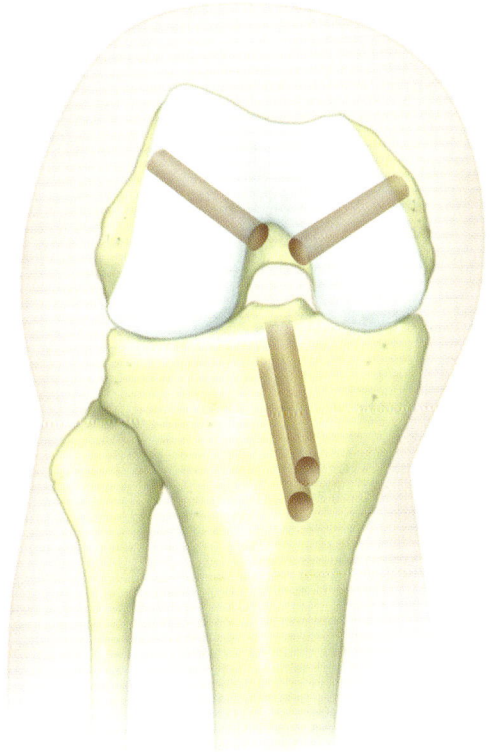

Figure 59-12. Anteroposterior knee schematic shows anterior cruciate ligament and posterior cruciate ligament femoral and tibial tunnels.

The Achilles allograft PCL graft is passed first. A long, looped 18-gauge wire is passed retrograde into the PCL tibial tunnel and is retrieved out the anterolateral arthroscopy portal with a pituitary rongeur. The draw suture of the graft is shuttled into the joint with the looped 18-gauge wire via the anterolateral portal and antegrade down the PCL tibial tunnel to exit on the anteromedial tibia. The draw suture securing the calcaneal portion of the graft is then passed out the anteromedial femur via a beath pin, through the PCL femoral tunnel, and out the anteromedial thigh. With arthroscopic assistance, a probe is used to direct the graft within the joint to facilitate passage of the graft.

The ACL graft is passed using the medial portal technique. A beath pin with a no. 5 suture attached to the eyelet is passed through the femoral tunnel via the medial portal. A pituitary rongeur is passed retrograde through the tibial tunnel, and the no. 5 suture is retrieved. The graft is then passed from the tibial tunnel into the femoral tunnel with arthroscopic assistance.

Femoral fixation of the PCL and ACL grafts is performed. Fixation at the tibia is performed after the collateral fixation is done. The PCL femoral grafts are fixed with a 4.5-mm AO screw and washer, or the grafts are tied and secured over a button. The anteromedial incision is extended proximally and distally adjacent to the exiting beath pins. The vastus medialis obliquus is split in line with its fibers, or a small subvastus approach is used to gain access to the graft sutures and the bone. Alternatively, an interference screw may be used for femoral fixation of the calcaneal bone plug for single-bundle reconstructions. For the ACL femoral fixation, a metal interference screw secures the femoral bone plug via the medial portal technique. Other types of fixation are feasible, and selection depends on the type of graft and the comfort level of the surgeon.

Cruciate and Medial-Sided Injury

If the cruciate ligaments are injured in combination with a medial-sided injury, a standard medial curvilinear incision is made. The PCL femoral tunnel, ACL and PCL tibial tunnels, medial meniscal repairs, or medial capsular repairs can be addressed through this incision. Peripheral meniscal tears can be repaired by standard meniscal repair techniques, and any capsular disruptions can be repaired with suture anchors. During the procedure, the infrapatellar branch of the saphenous nerve should be identified approximately 1 cm above the joint line and protected throughout the procedure.

The MCL should be repaired or reconstructed only for grade 3 injuries that open up with valgus stress testing in the extended knee. In the acute setting (<3 weeks), the MCL can be repaired at the time of cruciate reconstruction. MCL avulsions off of the tibial or femoral insertions are reattached to bone via suture anchors, and intrasubstance tears are repaired primarily with no. 2 braided nonabsorbable sutures using a modified Kessler stitch configuration. In the chronic setting, reconstruction may be required to augment the repair.

The posterior oblique ligament (POL), which is confluent with the posterior edge of the superficial MCL, is reinforced by the semimembranosus and is critical for medial knee stability. The plane between the posterior edge of the MCL and the POL is incised longitudinally, and the two flaps are elevated. Medial meniscal attachments to the POL must be

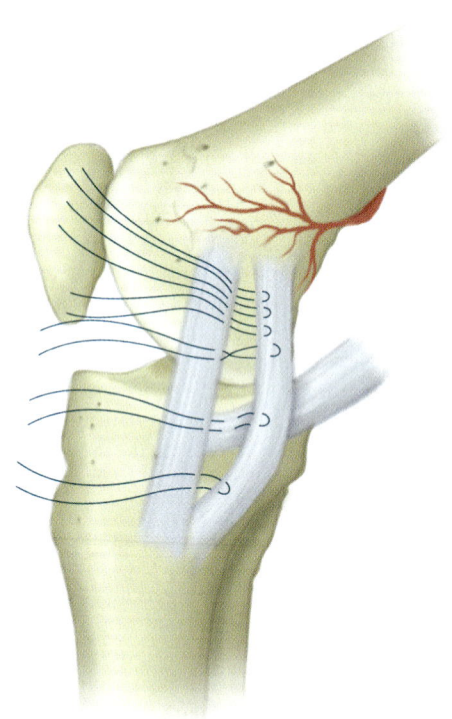

Figure 59-13. Schematic shows the posterior oblique ligament imbrication procedure.

released to the posteromedial corner of the knee. The peripheral border of the medial meniscus is rasped to prepare the tissue for eventual repair back to the POL. The medial meniscus is repaired to the anteriorly advanced POL with full-thickness outside-in no. 0 cottony Dacron sutures through the meniscus. The POL is advanced anteriorly and is imbricated to the MCL in a pants-over-vest fashion using no. 2 cottony Dacron sutures (Fig. 59-13). If needed, the repair can be augmented by a soft tissue graft at the anatomic origin and insertion of the MCL. The graft is inserted directly to bone on the femoral and tibial surfaces using suture anchors, and is reinforced to the native MCL in a side-to-side fashion.

Cruciate and Lateral-Sided Injury

Following femoral fixation of cruciate ligament reconstructions, a standard lateral "hockey-stick" incision is made. The plane between the posterior edge of the iliotibial band and the biceps femoris is incised longitudinally. The peroneal nerve is identified proximally as it travels posterior to the biceps femoris, and distally as it travels along the fibular neck and into the anterior tibialis muscle belly. A formal neurolysis generally is not performed unless evidence indicates compromise of the nerve at the time of surgery. The insertion of the iliotibial band at Gerdy's tubercle is partially released to enhance visibility of the LCL and popliteus insertions.

If reparable lateral meniscal tears or lateral capsular avulsions are visualized during diagnostic arthroscopy, a longitudinal capsular incision is made just posterior to the LCL, and

the lateral inferior geniculate artery is coagulated if encountered. The meniscus is repaired using standard meniscal repair techniques depending on the type and location of the tear. Capsular avulsions are repaired with suture anchors. The LCL and PFL are identified. If tissue quality allows, avulsions of the biceps, iliotibial band insertion, LCL, and/or popliteus are repaired directly and acutely with no. 2 braided nonabsorbable sutures (Fig. 59-14). If interstitial injury to these structures has occurred, or if the injury is chronic, reconstruction is usually necessary.

Our preferred method for LCL reconstruction involves a fibular-based reconstruction with Achilles tendon allograft and imbrication of the native LCL. The tendinous portion of the Achilles allograft is secured to the femoral LCL insertion by means of drill holes or suture anchors. The native LCL is imbricated to the tendinous portion of the allograft using a whipstitch technique. The injured LCL is then dissected free from its distal insertion on the fibular head, and a tunnel is drilled along the longitudinal axis of the fibula. The allograft calcaneal bone plug is tensioned and secured in the tunnel using a metal interference screw (Fig. 59-15). Alternatively, the calcaneal bone plug can be fixed initially into the fibular tunnel, and the tendinous portion recessed into the lateral femoral epicondyle via a small bone tunnel and tied over a post or a button on the medial femur.

The goal of reconstruction of the popliteus complex is to re-create its static component, the PFL.[39] We prefer a tibialis anterior allograft, although hamstring autograft can be used. The lateral epicondyle of the femur is exposed, and the popliteus tendon is dissected off of its anatomic insertion. A whipstitch is placed in the popliteus tendon with a no. 2 braided nonabsorbable suture. Verification of correct placement of the whipstitch is confirmed if the whole popliteus complex becomes taut when tension is placed on the suture. A 6-mm femoral tunnel is drilled at the lateral epicondyle, 18 mm away from the LCL, to a depth of 25 to 30 mm, and the tunnel is expanded to 7 mm in diameter with serial dilators. The posterior border of the fibula at the insertion of the PFL is exposed by incising horizontally just below the biceps insertion proximal to the peroneal nerve. The anterior border of the fibula also is exposed, and a guide wire is passed by hand (with it loaded on a chuck) from anterior to posterior across the fibular head in an attempt to match the oblique angle of the fibular head. The PFL tunnel rests more medial and closer to the proximal tibiofibular joint than the previously drilled LCL tunnel. The fibular head tunnel for the PFL graft is obliquely drilled over the guide wire by hand with a 6-mm drill and is dilated to a diameter of 7 mm. The graft is passed from posterior to anterior through the tunnel with a Hughson suture passer, but it is not fixed to the fibula until the graft is tensioned properly. The graft is passed underneath and medial to the LCL and into the previously drilled femoral tunnel. A beath pin is used to dock the graft into the femoral tunnel as it is pulled through to the medial side. Both the graft and the native popliteus tendon that was previously subperiosteally dissected are pulled into the tunnel together. Approximately 25 mm of the allograft and 10 mm of the popliteus tendon should be paralleled into the tunnel. Sutures from the graft and the popliteus tendon are tied over an AO screw with a washer or a button on the anteromedial distal femur. The reconstructed tendon is fixed to the fibula with a bioabsorbable interference screw, or over a button at the end

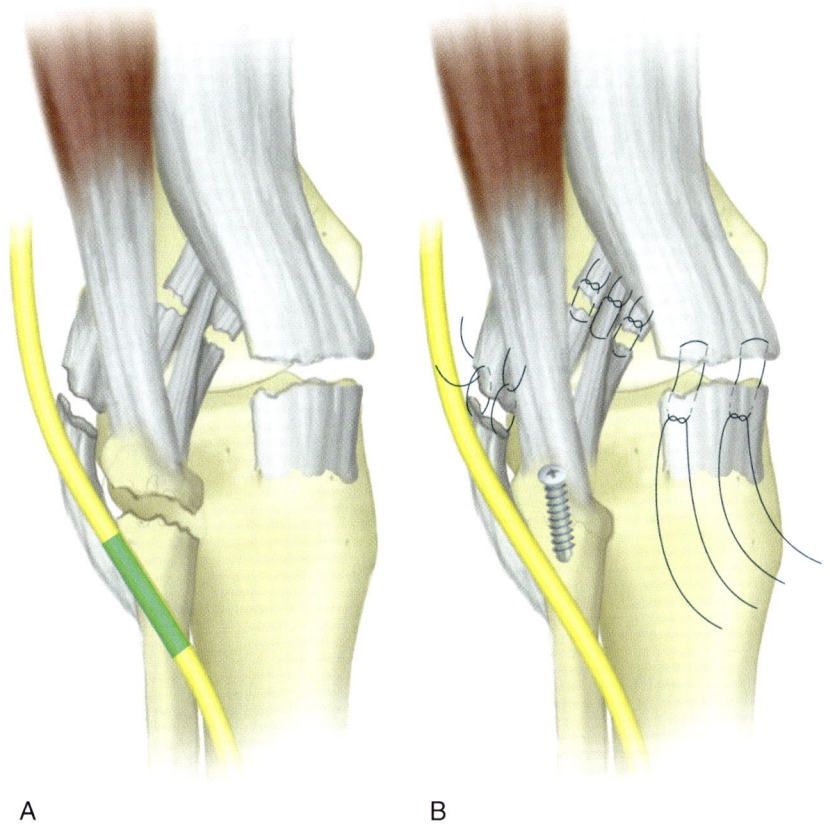

A   B

Figure 59-14. **A** and **B**, Schematic shows direct repair of the lateral structures.

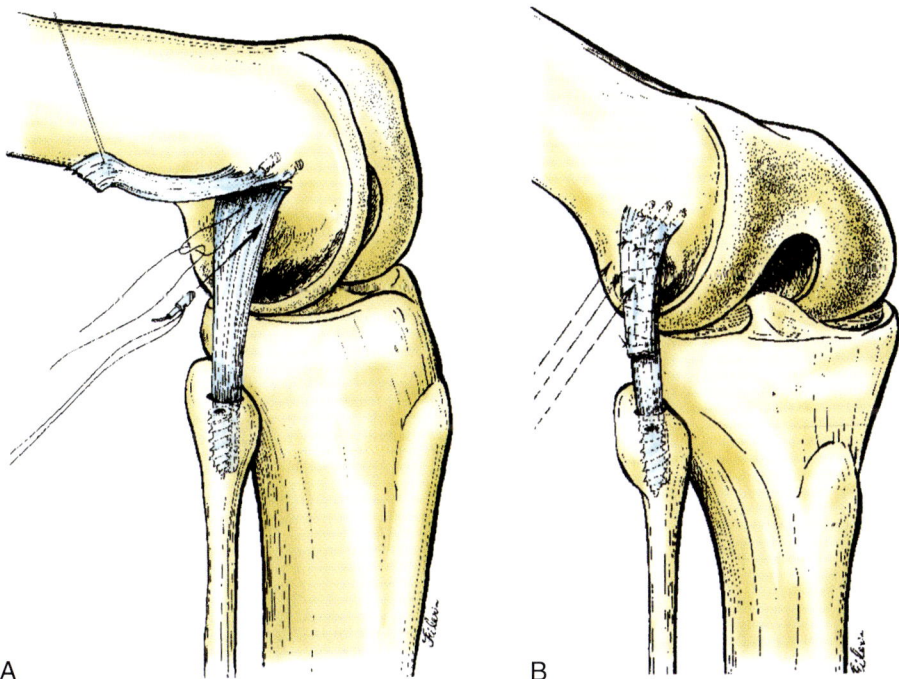

A   B

Figure 59-15. Schematic shows lateral collateral ligament (LCL) reconstruction with Achilles tendon allograft. **A**, The torn or stretched LCL is detached and elevated from its fibular insertion, and the allograft bone block is fixed in a tunnel in the proximal fibula using an interference screw. The tensioned graft is fixed at the lateral femoral epicondyle using multiple suture anchors. **B**, The native LCL is tensioned and sutured to the allograft.

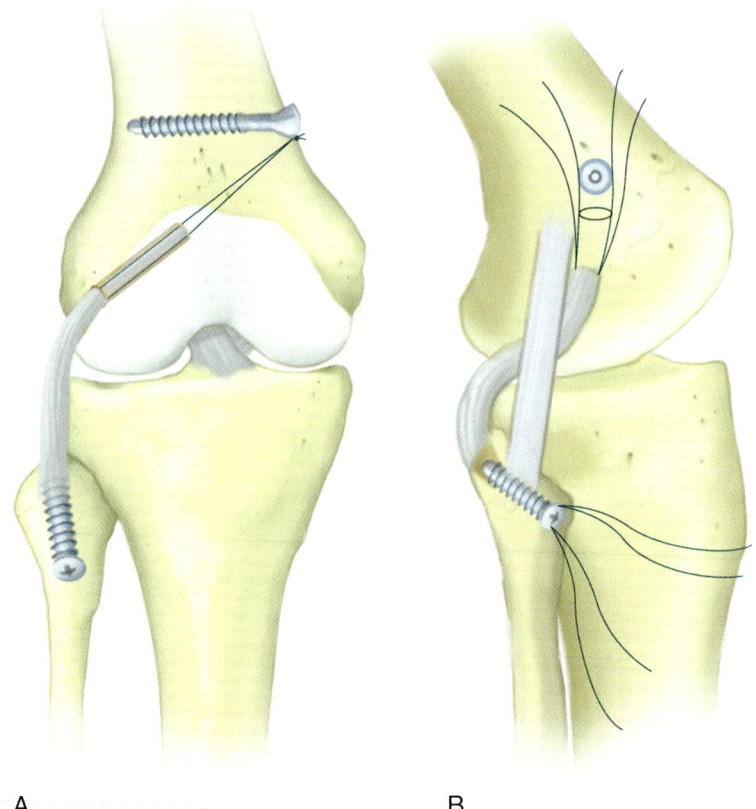

A   B

Figure 59-16. Schematic shows popliteofibular ligament reconstruction. The graft is fixed into a tunnel in the lateral femoral condyle over a post at the medial femoral condyle. It is passed deep to the lateral collateral ligament and through a tunnel in the fibula from posterior to anterior, where it is fixed with an interference screw. **A,** Anterior. **B,** Lateral.

of the case (Fig. 59-16). In certain cases, LCL and PFL complexes need to be reconstructed, and the techniques described here are used.

Cruciate, Medial, and Lateral-Sided Injuries

Combined cruciate, medial- and lateral-sided injuries are potentially the most unstable of injuries and are approached through medial and lateral "hockey-stick" incisions, as described earlier. Cruciate reconstruction is performed first, as described previously, followed by medial and lateral repair or reconstruction. Proximal fixation is performed first, followed by tensioning and distal fixation in a similar sequence.

Tensioning and Distal Fixation

After all grafts have been successfully passed and fixed on the femoral side, final tensioning and distal fixation of the grafts is performed. In a stepwise fashion, we prefer to tension and fix the PCL, ACL, lateral structures, and medial structures. For the PCL, the knee is brought to 90 degrees of flexion, and a bolster is placed under the tibia to support its weight against gravity. The medial step-off is reduced with an anterior drawer, so that the anterior edge of the medial tibial plateau rests approximately 10 mm anterior to the medial femoral condyle. The graft is fixed to the tibia with a bioabsorbable

interference screw, or an AO screw, and a soft tissue washer. The ACL graft is tensioned and fixed close to full extension with coaxial tension on the draw sutures and axial compression. We prefer a metal interference screw for the bone–patellar tendon–bone allograft fixation on the tibia. The PLC of the knee is reduced with an internal rotation force to the tibia relative to the fixed femur, and the LCL and the PFL are tensioned at 30 degrees of flexion. The LCL is fixed with a metal interference screw into the fibular head. The PFL is fixed with a bioabsorbable interference screw in the fibula, and the remaining graft is reapproximated to itself or over the insertion of the biceps in a figure-of-eight pattern with a no. 2 braided absorbable suture. Alternatively, the PFL graft is fixed to the fibula with sutures tied over a button. The MCL is fixed at 30 degrees of knee flexion, and the POL is fixed with the knee near full extension. This method prevents overconstraining of the knee during the repair/reconstruction. After all grafts are fixed, the knee should have a tension-free range of motion from 0 to 90 degrees.

Postoperative Regimen

In the early postoperative period, the main goals are to protect healing structures, maximize quadriceps recovery, and restore full passive extension. We place the limb locked in full extension for the first 4 weeks with a hinged knee brace. Exercises immediately after surgery include passive knee extension to neutral and isometric quadriceps sets with the knee in full extension. At 2 weeks postoperatively, physical therapy begins, with passive flexion limited to 90 degrees, and should prevent posterior tibial subluxation by applying an anterior force to the proximal tibia (can be performed prone). For the first 6 weeks, active flexion is avoided to prevent posterior tibial translation, which results from hamstring contraction. At 6 weeks, passive and active-assisted range of motion and stretching exercises are begun to increase knee flexion. The brace is discontinued after 6 weeks. Depending on the combination of injuries and the degree of instability, as determined by examination under anesthesia, a reasonable goal for range of motion is 0 to 120 degrees of flexion. Reports in the literature indicate that nearly half of patients require manipulation after reconstruction of all injured structures, despite aggressive postoperative rehabilitation.[34,46,50]

Quadriceps exercises are progressed to limited-arc, open-chain, knee-extension exercises only from 60 to 75 degrees of knee flexion as tolerated after 4 weeks. These exercises are performed to prevent excessive stress on the reconstructed grafts. Open-chain hamstring exercises are avoided for 12 weeks to prevent posterior tibial translation and excessive stress on the PCL graft. Crutch weight bearing is progressed from partial to total weight bearing as tolerated over the first 4 weeks, unless a lateral repair/reconstruction was performed. In this case, we maintain partial weight bearing until the patient has regained good quadriceps control, at which time the brace may be unlocked for controlled gait training. Running is permitted at 6 months if 80% of quadriceps strength has been achieved. Patients may return to sedentary work in 2 to 3 weeks, heavy labor in 6 to 9 months, and sports in 9 to 12 months.

CONCLUSION

Knee dislocations are serious injuries that require prompt evaluation and treatment to prevent major complications and poor results. The sequence of events includes (in this order) closed reduction and neurovascular evaluation with vascular repair where required. This is followed by evaluation and treatment of soft tissue injuries. Although the practicing orthopedist may encounter only a few of these injuries throughout a career, it is imperative that a high index of suspicion exist for a patient who presents with a multiple-ligament knee injury. As the approach toward isolated ligamentous injuries of the knee has continued to evolve, so has the treatment of knee dislocation. Treatment now involves early reconstruction of the cruciate ligaments combined with reconstruction or repair of collateral structures combined with aggressive rehabilitation. This approach has improved knee function with regard to stability and has improved the mobility of patients with knee dislocation. Further research is necessary to define appropriate timing and optimal types of reconstruction.

KEY REFERENCES

Dedmond BT, Almekinders LC: Operative versus nonoperative treatment of knee dislocations: a meta-analysis. Am J Knee Surg 14:33–38, 2001.

Harner CD, Waltrip RL, Bennett CH: Surgical management of knee dislocations. J Bone Joint Surg Am 86:262–273, 2004.

Kennedy JC: Complete dislocation of the knee. J Bone Joint Surg Am 45:889, 1963.

Klineberg EO, Crites BM, Flinn WR, et al: The role of arteriography in assessing popliteal artery injury in knee dislocations. J Trauma 56:786–790, 2004.

Levy BA, Fanelli GC, Whelan DB, et al: Controversies in the treatment of knee dislocations and multiligament reconstruction. J Am Acad Orthop Surg 17:197–206, 2009.

L'Insalata JC, Harner CD: The dislocated knee: approach to treatment. Pittsburgh Orthop J 7:32, 1996.

Liow RY, McNicholas MJ, Keating JF, Nutton RW: Ligament repair and reconstruction in traumatic dislocation of the knee. J Bone Joint Surg Br 85:845–851, 2003.

Mariani PP, Becker R, Rihn J, Margheritini F: Surgical treatment of posterior cruciate ligament and posterolateral corner injuries: an anatomical, biomechanical and clinical review. Knee 10:311–324, 2003.

Miller MD, Cooper DE, Fanelli GC, et al: Posterior cruciate ligament: current concepts. Instr Course Lect 51:347–351, 2002.

Mills WJ, Barei DP, McNair P: The value of the ankle-brachial index for diagnosing arterial injury after knee dislocation: a prospective study. J Trauma 24:403–407, 2004.

Mook WR, Miller MD, Diduch DR, et al: Multiple-ligament knee injuries: a systematic review of the timing of operative intervention and postoperative rehabilitation. J Bone Joint Surg Am 19:2946–2957, 2009.

Ranawat A, Baker CL III, Henry S, Harner CD: Posterolateral corner injury of the knee: evaluation and management. J Am Acad Orthop Surg 16:506–518, 2008.

Rihn JA, Cha PS, Groff YJ, Harner CD: The acutely dislocated knee: evaluation and management. J Am Acad Orthop Surg 12:334–346, 2004.

Seroyer ST, Musahl V, Harner CD: Management of the acute knee dislocation: the Pittsburgh experience. Injury 39:710–718, 2008.

Stannard JP, Sheils TM, Lopez-Ben RR, et al: Vascular injuries in knee dislocation: the role of physical examination in determining the need for arteriography. J Bone Joint Surg Am 86:910–915, 2004.

Full references for this chapter can be found on www.expertconsult.com.

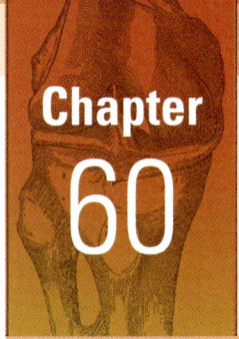

Chapter 60

Dislocation of the Proximal Tibiofibular Joint

Nathan Kopydlowski, Eric Tannenbaum, and Jon K. Sekiya

Dislocation of the proximal tibiofibular joint is a very rare condition that is easily misdiagnosed without suspicion of the injury. Proximal tibiofibular dislocation can be an idiopathic subluxation of the joint, more commonly seen in conjunction with high-energy tibia and ankle fractures. It is most common in sports that involve violent twisting of the knee such as wrestling, parachute jumping, mixed martial arts, gymnastics, skiing, rugby, football, soccer, snowboarding, long jumping, and baseball.* The pathology of the tibiofibular joint is a result of anatomic variations of the proximal joint, the biomechanical axis of the ankle, and training program errors.[39] Injury to this structure can be caused by ligaments that strengthen and support the proximal tibiofibular joint, as well as allow the functional structure and the biomechanics of the lower kinetic chain to influence movements at the joint, all of which increase the chance of instability.[29,30] Some physicians question the frequency of tibiofibular joint injury due to common misdiagnosis.[30,39] Diagnosis of this rare injury will be improved by a better understanding of the anatomy and biomechanics of the joint, the mechanisms leading to instability, and the symptoms that result from this injury.

ANATOMY

The chief function of the proximal tibiofibular joint is to dissipate some of the forces on the lower leg such as torsional stresses on the ankle, lateral tibial bending movements, and tensile weight bearing.[27] The proximal tibiofibular joint is a synovial membrane–lined, hyaline cartilage articulation that communicates with the knee joint in 10% of adults[†] and must be considered as the fourth compartment of the knee (Fig. 60-1A and B). The joint capsule is strengthened by ligamentous attachments that increase in strength and thickness from anterior to posterior.[‡] Responsibility for stabilization of the proximal tibiofibular joint falls on the anterosuperior and posterosuperior tibiofibular ligaments.[48] The joint capsule consists of the tibial facet and the fibular facet, located on the posterolateral aspect of the tibial condyle and the medial proximal surface of the head of the fibula, respectively.[39]

The anterior capsule of the joint is stabilized by the anterior tibiofibular ligament, which consists of three broad bands that pass obliquely distal from the fibular head and connect to the anterior aspect of the lateral tibial condyle. An extension of the deep layer of the biceps femoris tendon located anterior to the anterior proximal tibiofibular ligaments connects on Gerdy's tubercle and helps to stabilize the anterior joint capsule[8,25,28,32,35] (Fig. 60-2).

The posterior joint capsule is supported by the posterior proximal tibiofibular ligament, which consists of two thick bands that pass obliquely upward from the fibular head and connect to the posterior aspect of the lateral tibial condyle. The popliteus tendon covers and reinforces the posterior proximal tibiofibular ligament[8,28,32,35] (see Fig. 60-2).

Some physicians also believe that the posterolateral structures of the knee, including the arcuate ligament, the fabellofibular ligament, the popliteofibular ligament, the popliteus muscle, the interosseous membrane, and the lateral collateral ligament, stabilize the joint.[36,37,44] The lateral collateral ligament arises from the lateral femoral condyle in the midcoronal plane and runs distally and posteriorly to the posterolateral aspect of the fibular head[25,27,28] (see Fig. 60-2).

Ogden's historic 1974 article described two different anatomic variants based on the arbitrary determinant of a 20-degree angle with the horizontal plane.[27] The inclination angle for the proximal tibiofibular joint with respect to the horizontal plane is important when the anatomic stability of the joint is determined. The greater the slope that the joint makes with the horizontal plane, the more vulnerable it is to rotational forces.[48] Ogden described a horizontal variant as <20 degrees of joint inclination (Fig. 60-3A). It has been observed to have greater resistance to rotational forces because of its position behind the prominent ridge of the proximal tibia and its large planar, circular articular surface with an average surface area of 26 mm[2]. The horizontal variant was also observed to have greater external rotation compared with the oblique variant.[27-29] Ogden described an inclination of >20 degrees as an oblique variant (Fig. 60-3B). This increased angle of inclination can reach as high as 76 degrees and causes a highly variable surface area, averaging 17 mm[2], and configuration. The angle of inclination shows an inverse correlation with the surface area of the joint.[27,29,35] The oblique variant was found in 70% of the joint injuries described by Ogden and instability is thought to stem from the decreased surface area and increased angle of inclination found in oblique joints.[29,45]

The normal orientation of the proximal tibiofibular joint does not sit in a sagittal plane; as a result, it encounters normal movement in the anterolateral and posteromedial direction.[39] Anterior-posterior motion during flexion and extension, respectively, is increased in children and gradually decreases with age.[27] During anterior movement of the fibular head, the biceps femoris tendon, which inserts on the styloid process and the upper surface of the head of the fibula, adds support and stability.

When the knee is flexed between 0 degrees and 30 degrees, the lateral collateral ligament is tight and supports the joint. When the knee is flexed beyond 30 degrees, the lateral collateral ligament and the biceps femoris tendon relax, causing the proximal fibula to migrate anteriorly. Laxity in the joint capsule caused by the orientation of the knee in the flexed

---

*References 8, 13, 15, 19, 21, 24, 28, 29, 38, 40, and 45-46.
†References 7, 17, 27, 32, 35, and 38.

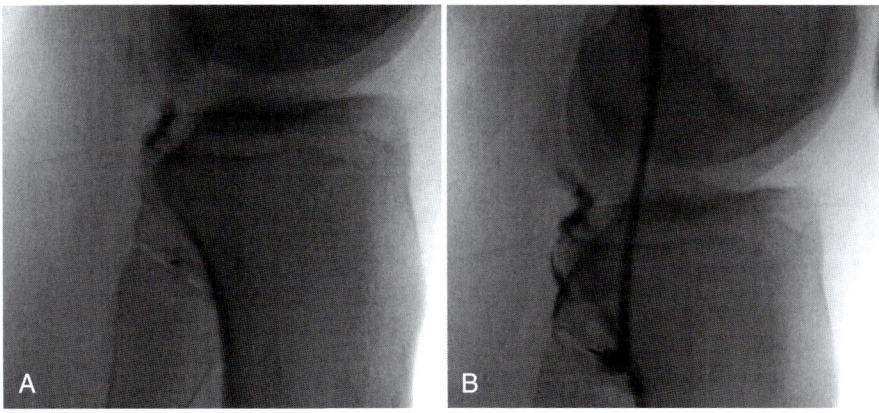

Figure 60-1. Arthrogram of diagnostic and therapeutic injections. **A,** Needle positioned in the proximal tibiofibular joint. **B,** Radiographic dye is used to verify that the needle is in the correct position. Note the communication of the proximal tibiofibular joint with the knee joint.

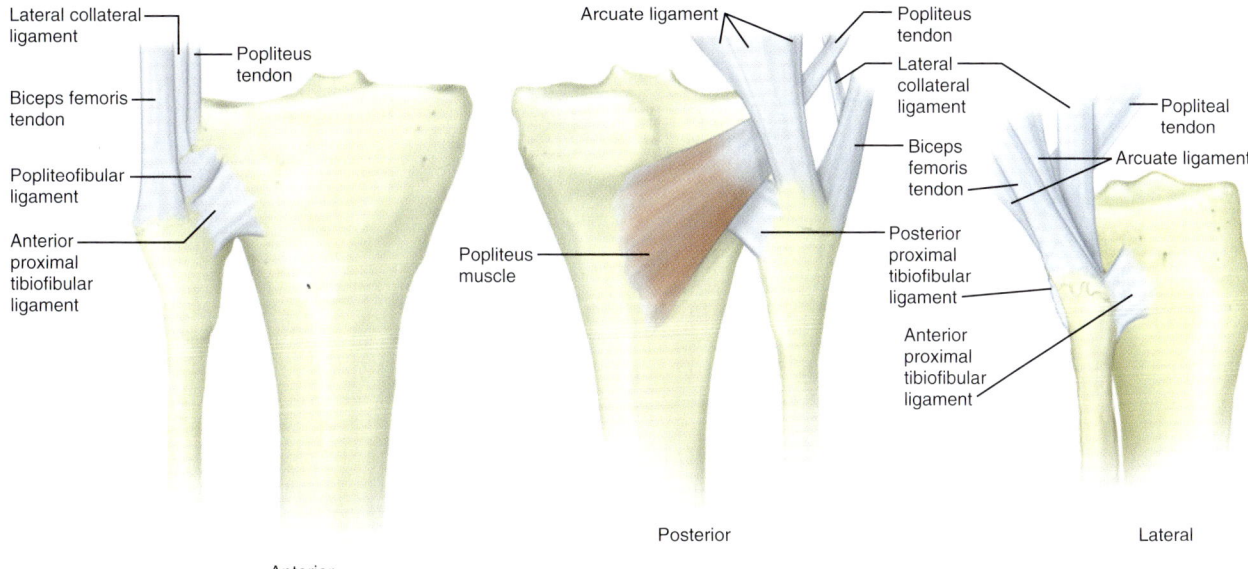

Figure 60-2. Anatomy of the proximal tibiofibular joint. (© Whiddon DR, Parker TA, Kuhn JE, Sekiya JK: Disorders of the proximal tibiofibular joint. In Scott NW [ed]: Surgery of the knee, ed 4, Philadelphia, 2006, Elsevier, pp 797–803.)

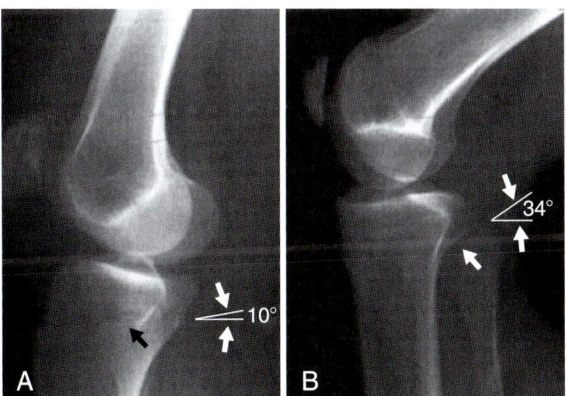

Figure 60-3. Lateral radiographs show the anatomic variations in the joint described by Ogden. An increased slope of the articulation causes instability in the joint by minimizing the surface area of the joint. **A,** Horizontal orientation (<20 degrees). **B,** Oblique orientation (>20 degrees) is more likely to develop instability. (© 2003 American Academy of Orthopaedic Surgeons. Reprinted from the Journal of the American Academy of Orthopaedic Surgeons, vol 11[2], pp 120–128, Figure 45-2, with permission.)

position increases the vulnerability of the proximal tibiofibular joint to injury.[27]

When the knee is extended, the same structures become tightened, causing the fibular head to return to its posterior position.[1,27] Because of the arrangement and tightening of the ligaments around the joint, the proximal tibiofibular joint is most stable when the knee is extended.[16,48]

The proximal tibiofibular joint is very important in the external rotation of the fibula with ankle dorsiflexion. It has been observed that during movement of the ankle, rotational movement can be observed in the proximal tibiofibular joint.[38] The oblique variant causes greater constraint in rotational mobility and is thought to increase torsional loads during forced ankle dorsiflexion, increasing the probability of fibular dislocation or fracture.[27]

Semonian et al reported that it is important to recognize the neurologic aspect of the lateral region of the knee owing to the fact that many diagnoses of joint instability go unnoticed until patients develop footdrop. The common peroneal nerve passes posteriorly over the head of the fibula and comes in close contact with the proximal tibiofibular joint. The peroneal nerve is palpable along the lateral aspect of the knee because of its path as it wraps around the fibular neck before the peroneus longus muscle overlaps it laterally.[39] Physicians diagnosing a patient with anterolateral, posteromedial, or superior dislocation must be aware of peroneal nerve injury.[48]

CLASSIFICATION OF INSTABILITY

Ogden described the four commonly used types of dislocation based on the direction of instability of the joint: atraumatic subluxation, anterolateral dislocation, posteromedial dislocation, and the rare superior dislocation.[29,35] In Ogden's study of 43 patients, 10 had subluxation, 29 anterolateral dislocation, 3 posteromedial dislocation, and 1 superior dislocation.[29] The literature also describes five cases of inferior dislocation.[11,26] Physicians diagnosing this type of injury should be aware of its association with a common peroneal nerve injury that most commonly occurs in patients diagnosed with anterolateral or posteromedial dislocation.[5,8]

Injury to the anterior and posterior capsular ligaments, and commonly the lateral collateral ligament, can lead to common anterolateral dislocation[29,30,35] (Fig. 60-4A). The main cause of this injury is a fall on a hyperflexed knee with the foot inverted and plantarflexed.* Flexion of the knee results in relaxation of the lateral collateral ligament and the biceps femoris tendon, and twisting of the body creates a torque that forces the fibular head laterally to the edge of the bone buttress of the lateral tibial metaphysis.[13,29] A reflex contracture of the peroneal, extensor hallucis longus, and extensor digitorum longus muscles, caused by forced plantar flexion and ankle inversion, forces the laterally displaced fibular head anteriorly.[4,28,29,32]

Posteromedial dislocation typically stems from direct trauma to the knee or from a twisting injury that puts torsional strain on supporting ligaments, causing them to tear[27,29,32,35] (Fig. 60-4B). The resulting loss of support causes tension in the biceps femoris tendon to displace the fibular head posteriorly and medially along the posterolateral tibial metaphysis.[29]

Subluxation typically occurs in patients who have no history of inciting trauma but may have generalized ligamentous laxity; it is not commonly bilateral.[29,30,35] The anterior capsule and the anterior ligament of the joint are thought to be involved in proximal tibiofibular joint subluxation.[39] Symptoms of subluxation include excessive anterior-posterior motion without actual dislocation of the joint.

Superior dislocations are caused by tearing of the tibiofibular interosseous membrane and result in dislocation of the entire fibula[29] (Fig. 60-4C). The superior migration of the entire fibula commonly results from high-energy ankle injuries.[35] They are commonly found in conjunction with lateral malleolar and tibial fractures.[29,32] Atraumatic superior dislocation of the proximal tibiofibular joint has been seen in conjunction with congenital dislocation of the knee.[29]

Five cases of inferior proximal tibiofibular dislocation have been described in the literature, and all were associated with severe neurovascular injury and fracture of the tibial

*References 9, 12, 22, 23, 27-29, 32, 33, 35, 38, 40, 45, and 46.

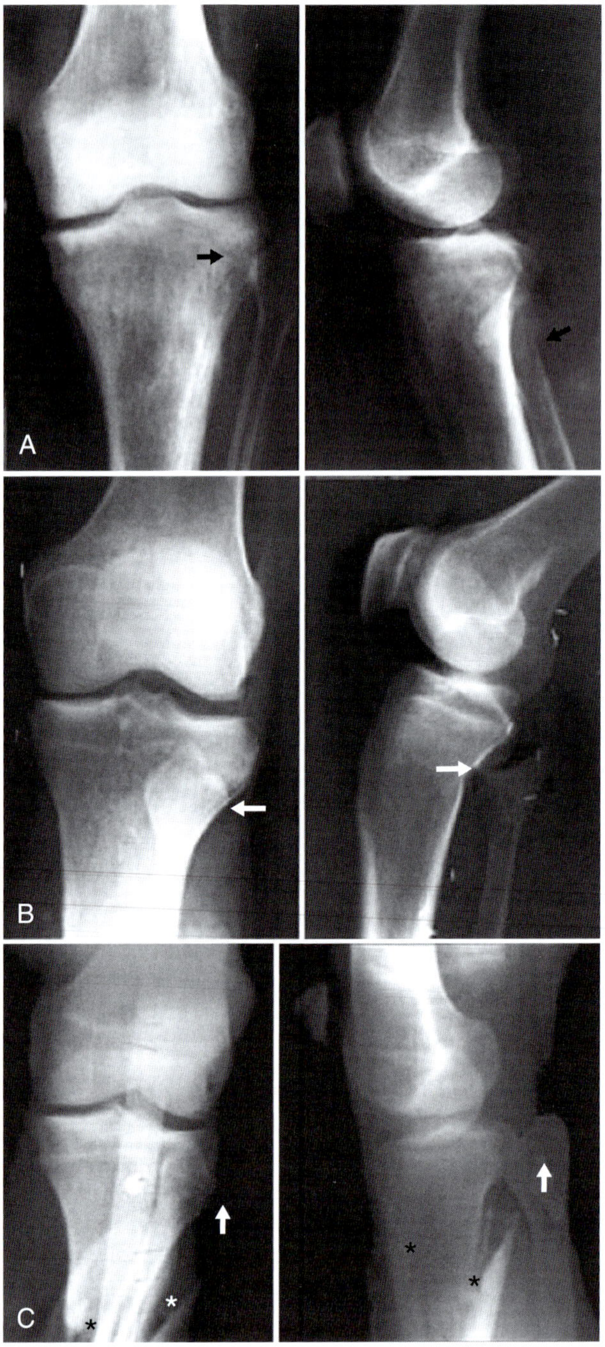

Figure 60-4. A, Anteroposterior and lateral radiographs of an anterolateral dislocation of the proximal tibiofibular joint. **B,** Posteromedial dislocation of the proximal tibiofibular joint. **C,** Superior dislocation. Note the tibia fracture *(asterisks)* associated with this high-energy injury. (© 2003 American Academy of Orthopaedic Surgeons. Reprinted from the Journal of the American Academy of Orthopaedic Surgeons, vol 11[2], pp 120–128, with permission.)

shaft.[11,26] In all cases, the common peroneal and tibial nerves were affected; all were high-energy motorcycle injuries.[11]

CLINICAL PRESENTATION

Early recognition of injury to the proximal tibiofibular joint is important to optimize management and avoid potential misdiagnosis.[36] Early treatment of these injuries may prevent this condition from developing into chronic or fixed subluxation, which is more difficult to treat.[39] Before a diagnosis of proximal tibiofibular joint instability is made, the integrity of surrounding ligamentous structures must be checked because of the common injuries that can present with the same symptoms.[48] When a patient presents with high-energy trauma, the proximal tibiofibular dislocation may be missed initially because of other traumatic injuries such as fracture of the tibial plateau or shaft, ipsilateral femoral head or shaft, distal femoral epiphysis, ankle fracture, or knee dislocation.[10,29]

Anterolateral injury usually occurs after a fall on a flexed knee or a violent twisting motion during an athletic activity, and prominent pain is common over the lateral aspect of the knee, along with a prominent fibular head.* Pain commonly causes the patient to be unable to bear weight on the affected leg; range of motion in the knee is limited, especially knee extension, and motion of the ankle may cause more pain.[46,51] Patients often present with pain along the biceps femoris tendon, which appears as a tense, curved cord. Pain that is increased by extending the flexed knee and by dorsiflexing and everting the foot is also seen.[29]

Posteromedial dislocations are common after direct trauma to the knee with pain secondary to that trauma. Common peroneal nerve injury can be seen with these injuries, even though symptoms are usually transient.[5]

Subluxation is seen most commonly in adolescents, can be bilateral, and usually presents with pain on the lateral side of the knee that is increased by direct pressure over the fibular head.[29,30] Instability of the knee can be demonstrated by moving the fibular head anteriorly and laterally by relaxing the lateral collateral ligament and the biceps femoris tendon with the knee flexed 90 degrees.[14] Muscular dystrophy, Ehlers-Danlos syndrome, and generalized ligamentous laxity can be associated with subluxation.[29,30,39,41] Prepubescent females commonly exhibit laxity and usually experience a decrease in symptoms as they reach skeletal maturity.[29-31,41,42] Other associated events include osteomyelitis, rheumatoid arthritis, septic arthritis, previous below-the-knee amputations, osteochondroma, and growth disturbances around the knee, as well as runners who have recently increased their mileage.[3,23,29,35,39]

Recurrence of chronic dislocation of the proximal tibiofibular joint is often missed because its symptoms mirror a wide range of other knee conditions. Most patients usually live their daily lives without symptoms until they become involved in activities that require sudden changes in direction, such as athletic movement.[12] It is common for patients to complain of sensations of knee instability or giving way, especially while climbing stairs.[42] The nature and location of this injury often mimic those of other knee pathologies, such as injury to the lateral collateral ligament or biceps femoris tendon, posterolateral rotatory instability, iliotibial band syndrome, or tendinitis of the popliteus tendon or biceps femoris tendon.[39] Associated symptoms of instability with clicking or popping also mimic a lateral meniscus injury, exostosis, or intra-articular loose bodies in the popliteus tendon sheath.†

Superior dislocations are rare and usually present after high-energy trauma with lateral knee pain and the displaced fibular head as a lateral mass.[29,35] They commonly occur with associated tibial and ankle fractures and often require surgery for correction.[29] Inferior dislocations have been described in the literature as having a very poor prognosis; four of five cases result in above-knee or below-knee amputation.[26] Posterolateral dislocation was described in the literature in one case and is not mentioned as one of the four types of dislocation by Ogden.[43] It is not uncommon for patients with chronic instability of the proximal tibiofibular joint to be diagnosed with Charcot-Marie-Tooth (CMT) disease or to undergo diagnostic knee arthroscopy for this problem, so this condition should be considered in the differential diagnosis in patients with lateral knee pain.

PHYSICAL EXAMINATION

Physical examination of a suspected injury to the proximal tibiofibular joint is very important as most patient histories do not reveal any specific mechanism of injury, and symptoms of lateral knee pain can be very misleading. Many patients present with pain along the lateral aspect of the knee that radiates proximally into the region of the iliotibial band and medially into the patellofemoral joint.[20] Side-to-side comparison is necessary in adolescents because of the mobility of the fibular head before skeletal maturity is reached.[30] The relative avascularity of tissues surrounding the joint reduces the likelihood that swelling may be present with an isolated proximal tibiofibular joint injury.[27,29,33,48] A prominent lateral mass with tenderness to palpation over this mass will be observed with any dislocation, along with a mobile fibular head with knee flexion. Also, locking and popping of the knee when mobilized can occur and can be confused with a lateral meniscal tear.[16] Some patients feel more intense pain when walking down a decline.[8] Patients have also been reported to have loss of sensation and a tingling feeling in the region of the fibular head after heavy activity.[15] It is necessary to examine the strength and functionality of the ankle and peroneal nerves because of the association of peroneal nerve damage with this injury. Examination of the ankle joint is important in determining functionality of syndesmotic ligaments and the interosseous membrane.[48]

Physical examination for chronic instability or atraumatic subluxation, in the absence of acute trauma, should first consist of assessment of the fibular head for tenderness while the knee is flexed to 90 degrees. Grasping the fibular head between the thumb and index finger should allow evaluation of anterior-posterior mobility; the patient should be asked if this motion reproduces the symptoms or causes any apprehension.[42] The Radulescu sign may be helpful; this is performed by having the patient lie prone with the knee flexed to 90 degrees. One hand stabilizes the thigh, while the other internally rotates the lower leg to see if the fibular head can be subluxated or dislocated anteriorly.[3]

IMAGING STUDIES

Plain radiographs should be taken of the injured knee in true anteroposterior and lateral views, and comparison views should be obtained from the uninjured knee or from preinjury radiographs if possible.[35,49] The anteroposterior view should show the medial aspect of the fibular head crossing the lateral border of the tibia. Using the lateral view, Resnick et al described a line that follows the lateral tibial spine distally

---

*References 9, 23, 28, 45, 46, and 51.
†References 3, 9, 31, 38, 40, 42, 45, 46, and 51.

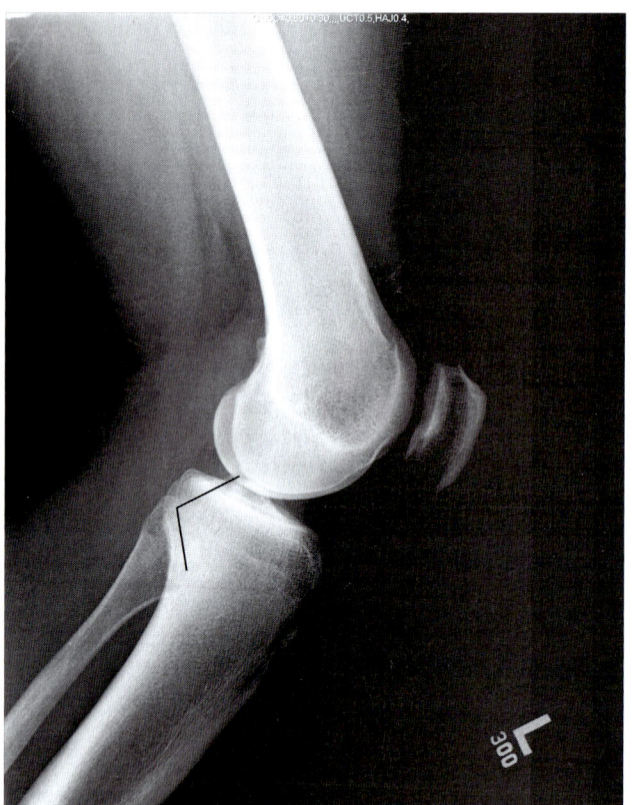

Figure 60-5. Resnick's line *(solid line)* depicted on the lateral radiograph of a normal knee is used to identify instability of the proximal tibiofibular joint. Resnick's line should intersect near the midpoint of the fibular head and defines the posterior border of the tibia. (© Whiddon DR, Parker TA, Kuhn JE, Sekiya JK: Disorders of the proximal tibiofibular joint. In Scott NW [ed]: Surgery of the knee, ed 4, Philadelphia, 2006, Elsevier, pp 797–803.)

along the posterior aspect of the tibia (Fig. 60-5). This important bony landmark for determining dislocation of the joint defines the most posteromedial portion of the lateral tibial condyle. In an uninjured knee, this line is observed over the midpoint of the fibular head because the fibular head extends over the posterior border of the tibia. The fibular head will be viewed as anterior to this line on the lateral view in radiographs of anterolateral dislocations. In a posteromedial dislocation, all or most of the fibular head is posterior to this line on the lateral radiograph.[35]

Resnick recommends an oblique view with the knee in 45 to 60 degrees of internal rotation for best visualization of the joint space, although much controversy surrounds this view. Internal rotation shows the proximal tibiofibular joint in profile and allows a view of the width of the articular space and appearance of the subchondral bone.[35] Veth et al described a view that demonstrated a change in the distance of the medial aspect of the fibular head from the lateral aspect of the tibia plateau, achieved by arranging the lower leg in a position of 30 to 90 degrees of internal rotation.[50]

If diagnosis is suspected but cannot be clearly established on a plain radiograph, axial computed tomography is a more accurate imaging modality in detecting injury to the joint.[18] Magnetic resonance imaging (MRI) has also confirmed the diagnosis of recent dislocation by the presence of pericapsular

edema of the joint, as well as edema of the soleus at its fibular origin of the popliteus muscle.[2] Other uses that can be very helpful are diagnostic and include therapeutic injection into the proximal tibiofibular joint using palpation or injection under fluoroscopic guidance; this topic will be discussed later under Treatment.

TREATMENT OF INSTABILITY

Symptomatic atraumatic subluxation of the proximal tibiofibular joint can commonly be treated successfully with nonsurgical treatment. Patients who present with generalized ligamentous laxity usually have self-limiting symptoms that resolve with skeletal maturity. Activity modification is important with avoidance of knee hyperflexion.[13,39] Placement in a cylinder cast for 2 to 3 weeks may help to reduce the substantial pain that some patients feel.[29,30]

An acute anterolaterally dislocated proximal tibiofibular joint should be treated by first trying a closed reduction under local anesthesia or intravenous sedation.[8,19] Closed reduction is most successful when the knee is in 80 to 110 degrees of flexion and pressure to the fibular head is applied in the posteromedial direction. Flexion of the knee relaxes the lateral collateral ligament and the biceps femoris tendon.[8,29,32,33,46] Closed reduction of the fibular head may fail if it is perched on the lateral tibial ridge by the lateral collateral ligament.[48] Controversy surrounds the orientation of the foot, although an externally rotated, everted, and dorsiflexed foot relaxes the peroneal, extensor hallucis longus, and extensor digitorium longus muscles, theoretically aiding in the reduction.[29,32,45] As the fibula is reduced, an audible pop may be heard, after which the posterolateral structures and the lateral collateral ligament should be assessed for strength and stability. Barring concomitant ligamentous injury, reductions are normally stable. Posteromedial dislocations can also be reduced using this method; however, the literature reports that long-term results may be poor.[29]

Postreduction management is controversial; some authors advocate a soft dressing without immobilization and crutch-assisted weight bearing progressing to full weight bearing over 6 weeks.[9,32,46] Some authors recommend immobilization for 3 weeks, with the knee in the neutral to slightly flexed position.[29,45,51] Other recommendations are that after closed reduction, patients are allowed to mobilize with a support bandage for 6 weeks, with sporting activities restricted for another 6 weeks, and can return to competitive athletics within 6 months of injury.[19] Ogden's study showed that immobilization following closed reduction later required surgical intervention for continuing symptoms in 57% of patients.[29]

When instability is not associated with self-limiting conditions, recurrent symptoms of proximal tibiofibular joint instability corrected by nonsurgical management may cause degenerative changes in the joint and necessitate surgical intervention. The most common symptoms of recurrent instability, such as pain that is felt within the joint,[29,30] can be corrected by several described procedures, such as arthrodesis, fibular head resection, and ligamentous reconstructions. Before any surgical intervention is attempted, an injection into the proximal tibiofibular joint in the office or under fluoroscopic guidance with local anesthetic and steroid can help to confirm the diagnosis and can potentially give some relief

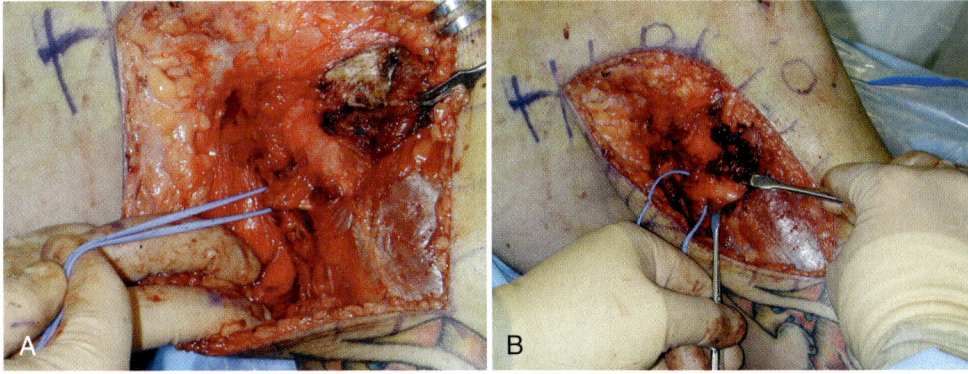

Figure 60-6. Isolation of the peroneal nerve during surgical reduction of the proximal tibiofibular joint.

of symptoms for even a long while (see Fig. 60-1). Recurrent symptoms of instability can be corrected by a supportive strap placed 1 cm below the fibular head, as well as by hamstring and gastrocnemius muscle strengthening. When the strap is placed too tightly, it can cause peroneal nerve palsy; thus, the strap should be worn only during activities that produce symptoms.[13,39,42,46]

In cases of irreducible dislocation in which closed reduction fails, surgical intervention, commonly open reduction, is advised.[1,4,32,46] Closed reduction can fail if the proximal fibula is caught anteriorly on the lateral tibial ridge and the lateral collateral ligament remains intact and taut.[4] Following open reduction, the joint should be stabilized using temporary cannulated screw fixation,[20] tricortical screw fixation,[36] Kirschner wires,[1,24,32,46] or a Steinmann pin,[29] combined with primary repair of the torn capsule and injured ligaments. Rajkumar described open reduction and internal fixation using bioabsorbable pins in a professional soccer player with good results.[34] In the presence of acute injury to the posterolateral structures, primary repair of these structures is associated with favorable outcomes.[50] Regardless of the surgical intervention, careful attention to avoidance of injury to the common peroneal nerve is important[5,9,18] (Fig. 60-6A and B).

MacGiobain et al described a surgical procedure performed to reduce an anterolateral dislocation after closed reduction failed. A short incision was made anterior to the joint, and the biceps femoris tendon was partly dissected off the fibular head. The reduction was maintained with a K wire that was removed electively 6 weeks following surgery, and the patient was found to have full function 12 weeks after surgery.[24]

Although arthrodesis is successful at reducing pain symptoms,[10] it predisposes the ankle joint to increased pain and instability by preventing rotation of the fibula, consequently transferring rotational forces to the ankle.[29,30] Arthrodesis is performed by isolating and protecting the peroneal nerve, after which the articular surfaces of the joint are denuded to bleeding subchondral bone (Fig. 60-7). The joint is reduced and fixed with cancellous lag screws (Fig. 60-8A through C). It is immobilized for 5 weeks; full weight bearing can be started after 8 weeks.[42] The authors recommend resecting 1.5 cm of the fibula at the junction of the proximal and middle thirds to reduce stress applied to the fibula and transferred to the ankle, which decreases the probability of further injury[3,12,29] (Fig. 60-9A through C).

Fibular head resection may be used when peroneal nerve symptoms or palsy associated with proximal tibiofibular

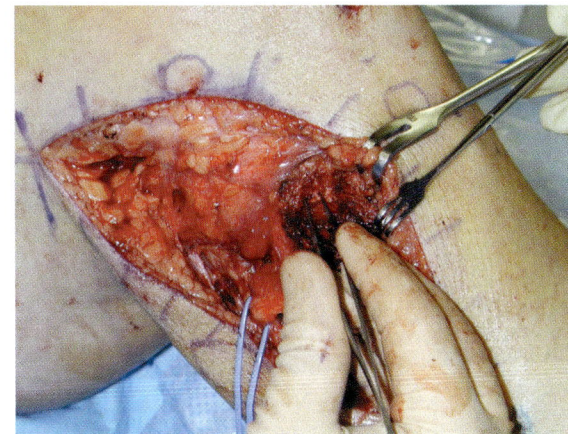

Figure 60-7. Identification of the proximal tibiofibular joint anteriorly.

subluxation or dislocations are present.[5,29,30] The head and neck of the fibula should be excised while the styloid process and the lateral collateral ligament are left intact. The lateral collateral ligament is then secured to the underlying tibia.[30,46] Scar tissue observed around the peroneal nerve should be treated with neurolysis.[30] This procedure successfully reduces pain symptoms but may cause chronic ankle pain and knee instability.[6,13] Fibular head resection is not recommended for children, whose physes are at risk for injury, or athletes, for whom instability can cause damage to the posterolateral structures of the knee. Both fibular head resection and arthrodesis could have negative effects on the epiphyseal plate of the proximal fibula, leading to unequal growth of the tibia and fibula.[48]

Patients experiencing recurrent instability have seen success in reconstruction of the ligamentous structures supporting the proximal tibiofibular joint in limited studies. Giachino[12] reported two cases of ligamentous reconstruction with good results, no recurrent pain or instability, and a return to previous activity levels. He described using one half of a posterior strip of biceps femoris tendon still attached distally to the fibular head and a 10-cm rolled strip of deep fascia of the anterolateral compartment of the leg still attached proximally to the fibular head. The common peroneal nerve is isolated, the lateral head of the gastrocnemius muscle is retracted, and the soleal attachment to the posterior part of the proximal tibiofibular joint is dissected to expose

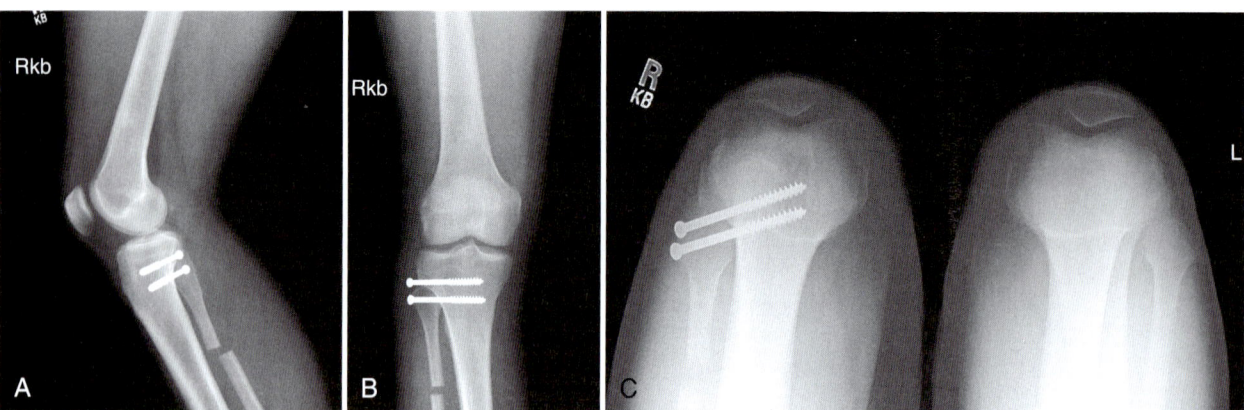

Figure 60-8. Radiographs taken during follow-up show fixation of the proximal tibiofibular joint using cancellous lag screws. **A,** Lateral. **B,** Anteroposterior. **C,** Merchant views.

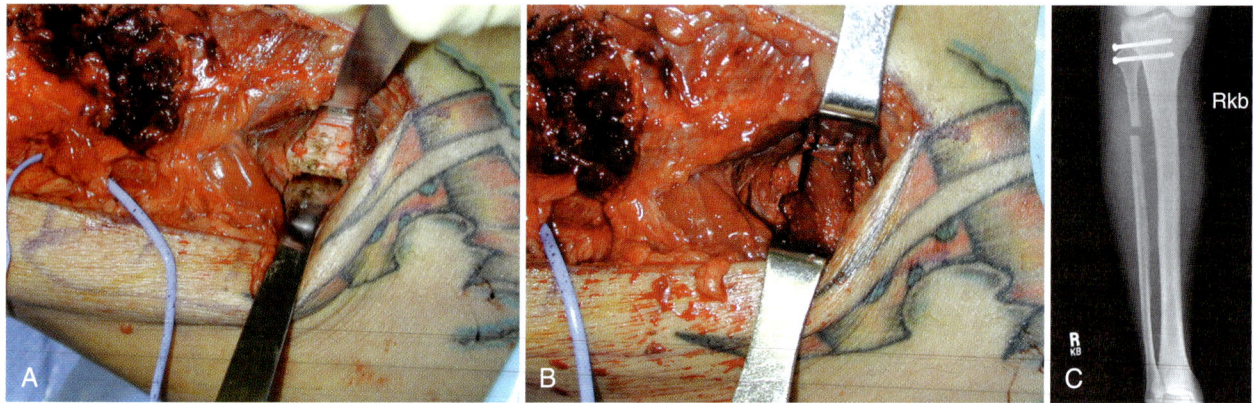

Figure 60-9. Surgical dissection during proximal tibiofibular joint stabilization. **A** and **B,** Before and after osteotomy. **C,** Anteroposterior radiograph depicting resection of the middle third of the fibula following arthrodesis.

the posterior surface of the proximal tibia. A hole is drilled from anterior to posterior in the tibia, and the two new ligaments are wrapped around the head of the fibula with the proximal tibiofibular joint held reduced. The grafts are passed through the tibial drill hole from posterior to anterior and are anchored to the fascia anteriorly. The knee is immobilized for 6 weeks with subsequent progressive weight bearing.

Alternatively, Shapiro[40] reported using a 20 × 2-cm strip of iliotibial band, still connected to its insertion on Gerdy's tubercle, that is tubularized and then passed through a drill hole in the tibia at a level just proximal to Gerdy's tubercle. The graft is passed through the posterior capsule and the arcuate complex, then through a drill hole from posterior to anterior in the reduced fibula at the fibular head/neck junction. The graft is placed deep to the lateral collateral ligament from anterior to posterior and tightened, then is secured to itself and the posterior capsule.

Van den Bekerom et al reviewed eight surgical stabilization procedures that produced highly successful results. The technique involved an open approach to the proximal tibiofibular joint, mobilization of the common peroneal nerve, fixation with one cancellous screw, and subsequent screw removal after 3 to 6 months.[47]

Nikolaides et al reported successful reduction of an inferior dislocation by open reduction and internal fixation with K wires. Fractures in the fibular shaft were fixed with plate fixation, and fractures in the ankle and fibular head were fixed with K wires. After 12 months, the patient was able to walk without crutches using a knee brace.[26]

Postsurgical management usually includes immobilization of the ankle and knee joints for 6 weeks in a non–weight-bearing status, with temporary fixation devices removed between 6 and 12 weeks. Gradual return to full weight-bearing status and initiation of muscle-strengthening and range-of-motion exercise can begin after fixation devices are removed.[32,46] Accurate diagnoses are very important, as strengthening of the lower leg muscles of a patient with anterolateral dislocation would enhance joint instability and increase symptoms.

CONCLUSION

We believe it is important to have a suspicion of a proximal tibiofibular dislocation/subluxation when a patient presents with lateral knee pain as part of the differential. Correct diagnosis of chronic subluxation of the joint versus acute injury is important to avoid long-term complications. Treatment of a proximal tibiofibular injury should be conservative when appropriate. When closed reduction fails, open reduction should be performed with capsular and ligamentous repairs ± surgical reconstruction versus surgical arthrodesis.

KEY REFERENCES

Baciu CC, Tudor A, Olaru I: Recurrent luxation of the superior tibio-fibular joint in the adult. Acta Orthop Scand 45:772–777, 1974.

Dennis JB, Rutledge BA: Bilateral recurrent dislocations of the superior tibiofibular joint with peroneal-nerve palsy. J Bone Joint Surg Am 40:1146–1148, 1958.

Falkenberg P, Nygaard H: Isolated anterior dislocation of the proximal tibiofibular joint. J Bone Joint Surg Br 65:310–311, 1983.

Ogden JA: Dislocation of the proximal fibula. Radiology 105:547–549, 1972.

Ogden JA: Subluxation and dislocation of the proximal tibiofibular joint. J Bone Joint Surg Am 56:145–154, 1974.

Ogden JA: Subluxation of the proximal tibiofibular joint. Clin Orthop Relat Res 101:192–197, 1974.

Ogden JA: The anatomy and function of the proximal tibiofibular joint. Clin Orthop Relat Res 101:186–191, 1974.

Parkes JC, 2nd, Zelko RR: Isolated acute dislocation of the proximal tibiofibular joint: case report. J Bone Joint Surg Am 55:177–183, 1973.

Resnick D, Newell JD, Guerra J, Jr, et al: Proximal tibiofibular joint: anatomic-pathologic-radiographic correlation. AJR Am J Roentgenol 131:133–138, 1978.

Sekiya JK, Kuhn JE: Instability of the proximal tibiofibular joint. J Am Acad Orthop Surg 11:120–128, 2003.

Turco VJ, Spinella AJ: Anterolateral dislocation of the head of the fibula in sports. Am J Sports Med 13:209–215, 1985.

Van Seymortier P, Ryckaert A, Verdonk P, et al: Traumatic proximal tibiofibular dislocation. Am J Sports Med 36:793–798, 2008.

Veltri DM, Warren RF: Treatment of acute and chronic injuries to the posterolateral and lateral knee. Oper Tech Sports Med 4:174–181, 1996.

Full references for this chapter can be found on www.expertconsult.com.

SECTION 6

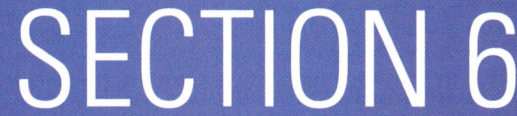

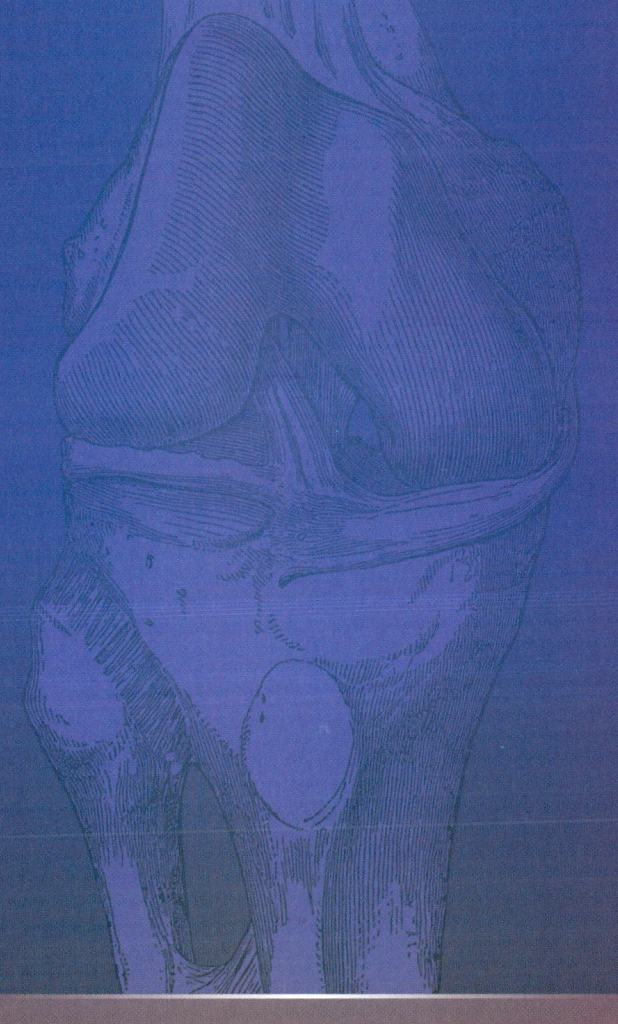

**Sports Medicine:
Patellar and
Extensor Mechanism
Disorders**

Disorders of the Patellofemoral Joint

David DeJour and Paulo R. F. Saggin

BASIC ANATOMY AND BIOMECHANICS

The patella is the biggest sesamoid bone in the human body. It is the link from the powerful quadriceps muscle to the patellar tendon. The patella is the connection element in the extensor mechanism, receiving the convergent quadriceps' fibers in its superior pole and the patellar tendon in its inferior pole.

Only the superior two thirds of the patella have an articular surface. The distal pole is extra-articular and serves as the patellar tendon insertion. Its anterior surface is convex, and on its articular side, the patella is divided by a longitudinal median ridge. This ridge divides the patella into medial and lateral facets, but overall, seven facets are described. A transverse ridge may also exist. In the most medial zone there is a secondary ridge, which delineates the odd facet. The cartilage in the articular surface of the patella is the thickest in the human body, reaching up to 7 mm.

Patellar shape, however, is not constant. Three different patellar types have been described by Wiberg,[110] and a type 4 was later described by Baumgartl, the "Jaegerhut" patella, with no medial facet and consequently no median ridge (Fig. 61-1).

A rich arterial plexus supply is present. A complex vascular anastomotic ring lying in the thin layer of loose connective tissue that covers the dense fibrous rectus expansions surrounds the patella. Six main arteries compound this ring. Two intraosseous systems were described by Scapinelli[93]: the mid patellar vessels, which enter the vascular foramina situated in the anterior surface; and a second system, which arises from the polar vessels, from the anastomosis behind the patellar ligament. Later, Bjorkstrom[8] described vessels entering from the quadriceps and from the medial and lateral retinacula.

The trochlea is situated in the distal part of the femur. The normal trochlea is formed by medial and lateral facets, divided by the trochlear groove (TG). The lateral facet is bigger and more prominent, and extends more proximally than the medial facet. Distally, in the transition from the trochlea to the femoral condyles, a groove can be observed in each side. The medial condylotrochlear groove is discrete and at times almost imperceptible; the lateral groove is more marked. The trochlear groove ends in the notch, and this can roughly serve as a reference for establishing surgical trochlear limits—distally from the notch, in a V-shaped form, going proximally through the grooves. Proximally, before the cartilage starts, cortical bone is covered by adipose tissue and synovium, which avoids patellar contact with the cortical femoral bone.

The TG deepens distally, and some controversy still exists regarding its orientation. If its deepest points are taken into account, the natural TG is most often aligned so that it deviates distally and laterally in relation to the femoral shaft axis.[97]

The quadriceps muscle is formed by four parts: rectus femoris, vastus medialis, vastus lateralis, and vastus intermedius. These muscles converge to a tendon 5 to 8 cm superior to the patella. Fibrous expansions arise from the vastus lateralis and medialis, blending with the lateral and medial retinacula, respectively. The most inferior part of the vastus medialis is known as the vastus medialis obliquus (VMO) and inserts in the patella at a mean of 47 ± 5 degrees from the femoral axis in the coronal plane.[34] Similarly, a vastus lateralis obliquus can be described, with a more vertical orientation (35 ± 4 degrees).

The patellar tendon arises from the inferior pole of the patella. Its average length is 4.6 cm (3.5 to 5.5 cm), and its width is between 24 and 33 mm.[87] It inserts in the tibial tubercle, which usually is a little lateralized in relation to the long axis of the tibia; thus the distal orientation of the patellar tendon is also lateralized (valgus). The posterior part of the patellar tendon is separated from the synovial membrane of the joint by the infra-patellar fat pad, and from the tibia, more distally, by a bursa.

Medially, the retinacular expansion of the vastus medialis merges with layers 1 and 2. Other portions of the middle layer persist as a separate layer, forming the medial patellofemoral ligament (MPFL), below the deep fascia and superficial to the joint capsule. The MPFL runs transversely from the patella to the femur. Some controversy exists about its femoral insertion, but it seems reasonable to define it as near the medial epicondyle, just proximal and posterior to it, distal to the adductor tubercle. The patellar attachment is wider than the femoral one, extending from the proximal and medial corner of the patella over approximately half of its length.[5] The mean length of the MPFL is 53 to 55 mm, and its width varies between studies, ranging from 3 to 30 mm and widening at its attachments.[5,19,87,106] As it approximates the patella, it is overlaid by the distal part of the VMO, and some of its fibers merge into the deep aspect of the muscle. Other bands with secondary functions have been described that link the patella to the tibia and the medial meniscus.

On the lateral side, the superficial oblique retinaculum runs from the iliotibial band (ITB) to the patella. The epicondylopatellar band, the transverse retinaculum (from the ITB to the patella), and the patellotibial band form the deep transverse retinaculum. This connection from the ITB may play a role in patellar lateral displacement and explains the contribution of a tight ITB to patellofemoral pathology.

Patellofemoral biomechanics can be understood as a complex interplay of factors that allow the quadriceps to exert its primary functions—knee extension and deceleration—especially during gait. To allow proper function, one must assume that the patella is located in the trochlear groove and that no instability is present. Continuity of the extensor mechanism should be mandatory to allow

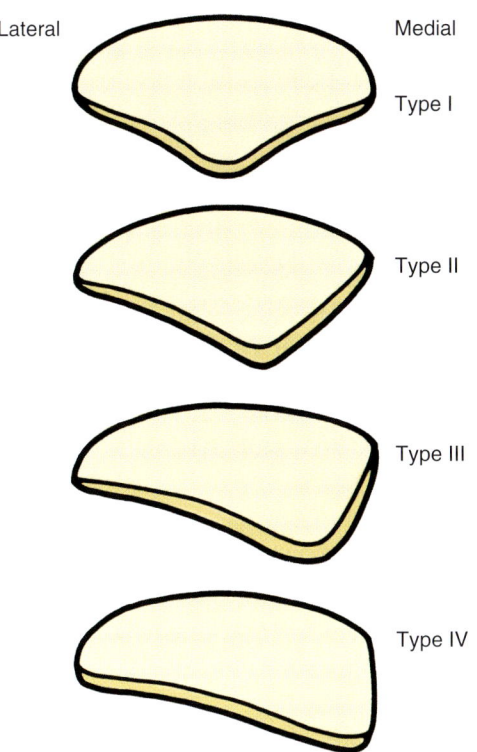

Figure 61-1. The four types of patella according to the Wiberg classification as seen on axial views are illustrated here.

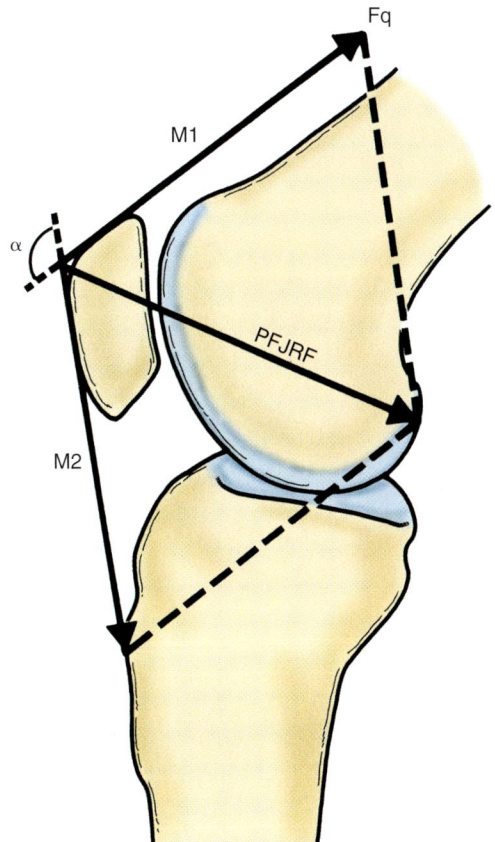

Figure 61-2. The patellofemoral joint reaction force (PFJRF) becomes higher as the knee flexion angle increases. In complete extension, M1 and M2 are in opposite directions, but in the same plane; the resultant PFJRF is almost zero. As flexion increases, M1 and M2 converge, and the vector PFJRF increases.

proper force transmission, and no pain should be present that would otherwise inhibit the quadriceps function.

The patella increases the moment arm of the extensor mechanism. It concentrates the tension of the converging quadriceps fibers and transmits it to the patellar tendon. In complete extension, a coronal result is produced, and no sagittal forces are expected (this is not completely true, as the retinacula exert some posterior displacement forces in the patella when the knee is near extension). As the knee flexes, however, a posteriorly directed force vector becomes clear, and this raises the patellofemoral joint reaction force. The greater the degree of flexion, the greater is the resultant force vector[53] (Fig. 61-2).

This posteriorly directed resultant vector is also important for patellar stability in the coronal plane. The trochlear lateral facet is deeper near the TG and becomes more prominent (higher) as it extends laterally. The patellar shape follows this principle: the crest is posterior, and the lateral facet more anterior. Thus, the articulation of the patellofemoral (PF) lateral facets is not in the coronal plane but is oblique in relation to it, with its more medial part posterior to its more lateral part. As a result, when the quadriceps contracts, the resultant posteriorly directed force vector tends to bring the mobile part of the articulation (the patella) medially.

Also in the coronal plane, multiple quadriceps insertions should be noted, along with their different angles of action. The VMO and the vastus lateralis obliquus (VLO) mainly act in an oblique manner in relation to the longitudinal direction. Based on this, malfunctioning of one (VMO) or hyperfunctioning of the other (VLO) can cause coronal displacement and, to a greater extent, instability. If the force-producing capacity of each muscle head is proportionate to its cross-sectional area, the VMO could contribute 10% to total quadriceps tension, and if completely relaxed, it can cause tension to swing laterally to approximately 6 degrees[34] (Fig. 61-3).

The angle of the quadriceps insertion and the angle difference of the patellar tendon insertion are other causes of a laterally directed force vector (valgus orientation of the extensor mechanism). This difference can be measured during the physical examination by tracing two lines that intersect each other in the center of the patella: one is traced from the patella to the anterior iliac spine, representing the quadriceps tension line; the other is traced from the patella to the tibial tubercle and represents the patellar tendon reaction force line. This is called the Q angle, and in normal subjects, it is expected to not exceed 15 or 20 degrees. Women have the greatest values.

Soft tissue restraints also play a fundamental role in coronal plane force balance. In complete extension, normal patellae are not engaged in the trochlear groove. This engagement starts at approximately 20 degrees of flexion, when the distal and lateral part of the patella touches the upper and proximal part of the trochlea, which comprises the lateral facet. Because the patella is not engaged before this point, only soft tissue stabilizers act to ensure its coronal location. On the lateral side, the retinaculum is directly linked to the ITB, and tension in the ITB causes the patella to track in a more lateral direction.[63] On the medial side, the MPFL contributes 50% to 60% of the restraint to patellar lateral displacement at 0 to 20 degrees of flexion, with a mean failure load of 208 N.[5,79] Although MPFL insufficiency is not the cause of lateral dislocation, one cannot assume lateral dislocation without its insufficiency or rupture.

With initial patellofemoral contact, as a result of the articular surface orientation, a medial patellar shift is produced when the patella engages and follows the trochlear groove. As the flexion angle of the knee is increased, the contact area of the patella progresses proximally, while the trochlear contact area progresses distally. From extension to 90 degrees of flexion, the patella holds the quadriceps tendon away from the femur, but with additional degrees of flexion, an extensive area of contact is formed between the tendon and the trochlea. At between 90 and 135 degrees of flexion, the patella rotates and the ridge that separates the medial and odd facets engages the femoral condyle. At 135 degrees, separate lateral and medial (limited to the odd facet) contact areas are formed[40,41] (Fig. 61-4).

PATELLOFEMORAL DISORDERS: ANALYSIS

Clinical Symptoms

Pain: In patellofemoral disorders, pain is usually anterior, not well localized, and diffuse. It may be referred to the medial retinaculum or, more rarely, to the lateral retinaculum. Sometimes the pain is located below the patella as a bar. Posterior knee pain, although rare, may also be possible, especially if an articular effusion is present. Usually, the pain is worse during or after activities that overload this joint, such as those that demand jumping, running, or vigorous quadriceps contraction. It can also be felt during stair climbing or descending. Patellofemoral joint reaction force reaches 3.3 times body weight in stair climbing or descending, and 7.6 times during squatting.[62,88] Prolonged sitting with the knees flexed is a classical situation that produces or increases patellofemoral pain; this is commonly known as the "movie sign" (or "theater sign"). Although classic, this sign is not specific.

Instability or feeling of instability: Instability is not the best definition for patellar dislocation. The word "instability" describes better the subjective feeling of an unstable knee.

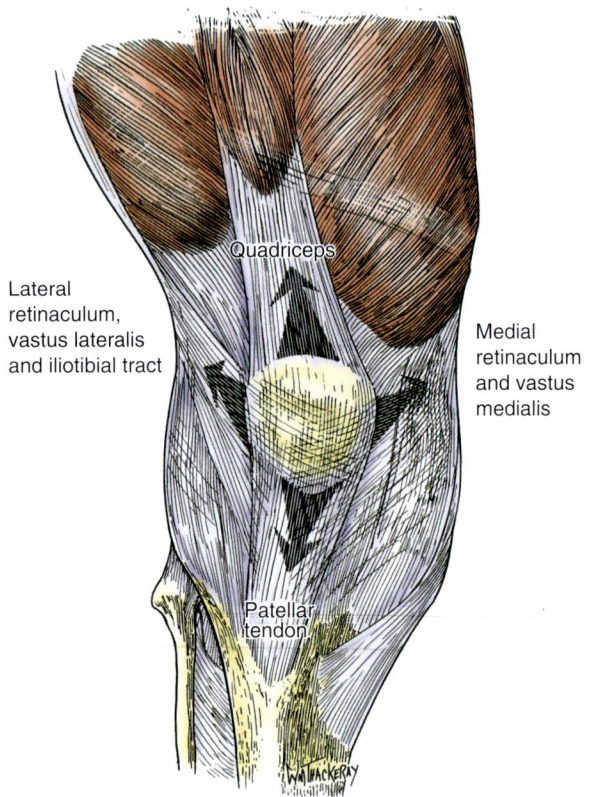

Figure 61-3. Anatomic view showing the valgus alignment of the extensor mechanism and the oblique contributions of medial retinaculum, vastus medialis, lateral retinaculum, vastus lateralis, and iliotibial tract.

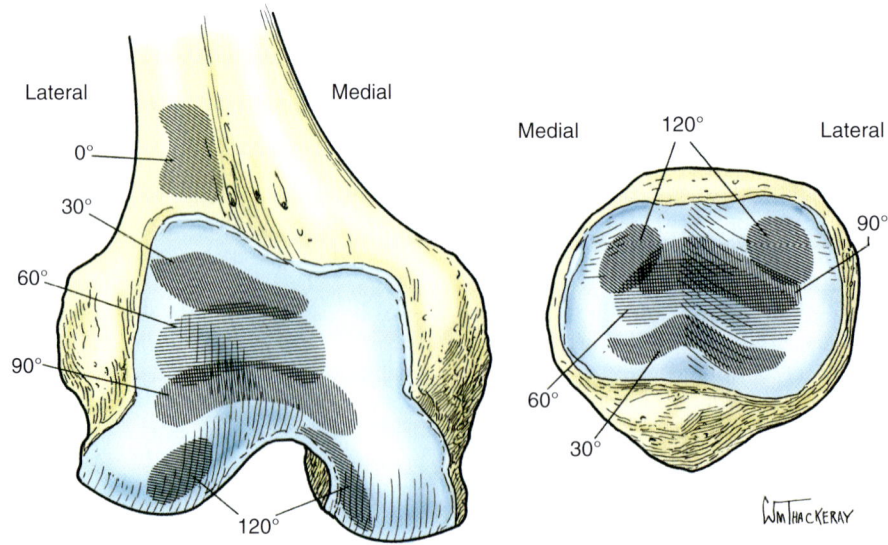

Figure 61-4. Illustration demonstrating the patellofemoral joint contact areas according to the knee flexion angle.

Instability may be objective, as found in patellar dislocation. It is a mechanical phenomenon whereby the patella loses contact with the trochlea. It first occurs during high-energy activity and is always followed by an effusion, hemarthrosis, or even sometimes hematoma, caused by capsule rupture and subcutaneous blood diffusion.

Instability may also be subjective, caused by quadriceps inhibition (reflex) as the result of pain, without loss of contact of the articulating surfaces. It occurs with low-energy activities, such as walking or ascending or descending stairs.

Careful analysis of the clinical history and the patient's description of the episode is useful in differentiating them. Objective instability is easy to diagnose when the patella is still dislocated, when a medical report indicates that a doctor relocated it, or when x-rays have been taken and show the dislocation or objective signs of it, such as a bone fracture (avulsion) on the medial part of the patella or on the lateral femoral condyle.

Locking or catching: This is the third great complaint and must be differentiated from those produced by meniscal tears. The main difference from meniscal locking is the fact that the knee is not able to flex or to extend, but in a bucket-handle tear the knee is able to flex. Sometimes, locking in extension may be produced by a reflex mechanism of quadriceps and hamstrings contracture due to pain to avoid contact of the opposed cartilage surfaces. Locking episodes are usually momentary, but in some cases can last for longer periods and can be really painful. Catching may be produced by cartilage lesions or by irregularities in the patella or trochlea as they glide over each other.

When collecting the clinical history, the physician should ask about associated conditions, which are common in patellofemoral disorders, such as global pathology—low back pain, hip catching, ankle pain or sprains—and, of course, symptoms in the opposite knee. Time from the onset of symptoms must be determined.

Physical Examination

Physical examination starts by looking at how the patient rises from their chair and walks into the physician's office. This information is interesting because the patient is acting naturally. In the office, evaluation starts with the patient standing. Asymmetry at the level of the shoulders or pelvis is noted when the patient is standing and sitting. The patellae should face forward. If femoral anteversion is present, they will face inward. Coronal and rotational alignments are observed. Genu valgum, tibial torsion, and limb discrepancy are also noted at this moment. The overall extensor mechanism alignment is checked, and the Q angle can be already estimated. From the back of the patient, subtalar eversion, which would produce compensatory internal tibial rotation, should be looked for.

The same observations done when the patient was standing should be done when he is walking. Rotational deformities are especially exacerbated during gait. Muscle hypotrophy can be noted. Any limp will become evident.

With the patient supine and the hips and knees extended, the Q angle measurement can be done effectively. Care should be taken because a laterally displaced patella will cause underestimation of its value. Knee flexion can correct this by bringing the patella into the center of the trochlear groove, but no agreement has been reached on the best Q angle measurement method (flexion or extension), or even on its applicability.[99] Normal individuals, in general, will not present with values greater than 20 degrees.

Asking the patient to contract both quadriceps will allow comparison of the contraction pattern and the muscular mass. The VMO bulk should also be noted at this moment. Active and passive movements of flexion and extension of the knee will allow patellar tracking assessment. The J sign, seen when the patella shifts abruptly medially, and then down in the trochlear groove as flexion progresses, similar to an inverted J, is sometimes found, meaning patellar lateral displacement in extension. Palpation and specific tests are then performed:

Palpation: Palpation should start in the less painful areas. The patella, patellar tendon, quadriceps tendon, and lateral and medial retinacula should be investigated for tenderness. The patellar facets may even be palpated and inspected for tenderness, but it should be noted that some structures (retinacula) are interposed, and this can confuse interpretation of the pain source. The distal-to-proximal position of the patella can be assessed by observation and palpation.

Glide test: Patellar medial and lateral glide should be tested at full extension and at 30 degrees of flexion. For this purpose, one can divide the patella into four vertical quadrants. Displacement of less than 1 quadrant or more than 3 is considered abnormal (Fig. 61-5).

Tilt test: The lateral and medial margins of the patella should be in the same horizontal plane, and its transverse axis should be elevated beyond the horizontal plane. Significant tilt in the physical examination correlates with magnetic resonance imaging (MRI)[46] or computed tomography (CT) scan tilt measures greater than 10 degrees. Anterior palpation should be done during the arc of movement in the search for pain and crepitus. The degree of flexion at the time the signals or symptoms are produced should be noted.

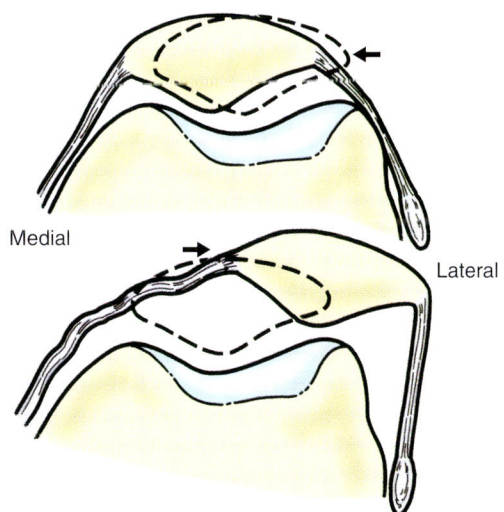

Figure 61-5. Clinical evaluation of mediolateral displacement of the patella. It should be tested at 0 degrees and 30 degrees of knee flexion and recorded in millimeters or quadrants.

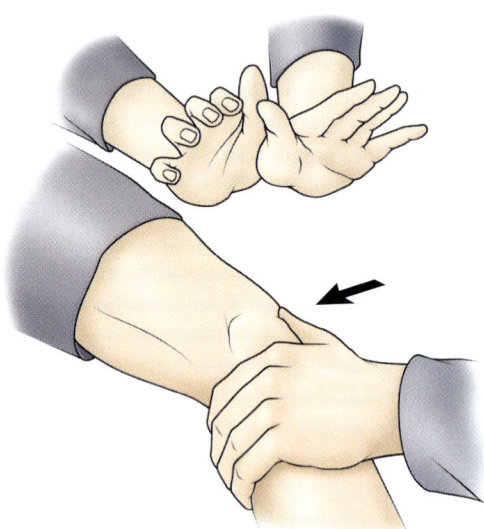

Figure 61-6. The Smillie or apprehension test. The physician displaces the patella laterally, and the patient shows apprehension and fear of dislocation. Test positivity is determined by the patient's reaction, not by the physician's ability to dislocate or sublux the patella.

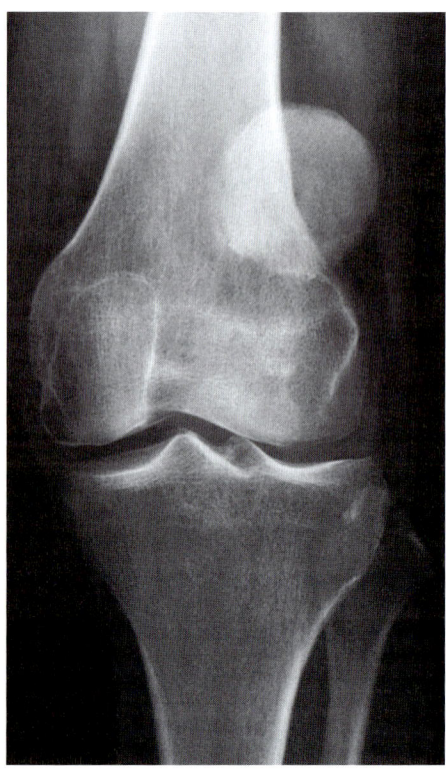

Figure 61-7. In rare cases, patellar tilt and subluxation are so pronounced that they can be evidenced even on anteroposterior (AP) views. In this case, note the high and tilted patella.

Smillie test[98] or **apprehension test:** This is performed with the knee extended. The examiner grasps the patella with his fingers and applies a laterally directed force, trying to dislocate it while holding the tibia with the other hand. This laterally directed force applied over the patella causes apprehension in the patient as he feels that the patella is about to dislocate. It is also called the apprehension test because it is the patient's positive reaction that will determine test positivity. For adequate examination, the quadriceps should be relaxed. The test should be performed bilaterally, and comparison with the opposite side may help. It is not useful in acute dislocations because pain and fear will be present even before the physical examination. In chronic cases, it reflects well the insufficiency of the patellar restraints (notably the MPFL) (Fig. 61-6).

Muscle stiffness: Hamstrings are tested with the patient supine and the opposite leg extended and flat over the table. The hip is flexed 90 degrees, and the knee is then extended as far as possible. The popliteal angle is observed and compared with the opposite side. The quadriceps is tested with the patient prone, and in most patients the heels should touch the buttocks. The ITB is tested with the Ober test: with the patient in lateral decubitus position (the side to be tested is up), the hip is extended and abducted, and the knee is extended. From this position, the thigh is released and is allowed to adduct. Most patients will be able to touch the examination table with the medial aspect of the knee.

IMAGING

X-ray Analysis

X-ray analysis is the first step before any other investigation of the knee is undertaken. Combined with the history and physical examination findings, it will guide and allow subsequent imaging procedures, and at times will even make them unnecessary. The basic protocol is almost uniform to the various situations, chronic or urgent. The only necessary condition is that the patient is able to stand up on the affected limb. Basic standard x-rays are described in the following paragraphs.

AP View

The anteroposterior (AP) view must be done in monopodal stance as long as the patient is able to do so. In younger patients (before 50 years old), it should be performed in 15 to 20 degrees of flexion; in older patients and in those who have antecedents of knee trauma or surgery, it should be done in 30 or 45 degrees of knee flexion (Schuss or Rosenberg). The AP analysis is not really helpful for patellofemoral problems. It will allow bone quality analysis, alignment assessment, and evaluation of femorotibial-associated pathology or arthritis. Gross patellar instability or displacement (Fig. 61-7) can also be observed in this view, along with malformations such as bipartite patella or fracture. A loose body in the lateral gutter may be found, representing a lateral condyle fracture that occurred during patellar dislocation.

In the AP view, we can observe a bipartite or a multipartite patella. It is the result of incomplete fusion of an ossification center and is described to have a frequency between 0.005% and 1.66%.[10,102] The accessory fragments commonly are located close to the superolateral border. The edges of the fragment are smooth, and this allows differentiation from fracture. Bipartite or multipartite patellae are often bilateral.

Lateral View

This is the most interesting view of the knee. The reliability of its interpretation depends on the technical quality of the image. It is essential to have a perfect superimposition of the two posterior condyles. The image is done in monopodal weight bearing with an angle of flexion between 15 and 20 degrees. Some authors propose to take the lateral view in full extension, but its accuracy in determining patellar height is controversial because different degrees of quadriceps contraction could modify the patellar height; also, if the patient has knee hyperextension, this could yield a false-positive patella alta and false information about patellar engagement. Nevertheless, the location of the patella in relation to the trochlea provides interesting data.

X-ray analysis has to be systematic and should follow the guidelines provided in the following sections.

Trochlea

In a normal knee, Blumensaat's line is continued anteriorly by the trochlear groove line, which should stay posterior to the projection of the femoral condyles (facets). In 1987, Henri Dejour described the crossing sign, which characterizes trochlear dysplasia on the sagittal view. The crossing point represents the exact location where the deepest point of the trochlear sulcus reaches the same height as the femoral condyles, meaning that the trochlea becomes flat in this location (Fig. 61-8).

The position of the trochlear sulcus line is abnormal in relation to the anterior femoral cortex. In a study performed by Dejour and associates,[30] in normal knees the trochlear sulcus line was at a mean distance of 0.8 mm posterior to a line projected from the anterior femoral cortex, and in those knees with dysplastic trochleae its mean position was 3.2 mm forward to the same line. This increases the contact force between the patella and the trochlea (anti-Maquet effect) (Fig. 61-9).

The crossing sign has been found in 96% of the population with antecedents of true patellar dislocation, and in only 3% of healthy controls.[29] The first published classification (Henri Dejour) divided dysplasia into three grades, according to the

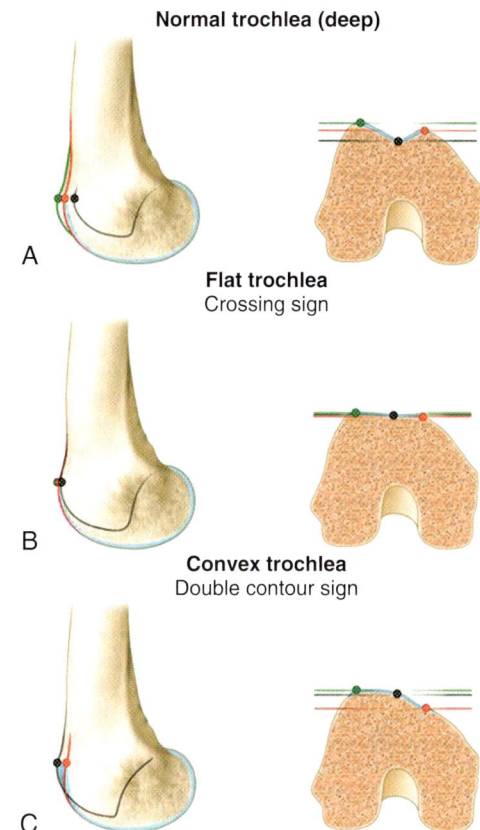

Figure 61-8. In a normal trochlea, the trochlear groove is posterior to the facets **(A)**. In a flat trochlea, the facets and the trochlear groove are in the same plane. In the lateral view, this is demonstrated by the crossing sign **(B)**. When the trochlea is convex, the "groove" does not exist, and the lateral part of the trochlea rests in front of the medial facet, which can be demonstrated in lateral view as the double-contour sign **(C)**.

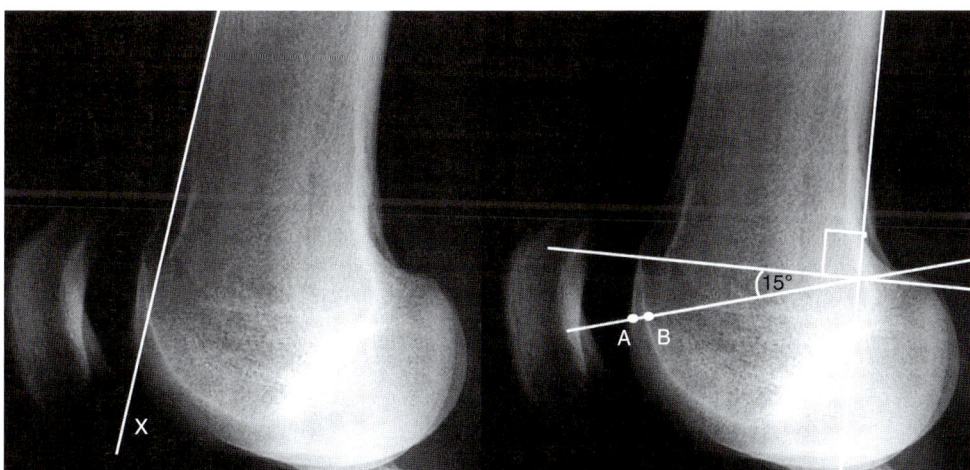

Figure 61-9. Trochlear groove position and depth in relation to the anterior femoral cortex. A line *(X)* is drawn tangential to the anterior femoral cortex along its most distal 10 cm, extending below the articular surface. The trochlear sulcus is anterior to this line *(left figure)*. The trochlear depth is the distance *A/B* (measured in millimeters) along a line subtended 15 degrees from the perpendicular to the tangent of the posterior femoral cortex *(right figure)*.

level of the crossing sign. Other noted signs included the following: (1) the deepness of the trochlea as measured by a line that traced 15 degrees from another one perpendicular to the femoral shaft and tangential to the posterior condyles (see Fig. 61-9), and (2) the "bump," which was defined as the distance between a line drawn tangential to the anterior femoral cortex and the highest point of the trochlea.

The classification in three grades has some limitations, as was corroborated by the work of Remy and colleagues.[89,90] They showed that interobserver reproducibility of trochlear analysis was low, especially for type II dysplasia. This led to a new study performed in 1996 by Dejour and Le Coultre, which analyzed 177 cases of patellar instability and included radiographs along with preoperative and postoperative CT scans. Based on this analysis, a new and more precise classification with four grades of trochlear dysplasia was defined.[26,28] Two new signs were added to the crossing sign. The first is the supratrochlear spur, which represents a global prominence of the trochlea and plays a role similar to a ski jump when the patella engages the trochlea. The second sign is the double contour, which is the radiographic line that ends below the crossing sign and represents the subchondral condensation of the hypoplastic medial facet on the lateral view. In 2002, the Lillois group conducted a new interobserver study[91] and concluded that "this new classification system is more reproducible than the former 3-type system proposed. The crossing sign and the supratrochlear spur are the most reproducible signs" (Fig. 61-10).

This classification system (Figs. 61-11 and 61-12) is based mainly in the lateral view, although CT may assist in differentiation between types. Four types, based on the three dysplastic signs described, are included:

- Type A: presence of crossing sign in the true lateral view. The trochlea is shallower than normal but is still symmetrical and concave.
- Type B: crossing sign and trochlear spur. The trochlea is flat in axial images. All of the trochlea is prominent.
- Type C: presence of crossing sign and the double-contour sign on the lateral view. No prominence is seen,

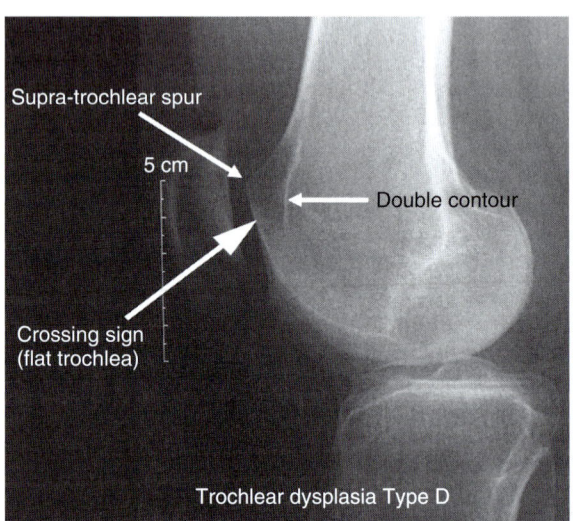

Figure 61-10. For analysis of trochlear dysplasia, a true profile is needed with a perfect superimposition of the posterior femoral condyles. The three trochlear dysplasia signs are the following: the crossing sign; the supratrochlear spur; and the double-contour sign, which goes below the crossing sign.

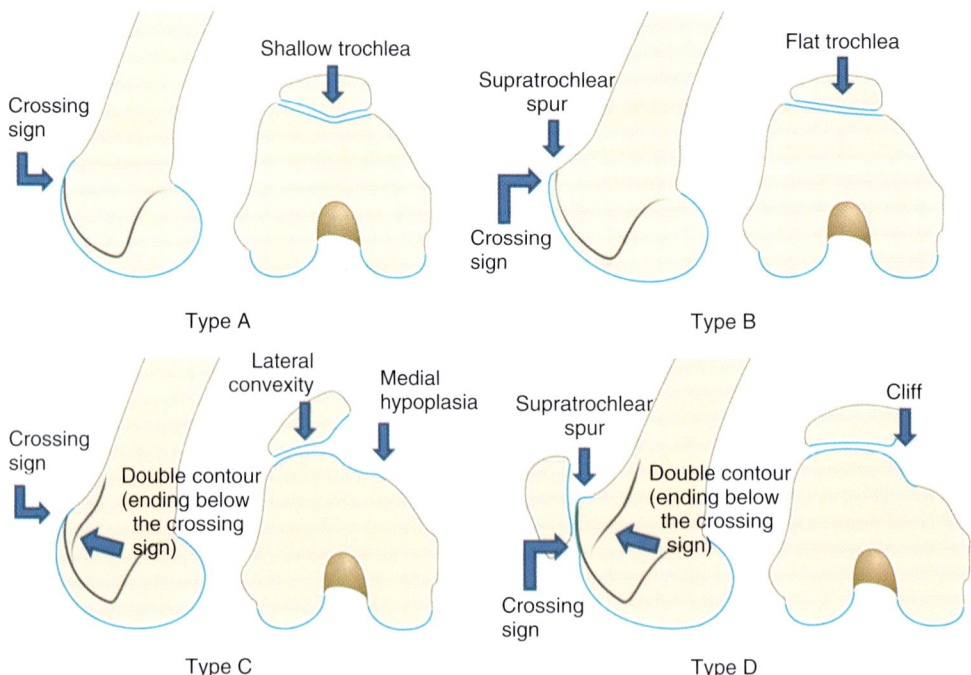

Figure 61-11. Trochlear dysplasia classification according to Dejour. Type A: crossing sign in lateral true view is present. The trochlea is shallower than normal but is still symmetrical and concave. Type B: crossing sign and trochlear spur. The trochlea is flat or convex on axial images. Type C: the crossing sign and the double-contour sign (the second representing the densification of the subchondral bone of the medial hypoplastic facet). On axial computed tomography (CT) scan views, the lateral facet is convex. Type D: all mentioned signs are combined, that is, crossing sign, supratrochlear spur, and double-contour sign that goes below the crossing sign. On axial CT scan views, a cliff pattern is seen.

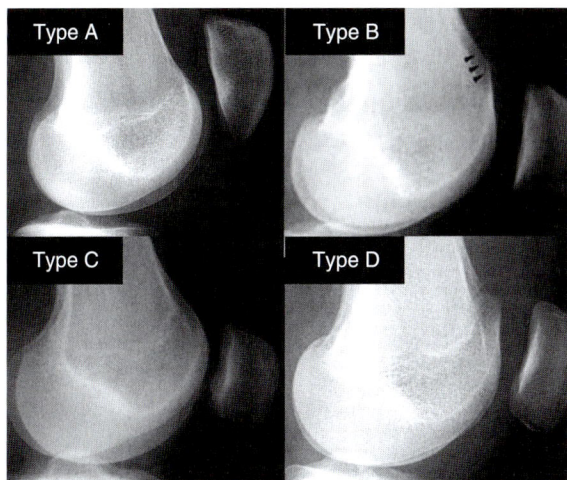

Figure 61-12. Trochlear dysplasia assessed in lateral views. The crossing sign, the supratrochlear spur, and the double-contour sign should be assessed to classify it. *Type A:* only crossing sign is present. *Type B:* crossing sign and trochlear spur can be seen. *Type C:* crossing sign and double-contour sign representing the medial hypoplastic facet are present. *Type D:* all the mentioned signs are combined: crossing sign, supratrochlear spur, and double-contour sign.

and in axial views, the lateral facet is convex and the medial facet hypoplastic.
- Type D: combines all previously mentioned signs, which are the crossing sign, supratrochlear spur, and double-contour sign. In the axial view, clear asymmetry of the height of the facets, also referred to as a cliff pattern, is evident.

Patella

Grelsamer et al[44] did a study describing three types of patella, based on the ratio between the length of the patella and the length of the articular surface. Most patellae exhibit a ratio between 1.2 and 1.5 and are classified as type I. Those with a ratio greater than 1.5 give the appearance of having a long nose; this is type II. Those with a ratio less than 1.2 (short nose) are type III (Fig. 61-13).

The shape of the patella on the lateral view is correlated with the tilt and with the global morphology of the patella. In a normal patella, with no tilt, the most posterior part visible in the lateral view should be the median longitudinal ridge. The lateral facet projection is located slightly anterior. In tilted patellae, these relations are lost, and the overall anteroposterior size of the patella appears increased (Fig. 61-14).

The tilt evaluation has been described by Maldague and Malghem.[69] Three positions are described: normal position, in which the lateral facet is in front of the crest; mild tilt, in which the two lines (lateral facet and crest) are on the same level; and severe tilt, which shows the lateral facet behind the crest (Fig. 61-15).

Patellar Height. Patella alta or infera is essentially diagnosed on the lateral view. Patellar height must be measured using an identified index. The main indexes used in the literature are listed here:
- The Caton-Deschamps index[14,15]: ratio between the distance from the lower edge of the patellar articular surface to the anterosuperior angle of the tibia outline

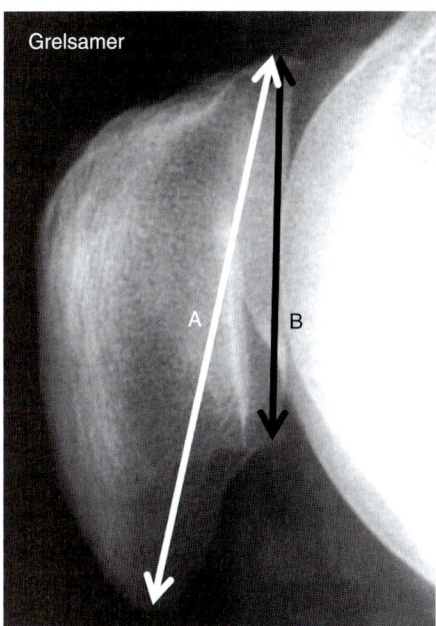

Figure 61-13. Patellar shape on lateral views according to Grelsamer. The ratio *(A/B)* between the length of the patella *(A)* and the length of its articular surface *(B)* is calculated. Most patellae exhibit ratios between 1.2 and 1.5.

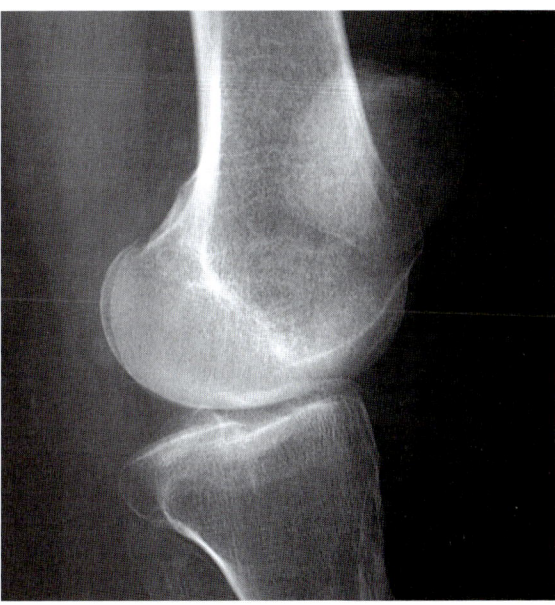

Figure 61-14. Lateral view of severe patellar tilt and subluxation. Note that the projection is a perfect lateral view (perfect posterior condyle superimposition). The patella, however, is not in front of the femur but it is lateral to it, and the patellar anteroposterior diameter is increased. Additionally, severe trochlear dysplasia can be noted.

(AT) and the length of the articular surface of the patella (AP). A ratio (AT/AP) of 0.6 or smaller reveals patella infera, and a ratio greater than 1.2 indicates patella alta (Fig. 61-16).
- The Insall-Salvati index[56]: ratio between the length of the patellar tendon (LT) and the longest sagittal diameter of the patella (LP). Insall determined that this ratio (LT/LP) is normally 1. A ratio smaller than 0.8 indicates

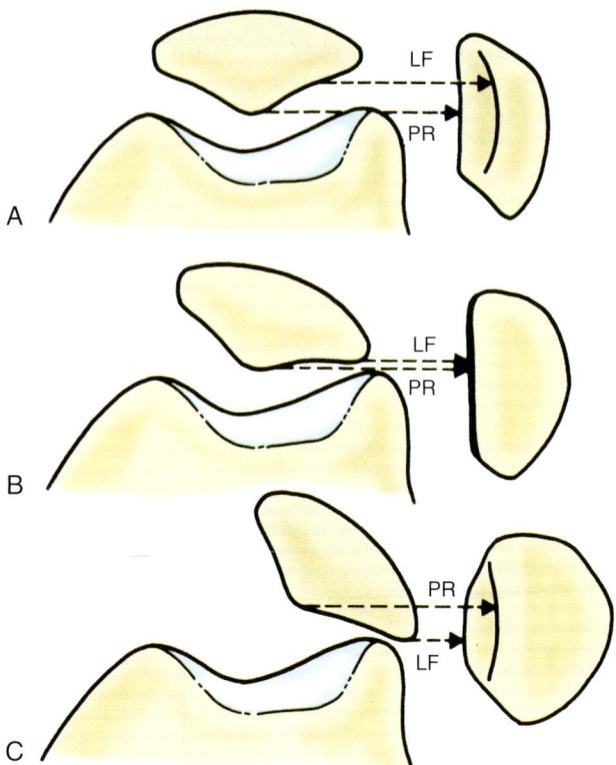

Figure 61-15. Tilt evaluation in lateral views as described by Maldague and Malghem. In the normal position, the lateral facet is in front of the crest. When mild tilt is present, the lateral facet and the crest are on the same level. When severe tilt occurs, the lateral facet is behind the crest.

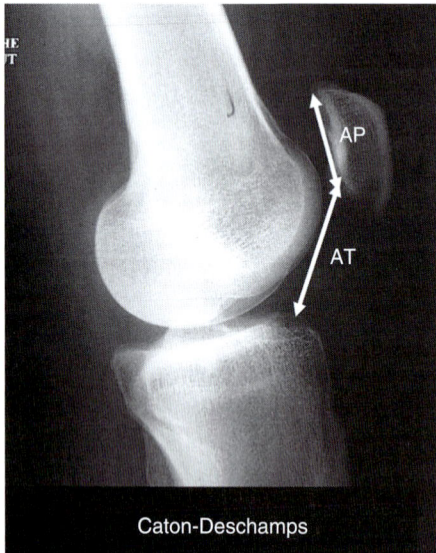

Figure 61-16. The Caton-Deschamps index *(AT/AP)* is the ratio between the distance from the lower edge of the patella's articular surface to the anterosuperior angle of the tibia outline *(AT)* and the length of the articular surface of the patella *(AP)*.

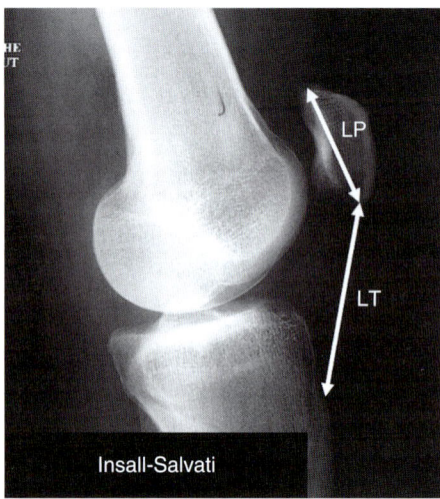

Figure 61-17. The Insall-Salvati index *(LT/LP)* is the ratio between the length of the patellar tendon *(LT)* and the longest sagittal diameter of the patella *(LP)*.

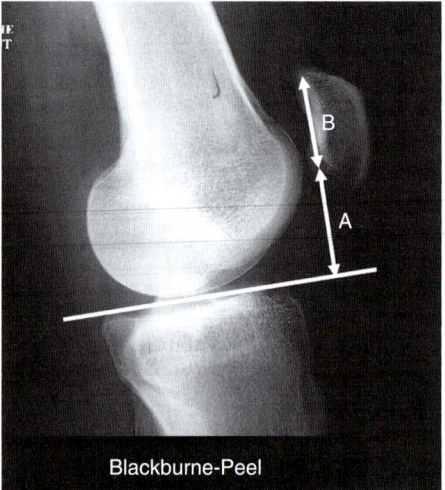

Figure 61-18. The Blackburne-Peel index *(A/B)* is the ratio between the length of the perpendicular line drawn from the tangent to the tibial plateau until the inferior pole of the articular surface of the patella *(A)* and the length of the articular surface of the patella *(B)*.

patella infera, and greater than 1.2 patella alta (Fig. 61-17).

- The Blackburne-Peel index[9]: ratio between the length of the perpendicular line drawn from the tangent to the tibial plateau to the inferior pole of the articular surface

of the patella (A) and the length of the articular surface of the patella (B). The normal ratio (A/B) was defined as 0.8. In patella infera it is smaller than 0.5, and in patella alta it is greater than 1.0 (Fig. 61-18).

Several factors must be considered when a decision is made regarding which index to use. Blackburne-Peel needs good superimposition of medial and lateral tibial plateaus. Insall-Salvati is not a good choice in the presence of Osgood-Schlatter disease or sequelae of it. Finally, the Caton-Deschamps method seems the easiest to use, especially for surgical planning.

Axial View

The axial view has been described at different angles of knee flexion and different positions of the x-ray cassette. Our common approach is to perform 30-degree axial views as described by Ficat, who also described axial views at 60

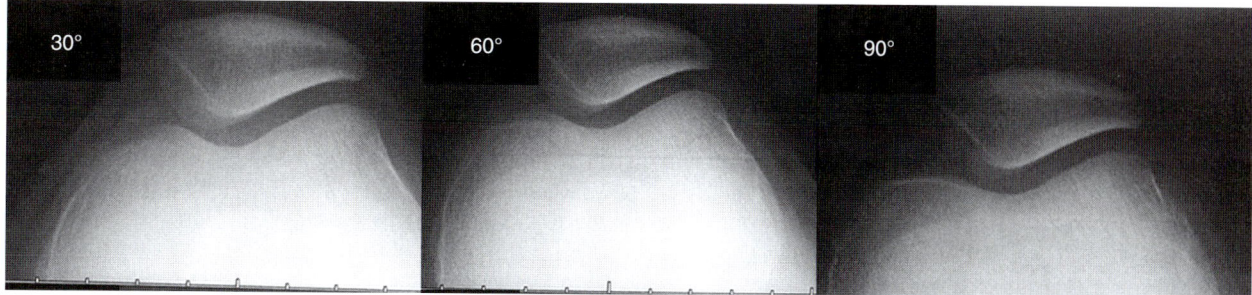

Figure 61-19. Axial views performed at 30, 60, and 90 degrees of knee flexion. Note how the trochlear shape changes as flexion increases and the medial facet seems bigger. It is not necessary to routinely perform 60-degree and 90-degree flexion x-rays in common patellofemoral (PF) disorders.

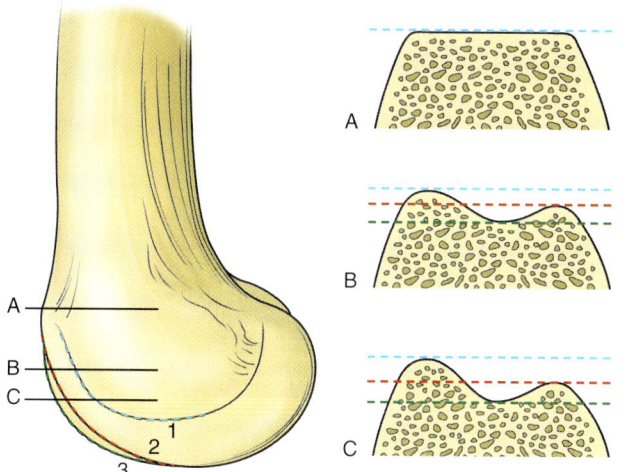

Figure 61-20. Sagittal model demonstrating how, in the same patient, different images can fail to show the abnormal trochlear shape. Proximally *(A)*, the trochlea is flat, but it deepens distally *(B* and *C)*. For this reason, it is important to have a full computed tomography (CT) scan acquisition of the trochlea. Axial views done with angles superior to 30 degrees could miss the proximal trochlear dysplasia.

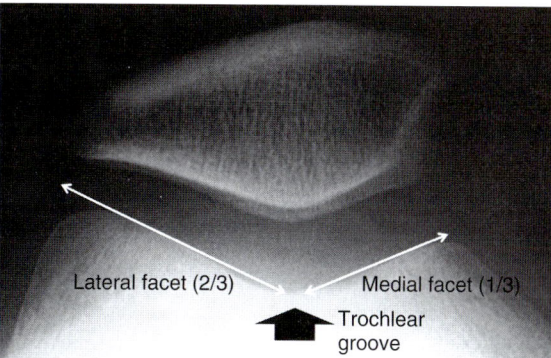

Figure 61-21. Axial view of the patellofemoral articulation at 30 degrees of knee flexion. The medial facet appears smaller and corresponds to one third of the trochlear width, while the lateral facet corresponds to two thirds of it. The patella is centered, and its long axis is horizontal, meaning that no tilt is present.

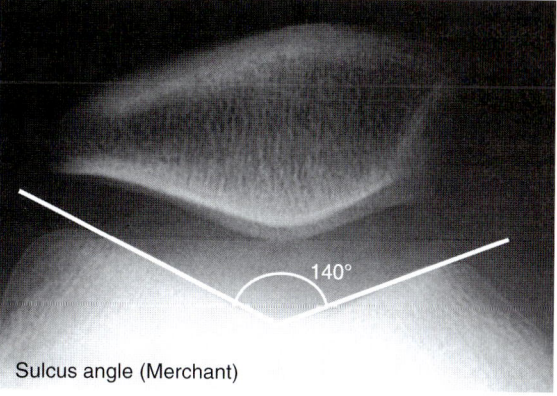

Figure 61-22. The sulcus angle defined by Brattström and popularized by Merchant is the angle formed by the two lines drawn from the deepest point of the trochlear groove to the highest point on the medial and lateral femoral condyles.

degrees and 90 degrees (Fig. 61-19). Radiographs are obtained with the knee flexed over the edge of the table, the beam directed proximally, and a perpendicular cassette in place. Images beyond 45 degrees of flexion, however, are less informative as they show the lower part of the trochlea and the patella as fully engaged, many times correcting tracking abnormalities (Fig. 61-20). These high–flexion angle images are not necessary.[23] Lower flexion angles, although capable of showing better the maltracking signs, are technically demanding and at times impossible. With a well done image, one can assess the relation between the femoral trochlea (at 30 degrees, the lateral facet should appear with two-thirds total trochlear width) (Fig. 61-21) and the patella (with the lateral facet also composing two thirds). Tilt, congruence, and cartilage thickness can also be appreciated.

Alternative methods have been proposed. The main choices are discussed in the following sections.

Merchant View[76]

The Merchant view is obtained with the patient in the supine position and the knees flexed at 45 degrees over the edge of the table. The lower limbs rest on an angled platform. The

x-ray beam is angled toward the feet, 30 degrees from horizontal, and the film cassette is positioned 30 cm below the knees. The x-ray beam strikes the cassette at a 90-degree angle, imaging both knees simultaneously. Two angles are measured on this view: the sulcus angle and the congruence angle.

• The sulcus angle (Fig. 61-22) (defined by Brattström) is the angle formed by two lines drawn from the deepest point of the trochlear groove to the highest point on the medial and lateral femoral condyles. This measurement reveals the shape of the groove; the greater the sulcus angle, the flatter is the trochlea. The average sulcus angle on the merchant view measures 138 degrees (standard deviation [SD] ± 6) and is equal in males and females. Values superior to 150 degrees are considered abnormal.

- The congruence angle (Fig. 61-23) is measured by bisecting the sulcus angle to construct a reference line, and then projecting a second line from the apex of the sulcus angle to the lower point of the subchondral articular surface of the patella (apex). If the line drawn from the patellar apex is lateral to the reference line, then the angle is positive; if the patellar apex is medial to this line, a negative value is assigned; –6 degrees (SD ± 11 degrees; abnormal if greater than +16 degrees).

Laurin View[64,65]

This image is obtained with the patient sitting and the knee flexed 20 degrees. The x-ray cassette is held approximately 12 cm proximal to the patellae and is pushed against the anterior thighs. The x-ray beam is directed cephalic and 20 degrees superior from the horizontal point. Two measurements are made on this view: the lateral patellofemoral angle and the patellofemoral index.

- The lateral patellofemoral angle (LPFA) (Fig. 61-24) is formed when one line connects the superior points of the medial and lateral trochlear facets and a second line is drawn tangent to the lateral facet of the patella. It measures tilt and subluxation and should open laterally in normal knees (97% open laterally and 3% are parallel; no LPFA opening medially was found in normal knees in Laurin's study).
- The patellofemoral index (Fig. 61-25) is the ratio (M/L) between the thickness of the medial joint space (M) and that of the lateral joint space (L). It should measure 1.6 or less (Fig. 61-26).

Malghem and Maldague Lateral Rotation View (30 Degrees LR)[70]

This view is obtained in 30 degrees of knee flexion while one examiner pulls the forefoot laterally. The cassette is held over the patient's thighs, and the x-ray beam is directed cranially. Patellar position (centered or subluxated) is defined according to Merchant's congruence angle. In the authors' series, the 30-degree lateral rotation (LR) view was superior to standard 45-degree axial views in detecting patellar subluxation. In 27 knees operated on for patellar instability, 45-degree routine views depicted subluxation in only seven cases, and 30-degree LR views demonstrated it in all cases. Additionally, when both views showed signs of instability, the degree of subluxation was greater in the 30-degree LR view.

In acute or chronic patellofemoral instability, medial patellar avulsions (Figs. 61-27 and 61-28) can be demonstrated and should not be confused with bipartite patella. Other important data provided by axial views include patellar shape and joint line thickness. Patellar shape is evaluated according to Wiberg's classification (Fig. 61-29). Joint space thickness is diminished in arthritis. Axial views at 30 degrees

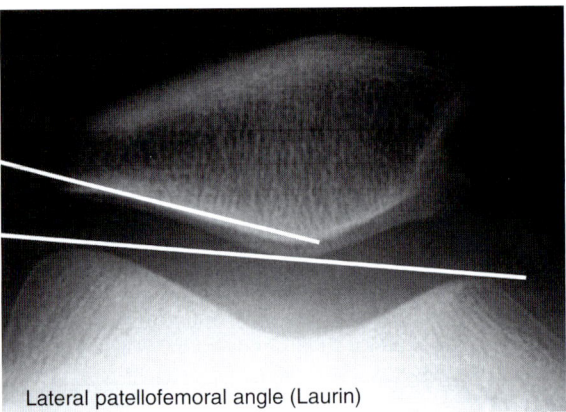

Lateral patellofemoral angle (Laurin)

Figure 61-24. The lateral patellofemoral angle (LPFA) is formed by one line connecting the superior points of medial and lateral trochlear facets and a second line tangent to the lateral facet of the patella.

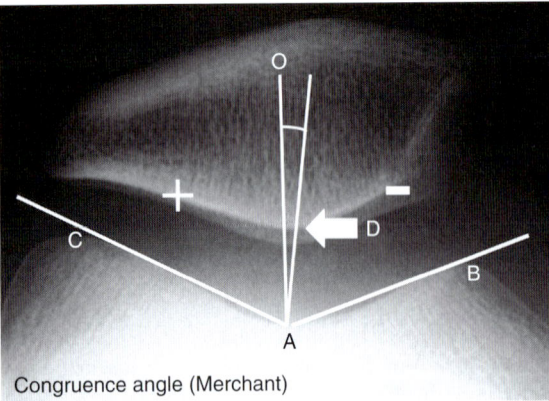

Congruence angle (Merchant)

Figure 61-23. The congruence angle is measured by bisecting the sulcus angle to construct a reference line and then projecting a second line from the apex of the sulcus angle to the lower point of the subchondral articular surface of the patella (apex). If the line drawn from the patellar apex is lateral to the reference line, then the angle is positive; if it is medial to this line, a negative value is assigned.

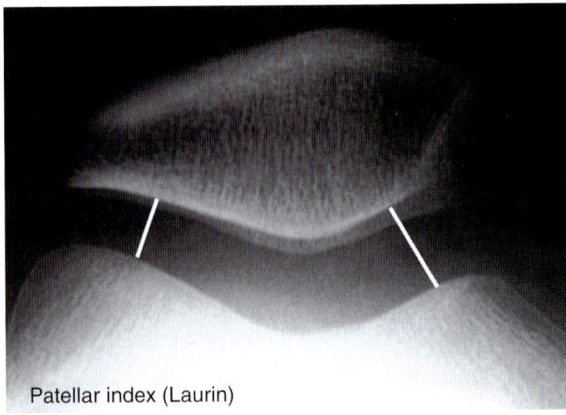

Patellar index (Laurin)

Figure 61-25. The patellofemoral index is the ratio (M/L) between the thickness of the medial joint space (M) and the lateral joint space (L).

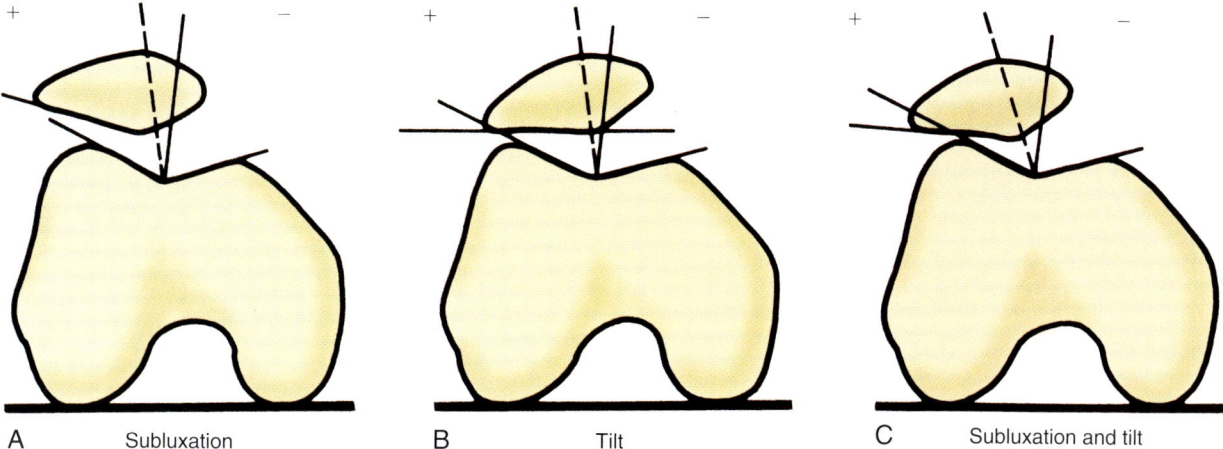

A   Subluxation   B   Tilt   C   Subluxation and tilt

Figure 61-26. **A-C,** Radiologic differentiation between tilt and subluxation. **A,** Subluxation can be detected using the congruence angle (the normal range is demonstrated in the figure). **B,** The congruence angle is within the normal range, but tilt is noted as the patellar transverse axis is lifted off from the horizontal. Another possible method of assessment could be the lateral patellofemoral angle (on computed tomography [CT] scans, the posterior femoral condyles could be used as reference). **C,** Both tilt and subluxation are present.

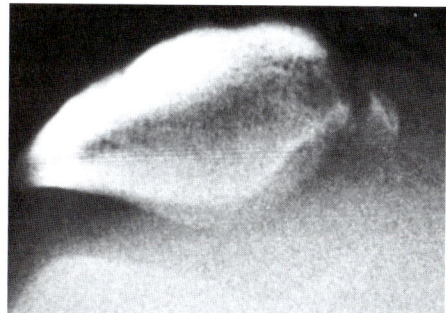

Figure 61-27. Avulsion of the medial aspect of the patella. Note the small osseous fragment corresponding to the patellar insertion of the medial patellofemoral ligament and retinaculum. In addition, a large effusion can be seen, which obscures structure individualization.

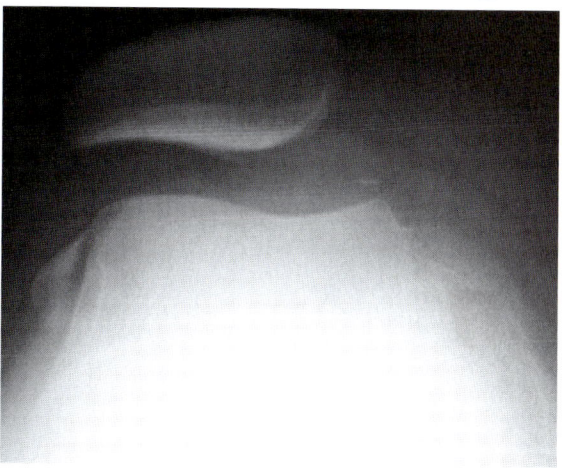

Figure 61-28. Axial view of patellar instability showing a fragment of the lateral femoral condyle fractured during the acute dislocation. Trochlear dysplasia can also be evidenced.

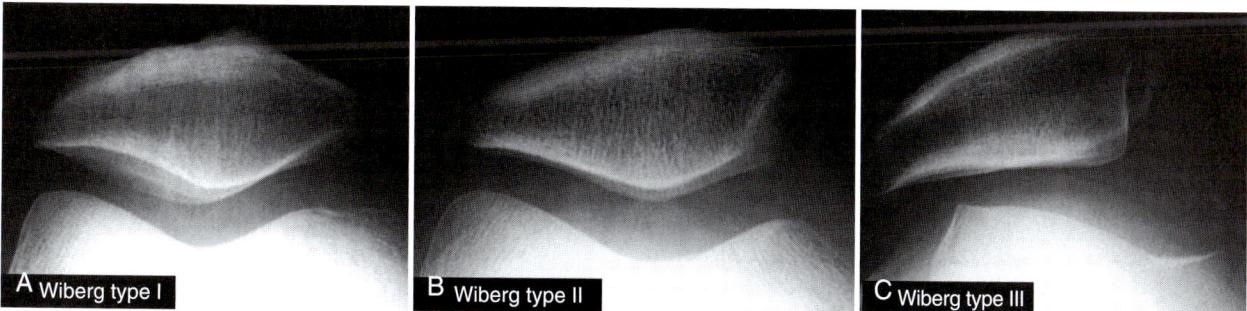

A Wiberg type I   B Wiberg type II   C Wiberg type III

Figure 61-29. **A-C,** Wiberg classification. Type I: medial and lateral facets are symmetrical and concave **(A)**. Type II: the lateral facet is bigger than the medial, accounting roughly for two thirds of patellar width **(B)**. Type III: the lateral facet is predominant; the medial facet is smaller than in type II and assumes a convex shape **(C)**.

allow assessment of which side of the articulation is affected (usually the lateral side). Information on the size of osteophytes and on joint line narrowing is provided. Iwano and coworkers[57] used the following simple staging system of lateral patellofemoral osteoarthritis (OA) (Fig. 61-30):

- Stage I, mild OA: joint space measures at least 3 mm.
- Stage II, moderate OA: joint space measures less than 3 mm, with no bony contact.
- Stage III, severe OA: bony contact in less than one quarter of the joint surface.
- Stage IV, very severe OA: joint surfaces entirely touch each other.

Computed Tomography

Many parameters observed in CT images are similar to those observed in axial views. The contribution of CT in this aspect, however, is its ability to produce such images in complete extension and perform measurements. This is particularly helpful when patellofemoral tilt or subluxation is considered, because flexion of the knee causes the patella to engage the trochlear sulcus, thus correcting (or at least reducing) these abnormalities[55,95] (Fig. 61-31). CT also provides a constant reference for measures: the posterior femoral condyles, otherwise not visualized in axial views.

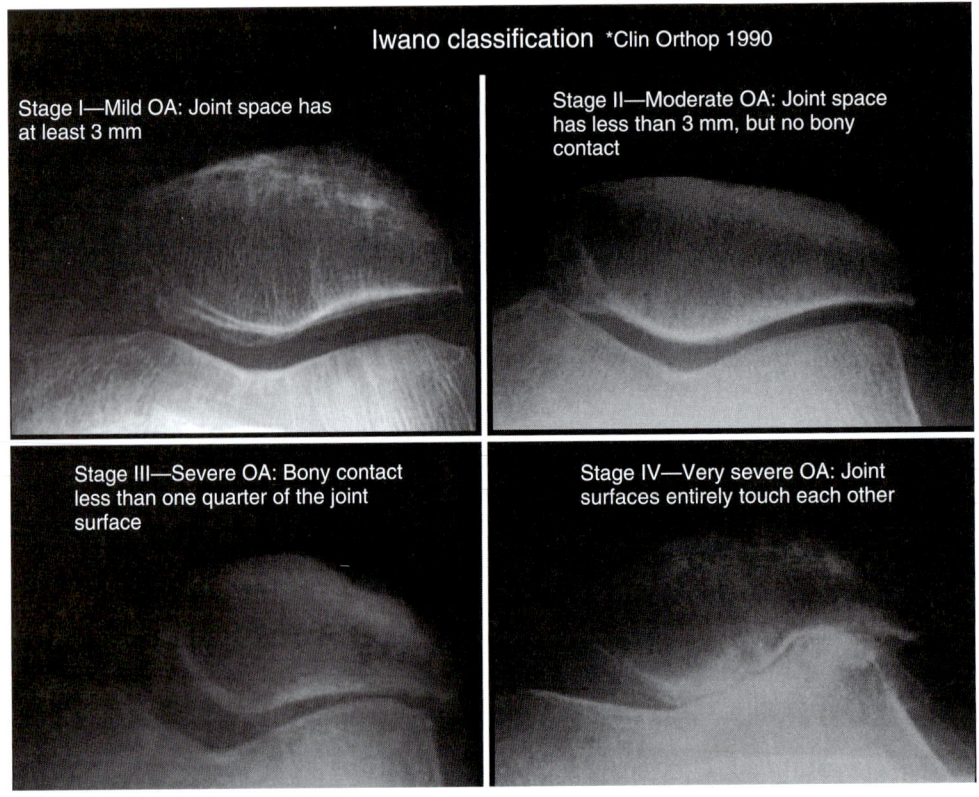

Figure 61-30. Iwano's osteoarthritis (OA) classification system, based on axial x-rays. Stage I is mild OA; the joint space measures at least 3 mm. Stage II is moderate OA; the joint space measures less than 3 mm, but no bony contact can be seen. Stage III is severe OA; patellar-trochlear bony contact occurs in less than one quarter of the joint surface. Stage IV is very severe OA; the joint surfaces entirely touch each other.

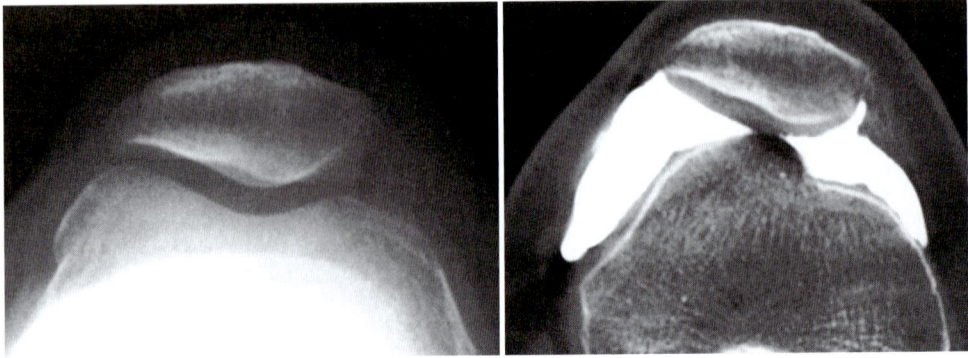

Figure 61-31. X-ray axial view and arthro–computed tomography (CT) of the same patient. Note how the trochlear dysplasia and the patellar subluxation are hidden on the x-ray and can be clearly identified in the arthro-CT performed in complete extension.

Another important contribution of CT is produced by the superimposition of images, allowing assessment of torsional deformities, such as femoral anteversion and external tibial torsion (always using the posterior condyles as a reference). By superimposing images, finally, one can assess the tibial tubercle–troclear groove (TT-TG) distance and patellar tilt (referenced to the posterior condyles, more reliable than the trochlear facets, which may change in dysplasia).

Henri Dejour and associates,[30] analyzing CT images of 143 knees operated on for symptomatic patellar instability and 27 control knee scans, determined the methods of measurement and normal and pathologic values considered in patellar instability. This protocol is known as Lyon's protocol.

The Protocol (Lyon's Protocol)

Image Acquisition (Volumic Acquisition)

The patient is imaged in the supine position, while lying on a rigid table with the knee in full extension and the patella strictly anterior—"looking to the roof." This usually places the feet in 15 degrees of external rotation. The feet are then fixed to the table with straps.

Image acquisition is performed for hip, ankle, and knee, the last with and without quadriceps contraction. The following protocol is applied:

Hip
- High-resolution filter
- Sequential acquisition
- 8 to 12 slices
- Slices thickness 2.5 mm
- 120 Kv, 200 mAs

Knee (±Quadriceps Contracted)
- High-resolution filter
- Sequential acquisition
- 8 to 12 slices
- Slices thickness 2.5 mm
- 120 Kv, 200 mAs

Ankle
- High-resolution filter
- Sequential acquisition
- 4 to 8 slices
- Slices thickness 2.5 mm
- 120 Kv, 200 mAs

Knee-Specific Volumic Acquisition

- High-resolution filter
- Slices thickness 1.4 mm/0.7 mm
- 140 Kv, 300 mAs

For measurements, some specific axial sections should be acquired:
- Section through both femoral necks at the top of the trochanteric fossa
- Section through the center of the patella, through its larger transverse axis
- Section through the proximal trochlea (where the intercondylar notch looks like a Roman arch, with slight condensation of the trochlear lateral facet subchondral bone)
- Section through the proximal tibial epiphysis, just beneath the articular surface
- Section through the proximal part of the tibial tuberosity

- Section near the ankle joint, at the base of the malleoli

Tibial Tubercle-Trochlear Groove Distance (TT-TG)

The resulting valgus vector of the extensor mechanism has been classically measured by the Q angle, with considerable heterogeneity of reported measurement methods and results. Also, lateral displacement of the patella underestimates this angle. This bias is not presented in CT measurements.

The TT-TG distance is a direct measure of the extensor mechanism valgus alignment. It is calculated from a CT scan protocol that superimposes two cuts: one through the bottom of the TG, in its most proximal part (where the notch looks like a Roman arch, with slight subchondral condensation seen in the trochlea), and the other through the most proximal part of the TT. Both cuts should be perpendicular to the long axis of the bones, and the two reference points are projected in the bicondylar line. The distance between their projections is the TT-TG value, expressed in millimeters. The average normal value in full extension is 12 mm, and 56% of knees with at least one episode of patellar dislocation will have values superior to 20 mm.[30] Thus, 20 mm is considered the uppermost limit (Figs. 61-32 and 61-33).

Patellar Tilt

Patellar tilt is assessed on CT views with and without quadriceps contraction. Its method of measurement is different

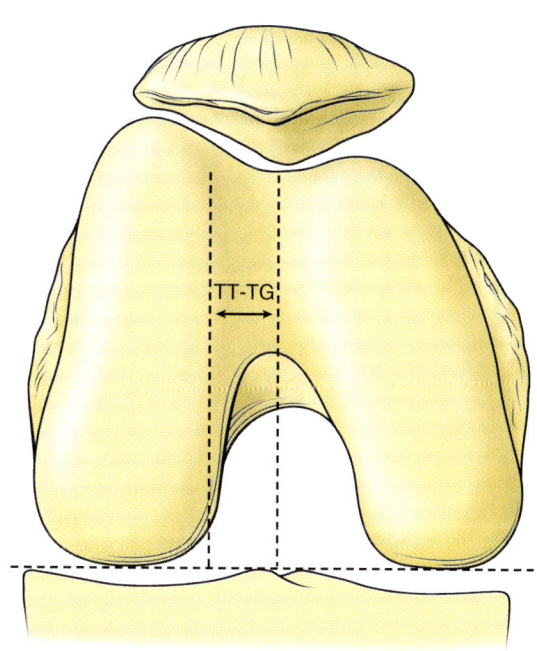

Figure 61-32. Tibial tubercle–trochlear groove distance *(TT-TG)*. Two computed tomography (CT) scan cuts are superimposed: one through the superior part of the trochlea and the other through the proximal patellar tendon tibial insertion. The deepest point of the trochlear groove and the tibial tubercle are projected on the posterior condylar line. The distance between them is the *TT-TG* value in millimeters.

from that used with x-ray views. Two lines are drawn: one tangent to the posterior femoral condyles, and another through the transverse axis of the patella (alternatively, one cut through the Roman arch level and another through the patella's longer transverse axis can be superimposed). The angle between the two lines is the patellar tilt measurement (Fig. 61-34). Eighty-three percent of patients presenting with patellofemoral instability with at least one episode of dislocation will present values over 20 degrees. If, instead of using only the relaxed quadriceps measure, a mean is calculated between the measures obtained relaxed and in contraction, and if the threshold value remains the same, sensitivity and specificity are improved. Ninety percent of patients with at least one previous patellar dislocation presented values higher than this, but only 3% of controls did the same[30] (Fig. 61-35).

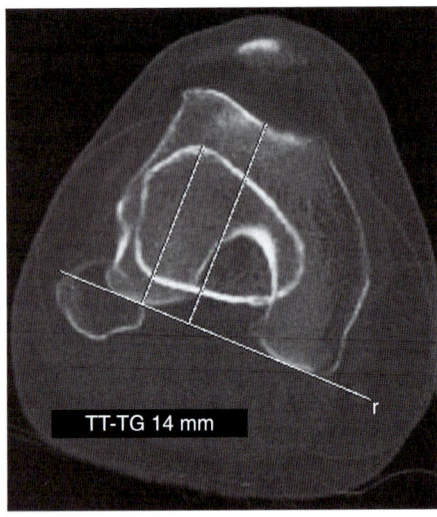

Figure 61-33. Tibial tubercle–trochlear groove (TT-TG) measurement.

Femoral Anteversion

Two cuts are superimposed. The trochlear reference cut and the posterior condylar tangent line are used again. In the femoral neck section, a line is drawn joining the center of the femoral head with the center of the femoral neck. This line and the posterior condylar line form the femoral anteversion angle[81,111] (Fig. 61-36).

In Dejour's study,[30] the femoral anteversion mean value was 10.8 ± 8.7 degrees in controls and 15.6 ± 9 degrees in patients with at least one patellar dislocation. Some overhanging of values was noted in both groups, and no statistical threshold could be set.

External Tibial Torsion

Two tibial cuts are superimposed—one proximal (beneath the articular surface) and one distal (ankle). One line is drawn tangent to the posterior aspect of the plateau, and another through the bimalleolar axis. The angle between them is measured.[58,59,112] In Dejour's study, mean tibial external rotation was 33 degrees in the patellar instability group and 35 degrees in the control group. Too much variation was present, and no particular significance could be demonstrated (Fig. 61-37).

Table 61-1 summarizes the CT scan protocol proposed by Dejour and colleagues (Lyon's protocol):

- CT plays an important role in the evaluation of anatomic abnormalities.
- Trochlear shape definition is essentially helped by its axial (Fig. 61-38) and sagittal views. Tridimensional reconstructions are also performed after image acquisition, and a precise judgment can be obtained. Finally, CT helps in the evaluation of joint line thickness (Fig. 61-39).
- Ordinary CT scans do not provide much information about cartilage status unless advanced osteoarthritis is established. However, cartilage can be well analyzed if

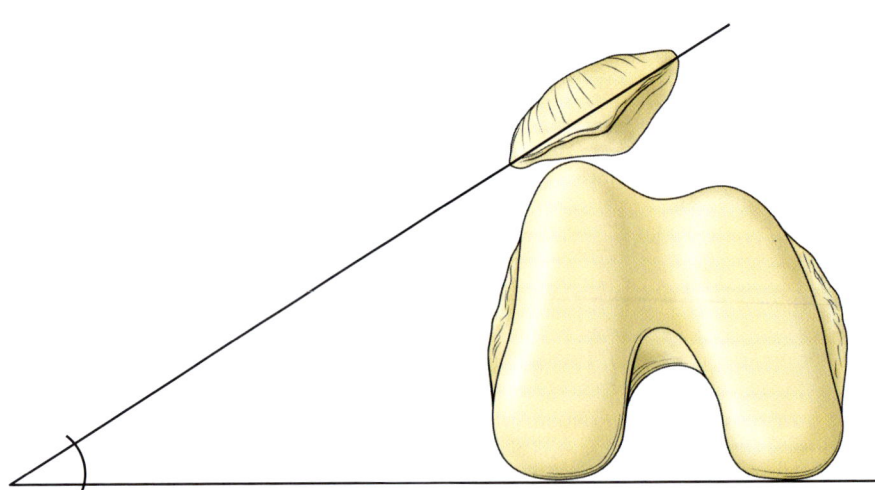

Figure 61-34. The patellar tilt measurement on computed tomography (CT) scans (in extension) is obtained by drawing two lines: one tangent to the posterior femoral condyles, and another through the patellar transverse axis. The angle formed between the two lines is the patellar tilt angle.

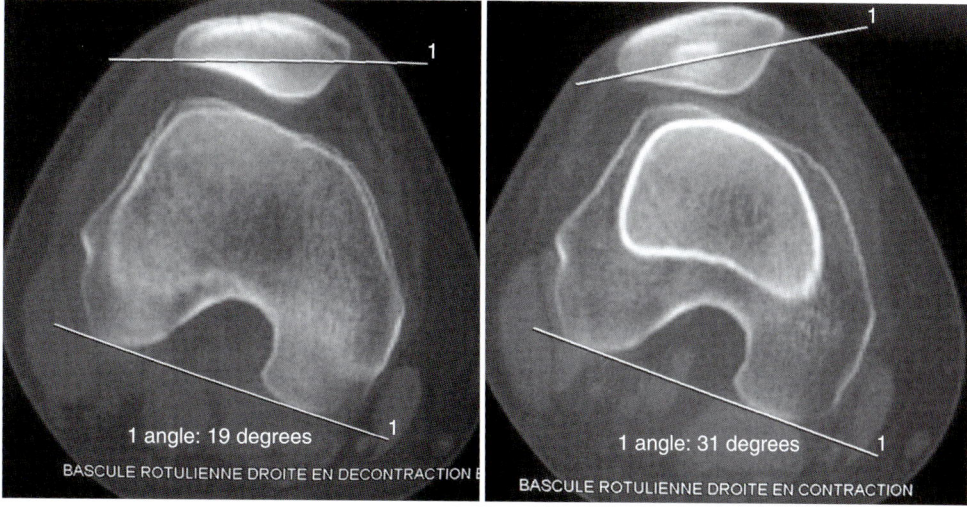

Figure 61-35. Patellar tilt measurement with and without quadriceps contraction. The value increases from 19 degrees (within the normal range) to 31 degrees (abnormal) after the patient effectively contracts his quadriceps.

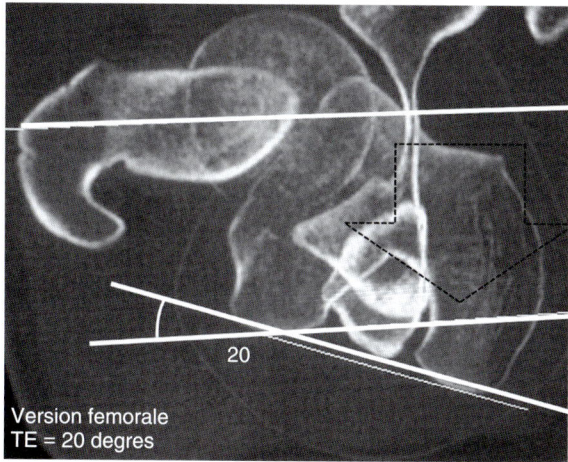

Figure 61-36. Femoral anteversion measurement. The trochlear reference cut provides the posterior condylar line. In a proximal cut through the femoral neck, a line is drawn joining the center of the femoral head and the center of the femoral neck. These cuts are superimposed, and the angle between the two lines is calculated.

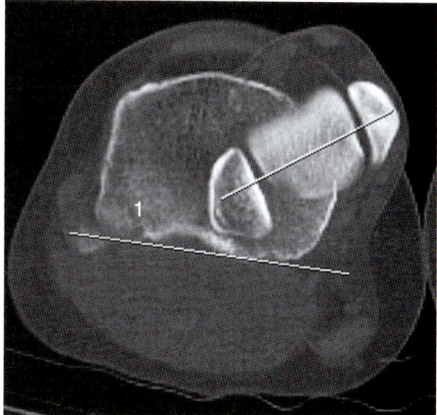

Figure 61-37. Tibial torsion measurement. Two cuts are superimposed: one through the proximal tibia, beneath the articular surface, and another through the ankle joint, at the base of the malleoli. The angle between the line tangent to the posterior plateau and the bimalleolar axis is the tibial torsion value, expressed in degrees.

intra-articular contrast is injected. Double-contrast methods use room air and positive contrast material. Two principles should be followed during double-contrast arthro-CT examination. First, an adequate amount of air is essential to separate the articular cartilage from surrounding soft tissues. Second, an adequate volume of positive contrast material is essential.

- Use of arthro-CT allows identification of several types of chondral lesions: fissures, fibrillation, ulcers, and erosion. Excessive amounts of positive contrast material have a tendency to make the edge of the cartilage obscure, thus making diagnosis of fibrillation very difficult. Conversely, if too little contrast is used, fibrillation and ulcers cannot be observed. Imbibition of contrast material is a sign of cartilage fibrillation. Decreased CT value of the cartilage, increased thickness at a noncontact area, and decreased thickness at a contact area may indicate the possibility of cartilage

softening. Overall cartilage thickness can also be assessed. Ihara[54] has shown that for patellofemoral cartilage, when arthro-CT findings were compared with arthroscopy or arthrotomy, CT diagnosis was accurate in 68 of 70 knees (97.1%). It is also useful for the diagnosis of plica syndromes and for detection of loose bodies.

Magnetic Resonance Imaging

Compared with CT scans, MRI provides superior anatomic and pathologic definition of soft tissue and articular cartilage. Conventional arthrography or arthro-CT allows visualization of surface anatomy but does not allow delineation of subchondral bone. In MRI, subchondral bone edema is a clue to cartilage damage.

On sagittal views, the entire extent of trochlear and patellar surfaces can be evaluated. The thickest part of the patella

Table 61-1 Lyon's Protocol

Measure	How to Measure (CT)	Patients With at Least One Episode of Patellar Dislocation (Mean ± SD)	Controls (Mean ± SD)	Comments
Femoral anteversion	Angle between center of femoral head/neck and posterior condyles	15.6 ± 9.0 degrees	10.8 ± 8.7 degrees	
TT-TG	Distance between trochlear groove and tibial tuberosity in two overlapped cuts	19.8 ± 1.6 degrees	12.7 ± 3.4 degrees	Pathologic threshold = 20 mm
External patellar tilt	Angle formed by the transverse axis of the patella and the posterior femoral condyles	28.8 ± 10.5 degrees; average increase of 6 degrees with quadriceps contraction	10 ± 5.8 degrees; average increase of 1.5 degrees with quad contraction	Pathologic threshold without quadriceps contraction = 20 degrees
External tibial torsion	Angle formed by the tangent to the posterior aspect of the plateau and the bimalleolar axis	33 degrees	35 degrees	Too much variation, no particular significance found

CT, Computed tomography; *TT-TG,* tibial tubercle-trochlear groove.

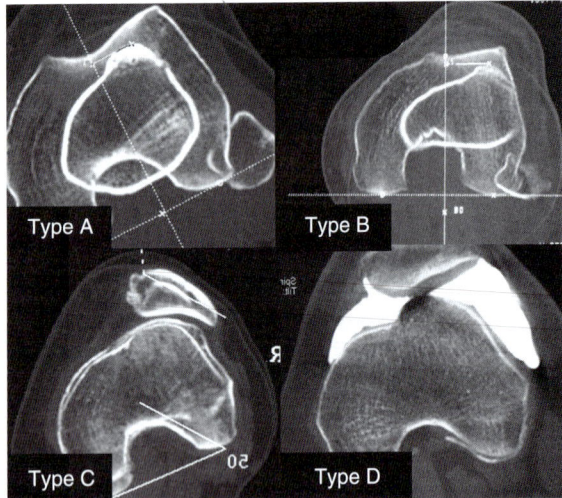

Figure 61-38. Trochlear dysplasia assessed on computed tomography (CT) axial views. *Type A:* mild flattening, but the groove is still present. *Type B:* flat trochlea, with no groove (if proximal cuts were performed, they would show the spur). *Type C:* the trochlea is convex (the patellar tilt is high). *Type D:* a cliff pattern (abrupt transition from lateral to medial facet) is present.

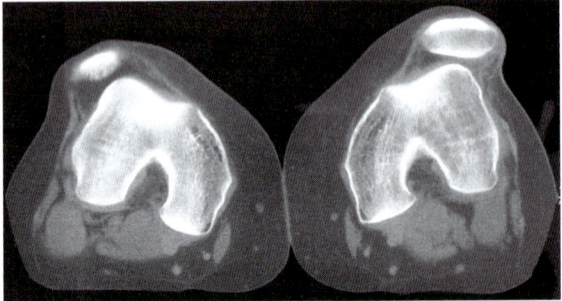

Figure 61-39. Computed tomography (CT) axial cuts of bilateral patellar instability. Note that on the right knee *(figure on the left),* only the distal part of the patella is shown, but on the other side, the patellar long axis is seen. Absence of the patella in front of the trochlear reference cut is an indirect and qualitative sign of patella alta.

corresponds to the median ridge, and images medial and lateral to it correspond, respectively, to medial and lateral patellar facets. The distal quadriceps and the entire patellar tendon are visualized with their anterior insertions on the patella. Tendon signal alterations should be examined for tendinosis or partial tears. Hoffa's infrapatellar fat pad lies posterior to the patellar tendon. The infrapatellar plica is identified in midline sagittal sections as a band linking the intercondylar notch to Hoffa's fat pad. In the presence of joint fluid, the suprapatellar bursa is seen proximal to the superior pole of the patella. The suprapatellar plica is identified in the superior aspect of the bursa.

On axial images, the patellofemoral osseous and cartilaginous relationships become evident. Trochlear groove cartilage can be assessed, but overlapping with Hoffa's fat pad and adjacent synovium may produce false-positive fissuring. The medial plica, extending from the medial capsule toward the medial patellar facet, is best visualized in the presence of joint fluid. The patellar and quadriceps tendons are visualized in their axial plane, and intrasubstantial signal intensity abnormalities are checked. Proximal to the patella, the vastus medialis and lateralis tendons are depicted, while distally, at the level of the patella, the medial and lateral retinacula are identified.

Intravenous gadolinium enhances areas of pannus in inflammatory arthritis; intra-articular contrast or distention with saline improves the identification of plicae.

Global and subjective evaluation of instability is facilitated by axial views, similar to CT, MRI produces axial images in full extension, but with thinner slices. Some of the measurements applied to x-ray or CT scanning can be applied to MRI when instability or maltracking is evaluated. Of great importance, MRI allows bony and cartilaginous shape assessment, and because in normal knees osseous and cartilaginous shapes do not match exactly,[100] this allows true articulating surface assessment. In fact, if the measures used for CT scanning are considered in MRI, a significant difference will be noted from those obtained using the subchondral bone and from those using the cartilaginous shape.[80] This is not so evident in trochlear dysplasia because the flat subchondral bone will be covered by equally flat cartilage (Fig. 61-40).

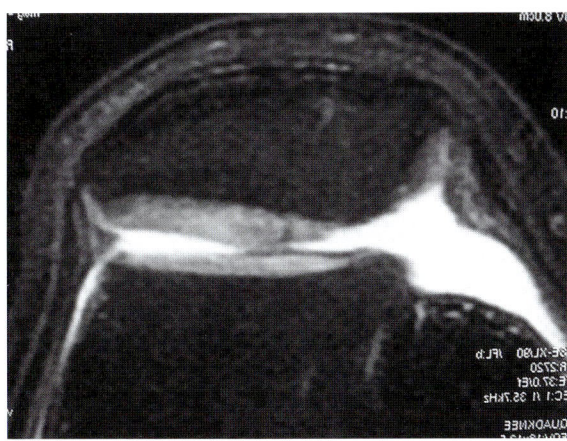

Figure 61-40. In dysplastic trochlea, matching between the cartilage and the bone is always perfect because the trochlea is flat or convex.

Some studies concerning patellofemoral instability have been performed and probably represent the future of approaches to this pathology. At this moment, however, no consensus has been reached on which indices and values could be commonly adopted in the measurement and differentiation of normal from abnormal patellofemoral joints.

Carrillon and coworkers[12] investigated the lateral trochlear inclination angle (LTI) calculated by means of a line tangential to the subchondral bone of the posterior aspect of the two femoral condyles crossed with a line tangential to the subchondral bone of the lateral trochlear facet in healthy and patellar instability patients. A significant difference between groups was recorded. The mean value in patellar instability patients was 6.17 degrees; in the control group, it was 16.9 degrees. When 11 degrees was chosen as the threshold value for LTI, results were excellent in discriminating between the two groups, with a sensitivity of 93%, a specificity of 87%, and an accuracy of 90%.

Schoettle and associates[94] evaluated the reliability of the TT-TG on MRI compared with CT scan in 12 knees with patellofemoral instability or anterior knee pain. The mean TT-TG referenced on bony landmarks was 14.4 ± 5.4 mm on CT scan, and 13.9 ± 4.5 mm on MRI. The mean TT-TG referenced on cartilaginous landmarks was 15.3 ± 4.1 mm on CT scan, and 13.5 ± 4.6 mm on MRI. Investigators found excellent interperiod (bony vs. cartilaginous TT-TG) and intermethod (CT vs. MRI measurement) reliabilities of 91% and 86%, respectively. They concluded that TT-TG can be determined reliably on MRI using cartilage or bony landmarks, and that additional CT scans are not necessary.

Miller and colleagues[77] analyzed patellar height on sagittal MRI of the knee. They applied the Insall-Salvati method to 46 knees and compared MRI and radiographs. Good to excellent correlation between values was found, and investigators concluded that patellar height can be assessed reliably on sagittal MRI using the patellar tendon-to-patella ratio. On sagittal MRI, patella alta is suggested at values greater than 1.3.

Neyret and coworkers[83] used radiography and MRI to measure patellar tendon length in 42 knees with a history of patellar dislocation and 51 control knees. On MRI, the mean length was 44 mm in controls and 52 mm in the dislocation group. The distance between the tibial plateau and the point

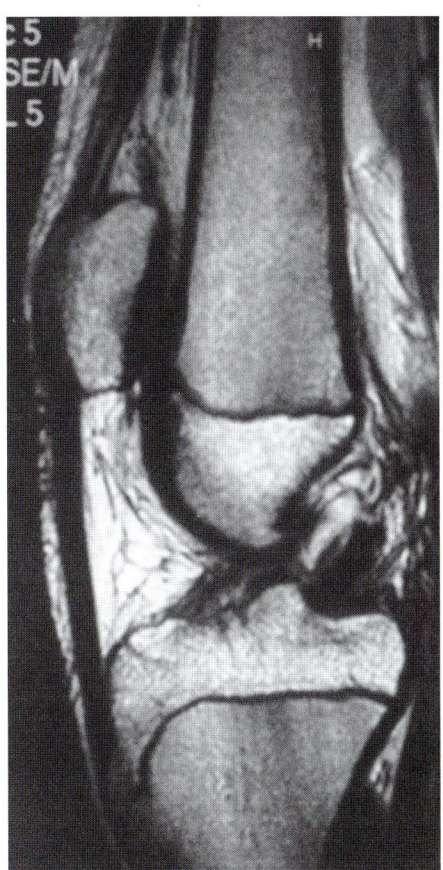

Figure 61-41. Sagittal magnetic resonance imaging (MRI) shows excessive length of the patellar tendon and consequent patella alta. The tibial insertion remains in its usual location.

of tendon insertion was also measured and was found to be 28 mm and 29 mm in the control and dislocation groups, respectively. Investigators concluded that patella alta is caused by a long patellar tendon rather than by a low insertion into the tibia. Additionally, they found no significant differences between x-ray and MRI tendon length measurements (Fig. 61-41).

Grelsamer and associates[46] described their results using an MRI tilt angle similar to that proposed by Dejour and colleagues[30]; they also used as a reference a line connecting the medial and lateral borders of the patella and the posterior femoral condyles. Thirty patients with tilt and 51 patients without tilt were evaluated. Patients with significant tilt on physical examination could be expected to have an MRI tilt angle of 10 degrees or greater, whereas an angle of less than 10 degrees was associated with absence of significant tilt on physical examination.

Dynamic MRI of the patellofemoral joint has been described to evaluate tracking during early flexion. Axial images are acquired sequentially with increments of flexion. These images can be analyzed individually or as a cine-loop display, thus facilitating interpretation and recognition of abnormal tracking. In normal tracking, the ridge of the patella is situated over the center of the trochlea (the groove), and this relation is maintained through increments of knee flexion as the patella moves distally in the vertical plane. Quantitative assessments have also been described, but

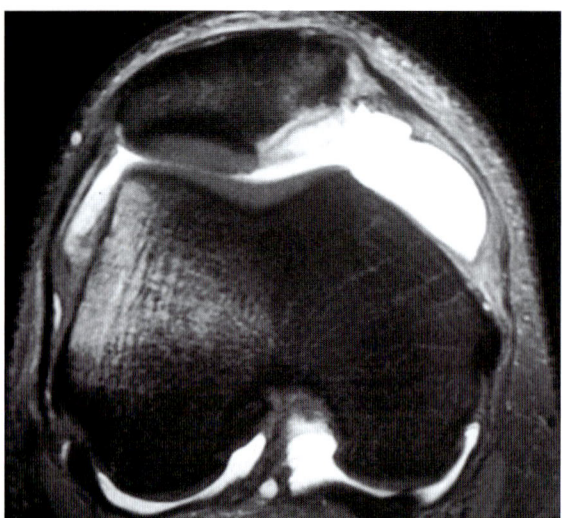

Figure 61-42. Magnetic resonance imaging (MRI) obtained after acute patellar dislocation. Lateral femoral condylar edema and the medial patellar osteochondral lesion can be clearly visualized and can make the diagnosis. Hemarthrosis is noted.

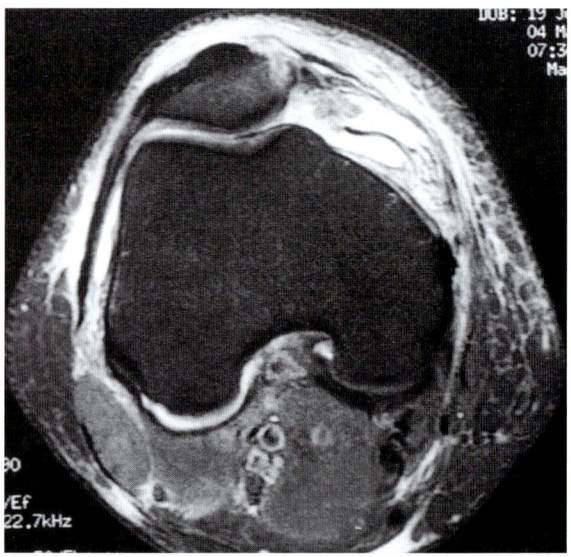

Figure 61-43. Magnetic resonance imaging (MRI) shows extensive medial retinaculum disruption and osseous avulsion from the patellar medial border. Associated effusion and edema of medial structures are evident.

despite all the studies produced, no consensus on measurement protocols and abnormal values exists. At the moment, dynamic MRI remains a promising procedure without a well-defined clinical application.

MRI is also particularly helpful in acute traumatic dislocation and in recognition and evaluation of associated lesions. Acute findings include the following:

- Lateral femoral condyle contusion and/or osteochondral lesion
- Medial patellar facet contusion and/or osteochondral lesion, sometimes with osteochondral fragment avulsion (Fig. 61-42)
- Injury of the medial retinaculum at its patellar attachments or midsubstance (Fig. 61-43); tearing of the distal belly of the VMO
- Injury of the MPFL at its femoral origin
- Patellar tilt and subluxation
- Joint effusion

PATELLOFEMORAL INSTABILITY

Patellofemoral joint stability is of great importance for proper functioning of the extensor mechanism of the knee, and of the knee joint as a whole. However, it has a low degree of congruency, as established by the balance of bony architecture and soft tissue restraints—active or passive. Anatomic aberrations are not unusual, and as a result of mechanical imbalance, instability may be overcome.

The clinical presentation of instability, however, contains a spectrum of manifestations. On this basis, it is important to differentiate patients who have symptoms but no anatomic abnormality from those who have subluxation and/or dislocation. Dislocation is defined as total loss of contact between the two articular surfaces; subluxation refers to partial loss of contact.

According to Henri Dejour, we can differentiate three major groups into which patients presenting with patellofemoral complaints may be classified:

- **Objective patellar instability (OPI) or objective patellar dislocation (OPD):** This group is composed of patients who have had at least one true dislocation of the patella. These patients will always present with at least one anatomic abnormality; otherwise they would not have the dislocation (rare cases of pure traumatic dislocation are excluded).
- **Potential patellar instability (PPI) or potential patellar dislocation (PPD):** These patients typically complain of knee pain and have anatomic abnormalities, but they have no history of patellar dislocation. Maltracking and subluxation are usually present in the affected knee and in the opposite knee.
- **Painful patellar syndrome (PPS):** These patients complain of knee pain but have no objective anatomic abnormalities or history of subluxation.

Patellar instability is more common among young females, 10 to 17 years old. The rate of subsequent dislocation after the first episode varies from 15% to 44% following conservative management; this rate is increased in those who have more than one episode.[18,36,48] In a natural history study, Fithian and associates[36] showed that only 17% of first-time dislocators suffered a second dislocation within the next 2 to 5 years. In contrast, patients who presented with recurrent patellar instability were much more likely to have subsequent dislocations than those who had had only one dislocation episode. The risk of an additional dislocation within 2 to 5 years was around 50% among patients with a history of prior patellar instability.

Complaints of pain and subjective instability are common following the initial episode and are frequently disabling. Macnab described a 33% rate of symptoms following first-time patellar dislocation, although the rate of redislocation was only 15%.[68] Hawkins and colleagues noted that at least 30% to 50% of all patients who sustained a primary patellar dislocation continued to have symptoms of instability and/or anterior knee pain.[48]

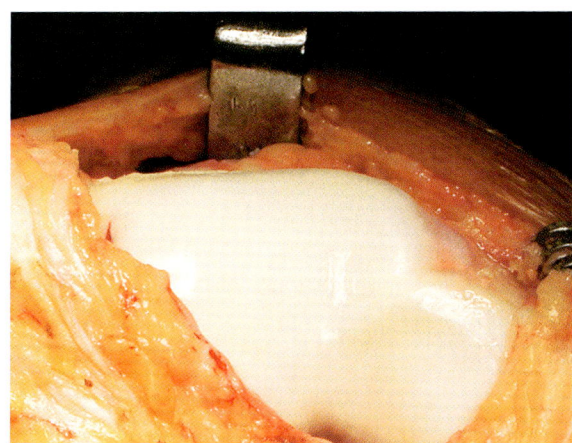

Figure 61-44. Trochlear dysplasia. Note that no sulcus and no distinct facets are present. The trochlea is flat (type B).

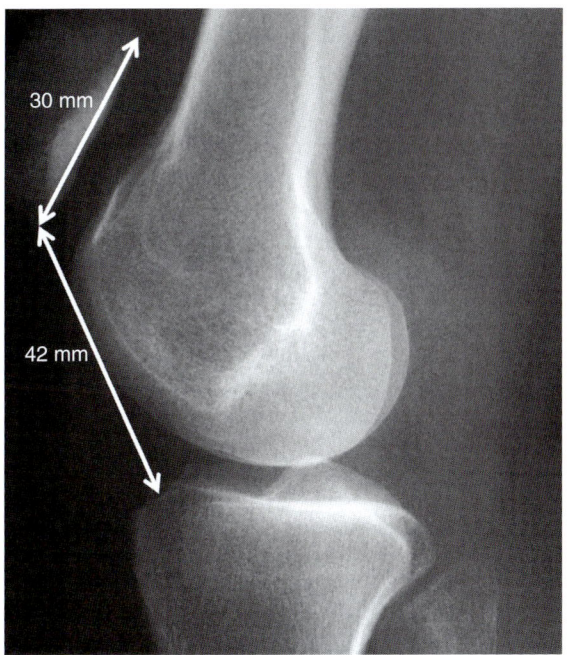

Figure 61-45. Patella alta. The Caton-Deschamps index is 1.4.

Figure 61-46. Axial view at 30 degrees of knee flexion shows patellar dislocation. The sulcus angle is abnormal, and the trochlea is completely flat.

Four major anatomic factors leading to instability were described by Henri Dejour et al[30]:

- **Trochlear dysplasia:** The shape of the trochlea is abnormal, and the osseous constraint to patellar tracking is lost (Fig. 61-44).
- **Excessive TT-TG distance:** This represents abnormal alignment of the extensor mechanism and a consequent valgus-displacing vector acting on the patella.
- **Patellar tilt:** This is due to insufficient medial restraints, but trochlear dysplasia also plays an important role in its genesis.
- **Patella alta:** The patella engages the femoral trochlea late in flexion, and this predisposes to instability (Fig. 61-45).

Trochlear dysplasia seems to be an inherited disorder. The asymmetrical orientation of the human trochlea seems to be acquired during hominid evolution and bipedal locomotion.[51,103,104] In apes, the femoral shaft is vertical (no obliquity) and the trochlear groove is wide and symmetrical, but the patella is flat. Different from apes, humans have asymmetrical trochlear grooves, and the lateral facets are higher and more prominent. This seems to occur in response to laterally directed forces acting on the patella created by the femoral shaft obliquity. This femoral obliquity is acquired with the process of learning to walk. Also, several authors* have demonstrated that fetal anatomy resembles that of adults and has an asymmetrical groove and facets. Because this asymmetrical trochlear shape is found in the fetus when no walking capacity is present, it seems reasonable to assume that trochlear dysplasia is an inherited condition and is primitive.

Minor or secondary instability factors include excessive femoral anteversion, excessive external tibial rotation, genu recurvatum, and genu valgum.

When the patient is evaluated, adequate interviewing will promptly reveal the most frequent symptoms, which are instability and pain. Subjective instability is usually reflexive, and objective instability may result from abnormal tracking and subluxation. True dislocation episodes must be searched, but usually gross anatomy disruption followed by important

swelling poses no difficulty for the diagnosis. Also of major importance is the quantification of previous dislocations experienced by the patient; this will guide treatment.

Imaging protocols (as described in earlier sections) are particularly rich in findings, allow the identification of major and minor anatomic abnormalities, and help in establishing the treatment plan. X-ray lateral views are indispensable for assessing and classifying trochlear dysplasia and for quantifying patella alta. Axial views allow measurement of the sulcus and of congruence angles (Fig. 61-46). CT images provide the TT-TG distance, the tilt value, and the rotational features. MRI is rich in acute dislocation and may show MPFL rupture, and osteochondral lesions, and bone bruises.

First Dislocation Management

For acute first time dislocations, the classic treatment is conservative. The more important exception to this is the presence of an osteochondral fracture. Some authors propose acute repair in cases of substantial medial structure disruption and a laterally subluxated patella with a normally aligned opposite knee.[101] The main goals of conservative treatment

*References 32, 38, 39, 43, 60, and 108.

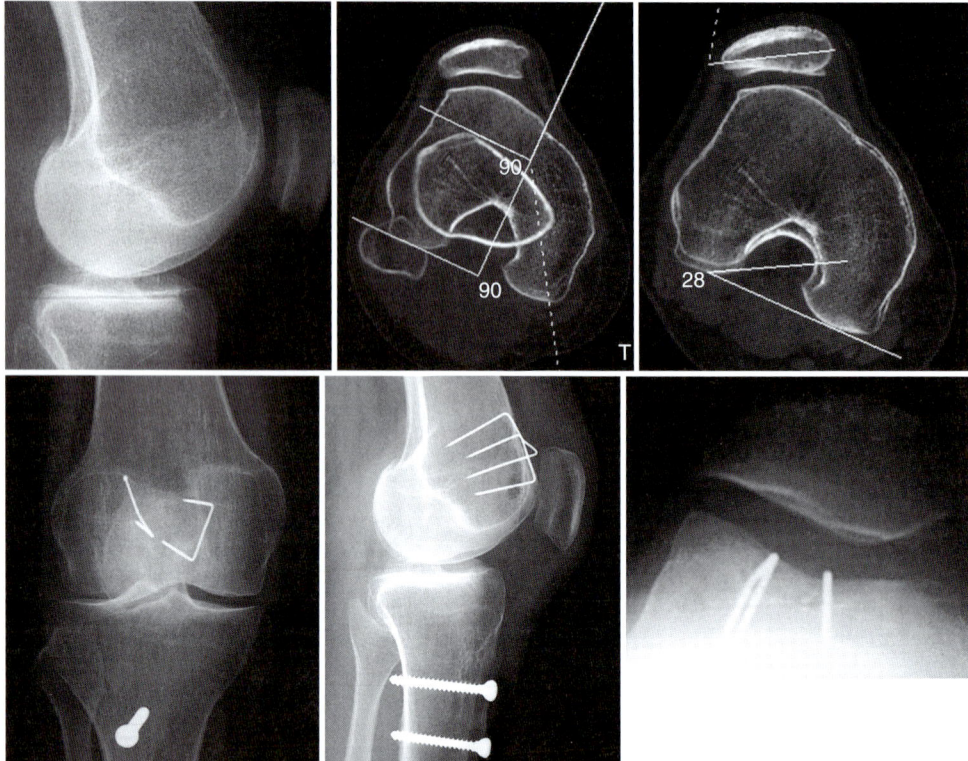

Figure 61-47. Series illustrating individual instability factor treatment. The patient presented with high-grade trochlear dysplasia (type D), increased tibial tubercle–trochlear groove (TT-TG) (23 mm), and increased patellar tilt (28 degrees). He was treated with sulcus-deepening trochleoplasty, tibial tubercle medial transfer, and medial patellofemoral ligament (MPFL) reconstruction. Postoperative images show correction of abnormalities and adequate patellar position. He presented no further dislocations.

are swelling and pain remission, as well as restoration of range of motion. Quadriceps strengthening is another goal of the conservative management strategy, and good quadriceps strength seems to alleviate symptoms, but whether it prevents further dislocation is unclear. Immobilization for up to 6 weeks may help in medial structure healing, but stiffness is a problem. If sequential dislocations occur, they will put the patient in a different category for treatment purposes: the chronic dislocation group. It is important to note that currently, some authors propose MPFL reconstruction or repair in acute dislocation cases, but this is yet to be validated because conflicting evidence exists.[84,85]

Chronic Dislocation Management

Surgical treatment is indicated in chronic dislocators, never for pain. Substantial controversy exists about procedure choice and usefulness. From a logical standpoint, the procedure (or the procedures) adopted should correct the observed root abnormalities, and it is more likely that a combination of procedures would correct those abnormalities one by one, rather than one standard procedure for every case. To remedy patellar instability, the surgeon will need to combine soft tissue and bony procedures to address all involved factors, each corrected individually (Fig. 61-47).

Soft Tissue Procedures

Soft tissue procedures used most often include lateral retinacular release, proximal VMO realignment, and MPFL reconstruction. Lateral retinacular release may be performed open

or arthroscopically to address lateral retinacular tightness. Variable amounts of release may be performed as it is extended proximally to the VL insertion, or distally along the patellar tendon. It has poor results if not associated with other procedures.[107] The absence of lateral tightness (assessed mainly on physical examination through the patellar glide) contraindicates the release, and caution should be taken in association with distal realignment because it could increase the possibility of iatrogenic medial dislocation[35] (Figs. 61-48 and 61-49).

VMO advancement, usually referred to as proximal realignment, is another possible method. The VMO insertion may be advanced in line with its fibers, or a medial plication may be performed, as part of the procedures described by Hughston or Elmslie and Trillat. Another option is complete overlap of the medial structures as described by Insall. Proximal realignments are commonly performed in conjunction with lateral release and distal realignments (tibial tubercle transfers). Alone, they are most probable to address patellar tilt and to exert medial traction and displacement on the patella (Fig. 61-50).

The MPFL, in conjunction with the VMO, opposes lateral patellar displacement. Although its tear is not the primary cause of instability, MPFL reconstruction effectively works and may alone avoid lateral patellar dislocation. Its rupture in previously abnormal but stable knees may predispose to subsequent dislocation. Several techniques have been proposed* with the use of different fixation methods and grafts,

---

*References 7, 11, 16, 18, 20, 24, and 66.

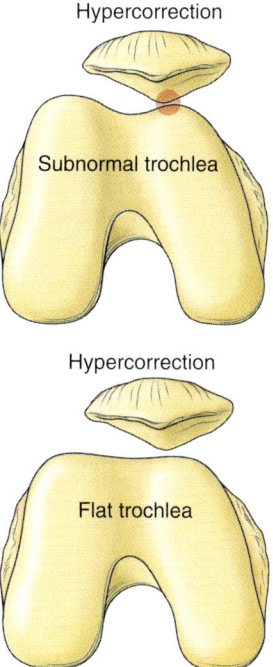

Hypercorrection

Subnormal trochlea

Hypercorrection

Flat trochlea

Figure 61-48. Hypermedialization is more probable to cause impingement in normal or subnormal trochlea. In flat or convex trochlea, absence of the prominence of the medial facet causes hypermedialization to be more tolerable. The amount of medialization has to take into account the trochlear shape.

but the overall principle remains the same: provide a check-rein to oppose lateral patellar displacement, especially in early flexion, although some degree of tilt correction is also achieved. MPFL reconstruction is an excellent alternative in patients with mild instability with no major abnormalities.

Our procedure of choice is reconstruction with gracilis tendon. Two convergent tunnels are performed from the anterior patella toward the articular surface, starting 1 cm from the medial border and approximately in the upper half of the patella. They should be 1.5 cm apart from each other and must converge before reaching the articular surface. After patellar tunnels are done, graft passage is performed in a loop. No fixation is needed there because its other end will be fixed in the femoral tunnel. A 1-cm window is performed in the medial retinaculum, 2 cm away from its free border. The graft will then pass through it from the deeper plane to continue in the subcutaneous tissue, and later enter the femoral tunnel. The femoral tunnel for graft fixation is drilled slightly superior and posterior to the medial femoral epicondyle using a 1-cm direct stab incision (Fig. 61-51). Before drilling, however, the graft is tied over the guide pin in the planned tunnel position to allow tunnel placement and isometricity testing. The graft is then passed in the femoral tunnel and is tensioned in 45 degrees of knee flexion. Proper tensioning should allow further flexion without overconstraining the knee but should also avoid patellar dislocation in extension. Finally, fixation in the femur is achieved with an absorbable interference screw (Fig. 61-52).

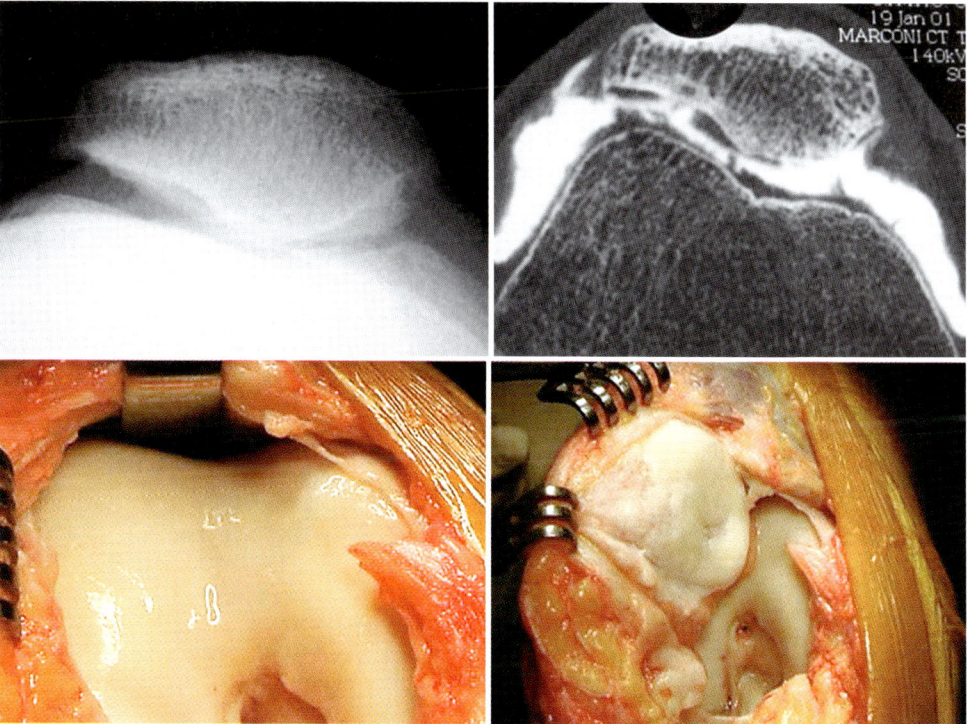

Figure 61-49. An example of hypermedialization with medial impingement. Note that cartilage damage predominates in the medial patellar aspect. The patient was submitted to lateral tibial tubercle transfer.

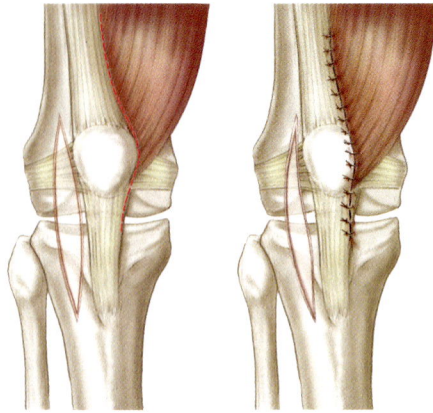

Figure 61-50. Medial advancement of the vastus medialis obliquus (VMO) and the medial retinaculum. Lateral release is also demonstrated. These procedures can be performed alone or as part of more complex procedures.

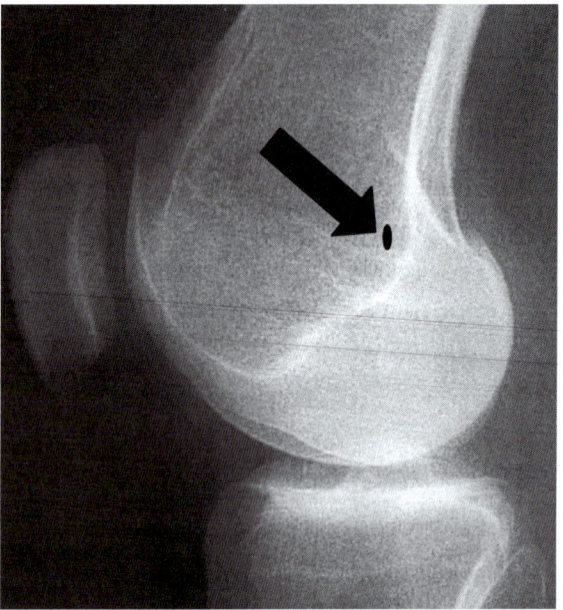

Figure 61-51. Adequate femoral insertion in medial patellofemoral ligament (MPFL) reconstruction.

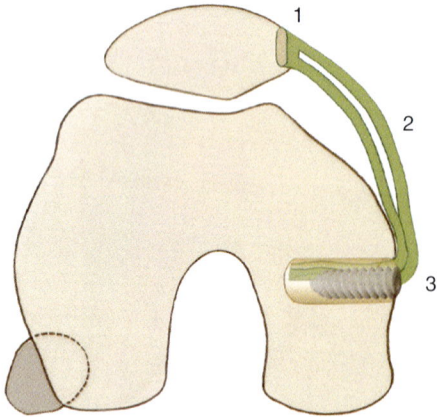

Figure 61-52. Schematic representation of medial patellofemoral ligament (MPFL) reconstruction. A two-strand gracilis tendon graft is passed in a loop through the patella and is fixated with an absorbable interference screw in the femur.

Bony Procedures

Tibial Tubercle Transfers

The first description of a tibial tubercle transfer was provided by Roux in 1888 and was modified by other authors such as Emslie and Trillat,[105] Maquet,[71] and Fulkerson.[37] This procedure involves displacing the insertion of the patellar tendon to realign the extensor mechanism and/or to correct patellar height. Medial tibial tubercle transfer is indicated in patients with extensor mechanism "malalignment." However, malalignment is somewhat difficult to define. The diagnosis may be made on clinical grounds, using the Q angle in flexion or extension as a criterion. More objective evidence will be provided by imaging techniques. The TT-TG is the most accurate and precise parameter. Therefore, the goal of tibial tubercle transfer is to reduce abnormal TT-TG (over 20 mm) to between 10 and 15 mm. Goutallier[42] stressed that the shape of the trochlea also has to be taken into account in correction of the TT-TG: the deeper the trochlea, the greater the risk of overmedialization, which would result in patellar impingement on the medial facet of the trochlea, and pain. If the patella is high, the tubercle should be distalized by the amount needed to correct the index. This would make it engage the trochlea earlier, opposing lateral displacement.

In earlier descriptions of tibial tubercle transfer, a lateral incision was used. Following the advances of patellofemoral surgery, and of knee arthroplasty in particular, an anteromedial incision is now the preferred approach. This allows the association of a medial soft tissue procedure such as VMO advancement or MPFL reconstruction with no additional incision. Complete exposure of the tibial tubercle must be attained, regardless of the type of transfer that is undertaken. The proximal limit of the insertion of the patellar tendon is identified, and the outline of the osteotomy is traced with a scalpel in the periosteum. An oscillating saw or an osteotome is used to fashion a 6-cm-long bone block. To decrease the risk of nonunion, the cut must be made sufficiently deep in cancellous bone.

Medial Tibial Tubercle Transfer. The principle of medial tibial tubercle transfer is credited to Emslie and was subsequently popularized by Trillat et al.[105] The tibial tubercle is fully detached on three sides only, leaving a distal bony hinge. Fixation is achieved with a single screw. The pilot hole for the screw is made prior to the osteotomy with a 3.2-mm drill bit and is overdrilled with a 4.5-mm drill bit to allow lagging. The bone bed to receive the block is prepared medially. The block must be trimmed to ensure that it can be medialized with sufficient ease, and that it will not sit proud of the tibia. The proximal portion of the tubercle is pried off using an osteotome and is medialized as planned. A hole is drilled in the opposite cortex with a 3.2-mm drill bit, and the tubercle is attached with a 4.5-mm screw (Fig. 61-53).

Distal Tibial Tubercle Transfer. For this transfer, the tibial tubercle is detached completely and therefore will require fixation with two screws. The screw sites are prepared prior to the actual osteotomy 2 cm apart. The block length should be increased by the amount of distal displacement planned. The proximal portion of the tibial tubercle is pried off and is grasped with bone-holding forceps, while the distal portion is being cut to the required length. The distal portion is tapered and trimmed to fit flush into its bone bed. It must not stand proud because any prominence would interfere with kneeling. The block is held in its distalized position, and fixation is started at the lower screw site. Screws are inserted perpendicular to the anterior border of the tibia to guard against movement of the tubercle back up the tibia during lagging, with loss of correction. Bicortical fixation is required for proper lagging of the tibial tubercle (Fig. 61-54).

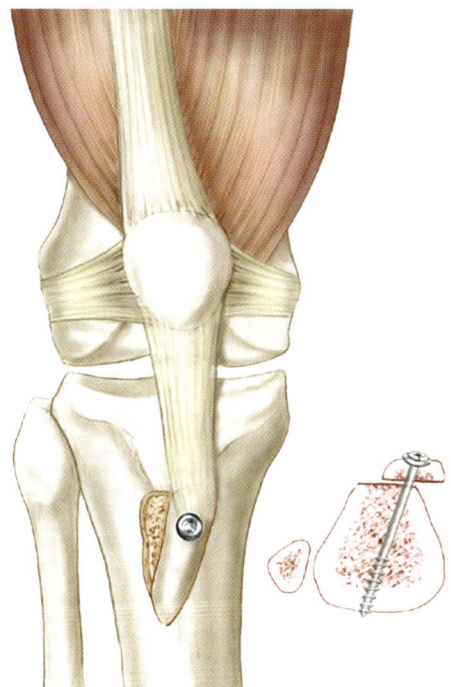

Figure 61-53. Medial tibial tubercle transfer. A distal bone–periosteum hinge is left, and one screw is used to fixate the osteotomy.

Tibial tubercle distal transfer induces medialization of 3 to 4 mm caused by tibial torsion. This phenomenon should be included in calculations for the desired correction as they could contribute to "over-medialization."[96] Additional medialization may be provided after the first screw has been inserted but not tightened. Once the desired amount of medialization has been attained, the second screw is inserted (Fig. 61-55).

Patellar Tendon Tenodesis. This is an adjuvant procedure to distal tibial tubercle transfer surgeries as described by Neyret et al.[83] It is indicated when the patient has a patellar tendon length superior to 52 mm, which represents a tendon that is too long. This measure can be found by radiographic examination, but it is far more reliable when MRI is used. After tibial tubercle osteotomy for distalization, as described previously, two anchors with sutures are fixed at both sides of the patellar tendon, about 29 mm distal to the tibial plateau level, at the normal tendon insertion. The sutures are tied, attaching the patellar tendon to the underlying bone and thus reducing the length of the patellar tendon, which can be assessed postsurgically through MRI.

Postoperative care is common to all tibial tubercle osteotomies. The patient wears a straight-leg splint and is allowed to walk with full weight bearing. Range-of-motion (ROM) exercises are started on the first postoperative day; to avoid excessive stress on the fixation of the tibial tubercle, flexion is limited to 100 degrees. After 45 days, the splint is removed and full flexion is allowed. Return to sports activities is permitted 6 months postoperatively.

Trochleoplasties

Trochleoplasty is indicated to correct severely dysplastic trochleae. Lateral-facet elevating trochleoplasty is indicated in patients with a flat or shallow trochlea, but without trochlear prominence. Care must be taken to ensure that the procedure does not result in greater trochlear prominence,

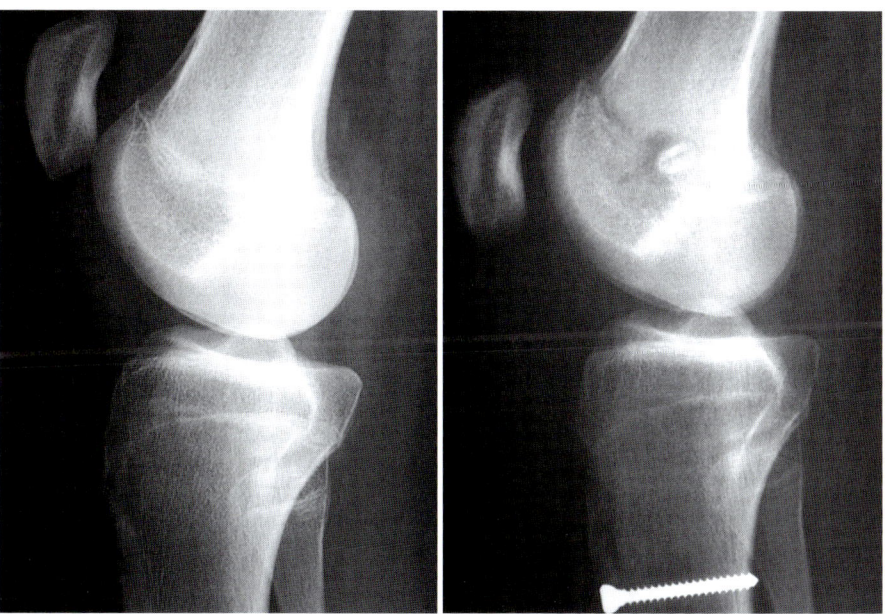

Figure 61-54. Preoperative and postoperative lateral views of patella alta. After distal tibial tubercle transfer, patellar height is corrected (1.5 preoperatively to 1 postoperatively). Associated medial patellofemoral ligament (MPFL) reconstruction was also performed, but note that the MPFL femoral insertion is too anterior and high.

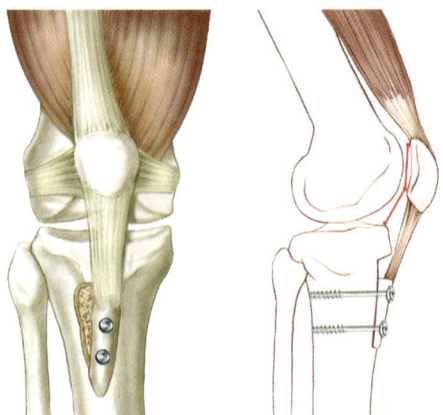

Figure 61-55. Medial and distal tibial tubercle transfer. Two screws are used. This procedure is used to increase tibial tubercle–trochlear groove (TT-TG) distance and patella alta. Caution should be taken to not overmedialize the tubercle, because the distalization procedure alone induces automatic medialization. Screws must be perpendicular to the tibial shaft to allow good compression.

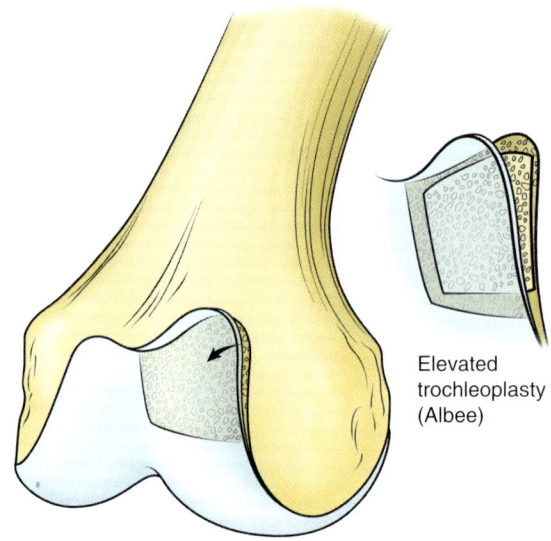

Elevated trochleoplasty (Albee)

Figure 61-56. Albee's lateral facet–elevating trochleoplasty. After the lateral facet osteotomy, a bone wedge is interposed, thus elevating the trochlear lateral facet and restraining patellar lateral displacement.

which might give rise to impingement in flexion. This procedure is certainly efficient in terms of stability but could lead to further patellofemoral arthritis by increasing compression forces. Sulcus-deepening trochleoplasty is more anatomic and is indicated in severe (type B or D) dysplasia, in which the trochlea is prominent and the patella impinges on the trochlea. The best indication is when the patient has abnormal patellar tracking with a J sign and a history of dislocations. The deepening trochleoplasty decreases the TT-TG because it redirects the trochlear groove; this must be considered when distal realignment procedures are added to the treatment plan.

Lateral Facet–Elevating Trochleoplasty. Described in 1915 by Albee,[3] this procedure consists of exposure of the trochlea, followed by an osteotomy of the lateral condyle to produce a hinge near the intercondylar groove. The osteotome enters the condyle at a distance of 5 mm from the cartilage, so as to preserve adequate thickness to prevent necrosis of the trochlea. The lateral condyle is pried open to create a 5-mm gap, and a wedge of corticocancellous bone (iliac crest, local bone graft) or of bone substitute is inserted. Fixation, if needed, is achieved with transosseous sutures. In this way, the lateral facet is elevated sufficiently to block any further tendency of the patella to dislocate (Fig. 61-56).

Sulcus-Deepening Trochleoplasty. This procedure was first described by Masse in 1978[75] and was subsequently modified and formalized by Dejour et al.[29] It is designed to abolish the prominence of the trochlear sulcus and to establish a groove of correct depth. After surgical exposure, the new trochlea is planned. Cancellous bone is removed from under the trochlea. Two osteochondral flaps, corresponding to the lateral and medial facets, are created and fixed in a way to re-create the trochlear shape, with a deeper central groove and higher facets diverging from it. The newly established trochlea is fixed with two small staples astride the osteochondral junction, one on either side of the groove (Figs. 61-57A and B and 61-58).

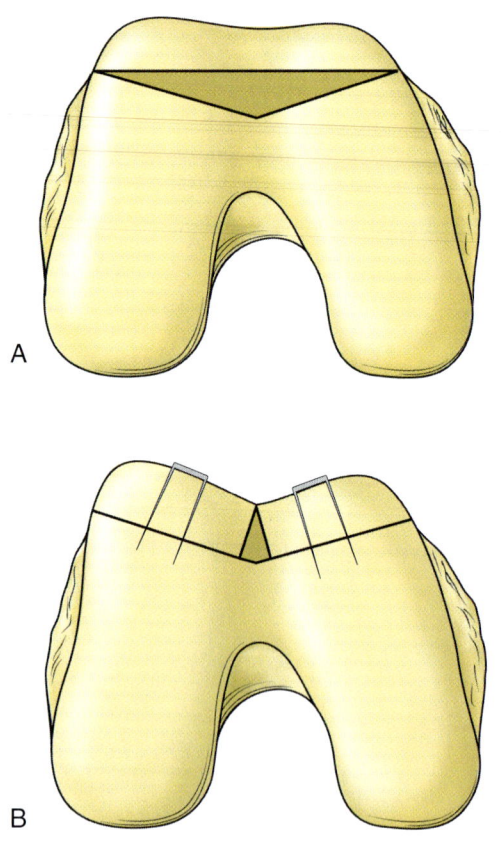

A

B

Figure 61-57. Sulcus-deepening trochleoplasty schematic model. **A,** Cancellous bone from the trochlear undersurface is removed to allow reshaping *(shaded zone).* **B,** The bone–cartilage flap is then modeled, and fixation is achieved with staples.

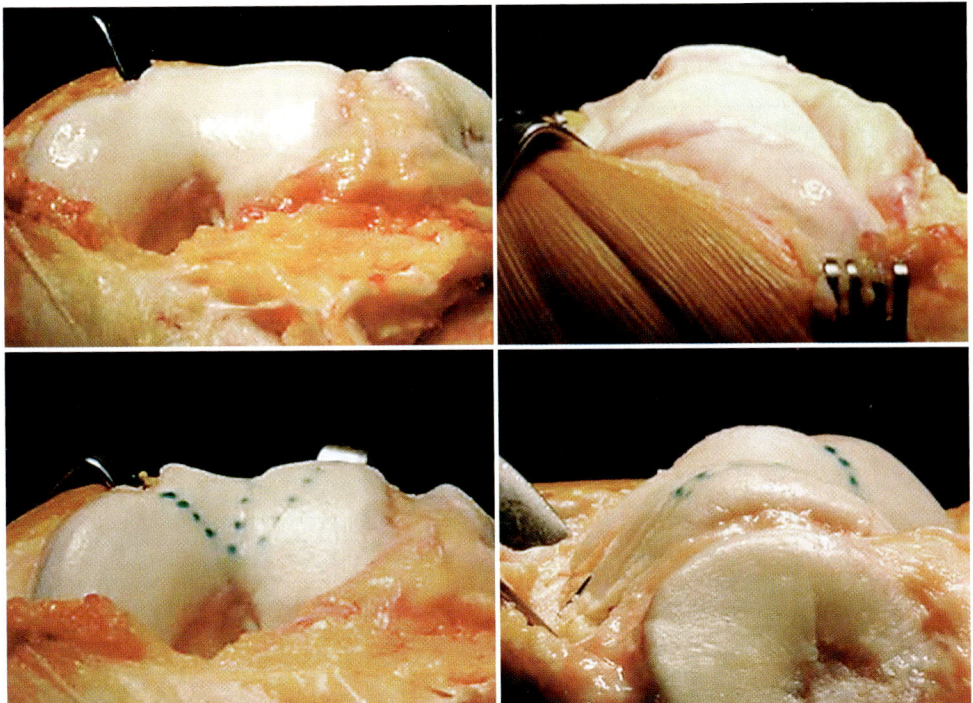

Figure 61-58. Trochlear shape before *(top)* and after *(bottom)* sulcus-deepening trochleoplasty. The trochlear sulcus is restored, and a more "anatomic" shape is achieved.

Bereiter's Trochleoplasty.[6] This is somewhat similar to the sulcus-deepening trochleoplasty but with a thinner and malleable osteochondral flap. After bone is removed from under the trochlea and the bone bed is prepared, the osteochondral flap is fixed to it with Vicryl strips.

In postoperative care, immediate weight bearing is permitted after trochleoplasty. No limitation is placed on range of motion. Knee movement is encouraged to restore the nutrition of the cartilage and to allow further molding of the trochlea by the patella.

Patellar Osteotomy

Morscher[78] described an anterior closing-wedge osteotomy fixed with transosseous sutures, designed to restore a patella with two facets. This procedure is technically demanding, in that the patella is a small, poorly vascularized structure with a high proportion of cortical bone. Also, it is difficult to decide how much space each facet should occupy and where exactly the ridge is to be placed. Major risks for necrosis and nonunion have been noted. Patellar osteotomy is indicated in patellar dysplasia such as Wiberg type III, in which the patella is flat. In such cases, reshaping of the patella is an adjunct to trochleoplasty. This is a highly theoretical indication. However, this procedure is not recommended because of the potential for numerous complications.

Femoral and Tibial Osteotomies. In a small number of cases, patellar instability will be found to be due to lower limb malalignment in excessive valgus or in torsion.

Valgus deformity increases the Q angle and enhances the dislocating pull on the patella. Valgus angulation should be considered abnormal if it is very pronounced (>10 degrees). The problem usually arises from the femur. This pattern may

be corrected by a lateral opening-wedge or a medial closing-wedge osteotomy performed in the distal femur.

Excessive femoral anteversion or tibial external rotation most likely will be seen in torsional deformities. Surgery should be considered in carefully selected cases only, with awareness that osteotomy is a major procedure. Femoral derotation osteotomy is best performed at the intertrochanteric level, and the preferred site for tibial derotation osteotomy is proximal to the tibial tubercle.

An algorithm to guide treatment is provided in Figure 61-59.

PAINFUL PATELLAR SYNDROME (PPS)— PATELLOFEMORAL PAIN SYNDROME

Anterior knee pain is one of the most common musculoskeletal disorders,[61] occurring in young and active patients. PPS is a syndrome characterized by peripatellar or retropatellar pain, resulting from physical and biomechanical abnormalities in the patellofemoral joint. It is a generic term that is usually used to describe anterior knee pain resulting from unknown (or controversial) causes. Differential diagnosis must be made with arthritis, chondral lesions, instability (dislocation), quadriceps or patellar tendon tendinitis, bursitis, plica, and neuropathic pain.

In PPS, activities that overload the patellofemoral compartment, such as squatting, descending or ascending stairs, and jumping, are most likely to produce or aggravate pain. Sitting for prolonged times with the knees flexed is also likely to cause pain; this is usually described as the "movie sign" (or theater sign) because patients may notice it in these situations. Reflex instability may occur when the pain is severe, and locking episodes have been reported.

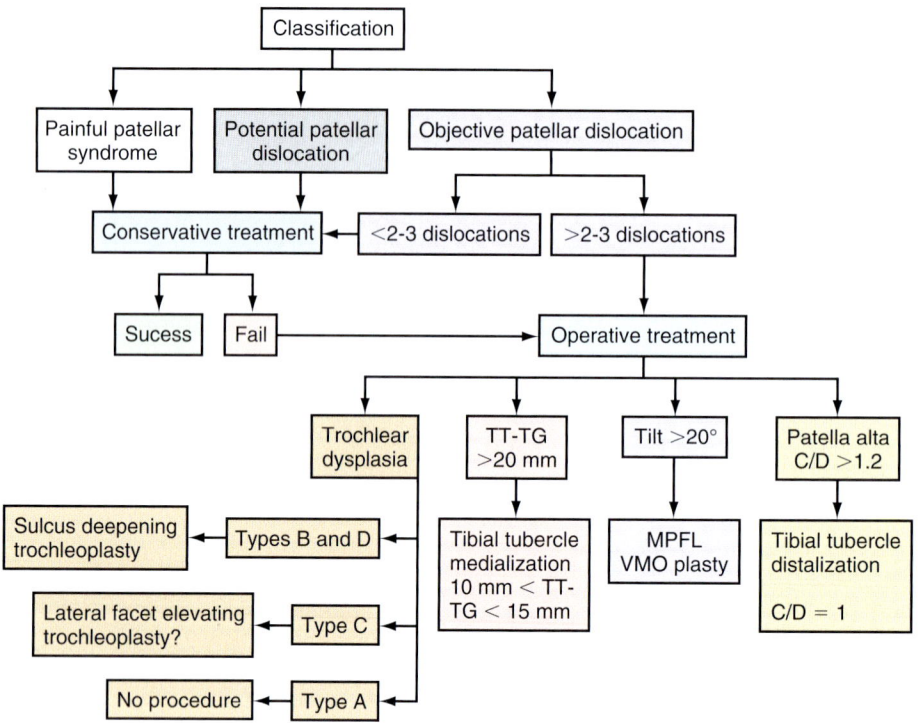

Figure 61-59. Algorithm for treatment of patellar instability.

Physical examination is the most important tool in the diagnosis of PPS. Post[86] has shown that increased Q angle, lateral and medial retinacular sensitivity, patellofemoral crepitus, squinting patella, and reduced mobility of the patella as assessed by the glide test were more frequent in the PPS group than in controls.

Imaging is usually normal, but the differential diagnosis relies on it. Several authors have shown that x-rays are not useful for PPS diagnosis, and the alignment parameters used for instability are within normal values in PPS patients. MRI findings (such as spin, tilt, or lateral translation) are also not useful in differentiating PPS patients from a control group.[67] Abnormal tilt, increased TT-TG, patella alta, and other abnormal tracking measurements, if present, would otherwise establish a diagnosis of potential patellar instability.

Several possible risk factors are known. Association between PPS and the following issues has been suggested: weakness in functional testing; gastrocnemius, hamstrings, quadriceps, or ITB tightness; generalized ligamentous laxity; deficient hamstrings or quadriceps strength; hip musculature weakness; excessive Q angle; patellar compression or tilting; and abnormal VMO reflex time compared to VL.[109] The relationship of causality, however, is not always clear, and some of these issues are actually consequences of the pain sensation. From the several factors included, two conclusions can be made. The first is that patellofemoral pain syndrome encompasses a range of possible pathologies distinct in origin but with similar presentation. The second is that some patients with mild features of patellar instability may be classified as PPS.

An interesting approach has been proposed by Dye,[33] in which loss of osseous and soft tissue homeostasis in anatomically normal patellofemoral structures culminates in the pain syndrome as a result of patients overcoming their functional limits. The range of painless loading of a joint compatible with tissue homeostasis is called "envelope of function." With such an approach, imbalances such as tightness or weakness could enhance or alter joint reaction forces, thus leading to loss of homeostasis. Objective loss of homeostasis in PPS patients has been shown by Naslund et al[82] through reduced pulsatile blood flow in the patella.

The mainstay of treatment for PPS is nonoperative. Patients usually improve with a conservative approach, including activity modification with load restriction and oral analgesics followed by stretching and strengthening exercises. Global balancing can be proposed. Spontaneous remission is also observed as patients reduce their activity levels unloading their painful knees.

A review from Cochrane (2004)[50] showed short-term pain reduction with nonsteroidal anti-inflammatory drugs, but overall pain did not improve after 3 months. This same review concluded that evidence on the effect of glycosaminoglycan polysulfate is conflicting. The anabolic steroid nandrolone may be effective, but its associated risks demand caution.

Another review from Cochrane (2003)[49] analyzed the effects of exercise on the patellofemoral pain syndrome. Trials included quadriceps strengthening. The authors found some evidence that exercise therapy might help to reduce pain in PPS. Evidence that exercise therapy is more effective than no exercise was limited with respect to pain reduction and was conflicting with respect to functional improvement. Another systematic review from 2001[21] concluded that consistent improvement in short-term pain and function appears to result from physiotherapy treatment, but comparison with a placebo group was needed to determine its efficacy. Patellar taping is another frequently used modality of treatment. A systematic review[4] concluded that it seemed to reduce pain and improve function with no detrimental effects; however, clinical evidence remains unclear.

Regarding orthotic treatment (foot or knee orthoses), one Cochrane review (2002)[22] concluded that the evidence analyzed at that time was too limited to allow definitive conclusions, but this review was withdrawn in 2009 because it was considered out-of-date. A recent study[17] demonstrated that foot orthoses may hasten recovery of the patient similarly to physiotherapy, but their addition to physiotherapy is not effective. Over the long term (52 weeks), no differences were found between patients submitted to orthoses, physiotherapy, or a combination of both, and a flat insert control group.

CHONDROMALACIA PATELLAE

Chondromalacia patellae is considered part of the patellofemoral pain syndrome. However, some authors have shown that many patients with PPS have no arthroscopic evidence of cartilage damage. Because the cartilage is aneural, pain is most likely to arise from the subchondral bone or the peripatellar soft tissues, and isolated cartilage abnormalities may not explain the development of PPS as it has been largely believed to occur. The great frequency of cartilage abnormalities found in nonsymptomatic individuals also supports the theory that chondromalacia patellae can be a different diagnosis from PPS.[1,13,40] Because it corresponds to an abnormality of the cartilage, chondromalacia can be understood as part of patellofemoral arthritis development, or as part of knee aging.

PATELLOFEMORAL ARTHRITIS

Arthritis affects the patellofemoral joint less frequently than the other compartments of the knee. The characteristics of this isolated arthritis remain badly understood, with few references in the literature. It is usually bilateral and predominates among females. Several causes have been proposed, such as

extensor mechanism malalignment, in particular with a valgus knee, hypermobile kneecap, excessive lateral hyperpression syndrome (ELHP), and a high- (patella alta) or low-riding (patella infera) patella. Two other causes often discussed are sequelae of articular fractures and rheumatoid disease (such as chondrocalcinosis).

Patients with patellofemoral arthritis (PFA) may present with the same complaints as those with PPS: anterior knee pain, frequently retropatellar but also around it. Posterior knee pain may be present less commonly. Pain is aggravated by activities that load the patellofemoral joint. Effusion is another feature that may be found. The typical age group is older than with patellar instability or PPS, and radiographic findings must be present to confirm a diagnosis.

Lateral x-ray views may allow the diagnosis of patellofemoral arthritis and the presence of trochlear dysplasia, but skyline views will be the most informative ones. Remodeling of subchondral bone, joint space narrowing, and osteophytes are the classical findings (Fig. 61-60). Malalignment is another feature to be looked for, and axial x-rays may show subluxation and tilt. The Iwano[57] classification system based on skyline views can be used. CT allows more precise alignment assessment, and arthro-CT is useful in assessing the cartilage. Finally, MRI shows the cartilage damage in detail, even in initial stages, and may also reveal subchondral bone edema.

In 2003, one of the authors (D.D.) organized a symposium[25,47] with the French Orthopedic Society (SOFCOT) to understand and to try to propose the best therapeutic solution to patients with isolated patellofemoral arthritis. Three hundred sixty-seven cases of isolated patellofemoral arthritis from several centers in France were reviewed. Similar to arthritis of the femorotibial compartment, osteoarthritis of the patellofemoral joint is found predominantly in females (72%), with 51% of patients having symptoms in the opposite knee. Average age at the time of first symptoms is 46

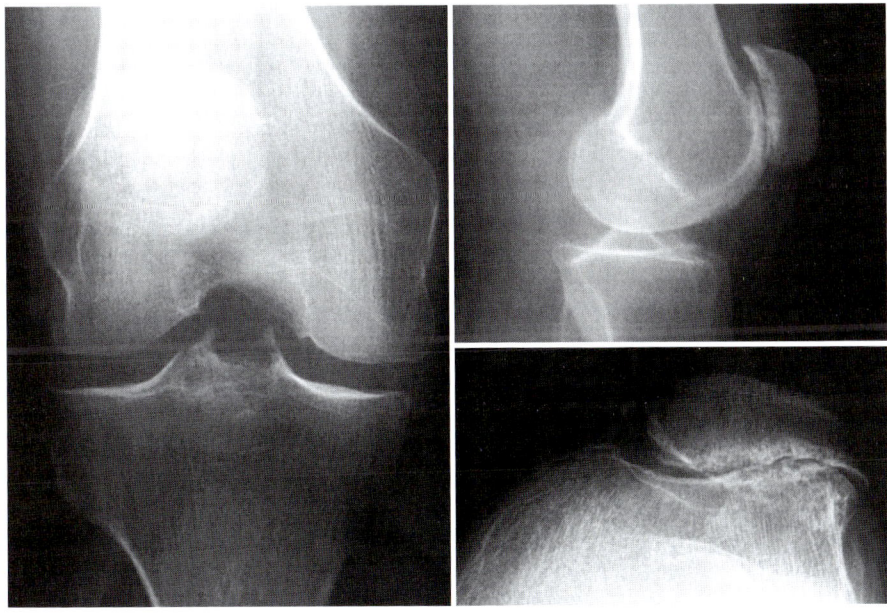

Figure 61-60. Isolated patellofemoral arthritis. The anteroposterior view is useful in assessing tibiofemoral involvement. The diagnosis can be made in the lateral view, but the axial view is the most informative. Note the trochlear dysplasia, which is present in 78% of cases of this type of arthritis.

years. The radiologic evolution is slower, with an average delay of 18 years to pass from Iwano stage I to stage IV. This type of arthritis was not statistically correlated with body mass index, but 29% of patients were obese, and 38% presented overweight. Activities that engage the patellofemoral joint are mainly altered. Ability to use the stairs was problematic in 65% of cases: 15% did not use stairs, and 92% needed aid to lift from a chair. Limitations on flat ground were also important, as 80% of patients reported that they could not walk more than 1 km.

In this symposium, four main causes were identified:

- Primary arthritis (49%): patients with no orthopedic antecedent, and especially no history of dislocation. Mean age at surgery was 58 years old.
- Post patellofemoral instability (33%): patients with a history of objective patellar dislocation (at least one dislocation). Mean age at surgery was 54 years old.
- Posttraumatic causes (9%): patients with a history of patellofemoral fractures. Mean age at surgery was 54 years old.
- Chondrocalcinosis (rheumatoid disease) (9%): mean age at surgery was 72 years old.

Trochlear dysplasia was identified as the principal factor in the series. Seventy-eight percent of all patients presented with trochlear dysplasia with the crossing sign. More dysplasia of higher grade was seen in the population with objective instability (66%) than within the primary arthritis group (38%). Absence of dislocations, however, does not exclude potential instability and maltracking as contributing factors in the primary arthritis group. Inversely, the high prevalence of trochlear dysplasia in these patients supports potential instability and the maltracking role in its genesis. Patellar dysplasia was also a significant factor.

Abnormal centering of the patella on the axial view is also correlated, but it must be understood as multifactorial: it may be a cause of arthritis, but it may also be a consequence of patellofemoral lateral compartment wear (tilt, however, is supported by Iwano as correlated with post instability arthritis). Patellar height was not a determining factor in the development of this arthritis. No correlation with axial deformity (varus or varus) of the lower legs was noted. Another interesting finding was the different rates of patients who progressed to tibiofemoral arthritis: 41% among primary cases and 32% in the post instability group.

Conservative treatment is the first option in patellofemoral arthritis. The same measures adopted for patellofemoral pain are used: analgesics, stretching, and, when pain subsides, strengthening of the lower limb muscles, especially the quadriceps.[31,45] Because most studies consider patients with osteoarthritis as a homogeneous group, little evidence is available to guide the pharmacologic treatment of isolated patellofemoral arthritis.[52] Taping and bracing may be used as well, also with unconfirmed efficacy.

When surgical treatment is planned, two main factors must be assessed: dysplasia (trochlea or patella) and malalignment. Nonprosthetic treatment is best suited for patellofemoral arthritis without dysplasia and malalignment, because the anatomic distortion is minimal, and this will favor achievement of postoperative tracking and its results. In patients without dysplasia but with malalignment, realignment procedures are helpful and may alleviate symptoms. Finally, in those who have dysplasia, prosthetic replacement seems to be

the most logical procedure, followed by realignment procedures as needed.

Lateral Retinacular Release and Vertical Lateral Patellectomy (Facetectomy)

Lateral release has been proposed as a method of treatment, but its indications and results are unclear. It seems more appropriate to perform it in patients with patellar tilt but no subluxation.[2,35,92] Lateral release is also helpful in decreasing patellofemoral joint reaction forces, especially in the presence of a tight retinaculum. It seems to be effective in pain relief, although inferior to realignment procedures, and for short-term results.[107] Vertical lateral patellectomy may also be an option that combines release with resection of lateral osteophytes and part of the degenerated lateral patellar facet (no more than 1.5 cm) (Fig. 61-61).

Tibial Tubercle Osteotomies

The rationale for anterior tibial tubercle transfer derives from biomechanical studies, which showed that this procedure reduces patellofemoral stress levels. This technique was first described by Maquet.[71-74] It involves anterior transfer of the tibial bone block and is designed to reduce compressive patellofemoral joint stresses. The procedure is similar to a medial transfer; however, an iliac crest graft is inserted between the tubercle and the tibia. Fulkerson's technique[37] involves anteromedialization without the use of a graft because an oblique osteotomy is performed and fixed with screws. It unloads the lateral and inferior parts of the patella; thus arthritis confined to these locations is best suited for the procedure. Also, anteromedialization promotes correction of malalignment, which should be taken in account when the procedure is selected.

Prosthetic Replacement

Absence of correction of patellofemoral dysplasia makes procedures such as tibial tubercle transfer or lateral facetectomy hazardous. The patellofemoral dysplasia will not be modified, and the imbalance of the patellofemoral joint will persist. In this situation, partial or total arthroplasty will be more interesting because it will permit substitution of the dysplastic

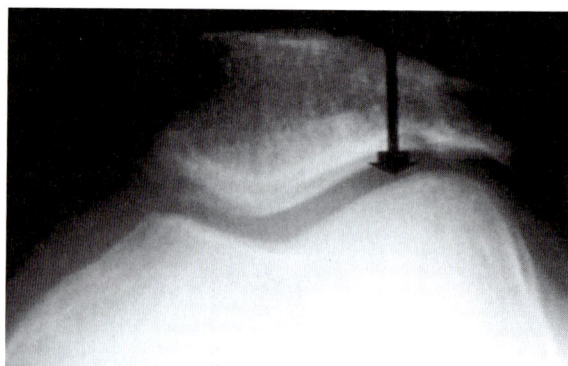

Figure 61-61. Axial view of isolated patellofemoral arthritis. Preoperative planning of vertical lateral facetectomy. A total of 15 mm of bone removal is necessary. The lateral retinaculum is not always released.

component. Therefore, trochlear prominence and orientation are corrected, and congruence is established between trochlea and patella. The TT-TG can be diminished by slight lateralization of the femoral component without touching the tibial tubercle. Regarding correction of the patella, it is necessary to pay attention to conserve a satisfactory bony thickness if possible with a minimum of 13 to 14 mm. Slightly undersized patellar components will allow mediolateral and distal to proximal positioning, aiding in correction of the alignment.

Prosthetic replacement may be complete (total knee arthroplasty [TKA]) or partial (patellofemoral arthroplasty [PFA]). TKA is an option in older patients with degenerative changes confined to the patellofemoral compartment, but its use in young patients in the same situation is debatable (Fig. 61-62). PFA seems better suited to these patients. Partial arthroplasty preserves bone stock and does not sacrifice a good tibiofemoral articulation. It also produces less surgical trauma, and for this reason, its use in older patients should be considered (Fig. 61-63).

Associated tibiofemoral disease should be ruled out, and failure to identify other causes of pain is a major reason for failure. The other great source of failure is arthritis progression in non-replaced compartments. Revision of an adequately performed PFA to a TKA is possible with no great technical challenge. Newer implants have compatibility with TKA implants, at times eliminating the need for patellar exchange.

PATELLA INFERA

Patella infera (or baja) is the opposite of patella alta. It represents the inferior (distal) position of the patella. Although it is usually assessed through profile x-ray views, its real importance lies in the biomechanical abnormality caused by the inferior situation of the patella in relation to the knee. In almost all cases, patella infera is acquired (trauma) or iatrogenic (postoperative, especially tibial tubercle transfer). Insufficiency of the quadriceps (rupture or insufficiency, as in paralytic poliomyelitis) is another known cause. Rarely, it may be of inflammatory origin.

This condition is frequently symptomatic. Knee stiffness and anterior knee pain are the usual complaints. Anterior knee pain may be perceived as a burning sensation, aggravated by effort. Patellofemoral arthritis is the main differential diagnosis, which is confirmed on profile views. Values equal to or less than 0.6 in the Caton-Deschamps method are diagnostic. If the Insall-Salvati method is preferred, values under 0.8 confirm the diagnosis. On adequate 30-degree axial views, the patella will have an unmistakable pattern: it appears superimposed on the trochlear groove, and the joint space cannot be seen. In contrast to the 30-degree "sunrise" view of the healthy side, the affected knee will show a "sunset" pattern (Fig. 61-64).

Conservative (symptomatic) treatment may be tried, but it is unlikely to change patellar height. The mainstay of treatment is operative. The technique will differ according to the cause of the condition. When the problem's origin is in the tibial tubercle, a proximal transfer will correct it. When the origin is in the quadriceps tendon, and especially when the patellar tendon is retracted, the procedure of choice is patellar tendon lengthening. In cases of inflammatory origin, an arthrolysis should be performed. In all cases, the medial and lateral retinacula must be released, and often also the fat pad. The postoperative goal is to reach a patellar index equal to 1 according to the Caton-Deschamps index.

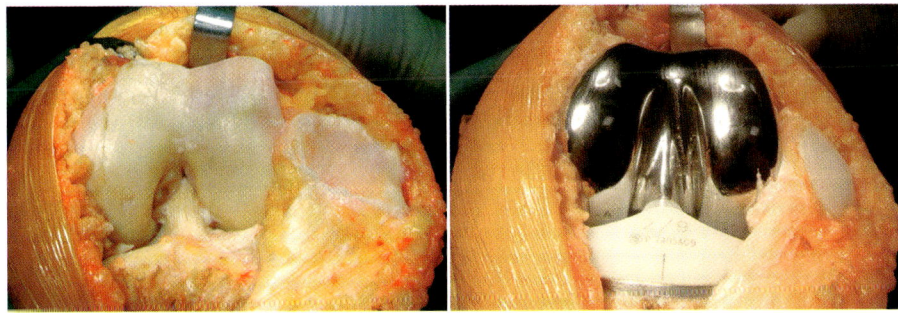

Figure 61-62. Advanced patellofemoral arthritis with no trochlear dysplasia (evolution to global arthritis is greater than in patellofemoral dysplasia) treated with total knee arthroplasty. No particular technical tricks are needed.

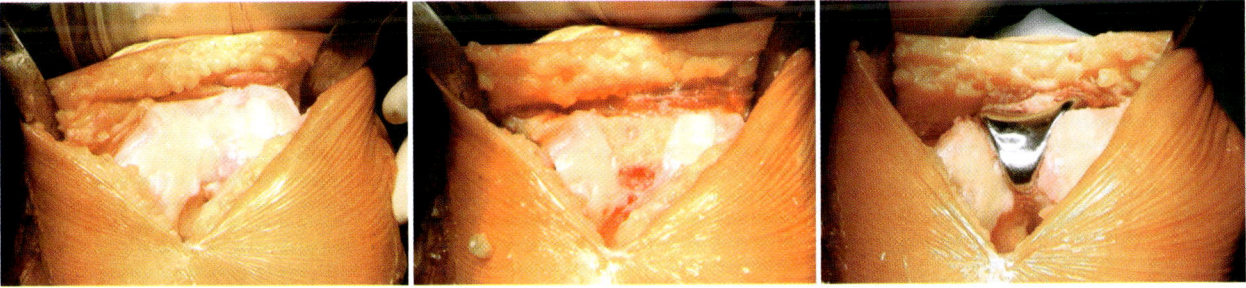

Figure 61-63. Isolated patellofemoral arthritis with a flat trochlea. Positioning of the patellofemoral arthroplasty is correlated with preoperative computed tomography (CT) scan planning to correct the wear and the patellofemoral dysplasia (trochlear dysplasia and malalignment).

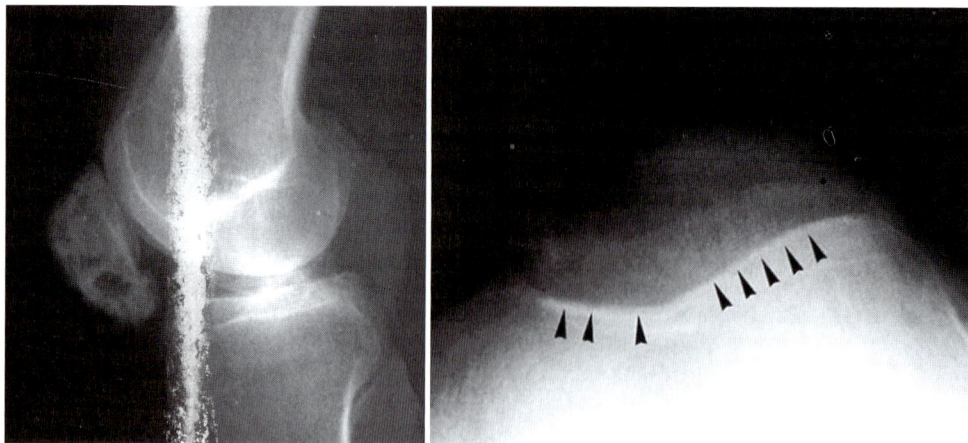

Figure 61-64. Patella infera. On the lateral view, the distance from the lower edge of the articular surface of the patella to the antero-superior angle of the tibia outline is almost zero. On the axial view, the "sunset pattern" is shown, as the articular space cannot be seen.

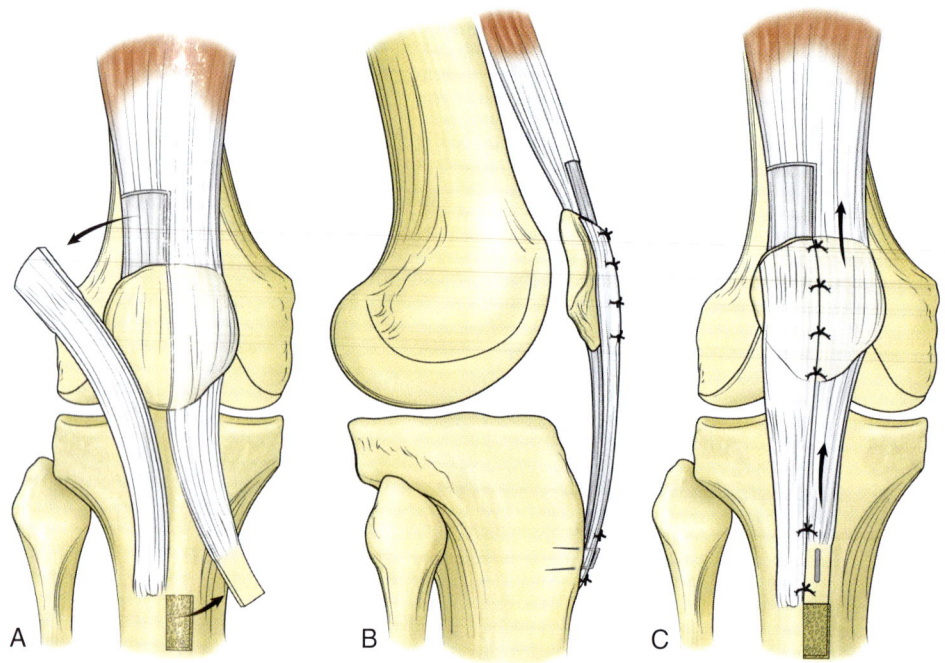

Figure 61-65. Patellar tendon lengthening (DeJour): The three steps include Z-plasty of the patellar tendon, perioperative x-ray evaluation of patellar height, and fixation with stitches protected with a metallic wire for 6 months.

Proximal Transfer of the Tibial Tubercle[15]

After an anteromedial approach, dissection of the patellar tendon and section of the peripatellar retinacular tissue are performed. An arthrotomy allowing arthrolysis of the knee and verification of the intra-articular space (this may also be done under arthroscopy) are then carried out. The tibial tubercle, after section of the medial and retinacular tissue, is detached with a hammer and chisel and is transferred upward according to preoperative planning, generally between 1 and 2 cm. It is fixed with two screws. The distal screw maintains

the height of the patella, while the second, more proximal screw allows correction of the lateral position of the patellar tendon, depending on the TT-TG preoperative measurement. The medial retinaculum is then closed, but the lateral is left open. One should take care that the patellar tendon is not folded when suturing the medial retinaculum. Postoperative care includes a splint or cast in 45 degrees of flexion. The patient is kept non–weight bearing for 3 weeks, and removal of the splint for ROM exercises is allowed. The goal of these exercises is to preserve knee mobility and good tension in the patellar tendon.

Treatment by Lengthening of the Patellar Tendon[27]

The procedure starts through an anteromedial approach from the superior part of the patellar tendon to the medial edge of the tibial tubercle, followed by extensive dissection of the medial and lateral aspects of the patellar tendon. It is often necessary to free the inferior and posterior aspects of the tendon and to perform an arthrolysis. Arthrotomy allows the surgeon to check the status of the patellar cartilage and to cut the fibrous adhesions of the suprapatellar pouch. Patellar tendon lengthening is then carried out by dividing it through the middle over its whole length (Z-plasty). The lateral portion remains anchored to the tibia, while the medial part remains anchored to the medial aspect of the patella. The patella should rise naturally, and the stumps of the tendon should slide over each other. The edges are then sutured and reinforced by an absorbable polydioxanone (PDS) band or a semitendinous tendon. The lateral retinaculum is left completely open, and the medial retinaculum is closed. Immobilization of the knee in the postoperative period is realized in a cast or a posterior plaster splint at more than 40 degrees of flexion, and ROM exercises are initiated as pain subsides. After 45 days, knee flexion can be undertaken beyond 90 degrees and the splint removed (Fig. 61-65).

KEY REFERENCES

Amis AA, Firer P, Mountney J, et al: Anatomy and biomechanics of the medial patellofemoral ligament. Knee 10:215–220, 2003.

Davies AP, Bayer J, Owen-Johnson S, et al: The optimum knee flexion angle for skyline radiography is thirty degrees. Clin Orthop Relat Res 423:166–171, 2004.

Dejour D, Le Coultre B: Osteotomies in patello-femoral instabilities. Sports Med Arthrosc 15:39–46, 2007.

Dejour D, Levigne C, Dejour H: [Postoperative low patella: treatment by lengthening of the patellar tendon.] Rev Chir Orthop Reparatrice Appar Mot 81:286–295, 1995.

Dejour H, Walch G, Nove-Josserand L, Guier C: Factors of patellar instability: an anatomic radiographic study. Knee Surg Sports Traumatol Arthrosc 2:19–26, 1994.

Dye SF: The pathophysiology of patellofemoral pain: a tissue homeostasis perspective. Clin Orthop Relat Res 436:100–110, 2005.

Fithian DC, Paxton EW, Stone ML, et al: Epidemiology and natural history of acute patellar dislocation. Am J Sports Med 32:1114–1121, 2004.

Heintjes E, Berger MY, Bierma-Zeinstra SM, et al: Exercise therapy for patellofemoral pain syndrome. Cochrane Database Syst Rev (4):CD003472, 2003.

Heintjes E, Berger MY, Bierma-Zeinstra SM, et al: Pharmacotherapy for patellofemoral pain syndrome. Cochrane Database Syst Rev (3):CD003470, 2004.

Iwano T, Kurosawa H, Tokuyama H, Hoshikawa Y: Roentgenographic and clinical findings of patellofemoral osteoarthrosis: with special reference to its relationship to femorotibial osteoarthrosis and etiologic factors. Clin Orthop Relat Res 252:190–197, 1990.

Jouve JL, Glard Y, Garron E, et al: Anatomical study of the proximal femur in the fetus. J Pediatr Orthop B 14:105–110, 2005.

Neyret P, Robinson AH, Le Coultre B, et al: Patellar tendon length—the factor in patellar instability? Knee 9:3–6, 2002.

Saleh KJ, Arendt EA, Eldridge J, et al: Symposium: operative treatment of patellofemoral arthritis. J Bone Joint Surg Am 87:659–671, 2005.

Schoettle PB, Zanetti M, Seifert B, et al: The tibial tuberosity-trochlear groove distance: a comparative study between CT and MRI scanning. Knee 13:26–31, 2006.

Smith TO, Hunt NJ, Donell ST: The reliability and validity of the Q-angle: a systematic review. Knee Surg Sports Traumatol Arthrosc 16:1068–1079, 2008.

Stefancin JJ, Parker RD: First-time traumatic patellar dislocation: a systematic review. Clin Orthop Relat Res 455:93–101, 2007.

Full references for this chapter can be found on www.expertconsult.com.

Distal Realignment of the Patellofemoral Joint: Indications, Effects, Results, and Recommendations

William R. Post and John P. Fulkerson

Effective surgical treatment of patellofemoral pain and/or instability depends on an accurate diagnosis, understanding of the pathophysiology of the condition, and knowledge of the effects of a given surgical treatment on the mechanics and biology of patellofemoral function. Anterior knee pain, often caused by a patellofemoral disorder, is a common disabling complaint in young adults, predominantly women. Fortunately, nonoperative treatment, including quadriceps strengthening, stretching, core stability training, McConnell taping, and bracing, is usually effective.* However, when conservative treatment fails, and a specific treatable cause of anterior knee pain can be identified after careful physical, radiographic, and, in some cases, arthroscopic examination, successful surgical treatment of patellofemoral disorders is likely. Likewise, in the event of recurrent patellar instability, when anatomic variables are correctly defined, a logical choice can be made for successful treatment. The purpose of this chapter is to define the situations in which tibial tubercle transfer is indicated for anterior knee pain and/or patellar instability and to present appropriate techniques for safe and reproducible treatment.

PATHOPHYSIOLOGY OF PATELLOFEMORAL PAIN AND INSTABILITY: IMPLICATIONS FOR TREATMENT

Patients with patellofemoral pain problems typically have various degrees of articular pain, soft tissue pain from overuse or chronic stretch, and mechanical instability from malalignment or dysplasia of the joint. Quadriceps weakness almost always accompanies anterior knee pain and may be a cause and/or result of knee pain. Restoration of quadriceps strength and flexibility is critical to improving load acceptance. A primary function of the quadriceps is to absorb energy during gait.[106] If the quadriceps is relatively weak and stiff, it can neither generate the desired force concentrically nor absorb the necessary energy eccentrically. In knees with a deficiency of muscular energy absorption as a result of eccentric quadriceps weakness, this energy must be absorbed elsewhere in the extensor mechanism, which may result in painful overload of patellar subchondral bone or excessive stretch of peripatellar soft tissues. Should the peripatellar soft tissues be less compliant and flexible than normal, such loads may be poorly tolerated. When the problem is viewed as a deficiency in energy absorption, one can imagine that nonoperative management must focus on improving strength and flexibility throughout the lower extremities. The rehabilitation regimen must not overload the system. The concept of staying within the

"envelope of function" during patellofemoral rehabilitation is especially critical to success.[27] Rehabilitation efforts that attempt to increase strength and function by working the knee as hard as possible are destined to fail in patients with patellofemoral disorders. The prime example is the effect of isokinetic exercise on patients with anterior knee pain. Because isokinetic equipment is designed to produce resistance proportional to the force applied, the joint is forced to work at its upper limits. Already overloaded tissue tolerates this situation poorly. Instead, flexibility, strengthening, judicious use of anti-inflammatory medication, and patience should be emphasized to allow overloaded tissues to heal.

Not every anterior knee pain patient with objective radiographic patellofemoral malalignment with or without arthrosis will need surgery. Only if a dedicated effort at nonoperative management of these patients fails *and* if malalignment is objectively present, surgery to realign the extensor mechanism and/or decrease patellofemoral joint reaction force may be appropriate. Although our discussion is limited to patellofemoral problems, it is important to remember that anterior knee pain does not necessarily come from patellofemoral disease. Other causes of pain to be considered before surgery on the patellofemoral joint itself is planned include symptomatic chondromalacia patellae, patellofemoral arthrosis, plica or fat pad syndrome, iliotibial band friction syndrome, vastus lateralis tendinitis, quadriceps or patellar tendinitis, retinacular strain,[42,94] referred pain, and chronic effusion from mechanical (meniscal and/or instability) or inflammatory problems. In addition, one must remember to examine the patient for posterior cruciate ligament deficiency, a condition sometimes associated with anterior knee pain.[61] Anterior cruciate ligament (ACL) deficiency has been reported to produce anterior knee pain in 20% to 27% of patients with chronic tears.[9,14] ACL reconstruction, particularly that performed with the use of a bone–patellar tendon–bone autograft, is well known to activate anterior knee pain in some cases.

Postoperative neuromas or reflex sympathetic dystrophy may further complicate the initial diagnosis. Referred, neoplastic, and nonorganic causes of knee pain must also be excluded.[66] Most diagnoses can be made on the basis of the history and physical examination and require only confirmation by radiographic and arthroscopic examination. Patients with patellofemoral problems, including recurrent dislocation, malalignment causing subluxation and/or tilt, osteoarthrosis, traumatic chondromalacia, and postpatellectomy pain, at times are candidates for surgery. It is imperative for the clinician to understand the pathophysiology of each diagnosis and whether the goal of surgery should be realignment, soft tissue débridement, and/or relief of pressure.

A rational approach to patellofemoral disorders requires the understanding that various problems are evidenced by different combinations of articular pain, soft tissue pain, and lateral instability of the joint. The search for the correct

*References 1, 11, 22, 39, 51, 80, and 86.

diagnosis therefore will require a search for the cause of the pain and/or instability. Of course, painful stimuli can originate only from tissues that contain pain receptors. Anatomic sources of pain in the patellofemoral joint include retinacular tissue, synovium, and subchondral bone (articular cartilage is devoid of nerve tissue).[28,87] In knees with patellofemoral degenerative disease, afferent pain-transmitting substance P–containing fibers were isolated in the retinaculum, fat pad, periosteum, and subchondral plate of the patella, thus suggesting that anterior knee pain may have multiple origins.[107] Conversely, a deficiency of such fibers has been seen in the case of congenital insensitivity to pain.[25]

In contrast, causes of patellar instability are less limited and may include both dynamic and static components. Dynamic (muscular) contributions to lateral instability may result from an increased Q angle or from an unbalanced quadriceps contraction (relative weakness of the vastus medialis obliquus [VMO], delayed VMO firing pattern, or relative hypertrophy of the vastus lateralis muscle). Anteversion of the femoral neck, poor muscular control of external rotation at the hip, pathologic tibial torsion, hindfoot pronation, contracture of the retinaculum and/or patellofemoral ligaments, and dysplasia of the patella or trochlea are examples of influences that may increase lateral patellar instability. While performing the history and physical examination on a patient who is suspected to be a surgical candidate, the physician must keep in mind the question of pain versus instability.

Careful examination is indispensable for proper diagnosis of patellofemoral disorders. The diagnosis of patellofemoral pain is dependent on the physician's ability to reproduce the patient's complaints by physical examination. The search for specific clues, such as an underlying malalignment pattern, abnormally tight soft tissue structures, generalized ligamentous laxity, and patterns of tenderness, is critical to understanding the pathophysiology of each individual.

Observation

Examine the patient while standing and ambulating for evidence of an increased Q angle, torsional deformities of the femur or tibia, knee varus/valgus, pronation of the hindfoot, leg length discrepancy, ankle deformity, scars, and other factors that may affect patellar alignment. Have the patient perform a single-leg knee bend as you watch from the front to see whether the knee rolls inward, thus suggesting weakness of external rotation at the hip. Quadriceps atrophy should also be noted, although we believe that apparent "isolated" VMO atrophy is not a true finding but rather is the superficial reflection of generalized quadriceps atrophy, as suggested by Lieb and Perry.[67,68]

The Q angle is classically measured in extension from the anterior superior iliac spine to the midpoint of the patella and onward to the tibial tuberosity (Fig. 62-1). An increased Q angle should be considered to potentially increase the lateral vector of quadriceps force, possibly causing at least a theoretical tendency toward lateral patellar translation (subluxation). Although the Q angle has always been part of the traditional evaluation of the patellofemoral joint, careful review of the available literature reveals that Q angle measurements have not been well standardized. Measurements of the Q angle have been made while the patient is supine and standing. We favor the standing measurement because it includes

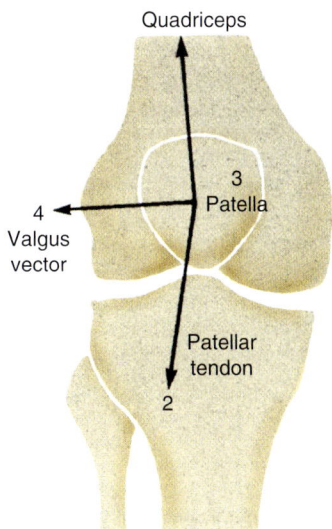

Figure 62-1. The Q angle. Lateralization of the proximal part of the quadriceps or the tibial tuberosity will increase the resultant valgus vector. (From Fulkerson JP: Disorders of the patellofemoral joint, Baltimore, 1990, Williams & Wilkins, p 36.)

physiologic loading. Unfortunately, the Q angle also has not been proved to correlate with the incidence of pain or the results of treatment.[85] Normal populations have been measured, and the results are summarized in Table 62-1. Although the importance of understanding the lateral extensor moment and its potential effects on patellar alignment is undeniable, the role of Q angle measurement is less clear.

At 90 degrees of flexion, the tuberosity is normally directly inferior to the patella. Lateral deviation of the tubercle can be measured in this position and recorded as the tubercle-sulcus angle.[62] Observation of these relationships allows the clinician to estimate the degree of valgus in the knee, as well as the position of the tibial tuberosity, which may be laterally displaced out of proportion to the tibiofemoral valgus. Lateral displacement of the tibial tubercle is more common in patients with patellofemoral pain and arthrosis and can be detected by physical examination and documented with computed tomography (CT).[78] The Q angle, as measured clinically, does not directly correlate with patellofemoral pain, and although it is related to patellofemoral mechanics, it is only one of the many factors that influence patellar balance. However, once nonoperative management maximizes dynamic factors, static alignment, including tubercle position relative to the trochlear groove, should be considered. Patellar tracking must be considered as well. Normally, the patella lies superior and lateral to the trochlea on the supratrochlear fat pad in full extension. One may recognize patella alta on examination by the abnormally proximal position of the patella, but it is more accurately diagnosed radiographically. The patella enters the trochlea smoothly from its superolateral position at 10 degrees of flexion and, with increasing flexion, is centered and drawn into the trochlea. If during early flexion the patella tracks laterally and then suddenly shifts medially into the trochlea with active or passive flexion, the J sign is positive. In a review of 210 asymptomatic adults, Johnson et al[59] found no subject with a positive J sign. Also, it should be kept in mind that the reverse J sign, in which

Table 62-1 Normal Population Q Angle Review

	SUPINE			STANDING	
Author	**Q Angle, Degrees**	**No. Knees/Age (Years)**	**Author**	**Q Angle, Degrees**	**No. Knees/Age (Years)**
Insall et al[a]	14	50/not specified	Woodland[d]	F 17.0 ± .072 M 13.6 ± .072	57/20.0 69/22.3
Aglietti et al[b]	F 17 ± 3 M 14 ± 3	75/23 75/23	Fairbank et al[e]	F 23 ± 1.2 M 20 ± 1.2	150/14.8 ± 0.1 160/14.6 ± 0.1
Hsu et al[c]	F 18.8 ± 4.7 M 15.6 ± 3.5	60/not specified 60/not specified	Horton & Hall[f]	F 15.8 ± 4.5 M 11.2 ± 3.0	
Woodland & Francis[d]	F 15.8 ± .072 M 12.7 ± .072	57/20.0 69/22.3			

From Fulkerson JP: Disorders of the patellofemoral joint, Baltimore, 1997, Williams & Wilkins.

F, Female; *M*, male.

[a]Insall J, Falvo KA, Wise DW: Chondromalacia patellae: a prospective study. J Bone Joint Surg Am 58:1, 1976.

[b]Aglietti P, Insall JN, Cerulli G: Patellar pain and incongruence. Clin Orthop Relat Res 122:217, 1983.

[c]Hsu RWW, Himeno S, Coventry MB, et al: Normal axial alignment of the lower extremity and load-bearing distribution at the knee. Clin Orthop Relat Res 255:215, 1990.

[d]Woodland LH, Francis RS: Parameters and comparisons of the quadriceps angle of college-aged men and women in the supine and standing positions. Am J Sports Med 20:208, 1992.

[e]Fairbank JCT, Pynsent PB, van Poortvliet JA, et al: Mechanical factors in the incidence of knee pain in adolescents and young adults. J Bone Joint Surg 66:685, 1984.

[f]Horton MG, Hall TI: Quadriceps femoris muscle angle: normal values and relationships with gender and selected skeletal measures. Phys Ther 69:897, 1989.

the patella of a patient with medial patella subluxation slides in a medial-to-lateral direction on knee flexion, is clearly an abnormal pattern, but often is very subtle. As with all tests of alignment, comparison with the other side is important.

Provocative Tests

Strong compression of the patella resulting in pain and crepitus during flexion and extension of the knee is helpful in determining whether the patient's pain syndrome has a significant patellofemoral component. Another method of provocative testing is isometric contraction of the quadriceps at different angles of flexion.[73] Isometric contractions, which should be sustained for 10 seconds, provide the advantage of avoiding direct palpation in patients who are particularly apprehensive. If one or both of these methods reproduce the patient's complaint, it is likely that the pain has a patellofemoral origin. These techniques of examination do not, however, distinguish between soft tissue and articular sources of pain because soft tissue stretch, as well as articular compression, is noted when the knee is moved or the quadriceps is fired during these examinations.

In an attempt to confirm whether a patient has medial patella subluxation, hold the patella slightly medial with one finger and the knee in extension, then abruptly flex the knee. If this maneuver reproduces the symptoms, the patient probably has a problem with medial subluxation, most commonly in the clinical setting of previous lateral release.[35]

Palpation

The subcutaneous position of the patellofemoral joint makes it uniquely available to careful examination. Palpation of the patellofemoral joint has two goals: (1) to differentiate between soft tissue and bony pain, and (2) to precisely localize the soft

tissue or articular area that reproduces the patient's complaint. Firm compression of the patella directly into the trochlea while the knee is held in various angles of flexion, combined with the knowledge that articulation starts distal on the patella and moves proximally with increasing flexion, can provide information to localize the articular disease. This can be accomplished by direct compression (with care taken to avoid compressing adjacent soft tissue structures). Meaningful specific palpation of medial or lateral patellar facets seems anatomically unlikely, given the interposition of innervated synovium and retinacular tissue. The degree of crepitus is more significant when absent or asymmetrical with the contralateral knee. When evaluating the presence or absence of crepitus, remember that Johnson et al found 94% of asymptomatic women to have crepitus.[59] It is more important to note whether articular compression reproduces the patient's pain. Also, knowledge of the character of the crepitus is helpful. Harsh, sustained grinding is different from the faint click that is common on flexion and extension of a normal knee.

Soft tissue palpation should systematically include the retinacular structures, the insertions of the quadriceps tendons into the superior pole of the patella, and the patellar tendon. Structures are generally best palpated in a position that places them on stretch and allows gentle palpation to achieve relative isolation from the underlying structures. This strategy allows discovery of specific points prone to overuse-type injury. We have previously described in detail a thorough anatomically and functionally oriented soft tissue examination, and the reader is encouraged to practice and master these techniques.[37,38,85] Points of intersection between structures, such as the junction of the medial patellar tendon, the inferior pole of the patella, and the medial retinaculum, seem particularly prone to tenderness, perhaps because of the stress concentration at locations where two or more different structures under load meet. These locations are frequently tender in patients with excessive lateral patellar tilt. A cautious search for such locations will often uncover the origin of a patient's soft tissue pain.

Such differentiation between soft tissue and articular pain helps in surgical planning. Stress-relieving anteriorization should be considered in patients with predominantly articular-based complaints and normal alignment. In contrast, coronal (medial/lateral) realignment may be adequate in cases of malalignment in which the articular surface has not degenerated. With severe articular degeneration, the patella may not tolerate even the relatively lower loads present after completion of a procedure that corrects alignment.

Stability Testing

Just as examination for ACL deficiency includes evaluation of the static stability of a joint in several planes, examination of the patellofemoral joint is not complete without evaluation of static constraints in both the sagittal (tilt) and coronal (medial/lateral) planes. Evaluation of patellar tilt and medial-to-lateral restraints provides important information.

The passive patellar tilt test is performed with the knee in full extension. While the patella is held in the center of the trochlea, the examiner attempts to correct the patellar tilt to neutral or beyond, if possible (Fig. 62-2). We agree with Kolowich et al[62] that normally the tilt should correct at least to neutral, although normal patellae often tilt up to 10 degrees or more past neutral. It is also possible to gain an impression of the nature of the resilience of the lateral retinaculum. Some patients seem to have a springy endpoint, whereas others have a very stiff and unyielding restraint. Comparison with the opposite knee often reveals relatively limited correction of lateral patellar tilt on the symptomatic side. Because the iliotibial band fibers contribute to the lateral retinacular tissue, poor iliotibial band flexibility frequently accompanies abnormal lateral tilt.

Medial and lateral patellar glide testing has been well described by McConnell[73] and by Kolowich et al.[62] It is similar to the passive hypermobility testing described by Hughston.[54] We believe that these tests should be performed with the patella in neutral tilt if possible to allow consistent comparison of the medial/lateral restraints. As described, medial patellar glide is tested with medially directed pressure on the patella and the knee in 20 to 30 degrees of flexion to effectively engage the patella in the trochlea (Fig. 62-3). This test is also effective with the knee in extension and earlier degrees of flexion. Near full extension, the ligamentous and muscular restraints may be more isolated because of less bony constraint before engagement of the patella in the trochlea. Through testing of lateral glide with the knee in extension, it is possible to palpate an endpoint to lateral translation similar to that palpable with the Lachman test. Absence of such an endpoint, together with increased translation, is highly suggestive of medial patellofemoral ligament (MPFL) deficiency. Any abnormal tightness found in the retinaculum at these lesser angles of flexion can affect the direction of patellar entry into the trochlea. Medial patellar glide is judged abnormal if medial translation is seen in less than one quadrant, as described by Kolowich and Paulos. Laterally directed pressure on the neutral patella that results in displacement of three quadrants or more is consistent with an abnormally lax medial restraint. Ligamentous laxity itself, as might be measured by quadrant displacement, should not be confused with actual subluxation and, if found, should generate caution if a realignment procedure is contemplated. Evidence of systemic ligamentous laxity should be sought in such patients before any conclusions are drawn regarding specific isolated incompetence of peripatellar restraints or malalignment. In hypermobile patients, dynamic muscular control of patellar position is even more critical. Emphasis should be placed on active muscular control and on being patient. Involuntary quadriceps contraction during positive lateral glide testing or the classic apprehension reaction to the perception of imminent dislocation is strong evidence of clinically relevant patellar instability.

Several tests have been developed to assist in the diagnosis of medial patellar instability, a condition that almost always occurs as a complication of patellar realignment. In patients with symptomatic medial patellar instability, one can displace the patella medially and then passively flex the knee, and the symptoms will be reproduced as the patella moves laterally from the subluxated position into the trochlea.[85] Although

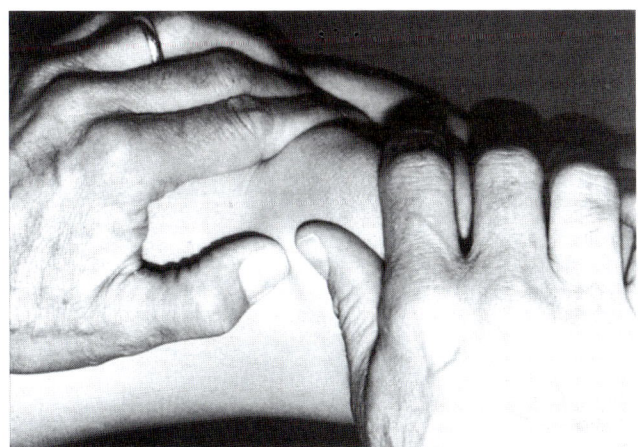

Figure 62-2. Physical examination for patellar tilt. Tilt should correct to neutral. (From Scott WN: The knee, vol 1, St Louis, 1994, Mosby-Year Book, p 445.)

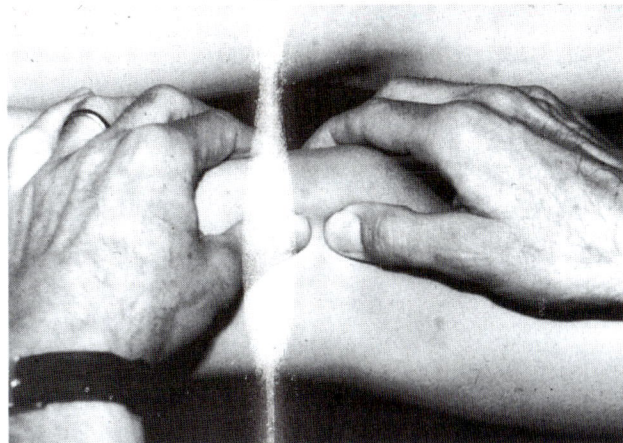

Figure 62-3. Physical examination for patellar glide. Medially directed force is applied to the lateral aspect of the patella. (From Scott WN: The knee, vol 1, St Louis, 1994, Mosby-Year Book, p 445.)

the patella is moving laterally, it is moving from a subluxated position into the trochlea, essentially a "reverse apprehension" test. Another helpful test in the setting of potential medial instability is the gravity subluxation test.[82] This test requires that the patient be placed in the lateral decubitus position. The patella is then manually displaced medially. Because of previous operative transection of the vastus lateralis, the patient cannot actively reduce the patella into the trochlea. Although provocative testing for medial patellar instability is not routinely necessary, these tests should be regularly included in the evaluation of patients after failed patellofemoral realignment.

Flexibility

Systematic evaluation of the quadriceps, hamstring, iliotibial band, and gastrocnemius/soleus muscle groups is important because each can contribute to anterior knee pain. Quadriceps tightness is often associated with patellar tendinitis and "failed" postoperative patellar pain patients. Quadriceps tightness is best tested with the patient prone, thereby stabilizing the pelvis. Hamstring contracture may result in abnormally increased knee flexion during the stance phase and, therefore, increased patellofemoral joint reaction force. Iliotibial band tightness has a more direct effect through its insertion into the lateral retinaculum and, consequently, abnormally increases posterolateral pull with increasing flexion. Increased hindfoot pronation is a result of gastrocnemius and/or soleus contracture in some patients. This causes the subtalar joint to compensate for the relative lack of tibiotalar dorsiflexion with increased hindfoot pronation. Increased subtalar pronation results in increased internal rotation of the tibia and femur and contributes to patellofemoral malalignment. When diminished flexibility is detected, nonoperative management must include stretching.

Radiologic Evaluation

Once a complete history and physical examination have been performed, radiologic studies are frequently indicated to confirm and document the clinical impression. Standing anteroposterior and lateral x-ray films are important to search for associated conditions and patella alta. A normal ratio of patellar ligament length to patellar length of less than 1.2 has been described by Insall and Salvati.[56] Blackburne and Peel[8]

described the ratio of the articular length of the patella to the height of the lower pole of the patellar articular cartilage above the tibial articular surface (normal, <1.0). These ratios can be used to quantify patella alta if desired. In cases in which patella alta is prominently abnormal, distal transfer of the tuberosity should be part of the surgical plan.

Axial tangential views of the patellofemoral joint, such as those described by Merchant et al[75] and Laurin et al,[65] may be used as screening tests for malalignment but can be difficult to interpret because of image overlap (unless the image is precisely tangential to the joint). The congruence angle of Merchant and Mercer and the lateral patellofemoral angle of Laurin and Dussault are estimations of lateral subluxation and tilt, respectively. The symmetry of subchondral sclerosis of the patellar facets should also be evaluated for signs of localized sclerosis (indicating unbalanced stress). These authors and their colleagues recognized the importance of imaging the patella early in flexion in the less constrained proximal femoral sulcus. Kujala and Kormano[64] emphasized imaging of the patellofemoral joint in early flexion. They found greater magnetic resonance imaging (MRI) differences in tilt and lateral subluxation on views with less than 30 degrees of flexion in a group of patients with recurrent patellar dislocations than in a normal control group. CT scans, first suggested by Delgado-Martins[24] in 1979, offer a significant advantage by providing imaging of earlier degrees of flexion with absolutely no image overlap. Advanced imaging studies such as CT scans assist in confirming the diagnosis and should be considered only in the evaluation of an unusual patient in whom nonoperative management fails.

Further work on CT technique, evaluation, and classification of patellofemoral disorders has been done by Schutzer and associates.[97,98] Several significant advantages of CT evaluation are now clear. Use of the posterior femoral condyles as a reference plane for measurement of the patellar tilt angle has proved significantly more consistent than use of the anterior intercondylar line, as reported by Laurin and Dussault. This increases the precision with which tilt can be measured and eliminates the variable of femoral rotation[40] (Fig. 62-4). Measurement of the congruence angle is also enhanced by the nature of the CT scan "slice" because it ensures that the trochlear and patellar images being measured are, in fact, at the same level and are not artifacts of image overlap (Fig. 62-5). Furthermore, a patellofemoral CT scan can be useful

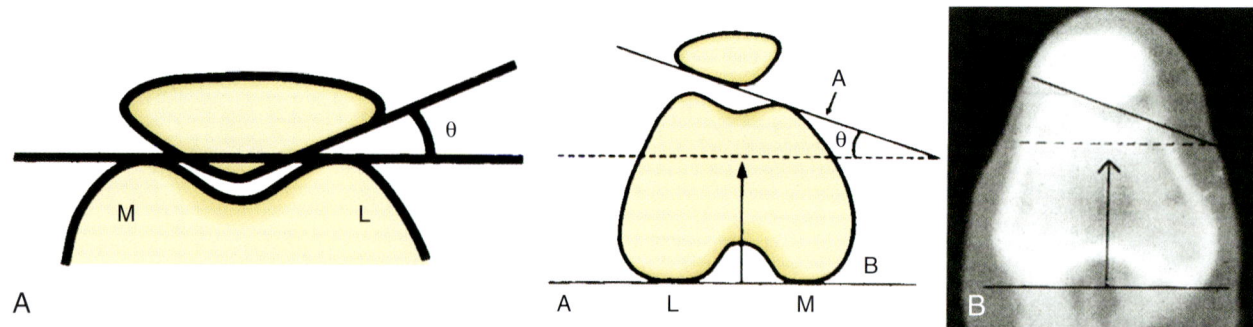

Figure 62-4. **A,** Patellar tilt angle of Laurin measured from an axial radiograph. **B,** Patellar tilt angle measured from a transverse midpatellar computed tomographic scan. (From Fulkerson JP: Disorders of the patellofemoral joint, Baltimore, 1990, Williams & Wilkins, pp 50, 60.)

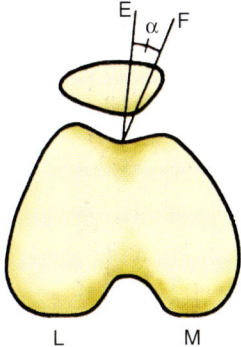

Figure 62-5. Congruence angle as measured on a midtransverse patellar computed tomographic scan. (From Scott WN: The knee, vol 1, St Louis, 1994, Mosby-Year Book, p 446.)

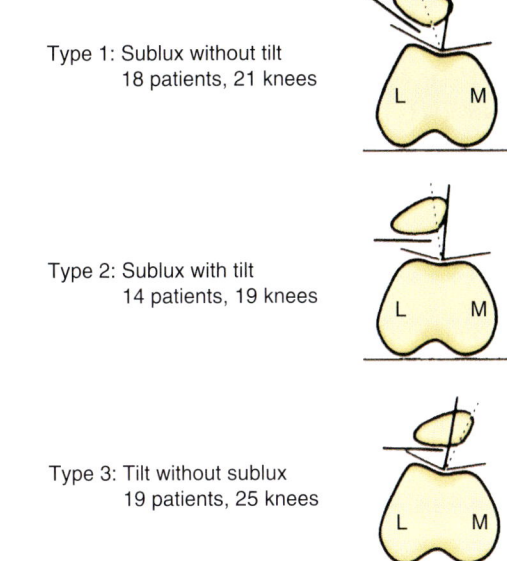

Type 1: Sublux without tilt
18 patients, 21 knees

Type 2: Sublux with tilt
14 patients, 19 knees

Type 3: Tilt without sublux
19 patients, 25 knees

Figure 62-6. Computed tomographic scan classification of patellofemoral malalignment. (From Schutzer SF, Ramsby GR: Computed tomographic classification of patellofemoral pain patients. Orthop Clin North Am 17:235, 1986.)

in detecting subtle patellar or trochlear dysplasia, such as a shallow trochlear groove in patients with lateral patellar subluxation. Moreover, limited CT evaluation of the patellofemoral joint can be accomplished quickly and at a cost similar to that of multiple conventional x-ray films. Patterns of patellofemoral malalignment on CT images are usually classified into three types. Type I is lateral subluxation, type II combines lateral subluxation and lateral tilt, and type III includes lateral tilt without subluxation (Fig. 62-6). Type IV has been defined as radiographically normal alignment.[41] This classification has been very helpful in confirming the clinical impression of specific patellar malalignment patterns (tilt and/or subluxation). Treatment selection is also dependent on accurate classification, as will be appreciated in the later discussion of our recommended surgical approach.

When distal realignment including tibial tuberosity transfer is considered, we believe it is wise to measure the position of the tuberosity relative to the trochlea. The most acceptable method for this consists of CT measurement of the tibial tuberosity–trochlear groove (TT-TG) distance (Fig. 62-7). Dejour and associates first described this measurement and found, upon comparing normal patients with those with patellar instability, that the threshold for normal was 20 mm.[23] This measurement is done by measuring the lateral distance of the tibial tuberosity from the most posterior point in the femoral sulcus, along a line parallel to the axis of the posterior femoral condyles. Schoetle et al showed that the MRI scan may be used for this measurement as well.[96] When the TT-TG distance is 20 mm or greater, available data suggest that such a measurement is abnormal on MRI or CT scan. Medialization of the tuberosity is then rational. The amount of medialization needed can also be estimated from this measurement, and the most often targeted goal for postoperative TT-TG distance is less than approximately 10 mm. Measurement of the TT-TG is helpful in confirming that tuberosity medialization is appropriate in a clinical situation that otherwise warrants medial or anteromedial transfer.

Nonoperative Management

Most patients with patellofemoral disorders improve without surgery. Dye has provided excellent reviews and a theoretical model that he calls the *envelope of load acceptance model* to enhance understanding of the mechanisms and reasons for improvement of patients with patellofemoral pain by rest and

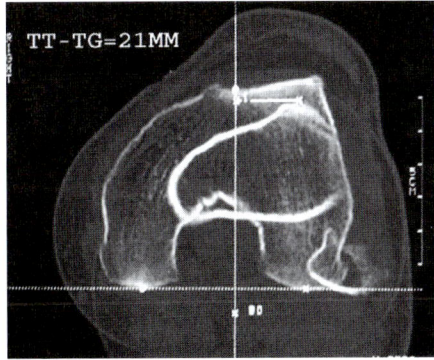

Figure 62-7. Tibial tuberosity–trochlear groove (TT-TG) distance. Axial image through the tibial tuberosity superimposed on a cut through the femoral trochlea at the level where the intercondylar notch appears to be a "Roman arch." TT-TG equals the lateral distance of the tibial tuberosity from the most posterior point in the femoral sulcus, along a line parallel to the axis of the posterior femoral condyles. Normal TT-TG distance should measure less than 20 mm. (Image courtesy of Dr. Rick Cautilli, Philadelphia, Pa.)

activity modification.[27] Initial management of patellofemoral disorders should include the goals of normal flexibility and balanced quadriceps strength. One should remember to include the entire extremity in rehabilitation, especially hip strengthening. This program should be directed by specific physical examination findings. Discussion of specific techniques exceeds the scope of this chapter. In addition to reassurance, strengthening, stretching, core stability training, taping techniques, anti-pronation orthotics, and patellar braces may be very beneficial in selected patients. Weight loss in obese patients is imperative in controlling patellofemoral pain. It is sometimes surprising how well patients, even those with severe radiographic findings, do without surgery. Therefore, before surgery, it is always important to confirm that a comprehensive nonoperative treatment program has been followed.

A RATIONAL APPROACH TO DISTAL REALIGNMENT

Realignment operations, including distal realignments, should be considered only when objective anatomic malalignment has been diagnosed AND nonoperative treatment has failed. Patients with malalignment may have pain and/or symptomatic patellar instability. It is very important to differentiate whether the goal of surgery is simply realignment with improvement in the balance of forces across the patellofemoral joint, or whether discrete episodes of patellar instability have occurred preoperatively. If dislocations have occurred, one must consider whether stabilization of the patella might be needed by medial patellofemoral ligament imbrication or reconstruction, along with correction of underlying malalignment. The decision to add imbrication or reconstruction must be made carefully and only after consideration of whether this would unwisely increase load on medial facet chondral lesions.

For patients who have severe symptomatic articular degeneration in a normally aligned patellofemoral joint, surgical choices include anteriorization, patellectomy, and patellofemoral arthroplasty. Patellofemoral resurfacing and patellectomy are rarely necessary unless no adequate articular cartilage remains. None of these operations restores the knee to "normal," and nonoperative management is often indicated. Frequently in such patients with severe arthrosis after blunt trauma, multiple localized foci of soft tissue inflammation and overload and of pain from articular degeneration are noted. Patient and persistent treatment directed at the soft tissues (e.g., stretching, strengthening, activity modification) can often produce satisfactory improvement without surgery. Distal realignment is NOT indicated in such patients, even as a "last resort."

Distal Realignment Procedures

Theory

Distal realignment of the patellofemoral joint by medial transposition of the patellar tendon insertion decreases the laterally directed moment that causes patellar subluxation upon quadriceps contraction. Ideal candidates for distal realignment have laterally displaced tibial tubercles, although this has not been proven to be a prerequisite. Lateral release usually accompanies the various methods of medialization and is important in relieving any lateral tether that is present. Alternatively, advancement of medial structures, or medial patellofemoral ligament (MPFL) reconstruction, might potentially create abnormally increased medial patellar facet pressure by attempting to counteract forceful, laterally directed pull on the patella using a posteromedially directed tether on the extensor mechanism. The concept that we wish to put forth here is that the extensor mechanism must be balanced first, before medial incompetent structures such as the MPFL are reconstructed. The biomechanics of posterior displacement of the tibial tuberosity dictates an increase in joint reaction force to accomplish the same work, and this should be avoided (Fig. 62-8). Distal transfer of the tuberosity

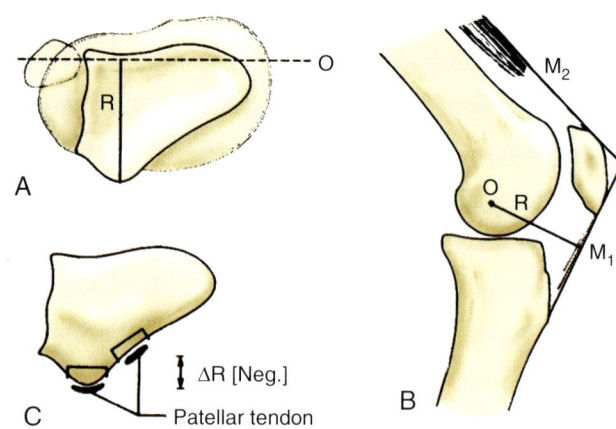

Figure 62-8. A, Note the lateral position of the tubercle with respect to the tibial plateau and the posteromedial slope of the anteromedial tibial cortex. Distance R illustrates the lever arm of the quadriceps. **B,** Lateral view illustrating the quadriceps lever R. **C,** Posterior displacement of the tibial tubercle as a result of medial transposition of the tibial tubercle (classic Hauser's procedure). The decreased mechanical advantage of the quadriceps mechanism in this situation results in the need to generate greater quadriceps muscle force to accomplish the same work, and this leads to increased patellofemoral joint reaction force. (From Fulkerson JP: Disorders of the patellofemoral joint, Baltimore, 1990, Williams & Wilkins, p 144.)

when pathologic patella alta is present helps the patella to enter the trochlea earlier in flexion and can be very helpful in some patients with patellar instability.

Clinical Data

Distal medialization procedures may be divided into two categories: (1) those involving soft tissue only, and (2) those involving transfer of the tibial tuberosity. Skeletal immaturity in a patient being considered for distal realignment mandates selection of a procedure that does not violate the proximal tibial physis or the apophysis of the tibial tubercle—a mistake that could cause complications such as genu recurvatum or continued distal migration of the tibial tuberosity with growth.*

Soft Tissue Medialization

Historically, options for distal realignment in a skeletally immature patient have included (1) the Roux-Goldthwait procedure, in which the lateral half of the patellar tendon is detached distally, passed behind the medial half of the tendon, and sutured to the pes anserinus insertion, and (2) the Galeazzi semitendinosus tenodesis. Each procedure normally would be done with a lateral release. Reports of the Roux-Goldthwait procedure vary from good success rates in two series[17,34] to a high failure rate in another.[10] Another, more recent study found a higher rate of patellofemoral osteoarthrosis when the Roux-Goldthwait procedure was compared with medial patellofemoral ligament reconstruction.[101] The mechanics of this operation, however, incurs the risk of inducing undesirable lateral patellar tilt, and this procedure is no longer recommended. The Galeazzi tenodesis procedure uses the distally attached semitendinosus tendon to pull the

---

*References 20, 21, 33, 47, 52, and 69.

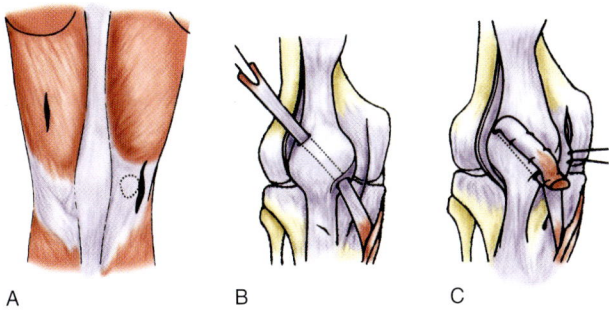

A   B   C

Figure 62-9. Galeazzi semitendinosus tenodesis, an option for soft tissue distal realignment in the skeletally immature patient. (From Baker RH, Carroll N: The semitendinosus tenodesis for recurrent dislocation of the patella. J Bone Joint Surg Br 54:103, 1972.)

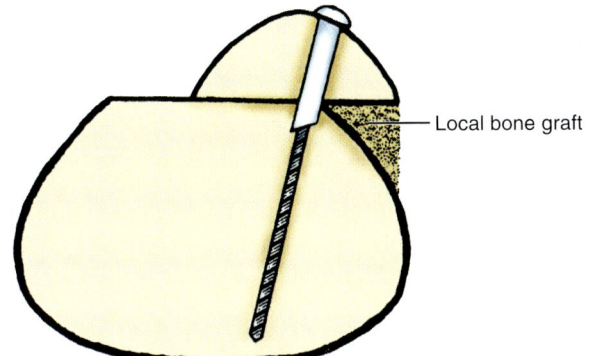

Local bone graft

Figure 62-10. Roux-Elmslie-Trillat procedure. Note that this medialization of the tibial tubercle results in no posterior displacement of the tuberosity. (From Cox JS: Evaluation of the Roux-Elmslie-Trillat procedure for knee extensor realignment. Am J Sports Med 10:303, 1982.)

patella distally and medially (Fig. 62-9). Baker et al,[2] when using this technique, achieved 81% good and excellent results with only 4% recurrent dislocations. In a small series of patients with malalignment reported by Hall et al,[44] 10 of 11 patients had good to excellent results. Perhaps it is not surprising that the authors also reported fair to poor results in 8 of 10 patients when this procedure was performed for dislocation or subluxation caused by ligamentous laxity or a direct blow. They noted no significant change in their results in patients in whom they combined a Roux-type patellar tendon transfer with a semitendinosus tenodesis. Pes anserinus transposition for lateral patellar instability has been reported by Baksi,[3,4] but we believe that additional studies are necessary before use of this technique becomes widespread. These procedures are rarely, if ever, necessary. Note that most authors include medial retinacular imbrication/VMO advancement, as well as soft tissue distal medialization, with each of these procedures. In analysis of these results, it is very difficult to justify distal medialization in skeletally immature patients. Judicious proximal realignment usually is most prudent.

Mini–proximal imbrication with MPFL and VMO advancement through a 2-inch incision can be very helpful in many patients and is preferable to alternative procedures when it can restore normal patellar tracking. MPFL reconstruction procedures that involve attaching a graft to the region of the medial femoral epicondyle are contraindicated in skeletally immature patients because of the risk of physeal damage. Immediate range of motion is imperative.

MPFL reconstruction by the technique of Deie and colleagues using a distally attached semitendinosus graft transferred to the medial proximal patella through a soft tissue attachment in the posterior part of the proximal medial cruciate ligament (MCL) provides good soft tissue stabilization in skeletally immature patients. We have rarely found that skeletally immature patients require management with distal realignment and recommend other management until skeletal maturity.

Tuberosity Transfers

The Hauser procedure, as described in 1938, includes medial and distal transplantation of the tibial tuberosity.[48] Several authors have noted only 67% to 74% rates of good to excellent pain relief and functional improvement after Hauser procedures for diagnoses of chondromalacia resulting from

malalignment,[55] recurrent patellar dislocation,[17] and acute and recurrent dislocations.[33] Recurrent dislocation has occurred at similarly steady rates of 17% to 20%.[17,21,60] Generalized ligamentous laxity has been strongly associated with poor results and recurrent dislocation.[21] Furthermore, in some series, a distressingly high percentage of patients (68% to 71%) have had evidence of progression to osteoarthrosis at average follow-up of 7.3 years,[21] 16 years,[46] and 18 years.[60] Unfortunately, because of the anatomy of the proximal end of the tibia, this procedure has resulted in posterior tuberosity displacement (see Fig. 62-8). The high incidence of articular degeneration is consistent with biomechanical theory, which predicts increased stress with distal and posterior transfer of the tuberosity. Posteromedial transfer of the tibial tubercle is rarely, if ever, justified.

Dougherty et al[26] and Grana and O'Donoghue[43] reported modifications of the Hauser procedure in which a slot-block method of fixation of the tibial tuberosity was used for lateral patellar instability. Both had 83% successful results, although Grana and O'Donoghue experienced a 26% rate of significant complications and labeled this procedure technically demanding. Dougherty and Wirth noted worse results in patients with more severe chondromalacia, although specific criteria were not cited. Again, this type of surgery is rarely appropriate and is primarily of historical interest.

Cox[18,19] successfully accomplished distal realignment by medial displacement of the tuberosity while avoiding any posterior displacement with the Roux-Elmslie-Trillat procedure (Fig. 62-10). This technique classically combines lateral release, medial capsular reefing, and medial displacement of the bony insertion of the patellar tendon with distal displacement titrated according to the degree of patella alta measured preoperatively. Excellent and good results were achieved in 77% of 116 patients, with only a 7% recurrence rate. Factors associated with poor outcomes included failure to adequately correct the Q angle or the patella alta, concomitant ACL deficiency, and preexisting patellar degeneration. Using the same procedure, Brown et al[12] found that adequate postoperative correction of the Q angle to 10 degrees or less correlated well with good to excellent results. Shelbourne et al[100] found that postoperative alignment (as measured radiographically by the congruence angle) correlated with the presence of recurrent instability. In their series, 26% (9/34) of patients with preoperative instability had postoperative subluxation. Although postoperative improvement in the congruence angle was the same for patients with stable patellae, these patients had higher preoperative and postoperative congruence angles. Durable results from tibial tubercle transfer have been reproducible with 10-year minimum follow-up in a number of reports.[16,21,58] No progression of osteoarthrosis was noted, and theoretically one would expect it to be less than with the Hauser procedure, which classically includes posterior tubercle displacement. The Elmslie-Trillat may be combined with arthroscopic lateral release and medial retinacular surgery to obtain results consistent with those described previously.[6]

In reviewing series of patients treated by distal realignment, one notes that the procedure is often modified in potentially important ways. Tomatsu et al[104] compared two groups of similar patients treated with Elmslie-Trillat procedures, but with omission of medial capsulorrhaphy in one group. Results were identical in both groups and were very similar to those reported by previous authors. The series of Shelbourne et al[100] also omitted medial capsulorrhaphy. Rantanen and Paananen[91] reported on 35 knees treated by medial transfer of the tibial tubercle; they omitted the lateral release in 14 patients. Their results were, again, practically identical to those reported by Cox. Rillmann et al[92] reported yet another modification in which only the medial third of the patellar tendon was transferred and lateral release was included in only 2 of 39 patients. Again, similar outcomes occurred with no redislocations and an 11% rate of postoperative subluxation. Some authors specifically measure patella alta and routinely include distal transfer of the tubercle.[12,18,19,91] Others specifically omit consideration of distal transfer to correct patella alta.[92,100,104] Although the data currently do not allow for definitive guidelines regarding specific operative procedures, we believe that factors such as systemic hypermobility, skeletal alignment, and articular surface condition should be considered when the best procedure to correct instability in any given patient is selected. Patients with severe radiographic malalignment may require medial imbrication, but based on previous studies, it is apparent that many patients do not require medial capsular imbrication.

Anteriorization

Theory

Anterior elevation of the tibial tuberosity, as proposed by Bandi[5] and Maquet,[70,71] enhances the efficiency of the quadriceps by increasing the lever arm while decreasing the patellofemoral joint reaction force. As illustrated in Figure 62-11, increasing the angle between the vector of quadriceps pull and the patellar tendon decreases the joint reaction force. The goal is to reduce articular stress by reducing the force and increasing the area of joint contact, thus further decreasing articular stress. Maquet's calculations of patellofemoral compressive force predict an approximately 50% reduction during the stance phase after a 2-cm elevation.

Laboratory Data

This hypothesis is generally confirmed by a progressive reduction in patellofemoral compressive force as cadaver tibial tubercles are advanced. Ferguson et al's comparison[31] of six

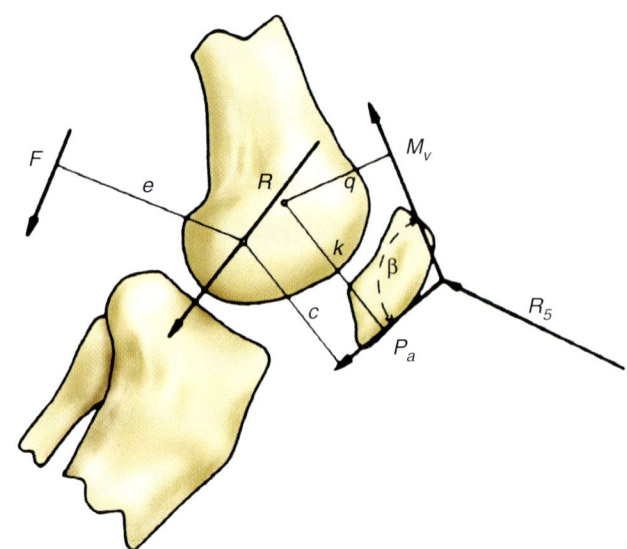

Figure 62-11. Anteriorization of the tibial tubercle decreases the angle β, thereby resulting in decreased patellofemoral joint reaction force. It also tips up the distal patella, thereby unloading distal patellar chondral lesions. (From Maquet P: Mechanics and osteoarthritis of the patellofemoral joint. Clin Orthop Relat Res 144:70, 1979.)

locations on the articular surface of the patella after 1.2-, 2.5-, and 3.7-cm anterior elevation demonstrated significant relief of stress. Overall stress relief with 1.2-cm advancement at 45 degrees of flexion was 57%. Further elevation to 2.5 and 3.7 cm resulted in additional progressive decreases in average stress of only 30% and 9%, respectively. In a review of these data, Radin[88] noted, however, that the absolute value of total contact stress after 1.2-cm elevation was more than twice that measured after an elevation of 2.5 cm. Ferguson and Brown's study used averaged values obtained from retropatellar sensors and assumed them to be equivalent to the overall average because their model did not permit measurement of contact areas. They concluded that most contact stress was relieved with the first 1.2 cm of tendon elevation, and that additional decreases were believed to represent decreasing returns in exchange for increasing risk of skin complications. In a similar study using retropatellar piezoelectric transducers, Ferrandez et al[32] confirmed close to a 50% decrease in pressure in the first 1 cm and a more gradual decline with further tubercle elevation.

Lewallen et al[66] used pressure-sensitive film to measure the joint contact force and area after 1.2-cm and 2.5-cm tubercle elevations in eight knees with variable degrees of chondromalacia (Outerbridge grades I to IV). They found significant decreases in joint contact force of 29% and 23% after 1.2-cm elevation at 60 and 90 degrees of flexion, respectively. Contrary to the findings of Ferguson et al's study,[31] elevation to 2.5 cm resulted in significant additional 60%, 53%, and 55% decreases in force in comparison with "preoperative" values at 30, 60, and 90 degrees. Patellar contact area was observed to shift proximally and laterally with progressive elevation. It is interesting to note that although force was reduced, joint contact area decreased significantly at 90 degrees of flexion with 1.2-cm elevation, and at 30, 60, and 90 degrees of flexion with 2.5-cm advancement.

Similar conclusions were reached by Nakamura et al,[79] who used silicone casting techniques to document progressive decreases in contact area with progressive elevations. Burke and Ahmed,[13] on the other hand, although confirming progressive significant load reduction with progressive advancement to 3 cm, did not find excessive superolateral peak pressures at high degrees of flexion. However, one must keep in mind that these experiments were performed in some normal knees, some with variable amounts of "chondromalacia," and possibly some with variable alignment patterns. With regard to the suggestion that anteriorization shifts the load proximally, this may occur secondary to the slight distal transfer that occurs as the shingle is rotated forward (and distally).[83] Logically, this effect is increased with shorter shingle length, which produces relatively more distal transfer for the same anteriorization as would a longer shingle. Overall, these findings substantiate the concept of further relief of joint reaction force with increasing elevation, even if these particular models do not specifically support or refute Maquet's contention that contact area is increased.

Clinical Experience

Maquet[70] reported on 37 patients with patellar arthrosis and chondromalacia an average of 4.7 years after 2- to 3-cm advancement of the tuberosity; 36 knees were stable with relief of pain and range of motion that approximated preoperative motion. His recommendations included medialization of the tubercle when the patella was subluxated, and osteoarthritis was limited to the lateral facet. Medialization was accomplished by notching the graft. Early postoperative motion was possible because of the stable geometry of the iliac graft (Fig. 62-12). In a report by Rozbruch et al[93] at the Hospital for Special Surgery, an additional 16 patients with various diagnoses experienced only 63% good results after Maquet procedures. Radin's[88] 36 patients had successful results from a modified Maquet procedure, including elevation of at least 2 cm, lateral release, and medialization of approximately 1 cm (as necessary to correct subluxation) in 94% with posttraumatic osteoarthrosis, in 88% with chronic patellar subluxation and osteoarthrosis, and in 66% with

postpatellectomy pain. Hirsh and Reddy[53] also reported successful results with elevation of 1.7 to 2.5 cm in a small series. Mendes et al,[74] in their series of 27 patients with primarily patellofemoral osteoarthritis, achieved 76% subjective satisfactory results at 5.5 years after a 2.5-cm elevation. Heatley et al[49] reported 65% excellent and good results in 29 patients. In a series of 184 patients treated by Ferguson[30] with anterior elevation of 1.25 cm and local bone grafting, satisfactory pain relief plus resumption of lost function were achieved in 92% of patients with "osteoarthrosis" (degree unspecified), 82% of patients with recurrent dislocations, 84% of patients with chondromalacia, 84% of patients with blunt patellar trauma, and 88% of patients with previous patellectomy. Medial transfer of 4 to 5 mm was regularly included in operations for recurrent dislocations and was performed as "desirable" in patients with other diagnoses. Lateral retinacular release was not performed routinely. No internal fixation was used, and patients were placed in a cast for 6 weeks and waited an average of 6 months for symptomatic relief. In general, these reports share a common theme of best results in patients with osteoarthrosis and less consistent results for other diagnoses.

Engebretsen et al's results[29] correlated with the pattern of articular degeneration; the best postoperative results were seen in patients with lateral facet degeneration. No improvement was noted in 18 of 20 patients with medial facet involvement. At long-term follow-up of 8 to 15 years, anteriorization has been found to be durable; Jenny et al[57] reported a 62% success rate. Silvello et al[102] treated patients with "chondromalacia" and patellofemoral arthritis with somewhat less anteriorization (1.2 to 1.5 cm) than the classic Maquet procedure and achieved only 53% good and excellent results. Conversely, emphasizing the importance of at least 2 cm of anteriorization, Schmid[95] found 80% good/very good results at a mean 16-year follow-up. When the use of anteriorization is considered for treatment of anterior knee pain, we believe it is important to recognize that the severity and the pattern of articular degeneration are critical. Distal lateral lesions are probably best suited for relief with this procedure; however, many successes have been reported in the literature with other lesions. Nonetheless, patients and surgeons must realize that this is generally a salvage procedure, and function is rarely truly normal after the procedure. Patients must also understand that the tubercle appears prominent after surgery and is usually uncomfortable when kneeling. It is wise preoperatively to show patients photographs of knees after anteriorization to avoid cosmetic dissatisfaction postoperatively.

Anteromedialization

Although anteriorization procedures have at times included medialization to control subluxation or recurrent dislocation, several procedures that routinely combine some degree of anteromedialization have been designed for patients with malalignment. Laboratory evaluation of this concept in a cadaver model with increased lateral facet overload induced by alteration of the proximal vector of the quadriceps showed excellent reduction of lateral facet pressure.[39] This study reported a 30% reduction in lateral facet pressure with anteriorization of 8.8 mm and medialization of 8.4 mm, and 65% relief after additional anteromedialization to 14.8/8.4 mm. By 20 to 30 degrees of knee flexion, reduction and equalization

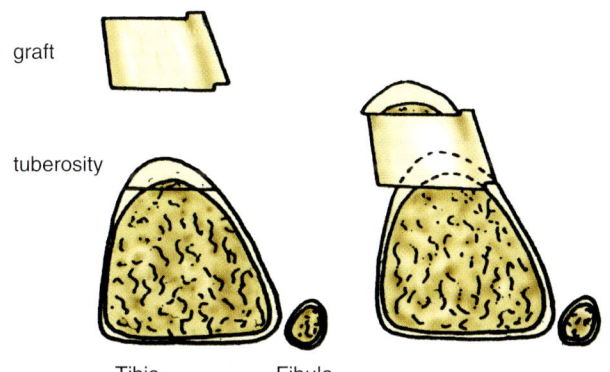

Figure 62-12. Maquet technique. A notched iliac crest graft is used to produce anterior and medial displacement of the tibial tuberosity. This procedure is rarely indicated. (From Maquet P: Advancement of the tibial tuberosity. Clin Orthop Relat Res 115:225, 1976.)

graft

tuberosity

Tibia   Fibula

of medial and lateral facet pressure were noted, with greater reduction in the more anteriorized group. When compared with previous studies of tubercle anteriorization, a similar slight proximal shift in contact area occurred, although no significant undesirable decrease in area was observed, as occurred with some previous laboratory evaluations of anterior tubercle transfer.[66,79]

Clinical Experience

Anteromedialization of the tibial tuberosity via an oblique osteotomy was introduced by John Fulkerson in 1983 (Fig. 62-13). This procedure allows variable anterior and medial displacement of the tubercle with rigid fixation and early motion, while maintaining a broad cancellous surface for primary bone healing.[36] The results of this procedure on 30 knees with patellofemoral pain, moderate articular degeneration, and clinical malalignment indicate excellent/good subjective results in 93%.[39] Objectively, 89% excellent/good results were documented, and 12 patients monitored for longer than 5 years showed no deterioration with time. Mean anteriorization was 10.6 mm. Even 75% of eight patients with advanced deterioration (Outerbridge grades III to IV) had good results, although excellent results were not achieved in this group. Morshuis et al[77] described a series of 25 similar osteotomies and reported 84% good and excellent short-term results. Anteriorization was less than 10 mm, and the best results were achieved in patients with mild articular degeneration. Bellemans et al[7] found consistent clinical improvement and correction of preoperative radiographic pathologic tilt and subluxation in 29 patients after anteromedialization by Fulkerson's technique. One noteworthy procedural modification was the omission of lateral release in 14 patients with CT-documented normal tilt angles preoperatively.

Pidoriano et al[84] studied the correlation between the pattern of articular degeneration and the result of anteromedialization and confirmed the theoretical and laboratory findings that distal and lateral lesions should respond best to anteromedialization. Distal lesions and lateral facet lesions, of varying severity, correlated with 87% good to excellent functional results (Fig. 62-14). Conversely, medial facet lesions had just 55% good to excellent functional results. Eight percent of patients with diffuse or proximal patellar

lesions did poorly. Patients with severe central trochlear lesions also did poorly. It is interesting to note that the location of the articular lesion correlated much better with the result than did the absolute degree of articular degeneration, as described by the Outerbridge classification, despite the fact that 28 of 36 patients in the series had grade III/IV articular cartilage degeneration. As predicted by patellofemoral mechanics, the location of the lesion is critical in selecting patients for anteromedialization.

In a later review, Buuck and Fulkerson established effective long-term success of the anteromedial tibial tubercle transfer procedure in a 4- to 12-year follow-up study.[15]

Other techniques of anteromedialization have also been studied. Combined rotation and elevation of the tibial tuberosity with lateral release was reported in 1986 by Miller and LaRochelle.[76] This technique, which uses a wedge-shaped graft rotated medially and fixed with a cortical lag screw, raises the tuberosity 9 to 11 mm and probably is less stable than that described by Fulkerson. Casts were maintained for 4 to 5 weeks postoperatively. Indications for surgery were refractory patellofemoral pain with normal or increased Q angles. Fifty-five percent of patients had a positive apprehension sign. Pain was decreased in 86% of 38 patients postoperatively, and no patient had residual patellar instability. Another potential problem with this method could be proximal shingle fracture caused by lack of support under the most proximal tip of the shingle.[88] Noll et al[81] reported a 1.25-cm elevation with transposition of the tubercle straight medially onto a tapered bony bed with fixation by a cancellous screw, thereby avoiding the need for bone grafting. Three weeks of cast immobilization followed. Patients had a variety of

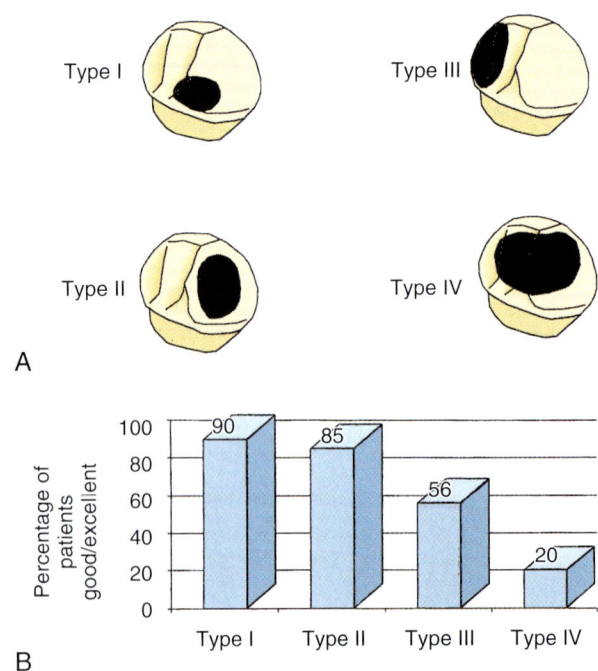

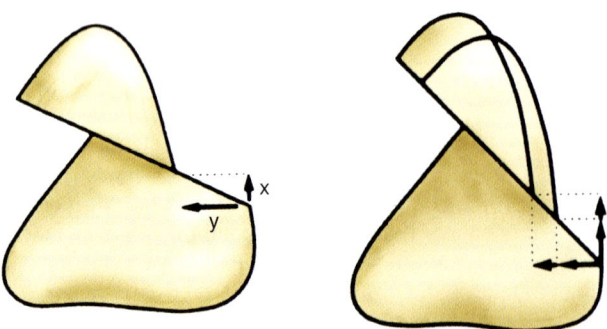

Figure 62-13. An oblique osteotomy allows anterior and medial displacement of the tibial tuberosity without a bone graft. A steeper osteotomy plane will produce increased anteriorization, along with medialization. (From Fulkerson JP: Anteromedialization of the tibial tuberosity for patellofemoral malalignment. Clin Orthop Relat Res 177:176, 1983.)

Figure 62-14. **A,** Classification of the location of patellar chondral lesions. **B,** Correlation of good/excellent results after anteromedialization with location of the chondral lesion. (From Pidoriano AJ, Weinstein RN: Correlation of patellar articular lesions with results from anteromedial tibial tubercle transfer. Am J Sports Med 25:533, 1997.)

diagnoses, primarily patellofemoral pain with an increased Q angle, but no patellar instability. Good to excellent relief was attained in 12 of 14 patients. Naranja and coworkers used a modified Maquet procedure with medialization of the tibial tubercle supported by a local bone graft in 55 knees (80% had preoperative subluxation or dislocation). They found only 53% good/excellent results based on the Fulkerson functional score, and 11% recurrent instability in 55 knees. Anteriorization was only 1 cm. The severity of articular cartilage changes was not noted, and some, but not all patients underwent medial reefing and VMO advancement.

In summary, although these series of distal realignment procedures differ in specific details, the results generally are good. If the clinician is certain to exhaust nonoperative treatment, document preoperative malalignment, reserve anteromedialization for patients with distal and lateral facet lesions, and avoid technical pitfalls, patient satisfaction is very high.

Complications of Distal Realignment

Upon review of the combined findings of six separate reports, potentially disastrous skin necrosis over the tibial tubercle was noted in 8.8% of 182 reported cases treated by a Maquet procedure with advancement of more than 2 cm.* In contrast, skin necrosis, to our knowledge, has not been reported with lesser advancements and has not been reported or seen by the authors after anteromedial tibial tubercle transfer. Other serious complications, including acute or stress fractures of the bony shingle, deep venous thrombosis, arthrofibrosis, and compartment syndrome, are less common but can

---

*References 50, 53, 70, 74, 88, and 93.

occur. Acute fracture of the proximal end of the tibia was reported in 6 of 234 patients who were encouraged to initiate immediate full weight bearing after anteromedialization; accordingly, patients should be gradually advanced to full weight bearing after about 6 weeks, with some radiographic evidence of consolidation of the tibial shingle.[103] Compartment syndrome occurred in 12 cases after the Hauser procedure,[105] but this procedure is no longer recommended. Emphasis has been placed on strict technique to avoid many of these complications, and indeed, several series have documented a decreased rate of complications as their experience with this procedure increased.[50,88] Radin and Labosky[90] wrote an important article on methods used to minimize complications associated with the Maquet procedure; clinicians planning this procedure would be well advised to study it. Special care should be taken in patients with multiple scars from previous surgery. Avoidance of complications entails careful handling of skin edges, techniques to minimize skin tension, postoperative use of suction drains, and early motion whenever possible.

Fulkerson's Technique of Anteromedialization

After arthroscopic confirmation of the preoperative diagnosis and examination of the medial and lateral joint compartments for associated disease, a straight incision, slightly lateral of midline, is made just lateral to the patellar tendon and tibial crest to a point approximately 5 cm distal to the tibial tuberosity (Fig. 62-15A). It is desirable to make this incision in such a way that a later midline or paramidline incision will be possible if arthroplasty or further surgery becomes necessary. Lateral retinacular release is almost always performed (either or open) in the patellofemoral ligaments (patellotibial and epicondylopatellar bands), synovium, and

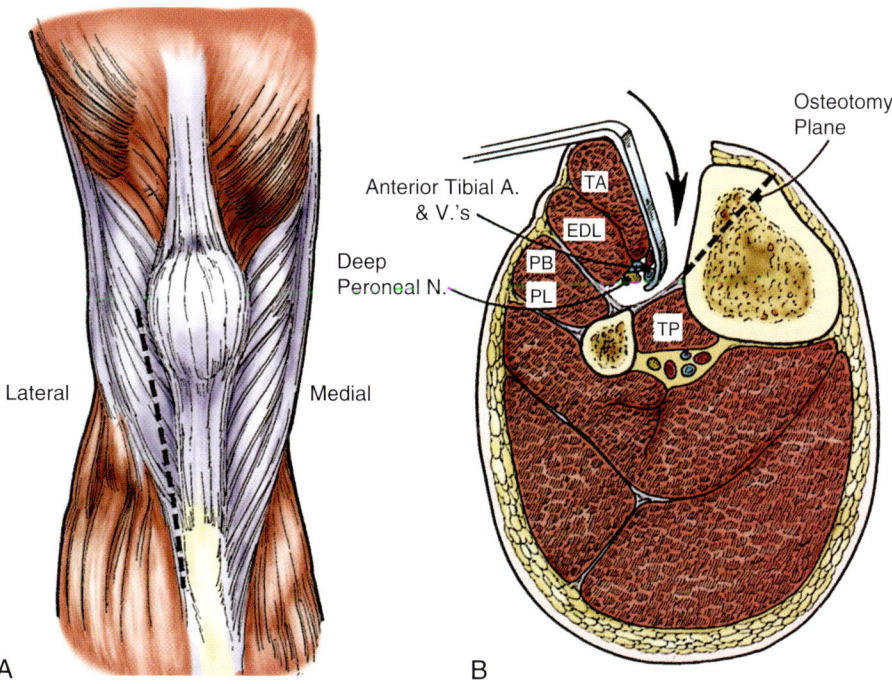

Figure 62-15. A, The *dotted line* indicates the suggested skin incision. (The surgeon must consider previous surgical scars and must modify the incision to prevent skin complications.) **B,** Plane of dissection. Note the potentially vulnerable position of the neurovascular bundle. During tibial drilling and osteotomy, these structures must be protected. (From Scott WN: The knee, vol 1, St Louis, 1994, Mosby-Year Book, p 458.)

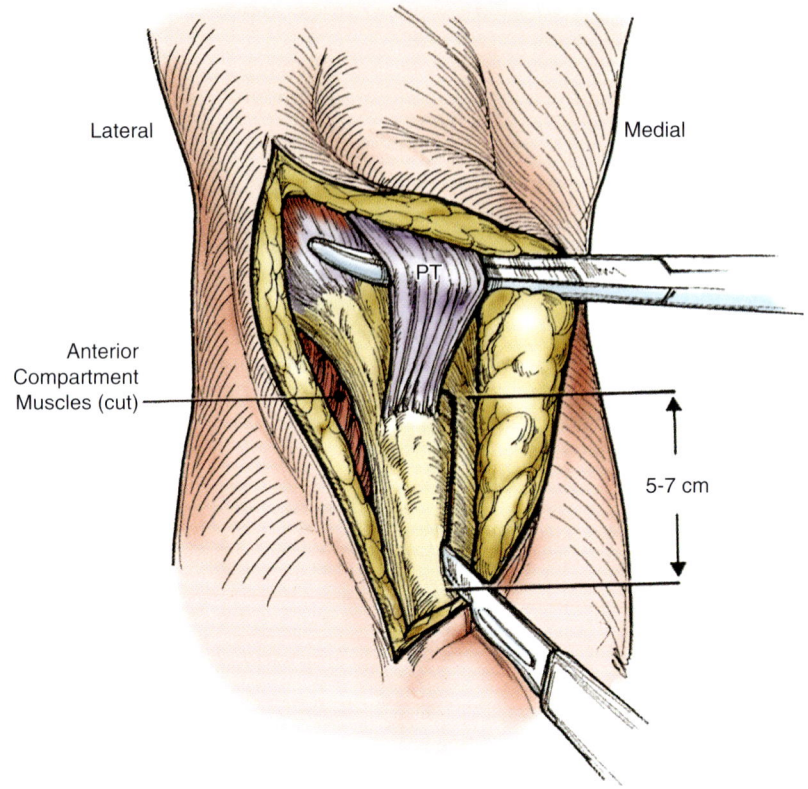

Lateral

Medial

Anterior
Compartment
Muscles (cut)

PT

5-7 cm

Figure 62-16. The patellar tendon is mobilized. The osteotomy plane is planned. (From Scott WN: The knee, vol 1, St Louis, 1994, Mosby-Year Book, p 459.)

vastus lateralis obliquus.[45] Proximally, the main tendon of the vastus lateralis is protected. Care is taken distally to avoid injury to the lateral meniscus, which is at the inferior extent of the release. If the release is adequate, 90 degrees of patellar eversion should be possible to allow direct examination and palpation of articular surfaces. Careful observation of the pattern and degree of articular changes and correlation with the patient's symptoms and preoperative evaluation are important in deciding the need for lateral release versus anteromedialization if the patient has an isolated tilt, or in deciding the degree of anteriorization appropriate for those undergoing anteromedial transfer.

Next, the musculature of the anterior compartment is sharply released from the tibial crest and is elevated atraumatically in a posterior direction to expose the posterolateral corner of the proximal end of the tibia. The anterior tibial artery and the peroneal nerve are at this level (Fig. 62-15B) and must be protected. The medial and lateral borders of the patellar tendon are then defined, with particular care taken to delineate the entire insertion into the tibial tuberosity (Fig. 62-16). Next, a longitudinal incision is made just medial to the tibial crest along the planned osteotomy (closer to the crest for a steeper osteotomy). The osteotomy plane is also tapered anteriorly at its distal extent to create a proximally based pie shape on the medial surface of the tibial narrowing down to a 2- to 3-mm apex 5 to 7 cm distal to the tuberosity (see Fig. 62-16). The periosteum is carefully elevated from the line of the planned osteotomy. Although exquisite care is taken to have the posterolateral aspect of the tibia under direct vision at all times, a series of 4.0-mm drill bits may be

placed parallel with use of the Hoffmann drill guide or a similar device in a plane from the anteromedial toward the posterolateral aspect of the tibia. Each drill bit should be carefully observed as it penetrates the lateral cortex to avoid injury to the anterior tibial vessels and peroneal nerve. Maintaining bicortical drill bits in the most superior and inferior positions along the drill guide helps place the remaining parallel drill holes accurately, but these bits must be checked frequently to prevent inadvertent and potentially dangerous advancement. A lateral osteotomy must then be made from the superior posterior drill hole to an anterior point proximal to the patellar tendon insertion to prevent propagation of the osteotomy into the proximal end of the tibia (Fig. 62-17). The cortical bone anterior and proximal to the tibial tuberosity is cut next with a half-inch osteotome, while care is taken to avoid injury to the tendon (Fig. 62-18). Alternatively, the Tracker AMZ Guide (Depuy Mitek, Raynham, Mass) may be used to design this osteotomy and make the cut. Arthrex (Naples, Fla) also makes a special guide for this procedure.

The main osteotomy is completed with an osteotome or a saw, while the superior and inferior drill bits are used as guides to the desired plane (Fig. 62-19). A perfectly flat osteotomy plane is critical to the ultimate apposition of the broad flat cancellous surfaces and the stability of fixation. Once the osteotomy is complete, the bone pedicle is hinged distally and is pushed up the inclined plane. Patellar tracking is then observed, and the optimal amount of medialization is maintained while two countersunk 3.2-mm AO cortical screws are placed into the posterior cortex (Fig. 62-20). Special care is exercised when drilling through the posterior cortex.

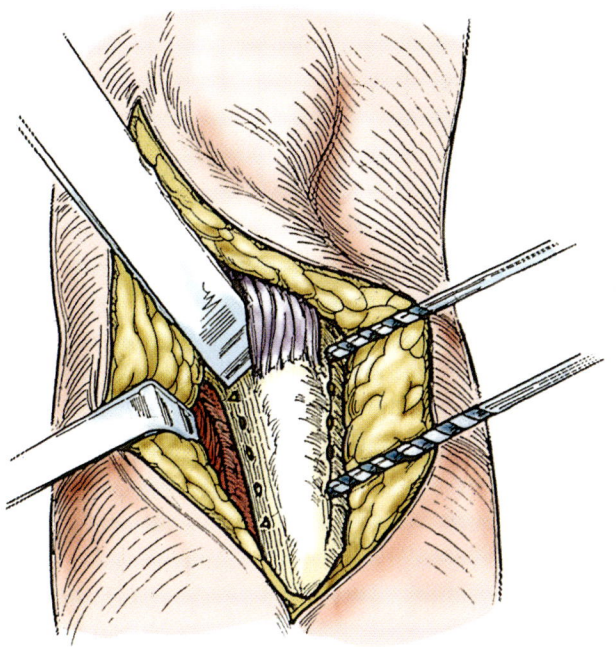

Figure 62-17. Lateral osteotomy frees the superior aspect of the tibial tubercle shingle and prevents propagation of the osteotomy into the proximal end of the tibia. (From Scott WN: The knee, vol 1, St Louis, 1994, Mosby-Year Book, p 460.)

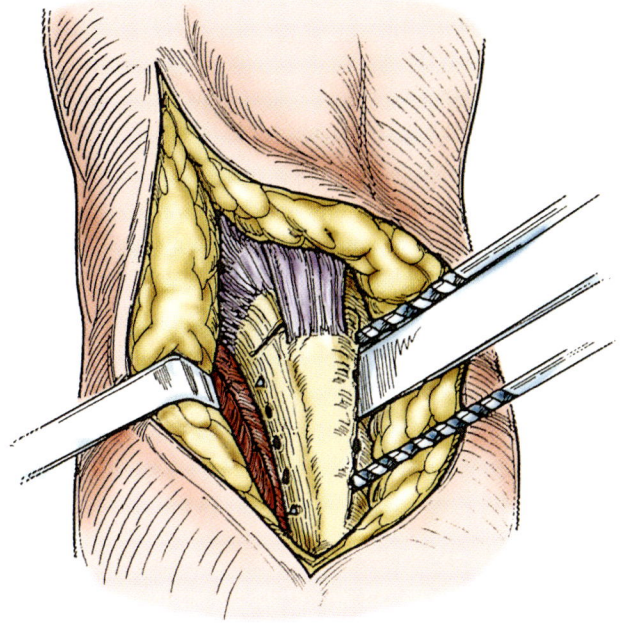

Figure 62-19. A wide osteotome is used to complete the oblique osteotomy along the plane defined by the drill bits previously placed with the parallel drill guide. Care should be taken to make sure that the osteotomy plane is completely flat to ensure good bony apposition. (From Scott WN: The knee, vol 1, St Louis, 1994, Mosby-Year Book, p 460.)

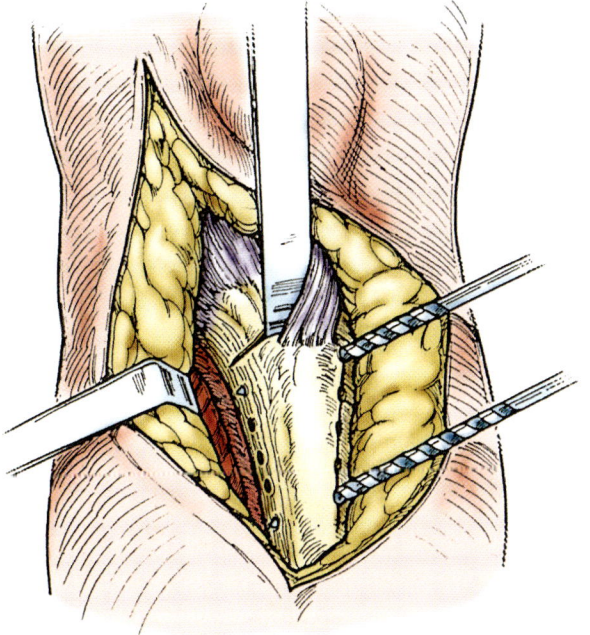

Figure 62-18. Completion of the superior aspect of the osteotomy. (From Scott WN: The knee, vol 1, St Louis, 1994, Mosby-Year Book, p 460.)

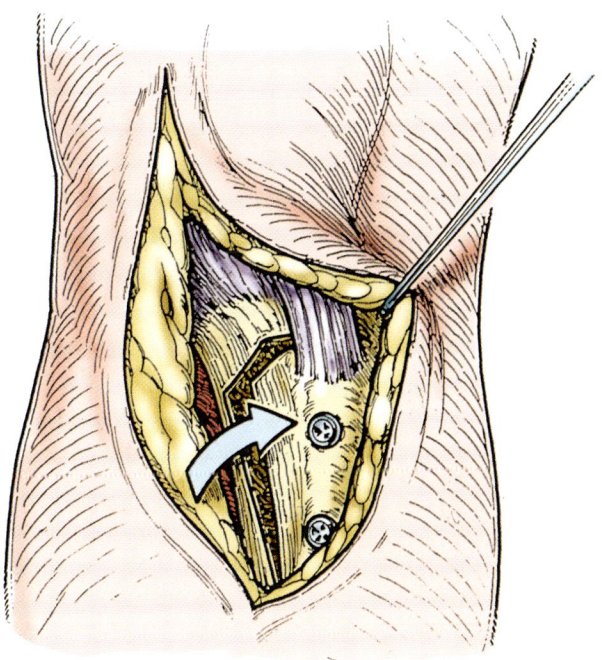

Figure 62-20. The tibial shingle is pushed anteromedially up the inclined plane and is rigidly fixed with two bicortical large-fragment AO cortical lag screws. (From Scott WN: The knee, vol 1, St Louis, 1994, Mosby-Year Book, p 460.)

Anteriorization of 12 to 15 mm is routine without a bone graft, although locally available bone (proximal lateral tibial metaphysis) can be used to neutralize the medialization and add anteriorization in selected rare cases. If pure medialization is desired, the osteotomy is simply modified to eliminate the anterior-to-posterior obliquity. The tourniquet is released and meticulous hemostasis ensured before placement of a suction drain and closure of the subcutaneous and skin layers.

Postoperative Care

A cooling device is placed over light bandages in the operating room to apply continuous cryotherapy and gentle compression. Drains, if used, are usually removed in the recovery room or within approximately 24 hours when the drainage diminishes. Quadriceps-setting exercises are encouraged on the day of surgery, and with the assumption of secure fixation of the shingle, early active and gentle passive motion is begun the next day. Toe-touch weight bearing is allowed with crutches and a knee immobilizer. At 4 to 6 weeks, quadriceps strength is improving, bony union has generally occurred, and crutches can be discontinued, usually with the help of a physical therapist, when the patient can perform a single-leg knee bend without support on the operated side. Full recovery generally is achieved between 3 and 4 months, but running and vigorous activity should be delayed until 8 to 12 months from the time of surgery to maximize bony recovery.

Anteriorization

Clinical Experience

Anteriorization of the tibial tubercle was reviewed in the previous section. Clinical results with this diagnosis are limited but encouraging. In articles that reported posttraumatic patients separately, successful results were achieved in at least 84%.[30,89] If a localized articular lesion has been identified, care should be taken that the anteriorization will effectively unload the lesion. It seems likely that the experience reported by Pidoriano et al[84] would apply equally well to straight anteriorization, with distal lesions being the best candidates for anteriorization. Although average retropatellar pressure is globally decreased after anteriorization, the physician, when contemplating this alternative, is urged to carefully consider the data presented previously with regard to specific local retropatellar effects of tibial tubercle anteriorization.

OUR RECOMMENDED TREATMENT APPROACH

Patellofemoral Malalignment

Patients with patellofemoral pain who have failed nonoperative management may have various degrees of articular pain, soft tissue pain, and instability. Preoperative history and physical examination findings, supplemented by x-ray film and, when necessary, CT evaluation, are used to assess the degree of articular degeneration and the degree of tilt and subluxation. An appropriate procedure can then be selected to address all components of the problem.

Tilt

Recognized on physical examination and confirmed by x-ray film or more reliably by CT, tilt, when isolated (no lateral subluxation or significant articular degeneration), can result in disabling soft tissue pain. A tight contracted lateral retinaculum draws the patella into increasing lateral tilt with knee flexion as a result of progressive posterior displacement of the iliotibial band (to which a strong portion of the retinaculum is anchored). Soft tissue pain can result from neuromatous degeneration in the lateral retinaculum under these conditions, or from tension overload in the medial tissues. Excessive pressure on the articular surface of the lateral facet is possible and may conceivably result in progressive

degeneration if not corrected in a symptomatic patient. Patients with pure tilt probably represent a subgroup of those labeled as having "chondromalacia" without subluxation in many series. Nonoperative management includes quadriceps strengthening, stretching of the tight lateral retinaculum and iliotibial band, McConnell taping, and bracing, and may be supplemented by nonsteroidal anti-inflammatory medication. Lateral release is our procedure of choice in this situation when surgery is necessary and has resulted in 92% excellent or good results in patients with CT-documented tilt and mild cartilage degeneration (Outerbridge grade II chondromalacia or less).[99] CT evaluation of tilt in patients with preoperative tilt and no lateral facet collapse showed consistent improvement to within the normal range 3 to 4 months after lateral release.[40] Medial imbrication has not been necessary to achieve this correction. When lateral patellar tilt is present with Outerbridge grade III to IV lateral facet arthrosis, anteromedialization with lateral release is a more dependable procedure than lateral release.

Lateral Translation (Subluxation) and Tilt Without Severe Chondral Damage

Patients whose knees fall into this category based on the history, physical examination findings, and radiographic studies respond less consistently to lateral release alone after failure of conservative care. Coronal malalignment related to the quadriceps vector and tibial tubercle position is not consistently improved by lateral release, as noted by unchanged postoperative Q angles[63] and by unchanged CT scans.[40] Medialization of the tibial tubercle helps decrease the Q angle, thus reducing the laterally directed component of the extensor force, which has been shown to contribute significantly to patellar subluxation. Thus, straight medialization of the tibial tubercle in conjunction with lateral release should be the appropriate procedure in the absence of significant articular damage. We have not found imbrication of the VMO to be routinely necessary.[104] This may be a clinical reflection of the findings of Mariani and Caruso,[72] who found electromyographic evidence of improved VMO function after lateral release and distal realignment.

When chronic lateral translation of the patella is seen radiographically, we do not believe MPFL reconstruction or medial imbrication alone should be used to pull the patella back into the trochlea. Such attempts at realignment by increasing medial soft tissue tension can produce increased medial facet pressure and increased patellofemoral pain. In cases of radiographically clear lateral translation on patellar axial films and/or CT scans, distal realignment is usually needed. In select patients with a discrete history of ongoing recurrent traumatic instability episodes, a procedure that includes restoration of medial ligament integrity is combined with distal realignment.

Lateral Translation (Subluxation) and Tilt With More Severe Chondral Damage or Arthrosis

In this situation, one must consider adding pressure relief to the procedure by including anteriorization to the lateral release and tuberosity medialization. In making this decision, one should recall the characteristic proximal and medial load transfer of anteromedialization in cadaver models and should not transfer increased loads onto damaged proximal articular surfaces. One must also remember that progressive elevation of the tubercle brings increasing relief of force but also increases the risk for complications. Anteriorization of up to 17 mm may be attained by using Fulkerson's technique of anteromedialization without the addition of an iliac graft. Advantages of the oblique osteotomy as described by Fulkerson over other techniques with similar goals include a broad flat surface for cancellous healing, rigid internal fixation allowing immediate motion, early functional recovery, and avoidance of skin complications.

Lateral Translation (Subluxation)

Without articular changes greater than Outerbridge I to II and in the absence of tilt, medialization is the primary goal. As noted earlier, a medial procedure is recommended to avoid pulling the patella into the trochlea. Patients with static lateral translation without tilt often seem to have some degree of systemic hypermobility. In such cases, careful evaluation by CT scan for evidence of skeletal dysplasia (excessive hip anteversion, trochlear dysplasia, lateralization of the tuberosity, external tibial torsion) is very important. Soft tissue tightening or lateral release in such cases, which include hypermobility, must be done cautiously to avoid iatrogenic medial instability. Most often in such cases, we would not include lateral release, but if the lateral retinaculum was tight intraoperatively, lateral lengthening would be preferred over release.

When necessary in a *skeletally mature* individual with severe subluxation, our preferred method is a Trillat-type procedure with medial rotation of a flat osteotomy, rigid fixation, and concomitant lateral release supplemented by MPFL advancement. Avoidance of posterior transposition of the tubercle is imperative to avoid increasing patellofemoral joint contact forces and the resultant high risk for osteoarthrosis.

Patella Alta

Fortunately, distal transfer of the tuberosity occurs with any distally based rotation of a shingle, whether the rotation is straight medial, anterior, or somewhere in between. With a longer tibial shingle, less distal displacement occurs. Thus, the degree of patella alta present can be a consideration in selecting the length of the tibial shingle. In patients with severe patella alta in the setting of patellar instability, one may want to be certain that the tubercle osteotomy allows adequate distal transfer for correction.

Medial Patellofemoral Ligament (MPFL) Reconstruction Without Tibial Tubercle Transfer

Suffice it to say for the purposes of this article that MPFL reconstruction by imbrication, advancement, or tendon graft reconstruction should be reserved for patients who have an otherwise balanced extensor mechanism. MPFL reconstruction should not be used to displace the structural tracking vector of the extensor mechanism, because this is likely to seriously alter articular pressures and increase the likelihood of failure.

SUMMARY

Most patients with patellofemoral disorders do not require surgery. Careful attention to the basics of restoring strength and flexibility and of correcting instigating factors in the patient's history often is all it takes to treat these problems successfully. When surgery is necessary, meticulous history and physical examination are invaluable. Diagnoses of malalignment should be documented radiographically before surgical realignment. The clinician should be patient during rehabilitation of deconditioned patients after patellofemoral surgery. As long as the clinician is careful to precisely define the indications for patellofemoral surgery, accurately perform the surgery, and rehabilitate the patient, successful results are possible in most cases.

KEY REFERENCES

Buuck D, Fulkerson J: Anteromedialization of the tibial tubercle: a 4-12 year follow up. Oper Tech Sports Med 8:131, 2000.

Dejour H, Walch G, Nove-Josserand L, Guier C: Factors of patellar instability: an anatomic radiographic study. Knee Surg Sports Traumatol Arthrosc 2:19–26, 1994.

Dye SF: The knee as a biologic transmission with an envelope of function: a theory. Clin Orthop Relat Res 325:10–18, 1996.

Dye SF, Vaupel GL, Dye CC: Conscious neurosensory mapping of the internal structures of the human knee without intraarticular anesthesia. Am J Sports Med 26:773–777, 1998.

Engebretsen L, Svenningsen S, Benum P: Advancement of the tibial tuberosity for patellar pain: a 5-year follow-up. Acta Orthop Scand 60:20–22, 1989.

Fulkerson JP: Evaluation of the peripatellar soft tissues and retinaculum in patients with patellofemoral pain. Clin Sports Med 8:197–202, 1989.

Fulkerson JP, Becker GJ, Meaney JA, et al: Anteromedial tibial tubercle transfer without bone graft. Am J Sports Med 18:490–496; discussion 496–497, 1990.

Fulkerson JP, Schutzer SF, Ramsby GR, Bernstein RA: Computerized tomography of the patellofemoral joint before and after lateral release or realignment. Arthroscopy 3:19–24, 1987.

Fulkerson JP, Shea KP: Disorders of patellofemoral alignment. J Bone Joint Surg Am 72:1424–1429, 1990.

Post W: History and physical examination of patients with patellofemoral disorders. In Fulkerson J, editor: Disorders of the patellofemoral joint, Baltimore, 1997, Williams & Wilkins.

Sanchis-Alfonso V, Rosello-Sastre E, Monteagudo-Castro C, Esquerdo J: Quantitative analysis of nerve changes in the lateral retinaculum in patients with isolated symptomatic patellofemoral malalignment: a preliminary study. Am J Sports Med 26:703–709, 1998.

Full references for this chapter can be found on www.expertconsult.com.

Surgery of the Patellofemoral Joint: Proximal Realignment

W. Norman Scott, Giles R. Scuderi, and Gabriel Levi

Disorders of the patellofemoral joint are numerous and are of great importance because they seriously limit patients' function. Treatment of these conditions is highly dependent on an accurate diagnosis and determination of the correct cause.[55] Within the spectrum of disorders of the patellofemoral joint, one of the more common is patellar instability, which will be the focus of this chapter. Instability can present with a variety of symptoms that mimic other pathology of the knee, such as pain, mechanical "clicking," feelings of instability or "giving out," weakness, and limited range of motion. We begin with a review of the presentation and pathophysiology of patellofemoral disorders, including patellofemoral instability. We then review physical examination of the patellofemoral joint, imaging modalities, and the surgical technique of proximal realignment.[80] The techniques of patellofemoral arthroplasty and distal patellar realignment are beyond the scope of this chapter and are discussed elsewhere in the text. A review of the biomechanics of the patellofemoral joint is recommended in conjunction with this chapter.

PATHOPHYSIOLOGY OF PATELLAR INSTABILITY

The stability of the patellofemoral joint is dependent on many factors. Specifically, it depends on the congruence of the trochlea and patella, static ligamentous stabilizers, and dynamic stabilizers. Bony and cartilaginous constraint is determined by the shape of the trochlea and the patella, which can be extremely variable. For example, a hypoplastic lateral condyle or a shallow trochlea can predispose to acute patellar dislocation after trauma, or can lead to chronic subluxation and dislocation. In addition to bony and cartilaginous constraints are the static ligamentous constraints. We now understand that the medial patellofemoral ligament (MPFL) is the greatest static stabilizer for lateral translation of the patella.[24,33,34,95] Finally, and perhaps most important, is the quadriceps mechanism. The coordinated contraction of the quadriceps mechanism centralizes the patella in the trochlea throughout a range of motion (Fig. 63-1). It is well known now that the vastus medialis obliquus (VMO) is the primary dynamic stabilizer of the patellofemoral joint (Fig. 63-2). Dysfunction of the VMO, whether by trauma or by atrophy, may lead to patellar instability. It is interesting to note that as we learn more about the anatomy of medial restraints, we are learning to appreciate the important relationship between the MPFL and the VMO.[91] The sum of these factors defines the ultimate stability of the joint. If any single factor or multiple factors are deficient or dysplastic, the remaining structures must compensate. The ability of these factors to collectively stabilize the joint determines the stability or instability of the joint. In the remainder of this chapter, we will describe how the history, physical findings, and radiographic studies are used to determine the relative contribution of each of these factors to the instability of the patellofemoral joint.

Presentation of Patellofemoral Disorders

Patellofemoral disorders, and especially instability, may present with a variety of symptoms. The history is important in determining the cause of the instability. Oftentimes, but not always, a patient with instability will present with a history of trauma. Commonly, a valgus and external rotational injury is the culprit. First-time dislocators may describe a traumatic event in which the patella dislocates and then self-reduces, or is reduced by the patient. Other first-time dislocators feel "their knee pop out of place." Recurrent dislocators often feel catching, locking, or a feeling of instability. However, many patients with patellar instability do not describe instability on presentation, and for this reason, it should be considered in all patients with patellofemoral discomfort and mechanical knee pain.

Pain

Typically, patients with patellar complaints have an aching pain situated behind the patella, often on the medial side of the joint, and sometimes located posteriorly in the popliteal fossa. The pain is aggravated by activities that require a strong quadriceps contraction, such as squatting, stair climbing, skiing, or riding a bike uphill. Descending stairs requires a strong eccentric quadriceps contraction to proceed to the next step smoothly. This is often more painful than ascending stairs, which requires a concentric quadriceps contraction. Prolonged periods with the knee flexed are usually painful (the movie sign). The reason for this phenomenon is not completely understood but may involve increased tension in the soft tissues or increased compression on the articular surfaces.

Pain may be bilateral, and the onset of symptoms is usually gradual and unrelated to any significant traumatic episode. At times, however, a bout of strenuous activity or a minor injury may seem to have initiated the complaint, although questioning generally demonstrates that such events merely served to worsen a preexisting disorder. Bilaterality and insidious onset are most characteristic of patellar pain.

Pain may begin in the soft tissues or in bone. Soft tissues include the retinacula, synovium, tendons, and nerves. Bone and subchondral bone are also richly innervated. Articular cartilage, however, is not so innervated.

The location of the pain can also produce diagnostic errors; the most common site is the anteromedial side of the knee, the same location as pain from a meniscal disorder—a fact that has contributed to the removal of many normal menisci. Less frequently, posterolateral pain may be felt, and when local tenderness is noted in this region as well, the diagnosis of bicipital or popliteal tendinitis may be entertained. Popliteal pain is a frequent symptom of patellofemoral arthritis; when an associated popliteal cyst is present, it might be assumed that the cyst is causing the pain, whereas in fact both are secondary to patellar arthritis.

Instability

Instability is the second major symptom of patellar dysfunction. Sometimes, instability represents an episode of dislocation or subluxation that can be documented by examination (objective instability), but on occasion, exactly similar episodes occur in patients in whom it is impossible, even under anesthesia, to displace the patella passively from the femoral sulcus (subjective instability). For this reason, the boundaries between subjective instability, subluxation, and dislocation should not be too fine, because other patients with passively dislocatable patellae will not complain of clinical instability. Instability of patellar origin may mimic the buckling caused by meniscal injury or ligamentous insufficiency, but most often it is a different sensation. Although instability may occur on pivoting or twisting movements, such as when "cutting" in sports, the patient is usually aware that it is the kneecap that has slipped. Otherwise, when the patient does not recognize the nature of the buckling, the event is described in such terms as the knee having "collapsed" or "gone forward." There is not the sensation of the joint "coming apart" or of "one bone sliding on the other" that is so typical of ligament insufficiency. Episodes of patellar instability may or may not be followed by pain and swelling lasting for a few days to several weeks.

Locking

A grating sensation, particularly when the patellofemoral joint is loaded as in stair climbing or arising from a chair, is a fairly common complaint and sometimes may be audible. It is usually an incidental finding and is rarely of great importance clinically. Momentary "catching" may also be experienced, and interruption of smooth patellar gliding may precipitate buckling or giving way. Actual locking of the knee sometimes happens, and it is curious that patellar locking is not always transient but may give the impression of a true mechanical block. In the case of patellar dislocation, it is not uncommon for a patient to present with an inability to extend the knee.

Swelling

Many patients with patellofemoral disease complain of swelling. Sometimes this is a subjective sensation because on

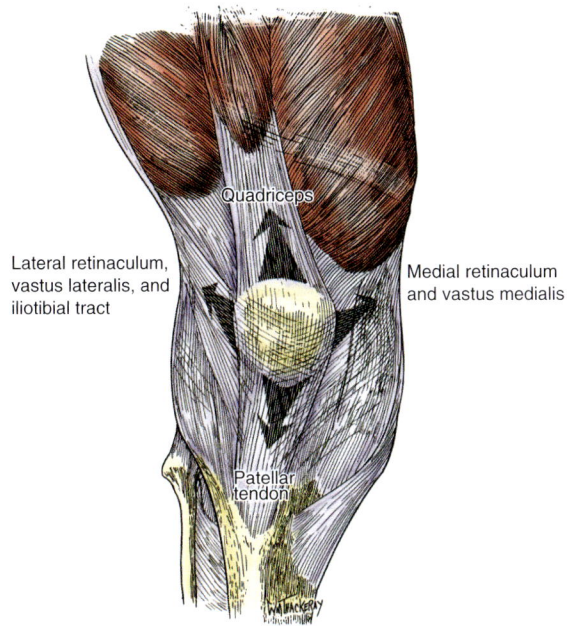

Figure 63-1. The patella is anchored and stabilized to the knee by four structures in a cruciform fashion: the patellar tendon inferiorly, the quadriceps tendon superiorly, and the retinacula medially and laterally.

Quadriceps

Lateral retinaculum, vastus lateralis, and iliotibial tract

Medial retinaculum and vastus medialis

Patellar tendon

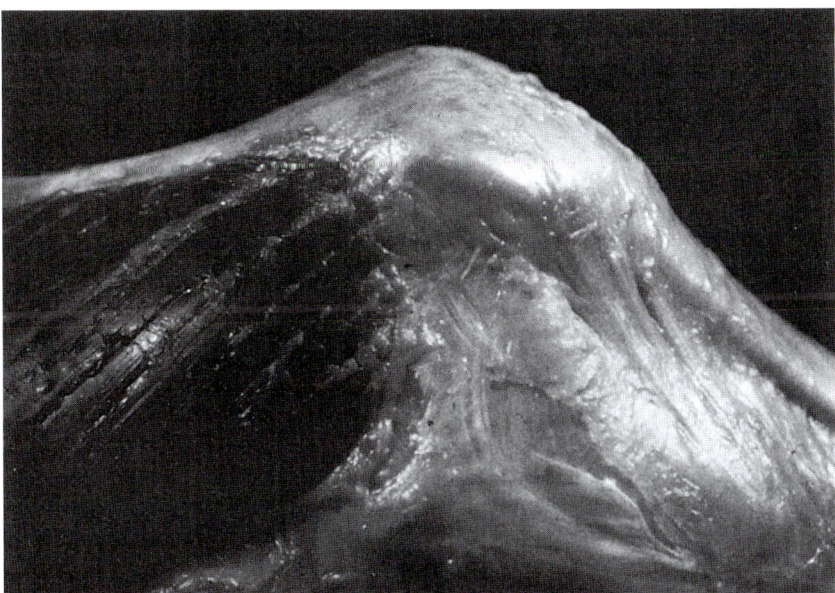

Figure 63-2. The vastus medialis obliquus becomes tendinous just a few millimeters proximal to the patella. Because of the oblique direction of its fibers, it is best suited to resist lateral displacement of the patella. The patellotibial ligament is visible as a distinct structure medial to the patellar tendon.

examination, an effusion is not found and circumferential measurement of the joint does not show an increase when compared with the opposite side. Synovitis with distention by synovial fluid or blood occurs after an episode of patellar subluxation and sometimes with chondromalacia or arthritis. Patients with acute patellar dislocations often present with a large hemarthrosis. Cartilaginous or osteocartilaginous loose bodies may be generated from the articular surfaces and may contribute to giving way and transient locking, although the patient is usually aware of a free body within the joint that may also be directly felt in the suprapatellar pouch. In this scenario, the aspirate of the joint typically contains fat droplets resulting from disruption of the subchondral bone.

Physical Examination

Thorough examination of the knee with a focus on the patellofemoral joint is essential to diagnosing patellofemoral instability or any associated patellofemoral or intra-articular pathology that often accompanies patellofemoral instability. During the physical examination, the patient should be examined sequentially while standing, walking, sitting, supine, and prone.

The examination begins with the patient standing with the feet together. Genu varum or valgum can be observed readily, as can rotatory malalignment such as in-facing or "squinting" of the patellae in patients with an increased quadriceps (Q) angle and hip anteversion (Fig. 63-3). Quadriceps

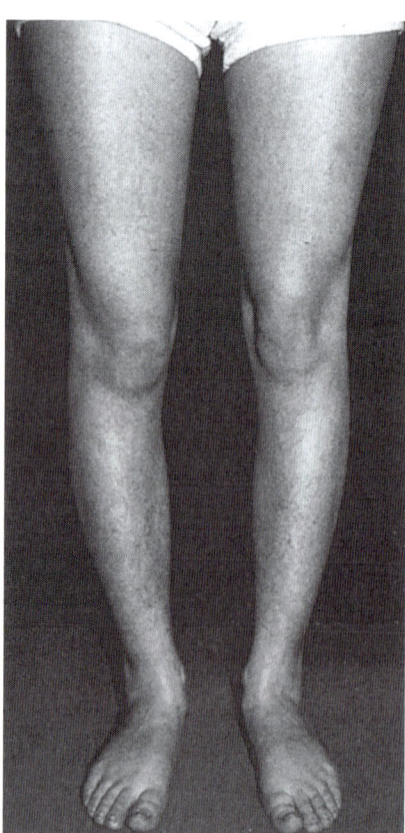

Figure 63-3. Squinting of the patellae caused by rotational malalignment of the limb. This phenomenon is accompanied by an increase in the Q angle.

tone and development can be appreciated in the standing position or during a half-squat. Hypoplasia of the VMO should be noted. Normally, the vastus medialis inserts on the upper third or half of the medial border of the patella. In knees with patellofemoral dysplasia, the muscle belly may end a few centimeters short of the superior patellar margin. The presence of quadriceps atrophy implies decreased dynamic muscle control on the patella.

The position of the foot also deserves attention. Eversion at the subtalar joint is accompanied by compensatory internal tibial torsion, which increases the Q angle and consequently stress on the patellofemoral joint. The subtalar joint is a single-axis joint that acts like a hinge connecting the talus to the calcaneus. The axis of the subtalar joint deviates an average of 23 degrees medially and anteriorly to the long axis of the foot and 41 degrees inferiorly and posteriorly in relation to the horizontal plane. Therefore, internal rotation of the leg causes eversion of the heel and depression of the medial side of the foot. External rotation of the leg produces the opposite effect.[22] Subtalar joint eversion may be primary or secondary, as in knees with varus alignment or tibia vara, wherein compensatory subtalar joint eversion is required to produce a plantigrade foot. This phenomenon is probably more important in long-distance runners.[62] Eversion of the heel (heel valgus) is readily appreciated by looking at the patient in the standing position from the back side. Abduction of the forefoot is evaluated in the standing position by palpation of the talar head on the anterior aspect of the ankle. The neutral position is defined when the head of the talus can be equally palpated on the medial and lateral sides. During weight bearing, a normal foot is in mild pronation, and additional pronation should still be possible.[18]

Gait is observed, and if possible, the patient is asked to squat and hold the halfway position briefly because pain in this position is usually patellar in origin (half-squat test). Whenever possible, stair climbing and descending should be observed because this activity also provokes patellar symptoms.

With the patient seated on the examining table, the position of the patella is first checked. Normally, it sinks between the femoral condyles with the knee at 90 degrees of flexion. If patella alta is present, its anterior surface points to the ceiling with the knee in the same 90-degree position. Active extension is observed, and the presence of patellar crepitus and painful catching, as well as abnormal patellar tracking, is recorded.

Ficat and Hungerford[36] stress the importance of observing the entrance and exit of the patella into and out of the sulcus between 10 and 30 degrees of flexion. They describe four common abnormalities in patellar tracking. Normal patellar tracking is present when the patella glides smoothly into the sulcus, and only minimal lateral displacement may be appreciated in the final extension when the patella exits the trochlear groove. We define more marked lateral displacement as lateralization, whereas greater degrees of pathologic tracking are defined as subluxation or dislocation. This finding is also called the J sign because the path resembles an upside-down J. (See video on the website.) Furthermore, evaluation of the tilt of the patella should be attempted. In normal knees, the medial border of the patella should be at the same level as the lateral border, with a minor lateral tilt in full extension. It should be noted that most abnormalities in patellar tracking involve lateral displacement and lateral tilt of the patella in extension, which reduces in flexion. Therefore, we find it useful to roughly estimate patellar subluxation and tilt during the physical examination (Fig. 63-4) and to verify this later with radiographic axial views or computed tomography (CT). Other abnormalities in patellar tracking, including medial dislocation or subluxation of the patella in flexion (after over-release of the lateral structures and excessive medial displacement of the tibial tuberosity) or lateral dislocation in flexion (as in habitual or permanent dislocation), may be encountered more rarely.

Patellar crepitation is appreciated during active extension and is recorded as absent, mild, moderate, or severe. It should be evaluated in the sitting position and is enhanced by the application of manual resistance on the lower part of leg. Because crepitation beyond 90 degrees of flexion cannot be evaluated in the sitting position, it is better assessed during a full squat.

Hughston and Walsh[51] described a lateral position of the patella in the flexed knee for which they coined the term *frog-eye* patella. This seems to be associated with patella alta, which can be suspected clinically when the fat pad is unusually prominent. In fact, the fat pad may, on inspection, be mistaken for the patella because it occupies the femoral sulcus

with the knee in extension while the patella is situated in the supracondylar pouch.

With the patient supine on the examining table, tenderness around the patella is evaluated systematically. Tenderness and swelling in the prepatellar area may be indicative of prepatellar bursitis. Evaluation of tenderness around the patella includes assessment of the medial and lateral retinacula, quadriceps, and patellar tendons, including their insertions. Joint line tenderness should also be evaluated.

The Q Angle (Quadriceps Angle)

The Q angle is measured by drawing an imaginary line connecting the center of the patella and the anterior superior iliac spine to produce a surface marking that approximates the line of pull of the quadriceps tendon (Fig. 63-5). A second line drawn from the center of the patella to the center of the tibial tubercle indicates the direction of the patellar tendon. The intersection of these two imaginary lines forms the Q angle. Because this measurement is affected by rotation of the hip, an effort is made to note the position of the medial border of the patient's foot during walking and to reproduce this position during measurement.

Active pronation or supination of the foot should be avoided because, as mentioned earlier, these movements are

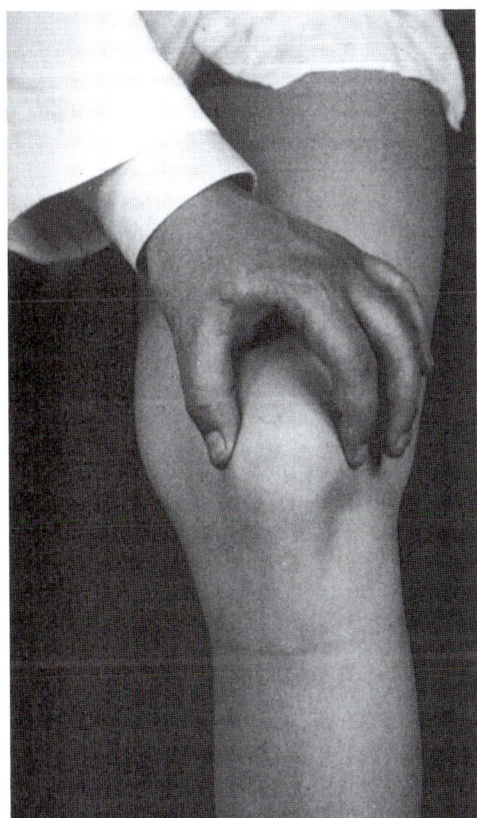

Figure 63-4. Clinical evaluation of patellar tracking. The patient is sitting on a firm examining table with the knee flexed at 90 degrees. The examiner places his hand on the knee so that the medial and lateral borders of the patella are palpated with the index finger and thumb. The patient is asked to actively extend the knee. An effort is made to detect the presence of lateral subluxation (displacement) or lateral tilt (lateral border of the patella lower than the medial border) during tracking.

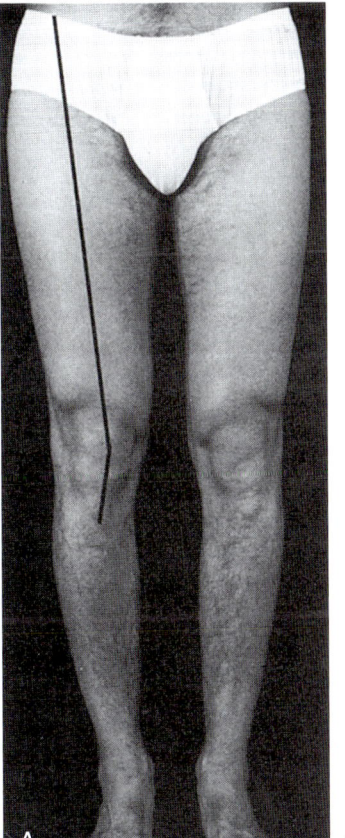
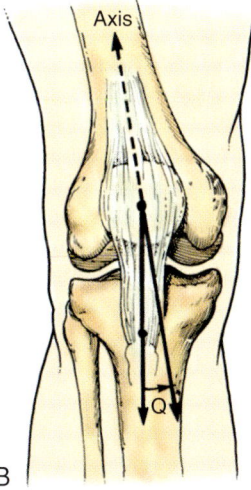

Figure 63-5. The quadriceps angle is measured by drawing two lines from the center of the patella. The first line is drawn up to the anterior superior iliac spine and represents the line of pull of the quadriceps muscle. The second line is drawn down to the tibial tubercle and indicates the line of the patellar tendon.

Table 63-1 Measurement of Quadriceps Angle and Radiographic Measurements of Patellar Height and Patellofemoral Congruence

	No. of Subjects	Q Angle, Deg	CONGRUENCE T/P Ratio*	A/B Ratio[†]	Sulcus Angle, Degrees	Angle Degrees
Normal knees[‡]	150	15 (3)	1.04 (0.11)	0.95 (0.13)	137 (6)	−8 (6)
Males	75	14	1.01	0.97	137	−6
Females	75	17 (P < .001)	1.06 (P < .05)	0.94 (NS)	137 (NS)	10 (P < .001)
Patella subluxation	37	15 (NS)	1.23 (P < .001)	1.08 (P < .001)	147 (P < .001)	16 (P < .001)
Males	16	13 (NS)	1.23 (P < .001)	1.07 (NS)	149 (P < .001)	15 (P < .001)
Females	21	16 (NS)	1.22 (P < .005)	1.08 (P < .001)	146 (P < .001)	17 (P < .001)
Patellar pain	53	20 (P < .001)	1.08 (P < .01)	1.91 (NS)	139 (P < .01)	−2 (P < .001)
Males	18	20 (P < .001)	1.11 (P < .001)	0.93 (NS)	140 (P < .005)	−1 (P < .005)
Females	35	19 (P < .001)	1.07 (NS)	0.90 (NS)	139 (NS)	−2 (P < .001)

The values of statistical significance reported in normal knees refer to the difference between males and females. The values reported in the pathologic groups (patellar pain and patellar subluxation) refer to the difference from normal knees.

Data from Aglietti P, Insall JN, Cerulli G: Patellar pain and incongruence. I. Measurements of incongruence. Clin Orthop Relat Res 176:217, 1983.

NS, Not significant.

*T/P ratio: tendon-patella ratio of Insall and Salvati[59] (see text).

[†]A/B ratio: Blackburne and Peel[38] ratio (see text).

[‡]Numbers in parentheses indicate standard deviation.

associated with internal and external rotation of the leg, respectively,[91] and consequently increase and decrease the Q angle.

Aglietti and associates measured the Q angle in 150 normal subjects and found it to be 15 degrees (range, 6 to 27 degrees; standard deviation [SD], 3 degrees) (Table 63-1).[3] It was lower in men (14 degrees; SD, 3 degrees) than in women (17 degrees; SD, 3 degrees), and the difference was significant (P = .001). Only 11 subjects, all women, had Q angles greater than 20 degrees (7%). Therefore, it seems that a Q angle greater than 20 degrees may reasonably be considered abnormal. The Q angle was also measured in a group of pathologic knees, including 53 patients with patellar pain and 37 with recurrent subluxation or dislocation. In the knees with patellar pain, the Q angle was significantly increased to 20 degrees; this was true for both men and women. In contrast, the Q angle was not significantly different from normal in knees with recurrent subluxation or dislocation (average, 15 degrees), and the same applied to both men and women. In patients with patellar subluxation or dislocation, the Q angle is usually underestimated for at least two reasons: first, the patella is displaced laterally in extension; second, the quadriceps tendon frequently lies more lateral than predicted when the superior iliac spine is used as the surface marking (Fig. 63-6).

To overcome the problem of lateral patellar displacement and consequent underestimation of the Q angle, Fithian and colleagues[37] measured the Q angle with the knee in 30 degrees of flexion. They simultaneously applied a posteriorly directed force so that the patella symmetrically contacted the trochlea. With this method, the Q angle was 12 degrees in control subjects (11.2 degrees in men and 13.4 degrees in women). A significantly higher value was found in a group of knees with patellar dislocation (average, 19.2 degrees). The contralateral knee of patients suffering from patellar dislocation also showed an increased value of the Q angle (average, 18.4 degrees).

It is debated whether the Q angle is better measured in the supine or the standing position. Woodland and Francis[118]

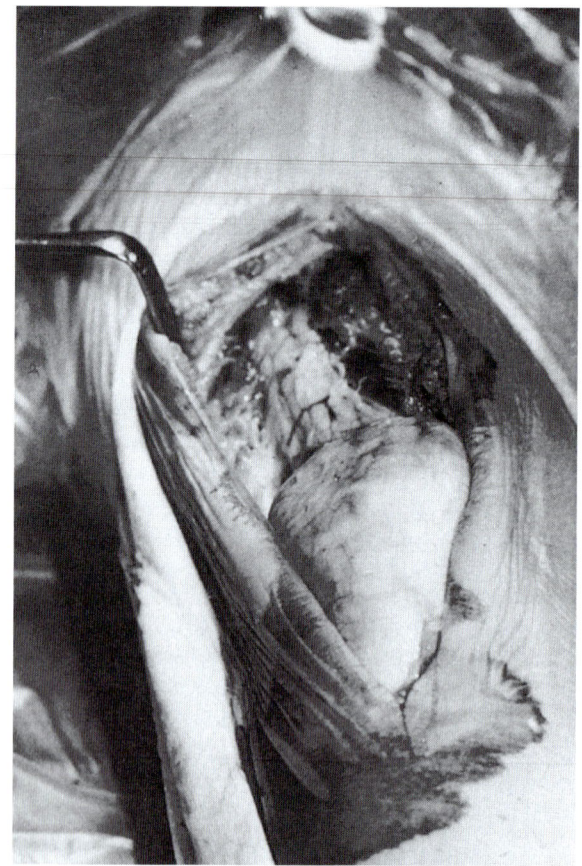

Figure 63-6. The quadriceps tendon often lies more laterally than the surface marking of the Q angle predicts.

measured the Q angle in the supine and standing positions in a large number of normal men[78] and women.[76] Average values in the supine position were 12.7 degrees for men and 15.8 degrees for women. Changing to the standing position increased the Q angle 0.9 degree in men and 1.2 degrees in women. The difference was statistically significant but probably is less significant clinically. It is relevant to note that the values determined by Woodland and Francis[118] are close to those detected by Aglietti and coworkers.[3]

It has been suggested that the Q angle should be measured at 30 degrees of knee flexion and with maximum external tibial rotation[107] because this position would give a more reliable measurement of the maximal valgus vector imposed on the patella. However, the difficulty involved in achieving standardized knee flexion and hip rotation makes the reproducibility of this measurement less reliable.

We recommend measurement of the tubercle-sulcus angle (TSA), as described by Kolowich and coworkers.[65] The TSA is measured with the knee at 90 degrees of flexion (Fig. 63-7). This allows the patella to engage in the sulcus and highlights any rotational abnormalities. It is defined as the angle formed by a line perpendicular to the transepicondylar axis and a line from the tibial tubercle to the center of the patella. The normal value for the TSA is 0 degrees, and values greater than 10 degrees are considered pathologic. However, consistent identification of the transepicondylar line is not easy, especially in obese patients.

In the supine position and with the knee in extension, the patient is asked to contract the quadriceps, and upward movement of the patella is noted (lateral pull test). In a normal knee, the patella is pulled predominantly upward with an associated minor lateral displacement. The lateral pull test result is considered abnormal if lateral displacement is excessive.[65]

Patellar mobility should be evaluated with the knee in full extension and at 30 degrees of flexion. With the knee in extension, the patella is out of the trochlear groove and may be easily displaced medially and laterally. Gross hypermobility, as seen in patients with patella alta and a dysplastic extensor apparatus, is easily detected in this position. With the knee flexed 20 to 30 degrees, the patella is normally drawn into the trochlear groove and stabilized. Excessive displacement in the lateral direction indicates laxity of the

medial retinaculum, or vice versa. On the other hand, reduced medial mobility indicates the presence of a tight lateral retinaculum. Kolowich and colleagues[65] suggested that patellar mobility is best evaluated by dividing the patella into longitudinal quadrants (Fig. 63-8). With the knee at 20 to 30 degrees of flexion, mobility in the medial or lateral direction should not exceed two quadrants. A medial glide of one quadrant or less suggests a tight lateral retinaculum, which may also be investigated by trying to lift the lateral border of the patella with the knee in extension (passive patellar tilt) (Fig. 63-9). If the transverse axis of the patella cannot be elevated beyond the horizontal plane, a tight lateral retinaculum is demonstrated.[65]

Medial and lateral displacement of the patella has been measured with a displacement transducer[37] or axial radiographs.[112] Fithian and associates[37] used a displacement sensor to record motion in the coronal plane with the knees bent at 30 degrees. Forces of 2.5 and 5 lb were applied with a handheld force applicator with a load cell. Under a 5-lb force, medial patellar displacement averaged 9.2 ± 3.5 mm, and lateral displacement was 7.7 ± 2.6 mm in a group of 188 normal knees. In a group of 22 patients with symptomatic lateral patellar dislocation, medial displacement at 5 lb was 8.3 ± 4.5 mm, and lateral displacement was 11.5 ± 4.7 mm. Using the lateral minus medial displacement index, control knees had an average value of −2.1 ± 2.8 mm. Symptomatic knees had a lateral minus medial displacement of 3.2 ± 3.4 mm. The difference was statistically significant. In summary, total mediolateral displacement of the patella in normal knees under a 5-lb force was close to 17 mm in normal knees and almost 20 mm in knees with patellar instability. The lateral minus medial displacement was useful for differentiating between normal and unstable patellae. Medial

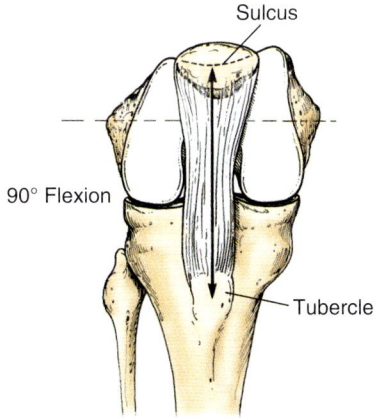

Figure 63-7. Tubercle-Sulcus Angle (TSA) is measured with the knee at 90 degrees of flexion. The patella is engaged in the sulcus. The angle is formed by a line perpendicular to the transepicondylar axis and a line form the tibal tubercle to the center of the patella. Normal TSA is 0 degrees and abnormal is greater than 10 degrees. (From Scuderi GR: The patella, New York, 1995, Springer-Verlag.)

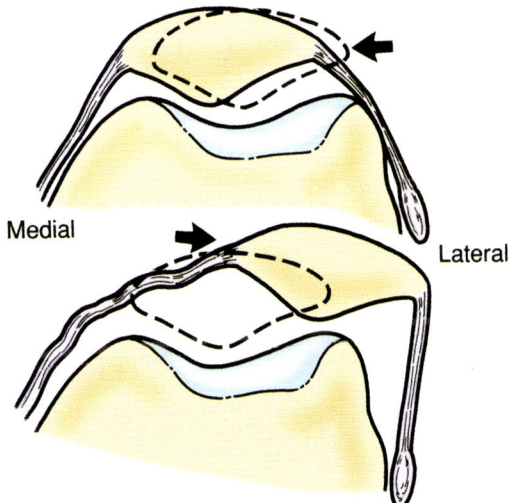

Figure 63-8. The mobility of the patella is best evaluated with the knee flexed to 20 to 30 degrees to engage the patella into the femoral sulcus. Displacement of the patella in the medial or lateral direction is best recorded in quadrants. Displacement in the medial direction of one quadrant or less indicates a tight lateral retinaculum. Displacement in the lateral direction over two quadrants indicates weakened medial stabilizers. (From Kolowich PA, Paulos LE, Rosenberg TD, Farnsworth S: Lateral release of the patella: indications and contraindications. Am J Sports Med 18:359, 1990.)

displacement was larger than lateral displacement in 81% of control subjects. In unstable patellae, lateral displacement was larger than medial displacement. Asymptomatic knees in patients with unilateral patellar dislocation could not be used as controls because they showed abnormal patellar mobility, similar to symptomatic knees. The authors offered the concept of balance between medial and lateral structures. A normal knee should have greater medial than lateral displacement. If lateral displacement exceeds medial displacement, the restraining structures are unbalanced.

Teitge and colleagues[112] evaluated medial and lateral patellar mobility with an axial radiograph at 30 to 40 degrees of flexion and a spring-loaded scale to apply a 16-lb force (7.3 kg). In a group of 20 asymptomatic knees, medial

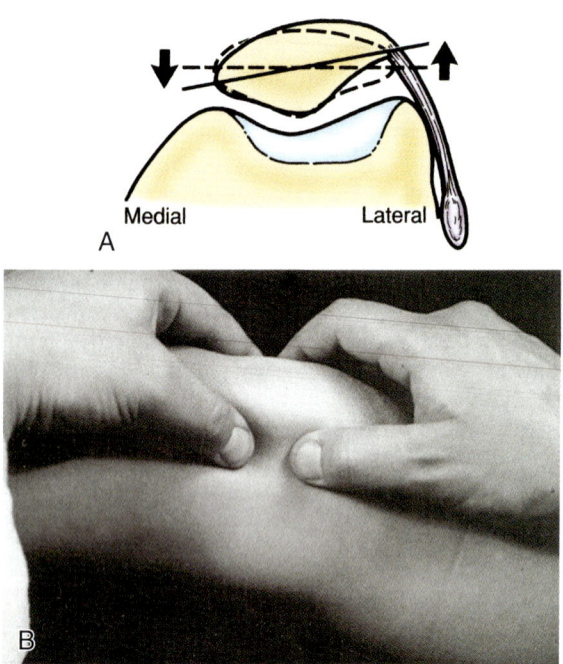

Figure 63-9. **A** and **B,** Passive patellar tilt test. In a normal knee in full extension, it is possible to lift the transverse axis of the patella beyond the horizontal. An inability to perform this maneuver indicates a tight lateral retinaculum. (From Kolowich PA, Paulos LE, Rosenberg TD, Farnsworth S: Lateral release of the patella: indications and contraindications. Am J Sports Med 18:359, 1990.)

displacement averaged 11.1 ± 3.6 mm, and lateral displacement was 11.6 ± 8.1 mm. These values are higher than those reported in the study by Fithian and coworkers,[37] but the displacing force was also greater (16 lb vs. 5 lb). In a group of knees with lateral instability, medial displacement was comparable (11.6 mm on average), whereas lateral displacement was highly increased to 21.9 mm on average.

Torsional abnormalities of the femur and tibia have been described as a possible factor leading to patellar pain or instability. The pattern would involve increased femoral neck anteversion so that the trochlear groove faces inward, the Q angle is increased, and the patellae are squinting. Compensatory external tibial torsion is required to produce a foot aligned in the sagittal plane.

Turner and Smillie[114] measured tibial torsion in 836 patients with a tropometer. They found an average lateral tibial torsion of 19 degrees in control knees, which was increased to 24.5 degrees in knees with patellofemoral instability, and to 24 degrees in those with chondromalacia. Because increased tibial rotation was also noted in Osgood-Schlatter disease, this finding does not seem to be specific for patellofemoral joint disorders.

The amount of femoral neck anteversion has often been indirectly estimated by measuring the proportion of internal to external rotation of the hips in extension (Fig. 63-10), which would be its major determinant.[9,109,110] Carson and colleagues[18] suggested that if internal rotation of the hip in extension exceeds external rotation by more than 30 degrees, femoral neck anteversion is increased. Insall and colleagues[58] suggested that increased femoral neck anteversion may be present in knees with patellofemoral malalignment. Hvid and Andersen[52] measured the Q angle and internal rotation of the hip in 29 patients with patellofemoral complaints. They found that both the Q angle and internal hip rotation were higher in women than in men. A significant correlation between the Q angle and hip rotation was noted, thus suggesting that the Q angle is in fact increased because of excessive femoral neck anteversion. Other authors,[35] however, have failed to identify any significant differences in Q angle, genu valgum, and anteversion of the femoral neck between normal adolescents and adolescents or adults with anterior knee pain. They concluded that because those affected by knee pain are also those most interested in sports activities, the probable cause is chronic overloading rather than faulty mechanics.

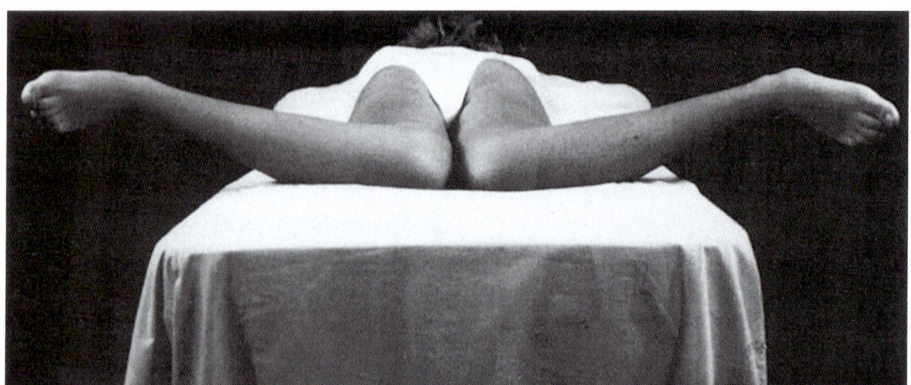

Figure 63-10. Excessive internal rotation of the hips in a patient with recurrent patellar dislocation. Increased femoral neck anteversion is usually present in these cases.

Dejour and associates[30] reported CT measurements of femoral anteversion and tibial torsion in normal controls and in knees with instability of the patella. They found that femoral neck anteversion was increased in knees with patellofemoral instability (15.6 degrees) as compared with controls (10.8 degrees). Tibial torsion was a less important factor. It was 33 degrees in the control group and 35 degrees in the knees with patellar instability.

In light of the data reported in the literature and our own clinical experience, we think that torsional abnormalities of the lower limb, including femoral neck anteversion and, less significantly, external tibial torsion, may contribute to and play a role in patellofemoral disorders by increasing lateral pull on the patella. However, because these deformities are often less marked and remote from the knee, their importance is minor from therapeutic and surgical points of view.

The ultimate goal, in addition to an accurate diagnosis, is to identify any malalignment, medial-lateral restraint imbalance, and patellofemoral articular disease. The history and physical examination, in combination with the correct imaging studies, are essential in developing an appropriate treatment plan for the patient with patellofemoral instability.

Summary of Physical Examination for Patellofemoral Instability

Alignment of the limb is examined in standing and supine positions. Special attention is paid to the Q angle, varus/valgus alignment, and rotation of the limb. Increased Q angle, excessive femoral anteversion, genu valgum, pronation of the foot, and external tibial rotation all lead to excessive lateral force on the patella.

The TSA is measured with the knee at 90 degrees of flexion. The patella is engaged in the sulcus. The angle is formed by a line perpendicular to the transepicondylar axis and a line from the tibial tubercle to the center of the patella. The normal TSA is 0 degrees, and an abnormal TSA measures greater than 10 degrees (see Fig. 63-7).[100]

Atrophy of the quadriceps muscle, especially the VMO, is noted.

Tightness and laxity of the medial and lateral soft tissue restraints are assessed. With the knee flexed to 20 to 30 degrees, the patella is displaced medially and laterally. Medial displacement of less than one quarter of the patella, or 5 mm, indicates a tight lateral retinaculum. Lateral displacement of more than three quadrants indicates medial soft tissue incompetence (see Figs. 63-8 and 63-9). Inability to tilt the patella past horizontal is indicative of a tight lateral retinaculum.[65]

A patella apprehension test is performed with the relaxed patient lying supine and the knee flexed to about 20 degrees. The examiner attempts to gently displace the patella laterally. Patients with instability will feel uncomfortable and apprehensive, and will inadvertently contract the quadriceps muscle to attempt to stabilize the patella.

Patellar tracking is assessed throughout a range of motion. A J sign,[36] in which the patella is tracking in an inverted J pattern, represents the patella that is tracking centrally and then shifts laterally as the knee is extended. (See video on the website.) At 90 degrees, the patella should be centered between the femoral condyles in a normal patellofemoral joint.

Crepitus in the patellofemoral joint should be noted throughout range of motion. Pain is noted with patellofemoral compression. Tenderness to palpation should be noted with direct palpation of the medial/lateral facets, medial/lateral retinacula, and medial and lateral femoral condyles.

Ligamentous examination of the entire knee, as well as provocative tests for meniscal injury, should be performed.

Radiographic Studies in the Diagnosis and Treatment of Patellofemoral Instability

Standard radiographic evaluation, including anteroposterior, lateral, and axial views, should be obtained in each patient with patellofemoral disorders to assess the height and congruence of the patella and to exclude other bone disorders. CT has been used widely to study the patellofemoral joint, as it provides substantially more detail about the bony anatomy. MRI has also been used to investigate the patellofemoral relationship in extension and early flexion, as well as to detect cartilage lesions and ligamentous injuries.

Radiography

Anteroposterior View

The anteroposterior view does not allow visualization of the patellofemoral joint; however, it does provide valuable information regarding overall alignment of the limb and the presence of degenerative changes in the tibiofemoral joint. Weight-bearing anteroposterior views of the knees, as well as standing full-length mechanical axis views, are recommended. In addition, because the outline of the patella is visible, abnormalities such as patella magna or parva, bipartite patellae, and fractures can be seen. Marked lateral subluxation of the patella can also be detected in the anteroposterior view.

Lateral View

The lateral view is taken with the knee in at least 30 degrees of flexion to place the patellar tendon under tension and to demonstrate the functional relationship between the patella and the femur. Excessive rotation should be avoided because it may obscure some of the bony landmarks, such as the tibial tubercle, and may make interpretation difficult. The patella is not visualized on the lateral view in rare cases of congenital absence and when it is completely displaced laterally, as in habitual dislocation. In children younger than 5 years, the ossific nucleus has not yet appeared, and thus the patella is invisible.

Patellar position is related to the length of the patellar tendon. Patella alta, in particular, is associated with patellar instability, dislocation, and abnormalities of the trochlear groove. Patella alta, in particular, has been identified as a strong contributor to patellofemoral instability. Several methods of measurement have been described, including those reported by Blumensaat,[15] Insall and Salvati,[59] Blackburne and Peel,[14] Caton et al,[20] Rünow,[93] and Grelsamer and Meadows.[42]

Blumensaat's Line. Blumensaat[15] states that on a lateral radiograph with the knee flexed 30 degrees, the lower pole of the patella should be on a line projected anteriorly from the intercondylar notch (Blumensaat's line). It is difficult to obtain routine radiographs with the knee flexed exactly the required number of degrees; this limits the usefulness of the method. Blumensaat's method is also inaccurate. Of 44 radiographs of the knee that were flexed exactly 30 degrees, in no case did the lower pole of the patella lie on Blumensaat's line; rather, the patella was positioned above this line (Fig. 63-11).

Insall-Salvati Method. Insall and Salvati[59] sought a method that would fit the following requirements: (1) simple and practical, as well as accurate; (2) applicable to the range of knee positions used during routine radiography, which in the lateral view is usually 20 to 70 degrees of flexion; and (3) independent of the size of the joint and the degree of magnification of the radiograph. Because the ligamentum patellae is not elastic, its length determines the position of the patella, provided that the point of insertion into the tibial tubercle is constant.

Insall and Salvati[59] describe an expression for normal patellar height in terms of the length of the patellar tendon. Measurements were made on 114 knees in which the diagnosis of a torn meniscus had been clearly established by clinical history and examination, by positive arthrographic results, and by the finding of a meniscal tear at arthrotomy. Any case in which the slightest doubt existed was excluded, and it was assumed that the joints examined were structurally normal before a traumatic episode produced a torn meniscus. All patients were adults, and none showed radiologic

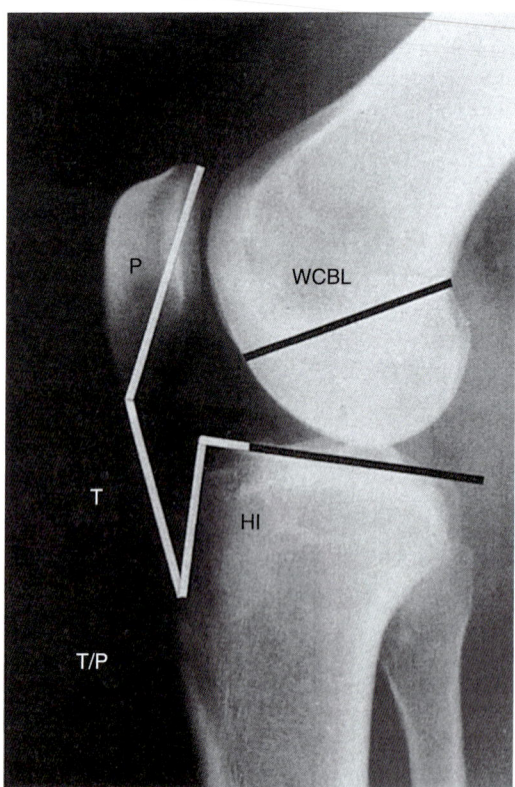

Figure 63-11. Insall-Salvati measurements to determine the height of the patella. *HI,* Height of insertion, or perpendicular distance between the joint line and the insertion of the patellar tendon; *P,* greatest diagonal length of the patella; *T,* length of the tendon measured on its deep posterior surface; *WCBL,* width of the femoral condyles at Blumensaat's line. (From Insall JN, Salvati E: Patella position in the normal knee joint. Radiology 101:101, 1971.)

evidence of osteoarthritis. The following measurements were taken (see Fig. 63-11):

1. T (length of tendon): The length of the patellar tendon was measured on its deep or posterior surface from its origin on the lower pole of the patella to its insertion into the tibial tubercle. The point of insertion is usually represented on the radiograph by a clearly defined notch.
2. P (length of patella): The greatest diagonal length of the patella was measured.
3. WCBL (width of the femoral condyles at Blumensaat's line): Both condyles were measured at the level of Blumensaat's line, and an average value was obtained. This measurement determined whether great variation in patellar size was present. Patellar size was considered to be acceptably constant.
4. HI (height of insertion): The perpendicular distance from the level of the tibial plateau surface to the point of insertion of the patellar tendon was measured to determine whether a constant relationship could be seen between the level of the tibial tubercle and the tibial plateau. Great variation in tendon insertion would have invalidated the measurements, but the insertion appeared to be acceptably constant. This measurement, therefore, may be disregarded in clinical evaluation.

The length of the patellar tendon (T) was found to be approximately equal to patellar length (P), and this was expressed as a ratio (because of variations in the size of individual knee joints and their projection on radiographs). The average value of the ratio T/P was 1.02, with a mean SD of 0.13. It was concluded that in a normal knee, the length of the patellar tendon should not differ from that of the patella by more than 20%.

Measurements were repeated on bilateral knee radiographs in 50 asymptomatic volunteers by Jacobsen and Bertheussen,[61] who confirmed a similar degree of accuracy. Agletti and associates also measured patellar height according to the Insall-Salvati method in a group of 150 normal knees[3] (see Table 63-1). The T/P ratio was found to be 1.04 on average (range, 0.8 to 1.38; SD, 0.11). The patella was significantly higher in women (1.06) than in men (1.01). In the same group of knees, the distance from the plateau level to the tibial tuberosity and the diagonal length of the patella varied only with sex, with larger values in men than in women. In 53 knees with patellar pain, the patella was slightly but significantly higher than in normal knees, with an average T/P ratio of 1.08 (range, 0.88 to 1.29; SD, 0.09). In a group of 37 knees with recurrent subluxation, the average T/P ratio was clearly increased to an average of 1.23 (range, 0.78 to 1.60; SD, 0.18). In conclusion, according to the Insall-Salvati method, an index over 1.2 indicates patella alta, whereas an index below 0.8 indicates a low patella.

Blackburne-Peel Ratio. Blackburne and Peel[14] criticized the T/P ratio on the basis of two observations:

1. The radiographic marking on the tibial tubercle may be indistinct or even unrecognizable when the tibial tuberosity has been affected by Osgood-Schlatter disease.
2. The nonarticular portion of the lower pole of the patella varies considerably in size; it is instead the

position of the articular surface that is of greatest clinical significance.

To overcome these difficulties, the authors suggested a ratio between the perpendicular distance from the lowest articular margin of the patella to the tibial plateau (A) and the length of the articular surface of the patella (B) as measured on a lateral view of the knee in at least 30 degrees of flexion (Fig. 63-12). The A/B ratio in 171 normal knees was 0.80 (SD, 0.14). No difference between the sexes was noted.

Aglietti and associates measured the A/B ratio in a group of 150 normal knees[3] and found a slightly higher value than the original authors did: an A/B ratio of 0.95 on average (range, 0.65 to 1.38; SD, 0.13), with an insignificant difference between men and women (see Table 63-1). In a group of patients with anterior knee pain, the A/B ratio was 0.91, an insignificant difference from the ratio in control knees. On the other hand, the A/B ratio was significantly increased in knees with recurrent subluxation (average, 1.08; range, 0.76 to 1.89; SD, 0.19).

Modified Insall-Salvati Ratio. Grelsamer and Meadows[42] observed that the Insall-Salvati index does not account for the shape of the patella. They found that patients with patella alta and a long distal nose may have a falsely normal Insall-Salvati index. The presence of patella alta in these patients can be easily verified by indices that use the patellar articular surface and the upper part of the tibia as landmarks (the Blackburne and Peel or the Caton ratio). The variable relationship between the length of the patella and the length of the articular surface as expressed by the morphology index[43] has been presented in the section on anatomy (Fig. 63-13).

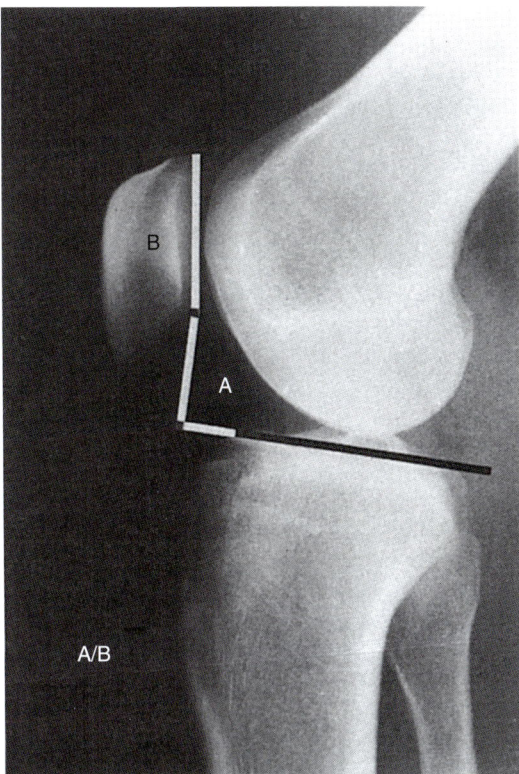

Figure 63-12. Blackburne and Peel method of measuring patellar height. Height is expressed as the ratio between *A* (perpendicular distance between the lowest part of the articular surface and the joint line level) and *B* (length of the articular surface of the patella). (From Blackburne JS, Peel TE: A new method of measuring patella height. J Bone Joint Surg Br 59:241, 1977.)

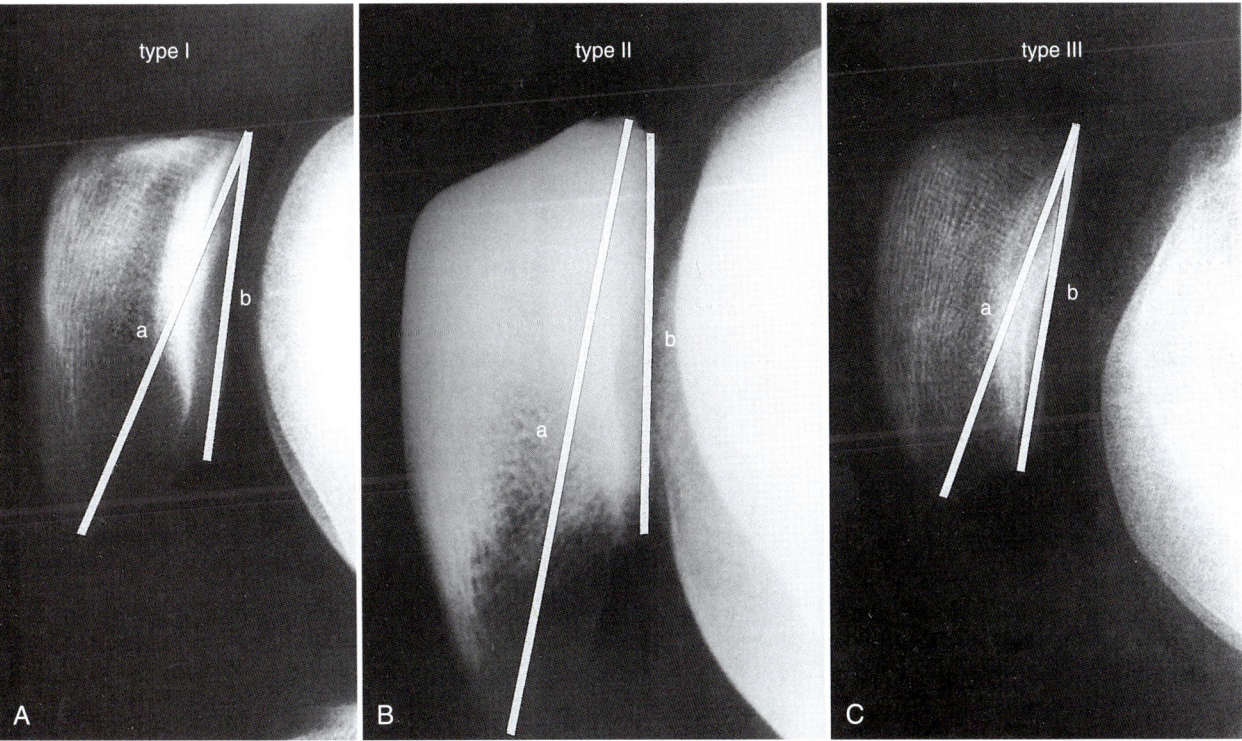

Figure 63-13. Different shapes of the patella in the sagittal plane according to Grelsamer and colleagues.[43] Patellar shape is described by the morphology ratio, that is, the ratio of patellar length to length of the articular surface. **A,** A normal type I patella has a morphology ratio between 1.2 and 1.5. **B,** Type II patella, with a morphology ratio greater than 1.5, that is, with a long inferior pole (Cyrano appearance). **C,** Type III patella with a morphology ratio below 1.2, that is, with a short inferior pole.

To overcome the problem of variable morphology of the patella, the Insall-Salvati ratio was modified. It was suggested that the ratio of the distance between the inferior articular facet of the patella and the tibial tuberosity and the length of the articular surface be used (Fig. 63-14). In other words, this method uses the same distal reference point as the Insall-Salvati method (the tibial tuberosity) and the same proximal reference point as the Caton method. In a group of 100 control knees, the modified Insall-Salvati ratio was 1.5 on average (range, 1.2 to 2.1). Ninety-seven percent of control knees had a ratio less than 2.0. Therefore, for practical purposes, a ratio of 2 or more can be used as an index of patella alta.

Lyon School. The Lyon School[20] criticized the previously existing methods of measuring the height of the patella. Members of this group found it difficult to define the insertion of the patellar tendon into the tibial tuberosity in knees with previous transposition of the tuberosity. They further observed that the use of a tangent to the tibial plateaus in the Blackburne and Peel method[14] may be a source of significant error. Perfect superimposition of the tibial plateaus is necessary to draw the line. The posterior slope of the tibial plateaus is not constant and may vary 15 degrees or more in subjects who have undergone anterior tibial epiphysiodesis. To overcome these difficulties, they tried to develop an easy method that could be used on lateral radiographs in flexion between 10 and 80 degrees and that was not influenced by radiographic magnification, by previous transposition of the tibial tuberosity, or by fractures of the tip of the patella. In this method, a ratio is calculated between the distance AT from the inferior point of the articular surface of the patella to the anterosuperior edge of the tibia and the length AP of the articular surface of the patella (Fig. 63-15). The AT/AP ratio was calculated in 141 normal subjects and was found to be 0.960[7] in 80 men and 0.990[6] in 61 women. Based on these findings, the authors considered the patella to be infera with a ratio of 0.6 or less and alta if 1.3 or more.

Norman Index. Norman and coworkers[89] observed that the Insall-Salvati method does not describe the relationship between the patella and the femoral sulcus, and that proximal or distal transposition of the tibial tuberosity may be performed without affecting the T/P ratio. To overcome these difficulties, Norman and associates described a method wherein a lateral radiograph is obtained with the knee in full extension (hyperextension) and in quadriceps contraction to straighten the patellar tendon. The film–focus distance should be kept constant (1 m) and the cassette placed in contact with the lateral aspect of the knee. Various parameters were measured in this radiograph, including the length of the tendon, patella, and articular facet and the vertical position of the patella—that is, the distance from the lowest point of the articular facet to the joint line. These measurements were related to the height of the patient, and it was found that the vertical position of the patella was constant without sex-related differences (Fig. 63-16). The Norman index, defined as the ratio between the vertical position of

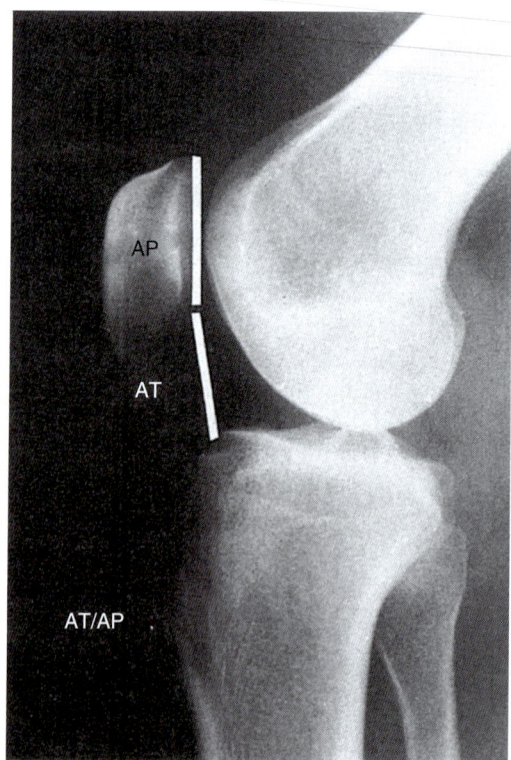

Figure 63-15. Caton's method to measure the height of the patella. Height is expressed as the ratio between the distance *(AT)* from the lowest point of the articular facet to the most prominent part of the tibial plateau and the length *(AP)* of the articular facet of the patella. See text for discussion of the ratio AT/AP. (From Caton G, Deschamps G, Chambat P, et al: Les routules basses: á propos de 128 observations. Rev Chir Orthop 68:317, 1982.)

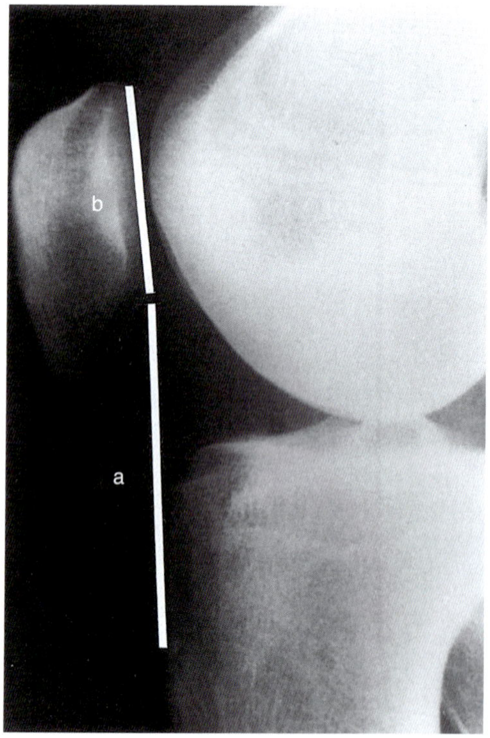

Figure 63-14. The modified Insall-Salvati method as described by Grelsamer and Meadows.[42] The distance between the lowest point of the articular surface of the patella and the tibial tuberosity (distance *a*) is divided by the length of the articular facet (distance *b*). A value of 2 or more indicates patella alta.

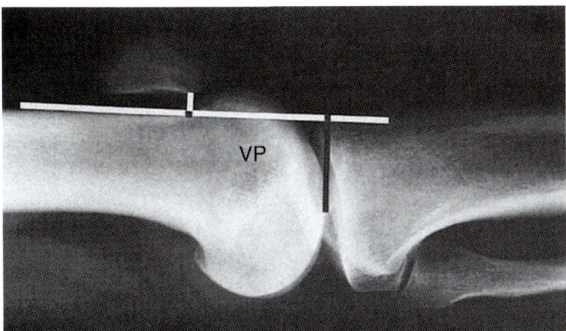

Figure 63-16. Norman's method to measure the height of the patella. A lateral radiograph is obtained with perfect superimposition of the femoral condyles, the knee hyperextended, and the quadriceps contracted to straighten the patellar tendon. A line is drawn tangential to the distal third of the anterior femoral cortex. Two perpendicular lines are then drawn that pass through the femoral–tibial contact point and through the inferior point of the articular facet. The distance between the two perpendicular lines, defined as the vertical position (VP) of the patella, is related to the height of the patient in centimeters. The Norman index is expressed as follows: Vertical position of the patella (mm)/Body height (cm). In a normal knee, its average value is 0.21. (From Norman O, Egund N, Ekelund L, Rünow A: The vertical position of the patella. Acta Orthop Scand 54:908, 1983.)

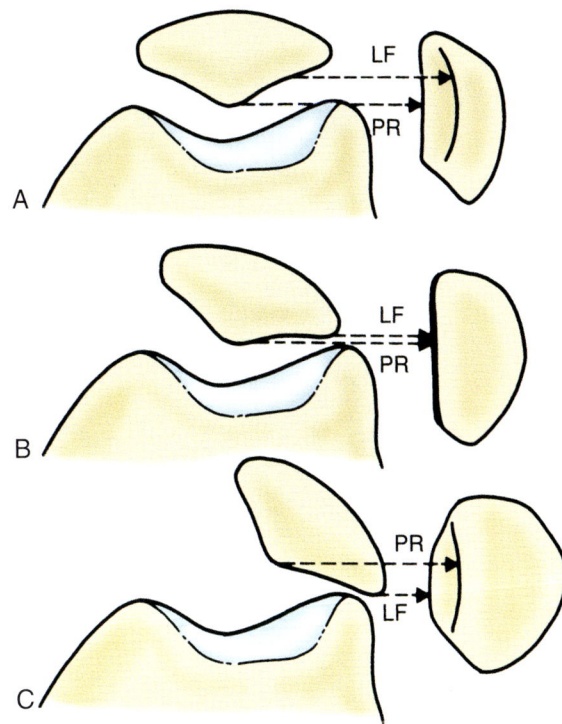

Figure 63-17. Patellar shape on lateral view with the knee flexed 10 to 15 degrees and good superimposition of the femoral condyles. **A,** In a normal knee, the posterior profile of the patella is represented by two lines: the most posterior one is the patellar ridge *(PR);* the anterior one is the lateral facet *(LF).* **B,** If the patella is slightly tilted laterally, the two lines superimpose. **C,** If the patella is severely tilted, the lateral facet overhangs the ridge line posteriorly, and the anteroposterior diameter of the patella is increased. (**A,** Modified from Maldague B, Malghem J: Apport du cliché de profil du genou dans le dépistage des instabilites rotuliennes: Rapport préliminaire. Rev Chir Orthop 71[Suppl 2]:5, 1985.)

the patella (in millimeters) and body length (in centimeters), is 0.21 in a normal knee (SD, 0.02). In patients with recurrent dislocation without associated generalized laxity, the index is 0.23 on average; in patients with associated generalized laxity, it is 0.25.

MRI Method. Biedert[13] proposed a different method by which to evaluate patellar height based on MRI scans in extension. Measurements are taken in the central or just lateral sagittal slice, where the articular cartilage is thicker. Patellar articular cartilage is projected on trochlear cartilage, and the height of its projection is calculated. The ratio between trochlear articular cartilage height and patellar articular cartilage height is deemed the patellar index. Normal values are 12.5% to 50%. An index less than 12.5% signifies patella alta, whereas an index higher than 50% indicates patella baja. The main advantage of this method is that it takes into consideration only the articular cartilage very precisely and is not affected by the patellar tendon.

Conclusions and Author's Recommendations. Various methods of measuring the height of the patella have been described. In our opinion, the Insall-Salvati T/P ratio remains a reliable and reproducible method. It does not require perfect alignment of the knee in the lateral view and does not need correction for magnification. Values greater than 1.2 are diagnostic of patella alta. The method may not be applicable in knees with previous Osgood-Schlatter disease, and the method is not suitable for evaluating patellar position after distal transfer of the tibial tuberosity. In this setting, one may use the Blackburne and Peel or the Caton method; these methods measure the height of the patella in relation to the tibial plateau and joint line. The main drawback of the Blackburne and Peel method is that it requires a lateral view with superimposition of the femoral condyles to accurately identify the joint line. An image amplifier is required to consistently obtain this degree of accuracy. The same problem is

encountered with the Norman technique, which has the additional difficulty of requiring an effective quadriceps contraction. Furthermore, the film–focus distance (1 m) must be kept constant, and the patient's height must be known. In the presence of abnormal patellar morphology with a long or short distal pole, the modified Insall-Salvati method should be used.

Evaluating for Patellofemoral Dysplasia

Attention has been drawn to evaluation of the anatomy of the trochlea and subluxation of the patella as seen on the lateral view. Maldague and Malghem[74] first described the radiographic appearance of the patella and trochlea femoralis on lateral views of normal knees and knees with patellar instability. It is necessary to obtain lateral views with satisfactory superimposition of the posterior and distal femoral condyles, which requires the use of an image amplifier. In the lateral view of a normal knee, the posterior aspect of the patella is represented by two lines: the most posterior one is the patellar ridge, the other is the lateral facet (Figs. 63-17 and 63-18). In knees with mild lateral tilt of the patella, the two lines superimpose. When the patella is more markedly tilted, the lateral facet overhangs the patellar ridge line posteriorly, and the anteroposterior diameter of the patella is greatly increased. The normal trochlea is composed of three

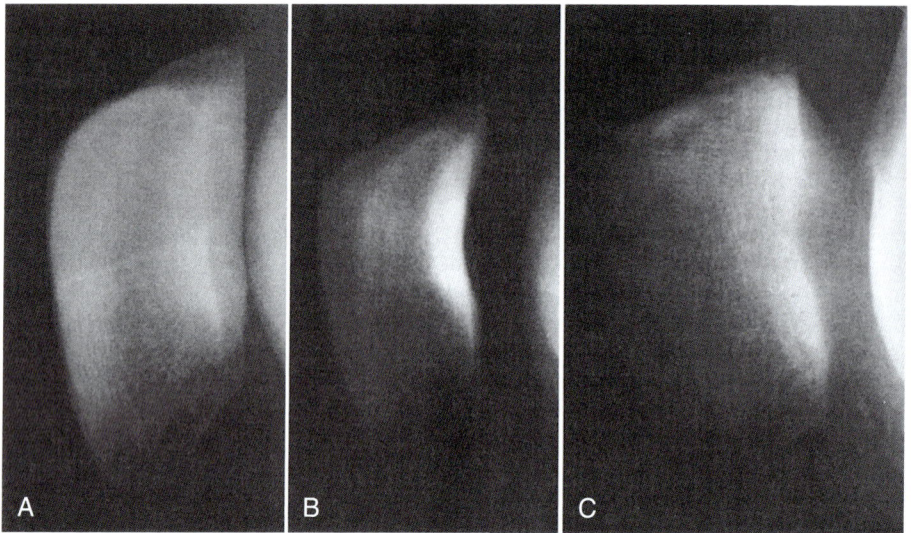

Figure 63-18. Lateral views. **A,** The patella in a normal knee. **B,** A knee with a mildly tilted patella. **C,** A knee with a markedly tilted patella.

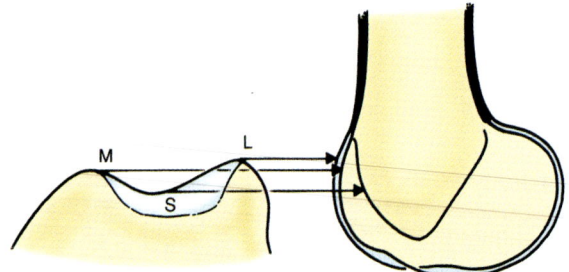

Figure 63-19. Morphology of the trochlea in a lateral radiograph with superimposition of the femoral condyles. The two anterior lines are the projection of the medial *(M)* and lateral *(L)* facets of the trochlea. The posterior line is in continuation with the intercondylar roof line and corresponds to the deepest part of the sulcus *(S)*. (Modified from Maldague B, Malghem J: Apport du cliché de profil du genou dans le dépistage des instabilites rotuliennes: rapport préliminaire. Rev Chir Orthop 71[Suppl 2]:5, 1985.)

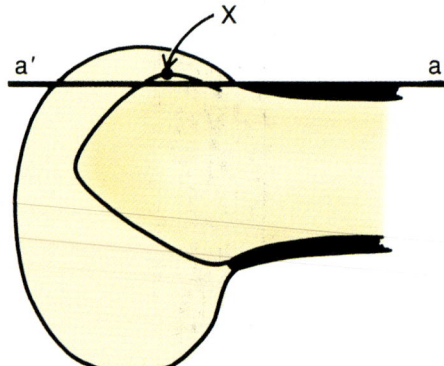

Figure 63-20. Quantification of the trochlear bump. A line (ac-a) is drawn tangential to the last 10 cm of the anterior femoral cortex. The line of the sulcus at its most anterior point *X* may pass in front of (positive value) or behind (negative value) the tangent line. The bump is measured as the distance between the femoral cortex line and the sulcus line in millimeters.

lines: the two anterior lines are projections of the top of the medial and lateral facets of the trochlea; the posterior line, in continuation with the intercondylar roof line, represents the deepest point of the sulcus (Fig. 63-19). The distance between the two anterior lines and the posterior line represents the depth of the sulcus. Maldague and Malghem observed that its depth is normally greater than 1 cm as it is measured 1 cm distal to the upper part of the trochlea. In knees with patellar instability, the depth of the trochlea is reduced throughout the length of the sulcus (totally deficient sulcus) or only in its upper part (focally deficient sulcus). The authors emphasized the importance of the lateral view in patients with clinically suspected patellar instability and axial views showing negative results. Because axial views are often obtained in more than 30 degrees of flexion, a lateral view taken at 15 degrees of flexion allows exploration of the patellofemoral congruence at a degree of flexion that cannot be visualized with conventional axial views.

These concepts have been carried a step farther by the Lyon School.[30] Members of this group examined the lateral views of 143 knees with recurrent or acute dislocation of the patella and compared these with the radiographs of 190 control knees. They studied two quantitative measurements—trochlear bump and trochlear depth—and one qualitative sign—the crossing sign.

On a lateral view with superimposition of the femoral condyles, a line is drawn tangent to the last 10 cm of the anterior cortex of the femur. The line of the femoral sulcus may end in front of (positive value), over, or behind (negative value) the line of the anterior cortex. The distance between the anterior cortex line and the sulcus (saille or bump) is measured in millimeters (Fig. 63-20). The bump of the sulcus line in relation to the anterior femoral cortex was found to be highly useful in differentiating between knees with instability (average, +3.2 mm) and normal knees (average, −0.8 mm). A pathologic threshold value for measurement of trochlear bump was identified: 3 mm. Sixty-six percent of knees with patellar instability had anterior trochlear translation of 3 mm or more as compared with only 6.5% of control knees.

The depth of the trochlea was measured as the distance between the floor of the trochlea and the most anterior condylar contour line. First, a line tangent to the posterior cortex of the femur was drawn. A second line was drawn perpendicular to the posterior femoral cortex line and tangent to

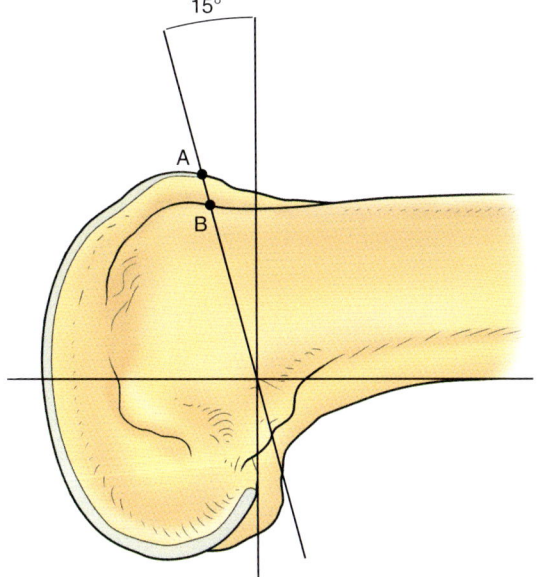

Figure 63-21. Quantification of trochlear depth. It is the distance *A-B* measured in millimeters along a line subtended 15 degrees from the perpendicular to the posterior femoral cortex line and crossing a line tangential to the posterior femoral condyles and perpendicular to the posterior cortex line.

the posterior aspect of the femoral condyles. A third line was finally drawn that subtended an angle of 15 degrees to the second line and passed through the intersection of the first and second lines. Trochlear depth was measured along this third line (Fig. 63-21). Trochlear depth was 7.8 mm in the control group and 2.3 mm in knees with patellar instability. A trochlear depth of 4 mm or less was considered pathologic. This value was found in 85% of knees with patellar instability and in only 3% of controls.

Dysplasia of the trochlea can be divided into three types according to the point at which the sulcus line crosses the lines of the condyles (the croisement, or crossing, sign) The crossing sign is a simple qualitative criterion defined as the crossing between the floor line and the lateral condylar line. At that level, the trochlea is considered flat (Figs. 63-22 and 63-23)[31]:

Type I dysplasia: This form is the mildest. The lines of the condyles are symmetrical, and they are crossed at the same point in the proximal part of the trochlea by the floor line. Only the very proximal part of the trochlea is flat.

Type II dysplasia: The lines of the condyles are not superimposed; the line of the sulcus crosses the medial condyle line first, and the lateral one crosses at a higher level. Separate crossing of the medial and lateral condyle lines is characteristic of this type.

Type III dysplasia: This form is the most severe. The condyle lines are superimposed, but they are crossed low on the trochlea by the sulcus line. Most of the trochlea is therefore flat.

Two types of normal trochlea were identified:

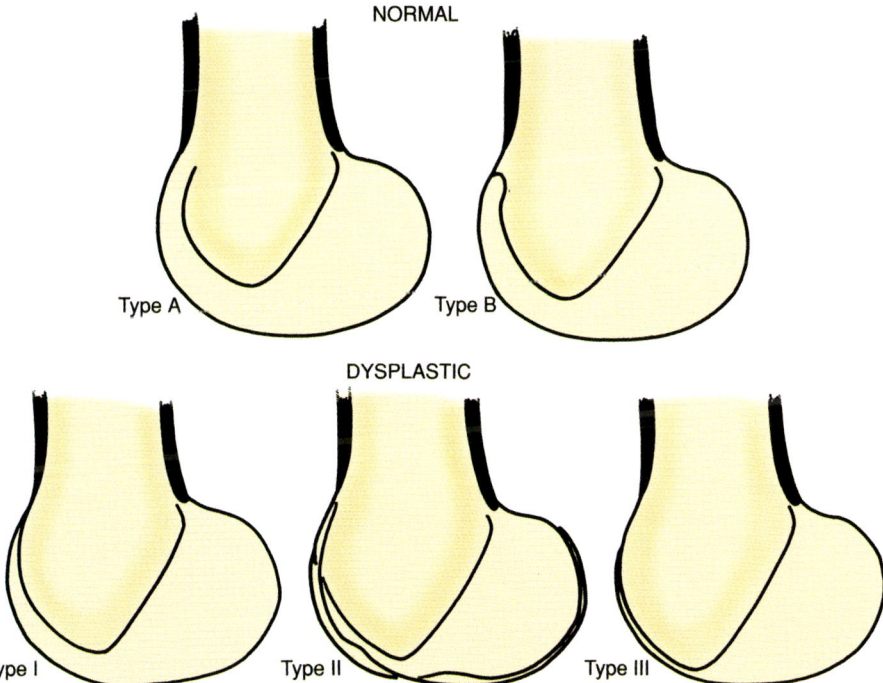

Figure 63-22. The croisement (crossing sign). In normal knees, the sulcus line may be posterior to the condyle lines throughout its length *(type A)* or may join the medial condyle line only in the upper part of the trochlea *(type B)*. Therefore, there is no crossing between the sulcus line and the condyle line in normal knees. The presence of the crossing sign indicates dysplasia of the femoral trochlea. See text for further discussion. (From Dejour H, Walch G, Neyret P, Adeleine P: La dysplasie de la trochlee femorale. Rev Chir Orthop 76:45, 1990.)

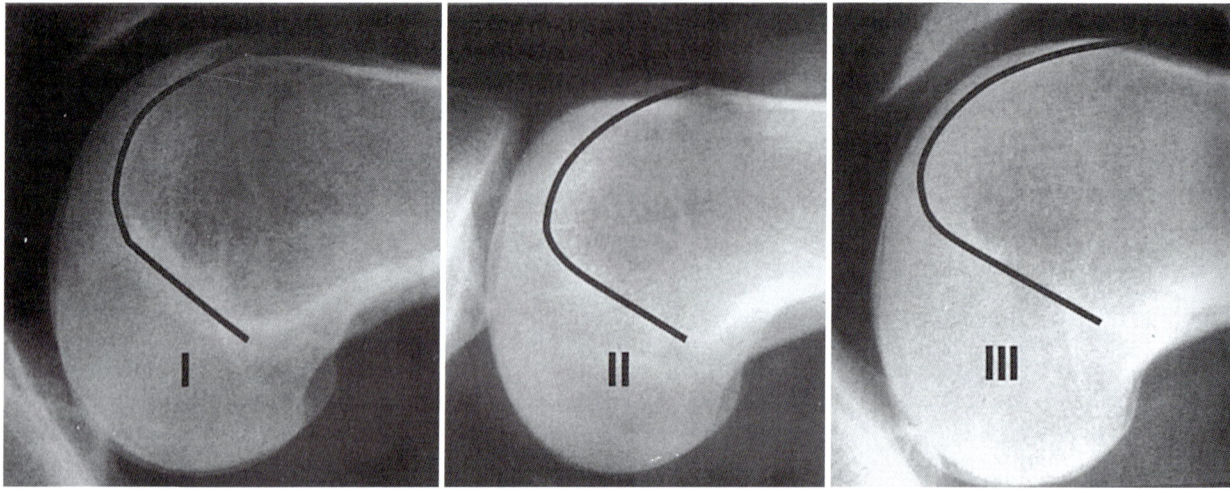

Figure 63-23. Trochlear dysplasia, types I, II, and III. See text for explanation. (From Dejour H, Walch G, Neyret P, Adeleine P: La dysplasie de la trochlee femorale. Rev Chir Orthop 76:45, 1990.)

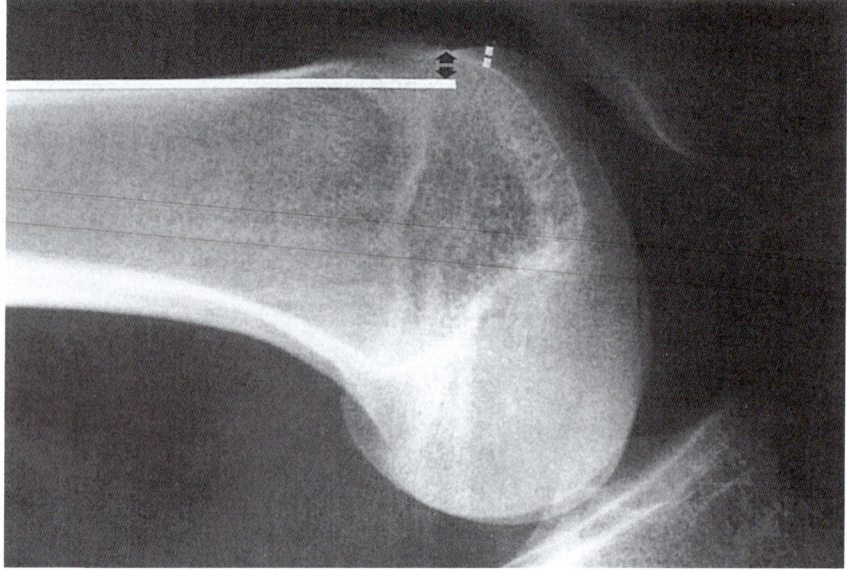

Figure 63-24. Lateral radiograph of a knee with recurrent patellar instability. The sulcus line is anterior to the femoral cortex line (bump of +4 mm), the sulcus depth is only 3 mm, and a crossing sign is present between the sulcus and condyle lines (type I dysplasia).

Type A (50%): The sulcus line is posterior to the condyle lines throughout its length (see Fig. 63-22).

Type B (50%): The sulcus line joins the line of the medial condyle, but only in the highest part of the trochlea.

Dysplasia of the femoral sulcus, as evidenced by the crossing sign, was present in the majority of knees with patellar instability (96%) (Fig. 63-24); the same was true in only 3% of control knees. In light of this study, the authors concluded that in trochlear dysplasia, the trochlea is flat in a zone of variable length and has a shallow groove more distally. According to the authors, trochlear dysplasia is better evaluated on a lateral radiograph than on CT. Such dysplasia is best recognized with the crossing sign, a qualitative factor that was present in 96% of knees with patellar instability. Two other quantitative measurements, trochlear bump (positive when ≥3 mm) and trochlear depth (positive when ≤4 mm), were both positive in 85% of cases.

The Lyon School[111] has modified this classification and has introduced new radiographic signs. The supratrochlear spur is located in the proximal aspect of the lateral trochlea in an attempt to keep the patella in the groove. The double-shape sign has been described as a vertical line of sclerosis that is the projection of the medial trochlea. Based on these new signs, trochlear dysplasia has been described as follows:

Grade A: crossing sign (symmetrical but less deep trochlea)

Grade B: crossing sign and trochlear spur (flat or convex trochlea)

Grade C: crossing and double-shape signs (asymmetrical trochlea, laterally convex and medially hypoplastic)

Grade D: crossing and double-shape signs, trochlear spur (asymmetrical trochlea with rapid mediolateral change)

It is suggested that treatment of instability of the patella should be based on recognized anatomic abnormalities.

Re-creation of a sulcus of normal depth is theoretically desirable to improve the stability of the patella. This may be achieved by elevating the lateral femoral condyle[6] or by depressing the central part of the trochlea.[79] Elevation of the lateral condyle is a logical approach if the saille of the sulcus is normal; it is contraindicated in knees with a positive saille. Deepening of the sulcus (trochleoplasty) seems to be more logical because it re-creates normal anatomy. However, the procedure is technically more demanding and involves violation of the articular cartilage.

Axial Views

An axial view of the patellofemoral joint adds considerably to our knowledge when performed in a correctly standardized manner. Unfortunately, all too often this portion of the examination is omitted or is performed haphazardly, so much useful information is lost. Various techniques are available.

In the method attributed to Settegast,[102] the patient lies prone with the knees acutely flexed. The x-ray plate is placed beneath the knees with the tube directed above so that the beam is at a right angle. This is an easy examination for the technician to perform. Unfortunately, it is also uninformative because if the angle of flexion is poorly controlled, the image of the patella is often distorted and the patella lies on the femoral condyles rather than in the sulcus, which is the most important and functional position.

Hughston and Walsh[51] advocate a modification of the Jaroschy technique.[63] The patient is placed prone with the cassette beneath the knees. The knees are flexed 55 degrees and rest on the tube, which is angled at about 45 degrees. Disadvantages of this method are that images are distorted because the beam strikes the plate at an angle, and the knees are flexed more than is desirable.

Ficat and Hungerford[36] describe a technique in which the patient's knees are flexed over the end of the x-ray table. The tube is placed at the patient's feet and the cassette is held proximally against the anterior of the thigh. In this position, the tube is perpendicular to the beam. Flexion views can be obtained at 30, 60, and 90 degrees. This technique is widely used in Europe but seems less popular in the United States, probably because of technical difficulties involved in obtaining good views.

Merchant and colleagues[83] describe a technique whereby the patient is positioned supine with the knees flexed 45 degrees over the end of the table. The knees are elevated slightly to keep the femurs horizontal and parallel with the table surface. The x-ray tube is kept proximally over the patient's head and angled down 30 degrees from the horizontal. The film cassette is placed about 30 cm below the knees, resting on the shins and perpendicular to the x-ray beam (Fig. 63-25). The legs are strapped together at about calf level to control rotation, and both knees are exposed simultaneously. It is important for the quadriceps muscle to be relaxed. The position of 45 degrees of knee flexion has been selected as the position of least flexion with which satisfactory results could be obtained.

Two angles are measured on the Merchant view: the sulcus angle and the congruence angle (Fig. 63-26). The congruence angle measures the relationship of the patella to the intercondylar sulcus. For this measurement, the sulcus angle is bisected to establish a zero reference line. A second line is then projected from the apex of the sulcus angle to the lowest point on the articular ridge of the patella. The angle measured between these two lines is the congruence angle. If the apex of the patellar articular ridge is lateral to the zero line, the congruence angle is designated positive. If it is medial, the congruence angle is negative. In a group of 100 normal knees, 50 males and 50 females, Merchant and colleagues[83] measured an average sulcus angle of 138 degrees (SD, 6 degrees) and an average congruence angle of −6 degrees (SD,

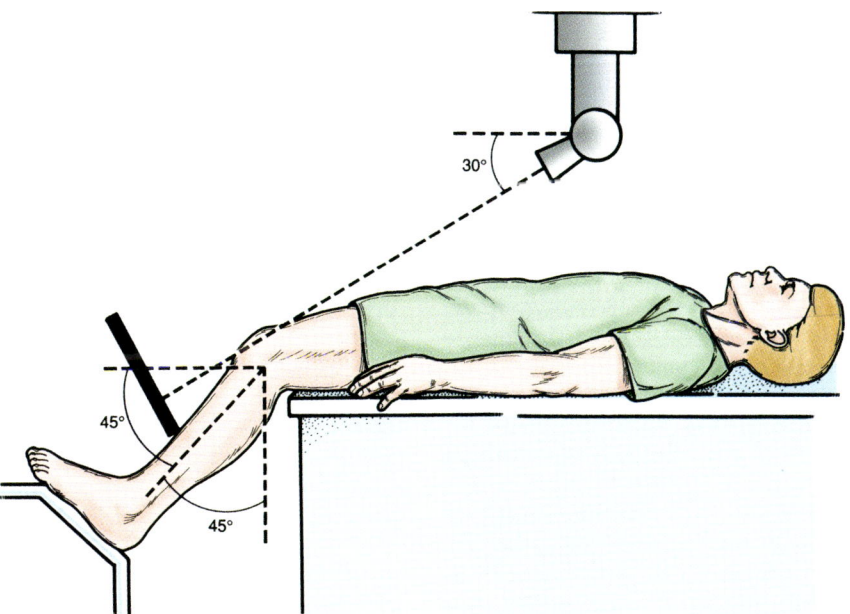

Figure 63-25. Merchant's technique to obtain axial views of the patella. The patient is supine with the knees flexed 45 degrees over the edge of the table and resting on a support. The cassette rests on the shins about 30 cm below the knees. It is struck at a right angle by the x-ray beam, which is angled 30 degrees down from the horizontal. (From Merchant AC, Mercer RL, Jacobsen RH, et al: Roentgenographic analysis of patello-femoral congruence. J Bone Joint Surg Am 56:1391, 1974.)

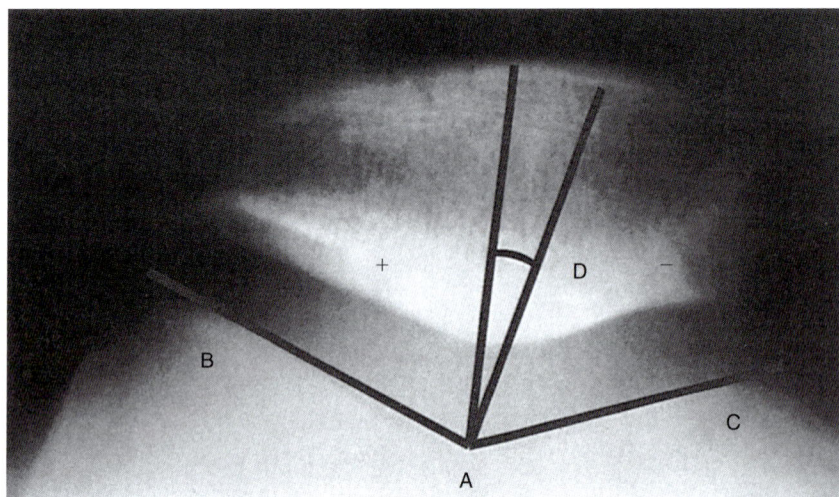

Figure 63-26. Measurement of the sulcus angle and the congruence angle on a Merchant view. The sulcus angle *(BAC)* is bisected by the reference line. A second line *(AD)* is drawn from the sulcus to the patellar ridge. If the apex of the patellar ridge is lateral to the reference line, the value of the angle is positive; if it is medial, the value of the angle is negative. (From Merchant AC, Mercer RL, Jacobsen RH, et al: Roentgenographic analysis of patello-femoral congruence. J Bone Joint Surg Am 56:1391, 1974.)

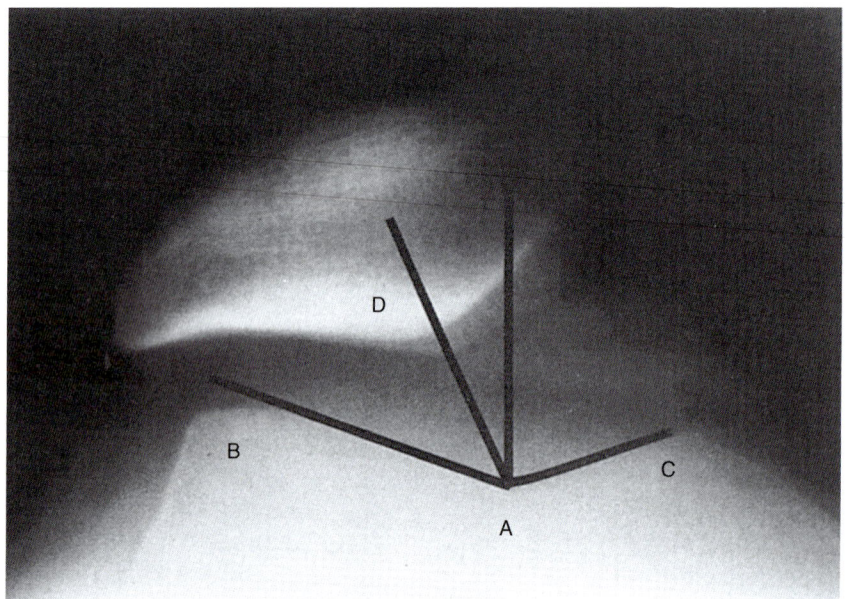

Figure 63-27. Merchant axial view in a patient with recurrent dislocation of the patella. Both the sulcus angle *(BAC)* and the congruence angle *(CAD)* were clearly increased over normal values.

11 degrees). Based on these data, it was suggested that any sulcus angle greater than 150 degrees and any congruence angle greater than 16 degrees is abnormal at the 95th percentile. In a group of patients with recurrent patellar dislocation (number not specified), the average congruence angle was +23 degrees, which is well beyond the 95th percentile of normal subjects.

Aglietti and coworkers repeated the measurements proposed by Merchant and associates in normal and pathologic knees.[3] In a group of 150 normal knees, the average sulcus angle was 137 degrees (SD, 6 degrees), with no differences noted between males and females. This is very close to the results of Merchant and associates. On the other hand, Aglietti and colleagues measured an average congruence angle of −8 degrees (SD, 6 degrees), thus suggesting a lower

upper limit in normal knees (+4 degrees) than that proposed by Merchant (+16). In 53 knees with anterior knee pain, the sulcus angle was similar to that of controls (average, 139; SD, 4 degrees), and the congruence angle was slightly increased (average, −2; SD, 9 degrees). In 37 knees with recurrent dislocation, both the sulcus angle (average, 147 degrees; SD, 7 degrees) and the congruence angle (average, −16; SD, 13 degrees) were clearly increased over those of controls (Fig. 63-27).

Laurin and coworkers[70,71] described a similar method in which the x-ray tube is positioned distally between the feet, and the cassette is held proximally against the anterior of the thighs (Fig. 63-28). The following details should be observed:

• The patient should be seated with the feet at the very edge of the table. The x-ray beam is directed parallel to

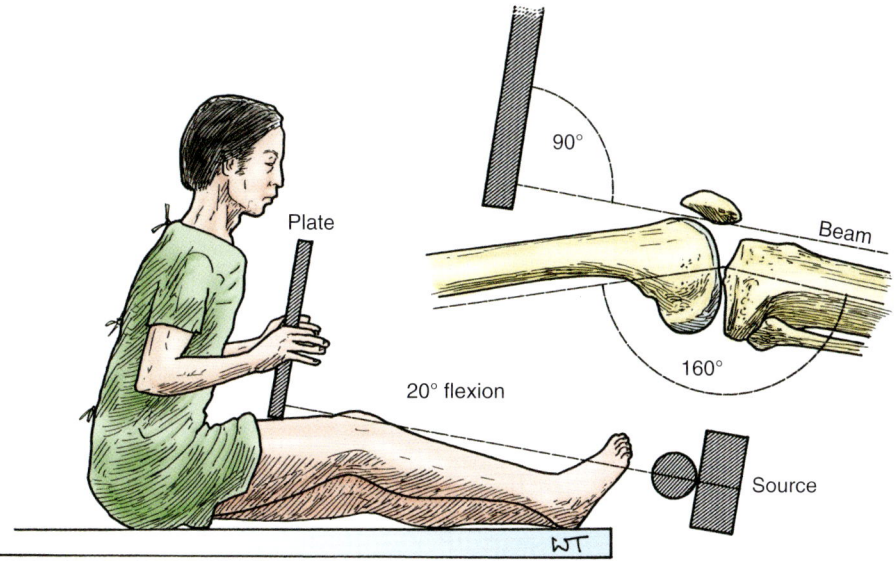

Figure 63-28. Laurin's method to obtain axial views of the patella. The patient is seated on the examining table with the feet near the edge. The x-ray beam is parallel to the anterior border of the tibia, and the knees are flexed 20 degrees. The cassette is held by the patient against the thighs and at 90 degrees to the beam. See text for further discussion. (From Laurin CA, Levesque HP, Dussault R, et al: The abnormal lateral patellofemoral angle: a diagnostic roentgenographic sign of recurrent patellar subluxation. J Bone Joint Surg Am 60:55, 1978.)

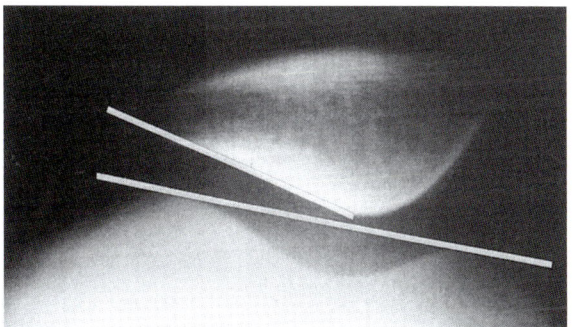

Figure 63-29. Measurement of the lateral patellofemoral angle (LPFA) on a Laurin view. The LPFA is measured by drawing a line tangential to the top of the medial and lateral condyle and a second line tangential to the lateral patellar facet. It is open laterally in normal knees.

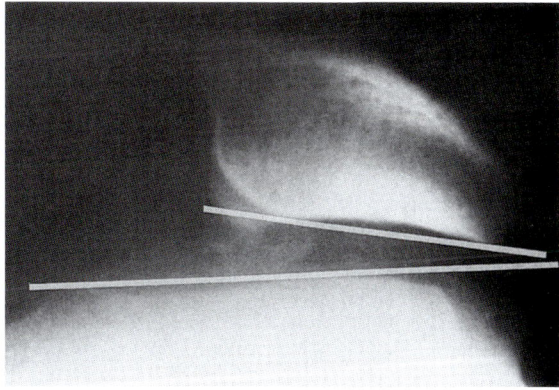

Figure 63-30. Laurin's view in a knee affected by recurrent dislocation of the patella. The lateral patellofemoral angle is open medially.

the anterior border of the tibia and the longitudinal axis of the patella. The x-ray beam is thus parallel to the specific proximal segment of the patellofemoral joint that must be visualized.

- The knees must be in a position of 20 degrees of knee flexion, and the quadriceps must be relaxed. A special adjustable support under the knees is recommended to maintain the position.
- The x-ray plate is held by the patient such that it is at 90 degrees to the long axis of the tibia and x-ray beam; it must not be laid flat against the thighs, nor should it be at 90 degrees to the tabletop. The patient must forcibly press the lower edge of the plate against the thighs. Otherwise, especially in muscular or obese patients, only the patella appears at the bottom of the x-ray film, and the femoral trochlea is not included. Under such circumstances, the radiographs must be repeated and the technique modified by pushing on the x-ray plate more forcibly or by holding the x-ray plate more

proximal on the thighs. The knees must not be flexed more than 20 degrees.

In a correctly obtained Laurin view, the patellofemoral compartment is clearly visualized. The lateral prominence of the trochlea has a rounded contour, whereas the medial prominence is sharp. The lateral patellofemoral angle (Fig. 63-29) can be measured by drawing a line tangent to the top of the medial and lateral femoral condyles and a second line tangent to the lateral facet of the patella.[71] The lateral facet of the patella was chosen as reference because given the wide variations in patellar morphology described by Wiberg[117] and Baumgartl,[10] it retains a relatively constant shape. In a group of 100 normal knees, the lateral patellofemoral angle was open laterally in the great majority (97%), whereas the lines were parallel in only 3%. In 30 knees with patellar subluxation, the lines were parallel in 60% and were open medially in 40% (Fig. 63-30). The lateral patellofemoral angle was of no assistance in the evaluation of knees with patellar pain because it was normal (open laterally) in 90%, and the lines were parallel in the remainder. In an effort to individuate a radiographic measurement diagnostic of chondromalacia, Laurin and coworkers[70] proposed the patellofemoral index (Fig. 63-31). The basic abnormality underlying patellar subluxation and patellar pain is the same, but it is less severe in the second condition. The lateral patellofemoral angle therefore is not altered, whereas the patellofemoral index may show a "mini-tilt" of the patella. The patellofemoral index is the ratio of the thickness of the medial to the lateral patellofemoral interspace. In normal knees, the medial interspace was equal or slightly wider than the lateral, and the patellofemoral index was 1.6 or less. In contrast, the patellofemoral index was higher than 1.6 in 97% of knees with patellar pain. An increased patellofemoral index with widening of the medial interspace indicates a mini-tilt of the patella.

Malghem and Maldague[75] suggested that axial views should be obtained at 30 degrees of flexion and external tibial rotation. This method takes advantage of the lateral pull of the patellar tendon to detect subluxability of the patella. Lateral rotation is produced manually by external rotation of the forefoot. Counterpressure on the lateral side of the thigh is necessary to keep the knee within the beam axis. The examination is performed sequentially for both knees. The tube is positioned between the feet of the patient, and the cassette rests against the thighs. In 27 knees that underwent surgery for patellar instability, the congruence angle was measured according to the method of Merchant and colleagues,[83] and a value greater than 16 degrees was considered evidence of subluxation. Subluxation was evident in 26% of cases by the 45-degree axial view and in 100% by the 30-degree lateral rotation view. Of these 27 knees, 13 had a centered patella in the 45-degree axial view and showed subluxation in the 30-degree lateral rotation view. In these knees, a 30-degree axial view without external rotation was added. This modification yielded a result (average congruence angle, +10.3 degrees) that was intermediate between the 45-degree (average congruence angle, +1.5 degrees) and the 30-degree (average congruence angle, +26.7 degrees) views with external rotation.

Toft[113] suggested that axial radiographs of the patella in the weight-bearing position can detect narrowing of the patellofemoral joint line.

An alternative method used to measure tilt of the patella was described by Grelsamer and associates.[41] They elected to use a line connecting the two edges of the patella (the corner-to-corner line) instead of the more usual line tangent to the subchondral bone of the lateral facet, as recommended by Laurin and colleagues.[71] They reasoned that the corner-to-corner line is independent of patellar morphology, it is easy to draw, and it corresponds more closely to clinical evaluation of the tilt. Patellar tilt was evaluated in relation to a horizontal line (Fig. 63-32) and not to a line tangent to the medial and lateral edges of the trochlea. Using a horizontal line as a reference has a drawback because it requires consistent rotational control of the leg and alignment of the cassette parallel to the ground. Rotational alignment of the leg was judged from the foot, which had to point directly upward. The purpose of using a horizontal line is to be independent of the morphology of the anterior trochlea, which is highly variable and may induce underestimation or overestimation of a tilt.

A second alternative is to use a line tangent to the posterior condyles, but this requires a CT scan. Axial views were obtained at 30 degrees of flexion via a Merchant technique. In a group of 100 knees with patellar malalignment, the average tilt angle was 12 ± 6 degrees, and 85% of cases had a tilt greater than 5 degrees. In a control group of 100 knees, the average tilt angle was 2 ± 1 degree ($P < .01$), and 92% of cases had a tilt of 5 degrees or less. Patellar tilt greater than 5 degrees is therefore 85% sensitive, 92% specific, and 89% accurate in the diagnosis of patellofemoral malalignment. This method of measuring patellar tilt may thus be advantageous if a dedicated radiologist is available to accurately position the patient and the cassette.

In conclusion, standard anteroposterior and lateral radiographs with a Merchant axial view can reasonably be accepted as a first step in the diagnosis of patellofemoral disorders. A lateral view with perfect superimposition of the femoral condyles is necessary to evaluate the morphology of the trochlea

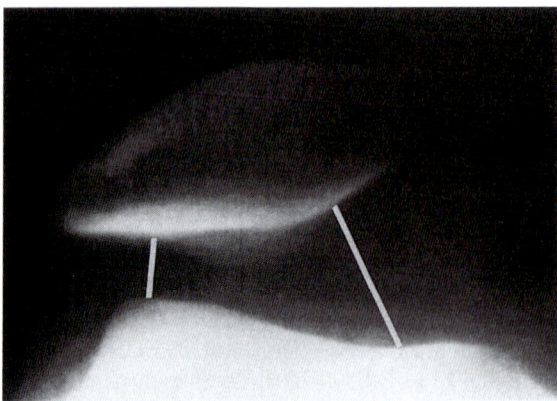

Figure 63-31. Measurement of the patellofemoral index on a Laurin view. The ratio of the medial interspace to the lateral interspace is up to 1.6 in normal knees. In this case, the measurement is clearly pathologic.

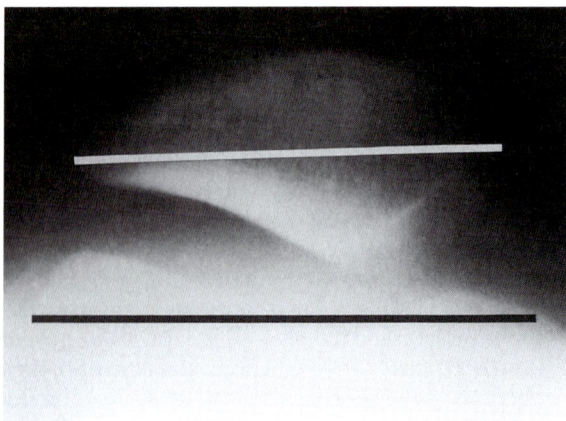

Figure 63-32. Tilt of the patella evaluated according to Grelsamer and colleagues.[41] The tilt is the angle joining the edges of the patella and the horizontal. The axial view is obtained with the knee flexed 30 degrees and with careful control of rotation of the leg with the foot pointing directly upward and the lower border of the film parallel to the ground.

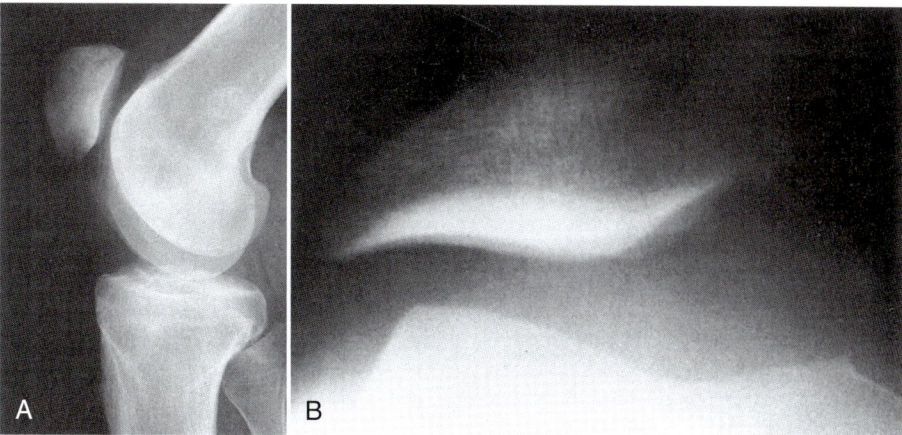

Figure 63-33. Lateral **(A)** and Merchant axial **(B)** views of a knee with recurrent dislocation of the patella. Clear anatomic abnormalities, including a high-riding patella, a flat sulcus, and a positive congruence angle, are evident.

for any evidence of dysplasia (flat trochlea). According to Aglietti et al (see Table 63-1),[3] a normal knee has, on average, a Q angle of 15 degrees, an Insall-Salvati T/P ratio of 1.04, a Blackburne and Peel A/B ratio of 0.95, a sulcus angle of 137 degrees, and a congruence angle of −8 degrees. Slightly but statistically significantly higher values for the Q angle and the T/P ratio have been found in females. For clinical purposes, we consider the following values to be pathologic: a Q angle greater than 20 degrees, a T/P ratio greater than 1.2 and certainly greater than 1.3, an A/B ratio greater than 1.2, a sulcus angle greater than 150 degrees, and a congruence angle greater than +4 degrees. Knees with patellar pain showed a clearly increased Q angle (average, 20 degrees), with minor and clinically insignificant differences in the T/P ratio, A/B ratio, and sulcus angle, as well as minor lateralization of the patella (average congruence angle, −2 degrees). Knees with recurrent subluxation or dislocation of the patella showed a high-riding patella with an average T/P ratio of 1.23 and an average A/B ratio of 1.08, a more open femoral sulcus (average sulcus angle, 147 degrees), and gross lateral displacement of the patella (average congruence angle, +16 degrees) (Fig. 63-33). In view of clear anatomic abnormalities in knees with recurrent dislocation of the patella, these simple radiographic measurements are diagnostic in most cases. Conversely, patients with anterior knee pain frequently have normal height of the patella and normal-appearing axial views at 45 degrees. In these cases, it is worthwhile to request an axial view at 20 degrees[71] or a CT scan of the patellofemoral joint to detect minor abnormalities in the first 30 degrees of flexion.

Computed Tomography

The introduction of CT in orthopedics has made it possible to investigate patellofemoral relationships in the arc between full extension and 45 degrees of flexion. Traditional axial views can be obtained in 20 degrees of flexion according to the method of Laurin and colleagues,[71] but the technique is not easy. Obese or muscular patients render the examination more difficult, and a skilled technician is required to obtain consistent results. Furthermore, the use of CT avoids image overlapping and distortion. For these reasons, CT has gained increasing popularity in the evaluation of patellofemoral disorders.

Delgado-Martins[32] first used CT to evaluate the patellofemoral joints of 12 normal subjects with the knee in extension and compared these images with traditional axial views at 30, 60, and 90 degrees. The patella was considered to be centered when the median crest fit exactly in the intercondylar groove. The author reported that the patella was centered in the groove in 96% of cases at 90 degrees, 63% at 60 degrees, 29% at 30 degrees, 13% in full extension with the quadriceps relaxed, and 4% in full extension with the quadriceps contracted. Although the images reported by Delgado-Martins suggest that some of these patients may suffer from subluxation of the patella, it is well emphasized that evaluation in the first degrees of flexion is far more informative than at 60 or 90 degrees.

Martinez and coworkers[78] made the same observation; they used CT to evaluate 10 normal volunteers and 5 patients with recurrent subluxation. Images were obtained at 0, 20, and 45 degrees of flexion with a special device used to position the knee.[77] The authors measured the sulcus angle and used a line tangent to the posterior condyles as a reference to evaluate patellar tilt angle, height of the lateral condyle, and centralization of the patella. In extension, 95% of normal patellae were centralized with the quadriceps relaxed, but this percentage decreased to 85% with quadriceps contraction. Centralization of the patella was maintained in most control subjects at 20 and 45 degrees of knee flexion. The patellar tilt angle was positive (open laterally) in all normal knees in extension (average, 11 degrees) and did not change with flexion. The sulcus angle was 143 degrees in extension and decreased with flexion. In the five knees with subluxation, the patella was clearly displaced laterally in extension but tended to reduce in flexion. The patellar tilt angle was negative (open medially) in extension but tended to reverse to a positive value (decreased patellar tilt) with flexion. The height of the lateral femoral condyle was decreased and the sulcus angle increased when compared with these values in controls. Martinez and colleagues concluded that axial or CT images at 20 and 45 degrees of flexion can falsely indicate a normal patellofemoral joint.

Sasaki and Yagi[96] used CT to investigate the patellofemoral joint with the knee in extension. They studied 24 knees with patellar subluxation and 24 controls. Lines tangent to the medial and lateral prominences of the trochlea and the transverse axis of the patella were used to measure tilt of the patella. Lateral shift of the patella was measured in relation to the most prominent aspect of the lateral femoral condyle. The results were compared with conventional axial views at 30 degrees of flexion. Mean patellar tilt angles in normal knees with the quadriceps relaxed and contracted were 15 degrees and 14 degrees, respectively. The same values in knees with patellar subluxation were 31 degrees and 40 degrees, respectively. The lateral shift of the patella measured in relation to the transverse diameter was 14% with the quadriceps relaxed and 28% with muscle contraction in the normal knees. These values increased to 31% and 59%, respectively, in knees with subluxation. Values of patellar tilt and shift were significantly higher in patients with subluxation than in controls, and the differences were more evident with the quadriceps contracted. Values of patellar tilt and shift in the knees with subluxation were higher on CT images in full extension than on axial views at 30 degrees. Among the 46 knees that underwent extensor mechanism realignment (proximal or distal), the values of patellar tilt and shift returned to nearly normal on postoperative CT scans. The 35 knees with satisfactory postoperative results showed greater improvement in patellar shift (14%) when compared with the 5 knees with unsatisfactory results (4.3%).

Fulkerson and colleagues have further progressed in CT evaluation of the patellofemoral joint by obtaining images at various degrees of flexion between 0 and 30 degrees and by emphasizing the importance of accurate and standardized scanning. They recommend the use of midtransverse patellar sections and a line tangent to the posterior condyles as reference for the measurements.[38,98,99] Care should be taken to position the patient in the gantry so that normal standing alignment is reproduced and to obtain the cuts through the same point of the patella. Fulkerson and coworkers use the Merchant method to measure the sulcus angle and the congruence angle,[83] tilt of the lateral patellar facet with respect to a line tangent to the posterior condyles (patellar tilt angle), and height of the lateral condyle from the deepest point of the sulcus.[98] These authors reported the measurement of 10 normal knees and 54 symptomatic knees, including 49 suffering from patellar pain and 5 from patellar dislocation. Evaluation of the congruence angle in the normal knees revealed that the patellae were slightly lateralized in extension (average congruence angle, +2.5 degrees); by 10 degrees of flexion, however, all were centered or slightly medial. Therefore, a patella can be considered subluxated if the congruence angle remains positive beyond 10 degrees of flexion. The patellar tilt angle of control knees was always positive (open laterally) in the first 30 degrees of flexion. None of the normal knees had a patellar tilt angle of less than 8 degrees in the first 30 degrees of flexion. Therefore, a patella was considered tilted if it showed a tilt of less than 8 degrees in any position between 0 and 30 degrees of flexion.

It should be remarked that both the congruence angle and the patellar tilt angle are necessary to describe an abnormal position of the patella. An abnormal congruence angle indicates lateral displacement of the patella (or lateral subluxation), whereas an abnormal patellar tilt angle indicates that the patella is tilted. These changes may occur independently. Based on measurements in normal knees, it was established that a normal patella should be centered by 10 degrees of flexion (congruence angle, 0 degrees or less), and that the

patellar tilt angle should be open laterally at least 8 degrees in the arc of motion between 0 and 30 degrees.

According to these criteria, three categories of abnormal patellar position were defined: subluxated, tilted, and tilted and subluxated (Fig. 63-34). Knees with subluxation showed a high congruence angle (average, +23 degrees) in extension, which progressively reduced (average, +8 degrees) at 30 degrees of flexion. Knees with subluxation could be further divided into those with an associated tilt and those without. The first group had a patellar tilt near 0 degrees throughout the range of motion, which is significantly different from controls. A third group included knees with an isolated patellar tilt. In these cases, the patellar tilt angle was slightly decreased in extension (10 degrees vs. 18 degrees in controls)

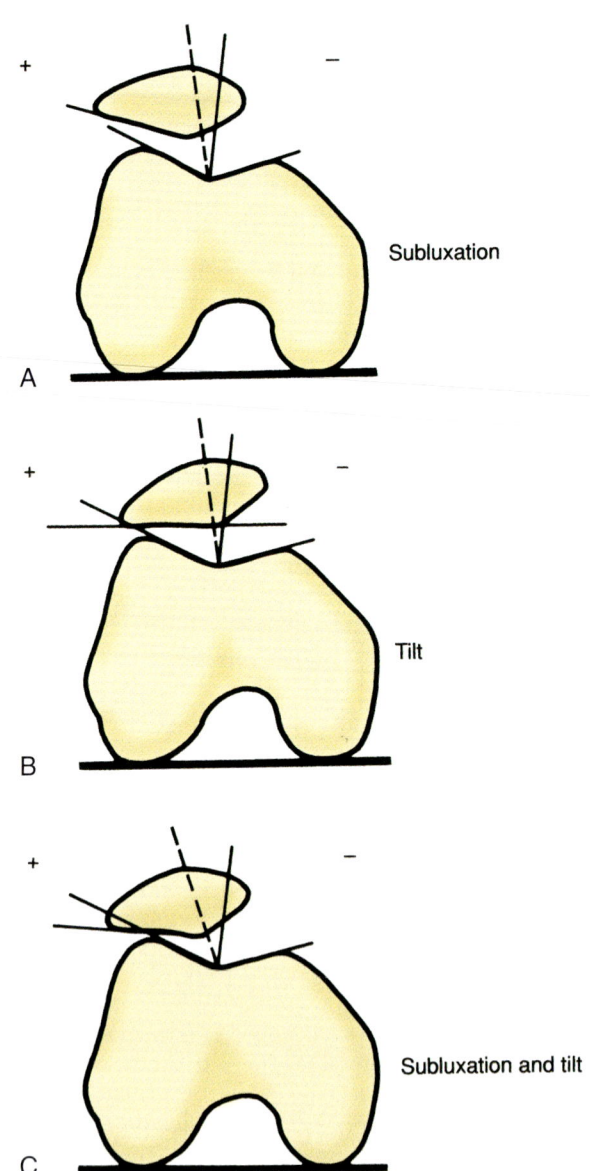

Figure 63-34. The position of the patella as visualized by computed tomography may present the following abnormalities: **A,** Subluxation with a positive congruence angle persisting beyond 10 degrees of flexion. **B,** Tilt with a lateral patellofemoral angle less than 8 degrees in the first 30 degrees of flexion. **C,** Subluxation and tilt when both abnormalities are present.

and was decreased further with flexion at 30 degrees (when it was 2 degrees vs. 16 degrees in controls).

The use of CT is recommended in patients with persistent knee symptoms and normal-appearing axial radiographic views at 30 and 45 degrees. Results from different centers seem to confirm that a normal patella is slightly displaced laterally in full extension (with a positive congruence angle), but that it reduces early in flexion, by 10 or 15 degrees of flexion. The patellar tilt angle, measured as the angle between the lateral patellar facet and either the tangent to the posterior condyles[38] or the tangent to the medial and lateral trochlear facets,[53] should be open laterally throughout the same arc of motion in normal knees. Knees affected by patellar subluxation or dislocation show excessive lateral displacement and lateral patellar tilt, which are more evident in extension but tend to reduce in flexion.

In 1978, Goutallier and Bernageau[40] described the method of radiologic measurement (with 30-degree axial views) of the distance between the apex of the tibial tuberosity and the deepest point of the trochlear groove. The tibial tuberosity–sulcus femoralis (TT-SF) distance gives a measure of the valgus vector that is imposed on the extensor mechanism at a given degree of flexion. Because the tibial tuberosity lies lateral to the sulcus femoralis, the greater the TT-SF distance, the higher the valgus vector. The TT-SF distance gives a true measure of the Q angle because it is independent of the position of the patella. It is well known that the clinical Q angle in extension may be normal in knees with recurrent subluxation or dislocation. This is due to the lateral displacement of the patella, which leads to an underestimate of the true Q angle. Goutallier and Bernageau[40] reported that the average value in a group of 16 normal knees was 13 mm (range, 7 to 17 mm). This distance was increased in most knees with patellofemoral osteoarthritis or recurrent subluxation of the patella. The introduction of CT offered the possibility of measuring the TT-SF distance in full extension by obtaining a first cut through the proximal part of the femoral sulcus and a second cut through the tibial tuberosity. Both should be perpendicular to the long axis of the bones. Dejour and colleagues[30] reported that the average TT-SF distance in normal knees in extension is 12.7 mm, whereas in knees with patellar instability, it is 19.8 mm. When 20 mm was used as the borderline value, the distance was greater than this value in 3% of control knees; the same was true in 56% of knees with patellar instability. The reproducibility of the measurement was fair, within 4 mm.

Aglietti used axial views according to Merchant and colleagues[83] and Laurin and coworkers[71] and CT in 20 and 30 degrees of flexion to evaluate patellofemoral congruence in a group of 86 knees.[4] Aglietti and associates included 20 controls, 25 knees with patellar instability, and 41 knees with patellar pain. In the patellar instability group, the height of the patella was significantly increased in comparison with controls when both the Insall-Salvati and Blackburne and Peel methods were used, whereas the group with patellar pain did not significantly differ from controls. In the Merchant view, the sulcus angle and the congruence angle of the patellar pain group were not significantly different from controls, whereas both values were significantly increased in the instability group. In the Laurin view, the lateral patellofemoral angle and the patellofemoral index were significantly increased in the instability group but not in the pain group.

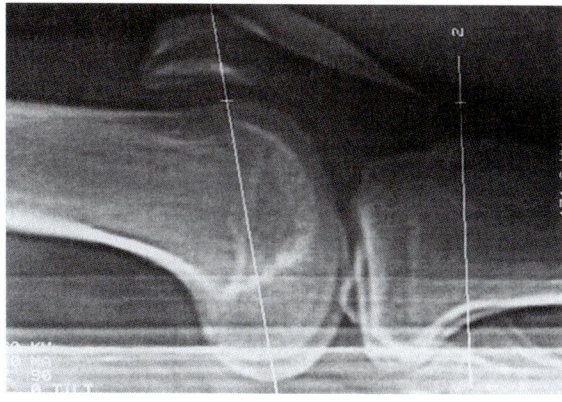

Figure 63-35. Orientation of the femoral cut passing through the middle of the patella, which corresponds to the lower third of the articular surface, and through the posterior aspect of the femoral condyles. Orientation of the tibial cut through the tibial tuberosity and at 90 degrees to the tibial axis.

In the CT scan at 30 degrees, values of the sulcus angle, congruence angle, patellar tilt angle, and sulcus depth were significantly different in the instability group, with a shallower sulcus, a subluxated and tilted patella, and reduced height of the lateral femoral condyle. The patellar pain group showed a significant difference (at the lowest level) from the control group in only congruence angle and sulcus depth. The average TT-SF distance was 8.7 mm in controls, 10.2 mm in the pain group, and 14.7 mm in the instability group. The difference between controls and the instability group was significant. Measurements of these parameters on scans with the knee at 20 degrees of flexion did not significantly differ from those at 30 degrees.

We continue to use CT in the evaluation of knees with patellofemoral disorders and have expanded its use to include four degrees of flexion: 0, 15, 30, and 45 degrees. At each angle of flexion, two cuts are made: through the tibia and through the patellofemoral joint. The tibial cut is made through the tibial tuberosity and at 90 degrees to the tibial axis (Fig. 63-35). The femoral cut is oriented to pass through the middle of the patella and the posterior femoral condyles. Because the apex of the patella is a nonarticular surface, a cut passing through the middle of the patellar height actually passes through the lower third of the articular surface. This is the part that contacts the femoral trochlea in the first 30 degrees of flexion. The femoral cut should pass posteriorly through the most posterior aspect of the femoral condyles, so that a reference line tangent to the condyles can be reliably identified. On the femoral cut, we measure the sulcus angle and the congruence angle,[83] the patellar tilt angle,[98] and the sulcus depth.[98] Furthermore, by superimposing the femoral and tibial cuts, the TT-SF distance can be measured (Fig. 63-36). Examples of CT at 0, 15, 30, and 45 degrees of flexion in a knee with recurrent dislocation and patellar pain are given in Figures 63-37 to 63-39, respectively.

Use of CT imaging for exploration of the patellofemoral relationship has led to a better understanding of the dynamics of this joint in normal and pathologic knees, and its usefulness for scientific purposes is widely accepted.[45,87] However, in knees with recurrent episodes of patellar dislocation, the degree of anatomic abnormality is such that it is promptly appreciated on a traditional axial view. If distal realignment

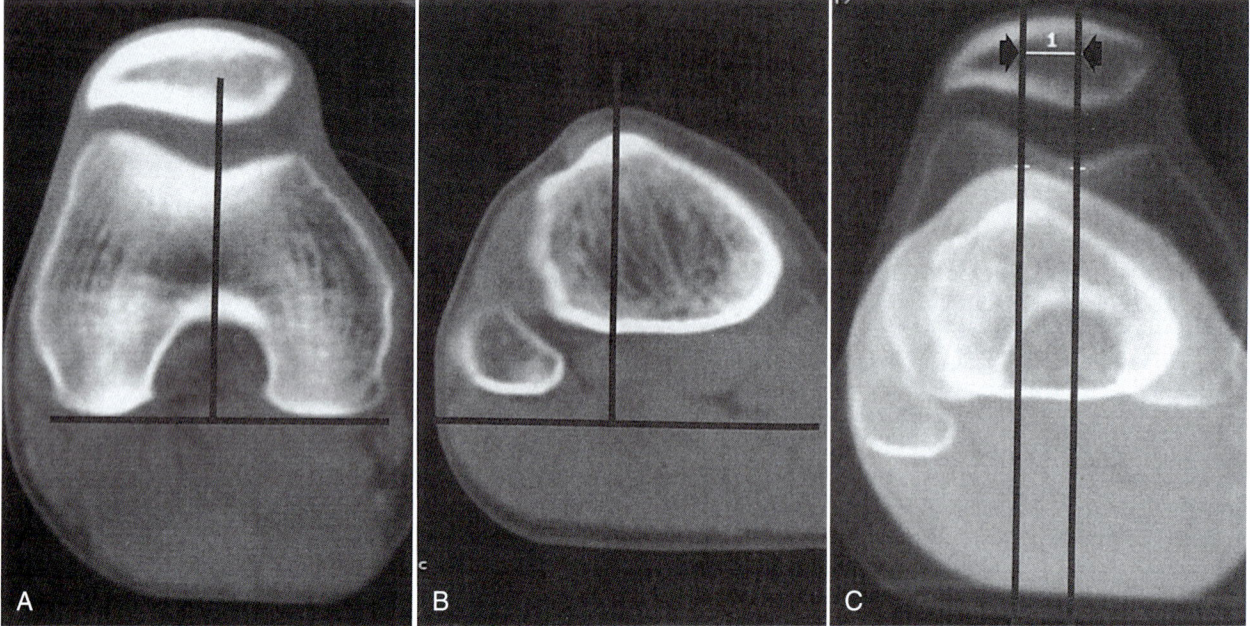

Figure 63-36. **A** through **C,** Measurement of the tibial tuberosity–sulcus femoralis (TT-SF) distance. By superimposing the femoral and tibial cuts, the distance between the deepest point of the sulcus and the tibial tuberosity can be measured. Values greater than 20 mm with the knee in extension are considered pathologic.

is being considered, knowledge of the TT-SF distance may allow more anatomic reconstruction of the joint and thus avoid overcorrection of the transposition itself in knees with a normal TT-SF distance. The usefulness of CT images is probably greatest in knees with patellofemoral disturbances and normal-appearing axial views if some abnormality can be disclosed in a more extended position.

Magnetic Resonance Imaging

MRI is a relatively new diagnostic modality for the knee.[60,86,108] It has been reported to be an accurate diagnostic tool for meniscal and cruciate ligament lesions. Because both osseous and soft tissue structures are visualized, it may be used to assess patellar tracking in the 0- to 30-degree arc of motion, as well as to evaluate lesions in patellar cartilage. MRI is also a valuable tool for detecting loose bodies in the knee after patellar dislocation.

Kujala and coworkers[66] used MRI to evaluate patellar tracking in the 0- to 30-degree arc of motion in 20 normal subjects (10 males and 10 females). Axial midpatellar images were obtained. They found that the sulcus angle became progressively sharper from full extension to 30 degrees of flexion and decreased 13 degrees on average. The lateral patellofemoral angle[71] increased an average of 6 ± 5 degrees during flexion, and lateral patellar displacement[70] decreased an average of 4 ± 3 mm with flexion. The congruence angle[83] shifted 31 degrees (±13 degrees) medially during flexion. In extension, the congruence angle was positive (open laterally) in all knees except in one male. At 30 degrees of flexion, the congruence angle was negative (open medially) in all knees except in one male and one female, where it was zero. Citing these data, Kujala and colleagues concluded that a normal knee (whether male or female) should be congruent (congruence angle, 0 degrees or negative) by 30 degrees of flexion (but not necessarily in a lesser degree of flexion). Females

were found to have significantly more laterally displaced patellae at 10 and 20 degrees of flexion, but the other differences were not significant.

Kujala and associates[67] compared the measurements obtained from normal knees and knees affected by recurrent patellar dislocation. For this study, 10 normal women and 11 women with recurrent subluxation were selected. Midpatellar sagittal and axial images were used to measure patellar length, patellar tendon length, Insall-Salvati ratio (T/P), sulcus angle, congruence angle, lateral patellofemoral angle, lateral patellar displacement, and depth of the femoral sulcus. Knees with recurrent patellar dislocation showed higher values for sulcus angle, lateral patellar displacement, and congruence angle, and lower values for the lateral patellofemoral angle, which indicates that dislocating patellae were more lateralized and were tilted laterally. The differences were more evident in extension and were gradually reduced when proceeding toward flexion. Statistical analysis showed that the two groups were most clearly differentiated by the sulcus angle at 10 degrees and by the lateral patellofemoral angle at 0 degrees. Kujala and colleagues concluded that in patients with recurrent dislocation, tilt and lateralization of the patella are more evident in early flexion. All control patellae were congruent at 30 degrees, but the same was true for most (77%) of the dislocating patellae. Therefore, differences between normal and dislocating patellae are most evident at the beginning of flexion (0 to 10 degrees).

MRI has been used to investigate knees with acute patellar dislocation.[94] This has led to a better understanding of the pathoanatomy of this condition. A series of 23 knees were examined with x-ray and MRI, followed by arthroscopy (19 knees) and open exploration of medial soft tissues (16 knees). Clinically, 83% of the knees exhibited moderate to large effusion, and 70% had tenderness over the posteromedial soft tissues and the adductor tubercle (Bassett's sign). Radiographs

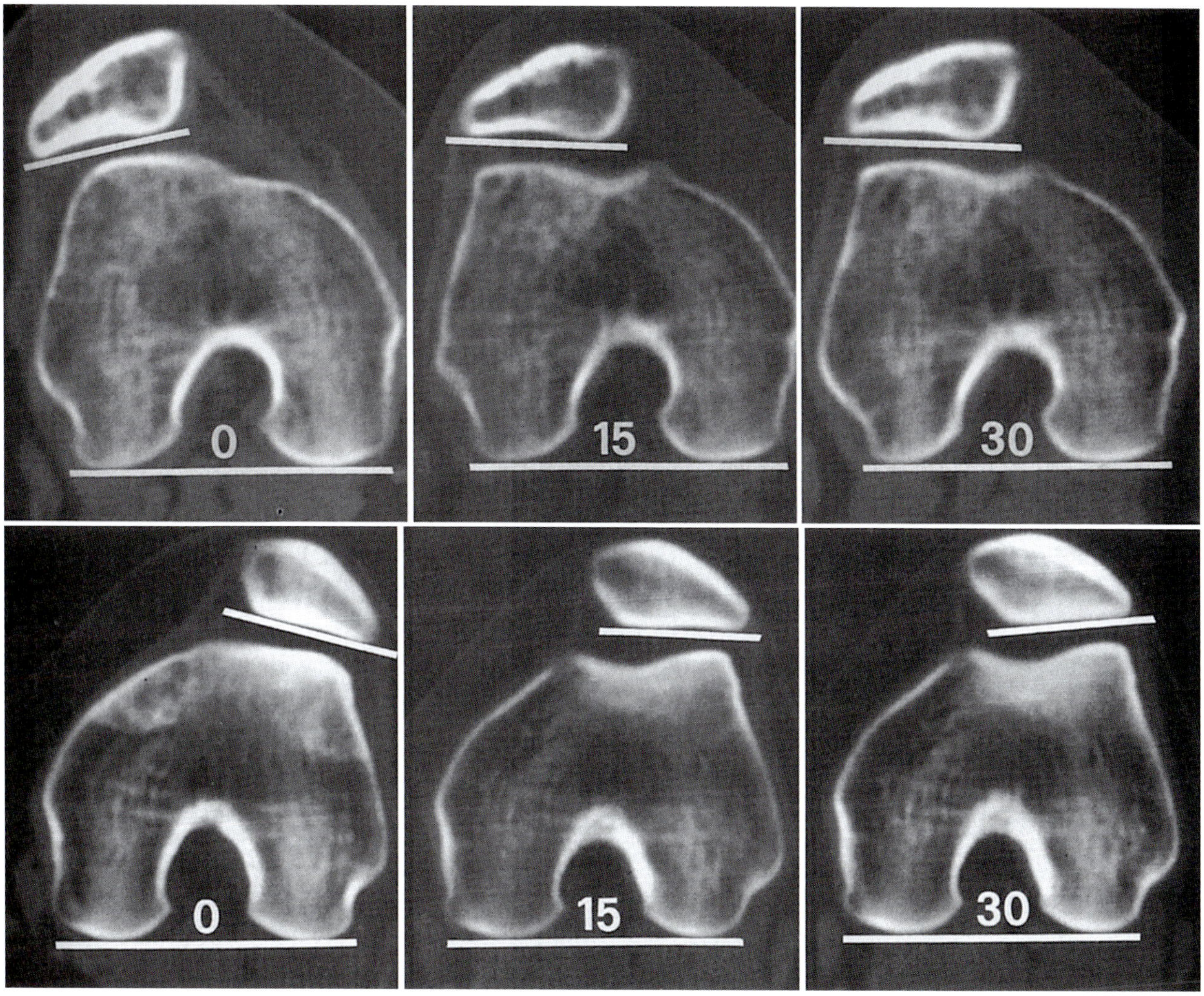

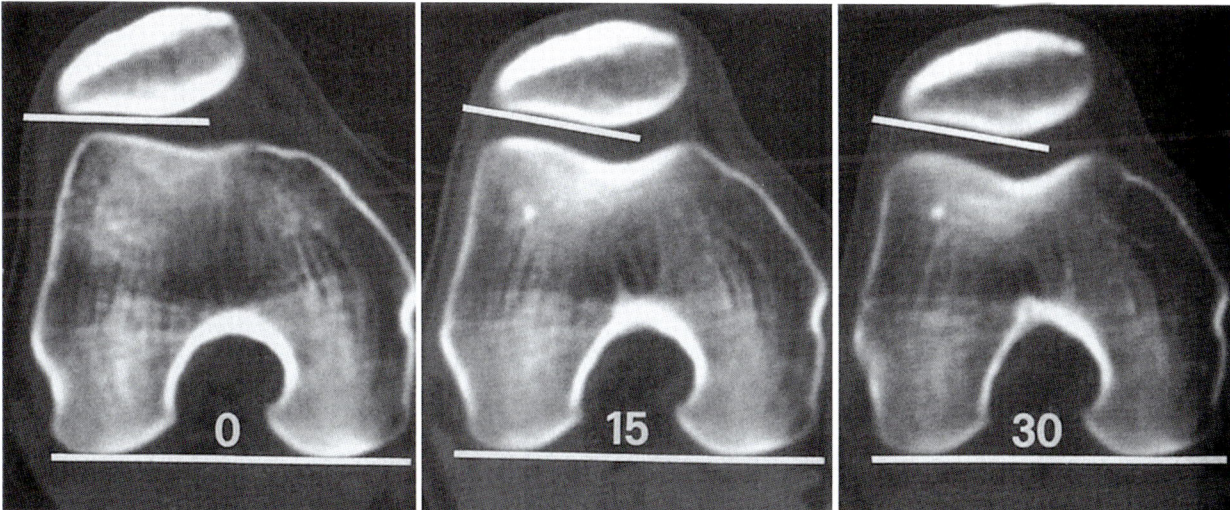

Figure 63-37. Computed tomography images at 0, 15, and 30 degrees of flexion in two knees affected by recurrent dislocation of the patella. Proceeding from extension to flexion, the congruence angle, the sulcus angle, and the patellar tilt angle are reduced, mainly between 0 and 15 degrees of flexion.

Figure 63-38. Computed tomography images of a knee affected by patellar pain. The patella is tilted laterally in extension, but almost normal congruence is restored by 15 degrees of flexion.

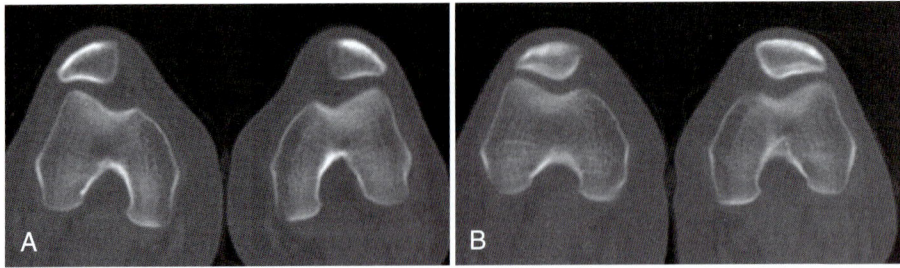

Figure 63-39. **A,** Computed tomography (CT) of patella at 30 degrees demonstrates that the patellae are subluxated laterally. **B,** CT of patella at 40 degrees demonstrates that the same patellae are tracking centrally in the sulcus.

revealed osteochondral fracture of the patella in 21% of cases and fracture of the lateral femoral condyle in 5%. MRI showed moderate to large effusion in all knees. A tear of the femoral insertion of the medial patellofemoral ligament (at the adductor tubercle) was present in 87% (20 knees). Two knees had a significant sprain of the medial patellofemoral ligament without detachment. One knee had a detachment of the medial retinaculum from the margin of the patella. Variable amounts of retraction of the VMO and increased signal were present in 78%. Bony injuries were noted in 87% of lateral femoral condyles near the sulcus terminalis and in 30% of patellae medially.

Nineteen knees with gross lateral instability underwent arthroscopy and evaluation under anesthesia. Medial soft tissue tears were not visualized by arthroscopy. Sixteen knees underwent open exploration. The fascia was found to be intact in all cases. After elevation of the vastus medialis, hemorrhage was common in the area of the adductor tubercle. A tear of the femoral insertion of the medial patellofemoral ligament was present in 15 of 16 knees. In some cases, this was a true avulsion. Repair of the torn medial patellofemoral ligament restored stability to the patella. None of the 12 patients with follow-up longer than 2 years experienced recurrent dislocation, although 4 had episodes of possible subluxation. It appears that detachment of the medial patellofemoral ligament from its insertion into the adductor tubercle is the most frequent lesion in acute dislocation of the patella. This is consistent with the biomechanical work of Conlan and colleagues,[24] who showed that the medial patellofemoral ligament was the primary restraint to lateral patellar dislocation and provided 53% of the total restraining force, followed by the patellomeniscal ligament, which contributed 22%. Detachment of the VMO from the adductor tubercle was also evident from MRI and surgical findings.

A predictable pattern of soft tissue injury and bony contusions can be seen in MRI studies of patients with prior dislocation of the patella. Soft tissue findings include joint effusion, disruption of the MPFL, injury to the medial retinaculum, and disruption of the VMO attachment. The typical osteochondral pattern of injury occurs when the medial facet of the patella impacts the lateral femoral condyle. This results in osteochondral fracture or contusion of the medial patellar facet and the lateral femoral condyle. Elias and associates[33,34] compared MRIs of 81 knees with previous lateral patellar dislocation versus 100 knees with no history of dislocation. In knees with prior lateral dislocation, investigators found contusions on the lateral femoral condyle in 80% and on the medial patella in 61%. They concluded that the specific finding of a concave impaction deformity in the inferomedial

aspect of the patella has 44% sensitivity but 100% specificity for lateral patellar dislocation. Furthermore, they found injury to the MPFL in only 49% of patellae in which the MPFL was visualized, and edema surrounding the VMO attachment in only 45% of knees with lateral patellar dislocation. The authors state that perhaps transverse images, as were used in this study, are not optimal for imaging these oblique structures, and that transverse oblique images may be of higher yield for detecting injury to these structures. This may account for their low rate of medial soft tissue injury compared with other studies.[24,94] It is important to note that the MPFL cannot always be visualized on MRI studies,[95] and in this study, it was visualized in only 87% of patients with dislocation and 80% of control subjects. The authors suggest that increased edema surrounding this structure after patellar dislocation may lead to higher rates of visualization in patients with prior dislocation compared with controls.

Sanders and colleagues[95] compared MRI findings in 14 knees with known dislocation versus surgical findings in these same knees. MPFL injury was detected in all 14 knees on MRI, and this was confirmed at the time of surgical exploration. MRI detected complete disruption of the MPFL in 57% and wavy or partial disruption in 43%. At the time of surgery, the MPFL was found to be completely disrupted in 50% of cases and partially disrupted in the other 50%. The authors concluded that the MPFL was injured in 100% of cases, and that MRI was 85% sensitive and 70% accurate in diagnosing MPFL injury. They also compared VMO findings in these 14 knees versus 100 control MRIs of knees that had no clinical or radiographic evidence of dislocation. The VMO was found to be elevated off the medial femoral condyle in 85% of injured knees, and edema was noted within the VMO tendon and muscle in 93% of all dislocators. No evidence of edema in the VMO was found in any of the 100 control knees. Furthermore, a significant difference was noted between the extent of elevation of the VMO in dislocators and in the 100 control knees. Average elevation of the VMO in dislocators was 1.7 cm compared with 0.18 cm in control knees.

MRI is frequently used to investigate patellar cartilage. Yulish and colleagues[120] compared the results of 23 MRI examinations with findings at arthroscopy: 3 patients were asymptomatic volunteers and 20 had patellar symptoms. Normal patellar cartilage appears uniformly smooth on axial and sagittal MRI views, with a signal intensity that is intermediate between that of cortical and cancellous bone. MRI alterations in patellar cartilage were classified as follows:

Stage 1: areas of swelling with decreased signal intensity
Stage 2: irregularity of the articular surface with focal thinning

Stage 3: absence of cartilage with exposure of subchondral bone or synovial fluid extending through the ulcer to subchondral bone

MRI correctly predicted arthroscopic findings in 20 of 22 knees (91%). It missed a knee with softening of the patella and diagnosed a chondral fracture that was not confirmed by arthroscopy. The presence of joint fluid visible on T2-weighted images was useful in detecting the presence of cartilage ulcers, through which fluid leaked to subchondral bone.

An experimental study[47] has compared the accuracy of CT-arthrography and MRI in detecting patellar cartilage lesions. Drill holes ranging from 0.8 to 5 mm in diameter and from 1 to 2 mm in depth were produced in cadaver knees. Double-contrast CT-arthrography easily detected 3- and 5-mm holes, but 50% of 1.5- and 2-mm lesions were missed. The 0.8-mm holes were not recognized at all. On the contrary, MRI detected the smallest 0.8-mm lesions because they were precisely delineated by intra-articular fluid, which appears bright on T2-weighted images.

In a clinical study, 54 knees were examined by MRI, and evidence of a cartilage lesion was found in 44 cases. At arthroscopy, however, the corresponding lesion was found in only 34 knees (77%), whereas no chondral lesion or softening was noted in the remaining 10 knees. When compared with arthroscopy, MRI had 81.5% accuracy, 100% sensitivity, and 50% specificity. As far as staging of the lesion, it was correctly predicted by MRI in 76% of cases, overrated in 5.8%, and underrated in 17.6%. Using these data, Handelberg and colleagues[47] proposed an MRI classification of chondral lesions. It is recognized that MRI yields a discrete incidence of false-positive results, possibly because of detection of early lesions in deep layers of cartilage that are not visualized at arthroscopy. They are evident as linear, dark areas in the gray signal of cartilage. Additional studies are needed to confirm whether these findings represent early lesions or a variation of normal anatomy.

Stage I lesions, described as softening at arthroscopy, are usually visible as round areas of low signal intensity on "proton density" and T2-weighted images.

Stage II lesions correspond to fissures that appear as zones of low signal surrounding the high signal of fluid leaking into the cleft.

Stage III lesions correspond to superficial or deep defects that appear as bright images because of the synovial fluid that fills them.

Stage IV lesions involve thinning and irregularity of cartilage, as found in degenerative arthritis.

In conclusion, we believe that MRI is an attractive diagnostic modality for the patellofemoral joint. It does not involve the use of ionizing radiation or contrast material and allows evaluation of both patellar tracking and cartilage lesions.

MRI is most useful in predicting the location and extent of articular cartilage disease, which is an important factor in determination of which surgical intervention is appropriate. Furthermore, MRI can be used to identify patellar congruence, patellar tilt, patellar morphology, trochlear morphology, and soft tissue injury such as MPFL and VMO injury. Osteochondral fractures of the medial facet of the patella and the lateral femoral condyle are commonly detected by MRI. Use of MRI in the treatment of patellar instability is increasing.

Our approach to imaging of patellofemoral instability begins with standing anteroposterior and lateral views, as well as a Merchant view of the patella. We evaluate the knee joint for coronal alignment and rotational alignment. Attention is paid to identifying patella alta and any trochlear or patellar dysplasia that would predispose to patellar instability. On the axial view of the patellofemoral joint, we pay particular attention to the congruence and sulcus angles. The lateral patellofemoral angle is assessed for evidence of lateral patellar tilt. CT scan may be used to better evaluate rotational abnormalities and the anatomy of the patellofemoral joint. MRI is used when cartilage injury or loose body is suspected, and to rule out other soft tissue and ligamentous injuries.

CLASSIFICATION OF PATELLAR SUBLUXATION AND DISLOCATION

Patellar subluxation and patellar dislocation can be grouped together as patellar instability. The difference is one of degree and not of nature. Subluxation is an alteration in the normal tracking of the patella, but with the patella still within the femoral sulcus. Dislocation means that the patella has been completely displaced out of the sulcus. Therefore, unless the patient has noted the patella lying on the lateral aspect of the knee, it appears that it may be impossible to know whether the patella was subluxated or dislocated during the single episode of instability. Furthermore, the patella may show lateralized tracking without episodes of instability (chronic subluxation of the patella).

Many classifications of patellofemoral disorders are known, all of which include several types of patellofemoral instability. These classification systems include the presence or absence of trauma, malalignment, and articular cartilage damage (Boxes 63-1 and 63-2). When classifying patellofemoral instability, we believe that it is important to consider three main factors: chronicity, presence or absence of malalignment, and the condition of the articular cartilage.[29] In doing so, we can define patellar instability as acute (generally traumatic) or recurrent (chronic). This classification system helps guide treatment tailored to the individual patient, as seen in Table 63-2.

Box 63-1   Insall's Classification of Patellofemoral Disorders

Presence of Cartilage Damage
Chondromalacia
Osteoarthritis
Osteochondral fractures
Osteochondritis dissecans

Variable Cartilage Damage
Malalignment syndromes
Synovial plicae

Usually Normal Cartilage
Peripatellar causes: bursitis, tendinitis
Overuse syndromes
Reflex sympathetic dystrophy
Patellar abnormalities

Data from Insall JN: Disorders of the patella. In Insall JN (ed): Surgery of the knee, New York, 1984, Churchill Livingstone, p 191.

Box 63-2 Merchant's Classification of Patellofemoral Disorders

I. Trauma (conditions caused by trauma in an otherwise normal knee)
  A. Acute trauma
    1. Contusion
    2. Fracture
      a. Patella
      b. Femoral trochlea
      c. Proximal tibial epiphysis (tubercle)
    3. Dislocation (rare in a normal knee)
    4. Rupture
      a. Quadriceps tendon
      b. Patellar tendon
  B. Repetitive trauma (overuse syndromes)
    1. Patellar tendinitis ("jumper's knee")
    2. Quadriceps tendinitis
    3. Peripatellar tendinitis (e.g., anterior knee pain in an adolescent as a result of hamstring contracture)
    4. Prepatellar bursitis ("housemaid's knee")
    5. Apophysitis
      a. Osgood-Schlatter disease
      b. Sinding-Larsen-Johansson disease
  C. Late effects of trauma
    1. Post-traumatic chondromalacia patellae
    2. Post-traumatic patellofemoral arthritis
    3. Anterior fat pad syndrome (post-traumatic fibrosis)
    4. Reflex sympathetic dystrophy of the patella
    5. Patellar osseous dystrophy
    6. Acquired patella infera
    7. Acquired quadriceps fibrosis
II. Patellofemoral dysplasia
  A. Lateral patellar compression syndrome
    1. Secondary chondromalacia patellae
    2. Secondary patellofemoral arthritis
  B. Chronic subluxation of the patella
    1. Secondary chondromalacia patellae
    2. Secondary patellofemoral arthritis
  C. Recurrent dislocation of the patella
    1. Associated fractures
      a. Osteochondral (intra-articular)
      b. Avulsion (extra-articular)
    2. Secondary chondromalacia patellae
    3. Secondary patellofemoral arthritis
  D. Chronic dislocation of the patella
    1. Congenital
    2. Acquired
III. Idiopathic chondromalacia patellae
IV. Osteochondritis dissecans
  A. Patella
  B. Femoral trochlea
V. Synovial plicae (anatomic variant made symptomatic by acute or repetitive trauma)
  A. Medial patellar ("shelf")
  B. Suprapatellar
  C. Lateral patellar

From Merchant AC: Classification of patellofemoral disorders. Arthroscopy 4:235, 1988.[82]

Table 63-2 Classification of Patellofemoral Diagnosis and Suggested Surgical Treatment

Diagnosis	Surgical Treatment
Lateral patellar compression syndrome	Lateral release
Patellar subluxation	Lateral release Proximal realignment Proximal and distal realignment
Acute patellar dislocation	Repair medial retinaculum and lateral release Proximal realignment
Recurrent patellar dislocation	Proximal realignment Proximal and distal realignment
Malalignment with severe chondromalacia	Fulkerson anteromedialization Maquet osteotomy Patellectomy

With kind permission of Springer Science+Business Media. From Scuderi GR: The patella, New York, 1995, Springer-Verlag, p 223 (Table 11.1).

Characteristics of Acute Patellar Dislocation

The diagnosis of acute dislocation of the patella is applied to knees seen after the first episode of dislocation. It often occurs after a traumatic event. The patient usually seeks treatment at the emergency department and reports that during a twisting movement of the knee, a snap was felt, the knee gave way, and the patient fell down onto the ground. The patient may have been able to observe the patella lying on the lateral side of the knee. At this time, the knee is straightened and the patella relocated in the sulcus. Swelling occurs rapidly. Therefore, it is unusual to observe the patella still in the dislocated position in the emergency department.

If the patient has observed abnormal lateral displacement of the patella, the diagnosis is straightforward. Otherwise, it can be difficult.[116] The physician is faced with a swollen and tender knee and a nonspecific history of giving way.[115] Aspiration of the joint demonstrates hemarthrosis, and fat droplets may be present if an associated osteochondral fracture has occurred. Careful inquiry about the mechanism of injury often reveals that the patient had the foot fixed on the ground, whereas the femur was internally rotated relative to the tibia and the quadriceps was contacted, as in the act of changing direction while running. In this position, the Q angle is increased, and contraction of the quadriceps pulls the patella laterally. This mechanism has also been described in baseball pitchers.[44] More rarely, a direct blow to the medial side of the knee may cause patellar dislocation in a knee with underlying malalignment.

Acute patellar dislocation rarely occurs in the absence of malalignment or dysplasia.[81] In addition, disruption of medial soft tissue restraints, such as the MPFL, is now thought to be almost obligatory.[34,94,95] Anatomic and radiologic studies have helped to better define the anatomic and biomechanical characteristics of this ligament. We now understand that the MPFL provides more than 50% of static restraint to lateral stability of the patella. Concomitant osteochondral injury is common and has a predictable pattern on the medial facet of the patella and the lateral femoral condyle[24,33,92] (Fig. 63-40).

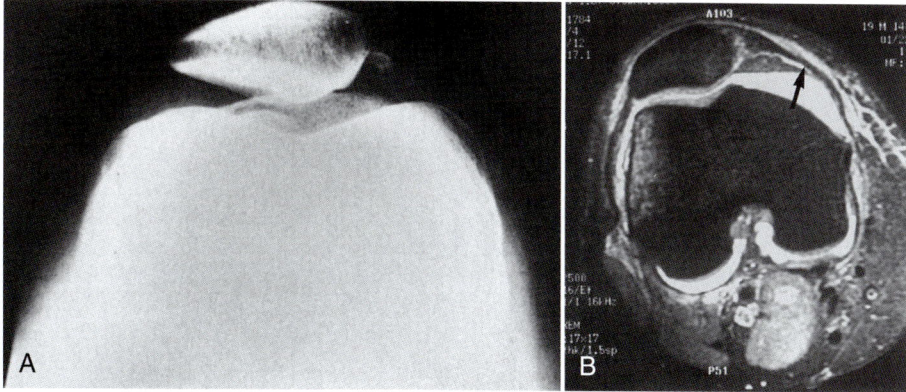

Figure 63-40. Lateral patellar dislocation. **A,** A tangential view of the patella demonstrates an osseous fragment at the medial margin of the patella, consistent with previous lateral patellar dislocation. **B,** An axial fat-suppressed magnetic resonance image shows a partial tear of the medial patellar retinaculum manifested as increased signal on either side of it *(arrow).* Signal is increased in the medial aspect of the patella and at the lateral margin of the lateral femoral condyle, indicative of bone contusions, and a large joint effusion is apparent. This constellation of findings is characteristic of a recent lateral patellar dislocation.

Conlan and colleagues[24] performed an anatomic study that helped to define the contribution of medial soft tissue structures to lateral restraint of the patella. A lateral displacing force was placed on the patella, and medial structures were sectioned. It was determined that the MPFL is responsible for 53% of static restraint against lateral translation of the patella. In a similar study, Hautamaa and coworkers[48] reported consistent results. After isolated section of the MPFL, they noted that the force required to displace the patella laterally was reduced by 50%.

Panagiotopoulos and associates[92] confirmed the findings of Conlan et al[24] and Hautamaa[48] in their cadaveric study. They also found that the MPFL contributes at least 50% of the static medial stability of the patella. Panagiotopoulos emphasized the importance of the finding of "meshing" of the MPFL to the undersurface of the VMO. Its femoral attachment is just anterior to the medial epicondyle, and distally its fibers blend with the undersurface of the VMO as it reaches the superior medial pole of the patella. Because of this meshing, they suggest that the MPFL shortens with contraction of the VMO, thus contributing more than 50% of the stability of the patellofemoral joint. The MPFL appears to work in concert with the dynamic restraint of the VMO in centralizing and stabilizing the patella.[48,92] It is now broadly accepted that the VMO is the primary dynamic restraint and the MPFL is the primary static restraint to lateral displacement of the patella.

Physical Examination of Acute Patellar Dislocation

If the knee is grossly swollen, physical examination is best performed after aspiration of the joint. Tenderness is easily evoked by palpation of the medial retinaculum and the medial femoral epicondyle. Attempts to displace the patella laterally are prevented by apprehension. Testing for ligamentous stability is rendered more difficult by muscle contracture, but with some patience one should be able to confirm the presence of an intact anterior cruciate ligament with a gentle Lachman test.

The differential diagnosis should include anterior cruciate ligament injury and rupture of the quadriceps or patellar tendon. The latter diagnosis can be excluded by asking the patient to perform a straight-leg raise. If the patient is unable to do this exercise and a defect that is proximal or distal to the patella is appreciated, the diagnosis is confirmed.

If an acute patellar dislocation is suspected, it is informative to examine the contralateral knee. Evidence of malalignment or maltracking of the patella may enhance the correct diagnosis.

Chronic Subluxations and Dislocations

Chronic dislocations or subluxations also almost always occur in the setting of dysplasia or misalignment or both. The combined contribution of increased Q angle, valgus alignment of the knee, increased femoral anteversion, and tibial external rotation leads to a lateral force vector on the patella. This results in chronic patellar subluxation and dislocation. The VMO is unable to function at its optimal angle and produces a dynamic stabilizing effect on the patellofemoral joint. History, physical examination, and imaging studies are necessary to determine the relative contributions of these factors to realign the vector of the VMO in a more appropriate direction, and to help stabilize the joint throughout a range of motion. Proximal and distal realignments can and oftentimes should be combined to achieve appropriate alignment and dynamic stability of the patellofemoral articulation.

Finally, the condition of the articular cartilage is important in that a distal realignment can be added to a proximal realignment in an attempt to unload the affected area of cartilage. However, a lesion in the proximal pole does not lend itself well to unloading because the zone of contact becomes more and more proximal as the knee flexes. Other cartilage restorative and reparative procedures have been described in the recent literature with some reports of promising results; however, in the presence of misalignment and improper mechanics, these procedures are unlikely to result in sustainable long-term results.

Treatments

Nonoperative Treatment

Conservative treatment should be attempted in knees with acute and recurrent patellar instability. It is based on strengthening of the quadriceps and VMO and stretching of the tight lateral structures, as previously described. The frequency of the episodes of instability may be reduced so that surgery is no longer necessary. If disabling symptoms persist, surgical treatment is indicated. Because of the high rate of recurrence and dissatisfaction, many are advocates for early surgical intervention.[16] Unfortunately, the results in the literature are mixed, and it is still unclear whether nonoperative treatment or early surgical intervention will lead to better long-term outcomes and more satisfied patients.

Several authors have attempted to define the prognosis after conservative treatment of acute patellar dislocation (Table 63-3). Cofield and Bryan[23] reported a discouraging experience in which 52% of their 50 cases were rated as failures. In light of their experience, they recommend selective immediate repair in patients with anatomic variants that would contribute to recurrence in high-level athletes and in knees with displaced intra-articular fractures. Larsen and Lauridsen[68] reviewed 79 acute patellar dislocations. A relevant primary trauma was reported in 41 cases (52%), whereas in 38 (48%), the trauma had been minor or absent. Patella alta and increased passive patellar mobility were more frequent in patients with atraumatic dislocations. Dislocation was more frequently atraumatic in females (57%) than in males (32%). Younger patients had a higher incidence of predisposing factors, which were present in 84% of patients younger than 14 years, in 69% between 15 and 19 years, and in 41% between 20 and 29 years. In agreement with this

finding, redislocation was more likely in younger patients (<20 years of age).

Mäenpää and Lehto[73] reviewed a series of 100 acute patellar dislocations with long-term follow-up (average, 13 years; range, 6 to 26 years). Patients were treated initially with a cast (60 knees), a splint (17 knees), or a bandage (23 knees), according to the physician's preference. At follow-up, 13% had restricted extension, 21% had restricted flexion, 61% had retropatellar crepitation, and the apprehension test yielded positive results in 52%. Redislocation had occurred in 44% of knees. The redislocation rate per follow-up year was 0.29 in the patellar bandage group, 0.12 in the cast group, and 0.08 in the splint group. Beyond the 44% incidence of recurrent dislocation, a 19% incidence of patellofemoral pain or subluxation was reported. Only 37% of patients had no complaints at the time of follow-up. This series suggests that application of a splint may be preferable to both cast and bandage. However, the duration of immobilization was different in each of the three groups. Therefore, redislocation rates are influenced by both type and length of immobilization. Furthermore, immobilization was found to result in a high rate of stiffness in this series.

Garth and coworkers[39] reported the results of 39 knees with acute patellar dislocation that were treated functionally. Treatment included immediate straight-leg–raising exercises followed by the application of a laterally padded knee sleeve and immediate mobilization. Average follow-up was 46 months (range, 24 to 71 months). Six patients (15%) experienced recurrent instability. Good or excellent results were achieved in 67% of knees subjectively and in 69% objectively. This means that results after functional treatment of acute patellar dislocation were not satisfactory in about a third of the knees. These results are similar to those achieved

Table 63-3 Prognosis After Conservative Treatment of Acute Patellar Dislocation

Author	Year	No. of Knees	Treatment	Avg. Follow-Up, Mo	Redislocation, %	Remarks
Cofield & Bryan[23]	1977	50	Conservative	44	High redislocation rate	52% of knees were considered unsatisfactory; 27% required further surgery
McManus et al[17]	1979	26	Cast for 6 weeks	31	19	Dislocations in children; 42% complained of instability without dislocation; 38% were asymptomatic
Larsen & Lauridsen[68]	1982	79	Cast or bandage	71	NA	Unable to define factors that may predispose to redislocation except age younger than 20 years
Hawkins et al[49]	1986	20	Arthroscopy (9), cast (11)	40	15	All patients who experienced redislocation had obvious lower limb malalignment; some degree of pain was present in 75% of cases
Cash & Hughston[19]	1988	74	Cast	96	36	Recurrence rate is higher in presence of signs of patellofemoral dysplasia of the opposite knee (43%) than when these are absent (20%); higher redislocation rate in younger patients
Garth et al[39]	1996	39	Functional padded sleeve	46	20	One third of cases remain unsatisfactory according to subjective and objective criteria
Mäenpää & Lehto[73]	1997	100	Cast (60), splint (17), bandage (23)	156	44	44% redislocation, 19% patellofemoral pain or subluxation; only 37% without complaints

NA, Not available.

with cast immobilization. However, functional treatment avoids the deleterious effects of immobilization and decreases the convalescence time.

A prospective nonrandomized study compared 40 patients with acute first-time patellar dislocation who were treated with nonoperative or acute operative repair of injured medial structures.[104] The nonoperative group was immobilized from 0 to 30 for 3 weeks, then from 0 to 90 until week 6, at which point full range of motion was permitted and a guided muscle strengthening program was initiated. The surgical group was treated with surgical stabilization at an average of 7 days after injury. Fourteen patients were treated with reefing of the medial soft tissues, and four patients were treated with the Roux-Goldthwait procedure, in which the lateral aspect of the patellar tendon was sutured to the medial aspect of the tibia. The surgical group had no redislocations and only two (12%) painful subluxations at 7 years' follow-up. The nonoperative group had six (29%) redislocations and four painful subluxations. Thus the nonoperative group had 10 (48%) patients with symptomatic instability.

A high rate of recurrent instability is clearly seen with nonoperative treatment; however, most of the authors would agree that a trial of nonoperative treatment should be attempted. A summary of the studies that have looked at nonoperative treatment of acute patellar dislocation is provided in Table 63-3.

Operative Treatment

Lateral Release and Proximal Realignment

Lateral Retinacular Release. Although the results of isolated lateral retinacular release for patellar instability have been notoriously poor, this procedure was popular for many years and is now falling out of favor. Results in knees affected by recurrent patellar subluxation and dislocation are reported in Table 63-4. The reported percentage of satisfactory results varies between 30% and 100%. However, rating systems used were not uniformly stringent. We think that any patient with persistent symptoms of instability cannot be included among satisfactory results. Dandy and Griffiths[28] reported on 41 knees that underwent lateral release for recurrent dislocation. Average follow-up was 4 years. Ninety percent of knees were classified as satisfactory according to the rating system of Crosby and Insall.[25] However, only 44% of the patellae were stable, 24% were occasionally insecure, and 32% underwent at least one redislocation.

Using an average follow-up of 8 years, Dandy and Desai[27] reviewed 33 knees in which the previous follow-up had been 4 years.[28] The percentage of satisfactory results decreased from 90% at 4 years to 72% at 8 years. Thirty-two percent of the patellae had dislocated at least once before the 4-year follow-up. Twenty-one percent (seven knees) continued to dislocate and underwent tibial tubercle transposition.

Table 63-4 Results of Lateral Retinacular Release for Recurrent Patellar Subluxation and Dislocation

Author	Year	No. of Knees	Avg. Follow-Up, Mo	Type of Release	Avg. % Satisfactory Result	Remarks
Metcalf[84]	1982	14	48	Arthroscopic	100	No redislocations
Chen & Ramanathan[65]	1984	39	72	Closed	86	Includes 15 acute dislocations, 9 recurrent subluxations, and 15 recurrent dislocations, with similar success rates in the 3 groups
Simpson & Barrett[105]	1984	32	15	Arthroscopic	86	Worse results with age <30 years, incomplete release, quadriceps weakness, and generalized laxity
Ogilvie-Harris & Jackson[90]	1984	46	60	Arthroscopic	44	Results correlate closely with degree of chondromalacia: 100% satisfactory with grade I chondromalacia but only 25% with grade III
Schonholtz et al[97]	1987	15	48	Closed	67	Better results than in pain syndromes
Betz et al[34]	1987	31	48	Closed	74	Knees with subluxation had a higher recurrence rate (64%) than those with dislocation (14%); one patient experienced medial subluxation
Sherman et al[103]	1987	45	28	Arthroscopic	75	One recurrence among 15 dislocations (6%); poor results more frequent in dislocators (39%) than in subluxers (15%)
Christensen et al[21]	1988	30	54	Open	30	Deterioration of satisfactory results from the 1-year (73%) to the 4-year (30%) follow-up
Dandy & Griffiths[28]	1989	41	48	Arthroscopic	90	44% of patellae were stable; 24% were occasionally insecure, and 32% had had at least one redislocation; worse results in hyperlaxity and knees with dislocation in flexion
Aglietti et al[5]	1989	20	66	Arthroscopic	65	35% experienced recurrent instability; worse results in females and knees with more than five preoperative dislocations
Dandy & Desai[27]	1994	33	96	Arthroscopic	72	

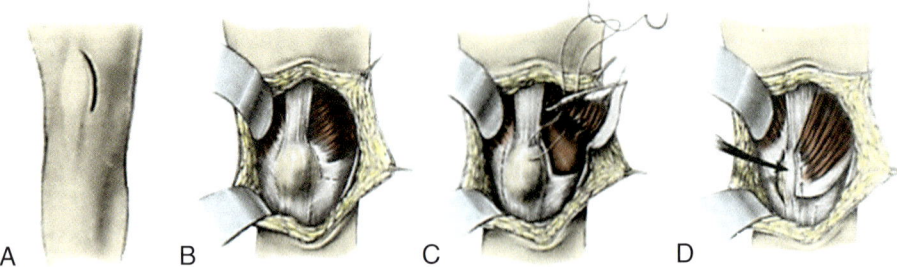

Figure 63-41. Technique of quadricepsplasty described by Madigan. **A,** Medial longitudinal incision. **B,** Interrupted line indicating capsular incision to mobilize vastus medialis obliquus. **C,** Interrupted line indicating lateral retinacular relaxing incision. **D,** Insertion of vastus medialis obliquus is transferred laterally and distally. (From Madigan R, Wissinger HA, Donaldson WF: Preliminary experience with a method of quadricepsplasty in recurrent subluxation of the patella. J Bone Joint Surg Am 57:602, 1975.)

Subluxation in extension and generalized ligamentous laxity correlated with an increased failure rate. The authors concluded that with these conditions, lateral release does not correct recurrent dislocation.

Aglietti and associates reported that their experience with lateral retinacular release for recurrent dislocation of the patella was not completely satisfactory either. They reviewed 21 knees.[2] The group included 12 females and 9 males whose age averaged 21 years (range, 12 to 48 years). The operation was performed with the arthroscopic technique described by Metcalf[84] in 18 cases, and with an open technique in 3 knees; 20 patients (95%) were reviewed with an average follow-up of 66 months (range, 22 to 101 months). Most patients (90%) had no pain or swelling at follow-up, but one knee (5%) showed instability during sports activity, and six knees (29%) during daily living activities. Therefore, only 66% of results could be considered satisfactory. On the axial view at 45 degrees of flexion,[83] the congruence angle was 19 degrees preoperatively and decreased to 3 degrees at follow-up, but it was still abnormal in 37% of cases. When satisfactory and unsatisfactory results were compared to identify predictive factors, investigators found that the prognosis was worse in females ($P = .05$) and in knees with more than five preoperative dislocations ($P = .05$). The persistence of lateral patellar tracking at follow-up was evaluated clinically ($P = .02$), and a deficit on the one-leg hop test for a distance greater than 15% ($P = .05$) correlated with an unsatisfactory result. No correlation was found between the results and generalized joint laxity, passive patellar tilt, congruence angle at follow-up, patellar height, and degree of chondromalacia.

Lattermann and colleagues[69] performed a recent review of the literature on lateral release. They found no level I evidence and only level V evidence in the literature. After review of these retrospective studies, they concluded that isolated lateral release had little or no place in the treatment of patellar instability. They recommend the use of isolated lateral release in cases of lateral patellar compression syndrome with a clearly tight lateral retinaculum. Lateral release is still indicated in proximal and distal realignment surgery.

In light of the high rates of failure and recurrent instability noted with lateral release alone, we have moved away from using this technique alone for the treatment of instability. We reserve the use of isolated lateral release for those patients with evidence of tight lateral retinaculum and with no evidence of malalignment and/or instability.

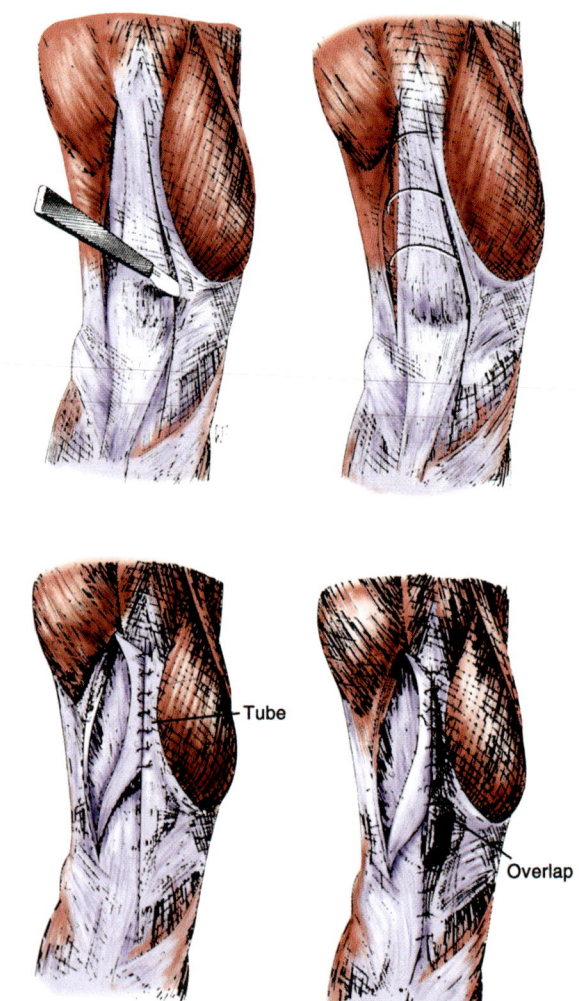

Figure 63-42. Proximal "tube" realignment as described by Insall. (From Insall J, Bullough PG, Burstein AH: Proximal "tube" realignment of the patella for chondromalacia patellae. Clin Orthop Relat Res 144:63, 1979.)

Insall's Proximal Realignment. The proximal realignment procedure was described by Insall et al in 1976[58] and again in 1979.[57] This was a modification of the quadricepsplasty procedure described by Madigan and coworkers in 1975[72] (Fig. 63-41). Insall originally described the "tube" realignment (Fig. 63-42), which he did not perform for very long before

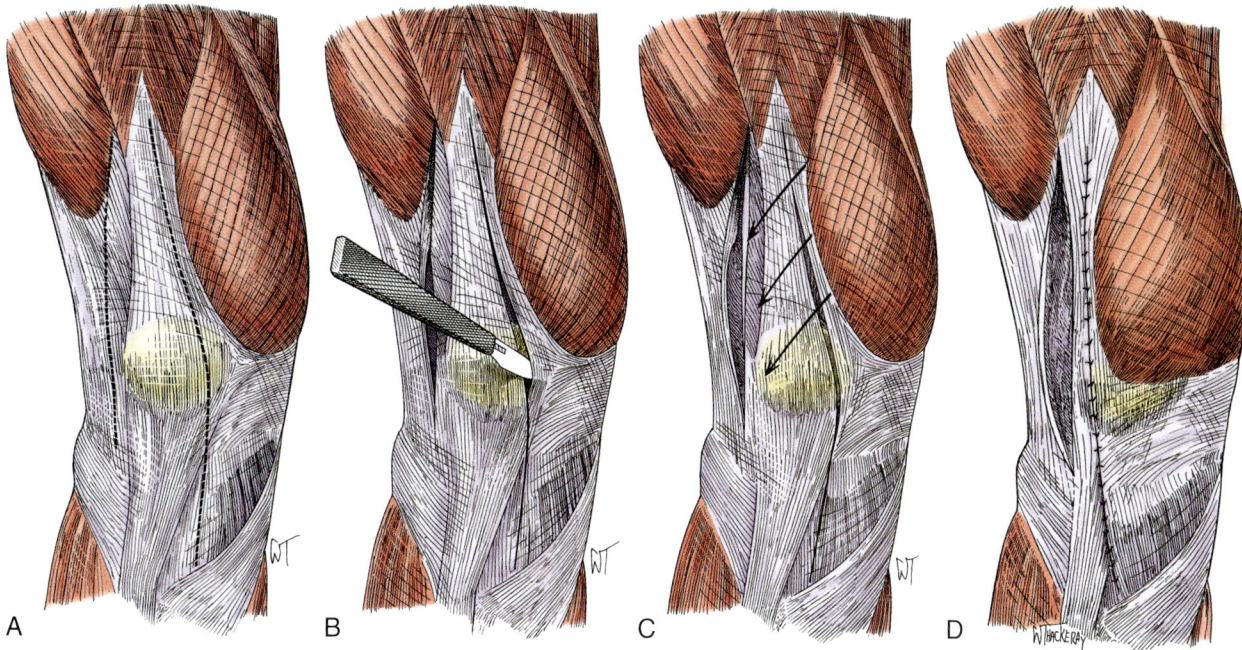

Figure 63-43. Insall's proximal realignment. **A,** After exposure of the quadriceps mechanism, two incisions are made. The first enters the knee joint by a capsular incision placed at the margin of the vastus medialis over the medial quarter of the patella and medial to the patellar tendon. The second is a lateral release extending into the fibers of the vastus lateralis. **B,** To preserve continuity of the medial flap, the quadriceps expansion crossing the patella must be carefully preserved and separated by sharp dissection. **C,** Realignment is effected by advancing the medial flap containing the vastus medialis laterally and distally in the line of the fibers of the oblique portion of the vastus medialis. **D,** After suturing, the incision lies in a straight line across the front of the patella, and the lateral release should open widely.

he modified it to the proximal realignment procedure that is now referred to as the Insall proximal realignment (Fig. 63-43). The procedure, as Insall stated, "…should not be considered merely a lateral retinacular release combined with a medial capsular reefing: it is in fact a quadricepsplasty in which the vastus lateralis is divided and the vastus medialis is advanced so that the line of pull of the quadriceps tendon is moved in a medial direction, thereby reducing the quadriceps angle…"[57,58] The procedure as Insall described it is in fact an extensive lateral retinacular release combined with lateralization of the insertion of the vastus medialis muscle.[57,58] Specifically, it improves the medial pull of the VMO, making it a more effective dynamic centralizing and stabilizing force on the patella. The method can be applied for both patellar pain and patellar dislocation syndromes.

The operation (see Figs. 63-43 and 63-44) is performed under tourniquet control after exsanguination of the limb by elevation or with a bandage. A midline skin incision is made over the patella and the extensor mechanism (see video on the website). The skin edges are undermined sufficiently to expose the patella and quadriceps expansions; the incision should be sufficiently extensive that the components of the quadriceps muscle are clearly visible (Figs. 63-45 and 63-46). We have modified our technique by creating a smaller skin incision; however, we maintain that adequate visualization should not be compromised for a smaller incision (see video on the website). Skin flaps should be raised deep to the fascia to make the skin flaps as thick as possible. Both the vastus medialis and the vastus lateralis must be exposed, as well as the proximal extent of the quadriceps tendon and the insertion of the fibers from the rectus femoris. The arthrotomy is

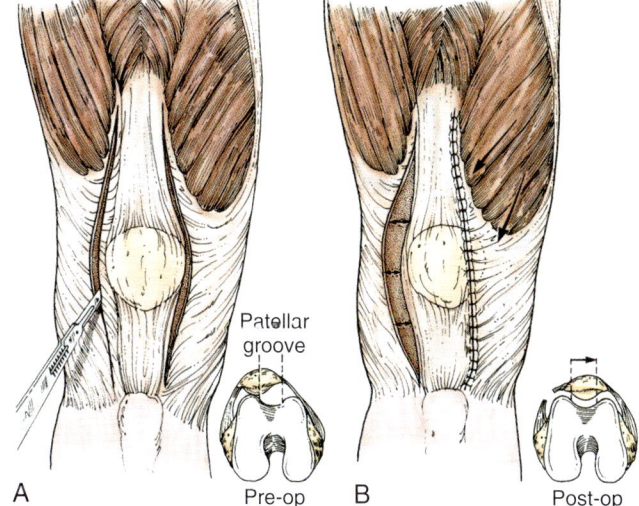

Figure 63-44. Proximal realignment. **A,** The medial parapatellar arthrotomy and lateral release. **B,** The medial flap is advanced laterally. (With kind permission of Springer Science+Business Media. From Scuderi GR: The patella, New York, 1995, Springer-Verlag, p 231.)

performed by making an incision beginning proximally at the apex of the quadriceps tendon and placed within the tendon close to the border of the vastus medialis. The incision is continued distally to the patella and is extended across the medial border of this bone, then distally medial to the patellar tendon. The incision described therefore is almost straight (see Fig. 63-43). The fibers of the quadriceps expansion

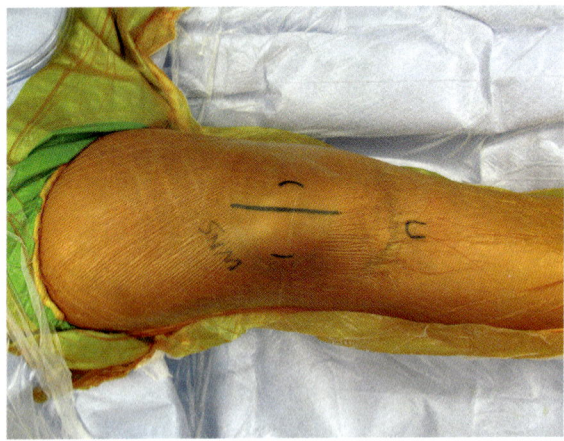

Figure 63-45. A midline incision is performed from the superior pole of the patella to about the level of the joint line. This incision may be extended to obtain adequate exposure.

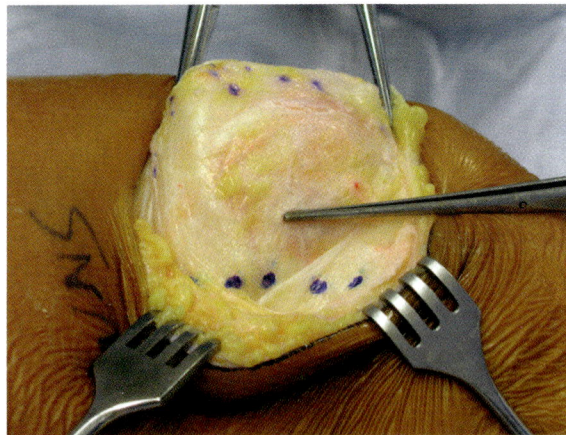

Figure 63-47. A capsular incision is made on the lateral side, beginning proximally in the muscle fibers of the vastus lateralis and extending distally to the tibial tubercle.

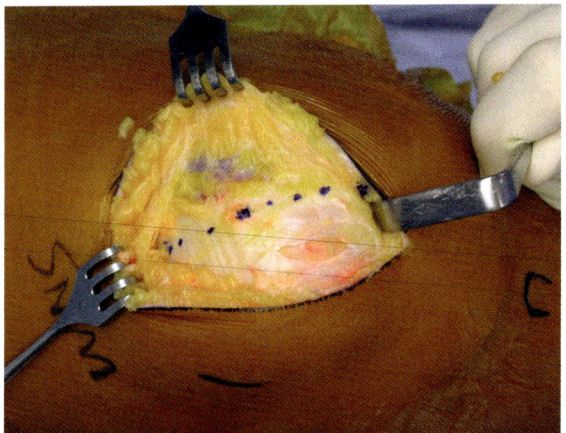
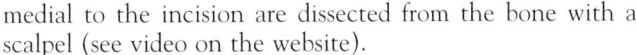

Figure 63-46. Thick skin flaps are made deep to the fascia over the extensor mechanism. A mobile window is created to keep the incision as small as possible so the procedure can be performed safely.

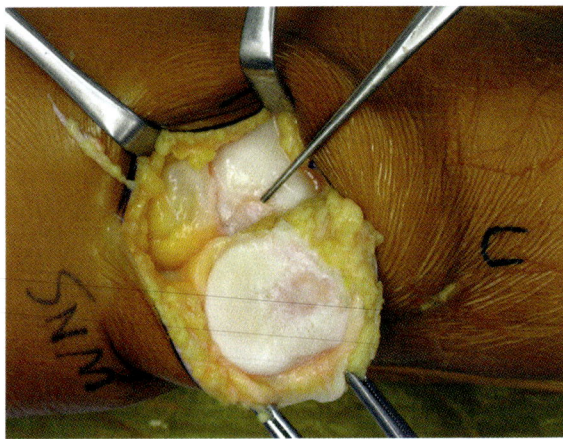

Figure 63-48. A common pattern of osteochondral injury seen on the medial facet of the patella and the lateral border of the femoral sulcus is caused by patellar dislocation.

medial to the incision are dissected from the bone with a scalpel (see video on the website).

Because of vertical ridges on the anterior surface of the patella, the incision can be difficult and should be performed with care to preserve the expansion intact without lacerations. This is necessary to obtain secure closure when the quadriceps repair is completed. The fibers of the expansion can be separated easily from the bone if the dissection proceeds from above and below alternately, thus forming a V and leaving the thinnest central part until last. When the procedure is performed in this manner, the central portion separates from the bone easily and can be fully preserved. Once the medial border of the patella is reached, the synovial lining is incised. Proceeding distally, the fat pad is divided in the line of the capsular incision until the patella can be everted for inspection of the joint. Partial excision of the fat pad may be performed to avoid bulging of the fat pad through the lateral release.

After the medial arthrotomy is completed, the lateral release must be performed to adequately realign the extensor mechanism (Fig. 63-47). A second capsular incision is made on the lateral side, beginning proximally in the muscle fibers

of the vastus lateralis and extending distally to the tibial tubercle (see video on the website). It is desirable, but not essential, to maintain the integrity of the synovium. Sometimes this is not possible because of tight fibrous bands in the substance of the synovium itself. A number of substantial vessels cross to the patella in the lateral retinaculum. At the level of the superior pole of the patella are two or three branches of the superior lateral geniculate vessels, which are large and bleed profusely if not ligated or coagulated. The branches of the inferior lateral geniculate vessels are smaller vessels that run beneath the retinaculum more distally at the lower pole of the patella; they are generally one or two in number. These vessels should also be identified and ligated or coagulated. Alternatively, an attempt can be made to preserve them.

The interior of the knee is thoroughly explored, and selective débridement is performed when necessary. In the malalignment syndrome, regardless of the extent of the patellar lesion, the femoral sulcus is usually normal. The exception is occasional evidence of an osteochondral fracture at the lateral border of the femoral sulcus caused by patellar dislocation (Fig. 63-48).

At this stage of the operation, the tourniquet should be released to enable coagulation of any bleeding points not previously identified. The knee should be flexed and slowly brought into extension while the bleeding vessels are systematically cauterized. Deflating the tourniquet ensures that the tourniquet does not alter the mechanics of the quadriceps muscle during realignment. The quadriceps must then be reconstructed in such a way that the subsequent line of pull will be in a more medial direction. This is the purpose of the operative procedure, and by altering the direction of quadriceps action, patellar congruence is restored and patellar instability prevented. Two critical sutures are placed: first at the proximal pole, then at the distal pole of the patella (see video on the website). The first suture is placed on an angle so that the most distal part of the vastus medialis is brought laterally and distally to overlap the upper pole of the patella and the adjoining quadriceps tendon (Fig. 63-49). Before the overlap is executed, the synovium should be removed from the deep surface of the medial flap, which includes the vastus medialis, the medial part of the quadriceps expansion, and distally the medial capsule of the knee. The amount of overlap that should be achieved depends on the preoperative laxity of the tissues. The suture is passed in a mattress fashion through the prepatellar tissue and the medial flap, then back through the flap and the prepatellar tissue. The point of penetration of the prepatellar tissue determines the amount of transposition of the medial flap over the patella (Fig. 63-50).

The amount of overlap is usually 10 to 15 mm, but if necessary it may be advanced as far as the lateral border of the patella. A second suture is inserted at the lower pole of the patella in the same fashion described previously. This suture will bring the medial flap across as tight as necessary, and often the tightness is determined by however much the soft tissue allows. The suture material may be absorbable or nonabsorbable, according to the surgeon's preference. The two initial sutures determine the remainder of the closure, and after they are placed, the knee should flex to 90 degrees without breakage of the sutures. The tension in these sutures is adjusted until the tracking of the patella is acceptable (see video on the website). The remaining closure is completed

distally by suturing the flap as it lies and proximally, with decreasing overlap of the vastus medialis over the quadriceps tendon. According to Insall, it is not possible to overtighten the medial structures; however, it appears that overtightening may lead to iatrogenic medial subluxation and a poor result.

Occasionally in patients with recurrent dislocation and an extreme lateral position of the patella, the medial flap is so stretched that overlapping to the lateral patellar border is still insufficient to hold the patella in the center of the femoral sulcus. In these circumstances, the medial flap, including the vastus medialis, should be everted and the free border rolled back on itself. A series of sutures are inserted, so that a tuck is made in the muscle. The reefed vastus medialis and the quadriceps expansion are sutured anterior to the patella and the quadriceps tendon. The tuck must be sufficient to keep the patella centralized. The resulting bulk of the muscle and capsule lying anterior to the patella may appear aesthetically unpleasant, but the tissue atrophies rapidly, so that within a few weeks the enlargement disappears.

Two features of the repair should be emphasized. First, the lateral incision into the vastus lateralis must extend proximally almost as far as the medial incision. The most common error is reluctance to make an adequate division of the vastus lateralis; unless this is done, proximal rearrangement of the quadriceps is not possible (Figs. 63-51 and 63-52). It might be expected that extensive division of the muscle would cause quadriceps weakness, but in practice this has not been observed. Insall emphasized that this was instrumental to the success of the procedure. In practice, the lateral release should extend as far proximal as necessary to centralize the patella.

Second, the more distal part of the closure must be snug but not excessively tight. In practice, it is almost impossible to overdo the overlapping in this area because it is prevented by soft tissue tension and the anatomy of the femoral sulcus.

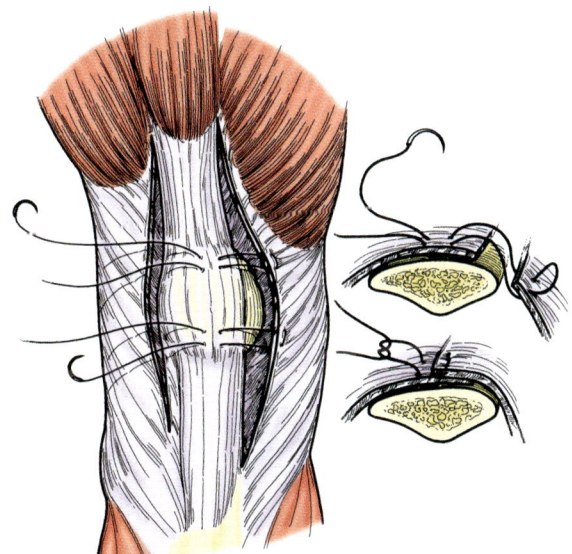

Figure 63-50. Suture of the medial arthrotomy after transposition of the tibial tuberosity in a combined proximal and distal realignment. Two critical stitches are placed at the upper and lower poles of the patella with nonabsorbable no. 5 Ethibond sutures. The suture is passed through the prepatellar tissues, the medial flap, and back through the flap and prepatellar tissues. The point of penetration through the prepatellar tissues determines the amount of overlap of the medial flap over the patella.

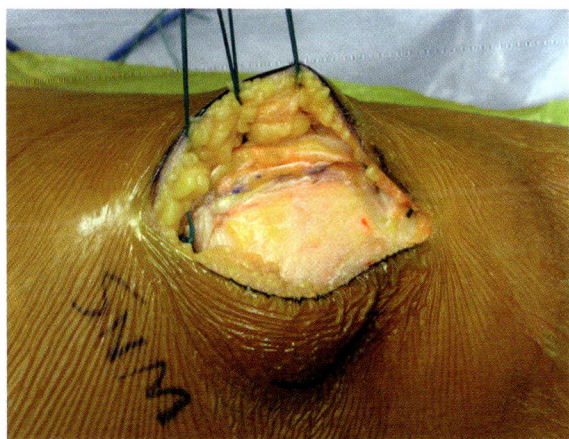

Figure 63-49. Two to three sutures are placed along the medial arthrotomy at the upper and lower poles of the patella. These sutures determine the extent of realignment of medial tissues. Proper patellar tracking is verified before the remaining sutures are placed.

Excessive tightness is revealed through observation of the behavior of the patella when the knee is flexed.

After routine closure of the subcutaneous tissue and skin, a compression dressing is applied. We no longer routinely close over a hemovac drain.

We are currently using an accelerated rehabilitation protocol. Full weight bearing as tolerated is permitted immediately postoperatively. The patient is discharged on the day of surgery. Continuous passive motion (CPM) is started the night of surgery at the patient's home. Physical therapy is started on postoperative day 1 with a focus on quadriceps strengthening and range of motion. We encourage full active and passive range-of-motion exercises.

RESULTS OF INSALL PROXIMAL REALIGNMENT PROCEDURE

Results of Insall's technique have been reported by different centers (Table 63-5). Insall[54] reviewed 75 realignments performed between 1969 and 1979 for patellar pain and instability. Ten operations were bilateral. The procedures were performed in 40 female and 25 male patients, and the average patient age was 20 years (range, 13 to 32 years). Patients were selected for surgery very carefully. All had dysplasia of the extensor mechanism and serious complaints of pain or instability for a long time, ranging from 1 to 5 years. All had undergone lengthy conservative treatment. Symptoms were always severe enough to interfere with everyday activity, not only with sports. Absence from school was a frequent problem in younger patients.

Of 75 knees, 36 had an increased quadriceps angle (at least 20 degrees), 21 had a high-riding patella (average T/P ratio, 1.19), and 18 had both conditions (quadriceps angle, >20 degrees; average T/P ratio, 1.23); a preoperative Merchant view had been obtained in 20 knees, and findings for the sulcus and congruence angles were in accord with measurements reported by Aglietti and associates.[3] Thus, the 10 knees with an increased quadriceps angle had an average sulcus angle of 138 degrees and an average congruence angle of 0 degrees. The six knees with a high-riding patella had a sulcus angle averaging 161 degrees and a congruence angle that averaged 25 degrees. The four knees with both variants had an average sulcus angle of 143 degrees and a congruence angle of 19 degrees. The 75 knees were divided according to primary symptoms into 40 knees with patellar pain (32 with an increased quadriceps angle, 3 with a high-riding patella, and 5 with both), 29 knees with subluxation (18 with a high-riding patella, 4 with an increased quadriceps angle, and 7 with both), and 6 knees with both pain and subluxation (all with an increased quadriceps angle and a high-riding patella).

The findings at surgery for patellar surface lesions were normal or grade I in 76%, grade II in 12%, grade III in 4%, and grade IV in 8% of cases. Pain was moderate to severe in 32 of 57 grade I lesions (56%), in 7 of 9 grade II lesions

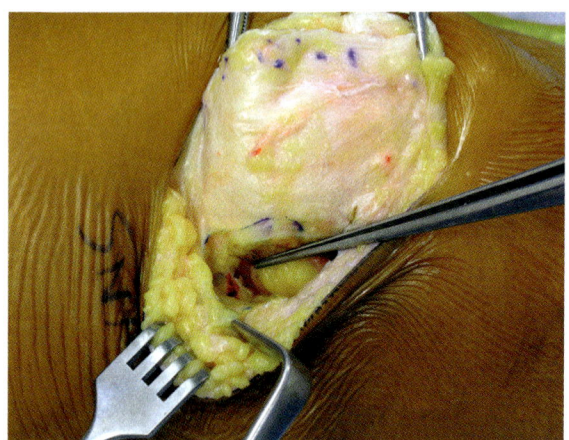

Figure 63-51. The lateral release should extend proximally into the muscle fibers of the vastus lateralis.

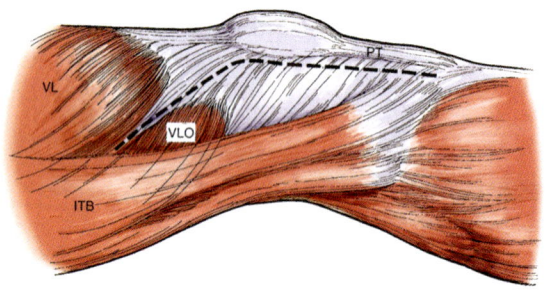

Figure 63-52. The dotted line indicates the extent of lateral release recommended. Note that it extends proximally between the vastus lateralis *(VL)* and the vastus lateralis obliquus *(VLO)*. *PT,* Patellar tendon. (From Scott WN: The knee, vol 1, St Louis, 1994, Mosby–Year Book, p 451.)

Table 63-5 Results of Proximal Realignment With Insall's Technique

Author	Year	No. Of Knees	Diagnosis	Follow-Up, Mo	Avg. % Satisfactory Result	Remarks
Insall et al[56]	1983	75	Pain and subluxation	48	91	Better results when the patella is centered in the sulcus after the operation; no correlation with the severity of chondromalacia
Scuderi et al[101]	1988	60	Subluxation and dislocation	42	81	Only one redislocation (1.7%); females and older patients had inferior results; better results with patellar centralization
Abraham et al[1]	1989	35	Pain and dislocation	76	62	Less satisfactory results in knees with patellofemoral pain (53%) than in knees with recurrent dislocation (78%)
Aglietti et al[5]	1989	11	Dislocation	102	91	Only one case was unsatisfactory because of insufficient quadriceps rehabilitation

(78%), in no grade III lesions, and in 4 of 6 grade IV lesions (67%). At surgery, 14 patellae were shaved, and 7 were shaved and drilled.

The grading system was similar to that described by Bentley.[11] At follow-up ranging from 2 to 10 years with an average of 4 years, the results were as follows: excellent in 37%, good in 54%, fair in 5%, and poor in 4%. Excellent and good results were obtained in 93% of stage I cartilage lesions, 100% of stage II lesions, 33% of stage III lesions, and 83% of stage IV lesions. Of 21 knees in which the patella was shaved or drilled, 86% had satisfactory results. Postoperatively, only 14 patients could not participate in sports.

In 57 knees, a postoperative Merchant view was obtained. Among 52 satisfactory knees, the average congruence angle was −11 degrees; 35 knees had a negative angle, 5 measured 0 degrees, and 12 had a positive congruence angle. Five knees were rated fair or poor, and in these knees the average congruence angle was 0 degrees. (Two knees had a positive congruence angle, 2 measured 0 degrees, and 1 had a negative angle.) Naturally, one must not put too much store in radiographic measurements of any kind, and some inconsistencies are to be expected. However, these findings suggested a trend, in that clinical improvement correlated with correct alignment, whereas no such correlation existed with the severity of chondromalacia or with its treatment by patellar shaving.

The complications of proximal realignment were relatively few and minor. They included superficial phlebitis, hematoma, delayed wound healing, and culture-negative drainage. Five knees (7%) required manipulation under anesthesia to allow better range of motion. One subsequent patellectomy was performed because of persistent patellar pain.

Scuderi and colleagues[101] reported the results of a group of 60 knees with patellar subluxation (34 knees) or dislocation (26 knees) that were treated by Insall's proximal realignment. In this study, 20 knees had undergone previous surgery (33%), including proximal and distal realignment, lateral retinacular release, anterior cruciate ligament surgery, meniscectomy, and removal of loose bodies. Postoperatively, a cast was applied for 1 month. The follow-up period was 3.5 years (range, 2 to 9 years). Results were excellent in 30%, good in 52%, fair in 10%, and poor in 8%. Results were significantly better in males and in younger patients. No patients younger than 20 years had an unsatisfactory result. The preoperative diagnosis (subluxation or dislocation), the length of follow-up, and the severity of chondromalacia did not correlate with the result. Knees with a satisfactory result showed a greater change in the congruence angle (medial displacement of the patella) than did those with an unsatisfactory grading. The complications were as follows: seven patients (12%) needed postoperative manipulation to increase range of motion, one patient experienced a single episode of recurrent dislocation, three patients underwent arthroscopy for recurrent patellofemoral pain, and one patient underwent bilateral patellectomy for degenerative joint disease. Although the overall results did not correlate with the severity of chondromalacia, it is noteworthy that all patients who needed a reoperation had severe, degenerative osteoarthritis.

Abraham and colleagues[1] reported the results of Insall's proximal realignment in 15 knees with patellofemoral pain and 9 knees with recurrent dislocation with an average follow-up period of 6.3 years. Satisfactory results in the group of knees with patellofemoral pain decreased from 87% at 2 years to 53% at 5 years. It should be noted that a quarter of these patients had severe grade IV chondromalacia at the time of the operation: none of these knees obtained a satisfactory result. Better results were achieved in knees with recurrent patellar dislocation: 92% were satisfactory at 2 years, and 78% remained so at 5 years. Two knees required additional surgery for recurrence of dislocation. An anatomic study in cadaver knees was undertaken to define the innervation of the patella. It was noted that branches of the femoral and lateral femoral cutaneous nerves innervated the patella. All these branches are cut by the skin and subcutaneous incisions and by the medial capsulotomy plus lateral release. In light of these findings, Abraham and coworkers suggested that pain relief may be attributed in part to denervation. No radiographic data were presented to describe the relationship between clinical results and restoration of congruence.

Aglietti and coworkers[2] reported the results of proximal realignment in 11 knees affected by recurrent patellar dislocation that were reviewed with a long average follow-up of 102 months. Only one case was considered unsatisfactory because of poor quadriceps rehabilitation. No recurrences of dislocation were reported. Eight of these patients (73%) were interested in sports preoperatively, and all returned to their desired sport, including soccer (2), running (3), and aerobics (3). Analysis of Merchant axial views revealed that preoperatively, the average congruence angle was +16 degrees, with 80% of knees considered abnormal. At follow-up, only one knee was still abnormal (9%), and the average congruence angle was reduced to −8 degrees. No signs of degenerative arthritis were seen during the long period of follow-up.

There is a paucity of new literature on isolated proximal realignment procedures. Most of the current literature reports results of proximal and distal combined procedures or of medial patellofemoral ligament reconstruction. Because no new comparative studies have been done, it is difficult to compare these newer techniques with the results of proximal realignment alone. Therefore, we conclude that proximal realignment remains a good surgical intervention for patients with patellar instability. It appears to improve the congruence of the patellofemoral joint by redirecting the pull of the quadriceps mechanism. Some evidence suggests that the procedure is more successful when performed for instability as opposed to advanced articular degeneration. In the face of severe deformity with large Q angles or rotational abnormalities, this procedure may be combined with a distal bony procedure to improve patellofemoral mechanics.

Arthroscopically Assisted Proximal Soft Tissue Plication Procedures

Arthroscopically assisted procedures have been described in the literature.* Basically, they include lateral retinacular release and plication of the medial capsule. Plication is achieved percutaneously or through short skin incisions with the use of spinal needles, straight or curved, which are used to deliver sutures into the joint and are then extracted and tied over the capsule.

These procedures are not simply less invasive forms of the same proximal realignment procedure that Insall described in

---

*References 3, 4, 7, 8, 12, 46, 50, 64, 85, 88, 106, and 119.

1976.[58] The procedures do not realign or advance the VMO. By including plication of the medial capsule and remaining soft tissue without advancement of the VMO, these procedures functionally shorten the medial restraints on the patella. In theory, these techniques may shorten the MPFL, which is the primary restraint to lateral displacement of the patella.[24] Distal extension of the plication to the tibial tuberosity (through a short incision) may give additional support by shortening the patellomeniscal and patellotibial ligaments.

We favor traditional proximal realignment over the arthroscopic approach. Our concern is that exact tensioning of medial structures and secure repair may be more difficult to achieve by arthroscopic than by more traditional open techniques. Results from small series of arthroscopically assisted repairs are encouraging.[7,17,46,88,106] However, we think that larger series with longer follow-up are needed.

Ali and associates[8] published medium-term results of 7 years' follow-up in 36 patients treated with their technique of arthroscopic medial plication and lateral release. The results are promising, with excellent outcomes in 50%, good results in 28%, and poor results in only four knees (11%). Investigators reported two (5%) cases of recurrent instability that improved with reoperation. Overall, 89% of patients were satisfied with the operation, and only three (8%) patients were disappointed at follow-up. Of note, the authors reported no radiographic measurements on these patients because it is their belief that the best assessment of patellar instability is arthroscopic visualization of the patellofemoral joint.

Halbrecht[46] described a technique of all-inside arthroscopic medial plication and arthroscopic lateral release performed on 45 knees with recurrent patellar instability. His technique involves percutaneous passage of sutures and arthroscopic knot tying within the joint to reef the medial soft tissues. Halbrecht reports that at 2 years' follow-up, 93% of patients experienced significant improvement. Significant improvement was observed in all radiographic measures such as congruence angle and lateral patellofemoral angle. In this series, no complications such as dislocation or recurrent instability were reported.

CONCLUSION/SUMMARY OF CHAPTER

Treatment of patellofemoral instability with proximal realignment dates back to at least 1975, with Madigan's description of the quadricepsplasty.[72] Insall then described the proximal realignment procedure, which consisted of lateral and distal translation of the vastus medialis, as well as an obligatory lateral retinacular release.[57,58] The combination of translation of the vastus medialis and lateral retinacular release is what is now referred to as the Insall proximal realignment procedure. This technique can be combined with distal realignment procedures when the malalignment is severe. We have seen very good results with this technique over the years, although similar to many other treatments for patellar instability, this technique is not perfect, and some recurrence of symptoms is seen.

In recent years, many attempts have been made to modify the original technique. Most of these modifications involve arthroscopic assistance or smaller incisions. It is important to remember that all of the described arthroscopic techniques to date omit a very important aspect of the procedure, that is, transposition of the medial tissue. For this reason, we do not advocate the use of these arthroscopic techniques. We have modified our technique by performing the procedure through a much smaller incision than was originally described. However, we must emphasize that adequate exposure should not be compromised for a smaller incision. We have also maintained the two main tenets of this procedure: redirecting the pull of the vastus medialis and performing an adequate lateral retinacular release.

An accurate diagnosis is paramount in the treatment of patellofemoral instability. The combination of a thorough physical examination and multiple imaging studies is essential for determining the cause of the instability. Patellofemoral anatomy, as well as angular and rotational malalignment, may contribute to the instability. Only after all of these factors have been identified can the appropriate treatment be provided. Ultimately, the sum of these factors produces an abnormal, laterally directed force on the patella, and treatment must be directed at restoring patellofemoral congruency by re-establishing a centralizing force vector on the patella. The proximal realignment procedure, as described by Insall, restores patellofemoral congruency and centralizing force by combining lateral translation of the vastus medialis insertion on the patella with extensive lateral release.

Acknowledgment. The authors would like to thank Paolo Aglietti, Francesco Giron, and Pierluigi Cuomo for their work on the previous edition of this chapter.

KEY REFERENCES

Abraham E, Washington E, Huang TL: Insall proximal realignment for disorders of the patella. Clin Orthop Relat Res 248:61, 1989.

Aglietti P, Buzzi R, De Biase P, Giron F: Surgical treatment of recurrent dislocation of the patella. Clin Orthop Relat Res 308:8, 1994.

Aglietti P, Insall JN, Cerulli G: Patellar pain and incongruence. I: Measurements of incongruence. Clin Orthop Relat Res 176:217, 1983.

Conlan T, Garth WP, Lemons JE: Evaluations of the medial soft-tissue restraints of the extensor mechanism of the knee. J Bone Joint Surg Am 75:682, 1993.

Crosby BE, Insall JN: Recurrent dislocation of the patella: relation of treatment to osteoarthritis. J Bone Joint Surg Am 58:9, 1976.

Elias DA, White LM, Fithian DC: Acute lateral patellar dislocation at MR imaging: injury patterns of medial patellar soft-tissue restraints and osteochondral injuries of the inferomedial patella. Radiology 225:736, 2002.

Hautamaa PV, Fithian DC, Kaufman KR, et al: Medial soft tissue restraints in lateral patellar instability and repair. Clin Orthop Relat Res 349:174, 1998.

Insall JN, Aglietti P, Tria AJ: Patellar pain and incongruence. II: Clinical application. Clin Orthop Relat Res 176:225, 1983.

Insall JN, Bullough PG, Burstein AH: Proximal "tube" realignment of the patella for chondromalacia patellae. Clin Orthop Relat Res 144:63, 1979.

Insall JN, Falvo KA, Wise DW: Chondromalacia patellae: a prospective study. J Bone Joint Surg Am 58:1, 1976.

Madigan R, Wissinger HA, Donaldson WF: Preliminary experience with a method of quadricepsplasty in recurrent subluxation of the patella. J Bone Joint Surg Am 57:600, 1975.

Panagiotopoulos E, Strzelczyk P, Herrmann M, et al: Cadaveric study on static medial patellar stabilizers: dynamizing role of the vastus medialis obliquus on medial patellofemoral ligament. Knee Surg Sports Traumatol Arthrosc 14:7, 2006.

Sanders TG, Morrison WB, Singleton BA, et al: Medial patellofemoral ligament injury following acute transient dislocation of the patella: MR findings with surgical correlation in 14 patients. J Comput Assist Tomogr 25:957, 2001.

Scuderi G, Cuomo F, Scott NW: Lateral release and proximal realignment for patellar subluxation and dislocation: a long-term follow-up. J Bone Joint Surg Am 70:856, 1988.

Full references for this chapter can be found on www.expertconsult.com.

Chapter 64

Repair and Reconstruction of the Medial Patellofemoral Ligament for Treatment of Lateral Patellar Dislocations: Surgical Techniques and Clinical Results

Julian Feller, Martin Lind, Joshua Nelson, David R. Diduch, and Elizabeth Arendt

SURGICAL INDICATIONS

The medial patellofemoral ligament (MPFL) is the primary soft tissue restraint to lateral patellar displacement in early flexion[6]; it is in early knee flexion that almost all noncontact lateral patellar dislocations occur. The biomechanical role of the MPFL is to contain the patella when it is subjected to the extremes of motion secondary to a lateralizing force. The goal of an MPFL repair or reconstruction is to restore the loss of the medial patellar soft tissue stabilizer that has been torn and may be chronically lax because of recurrent lateral patellar dislocations.

MPFL tearing is a consequence of patellar dislocation and not a cause of instability. Surgical intervention should be aimed at treating specific injuries, including a torn MPFL, and correcting relevant risk factors. An MPFL reconstruction is most often used alone when the bony morphology is normal or near-normal. In situations in which there is trochlear dysplasia and/or patella alta, the MPFL may play an even greater role as a biomechanical restraint than when the trochlear groove and patellar height are normal. However, the current literature does not provide any clear indications of when risk factor(s) need to be corrected in addition to an MPFL reconstruction.

An ideal candidate for an isolated MPFL repair or reconstruction might have the following profile with regard to potential risk factors for recurrent patellar dislocation:

- Trochlear morphology; normal or type A dysplasia[9,41]
- Tibial tuberosity–trochlear sulcus angle of 0 to 5 degrees valgus or a tibial tuberosity trochlear groove distance less than 20 mm with the knee at 0 degree flexion
- No excessive increase in the patellar height ratio (Caton-Deschamps index <1.2 or Insall-Salvati index <1.4)
- Patellar tilt less than 20 degrees when measured on an axial image, using the posterior femoral condyles as a reference line, or some tilt but no lateral tightness on physical examination with the patella reduced

ANATOMY OF THE MEDIAL SIDE OF THE KNEE: SURGICAL IMPLICATIONS

Knowledge of the medial side knee anatomy is necessary for proper surgical execution of MPFL reconstruction techniques. The capsuloligamentous structures on the medial aspect of the knee have been described as being in three layers.[46] Layer 2 is the ligament layer in which the MPFL and superficial medial collateral ligament (MCL) are situated.

The MPFL runs transversely from the proximal half of the medial patellar border to the femur, near the medial epicondyle. Although some fibers of the MPFL fan out and have a broad attachment, the most consistent attachment site is the saddle between the epicondyle and the adductor tubercle.

The patellar attachment of the MPFL is wider than the femoral attachment and approximates the upper third of the medial border of the patella, typically at the location where the perimeter of the patella becomes more vertical. As a percentage of the longitudinal length of the patella, Nomura and colleagues[30] have reported that the MPFL insertion is 27% ± 10% from the proximal extent of the patella. The MPFL acts as a check rein restraint to lateral deviation of the patella. As the knee progresses into flexion, patellofemoral congruence, and trochlear geometry, in particular the slope angle of the lateral trochlear facet, provide the major restraints to lateral patellar displacement.[14]

The medial patellotibial ligament (MPTL) is in a more superficial plane than the MPFL and is an oblique condensation of the medial patellar retinaculum. It attaches to the tibia approximately 1.5 cm below the joint line, close to the insertion of the medial collateral ligament, although individual components of the medial retinaculum are more difficult to assess as dissection extends distally.[46] The MPTL is uniquely positioned to help resist superior and superolateral translation of the patella because of the oblique orientation of its fibers. However, the role of the MPTL in resisting lateral patellar displacement is debated, ranging from being an important secondary stabilizer[21] to being functionally unimportant.[6]

MEDIAL PATELLOFEMORAL LIGAMENT REPAIR

Primary Repair of the Medial Patellofemoral Ligament

Imbrication of the medial retinaculum has long been a component of surgical procedures for lateral patellar dislocations. However, with the increasing focus on MPFL reconstruction, there has also been greater scrutiny of the results of primary and secondary repair of the ligament itself. Unfortunately there are many variations in the techniques of MPFL repair, making it difficult to compare one surgeon's experience with another's. Moreover, it has recently been demonstrated that the location of MPFL injury may further stratify patients into risk categories for recurrent dislocation. In a 7-year follow-up study[37] of patients with a primary traumatic patellar dislocation treated nonoperatively, those with a femoral avulsion of the MPFL were at significantly greater risk of developing patellar instability than those with midsubstance tears or disruption at the patellar insertion.

Some authors have recommended against medial repair for first time patellar dislocations. In a randomized controlled study of non-operative management versus repair undertaken at a mean of 50 days after presentation to an emergency department, Christiansen and associates[4] have reported a 17.5% redislocation rate in the operative group compared with 20% in the nonoperative group. In another level 1 study,

Nikku and coworkers[27] have reported the 7-year results of a variety of medial repair procedures compared with nonoperative treatment. The outcomes were similar between the two groups both in regard to patients' self-assessed outcomes and patellar redislocation.

On the other hand, there also are studies that support medial repair. A recent level 1 study[36] compared nonoperative treatment versus open medial surgery in younger, mostly male patients. Preoperative MRI in the operatively treated group helped define the location of the MPFL lesion. Fourteen of 18 operatively treated subjects had a medial reefing at the imaged site of injury and 4 had a Roux-Goldthwait procedure. The surgical decision was based on surgeon preference. At 7-year follow-up there were no redislocations in the operative group compared with further dislocations in 6 of 21 patients in the nonoperative group. However, there were no subjective differences between the two groups. A level 2 study[3] also reported improved outcomes for acute patellar dislocations treated surgically. Preoperative magnetic resonance imaging (MRI) was again used to determine the location of MPFL injury. Lesions close to the patella were repaired arthroscopically with an outside to inside technique, whereas femoral avulsion injuries were repaired with suture anchors in the epicondyle. At an average of 40 months follow-up, there were no redislocations in the 17 patients in the operative group compared with 8 redislocations in the 16 patients in the nonoperative group.

A variety of arthroscopic techniques of medial soft tissue repair have been developed over recent years.[10,18-20] There are numerous studies both supporting and discouraging arthroscopic repair techniques for patellar instability,[2,10,19,20,35] but the results are confounded by various combinations of open and arthroscopic techniques. In one such prospective but nonrandomized study, the results of initial arthroscopic medial repair of the MPFL were compared with those of nonoperative management. At a median 7-year follow-up, initial arthroscopic repair was not associated with a reduced incidence of redislocation. Further detailed outcome studies are needed to clarify the role of arthroscopic repair and to endorse any particular arthroscopic procedure over another.

Thus, the indications for repair of the MPFL have not as yet been clearly defined. Taking a relatively conservative standpoint, an avulsion of the ligament from the patella or the femur may represent an indication for repair, particularly if open surgery is already planned to address an osteochondral lesion of the patella or trochlear groove. The situation for midsubstance ruptures of the ligament is more controversial. Surgical techniques will continue to develop, and the relative merits of MPFL repair versus MPFL reconstruction or nonoperative management will become clear as more outcome data becomes available. In the meantime, there are certain principles to which the orthopedic surgeon should adhere if performing an MPFL repair:

1. Evaluate each patient for factors that predispose to patellar instability, even though at this time the literature does not provide clear evidence about which predisposing factors should be corrected nor at what threshold value.
2. The location of injury to the MPFL should be identified when possible (e.g., femoral avulsion, midsubstance, patellar avulsion) and the repair should be focused on this site.

3. Based on the available literature, open repair techniques seem to outperform current arthroscopic techniques. Proper tensioning of the MPFL is critical. Intraoperatively, the knee should easily flex to 90 degrees after repair. Overtightening of the MPFL should be avoided.
4. Suture repairs should be stout and anchors used to further strengthen the repair when feasible. In a biomechanical evaluation, MPFL repairs using suture anchors plus sutures failed at 142 N, whereas suture repair alone failed at 37 N.[24]

Medial Patellofemoral Ligament Repair Technique

Diagnostic arthroscopy is first performed to address any associated intra-articular pathology. Occasionally, the point of disruption to the medial patellofemoral ligament can be visualized arthroscopically. If a distal realignment procedure is to be performed, it should be done prior to the repair of the medial patellofemoral ligament to allow for proper tensioning. The following repair technique is offered as one option for surgical management.

Most commonly, the medial patellofemoral ligament is torn from its femoral origin. For primary repair to the adductor tubercle region, a longitudinal incision is made in the deep fascia and periosteum just proximal to the medial epicondyle. In the initial dissection, the MPFL may be more readily palpated than seen. By holding tension on the tissue with forceps, the patella is translated laterally and the MPFL is identified as that tissue resisting translation (Fig. 64-1). Two suture anchors are then placed into the femur at the attachment site of the MPFL, and mattress sutures are used to repair the ligament with the knee in 30 to 40 degrees of flexion (Figs. 64-2 and 64-3).

If the MPFL is torn off the patella, traction on the medial end of the ligament will not restore patellar stability. In these cases, the MPFL is repaired back to the patella with the use of nonabsorbable sutures placed through drill holes or suture anchors in the patella, in a similar fashion to reconstruction techniques[18,20] (see later).

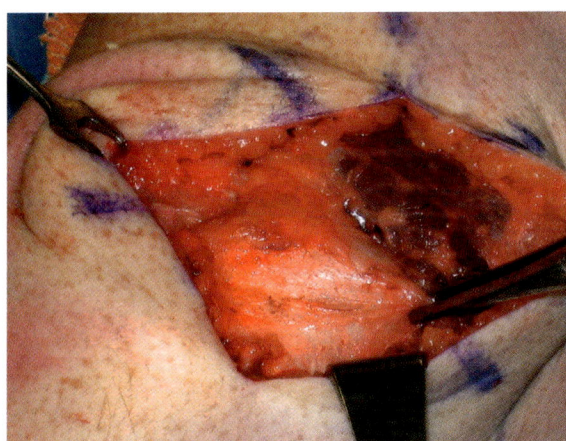

Figure 64-1. MPFL repair. The MPFL has been localized deep and distal to the vastus medialis obliquus. Traction is applied to the patella to determine the point of ligament disruption. (From Redziniak DE, Diduch DR, Mihalko WM et al: Patellar instability. J Bone Joint Surg Am 91:2264, 2009.)

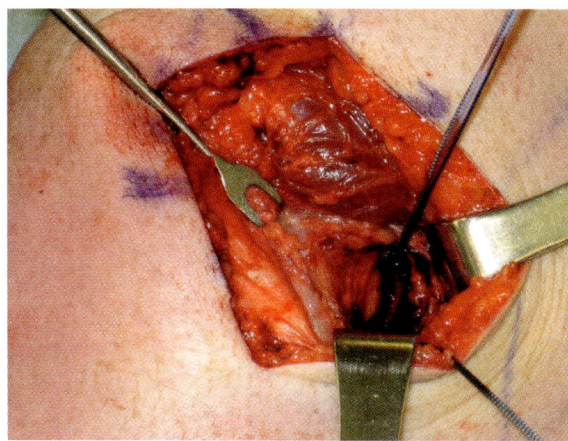

Figure 64-2. MPFL repair. A longitudinal incision in the deep fascia and periosteum permits exposure of the MPFL origin for the placement of two suture anchors in the femur. (From Redziniak DE, Diduch DR, Mihalko WM et al: Patellar instability. J Bone Joint Surg Am 91:2264, 2009.)

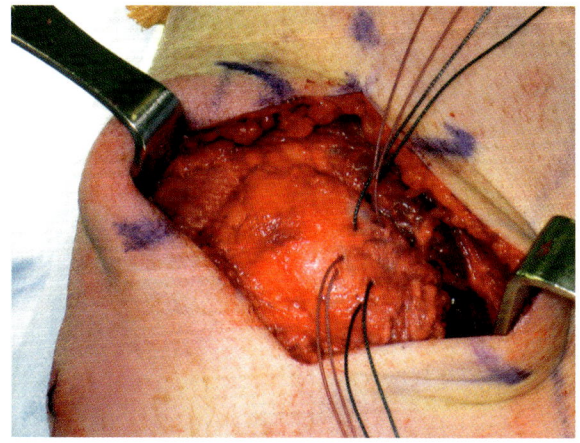

Figure 64-3. MPFL repair. Horizontal mattress sutures are placed through the medial patellofemoral ligament origin and tied at 30 to 40 degrees of knee flexion. (From Redziniak DE, Diduch DR, Mihalko WM et al: Patellar instability. J Bone Joint Surg Am 91:2264, 2009.)

In situations involving midsubstance tears of the MPFL or when there is redundant medial tissue with attenuation, an imbrication of the ligament may be performed.[45] A longitudinal incision is made in the MPFL at the point of midsubstance disruption. This incision includes the joint capsule but does not penetrate the synovium. Once the edges are appropriately identified and tension on the anterior end of the medial portion of the ligament confirms a solid femoral attachment, nonabsorbable sutures are passed in a pants over vest fashion. Optimal tensioning of the MPFL is confirmed by ensuring that at least 90 degrees of knee flexion is easily possible with the sutures in place and by tying the sutures with the knee at 20 to 30 degrees flexion. Occasionally, an arthroscopic lateral release may be warranted if there is excessive lateral patellar tilt that cannot be restored to neutral. If performed, the lateral release should be completed prior to tensioning of the medial structures. After the sutures have been tied, patellar tracking is again assessed and a firm end point to lateral patellar displacement should be appreciated. The investing fascia is repaired prior to skin closure.

Rehabilitation After Medial Patellofemoral Ligament Repair

There is presently no evidence to support any specific postoperative rehabilitation regimen after MPFL repair. The published series rarely include a description of postoperative management. Those studies that report their rehabilitation regimen describe a period of restricted range of motion using a knee immobilizer or a hinged brace from 2 to 6 weeks. Typically, the range of motion is limited to 0, or 0 to 30 degrees, with the rationale being that the repaired MPFL may be under greater tension at higher angles of knee flexion. However the MPFL tissue is also stressed with full quadriceps contraction, particularly in early flexion, and the basis for limiting motion may not match known patellofemoral biomechanics. Weight-bearing status also varies considerably in the published series, ranging from minimal to full weight bearing.

Increasing the range of motion and weight bearing should be based on the surgeon's confidence in the quality of the repair tissue and repair fixation, coupled with an appropriate progression to full strength and agility before a full return to sports. Most authors advocate introducing more demanding rehabilitation tasks from the 10- to 12-week mark, with unrestricted activities commencing from 4 months onward.

MEDIAL PATELLOFEMORAL LIGAMENT RECONSTRUCTION

Basic Principles

Documenting an increase in passive lateral patellar translation beyond the confines of the trochlear groove is a necessary first step because it implies laxity of the MPFL. This is most often established by physical examination with the knee at 20 to 30 degrees flexion, but stress radiographs can also be used.[42] If the diagnosis is in question, an examination under anesthesia can be used to document laxity without guarding or apprehension confounding the findings. Arthroscopy is used to identify and address articular cartilage lesions. However, because distention of the joint during arthroscopy usually results in lateral tilt and translation of the patella, one should not attempt to assess lateral patellar tilt and translation based on arthroscopic appearances alone.

Numerous techniques for MPFL reconstruction have been described. All reconstruction techniques aim to re-create the absent or insufficient ligamentous tissue between the proximal medial aspect of the patella and the attachment site of the MPFL to the femur. Various autologous grafts, such as the semitendinosus, gracilis, quadriceps, and semimembranosus tendons, as well as the medial retinacular tissues, have been used. The use of allograft tendon and synthetic grafts has also been described. Regardless of the technique used, the surgical principles are the same and should be followed to produce an effective reconstruction that does not impair normal knee function.

The selection of graft type will in part dictate the site and method of fixation of the reconstruction. Free tendon grafts are the most frequently used, usually the gracilis or semitendinosus tendons. The attachment sites of free grafts can be selected based on the anatomy of the native MPFL. Alternatively, tendon grafts may be left attached at one end—for example, semitendinosus or gracilis tendons left attached to the tibia, a strip of quadriceps tendon left attached to the patella or a strip of adductor magnus tendon left attached to the femur. In the case of the quadriceps and adductor magnus tendons, the retained attachment will dictate one of the attachment sites of the reconstructed ligament.

When selecting a graft type, consideration should be given to the biomechanical properties of the native MPFL. The ideal tissue for the graft would have similar stiffness, but greater strength, than the native MPFL. All current grafts have both strength and stiffness that are significantly greater than those of the native MPFL. Given this, it seems preferable to use a graft with stiffness that is closest to the native ligament. For this reason, the gracilis tendon may be preferable to the stiffer semitendinosus tendon.[16]

The incisions used will also in part depend on the tendon being harvested. However, for the placement of the graft, access to the medial aspect of the patella and the region between the adductor tubercle and medial femoral epicondyle is required. This can be accomplished with a single incision or two separate smaller incisions. The orientation of the incision(s) can be longitudinal, oblique, or transverse. Oblique and transverse incisions may be associated with less sensory disturbance from injury to the prepatellar and infrapatellar branches of the saphenous nerve and may leave a more cosmetically acceptable scar. Longitudinal incisions are, however, more versatile for potential future surgical procedures.

The graft can be fixed to the patella by suturing it to the periosteum with bone anchors or by using one or two bone tunnels. If there are two strands of tendon, the fixation sites are at the superomedial corner of the patella and at or just distal to the junction of the upper and middle thirds of the medial border of the patella. If bone tunnels are used, they should be just large enough to allow passage of the graft. If two tunnels are used, the graft can be passed through one and into the other to create a sling (Fig. 64-4). Some authors believe that to reduce the risk of fracture, it is important not to breach the anterior cortex of the patella, whereas some techniques deliberately have the tunnel exit the bone anteriorly rather than laterally. Whatever the case, the reconstructed ligament should be placed in layer 2. It should lie deep to the distal end of the vastus medialis anteriorly and deep to the deep fascia more medially, superficial to the capsule of the joint.

The femoral attachment site can be referenced from the medial femoral epicondyle, 10 mm proximal and 2 mm posterior; or from the adductor tubercle, 4 mm distal and 2 mm anterior. The femoral insertion point can also be identified with fluoroscopic imaging of a true lateral view of the knee[33] (Fig. 64-5). However, a critical aspect of MPFL reconstruction is to reproduce the normal tightening of the ligament in extension and relaxation in flexion. The ligament functions as a check rein in early flexion (0 to 30 degrees) and is therefore under the greatest tension in this range of knee flexion. Excessive tension in flexion can lead to painful restriction of knee flexion and articular cartilage overload in the medial half of the patellofemoral compartment. This can mean that the ideal femoral attachment site of the reconstructed ligament needs to be adjusted rather than be based purely on bony landmarks. In techniques in which the femoral attachment is fixed before the patellar attachment, it may be

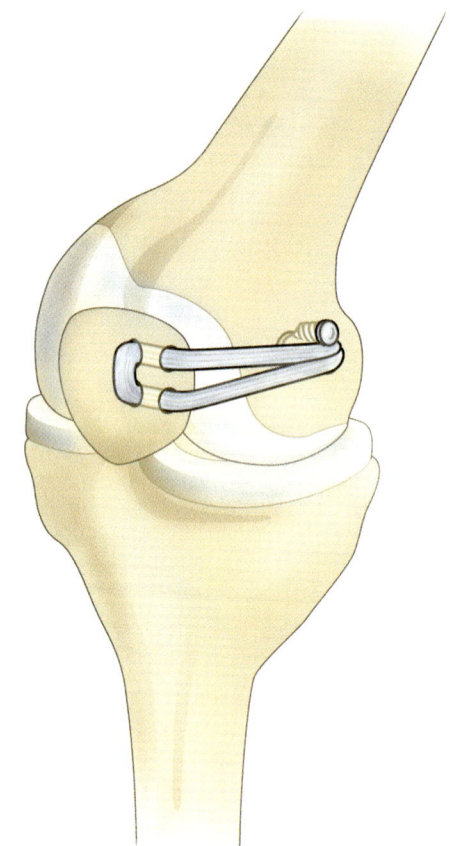

Figure 64-4. MPFL reconstruction using a gracilis tendon that is looped through two tunnels in the medial half of the patella. The tunnels exit in the midline of the patella, avoiding tunnels that pass across the full width of the bone. The femoral fixation at the adductor tubercle is by a means of an interference screw. (Courtesy M. Lind.)

necessary to lengthen the reconstructed ligament to reduce tension in deeper flexion, although this can lead to an undesirable increase in lateral laxity of the patella in early flexion.

A useful method of assessing the length-tension behavior of the planned femoral attachment site is to insert a Kirschner wire (K wire) into the planned site. The ends of the graft itself or the ends of temporary sutures or wires attached the patella are reflected around the K wire. The knee is then cycled through flexion and extension and the movement of the graft relative to the K wire is assessed to ensure that the distance between the patellar and femoral attachment sites of the graft decreases or does not change with increasing knee flexion.

The ideal tension at the time of fixation of the graft is unknown. Based on the aim of restoring a check rein in early flexion, it is logical to fix the graft with the knee at 30 to 40 degrees flexion. The patella should not be pulled medially by the reconstructed ligament but lateral translation beyond the lateral margin of the trochlear should be prevented. The tension of the graft can be adjusted to achieve this balance prior to fixation. Cycling of the knee through flexion and extension prior to fixation may help reduce subsequent creep in the construct.

As with the patella, there are many options for graft fixation to the femur. These include suture anchor fixation and

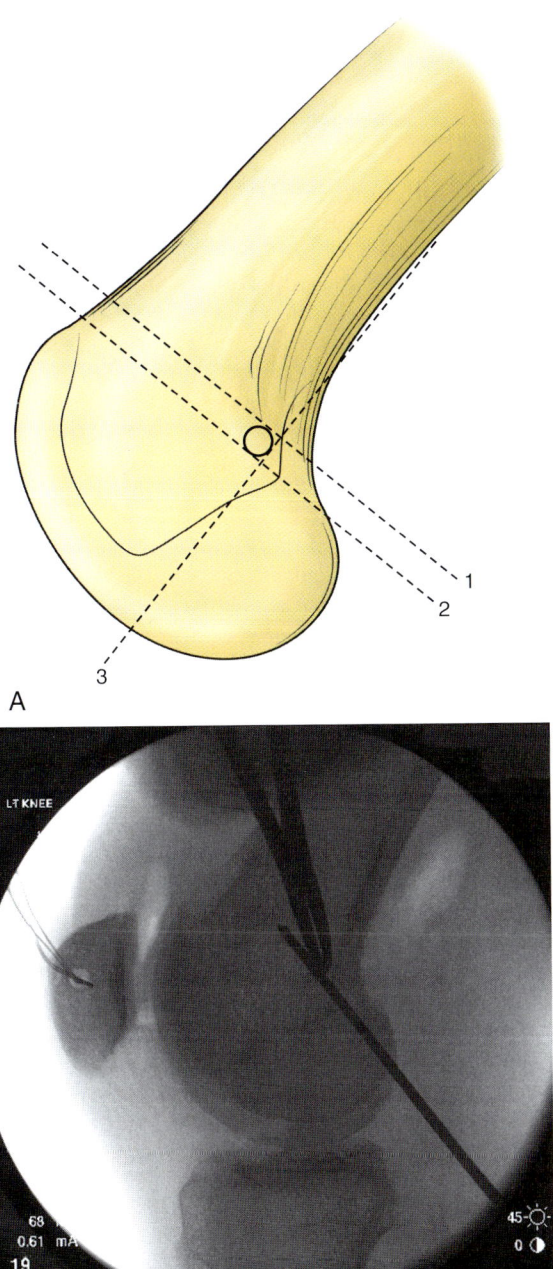

A

B LT KNEE

68
0.61 mA
19

45
0

OEC

Figure 64-5. A, Two lines are drawn perpendicular to line 3, the first intersecting the point where the margin of the medial condyle meets the posterior cortex (line 1) and the second intersecting the most posterior point of Blumensaat's line (line 2). A line is drawn extending distally from the posterior femoral cortex (line 3). A circle of 5-mm diameter is drawn contacting the line drawn from the posterior cortex. The MPFL femoral insertion should fall within this circle. **B,** A fluoroscopic intraoperative image of a knee marking the insertion point of a K wire entering the femur, identifying the position of the femoral tunnel for the MPFL reconstruction. (Courtesy E. Arendt.)

direct soft tissue fixation by looping the graft around the adductor magnus tendon or by looping it around the proximal MCL. If a bone tunnel is created, interference screw fixation is commonly used. This can be augmented or even replaced by securing the trailing ends of the tendon to the lateral side of the femur, usually by means of whipstitches in the tendon and a fixation post or button.

Procedures

Double-Strand Gracilis Autograft

This technique uses two transverse tunnels in the patella through which a gracilis tendon autograft is passed to create a double-stranded MPFL reconstruction (see Fig. 64-4). The two strands of tendon are inserted into a tunnel in the femur in the region of the adductor tubercle and fixed with an interference screw. This technique secures the graft to the patella first and makes adjustments in the length-tension relationship by adjusting the location of the femoral fixation point.

The gracilis tendon is harvested in a standard fashion through a 2- to 3-cm incision over the pes anserinus. The ends of the gracilis tendon are secured with an absorbable no. 1 whipstitch. Two transverse incisions, 2 cm in length, are made over the medial border of the patella at the junction of the upper and middle thirds of the bone and over the adductor tubercle.

Via the more anterior incision, the medial border and anterior aspect of the patella are exposed. This involves retracting the distal end of the vastus medialis muscle proximally and sharply dissecting into the attachment of the native MPFL. Two transverse tunnels, 3.5 to 4.5 mm diameter, depending on the size of the graft, are then drilled over guide wires through the patella. The two tunnels commence on the medial border of the patella, one at the superomedial corner of the bone and the other at the junction of the upper and middle thirds of the medial border. It is important to commence both tunnels in the deeper half of the medial border but care should be taken not to violate the articular surface. Both tunnels exit anteriorly in the midline of the patella. Slight divergence of the tunnels anteriorly may reduce the risk of fracture of the intervening patellar segment. A variation of this technique is to drill the patellar tunnels to exit on the lateral side of the bone (Fig. 64-6). This requires an additional exposure of the lateral aspect of the patella.[5]

The adductor tubercle of the medial femoral condyle is then identified through the more medial incision. The gracilis tendon is passed through the patellar bone tunnels using a suture-passing loop. The tendon is first passed through one tunnel from medial to lateral and then back through the other tunnel from lateral to medial. This results in two free tendon ends on the medial side of the patella (Fig. 64-7). Using a hemostat or similar clamp to create a soft tissue tunnel, these tendon ends are then passed deep to the deep fascia to the adductor tubercle, exiting through the more medially placed incision (Fig. 64-8). The path of the most anterior portion of the graft is through the anterior aspect of the vastus medialis aponeurosis.

A K wire is used to find the best point at which to commence the femoral tunnel. Initially, this is placed at the anatomic site of attachment of the MPFL, 2 mm anterior and 4 mm distal to the adductor tubercle. The tendon ends are then reflected around the K wire. The knee is taken through flexion and extension and the movement of the graft relative to the K wire is assessed. The aim is to ensure that the distance between the patellar and a femoral attachment site of the graft decreases or does not change with increasing knee flexion. The position of the K wire is adjusted until this is achieved. The K wire needs to be aimed transversely or slightly proximally to avoid the intercondylar notch. A 6- or 7-mm drill is then passed over the wire to a depth that will comfortably accommodate the free tendon ends. For ease of insertion of the tendons, the tunnel can be continued laterally through the cortex of the femur.

Using a Beath pin, the tendon ends are then passed into the femoral tunnels, with the whipstitches exiting through a small stab incision over the lateral femoral condyle. With traction applied to the whipstitches, the knee is cycled through flexion and extension to reduce subsequent creep of the construct. With the knee in 20 to 30 degrees flexion, enough traction is applied to the whipstitches to allow the patella to be laterally displaced, up to 5 mm. The graft is then fixed with an interference screw 6 or 7 mm in diameter, depending on the bone quality (see Fig. 64-4). It is important to bury the head of the screw subcortically to avoid local irritation of the soft tissues.

There are variations of this technique that avoid drilling through the anterior patellar cortex but use essentially the same attachment points of the graft. One is to use anchor fixation of a semitendinosus graft on the medial aspect of the patella and an interference screw in the medial femoral condyle[15] (Fig. 64-9). The same technique has been modified to use small-diameter biotenodesis screws in the patella instead of anchors.[32]

A similar technique is to use a gracilis graft and secure it first on the femur with a bone anchor and then to pass the free ends through two 2.5-mm very oblique (deep to superficial) tunnels in the medial border of the patella. As they exit the anterior aperture of the patellar tunnels, the tendon ends are folded back on themselves and secured with a suture technique.[17,44] If all bone tunnels are to be avoided, the patellar tunnels can be replaced with bone anchors.

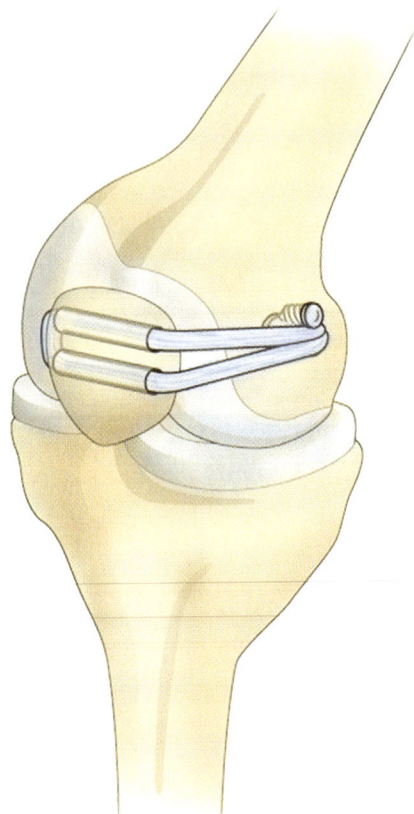

Figure 64-6. MPFL reconstruction using a free gracilis tendon that is passed through two transverse tunnels in the proximal part of the patella. The femoral fixation at the adductor tubercle is by a means of an interference screw. (From Christiansen SE, Jacobsen BW, Lund B, et al: Reconstruction of the medial patellofemoral ligament with gracilis tendon autograft in transverse patellar drill holes. Arthroscopy 24:82, 2008.)

Combined Medial Patellofemoral Ligament Repair and Medial Patellotibial Ligament Reconstruction

This technique combines reconstruction of MPFL and the MPTL. Either the semitendinosus or gracilis tendon alone or both tendons are harvested but left attached distally. The

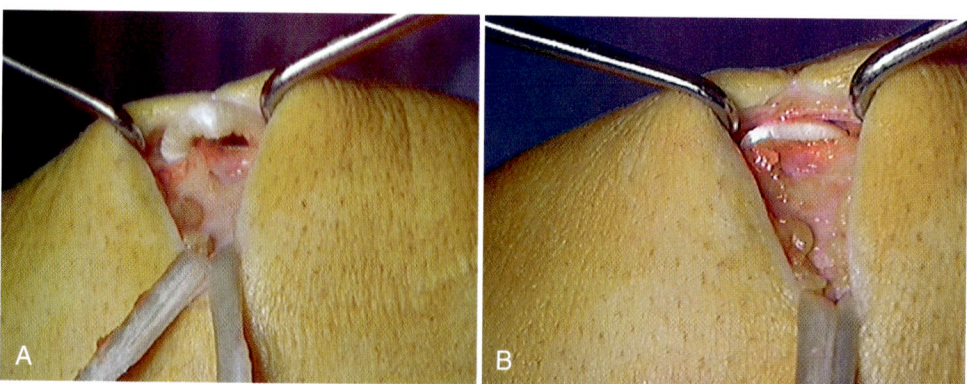

Figure 64-7. A, Photograph of the anterior incision of the right knee during MPFL reconstruction using a free gracilis tendon graft that is looped through two tunnels in the patella. The free ends of the graft can be seen at the bottom of the picture. **B,** Photograph of the anterior incision of the right knee during MPFL reconstruction using a free gracilis tendon graft that is looped through two tunnels in the patella. The loop of tendon has been snugged down onto the anterior aspect of the patella. (Courtesy J. Feller.)

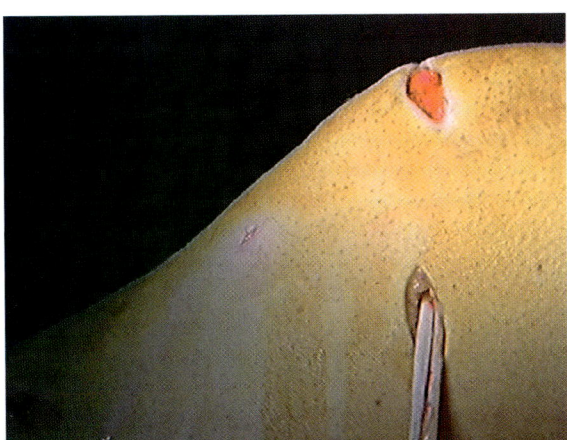

Figure 64-8. Photograph of the medial aspect of the right knee during MPFL reconstruction using a free gracilis tendon graft that is looped through two tunnels in the patella. The free ends of the graft have been passed medially deep to the deep fascia to exit through the more medial wound before being passed into a tunnel in the femur. (Courtesy J. Feller.)

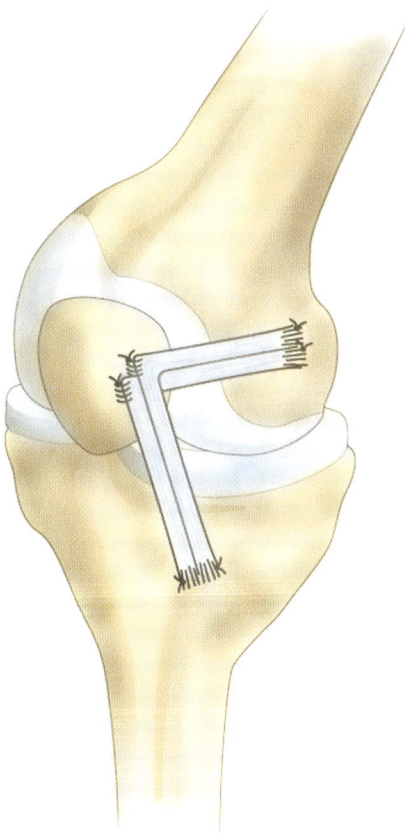

Figure 64-10. Technique that combines reconstruction of the MPFL with reconstruction of the medial patellotibial ligament. The semitendinosus and gracilis tendons are sutured to the medial border of the patella and medial femoral condyle. The distal limb of the tendon grafts is sutured to the proximal medial tibial periosteum to reconstruct the medial patellotibial ligament. (From Acta Orthop Scand.)

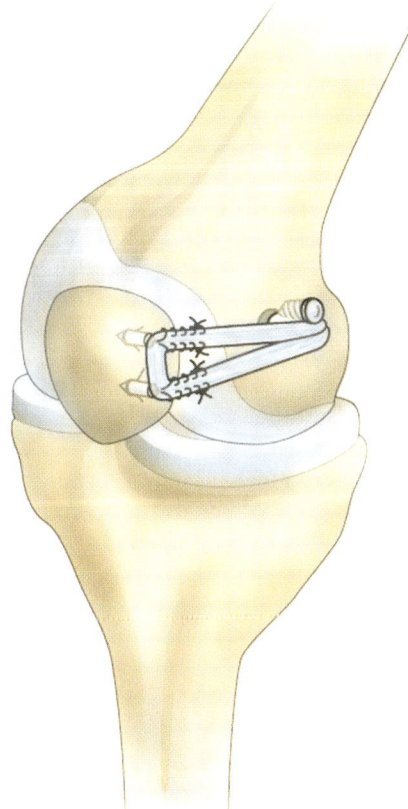

Figure 64-9. MPFL reconstruction that avoids creating tunnels in the patella by using anchor fixation of the free tendon graft to the medial aspect of the patella, combined with interference screw fixation of the graft to the medial femoral condyle. (From Acta Orthop Scand.)

suture the distal end to the tibial periosteum approximately 1.5 cm distal to the joint line[11,26] (Fig. 64-10). The disadvantage of this technique is that one must tension two arms of the graft in an attempt to duplicate both the MPFL and MPTL. Little is known about the length-tension characteristics of the MPTL.

Single-Strand Middle Third Quadriceps Tendon Autograft

An alternative graft is the central portion of the quadriceps tendon.[38] A 5-cm midline incision is made over the distal quadriceps tendon and another 2-cm vertical incision is made over the medial femoral condyle. A 10- to 11-cm-long and 10-mm-wide graft is harvested. Only half the thickness of the tendon needs to be harvested. The distal end of the graft is left attached to the patella. The released tendon is reflected 90 degrees toward the medial condyle and is passed subcutaneously to the MPFL attachment site on the medial femoral condyle (Fig. 64-11). It can be fixed by any of the techniques already described. The disadvantage of this technique is that one cannot always predict the length of the tendon able to be harvested, which may compromise the femoral fixation point. Typically, a longer anterior incision than with other techniques is required to harvest the distal quadriceps tendon.

graft is then passed to the medial border of the patella, where it is passed through a bone tunnel or sutured to periosteum before being passed in layer 2 to the standard attachment point on the femur. Here it can be fixed by any of the methods already described. A variation is to use a free graft and to

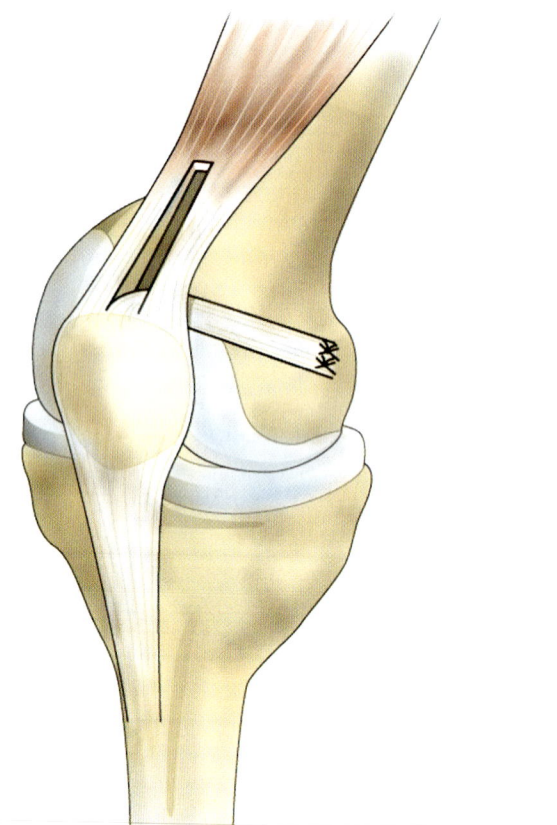

Figure 64-11. MPFL reconstruction using the central portion of the quadriceps tendon. The tendon is released proximally and the patellar insertion left intact. The tendon flap is passed subcutaneously to the medial femoral condyle. (From Acta Orthop Scand.)

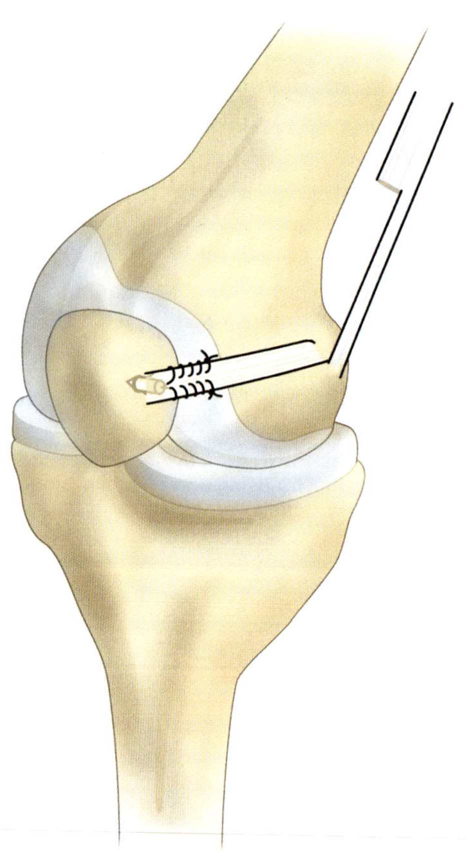

Figure 64-12. MPFL reconstruction using the anterior two thirds of the adductor tendon. The tendon is released proximally and the femoral insertion left intact. The tendon flap is passed subcutaneously to the proximal patellar edge. (Courtesy M. Lind.)

Single-Strand Adductor Magnus Split Tendon Transfer

This technique uses an adductor magnus tendon autograft left attached to the femur.[34] A 3- to 4-cm skin incision is made between the adductor tubercle and proximal half of the patella. The adductor magnus tendon is exposed and split at the junction of its middle and posterior thirds. The split is continued proximally with a tendon harvester to a length of 12 to 14 cm, where the anterior two thirds are released. The free end of the graft is passed through a soft tissue tunnel created in layer 2, deep to the distal part of vastus medialis and superficial to the joint capsule. The graft is then fixed with two suture anchors to the superomedial aspect of the patella, with the knee in 30 degrees flexion (Fig. 64-12). The disadvantage of this technique is also that one cannot always predict the length of the tendon able to be harvested, which may compromise the ultimate patellar fixation.

Adductor Sling Technique

A 2- to 3-cm incision is made along the medial border of the patella. A K wire is passed transversely through the patella from medial to lateral, starting at the junction of upper and middle thirds of the patella and exiting at the lateral border of the patella, passing through a small stab incision in the skin. This K wire is overdrilled with a 4.0- or 4.5-mm cannulated reamer to a depth of 10 to 15 mm, 10 mm for a small

patella (less than 35 mm in width) and 15 mm for most patellae.

A looped passer is used to pass a single-strand gracilis graft through the patella from medial to lateral using the ends of a whipstitch in the graft. The graft is secured on the lateral side using the two ends of the whipstitch. One limb of the stitch is passed through the lateral retinaculum with a free needle. It is then tied to the other limb. On the medial side of the patella, a cuff of medial retinaculum is sutured to the graft as it exits the medial border.

The adductor magnus tendon is approached through a separate 3-cm-long incision that extends proximally from a point slightly superior and posterior to the medial femoral epicondyle. The adductor magnus tendon is identified; it can often be palpated before it can be seen. Dissection of the distal tendon insertion includes freeing all interdigitations of the tendon down to its insertion to allow the graft subsequently to lie as distal as possible, approaching the MPFL's anatomic insertion.

The free end of the graft is passed medially from the patella, deep to the deep fascia. It is then passed distal to the adductor tubercle and reflected proximally around and deep to distal adductor magnus tendon. From here, the free end of the graft is passed anteriorly, again deep to the deep fascia, to reach the midpoint of the medial aspect of the patella. The knee is flexed to 30 to 40 degrees, locating the patella in the trochlear groove. The graft is tensioned just enough to

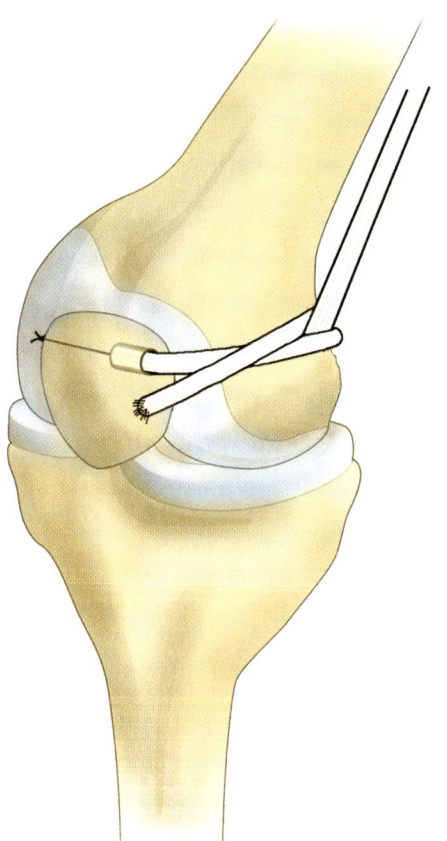

Figure 64-13. MPFL reconstruction using the free semitendinosus and gracilis tendons looped around the adductor magnus femoral insertion and fixed to the patella via a short tunnel proximally and a direct suturing to the middle third of the patella. (Courtesy M. Lind.)

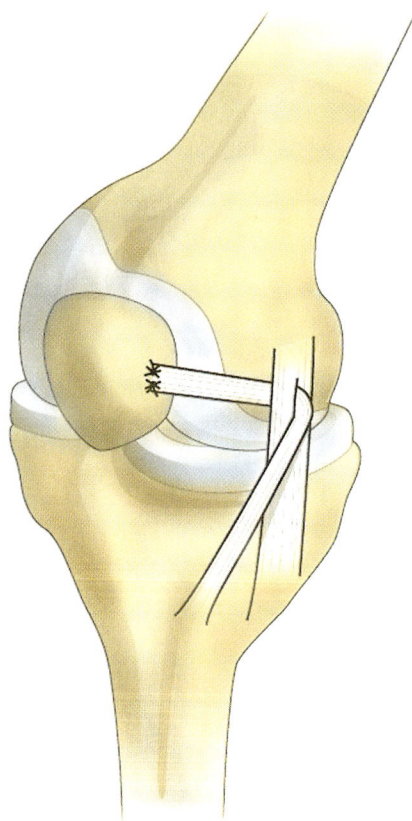

Figure 64-14. MPFL reconstruction using the semitendinosus tendon and soft tissue fixation. The tendon insertion is retained and the proximal end of the tendon is transferred to the femoral insertion of the medial collateral ligament (MCL). The graft is passed through a split in the proximal MCL and then sutured to the medial aspect of the patella. (From Lind M, Jakobsen BW, Lund B, et al: Reconstruction of the medial patello-femerol ligament; a new treatment for chronic patella instability. Acta Orthop Scand 79:354–360, 2008.)

eliminate redundancy in the graft. Where the two arms of the graft pass over one another, just anterior to the adductor insertion, a single stitch is used to secure them to each other. Finally, the free end of the graft is sutured to the periosteum over the middle third of the medial border of the patella (Fig. 64-13).

Medial Collateral Ligament Sling Technique

This technique uses a semitendinosus autograft tendon to reconstruct the MPFL[8] (Fig. 64-14). The tendon is harvested and the tibial attachment at the pes anserinus is retained. The proximal end of the tendon is transferred to the femoral insertion of the medial collateral ligament.

A 2-cm incision is made over the medial femoral epicondyle and a short longitudinal split is made in the posterior third of the proximal end of the medial collateral ligament. This split subsequently acts as a pulley through which the free end of the semitendinosus graft is passed. The free end of the graft is then passed to the anteromedial aspect of the patella. The transferred tendon is sutured to the anterior surface of the patella with the knee flexed to 30 degrees. The criticism of this technique is that it places the femoral insertion of the MPFL lower than its anatomic location. In addition, the more vertical arm does not anatomically duplicate the MPTL.

REHABILITATION AFTER MEDIAL PATELLOFEMORAL LIGAMENT REPAIR RECONSTRUCTION

As with MPFL repair, there is at present no evidence that supports any specific postoperative rehabilitation regimen after MPFL reconstruction. Most of the published series have described a period of restricted range of motion using a knee immobilizer or a hinged brace for from 2 to 6 weeks. Typically, the range of motion is limited to 0 to 60 degrees, although the rationale for this is not entirely clear, given that the reconstruction should be under maximum tension in early knee flexion. Weight-bearing status also varies considerably in the published series, ranging from minimal to full weight bearing.

Using interference screw femoral fixation of a gracilis tendon graft that has been looped through two patellar bone tunnels, we have not experienced problems with a less restrictive regimen, in which a full range of motion and full weight bearing are allowed within the limits of comfort. However, if direct soft tissue fixation is used, some limitation of range of motion and reduced weight bearing may be appropriate until sufficient healing can be expected to have taken place.

With regard to a return to sports activities, it is suggested that closed kinetic chain quadriceps strengthening be introduced from between 3 and 6 weeks and controlled open kinetic strengthening from 3 months. This is followed by a return to noncontact sports, with a resumption of contact sports being considered from 4 to 6 months, depending on individual strength, agility, and confidence.

SKELETALLY IMMATURE PATIENTS

In the skeletally immature, it is preferable not to create bone tunnels or dissect the periosteum in the region of the distal femoral physeal plate. This may require a modification of the femoral fixation method used. Some of the techniques described are suitable for patients with open growth plates. These include the adductor magnus tendon transfer, adductor sling technique, and medial collateral ligament sling technique. The combined MPFL and MPTL reconstruction can also be safely used, provided appropriate fixation is used at the femoral attachment.

COMPLICATIONS

As with all surgical procedures, there are nonspecific complications such as infection and hematoma formation, as well complications such as the morbidity of harvesting a tendon autograft and sensory disturbances related to the location of incisions. In particular, the prepatellar and infrapatellar branches of the saphenous nerve can be damaged, with resultant alteration of sensation over the anterior aspect of the knee and proximal leg.[25,31] Another issue relating to the incisions is the potential for widened and unsightly scars on the medial aspect of the knee.[11]

Complications related specifically to the reconstructive procedure include recurrent lateral patellar dislocation, pain and stiffness, and patellar fracture. The rate of redislocation can be affected not only by the surgical technique, but also by the presence of predisposing factors such as patellar alta, trochlear dysplasia, and lateralization of the tibial tuberosity, as well as the overall alignment of the lower limb.

Pain and stiffness can have a number of causes. They may be transient and simply to the result of surgical intervention on the highly innervated medial aspect of the knee.[1,25] Painful restriction in the immediate postoperative period may lead to adhesion formation and a persisting loss of flexion,[11,44] which may occasionally require manipulation under anesthesia to restore a satisfactory range of motion.[4,31] Prominence of fixation hardware on the medial aspect of the medial femoral condyle may also cause local irritation and potentially restrict motion.[7,28,39,40] Even in the absence of prominent hardware, a tunnel in the medial femoral condyle can be a source of ongoing pain. Pain and stiffness may also relate to underlying damage to the articular surfaces of the patellofemoral compartment. As noted, all injuries to the knee need to be addressed, not just the deficient MPFL.

From a surgical point of view, an important cause of postoperative pain and/or stiffness is inappropriate positioning of the graft.[15,43] A graft that is positioned so that it is tighter in flexion than extension can cause anteromedial pain and a restriction of flexion as well as an increase in the force on the articular surface of the medial half of the patellofemoral compartment as the knee moves into greater flexion.[12] Overtensioning the graft will exacerbate these problems.

Patellar fracture is uncommon but usually relates to the use of bone tunnels for graft positioning and attachment.[44] Excessively large tunnels may increase the risk of fracture.[22] Some authors believe that penetration of the anterior cortex of the bone may also increase the risk.[4] When a transverse tunnel is used, a displaced transverse fracture of the patella may occur, a disabling complication. For those techniques using tunnels that breach the anterior cortex, the fracture is typically an oblique or vertical fracture of the medial border of the patella.

SUPPLEMENTARY SURGICAL PROCEDURES

In the presence of predisposing factors such as trochlear dysplasia, patella alta, and an increased tibial tuberosity–trochlear groove distance, additional procedures may be undertaken to help stabilize the patella. Despite various published protocols, at present there is no evidence to indicate when a supplementary procedure should be performed in conjunction with an MPFL reconstruction. It should, however, be kept in mind that a successful MPFL reconstruction effectively restores the stabilizing anatomy of the individual back to the predislocation state. The decision to use one or more supplementary procedures needs to be based on the perceived risk of further challenges to patellar stability in a given individual.

CLINICAL RESULTS

Reconstruction of the MPFL is a relatively new surgical solution for recurrent lateral patellar dislocation. There have been no level 1 or level 2 studies that report the outcome of this type of surgery. The evidence for clinical outcome results after MPFL reconstruction is based purely on level IV case series of up to 50 patients, and with up to 4 years follow-up. Moreover, a variety of clinical outcome tools and follow-up examination parameters have been used, making comparison among studies difficult. The published studies that present clinical outcomes in more than 20 patients are summarized in Table 64-1.

In general, MPFL reconstruction results in very good patellar stability, with no redislocations in seven of nine studies and a less than 5% redislocation rate in two studies. The incidence of further episodes of patellar subluxation, as opposed to dislocation, has been inconsistently reported and no conclusions can be drawn about this entity. This is in part also to the result of the lack of consistency in terminology and clinical assessment of patellar subluxation.

Success rates based on clinical scores have generally been good, with increases in Kujala scores from approximately 50 to 90 and Lysholm scores to more than 90. The Crosby-Insall scores reported in earlier studies also showed promising results, with approximately 90% of patients having good or excellent results. Although a variety of operative techniques and graft choices have been evaluated, graft type and surgical technique do not seem to have influenced the clinical results. Several studies did, however, demonstrate poorer clinical outcome in patients with patellofemoral articular cartilage lesions at the time of surgery.

Table 64-1 Results from Clinical Studies of Medial Patellofemoral Ligament Reconstruction

Study (Year)	Graft Technique	Fixation Methods	N	Follow-up (Yr)	Redislocation Rate (%)	Clinical Outcome Tool and Mean Score
Ellera Gomes (1992)[13]	Synthetic ligament	Patella—bone tunnel Femur—metal screw	30	3.25	0	Crosby-Insall, 84% good-excellent; poorer results with articular cartilage damage
Nomura and Inoue (2003)[29]	Synthetic ligament	Patella—bone tunnel Femur—staple	27	5-9	4	Crosby-Insall, 96% good-excellent
Deie et al (2005)[8]	Semitendinosus; concomitant tibial tuberosity transfer, lateral release and VMO advancement	Patella—sutures Femur—sutures	39	5	0	Kujala, 92
Steiner et al (2006)[40]	Adductor magnus	Patella—bone tunnel Femur—sutures	34	2-10	0	Kujala, 90
Mikashima et al (2006)[23]	Semitendinosus	Patella—suture, bone tunnels Femur—screw	24	2	0	No difference between suture and tunnel fixation at the patella
Watanabe et al (2008)[47]	Semitendinosus; concomitant tibial tuberosity transfer	Patella—sutures Femur—EndoButton	42	4.3	Not provided	Lysholm, 92 (without tibial tuberosity transfer); 90 (with tibial tuberosity transfer)
Christiansen et al (2008)[4,5]	Gracilis	Patella—bone tunnels Femur—IF screw	45	2	2	Kujala, 86

CONCLUSIONS

In general terms, there are three surgical approaches to the restoration of function of the MPFL:

1. Acute repair. At this time the literature yields a mixed picture of results. Using redislocation rate as an end point, the literature does not support acute MPFL repair as a best practice option. However, in the setting of a surgical intervention to stabilize an osteochondral fracture of the patella or trochlea, MRI localization of the site of an MPFL tear that may be amenable to repair seems prudent. A decision regarding repair can then be made at the time of surgery.

2. Delayed tightening of the MPFL (for chronic laxity). This is not recommended as a best practice option at this time.

3. Reconstruction of MPFL with graft. This has been shown to produce the most consistent results, even in the presence of risk factors. There is currently no consensus regarding which surgical technique provides the best clinical results. Graft and technique choice do not seem to influence the clinical results, as long as key surgical principles are followed.

KEY REFERENCES

Christiansen SE, Jakobsen BW, Lund B, et al: Isolated repair of the medial patellofemoral ligament in primary dislocation of the patella: a prospective randomized study. Arthroscopy 24:881, 2008.

Conlan T, Garth WP, Lemons JE: Evaluation of the medial soft-tissue restraints of the extensor mechanism of the knee. J Bone Joint Surg Am 75:682, 1993.

Elias JJ, Cosgarea AJ: Technical errors during medial patellofemoral ligament reconstruction could overload the medial patellofemoral cartilage: a computational analysis. Am J Sports Med 34:1478, 2006.

Farr J, Schepsis AA: Reconstruction of the medial patellofemoral ligament for recurrent patellar instability. J Knee Surg 19:307, 2006.

Feller JA, Amis AA, Andrish JT, et al: Surgical biomechanics of the patellofemoral joint. Arthroscopy 23:542, 2007.

Fithian DC, Gupta N: Patellar instability: principles of soft tissue repair and reconstruction. Tech Knee Surg 5:19, 2006.

Hautamaa PV, Fithian DC, Pohlmeyer AM, et al: The medial soft tissue restraints in lateral patellar instability and repair. Clin Orthop Relat Res 349:174, 1998.

Lind M, Jakobsen BW, Lund B, et al: Reconstruction of the medial patellofemoral ligament for treatment of patellar instability. Acta Orthop 79:354, 2008.

Mountney J, Senavongse W, Amis AA, et al: Tensile strength of the medial patellofemoral ligament before and after repair or reconstruction. J Bone Joint Surg Br 87:36, 2005.

Nomura E, Inoue M, Osada N: Anatomical analysis of the medial patellofemoral ligament of the knee, especially the femoral attachment. Knee Surg Sports Traumatol Arthrosc 13:510, 2005.

Schottle PB, Schmeling A, Rosenstiel N, et al: Radiographic landmarks for femoral tunnel placement in medial patellofemoral ligament reconstruction. Am J Sports Med 35:801, 2007.

Sillanpaa PJ, Peltola E, Mattila VM, et al: Femoral avulsion of the medial patellofemoral ligament after primary traumatic patellar dislocation predicts subsequent instability in men: a mean 7-year nonoperative follow-up study. Am J Sports Med 37:1513, 2009.

Steiner TM, Torga-Spak R, Teitge RA: Medial patellofemoral ligament reconstruction in patients with lateral patellar instability and trochlear dysplasia. Am J Sports Med 34:1254, 2006.

Tecklenburg K, Dejour D, Hoser C, et al: Bony and cartilaginous anatomy of the patellofemoral joint. Knee Surg Sports Traumatol Arthrosc 14:235, 2006.

Warren RF, Marshall JL: The supporting structures and layers on the medial side of the knee. J Bone Joint Surg Am 61:56, 1979.

Full references for this chapter can be found on www.expertconsult.com.

Chapter 65

Sulcus-Deepening Trochleoplasty

David DeJour and Paulo R. F. Saggin

NORMAL AND PATHOLOGIC ANATOMY

The normal trochlea is located in the anterior aspect of the distal femur. It is composed of two facets divided by a longitudinal groove, the trochlear sulcus. The lateral facet is the largest; it extends more proximally than the medial one, and is more protuberant in the anteroposterior aspect (also referred to as higher). Proximally, the trochlea extends until the junction of the articular cartilage with the femoral anterior cortex, which is covered by adipose tissue and synovium. Distally, it is limited by the condylotrochlear grooves, one in each division of the facets with the correspondent femoral condyle. The trochlear groove extends distally and slightly laterally from the femoral axis.[16]

Dysplastic trochleae are shallow, flat, or even convex. It is easier to consider and define their abnormality in terms of function or deviation from the normal pattern. Radiologic features are also easier to define and measure than those observed during surgical procedures. It is common sense, however, that the surgical mark of these trochleae is their abnormal shape. A bump in the superolateral aspect is common (Fig. 65-1).

Radiographic lateral projections of normal trochleae, obtained with perfect superimposition of both femoral condyles, will typically show the contour of the facets and, posterior to them, the line representing the deepest points of the sulcus.[11,12] The lateral facet is distinguished from the medial one by its more visible condylotrochlear groove and by the greater opacity to the rays of the lateral condyle, which is more perpendicular than the medial one to the x-ray beam in the lateral projection. The line representing the bottom of the groove is continuous with the intercondylar notch line, and extends anteriorly and proximally. It may end posteriorly to the condyle line (type A) or join the medial condyle line in the superior part of the trochlea (type B).[7]

On lateral projections, trochlear dysplasia is defined by the crossing sign, where the radiographic line of the trochlear sulcus crosses (or reaches) the projection of the femoral condyles. The crossing point represents the exact location at which the floor of the trochlear sulcus reaches the same height as that of the femoral condyles, meaning that the trochlea becomes flat in this exact location. The position of the trochlear sulcus floor is also abnormal in relation to the anterior femoral cortex. Although in normal knees it is usually at a mean distance of 0.8 mm posterior to a line tangent to the anterior femoral cortex, in knees with dysplastic trochlea its mean position is 3.2 mm in front of this same line[8] (Fig. 65-2).

Two other features are typical of dysplastic trochleae in lateral views, the supratrochlear spur and the double-contour sign. The supratrochlear spur is the same as

sometimes visualized during surgical exposure located in the superolateral aspect. It corresponds to an attempt at containing the lateral displacement of the patella. The double contour represents the medial hypoplastic facet, seen posterior to the lateral one in this projection. Based on these signs, trochlear dysplasia may be classified into four types[6,18]:

- Type A: Presence of crossing sign in the true lateral view. The trochlea is shallower than normal, but still symmetrical and concave.
- Type B: Crossing sign and trochlear spur. The trochlea is flat or convex in axial images.
- Type C: There is the presence of crossing sign and, in addition, the double-contour sign can be found on the lateral view, representing the medial hypoplastic facet. There is no spur and, in axial views, the lateral facet is convex and the medial hypoplastic.
- Type D: Combines all the mentioned signs—crossing sign, supratrochlear spur, and double-contour sign. In the axial view, there is clear asymmetry of the facet's height, also referred as a cliff pattern (Fig. 65-3).

Axial views obtained at 45 degrees (Merchant view) will allow the measurement of the sulcus angle. From the point of the bottom of the groove, two lines are drawn, connecting it with the most superior point of each facet. The mean normal value defined by Merchant was 138 degrees (standard deviation [SD] ± 6), and angles superior to 150 degrees are considered abnormal. Dysplastic trochleae will show higher angles, some of which cannot be measured because there is no sulcus. Alternatively, 30-degree flexion axial views will provide those measurements with better trochlear shape assessment.[5] The subjective impression of the trochlear shape is important and should be taken in no more than 45 degrees of knee flexion. Greater flexion angles show the lower part of the trochlea, which is more normal. Finally, any signs of patellar instability, such as those evidenced in other projections and with other methods, serve as clues to the dysplasia diagnosis, because 96% of patients with a true patellar dislocation will present with it.[8]

The computed tomography (CT) scan will aid in visualizing the axial views. Three-dimensional reconstruction can also be obtained for global shape assessment. Magnetic resonance imaging (MRI) is another modality in which dysplasia is well documented. The cartilaginous shape of the sulcus can be evaluated; this is particularly interesting because the cartilaginous anatomy does not follow the underlying bony anatomy exactly.[17] In dysplastic trochleae, however, bony and cartilaginous anatomies do match. Another interesting point of view is demonstrated by condylar and sulcus height measurements from the posterior condyles in axial views: the lateral facet seems to have a normal height, whereas the groove and medial facet are protuberant.[4]

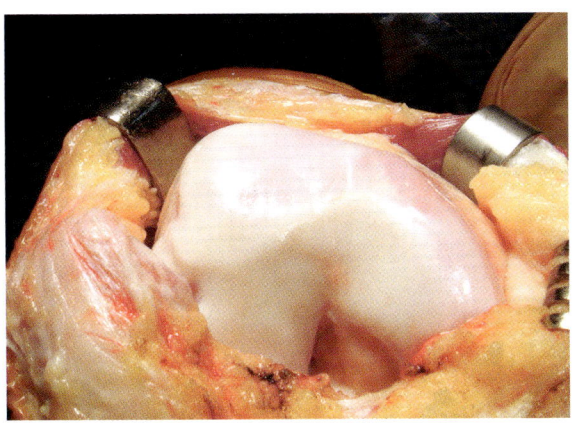

Figure 65-1. High-grade trochlear dysplasia (anterior view of a right knee). There is no sulcus and in the lateral aspect *(right)* a big bump can be observed.

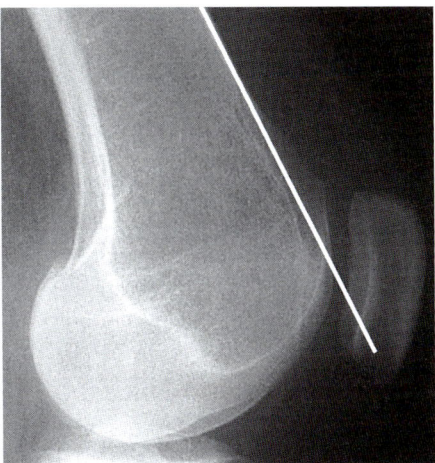

Figure 65-2. The trochlear bump is calculated as the amount of trochlea that is in front of a line parallel to the anterior femoral cortex. Alternatively, the sulcus floor position can also be calculated from this line.

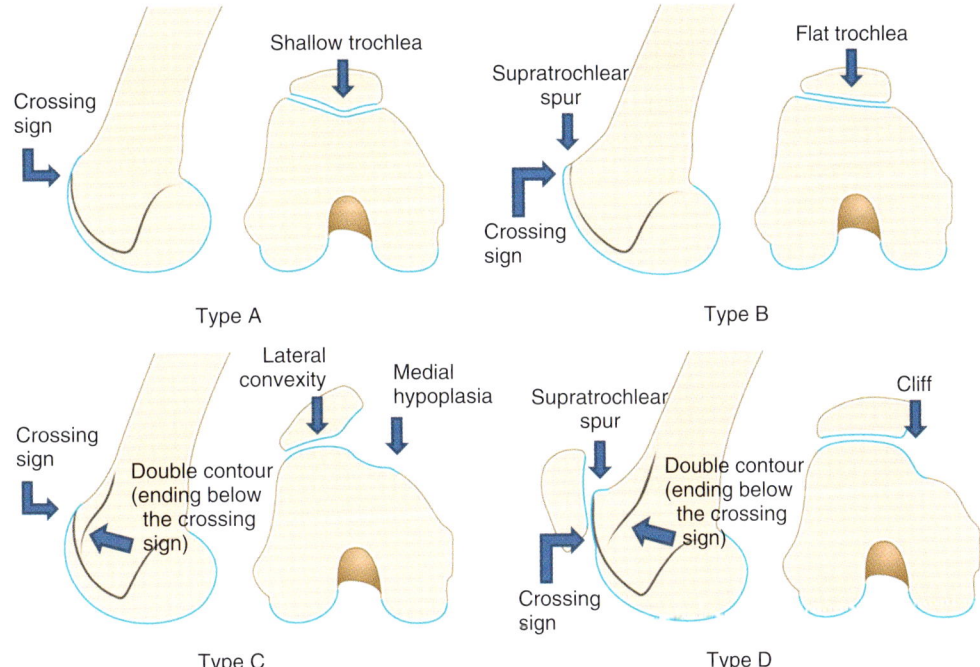

Figure 65-3. Trochlear dysplasia according to the senior author (DD). Trochlear dysplasia, *type A,* with the crossing sign in the lateral view. The trochlea is shallower than normal, but still symmetrical and concave. Trochlear dysplasia, *type B,* with the crossing sign and trochlear spur. The trochlea is flat on axial images, with prominence of all of the trochlea. Trochlear dysplasia, *type C,* with the crossing sign and double-contour sign on the lateral view. There is no prominence and, in axial views, the lateral facet is convex and the medial is hypoplastic. Trochlear dysplasia, *type D,* with the crossing sign, supratrochlear spur, and double-contour sign. In the axial view, there is clear asymmetry of the height of the facets, also referred to as a cliff pattern.

FUNCTION AND BIOMECHANICS

To understand the principles of modifying trochlear shape, its function must be well understood. The lateral facet of the trochlea is oriented obliquely in both the sagittal and coronal planes. It deviates anteriorly and laterally from the bottom of the groove. The articulating opposed lateral patellar surface follows this orientation. The patella rests in front of the femoral cortex in total extension, but engages the trochlea in early flexion. A posteriorly directed force, the patellofemoral reaction force, pushes the patella against the trochlea and, as a result of the articulating surfaces' configuration a medial vector is created, directing patellar tracking.[2]

From this brief biomechanical explanation, one conclusion is obvious—the trochlea guides patellar tracking. Not only is patellar subluxation or lateral displacement dependent on trochlear shape, but also patellar tilt. There is a high statistical correlation between patellar tilt and the type of trochlear dysplasia.[18] The higher the degree of dysplasia, the higher the patellar tilt.

Another feature not included in trochlear function but derived from the same principle is that the patellofemoral reaction force depends on the trochlear prominence. The bigger the trochlear prominence, the greater the reaction force. Inversely, by diminishing the protrusion, the reaction force is also expected to be diminished.

INDICATIONS

Trochleoplasty indications are precise—high-grade trochlear dysplasia with patellar instability and/or abnormal patellar tracking in the absence of established osteoarthritis, which would otherwise indicate a patellofemoral arthroplasty. Open growth plates are a contraindication to trochleoplasty.

The type of dysplasia should be observed when determining the procedure, because not all procedures fit all deformities. Types B and D are the most suitable to deepening trochleoplasty. Lateral facet elevating trochleoplasty is proposed by some authors and, although no consensus of indication exists, type C dysplasia would be the best candidate for this.

Type A dysplasia, in our opinion, does not fit any procedure. It is also not considered severe trochlear dysplasia. Major instability or maltracking, if present, should be attributed to other anatomic abnormalities (e.g., tibial tubercle–trochlear groove distance [TT-TG], patellar tilt, patella alta).

The degree of instability should also be taken into account. Trochleoplasty, like any other surgical procedure, is liable to failure. This should be known when discussing the procedure with the patient with mild symptoms and when no conservative treatment has yet been proposed.

As important as a precise indication, the evaluation and correction of associated abnormalities have to be accomplished. No procedure will be successful if there are other important issues neglected. The TT-TG should be assessed preoperatively. Its correction is not always necessary because the trochleoplasty procedure lateralizes the groove, thus diminishing the TT-TG. The sulcus-deepening trochleoplasty is only one of several specific procedures for addressing each of the main factors in patellar instability.

PROCEDURES AND OPTIONS

Three main techniques are described.

Lateral Facet–Elevating Trochleoplasty

This procedure was pioneered by Albee in 1915.[1] It consists of an oblique osteotomy under the lateral facet, where a corticocancellous bone wedge is interposed, with the apex medial and the base lateral. The osteotomy advances to the base of the trochlear groove, but does not disrupt it, producing a hinge in its medial aspect. The result is that it elevates the more lateral aspect of the trochlear lateral facet and also increases its obliquity, thus increasing the containment force acting on the patella. At least 5 mm of subchondral bone should be maintained to avoid trochlear necrosis (Fig. 65-4).

It is effective for patellar containment, but at the same time it increases the patellofemoral reaction force when it increases the trochlear protuberance. Pain and arthritis may result from this.

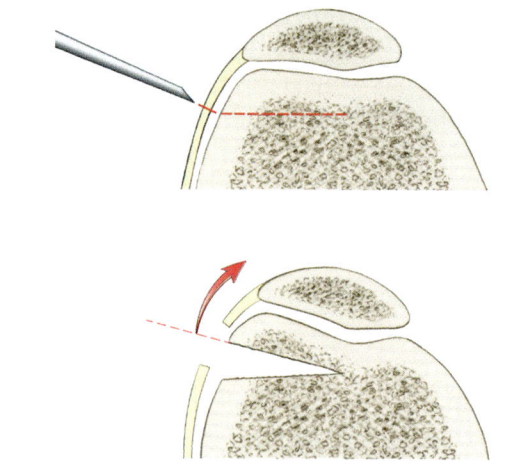

Figure 65-4. Albee's lateral facet–elevating trochleoplasty. The osteotomy is performed under the lateral facet. The medial osteochondral hinge is preserved intact and subsequent grafting under the flap will increase the lateral facet height.

Sulcus-Deepening Trochleoplasty

This procedure was first described by Masse in 1978[13]; it was modified and standardized by Dejour and colleagues in 1987.[7] The main goal is to decrease the prominence of the trochlea and create a new groove with a normal depth. This procedure is technically more demanding than a lateral facet–elevating trochleoplasty, but is more anatomic and it acts on the essential cause of the problem. It has the advantage of treating the cause of the dislocation by correcting the abnormal patterns underlying the different grades of trochlear dysplasia.

The procedure can be performed under regional anesthesia and with patient sedation. The patient is positioned supine. The entire extremity is prepared and draped, and the incision is performed with the extremity flexed to 90 degrees. A straight midline skin incision is carried out from the superior patellar margin to the tibiofemoral articulation. The extremity is then positioned in extension and a medial full-thickness skin flap is developed. The arthrotomy is performed through a mid–vastus-adapted approach: medial retinaculum sharp dissection starting over the 1- to 2-cm medial border of the patella and blunt dissection of vastus medialis oblique (VMO) fibers starting distally at the superomedial pole of the patella, extending approximately 4 cm into the muscle belly (Fig. 65-5).

The patella is briefly everted for inspection of chondral injuries and proper treatment (flap resection, microfracture, autologous chondrocyte implantation), if needed, and then retracted laterally. The trochlea is exposed and the peritrochlear synovium and periosteum are incised along their osteochondral junction and reflected from the field using a periosteal elevator (Fig. 65-6). The anterior femoral cortex should be visible to determine the amount of deepening. Changing the knee degree of flexion allows a better view of the complete operative field and avoids extending the incision.

Once the trochlea is fully exposed, the new one is planned and drawn with a sterile pen. The new trochlear groove is marked, using the intercondylar notch as a starting point. From there, a straight line representing it is directed proximally and 3 to 6 degrees laterally. The superior limit is the

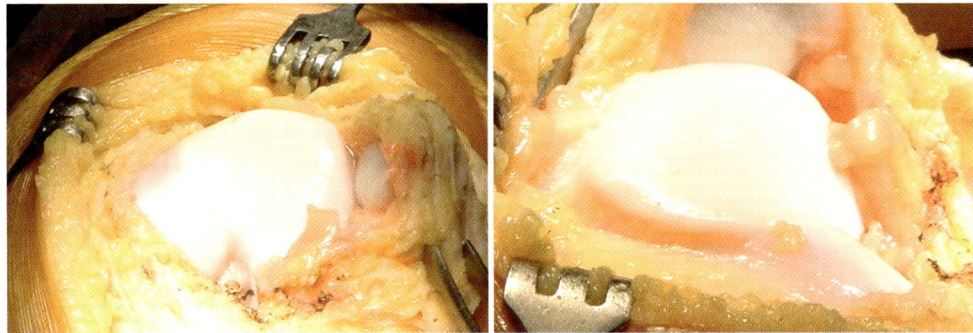

Figure 65-5. Trochlear dysplasia. Anterior *(left)* and lateral *(right)* views during surgical exposure show the absence of the sulcus and the prominence of the trochlea in relation to the anterior femoral cortex.

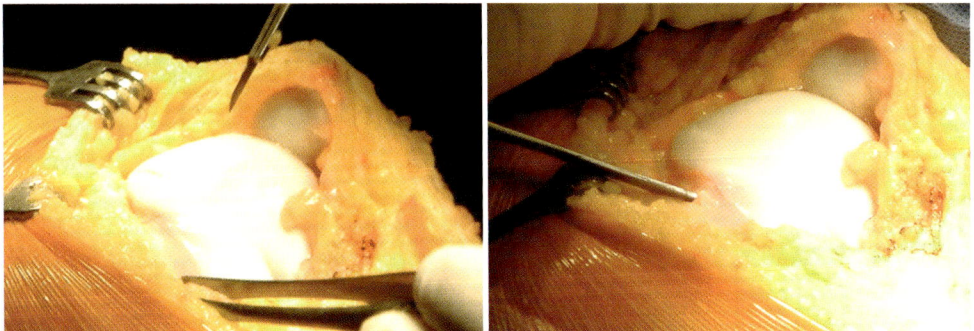

Figure 65-6. Surgical exposure. The periosteum is incised along the osteochondral edge and reflected away from the trochlear margin. The anterior femoral cortex should be visible to guide the bone resection.

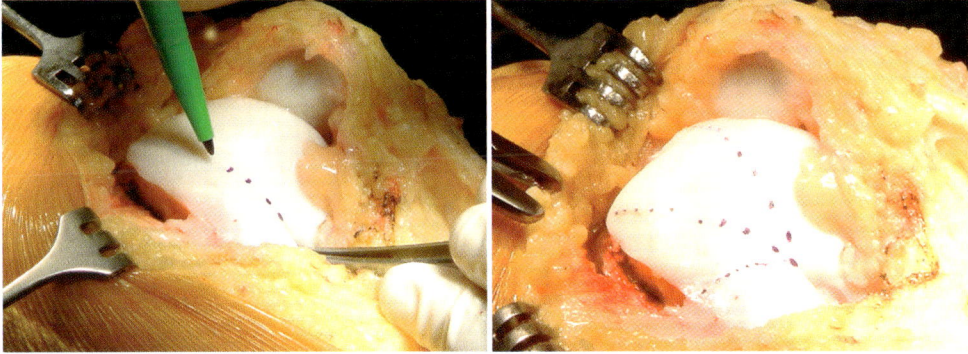

Figure 65-7. After the surgical exposure, the new trochlea is drawn. From the intercondylar notch, the bottom of the sulcus and facets are planned.

osteochondral edge. Two divergent lines are also drawn, starting at the notch and going proximally through the condylotrochlear grooves (sulcus terminalis), representing the lateral and medial facet limits. They should not enter the tibiofemoral articulation (Fig. 65-7).

The next step is accessing the undersurface of the femoral trochlea. For this purpose, a thin strip of cortical bone is removed all around the trochlea. The width of the strip is equal to the prominence of the trochlea from the anterior femoral cortex—that is, the bump formed. A sharp osteotome is used and gently tapped. A rongeur is used next to remove the bone.

Subsequently, cancellous bone must be removed from the undersurface of the trochlea. A drill with a depth guide set at 5 mm is used to ensure uniform thickness of the osteochondral flap, thus maintaining an adequate amount of bone

attached to the cartilage (Fig. 65-8). The guide also avoids injuring the cartilage or getting too close to it, which could result in thermal injury. The shell produced must be sufficiently compliant to allow modeling without being fractured. Cancellous bone removal is extended until the notch. More bone is removed from the central portion, where the new trochlear groove will rest.

Light pressure should be able to model the flap to the underlying cancellous bone bed in the distal femur (Fig. 65-9). The groove, and sometimes the lateral facet external margin, should be cut to allow further modeling, which is done by gently tapping over a scalpel (Fig. 65-10). If the correction obtained is satisfactory, the new trochlea is fixed with two staples (Kirschner wire [K wire] of 1-mm diameter modeled on the trochlear shape), one in each side of the groove. The staples are fixed with one arm in the cartilaginous upper part of each facet and the other arm in the anterior femoral cortex (Fig. 65-11). Patellar tracking is tested. Periosteum and synovial tissue are sutured to the osteochondral edge and anchored to the staples.

We routinely associate a soft tissue procedure to the trochleoplasty. Formerly, a VMO-plasty was added. However, since 2003, medial patellofemoral ligament (MPFL) reconstruction has been our procedure of choice.

Deepening trochleoplasty plays a triple role in cases of trochlear dysplasia. It creates a new trochlear shape with a central groove and oblique facets, it reduces the patellofemoral joint reaction force by decreasing the trochlear prominence (Fig. 65-12), and it does a proximal realignment, reducing the TT-TG. It is recommended for patients with types B and D dysplasia, in which the prominence of the trochlea is important. This procedure is not adequate for type C patients, in which there is no prominence.

Bereiter Trochleoplasty

This technique was described by Bereiter and Gautier in 1994.[3] In this method, a lateral parapatellar approach is performed, the trochlea exposed, and the synovium dissected away from it. Then, a thin osteochondral flake with 2 mm of subchondral bone is elevated from the trochlea, extending to the intercondylar notch. The distal femoral subchondral bone is deepened and refashioned with osteotomes and a high-speed burr. Next, the osteochondral flap is seated in the refashioned bed and fixed with 3-mm-wide Vicryl bands, passing through the center of the groove and exiting in the lateral femoral condyle. The periosteum is reattached to the edge of the cartilage and the wound is closed.

POSTOPERATIVE CARE

Trochleoplasty does not need weight protection or range of motion limitation. Movement such as CPM (continuous passive motion) may also improve cartilage healing. Quadriceps wasting is another negative outcome of immobilization. The main principles guiding trochleoplasty rehabilitation are presented here, but the associated procedures have to be taken into account and rehabilitation also has to apply to them.

The rehabilitation is divided into three phases. There are at least three physiotherapy sessions each week but specific goals depend on the phase. Phase 1 starts the day after the surgery and ends on day 45. Knee movement is encouraged to improve the nutrition of the cartilage and to allow further modeling of the trochlea by patellar tracking. Immediate weight bearing is allowed with crutches and an extension brace for 4 weeks. Walking without the brace is allowed, generally after 1 month. Range of motion is gradually

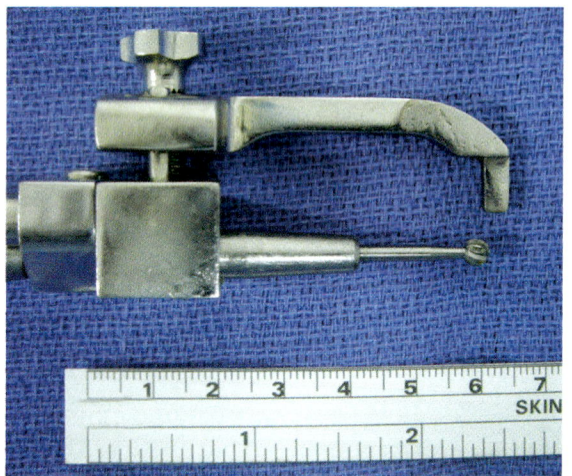

Figure 65-8. Drill with depth guide used to remove cancellous bone from the trochlear undersurface.

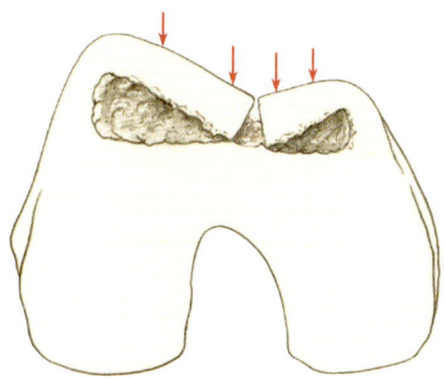

Figure 65-9. After the cancellous bone has been removed, the osteochondral flaps can lie over the new bone bed and the sulcus shape can be corrected.

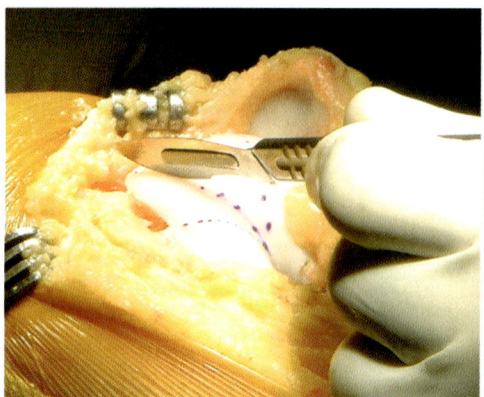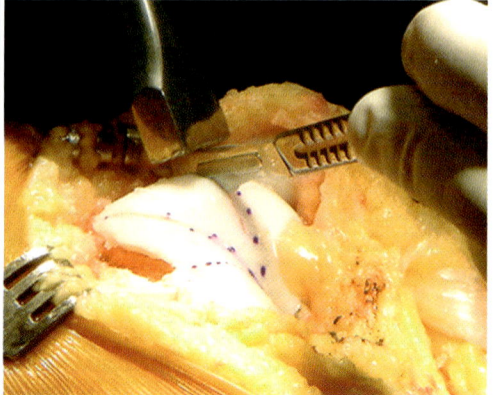

Figure 65-10. To allow further modeling to the underlying bone bed, the osteochondral flaps may be cut in the sulcus and facet lines.

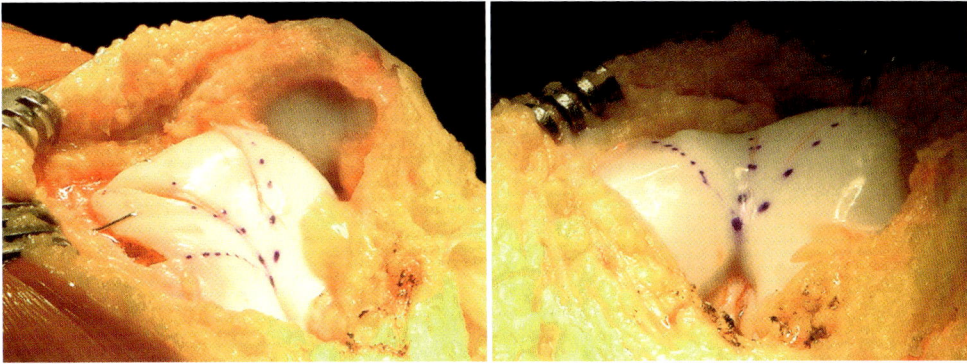

Figure 65-11. Lateral and anterior views of dysplastic trochlea after trochleoplasty (same patient as in prior figures). Notice that the sulcus and facet relationship resembles a normal trochlea.

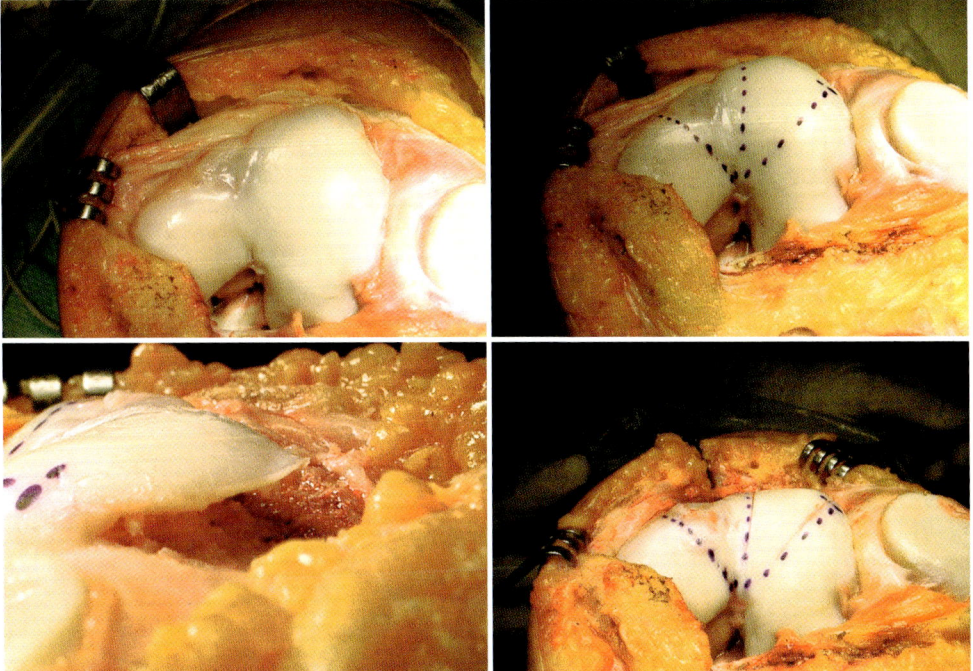

Figure 65-12. High-grade trochlear dysplasia in a different patient after exposure *(top left)*. The new trochlea is drawn *(top right)*. Bone is removed from the trochlear inferior surface allowing the trochlear modeling and the bump resection *(botttom left)*. Anterior view after the procedure before closing *(botttom right)*.

regained, avoiding passive, forced, or painful postures. Dynamic and isometric quadriceps strengthening with weights on the feet or tibial tubercle is prohibited.

Phase 2 goes from day 46 until day 90. Cycling is possible, with weak resistance initially. Active ascension of the patella can be performed seated, with the leg stretched and the knee unlocked, by static and isometric quadriceps contractions. Active exercises are added but dynamic and isometric quadriceps strengthening with weights on the feet or tibial tubercle are still forbidden. The anterior and posterior muscular chains are stretched. Weight bearing proprioception exercises are started when full extension is complete, first in bipodal stance and later in monopodal stance when there is no pain.

Phase 3 continues from month 4 until month 6; this is the sports phase. Running can be initiated on a straight line. Closed kinetic chain muscular reinforcement between 0 and 60 degrees with minor loads but long series are allowed. Stretching of the anterior and posterior muscular chains is

continued. The patient is encouraged to proceed with the rehabilitation on his or her own. After 6 months, sports on a recreational or competitive level can be resumed.

Six weeks postoperatively, radiographs, including AP and lateral views (Fig. 65-13) and an axial view in 30 degrees of flexion, are taken. After 6 months, a CT scan is obtained to document the obtained correction (Fig. 65-14).

RESULTS

Two series reviewing deepening trochleoplasty were presented in the I0èmes Journées Lyonnaises de Chirurgie du Genou in 2002.

Group I

The first group included 18 patients who had failed patellar surgery for instability. The mean age at surgery was 24 years.

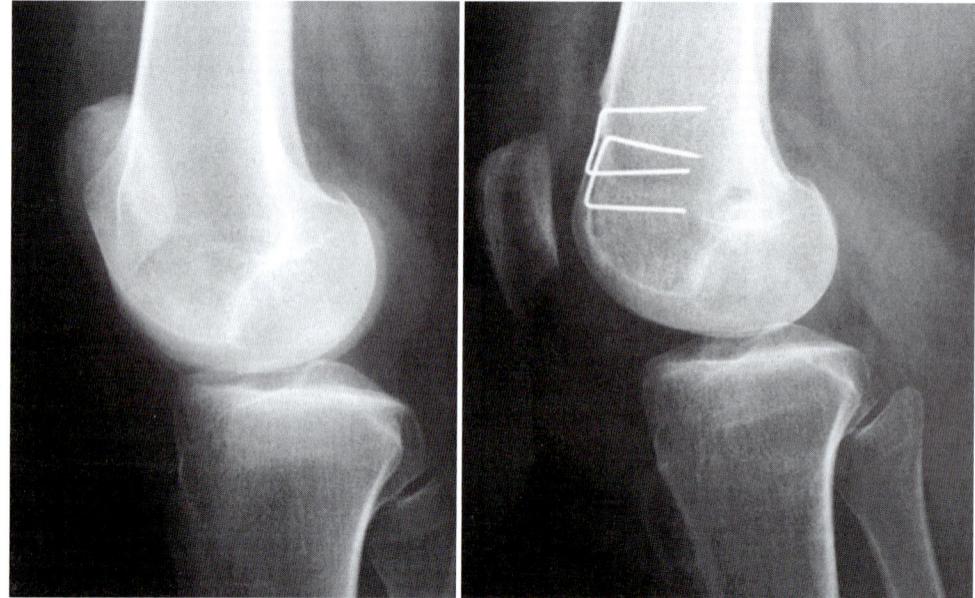

Figure 65-13. Preoperative and postoperative lateral x-rays for patient in Figure 65-12 showing the resection of the supratrochlear bump and trochlear prominence correction. Also, patellar tilt is clearly improved.

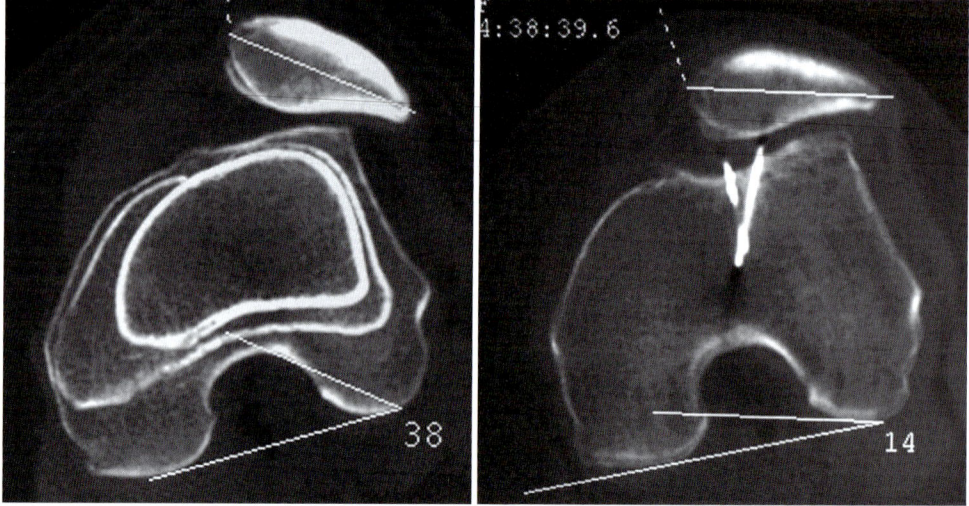

Figure 65-14. CT scans before and after trochleoplasty for the patient in Figure 65-12, axial views. The trochlear sulcus is restored and patellar tilt is corrected. Patellar subluxation is also improved.

There were no patients lost to follow-up. The mean follow-up was 6 years (range, 2 to 8 years). The new surgery was indicated 6 times for pain and 12 times for recurrence of instability. The average number of surgeries before the trochleoplasty was two (e.g., tibial tubercle medialization, distalization, arthroscopy, lateral release). The deepening trochleoplasty was combined with a tibial tubercle medialization in 8 patients, in 6 with a tibial tubercle distalization, and in 18 with a VMO-plasty. All patients were reviewed clinically with the International Knee Documentation Committee (IKDC) form and radiographically. Of these, 65% were satisfied or very satisfied. Knee stability was rated 13 times as very good and five times as good. Twenty-eight percent of the patients had residual pain, and this was correlated to the cartilage status at surgery. Two patients developed patellofemoral arthritis. The mean patellar tilt was 35 degrees (18

to 48 degrees) in the preoperative setting and improved to 21 degrees (11 to 28 degrees) with the quadriceps relaxed and 24 degrees (16 to 32 degrees) with the quadriceps contracted postoperatively.

Group II

In the second group, there were 44 patients. They all had had no previous patellofemoral surgery. The mean age at surgery was 23 years old. The mean follow-up was 7 years (range, 2 to 9 years). The procedure was combined with 22 tibial tubercle medializations, 26 distalizations, and 32 VMO-plasties at the time of surgery. These patients were also reviewed clinically with the IKDC form and radiographically; 85% were satisfied or very satisfied. The knee stability was rated 31 times as very good and 13 times as good. Five percent had residual pain, but this was not correlated with the cartilage status at surgery. No patellofemoral arthritis was noted. The mean patellar tilt preoperatively was 33 degrees (24 to 52 degrees), and improved postoperatively to 18 degrees (9 to 30 degrees) with the quadriceps relaxed and 22 degrees (14 to 34 degrees) with the quadriceps contracted.

Verdonk and colleagues[19] have described 13 procedures (deepening trochleoplasty), with a mean follow-up of 18 months. Patients were assessed using the Larsen-Lauridsen score considering pain, stiffness, osteopatellar crepitus, flexion, and loss of function. Seven patients scored poorly, three fairly well, and three well. On a subjective scoring system, however, six patients rated the result as very good, four as good, and one as satisfactory. Only two patients found the result inadequate and would never undergo the procedure again. Thus, 77% were satisfied with the procedure.

Donell and associates[9] have described 15 patients (17 knees) submitted to deepening trochleoplasty, with a mean follow-up of 3 years. Trochleoplasty was indicated if there was a boss larger than 6 mm, and associated procedures were performed as required. Of the 17 knees, 9 had undergone previous surgery for patellar instability. The boss height was reduced postoperatively from an average of 7.5 to 0.7 mm. Tracking became normal in 11 knees and 6 had a slight J sign. Seven knees had mild residual apprehension. Seven patients were very satisfied, six were satisfied, and two were disappointed. The Kujala score improved from an average of 48 to 75 out of 100.

von Knoch and coworkers[20] have described 45 knees that underwent Bereiter's trochleoplasty, with a mean follow-up of 8.3 years; 15 had undergone previous surgery. None of them had recurrence of dislocation after the trochleoplasty. Thirty-five knees had pain preoperatively. Postoperatively, pain became worse in 15 (33.4%), remained unchanged in 4 (8.8%), and improved in 22 (49%). Four knees that had no pain preoperatively (8.8%) continued to have no pain. Of 33 knees available for radiologic assessment postoperatively, all but 2 knees (93.9%) had correction of trochlear dysplasia radiologically. Degenerative changes of the patellofemoral joint developed in 30% (10) of the knees.

Schottle and colleagues[14] have reported 19 knees that underwent trochleoplasty (Bereiter) in 16 patients, with a mean follow-up of 3 years. None of the patients sustained a redislocation. Sixteen of 19 knees improved subjectively. The mean Kujala score improved from 56 points preoperatively to 80 points in the latest visit. In 12 knees, the pain level became reduced, whereas there was increased pain in 2 knees postoperatively. Four patients reported persistent apprehension while the examiner attempted to lateralize the patella in the extended leg.

COMPLICATIONS

Patients submitted to trochleoplasty are at risk of the same complications inherent to any surgical procedure (e.g., infection, deep venous thrombosis). Specific complications include trochlear necrosis, cartilage damage, incongruence with the patella, and hypo- or hypercorrection. Schottle and coworkers[15] have performed biopsies in three patients after trochleoplasty, showing cartilage cell viability and flap healing, and concluded that the risk of cartilage damage is low.

Incongruence with the patella is another concern. Studies with longer follow-ups are needed before any assumptions can be made about its consequences. Also, osteoarthritis development is multifactorial. Patients with patellofemoral instability are prone to develop osteoarthritis, and those patients operated on for patellofemoral instability seem even more prone to degeneration than those treated conservatively.[10]

Arthrofibrosis incidence varies among series but is always a possibility in patellofemoral surgery. Verdonk and associates[19] have reported 5 cases in 13 patients, and von Knoch and colleagues[20] have reported that all patients had full range of motion at their final visit. The number of previous or associated procedures is variable, which could interfere with data interpretation.

Recurrence of instability is very rare after such a procedure and is more likely to result from missed associated abnormalities. The procedure results for pain are not consistent and, although it seems to improve, some patients may complain of worsening.

CONCLUSION

Sulcus-deepening trochleoplasty is a demanding procedure that is indicated for a few cases of patellofemoral dislocation. It has the advantage of treating its essential cause, but trochleoplasty indications are selective. It should not be performed in cases of pain, arthritis, or open growth plates. As with any surgical procedure, it carries a risk of complications. In recurrent patellar instability, it is a salvage procedure.

KEY REFERENCES

Amis AA: Current concepts on anatomy and biomechanics of patellar stability. Sports Med Arthrosc 15:48–56, 2007.

Dejour D, Le Coultre B: Osteotomies in patello-femoral instabilities. Sports Med Arthrosc 15:39–46, 2007.

Dejour H, Walch G, Neyret P, Adeleine P: [Dysplasia of the femoral trochlea.] Rev Chir Orthop Reparatrice Appar Mot 76:45–54, 1990.

Dejour H, Walch G, Nove-Josserand L, Guier C: Factors of patellar instability: an anatomic radiographic study. Knee Surg Sports Traumatol Arthrosc 2:19–26, 1994.

Donell ST, Joseph G, Hing CB, Marshall TJ: Modified Dejour trochleoplasty for severe dysplasia: Operative technique and early clinical results. Knee 13:266–273, 2006.

Schottle PB, Schell H, Duda G, Weiler A: Cartilage viability after trochleoplasty. Knee Surg Sports Traumatol Arthrosc 15:161–1617, 2007.

Shih YF, Bull AM, Amis AA: The cartilaginous and osseous geometry of the femoral trochlear groove. Knee Surg Sports Traumatol Arthrosc 12:300–306, 2004.

von Knoch F, Bohm T, Burgi ML, et al: Trochleaplasty for recurrent patellar dislocation in association with trochlear dysplasia. A 4- to 14-year follow-up study. J Bone Joint Surg Br 88:1331–1335, 2006.

Full references for this chapter can be found on www.expertconsult.com.

Quadriceps and Patellar Tendon Disruption*

Ari D. Seidenstein, Christopher M. Farrell, Giles R. Scuderi, and Mark E. Easley

ANATOMY

The extensor mechanism of the knee consists of the quadriceps musculature, quadriceps tendon, patella, and patellar tendon. The quadriceps musculature is composed of the rectus femoris, vastus medialis, vastus lateralis, and vastus intermedius, which coalesce in a trilaminar fashion to form the quadriceps tendon. The direct head of the rectus femoris takes origin from the anterior inferior iliac spine and the indirect head from the anterior hip capsule. These muscle heads unite distally and form the rectus femoris muscle, the most superficial component of the quadriceps musculature. The muscle bodies narrow to a tendon approximately 3 to 5 cm superior to the patella. The fibers of the quadriceps tendon continue over the anterior surface of the patella and into the patellar tendon. The vastus medialis is divided into two groups, the vastus medialis obliquus and the vastus medialis longus. The muscle fibers of the vastus medialis continue toward the superomedial border of the patella and become tendinous a few millimeters before their insertion. The muscle fibers of the vastus lateralis terminate more proximally than those of the vastus medialis and become tendinous approximately 3 cm from the superolateral border of the patella. The vastus intermedius lies deep to the other three muscles, and its tendinous fibers insert directly into the superior border of the patella and blend medially and laterally with the vastus medialis and vastus lateralis. Aponeurotic fibers from the vastus lateralis and vastus medialis contribute to the lateral and medial retinaculum.

The patellar tendon is primarily derived from the central fibers of the rectus femoris, which extend over the anterior surface of the patella and form a flat tendinous structure that inserts into the tibial tubercle. It continues past the tubercle and blends with the iliotibial band on the anterolateral surface of the tibia. The average length of the patellar tendon is 4.6 cm (range, 3.5 to 5.5).[109]

CAUSES OF EXTENSOR MECHANISM DISRUPTION

Experimental studies have shown that a normal tendon will not rupture when a longitudinal stress is applied but, instead, the disruption will occur at the musculotendinous junction, muscle belly, or tendinous insertion into the bone. It has been shown that the normal quadriceps tendon may be able to tolerate up to 30 kg/mm of longitudinal stress before failing. Patellar and quadriceps tendon ruptures therefore occur

through a pathologic area of the tendon. The estimated force required to disrupt the extensor mechanism of the knee is 17.5 times body weight and usually occurs during a sudden eccentric contraction of the extensor mechanism with the foot planted and the knee flexed as the person falls. With this in mind, many pathologic conditions can affect the extensor mechanism, including renal disease, diabetes mellitus, hyperparathyroidism, rheumatoid arthritis, systemic lupus erythematosus, gout, osteomalacia, infection, obesity, steroid use,[71,86] and other metabolic diseases. These metabolic diseases cause microscopic damage to the vascular supply to the tendons or alter the architecture of the tendon. Diabetes has been shown to cause arteriosclerotic changes in the tendon vessels, whereas chronic synovitis causes fibrinoid reactions within the tendon. Muscle fiber atrophy secondary to renal disease and uremia will also weaken the tendon. Pathologic changes from advancing age include fatty and cystic degeneration, myxoid degeneration, and calcification, all of which alter tendon architecture. Bone resorption and osteopenia can also occur at the osteotendinous junction with advancing age. A report of spontaneous patellar tendon rupture in identical twins has further supported the concept that predisposing factors for extensor mechanism rupture exist.[41] Although quadriceps tendon rupture tends to occur in older patients or those with systemic disease or degenerative changes, patellar tendon rupture or avulsion is more common in patients younger than 40 years.[62,120] Most spontaneous ruptures of the quadriceps tendon occur within 1 to 2 cm of the patella through the pathologic areas mentioned, leaving the periosteal attachment intact. This also correlates to the zone of the quadriceps tendon with the poorest vascularity.[131] Numerous cases of bilateral extensor mechanism rupture have been reported. Although most ruptures occur in patients with predisposing conditions such as obesity, systemic illness,* and use of anabolic steroids, several reports have noted simultaneous bilateral extensor mechanism rupture in healthy patients without predisposing factors.† In a retrospective review of bilateral and unilateral quadriceps tendon rupture, Konrath and associates[60] have noted a significant correlation between bilateral simultaneous rupture and systemic disease.

Iatrogenic conditions that may alter the local properties of the extensor mechanism include total knee arthroplasty (TKA),[74] lateral retinacular release,[9,29,118] and harvesting of the central third of the patellar tendon for ligament reconstruction.[10,64,78] Local steroid injection has similarly been implicated as a cause of tendon rupture. Rupture of the quadriceps tendon has been reported after patellar dislocation.[92] Partial patellar tendon rupture may occur with tibiofemoral dislocations.[130]

---

*This chapter was modified from Scuderi GR, Easley ME, Farrell CM: Quadriceps and patellar tendon disruptions. In Insall JN, Scott WN (eds): Surgery of the knee, ed 4, New York, 2006, Churchill Livingstone, pp 967–985.

*References 1, 17, 20, 41, 43, 77, 90, 94, 119, and 127.
†References 3, 17, 26, 42, 53, 65, 102, 108, 119, 122, and 127.

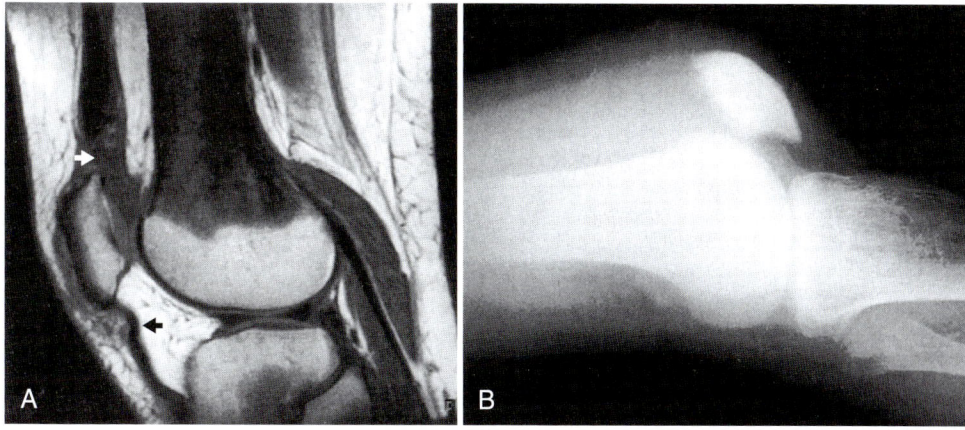

Figure 66-1. **A,** MRI scan of a torn quadriceps tendon *(white arrow).* Note the laxity of the patellar tendon *(black arrow).* **B,** Radiograph showing the low position of the patella associated with quadriceps tendon rupture. This patient has chronic renal failure and hyperparathyroidism. (From Scott WN [ed]: The knee, vol 1, St. Louis, 1994, Mosby–Year Book, p 470.)

Disruption of the extensor mechanism is a significant disabling injury and should be diagnosed early.[104,116] Patients usually have an acute onset of knee pain, swelling, and loss of function after a stumble or fall. Although rare, acute compartment syndrome of the thigh secondary to a quadriceps rupture has also been reported.[63] The physical examination generally reveals a palpable defect in the quadriceps tendon with a low-lying patella. When asked to perform a straight-leg raise, the patient may be unable to do so or will demonstrate an extensor lag. A patellar tendon rupture has similar findings; however, the palpable gap is in the patellar tendon with a proximally retracted patella.

Although extensor mechanism disruptions are typically diagnosed from the history and physical examination, imaging studies often prove useful in confirming the diagnosis of quadriceps and patellar tendon tears or differentiating complete from incomplete tears.[103] Radiographs provide supporting information, especially on the lateral view. A low position of the patella and disruption of the quadriceps tendon shadow are associated with quadriceps tendon rupture (Fig. 66-1), whereas a high patellar position and disruption of the patellar tendon shadow or the infrapatellar fat pad contour are associated with patellar tendon rupture.[19,51,56,91] Despite relatively obvious findings on physical examination and standard radiographs, delay in diagnosis of extensor mechanism rupture still occurs.[70,81,112,120] Several diagnostic imaging modalities may be used in addition to standard radiographs to confirm the diagnosis, including arthrography, ultrasound, and magnetic resonance imaging (MRI). Before the advent of MRI, arthrography was widely used. In the presence of an extensor mechanism tendon rupture, extravasation of radiopaque dye into the defect occurs.[2] However, arthrography has been largely replaced by noninvasive methods such as ultrasound and, more commonly, MRI for evaluation of this problem. High-resolution ultrasonography* may reveal a hypoechogenicity across the entire thickness of the tendon with an acute rupture or tendon thickening and alteration of the normal echo signal with chronic tears. Advantages of ultrasonography include collection of images in real time without exposure to ionizing radiation and relatively limited expense.

However, operation of the ultrasound equipment plus interpretation of the images require the skills of a highly trained and experienced technician and radiologist. Hence, the reliability is highly operator-dependent. MRI is the imaging study of choice if the diagnosis cannot be established from the clinical and radiographic examination alone.[10,29,117,121,126] In addition, MRI may be useful to identify other problems within the knee.[132]

QUADRICEPS TENDON RUPTURE

Quadriceps tendon rupture may be complete or incomplete. Whereas incomplete tears may be treated nonoperatively, complete tears are best treated with surgery. These ruptures usually occur at the osteotendinous junction or through an area of degenerate tendon. The rupture originates in the tendon of the rectus femoris, often extending into the vastus intermedius tendon or transversely into the medial and lateral retinacula.

Overview of Surgical Management

Numerous techniques have been described in the literature for repair of acute and chronic rupture of the quadriceps tendon.[†] Over the years, the repair techniques have progressed from simple suture with catgut or silk[80] to wire-reinforced repairs, suture anchors,[110] autografts,[40] xenografts, allografts, and the use of synthetic material.[37,87] McLaughlin[82,83] and McLaughlin and Francis[84] have even recommended a two-stage procedure with traction for better approximation of the tendon. With an acute intrasubstance rupture, direct repair may be performed. A straight midline incision will expose the quadriceps tendon rupture, which is then irrigated of hematoma. The tendon edges are débrided and cut fresh to normal-appearing tendon. If there is sufficient tendon proximally and distally, an end to end repair is performed with multiple interrupted no. 2 nonabsorbable sutures, and the retinaculum is repaired with multiple interrupted no. 0 absorbable sutures. Once the repair is complete, careful assessment of patellar rotation and tracking should be

*References 8, 25, 26, 69, 77, and 101.

†References 24, 46, 56, 65, 69, 96, 102, and 120.

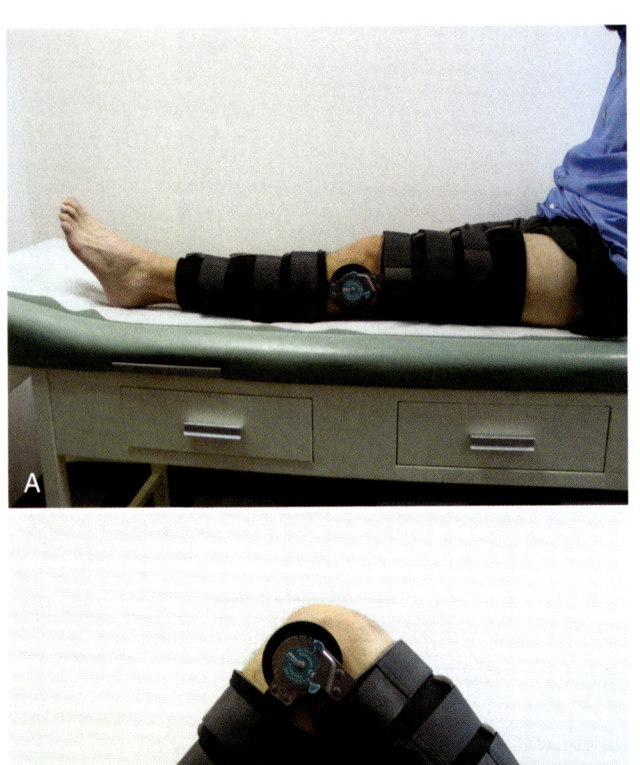

Figure 66-2. A control dial hinged-knee orthosis with a drop lock to keep the knee in extension **(A)** during early ambulation and allow flexion when exercising **(B)**. (Courtesy Breg, Vista, Calif.)

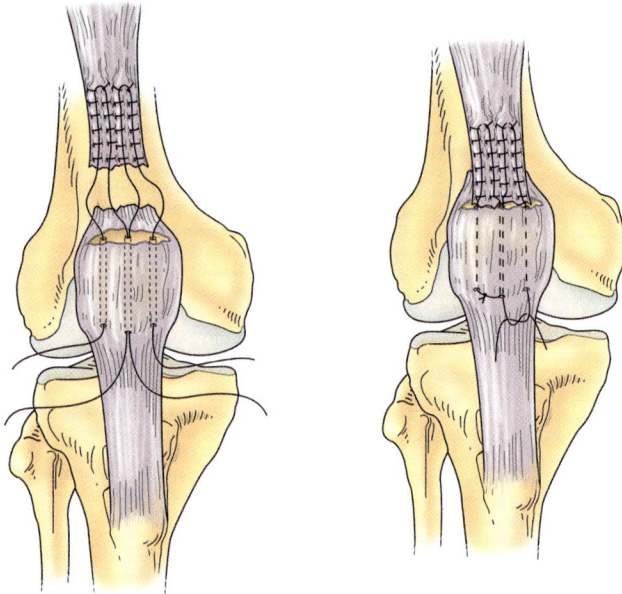

Figure 66-3. Acute repair of the quadriceps tendon into a bony trough. (Redrawn from Scott WN [ed]: The knee, vol 1, St. Louis, 1994, Mosby–Year Book, p 472.)

performed. The knee is then extended and the repair may be protected with a cerclage wire or nonabsorbable suture. The wound is closed in layers and the leg placed in a cylinder cast for 6 weeks. When the cast is removed, a control dial hinged-knee orthosis (Fig. 66-2) is used so that flexion can be gradually increased. The brace is discontinued when more than 90 degrees of flexion has been achieved and quadriceps strength is sufficient to support the limb.

Procedures

Acute Disruption

When the rupture occurs at the osteotendinous junction, we prefer to repair the tendon with transosseous sutures (Fig. 66-3). The MRI and repair technique are illustrated in Figure 66-4. A straight midline incision will expose the quadriceps tendon rupture (see Fig. 66-4C). The hematoma is evacuated (see Fig. 66-4D), the proximal end of the rectus femoris and vastus intermedius tendon is cut fresh to normal tendon, and the superior pole of the patella is débrided of residual tendon (see Fig. 66-4E). A no. 5 nonabsorbable suture is secured with an interlocking stitch along the lateral portion of the tendon.[61] A second no. 5 nonabsorbable suture is placed in similar fashion along the medial portion of the tendon (see Fig.

66-4F). A transverse trough is then made in the superior pole of the patella with a high-speed bur (see Fig. 66-4G). To avoid patellar tilt, the trough should be placed as posterior as possible in the patella. Next, three marks are made with a methylene blue pen approximately 1.0 to 1.5 cm apart in the trough (see Fig. 66-4H). A Beath pin is used to drill through the medial mark, exiting at the inferior pole of the patella (see Fig. 66-4I). An anterior cruciate ligament (ACL) drill guide may be used to facilitate precise placement of the drill holes.[95] The medial free end of suture is next placed through the eyelet of the Beath pin and the pin is pulled distally (see Fig. 66-4I). The Beath pin is then used to drill and pass the sutures in the central and lateral transosseous patellar tunnels (see Fig. 66-4J). The proximal end of the tendon is pulled into the trough and the sutures are held provisionally with a hemostat. The knee is then flexed so that patellar tracking and rotation can be assessed. The repair is completed by tying the no. 5 nonabsorbable suture distally with the knee in full extension (see Fig. 66-4K). Because the medial and lateral retinacula act as frontal plane stabilizers and play a complementary load-sharing role with respect to the patellar tendon, they are both repaired with multiple interrupted no. 0 absorbable sutures (see Fig. 66-4L).[100] The repair is then checked to ensure that gapping at the repair site does not occur at 20 to 30 degrees of flexion (see Fig. 66-4M). Augmentation is typically not necessary.[60,75,120] However, if the strength of the repair is in doubt, augmentation may be achieved with wire or Mersilene tape.[83,87] Satisfactory results have also been obtained with suture anchors in lieu of transosseous sutures.[110] After closure of the subcutaneous layer and skin, a cylinder cast is applied with the knee in full extension. Postoperatively, the cylinder cast is maintained for 6 weeks and the patient is allowed weight bearing as tolerated with a walker or crutches. Once the cast is removed, a control dial hinged-knee orthosis is used until 90 degrees of flexion is achieved and quadriceps strength returns. Although we prefer

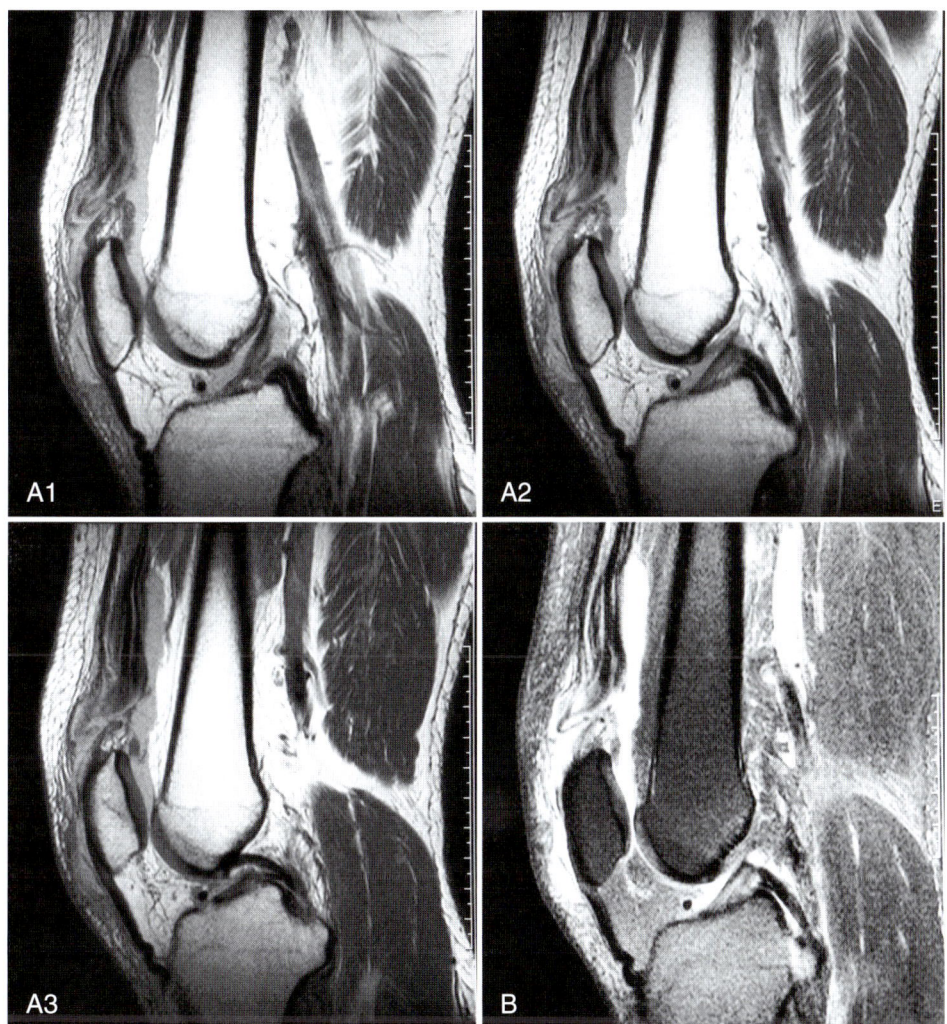

Figure 66-4. Technique for repair of a quadriceps tendon tear. **A, B,** Sagittal MRI scans demonstrating a quadriceps tendon tear at the osteotendinous junction.

Continued

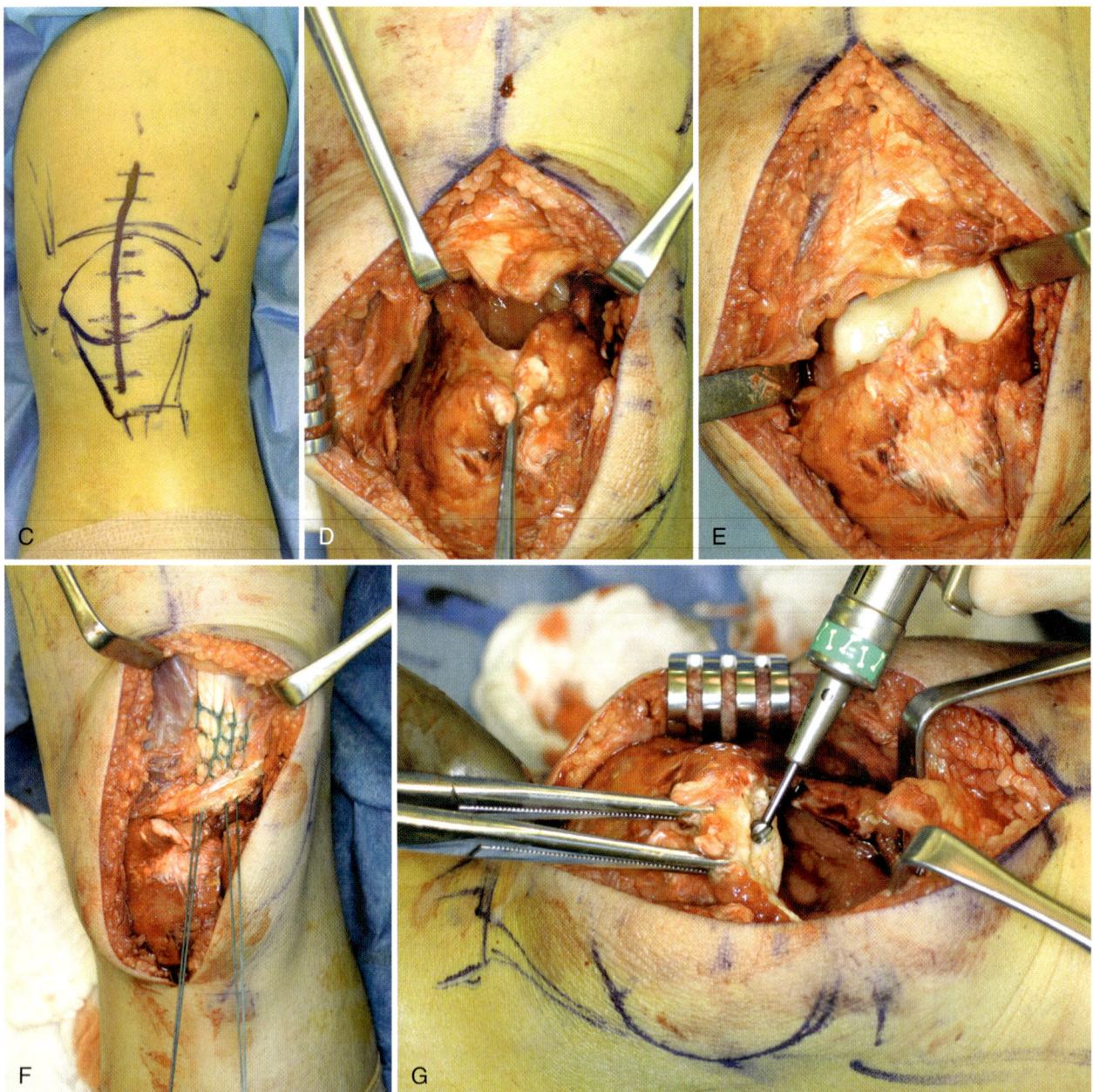

Figure 66-4, cont'd. C, Straight midline incision for exposure of the quadriceps tendon rupture. **D,** Hematoma is evacuated and the free tendon ends exposed. **E,** The proximal rectus femoris and vastus intermedius tendon edges are débrided to healthy tendon and the superior pole of the patella is débrided of residual tendon. **F,** Two no. 5 nonabsorbable sutures are placed along the medial and lateral borders of the quadriceps tendon in an interlocking fashion. **G,** A bur is used to create a transverse trough in the superior pole of the patella near the chondral surface.

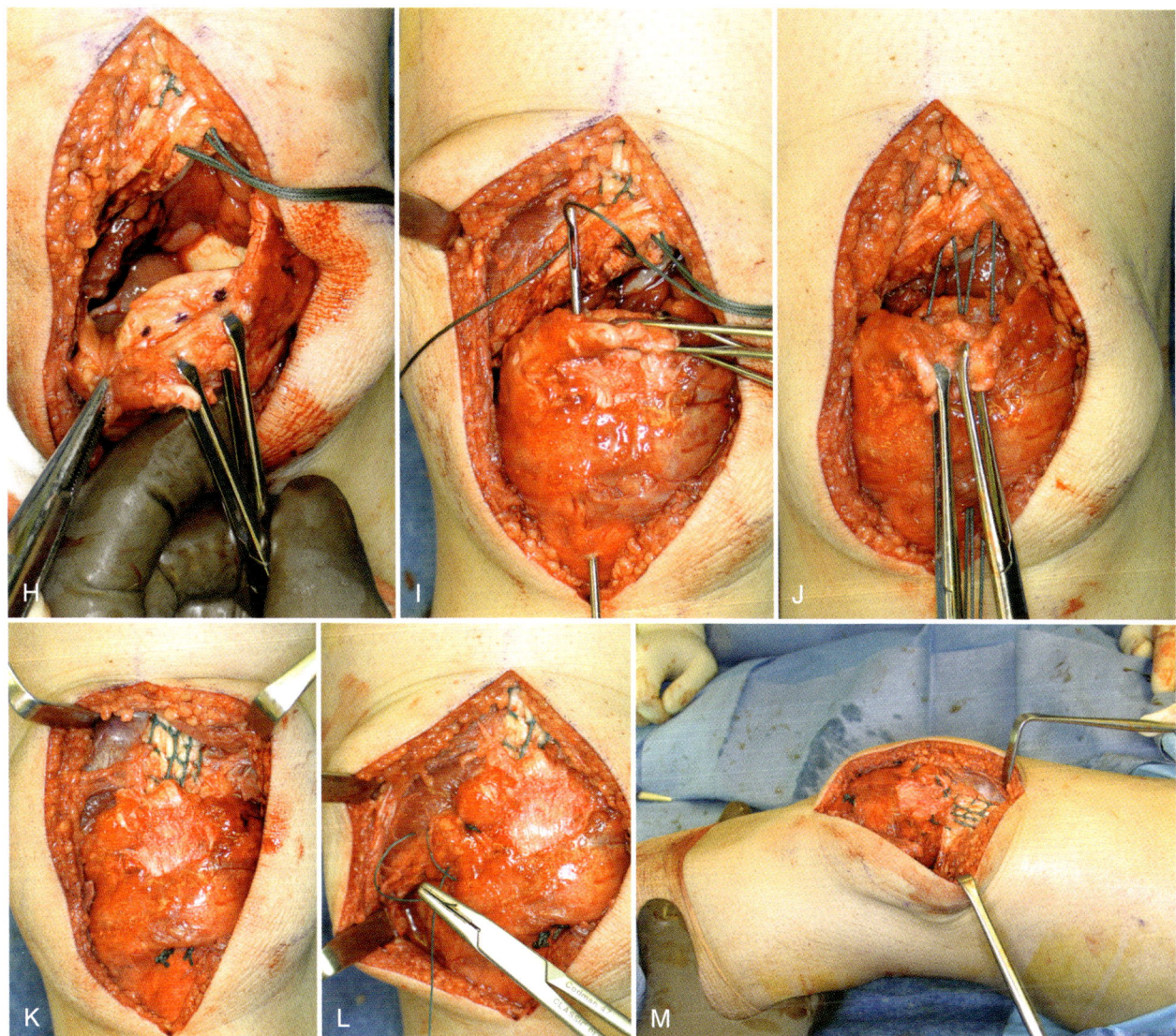

Figure 66-4, cont'd. H, A methylene blue pen is used to mark the site for transosseous drill holes to be placed 1.0 to 1.5 cm apart in the trough. **I,** A Beath pin is used here to drill and pass the suture through the medial tunnel. **J,** The step is repeated for the central and lateral tunnels so that the central two suture ends are passed through one central tunnel. **K,** The sutures are tied with the knee in full extension. **L,** The medial and lateral retinacula are closed. **M,** The repair is checked to ensure that no gapping at the repair site occurs with 20 to 30 degrees of flexion.

immobilization in the immediate postoperative period, some authors advocate early passive and active assisted range of motion of the knee after quadriceps tendon repair.[69]

Alternatively, the quadriceps tendon may be repaired using suture anchors rather than with this transosseous technique. The sutures may still be placed along the medial and lateral halves of the quadriceps tendon with an interlocking technique (modified Mason-Allen, Kessler, Krackow, or Bunnell technique).[15]

The Scuderi technique[48,50,114,115] for repairing acute rupture of the quadriceps tendon has been widely used (Fig. 66-5). Using a midline longitudinal incision, the tendon rupture is exposed and the tendon edges are débrided until solid tendinous material is achieved. The knee is extended and the tendon edges are pulled with clamps, overlapped, and repaired with interrupted absorbable suture. A triangular flap 2.4 to 3.2 mm thick, 7.5 cm long on each side, and 5.0 cm at the base is fabricated from the anterior surface of the proximal part of the tendon. The base of the flap is left attached about 5.0 cm proximal to the rupture. The flap is folded distally over the rupture and sutured in place. A Bunnell pullout wire is placed along the medial and lateral side of the quadriceps tendon, patella, and patellar tendon. The wound is closed in layers and the leg placed in a cylinder cast, with the knee in the extended position. Postoperatively, the cylinder cast is maintained for 6 weeks and, at 3 weeks, the pullout wires are removed. When the cast is removed, a control dial hinged-knee orthosis is used so that flexion can be gradually increased. It is also recommended that the patient undergo physiotherapy, especially a quadriceps-strengthening program.

Chronic (Neglected) Disruption

Neglected or chronic rupture of the quadriceps tendon presents a difficult reconstruction, and the results after repair of

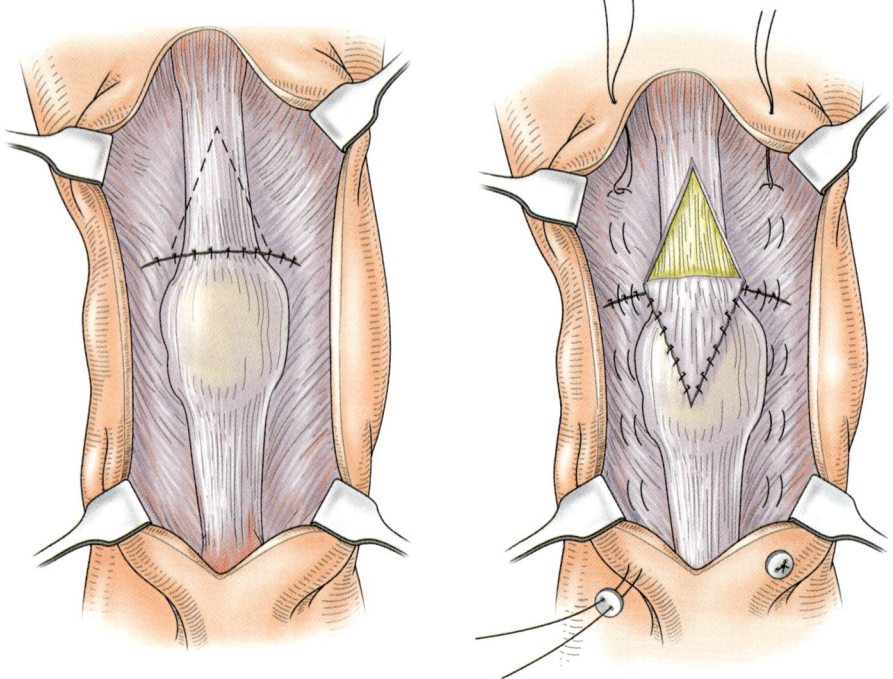

Figure 66-5. Scuderi technique for repairing acute tears of the quadriceps tendon. (Redrawn from Scuderi GR: Extensor mechanism injuries: treatment. In Scott WN [ed]: Ligament and extension mechanism injuries of the knee, St. Louis, 1991, Mosby–Year Book, p 190.)

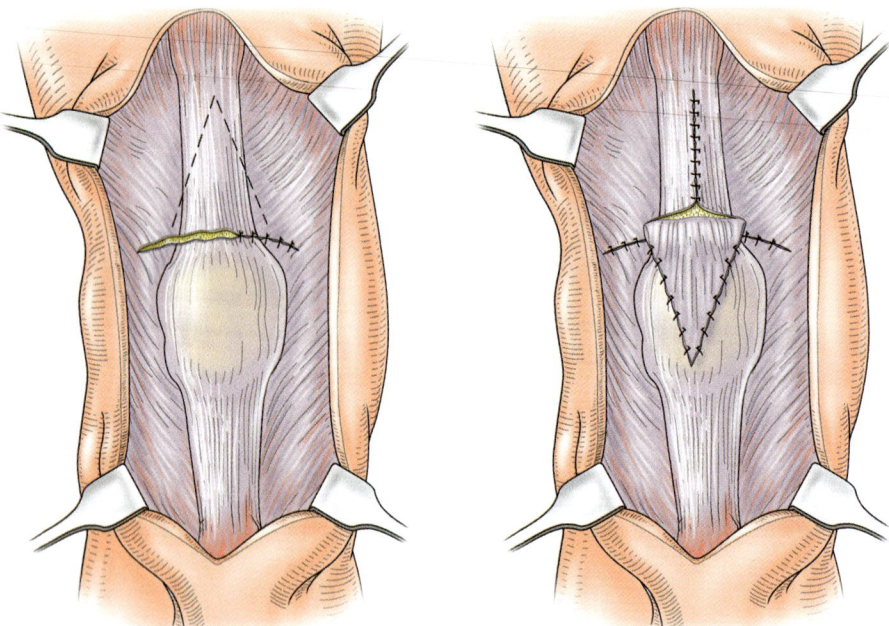

Figure 66-6. Codivilla quadriceps tendon lengthening and repair for chronic ruptures. (Redrawn from Scott WN [ed]: The knee, vol 1, St. Louis, 1994, Mosby–Year Book, p 473.)

such tears are less satisfactory than after treatment of acute tears.[112] A longitudinal midline incision is the preferred approach and the exposure may reveal a large gap between the tendon edges. When the tendon edges can be apposed, the ends are débrided and repaired with the Scuderi technique, as described earlier. However, when there is contraction of the tendon and a large gap, a Codivilla tendon-lengthening and repair procedure is recommended (Fig. 66-6). An inverted V is cut through the full thickness

of the proximal part of the quadriceps tendon, with the lower margin of the V ending approximately 1.3 cm proximal to the rupture. The tendon ends are apposed and repaired with multiple no. 0 nonabsorbable sutures. The medial and lateral retinacula are also repaired at this time with multiple interrupted no. 0 absorbable sutures. The flap is brought distally and sutured in place. The open upper portion of the V is closed with interrupted no. 0 absorbable sutures. The reconstruction should be protected with a pullout cerclage wire.

Postoperative treatment is similar to that after the Scuderi procedure.

Results of Surgical Management of Quadriceps Tendon Rupture

Results of repair and/or reconstruction of acute quadriceps tendon disruptions are generally favorable, irrespective of the type of repair or location of the tear (avulsion from the patella versus midsubstance tendon disruption).[60,69,104,106,112] Results are comparable between unilateral and simultaneous bilateral disruption. Although 15% to 53% of patients may have quadriceps tendon deficits based on isokinetic testing postoperatively,[27] most are able to return to their preinjury occupations. However, fewer than half of patients reach their preinjury recreational activity level. Range of motion is typically recovered postoperatively and approaches the motion of the contralateral extremity. Although Konrath and coworkers[60] found no detrimental effect of delay in repair, others have shown a delay in surgical repair to be the single most important factor predictive of a poor outcome. Rougraff and colleagues[112] have suggested that a delay of 1 week compromises the outcome of quadriceps tendon repair, with significantly worse functional results and lower satisfaction scores. These findings are supported by Siwek and Rao[120] and Scuderi,[114] who observed worse results with a delay in surgical repair of 2 weeks and 3 days, respectively. In a study of 29 quadriceps tendon repairs, Wenzl and associates[128] have demonstrated a significantly higher probability of a successful outcome with repairs performed within 2 weeks from the time of injury. Levy and coworkers[69] have also noted the best results in patients managed acutely with a Dacron graft. Surgical débridement of scar tissue plus direct repair of the quadriceps tendon are effective in the management of partial quadriceps rupture. Complications include rerupture and wound compromise. In a series of 53 repairs, Rougraff and colleagues[112] have observed two reruptures; in Konrath and associates' series[60] of 51 patients, one rerupture was noted. No large series of surgical repair of chronic or neglected quadriceps tendon rupture is available; however, a number of case reports have suggested favorable results with several different reconstruction methods.

Quadriceps Tendon Disruption Associated With Total Knee Arthroplasty

Tears of the quadriceps tendon after TKA are rare, with a reported incidence ranging from 0.1% to 1.1%.[28,74] Although a traumatic event may result in a quadriceps tendon tear, the contribution of other factors such as systemic disease, local injury, and factors related to the TKA technique may predispose an individual. With only a few series in the literature, these factors may only be speculated on; they may include rheumatoid and other inflammatory arthritides, diabetes mellitus, chronic renal failure, hyperthyroidism, and systemic and local steroid use. Possible factors related to the arthroplasty include overresection of the patella with subsequent quadriceps tendon injury, vascular injury to the tendon resulting from lateral retinacular release, incomplete healing after extensile approaches, and manipulation.[98]

As in the case of the native knee, incomplete tears of the quadriceps tendon in patients with a TKA generally do well with nonoperative treatment. In a series from Dobbs and coworkers,[28] seven partial quadriceps tendon ruptures were treated nonoperatively, all with a satisfactory outcome. One of these seven ruptures was diagnosed 1 year after partial rupture and had no further treatment. This patient had a persistent extensor lag of 10 degrees and a palpable defect in the quadriceps tendon. Sixteen patients with a partial quadriceps tendon rupture underwent primary repair. These patients had a high complication rate (5 of 16), and 4 ultimately had an unsatisfactory result. This suggests that early diagnosis is imperative and nonoperative management, consisting of immobilization of the knee in extension for 4 to 6 weeks with weight bearing as tolerated, can yield good results for partial quadriceps tendon tears.

In contrast to the native knee, the results of complete quadriceps tendon tears in patients with a TKA are less predictable. In the series of Dobbs and colleagues,[28] 11 patients were identified with a complete quadriceps tendon tear. Ten underwent primary repair and only four had a satisfactory result. Complications included four reruptures, two infections, and one patient with symptomatic recurvatum and instability. Similarly, Lynch and associates[74] have reported unsatisfactory results with direct suture repair for three quadriceps tendon ruptures, with one sustaining a rerupture and the other two demonstrating limited knee flexion and significant extensor lag. Because of the discouraging results of operative treatment by direct suture repair, augmentation with autogenous graft material such as semitendinosus tendon or graft material such as Marlex mesh should be considered.

PATELLAR TENDON RUPTURE

Overview

Rupture of the patellar tendon is less common than rupture of the quadriceps tendon and generally occurs in patients younger than 40 years.[55,120] Systemic inflammatory diseases, chronic metabolic disorders, anabolic steroid abuse, local steroid injections and, most commonly, progressive degenerative processes of the tendon have all been implicated as potential factors associated with an increased risk for tendon rupture.[21,52,86,89,111] Rarely, patella tendon rupture occurs following anterior cruciate ligament reconstruction using bone-patellar tendon-bone (BPTB) autograft, predominantly in the early postoperative period.[44] Most of these ruptures occur at the inferior pole of the patella, but may also take place in the midsubstance of the tendon or, rarely, at the insertion of the tubercle.[22,76] The patella may be displaced 5 cm proximally as a result of associated retinacular and capsular disruption caused by the strong pull of the quadriceps mechanism. Disruptions through the substance of the patellar tendon can occur spontaneously but are more often caused by trauma or laceration. Early diagnosis and treatment provide the best results.

Historically, McLaughlin[83] and McLaughlin and Francis[84] recommended that repair of the patellar tendon be reinforced with the use of stainless steel wire anchored to a bolt placed in the tibial tubercle. Hsu and colleagues[47] have reported a technique of primary repair reinforced with a neutralization wire. Siwek and Rao[120] also recommended that all immediate repairs of the patellar tendon be reinforced by external devices. Several reports have described reinforcing the repair with various augmentation grafts, including autografts, allografts[30,54] (fascia lata, semitendinosus, gracilis), and synthetic grafts (Mersilene,[87] Dacron,[35,36,69] carbon fiber,[33] and a poly-p-dioxannone cord[59]). In a study by Ravalin and associates,[107] 12 fresh-frozen cadaveric specimens were used to compare standard repair with transosseous sutures without augmentation, with augmentation using a no. 5 Ethibond suture and with augmentation using 2.0-mm Dall-Miles cable. Gap formation at the repair site was assessed after cycling the knees in a custom knee jig; it was greatest in the repairs without augmentation and least in the group augmented with the cable. However, clinical reports have demonstrated satisfactory results of acute patellar tendon disruption repaired without augmentation. In a series of 15 consecutive patients, Marder and Timmerman[76] published excellent results with primary repair of acute patellar tendon disruption treated by suture repair alone.

Procedures

Acute Disruption

Complete patellar tendon rupture requires surgical intervention to restore extensor mechanism function. A straight midline incision is made, and small full-thickness medial and lateral subcutaneous skin flaps are developed. The paratenon overlying the patellar tendon is identified and carefully incised longitudinally. The paratenon is elevated medially and laterally and preserved for subsequent repair at the time of closure. Hematoma within the disrupted tendon is evacuated. In situations in which rupture of the patellar tendon occurs at the osteotendinous junction, the free tendon is freshened and a horizontal trough is then made along the posterior half of the inferior pole of the patella (Fig. 66-7).

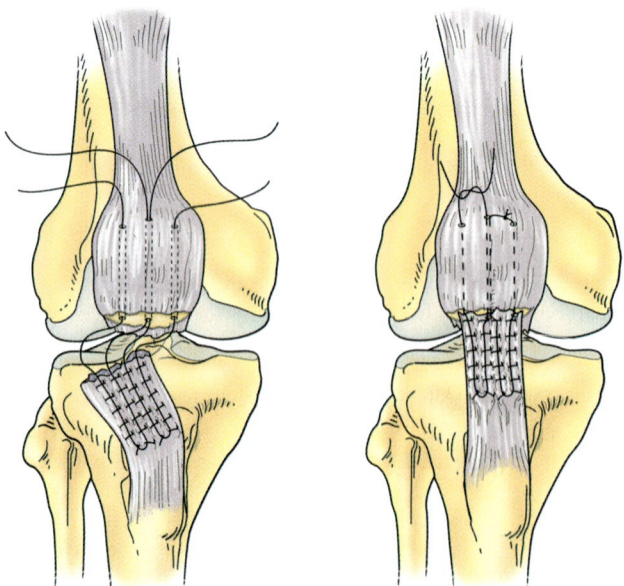

Figure 66-7. Acute repair of the patellar tendon into a bony trough. (Redrawn from Scott WN [ed]: The knee, vol 1, St. Louis, 1994, Mosby–Year Book, p 474.)

In a study by Lu and coworkers,[73] 32 rabbits underwent a partial inferior patellectomy and patellar tendon reattachment. Histologic evaluation was done at 2, 4, 8, and 16 weeks postoperatively comparing both cartilage-tendon and bone-tendon interfaces, which showed that greater healing occurred at the cartilage-tendon interface in the 2- to 4-week period. These results may support the idea of creating the trough closer to the articular cartilage for facilitating earlier biologic repair for the patella–patellar tendon complex. Two no. 5 nonabsorbable sutures are then placed along the medial and lateral halves of the patellar tendon with an interlocking (Krackow[61]) stitch such that the four free ends of suture are left emanating from the proximal portion of the tendon. Using a Beath pin, a longitudinal drill hole is placed centrally in the patella at the base of the trough, exiting at the superior pole of the patella. An ACL drill guide may be used to place the patellar drill holes precisely.[95]

The two central free ends of suture are then placed through the eyelet of the Beath pin, and the pin is pulled proximally. The Beath pin is used to drill and pass the sutures on the medial and lateral sides of the patella approximately 1.0 to 1.5 cm apart. The sutures are pulled taut and the free end of the patellar tendon should be seated within the trough. The sutures are held provisionally with a hemostat to assess patellar tracking and rotation. It is important to ensure that the repair has not produced patella baja. At 45 degrees of flexion, the inferior pole of the patella should be above the roof of the intercondylar notch. A mosquito clamp is used to pass one of the central sutures medially and the other laterally so that the suture knots may be placed over bone rather than the quadriceps tendon. The medial and lateral retinacula are repaired with no. 0 absorbable sutures. In most cases, we prefer to tie the sutures with the knee in full extension and augment the repair with Mersilene tape placed circumferentially around the repair through drill holes in the patella and the anterior cortex of the proximal end of the tibia.

Alternatively, the patellar tendon may be repaired with suture anchors rather than with this transosseous technique. The sutures may still be placed along the medial and lateral halves of the patellar tendon with an interlocking technique (Bunnell or Krackow-Bunnell).[14,39]

The wound is then closed in layers and a cylinder cast with the knee in extension is applied and maintained for 6 weeks. The patient may ambulate with full weight bearing, as tolerated, with crutches. When the cast is removed, the control dial hinged-knee orthosis allowing progressive flexion of the knee is used. When the patient has achieved more than 90 degrees of flexion and sufficient quadriceps strength to support the limb, the orthosis is discontinued.

Acute ruptures that occur within the substance of the patellar tendon can be repaired with running interlocking sutures of no. 2 nonabsorbable suture material (Fig. 66-8). The distally based tendon is reinforced through longitudinal drill holes in the patella, whereas the proximally based tendon is repaired through a horizontal drill hole in the tibial tubercle. Each flap is repaired side to side with interrupted no. 0 absorbable sutures. The medial and lateral retinacula are also repaired with no. 0 absorbable sutures at this time. The postoperative course is similar to that described earlier.

If secure repair of the patellar tendon cannot be achieved with either of the repairs described earlier, augmentation with the semitendinosus or gracilis tendon is recommended (Fig.

66-9).[54,66] The insertion sites of the semitendinosus and gracilis are identified through the original midline incision. While preserving the distal insertion, a tendon stripper is used to divide the tendon proximally. If only the semitendinosus is used for augmentation, it should be passed through an oblique drill hole at the tibial tubercle in a medial to lateral direction. The graft is pulled superiorly, passing laterally to medially

through a transverse drill hole in the inferior aspect of the patella, and then sutured to the origin of the semitendinosus with no. 0 nonabsorbable sutures. This technique creates a box around the patellar tendon. The corners of the graft are sutured with nonabsorbable sutures to prevent slippage. If the semitendinosus tendon is thin and further augmentation is needed, the gracilis tendon can also be used. The insertion of the gracilis tendon is maintained distally, and the tendon is passed in a medial to lateral direction through a second horizontal drill hole in the patella; it then circles the patellar tendon and returns in a lateral to medial direction through the oblique tibial drill hole.

The postoperative course is similar to that described earlier, with 6 weeks of immobilization in a cylinder cast. We prefer a postoperative course of immobilization in a cylinder cast before initiation of a physical therapy program. However, Larson and Simonian[66] have suggested that immediate mobilization with initial passive and active-assisted exercises after reconstruction of the patellar tendon with semitendinosus augmentation may be beneficial. Bhargava and colleagues[6] have reported on 11 patients treated with primary repair protected by a cerclage wire and early mobilization, and all did well. However, patients with a history of systemic collagen vascular disorders or previous steroid injection were excluded. Levy and associates[69] have also recommended immediate postoperative mobilization after reconstruction with a Dacron graft. Marder and Timmerman[76] have used early mobilization in athletes younger than 40 years after primary repair without augmentation.

Fulkerson and Langeland's technique,[38] in which the central quadriceps tendon is harvested with a patellar bone graft for ACL reconstruction, has also been applied to repair or reconstruct patellar tendon disruptions. Williams and

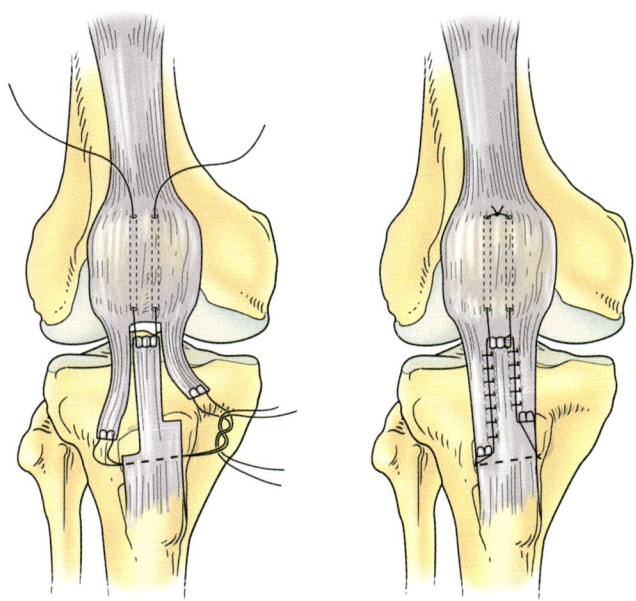

Figure 66-8. Acute repair of intrasubstance tears of the patellar tendon. (Redrawn from Scott WN [ed]: The knee, vol 1, St. Louis, 1994, Mosby–Year Book, p 475.)

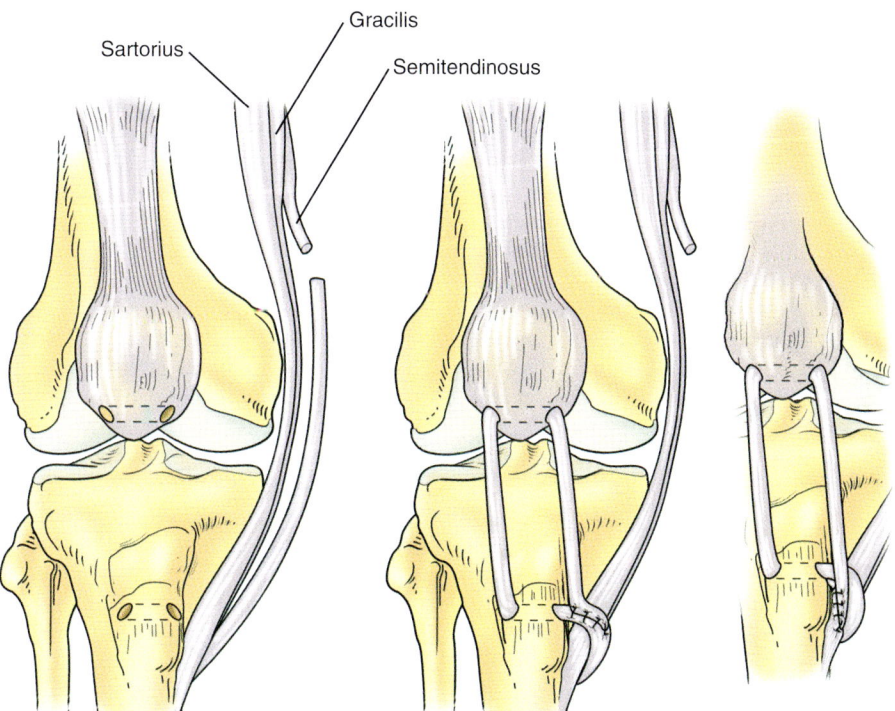

Sartorius Gracilis Semitendinosus

Figure 66-9. Augmentation of a patellar tendon repair with the semitendinosus tendon. (Redrawn from Scuderi GR: Extensor mechanism injuries: treatment. In Scott WN [ed]: Ligament and extension mechanism injuries of the knee, St. Louis, 1991, Mosby–Year Book, p 191.)

coworkers[129] have reported success with this technique in three cases of patellar tendon compromise—one acute, one chronic, and one with patella infera. The patellar bone graft is inset into the tibial tubercle and the quadriceps tendon graft is secured with sutures passed through the patella in a distal to proximal direction. In a case report, Edwards and colleagues[31] used this technique to reconstruct an acute patellar tendon disruption associated with bony compromise of the tibial tubercle.

Chronic (Neglected) Disruption

Chronic rupture of the patellar tendon poses a particular problem, especially if there is retraction of the quadriceps tendon with proximal migration of the patella. Previously, a two-stage reconstruction with preoperative traction through a transverse Steinmann pin placed in the patella was described. Currently, mobilization of the patella and quadriceps tendon can be achieved by clearing the medial and lateral gutters into the suprapatellar pouch and subperiosteally elevating the vastus intermedius from the anterior aspect of the femur.[124] A lateral retinacular release is also performed. If necessary, a medial retinacular release can be done, but this may increase the risk for avascular necrosis of the patella.[116,117] Several techniques have been described for reconstruction of chronic tears of the patellar tendon, including direct repair with augmentation using cerclage wires, autograft, allograft, and synthetic grafts. Direct repair may be performed with transosseous sutures or the more recently described suture anchors.[45] Regardless of the technique performed, it is important that care be taken to maintain normal patellar tracking, rotation, and height. Preoperative planning should include a lateral radiograph of the contralateral knee to determine patellar height. Intraoperatively, the inferior pole of the patella should be above the roof of the intercondylar notch at 45 degrees of flexion. The knee should be able to achieve 90 degrees of flexion and, when in full extension, the patellar tendon should be lax, approximately 1.0 to 1.5 cm.

Reconstruction of chronic patellar tendon rupture is performed through a longitudinal midline incision. The paratenon is incised longitudinally to expose the patellar tendon. If sufficient tendon is available, the ends are cut fresh and sutured, as described earlier for the acute repair, but augmentation with a semitendinosus and/or gracilis autograft is typically recommended. A bone tenaculum can be used to pull the patella distally, and the semitendinosus and gracilis are sutured under tension. Casey and Tietjens[18] have reported on their series of four patients with neglected patellar tendon rupture repaired primarily and augmented with three 1.5-mm cerclage wires in a figure-of-eight pattern from the quadriceps tendon to the tibial tubercle. All underwent a supervised therapy program and immediate mobilization in a brace. Average range of motion was 112 degrees, and no extensor lag was reported. All patients had the hardware removed between 3 and 13 months postoperatively.

When there is a deficiency of remaining tendon or the remaining tendon is attenuated and scarred, a Z-shortening of the patellar tendon and a Z-lengthening of the quadriceps tendon can be performed (Fig. 66-10). This technique requires intraoperative radiographs to determine appropriate patellar height and position because of the increased tendency for patella infra with this reconstruction. Once the proper position of the patella has been determined, the

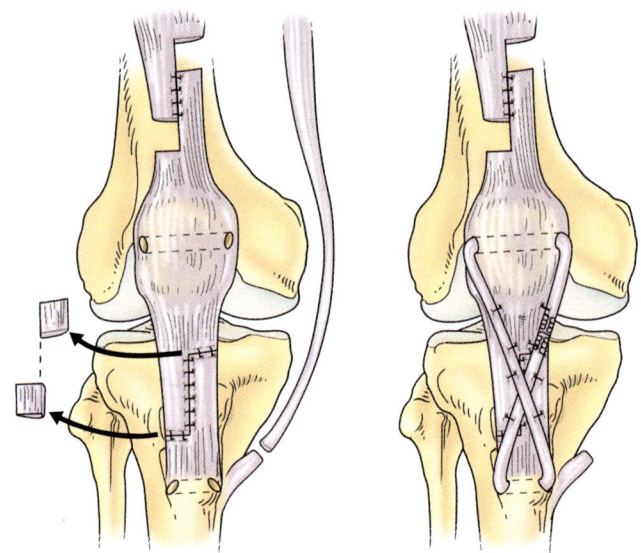

Figure 66-10. Repair of a chronic patellar tendon rupture with a Z-shortening of the patellar tendon and a Z-lengthening of the quadriceps tendon plus augmentation with the semitendinosus and gracilis tendons sutured end to end. (Redrawn from Scott WN [ed]: The knee, vol 1, St. Louis, 1994, Mosby–Year Book, p 476.)

Z-plasty is reinforced with multiple interrupted no. 0 nonabsorbable sutures. This reconstruction requires augmentation with the semitendinosus and gracilis tendons, which are harvested as two free tendons and sutured end to end. The hamstring tendons pass through a transverse drill hole in the midportion of the patella and then through a transverse hole in the tibial tubercle in a figure-of-eight fashion. The semitendinosus and gracilis grafts are secured to the patellar tendon with absorbable suture. Alternatively, the quadriceps tendon–patellar bone graft technique described earlier may be applied.[38,129] The postoperative course is similar to that described previously. Some authors have suggested that a judicious program of immediate postoperative mobilization is possible when the repair is augmented with the semitendinosus tendon or a Dacron graft.[66,69]

Allografts[34,85,99] have been used for reconstruction of neglected patellar tendon rupture (Fig. 66-11). The Achilles tendon with a corticocancellous calcaneal bone block is a convenient allograft. The tibial tubercle is prepared with an oscillating saw or bur to create a trough measuring 2.5 to 3.0 cm long, 1.5 to 2.0 cm wide, and 1.5 cm deep. The bone block is contoured and press-fit into the trough. It is then secured with two 4.0-mm cancellous screws. The Achilles tendon graft is divided into thirds. The central third, which should measure 8 to 9 mm in width, is pulled through a slit in the residual patellar tendon. The graft is then passed through a longitudinal 8- to 9-mm-wide drill hole in the patella. This drill hole enters the inferior pole of the patella and exits at the superior border proximally, 3 mm posterior to the central portion of the quadriceps tendon. The tendon is then pulled through a vertical slit in the quadriceps tendon. The tendon is sutured at the inferior pole of the patella and at the quadriceps tendon with multiple interrupted no. 0 nonabsorbable sutures. Patellar height should be determined at this time. The knee should flex to 90 degrees and, at 45 degrees of flexion, the inferior pole of the patella should be

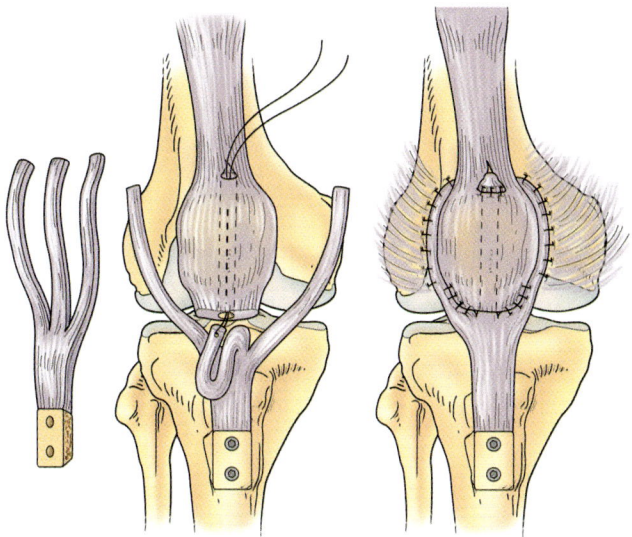

Figure 66-11. Allograft reconstruction for neglected patellar tendon rupture. (Redrawn from Scott WN [ed]: The knee, vol 1, St. Louis, 1994, Mosby–Year Book, p 476.)

superior to the roof of the intercondylar notch. Once the patellar position has been determined to be correct, the medial and lateral flaps are sutured to the medial and lateral retinacula with multiple no. 0 nonabsorbable sutures. If the paratenon is present, it should be closed over the graft with 2-0 absorbable sutures.

The wound is closed in layers and a cylinder cast is applied. The cast is worn for 5 weeks and then a control dial hinged-knee orthosis is worn until 90 degrees of flexion has been achieved and quadriceps strength is sufficient to support the limb during ambulation. Wascher and Summa[126] have described a technique in which an Achilles tendon allograft is used to reconstruct a ruptured extensor mechanism after patellectomy that had failed two previous attempts at primary repair. Bermúdez and colleagues[5] have described a similar technique in which an Achilles tendon allograft was used to reconstruct a ruptured extensor mechanism in a 20-year-old woman 6 months status post–partial patellectomy. Park and associates[97] have described reconstructing the extensor mechanism of a patient with a large patella and patellar tendon defect with an extended medial gastrocnemius flap, including a tendinous portion of the Achilles, while simultaneously using a saphenous neurocutaneous flap for additional soft tissue coverage.

Results of Surgical Repair of Patellar Tendon Disruption

As for quadriceps tendons, the results of patellar tendon repair are favorable, regardless of the location of the rupture or the method of repair.[47,62,66,79,120] Again, delayed repairs have worse outcomes than repairs performed in the acute setting. When the patellar tendon is repaired in the acute setting, range of motion approaching that of the contralateral knee is typically regained and, in athletic individuals, premorbid activity levels and strength can be expected. No large series of neglected patellar tendon ruptures managed with patellar ligament reconstruction have been published. Complications

include rerupture, wound problems, and patellofemoral symptoms. Rerupture is generally related to return to rigorous activity before completion of proper physical therapy. Wound complications are more common than with quadriceps tendon disruption because of the thinner skin at the tibial tubercle; therefore, it is recommended that the skin incision be made adjacent to, but not directly over, the tubercle. Patellofemoral symptoms have been managed with lateral release.[60] Obtaining an intraoperative radiograph at completion of the patellar tendon repair is prudent to ensure that patella baja has not been created.

Patellar Tendon Disruption Associated With Total Knee Arthroplasty

Rupture of the patellar tendon after TKA is a rare but devastating complication, with a reported prevalence ranging from 0.17% to 2.5%.[74,105] Ruptures may occur intraoperatively, in the immediate postoperative period or at some time after the postoperative period. Intraoperative ruptures can occur during exposure, especially while trying to evert the patella in a stiff knee. Patients with multiple operated knees are at a significant risk, probably because of soft tissue scarring, stiffness, and devascularization of tissues. Previous distal alignment procedures, excessive patellar resection,[32] and hinged implants[88] have all been implicated as potential contributors to patellar tendon rupture after TKA. Postoperatively, rupture can occur during manipulation of a stiff knee, from trauma, or as a delayed complication such as chronic attrition from impingement against the tibial insert or an anteriorly overhanging tibial tray.

Prevention is of paramount importance. Awareness of this potential problem should be raised preoperatively in patients with a stiff or multiple operated knee. Intraoperatively, if difficulty with exposure is encountered, several techniques may aid in safely performing a TKA. Posteromedial dissection from the tibia may help allow external rotation of the tibia, which can markedly relieve tension on the patellar tendon. Incising the lateral patellofemoral ligament in primary TKA and excision of scar tissue in the lateral gutter and beneath the patellar tendon in revision TKA can often allow the extensor mechanism to sublux laterally more easily. A quadriceps snip should be performed if there is still significant tension. Finally, if none of these measures adequately decrease tension on the patellar tendon, a tibial tubercle osteotomy or quadriceps turndown may be required to expose the knee safely.[98]

Management of patellar tendon rupture after TKA is considerably more difficult than management of rupture arising in the native knee. Patellar tendon avulsions that occur intraoperatively and have an intact periosteal sleeve may be reattached with staples, transosseous sutures,[1] or suture anchors. However, late ruptures are much more difficult to treat. Rand and coworkers[105] have reviewed 18 patients with patellar tendon rupture. Nine patients underwent primary suture repair and, in all nine cases, the repair failed.

As a result, late rupture of the patellar tendon in patients after TKA generally requires a more extensive reconstruction to restore extensor mechanism function. Options for reconstruction include primary repair augmented with semitendinosus tendon autograft, Achilles tendon allograft,[23] and quadriceps tendon–patella–patellar tendon–tibial tubercle allograft.[12,68,105] Cadambi and Engh[16] have described a technique for primary repair augmented with an autogenous semitendinosus tendon. In this procedure, the semitendinosus tendon is harvested at the musculotendinous junction, with the distal insertion left intact. The tendon is routed medially through a drill hole in the distal pole of the patella and then sutured to itself at its distal insertion. The knee was immobilized for 6 weeks and patients were permitted to bear weight as tolerated. In their series of seven patients, the average extensor lag was 10 degrees, with an average flexion of 79 degrees. The authors concluded that the use of autogenous semitendinosus tendon augmentation of primary patellar tendon repairs could restore sufficient quadriceps strength and motion.

Achilles tendon allograft has also been used to reconstruct chronic patellar tendon rupture after TKA. Crossett and coworkers[23] have reviewed their experience with fresh-frozen Achilles tendon allograft with an attached calcaneal bone graft in nine knees. The calcaneal bone block is cut to match a defect created in the tibia and the bone block is impacted with an interference fit. The bone block is secured with a screw or wires. The allograft tendon is then sewn to the underlying extensor mechanism with nonabsorbable suture while the knee is in full extension. Postoperatively, the knees were immobilized in extension for 4 weeks and then progressive flexion was allowed. The average extensor lag improved from 44 degrees preoperatively to 3 degrees postoperatively and, although two grafts had failed, both were repaired successfully.

Emerson and colleagues[32] were the first to describe an allograft reconstruction using the quadriceps tendon, a patella with a cemented prosthesis, the patellar tendon, and the tibial tubercle. In their description, the allograft tubercle is fixed to the host tibia with screws or wire and the patella is placed on the anterior flange of the femoral component. The allograft quadriceps tendon is then sutured to the host tendon with nonabsorbable sutures while the extensor mechanism construct is placed under slight tension. There was a high complication rate, with one third of patients demonstrating an extensor lag of 20 to 40 degrees. Leopold and associates[68] reconstructed seven extensor mechanisms with Emerson's technique and rated all seven as failures based on persistent extensor lag of more than 30 degrees.

Nazarian and Booth[93] have studied a larger series of 36 patients with chronic extensor mechanism disruption and used a modification of Emerson's technique. In their technique, the distal extensor allograft was tensioned with the knee in full extension. The average extensor lag was 13 degrees; 23 achieved full active extension that equaled passive extension. However, eight knees required a repeat allograft reconstruction. This modification seems to provide improved active knee extension, a finding supported by Burnett and associates,[11] who evaluated 20 extensor mechanism allografts: group I consisted of 7 knees reconstructed with the allograft slightly tensioned and group II consisted of 13 knees with the allograft tightly tensioned in full extension. The average postoperative extensor lag was 59 degrees in group I and 4.3 degrees in group 2. All 7 knees reconstructed with the graft slightly tensioned were clinical failures, whereas all 13 reconstructed with the allograft tightly tensioned in full extension were clinical successes.

Other techniques described include a medial gastrocnemius flap,[13] the use of synthetic ligament augmentation,[4] and patellotibial fusion.[57] Itälä and coworkers[49] have conducted a canine study reattaching distal patellar tendons to porous tantalum washers that suggested that tendon healing into a prosthetic material can be achieved with sufficient soft tissue ingrowth and mechanical strength to withstand physiologic loading. In a study by Sundar and colleagues,[123] the patella tendons of six ewes were reattached to a hydroxyapatite-coated titanium implant (attached to the proximal tibia) using a four-ply Vycryl mesh and then augmented the construct with DBM, cancellous autograft, and iliac crest autologous bone marrow. The study results demonstrated good functional outcomes at 6 weeks and a direct-type enthesis at 12 weeks.

The technique for extensor mechanism allograft that we prefer (Fig. 66-12) is similar to that described by Nazarian and Booth.[93] A long midline incision is used to provide wide exposure and preserve as much of the residual extensor mechanism tissue as possible. The host tibia is exposed by subperiosteal dissection. Full passive extension of the knee is achieved. The allograft tibial tubercle is then prepared with a microsagittal saw to fashion a bone block approximately 3 cm long, 1.5 cm wide, and 1cm deep and an oblique dovetail proximal cut.[16] The host tibia is then prepared to create a lock and key fit. The allograft tibia is secured with screws or wires. Two nonabsorbable no. 5 sutures are then secured to the allograft quadriceps tendon with a locking Krackow stitch. The residual extensor mechanism tendon is sewn over the extensor mechanism allograft construct in a pants over vest technique. As emphasized by Nazarian and Booth[93] and Burnett and colleagues,[11,12] the graft is tensioned with the knee in full extension. Marlex mesh is used to reinforce the repair. This is just one method to reconstruct the extensor mechanism in TKA. A more comprehensive review of this problem is found elsewhere in this text.

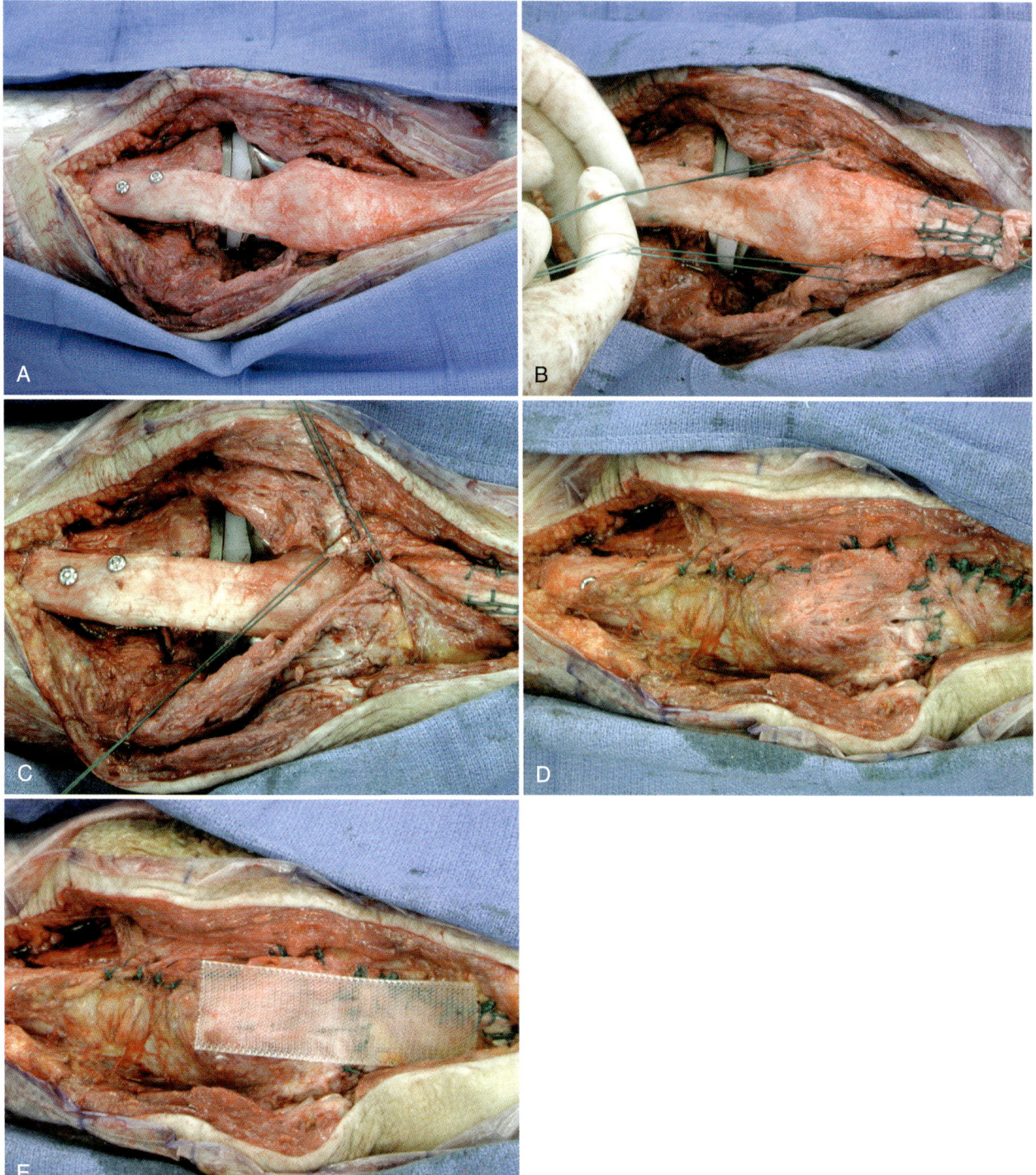

Figure 66-12. Extensor mechanism allograft reconstruction for patellar tendon disruption in a total knee arthroplasty. **A,** An allograft tibial tubercle is fixed to host bone through an interference fit of the allograft-host junction and the use of two 4.5-mm bicortical screws. The allograft quadriceps tendon is secured proximally with two no. 5 nonabsorbable sutures in the Krackow method, with the knee in full extension. The length of the allograft is adjusted to ensure that the allograft patella lies in the trochlear groove. **B,** Two sutures are then placed in the host retinacular tissue. **C** and **D,** The residual host extensor tissue is then sewn over the allograft reconstruction in a pants over vest method. **E,** Marlex mesh is used to reinforce the repair. (Adapted from Scuderi GR, Easley ME: Quadriceps and patellar tendon disruptions. In Insall JN, Scott WN [eds]: Surgery of the knee, vol 1, New York, 2001,Churchill Livingstone, pp 1074–1086.)

KEY REFERENCES

Anderson WE, Habermann ET: Spontaneous bilateral quadriceps tendon rupture in a patient on hemodialysis. Orthop Rev 17:411, 1988.

Bhole R, Johnson JC: Bilateral simultaneous spontaneous rupture of quadriceps tendons in a diabetic patient. South Med J 78:486, 1985.

Goodrich A, Difiore RJ, Tippens JK: Bilateral simultaneous rupture of the infrapatellar tendon: a case report and literature review. Orthopedics 6:1472, 1983.

Kamali M: Bilateral traumatic rupture of the infrapatellar tendon. Clin Orthop 142:131, 1979.

Keogh P, Shanker SJ, Burke T, et al: Bilateral simultaneous rupture of the quadriceps tendons. Clin Orthop Relat Res 234:139, 1988.

Lavalle C, Aparicio LA, Moreno J, et al: Bilateral avulsion of quadriceps tendons in primary hyperparathyroidism. J Rheumatol 12:596, 1985.

Lombardi LJ, Cleri DJ, Epstein E: Bilateral spontaneous quadriceps tendon rupture in a patient with renal failure. Orthopedics 18:187, 1995.

MacEachern AG, Plewes JL: Bilateral simultaneous spontaneous rupture of the quadriceps tendons: five case reports and a review of the literature. J Bone Joint Surg Br 66:81, 1984.

Margles SW, Lewis MM: Bilateral spontaneous concurrent rupture of the patellar tendon without apparent associated systemic disease: a case report. Clin Orthop 136:186, 1978.

Preston ET: Avulsions of both quadriceps tendons in hyperparathyroidism. JAMA 221:406, 1972.

Razzano CD, Wilde AH, Phalen GH: Bilateral rupture of the infrapatellar tendon in rheumatoid arthritis. Clin Orthop 91:158, 1973.

Rose PS, Frassica FJ: Atraumatic bilateral patellar tendon rupture: a case report and review of the literature. J Bone Joint Surg Am 83:1382, 2001.

Schwartzberg RS, Csencsitz TA: Bilateral spontaneous patellar tendon rupture. Am J Orthop 25:369, 1996.

Stern RE, Harwin SF: Spontaneous and simultaneous rupture of both quadriceps tendons. Clin Orthop Relat Res 147:188, 1980.

Walker LG, Glick H: Bilateral spontaneous quadriceps tendon ruptures: a case report and review of the literature. Orthop Rev 18:867, 1989.

Full references for this chapter can be found on www.expertconsult.com.

SECTION 7

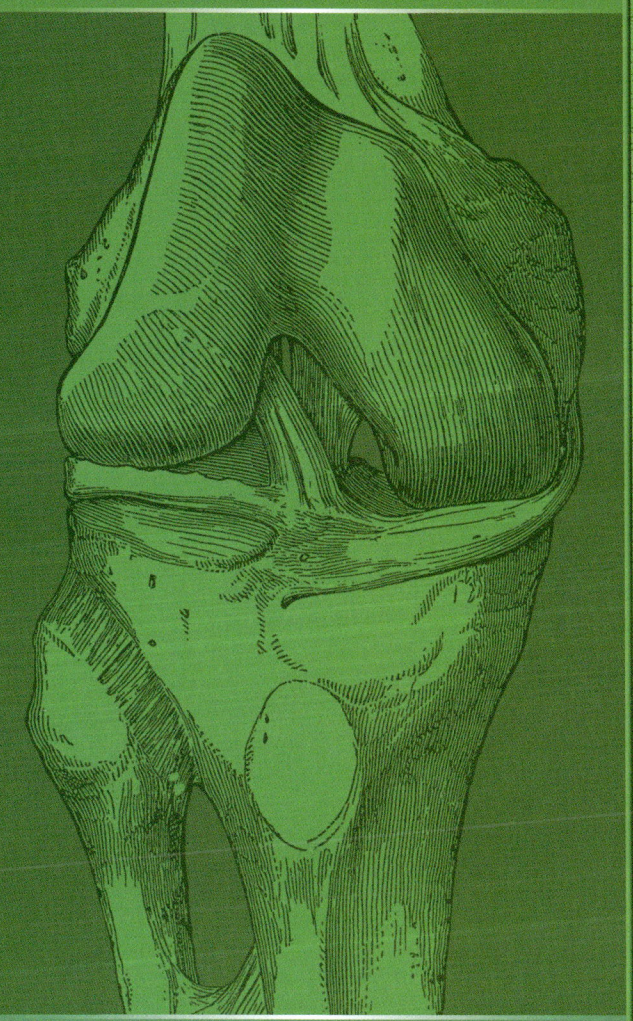

Knee Arthritis

Gout and Other Crystalline Arthropathies

Aryeh M. Abeles and Michael H. Pillinger

CRYSTALLINE ARTHROPATHIES

Although there are a number of crystal-related arthropathies, the most common are gout and pseudogout, caused by urate and calcium pyrophosphate crystals, respectively. In this chapter, we will focus on gout, with a brief discussion of calcium pyrophosphate and other crystalline diseases.

Gout

Gout, first described in antiquity by Hippocrates, is becoming increasingly prevalent,[10] yet remains underdiagnosed and poorly managed in the clinic.

Gout is an end result of sodium urate crystal deposition in joints and soft tissues as a consequence of chronic hyperuricemia. Uric acid is produced via the metabolism of purines. The breakdown of guanine and adenine converges at an intermediate product, xanthine, which is then converted to uric acid via xanthine oxidase. In most mammals, the enzyme uricase then breaks uric acid down to allantoin, a highly soluble, easily excreted molecule. However, humans, great apes, and some New World monkeys developed mutations in the uricase gene approximately 8 to 24 million years ago, leading to gene silencing.[21] The result has been an inactive uricase, the accumulation of uric acid, and serum urate levels higher than those seen in other mammals.[19] Although much of the uric acid is excreted by the gut, a significant portion is renally excreted; accordingly, any failure of renal urate excretion may result in absolute hyperuricemia.[17]

Uric acid is soluble in serum up to a concentration of approximately 6.8 mg/dL, above which deposition of urate crystals can occur. Peripheral joints are typically the sites of urate deposition because of the effects of temperature on crystal solubility—namely, at lower temperatures (e.g., in the peripheral joints, which are several degrees cooler than core body temperature), urate crystals are less soluble in serum and precipitate out of solution into joints and soft tissues. Other factors promoting crystal formation in joints, such as differences in synovial fluid protein concentrations, may also play a role. Although serum uric acid concentrations greater than 6.8 to 7.0 mg/dL predispose to developing gout,[8] only a minority of patients with elevated uric acid levels actually go on to frank gout, and the diagnosis of gout should never be made on the basis of elevated serum uric acid levels alone. The higher the serum uric acid level, however, the more likely a given patient will be suffering, or will eventually go on to suffer, gouty arthropathy.

Most patients suffering their first gouty attack are men between the ages 30 to 60 years. Male sex hormones may contribute to rising uric acid levels (by reducing uric acid renal excretion), and therefore gout in males is typically delayed, at least until after puberty. Conversely, estrogen is uricosuric (i.e., helps maintain low serum urate levels),[16] so women rarely have hyperuricemia or gout before menopause. Aside from androgens and estrogen, other factors influencing serum uric acid concentration include diet and renal function. As expected, a diet rich in purines increases the risk of gout. Purine-rich foods include oily fish (e.g., sardines, herring, mackerel), shellfish, beer, and organ meats such as sweet bread and liver. Although many of these foods are also high in protein, protein consumption per se does not increase serum urate levels and may actually stimulate renal urate excretion. Alcohol consumption also raises serum urate levels and some alcoholic beverages (e.g., beer, ale) are simultaneously high in purines. Often, patients with gout present with an acute arthritic attack shortly after ingestion of a large purine load (e.g., heavy beer consumption, shrimp), which leads to a sudden and precipitous rise in serum uric acid levels. Some investigators have suggested that excessive consumption of fructose, a common food additive, also contributes to hyperuricemia.[5] Urate clearance declines with kidney function, so that patients with impaired renal function have elevated serum uric acid levels and a higher incidence of gout. Some medications block urate excretion, such as thiazide diuretics used for hypertension. Probably because a number of these secondary risk factors for hyperuricemia are increasing, the prevalence of gout has increased by as much as fourfold in the past few decades.[4]

Acute Gout: Presentation and Evaluation

As a rule, gout attacks occur acutely and, although gout attacks can occur at any time of day, patients typically are awakened by the onset of symptoms. Patients describe severe localized pain in combination with marked tenderness, as well as swelling and redness. The peak of an attack generally occurs within hours of onset, and the attack can last from days, in the case of early gout, to weeks or even months in established gout. First attacks of gout most typically occur in the first metatarsophalangeal (MTP) joint, although there are many exceptions to this. Diagnostic clues in the history include recent dietary indiscretions (see earlier) or systemic insults, such as surgery, physical trauma (which may liberate crystals from preestablished deposits), or infection; it is very common for patients with a crystalline arthropathy to have a disease flare with these precipitants.

On examination, the involved joint(s) is generally warm, red, swollen, and markedly tender. Loss of motion because of pain and swelling is the norm. Signs of systemic inflammation may be present, including fever and tachycardia. Joint effusions are usually noted with knee involvement and, if the diagnosis has not already been definitively been made, fluid should be withdrawn not only for therapy, but also for cell count, which in gout will be inflammatory and neutrophil-predominant, crystal identification, and Gram stain and culture. The key to diagnosis is the identification of urate crystals under a polarizing microscope (Table 67-1). Urate

Table 67-1 Common Crystal-Associated Arthropathies

Parameter	Gout	Pseudogout
Crystal	Sodium urate	Calcium pyrophosphate
Radiograph	Early: Soft tissue swelling Later: Radiolucent erosions around edge of articular cartilage	Fine, radiopaque, linear deposits in the menisci and articular cartilage
Frequency of occurrence in knee	Common	Very common; increases with age, DJD
Laboratory studies	Elevated serum uric acid	None
Crystal shape	Needle-shaped	Rhomboid
Crystal character with compensated polarized light	Parallel, yellow; perpendicular, blue (negatively birefringent)	Parallel, blue; perpendicular, yellow (positively birefringent)

From Vigorita VJ: The synovium. In Vigorita VJ, Ghelman B (eds): Orthopaedic pathology, Philadelphia, 1999, Lippincott Williams & Wilkins, p 596.

DJD, Degenerative joint disease.

crystals are negatively birefringent, so the needle-shaped crystals should appear yellow when viewed parallel to the optical axis and blue when perpendicular (Fig. 67-1). Extracellular urate crystals confirm that the patient has gout, but may persist in the joint long after prior attacks; consequently, only intracellular crystals in neutrophils unequivocally confirm that the patient is in the midst of a gouty attack (i.e., that the crystals are activating neutrophils).

In addition to crystal analysis, laboratory evaluation should also include assessment of inflammatory markers (e.g., erythrocyte sedimentation rate, C-reactive protein [CRP] to confirm that the problem is inflammatory), renal function (to identify possible and perhaps remediable risk factors for hyperuricemia), and serum uric acid concentration. Checking the serum uric acid concentration is not as straightforward as it might seem, however. Because serum uric acid concentration can actually drop during an acute gouty attack because of inflammatory effects, serum urate measured during that period may sometimes be normal or even low, leading the clinician to rule out gouty arthritis incorrectly. We therefore recommend rechecking the uric acid 2 or 3 weeks until after an attack has subsided to assess the true baseline level. Radiographs are not particularly useful early in the course of disease, unless they are needed to rule out alternative diagnoses.

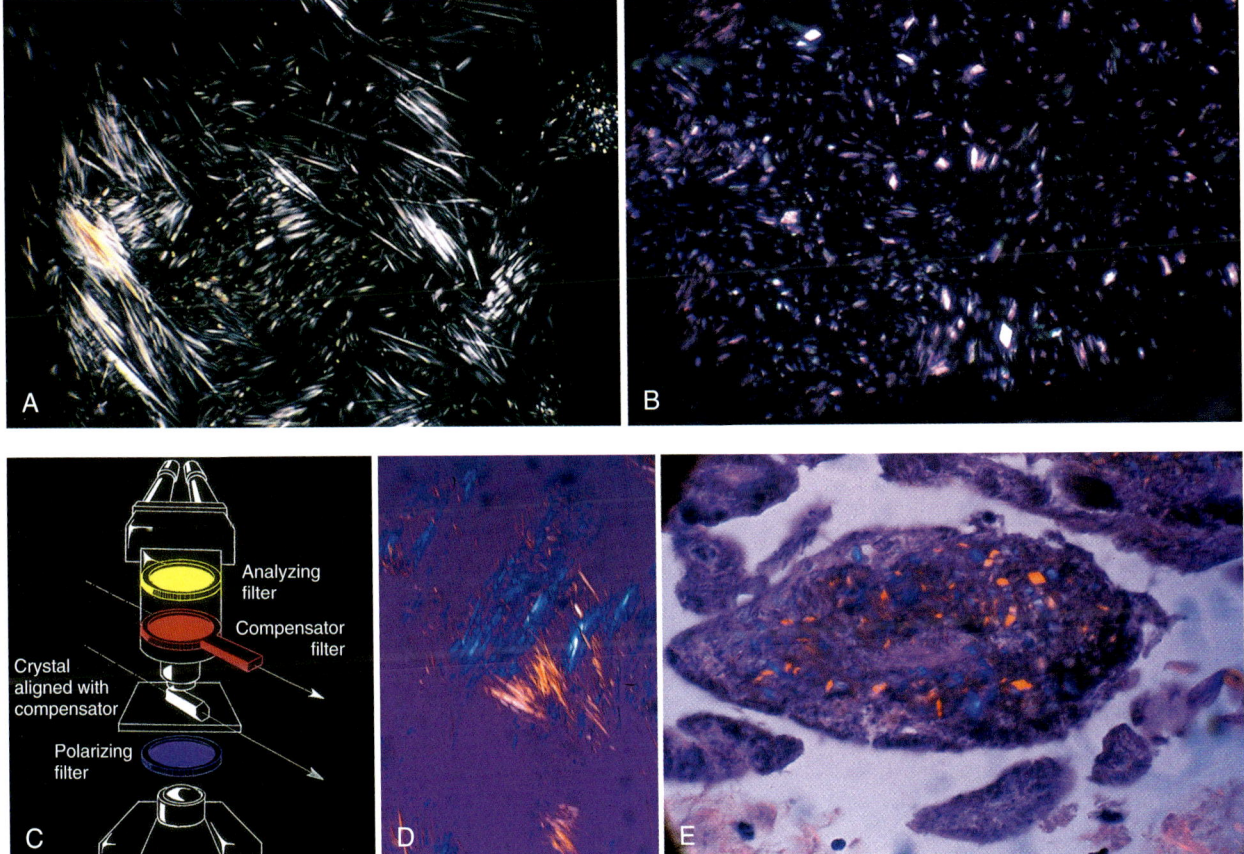

Figure 67-1. Gout versus calcium pyrophosphate crystals. **A,** On polarized light microscopy, sodium urate crystals appear needle-shaped and brilliantly refractive. **B,** Calcium pyrophosphate crystals are less refractile, and crystals are rhomboid in shape. **C,** On polarized light microscopy with a red compensator filter, gout (urate) crystals **(D)** appear yellow when oriented parallel to the axis of compensation and blue when perpendicular (negatively birefringent). **E,** Conversely, CPPD crystals appear blue when parallel to the axis of compensation and yellow when perpendicular (positively birefringent). (From Vigorita VJ: The synovium. In Vigorita VJ: Orthopedic pathology, Philadelphia, 1999, Lippincott Williams & Wilkins, pp 516–576.)

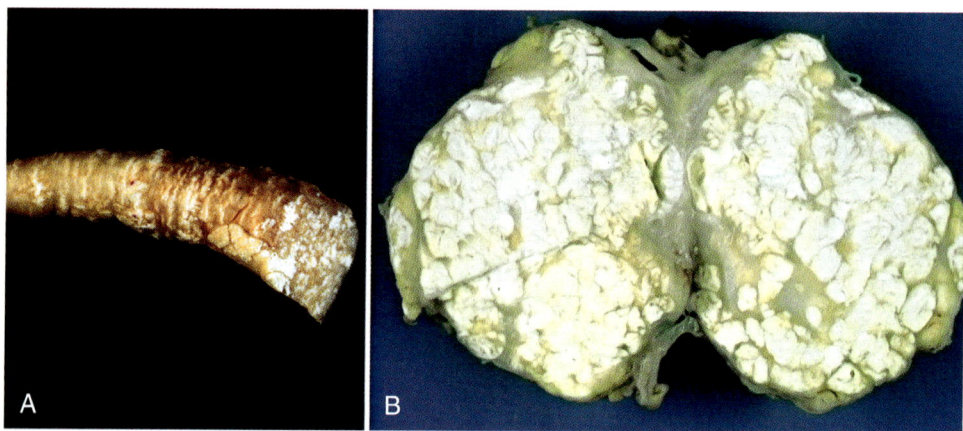

Figure 67-2. Urate crystals seen grossly involving the Achilles tendon **(A)** and synovium **(B)**. The chalk white deposits have a pastelike consistency. (From Vigorita VJ: The synovium. In Vigorita VJ: Orthopedic pathology, Philadelphia, 1999, Lippincott Williams & Wilkins, pp 516–576.)

Chronic Gout

Patients whose gout has persisted for many years, typically with excessive hyperuricemia and multiple episodic acute attacks annually, may proceed to a more chronic phase characterized not only by continued episodic attacks, but by a persistent, smoldering inflammatory arthritis in the affected joints. In addition, such individuals may go on to develop tophi (Latin for "stone")—the deposition of crystal aggregates, many large and surrounded by a corona of inflammatory cells. These tophi are most visible in soft tissue areas such as the olecranon bursa but may be present in almost any tissue (Fig. 67-2). In the bone and cartilage, they may invade and contribute to joint destruction. On plain x-ray, patients with chronic tophaceous gout may have typical erosive changes, particularly of the feet and hands (see Table 67-1). These distinctive erosive changes appear as punched-out lesions, with overhanging edges of bony cortex, and are diagnostic.[20]

Diagnosing Gout

Diagnosing gout can be straightforward, but a few caveats deserve mention. Although an acute gouty attack involving the first MTP joint is typical enough to merit its own name, podagra, acute gouty arthritis can presents in a multitude of ways. In men, initial attacks can occur in the ankles, knees, olecranon bursae, hands, or soft tissue of the feet—almost anywhere—and can be mono- or polyarticular. Polyarticular gout attacks become more common as the disease progresses. As noted earlier, women rarely develop the disease until several years after menopause, and women do not typically experience podagra. In contrast to men, women may more commonly experience initial and/or subsequent attacks in the upper extremities and, in particular, in small joints affected by osteoarthritis, because urate crystals have a predilection to deposit in previously damaged joints.[6] Older women with gout not uncommonly have tophaceous deposits in osteoarthritic nodes in their distal interphalangeal (DIP) joints, and an examiner should look for chalky white subcutaneous deposits in the DIP joints in this patient population.

Because some patients with gout do not present to a physician until late in the disease course, or have been misdiagnosed with another condition, patients should always be examined for subcutaneous tophi, even on the first visit. Common areas for examination include the olecranon processes, Achilles tendons, and first MTP joint.

Because active gouty arthritis can occur concurrently with septic arthritis, appropriate diagnostic and therapeutic measures are necessary if the clinical picture is compatible with infectious arthritis. Although uncommon, gout and infection can coexist; therefore, a diagnosis of gout does not unequivocally preclude the possibility of a septic joint.

Treatment

In treating gout, one must consider three separate aspects of addressing the disease: (1) treating acute gouty attacks; (2) prophylaxis of future attacks; and (3) addressing the underlying cause of gout, which is to say, treating the hyperuricemia.

Treating Acute Gouty Arthropathy

A patient presenting with an acute gouty attack can be treated in a number of ways. A patient with a monoarticular presentation is most easily and effectively managed with an intra-articular steroid injection. However, intra-articular steroid injections should be given only after complete drainage of joint fluid (if the fluid is not drained, the injection will be less efficacious) and, if necessary, confirmation that the joint is not infected. Intra-articular injection is a poor option for patients with a polyarticular presentation or soft tissue involvement, or who decline an intra-articular injection. In such cases several options remain, including the following: (1) a several-day course of a nonsteroidal anti-inflammatory drug (NSAID); (2) a single intramuscular injection of methylprednisolone (80 to 120 mg); or (3) a short course of systemic steroids (e.g., 40 mg daily for 5 days).

NSAIDs are anti-inflammatory and have the added benefit of providing analgesia. However, they have multiple potential risks and side effects that could preclude their use in a number of conditions common to gout patients. Contraindications to NSAIDs include concomitant warfarin therapy, renal insufficiency, congestive heart failure, and a history of upper gastrointestinal GI bleeding. Relative contraindications include age older than 65 years, history of lower GI bleed, chronic liver disease, hypertension, and coronary artery disease. As one might suspect, these are relative contraindications in older patients and we tend to reserve NSAID therapy for younger patients without comorbid conditions.

It must also be noted that all NSAIDs are effective for treating gout. Although indomethacin is the classic NSAID for treating gout, its superiority to other NSAIDs has been repeatedly questioned, although its relatively high potential for side effects (e.g., GI bleeding, nephrotoxicity, hepatotoxicity, central nervous system [CNS] symptoms) are universally recognized. Consideration should therefore be given to using other NSAIDs, as tailored to the comorbidities of the individual patient. For older patients (>65 years) or those with the comorbid conditions listed, we recommend either a single intramuscular methylprednisolone acetate (Depo-Medrol) injection or a short course of oral steroids, with the caveat that polyarticular attacks often require more prolonged treatment, generally 3 weeks or less, depending on the severity of the attack and severity of the patient's underlying disease.

Colchicine, derived from the autumn crocus, was previously the drug of choice for acute attacks. The use of one or two doses may prevent an attack in patients sensing very early symptoms. However, colchicine is not an ideal choice for aborting an established gout attack. A recently presented randomized controlled study demonstrated that both low-dose (1.2 mg PO initially; 0.6 mg PO 1 hour later) and high-dose colchicine (1.2 mg PO initially; 0.6 mg every hour × 6) effectively reduce pain in only approximately 40% of patients; the low dose was actually more effective, but much less toxic.[18] The U.S. Food and Drug Administration (FDA) banned IV colchicine in 2008 because of its narrow therapeutic range and potential for severe toxicity (e.g., severe bone marrow suppression, sloughing of the GI lining, death).

Prophylaxis of Attacks

Patients who have had a single attack, or whose gout attacks are rare, may not require prophylaxis. Others deserve prevention.

Although colchicine is generally not ideal for managing acute gout, it remains the anti-inflammatory treatment of choice for the prevention of future gouty attacks. In a subset of patients, colchicine alone may be sufficient. The standard dose of colchicine for prophylaxis is 0.6 mg twice daily. Although this dose is typically well tolerated, occasional patients may experience diarrhea and require a once-daily regimen. Colchicine dosing must be renally adjusted and, for patients with an estimated glomerular filtration rate (eGFR) of 30 to 50 mL/min, the dose should be 0.6 mg daily. Patients with an eGFR between 10 and 30 mL/min should receive alternate-day dosing, and those with an eGFR lower than 10 mL/min should not receive colchicine. Those who are intolerant of colchicine, or who experience recurrent gouty attacks despite it, may be considered for prophylaxis with a daily NSAID or low-dose prednisone, though these strategies are not well studied.

Urate Lowering: Addressing the Root of the Problem

Although colchicine can provide effective prophylaxis, many individuals who need prophylaxis probably also warrant urate-lowering therapy. Although no official recommendations exist, this would probably include patients who average more than two attacks/year, have a history of any polyarticular attack (or a severe and difficult to treat monoarticular attack), or have a serum uric acid level higher than 9.0 mg/dL.

There are currently two methods available for lowering the serum uric acid level. One is by increasing urate excretion through the use of uricosuric agents and the other is by preventing the production of uric acid via xanthine oxidase inhibitors.

The only approved uricosuric agent in the United States is probenecid, a urate transporter-1 (URAT1) inhibitor, which inhibits urate resorption in the proximal renal tubule. Although safe and effective in the right setting, the drug is uncommonly used for pragmatic reasons, because it requires intact renal function, twice-daily dosing, and adequate hydration to prevent formation of renal urate stones. Moreover, probenecid is only effective in those whose hyperuricemia is caused by renal tubular defects that lead to uric acid underexcretion, which is the case in 90% of patients with gout. The effective dose of probenecid is 500 to 1000 mg twice daily; prior to initiating probenecid, a 24-hour urine collection must be performed to confirm underexcretion. If the 24-hour uric acid excretion is more than approximately 750 mg, probenecid will be ineffective and should be avoided—the patient's kidneys are already excreting as much urate as possible. Benzbromarone, a URAT-1 inhibitor that is more potent than probenecid (and was recently demonstrated as such in a head to head trial),[12] is not available in the United States because of concerns over hepatotoxicity.

Allopurinol has long been, and still remains, the principal agent used to lower hyperuricemia. Allopurinol is a purine analogue that lowers urate levels by inhibiting xanthine oxidase, thus blocking the conversion of hypoxanthine to xanthine and of xanthine to uric acid. Allopurinol use is convenient for both physicians and patients. It is most commonly used once or (at higher doses) twice daily and is effective for both underexcreters and overproducers. Dosing of allopurinol should be titrated to achieve a target serum urate level (usually defined as <6.0 mg/dL in patients without tophi and <5.0 mg/dL in patients with tophi). Dosing should begin at 100 to 300 mg daily, depending on factors such as patient urate level and renal function, but may go as high as 800 mg daily for some resistant patients. During allopurinol titration, we recommend checking urate levels frequently (every 2 to 4 weeks) and adjusting the allopurinol dose by 100 mg after each assessment. Of note, one consequence of lowering the serum urate level by any means is a paradoxical transient period of increased risk for gouty attack. Accordingly, in most cases, neither allopurinol nor probenecid should be initiated until 1 to 2 weeks after colchicine or another anti-inflammatory prophylactic agent is initiated. Barring any contraindications, the colchicine or other anti-inflammatory drug should be continued for at least 6 to 12 months after the target serum urate is achieved.

Generally well tolerated, allopurinol nonetheless carries a less than 1% risk of causing a hypersensitivity syndrome characterized by a morbilliform rash, Stevens-Johnson syndrome, fever, eosinophilia, and bone marrow and renal failure.[2] If allowed to continue, the allopurinol hypersensitivity syndrome may carry as high as a 50% mortality. Physicians should therefore warn patients about the symptoms of hypersensitivity when initiating allopurinol therapy; should a rash or other symptoms occur, the patient must discontinue the drug at once and seek medical advice.

Using allopurinol in patients with renal insufficiency is controversial, because rigorous evaluation has not been performed, and we prescribe it judiciously. Although experts previously expressed concern that the risk of allopurinol hypersensitivity was higher in these patients, some recent small studies have suggested that allopurinol may be safe in patients with renal insufficiency as long as the dose is titrated to the target serum urate level. In patients with an eGFR less than 60 mL/min, we therefore recommend starting low (initiating 100 mg daily), checking the serum urate levels in 2 weeks, and then increasing to 200 mg daily if target levels have not been achieved. This process should be repeated until the target has been achieved, within the limits of physician comfort. It may be reasonable for nonexperts to seek advice before going above the 300-mg dose in these patients.

As simple as it seems to prescribe allopurinol, the drug is frequently prescribed, and taken, incorrectly. Allopurinol should not be initiated, stopped, increased, or decreased during or shortly after a gout attack, because any shift in serum urate levels can prolong an existing flare of disease. Patients must be made aware that the drug is not to be taken on an as-needed basis, but rather is intended as chronic daily therapy. Finally, allopurinol should not be discontinued when the serum urate target level has been reached, any more than antihypertensives should be discontinued once a patient is normotensive.

Febuxostat, a xanthine oxidase inhibitor that is not a purine analogue, gained FDA approval for treating gout in February 2009. Two daily dosage forms are available, 40 and 80 mg. In three head to head trials with allopurinol, 300 mg daily, significantly more patients achieved a serum urate of less than 6.0 mg/dL with the higher dose of febuxostat.[3,15] Febuxostat therefore represents a welcome treatment option whose best practices for use are currently being determined.

Gout therapeutics are enjoying a renaissance after a fallow period of over 40 years. Febuxostat was approved in early 2009 and several other treatments are in development, including a novel uricosuric agent, interleukin-1 (IL-1) inhibitors (to treat acute gout), and recombinant uricase.

Pseudogout

The clinical presentation of pseudogout, calcium pyrophosphate dehydrate (CPPD) deposition disease, is similar to acute gout; attacks are highly inflammatory, occur acutely, and may be mono- or polyarticular. In contrast to gout, attacks are most often seen in the knee, followed by the wrist.[1] The results of laboratory studies are often similar to gout and infection, with elevated erythrocyte sedimentation rates, CRP levels, and white counts. In contrast to gout, which is more or less a systemic disease characterized by elevated serum urate levels, pseudogout is almost invariably a local disease that may develop from local production of calcium pyrophosphate in a joint with abnormally functioning cartilage (e.g., pseudogout is not uncommonly seen in joints affected by osteoarthritis).[14] X-rays of an affected joint often demonstrate chondrocalcinosis, the hallmark of CPPD deposition, appearing as a thin white line running parallel to and just beneath the surface of the cartilage (Fig. 67-3).[13] However, calcium pyrophosphate crystals may appear, and pseudogout attacks may occur, in the absence of radiographic chondrocalcinosis. Conversely, radiographic chondrocalcinosis is often incidentally observed in patients with no clinical pseudogout.

As with gout, definitive diagnosis is made via crystal identification under polarizing microscopy (see Fig. 67-1). In contrast to uric acid, calcium pyrophosphate crystals are positively birefringent and most typically rhomboid-shaped (see Table 67-1). These crystals are smaller, paler, and more difficult to appreciate than urate crystals, and are therefore easily missed. Cell counts from joint fluid are inflammatory, although often less inflammatory than in gout, with neutrophil predominance. As in gout, the presence of intracellular crystals unequivocally confirms that an inflammatory attack is crystal-driven. Also as in gout, pseudogout and infection may occasionally coexist, so vigilance is warranted.

The therapy for acute pseudogout is similar to that for acute gout. NSAIDs and intramuscular, oral, or intra-articular glucocorticoids are effective. Long-term treatment of pseudogout can be difficult, because no known therapies regulate the deposition of the calcium pyrophosphate crystals. However, most patients with pseudogout experience rare attacks and only a very small percentage develop chronic pseudogouty

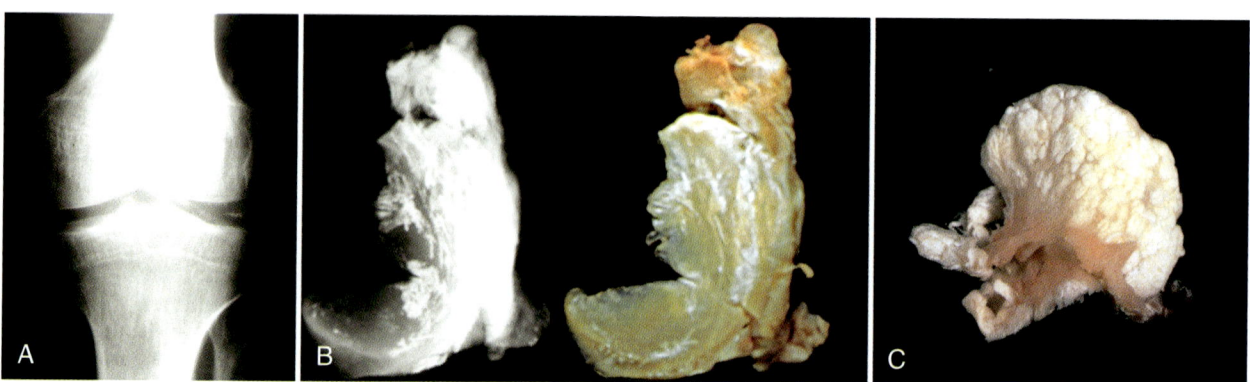

Figure 67-3. Radiograph of the knee in calcium pyrophosphate deposition **(A)**, meniscus gross and specimen x-ray film **(B)**, and synovium **(C)**. (From Vigorita VJ: The synovium. In Vigorita VJ: Orthopedic pathology, Philadelphia, 1999, Lippincott Williams & Wilkins, pp 516–576.)

arthropathy. Low-dose colchicine may be used prophylactically in patients who experience frequent attacks, and NSAIDs may also afford prophylaxis in patients with coexistent osteoarthritis. A small number of patients with pseudogout may have underlying conditions that contribute to the condition (e.g., hypomagnesemia, hypothyroidism, hyperparathyroidism, hemochromatosis). These should be addressed, although it is unclear that such treatment ameliorates the risk of crystal arthritis.

OTHER CRYSTAL DEPOSITION DISEASES

A number of other crystal diseases may occur more rarely, and more sporadically, than gout or pseudogout. Most common of these is basic calcium phosphate (hydroxyapatite) deposition. Hydroxyapatite deposition is seen most typically in older individuals; women may be more commonly affected. Characteristically, hydroxyapatite disease presents as an acute periarthritis or peritendinitis; x-rays of the affected region may reveal calcium deposition in the tendons or capsular structures.[9] Hydroxyapatite disease can also affect the joint itself. Shoulder involvement (Milwaukee shoulder) is perhaps the most common presentation. Aspiration of the joint characteristically reveals a neutrophilic infiltrate; because the crystals are not birefringent, they may be difficult to see on microscopy but can be seen after staining with alizarin red S or when viewed under electron microscopy.[7] The condition may resolve spontaneously, persist or, in some cases, result in a severe destructive arthropathy. Treatment includes rest and anti-inflammatory agents, including oral or intra-articular steroid injections.

Calcium oxalate crystals may produce arthritis in patients with renal disease, particularly those on dialysis or with familial forms of early onset renal failure.[11] Attacks tend to be acute and resemble those of gout or pseudogout. Examination of joint fluid under polarizing microscopy reveals bipyramidal-shaped birefringent crystals. Given the toxicities of NSAIDs and colchicines in renal failure, these attacks may be best managed with low-dose oral steroids; some experts express concern about using intrarticular injections because of the risk of infection.

In patients with chronic arthritis, particularly in long-standing rheumatoid arthritis and osteoarthritis, cholesterol crystals may be identified in joints or, more typically, in the olecranon bursa. These birefringent platelike crystals appear to have no inflammatory potential and do not require therapy beyond appropriate management of the underlying condition.

KEY REFERENCES

Agudelo CA, Wise CM: Crystal-associated arthritis in the elderly. Rheum Dis Clin North Am 26:527–546, 2000.

Arellano F, Sacristan JA: Allopurinol hypersensitivity syndrome: a review. Ann Pharmacother 27: 337–343, 1993.

Becker MA, Schumacher HR, Jr, Wortmann RL, et al: Febuxostat compared with allopurinol in patients with hyperuricemia and gout. N Engl J Med 353:2450–2461, 2005.

Choi HK, Curhan G: Gout: epidemiology and lifestyle choices. Curr Opin Rheumatol 17:341–345, 2005.

Choi HK, Curhan G: Soft drinks, fructose consumption, and the risk of gout in men: prospective cohort study. BMJ 336:309–312, 2008.

De Leonardis F, Govoni M, Colina M, et al: Elderly-onset gout: a review. Rheumatol Int 28:1–6, 2007.

Mikuls TR, Saag KG: New insights into gout epidemiology. Curr Opin Rheumatol 18:199–203, 2006.

Rosenthal AK: Pathogenesis of calcium pyrophosphate crystal deposition disease. Curr Rheumatol Rep 3:17–23, 2001.

Taniguchi A, Kamatani N: Control of renal uric acid excretion and gout. Curr Opin Rheumatol 20:192–197, 2008.

Terkeltaub R, Bennett FD, Kook K, et al: Colchicine efficacy assessed by time to 50% reduction of pain is comparable in low dose and high dose regimens: secondary analyses of the AGREE trial. Arthritis Rheum 60:S413, 2009.

Watt I: Radiology of the crystal-associated arthritides. Ann Rheum Dis 42(Suppl 1):73–80, 1983.

Full references for this chapter can be found on www.expertconsult.com.

Chapter 68

Knee Osteoarthritis

Pamela B. Rosenthal

Osteoarthritis (OA) is the leading cause of musculoskeletal disability worldwide. The incidence and prevalence of OA increase with aging. Already over a decade ago, in 1996 the estimate was that 9.6% of men and 18% of women 60 years of age and older worldwide suffered from symptomatic OA.[27] Osteoarthritis is thought to be more prevalent in developed than in developing regions of the world.[47] In the United States, estimates indicate that 85% of the population 75 years of age and older are afflicted.[14] Osteoarthritis of the knee represents an important subset of the overall OA burden and is the leading cause of functional disability. A European study estimated that the prevalence of radiographic knee OA is 13% for women and 8% for men between the ages of 45 and 49, rising to 55% and 22%, respectively, for persons 80 years of age and older.[44] These data were corroborated by a groundbreaking study in Johnston County, North Carolina, which concluded that the lifetime risk of symptomatic knee OA was 44.7%.[26] In the United States in 2004, hospital and associated costs of total knee replacement were estimated at $14.3 billion.[2]

Osteoarthritis presents with a complaint of pain and swelling resulting in decreased joint mobility. Traditionally, diagnostic criteria include characteristic radiologic changes inclusive of joint space narrowing and associated bone changes. This diarthrodial joint is a complex organ that comprises a variety of tissue and cell types, all of which are modified in the setting of active OA.

Hominid knees have evolved in response to constraints and requirements of a bipedal gait. Our earlier hominid ancestors were arboreal. Obligate hominid bipedalism evolved approximately 4 million years ago, with resultant skeletal changes to accommodate the increased demands of weight bearing across two rather than four limbs. The vertebral column assumed its characteristic curve and the pelvis evolved a dorsal projection, resulting in the placement of our center of mass above our hips and allowing for translation of forces through our knees and feet.[45] Many intriguing theories have been proposed as to the evolutionary selection pressures that resulted in this transformative stance and gait, including the secondary benefits of an upright head and the advantages of liberated upper extremities. It is also suggested that the elongated lower limb and upright posture allow for an energetically more efficient gait than a quadruped gait.[36] Although OA is a general cost of a vertebral skeleton, the vulnerability of our lower lumbar spine, hips, and knees to OA processes may be a consequence of the unique mechanical forces associated with a bipedal gait.

The knee, which is the largest joint in the body, is routinely subjected to forces that are three to five times body weight during normal gait. The added weight-bearing and stability requirements of the human knee have resulted in expanded femoral and tibial condyles relative to the knees of other vertebrates. In addition, the human patella is notable for its large size and its concomitant role in knee stabilization. The menisci of human knees are much larger than those of other vertebrates.[16]

LESSONS FROM EPIDEMIOLOGY/ROLE OF JOINT STRESS

Osteoarthritis is conceived of as a process that is initiated and perpetuated by mechanical stress. Normal healthy joints are defined by their nearly frictionless excursion and physiologic loading, as maintained and limited by constraints on joint range of motion. Increased mechanical stress resulting from traumatic ligamentous and cartilage injuries and from increased mechanical forces associated with obesity is a prominent risk factor for the development of knee OA. Interest in the role of gait variance as an OA risk factor is evolving. Yet OA is a tissue-based process. The mechanical forces that result in OA are translated into biochemical and cellular perturbation that manifests as and is a consequence of focal loading defects.

As with all disease, OA is a consequence of the interplay between host and environmental factors. Lifestyle and life cycle events influence the natural history of OA. Osteoarthritis is described as primary (idiopathic) or secondary, localized or generalized. Osteoarthritis that is associated with trauma, congenital defects, inflammatory arthritis, or neuropathic or metabolic disease is conceived of as secondary.[32] Knee OA can present in isolation or in association with polyarticular OA, especially OA of the hands.[17]

Aging and female gender are invariant risk factors associated with increased incidence of knee OA. By contrast, obesity and trauma are life experience variables that correlate with knee OA incidence and progression. In all cases, knee OA can be conceived of as resulting from excessive joint loading caused by perturbations of joint biomechanics.

Explanations for the increased incidence and prevalence of OA with aging include factors attributable to events earlier in life and special circumstances of aging. For example, radiographic knee OA may present in old age, but events that initiated the OA may have occurred years earlier. The natural history of OA is such that it likely takes years to manifest as radiographic damage. The initial radiographic marker of OA is uncertain; once established radiographically, detectable cartilage volume loss seen on x-ray may be as little as less than 2% per year.[19] Muscle strength, reaction time, and proprioception are factors implicated in joint stability and health; all are impaired with aging. As a consequence, aging is characterized by an increased inclination to injury. The risk of OA in aging is magnified by a decreased capacity for cellular repair. These two characteristics of the aging process alone may contribute to increased risk of knee OA incidence and progression,[32] although microscopic and subcellular changes of aging are also likely to play a role.

The predilection of women's joints to OA is not well understood. In the Framingham cohort, women developed symptomatic radiographic OA at a rate of 1% per year as compared with 0.7% per year for men. At baseline, the women in this cohort had a mean age of 71 years. Estrogens are presumed to be protective, and in the postmenopausal state their relative deficiency may correlate with accelerated cartilage loss. However, no clear consensus has been reached with respect to the role of estrogen biology as it pertains to the risk of incidence or progression of OA. Instead, the reported increased risk may correlate with other genetic and phenotypic variables. A Dutch study reported the protective effects of an allelic variation of one of the bone morphogenetic proteins—growth differentiation factor 5 (GDF5)—on the incidence of hand and knee OA in women, but not in men, suggesting that as yet unidentified biochemical variables may influence the observed OA gender dimorphism.[40,43] Equally straightforward and well-documented differences in life expectancy, adiposity, muscle mass, ligamentous laxity, joint stability, and propensity to obesity may influence OA risk.

The obesity epidemic has wide-ranging implications for public health. A recent analysis demonstrated that if current obesity trends continue, the deleterious effects of weight gain on life expectancy will shortly outweigh the positive impact on life expectancy of decreased rates of smoking. Estimates suggest that in the United States, obesity currently accounts for 5% to 15% of deaths each year. It is projected that nearly half the population (45%) will be obese (body mass index [BMI] > 30) by the year 2020.[38]

Obesity has a profound impact on joint health. The incidence of knee OA across all population studies is highly correlated with BMI. Initial observations in the Framingham study correlating knee OA with obesity continue to be substantiated.[8] The Johnston County, North Carolina, cohort study concluded that lifetime risk of knee OA for obese (BMI ≥30) persons is 60.5% versus 46.9% for the overweight (BMI, 25 to <30) and 30.2% for those with BMI <25.[26] An influence of childhood obesity on lifetime OA risk is likely. Several studies have demonstrated a correlation between increased BMI early in life and the development of subsequent knee OA.[11] However, the Johnston County cohort showed that obesity at baseline and follow-up visits more strongly correlates with lifetime OA risk than BMI at 18 years of age. Equally, although obesity is clearly and strongly correlated with risk for OA, several studies have suggested that obesity does not necessarily correlate with OA progression. In a study of 60 obese and 81 nonobese women followed by x-ray over 12 months, although the obese women demonstrated greater initial radiographic OA severity, their joint space widths did not diminish.[22] Another study showed a correlation between radiographic progression and obesity among patients with a neutral or valgus alignment, but not a varus alignment, lending further insight into the complexity of the relationship between obesity and knee OA progression.[6]

Obesity in combination with cardiovascular risk factors may enrich a patient's risk for knee OA. In an intriguing analysis, Sowers and associates evaluated 482 women (mean age, 47 years) using knee films for evidence of diabetes mellitus and/or dyslipidemia and hypertension, with the result that obese patients with cardiometabolic clustering had a knee OA prevalence of 23.2% versus 12.8% among obese women without cardiometabolic clustering. In addition, women with the cardiometabolic syndrome reported more knee pain than those without the cardiometabolic syndrome. These data point to the influence of metabolic factors on joint health.[37]

The medial and lateral compartments of the tibial-femoral knee joint do not bear load equally. In neutrally aligned knees, the medial compartment bears 60% to 70% of the force across the knee in weight-bearing activities. Therefore, it is not surprising that the medial compartment of the knee is disproportionately afflicted with OA, with medial OA representing up to 75% of the disease burden. Equally patellar-femoral osteoarthritis is also disproportionately medial.[20]

By extension, knee malalignment is the single biggest risk factor in OA disease progression. Varus-valgus malalignment correlates with OA progression in isolation and/or in synergy with other risk factors. Varus malalignment increases the predisposition to OA disease progression by upward of four-fold, and valgus malalignment by as much as fivefold in some studies.[33] Data on the role of malalignment as a risk factor for initiation of disease are not as consistent as for progression. Traditionally, mechanical knee malalignment is assessed with static limb x-rays. Mechanical axis and dynamic adduction moments are highly correlated. Yet forces across the joint during the dynamic phase of gait may have an even more powerful effect on disease progression than malalignment measured during a static stance. During normal gait, the adduction moment is approximately 3.3% of body weight × height, compared with 4.2% body weight × height in patients with medial knee OA.[31] The degree of joint space loss has been shown to correlate with the degree of adduction moment. Persons with greater adduction moment lost joint space more quickly.[25]

Static knee alignment is determined by a variety of biomechanical factors. Tibiofemoral congruence, integrity of the anterior cruciate ligament (ACL) and the meniscus, and supporting muscular strength all influence joint alignment.[20] Torn ACLs and damaged and extruding menisci have long been known to be associated with progression of knee OA. The standard of care for debilitating knee pain used to include total meniscectomy, until it was learned that surgical meniscal resection correlates with accelerated OA. Menisci tear both as a consequence of trauma, a very common athletic injury, and secondary to degenerative change. The advent of magnetic resonance imaging (MRI) as an OA investigational tool allowed for the prospective examination of 121 cases and 294 control knees over a 30-month period as part of the Observational Multicenter Osteoarthritis Study. Patient age ranged from 50 to 79 years, and all were determined to be at high risk for OA because they were overweight, had persistent knee pain, or had a history of knee trauma. Patients were followed in two cohorts: one with incident OA, and the other studied as controls. Meniscal damage at baseline was more frequent in knees with progressive joint space loss/cartilage degeneration than in radiographically stable knees (54% vs. 18%; $P < .001$). A dose effect of meniscal damage with more severe baseline meniscal disease was noted to correlate with increased progressive radiologic OA. It was no surprise that 30-month MRIs captured new meniscal tears in both cohorts, although more frequently in the OA than in the non-OA group. Taken together, these data show the pivotal role that meniscal integrity plays in knee health; they also raise compelling questions about the pathoetiologic role of meniscal deformities. Do they initiate or propagate OA? No doubt their role is complex, with meniscal injuries at once resulting in and signifying the biomechanical derangement and modification of associated joint structures.[6]

LESSONS FROM RADIOLOGY

Adapting to changing load is a requirement of a healthy joint. Each tissue and cell type contributes. Osteoarthritis results when the capacity to adapt is exceeded, resulting in structure modifications that cause characteristic tissue changes. In recent years, insights provided by MRI study of knee OA have expanded our understanding of the pathophysiology. Historically, OA was thought of as a primary condition of articular hyaline cartilage. Now it is appreciated that all joint tissues are concurrently involved—cartilage, synovium, and bone together—and that tissue inflammation and inflammatory pathways play a prominent role in the pathophysiology of OA. Enthesitis, synovitis, bone marrow lesions, and cartilage loss are all lesions of evolving interest in OA. In particular, evolving evidence suggests that synovitis and bone marrow lesions may correlate with joint pain and progression of OA.[30]

Bone is the defining characteristic of skeletal anatomy. Bone is at once brittle and resilient. It is characterized by its ability to respond to mechanical stress with upregulation of bone formation with osteoblast activation, and resorption with osteoclast activation, allowing for the dynamic response of the skeleton to environmental forces. This homeostatic remodeling process is perturbed in OA, resulting in characteristic subchondral sclerosis and subchondral plate thickening. In several studies, these changes have preceded cartilage volume loss.[4]

Subchondral bone is the interface between overlying articular cartilage and underlying cortical and trabecular bone. Although the volume of trabecular bone may increase in OA, paradoxically, perhaps in response to altered mineralization kinetics, the stiffness of this new bone may actually decrease.[13]

Bone marrow lesions first came to the attention of investigators more than 20 years ago and were originally described as bone marrow edema.[46] Nearly a decade ago, the correlation between bone marrow lesions and OA progression and pain was first identified.[10] More recently, 70% of patients with bone marrow lesions were found to have pseudocysts on histopathologic examination of surgical specimens.[39] These lesions corresponded to the areas of most severe damage in the overlying cartilage and likely correlated with areas of focal bone necrosis.

Bone marrow lesions are of interest not only because of their pathophysiologic significance, but also because they correlate with knee pain. In a 2001 study, Felson and colleagues showed that 37% of patients with documented x-ray OA with knee pain had bone marrow lesions versus only 2% of patients with x-ray OA but without knee pain ($P < .001$).[9]

Osteophytes are a pathopneumonic radiologic finding of OA. They are known to precede joint space narrowing and cartilage degradation. It has been suggested that they may represent a compensatory response to ligamentous injury or laxity. Anterior and posterior osteophytes form in response to ACL tear and limit tibial-femoral excursion.[42] Thus although conceived of as pathogenic, they may contribute to

joint stability. Osteophytes form in areas of active joint loading as a result of endochondral ossification. Periosteal cells first proliferate then differentiate into chondrocytes, which, in turn, hypertrophy and ossify.[13]

Synovial hypertrophy is a hallmark of advanced OA; on MRI, it strongly correlates with knee pain. Synovial lining hypertrophy correlates topographically with areas of underlying cartilage denudation and bone damage. Several prospective MRI studies of OA cohorts have concluded that a decrease in synovitis on MRI correlates with a decrease in pain score. Synovitis is often correlated with joint effusions and joint capsular swelling. The size of a joint effusion itself correlates with the degree of knee pain. The synovium is an extremely bioactive tissue. In addition to playing the role of synovial-like fibroblasts in the production of synovial fluid, it is home to various monocytes and macrophages, which, when activated, assume an inflammatory phenotype. The relevance of inflammation to osteoarthritis has taken on new importance as the role of synovium in OA has become better appreciated with the advent of newer radiologic techniques.[30]

LESSONS FROM CELL BIOLOGY AND GENETICS

Osteoarthritis is a heterogeneous disorder. Age, trauma, obesity, and gender are independent risk factors for knee OA. Although they share the common pathway of disruption of biomechanical joint integrity, the mechanism by which aberrant loading is translated into a biochemical event is less well understood. On a macromolecular level, OA cartilage demonstrates fibrillation, fissuring, neovascularization, areas of focal necrosis, and other hallmarks of stress. On a molecular level, OA is characterized by disruption of the extracellular cartilaginous matrix associated with upregulation of matrix metalloproteinases (MMPs) and proinflammatory and counterregulatory signaling molecules.

Chondrocytes live in an avascular environment. Presumably the avascular setting is an adaptive constraint to the biomechanical demand placed on cartilage. No doubt the regular sheer forces experienced by joints and their shock-buffering cartilage would result in routine vessel sheer. Consequently, chondrocytes have a low metabolic rate, yet are responsible for production of the extremely elaborate and long-lived extracellular matrix. The dominant molecule of the extracellular matrix is type II collagen. The stability of this molecule is marked by its exceptional half-life of 100 years, making it among the few macromolecules that journey with us from cradle to grave.[34] The chondrocyte is also charged with cartilage remodeling and repair. When the demands of repair outpace the reparative capacity of the chondrocytes, OA ensues.

Chondrocytes have the capacity to respond to mechanical stress via integrin and related surface receptors. Many of these receptors also engage type II collagen fragments and glycoprotein fragments. Once activated, receptors trigger the production of MMPs, as well as chemokines and cytokines. MMP-13 is of particular interest in the degradative processes that characterize degradation of type II collagen in OA. Chondrocytes located closer to the cartilage surface assume a more activated catabolic phenotype; deeper in the matrix, close to the bone margin, they assume a more regenerative phenotype and synthesize additional extracellular matrix proteins. In OA, the catabolic phenotype outpaces the regenerative/anabolic phenotype. Type II collagen fragments themselves provide feedback to activate the production of additional metalloproteinases. Type II collagen fragments bind to discoidin domain receptor-2 (DDR-2), upregulating MMP-13.[12]

Collagens provide tensile strength to the cartilage matrix. Matrix proteoglycans and glycoproteins help to stabilize the collagen matrix and contribute to the biomechanical properties of cartilage. For example, the hydroscopic properties of aggrecans contribute compressive strength to cartilage. In addition to collagen degradation by MMPs, collagen-associated glycoproteins and proteoglycans are actively degraded in OA. Increased expression of ADAMTS, a specific aggrecan proteinase, is a hallmark of OA.[21] Not only do increased levels of glycoprotein break down proteins found in OA joint tissues, they also are found in the circulation. COMP (thrombospondin 5) circulates in high levels in OA serum and is associated with radiographic progression and increased OA-associated joint pain.[28] Structurally compromised extracellular matrix perpetuates the OA cycle, in part through binding of constituent breakdown products to cell surface receptors.

Osteoarthritis traditionally is not considered an inflammatory arthritis because of the dearth of neutrophilic infiltrate and the absence of systemic inflammatory biomarkers. Yet the key regulatory role played by inflammatory mediators has gained appreciation over the past decade. Chondrocytes and synoviocytes respond to and themselves synthesize proinflammatory cytokines such as interleukin (IL)-1 and tumor necrosis factor (TNF); this, in turn, leads to upregulation of MMPs, MMP-13 in particular, as well as upregulation of cyclooxygenase (COX)-2 genes.[15,24]

The role of complement activation in OA is not well appreciated. However, recent work has revealed that the extracellular matrix proteins fibromodulin, osteoadherin, and lumican can activate the classical complement pathway, and that biglycan and decorin can act as counterregulatory elements and can inhibit complement activation.[35]

Nitrite oxide (NO), traditionally thought of as a proinflammatory mediator, also acts in a counterregulatory fashion, limiting catabolism. The functional effects of NO may act along a gradient in part contingent on the topographic location of the chondrocyte in the matrix. NO can inhibit the synthesis of proteoglycans and collagens and can accelerate their degeneration through upregulation of MMPs. NO stimulates proinflammatory cytokines and their upstream activating enzymes, such as IL-1 converting enzyme. NO induces prostaglandin (PG)E$_2$ and COX-2 synthesis through the activation of nuclear factor kappa B (NFκB). NO can also induce apoptosis. However, NO is part of a complex system of reactive species that includes superoxide and its reactive product with NO, peroxynitrite. Peroxynitrite and NO themselves demonstrate discrete functions. NO has been demonstrated to increase collagen synthesis in tendons, although a dose-dependent response may be seen with moderate amounts of NO, yielding increased collagen synthesis; higher doses result in a net collagen loss.[5] NO and other reactive oxygen species (ROS) are important mediators of pain. Peroxynitrite in particular is known to induce hyperalgesia through the COX–PGE$_2$ pathway. Taken together, these data point to the complex role of NO and its associated reactive oxygen species in OA.[1]

The Wnt signaling pathway is the central signaling pathway that controls bone morphogenesis. Mechanical loading results in Wnt signaling through frizzled receptors (LRP5), which leads to activation of the nuclear transcription factor β-catenin; this causes increased production of osteoprotegerin (OPG), bone morphogenetic proteins (BMPs), osteocalcin, and insulin-like growth factor (IGF). Wnt-stimulated osteoblasts are apoptosis resistant. In addition, OPG binds receptor activator of nuclear factor kappa B ligand (RANKL), which results in downregulation of osteoclast activation. Another protein in this system is sclerostin (SOST), which is an inhibitor of Wnt signaling. SOST provides another link between mechanical stimuli and cellular response. Under mechanical loading conditions, SOST expression is diminished, favoring osteoblast activity.[29] It is presumed that this system plays a role in the pathophysiology of OA. However, evidence supporting this contention is largely genetic. Frizzled-related proteins, sFRP3 and FRZB among them, are direct antagonists of Wnt; this can lead to osteoblast apoptosis. Polymorphisms in these genes are of interest with respect to contributing to OA risk.[12]

Osteoarthritis is polygenetic. The effect size of any one gene in contributing to the propensity to OA is small. Yet OA runs in families, and twin studies have suggested that genetic factors may contribute as much as 70% of OA risk. To date, as many as 95 different genes have been proposed to contribute to this risk. Polymorphisms in extracellular matrix component molecules, such as type II and type IX collagens and aggrecan, have been proposed, as have polymorphisms in signaling molecules such as estrogen receptors and the IL-1 gene cluster.[3,12] Insight into the contribution of genes to OA risk is just beginning to be gained. Data from large-population genome-wide association scans are awaited.[23] Yet a pattern is emerging that confirms what is known epidemiologically, namely, that OA at different anatomic sights represents variations on the OA pathway theme. For example, a recent study found that polymorphisms in the growth differentiation factor 5 gene (GDF5), a member of the transforming growth factor superfamily implicated in regulating proteoglycan synthesis, are more strongly correlated with risk for knee OA than OA at any other site.[7] As previously mentioned, another polymorphism in this gene may reduce OA risk for women.[40]

THERAPY

Osteoarthritis of the knee is a debilitating and complex medical problem. Research into its epidemiology and associated pathophysiology is rapidly advancing, with the implicit goal that research insights will lead to better therapies. Ideally, strategies will be found that can blunt progressive joint damage and promote healing. Although many pipeline compounds are based on the biologic insights discussed previously, to date disease-modifying compounds remain elusive. Instead, American College of Rheumatology (ACR) 2009 revised recommendations for the treatment of osteoarthritis are significant for reliance on traditional analgesics and nonpharmacologic interventions. Two categories of advice are based on the strength of the evidence. Recommended interventions are based on stronger evidence than suggestions. For knee OA, recommendations include land-based aerobic and resistance exercise, as well as aquatic exercise and weight loss in the setting of overweight and obese patients. Suggestions include a variety of strategies to improve joint angulation, including medially wedged insoles for valgus knee, medially directed patellar taping, and subtalar strapped lateral insoles for varus knees. Additionally, self-management program participation, psychosocial intervention, manual therapy in combination with supervised exercise programs, walking aids, and instruction in the use of thermal agents are recommended. With respect to pharmacologic recommendations, if the patient is older than 75 years of age, topical nonsteroidal anti-inflammatory drugs (NSAIDs) are recommended, or an oral NSAID if the patient is younger than 75. Intra-articular steroids are also recommended. Tramadol, opioid analgesics, and intra-articular hyaluronate injections are suggested.[18]

In addition, various nutraceuticals formulations are marketed for the treatment of knee pain. Among the most widely consumed and best known are the glucosamine and chondroitin sulfate products. Despite considerable and thoughtful effort on the part of many investigative bodies, including the GAIT trial supported by the NIH division National Center for Complementary and Alternative Medicine, there is no clear evidence that these compounds are effective at reducing osteoarthritis progression, although in some cases they may help ameliorate pain. In addition there are ongoing tissue-engineering efforts, which are slowly meeting with some success.[4a]

CONCLUSION

Osteoarthritis is common to all vertebrates, and we share with all vertebrates this problem as a condition of aging. The biology of aging is itself complex. Senescence and its associated biology are thought to be independent of evolutionary selection pressure. Selective forces are meant to act on maximizing reproductive fitness. Whatever happens to individuals after their peak reproductive period is merely a consequence of the biologic tradeoffs and optimizations selected for the benefit of propagating one's genes into the next generation. Historically, the human life span was considerably shorter than it is now, approximately 35 years versus 78 years in the United States as of 2009. It is not a coincidence that OA starts to emerge just past the limit of our historical life span, around 40 to 45 years of age. Yet as we have seen, the risk factors for OA are diverse and do not consist of aging alone.

Age-related changes in the joint may predispose to vulnerability to OA, even if the more discrete risk factor might be trauma and/or even obesity. In other words, the effects of aging and abnormal joint loading are likely synergistic. It may be that some age-related cartilage changes sensitize the joint to mechanical stimuli. Cartilage may lose its resiliency as a consequence of the aging-related breakdown of aggrecan and an age-related increase in type II cartilage cross-links. Aging is also associated with accumulation of glycation end products in articular cartilage, which results in increased stiffness of the extracellular matrix. Natural history reveals that chondrocytes may themselves switch to an aging phenotype, resulting in modification of signaling pathway thresholds.[41] Human knees may be especially vulnerable to OA as a consequence of our unique bipedal gait.

Regardless of the cause of OA, it needs to be treated. Pain and disability associated with knee arthritis result in substantive disability. The OA research community will continue to investigate causality in an effort to improve therapy and patient outcomes.

KEY REFERENCES

Abramson SB: Osteoarthritis and nitric oxide. Osteoarthritis Cartilage 16(Suppl 2):S15–S20, 2008.

Englund M, Guermazi A, Roemer FW, et al: Meniscal tear in knees without surgery and the development of radiographic osteoarthritis among middle-aged and elderly persons: the Multicenter Osteoarthritis Study. Arthritis Rheum 60:831–839, 2009.

Felson DT, Anderson JJ, Naimark A, et al: Obesity and knee osteoarthritis: the Framingham study. Ann Intern Med 109:18–24, 1988.

Felson DT, Chaisson CE, Hill CL, et al: The association of bone marrow lesions with pain in knee osteoarthritis. Ann Intern Med 134:541–549, 2001.

Felson DT, McLaughlin S, Goggins J, et al: Bone marrow edema and its relation to progression of knee osteoarthritis. Ann Intern Med 139(5 Pt 1):330–336, 2003.

Gelber AC, Hochberg MC, Mead LA, et al: Body mass index in young men and the risk of subsequent knee and hip osteoarthritis. Am J Med 107:542–548, 1999.

Goldring MB, Goldring SR: Osteoarthritis. J Cell Physiol 213:626–634, 2007.

Herzmark MH: The evolution of the knee joint. J Bone Joint Surg Am 20:77–84, 1938.

Hochberg MC: Development of the 2009 revised ACR recommendations for the management of osteoarthritis. Paper presented at the American College of Rheumatology Annual Meeting, Philadelphia, Pa, October 16–21, 2009.

Hunter DJ, Sharma L, Skaife T: Alignment and osteoarthritis of the knee. J Bone Joint Surg Am 91(Suppl 1):85–89, 2009.

Murphy L, Schwartz TA, Helmick CG, et al: Lifetime risk of symptomatic knee osteoarthritis. Arthritis Rheum 59:1207–1213, 2008.

Schipplein OD, Andriacchi TP: Interaction between active and passive knee stabilizers during level walking. J Orthop Res 9:113–119, 2001.

Sharma L, Kapoor D, Issa S: Epidemiology of osteoarthritis: an update. Curr Opin Rheumatol 18:147–156, 2006.

Sharma L, Song J, Felson DT, et al: The role of knee alignment in disease progression and functional decline in knee osteoarthritis. JAMA 286:188–195, 2001.

van der Kraan PM, van den Berg WB: Osteoarthritis in the context of ageing and evolution: loss of chondrocyte differentiation block during ageing. Ageing Res Rev 7:106–113, 2008.

Full references for this chapter can be found on www.expertconsult.com.

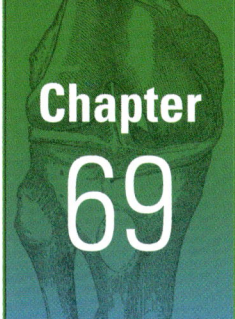

Chapter 69

Overview of Psoriatic Arthritis

Gary E. Solomon

Psoriatic arthritis (PsA) is a chronic inflammatory disorder with clinical features that overlap with those of rheumatoid arthritis. There are, however, important differences in pathophysiology and clinical course, which has implications for the medical and surgical management of patients with this disorder. This chapter will review the epidemiology, genetics, pathophysiology, and immunopathogenesis of PSA in an effort to provide the orthopedist treating a patient with this disorder a firm understanding of unique treatment issues.

GENERAL CONSIDERATIONS

Psoriatic arthritis is defined as arthritis, spondylitis, or dactylitis occurring in association with the skin disease psoriasis (PsO). The recent CASPAR criteria for PsA (Box 69-1) dramatically explain the spectrum of this disorder by allowing the inclusion of patients who do not currently have psoriasis, but have a past history of psoriasis or a family history of psoriasis.[7] The criteria also recognize the importance of changes in the nails, as well as changes in the skin.

Epidemiology

The National Psoriasis Foundation has estimated that PsO affects 1% to 3% of the population.[3,4] Estimates of the prevalence of PsA in patients with PsO are 15% to 39%, with the higher estimates being based on patient series in which patients have actually been examined. As a consequence, PsA is likely a more common disorder than rheumatoid arthritis.

Unlike rheumatoid arthritis, which affects women more frequently than men, the incidence of PsA is equal between men and women and the disorder may present at any age. PsO usually precedes the appearance of PsA, but, in up to 15%, the arthritis may precede the psoriasis, making the diagnosis more difficult. In patients in whom the skin disease occurs first, the mean delay until the onset of PsA is 10 years.

Although there is no linear correlation between severity of skin disease and severity of arthritis, patients with more severe psoriasis are more likely to develop arthritis. Patients with psoriatic nail changes often have distal interphalangeal joint (DIP) arthritis.

Patterns of Arthritis

Moll and Wright have described five patterns of PsA, which are listed in Box 69-2.[5] Any given patient may present with a combination of arthritis, spondylitis, dactylitis, and enthesitis (insertional tendinitis).

The arthritis itself tends to be preferentially involves large joint, is lower extremity predominant, and is often asymmetrical (Fig. 69-1). It frequently involves the foot and ankle and may involve the axial skeleton. The arthritis is often palindromic, unlike the additive pattern seen in rheumatoid arthritis (RA). Spine involvement often begins in the cervical spine rather than the lumbar spine, which serves to distinguish it from ankylosing spondylitis. Insertional tendinitis is a prominent feature that may dominate the clinical presentation. The net effect of the disease is to cause stiffening rather than gnarling and the end result may be ankylosis of the spine or arthrofibrosis of the knee. Each of these criteria serve to distinguish it from rheumatoid arthritis. (Table 69-1).

Radiographic Features

PsA may be distinguished from RA by its radiographic findings. These are summarized in Table 69-2. The earliest lesion of PsA is bone marrow edema, best demonstrated on T2 images. Figure 69-2 contrasts the magnetic resonance imaging (MRI) appearance of PsA with that of RA. As expected, the inflammation in PsA centers on the enthesis rather than the synovium as seen in RA.

Unique radiographic features of PsA include osteolysis (Fig. 69-3) and pencil in cup deformities, as well as asymmetrical sacroiliitis (Fig. 69-4).

Immunogenetics

Rheumatoid arthritis is associated with class II major histocompatibility complex (MHC) loci, most notably human leukocyte antigen (HLA)-DR4. PsA is associated with class I MHC loci, most notably HLA-Cw6. Other associations for PsA include B13, B38, B39, B41, and HLA-B27 with psoriatic spondylitis and all forms of PsA associated with human immunodeficiency virus (HIV).

Because of the strong MHC associations, PsA tends to run in families, unlike RA, which usually is sporadic. Families that have members with PsA often also have members with PsO, inflammatory bowel disease, uveitis, and aphthous stomatitis.

Immunopathogenesis and Synovial Histology

PsA likely involves the interplay between genetic predisposition (most notably in the form of HLA) and environmental events, including infection and physical trauma. Up to half of all cases of psoriasis follow streptococcal infections and other bacterial infections may also precipitate the first appearance of PsO or PsA. The Koebner phenomenon refers to PsO occurring at sties of skin trauma, including surgical incision sites, burns, and abrasions. A similar musculoskeletal Koebner phenomenon may result in response to skeletal trauma such as sports impact or accidents and may explain the acute appearance of PsA following significant trauma.[8] It may also explain the prominent foot and ankle involvement, as well as the frequency of common sports injuries, such as rotator cuff tendinitis and epicondylitis, which often recur in the absence of significant risk factors (Table 69-3).

Although psoriatic synovium is indistinguishable under light microscopy from rheumatoid synovium, there are ultrastructural and immunohistochemical differences between the two conditions. Compared with RA, there is more vascularity, lymphocyte rather than neutrophil predominance, and less lining cell hyperplasic. The cytokine profile is Thy-1 predominant, with elevated levels of both tumor necrosis factor-alpha (TNF-α) and interleukin-1. A unique feature of

---

Box 69-1 Caspar Criteria for Psoriatic Arthritis

Established inflammatory articular disease (joint, spine, or entheseal) with three or more of the following:

1. Psoriasis
   - Current: Psoriatic skin or scalp disease present today as judged by a physician
   - History: History of psoriasis that may be obtained from patient, family physician, dermatologist, or rheumatologist
   - Family history: History of psoriasis in a first- or second-degree relative according to patient report
2. Psoriasis: Typical psoriatic nail dystrophy including onycholysis, pitting, and hyperkeratosis observed on current physical examination
3. Negative test for rheumatoid factor (RF): By any method except latex but preferably by enzyme-linked immunosorbent assay (ELISA) or nephelometry, according to the local laboratory reference range
4. Dactylitis
   - Current: Swelling of an entire digit
   - History: History of dactylitis recorded by a rheumatologist
5. Radiologic evidence of juxta-articular new bone formation: Ill-defined ossification near joint margins (but excluding osteophyte formation) on plain radiographs of hand or foot

From Taylor WJ, Gladman D, Helliwwell P et al: Classification criteria for psoriatic arthritis; development of new criteria from a large international study. Arth Rheum 54(8):2665–2673, 2006.

Box 69-2 Moll and Wright Classification of Psoriatic Arthritis*

- Symmetrical polyarticular pattern—RA-like (small joints of hands, metacarpophalangeal joint, proximal interphalangeal joint [sparing DIP], symmetrical)
- Asymmetrical oligoarticular pattern—Four joints or less
- DIP-predominant pattern (nail and distal involvement predominate)
- Spondylitis predominant pattern (progressive low back pain, morning stiffness, sacroiliac and axial joint involvement)
- Arthritis mutilans (destructive form of arthritis, telescoping, joint lysis, typically in phalanges and metacarpals)

*These subtypes are not fixed and patients can change over time to different patterns.

Table 69-1 Contrasting Clinical Features of Rheumatoid Arthritis and Psoriatic Arthritis

Rheumatoid Arthritis	Psoriatic Arthritis
Female predominance	No gender predominance
Peak onset at 45-55 yr	Variable age of onset
Sporadic	Familial occurrence
Symmetrical	Asymmetrical
Upper extremity	Lower extremity
Small joint	Large joint
Polyarticular	Oligoarticular
No axial disease	Axial disease
Synovitis	Enthesitis

Table 69-2 Radiographic Differences Between Rheumatoid Arthritis and Psoriatic Arthritis

Rheumatoid Arthritis	Psoriatic Arthritis
Periarticular osteoporosis	Periarticular osteosclerosis
Small marginal erosions	Atypical, large erosions
No periostitis	Periostitis
MCP, PIP changes; no DIP changes	DIP common
Bone resorption	Proliferative changes
Spine changes limited to C1-2	Sacroiliitis, spondylitis

Table 69-3 Enthesitis by Anatomic Site

Site	Features
Shoulder	Rotator cuff tendinitis
Elbow	Medial and lateral epicondylitis
Wrist	De Quervain tendinitis, flexor carpi ulnaris tendinitis
Hand	Trigger fingers
Hip	Trochanteric tendinitis, anterior quadriceps tendinitis
Knee	Pes anserine tendinitis, patellar tendinitis, hamstring tendinitis
Foot and ankle	Achilles tendinitis, plantar fasciitis, anterior and posterior tibial tendinitis, peroneal tendinitis

---

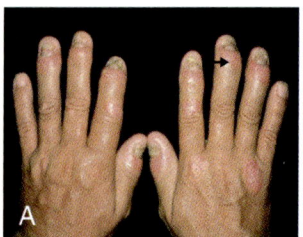 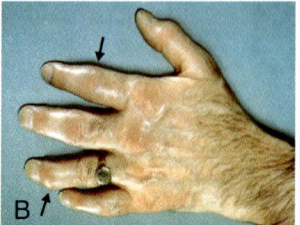 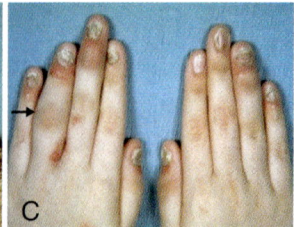 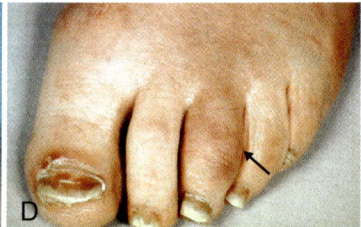

Figure 69-1. Psoriatic arthritis: joint inflammation. **A,** Distal interphalangeal synovitis. **B,** Proximal interphalangeal and distal interphalangeal synovitis. **C,** Asymmetrical oligoarthritis. **D,** Dactylitis with nail changes.

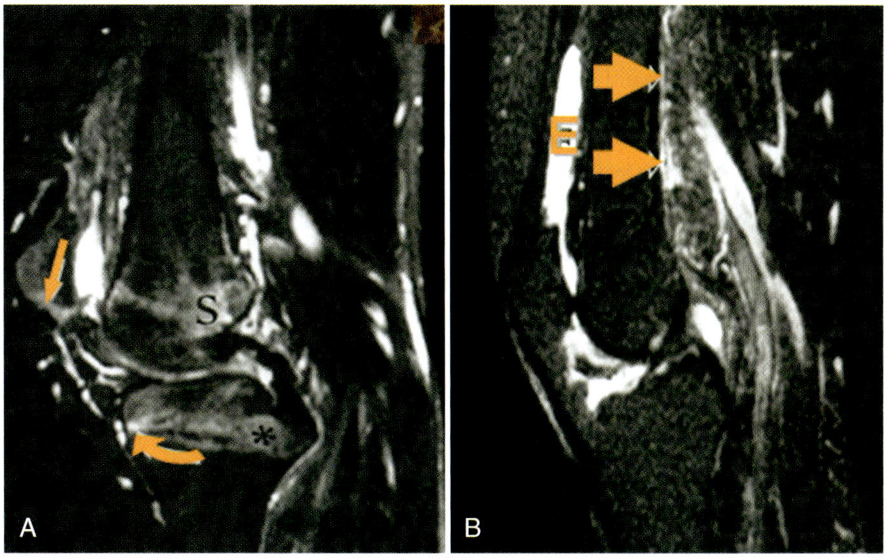

Figure 69-2. Fat-suppressed MRI scan of psoriatic arthritis, enthesitis. **A,** Psoriatic arthritis (*straight arrow,* anterior patella; *curved arrow,* patellar tendon insertion; *S,* superior insertion of the posterior cruciate ligament; *,* inferior insertion of the posterior cruciate ligament). **B,** Rheumatoid arthritis (*E,* knee effusion; *arrows,* vessels posterior to the distal femoral diaphysis). (From McGonagle D, Gibbon W, O'Connor P, et al: Characteristic magnetic resonance imaging entheseal changes of knee synovitis in spondylarthropathy. Arthritis Rheum 1998;41:694–700.)

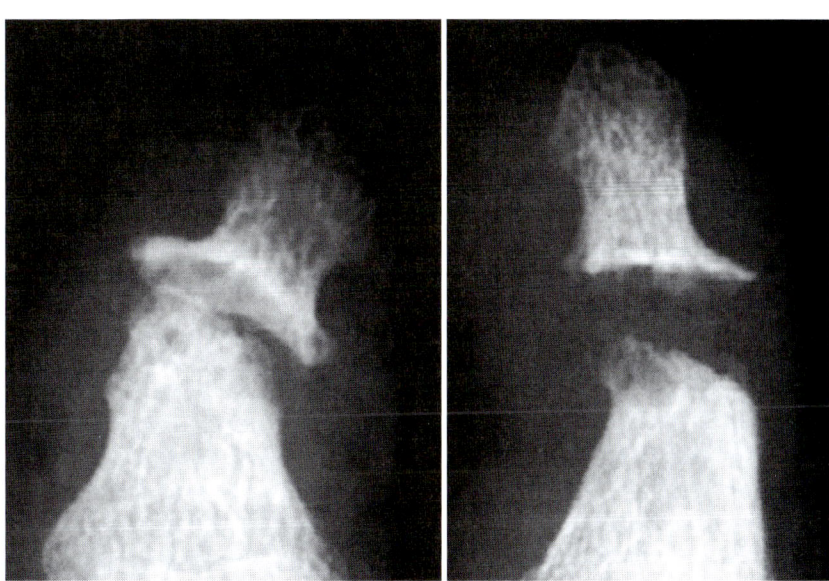

Figure 69-3. Osteolysis. *Left,* Pencil cup osteolysis (erosions = 6; joint space narrowing [JSN] = 5). *Right,* Gross osteolysis (erosions = 7; JSN = 5).

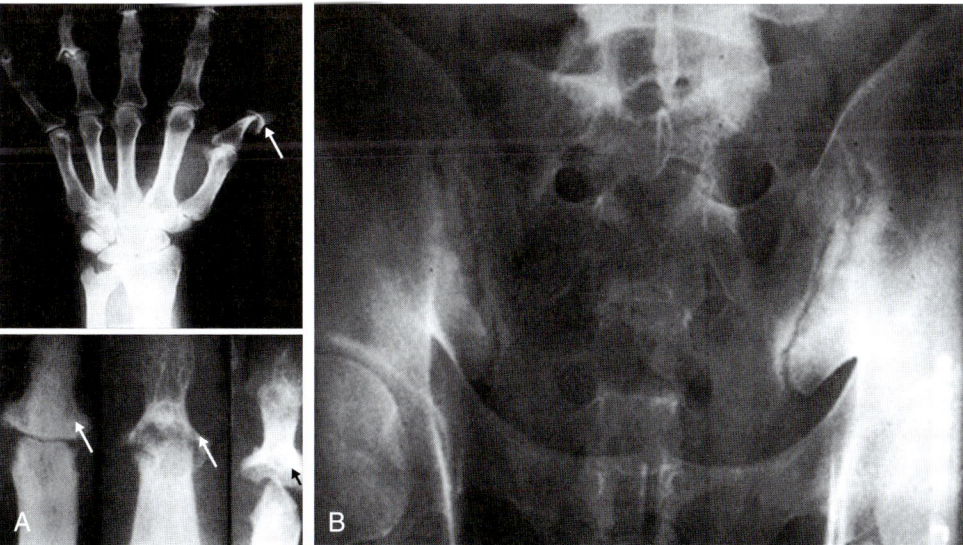

Figure 69-4. Psoriatic arthritis, radiologic features. **A,** Productive pencil in cup joint erosions. **B,** Sacroiliitis.

PsA is large numbers of activated macrophages that differentiate in the presence of TNF-α or receptor activator of nuclear factor κB (RANK) ligand into activated osteoclasts, which serve to digest subchondral bone. Joint destruction in PsA occurs from the outside (proliferative synovitis) and from the inside (activated osteoclasts).[6] Both processes may be interrupted with aggressive treatment with biologic agents directed at TNF-α or other cytokines.

Medical Comorbidities

In contrast to RA, patients with PsA tend to be male, heavier, with a higher prevalence of serious medical comorbidities, including diabetes, hypertension, hyperlipidemia, and coronary artery disease. They are far more likely to be smokers and to consume excess alcohol. Many will have full-blown metabolic syndrome (Box 69-3). These medical issues need to be addressed prior to surgical intervention to ensure a good surgical outcome and minimize the risk of surgical complications.

Agents Used to Treat Psoriasis and Psoriatic Arthritis

PsA and PsO are treated with a diverse array of medications, including topical therapies, retinoids, nonbiologic disease-modifying antirheumatic drugs (DMARDs) and, increasingly, with a growing array of biologic agents directed against specific cytokine pathways that are relevant to the pathogenesis of these disorders. Whereas a review of these agents is beyond the scope of this chapter, it is important to understand the risks associated with each of these agents, their effective half-life and, by extension, the appropriate time interval that these drugs should be held before total joint replacement. This is summarized in Table 69-4.

UNIQUE MANAGEMENT ISSUES

Surgical Problems

Psoriasis at Incision Site

Psoriasis at the proposed incision site poses an increased risk of infection because the psoriatic plaque is frequently colonized with bacteria. Every effort should be made to have the proposed incision site clear of psoriatic plaque. When this cannot be accomplished with the use of topical steroids, the patient should be referred to the dermatologist or rheumatologist to address this issue with systemic medications and/or light therapy. Refractory cases can be treated with an excimer laser, which can clear selected areas of the skin for weeks to months.

Heterotopic Ossification

Patients with PsA are at high risk for heterotopic ossification.[1] This can be prevented with the administration of radiation to the joint immediately before surgery or the postoperative administration of NSAIDs for 6 months after surgery. Indomethacin is the best-studied NSAID for this purpose but there is no reason to believe that newer NSAIDs will not be similarly efficacious and likely better tolerated.

Other Issues

Immunosuppressive Therapy

For patients on biologic and nonbiologic immunosuppressive therapy, similar guidelines should be followed as those used for RA. Methotrexate or leflunomide should be discontinued for at least 2 weeks prior to surgery and may be reinstituted 1 to 2 weeks postoperatively, provided that the wound is healing without complication. For patients on biologic therapy, it is reasonable to hold a drug for at least four half-lives. The half-lives of the common agents are listed in Table 69-4. These agents can also be restarted at 1 week if the patient is healing well. Withholding drugs for longer periods of time may result in arthritis flares, which compromise the patient's ability to rehabilitate following total joint replacement. There is no evidence that either methotrexate or anti–TNF-α agents have any impact on wound healing and there is no need to withhold these agents for long periods.

Thromboembolic Disease

Patients with inflammatory diseases are more prone to thromboembolic disorders than patients without evidence of

---

Box 69-3   Definition of Metabolic Syndrome

The presence of at least three of the following five:
- Increased waist circumference or abdominal obesity
- Hypertension
- Hypertriglyceridemia
- Reduced high-density lipoprotein (HDL)
- Insulin resistance
- Chronic inflammatory state
- Associated with markedly increased cardiovascular mortality
- United States = 25% of the population; Australia = 20%; France = 10%

Data from National Cholesterol Education Program (NCEP) Expert Panel on Detection, Evaluation, and Treatment of High Blood Cholesterol in Adults (Adult Treatment Panel III): Third Report of the National Cholesterol Education Program (NCEP) Expert Panel on Detection, Evaluation, and Treatment of High Blood Cholesterol in Adults (Adult Treatment Panel III) final report. Circulation 106:3143–3421, 2002; and Eckel RH, Grundy SM, Zimmet PZ: The metabolic syndrome. Lancet 365:1415–1428, 2005.

Table 69-4 Agents Used to Treat Psoriatic Arthritis

Agent	Half-Life
Topical steroids	NA
Topical tacrolimus and picrolimus	NA
Topical retinoids	NA
Oral retinoids (soriatane [Acitretin])	NA
Methotrexate	Hours
Cyclosporine	Hours
Azathioprine (Imuran) and mercaptopurine (Purinethol)	Hours
Etanercept (Enbrel)	4 days
Adalimumab (Humira)	14 days
Infliximab (Remicade)	8-9.5 days
Golimumab (Simponi)	14 days
Certolizumab (Cimzia)	14 days
Ustekinumab (Stelara)	14.9-45.6 days

NA, Not applicable.

inflammation. Comorbidities such as obesity or diabetes may further predispose to vascular problems. All patients with PsA should be anticoagulated according to current guidelines from the American Academy of Chest Physicians. Acceptable modalities would include coumadin, enoxaparin (Lovenox), and fondaparinux (Arixtra).[2]

Arthrofibrosis

Patients with PsA often develop arthrofibrosis and may achieve a lesser degree of range of motion than patients who have similar surgical procedures for OA and RA. The intensity of physical therapy should be adjusted accordingly and the orthopedist should pay close attention to postoperative milestones. Modalities such as the use of a Dynasplint or postoperative manipulation under anesthesia may be needed to ensure that a satisfactory range of motion is achieved.

Enthesitis

Patients with PsA may present with postoperative pain that is not to the result of failure of the surgical procedure but rather of acute enthesitis of the tendons attaching to the knee. The pes anserine complex is particularly vulnerable and inflammation at this site can create severe pain that limits postoperative physical therapy. Prompt identification and treatment of this problem is essential.

Postoperative Inflammation of the Operative Site

Koebnerization (see earlier) of the surgical incision site may mimic wound infection or tape allergy and should be treated promptly to prevent secondary bacterial superinfection. The dermatologist may need to be consulted for diagnosis and treatment of this condition.

KEY REFERENCES

1. Baird EO, Kang QK: Prophylaxis of heterotopic ossification—an updated review. J Orthop Surg Res 4:12, 2009 Apr 20.
2. Geerts WH, Bergvist D, Pineo GF, et al: Prevention of venous thromboembolism: American College of Chest Physicians evidence based practice guidelines (8th edition). Chest 122:381S, 2004.
3. Gelfand JM, Gladman DD, Mease PJ, et al: Epidemiology of psoriatic arthritis in the population of the United States. J AM Acad Dermatol 53(4):573, 2005.
4. Gladmann DD: Psoriatic arthritis. Rheum Dis Clin North Am 24(4):829–844, 1998.
5. Moll J, Wright V: Psoriatic arthritis. Sem Arth Rheum 3(1):55–78, 1973.
6. Ritchlin CT, Haas-Smith SA, Li P, et al: Mechanisms of TNF-alpha and Rank L mediated osteoclastogenesis and bone resorption in psoriatic arthritis. J Clin Invest 111(6):821–831, 2003.
7. Taylor WJ, Gladman D, Helliwell P, et al: Classification criteria for psoriatic arthritis; development of new criteria from a large international study. Arth Rheum 54(8):2665–2673, 2006.
8. Thappa DM: The isomorphic phenomenon of Koebner. IJDVL 70(3):187–189, 200.

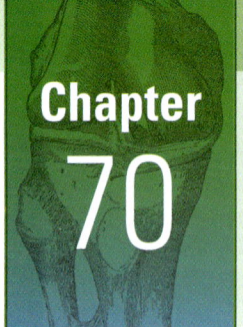

Chapter 70

Systemic Allergic Dermatitis in Total Knee Arthroplasty

Gideon P. Smith, Andrew G. Franks, Jr, and David E. Cohen

Metal sensitivity in orthopedics was first reported in 1966 by Foussereau and Laugier. Sensitivity to nickel, stainless steel, cobalt, chromium, as well as titanium-containing implants, has been well documented and remains a consideration in the differential diagnosis of osteolysis and aseptic joint loosening. This chapter focuses on the systemic allergic dermatitis—type reactions that may be associated in some patients with these events.

SYSTEMIC ALLERGIC DERMATITIS

Systemic allergic (contact) dermatitis (SAD or SCD) is a type IV or delayed cell-mediated hypersensitivity in the skin.[81] It is caused by systemic exposure to a specific allergen to which the patient has a prior exposure and preexisting sensitization. This systemic reexposure may come from ongoing contact with an internal substance, either consumed, such as foodstuffs or medications, or implanted, such as prostheses. Although traditionally described following topical exposure, in the case of medications the primary exposure may also be systemic, such as prior exposure to the same drug or a cross-reacting medication.[102] With implants, although it is theoretically possible for the primary exposure to be from a systemic exposure, it is believed that usually these sensitizing exposures occur first in the skin from environmental exposure to components of the implant or a cross-allergen.[36] In such cases, the patient may report a prior history of dermatitis occurring in localized areas from contact with external allergens, a syndrome termed *allergic contact dermatitis* (ACD). SAD is also known by other names, including mercury exanthema, internal-external contact-type hypersensitivity, systemically induced allergic contact dermatitis, baboon syndrome, paraptic eczema, nonpigmented fixed drug eruption, symmetrical psychotropic and nonpigmented drug eruption, intertriginous drug eruption, drug-induced intertrigo, and flexural eruptions,[50] although some of these syndromes may have been erroneously classified as SAD.

In orthopedic patients, this syndrome is important because it not only may lead to a chronic and debilitating skin condition, but also may be associated with failure of joint prosthesis. The latter remains somewhat controversial but is supported by observations of a high rate of metal sensitivities in patients with prosthetic loosening,[45] shorter joint life span in patients with positive patch tests,[41] and common finding of hypersensitivity-like reactions on histopathologic testing of the tissue surrounding loosened joints.[112]

Pathophysiology

The pathophysiology of a dermatitis becoming systemic is poorly understood. However, in SAD, the initial sensitization is traditionally described as coming from external exposure and thus the pathomechanism of this stage is identical to that of ACD. On primary exposure to a chemical or contact allergen responsible for SAD or ACD, haptens from these allergens bind to proteins found on epidermal Langerhans cells.[74] This is termed the *afferent stage* of sensitization. Subsequently, these Langerhans cells migrate to the lymph nodes, where they present haptenated peptides on major histocompatibility complex class I and II molecules, resulting in the induction of hapten-specific CD8+ and CD4+ T cells, respectively.[14,57] This initial sensitization stage takes approximately 10 to 14 days. However, on reexposure, the response is much quicker, typically taking between 12 and 48 hours. During this latter efferent, stage, cloned memory Th1 cells are activated, releasing a cascade of inflammatory cytokines, promoting spongiosis and dermal edema. In ACD, the reexposure is from direct skin contact, whereas in SAD the hapten must be distributed hematogenously from its site of origin to the skin site to elicit a cutaneous response. Conversely, response at the site of implant may cause inflammation, leading to implant complications (see later).

Histopathologic immunophenotyping of cutaneous SAD to systemic nickel reveals CD4+ and CD8+ T lymphocytes in the epidermis and dermis,[37] but decreased CD4+ and CD8+ T cells, along with decreased CD3+, CD45RO+, and CD19+ T and B cells in peripheral blood.[12] Similarly, in the gastrointestinal mucosa of nickel-sensitive patients, CD4+, CD45RO+, and CD8+ lymphocytes are increased when orally challenged.[27] Nickel-sensitive patients have also been shown to have a higher fraction of skin-homing CLA+ (cutaneous lymphocyte antigen) CD3+ CD45RO, CD4+ CD45RO, and CD8+ CD45RO T cells when compared with healthy controls, but a decrease in blood CLA+ CD8+ CD45RO memory T cells after nickel provocation. This suggests that these cells may have migrated to the skin and is consistent with a delayed cell-mediated hypersensitivity.[54]

Cytokine dysregulation is also consistent with a Th1–driven delayed-type hypersensitivity. Tumor necrosis factor-alpha (TNF-α), soluble TNF receptor type 1 (sTNF-R1), interleukin-1 (IL-1 receptor antagonist, and neutrophil gelatinase-associated lipocalin (NGAL) have been shown to be upregulated in gold-sensitive patients when challenged.[70] In nickel-sensitive patients, similar challenge only provoked increases in sTNF-R1,[71] although other studies using high-dose nickel also noted upregulated IL-2, IL-5,[12] IL-6, and IL-10.[54] In a zinc-sensitive patient, both TNF-α and migration inhibitory factor (MIF), which upregulates TNF-α, were found to be increased.[113] In addition, upregulation of IL-1β, TNF-α, IL-6, and prostaglandin E2 (PGE2) have been associated with proinflammatory cytokine–induced bone resorption via activation of osteoclasts and suppression of osteoblasts,[79] providing a mechanism for the observed aseptic loosening.

Other Types of Reaction to Implants

This type of reaction should be distinguished from other forms of inflammation that may exist, at times ranging from during surgery to months or years afterward. One such reaction is IgE-mediated immediate hypersensitivity response, which presents with a variety of clinical signs including contact urticaria, angioedema, asthma, and anaphylaxis within minutes of exposure and is most commonly associated in the clinical setting with natural rubber latex allergy. A second type is a granulomatous reaction, which often occurs in response to a foreign body such as plastic particulate matter from a worn prosthesis or talc from surgical gloves. This type of reaction is also associated with joint loosening.[7] Although starting immediately, this reaction may not show clinical significance for weeks to months after particle deposition. The normal healing and repair response also invokes significant stages of inflammation and repair in the weeks to months after surgery. Finally, an autoimmune reaction, in which the body produces antibodies against itself, is theoretically also possible to trigger with prosthesis placement. A humoral type 3 immune reaction mediated by circulating antigen-antibody complexes that cause inflammation on tissue deposition has been postulated; it is supported by the identification of antibodies against hapten-albumin complexes in the blood.[80,107]

Epidemiology

More than 3000 environmental chemicals have been identified as causing SAD or ACD. However, although one contact dermatitis is a risk factor for developing another, it is important to assess the clinical relevance of allergies identified because only some of these are relevant to orthopedic implants.

Allergenic Substances Used in Orthopedics

There are a variety of designs of knee prosthesis used throughout the world. However, as their components generally do not vary greatly, we will review here standard constituents and not specific designs. In orthopedic prostheses, the metals used are alloys, or combinations of metals, very rarely pure metals. It is often the minor impurities that are the common allergens.

Vitallium, a commonly used alloy, is composed of 70% cobalt, 25% to 30% chromium, and 6% to 7% molybdenum, with trace amounts of nickel. Austenitic stainless steel, which is also commonly used, occasionally contains up to 35% nickel, but generally contains 8.5% to 14% nickel, 17% to 20% chromium, 2% to 3% molybdenum, and less than 1% carbon, nitrogen, manganese, silicon, sulfur, phosphorus, and niobium. Alloys of cobalt-chromium-tungsten-nickel with 9% to 11% nickel and cobalt-chromium-molybdenum with 2% nickel are also sometimes used. Titanium is used in its pure form and alloyed with 6% aluminum or 4% vanadium for improved tensile strength.[36]

In addition to the metals in prosthesis, bone cement is sometimes used. The most common bone cement is polymethylmethacrylate (PMMA)-based, but this and others may have allergenic additives, the most common of which are gentamicin and benzoyl peroxide.[94,95] These allergens are likely less significant than the metal sensitivities, given the lower prevalence of these allergies in the general population

and the lower amounts of these substances in prostheses. The allergenicity of all these standard components is reviewed below.

Genetics of Contact Sensitization

In general, there is no known genetic predilection for the development of contact sensitization to prosthesis components. The exception to this is in nickel sensitivity. The increased prevalence of nickel allergy in monozygotic over dizygotic twins in epidemiologic studies suggests a possible genetic component to nickel allergy,[67] although these results have not been consistently reproduced.[18] Null mutations in filaggrin have been found to be associated with nickel allergy.[77] Filaggrin is a highly phosphorylated, histidine-rich polypeptide important in keratin filament aggregation and formation of the skin barrier.[23] This may be particularly important in nickel-sensitive patients because histidine-rich polypeptides are strong nickel-chelating agents and thus may also cause the accumulation of nickel in the stratum corneum.[97] The discrepancy in epidemiologic study findings noted earlier may therefore partly be explained by the fact that the study showing no correlation included a significant number of patients exposed via ear piercing, thus circumventing the need for a genetic basis for barrier disruption, whereas the earlier study looked primarily at patients with topical clothing-based exposures.

Prevalence of Contact Sensitization

Risk factors for the development of SAD are directly linked to the risk factors for developing an initial cutaneous sensitization. These will therefore be reviewed to facilitate patient risk stratification for SAD. Because exposure risk is controlled by the environment, prevalence data and risk factors vary by geographic location and therefore need to be assessed based on the patient population. For example, nickel allergy rates are lower in Denmark and Germany than in the United States, presumably because nickel content for clothing (buttons, fasteners) and piercings is more stringently regulated in these countries.[68,88,98,99] The effects of such local restrictions on prevalence can be seen by the decline in nickel allergies after these nickel content regulations were introduced in these countries.

Nickel allergy is among the most common contact allergies, with an estimated prevalence based on positive patch testing of 16.7%[61] to 19%[116] in the United States. In Thailand, this figure is reported to be as high as 33.8%,[111] whereas in Europe a similar incidence has been reported but with a clear disparity between women (17%) and men (3%).[29,101] This gender discrepancy may be explained by a discrepancy in the rates of ear piercings,[75] with 80% of women and 10% of men estimated to have piercings in this population. As noted, however, the prevalence of nickel allergy in Denmark is reported to have dropped to 6.9% ($P = .004$) in piercings in women since the introduction in 1990 of more stringent nickel content restrictions.[98,99] Cobalt and chromium sensitivity are estimated to be approximately 1% to 3% range,[68,88] although chromium sensitivity is believed to be increasing in Denmark, Singapore,[39] and the United States.[73]

When the results of 10 European patch-testing centers were pooled, cobalt sensitivity was seen to have an age-dependent prevalence of 6.2% to 8.8% and chromium of 2.4% to 5.9%. Gold[11,82] and palladium[1] allergies are seen in about 10% of dermatitis patients, although gold sensitivity increases to 30% in patient with gold dental[2] and cardiac[31] implants. In contrast, aluminum sensitivity is rarely reported.[56]

Titanium hypersensitivity is regarded as extremely rare.[60] However, it has been reported in hip replacement[59] and with a static titanium implant in which dermatitis was observed overlying the site and a positive lymphocyte transformation test result was obtained.[93]

Coreactivity to metals is common, with one study showing nickel reactivity in 79% of cobalt-sensitive patients, 39% of chromium-sensitive patients and 95% of palladium-sensitive patients.[56] This high rate of coreactivity between nickel and palladium, and the low rate of palladium exposure outside the electronics and chemicals industry, has led many to question whether this is in fact simply a cross reaction to a nickel allergy.[105] In contrast, the high rate of concordance of cobalt and nickel sensitization is believed to be caused by concomitant sensitization rather than cross sensitization because of the prevalence of cobalt in consumer products, and is thus clinically relevant.

Risk Factors

For Nickel Sensitivity

Nickel allergy has been identified in a variety of occupational exposures. These include plating industry workers,[103] retail clerks, hairdressers, domestic cleaners, metal workers, caterers,[90] locksmiths, and carpenters.[62] Nickel dermatitis has also been reported as being caused by clothing, ranging from suspenders[22] to jeans' buttons and zippers.[16] Other sources include headsets and mobile phones.[100] Jewelry and body piercings are a common cause in women[13,32] and in men the number of body piercings has been shown to correlate positively with the risk of nickel allergy.[30] Significant long-time exposure to metals that release nickel are also likely to be a risk factor. These include white gold, gold plating, German silver, Monel solder, nickel plating, and stainless steel. Finally, some reports have implicated nickel-containing cosmetics and devices such as eye shadow,[38] mascara,[106] eyeliner pencils,[115] and eyelash curlers.[15]

For Chromium Sensitivity

Occupational exposure to chromium is possible in locksmiths and carpenters[62] and those working with cement,[114] dyeing agents, metal alloys, pottery, colorant, and antirust agents in coolants, such as mechanics.[4] Although cement workers have historically been the most important of these, addition of iron sulfate to reduce the amount of water-soluble hexavalent chromium reduced chromium sensitivity from 12.7% in 1989 to 1994, prior to its addition, to 3.0% in 1995 to 2007. In contrast, in the same time period, chromium sensitivity from consumer exposure to leather has increased from 24.1% to 45.5%.[34,89,96]

For Cobalt Sensitivity

Occupational exposures to cobalt include hard metal workers, painters in the glass and pottery industry,[33,86] locksmiths, carpenters, cashiers, and secretaries.[62] In consumer exposure many of the same risk factors are present as in nickel as chromium has historically often been mixed with nickel. These include jewelry and piercings.[65,75]

SENSITIVITY TO IMPLANTS

Systemic Allergic Dermatitis to Implants

Metal implants have been used for the repair of fractures since the 1950s and in joint replacements since 1962, with the first prosthetic hip. All metal implants, even static ones such as those used to repair fractures or in pacemaker devices, are inevitably in contact with body fluids. Therefore, they will corrode and release metal ions, which have the potential to bind proteins and activate T cells[46,69] and macrophages.[21] As noted, T-cell activation can lead to an allergic contact dermatitis in the overlying skin in pacemakers[19] and joints,[85] or to a more extensive SAD. In contrast, macrophage activation has been associated with device failure.

The degree of allergenicity in stainless steel implants has been shown to be directly related to the sulfur content, which reflects the alloy's ability to liberate nickel ions. High-sulfur (0.3%) stainless steel AISI 303 can release up to 1.5 $\mu g/cm^2$/week, sufficient to induce dermatitis in nickel-sensitive patients.[48,66] In contrast, stainless steel with less than 0.03% sulfur release only 0.03 $\mu g/cm^2$/week and does not result in nickel dermatitis. Despite multiple reports of localized dermatitis over a static implant[64,83] in a prospective study of 48 subjects receiving static stainless steel orthopedic implants, none developed dermatitis, even the three subjects shown by patch testing prior to implantation to have a nickel allergy.[36] However, restenosis of stainless steel stents, which contain nickel, cobalt, and molybdenum, have been associated with the presence of a nickel allergy,[52,55,87] although this association continues to be debated.[51,91] In contrast, coronary artery stent restenosis is strongly associated with gold allergy in gold-plated stents.[31]

In nonstatic implants, there is an even greater theoretical potential for metal ion exposure because of the mechanical wear inherent in the device's function. Today, the most commonly reported systemic allergic dermatitis associated with an implanted orthopedic joint prosthesis is that following hip replacement. This may be caused by combination of factors, including the fact that hip replacement is the most common type of implanted joint prosthesis performed, the high load and frictional forces of this joint contributing to high wear and particulate production, and the materials and design used, most especially in early hip prostheses, which were more prone to allergenic particulate production. Early prosthetic hips consisted of metal on metal components resulting in much higher frictional wear, subsequent release of particulate metals and metallic ions, and eventual loosening in up to one quarter of cases.[36]

Subsequent to this, hips with metal femoral but plastic acetabular components were introduced. Currently, the former is most commonly austenitic stainless steel and the latter is composed of high or ultra–high-molecular-weight polyethylene (UHMWPE), ceramic, or carbon fiber. In younger patients, porous-coated implants are sometimes used that require no cement but in older, and other higher risk patients, PMMA bone cement is used. Because acrylic bone cements are not easily biodegraded, inflammatory reactions to PMMA and other bone cements have been reported.[42] In addition, additives such as benzoyl peroxide[104] and gentamicin[43,63] can be allergenic. In one study, 28 of 113 patients with cemented prostheses had a sensitivity to bone cement components[94]; 16.8% were sensitive to gentamicin and 8.0% to benzoyl peroxide, although N,N-dimethyl-p-toluidine and hydroquinone sensitivities were also identified in a minority of patients. With the metal on plastic hips, many reports exist of patch test–confirmed metal-sensitive patients receiving implants with no development of cutaneous problems or loosening.[6,20] The downside of these metal on plastic hips is that although they release less metal, they do produce greater overall wear, losing 0.2 mm/year from the polyethylene surface,[109] in comparison to 0.1 10 µm/year for the ball and 0.2 to 6 µm/year for the cup in all-metal prosthesis. The polyethylene particles also tend to be larger, inducing greater tissue reaction and thus more osteolysis. For this reason, metal on metal hips consisting of a cobalt alloy femoral stem and a titanium acetabular cup were reintroduced in the 1980s. Three years after prosthesis insertion, serum levels of titanium were found to be threefold higher and that of chromium fivefold higher,[17,53] leading to the potential for development of SAD long after implantation.

The knee, after the hip, is the next most common prosthetic joint replacement. Although many of the same concerns that exist for hip replacement could be extended to knee prosthesis, the design and biomechanics of the two joints are different. In particular, in knee prostheses, the articulation in more commonly metal on plastic, leading to decreased metal debris. Despite this, SAD cases have been reported in nickel- and cobalt-sensitive patients even after preoperative patch testing.[8] Localized dermatitis over an artificial knee joint has also been reported occurring 2 months after the use of a condylar knee joint replacement.[47] This prosthesis contained a Cu^{2+}-Cr^{3+} alloy femoral component. The patient did not go on to SAD and serum levels of copper, nickel, and chromium were shown to be normal, but the patient had a positive patch test result to copper sulfate and cobalt chloride, but not to nickel. An 80-year-old Japanese patient also developed knee dermatitis after total knee arthroplasty (TKA) with a Co-Cr alloy knee.[78] The patient patch-tested positive to Co, Ni, Cr, Mn, Pt, Ir, In, Hg, Sn, and Zn; the dermatitis was resolved when the prosthesis was replaced with a titanium-ceramic device.

In one case series, 30 patients were observed to develop localized dermatitis around the knee 1 to 3 months after joint revision with a total condylar knee prosthesis (DePuy Orthopaedics, Warsaw, Ind).[108] This prosthesis contains a femoral component consisting of a cobalt-chrome alloy made up of 27% to 30% chromium, 5% to 7% molybdenum, 0.7% nickel, 59% to 64% cobalt, and 4% other elements. The tibial component was a titanium alloy containing 5.5% to 6.5% aluminum, 3.5% to 4.5% vanadium, and 88% to 91% titanium. Of the 30 original patients, 15 consented to patch testing. Testing was performed to nickel sulfate (5% in pet), cobalt chloride (1% pet), and potassium dichromate (0.5% pet). At 3 days, 7 of 15 patients showed a positive metal sensitivity, 4 to nickel, 2 to chromium, and 1 to cobalt.

In a different case series, four German female patients were reported to have persistent dermatitis after a Co-Cr alloy TKA.[28] Each patient underwent a lymphocyte transformation test (LTT) to Ni, Cr, Co, Mo, Mn, and Ti and patch testing to a standard series containing Ni, Cr, and Co, an expanded metal series, including Mn, Mo, V, and Ti, and a bone cement series, comprised of 2-hydroxyethylmethacrylate, PMMA, copper sulfate pentahydrate, benzoyl peroxide, gentamicin sulfate, hydroquinone and N,N-dimethyl-p-toluidine. The first patient in the series had a positive nickel sensitivity. The second patient in the series was sensitive to both cobalt and nickel. In the third patient, patch testing was positive to cobalt and the LTT showed elevated sensitivity to both nickel and cobalt. The final patient was sensitive to nickel and cobalt but was also sensitive to ethylene glycol dimethacrylate, 2-hydroxyethylmethacrylate, and 2-hydroxypropylmethacrylate. Resolution of all symptoms in all four patients, including joint effusion and dermatitis, was achieved after switching to a titanium-plated prosthesis and, in the case of the final patient, removal of residual cement at the time of titanium prosthesis implantation.

In a prospective study of 92 patients undergoing TKA between 2000 and 2002, preoperative modified lymphocyte stimulation tests (mLSTs) to Ni, Co, Cr, and Fe were performed.[76] Of these, 26% showed positive sensitivity to at least one of these metals. Five of the patients with preoperative metal sensitivity went on to develop implant-related dermatitis, although the only association reaching statistical significance was with Cr ($P < .05$). Two of the metal-sensitive patients had TKA revision, with resolution of the dermatitis.

In a different study, 94 subjects were recruited, 20 prior to TKA, 27 with a well-functioning TKA, and 47 with loosening of the joint after revision.[40] Patch testing for 5% nickel sulfate, 1% cobalt chloride, 2% chromium trichloride, 0.5% potassium dichromate, 2% ferric chloride, 2% molybdenum chloride, 1% niobium chloride, 2% titanium dioxide, 5% PMMA, 2% butyl methacrylate, 2% triethylene glycol dimethacrylate, 2% ethylene glycol dimethacrylate, 2% N,N-dimethyl-p-toluidine, 5% hydroxylethylmethacrylate, 2% benzoyl peroxide, and 1% hydroquinone monobenzyl ether was performed. In preimplant patients, a positive patch test result was seen in 20% of patients. In postimplant patients, positive patch tests were shown to be higher in both groups tested after TKA, with a slight increase in patch test positives in patients with TKA loosening (59.6%) over those with stable TKA (48.1%). The most important factor identified in this study in predicting joint loosening was a prior history of contact allergy to metals. This single item in the history increased the risk of failure fourfold.

Finally, one case has been reported in which TKA failure was attributed to a preexisting contact sensitivity to PMMA.[49] The patient had previously had a periungual dermatitis believed to be from acrylic nail use, which resolved with the avoidance of acrylic nails and glues. She subsequently underwent TKA with a PMMA-containing bone cement. The patient went on to experience significant early joint loosening and was patch-tested to both the bone cement and metals. PMMA was positive but metal patch testing was negative. The patient subsequently underwent joint revision with a cementless prosthesis, with no recurrence of the problem.

Development of a New Hapten Sensitization from Prosthesis Implantation

Although the initial sensitization event is classically described as coming from topical exposure, it is theoretically possible that the initial exposure could be from a systemic event. In this regard, a metal orthopedic implant could theoretically serve as the sensitizer for a new dermatitis in a patient. In retrospective studies of 112 patients after metal on metal hip replacement, 1 was found to have a new nickel allergy and 2 a new cobalt allergy.[24] In another series of 85 patients post–hip replacement, 2 nickel, 5 cobalt, and 1 chromate nickel allergy were documented after surgery.[110] In addition, 3 nickel and 1 new cobalt allergy were documented in 66 hip surgeries.[26] Of 1400 patients receiving joint replacement and 200 internal fixations, only 2 of 13 with a persistent eczematous dermatitis patch tested positive to a metal.[58]

However, to assess this rigorously, patchtesting has to be prospectively examined and needs to be performed before and after prosthesis implantation. Interestingly, in one study in which 69 patients were patch tested before and after prosthesis implantation, 5 subjects who initially tested positive to nickel, chromium, or cobalt tested negative postsurgery.[84] This may reflect the sensitivity of the test or induction of immunologic tolerance after prosthesis insertion, although another study of 85 patients did show induction of sensitivity to cobalt (4 patients), PMMA, nickel, cobalt, and chromium postimplantation.[1,2,110] The very fact that studies are equivocal, with some supporting a low rate of induction of tolerance and some supporting a low rate of induction of sensitivity, demonstrates that this is probably not of high clinical concern. It is important to assure patients with other contact allergens that although this is theoretically possible, and the presence of one contact allergy is a risk factor for a second, the evidence of development of new sensitivity from an orthopedic prosthesis is low.

WORKUP PRIOR TO IMPLANTATION

History and Physical Examination

Although SAD from knee prostheses therefore appears rare, because of its serious potential consequences, including morbidity from skin involvement and joint loosening, screening may be considered for highly suspect patients prior to prosthesis implantation. As noted, the most significant historical factor is a known clinical sensitivity or prior positive patch test to metals, but any type of prior contact sensitivity suggests that the patient may be more prone to the development of SAD. Patients may not be specifically aware of contact sensitivities and the physical examination should also assess for any unexplained exanthemas, especially if located in proximity to a likely contactant, such as a nickel-containing jeans' stud or button. In such a case, the patient should be referred to a dermatologist for full evaluation. Other important historical factors are history and number of piercings, occupational exposures—including metal workers, retail clerks, hairdressers, domestic cleaners, caterers, locksmiths, and carpenters, and those exposed to cements, dyeing agents, metal alloys, pottery, colorants, and antirust agents in coolants (e.g., mechanics, painters in the glass or pottery industry). In addition, although atopic dermatitis has variably been described as both a risk and protective factor for the development of contact dermatitis, contact dermatitis can sometimes be incorrectly diagnosed as atopic dermatitis or another skin rash. Thus, any patient with an ongoing or history of recurrent rash should be evaluated by a dermatologist.

Patch Testing

Patch testing is seen as the gold standard for the evaluation of ACD. The usefulness of the test, however, is affected by a number of factors. The testing must be performed by someone experienced in appropriate patient selection, selection of allergens, patch application, appropriate reading of the skin reactions to patches, and interpretation of the clinical relevance of the results.[72]

Patch testing consists of the application of nonirritating concentrations of allergens suspected of causing ACD in the particular patient. The skin must be intact and noninflamed prior to application. The upper back is the most common site chosen because it provides a large surface area for the application of series of patches. The patches should remain on for 48 hours; during this period; the patient is unable to bathe her or his back because this would risk washing away allergens, moving patches, or erasing marks identifying patches. The first read is performed on removal of the patches at 48 hours. Different scales exist for this initial read but generally include no reaction, weak reaction (e.g., mild macular erythema), positive reaction (e.g., edema with erythema), strong reaction (e.g., bullae), and irritant. The locations of the patches are marked on the skin with tape or surgical marker. To differentiate between allergic and irritant reactions, a second read is performed at day 4 or 5. Very strong positive patch test results may imply negative tests to appear mildly positive; thus, repeat isolated testing of the weaker positive may be required in this case. Because the patch test relies on the patient being able to mount an immune response to the applied patches, the patient cannot have ongoing treatments or engage in activities that would interfere with this testing, such as treatment with systemic steroids or other immunosuppressive drugs and activities such as tanning.

In the United States, the most common patch testing performed is the thin-layer rapid-use epicutaneous (TRUE) test, which consists of 28 common skin sensitizers and one negative control. Unfortunately, of the substances relevant to prosthesis, this only contains nickel sulfate and cobalt dichloride. Ideally, therefore, the examiner will use a nonstandard test patch series, sometimes individually prepared in aluminum (Finn) chambers mounted on hypoallergenic paper tape (Scanpor).[9] This often requires referral to a dermatologist specializing in contact dermatology. When clinical concern is particularly high, such as in a patient with known metal allergies, samples of the materials and alloys specifically used in the prosthesis being considered can be obtained from the manufacturer and the patient can be patch-tested to these.

In SAD, the use of patch testing is less conclusive than in ACD, in part because the epicutaneous application of metal salts is likely biologically distinct from exposure to metal ions within the joint. Use of subcutaneous metal implants prior to prosthesis implantation has been attempted but has its own dissimilarities to the long-term joint environment.[8] Because contact sensitivity is more prevalent than postprosthesis SAD, patch testing will also likely overpredict sensitivities. Finally, metal allergens likely to be the most significant allergens in prostheses are notoriously difficult to reproduce. Despite this, patch testing should theoretically be able to provide some level of reassurance when a negative result is obtained requiring, like SAD, prior cutaneous sensitization.

It also allows for rapid screening of a large number of potential allergens. Thus, it remains probably the best and certainly most cost-effective screening tool for determining sensitivity to prosthesis components.

POST–KNEE ARTHROPLASTY

Clinical Cutaneous Signs of Sensitivity

Clinical features of patients with hypersensitivity to their prosthetic implant are variable but often reflect the standard symptoms of prosthetic failure, including loosening, pain, and instability. Local inflammatory reactions are possible, such as warmth and erythema, and skin dermatitis may be localized or, more commonly, generalized. The exact appearance of SAD lesions will vary, depending on the stage of the disease. During the early acute phase, like other dermatitides, lesions are often edematous and/or erythematous and may produce papular or vesicular lesions. If vesicles rupture, oozing ensues and patients may develop secondary bacterial infection. In the chronic stage, scaling, lichenification, and excoriations predominate. The initial site of the dermatitis in SAD may often provide the best clue regarding the allergic origin because reactivation often occurs first at sites of prior ACD. For example, the ears are susceptible to metals from earrings.

Workup After Implantation

If, after implantation, a rash fitting the clinical characteristics of SAD should occur, especially if the patient had risk factors, postimplantation patch testing may be performed. This is important because no curative medical therapy exists; if the artificial joint is the cause, prosthetic revision might be considered prior to joint failure. Patch testing may also be considered in a patient subsequently presenting with symptoms of joint loosening who has risk factors for sensitivity to allow adequate selection of the replacement prosthesis. In either case, x-rays of the joint should be obtained.[3,10] Signs that may be attributable to loosening from hypersensitivity include radiolucencies around the implant, screw migration, or change in implant position. In hypersensitivity-induced osteolysis, cystic changes may also be seen. Magnetic resonance imaging (MRI) and computed tomography (CT) scans have not proven additionally helpful in the assessment and bone scans, although sometimes positive, are nonspecific. Although serum levels of different suspected allergens may be determined, standard levels above which an allergic event is likely have not been established because sensitivity depends on the individual patient, making clinically significant interpretation impossible.[35] In addition, a high serum level does not necessarily prove causation because a preexisting sensitization must still exist. This may be seen in the lack of prognostic significance of elevated serum metal levels.[25]

The list of medications causing SAD is long. It includes many common medications, including antibiotics, antihistamines, and heart medications, which the patient may not think are related to the exanthema. The list of such agents has recently been updated,[102] but new medications are continually being identified; the list should be reviewed on an ongoing basis when clinical suspicion is high—for example, because of the timing of the exanthema in relation to the administration of new medications. Medications should always be excluded because this does not affect the prognosis of the joint and elimination of the drug is curative. Therefore, SAD is best assessed by an experienced dermatologist who can evaluate all its potential causes.

CONCLUSIONS

In conclusion, SAD after knee arthroplasty is a rare but serious condition. Consequences include chronic systemic dermatitis and joint prosthesis failure secondary to the hypersensitivity reaction and chronic inflammation. In patients with an identified risk of SAD, or SAD itself, alternative knee prosthesis components may be tried. These include prostheses with ceramic rather than metal components, use of nonallergenic metallic implants such as titanium or Zn-Nb alloys, or a prosthesis with a suitable coating to mask the allergenic components.[5] SAD is therefore a syndrome of which generalists and specialists dealing with these patients, such as orthopedists, dermatologists, and rheumatologists, should be well aware—in the preimplant screening, in the clinical findings, and in the workup and treatment of this condition in the post-TKA patient.

KEY REFERENCES

Berquist TH: Imaging of joint replacement procedures. Radiol Clin North Am 44:419–437, 2006.

Dahlstrand H, Stark A, et al: Elevated serum concentrations of cobalt, chromium, nickel, and manganese after metal-on-metal alloarthroplasty of the hip: a prospective randomized study. J Arthroplasty 24:837–845, 2009.

Dietrich KA, Mazoochian F, Summer B, et al: Intolerance reactions to knee arthroplasty in patients with nickel/cobalt allergy and disappearance of symptoms after revision surgery with titanium-based endoprostheses. J Dtsch Dermatol Ges 7:410–413, 2009.

Gawkrodger DJ: Metal sensitivities and orthopaedic implants revisited: the potential for metal allergy with the new metal-on-metal joint prostheses. Br J Dermatol 148:1089–1093, 2003.

Granchi D, Cenni E, Tigani D, et al: "Sensitivity to implant materials in patients with total knee arthroplasties. Biomaterials 29:1494–1500, 2008.

Hallab N, Merritt K, Jacobs JJ: Metal sensitivity in patients with orthopaedic implants. J Bone Joint Surg Am 83:428–436, 2001.

Haudrechy P, Foussereau J, Mantout B, Baroux B: Nickel release from nickel-plated metals and stainless steels. Contact Dermatitis 31:(4)249–255, 1994.

Kranke B, Aberer W: Multiple sensitivities to metals. Contact Dermatitis 34:225, 1996.

Lalor PA, Revell PA, et al: Sensitivity to titanium. A cause of implant failure? J Bone Joint Surg Br 73:25–28, 1991.

Merritt K, Rodrigo JJ: Immune response to synthetic materials. Sensitization of patients receiving orthopaedic implants. Clin Orthop Relat Res (326): 71–79, 1996.

Niki Y, Matsumoto H, Otani T, et al: Screening for symptomatic metal sensitivity: a prospective study of 92 patients undergoing total knee arthroplasty. Biomaterials 26:1019–1026, 2005.

Otto M, Kriegsmann J, Gehrke T, Bertz S: [Wear particles: key to aseptic prosthetic loosening?] Pathologe 27:447–460, 2006.

Thomas P, Schuh A, Ring J, Thomsen M: [Orthopedic surgical implants and allergies: joint statement by the implant allergy working group (AK 20) of the DGOOC (German association of orthopedics and orthopedic surgery), DKG (German contact dermatitis research group) and dgaki (German society for allergology and clinical immunology).] Orthopade 37:75–88, 2008.

Willert HG, Buchhorn GH, Fayyazi A, et al: Metal-on-metal bearings and hypersensitivity in patients with artificial hip joints. A clinical and histomorphological study. J Bone Joint Surg Am 87:28–36, 2005.

Full references for this chapter can be found on www.expertconsult.com.

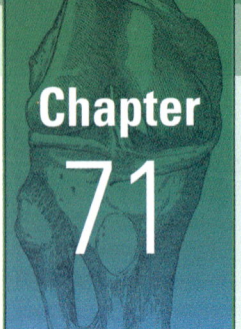

Chapter 71

Rheumatoid Arthritis of the Knee: Current Medical Management

Andrew G. Franks, Jr.

There has been substantial transformation, not without controversy, in the suggested algorithms for the treatment of rheumatoid arthritis (RA) over the past decade.[4,6,23] This has been accelerated by increasing understanding of the immune pathways of the disease itself (Fig. 71-1). Most of the nonsteroidal anti-inflammatory drugs (NSAIDs) have more limited use than in the past because of their cardiovascular risks through cyclooxygenase-2 (COX-2) inhibition[15] or their risk for gastrointestinal intolerance[16] and, in fact, have never appreciably affected the disease process. Corticosteroids reduce symptoms and systemic manifestations of RA, but chronic use is associated with frequent side effects and also does not appreciably prevent disease progression.[17] Methotrexate and other disease-modifying antirheumatic drugs (DMARDs; Fig. 71-2) usually yield no immediate relief, but over time can control symptoms and are thought to delay progression of the disease. These remain the most often used agents by rheumatologists throughout the world for the treatment of RA.[1]

Nevertheless, recent advances by the novel biologic agents (biologics; Fig. 71-3), such as the tumor necrosis factor-alpha (TNF-α) inhibitors and anti-CD20 monoclonal antibodies, have allowed many patients with RA to experience improvement in symptoms, function, and quality of life to a degree they might not have achieved in the past. Etanercept, infliximab, adalimumab, anakinra, golimumab, certolizumab pegol, rituximab, abatacept and most recently, tocilizumab are currently U.S. Food and Drug Administration (FDA) approved for the treatment of rheumatoid arthritis. Thus, therapeutic decision making for this disease has become more complex for clinicians, with many conflicting factors playing increasingly important roles. According to the most objective measures of RA progression, very early intervention with conventional DMARDs is cost-effective whereas that of very early intervention with biologics remains unclear.[13] However, more recent data indicate that biologic therapy is associated with increases in workforce participation in patients typically expected to experience progressively deteriorating ability, which could result in significant indirect cost benefits to society.[3]

In addition to cost, the overall safety profile of the biologics remains a central issue and a number of disturbing side effects have been reported.[8,19] Reactivation of tuberculosis and other opportunistic infections has occurred after introduction of these agents.[12] Data suggest that anti-TNF therapy may be safe in chronic hepatitis C[20]; however, TNF-α antagonists have resulted in reactivation of chronic hepatitis B if not given concurrently with antiviral therapy.[9] Solid tumors do not appear to be increased with anti-TNF therapy.[19] Although variable rates of increased lymphoma risk have been described compared with those in the general population, no increase over patients with RA in general has been reported.[17] Use of TNF-α antagonists in advanced heart failure has shown a worse prognosis and should be avoided, if possible.[10] The formation of autoantibodies may occur, including antinuclear antibody (ANA) and anti–double-stranded DNA (anti-dsDNA), but fortunately these autoantibodies are only rarely associated with clinical syndromes.[2,21] Rare cases of aplastic anemia, pancytopenia, vasculitis, and demyelinating disorders have also been reported.[11] Most recently, progressive multifocal leukoencephalopathy (PML), a lethal rare brain disease caused by reactivation of the JC virus, has been described with anti-TNF therapy.[14,24] Finally, whether adverse events after orthopedic intervention are higher with these agents than with conventional DMARDs remains inconclusive, although recent data suggest that they are equally safe.[18] It is generally suggested they be discontinued 1 week prior to surgery and reinstituted 1 week thereafter or, depending on the frequency of administration of the agent itself, that surgery be performed at the latter end of the biologic half-life of the drug.

Despite recent advances with the biologic therapies and combination DMARD strategies, remission rates still remain suboptimal and patients with RA are still missing a considerable number of work days. Early diagnostic criteria are needed to ensure that appropriate treatment is initiated early to prevent joint damage. Better prognostic markers are also needed to identify patients with the potential for poor outcomes, for whom more aggressive strategies can be applied at the outset.[7] Patient preference is also important and may depend on mode and frequency of administration and, finally but very importantly, the risks versus benefits as they continue to unfold.[5] The current guidelines of the American College of Rheumatology clearly define the role of the biologics in RA related to DMARDs and NSAIDs, and combinations thereof, as they relate to onset and severity of disease, and to early versus late intervention and prior treatment failures.[22] Continued discussion and controversy will remain very much the norm as more of these agents are introduced for the treatment of RA around the world, and it will remain the clinician's task to keep their patients wisely informed.

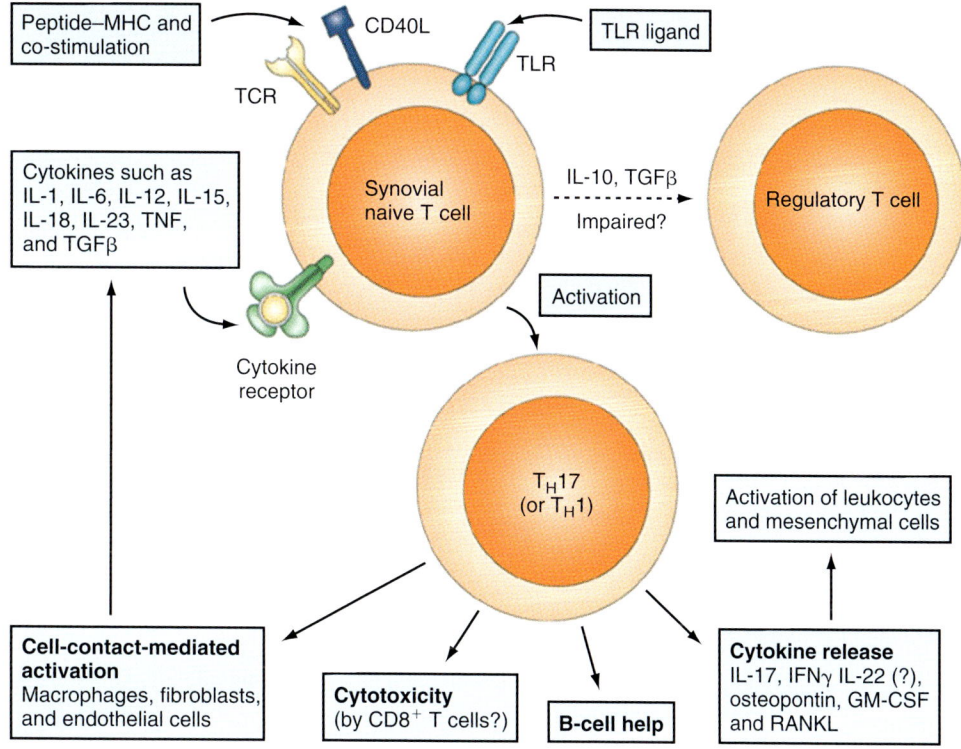

Figure 71-1. Synovial T cells may be activated by a T-cell receptor (TCR) and costimulation pathways and by cytokine- or Toll-like receptor (TLR)–driven stimuli. In particular, the synovial milieu contains interleukin-12 (IL-12), IL-23, IL-6, and transforming growth factor beta (TGFβ) and, as such, promotes the differentiation of T-helper 1 (TH1) and TH17 cells. Regulatory T cells, although present, may not exhibit optimal regulatory activity. In rodent models, regulatory T cells are present in high numbers in the joints, whereas in human disease the relative contribution of these subsets remains unknown. Activated T cells mediate effector function in rheumatoid arthritis through the release of cytokines to promote downstream leukocyte and mesenchymal cell activation, through the provision of help to B cells and, in the case of CD8+ effector T cells, cytotoxic activity. They also activate macrophages, fibroblasts, and endothelial cells through direct cell contact. CD40L, CD40 ligand; GM-CSF, granulocyte-macrophage colony-stimulating factor; IFNγ, interferon-γ; RANKL, receptor activator of nuclear factor-κB (RANK) ligand; TNF, tumor-necrosis factor. (From McInnes IB, Schett G: Cytokines in the pathogenesis of rheumatoid arthritis. Nat Rev Immunol 2007;7:429–442.)

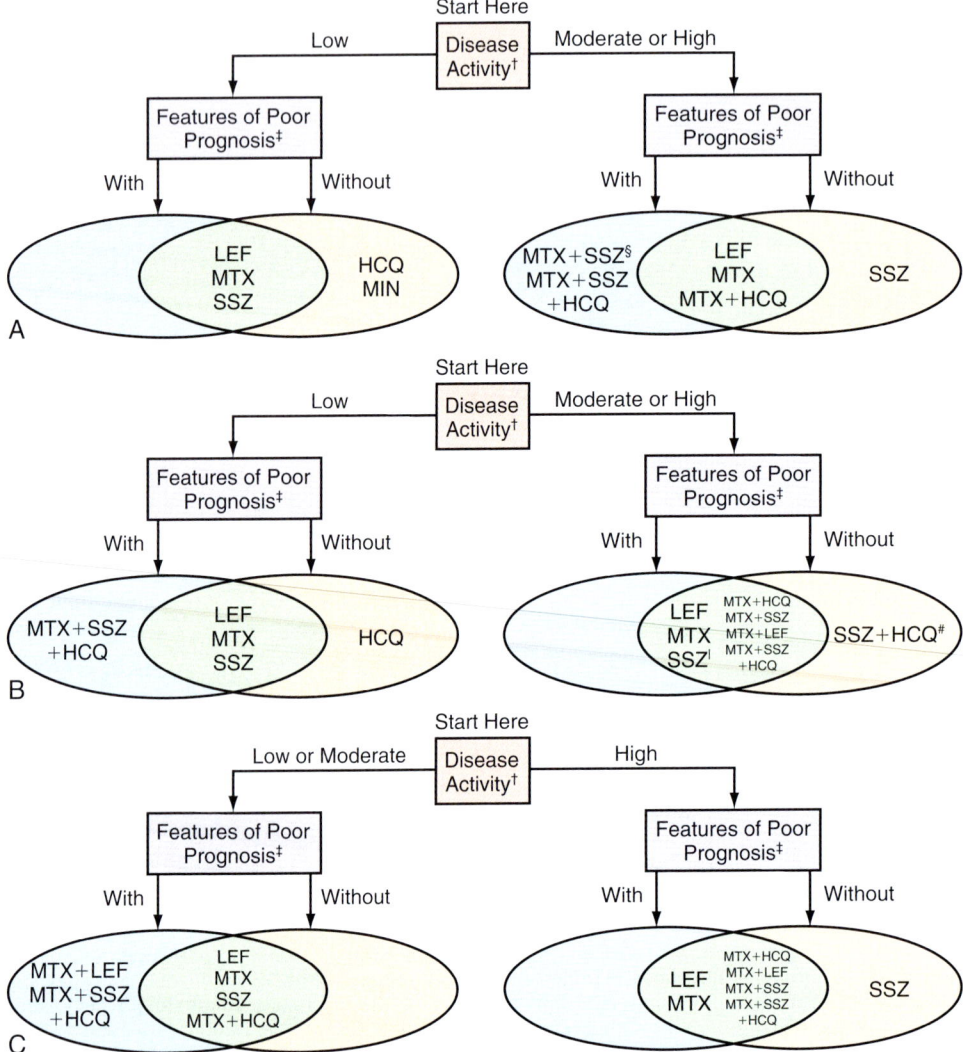

Figure 71-2. Recommendations of indications for the use of nonbiologic DMARDs in RA patients who have never received DMARDs. These recommendations do not specifically include the potential role of glucocorticoids or NSAIDs in the management of patients with RA. Therapies are listed alphabetically. **A,** Disease duration <6 months. **B,** Disease duration of 6 to 24 months. **C,** Disease duration >24 months. ‡, Includes functional limitation (defined using standard measurement scales such as Health Assessment Questionnaire score or variations of this scale), extra-articular disease (e.g., presence of rheumatoid nodules, secondary Sjögren's syndrome, RA vasculitis, Felty's syndrome, and RA lung disease), rheumatoid factor positivity, positive anticyclic citrullinated peptide antibodies, or bony erosions by radiography, §, only recommended for patients with high disease activity with features of poor prognosis; ‖, only recommended for patients with moderate disease activity irrespective of prognostic features and patients with high disease activity without features of poor prognosis; #, only recommended for patients with high disease activity without features of poor prognosis; *HCQ,* hydroxychloroquine; *LEF,* leflunomide; *MTX,* methotrexate; *MIN,* minocycline; *SSZ,* sulfasalazine. (From Saag K, Teng G, Patkar N, et al: American College of Rheumatology 2008 recommendations for the use of nonbiologic and biologic disease-modifying antirheumatic drugs in rheumatoid arthritis. Arthritis Rheum 2008;59:762–784.)

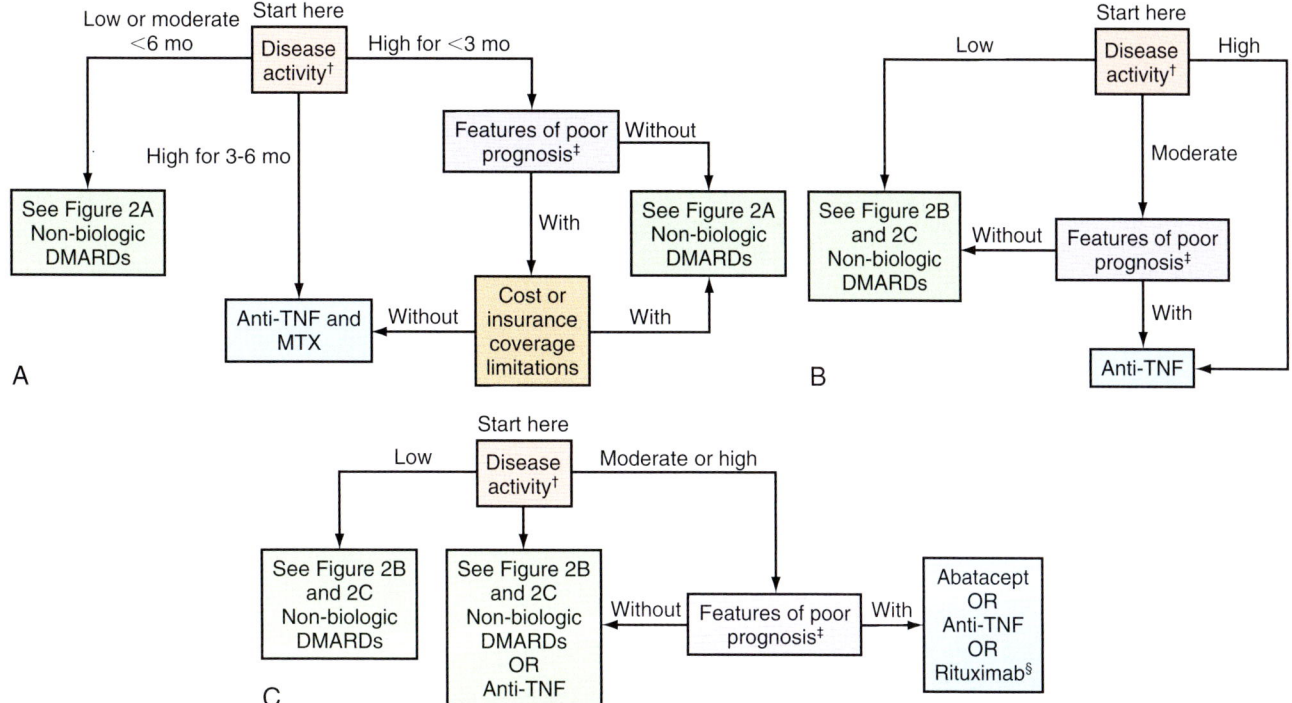

Figure 71-3. Recommendations of indications for the use of biologic (DMARDs in patients with RA). These recommendations do not specifically include the potential role of glucocorticoids or NSAIDs in the management of patients with RA. Therapies are listed alphabetically. **A,** Patients with RA <6 months, **B,** patients with RA ≥6 months who failed prior MTX monotherapy, **C,** patients with RA disease duration of ≥6 months who failed prior MTX combination therapy or after sequential administration of other nonbiologic DMARDs. [†], Includes functional limitation (defined using standard measurement scales such as Health Assessment Questionnaire score or variations of this scale), extra-articular disease (e.g., presence of rheumatoid nodules, secondary Sjögren's syndrome, RA vasculitis, Felty's syndrome, and RA lung disease), rheumatoid factor positivity, positive anticyclic citrullinated peptide antibodies, or bony erosions by radiography; [§], only recommended for patients with high disease activity with features of poor prognosis; *MTX,* methotrexate; *TNF,* tumor necrosis factor. (From Saag K, Teng G, Patkar N, et al: American College of Rheumatology 2008 recommendations for the use of nonbiologic and biologic disease-modifying antirheumatic drugs in rheumatoid arthritis. Arthritis Rheum 2008;59:762–784.)

KEY REFERENCES

Agarwal S, Zaman T, Handa R: Retention rates of disease-modifying antirheumatic drugs in patients with rheumatoid arthritis. Singapore Med J 50:686–692, 2009.

Augustsson J, Neovius M, Cullinane-Carli C, et al: Patients with rheumatoid arthritis treated with tumour necrosis factor antagonists increase their participation in the workforce: potential for significant long-term indirect cost gains (data from a population-based registry). Ann Rheum Dis 69:126–131, 2010.

Barton J: Patient preferences and satisfaction in the treatment of rheumatoid arthritis with biologic therapy. Patient Prefer Adherence 3:335–344, 2009.

Braun J, Kalden J: Biologics in the treatment of rheumatoid arthritis and ankylosing spondylitis. Clin Exp Rheumatol 27(Suppl 55):S164–S167, 2009.

Bykerk V: Unmet needs in rheumatoid arthritis. J Rheumatol Suppl 82:42–46, 2009.

Caporali R, Caprioli M, Bobbio-Pallavicini F, et al: Long-term treatment of rheumatoid arthritis with rituximab. Autoimmun Rev 8:591–594, 2009.

Cuchacovich R, Espinoza L: Does TNF-alpha blockade play any role in cardiovascular risk among rheumatoid arthritis (RA) patients? Clin Rheumatol 28:1217–1220, 2009.

Desai S, Furst D: Problems encountered during anti-tumour necrosis factor therapy. Best Pract Res Clin Rheumatol 20:757–790, 2006.

Dixon W, Hyrich K, Watson K, et al: Drug-specific risk of tuberculosis in patients with rheumatoid arthritis treated with anti-TNF therapy: results from the British Society for Rheumatology Biologics Register (BSRBR). Ann Rheum Dis Ann Rheum Dis 69:522–528, 2010

Finckh A, Bansback N, Marra C, et al: Treatment of very early rheumatoid arthritis with symptomatic therapy, disease-modifying antirheumatic drugs, or biologic agents: a cost-effectiveness analysis. Ann Intern Med 151:612–621, 2009.

Gupta M, Eisen G: NSAIDs and the gastrointestinal tract. Curr Gastroenterol Rep 11;345-353, 2009.

Li S, Kaur P, Chan V, et al: Use of tumor necrosis factor-alpha (TNF-alpha) antagonists infliximab, etanercept, and adalimumab in patients with concurrent rheumatoid arthritis and hepatitis B or hepatitis C: a retrospective record review of 11 patients. Clin Rheumatol 28:787–791, 2009.

Saag K, Teng G, Patkar N, et al: American College of Rheumatology 2008 recommendations for the use of nonbiologic and biologic disease-modifying antirheumatic drugs in rheumatoid arthritis. Arthritis Rheum 59:762–784, 2008.

Yazici Y: Treatment of rheumatoid arthritis: we are getting there. Lancet 374:178–180, 2009.

Yurube T, Takahi K, Owaki H, et al: Late infection of total knee arthroplasty inflamed by anti-TNF alpha, Infliximab therapy in rheumatoid arthritis. Rheumatol Int 30:405–408, 2010.

Full references for this chapter can be found on www.expertconsult.com.

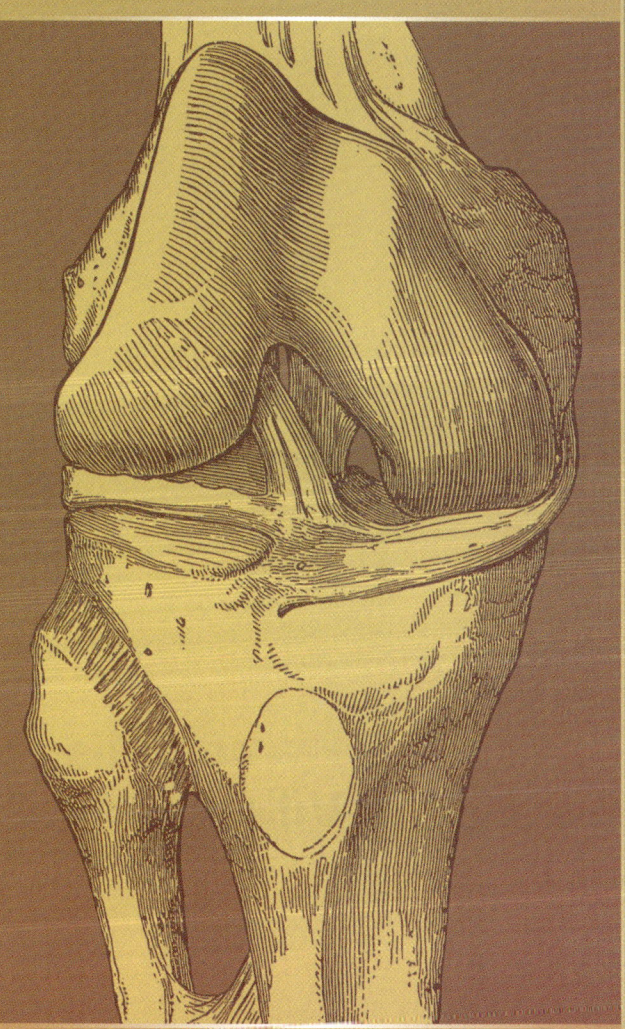

SECTION 8

Miscellaneous Conditions and Treatments

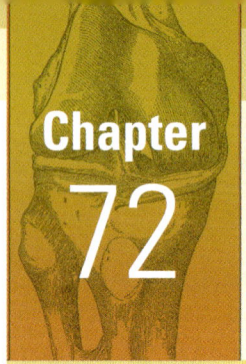

Chapter 72

The Synovium: Normal and Pathologic Conditions

Vincent J. Vigorita and Douglas Mintz

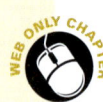

Chapter 73

Hemophilia and Pigmented Villonodular Synovitis

Anthony S. Unger, Craig Kessler, and Randall J. Lewis

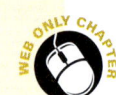

Chapter 74

Anesthesia for Knee Surgery

Terese T. Horlocker and Sandra L. Kopp

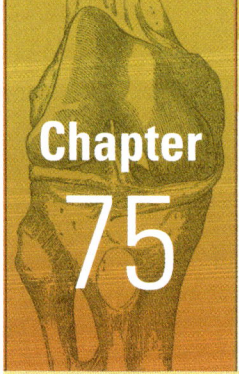

Chapter 75

Complex Regional Pain Syndrome of the Knee

Donna R. Kesselman

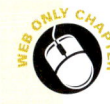

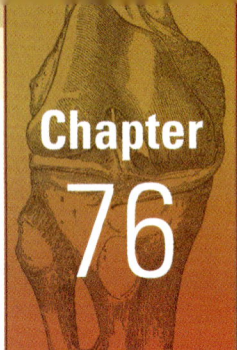

Chapter 76

Partial Denervation for the Treatment of Painful Neuromas Complicating Total Knee Replacement

A. Lee Dellon and Michael A. Mont

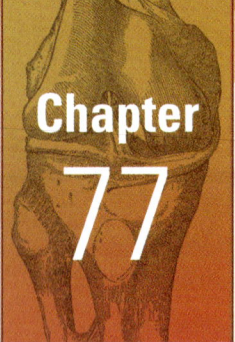

Chapter 77

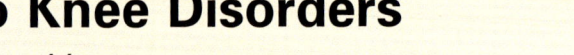

HIV Infection and Its Relationship to Knee Disorders

Henry Masur

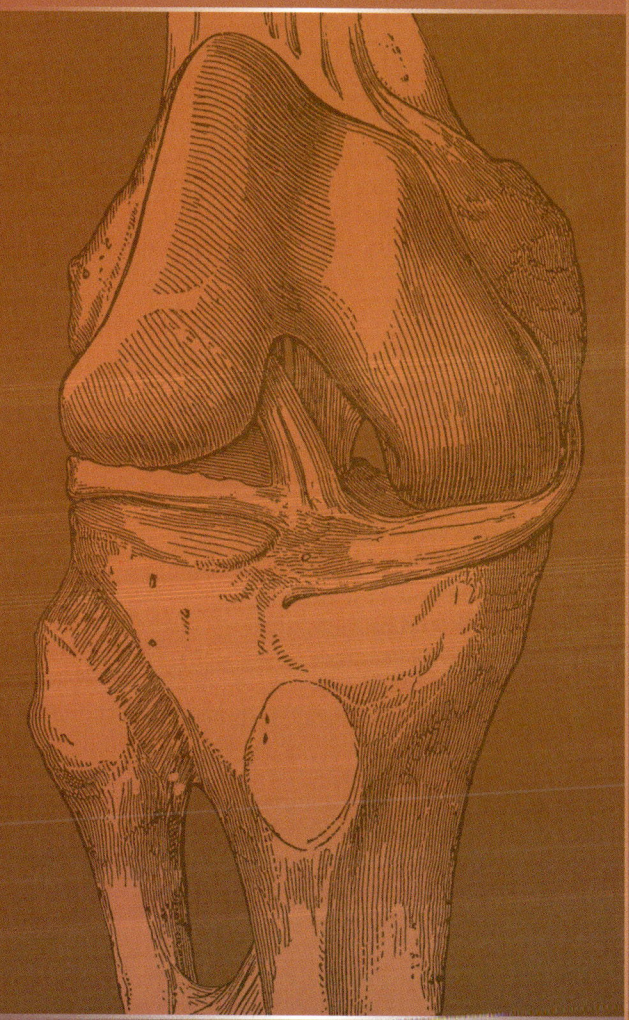

Plastic Surgery

Chapter 78

Soft Tissue Healing

Susan Craig Scott and Robert S. Reiffel

A patient who is to undergo total knee arthroplasty is focused on relief of pain and increased mobility, major quality of life issues that the operation reliably provides. Considerations of soft tissue healing are not ordinarily present in the patient's mind at the time of initial evaluation. That there might be difficulty with soft tissue healing may well be the farthest thing from a patient's thoughts. It is not unusual for a physician who introduces the subject of wound healing to be met with surprise, disbelief, or even suspicion. Only those who have had difficulty with soft tissue healing in the past are even aware that healing might be an issue. Unfortunately, patients who are likely to have difficulty with soft tissue healing are not limited to those with difficulty in the past.

Responsibility for assessing the condition of the soft tissues and systemic and local factors that might cause difficulty with healing lies with the treating physician. In the past 30 to 40 years, encompassing the modern era of total knee replacement, our knowledge of these wound-compromising factors has allowed us to predict with some degree of accuracy those who might have trouble and what we might do preoperatively, intraoperatively, and postoperatively to maximize healing. This chapter is a summary of our current knowledge and approach to soft tissue healing. A basic understanding of the biochemical and cellular processes of wound healing helps us appreciate the complexity of a process that we sometimes take for granted. In addition, in exploring factors that influence wound healing, we can better realize at which points interruption of normal healing might occur. Finally, steps that might be taken before and after surgery to influence the wound-healing process favorably become clear if we know where normal healing might go wrong.

Uncomplicated wound healing is a beautiful and precise series of events. A troublesome wound can cause significant disability and prolonged recovery and result in prosthesis loss, amputation and, in extreme circumstances, death. In the last 15 years, there has been an explosion of research and information about the biochemical aspects of healing, chemoattractants, cytokines, growth factors, and recombinant DNA technology, all of which hold promise for furthering our understanding of soft tissue healing. Although this exciting research has not yet led to acceleration of the normal healing of a wound in a healthy patient, it shows great promise in treating difficult wounds, as this chapter will outline. The normal healing phases will be described and factors that might enhance these phases in a wound that is healing poorly will be identified.

HISTORY

As long as there have been medical writings, attention has been directed to wound healing and attempts to enhance and accelerate it. The use of plant extracts, even bread mold, in healing is at least 2000 years old by written record.[9,52] Both the Edwin Smith Surgical Papyrus from 3000 to 2500 BC and the Ebers Papyrus described certain of the earliest known wound manipulations—splinting and honey—to influence outcome.[6,19] Among the contributions of Hippocrates, who lived around 400 BC, was his insistence on cleanliness and irrigation of wounds with boiled water. In addition, his prescient emphasis on documentation and accurate recording of events is a primary characteristic of good medical practice to this day. Hippocrates' scholarship was followed 300 years later by the Roman Celcus and about 100 years after that by Galen, whose work on wounded gladiators of Asia Minor led to his understanding of the venous and arterial systems, wound care dressings, and meticulous follow-up. Descartes wrote the first Western physiology text, and Ambroise Paré deserves credit for one of the most significant contributions to our current approach today, the emphasis on gentle handling of tissues and on the harmful effects of trauma on tissue.[26,42] This concept, crucial today in the handling of all surgical wounds, such as avoidance of crushing clamps and prolonged vigorous retraction, is all the more remarkable because it was introduced into a medical world in which wounds were being treated with boiling oil and "laudable pus" was the ideal. Paré insisted that careful tissue handling was the first step to uncomplicated tissue healing, a point we will emphasize.

The late 19th and early 20th centuries saw rapid progress in our understanding of the causes of healing difficulties. Joseph Lister's practical acceptance of Pasteur's germ theory of infection, controversial at the time, bore fruit in his description of aseptic technique and the use of carbolic acid as a topical disinfectant in hospitals in which infection was rampant.[9] His practical application of this sound principle, coupled with the discovery of antibiotics, sulfanilamide in the late 1930s and penicillin soon after, which resulted in Alexander Fleming's shared Nobel Prize in 1945, put in place the last essential component of normal wound healing, control of infection, as the second half of the 20th century began.[17]

The latter part of the 20th century saw dramatic technologic advances and advances in molecular biology, biochemistry, and immunology. At the same time, surgical techniques and scholarship have produced real replacements for knees, hips, wrists, and elbows and functional replacements for kidneys, lungs and, even, for short periods, hearts. There is no limit to our ingenuity and to what the confluence of ingenuity, adequate resources, and need might produce. Our challenge remains to follow where these advances lead without losing sight of the basic precepts that have brought us here.

PHASES OF WOUND HEALING

Wound healing may be separated chronologically into three phases. Although these phases overlap, the events that

744

predominate in each phase are different and together produce the strong, substantial, protective, resilient end point that we called the healed wound.[7]

Inflammation Phase

Initiation of the inflammatory phase of healing may be nonspecific—infection, laceration, or trauma—but the surgical wound is the inciting factor that we deal with here. The first component of the inflammatory phase, vasoconstriction, occurs even before the wound is closed. Lasting roughly 10 minutes, this phase is followed rapidly by vasodilation, whose purpose is to allow the influx of cellular elements responsible for cleaning debris from the wound in preparation for the structural events that result in wound closure. An influx of platelets is followed by polymorphonuclear leukocytes, lymphocytes, and macrophages. Vascular permeability increases dramatically at the wound site, most likely moderated by histamine. These cellular events, especially the influx of platelets, result in the release of multiple factors—cytokines, platelet-derived factors, complement, and possibly even prostaglandins—that enhance the local cellular response in preparation for healing.

The elements of this first healing phase result in local control, hemostasis, protection against infection, and preparation for the series of structural events that will ultimately close the soft tissue in a healed wound.

Fibroblastic Proliferative Phase

The cellular elements and chemotactants that rapidly accumulate in the wound during the first phase of healing prepare the wound for the migration of fibroblasts, which are the primary synthesizers of collagen, the substance responsible for the healed wound's strength and durability. This second phase of healing begins at approximately 48 hours after the wound occurs. Fibroblasts climb along the fibrin matrix that has been deposited during the inflammatory phase of platelet aggregation and hemostasis. This crucially important matrix can be interfered with and can be a cause of wound-healing delay.[80] As fibroblasts migrate in and provide the predominant cell type present in the healing wound at approximately day 5, they produce ground substance, a gel-like combination of hyaluronic acid and chondroitin 4-sulfate, the glycosaminoglycans. This substrate will act as a matrix for the collagen fibrils synthesized most rapidly during the first few days of wound healing. This first collagen synthesized, tropocollagen, is converted to collagen fibrils, which assume structural and biochemical integrity and on which wound strength is based; it is in the first 3 or so weeks after healing that we see the most rapid rise in wound strength gains.[56] Collagen homeostasis is reached at approximately 3 weeks as collagen synthesis and degradation rates approach one another. This stage leads to the last and most prolonged phase of wound healing, the phase of remodeling, or the phase of collagen maturation.

Wound Maturation Phase

In this last phase, the cellular elements producing collagen within the wound are markedly diminished; the collagen fibrils deposited become dramatically more organized and structured in response to a variety of factors, including local mechanical demands. The water content of the wound, along with measurable ground substance, diminishes and is manifested as local induration. The amount of type III collagen, initially present in large amounts, is reduced and replaced by type I collagen as the tissue strength–providing elements much more closely approach the elements that give strength to normal skin. Stronger collagen cross links create mechanical resistance to disruption in the now-maturing wound. This process continues for many months, even years, after the initiating event.[68,69]

CELLULAR ELEMENTS OF HEALING

Specific cellular elements in wound healing are responsible for stimulation of fibroblasts, ingrowth of new and essential blood vessels, and clearing out debris in preparation for healing. Some medical illnesses, certain medications, and environmental factors can challenge the ability of these cellular elements to perform their essential functions.

T lymphocytes produce a sustained response to injury in the wound. They generate local influences on the vascular endothelial lining in preparation for regrowth of new vessels. In addition, they produce fibroblast-activating factor, which encourages and regulates fibroblastic activity in the healing wound. T-cell depletion at the time that a wound occurs can significantly deter breaking strength in the healing wound.[4,70]

Macrophages migrate into the healing wound and are activated as they participate in the initial inflammatory phase. These cells remain in the wound much longer than other responders, such as polymorphonuclear leukocytes, and release cytokines responsible for angiogenesis and for stimulating fibroblast proliferation.[55] Some studies have noted significant loss of the essential early functions of fibroplasia and debris clearance if the accumulation or availability of macrophages or their active migration into a wound is interfered with.[98]

FACTORS AFFECTING SOFT TISSUE HEALING

With a clear understanding of the normal unfolding of events from wounding to a strong stable healed wound, a variety of factors that have some bearing on tissue healing, which are always present and might be manipulated to benefit or deter tissue healing, can be examined for their influence before, during, and after surgery.

In the practical reality of the daily care of a surgical patient, environmental and physical factors, patient-related factors, and nutrition-related factors, as well as factors related to underlying medical illnesses, can all affect the progress of wound healing. A thorough understanding of the role of these factors in wound healing helps the physician avoid healing difficulties, encourages patient participation in recovery, and mitigates the effects when healing does not progress as expected.

Scarring and Tissue Perfusion

Adequate levels of PO_2 in the healing wound are essential. The oxygen delivery system, whereby inspired oxygen traverses the pulmonary vessels, binds to hemoglobin, and is subsequently released in response to tissue demands, can be subject to breakdown at several points.[50] Local scarring, irradiated tissue, diabetes, and chronic exposure to cigarette smoke can all interfere with the ability of small vessels to provide sufficient oxygen to the healing wound. Even local swelling or increased tissue pressure, such as that created by a hematoma, can so reduce perfusion that ischemia results.[90] Preparation for surgery requires attention to all these factors. At the molecular level, collagen synthesis by fibroblasts will not occur if tissue oxygenation is not adequate.

The mechanism whereby the destructive effect of tissue ischemia occurs, whether the result of poor perfusion, radiation injury, or even small-vessel disease such as seen in diabetes mellitus, is believed to be the production of oxygen free radicals. These free radicals may be a factor in aging skin and its loss of elasticity. Free radicals are in fact cytotoxic to cells, both to cell membranes and to their internal components.[58,101] In addition, free radicals can disrupt protein components such as enzymes and cause collagen to degrade prematurely.[93] Minimizing free radical production by ensuring adequate tissue oxygenation is one way of minimizing or even reversing these detrimental effects.

When local factors dramatically reduce wound perfusion and create severe local ischemia, the only solution is a dramatic increase in local tissue oxygenation or the local blood supply. One treatment option here is the use of hyperbaric oxygenation therapy. This modality increases the partial pressure of oxygen in plasma by subjecting the patient and wound to an atmosphere of 100% oxygen at twice the normal atmospheric pressure at sea level.[103] This creates an elevated PO_2 level in the arterioles, thereby forcing increased amounts of oxygen into compromised tissue (Fig. 78-1). For this treatment to be effective, there must be no local infection nor any local perfusion problems. Most notably, hyperbaric oxygenation therapy is not effective in the presence of frank tissue necrosis. Also, the requirement for specialized equipment is an additional economic factor in this choice of treatment. Tissue that is severely ischemic in the postoperative period is treated by local or distant flap transfer, which allows removal of tissue with circulatory compromise and the introduction of healthy, well-vascularized tissue to deliver oxygen so that healing may progress.[60]

Smoking

Although cigarette smoking has an unhealthy effect on almost every organ system of the body, the detrimental effects on wound healing can, unfortunately, be manifest in the postoperative period as progressing wound ischemia and marginal necrosis. Absorbed nicotine and its breakdown product, cotinine, have an inhibiting effect on capillary circulation and cause necrosis of skin margins to an unpredictable degree. Moreover, in a cigarette smoker, the addition of even a small degree of overzealous traction may cause wound compromise because the effect is additive to the peripheral circulatory effect of inhaled cigarette smoke. In addition, the carbon monoxide contained in cigarette smoke forms carboxyhemoglobin, a form of hemoglobin that shifts the oxygen dissociation curve to the left, which makes oxygen release to ischemic tissue more difficult.[25,32,51,82] This twofold effect of cigarette smoking on tissue oxygenation puts a patient who smokes at risk for wound-healing difficulties. Although there is no hard evidence regarding a well-defined preoperative period of discontinuation of smoking that would ensure uncompromised healing, we insist on at least 3 weeks' abstention from smoking or from exposure to second-hand smoke and require such abstention until skin sutures are removed in the postoperative period.[57] In our practice, smokers are required to sign an additional consent form (Fig. 78-2).

Diabetes Mellitus

The fact that a diabetic patient is prone to a variety of secondary vascular, neurologic, and wound-healing difficulties is well known to surgeons. However, the concept of small-vessel occlusive disease as the primary reason for these secondary illnesses, as well as for the wound-healing difficulties sometimes experienced by diabetic patients, has not been borne out in multiple studies of ischemia in the diabetic wound; other factors seem to play a larger role.[54]

Diabetic patients have increased blood viscosity secondary to a stiffer, less deformable red blood cell, thus making it more difficult for the red cells to pass through the tiny capillaries supplying oxygen to local tissue.[91] The high serum glucose level in a poorly controlled diabetic patient shifts the

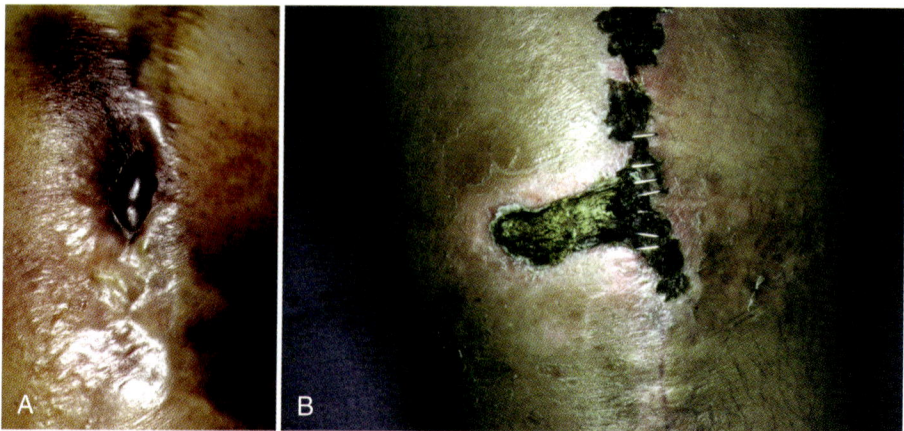

Figure 78-1. **A,** Circulation present but compromised. Hyperbaric O_2 therapy is indicated. **B,** Eschar indicates full-thickness tissue loss, with no circulation. Hyperbaric O_2 therapy is contraindicated.

CONSENT FOR SURGICAL PROCEDURES FOR SMOKERS

Patient ______________________ Age ______

Dr. ____________ and her staff have advised me that I must not smoke or use nicotine substitutes for a **minimum** of three weeks before surgery and after my surgery.

It has been explained to me that the risks of surgery are much greater for smokers, and even if I am refraining from the use of nicotine for three weeks before and after surgery, I may still experience the effects of nicotine in my bloodstream.

There is a greater risk in smokers of bad scarring, hematoma formation, intraoperative bleeding, poor or delayed healing, hair loss, sloughing of the skin (skin loss), infection, increased or prolonged bruising, and hyperpigmentation.

I ACKNOWLEDGE THAT I HAVE READ AND FULLY UNDERSTAND THE ABOVE CONSENT TO OPERATION AND THAT THE RISKS HAVE BEEN FULLY EXPLAINED TO ME, AND I WISH TO PROCEED WITH SURGERY.

Patient signature ____________________ Date ____________

Figure 78-2. Consent form used for patients who smoke cigarettes.

hemoglobin dissociation curve and inhibits oxygen delivery to the capillaries, thereby causing lower tissue PO_2 and resulting in impaired healing.[16]

Finally, the tibial and peroneal arteries in a diabetic patient seem to be particularly prone to atherosclerotic peripheral vascular disease.[65] Preventive measures regarding these vulnerable patients include preoperative vascular examination of the lower extremities, with palpation of the peripheral pulses, and further evaluation if abnormalities are noted, meticulous control of the serum glucose level in the perioperative period, and avoidance of extremity edema and the local compounding of a diabetic's rheologic changes that edema increases.

Other Factors

Anemia

The evidence regarding anemia as a contributing factor in the failure of wounds to heal is inconclusive. Hemoglobinopathies and extreme drops in the hematocrit level, both of which can compromise delivery of oxygen, have not been proved to compromise soft tissue healing.[3,35,43,85]

Radiation Exposure

Ionizing radiation causes injury, not just to the target tissue but also to the tissue that surrounds the target. Radiation was at one time used to aid in wound healing and treat scar formation, for keloid control in particular; there are patients today who have had such exposure (Fig. 78-3). The damage caused by ionizing radiation is permanent, progressive, and irreversible. Radiation causes an obliterative endarteritis that results in local tissue ischemia and permanent difficulty with wound healing, normal wound contracture, and the formation of healthy granulation tissue. There is some evidence that these healing difficulties in irradiated tissue are caused by collateral damage to local fibroblasts and their proliferation, on which tissue healing is dependent.[30,31,86]

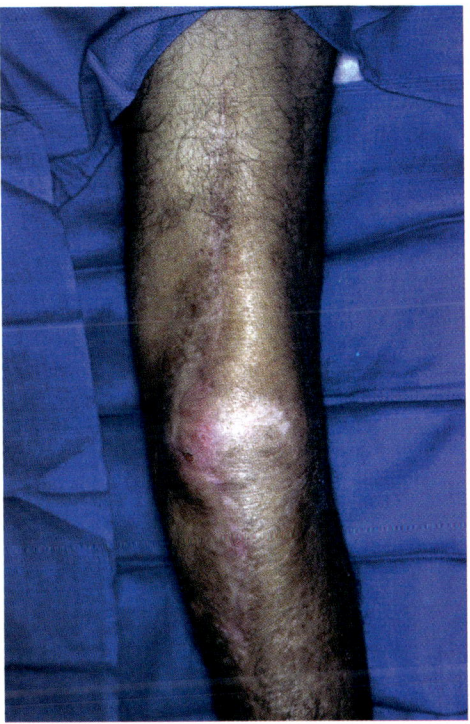

Figure 78-3. Radiation therapy in childhood caused profound scarring. Tissue must be replaced by well-vascularized coverage.

Steroids

It becomes obvious from a discussion of the phases of wound healing that corticosteroids, which inhibit fibrin synthesis, macrophage migration, wound contracture, and the events that lead to the formation and ingrowth of new blood vessels, are responsible for the poor progression in wound healing that we see in patients receiving corticosteroid therapy. Early and late effects, including loss of tensile strength and failure to gain strength in the healing wound, can both be attributed to steroid intake.

The effect of steroids on wound healing can be minimized by the administration of vitamin A, topically or orally. Collagen deposition, increase in wound strength, and functional macrophage support are documented effects of oral vitamin A in a steroid-dependent patient.[21,37,38]

Aspirin and Nonsteroidal Medications

Many prospective total knee replacement patients take nonsteroidal anti-inflammatory drugs (NSAIDs) for pain relief, and a large number of adults take one or more aspirin tablets daily as a cardioprotective regimen. There is some evidence that collagen synthesis is inhibited by normal therapeutic dosages of these medications, even in the normal population, and discontinuation of these medications in the perioperative and postoperative periods is recommended, in part because of this effect.[47]

Chemotherapy

Medications used to fight cancer inhibit wound healing. Although there is variation in the category and mechanism of action of this group of drugs, they are all designed to target rapidly dividing cells in some fashion. None are selective enough to protect healing tissue while continuing antineoplastic activity elsewhere. It is recommended, when possible, that the perioperative period provide a break in the administration of chemotherapeutic agents.[102] The harmful effects seem to be most evident in the early phases of wound healing; a 2-week postoperative delay in administration can mitigate these harmful effects.[23,24]

Age

It is unclear whether advancing age alone inhibits wound healing. There is ample anecdotal evidence that whereas very young patients heal with scars that remain hyperemic and indurated for prolonged periods, older patients seem much less prone to this type of healing, a fact that is to their advantage when incisions are placed in cosmetically obvious areas such as the face.[2,18,27,49,100] There is certainly no evidence that the final results of wound healing in terms of ultimate closure and tensile strength are inhibited or influenced by age. It may simply be that aging produces a slowing in the processes that lead to wound healing and that a more protracted course of collagen synthesis and cross linking is normal in an older patient.

Nutrition

Nutritional factors play a role in wound healing; a serum protein level below 2 g/dL is indicative of severe nutritional deficiency and can result in a prolonged inflammatory phase and impaired fibroplasia.[73,77,97] Nutritional factors seem to be most important in the early phases of wound healing, when the local inflammatory response and early fibroplasia are most active. Only when profound malnutrition is present are the phases of wound healing impaired. Although it is most unlikely to encounter this problem in today's surgical environment, many older patients are at least mildly deficient in one or more vitamins essential to healing; obtaining a nutritional consultation plus supplementing these patients with certain essential elements is an excellent idea.

Vitamin C

An essential element of wound healing, vitamin C, is required for the maintenance of tissue integrity in a normal healthy patient.[72] Even a completely healed wound will lose strength over time if vitamin C intake is not adequate. Ascorbic acid is an absolute requirement for the normal synthesis of collagen, so stable structural elements, including the vessel wall, skin integrity, and the type III collagen of healing tissue, are affected when vitamin C intake is deficient. A truly vitamin C–deficient wound can be separated with only the smallest amount of manual pressure and hemorrhage from weakened capillaries is common. Rarely seen today, vitamin C deficiency is easily remedied when recognized.[10]

Zinc

Zinc is a trace element present in all human tissue and is required in almost every enzymic reaction. Administration of exogenous zinc increases the rate of wound healing only when there is a zinc deficiency; the surgeon may encounter deficiencies of this trace element in patients with chronic alcoholism, cirrhosis, and gastrointestinal absorption problems, such as short bowel syndrome. Zinc is required in such minute amounts for normal healing that only a dramatic loss of absorptive surface will produce a deficiency; in such cases, zinc administration can rapidly and markedly accelerate healing when provided as a supplement.[53,76]

Delay in the early phases of wound healing has been demonstrated in animal studies of zinc deficiency. Compromise in the cellular and humeral immune systems occurs as well.[78,79]

Vitamin E

Vitamin E, tocopherol, has achieved almost mythical properties in our popular culture for preserving healthy tissue, particularly for minimizing scar overhealing and keloid formation. The best evidence for vitamin E's beneficial effect indicates that it is a membrane-stabilizing antioxidant that counters the damaging cumulative effect of preoperative irradiation on wounds. In large doses, vitamin E has an inhibitory effect on wound healing that can be reversed by vitamin A.[96]

Several studies demonstrating a beneficial effect of vitamin E supplementation in lowering the risk for coronary artery disease have made this vitamin an extremely popular supplement.[83] It should, however, be discontinued before surgery because of its inhibiting effect on platelet adhesion.[40,92] In addition, there is evidence that supplementing a normal diet with vitamin E can cause impaired collagen synthesis and impaired wound healing.[20]

Mechanical Stress of Healing

All healing tissue responds to mechanical stress. Expanded tissue gains strength and its collagen is more precisely oriented to resist disruption than nonexpanded tissue. More specifically, forces on a healing wound, depending on their magnitude and direction, will affect the orientation, amount, and strength of collagen fibers that create healing. The benefits of controlled passive motion on the postoperative wound are not just a rapid and early gain in range of motion. Provided that swelling is controlled, hematoma and the potential for wound necrosis are avoided, and stress across the wound is gradual, so the benefit for short- and long-term wound healing is evident.[28,99]

Skin Closure

An assessment of the available and commonly used wound closure materials is appropriate at this point. The purpose of closure is to provide sufficient local support for the evolution of wound healing and strength gain for enough time that the mechanical support afforded by sutures is no longer needed. Primary suturing of a wound provides skin closure as a temporary barrier between contamination from the skin surface and the outside world and replicates the function of the skin as an organ. To this end, an evaluation of closure techniques and materials is in order.

A variety of options exist to effect skin closure—staples, skin sutures, skin tape, skin glue—all of which will coapt the skin margins appropriately. As they contribute to wound healing, sutures also have a number of less desirable effects. By penetrating local intact skin to a variable degree, sutures introduce an additional source of local contamination. When tied tightly, sutures can impede local blood supply and, if left in place for a long period, cosmetically unsatisfactory cutaneous marks ("railroad tracks") can be the result (Fig. 78-4).

Suturing of a wound can be accomplished with material that is braided or monofilament, permanent or nonpermanent. Closure can also be achieved with skin staples, which are stainless steel and smooth-surfaced. Skin tape made of a variety of materials—plastic, fabric, paper—is bonded to an adhesive and applied to dry skin, where appropriate.

Several important facts are known regarding the materials that we use for skin closure. First, there is excellent evidence that stapled wounds provide superior resistance to infection when compared with sutured wounds. Particularly at lower levels of bacterial contamination, skin staples have a lower infection rate than even the least reactive nonabsorbable suture, monofilament nylon.[41,94]

Second, skin tapes used to close a wound that is dry (but not when continuous oozing loosens the tape) seem to provide the greatest resistance to infection, especially from surface contamination, when compared with other closure techniques.[12] Perfect skin edge to edge coaptation is essential for uneventful wound healing. Although manual suturing is perhaps best suited to compensate for the inequalities in skin thickness that result in surface overlap or override, if the deep tissues are accurately approximated, skin staples appear to be an excellent choice for skin closure in total knee arthroplasty. Concern regarding compressive ischemia between the legs of the skin staples is unfounded.

SKIN HEALING

Faced with the possible loss of skin coverage and the need to promote healing and provide a barrier, surgeons dealing with wound problems about the knee have the added concern of protecting the prosthesis from infection. There are several steps involved in assessing the progress of healing; determining tissue viability and therefore the propensity for healing is essential. Tissue whose blood supply is clearly compromised is treated differently from tissue in which viability is questionable or marginal or is robustly adequate. In the postoperative period, cutaneous blistering of the skin is an indication of superficial loss (Fig. 78-5).

Preoperative Preparation

The largest organ in the body, the skin, has certain nutritional and metabolic requirements and physical characteristics

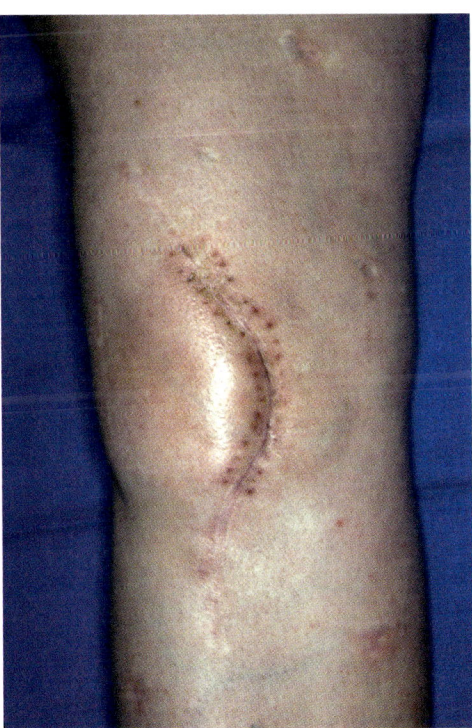

Figure 78-4. Cutaneous sutures in place for 3 weeks epithelialize along suture tracks. Permanent scarring results.

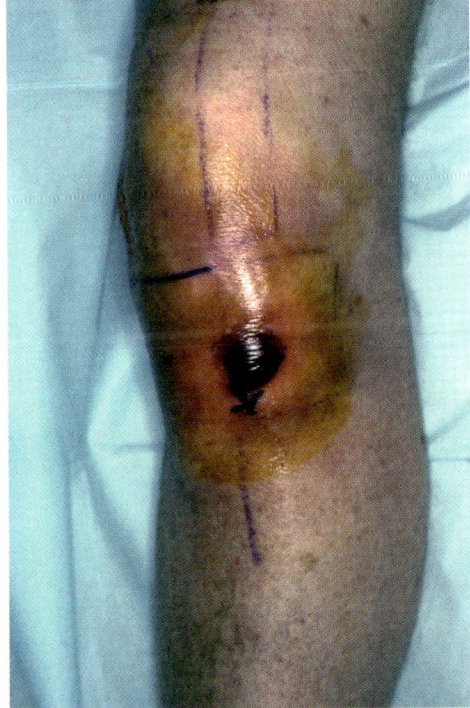

Figure 78-5. Partial-thickness skin circulatory compromise is indicated by skin blistering.

that must be respected and supported if optimal healing is desired. Any discussion regarding treatment of a nonhealing surgical wound must begin with an analysis of the cause of the healing problem. The final common denominator for most wound-healing issues is insufficient blood flow at the cellular level. Circulation must be adequate to provide for routine cellular metabolic requirements and for the additional demands of tissue repair and bacterial defense. Factors such as anemia, malnutrition, circulatory inadequacy from large- or small-vessel disease, hypotension with vasoconstriction, cigarette smoking, and other issues must be recognized in the preoperative period. They must be addressed if wound-healing problems occur.

What matters in wound closure is the ability of the dermal and epidermal cells to replicate and seal the wound, thereby restoring the body's normal protective barrier against a dry hostile environment and against infection caused by the bacterial invasion. In addition, there must be optimal circulation for the mobilization and effectiveness of the macrophages, phagocytes, leukocytes, and other cells associated with the process. Any chemical or physical condition that compromises the environment at the cellular level will have a negative impact on the process.

Prevention of healing problems before they occur is frequently easier to accomplish than treating established complications.[5] For the most favorable healing, one must minimize the amount of trauma to which the wound is subjected and optimize the wound environment before, during, and after surgery. The most onerous of the detrimental factors mentioned interfere with the delivery of oxygen and nutrients to the skin and healing wound and alter the ability of the dermal and epidermal cells to multiply and heal.

Preoperatively, bacteria embedded in the dermis will contaminate skin that is traumatized in any way. Dry, cracked, or crusted skin should be treated by daily cleansing and moisturization with a suitable emollient cream such as Eucerin to promote restoration of an intact epidermal barrier and lessen the bioburden to which the wound will be exposed.

Hair removal should be done in the manner that least injures the skin. Shaving with a razor may injure the skin and allow for bacterial contamination, especially if performed the night before surgery. Therefore, hair removal should be done immediately preoperatively, by clipping, depilatory cream, or extremely gentle shaving immediately prior to surgery.[1,14,45,59,89]

Bacterial contamination at the time of surgery is inevitable in every operation. It is impossible to achieve absolute sterility, no matter what type of preparation is used. A key to reducing the incidence of surgical site infection is reducing the bacterial inoculum to a size that the tissue can handle. For ordinary tissue, this has been calculated to be 10^5 μm for *Staphylococcus aureus*.[34,46,62,84] This allows for two approaches to minimizing the chance of infection—reducing significantly the surface bacterial count and improving tissue resistance.

There is excellent clinical and experimental evidence about the importance of the type of preparation used to lower surface bacterial count. The skin is colonized primarily by gram-positive organisms. They live on any surface covered by skin cells, even down along the cells lining subcutaneous structures, such as hair follicles and sebaceous glands. The chosen skin preparation should remove skin oils and dead skin cells; in addition, it must selectively target the type of

bacteria residing on the skin.[81,87,88] Other factors, such as how long a particular agent takes to achieve bacterial death, its duration of action, its allergic potential, and the likelihood that it will cause skin irritation, are important. Most surgeons paint a topical solution on the skin surface in preparation for surgery; unfortunately, this does not remove skin oils or dead cells. Thus, a surgical scrub is preferred.

The choice of surgical site preparation method may also affect the healing of the wound. Alcohol-containing preparations, especially those with a higher concentration (60% to 70%), are highly effective against a broad spectrum of microorganisms. However, these agents are drying and therefore damaging to the skin. Also, although they have a rapid onset of action, they do not have a prolonged duration of activity.

Chlorhexidine (e.g., Hibiclens), in a concentration of 4%, has a broad spectrum of activity against gram-positive and gram-negative bacteria. Blood and other organic matter do not reduce its lengthy 6-hour duration of activity or its effectiveness, and this effectiveness increases when chlorhexidine is combined with alcohol. When chlorhexidine used as a scrub in the hours or days prior to surgery is added to its use as a scrub at the time of surgery, a further reduction in the level of bacterial skin contamination can be achieved.[13,22]

Iodophor-containing preparations (e.g., Betadine), although popular, have drawbacks in effectiveness and duration. To exert their full antibacterial effect, they must be allowed to dry on the skin; blood or other organic matter may diminish their antibacterial impact, and their duration of activity is shorter than that of chlorhexidine.[104] A newer, water-insoluble, iodophor alcohol solution (DuraPrep [iodine povacrylex]) has been shown to be as effective as and longer lasting than the standard two-step iodophor scrub and then paint regimen.[95]

Chloroxylenol 3.0% (Technicare) has the advantage of killing 99.9% of a broad range of bacteria in 30 seconds, with a long duration of activity. It is not drying and has no alcohol; terefore, it is not toxic to mucous membranes and corneas.

These recommendations are based on the assessment of bacterial counts at varying times before, during, or after surgery. It must be remembered that although some studies have shown reduced rates of surgical site infections using newer methods, the conclusion that reducing wound infections by improving the method of skin preparation is largely intuitive and applies only to those infections that are a direct result of inadequate skin decontamination.

Intraoperative Factors

Improving tissue resistance, by definition, means preserving the nutrient circulation by limiting tissue damage with gentle handling, proper planning of incisions to minimize ischemia, use of prophylactic antibiotics, and limiting the amount of foreign material left in the wound. An important step in reducing the degree of bacterial contamination of the wound is the use of prophylactic antibiotics; the timing of antibiotic administration seems to be at least as important as the antibiotic itself. Administration within the 2-hour period before the incision is made, and maintenance of tissue levels with supplementary doses during longer surgery, is more effective than commencing therapy after the surgery has begun.[5]

Intraoperative hypothermia diminishes skin perfusion and increases the rate of wound infection. There are several reasons for this well-documented effect. First, hypothermia causes peripheral vasoconstriction, decreasing tissue perfusion and with it decreasing tissue oxygen tension and tissue antibiotic levels. Next, hypothermia diminishes the bactericidal capability of infection-fighting cells such as polymorphonuclear leukocytes and T cells.[11,36,48,61] Therefore, maintenance of normothermia during surgery is essential. Small preoperative and intraoperative details such as the use of alcohol-based skin preparations, which cool as they evaporate, will contribute to hypothermia. The careful use of underbody-type warmers, using the natural tendency of heat to rise, may be more effective than warmers placed on top of the patient.

The entire surgical procedure includes multiple opportunities to enhance or endanger wound healing by rendering the skin and subcutaneous tissue more susceptible to poor healing and possible infection. Proper tissue handling leaves the skin flaps and wound edges better able to meet the demands of the healing process. In healthy individuals, with surgery on well-vascularized areas, these issues may be of little importance. However, in or around the knee. in a patient with local or systemic comorbid conditions, such factors may rise to a level of significance.

Although it is rare for a surgeon to make the skin incision with the electrocautery, the use of that instrument for deeper dissection is common. It should be remembered that the cautery not only incises the tissues on which it is used, but it damages the tissue left in place on either side of the wound. This creates a sizeable and expanded zone of injury that can easily lead to seroma formation, poor healing, or wound infection. As a method of hemostasis, the unipolar current spreads from the point of contact beyond the tissue being treated, creating widespread damage. The choice of a bipolar cautery as a method of hemostasis, in contrast, mitigates collateral damage, because a bipolar cautery only affects tissue between the cautery tips.

Excessive traction on skin flaps can easily damage the soft tissues during the exposure of the wound or the application of sutures. Wound edges may be further crushed by the use of surgical instruments or the application of staples, which can crush the tissue enclosed within the staples. Even the type of suture material used is important, because a single silk suture, a braided construct composed of a foreign protein, can make the tissue more vulnerable to infection by significantly reducing the concentration of bacteria required to cause an infection.[64]

For areas of thin or tenuous soft tissue coverage, acellular tissue matrices such as Alloderm or Strattice have been used internally for support and tissue reinforcement. These aseptically harvested materials provide an additional layer that acts as a scaffold for the ingrowth of collagen-producing fibroblasts essential for soft tissue healing.

Postoperative Factors

Once the wound is closed, the dressing must provide an optimal environment for tissue repair and regeneration. Because the epidermis is missing along the length of the wound, the maintenance of proper hydration of the underlying epidermal and dermal cells as they heal becomes one of several functions of a properly chosen and applied dressing. Petrolatum-based ointments, with or without antibiotics, should be used until epithelialization is complete along the length of the incision.

The ointment used can contain antimicrobials, such as bacitracin, with its effectiveness against gram-positive organisms. Neosporin contains bacitracin in addition to neomycin, which is effective against a broad spectrum of gram-negative and a few gram-positive bacteria, and polymyxin B, which adds to the gram-negative coverage. Alternatively, mupirocin (Bactroban) is an effective choice against numerous gram-positive bacteria, including methicillin-resistant *Staphylococcus aureus* (MRSA). It should be remembered that topical allergies exist or may develop against any medication, particularly the neomycin component of Neosporin, so its routine use should be limited.

The epidermis functions to keep the underlying dermis protected and moist. When an incision is made, the epidermis is lost. Using an ointment can speed the growth of epidermal cells across the healing incision. A fresh wound should be washed with soap and water once or twice daily to remove any debris and residual ointment; it should then be dried thoroughly. A fresh layer of ointment and a dry sterile dressing should be applied. Getting a wound wet with soap and water is not equivalent to leaving it wet; wet bandages and waterproof tape (and others of a similar nature) should absolutely be avoided because they can lead to maceration, which leads to skin breakdown and infection.

It is essential to recognize that wounds swell for a period of roughly 48 hours after surgery; the physical dressing must allow for this or risk compromising cutaneous circulation and causing skin necrosis. Tight dressings can impede lymphatic and/or venous blood flow. The muscles of the lower leg provide significant pumping action during ambulation; in a patient whose ambulation is limited, the addition of a tight wound dressing can contribute to peripheral edema in the involved extremity. Any degree of right-sided heart failure can also exacerbate the problem of peripheral edema. The presence of edema within soft tissue reduces cellular nutrition; as a result, healing is compromised.

If tape is used, the same tendency to swell may cause a shearing effect at the tape-skin interface; blistering from damage to the epidermis when tape constricts the skin's ability to expand in response to postoperative swelling may also occur. Allergies to the type of tape used, or to topical medication applied, perhaps to improve tape adherence, can cause a skin reaction and may result in contamination and infection of the wound.

Postoperatively, other issues may develop that compromise wound healing. Steroid use topically, or systemically, or as a recent depot injection, will inhibit the normal postoperative inflammatory response and slow the rate of white blood cell and macrophage activity, thereby lessening the ability to fight infection and produce cytokines and other factors necessary for healing. Collagen synthesis by fibroblasts is impeded and strength gains on which adequate healing depends is delayed or inhibited.

Localized bluish discoloration along the incision can mean vascular compromise to the skin. Removing staples or sutures may help. If the surgical area is swollen and bluish in color, a hematoma may be present. Only noninvasive diagnostic techniques should be used to clarify this diagnosis in situations in which there is doubt.[67] In the first 2 weeks after surgery, any hematoma present is usually too gelatinous to aspirate; when a large hematoma is suspected, immediate surgical exploration is warranted. The hematoma must be thoroughly evacuated and the wound irrigated[29]; the presence of a large hematoma may cause necrosis of the overlying skin flaps or may become infected by direct contamination or seeded by a bacterial shower. Following total knee replacement, the temptation to aspirate a hematoma as a diagnostic maneuver or as a form of treatment once the hematoma has liquefied and softened must be resisted, because the underlying prosthesis is at significant risk for infection from bacterial seeding when an aspirating needle is introduced through the skin.

ELEMENTS OF WOUND CARE

The function of the intact epidermis is to keep the underlying organism infection-free and moist in a dry hostile environment. The skin's barrier function keeps bacteria and other pathogens out, yet the skin's flexibility and the ability to deform without loss of continuity is to be maintained. Epidermal cells begin as a living layer at the dermoepidermal junction, where they grow and start a 6-week migration to the skin surface. By the time the journey is complete, they have formed a flat and dry but flexible layer. If the epidermal layer has been lost but the dermis is preserved, a new epidermal layer will regenerate from skin cells lining the adnexae. Functioning epidermis will usually develop within approximately 2 weeks, although it will take 6 weeks for a mature layer to form that can withstand the usual traumas of daily life.

One of the goals of wound care is to provide a substitute for epidermal function while the epidermis is regenerating, a moist environment that simulates the isotonic properties of normal tissue and prevents bacterial colonization. A large selection of agents is available for this purpose. When choosing one, effectiveness, ease of use, cost, and any requirements particular to the wound being cared for, such as treatment for or prevention of infection, must be considered. Any of the various medicated and nonmedicated petrolatum-based ointments described earlier may be used, depending on the presumed or identified bacterial species present.

Another alternative to treatment of superficial skin loss involves the use of an aloe vera–based hydrogel, Carrasyn Gel, which not only increases the rate of skin cell growth but also decreases the rate of bacterial growth.[75] Carrasyn has been compared with silver sulfadiazine (Silvadene), which is extremely effective in preventing bacterial growth but slows skin cell growth, and to salicylic acid cream, which increases skin cell growth but has no antibacterial activity. Carrasyn requires two or three daily dressing changes, but usually works well when an agent that fights infection and encourages cell growth is needed. Many other hydrogel products are available. Some are thicker and some may be easier to use. However, none have been shown to increase the rate of skin cell growth or decrease the rate of bacterial growth when compared with Carrasyn.

If the wound edges are discolored but retain capillary refill, the underlying dermis may still be viable. However, if blistering develops, indicating separation at the dermal-epidermal interface, underlying dermal necrosis is a near-certainty.

When this occurs, the focus of attention must be to limit additional damage and expedite wound closure.

The cause of the damage must be accurately identified and treated, as described. Remember that dead skin has no circulation; therefore, it has no ability to fight infection and should be removed. Patience is required because the extent of tissue necrosis may not be evident early on; it is generally best to wait for necrotic skin to demarcate clearly before proceeding with débridement and coverage.

Use of a topical débriding enzyme such as collagenase (Santyl) can be highly effective and may eliminate the need for surgical débridement if the extent of necrosis proves to be limited. Used once or twice daily, it can be combined with a topical antimicrobial ointment or powder; exposure to metal ions such as silver or iodine (as in povidone-iodine or Silvadene) must be avoided because such exposure inactivates the active enzyme. Detergents and any cleansing or rinsing agents with a pH above or below neutral also cause inactivation of enzymatic débriding agents. When the dressing is changed and the wound is cleaned, the area must be rinsed well with saline prior to application of the ointment to ensure that all traces of loosened débrided material have been removed and to restore the pH to neutral actively.

If a hard dry eschar develops, it will generally need sharp debridement. On occasion, a negative-pressure wound dressing (V.A.C.; KCI, San Antonio, Tex) will then be needed until wound closure can be accomplished.

Once necrotic tissue begins to separate, a considerable amount of drainage may be associated with the open wound. A number of absorptive dressings are available to address this problem; these agents aid healing by removing exudates and preventing wound maceration and further tissue destruction from potentially toxic enzymes.[15,33]

Calcium or sodium alginate dressings such as Sorbsan (calcium alginate) may be placed on the wound after cleaning with saline. These must be changed at least once daily, athough if drainage is excessive, more frequent dressing changes may be required. Although more costly than calcium alginate dressings, hydrofiber dressings (Aquacel) or polyurethane dressings (PolyMem) offer the advantage of being more absorptive; they also tend to fragment less on removal. In addition, all these absorptive dressings are available impregnated with silver ions; silver is a potent barrier to bacterial invasion and acts as a broad-spectrum antibiotic. In the initial stages of wound treatment, a silver-containing dressing or topical agent can be most beneficial. Other highly absorptive and antibacterial dressings, also available as gels, include iodine-containing Iodosorb and silver-containing Silvasorb. When a dressing is needed primarily for its antibacterial effect, and an absorptive function is not required, silver-containing dressings such as Acticoat, a knitted polyester that allows drainage to pass through to an overlying absorptive layer are also available.

During this phase of achieving secondary wound closure, efforts must be made to preserve as much viable tissue as possible. We recommend that treatments such as wet to dry dressings be avoided. Although they adhere to necrotic tissue and remove it, the process of removal damages fragile healthy tissue and can be painful. Wet to moist dressings with dilute povidone-iodine and hydrogen peroxide may be useful in the initial phases of treatment of heavily draining wounds contaminated with anaerobic bacteria, but these topical treatments are severely toxic to replicating skin cells and to vascular endothelium when used in concentrated solutions. Their use should be discontinued as rapidly as possible.[66]

The appearance of granulation tissue is usually an encouraging sign. It is primarily composed of new blood vessels, at least when it first appears, and is a good barometer of the decline of necrotic tissue in the wound. Granulation tissue may be contaminated, but rarely is it infected. However, granulation tissue becomes increasingly fibrotic with time; as a result, the amount of systemic antibiotic that penetrates it is limited. Topical application of antibiotics may need to be used if some areas of the wound persist in exhibiting necrotic material or are slow to granulate.

Because granulation tissue contains myofibroblasts, which exhibit contractile properties similar to smooth muscle cells, granulating wounds will generally become smaller as wound contraction and epidermal regeneration at the periphery combine to minimize the size of the open wound. The goal of treatment is a clean closed wound with no contamination or infection of the deeper joint capsule or implant, so a wound that shows daily progress and improvement in color, reduction in size and drainage, decreased swelling, and erythema can continue with topical treatments. If, however, drainage is out of proportion to the size of the wound or is purulent, or if the wound does not show steady signs of improvement, consideration must be given to surgical exploration because there may be a deeper source of necrotic or infected subcutaneous tissue not visible on the surface. Until that situation is corrected, the danger of joint infection persists.

INFLUENCE OF GROWTH FACTORS

A complete discussion of the topical treatment of healing wounds must include a discussion of cytokines, or polypeptides, whose function is to facilitate the cellular, biochemical, and mechanical stages of normal wound healing and regulate many of these processes.[63] Among these cytokines are growth factors, which have been explored as topical applications to the open wound to aid in healing. The nomenclature of growth factors is confusing; some are named for the cell from which they are derived, some for the cell that is their target or, in some cases, even for the function for which they are responsible. Growth factors are large polypeptides that function to facilitate the various stages of wound healing. Certain growth factors encourage angiogenesis, others are responsible for cell mitosis, and still others influence the cellular elements in surrounding soft tissue to mobilize in response to injury.

The literature over the last 15 years contains many studies using growth factors to aid in wound healing; the evidence for their use to benefit normal wound healing in terms of speed of healing, strength gain, or ultimate satisfactory cosmesis is conflicting.[8,44,71] Some clinical trials have supported evidence for more rapid shrinkage of an opened wound to which growth factors are applied, whereas other evidence has indicated that the ultimate outcome regarding time to closure and strength gain is unaffected. Considering these agents as an early step in influencing more rapid wound closure is useful because evidence exists to support their importance in aiding the closure of difficult wounds. There is some evidence that growth factors can influence events in disorders of healing skin, such as keloid and hypertrophic scar formation.[39,74,105] Whether this information will ultimately lead to topical agents that accelerate wound healing, in addition to agents that are useful adjuncts to the basic surgical principles of adequate débridement and edema control in local wound care, is hoped for but not yet ensured.

KEY REFERENCES

Bosco JA 3rd, Slover JD, Haas JP: Perioperative strategies for decreasing infection: a comprehensive evidence-based approach. Instr Course Lect 59:619–628, 2010.

Broughton, G II, Janis, JE, Attinger, CE: Wound healing: an overview. Plast Reconstr Surg 117:1eS–32eS, 2006.

Burns JL, Mancoll JS, Phillips LG: Impairments to wound healing. Clin Plast Surg 30:47–56, 2003.

Carli F, Emery PW, Freemantle CA: Effect of peroperative normothermia on postoperative protein metabolism in elderly patients undergoing hip arthroplasty. Br J Anaesth 63:276–282, 1989.

Darouiche RO, Wall MJ Jr, Itani KM, et al: Chlorhexidine-alcohol versus povidone-iodine for surgical-site antisepsis. N Engl J Med 362:18–26, 2010.

Disa JJ, Alizadeh K, Smith JW, et al: Evaluation of a combined calcium sodium alginate and bio-occlusive membrane dressing in the management of split-thickness skin graft donor sites. Ann Plast Surg 2001:405–408, 2001.

Krizek TJ, Robson MC: Evolution of quantitative bacteriology in wound management. Am J Surg 130:579–584, 1975.

Kurz A, Sessler DI, Lenhardt R: Perioperative normothermia to reduce the incidence of surgical-wound infection and shorten hospitalization. N Engl J Med 334:1209–1215, 1996.

Manchio JV, Litchfield CR, Sati S, Bryan DJ: Duration of smoking cessation and its impact on skin flap survival. Plast Reconstr Surg 124:1105–1117, 2009.

Mauermann WJ, Nemergut EC: The anesthesiologist's role in the prevention of surgical site infections. Anesthesiology 105:413–421, 2006.

Omonbude D, El Masry MA, O'Connor PJ, et al: Measurement of joint effusion and haematoma formation by ultrasound in assessing the effectiveness of drains after total knee replacement: a prospective randomized study. J Bone Joint Surg Br 92:51–55, 2010.

Saltzman MD, Nuber GW, Gryzlo SM, et al: Efficacy of surgical preparation solutions in shoulder surgery. J Bone Joint Surg Am 91:1949–1953, 2009.

Yule GJ, Concannon MJ, Croll GH, Puckett CL: Is there liability with chemotherapy following immediate breast reconstruction? Plast Reconstr Surg 97:969–973, 1996.

Full references for this chapter can be found on www.expertconsult.com.

The Problem Wound: Coverage Options

Susan Craig Scott

In assessing the approach to soft tissue healing in patients who are candidates for total knee arthroplasty, ideal circumstances allow sufficient preoperative planning to provide optimal skin conditions for wound healing. Such planning involves assessment of factors in the patient's history that might inhibit healing, as well as manipulation of the operative area in an attempt to ensure primary healing.

LOCAL SOFT TISSUE MANIPULATION

Certain patients have multiple existing incisions or other local conditions that might portend primary wound-healing difficulties after total knee arthroplasty (Fig. 79-1). Anticipating which patients will have healing difficulties allows us to plan preoperatively for primary healing and to provide healthy soft tissue coverage; consequently, wound compromise is avoided, and long months of recovery, delay in motion gains, and other complications that occur when healing fails to progress as expected are avoided. In these patients, we will use a sham incision, tissue expansion, or flap coverage from a local or distant source.

Sham Incision

A sham incision creates the skin incision and subcutaneous tissue elevation for total knee arthroplasty; this incision is then closed. The usefulness of this approach is that it informs us regarding the health and vascularity of local tissue. Primary healing of this incision allows us to anticipate no wound complications when the joint is replaced. The sham procedure acts as a kind of delay; by interrupting the blood supply that traverses the incision and increasing demand from the periphery, we anticipate a local response augmenting the existing supply. In fact, the primary benefit of the sham incision is its effect on local tissue in stimulating increased blood supply.

The sham incision, and probably tissue expansion as well, makes use of the delay phenomenon to increase tissue survival. Despite some controversy regarding the actual mechanism for effecting delay, there is no doubt that delay works when planned with care. When a surgical wound is incised with a plan to delay, hypertrophy and reorganization of vessels along the axis of the delayed tissue occur and result in improved surviving length.[2] Whether the success of the delay technique is due to vascular ingrowth in response to ischemia, enlargement of existing vessels, or conditioning of tissue to ischemia is unknown.[7] One week is sufficient time for the delay phenomenon to occur; longer time provides no advantage in the number or size of improved vasculature.[10,21,23]

The indication for a sham incision is a situation wherein the likelihood of primary healing is reasonable but some question remains regarding the health and vascularity of the local soft tissue. The disadvantage of this approach is the potential for tissue loss in the wound created by the sham incision. Although it is certainly preferable to have tissue loss occur in the knee before placement of a prosthesis, if tissue necrosis occurs after a sham incision, the surgeon is now faced with addressing a nonhealing wound in a patient who has yet to undergo total knee arthroplasty. In an attempt to avoid this situation, to provide adequate soft tissue coverage, and to increase vascular supply to the skin over the knee before joint replacement in situations of marginal supply, tissue expansion has proved to be an excellent technique (Fig. 79-2). Our indications for its use have evolved over the last decade, as have our contraindications. We now find that this coordinated approach serves as a satisfactory solution in selected patients.

Soft Tissue Expansion

The tissue expander is inserted about 8 weeks before the planned total knee arthroplasty is performed. To insert the expander, a pocket is created in the area and adjacent to the area of questionable blood supply; an expander as large as can be accommodated by the space is inserted. The expander is completely buried, as is its access port. Weekly or biweekly injections follow until adequate expansion is achieved.

The expander access port is always placed proximally, and injections are carried out with a needle no larger than 23 gauge. A well-vascularized pseudocapsule develops around the expander tubing and port; this pseudocapsule will generate a small amount of fluid. If the port is placed distal or inferior to the expander in a dependent position, leakage may occur around the injection site for a prolonged period when weekly injections are performed.

When the expander is inserted, the planned arthroplasty incision is drawn. In a proximal section of this incision, a 1.5-inch segment is selected for access. A syringe with 250 to 350 mL of very dilute lidocaine is injected into the areolar plane between the skin/subcutaneous tissue and the deeper retinacular layers. This hydrodissection follows the plane and atraumatically creates a pocket to receive the expander.

The expander is removed at the time of total knee arthroplasty; at closure, the expander pocket is always drained separately with a large-bore drain. This drain is removed when it returns less than 10 mL per shift. At the time of expander removal and joint arthroplasty, it is critically important to keep the capsular attachment at the perimeter of the expander pocket in continuity with the anterior and posterior capsular surfaces, because this region is the source of plentiful vessels in the vascular layer of the pseudocapsule.

It is our preference to place one or more rectangular expanders oriented longitudinally or transversely on the anterior aspect of the knee. Tissue expanders are available in a wide variety of shapes and sizes.

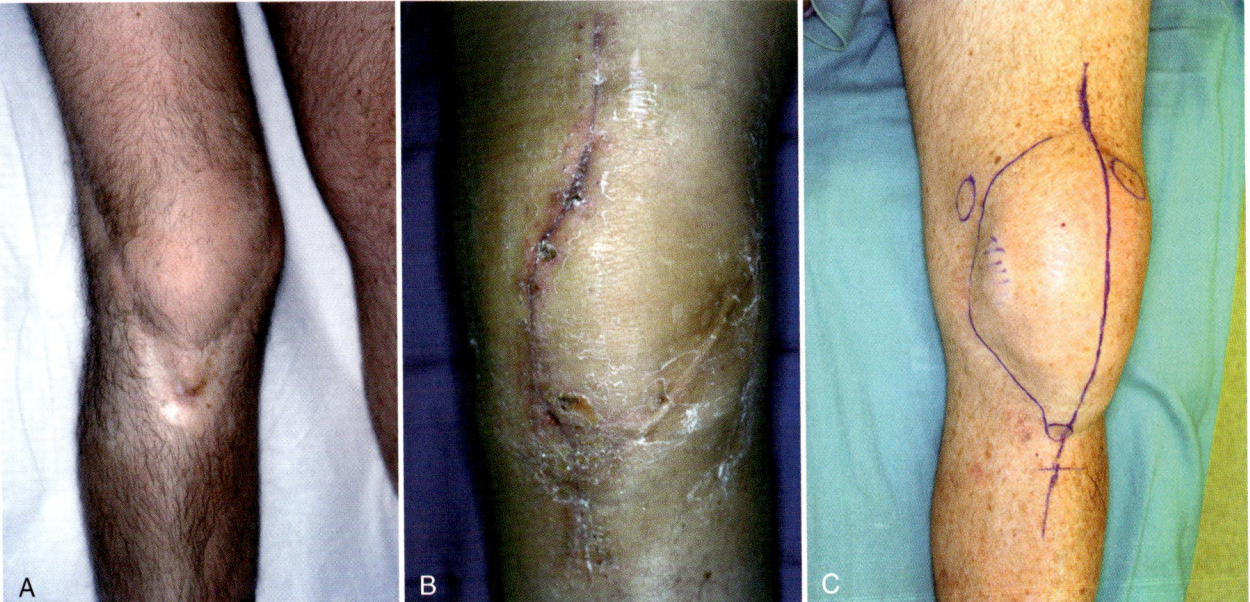

Figure 79-1. **A** through **C**, Patients who have undergone multiple previous surgical procedures through a variety of incisions may be at risk for healing compromise after total knee arthroplasty.

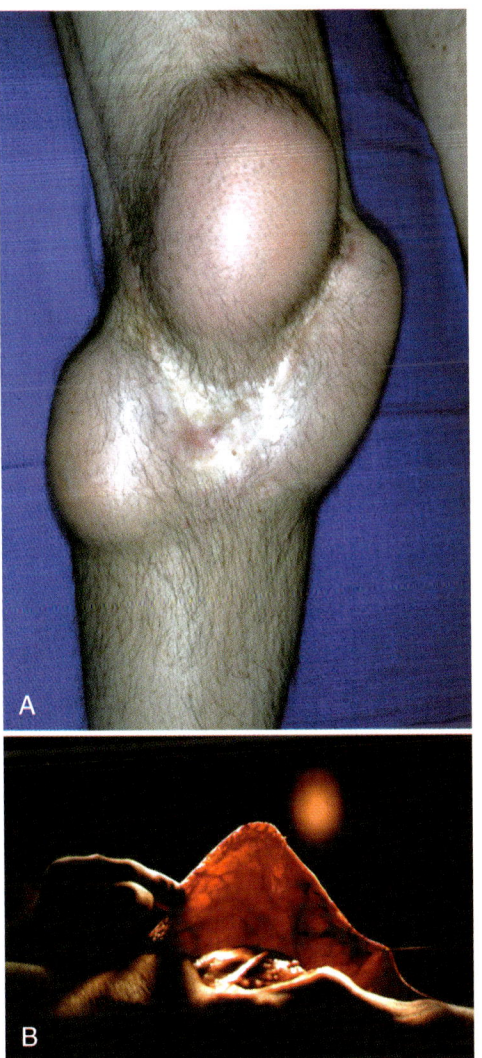

Figure 79-2. **A** and **B**, Tissue expansion can improve the local blood supply in patients with potential healing compromise.

THE PROBLEM WOUND

Skin Grafting

When full-thickness tissue has been lost, meticulous wound care after débridement will provide a bed that is satisfactory for the least complex form of coverage: skin grafting. This approach is used when the joint capsule is completely intact and there is no threat of prosthesis exposure.

Skin grafting removes a dermal-epidermal layer of skin from a donor site and applies it to a suitably prepared recipient bed. The bed must have appropriate vascularity to allow the skin graft to survive initially by serum imbibition for 48 hours, after which the skin graft is penetrated by ingrowth of vascular channels; by about day 5 or 6 after grafting, circulation is reestablished.[1,4,5] The bed on which the graft is placed must be free of infection with excellent hemostasis (Fig. 79-3). Once in place, the graft must be well fixed with suture, a compressive dressing, or application of the wound vacuum-assisted closure (V.A.C. Kinetec Concepts, Inc., San Antonio, Tex). Stability will allow revascularization.

At about 5 days, the skin graft dressing may be removed and dependence of the limb gradually initiated. Topical ointment should be applied to the graft until all crusted areas are gone, whether in the interstices if a meshed graft is used, or at the perimeter of the grafted area. Depending on thickness, the graft in the long term is likely to be dry and to require some assistance with moisturizing because its limited thickness does not bring with it sebaceous glands normally located in the deep dermis or subdermis to maintain adequate surface moisture.

The skin graft donor site ordinarily heals by secondary intention and must be protected from trauma and invasion of bacteria until healing occurs. It may be dressed with Xeroform (Covidien, Mansfield, Mass) and allowed to air-dry, or it may be dressed with an occlusive dressing, as the surgeon prefers. Some evidence suggests that occlusion until the donor site heals is more comfortable for the patient.[27] Once

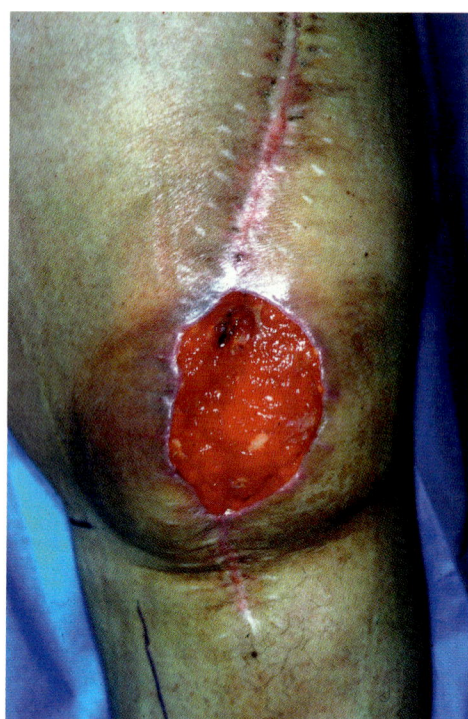

Figure 79-3. A healthy bed with excellent vascularity will support a split-thickness skin graft.

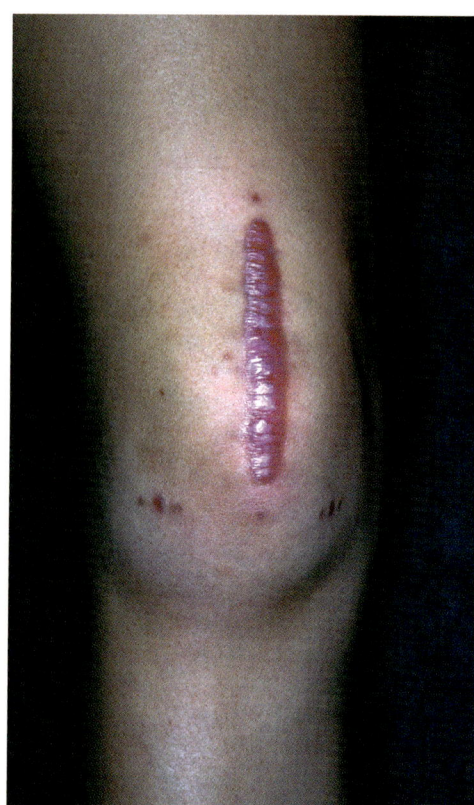

Figure 79-4. Scar hypertrophy will respond to the application of topical silicone sheeting.

the donor site has epithelialized, long-term effects such as pruritus, sensitivity, pigment changes, and even scar hypertrophy may occur. These conditions are ordinarily self-limited, but if persistently troublesome, they may be addressed with antipruritics, antihistamines, lubricants, or topical silicone sheeting such as Mepiform (Molnlycke Health Care, Oldham, United Kingdom) or Cica-Care (Smith & Nephew, Hull, United Kingdom) (Fig. 79-4). Corticosteroid injection and even irradiation may be indicated in situations where true keloid formation occurs, although these instances are rare.[19]

Muscle and Myocutaneous Flaps

When tissue loss is more extensive than simply skin and subcutaneous tissue, when the prosthesis is exposed or exposure is threatened, or when cutaneous cover is lost in a situation of incomplete joint capsular closure, as is sometimes the case, more robust coverage that brings with it its own vascular supply and is relatively independent of local tissue conditions is the treatment of choice. This option includes local rotation flaps composed of skin and muscle, muscle alone, skin and fascia, or fascia alone. The location and precise coverage requirements of the recipient bed determine the choice of coverage. These tissues are most expeditiously raised as a pedicle that is rotated or as an island that is transposed into position, as required. In a multiple operated knee, the surgeon may face a situation in which no suitable local donor site is available. In such cases, a free flap of muscle and skin or muscle alone from a distant part of the body is the solution of choice.

The local workhorse for coverage of defects about the knee is the gastrocnemius muscle or myocutaneous flap. The most

superficial muscle layer of the posterior region of the calf, this muscle has a medial and a lateral head, each of which is usually supplied by an independent artery.[18] Each head of the muscle originates on its respective posterior surface of the femoral condyle, with the medial head originating medially and the lateral head laterally. The medial head is usually the longer of the two heads and extends farther distal than the lateral head does; the two heads are divided by a median raphe, which also marks a clear division of their separate vascular territories. The raphe transitions to the musculotendinous junction as the gastrocnemius contributes to the broad, substantial Achilles tendon. Each gastrocnemius muscle head is a type II flap anatomically, with a single arterial pedicle providing blood supply supported by at least one secondary pedicle from the posterior tibial and peroneal arteries.[25] The medial and lateral heads are supplied by the medial and lateral sural arteries, respectively. The arteries arise at (60%) or above (32%) the joint line of the knee.[22] Most commonly, the medial sural artery arises slightly more proximally than the lateral artery; few, if any, arterial communications occur between the medial and lateral heads within or across the median raphe.[25] Because of this independent and very reliable blood supply, each head can be taken separately with or without overlying skin for coverage. Each sural artery has a 6- to 8-cm course before it penetrates the deep surface of the muscle and then arborizes and divides within that muscle.

This muscle provides a number of perforators to the skin overlying the muscle and distal to it and can be taken with a sizable skin paddle when needed. The perforators are located

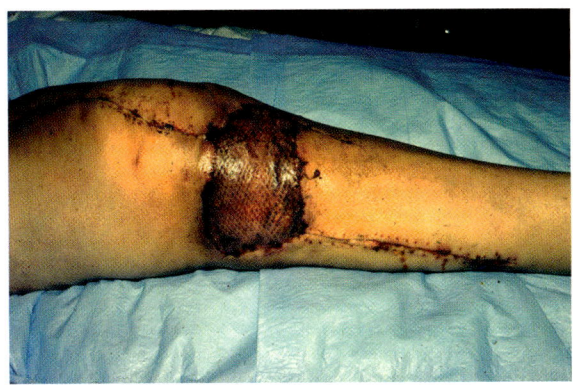

Figure 79-5. The gastrocnemius muscle flap provides reliable soft tissue coverage when needed.

just off the midline of the posterior of the calf. The first of those over the medial head is approximately at the level of the tibial plateau, the next is about 3 cm lower, and the last perforating branch is close to but above the musculotendinous insertion into the Achilles tendon.[3,6,26] Provided that these perforators are identified and protected, a medial gastrocnemius flap can be harvested with overlying skin to within 5 cm of the medial malleolus with continuous Doppler assessment of perforators to verify viability as the flap is manipulated.[8] The arc of rotation of the medial gastrocnemius muscle flap allows coverage of the proximal third of the tibia, the medial knee joint, the tibial tubercle, and the patella (Fig. 79-5). When taken as an extended flap with overlying skin, coverage can be achieved from the middle third of the tibia to the suprapatellar region. If more extensive reach is needed, the muscle origin can be taken down from the posterior surface of the medial femoral condyle. This technique provides adequate release if there is any tension on the closure and can add almost 2 cm of flap advancement when needed. If the required coverage is deficient in width rather than length, the deep muscle surface can be incised through its fascia and the muscle spread to increase its width of coverage.[17]

The lateral head of the gastrocnemius is shorter than the medial head and can be used to cover the lateral knee joint and the lateral aspect of the fibula; it, too, can be taken with overlying skin while the perforators are carefully identified to provide more extensive coverage. Proximal dissection and transposition must be done with great care, as the peroneal nerve is in a vulnerable subcutaneous position as it travels distally around the head the fibula.[17]

The major drawback to the use of a gastrocnemius myocutaneous flap is the cosmetic deformity that is created at the donor site. Some patients have a thick superficial and deep adipose layer over the muscle, which adds to the significant donor deformity when this flap is used. This can result in a sizable disparity in thickness between the flap and skin edges in the thin recipient area of the anterior aspect of the knee, which is often lacking in subcutaneous fat. We prefer to address this issue by having a thorough discussion with the patient before surgery, by transposing muscle alone when possible, by elevating skin margins in the recipient area and tucking the flap margin beneath, and of course by meticulously repairing the donor site.

Fascial and Fasciocutaneous Flaps

Our understanding of the blood supply to the skin and subcutaneous tissues of the leg is a direct result of original work by Pontén, Haertsch, Cormack, and Lamberty, whose descriptions of blood supply and fascial organization outlined the essential foundation for the more recent development of fasciocutaneous flaps for knee coverage.[6,11,20] Expansion of our understanding of these flaps and their clinical application is due primarily to Hallock's elegant and original descriptions of fasciocutaneous flap procedures.[12,13] Varied flap design allows satisfactory coverage while minimizing the cosmetic deformity resulting from harvesting the gastrocnemius muscle and overlying skin. When carefully designed, these flaps can provide hardy coverage of the exposed knee joint and a satisfactory bed for skin grafting. Only the reliability of their vascular pedicle, which is not present in all patients and must be meticulously defined, prevents them from being adapted universally as the most satisfactory local coverage option about the knee joint.

The fasciocutaneous system of the lower extremity has been clearly outlined in several studies.[14,28,29] This system, similar in concept to the system of angiosomes, which informs our understanding of musculocutaneous flaps, allows harvest and transposition of a variety of thin flaps in the lower extremity. Although the basis for this work is almost 25 years old, clinical application is still evolving as our experience grows and fascial flap reliability is reinforced.

Several local fasciocutaneous flaps may be used to cover the variety of defects seen around the knee. Among these flaps is the posterior calf fasciocutaneous flap supplied directly by the descending cutaneous branch of the popliteal artery, called the median sural artery by Cormack and Lamberty.[6] When the artery is present, this fascial or fasciocutaneous flap extends from the popliteal crease to the junction of the middle and distal thirds of the posterior aspect of the calf. Harvest of the flap requires careful preoperative Doppler outlining of the vascular supply, because in about a third of cases the aforementioned artery is small or absent.[28] This flap is available for thin coverage about the knee or as a free flap donor for distant sites.

The second fasciocutaneous flap coverage option in this area is the saphenous fasciocutaneous flap. The saphenous artery, a branch of the descending genicular artery from the superficial femoral artery, supplies the skin of the medial aspect of the thigh and the superior anteromedial aspect of the leg. It is very reliably present, originating deep to the sartorius muscle and becoming superficial distal and medial to the insertion of this muscle; this course makes the artery vulnerable to injury during total knee arthroplasty, particularly if wound-healing complications follow. In addition, the artery, its fasciocutaneous course, and its cutaneous perforators must be dissected with meticulous care before flap incision because adequate anterior perforators are present in only about 45% of dissections.[28] Its arc of rotation limits its use to defects in the proximal third of the knee and distal femur—two areas where wound healing difficulties rarely occur.

Our evolving knowledge of and experience with subcutaneous and fascial blood supply make use of these flaps possible for local coverage of the knee.

Free Flap Coverage

When local tissue is not available or has been used in previous surgical procedures, a flap from a distant part of the body is used for coverage of full-thickness defects in which there is threatened exposure of the joint or prosthesis. Although more than one potential donor site can be used for free flap coverage of the knee, local requirements mean that a flap of adequate dimension to cover the exposed area and allow excision of compromised soft tissue is required. In ideal circumstances, the flap must bring with it a pedicle of adequate length to allow a vascular anastomosis outside the area of immediate surgical involvement.

Patients requiring free flap coverage of wounds about the knee often have been hospitalized for a prolonged period. Not infrequently, more conservative wound care approaches have been tried for a number of weeks and have been unsuccessful. One or more attempts at coverage may have been made, perhaps with a skin graft or a local flap that was not successful. Patients approach total knee arthroplasty with the expectation that within a few short weeks after surgery, they will be fully ambulatory and able to resume a normal life. A great deal of disappointment and frustration is always involved in these relatively rare instances when healing does not progress as expected. When healing problems occur, our approach is one of watchful waiting, provided that we have full control of local tissue conditions, no infection is present, and most important, there is no threat of exposure of the prosthesis. When such is the case, we are extremely aggressive in our approach.

Our choice of free flap donor for coverage of the anterior knee focuses on several requirements. First, the flap pedicle must be of adequate length, so that the vascular anastomosis is done well out of the zone of injury. This required length might be as long as 12 cm to reach the superficial femoral artery in the adductor (Hunter's) canal. Next, the blood supply of the donor flap must be predictable with only rare anatomic variants. This minimizes the need for preoperative angiographic study of the donor flap and requires only study of potential recipient vessels. Third, although coverage is not performed for aesthetic reasons, a relatively thin flap is preferred, as normal soft tissue coverage of the knee is thin, pliable, and elastic. Fourth, the shape and volume of the defect dictate flap choice. A wide area of tissue loss may easily accept a latissimus flap that offers the advantage of a very reliable and lengthy vascular pedicle of type I variety. Narrow defects may not accommodate this large musculocutaneous flap and may be better suited to coverage with a free fasciocutaneous or adipofascial flap. Experience gained in a wide variety of reconstructive situations has expanded our knowledge of flap anatomy and our technical expertise in solving these difficult problems.[15,16]

We make every effort to thoroughly evaluate the soft tissues prior to knee replacement, and we try to anticipate which patients will have healing difficulties. Patients who present for revision total knee arthroplasty necessarily have scars present in the surgical area. Some of these patients have had extensive local soft tissue damage and a sizable zone of injury, which makes the preferred use of local soft tissue coverage impossible. Some have skin grafts that are densely adherent to retinaculum such that even a sham incision with local elevation is not a viable option and the use of tissue expansion is not possible. When such a patient presents for total knee arthroplasty or requires revision of an existing joint, free flap coverage is an ideal solution and in some instances precedes joint replacement by weeks to months, which allows sufficient time for soft tissues to heal adequately. Simultaneous total knee arthroplasty and flap transfer may be done successfully in very experienced hands. Such an effort accomplishes the goal of joint replacement with its life-altering benefits and avoids delays in rehabilitation and mobilization.

When distant tissue coverage is required, our preferred donor site to cover the anterior surface of the knee is the latissimus dorsi muscle with its long thoracodorsal pedicle (Fig. 79-6). The flap offers several advantages over other choices. First, the latissimus dorsi muscle is broad and relatively flat and provides an excellent and large surface area of coverage. Second, the blood supply to this flap, the thoracodorsal artery, is extremely reliable. It is a terminal branch of the subscapular artery, which originates from the axillary artery. The thoracodorsal pedicle can be as long as 12 cm, thus allowing its anastomosis to be placed proximal to the knee. In our hands, the preferred recipient vessel is the descending genicular branch of the superficial femoral artery, which is commonly found after the adductor canal is exposed, with one or two accompanying veins. When this vessel is not satisfactory, an end-to-side juncture with the superficial femoral artery and/or the superficial femoral vein can be created via this exposure. Third, use of this particular muscle allows for a two-team approach. The flap can be dissected from the back on the side opposite the involved knee by one team, while the second team exposes and prepares the recipient vessels.

The liability of the latissimus donor is the other side of its size advantage: although it is a wide, relatively thin muscle,

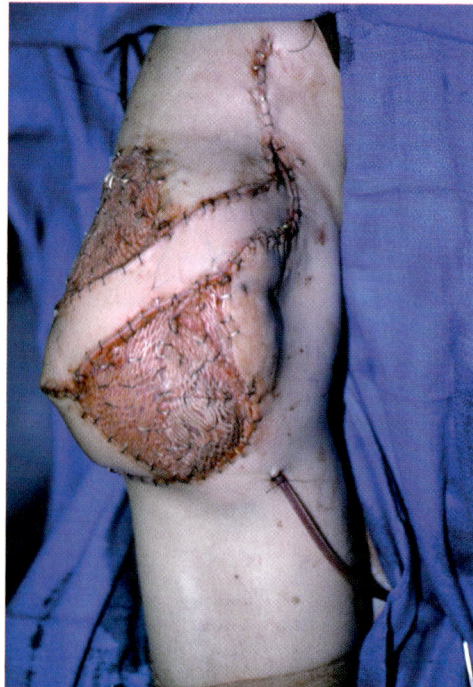

Figure 79-6. Free myocutaneous flap coverage is the ideal solution when local coverage is not available.

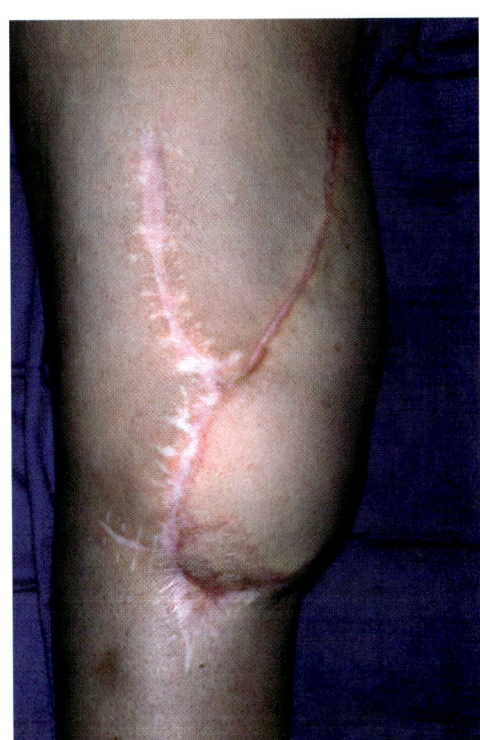

Figure 79-7. The transverse rectus abdominis flap provides thin suitable coverage in selected patients.

in some patients it can be bulky in this recipient area of limited anatomic dimension.

Other options are available for free flap donor coverage of the knee. The anterolateral thigh flap described by Song et al in 1984 is in a nearby operative field and can be taken as a fasciocutaneous flap; the donor site sometimes can be closed primarily as a linear scar.[24]

Other potential donor options include gracilis muscle, the rectus abdominis musculocutaneous or perforator flap, and the radial forearm fascial flap. All offer the advantage of not requiring a change in body position; each has its own disadvantages. The gracilis requires extended local fascial harvest for its skin paddle to reliably survive.[30] The rectus abdominis muscle, although a satisfactory donor in slender patients (Fig. 79-7), can be extremely bulky when combined with skin and subcutaneous tissue. The radial forearm flap, a thin pliable septocutaneous flap, has the disadvantage of being an unsightly donor, and its lack of carrier muscle can be a drawback when there is dead space to fill.

Newer vascular evaluation techniques such as computed tomography (CT) angiography have enhanced preoperative planning and significantly reduced intraoperative surprises requiring changes in operative plans.[9]

CONCLUSION

Extensive experience with these difficult wounds can dictate the most satisfying conclusion for patient and doctor. Salvage of the prosthesis and of the limb, maintenance of the ability to ambulate, diminution of pain, and gain in motion are all worthy goals.

KEY REFERENCES

Hallock GG: Lower extremity muscle perforator flaps for lower extremity reconstruction. Plast Reconstr Surg 114:1123–1130, 2004.

Hong JP: The use of supermicrosurgery in lower extremity reconstruction: the next step in evolution. Plast Reconstr Surg 123:230–235, 2009.

Ogawa R: The most current algorithms for the treatment and prevention of hypertrophic scars and keloids. Plast Reconstr Surg 125:557–568, 2010.

Song Y-G, Chen G-Z, Song Y-L: The free thigh flap: a new free flap concept based on the septocutaneous artery. Br J Plast Surg 37:149–159, 1984.

Whetzel TP, Barnard MA, Stokes RB: Arterial fasciocutaneous vascular territories of the lower leg. Plast Reconstr Surg 100:1172–1183, 1997.

Full references for this chapter can be found on www.expertconsult.com.

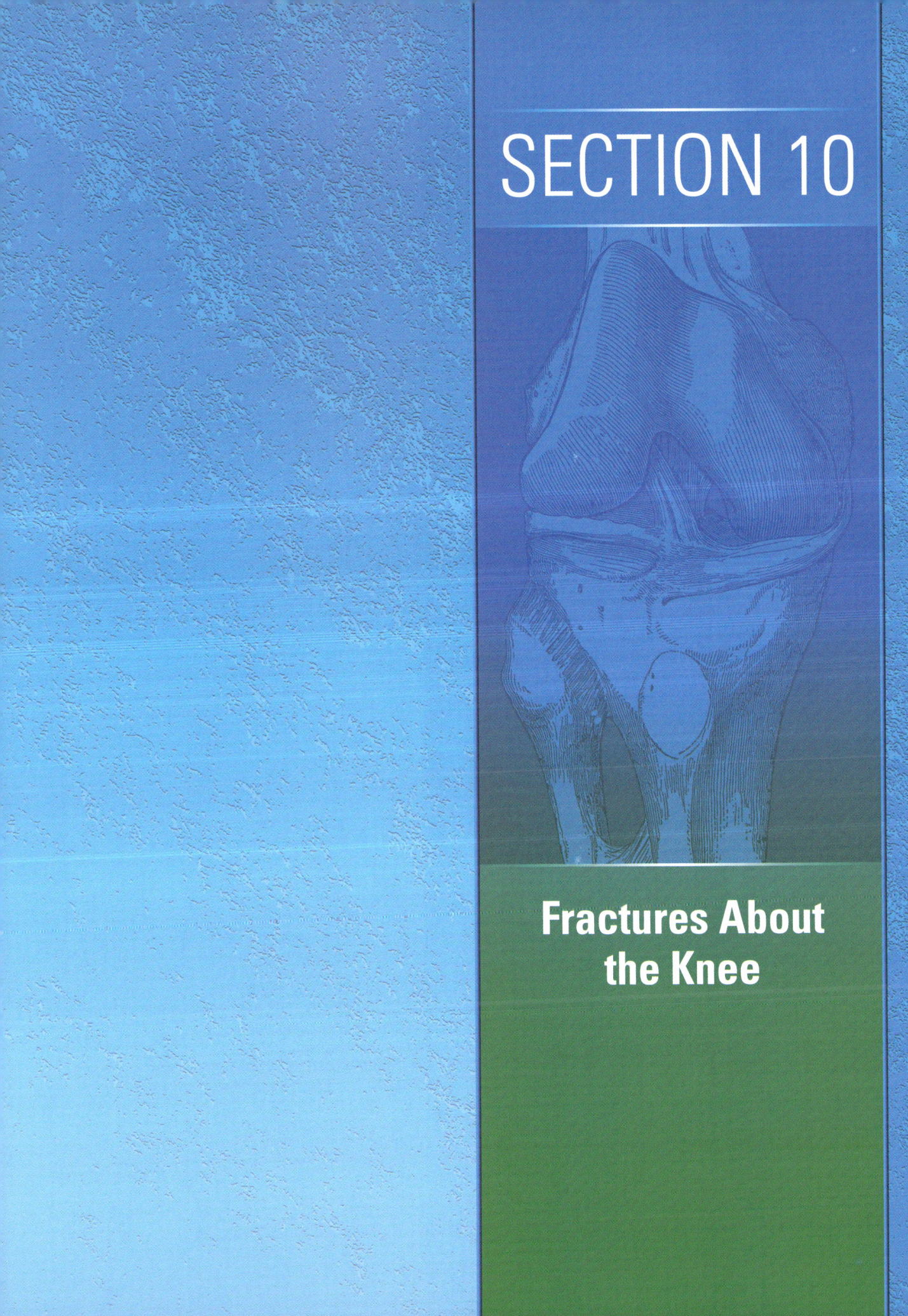

SECTION 10

Fractures About the Knee

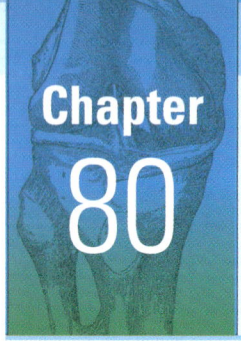

Distal Femur Fractures

Eric M. Lindvall, Anthony F. Infante, Jr., and Roy Sanders

ANATOMY

General Anatomy

The distal femur extends for approximately the distal third of the femur.[23,28,70] It begins as the canal gradually widens and the cortices thin and continues distally to the joint line. The supracondylar region (distal metaphysis) flares medially greater than laterally in the coronal plane and broadens laterally greater than medially in the sagittal plane. The anterior and distal trochlear groove allows patellar articulation with the distal end of the femur. The intercondylar notch is posteriorly based and houses the cruciate ligaments.

An axial cut through the distal articular surface reveals a trapezoidal shape with the greatest dimension located posteriorly in a lateral-to-medial direction and the narrowest dimension located medially in an anterior-to-posterior direction. The medial side slopes approximately 25 degrees in a posteromedial-to-anterolateral direction. The lateral side slopes approximately 15 degrees in a posterolateral-to-anteromedial direction (Fig. 80-1).[54] The shaft lies in the anterior two thirds of the condyles in the sagittal plane and slightly lateral, with a 9-degree valgus orientation in the coronal plane.[28,54,61,87]

The joint capsule has greater space anteriorly than posteriorly and extends more than 2 cm proximal to the superior pole of the patella along the anterior aspect of the distal femur. Posteriorly, the joint space extends only to the condyle–shaft junction.

The articular surface involves the entire medial and lateral condyles and is thickest along the distal articular curvature and within the trochlear groove, the regions with the highest contact pressure. Anteriorly, the articular cartilage extends more proximally on the lateral condyle than on the medial condyle.

The critical nervous and arterial anatomy of the distal end of the femur includes the sciatic nerve and the femoral artery. The femoral artery proceeds distally beneath the sartorius to lie between the adductors and the vastus medialis before entering the adductor canal. It then courses posteriorly through the adductor hiatus and into the popliteal fossa, where it changes name and becomes the popliteal artery until its trifurcation. The sciatic nerve lies posterior in the thigh between the long head of the biceps femoris and the semimembranosus. It then divides into the tibial and common peroneal branches before it emerges from the popliteal fossa.

Radiographic Anatomy

The anteroposterior (AP) radiograph demonstrates the 9-degree valgus angle created between the femoral shaft and the distal joint line. It also shows the greater medial condyle flare but does not reveal the trapezoidal shape as seen on an axial computed tomography (CT) image. The lateral radiograph demonstrates an anterior curvilinear sclerotic line representing the trochlear groove and a convergent posterior sclerotic line representing the intercondylar notch (Blumensaat's line), both of which end as they meet distally (Fig. 80-2). In addition, a true lateral radiograph of the knee allows identification of the medial femoral condyle as it articulates with the concave medial tibial plateau, and the lateral femoral condyle as it articulates with the convex lateral tibial plateau (see Fig. 80-2). Flexion of the knee during the AP radiograph allows visualization of the intercondylar notch.

Surface Anatomy

Palpation of the distal femur demonstrates a medial prominence, the adductor tubercle, which allows for muscle and ligament attachment. A lesser lateral prominence slightly more proximal represents the lateral tubercle. With the knee in the extended position, the inferior pole of the patella corresponds to the level of the tibiofemoral joint line. Approximately two to three fingerbreadths proximal to the superior pole of the patella is the proximal extension of the suprapatellar pouch. Four fingerbreadths proximal to the adductor tubercle is the level where the femoral artery traverses from the anterior half of the femur to the posterior half.

INCIDENCE AND ETIOLOGY

The incidence of supracondylar femoral fractures has a bimodal distribution—young adult patients with higher-energy injuries and elderly patients with lower-energy injuries.[3,23,38] The supracondylar femoral fracture is typically the result of an external force, but the amount of force required to cause the fracture can vary significantly and is dependent on bone quality. In a 2000 report on 2165 distal femoral fractures, the distribution of such fractures was found to be bimodal, occurring in young men and elderly women.[47] Lower-energy injuries are generally the result of ground-level falls or torsional injuries in patients with osteopenic or osteoporotic bone. Periprosthetic fractures are usually low-energy injuries that are encountered most commonly in the elderly as a result of disuse osteopenia, osteoporosis, and/or stress shielding around a prosthetic device or other metallic implant. A stress riser is created in the transition area between the prosthesis and routine bone. Examples include the area distal to a hip stem, proximal to a short supracondylar nail, and proximal to a total knee prosthesis.

Paraplegics and quadriplegics have weakened bone and, because of the resultant osteopenia and frequent contractures, are at increased risk for distal femoral fracture through falls from a wheelchair or transfer of the patient.

The amount of energy required to cause a supracondylar or distal femoral fracture in young patients with no existing

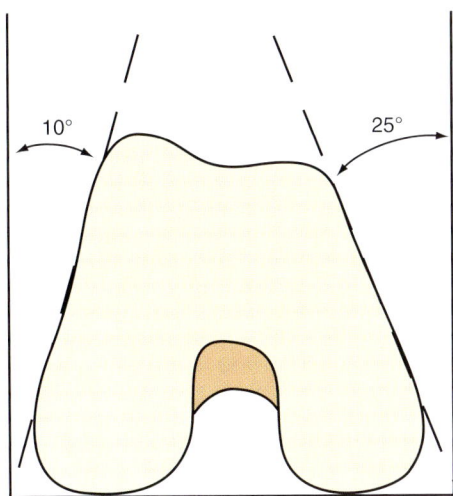

Figure 80-1. Diagram depicting the trapezoidal shape of the distal end of the femur. The 10-degree slope is shown laterally, and the 25-degree slope is shown medially.

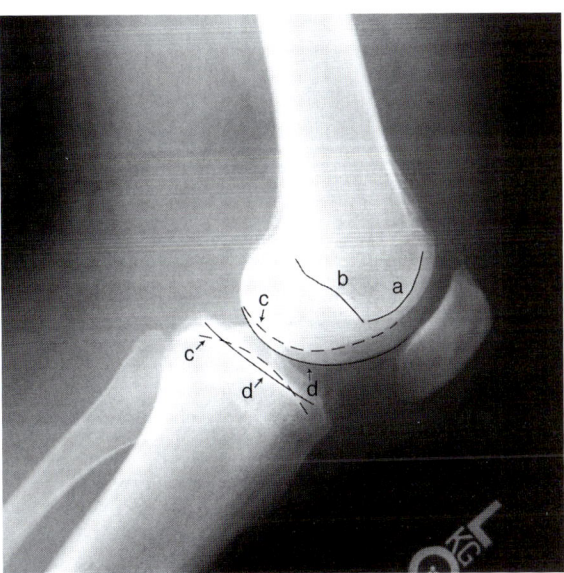

Figure 80-2. Lateral radiograph of the knee showing the trochlear groove *(a)*, the intercondylar notch (Blumensaat's line) *(b)*, the lateral distal femoral condylar articular surface with matching lateral tibial convex surface *(c)*, and the medial femoral condylar articular surface with matching medial tibial concave surface *(d)*.

bone pathology is usually significant, and this fracture is often seen in conjunction with other associated fractures.[4,6,8,14,81] Knee ligament injuries and intra-articular pathology have been reported in approximately 20% to 70% of ipsilateral femoral fractures.[6,14,81] Motor vehicle or motorcycle accidents, falls from heights, pedestrian versus auto accidents, and other heavy industrial accidents are common mechanisms of injury.[47]

CLASSIFICATION

A number of classification systems have been proposed for fractures of the distal femur. In 1967, Neer and associates described a classification system that divided fractures into three main categories: minimal displacement,

condylar displacement from the shaft, and supracondylar or shaft comminution.[57] Seinsheimer later published a more detailed system.[70] The Swiss Arbeitsgemeinschaft für Osteosynthesefragen/Association for the Study of Internal Fixation (AO/ASIF) group has since developed a comprehensive fracture classification scheme that has become accepted in the trauma community: type A, extra-articular; type B, unicondylar; and type C, bicondylar (Fig. 80-3). This classification is further subdivided by the degree of comminution.[56] The Orthopaedic Trauma Association (OTA) has developed a similar detailed and well-accepted classification system that encompasses the entire axial skeleton.[19]

DIAGNOSIS

History and Physical Examination

As with any traumatized patient, a complete history and detailed physical examination should be conducted. The pre-injury level of function and additional medical conditions should be recorded because such knowledge will aid in determining whether conservative or operative treatment should be performed. The mechanism of injury must also be ascertained to help determine the severity of the injury and other associated injuries. The physical examination should include a detailed evaluation of the entire limb and other extremities to rule out ipsilateral and associated fractures.[8] The skin must be circumferentially inspected for open wounds, and a detailed neurologic and vascular examination of the entire extremity should be documented. Higher-energy injuries can result in laceration or rupture of the quadriceps tendon, the femoral artery as it exits the adductor hiatus, the popliteal artery, and knee ligaments.[4,6,81] The knee joint itself should be evaluated for an effusion because an effusion often represents a radiographically unnoticed intercondylar split, an associated tibial plateau or patellar fracture, and/or anterior or posterior cruciate ligament rupture.

In higher-energy fractures, the ankle-brachial index should be documented even if palpable pulses are present. A ratio less than 0.9 has been shown to correlate with a high incidence of arterial injury, whereas ratios greater than 0.9 show that vascular intervention was not required. If abnormal, angiography and vascular surgery consultation should be performed.[37,51]

Radiographic Examination

As with any fracture, orthogonal views (AP and lateral) are indicated. Both knee and femur radiographs are necessary to fully evaluate the fracture and the entire femoral shaft. A traction radiograph may be helpful to better delineate all fracture fragments. Knee views will better diagnose intra-articular extension or comminution and associated patellar or tibial plateau fractures. Coronal condylar fractures (the so-called Hoffa fragment) seen in the lateral view must not be missed because the presence of such coronal splits will influence the selection of fixation devices.[4,30] Femoral shaft radiographs will reveal the proximal extent of the fracture, segmental fracture patterns, or possibly ipsilateral femoral neck fractures. If femoral neck involvement is at all suspected, dedicated hip radiographs must be obtained, because intraoperative discovery of this associated fracture can lead

33-Femur Distal

Location

Essence: The fractures of the distal segment are divided into 3 types:
A, extra-articular; B, partial articular; C, complete articular

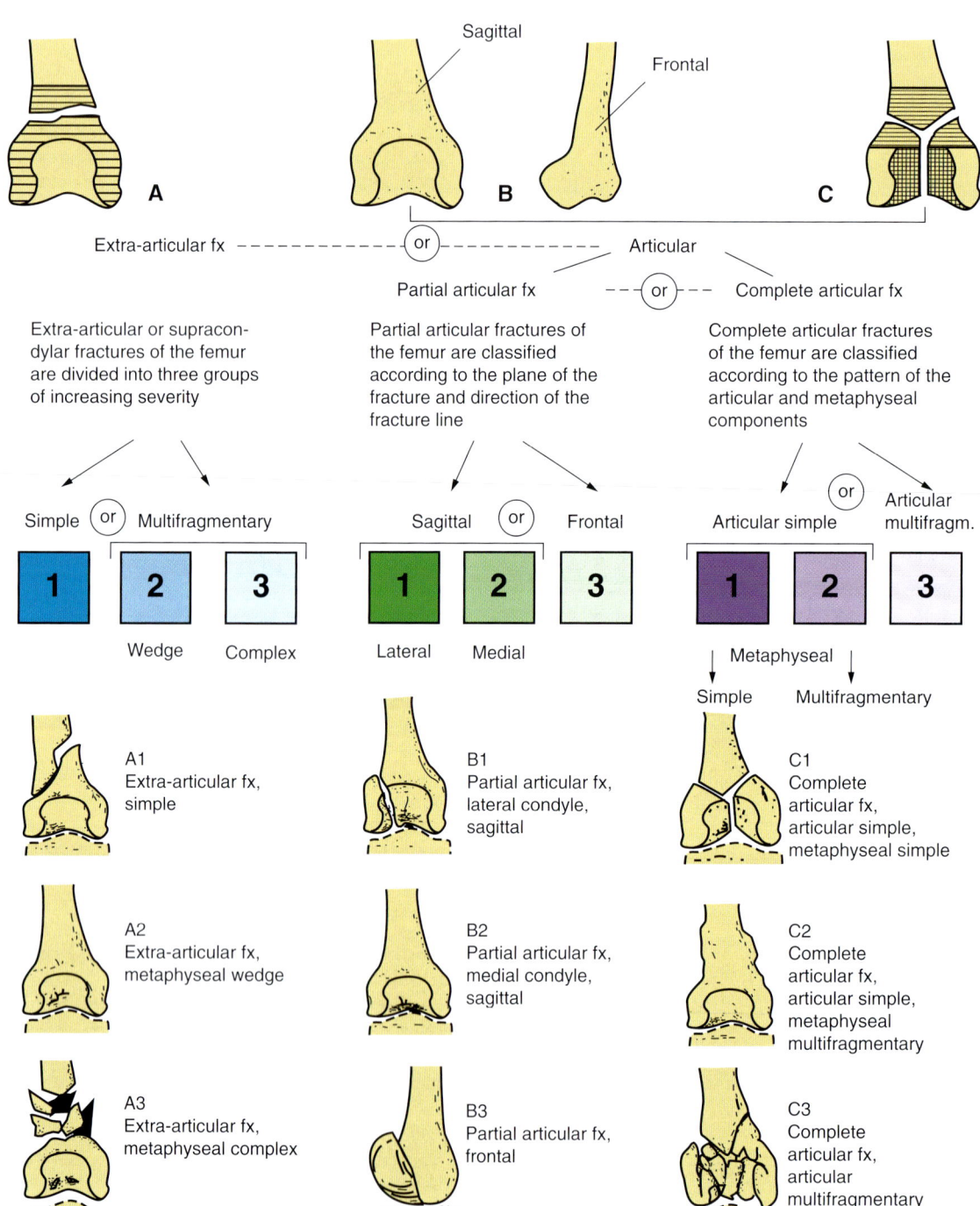

Figure 80-3. Arbeitsgemeinschaft für Osteosynthesefragen/Association for the Study of Internal Fixation (AO/ASIF) classification. (From Müller ME, Nazarian S, Koch P, et al: The comprehensive classification of fractures of long bones, Bern, Switzerland, 1995, M.E. Müller Foundation.)

to different instrumentation and patient positioning. CT is indicated for comminuted fractures, or if absolute certainty of all fracture lines cannot be gained from plain radiographs. Once all fracture planes are determined, more optimal fixation can be applied. The authors routinely obtain CT scans when planning definitive internal fixation.

MANAGEMENT

Conservative versus Operative Management

Nonoperative management should be reserved for patients who are too debilitated and/or bedridden, or who have prohibitive medical comorbid conditions. Other indications for conservative treatment may include nondisplaced, incomplete, and/or avulsion fractures. These situations are extremely rare.

The overwhelming majority of distal femoral fractures should be treated surgically. Operative stabilization allows increased mobility and early knee range of motion. The goals of surgical treatment are to reduce the joint anatomically, restore condyle–shaft alignment, and provide fracture stability to permit uneventful fracture healing and regain early knee range of motion.

Surgical Approaches

Lateral

The lateral approach, the most commonly used approach for supracondylar and distal femoral fractures, is an extension of the lateral approach to the femoral shaft. The patient is positioned supine, and the incision begins along the midlateral aspect of the thigh and extends distally to the lateral femoral epicondyle. If joint visualization is necessary, the incision is extended distally and curved anteriorly toward the midportion of the patellar tendon. The iliotibial band is then incised in line with the skin incision. Distally, the joint capsule is incised as distal as necessary, and medial subluxation of the patella allows intercondylar inspection. Proximally, the fascia of the vastus lateralis is incised and the muscle is dissected in a distal-to-proximal direction from the lateral intermuscular septum and posterior fascia, with ligation of any perforating arteries encountered. The muscle is then retracted anteriorly to expose the distal femoral shaft. The periosteum should be carefully preserved and no medial dissection should be performed to avoid devascularization of fracture fragments.

Alternative Exposures

Medial

The medial approach is less commonly used because essentially all anatomically designed plates have been created for the lateral aspect of the distal femur. If necessary, however, the medial approach also offers adequate distal femur exposure. The incision is made along the medial aspect of the distal femur, just anterior to the sartorius, while avoiding the saphenous vein. The fascia is incised in line with the skin incision to expose the vastus medialis. The vastus medialis

fascia is then incised at the medial intermuscular septum. As with the lateral approach, the muscle is dissected in a distal-to-proximal direction off the fascia (medial intermuscular septum), and any perforating arteries encountered are ligated. The muscle is retracted anteriorly to expose the medial aspect of the distal femur. The femoral artery remains posterior and proximal to the dissection. This approach may be useful for isolated medial condylar fractures or for corrective distal femur osteotomies.

Anteromedial and Anterolateral

The anteromedial and anterolateral approaches are rarely used because of additional adhesions that are created by dissection through the vastus intermedius. The adhesions often lead to decreased knee range of motion; therefore these approaches should be reserved for fractures that do not extend into the midshaft of the femur, or that do not already have a large open wound through this region.

The anteromedial approach involves dissection between the rectus femoris and vastus medialis. The fascia is incised over this palpable interval, and the distal portion of the incision includes the medial border of the patellar tendon to facilitate later closure. The vastus intermedius is then visualized, and splitting these fibers longitudinally allows exposure of the distal femur. The anterolateral approach involves dissection between the rectus femoris and vastus lateralis. Separation of these two muscles exposes the vastus intermedius. As with the anteromedial approach, the vastus intermedius must now be split longitudinally to allow visualization of the distal femoral shaft.

Anterior

The anterior approach requires a midline incision and a parapatellar arthrotomy. It allows excellent joint exposure but also requires separation of the vastus intermedius as the approach is extended proximally from the knee joint. A variation of the anterior approach described as the "swashbuckler" also allows for excellent joint exposure and is basically a lateral approach with an anteriorly placed incision.[75] Other variations of the aforementioned standard approaches have also been described.[52,58]

IMPLANTS—DESIGN AND FUNCTION

Numerous implants have been described and designed for supracondylar and distal femoral fractures. Implant types include short and long retrograde nails, various fixed-angled devices, and standard compression and buttress plates. Specific examples include Zickel, GSH, and standard retrograde nails; the AO angled blade plate; the dynamic condylar screw; the condylar buttress plate; and, more recently, locked plates.*

Intramedullary nails are available as shorter-length nails with multiple holes for interlocking, or as longer "retrograde" nails that typically provide multiple distal locking options. If sufficient distal bone is available, retrograde nailing is an excellent fixation option, especially for extra-articular fractures. Careful attention to distal fragment alignment is critical during reaming and nailing.

*References 24, 29, 33, 55, 63, 65, 69, 71, 73, 90.

Plates initially consisted of a condylar buttress-type plate and standard compression plates. The AO angled blade plate and condylar compression screw were the early forms of "fixed"-angle devices; the condylar compression screw allowed an additional degree of freedom and therefore easier insertion. Although the 95-degree angled blade plate does not anatomically match the medial distal femoral angle (99 degrees), the design allows for slight overbending of the plate to create compression of the opposite medial cortex. As the blade is inserted parallel to the joint line, the femoral shaft is reduced to the plate, which causes the "preloaded" plate to compress the opposite cortex. The 95-degree condylar compression screw, however, is extremely rigid and therefore can create a slight varus deformity if inserted improperly.

Additional fixed-angle devices have become available in the form of anatomically designed plates with locking screw technology that can be inserted through a traditional open approach or percutaneously.[17,41] The locking plate design also creates a 95-degree angle between the distal screws and the plate. Proper insertion is achieved with the distal screws parallel to the joint line; this is followed by reduction of the femoral shaft to the plate.[20,65] The advantage of locked plates over the traditional angled blade plate is seen with intercondylar split fractures. Insertion of an angled blade generates significantly more force than is generated by insertion of a threaded locked screw, and can therefore displace an undisplaced or previously reduced and compressed intercondylar split. In addition, rotational freedom during insertion is present with locked plates, as with the condylar screw, and the advantage of a fixed-angle device is gained. Newer anatomically designed locking plates may also allow for variable-angle locked screws that are inserted at the surgeon's preferred angle and then locked to the plate once fully seated.[86]

In cases of extreme osteopenia, osteoporosis, tumor, or other conditions with poor bone quality, a second medial implant has been described to add to construct stability.[26,35,48,49,64] The addition of bone cement has been advocated in similar situations to achieve increased screw purchase.[5,77] With the advent of modern locking plate technology, the need for adjunctive medial fixation or cement augmentation has essentially been eliminated.

The choice of implant is dependent on the location of the fracture, the fracture pattern, existing hardware, bone quality, and surgeon preference. It must also be stated that great care must be instituted when using locking plate technology as there is early evidence that these constructs may actually be too rigid, thereby increasing the risk of nonunion if not used properly.[8]

TREATMENT

Initially, as with all fractures, splinting and immobilization were favored over internal fixation. In the 1940s and 1950s, internal fixation was reported, but without overwhelming success.[1,79,85] As technology advanced and techniques improved, success rates with internal fixation began to increase. The Swiss AO group in 1958 defined the goals of open reduction and internal fixation as follows: (1) anatomic reduction, (2) preservation of the blood supply, (3) stable internal fixation, and (4) early mobilization.[55] Schatzker and Wenzl began documenting improved results with the AO

principles and showed open reduction and internal fixation to be superior to conservative management.[66-68,84] Other authors soon reported similar findings.* Today, although slightly modified, the AO principles are still being used, and the results of surgical treatment remain superior to those of nonoperative management for displaced fractures.

Conservative Treatment

Conservative management of distal femoral and supracondylar fractures has fallen out of favor as surgical techniques, implant designs, and rehabilitation protocols have continued to progress and yield outcomes superior to those of nonoperative treatment.† Certain situations, however, still require nonoperative management; it is therefore necessary to remain familiar with conservative treatment options.

For patients with low-energy, extra-articular, nondisplaced fractures who refuse or cannot medically tolerate a surgical procedure, cast bracing or casting is recommended. Non–weight bearing must be enforced until adequate healing is achieved to avoid creating a deformity or unstable fracture. Knee joint stiffness typically becomes problematic with longer than 6 weeks of immobilization.[21]

Special attention must be paid to the skin condition during casting or bracing. Paraplegics and quadriplegics also present a treatment challenge because skin breakdown can occur without warning, leading to additional setbacks.

Operative Management

Operative stabilization of low-energy, nondisplaced, or minimally displaced fractures is similar to operative stabilization of displaced or high-energy fractures, but usually involves less difficulty in achieving anatomic alignment. For extra-articular fractures, anatomic reduction is less important than anatomic alignment. Intra-articular fractures, however, should undergo anatomic reduction to decrease the chance of later arthritis. The more distal the fracture and the greater the mechanism of injury, the greater the likelihood of an unrecognized intra-articular split. Depending on the location of the fracture, an intramedullary device or a plate is typically used to achieve fracture stability. The ideal implant would be inserted with minimal dissection and would allow immediate knee range of motion and early weight bearing.

High-energy injuries involving the distal femur are frequently comminuted and have significant intra-articular involvement (Fig. 80-4A through D). If the fracture is an open fracture, adequate initial débridement must be performed, followed by thorough irrigation and temporary or definitive stabilization. If temporary stabilization is chosen, a spanning external fixator can be used, with the pins for the fixator placed away from the region of future definitive fixation. Two pins are typically inserted anteriorly or laterally into the femur, and two pins into the proximal end of the tibia, with the frame then spanning the knee joint (Fig. 80-5). If the soft tissues appear stable and appropriate studies and implants are available, definitive fixation may be performed at the time of

---

*References 11, 27, 52, 58, 72, 73, and 76.
†References 11, 27, 52, 57, 58, 66-68, 72, 73, 76, 84.

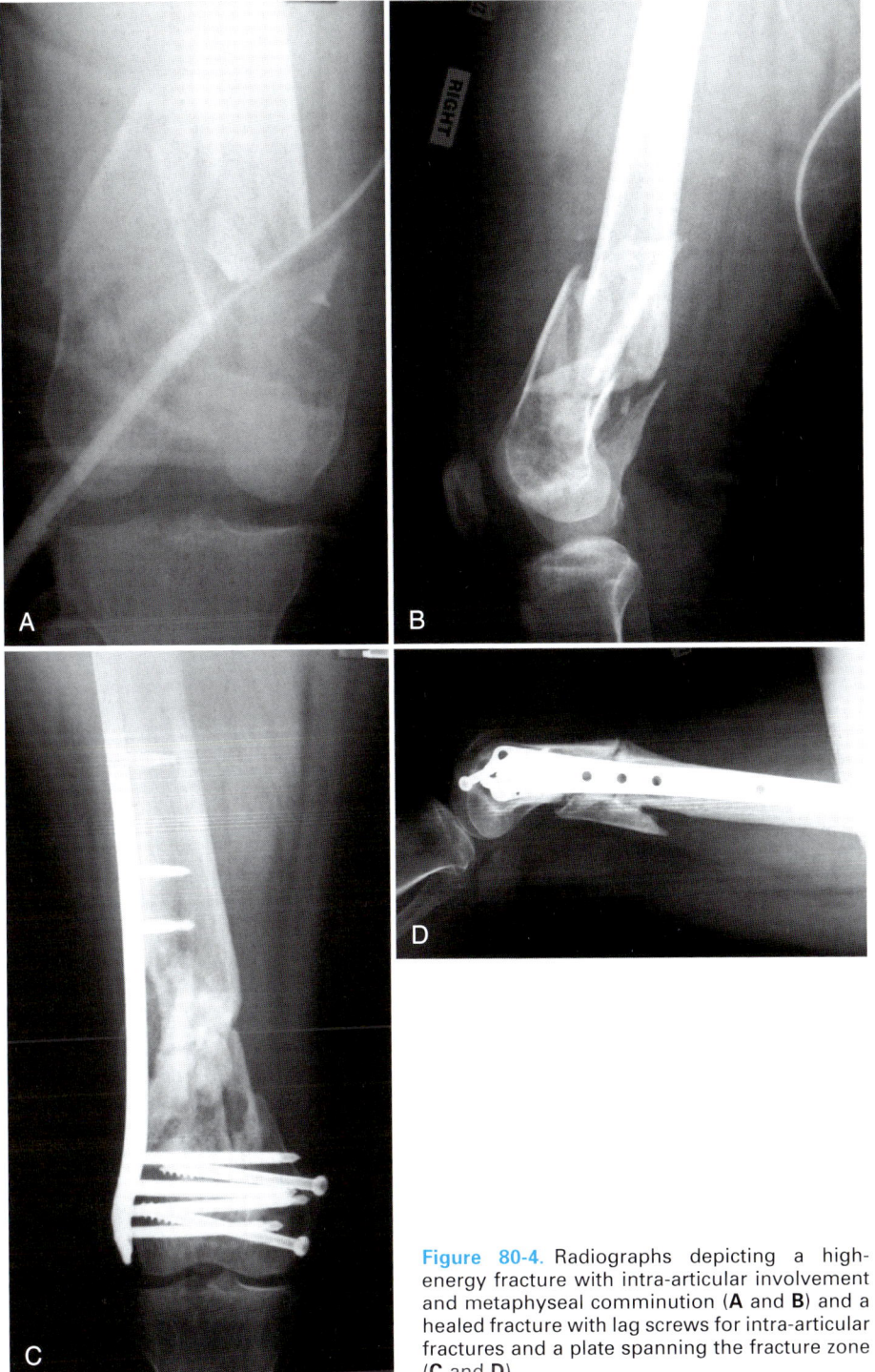

Figure 80-4. Radiographs depicting a high-energy fracture with intra-articular involvement and metaphyseal comminution (**A** and **B**) and a healed fracture with lag screws for intra-articular fractures and a plate spanning the fracture zone (**C** and **D**).

initial débridement. When significant intra-articular comminution warrants a CT scan, a staged approach must be adopted if the CT scan is not available prior to the initial open fracture débridement. The distal femur has better soft tissue coverage than the tibia, so plate application can be safely performed acutely unless significant soft tissue loss and/or excessive gross contamination is present. If tissue transfer is required for bone or plate coverage, or for both, initial spanning external fixation would be more appropriate. Intravenous antibiotic coverage based on the type and degree of soft tissue wounds is necessary, as in all long-bone open fractures. Initial bone grafting of open fractures is not recommended because of the increased risk of infection, although the literature mostly pertains to open tibia rather than open femur fractures. Intraoperative techniques that can assist in achieving adequate length or fracture reduction include manual traction, application of the AO femoral distractor, and use of the AO articulating tensioning device.

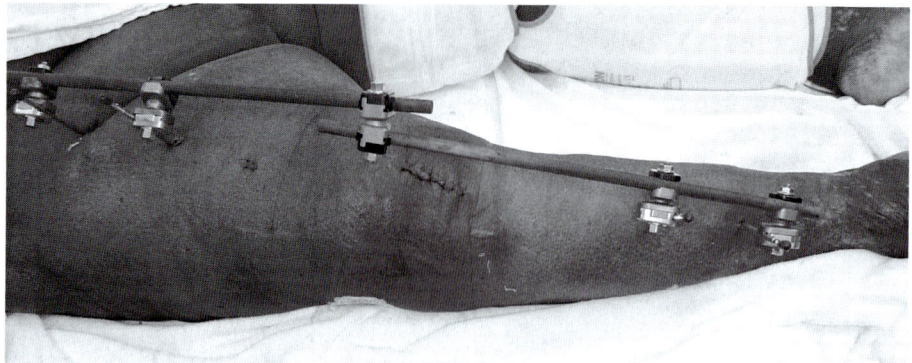

Figure 80-5. Photograph demonstrating a temporary spanning external fixator for an open fracture of the distal end of the femur.

Operative Treatment: General Principles

Regardless of whether a plate or nail is chosen to stabilize an intra-articular distal femoral fracture, adherence to the following principles is essential:

1. Achieving anatomic reduction with lag screw fixation of the articular surface
2. Maximizing distal fragment fixation
3. Obtaining correct coronal and sagittal plane alignment (5 to 7 degrees valgus)
4. Obtaining correct leg length
5. Obtaining correct leg rotation
6. Achieving stable proximal fragment fixation
7. Preserving fracture fragment viability by avoiding periosteal stripping and medial dissection

Intramedullary Devices

Once the "personality" of the fracture has been defined, the surgeon can decide on the most appropriate implant. The authors find retrograde nailing useful for extra-articular fractures with a distal fragment of sufficient length to allow stable distal fixation. Occasionally, a fracture with extensive femoral shaft extension and simple or nondisplaced intra-articular involvement can be managed effectively with lag screws and a retrograde nail. If a retrograde intramedullary nail is selected, an anterior incision is made over the patellar tendon and a medial miniarthrotomy performed on the medial border of the tendon. The entry point in the trochlear groove must be accurately placed to avoid injury to the anterior cruciate ligament and patella. Ideally, the entry point should cheat a few millimeters medial to center on the AP view and at the intersection of Blumensaat's line and the sclerotic line representing the femoral notch on the lateral view.[10] If the nail is inserted in the center and is not directed slightly lateral to remain in line with the anatomic femoral axis, a varus deformity will result when the nail enters the isthmus of the femoral canal. Because there is no canal fill in the metaphyseal flare of the distal femur, it is easy to create an angular deformity during nail insertion. A flexion or extension deformity can also be created if reduction in the sagittal plane is not obtained and maintained before reaming and insertion of the nail. Vigilance is required to avoid malalignment. It is important to understand that the nail will not reduce the fracture in this situation.

Early treatment of supracondylar femoral fractures with a retrograde intramedullary device was reported by Zickel and associates in 1977.[90] Difficulty was noted in achieving stability in patients with intra-articular comminution. A subsequent report by Zickel and colleagues showed improved results with the Zickel nail, but half the patients with intra-articular fractures did not regain more than 90 degrees of knee motion.[91]

Antegrade nailing of supracondylar femoral fractures has also been reported as a successful procedure.[44] Its effectiveness is limited with intercondylar fractures unless adjunctive fixation is used.[44,78] Adequate distal fragment length is necessary to achieve stable distal fixation, which in reality is rare.

Tornetta and Tiburzi achieved a 100% union rate with antegrade nailing of supracondylar femoral fractures but reported a 50% incidence of valgus malunion in patients in whom nailing was performed in the lateral position.[78] Dominquez and associates also noted successful results with antegrade nailing of distal femoral fractures and had only 1 nonunion in a series of 20 fractures.[15]

Retrograde nailing continues to be more popular than antegrade nailing because it is easier to control the distal fragment. The so-called supracondylar nail was inserted through the knee joint and not through the condyles.[29] Lucas and colleagues reported union of all 25 fractures in their series with use of the GSH nail, although four fractures did require bone grafting.[45] Danziger and associates also demonstrated successful treatment with the GSH nail, with healing of all but 1 of 16 fractures in their series.[12] Iannacone and associates, however, reported 4 nonunions, 5 delayed unions, and 4 stress nail fatigue fractures in 41 patients.[32] During their series, the nail was changed from an 11-mm nail with 6.4-mm locking screws to 12- and 13-mm nails with 5.0-mm locking screws. All device failures were noted with the 11-mm nail. In a series of fractures in elderly patients that involved the supracondylar region, Janzing and coauthors reported 89% good or excellent results with use of the GSH nail.[34] However, these investigators did comment on poor fixation distally with locking screws in osteoporotic bone.

Mechanical testing to evaluate various fixation constructs has been reported. Firoozbaksh and associates tested retrograde nailing versus DCS plate fixation in a synthetic bone model.[18] The DCS plate was found to be stiffer in lateral bending and torsion, but no significant difference was found with respect to bending stiffness in varus and flexion. Because the most common clinical forms of failure occurred in varus and flexion, both devices were deemed biomechanically adequate fixation for these fractures.[18] Koval and coworkers compared a short retrograde nail, an antegrade nail, and a DCS plate in a cadaveric model.[40] They demonstrated that the antegrade nail was the least stable and recommended use of the DCS plate when maximum stiffness is desired. In a comparison of a locked intramedullary nail versus a 95-degree angled plate, David and associates also concluded that the plate provided greater stiffness.[13] Ito and colleagues similarly compared the 95-degree angled plate with both the GSH and the AO supracondylar nail and concluded that the nails were inferior in torsion and varus loading.[33] With respect to specific nail comparison, Voor and associates compared fatigue testing on 5- and 12-hole supracondylar nails and found better fatigue strength in 5-hole nails because of fewer stress risers and therefore recommended their use.[80] More recently, biomechanical comparisons of modern retrograde nails have even been reported.[31] The authors routinely use long retrograde nails when treating these fractures. Long nails allow the fit in the femoral diaphysis to assist with proximal fixation and alignment and avoid the need for interlocking screws in the femoral diaphysis; instead, locking screws are inserted more proximally in the femur than short retrograde nails. The authors currently have no indication for short retrograde nails.

Plates

Plate insertion requires knowledge of femoral condylar anatomy in the coronal, sagittal, and axial planes. Although most distal femoral or supracondylar plates are anatomically designed, they still require correct placement to achieve anatomically aligned reduction. The need for double plating and intramedullary plating for medially comminuted fractures has essentially been eliminated with the advent of locked plating.[45,83,92] The locked plate has replaced the traditional condylar plate and, to a large extent, the condylar screw and blade plate (Fig. 80-6).* Four locked screws distally have been shown to be equivalent in fixation to the standard blade of a 95-degree blade plate.[39] The locked plates can be inserted percutaneously, thus allowing easier insertion and enhanced stability, especially in comminuted fractures of the medial and lateral columns (Fig. 80-7).[83] The locked plate must be correctly placed on the distal end of the femur to allow precise placement of the locked screws, because the angle of screw insertion is not variable and the screws will lock into the plate only at the predetermined angle. Once correct plate location is achieved in the AP and lateral views, the appropriate femoral length and alignment must be restored before proximal plate fixation.[36,88] As with intramedullary nailing, flexion or extension deformities can occur and are often difficult to assess intraoperatively if an external locking handle of the plate partially obstructs a fluoroscopic image.[43] Provisional fixation of the plate both distally and proximally is encouraged to avoid extensive revision of screw or plate placement should adjustments be necessary. If the plate is fixed distally first, a small amount of anterior or posterior plate angulation will translate into an increasing amount of plate–shaft mismatch as one progresses proximally. Therefore, a flexion or extension deformity will result as one reduces the plate to the shaft. To avoid extensive intraoperative revision, a single initial locked screw can be inserted distally without seating the head to allow rotational freedom of the plate. Once appropriate length is restored through gentle

manual traction or the use of a femoral distractor, the plate can be fixed proximally to the shaft. The distal screw is then seated and locked to achieve rotational control. If adjustments are required, distal screw revision is simplified because only a single screw needs to be removed. The surgeon must be extremely vigilant to avoid plate malposition or fracture malalignment, typically valgus of the distal fragment.

Plate fixation of the distal femur with a condylar screw, angled blade plate, or lateral condylar buttress plate is a well-established procedure described in detail elsewhere.* Fixation of intra-articular distal femoral fractures with a DCS plate has been compared with nonoperative treatment in elderly patients and has been shown to result in fewer malunions, fewer nonunions, and a decrease in complications such as respiratory infection, deep vein thrombosis, and pressure sores.[9] Other forms of plate fixation have also provided satisfactory results.[1,7,50,60,84] Wenzl documented the first series of supracondylar femoral fractures stabilized with the angled blade plate and reported 73.5% good to excellent results.[84] Indirect reduction, pioneered by Mast and associates,[48] has changed fracture fixation techniques and continues to evolve. The lateral condylar buttress plate and angled blade plate combined with indirect reduction techniques have provided 84% to 87% good to excellent results in treating supracondylar femoral fracture with intra-articular comminution.[7,60] It has been shown that malunion and nonunion are often the result of bone loss, severe osteoporosis, and/or medial column comminution.[2] Because of medial comminution, osteoporosis, and/or bone loss, double plating, intramedullary plating, bone grafting, and the use of bone cement are some of the techniques described to add additional medial stability and avoid varus collapse or fixation failure.†

The locked plated construct, even in osteoporotic bone, has been shown to provide enhanced stability and rarely requires additional fixation.‡ Locked plating has evolved as an extension of indirect reduction techniques, and results appear to be better than those of traditional techniques.[42,43,69,83] Weight and Collinge reported on 22 patients with unstable distal femoral fractures (AO/OTA types A2, A3, C2, and C3) stabilized with percutaneous locked plating and documented a 100% union rate.[83] All fractures healed without the need for bone grafting, and no hardware failures were noted. Average knee range of motion was 5 to 114 degrees. Kregor and colleagues documented similar results in 103 distal femoral fractures stabilized with percutaneous locked plating.[43] They reported a 93% union rate after the initial procedure and average knee motion of 1 to 109 degrees. Only 1 of 68 closed fractures required later bone grafting, whereas 6 of 35 open fractures needed later bone grafting (because of bone loss) to eventually achieve union in all fractures. Of importance was the fact that no fracture sustained loss of distal fixation. Schutz and associates reported early healing in 37 of 40 patients treated with locked percutaneous plating of the distal femur.[69] As previously stated, although locked plating provides documented advantages, it must be used properly to avoid the increased risk of nonunion due to its increased construct stiffness.[8]

---

*References 42, 43, 45, 62, 69, and 74.

*References 1, 7, 50, 60, 63, 71, 79, and 84.
†References 5, 26, 35, 48, 49, 64, and 77.
‡References 16, 22, 46, 74, 83, and 92.

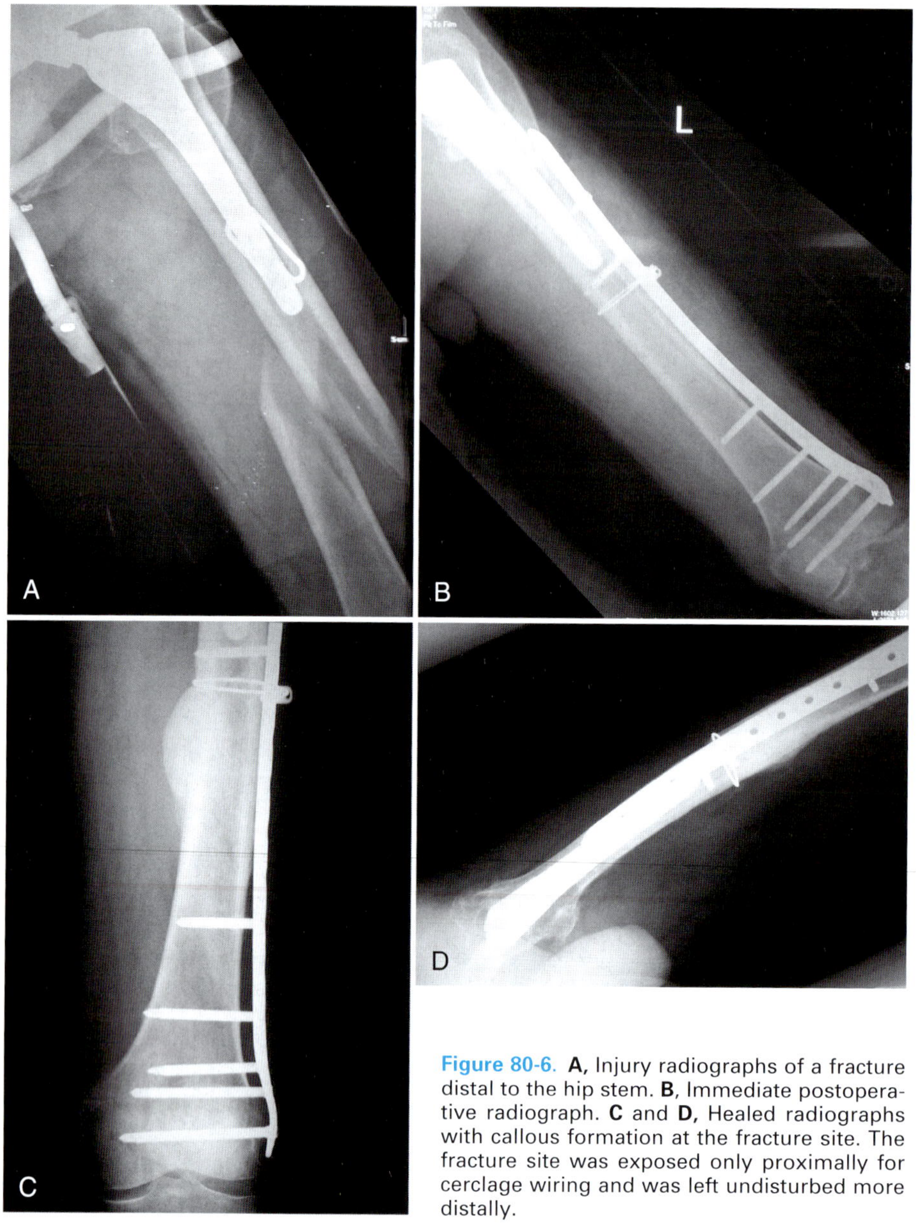

Figure 80-6. A, Injury radiographs of a fracture distal to the hip stem. **B,** Immediate postoperative radiograph. **C** and **D,** Healed radiographs with callous formation at the fracture site. The fracture site was exposed only proximally for cerclage wiring and was left undisturbed more distally.

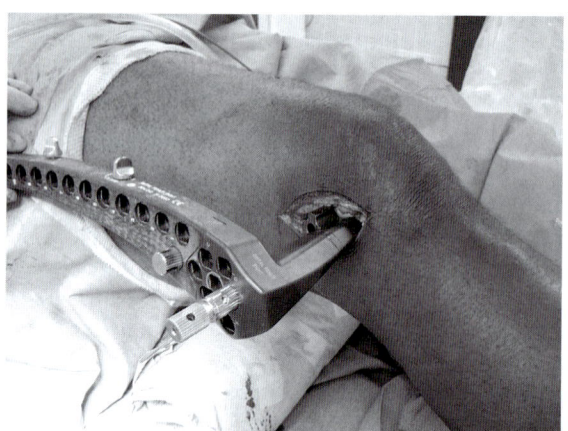

Figure 80-7. Photograph demonstrating percutaneous insertion of a locked plate on the distal end of the femur with a guide for insertion of screws. (Photograph courtesy L.I.S.S. Synthes, Paoli, Pa.)

COMPLICATIONS

Complications of nonoperative treatment include skin breakdown from casting, stiffness from prolonged immobilization, malunion, and nonunion. Skin breakdown often occurs in patients who are bedridden and may not be surgical candidates. Knee stiffness is seen more frequently in nonoperatively treated patients than in operatively stabilized patients because early motion will occur through the fracture site, and therefore lengthier immobilization is required. Malunion is also more common with closed treatment because achieving fracture stability is more difficult without internal fixation (Fig. 80-8A and B).[9] Although nonunion can also occur, some bedridden patients fare better with nonunion than with a postoperative infection or wound complication. Other complications with conservative care include deep vein thrombosis, respiratory infection, and pressure sores.[9]

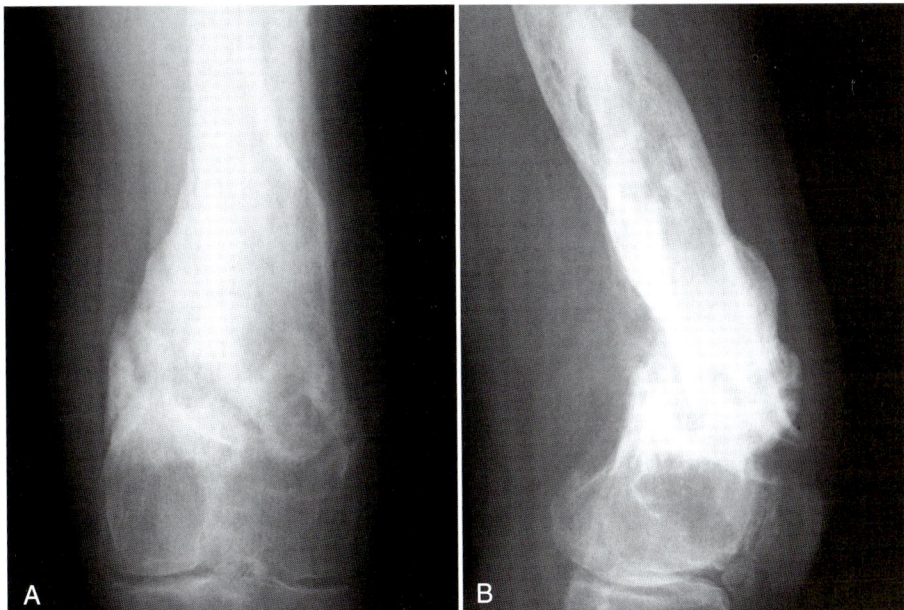

Figure 80-8. A and **B,** Radiographs showing malunion of a supracondylar femoral fracture treated 12 years earlier by skeletal traction.

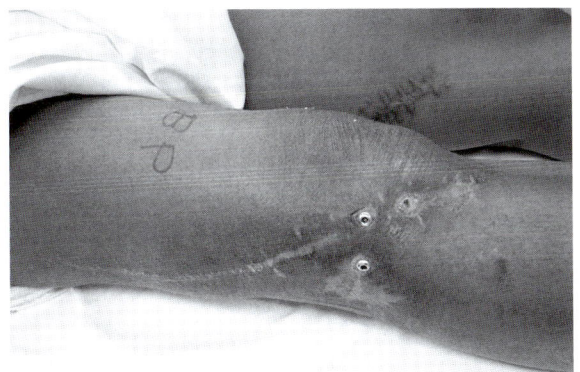

Figure 80-9. Clinical photograph revealing exposed hardware with active drainage from wounds.

Infection remains the most significant complication of operative treatment (Fig. 80-9). Although the infection rate was previously reported to be as high as 20%, advances in surgical technique, patient selection, and perioperative antibiotic therapy have continued to decrease infection rates to below 7%.* Factors that contribute to increased risk for infection include open fractures, high-energy trauma, lengthy and extensive surgical dissection, and inadequate surgical stabilization.[28]

Mast and associates pioneered the technique of indirect reduction and biologic, balanced, stable internal fixation.[48] Bolhofner and colleagues and Ostrum and Geel applied these concepts and reported much improved results when compared with older techniques described in the literature.[7,60] More recent techniques involving percutaneous locked plating have decreased infection rates to 0% to 3%.[43,83]

Open fracture management continues to improve. The tenets of open fracture care include immediate tetanus prophylaxis and appropriate antibiotic administration, followed by initial immediate surgical wound irrigation and débridement. Controversy continues regarding the number of débridement sessions required and the optimal timing of wound closure. These issues must be individualized by the surgeon and should take into account the mechanism of injury, the quality of local tissue at the time of initial surgery, and the presence or absence of any gross contamination. Once the tissues are judged to be healthy and clean, definitive wound closure should be performed. The sooner the traumatized region can resume its previous biologic environment, the sooner the healing process can occur. Ostermann and associates demonstrated decreased infection rates in open fractures when antibiotic polymethylmethacrylate beads were inserted into the fracture zone, but no prospective, randomized study has evaluated the routine use of beads in open distal femoral fractures.[59] The senior author uses beads routinely in high-energy open fractures with bone loss. These beads not only provide high local concentrations of antibiotic but also make subsequent bone grafting easier by "keeping the space open."

Nonunion, which is a possible complication of any fracture, initially occurred in 10% to 19% of patients in early reports of open reduction and internal fixation of supracondylar femoral fractures (Fig. 80-10A and B).[53,57,72,89] The current literature describes a significant improvement in the nonunion rate of operatively stabilized supracondylar femoral fractures, which is now reported to be between 0% and 5%.* Two recent studies have documented successful treatment of distal femoral nonunion with union rates of 95% to 100%.[25,82] Haidukewych and associates reported on distal femoral nonunion in 22 patients and achieved union in 21 with repeat open reduction and internal fixation and bone grafting.[25] Achieving stable fixation of the distal fragment was critical to successful union. Autogenous bone grafting was used in the vast majority of cases. Wang and Weng documented a 100%

*References 7, 11, 43, 57, 59, 60, 63, 72, and 83.

*References 23, 42, 43, 57, 68, 83, 84, and 89.

Stiffness, however, remains the most common complication following intraarticular distal femur fractures.[61] Patellofemoral arthrofibrosis and patella baja are especially problematic with open fractures.

SUMMARY AND FUTURE DIRECTIONS

Internal fixation techniques for distal femoral fractures continue to evolve. More biologically friendly plating techniques using locked screw technology for improved mechanical performance, percutaneous plate insertion, and screw targeting for preservation of fracture vascularity have improved union rates and essentially eliminated varus collapse and the need for bone grafting. Newer-generation locking plates offer polyaxial locking screws in conjunction with fixed locking screws. Such "hybrid plate" technology will offer even greater versatility in achieving maximal distal fragment fixation. The role of orthobiologic agents remains undefined.

KEY REFERENCES

Chiron HS, Casey P: Fractures of the distal third of the femur treated by internal fixation. Clin Orthop Relat Res 100:160, 1974.

Goesling T, Frenk A, Appenzeller A, et al: LISS plate: design, mechanical and biomechanical characteristics. Injury 34(Suppl 1):A11, 2003.

Healy WL, Brooker AF: Distal femoral fractures: comparison of open and closed methods of treatment. Clin Orthop Relat Res 174:166, 1983.

Henry S, Trager S, Green S, et al: Management of supracondylar fractures of the femur with the GSH supracondylar nail. Contemp Orthop 22:631, 1991.

Ito K, Grass R, Zwipp H: Internal fixation of supracondylar femur fractures: comparative biomechanical performance of the 95-degree angled blade and retrograde nails. J Orthop Trauma 12:259, 1998.

Müller ME, Allgower M, Schneider R, Willenegger H: Manual of internal fixation, ed 3, New York, 1991, Springer-Verlag.

Neer CS, Grantham SA, Shelton ML: Supracondylar fracture of the adult femur. J Bone Joint Surg Am 49:591, 1967.

Olerud S: Operative treatment of supracondylar fractures of the femur: technique and results in fifteen cases. J Bone Joint Surg Am 54:1015, 1972.

Sanders R, Regazzoni P, Reudi T: Treatment of supracondylar-intraarticular fractures of the femur using the dynamic condylar screw. J Orthop Trauma 3:214, 1989.

Schandelmaier P, Partenheimer A, Koenemann B, et al: Distal femoral fractures and LISS stabilization. Injury 32(Suppl 3):SC55, 2001.

Schatzker J: Fractures of the distal femur revisited. Clin Orthop Relat Res 347:43, 1998.

Schatzker J, Horne G, Waddell J: The Toronto experience with the supracondylar fracture of the femur, 1966-1972. Injury 6:113, 1975.

Schatzker J, Lambert DC: Supracondylar fractures of the distal femur. Clin Orthop Relat Res 138:77, 1979.

Schutz M, Muller M, Krettek C, et al: Minimally invasive fracture stabilization of distal femoral fractures with the LISS: a prospective multicenter study. Results of a clinical study with special emphasis on difficult cases. Injury 32(Suppl 3):SC48, 2001.

Shewring DJ, Meggitt BF: Fractures of the distal femur treated with the AO dynamic condylar screw. J Bone Joint Surg Am 74:122, 1992.

Siliski JM, Mahring M, Hofer HP: Supracondylar-intercondylar fractures of the femur: treatment by internal fixation. J Bone Joint Surg Am 71:95, 1989.

Slatis P, Ryoppy S, Huttinen V: AO osteosynthesis of fractures of the distal third of the femur. Acta Orthop Scand 42:162, 1971.

Stewart MJ, Sisk TD, Wallace SL: Fractures of the distal third of the femur: a comparison of methods of treatment. J Bone Joint Surg Am 48:784, 1966.

Wenzl H: [Results in 112 surgically treated distal femoral fractures.] Hefte Unfallheilkd 120:15, 1975.

Zickel RE, Fietti VG, Lawsing JF, et al: A new intramedullary fixation device for the distal third of the femur: Clin Orthop Relat Res 125:185, 1977.

Full references for this chapter can be found on www.expertconsult.com.

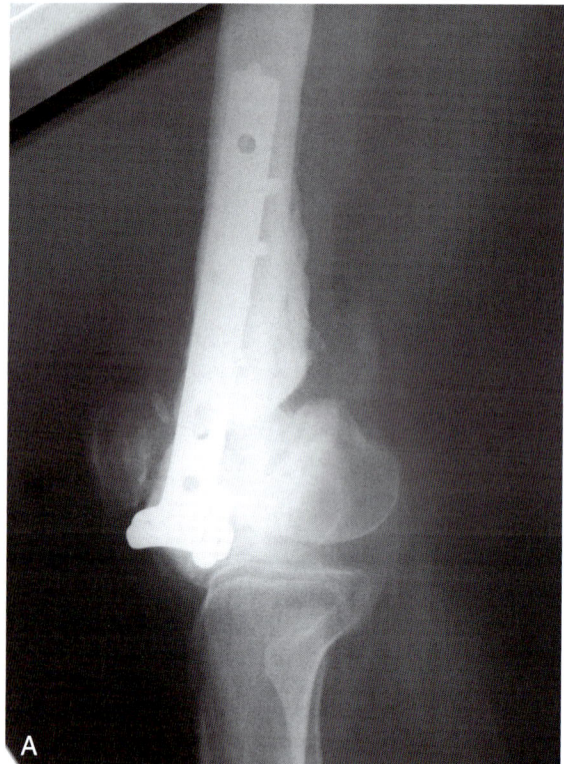

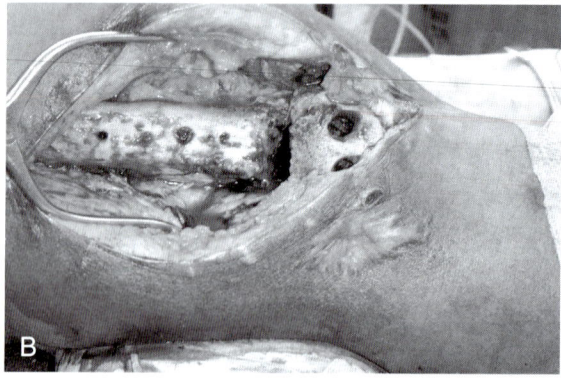

Figure 80-10. **A,** Radiograph of fracture nonunion and hardware migration. **B,** Intraoperative photograph demonstrating fracture nonunion and enlarged screw holes secondary to loosening and bone absorption.

union rate in 13 distal femoral nonunions treated with cortical strut allografting, autogenous bone grafting, and internal fixation with angled blade plates and intramedullary nails.[82]

Malunion, another complication, was initially seen most commonly in fractures with significant medial comminution treated with conventional nonlocking plates. Traditional plating techniques have been associated with malunion greater than 5 degrees in the frontal plane in as many as 26% of patients.[88] Newer plating techniques with anatomically designed locked plates also initially resulted in higher than expected rates of malunion greater than 5 degrees in the frontal plane, with rates reported to be as high as 20%.[69] Percutaneous techniques require vigilance to avoid plate malposition and fracture malalignment. As our experience with and understanding of the newer implants advances, percutaneous locked plating continues to improve and most recently has resulted in malunion rates as low as 4.5% to 6%.[42,83]

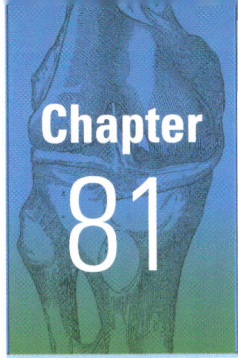

Chapter 81

Tibial Plateau Fractures

Joshua R. Langford, David J. Jacofsky, and George J. Haidukewych

Fractures of the tibial plateau represent only 1% to 2% of all fractures but account for approximately 8% of fractures occurring in older adults.[18] As our understanding of the importance of soft tissue injury has evolved concurrently with the evolution of internal fixation devices and techniques, management of these difficult injuries has slowly shifted from primarily a nonoperative course to one of restoration of the articular surface with internal or external fixation and early motion, when possible. Additionally, classification systems and clinical outcome data have dramatically improved our ability to understand and manage these fractures.

Articular fractures of the proximal end of the tibia not only involve the articular cartilage itself but can also involve the epiphysis, metaphysis and, in more severe injuries, the diaphysis. At times, associated injuries of the tibial spine, tibial tuberosity, menisci, and ligamentous structures can make management of these injuries all the more difficult. Furthermore, to the frustration of orthopedic traumatologists, even the anatomic reduction of high-energy injuries often results in the development of post-traumatic arthritis because of damage to the chondral surface.

RELEVANT ANATOMY

The proximal surface of the tibia contains the medial and lateral tibial plateaus, which are separated by the intercondylar tibial eminences. The articular cartilage on the lateral plateau is slightly thicker than that on the medial side. The lateral tibial plateau is convex in the sagittal plane and almost flat to slightly convex in the coronal plane. The medial tibial plateau is larger than the lateral plateau and is gently concave in both the sagittal and coronal planes. In the frontal plane, the tibial articular surface forms an angle of approximately 3 degrees of varus with the long axis of the tibia. This varus, as well as the slight difference in cartilaginous thickness between the medial and lateral plateaus, results in the lateral plateau being slightly higher than the medial plateau. This difference is further exacerbated by the convexity of the lateral side and the concavity of the medial side. Such knowledge is extremely important during placement of screws from the lateral to the medial side of the proximal end of the tibia because, if not cognizant of this anatomy, one can easily place a subchondral lateral screw through the articular cartilage of the lower medial side.

Between the plateaus lies a nonarticular area that contains the anterior and posterior tibial spines. The anterior spine is more medial and lies just posterior to the insertion of the anterior cruciate ligament (ACL). This area is often comminuted in high-energy injuries involving the tibial plateau and although nonarticular, it is important to restore the general width of the intercondylar eminence to restore the anatomic width of the proximal end of the tibia as a whole appropriately. In a normal knee, load is predominantly borne on the medial side. Consequently, the trabecular bone on the medial tibial condyle is stronger and more sclerotic than that on the lateral side, perhaps explaining why lateral-sided fractures are far more common, except in higher energy injuries.

The medial and lateral menisci are both semilunar, triangular-shaped fibrocartilage that rest between the femoral condyles and tibial plateaus. They serve an important function in load sharing by protecting the articular cartilage from up to 60% of the load encountered by the knee.[20] The lateral meniscus is larger than the medial meniscus and covers a larger percentage of the lateral plateau. The intermeniscal ligament anteriorly connects the anterior horns of the two menisci, and the menisci are attached peripherally by the coronary ligaments to the peripheral rim of their respective tibial plateaus. The anterior attachment of the lateral meniscus is slightly posterior to that of the medial meniscus. It is important to recognize the normal anatomy of these structures because they are often damaged and require repair in the management of tibial plateau fractures.

MECHANISM OF INJURY

The predominant pattern producing tibial plateau fractures is a varus or valgus stress, with concomitant axial loading. This combination may be seen with low-energy injuries, such as falls from a standing height, or with high-energy injuries, such as motor vehicle accidents. Isolated valgus or varus loading tends to cause an isolated lateral or medial injury, respectively. The more an axial load predominates, the more likely a patient is to sustain a bicondylar injury. The lateral plateau is involved in 55% to 70% of cases, with medial plateau or bicondylar involvement occurring in 10% to 30% of cases.[18] Simple central depression–type injuries are often the result of low-energy injuries in older patients with osteoporotic bone and, conversely, bicondylar fractures with axial loading and shearing injuries tend to be seen in high-energy injuries in younger patients.

CLASSIFICATION

Comprehensive anatomic classifications such as the AO (*Arbeitsgemeinschaft fur Osteosynthesefragen*) classification or the Orthopaedic Trauma Association classification may be useful for research purposes (Fig. 81-1). However, they are somewhat cumbersome and may be difficult for surgeons to use for clinical communication. The most commonly used classification system in clinical practice is the Schatzker classification system (Fig. 81-2).[19]

In the Schatzker classification system, a type I injury is a "pure" split fracture of the lateral tibial plateau. It is typically seen in young patients with strong cancellous bone and, by definition, there is no associated articular depression. With

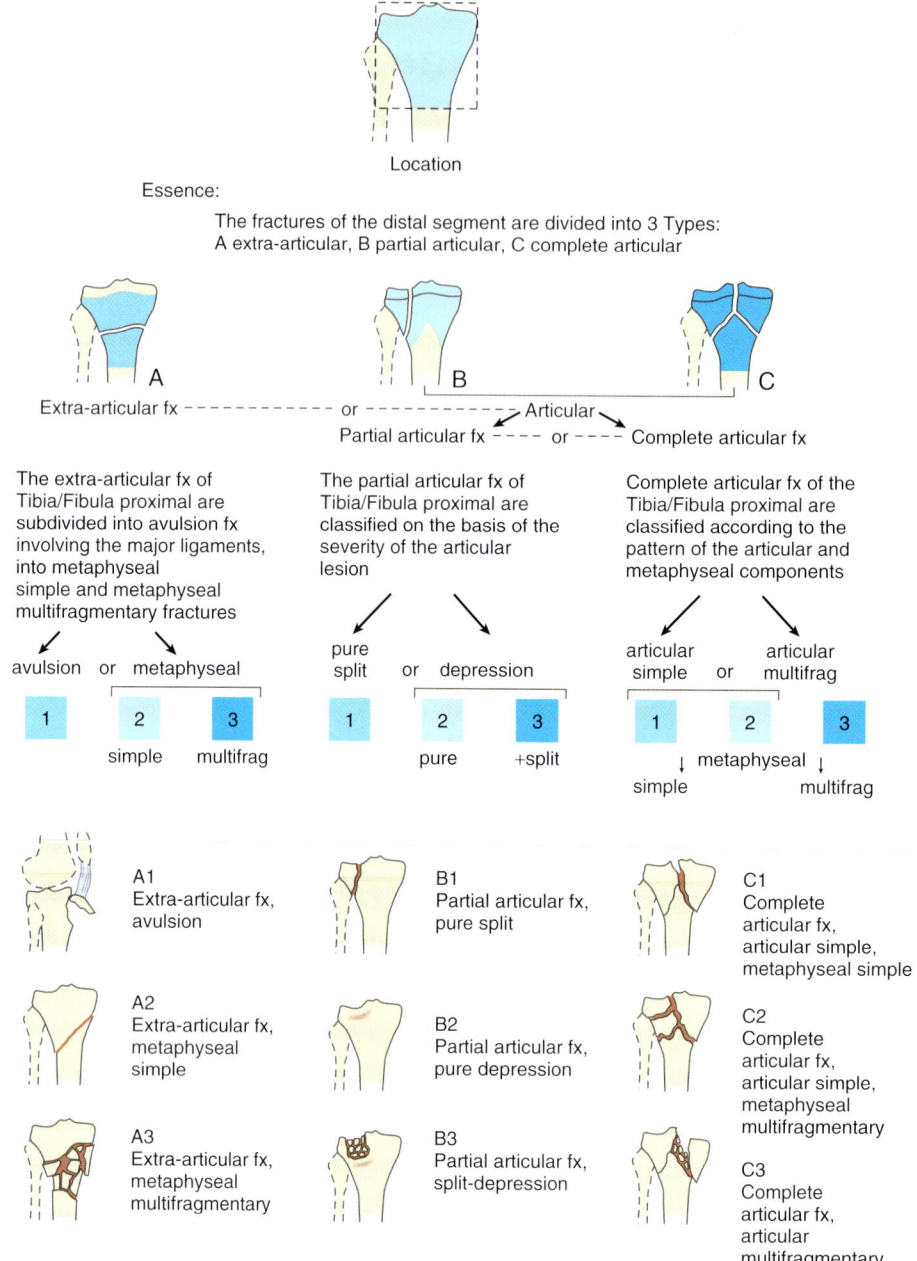

Figure 81-1. AO-ASIF classification of tibial plateau fractures. (From Müller ME, Nazarian S, Koch P, Schatzker J: The comprehensive classification of fractures of long bones, Bern, Switzerland, 1995, ME Müller Foundation.)

significant displacement, it is frequently associated with a peripheral tear of the lateral meniscus. Type II fractures are combined split depression fractures of the lateral tibial plateau. Similar to a type I injury, this injury is most commonly caused by a lateral bending force combined with axial loading. Type III fractures, the most common fracture pattern in Schatzker's series (accounting for 36% of injuries), are pure depression fractures of the lateral plateau and are primarily seen in older osteoporotic individuals sustaining lower energy injuries. The type IV fracture pattern is a fracture of the medial tibial plateau. Because the medial plateau is stronger than the lateral side, these fractures are typically secondary to higher energy injuries and, as such, have commonly associated ligamentous and soft tissue damage. Type V injuries are

bicondylar fractures involving both the medial and lateral plateaus and are often the result of a pure axial load applied while the knee is in full extension, such as may be seen in a driver pressing on the brake before impact during a motor vehicle accident. Type VI injuries are the highest energy injuries; they involve both the medial and lateral plateaus and are associated with metaphyseal-diaphyseal dissociation.

Experienced surgeons know that it is the status of the soft tissues and classification of the soft tissue envelope injury that are as important, if not more important, than the underlying osseous injury. The Tscherne classification of soft tissue damage in closed fractures is an excellent means whereby surgeons can evaluate associated soft tissue injuries.[16] A grade

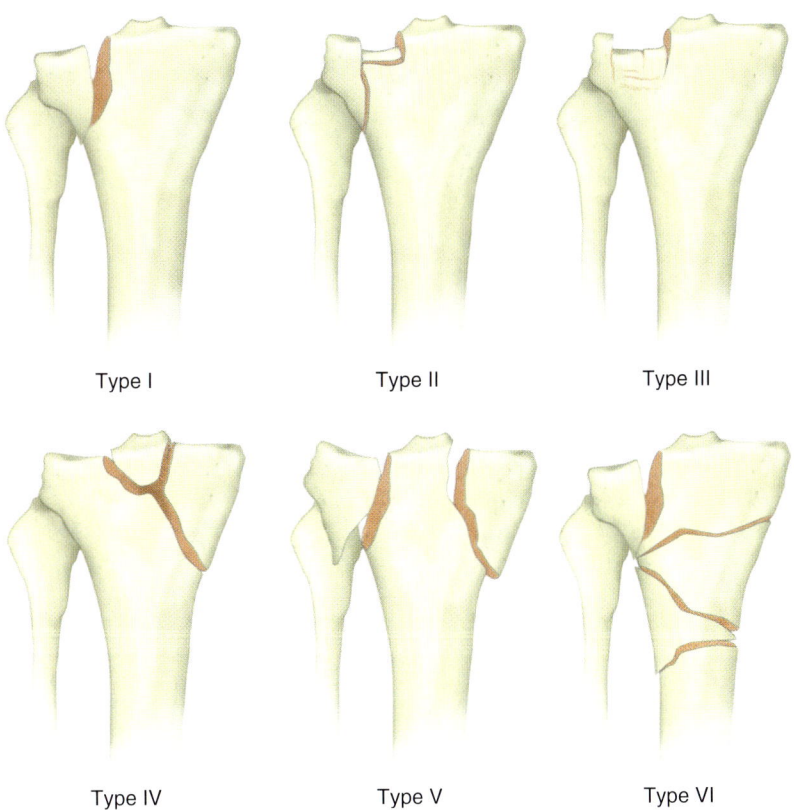

Type I   Type II   Type III

Type IV   Type V   Type VI

Figure 81-2. Schatzker classification tibial plateau fractures.

0 injury results from indirect trauma and is associated with negligible soft tissue damage. A grade I injury typically results from low or moderate energy and is identified by superficial abrasions or overlying contusions. In grade II injuries, significant muscle contusion and possible deep contaminated abrasions may be seen. Grade II injuries may be the result of a bumper strike and are often associated with marked fracture comminution. The highest grade in the classification system is grade III soft tissue injury, which is frequently associated with extensive crushing of soft tissues and subcutaneous degloving. There may be concomitant arterial injury. Patients with compartment syndrome automatically fall into the grade III category.

CLINICAL EVALUATION

History

The type of knee injury that has occurred can usually be inferred from a thorough patient history. Establishing the magnitude and direction of the force that was applied to the knee, when possible, is extremely helpful. The force from high-velocity motor vehicle accidents will certainly create a different and often more obvious injury pattern than the noncontact injuries that may occur with sudden stops or pivoting movements during sports. In polytraumatized patients, especially those with high-energy injuries to the lower extremities, the physician must expect and exclude knee injuries. Often, these polytraumatized patients are unable to give any history at all because they may have a closed head injury, be intubated, or suffer distracting injuries.

The time at which the injury occurred can be of paramount importance in the event of vascular injury or impending compartment syndrome.

Physical Examination

Clearly, in a polytraumatized patient, primary advanced trauma life support survey protocols and examination to stabilize the patient should be undertaken. During the secondary survey, the entire skeleton should be examined as indicated and, if a tibial plateau fracture is present, it is mandatory that the entire affected limb be examined fully.

Careful circumferential inspection to rule out open fractures is mandatory and visual inspection can reveal abrasions, contusions, or early fracture blisters that must be considered because they may markedly alter the recommended surgical management. Visual inspection may also reveal an effusion or hemarthrosis.

Although examination of the ligaments and menisci is of paramount importance, it is typically too painful for the patient in the acute setting and needs to be performed under anesthesia. Similarly, without the concomitant use of fluoroscopy, it is difficult to determine whether fracture or ligamentous insufficiency has led to perceived instability on physical examination.

One cannot overemphasize the importance of a complete neurologic and vascular examination. Knee dislocations leading to vascular or neurologic injury in association with tibial plateau fractures have been reported to reduce spontaneously and may be missed without careful examination. If pulses are not equal on palpation, arteriography may be performed.[15] Use of the ankle-brachial index (ABI) to compare blood pressure in the arm and ankle can help evaluate the vascular status of the limb further. Neurologic injury, most commonly in the form of peroneal nerve palsy, is not uncommon.[19] Careful motor and sensory evaluation of the lower part of the leg must be undertaken arduously.

Careful evaluation for compartment syndrome should be performed in all patients with tibial plateau fractures. The index of suspicion should be high for Schatzker types IV, V, and VI, but compartment syndrome can also occur in simple fracture patterns associated with high-energy injury. Patients who are at risk for compartment syndrome should be monitored carefully for at least the first 24 to 48 hours after injury and for a similar period after each closed reduction or surgical intervention. If any question about compartment syndrome exists as a result of clinical evaluation, compartment pressures should be measured and fasciotomies performed, as indicated.

Imaging Studies

Radiographs should be obtained after all acute knee injuries. The standard knee trauma series should include anteroposterior, lateral, and patellar tangential views. Oblique radiographs can be extremely helpful in diagnosing minimally displaced fractures of the proximal end of the tibia. Alignment, the presence of bony injury, and the details of the soft tissue should all be examined on radiographs. Stress radiographs may occasionally be helpful to define the severity and stability of tibial plateau fractures and associated collateral ligament injuries better. However, we rarely find them helpful. Moreover, stress radiographs have not been shown to increase diagnostic accuracy over examination under anesthesia and/or arthroscopy.

Computed tomography (CT) is perhaps the most valuable test because it helps rule out the possibility of occult plateau fractures that are missed on plain radiographs and helps define the nature of these complex intra-articular fractures. Surgical planning of tibial plateau fractures is largely aided by two-dimensional and, occasionally, three-dimensional reconstructions from CT scans. CT, however, is an adjuvant test that should be performed with, and not in place of, plain radiography. Soft tissue structures such as the menisci and collateral ligaments are poorly visualized on a CT scan. Magnetic resonance imaging (MRI) is superior for determining the status of such structures.

The use of MRI for the evaluation of acute knee injuries continues to improve and evolve. The sensitivity and specificity of MRI for meniscal and cruciate ligament injury are greater than 90% when correlated with arthroscopic or intraoperative findings.[5] MRI should not be used indiscriminately in place of a careful clinical evaluation, routine plain films, and CT scanning. Its benefit in tibial plateau fractures lies largely in the exclusion of significant meniscal tears or ligamentous injuries in patients who would otherwise be treated nonoperatively or in a percutaneous fashion such that these injuries would then perhaps be missed. Studies in which MRI was performed on tibial plateau fractures have shown associated soft tissue injuries in greater than 45% of patients.[11] The role of MRI in the preoperative evaluation of these injuries remains undefined.

Angiography

Angiography is indicated when the vascularity of the lower part of the leg is in question. Asymmetrical distal pulses or an ABI below 0.9 should prompt angiographic examination.[15] It is important to recognize that if a leg is obviously ischemic, angiography may be helpful in localizing the injured area but it must not delay vascular exploration and subsequent revascularization to the point that viability of the limb will potentially be compromised. "On the table" angiography by the vascular team in the operating room while spanning external fixation is being performed may help expedite the overall care of the patient in such circumstances. Prolonged ischemia may cause a reperfusion compartment syndrome after perfusion is restored. Therefore, prophylactic fasciotomies may be indicated.

TREATMENT

Initial Management

In all tibial plateau fractures, the status of the soft tissues is of paramount importance in determining the timing of internal fixation. Patients with higher energy injuries and significant soft tissue damage should typically undergo temporizing knee-spanning external fixation until the soft tissues have recovered to a state in which a surgical incision can safely be made. Surgical incisions made through acutely traumatized tissue portend a high rate of wound dehiscence, wound infection, and subsequent soft tissue complications. It is not uncommon in higher energy injuries for it to take several weeks for the soft tissue envelope to become amenable to surgical intervention. At times, it may be estimated by an experienced physician that the soft tissue envelope will not become amenable to surgical incision for more than 3 to 4 weeks. In such situations, methods other than formal internal fixation will probably need to be used. Delayed definitive internal fixation with the use of temporizing spanning external fixation (Fig. 81-3) has markedly decreased the rate of complications in this difficult patient population. Lower energy injuries, such as those seen after a simple fall that

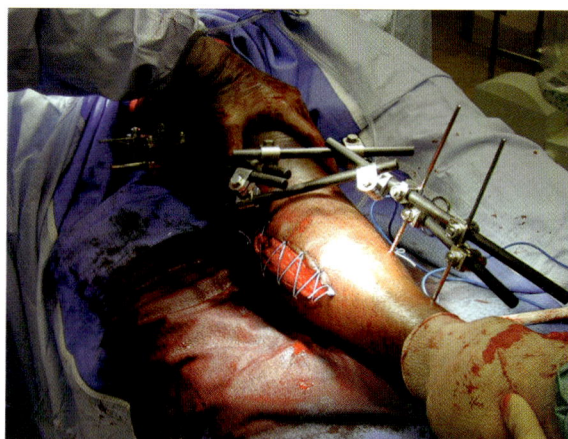

Figure 81-3. Clinical postoperative photograph taken in the operating room after a patient with a tibial plateau fracture and compartment syndrome underwent fasciotomies and spanning external fixation.

results in a depression fracture in an osteoporotic patient, may often be fixed relatively acutely because the associated soft tissue injury is minor. Obviously, the surgeon's judgment is paramount when evaluating the character of the osseous and soft tissue injuries.

Nonoperative Management

Although no clear-cut guidelines have been established across all patient ages and activity levels regarding what is acceptable to treat nonoperatively, some general rules can be applied. An articular step-off of less than 3 mm or condylar widening of less than 5 mm tends to have an acceptably low rate of adverse long-term effects if treated nonoperatively. Function deteriorates, however, with varus tilt, whereas mild valgus tilt up to 5 degrees is generally well tolerated.[8] Nonoperative management would be poorly advised if a tibial plateau fracture were associated with varus or valgus instability in a fully extended knee joint. Age alone is not an absolute contraindication to surgical management because older patients do well functionally with proper treatment.[10] However, surgeons must clearly use their judgment about the expectations, functional demands, medical comorbid conditions, and surgical risks of the specific patient being treated when making a decision regarding the most appropriate intervention. The goal of nonoperative treatment is still to allow early range of motion to include full extension and 120 degrees of flexion. It is known that permanent knee stiffness will probably develop if fractures treated nonoperatively are immobilized for longer than 6 weeks.[6]

Nonoperative management can include a period of traction and/or casting, followed by early range of motion in a cast brace or functional brace. Cast brace treatment of minimally displaced unicondylar fractures tends to yield good results, but outcomes are far less predictable with bicondylar fractures.[2] In general, nonoperative treatment is typically reserved for stable, well-aligned, minimally displaced fractures or fractures in patients with prohibitive medical comorbidity.

Operative Management

Schatzker Injuries

Type I

A displaced wedge or split fracture of the lateral plateau will be unstable and, in most cases, is an absolute indication for open reduction and internal fixation. In general, reduction may be achieved by applying a varus force manually or by using a laterally based femoral distractor, or reduction may be performed with the use of a large "King-Tong" or pelvic-type reduction forceps placed percutaneously through small stab incisions (Fig. 81-4). Clamps that are curved may be beneficial in protecting the soft tissues around the anterior face of the tibia from becoming crushed during compression of the fracture. It is important to note that if compression of the fracture site appears to be difficult in that the fracture seems to require significant force to close down completely, the lateral meniscus may be incarcerated in this fracture fragment and arthroscopic or open removal of the meniscus from the fracture site must be undertaken. It is possible to place so much force on the reduction forceps that the meniscus will simply be crushed within the trabecular bone and the fracture will appear reduced under fluoroscopy. If the split does not close down easily, a miniopen, arthroscopic, or formal open reduction is indicated.

Fixation is typically accomplished with two or three large cannulated screws inserted percutaneously. As with all

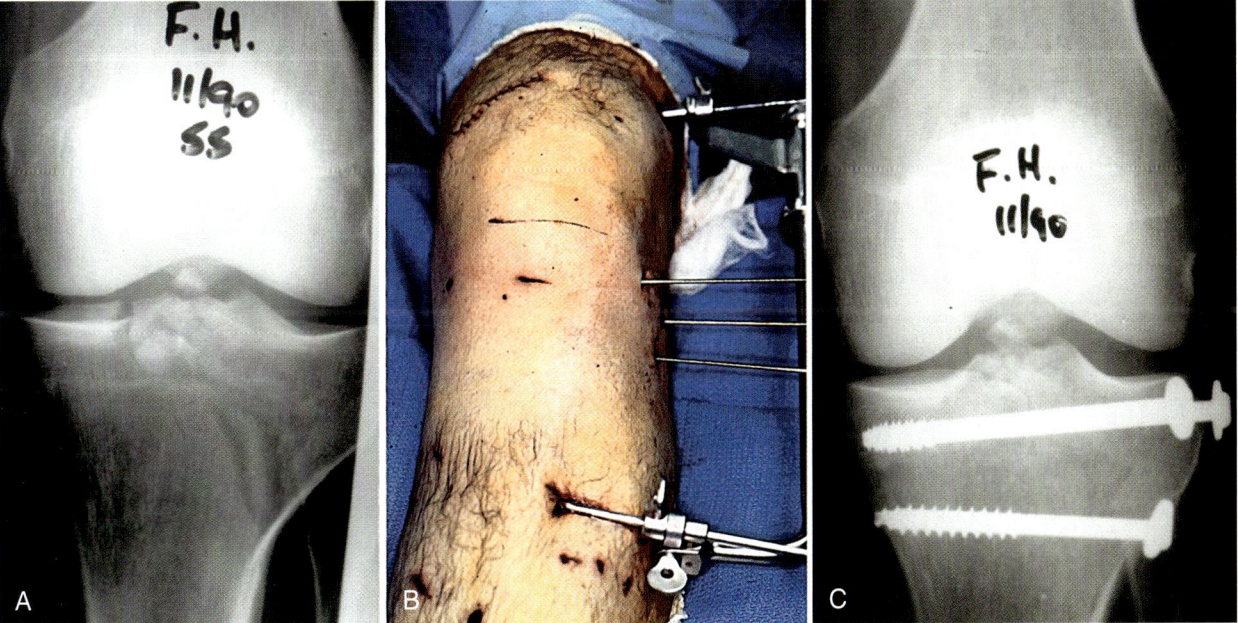

Figure 81-4. Schatzker type I tibial plateau fracture in a 30-year-old man who fell from a ladder. **A,** Preoperative anteroposterior radiograph. **B,** Intraoperative photograph showing a femoral distractor being used to obtain indirect reduction, with guide wires for the cannulated screws in place. **C,** Postoperative anteroposterior radiograph showing anatomic reduction of the tibial plateau.

fractures, the screws should be placed perpendicular to the major fracture lines to achieve compression of the fracture without displacing it when the screws are tightened.[12,14]

In general, two to three solitary lag screws are adequate for fixation,[13] although an antiglide plate or a buttress plate may be necessary in patients with poor bone quality, especially in the face of a vertically orientated condylar fracture. A gentle varus-valgus stress under real-time fluoroscopy can help determine whether screw fixation alone is adequate. If instability is noted and the screws toggle, buttress plate fixation is indicated. In general, we would use a lag screw–only approach in younger patients with excellent bone quality and routinely add a buttress plate in patients with poor bone quality.

Type II

Schatzker type II injuries are more difficult to treat than type I injuries because of the associated joint depression and, at times, more severe instability than seen with a simple split fracture of the lateral condyle (Fig. 81-5). Minimally invasive techniques such as arthroscopically assisted fixation are rarely indicated but, at times, may be feasible when the lateral cortical disruption is nondisplaced or minimally displaced and the peripheral rim of cortical bone laterally is functionally competent. In this situation, arthroscopically assisted reduction of the joint surface can be performed. The arthroscope is placed in the joint and a hole is drilled in the medial face of the tibia through a stab incision in a location that will allow curved or straight bone tamps to reach the area of the depressed lateral plateau. An ACL drill guide may be helpful to position the drill precisely. Bone graft or a bone graft substitute can then be impacted or injected through the tunnel from the medial aspect of the tibia to beneath the area of

reduced subchondral bone. The arthroscope can assist in determining when appropriate reduction has been achieved. Overreduction by 0.5 to 1 mm may be beneficial because subsidence occurs in most cases, despite the best efforts of the surgeon. Injectable bioresorbable cement may help alleviate this problem, but long-term data are not yet available. After articular reduction has been achieved, multiple 3.5-mm screws may be placed just under the subchondral bone to help prevent settling and fracture of the lateral condyle. Smaller diameter screws can be placed in close proximity to subchondral bone in a so-called raft fashion.

More commonly, however, open reduction with internal fixation is required for most type II injuries. In this situation, we prefer a straight, lateral, parapatellar arthrotomy to allow improved visualization of the joint line. The lateral aspect of the joint may be visualized through a submeniscal approach or by splitting the intermeniscal and anterior coronary ligaments of the lateral meniscus and reflecting the lateral meniscus posteriorly to expose the lateral side of the joint. In almost all cases, a plate is required and, as such, the distal aspect of the lateral parapatellar arthrotomy at the lateral aspect of the tibial tubercle can typically be extended laterally and inferiorly to dissect the anterior compartment muscles extraperiosteally from the proximal end of the tibia and allow placement of a traditional or percutaneous plate. For simpler fracture patterns requiring a plate, a laterally based submeniscal approach may be adequate (Fig. 81-6). It is important to not strip all the musculature from the lateral condylar fragment, but rather strip only what is required to allow placement of the plate. The fracture itself will actually act as access to the subchondral and posterior regions of the lateral plateau in that reduction and grafting can be performed through a fracture line that has been booked open. A femoral distractor and lamina spreader are often helpful for visualizing the joint space and allowing enough space to be created so that the depressed joint line can be elevated without competing with the lateral femoral condyle. Flexion of the knee to force femoral rollback posteriorly also assists with reduction of the joint, especially anteriorly and centrally.

After the fracture has been booked open, the joint line is reduced with an impactor. The impactor is used to scrape metaphyseal cancellous bone from beneath the

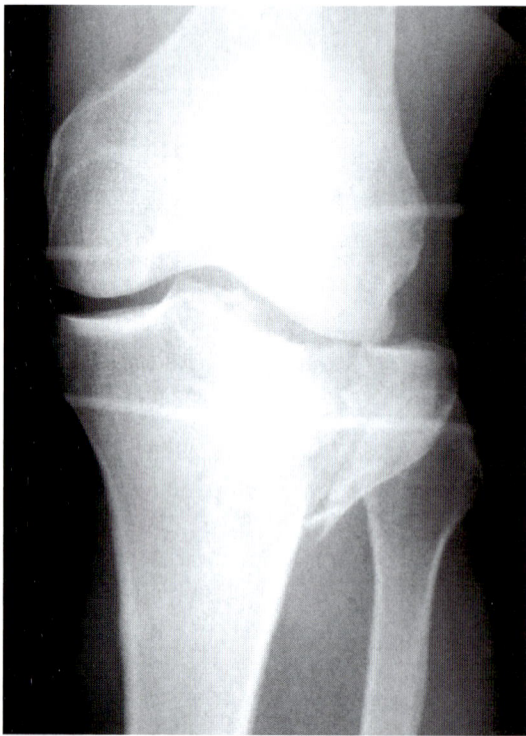

Figure 81-5. Anteroposterior radiograph of a patient with a Schatzker type II tibial plateau fracture.

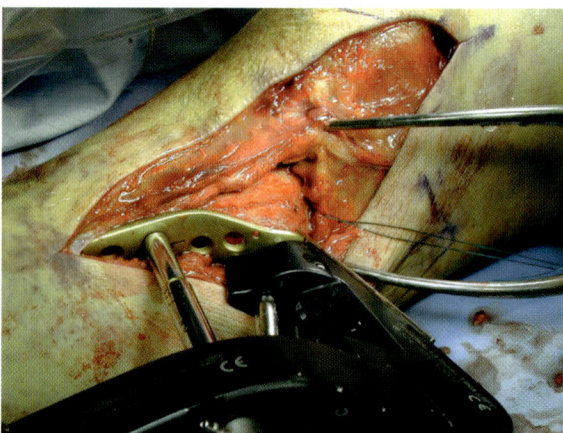

Figure 81-6. Intraoperative clinical photograph of a lateral submeniscal exposure with placement of a lateral submuscular plate.

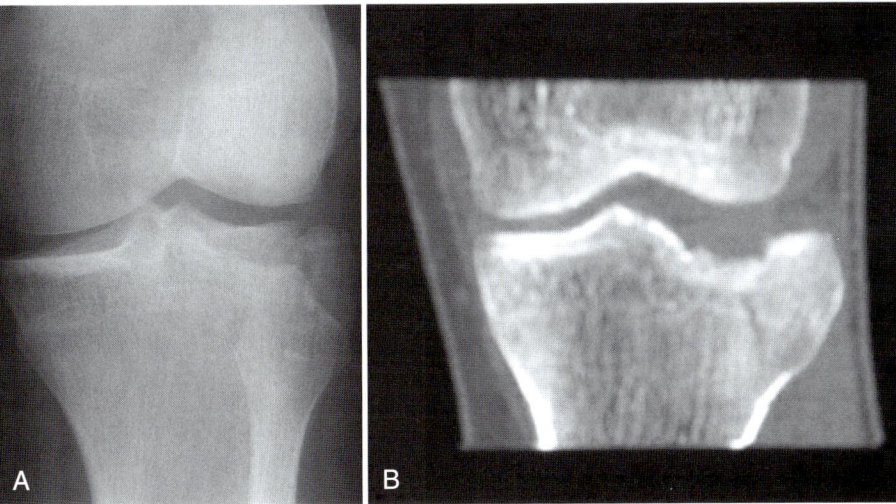

Figure 81-7. A and **B,** Preoperative two-dimensional coronal reconstruction of a Schatzker type III tibial plateau fracture amenable to percutaneous treatment.

articular fragments so that the articular fragments are reduced indirectly with this metaphyseal cancellous bone. Placing the impactor directly on subchondral bone, although tempting, can often lead to complete cracking of incompletely cracked articular cartilage as a result of overzealous force. Additionally, this metaphyseal cancellous bone makes excellent autograft for the subchondral grafting portion of the procedure. Once the depressed articular surface has been anatomically elevated under direct vision, additional graft material can be placed in the defect, which typically remains inferior to the area that has been reduced. Grafting can be performed with autograft but is commonly performed with allograft or a bone graft substitute (see later). The split condyle is then reduced and held with a large reduction clamp. Fixation of the condyles should be achieved with a periarticular buttress plate. More recently developed locked plates may have advantages in osteoporotic bone, but in general are reserved for more unstable bicondylar injuries that require more coronal plane stability.

Type III

Type III fractures of the lateral plateau are pure depression fractures usually found in osteoporotic patients after sustaining a valgus stress; however, they can occur as a result of athletic trauma in younger individuals. Valgus instability of more than 5 to 8 degrees in a patient without significant preexisting arthritis is typically an indication for surgical intervention.

Treatment of this injury in general is performed with arthroscopic or fluoroscopic assistance in a percutaneous fashion (Figs. 81-7 to 81-11). The arthroscope is placed in the joint, as previously described for type II injuries. A cortical window is made distally on the medial or lateral face of the metadiaphysis to allow percutaneous bone tamps to be placed through a tunnel to reduce the depressed fracture fragments under arthroscopic visualization. The location of this window can best be determined by the location of the depression needing to be accessed, which is best determined with a CT scan. Very anterior depressions are usually best managed through a medial corticotomy, whereas posterolateral depressions are often best managed from the distal aspect of the

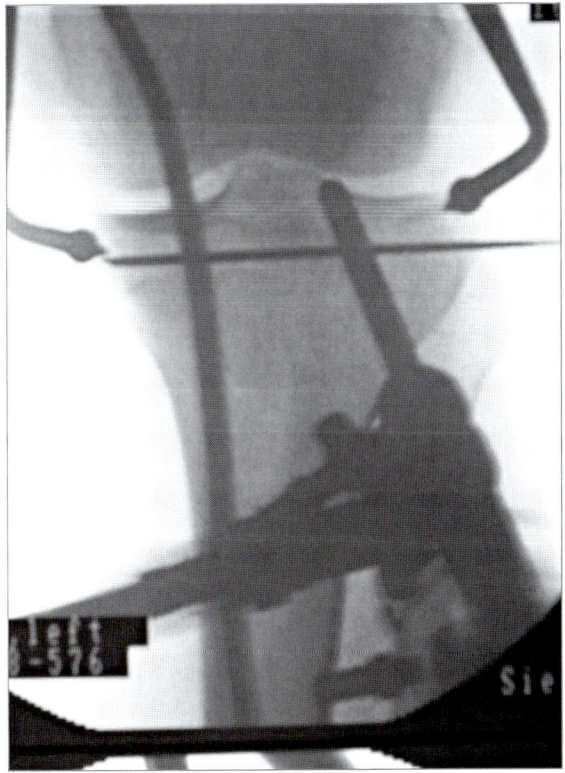

Figure 81-8. Intraoperative fluoroscopic image of reduction of the cortical rim and placement of the arthroscope.

lateral tibial metaphysis. An ACL drill guide can be used to place the tunnel more accurately. After the tunnel is then completely packed with graft, screws are placed across the joint just under subchondral bone to prevent collapse of the elevated joint surface.

Type IV

Nonoperative management of type IV injuries has been associated with a high incidence of varus malunion and is indicated only for nondisplaced stable injuries.[3,4] In general,

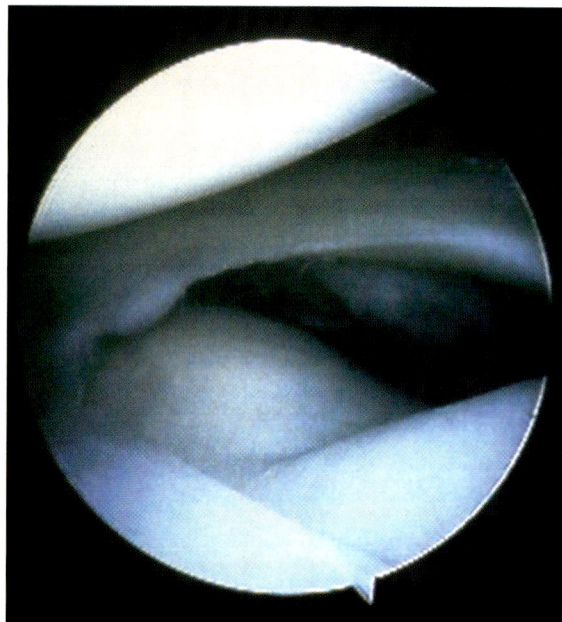

Figure 81-9. Intra-articular view through the arthroscope of the articular depression present before reduction of the articular surface.

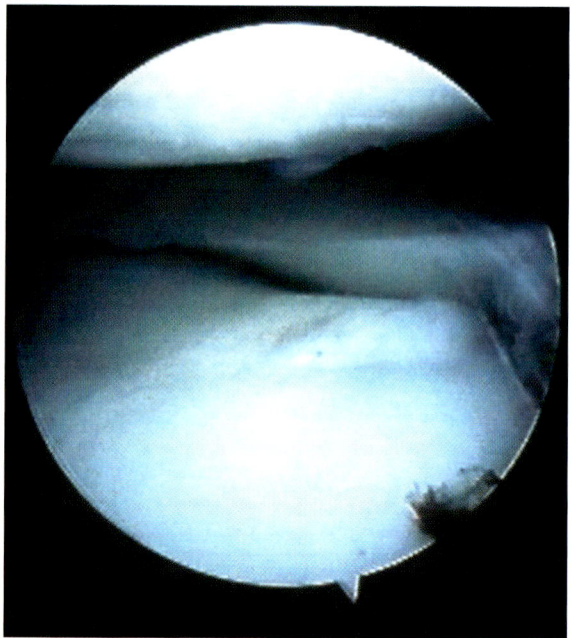

Figure 81-10. Intra-articular view through the arthroscope of the articular surface after reduction.

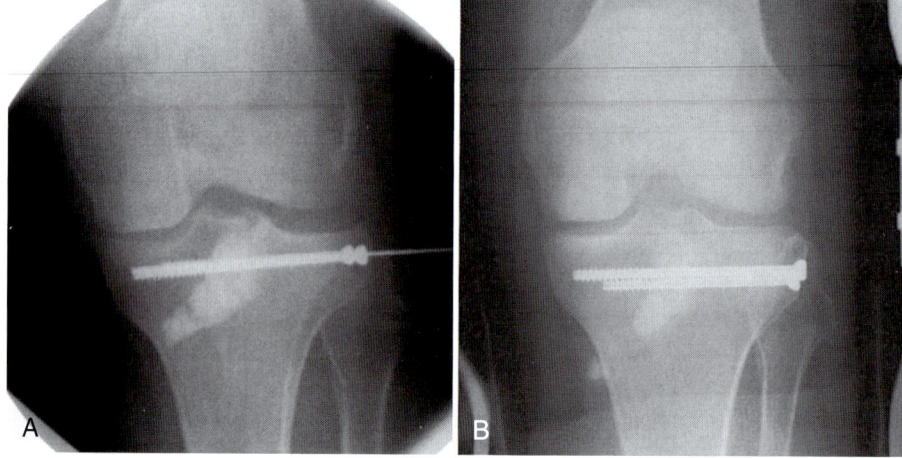

Figure 81-11. A, Intraoperative anteroposterior radiograph of a reduction achieved through a metaphyseal tunnel that was back-filled with calcium sulfate cement. **B,** Anteroposterior radiograph of the same patient 6 weeks after surgery showing resorption of the calcium sulfate cement.

however, because that these injuries are typically caused by very high energy, nondisplaced fractures of the medial plateau are exceedingly rare. It is extremely important to remember that these fractures are often associated with disruption of the lateral collateral ligament complex and, as such, should often be thought of as fracture-dislocation variants of knee dislocations. Therefore, neurovascular examination is of the utmost importance (see earlier). It is the magnitude of the soft tissue injuries associated with medial plateau fractures that portend the higher complication rates and the poorer prognosis, more so than the osseous injury itself.

Because these fractures are typically displaced and comminuted to some degree, open reduction plus internal fixation is generally the preferred method of treatment. One cannot, however, overemphasize the importance of delaying definitive open reduction and internal fixation in the face of a

high-energy fracture. Temporizing spanning external fixation until the soft tissue envelope has recovered adequately is recommended to minimize complications. In general, definitive surgery is carried out through a medial parapatellar arthrotomy and, after adequate reduction, fixation is achieved with a plate and screws. The plate is typically placed medially, and exposure of an isolated medial condylar fracture requires elevation of the pes anserinus and the superficial medial collateral ligament in an extraperiosteal fashion. Some authors have advocated placing the plate superficial to this complex; fixation can occasionally be performed in such a manner if the condylar split is near the location of the incision and the entire exposure can be accomplished by booking open the fracture. Placing the plate outside the superficial medial collateral ligament complex helps preserve the vascularity to the area of the fracture but also, in theory, may lead to increased wound healing complications because the flap that is created will be subcutaneous in nature (Figs. 81-12 and 81-13).

In the rare situation of an isolated posteromedial fracture fragment, a posteromedial incision may be adequate for reduction and fixation. The complexity of the posteromedial fragment as determined by CT scan will best establish whether a single medially based plate will be adequate. A significant posteromedial fragment that is separate and displaced from the medial condyle proper may require a second posteromedial incision and placement of a posteromedial buttress plate to prevent displacement and subsidence of the posteromedial fragment, which can lead to posterior subluxation of the medial femoral condyle, subsequent instability, and poor results.[7]

Types V and VI

All types V and VI injuries are high-energy injuries. Both are bicondylar tibial plateau fractures, with type VI injury being complicated by metadiaphyseal dissociation and, often, shaft extension (Figs. 81-14 and 81-15).

These injuries should always be considered high-energy injuries and, as such, immediate definitive incision and

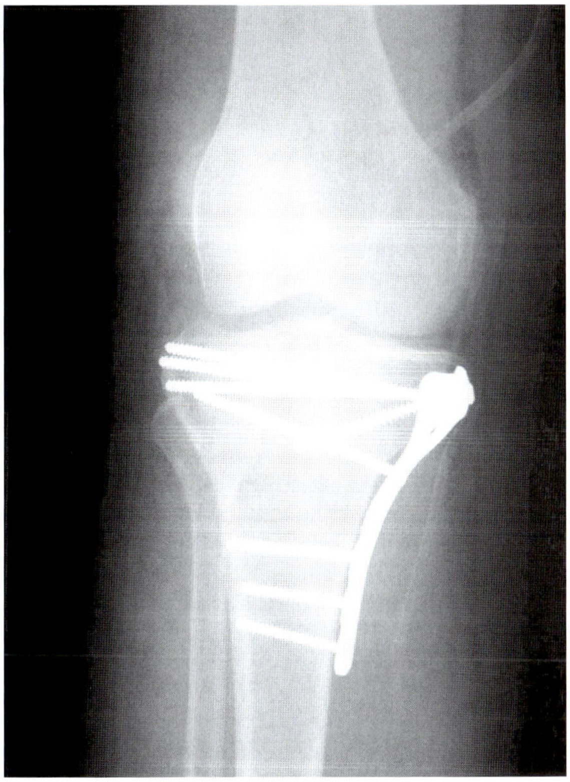

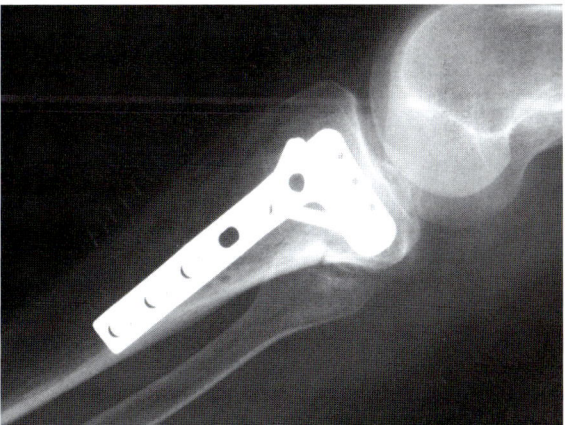

Figure 81-12. Anteroposterior radiograph after open reduction and internal fixation of a Schatzker type IV tibial plateau fracture with a medial buttress plate.

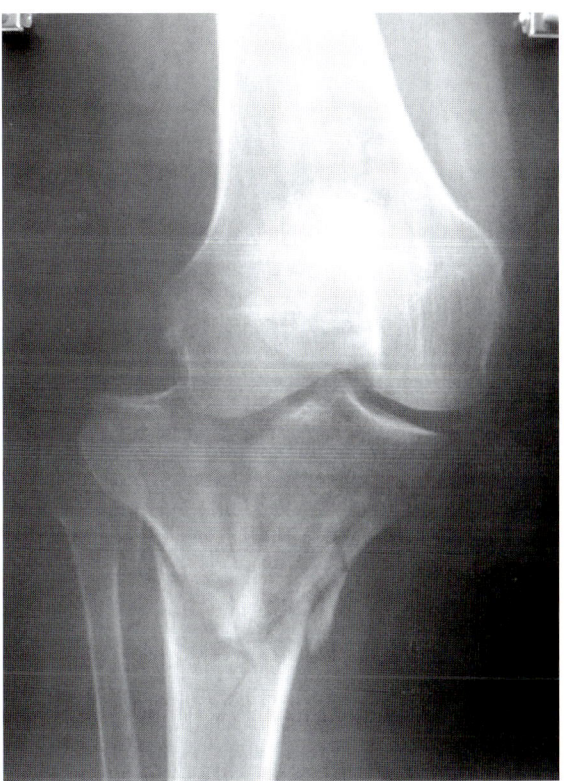

Figure 81-14. Anteroposterior radiograph of a Schatzker type VI tibial plateau fracture.

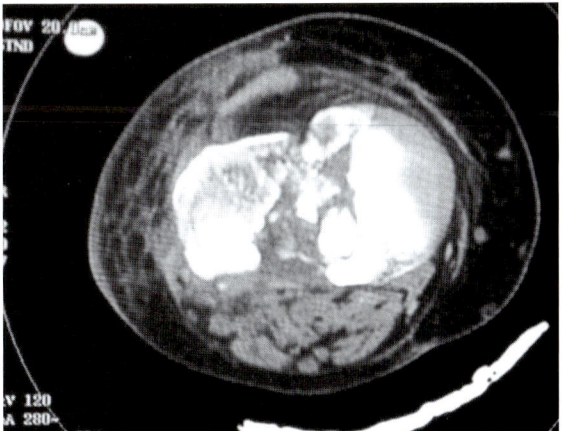

Figure 81-13. Lateral radiograph after open reduction and internal fixation of a Schatzker type IV tibial plateau fracture with a medial buttress plate.

Figure 81-15. Axial CT scan of a Schatzker type VI tibial plateau fracture showing a split of the condyles and comminution in the region of the tibial spines.

internal fixation are generally contraindicated. Temporizing spanning external fixation, as well as fasciotomies when indicated for compartment syndrome, is typically the mainstay of initial treatment (Fig. 81-16). As noted, definitive internal fixation should be carried out only when the soft tissue envelope has recovered to the point at which such fixation is safe and reasonable, typically 7 to 10 days after injury but, in more severe injuries, weeks later. We prefer to wait until skin wrinkles return and all blister area have been epithelialized.

Open reduction plus internal fixation of these injuries generally requires a standard parapatellar arthrotomy. One can split the intermeniscal ligament centrally and then the coronary ligaments peripherally so that the menisci can be tagged and lifted to expose and visualize both condylar surfaces. Traditionally, plating both condyles had been required for most of these bicondylar injuries. However, if the medial condylar component is large and relatively simple, a laterally based locked plate may be adequate for maintenance of medial reduction (Fig. 81-17). Early data have been encouraging; however, long-term data on the ability of laterally based locked plates to maintain reduction of the medial side

are still unavailable.[11] Locked screws in a plate prevent screw toggle and can therefore prevent varus collapse of coronally unstable fractures without the need for adjuvant medial plating. This concept, of course, depends on a medial condylar fragment of sufficient size to be able to be controlled with laterally inserted screws. The biologic advantage of avoiding double plating and the inevitable soft tissue dissection necessary for double plating is intuitive. Gentle varus-valgus stress testing under real-time fluoroscopy can assist the surgeon in deciding whether a lateral locking plate is sufficient fixation. If double plating is to be performed, it is recommended that the medial plate be placed superficial to the superficial medial collateral ligament and pes anserinus to prevent what has become to be known as the "dead bone sandwich," which results from stripping of both the lateral and medial aspects of the tibial metaphysis (Figs. 81-18 and 81-19).

In general, CT scans to evaluate the complexity of the medial condylar component can help determine whether a lateral locked plate will suffice or whether a medial plate will be necessary. Typically, the more complex the medial fracture, the more likely that a medial plate will be needed. For the posteromedial fragment, a posteromedial approach and plating are necessary for adequate stability. In general, if the medial split is sagittal and the fragment is large, a lateral locked plate will suffice. If the split medially is coronal or the fragment is complex, a two-incision, two-plate strategy is preferred.

In patients whose soft tissue envelope the surgeon deems will not be amenable to formal open reduction and internal fixation within 14 to 21 days, or in those with a markedly comminuted metaphysis and minimal involvement of the articular surfaces, hybrid or fine wire external fixation may be the best option (Fig. 81-20). Multiple percutaneous screws can be placed to lag large fragments at the joint and fine wires and/or half-pins can be placed proximally to achieve adequate proximal fixation. It is important to remember that wires and half-pins should be placed at least 15 mm distal to the joint line to prevent penetration of the synovial capsular reflections and thereby lead to intra-articular hardware and possible septic arthritis.[1] Olive wires can be helpful for achieving and maintaining reduction. Additionally, external

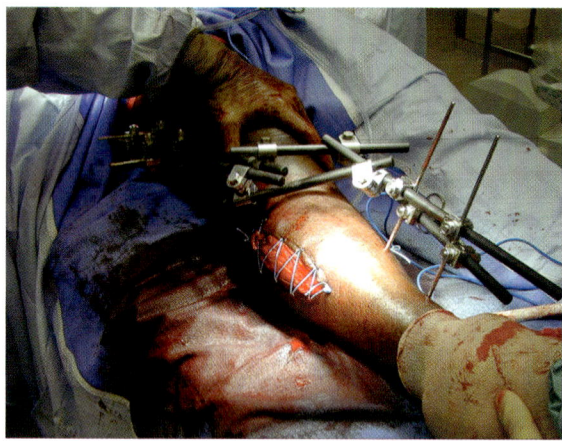

Figure 81-16. Clinical postoperative photograph taken in the operating room after a patient with a tibial plateau fracture and compartment syndrome underwent fasciotomies and spanning external fixation.

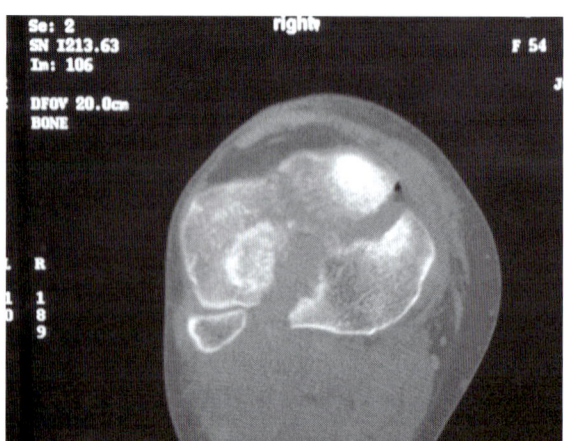

Figure 81-17. Axial CT scan showing a large posteromedial fracture fragment in a Schatzker type VI tibial plateau fracture.

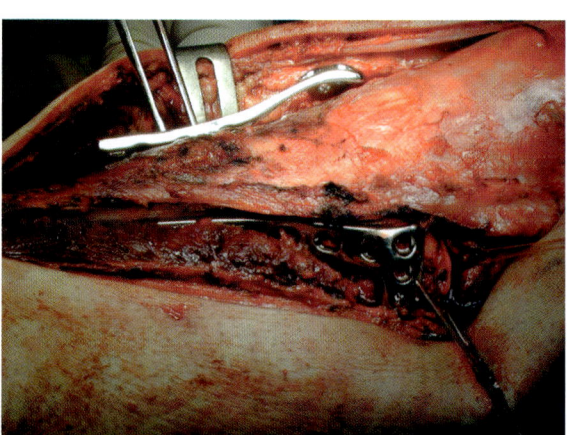

Figure 81-18. Intraoperative photograph showing the exposure for double plating through a midline incision. Note that the medial plate should be placed superficial to the superficial medial collateral ligament.

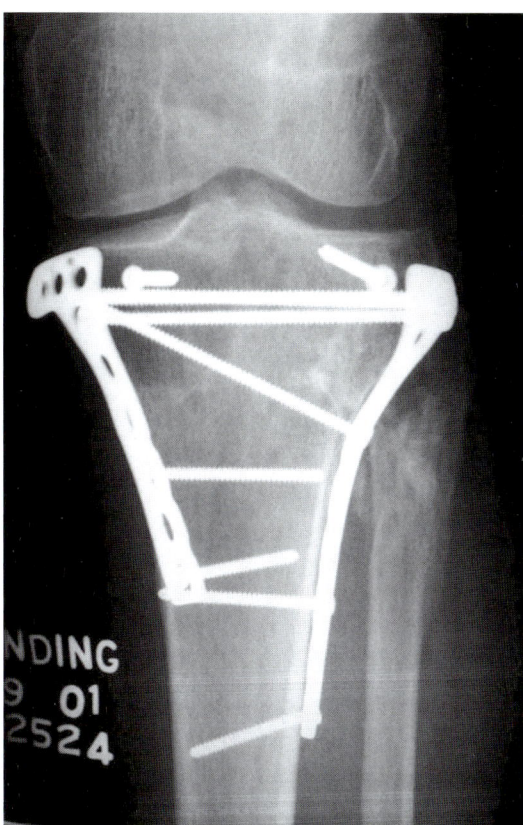

Figure 81-19. Anteroposterior radiograph showing double plating in the same patient seen in Figure 81-18.

fixation can be used definitively for patients with extensive metadiaphyseal comminution, especially those with associated significant soft tissue injury (Fig. 81-21).

Open Fractures

Open fractures of the tibial plateau require emergency irrigation and débridement. Spanning external fixation is very useful in this setting. Extensions of incisions to expose and débride the fracture and/or fasciotomy incisions should be undertaken with consideration for the location of future incisions that will probably be needed for the reconstruction. General principles of open fracture management apply and definitive internal fixation, when indicated, should commence only after the soft tissue envelope permits and the wounds are deemed to be clean. Grossly contaminated wounds may require multiple débridement to achieve this end. When using temporizing external fixators, pins should be placed well away from the area of planned future incisions to avoid potential bacterial contamination and infection. We typically will not perform the definitive fixation until the soft tissues have recovered.

Orthobiologic Agents

Injectable resorbable cement has now become popular, especially for the percutaneous injection of contained defects in periarticular areas. In 2004, Watson reported a series of eight comminuted tibial plateau or tibial pilon fractures treated with calcium sulfate injectable cement. Although one with a large defect required additional grafting, the other seven

healed. At 3 months, over 90% of the graft was resorbed radiographically. The same technique has been used for distal radius fractures in an effort to assist with stability by percutaneous grafting after closed reduction or external fixation. Russell and colleagues and others have reported similar findings in prospective randomized trials, even showing calcium phosphate cement to be superior to autograft impaction for subchondral support in tibial plateau fractures. Such agents avoid the donor site morbidity associated with autografts and the risk of disease transmission associated with allografts. We prefer injectables for the support of comminuted fragments in osteopenic patients. More simple defects can be managed effectively with allograft croutons.

COMPLICATIONS

Infection

Deep infections in tibial plateau fractures often result from surgical procedures performed through tenuous soft tissue envelopes, with subsequent poor wound healing and bacterial colonization. Superficial wound infections that occur early should be aggressively treated with antibiotics and surgeons should have a low threshold for surgical débridement. Deep infections may also require irrigation and débridement with arthrotomy and irrigation of the knee joint. Stable implants are typically retained if the fracture has not yet united and it may be beneficial, when an organism has been isolated, to suppress the infection with antibiotics until union has occurred. Hardware can subsequently be removed as indicated. Loose hardware should be removed. Consultation and comanagement with an infectious disease specialist and plastic surgeon may be beneficial.

Arthrofibrosis

Stiffness is one of the most common complications after tibial plateau fractures, especially in more severe injuries. The best treatment is prevention, which can be achieved through stable fixation and early range of motion. Early range of motion requires that the surgeon obtain fixation as stable as possible. Closed manipulation in conjunction with arthroscopic lysis of adhesions in appropriately chosen patients who do not respond to physical therapy may be performed, but one must be cautious with manipulation in patients with existing fractures; we have found that such treatment is rarely indicated. It may be preferable, after fracture union has been achieved, to consider open lysis of adhesions, with or without quadricepsplasty, followed by physical therapy with epidural anesthesia.

Post-Traumatic Complications

The articular cartilage and meniscal damage that occur at the time of tibial plateau fracture predisposes the joint to arthrosis, often regardless of the adequacy of the reduction. Honkonen[9] has reported that 44% of patients had arthrosis at a mean of 7.6 years after injury. In patients who underwent total meniscectomy on the affected plateau, this percentage rose to 74%. However, it is difficult to determine whether it was the meniscectomy or perhaps the increased magnitude of the injury causing the meniscal pathology that led to this

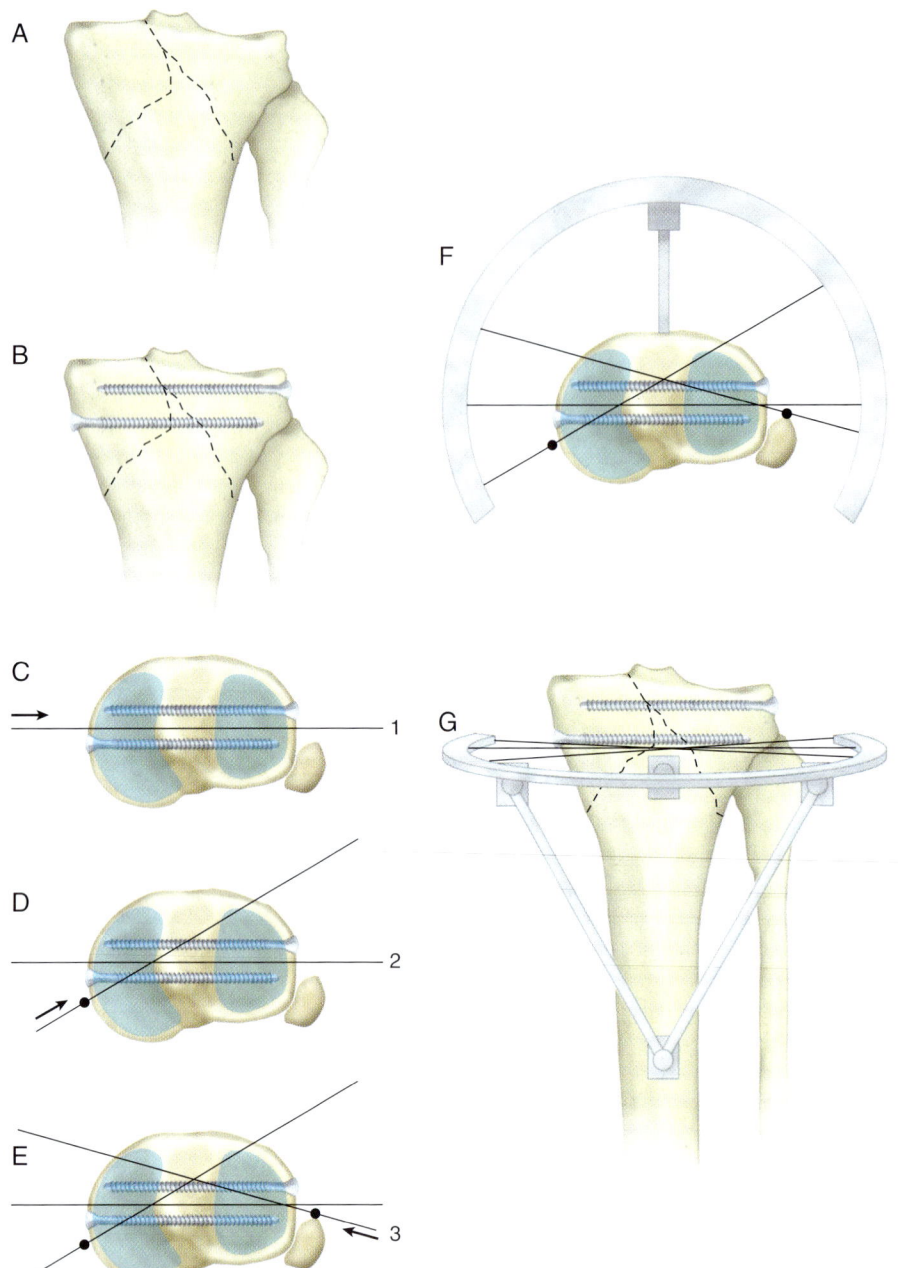

Figure 81-20. Technique for reduction and fixation of a Schatzker type V tibial plateau fracture with cannulated screws and a hybrid external fixator. **A,** Reduction is obtained via open or closed methods and held with a reduction clamp. **B,** Cannulated screws are placed to hold the articular reduction. **C,** A smooth guide wire for the external fixator is placed in the coronal plane, at least 14 mm distal to the joint line. **D,** The second wire, with a bead or olive, is passed posteromedially to anterolaterally. **E,** A third wire, also beaded, is passed posterolaterally to anteromedially. **F,** The wires are appropriately tensioned and fixed to the ring. An optional half-pin can be placed from the anterior to the posterior aspect and attached to the ring for increased stability. **G,** Half-pins are inserted into the tibial shaft, and the distal pins are connected to the ring with the appropriate clamps and bars.

change. The best prognosis was seen in patients with normal or slight valgus limb alignment and an intact meniscus on the affected side. It is important to remember, however, that many studies have found little correlation between radiographic arthrosis and clinical symptoms.[14,17] Corrective osteotomy, total knee arthroplasty, unicompartmental arthroplasty, and arthrodesis are potentially viable options for the management of symptomatic post-traumatic arthritis that is refractory to conservative management. Decision making is

based on the underlying pathology, patient age, and activity. However, a full discussion of reconstructive options is beyond the scope of this chapter.

Nonunion

Nonunion of tibial plateau fractures is relatively rare. It is typically associated with open fractures or higher energy injuries with significant soft tissue damage and typically occurs

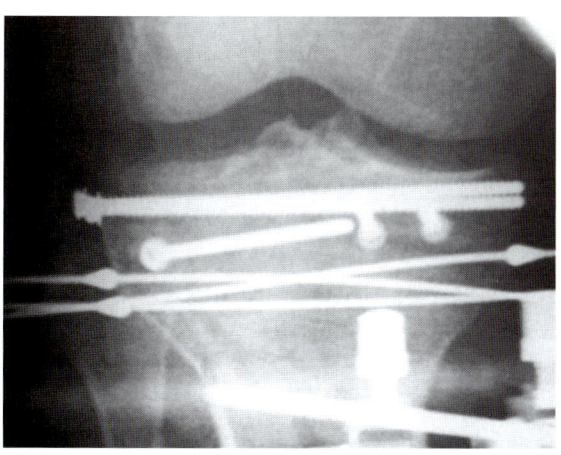

Figure 81-21. Anteroposterior radiograph of a patient with a Schatzker type VI tibial plateau fracture. Extensive metaphyseal comminution and a simple articular fracture are seen. A fine wire fixator and lag screw fixation at the subchondral region were used in this patient because of significant soft tissue injury.

surgeons, the injuries sustained by the cartilage may cause the development of arthrosis, even when a seemingly perfect postoperative radiograph is obtained. Minimally invasive treatment modalities and locked plating technologies have continued to evolve and these advances, as well as the development of improved bone graft substitutes that could minimize articular loss of reduction, may translate into improvements in outcome. Our recognition of the importance of the soft tissue envelope in higher energy injuries and understanding the use of temporizing external fixation before definitive internal fixation have markedly reduced the complication rate in the management of these injuries.

at the metadiaphyseal junction of bicondylar fractures. In patients who appear to be acutely at risk for nonunion secondary to significant bone loss or a poor soft tissue envelope, bone grafting can be performed at the time of the index definitive procedure, if feasible. If, however, healing appears to be delayed in the postoperative course, early bone grafting should be performed. If nonunion has led to fixation failure, revision of this fixation is typically indicated. In some cases, arthroplasty may be a better option.

CONCLUSIONS

Tibial plateau fractures are severe injuries that continue to pose a significant challenge to even the most highly trained orthopedic traumatologists. To the frustration of many

KEY REFERENCES

DeCoster TA, Nepola JV, el-Khoury GY: Cast brace treatment of proximal tibia fractures. A 10-year follow-up study. Clin Orthop Relat Res 231:196–204, 1988.

Drennan DB, Locker FG, Maylahn D: Fractures of the tibial plateau: treatment by closed reduction and spica cast. J Bone Joint Surg Am 61:989–995, 1979.

Gausewitz S, Hohl M: The significance of early motion in the treatment of tibial plateau fractures. Clin Orthop Relat Res 202:135–138, 1986.

Honkonen SE: Indications for surgical treatment of tibial condyle fractures. Clin Orthop Relat Res 302:199–205, 1994.

Honkonen SE: Degenerative arthritis after tibial plateau fractures. J Orthop Trauma 9:273–277, 1995.

Koval KJ, Helfet DL: Tibial plateau fractures: evaluation and treatment. J Am Acad Orthop Surg 3:86–94, 1995.

Koval K, Polatsch D, Kummer FJ, et al: Split fractures of the lateral tibial plateau: evaluation of three fixation methods. J Orthop Trauma 10:304–308, 1996.

Koval K, Sanders R, Borrelli J, et al: Indirect reduction and percutaneous screw fixation of displaced tibial plateau fractures. J Orthop Trauma 6:340–346, 1992.

Roberts JM: Fractures of the condyles of the tibia: an anatomical and clinical end-result study of 100 cases. J Bone Joint Surg 50:1505–1521, 1968.

Schatzker J, McBroom R: Tibial plateau fractures: the Toronto experience, 1968–1975. Clin Orthop Relat Res 138:94–104, 1979.

Full references for this chapter can be found on www.expertconsult.com.

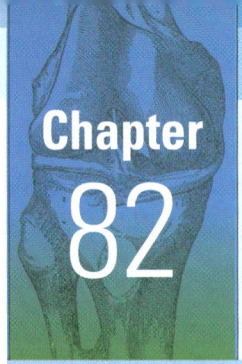

Chapter 82

Fractures of the Patella

Frank A. Liporace, Joshua R. Langford, and George J. Haidukewych

Patellar fractures constitute approximately 1% of all bony injuries, with traffic accidents and falls being the most common causes.[16] Fractures have also been associated with excessive extensor mechanism contraction, total knee arthroplasty, post–anterior cruciate ligament (ACL) reconstruction, postsurgical stabilization, chronic disease (e.g., gout), and severe squatting with weight lifting. Because of its subcutaneous location and the significant joint reactive forces to which it is subjected, the patella is prone to injury.[2,52,66,74,100] Post-traumatic complications include knee stiffness, extensor mechanism weakness, and symptomatic arthritis. Compared with other orthopedic injuries, a paucity of literature on treatment is available along with a limited consensus on which treatment options are best. Even so, the goals of treatment remain constant: reconstitution of the extensor mechanism and restoration of articular congruity.

ANATOMY

The patella lies deep to the fascia lata and tendinous rectus femoris, making it the largest sesamoid bone in the body.[84] Its distal-most aspect is termed the *apex*, and its proximal end is known as the *basis*.[84] Seven facets are separated by a major and minor vertical ridge, and two transverse ridges traverse the major vertical ridge[84] (Fig. 82-1).

The ossification center of the patella most commonly presents between 3 and 5 years of age. As this center enlarges, it may be associated with multiple accessory ossification centers, most commonly superolateral—the bipartite patella.[77] These accessory ossification centers usually have a nonossified cartilaginous connection to the central ossification center.

The Wiberg classification and the Baumgartl modification have been used to classify the patella. Type I has equal medial and lateral facets, and progressive types have smaller medial facets finally leading to no medial facet, also known as the Jaegerhut patella.[7,111] Proximally, the undersurface of the patella is covered with the thickest articular cartilage in the body, and the distal 25% is devoid of articular cartilage.[29]

The four muscles of the extensor mechanism (rectus femoris, vastus medialis, vastus lateralis, and vastus intermedius), the fascia lata, the patellar tendon, and the retinaculum of the knee all attach to the patella (Fig. 82-2). The rectus femoris is most superficial and central, with its fibers running approximately 7 to 10 degrees medial relative to the femur. The vastus medialis has two portions (longus—proximal attachment to patella, obliquus—distal attachment to patella) that attach to the patella at angles of approximately 15 and 50 degrees, respectively. The vastus lateralis attaches proximally on the patella at an angle of approximately 30 degrees. Laterally, it fuses with the iliotibial band and the lateral retinaculum. The vastus intermedius is the deepest portion of the

quadriceps, attaching directly superiorly into the patella. The retinaculum of the knee is composed of the overlying fascia lata anteriorly, which blends with the vastus medialis and lateralis, as well as with the capsule. The patellar tendon is the terminal soft tissue extension of the extensor mechanism that inserts into the tibial tubercle. It is approximately 5 cm long and is formed by central fibers of the rectus femoris, fascial expansions of the iliotibial band, and the patellar retinaculum.[16,59,84] Thickenings of the capsule connect the patella to the femoral epicondyles and aid in appropriate tracking, with the medial patellofemoral ligament contributing 53% to the lateral stability of the patella.[28]

The blood supply of the patella is composed of the peripatellar plexus, which is derived from six separate arteries (Fig. 82-3). The supreme geniculate artery is derived from the superficial femoral artery at the adductor canal. The four geniculate arteries (superolateral, superomedial, inferolateral, and inferomedial arteries) are derived from the popliteal artery. Finally, the recurrent anterior tibial artery is derived from a branch of the anterior tibial artery at the interosseous membrane.[6,89] The net functional blood supply of the patella moves in a distal-to-proximal direction[96] (Fig. 82-4).

BIOMECHANICS

From full flexion to 45 degrees, the load is shared between the patella and the tendinous portion of the extensor mechanism. At less than 45 degrees of flexion, the only component of the extensor mechanism in contact with the distal femur is the patella. The patella causes an increase in the moment arm of the extensor mechanism by displacing it anteriorly from the knee's center of rotation (Fig. 82-5). This increases the force of the extensor mechanism by up to 50%. The terminal 15 degrees of extension require twice the torque required to extend the knee from full flexion to 15 degrees.[51,59] Thus, the patella functions as a pulley. With total patellectomy, numerous studies have documented up to a 50% decrease in isokinetic strength testing of the extensor mechanism.[82,102,108]

Because of the small area of contact at the patellofemoral articulation, the undersurface of the patella is subjected to some of the highest joint reactive forces in the body—up to 7.6 times body weight—even though overall tibiofemoral forces are greater.[40,85]

At any point within the knee's range of motion, a maximum of 13% to 38% of contact of the patella occurs with the femur.[65] Throughout flexion, the area of patellofemoral contact changes. At 20 degrees of flexion, the patella centers within the trochlear groove. As greater angles of flexion are achieved, the area of contact moves proximally on the patella's undersurface and distally on the trochlea[36] (Fig. 82-6).

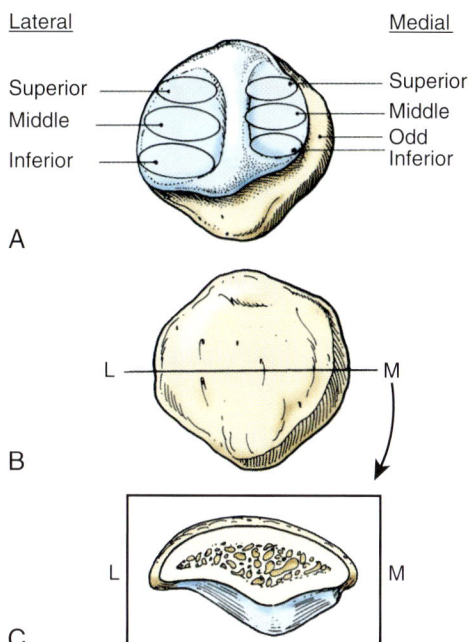

Figure 82-1. **A,** The seven patellar facets. **B,** The anterior surface. **C,** Cross-section of a Wiberg II patella. (From Scuderi G: *The patella,* New York, 1995, Springer-Verlag.)

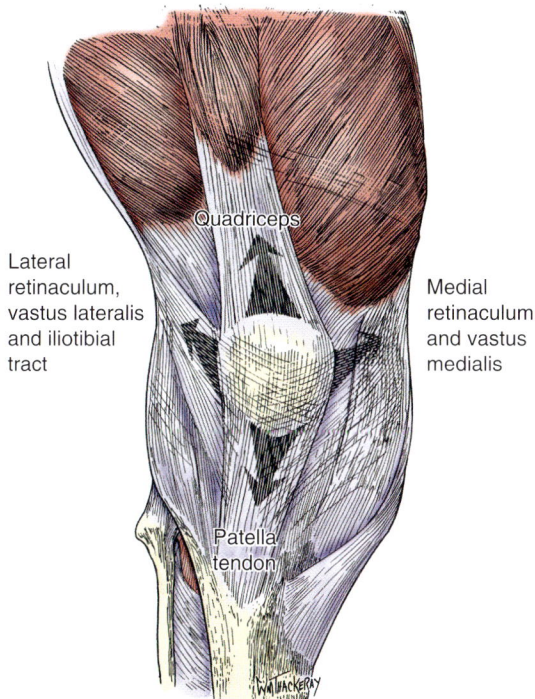

Figure 82-2. The patella is anchored and stabilized to the knee by four structures in a cruciform fashion: the patellar tendon inferiorly, the quadriceps tendon superiorly, and the retinaculum medially and laterally.

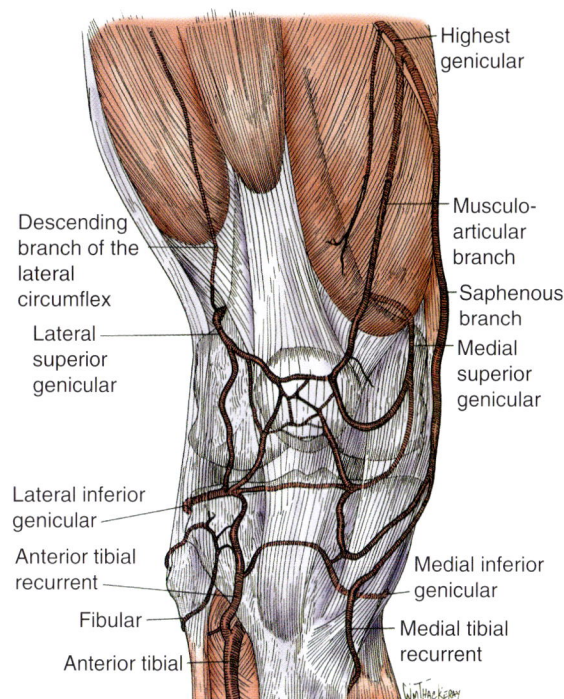

Figure 82-3. Anastomosis at the front of the knee formed by genicular branches from the popliteal artery and descending branches, which connect the femoral artery proximally with the popliteal and anterior tibial arteries distally.

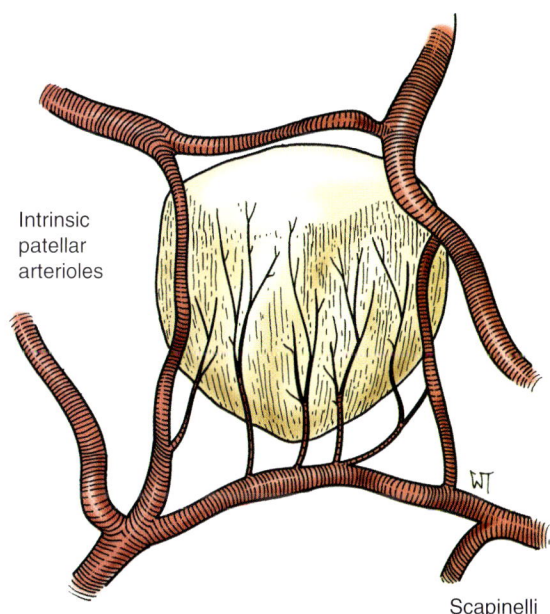

Figure 82-4. Vascular circle around the patella, which, according to Scapinelli,[20] supplies the patella by nutrient arteries that enter predominantly at the inferior pole. The genicular arteries and their branches lie in the most superficial layer of the deep fascia.

DIAGNOSIS

History and Physical Examination

Usually the patient will describe a fall or a direct blow to the anterior knee that represents direct force. Indirect force may be represented by a severe eccentric contraction resulting in a transverse patellar fracture. This may occur in the flexed knee with severe quadriceps contraction that literally results in transverse tearing of the patella and the retinaculum. Historically, classification systems involved stratifying injury patterns according to mechanisms.[6,15,16] Frequently, injuries represent a combination of direct and indirect forces.

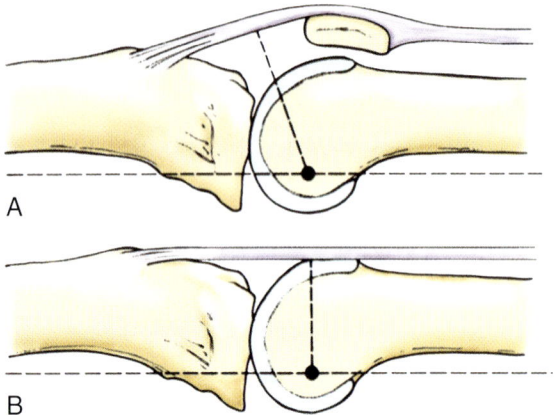

Figure 82-5. In **(A)**, the patella increases the effective moment arm. In **(B)**, after patellectomy, the moment arm is decreased, thereby diminishing extensor force. (From Sanders R: Patella fractures and extensor mechanism injuries. In Browner B [ed]: Skeletal trauma, Philadelphia, 1992, WB Saunders.)

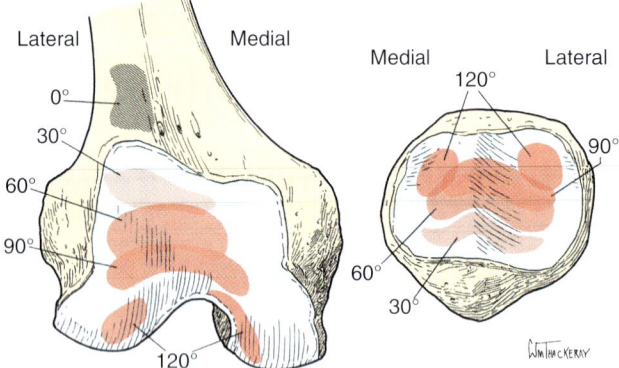

Figure 82-6. Patellofemoral contact zones. (From Aglietti P, Insall JN, Walker PS, et al: A new patella prosthesis. Clin Orthop Relat Res 107:175, 1975.)

The patient often presents with pain, a large effusion, inability to walk, and inability to straight-leg raise or extend the bent knee. It is important to examine for other associated injuries that may be present in high-energy trauma. Also, the quality of the surrounding soft tissues is important when any patient with an orthopedic injury is evaluated and treated. If traumatic arthrotomy or open patellar fracture is suspected, diagnostic injection may facilitate making the diagnosis. Also, sterile local anesthetic injection following needle aspiration of hematoma may allow for more accurate physical examination. A persistent inability to actively extend the knee implies concomitant injury to the medial and lateral quadriceps expansions.[16,94]

Diagnostic Studies

Plain radiographs may be useful in determining the type and degree of patellar injury. In subtle extensor mechanism injuries, computed tomography or magnetic resonance imaging may prove helpful. The standard plain radiographic series for evaluating the patella includes anteroposterior (AP), lateral, and tangential views of the patellofemoral joint. Use of large cassettes (14 × 17 inch) can facilitate evaluation of concomitant ipsilateral knee injuries.

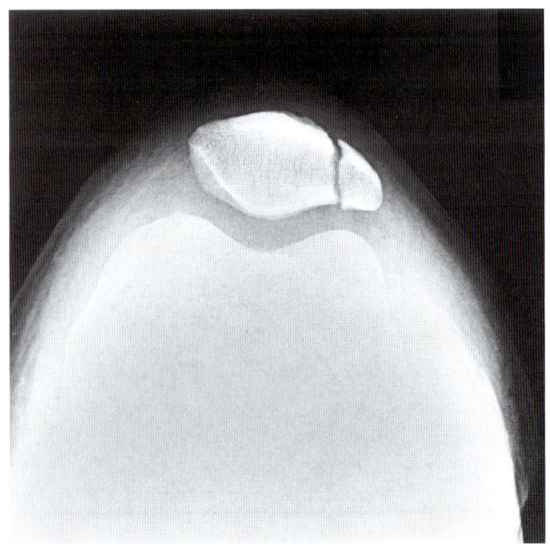

Figure 82-7. Merchant view clearly demonstrates a displaced longitudinal fracture.

The AP view should reveal the position of the patella relative to the femoral sulcus and the relation of the distal pole of the patella to the distal femoral condyles. At times, the presence of an accessory ossification center (e.g., bipartite patella) may be confused for a fracture. Frequently, bipartite patellae are bilateral and are found at the superolateral aspect of the patella. Usually, a bipartite patella is asymptomatic and does not affect extensor mechanism function. Contralateral radiographs may be useful in confirming this diagnosis.[68] Unilateral bipartite patellae are rare and often represent an old marginal patellar fracture.[30] Recent reports in the literature have documented cases of painful bipartite patella after injury. These have been treated nonoperatively, with excision, or with lateral release.[22,46,71,78]

Lateral radiographs help define displacement and articular step-off with patellar fractures. Also, avulsion fractures of the tibial tubercle can be identified. These views should be acquired with 30 degrees of knee flexion to allow calculation of the height of the patella relative to the long bones of the knee. The Insall-Salvati ratio, that is, the length of the patellar tendon to the length of the patella (distal pole should be at a level tangential to Blumensaat's line—distal physeal scar remnant) can be calculated. Approximately 1.0 is normal, >1.2 indicates patella alta, and <0.8 indicates patella baja.[44,48,86] This method has been criticized because patellar shape is known to be variable—a fact that may influence classification of patellar height.[38,48] Alternatively, the Blackburne-Peel index (ratio of the distance from the tibial plateau to the inferior articular surface of the patella to the length of the patella articular surface) can be calculated. Normally, this is approximately 0.8, with a value >1.0 indicating patella alta.[11,12,93]

The tangential view (Merchant view) is taken with the patient supine and with passive positioning of the limb at 45 degrees of flexion.[70] This view may help define vertical fractures, osteochondral fractures, and marginal fractures (Fig. 82-7).

Computed tomography (CT) has been used to identify stress fractures, especially in patients with osteopenia and hemarthrosis.[4] CT scans have been shown to have a 71%

detection rate of these fractures as opposed to a 30% detection rate with bone scans in the setting of negative plain radiographs.[4] With patellar pathology, bone scans ± indium-labeled leukocytes or gallium scanning may be helpful in evaluating patellar osteomyelitis, tumors, and ischemia.[1,32,34,49] CT scans may also be used to evaluate cases of nonunion and malunion, as well as patellofemoral alignment disorders.

Magnetic resonance imaging (MRI) has been used in evaluation of quadriceps tendon injury, patellar tendon injury, and post patellar dislocation. With tendon rupture, the normal low-intensity signal of the tendon will be interrupted and the tendon edges obscured.[113] Even after relocation of a dislocated patella, a set of concomitant injuries is often present (e.g., contusion of the lateral femoral condyle, tear of the medial retinaculum, and a joint effusion).[107]

CLASSIFICATION

No specific classification system has proved effective in determining outcomes based on degree of displacement, fracture pattern, or proposed mechanism of injury. Therefore, long-term results most commonly have been associated with the type of treatment.* Reasons for selecting operative

*References 6, 15-17, 69, 76, 80, 95, and 115.

treatment have included fractures with a ≥3-mm fracture gap, ≥2 mm articular incongruity, and extensor mechanism dysfunction.[15,16,68,94]

Evaluation of a fracture according to its pattern (transverse, vertical, stellate, apical, marginal, osteochondral), the patient's functional capacity, and the surrounding soft tissue envelope provides the surgeon with the most helpful information when choosing appropriate treatment (Fig. 82-8).

NONOPERATIVE TREATMENT

Nonoperative treatment is traditionally chosen when there is lack of significant displacement or articular incongruity and the extensor mechanism is confluent after careful physical examination. Also, it is used when the extensor mechanism forces are perpendicular to the direction of displacement in vertical patellar fractures, thus making nonoperative treatment appropriate.

Typically, nonoperative treatment involves application of well-padded immobilization (cast, splint, knee immobilizer) in nearly full extension for 4 to 6 weeks. Weight bearing as tolerated is permitted, and isometric quadriceps exercises along with straight-leg raises are begun within 1 week of injury.[16,18,39] When consolidation is evident on follow-up radiographs, active range-of-motion exercises are encouraged.

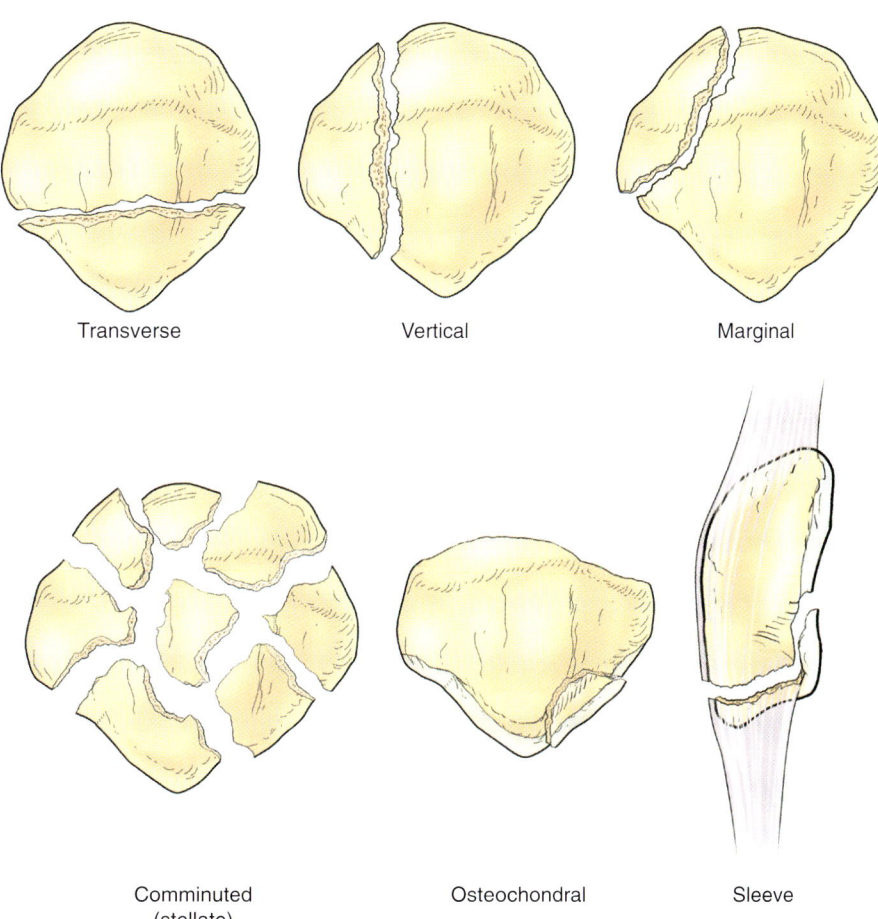

Transverse   Vertical   Marginal

Comminuted   Osteochondral   Sleeve
(stellate)

Figure 82-8. Classification of patellar fractures based on fracture configuration. (Redrawn from Cramer K, Moed B: Patellar fractures: contemporary approach to treatment. J Am Acad Orthop Surg 5:323, 1997.)

Historically, nonoperative treatment has yielded 90% good to excellent results, with only 1% of treatments leading to a poor result.[16] A more modern series reviewing nonoperative treatment of 40 patellar fractures revealed that 80% of patients were pain free and 90% had full knee range of motion at an average follow-up of 30.5 months.[18] The importance of timely, controlled physical therapy is imperative for avoiding arthrofibrosis and patella infera.[63] One case report describes patella infera following nonoperative treatment; a tibial tubercle osteotomy was required that yielded only partial correction and resulted in symptomatic recurrence.[72]

OPERATIVE TREATMENT

Operative intervention has been indicated in patellar fractures that are open, with a ≥3-mm fracture gap, ≥2 mm articular incongruity, or extensor mechanism dysfunction.[15,16,68,94,104] The goals are to provide adequate reduction with stable fixation while preserving a viable soft tissue envelope to allow early rehabilitation and uneventful healing.

Surgical intervention involves internal fixation, external fixation, or patellectomy (partial or complete). The patient is placed supine with a small bolster under the ipsilateral buttock to allow the patella to face directly anteriorly. A nonsterile tourniquet is applied to the proximal aspect of the ipsilateral thigh. Esmarch exsanguination and tourniquet inflation are conducted just prior to incision unless a grossly contaminated open injury is present. Prior to inflation, the quadriceps mechanism must be pulled distally manually or with knee flexion.

If the surrounding soft tissue allows, a midline vertical incision extending from the proximal pole of the patella to the tibial tubercle will provide adequate exposure while not limiting reoperation in the area. Full-thickness subcutaneous flaps can be made to the mid-axis both medially and laterally.

Alternatively, a transverse incision can be used in cases of transverse fracture to allow limited soft tissue stripping and to obtain a cosmetically pleasing result.[6,73] Before this approach is chosen, careful consideration must be given to the potential for subsequent procedures.

In young patients with severely comminuted fractures and good bone quality with an intact soft tissue envelope, extensile exposure through a tibial tubercle osteotomy has been described. After a midline longitudinal incision through skin and subcutaneous tissue, a lateral parapatellar incision is made. The tibial tubercle is predrilled and tapped for eventual large fragment screw fixation. Then it is osteotomized 1.5 cm deep to a healthy bed of dense cancellous bone.[9] Six patients with an average of 31 months' follow-up had four good results, one fair, and one poor with this technique. Clinical union of the osteotomy occurred at an average of 8 weeks, and clinical union of the patella was noted at an average of 11 weeks.[9]

After the surgical approach is selected, the following steps should be followed. In the case of open fractures, all foreign material and nonviable tissue should be debrided; this should be followed by copious lavage. Careful assessment of the entire extensor mechanism is necessary to avoid neglecting tendinous or retinacular injury. The distal femoral condyles should also be evaluated. Bone fragments that lack soft tissue attachments and are too comminuted for fixation should be removed. Prior to fixation, articular reduction, including

reduction of impacted fragments, should be performed. Provisional reduction with Kirschner wires, large pointed bone reduction forceps, and patellar forceps should be completed before definitive fixation is begun. Throughout the procedure, reduction should be assessed via palpation through a retinacular defect, surgical arthrotomy, and orthogonal fluoroscopy.

Internal Fixation

Original wiring techniques used circumferential cerclage wires, or wires passed through drill holes were used; this was followed by 4 to 6 weeks of cast immobilization. These techniques did not incorporate tension band principles. Results were often suboptimal as noted in the inability to start early motion, lack of articular compression, and lack of stable fixation.[13,16,92]

In the 1950s, the tension band concept was popularized by the Arbeitsgemeinschaft für Osteosynthesefragen/Association for the Study of Internal Fixation (AO/ASIF) group. Two 18-gauge stainless steel wires are used. One is placed through the quadriceps and patellar tendons in a figure-of-eight configuration anterior to the patella; the other is placed in a cerclage fashion around the patella.[73] Weber showed that these techniques yielded improved results and were stable enough to allow early range of motion.[110] Modifications to this technique have evolved. The addition of two parallel longitudinal Kirschner wires placed through the patella can prevent toggling of fragments (Figs. 82-9 and 82-10). The Kirschner wires may be placed retrograde through the transverse component of the main proximal and distal fragments and then advanced antegrade once reduction has been attained. The proximal ends of the Kirschner wires are bent into a "hook" that is bent over the tension band wire into the proximal pole of the patella. To be effective, the figure-of-eight tension band wire must be free of slack and must come in contact with the posterior aspect of the Kirschner wires and the bone, both proximally and distally (Fig. 82-11A and B).

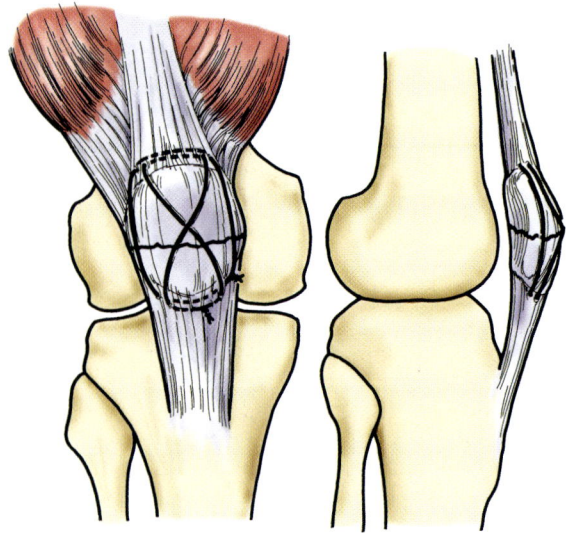

Figure 82-9. Tension cerclage of patellar fractures.

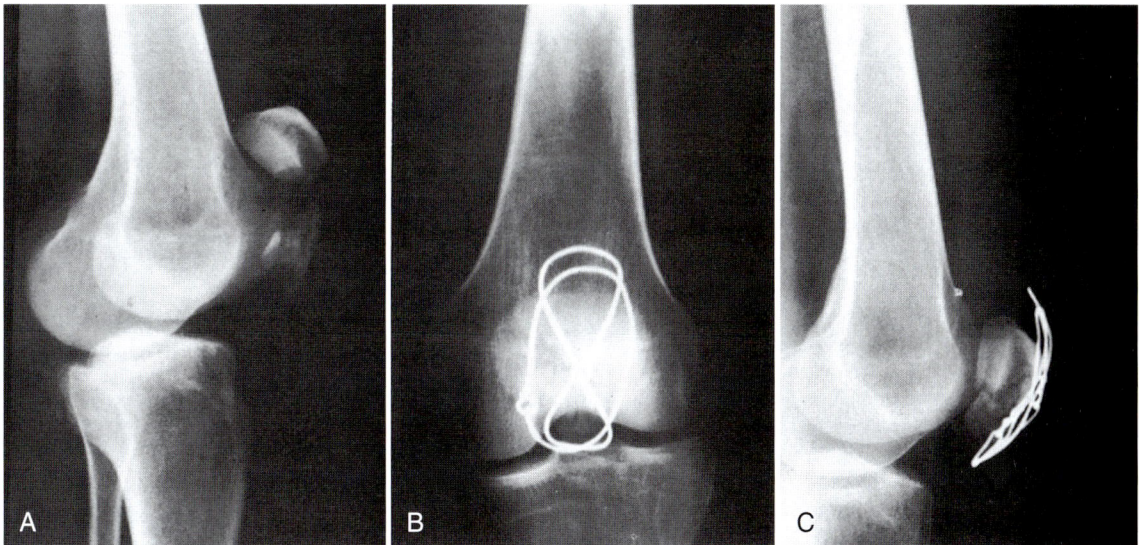

Figure 82-10. **A,** Transverse fracture of the patella with some distal fragment comminution. **B** and **C,** Treatment by tension band cerclage with two wires; after 1 month, the fracture showed good healing, with a little step on the articular surface.

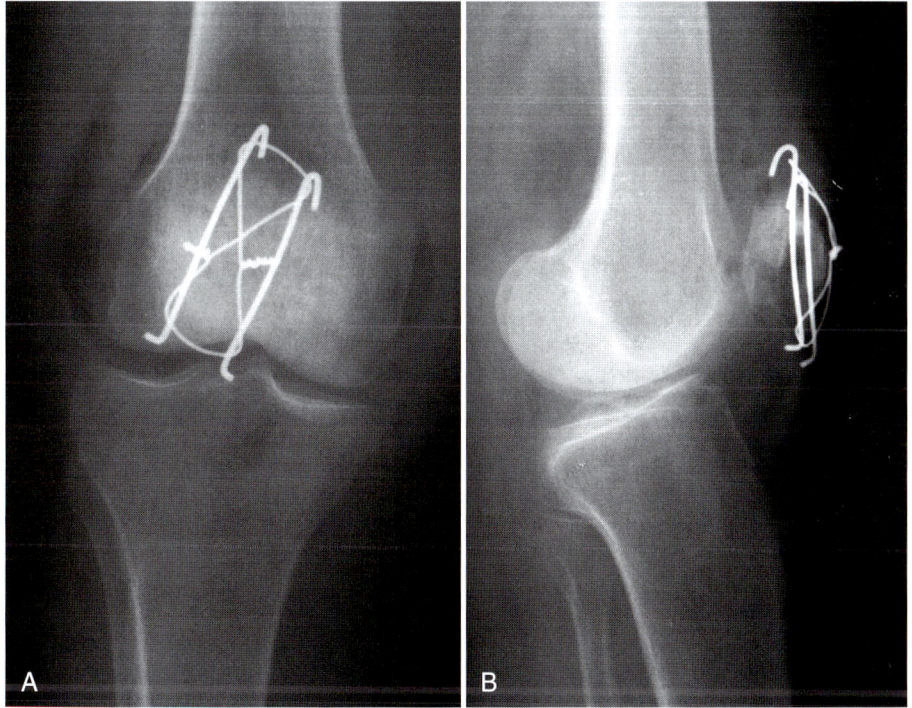

Figure 82-11. **A,** Postoperative anteroposterior radiograph of the patella demonstrating a tension band construct. **B,** Postoperative lateral radiograph of the patella demonstrating a tension band construct.

Horizontal wiring versus standard vertical wiring in tension banding has been evaluated biomechanically. With this method, K-wires are inserted in standard fashion, but the 8 created by the wire around the K-wires lies horizontally versus its classical vertical position. In biomechanical testing, permanent fracture displacement was 67% lower with a horizontal orientation than with the standard vertical orientation.[47]

Lotke and associates described a modified technique for transverse patellar fractures called longitudinal anterior band plus cerclage wiring (LABC). Two vertical holes separated by a 1-cm bone bridge are drilled longitudinally with a Beath-Steinmann pin through the reduced patella. A single wire is threaded on the pins and drawn through the patella. The midportion of the wire is folded over the anterior surface of the patella, while one end of the wire is passed through this loop and tied. If necessary, a supplementary cerclage wire can be added[6] (Figs. 82-12 and 82-13A and B). In the original series of 16 patients, 13 were asymptomatic, and 3 noted some discomfort with stairs or prolonged activity. All patients had ≥90 degrees of motion within 6 weeks of the procedure.[6]

When four wiring techniques—circumferential wiring, tension band cerclage, cerclage over Kirschner wires, and LABC—were compared, the latter two showed the most stable fixation with displacements of less than 1 mm when subjected to a 90-degree arc of knee motion.[20] This enforces the importance of the tension band principle combined with transosseous fixation.

Braided cable has been proposed as an alternative to monofilament wire loop.[91] A retrospective review of 51 patellar fractures treated with tension band wiring and early motion showed a 22% rate of displacement ≥2 mm in the early postoperative period when monofilament wire was used.[98] It is speculated that the braided cable acts as a wire rope, allowing it to conform better to bone surfaces without kinking. Also, its ends are secured with a crimp sleeve that cannot unravel, like a twisted monofilament wire knot. In a biomechanical comparison of transverse patellar fractures treated by a modified tension loop with monofilament or

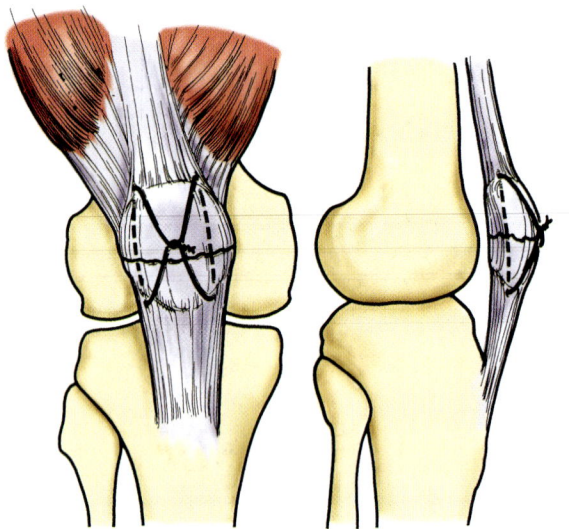

Figure 82-12. Internal fixation of a transverse fracture of the patella according to the method of Lotke and Ecker.

braided wire of equal diameter (1.0 mm), the specimens fixed with braided wire showed approximately one third the displacement of those fixed with monofilament wire after cyclical loading.[91]

In an effort to avoid the reported 30% to 50% need for removal of hardware in these fractures,[42,43,75] alternative fixation with suture has been investigated. A biomechanical study compared tension band and LABC fixation of transverse patellar fractures with 1.25 mm (18 gauge) stainless steel wire or braided polyester suture (no. 5 Ethibond). Through a 90-degree arc of knee motion, no significant difference in failure or fracture gapping was appreciated after 1000 cycles.[81] In a similar dynamic model that involved 2000 cycles per specimen, similar results were acquired when a modified tension band technique was used.[67] Tensile testing of each material showed that polyester was 75% as strong, but this did not affect dynamic testing.[67]

Clinically, suture fixation has been shown to be adequate. A clinical review of seven patients treated with a modified tension band of no.5 TiCron suture reported 100% union with good restoration of knee function.[25] In a pediatric case report, no. 1 polydioxanone (PDS) absorbable suture was used, and the patient was allowed range of motion in 2 months with uneventful healing and full, asymptomatic function by 1 year.[101] The authors attributed the accelerated healing without displacement after such early range of motion to the fact that pediatric patients have accelerated healing potential compared with adults.[101] A recent biomechanical study in which braided suture with a special knot configuration was used also showed that knot configuration helps to decrease displacement with cyclical loading.[41]

A randomized clinical trial compared the modified tension band technique in 18 patients using biodegradable implants (polyglycolide [PGA] or poly-l-lactide [PLLA] plugs with polyester ligament) versus 20 patients using stainless steel fixation.[26] All fractures healed within a mean time of 8 weeks. At an average 2-year follow-up, 72% of patients treated with biodegradable implants had a good result compared with 75% in the metallic group. No clinical or radiographic differences were noted between groups.[23,26]

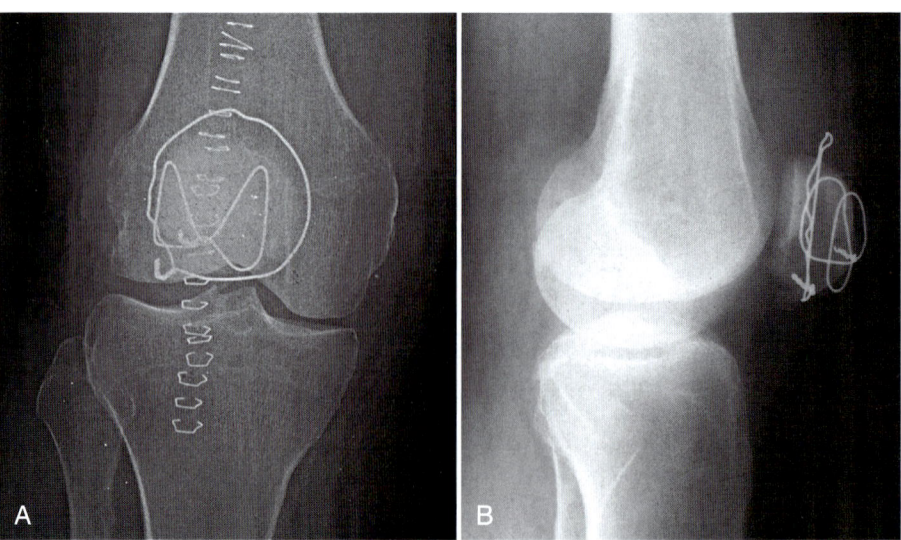

Figure 82-13. A, Postoperative anteroposterior radiograph of the patella demonstrating longitudinal anterior banding with cerclage (LABC). **B,** Postoperative lateral radiograph of the patella demonstrating LABC.

An alternative to the modified tension band technique replaces the two Kirschner wires with cannulated screws.[10] Screws alone may be used in vertical fracture patterns, in fractures with a simple transverse component in patients with good bone quality, or in fixing multiple fragments to create two main fragments that can be addressed with any of the techniques mentioned in this chapter. Cannulated screws may be inserted antegrade or retrograde with the wire tension band loop inserted through the screws. It is important to have the distal aspect of the screw recessed deep to the bony margin. If the screw is prominent, fretting of the wire at the wire–screw interface can result in fixation failure. Also, if one end of the wire is against the screw head and the other end is around the distal aspect of the screw, not against bone, additional compression of fragments cannot be achieved and the tension band is ineffective through range of motion (Figs. 82-14 and 82-15A and B). In a biomechanical study comparing screws with tension band versus screws alone or versus a modified tension band with Kirschner wires, the screws with tension band failed at significantly higher loads than the other two techniques. Although screws alone were more stable than the modified tension band with Kirschner wires, this was not statistically significant.[23] A clinical study evaluating 10 patients (3 smokers and 7 with severe osteopenia) with patellar fracture treated with cannulated screws and wire

tension band reported 100% clinical union at a mean of 8 weeks and radiographic union at a mean of 13 weeks. Seventy percent had excellent and good results at an average 24-month follow-up.[10]

Arthroscopically assisted reduction and fixation with cannulated screws has also been described.[62,103] With an infrapatellar arthroscope inserted, percutaneous reduction with pointed reduction clamps can be achieved and provisionally maintained with guide wires for cannulated screws. Screws are inserted over the guide wires, which are subsequently replaced with a wire loop as previously described.[62,103] Tandogan and coworkers used this technique on five patients, including two with severe osteopenia. All patients had uneventful healing, and 80% had full knee range of motion at 28-month follow-up.[103] Makino and associates evaluated five patients treated with this technique at a mean 24-month follow-up. All had uneventful healing and full return of range of motion and preinjury activity level.[62]

Although techniques have continued to evolve, return of completely normal knee function following displaced patellar fracture remains elusive. In a recent study, at a mean of 6.5 years' follow-up, 20% of patients had an extensor lag greater than 5 degrees. Compared with the normal knee, Biodex testing of these patients revealed a mean isometric extension deficit of 25.5%, an extension power deficit of 31% at an

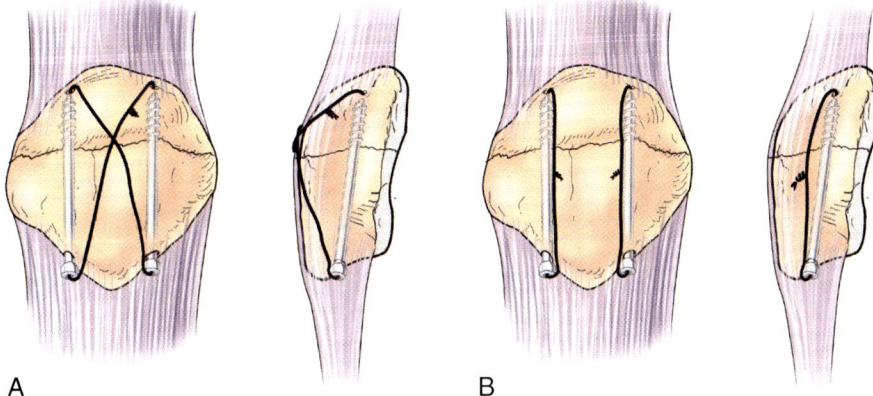

Figure 82-14. A, Cannulated screws augmented with a figure-of-eight tension band anteriorly. Note that the threads of the screw do not cross the fracture site. **B,** The separate tension bands are applied vertically. (Redrawn from Cramer K, Moed B: Patellar fractures: contemporary approach to treatment. J Am Acad Orthop Surg 5:323, 1997.)

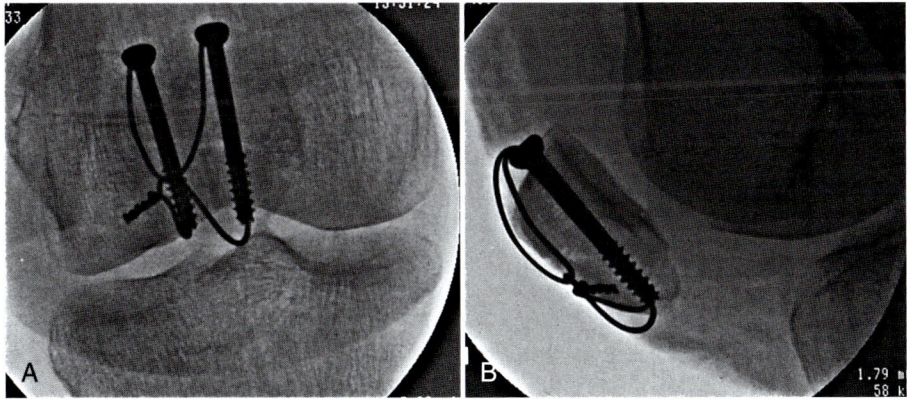

Figure 82-15. A, Intraoperative anteroposterior radiograph of the patella demonstrating a cannulated screw tension band (CSTB) construct. **B,** Intraoperative lateral radiograph of the patella demonstrating a CSTB construct.

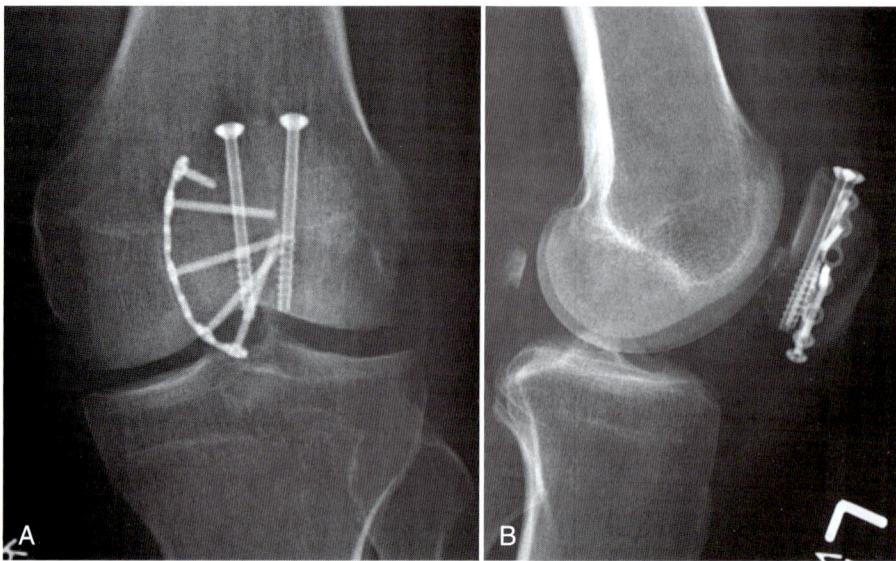

Figure 82-16. **A,** Postoperative anteroposterior radiograph of the patella demonstrating the addition of a minifragment locking plate medially to augment fixation. **B,** Postoperative lateral radiograph of the patella demonstrating the addition of a minifragment locking plate medially to augment fixation.

angular velocity of 90 degrees/sec, and an extension power deficit of 28.9% at an angular velocity of 180 degrees/sec on the side of the patellar fracture.[55]

Future directions for internal fixation will likely focus on materials that are less prone to failure. One such device uses nitinol compression staples for transverse fractures. Under cadaveric testing, this method showed much less displacement than standard tension band techniques and was highly resistant to implant failure.[90]

Another promising technique is the use of minifragment locking plate fixation for fractures that have comminution or for revision of failed patellar fixation. In this situation, the minifragment locking plate is precontoured on the back table and may be placed inferiorly, medially, and/or laterally (Fig. 82-16A and B). These plates may be used in conjunction with lag screws, thus neutralizing compression, as in other fractures. Another recently released device offers cannulated locking bolt fixation. The bolt and nut achieve acute compression, which is then locked in place using a set screw in the nut.

External Fixation

The use of external fixator techniques with patellar fracture has been described in cases of a compromised soft tissue envelope and open injury with contamination.[5,53,54,58,114] In such severe circumstances, standard internal fixation may result in septic arthritis, failure of fixation, or further soft tissue compromise.

A four-hook external fixation compression clamp has been designed. In its first clinical trial on five patients with open patellar fractures (grades II and III), reduction was percutaneously obtained and the compression clamp applied percutaneously. Union occurred at an average of 13 weeks. At an average follow-up of 25.6 months, four of five patients returned to their previous level of activity and had mild to no pain with an average range of motion of 0 to 120 degrees.

One patient had recurrent septic arthritis with moderate pain and a range of motion of 10 to 45 degrees.[53]

Alternatively, limited open reduction with external fixator application has been used.[58] One series of 27 cases evaluating open reduction with subsequent application of two external compressive clamps over wires yielded 24 of 27 patients with excellent and good results. These 24 patients returned to full activity and knee range of motion comparable with the contralateral, uninjured extremity.[58]

Reduction with the external fixation techniques of Ilizarov has been combined with limited percutaneous screw fixation.[5] With this technique, percutaneous olive wires are inserted across the fracture with one olive on either side. Compression across the fracture is then achieved with a tension bow. When the reduction is deemed acceptable, guide wires for percutaneous screws are inserted parallel to the olive wires, and screws are placed. When stable screw fixation is achieved, the olive wires may be removed. A description of the technique with a presentation of four cases has been published. Although the authors cite uneventful healing, no specific evaluation of functional outcome was discussed.[5] Another series examined use of only circular external fixation in comminuted patellar fracture in conjunction with arthroscopic evaluation. Although this series consisted of only five patients, the mean Lysholm score at follow-up was 94.[112]

Partial Patellectomy

In cases of polar fracture in which the fracture fragments are not of adequate size to support internal fixation, partial patellectomy and extensor mechanism advancement are indicated after stable fixation of any large fragments.* Once excision of irreparable fragments is completed, a bony trough should

---

*References 3, 29, 43, 73, 80, 87, and 105.

be made in the remaining patella. Then two locking stitches with nonabsorbable braided suture (e.g., no. 5 Ethibond) should be placed in the tendon, resulting in one suture tail medially, one laterally, and two centrally. Three holes can be drilled longitudinally through the patella—one centrally and one on each side. The two central suture tails should be placed through the central hole and the medial and lateral suture tails passed through their corresponding holes. Finally, the appropriate sutures should be tied to each other at the far end of the patella. A medial and lateral retinacular repair is then achieved (Fig. 82-17). A reinforcing wire or cable may be placed around the patella and through the tibial tubercle. This has been shown to improve the overall strength of the repair.[83]

With partial patellectomy, outcomes comparable with those of internal fixation, with up to 88% good to excellent results, have been reported.[14-16,80,87] Saltzman and colleagues evaluated 40 patients with partial patellectomy, with a mean follow-up of 8 years. Seventy-eight percent had good to excellent results; mean range of motion was 94%, and mean quadriceps strength was 85%.[87] Most reports cite results with distal pole excision and tendon advancement.[14,15,80,87]

No specific correlation has been shown between the size of the retained fragment and the functional outcome.[87] Pandey and coworkers suggested that retaining any amount of patellar fragment potentially contributes to a biomechanical advantage over total patellectomy.[80] This argument was strengthened by an article looking at distal pole preservation using a basket plate. The group treated with basket plate fixation had less pain, an increased level of activity, and better range of motion than the control partial patellectomy group.[50] Another study confirmed these results with a series of 120 patients comparing partial patellectomy (n = 49) versus basket plate fixation (n = 71). Using validated outcome tools, investigators found statistically significant improvement in patellofemoral function with distal pole preservation.[64]

Total Patellectomy

Total patellectomy should be reserved as a salvage procedure when comminution is so severe that it is technically impossible to retain any congruous fragments of patella at the articulation with the trochlea. Functionally, the soft tissue contribution of the extensor mechanism is lengthened with total patellectomy. Therefore, some imbrication is indicated in an attempt to avoid future extensor lag.[88] Soft tissue repair should proceed with multiple nonabsorbable tendon-grabbing stitches once all bone fragments have been removed. It is imperative that intraoperative flexion of 90 degrees be attained. If inadequate soft tissue is present for primary repair, or if augmentation is needed, an inverted V-plasty "turndown" should be performed.[97] Mobilization may begin within 3 to 6 weeks postoperatively if the repair allows. Up to 2 years may be required before maximal rehabilitation is achieved.[56]

When adequate soft tissue is available, the remaining extensor mechanism can be "tubularized," as described by Compere and associates (Fig. 82-18). At times, ossification will develop within the "tube," forming a "pseudo-patella" to help restore some of the mechanics of the extensor mechanism.[27]

Overall results with total patellectomy are poor when compared with other treatment options. Sutton and colleagues reported a 49% reduction in extensor mechanism strength in patients who underwent total as opposed to partial patellectomy.[102] Severe quadriceps atrophy, difficulty with stair climbing, and pain with activity have been reported.[31] Levack and coworkers postulated that good results were attainable if patients maintained 70% quadriceps function of the contralateral limb. However, 27 of 34 patients in that series maintained less than 70% of quadriceps strength and did not have a good result.[56] At 7.5 years' follow-up, Einola and associates had only 21% of 28 patients with good results and maintenance of 75% quadriceps power.[31]

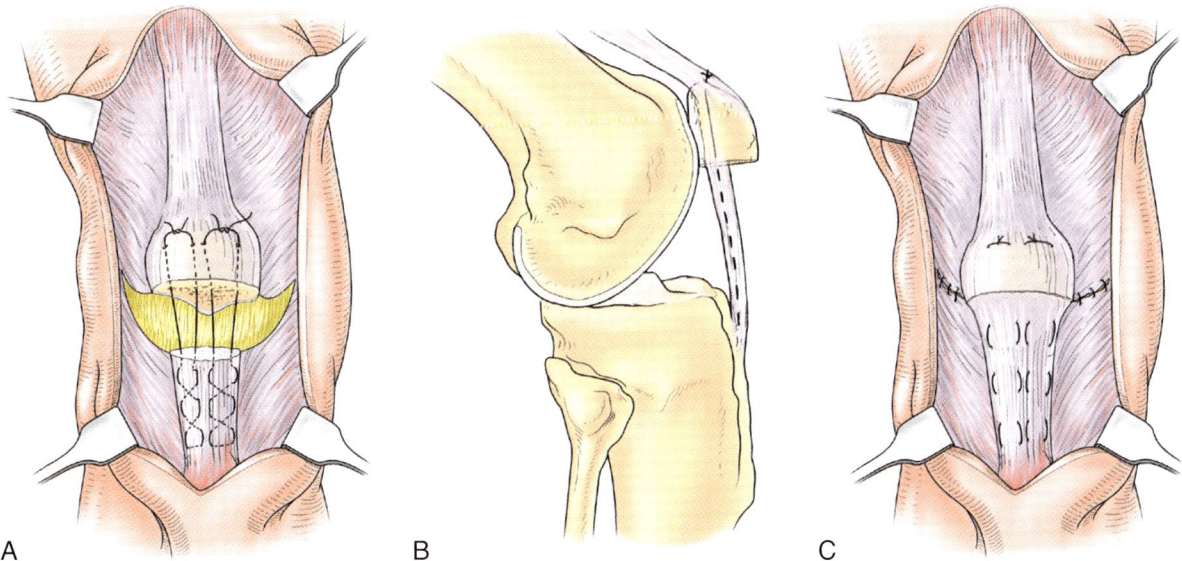

A   B   C

Figure 82-17. Technique of partial patellectomy. Note the placement of the patellar tendon at the articular surface of the remaining patella. (Redrawn from Cramer K, Moed B: Patellar fractures: contemporary approach to treatment. J Am Acad Orthop Surg 5:323, 1997.)

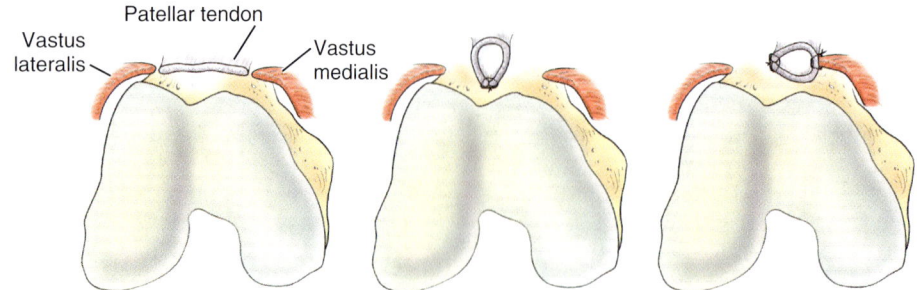

Vastus lateralis   Patellar tendon   Vastus medialis

Figure 82-18. Compere's technique for patellectomy (see text). Ossification will occur within the tube.

COMPLICATIONS

Loss of Knee Motion

This may be the most common complication with loss of terminal knee flexion.[29] Usually this does not affect daily function. If severe, manipulation under anesthesia, arthroscopic lysis of adhesions, or quadricepsplasty may be considered. To date, widely accepted standard protocols do not exist for specific interventions.

Although some authors have not reported long-term effects of immobilization up to 6 weeks,[15,16] early motion is generally instituted to promote cartilage healing and potentially decrease short-term stiffness.

Infection

Postsurgical infection of patellar fracture ranges from 3% to 10%.[15,42,98] Because of the limited soft tissue envelope around the patella, surgical handling must be done carefully. In cases of concomitant soft tissue injury, attempts should be made to avoid the zone of injury. Additionally, adequate débridement of all necrotic and nonviable tissue, as well as foreign material, should be conducted with open injuries. If suspected deep infection is present, appropriate antibiotics and thorough débridement should be provided. If healing has not occurred, implants should remain in place with plans for a staged removal after union if risk of infection persists.

Loss of Reduction

Loss of reduction after operative fixation has ranged from 0% to 20%.[15,16,42,98] This may be related to technical errors, unrecognized injury, or patient noncompliance.[56,98] If displacement is minimal, a period of immobilization may be indicated to allow the remaining reduction to heal. If displacement is severe or discontinuity of the extensor mechanism is noted, revision surgery is indicated.

Osteoarthrosis

Long-term follow-up has indicated that rates of osteoarthrosis in a knee that has sustained a patellar fracture are greater than in the contralateral, uninjured extremity.[42,99] Severe articular damage at the time of injury may result in osteoarthritis, even with anatomic reduction. Exuberant callus during healing may also contribute to degenerative joint disease.[88] Finally, inadequate restoration of the articular surface may result in osteoarthritis after surgery for patellar fracture.

Hardware Irritation

Two separate studies have indicated that subcutaneous hardware may become symptomatic in 15% of cases.[42,98] When necessary, it should be removed on an elective basis after full healing has occurred.

Delayed Union and Nonunion

With modern fixation, this complication is extremely rare. Frequently, it is an asymptomatic fibrous nonunion with an intact extensor mechanism that does not necessitate further treatment. Bostrom reported a 3% incidence of asymptomatic pseudoarthrosis, regardless of whether operative or nonoperative treatment was provided.[16] Carpenter and associates described a 1% incidence of nonunion.[24] If delayed union is present, a period of immobilization will often allow healing to progress. If this fails, revision fixation with bone grafting should be considered. With revision surgery, Weber and Cech reported a 100% healing rate.[109]

Patellar Fracture in Total Knee Arthroplasty

Although overall it is a rare complication of total knee arthroplasty, patellar fracture may be the most frequently occurring periprosthetic knee fracture.[88] The frequency range of this complication is 0.33% to 6.3%.[21,37]

Many risk factors have been associated with patellar fracture in total knee arthroplasty. These include patient factors (osteoporosis, rheumatoid arthritis, male sex, overactivity, excessive knee motion), implant factors (central peg, cementless implants, posterior cruciate ligament [PCL]-substituting prosthesis, inset design, osteolysis), and technical factors (excessive resection, inadequate resection, anterior patellar perforation, revision surgery, cement usage, malalignment, patellar blood supply disruption).[57]

Insall classified these injuries according to the configuration of the fracture (horizontal, vertical, and comminuted) and as traumatic or fatigue fracture. He recommended that traumatic, displaced injuries should be treated operatively, and nondisplaced fatigue fractures with adequate component stability should be treated nonoperatively.[45]

TYPE   DESCRIPTION

EXAMPLE/DIAGRAM

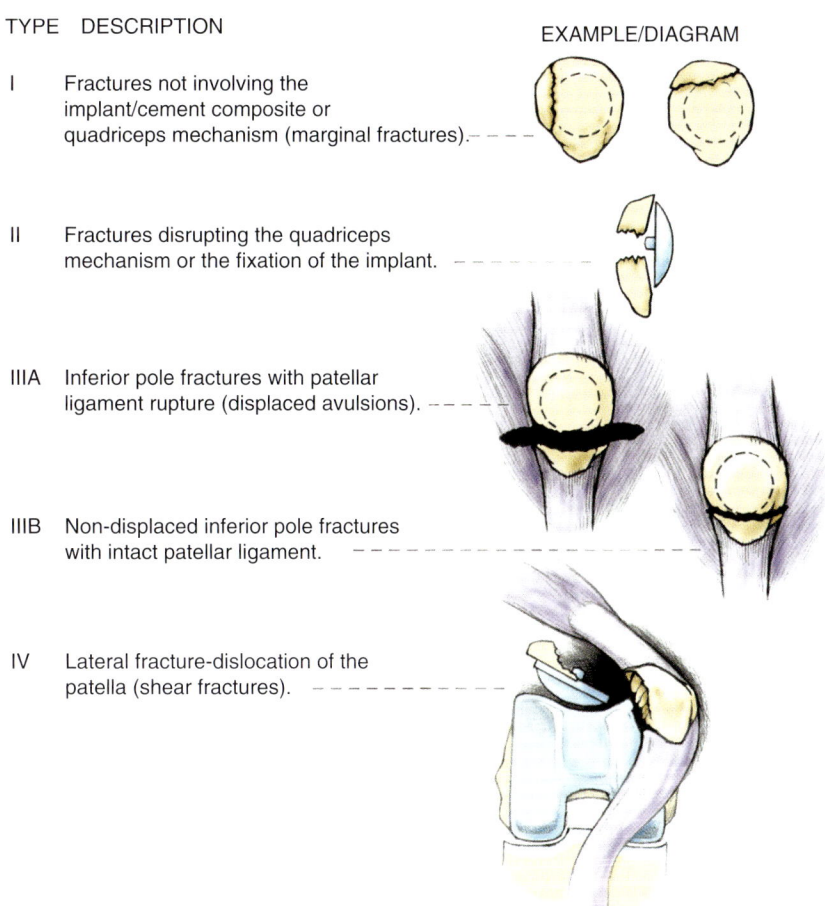

I   Fractures not involving the implant/cement composite or quadriceps mechanism (marginal fractures).

II   Fractures disrupting the quadriceps mechanism or the fixation of the implant.

IIIA   Inferior pole fractures with patellar ligament rupture (displaced avulsions).

IIIB   Non-displaced inferior pole fractures with intact patellar ligament.

IV   Lateral fracture-dislocation of the patella (shear fractures).

Figure 82-19. Goldberg's classification[48] of patellar fractures after total knee arthroplasty. (From Kolessar D, Rand J: Extensor mechanism problems following total knee arthroplasty. In Morrey B [ed]: Reconstructive surgery of the joints, ed 2, New York, 1996, Churchill Livingstone.)

Goldberg classified patellar fractures according to concomitant extensor mechanism injury. Type I consists of marginal fractures without component involvement or extensor injury. Type II injuries have disruption of the extensor mechanism or the implant–bone interface. Type III fractures involve the inferior pole; type IIIA injuries have patellar tendon disruption, and type IIIB fractures include a competent patellar tendon. Type IV fractures exhibit concomitant patellofemoral dislocation[35] (Fig. 82-19).

Treatment is based on the competence of the extensor mechanism and the stability of the prosthetic component. For Goldberg type I fractures, nonoperative treatment is appropriate. With extensor mechanism incompetence (types II and IIIA), surgical repair must be undertaken. Fractures with excessive displacement or extreme component loosening also require operative intervention.[19,35,37] If standard fixation techniques are technically impossible, cerclage fixation or partial patellectomy with delayed postoperative range of motion may be necessary.[8,33,60,106]

A retrospective study reviewed 85 periprosthetic patellar fractures with a mean follow-up of 3.6 years. Of 38 fractures without extensor mechanism dysfunction or component loosening, 37 were treated successfully using a nonoperative approach. Of 12 fractures with extensor mechanism disruption, 11 were treated operatively. Postoperative complications were reported in six cases, five of which required reoperation. Of 28 fractures with a loose patellar component, 20 were treated operatively and 9 had complications. This highlights that periprosthetic patellar fractures in the setting of a total knee arthroplasty that require operative intervention have a high complication rate.[79]

SUMMARY

Patellar fractures are fairly common injuries. Current classification schemes based on fracture pattern and mechanism of injury do not correlate with functional outcomes. It is relatively clear that maintenance of the patella when possible is superior to total patellectomy. Results of treatment seem to be based on maintenance and adequacy of reduction and fixation. Currently, modified tension band techniques with or without screw fixation appear to provide the best results. Biomechanically, cannulated screws and braided wire have added to the stability of repairs but have not been proven to improve clinical results.

Because of the subcutaneous location and potential for anterior soft tissue injury associated with patellar fracture, treatment may be dictated by these factors. With an intact soft tissue envelope, treatment must be based on surgeon experience and comfort with techniques required to obtain the treatment goals presented in this chapter. Postoperative protocols for initiation of range of motion and strengthening are personalized to patient needs and the stability of the fixation.

KEY REFERENCES

Berg EE: Open reduction internal fixation of displaced transverse patella fractures with figure-eight wiring through parallel cannulated compression screws. J Orthop Trauma 11:573–576, 1997.

Bostman O, et al: Fractures of the patella treated by operation. Arch Orthop Trauma Surg 102:78–81, 1983.

Bostman O, Kiviluoto O, Nirhamo J: Comminuted displaced fractures of the patella. Injury 13:196–202, 1983.

Bostrom A: Fracture of the patella: a study of 422 patellar fractures. Acta Orthop Scand Suppl 143:1–80, 1972.

Braun W, et al: Indications and results of nonoperative treatment of patellar fractures. Clin Orthop Relat Res 289:197–201, 1993.

Carpenter JE, et al: Biomechanical evaluation of current patella fracture fixation techniques. J Orthop Trauma 11:351–356, 1997.

Cramer KE, Moed BR: Patellar fractures: contemporary approach to treatment. J Am Acad Orthop Surg 5:323–331, 1997.

Kastelec M, Veselko M: Inferior patellar pole avulsion fractures: osteosynthesis compared with pole resection. J Bone Joint Surg Am 86:696–701, 2004.

Lotke PA, Ecker ML: Transverse fractures of the patella. Clin Orthop Relat Res 158:180–184, 1981.

Matejcic A, et al: Multifragment fracture of the patellar apex: basket plate osteosynthesis compared with partial patellectomy. Arch Orthop Trauma Surg 128:403–408, 2008.

Nummi J: Fracture of the patella: a clinical study of 707 patellar fractures. Ann Chir Gynaecol (Fenn Suppl) 179:1–85, 1971.

Nummi J: Operative treatment of patellar fractures. Acta Orthop Scand 42:437–438, 1971.

Seligo W: Fractures of the patella: treatment and results. Reconstr Surg Traumatol 12:84–102, 1971.

Shabat S, et al: Functional results after patellar fractures in elderly patients. Arch Gerontol Geriatr 37:93–98, 2003.

Smith ST, et al: Early complications in the operative treatment of patella fractures. J Orthop Trauma 11:183–187, 1997.

Sorensen KH: The late prognosis after fracture of the patella. Acta Orthop Scand 34:198–212, 1964.

Torchia ME, Lewallen DG: Open fractures of the patella. J Orthop Trauma 10:403–409, 1996.

Watkins MP, et al: Effect of patellectomy on the function of the quadriceps and hamstrings. J Bone Joint Surg Am 65:390–395, 1983.

Full references for this chapter can be found on www.expertconsult.com.

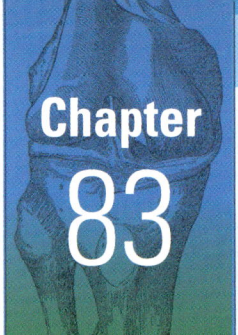

Treatment of Periprosthetic Fractures Around a Total Knee Arthroplasty

George J. Haidukewych, Steven Lyons, and Thomas Bernasek

Periprosthetic fractures remain common complications after total knee arthroplasty. The number of knee arthroplasties performed worldwide continues to increase, and with the ever-growing older population, the number of periprosthetic fractures will continue to increase as well. Decision making regarding the management of these fractures is divided according to whether the fracture has occurred in the femur or the tibia or whether the arthroplasty is loose or well fixed. Fractures of the distal end of the femur above a well-fixed arthroplasty are typically treated with some form of internal fixation. The use of fixed-angled, locked, percutaneously inserted plates has revolutionized the treatment of these fractures. Early clinical and biomechanical data are encouraging. For loose implants, revision is typically considered. Bony defects, areas of osteolysis, osteopenia, and short periarticular fragments all pose challenges to a successful revision arthroplasty in this setting. In older patients, distal femoral replacement tumor prostheses are often required to reconstruct massive bony defects. Attention to specific technical details is necessary for a successful result, and surgeons undertaking such reconstructions should be experienced in arthroplasty and fracture management techniques.

The number of primary knee arthroplasties performed annually in the United States continues to increase. It is estimated that 0.3% to 2.5% of patients will sustain a periprosthetic fracture as a complication of total knee arthroplasty.[1,11,31] Patient-specific risk factors such as rheumatoid arthritis, osteolysis, osteopenic bone, and frequent falls, common in the older population, and technique-specific risk factors such as anterior femoral cortical notching have all been implicated as potential causes of periprosthetic fractures. The economic impact and disability associated with these fractures is substantial; therefore, having an effective strategy to manage these challenging injuries is important. Typically, fractures occur in the supracondylar area of the femur above a well-fixed total knee arthroplasty (Fig. 83-1).[2,18,24] Fractures of the tibia are much less common and are frequently associated with implant loosening.[12,17] Decision making regarding the treatment of periprosthetic fractures around a total knee arthroplasty is divided, as noted earlier. In general, patients with fractures around loose implants are considered candidates for revision total knee arthroplasty, whereas fractures around well-fixed implants are candidates for open reduction and internal fixation. Various methods of internal fixation have been described for the treatment of these injuries.[5,33] There has been recent enthusiasm for minimally invasive osteosynthesis of these injuries with the use of locked plates. Revision arthroplasty in this setting can be very demanding, with a unique set of technical challenges. The purpose of this chapter is to review the decision making, contemporary techniques, and potential complications of the management of periprosthetic fractures of the femur and tibia around a total knee arthroplasty. Periprosthetic fractures of the patella are discussed in Chapter 67.

PATIENT EVALUATION

Patients with fractures around asymptomatic, well-fixed implants do not usually require an infection workup. However, in patients with a loose implant or history of prefracture knee pain, routine preoperative evaluation of these patients should include a complete blood count with manual differential, sedimentation rate, C-reactive protein serology, and knee aspiration to exclude occult infection. Medical optimization for these frequently frail older patients is recommended.

High-quality radiographs are necessary to evaluate the fixation status of the arthroplasty and the amount and quality of remaining periarticular bone stock. The history and physical examination should focus on prefracture knee symptoms such as pain, instability, and stiffness. If available, the operative notes from the original arthroplasty should be obtained. This is especially important if isolated component revision is contemplated. Older implant designs may not offer varying degrees of constraint, augmentation, polyethylene insert sizes, and other factors, and thus compatibility issues may necessitate complete arthroplasty revision. Previous incisions and the status of the soft tissues should be circumferentially evaluated. The neurovascular status of the limb should be carefully documented.

OPEN REDUCTION AND INTERNAL FIXATION

Supracondylar Periprosthetic Fractures

The typical clinical situation that the orthopedic surgeon will encounter is a supracondylar femoral fracture above a well-fixed, well-functioning, total knee arthroplasty (Figs. 83-2 and 83-3).[1,11] Minimally displaced stable fractures and those impacted in good alignment may be candidates for nonoperative treatment. In our experience, however, these situations are rare. Long-leg casting with or without incorporation of a hip guide brace to control leg rotation is recommended. Close radiographic follow-up is indicated, with early surgical intervention if fracture instability is noted. Prolonged attempts at managing unstable fractures with casting may result in further erosion of the distal bone stock and potentially compromise the success of any future reconstruction.

The principles of treatment of these injuries include obtaining bony union, maintaining correct limb alignment, length, and rotation, and avoiding complications. Surgical challenges to achieving these goals include the often short, osteopenic distal bony fragments, fracture comminution, areas of osteolysis, and parts of the femoral component that

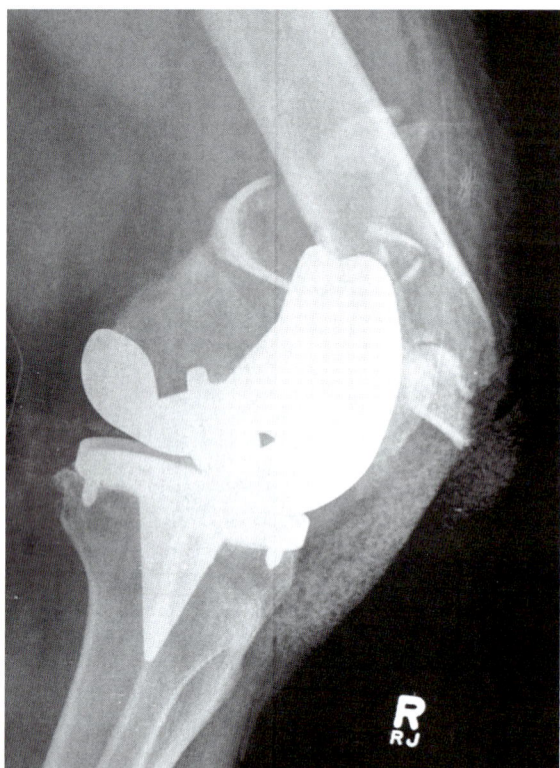

Figure 83-1. Displaced comminuted periprosthetic distal femoral fracture.

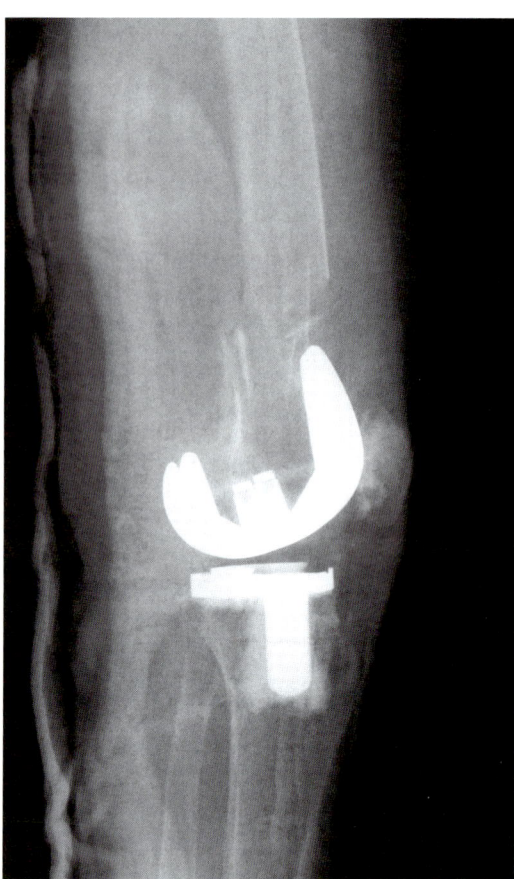

Figure 83-3. Lateral view of the patient in Figure 86-2. Note the fracture at the level of the anterior femoral flange, the most common fracture location.

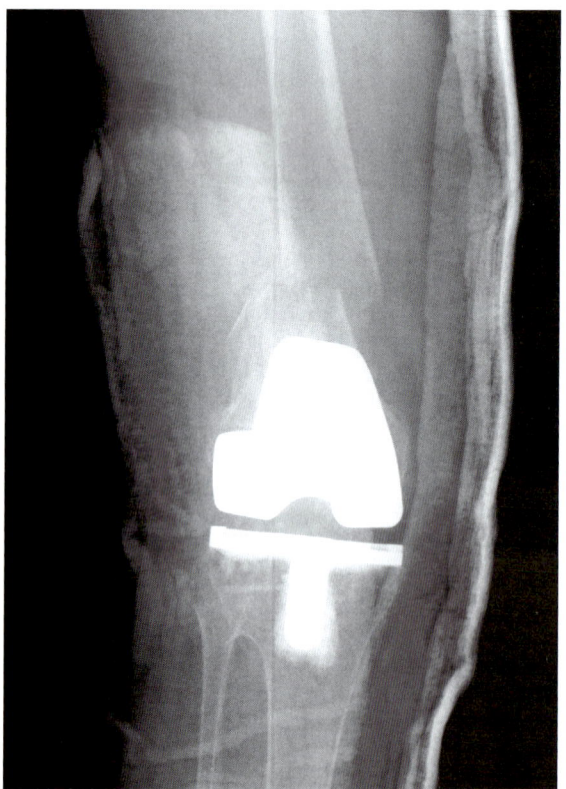

Figure 83-2. Anteroposterior view of a typical distal femoral periprosthetic fracture above a well-fixed total knee arthroplasty.

can make obtaining stable distal fixation difficult, such as lugs, boxes, and stems. Such fractures usually require an internal fixation device that provides coronal plane stability to avoid the deformity, typically varus collapse, that can occur during the healing process. In the past, devices such as the 95-degree angled blade plate and dynamic condylar screw have been used, with mixed results.*

Because of the extremely distal nature of these fractures, the blade of the blade plate or the lag screw of the dynamic condylar screw must often be inserted more proximally to avoid portions of the femoral component, and thus distal fixation is often suboptimal. The traditional condylar buttress plate offers more freedom of angulation of distal screws but provides no coronal plane stability. Unacceptable rates of varus collapse have been reported when this device was used for unstable fractures.[10]

Retrograde intramedullary nailing has been used successfully in many series to manage these fractures and offers the advantage of soft tissue–friendly, minimally invasive stability for complex periprosthetic fractures.[1,5,11,18-20] Challenges to successful union with intramedullary techniques include the marginal distal fixation provided by locking screws for the typically comminuted, osteopenic distal bony fragments (Figs. 83-4 and 83-5). Also, intramedullary nailing is not

_____
*References 1-3, 5, 8, 18, 31, and 33.

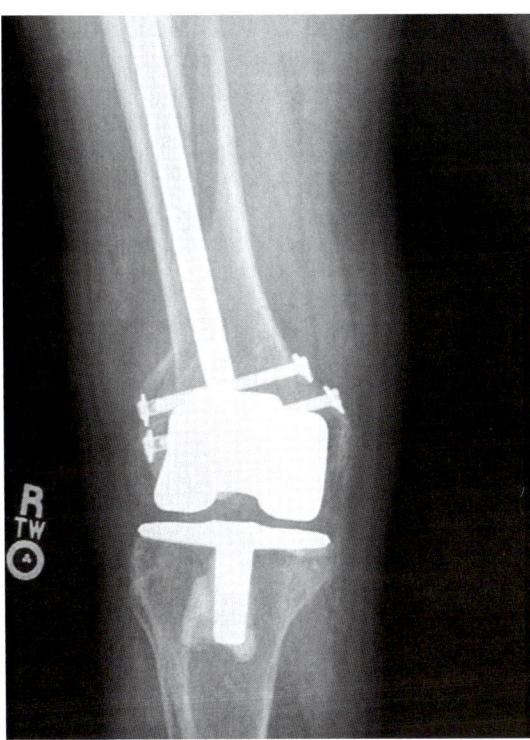

Figure 83-4. Loss of fixation after retrograde nailing because of inadequate distal fixation.

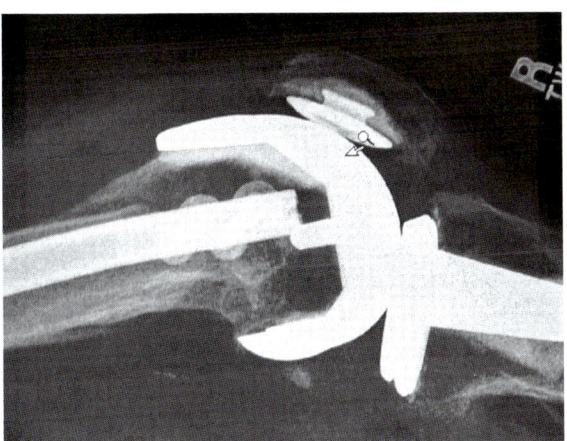

Figure 83-5. Lateral view of the patient in Figure 86-4.

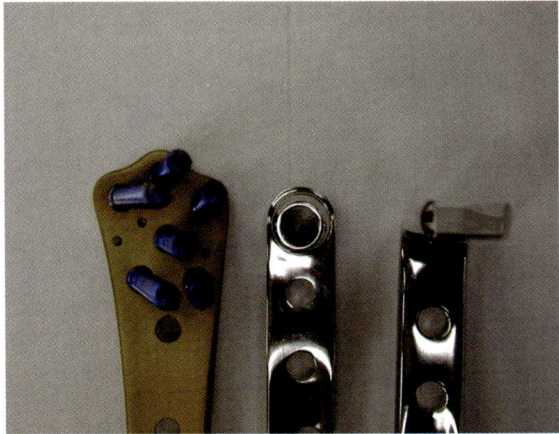

Figure 83-6. En face view of a locked plate, dynamic condylar screw, and blade plate. The versatility and superior ability to obtain distal fixation with the locked plate are obvious.

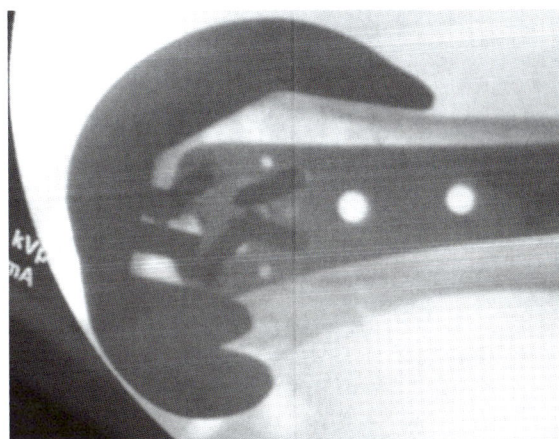

Figure 83-7. Internal fixation with the LISS device (Synthes, West Chester, Pa). Note the positioning of the screws around distal obstacles such as femoral lugs.

practical with implants that substitute for the posterior cruciate ligament because the femoral housing precludes access to the intramedullary canal. We currently reserve intramedullary techniques for fractures above cruciate-retaining designs with sufficient distal bone to allow purchase with a minimum of two distal locking screws. Furthermore, biomechanical evidence has suggested that in the presence of medial comminution, retrograde intramedullary nails may be mechanically more stable than laterally placed locking plates.[4] Occasionally, antegrade femoral nailing can be used for periprosthetic distal femoral fractures as well, provided that a sufficiently long distal fragment is present. In our experience, such fractures are extremely rare. The main challenge with antegrade techniques is obtaining appropriate alignment and stable distal fixation. Additionally, with antegrade techniques, an area of high-stress concentration is created between the distal end of the nail and the femoral component.

Locking plate technology has gained popularity for the management of complex periarticular fractures about the knee.* Threads on the screw heads are threaded into corresponding threads in the plate holes, thereby forming a fixed-angle construct and providing coronal plane stability.[15] These devices have been used with excellent results for the management of complex periarticular injuries and have an excellent track record for providing reliable distal fixation. Additionally, such devices allow multiple locked screws to be placed around and between portions of the femoral component to improve distal fixation (Figs. 83-6 to 83-8).[38] Kregor and colleagues[24,25] have reported a series of 38 periprosthetic fractures treated with the Less Invasive Stabilization System (LISS) device (Synthes, West Chester, Pa). There were only two failures (5%). One patient required revision knee arthroplasty and one required bone grafting to achieve solid union.

*References 7, 16, 21, 23-26, 28, 30, 34, and 35.

Ultimately, 37 of 38 fractures (97%) healed. Medical and orthopedic complications were uncommon. Leaving metaphyseal comminution undisturbed, thereby preserving vascularity to the fragments, is critical to predictable healing with this technique.

In addition to providing excellent mechanical stability, several locked plating designs also offer the added theoretical biologic advantage of allowing percutaneous insertion.[23] This type of insertion minimizes the need for additional large incisions around the knee and potentially minimizes the soft

tissue complications and stiffness associated with the traditional exposures used for open reduction and internal fixation.[16] When percutaneous techniques are used, vigilance is required to avoid malalignment, typically valgus deformity and hyperextension of the distal fragment. Many commercially available locked plating designs offer the surgeon the option of open or percutaneous insertion. When possible, we perform the internal fixation percutaneously to take advantage of the mechanical stability provided by these devices, as well as the advantages that percutaneous insertion allows.[12]

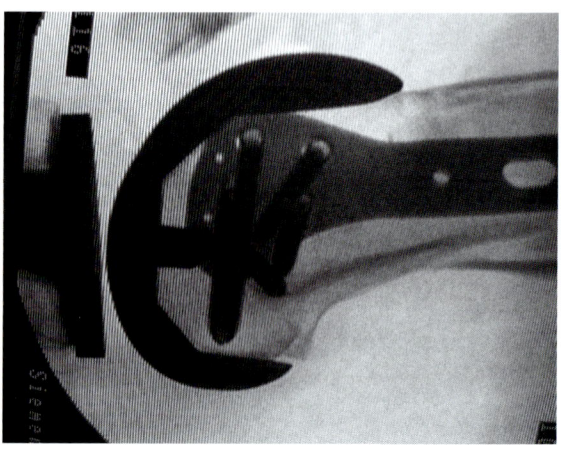

Figure 83-8. Internal fixation with the PolyAx device (DePuy, Warsaw, Ind), which allows angled polyaxial screws and fixed-angle locking screws as well.

Percutaneous Technique of Distal End of the Femur Using Locked Plating Designs

The patient is positioned supine on a radiolucent table and intravenous antibiotics are administered. Excellent muscle relaxation and fluoroscopic images are essential. Preparing both legs in the operative field can make it easier to obtain a lateral view of the fractured extremity by lifting the normal extremity out of the C-arm beam (Fig. 83-9). A lateral incision is made at the flare of the lateral condyle. A plate of appropriate length is then inserted in a submuscular extraperiosteal fashion under fluoroscopic control. The plate is positioned as distally as possible on the distal fragment and provisionally held with a guide pin. It is critical to place this guide pin parallel to the knee joint to ensure excellent alignment. Limb length and rotation are then adjusted, and a second guide pin is placed proximally into the femoral shaft. Leaving metaphyseal comminution undisturbed by bridging

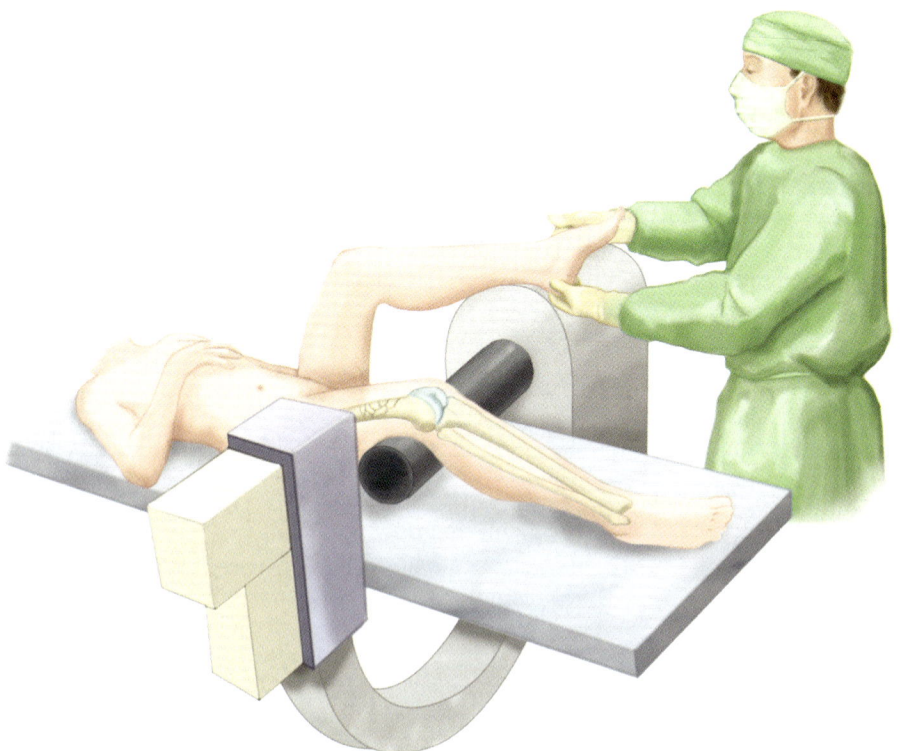

Figure 83-9. Patient positioning with the fluoroscope from the opposite side and inclusion of both lower extremities in the surgical draping. Such positioning allows simple lifting of the well leg to obtain a true lateral view. (Courtesy Mayo Foundation for Medical Education and Research, Rochester, Minn.)

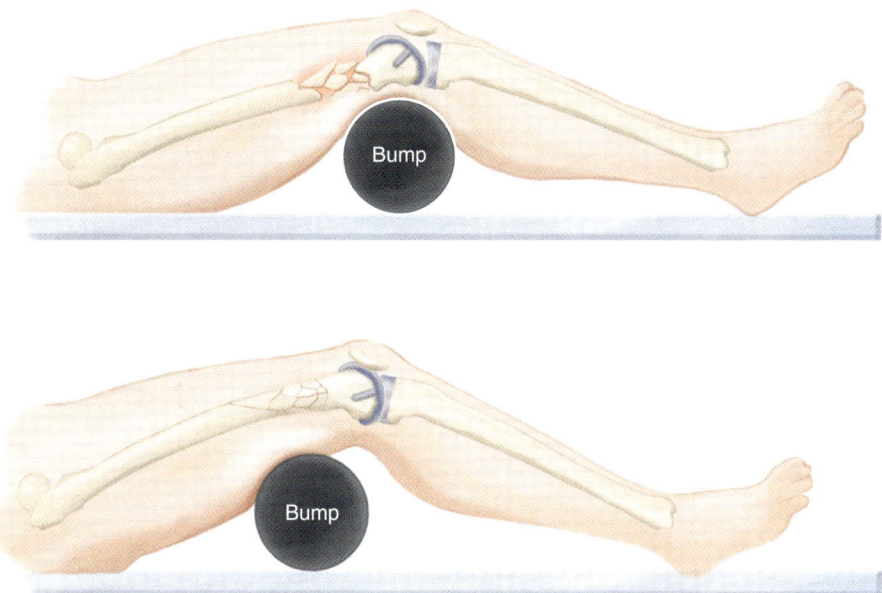

Figure 83-10. Use of a bump to assist in avoiding hyperextension of the distal fragment. A more proximal bump location allows the distal fragment to flex into the appropriate position. Often, multiple attempts with bumps of various sizes and positions are necessary to determine which will reduce the fracture best.

this area is critical to the success of this technique. A combination of gentle manual traction and placement of a small bump under the fracture site can assist with closed reduction, the most difficult portion of the procedure. There is a strong tendency for the distal fragment to tip into hyperextension because of pull of the gastrocnemius muscles (Figs. 83-10 to 83-15). With first-generation locking plates, it is critical to have the plate positioned accurately and have all aspects of the reduction complete before placing any locking screws. These screws will not pull the plate down to bone, nor will they allow fine adjustments in alignment once they are inserted. Newer locking plate designs offer so-called hybrid fixation that allows the surgeon a choice of locked, traditional unlocked, or polyaxial angled locked screws (PolyAx, DePuy, Warsaw, Ind). Distal fixation should be optimized by placing as many distal screws as possible. Typically, screws can pass just posterior to the anterior flange of the femoral component or just above the box of a posterior-stabilized housing. We attempt to use all distal screws and at least four proximal screws.

Fracture stability is assessed by intraoperatively testing flexion and varus-valgus stability under live fluoroscopy. The wound is closed in a routine layered fashion over a suction drain. Generally, a hinged knee brace is used postoperatively and knee motion is started when the wound is dry. Toe-touch weight bearing is maintained until healing is evident, typically at 10 to 12 weeks postprocedure (Fig. 83-16).

Periprosthetic Tibial Fractures

Periprosthetic fractures of the proximal tibia are rare, and no specific incidence has been reported. They typically occur around loose tibial components. Felix and associates[13] have reported on 102 periprosthetic tibial fractures below a total knee arthroplasty. Of these, 83 fractures occurred postoperatively and 19 occurred intraoperatively. The authors of this study developed a treatment-based classification system in which fractures were classified into three types based on the fixation status of the implant and four types based on the location of the fracture. Type A fractures occurred around implants that were radiographically well fixed, type B occurred in those that were radiographically loose, and type C fractures occurred intraoperatively. Type I fractures occurred at the tibial plateau, type II were located adjacent to the prosthetic stem, type III occurred distal to the prosthetic stem, and type IV involved the tibial tubercle. Type I fractures were the most common, accounting for 61 fractures. Type II fractures were the second most common, accounting for 22 fractures. Only 17 fractures occurred distal to the prosthetic stem. Most proximal fractures were associated with a loose prosthesis, and these were managed successfully with revision surgery, typically involving stems to bypass the deficient bone. Fractures around a stable implant were managed successfully by the standard principles for tibial fracture management. No large series has evaluated the outcomes of open reduction and internal fixation of periprosthetic fractures of the tibia below a total knee arthroplasty. Therefore, treatment of fractures of the tibia below a total knee arthroplasty is dictated by the location and stability of the fracture and the fixation status of the implant.[1,8,11,17,31] For example, closed reduction and casting may be very successful for spiral, "boot top"–type distal tibial fractures; however, a comminuted midshaft, same-level tibiofibular fracture would probably be difficult to manage nonoperatively.

Fractures of the tibia distal to the arthroplasty can often be managed by closed reduction and casting if appropriate alignment can be obtained. The tibial component obviously precludes the use of routine locked intramedullary nails, and therefore plating may be the best choice for unstable fractures with a healthy soft tissue envelope. Contemporary locked plate technology allows long, fixed-angle plates to be applied percutaneously, thus minimizing soft tissue dissection and the

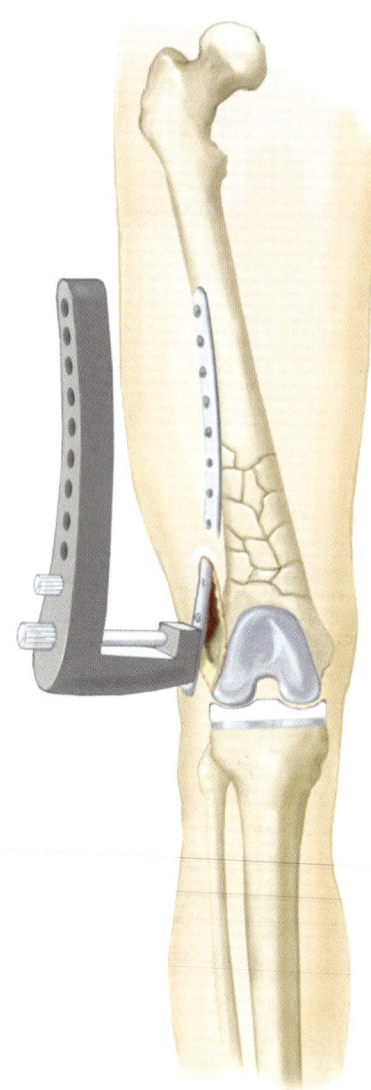

Figure 83-11. Percutaneous, submuscular, extraperiosteal insertion of a locked plate. (Courtesy Mayo Foundation for Medical Education and Research, Rochester, Minn.)

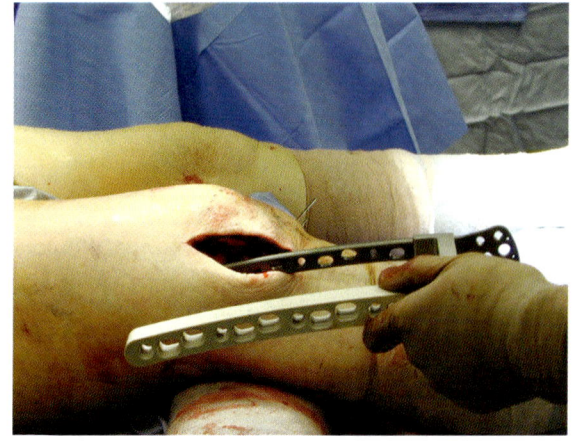

Figure 83-12. Clinical photograph of percutaneous plating.

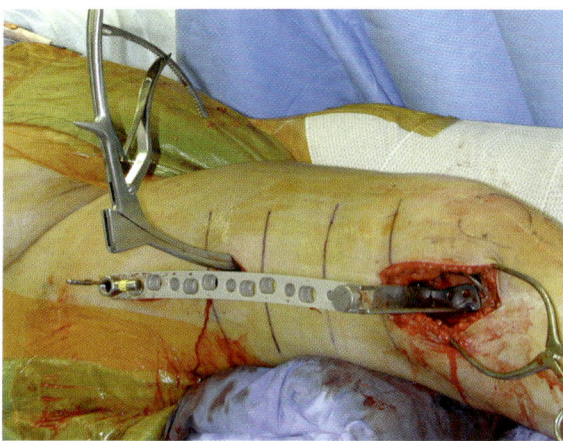

Figure 83-13. Use of percutaneous clamps for reduction and an aiming arm to target percutaneous screws.

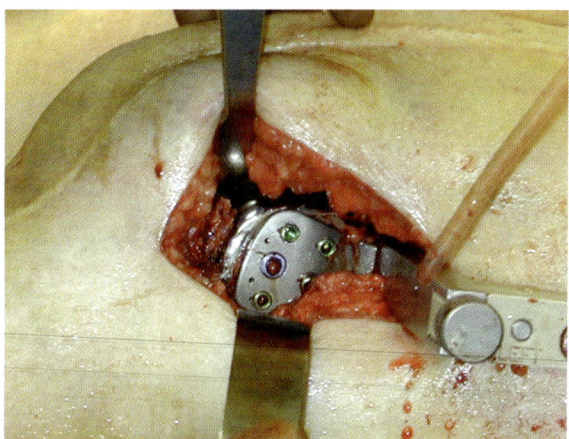

Figure 83-14. Clinical photograph demonstrating the minimally invasive nature of the internal fixation.

potential disastrous risk of wound infection. Additionally, excellent proximal fixation can be obtained with multiple locked screws placed around stems or keels of the tibial component.[7]

Fractures of the proximal end of the tibia in contact with the tibial component are typically associated with loosening of the tibial component and are usually managed with revision arthroplasty in which the deficient proximal bone is bypassed with an intramedullary stem.[1,11,13] The use of metal augmentation or structural bone grafting may be required if insufficient host bone support for the tibial component is available.

The use of external fixation is discouraged because of concern for pin site sepsis and potential contamination of the total knee arthroplasty. When external fixation is unavoidable, meticulous pin site care and extreme vigilance are recommended to minimize pin site infections. Because of this concern, we reserve the use of external fixation as a last resort when treating these injuries.

ROLE OF REVISION ARTHROPLASTY

The need to revise a total knee arthroplasty secondary to a periprosthetic fracture has become less common in our

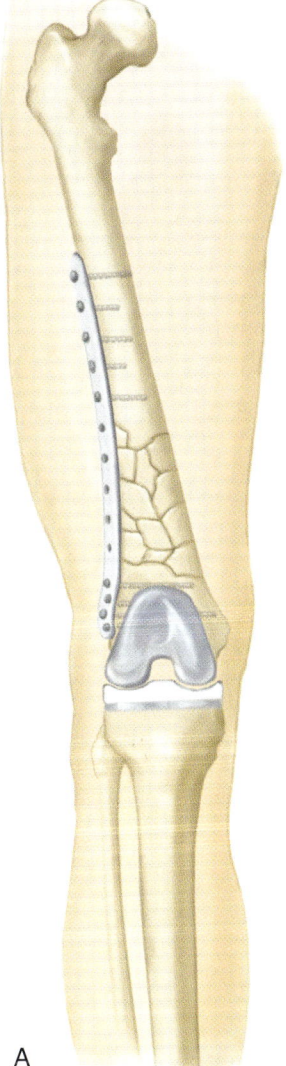

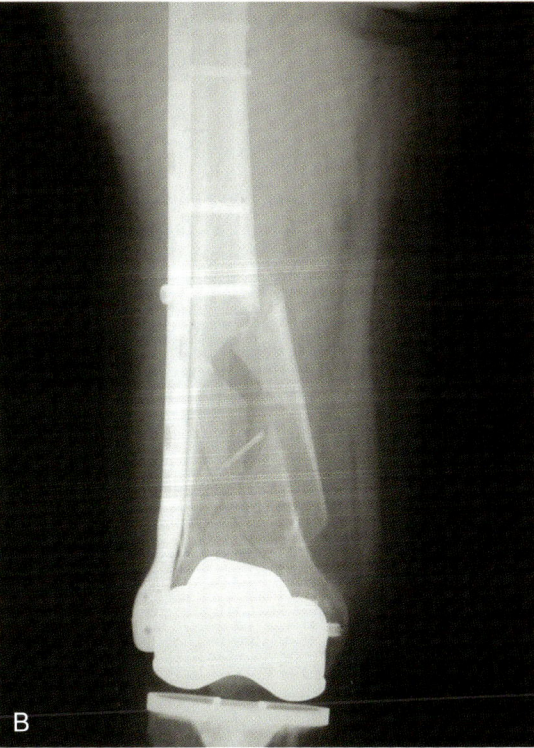

Figure 83-15. **A, B,** Bridge plating, leaving the metaphyseal comminution undisturbed and thereby preserving its vascularity. (Courtesy Mayo Foundation for Medical Education and Research, Rochester, Minn.)

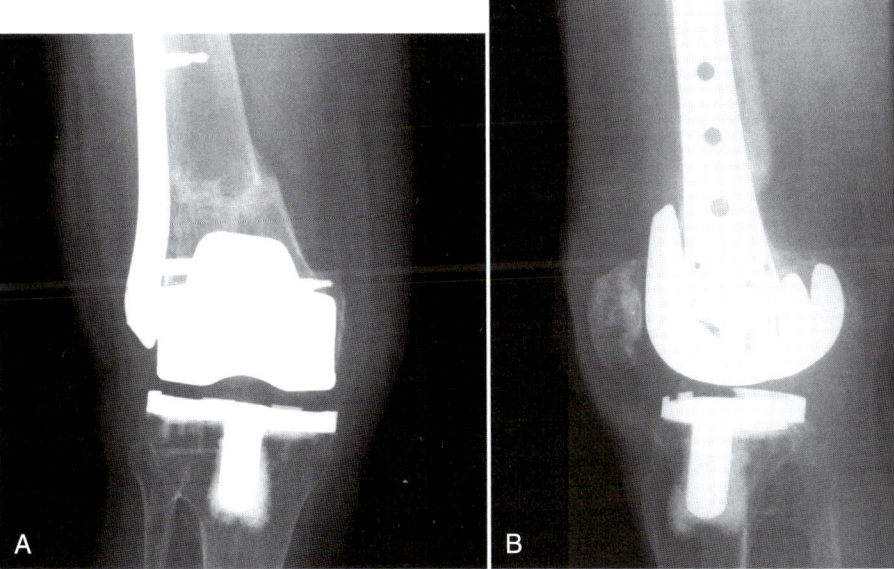

Figure 83-16. Anteroposterior **(A)** and lateral **(B)** views at follow-up after locked plating of a periprosthetic fracture. Note the slight valgus malalignment. Careful vigilance and fluoroscopic scrutiny are necessary to avoid malalignment when using percutaneous techniques.

practices with the advent of improved internal fixation devices such as locked plates. Typically, revision arthroplasty is reserved for fractures around a loose prosthesis, fractures with inadequate bone stock to allow for stable internal fixation, or recalcitrant supracondylar nonunion that requires resection and implantation of a so-called tumor prosthesis. Surgeons who treat periprosthetic fractures around a total knee arthroplasty must have the expertise and technical support to be able to perform long-stemmed, revision total knee arthroplasty because one is often unable to determine which reconstructive option is necessary until the fracture has been exposed in the operating room. Bony defects secondary to comminution, multiple previous procedures, presence of broken hardware, and presence of deformity may all present technical challenges to a successful outcome.

Supracondylar Fractures

Revision total knee arthroplasty with intramedullary femoral stems that engage the diaphysis and simultaneously stabilize the fracture can be effective. Cemented stems may be used, but care must be taken to prevent extrusion of cement into the fracture site. Allograft struts with cerclage wiring can be used to reinforce the stability provided by a long-stemmed prosthesis. It is unusual, however, to have distal femoral bone stock that is inadequate for internal fixation yet adequate for formal revision. The ideal indication for long-stemmed revision total knee arthroplasty would be the presence of adequate bone stock in the face of a supracondylar fracture with a grossly loose femoral component.[1,11] Most of the clinical data evaluating the outcomes of a simultaneous revision arthroplasty with intramedullary stem fixation of a supracondylar fracture have been gathered from the treatment of distal femoral nonunion in this situation. Kress and coworkers[27] have reported a small series of nonunions about the knee treated successfully with revision and uncemented femoral stems with bone grafting. Union was achieved in 6 months.

Distal femoral replacement tumor prostheses have been used for salvage of failed internal fixation of supracondylar periprosthetic femoral fractures. The long-term results of the kinematic rotating hinge prosthesis for oncologic resections about the knee have been good, with a 10-year survivorship of approximately 90%.[36] As their success becomes more predictable, the indications for such megaprostheses are expanding. Older patients with refractory periprosthetic supracondylar nonunion or those with acute fractures and bone stock inadequate for internal fixation are reasonable candidates for megaprostheses. Davila and colleagues[9] have reported a small series of supracondylar distal femoral nonunions treated with a megaprosthesis in older patients. They indicated that a cemented megaprosthesis in this patient population permits early ambulation and return to activities of daily living. Freedman and associates[14] have performed distal femoral replacement in five older patients with acute fractures and reported four good results and one poor result secondary to infection. The four patients with good results regained ambulation in less than 1 month and had an average arc of motion of 99 degrees. All patients had some degree of extension lag.

For a younger, active patient, an allograft prosthetic composite may be a better alternative. Distal femoral reconstruction with an allograft prosthetic composite to provide a biologic interface can help restore bone stock and potentially make future revision easier.[11,16] Kraay and coworkers[22] have reported a series of allograft prosthetic reconstructions for the treatment of supracondylar fractures in patients with total knee arthroplasties. At a minimum 2-year follow-up, the mean Knee Society score was 71 and the mean arc of motion was 96 degrees. All femoral components were well fixed at follow-up. The results of this study indicate that large segmental distal femoral allograft prosthetic composites can be a reasonable treatment method in this setting. In our experience, when revision is required because of fracture and distal bone loss, a tumor prosthesis is usually required.

Periprosthetic Fractures of the Tibia

Periprosthetic fractures of the tibia associated with total knee arthroplasty are extremely uncommon. Tibial fractures associated with loose components are best treated with revision arthroplasty, frequently with the use of a long stem to bypass the fracture.[1,11,13] Often, these fractures are associated with extensive osteolysis and may therefore require structural or morselized bone grafting, the use of metal wedges, metaphyseal filling sleeves or, in the most severe cases, a proximal tibial megaprosthesis or allograft prosthetic composite. Maximizing host bone support is critical for a good result. The largest series of periprosthetic tibial fractures around loose prostheses was reported by Rand and Coventry.[32] In their series, all 15 knees had varus axial malalignment when compared with those of a control group. Similar studies have confirmed that varus malalignment may be a potential risk factor for periprosthetic tibial fractures.[29,37] Specific technical considerations include careful soft tissue dissection and retraction to minimize soft tissue trauma to the already compromised skin flaps. It is important that surgeons undertaking these reconstructions be experienced in revision arthroplasty and fracture management techniques to achieve a successful outcome.

CONCLUSIONS

Periprosthetic fractures around total knee arthroplasty remain difficult injuries to treat. With the ever-growing older population, the incidence of these fractures will increase. Decision making regarding open reduction and internal fixation or revision arthroplasty is based on the fixation status of the implant, remaining bone quality, physiologic age of the patient, and location and stability of the fracture. Advances in locked plate technology show promise for improved fixation of such complex fractures, with minimal additional soft tissue trauma. More data are needed to define fully the role of this exciting technology along with traditional techniques of internal fixation of these fractures. Revision arthroplasty frequently requires modular distal femoral replacement, metal or allograft augmentation of bone deficiency, and long stems to bypass deficient bone. These reconstructions are demanding and fraught with complications. Attention to specific technical details is essential for a successful result.

KEY REFERENCES

Bolhofner BR, Carmen B, Clifford P: The results of open reduction and internal fixation of distal femur fractures using a biologic (indirect) reduction technique. J Orthop Trauma 10:372–377, 1996.

Davison BL: Varus collapse of comminuted distal femur fractures after ORIF with a lateral condylar buttress plate. Am J Orthop 32:27–30, 2003.

Felix N, Stuart M, Hanssen A: Periprosthetic fractures of the tibia associated with total knee arthroplasty. Clin Orthop Relat Res 345:113–124, 1997.

Freedman DL, Hak DJ, Johnson EE, et al: Total knee arthroplasty including a modular distal femoral component in elderly patients with acute fracture or nonunion. J Orthop Trauma 9:231–237, 1995.

Haidukewych GJ: Innovations in locking plate technology for orthopedic trauma. J Am Acad Orthop Surg 12:205–212, 2004.

Henry SL, Busconi B, Gold S, et al: Management of supracondylar femur fractures proximal to total knee prostheses with the GSH supracondylar intramedullary nail. Orthop Trans 19:153, 1995.

Koval KJ, Hoehl JJ, Kummer FJ, Simon JA: Distal femoral fixation: a biomechanical comparison of the standard condylar buttress plate, a locked buttress plate, and the 95-degree blade plate. J Orthop Trauma 11:521–524, 1997.

Kregor PJ, Hughes JL, Cole PA: Fixation of distal femoral fractures above total knee arthroplasty utilizing the Less Invasive Stabilization System (LISS). Injury 32:SC64–SC75, 2001.

Full references for this chapter can be found on www.expertconsult.com.

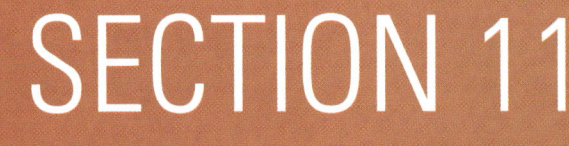

SECTION 11

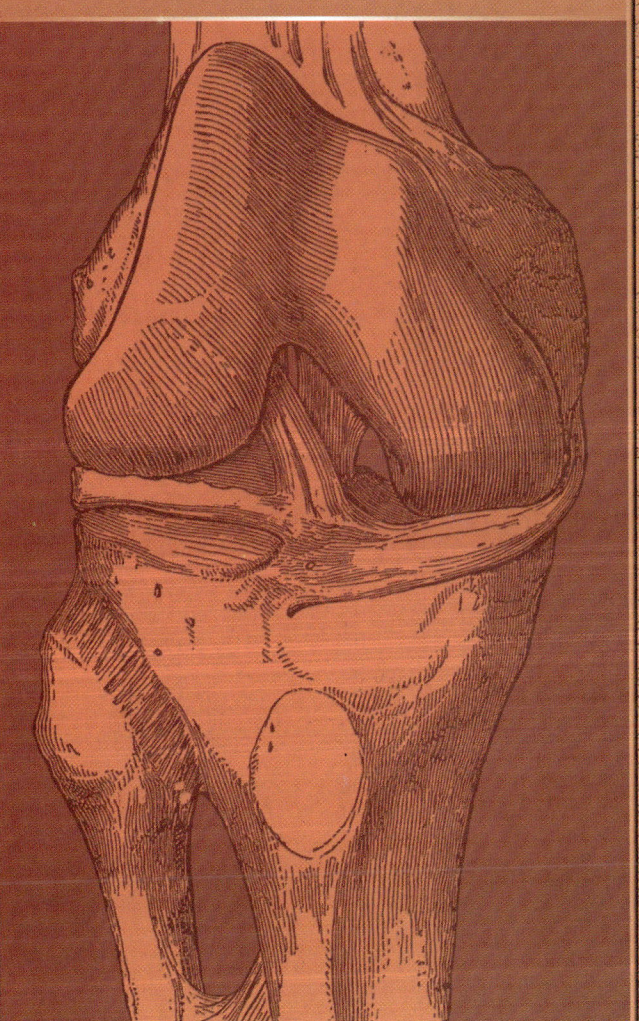

Pediatric Knee

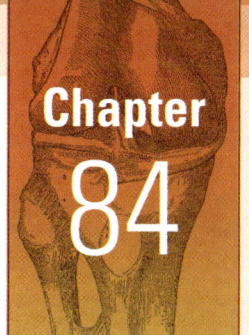

Chapter 84

Normal Knee Embryology and Development

James G. Jarvis and Hans K. Uhthoff

The term *embryology* infers the study of embryos. Today, embryology generally refers to the entire period of prenatal development, however, and includes the study of embryos and fetuses. Although prenatal development is more rapid than postnatal development and results in striking changes, the developmental mechanisms of the two periods are the same. "Embryology provides a mechanism to help understand the causes of variations in human structure. It illuminates gross anatomy and explains how both normal relations and abnormalities develop."[20]

OVERVIEW OF EMBRYOLOGY

Prenatal development consists of four sequential stages:
1. *Gametogenesis.* Gametogenesis is the process of formation and development of specialized generative cells called gametes, which unite at fertilization to form a single cell called a zygote.
2. *Early embryonic period (weeks 1 and 2).* The early embryonic phase encompasses the 2-week period from fertilization to implantation of the embryo, during which the zygote repeatedly divides. During week 2, the amniotic cavity and trilaminar embryonic disk are formed. The early embryo usually is aborted if a lethal or serious genetic defect is present, although at this time, the early embryo is less susceptible to teratogens than during the remainder of the embryonic period.
3. *Embryo (weeks 3 to 8).* Week 3 is the first week of organogenesis. The trilaminar embryonic disk develops, somites begin to form, and the neuroplate closes to form a neural tube (Fig. 84-1).[37] At week 4, the limb buds become recognizable, and the somites differentiate into three segments. The dermatome becomes skin, the myotome becomes muscle, and the sclerotome becomes cartilage and bone. Serious defects in limb development may originate at this time (Fig. 84-2).[36] By week 8, the basic organ systems are complete.
4. *Fetus (week 8 to term).* The first half of the fetal period is characterized by rapid growth and changes in body proportions. The lower limbs become proportionate, and most bones start to ossify. During the second half of gestation, growth continues, and body proportions become more infant-like (see Fig. 84-2).

Timing and Staging of Development

Gestational age based on the date of the mother's last menstrual period overestimates the actual gestational age by more than 2 weeks. To estimate age more accurately, embryos are staged according to the method of Streeter.[39] This system, a derivative of the Carnegie Embryonic Staging System, divides the embryonic period into 23 stages based on clearly defined details of either external form or the development of

structures.[26,27] The maturity of older embryos and fetuses is based on measurement of the crown-rump length.[28]

NORMAL SEQUENTIAL EMBRYOLOGIC DEVELOPMENT OF THE KNEE*

Week 6

Figure 84-3 shows an embryo at 6 weeks old, Streeter stage 17. The cartilaginous anlagen of femur and tibia are separated by cells of uniform density, the future femorotibial joint. Early evidence of cavitation, a sign of beginning joint formation, in the otherwise homogeneous, uniform interzone is easily recognizable.

Week 7

Figure 84-4 shows an embryo at 7 weeks old, Streeter stage 19. Already at this stage, the lateral femoral condyle and medial femoral condyle are well formed. The lateral collateral ligament spans from the femur to the fibular head, and the medial collateral ligament connects the femur to the tibia.

Week 8

Figure 84-5 shows an embryo at 8 weeks old. Not only is the posterior cruciate ligament seen, but also the multiple sites of beginning cavitation. Persistence of some of these intra-articular strands may lead to the development of plicae.

Week 10

Figure 84-6 shows a fetus 10 at weeks old. Between the medial femoral condyle and tibia, the medial meniscus can be seen. A small plica connects the midpart of the medial meniscus with the medial femoral condyle.

Figure 84-7 also shows a fetus at 10 weeks old. Not only the femur, tibia, and fibular head but also the anterior cruciate ligament are seen in the figure. At this stage, no vascular channels are present in the epiphyses.

Week 12.5

Figure 84-8 shows a fetus at 12.5 weeks old. A dense layer of cells covers the articular surfaces of the femur and tibia. Lateral to the lateral femoral condyle, the popliteus muscle is seen. Both menisci are well formed. Vessels are present at their periphery. Vascular channels are present in the femoral epiphysis. The posterior cruciate ligament inserts into the tibia.

Week 15.5

Figure 84-9 shows a fetus at 15.5 weeks old. The much longer lateral facet of the patella helps distinguish it from the medial

*NOTE: All specimens are from spontaneous abortions because no therapeutic abortions are permitted in our Catholic institution.

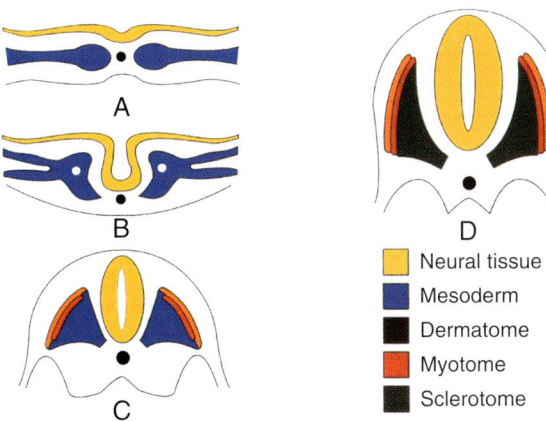

Figure 84-1. **A-D,** Trilaminar disk. **A,** The neural tube closes. The mesoderm differentiates into dermatome **(B)**, myotome **(C)**, and sclerotome **(D)**. (From Staheli L: Growth. In Staheli L: Practice of pediatric orthopedics, Philadelphia, 2001, Lippincott Williams & Wilkins.)

facet. The lateral retinaculum is much denser than the medial retinaculum.

Week 16.5

Figure 84-10 shows a fetus at 16.5 weeks old. The ossification processes that started in the diaphyses of the femur and tibia are progressing toward the metaphyses. At this stage, blood vessels still cross the growth plate. The suprapatellar bursa extends under the quadriceps muscle. The posterior cruciate ligament originates in the intercondylar fossa and infrapatellar fat pad.

Week 18

Figure 84-11 shows a fetus at 18 weeks old. The formation of the tibial tuberosity (TT) that had started at 14 weeks has continued to separate this apophysis from the tibial epiphysis as a result of an advancing ingrowth of vessels. A thick periosteum (PE) spans from the tuberosity to the tibial metaphysis.

	Age (wks)	Size (mm)	Shape	Form	Bones	Muscles	Nerves
Embryo			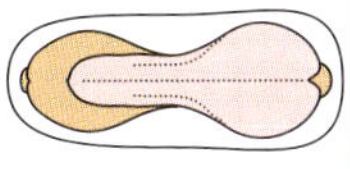	Trilaminar notochord			Neural plate
			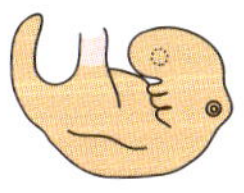	Limb buds	Sclerotomes	Somites	Neural tube
			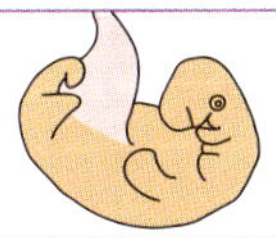	Hand plate	Mesenchyme condenses	Premuscle	
	12		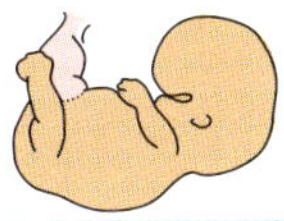	Digits	Chondrification	Fusion myotomes	
	17		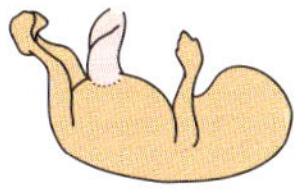	Limbs rotate	Early ossification	Differentiation	
	23		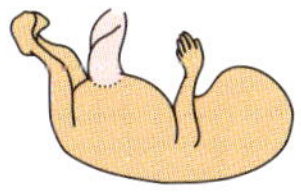	Fingers separate		Definite muscles	Cord equals vertebral length
Fetus	12	156	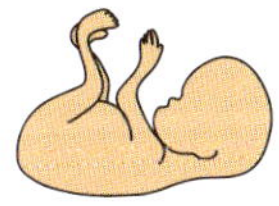	Sex determined	Ossification spreading		
	16	112	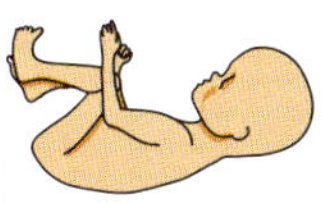	Face human	Joint cavities	Spontaneous activity	
	20 40	160– 350	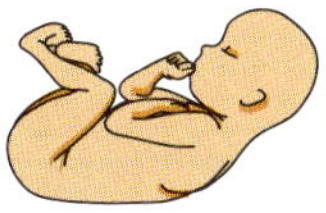	Body more proportional			Myelin sheath forms; cord ends L3

Figure 84-2. Prenatal development. This chart summarizes musculoskeletal development during embryonic and fetal life. (From Staheli L: Growth. In Staheli L: Practice of pediatric orthopedics, Philadelphia, 2001, Lippincott Williams & Wilkins.)

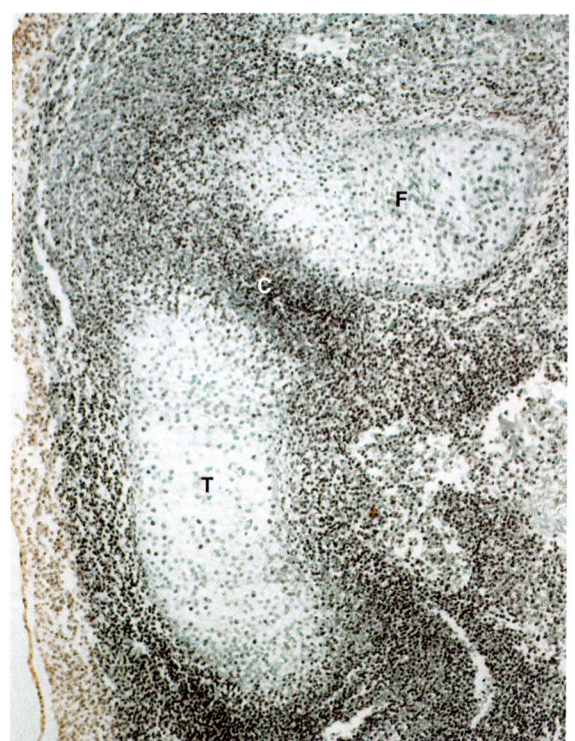

Figure 84-3. Embryo 117N, 6 weeks old, Streeter stage 17, sagittal section (see text). *C,* Cavitation; *F,* femur; *T,* tibia (Goldner, ×100).

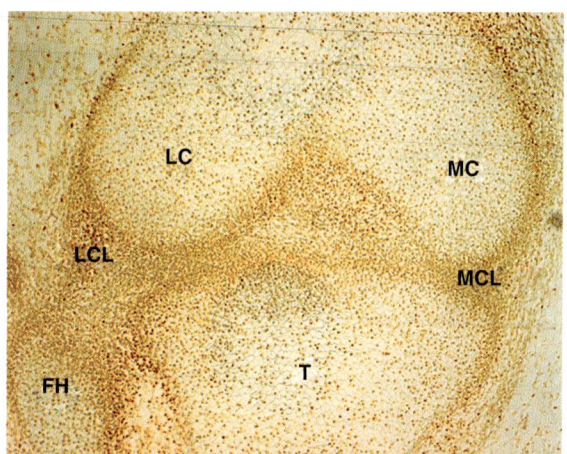

Figure 84-4. Embryo 123N, 7 weeks old, Streeter stage 19, frontal section (see text). *FH,* Fibular head; *LC,* lateral femoral condyle; *LCL,* lateral collateral ligament; *MC,* medial femoral condyle; *MCL,* medial collateral ligament; *T,* tibia (Azan, ×100).

Week 19

Figure 84-12 shows a fetus at 19 weeks old. Intra-articular tissues at the level of the intercondylar notch are visible in the figure. The fat pad is well developed. The posterior cruciate ligament is extra-articular.

Week 20

Figure 84-13 shows a fetus 20 at weeks old. Although vessels are seen at the periphery of the medial meniscus (MM), no vascular structures can be identified at its inner border.

Figure 84-14 also shows a fetus at 20 weeks old. The enchondral ossification of the tibia has almost reached its

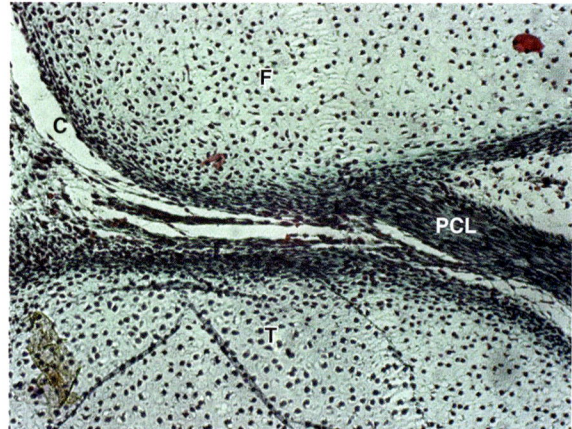

Figure 84-5. Embryo 50N, 8 weeks old, Streeter stage 23, sagittal section (see text). *C,* Area of cavitation; *F,* femur; *PCL,* posterior cruciate ligament; *T,* tibia (Azan, ×100).

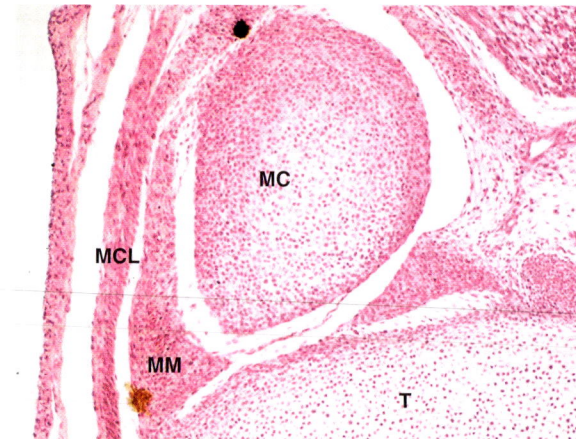

Figure 84-6. Fetus HHF2, 10 weeks old, frontal, slightly oblique section going through the posterior part of the medial compartment (see text). *MC,* Medial femoral condyle; *MCL,* medial collateral ligament; *MM,* medial meniscus; *T,* tibia (Azan, ×100).

final destination between the metaphysis and epiphysis. Ossification of the tibial tuberosity occurs late and is a postnatal event.[25,33] Strong collagenous tissue binds this apophysis to the periosteum of the tibia.

Week 40 (Full Term)

Figure 84-15 shows the knee of a full-term specimen. Rich vascularity is present at the base of the meniscus. The medial meniscus is attached to the medial collateral ligament (not separate).

EMBRYOLOGIC DEVELOPMENT OF VARIANTS AND SPECIFIC ABNORMALITIES

Discoid Lateral Meniscus

Discoid lateral meniscus initially was believed to be a failure of the embryologic degeneration of the center of the meniscus[35]; however, this subsequently was shown not to be the case.[15] It is now known that the lateral meniscus is semilunar

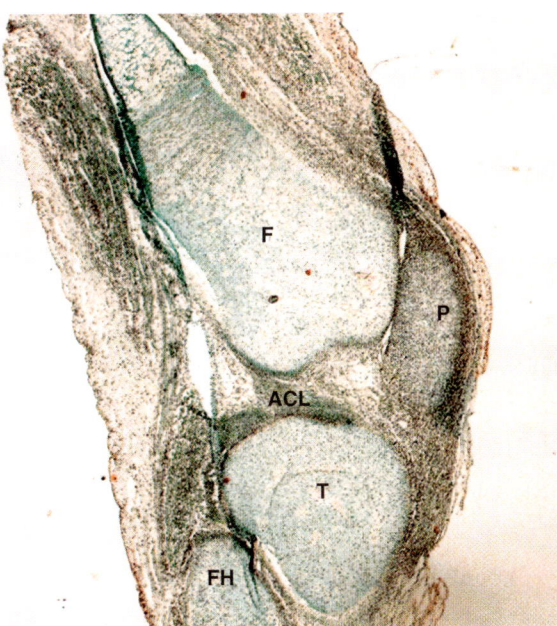

Figure 84-7. Fetus HKSAG3, 10 weeks old, sagittal section (see text). *ACL,* Anterior cruciate ligament; *F,* femur; *FH,* fibular head; *T,* tibia; *P,* patella (Goldner, ×20).

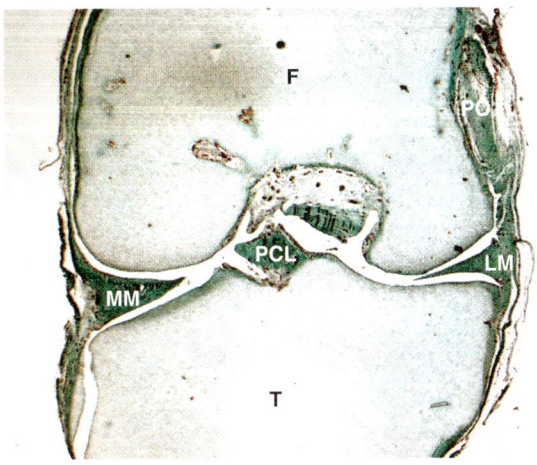

Figure 84-8. Fetus HK24F, 12.5 weeks old, frontal section (see text). *F,* Femur; *LM,* lateral meniscus; *MM,* medial meniscus; *PCL,* posterior cruciate ligament; *PO,* popliteus muscle; *T,* tibia (Goldner, ×20).

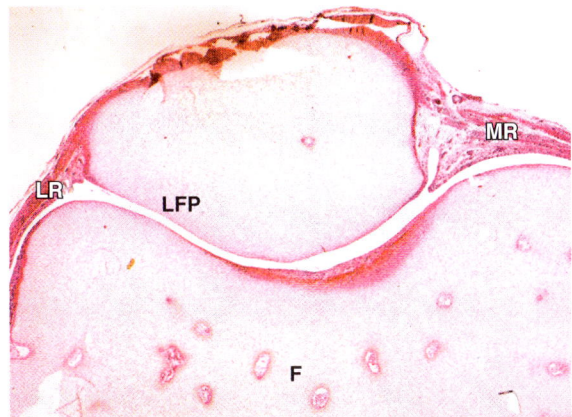

Figure 84-9. Fetus 130N, HKFr, 15.5 weeks old, frontal section going through the patellofemoral joint (see text). *F,* Femur; *LFP,* lateral facet of the patella; *LR,* lateral retinaculum; *MR,* medial retinaculum (Azan, ×20).

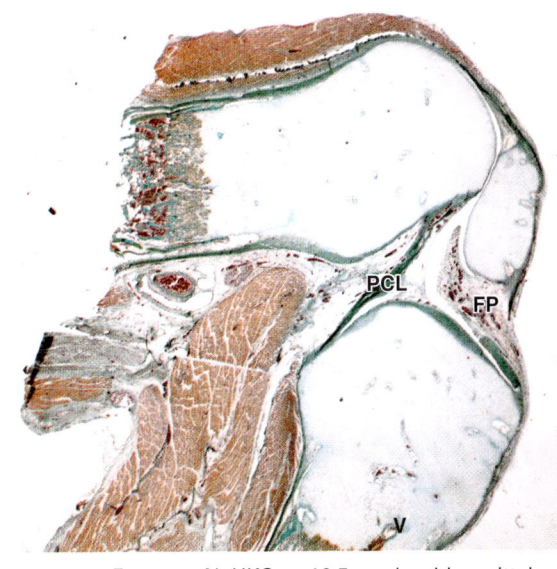

Figure 84-10. Fetus 147N, HKSag, 16.5 weeks old, sagittal section (see text). *FP,* Infrapatellar fat pad; *PCL,* posterior cruciate ligament; *V,* blood vessels (Goldner, ×5).

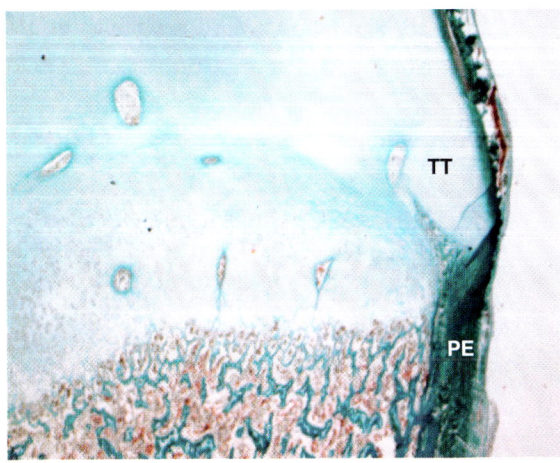

Figure 84-11. Fetus 73N, 18 weeks old, sagittal section (see text). *PE,* Periosteum; *TT,* tibial tuberosity (Goldner, ×20).

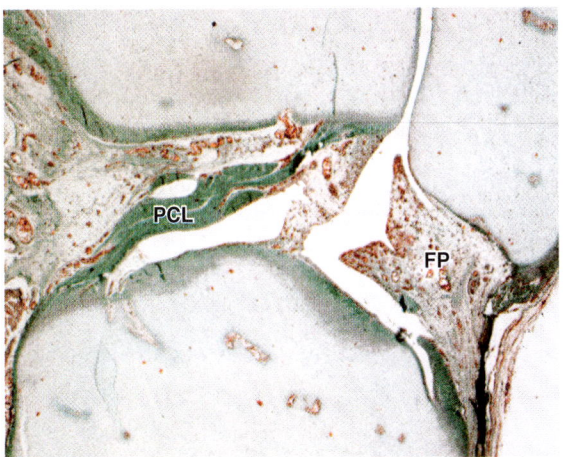

Figure 84-12. Fetus 28N, 19 weeks old, sagittal section (see text). *FP,* Fat pad; *PCL,* posterior cruciate ligament (Goldner, ×20).

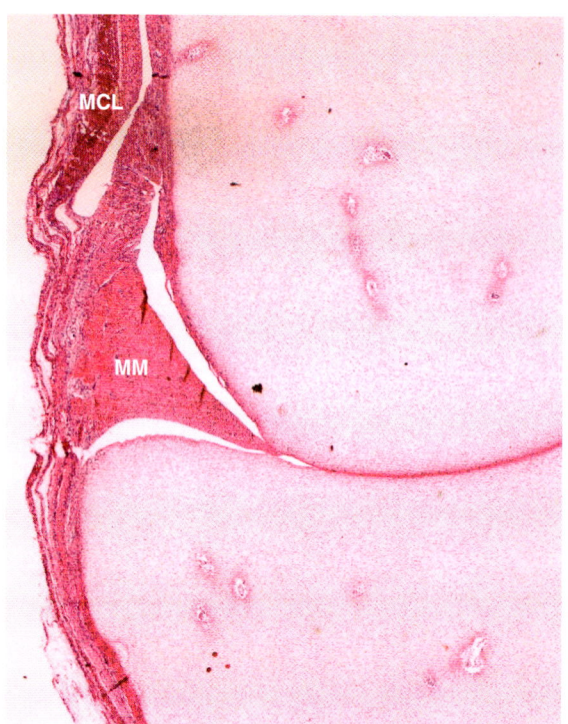

Figure 84-13. Fetus 132N, HKF, 20 weeks old, frontal section of the medial compartment (see text). *MCL,* Medial collateral ligament; *MM,* medial meniscus (Azan, ×20).

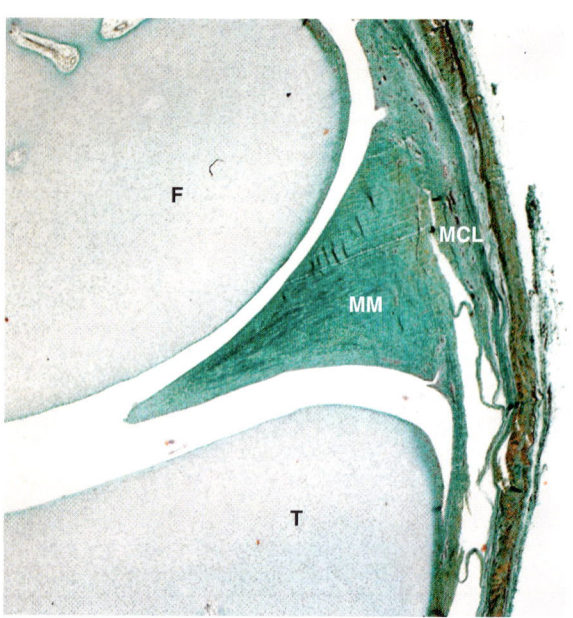

Figure 84-15. Fetus A10917, term, frontal section showing the medial meniscus (see text). *F,* Femur; *MCL,* medial collateral ligament; *MM,* medial meniscus; *T,* tibia (Goldner, ×20).

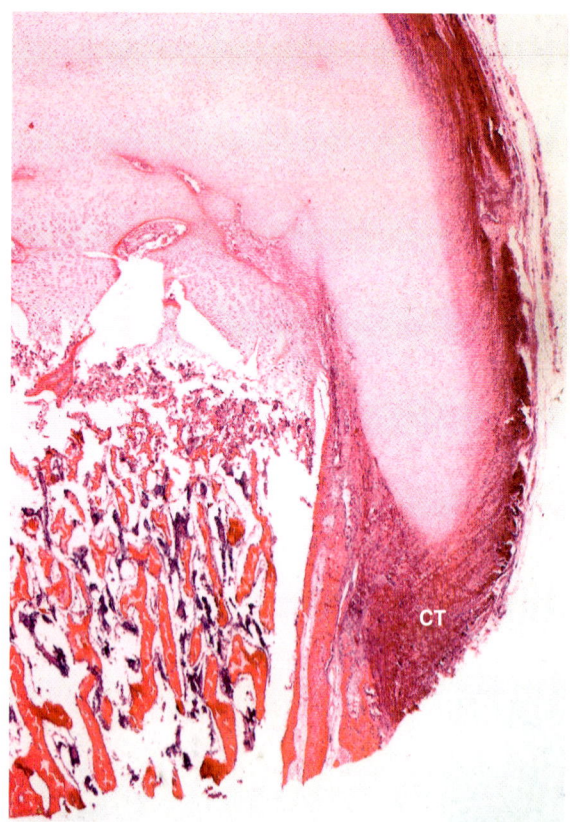

Figure 84-14. Fetus 116N, 20 weeks old, sagittal section at the level of the tibial tuberosity (see text). *CT,* Collagenous tissue (Azan, ×20).

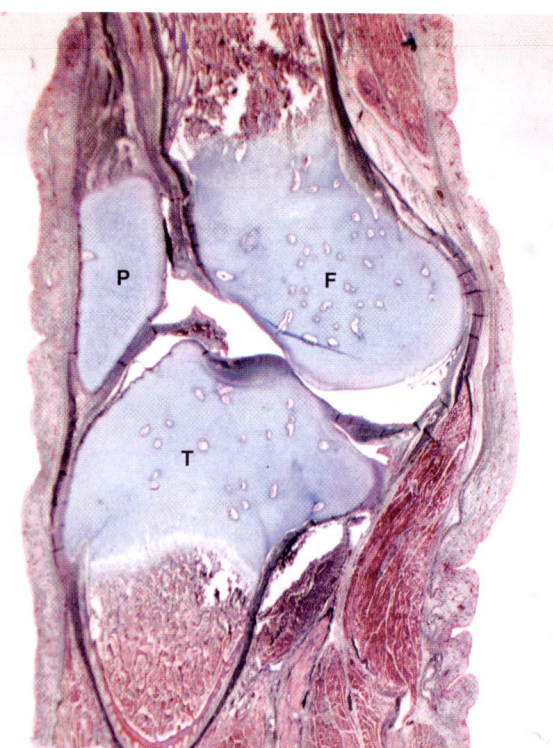

Figure 84-16. Fetus 71N, 19.5 weeks old, sagittal section (see text). *F,* Femur; *P,* patella; *T,* tibia (Azan, ×5).

in shape from its earliest development.[10,14,31] Although some discoid menisci (Wrisberg type 1) may be caused by abnormal meniscal attachments, because discoid menisci have been reported in very young children, the condition is likely the result of early development.[1,22]

Morphometric analyses have revealed that in the developing meniscus, the proportion of the area of meniscus to that of plateau is consistently higher in the lateral, compared with the medial, side.[9] Similarly, the layered structure of fibers developed earlier in the lateral meniscus than in the medial. The differential development of the lateral and medial sides of the meniscus may be involved in the early development of discoid meniscus.

Congenital Dislocation of the Knee

First described in the early 1800s,[4,30] congenital dislocation of the knee now can be diagnosed in the prenatal period using ultrasound.[6] Although congenital dislocation is seen frequently in association with other hereditary conditions (e.g., Larsen's syndrome), it is not believed to be genetic.[5,13,16,18] Uhthoff and Ogata[42] have reported congenital dislocation in a fetus of 19.5 weeks' gestation (see Fig. 84-16).

Figure 84-16 shows a fetus at 19.5 weeks old. This fetus presented with a bilateral (congenital) dislocation of the knee accompanied by rotation. Not only is the knee in hyperextension, but also the tibia is displaced anteriorly; it rides on the anterior surface of the femur. The joint cavity barely reaches under the patella. Despite more than 200 serial sections, we could not detect any trace of a cruciate ligament going from femur to tibia. An unusually strong component of fibrous tissue was noted in the quadriceps muscle.

Multiple causative theories involving intrauterine events have been proposed, including abnormal fetal position of hyperextension,[34] congenital absence of the cruciate ligaments,[16] fibrosis of quadriceps,[19] and intrauterine ischemia causing compartment syndrome–like fibrosis.[7] It has not always been possible to separate cause and effect, but these findings are most likely to be secondary adaptive changes.[42]

Bipartite Patella

Bipartite patella is a phenomenon of secondary ossification and probably a postnatal event.

Synovial Plica

The embryonic knee is partitioned into suprapatellar, medial, and lateral compartments by synovial septa. Synovial plicae are regarded as remnants of the divisions between these compartments that were present in the knee during embryologic development.[29] Although more typically seen in adults than children, residual synovial plicae have been noted in the fetus between 11 and 20 weeks of gestation (see Fig. 84-6).[24]

The suprapatellar plica can be explained as a septum between the suprapatellar bursa and patellofemoral cavitation. The infrapatellar plica may be considered a septum of the medial and lateral femorotibial cavitations. The mediopatellar plica is not a remnant of a septum of a distinct compartment present during the developmental stage, but

probably constitutes a remnant of mesenchymal tissue caused by developmental circumstances.[24]

Patellofemoral Instability and Congenital Dislocation of the Patella

Recurrent dislocation of the patella usually is caused by lateral malalignment of the quadriceps mechanism. Associated contributing factors, including ligamentous laxity, lateral soft tissue contractures, external tibial torsion, shallow intercondylar notch of the femur, patella alta, and vastus medialis insufficiency, play a role but mainly develop in the postnatal period.

In congenital dislocation of the patella, the patella is dislocated at birth and there is usually deformity of the knee. Although the condition has been reported within families,[21] it also is seen in association with other conditions, most notably arthrogryposis and Down syndrome.[17] Stanisavljevic and colleagues[38] have suggested that dislocation occurs during the first trimester as a result of failure of medial rotation of the myotome that contains the quadriceps mechanism.

Both patellar retinacula can be recognized in the fetus by 9.5 weeks. The lateral retinaculum is dense and fibrous, whereas the medial retinaculum is loosely arranged. The patella is not completely centered in the femoral groove and tends to ride more laterally. These two features may predispose to lateral tracking or dislocation of the patella or both (see Fig. 84-9).[8,42]

Congenital Absence of the Anterior Cruciate Ligament

Although typically described in association with congenital dislocation of the knee, congenital absence of the anterior cruciate ligament also has been reported as an isolated finding.[11] Associations with other abnormalities include congenital short femur,[2,12] congenital absence of the menisci,[40] congenital ring menisci,[3,23] and thrombocytopenic absent radius syndrome.[32,41]

KEY REFERENCES

Basmajian JV: A ring-shaped medial semi-lunar cartilage. J Bone Joint Surg Br 34:638, 1952.

Curtis B, Fisher R: Congenital hyperextension with anterior subluxation of the knee: surgical treatment and long-term observation. J Bone Joint Surg Am 51:255, 1969.

Finnegan M, Uhthoff H: The development of the knee. In Uhthoff HK, editor: The embryology of the human locomotor system, New York, 1990, Springer-Verlag, pp 129–140.

Gardner E, O'Rahilly R: The early development of the knee joint in staged human embryos. J Anat 102:289, 1968.

Johnson E, Audell R, Oppenheim WL: Congenital dislocation of the knee. J Pediatr Orthop 7:194, 1987.

Ogata S, Uhthoff HK: The development of synovial plicae in human knee joints: an embryologic study. Arthroscopy 6:315, 1990.

O'Rahilly R, Muller F: Developmental stages in human embryos, Washington, DC, 1987, Carnegie Institute of Washington.

Streeter GH: Developmental horizons in human embryos, Washington, DC, 1951, Carnegie Institution of Washington.

Uhthoff HK, Ogata S: Early intrauterine presence of congenital dislocation of the knee. J Pediatr Orthop 14:254, 1994.

Full references for this chapter can be found on www.expertconsult.com.

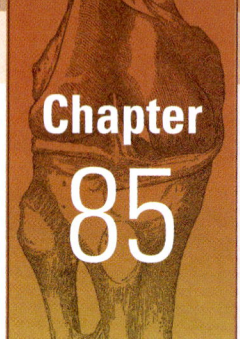

Chapter 85

Congenital Deformities of the Knee

Charles E. Johnston, II and Matthew E. Oetgen

Congenital deformities of the knee include hyperextension and flexion deformities, present at birth, whose severity at first glance may appear to be incompatible with functional ambulation. With the exception of patellar dislocation, which may not be apparent at birth, these deformities differ from acquired or developmental angular, torsional, or internal derangement problems in that they are usually obvious in the newborn or toddler. Once the diagnosis is made and the prognosis defined, rational early treatment can significantly improve the outlook for functional ambulation. In this chapter, we will describe and review treatment options for these relatively rare but dramatic congenital knee abnormalities.

CONGENITAL DISLOCATION OF THE KNEE

Few orthopedic birth abnormalities are as dramatic and obvious as congenital dislocation of the knee (CDK; Fig. 85-1A). Those unfamiliar with the deformity may describe the extremity as having the knee on backward because of the unstable excessive hyperextension combined with an element of angular deformity. CDK is rare, being only about 1% as common as congenital hip dislocation.[28] Even if the milder form of congenital hyperextension deformity is included as CDK, the incidence is still less than 0.1%.[8] It can be diagnosed prenatally by ultrasound.[15]

Clinically, the hyperextension deformity is unmistakable, with the femoral condyles often being prominent on the posterior distal thigh. The foot may present at the baby's face or shoulders, and this marked hyperflexion of the hip (see Fig. 85-1B), reflecting the positioning in utero,[48] raises the suspicion of concomitant congenital hip instability. Radiographically, the relationship between the distal femur and proximal tibia should be determined on a true lateral radiograph of the knee, defining that relationship as hyperextended, subluxated, or dislocated (Fig. 85-2). Next, the degree of passive flexion of the knee is important to determine prognosis, because it may be immediately apparent that the knee will flex and reduce with gentle stretching of the quadriceps, in which case the deformity can be classified clinically as grade 1 congenital hyperextension.[10,39] On the other hand, any flexion of the knee may be impossible, and the tibia, which is anteriorly translated in the resting position, may subluxate laterally on the femur when more vigorous flexion is attempted, indicating a grade 3 irreducible dislocation. (Fig. 85-3). The latter is always associated with significant quadriceps fibrosis and shortening, which may be the cause of the deformity.[43] An intermediate degree of contracture, a grade 2 subluxation, may be noted when the knee will not flex beyond neutral extension, but the femoral and tibial epiphyses are in contact and do not subluxate readily when flexion is attempted.

Equally important at the initial evaluation is the search for associated anomalies and syndromes. Both ipsilateral hip dysplasia and clubfoot are present 70% and 50% of the time, respectively,[5,29] with other anomalies of the upper extremity, face, gastrointestinal (GI), and genitourinary (GU) systems not uncommon. Bilateral CDK is almost always syndromic, most commonly associated with laxity syndromes such as Larsen, Beals, or Ehlers-Danlos syndrome. Neurologic conditions, such as arthrogryposis or spinal dysraphism, may have bilateral CDK, or may have one extended (dislocated) knee and one with a flexion deformity. Whether isolated or syndromic, abnormal fetal positioning is likely the common mechanical cause. Lack of movement because of neuromuscular conditions (e.g., arthrogryposis), or hyperlaxity can easily be invoked as causative once the abnormal position (see Fig. 85-1B) occurs, with quadriceps fibrosis and atrophy developing when the knee cannot move and the muscle shortens in the extended position. Hypoplasia of the patella and contracture of the iliotibial band probably result from the same lack of joint and muscle movement.

Ligamentous laxity, with elongation, insufficiency, or absence of the cruciate ligaments, has long been known as a complicating feature of CDK,[4,10,32,50] although it has been downplayed in importance in some reports.[5,55] Cruciate absence is actually typical of bilateral, syndromic cases (see Fig. 85-3D), and should be addressed as part of the comprehensive surgical management (see later). Conversely, isolated CDK (with or without ipsilateral hip or foot deformity) is often unilateral, and once reduced the knee is relatively stable (anterior cruciate ligament [ACL] present), and thus can been termed *stiff* CDK as opposed to the lax syndromic variety.

Other pathologic findings in grade 3 CDK include anterior subluxation of the posterolateral and posteromedial periarticular tissues, including hamstring tendons and the iliotibial (IT) band, because of the chronic hyperextension and anterior translation of the tibia on the femur (Fig. 85-4).[5,10,29,64] The suprapatellar pouch may be atrophic or obliterated, with adhesions between the hypoplastic patella and the femur and IT band. All these intra-articular abnormalities will need to be addressed surgically in the irreducible CDK.

Treatment

Nonoperative Management

Nonoperative treatment should begin as soon as possible in infancy. After determining the radiographic position (see Fig. 85-2A), initial flexibility of the quadriceps contracture is assessed by applying gentle traction to the tibia and attempting flexion of the knee.[34] The tibia, if anteriorly located, engages the distal femur and translates posteriorly with traction and, as the knee is flexed, a stable articulation can be palpated. In simple hyperextension cases, this may be readily

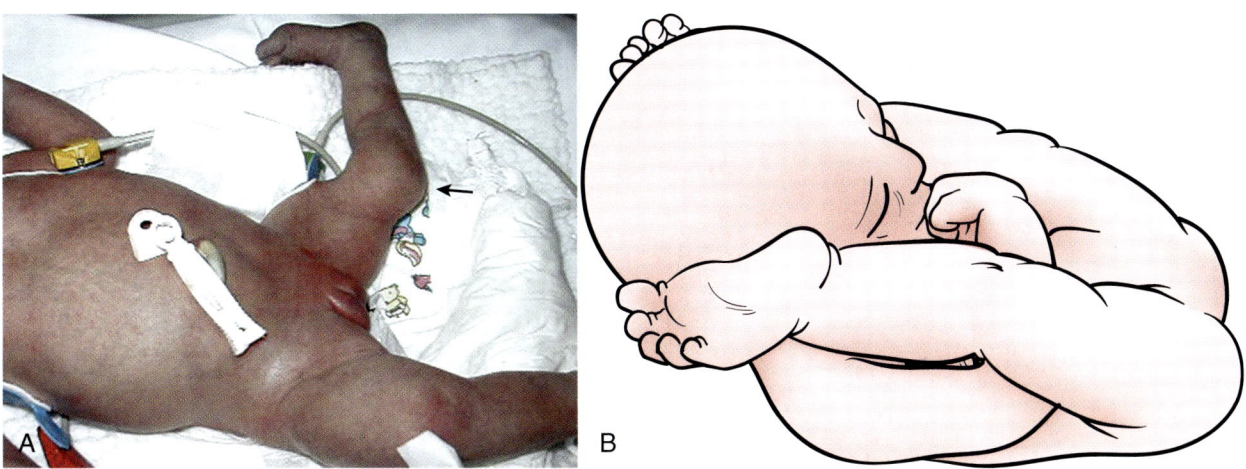

Figure 85-1. A, Left CDK in a newborn. The femoral condyles in the popliteal fossa are prominent *(arrow)*. **B,** Typical intrauterine position associated with CDK, hyperflexion of hips with hyperextended knees. (Redrawn from Niebauer JJ, King D: Congenital dislocation of the knee. J Bone Joint Surg Am 42:207, 1960.)

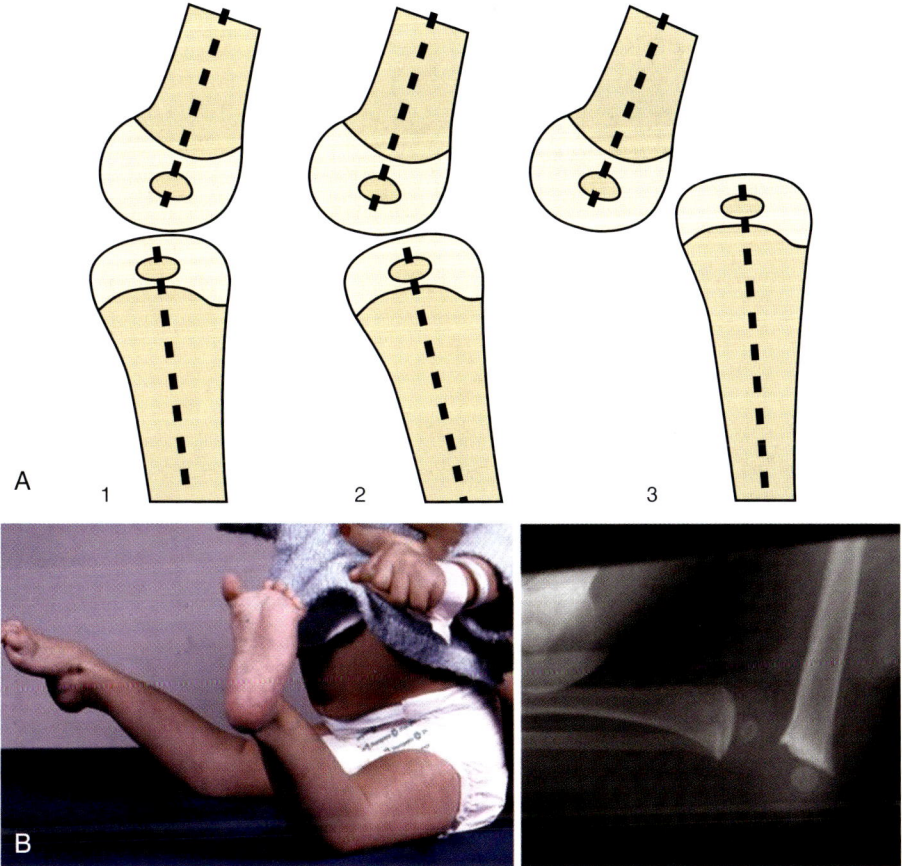

Figure 85-2. A, Degrees of congenital knee instability: *1,* hyperextension; *2,* subluxation; *3,* dislocation. **B,** Clinical and radiographic views of a grade 3 dislocation.

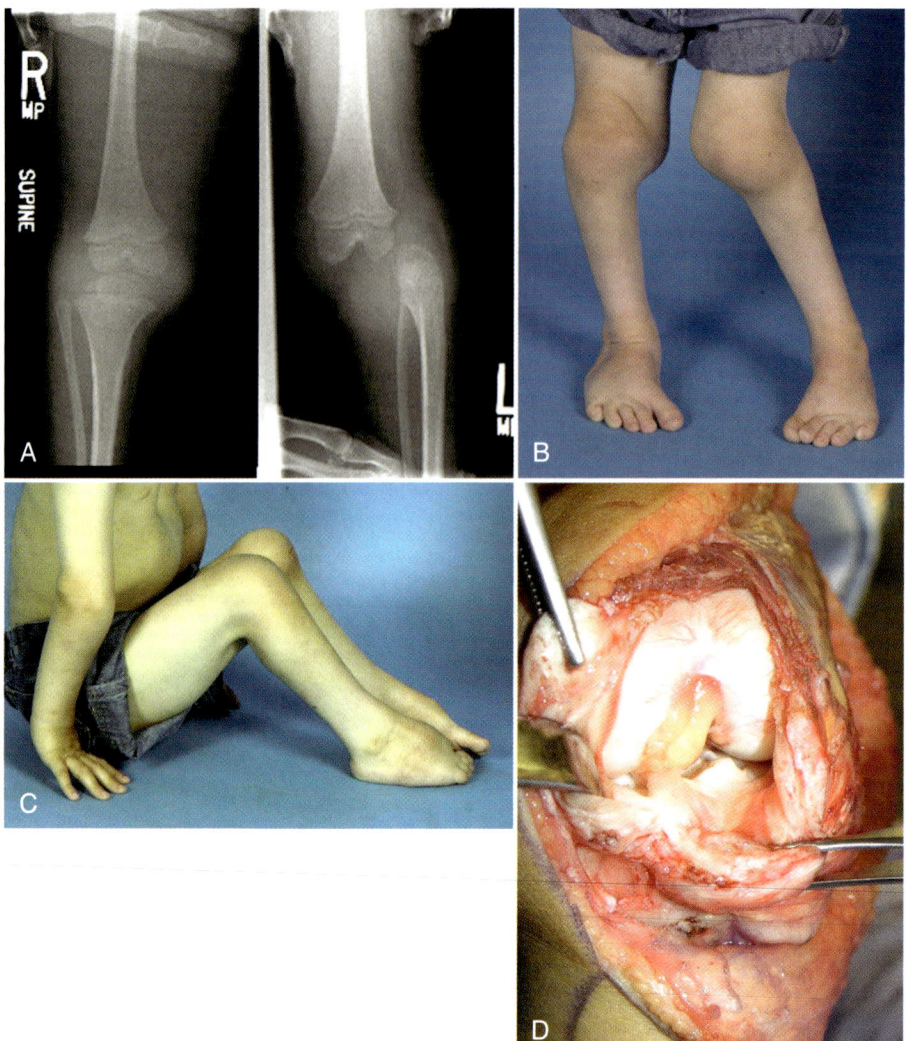

Figure 85-3. **A**, Anteroposterior radiographs of a 3-year-old boy with Larsen syndrome and bilateral CDK. **B**, Clinical appearance, grade 3 dislocation on the left. **C**, The right knee reduces with flexion, grade 1 (see Fig. 85-14). **D**, The ACL is congenitally absent.

achievable and usually maintained with an anterior plaster slab or a long-leg cast. The latter is actually more difficult to apply in the infant and maintain reduction. Obviously, forceful manipulation is contraindicated because of risk of pressure damage to cartilaginous epiphyses or fracture-separation of the proximal tibial physis (Fig. 85-5).[59] Serial manipulations and splinting in increasing flexion proceed until the knee will flex more than 90 degrees, at which time a removable plastic splint can be used to maintain reduction while allowing some active motion. Alternatively, if the patient also has an ipsilateral CDH, the knee can be maintained in a Pavlik harness while the hip is simultaneously addressed.

In knees with more severe quadriceps contracture preventing effective gradual flexion, femoral nerve block or botulinum toxin can been effective. Botox injection of the quadriceps has the added advantage of longer term paralysis of the quadriceps, allowing gradual stretching to occur, even when initial flexibility seemed unfavorable for nonoperative reduction (Fig. 85-6). A trial of nonoperative management, with or without adjunctive neuromuscular blockade, is appropriate initial treatment in infants up to 12 months of age.

Surgical Management

Surgical treatment is indicated for cases not responding to nonoperative means, and has been advocated for infants as early as 6 months of age.[4,5] Although earlier reduction of the knee may provide greater potential for remodeling of articular surfaces, patients as old as 4 years have had successful initial reduction, and patients as old as 16 years have had late gross instability with reducible but recurrent dislocation addressed. Considering the current use of femoral shortening to achieve reduction (see later), the earliest age for surgery should be when the surgeon thinks that the femur is robust enough to accept meaningful internal fixation to stabilize a shortening osteotomy.

Reduction and Flexion With Femoral Shortening

Classic surgical treatment of CDK has invariably used extensive V-Y quadriceps tendon lengthening (Fig. 85-7; see Fig. 85-4) to gain flexion, and hence reduction, of the joint. Outcomes of such lengthenings are poorly documented in many series, because simple documentation of reduction and

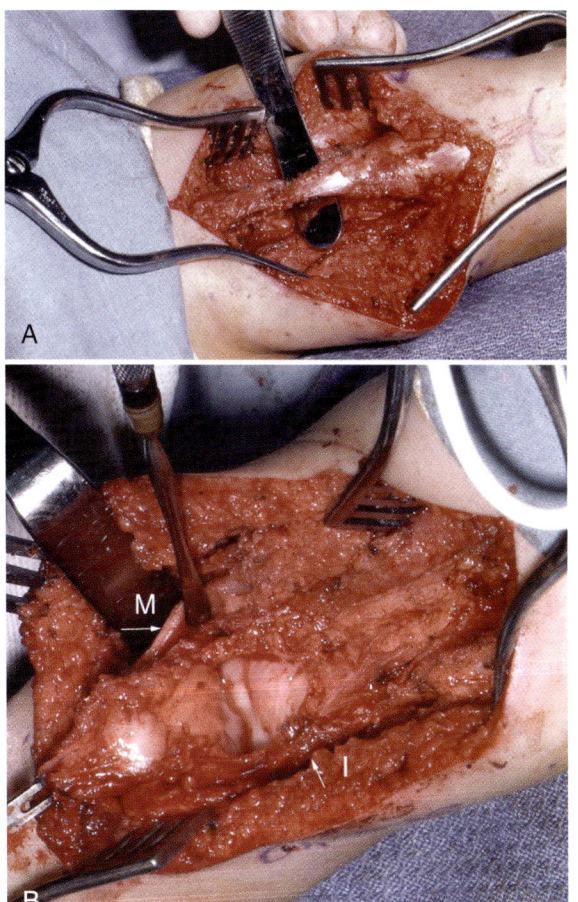

Figure 85-4. **A,** Contracted quadriceps tendon prior to V-Y lengthening (not recommended during open reduction). The hip is to the right. **B,** Medial hamstrings *(M)* and IT band *(I)* both subluxated anterior to the distal femur (note physis). The patella has been reflected distally with the quadriceps tendon.

reporting of passive range of motion is sometimes all that is recorded. Because many patients have other anomalies and comorbidities affecting outcome, the functional results of the knees themselves have rarely been reported. Actually, the extensive lengthening invariably leads to weakness and an extensor lag, and the extensive dissection required to obtain such length produces additional fibrosis, limiting flexion. Finally, wound healing over the anterior knee surface may be compromised because of ischemia produced by the flexion stretching the contracted anterior skin (see Fig. 85-7C).

In addition to the quadricepsplasty, arthrotomy must be performed to mobilize the anteriorly subluxated medial and lateral periarticular structures and allow them to relocate to their normal anatomic position as the knee is flexed (see Fig. 85-4B). However, once the knee is reduced in flexion, the redundant posterior capsule resulting from that maneuver has rarely been addressed (by capsulorrhaphy), thus inviting a redislocation into the same incompetent posterior space. The irrationale of this oversight can be easily appreciated if one considers that a late open reduction of a congenital hip dislocation would never be completed without performing a capsulorrhaphy to obliterate a potential space into which the femoral head could redislocate. Thus, if the ACL is also

congenitally absent in a CDK reduced without capsulorrhaphy, it is hardly surprising that chronic hyperlaxity-instability of the knee at a minimum, and frank redislocation at the other extreme, would be the common outcome of knees treated by such an approach, especially if flexion is limited by the scarred fibrotic quadriceps muscle, which has been extensively dissected.

As a result, we strongly recommend that V-Y quadricepsplasty should be abandoned in favor of femoral shortening to minimize quadriceps dissection and weakening (Fig. 85-8). Acute femoral shortening decompresses the anterior skin and allows knee flexion without surgical lengthening of the muscle. The operative procedure begins with a lateral parapatellar arthrotomy incision that is extended proximally along the lateral femur to allow mobilization of the distal contracted lateral tissues (IT band, released from its distal insertion, and vastus lateralis from intermuscular septum) and provide subperiosteal access to the supracondylar region for the bone shortening (Fig. 85-9). The quadriceps tendon, patella, and patellar tendon are mobilized (skeletonized) as a continuous longitudinal structure via a medial arthrotomy to allow sharp dissection and elevation of medial periarticular structures (pes tendons), which are subluxated anteriorly. The intercondylar notch is inspected for the presence or absence of the anterior cruciate ligament. Once the femur is acutely shortened and plated—usually approximately 2.0 to 2.5 cm is removed—the knee will usually reduce with flexion, and the only repair necessary is to stabilize the patellar mechanism in the intercondylar groove, generaally by medial imbrication and advancement of the vastus medialis obliquus (see Fig. 85-9E and F). The lateral release is repaired only to the extent of covering the internal fixation.

Capsulorrhaphy is performed at the posterolateral corner of the lateral femoral condyle by bluntly dissecting the capsule, with the knee flexed, from the more superficial tissues with an elevator. The dissection is simplified once the it band and vastus lateralis have been released and mobilized. The lateral half of the posterior capsule is imbricated proximal to the distal edges following excision of 1 to 1.5 cm of redundant patulous capsule (Fig. 85-10). Shortening of the hamstrings[4,5,29] may be done in conjunction with the capsulorrhaphy (and ACL reconstruction, if necessary; see later), but should not be considered a replacement for it.

The posteromedial capsulorrhaphy is performed through a separate 3- to 4-cm incision behind the medial femoral condyle (Fig. 85-11). This incision can be located by placing a blunt instrument from inside the arthrotomy to the posteromedial corner and then cutting down on the instrument tenting the skin. The redundant capsule is dissected free of superficial tissues with the knee flexed, a segment excised, and the imbrication performed (see Fig. 85-11B-D). Following the medial-lateral capsulorrhaphies, the knee should lack 30 degrees or more from full extension; the patient will eventually stretch this iatrogenic flexion contracture in 4 to 6 months.

At this point, the knee must be assessed for ligamentous instability, especially anterior drawer with the knee flexed; the posterior capsulorrhaphy should prevent significant drawer in maximum extension. The surgeon must decide whether the ACL should be reconstructed if congenitally absent or severely attenuated. If anterior drawer is unacceptable, the ligament should be reconstructed, if not during this

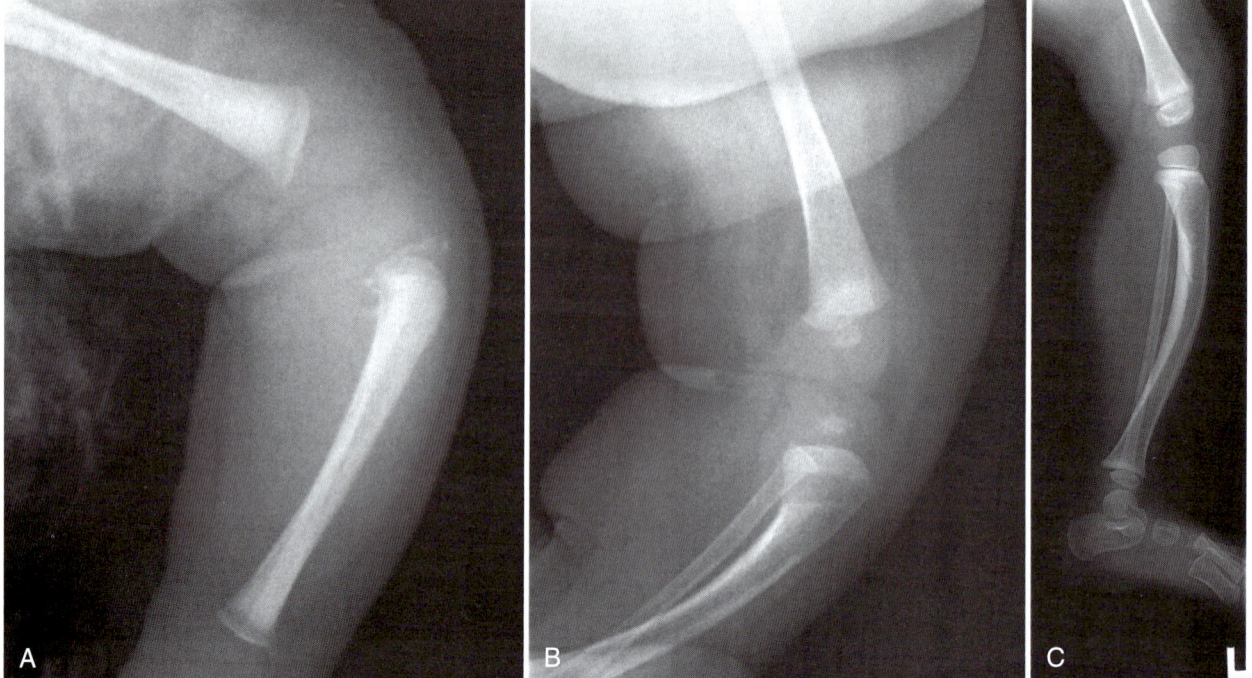

Figure 85-5. **A,** Fracture-separation of the proximal tibial epiphysis in a 2-week-old infant initially with a hyperextended knee. **B,** Healed fracture at age 4 months. The limb was splinted in the degree of flexion obtained in **A. C,** Residual antecurvatum deformity with otherwise normal growth of the tibia, age 3 years.

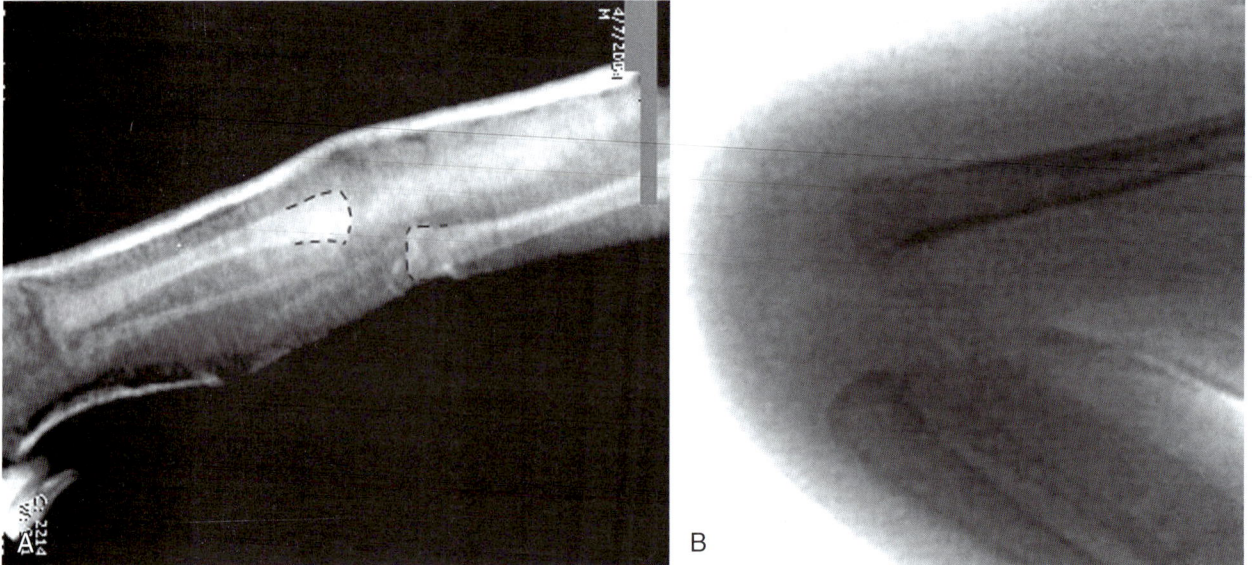

Figure 85-6. **A,** Right knee, failed closed reduction in a 2-month-old infant. **B,** Botox injection was performed twice, at 1-month intervals, and daily manipulations carried out. Full flexion-reduction was achieved 2 months later.

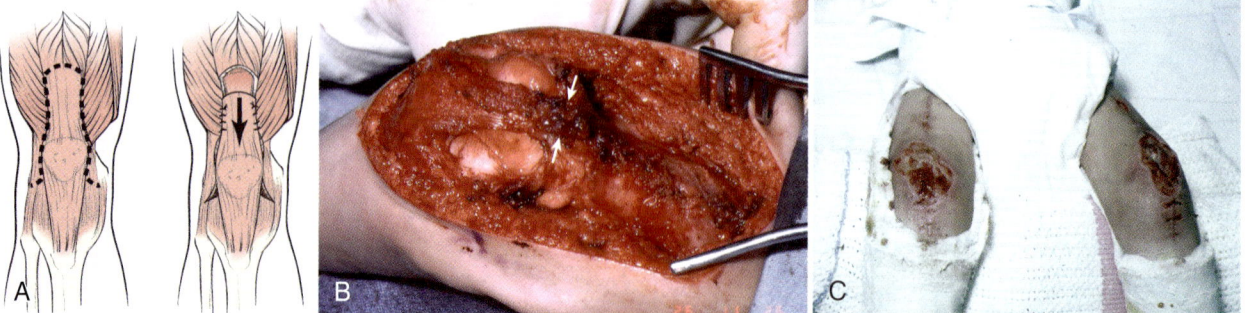

Figure 85-7. **A,** Classic V-Y quadricepsplasty. **B,** The resulting repair of the quadriceps tendon *(arrows)* is tenuous at best because of the extensive lengthening required to gain knee reduction (same patient as in Fig. 85-4). **C,** Wound dehiscence-slough as a result of skin necrosis from knee flexion. (**A** from Curtis B, Fisher R: Congenital hyperextension with anterior subluxation of the knee; surgical treatment and long-term observations. J Bone Joint Surg Am 41: 255, 1969.)

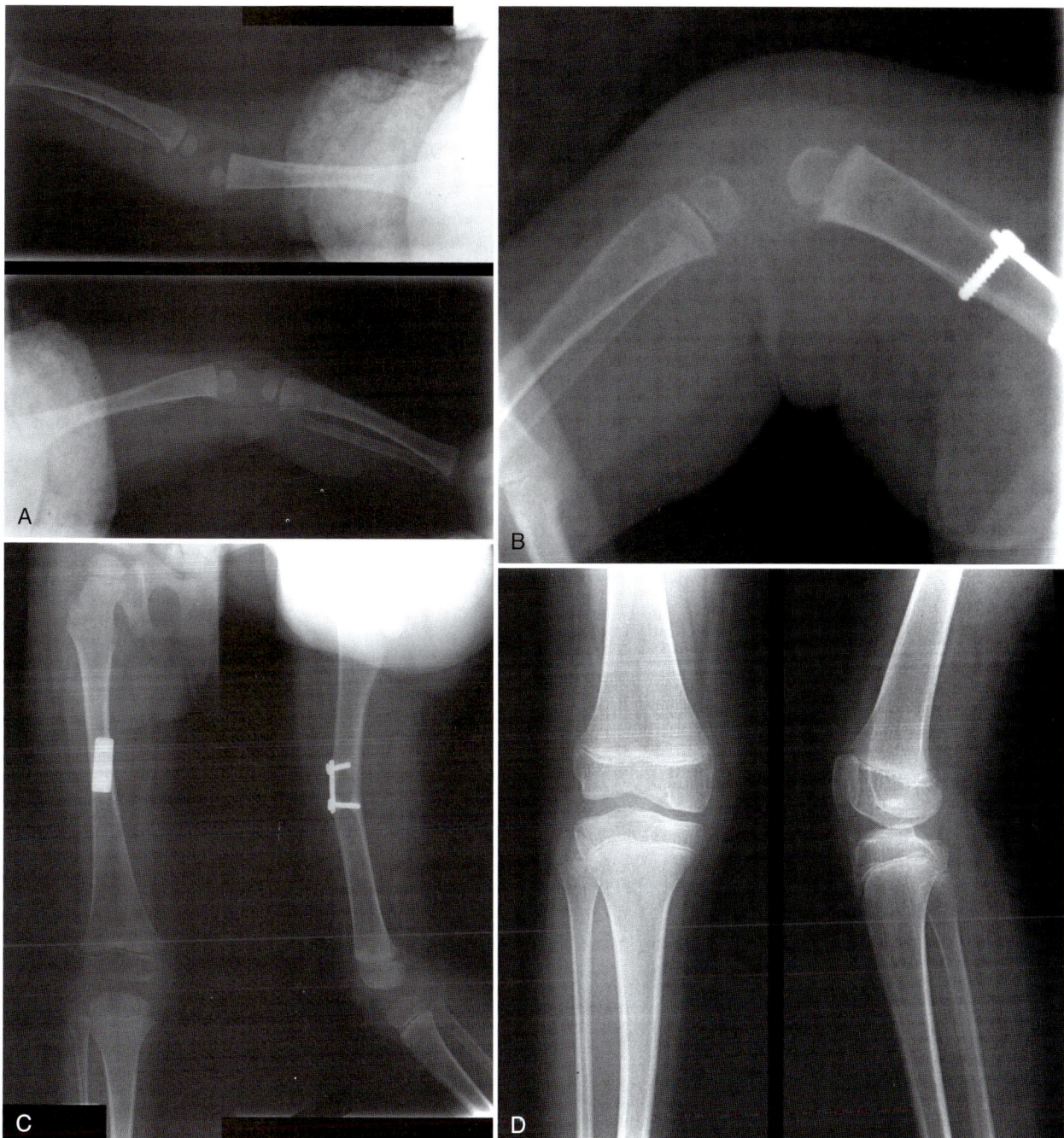

Figure 85-8. A, Lateral radiographs of a 6-month-old female with persistent subluxation and inadequate flexion. **B,** Four months following limited open reduction (no quadriceps tendon lengthening) with femoral shortening. **C,** Three years postoperatively. **D,** 12 years postoperatively. Range of motion is 5 to 70 degrees of flexion, with normal quadriceps strength. Note the hypoplastic patella. She is completely asymptomatic other than the limited flexion.

procedure, then as a staged procedure later. If ACL competence is satisfactory, the wounds are closed and the knee casted in 45 to 60 degrees of flexion for 8 weeks, followed by gradual active range of motion exercises, with full extension limited by a brace for the first 4 months.

We have recently determined[49] the long-term outcomes of seven patients (nine knees) who underwent surgical correction of CDK, with objective criteria that included functional outcome assessment (Lysholm knee questionnaire, Pediatric Outcomes Data Collection Instrument [PODCI]) and three-dimensional kinematic and kinetic gait evaluation. The

patients were evaluated as a group and compared based on surgical approach (femoral shortening vs. V-Y quadricepsplasty) at an average of 12-year follow-up. A fairly normal total arc of knee motion (112 degrees) was found, with only one patient from each group demonstrating an extensor lag. Although not statistically significant, the femoral shortening group did demonstrate a better range of motion and Lysholm knee scores when compared with the V-Y quadricepsplasty group. Gait analysis of these patients demonstrated that they walked with more flexion during stance and achieved less peak knee flexion during swing as compared with normal

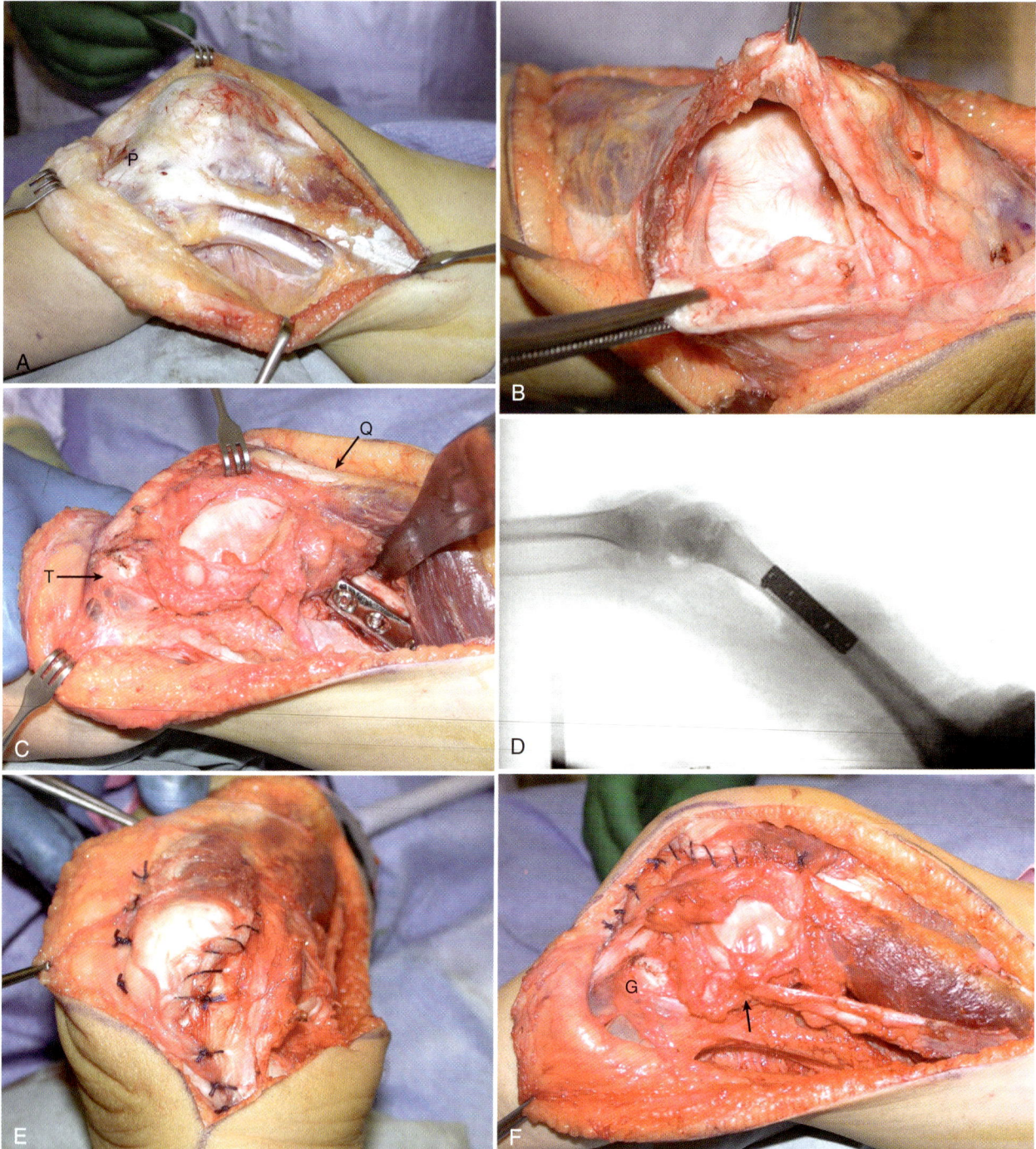

Figure 85-9. A, Lateral knee, distal femoral exposure. The tibia is dislocated posterolaterally (same patient as in Fig. 85-3, left knee). The IT band and biceps are seen prior to release of the former from its insertion. Anteriorly, the patellar tendon is marked. **B,** Medial arthrotomy. The vastus medialis and medial retinaculum are being separated from the quadriceps tendon (inferior clamp). **C,** The femur has been shortened and plated. The tibia *(T)* now reduces under direct vision. The quadriceps mechanism *(Q)* is in continuity. **D,** Intraoperative radiograph confirming reduction. **E,** Anterior view of advancement-imbrication of vastus medialis to hold patella centralized (medial to right). **F,** Lateral view of the imbrication. No attempt has been made to close the lateral arthrotomy. The vastus lateralis covers the plate. Posterolateral capsulorrhaphy has been performed deep to the IT band, which has been reattached to the posterolateral condyle *(arrow)*. Reattachment to Gerdy's tubercle *(G)* is both impossible and contraindicated.

controls (Fig. 85-12). Comparison of the gait between the patients with femoral shortening and V-Y quadricepsplasty showed minor differences in the sagittal plane of the knee, which were consistent with increased stiffness in the quadriceps muscle in the V-Y quadricepsplasty group, consistent

with more extensive dissection and resultant fibrosis (Fig. 85-13). Because of the small number of patients, caution must be used in drawing definitive conclusions, but overall it does appear that patients treated surgically for CDK maintain functionality fairly well, with femoral shortening providing

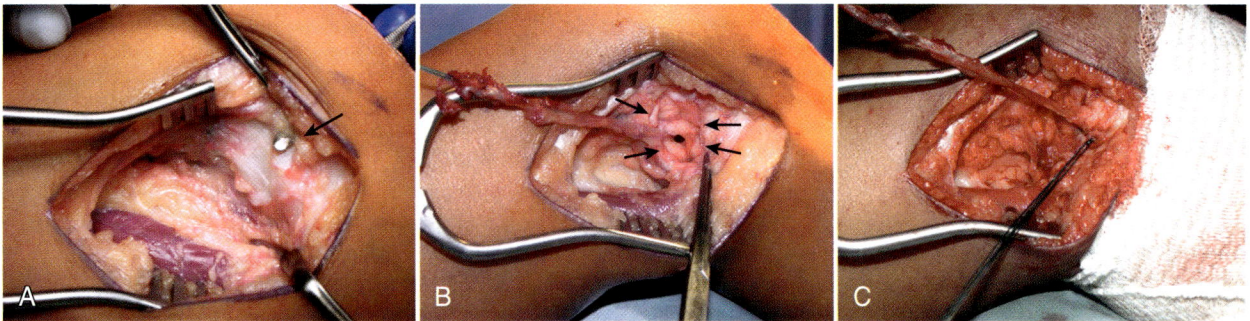

Figure 85-10. **A,** Exposure of posterolateral capsule (hip to left). A Freear elevator *(arrow)* has been inserted through the anterior arthrotomy to localize site of capsular incision. **B,** Excision of posterolateral capsule (*arrows* indicating capsule edges) with semitendinosus graft inserted through capsular window. **C,** Completed posterolateral capsulorrhaphy.

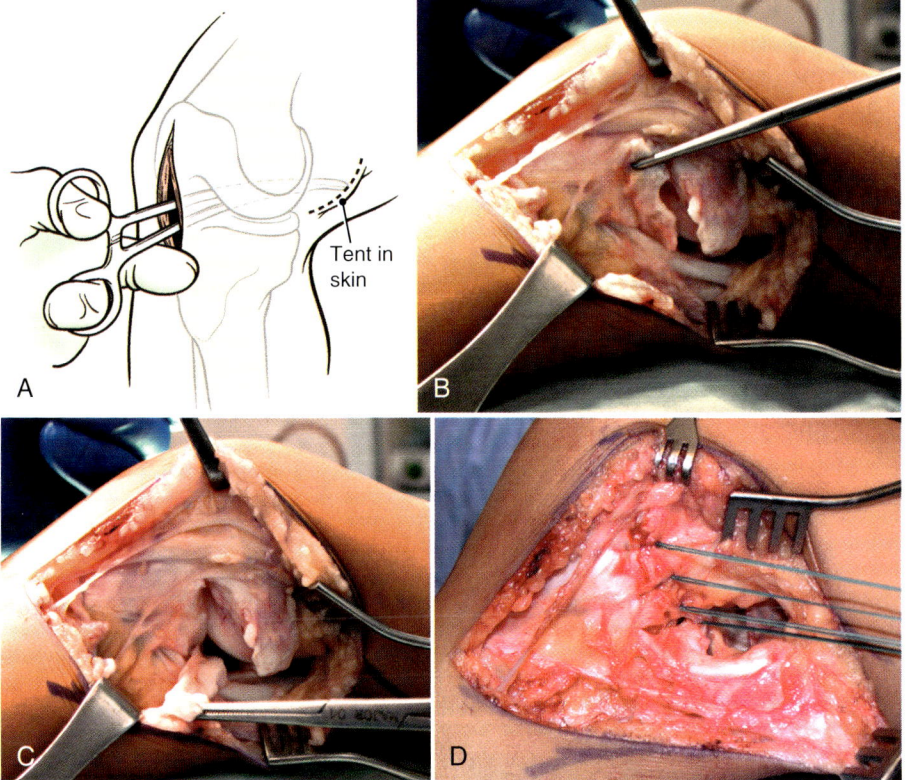

Figure 85-11. **A,** Skin incision for the posteromedial capsulorrhaphy. **B,** Exposure of posteromedial joint with posteriomedial arthrotomy. **C,** Excision of redundant capsule (in clamp). **D,** Completed capsulorrhaphy.

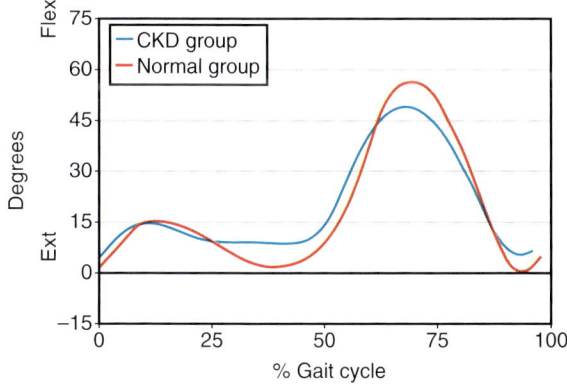

Figure 85-12. Gait plot for the sagittal plane of the knee for the normal controls and CDK group.

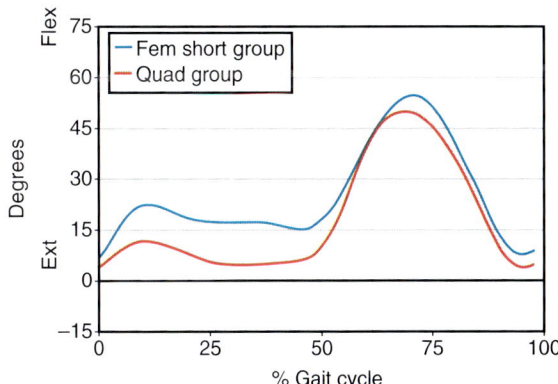

Figure 85-13. Gait plot for the sagittal plane of the knee for the quadricepsplasty and femoral shortening groups.

improved knee motion and self-reported knee function as compared with V-Y quadricepsplasty.

Anterior Cruciate Ligament Reconstruction

The issue of ACL reconstruction in a young child is controversial, to say the least, but in an unpublished review of 22 knees (14 patients) treated at our institution, with up to 15-year follow-up, the 9 knees that underwent reduction by V-Y quadricepsplasty and no ligament reconstruction were uniformly unstable, had poor quadriceps strength, and required full-time bracing or assistive devices (crutches, wheelchair) for community ambulation. Of these 9 unsatisfactory knees, 8 were in patients with laxity syndromes (predominantly Larsen). The instability was dramatic in that unbraced knees dislocated in the extended position (Fig. 85-14) and, even with bracing, were still unstable, although were usually capable of weight bearing. As a result of this review, an attempt to reconstruct the ACL-deficient knee in the laxity syndrome group seemed justified in an attempt to improve the uniformly unacceptable results of the earlier cases.

Although historically there has been reluctance to attempt intra-articular ACL reconstruction in children, because of fear of physeal injury producing deformity and growth arrest from transphyseal procedures, these concerns are gradually relenting because both clinical and experimental studies have shown that this risk may be overplayed. Options include

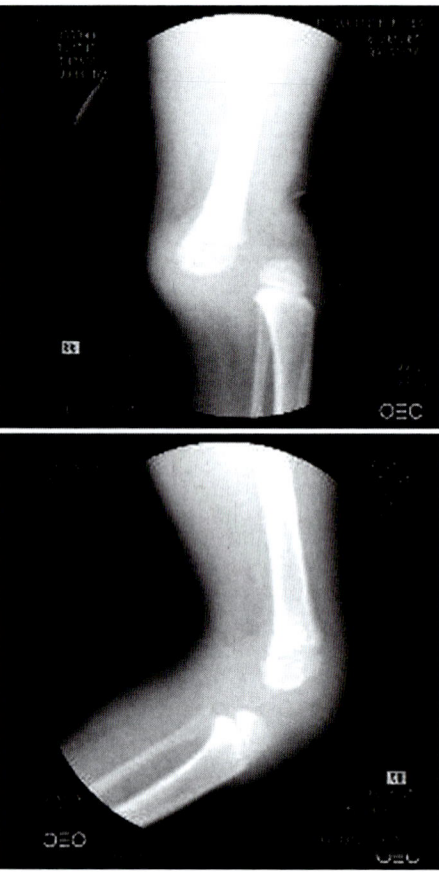

Figure 85-14. Right knee of patient in Figure 85-3 showing dislocation in extension and reduction in flexion.

transphyseal and physeal-sparing techniques. Although drilling an anchoring hole across any physis potentially risks injury, the practice of placing smooth pins across physes for periarticular and physeal trauma is well accepted, especially if the fixation is temporary. Logically, a smooth, centrally placed hole across a physis that is filled with a nonosseous (e.g., tendon) material is no more likely to produce growth disturbance than temporary pin fixation because it is an interposition material. Both animal[23,61] and clinical studies[52] using hamstrings, IT band, or patellar tendon as transphyseal ligament reconstructions have demonstrated knee stability without limb length or angular deformity.

The pes anserine tendons are conveniently used for ACL reconstruction by physis-sparing or physis-crossing techniques.[2,40,52,54] In the former, the tendon(s) are left attached at their insertion, detached proximally in the posteromedial thigh, pulled distally and rerouted superficially over the anterior tibial surface, passed under the transverse meniscal ligament to penetrate the knee joint, and passed through the intercondylar notch and over the top of the lateral femoral condyle to be anchored to bone and lateral intermuscular septum (Fig. 85-15A). To place such an ACL substitution closer to anatomic position, the tendon(s) may be passed through a transphyseal drill hole exiting the tibial articular surface at the normal ACL insertion point (see Fig. 85-15B). This method is currently our treatment of choice, regardless of patient age (see later). A 6-mm drill hole has proven technically adequate and noninjurious, with the tendons again anchored over the top of the lateral femoral condyle after traversing the notch. In either technique, care in drilling or passing tendons near the tibial tubercle is most important, because this part of the physis seems most vulnerable. For the same reason, use of the patellar tendon as a ligament substitution is not recommended because of the dissection near this portion of the physis. Several small series[2,40,54] have reported restoration of stability, as documented by KT-1000 instrumentation, improvement in Lachman test, and return to previous levels of sport, without physeal injury in immature patients followed up to 5 years.

An alternative ACL reconstruction involves the use of the IT band in a combined intra-articular and extra-articular technique (see Figs. 85-9 and 85-15C). This method, a modification of the procedure described by McIntosh and Darby, has been popularized by Kocher and collagues.[35] The technique involves rerouting a central slip of IT band, which is left attached distally to Gerdy's tubercle, in an over the top position. The tendon is sutured to the lateral femoral condyle to secure its position and routed through the intracondylar notch. The tendon can then exit the knee in the over the front position under the transverse meniscal ligament or it can be routed through a more anatomically positioned drill hole through the tibial articular surface, as described earlier. Good results were reported with this technique in their series of 44 skeletally immature patients, with a 95% graft survival at an average follow-up of 5.3 years. If this technique is used in a child with CDK, it may be helpful to use the anterior third instead of the middle third of the IT band for the reconstruction. This minor modification would allow the most anterior aspect of the IT band to be detached, eliminating this deforming structure of the knee dislocation.

We have previously used the IT band transfer rerouted through the intercondylar notch, as described by Insall and associates.[27,58,65] It is readily detached from Gerdy's tubercle during the approach described for the open reduction of the knee (see Figs. 85-9 and 85-15D), and mobilized proximally to be passed antegrade over the top of the lateral femoral condyle and through the notch prior to completing the capsulorrhaphy. The tubed tendon is then anchored in the proximal tibia through a drill hole within the epiphysis (see Fig. 85-15E), and is tensioned prior to wound closure with the tibia in maximum posterior drawer and the suture tied over a button on the anterior tibial skin or over a suture staple in the tibial metaphysis. The drill hole should be placed with radiographic control to minimize the possibility of oblique transphyseal placement; the tunnel must include the ossification center to provide tendon to bone anchorage. Alternative transphyseal placement through a more vertical, centrally placed tunnel can be attempted if enough length of tendon is available. The postoperative care is the same as for the knee reduction procedure.

The advantage of the Insall technique, as opposed to other ACL substitution procedures, in which the IT band is left attached at its insertion and rerouted as a passive restraint,[44,47]

is that it is an active transfer in which only the insertion of the tendon is being rerouted. The structure being transferred is also probably one of the deforming forces maintaining the CDK in the first place, so its rerouting should be beneficial. In any case, it will be dissected and mobilized as part of the open reduction-shortening procedure. The disadvantage of the antegrade transfer is poor maintenance of adequate anchorage of the insertion in a diminutive, mostly cartilaginous tibial epiphysis. This has been noted visually in two cases of revision performed for recurrent anterior instability, in which the IT band insertion was severely attenuated 2 to 3 years after the initial transfer. Also, this transfer retains the possibility of physeal injury at the proximal tibia, a feared complication that has restrained the use of transphyseal ACL substitutions, except in adolescents nearing skeletal maturity. Three knees in two children younger than 5 years have undergone this reconstruction simultaneously with the index open reduction procedure, with one physeal arrest (Fig. 85-16). This complication occurred in the first of bilateral reconstructions in a boy with Larsen syndrome, operated at age 18 months. He underwent the identical procedure on the

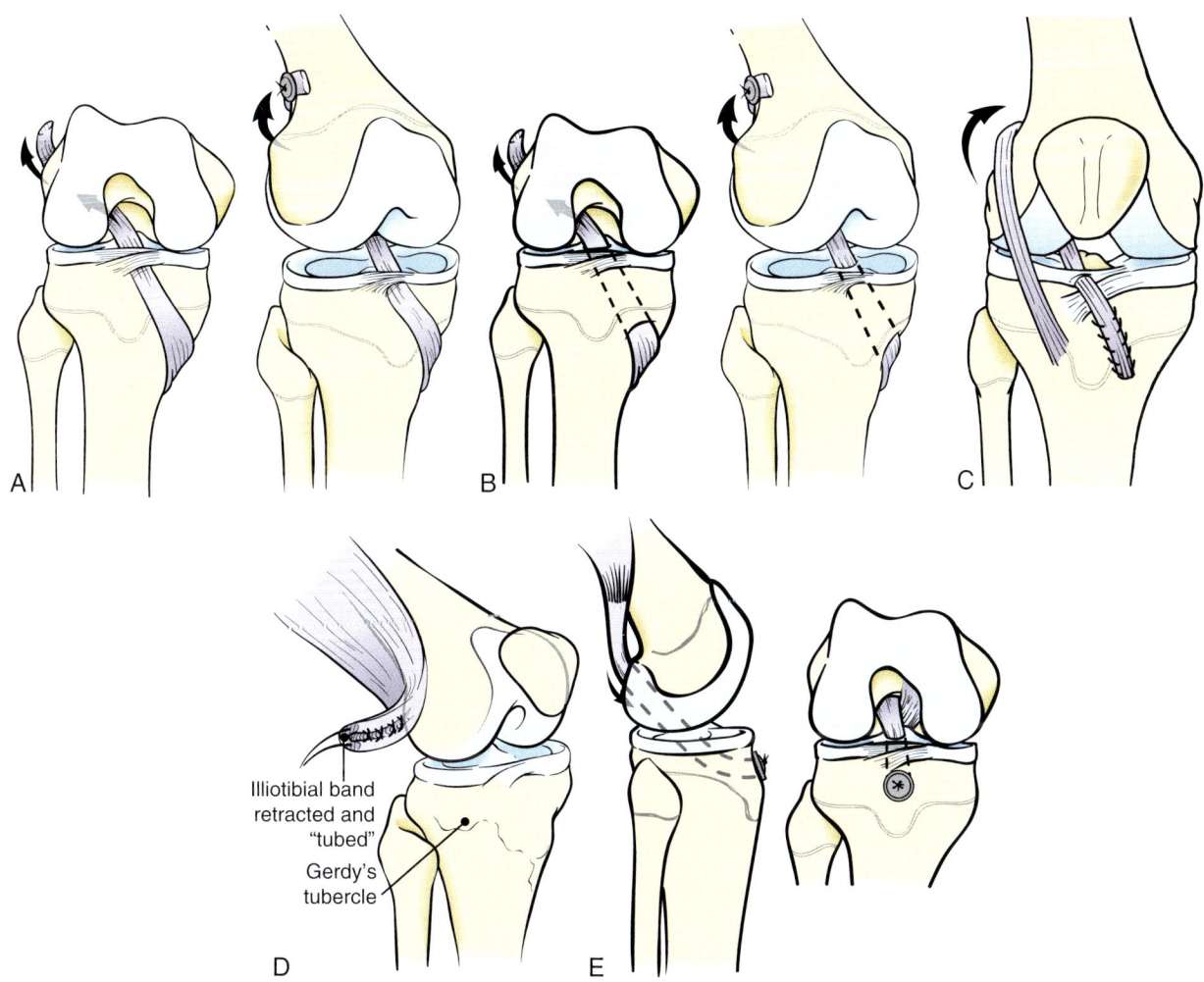

Figure 85-15.　A, Complete physeal-sparing ACL reconstruction using pes tendon(s). No drill holes cross any physes. **B,** Transtibial physis reconstruction using pes tendon(s). **C,** McIntosh ACL reconstruction using IT band. **D, E,** Insall-type reconstruction using IT band, rerouted antegrade over the top of the femoral condyle, anchored within the proximal tibial epiphysis (physeal-sparing).

Continued

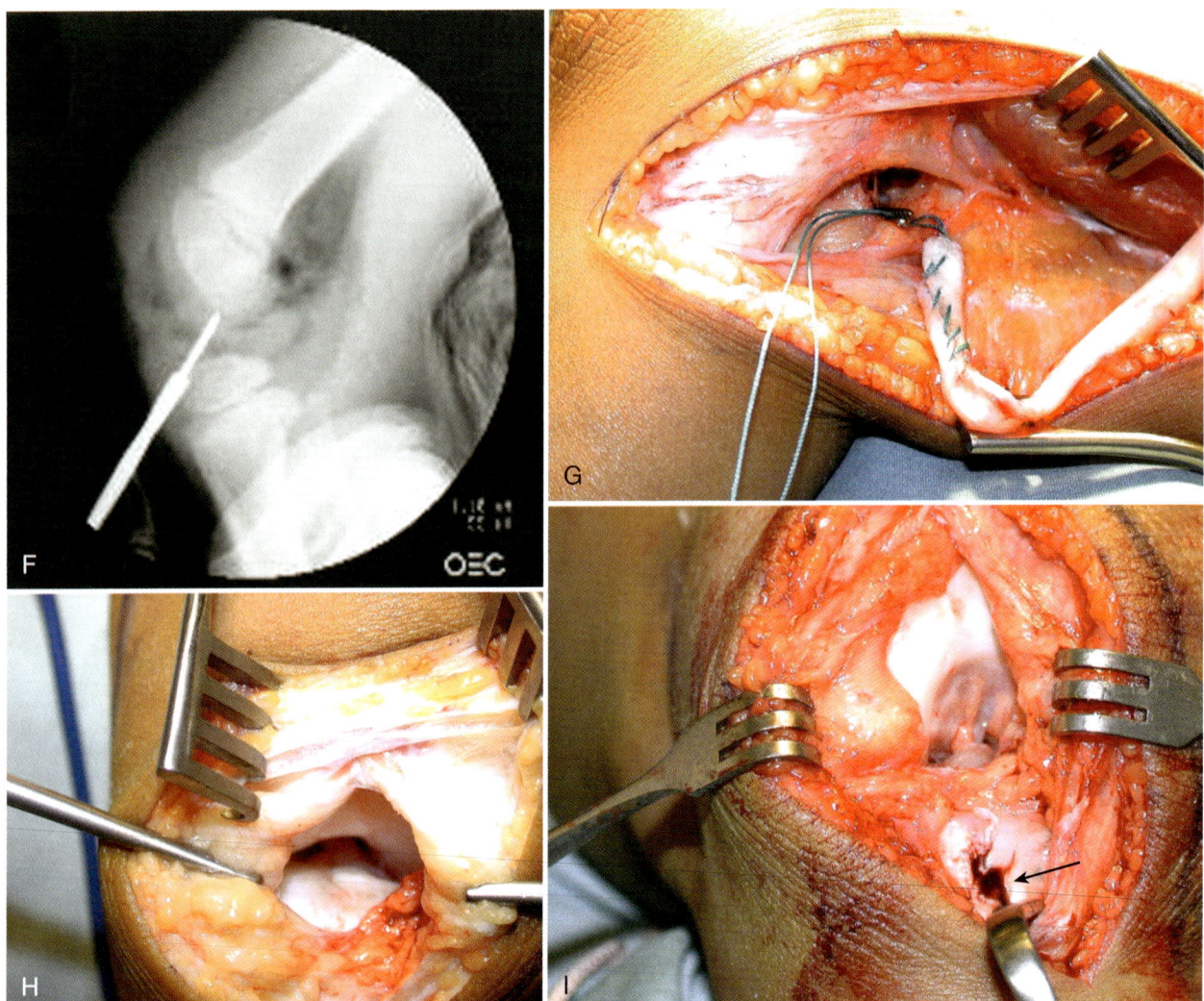

Figure 85-15, cont'd. F, Intraoperative placement of epiphyseal tunnel for IT band transfer. A guide wire is placed entirely within the epiphysis, followed by cannulated drill. G, Tubed IT band tendon ready for rerouting over the top of the lateral femoral condyle. H, Congenital absence of ACL. I, Transferred IT band has been anchored in epiphyseal hole (arrow) created in E.

second knee at age 3, with no physeal injury apparent at 9-year followup. The first side eventually developed a varus-flexion deformity, corrected uneventfully by a simple open wedge proximal tibia osteotomy at age 12. Both knees are painless and stable, with 0- to 120-degree range of motion and normal quadriceps strength. The third knee in the series, in a second child with fibular hemimelia, is stable and painless, and the patient actively runs and plays using a Syme's amputation prosthesis on the operated side. Although other investigators[47] have reported satisfactory stability without physeal injury using this technique in older children (age 12 years), the combined problems of gradual stretching out of the insertion and possibility of physeal injury has led us to use transphyseal hamstring reconstruction more frequently.

Summary

This imposing birth deformity should no longer present as a disabling or unreconstructable problem as a result of joint instability and quadriceps insufficiency. Early treatment (newborn) often succeeds in gaining closed reduction[55] and, with the use of adjunctive nerve block or Botox, even grade 3 dislocations can be successfully reduced nonoperatively. Late reduction in syndromic knees (after walking age) using femoral shortening to minimize quadriceps weakening and scarring by extensive dissection and early ACL reconstruction, either simultaneous with the open reduction or staged, can still provide a stable and functional outcome if the treatment approach described here is effectively applied. Although transphyseal ACL reconstruction will remain controversial, especially in children younger than 5 years undergoing CDK reduction, we are convinced that at least a physeal-sparing reconstruction is indicated to provide a functional knee to a patient with perhaps other syndromic orthopedic disabilities as well. The stability provided by the early ACL reconstruction is invaluable to the function of such syndromic patients and, should a physeal growth disturbance occur, it can always be reconstructed later by appropriate osteotomy and/or lengthening.

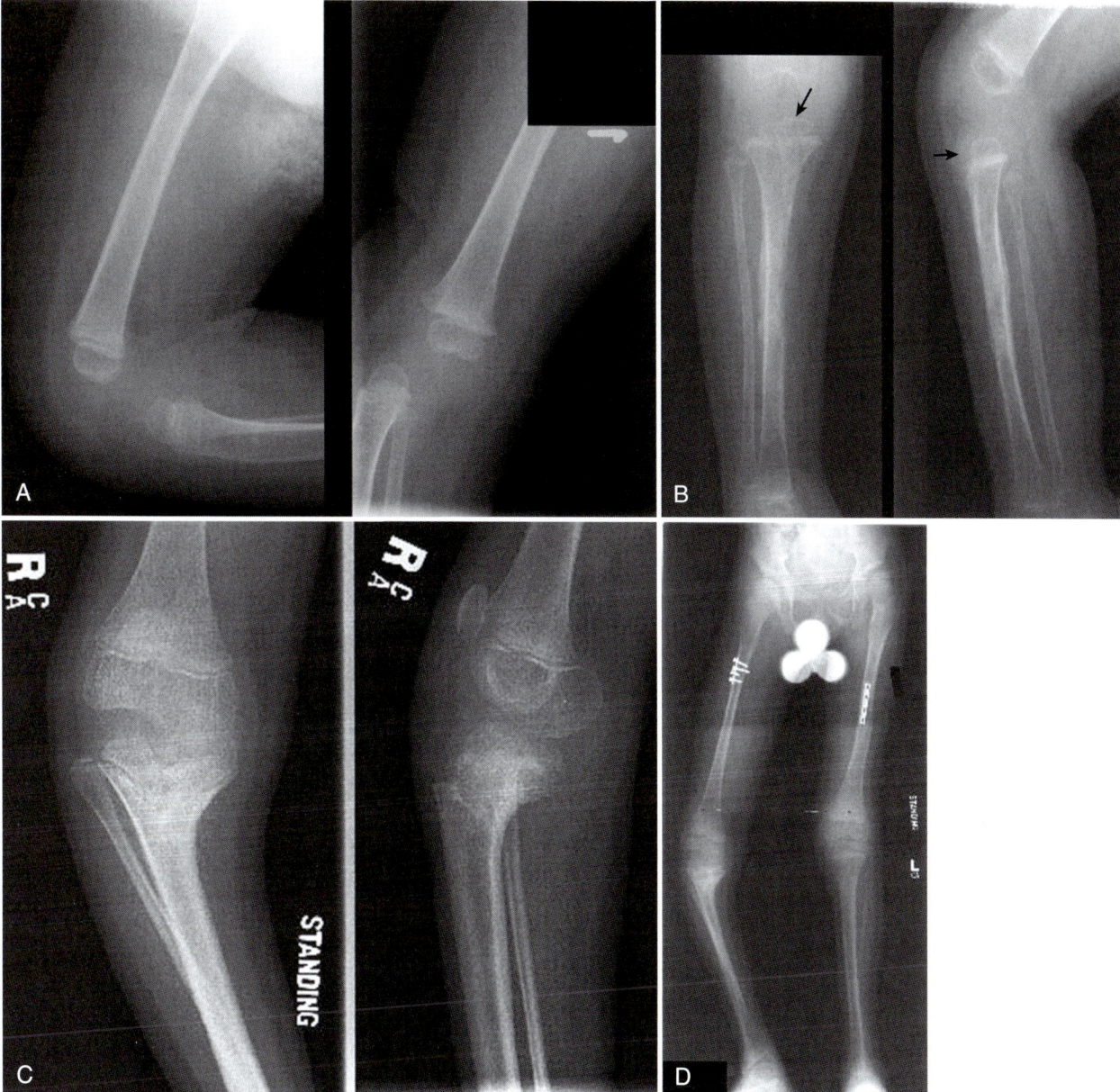

Figure 85-16. A, Radiographs of an unstable right knee in an 18-month-old boy with Larsen syndrome after closed reduction of CDK. **B,** Five months after ACL reconstruction using IT band (tunnel visible in epiphysis). A tibial diaphyseal bone graft had been harvested previously for a cervical fusion. **C, D,** At age 12, a flexion-varus deformity has developed, subsequently corrected by osteotomy. No deformity is seen in the left knee, which had an identical procedure performed at age 3.

CONGENITAL DISLOCATION OF THE PATELLA

Patellofemoral instability is a common and well-known problem familiar to all orthopedists. The term describes a continuum of deformities, which in the severest form is a congenital dislocation of the patella. This should be defined as a laterally displaced, hypoplastic patella, present at birth, diagnosed by age 10, associated with a flexion contracture of the knee and a valgus and external rotation deformity of the leg, and basically irreducible (fixed dislocation) by closed means.[16,62] The continuum or grades of congenital patellar dislocation and dysplasia are also described as

recurrent, habitual, or obligatory dislocations,[14] in which the patella is sometimes reducible in extension but unstable in flexion, resuming its laterally displaced position as the knee is flexed (Fig. 85-17), because of a variety of soft tissue contractures and/or deficient lateral femoral condyle. Regardless, an attempt to discuss all grades and types of patellofemoral instability, such as those associated with adolescence, including developmental, rotational (miserable malalignment) and possibly traumatic causes, is a monumental task fraught with confusing terms and a myriad of treatment approaches. Thus, this chapter will limit the discussion to the irreducible or obligatory congenital lesion described earlier.

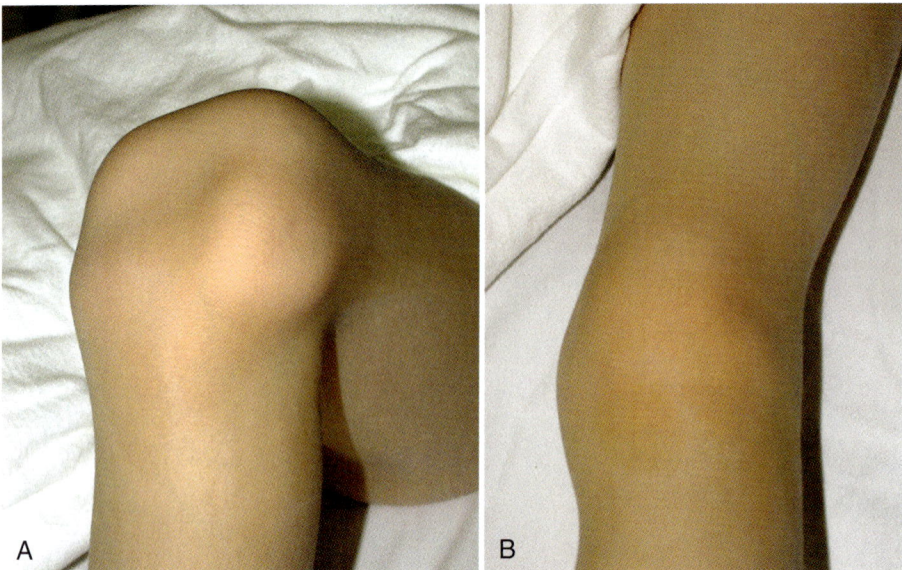

Figure 85-17. A, Obligatory patellar dislocation when the knee is flexed in a 5-year-old. **B,** Reduction in extension.

Clinical Features

Goldthwait[20] first described the surgical treatment of a permanent dislocation of the patella in 1899, and Conn[9] described the release of the contracted lateral soft tissues and advancement of the vastus medialis in 1925. However, the true cause and pathoanatomy for the dislocated patella was probably not described until Stanisavljevic and colleagues,[62] in 1976, described the failure of the internal rotation of the quadriceps myotome in the fetus. They noted that the laterally placed thigh structures normally rotate internally in the first trimester of fetal development and that when this fails to occur, the patella remains laterally displaced on the lateral femoral condyle and the entire quadriceps mechanism remains rotated anterolaterally. The actual diagnosis of this situation may be delayed because of the inability to palpate the true position of the patella in the newborn or young child and inability to document its position radiographically until later. Normal ossification of the patella occurs at around age 3 but is often delayed further when the patella is hypoplastic, as in congenital dislocation.

Diagnosis of the condition may not occur until the child presents for a disability of the leg, including delayed weight bearing.[17,41] There may be a valgus and flexion deformity with external tibial torsion, with seeming lateral instability during weight bearing. An empty intercondylar space at the anterior distal femur when the knee is flexed is seen. The patella may not be palpable, as noted, because of its hypoplasia and fixation to the lateral femoral condyle; therefore, it is mistaken for the latter structure. Quadriceps insufficiency, denoted by an extension lag (and thus the flexion contracture deformity), may be the most obvious physical finding, suggesting the diagnosis in the infant. On the other hand, in patients with less quadriceps insufficiency and a mobile patella reducible in extension, the lateral dislocation of the patella with flexion will confirm the diagnosis (Fig. 85-17). It may be possible to demonstrate inability to extend the knee against resistance from a flexed position, when the patella is dislocated, while strength-tested in extension, when the patella is more normally positioned, is almost normal. Depending on

the degree of quadriceps dysfunction, the child may do relatively well in the first decade, only to begin falling or have increasing relative weakness or loss of ability to keep up with peers as increasing body size overstresses the quadriceps mechanism. This scenario is often seen in patients with syndromic associations underlying their patellar dislocation, such as children with Down, Rubinstein-Taybi, or nail-patella syndrome. It may be necessary to resort to ultrasonography, computed tomography (CT), magnetic resonance imaging (MRI) or, rarely, open exploration, to make the diagnosis in some cases.[17,36]

Treatment

Treatment for congenital dislocation of the patella is surgical, because this dislocation is by definition irreducible or unstable. The goal is to realign the quadriceps mechanism and place the patella in the intercondylar groove, balancing the muscle insertions so that the reduction is stable. The groove, congenitally hypoplastic because of anterior flattening of the lateral femoral condyle, should deepen as normal patellar tracking ensues.[14] The classic procedure involves the concepts of Judet[31] and Stanisavljevic and associates[62] in dissecting the vastus lateralis from the lateral intermuscular septum from origin to insertion and subperiosteally rotating the entire quadriceps muscle mass medially. Thus, the skin incision basically extends from the greater trochanter to the lateral parapatellar area and distally to just beyond the tibial tubercle if infrapatellar realignment is necessary (Fig. 85-18). Distally, in the thigh, the lateral retinaculum and muscle insertions are abnormally contracted and must be divided to free the patella from these tethering structures (see Fig. 85-18C), which actually produce the flexion deformity by being displaced posterior to the axis of knee motion. Transversely dividing the iliotibial band corrects the external tibial rotation, genu valgum, and knee flexion deformity. Lengthening the quadriceps tendon by Z- or V-Y plasty has been advocated, if necessary, to remedy the obligatory dislocation caused by quadriceps contracture.[14] Femoral shortening (see

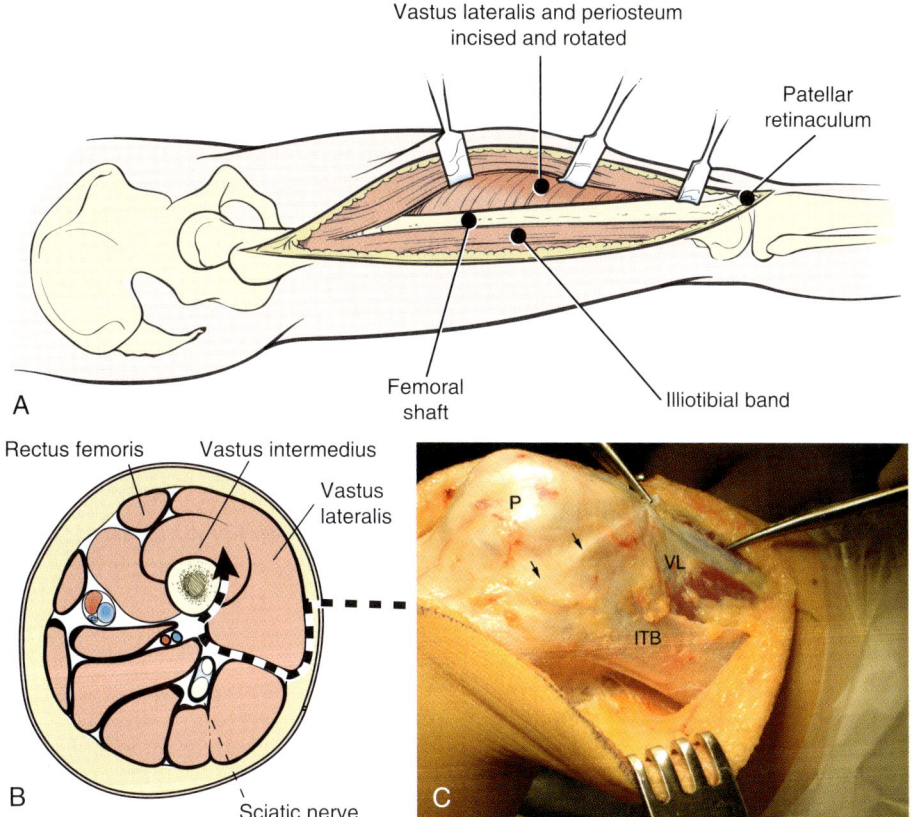

Figure 85-18. **A,** Incision and mobilization of vastus lateralis, intermedius, and rectus for Judet-Stanisvljevic quadricepsplasty. **B,** Dissection posterior to vastus lateralis with subperiosteal mobilization of vasti lateralis and intermedius. **C,** Abnormal lateral insertions of vastus lateralis (VL) and IT band into patellar retinaculum (P).

earlier) may be a better solution if the quadriceps is that severely contracted. The biceps may also require division to completely reduce the tibial subluxation-valgus.[38] Once the patella and quadriceps can be centralized, a medial imbrication is necessary to maintain the reduction. A medial arthrotomy is performed to mobilize the vastus medialis insertion, which is then advanced distally and laterally to maintain centralization of the patella (see Fig. 85-9E and F). There is no need to close or otherwise repair the large lateral retinacular defect, although some have described excising the fascia lata and using it as a graft to cover the defect and close the joint.

The final step is to realign the patellar tendon insertion if it remains too lateral. The classic Goldthwait transfer of the lateral half of the patellar tendon, split longitudinally from the medial half, sharply dissected from its insertion, and passed medially under the intact medial portion to be reattached to bone-periosteum for distal medial advancement, is generally used in immature patients for this purpose.[20] Others prefer complete release and reinsertion of the entire patellar tendon,[14,38] although the risk of tibial tubercle physeal injury[22] or excessive patellofemoral joint compression[42] may be increased by this method. Prior to closure, the knee is ranged to ascertain whether the suprapatellar or infrapatellar imbrications are too tight, preventing passive flexion to at least 45 degrees. Alternatively, if the patella continues to dislocate laterally, additional proximal lateral release (see later) and/or a revision of the medial imbrication is indicated. In the most

severe cases, a semitendinosus transfer[3,14] may be added as an additional checkrein to continued lateral subluxation. Normally, 6 to 8 weeks of cast immobilization in slight flexion is required to achieve stability following the medial imbrication and Goldthwait and Dewar procedures, followed by vigorous rehabilitation.

Often, the extensive quadriceps dissection and mobilization into the proximal thigh described earlier are unnecessary. Although it may seem logical to perform this dissection to address the pathoanatomy completely, the dissection can often be limited to the distal third of the thigh, avoiding filleting the thigh from trochanter to knee to rotate the entire quadriceps. We have found that a competent and adequately tensioned medial imbrication is stable, even if there appears to be some persistent lateralization of the proximal thigh musculature. If intraoperative stability through 45 to 60 degrees of flexion is documented, additional dissection of the intermuscular septum proximally is unnecessary. Furthermore, early range of motion exercises can be started after 2 to 3 weeks for wound healing if the medial imbrication is competent and the patella stable. Similar experiences have been reported.[17]

Results and Comments

Unfortunately, the results of quadriceps realignment are not that well documented, with many classic procedures and recent advancements in technique being reported in individual case reports or small case series with little outcome data. A 10% incidence of recurrent dislocation has been reported[16,21,30] at an average 5-year follow-up, and extension lag is generally improved, although not always in the more severe arthrogrypotic or skeletal dysplasia patients.[38] Other complications include medial dislocation, presumably from overzealous vastus medialis advancement, and peroneal nerve palsy. In patients with Down syndrome, in whom patellar instability occurs in 5% to 8% of affected persons, and includes fixed persistent dislocation and frank obligatory instability, the indication for patellar stabilization has been questioned because of the frequent absence of symptoms or functional deficit.[13,63] Operative treatment for patients with poor function secondary to instability has been reported successful in up to 86% of patients[42] and in patients followed up to 15 years, although most series have been small, with short follow-up. Readers can draw their own conclusions concerning the effectiveness of patellar stabilization in this group of patients with notorious laxity and consequent risk of recurrence.

Because the main indication for patellar stabilization surgery is the local functional deficit caused by the impaired quadriceps function and the flexion–valgus–external rotation deformity, any outcome that improves the extension lag, instability in gait, and overall function with a range of knee motion compatible with normal activities (generally 0 to 90 degrees of motion) should be considered worthwhile, even if a repeat operation is necessary later to deal with recurrence. Ultimately, it is assumed that chronic patellar dislocation, fixed or recurrent-obligatory, will degenerate into significant painful arthritis, at which time other reconstructive procedures, including patellectomy or total arthroplasty, may not be attractive because of long-standing quadriceps and periarticular soft tissue laxity or insufficiency. Thus, surgical reduction of congenital patellar dislocation with any functional impairment should always be attempted, except in cases such as Down syndrome, in which symptoms and long-term disability have been documented not to occur with significant frequency.

FLEXION DEFORMITY OF THE KNEE

A knee flexion contracture (KFC) of up to 45 degrees is a normal finding in the neonate, with further flexion to 160 degrees, the normal intrauterine position of the knee at term, also possible. As long as the quadriceps function is normal and there are no other neurologic or dysmorphic features, this congenital contracture gradually resolves in the first few months of life. By age 6 months, a significant amount of fixed knee flexion (45 degrees or more), with or without limitation of further flexion, will probably have been noted if there is a local or syndromic condition affecting the extremity. In general, such a knee deformity would be a manifestation of one of the underlying conditions in Box 85-1, which would probably have been recognized because of other orthopedic deformities or syndromic features.

Establishing the associated diagnosis underlying the knee flexion deformity has important prognostic and therapeutic value. In conditions in which femoral-tibial extension is blocked by intrinsic bony deformity (e.g., skeletal dysplasias), early soft tissue releases are probably of little value to increase extension, and thus correction by osteotomy or growth

---

Box 85-1 Conditions Associated With Congenital Knee Flexion Deformity

Localized Dysplasia Affecting the Extremity Only
Congenital femoral deficiency
Tibial hemimelia type 1a, 1b
Congenital quadriceps/patellar tendon dysplasia
Congenital dislocation (fixed) of the patella

Syndromes With Soft Tissue Contracture
Arthrogryposis
Popliteal pterygium syndrome
Escobar (multiple pterygium) syndrome
Beals syndrome (congenital contractural arachnodactyly)
Paralytic (sacral agenesis, myelodysplasia)

Skeletal Dysplasia With Bony Flexion Deformity
Diastrophic dysplasia
Metatropic dysplasia
Miscellaneous skeletal dysplasias

---

manipulation will be considered and probably delayed until technical considerations and ambulatory status indicate treatment. On the other hand, in soft tissue contracture syndromes, early aggressive treatment may be important to prevent development of secondary joint deformity precluding full extension and irreversible quadriceps dysfunction, which will impede ambulatory capability. Finally, treatment of the knee in the limb reduction anomalies (e.g., femoral deficiency, tibial hemimelia) is dictated by overall function, knee stability, and limb length considerations, and whether the involvement is unilateral or bilateral. This section will focus on soft tissue webbing syndromes, in which early reconstructive knee surgery may be of benefit; the skeletal dysplasias and limb reduction anomalies, requiring a combination of angular and growth manipulations of the entire extremity, will not be discussed further here.

Correcting a congenital KFC, or any significant KFC, is often a frustrating and complication-riddled proposition. The decision to proceed must involve an overall evaluation of the prognosis for functional ambulation, appreciating the extent of involvement of the ipsilateral hip and foot as well as any neurodevelopmental implications for function. A KFC exceeding 30 degrees alters gait adversely because of overstressing of the quadriceps.[56] It is often problematic to determine the pretreatment status of the quadriceps when a significant KFC is present. Furthermore, significant hip flexion deformity or severe equinus may have to be corrected simultaneously, or else these uncorrected deformities will induce recurrent knee flexion to maintain overall sagittal alignment for upright posture. The absolute prerequisite for KFC treatment is the identification of a functional quadriceps, without which any extension obtained through treatment will be certainly lost as the unopposed forces producing the original contracture persist.

PTERYGIUM SYNDROMES

These congenital syndromic deformities produce soft tissue webbing on the flexion side of various joints. The popliteal pterygium syndrome (PPS, also known as faciogenitopopliteal syndrome) includes, in addition to the popliteal web restricting extension, cleft lip and palate, intraoral webbing sometimes requiring surgical release to open the mouth, intercrural webs distorting the external genitalia, and finger and toe syndactylies with nail abnormalities (Fig. 85-19). Patients have normal intelligence and development. In multiple pterygium (Escobar) syndrome, webs occur across every flexion area, with particular involvement of the neck (85%) and popliteal (60%) areas, and with less common involvement of the axilla, antecubital area, and fingers. Severe kyphoscoliosis and short stature (adult height, 135 cm [53 inches]) are typical of Escobar patients, who may also show little abnormality at birth but then the webs develop with

growth. In arthrogryposis and Beals syndrome (Fig. 85-20), multiple joints are typically involved, with stiffness, lack of active motion, and absence of flexion creases noted, especially in classic arthrogryposis. In sacral agenesis and myelodysplasia, lack of motion is also obvious, related to the neurologic deficit of spinal cord origin.

Pathoanatomy

The hallmark of popliteal pterygia is the extension of a fibrous band from the ischium to the calcaneus, with a subcutaneous cord (the calcaneoischiadicus muscle) and the sciatic nerve,

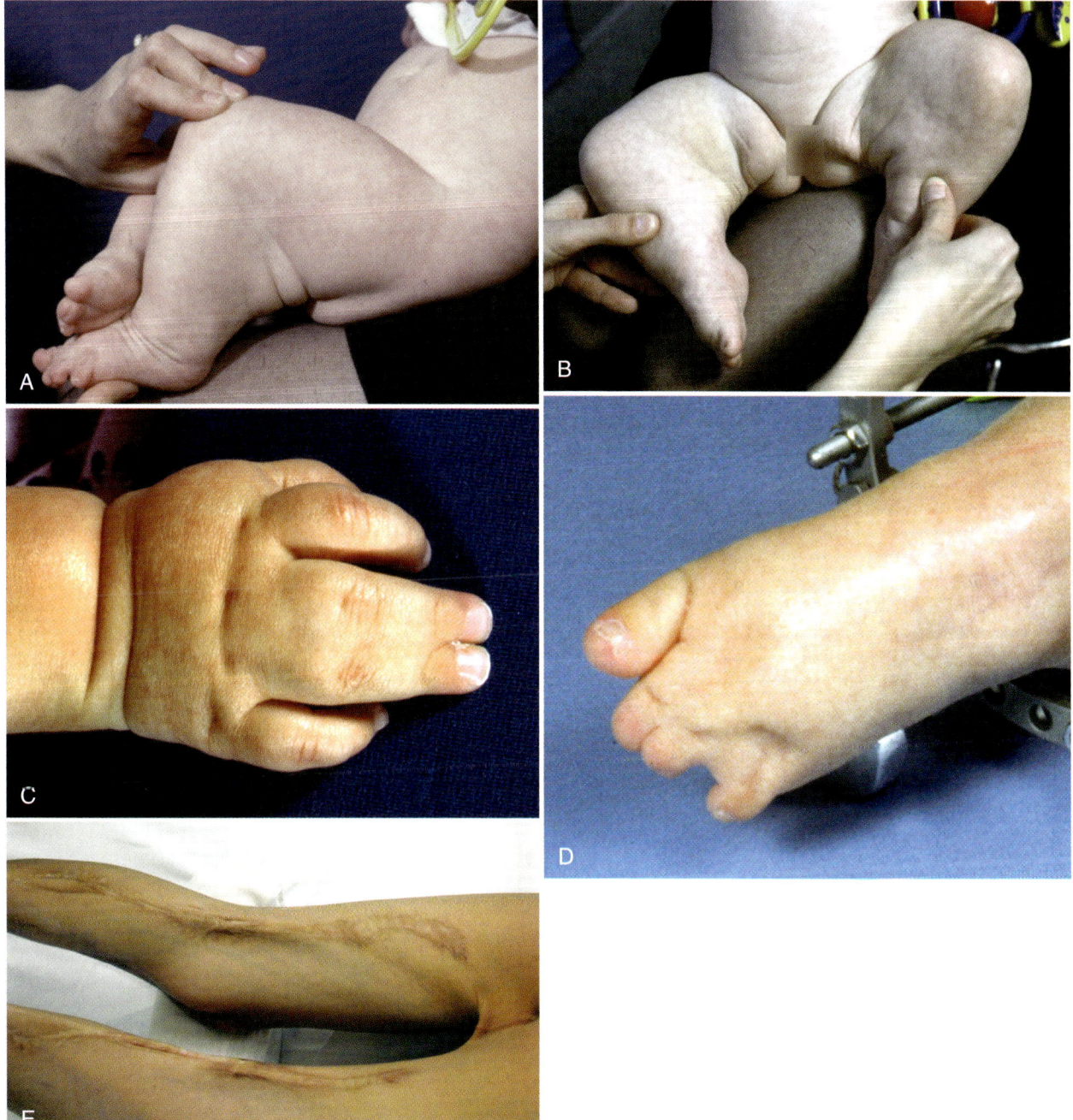

Figure 85-19. **A, B,** Clinical appearance of lower extremities in PPS in an infant. **C, D,** Syndactyly and toe deformities in PPS. **E,** Intercrural webbing affecting perineal area (buttocks to *right*).

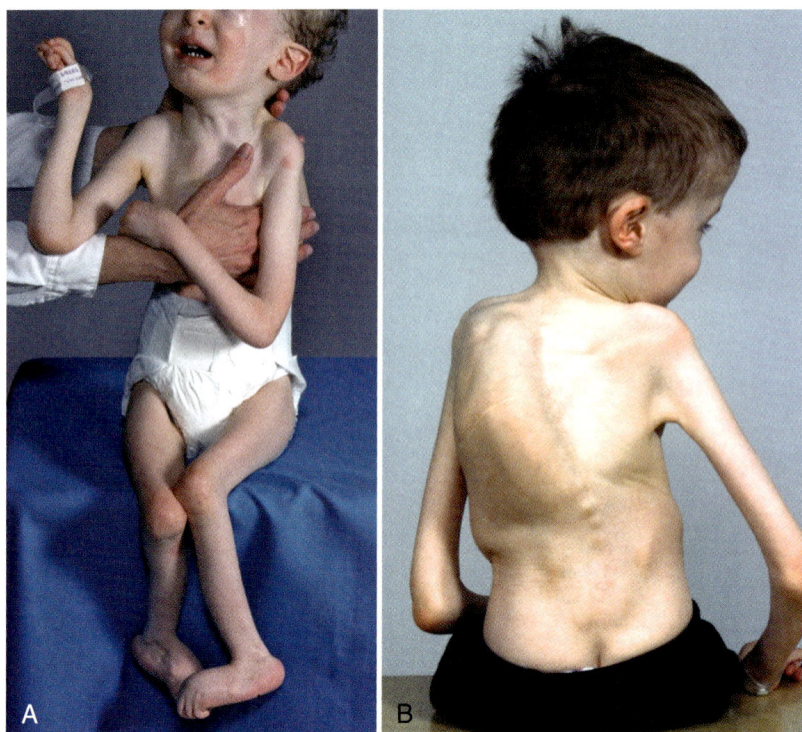

Figure 85-20. **A,** Congenital contractural arachnodactyly (Beals syndrome)—elbow and knee flexion contractures in a 1-year-old. **B,** Spinal deformity in Beals syndrome.

or one of its divisions (usually tibial), intimately adherent within the web (Fig. 85-21). There is often a longitudinal skin marking of a lighter color outlining the path of the subcutaneous cord. The cord is covered by a tent of muscle or fascia that fills the web and connects to the medial and lateral intramuscular septae of the thigh and leg. Abnormal muscle bellies and aberrant nerve paths piercing the pterygium fascia should be expected in any surgical dissection.

The obstacles to correction of a pterygium contracture include the following: (1) the calcaneoischial cord, which is generally not flexible and intuitively invites excision, usually with a Z-plasty of the skin; (2) the shortness of the sciatic or tibial nerve division accompanying the cord,[24,51] which cannot be stretched acutely; and (3) intra-articular incongruity, secondary to flattening of the femoral condyles caused by persistence of growth in flexion. The latter is an important argument for early surgical correction before the joint deformity per se prevents full extension because of misshapen articular surfaces. Recurrence of the contracture is extremely frequent because of reconstitution of the calcaneoischial cord and popliteal scar formation, and secondarily by ankle equinus from the calcaneal insertion; the knee must flex to accommodate the persistent or recurrent equinus. The role of a weak quadriceps is obvious, although in practice the actual strength is difficult, if not impossible, to test or document—the pretreatment strength of the muscle cannot be determined in an infant or toddler with a rigid flexion deformity that prevents extension. About all that can be determined is whether the muscle contracts when the leg is stimulated.

In arthrogryposis and similar conditions, the obstacles to correction are mainly the periarticular fibrosis and underlying muscle paralysis. These joints are congenitally rigid, because of lack of intrauterine movement—for example, as evidenced

by absence of flexion creases. Periarticular tissue and joint capsules are contracted as a result. Early attempts to mobilize these joints with physical therapy are usually unrewarding because of lack of active movement, but should always be attempted. At some point, in the 12- to 24-month old patient, a decision must be made about prognosis for ambulation based on active movements of the lower extremities and, in particular, the presence of quadriceps function. In cases of total absence of quadriceps function, the decision to accept the flexed knee position and consequent nonambulatory status, and thus forego knee flexion deformity treatment, is completely justified.

The prognosis for obtaining and maintaining correction of congenital KFC of these causes, and thus useful ambulation, is guarded, at best, because of the often insurmountable problem of recurrence. Treatment must anticipate that recurrence to some degree is inevitable and that functional gains are elusive because of numerous possible complications, including nerve stretching and neuropathic pain, joint damage from extensive dissection producing avascular necrosis of epiphysis and physis, incongruity and cartilage necrosis (Fig. 85-22), and inadequate muscle strength to allow nonsupported knee extension.

Treatment

Acute Correction: Pterygium and Arthrogryposis

Correction by surgical release of popliteal structures, combined with femoral and possibly tibial shortening, is first-line treatment for deformities of moderate severity, up to perhaps 60 degrees. The popliteal release may be best accomplished with the patient prone although, if hip mobility is normal

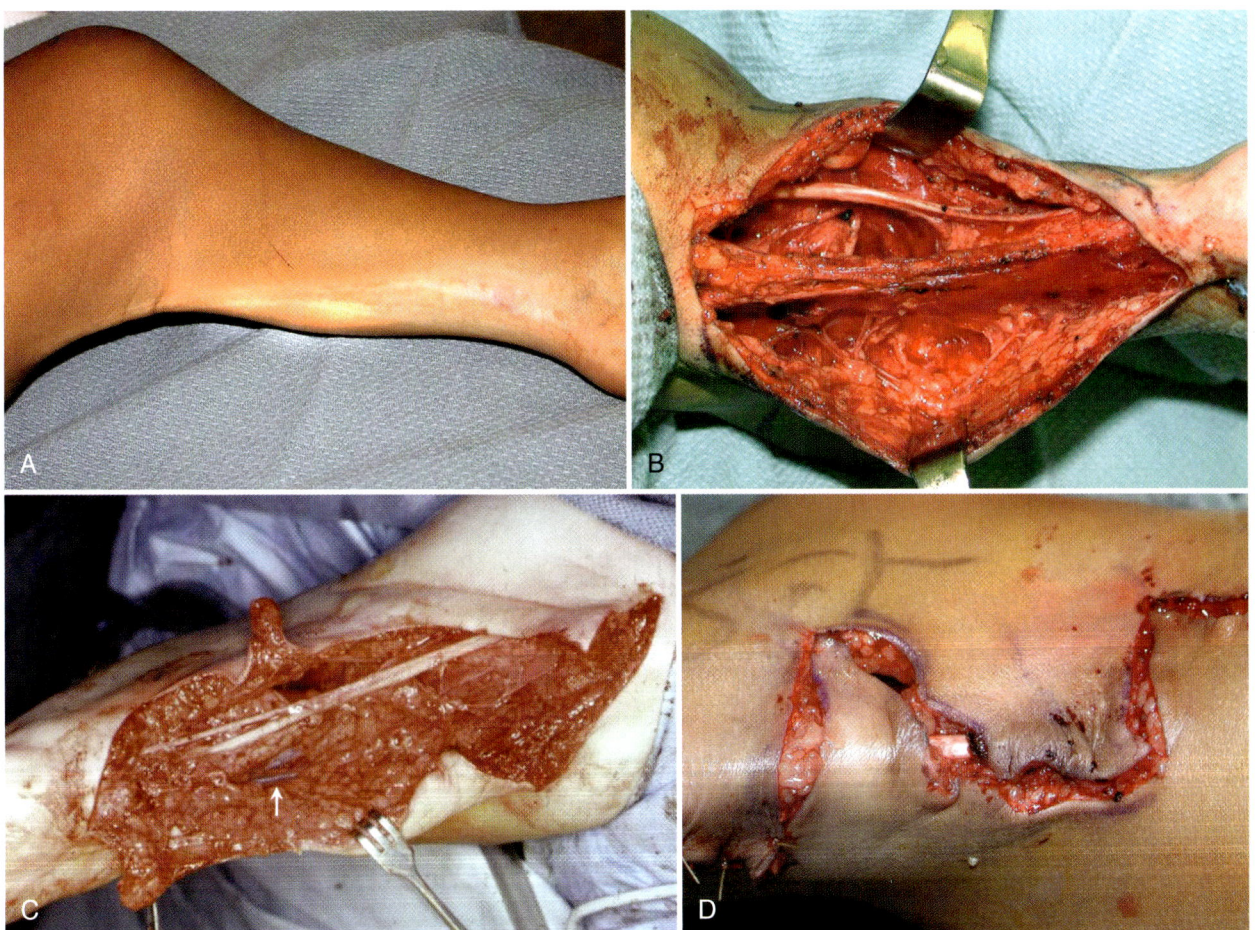

Figure 85-21. **A,** Superficial band with skin discoloration overlying the ischiocalcaneal structure (foot to *right*). **B,** Ischiocalcaneal muscle and band, with the sciatic nerve isolated. **C,** All popliteal soft tissue structures have been released except the major nerve divisions and the vascular bundle *(arrow)*. **D,** Following wound closure, the sciatic nerve is bowstrung directly under the skin.

and allows full internal and external rotation, the patient can be positioned supine, allowing access to anterior and posterior structures simultaneously. Anterior exposure is needed to inspect the intercondylar notch and patellofemoral joint following posterior release, because there is often a soft tissue pulvinar in the notch blocking full extension, which must be excised. In arthrogrypotic patients, the patellofemoral joint is often scarred or obliterated and the quadriceps mechanism must be freed from the femur and a suprapatellar pouch created (Fig. 85-23).

Regardless of the patient position, the skin over the ischiocalcaneal band must be incised longitudinally with multiple Z-plasties and the actual cord exposed circumferentially from ischial tuberosity to calcaneal tuberosity. The exposure of the cord will encounter the sciatic nerve and its tibial, peroneal and sural components, which should be completely dissected, mobilized, and protected (see Fig. 85-21). The ischiocalcaneal structure is excised. The arcade of fascia enveloping the band can then be safely followed to the medial and lateral intermuscular septae and divided transversely, just like a fasciotomy of the leg or plantar surface of the foot. This fascial division is best accomplished close to the joint, near the axis of rotation, but can also be accomplished at points proximal and distal to the knee. Deeper structures in the popliteal fossa can then be dissected and released sharply, obviously

protecting the vascular structures deep midline, which are in the normal anatomic location (see Fig. 85-21C). Beginning laterally, the biceps and iliotibial band are released (Henry approach); posterior capsulotomy of the knee is the ultimate goal of the dissection. Medially, the hamstring tendons are released, leading to complete posteromedial capsulotomy. However, in spite of what appears to be a comprehensive, thorough posterior knee release, the limiting factor—the sciatic nerve or its tibial component—usually prevents adequate extension, and bowstrings in the popliteal area so severely that skin closure over the nerve may be an issue (see Fig. 85-21D).

The femur should then be shortened,[51,57] as much as 3 to 4 cm if necessary, to achieve as much extension as possible (see Figs. 85-22A and 85-23E and F). This effectively decompresses the tissue around the knee, much like femoral shortening applied to the reduction of a late-diagnosed congenital dislocation of the hip,[6] allowing extension without undue tension on the nerves. This can be accomplished in the distal diaphysis by plating the femur laterally or posteriorly; the latter is theoretically preferable because the plate will then be on the tension side of the osteotomy when the knee is extended with some force. An overly aggressive popliteal soft tissue release combined with a distal femoral shortening can result in avascular injury to the distal femoral physis (see

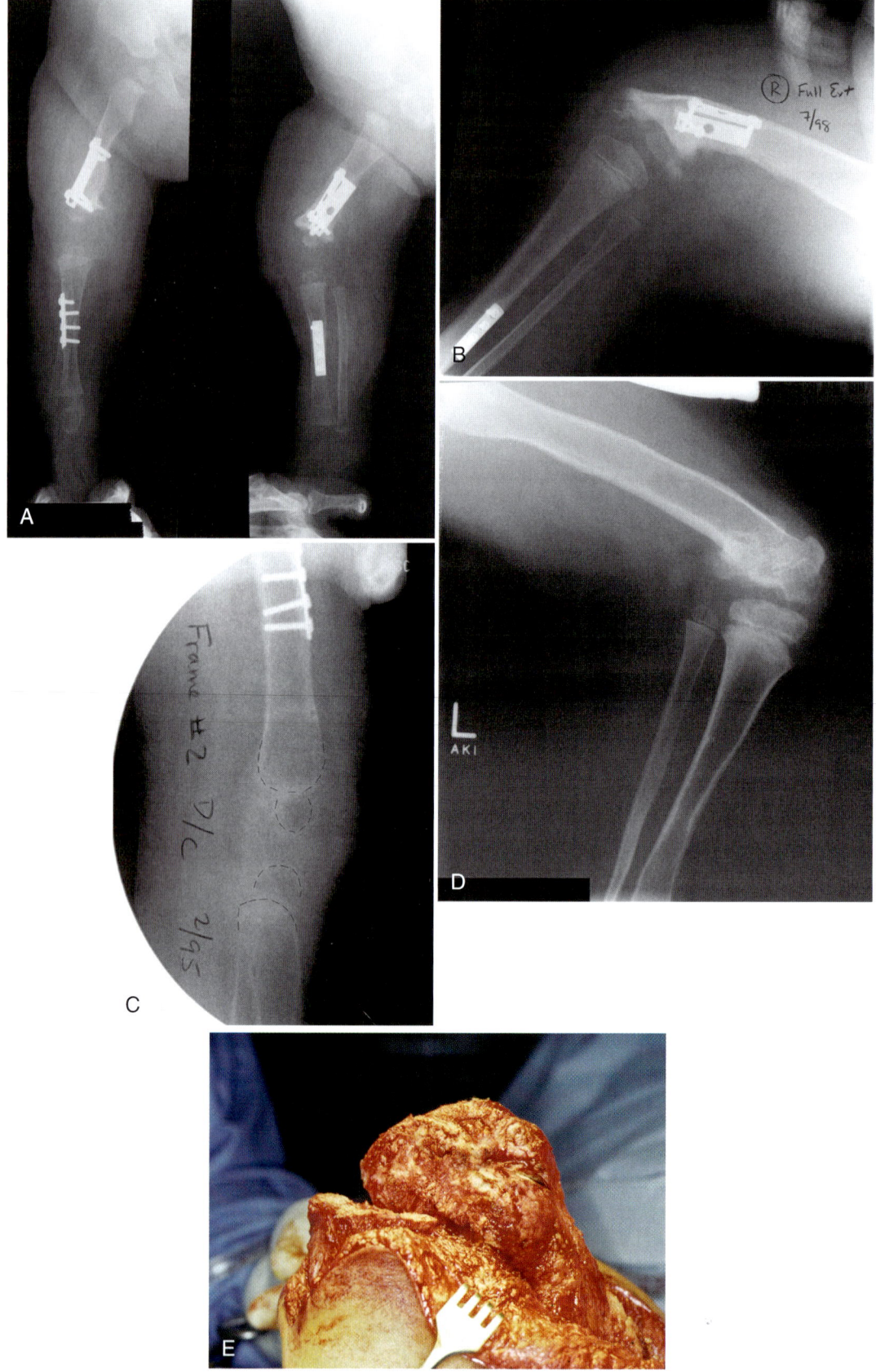

Figure 85-22. A, Radiograph 4 months after extensive popliteal release and femoral and tibial shortening were performed on the right lower extremity of the patient in Figure 85-16. **B,** Avascular necrosis of the distal femoral epiphysis and physis resulted. **C,** Left knee radiograph, showing full extension, of the same patient after second attempt at distraction arthrodiastasis correction with Ilizarov method (see also Fig. 85-25). Soft tissue release and femoral shortening followed the second frame correction. **D,** The result was recurrent deformity with severe degenerative changes 2 years later. **E,** Intraoperative view of destroyed distal femur in **D**. The articular surface is covered with pannus and cartilage cannot be identified. Knee fusion with rotationplasty was performed.

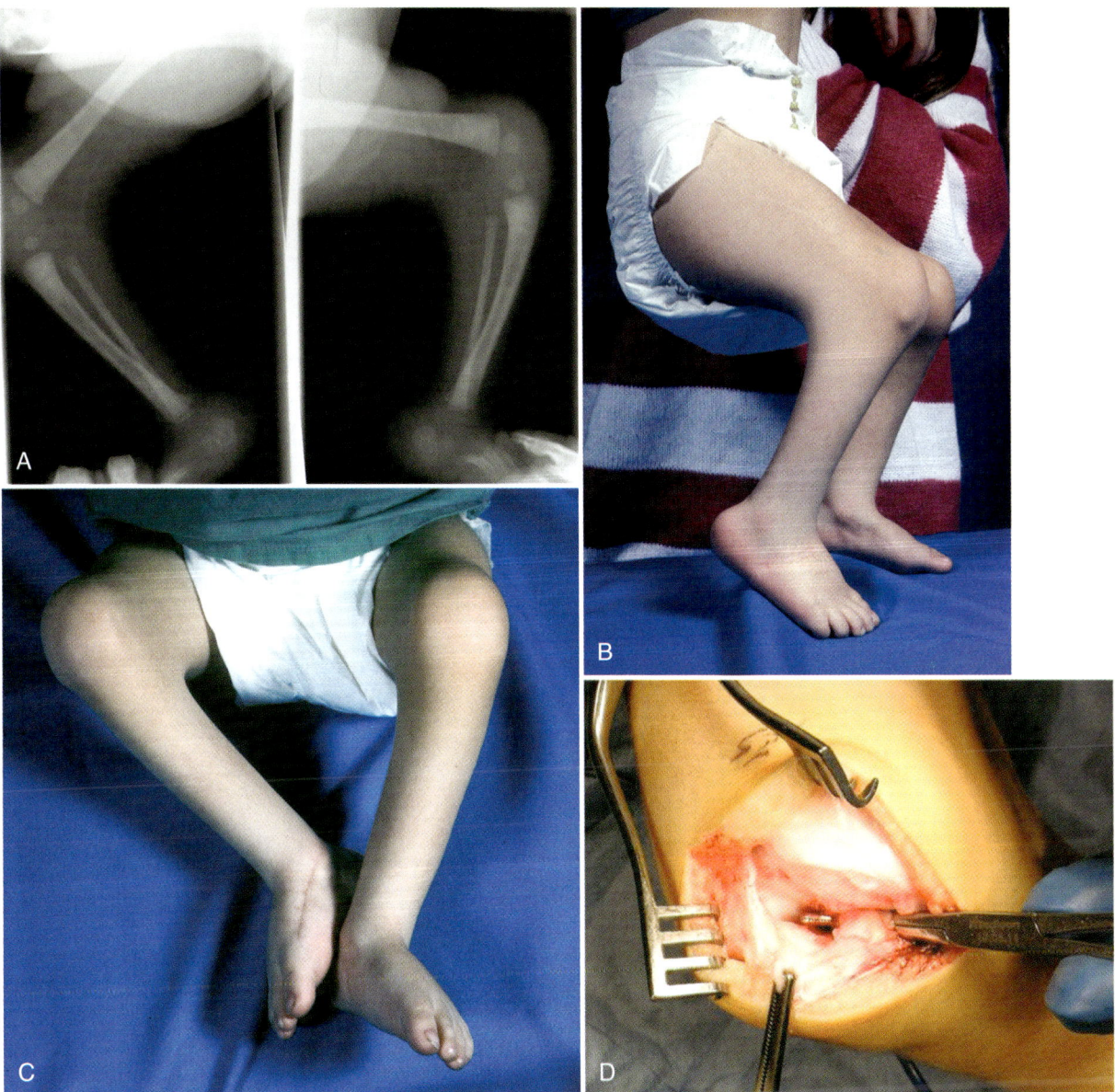

Figure 85-23. **A,** Knee radiographs of an infant boy with multiple pterygia (Escobar syndrome). **B** and **C,** Clinical appearance of lower extremities. **D,** Anterior arthrotomy to excise fibrofatty soft tissue obstructing the intercondylar notch, blocking full extension.

Continued

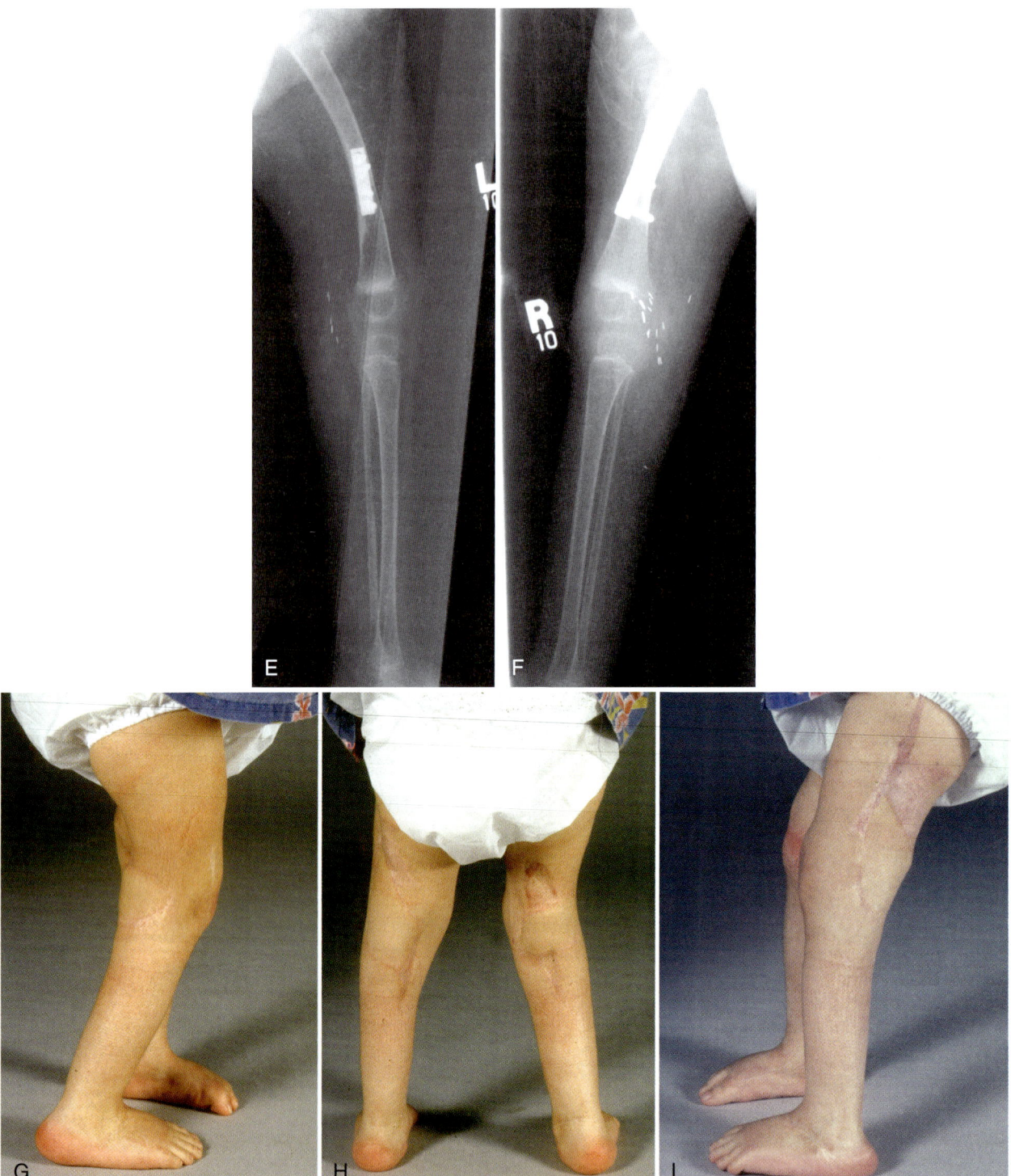

Figure 85-23, cont'd. E and **F,** Radiographs at age 3½ years after staged popliteal releases, femoral shortening, and anterior arthrotomy, with latissimus dorsi free flaps for soft tissue closure of the popliteal fossae. **G-I,** Clinical appearance at age 3½ years.

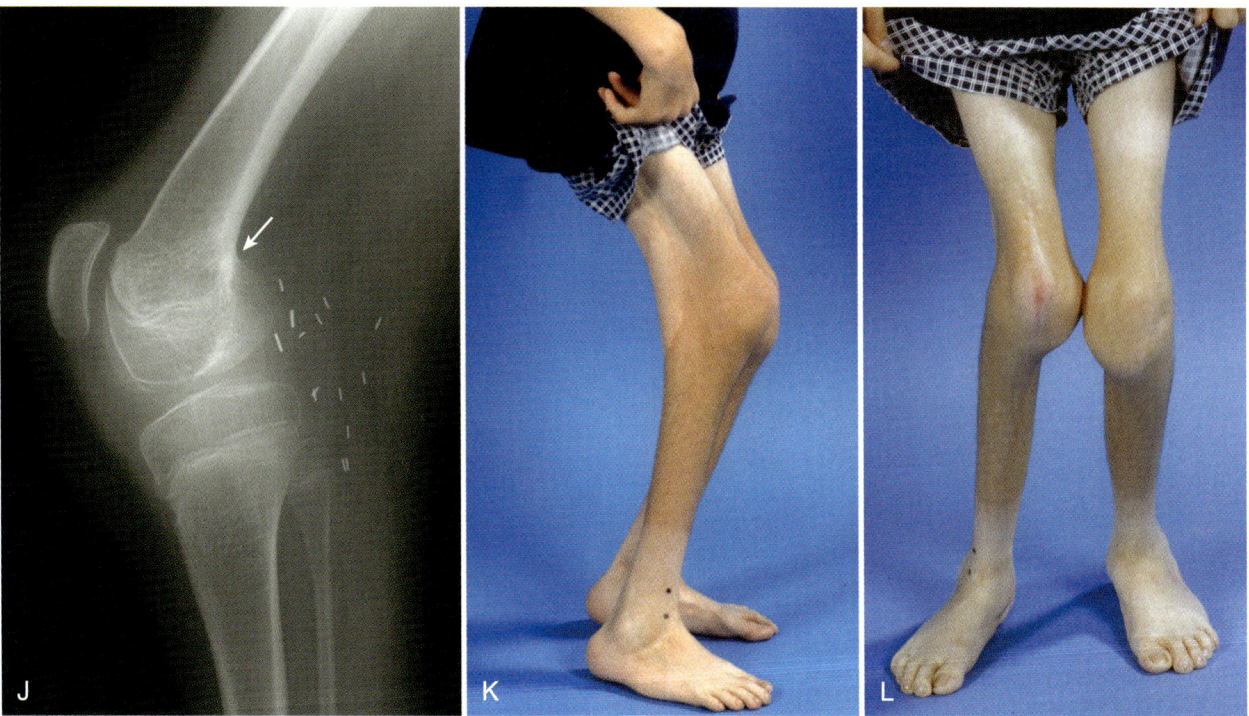

Figure 85-23, cont'd. J, Ten years postoperatively, a significant flexion deformity has recurred on the right. Premature growth arrest at the posterior physis is suspected *(arrow)*. Joint incongruity is also apparent. **K** and **L,** Clinical appearance at age 14.

Fig. 85-22B). The tibia can also be shortened to benefit the ankle equinus and decompress the popliteal structures further. Hyperextension osteotomy of the distal femur has been used to correct KFC[12] but, in a young child, provides only temporary improvement because of remodeling by the distal physeal growth.

As suggested earlier, anterior arthrotomy must be considered for removal of fibrofatty soft tissue, which often fills the intercondylar notch and prevents the final 10 to 15 degrees of extension (see Fig. 85-23D). The patellofemoral joint may need to be inspected to assess whether full passive extension is possible. Finally, plication of the patellar tendon should be considered following the femoral shortening to remove excessive redundancy, which will compromise eventual quadriceps strength. In children younger than 2 years this may not be necessary, but one will never be criticized for this final step in attempting to balance and augment the extension function in this deformity, in which such function is often lacking.

Once maximum extension has been achieved, the incisions are closed and a spica cast is applied to control the proximal thigh, because a long-leg cast has inadequate purchase on the thigh following femoral shortening. Once the osteotomies are healed (5 to 6 weeks), the patient is actively mobilized, concentrating on active extension and unencumbered weight bearing. Bracing in full extension can be used if quadriceps weakness appears to be allowing excessive flexion. Long-term night bracing in full extension is often recommended, but its efficacy is unknown. As noted, the tendency for recurrence is overwhelming, so attempts to delay it by long term bracing are appropriate.

In spite of vigorous treatment of KFC in arthrogryposis, over half of patients lose ambulatory ability because of ineffective correction or recurrence, and thus do not remain community ambulators.[46,60] A recent report[26] of functional outcomes following knee release in patients with arthrogryposis found only 31% of patients to be independent ambulators, with the remainder being wheelchair-bound for community mobility at a mean follow-up of 12 years after surgical release. Despite the observation of increased recurrence rate of flexion contracture with extended follow-up, improved functional mobility scores, functional independence scores, and self-reported sports and physical functioning scores with increased knee extension were documented. This study reinforces the difficulty in treating KFC in arthrogryposis. Although short- and intermediate-term function may be significantly improved with aggressive surgical management, long-term ambulatory ability invariably declines as the knee contracture recurs, despite early intervention. For PPS patients, many will remain community ambulators with repetitive surgery, depending on initial severity,[51,53] provided that the knees do not succumb to painful degenerative arthritis (see Fig. 85-22). Knee fusion or amputation may be resorted to in the latter situation.

Microvascular free tissue transfer has been used in place of Z-plasty in an attempt to decompress the popliteal scarring further, which contributes to recurrence. Limited experience with latissimus dorsi free transfer (see Fig. 85-23) has shown that KFC recurrence can be delayed to some degree, but cannot be prevented simply by supplying noninvolved healthy tissue to cover the popliteal space. Because of the possible untoward effects of bilateral free latissimus flaps on development of spinal deformity, this method may be appropriate only for patients nearing skeletal maturity, in whom the risk of progressive spinal deformity is minimal.

Full passive extension is almost never achieved in spite of comprehensive surgery, usually because of incomplete

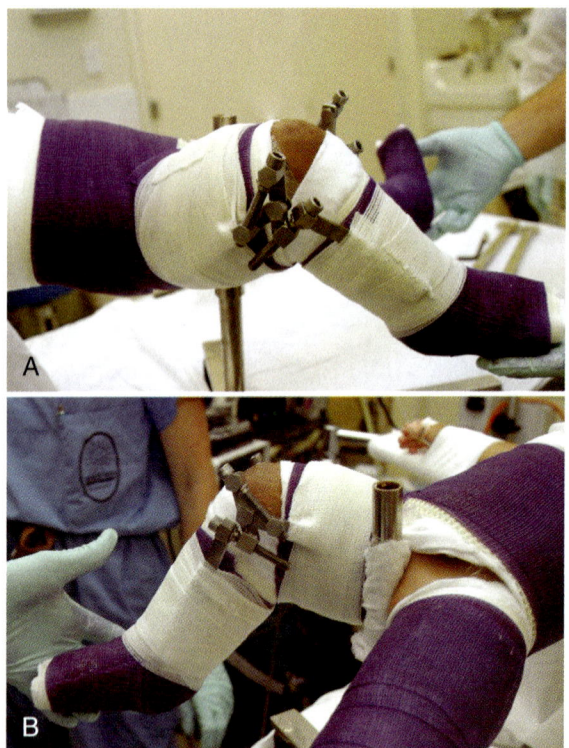

Figure 85-24. **A, B,** Extension-desubluxation hinge cast applied immediately following acute correction surgery. The proximal threaded screw extends the knee and the distal one translates the tibia anteriorly to prevent posterior subluxation.

decompression of neurovascular structures, but also because of early joint incongruity. A form of gradual extension improvement can then be attempted postoperatively with serial casts in progressively more extension or with the use of an extension-desubluxation hinge cast (Quengel hinges; Fig. 85-24). The latter allow casting in flexion, with progressive extension produced once early wound healing has occurred, retaining the ability to translate the tibia anteriorly during correction to avoid knee subluxation. Care is required to avoid decubiti at the anterior distal thigh, where careful padding and judicious cast trimming are crucial to prevent skin complications as progressive extension is achieved. A spica cast is recommended to avoid posterior proximal thigh skin pressure caused by the Quengel technique when a long-leg–only cast is placed.

Gradual Correction: Ilizarov Technique

Gradual correction of joint contracture with an external fixator is an attractive option for severe congenital KFCs. The amount of corrective force that can be applied to the bony skeleton is not limited by skin tolerance and, because the skeletal elements are controlled directly by the external fixation, joint subluxation can be avoided. The sciatic nerve and its branches, the structures directly limiting the amount of acute correction, tolerate slow stretching well. Both circular and monolateral devices using a hinge distractor method have been reported.[7,45] Improvement in extension and total arc range of motion, changed to a more functional range, can be achieved. The problem, as with acute correction, remains maintenance of correction whether or not soft tissue release has been performed simultaneously.[11,18,25]

Loss of correction with recurrence of deformity and stiffness are common in our limited experience (Fig. 85-25; see Fig. 85-22). Although gradual correction remains attractive, it still does not eliminate the problem of recurrences following Ilizarov correction of pterygia. The question arises as to whether a soft tissue release prior to frame correction is advisable. The reasoning might be that the distraction arthrodiastasis actually induces increased fibrous tissue as the surgically treated popliteal structures are lengthened, in the same way that bone is created by distraction forces after osteotomy. Such distraction histogenesis invites recurrence by the stimulation of new popliteal fibrous tissue, becoming apparent after frame removal. Thus, it is probable that Ilizarov correction of pterygia should not be preceded by soft tissue release; instead, the deformity should be addressed by external fixation–arthrodiastasis alone. At first sign of recurrence (loss of extension), following healing of pin tracts, it can be subjected to formal soft tissue release and femoral shortening, as described for acute correction.

The frame is constructed with double points of fixation on the femur and tibia, usually with an arch proximally and a ring distally on the femur, and two rings for the tibia (see Fig. 85-25A). The foot should be included in a static frame, fixed to the tibia in neutral position, whenever there is potential for significant equinus during correction, which in practice means essentially every case of KFC. An extra point of fixation to the distal femoral ring is a transverse wire through the femoral epiphysis to protect this physis from separation during correction,[11] although this is not mandatory; monolateral fixators have successfully corrected KFCs,[45] obviously without such a protective wire for the distal femoral epiphysis. The hinge must be placed as a distraction hinge, with the axis of rotation being just distal to the anterior distal edge of the distal femoral condyle (see Fig. 85-25D). This is intended to prevent articular cartilage pressure damage, but this is probably the least controllable complication of the procedure. The rate of angular correction can be calculated using the triangulation formula or concentric radii,[25] but in practice is generally tailored to the patient's tolerance and the appearance of any neuropraxic complications. Empirically, 4 mm/day distraction on the motor rod seems to correct the deformity efficiently. Distal neuropathy, as evidenced by hyperesthesia or dysesthesia of the foot, warrants a temporary slowing or pause from correction and consideration of the use of gabapentin (Neurontin) if it does not resolve.

Once full extension is achieved, it is generally recommended to maintain the frame locked in full extension for 4 to 6 weeks.[45] Rapid flexion and extension through an arc of 30 degrees or more can be attempted during this period to mobilize the periarticular tissues once full extension is reached. The frame should then be removed and the knee casted for an additional 4 to 6 weeks to help maintain correction and allow pin tracts to heal in preparation for possible additional surgery, such as ischiocalcaneal cord excision and femoral shortening, to decompress the correction. Such surgery should be considered as soon as recurrence or loss of extension becomes apparent. Although long-leg bracing is commonly recommended once the final cast is removed, this is mechanically ineffective in young children because of the limited control of the thigh, especially if the femur has been shortened. A nighttime extension orthosis may be the most practical for post-treatment splinting.

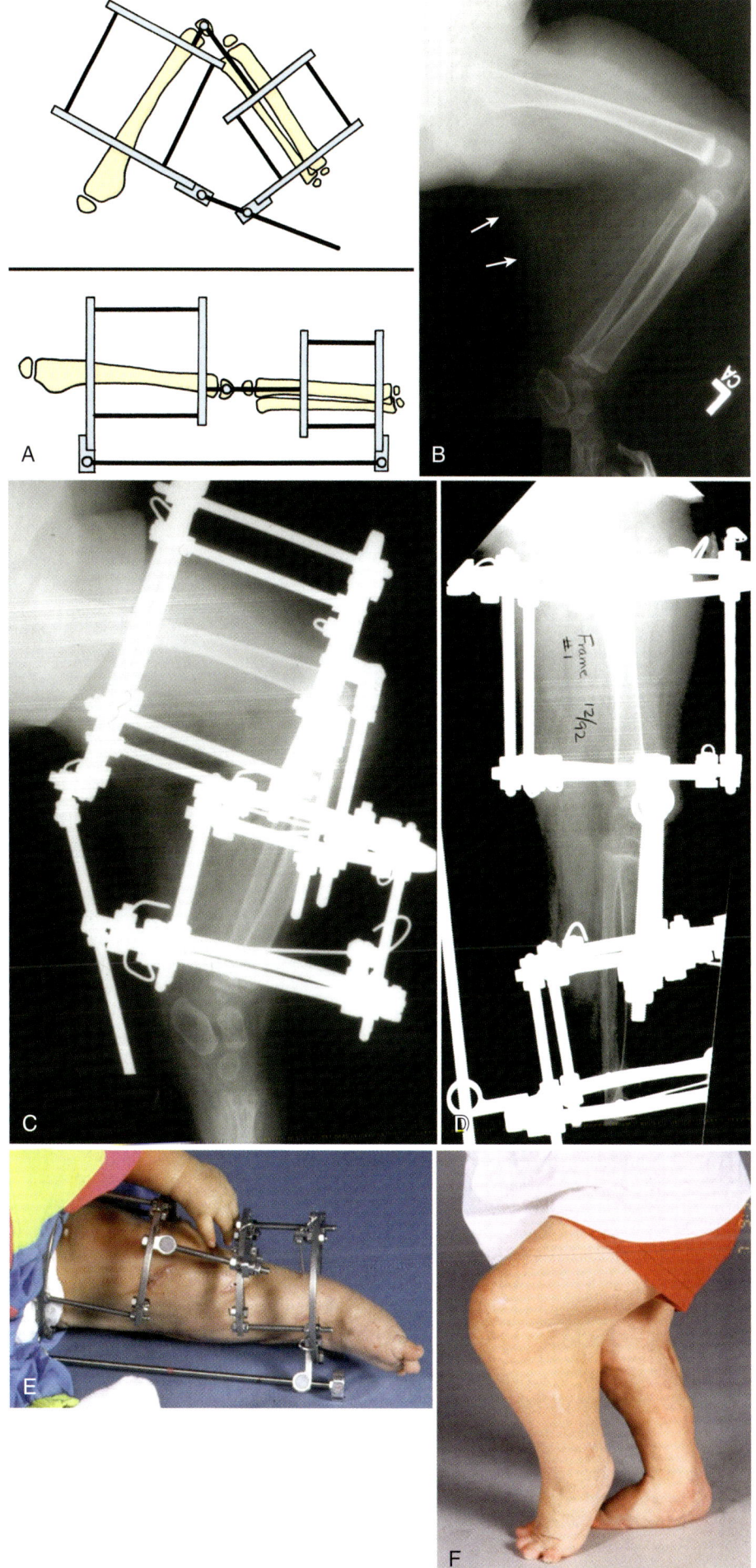

Figure 85-25. A, Diagram of frame for correction of KFC by distraction hinge method. **B,** Radiograph of left lower extremity (patient in Fig. 85-19) prior to frame application. The soft tissue edge of the pterygium can be seen *(arrows).* **C,** Radiograph of initial position in frame. **D,** Full extension achieved. Note position of the knee hinge at the anterior edge of the distal femur to accomplish joint distraction with extension. **E,** Clinical appearance with knee extended. Failure to incorporate the foot allowed uncontrolled equinus, contributing to recurrence. **F,** Recurrent deformity 1 year later. This extremity was treated a second time (see Fig. 85-22*C*), with a similar outcome.

Results of Ilizarov correction of KFCs are far more encouraging than for acute correction, except for PPS patients, for whom recurrence is almost expected. The results indicate that 60% to 85% of knees gain significant correction and maintain it at up to 5-year follow-up. Brunner and associates[7] have corrected 11 of 13 knees from 39 degrees flexion to 17 degrees at follow-up, without frame-related complications. Herzenberg and coworkers[25] have achieved good to excellent results in 9 of 14 knees, starting from an average 60-degree contracture, corrected to 16 degrees at follow-up without complications. Damsin and Ghanem[11] have reported 13 corrections of more than 90-degree contracture—by far the most severe contractures ever reported—to an average of 10 degrees at follow-up, excluding two cases with multiple pterygia syndrome that recurred and needed further treatment. Damsin and Ghanem encountered three fractures and one nerve palsy in their series, and 5 of 13 knees remained stiff after treatment, more a reflection of the severity of the joint pathology than a complication per se.

Perhaps the most discouraging aspect of severe KFC correction by the Ilizarov technique is the potential joint damage from cartilage pressure necrosis (see Fig. 85-22). There is no agreed method to avoid this complication, other than to proceed slowly and to ensure that the joint is distracted during the extension period. The recurrence of flexion deformity after correction to full extension may also be related to an inadequate quadriceps, which has not been addressed by patellar tendon plication, for example, in any series of Ilizarov corrections to date.

Anterior Femoral Guided Growth (Hemiepiphysiodesis)

Mild (10- to 25-degree) flexion deformities are amenable to nonoperative management, soft tissue releases with casting, or anterior distal femoral hemiepiphysiodesis.[37] The latter is a minimally invasive method to obtain correction via a hemiepiphysiodesis effect using an anterior distal femoral tethering device. It requires only that the distal femoral physis be functional and have sufficient growth potential remain to obtain adequate correction, typically more than 2 years of growth remaining. Kramer and Stevens[37] have reported their experience with this technique, first using traditional epiphyseal staples and more recently using nonlocking eight-plates.[33] They found promising results using the eight-plates for fixed knee flexion deformities, with 17 of 18 patients having significant improvement of their deformities (total mean correction, 15 degrees). They calculated a mean correction of 1.4 degrees/month, with few complications (one wound breakdown, one knee effusion, one rebound deformity after plate removal). Comparing these results with their results using epiphyseal staples, they believe that the eight-plates offer a more reliable and faster correction of the flexion deformity.

Despite these promising early results, long-term data are needed to determine whether rebound deformity will be problematic once the hardware is removed. Additionally, we have found anterior femoral hardware to be prominent, with potential for soft tissue problems when used in very young or small children, who are typically the population with less severe deformity in whom this technique may be most successful. This technique is worth considering when an extensive surgical release or osteotomy is being considered for a less

severe deformity, or with younger children with more severe deformities if significant growth potential is remaining and anterior femoral soft tissue coverage is deemed sufficient.

Amputation, Arthrodesis, and Rotationplasty

Failure to achieve a functional knee position, especially if accompanied by pain not amenable to bracing or medication, after perhaps two attempts to correct a severe KFC, is an indication for knee fusion or disarticulation. Any discussion of treatment of severe KFC must include a realization that especially if the failure is primarily unilateral, these are appropriate and useful alternatives. Because most congenital KFC cases are bilateral, these salvage procedures are usually considered when one knee is considerably worse than the other. The decision to proceed with this type of salvage surgery must obviously be individualized.

Knee fusion with rotationplasty[1,19] should also be considered if the foot and ankle are functional in spite of the failed knee correction. The procedure simulates an internal knee amputation, with the limb being rotated 180 degrees externally after excising the distal femur and proximal tibia. This converts the ankle to a functional knee and, with a below-knee prosthesis fitted to the foot, ankle plantarflexion becomes knee extension, with dorsiflexion becoming knee flexion. The rotated foot should be at the level of the contralateral knee, so use of this salvage method generally is limited to patients with one sound limb and one requiring knee ablation.

Summary and Comments

Congenital KFC presents some of the most challenging treatment problems in orthopedics. In deformities more than 45 degrees, with a functional quadriceps, treatment to improve extension is indicated to avoid gait deterioration from quadriceps mechanical insufficiency. In young children, treatment may be important to achieve ambulation if the contracture is severe and, in patients with multiple syndromic deformities (arthrogryposis is the classic example) the decision to treat is difficult if the prognosis for functional ambulation is uncertain or poor.

Milder deformities are generally amenable to nonoperative management (bracing), soft tissue releases with casting (including extension-desubluxation hinges), or possibly growth-modulating hemiepiphysiodesis. In the more severe cases described in this chapter, extensive surgical approaches are indicated but unfortunately are fraught with recurrence as well as complications. Gradual correction by arthrodiastasis-extension (Ilizarov) methods are more effective, with or without soft tissue release, and appear to be the treatment of choice for deformities greater than 60 degrees. Frame correction, however, is no panacea, because the potential for complications is just as great as with acute correction, and experience and attention to correction details are mandatory if there is to be a moderate chance of lasting success.

KEY REFERENCES

Curtis B, Fisher R: Congenital hyperextension with anterior subluxation of the knee; surgical treatment and long-term observations. J Bone Joint Surg Am 41:255, 1969.

Ghanem I, Wattincourt L, Seringe R: Congenital dislocation of the patella. Part I: Pathologic anatomy. Part II: Orthopedic management. J Pediatr Orthop 20:812, 2000.

Herzenberg JE, Davis JR, Paley D, Bhave A: Mechanical distraction for treatment of severe flexion contractures. Clin Orthop Clin Orthop Relat Res (301):80, 1994.

Ho CA, Karol LA: The utility of knee releases in arthrogryposis. J Pediatr Orthop 28:307, 2008.

Klatt J, Stevens PM: Guided growth for fixed knee flexion deformity. J Pediatr Orthop 28:626, 2008.

Kocher MS, Garg S, Micheli LJ: Physeal sparing reconstruction of the anterior cruciate ligament in skeletally immature prepubescent children and adolescents. J Bone Joint Surg Am 87:2371, 2005.

Paletta GA, Jr: Special considerations. Anterior cruciate ligament reconstruction in the skeletally immature. Orthop Clin N Am 34:65, 2003.

Full references for this chapter can be found on www.expertconsult.com.

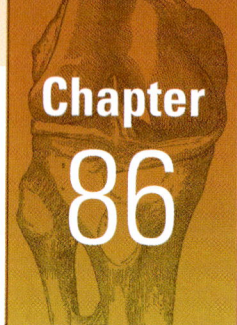

Chapter 86

Meniscal Disorders

Kevin Klingele, Dennis Kramer, and Mininder S. Kocher

MENISCAL TEARS

Meniscal tears are being seen with increasing frequency in the pediatric population.[9] Potential causes of this include a rise in organized sports participation in younger children, an improved awareness of this diagnosis among common practitioners, and wider availability and improved quality of magnetic resonance imaging (MRI).[33]

Anatomy and Classification

Pediatric meniscal tears are believed to have a greater healing potential as compared with adult tears.[10] This may be in part to the result of the vascularity of the developing meniscus. The meniscus is completely vascular at birth, and its vascularity gradually diminishes over time, resembling the adult meniscus by age 10.[21] The peripheral 25% to 30% of the adult meniscus has direct vascular supply from the perimeniscal capillary plexus and so is termed the *red-red zone*. This area is thought to have the greatest potential for repair. The remainder of the meniscus obtains its nutrition through synovial diffusion with the middle third, termed the *red-white zone,* and the central third, termed the *white-white zone* to emphasize diminishing vascular supply.

Other factors may also contribute to the healing potential of pediatric and adolescent meniscal tears. Pediatric meniscal tears usually occur following a specific injury to a previously normal meniscus. Simple nondegenerative tear patterns are most common and include longitudinal and bucket handle tears in the red-red zone.[14] Degenerative tear patterns such as parrot beak, horizontal cleavage, and complex tears are more often seen in the adult population and have lower healing potential. Additionally, many pediatric meniscal injuries occur in the setting of anterior cruciate ligament (ACL) tears.[56] The highest healing rates for meniscal repair have traditionally been seen in the setting of ACL reconstruction.

Diagnosis

Meniscal tears in children younger than 10 years generally occur in the setting of a discoid meniscus. Nondiscoid tears most commonly occur in the adolescent age group following a twisting knee injury during sports activities. Children often present with knee pain and swelling. Mechanical symptoms such as locking or catching suggest meniscal tear instability. A locked knee (unable to be fully extended or flexed) is highly suggestive of a displaced bucket handle meniscal tear. In these cases, displaced meniscal tissue occupies the intercondylar notch area to block motion. A hemarthrosis is a strong indicator of potential meniscal pathology. In one report, meniscal tears were identified in approximately 45% of children ages 7 to 18 years who presented with an acute knee hemarthrosis.[56] In this series, the medial meniscus was more commonly torn (70% to 88%) and a concurrent ACL tear was noted in 36% of the adolescents.

On physical examination, a knee effusion is often accompanied by joint line tenderness. Range of motion should be carefully assessed to identify mechanical blocks to motion. Provocative physical examination maneuvers on children may be difficult and limited by pain and apprehension. The traditional McMurray test for meniscal pathology in adults requires 90 degrees of knee flexion, which may be uncomfortable for children following a knee injury. The test has been modified for children: the knee is flexed to 30 to 40 degrees and a rotational varus or valgus stress is placed on the knee.[9,11] Joint line pain following this maneuver is indicative of meniscal pathology. When performed by an experienced examiner, the physical examination can be used to diagnose both medial (62% sensitivity, 80% specificity) and lateral (50% sensitivity, 89% specificity) meniscal tears in children reliably.[30] Other potential diagnoses must be considered in this population, including patellar dislocation, osteochondritis dissecans (OCD), osteochondral injury, and plica syndrome. The ipsilateral hip should be assessed because knee pain may be indicative of hip pathology (e.g., slipped capital femoral epiphysis) in this age group.

A meticulous ligamentous examination of the knee is necessary for children with suspected meniscal tears. Concurrent injuries such as ACL tears are common.[56] The Lachman test is reliable in the pediatric population for the diagnosis of ACL insufficiency but the test findings must be compared with those of the contralateral knee because normal tibial translation is increased in younger patients.[16] Knee radiographs are standard following knee injuries in children. A complete radiographic series in children includes an anteroposterior (AP), lateral, intercondylar notch (tunnel), and Merchant (sunrise) views. Tunnel views are helpful to identify OCD lesions located posteriorly on the femoral condyles whereas sunrise views can show patellar subluxation or osteochondral loose bodies indicative of patellar dislocation.

(MRI, when used appropriately, can aid in the diagnosis of meniscal pathology. In the proper clinical setting, MRI findings can support a presumptive diagnosis of meniscal pathology in children. Overuse of MRI in children, however, has its drawbacks. A high rate of false-positive MRI findings has been noted in the pediatric population.[40] The increased vascularity of the pediatric meniscus causes intrameniscal signal change, which can be misinterpreted as a meniscal tear (Fig. 86-1). MRI has lower sensitivity and specificity when used to evaluate meniscal pathology in children compared with adults and in younger children compared with older children.[56] MRI sensitivity (61.7%) and specificity (90.2%) for the diagnosis of meniscal tears in children younger than 12 years has been reported and compared unfavorably with children aged 12 to 16 years old (sensitivity 78.2%;

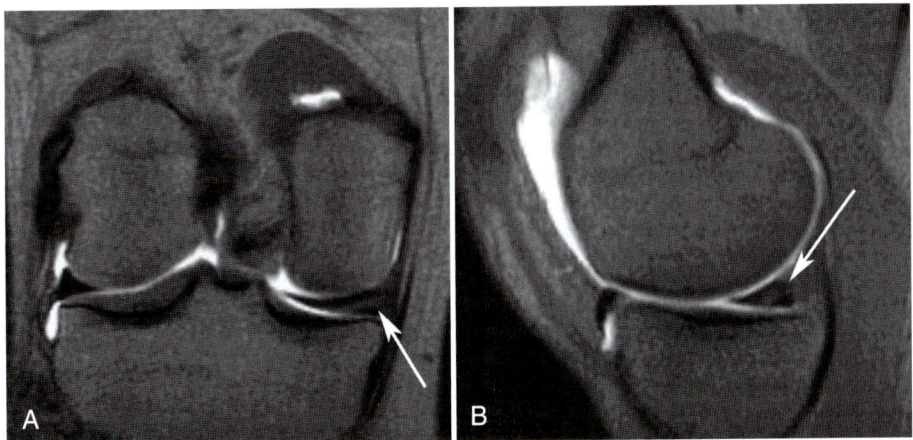

Figure 86-1. Coronal **(A)** and sagittal **(B)** T1-weighted MRI images of the knee showing intrameniscal signal abnormality *(white arrow)* consistent with the high vascularity of the meniscus in the skeletally immature child. This can easily be mistaken for a meniscal tear.

specificity 95.5%).[30] Advances in MRI have improved these percentages in the adolescent age group.[38]

Treatment

Asymptomatic meniscal tears noted incidentally on MRI can be observed over time for healing. Small symptomatic meniscal tears noted on physical examination or MRI scans may be initially treated with a trial of conservative management but persistent symptoms warrant surgical intervention. Large tears should be addressed surgically in a prompt fashion because higher healing rates have been reported when the tear is repaired within 3 months of the injury.[60] Meniscal tears identified during arthroscopy should be assessed for stability. Small tears (<10 mm) that are stable (manually displaceable less than 3 mm) may heal without repair. Meniscal trephination and synovial rasping are commonly used techniques to stimulate bleeding near the tear site.

In most cases, arthroscopic meniscal repair is favored over partial or total meniscectomy in children. Most pediatric tear patterns are amenable to repair. Removal of part or all of the meniscus may accelerate degenerative changes in the knee.[41] Contact forces in the knee increase significantly following partial meniscectomy in proportion to the amount of meniscal tissue removed.[36] Removal of a small bucket handle medial meniscal tear increases contact stresses by 65% and débridement of the posterior horn of the medial meniscus increases contact stresses to near-total meniscectomy.[7,17] Total meniscectomy increases contact stresses by 235% and should be avoided in the pediatric population. One group reported that at 5-year follow-up after partial or total meniscectomy in 20 children, mean age 15 years, 75% of patients continued to have symptoms, 80% had radiographic changes consistent with early osteoarthritis, and 60% were dissatisfied with their results.[39] A recent review has noted that 50% of patients who underwent total meniscectomy had radiographic changes, symptoms, and functional loss consistent with osteoarthritis at 10- to 20-year follow-up.[37] Unfortunately, no studies to date have demonstrated whether meniscal preservation through repair lowers the incidence of early osteoarthritis in this young and active population.

Fortunately, most pediatric meniscal tears are amenable to repair. Longitudinal peripheral tears in the red-red zone are

the most common tear type (50% to 90%) and are ideal tears to repair.[17] Other repairable tear types include bucket handle tears, meniscal root tears, and most tears that extend into the red-red or red-white zones. Many meniscal repairs in children are done in the setting of ACL reconstruction, which increases the potential for success.[35] Complex, degenerative, adult-type meniscal tear patterns, such as horizontal cleavage tears and radial tears, are less commonly seen in the pediatric population and may reflect a genetic or structural weakness of meniscal tissue.[33] These tears are generally treated with partial meniscectomy, with an attempt to preserve as much meniscal tissue as possible.

Arthroscopic techniques for meniscal repair can be divided into three groups—inside-out, outside-in, and all-inside repair. For all techniques, the tear is first identified and probed to evaluated size, location, tear pattern, and instability. Repairable tears are then reduced and the tear site is prepared for repair through rasping of the nearby synovium to create a bleeding surface for repair. Inside-out arthroscopic techniques have traditionally been the gold standard method of repair for most midbody and posterior horn tears. This technique relies on the use of double-armed absorbable or nonabsorbable repair sutures linking long flexible needles. The flexible needles are placed through curved cannulas and across the meniscal tear in a horizontal or vertical mattress fashion. The sutures are spaced approximately 3 to 5 mm apart and must be tied down to the capsule through a separate incision (Fig. 86-2).[20] An open incision may be necessary to protect posterior neurovascular structures for inside-out repair of posterior horn tears. Outside-in repair is a similar technique used mostly for anterior horn tears that relies on sutures fed through spinal needles percutaneously placed across the tear site. After passing through the tear, the sutures are retrieved and tied down to the capsule anteriorly.

Recently, arthroscopic all-inside meniscal repair techniques have gained in popularity. These techniques rely on newer generation implants that are suture-based, flexible, and low profile and provide secure fixation across the tear site while minimizing risk of adjacent chondral injury (Fig. 86-3). These implants rely on capsular penetration for deployment during repair of tears. In younger children and smaller knees, the posterior neurovascular structures lie near the posterior capsule, which may preclude the use of these implants for

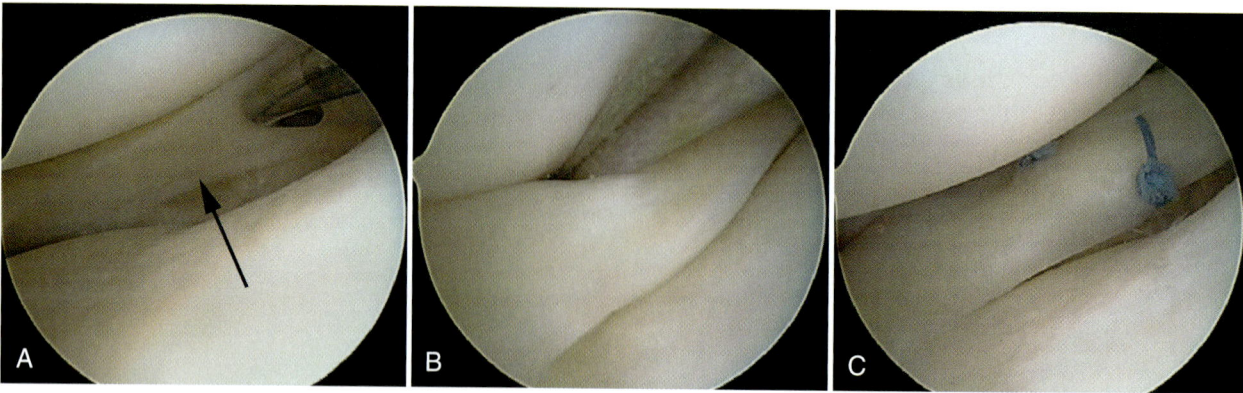

Figure 86-2. Reduction and repair of a bucket handle meniscal tear using an inside-out technique. **A,** Bucket handle meniscal tear is identified *(black arrow).* **B,** Meniscal fragment is reduced with probe and tear is identified. **C,** Meniscal repair using inside-out technique with horizontal mattress suture.

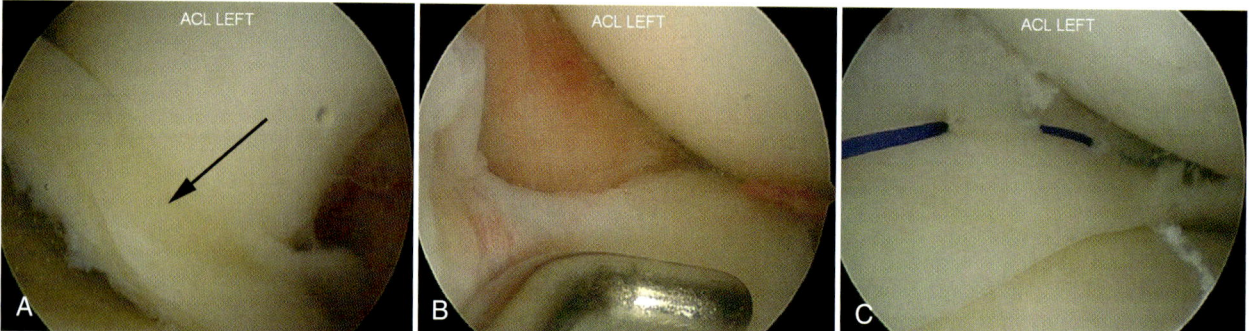

Figure 86-3. All-inside meniscal repair. **A,** Meniscal tear is identified *(black arrow).* **B,** Tear is assessed for stability with a probe. Note the displacement of the meniscus. **C,** All-inside meniscal repair with two sutures.

posterior horn tears. In these cases, a standard inside-out repair with protection of the posterior neurovascular structures is safest.

Postoperative protocols vary following meniscal repair. In most cases, a combination of limited weight bearing, bracing, and restricted motion is used for a period of 4 to 6 weeks. Physical therapy is prescribed with the goal of obtaining full knee range of motion and strength. Return to sports occurs over 3 to 6 months. Patients are clinically assessed for meniscal healing and the routine use of postoperative MRI is not recommended unless warranted by patient symptoms.

Outcome

Prior studies have published promising results on meniscal repair in children as part of a larger cohort of adult patients.[13,58] There is a paucity of data on success rates of meniscal repairs in an exclusively adolescent population. In the first published report, 26 patients, mean age 15.3 years (range, 11 to 17 years), underwent 29 meniscal repairs (12 medial and 17 lateral), with 15 of the patients (58%) undergoing simultaneous ACL reconstruction.[42] All repairs were performed arthroscopically, 25 with an inside-out technique and 4 with an all-inside technique. At mean 5-year follow-up, no meniscal symptoms were noted, all meniscal repairs were believed to have healed, and 27 of 29 patients returned to preinjury level sports. Another series reported results on 71 children and adolescents, mean age 16 years (range, 9 to 19 years), following repair of complex meniscal tears extending into the

central avascular region.[1] At a mean 51-month follow-up, 53 of 71 patients (75%) were deemed clinically healed. Notably, an 87% healing rate (39 of 45 patients) was noted in patients who were simultaneously undergoing ACL reconstruction.[45]

A retrospective case series of 45 isolated meniscal repairs in children, mean age 16 years (range, 10 to 18 years), reported clinical success in 80% of simple tears, 68% of displaced bucket handle tears, and 13% of complex tears at a mean follow-up of 5.8 years.[65] Of these, 17 repairs (38%) failed at a mean time of 17 months (range, 3 to 61 months) and required reoperation. Failure was associated with a rim width of 3 to 6 mm from the meniscosynovial junction, suggesting a tear location outside the red-red zone. The same group later reported improved meniscal repair results in the setting of ACL reconstruction. In 96 children, mean age 16 years (range, 13 to 18 years), clinical success was 84% for simple tears, 59% for displaced bucket handle tears, and 57% for complex tears. Another group included adolescents in a larger adult series and reported an 82% healing rate (based on second-look arthroscopic evaluation) for bucket handle meniscal repairs done in the setting of ACL reconstruction.[14]

Complications of meniscal repair in children are rare but can include neurovascular injury, arthrofibrosis, complex regional pain syndrome, and chondral injury from a protruding implant. In the studies noted, only two cases of arthrofibrosis and one painful neuroma of the infrapatellar branch of the saphenous nerve following inside-out repair were reported.[42] Although success rates following meniscal repair in the adolescent population are encouraging, long-term data are lacking and it remains to be seen whether meniscal preservation through repair will translate into lower rates of early osteoarthritis for these young active patients.

DISCOID MENISCUS

Since its first description in a cadaveric specimen by Young in 1889,[65] discoid lateral meniscus has become a well-documented meniscal abnormality seen in children. Although often synonymous with so-called snapping knee syndrome, discoid lateral menisci may manifest in a variety of ways. The true incidence of discoid lateral meniscus is unknown. Many children may remain asymptomatic, and few present with a true snapping knee. Nonetheless, the incidence is thought to be 3% to 5% in the general population and the incidence is slightly higher in Asian populations.[12,26,27,31] Discoid morphology almost exclusively occurs within the lateral meniscus, but medial discoid menisci also have been reported.[10] In addition, the incidence of bilateral abnormality has been reported to be 20%.[4,8,49,54]

Cause

Debate exists over the exact cause of a discoid lateral meniscus. Smillie[55] has hypothesized that discoid morphology represents an arrest in embryologic development, causing failure of central resorption within the meniscus. This theory has been disputed, however. During no stage of meniscal development is the meniscus found to be discoid in shape.[28] Further theories have claimed that increased mobility and subsequent repetitive microtrauma to the meniscus lead to its morphology and degenerative changes within its substance.[43] Early studies have shown that discoid menisci are more prone to mechanical stresses because of a thicker, less vascular structure, which often lacks peripheral attachments.[10] Other studies have noted that hypermobility does not explain the formation of the commonly seen stable discoid meniscus with intact peripheral attachments.[62] Many authors consider discoid meniscus as an anatomic variant, with a propensity for tearing because of mechanical stresses and hypermobility as a result of meniscocapsular separation secondary to increased shear stress.[31,41] Recent studies have reported a different ultrastructure of discoid menisci compared with normal menisci, including a decreased number of collagen fibers and a disorganization and discontinuity of the collagen network.[6,47] Reports of familial transmission and occurrence among identical twins support the congenital theory.[26]

Classification

The most widely documented classification system is that of Watanabe and associates,[61] who have described three types of discoid lateral menisci based on arthroscopic appearance (Fig. 86-4). Discoid menisci with intact peripheral attachments are complete (type I), covering the entire tibial plateau, or incomplete (type II). Type III discoid lateral menisci, the so-called Wrisberg ligament type, are complete or incomplete in morphology and lack posterior capsular attachments, with the exception of the posterior meniscofemoral ligament (ligament of Wrisberg). This type of discoid meniscus is thought to produce the classic snapping knee syndrome.[12]

More recent reports have described variability, not only in the size and shape of lateral menisci, but also in the peripheral rim stability and attachment.* As a result, newer classification systems have been proposed. Jordan and colleagues[26,27] have suggested a system based on peripheral stability, type of discoid meniscus (complete or incomplete), presence of associated meniscal tear, and presence or lack of clinical symptoms (Table 86-1).

The true incidence of the Wrisberg-type, or unstable, discoid meniscus is difficult to assess. Previous series have documented between 0% and 33% of symptomatic discoid menisci as unstable.[24,25,28,49,59] With variability in the morphology and the subjective nature of assessing hypermobility, reporting stability is problematic. In a review of 128

---

*References 6, 7, 19, 29, 44, and 67.

Table 86-1 Jordan Classification of Discoid Lateral Meniscus

Classification	Correlation	Tear	Symptoms
Stable	Complete, incomplete	Yes, no	Yes, no
Unstable with discoid shape	Wrisberg type	Yes, no	Yes, no
Unstable with normal shape	Wrisberg variant	Yes, no	Yes, no

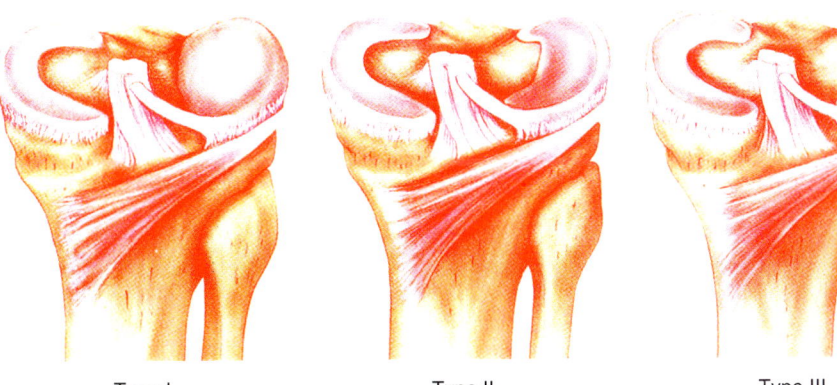

Type I   Type II   Type III

Figure 86-4. Watanabe classification of discoid lateral meniscus. Type I is a complete variant, type II is a partial variant, and type III is a Wrisberg variant.

cases of discoid menisci, Klingele and coworkers[29] have reported a 28% prevalence of peripheral rim instability, almost 47% of which were detached along the anterior third peripheral attachment, 11% at the middle third, and almost 39% at the posterior third peripheral attachment. Good and colleagues[19] have reported a 77% prevalence of meniscal instability, documenting a 53% prevalence of anterior horn detachment or hypermobility, defined as the ability to evert the meniscus or translate the anterior horn to the posterior half of the tibial plateau. Such studies suggest that the classification of discoid menisci should be based on shape (complete or incomplete), stability (stable or unstable), and presence or absence of a meniscal tear. The assumption that an unstable discoid meniscus, or what many describe as a Wrisberg type, is present at birth may not hold true. With varying locations of instability identified, discoid menisci may begin as stable and become unstable, or hypermobile, because of the repetitive stress placed on a thicker, histologically abnormal meniscus.

Diagnosis

The clinical presentation of a discoid lateral meniscus varies. Symptoms often are related to the type of discoid present, peripheral stability of the meniscus, and presence or absence of an associated meniscal tear.* Stable discoid menisci without associated tears often remain asymptomatic, identified only as incidental findings during MRI or arthroscopy. Unstable discoid menisci more commonly occur in younger children and in those with complete discoid menisci.[29] Peripheral rim detachment or hypermobility may produce the so-called snapping knee syndrome. In such cases, a painless and palpable audible or visible snap is produced with knee range of motion, especially near terminal extension. This snap is thought to be secondary to reduction of the subluxed unstable meniscus as the joint space widens with knee extension. Limitation of knee extension by 10 degrees or more has been shown to correlate with unstable and complete discoid menisci.

In children with stable discoid lateral menisci, symptoms often present when an associated tear is present. In contrast to acute meniscal tears, such symptoms may present insidiously without previous trauma. Signs and symptoms of a meniscal tear may exist, including pain, swelling, catching, locking, and limited motion. On physical examination, there may be joint line tenderness, popping, limited motion, effusion, terminal motion pain, and positive provocative test results (e.g., McMurray maneuvers, Apley test). Degenerative horizontal cleavage tears are the most common type of tear seen, reported in the largest series to occur in 58% to 98% of symptomatic discoid menisci.[4,8,49]

Imaging Studies

Radiographic evaluation is often helpful to aid in diagnosis. Standard plain radiographs of both knees should be obtained, including anteroposterior, lateral, Merchant, and tunnel views. Characteristic findings on plain radiographs are often subtle, but include a widened lateral joint line, calcification

of the lateral meniscus, squaring of the lateral condyle with concomitant cupping of the lateral tibial plateau, mild hypoplasia of the tibial spine, and an elevated fibular head. Ha et al. have described hypoplasia of the lateral femoral condyle as seen on a tunnel view radiograph, terming this the condylar cutoff sign.[22] This is seen as a decreased prominence on the lateral femoral condyle adjacent to the intercondylar notch.

On MRI, discoid meniscus is seen as three or more successive sagittal slices with continuity between the anterior and posterior meniscal horns or a transverse meniscal diameter of greater than 15 mm or greater than 20% of the tibial width on transverse images. In addition, MRI can detect the presence of an associated meniscal tear. MRI has a high positive predictive value for discoid meniscus.[30] That is, when MRI is positive, discoid meniscus is almost always present. MRI has low sensitivity for discoid meniscus, however. That is, discoid meniscus still may be present despite negative MRI. When there is strong clinical suspicion for discoid meniscus despite negative MRI, the diagnosis still should be considered, and diagnostic arthroscopy may be necessary. Complete discoid menisci are detected more easily than partial discoid menisci. Normal morphology with detachment or hypermobility can be difficult to detect on MRI. Techniques to improve the detection of discoid meniscus include newer meniscal sequences, finer cuts, and increased MRI and pediatric imaging experience. Ahn and associates[3] have proposed a classification of discoid menisci based on MRI visualization of peripheral attachments.

Treatment

If the diagnosis of a symptomatic, discoid lateral meniscus is confirmed, surgical intervention is indicated. For stable, complete, or incomplete discoid menisci, partial meniscectomy, or so-called saucerization, is the technique of choice. If meniscal instability with detachment also exists, meniscal repair can be performed in addition. Traditionally, complete meniscectomy via open or arthroscopic means was suggested for such lesions. The long-term results of complete meniscectomy and near-total meniscectomy in children are poor, however, with early degenerative changes.*

Although there may be a rare case in which salvage of a discoid meniscus may seem unobtainable, better arthroscopic technology and techniques have made meniscal preservation the ideal treatment through saucerization and repair.

Arthroscopic saucerization should débride the discoid meniscus to a peripheral rim of 6 to 8 mm (Figs. 86-5 and 86-6).† Often, an indentation on the lateral femoral condyle guides the depth of resection needed. If a meniscal tear is present, incorporation of its débridement into saucerization is most commonly performed. Most tears are of the horizontal cleavage variety, seen primarily in the posterior central area. Such tears can be débrided with adequate saucerization. If the tear extends into the peripheral vascular zone, repair should be attempted. Arthroscopic saucerization can be challenging to an inexperienced surgeon because visualization and performance within the lateral joint space can

---

*References 5, 12, 14, 15, 26, 44, 52, 62, and 64.

*References 1, 13, 23, 32, 39, 41, 50, 51, 53, and 63.
†References 18, 24, 25, 32, 46, 48, and 57.

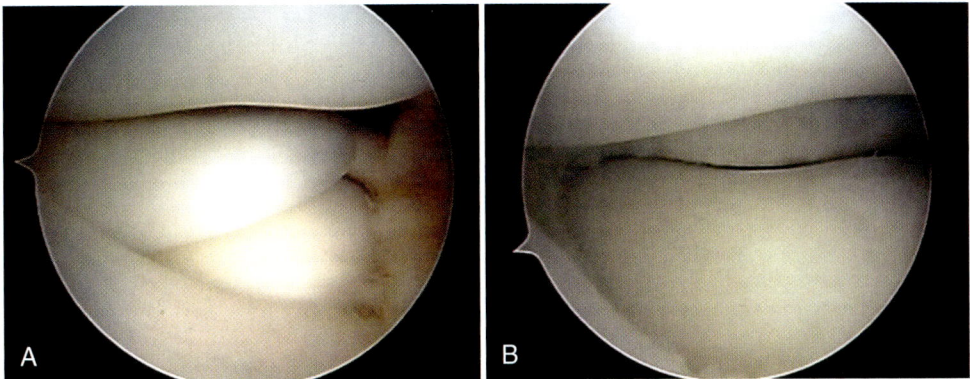

Figure 86-5. Saucerization of a partial discoid lateral meniscus. **A,** Presaucerization. **B,** Postsaucerization.

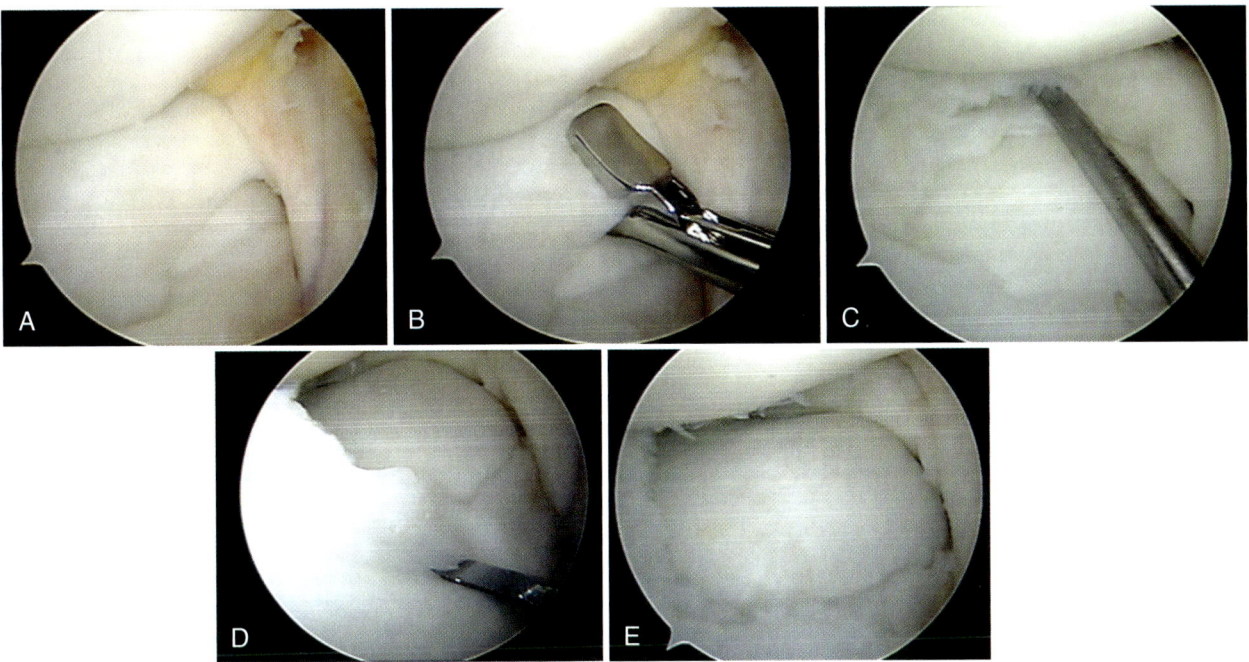

Figure 86-6. Saucerization of a complete discoid lateral meniscus. **A,** Presaucerization. **B,** Excision of the central portion in the flexed knee position. **C,** Probe within the horizontal cleavage tear. **D,** Arthroscopic knife excision of the excess anterior horn. **E,** Postsaucerization.

be limited by the thickened meniscus and small size of the knee in pediatric patients. Saucerization is best begun with the knee in flexion by the aid of a straight biter, or scissor punch. Smaller baskets are available and are more appropriate for pediatric knees. A meniscal or cartilage knife can aid in contouring the abnormal meniscus, especially the anterior horn. The knee can be placed in the figure-four position for further work. A combination of small arthroscopic shavers and biters further facilitates saucerization. With horizontal cleavage tears, often the smaller of the present meniscal flaps is débrided, leaving an intact peripheral rim to the remaining flap. Resection to widths more than 8 mm is thought to increase the risk of recurrent tear.

A careful and methodical assessment of peripheral rim stability and attachment must be carried out after saucerization.[19,29] The frequency of peripheral rim instability mandates a systematic probing of the remnant meniscus at all peripheral attachments. In contrast to the posteriorly unstable Wrisberg type of discoid meniscus, anterior or middle horn

peripheral detachment also can be seen. If peripheral instability is identified, meniscal repair is indicated. We prefer to perform meniscal repair using numerous inside-out sutures, zone-specific cannulas, and an open posterolateral incision to retrieve and tie the sutures, protecting the peroneal nerve. All-inside devices may be inappropriate for discoid lateral meniscus repair, given the extreme meniscal instability and the size of the implants. For anterior horn instability, outside-in techniques are useful (see Fig. 86-6).

Postoperatively, protected motion and weight bearing followed by progressive mobilization and rehabilitation are necessary. Younger children may be unable to ambulate effectively with crutches or comply with motion and weight-bearing restrictions.

The results of arthroscopic saucerization with or without repair have not been established. Ahn and coworkers[2] have reported on 28 knees that underwent saucerization and peripheral rim repair. At minimum 2-year follow-up, all patients were able to return to full activity with improved

Lysholm and Hospital for Special Surgery (HSS) knee scores. Rosenberg and colleagues[52] have presented a case report of arthroscopic attachment of a free posterior edge in a normal-shaped, Wrisberg-type lateral meniscus, with good results at 1-year follow-up. Woods and Whelan[62] have described four patients with unstable, discoid lateral menisci and lack of posterior attachment. All patients underwent repair; three of four had good results at 37.5-month follow-up. Similarly, Neuschwander and coworkers[44] have identified six patients with lateral meniscal variants who underwent arthroscopic repair of posterior detachment, and four had an excellent result.

With further understanding of discoid menisci and the potential for developing peripheral rim instability, treatment of a stable asymptomatic discoid is now debatable. Classic teaching has been to treat asymptomatic discoids or those found incidentally without surgical intervention.

Unstable discoid menisci, which may be harder to salvage, more commonly present in younger patients with complete discoid morphology. Saucerization prior to symptoms and/or peripheral rim detachment may prevent future instability or the development of degenerative cleavage meniscal tears.

KEY REFERENCES

Aichroth PM, Patel DV, Marx CL: Congenital discoid lateral meniscus in children. A follow-up study and evolution of management. J Bone Joint Surg Br 73:932–936, 1991.

Clark CR, Ogden JA: Development of the menisci of the human knee joint. Morphological changes and their potential role in childhood meniscal injury. J Bone Joint Surg Am 65:538–547, 1983.

Dickhaut SC, DeLee JC: The discoid lateral-meniscus syndrome. J Bone Joint Surg Am 64:1068–1073, 1982.

Ikeuchi H: Arthroscopic treatment of the discoid lateral meniscus. Technique and long-term results. Clin Orthop Relat Res 1982 67:19–28, 1982.

Jordan MR: Lateral meniscal variants: evaluation and treatment. J Am Acad Orthop Surg 4:191–200, 1996.

Kaplan EB: Discoid lateral meniscus of the knee join: nature, mechanism, and operative treatment. J Bone Joint Surg Am 39-A:77–87, 1957.

Klingele KE, Kocher MS, Hresko MT, Gerbino P, Micheli LJ, et al: Discoid lateral meniscus: prevalence of peripheral rim instability. J Pediatr Orthop 24:79–82, 2004.

Kramer DE, Micheli LJ: Meniscal tears and discoid meniscus in children: diagnosis and treatment. J Am Acad Orthop Surg 17:698–707, 2009.

Manzione M, Pizzutillo PD, Peoples AB, Schweizer PA: Meniscectomy in children: a long-term follow-up study. Am J Sports Med 11:111–115, 1983.

Medlar RC, Mandiberg JJ, Lyne ED: Meniscectomies in children. Report of long-term results (mean, 8.3 years) of 26 children. Am J Sports Med 8:87–92, 1980.

Mintzer CM, Richmond JC, Taylor J: Meniscal repair in the young athlete. Am J Sports Med 26:630–633, 1998.

Raber DA, Friederich NF, Hefti F: Discoid lateral meniscus in children. Long-term follow-up after total meniscectomy. J Bone Joint Surg Am 80:1579–1586, 1998.

Smillie IS: The congenital discoid meniscus. J Bone Joint Surg Am Br 30B:671–682, 1948.

Vandermeer RD, Cunningham FK: Arthroscopic treatment of the discoid lateral meniscus: results of long-term follow-up. Arthroscopy 5:101–109, 1989.

Wroble RR, Henderson RC, Campion ER, et al: el-Khoury GY, Albright JP: Meniscectomy in children and adolescents. A long-term follow-up study. Clin Orthop Relat Res 279:180–189, 1992.

Full references for this chapter can be found on www.expertconsult.com.

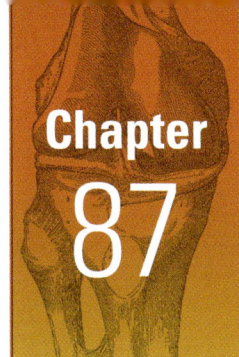

Chapter
87

Osteochondritis Dissecans

Theodore J. Ganley and John M. Flynn

Osteochondritis dissecans (OCD) is an acquired, potentially reversible disorder of the subchondral bone and of the overlying articular cartilage. Initially, softening of the overlying articular cartilage is noted with an intact articular surface (Fig. 87-1), which can progress to early articular cartilage separation, partial detachment of an articular lesion, and eventual osteochondral separation with loose bodies.* Osteochondritis dissecans is a relatively common cause of knee pain and dysfunction in the child and adolescent. The cause of OCD is unknown; however, repetitive microtrauma is often implicated.[13,17,30,58,74] OCD of the knee is subcategorized into a juvenile form and an adult form, depending on the status of the distal femoral physis, and is classified on the basis of anatomic location, surgical appearance, scintigraphic findings, and age.[†] Juvenile OCD (JOCD) has a much better prognosis than adult OCD, with more than 50% of cases demonstrating healing within 6 to 18 months from nonoperative treatment.[15,31,34,66,70] Adult OCD, on the other hand, frequently requires operative intervention for healing.[6,15] Adult OCD and juvenile OCD lesions that do not heal have the potential for later sequelae, including osteoarthritis.[48,69]

HISTORY AND CAUSES OF JOCD AND OCD

Several factors have been implicated in the origin of OCD: inflammation, genetics, ischemia, accessory centers of ossification, and repetitive trauma. In 1887, König suggested an inflammatory origin, using the name "osteochondritis dissecans."[44] Further study, however, did not support inflammation as a primary cause of OCD. Ribbing ascribed OCD to an ossification abnormality of the distal femoral epiphysis in 1955.[64] Although abnormalities in ossification do not account for most cases of OCD, some incidentally found lateral femoral condylar lesions in younger children that resolve spontaneously may represent an ossification variant. Based on their anatomic and histologic findings, Green and Banks[31] proposed that ischemia was implicated in OCD, although additional studies have failed to find avascular necrosis of the OCD fragment or a relative ischemic watershed of the lateral aspect of the medial femoral condyle.[16,40,62,65] Some investigators have suggested a genetic predisposition to OCD. Petrie[60] found OCD in only one of 86 first-degree relatives, although as many as 12 instances of family members with OCD over the course of four generations have been reported by Mubarak and Carroll.[54] It is widely believed that the common form of OCD is not familial. Endocrinopathies, ligamentous laxity, malalignment, apophysitis, epiphyseal dysplasia, and other osteochondropathies have not been described in association with OCD.

In 1933, Fairbanks[24] suggested that OCD might be due to a "violent rotation inwards of the tibia, driving the tibial spine against the inner condyle." Although anterior tibial spine impingement may not be the cause of lesions in the most common location of the posterolateral aspect of the medial femoral condyle, the frequent occurrence of OCD in patients who are involved in sports with repetitive impact supports a repetitive trauma etiology.[25] OCD may begin after repetitive trauma causes a stress reaction, which then may further progress to a stress fracture of the underlying subchondral bone. Without a reduction in repetitive loading, the ability of the subchondral bone to heal is exceeded, necrosis of the fragment occurs, and eventual fragment dissection and separation develop.

OCD lesions may resemble acute osteochondral fracture, chondral injury, or osteonecrosis. The estimated incidence of OCD ranges from 15 to 29 cases per 100,000.[35,47] The mean age of patients with OCD appears to be decreasing, and more girls seem to have involvement.[13] The widespread use of magnetic resonance imaging (MRI) and arthroscopy in the pediatric population has likely resulted in greater recognition of OCD lesions. Trends in youth sports such as loss of free play, early sport specialization, multiple leagues in a single sport, and intensive training may be contributing factors.

DIAGNOSIS

Clinical Presentation

The presenting complaints of most children and adolescents with OCD are nonspecific. Because most patients have a stable lesion, aching and activity-related knee pain localized to the anterior aspect of the knee are the most common complaints. Symptoms resemble those produced by chondromalacia patellae and subtle forms of patellofemoral malalignment. In both patellofemoral pain and OCD, climbing hills or stairs may produce symptoms. Children with OCD usually do not complain of knee instability.

Physical examination findings are often subtle. Children and adolescents with stable OCD lesions may walk with a slight antalgic gait. With careful palpation through varying amounts of knee flexion, a point of maximum tenderness can often be located over the anterior medial aspect of the knee. The tender area will correspond to the lesion, usually on the lateral aspect of the distal medial femoral condyle. With stable lesions, knee effusion, crepitus, and extreme pain are rarely observed through a normal range of motion. Wilson's sign may be helpful but often is not present.[18,76] Wilson's test is performed by starting with the knee flexed to 90 degrees. The tibia is then internally rotated as the knee is extended

---

*References 5, 13, 17, 30, 36, 42, 58, and 74.
[†]References 13, 14, 17, 30, 34, and 58.

from 90 degrees toward full extension. A positive Wilson's test will elicit pain at about 30 degrees of knee flexion located over the anterior aspect of the medial femoral condyle. This pain is thought to result from contact of the medial tibial eminence with the OCD lesion. Ipsilateral quadriceps atrophy may be noted if the patient has been having pain for longer than a few months.

Mechanical symptoms are more pronounced in the unusual circumstance in which the child or adolescent presents with an unstable lesion. An antalgic gait is common, as is a knee effusion, possibly associated with crepitus, as the knee is taken through a range of motion. In the case of both stable and unstable presentations, both knees should be examined to determine whether or not the condition is bilateral.

Imaging Studies

Imaging protocols have received close attention in the literature because of the varied success of nonoperative treatment. The goals of imaging are to characterize the lesion, determine the prognosis of nonoperative management, and monitor healing of the lesion (Fig. 87-2A through C).

Imaging workup begins with plain radiographs: anteroposterior (Fig. 87-3A), lateral, and tunnel views. The tunnel view is particularly valuable because the typical OCD lesion is located on the lateral portion of the medial femoral condyle (see Fig. 87-3B). Because patellar OCD lesions also occur, a Merchant or skyline view should be included as well. Plain radiographs usually characterize and localize the lesion and rule out other bony pathology of the knee region. In children 6 and younger, the distal femoral epiphyseal ossification center may exhibit irregularities that simulate the appearance of an OCD. In older children, the status of the physis (open, closing, or closed) should be assessed, as this has major implications in the prognosis for healing. Cahill and Berg[14] developed a classification system based on lesion location and size, such that the type of lesion can be determined on plain films.

MRI is most useful for determining the size of the lesion and the status of the cartilage in the subchondral bone.[41,73] The extent of bony edema, the presence of a high signal zone beneath the fragment (Fig. 87-4A through C), and the presence of other loose bodies are important findings on the initial MRI (Table 87-1). Routine imaging studies performed

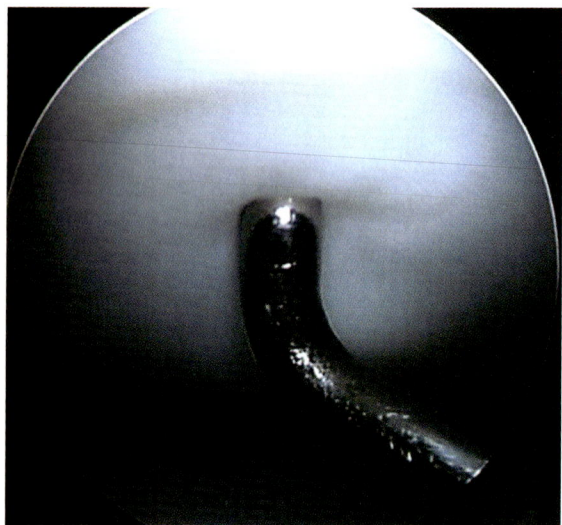

Figure 87-1. Probe demonstrates softening of a femoral condyle osteochondritis dissecans (OCD) lesion.

Table 87-1 MRI Classification of Juvenile Osteochondritis Dissecans

Stage	MRI Finding
I	Small change of signal without clear margins of fragment
II	Osteochondral fragment with clear margins, but without fluid between fragment and underlying bone
III	Fluid visible partially between fragment and underlying bone
IV	Fluid completely surrounding the fragment, but the fragment is still in situ
V	Fragment completely detached and displaced (loose body)

Data from Hefti F, Berguiristain J, Krauspe R, et al: Osteochondritis dissecans: a multicenter study of the European Pediatric Orthopedic Society. J Pediatr Orthop 8B:231–245, 1999.

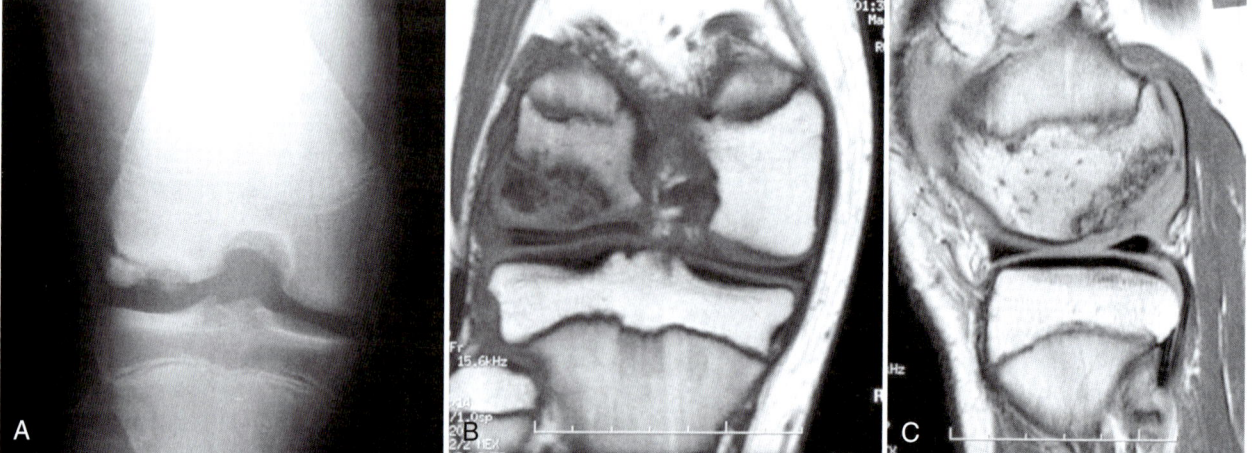

Figure 87-2. A, Anteroposterior x-ray of a large osteochondritis dissecans (OCD) of the lateral femoral condyle in an adolescent patient. **B,** Anteroposterior and **(C)** lateral T1-weighted images of a large OCD lesion in the posterolateral aspect of the lateral femoral condyle.

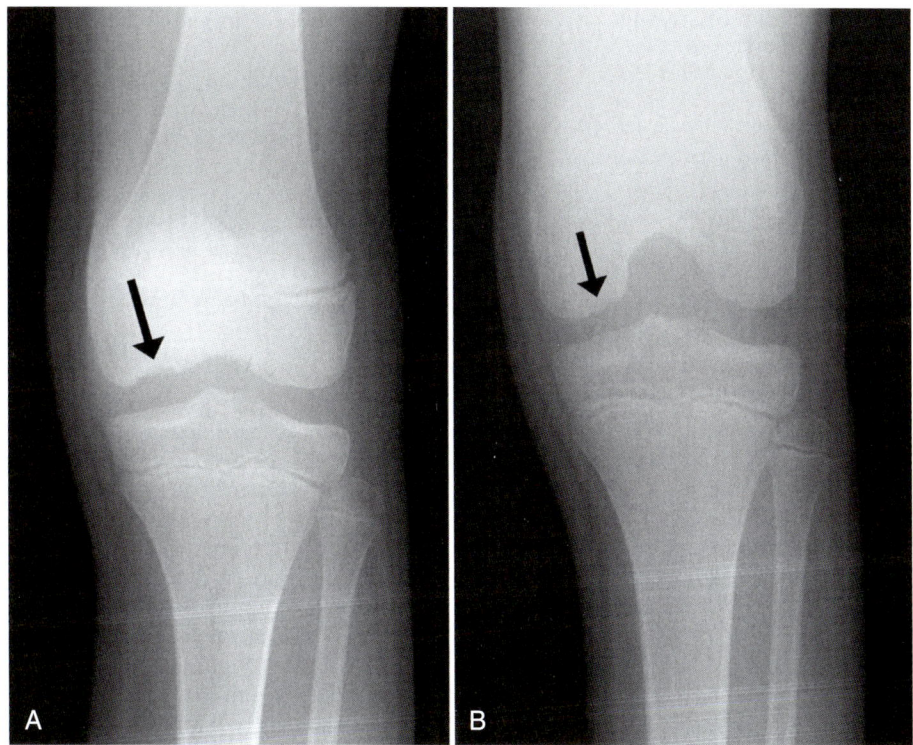

Figure 87-3. **A,** Anteroposterior and **(B)** tunnel plain radiographs demonstrating osteochondritis dissecans (OCD) of the lateral aspect of the medial femoral condyle.

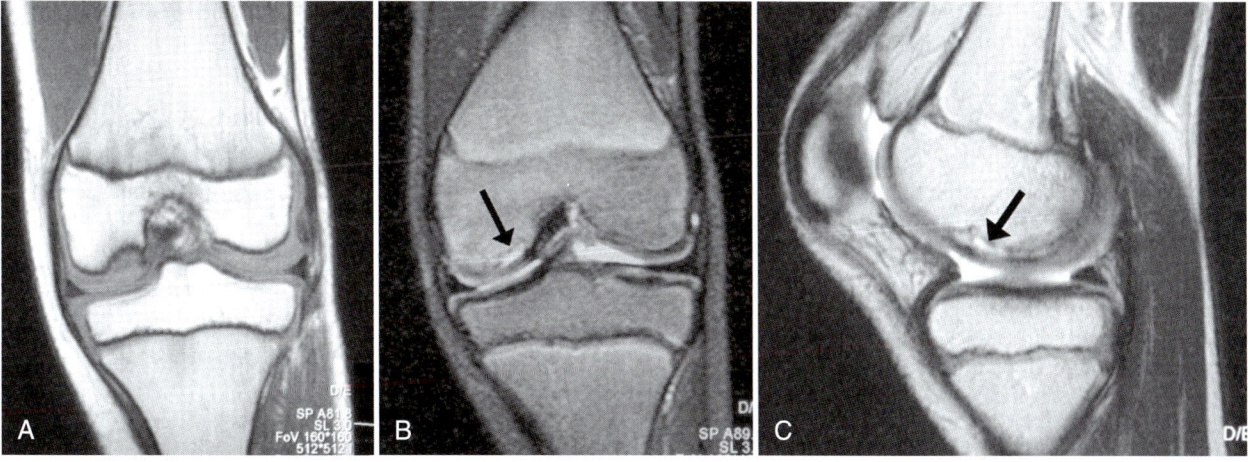

Figure 87-4. **A,** Anteroposterior T1-weighted image, **(B)** anteroposterior T2-weighted image, and **(C)** lateral T1-weighted image show classic location of an osteochondritis dissecans (OCD) lesion at the lateral aspect of the medial femoral condyle with fluid shown beneath the lesion *(arrows)*.

during the course of nonoperative treatment in skeletally immature patients can help identify patients at risk for treatment failure. Evidence suggests that a high signal line on T2-weighted images, representing healing vascular granulation tissue or articular fluid beneath the subchondral bone, is a predictor of instability.[11,20,56,61] A breach in the cartilage seen on T1-weighted MRI may help predict treatment failure, particularly when seen in conjunction with a high signal line on T2-weighted images.[56] Recent investigations of the relationship between gadolinium enhancement and healing have been inconclusive.[11,45,72] The healing potential of stable

JOCD was studied recently, and it was found that after 6 months of nonoperative treatment, 16 (34%) of 47 stable lesions did not progress to healing. The size of the lesion determined by MRI was the strongest prognostic variable.[75]

Technetium bone scans have been used to obtain information about the biologic capacity of an OCD lesion to heal (Table 87-2).[14,48,57] Although some authors have found that serial bone scans indicate the extent of healing, this imaging technique has not been widely accepted, most likely because of the length of the test, the need for intravenous access, and the perceived risk of the radiotracer injection.

Table 87-2 Bone Scan Classification of Juvenile Osteochondritis Dissecans Lesions

Stage	Bone Scan Finding
0	Normal radiographic and scintigraphic appearance
I	Lesion visible on plain radiographs, but bone scan reveals normal findings
II	Bone scan reveals increased uptake in the area of the lesion
III	Increased isotopic uptake in the entire femoral condyle
IV	Uptake in the tibial plateau opposite the lesion

Data from Cahill BR: Osteochondritis dissecans of the knee: treatment of juvenile and adult forms. J Am Acad Orthop Surg 3:237–247, 1995.

NONOPERATIVE MANAGEMENT

Nonoperative management is the treatment of choice for skeletally immature children.[70] Because of the vague origin of OCD, debate is ongoing about whether immobilization or bracing is therapeutic or detrimental. Because a primary goal is regeneration of injured subchondral bone, casting or knee bracing is favored by many to provide immobilization or to help unload an affected area. Other clinicians have sought to reach the same goals by using algorithms that include lesser forms of intervention such as restriction from high-impact sports; others have used partial weight-bearing or non–weight-bearing treatments. The common denominator in all programs is a structured therapy regimen to ensure the return of appropriate strength and flexibility.

Options for immobilization include casting, bracing, and standard knee immobilization. Partial weight bearing in slight flexion minimizes shear, while preserving a limited amount of compression across the lesion. Selecting an immobilization protocol can be difficult. Casts present children with the inconvenience of more restricted range of motion, but can be useful in children who are noncompliant with bracing. Recent data have shown that casts are efficacious for healing and allow maintenance of motion and strength during treatment.[71]

The authors recommend a three-phase approach to the nonoperative management of OCD lesions. In phase I, knee bracing is recommended. Unloader bracing allows for range of motion, and weight bearing with hinged knee bracing requires that the knee be locked in extension for weight-bearing activities. However, a hinged brace can be unlocked to allow the patient to perform range-of-motion exercises as well. If the patient is pain free and radiographs show signs of healing after 6 weeks, he or she is allowed to begin weight bearing without bracing and to begin a physical therapy protocol to improve knee range of motion and quadriceps and hamstring strength (phase II, weeks 6 to 12). Three months after diagnosis, a patient who has remained pain free and shows radiographic evidence of healing begins phase III, in which running, jumping, and cutting sports are permitted under close observation. High-impact activities and activities that might involve shear stress to the knee should be restricted until the child has been pain free for several months and radiographs show a healed lesion. Although patients with JOCD have a better prognosis for healing than those with adult OCD, not all lesions in skeletally immature knees heal. Repeat nonoperative treatment can be considered if radiographs show progression of the lesion, or if symptoms return.

Although immobilization is often successful in JOCD, it may not be the ideal treatment option for a young athlete and his or her parents. Patients and their parents should be informed of the risks and benefits of nonoperative treatment relative to those presented by surgical management (Fig. 87-5).

OPERATIVE MANAGEMENT

It is widely accepted that operative treatment should be considered for patients with unstable or detached lesions, in patients approaching skeletal maturity, and in patients whose lesions have not resolved after an appropriate period of nonoperative management.[6,13,23,33,36] The goals of operative treatment are to promote healing of subchondral bone, to maintain joint congruity, to rigidly fix unstable fragments, and to replace osteochondral defects with cells that can replace and grow cartilage.[29,66] Optimal surgical treatment will provide a stable construct of subchondral bone, calcified tidemark, and repair cartilage with viability and biomechanical properties similar to those of native hyaline cartilage.

Arthroscopic drilling is indicated for stable lesions with an intact articular surface. Drilling creates channels to promote revascularization and healing (Fig. 87-6). Although more technically challenging, antegrade or retroarticular drilling (proximal to distal) precludes disruption of the articular surface. This technique has been reported as an effective alternative to promote bone healing and protection of the articular surface as well.[22] Conversely, a transarticular technique is more straightforward from a surgical perspective, but it creates small articular cartilage channels that can heal with fibrocartilage.[8]

Arthroscopic transarticular drilling is effective in the treatment of OCD lesions in skeletally immature patients. A number of authors have reported radiographic resolution and increases in Lysholm score throughout postoperative follow-up.[1,3,8,12] Adachi and associates recently studied 20 stable lesions in 12 skeletally immature patients (mean age, 12 years) and found that with transarticular drilling, 19 of the 20 showed successful healing.[1] Treatment success is much better for children with open physes than for skeletally mature patients. Anderson and colleagues[8] noted healing in 18 of 20 lesions in a skeletally immature group, and only 2 of 4 healed at an average follow-up of 5 years in a skeletally mature group. Younger age has also been shown to be a predictor of a more favorable Lysholm score.[43] Factors associated with inadequate healing after drilling include lesions in atypical locations, multiple lesions, and patients with underlying medical conditions.[26]

The goal of operative treatment of flap lesions is removal of the fibrous tissue found between the fragments and underlying bone without disruption of the underlying bone from the fragment or the subchondral bone at the base of the lesion. In patients with partially unstable lesions or unstable lesions with adequate subchondral bone to match the defect and the fragment, open or arthroscopic fixation can be performed. For cases in which subchondral bone loss has occurred, autogenous bone graft can be packed into the crater prior to reduction and fixation. Rapid relief of discomfort upon reduction has led some authors to theorize that pain is the result

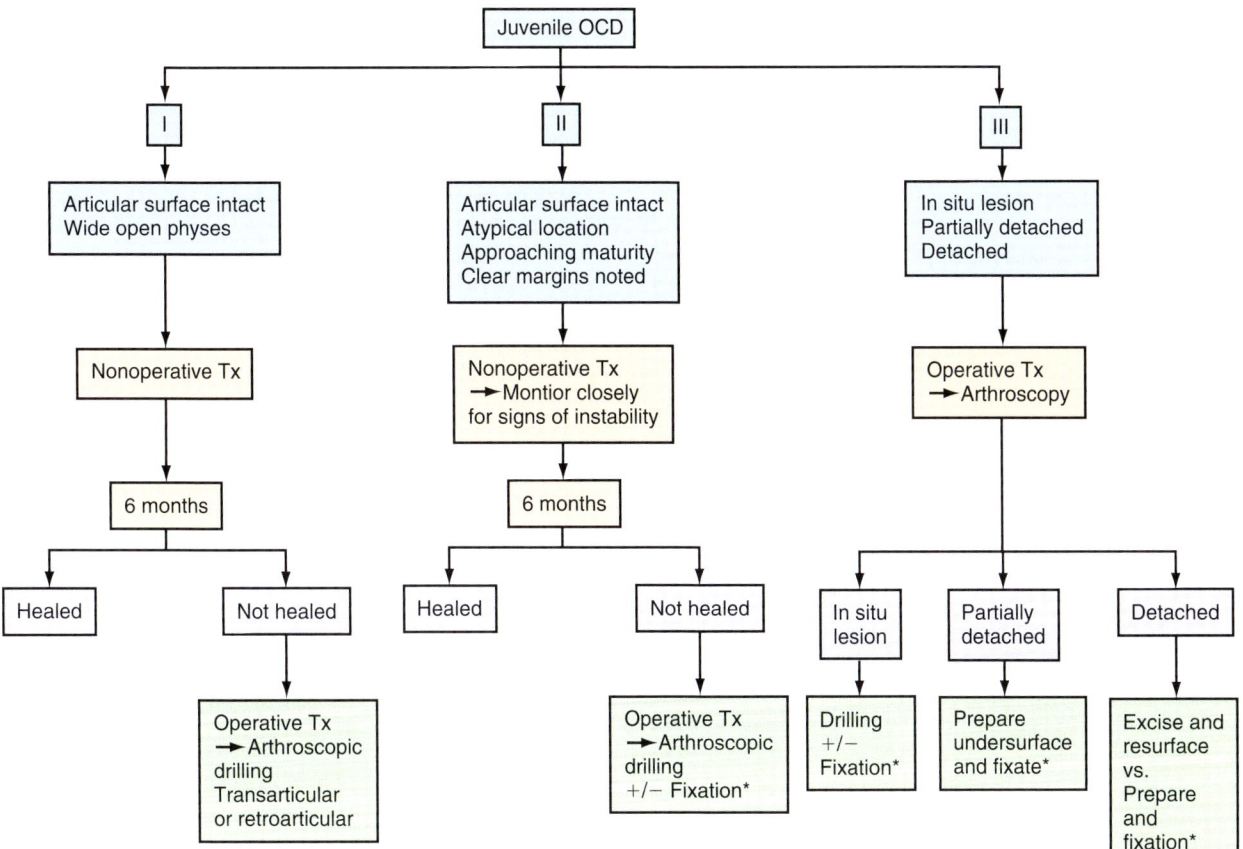

Figure 87-5. Algorithm for the treatment of osteochondritis dissecans in the pediatric patient.

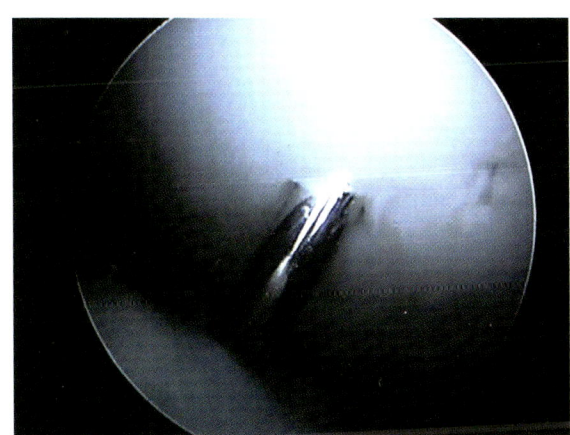

Figure 87-6. Drilling osteochondritis dissecans (OCD) lesion with smooth K-wire.

of increased pressure at the line of separation between the fragment and the epiphysis.[12,37,68]

Poor long-term results following excision of a loose OCD fragment in skeletally mature patients have led authors to recommend more aggressive attempts to preserve the articular cartilage and avoid excision of the fragments.[77] Cortical strips of bone from the metaphysis of the tibia have also been used.[29,55] Although Herbert screws and cannulated screws have been used successfully,[51] second surgeries may be required for removal.[19,63] A review of Herbert screw fixation performed in 15 knees (14 patients, ages 12 to 35) with 50-month

follow-up showed that 14 of 15 knees had stable fragments at second-look arthroscopy.[51] Screw fixation is also reported to have successful functional outcomes. A recent case series of 12 patients with grade IV loose bodies treated with screw fixation showed that at an average 9 years after surgery, no incidences of osteoarthritis pain were reported and all patients described normal knee function.[50] More recently, authors have reported good results with bioabsorbable pin fixation as an alternative to metal fixation.[7,21] A study of 11 patients with bioabsorbable Pla pin fixation reported union in all patients as noted by MRI, and one case of early synovitis was treated with nonsteroidal anti-inflammatory drugs (NSAIDs).[21] Adachi and coworkers evaluated the histology of 10 unstable lesions (mean age, 15 years) treated with bioabsorbable pins alone or with pins and grafting and found that postoperative specimens had both significantly improved grading scores and signs of regeneration of the articular cartilage.[2]

In a large unsalvageable fragment, the goal is to replace the defect with subchondral bone, calcified tidemark, and overlying cartilage. Drilling, abrasion arthroplasty, and microfracturing with awls as well as picks recruit pluripotential cells from marrow that preferentially differentiate into fibrocartilage.[67] These techniques are used primarily for smaller lesions because fibrocartilage does not respond to shear stress as effectively as native hyaline cartilage, and deterioration of the repaired site over time has been reported.[52] An alternative treatment option reported in the literature consists of removal of the fragment and simple débridement of the crater.[4]

However, results of long-term follow-up with weight-bearing anteroposterior (AP) radiographs have shown the progression of Fairbanks changes and suggest a poor prognosis for lesions larger than 2 cm.[7]

A cartilaginous extracellular matrix can be generated in the defect with periosteum and transplant of the cambium layer. Results of studies with long-term follow-up suggest that this operative technique is not ideal because of the incidence of reoperation and persistent knee pain.[49,61] Concerns about the durability of reparative fibrocartilage have provided the impetus for the development of alternative techniques. Autologous osteochondral plugs obtained from non–weight bearing regions of the knee (e.g., the edge of the intercondylar notch or upper outer trochlea) have also been transplanted to replace defects.[9,10,28,46] Good results have been reported in recent studies, both in patients with open growth plates and in those who have reached skeletal maturity.[57,78] A recent prospective, randomized study of 47 patients compared outcomes of patients treated with microfracture versus those treated with autologous osteochondral plugs. Both microfracture and osteochondral autografts gave encouraging clinical results; however, lesions treated with osteochondral plugs showed superior outcomes at 4.2-year follow-up.[32] Potential disadvantages of osteochondral grafts, including donor site morbidity, are balanced by the advantages of biologic internal fixation.[38] Secondary reconstruction with bone–articular surface allografts has been described with success in patients with significant surface defects in OCD, although no long-term results in skeletally immature patients are yet available.[27]

Autologous chondrocyte implantation has been used in younger patients with no lower extremity malalignment to repair large, isolated femoral defects. Recent studies have reported high rates of successful repair, although information about long-term prognosis is not yet available.[9,59] King and associates[39] noted slightly better outcomes of autologous chondrocyte transplantation for large defects in articular cartilage of the distal femur in adolescent patients than were previously reported in adult patients, probably caused by superior articular substance in adjacent regions of the knee.[53]

SUMMARY

The prevalence of OCD of the knee is increasing among children. Careful attention to presenting symptoms accompanied by successful imaging is an integral part of making the diagnosis. Timely recognition is essential, because stable lesions with an intact articular surface can usually be treated successfully with a three-stage nonoperative management protocol. The fundamental principle of this protocol is the cessation of repetitive impact loading followed by gradual return to normal activity, usually facilitated by some form of adjunctive bracing. MRI may aid in the early prediction of a lesion's healing potential. For stable lesions that do not show signs of resolution after the nonoperative protocol has been followed for 6 months, arthroscopic drilling should be considered to prevent progression to an unstable lesion. Excision of large lesions generally yields poor results, but chondral resurfacing techniques may decrease the risk of subsequent arthrosis. Fixation and bone grafting for unstable lesions and cartilage resurfacing techniques for full-thickness defects have evolved and show encouraging results; however, further study is required before definitive statements can be made regarding long-term prognosis in children and adolescents. Overall, early recognition and treatment of these lesions when patients are younger helps to minimize the degree of intervention required to promote lesion healing.

KEY REFERENCES

Adachi N, Motoyama M, Deie M, et al: Histological evaluation of internally-fixed osteochondral lesions of the knee. J Bone Joint Surg Br 91:823–829, 2009.

Anderson AF, Pagnani MJ: Osteochondritis dissecans of the femoral condyles: long-term results of excision of the fragment. Am J Sports Med 25:830–834, 1997.

Bentley G, Biant LC, Carrington RW, et al: A prospective, randomised comparison of autologous chondrocyte implantation versus mosaicplasty for osteochondral defects in the knee. J Bone Joint Surg Br 85:223–230, 2003.

Conrad JM, Stanitski CL: Osteochondritis dissecans: Wilson's sign revisited. Am J Sports Med 31:777–778, 2003.

Donaldson LD, Wojtys EM: Extraarticular drilling for stable osteochondritis dissecans in the skeletally immature knee. J Pediatr Orthop 28:831–835, 2008.

Flynn JM, Kocher MS, Ganley TJ: Osteochondritis dissecans of the knee. J Pediatr Orthop 24:434–443, 2004.

Gudas R, Simonaityte R, Cekanauskas E, Tamosiunas R: A prospective, randomized clinical study of osteochondral autologous transplantation versus microfracture for the treatment of osteochondritis dissecans in the knee joint in children. J Pediatr Orthop 29:741–748, 2009.

Hefti F, Beguiristain J, Krauspe R, et al: Osteochondritis dissecans: a multicenter study of the European Pediatric Orthopedic Society. J Pediatr Orthop B 8:231–245, 1999.

Kocher MS, Micheli LJ, Yaniv M, et al: Functional and radiographic outcome of juvenile osteochondritis dissecans of the knee treated with transarticular arthroscopic drilling. Am J Sports Med 29:562–566, 2001.

Magnussen RA, Carey JL, Spindler KP: Does operative fixation of an osteochondritis dissecans loose body result in healing and long-term maintenance of knee function? Am J Sports Med 37:754–759, 2009.

Makino A, Muscolo DL, Puigdevall M, et al: Arthroscopic fixation of osteochondritis dissecans of the knee: clinical, magnetic resonance imaging, and arthroscopic follow-up. Am J Sports Med 33:1499–1504, 2005.

Micheli LJ, Moseley JB, Anderson AF, et al: Articular cartilage defects of the distal femur in children and adolescents: treatment with autologous chondrocyte implantation. J Pediatr Orthop 26:455–460, 2006.

Pill SG, Ganley TJ, Milam RA, et al: Role of magnetic resonance imaging and clinical criteria in predicting successful nonoperative treatment of osteochondritis dissecans in children. J Pediatr Orthop 23:102–108, 2003.

Wall EJ, Vourazeris J, Myer GD, et al: The healing potential of stable juvenile osteochondritis dissecans knee lesions. J Bone Joint Surg Am 90:2655–2664, 2008.

Wright RW, McLean M, Matava MJ, Shively RA: Osteochondritis dissecans of the knee: long-term results of excision of the fragment. Clin Orthop Relat Res 424:239–243, 2004.

Full references for this chapter can be found on www.expertconsult.com.

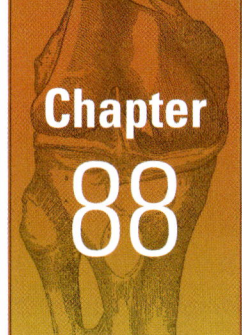

Reconstructing the Anterior Cruciate Ligament in Pediatric Patients

Allen F. Anderson and Christian Noel Anderson

An intrasubstance tear of the anterior cruciate ligament (ACL) is rare in pediatric patients, although it is a common injury in adults. Typically, knee trauma in a child or adolescent results in a bone or a physeal injury.[41] However, the reported incidence of debilitating ACL injury in children has risen because of their increased participation in competitive sports and improved ACL diagnostic techniques.[*]

A torn ACL in a skeletally immature patient is a treatment dilemma for the physician. In such cases, two basic treatment options are available: nonoperative and operative. Each option has its own set of challenges and possible long-term consequences for the child. The nonoperative approach can lead to instability, meniscal tears, and cumulative degenerative changes,[1,15,23,27,31] while operative treatment can result in iatrogenic leg length discrepancy or angular deformity.[4,24-27,32,39]

No consensus has been reached on the best method of treatment for a torn ACL in children and adolescents, primarily because of the paucity of basic science research on physeal growth and its response to injury. Although several retrospective studies on ACL tears in children have been conducted, the methods of the studies and the quality of the data have been inadequate.[†] Consequently, the treatment of ACL tears remains controversial in the pediatric population. Despite the lack of consensus, by using the current pediatric literature on the natural history of ACL tears, average growth and development patterns, and the response of the physis to injury, a reasonable treatment plan can be developed that is based on the consequences of iatrogenic growth disturbance. This chapter presents an evaluative approach to ACL reconstruction and describes three surgical techniques that may be used in the pediatric population.

THE NATURAL HISTORY OF ACL INJURY

The natural history of ACL tears in pediatric patients is not fully understood. However, evaluating the results of nonoperative treatment of ACL tears leads to some understanding of it. Physicians often favor nonoperative treatment for ACL injury because of the risks involved in operating on a skeletally immature patient. Nonoperative treatment may include activity modification, bracing, and rehabilitation. However, studies have shown that these nonoperative approaches have poor efficacy,[‡] predominantly because pediatric patients are noncompliant, especially with modification of sports activity, and patients may be injured during free play. Noncompliance often leads to recurrent and sports-related instability and damage to the menisci.

Evidence suggests that the efficacy of nonoperative treatment is related to the severity of the ACL tear. Kannus and Jarvinen[23] treated 32 patients nonoperatively with grade II (partial) and grade III (complete) ACL tears. At 8-year (on average) follow-up, 25 patients in this series with grade II tears had good to excellent outcomes. Seven patients with complete grade III tears had poor outcomes that included chronic instability and posttraumatic arthritis. These outcomes led the authors to reject nonoperative treatment of grade III ACL tears in pediatric patients. Angel and Hall also reported poor outcomes, including pain and limited activity, with nonoperative treatment of 27 pediatric patients with grade III ACL tears.[5] Most children younger than 14 years of age (92%) had functional knee disability at follow-up evaluation. Graf and associates found new meniscal tears after 15 months of nonoperative treatment in 87.5% of pediatric patients.[15] In a study of 38 adolescent patients, McCarroll and coworkers reported that 97% of patients experienced episodes of instability, and 71% had symptomatic meniscal tears.[31] Mizuta and colleagues found degenerative changes in 61% (11/18) of patients within 51 treatment months[35] and concluded that these outcomes were unacceptable. A study by Millet and associates found significantly increased meniscal injuries in chronic cases.[34] Finally, T. J. Ganley, M.D. (personal communication, July 2009) evaluated 70 pediatric patients with ACL tears to determine independent risk factors for and relative risk of meniscal and chondral injuries. Despite activity modification, bracing, and rehabilitation, patients who delayed surgical reconstruction for longer than 12 weeks had a fourfold increase in irreparable medial meniscal tears, an 11-fold increase in lateral compartment chondral injuries, and a threefold increase in patella-trochlear injuries. A single episode of instability was associated with an 11-fold increase in irreparable medial meniscal tears. This large body of evidence strongly suggests that nonoperative treatment of an ACL injury in children carries a high probability of long-term knee disability.

Although operative treatment has serious risks, these risks can be mitigated by careful evaluation of skeletal and sexual maturity of the patient and by selection of the appropriate surgical technique based on these presurgical evaluations.

SKELETAL MATURITY

Although chronological age is a good indicator of mean skeletal maturity in large populations, an individual child can vary widely from the mean. The skeletal age of the pediatric patient is a key factor in determining appropriate treatment for an ACL tear. By estimating the skeletal age of the patient, the physician can gauge the potential risks and consequences of iatrogenic injury to the physis. As a rule, the younger the skeletal age (i.e., the more growth remains in the distal femur

*References 1, 4-6, 8, 9, 15, 23-28, 31-33, 35, 36, 39, and 44.
†References 4, 8, 9, 26, 28, 31-33, 36, and 39.
‡References 5, 15, 23, 31, 34, and 35.

855

Table 88-1 Tanner Stages of Development

| Tanner Stage | Sexual Characteristics | |
	Boys	Girls
I (prepubescent)	No pubic hair Testes <4 mL or <2.5 cm	No pubic hair No breast development

II	Minimal pubic hair
	  at base of penis
	Testes 4 mL or
	  2.5-3.2 cm
		Minimal pubic hair
		  on labia
		Breast buds

III (pubescent)	Testes 12 mL or
	  3.6 cm
	Public hair over
	  pubis
	Voice changes
	Muscle mass
	  increases
		Pubic hair on mons
		  pubis
		Elevation of breast;
		  enlargement of
		  areolae
		Axillary hair
		Acne

IV	Adult pubic hair Testes 4.1-4.5 cm Axillary hair Acne	Adult pubic hair Areolae enlargement
V (postpubescent)	No growth Adult testes Adult facial hair Adult physique	No growth Adult breast shape Adult pubic hair

and proximal tibial physes), the greater the risk of severe treatment-related growth disturbances.

Skeletal age is determined with radiographs. The most common method of determining skeletal age is to compare an anteroposterior radiograph of the patient's left hand and wrist with the age-specific radiograph in the Greulich and Pyle atlas.[16]

Although skeletal age is essential to determining the relative risk of ACL reconstruction, the physiologic age of the patient is also important and should be considered when the treatment planning. Physiologic age can be determined using the Tanner staging of sexual maturation.[45] Tanner stages can determine whether the child is prepubescent (stages I and II), pubescent (stage III), or postpubescent (stages IV and V) through the presence or absence of secondary sexual characteristics (i.e., pubic and axillary hair and development of breasts and genitalia) (Table 88-1).

Preliminary staging should be assigned before surgery by asking the patient about the onset of menarche or the growth of axillary hair. To spare the child the trauma of genital examination, a thorough examination should be completed after the child is under anesthesia, but before surgery, for precise determination of the Tanner stage.

GROWTH AND DEVELOPMENT

The most rapidly growing physes in the body are located on the distal femur and the proximal tibia. The distal femoral physis contributes about 40% of the overall lower extremity length, and the proximal tibial physis contributes about 27%.[3] The distal femur grows at the annual rate of 1.3 cm, but slows in the last 2 years of growth to an annual rate of 0.65 cm.[40] In boys, the mean peak height velocity occurs at age 13.5 years, with a range from 13 to 15 years of age. Peak height velocity in boys usually occurs at Tanner stage IV. However, about 20% of boys do not reach peak height velocity before Tanner stage V. Girls reach peak height velocity

earlier than boys. The mean age for girls is age 11.5 years, with a range from 11 to 13 years of age. Onset of menarche typically occurs 1 year after peak height velocity is reached.

The severity of iatrogenic growth disturbance can be predicted by the skeletal maturity of the patient at the time that injury occurred. A 3-cm discrepancy in leg length—nearly three times normal variance—is estimated to occur from complete closure of the proximal tibial physis in an average 12-year-old boy, complete closure of the distal femoral physes in a 13-year-old boy, or complete closure of the femoral and tibial physes in a 14-year-old boy.

Although leg length discrepancy is an undesirable result of surgery, angular deformity is the more serious surgical complication. A valgus/flexion deformity of the distal femur can be caused by an over-the-top femoral groove if the perichondral ring of LaCroix is damaged, and recurvatum of the knee can occur if the anterior tibial physis is damaged. Webster and colleagues estimated that partial tibial physeal arrest in a 14-year-old boy with 2 cm of growth remaining in the distal femur could result in a 14-degree valgus deformity with a lateral femoral epiphysiodesis, or 11-degree recurvatum with a partial tibial physeal arrest.[46]

Each of the studies reviewed in the following section illustrates the potential consequences of iatrogenic injury to the physis during surgical treatment. Patients at greatest risk are prepubescent (Tanner stages I and II), followed by pubescent patients (Tanner stage III). Patients at least risk are those nearing and those who have reached sexual maturity (Tanner stages IV and V).

BASIC RESEARCH ON PHYSEAL INJURY

Although there is a dearth of basic research on physeal injury in pediatric patients, several animal studies have evaluated the consequences of drill hole damage to the physis and of insertion of a soft tissue graft through a transphyseal hole. In 1988, Makela and coworkers studied the effects of 2.0- and 3.2-mm transphyseal femoral drill holes in rabbits.[29] The cross-sectional area of the physis destroyed was 3% for the 2-mm drill hole and 7% for the 3.2-mm drill hole. Results showed that 7% cross-sectional destruction of the physis resulted in permanent disruption of growth.

Guzzanti and colleagues evaluated the effects of placing a soft tissue graft across the physis in immature rabbits.[17] ACL reconstruction was performed with the semitendinosus tendon using 2-mm transphyseal femoral and tibial holes. Drill hole damage to the femoral physis was seen in 11% of the transverse diameter and 3% of the cross-sectional diameter. The extent of damage to the tibial physis was 12% of the transverse diameter and 4% of the cross-sectional area. A valgus deformity developed in about 9% (2/21) of tibiae, and one incident of tibial growth disruption was noted. Based on these data, the authors recommended extreme caution when transphyseal reconstruction is considered in pediatric patients.

Transphyseal ACL reconstruction in a rabbit model using four tunnel diameters ranging from 1.95 to 3.97 mm was conducted by Houle and associates.[20] Larger drill hole size was associated with increased and substantial deformity, and physeal arrest occurred despite the soft tissue graft. This study suggests that no more than 1% of the physis should be disrupted in children during an ACL reconstruction. In a rabbit model, Babb and coworkers evaluated the potential for growth arrest in three groups.[7] Group 1 was the control group; tunnels were drilled in the femur and tibia and were left open. In group 2, the tunnels were filled with a soft tissue autograft, and in group 3, the autograft was seeded with mesenchymal stem cells. Angular deformity and growth arrest were prevented only in group 3.

In contrast to these three studies, which found that soft tissue provided no protection, the following two studies demonstrated that a soft tissue graft across the physis prevents growth disturbance. In rabbit femurs, drill holes of 1.7, 2.5, and 3.4 mm were evaluated, where one hole was left empty and the contralateral one was filled with an autograft of soft tissue.[22] Growth was retarded when 7% to 9% of the distal femoral physis was destroyed, but not when 4% to 5% of the cross-sectional area of the physis was destroyed. Bone cylinders were observed around the soft tissue grafts, but solid bone bridging did not occur. Prevention of bony bridge development followed by growth disturbance was also found in a canine model subsequent to a soft tissue graft placement in transphyseal drill holes.[43]

Other researchers have evaluated the effects of graft tension. Edwards studied the effect of tensioning a graft across open physes in a canine model at 80 N.[13] This technique resulted in the development of valgus femoral and varus tibial deformities without radiographic or histologic evidence of physeal bar formation. Chudik and colleagues also tensioned autografts at 80 N using transepiphyseal, transphyseal, and over-the-top femoral positions.[10] They found growth disturbances with each technique. However, the transepiphyseal technique was more anatomic and caused less growth disturbance. These results are predicted by the Hueter-Volkman principle, that is, when compressive force is applied perpendicular to the physes, longitudinal growth is inhibited. This suggests that even physeal-sparing procedures pose a risk for ACL reconstruction in pediatric patients.

CAUSES OF IATROGENIC GROWTH DISTURBANCE

Decisions about the surgical technique used in ACL reconstruction of a skeletally immature knee should be made after the potential for growth disturbance is weighed. Basic research, although incomplete and not entirely generalizable to humans, provides some evidence to assess the risk factors. Studies by Guzzanti and coworkers[17] and by Houle and associates[20] found that the risk for arrested growth is greater in the proximal tibial physis than in the femoral physis.

The risk of growth disturbance is generally associated with the extent of damage to the cross-sectional area of the physis. It is not completely understood, in animal models or in children, which drill hole size and orientation can be used without risk of disturbing growth. In animal models, the threshold for drill size growth disturbance appears to be between 1% and 7% of the cross-sectional area of the physis.[7,17,20,22,29] Damage to the cross-sectional area of the physis can be diminished by making drill holes perpendicular rather than oblique to the surface of the physis. Although study results are not uniform, soft tissue grafts placed across the physis are probably protective against bone bridging and arrested growth. The physes are sensitive to compression forces,[13] so excessive ACL graft tension should be avoided.

Rare complications, such as angular deformity and significant leg length discrepancies, have been reported in children who underwent ACL reconstruction.[24,26,27] Kocher and colleagues found 15 cases of growth disturbance in a survey of 140 physicians.[24] Lipscomb and Anderson[27] had one case of valgus deformity following ACL reconstruction in skeletally immature patients. One patient's deformity followed placement of a staple across the lateral femoral physis. The authors evaluated another patient in consultation—a 12-year-old boy who had undergone transphyseal ACL reconstruction with an Achilles tendon allograft. At the 6-month follow-up, the graft had failed, resulting in a 3-degree valgus alignment of the nonoperative knee and a 7-degree valgus alignment of the ACL-reconstructed knee without physeal arrest.

TREATMENT OPTIONS

Reports of iatrogenic growth disturbance following intra-articular transphyseal replacement in both basic research and case studies illustrate the risks of using adult ACL reconstruction techniques on pediatric patients. Delaying surgery with nonoperative treatment in immature patients has some appeal and benefits. A more physically and psychologically mature patient is typically more compliant with postoperative rehabilitation. Additionally, delaying surgery until the patient reaches skeletal maturity allows the physician to use traditional surgical procedures. However, as discussed earlier, nonoperative treatments usually have undesirable outcomes.[4,14,26,32]

Some operative approaches in pediatric patients, such as primary repair[11,13] and extra-articular replacements,[15,31] have also resulted in poor outcomes. It is possible to minimize the risk of physeal injury using a modified physeal-sparing intra-articular replacement.[36] Parker and coworkers reconstructed an ACL by passing hamstring tendons through a groove in the anterior aspect of the tibia and over the top of the lateral femoral condyle.[38] In 44 Tanner stage I or II patients, Kocher and associates used a combined intra-articular/extra-articular ACL reconstruction technique.[25,33] This technique places the iliotibial band around the lateral femoral condyle extra-articularly and passes it through the intercondylar notch. It is then sutured to the periosteum of the proximal tibia. In 42 of the 44 patients, a mean International Knee Documentation Committee (IKDC) subjective score of 96.7 was reported. Mean growth from surgery to follow-up was 21 cm. Lachman examinations were normal in 23 patients, nearly normal in 18, and abnormal in one patient. Pivot-shift test results were normal in 31 patients. Functional outcomes were excellent, and growth disturbance was minimal. Two patients had graft failure and subsequent reconstruction. Transphyseal tibial holes and over-the-top femoral positions with autografts[8,28] and allografts[4] have also been used.

In Tanner stage I patients, Guzzanti and colleagues suggested reconstructing the ACL using single-stranded semitendinosus and gracilis tendon grafts with a transepiphyseal tibial hole and an over-the-top femoral position.[18] No growth disturbances have been reported with over-the-top procedures, but lack of isometry can be an issue with this technique. The femoral over-the-top position has resulted in a mean graft elongation of 10 mm as the knee approaches full extension.[37] Avoid rasping with the over-the-top femoral position, as this may damage the perichondral ring of LaCroix.

Controversy continues over ACL replacement procedures that use intra-articular transphyseal graft placement, because of deficiencies in basic science and clinical literature. Clinical studies that demonstrate the safety of transphyseal replacements have included postmenarchal girls and postpubescent boys with physes near closure.[4,6,12,30,31] Intra-articular replacements were performed by Pressman and coworkers in a series of 18 patients, 7 with open physes and 11 with closed or nearly closed physes.[39] Other surgeons have performed intra-articular ACL replacements as well, but patients in these cohorts had only 2.3 cm to 4.5 cm of postoperative growth.[4,32] In other case series, average patient age was greater than 14 years at the time of surgery, so the risks of angular deformity and leg length discrepancy were low compared with those in younger children.[6,30,42]

Children in Tanner I and II stages are at greatest risk for growth disturbance as a consequence of ACL surgery. Few patients in the early Tanner stages have participated in studies of transphyseal procedures; therefore, the safety of these procedures in preadolescent patients is not documented in the clinical literature. Further, basic research has not proven the safety of drilling across the physis, or of placing a soft tissue graft across the physis.

In an effort to minimize physeal trauma in Tanner stage II and III patients, Guzzanti and associates used a semitendinosus graft passed through 6-mm or smaller transphyseal femoral holes and transepiphyseal tibial holes.[19]

Anderson performed transepiphyseal replacement in a series of 12 patients (Tanner stage I, n = 3; Tanner stage II, n = 4; Tanner stage III, n = 5) using a modified adult ACL reconstruction procedure that did not transgress the physes of the tibia or the femur.[2] At the 4-year follow-up, mean growth from surgery was 16.5 cm. No clinically significant differences were noted in lower leg lengths, as determined by long leg radiographs. The mean IKDC Subjective Knee Form score was 96.5. The ligament laxity testing performed using a KT-1000 arthrometer showed a mean side-to-side difference of 1.5 mm at 134 N. According to the criteria of the Objective 2001 IKDC Knee Form,[21] the rating was normal for seven patients and nearly normal for the remaining five. At 4 years post surgery, one patient, who rated 100 on the IKDC Subjective Score at follow-up year 2, ruptured his ACL graft during a sporting event.

This technique was subsequently performed on an additional 26 patients (Tanner stage I, n = 6; Tanner stage II, n = 7; Tanner stage III, n = 13). Two patients re-ruptured their ACL grafts. One was in a motorcycle accident 8 weeks post surgery, sustaining a grade III injury to the ACL graft, as well as an injury to the medial collateral ligament. In the other patient, the graft failed, and no history of trauma was reported. The only other complication was seen in a patient who had a break in the EndoButton continuous loop 1 year after surgery. This patient had an excellent recovery after removal of the washer without residual pathologic laxity.

ACL RECONSTRUCTION RECOMMENDATIONS

Determining the best treatment for skeletally immature patients is not always easy or straightforward. The surgical literature is the most important factor in determining the best treatment. Unfortunately, the literature is often contradictory, leading to inconsistent treatment recommendations. Increased scientific rigor provided by multicenter research is necessary to clarify the contradictions in the literature and to help in determining the best method of treatment for pediatric patients with ACL injuries. Until a higher level of evidence is available, our bias is to modify the surgical procedure based on the patient's physiologic and skeletal age; this approach identifies the consequences should a growth disturbance occur.

For patients at highest risk—those in Tanner stages I and II (prepubescent males younger than 12 and females younger than 11 years)—a transepiphyseal ACL reconstruction procedure is recommended because it does not transgress the tibial or femoral physis, thus minimizing the risk of physeal injury, but follows the accepted principles of adult ACL reconstruction. Some surgeons concerned about the technical difficulty of this procedure prefer the physeal-sparing procedure described by Kocher and colleagues, which utilizes an iliotibial graft.[25] The functional results of this procedure are also good, although the iliotibial band is a weaker graft and is not isometrically placed on the tibia or the femur.

Intermediate-risk patients in early Tanner stage III (pubescent boys 13 to 16 years old and girls 12 to 14 years old) may be treated with the same procedures.

For lower-risk patients in later Tanner stage III or IV, the recommended procedure is a transphyseal replacement using quadruple hamstring grafts fixed with a proximal EndoButton and a distal screw and post. The recommended procedure for Tanner stage V patients (i.e., boys older than 16 years and girls older than 14 years) is a standard adult ACL replacement procedure.

SURGICAL TECHNIQUES AND POSTOPERATIVE REHABILITATION PROCEDURES

Transepiphyseal ACL Reconstruction

Place the injured leg in an arthroscopic leg holder, and flex the hip to 20 degrees to facilitate visualization of the knee in the lateral plane using the C-arm fluoroscope. Position the C-arm on the side of the table opposite the injured leg, and place the monitor at the head of the table on the same side as the injured knee. Before the leg is prepared and draped, visualize the tibial and femoral physes in both lateral and anteroposterior planes. Adjust the C-arm to precisely align the medial and lateral femoral condyles in the lateral plane. Then, rotate the C-arm 30 degrees internally to visualize the extension of the tibial physis into the tibial tubercle on the lateral view of the tibia.

Make an oblique incision 4 cm long, and dissect the semitendinosus and gracilis tendons free. Then, transect the tendons at the musculotendinous junction using a standard tendon stripper, and detach them distally. Next, double the tendons and place a no. 2 FiberWire suture (Anthrex, Naples, Fla) in their ends using a locking whipstitch. Place the doubled tendons on the back table under 4.5 kg (10 lb) of tension using the Graft Master device (Acufex-Smith Nephew, Andover, Mass). Insert the arthroscope into the anterolateral portal, and insert the probe through the anteromedial portal. Perform an intra-articular examination in the standard manner. Remove the debris from the intercondylar

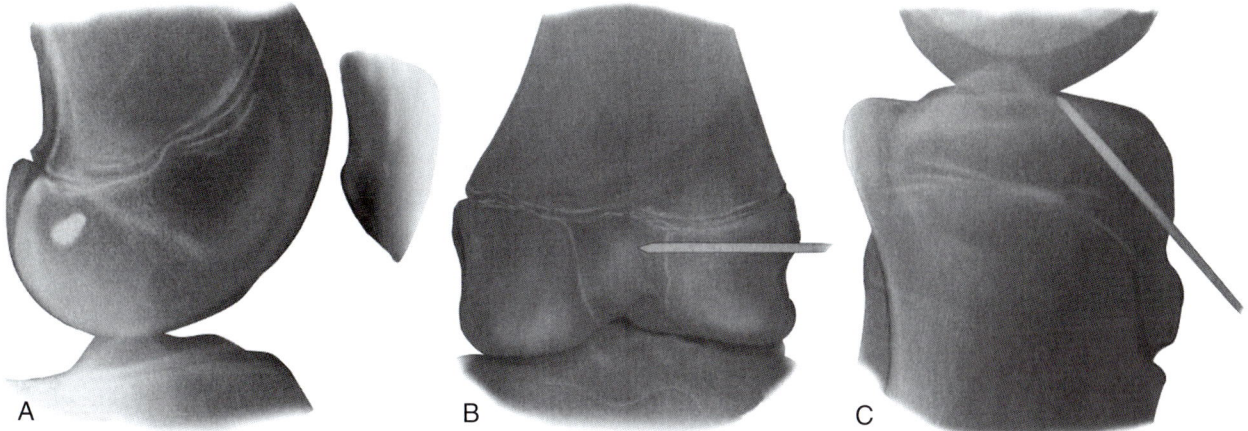

A   B   C

Figure 88-1. Lateral **(A)** and anterior posterior **(B)** views demonstrate the position of the femoral transepiphyseal guide wire. Lateral view **(C)** of the tibia shows the position of the tibial guide wire. This guide wire enters the epiphysis medial to the tibial tubercle.

notch and perform a minimal notchplasty, so that the anatomic footprint of the ACL on the femur can be visualized. At this point in the procedure, repair any extensive tears of the meniscus.

Adjust the C-arm to the lateral position to get a precise lateral view of the knee, then place the point of the guide wire on the skin over the lateral femoral condyle that corresponds with the footprint of the ACL on the femur. It is located about one quarter of the distance from posterior to anterior along Blumensaat's line and one quarter of the distance down from Blumensaat's line (Fig. 88-1A). At this point, make a lateral incision 2 cm long, and longitudinally incise the iliotibial tract; then strip the periosteum from a small area of the lateral femoral condyle. Use the C-arm to visualize the entry point of the guide wire in the lateral plane. Use a freehand technique to introduce the point of the guide wire 2 to 3 mm into the femoral epiphysis. The pin should remain perpendicular to the femur in the coronal plane. Rotate the C-arm to the anteroposterior plane to ensure that the guide wire has not become angulated proximally or distally. The next step is to drive the guide wire across the femoral epiphysis, keeping it perpendicular to the femur and distal to the physis (Fig. 88-1A and B). Using the arthroscope, visualize the entrance of the guide wire into the intercondylar notch. The proper entry point is at the center of the anatomic footprint of the ACL on the femur. Alternatively, the femoral guide wire may be inserted with the use of an ACL guide placed through the anterolateral portal and visualization with the arthroscope in the medial portal. With the femoral guide wire in place, insert a second guide wire into the anteromedial aspect of the tibia, passing through the epiphysis, with the aid of a tibial drill guide. From the direct lateral position, externally rotate the C-arm to about 30 degrees to reveal the physis extending into the tibial tubercle. Then drill the guide wire into the tibial epiphysis using real-time fluoroscopic imaging (see Fig. 88-1C). Lift the handle of the drill guide so that the pin clears the anterior portion of the tibial physis. Ensure that the pin enters the joint at the free edge of lateral meniscus and in the posterior footprint of the ACL on the tibia.

Before proceeding, confirm that both guide wires are in the correct position. Measure the diameter of the quadruple tendon graft using tendon sizers; these grafts typically range

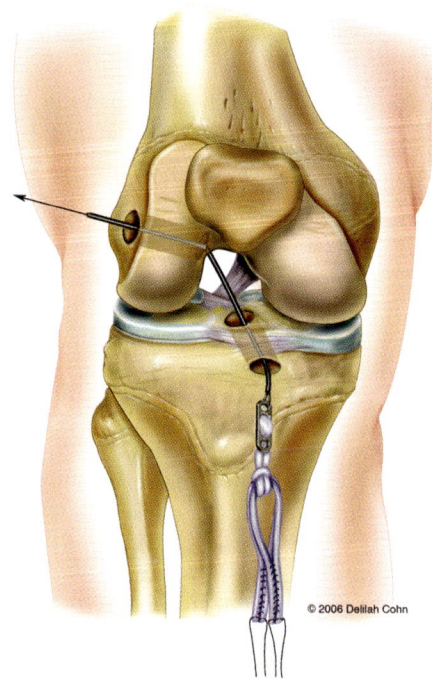

© 2006 Delilah Cohn

Figure 88-2. The semitendinosus and gracilis tendons are pulled up through the tibia and out the lateral femoral condyle with a no. 5 suture in the EndoButton.

from 6 to 8 mm in diameter. Because a tight fit is essential, use the smallest drill possible to ream over the guide wires. Chamfer the edge of the femoral hole intra-articularly, and measure the width of the lateral femoral condyle. Choose an EndoButton continuous loop (Acufex-Smith Nephew; 2 to 3 cm) that allows about 2 cm of the quadruple hamstring tendon graft to remain within the lateral femoral condyle. Pass the EndoButton continuous loop around the middle of the double tendons, and loop it inside itself to proximally secure the tendons (Fig. 88-2). An alternative method is to place the tendons through the continuous loop before suturing the tendon ends together. This method requires drilling and measuring the length of the femoral hole to determine the appropriate length of the EndoButton continuous loop before the graft is prepared.

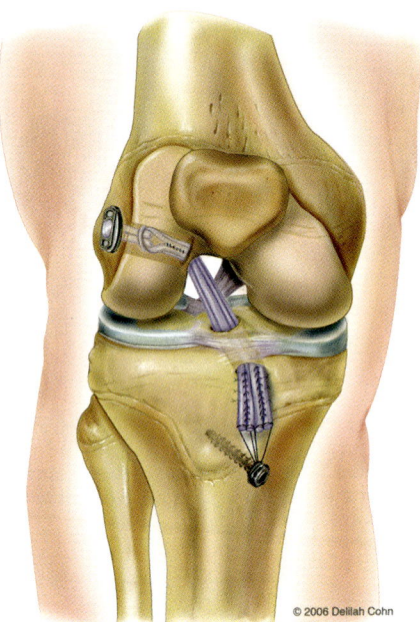

Figure 88-3. The EndoButton washer is placed over the EndoButton, and the washer is pulled back to the surface of the lateral femoral condyle. The quadruple hamstring grafts are secured distally by tying the no. 2 FiberWire sutures over a tibial screw and post.

In one end of the EndoButton, place a no. 5 FiberWire suture. Pass the suture from anterior to posterior through the tibia and out the lateral femoral condyle using a suture passer (see Fig. 88-2). Then pull the EndoButton and tendons up through the tibia and out the femoral hole using the suture. Place an AO washer that is 3 to 4 mm larger than the femoral hole over the EndoButton. Apply tension to the tendons distally and pull both the EndoButton and the washer up to the surface of the lateral femoral condyle. The washer anchors the graft proximally, so the EndoButton does not get pulled through the hole in the lateral femoral condyle. Place the graft under tension and extend the knee to arthroscopically ensure that the graft is not impinging on the intercondylar notch. It is usually unnecessary to perform an anterior notchplasty with this technique; however, a small anterior area of the intercondylar notch may be removed if it comes in contact with the graft in terminal extension. Place the knee in 20 degrees of flexion and secure the quadruple hamstring graft distally by tying the no. 5 FiberWire sutures over a tibial screw and post located medial to the tibial tubercle apophysis and distal to the proximal tibial physis (Fig. 88-3). Figure 88-4 shows an arthroscopic view of the graft. Using standard procedure, close the subcutaneous tissue and skin. Place the knee in a hinged brace. Postoperative radiographs show the drill holes and fixation in a 9-year–5-month-old male (Fig. 88-5).

Postoperative Rehabilitation

Rehabilitation following the transepiphyseal ACL reconstruction procedure has three phases. Phase I begins when the patient awakens from surgery. Encourage the patient to perform straight-leg raises and to contract the quadriceps muscle. Use cryotherapy for 5 to 10 minutes each hour. The day after surgery, the patient performs range-of-motion exercises and hamstring stretches from a prone position. Patients

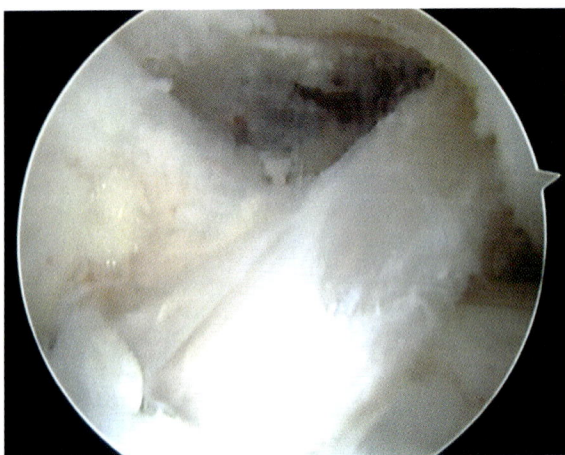

Figure 88-4. An arthroscopic view of a quadruple hamstring graft after transepiphyseal anterior cruciate ligament (ACL) reconstruction.

without meniscal repairs may ambulate with crutches and partial bearing weight for 4 weeks. For patients who required meniscal repair, only toe-touch weight bearing is allowed for the first 6 weeks. The 1-week postsurgical goal is to have a range of motion from 0 degrees of extension to 90 degrees of flexion.

Rehabilitation phase II is the strengthening phase and may last for 2 to 11 weeks. During this phase, patients perform active range-of-motion exercises and patellar mobilization and undergo electrical muscle stimulation. Patients should work at a comfortable pace. At postsurgical week 2, the patient is fitted with a functional knee brace and is encouraged to bear weight. Exercises should be introduced in order of increasing difficulty, including hamstring stretches, quadriceps muscle stretches and strengthening, proprioception exercises, and functional strengthening. Finally, strengthening exercises are performed in a pool. The goal is for the operative knee to have the same range of motion as the normal knee by postsurgical week 6.

The goal of the final rehabilitation phase is regaining full functional ability of the knee. This phase lasts from 12 to 20 weeks. Rehabilitation activities during this phase include functional strengthening exercises, straight-line jogging, plyometric exercises, sport cord exercises for jogging, lateral movement, and foot agility exercises. Between postsurgical weeks 16 and 20, patients may resume functional activities (e.g., full-speed running) while wearing the brace. At postsurgical week 32, patients may fully engage in all activities, including competitive sports.

Physeal-Sparing ACL Reconstruction With the Iliotibial Band

This iliotibial band technique was previously described by Kocher and associates,[24] who modified it from the McIntosh and Darby intra-articular and extra-articular ACL reconstruction.[43,45] Kocher had good functional results despite the fact that this is not an anatomic ACL replacement. One cautionary note: this technique causes a defect in the iliotibial band over the vastus lateralis muscle that should be closed to prevent a cosmetic problem caused by herniation of the muscle.

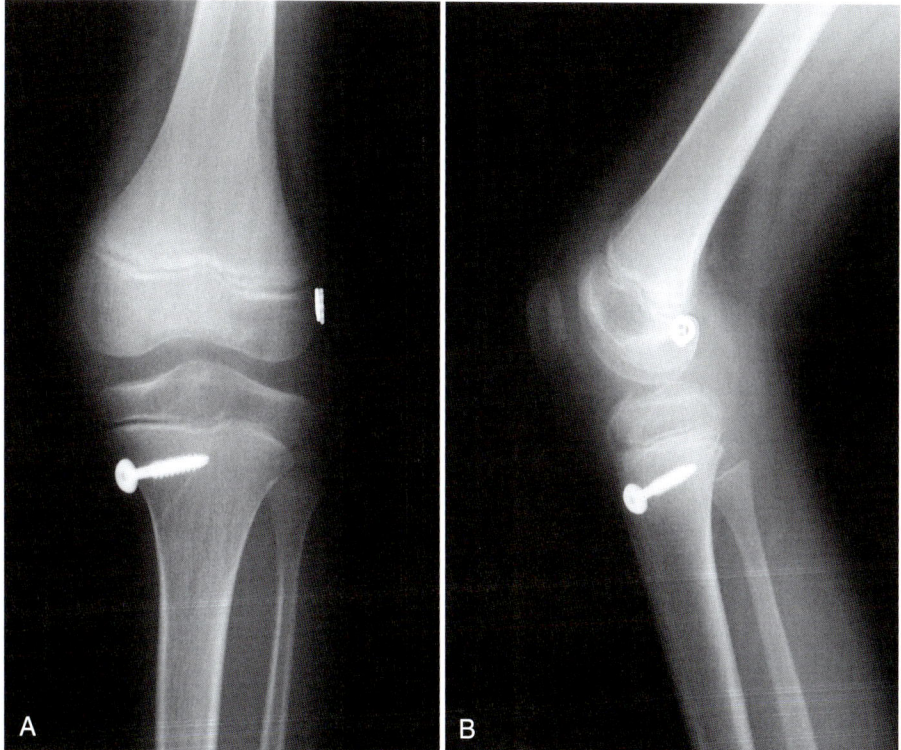

Figure 88-5. Anteroposterior and lateral radiographs of a transepiphyseal anterior cruciate ligament (ACL) reconstruction in a boy 9 years 6 months of age (Tanner stage I) who is 4 months post surgery.

The procedure begins with the patient in a supine position with a tourniquet on the proximal thigh. Make a 6- to 10-cm-long incision from the lateral joint line along the superior border of the iliotibial band. Expose the band and make incisions along its superior and inferior margins from Gerdy's tubercle to 15 to 20 cm proximal to the joint line, depending on the size of the patient. Detach the iliotibial band proximally and dissect it free from the lateral capsule; tabularize it with a whipstitch using a no. 5 Ethibond suture. Using the arthroscope through the anteromedial and anterolateral portals, resect remnants of the torn ACL and fat pad and perform a small notchplasty. Remove soft tissue from the over-the-top position of the lateral femoral condyle, taking care to avoid injury to the perichondral ring. Make a second incision parallel to the medial border of the patellar tendon, extending 4 cm distally from the joint line, and carry the dissection down to the periosteum. Use a Keith needle to identify the physis. Place a curved clamp under the intermeniscal ligament and make a groove in the proximal tibial epiphysis using a small curved rasp; be careful not to damage the anterior tibial physis. Pull the iliotibial band graft into the knee using a full-length clamp or a tendon passer. Pass it through the anteromedial portal, over the top of the lateral femoral condyle, and out the lateral capsule. Then, pass the clamp under the intermeniscal ligament, grasp the graft again, and pull it into the medial incision. The graft can now be seated into the groove in the tibial epiphyses. After placing it under tension, suture it to the lateral femoral condyle at the insertion of the lateral intermuscular septum with the knee placed in 90 degrees of flexion and 15 degrees of external rotation (Fig. 88-6). Incise the periosteum distal to the physis and make a trough into the metaphysis. Next, with the

knee placed in 20 degrees of flexion, place the graft under tension and suture it to the periosteum. Close the defect over the vastus lateralis muscle that was created when the iliotibial band was harvested. Leave the lateral patellar reticulum open to avoid excessive pressure on the lateral facet of the patella. Close the wounds using standard technique and place the knee in a hinged knee brace.

Postoperative Rehabilitation

Keep the knee in the hinged knee brace for the first 6 postoperative weeks. For the first 2 postoperative weeks, a continuous passive motion (CPM) machine is used with the range of motion set at 0 to 90 degrees. The patient should be maintained on partial weight bearing for 6 weeks. Rehabilitation otherwise should proceed in the same manner as that for the transepiphyseal ACL reconstruction.

Transphyseal ACL Reconstruction

Place the lower limb in an arthroscopic leg holder at 60 degrees flexion. Make an oblique incision 4 cm long over the semitendinosus and gracilis tendons and dissect the tendons free. Transect the tendons at the musculotendinous junction using a standard tendon stripper, and detach them at the distal end. Place a no. 2 FiberWire suture in each end of the tendons, using an interlocking whipstitch. Measure the diameter of the quadruple hamstring grafts with tendon sizers; they typically range in size from 6 to 8 mm. Double the tendons and place them under 4.5 kg (10 lb) of tension on the back table with the Graft Master device (Acufex-Smith Nephew). Next, insert the arthroscope into the anterolateral portal and insert a probe through the anteromedial portal. Perform a

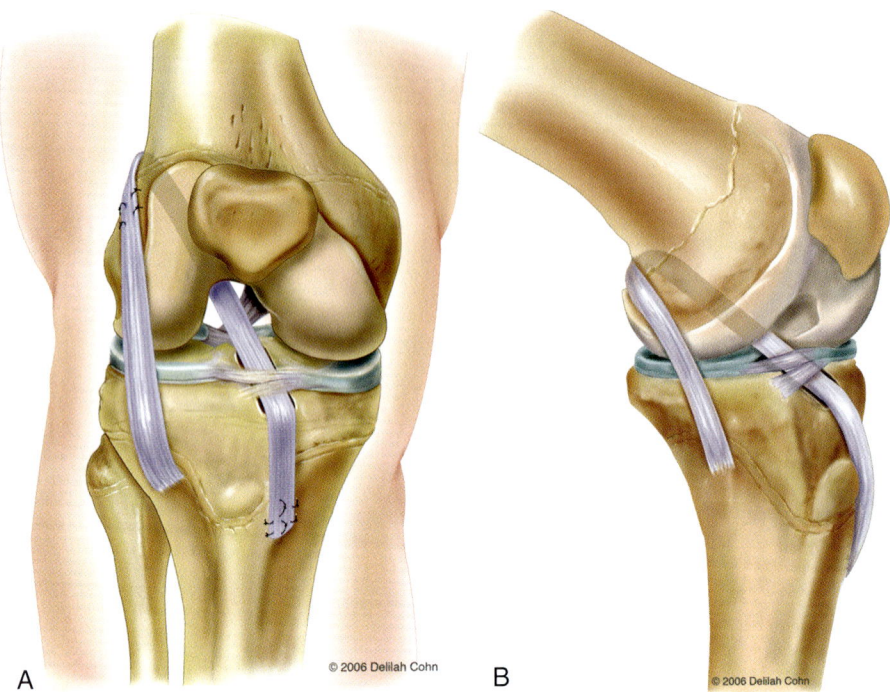

A   © 2006 Delilah Cohn   B   © 2006 Delilah Cohn

Figure 88-6. The iliotibial band graft is passed over the top of the lateral femoral condyle, through the knee, under the intermeniscal ligament, and into the groove in the proximal tibia. The graft is sutured to the lateral femoral condyle with the knee in 90 degrees of flexion and 15 degrees of external rotation. It is then sutured to the periosteum of the proximal tibia with the knee in 20 degrees of flexion.

systematic intra-articular examination using standard methods. Remove any debris found in the intercondylar notch, and perform a minimal notchplasty to visualize the anatomic footprint of the ACL on the femur. Note that the femoral physis is in close proximity, and be careful to avoid enlarging the posterior arch of the intercondylar notch. At this point in the procedure, repair any significant tears in the meniscus.

Insert the point of the tibial drill guide through the antero-medial portal. With the guide set at a 55-degree angle, orient it so that the guide pin enters the anteromedial aspect of the tibia at a 65- to 70-degree angle in the coronal plane. Ensure that the pin enters the joint at the level of the free edge of the lateral meniscus and in the posterior footprint of the ACL on the tibia. Ream the tibial hole over the guide wire with a standard cannulated drill bit. Ensure that the fit of the graft is tight within the tibial tunnel by using the smallest drill bit possible to ream the tibial hole. Once drilling is complete, remove debris using a shaver.

Before inserting the femoral guide wire, flex the knee to at least 90 degrees. Use an over-the-top femoral guide, leaving 2 mm of bone between the drill hole and the posterior cortex of the lateral femoral condyle. Advance a 2.7-mm passing pin through the offset guide and the lateral femoral condyle, penetrating the lateral femoral cortex. It should be possible to palpate the pin under the skin just distal to the tourniquet. Using an acorn reamer matched to the diameter of the graft, create the femoral tunnel. Drill a 30- to 35-mm hole in the femur at the 10 o'clock position to the left knee and the 2 o'clock position to the right knee. The depth of the femoral hole should be 10 mm greater than the desired graft insertion in the lateral femoral condyle to allow for rotation of the EndoButton. Drill the 4.5-mm EndoButton reamer over the

guide wire and out the lateral femoral cortex. Chamfer the hole to minimize fraying of the graft. Measure the length of the femoral tunnel using the EndoButton depth gauge from the anterolateral femoral cortex to the opening of the inter-condylar notch. Use the EndoButton continuous loop that leaves 20 to 25 mm of graft within the femoral tunnel. Pass a no. 5 Ethibond suture through one of the outside holes of the EndoButton to facilitate its passage through both the tibia and the femur. Then, use a no. 2 Ethibond suture through the other outside EndoButton hole to rotate the EndoButton after it exits the anterolateral femoral cortex (Fig. 88-7). Pass the hamstring grafts through the EndoButton continuous loop, thus creating a quadruple graft. Thread both suture strands through the eye of a 2.7-mm passing pin. Insert the pin up through the tibial and femoral holes, piecing the quadriceps and the skin proximal to the knee (see Fig. 88-7). Pass the suture by pulling the pin out of the femur. Pull the no. 5 suture first, and advance both the EndoButton and the graft into the femoral hole (Fig. 88-8). To lock the Endo-Button on the outside of the femoral cortex, pull the graft distally. It should feel securely fixed in place.

At this point, remove both sutures from the EndoButton. Pretension the graft by cycling the knee through the ranges of motion several times. Next, place the graft under tension and extend the knee. Using the arthroscope, ensure that the graft is not being impinged by the intercondylar notch. It may be necessary to remove a small portion of the anterior outlet of the intercondylar notch. Place a tibial Bioscrew and post medial to the tibial tubercle apophysis and distal to the proximal tibial physis. With the knee in 20 degrees of flexion, secure the quadruple hamstring graft distally by tying the no. 5 FiberWire sutures over the Bioscrew and post (Fig. 88-9). A graft that extends through the tibial drill hole should also

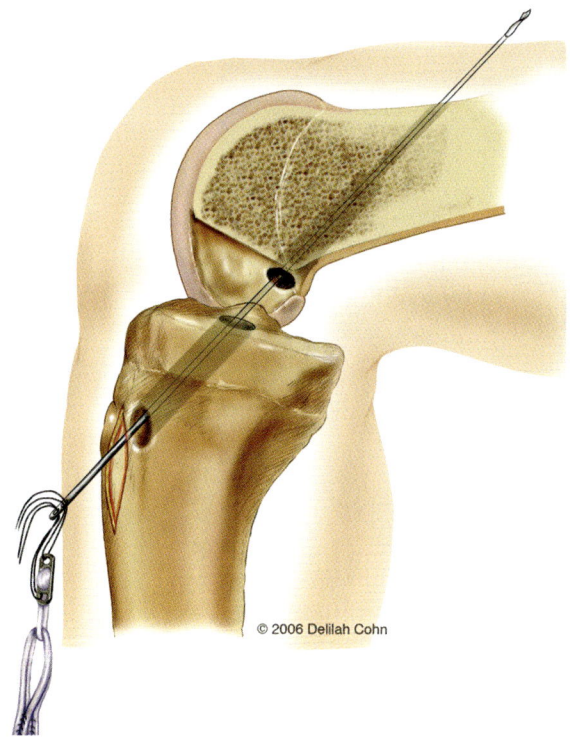

Figure 88-7. No. 2 and no. 5 Ethibond sutures are threaded through the eye of a 2.7-mm passing pin. The pin is inserted through both tibial and femoral holes, piercing the quadriceps and the skin.

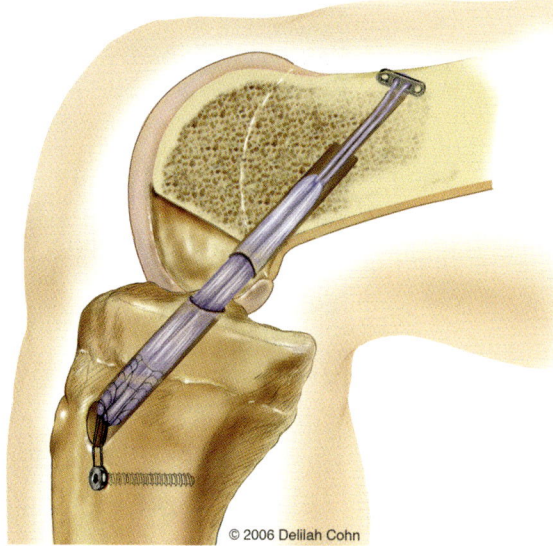

Figure 88-9. The graft is pulled distally to lock the EndoButton on the outside of the femoral cortex. The quadruple hamstring graft is secured using a no. 5 FiberWire suture tied over a screw and post in the distal tibia.

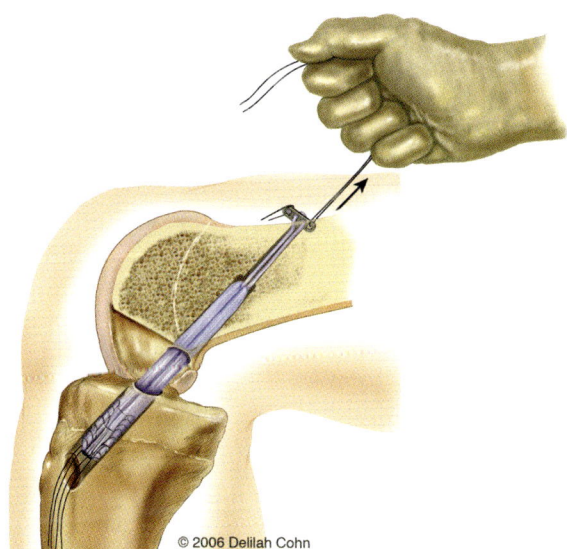

Figure 88-8. First, the no. 5 suture is pulled to advance the Endo-Button and graft. Then, the no. 2 suture is pulled to rotate the EndoButton external to the femur.

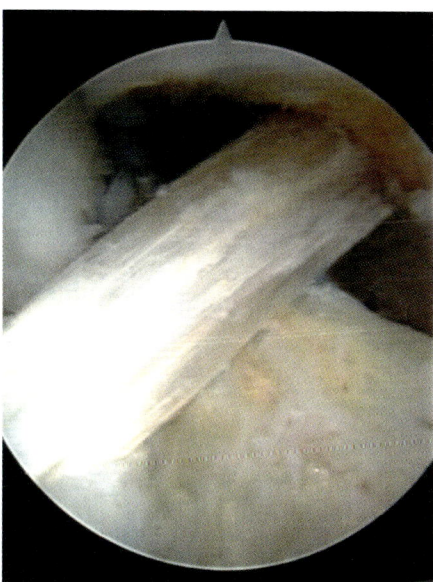

Figure 88-10. This arthroscopic view shows the position of the quadruple hamstring graft after physeal anterior cruciate ligament (ACL) reconstruction.

be secured to the periosteum of the anterior tibia with several no. 1 Ethibond sutures using a figure-of-eight pattern. After closing the subcutaneous tissue and the skin with standard methods, apply a hinged brace. Figure 88-10 shows a more vertical graft position when the transtibial hole is used to create the femoral hole compared with the transepiphyseal technique. Postoperative radiographs show the drill holes and fixation in a male with a chronological age of 12 years 9 months, and a bone age of 14 years (Fig. 88-11).

Postoperative Rehabilitation

The postoperative rehabilitation protocol for the transepiphyseal ACL reconstruction should be used following this surgery.

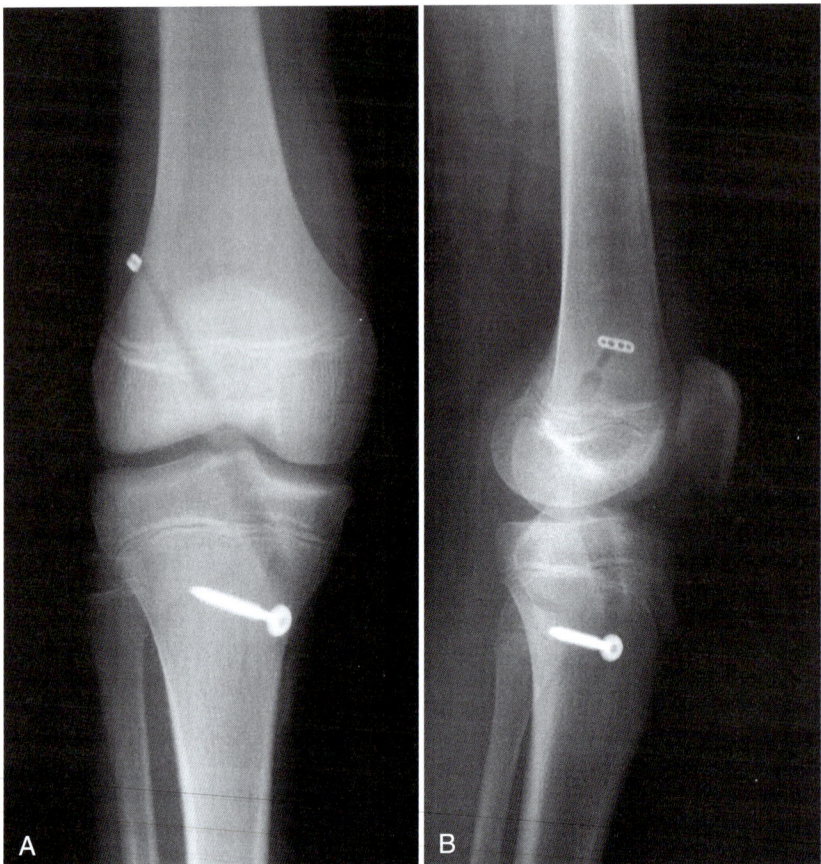

Figure 88-11. Anteroposterior and lateral radiographs show the positions of the drill holes 6 months after transphyseal anterior cruciate ligament (ACL) reconstruction in a 12-year–9-month-old male with a bone age of 14. He was in late Tanner stage III of sexual maturity.

KEY REFERENCES

Anderson AF: Transepiphyseal replacement of the anterior cruciate ligament in skeletally immature patients: a preliminary report. J Bone Joint Surg Am 85:1255–1263, 2003.

Babb JR, Ahn JI, Azar FM, et al: Transphyseal anterior cruciate ligament reconstruction using mesenchymal stem cells. Am J Sports Med 36:1164–1170, 2008.

Chudik S, Beasley L, Potter H, et al: The influence of femoral technique for graft placement on anterior cruciate ligament reconstruction using a skeletally immature canine model with a rapidly growing physis. Arthroscopy 23:1309–1319, 2007.

Edwards TB, Greene CC, Baratta RV, et al: The effect of placing a tensioned graft across open growth plates: a gross and histologic analysis. J Bone Joint Surg Am 83:725–734, 2001.

Graf BK, Lange RH, Rujisaki CK, et al: Anterior cruciate ligament tears in skeletally immature patients: meniscal pathology at presentation and after attempted conservative treatment. Arthroscopy 8:229–233, 1992.

Houle JB, Letts M, Yang J: Effects of a tensioned tendon graft in a bone tunnel across the rabbit physis. Clin Orthop 391:275–281, 2001.

Janarv PM, Wikstrom B, Hirsch G: The influence of transphyseal drilling and tendon grafting on bone growth: an experimental study in the rabbit. J Pediatr Orthop 18:149–154, 1998.

Kannus P, Jarvinen M: Knee ligament injuries in adolescents: eight year follow-up of conservative management. J Bone Joint Surg Br 70:772–776, 1988.

Kocher MS, Saxon HS, Hovis WD, Hawkins RJ: Management and complications of anterior cruciate ligament injuries in skeletally immature patients: survey of the Herodicus Society and the ACL Study Group. J Pediatr Orthop 22:452–457, 2002.

Kocher MS, Sumeet G, Micheli L: Physeal sparing reconstruction of the anterior cruciate ligament in skeletally immature prepubescent children and adolescents. J Bone Joint Surg Am 87:2371–2379, 2005.

Lipscomb AB, Anderson AF: Tears of the anterior cruciate ligament in adolescents. J Bone Joint Surg Am 68:19–28, 1986.

Makela EA, Vainionpaa S, Vihtonen K, et al: The effect of trauma to the lower femoral epiphyseal plate: an experimental study in rabbits. J Bone Joint Surg Br 70:187–191, 1988.

Millett PJ, Willis AA, Warren RF: Associated injuries in pediatric and adolescent anterior cruciate ligament tears: does a delay in treatment increase the risks of meniscal tear? Arthroscopy 18:955–999, 2002.

Mizuta H, Kubota K, Shiraishi M, et al: The conservative treatment of complete tears of the anterior cruciate ligament in skeletally immature patients. J Bone Joint Surg Br 77:890–894, 1995.

Stadelmaier D, Arnoczky S, Dodds J, Ross H: The effects of drilling and soft tissue grafting across open growth plates. Am J Sports Med 23:431–435, 1995.

Full references for this chapter can be found on www.expertconsult.com.

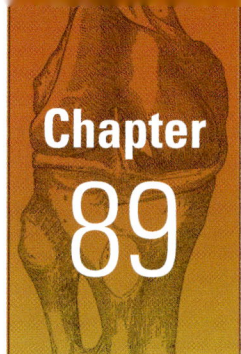

Chapter 89

Tibial Spine Fractures

Yi-Meng Yen and Mininder S. Kocher

An avulsion fracture of the tibial intercondylar eminence usually occurs in individuals between the ages of 8 and 14 with no predilection for gender. This is still a relatively rare injury, accounting for about 2% of knee injuries and occurring in 3 per 100,000 children per year.[29,48] Classically, pediatric tibial spine fractures have resulted from bicycling accidents, although they have also been seen with pedestrian–motor vehicle accidents (MVAs) or sports injuries.[36,41,42] Although far less common, tibial spine fractures can occur in adults and frequently involve lesions of the meniscus, capsule, or collateral ligaments because they are associated with higher-energy mechanisms.*

Fractures of the tibial spine are avulsion fractures of the anterior cruciate ligament (ACL) insertion; in addition to disrupting ACL continuity, these fractures may, depending on their size, involve the articular surface of the tibia.[40,58] Noyes has shown that as the subchondral bone fails, elongation or stretch of the ACL occurs.[40] This has led many authors to equate this injury to midsubstance ACL rupture in adults.†

Historically, treatment has evolved from closed treatment of all fractures to operative treatment of certain types. Garcia and Neer[12] reported 42 fractures of the tibial spine in patients ranging in age from 7 to 60 years with successful closed management in half their patients. Meyers and McKeever[36] recommended arthrotomy and open reduction for all displaced fractures, followed by cast immobilization with the knee in 20 degrees of flexion. Gronkvist and associates[14] reported late instability in 16 of 32 children with tibial spine fractures, and recommended surgery for all displaced tibial spine fractures, particularly in children older than 10 years of age, because of increased demand on the ACL–tibial spine complex. In a comparison of displaced tibial spine fractures, McLennan[32] reported on 10 patients treated with closed reduction or with arthroscopic reduction with or without internal fixation. After a second-look arthroscopy at 6 years, those treated with closed reduction had greater knee laxity than those treated arthroscopically.

Modern treatment is based on fracture type. Fractures that are able to be reduced can be treated closed. Hinged and displaced fractures that do not reduce require open or arthroscopic reduction with internal fixation. A variety of treatment options have been reported with the goal of treatment to obtain a stable, pain-free knee. The prognosis for closed treatment of nondisplaced and reduced tibial spine fractures and for operative treatment of displaced fractures is good. Most series report healing with an excellent functional outcome despite some residual knee laxity.* Potential complications include nonunion, malunion, arthrofibrosis, residual knee laxity, and growth disturbance.†

MECHANISM OF INJURY

The most common mechanism of tibial eminence fracture in children has been a fall from a bicycle. However, with increased participation in youth sports at earlier ages and higher competitive levels, fractures resulting from sporting activities are being seen with increased frequency. The differential injury patterns of an ACL tear versus a tibial eminence fracture in the skeletally immature knee may be due to loading conditions, biomechanical properties, and anatomic differences.[22,40,55,58] The most common mechanism of tibial eminence fracture is forced valgus and external rotation of the tibia, although tibial spine avulsion fractures can also occur from hyperflexion, hyperextension, or tibial internal rotation. Slower loading rates, relative weakness of the incompletely ossified intercondylar eminence compared with the ligament midsubstance, greater elasticity of the ACL, and a wider intercondylar notch are believed to preferentially result in tibial spine avulsion fracture.[22,40,55,58]

In a biomechanical cadaver study, a fracture of the anterior tibial eminence was simulated by an oblique osteotomy beneath the eminence and traction on the ACL. In each specimen, the displaced fragment could be reduced into its bed by extension of the knee, likely affected by the lateral femoral condyle.[49] In experimental models, midsubstance ACL injuries tend to occur under rapid loading rates, whereas tibial eminence avulsion fractures tend to occur under slower loading rates.[40]

Additionally, intercondylar notch morphology may influence injury patterns. In a retrospective study of 25 skeletally immature patients with tibial spine fractures and midsubstance ACL injuries, Kocher and colleagues found narrower intercondylar notches in those patients sustaining midsubstance ACL injuries.[22]

PHYSICAL EXAMINATION

Similar to patients with fractures around the knee joint, patients with tibial spine fractures present with a painful swollen knee (hemarthrosis), limited knee motion, and difficulty with weight bearing. Evaluation should consist of a thorough history and physical examination. Sagittal plane laxity is often present, but the contralateral knee should be assessed for physiologic laxity. Pain may make thorough examination of the ligaments difficult. If possible, gentle

---

*References 1, 9, 10, 19, 43, and 52.
†References 4, 5, 8, 14, 17, 41, 42, 55, and 57.

*References 3-5, 18, 21, 24, 30, 32, 37, 38, 50, 55, and 57.
†References 3-5, 13, 18, 21, 24, 26, 30, 32, 37-39, 50, 53, 55, and 57.

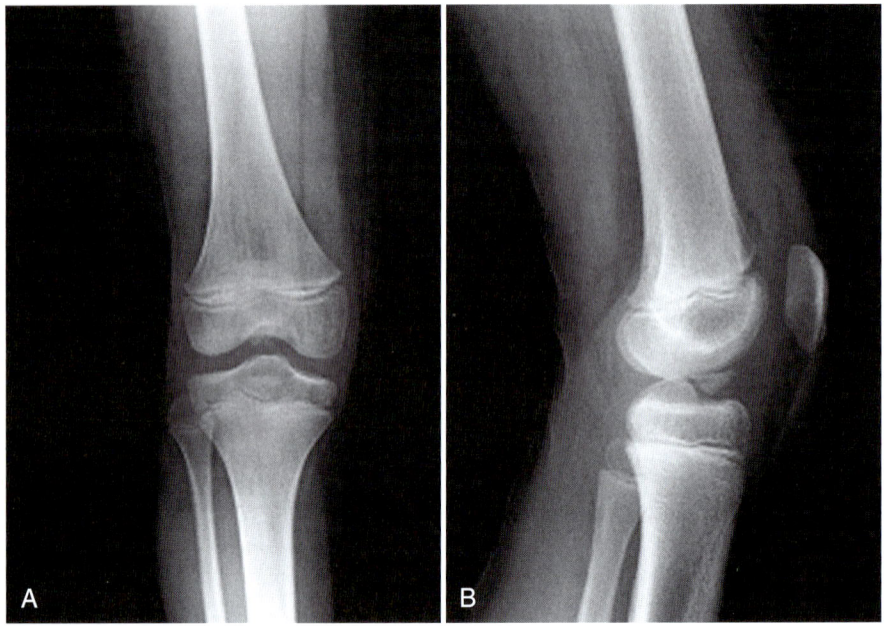

A

B

Figure 89-1. **A,** Anteroposterior radiograph of displaced tibial spine fracture. **B,** Lateral radiograph of displaced tibial spine fracture.

stress testing should be performed to detect any tear of the medial collateral ligament (MCL) or lateral collateral ligament (LCL). Patients with late malunion of a displaced tibial spine fracture may lack full extension because of a bony block. Patients with late nonunion of a displaced tibial spine fracture may have increased knee laxity and positive Lachman and pivot-shift examinations. A complete neurologic and vascular examination should be performed.

IMAGING

Standard roentgenograms and anteroposterior, lateral, and notch radiographic views are usually diagnostic. The fracture is best seen on lateral and notch views (Fig. 89-1). Radiographs should be carefully scrutinized, as the avulsed fragment may be mostly nonossified cartilage with only a small, thin ossified portion visible on the lateral view. If necessary, computed tomography (CT) scanning allows refined definition of the fracture anatomy.

Magnetic resonance imaging (MRI) typically is not needed in the diagnosis and management of tibial eminence fractures in children. However, MRI may be helpful in confirming the diagnosis in cases with a very thin ossified portion of the avulsed fragment, and in evaluating associated collateral ligament, chondral, meniscal, or physeal pathology, although these events are uncommon. If distal pulses are abnormal or a dislocation is suspected, an arteriogram should be obtained.

ASSOCIATED INJURIES

Associated intra-articular injuries are relatively uncommon. Intercondylar eminence fractures may include or may be associated with any combination of bone, chondral, meniscal, and ligamentous injuries.[10] However, in a series of 80 skeletally immature patients who underwent surgical fixation of tibial eminence fractures, Kocher and coworkers found no associated chondral injuries and associated meniscal tear in only 3.8% (3/80) of patients (Fig. 89-2).[23] Associated col-

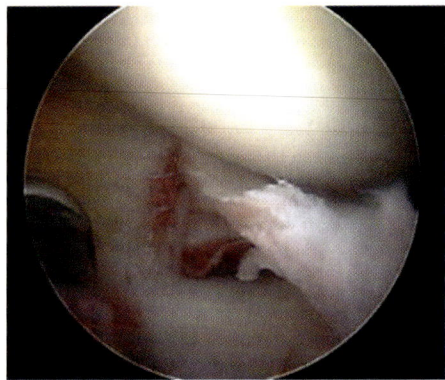

Figure 89-2. Meniscal tear in conjunction with a tibial spine fracture.

lateral ligament injury or proximal ACL avulsion in conjunction with a tibial spine fracture has also been reported.[15,45]

CLASSIFICATION

The classification system of Meyers and McKeever is based on the degree of displacement and is widely used to classify fractures and to guide treatment (Fig. 89-3).[35,36] Zaricznyj later modified this classification to include a fourth type—comminuted fractures of the tibial spine[59]:

1. Type 1: minimal displacement of the tibial spine fragment from the rest of the proximal tibial epiphysis
2. Type 2: displacement of the anterior third to half of the avulsed fragment, which is lifted upward but remains hinged on its posterior border, which is in contact with the proximal tibial epiphysis
3. Type 3: complete separation of the avulsed fragment from the proximal tibial epiphysis, usually associated with upward displacement and rotation

Interobserver reliability with type 1 and type 2/3 fractures is good; however, differentiation between type 2 and 3 fractures may be difficult.[22]

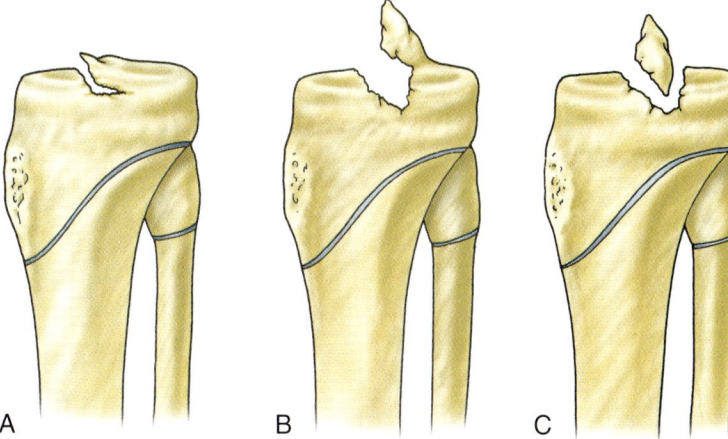

Figure 89-3. Meyers and McKeever classification system of tibial spine fracture in children. **A,** Type 1: minimal displacement. **B,** Type 2: displaced and hinged posteriorly. **C,** Type 3: complete displacement.

SURGICAL AND APPLIED ANATOMY

Between the condyles, the intercondylar eminence or the spine is the insertion point for portions of the menisci and the anterior and posterior cruciate ligaments. The tibial eminence is triangular and refers to the portion of the proximal tibia that includes two ridges of bone and cartilage. In the immature skeleton, the proximal surface of the eminence is covered entirely with cartilage. The ACL attaches distally to the anteromedial portion of the tibial intercondylar eminence (Fig. 89-4). The posterior cruciate ligament (PCL) inserts on the posterior aspect of the proximal tibia, distal to the joint line. Both menisci insert into the tibia in the region between the lateral and medial eminences, but no direct connection exists between the ACL and the menisci. In 12 patients with displaced tibial spine fractures that were unable to be reduced closed, Lowe and colleagues reported that the anterior horn of the lateral meniscus and the ACL were attached simultaneously and were pulling in different directions.[27]

Meniscal or intermeniscal ligament entrapment under the displaced tibial eminence fragment can be common and may be a rationale for considering arthroscopic or open reduction in displaced tibial spine fractures (Fig. 89-5).[6,7,10,23] Meniscal entrapment can prevent anatomic reduction of the tibial spine fragment, which may result in increased anterior laxity or a block to extension and knee pain after the fracture has healed.[14,17,32,41,42] Mah and coworkers found medial meniscal entrapment preventing reduction in 8 of 10 children with type 3 fractures undergoing arthroscopic treatment.[31] In a consecutive series of 80 patients who underwent surgical fixation of tibial eminence fractures that were not able to be reduced closed, Kocher and associates reported entrapment of the anterior horn medial meniscus (n = 36), the intermeniscal ligament (n = 6), or the anterior horn lateral meniscus (n = 1) in 26% of type 2 fractures and 65% of type 3 fractures.[23] The entrapped meniscus typically can be extracted with an arthroscopic probe and retracted with a retaining suture (Fig. 89-6).

CURRENT TREATMENT OPTIONS

Current treatment options include cast immobilization,[24,37] closed reduction with immobilization,[41,57] open reduction

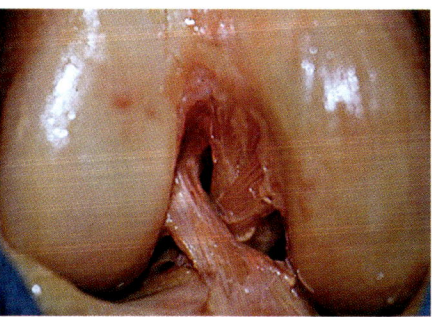

Figure 89-4. Anterior cruciate ligament (ACL) insertion onto the anteromedial portion of the tibial eminence.

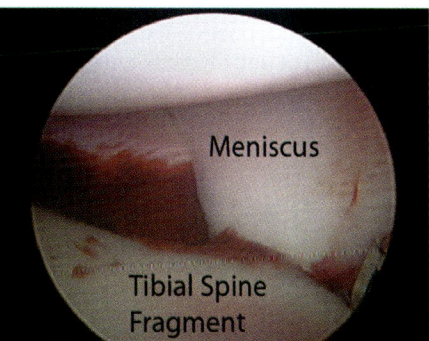

Figure 89-5. Anterior horn of the medial meniscus entrapped under the tibial spine fragment.

with immobilization,[37] open reduction with internal fixation,[38,57] arthroscopic reduction with immobilization,[33] and arthroscopic reduction with a variety of fixation methods, including suture fixation,* wire[3] and screw fixation,[5,24,33,44] anchor fixation,[54] and bioabsorbable nail fixation.[46] Many options regarding fixation of the fracture are available, and all have been used with good success, most commonly, suture and screw fixation. Study findings are equivocal in terms of strength of fixation, although suture fixation may be favored because it offers the advantages of eliminating the risks of

_____

*References 16, 18, 24, 25, 31, and 47.

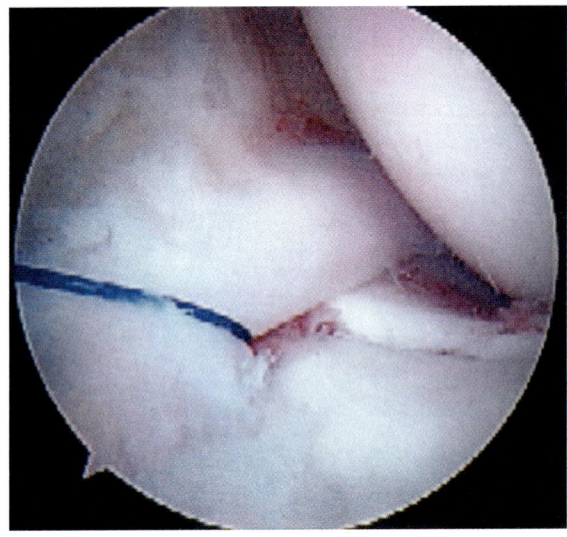

Figure 89-6. Use of a retention suture to retract the anterior horn of the medial meniscus.

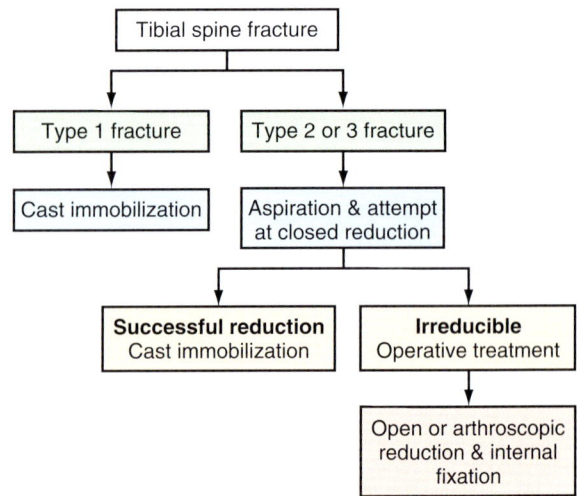

Figure 89-7. Authors' preferred treatment algorithm for tibial spine fractures in children.

comminution of the fracture fragment and posterior neurovascular injury and the need for hardware removal.[2,25,46,47]

The goal of treatment of a tibial spine avulsion is anatomic reduction; however, controversy continues regarding whether the tibial spine should be over-reduced. Theoretically, over-reduction may lead to excessive tightening of the ACL and limited knee motion.[28] On the other hand, it is likely that permanent intersubstance stretching of the ACL occurs before the fracture[40]; therefore, over-reduction could be considered. Although further clinical or in vitro research is required, long-term evaluation of well-reduced tibial eminence fractures shows subtle increases in anteroposterior knee laxity without functional deficit.*

Closed treatment is typically used for type 1 fractures and for type 2 or 3 fractures that can be successfully reduced closed. Aspiration of the hematoma is performed first, and closed reduction is achieved by placement of the knee in full extension or 20 to 30 degrees of flexion. If the fracture fragment extends into the medial or lateral tibial plateaus, full extension may aid reduction through pressure applied by medial or lateral femoral condyle congruence, whereas fractures confined completely within the intercondylar notch may not reduce. Portions of the ACL are tight in all knee positions; therefore, no single position that exists without application of traction by the ACL may prevent anatomic reduction. Radiographs are used to assess adequacy of reduction.

Closed reduction can be successful for some type 2 fractures but frequently is not successful for type 3 fractures. In their series, Kocher and associates reported closed reduction in approximately 50% of type 2 fractures (26/49) and unsuccessful closed reduction in all 57 type 3 fractures.[23] Arthroscopic or open reduction with internal fixation of type 2 and 3 tibial eminence fractures, which do not reduce, has been advocated because of the potential for clinical instability and loss of extension associated with closed reduction and immobilization, the ability to evaluate and treat injuries, and

the opportunity for early mobilization.[6,7,21,31] For displaced type 2 and 3 fractures, Wiley and Baxter found a correlation between fracture displacement and measured knee laxity despite good patient function.[55]

AUTHORS' PREFERRED TREATMENT

The authors' algorithm for treatment of tibial spine fractures is shown in Figure 89-7.

Type 1 fractures are treated with cast immobilization after aspiration of the hematoma. A local anesthetic can be injected into the joint under sterile conditions if the patient is in severe pain. A long leg cast is applied in 0 to 20 degrees of flexion; we usually avoid a cylinder cast to avoid slippage and malleolar irritation. The patient and the family are cautioned to elevate the leg to avoid swelling. Radiographs are repeated in 1 to 2 weeks to ensure that the fragment has not displaced and that alignment is adequate. The cast is removed 6 weeks after injury. A hinged knee brace or a custom ACL brace is used and physical therapy is initiated to regain motion and strength. Patients typically are allowed to return to sports at 3 months after injury if they demonstrate fracture healing and adequate motion and strength; use of the ACL brace for 6 months is encouraged.

Type 2 fractures are treated initially with an attempt at closed reduction. The hematoma is aspirated, and local anesthetic is injected into the knee under sterile conditions. Reduction is attempted at full extension and at 20 degrees of flexion. Radiographs are taken to assess reduction. If anatomic reduction is attained, a long-leg cast is applied in the position of reduction, and the protocol for type 1 fractures is followed. If the fracture does not reduce adequately or if the fracture displaces later, operative treatment is performed.

Type 3 fractures may be treated with attempted closed reduction; however, this is usually unsuccessful, and operative treatment is typically performed.

The authors' preferred operative treatment is arthroscopic reduction and internal fixation. Open reduction through a medial parapatellar incision can also be performed per surgeon preference and/or experience, or if arthroscopic visualization is difficult.

*References 4, 14, 21, 27, 44, 50, and 55.

ARTHROSCOPIC REDUCTION AND INTERNAL FIXATION WITH EPIPHYSEAL CANNULATED SCREWS

A standard arthroscopic operating room setup is used. The patient is placed supine, and general anesthesia is typically used. A standard arthroscope can be used in most patients, and a small (2.7 mm) arthroscope is used in younger children. An arthroscopic fluid pump is used at 35 mm Hg to prevent excess bleeding, and a tourniquet is used routinely. Standard anteromedial and anterolateral portals are established and accessory superomedial and superolateral portals are used for screw insertion. The hematoma is evacuated prior to insertion of the arthroscope.

A thorough arthroscopic examination of the entire knee joint is conducted to evaluate for concomitant injuries. Frequently, we excise some portion of the anterior fat pad and ligamentum mucosum with an arthroscopic shaver for complete visualization of the intercondylar eminence fragment. An entrapped meniscus or intermeniscal ligament can be extracted with an arthroscopic probe and retracted with a retention suture inserted from outside in (see Fig. 89-6). The base of the tibial eminence fragment is elevated (Fig. 89-8A), and the entire fracture bed débrided with an arthroscopic shaver and hand curette (Fig. 89-8B). Anatomic reduction is obtained using a probe, microfracture pick, or Kirschner wire with the knee in 30 to 90 degrees of flexion (Fig. 89-8C). Cannulated guide wires are placed through portals just off the superomedial and superolateral borders of the patella through the accessory portals at the base of the ACL. Fluoroscopic assistance is used to confirm anatomic reduction, guide correct wire orientation, and avoid the proximal tibial physis. A cannulated drill is used over the guide wires, and one or two screws are inserted, based on the size of the

tibial eminence fragment (Fig. 89-8D). Partially threaded 3.5-mm-diameter screws (Fig. 89-8E) are used in children, and 4.5-mm-diameter screws are used in adolescents. The knee is evaluated through a full range of motion to ensure rigid fixation without fracture displacement, and to ensure that there is no impingement of the screw heads in extension.

Postoperatively, patients are placed in a hinged knee brace and are maintained at touch-down weight bearing for 6 weeks. Motion is restricted to 0 to 30 degrees for the first 2 weeks, 0 to 90 degrees for the next 2 weeks, followed by full range of motion. The brace is kept locked in extension at night. Radiographs are obtained to evaluate maintenance of reduction and fracture healing at 2 and 6 weeks (Fig. 89-9). Cast immobilization in 20 to 30 degrees of flexion for 4 weeks postoperatively may be necessary in younger children who are unable to comply with protected weight bearing and brace immobilization. Physical therapy is used to achieve motion, strength, and sport-specific training. Patients typically are allowed to return to sports at 12 to 16 weeks postoperatively, depending on knee function and strength. Screws are not routinely removed. Functional ACL bracing is used when residual knee laxity is observed.

ARTHROSCOPIC REDUCTION AND INTERNAL FIXATION WITH SUTURE

Arthroscopic setup and examinations are similar to the techniques described for epiphyseal screw fixation. Accessory superomedial and superolateral portals typically are not used. A small incision is made just medial and distal to the tibial tubercle, as would be performed for an ACL reconstruction. After the fracture is débrided and slightly over-reduced, a tibial ACL guide system with the tibial aimer set at 55 degrees

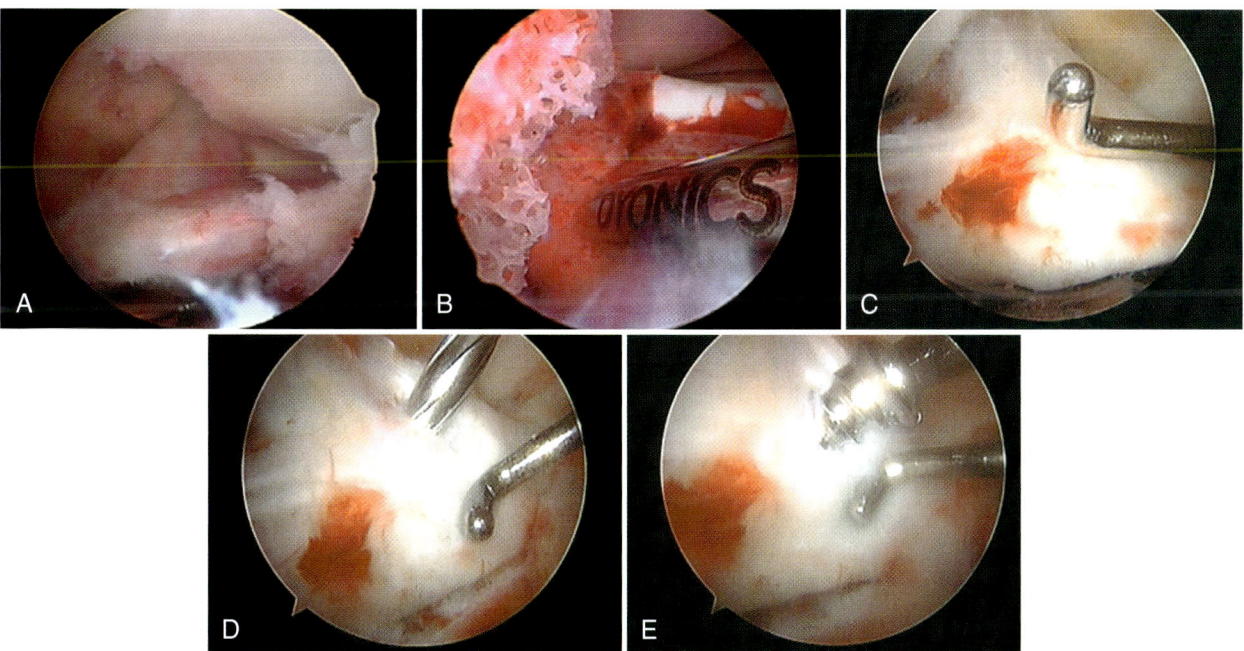

Figure 89-8. Arthroscopic reduction and insertion of cannulated screw internal fixation for a displaced tibial spine fracture. **A,** Tibial spine fragment. **B,** Elevation and débridement of the fracture bed. **C,** Reduction of tibial spine fragment. **D,** Drilling with a cannulated screw system. **E,** Insertion of a 3.5-mm screw.

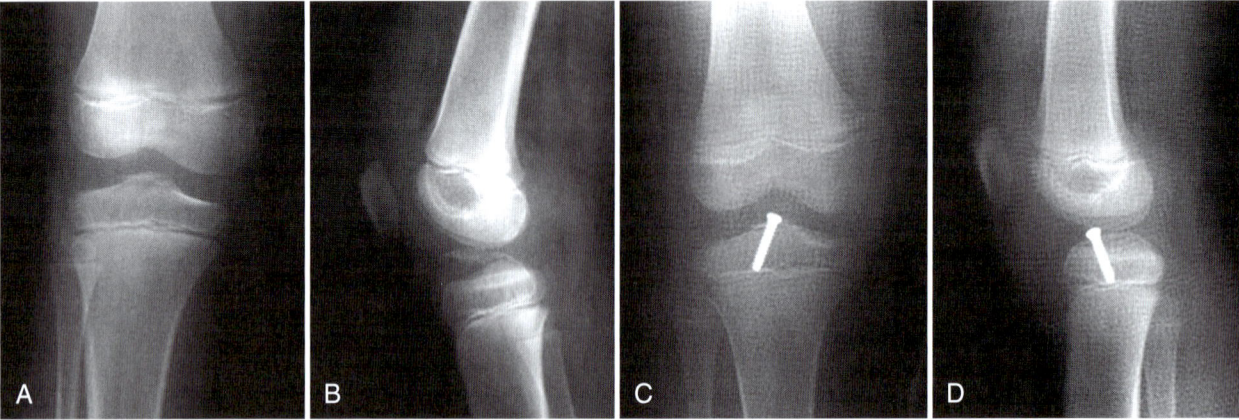

Figure 89-9. Type 3 tibial spine fracture treated with arthroscopic reduction and screw fixation. **A,** Preoperative anteroposterior radiograph. **B,** Preoperative lateral radiograph. **C,** Postoperative anteroposterior radiograph. **D,** Postoperative lateral radiograph.

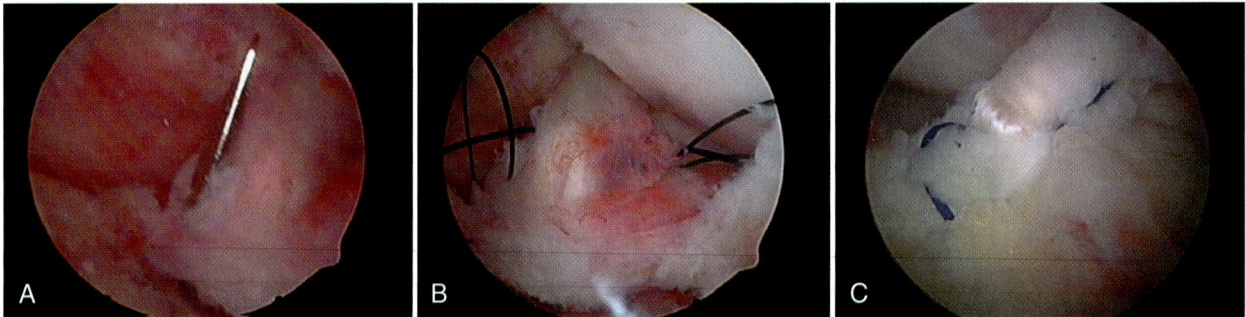

Figure 89-10. Treatment of a type 2 tibial spine fracture with arthroscopic reduction and suture fixation. **A,** Drilling of guide wire with anterior cruciate ligament (ACL) guide system. **B,** Hewson suture passers on either side of the ACL and passage of absorbable sutures through the ACL. **C,** Final appearance after suture fixation.

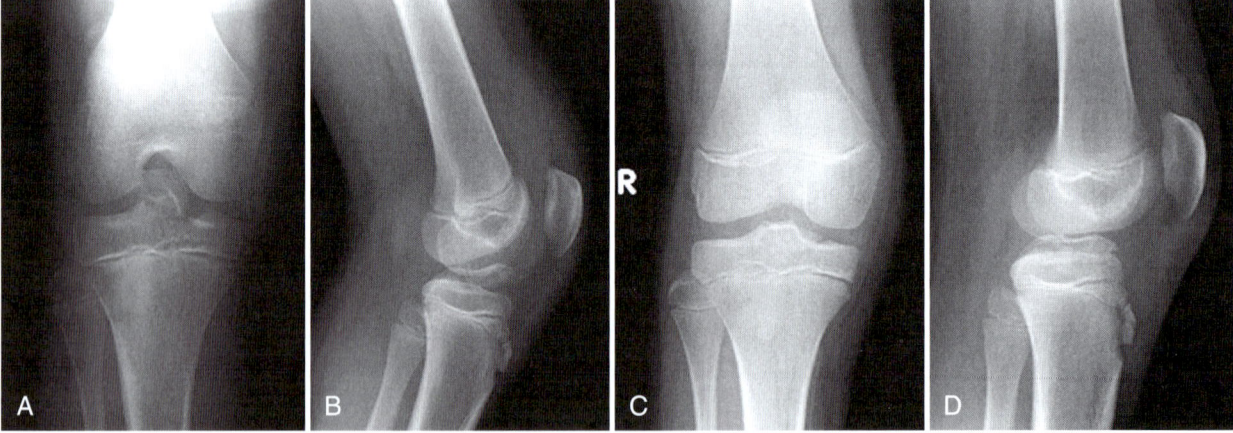

Figure 89-11. Type 2 tibial spine fracture treated with arthroscopic reduction and suture fixation. **A,** Preoperative anteroposterior radiograph. **B,** Preoperative lateral radiograph. **C,** Postoperative anteroposterior radiograph. **D,** Postoperative lateral radiograph.

is used to place two guide wires through the base of the ACL. These guide wires will traverse the tibial physis, but no cases of growth arrest after suture fixation have been reported. The guide wires are exchanged for Hewson suture passers, and two heavy absorbable sutures are passed through the Hewson suture passers and the base of the ACL using a suture punch (Fig. 89-10) or a suture lasso. The sutures are retrieved through the tibial tubercle incision and are tied down onto

the tibia. This procedure may be repeated for additional sutures. The postoperative protocol is the same (Fig. 89-11).

PEARLS AND PITFALLS

When tibial eminence fractures are managed with closed reduction, follow-up radiographs must be obtained at 1 and 2 weeks post injury to verify maintenance of reduction. Late displacement and malunion can occur, particularly for type 2 fractures. Injection of local anesthetic under sterile conditions can be helpful in minimizing pain and allowing for full knee extension in attempts at closed reduction.

During arthroscopic reduction and fixation of tibial spine fractures, visualization can be difficult unless the large hematoma is evacuated before the arthroscope is introduced and bleeding from the fracture is controlled. Adequate inflow and outflow is essential for proper visualization; we routinely use an arthroscopic pump and a tourniquet to achieve this. Careful attention should be paid to preparing the fracture bed to provide optimal conditions for bony healing. A slight over-reduction of the fracture is attempted.

Epiphyseal cannulated screw fixation of small or comminuted tibial eminence fragments can fail owing to inadequate bony purchase or further comminution; in these cases, suture fixation is preferred. If epiphyseal cannulated screw fixation is used, fluoroscopy is necessary to ensure that the screw does not traverse the proximal tibial physis, which may result in a proximal tibial physeal growth arrest.[39]

Early mobilization is useful for avoiding arthrofibrosis, which can occur with immobilization. However, in younger children, compliance with protected weight bearing and brace use can be problematic, and these patients must be casted.

PROGNOSIS AND COMPLICATIONS

Most studies have shown that the overall prognosis of tibial eminence fractures is good to excellent if satisfactory reduction is achieved. However, some studies have reported no difference in outcome of displaced tibial spine fractures treated closed versus open or arthroscopically.[4,14,40,55-57] A majority of studies have found residual laxity of the knee after open or closed treatment for all tibial eminence fracture types up to 6 mm compared with the contralateral side.* Baxter and Wiley found excellent functional results without symptomatic instability in 17 pediatric knees with displaced tibial spine fractures, despite a positive Lachman examination in 51% of patients and increased measured mean knee laxity up to 3.5 mm.[4,55] In a study of 12 pediatric knees undergoing open reduction and internal fixation, Smith found subluxation symptoms in two patients despite positive Lachman examinations in 87% of patients.[50] Willis and associates reported excellent clinical stability in all 50 children treated closed or open, despite a positive Lachman examination in 64% of patients and instrumented (KT-1000) knee laxity of 3.5 mm for type 2 fractures and 4.5 mm for type 3 fractures.[57] Similarly, Janarv and colleagues and Kocher and coworkers found excellent functional results despite persistent laxity in up to 80% of patients even with an anatomic reduction.[17,21]

This laxity is worse with type 3 injuries, with pedestrian–MVA trauma, and with other associated ligament tears.† Increased laxity is likely due to intrasubstance stretching of the ACL during injury. At the time of tibial spine fixation, the ACL often appears hemorrhagic within its sheath, but grossly intact and in continuity with the bony bed of the tibia. However, ACL injury after previous tibial spine fracture is rare.

Poor results may occur after eminence fractures associated with unrecognized injuries to the collateral ligaments or physeal fracture.[34,50,51] In addition, hardware across the proximal tibial physis may result in a growth disturbance with a recurvatum deformity.[39] Malunion of type 2 and 3 fractures may cause bony impingement of the knee during full extension.[11,30] This can be corrected by excision of the malunited fragment and anatomic reinsertion of the ACL, or excision of the fragment and ACL reconstruction can be considered in adults and older adolescents.

Nonunion of type 2 and 3 tibial spine fractures treated closed usually can be managed by arthroscopic or open reduction with internal fixation with or without bone graft.[20,26,53] Débridement of the fracture bed and of the fracture fragment to bleeding bone is essential to optimize bony healing; bone graft may be required in some cases. Excision of the fragment and ACL reconstruction can be considered in adults and older adolescents.

Arthrofibrosis, particularly loss of extension, can occur after tibial spine fracture, even after anatomic reduction.[13] It is thought to be due to the local increase in blood supply during healing; this leads to spine enlargement or arthrofibrosis, which can cause a mechanical block to extension. Early range of motion and mobilization are essential in attempts to prevent loss of motion. Dynamic splinting and aggressive physical therapy can be used during the first 3 months after fracture if stiffness is present. If stiffness persists after 3 months, manipulation under anesthesia and lysis of adhesions can be performed. Overly vigorous manipulation should be avoided to avert injury to the proximal tibial or distal femoral physis. A notchplasty can be performed if near skeletal maturity to regain extension.

KEY REFERENCES

Ahmad CS, Stein BE, Jeshuran W, et al: Anterior cruciate ligament function after tibial eminence fracture in skeletally mature patients. Am J Sports Med 29:339–345, 2001.

Baxter MP, Wiley JJ: Fractures of the tibial spine in children: an evaluation of knee stability. J Bone Joint Surg Br 70:228–230, 1988.

Burstein DB, Viola A, Fulkerson JP: Entrapment of the medial meniscus in a fracture of the tibial eminence. Arthroscopy 4:47–50, 1988.

Gronkvist H, Hirsch G, Johansson L: Fracture of the anterior tibial spine in children. J Pediatr Orthop 4:465–468, 1984.

Kocher MS, Foreman ES, Micheli LJ: Laxity and functional outcome after arthroscopic reduction and internal fixation of displaced tibial spine fractures in children. Arthroscopy 19:1085–1090, 2003.

Lubowitz JH, Grauer JD: Arthroscopic treatment of anterior cruciate ligament avulsion. Clin Orthop Relat Res 294:242–246, 1993.

McLennan JG: Lessons learned after second-look arthroscopy in type III fractures of the tibial spine. J Pediatr Orthop 15:59–62, 1995.

Meyers MH, McKeever FM: Fracture of the intercondylar eminence of the tibia. J Bone Joint Surg Am 41:209–220, 1959; discussion 220–202.

Molander ML, Wallin G, Wikstad I: Fracture of the intercondylar eminence of the tibia: a review of 35 patients. J Bone Joint Surg Br 63:89–91, 1981.

Noyes FR, DeLucas JL, Torvik PJ: Biomechanics of anterior cruciate ligament failure: an analysis of strain-rate sensitivity and mechanisms of failure in primates. J Bone Joint Surg Am 56:236–253, 1974.

Rademakers MV, Kerkhoffs GM, Kager J, et al: Tibial spine fractures: a long-term follow-up study of open reduction and internal fixation. J Orthop Trauma 23:203–207, 2009.

Wiley JJ, Baxter MP: Tibial spine fractures in children. Clin Orthop Relat Res 255:54–60, 1990.

Willis RB, Blokker C, Stoll TM, et al: Long-term follow-up of anterior tibial eminence fractures. J Pediatr Orthop 13:361–364, 1993.

---

*References 4, 5, 21, 24, 30, 41-43, 56, and 57.
†References 4, 5, 21, 24, 30, 41-43, 56, and 57.

Full references for this chapter can be found on www.expertconsult.com.

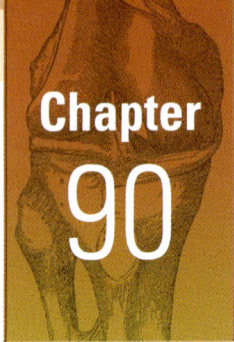

Chapter 90

Physeal Fractures About the Knee

Jennifer Weiss and David L. Skaggs

BACKGROUND

Physeal fractures about the knee can occur in the form of distal femoral physeal fractures, proximal tibial physeal fractures, tibial tubercle fractures, tibial eminence fractures, and patellar sleeve fractures. Diagnosis and treatment of these fractures and their complications can be challenging. Even physeal fractures that are not displaced can lead to complications of physeal arrest, making proper treatment and long term follow-up essential.

DISTAL FEMUR

Distal femoral physeal fractures are most common in older children and tend to occur from high-energy trauma.[27] Most commonly, these fractures are Salter-Harris II fractures.[18] The most common mechanisms of injury are motor vehicle accidents and falls.[18] Most commonly, a valgus force leads to medial physeal separation extending into an oblique fracture through the lateral metaphysis.[6] Less commonly, a hyperextension injury is responsible, with risk of neurovascular injury.[6] The distal femoral physis is at risk for fracture in this scenario because of the fact that the anterior cruciate ligament (ACL), posterior cruciate ligament (PCL), lateral collateral ligament (LCL), and medial collateral ligament (MCL) do not span or protect it.

This fracture is four times more common in boys than in girls.[18]

Imaging should begin with anteroposterior, lateral, and oblique radiographs. Stress radiographs may provide a definitive diagnosis but risk further physeal damage. If nonstress radiographs are inconclusive, magnetic resonance imaging (MRI) is less painful for the patient and can provide more information.[1]

Suspicion for popliteal vascular injury should be high, with the incidence of popliteal artery injury reported at 3%.[8] Angiography is the gold standard for evaluation of arterial injury in the setting of a fracture about the knee.[8] Prompt recognition and intervention for vascular injury in this scenario decreases the risk of catastrophic complications such as loss of limb.

At least 20% of distal femoral physeal fractures lead to angular deformity and growth arrest requiring reconstructive surgery.[18] Factors that predict outcome include type of fracture, initial fracture displacement, and exactness of reduction.[18] Growth disturbances are usually evident within 6 months to 1 year, but follow-up may be considered until skeletal maturity.[28]

Anatomic reduction of extra-articular distal femoral physeal fractures (Salter-Harris types I and II) usually can be done via closed reduction. To address the flexion deformity, the knee may be flexed to relax the gastrocnemius muscle. Once the knee is flexed, assessment of coronal plane alignment can be challenging. Closed reduction attempts should be gentle and repeated attempts minimized, as these may exacerbate trauma to the physis. The reduction maneuver should consist of 90% traction and 10% manipulation to minimize iatrogenic damage to the physis. Open reduction may be necessary, as periosteum may be interposed.

At times, interposed periosteum may be removed through a relatively small incision with a skin hook. If the Thurston-Holland fragment is large enough, lag screws may be placed for relatively rigid fixation (Figs. 90-1 through 90-4). Thompson and associates demonstrated that 43% of fractures reduced without fixation displaced during cast treatment, whereas no fractures treated with internal fixation displaced.[29] Smooth pins can be placed percutaneously to maintain reduction with little risk to the physis. Once the fracture reduction is maintained, the knee can be extended again to assess coronal plane alignment.

Anatomic reduction of intra-articular distal femoral physeal fractures (Salter-Harris types III and IV) frequently requires open reduction. Visualization of the articular surface is encouraged if there is any doubt about the reduction. When a large metaphyseal fragment permits, cannulated screws can be used for secure fixation in both extra-articular and intra-articular physeal fractures of the distal femur. Titanium screws should be considered, as these can facilitate future MRI scanning. MRI may be of interest, because these patients can have concomitant intra-articular injury to the ligaments or meniscus. MRI can also be useful in evaluating for physeal bar formation.

Postoperative care of these fractures should include a long-leg cast or brace applied with the knee in 0 to 30 degrees of flexion. In patients with short, thick thighs, a waist band may be considered. Non–weight bearing is recommended for 3 weeks. When pins are used, the pins are removed at 4 weeks post surgery, as pin tract infection can lead to a septic knee. Immobilization then should be continued until 6 weeks postoperatively. Screw removal is not mandatory, and no studies have compared outcomes in patients with retained versus removed hardware in this location.

Figures 90-1 through 90-4 illustrate a distal femoral Salter-Harris III fracture treated with closed reduction and internal fixation.

PROXIMAL TIBIA

Physeal fractures of the proximal tibia are extremely rare. The stabilizing anatomy of the hamstrings, MCL, and LCL protects this region, and high energy is required to disturb the area. Peak incidence of proximal tibia physeal fractures occurs between the ages of 10 and 12 years. Extension is the predominant mechanism of injury for these fractures.[21] Salter-Harris type I and II fractures predominate in this age group, and Salter-Harris type III and IV fractures tend to occur at a

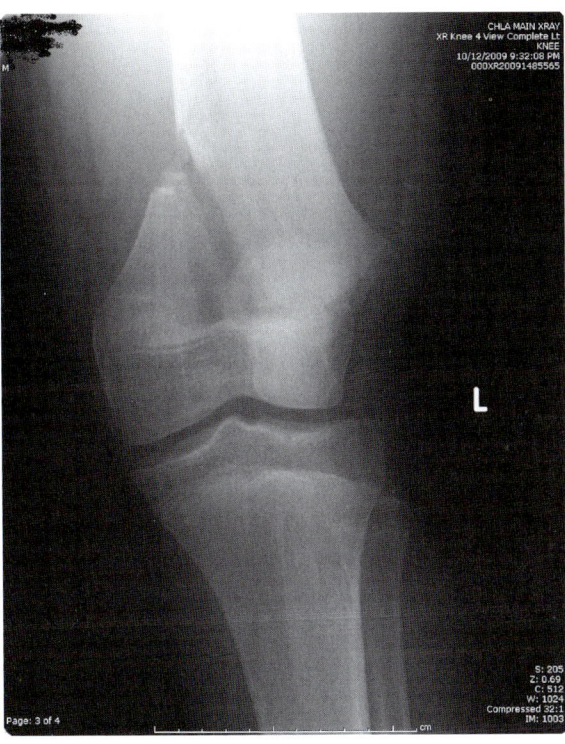

Figure 90-1. Anteroposterior (AP) radiograph of distal femoral physeal fracture. (Image property of Children's Orthopedic Center.)

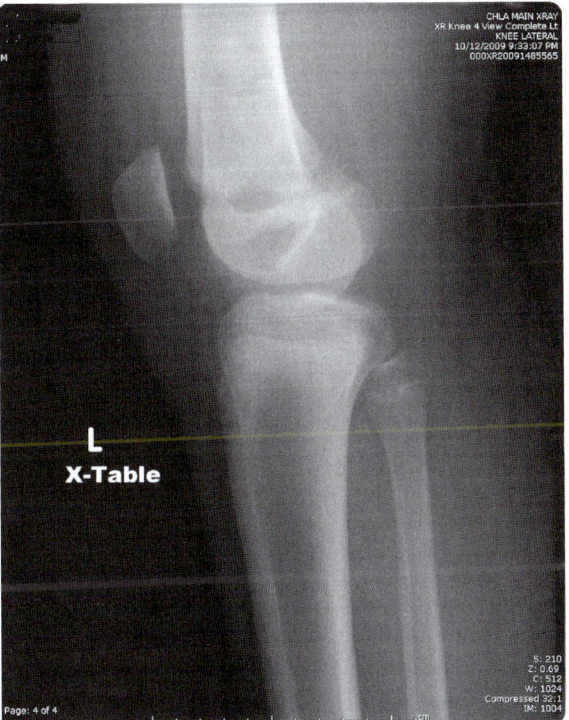

Figure 90-2. Lateral radiograph of distal femoral physeal fracture. (Image property of Children's Orthopedic Center.)

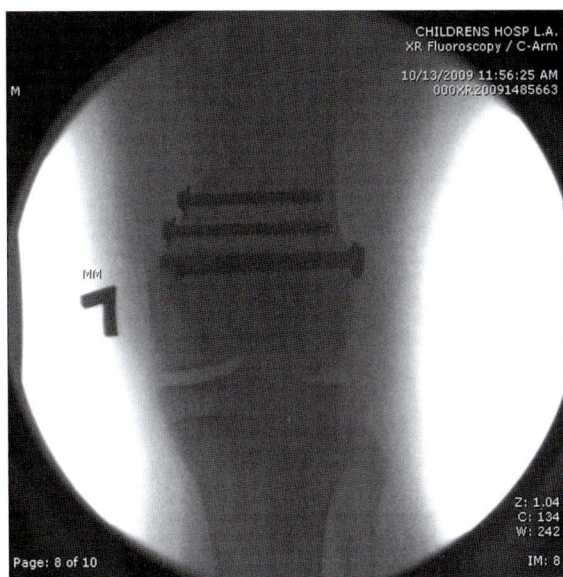

Figure 90-3. Anteroposterior (AP) radiograph post closed reduction internal fixation distal femur physeal fracture. (Image property of Children's Orthopedic Center.)

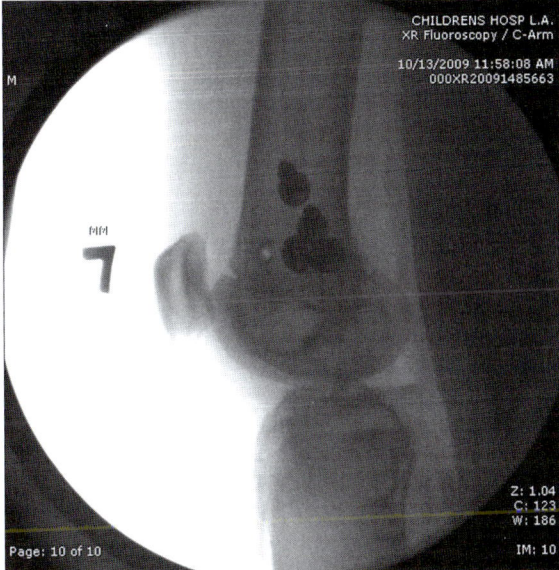

Figure 90-4. Lateral radiograph post closed reduction internal fixation distal femoral physeal. (Image property of Children's Orthopedic Center.)

later age (14 years).[21,23] Proximal tibial triplane fractures have also been described, but these occur rarely.[26]

When injury to the proximal tibia is suspected, imaging consists of anteroposterior and lateral radiographs of the knee. Stress views should be avoided, as they may cause further physeal damage. If radiographs are inconclusive, MRI can be used to further investigate for physeal injury.[1]

As in fractures of the distal femur and in knee dislocations when there is posterior placement of the tibia, suspicion for injury to the popliteal artery should be high. Angiography is the standard of care in diagnosing popliteal injury, and vascular consultation should be obtained promptly.[8] Shelton and Canale reported popliteal artery injuries resulting in vascular insufficiency in 2 of 39 patients.[25]

Anatomic reduction of proximal tibial fractures is necessary to protect both the articular surface and the physis. Direct visualization may augment radiographic evaluation of the articular surface and is recommended if there is any doubt

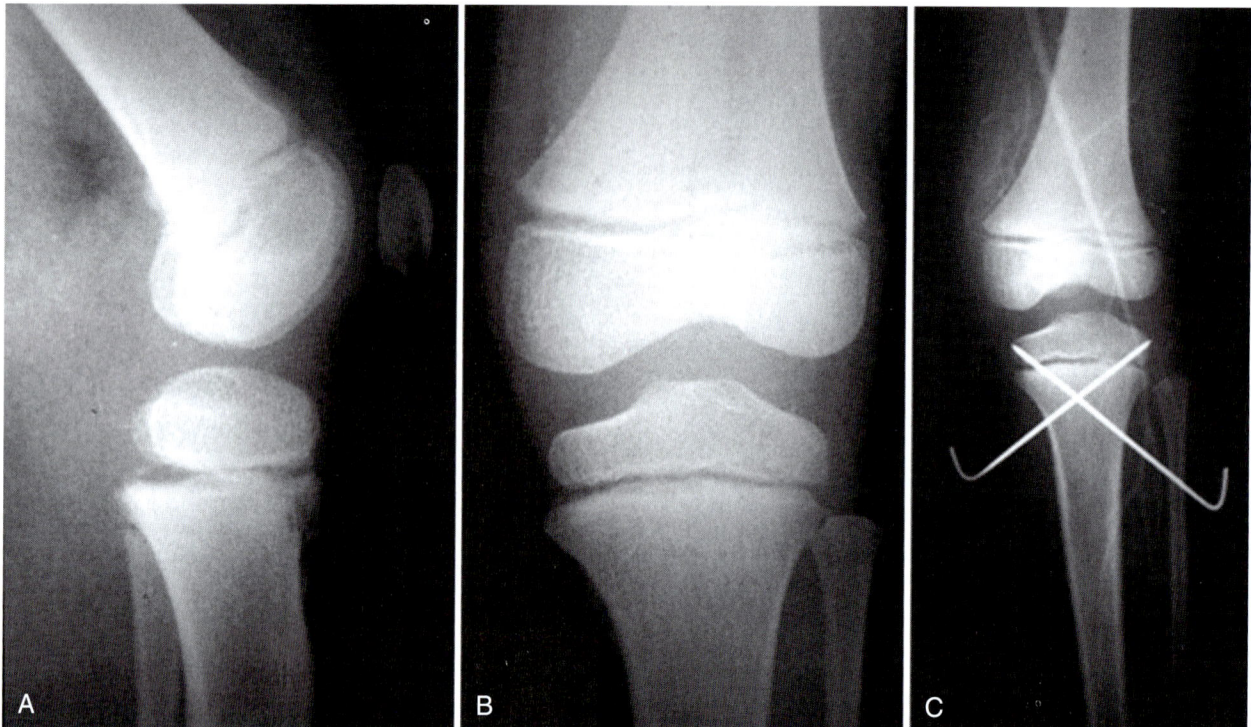

Figure 90-5. **A** and **B,** Proximal tibial physeal fracture that is minimally displaced. **C,** Fixation of this fracture with percutaneous pins.

about articular congruity. Arthroscopic assistance to assess the reduction is well reported in the adult literature and can be considered for adolescents.[5] If a large metaphyseal fragment is present, cannulated screws can be used as fixation. If the physis must be crossed, smooth pins should be used. Because they may need to enter the knee joint itself, early removal of these pins is recommended to prevent infection. Figure 90-5 shows operative fixation of a proximal tibial physeal fracture with K-wires.

Complications of proximal tibial physeal fractures include popliteal artery injury (associated with posterior displacement of the tibial shaft), compartment syndrome, peroneal nerve palsy, growth disturbance, and traumatic arthritis.[25] Because of the high energy required to cause this fracture, and the risk of compartment syndrome, inpatient admission for observation should be considered for even minimally displaced proximal tibial physeal fractures. Initially, regaining range of motion can be challenging. Vigilant follow-up to evaluate for growth plate injury in the form of angular deformity or leg length discrepancy should continue for at least a year post surgery. Standing radiographs from hip to ankle should be reviewed at 6 months and 1 year postoperatively.

Tibial Tubercle Fractures

Tibial tubercle fractures occur when the tibial tubercle physis is closing at the age of 11 or 12. These fractures occur much more frequently in boys than in girls.[3] They are classified according to the Watson-Jones classification, which was modified by Ogden in 1980 to include "A" and "B" subsets.[22] A type I fracture is a small fragment of the tuberosity, which is avulsed and displaced upward. Type IA is an incomplete separation of the fragment from the metaphysis, and type IB

is a complete separation. In a type II fracture, the entire lip of the tibial tuberosity is displaced upward. A type IIA fracture has no comminution, and a type IIB fracture has comminution. A type III fracture is one in which the entire tuberosity is fractured at its base, and the fracture line extends superiorly into the proximal tibial intra-articular surface. A type IIIA fracture has a single displaced fragment, and a type IIIB fracture includes comminuted displaced fragments. This classification system was further expanded by Ryu and Debenham[24]: They added a type IV fracture, which is an avulsion fracture of the proximal tibial epiphysis that extends into the posterior cortex of the tibia.[13] This type of flexion avulsion fracture of the proximal tibia is seen most commonly in the prepubescent patient age 13 or older.[21] Jumping with eccentric contraction of the quadriceps mechanism is the most common mechanism of injury.

Physical examination reveals point tenderness at the tibial tubercle, and the bony fragment can be palpated frequently. The extensor mechanism may not be intact, and the patient may not be able to initiate or maintain a straight-leg raise. A clinical pearl: any time an injured patient cannot actively bring their knee into full extension, consider the possibility of an injury somewhere along the extensor mechanism (quadriceps tendon, patella, patellar sleeve, patellar tendon, or tibial tubercle). The injury is most evident on the lateral radiograph.

Operative indications for tibial tubercle fracture include displacement or intra-articular extension into the proximal tibia.[22] Because these fractures usually occur when the tibial tubercle physis is beginning to close, treatment involves screw fixation across the fracture and physis without concern for growth disturbance in those approaching the end of growth. Type IV tibial tubercle fractures that extend to the posterior aspect of the tibia must also be fixed by securing the tibial tubercle. Although these fractures may appear similar to proximal tibial physeal fractures, they are on a continuum with tibial tubercle fractures (particularly in terms of mechanism and energy of injury) and should be treated as such.

Complications

Compartment syndrome can occur in displaced tibial tubercle fractures as the result of damage to the recurrent branch of the anterior tibial artery. Because this physis is beginning to close, genu recurvatum is actually a rare complication.[22] Genu recurvatum may occur, however, in the rare patient below the age of 11 or 12 who sustains a tibial tubercle fracture. Avulsion of the tibialis anterior muscle has been reported in concert with a type III tibial tubercle fracture.[14]

The case pictured in Figures 90-6 through 90-12 illustrates a type IV tibial tubercle fracture that was treated incorrectly. The proximal tibial physeal fracture was secured with smooth pins, and this portion of the fracture did in fact heal. However, the tibial tubercle component did not heal. The patient thus went on to sustain a tibial tubercle fracture. This was subsequently appropriately treated with open reduction and screw fixation.

Patellar Sleeve Fractures

Although proximal patellar sleeve fracture has been reported as a rarity, almost all patellar sleeve fractures are of the distal

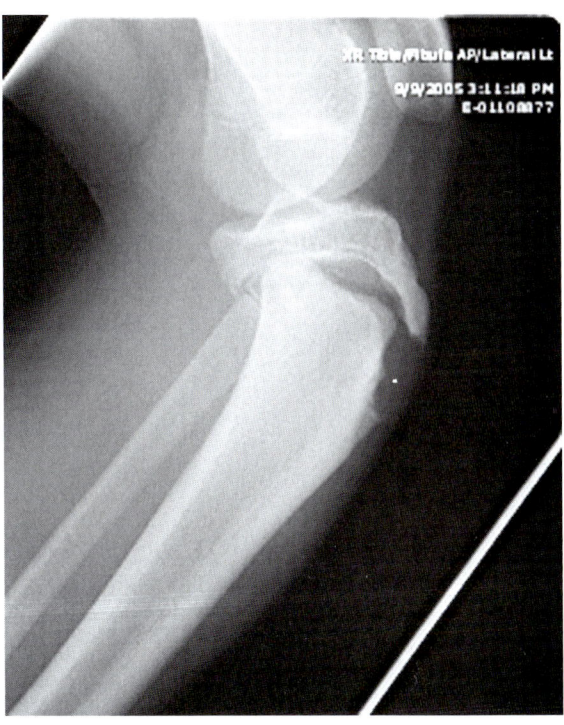

Figure 90-7. Lateral radiograph of type IV tibial tubercle fracture. (Image property of Children's Orthopedic Center.)

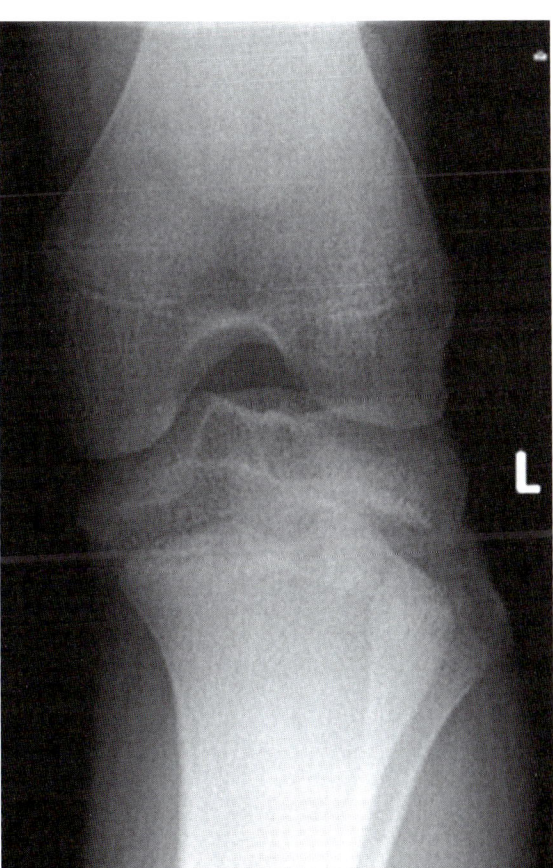

Figure 90-6. Anteroposterior (AP) radiograph of type IV tibial tubercle fracture. (Image property of Children's Orthopedic Center.)

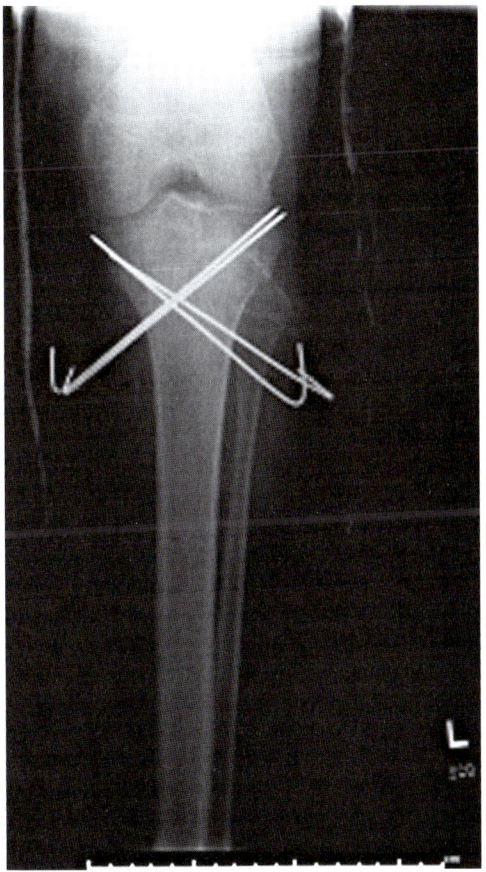

Figure 90-8. Anteroposterior (AP) radiograph post smooth pin fixation of type IV tibial tubercle fracture. (Image property of Children's Orthopedic Center.)

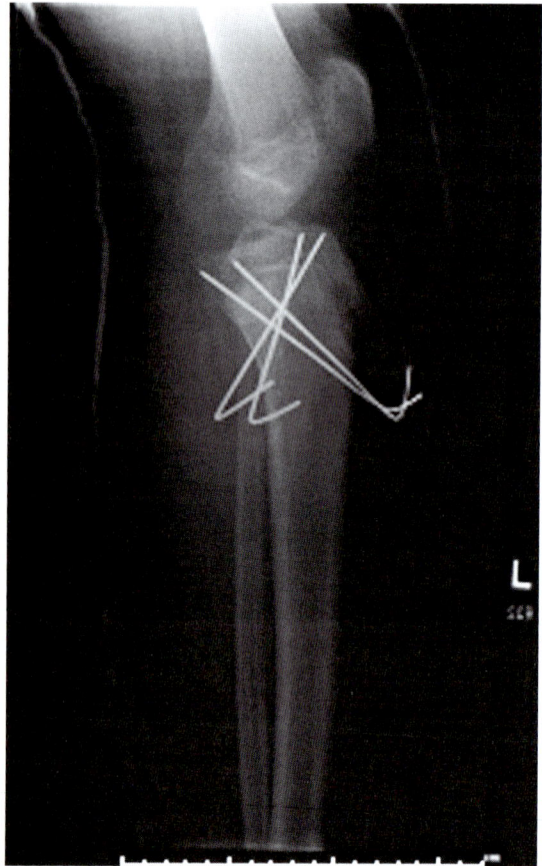

Figure 90-9. Lateral radiograph post smooth pin fixation of type IV tibial tubercle fracture. (Image property of Children's Orthopedic Center.)

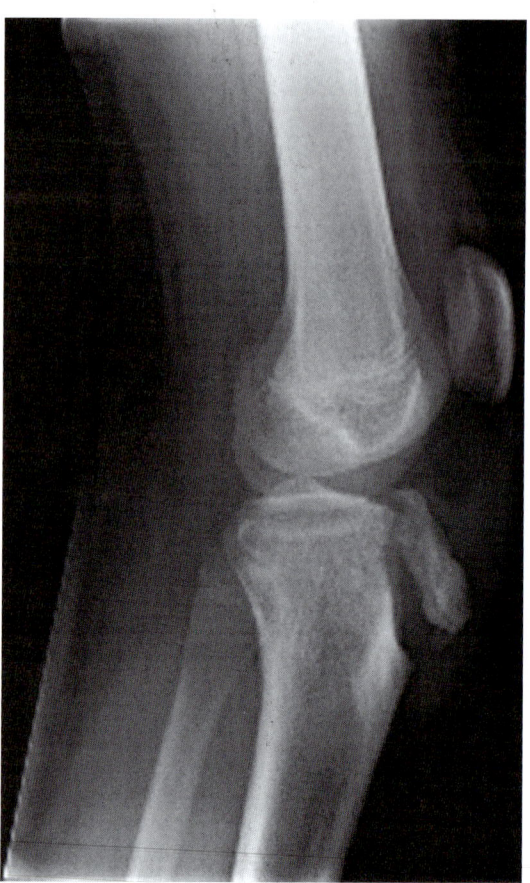

Figure 90-10. Lateral radiograph after refracture of tibial tubercle following incorrect treatment with smooth pins. (Image property of Children's Orthopedic Center.)

pole of the patella.[2,4,19] Patellar sleeve fractures are the most common type of patellar fracture in children.[11] Because the distal fragment of bone can be small, it is easy to overlook this entity on radiographs. MRI is helpful when physical examination and radiographs are inconclusive. Figure 90-12 shows that the distal fragment may be very subtle, and that the fracture can be easy to overlook. Suspicion of this injury should be great after a mechanism of eccentric contraction of the quadriceps is noted. Physical examination may reveal an absent extensor mechanism. Point tenderness will be present over the distal or proximal pole of the patella, and a defect may even be palpable (pictured in Fig. 90-13). In truly nondisplaced patellar sleeve fractures, cylinder casting is the treatment of choice. When the fracture is displaced, treatment consists of open reduction with internal fixation in the form of tension band fixation.[7] If reduction and fixation are not achieved in a timely fashion, there is risk of patellar elongation and disruption of patellofemoral joint mechanics.

Figure 90-14 shows the intraoperative appearance of the patellar sleeve fragment. Note the large size of the distal fragment that was difficult to appreciate on the radiograph. Figure 90-15 shows the postoperative appearance of a healing patellar sleeve fracture after open reduction and internal fixation.

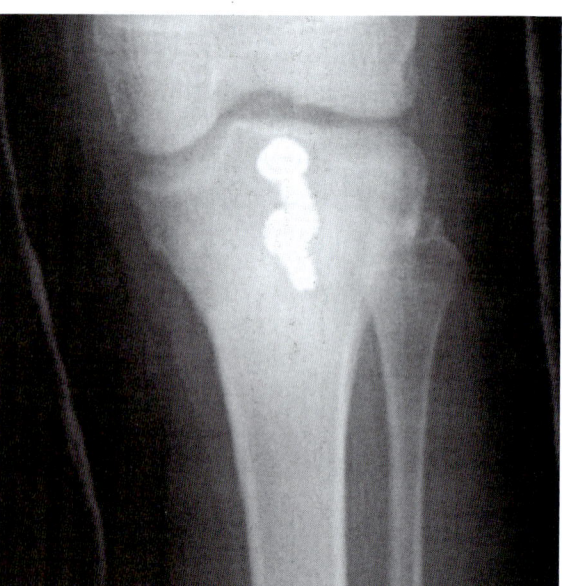

Figure 90-11. Anteroposterior (AP) radiograph of correct treatment of tibial tubercle fracture with screw fixation. (Image property of Children's Orthopedic Center.)

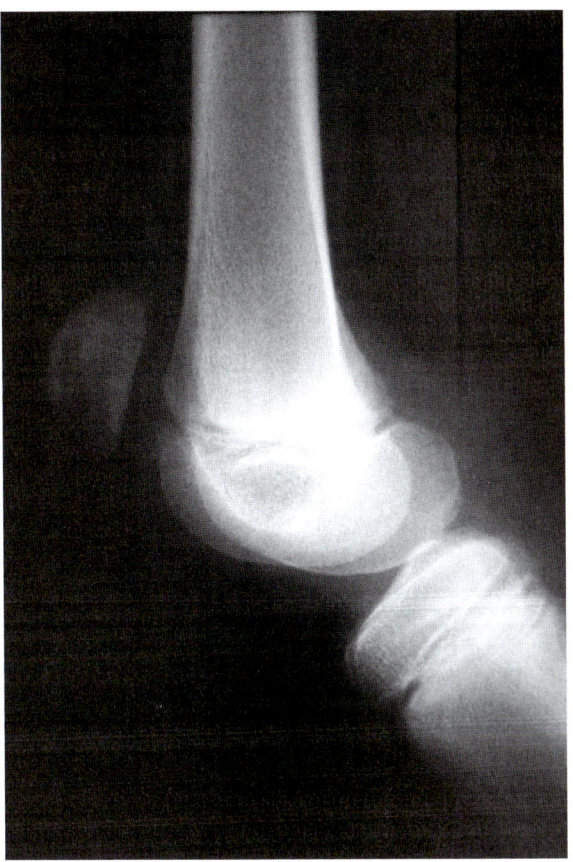

Figure 90-12. Lateral radiograph of correct treatment of tibial tubercle fracture with screw fixation. (Image property of Children's Orthopedic Center.)

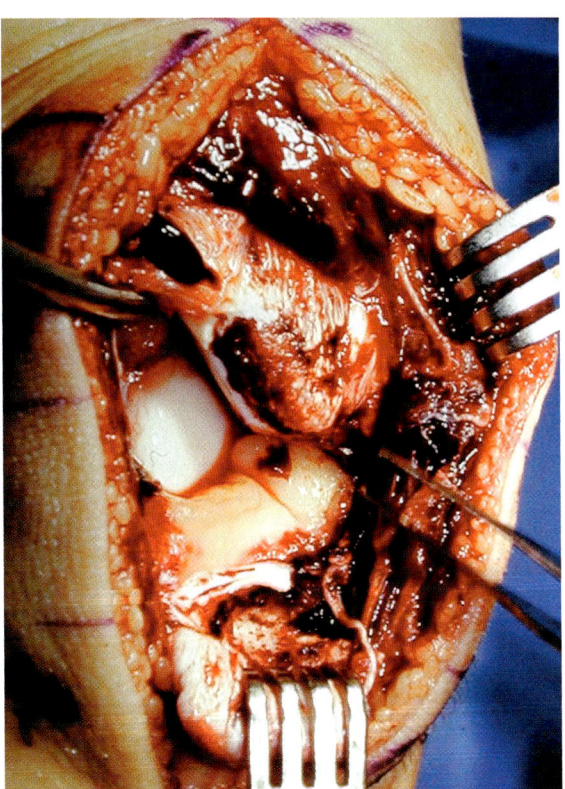

Figure 90-14. Intraoperative photograph demonstrating patellar sleeve fracture. (Photograph property of Children's Orthopedic Center.)

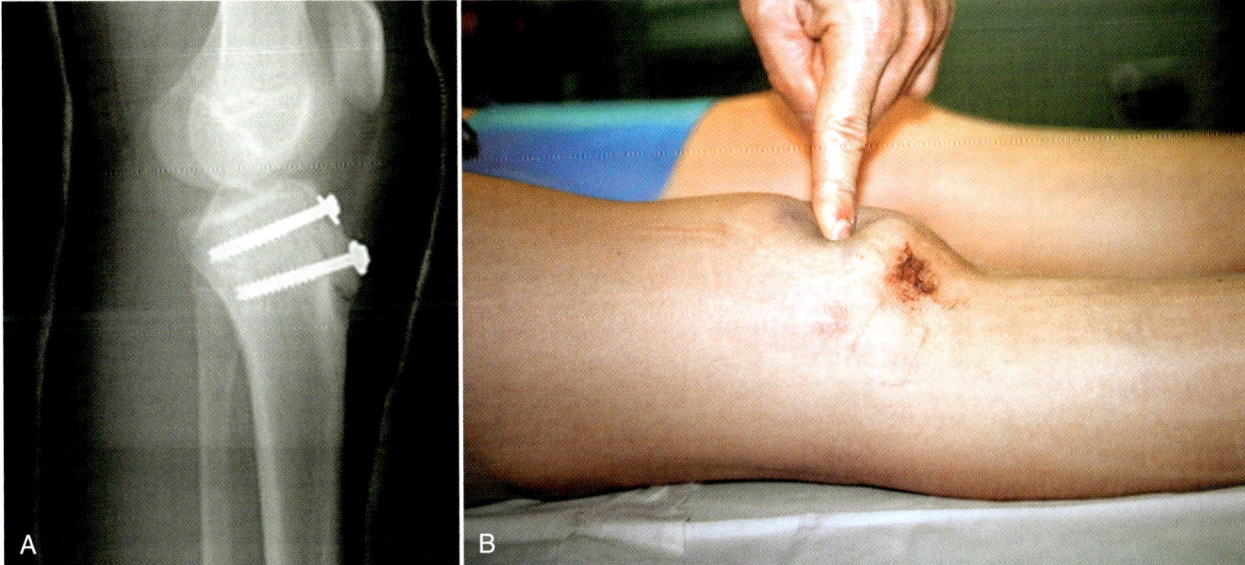

Figure 90-13. A, Lateral radiograph of displaced patellar sleeve fracture. **B,** Physical examination of patellar sleeve fracture demonstrating palpable defect at fracture site. (Images property of Children's Orthopedic Center.)

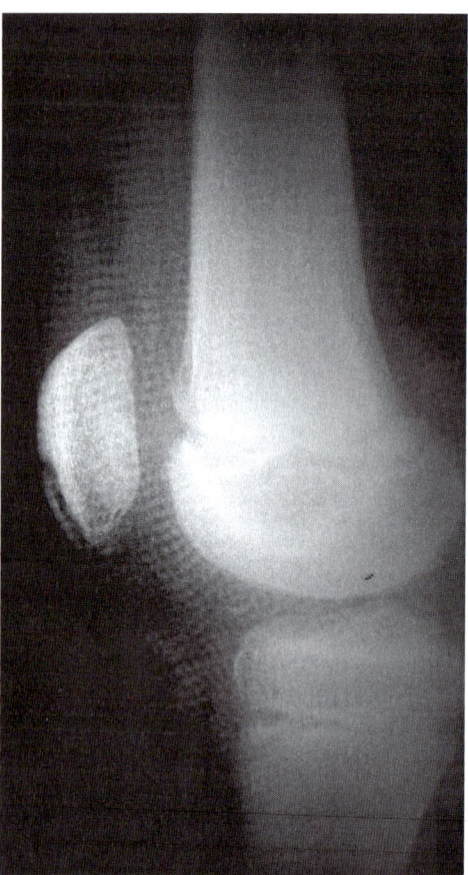

Figure 90-15. Postoperative radiograph after fixation of patellar sleeve fracture demonstrating healing. (Image property of Children's Orthopedic Center.)

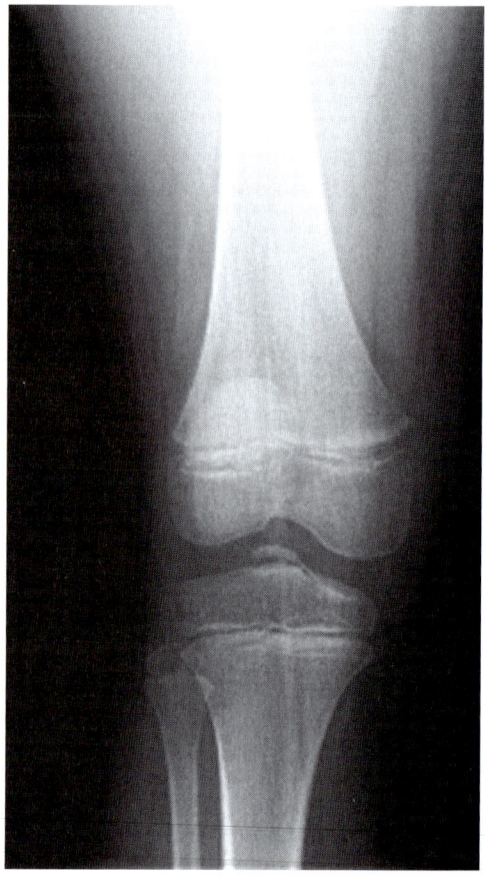

Figure 90-16. Anteroposterior (AP) radiograph of displaced tibial spine fracture. (Image property of Children's Orthopedic Center.)

Tibial Eminence Fractures

The mechanism of injury for a tibial eminence fracture is hyperextension coupled with lateral loading. Patients with a narrow intercondylar notch may be more susceptible to ACL tears, whereas those who sustain a tibial eminence fracture are thought to have a slightly wider notch index.[16] The peak age for tibial eminence fracture is 10 years.[21] Most frequently, tibial eminence fractures in the skeletally immature knee occur as an isolated injury. However, reports have described concomitant MCL injury.[9]

Tibial eminence fractures are classified by the Myers and McKeever system.[20] Type I fractures are nondisplaced. Type II fractures are displaced, with elevation of the anterior portion of the spine and hinging of the posterior aspect of the spine (Figs. 90-16 and 90-17). Type III fractures are displaced and detached.

Nondisplaced fractures are treated with a long-leg cast with the leg in extension. Type II, or hinged, fractures may be reduced with knee extension to 30 degrees or full extension. The intermeniscal ligament may prevent reduction, in which case open or arthroscopic reduction with fixation is indicated. Type III, or detached and displaced, fractures require reduction and fixation.

Concomitant meniscal tears can occur with tibial spine fractures. Unstable torn menisci and the intermeniscal

ligament can become entrapped under a displaced tibial spine fracture. MRI can be used to evaluate for concomitant meniscal pathology. A benefit of arthroscopic treatment of these fractures is the ability to evaluate the menisci and treat tears at the same time.

Arthroscopically assisted reduction and fixation is an excellent alternative to open reduction and internal fixation for these fractures. Different techniques have been described for fixation, including suture fixation, metallic screw fixation, and absorbable implant fixation.[12,17] A physeal-sparing arthroscopically assisted technique has been reported with good results.[10] In 2003, Kocher and associates reported on six patients who underwent this surgery. They indicated that five of their six patients had an abnormal Lachman examination, and two of the six had an abnormal pivot-shift examination. Functional outcomes, which were evaluated by Lysholm, Marshall, and Tegner scores, were excellent.[15] Because laxity may result from interstitial damage to the ACL, these authors recommend slight countersinking of the fragment to combat this laxity. Wiley and colleagues reported objective loss of extension in 100% of patients treated operatively and nonoperatively for tibial spine fractures. Subjective stiffness was noted in 65% of patients.[30] Figures 90-18 and 90-19 depict fractures after arthroscopically aided reduction and fixation.

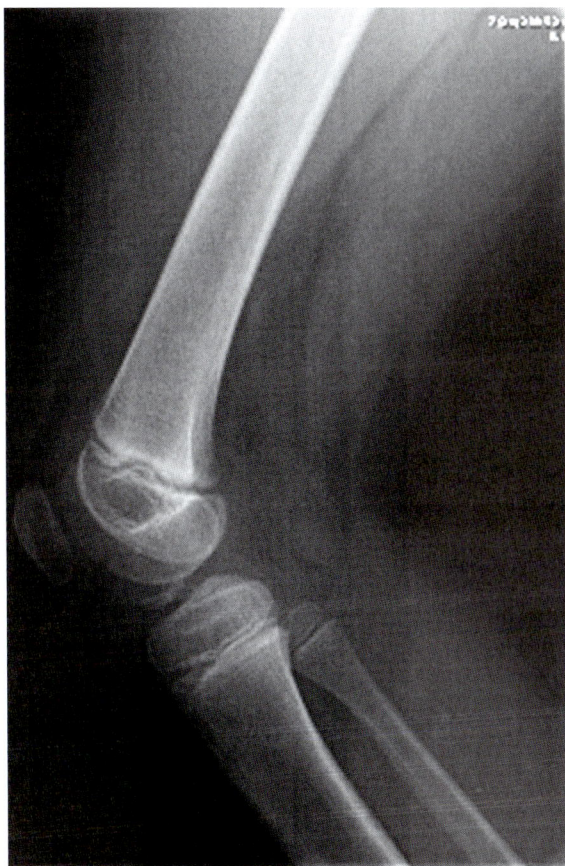

Figure 90-17. Lateral radiograph of displaced tibial spine fracture. (Image property of Children's Orthopedic Center.)

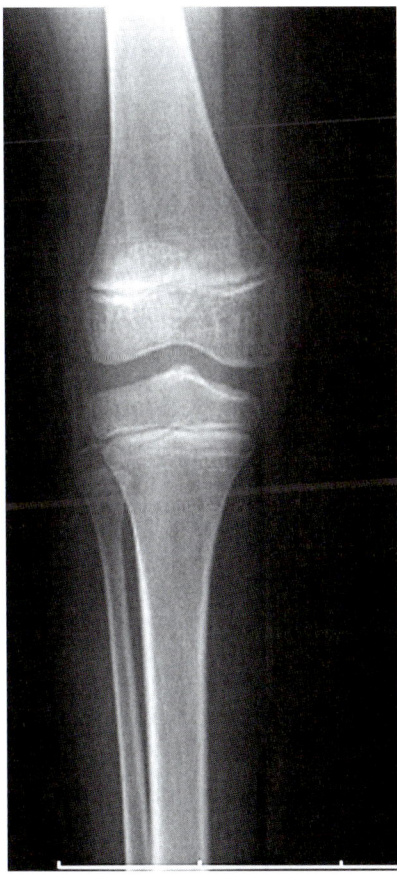

Figure 90-18. Anteroposterior (AP) radiograph after surgical fixation of displaced tibial spine fracture. (Image property of Children's Orthopedic Center.)

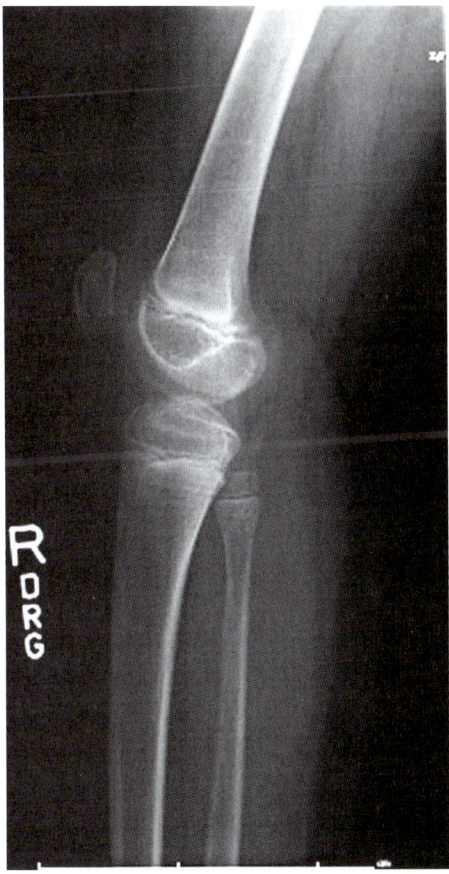

Figure 90-19. Anteroposterior (AP) radiograph after surgical fixation of displaced tibial spine fracture. (Image property of Children's Orthopedic Center.)

KEY REFERENCES

Berquist TH: Osseous and myotendinous injuries about the knee. Magn Reson Imaging Clin N Am 15:25–38, 2007.

Bolesta MJ, Fitch RD: Tibial tubercle avulsions. J Pediatr Orthop 6:186–192, 1986.

Edwards PH Jr, Grana WA: Physeal fractures about the knee. J Am Acad Orthop Surg 3:63–69, 1995.

Gao GX, Mahadev A, Lee EH: Sleeve fracture of the patella in children. J Orthop Surg (Hong Kong) 16:43–46, 2008.

Harrell DJ, Spain DA, Bergamini TM, et al: Blunt popliteal artery trauma: a challenging injury. Am Surg 63:228–231, 1997; discussion 231–232.

Hunt DM, Somashekar N: A review of sleeve fractures of the patella in children. Knee 12:3–7, 2005.

Kocher MS, Foreman ES, Micheli LJ: Laxity and functional outcome after arthroscopic reduction and internal fixation of displaced tibial spine fractures in children. Arthroscopy 19:1085–1090, 2003.

Lombardo SJ, Harvey JP Jr: Fractures of the distal femoral epiphyses: factors influencing prognosis: a review of thirty-four cases. J Bone Joint Surg Am 59:742–751, 1977.

Meyers MH, McKeever FM: Fracture of the intercondylar eminence of the tibia. J Bone Joint Surg Am 52:1677–1684, 1970.

Mubarak SJ, Kim JR, Edmonds EW, et al: Classification of proximal tibial fractures in children. J Child Orthop 3:191–197, 2009.

Ogden JA, Tross RB, Murphy MJ: Fractures of the tibial tuberosity in adolescents. J Bone Joint Surg Am 62:205–215, 1980.

Shelton WR, Canale ST: Fractures of the tibia through the proximal tibial epiphyseal cartilage. J Bone Joint Surg Am 61:167–173, 1979.

Skak SV, Jensen TT, Poulsen TD, Sturup J: Epidemiology of knee injuries in children. Acta Orthop Scand 58:78–81, 1987.

Thomson JD, Stricker SJ, Williams MM: Fractures of the distal femoral epiphyseal plate. J Pediatr Orthop 15:474–478, 1995.

Wiley JJ, Baxter MP: Tibial spine fractures in children. Clin Orthop Relat Res 255:54–60, 1990.

Full references for this chapter can be found on www.expertconsult.com.

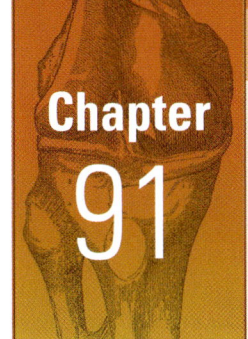

Chapter 91

Patellar Instability

Richard Y. Hinton and Robert Kyle Fullick

Patellofemoral instability is a common cause of subjective complaints and activity impairment in the pediatric population. Conditions may vary from fixed, in utero dislocations to macrotraumatic injuries in previously asymptomatic, scholastic athletes. As discrepant as these scenarios may seem, they have in common a "relative" imbalance of the extensor mechanism of the knee. Effective evaluation and treatment of patellofemoral instability is based on an understanding of the "normal envelope"[29] of extensor mechanism function and the multitude of factors that may disrupt its complex activity.

This chapter focuses primarily on patellofemoral instability in young, athletically active patients. We discuss the host, agent, and environmental risk factors that contribute to patellofemoral instability with a focus on age-specific information, a review of the pertinent literature, and a discussion of current treatment concepts.

EMBRYOLOGY

The appendicular skeleton appears very early in embryologic development. By the fourth week of gestation, the limb buds are easily identifiable, with maturation of the lower extremities trailing the upper ones by several days. The leg buds begin to bend anteriorly at the developing knee during the fifth week. By week 7, the distal end of the femur and the patella have undergone chondrification, and the patellofemoral articulation is recognizable in its adult form. Initially, the lower limbs extend from the torso with the soles of the feet facing medially, toward one another. By the eighth week of gestation, the lower limbs complete a 90-degree, internal rotation, which brings them into their adult orientation.[32,67,84,94] It is thought that failure of the quadriceps myotome to complete this internal rotation is the most probable cause of in utero, congenital patellofemoral dislocation.[40,41,98] Failure of rotation leaves the extensor mechanism in a contracted, laterally dislocated position relative to the distal end of the femur.

Initial formation or malformation of the patellofemoral joint and other knee structures appears to be genetically driven without dependence on function.[32,50] However, abnormal motion and stress across the articulation appear to play a role in progressive, developmental dysplasia. Individual abnormalities such as a shallow femoral sulcus, patellar hypoplasia, and patella alta tend to appear in relative amounts within a constellation of dysplastic changes. In cases of congenital, developmental, and habitual dislocation, early surgical restoration toward more normal extensor mechanism biomechanics may lead to partial normalization of patellofemoral architecture.[38,41,52]

ANATOMY AND BIOMECHANICS

The patella lies within the trochlea of the femur, bounded by the medial and lateral femoral condyles. Cartilaginous at birth, the patella begins ossification from multiple centers during early childhood. The relatively cartilaginous composition of the immature patella has diagnostic and clinical implications. Apparent lack of patellofemoral congruity and excessive shallowness of the femoral sulcus in the child's knee are in large part an illusion (Fig. 91-1). Nietosvaara[71] has shown that although the osseous patellofemoral sulcus angle is inversely proportional to age, ultrasound measurements of the cartilaginous sulcus are nearly constant throughout growth. Gradual thinning of the articular cartilage from the outer areas of the sulcus and retropatellar facets leads to apparent deepening of the sulcus with age.[77] Even in a mature knee, a significant mismatch is seen between the osseous outlines of the patellofemoral articulation and the geometry of the true articular cartilage surfaces (Fig. 91-2).[97] For these reasons, congenital and acquired patellofemoral dysplasia may be better represented on magnetic resonance imaging (MRI) than on plain radiographs.

Patellar height is an important factor to consider during the evaluation of patellofemoral disorders. Patella alta is one of the best substantiated radiographic risk factors for patellar instability.* However, reliable measurement of this condition is limited by the cartilaginous nature of the patella and the tibial tubercle in the younger knee.[102] Alternatives to the traditional Insall-Salvati method aim to minimize these effects (Fig. 91-3). Koshino and Sugimoto's method[51] uses relationships of the midpatella to the midepiphyseal lines of the tibia and femur. This scheme may be most appropriate for younger children. The Blackburne-Peel[12] modification uses the relationship between posterior facet length and the distance to the tibial articular surface. This method is helpful in adolescents, in whom the inferior pole of the patella is not fully ossified, or who have secondary tibial tubercle changes associated with Osgood-Schlatter disease.

The tibial tubercle also undergoes gradual ossification during childhood. Genu recurvatum is a potential complication with tubercle osteotomies and distal extensor realignment procedures. The appropriate age cutoff is not well described. However, older case series[45,57] report such complications in patients younger than but not older than 14.

The femoral origin of the medial patellofemoral ligament (MPFL) is just distal to the femoral physis. The femoral physis is cup shaped at its periphery, and the MPFL attachment on the medial epiphyseal bone is actually superior to the more central physeal plate. This must be taken into consideration when drilling tunnels or using various fixation devices for the femoral side of MPFL reconstructions. These must be angled downward and parallel to the physis, not perpendicular and inadvertently into the physeal plate. As will be discussed in later text, erring slightly more distal in the femoral insertion

---

*References 8, 34, 47, 59, 64, and 87.

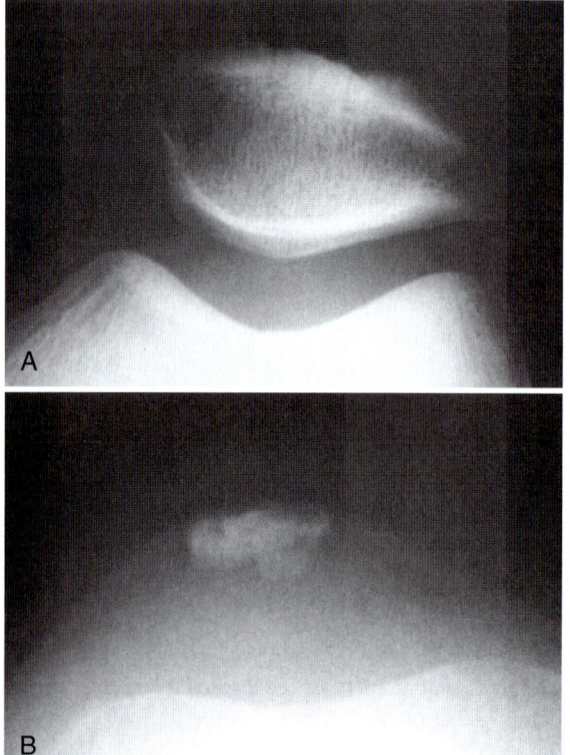

Figure 91-1. Sunrise view of the patellofemoral joint in an adult man **(A)** and an 8-year-old boy **(B)**. (From Hinton RY, Sharma KM: Acute and recurrent patellar instability in the young athlete. Orthop Clin North Am 34:285–396, 2003.)

of an MPFL reconstruction has fewer adverse consequences for the biomechanics of the graft within its functional range of full extension to 40 degrees of flexion. This distal "malposition" can help to protect the physis (Fig. 91-4).

The multilayer soft tissue envelope about the patellofemoral joint has been described as having three layers on both medial and lateral sides.[25,95,96,103] Medially, the superficial layer is the investing fascia over the sartorius muscle. The second layer includes the MPFL, the parapatellar retinaculum, and the superficial medial collateral ligament (MCL). The third medial layer contains the deep MCL and joint capsule. This arrangement places the MPFL in the same extracapsular environment as the MCL (Fig. 91-5). Such an environment is one that may promote ligamentous healing, as seen by the ability of the MCL to regain function and structure even after major injury. Laterally, fascial interconnections are seen between the fibers of the iliotibial band, lateral hamstrings, lateral patellofemoral ligaments, and lateral quadriceps retinaculum that feed into the lateral aspect of the patella. Tightness in these structures may cause excessive posterior and lateral pull, thereby contributing to lateral patellar tilt and increased retropatellar pressure.

The MPFL is an hourglass-shaped, ligamentous structure that runs transversely from the posterior part of the medial epicondyle, approximately 1 cm distal to the adductor tubercle, to the superomedial part of the patella. Although present as a distinct structure in 90% of specimens, this ligament can vary greatly in size and strength.[14,25,46] The femoral origin is intimately associated with insertions of the adductor tendon and the superficial MCL (Fig. 91-6). The MPFL originates in the saddle area distal to the adductor tubercle, just superior to the MCL origin and posterior to both.[76,80,95] Radiographically, on a true lateral, the center of femoral origin is 1 mm anterior to an extension line from the posterior cortex,

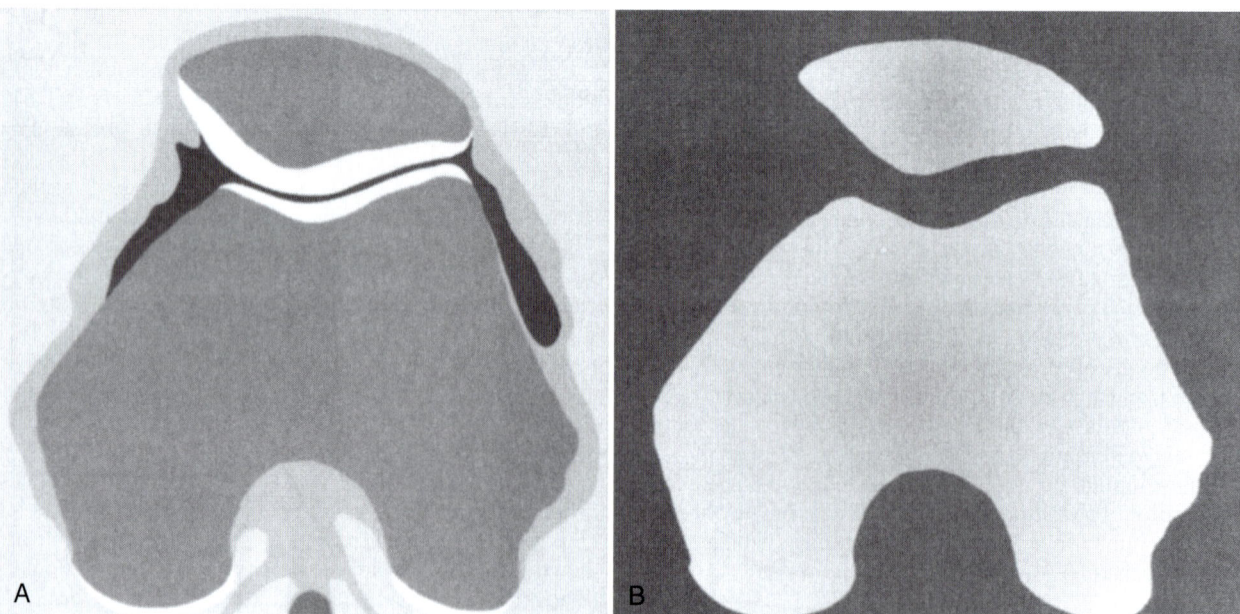

Figure 91-2. A, Diagram of a magnetic resonance arthrotomogram of the left knee in the axial plane shows articular cartilage congruence of the patellofemoral joint. **B,** Diagram shows the osseous contour of same knee with "apparent" incongruence. (From Staeubli HU, Bosshard C, Porcellini P, Rauschning W: Magnetic resonance imaging for articular cartilage: cartilage-bone mismatch. Clin Sports Med 21:417–433, viii–ix, 2002.)

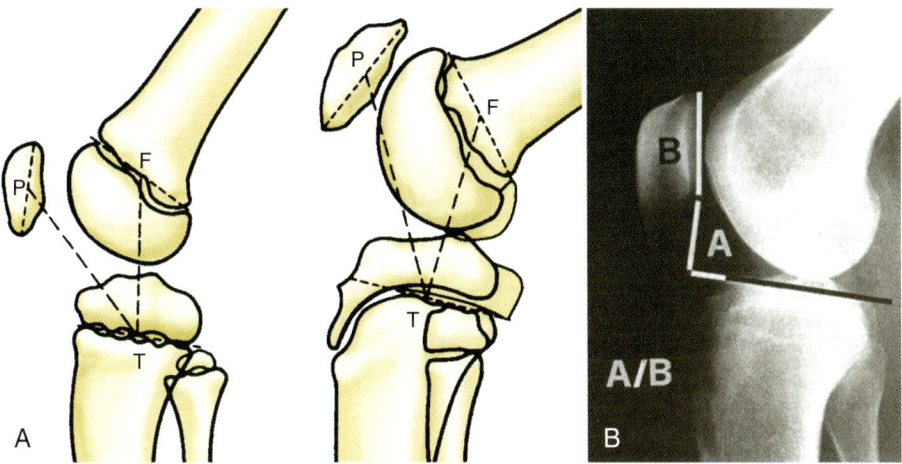

Figure 91-3. **A,** Epiphyseal line midpoint method of determining patella alta in skeletally immature patients. **B,** Method of determining patella alta. (**A,** From Koshino T, Sigimoto K: New measurement of patellar height in the knees of children using the epiphyseal line midpoint. J Pediatr Orthop 9:216–218, 1989. **B,** From Blackburne JS, Peel TE: A new method of measuring patellar height. J Bone Joint Surg Br 59:241–242, 1977.)

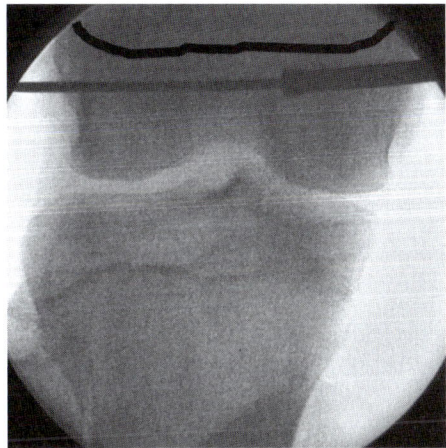

Figure 91-4. Anteroposterior view of the knee showing the guide wire and acorn drill entering distal to the physis. The distal femoral physis is outlined by a bold black line.

2.5 mm distal to the origin of the medial femoral condyle, and proximal to the level of the posterior point of Blumensaat's line (Fig. 91-7).[91] The ligament courses from its femoral origin to attach to the superior medial border of the patella and the undersurface of the vastus medialis. Several studies[14,25,39,46,75] undertaken to compare the roles of the MPFL, medial patellar retinaculum, patellotibial ligament, patellomeniscal ligament, and lateral retinaculum have found that the MPFL provides between 50% and 80% of soft tissue restraint to lateral patellar displacement in functional positions of slight knee flexion. Several authors[31,95] have investigated the isometricity of various origin and insertion positions for MPFL reconstruction. The best results were obtained by using the anatomic femoral and patellar attachments (Fig. 91-8). Superior displacement of the femoral attachment resulted in increased distance between insertion sites as the knee moved into greater flexion, which could lead to loss of knee flexion or disruption of the graft after MPFL reconstruction. Proximal malposition coupled with a shorter than anatomic MPFL graft substitute appears to result in significantly increased medial patellar tilt and retropatellar pressure.[31]

Inferior displacement of the femoral insertion (see Fig. 91-5, position F3) results in minimal changes in graft length and tension during the first 40 degrees of knee flexion, followed by decreased graft tension with continued flexion, at which point the bony architecture has taken on a primary stabilizing role.

Imaging and surgical exploration studies[60,88,89] have found the MPFL to be routinely injured at the time of patellar dislocation. Disruption appears to occur most often at the adductor tubercle, but it may take place along the length of the ligament or its patellar attachment. In patients with chronic dislocation, Nomura[75] reported that the MPFL is healed throughout its course with scar tissue, unhealed with femoral avulsion, or atrophied throughout its course. Laboratory studies and clinical reports* have indicated that repair or reconstruction of the MPFL is integral to reestablishing lateral patellar stability.

Muscle contraction may affect patellofemoral stability by "seating" the articulation as a result of increased joint reaction forces, or by generating dynamic medial or lateral displacement forces.[96] Relative vectors of the individual quadriceps muscular components are determined by their level of attachment, angle of pull, and cross-sectional area. The vastus medialis obliquus (VMO) is a primary dynamic stabilizer. It is intimately associated with the MPFL and the adductor musculature. Although conceptually interesting, independent function, disuse, or rehabilitation of the VMO separate from the remaining quadriceps has not been proved.[1,53,83] Musculotendinous units are primarily dynamic actors, and advancement of the VMO to increase passive restraint to lateral patellar dislocation is unpredictable.[96]

The bony architecture of the patellofemoral joint also plays a role in stability. Trochlear dysplasia, altered convexity of the retropatellar surface, patella alta, and patellar hypoplasia all have been found to be risk factors for initial and recurrent patellar instability.[34,47,50] The normal sulcus angle for young normal individuals has been reported to be 138 ± 3 degrees.[86,103] Mild trochlear dysplasia corresponds to a sulcus

---

*References 14, 25, 33, 60, 75, and 89.

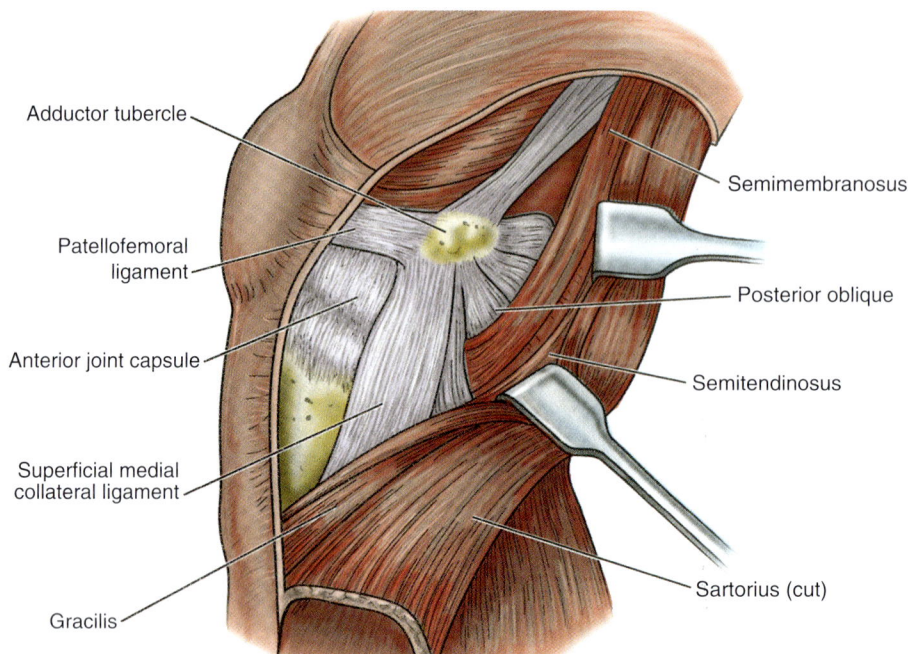

Figure 91-5. Diagram of layer II medial-side knee structures. (From Clarke HD, Scott WN, Insall JN, et al: Anatomy. In Insall JN, Scott WN [eds]: Surgery of the knee, Philadelphia, 2001, WB Saunders, p 52.)

angle of 143 degrees, moderate dysplasia to an angle of 149 degrees, and severe dysplasia to an angle of 171 degrees.[22] Runow[87] found the average sulcus angle in a large group of young patients with documented patellar dislocation to be increased to 146 ± 6 degrees. A very similar increase to 147 degrees has been reported by Aglietti and associates[2] in symptomatic patellar subluxers.

With the knee in full extension, the patella rests lateral and superior to the trochlea. Engagement occurs between 10 and 30 degrees of flexion. This is dependent on relative patellar tendon length, and in individuals with patella alta, engagement will occur later in flexion. This condition leads to less stability in early degrees of knee flexion, in which most sporting activity occurs. For the adolescent and young adult population, the Insall ratio has been measured as 0.98 ± 0.13 for males and 1.08 ± 0.15 for females.[87] In a study of 104 patellar dislocators, Runow[87] found that the average Insall ratio was greater than 1.0 in all patients, and that a ratio greater than 1.3 was significantly correlated with recurrent and bilateral dislocation. Several other studies have reported that patella alta is a significant risk factor for initial and recurrent patellar instability.*

The Q angle is subtended by a line drawn from the anterior superior iliac spine to the center of the patella or the trochlear groove, and a second line drawn from the center of the tibial tubercle. An increased Q angle suggests a greater lateralizing vector on the patella. Unfortunately, no agreed-on standards are available for Q angle measurement with regard to the most appropriate degree of knee flexion, weight-bearing status, and quadriceps activity. Axial computed tomography (CT) scans can be used to generate more reproducible measurements of relative tibial tubercle "lateralization" by

providing anterior tibial tuberosity–trochlear groove (TT-TG) distances[9] and tibial tubercle–lateral condylar (TT-LC) angles.[68] An increased Q angle is often discussed as a risk factor for instability, but it has not been reliably associated with patellar instability in many large-group studies.[8,18,33,56] This may reflect the inability of a static measurement, made in a static situation, to capture dynamic, functional impairment. However, we do incorporate TT-TG and TT-LC measurement data when considering the need for distal realignment in combination with MPFL repair or reconstruction.

RISK FACTORS

As with other musculoskeletal injuries, risk factors for patellofemoral instability are best viewed within the disease triad of *host* (patient characteristics), *agent* (macrotraumatic or repetitive microtraumatic energy exchange), and *environmental* (physical and social milieu of athletic participation) risk factors.[47,61] We classify young patients with patellofemoral instability into two large, somewhat overlapping groups (TONES and LAACS) based on "relative" risk factors, natural history, and characteristics (Table 91-1).

Host factors that may play an important role in patellar instability include age, gender, previous history of patellar instability, generalized ligamentous laxity, and patellofemoral dysplasia. Patellar dislocation rates are highest during the second decade of life,[8,34,87] probably because of higher athletic activity during this period and an underlying musculoskeletal predisposition in this age group. During a period of rapid growth, children and early adolescents are in the seemingly dichotomous situation of simultaneous musculotendinous tightness and relative ligamentous laxity. This is particularly apparent with the straplike, two-joint musculotendinous units crossing the knee. Tightness in the iliotibial band, abductors, and lateral hamstrings may lead to increased valgus

---

*References 8, 34, 47, 59, 64, and 87.

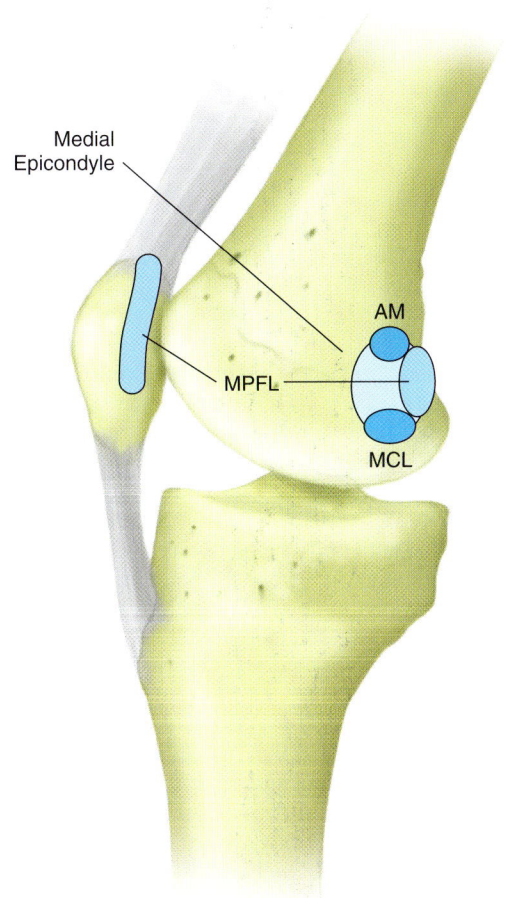

Figure 91-6. Schematic diagram shows the medial femoral epicondyle and its attachments for the adductor magnus tendon (AM), the medial patellofemoral ligament (MPFL), and the medial collateral ligament (MCL). (From Smirk C, Morris H: The anatomy and reconstruction of the medial patellofemoral ligament. Knee 10:221–227, 2003.)

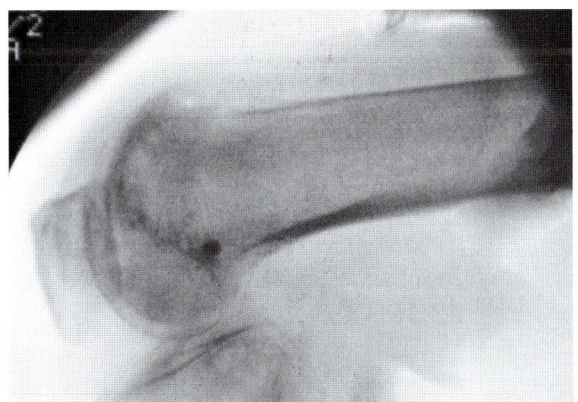

Figure 91-7. Lateral radiograph of the distal femur confirming guide wire placement at the femoral origin of the medial patellofemoral ligament.

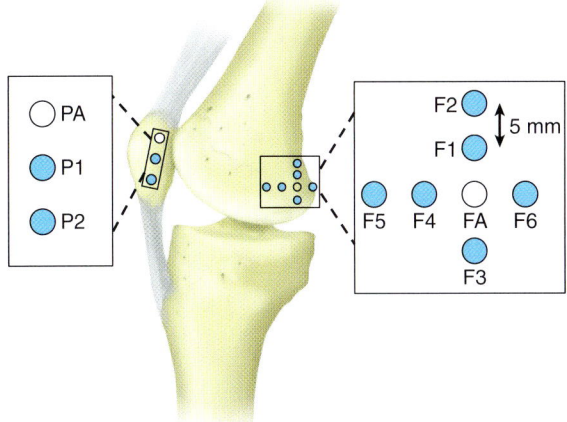

Figure 91-8. Potential graft attachment sites. *FA,* Normal femoral attachment, 1 cm distal to the adductor tubercle. All femoral sites were 5 mm apart. *PA,* Normal patellar attachment in the superior third of the patella. (From Smirk C, Morris H: The anatomy and reconstruction of the medial patellofemoral ligament. Knee 10:221–227, 2003.)

Table 91-1 Classification of Patellofemoral Instability in Young Patients: TONES and LAACS

T	**T**raumatic, sports-related injury mechanisms
O	**O**lder at initial dislocation, **O**steochondral fractures more common
N	**N**ormal patellofemoral architecture, **N**ormal ligamentous function
E	**E**qual sex distribution
S	**S**ingle occurrence, **S**ingle-leg involvement
L	**L**axity, generalized, **Lower** age at onset
A	**A**traumatic in nature
A	**A**bnormal patellofemoral architecture, **A**bnormal ligamentous laxity
C	**C**hronic in nature, **C**ontralateral involvement
S	**S**ex dependent, with greater number of females

vector on the patella, which may be poorly balanced by lax medial ligamentous restraints and poorly developed quadriceps musculature. Age is also a significant risk factor for recurrence, with earlier initial dislocation being a positive predictor of higher recurrence rates.* Generalized ligamentous laxity is correlated with earlier onset, more frequent recurrence, and dislocations that occur with lesser trauma.[87] However, patellar dislocation in a hyperlax patient carries a significantly lower risk of concurrent osteochondral fracture.[87,99] Patellofemoral markers that have been linked most reliably to increased dislocation and recurrence risk are patella alta, increased sulcus angle, and lateral dominance of the retropatellar surface. These dysplastic changes usually occur as a constellation and are more often seen in younger, hyperlax female LAACS-type patients (see Table 91-1). However, subtle abnormalities in these measurements are often noted among TONES-type patients as well (see Table 91-1). A key host characteristic of recurrent dislocation is a history of previous dislocation.[34]

---

*References 17, 34, 36, 64, 65, and 87.

Table 91-2 Classification of Patellar Instability

Instability Grade	Joint Laxity	Insall Index >1.3	Percent of Total Group	Age At Onset, yr	Frequent Dislocations (Fraction)	Bilateral Dislocations (Fraction)	Moderate Trauma (Fraction)	Fracture(s) (Fraction)	Instability Score
0	—	—	—	—	—	—	—	—	—
I	—	—	16	19	0.13	0.13	0.76	0.63	2.1
II	+	—	35	15	0.26	0.19	0.69	0.38	2.7
III	—	+	19	15	0.60	0.35	0.55	0.33	3.6
IV	+	+	30	13	0.74	0.68	0.26	0.17	5.0
Total/average			100	15	0.46	0.37	0.55	0.33	3.6

From Runow A: The dislocating patella: etiology and prognosis in relation to generalized joint laxity and anatomy of the patellar articulation. Acta Orthop Scand Suppl 201:1–53, 1983.

Trauma, in varying degrees, is almost always associated with patellar dislocation. A large population-based study conducted by Atkin and colleagues[8] points to the "agent" of high sports participation as the major risk factor for first-time, acute patellofemoral dislocators. The most common mechanism of patellar dislocation—noncontact external rotation of the lower part of the leg on a planted foot, resulting in valgus overload of the extensor mechanism—is common in sports participation. In their group of TONES-type patients, investigators reported no predictive role for gender, family history, increased Q angle, or excessive hip rotation. Patella alta was the one traditional factor associated with higher risk in this patient group. In TONES patients, patellar dislocation is a more traumatic event, with higher rates of magnetic resonance imaging (MRI)-documented disruption of the MPFL, VMO, and medial retinaculum. Fithian and coworkers[34] suggested that increased soft tissue trauma is a sign of macrotrauma to normal structures, and that given adequate chance to heal, a lower risk of recurrence will be seen than in cases in which the patella dislocates with less trauma. Osteochondral fracture rates are significantly higher in TONES patients as a result of the greater stress required to dislocate the patellofemoral joint in patients with more normal soft tissue function. It is interesting to note that fractures tend to be avulsion-type or intra-articular osteochondral in nature, but the two rarely occur concurrently.[103] An initial avulsion may serve to decompress the patellofemoral joint, thus decreasing stress between the retropatellar surface and the lateral femoral condyle. Sports, dance, and other high-demand activities are often the primary cause of injury in initial dislocators. Even most LAACS-type patients will report some level of trauma as precipitating a recurrent event. Only in the small group of "habitual" dislocators does the patella routinely dislocate with normal gait.

Today's young athletes are playing sports in an environment of relatively more game to practice time, consistently higher competitive levels, and early specialization in single sports. These factors combine to significantly increase injury exposure and risk. Also, increasing social pressure is pushing the young athlete back to play before adequate postoperative or postinjury rehabilitation is completed.

CLASSIFICATION

A myriad of classification systems for patellofemoral instability and maltracking have been devised. In his classic treatise on patellofemoral instability, Anders Runow[87] grouped initial

dislocators into four groups. Group I had only minimal patella alta (Insall ratio of 1.0 to 1.3), minimal trochlear dysplasia, and no generalized hyperlaxity. Seventy-six percent of these patients experienced significant trauma causing the dislocation; they had an average age at initial onset of 19 and a low rate of recurrence, and osteochondral fractures occurred in 63%. Group II had generalized hyperlaxity and an Insall ratio of 1.0 to 1.3, whereas group III had normal soft tissue function but an Insall ratio greater than 1.3. Group IV demonstrated both hyperlaxity and severe patella alta. Among group IV patients, the age at onset was 13, the recurrence rate was 74%, bilateral involvement occurred in 68%, significant trauma played a role in only 28%, and osteochondral fractures occurred in only 17% (Table 91-2). In a recent comprehensive population study, Fithian and coworkers[34] classified acute dislocators into those with and without a history of previous dislocation. Those with a history of previous dislocation were more likely female and had a higher risk of future dislocation, a positive family history for patellar instability, higher rates of dysplastic hip disease, and increases in patella alta, patellar tilt, and patellar subluxation. As discussed earlier, we have found that grouping patients generally into the TONES and LAACS classifications is useful in assessing risk factors, discussing the natural history, and guiding treatment options.

In getting one's "clinical hands" around a patient with supposed patellofemoral instability, the following questions are important to answer: (1) What is the personality of the injury? Is the situation one of a mechanically normal knee subjected to macrotrauma, or did the dislocation occur with minimal trauma in a patient with significant underlying mechanical risk factors? (2) Is this problem an aggravation or a disability, as gauged by lost play/practice time, the presence of chronic quadriceps atrophy, or loss of explosive jumping ability? (3) Has truly adequate nonoperative care been provided, and what was the response? (4) Are signs or symptoms of concurrent knee injury present, such as osteochondral fractures, other extensor mechanism overuse syndromes, or missed ligamentous injuries? (5) Is the instability truly first-time, acute recurrent, or chronic? (6) Is the patella grossly unstable during clinical examination or daily activities? (7) What are the age, activity level, and athletic potential of the patient?

NATURAL HISTORY

Well-controlled, population-based studies have estimated the per capita risk for first-time dislocation in children and adolescents to be between 29 and 43 per 100,000.[8,34,71] The natural history of this fairly common major knee malady is not benign. A significant number of patients experience recurrent instability and/or patellofemoral pain related to maltracking or osteochondral injury. For nonoperative patients, reported redislocation rates vary widely from 15% to 45%, and 30% to 50% may be expected to suffer anterior knee pain.[10,47] Less than perfect outcomes after nonoperative care suggest the need for early surgical intervention. However, the results of early operative repair have been mixed.* Results of early surgical intervention appear to decline over time and may be less favorable in LAACS-type patients.[101] As discussed earlier, the natural history after an acute dislocation is dependent on host, agent, and environmental risk factors for the individual patient. Fithian and associates,[34] in their group of first-time dislocators, reported recurrent instability in 49% of patients with a previous history of instability and only a 17% recurrence rate. Runow[87] reported a redislocation rate of only 13% in his group I patients without laxity or patellofemoral dysplasia. However, the rate jumped to 74% in group IV patients with both generalized hypermobility and patellofemoral dysplasia. In their study of 100 young acute dislocators, Mäenpää and colleagues[58] found a redislocation rate of 44%, patellofemoral pain in 19%, and no complaints after nonoperative treatment in only 37% of patients. However, of 14 patients who underwent surgical reconstruction, 47% continued to have a positive apprehension sign and 79% had significant retropatellar crepitance. In a randomized study of nonoperative and operative treatment, Nikku and coworkers reported recurrent instability rates of 20% in their nonoperative group and 18% in their operative group and overall better function in their nonoperative patients.[74] In a large group of male Army conscripts with an average age of 20 years who underwent surgery for acute or recurrent patellar dislocation, Mäenpää and associates[58] found that only 19% had excellent results. Just 35% were able to finish their military service normally after surgical intervention.

A systematic review of 70 articles on first-time dislocators speaks to the lack of a definitive treatment algorithm for treating young patients with acute patellar dislocation.[100] Many studies are retrospective in nature, are short term in follow-up, use various and sometimes dated surgical interventions, suffer from subject/treatment selection bias, and lack defined outcomes variables. This review recommended nonoperative care for the first-time dislocator except in cases of comorbid osteochondral injury, early recurrent dislocation, substantial disruption of the MPFL-VMO-adductor mechanism, or failure to progress with nonoperative care. We follow similar guidelines but would also offer early operative intervention to LAACS-type patients who have had contralateral repetitive dislocation (often proximal and distal reconstruction) and to high-demand athletes whose competitive schedules will not tolerate downtime or future dislocation.

INJURY HISTORY

The history of an acute patellar dislocation is not always as straightforward as it may seem. The young athlete is able to recount a major injury, but rarely the details. The athlete has

a painful, swollen, guarded knee, but rarely a fixed dislocation. Although injuries can occur as the result of a direct fall onto the patella, most occur through the noncontact mechanisms previously described. Children and younger adolescents can have a hard time differentiating this plant-twist mechanism from that leading to a noncontact anterior cruciate ligament (ACL) injury. Both result in a sense of traumatic giving way, pain, hemarthrosis, and significant impairment. Both diagnoses must be considered and carefully ruled out in an acutely injured knee. A patient with recurrent, acute dislocation usually is able to relate an appropriate history and a feeling of "sameness" to the current dislocation episode. Symptomatic osteochondral fractures may result in complaints of mechanical locking and persistent effusion. Complaints associated with chronic subluxation are often vague. The child often complains of generalized anterior knee pain or burning and a sense of the knee giving way with quick stops, jumping, or change of direction. A history of multiple physician consultations and sporadic efforts at rehabilitation is often reported.

PHYSICAL EXAMINATION

Fortunately, the patellofemoral articulation is very accessible for physical examination. Efforts should be made to specifically correlate underlying anatomic structures with superficial palpation. For example, injury to the MPFL can be inferred from tenderness at its origin at the adductor tubercle or a rent at its patellar attachment.

In the acute setting, arthrocentesis is both diagnostic and therapeutic. Hemarthrosis and fatty globules can be documented. Instillation of a local anesthetic and decompression of the joint may improve the quality of the examination. Pain is decreased and early range-of-motion and quadriceps activities are improved. A standard ligamentous examination of the knee should be performed to rule out concurrent injury. A sense of the overall tissue trauma should be established. Large palpable rents in the VMO, adductors, or MPFL and a grossly dislocatable patella are relative indicators for surgical intervention in a TONES-type patient. Generalized hypermobility is assessed, and mechanical and alignment risk factors in the contralateral leg are evaluated.

A LAACS patient with chronic patellar instability deserves an inclusive examination.[82] Overall alignment of the lower extremities should be determined in a weight-bearing position. This examination includes an assessment of generalized joint laxity, knee valgus, femoral/tibial rotation, and foot posture. Walking, jogging, jumping, and other sport-specific activity should be evaluated. Total lower extremity flexibility/strength and core strength should be assessed. Particular emphasis is placed on the following: hip abductor/adductor strength balance, iliotibial band and hip flexor tightness, quadriceps atrophy, and painful arcs of resisted knee motion. The patient should be assessed for excessive guarding of the knee, hypersensitivity to light touch, and other signs of saphenous nerve irritation or early reflex sympathetic dystrophy.

More specific evaluation of the patellofemoral joint can then be carried out. Evaluation includes assessing the Q angle in full extension and at 20 degrees of flexion. Patellar apprehension testing is then performed by attempting to displace the patella laterally over the lateral femoral condyle while

---

*References 16, 70, 73, 74, 79, 92, and 93.

observing the patient for signs of apprehension or discomfort. Medial and lateral patellar translation and endpoint compliance are assessed. The patella normally can be displaced both medially and laterally between 25% and 50% of the width of the patella. Patellar tilt should be evaluated. Lateral retinacular tightness may prevent the lateral facet from being tilted above the horizontal. Patellar tracking is evaluated through a full range of motion with and without patellofemoral compression. Late engagement, patella alta or baja, lateralization, and painful arcs of motion are documented.

PATELLOFEMORAL IMAGING

With regard to patellofemoral instability, diagnostic imaging serves two broad functions. It provides information on extensor mechanisms and concurrent knee injury, and it assesses architectural characteristics of the knee that may predispose to patellofemoral maltracking and instability. Unfortunately, most imaging studies are static and give little indication about the dynamic nature of the patellofemoral joint. As discussed earlier, the relative cartilaginous nature of a child's patellofemoral articulation also limits the usefulness of standard radiographs.

Radiographs should begin with standard anteroposterior, bent-knee weight-bearing, true lateral views at 20 to 30 degrees, and sunrise views at 20 degrees. A true lateral radiograph can be helpful in assessing patellar tilt, trochlea depth, dysplastic changes, and patella alta.[59] Some time should be devoted to assessment of patella alta because it is one of the radiographic risk factors that is most correlated with symptomatic instability.[8,54,64,87] Many different methods and standard ratios are used. For young children, we recommend the method of Koshino and Sugimoto[51] (see Fig. 91-3A); for adolescents, the Blackburne-Peel method (see Fig. 91-3B)[12]; and for a skeletally mature patient, the modified or standard Insall-Salvati method.[48] Walker and associates[102] generated age-specific data for patella-to-patellar tendon ratios with the Insall-Salvati method. We use the sunrise view at 20 degrees to determine a lateral patellofemoral angle by drawing a line across the top of the lateral and medial condyles and an intersecting line along the posterior face of the lateral facet. This angle should be open to the lateral side.[54] The degree of subluxation can also be assessed.

The Merchant view[66] is taken at 45 degrees of knee flexion and yields information on the patellofemoral relationship in a more seated position. The congruence angle defines the relationship of the patellar apex to the bisected femoral trochlea, and the sulcus angle defines the depth of the trochlear groove. A CT scan can be used to evaluate tilt, translation, and congruence in varying degrees of knee flexion. Superimposed axial cuts may be used to evaluate long-bone torsional deformities and to determine the rotational relationship between the tibial tubercle and the femoral sulcus in varying degrees of flexion. Lateral radiographs can also be used to project trochlear dysplastic patterns.[9]

Plain radiographs miss a high percentage of osteochondral fractures that occur at the time of patellofemoral dislocation. Dainer and colleagues[21] found that 40% of arthroscopically documented lesions were missed on initial films. In a group of adolescent dislocators, Stanitski[99] found that only 34% of arthroscopically diagnosed osteochondral injuries were apparent on standard radiographs. The correlation of

MRI with arthroscopic findings has also been questioned. However, newer articular cartilage imaging techniques promise better resolution and more accurate scans. Discussion of current and future techniques for patellofemoral imaging, including specific sequences, magnetic resonance arthrography, and dynamic MRI, can be found in review articles by Recht and coworkers,[85] McCauley and Disler,[63] and Witonski.[104]

MRI also has an important role in determining the extent and location of injury to the MPFL.[60,88,96] The most common MRI findings associated with acute patellar dislocation include disruption of the MPFL and medial retinaculum and edema at the inferior border of the VMO. Although it is most commonly avulsed from its femoral attachment, the MPFL may be disrupted at any point along its course, and the disruption may be partial or complete. Hard tissue abnormalities also are commonly seen. Medial patellar avulsion fractures and osteochondral fractures from the retropatellar surface or lateral condyle are common. Runow[87] found 46 fractures in his series of 140 dislocated knees. He and Stanitski[99] pointed out the significantly lower rate of osteochondral fracture in LAACS- versus TONES-type patients. Scheller and Martenson[90] and Rünow[87] have detailed the distribution of dislocation-related fractures and the infrequent occurrence of concurrent avulsion and osteochondral fractures.

TREATMENT

A number of factors must be considered in deciding on treatment of patellofemoral instability in a young patient, including the chronicity of the instability, the presence of predisposing mechanical risk factors, the degree of instability, the existence of concurrent injury, the age and activity level of the athlete, progression with nonoperative care, and the desires of the athlete and family. Most patients with patellofemoral instability should be treated initially with a comprehensive, well-monitored nonoperative program. However, the indications for initial surgical intervention and earlier reconstruction are evolving.

Nonoperative Care

Most dislocations will spontaneously reduce on the field with terminal knee extension. If this does not happen, reduction should be done in a controlled setting. Usually, intra-articular lidocaine injection, full passive extension, and gentle pressure are adequate for successful relocation. Although uncommon, sedation is reserved for difficult cases. As discussed earlier, arthrocentesis is preformed for diagnostic and therapeutic benefit. Early immobilization in full extension is used for comfort and to let injured soft tissues quiet down. However, quad sets, straight-leg raises, and single-plane motion are begun early and are progressed as tolerated. Conceptually, early nonoperative treatment is similar to that for initial MCL sprain. Early guarded motion and exercise are beneficial. It is unlikely that single-plane motion, particularly mid flexion to full extension, will stretch the healing MPFL or cause recurrent instability. It is repetition of the injury mechanism or mechanically similar activities that must be avoided in the healing period. The MPFL is in the same layer II environment as the MCL. Although this is not known for certain, its healing potential may be similar.[96]

As strength and symptoms allow, patients progress out of their brace in the protected environment of physical therapy to single-plane walking, running, cutting, and finally sport-specific activity. Early modalities and exercise are aimed at decreasing pain and effusion while triggering quadriceps activity. It is much easier to maintain quadriceps function than to retrieve it after a period of complete immobilization and inactivity. Early motion also helps maintain articular cartilage health.

Rehabilitation involves optimizing the environment for quadriceps activity, restoring extensor mechanism balance, and improving lower extremity alignment. Long-term maintenance and preventive training programs are geared toward raising the level of extensor mechanism function to meet the demands of the sports environment without subsequent injury. Retropatellar irritation is a potential source of problems during extensor mechanism rehabilitation. Pain leads to significant quadriceps inhibition and may indicate increasing articular cartilage damage. Exercises should be done in a pain-free range and manner. In closed-chain exercises, patellofemoral stress increases as flexion increases. In open-chain exercises, the opposite is true. We have found that open-chain resistive exercises done in early to mid flexion are well tolerated. The patella is well seated, and areas of articular damage incurred at the time of dislocation in relatively greater extension may not be weight bearing. Strengthening in more terminal extension is done with functional closed-chain exercises. Variable-arc isometrics is another way to avoid painful areas of patellofemoral compression. Despite traditional thought, selected VMO recruitment or strengthening has not been supported in the research.[1,53,83] It appears that the quadriceps weaken and must be strengthened as a whole. However, quadriceps activity should be incorporated into functional patterns as soon as possible. Examples include working lateral pelvic tilts (hip abduction) or hip adduction (ball squeezes) with concurrent quadriceps contraction. Trampoline activities and multijoint exercises, such as short-arc squats, also require the quadriceps to work in a sport-specific manner. Core strengthening of the abdominals, hips, and low back is an essential part of the rehabilitation/prevention program.

Patellar taping as described by Gilleard and associates[42] has been shown to decrease pain, allow increased quadriceps activity, and improve weight acceptance in functional activities during the early rehabilitation period. The exact mechanism of the beneficial effects is unclear, but does not appear to involve a significant change in static patellar position. Potential reasons include changes in patellofemoral compressive forces possibly resulting from increasing rather than decreasing the area bearing weight and thereby decreasing force per unit area, proprioceptive feedback to improve recruitment of quadriceps activity, and subtle improvements in dynamic patellar tracking. Patellar knee sleeves appear to serve a similar function on a more long-term basis.

Although quadriceps strengthening is paramount, selective stretching is required to achieve a balanced extensor mechanism. Stretching of the upper and lower iliotibial band, hamstrings, gastrocnemius, and hip flexors is preformed by the patient. Patellar mobilization can be done by the therapist to stretch a tight lateral retinaculum. Relative internal rotation of the lower extremity increases the lateralizing vector on the patella. Excessive or prolonged midfoot pronation may be a contributor, and semirigid orthotic devices are helpful in selected patients. Dynamic hip anteversion may also be improved by proximal strengthening.

Operative Care

Surgical interventions for patellofemoral instability are numerous. The phrase "over 100 procedures" has become synonymous with any discussion of surgery to address patellofemoral instability. In considering repair versus reconstruction, surgical approaches, graft options, fixation techniques, origin and insertion points, and dynamic versus static constructs, the "over 100 procedures" may soon apply to MPFL surgeries alone.

Surgical care may involve acute repair or later reconstruction, bony or soft tissue procedures, or proximal or distal realignment. Surgery may be aimed at anatomic restoration or compensatory realignment. Historically, many of the "nonanatomic" soft tissue procedures have met with success probably because of the "healing" layer II environment of the medial aspect of the knee in which the MPFL is located. Lateral advancement of medial soft tissues containing a healed, but somewhat stretched, MPFL may provide adequate restraint to patellar dislocation in some cases. However, a recent trend has been noted toward anatomic restoration of the primary soft tissue restraints to lateral patellar dislocation, specifically, the MPFL. This development reflects trends in ACL reconstruction and shoulder instability surgery, which now incorporate anatomic restoration of the ACL or labrum rather than compensatory extra-articular, musculotendinous procedures.

Several relative indications for operative intervention after patellar dislocation have been identified: (1) failure to progress with initial nonoperative care, (2) concurrent osteochondral injury that necessitates operative intervention, (3) continued gross patellar instability, (4) grossly palpable disruption of the MPFL-VMO-adductor mechanism, (5) high-level athletic demands coupled with mechanical risk factors and an initial mechanism not related to contact injury, and (6) recurrent dislocation and failure of a long-term nonoperative program. In general, TONES-type patients will get by with less surgery, most commonly, repair or reconstruction of the MPFL. LAACS patients may often require combined proximal and distal realignment to address their chronic maltracking.

Osteochondral fractures must be suspected with all patellar dislocations. They may show up on diagnostic imaging or may manifest as mechanical symptoms and disproportionate pain during the early rehabilitation period. These fractures are rarely large or intact enough and do not have sufficient bony backing to warrant open reduction and fixation. Most are treated by loose-body removal, débridement of unstable shoulders, microfracture, and assessment for future chondral restoration procedures. Arthroscopic or open techniques may be used for the few fractures amenable to fixation.

Surgery Addressing the Medial Patellofemoral Ligament

Surgery addressing the MPFL is appropriate when the primary deficiency is of medial soft tissue restraints. If significant malalignment and functionally increased Q angle are present, a distal realignment is required. In a combined deficiency,

MPFL repair or reconstruction may be used in combination with distal realignment. The safe age for tibial tubercle osteotomy is not well defined. However, a bone age of 14 to 15 years for boys and 12 to 13 years for girls should avoid any significant iatrogenic recurvatum.[45,57]

An injured MPFL may be addressed by acute repair, repair with augmentation, or reconstruction. A variety of graft options, fixation devices, and surgical techniques have been described* and the timing of surgery may vary, depending on numerous patient and clinical factors. In a patient with acute or early recurrent dislocation, the primary surgery is repair of the MPFL. Adjunctive reconstruction may be required if the native tissue is judged to be insufficient. With more chronic instability patterns, reconstruction of the MPFL is required more routinely. If preexisting lateral facet syndrome or significant lateral patellar tilt is present, concurrent lateral release may be performed. However, release is not routinely required. If distal realignment is required, posterior medialization or distal displacement of the tubercle should be avoided because of a significant risk for secondary retropatellar arthritis. Unfortunately, straight medialization and even anteromedialization may also increase medial retropatellar loading.[81] In a more immature patient with a significantly increased Q angle or patella alta, reconstruction of the MPFL may be augmented by using a limb of the hamstring graft to reconstruct the patellotibial ligament, or by performing a patellar tendon split and turn-under.[7,72] Andrish[7] has described a soft tissue, patellar tendon imbrication to address patella alta in the skeletally immature who are not candidates for tubercle osteotomy.

Medial Patellofemoral Ligament Repair/Reconstruction

Repair may be done acutely or after a period of initial healing. Acute repairs may be performed with suture to periosteum or by using suture anchors on the patellar or femoral sides. Acute repair must be accomplished at the site of MPFL disruption, most commonly at its femoral attachment, but it may also be accomplished at the superior medial patellar attachment or within its interstitial substance. MRI is useful in localizing areas of MPFL damage. If the area of injury is uncertain, or if initial repair at a particular site does not result in adequate tensioning, the ligament should be directly evaluated throughout its length. Ahmad and colleagues[5] emphasized the importance of concurrently assessing the femoral attachment of the VMO, which may be ruptured. Specific repair techniques and the necessary anatomic dissection have been described by previous authors.[5,39,96] The repair must be appropriately tensioned. Some laxity should be seen in the repaired MPFL in terminal knee extension. A normal patella can be translated 25% to 50% at full extension. The operative knee may be matched to an asymptomatic, contralateral knee with regard to medial/lateral translation and tilt. With lateralization of the patella, the repair should have a firm endpoint. Full range of motion should be possible without undue force or tension on the repair. If the native tissue is judged to be insufficient or inherently lax, the repair may be supplemented with a partial turndown of the adductor magnus tendon to increase the bulk of repaired tissue.

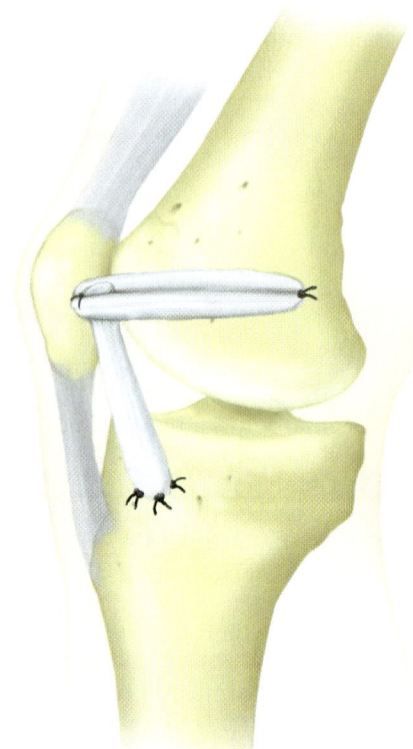

Figure 91-9. Reconstructed medial patellofemoral ligament and medial patellotibial ligament. (From Drez D Jr, Edwards TB, Williams CS: Results of medial patellofemoral ligament reconstruction in the treatment of patellar dislocation. Arthroscopy 17:298–306, 2001.)

In patients with recurrent instability, deficient bony stabilizers, native soft tissue laxity or insufficiency, or more pronounced dislocation, formal reconstruction of the MPFL is required. Numerous tissues, including free and distally attached hamstring autografts, a slip of adductor tendon, quadriceps tendon, iliotibial band, and allograft materials, have been described (Figs. 91-9 through 91-11).* The MPFL may be reconstructed alone or in combination with the medial patellotibial ligament. Fixation on the patellar side can be achieved with the use of bone tunnels, suturing, or suture anchors. On the femoral side, tunnel with interference screw fixation, direct suturing, a post with a washer, suture anchors or punch lock devices, and sling fabrication from the MCL, adductor tendon, or intermuscular septum have been described. In a skeletally immature patient, hardware and graft tunnels must be kept out of the femoral growth plate and excessive dissection about the peripheral growth plate avoided. The undulating anatomy of the distal femoral physis was discussed earlier. Live-time x-ray should be available for all MPFL cases.

Preferred MPFL Reconstruction Technique. For MPFL reconstruction, we currently use three small incisions: one over the superomedial border of the patella, one over the

---

*References 3, 7, 15, 20, 26, 27, 35, 72, and 78.

*References 3, 7, 15, 20, 23, 26, 27, 35, 72, and 78.

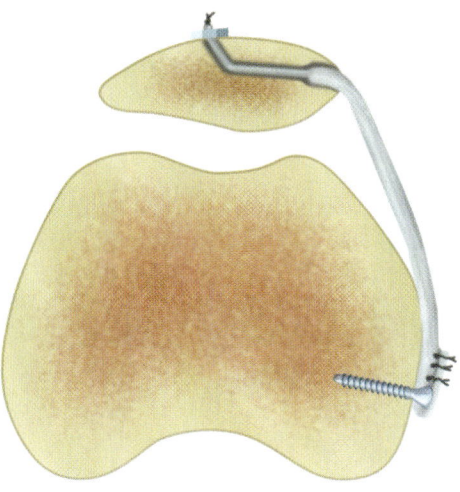

Figure 91-10. Drawing of patellofemoral fixation with a graft passing into the tunnel and fixed with a button. (From Muneta T, Sekiya I, Tsuchiya M, Shinomiya K: A technique for reconstruction of the medial patellofemoral ligament. Clin Orthop Relat Res 359:151–155, 1999.)

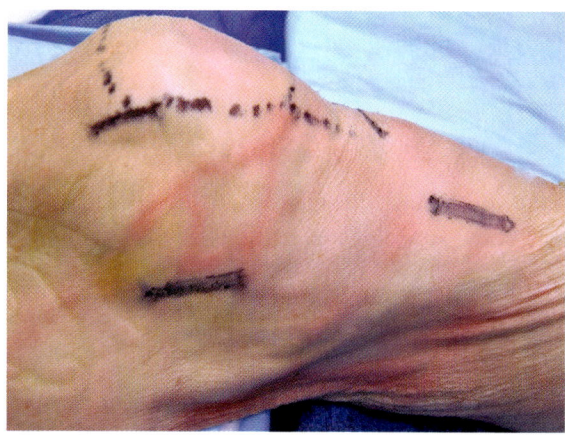

Figure 91-12. View of the medial knee showing the planned operative incisions for medial patellofemoral ligament reconstruction. These are located at the superomedial patella, over the medial epicondyle of the femur, and distally at the autograft hamstring harvest site.

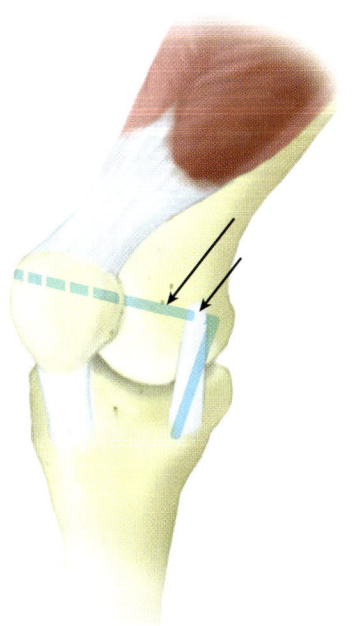

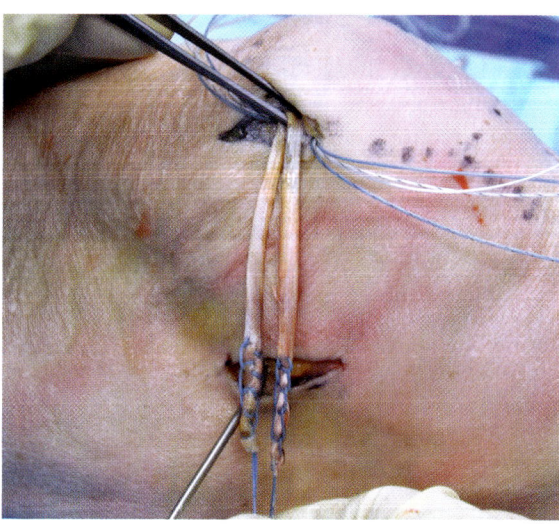

Figure 91-13. Prepared gracilis autograft: This confirms adequate length for final fixation of the doubled gracilis autograft.

Figure 91-11. Reconstruction of the medial patellofemoral ligament. The semitendinosus tendon *(large arrow)* is transferred to the patella with a pulley in the posterior third of the proximal aspect of the medial collateral ligament *(small arrow)*. (From Deie M, Ochi M, Sumen Y, et al: Reconstruction of the medial patellofemoral ligament for the treatment of habitual or recurrent dislocation of the patella in children. J Bone Joint Surg Br 85:887–890, 2003.)

medial epicondyle, and one for hamstring graft harvest (Fig. 91-12). For acute repairs, we use a single, larger vertical incision midway between the origin and insertion of the MPFL. This technique allows full inspection of the origin, insertion, and intraligament substance. Our graft of choice is a doubled gracilis autograft, which provides adequate length and bulk. On occasion, we have also gone to the semitendinosus if the gracilis was not adequate. Before prepping and draping, an

examination of the involved and contralateral patellofemoral articulations is performed. Special emphasis is given to the amount of lateralization noted at 30 degrees of flexion/full extension and to the endpoint quality. The need for distal realignment has been observed preoperatively based on a combination of diagnostic imaging findings, Q angle determination, patellofemoral architecture, and soft tissue quality. We first take a free hamstring tendon in standard fashion. An estimate is made of required graft length (distance from posterior femoral epicondylar origin to superior medial patella plus at least 20 mm of graft tails in femoral tunnel). The hamstring graft is prepared on the back table with locking stitches in both ends of the graft. The tails of the graft are tapered to ease passage into the femoral tunnel. The prepared graft is now ready for later use (Fig. 91-13). Following graft preparation, diagnostic/therapeutic arthroscopy is undertaken (Fig. 91-14A). A one-half inch, vertical incision is then made over the superior medial patella. Soft tissue is dissected along the border of the patella, and layers I, II, and III

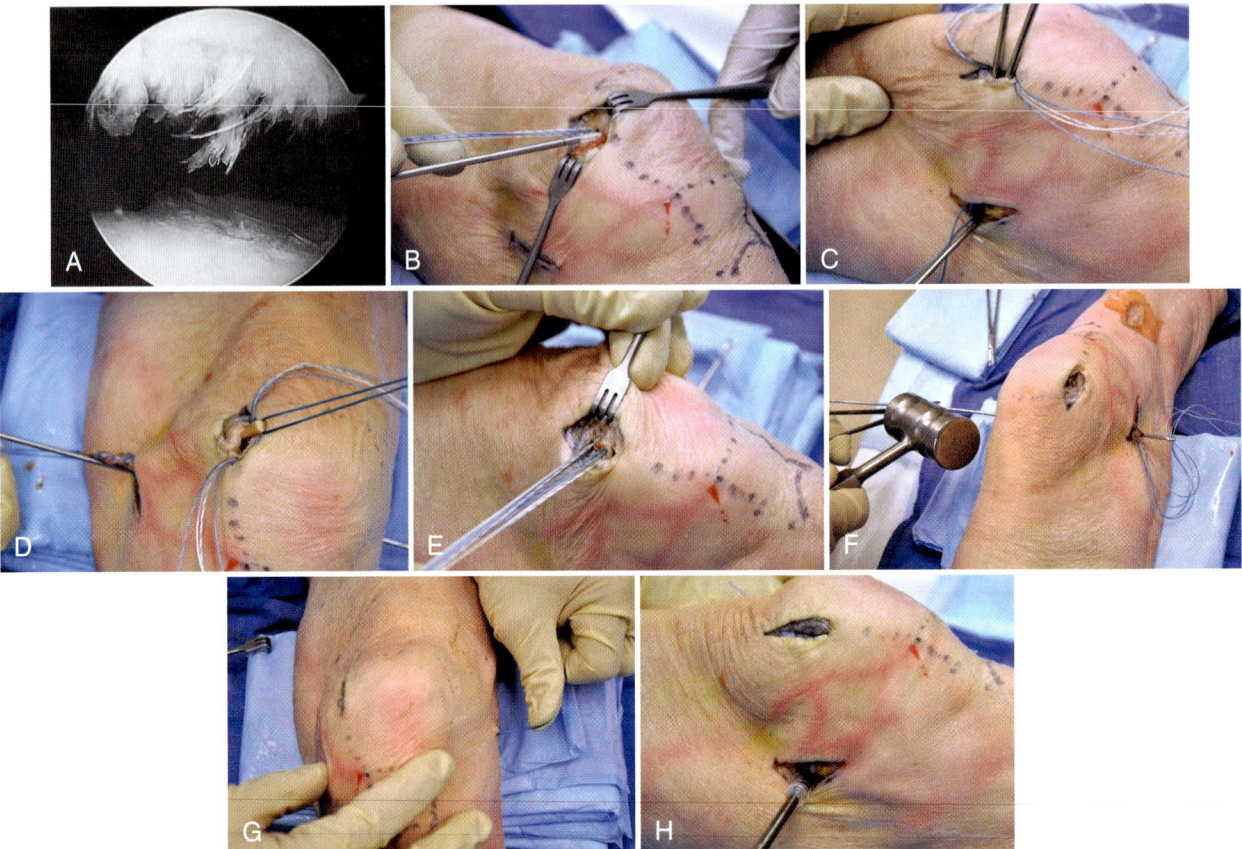

Figure 91-14. A, Arthroscopic view shows posttraumatic retropatellar changes in the adolescent recurrent dislocator. **B,** Doubly loaded suture anchors are inserted at the superomedial patella. **C** and **D,** A path is developed bluntly under layer II, and the graft is shuttled with a looped passing suture. **E,** Sutures are spaced in the graft to re-create the broad patellar attachment of the medial patellofemoral ligament. **F,** The Beath pin is used to shuttle the sutures and the graft into the femoral tunnel. **G,** Sutures are pulled laterally to effectively tension the graft. **H,** The graft is secured on the femoral side by soft tissue interference screw fixation.

of the medial soft tissues are defined. A 1-inch incision is made over the medial epicondyle, and the saddle area between the adductor tubercle and the epicondyle is identified. A C-arm is used to check the relative position of the growth plate. We bluntly dissect a tunnel under layer II from the superior medial patella to the epicondylar attachment of the MPFL (see Fig. 91-14B). At the patella, a shallow trough is burred in the medial superior shoulder of the patella at its midlevel (see Fig. 91-14C). Two or three 2.3-mm biodegradable suture anchors are used to fix the crotch (folded) portion of the hamstring graft to the patella (see Fig. 91-14D). This provides a wide area of attachment, simulating the native insertion (see Fig. 91-14E). Small, biodegradable anchors provide stronger fixation than suturing alone and avoid fracture risk, which has been reported with intrapatellar tunnels.

On the femoral side, we place a Beath needle from medial to lateral. The needle is checked under fluoroscopy for its proximal/distal and anterior/posterior position.[91] Sutures from the two tails of the graft are placed in the eyelet of the needle and are brought out the lateral side of the knee, while the graft is pulled into the tunnel. With pulling on these sutures from the lateral side, the graft can be tensioned easily (see Fig. 91-14F). We have tried various femoral fixation techniques, and interference screw fixation has provided the easiest and most reliable tensioning of the graft. Before

placement of the interference screw, the knee can be taken through a full range of motion and tension checked. We use a soft tissue interference screw 1 or 2 mm larger than the tunnel because the metaphyseal bone in this area tends to be soft (see Fig. 91-14G). We have not routinely reconstructed the medial tibiopatellar ligament. We usually fix the graft at approximately 20 to 30 degrees of flexion and allow 25% to 50% lateral translation and a crisp endpoint. We also use the mobility of the asymptomatic patella as a template.

Postoperatively, extended immobilization must be avoided. The soft tissues are given a week to quiet down, then progressive range of motion is begun. Maintaining quadriceps function is essential to success, and an adjustable hinged brace is used to prevent valgus stress on the knee. Postoperative rehabilitation follows the nonoperative program as outlined earlier. Return to sporting activity can be anticipated within 6 months after reconstruction. Studies have reported a wide range of success with MPFL repair and reconstruction.* This variability may be related to selection bias, definition of the injury, concurrent osteochondral injuries, and the varied use of simultaneous procedures such as lateral release and/or distal realignment. In general, poor and fair results appear to

---

*References 5, 23, 24, 28, 39, 69, 74, and 87.

be related more to retropatellar pain than to recurrent instability.

Non–Medial Patellofemoral Ligament Reconstruction in Younger Patients

Historically, the same type of nonanatomic procedures applied to patellofemoral instability in adult patients has been used in children, but with some modification to accommodate the immature tibial tubercle. These procedures are aimed at realigning or advancing the medial extensor mechanism and/or the distal patellar tendon attachment to reduce lateralizing forces on the patella. McCall and Ratts[62] reported the successful use of extensive proximal and distal soft tissue advancement coupled with lateral release in a large group of young patents with patellofemoral instability. Although it is effective in controlling instability, this procedure requires extensive dissection and may increase retropatellar contact force. Letts and colleagues[55] reported on the use of semitendinosus tenodesis as first described by Galeazzi.[37] A semitendinosus graft left attached distally is placed through an obliquely drilled tunnel in the patella and is sewn back on itself. This technique may be combined with medial reefing and/or lateral release. Good to excellent results in a skeletally immature population have been achieved in 62% to 82% of cases. However, routing of the graft does not duplicate that of the native MPFL. Dislocation recurrence rates may be as high as 10%, and the results may be compromised by persistent patellofemoral pain or chondromalacia.[55] In the Roux-Goldthwait procedure,[19] distal realignment is attempted by detaching the lateral half of the patella and transferring it medially under the remaining attached tendon. This may result in initial weakening of the patellar tendon and increased patellar tilt. The transferred tendon often atrophies and becomes of little biomechanical importance over time.

Several arthroscopic soft tissue balancing techniques for lateral patellar instability have been reported. These are essentially medial advancements coupled with an arthroscopic lateral release.[4,13,44] They offer the advantages of being minimally invasive and seemingly as effective as similar open surgeries, and of not burning any treatment bridges for young patients. Ahmad and Lee[4] described making an incision in the medial retinaculum, which is then repaired in a pants-over-vest fashion. The distance that sutures are passed from the edge of the incision will determine the degree of imbrication. Halbrecht[44] reported the use of suturing to bunch and tighten the medial retinaculum without incising it. These authors combined medial reefing with arthroscopic lateral release. The procedures that they describe may be best performed in patients with more subtle instability, good soft tissue quality, and relatively normal patellofemoral bony architecture. These procedures may also be used as an adjunct to distal realignment.

CONGENITAL, DEVELOPMENTAL, AND HABITUAL DISLOCATION

Significant confusion has arisen concerning the terminology of the early-onset, more involved forms of patellofemoral instability. After a thorough review of the pertinent literature, we suggest the following guidelines to be helpful:

Congenital dislocation: Persistent or fixed lateral dislocation of the patella detected at or near birth. It is manifested as knee flexion contracture with the patella tethered lateral to the femoral condyles. The probable cause is failure of normal embryologic rotation of the quadriceps myotome during lower extremity development.

Developmental dislocation: Significant maltracking or dislocation resulting from abnormal growth and development and stress across the extensor mechanism. It is often associated with systemic or generalized syndromes.

Habitual dislocation: Dislocation with spontaneous reduction that occurs with every flexion-extension cycle. It is atraumatic and occurs with normal activities of daily living. Habitual dislocation is usually associated with significant patellofemoral dysplasia and tightness of the extensor mechanism.

Ghanem and coworkers[40,41] pointed out that true congenital, in utero fixed dislocation of the patella is rare. It may occur as a result of arthrogryposis, skeletal dysplasia, and other related abnormalities. However, it should be differentiated from developmental dislocation, in which the extensor mechanism is located normally at birth but progressively moves toward a fixed dislocation later in childhood. The probable cause of congenital dislocation is failure of normal medial rotation of the quadriceps myotome during in utero development.[40,98] In contrast, the patellar dislocation often associated with Down syndrome, as well as nail-patella syndrome, acquired quadriceps fibrosis, and various neuromuscular conditions, is related to abnormal biomechanical forces on an initially normally located patella. Although congenital dislocation is usually associated with more severe deformity, developmental dislocation can progress to a similar phenotypic manifestation of fixed lateral patellar dislocation, severe quadriceps contracture, and functional disability. It appears that early, comprehensive surgical realignment affords the best chance to normalize lower extremity function.[30,41,43,49] Such realignment involves aggressive mobilization of the entire patella/quadriceps mechanism, division of the lateral soft tissues, imbrication of the medial soft tissues, and possible transfer of the insertion of the patellar ligament.

Habitual dislocators present a significantly different picture. Their problem involves spontaneous dislocation and reduction of the patella with every flexion-extension cycle of the knee. This condition does not significantly delay the age or ability of early ambulation. Consequently, it is usually diagnosed later, at 5 to 10 years of age. It is relatively painless and is not voluntary in nature. In contrast, recurrent dislocation is typically episodic, is often a result of minor trauma, is painful, and can lead to swelling. Some degree of extensor mechanism contracture is usually seen, so full range of motion is possible once the patella dislocates; however, with the patella held in place, flexion is limited. Several authors describe the underlying pathology as quadriceps muscle contracture, which is often thought to result from local trauma.[6,11] In contrast to the more common recurrent dislocation, treatment of habitual dislocation would routinely require quadriceps lengthening and lateral release.

SUMMARY

Many reports on patellofemoral instability suffer from the same flaws found in other areas of the orthopedic literature, namely, inappropriate patient selection, poor definition of injury, and insufficient assessment of activity. A number of "truths" concerning risk factors and treatment interventions have seemingly been recycled through the literature without adequate substantiation. Two large groups of young patellar dislocators have been identified; they are defined as TONES and LAACS based on their risk factors and natural history. Traditionally, patellar instability has been treated with variable periods of immobilization and sporadic rehabilitation, with anticipated full return to sports activity. The reality is that many young athletes suffer long-term retropatellar pain and sport-limiting extensor mechanism impairment. Although most athletes still benefit from an initial nonoperative program, the care provided must be aggressive, comprehensive, and responsive to early treatment outcomes. Concurrent osteochondral injuries are common and are a major contributor to adverse outcomes. Diagnostically, MRI is improving in its ability to detail osteochondral injury, and it plays an important role in determining the location and extent of MPFL injury. The primary stabilizing role of the MPFL and its injury as the essential lesion in patellar instability is just now being appreciated. Increased interest has focused on replacing the myriad of nonanatomic extensor mechanism reconstructions with more anatomically based MPFL-based surgeries.

Acknowledgment. *Krishn M. Sharma contributed to the previous version of this chapter.*

KEY REFERENCES

Ahmad CS, Lee FY: An all-arthroscopic soft-tissue balancing technique for lateral patellar instability. Arthroscopy 17:555–557, 2001.

Andrish J: Surgical options for patellar stabilization in the skeletally immature patient. Sports Med Arthrosc 15:82–88, 2007.

Beaconsfield T, Pintore E, Maffulli N, Petri GJ: Radiological measurements in patellofemoral disorders: a review. Clin Orthop Relat Res 308:18–28, 1994.

Beasley LS, Vidal AF: Traumatic patellar dislocation in children and adolescents: treatment update and literature review. Curr Opin Pediatr 16:29–36, 2004.

Cash JD, Hughston JC: Treatment of acute patellar dislocation. Am J Sports Med 16:244–249, 1988.

Colvin AC, West RV: Patellar instability. J Bone Joint Surg Am 90:2751–2762, 2008.

Fithian DC, Paxton EW, Stone ML, et al: Epidemiology and natural history of acute patellar dislocation. Am J Sports Med 32:1114–1121, 2004.

Froelke BM, Elias JJ, Cosgarea AJ: Surgical options for treating injuries to the medial patellofemoral ligament. J Knee Surg 19:296–306, 2006.

Nomura E, Inoue M, Osada N: Anatomical analysis of the medial patellofemoral ligament of the knee, especially the femoral attachment. Knee Surg Sports Traumatol Arthrosc 13:510–515, 2005.

Palmu S, Kallio PE, Donell ST, et al: Acute patellar dislocation in children and adolescents: a randomized clinical trial. J Bone Joint Surg Am 90:463–470, 2008.

Philippot R, Chouteau J, Wegrzyn J, et al: Medial patellofemoral ligament anatomy: implications for its surgical reconstruction. Knee Surg Sports Traumatol Arthrosc 17:475–479, 2009.

Schottle PB, Schmeling A, Rosenstiel N, Weiler A: Radiographic landmarks for femoral tunnel placement in medial patellofemoral ligament reconstruction. Am J Sports Med 35:801–804, 2007.

Smirk C, Morris H: The anatomy and reconstruction of the medial patellofemoral ligament. Knee 10:221–227, 2003.

Stefancin JJ, Parker RD: First-time traumatic patellar dislocation: a systematic review. Clin Orthop Relat Res 455:93–101, 2007.

Full references for this chapter can be found on www.expertconsult.com.

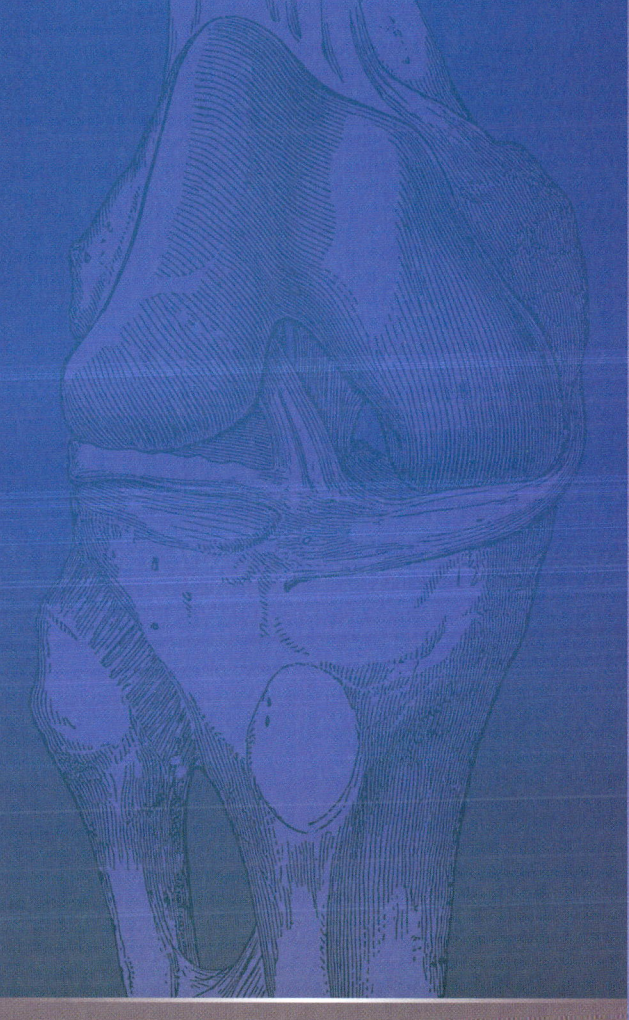

Joint Replacement and Its Alternatives

Nonoperative Treatment of Knee Arthritis

Harpal S. Khanuja, Marc W. Hungerford, Stephen R. Thompson, Maria S. Goddard, and Michael A. Mont

Osteoarthritis is one of the most common musculoskeletal ailments[288] affecting an estimated 26.9 million adults in the United States.[159] The overall prevalence of osteoarthritis is 13.9% in adults aged 25 years and older and 33.6% in those 65 and older. Symptomatic osteoarthritis of the knee is present in 16% of adults age 45 and older, affecting approximately 18.7% of women and 13.5% of men in this age group.[138]

Nonoperative management of knee arthritis is currently aimed at symptomatic treatment. As our understanding of the disease process continues to grow, interventions will be aimed at earlier stages with the goals of repair and prevention. This chapter will review the nonoperative treatment currently available for knee osteoarthritis.

There are many treatment options available for osteoarthritis of the knee. The choice depends on the severity of symptoms. Although a radiographic diagnosis of osteoarthritis is relatively straightforward, these findings can commonly be seen in asymptomatic individuals. Therefore, radiographic changes do not warrant treatment. It is important to exclude other sources of knee pain, such as hip and spinal pathology. Before deciding on a course of therapy, the question of whether the patient has osteoarthritis and whether the disease accounts for the patient's symptoms should be carefully considered.

The differential diagnosis for joint pain covers the spectrum of rheumatologic, orthopedic, neurologic, and vascular diseases. It includes soft tissue disorders ranging from muscle and ligament strains to pes anserine bursitis or meniscal problems. Inflammatory arthropathies can mimic osteoarthritis and include crystal arthropathy, which has a predilection for the knees and other large joints, rheumatoid arthritis, and systemic lupus erythematosus. Spontaneous osteonecrosis of the knee (SPONK) is typically present in patients older than 55 years. Secondary or idiopathic osteonecrosis may present in younger patients, especially those with relevant risk factors (e.g., corticosteroids or alcohol). Other causes of knee pain include neurologic (radiculopathy, peripheral neuropathy, spinal stenosis), vascular (claudication, insufficiency), malignancy, and infection.

Knowledge of the natural history of osteoarthritis influences the aggressiveness of treatment. Although end-stage disease can be extremely painful and debilitating, osteoarthritis in general is not relentlessly progressive. In a survey of 682 older people, the prevalence and severity signs and symptoms of osteoarthritis about the knee remained constant through the seventh, eighth, and ninth decades.[87] In another study documenting radiographic progression in patients older than 54 years, the percentage of patients with the most severe changes did not increase with age.[158] Following symptomatic osteoarthritic defects with magnetic resonance imaging (MRI) over 2 years, it was found that 81% of the defects increased, 15% remained unchanged, and 4% regressed. Age and the area of bone affected were predictors of progression.[54] Osteoarthritis is a chronic disease, with a waxing and waning course. With proper management, many patients can maintain reasonable comfort and function.

The source of pain in osteoarthritis is not completely understood. Cartilage itself is avascular and aneural. Proposed causes of pain include muscle strain caused by overuse, microfractures in the subchondral trabeculae, irritation of periosteal nerve endings, ligamentous stress caused by bone deformity or effusion, and venous congestion caused by remodeling of subchondral bone. Various mechanisms likely play a role in different patients. This probability helps explain the inconsistency in patient response to a given treatment regimen. It also underscores the need to define the sources of pain more thoroughly so that the most effective treatment modalities can be selected.

Synovitis is a prime candidate for pain generation in osteoarthritis. Synovium is richly innervated.[145] Patients with early-stage osteoarthritis may not show much evidence of synovial inflammation. However, in patients with more advanced disease, synovial inflammation is common and may be a significant source of pain. Inflammation in osteoarthritis may be induced by cartilage fragments[72] or proteoglycans[26] released by damaged cartilage. Synovitis leads to the release of inflammatory mediators sensitizing nociceptive cells and damaging cartilage directly. If synovial inflammation is the predominant source of pain, then corticosteroids and anti-inflammatory medications represent a rational therapy. However, inflammation in osteoarthritis is much less intense than in rheumatoid arthritis. In an arthroscopic study of patients with mild or moderate radiographic disease of the knee, almost 50% of those examined had no appreciable synovitis. No relation among severity, size or location of lesion, and synovitis was noted.[203]

Pain fibers have been found in multiple locations in the knee by a variety of methods. Immunohistochemistry stains identify substance P fibers in structures that include the periosteum, subchondral bone, fat pad, and capsule.[77,304] Evidence also demonstrates the possibility that there is a decreased threshold to noxious stimuli in limbs affected by osteoarthritis.[212]

The understanding of the pathophysiology of osteoarthritis remains limited and treatment options will change and improve as our knowledge grows. A clinical practice guideline for the nonarthroplasty treatment of osteoarthritis of the knee has recently been published by the American Academy of Orthopaedic Surgeons (AAOS).[2] This is based on an extensive systematic review of the published literature. The Osteoarthritis Research Society International (OARSI) has published similar guidelines.[155,298]

EDUCATION

The goals of education are to reduce anxiety and make patients aware of treatment and activity modifications so they can participate in their care proactively. Patient education and self-management programs have proven beneficial in reducing pain[47] associated with knee arthritis. Regular contact with patients pertaining to their arthritis may be beneficial. A large randomized control trial has demonstrated that telephone contact leads to improvements in pain and functional status, and is cost-effective.[155,298]

A meta-analysis of studies contrasting patient education with ibuprofen therapy has concluded that there is a significant reduction of pain with education, but not disability. There was some evidence for a synergistic effect of both interventions.[272]

Education allows for a better understanding of activity modification. As examples, activities that lead to excessive loading of the knee should be avoided when possible.[166] Loading activities are better performed in short periods; rest periods for 30 minutes between periods of activity may help reduce pain and allow greater overall productivity. Several shorter periods of standing are preferable to a single prolonged period.

PHYSICAL THERAPY AND MODALITIES

The proven benefit of physical therapy coupled with the absence of side effects argues for a prominent role of these modalities in the treatment of osteoarthritis. The advantageous risk-benefit ratio is further amplified in older adults, a population at greater risk of side effects from pharmacologic intervention. The general rehabilitation goals in treating patients with osteoarthritis of the knee are to increase and maintain current function and prevent further joint deterioration. There are multiple modalities that physical therapy uses to achieve these goals, including braces, orthoses, exercises, educational plans, and physical (e.g., temperature, electrical stimulation, ultrasound) modalities. In general, a physical therapy program involves the use of heat, cold, or other modalities followed by an exercise program. This section will provide a brief description of these and review the literature regarding their efficacy and indications.

Exercise

Exercise programs have been devised with diverse goals, including increasing strength, endurance, and/or range of motion (ROM) in patients with knee arthritis. Most (but not all) of the published and ongoing research is directed at the quadriceps mechanism.* Different types of exercise include passive exercises, in which the joint and thus muscles are moved by the therapist, and include the use of a continuous passive motion machine, without active input by the patient. Active or active-assisted exercises are performed by active contraction of muscles with assistance by the therapist. Resistive exercises are accomplished by active contraction of muscles by the patient against resistance (mechanical or manual). Isometric, isotonic, and isokinetic contractions may all be used. Stretching exercises to increase joint motion and flexibility are frequently added to the regimen.

Range of Motion and Stretching Exercises

ROM and stretching exercises should be part of every osteoarthritis patient's daily routine. Beneficial effects reported

include maintenance of function, decreased edema, stimulation of flexion-extension reflexes, and preparation of the limb for active exercise. Stretching exercises can restore or maintain ROM. Care should be taken with inflamed joints, because passive ROM exercise has been shown to increase joint inflammation. Although almost universally recommended, there is little scientific evidence for the use of stretching in the treatment of OA.

Strengthening Exercises

In knee arthritis, loss of strength and function occurs rapidly. A muscle can atrophy up to 30% in 1 week. A muscle at complete rest will lose strength at a rate of 3%/day.[81,82,198]

Despite a wealth of published literature, consensus regarding optimum dosage, modality, and frequency of exercise for strengthening the quadriceps is lacking. In one case study,[177] isometric strengthening of the quadriceps muscles led to improvements in quadriceps torque, clinical status, and pain after walking. This program consisted of exercises performed three times weekly for 6 weeks with the knee flexed to 60 degrees. Other studies have demonstrated improvement in function of quadriceps-trained individuals, but most of these studies failed to compare the results to patients who rested. Three randomized controlled trials (RCTs)[70,76,133] in patients with knee osteoarthritis who underwent quadriceps strengthening with isometric, isotonic, or resistive exercises showed significant improvements in quadriceps strength, knee pain, and function when compared with controls. A recent meta-analysis of 10 RCTs has concluded that quadriceps strengthening has statistically significant treatment effects on pain and function in patients with osteoarthritis of the knee.[242]

Nevertheless, strengthening exercises must be used with caution. Exercises that use repetitive joint motion or require a full ROM may increase inflammation and pain, and thus fail to achieve muscle strengthening. Isometric contraction is less likely to increase joint pain or inflammation. Dynamic (repetitive) exercises are appropriate using isotonic or isokinetic muscle contraction after pain is controlled. Isokinetic exercises can be used for patients with ligamentous stability and no internal derangement. Deep knee bends, however, may increase intra-articular pressure and should be avoided.[41]

Aerobic Conditioning

In addition to weakness, patients with osteoarthritis often suffer from decreased cardiovascular endurance.[124] Aerobic exercise can increase the overall vitality, activity, and feeling of well-being in these patients. Suitable endurance exercises include cycling, swimming, and low-impact aerobics. High-impact loading activities, such as jogging, should probably be avoided.

Increased aerobic fitness not only improves the patients overall health, but specifically improves their arthritic symptoms. Kovar and coworkers,[152] in an 8-week supervised fitness walking program in 102 patients with knee osteoarthritis, found improvements in 6-minute walking distance and reductions in pain and the use of medications in the exercise group when compared with controls. In another study, 12 weeks of aerobic walking or aquatic exercises improved overall exercise capacity, with aerobic gains maintained at 9 months. In the Fitness, Arthritis and Seniors Trial,[71] 439 subjects with radiographically confirmed osteoarthritis of the knee, pain, and disability were randomized to a program of aerobic

---

*References 60, 70, 71, 76, 80-82, 124, 133, 152, 177, 178, 190, 191, 198, 208, 230, 266, 274, and 279.

exercise, resistance exercise, or health education. In this 18-month trial, those in the exercise groups showed improvements in tests of physical performance (climbing and descending stairs, lifting and carrying 10 pounds) compared with the education group. Pain and disability self-reported scores improved in the exercise groups.

Roddy and colleagues have published a systematic review of 13 RCTs. They reported a significant treatment effect for aerobic conditioning and quadriceps strengthening in patients with osteoarthritis of the knee.[242]

Weight Loss

Weight reduction should also be encouraged on principal. A 1-pound weight loss translates into a 3- to 4-pound decrease in load across the joint. One study has shown that weight loss in middle-aged and older women significantly reduces the incidence of symptomatic osteoarthritis in the knee.[79] OARSI guidelines published in 2007 recommended at least a 5% reduction in overall body weight for patients with a body mass index (BMI) more than 25.[308,309] Although this seems rational, few controlled data exist to demonstrate reduction in joint pain or slowed progression of arthrosis with weight loss.[78]

Therapy regimens are generally prescribed in a programmatic fashion rather than in isolation. The Arthritis, Diet and Activity Promotion Trial (ADAPT) has tried to estimate the relative contribution of each of the following modalities.[188] In this trial, 316 overweight patients with knee OA were randomized into four groups: healthy lifestyle (education), diet only, exercise only, and diet plus exercise. At the end of the 18-month trial, the diet plus exercise group showed improvement in self-reported function, 6-minute walk distance, stair climb time, and knee pain. The exercise-only group showed improvement in walk distance. The diet-only group was no better than the education group. Whether the benefits persist over the long term remains questionable.[285]

Biomechanical Treatment

Taping

Appliances that alter the biomechanics of the knee joint may be helpful. Cushnaghan and associates[50] have found that taping the patella medially is effective in reducing knee pain in patients with patellofemoral arthritis. In this randomized, single-blind, crossover trial with 14 subjects, medial taping was superior to lateral or neutral taping for pain scores, symptomatology, and patient preference. Others have used taping before quadriceps exercises for chondromalacia patellae.[186]

Knee Bracing and Orthotics

The usefulness of bracing for the treatment of knee osteoarthritis has been controversial.[88,146,250,266] Most clinical and biomechanical studies have shown little or no benefit from these devices. The primary goal of knee brace designs is to assist in the restoration of normal mechanical stability. The first step in fitting for a brace is to define abnormal motion that the brace should control.

A Swedish knee cage or a hinged knee brace may provide support in limiting extension and may help decrease pain.[250] There are a number of three-point pressure braces to control

medial or lateral instability.[266] In selected patients, these devices can be effective. In one study, Kirkley and associates[146] found that valgus-producing functional knee braces were much more effective for the treatment of medial compartment osteoarthritis of the knee than a simple neoprene sleeve. Furthermore, quality of life (Western Ontario and McMaster Universities Osteoarthritis Index [WOMAC]) scores of both braced groups exceeded those of a control group receiving standard medical treatment in a prospective, parallel group, randomized clinical trial.

Immobilization of the knee during periods of increased pain or inflammation may be useful. This may be done with a knee immobilizer or posterior splint. These support the knee in extension and permit relaxation of the flexor muscles. An elastic bandage may control knee swelling but is actually not a knee orthosis.

Assistive Devices: Cane or Walker

The cane can successfully unload the knee joint.[23] Assistive devices to unload the knee joint are most effectively used on the side opposite the pathologic condition. The use of a crutch or cane will reduce the joint load on the opposite limb by about 50%. A quadriceps cane can be used instead of a straight cane when balance is a problem.

Hydrotherapy

The buoyancy of water is useful to minimize stress on the knee joint by effectively neutralizing the force of gravity. This is especially useful when ROM and strengthening exercises are prescribed for the obese patient. The external application of water for therapeutic purposes can provide heat or cold. There are many physiologic effects that have been reported in patients treated with warm water hydrotherapy. These include a rise in body temperature, increased sweating, superficial vasodilation, increase in peripheral circulation, decrease in blood pressure after immersion, sedative effect on nerve endings, and muscle relaxation. The water temperature should be between 34° C and 37° C. Contraindications to hydrotherapy include skin infections or lesions, open wounds, and cardiovascular disorders.

The efficacy of hydrotherapy has been questioned. One study of hydrotherapy and home exercises compared with home exercises alone found no differences in osteoarthritis of the hip.[112] More research needs to be conducted in patients with knee osteoarthritis to ascertain the efficacy of this modality.

Electrical and Related Energy Treatments

Heat Modalities

Therapeutic heat can be applied superficially or to a deep location. Heat is usually applied at temperatures of 41° C to 45° C. Superficial heat is capable of elevating the soft tissue temperatures by 3° C at a depth of 1 cm without penetrating deeper depths and thus penetrates the knee joint.[128] Some studies have demonstrated that the threshold for pain can be raised in humans as well as in animals by the application of superficial or deep heat.[163] The effect is produced by analgesia of free nerve endings (peripheral nerves and gamma fibers of muscle spindles) and muscle relaxation is produced.[164] Local heat may also relieve pain by acting on sensory afferents and closing the pain gate, or increasing local blood flow and thus washing out pain-inducing metabolites and inflammatory mediators produced in osteoarthritis.

The four general methods that produce superficial heat include diathermy (shortwaves) microwaves, ultrasound, radiation (infrared), conduction (heating pad, water bottle), and convection (sauna, steam room).[57,66,211,234] Moist heat produces a greater temperature elevation than dry heat and may be preferable for clinical applications.[128] For all these modalities, care must be exercised to avoid burns, especially with uneven application. A towel-wrapped hot water bottle, gel-filled hot pack, or thermostatically controlled electric heating pad provides a simple method for the patient to benefit from superficial heat application at home.

Diathermy

Deep heat can be used as a modality that affects the visco-elastic properties of collagen.[287] Diathermy can use shortwave (11.062-m wavelength, 27.12 MHz frequency) radiation delivered via two electrodes or an induction cable for approximately 20 minutes.[234] This treatment leads to an increase in skin temperature, blood flow, and pain threshold. The effects are maintained for 15 to 30 minutes after cessation of treatment.

Diathermy has demonstrated clinical benefit when used in combination with exercise but should not be used indescriminantly.[234] Shortwave diathermy can exacerbate knee arthritis caused by the heat-induced proliferation of collagenous tissue, leading to the development of adhesions and thus a decreased range of motion. Microwave electromagnetic radiation (12.2 cm at 2456-, 915-, and 433.9-MHz frequencies) is used less frequently, probably because of safety concerns.[57]

Ultrasound

Ultrasound is a well-established deep-heating modality that can have greater depth of penetration than that of shortwave or microwave diathermy.[274] Several early studies have demonstrated the efficacy of this modality in relieving osteoarthritic pain.[66,163] Its effects are attributed to thermal and mechanical mechanisms. Ultrasound is absorbed and creates heat in structures with high protein content. The physiologic effects of local tissue heating, as described earlier, include increase in pain threshold, reduction of muscle spasm, and promotion of the healing process. The nonthermal or mechanical effects include microstreaming, or small fluid movements around cells that alter cell membrane permeability, promote collagen synthesis, and alter electrical activity in painful nerve afferents.

Ultrasound therapy requires the use of a coupling agent (water or mineral oil) to prevent attenuation of the sound waves in air. Energy exposures of 0.5 to 4.0 W/cm^2 for 5 to 10 minutes are commonly used. The therapist must keep the ultrasound applicator in constant motion to decrease excessive focal heating. The effects of ultrasound have also been found to be additive with a nonsteroidal anti-inflammatory drug (NSAID) treatment.

There is still little documented, well-controlled evidence of the effectiveness of ultrasound as well as its optimal dosage. In fact, two meta-analyses have concluded there is little evidence to support the use of ultrasound to treat pain in various musculoskeletal conditions.[96,286] Significant response rates to ultrasound treatment are only seen in approximately 40% of cases.[153] Ultrasound may be a useful adjunct to other modes of treatment, but should not be a mainstay of therapy.

Summary of Heat Treatment Modalities

All these heat treatment modalities should be used as adjuncts or precursors to other treatment regimens, such as before exercise, mobilization, or stretching. They should be used cautiously, because the use of heat may increase inflammation or joint damage. Use of heat therapy in patients with inadequate thermal sensation is contraindicated.

Interferential Therapy

Interferential therapy uses two medium-frequency (approximately 4 KHz) alternating currents applied to the skin through suction cups or adhesive padding. The resultant current has a low frequency that is the difference between the two original frequencies applied. This current is usually applied for about 15 minutes for the knee and is experienced as a prickling sensation. Various pain-relieving mechanisms, which block nonmyelinated nociceptive fibers, activate delta A and C fibers, releasing encephalins and endorphins, or activatef the opioid system, have been proposed for the pain relief that this technique provides.[234]

Transcutaneous Electrical Neuromuscular Stimulation

Transcutaneous electrical nerve stimulation (TENS) delivers short pulse width (50 to 250 microsecond), low-frequency waves (2 to 150 Hz) that are used specifically for pain relief.[134] As with interferometry, a prickly sensation is produced. Carbon-rubber electrodes with a coupling gel on the skin or with self-adhesive electrodes are used to deliver pulses for 30 to 60 minutes once or twice daily. The finding that large-diameter, cutaneous nerve fibers are preferentially stimulated by TENS is thought to account for its efficacy. These fibers inhibit the transmission of painful stimuli to the spinal cord. Double-blind studies using TENS for the control of pain in osteoarthritis (OA) of the knee have yielded conflicting results. One study concluded that it provides no greater benefit than placebo whereas the other study demonstrated improvement over placebo.[115] A recent meta-analysis was inconclusive; it found only small, poorly constructed studies.[251] More research is needed to demonstrate the effectiveness of this modality and define optimum parameters for its use.

Acupuncture

Interest in traditional Chinese medicine in general, and acupuncture specifically, has been increasing steadily since the 1970s. Information from the 2007 National Health Interview Survey[13] showed that approximately 3 million patients receive acupuncture treatments in the United States annually, many of them for musculoskeletal ailments. The technique has been applied to a wide variety of conditions. including postoperative pain, arthritis, obesity, and nicotine addiction.

Although interest remains strong, science evidence for efficacy is frequently lacking. Studies involving acupuncture frequently suffer significant methodologic deficiencies, such as lack of placebo control and lack of blinding. Most of the studies also reported small sample sizes.

Ezzo and colleagues[73] have performed a systematic review of studies specific to OA of the knee. Of the seven studies identified, there was limited evidence that acupuncture is more effective in improving pain and function than treatment as usual. It was found several of these studies showed significant improvement in pain scores, an effect that lasted more than 1 month after the cessation of treatment. This improvement was not seen in two of three studies in which sham acupuncture was used.

The AAOS work group has performed a meta-analysis of nine RCTs on the effectiveness of acupuncture for the treatment of OA.[2] They found that the treatment effect on pain and function was much smaller in studies in which the patient was blinded and the blinding was confirmed. They therefore gave it an equivocal recommendation.

Cryotherapy

Cold can be used to decrease pain. Joints are cooled by the application of ice packs or commercial gel hydropacks.[211] The pack should be applied for 15 to 20 minutes and be separated from the skin by a towel to prevent freezing of the skin. Decreasing skin and muscle temperature may reduce muscle spasm by reducing muscle spindle activity and raising the pain threshold. Cryotherapy may also provide functional improvements. One study has shown that cryotherapy leads to improvements in passive ROM and joint stiffness in osteoarthritis.[161] Cold therapy is contraindicated in patients with Raynaud's disease and should be used cautiously in patients with cardiovascular disease.

Other Methods

Magnetism, Electrical Stimulation, and Low-Intensity Pulsed Ultrasound

Magnetism, electrical stimulation, and low-intensity pulsed ultrasound use low-energy fields to achieve their effects. The device that delivers a pulsed electrical signal has been approved by the U.S. Food and Drug Administration (FDA) for the treatment of OA of the knee and rheumatoid arthriis (RA) of the hand. Zizic and associates[310] have published a short-term clinical study comparing patients with OA of the knee treated with this device versus those treated with placebo. The treatment group had statistically significant improvement in pain and function scores over the 4-week treatment period. There is even some indication that these modalities have a disease-modifying effect. Low-intensity pulsed ultrasound was recently shown to yield more hyaline-like cartilage in a rabbit model when compared with non-treated controls in a study by Cook and coworkers.[48] Lippiello and colleagues,[168] using this device, also reported improved hyaline cartilage repair in a ulcerative and bone defect model in rabbits when the animals were treated with electromagnetic stimulation. In a recent Cochrane database review of TENS for OA of the knee, the efficacy could not be confirmed, given the small number of clinical studies of questionable quality.[251]

PHARMACOLOGIC MEASURES

Analgesics

Acetaminophen is the sole representative of the class of simple, non-narcotic analgesics available in the United States. Alternately classified as a peripheral or central analgesic, its mode of action is poorly understood. Acetaminophen readily penetrates the central nervous system. Its analgesic action may be mediated through the diffuse noxious inhibitory control pathway.[276] It has no significant effect on cyclooxygenase (COX) and thus does not demonstrate the toxicity plaguing NSAIDs (see later). Acetaminophen can cause interstitial nephritis when consumed in large quantities over a long period of time. The maximum dose should not exceed 4 g/day. Dosage should be lowered in patients with renal or hepatic impairment.[225,253] A number of randomized control studies have demonstrated decreased pain in OA patients taking acetaminophen compared with placebo, with no increase in toxicity.[278] The clinical significance of this pain reduction, however, cannot be quantified.

Acetaminophen is inexpensive, readily available, well tolerated, and effective. It is often recommended as first-line treatment for mild to moderate OA of the hip and knee in doses up to 4 g/day.[307] There are increasing reports of risks associated with acetaminophen that were not previously highlighted. A population-based cohort study from the United Kingdom of 958,397 people has demonstrated a relative risk of 3.6 for upper gastrointestinal (GI) complications from acetaminophen at doses higher than 2 g/day.[100] The relative risk of these complications was 2.4 and 4.9 for low to medium and high doses of NSAIDs, respectively. Other studies have shown that patients on higher dosages of acetaminophen are at increased risk for GI events, including hospitalizations, ulcers, and dyspepsia, compared with those on lower doses.[235] In patients with early renal failure, acetaminophen has been associated with further decline.[84] This drug has also been associated with an increase in hypertension in both men and women.[85,86]

Nonsteroidal Anti-Inflammatory Drugs

NSAIDs are commonly prescribed for osteoarthritis. NSAIDs bind to the COX enzyme, thereby blocking the conversion of arachodonic acid to prostaglandins. This is likely the main mechanism for their anti-inflammatory and analgesic effects.[14] The COX-1 isoform of the enzyme is expressed in many normal tissues. Prostaglandins produced by COX-1 play a role in normal tissue hemostasis, such as mucosal defense and repair in the GI system as well as renal perfusion.[179,254] COX-1 is also found in platelets and plays a role in platelet aggregation.[132,179] The COX-2 isoform, although found in normal tissue, is also an inducible enzyme and appears in areas of inflammation and injury.[139]

Traditional NSAIDs were nonselective in that they bound to and inhibited the COX-1 and COX-2 isoforms. Isolated COX-2 inhibitors, commonly called coxibs, were developed to avoid the side effects associated with nonspecific COX inhibition.

Nonselective Nonsteroidal Anti-inflammatory Drugs

Inhibition of prostaglandin synthesis has detrimental effects. Prostacyclin (PGI2) and prostaglandin E2 (PGE2) are both vasodilators important in maintaining renal perfusion during hypovolemia. Prostaglandin inhibition leads to sodium retention in the kidney, which may worsen congestive heart failure. A number of medical conditions depend on renal prostaglandins to maintain renal profusion, including congestive heart failure, cirrhosis, certain forms of hypertension, and dehydration. In these patients, exposure to NSAIDs will lead to a decline in renal function, even if creatinine clearance was normal before treatment.[46,202] This decline is usually reversible. NSAIDs may increase the overall risk of chronic renal failure.[225] Acute interstitial nephritis has also been noted with most of the NSAIDs, but is seen most commonly with fenoprofen.[37,176] sulindac,[299,300] and nabumatone[5] are purported to be less likely to cause deterioration in renal function.[38]

The most common toxic side effect of traditional NSAIDs occurs in the GI tract. It has been estimated that 15% to 35% of all peptic ulcer complications are attributable to these drugs.[113,114,116,120,156]

Morbidity includes 107,000 hospitalizations and 16,500 deaths annually in the United States alone.[264] Upper GI symptoms caused by NSAIDs include dyspepsia, ulceration, hemorrhage, perforation, and death.[94,99,265] There is an estimated three- to fivefold increased relative risk of GI bleeding from the use of NSAIDs.[119] Risk factors for developing a bleeding complication with the use of these medications include a history of prior peptic ulcer disease, concomitant use of corticosteroids or anticoagulants, and poor general health.[92,98,261,263] Toxicity from NSAIDs is additive, so the use of more than one NSAID at a time is contraindicated.[40,189] The concomitant use of NSAIDs in patients who are also taking systemic corticosteroids should be avoided, if possible, because the incidence of bleeding complications and mortality is significantly elevated.

Selective COX-2 Inhibition

COX-2 inhibitors, also called coxibs, reduce GI adverse events and complications.[56,67,254] Two large, prospective, randomized outcome studies were performed for celecoxib and rofecoxib.[25,262] Celecoxib was compared with diclofenac and ibuprofen and rofecoxib was compared with naproxen. The risk of symptomatic ulcers or ulcer complications was lower with the selective COX-2 inhibitors.

The selectivity of COX 2 inhibitors, although beneficial to the GI mucosa, may lead to problems with thrombosis as well as salt and fluid imbalance.[305] The incidence of acute myocardial infarction was significantly higher for rofecoxib than naproxen in this study. The celecoxib did not demonstrate increased risk or cardiac events compared with ibuprofen or diclofenac. An independent reanalysis of the celecoxib data confirmed that there was no increased risk of myocardial infarction with celecoxib.[301] Two large chemoprevention trials for adenomatous polyps, one with celecoxib and one with rofecoxib, were discontinued after demonstrating increased cardiovascular risk.[75,187] The dosages of the medications in these studies were far greater than those used to treat arthritis. As a result of its increased cardiac risk profile, rofecoxib was removed from the market.

The exact mechanism for increased cardiac risk has not been elucidated. In addition to vasoconstriction, which can be associated with COX-2 inhibition, a number of other factors may cause increased cardiac risk. The COX-2 enzyme expression is found in endothelial cells in response to injury.[139] It is also found in atheromatous plaques and may play a role in decreasing vascular inflammation.[258] Furthermore, there is no COX-2 expression on platelets. COX-2 inhibitors, unlike their nonselective counterparts, do not block formation of thromboxane, which plays an important role in platelet aggregation and vasoconstriction. This may explain the apparent increased cardiovascular risk of coxibs over traditional NSAIDs. A recent trial of anti-inflammatory drugs in patients with Alzheimer's disease indicated that naprosyn, 220 mg, had an increased risk of cardiovascular risk that was higher than celebrex, 200 mg, in older patients.[1] In a report of population-based National Health Insurance data from Taiwan, four NSAIDs were examined.[130] In patients 18 years of age or older, there was no difference in the risk of serious long-term events in patients treated with etodolac, ibuprofen, naproxen, nambutone, or celebrex for an 180-day period. In this study, a previous history of cardiovascular disease was the greatest predictor of risk.

Hypertensive effects of COXIBs enzymes seem equal to those of nonselective NSAIDs. It appears that COX-2 enzyme is responsible for prostaglandin production, which is important for fluid balance. Blocking its production affects fluid retention, which can result in hypertension.[139] The COX-2 enzyme is also responsible for the production of PGI2, which is a vasodilator.[83] A number of products of the COX-1 enzyme have vasoconstrictive effects. Therefore, selective inhibition of COX-2 favors vasoconstriction, which plays a role in hypertension and heart disease.

Nonsteroidal Anti-Inflammatory Drugs versus Analgesics

Although a number of studies have shown that NSAIDs are more effective than placebo, evidence that they are more effective than simple analgesics (such as acetaminophen) in osteoarthritis is not consistent. Several studies have demonstrated a 10% to 20% improvement in scores of pain and stiffness when NSAIDs were compared with placebo.[17,20,280] In a large comparative trial, slightly less than 50% of patients exhibited a favorable response to treatment. No difference in response rates among drugs was noted.[170]

A 4-week randomized, prospective, blinded study comparing an anti-inflammatory dose of ibuprofen, an analgesic dose of ibuprofen, and acetaminophen failed to show any significant difference among the three treatment groups.[28] Another study comparing ketaprofen with dextropropoxyphenacetaminophen (a non-narcotic analgesic) failed to show any difference between the regimens.[63] Consistent with these findings have been several studies in which ibuprofen given in an analgesic dose (1200 mg) was equivalent to several other NSAIDs for the treatment of osteoarthritic joint pain.[32,44,55,197,249] Given the evidence, one might consider that the efficacy of NSAIDs lies in their analgesic effect rather than in the anti-inflammatory one. Schumacher and associates have shown that high-dose ibuprofen is superior to acetaminophen in patients with knee arthritis and a synovial effusion. Therefore, there may be a subset of patients with

OA and an inflammatory component who benefit additionally from NSAIDs.[259]

A recent study has compared an extended-release acetaminophen, 1300 mg three times daily, to rofecoxib 12.5 and 25 mg once daily.[257] Acetaminophen was noninferior to rofecixib at the 12.5-mg dose. Some studies have shown some potential benefit of NSAIDs over acetaminophen. In a 6-week trial comparing acetaminophen with diclofenac and misoprostol, the latter had a statistically higher response to treatment for OA of the hip and knee.[227]

NSAIDs are considered more effective for symptomatic treatment than acetaminophen. In a meta-analysis of 10 randomized control trials including 1712 patients,[307] NSAIDs were more effective for pain relief and had a better clinical response rate than acetaminophen. Twice as many patients preferred NSAIDs to acetaminophen. However, NSAIDs were more commonly associated with GI side effects, including nausea, vomiting, distress, abdominal pain, and diarrhea.

Another meta-analysis of 23 randomized, placebo-controlled studies has demonstrated that NSAIDs are effective in pain reduction in osteoarthritic knees over short periods.[22] This analysis included selective COX-2 inhibitors. Although the reduction in pain with NSAIDs is overall greater than that seen with acetaminophen, the difference may not be enough for clinical significance.[307] NSAIDs are associated with higher rates of GI discomfort than Tylenol.[278]

There is some evidence to suggest that NSAIDs interfere with synovial blood flow or repair of microfractures of subchondral bone.[270,271] Furthermore, various animal models have shown that the most commonly used NSAID, aspirin, inhibits proteoglycan synthesis and leads to enhanced cartilage destruction.[29,30,213-215] Early clinical studies implied that NSAIDs were associated with more rapid degeneration of the osteoarthritic joint and quicker presentation for surgery. A retrospective analysis of radiographic progression of osteoarthritis of the hip has concluded that indomethacin is associated with greater joint destruction than that seen in control patients.[246] In another study, patients with advanced hip OA awaiting arthroplasty were treated with indomethacin or azapropazone.[236] Azapropazone is a nonselective NSAID available for use in Britain. It was concluded that the indomethacin group showed more rapid radiographic deterioration and presented to surgery earlier then the azapropazone group. However, the results of this study have been called into question,[62] and a double-blind study of indomethacin versus placebo showed no increase in disease progression.[125]

Possible Chondroprotective Action of Nonsteroidal Anti-Inflammatory Drugs

The traditional view that osteoarthritis is an inevitably progressive disease and results from wear and tear of the cartilage has been replaced by an understanding of the biochemical and biomechanical factors in the cause and progression of the disease. Because cartilage is continuously undergoing degradation and renewal, it appears logical to design a medication that promotes anabolic activity of cartilage while inhibiting its degradation. The evidence for these beneficial activities of NSAIDs is mixed.[123]

A chondroprotective effect of NSAIDs has been postulated.[61] Proposed mechanisms include improved biomechanics by decreasing arthralgia and inhibition of cartilage catabolism. Cartilage matrix proteoglycans are degraded by enzymes such as metalloproteases and serine proteases. Some NSAIDs are effective inhibitors of these enzymes.[34,101,165] Release of oxygen free radicals and other inflammatory mediators may also be suppressed by NSAIDs.[122,221,224] Other NSAIDs may actually stimulate glycosaminoglycan production, as indicated by increased sulfate incorporation.

The net effect of NSAIDs on cartilage remains to be determined and may vary among NSAIDs.[214] The effects of COX-2 inhibitors on articular cartilage have not been extensively studied. Celecoxib and diclofenac on human chondrocyte metabolism were compared in an in vitro model. Celecoxib increased the synthesis of hyaluronan and proteoglycans in these explanted cells, whereas diclofenac did not have such an effect.[69]

Other studies have also demonstrated a potential chondroprotective effect of COX-2 inhibitors in vitro. Human articular cartilage cells exposed to celecoxib in culture have demonstrated increased proteoglycan synthesis and decreased proteoglycan release.[180]

Future Medications

COX-inhibiting nitric oxide donators (CINODs) are a recently developed group of analgesic and anti-inflammatory medications. It is theorized that the addition of the nitrogen oxide (NO) will counteract some of the known complications seen with COX-inhibitors, specifically elevated blood pressure and gastrointestinal upset.[295] The release of NO causes vasodilation of blood vessels, which decreases systemic blood pressure and decreases platelet aggregation. The first drug in this class is AZD3582 or naproxcinod, a combination of naproxen and nitric oxide.

White and coworkers[302] have recently conducted a study to compare the effects of naproxen alone versus naproxcinod on blood pressure. The treatment protocols for the four comparison groups were as follows: (1) 750 mg naproxcinod twice daily; (2) 375 mg naproxcinod twice daily; (3) naproxen 500 mg twice daily; and (4) placebo twice daily. The authors found that neither dose of naproxcinod resulted in increased blood pressure compared with the naproxen group. Also, patients who had a known diagnosis of hypertension prior to beginning the study who were treated with naproxen alone had an elevated blood pressure, 6.5 mm Hg higher than those hypertensive patients in the 500-mg naproxcinod treatment arm.

Karlsson and associates,[140] in a phase 2, randomized, double-blind study, found the most efficacious dose of naproxcinod to be 750 mg twice daily. Included in the study were patients treated with 25 mg daily of the COX-II inhibitor rofecoxib. This study found that no statistically significant difference in WOMAC pain score for those treated with naproxcinod, 750 mg twice daily; naproxcinod, 1125 mg twice daily; and rofecoxib, 25 mg daily. However, patients on these regimens had better pain relief than those taking a once-daily dose of naproxcinod, 750 mg, or placebo. The authors also reported decreased systolic blood pressure in the cohort being treated with rofecoxib.

Although these early results are promising, long-term follow-up of the CINOD group of drugs must be conducted to identify possible idiosyncratic side effects that have not been as yet identified.

Summary

If nonpharmacologic measures fail, acetaminophen should probably be tried as a first-line measure. In the subset of patients in whom analgesic therapy is not effective, a low dose (less than 1200 mg/day) of ibuprofen often provides effective therapy. Low-dose ibuprofen is not anti-inflammatory and is very inexpensive. If the ibuprofen is not effective in an analgesic dose, anti-inflammatory doses of ibuprofen or other nonselective NSAIDs may be tried. As a first-line pharmacologic treatment, the AAOS clinical practice guideline recommends acetaminophen or NSAIDs.[2]

In patients with GI risk, acetaminophen, COX-2 inhibitors, or nonselective NSAIDs with a gastroprotective agent such as a protein pump inhibitor may be used.[2,309] All NSAIDs should be used cautiously in patients with hypertension, a history of cardiac or renal disease, and in older adult. Scheiman and Fendrick[255] have provided an algorithm to help determine the appropriate NSAID based on gastrointestinal and cardiovascular risk (Table 92-1).

Once relief is achieved with NSAIDs, periodic withdrawal of therapy with substitution of a simple analgesic is prudent, especially in the older population. NSAIDs should be avoided in high-risk patients, such as those with a history of ulcer disease, those on concurrent oral corticosteroids, history of gastrointestinal bleeding, congestive heart failure, or renal insufficiency. Nonacetylated salicylates (Arthropan), salsalate (Disalcid), choline magnesium trisalicylate (Trilisate), or renal-sparing NSAIDs such as sulindac may have a role in the treatment of these patients.

Injectable Corticosteroids

Injectable corticosteroids have been a part of the therapeutic armamentarium since they were introduced by Hollander and colleagues in the 1950s.[129] Despite the frequency of their use and the length of experience with them, there is little literature to guide the physician about the optimal corticosteroid preparation, appropriate frequency of dosage, and length of treatment. In addition, there are few well-controlled studies documenting their efficacy. Concern also persists about the possible deleterious effects of these medications on cartilage.

Corticosteroids inhibit phospholipase A2 expression, which blocks the cyclooxygenase and lipoxygenase pathways.[74] This is likely their main mechanism of action, although they also affect ribonucleic acid protein synthesis and cellular metabolism.[15]

A variety of injectable corticosteroids are available. Their duration of action appears to be related to the solubility of the compound.[15] Hydrocortisone acetate is absorbed rapidly from the knee (half-life, 1 to 2 hours) and provides only a few days of relief; triamcinolone hexacetonide is the longest acting, with a half-life of several weeks.[58]

Systemic absorption of these compounds from the joint can occur. Suppression of the hypothalamic-pituitary axis is possible if multiple joints are injected or if injections are given at close intervals.[210] Decreased serum cortisol levels have been noted from even a single intra-articular injection.[160] Suppression of the hypothalamic-pituitary axis does not persist for more than 2 days and adrenocorticosteroid secretion returns to normal in 3 to 6 days.[149] Systemic absorption is rarely a clinical problem.

Hollander[126] originally reported on 231 patients who received corticosteroid injections over a period of 20 years in 1953. Of those patients, 87% reported complete relief of pain. Since then, a recent systematic review[121] has found only six level I trials in five reports (279 total knees)[59,91,95,136,237] comparing intra-articular corticosteroid injections with placebo. A more broadly defined Cochrane review has found 28 trials (1973 total knees) comparing intra-articular corticosteroid against placebo, intra-articular hyaluronan and hylan (HA) products, joint lavage, and other intra-articular corticosteroids.[18]

The results of both reviews demonstrated a short-term benefit to intra-articular corticosteroid injections versus placebo. At week 1, all studies demonstrated approximately a one-third decrease in pain as measured by the Visual Analogue Scale (VAS) that was statistically significant. Functional improvement was also noted in the corticosteroid group. Between 2 and 3 weeks, there was inconsistent evidence for pain reduction. At 4 to 24 weeks, no statistically significant difference in pain or functional status was noted in any of the analyzed studies. Both reviews concluded that intra-articular corticosteroid injections were associated with a clinically important improvement in pain 1 week after injection, but with little evidence for longer term benefit. Triamcinolone was used in most trials, but methylprednisolone and betamethasone were also used. Data were inconclusive with regard to the efficacy of one form of corticosteroid over another.

Recognized complications from corticosteroid injections include intra-articular infection and inflammatory flair.[110,111] Intra-articular infection is extremely rare, even when rigorous aseptic technique is not used. The incidence is estimated at 0.01% to 0.005%.[256] Postinjection flair is far more common, with an incidence of 2% to 5%. Inflammation occurs within hours of injection. It is a neutrophil-dependent inflammatory

Table 92-1 Clinicians Guide to Anti-Inflammatory Therapy

Cardiovascular Risk	NSAID GASTROINTESTINAL RISK	
	None or Low	**Risk Present**
None (without aspirin)	Nonselective NSAID (cost consideration)	COX-2 selective or nonselective inhibitor; NSAID + proton pump inhibitor; COX-2 selective inhibitor + proton pump inhibitor for those with prior GI bleeding
Cardiovascular risk (with aspirin)	Naproxen*; addition of proton pump inhibitor if GI risk of aspirin-NSAID combination warrants gastroprotection	Proton-pump inhibitor irrespective of NSAID; naproxen if cardiovascular risk outweights GI risk; COX-2 selective inhibitor + proton pump inhibitor for those with previous GI bleeding

Adapted from Scheiman JM, Fendrick AM: Summing the risk of NSAID therapy. Lancet 369:1580–1581, 2007.

response, most likely caused by the corticosteroid crystals themselves.[184] It is almost always self-limited, resolving within 1 to 3 days.

Dark-skinned individuals may have local discoloration of the skin from subcutaneous injection, which may be permanent.[206] This cosmetic discoloration is not serious, but can lead to considerable consternation on the part of the patient and therefore should be a part of informed consent. Temporary disturbances may include an elevated blood sugar level, arterial hypertension, and facial flushing.[137,216] One should caution diabetic patients about the potential glucose level elevations to heighten their vigilance after injection.

Effects on Cartilage

The evidence for the effects of injected corticosteroids on cartilage metabolism is mixed. Corticosteroids are potent inhibitors of anabolic and catabolic processes in cartilage. As with NSAIDs, interpretation of animal data is difficult because of the species-specific response to these compounds. Weekly injections into rabbit joints has produced histologic and macroscopic evidence of cartilage degeneration and depressed synthesis of collagen and proteoglycan.[16,195] Weight-bearing joints were more strongly affected. On the other hand, injection of corticosteroid provided significant protection from cartilage breakdown in secondary arthritis in rabbits.[36,196] Similar protective effects have been noted in primates and dogs.[107,220,222,303] An in vitro study of human chondrocytes has demonstrated that dexamethasone administration decreases proteoglycan concentration.[269] Whether inhibition of anabolic or catabolic functions predominates in humans is unknown.

Anecdotal reports linking intra-articular corticosteroid therapy with accelerated joint destruction have not been substantiated by clinical experience or historical data. Even in those uncontrolled reports, this was a rare occurrence.[109,110,144,306] Historical data covering over 330,000 injections have put the incidence of this complication at less than 1%, which is well within the realm of coincidence.[10] Nevertheless, given the possibility of a deleterious effect on the joint, most practitioners are reluctant to inject a joint more frequently than every 4 to 6 weeks. Our current practice is, at most, every 3 months.

Theoretically, pain masking may lead to overuse and subsequent accelerated breakdown. Therefore, some recommend a period of joint rest after corticosteroid injection.[127,183,205] In rheumatoid arthritis patients, those who had a period of rest after triamcinolone hexacetonide injection experienced a longer period of relief than ambulatory patients. In animal studies, articular cartilage damage produced by corticosteroids in meniscectomized rabbits seemed to be potentiated by exercise.[195]

In summary, intra-articular corticosteroid therapy is appropriate as a stopgap measure for acute pain in osteoarthritis. It should only be considered as a long-term treatment for patients in whom it is effective and other regimens have failed. It appears prudent for patients to rest for a time immediately following injection.

Chondroprotective Agents

Attention has focused on the development of agents or interventions that could actually slow or reverse the progression of disease. Such agents are called chondroprotective agents, or disease-modifying osteoarthritis drugs (DMOADs). Although no agreed on definition exits, Ghosh and Brooks have proposed that a chondroprotective agent should do the following: (1) enhance chondrocyte macromolecule synthesis; (2) enhance synthesis of hyaluronan; (3) inhibit degradative enzymes; (4) mobilize deposits of thrombin, fibrin, lipids, and cholesterol in vessels surrounding the joint; (5) reduce joint pain; and (6) reduce joint synovitis.[105] With these guidelines in mind, we will examine the scientific evidence for several agents.

Hyaluronic Acid

Hyaluronic acid (HA), also referred to as hyaluronate or hyaluronan, is a key constituent of cartilage ground substance and synovial fluid. It is composed of continuously repeating sequences of glucuronic acid and N-acetylglucosamine. Type B synovial cells synthesize and secrete it into the joint space. It has several important roles in the viscous and elastic properties of synovial fluid. The precise mechanism of action remains elusive. HA is believed to provide joint lubrication and shock absorbancy,[223] promote chondrocyte proliferation and differentiation,[143] and stabilize proteoglycan structure.[131,267]

Early OA is characterized by loss and degradation of hyaluronic acid from cartilage and synthesis of lower molecular weight hyaluronic acid by synoviocytes.[297] As a pharmacologic agent, anti-inflammatory, antinociceptive, and cartilage anabolic effects have been ascribed to hyaluronic acid.[102,103] Thus, the purpose of HA injection in patients with mild to moderate OA is not only to act as an analgesic, but also to increase the viscosity of synovial fluid and promote endogenous HA production.[8]

Intra-articular hyaluronic acid has been used in veterinary practice for at least 30 years. Beneficial effects have been noted in several different species, including horses and dogs.[7,35,97,247] Experience in human subjects began in 1974, when Peyron and Balazs[226] reported a beneficial effect of intra-articular hyaluronic acid in a double-blind, placebo-controlled study of 28 patients. Since then, many clinical studies, including some prospective, randomized, controlled studies, have lent credence to the assertion that injected hyaluronic acid has a beneficial effect in OA. Despite this lengthy and sustained clinical and laboratory interest in hyaluronate as a possible treatment for osteoarthritis, its use and efficacy remain controversial.[51-53,103,147] The AAOS guidelines for nonarthroplasty treatment of OA of the knee failed to recommend for or against the use of intra-articular HA, citing inconclusive evidence.[240]

Human data on the efficacy of HA injection can be divided into basic science and clinical efficacy studies. Several basic science studies have tried to investigate the tissue and disease-modifying properties of injected hyaluronic acid. In a pilot study of 40 patients treated with 20 mg of Hyalgan interarticularly, once weekly for 5 weeks, Frizziero and coworkers[93] found that 30% of patients had morphologic improvement in cartilage and synovial membranes as compared with baseline. Improvements included reconstitution of the superficial amorphous layer, improvements in chondrocyte density and vitality, and reduction in synovial inflammation. However, 60% of patients showed no improvement, 7% worsened, and there was no placebo control group in the study. In a small randomized but unblinded study of hyaluronan injection versus standard therapies, Listrat and associates[171] found less deterioration in structural parameters of cartilage evaluated by arthroscopy in the study group. Bagga and coworkers[8] demonstrated a 13% increase in synovial fluid HA and a 16% increase in the complex shear modulus 3 months after injection of Hylan GF-20, suggesting a stimulating effect of HA injection on endogenous HA production.

Interpretation of clinical efficacy studies on HA injection is confounded by differing study designs, injection regimens, outcomes evaluation criteria and, importantly, failure to control for concurrent NSAID use. Furthermore, it is well recognized that the placebo effect becomes more pronounced as the therapy becomes more invasive. Given that there are more than 75 RCTs investigating the effects of hyaluronic acid and hylan derivatives in the treatment of knee OA, the use of meta-analyses becomes an important tool to determine the efficacy of HA. Presently, there are five published meta-analyses that review the literature.[6,19,172,192,296]

Each meta-analysis reviewed similar papers and many of the same trials were used in each analysis. All levels of OA severity were included in patients between 55 and 75 years of age. A validated outcome measure was used, such as the VAS, WOMAC, Lequesne, or numeric rating scale. Observation periods varied, but typically did not exceed 52 weeks. Most studies analyzed in the meta-analyses used lower molecular weight Hyalgan, but all FDA-approved HA products were included in the analysis.

Lo and associates[172] performed the first meta-analysis evaluating the efficacy of HA. They observed a small improvement in pain compared with placebo; the effect size was comparable to that observed with NSAID administration. Wang and coworkers[296] performed a similar analysis and came to the same conclusions as Lo's group. They also noted that studies with lower methodologic quality resulted in higher estimates of HA efficacy. In the analysis by Arrich and colleagues,[6] significant improvement in rest pain and exercise pain were noted between 10 and 30 weeks post-treatment, but the authors suggested that the findings were inconclusive because of excessive heterogeneity in the data. Modawal and colleagues[192] determined the causes of heterogeneity among the data in their meta-analysis using random effect regression models. Quality of the study, pain, and form of HA used were the three causes, with study quality being predominant. The lowest quality studies were eliminated and heterogeneity was improved, allowing the authors to conclude that HA is moderately effective in relieving rest pain between 5 to 12 weeks when compared with placebo. Bellamy and associates[19] performed the largest meta-analysis and obtained similar results to the previous meta-analysis, with improvements in rest and weight-bearing pain, particularly between 5 and 13 weeks. Notably, no meta-analysis was able to differentiate between lower and higher molecular weight HA preparations.

Intra-articular HA is generally well tolerated, but problems may arise occasionally. Infection is a small risk and, although not specifically reported, may be assumed to be of the same magnitude as that reported for corticosteroid injection. A local inflammatory reaction is a more frequent occurrence.[3,209] The incidence can be as low as 3%.[174] One study reported local inflammation with 11% of injections and 27% of patients; occurrence was unpredictable and symptoms lasted up to 3 weeks.[232] Three of the five meta-analysis

discussed adverse effects. Wang and coworkers[296] noted three major adverse effects among the 1002 injected knees—an episode of severe knee swelling, a vasculitis, and a hypersensitivity reaction. The relative risk of minor adverse events was 1.19 and included transient mild increases in local pain or swelling.

Despite the wealth of positive clinical and laboratory evidence, the question of the efficacy of injected hyaluronates remains to be resolved. No evidence exists to support the use of one commercially available preparation over another, nor is the optimal dosage, injection regimen, or patient selection criteria known at this time.

Glucosamine

Popular books[275] and media articles have drawn attention to the use of oral glucosamine sulfate as treatment for osteoarthritis. Glucosamine has been shown in culture studies dating back to the 1950s to enhance secretion of mucopolysaccharides in cartilage-derived fibroblasts. As early as 1994, McCarty[185] advocated intensified research into the use of glucosamine as a treatment for arthritis, citing animal and human studies that demonstrated a beneficial effect on the prevention and treatment of arthritis. Support for the use of glucosamine increased in the popular media and scientific circles, culminating in the glucosamine-chondroitin Arthritis Intervention Trial of 2006, a blinded, randomized, and placebo-controlled trial.[45]

Rationale for Glucosamine

Glucosamine is a simple amino sugar that serves as a substrate for the synthesis of glycosaminoglycans and hyaluronic acid. Glucosamine is synthesized directly by the chondrocyte but, when supplemented, can be used directly to synthesize larger macromolecules. Most preparations are derived from chitin in crustacean shells. In in vitro and animal models, a wide variety of effects have been documented. These can be broadly classified as substrate, transcriptional, antireactive, and antiarthritic effects.

As far back as 1956, Roden[243] noted an increased production of glycosaminoglycans and collagen when glucosamine sulfate was added to cartilage-derived fibroblast cell cultures. Other studies have confirmed this effect.[293,294] Karzel and Domenjoz[141] later demonstrated that glucosamine sulfate was efficiently incorporated into mucopolysaccharides. These studies demonstrated a specific effect; N-acetylglucosamine was far less active and glucuronic acid had no effect.[154]

In addition to functioning as a simple substrate, other studies have shown glucosamine to affect gene transcription within the chondrocyte. Jimenez and coworkers[135] have demonstrated a twofold increase in perlecan and aggrecan mRNA levels and a moderate increase in stromelysine mRNA in chondrocyte cultures incubated with 50 μM glucosamine. They also found a dose-dependent downregulation of metalloproteinase I and II (enzymes important in the degradation of cartilage) mRNA in the same model.

Glucosamine may be more effective in upregulating cartilage metabolism in arthritic or stressed cartilage. Lippiello and colleagues[167] found an increase in GAG synthesis in arthritic cartilage explants under various types of stress when exposed to glucosamine compared with young or nonstressed explants. Looking at a biologic marker of type II cartilage degradation, Christgau and associates[43] determined that those patients with higher rates of cartilage turnover (higher levels of cross-linked telopeptide type II collagen [CTX-II] in the urine) benefited the most from glucosamine supplementation.

Glucosamine increases the synovial production of HA, which has itself been shown to have anti-inflammatory effects, induce anabolic activity in chondrocytes, decrease joint pain, and increase mobility in vivo and in clinical studies.[185] Animal studies have demonstrated an antireactive effect of glucosamine, finding that glucosamine prevents an inflammatory response to certain irritants known to cause inflammation in rats, but has no inhibitory effects on inflammation caused by inflammatory mediators such as bradykinin, serotonin, or histamine.[260] Specifically, and importantly, glucosamine did not show any inhibition of the cyclooxygenase system, thus lending some credibility to the claim of GI tolerability. In fact, glucosamine may stimulate the production of protective mucopolysaccharides in the gastric mucosa and therefore may be useful in ulcer therapy.[193]

An antiarthritic effect of glucosamine has been demonstrated in animal models for inflammatory arthritis, mechanical arthritis, immunoreactive arthritis, and generalized inflammation. Efficacy in these models was lower than with indomethacin, but toxicity was significantly lower, so the overall therapeutic margin was much more favorable. Therefore, glucosamine may have a place in the therapy of inflammatory arthritis in addition to OA.[260]

Human Studies

Contrary to belief in the United States, glucosamine sulfate has been heavily studied in human arthritis sufferers over the past 30 years. Studies have been performed in many countries, including Italy,[49] Germany,[24,65,68,201] Spain,[173] Portugal,[273] China,[233] and the Philippines.[231] Subjects suffered from arthritis of the hand, spine, shoulders, hips, and knees. The results were consistent; all studies showed a beneficial effect of the study drug. Improvement in pain occurred slowly over a period of several weeks. Subjects continued to improve while taking the study drug as compared with patients taking placebo, who did not. Subjects also maintained improvement for weeks to months after the drug was discontinued. Response to treatment was high, ranging from 56% to over 90%. Equally important, no study encountered significant side effects with glucosamine. Early clinical uncontrolled trials performed in Germany beginning in 1969 used an injectable form, and a dosage of 400 mg/day. Injections were intra-articular, intramuscular, or intravenous. All studies reported diminution of pain, some improvement of mobility, and no significant side effects.[284] Interest in glucosamine accelerated in Europe with the synthesis of an easily absorbable oral preparation. Since the early 1980s, numerous controlled studies, including a number of double-blind studies,* have been carried out. Of these, at least five double-blind, single-joint, placebo-controlled studies using a validated outcome tool have been performed.[200,207,217,238,239]

Criticism of the older literature on glucosamine has centered on the small numbers of patients studied, short time periods of those studies, and relative lack of studies independent of corporate sponsorship. Methodologic concerns,

specifically the failure of most studies to control for NSAID use specifically, have also been raised.[148] Meta-analyses have generally supported the use of glucosamine. Towheed and coworkers[277] evaluated 16 RCTs, 12 comparing glucosamine to placebo and 4 comparing it to an NSAID. It was concluded that glucosamine is both safe and effective. McAlindon and colleagues[182] reviewed six studies of glucosamine involving 911 patients. Quality scores for these studies ranged from 12% to 52%. Combined results showed a moderate treatment effect of glucosamine. Of the six meta-analyses published on the subject, five supported a mild treatment effect[162,182,229,241,278] and one reported no difference to placebo.[21]

Interest in glucosamine has been tempered somewhat since the publication of the GAIT study.[45] In this large, multicenter, randomized, placebo-controlled study, 1583 patients suffering with osteoarthritis of the knee were randomized to glucosamine, 1500 mg/day; chondroitin, 1200 mg/day; glucosamine-chondroitin in combination, celecoxib, 200 mg/day; or placebo. Aceteominophen, up to 4000 mg/day, was used as a rescue medication. Both glucosamine and chondroitin showed a decrease in pain levels from baseline, but not significantly greater than placebo and not as much as celecoxib, which was significantly greater than placebo. However, in patients with moderate to severe pain, the response to combined glucosamine-chondroitin therapy was significantly greater than placebo (79.2% vs. 54.3%; $P > .002$)

Chondroitin

Several other amino sugars or glycosaminoglycans are commercially available for the treatment of osteoarthritis. These include chondroitin sulfate, glycosaminoglycan-peptide association complex (Rumalon), glycosaminoglycan (GAG) polysulfuric acid (GAGPS; Arteparon), and sodium pentosan polysulfate (Cartrofen). Although these compounds enjoy some laboratory and clinical support, they have not gained the popularity, nor been as well studied as glucosamine or hyaluronic acid.

Chondroitin sulfate (galactosaminoglycuronoglycan sulfate) is a mucopolysaccharide, which together with keratan sulfate and a protein core forms aggrecan. Aggrecan, in turn, associates with hyaluronan to form a hydroscopic macromolecule largely responsible for the physical elasticity of cartilage. During aging, the ratio of keratan sulfate to chondroitin sulfate in aggrecan increases, reflecting a relative loss of chondroitin. Also, chondroitin sulfate from diseased cartilage is shorter in length than normal.[31]

As a pharmaceutical, chondroitin exhibits anti-inflammatory properties similar to those of other glycosaminoglycans and GAG precursors.[9] In humans it is well tolerated and has few side effects and reasonable bioavailability.[245] Also, like other GAG precursors, stimulatory effects on cartilage have been reported.[142] Chondroitin sulfate has also been shown to neutralize catabolic processes, such as interleukin-1 (IL-1) production and metalloprotease activation in human OA chondrocyte tissue culture.[181]

Several RCTs demonstrating a beneficial effect of chondroitin sulfate have been published.*

Morreale and associates,[194] in a rigorous study comparing chondroitin to diclofenac, found a more rapid response to

---

*References 49, 64, 118, 173, 231, 233, and 284.

*References 27, 33, 248, 282, 283, and 289.

diclofenac, but a more profound and long-lasting response to chondroitin. The chondroitin group maintained their symptomatic improvement 3 weeks after discontinuation of the drug, whereas symptoms in patients treated with diclofenac returned immediately after cessation of therapy.

There is even some credible evidence that chondroitin alters the course of disease in humans. Studying 120 patients with knee OA, Uebelhart and coworkers[281] found the group given chondroitin sulfate had better functional outcomes and less joint space narrowing on standard radiographs at 1 year compared with controls. Verbruggen and colleagues[290] have also reported on two studies in which patients with erosive arthritis of the hand suffered less progression and fewer new lesions when given chondroitin than the control group.

Glucosamine-Chondroitin Synergy

Looking back to the definition of a chondroprotective agent supplied by Ghosh and Brooks,[105] it is clear that neither glucosamine alone nor chondroitin alone satisfy all the criteria. Because they both act through different mechanisms, it is reasonable to suppose that they could have a synergistic effect (Table 92-2). Lippiello and associates[169] published a dramatic study of a rabbit instability model of knee OA. They compared glucosamine alone, chondroitin alone, the combination, and the carrier. Although a chondroprotective effect of both glucosamine and chondroitin was noted, the combination almost completely prevented the onset of OA (Figs. 92-1 to 92-3).

For the same reasons as glucosamine, enthusiasm for chondroitin waned after publication of the GAIT trial. Recently, in its treatment guidelines for the nonoperative management of osteoarthritis, the AAOS has recommended against the use of both glucosamine and chondroitin.[2]

Dangers of "Nutraceuticals"

Most of the studies cited were performed in countries in which glucosamine and chondroitin are considered pharmaceuticals and are regulated accordingly. In the United States, these substances are considered nutritional supplements and

Table 92-2 Postulated Synergistic Mechanism Between Glucosamine and Chondroitin Sulfate

Chondroprotective Agent	Characteristics
Glucosamine	Stimulates chondrocyte and synoviocyte metabolism
Chondroitin sulfate	Inhibits degradative enzymes; prevents fibrin thrombi in periarticular tissues

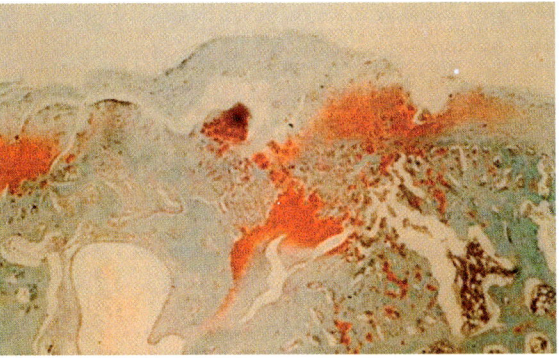
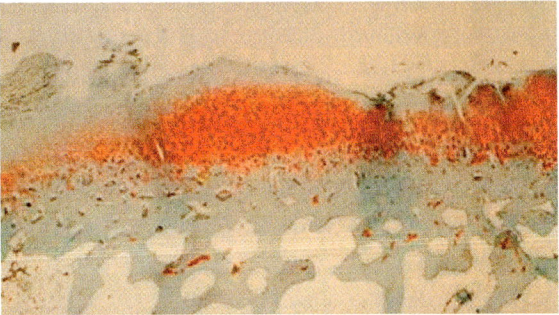
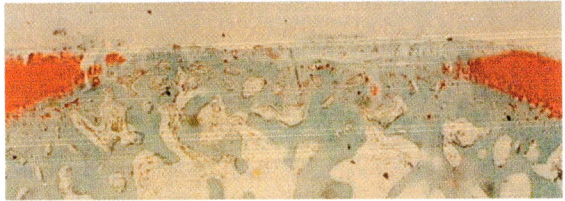

Figure 92-2. Cross section of an experimental animal treated with placebo. Extensive loss of glycosaminoglycan and cartilage destruction can be noted (safranin O).

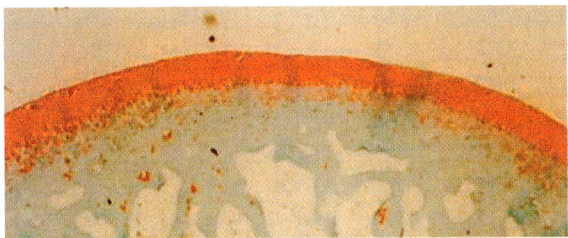

Figure 92-1. Cross section of normal rabbit femoral condyle. Cartilage is of normal thickness and shows normal glycosaminoglycan staining (safranin O).

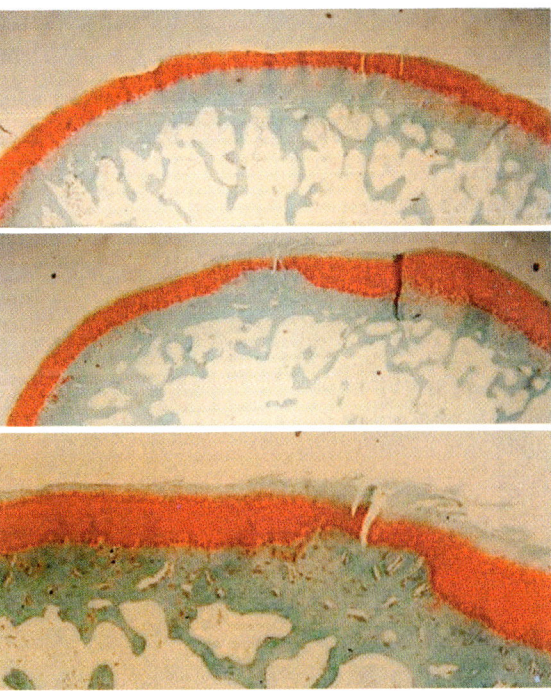

Figure 92-3. Experimental animal treated with a glucosamine-chondroitin combination. Cartilage shows near-perfect preservation (safranin O).

are therefore not regulated by the FDA. The nutritional supplement industry is regulated by the Dietary Supplement Health Education Act, which simply requires that the percentage of active ingredients match claims on the label. There is no requirement for safety, efficacy, or bioavailability of the product. Reports have cast doubt that even the percentage claimed on the label is accurate. Furthermore, two studies have shown that high-molecular-weight chondroitin sulfate is poorly absorbed and much less permeable into the chondrocyte.[4,42] Until the FDA takes a more serious position on these agents, it will be incumbent on the physician to investigate the purity and efficacy of individual formulations before recommending them to patients.

Other agents primarily directed at inhibiting enzymatic or inflammatory cartilage destruction are being investigated. These include bovine superoxide dismutase (Orgotein), IL-1receptor antagonists, S-adenosyl methionine,* and sodium pentosan polysulfate (Cartrofen). Although some encouraging data have been presented,[†] these compounds should be considered investigational at this time.

KEY REFERENCES

American Academy of Orthopaedic Surgeons (AAOS): Treatment of osteoarthritis of the knee (nonarthroplasty), Rosemont, Ill, 2008, American Academy of Orthopaedic Surgeons.

Bellamy N, Campbell J, Robinson V, et al: Intra-articular corticosteroid for treatment of osteoarthritis of the knee. Cochrane Database Syst Rev, (2):CD005328, 2006.

Bellamy N, Campbell J, Robinson V, et al: Viscosupplementation for the treatment of osteoarthritis of the knee. Cochrane Database Syst Rev, (2):CD005321, 2006.

---

*References 12, 108, 117, 151, 157, 175, 199, 218, 228, and 292.
†References 11, 39, 89, 90, 104, 106, 150, 204, 219, 244, 252, 268, and 291.

Brandt KD, Palmoski MJ: Effects of salicylates and other nonsteroidal anti-inflammatory drugs on articular cartilage. Am J Med 77:65–69, 1984.

Davies-Tuck ML, Wluka AE, Wang Y, et al: The natural history of cartilage defects in people with knee osteoarthritis. Osteoarthritis Cartilage 16:337–342, 2008.

Felson DT, Anderson JJ, Naimarck A, et al: Obesity and knee osteoarthritis-the Framingham study. Ann Intern Med 109:18–24, 1988.

Hepper CT, Halvorson JJ, Duncan ST, et al: The efficacy and duration of intra-articular corticosteroid injection for knee osteoarthritis: a systematic review of level I studies. J Am Acad Orthop Surg 17:638–646, 2009.

Huang WF, Hsiao FY, Wen YW, Tsai YW: Cardiovascular events associated with the use of four nonselective NSAIDs (etodolac, nabumetone, ibuprofen, or naproxen) versus a cyclooxygenase-2 inhibitor (celecoxib): a population-based analysis in Taiwanese adults. Clin Ther 28:1827–1836, 2006.

Lawrence RC., Felson DT, Helmick CG, et al: Estimates of the prevalence of arthritis and other rheumatic conditions in the United States. Part II. Arthritis Rheumatism 58:26–35, 2008.

Pelletier JP, Martel-Pelletier J: The pathophysiology of osteoarthritis and the implication of the use of hyaluronan and hylan as therapeutic agents in viscosupplementation. J Rheumatol Suppl 39:19–24, 1993.

Smalley WE, Ray WA, Daugherty J, Griffin MR: Nonsteroidal anti-inflammatory drugs and the incidence of hospitalizations for peptic ulcer disease in older persons. Am J Epidemiol 141:539–545, 1995.

Superio-Cabuslay E, Ward MM, Lorig KR: Patient education interventions in osteoarthritis and rheumatoid arthritis: a meta-analytic comparison with nonsteroidal antiinflammatory drug treatment. Arthritis Care Res 9:292–301, 1996.

Wang CT, Lin J, Chang CJ, et al: Therapeutic effects of hyaluronic acid on osteoarthritis of the knee. A meta-analysis of randomized controlled trials. J Bone Joint Surg Am 86:538–545, 2004.

Zhang W, Moskowitz RW, Nuki G, et al: OARSI recommendations for the management of hip and knee osteoarthritis. Part I: Critical appraisal of existing treatment guidelines and systematic review of current research evidence. Osteoarthritis Cartilage 15:981–1000, 2007.

Zhang W, Moskowitz RW, Nuki G, et al: OARSI recommendations for the management of hip and knee osteoarthritis. Part II: OARSI evidence-based, expert consensus guidelines. Osteoarthritis Cartilage 16:137–162, 2008.

Full references for this chapter can be found on www.expertconsult.com.

Chapter 93

Scoring Systems and Their Validation for the Arthritic Knee

Adam C. Brekke, Philip C. Noble, Brian S. Parsley, and Kennith B. Mathis

Chapter 94

Osteotomy About the Knee: American Perspective

James M. Leone and Arlen D. Hanssen

The purpose of realignment osteotomy about an arthritic knee is to transfer weight-bearing forces from the arthritic portion of the knee to a healthier location in the knee joint.[21] This redistribution of mechanical force to increase the life span of the knee joint distinguishes osteotomy from other treatment modalities of arthritic knees.[37] The prevalence of realignment osteotomy has steadily declined because of the success of total knee replacement (TKR) and the recent resurgence of enthusiasm for unicompartmental knee replacement.[13,67,97] Despite this rather significant decline, osteotomy about the knee remains a viable treatment option in carefully selected patients with knee arthritis.[6,40,83,84] The use of osteotomy has increased in patients who are undergoing other surgical procedures such as cartilage or meniscal transplantation or ligamentous reconstruction.[12,17,62,94] Over the past decade, interest has exploded in the areas of developing modifications of surgical technique,[7,49,52] new surgical instrumentation,[16,31] and new fixation devices,[93,95] along with the use of external fixation devices[1,85,104] and computed tomography (CT)-free navigation systems aimed at improving the accuracy, reliability, and safety of realignment osteotomy.[47]

Goals of osteotomy include pain relief, functional improvement, and the capacity to maintain heavy functional demands otherwise precluded by prosthetic replacement. Alternative procedures should be compared with current standards of osteotomy and not with historical controls, because patients currently undergoing osteotomy are generally considered worst-case scenarios for a successful long-term outcome with prosthetic replacement. The key to success after osteotomy is careful patient selection combined with skillful surgical technique.

PATIENT SELECTION PROCESS

The process of patient selection is possibly the single most important factor in obtaining a successful result after osteotomy. Thorough synthesis of multiple variables is required to formulate the decision to proceed with osteotomy (Box 94-1). The primary indications for osteotomy include pain relief for degenerative arthritis associated with malalignment or the need for mechanical axis correction in conjunction with ligamentous reconstruction or transplantation of cartilage or meniscal allografts. It is often helpful to start by focusing on the relative and absolute contraindications to corrective osteotomy during the patient selection process (Box 94-2).

Historical Variables

The ideal candidate for osteotomy is a thin, active individual in the fifth or sixth decade of life with localized, activity-related unicompartmental knee pain, no patellofemoral symptoms, a stable knee, and full knee extension with flexion of at least 90 degrees.[37,72] Although many patients do not meet all of these ideal guidelines, a careful selection process will optimize clinical outcomes.

Emphasis on the location and character of pain, the desired activity level, and appropriate patient expectations is particularly important when osteotomy is considered. Diffuse and nonspecific knee pain reduces the chance for a successful outcome after osteotomy. Although it was previously believed that symptoms related to knee instability precluded osteotomy, the practice of treating malalignment in conjunction with concomitant ligamentous reconstruction is becoming increasingly common. Interested readers are referred elsewhere in this textbook for more information on the treatment of young active patients with malalignment and instability. An elderly patient with degenerative arthritis and instability would be optimally treated by TKR rather than osteotomy.[42]

Patients with osteoarthritis fare better than those with rheumatoid arthritis, and realignment osteotomy for inflammatory disorders is not recommended.[23] In the presence of secondary degenerative arthritis from a previous fracture, osteochondritis dissecans, or a prior medial meniscectomy, the results of osteotomy do not seem to be adversely affected, whereas patients who have undergone combined medial and lateral meniscectomy have disappointing outcomes.[68,87]

Degenerative arthritis of the patellofemoral joint has long been cited as a cause of failure after corrective osteotomy.[42] Conversely, long-term studies have shown a low incidence of unsatisfactory results attributed to the patellofemoral joint, and it is possible that realignment of the extremity may favorably alter patellofemoral mechanics inasmuch as it has been demonstrated that patellofemoral pain can improve after upper tibial osteotomy.[27,35] Significant retropatellar pain should be a cautionary factor during patient selection, but mild retropatellar pain should not preclude osteotomy if the primary indication for osteotomy is unicompartmental tibiofemoral pain.[35]

Age assessment requires consideration of physiologic status and lifestyle requirements. Many younger and sedentary patients may be better served by arthroplasty, whereas some elderly and active patients may be better suited for osteotomy. Arthroplasty provides more complete pain relief and shorter rehabilitation and is more reliable than osteotomy in most individuals older than 60 years.[42] It has been proposed that unicompartmental knee replacement is an ideal temporizing procedure for middle-aged patients in preference to osteotomy.[78,97] Others who believe that unicompartmental knee replacement remains a prosthetic arthroplasty option that should not be considered a direct alternative to osteotomy are concerned about increased complications in young, active patients with prosthetic implants.[37,82,84,100]

Box 94-1 Selection Factors for Realignment Osteotomy

Historical

Age
  Chronological
  Physiologic
Patient's desired activity level
Pain
  Location
  Character
    • Patellofemoral?
Rheumatologic status
Previous meniscectomy
Infection history

Radiologic

Anatomic axis
Mechanical axis
Severity of arthrosis
Magnitude of deformity
Tibiofemoral subluxation
Status of other compartments
Joint space opening
Amount of articular cartilage
  loss
Calcium pyrophosphate
  deposition
Osseous defects
Deformities away from the joint
Joint line obliquity

Examination

Malalignment
  Magnitude
  Direction
Previous incisions
Body habitus
Range of motion
  Total arc
  Flexion contracture
Ligamentous deficiencies
Patellofemoral mechanics
Adductor thrust

Miscellaneous

Patient expectations
Surgeon capabilities
Dynamic gait factors
  Soft tissue tension
  Upper body shift
Potential complications
Postoperative recovery
Immobilization time
Durability of the procedure
Ease of revision to total knee
  arthroplasty

Box 94-2 Contraindications to Corrective Osteotomy

Absolute

Diffuse, nonspecific knee pain
Primary complaint of patellofemoral pain
Meniscectomy in the compartment intended for weight bearing
Arthrosis in the compartment intended for weight bearing
Underlying diagnosis of inflammatory disease
Unrealistic patient expectations

Relative

Age older than 60 years
Range-of-motion arc less than 90 degrees
Obesity (1.3 × ideal body weight)
Severe arthrosis
Tibiofemoral subluxation
Moderate or severe ligamentous instability

Examination

Ipsilateral hip function should always be assessed, and if hip surgery is required, it should be completed before realignment osteotomy. Limb inspection should confirm the presence of axial malalignment and should assess for the presence of lateral thrust because it is a potential risk factor for a poor clinical outcome.[77] In patients with high adduction moments, if sufficient correction of alignment is achieved at surgery, these moments of the knee do not seem to correlate with the clinical outcome.[102]

Previous skin incisions, which may affect the intended surgical exposure, should be noted. Knee motion should reveal a flexion arc of at least 90 degrees with less than 10 to 20 degrees of flexion contracture; however, these criteria have been established only by clinical convention. Patellofemoral symptoms or significant meniscal pathology should not be the primary cause of the patient's complaints, and every effort must be pursued to differentiate the potential sources of pain. It is imperative that the neurovascular status of the intended surgical limb be accurately assessed preoperatively and documented accordingly.

It cannot be overemphasized that osteotomy is technically more difficult in obese patients, particularly those with peripheral dystrophic weight distribution. Obesity has been associated with lower success rates after high tibial osteotomy (HTO) because the surgical technique and postoperative immobilization are more difficult in these individuals.[27] The long-term clinical results are worse in individuals who exceed

their ideal body weight by 1.32 times.[27] The activity level of these patients should be carefully assessed because sedentary, overweight individuals of any age may be better served by prosthetic replacement. It should be stressed that significant weight loss may provide enough symptomatic relief to defer any operative intervention.

Counseling

The surgeon needs to discuss all treatment alternatives and to convey that neither osteotomy nor arthroplasty provides a "normal joint." The long-term results, rehabilitation, pain relief, and durability of realignment osteotomy and arthroplasty should be specified for the patient. A longer postoperative recovery period with less pain relief after rehabilitation is expected after osteotomy. These disadvantages need to be balanced against the possible catastrophic complications of infection or prosthetic failure with arthroplasty in a young and active patient.[6,90,100]

Specifically, realignment osteotomy is based on the concept that certain high-impact and excessive loading activities are not sanctioned with prosthetic arthroplasty.[37] Functional analysis of young patients after osteotomy reveals that many are able to participate in running and jumping activities that probably would damage a knee prosthesis.[6,69,75] Many patients also value the real potential for technological advances in arthroplasty over the expected survival period of an osteotomy and recognize that "buying time" with an osteotomy is a viable concept.

The expected results of TKR after osteotomy should be considered and discussed with the patient. Potential technical obstacles encountered include difficulty with exposure,[106] bony deficiencies necessitating grafts or wedges, difficulty in attaining ligament balance,[73] prolonged operative times,[36] and increased blood loss.[44,45,54] Other authors have noted no significant differences in the technical difficulty or outcome of TKR after HTO.[64,79,91] Poorer long-term radiographic results of TKR after HTO occur in a specific subset of patients.[76] These patients are younger, heavier, and more active males who are also at risk for early wear of prosthetic components. A well-performed osteotomy in these patients seems reasonable if the goal is to postpone prosthetic replacement to a later stage in their lives, when their activity level and age favor a decrease in the likelihood that they will require multiple revision surgeries. The literature detailing poor results of arthroplasty after osteotomy clearly indicates that technical difficulties or complications associated with osteotomy produce worse results with the subsequent arthroplasty.[15,106] Surgeons with only occasional experience performing corrective osteotomy should consider referral because a suboptimal surgical technique that may compromise subsequent procedures should not be the sole criterion used to abandon osteotomy.

Other important variables in this patient population also portend a poor result. Factors that prognosticate a worse outcome in HTO patients ($P < .01$) include (1) workers' compensation claim, (2) history of reflex sympathetic dystrophy after HTO, (3) early onset (within 1 year) or no period of relief of pain after HTO, (4) multiple surgeries before HTO, and (5) occupation as a laborer.[66]

Radiographic Evaluation

The location and severity of arthritis are determined by standing anteroposterior, lateral, intercondylar notch, and skyline patellar views. One should carefully inspect the contralateral tibiofemoral compartment for marginal osteophytes, which indicate the presence of diffuse arthritis. Tibiofemoral subluxation, excessive bony erosion, and diffuse arthritic involvement are associated with poorer outcomes. A full-length, 51×14-inch, weight-bearing radiograph is necessary to determine the mechanical axis.[89] Although high correlation between anatomic and mechanical axes is generally noted, long films are also helpful in determining whether deformities of the tibia or femur exist, and in revealing the effect that these deformities have on overall mechanical alignment.

Preoperative Planning

The principal considerations in osteotomy planning include the location, direction, and magnitude of malalignment (Box 94-3). These variables need to be weighed concurrently during the planning phase to achieve appropriate angular correction. One of the reasons for premature failure after osteotomy is undercorrection or overcorrection of the deformity, which may be due to deficiencies in the preoperative planning process or the surgical technique.[27,80,89] Clearly, philosophy, training, and experience heavily bias preference for a specific osteotomy technique. The rationale for choosing between one of these options is delineated in the discussion of these various techniques (Box 94-4). In recent times, varus deformities have been corrected by HTO, whereas most valgus deformities are corrected by distal femoral osteotomy. Previously, the most pragmatic approach for most surgeons was a closing wedge osteotomy; however, opening wedge techniques are becoming more popular.[28,38,49,55]

Intra-articular deficiencies require special consideration when the degree of desired angular correction is calculated. Slack collateral ligamentous restraint causes angular deformity, and tibiofemoral separation requires subtraction of roughly 1 degree per millimeter to avoid overcorrection (the correction factor will change depending on the actual width of the proximal tibia).[29] It is important to remember

that ligamentous laxity will not be detected on standing radiographs when laxity exists in the same compartment that is being overloaded. For example, lateral ligament laxity in a valgus knee or medial collateral ligament (MCL) laxity in a varus knee, not observed on radiographs, may cause overcorrection of alignment after realignment osteotomy once the load has been shifted toward the opposite compartment of the knee.

Some patients with proximal tibial varus deformity have excessive valgus angulation of the distal femoral articular surface. This obliquity of the distal femoral surface affects the magnitude of alignment correction and requires special consideration during preoperative planning because patients with femoral shaft–transcondylar angles less than 9 degrees have an

---

Box 94-3   Components of Malalignment

Location

Extra-articular
  Femur
  Tibia
Intra-articular
  Joint line obliquity
  Ligamentous laxity
  Articular cartilage deficiency
  Osseous deficiencies

Direction

Sagittal
  Flexion
  Extension
Coronal
  Varus
  Valgus
Rotational

Magnitude

Mild (<10 degrees)
Moderate (10 to 20 degrees)
Severe (>20 degrees)

Box 94-4   Corrective Osteotomy Techniques

Tibial

Lateral closing wedge
Medial closing wedge
Medial opening wedge
  Graft
  Staple
Distraction histogenesis
Barrel vault (dome) osteotomy
Oblique metaphyseal wedge

Femoral

Medial closing wedge
  Medial fixation
  Lateral fixation
Oblique metaphyseal wedge
Lateral opening wedge
Lateral closing wedge

increased incidence of undercorrection.[81] Increased valgus orientation of the distal end of the femur can result in deleterious overcorrection after HTO.[80] Extra-articular deformities distant from the knee joint may need to be addressed at the apex of the deformity, rather than by periarticular correction.

The magnitude of coronal plane malalignment may dictate the location of the osteotomy or may suggest the use of a particular technique. For example, excessive malalignment may contraindicate HTO if the tibial articular surface will be adversely tilted, and for malalignment exceeding 12 to 15 degrees, a supracondylar femoral osteotomy is recommended.[26] Alternatively, a dome or barrel vault osteotomy allows greater correction with less effect on the resultant joint line obliquity and should potentially be considered for varus deformities exceeding 20 degrees.[9] For severe deformities, a dual (double) osteotomy of the distal femur and the proximal tibia may be deemed necessary.[11] Sagittal plane deformities can be corrected with proper planning and appropriate adjustment of the osteotomy technique. As HTO techniques are becoming more refined, more attention is being directed to the sagittal plane of correction in an attempt to better offload areas with significant cartilage damage.[4,59]

Historically, axial limb alignment was determined by measuring the femoral–tibial (anatomic) angle from standing radiographs and then judging the amount of correction required to restore this angle to normal, which typically averages 5 degrees of valgus (Fig. 94-1). The height of a tibial osteotomy wedge was then estimated by the rule of thumb, so that each millimeter provided roughly 1 degree of angular correction. This method of calculation is accurate only when the actual width of the tibial flare is 56 mm, and it is significantly altered by differences in tibial width or distortion that may result from radiographic magnification.[24] Use of this method without consideration of actual tibial width invariably leads to undercorrection because the mean tibial width is 80 mm in men and 70 mm in women (Fig. 94-2). The mechanical axis averages 1.2 degrees of varus and is based on a line connecting the centers of the femoral head and the tibiotalar joint (see Fig. 94-1). This axis is more accurate than the anatomic axis when load transmission forces across the knee joint are defined, particularly when femoral or tibial deformities are contributing to malalignment.

One measurement method for HTO uses the mechanical axis on a full-length standing radiograph with radiographic markers to adjust for magnification. By using trigonometric principles and adjusting for radiographic magnification, the intended wedge height is determined by ascertaining the amount of angular correction required to place the mechanical axis at the desired location within the knee joint. The formula for these calculations is shown in Figure 94-3. A similar method, the weight-bearing line method, divides the tibial plateau from 0% to 100% (medial to lateral) to determine the appropriate coordinate for the mechanical axis to intersect the knee joint (Fig. 94-4).[29] Lines to the center of the femoral head and the talar dome connect this coordinate, and the angle formed by these lines is the angle of desired correction. This angle is adjusted accordingly for distraction of the tibiofemoral joint surfaces allowed by ligamentous laxity and articular cartilage deficiency. The height of the wedge is then calculated by tracing the wedge on the radiograph and normalizing the measured height of the wedge by the amount of radiographic magnification. Both of these

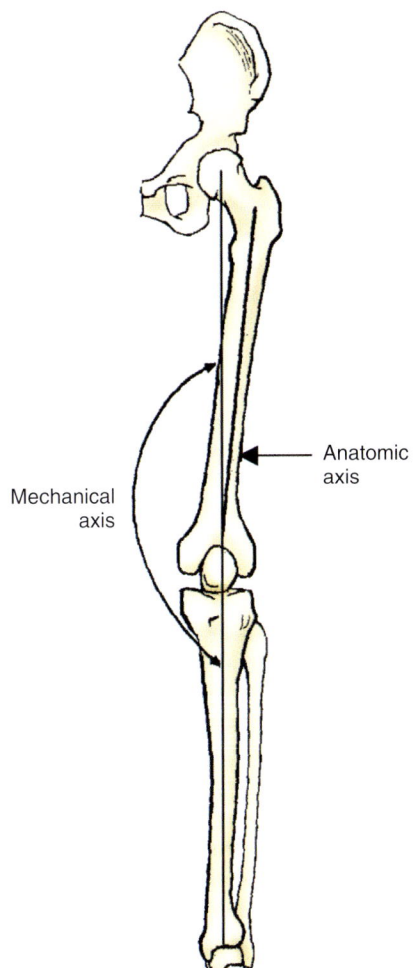

Figure 94-1. The mechanical axis, based on a line connecting the centers of the femoral head and the tibiotalar joint, averages 1.2 degrees of varus, whereas the femoral–tibial (anatomic) angle normally averages 5 degrees of valgus.

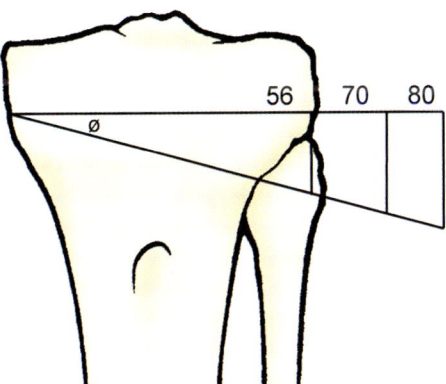

Figure 94-2. Given the same desired angle of correction (ø), the wedge height measurement progressively increases with increasing tibial width. The rule of thumb that 1 mm of wedge height equals 1 degree of angular correction results in undercorrection for tibial widths exceeding 56 mm.

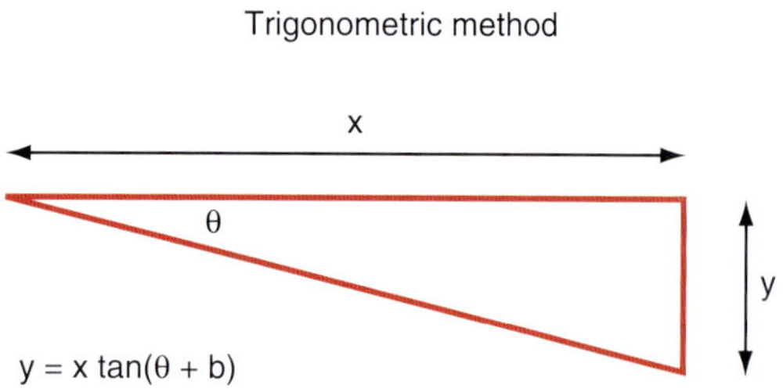

Trigonometric method

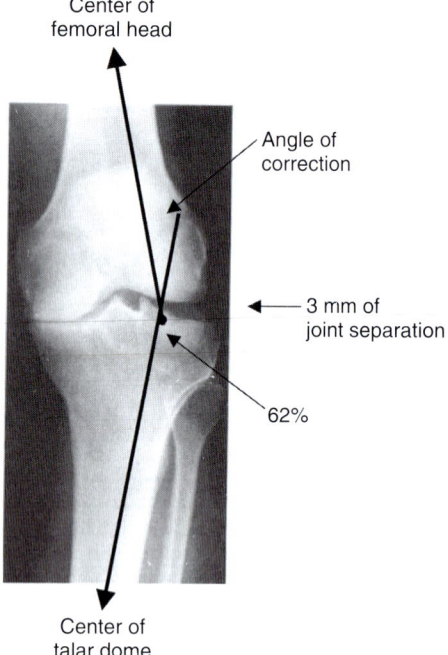

$$y = x \tan(\theta + b)$$

Figure 94-3. The trigonometric method of determining actual wedge height *(y)* is calculated with a trigonometric formula using known values of the desired angle of correction *(ø)* and actual tibial width *(x)*. Direct measurement of tibial width at a point 2.0 to 2.5 cm distal to the joint line, on radiographs incorporating radiographic markers, is normalized by the amount of magnification present to obtain the actual tibial wedge height *(y)*.

Figure 94-4. The weight-bearing line method divides the tibial plateau from 0% to 100% (medial to lateral) to determine the desired intersection coordinate of the mechanical axis through the knee joint. The angle formed by lines drawn from this coordinate to the center of the femoral head and talar dome is corrected for tibiofemoral joint surface distraction allowed by ligamentous laxity to establish the desired angle of correction. Wedge height is calculated by tracing the wedge on the radiograph with the desired angle of correction. The wedge height measurement on the radiograph is then normalized by the radiographic magnification present.

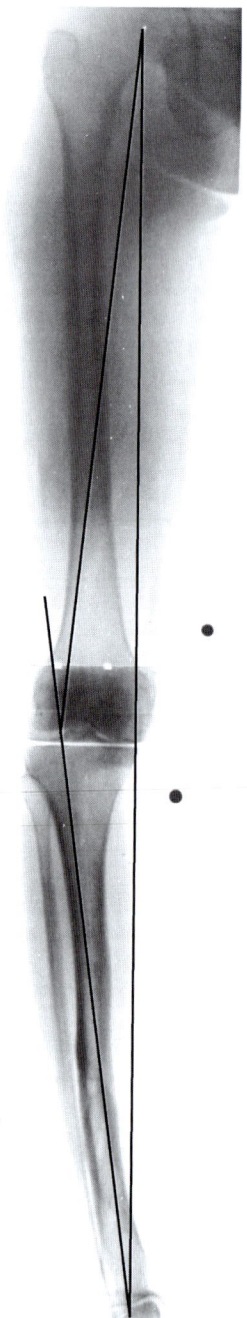

Figure 94-5. Standing full-length radiograph of an active 46-year-old woman with localized medial compartment knee pain. Note the tibial distal malunion.

measurement methods account for the actual width of the tibial plateau.

A full-length radiograph used for measurement of mechanical alignment is a static measurement only. Soft tissue tension, joint line obliquity, and upper body gravity shift also affect tibiofemoral plateau pressure distribution during dynamic gait. Software programs are emerging to help with preoperative assessment of these factors and to assist the surgeon's in final determination of the location, magnitude, and type of knee osteotomy.[31,47] The data printout generated by these programs details various osteotomy options and seems most useful for several specific circumstances: (1) in

deciding whether to perform a periarticular osteotomy or an osteotomy at the apex of the deformity away from the knee joint, and (2) in determining whether joint line obliquity may be adversely affected after correction of severe malalignment with a particular technique, thereby suggesting the need for a combined dual osteotomy of the tibia and femur. Currently, no data suggest the upper limit of acceptance for resultant joint line obliquity, and we often accept up to 10 degrees of joint line obliquity before proceeding with a dual osteotomy (Figs. 94-5 to 94-9).

For patients with mild or moderate deformity, static measurement planning methods seem sufficient. Although these

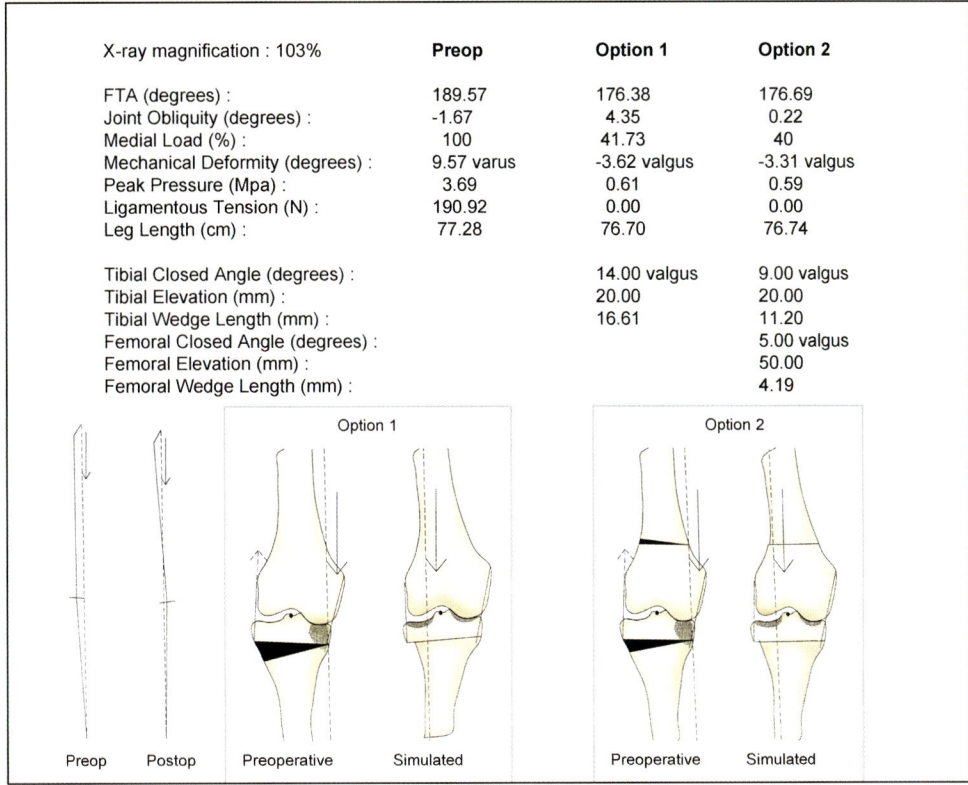

X-ray magnification : 103%	**Preop**	**Option 1**	**Option 2**
FTA (degrees) :	189.57	176.38	176.69
Joint Obliquity (degrees) :	-1.67	4.35	0.22
Medial Load (%) :	100	41.73	40
Mechanical Deformity (degrees) :	9.57 varus	-3.62 valgus	-3.31 valgus
Peak Pressure (Mpa) :	3.69	0.61	0.59
Ligamentous Tension (N) :	190.92	0.00	0.00
Leg Length (cm) :	77.28	76.70	76.74
Tibial Closed Angle (degrees) :		14.00 valgus	9.00 valgus
Tibial Elevation (mm) :		20.00	20.00
Tibial Wedge Length (mm) :		16.61	11.20
Femoral Closed Angle (degrees) :			5.00 valgus
Femoral Elevation (mm) :			50.00
Femoral Wedge Length (mm) :			4.19

Figure 94-6. An OASIS data printout obtained from the full-length radiograph in Figure 94-5 details several corrective osteotomy options. Option 1, with a proximal tibial wedge resection of 16.61 mm, is calculated to leave 4.35 degrees of resultant joint line obliquity. Option 2 describes a dual osteotomy designed to minimize resultant joint line obliquity. *FTA*, Femorotibial angle.

preoperative planning schemes provide objective criteria to guide surgery, even the most detailed plans rely on the ability of the surgeon to carry out the procedure accurately.

SURGICAL TECHNIQUES

Principles inherent in these techniques include appropriate placement of skin incisions, careful handling of soft tissues, respect for neurovascular structures, accurate execution of the osteotomy, and adequate skeletal fixation. Options for fixation and a discussion of complications associated with osteotomy are presented later in this chapter. Preparation for a skin incision should include forethought regarding an eventual TKR, and longitudinal incisions on the lateral or medial side of the knee should provide large bridges of skin to accommodate for any future midline or parapatellar approach. Incisions carelessly placed for the osteotomy may lead to catastrophic complications of wound healing and infection at a later arthroplasty.

The accuracy of the osteotomy based on preoperative planning and intraoperative technique cannot be overemphasized. With closing wedge techniques, apposition of bone surfaces facilitates prompt healing, whereas proper orientation and resection of bone ultimately determine final mechanical alignment. Opening wedge techniques provide greater versatility intraoperatively, with the surgeon able to manipulate the osteotomy site after the initial bone cut, although this technique also requires special attention to detail and must be carried out meticulously. Jig systems to assist in achieving correct placement and orientation of the

osteotomy appear to be particularly useful for many surgeons who have limited experience performing these osteotomies.[16,41] The use of intraoperative radiographs and fluoroscopy to document that appropriate alignment has been achieved is recommended.

Historically, loss of patellar height was often seen with closing wedge osteotomy techniques because the knee was subsequently immobilized in a postoperative cast with resultant contracture of the patellar ligament. This complication has become less common because surgeons are now using more rigid fixation methods that allow earlier knee mobilization during the immediate postoperative period.[2,16,105] Although loss of patellar height has been seen with opening wedge techniques, the cause of this phenomenon differs in that the opening wedge technique causes an elevation of the joint line that results in patellar migration distally relative to the femoral trochlea rather than patellar ligament contracture.[108] The clinical implications of patella infera associated with HTO remain poorly understood.

Varus Deformity

For varus malalignment about the knee, many surgeons continue to prefer a lateral closing wedge osteotomy of the proximal tibia.* Because of its perceived simplicity, medial opening wedge osteotomy is becoming more popular.† Both techniques

---

*References 16, 20, 37, 51, 56, and 72.
†References 7, 28, 38, 49, 55, and 71.

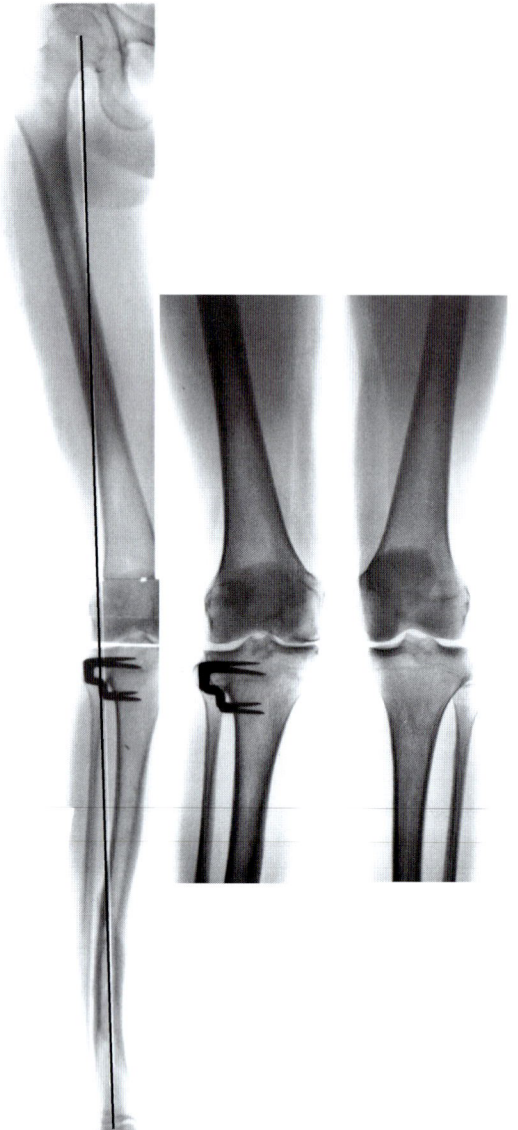

Figure 94-7. Postoperative full-length radiograph of a patient after a 16-mm lateral wedge resection osteotomy of the proximal end of the tibia demonstrating that the mechanical axis now intersects the lateral tibial compartment at the 75% coordinate. The inset standing radiograph demonstrates symmetry of the lower extremities.

are used to address varus malalignment with medial compartment arthritis, and each technique has inherent advantages and disadvantages. The decision to use one over the other must be based on the surgeon's philosophy and clinical experience (Table 94-1). Although they are less commonly performed, dome osteotomies and double osteotomies are viable treatment options in selected individuals.[11,48,53]

Lateral Closing Tibial Wedge Osteotomy

The following description, modified from the original report, is currently the preferred technique for a closing wedge osteotomy at our institution and is relatively straightforward when compared with some other techniques.[21] The primary modification of this technique is partial resection of the fibular head rather than total fibular head resection combined with advancement of lateral ligamentous structures.

The patient is positioned supine with a sandbag beneath the ipsilateral trochanteric region to place the extremity in neutral rotation. The extremity is exsanguinated and under tourniquet control, and the procedure is typically performed with the knee flexed to 90 degrees, although such flexure does not protect the popliteal artery from injury when compared with the fully extended position.[109] Although a long curvilinear incision was originally described, a short oblique incision coursing from the fibular head toward the tibial tubercle is currently preferred. The iliotibial band is split longitudinally just anterior and parallel to the fibular collateral ligament, and the peroneal nerve is located by palpation only. The anterior tibial musculature is then subperiosteally from the proximal end of the tibia.

Removal of the inner third of the fibular head and cartilage is accomplished with an osteotome. The posterior portion of the tibia is subperiosteally exposed to allow insertion of a broad malleable retractor to protect the neurovascular structures. An anterior retractor is placed between the patellar ligament and the tibia just proximal to the tibial tubercle. The location of the joint line can be established with a small arthrotomy or by placement of medial and lateral Kirschner wires. At a point 2.0 to 2.5 cm below the joint line, a guide wire is inserted in a lateral-to-medial direction parallel to the tibial articular surface (Fig. 94-10A). The second pin is inserted at a point measured distally from pin no. 1 based on preoperative calculation of tibial wedge height. This pin is advanced obliquely to intersect with the first pin at the

Table 94-1 Comparison Between High Tibial Osteotomy Techniques

HTO Type	Fixation	Advantages	Disadvantages
Opening wedge	Plate system External fixator or spatial frame (larger correction) Bone grafting (alone)	Potentially simpler Avoids the proximal tibiofibular joint Avoids the peroneal nerve More control of multiplanar correction (sagittal/coronal) Avoids the anterior compartment No bone loss	Less aggressive weight bearing/rehabilitation Often requires a graft with potential implications of healing/union May overlengthen the extremity May alter patellar height
Closing wedge	Plate system Staples	More aggressive weight bearing/rehabilitation Does not require a graft	More difficult to control tibial slope (often inadvertently decreased) Intraoperative adjustments more difficult Proximal tibiofibular joint violated Increased risk to the peroneal nerve Alters the shape of the upper part of the tibia with implications for joint reconstruction Bone loss/shortening May alter patellar height

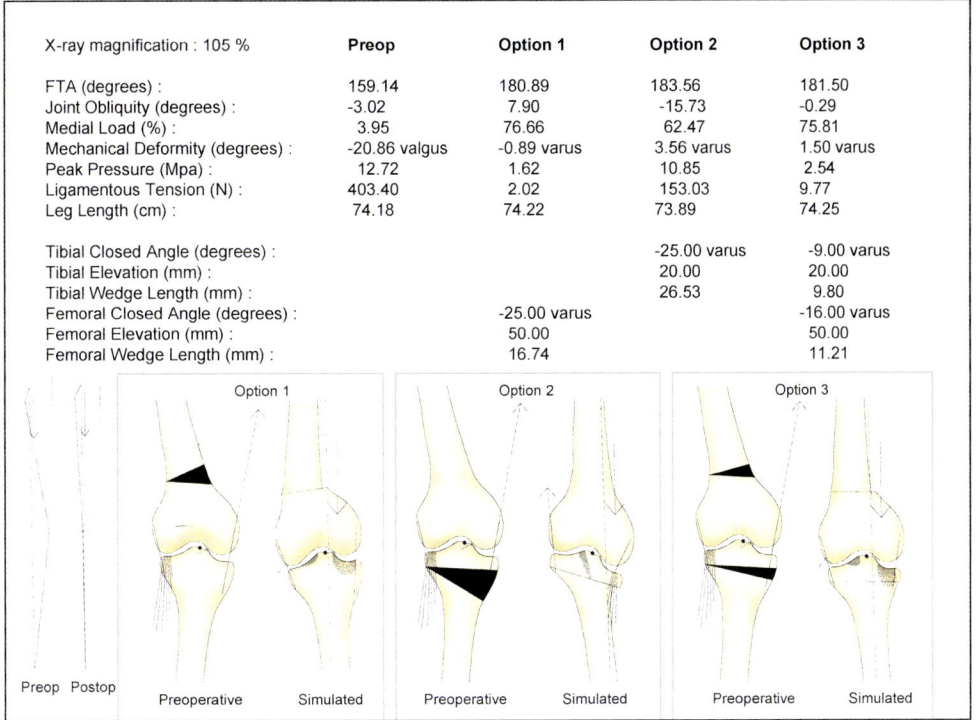

X-ray magnification : 105 %	Preop	Option 1	Option 2	Option 3
FTA (degrees) :	159.14	180.89	183.56	181.50
Joint Obliquity (degrees) :	-3.02	7.90	-15.73	-0.29
Medial Load (%) :	3.95	76.66	62.47	75.81
Mechanical Deformity (degrees) :	-20.86 valgus	-0.89 varus	3.56 varus	1.50 varus
Peak Pressure (Mpa) :	12.72	1.62	10.85	2.54
Ligamentous Tension (N) :	403.40	2.02	153.03	9.77
Leg Length (cm) :	74.18	74.22	73.89	74.25
Tibial Closed Angle (degrees) :			-25.00 varus	-9.00 varus
Tibial Elevation (mm) :			20.00	20.00
Tibial Wedge Length (mm) :			26.53	9.80
Femoral Closed Angle (degrees) :		-25.00 varus		-16.00 varus
Femoral Elevation (mm) :		50.00		50.00
Femoral Wedge Length (mm) :		16.74		11.21

Figure 94-8. OASIS data printout obtained from a full-length standing radiograph of a 42-year-old active woman with painful genu valgum and osteoarthritis of the lateral compartment of her right knee. Option 2 demonstrates the anticipated resultant joint line obliquity created by a varus-producing osteotomy of the proximal end of the tibia. *FTA,* Femorotibial angle.

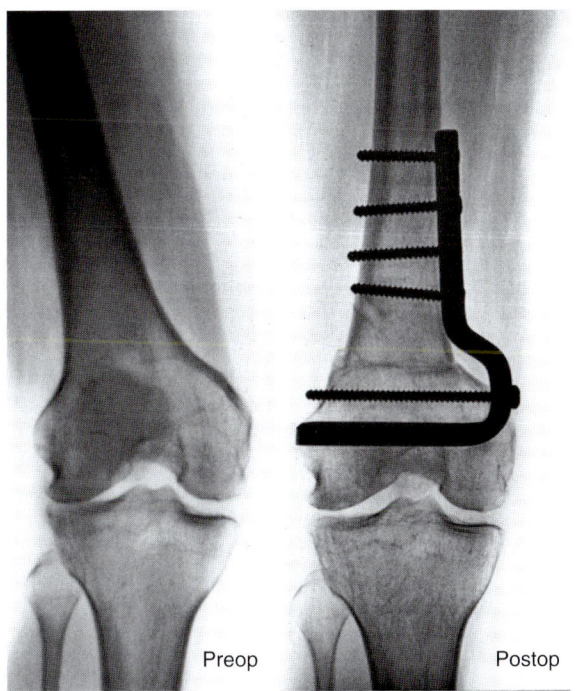

Figure 94-9. Spot views of the full-length radiographs presented in Figure 94-8. Note the correction of the mechanical axis from the 95% coordinate in the preoperative radiograph to the 50% coordinate (neutral position) in the postoperative radiograph.

medial tibial cortex. Pin placement should be confirmed radiographically.

The osteotomy is performed parallel to the posterior slope of the tibial articular surface in the sagittal plane with a broad osteotome or an oscillating saw. The tibia is transected on the undersurface of pin no. 1 and the upper surface of pin no. 2. The width of the wedge can be adjusted to correct for flexion or extension deformity by altering the height of the wedge in the anteroposterior plane. Initially, the osteotomy traverses approximately 50% to 75% of the tibial width, so that the outer wedge of bone can be removed to facilitate completion of the osteotomy with small osteotomes (see Fig. 94-10B). It is important that the medial cortex not be transected, but rather should be perforated four to five times with a long drill bit or a small osteotome, to maintain an intact periosteal hinge. The bone from the inner wedge is removed with small curettes while great care is taken to ensure removal of all cortical bone, especially in the posteromedial tibial corner.

Osteoclasis is achieved by applying valgus stress to the extremity with the knee in full extension. The fibular head is inspected to verify that it is not preventing complete closure of the osteotomy. Mechanical alignment is verified by fluoroscopy with a rod extending from the femoral head to the talar dome. Fixation is then accomplished by inserting two stepped staples, with the first staple positioned just anterior to the fibular head and the second staple yet more anterior (see Fig. 94-10C). During staple insertion, it is helpful to start advancing the proximal tine into the tibial plateau until the distal tine rests against the tibial cortex. Using a 3.2-mm drill bit, a starter hole is made just distal to the tine to facilitate compression at the osteotomy site and avoid propagation of a fracture through the thick tibial cortex.

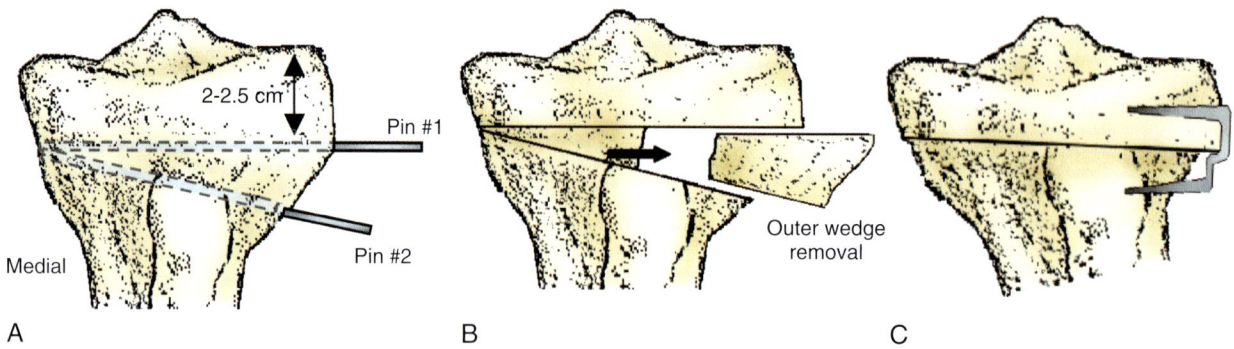

Figure 94-10. **A,** The first guide wire is inserted parallel to the tibial articular surface approximately 2.0 to 2.5 cm below the joint line. The second guide wire, inserted at a point distally based on the preoperative calculation of actual tibial wedge height, is advanced obliquely to intersect at the medial tibial cortex with the first guide wire. **B,** The outer 50% to 75% of the wedge is initially removed to allow completion of the inner portion of the wedge. **C,** The tibia is stabilized by the insertion of two stepped staples bridging the osteotomy site.

Counterpressure against the medial portion of the tibia by a surgical assistant during final staple insertion helps prevent tibial translation and disruption of the medial periosteum. In overweight individuals, it is often difficult to provide adequate medial tibia counterpressure because of the thickness of the subcutaneous tissue. A large provisional pin inserted obliquely across the osteotomy site helps stabilize the tibia during staple insertion in these patients. The accuracy of apposition and the integrity of the medial periosteal hinge are then assessed dynamically with fluoroscopy. Bone graft from the removed wedge of bone is placed adjacent to the staples. After tourniquet release, careful hemostasis is achieved, with particular attention paid to the region of the anterior tibial musculature. Deep drains are inserted along the posterior aspect of the tibia and beneath the anterior compartment musculature. The wound is closed in layers and the extremity placed in a compressive dressing.

Postoperatively, the patient wears a hinged knee brace to allow early range of motion. Partial weight bearing is allowed for the first 6 to 8 weeks and is followed by progression to full weight bearing.

Because two-dimensional planning (based on preoperative and intraoperative radiographs or imaging) is used to execute a three-dimensional procedure, the role of computer-assisted surgery has been explored with the hope of improving the placement and orientation of osteotomy resection planes for closing wedge techniques.[31,47] The role of computer-aided surgery is presently evolving; this approach may ultimately provide significant benefits in realignment surgery, particularly for surgeons with limited experience.

Medial Opening Tibial Wedge Osteotomy

Correction of malalignment with an opening medial wedge osteotomy has been reported to be successful (Fig. 94-11).[28,38,49,55] A number of technical improvements have contributed to the safety and reproducibility of this technique.[52] Advantages of this technique include the requirement for only a single osteotomy with surgical dissection away from the peroneal nerve, no violation of the fibula and tibiofibular joint, and the capability for intraoperative adjustment of the correction. Inherent disadvantages include the potential need to procure an autogenous bone graft and the use of an alternative bone graft source such as an allograft or a synthetic bone graft substitute.[49] New fixation devices, such

as the Puddhu plate[95] and the TomoFix,[93,95] have been specifically developed for medial opening wedge osteotomies.

Operative details of the procedure include positioning the patient supine with a sandbag beneath the ipsilateral trochanteric region to place the extremity in neutral rotation. A small vertical incision is made over the pes anserinus insertion halfway between the medial border of the patellar ligament and the posterior margin of the tibia to expose the sartorial fascia. This fascia is incised to expose the hamstring tendons. The osteotomy is often planned above the tibial tubercle. Retractors are carefully placed anterior and posterior to protect the patellar tendon and posterior neurovascular structures, along with the hamstring tendons and the MCL. The superficial MCL inserts 5 to 7 cm distal to the joint and usually is retracted out of harm's way.

Under fluoroscopic imaging, a guide wire is drilled across the proximal tibia in a medial-to-lateral direction. The guide is positioned at the level of the superior aspect of the tibial tubercle and is oriented obliquely to end approximately 1 cm below the joint line at the lateral tibial cortex. The tip of the fibular head can be used as a reference point. The starting point on the medial cortex is usually about 4 cm below the joint line. The guide pin should be repositioned until placement is optimal. The saw cut then is made on the underside of the pin and is advanced to within 1 cm of the lateral edge of the tibia. Oftentimes, the cortical cut is made with a small sagittal saw, and flexible osteotomes are used to deepen the osteotomy. Continuous or frequent imaging should be performed to protect the lateral cortex. Once the osteotomy is completed (i.e., the anterior and posterior cortices are penetrated), the medial opening is created with an osteotomy wedge in a slow and careful fashion to the predetermined size. The anteroposterior slope can be matched or changed depending on the amount of deformity present and the preoperative goals. If replicating the native slope, it is important to understand that the distraction anteriorly at the tubercle should be less than that at the posteromedial corner; otherwise, the slope will be increased. In cases in which the anterior opening is greater than 1 cm, a tibial tubercle osteotomy can be performed to advance the tubercle to the same height as the osteotomy.[71]

Fluoroscopic imaging is used intraoperatively to evaluate the mechanical axis and ensure that it is appropriate. When the desired opening is achieved, the osteotomy is secured

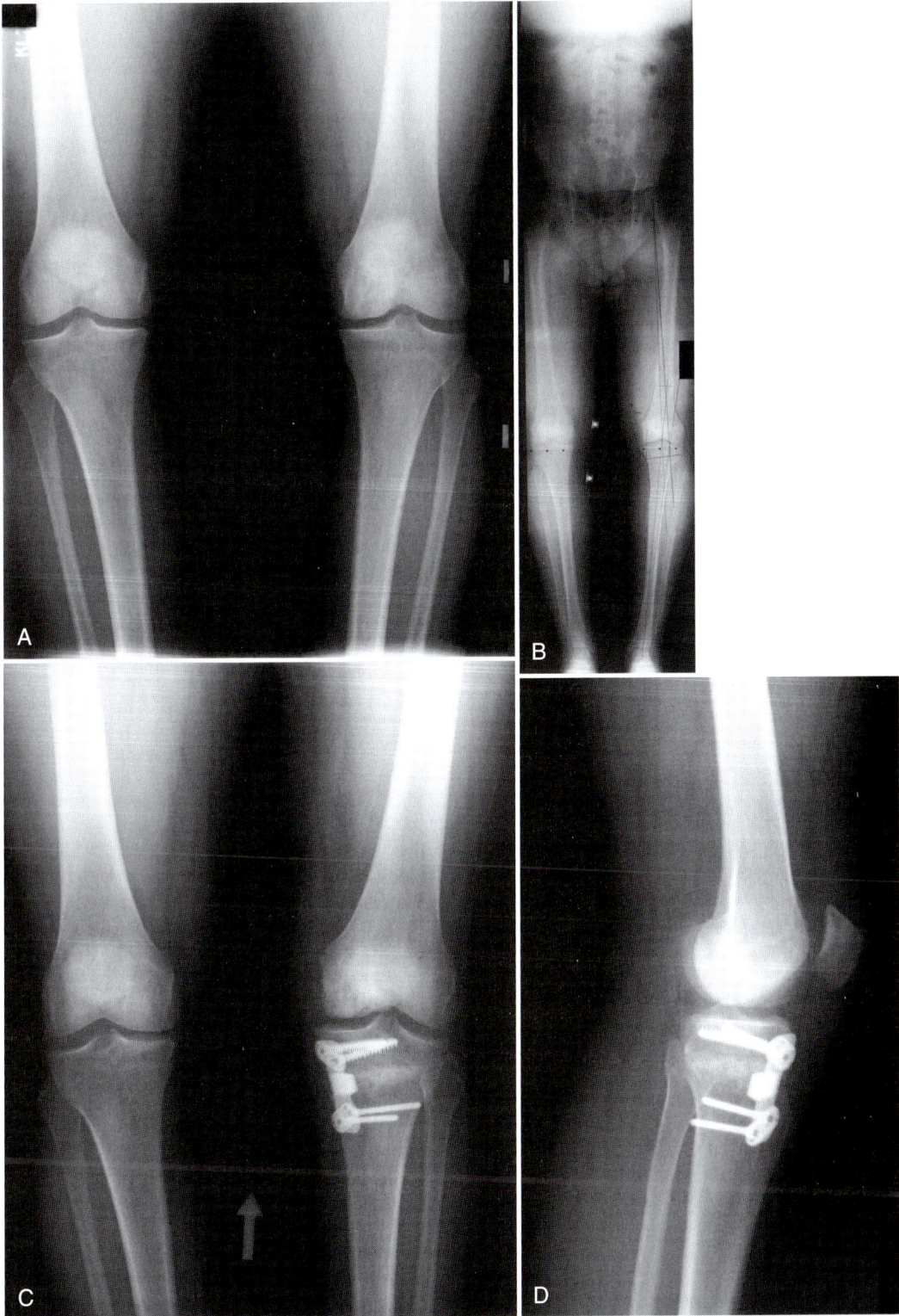

Figure 94-11. **A,** Patient with left knee medial compartment osteochondritis dissecans and posttraumatic medial compartment degenerative arthritis with varus malalignment. **B,** Preoperative templating for a planned left knee valgus-producing, medial tibial opening wedge osteotomy. Lines to the center of the femoral head and the talar dome connect at the 50% coordinate and the 62.5% coordinate along the tibial plateau. The angle formed by the lines that connect at the 62% coordinate (lateral transection on the radiograph) outlines the desired correction to unload the medial compartment. **C,** Postoperative anteroposterior radiograph outlining the opening wedge osteotomy, which was fixed with an Arthrex opening wedge osteotomy locking plate. The osteotomy site was bone-grafted with cancellous allograft mixed with bone graft substitute. **D,** Postoperative lateral radiograph outlining the opening wedge osteotomy.

with a plate with the leg in extension (using two 6.5-mm cancellous screws proximally and two 4.5-mm cortical screws distally) and usually a bone graft or a bone graft substitute. Before closing, the MCL can be fenestrated and allowed to slide if it is too taut. Fluoroscopy is used at this stage to ensure that the graft is adequately seated. A drain is then inserted and the wound closed in layers. Postoperatively, the leg is placed in a hinged knee brace with toe-touch weight bearing for 6 to 8 weeks. Progression of weight bearing at that time is dependent on radiologic evidence of bony union.

An alternative approach includes gradually opening the medial wedge with a variety of external fixation devices, including biplanar external fixators, semicircular external fixators, or small wire frames.[55,70,85] Advantages of these external fixation distraction histogenesis techniques include accurate correction of the desired mechanical axis at termination of distraction, ability to continuously adjust the correction over time, potentially less effect on patellar height, rapid mobilization of the patient, absence of limb length shortening, and maintenance of soft tissue tension about the knee. In a matched-pair comparative analysis contrasting outcomes between a Coventry-type closing wedge valgus HTO and an HTO using an Ilizarov apparatus, a significantly greater decrease in pain and increase in function were seen in the Ilizarov group at a mean follow-up of greater than 2 years.[1] Disadvantages of distraction histogenesis techniques include the use of an external fixation device, which can be cumbersome and poorly tolerated by patients. Pin site difficulties are the primary concern because many old pin tracts become colonized, with potential implications for deep infection if the knee is ultimately converted to a TKR.

Barrel Vault (Dome) Tibial Osteotomy

A dome osteotomy involves the use of a curved osteotomy that allows rotation or translation of the distal end of the tibia on the proximal fragment.[9,57] A fundamental aspect of this procedure is that a portion of the fibula must be resected to allow correction of the malalignment.[57] Advantages of this method include avoidance of limb length alteration, the potential for anterior displacement of the tibial tubercle to decrease patellofemoral joint reaction forces, and the capacity to address large corrections of malalignment without adversely affecting the resultant joint line obliquity. This procedure is technically demanding, yet when the practitioner has adequate experience, proponents prefer this procedure because of the ability to adjust the mechanical axis exactly. Disadvantages of this technique include an increased incidence of complications, including pin tract infection, loss of correction after fixator removal, and peroneal palsy.[8]

Dual (Double) Osteotomy

A dual osteotomy is another alternative for patients with severe deformity in whom osteotomy would potentially and adversely alter the obliquity of the joint line. This procedure involves osteotomy of both the femur and the tibia to correct malalignment.[11] Typically, the femoral wedge is performed as a lateral closing wedge when varus malalignment is corrected, and as a medial closing wedge when valgus malalignment is corrected. A published study of 29 double-level osteotomies reported a 96% cumulative rate of survival at 100 months.[11] These authors attribute their high rate of success to proper selection of patients, careful preoperative planning with

biomechanical analysis that accounted for redistribution of the joint load, limited exposure of the knee joint, and modern techniques of internal fixation that allowed for early motion. Overall, the potential additional morbidity previously thought to be associated with double-osteotomy techniques should be considered and weighed against the disadvantages of slight joint line obliquity.

Valgus Deformity

Genu valgum is a much rarer entity than varus deformity of the knee. The biomechanical characteristics of varus and valgus knees are also different because most valgus knees have inherent superolateral obliquity of the joint line. Classically, distal femoral osteotomy has been recommended for valgus deformities exceeding 12 to 15 degrees, or when joint line obliquity would exceed 10 degrees after correction.[22] Although genu valgum may be corrected by a varus-producing proximal tibial osteotomy, the magnitude of the joint line obliquity is increased by the wedge resection and may be a cause of clinical failure. Excessive joint line obliquity produces ineffective weight transfer because some weight is applied as shear force against the intercondylar eminence when the femur subluxes on the tibia. In the current era, the use of a varus closing wedge osteotomy of the proximal tibia for correction of valgus malalignment is virtually obsolete. The reader is referred to Coventry's description of a closing wedge, varus-producing proximal tibial osteotomy.[22] Although dome osteotomy of the proximal tibia does not increase joint line obliquity, the superolateral obliquity of the distal femur associated with a valgus deformity is not corrected, and the persistent femoral valgus angulation continues to exert valgus force on the knee joint.

Osteotomy in the supracondylar region is the most effective method of addressing valgus deformity because the transcondylar line becomes perpendicular with the mechanical axis and MCL laxity is minimized.[60] For most surgeons today, valgus malalignment about the knee of any magnitude is best managed by femoral osteotomy, and a medial closing wedge osteotomy with lateral or medial fixation seems to be the preferred technique.* Valgus deformity can also be corrected by an opening wedge osteotomy of the distal femur with insertion of tricortical autograft wedges supplemented by lateral plate fixation.[98]

Supracondylar femoral osteotomy is an "unforgiving" procedure for three specific reasons: (1) difficulty cutting the wedge effectively, (2) difficulty establishing effective stabilization of the closed osteotomy, and (3) difficulty predicting the wedge size necessary to ensure proper correction of the limb. In many respects, it is clear that the biomechanics, preoperative planning, and operative technique of a supracondylar femoral osteotomy are different from those of a proximal tibial osteotomy. These three concerns are adequately addressed by the following surgical technique, which is characterized by a simple preoperative planning process and a straightforward surgical approach that minimizes wedge removal difficulties and reproducibly allows accurate extremity realignment.

---

*References 3, 18, 30, 32, 58, and 92.

Medial Closing Femoral Wedge Osteotomy

This technique, which can be performed with medial or lateral fixation, has been modified from the original description.[61] Essentially, this method uses the transcondylar line and a 90-degree AO blade plate to correct the mechanical axis to neutral. The patient is placed in the supine position; tourniquet control is optional. A 12- to 15-cm longitudinal incision extending from the joint line proximally can be placed anywhere from the midline to the medial side of the thigh. The vastus medialis obliquus is elevated from the medial septum and retracted anteriorly to expose the medial femoral condyle and the femoral cortex. The joint line is located with a small arthrotomy or with the use of a large needle.

With the knee flexed to 90 degrees, a guide wire is placed across the joint parallel to the articular surface of the distal end of the femur (Fig. 94-12). A second guide wire, inserted approximately 2.0 cm proximal and parallel to the first pin, is directed in an anteromedial-to-posterolateral direction to aid insertion of the blade plate chisel at the correct angle (Fig. 94-13). It is imperative that radiographs be used to confirm a truly parallel position of these pins with the transcondylar line. The guide wire is inserted up to the lateral cortex of the femur to allow measurement of proper blade plate length, which is usually 50 to 70 mm.

Three 4.5-mm holes are drilled just above the second pin in the medial femoral condyle to prevent cortical comminution during chisel penetration. The chisel is impacted along the upper surface of pin no. 2 to the desired depth. The plate holder attached to the box chisel facilitates proper chisel entry and ensures correct apposition of the blade plate against the proximal end of the femur. Radiographs taken at this point document the proper chisel angle and ascertain that the chisel has not penetrated the intercondylar notch or the anterior femoral surface. Large malleable retractors are placed medially and posteriorly to protect neurovascular structures.

Guide wires, placed in a medial-to-lateral direction and converging at the lateral cortex, are used to perform the osteotomy. The inferior guide wire is placed parallel to the transcondylar pin in the supracondylar region just proximal to the adductor tubercle (see Fig. 94-12). A longitudinal line extending above and below the site of the osteotomy is placed on the femur with a marking pencil to ensure proper rotation of the limb at the time of osteotomy closure. The medial portion of the osteotomy is performed with an oscillating saw so that the outer 50% to 75% of the wedge can be removed before the lateral cortex is perforated with several drill holes. Great care is taken to avoid transection of the lateral cortex and overlying periosteum with the saw. The height of the wedge can be a predetermined measurement, but preferably removal of only a 5- to 10-mm wedge allows impaction of the proximal fragment into the metaphysis of the distal fragment (Fig. 94-14). Such impaction promotes maximal bone apposition and improves the stability of the osteotomy site.

Use of preoperative templates to determine proper plate size is prudent. The proper 90-degree AO blade plate, selected by length of the blade and one of three sizes of offset, is inserted into the femur. Osteoclasis is performed with a varus force applied to the extremity to close the osteotomy site, impact the proximal fragment, and enable application of the plate along the medial femoral cortex proximally. Multiple cortical screws are used to secure the plate to the femur via the dynamic compression technique; however, the AO outrigger compression device should be avoided because of the proximity of the vascular structures in the adductor canal. The medial femoral cortex and the distal femoral articular surface should now be perpendicularly aligned, and the resultant mechanical axis should be approximately neutral (see Fig. 94-9). The removed bone wedge is morselized and is placed medially and posteriorly along the osteotomy site (see Fig. 94-14). The vastus medialis obliquus is reattached to the medial septum with several interrupted sutures over a drain placed at the osteotomy site. The wound is closed in layers and the limb placed in a compressive dressing.

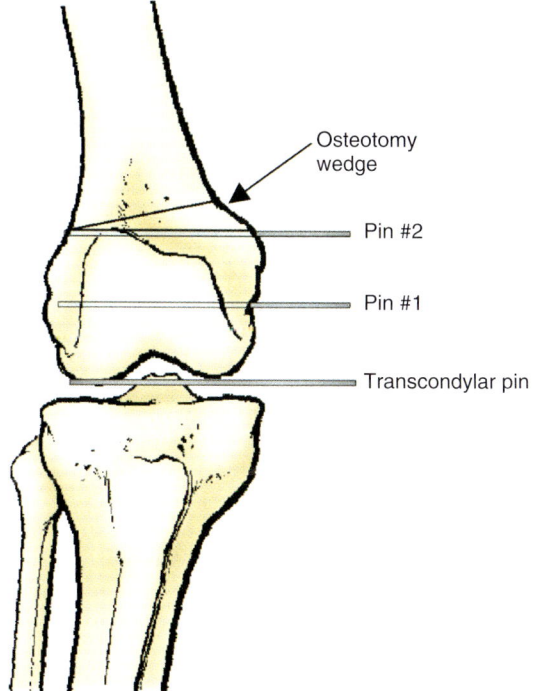

Figure 94-12. Diagram depicting placement of the transcondylar pin, the location of pin no. 1 for entry of the blade plate, and the location of pin no. 2 used for the inferior portion of the osteotomy wedge. A truly parallel position of the transcondylar pin and blade plate entry is essential to obtain a neutral mechanical axis.

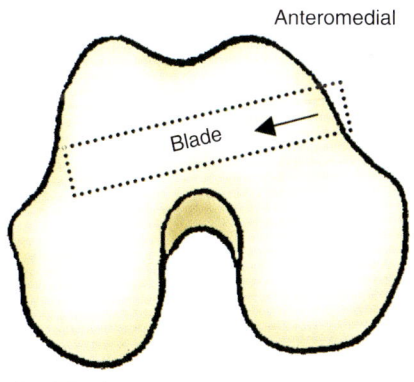

Figure 94-13. The blade plate should be inserted obliquely in an anteromedial-to-posterolateral direction to avoid penetration of the intercondylar notch or the anterior femoral articular surface.

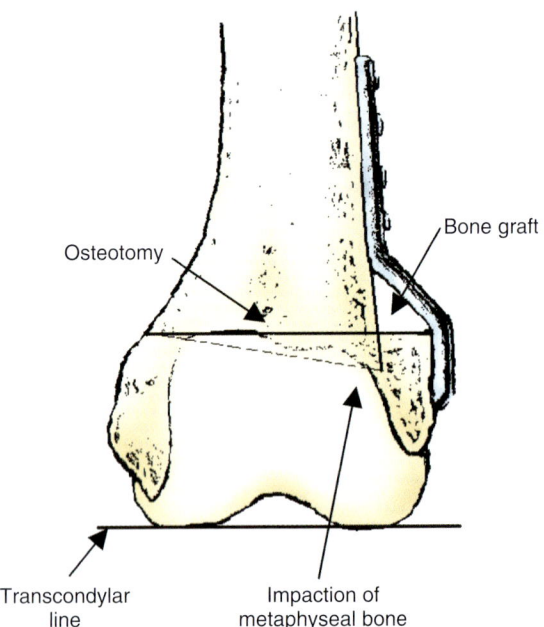

Figure 94-14. After osteotomy closure and impaction of the proximal fragment, the 90-degree AO osteotomy blade plate is secured to the proximal end of the femur, which is now perpendicular to the transcondylar line.

Postoperatively, the patient should remain toe-touch weight bearing for 4 to 6 weeks. The patient then begins partial weight bearing in a hinged knee brace locked in extension for an additional 6 weeks. Weight bearing as tolerated is allowed at 3-month follow-up if radiologic evidence of bony union is found. Adequate fixation plus intraoperative stability of the osteotomy site is a prerequisite for early active range of motion.

Because of concern regarding delayed union, nonunion, and hardware failure after supracondylar osteotomy with medially based fixation, a method of closing wedge osteotomy involving lateral fixation has been proposed.[65] This technique is based on the rationale that the lateral aspect of the femur becomes the tensile side of the knee after osteotomy, and, under these circumstances, laterally based fixation is superior to fixation inserted medially. Indeed, these authors report a higher incidence of implant failure or nonunion with medial fixation than with lateral fixation. It is important to note that the technique described in this study incorporates more than just fixation location because the osteotomy is performed obliquely and is stabilized with an interfragmentary screw. Undoubtedly, these technical aspects contribute to differences observed between the two techniques.

ARTHROSCOPY: DIAGNOSTIC VERSUS THERAPEUTIC

It is commonly believed that some patients might benefit from arthroscopic débridement performed in conjunction with corrective osteotomy. In one study, osteotomy patients undergoing simultaneous arthroscopic abrasion arthroplasty (group A) were compared with patients who underwent osteotomy alone (group B).[5] At 12-month follow-up, arthroscopic evaluation of group A knees revealed a significantly higher incidence of grade II cartilage repair; however, no difference

in clinical outcome was noted between the two groups at 2- to 9-year follow-up.

Another reason for considering arthroscopy might be to evaluate the stage of arthritis in the knee to predict the potential efficacy of osteotomy. Prognostic value has not been demonstrated when arthroscopy is used to evaluate the joint before corrective osteotomy.[46] The observation of moderate or severe degenerative patellofemoral joint changes has not adversely affected the eventual clinical results.[46] Proliferation of fibrocartilage and regeneration of articular cartilage have been documented by comparing findings at second-look arthroscopy with those visualized preoperatively.[43,50,103] These data support the concept of mechanical realignment to enhance the reparative capacity of the knee joint once unloaded, with one second-look study demonstrating a correlation between visible improvement of the articular surface, clinical outcome (functional score), and the degree of correction achieved.[43]

FIXATION

Skeletal fixation should be sufficiently rigid to allow early knee motion if desired and yet promote bone healing. Many options are available for fixation, and most are used in conjunction with a specific osteotomy technique. It is generally accepted that fixation of a distal femoral osteotomy requires a more rigid construct than is required for fixation of a proximal tibial osteotomy. Difficulties in fixation are more frequently reported with supracondylar osteotomy, and most authors agree that rigid internal fixation is required.

Various methods of fixation have been described for closing wedge techniques, including (1) cast immobilization without internal fixation, (2) external fixation devices, (3) staple fixation, (4) screw fixation, (5) buttress plates, (6) tension band plates, (7) "L"-plates, and (8) blade plate fixation.[33] Because of difficulty associated with loss of correction, the use of internal or external fixation is preferable to cast immobilization without internal fixation. A cadaveric study comparing mechanical stability between blade plates, one-third tubular plates, bone staples, and an external fixator (Orthofix) after a closing wedge osteotomy showed greater stability with the use of external fixators or bone staples.[33] In our hands, although staple fixation has been inadequate for distal femoral osteotomy, it remains the preferred method of fixation for a closing wedge HTO. The benefits of using staple fixation compared with plate fixation include less soft tissue dissection, less likelihood of hardware removal at subsequent TKR, and fewer problems with conformity. Fixation for opening wedge techniques can be accomplished successfully with specialized plates, as discussed earlier in this chapter, but buttress plates and fixed-angle devices are other options. The blade plate remains a favorable option for fixation of distal femoral osteotomies, although other techniques have been described, such as fixation with a malleable plate.[92] Favorable rates of osteosynthesis have been reported with this technique.[92]

One of the stated advantages of external fixation devices includes the absence of internal hardware. Although this is undoubtedly true, premature removal of external fixation is often dictated by pin site difficulties, and loss of correction may occur in these patients. Pin site difficulties are definitely more common when external fixation techniques are used in the distal femur, and their use in this setting cannot be recommended.[30] Potentially serious complications of septic arthritis of the knee joint or of an infected total knee arthroplasty after previous pin site infection must be considered, especially in cases in which the treating surgeon does not have adequate experience with external fixation techniques. Although the incidence of this phenomenon is unknown, concern about the prognosis of these patients is warranted.

COMPLICATIONS

Technical difficulties and potentially severe complications associated with realignment osteotomy have undoubtedly biased the occasional surgeon to favor prosthetic treatment options. In general, complications can be categorized as major and minor (Box 94-5). Clearly, many complications arise from errors involved in selecting the appropriate patient, preoperative planning, surgical technique, and postoperative regimen. Patient selection factors and poor postoperative alignment, probably the most common complications of corrective osteotomy, are discussed in the section in which results are detailed. Some of the other complications such as pin site infection, fixation problems, and adverse joint line obliquity have already been discussed.

Neurologic injury after osteotomy ranks as one of the most adverse consequences of HTO. Causative factors include intraoperative injury (as a result of traction, compression, laceration, or penetration by an external fixation pin), tight postoperative dressings or casts, and progressive development of postoperative edema or hematoma. Some of these risks are technique specific; the incidence of neurologic injury is lower with opening wedge techniques. Avoidance of dissection of the peroneal nerve, careful placement of retractors, and maintenance of flexion of the knee during the operative procedure are useful adjuncts that help safeguard the nerve. Postoperative dressings should be well padded with the knee in a slightly flexed position.

The occurrence of a neurologic deficit is clearly related to the performance and level of a concomitant fibular osteotomy.[107] A safe area for proximal fibular osteotomy is up to 20.5 mm distal to the tip of the fibular head.[88] When applicable, a distal fibular osteotomy should be performed at the junction of the middle and distal thirds of the fibula.[10] Injury to the posterior tibial nerve has also been described.[63] Vascular injury associated with HTO is fortunately rare, and most reported cases involved the popliteal artery.[109] As shown in 20 cadaveric dissections, flexion of the knee joint as compared with full knee extension does not protect the knee from popliteal artery injury.[109] The more extensive dissection required for plate and screw fixation with closing wedge techniques predisposes to anterior tibial artery compromise.[24]

Compartment syndrome is a rare, yet devastating complication after osteotomy. It has been demonstrated that suction drainage of the anterior compartment is helpful inasmuch as 8 of 10 patients with drains had postoperative compartment pressures of less than 30 mm Hg versus pressure elevation greater than 50 mm Hg in 7 of 10 patients without drains.[34] The importance of rapid diagnosis and the potential to avert an impending compartment syndrome before the onset of an established compartment syndrome must be emphasized to all members of the health care team when they are participating in the patient's care.

Deep infection is rare after corrective osteotomy, but the risk is greater when external fixation devices are used. Thromboembolic disease occurs with lower frequency after osteotomy than after total knee arthroplasty, and the ideal method of prophylaxis is controversial. We prefer to use the same anticoagulation protocol for both osteotomy and arthroplasty.

Intra-articular fracture of the tibial plateau, which may occur during manipulation of the osteotomy, can be minimized by maintaining an adequate thickness of the proximal tibial fragment (usually 2 cm), removing the entire bone wedge (for a closing wedge technique), or extending the osteotomy bone cuts far enough laterally (for an opening wedge technique), allowing for plastic deformation of bone while slowly and carefully applying a directional force to the extremity, and carefully perforating the apical portion of the osteotomy when necessary. When guide wires are used to direct a tibial osteotomy, one should cut on the undersurface of the most proximal wire. Evaluation of the osteotomy site by fluoroscopy before and intermittently during the manipulation will ensure that the osteotomy is adequately fashioned and is responding appropriately to external realignment forces. The lateral tibial cortex (opening wedge) or the medial tibial cortex (closing wedge) may also fracture through and destabilize the proximal osteotomy fragment during manipulation. If this complication occurs, the surgeon will need to apply supplemental fixation (usually staples) to address the resultant instability on that side. Fluoroscopy is also required to ensure that the hardware has not penetrated the joint itself. Excessive medial bone loss can cause an errant direction of the osteotome or saw, leading to direct osteotomy of the joint surface. Any plateau fracture should be reduced and adequately stabilized to maintain the proper position of the plateau for weight distribution and early range of motion. Osteonecrosis of the tibial plateau can occur when the proximal tibial fragment is fashioned too thin.[25]

Joint stiffness has been reported rarely after HTO, whereas this phenomenon has been reported frequently after supracondylar osteotomy.[19,30,60] Rigid fixation and early range of motion minimize the prevalence of stiffness, but rapid healing of the osteotomy and maintenance of postoperative

---

Box 94-5   Complications Associated With Realignment Osteotomy

Major	Minor
Neurologic injury	Superficial wound healing
Vascular injury	Pin site infection
Compartment syndrome	Skin numbness
Deep infection	Neuroma formation
Thromboembolic disease	Arthrofibrosis
Intra-articular fracture	Knee instability
Hardware failure	Adverse joint line obliquity
Nonunion	Patella infera
Malunion	Delayed union
Loss of correction	Inadequate pain relief
Undercorrection	Painful hardware
Overcorrection	Flare-up chondrocalcinosis
	Osteonecrosis of the tibial plateau

alignment should take priority. Stiffness associated with supracondylar osteotomy does make surgical exposure more difficult for subsequent knee arthroplasty in some patients.[15] Early range of motion also helps avoid quadriceps atrophy and may aid in the prevention of patellar ligament shortening after osteotomy.[105] It has been questioned whether patellar position is actually lowered after HTO.[101]

An acute postoperative flare-up of joint pain may be due to calcium pyrophosphate deposition and has been reported to occur in 4.6% of cases.[24] These flare-ups generally are documented by analysis of synovial fluid and radiographic evidence of crystalline deposition. Management with anti-inflammatory medications or intra-articular injection of corticosteroids is usually sufficient. It has been proposed that preoperative evidence of calcium pyrophosphate deposition, with the attendant generalized joint inflammation, should be a contraindication to corrective osteotomy.[24]

A cadaveric study suggests that conventional closing wedge HTO carried out without lateral collateral imbrication or advancement probably accounts for recurrence of varus deformity.[86] Recurrence of preoperative deformity over time has been correlated with clinical deterioration.[96] This study showed that most patients had some recurrence of varus at a minimum of 5 years of follow-up, but that only 18% had more than 5 degrees of recurrence.[96] In contrast, 83% had significant progression of lateral compartment arthritis.

Discussions regarding difficulty with successful union are ubiquitous in all reports of corrective osteotomy. Potential causes include the location of the osteotomy, the fixation method used, bone necrosis (secondary to heat generated by the power saw), fibular impingement against the proximal tibial fragment, and poorly performed osteotomy cuts. Tibial osteotomy below the tibial tubercle is associated with a four-fold increase in delayed union when compared with tibial osteotomy performed above the tibial tubercle.[99] The rate of nonunion after HTO performed above the tubercle ranges from 2% to 4% in the literature, which is distinctly less than rates reported for supracondylar osteotomy (between 4.2% and 19%).[30,101] The opportunity to remove a section of bone

and compress the opposing vascularized bone fragments in a closing wedge HTO has a clear advantage for establishing union versus an opening wedge technique, wherein an osteotomy is made and the wedge-shaped space created by distractive methods is commonly filled with nonvascularized bone graft or bone graft substitute.

RESULTS

High Tibial Osteotomy

It is clear that reported outcomes of HTO are variable. Factors that affect outcome, such as patient selection and surgical technique, have been clarified over the past 4 decades. Recent literature suggests that HTO provides durable and satisfactory long-term clinical results if the procedure is performed accurately in carefully selected patients, who typically are younger than 60 years and have less than a 12-degree angular deformity, pure unicompartmental disease, ligamentous stability, and a preoperative range-of-motion arc of at least 90 degrees.[14] The importance of patient selection is underscored by the results obtained in 39 osteotomies, many of which were performed without precise indications.[14] Among the 10 poor results, preoperative diagnoses included four cases of diffuse degenerative arthritis, two cases of inflammatory disease, one case of previous septic arthritis, and one case of posttraumatic arthritis with severe deformity. If these 10 patients were excluded from analysis, the percentage of overall satisfactory results would be 79% at 12 years' follow-up.

An equally important consideration for a successful clinical outcome includes the quality of the surgical technique. It is often difficult to ascertain the effects of patient selection and technical errors on the long-term outcome while evaluating many of these clinical series. Many HTO series reveal satisfactory results at 5 to 7 years' follow-up; the percentage of satisfactory clinical results then diminishes significantly (Table 94-2). A meta-analysis reviewing 19 previous HTO publications reported good or excellent results in 75.3% of patients at 60 months' follow-up and in 60.3% at 100 months'

Table 94-2 Survival Success of Selected Series of High Tibial Osteotomy

Author	Year	N	2 yr	5 yr	7 yr	10 yr	15 yr
Aglietti et al[2]	2003	102	—	96%	88%	78%	57%
Berman et al[14]	1991	39	87%	—	—	—	57%*
Billings et al[16]	2000	64	—	85%	—	53%	—
Cass and Bryan[19]	1988	86	94%	87%	—	69%	—
Coventry et al[27]	1993	87	—	87%	—	66%	—
				(96%)[†]		(91%)[†]	
				(94%)[‡]		(94%)[‡]	
Hernigou and Ma[38]	2001	245	—	94%	—	85%	68%
Majima et al[56]	2000	48	91%[§]	—	—	61%	—
Naudie et al[72]	1999	85	—	95%	—	80%	60%
Ritter and Fechtman[79]	1988	78	95%	80%	58%	58%	58%*
Rudan and Simurda[82]	1991	128	—	—	—	80%	70%
Sprenger and Doerzbacher[90]	2003	66	—	86%	—	74%	56%

*Twelve to 13 years.
[†]Body weight less than 1.17 times normal.
[‡]Postoperative alignment in 8 degrees or more of valgus.
[§]One year.

follow-up.[101] Several of these studies carefully analyzed sub-groups of patients to further refine the prognostic factors associated with long-term success. The following quote requires careful consideration: "The passage of time seemed to influence the result only in knees that were undercorrected or overcorrected."[39] This quote can be appreciated in a series of 93 osteotomies in which the overall 5-year survival rate was 90%, which then diminished to 45% at 10 years, thus hiding the results obtained in patients with good postoperative alignment. Favorable alignment was noted in 20 patients, and no failures were observed at 11.5 years after the index surgery. This result sharply contrasts with the observed deterioration noted in 51 of 68 knees (75%) with postoperative undercorrection.

Excluding patient selection, the accuracy of postoperative alignment clearly appears to be a primary factor in success with the passage of time. The difficulty lies in determining the "appropriate postoperative alignment" because recommendations vary between reports. Some recommend 3 to 6 degrees of valgus,[39] others suggest 10 to 12 degrees,[19] and 6 to 14 degrees of anatomic valgus has even been advocated.[81] Coventry reported that for knees with 8 degrees or more of postoperative valgus, the survival rate was 94% at 5 and 10 years' follow-up versus 63% at 5 and 10 years' follow-up for knees corrected to 5 degrees or less of valgus angulation.[22]

Finally, among 314 patients monitored for 10 to 19 years, of 170 patients who had undercorrection, 54 subsequently required additional revision surgery for clinical deterioration, whereas of 144 patients with a normalized or overcorrected alignment, only 8 required surgical revision.[74] Based on this long-term experience, these surgeons suggest that a properly performed HTO rivals the longevity of current prosthetic replacements.

Distal Femoral Osteotomy

As with HTO, reported success with distal femoral osteotomy has been variable (Table 94-3). Patient selection factors,

good surgical technique, appropriate postoperative alignment, and the passage of time all affect the final clinical outcome. Many studies comment on the fact that some clinical failures were poor candidates for distal femoral osteotomy and report better success in patients meeting strict selection criteria.[30] In general, patients should be younger than 65 years and should have good bone stock and isolated osteoarthritis of the lateral compartment, minimal ligamentous laxity, a range-of-motion arc greater than 90 degrees, and flexion contracture less than 20 degrees.

Proper postoperative alignment appears to be an essential factor for a good long-term result, and again, the optimum range of alignment has not been determined. In one study, the success rate was 77% if the alignment was corrected to neutral or varus, as opposed to 60% success in patients left in some degree of valgus.[30] We would agree with others that a tibiofemoral angle of approximately 0 degrees (neutral alignment) is the desired correction for a supracondylar osteotomy.[61]

SUMMARY

Realignment osteotomy about the knee continues to meet many of the original expectations. Although the current indications are relatively narrow, the surgeon should be confident in choosing corrective osteotomy when appropriate criteria are met. Long-term results linked with careful patient selection, accurate surgical technique, and appropriate postoperative alignment portray a favorable outlook for these procedures, particularly because the population at large is more active and is expected to have increasing longevity.

KEY REFERENCES

Aglietti P, Buzzi R, Vena LM, et al: High tibial valgus osteotomy for medial gonarthrosis: a 10- to 21-year study. J Knee Surg 16:21–26, 2003.

Aglietti P, Menchetti PP: Distal femoral varus osteotomy in the valgus osteoarthritic knee. Am J Knee Surg 13:89–95, 2000.

Amendola A, Fowler PJ, Litchfield R, et al: Opening wedge high tibial osteotomy using a novel technique: early results and complications. J Knee Surg 17:164–169, 2004.

Babis GC, An KN, Chao EY, et al: Double level osteotomy of the knee: a method to retain joint-line obliquity. Clinical results. J Bone Joint Surg Am 84:1380–1388, 2002.

Edgerton BC, Mariani EM, Morrey BF: Distal femoral varus osteotomy for painful genu valgum: a five-to-11-year follow-up study. Clin Orthop Relat Res 288:263–269, 1993.

Hernigou P, Ma W: Open wedge tibial osteotomy with acrylic bone cement as bone substitute. Knee 8:103–110, 2001.

Koshino T, Yoshida T, Ara Y, et al: Fifteen to twenty-eight years' follow-up results of high tibial valgus osteotomy for osteoarthritic knee. Knee 11:439–444, 2004.

Marti CB, Gautier E, Wachtl SW, Jakob RP: Accuracy of frontal and sagittal plane correction in open-wedge high tibial osteotomy. Arthroscopy 20:366–372, 2004.

Parvizi J, Hanssen AD, Spangehl MJ: Total knee arthroplasty following proximal tibial osteotomy: risk factors for failure. J Bone Joint Surg Am 86:474–479, 2004.

Sprenger TR, Doerzbacher JF: Tibial osteotomy for the treatment of varus gonarthrosis: survival and failure analysis to twenty-two years. J Bone Joint Surg Am 85:469–474, 2003.

Full references for this chapter can be found on www.expertconsult.com.

Table 94-3 Results of Distal Femoral Osteotomy

Author	Year	N	Success, %	Follow-up, yr
Aglietti and Menchetti[3]	2000	18	77	9
Cameron et al[18]	1997	49	87	7*
Edgerton et al[30]	1993	24	71 (86)[†]	8.3 (5-11)
Finkelstein et al[32]	1996	21	64	11 (8-20)
Marin Morales et al[58]	2000	17	75	6.5
Mathews et al[60]	1998	21	57	3 (1-8)
McDermott et al[61]	1988	24	92	4 (2-11.5)
Miniaci et al[65]	1989	35	86 (100)[‡]	5.4 (2-16.7)
Terry and Cimino[98]	1992	35	60	5.4 (2-19)

*Endpoint of survival analysis.
[†]Isolated compartment disease.
[‡]Valgus deformity without arthrosis.

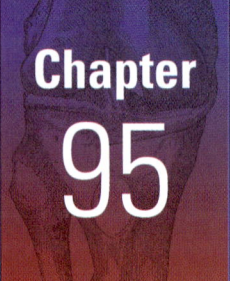

Chapter 95

Osteotomy for the Arthritic Knee: A European Perspective

Sébastien Lustig, Elvire Servien, Guillaume Demey, and Philippe Neyret

OSTEOTOMY: GENERAL PRINCIPLES AND INDICATIONS

Before the introduction of unicompartmental* and total knee arthroplasty,[22,26,73] an osteotomy of the knee was the treatment of choice for gonarthrosis.[16,20,40,57] It has a long past, dating back to the 19th century.[90] Today, however, an osteotomy is considered technically difficult for many surgeons and demanding for the patient. Nevertheless, osteotomies remain an important treatment option for arthritis of the knee in our daily practice because they authorize a return to a high level of activities, including sports, and can delay the need for a total knee prosthesis in young and active patients.

The indications for osteotomy should be defined. Many factors have to be taken into account, such as the type of arthritis, clinical and radiologic criteria, and level of patient expectations.

Why an Osteotomy?

The surgical management of gonarthrosis includes three types of interventions—osteotomies, unicompartmental arthroplasty (UKA), and total knee arthroplasty (TKA). Considering the improvement of the outcome of total[22,26,73] and unicompartmental[12,44,65] knee arthroplasties reported in recent years, the legitimate question arises about the necessity of osteotomies. The final choice of interventions will largely depend on the history of the patient, functional complaints, motivations, clinical examination, and radiologic findings.

Anatomic and Clinical Findings

Anatomic findings have to be considered, such as the stage of osteoarthritis, analysis of the deformity and its reducibility, ligamentous status (frontal and sagittal laxity), and range of motion. Clinical findings are also essential, such as weight, age, level of activity, autonomy, general conditions (e.g., diabetes, rheumatoid arthritis, use of anticoagulants), and surgical history. The decision to perform a certain type of intervention is also sometimes influenced by geographic factors (e.g., an osteotomy is more frequently performed in regions close to the pole, whereas a prosthesis is more common in regions away from the poles), cultural factors (e.g., osteotomy more common in Asia and the Middle East, prosthetic surgery more common in English speaking countries), economic factors (e.g., UKA is not recognized and taught as a treatment option in some countries).

Patient Expectations

Patient satisfaction after an intervention is the result of the difference between the patient's expectations (functional result expected), and functional result obtained. This means that vital information has to be given to the patient, which has to be adapted to the level of the patient's understanding. If not done, this will sometimes lead to the patient's misconceptions about the procedure and its results.

Concept of Functional Envelope Applied to Gonarthrosis

The x axis shown in Figure 95-1 represents the frequency of the applied forces or load and the y axis represents the intensity of the applied forces or load.[23] The surface under the curve defines the functional envelope of the knee. The upper limit thus defines the threshold above which a clinical reaction may be observed (e.g., discomfort, pain, swelling, stress fracture). The definition of the functional envelope remains a theoretical concept, with a large variation among individuals and over time. It remains difficult to determine the individual upper and lower thresholds.

Nevertheless, the profile of the functional envelope will be modified by medication, surgery, and rehabilitation. Each type of intervention will modify the functional envelope in a specific way; for example, total knee arthroplasty will change the aspect of the curve differently than an osteotomy.

These considerations must be taken into account:

1. The patient has the possibility to modify his or her activity (or body weight) to re-enter the functional envelope.
2. The aim of surgery is to enlarge this envelope. If a zone of the envelope will be reduced, it has to be clearly explained to the patient.

If the patient applies excessive force, above the threshold, the risk for failure is increased.

Functional Results of an Osteotomy

- Pain-free (95%), forgotten knee (80%), stability (90%), unlimited walking distance, normal stair climbing and descent, no limp, no use of cruches, no swelling
- All sports (impact and contact) possible, but not recommended
- Full extension, flexion to 145 degrees
- Limiting intervention—weight bearing not allowed until 2 months postsurgery, 5 days hospitalization, return to home, functional autonomy and driving (75 days); takes 4 to 6 months to adapt to the modified biomechanics and degree of valgu
- Revision total knee arthroplasty not difficult

The survival rate is 70% at 10 years[33] and the infection rate is less than 0.5%.

---

*References 12, 15, 44, 65, 75, and 81.

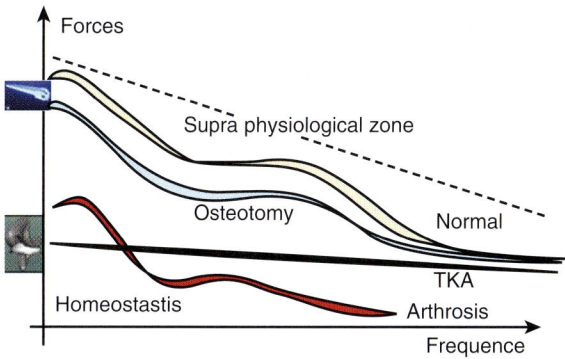

Figure 95-1. Functional envelope according to Dye. (From Dye SF: The knee as a biologic transmission with an envelope of function: a theory. Clin Orthop Relat Res [325]:10–18, 1996.)

Radiologic Workup

The radiologic workup is the same for all types of osteotomies and in our daily practice is no different from that for UHKs and total knee protheses. It includes the following:

- Unipodal weight bearing: Type of arthrosis, localization, presence of osteophytes, cysts, foreign bodies, obliquity of joint line
- Unipodal stance profile at 30 degrees of flexion: Presence of a cupule, patellar height, tibial slope, anterior tibial translation, malunion with flexion deformity (this view is the most important view for antirecurvatum osteotomies)
- Skyline view of patella in 30 degrees of flexion to examine the patellofemoral joint
- Bipodal stance at 45 degrees of flexion view (schuss view; this view excellent to evaluate femorotibial joint space width narrowing that is frequently underestimated on the above-mentioned views)

Prior to the intervention, preoperative radiographic evaluation is essential. It includes a bipodal stance full leg film that allows measuring of the different angles and axes. The mechanical femoral axis is represented by a line connecting the center of the femoral head and middle of the tibial spine. The mechanical tibial axis connects the middle of the tibial spine and middle of the ankle joint. The mechanical femorotibial axis represents the overall deformity of the lower limb. This view will define the origin of the deformity (at the level of the femur or tibia) and will thus indicate the level at which to perform the osteotomy, importance of the overall deformity, and amount of correction that will have to be performed.

Stress x-rays in varus and valgus will illustrate articular laxity and reducibility of the deformity. Measurement of the constitutional varus is the epiphyseal axis as defined by Levigne[47]—a line connecting the middle of the tibial joint line and the middle of the line connecting the tibial epiphesis. This axis forms a constant angle of 90 ± 2 degrees to the lateral tibial plateau (Fig. 95-2). The constitutional deformity of the tibia is defined as the angle between the epiphyseal and tibial mechanical axes (Fig. 95-3).

Sometimes, it is difficult to determine the middle of the tibial joint line and where to perform the measurement. Therefore, we prefer to determine the level of the original tibial plateau by the line tangent to the normal contralateral tibial plateau. Subsequently, the mechanical tibial axis is

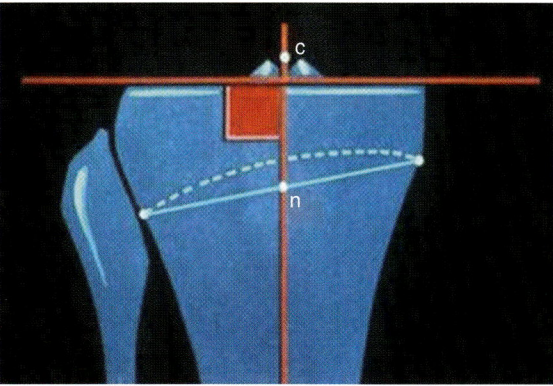

Figure 95-2. Epiphyseal axis, as defined by Levigne. This is a line connecting the middle of the tibial joint line and the middle of the line connecting the tibial epiphesis. This axis forms a constant angle of 90 ± 2 degrees to the lateral tibial plateau. (Adapted from Levigne CH: Interêt de l'axe épiphysaire dans l'arthrose. In Neyret P, Dejour H [eds]: Journées Lyonnaises de chirurgie du genou, Lyon,1991, Hôpital de Lyon Sud, pp 127–141.)

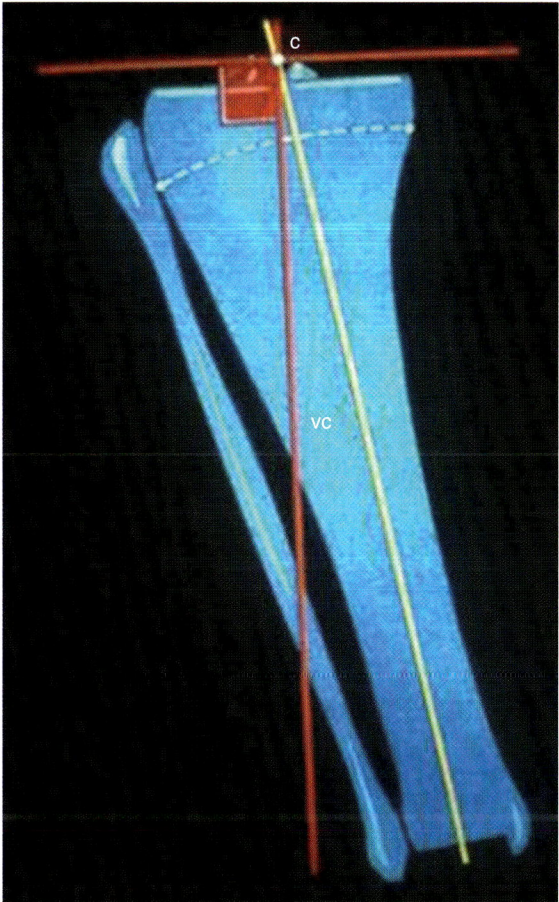

Figure 95-3. Constitutional deformity of the tibia—defined as angle between epiphyseal axis and tibial mechanical axis. (Adapted from Levigne CH: Interêt de l'axe épiphysaire dans l'arthrose. In Neyret P, Dejour H [eds]: Journées Lyonnaises de chirurgie du genou, Lyon,1991, Hôpital de Lyon Sud, pp 127–141.)

drawn. The angle between both axes is the angle α. The constitutional varus is defined by the complementary angle 90α (Fig. 95-4).

Additional radiologic investigations also include a computed tomography (CT) scan to determine the presence of

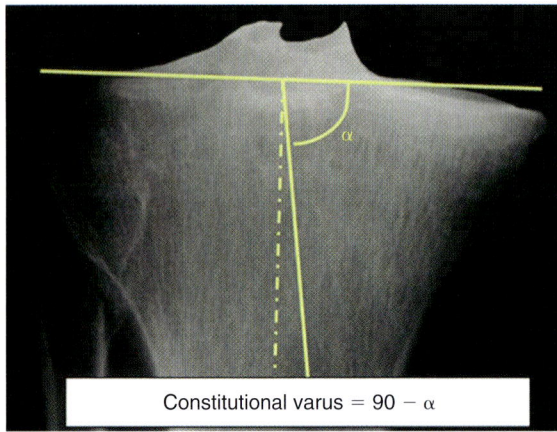

Constitutional varus = 90 − α

Figure 95-4. The level of the native tibial plateau is determined by the line tangent to the normal contralateral tibial plateau. The mechanical tibal axes are then drawn. The angle between both axes is the angle and the constitutional varus is defined by the complementary angle 90 − α.

rotational problems. Certain patients with a frontal valgus or varus deformity can develop a unilateral arthritis at the side of the convexity of the malunion. This lateralization of the degenerative process can be explained by the rotational problem. An internal medial rotation will cause a lateral femorotibial arthrosis, whereas an external rotation of the femur will cause a medial femorotibial arthrosis.

Indications

The indication is often a compromise and represents a choice made by the patient and surgeon. For teaching purposes, we would like to note that it is not always possible to have ideal indications. Sometimes, one or more criteria will make the indications limited or disputable.

Physical Indications

- Pain localized on femorotibial joint line
- Normal range of motion
- Normal ligamentous status (but anterior cruciate ligament [ACL] or posterior cruciate ligament [PCL] insufficiency is not a contraindication)
- Nonreducible deformity
- No inflammatory arthritis
- Younger than 70 years
- No obesity

Radiologic Indications

- Partial or complete joints space width narrowing in one compartment
- No contralateral femorotibial joints space width narrowing or patellofemoral joint space width narrowing
- Extra-articular deformity more than 5 degrees

Disputable Indications

- Patellofemoral arthritis
- Flexion less than 100 degrees or fixed flexum deformity
- Extra-articular deformity
- Older than 70 years
- Obese female

Activity Level

The preoperative level of activity and expected postoperative level of activity of the patient will influence the indications of osteotomy. We are more likely to treat even an older patient with a high level of activity, including sports, by an osteotomy.

Factors Influencing Choice of Osteotomy

Type of Arthritis

Medial Gonarthritis

Some factors support an osteotomy:
- The origin of the medial gonarthrosis is most likely on the tibial site and usually in the proximal metaphyseal region. The result of a high tibial osteotomy (HTO) remains an important surgical option. The long-term clinical outcome at 10 years is better for a varus deformity mainly caused by bowing than a deformity essentially caused by wear.[9,50]
- The clinical outcome of an osteotomy in medial gonarthrosis is reported to be good, reliable, and durable, with a survivorship of approximately 70% at 10 years.[5]
- An osteotomy restores the morphology with a horizontal joint line.
- Technically, the objective of this procedure is to obtain a hypercorrection between 3 to 6 degrees of valgus, as measured on the mechanical femorotibial angle between 183 and 186 degrees.[1,7,31,35,39]

Opening Wedge Osteotomy. There are many advantages in comparison with a closing wedge osteotomy: a more accurate correction; no peroneal nerve injury (palsy); and can be combined with an ACL reconstruction through the same incision.[72] The disadvantages are that a graft is needed (e.g., bone graft, ceramic), the consolidation may be longer (8 to 10 weeks), and the tensioning of the extensor system (and, to a lesser degree, the medial collateral ligament and medial tendinous structures). We prefer an opening wedge high tibial osteotomy for the younger patient with preosteoarthritis or limited osteoarthritis.

Closing Wedge Osteotomy. Its advantages are a shorter consolidation (7 to 8 weeks) and a natural tendency to decrease the tibial slope angle. The disadvantages are the risk for damaging the peroneal nerve and more variability in the obtained correction.

We prefer a closing wedge high tibial osteotomy for the somewhat older patient with advanced osteoarthritis. In case of evolved osteoarthritis (OA) secondary to chronic anterior laxity, this is the technique of choice.

Lateral Gonarthrosis

This type of OA, with valgus deformity, is of mixed origin, both on the femur and tibia, and in our experience the clinical outcome is less reproducible. We attempt to achieve a normal correction between 0 and 2 degrees of varus.

Opening Wedge Distal Femoral Osteotomy. Because the origin of the valgus knee is situated in the distal femur, an osteotomy of the distal femur seems logical. Nevertheless, we have to understand that a correction by osteotomy is only obtained in the frontal plane, in extension (Fig. 95-5). The anatomy and alignment are not changed in flexion and thus a valgus knee will persist in flexion after a distal femoral osteotomy. Therefore, the indication for a distal femoral osteotomy is a valgus knee in extension (Fig. 95-6). We currently believe that the classification of the valgus knee according to

the origin of the deformations is not yet well understood and that the deformities at a level of the diaphysis are still not yet included. A distal femoral osteotomy requires a rigid fixation and is associated with more blood loss and a high risk for arthrofibrosis.

We have generally performed a distal femoral osteotomy in the younger patient with a valgus of distal femoral origin. The patient should be well motivated.

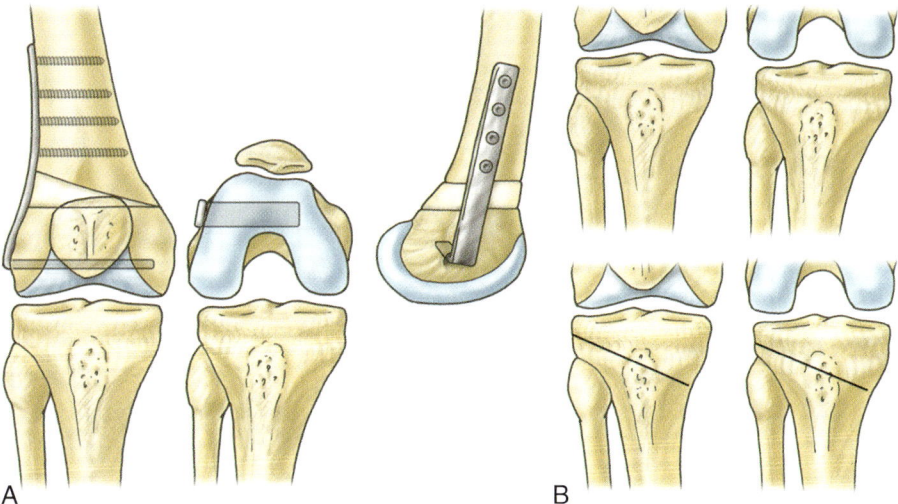

Figure 95-5. **A,** Correction by femoral osteotomy is only obtained in the frontal plane, in extension. **B,** HTO for varisation (medial closing wedge high tibial osteotomy), on the contrary, will have an effect both in extension and flexion. (Courtesy Dr. P. Chambat.)

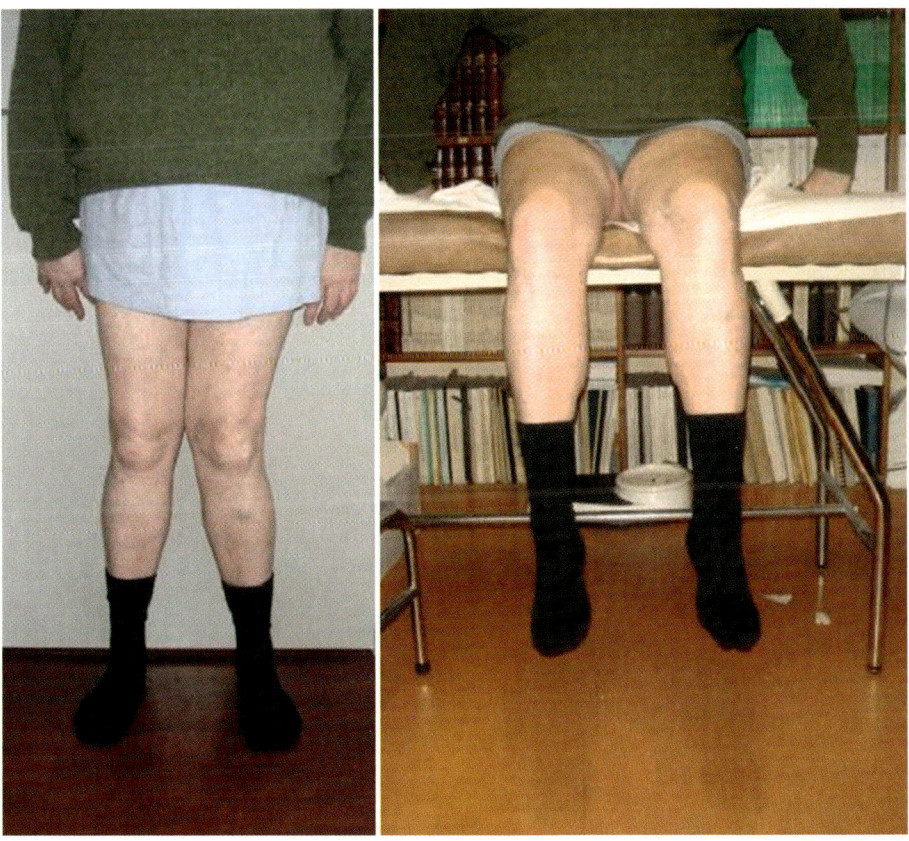

Figure 95-6. Typical indication for a distal femoral osteotomy—valgus knee in extension and no valgus in flexion.

High Tibial Osteotomy for Varisation (Medial Closing Wedge High Tibial Osteotomy). This type of osteotomy, on the contrary, will have an effect in extension and in flexion, and is the only one with an action in flexion. It is indicated and justified in those valgus knees of mixed origin. However, it is accompanied by a risk for an important obliquity in the joint line. This obliquity, if greater than 10 degrees, can lead to excessive stress on the patellofemoral joint, especially on the medial side. We propose a medial closing wedge high tibial osteotomy for the patient who is 60 years old (average age) with a high activity level, including sports, with a valgus knee of mixed origin or of tibial origin that is less than 8 degrees.

Clinical Criteria

The age of the patient has to be taken into account. In a young patient with limited or early medial OA, we prefer an opening wedge high tibial osteotomy. The patient's weight can also influence the decision; morbid obesity has a negative influence because of loss of correction in the osteotomy on one side and because of difficulties during the non–weight-bearing period on the other side.

Arthritis secondary to ACL rupture can influence the choice of the technique. Because of the wear pattern located more posteriorly on the tibial plateau as a result of the ACL rupture, decreasing the tibial slope will limit the anterior tibial translation. Therefore, a closing wedge high tibial osteotomy seems to be more appropriate.

Radiologic Criteria

The origin of the deformation can be determined radiographically:
- If extra-articular constitutional or malunion is seen, the osteotomy will be considered corrective because it will correct the bony deformity.
- If intra-articular wear is noted, the osteotomy is considered palliative because the wear deformation will be compensated by creating a bony deformity.

HIGH TIBIAL OSTEOTOMY

In case of medial OA in association with a genu varum morphotype, a high tibial osteotomy remains an important surgical option. The long-term clinical outcome at 10 years continues to be favorable in more than 70% of patients if the frontal angular malalignment has been corrected to 3 to 6 degrees of valgus.

The main reasons for failure are the following:
1. A hypocorrection with the presence of a residual varus deformity
2. An overcorrection with progressive lateral gonarthrosis
3. Development of patellofemoral arthritis

Despite the progression in cartilage degeneration overtime, this type of intervention remains indicated, especially for middle-aged individuals.

Two surgical techniques are available. First is the opening wedge medial HTO, which should be associated with the use of a bone graft. Second is the lateral closing wedge high tibial osteotomy associated with a fibular neck osteotomy. The clinical outcome is more predictable in nonobese patients. Therefore, we generally provide information preoperatively on hygiene, smoking cessation, and caloric intake.

If we have a young, sports-minded patient, an osteotomy still remains the option of choice before an arthroplasty.

Radiologic Workup

The height of the opening wedge to obtain a valgus correction of 3 to 6 degrees is calculated as a function of the width of the tibia at the level of the osteotomy and the angular correction needed.

Lateral Closing Wedge High Tibial Osteotomy

Patient Preparation

The patient is in a supine position. A tourniquet is generally used. The patient is draped using an extremity sheet and the image intensifier is installed. A slightly oblique, almost horizontal anterolateral skin incision is made. It starts 1 cm above the anterior tibial tuberosity and goes laterally 1 cm below the fibular head. The insertion of the tibialis anterior is released as a Z-plasty. Subsequently, the tibialis anterior muscle and long toe extensor muscle are released from the tibial metaphysis using a large periosteal elevator.

Osteotomy of the Neck of the Fibula

The neck of the fibula is identified and presented. A periosteal elevator is slid around the neck, always staying in contact with the bone. This protects the peroneal nerve. Four holes are now drilled in the neck using a 3.2-mm drill. With the use of the osteotome, the four holes are interconnected and the segment is removed using a large grasper. The fibular shaft should be mobile. Care is taken that the peroneal nerve is not entrapped in the osteotomy.

Peroneal Nerve Protection

- Release the tibialis anterior muscle distally enough.
- Distally, the fibular neck is identified and presented. A periosteal elevator is slid laterally around the neck, always staying in contact with the bone.
- Four drill holes are made in the neck.
- The two distal drill holes are first interconnected with the osteotome and then the proximal drill holes.
- The bone segment can be removed using a large grasper.

Closing Wedge Osteotomy of the Tibia

Specific instruments are available to perform the HTO and its fixation reproducibly. The osteotomy is done proximal to the tibial tubercle in an oblique direction. Imaging identifier control of the pin position is unnecessary if the following guidelines are followed:
- Laterally, the osteotomy should start distally from the peroneotibial joint and should cross the tibial tubercle proximally. In this direction, there is no danger to the tibial plateau.
- The patellar tendon should be protected during the procedure and should not be damaged.
- Always check the obtained alignment correction during the operation with an imaging identifier control.

We use the HTO Intrasoft device (Tornier Orthopedics, Montbonnot, France) for the fixation.. This blade plate–screw system has been specifically designed to minimize subcutaneous irritation. Different lengths of blade and screws are available to adapt to the different widths of the tibia.

A small guide pin is introduced at the level of the joint line and an alignment guide is subsequently introduced over this guide pin. The alignment guide will now automatically give the position and direction of a second guide pin parallel with the joint line and 1 cm distal to it.

We then introduce the blade reamer over the second guide pin. The length of the blade should be 1 cm shorter than the total width of the tibia. The box preparation guide is introduced over the guide pin and impacted. Four 6-mm diameter drill holes are made. The HTO blade is introduced and impacted into the box (Fig. 95-7).

Then we perform the distal cut of the closing wedge osteotomy. Many surgeons use a guide pin for the distal cut of the osteotomy but we do not believe that this is necessary. The posterior surface of the tibia is protected by a large periosteal elevator and the patellar tendon is retracted anteriorly. An oscillating saw is used to make the distal cut.

An angled cutting guide (6, 8, or 10 degrees) is introduced in the distal cut of the osteotomy and the proximal cut is now made using this angle. The cutting guide should be introduced and impacted on the medial cortex. An oscillating saw is used. The bone wedge is removed (Fig. 95-8).

The medial cortex is weakened with a 3.2-mm drill. A provisional unicortical screw is positioned distally from the osteotomy. This will be used as support for the reduction clamp. The wedge is closed with the reduction clamp (Fig. 95-9). Using a long metal bar positioned on the center of the femur head and in the middle of the ankle joint, the mechanical femorotibial axis is evaluated. The metal bar should pass just laterally to the lateral tibial spine (Fig. 95-10). The osteotomy is fixed with two bicortical long screws that are introduced through the blade into the distal tibia. The muscle insertions are now closed over a drain. The skin is closed with separate sutures.

Other fixation devices and guiding jigs are available, such as the swan neck blade plate,[21,50] classic blade plates,[43,64] and staples.[6,17,30,87,93] One study has shown the biomechanical superiority of plate fixation for proximal tibial osteotomy.[28] There is no advantage in using staples as a means of fixation because the plates and blade plates that are now available are more stable and do not carry additional risks of complications.

Medial Opening Wedge High Tibial Osteotomy

Patient Preparation and Skin Incision

The patient is placed in a supine position. A tourniquet is applied. An extremity sheet is used for the knee and a small square field is applied on the ipsilateral iliac crest. A small cushion is positioned underneath the buttocks to obtain a better exposure of the iliac crest. An 8-cm-long horizontal

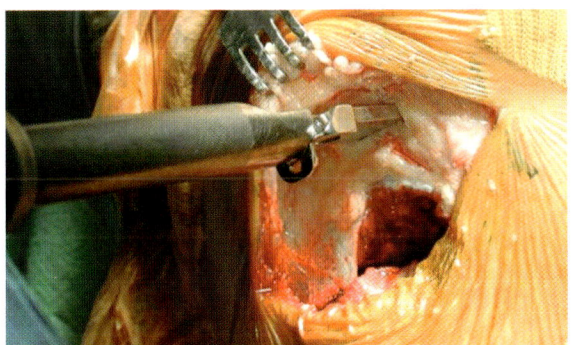

Figure 95-7. Introduction and impaction of the blade.

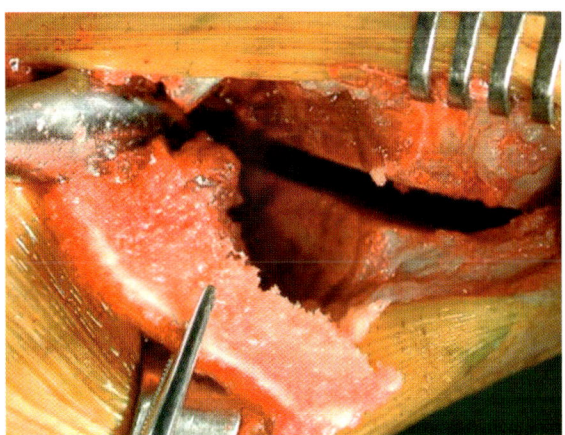

Figure 95-8. Removal of the bone wedge.

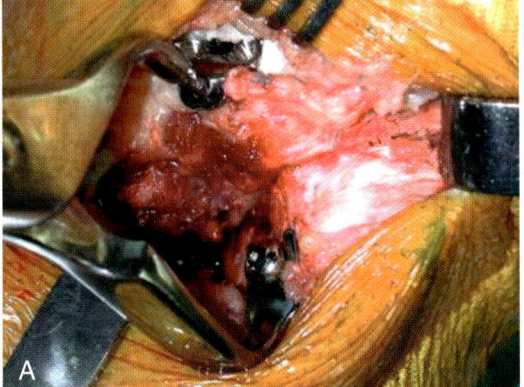

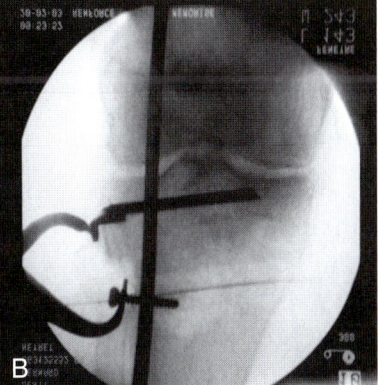

Figure 95-9. **A,** Closing of the wedge with the reduction clamp. **B,** Using a long metal bar positioned from the center of the femur head to the middle of the ankle joint, the mechanical femorotibial axis is evaluated. The metal bar should pass just laterally to the lateral tibial spine.

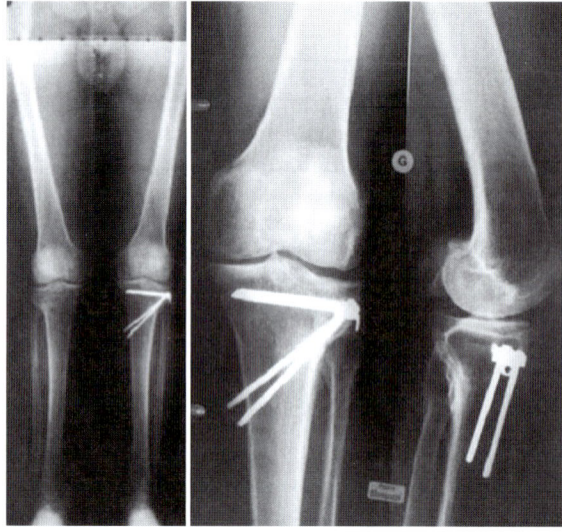

Figure 95-10. Closing wedge high osteotomy of the tibia, with 5-year follow-up.

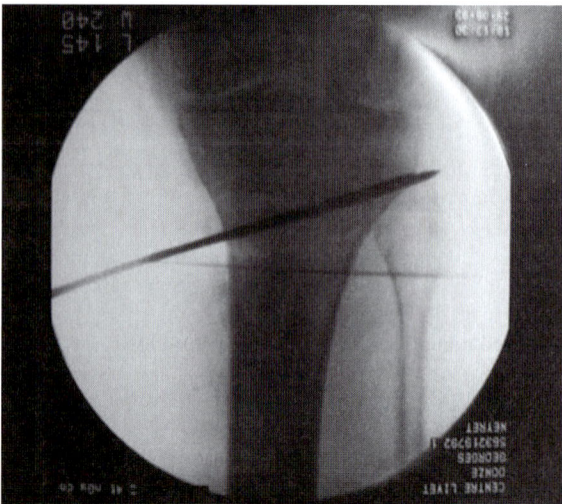

Figure 95-12. Control of the correct position of the guide pins with imaging identifier. The pins should be introduced from a medial direction and be just superior to the head of the fibula laterally.

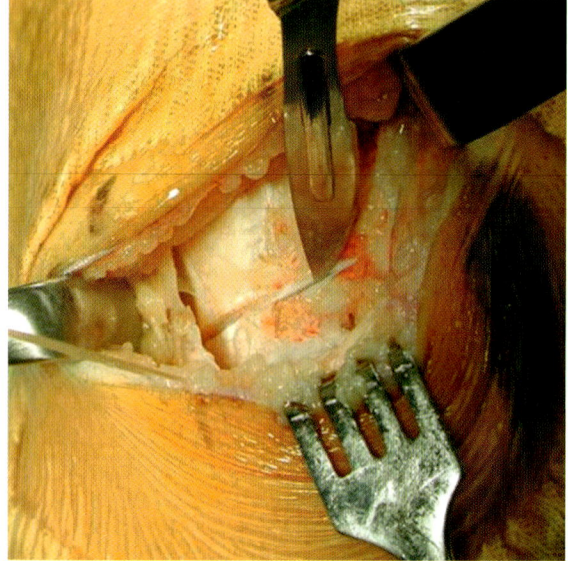

Figure 95-11. Incision of the superficial medial collateral ligament at the level of the osteotomy.

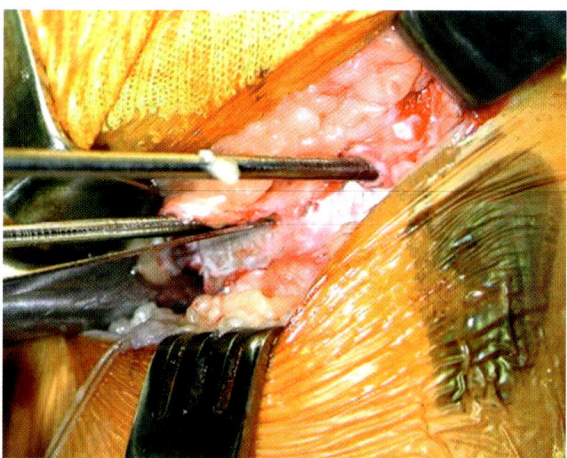

Figure 95-13. The tibial cut is performed underneath two guide pins introduced medially.

anteromedial skin incision is made, starting anteriorly just proximally to the tibial tubercle. The pes anserinus tendons are retracted. The superficial medial collateral ligament is incised at the level of the osteotomy (Fig. 95-11). The posterior surface of the tibia is exposed using a large periostal elevator.

During the osteotomy, this periosteal elevator is left in place. Anteriorly, the patellar tendon is retracted using a Farabeuf retractor.

Procedure

The osteotomy is performed proximally to the tibial tubercle and through the superficial medial collateral ligament, which has previously been incised. The plane of the osteotomy is horizontal, slightly different from the closing wedge medial HTO, which is more oblique. First, two Kirschner 20/10

guide pins are introduced medially. Laterally, these guide pins should be just superior to the head of the fibula.

An imaging identifier control is now performed to evaluate the correct position of the guide pins. The direction can be adjusted, if necessary (Fig. 95-12). Using an oscillating saw, the tibial cut is made underneath these guide pins, but always staying in contact with them (Fig. 95-13). First, the center of the tibia is cut, followed by the anterior and posterior cortex. The cuts are completed using an osteotome, especially on the anterior cortex, where the patellar tendon is in danger.

It is necessary to have an intact lateral hinge for this type of osteotomy. This hinge can be damaged by a number of drill holes.

Subsequently, a Lambotte osteotome (thickness, 2 mm, corresponding with approximately 2 degrees of angular correction) is introduced into the osteotomy. A second osteotome is now introduced below the first. To open up the osteotomy gently, several more osteotomes are introduced between the first two (Fig. 95-14).

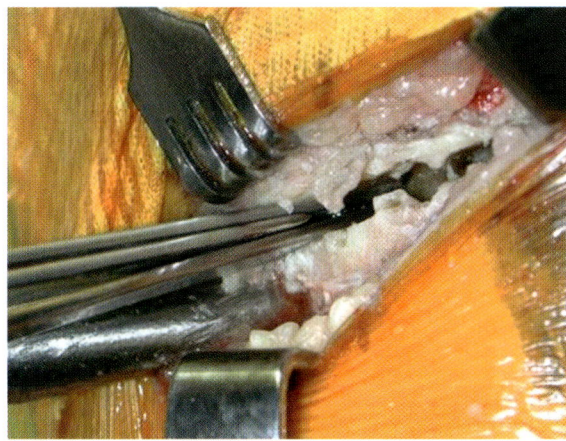

Figure 95-14. Progressive and controlled opening up of the osteotomy with several osteotomes introduced between the first two.

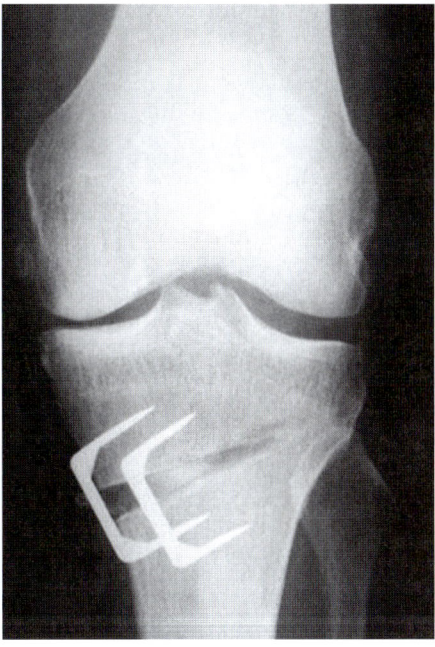

Figure 95-15. Fixation with staples.

If an insufficient opening of the osteotomy is made, the bony bridges anteriorly and posteriorly should be carefully fragilized using an additional osteotome. In general, the opening is more important anteriorly than posteriorly.

Two complications can be encountered during this type of osteotomy:

- Fracture of the lateral hinge. This is fequently observed in important corrections and results in a surgical undercorrection of the deformity.
- Fracture of the lateral tibial plateau. This is observed if the lateral hinge has been insufficiently fragilized, if one forcefully tries to open the osteotomy with a valgus maneuver, or if the osteotomes are impacted too deeply. Usually, plate and screw fixation suffice to overcome this complication.

The obtained angle of correction is evaluated using a long metal bar centered on the hip and ankle. The angular correction is evaluated at the level of the joint line. If necessary, an additional osteotome is introduced or removed.

Osteosynthesis

To avoid loss of correction in the postoperative period, the fixation should be strong and stable. We use two or three Blount or Orthomed staples (Fig. 95-15) to ensure the fixation.

We have used a TomoFix locking plate (Synthes, West Chester, Pa; Fig. 95-16) for several years. This is a plate fixator based on the internal fixator principle and allowing secure fixation of locking head screws in the plate. Plates are adapted to the anatomy of the lateral femur and of the medial or lateral tibia. Lobenhoffer and colleagues[48,49] and Staubli and associates[80] reported good results of opening high tibial osteotomy (without bone graft) using TOMOFIX medial plate. Other types of fixation can also be used (e.g., Surfix plate, Surfix Technologies, Saint Sébastien sur Loire, France; Puddu-Chambat plate, Tornier; Fig. 95-17).

The opening wedge is filled up by tricortical bone graft harvested from the ipsilateral anterior iliac crest (Fig. 95-18). Bone substitutes are also available and can be used instead of the bone graft. These grafts are impacted, taking care not to overcorrect. The superficial medial collateral ligament is then approximated over the staples.

Postoperative Guidelines

The postoperative guidelines are identical for the closing wedge and opening wedge HTO.

- No weight bearing for 2 months
- Walking protected by two crutches
- Thromboprophylaxis for 1 month
- Bracing in extension for 2 months
- Flexion is limited to 120 degrees for the first 15 days. After that, flexion can be progressively augmented.
- The drain is removed between days 2 and 4.
- Hospital stay is 4 or 5 days.
- Skin sutures are removed around day 12.
- Driving a car with a manual transmission is not allowed for 10 weeks, but is allowed if the car has an automatic transmission.
- Physical work is not allowed for 3 to 4 months.
- Strenuous sports are allowed after 6 months.

The patient is invited for a clinical visit 2 months after the intervention. Radiographs should be taken. If bone healing is observed, weight bearing can be started. If delayed union is suspected, weight bearing is allowed and the patient is invited to come back in 1 month.

Results

The results of high tibial osteotomy have been studied and reported extensively since the 1960s. Insall[37] and Healy and coworkers[29] have reviewed studies from the 1960s through the 1990s. They have drawn several conclusions from these reviews:

1. After a high tibial osteotomy, pain recurs in most knees, and most knees eventually require TKA.[60]
2. Younger patients with moderate varus deformities have the best results; obesity, undercorrection, and overcorrection[15,60] are adverse predictive factors.
3. The overall preoperative state of the knee is the most important determinant of an eventual good result.[34]

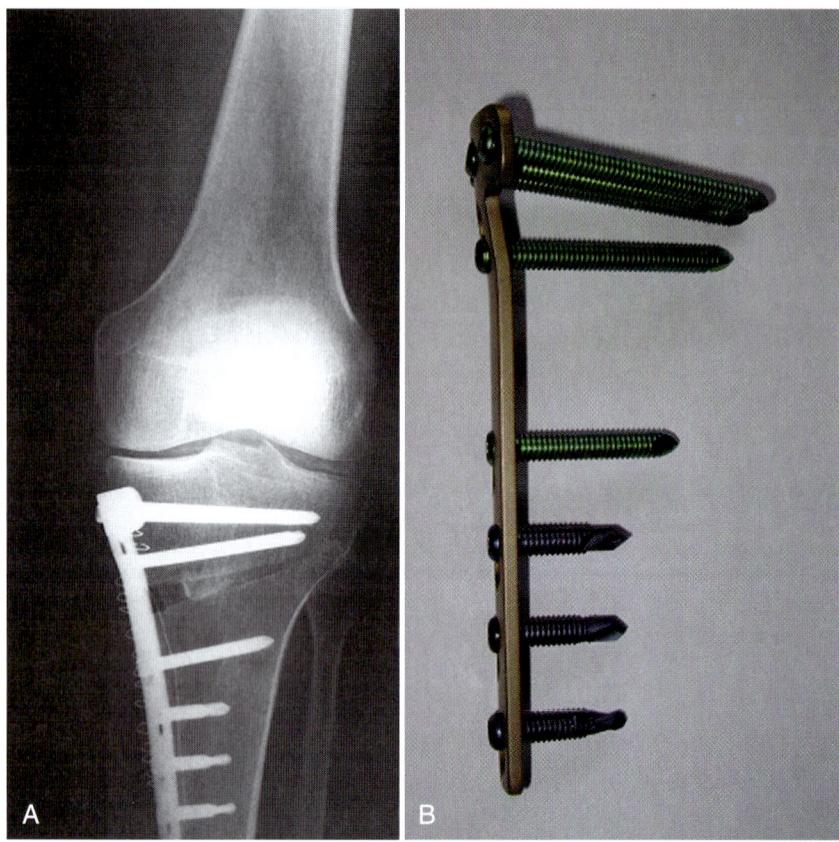

Figure 95-16. TomoFix plate.

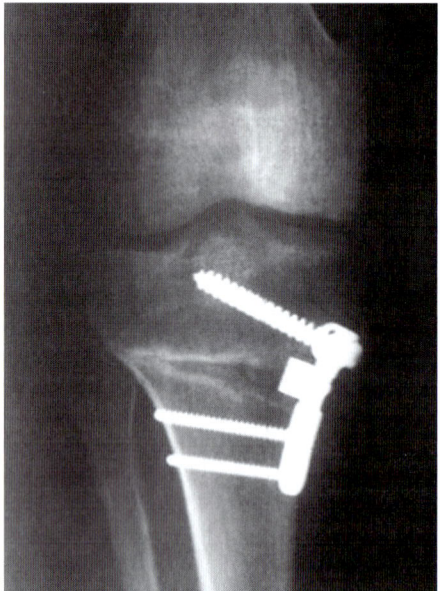

Figure 95-17. Fixation with Puddu-Chambat Plate.

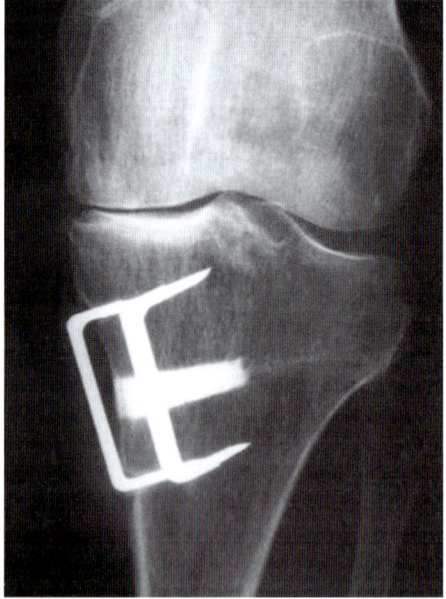

Figure 95-18. Orthomed staples and bone substitute.

4. Preoperative arthroscopic assessment of the knee is not useful.[41]
5. Previous medial meniscectomy[71] and ACL deficiency are not contraindications, but a previous lateral meniscectomy may be.
6. The addition of tibial tubercule elevation to the osteotomy in the case of associated patellofemoral arthritis is unnecessary and increases the complication rate.[35,68]

Some additional information has been given in recently published results. Reported outcomes are variable, but suggest that HTO provides satisfactory and durable results if the procedure is accurately performed in select patients.

The negative influence of the passage of time on the results of HTO has been confirmed repeatedly. Many HTO series reveal satisfactory results at 5 to 7 years of follow-up, but the rate of satisfactory clinical results then diminishes

Table 95-1 Survival Rates in High Tibial Osteotomy Series

Study (Year)	N	10-Year Survival Rate (%)
Aglietti et al (2003)[2]	102	78
Billings et al (2000)[8]	64	53
Cass and Bryan (1988)[13]	86	69
Coventry et al (1993)[18]	87	66
Hernigou and Ma (2001)[32]	245	85
Majima et al (2000)[52]	48	61
Naudie et al (1999)[66]	85	80
Ritter and Fechtman (1988)[74]	78	58
Rudan and Simurda (1991)[77]	128	80
Sprenger and Doerzbacher (2003)[79]	66	74

significantly (Table 95-1). A meta-analysis reviewing 19 previous HTO studies has reported good or excellent results in 75.3% of patients at 60-month follow-up and in 60.3% at 100-months follow-up,[89] but we would like to emphasize that the results were influenced by the quality of the selection criteria.

The importance of precise postoperative alignment has been stressed in many reports.* There is no general agreement, however, about the optimal postoperative femorotibial alignment. If one tries to define a consensual ideal postoperative hip-knee-angle, the obtained value approximates 3 to 6 degrees valgus, although Yasuda and colleagues[91,92] have recommended a larger overcorrection of up to 10 degrees valgus.

The importance of the preoperative grade of osteoarthritis on the long-term result of HTO also has been confirmed.† A preoperative Ahlback grade I or II is predictive for a good long-term result.

HTO for medial OA is a successful procedure for select patients. The ideal patient would typically be younger than 65 years, have less than 12-degree angular deformity, ligamentous stability, unicompartmental disease, and a preoperative range of motion arc of at least 90 degrees.[7] The axial correction should be accurate, and stable internal fixation with an early range of motion is advisable. Despite the remarkable results of knee arthroplasty, a place should remain for this surgical procedure, aimed at maintaining the natural knee.

Complications

Infection

Deep infection is rare after an HTO. Compiling the complications of 10 clinical series for a total of 804 osteotomies, Insall conducted a census of 5 deep and 55 superficial infections; 37 occurred when an external fixator was used.[38] Maquet and colleagues,[55] in a series of 700 osteotomies, noted a 2.8% rate of skin necrosis and a 7.7% infection rate.

Lortat-Jacob and coworkers[51] reported six cases of early reintervention for infection after high tibial osteotomy. In

four cases, the internal fixation was left in place, with a good end result. One patient with gas gangrene required amputation and another died from septic shock.

Lemaire,[46] in a series of 201 dome osteotomies, reported three infections. One was treated successfully by general antibiotics and two were treated by curettage and antibiotic-impregnated polymethylmethacrylate (PMMA) beads left temporarily in the wound. The infection rate after high tibial osteotomy justifies routine antibiotic prophylaxis.

Nonunion

Delayed union or nonunion of the osteotomy is rare. The reported rate of nonunion ranges from 0% to 3%.[13,37,84,85] Jackson and Waugh[40] reported a threefold increase in the nonunion rate when the osteotomy was performed below the tuberosity rather than above it. Insall[38] has noted that a thin proximal fragment is a risk factor for nonunion, perhaps because of avascular necrosis.

Treatment of nonunion after osteotomy usually requires a bone graft and compression fixation in cases for which rigid fixation was not used initially.[29] This fixation may be internal. Some recommend use of an external fixator.[11,17,75]

Peroneal Nerve Dysfunction

Fibular osteotomy or resection of the fibular head can induce a common peroneal nerve palsy[19] or an isolated weakness of the extensor hallucis longus muscle. Kirgis and Albrecht[42] have defined two high-risk regions for an isolated injury of the motor branches to the extensor hallucis longus, the first one about 30 mm and the second one 68 to 153 mm distal to the fibular head.

Maquet[53] has recorded a 3.1% rate of motor deficits and a 4.1% rate of sensory deficits, of which 1.2% and 1.5% were definitive. Idusuyi and Morrey[36] have documented 32 postoperative peroneal nerve palsies in a retrospective review of 10,361 consecutive total knee arthroplasties performed at the Mayo Clinic. They have shown that epidural anesthesia for postoperative control of pain is significantly associated with peroneal nerve palsy. The anesthesia should not produce prolonged sensory and motor blockade.

Compartment Syndrome

The exact incidence of compartment syndrome after high tibial osteotomy is unknown.[27] Some technical precautions can help decrease this risk. The fascial incision should not be closed tightly. A suction drain should be left in place.[27,45,54,86] The tourniquet should be released before closure and careful hemostasis should be performed. Epidural anesthesia can mask the signs of an impending ischemia. If epidural anesthesia is used, the amount of local anesthetic given should be sufficient to make the patient comfortable without producing prolonged sensory and motor blockade, and the status of the leg should be observed even more closely. If in doubt, the tissue pressure should be monitored; a high pressure is a strong indication that fasciotomy should be performed.

Future Improvements

Several considerations may improve our results in the future:
- Inclusion of the femoral rotation component in the preoperative planning for the desired angle of correction.

*References 1, 7, 18, 31, 35, 39, 41, 50, 66-70, 76-79, 88, 91, and 92.
†References 7, 31, 39, 50, 70, 76, and 77.

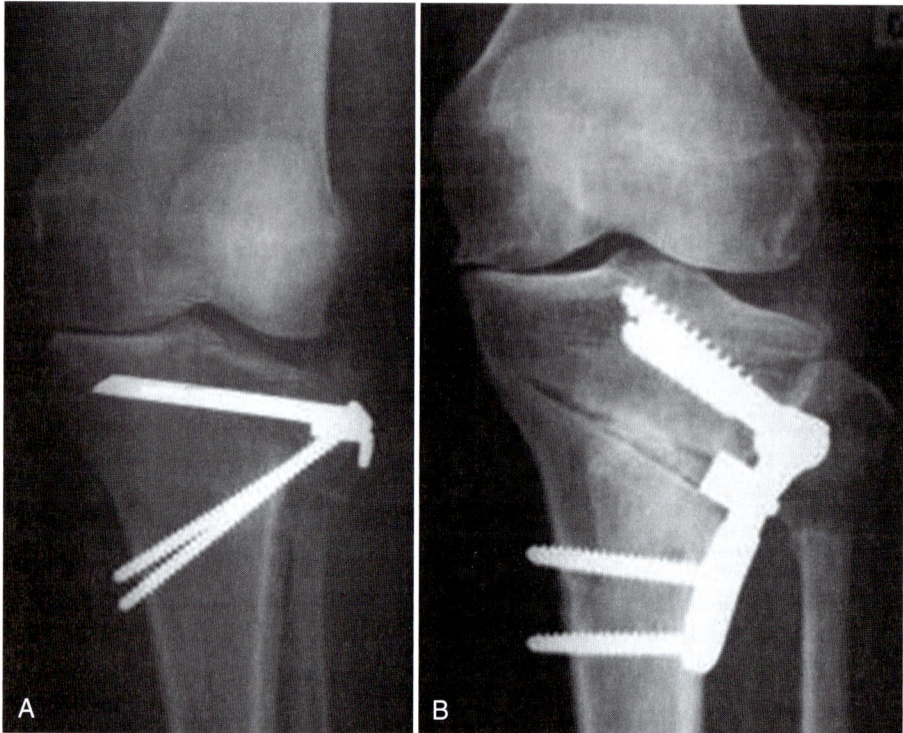

Figure 95-19. Lateral opening wedge osteotomy occasionally performed to correct excessive hypercorrection of closing wedge HTO. **A,** Preoperative x-ray. **B,** Postoperative x-ray.

- Computer-assisted surgery to achieve and evaluate the obtained mechanical femorotibial axis (currently under investigation)
- Better accuracy to reach this target (with computer-assisted surgery)
- Gait analysis probably should become part of the preoperative assessment for all HTO patients (to adapt amount of overcorrection according to importance of the adduction moment)

High Tibial Varus Osteotomy

The high tibial varus osteotomy is indicated for the young and active patient with lateral arthritis of the knee and a moderate valgus knee. This surgical procedure results in a durable and satisfying clinical outcome for up to 8 to 12 years if the lower limb has been corrected to neutral.[58] This procedure addresses the valgus in extension and in flexion. It frequently results in an obliquity of the joint line.

This surgery should be conceived as an alternative to a knee prosthesis (TKA or UKA). The surgical technique consists of a closing wedge osteotomy on the medial side of the tibia. Occasionally, a lateral opening wedge osteotomy is done to correct an initial hypercorrection of a closing wedge high tibial osteotomy (Fig. 95-19).

Radiologic Workup

The amount of correction needed to obtain a mechanical femorotibial axis of approximately 180 degrees is calculated as a function of the width of the metaphyseal area of the tibia. The evaluation of a valgus deformity remains more difficult than the evaluation of a varus deformity.

Medial Closing Wedge High Tibial Osteotomy

Patient Preparation

The patient is placed in a supine position and a tourniquet is used. The lower limb is covered with an extremity sheet. The image intensifier should be available. The surgical approach is identical to the surgical approach for an opening wedge high tibial osteotomy. The anteromedial, slightly oblique, almost horizontal skin incision starts 1 cm proximal to the tibial tubercle and continues medially over a distance of 8 cm. The hamstring tendons are identified and retracted.

The superficial medial collateral ligament is incised horizontally at the level of the osteotomy . The proximal fibers of the superficial medial collateral ligament are elevated proximal and distal to the incision over a distance of several millimeters (as a function of the height of the wedge that will be resected). A periosteal elevator is introduced posterior to the metaphyseal area of the tibia, always staying in contact with the bone. The periosteal elevator is kept in place once the lateral side of the posterior tibia is reached. It will protect the posterior structures during the osteotomy. A Farabeuf retractor is introduced underneath the patellar tendon to retract and protect it during the osteotomy.

Procedure

The tibial osteotomy is performed just proximally to the level of the tibial tubercle. It is almost horizontal in the coronal plane, slightly oblique and upsloped from medial to lateral. Two Kirschner wires will serve as guide pins for the proximal cut of the osteotomy. The pins are introduced medially and will emerge laterally just proximal to the fibulotibial joint.

After the introduction of two guide pins, their correct position is verified using an image intensifier.

The proximal cut of the osteotomy is done with an oscillating saw on the two guide pins. First the midsection of the tibial is done and then the anterior and posterior cortex; the lateral cortex should not be transected. This will serve as a hinge during the procedure.

Subsequently, the distal cut is performed. In the sagittal plane, it should be parallel to the proximal cut and, in the frontal plane, it should converge on the lateral side. The distance between both cuts at the level of the medial cortex has been defined preoperatively, during the surgical planning. The wedge is removed using a large grasper. The lateral hinge is now gently perforated with a drill to fragilize it. Subsequently, the osteotomy will progressively be closed by introducing an osteotome into the osteotomy and gently fragilizing the lateral hinge further.

An intraoperative evaluation of the correction is mandatory. A long metal bar is placed, projected from the center of the femoral head and to the center of the ankle joint. At the level of the knee, this bar should pass through the center of the knee. An overcorrection should be avoided. Therefore, the height of the resected wedge should not be excessive. A frequent error of overcorrection is that the surgeon did not include the thickness of the saw blade into the resection width.

The osteotomy is fixed using two or three Blount or Orthomed staples on the medial side (Fig. 95-20). Use of other fixation devices, such as plate and screw fixation, are possible but we prefer to use less space-filling types of fixation in this area of the knee.

The pes anserinus is closed over the staples. A drain is positioned near the osteotomy and the skin is closed using interrupted sutures.

Postoperative Recommendations

The patient should receive information on the postoperative guidelines prior to the surgery. These are identical to those for an opening wedge osteotomy.

Complications

These include the following:
- Errors of correction—hypocorrection is more frequent than hypocorrection.
- Nonunion and fixation failures are rare.
- Delayed union can be observed in case of an imperfect fit between the osteotomy cuts.
- The osteosynthesis material can cause pain or discomfort; its removal is often sufficient.
- The clinical outcome of a medial closing wedge high tibial osteotomy can decline after approximately 7 to 20 years (Fig. 95-21). In those cases, a TKA can be performed without any major difficulties.

Future Considerations

The following are future improvements:
- Exact calculation of the correction
- Better reproducibility of the desired correction (computer-assisted surgery and navigation could result in more precise evaluation of mechanical femorotibial axis)
- Improvements to fixation of the osteotomy, allowing earlier weight bearing
- Applications of specific growth factors to improve early consolidation

DISTAL OPENING WEDGE FEMORAL OSTEOTOMY FOR TREATMENT OF VALGUS DEFORMITY

The overall aim of this osteotomy is to correct the mechanical axis of the lower limb to a normal varus (0 to 3 degrees). In general, it is better to overcorrect slightly than to undercorrect. During the preoperative planning, one can determine the desired angle of correction and the opening that will be needed to obtain this correction. Radiographs help determine the proper indications but also can measure the correction needed.

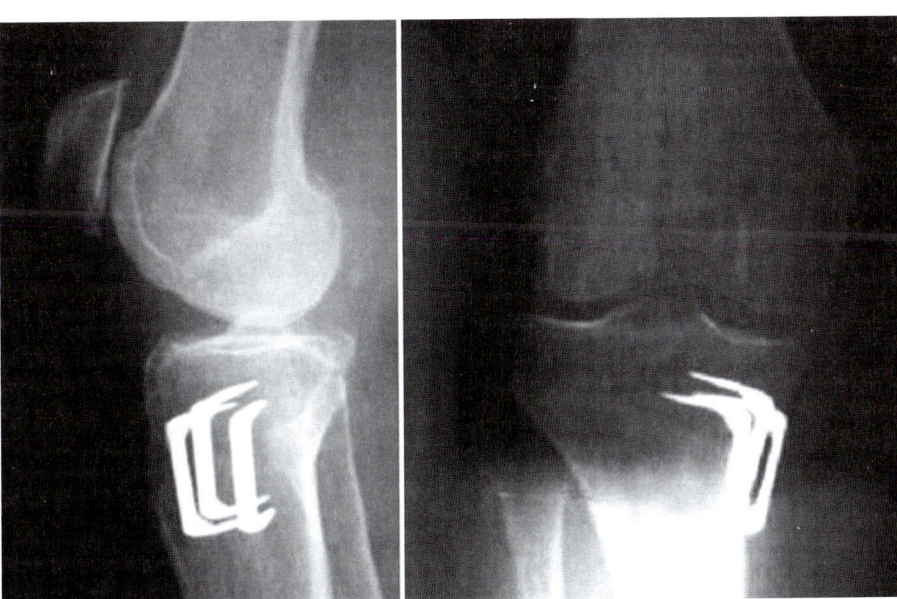

Figure 95-20. Medial closing wedge HTO using two or three Blount or Orthomed staples on the medial side.

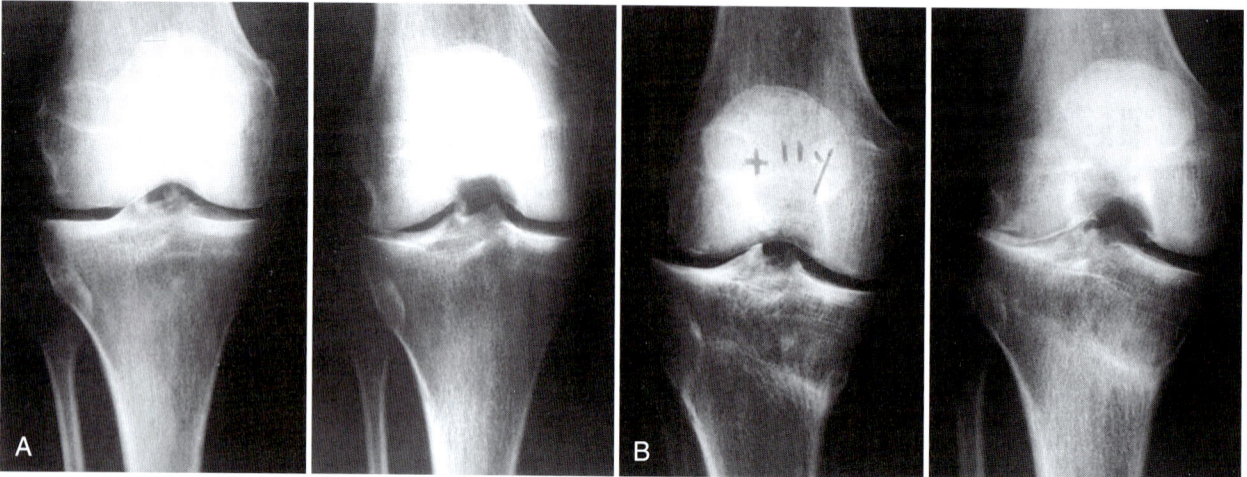

Figure 95-21. Same patient as in Figure 95-20. **A**, Preoperative x-rays. **B**, 11-year follow-up x-rays.

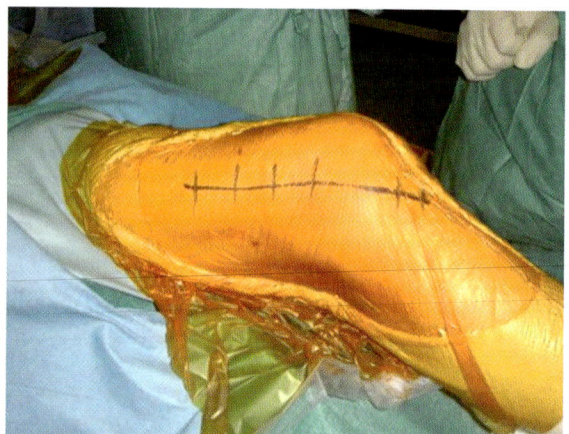

Figure 95-22. Lateral skin incision for distal opening wedge femoral osteotomy. It starts 1 cm proximal to the joint line and ends at the level of Gerdy's tubercle.

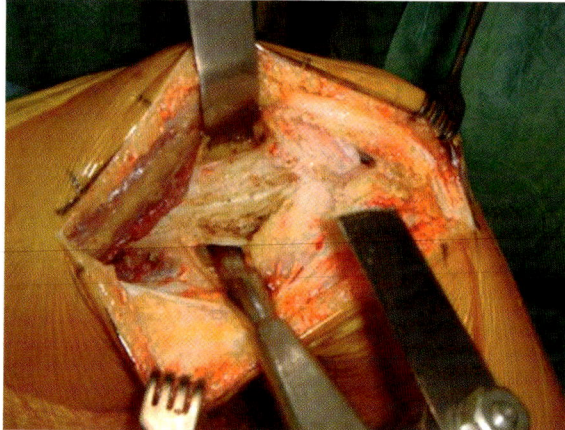

Figure 95-23. Exposure of the lateral distal part of the femoral diaphysis with elevation of the vastus lateralis. With the knee at 90 degrees of flexion, the posterior side of the metaphyseal region is exposed. A landmark is made with the oscillating saw; this will serve as a guide to determine the rotation.

Surgical Technique

With the knee in 90 degrees of flexion, a lateral skin incision starts 15 cm proximal to the joint line and ends at the level of Gerdy's tubercle (Fig. 95-22). The fascia lata is incised slightly anteriorly in the direction of its fibers and the lateral vastus muscle is elevated. The perforating arteries of the vastus lateralis are carefully coagulated or ligated. Subsequently, the vastus lateralis is elevated from the lateral border of the femoral diaphysis using a periosteal elevator. The patellar tendon is identified and a limited lateral arthrotomy is performed; this exposes the orientation of the trochlea and condyles. Two guide pins are inserted into the joint, one at the femorotibial joint line and the other in the patella femoral joint. The guide pins help guide the blade plate and reduce the radiation caused by image amplification.

Next, the zone of the osteotomy is prepared. The osteotomy is horizontal, just proximal to the lateral part of the trochlea. With the knee in extension, the suprapatellar approach is elevated and, with the knee at 90 degrees of flexion, the posterior side of the metaphyseal region is elevated. A landmark is made on the lateral side of the femur with the oscillating saw, perpendicular to the horizontal

osteotomy. This will serve as a guide to determine the rotation (Fig. 95-23).

Introduction of the Blade

The blade should be introduced into the epiphyseal region, 30 mm proximal to the joint line (Fig. 95-24). The blade plate is 5.6 mm thick and 16 mm wide, and the distance between the screw holes is 16 mm.

The guide for the blade plate should be introduced ventrally and proximally to the femoral insertion of the lateral collateral ligament. The angle of insertion depends on the level of the deformation. If the deformation is located at the diaphyseal level, the blade should be introduced oblique to the joint line. To obtain a varisation of 10 degrees, the angle should be set at 75 degrees (85–10 degrees) at a complementary angle to the anatomic distal femoral angle (95 degrees; angle of correction). If the deformation is situated at the metaphyseal level, the blade should be introduced parallel to the joint line (this is the most common situation). When introducing the blade parallel to the joint line, a correction to a normal anatomic femoral valgus of 5 degrees is

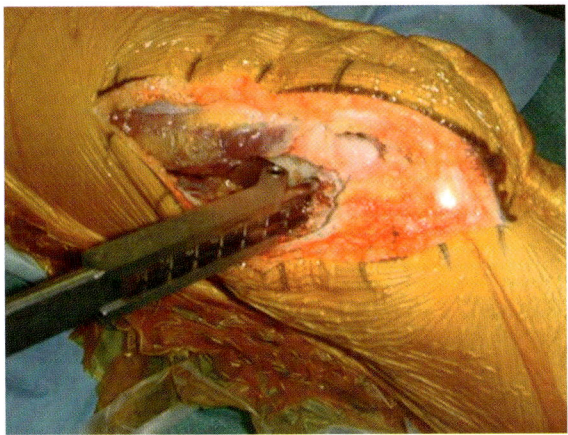

Figure 95-24. Introduction of the blade into the epiphyseal region.

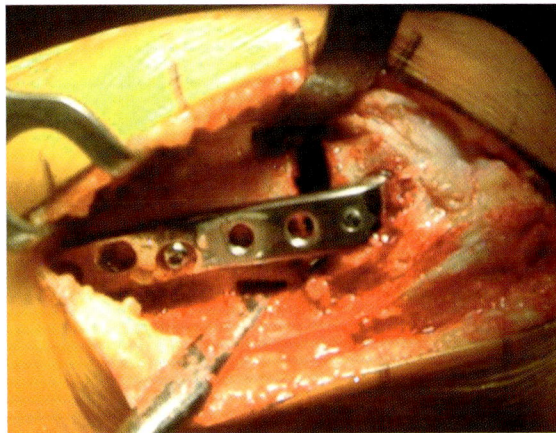

Figure 95-26. Impaction of the blade plate and progressive opening up of the osteotomy.

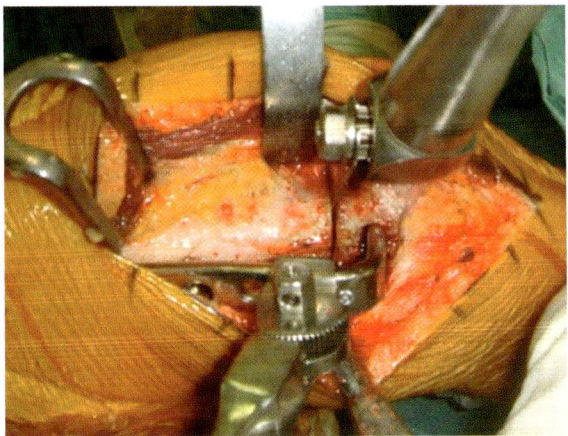

Figure 95-25. Femoral osteotomy performed with an oscillating saw. The blade plate is introduced.

automatically obtained by introducing a 95-degree angled blade plate. In other words, if the femur were to be normal, no correction would be obtained if the blade plate would have been introduced parallel to the joint line. If we are confronted with a combined deformation or with a mixed metaphyseal component (lateral condyle hypoplasia or diaphyseal malunion), the angle of introduction should be even smaller and the blade plate should be introduced at a smaller angle. Preoperative planning is essential to evaluate the correction needed.

The position of the blade can be checked using the imaging intensifier. The angle of correction can now be measured on a printout by drawing a line tangent to the medial and lateral condyles and another line tangent to the blade.

Procedure

The femoral osteotomy is performed with an oscillating saw. The medial cortex should not be cut. Once the blade plate is introduced, the medial cortex is fragilized using a drill bit (Fig. 95-25). Two or more osteotomes are then introduced into the osteotomy but it is the impaction of the blade plate that will progressively open up the osteotomy once in contact with the diaphysis (Fig. 95-26). A screw is temporarily placed in the distal oval screw hole, in the proximal zone of the hole.

The blade plate is now impacted. Subsequently, a screw is introduced into another screw hole while the former screw is taken out. The impaction of the blade plate is continued and the osteotomy will progressively open up until the blade plate is in full contact with the lateral side of the femoral diaphysis.

Progressive impaction allows opening of the osteotomy. Provisional fixation with one screw helps control the correction and provides additional stability. By playing with the impaction and positioning of the screws, one can increase or decrease the amount of opening. If the blade plate is impacted with the screw left in place, the correction will be halted. Conversely, if an additional screw is again placed in the distal part of the screw hole and the former screw is taken out, the correction can be increased.

Final fixation of the blade plate is achieved by four of 4.5-mm-diameter cortical screws (Fig. 95-27). Cortical and cancellous iliac crest bone grafts are used to fill up the opening wedge osteotomy. The soft tissues and skins are closed over a drain, which is introduced underneath the fascia lata.

Postoperative Guidelines

Continuous passive motion is allowed immediately postoperatively. The flexion should be limited to 120 degrees during the first 15 postoperative days.

Nonweight bearing is continued for 2 months and an extension brace is applied. Complications are observed somewhat more frequently than after a tibial osteotomy. Postoperative blood loss can occur, and stiffness of the knee and delayed union occur more frequently. Possible complications should be avoided using strict surgical technique and a specific postoperative rehabilitation protocol.

Complications

Supracondylar femoral osteotomy is technically demanding and is not performed frequently. It has a high rate of complications.

Cameron and colleagues[10] reported on 49 consecutive patients treated by supracondylar varus closing wedge osteotomy stabilized with a blade plate and had six cases of delayed union, one case of loss of fixation, and one case of

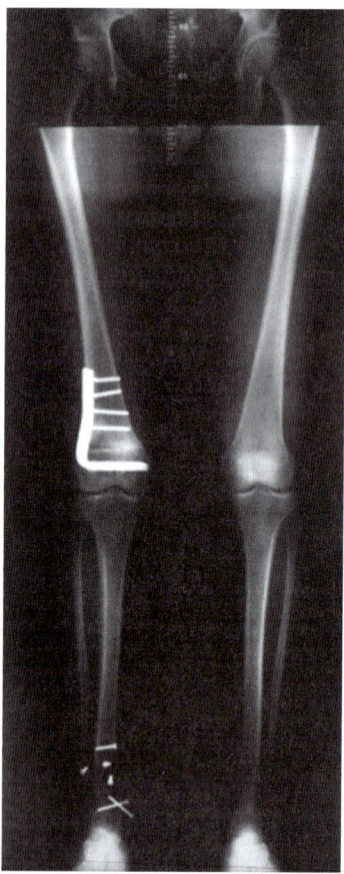

Figure 95-27. Lateral opening wedge osteotomy with blade plate, 6-month follow-up.

Table 95-2 Results of Distal Femoral Osteotomy

Study (Year)	N	Follow-Up (Yr)	Survival Rate (%)
Marin Morales et al (2000)[56]	17	6.5	75
Aglietti and Menchetti (2000)[3]	18	9	77
Mathews et al (2000)[59]	21	3	57
Cameron et al (1997)[10]	49	7	87
Finkelstein et al (1996)[25]	21	11	64
Edgerton et al (1993)[24]	24	8.3	71
Terry and Cimino (1992)[83]	35	5.4	60
Miniaci et al (1989)[62]	35	5.4	86
McDermott et al (1988)[61]	24	4	92

Our goal of postoperative alignment is a tibiofemoral angle of approximately 0 degrees (neutral alignment) for a supracondylar osteotomy.

The ideal candidate should be younger than 65 years and have good bone stock and isolated osteoarthritis of the lateral compartment (Ahlback stage I or II), minimal ligamentous laxity, range of motion arc of more than 90 degrees, and flexion contracture of less than 20 degrees.

DOUBLE OSTEOTOMY

Indications

There are two different types of indications for a double osteotomy. The first is when a unipolar osteotomy (on the femur or on the tibia) will result in an oblique joint line to address a major angular deformity (10 degrees or more) in the frontal plane, in valgus or varus (Fig. 95-28). This obliquity creates shear forces across the knee joint, which could lead to early failure. Also, in case of a unipolar correction by an opening wedge osteotomy, the stability of the osteotomy is compromised. In the case of a closing wedge unipolar osteotomy, the proximal and distal ends will not adapt sufficiently, which can cause problems for future total knee arthroplasty. A distal femoral osteotomy combined with a proximal tibial osteotomy is able to correct the axis of the lower limb while maintaining an acceptable obliquity of the joint line (Fig. 95-29).

The second is for treatment of an OA secondary to a malunion of the femur. In these cases, the aim of the procedure is to address the frontal or torsional malunion on the femur by a normal correction and address the arthritis with a tibial osteotomy. It is important to note that a femoral malunion situated close to the knee joint is more severe than other types. A femoral osteotomy can only correct a deformation in extension and not in flexion.

Double osteotomy has certain difficulties and complications:

1. The risk for a delayed union or malunion is increased compared with a normal osteotomy.
2. Calculation of the correction remains difficult and complicated. In case of a femoral malunion, one could perform both interventions separately, starting with the femoral derotation and then performing the tibial osteotomy. If computer-assisted navigation is available,

rotational deformity. Teinturier and associates,[82] in a series of 131 lateral supracondylar osteotomies, reported 4 infections, 1 nonunion, and 5 deep vein thromboses. Mironneau[63] has analyzed the results of 28 supracondylar osteotomies, all fixed with a blade plate. The morbidity was high, with three losses of fixation, one fracture, one nonunion, and one arthrofibrosis.

The reported complication rate varies. As noted by Aglietti and coworkers,[4] avoidance of entering into the knee joint should reduce the incidence of stiffness. A rigid internal fixation is mandatory, given the high rate of loss of fixation and nonunion when staples are used.

Results

As with an HTO, variable success with a distal femoral osteotomy has been reported (Table 95-2). Patient selection factors, good surgical technique, appropriate postoperative alignment, and the passage of time all affect the final clinical outcome.

Cognet and Mousselard[14] reported the results of 75 closing wedge supracondylar osteotomies fixed by a guided blade plate, with an average follow-up of 8.7 years (range, 5 to 14 years). The mechanical axis at follow-up was 0.1 degree varus. Of all the patients, 77% were satisfied or very satisfied. In one study with 5- to 11-year follow-up,[24] the success rate was 77% if the alignment was corrected to neutral or varus, as opposed to a 60% success rate in patients left in some degree of valgus.

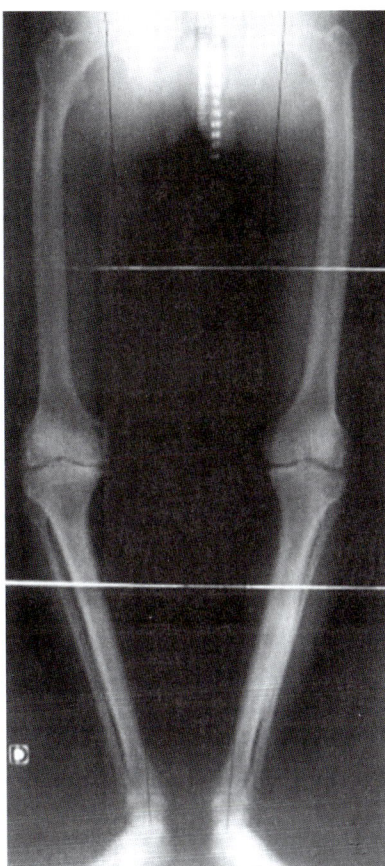

Figure 95-28. Preoperative x-rays of major angular deformity in varus.

correction in the frontal and horizontal planes can be combined during the same intervention.

Nevertheless, indications for a double osteotomy remain rare.

Varus Knee

In case of a varus knee with a mechanical axis less than 165 degrees, the combination of a lateral closing wedge distal femoral osteotomy with a lateral closing wedge HTO or medial opening wedge HTO is indicated. The advantage of an opening wedge HTO is the preservation of the length of the lower limb. In that case, the skin incision is laterally placed on the femur, crosses the midline at the level of the tibial tubercle, and continues medially on the tibia.

An isolated lateral femoral incision can be combined with an isolated medial tibial incision. Commonly, however, in the case of a closing wedge high tibial osteotomy, a laterally based long skin incision is used.

Valgus Knee

In case of a valgus knee with a mechanical axis more than 190 degrees, a combination of an opening wedge lateral distal femoral osteotomy with a closing wedge medial high tibial osteotomy is indicated. This combination results in an acceptable orientation of the joint line and the risk for neuropraxia of the peroneal nerve remains low.

Malunion With Torsional Problem

In case of OA secondary to a femoral malunion with a torsional problem more than 15 degrees and a frontal deviation more than 10 degrees, we advise combining with a derotation osteotomy on the femur.

Surgical Technique

On the Femur

This approach has been described in detail in the chapter on femoral osteotomy for varisation.

Lateral Opening Wedge Osteotomy for Valgus Knee

See the surgical technique previously described in this chapter.

Closing Wedge Osteotomy for Varus Knee

The area for the osteotomy is prepared. Two additional Kirschner guide pins are introduced in the femur as guide pins for the future osteotomy. One pin is introduced parallel to the joint line, approximately 50 mm proximal to the joint line. The second pin is introduced proximally to the first on the lateral cortex but converging with the first medially. This represents the angle and wedge that will be resected. The quadriceps muscle is retracted at a level proximal to the trochlea with the knee in extension; the posterior side of the knee is cleared. A superficial mark with the oscillating saw on the lateral cortex of the femur can serve as a landmark for determining the rotation.

The blade plate has to be introduced into the epiphyseal area approximately 30 mm proximal to the joint line. The blade is 5.6 mm thick and 16 mm in wide and the distance between the holes is 16 mm.

Its entry point is ventral and proximal to the lateral collateral ligament; the entry angle has been determined by the specific instruments and reamer used. For a calculated valgus correction of 8 degrees, the guide instrument is set at 93 degrees (85 + 8 degrees), which is the complementary angle to the desired anatomic angle of 95 degrees plus the angle of correction.

The blade is subsequently introduced into the femur. The correct angulations are again checked using the image intensifier.

Derotation Osteotomy in Case of Femoral Malrotation

The area of the osteotomy is prepared in the same manner. Two superficial saw marks are made on the lateral cortex, indicating the desired angle of the derotation. Thus, an isolated derotation osteotomy can be performed as well as a derotation osteotomy in combination with an opening or closing wedge femoral osteotomy. The derotation osteotomy should not interfere with patellar tracking or create a step on the anterior cortex.

On the Tibia

The bone graft obtained in the procedure for a closing wedge femoral osteotomy is used to fill the opening wedge tibial osteotomy.

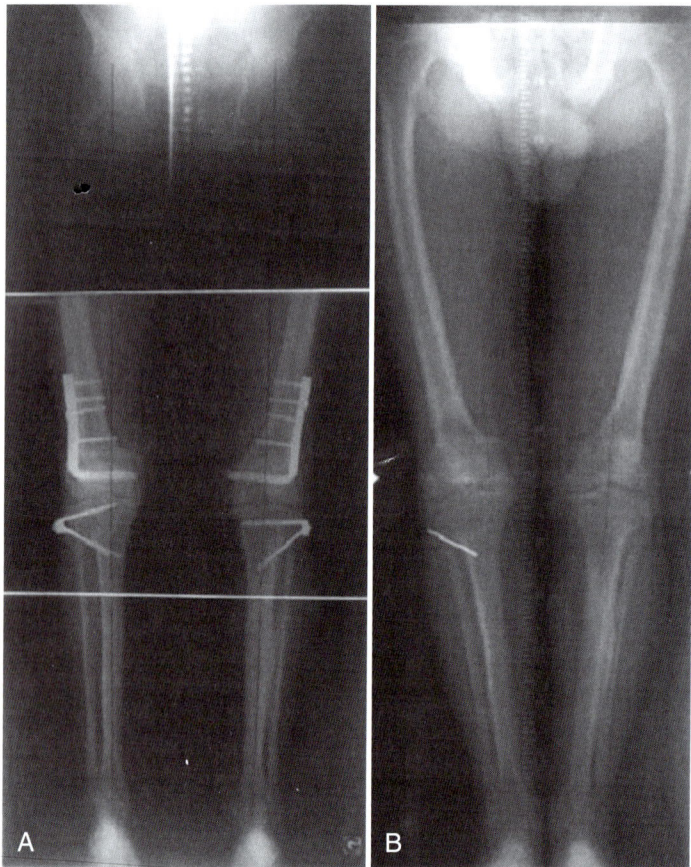

Figure 95-29. Double osteotomy for major angular deformity in varus. **A,** Postoperative x-rays. **B,** 15-Year follow-up, with excellent results.

CONCLUSION

In conclusion, osteotomy is still a treatment of choice for OA. For a medial femorotibial arthrosis, the main indications are as follows:

- Opening wedge high tibial osteotomy:
  - Younger patient
  - Early OA, stage 1 or 2
  - Extended indication—combination ACL reconstruction and osteotomy
  - In the exceptional case of a constitutional varus knee without OA (constitutional varus >8 degrees, if bilateral or with more than four fingerwidths of space between the condyles). In these rare cases, the aim is to leave some residual varus (2 to 3 degrees)
- Closing wedge high tibial osteotomy:
  - Older patient but still active
  - Stage 3 or 4
  - Associated patella infera
  - Chronic anterior laxity with posterior wear on the tibial plateau
  - Femoral osteotomy and double osteotomy are exceptional; these techniques indicated in certain cases (e.g., arthritis secondary to malunion, vitamin D deficiency)

For a lateral femorotibial arthrosis, the main indications are as follows:

- Tibial osteotomy
  - We prefer a medial closing wedge osteotomy.

- To correct abnormalities of mixed origin (femoral and tibial), but only if the obliquity of the joint line will not be more than 10 degrees after osteotomy and, in a valgus knee, less than 8 degrees
  - Lateral opening wedge HTO with a re-osteotomy of the fibula is only indicated secondary to an excessive closing wedge HTO with an overcorrection.
- Femoral osteotomy
  - If valgus knee is of femoral origin
  - If valgus with a fixed flexion deformity or a hyperextension of more than 20 degrees. This pathology can be addressed more appropriately with a femoral osteotomy than with a tibial osteotomy. However, the morbidity of the femoral osteotomy is more important and has to be integrated into the flow chart of indications to prevent complications.
- Large deformation—double osteotomy combining a lateral distal femoral opening wedge osteotomy and a medial closing wedge HTO

KEY REFERENCES

Aglietti P, Menchetti PP: Distal femoral varus osteotomy in the valgus osteoarthritic knee. Am J Knee Surg 13:89–95, 2000.

Aglietti P, Stringa G, Buzzi R, et al: Correction of valgus knee deformity with a supracondylar V osteotomy. Clin Orthop Relat Res, (217):214–220, 1987.

Coventry MB: Osteotomy about the knee for degenerative and rheumatoid arthritis. J Bone Joint Surg Am 55:23–48, 1973.

Coventry MB: Upper tibial osteotomy for osteoarthritis. J Bone Joint Surg Am 67:1136–1140, 1985.

Hernigou P, Medevielle D, Debeyre J, Goutallier D: Proximal tibial osteotomy for osteoarthritis with varus deformity. A ten- to thirteen-year follow-up study. J Bone Joint Surg Am 69:332–354, 1987.

Holden DL, James SL, Larson RL, Slocum DB: Proximal tibial osteotomy in patients who are fifty years old or less. A long-term follow-up study. J Bone Joint Surg Am 70:977–982, 1988.

Ivarsson I, Myrnerts R, Gillquist J: High tibial osteotomy for medial osteoarthritis of the knee. A 5- to 7- and 11-year follow-up. J Bone Joint Surg Br 72:238–244, 1990.

Jackson JP, Waugh W: The technique and complications of upper tibial osteotomy. A review of 226 operations. J Bone Joint Surg Br 56:236–245, 1974.

Keene JS, Monson DK, Roberts JM, Dyreby JR, Jr: Evaluation of patients for high tibial osteotomy. Clin Orthop Relat Res, (243):157–165, 1989.

Lobenhoffer P, Agneskirchner JD: Improvements in surgical technique of valgus high tibial osteotomy. Knee Surg Sports Traumatol Arthrosc 11:132–138, 2003.

Maquet P: The treatment of choice in osteoarthritis of the knee. Clin Orthop Relat Res, (192):108–112, 1985.

Matthews LS, Goldstein SA, Malvitz TA, et al: Proximal tibial osteotomy. Factors that influence the duration of satisfactory function. Clin Orthop Relat Res, (229):193–200, 1988.

Neyret P, Deroche P, Deschamps G, Dejour H: [Total knee replacement after valgus tibial osteotomy. Technical problems.] Rev Chir Orthop Reparatrice Appar Mot 78:438–448, 1992.

Rudan JF, Simurda MA: High tibial osteotomy. A prospective clinical and roentgenographic review. Clin Orthop Relat Res, (255):251–256, 1990.

Rudan JF, Simurda MA: Valgus high tibial osteotomy. A long-term follow-up study. Clin Orthop Relat Res, (268):157–160, 1991.

Full references for this chapter can be found on www.expertconsult.com.

Chapter 96

Osteotomy About the Knee: International Roundtable Discussion

Michael Stuart, David Backstein, Martin Logan, and Thomas Muellner

Osteotomy about the knee has traditionally been used to treat the middle-aged patient with gonarthrosis, but the indications have broadened to include the younger patient or athlete with ligament deficiencies, chondral defects, absent menisci, or posttraumatic degenerative arthritis. We have assembled a panel of experts that includes Michael Stuart (moderator), David Backstein, Martin Logan, and Thomas Muellner, who will share their personal ideas and preferences based on extensive experience with this procedure.

Michael Stuart

For many orthopedic surgeons, unicompartmental or total knee arthroplasty has supplanted realignment osteotomy as their primary treatment for gonarthrosis.

Is there a role for osteotomy in treating isolated medial or lateral compartment arthritis in your practice, and what specific factors affect your treatment decision making?

David Backstein

The frequency of osteotomy for unicompartmental arthritis of the knee has declined somewhat in my practice over the past 5 to 10 years; however, I strongly believe that there are still several excellent indications for osteotomy around the knee. In addition to unicompartmental arthritis, other indications include osteonecrosis, adult osteochondritis dissecans, and osteotomy in combination with osteochondral grafting to off-load the involved compartment.

Candidates must have adequate bone stock to allow effective fixation and early range of motion, a preoperative range of motion arc of at least 90 degrees, and less than 15 degrees flexion-contracture. Because of osteoporosis and its impact on fixation, it is my practice to avoid performing an osteotomy on males older than 65 years and females older than 60 years.

Martin Logan

Undoubtedly, osteotomy has a role in patients with isolated unicompartmental osteoarthritis. Our improved understanding of knee kinematics and joint implant design makes unicompartmental arthroplasty a more attractive option than ever before. That said, the joint registry data on unicompartmental arthroplasty around the world show a higher failure rate in patients younger than 55 years of age.

Factors that affect decision making include patient motivation, understanding, compliance, and occupation. For example, a manual laborer in his mid 40s is a better candidate for osteotomy rather than unicompartmental arthroplasty. A sedentary female with isolated medial osteoarthritis and normal preoperative alignment is unlikely to be satisfied functionally and cosmetically with an osteotomy; therefore, I would prefer a unicompartmental arthroplasty.

Michael Stuart

We all agree that osteotomy still has a role in selected patients with unicompartmental arthritis and malalignment.

Thomas, in your opinion, who is the "ideal candidate" for an osteotomy?

Thomas Muellner

There is absolutely a role for realignment osteotomies in treating isolated medial or lateral compartment arthritis in patients with varus or valgus malalignment. In my practice, the ideal candidate for a realignment procedure is the middle-aged patient who has pain during heavy work or recreational sports activities. If instability is an accompanying symptom, combined realignment and ligament reconstruction should be considered.

David Backstein

Yes, the ideal candidate for a proximal tibial valgus osteotomy is a young, physically active patient with medial compartment osteoarthritis of the knee and varus tibiofemoral alignment, for example, the young patient with a highly physical job such as a firefighter or construction worker, who possesses the capacity for a fairly prolonged and at times arduous rehabilitation process. Although this is not commonly encountered, young and active individuals with isolated lateral compartment arthritis and valgus alignment are similarly excellent candidates for osteotomy and are treated with distal femoral varus osteotomy.

Martin Logan

In my mind, the ideal candidate is a male in his early 50s with normal BMI—a highly motivated nonsmoker who has isolated medial osteoarthritis with normal patellofemoral articulation, intact lateral meniscus, normal cruciate ligaments, and a preserved lateral tibiofemoral joint. The knee would be in 5 to 10 degrees of varus compared with the normal contralateral limb and would have a full range of motion without a fixed flexion deformity.

Michael Stuart

The consensus seems to be that an osteotomy is a good option for the young, active patient with a stable, arthritic knee and good bone stock.

Who would you consider to be an "unacceptable candidate" for an osteotomy?

David Backstein

Contraindications for a proximal tibial valgus osteotomy include moderate to severe lateral compartment arthritis or significant and symptomatic patellofemoral arthritis. In particular, I avoid an osteotomy if the patient experiences anterior knee pain when climbing or descending stairs, after prolonged sitting, or when getting up from a chair. Osteotomy is also contraindicated in patients with an arc of motion less than 90 degrees, a flexion deformity greater than 15 degrees, and maximum flexion less than 90 to 100 degrees. Inflammatory arthritis, which by its very nature affects the entire joint in a congruous manner, is considered unacceptable for this operation. Two additional situations that are relative contraindications to osteotomy include (1) a high adductor moment (varus thrust), because it is associated with poorer results and recurrence of varus deformity after tibial osteotomy; and (2) obesity, which has been shown to be a risk factor for early failure of high tibial osteotomy.

Martin Logan

Absolute contraindications in my practice include inflammatory arthropathy, previous meniscectomy or arthritis in the compartment intended for weight bearing, gross obesity with BMI over 50, and a patient who is a smoker or a noncompliant patient.

Thomas Muellner

I would add the uncooperative patient, loss of bone with "teeter effect," and an associated hip flexion contracture.

Michael Stuart

The orthopedic literature has taught us that the success of an osteotomy is dependent on adequate correction of limb malalignment (see Coventry M, Ilstrup D, Wallrichs S: Proximal tibial osteotomy: a critical long-term study of eighty-seven cases. J Bone Joint Surg Am 75:196–201, 1993). Therefore, it is essential to accurately determine the desired amount of correction before surgery and then employ meticulous surgical technique.

What is your typical routine for preoperative planning? Is there a role in your practice for gait analysis?

Martin Logan

I always get long-leg weight-bearing films and use the Miniaci technique, usually aiming to overcorrect by around 2 degrees and taking into consideration the natural alignment of the contralateral limb (see Miniaci A, Ballmer FT, Ballmer PM, Jakob RP: Proximal tibial osteotomy: a new fixation device. Clin Orthop Relat Res 246:250–259, 1989).

I don't routinely use gait analysis for osteotomy.

David Backstein

I also get full-length anterior-posterior weight-bearing radiographs of the lower limbs, including the hips, ankles, and knees, to establish the mechanical axis, the anatomic axis, and the point of intersection of the weight-bearing line at the joint line. I aim for a correction that results in passage of the weight-bearing line through the 62% coordinate of the tibia articular surface (medial border of tibia articular surface is 0%, and lateral border is 100%), resulting in preferential loading of the lateral tibiofemoral compartment. The angular correction is calculated by drawing a line from the center of the femoral head to the 62% coordinate of the tibia at the knee. A second line is then drawn from the center of the ankle to the 62% coordinate. The angle between the first and second lines represents the angle of correction required.

I don't use gait analysis: however, I do examine the patient's gait, and I consider a severe varus thrust as a relative contraindication to HTO.

Thomas Muellner

In patients who are potential candidates for a realignment procedure, it is essential to assess the alignment on long-standing radiographs (femorotibial angle, LDFA, MPTA, Mikulicz's line), lateral radiographs of the knee in 90 degrees of flexion, patella tangential, and MRI of the knee. I also use intraoperative control with the image intensifier, which allows accuracy of about ±2 degrees.

Unfortunately, I have only restricted access for gait analysis in my patients to study the adduction moments.

Michael Stuart

I don't have any experience with osteotomy computer navigation, but it may be helpful for intraoperative verification of multiplanar corrections in complex cases. I routinely use the weight-bearing line method because it is a simple and reproducible technique for determining the desired coronal plane correction angle (Fig. 96-1) (see Dugdale TW, Noyes FR, Styer D: Preoperative planning for high tibial osteotomy: the effect of lateral tibiofemoral separation and tibiofemoral length. Clin Orthop Relat Res 274:248–264, 1992). The surgeon chooses the desired coordinate, which equals the angle of correction according to the specific clinical situation

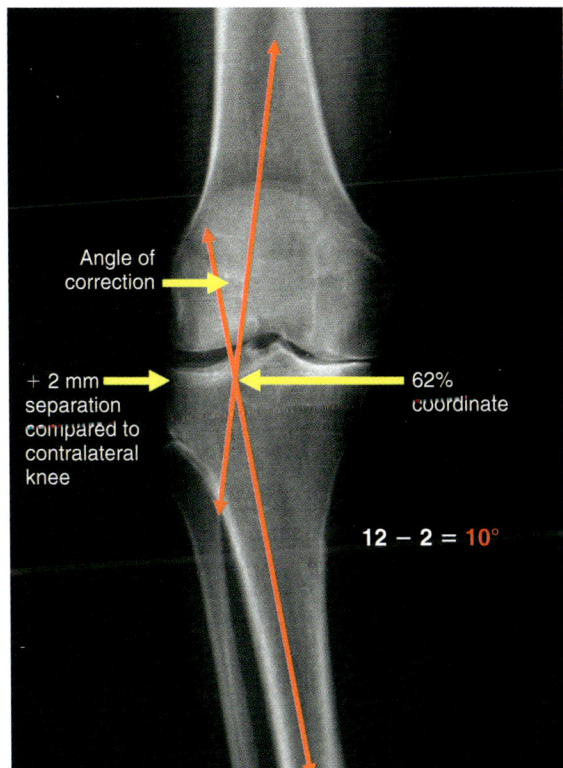

Angle of correction

+ 2 mm separation compared to contralateral knee

62% coordinate

12 − 2 = 10°

Figure 96-1. The weight-bearing line method is a simple technique for determining the coronal plane correction angle. (From Stuart MJ: Opening wedge-proximal tibial osteotomy. In Lotke PA, Lonner JH [eds]: Knee arthroplasty, ed 3, Baltimore, 2009, Wolters Kluwer Health/Lippincott William & Wilkins [Master Techniques in Orthopaedic Surgery], pp 361–371.)

(typically 62%; range, 50% to 75%). Remember that standing radiographs can overestimate the magnitude of correction as the result of osseous defects and/or attenuated ligaments. Compare the amount of lateral joint space opening (in millimeters) with the contralateral knee and subtract the difference from the calculated angle (1 degree per millimeter) to avoid overcorrection.

The lateral closing wedge osteotomy of the proximal tibia was the procedure of choice in the past to correct a varus deformity. In recent years with the advent of new implant designs, the medial opening wedge technique has become popular.

Please describe your preferred surgical technique for correcting varus malalignment. Do you have any technical pearls for surgeons who are learning this technique?

David Backstein

My preference for varus deformity correction of less than 15 degrees is a medial, opening wedge osteotomy. For situations in which the deformity is 15 to 20 degrees, I perform a closing wedge lateral osteotomy because of the lesser risk of nonunion by opposing and compressing host bone. A fixed varus deformity greater than 20 degrees may necessitate an osteotomy of both the proximal tibia and the distal femur to achieve correction.

Pearls

- Position the patient supine on a radiolucent table to allow intraoperative visualization of the hip, knee, and ankle with fluoroscopy.
- Make a 10-cm longitudinal, midline incision that can be easily used for TKA at a later date.
- Prevent an overly large lateral hinge, which can result in fracture propagation into the tibial articular surface when the osteotomy is opened.
- Regardless of technique, don't allow *undercorrection*, because this has been associated with poorer survival results. I aim for a 3-degree *overcorrection*.
- Place the plate and the "wide portion" of its block as posterior as possible to avoid increasing the posterior tibial slope.

Thomas Muellner

In patients with an extra-articular tibial varus deformity, I prefer an opening wedge osteotomy. In patients with a combined deformity of the distal femur and the proximal tibia, combined osteotomies have to be considered to avoid an oblique joint line.

Pearls

- Patients with ligament instability should also have correction of the tibial slope when ligament reconstruction is not planned at the index operation. In ACL-deficient patients, the slope is decreased. In PCL-deficient patients, the slope is increased.
- The osteotomy should be biplanar to increase the amount of bone contact and to prevent possible rotational deformity.

Michael Stuart

I also prefer the opening wedge osteotomy for most patients because it avoids violation of the proximal tibiofibular joint,

does not change the fibular collateral ligament length, and allows for more precise intraoperative correction and an easier biplanar correction, and you can use the same incision for concomitant procedures (ACL reconstruction, osteochondral allografts, etc.) or for subsequent knee arthroplasty.

For a severe deformity, a combined distal femoral and proximal tibial osteotomy may be necessary to achieve adequate correction and avoid excessive joint line obliquity (Fig. 96-2).

Pearls

- Protect the patellar tendon and neurovascular structures by flexing the knee when using the saw and osteotome and placing malleable retractors along the anterior and posterior tibial cortices (Fig. 96-3).
- Prevent intra-articular fracture with the use of fluoroscopic guidance to determine the depth of osteotome penetration while maintaining 1 cm of intact lateral tibial bone, and gradually open the osteotomy. If the osteotomy does not open, use an osteotome to ensure that the anterior and posterior tibial cortices have been cut.
- Avoid increased posterior slope (unless desired for a posterior cruciate–deficient knee), place the plate as posterior as possible, and create an anterior tibial gap that is approximately ⅔ of the posterior tibial gap.

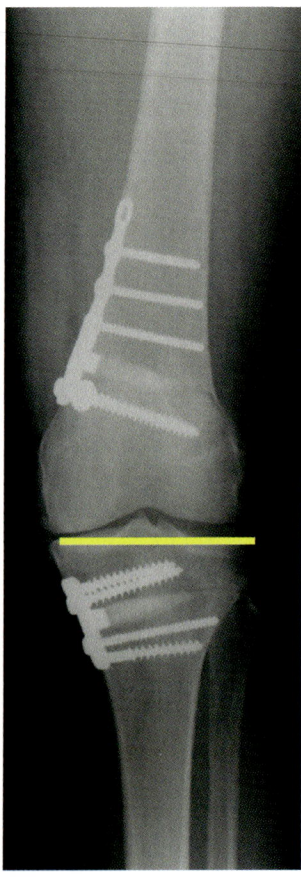

Figure 96-2. Anteroposterior radiograph following combined distal femoral and proximal tibial valgus-producing osteotomies to achieve the desired correction and maintain a level joint line.

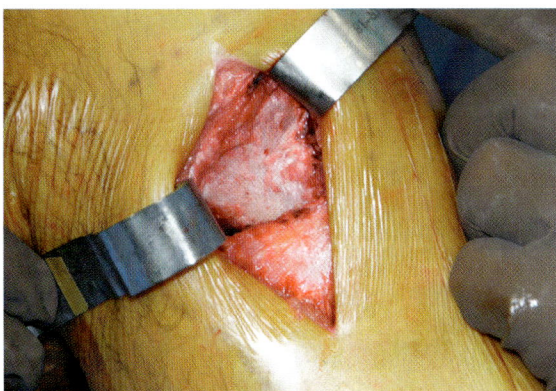

Figure 96-3. Malleable retractors placed along anterior and posterior tibia to protect the patellar tendon and neurovascular structures. (From Stuart MJ: Opening wedge-proximal tibial osteotomy. In Lotke PA, Lonner JH [eds]: Knee arthroplasty, ed 3, Baltimore, 2009, Wolters Kluwer Health/Lippincott William & Wilkins [Master Techniques in Orthopaedic Surgery], pp 361–371.)

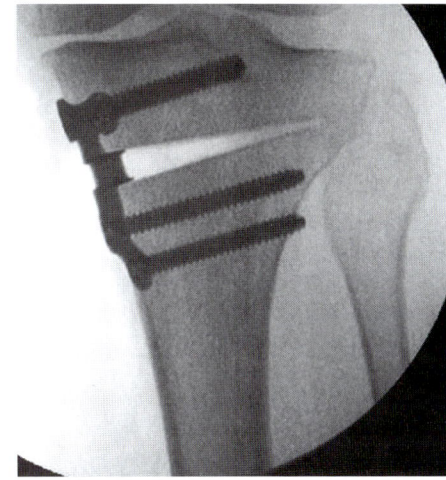

Figure 96-4. Anteroposterior fluoroscopic view prior to bone graft insertion, demonstrating osteoclasis of the lateral tibial cortex with an intact periosteal hinge and preservation of the medial tibial cortex at the site of the plate tines. (From Stuart MJ: Opening wedge-proximal tibial osteotomy. In Lotke PA, Lonner JH [eds]: Knee arthroplasty, ed 3, Baltimore, 2009, Wolters Kluwer Health/Lippincott William & Wilkins [Master Techniques in Orthopaedic Surgery], pp 361–371.)

- Ensure a stable construct by osteoclasis of the lateral tibial cortex to maintain an intact periosteal hinge and to preserve the medial tibial cortex at the site of the plate tines; consider bicortical autograft or allograft wedges for added stability if large correction is required.
- Avoid hematoma or compartment syndrome by releasing the tourniquet prior to bone grafting to attain hemostasis; place a drain if necessary.
- Prevent loss of correction or nonunion by irrigating the bone when using an oscillating saw and by achieving stable internal fixation (Fig. 96-4).

Martin Logan

I prefer a lateral closing wedge osteotomy for the young patient with varus malalignment. Opening wedge osteotomy is associated with a higher complication rate, including nonunion, and the plate often requires removal because of pain. If autograft is used, the added morbidity of the bone graft donor site is significant. I wouldn't do an opening wedge tibial osteotomy in an obese patient or in a smoker (see Hernigou P, Medevielle D, Debeyre J, Goutallier D: Proximal tibial osteotomy for osteoarthritis with varus deformity: a ten- to thirteen-year follow-up study. J Bone Joint Surg Am 69:332–354, 1987; Brouwer RW, Bierma-Zeinstra SMA, van Koeveringe AJ, Verhaar JAN: Patellar height and the inclination of the tibial plateau after high tibial osteotomy: the open versus the closed-wedge technique. J Bone Joint Surg Br 87:1227–1232, 2005; Hart JAL, Sekel R: Osteotomy of the knee: is there a seat at the table? J Arthroplasty 17[Suppl 1]:45–49, 2002).

Pearls

Lateral Tibial Closing Wedge Technique
- Make an 8- to 10-cm longitudinal, anterolateral incision centered between the fibula head and the tibial tuberosity without exposing the peroneal nerve.
- Use an osteotome to remove only the anteromedial aspect of the fibular head (Fig. 96-5).
- Insert a drill bit at the level of the lateral flare of the tibia, parallel to the joint under fluoroscopic control, stopping 1 cm before the medial cortex.

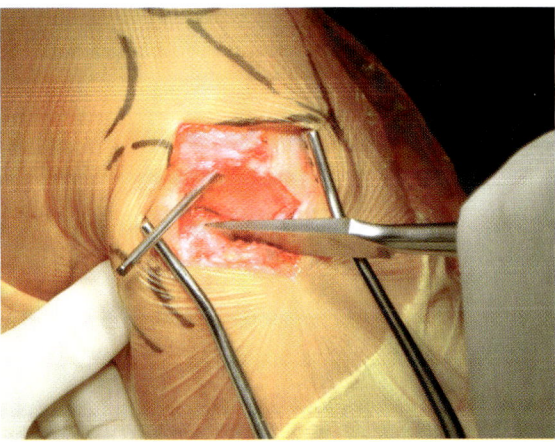

Figure 96-5. Identification of the superior tibiofibular joint and then osteotomy of the anteromedial part of the fibular head. Note that the drill bit has been inserted parallel to the joint.

- Use a jig system to place a second drill bit at the chosen angle (Fig. 96-6).
- Tilt the plane of the first proximal tibial cut around 10 to 15 degrees to the shaft of the tibia to ensure that the cut is parallel to the tibial slope, and that the posterior cortex is cut in the "curve" of the tibia safely away from the artery.
- Make a second parallel cut along the inferior drill bit and parallel to the first cut to correct a fixed flexion deformity or anterior cruciate ligament laxity and remove more bone anteriorly. To correct hyperextension or posterior cruciate ligament laxity, remove more bone posteriorly.
- Do not cut the medial cortex. The blade can be palpated subcutaneously on the anteromedial aspect and a measurement made of the length of the saw blade. This is the length of the saw cut along the posterior cortex, where the cutting edge of the blade cannot be palpated.

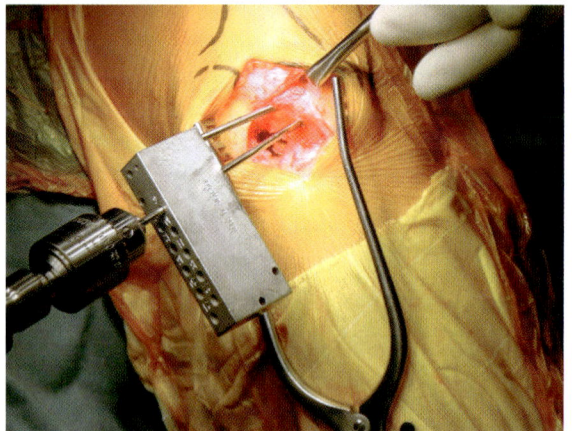

Figure 96-6. A second drill bit is placed through the jigging system, ensuring an accurate resection angle.

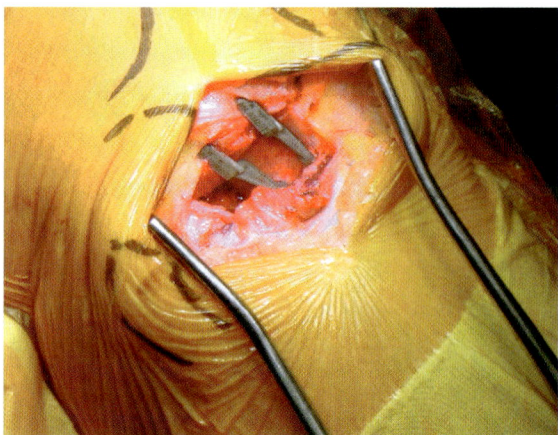

Figure 96-7. Two stepped staples have been inserted to stabilize the fixation of the closed wedge osteotomy.

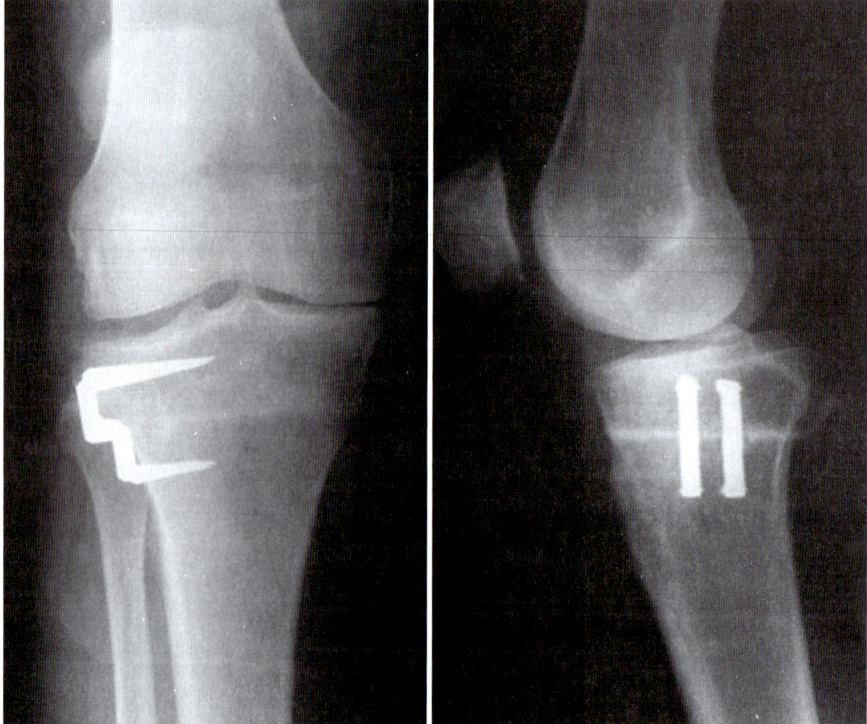

Figure 96-8. Postoperative check radiograph of a closing wedge high tibial osteotomy.

Alternatively, fluoroscopy can be used to follow the saw cuts to ensure that the medial cortex is not breached. Also the length of the drill in the tibia can be used as a guide to the length of the saw cut.

- One or two stepped staples usually provide sufficient fixation (Figs. 96-7 and 96-8).

Michael Stuart

Do you use computer navigation in the operating room when performing an osteotomy about the knee?

Martin Logan

I think that computer navigation is not necessary.

David Backstein

I have no experience with computer navigation in conjunction with osteotomy around the knee.

Thomas Muellner

Computer navigation will be as reliable and cost-effective as it is in total knee arthroplasty.

Michael Stuart

A variety of void fillers have been used when performing an opening wedge osteotomy, including iliac crest autograft, cancellous or structural allograft wedges, and synthetics. I routinely use densely packed cancellous allograft mixed with platelet-rich fibrin matrix. The healing rate is excellent, but I am unaware of any studies that show a faster or more reliable union rate using this blend. I prefer to use autograft for a large defect, and I don't consider a smoker a candidate for an opening wedge osteotomy.

What is your preferred material to fill the defect? Does your preference change for a high-risk patient: obese, smoker, large correction, etc.? Is there a role for platelet-rich plasma?

David Backstein

I use local autologous bone mixed with allograft, which provides both structural and biologic characteristics. Morcellized cancellous allograft bone from a young donor is used only for large corrections that involve a wedge greater than 15 mm. I have no experience with bone graft substitutes in this context.

Martin Logan

When performing an opening wedge tibial osteotomy to increase the posterior tibial slope in the setting of posterolateral corner insufficiency, I always use iliac crest autograft. I have no experience using platelet-rich plasma for osteotomies.

Thomas Muellner

So far, I use only iliac crest autografts and only in patients with an opening tibial wedge greater than 12 mm. This may change because bone allografts cleaned and processed with supercritical CO_2 are now available in my country.

I have not yet used platelet-rich plasma. The studies that I am aware of have small sample sizes, and the results are not so clear regarding whether the use of platelet-rich plasma made any difference. I think that further research is needed.

Michael Stuart

Although this is not frequently encountered, lateral compartment arthritis and valgus deformity can be treated with a distal femoral varus-producing osteotomy.

Please describe your preferred surgical technique for correcting valgus malalignment.

David Backstein

In my practice, knees with lateral tibiofemoral compartment disease resulting in valgus deformity are treated with DFVO. I rarely use a tibial osteotomy for lateral compartment arthritis. These knees tend to have a superolateral tilt to the joint line, and medial closing or lateral opening wedge osteotomy of the tibia tends to worsen this obliquity. Furthermore, most valgus deformities are associated with a hypoplastic lateral femoral condyle; thus a femoral osteotomy addresses the problem more directly.

We recently published our long-term results of DFVO and reported very satisfactory outcomes (Int Orthop 2009 May 26 [Epub ahead of print]). Thirty-three consecutive DFVOs (31 patients) with a minimum follow-up of 10 years (mean, 15.1; range, 10 to 25) had a survivorship of 89.9% at 10 years and 78.9% at 15 years.

My preference is to use a medial, *femoral*, closing wedge technique for correction of valgus knees. Fixation is achieved with a 90-degree offset dynamic compression blade plate. If the plate cannot be brought into contact with the medial

femoral diaphyseal cortex after the blade is inserted, a slot can be created to better accommodate the shoulder of the blade plate until satisfactory contact is achieved. The osteotomized bone wedge is morcellized and used as an autograft along the medial aspect of the osteotomy. This technique ensures that the medial part of the femoral cortex and the transepicondylar femoral line are 90 degrees to each other, resulting in an anatomic tibiofemoral angle of approximately 0 degrees.

Martin Logan

My preferred technique is to perform a lateral-based, varus-producing, opening wedge distal femoral osteotomy. In my experience, locking distal femoral osteotomy plates that use bicortical locking screws proximally are essential for this procedure. I routinely use iliac crest autograft for this operation.

Thomas Muellner

Usually, I perform a lateral femoral opening wedge osteotomy in patients with a femoral valgus malalignment.

Michael Stuart

Intra-articular problems that are amenable to arthroscopic treatment may coexist. I will evaluate the intra-articular structures only if the patient has symptoms or MRI findings consistent with an unstable meniscus tear, chondral flap, or loose body.

Do you routinely perform arthroscopy at the time of osteotomy? If not, what are your indications for concomitant arthroscopy?

David Backstein

I do not perform arthroscopy for any of my osteotomy patients. My intra-articular assessment is based on the history and physical examination. If I am in doubt about the status of one or more compartments, I obtain a preoperative MRI.

Martin Logan

I always perform an arthroscopy before proceeding to the osteotomy.

Thomas Muellner

I routinely perform an arthroscopy at the time of osteotomy, not only to treat coexisting intra-articular problems, but also to evaluate the integrity of the contralateral compartment.

Michael Stuart

The specific surgical technique, type of implant, and amount of correction can affect the stability of the construct and the postoperative regimen.

What is your typical postoperative protocol, including weight-bearing status, use of a brace, and physical therapy instructions?

David Backstein

I prescribe non–weight bearing for 6 to 8 weeks after surgery until early evidence of osteotomy healing is seen. Range-of-motion exercises are initiated at 7 to 10 days, along with isometric quadriceps exercises. At 6 weeks, partial weight bearing usually commences, as do light resistance exercises. If radiographic and clinical evidence of union is apparent, full weight bearing is usually allowed by 10 to 12 weeks postoperatively.

I do not use any braces.

Martin Logan

Postoperatively, the patient is touch-weight bearing on crutches for 2 weeks. Weight bearing is progressed with the aim of full weight bearing with crutches by 6 weeks. Range-of-motion exercises begin at 2 weeks with the brace off. The patient progresses to independent weight bearing over the next 2 to 4 weeks. Rehabilitation is continued for an additional 6 to 8 weeks, and home exercises for 3 months.

Thomas Muellner

My patients wear a brace for 6 weeks, bear partial weight after 2 weeks, and initially use a continuous passive motion machine, then a stationary bike and a muscle-strengthening program.

Michael Stuart

The risk of deep vein thrombosis and pulmonary embolus may be less after osteotomy as compared with total knee arthroplasty, but nonetheless remains a concern. I prescribe enteric-coated aspirin twice daily for 6 weeks after surgery, but I recommend low-molecular-weight heparin for 10 days followed by aspirin for those patients at higher risk (history of deep vein thrombosis, steroid use).

> *Do you routinely use any methods for thromboembolic prophylaxis before, during, or after osteotomy?*

David Backstein

Yes, I prescribe low-molecular-weight heparin for 10 days postoperatively.

Martin Logan

The patient wears compression stockings for 6 weeks. I give the patient a perioperative single injection of low-molecular-weight heparin, and postoperatively they are commenced on low-dose aspirin for the first 6 weeks.

Thomas Muellner

Following the osteotomy, patients are given low-molecular-weight heparin for at least 2 weeks. In case of any additional risk factors, the LMWH is continued for a total of 6 weeks.

Michael Stuart

In my practice, the indications for an osteotomy have actually expanded in recent years to include patients with a misaligned knee who require ACL/PCL reconstruction, meniscus transplantation, osteochondral transplantation, microfracture, or autologous chondrocyte implantation.

> *What criteria do you use to determine the need for an osteotomy in these patients? Is there a role for an osteotomy in the acute setting when a patient with a varus knee requires an ACL reconstruction or a multiligament reconstruction (ACL combined with FCL and posterolateral repair or reconstruction)?*

David Backstein

Our center has extensive experience with proximal tibial and distal femoral osteotomy in combination with a fresh osteochondral allograft. A distal femoral osteotomy in conjunction

Table 96-1 Osteotomy

Osteotomy Timing	Mean HSS Score	Time to TKR Conversion
Prior osteotomy	95.0 ± 6.2	NA
Coincident w/graft	85.4 ± 11.9	115.8 months
Delayed osteotomy	76.8 ± 6.7	83.2 months

HSS, Hospital for Special Surgery; *NA*, not applicable; *TKR*, total knee replacement.

with lateral osteochondral tibial grafts and a proximal tibial osteotomy with medial osteochondral femoral grafts have improved survivorship. Our series of tibial grafts published in 2003 (J Bone Joint Surg Am 85:33–39, 2003) demonstrated that realignment osteotomy should be conducted concomitant with fresh osteochondral allograft procedures whenever the final alignment will be less than overcorrected. Table 96-1 reflects our experience.

Martin Logan

If a patient has malalignment and requires articular cartilage grafting, it is sensible to combine this procedure with an osteotomy. I don't think an osteotomy should ever be used to overcorrect a normal knee just to protect an articular cartilage procedure or a meniscus transplantation.

If a varus knee requires ACL reconstruction, as long as the medial meniscus is intact or repairable, I would not do an osteotomy. My only indication for osteotomy in the context of ligament reconstruction is to address posterolateral instability and a varus thrust. In these patients, I perform a medially based, opening wedge, proximal tibial osteotomy, aiming to increase the posterior tibial slope. My personal preference is to use a locking plate with iliac crest autograft.

Thomas Muellner

In the acute setting of an ACL reconstruction, I would not perform an osteotomy at the same time if no other changes indicate that the medial compartment will deteriorate soon. In an active professional soccer player, an osteotomy is a contraindication unless he or she is willing to finish his or her career. In a patient with a varus thrust and lateral instability, an osteotomy has to be performed prior to ligament reconstruction.

Michael Stuart

Chronic anterior cruciate deficiency has been considered to be a relative contraindication for medial unicompartmental arthroplasty.

> *Do you think there is a role for simultaneous anterior cruciate ligament reconstruction and opening wedge high tibial osteotomy?*

David Backstein

Young, active patients with ACL deficiency in combination with medial arthritis and a varus deformity are treated with proximal tibial osteotomy alone. Before ACL reconstruction is considered in this scenario, an osteotomy is performed and the posterior tibial slope is increased slightly.

Patients with instability and varus deformity in the absence of medial arthritis are treated with ACL reconstruction alone as a first step. If they remain symptomatic, an osteotomy is conducted as a second procedure.

Martin Logan

No, I think if you are going to do an ACL reconstruction and a proximal tibial osteotomy, then the closing wedge technique is by far the best option. It is all too easy to increase the posterior tibial slope with an opening wedge; this will not help the longevity of the ACL graft (see Rodner CM, Adams DJ, Diaz-Doran V, et al: Medial opening wedge tibial osteotomy and the sagittal plane: the effect of increasing tibial slope on tibiofemoral contact pressure. Am J Sports Med 34:1431–1441, 2006). ACL reconstruction does not restore normal tibiofemoral kinematics in the lateral compartment, and ACL reconstruction combined with a unicompartmental arthroplasty is less satisfactory than a total knee arthroplasty (see Logan MC, Williams A, Lavelle J, et al: Tibiofemoral kinematics following successful anterior cruciate ligament reconstruction using dynamic magnetic resonance imaging. Am J Sports Med 32:984–992, 2004).

Thomas Muellner

ACL deficiency for me is an absolute contraindication for unicompartmental arthroplasty. ACL reconstruction with simultaneous opening wedge osteotomy has a role in ACL-deficient patients with cartilage damage and/or medial meniscus tears.

Michael Stuart

I would like to thank each of you for your insightful comments regarding patient selection for an osteotomy about the knee. The technical pearls are pragmatic and will definitely come in handy in the operating room. It is clear from your discussion that osteotomy of the proximal tibia and of the distal femur continues to play an important role. These procedures are typically successful, provided that we choose patients carefully, plan precisely before surgery, and use fastidious surgical technique.

KEY REFERENCES

Brouwer RW, Bierma-Zeinstra SMA, van Koeveringe AJ, Verhaar JAN: Patellar height and the inclination of the tibial plateau after high tibial osteotomy: the open- versus the closed-wedge technique. J Bone Joint Surg Br 87:1227–1232, 2005.

Coventry M, Ilstrup D, Wallrichs S: Proximal tibial osteotomy: a critical long-term study of eighty-seven cases. J Bone Joint Surg Am 75:196–201, 1993.

Dugdale TW, Noyes FR, Styer D: Preoperative planning for high tibial osteotomy: the effect of lateral tibiofemoral separation and tibiofemoral length. Clin Orthop Relat Res 274:248–264, 1992.

Hart JAL, Sekel R: Osteotomy of the knee: is there a seat at the table? J Arthroplasty 17(Suppl 1):45–49, 2002.

Hernigou P, Medevielle D, Debeyre J, Goutallier D: Proximal tibial osteotomy for osteoarthritis with varus deformity: a ten to thirteen-year follow-up study. J Bone Joint Surg Am 69:332–354, 1987.

Logan MC, Williams A, Lavelle J, et al: Tibiofemoral kinematics following successful anterior cruciate reconstruction using dynamic magnetic resonance imaging. Am J Sports Med 32:984–992, 2004.

Miniaci A, Ballmer FT, Ballmer PM, Jakob RP: Proximal tibial osteotomy: a new fixation device. Clin Orthop Relat Res 246:250–259, 1989.

Rodner CM, Adams DJ, Diaz-Doran V, et al: ACL reconstruction does not restore normal tibiofemoral kinematics in the lateral compartment and combined ACL reconstruction with a unicompartmental arthroplasty is less satisfactory than a total knee arthroplasty. Am J Sports Med 34:1431–1441, 2006.

Shasha N, Krywulak S, Backstein D, et al: Long-term follow-up of fresh tibial osteochondral allografts for failed tibial plateau fractures. J Bone Joint Surg Am 85(Suppl 2):33–39, 2003.

Chapter 97

Historic Development, Classification, and Characteristics of Knee Prostheses

John N. Insall and Henry D. Clarke

The evolution of modern total knee replacement (TKR) over the past 40 years is not merely of historic interest. Surgeons with some years of experience will have noticed that fashion tends to repeat itself. For example, in the early years (1970 to 1974), a range of prostheses (unicondylar, bicondylar, and hinged) were used, depending on the preoperative condition and deformity. Many of these devices and concepts fell out of favor and, for a while, except in select centers, tricondylar resurfacing prostheses were in vogue for almost all procedures. In the past 10 years, we have witnessed renewed interest in a graduated approach to knee replacement, with increased use of unicondylar and bicondylar prostheses for the femorotibial and patellofemoral compartments. Growth in the use of these devices has been in large part the result of the increased emphasis on less invasive surgical techniques fueled by ever-increasing patient desires to shorten postoperative recovery. In addition to the resurrection of partial knee replacements, we have seen increased use and acceptance of constrained condylar and hinged knee prostheses for a variety of difficult cases. As the problems encountered in revision TKR have become more challenging because of osteolysis and bone loss, these devices have assumed an important place in our surgical armamentarium. In addition, during the past 10 years, interest in mobile-bearing prostheses has been rekindled as the theoretical limits of current fixed-bearing prostheses are defined. Yet another example of a trend that is reemerging is the concept of uncemented fixation in TKR. After more than a decade of limited application of this form of fixation, new materials that mimic the structure of natural cancellous bone, and increasing success with this mode of fixation in total hip replacement, have prompted renewed interest.

The resurrection of the concepts and devices noted, which have been investigated in one form or another, is often fueled by promises from the device manufacturers for design improvements that will theoretically eliminate the less desirable outcomes seen with previous generations of implants (and surgeons). Whether these developments will provide significant advantages at this time still remain to be definitively proven. The proliferation of newer materials, such as ceramics and cross-linked polyethylene, as well as prosthesis design changes to maximize flexion, minimize potential backside wear, optimize kinematics, better accommodate gender and racial anatomic variation, and allow prosthesis insertion through minimally invasive approaches, has led to more unanswered questions in the field of TKR.

It is concerning that many of these concepts have been embraced in widespread clinical use prior to the publication of scientific results to support these changes. It is also of concern that this behavior appears to be partly caused by patient demand, which has been driven by the fairly recent use of direct advertising to consumers by the implant manufacturers. Therefore, at this important time in the field of TKR, as the original pioneers are succeeded by a new generation of joint replacement surgeons, it is important to emphasize that change should only be embraced once three criteria have been met:

1. A problem that needs a solution should exist.
2. The solution should be based on solid basic science research.
3. Improvements in clinical outcomes should be documented by independent centers.

To help guide this pursuit of continuing improvement in TKR, we believe that it is useful to look at what has not worked in the past. Finally, it is important to note that although the manufacturers of current systems are acknowledged, only the names of earlier devices are used. In some cases, early prostheses were manufactured by more than one company and, in other cases, the original manufacturers have vanished or merged, which makes accurate acknowledgment difficult at times and often meaningless in the context of this review.

EARLY PROSTHETIC MODELS

Interposition and Resurfacing Prostheses

The concept of improving knee joint function by modifying the articular surfaces has received attention since the 19th century. In 1860, Verneuil[295] suggested the interposition of soft tissues to reconstruct the articular surface of a joint. Subsequently, pig bladder, nylon, fascia lata, prepatellar bursa, and cellophane were some of the materials used for this purpose. The results were disappointing. In 1860, Ferguson[82] resected the entire knee joint, which resulted in mobility of the newly created subchondral surfaces (Fig. 97-1). When more bone was removed, the patients enjoyed good motion but lacked the necessary stability, whereas with less bone resection, spontaneous fusion often resulted. These early attempts were usually performed on knees damaged by tuberculosis or other infectious processes, along with concomitant ankylosis and deformity. The results of this procedure were sufficiently poor to discourage anything more than occasional attempts in severe cases.

Encouraged by the relative success of hip cup arthroplasty, Campbell[50] reported the successful use of a metallic interposition femoral mold in 1940. A similar type of arthroplasty was developed and used at Massachusetts General Hospital. The results, published by Speed and Trout[280] in 1949 and by Miller and Friedman[209] in 1952, were not very good, and this type of knee arthroplasty never achieved wide recognition.

In 1958, MacIntosh[191] described a different type of hemiarthroplasty that he had used in treating painful varus or valgus deformities of the knee. An acrylic tibial plateau prosthesis was inserted into the affected side to correct deformity, restore stability, and relieve pain. Later versions of this prosthesis[190] were made of metal (Fig. 97-2), and the somewhat similar McKeever prosthesis[75,205,253] showed considerably more success and was extensively used, particularly in patients with rheumatoid arthritis. Gunston[113] carried MacIntosh's

ideas a step further and, instead of using a simple metal disk interposed within the joint, substituted metallic runners embedded in the femoral condyles that articulated against polyethylene troughs attached to the tibial plateau. To make a four-part system of this type feasible, it was necessary to find a means of fixing the components rigidly to the bone. The solution was provided by acrylic cement.

Although the Gunston polycentric prosthesis[113] was the first cemented surface arthroplasty of the knee joint, the work of Freeman and colleagues[90,97] has had an even greater influence on the direction of both prosthetic design and surgical technique. The design objectives for a prosthesis (Fig. 97-3) were outlined in 1973 by Freeman and colleagues.[97] The most important of these objectives are the following:

1. A salvage procedure should be readily available. Implantation of the prosthesis should require the removal of no more bone than for primary arthrodesis and should leave large, flat surfaces of cancellous bone.
2. The chances of loosening should be minimized.
   a. The femoral and tibial components should be incompletely constrained relative to each other so that twisting, varus, or valgus moments cannot be transmitted to the bonds between the prosthesis and skeleton.
   b. The friction between components should be minimized.
   c. Any hyperextension-limiting arrangement should be progressive and not sudden in action.
   d. The prosthetic component should be fitted to the bone by means that spread the loads over the largest possible area of the bone-prosthesis interface.
3. The rate of production of wear debris should be minimized, and the debris produced should be as innocuous as possible. This objective leads to a preference for metal-on-plastic bearing surfaces, which should be as large as possible to keep the surface stress low.
4. The probability of infection should be minimized by having compact prosthetic components with few dead spaces.

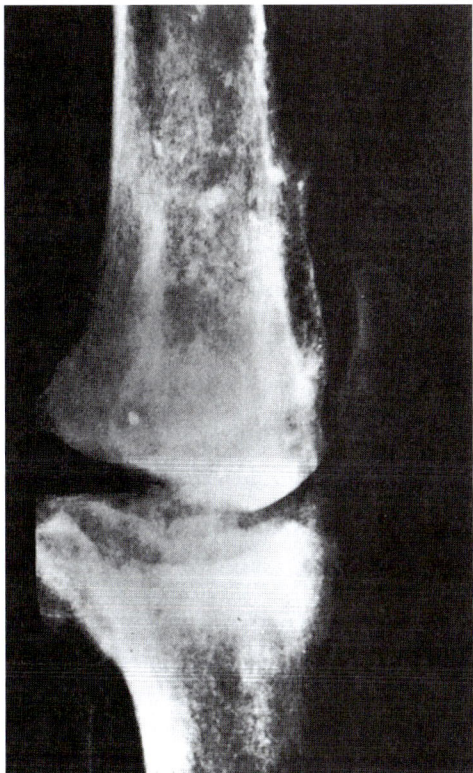

Figure 97-1. Resection arthroplasty creates a mobile but usually unstable joint.

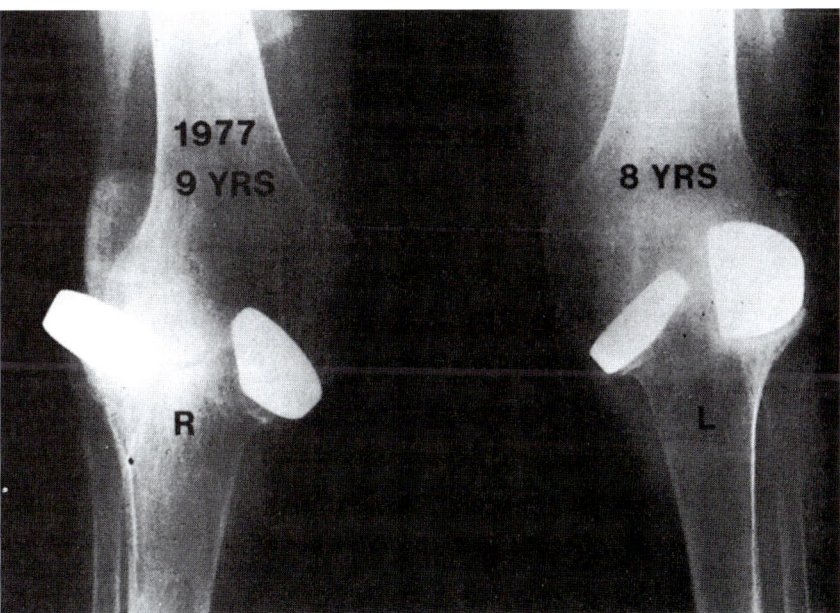

Figure 97-2. Use of the MacIntosh hemiarthroplasty in patients with rheumatoid arthritis often restored alignment and stability for a few years. However, as in this bilateral case, late dislocation and sinkage were common.

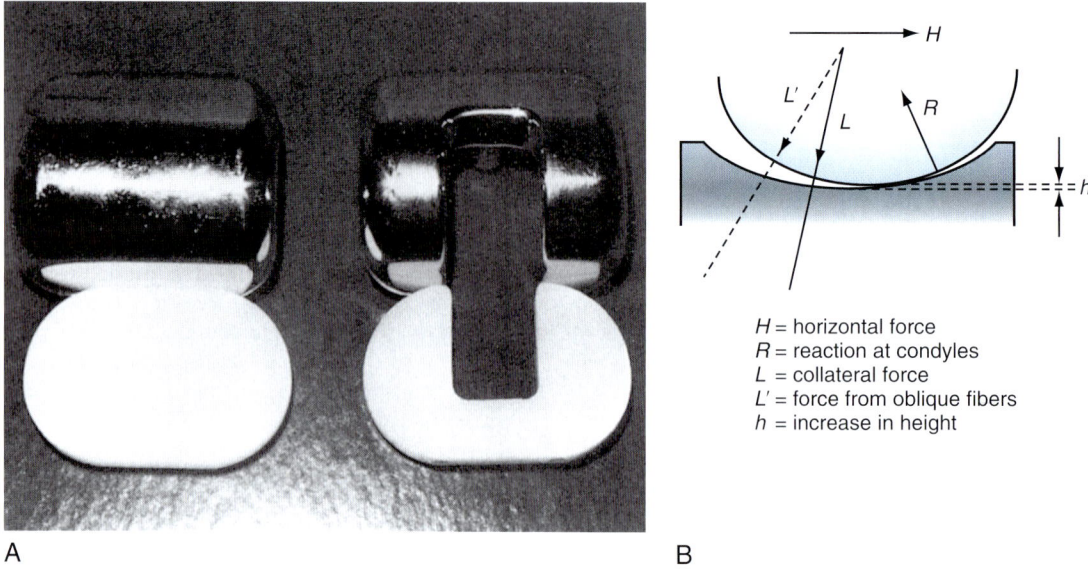

H = horizontal force
R = reaction at condyles
L = collateral force
L' = force from oblique fibers
h = increase in height

Figure 97-3. A, The original Freeman-Swanson prosthesis used two one-piece components. **B,** Stability was obtained by the roller-in-trough concept; dislocation could occur only if one component ran uphill on the other. Distraction was resisted by capsular and collateral ligament tension.

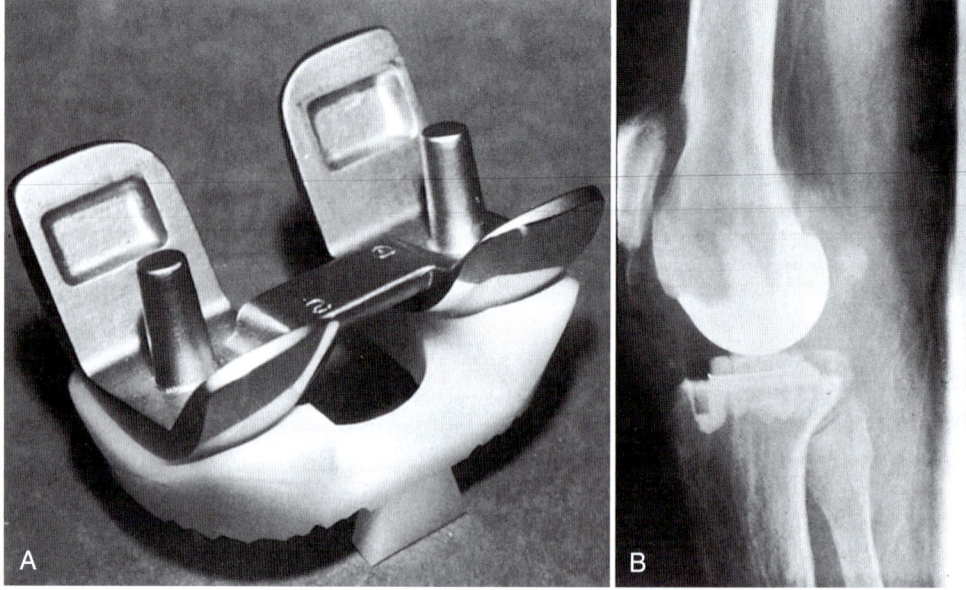

Figure 97-4. A, B, An early and widely used surface replacement was the Geometric prosthesis.

5. The consequences of infection should be minimized by avoiding long intramedullary stems and intramedullary cement.
6. A standard insertion procedure should be available.
7. The prosthesis should give motion from 5 degrees of hyperextension to at least 90 degrees of flexion.
8. Some freedom of rotation should be resisted.
9. Excessive movements in any direction should be resisted by the soft tissues, particularly the collateral ligaments.

Most of these objectives remain valid today, although two additional points cited in the Freeman report remain issues for debate: (1) the place of the cruciate ligaments in TKA;

and (2) the need to replace the patellofemoral joint and the desirability of patellar resurfacing.

Other early examples of resurfacing prostheses (Figs. 97-4 and 97-5) were the Geometric,[61,62,292] Duocondylar,[234,274] UCI (University of California at Irvine),[308] and Marmor.[197-201]

Constrained Prostheses

A second line of development in knee arthroplasty occurred parallel to the concepts of interposition and, later, surface replacement. In 1951, Walldius[302] developed the hinged prosthesis that bears his name. The device was initially made of acrylic and later of metal.

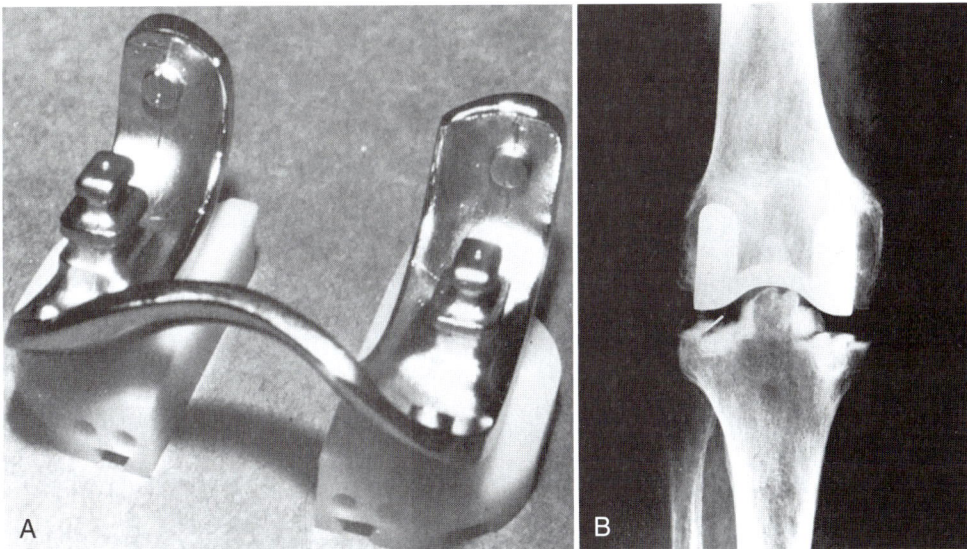

Figure 97-5. **A,** The Duocondylar prosthesis was anatomic in concept and retained both cruciate ligaments when present, but did not resurface the patellofemoral joint. Sinkage and loosening of the tibial components were an eventual problem with this design. **B,** Anteroposterior radiograph with the Duocondylar prosthesis inserted. Radiolucent lines around both tibial components are visible.

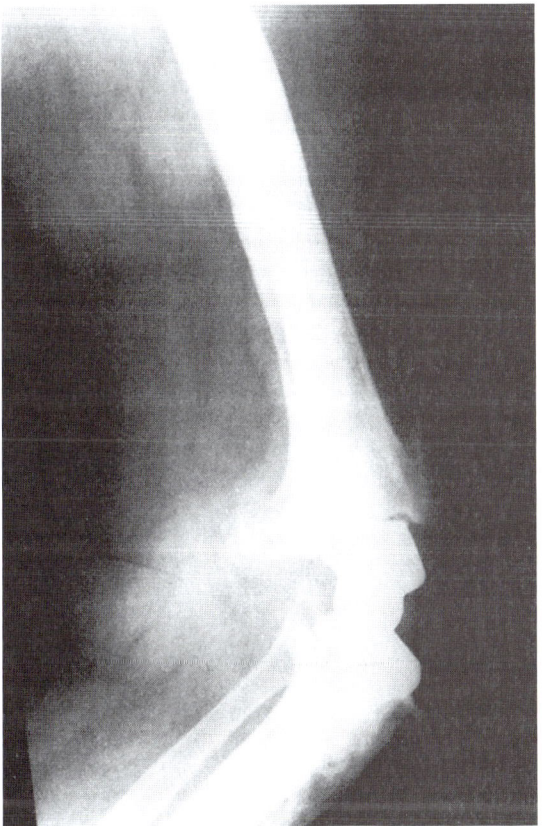

Figure 97-6. The Shiers prosthesis was a simple uniaxial metallic hinge.

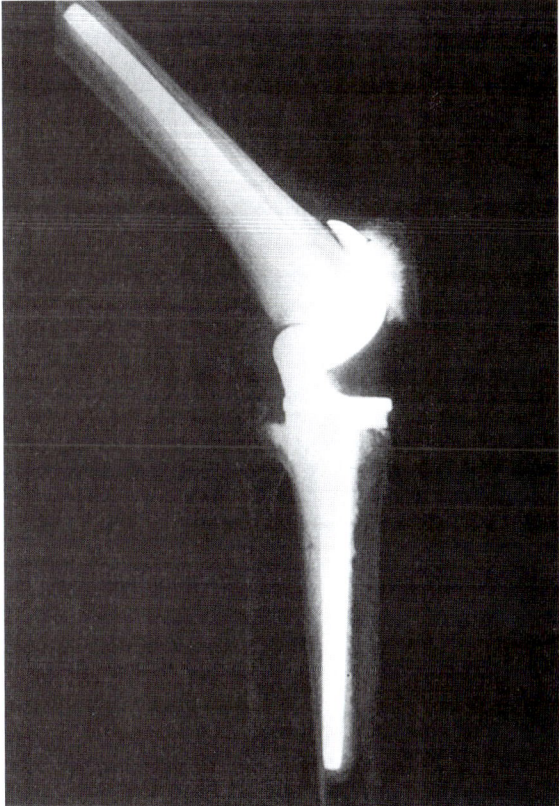

Figure 97-7. The GUEPAR hinge was similar to the Shiers uniaxial metallic hinge, but with the axis placed more posteriorly and femoral resurfacing for the patellar articulation.

Shortly thereafter, Shiers[266] described a similar device with even simpler mechanical characteristics (Fig. 97-6). A hinged prosthesis has considerable appeal. Technically, it is easy to use because the intramedullary stems make the prosthesis largely self-aligning and all the ligaments and other soft tissue constraints can be sacrificed because the prosthesis is self-stabilizing. The extent of damage to the knee is therefore of no consequence, and even the most extreme deformities can be corrected by dividing the soft tissues and resecting sufficient bone. Of course, the early hinged designs were uncemented, although later developments such as the GUEPAR (Fig. 97-7) were designed from the outset to be used with

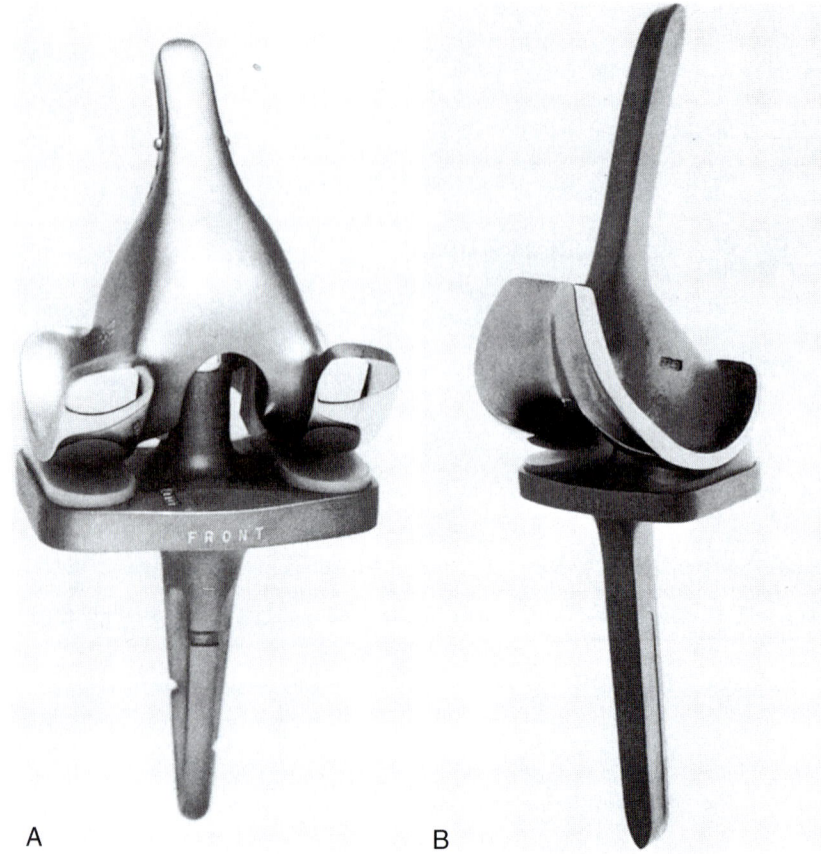

A   B

Figure 97-8. Spherocentric prosthesis. **A,** Standard version. **B,** Long-stemmed variant with a patellar flange. (Courtesy Dr. H. Kauffer and Dr. L.S. Matthews.)

methylmethacrylate cement. Because of inherent limitations with a simple hinge, including limited range of motion and transmission of stress to the prosthesis-cement interface, the early hinged prostheses were supplanted by rotating hinge devices that constrain the prosthesis in the coronal and sagittal planes, but allow rotation in the axial plane. Early designs included the Spherocentric (Fig. 97-8) prosthesis; current models include the Zimmer Rotating Hinge Knee and the DePuy SROM-Noiles prosthesis. In cases in which the maximal constraint offered by a linked hinge is not required, unlinked but constrained devices have been extensively used in revision and complex primary TKR. Historical devices include the Total Condylar Prosthesis III (TCP III; Fig. 97-9)[68] and the Constrained Condylar Knee (CCK)[168]; their modern counterparts include the DePuy PFC Sigma TC3 and Zimmer Legacy Constrained Condylar Knee (LCCK). The primary characteristic of these devices is a cam and post mechanism, similar to that found in a posterior-stabilized (PS) prosthesis, but thicker and taller, and it provides resistance not only to posterior translation but also to varus and valgus stress. At the present time, the use of cemented or uncemented stems with both hinged and constrained but unlinked devices is based on surgeon preference.

EVOLUTION OF PROSTHETIC DESIGN

The prostheses discussed up to this point are now more or less obsolete. Although the early results were encouraging, further follow-up demonstrated various problems. The litera-

ture relevant to TKR includes many articles that report the clinical results of designs no longer in common use.*

These published reports on early models are somewhat difficult to compare because different rating methods were used. A review conducted at the Hospital for Special Surgery (HSS) between 1971 and 1973 is probably representative. This review[136] compared four different models (Fig. 97-10): the unicondylar (Fig. 97-11), Duocondylar, Geometric, and GUEPAR (see Fig. 97-7). The results were expressed by using the HSS 100-point knee rating scale.

Postoperative knees were classified into four groups according to their scores on the HSS scale:

Excellent: 85+. These knees approached the normal and were obviously much improved in the opinion of both the patient and the examiner.

Good: 70 to 84. These knees showed obvious improvement after arthroplasty, but the result was not as good as in the excellent group.

Fair: 60 to 69. This group mostly consisted of knees in which the result of arthroplasty was deficient in some way (e.g., persistent pain, moderate instability, unsatisfactory range of motion), but also included some in

---

*References 5, 11,12,14-16, 18, 28, 40, 42, 49, 52, 53, 57, 63, 64, 68, 70, 79-81, 86, 89, 91, 95, 96, 98, 101, 104, 110, 114, 123, 128, 131-133, 136, 139, 141-144, 146, 147, 151, 174, 175, 183-185, 195, 202, 203, 214, 215, 225, 227, 238, 240, 241, 243, 250, 264, 265, 267, 268, 270, 272, 273, 276, 286, 290, 294, 309, 310, 317, 319, and 326.

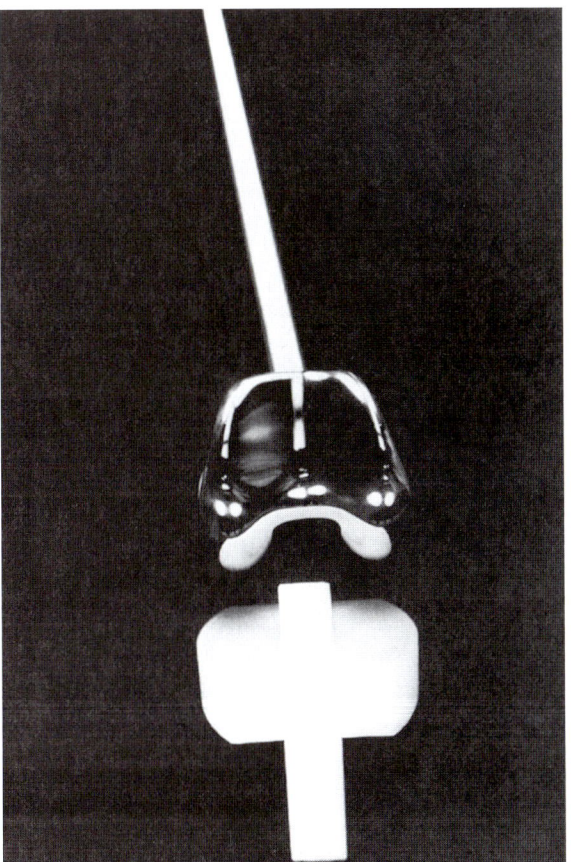

Figure 97-9. The constrained but unlinked TCP III. Varus and valgus constraint were provided by the rectangular central peg on the tibial component.

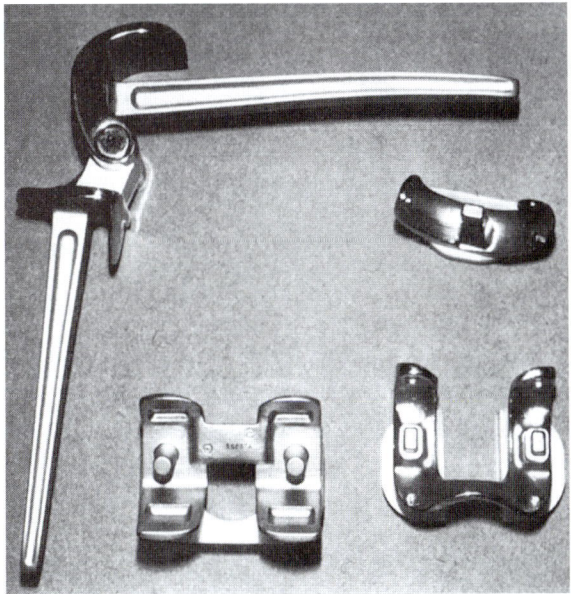

Figure 97-10. The graduated system concept selected the prosthesis according to the degree and extent of damage. The prostheses shown here in a clockwise direction are the unicondylar, Duocondylar, Geometric, and GUEPAR prostheses.

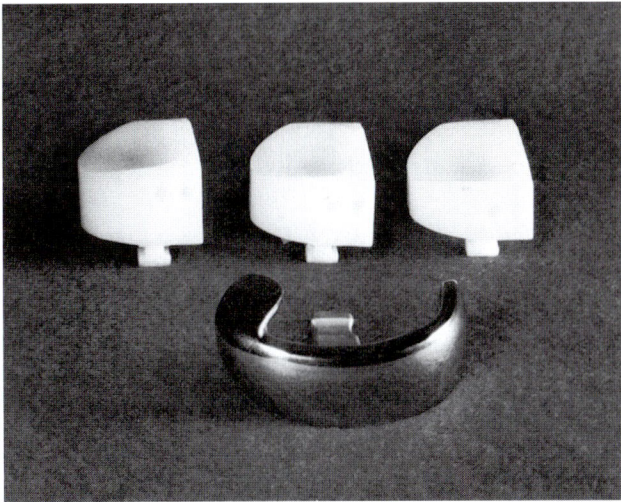

Figure 97-11. The unicondylar prosthesis was designed to resurface only the affected femorotibial compartment. The shape and curvature of the component were similar to that of the Duocondylar design.

which the rating of the arthroplasty was downgraded by the patient's general condition (e.g., multiple joint involvement in rheumatoid arthritis or systemic disease).

Failure: Less than 60. These knees were evidently unsatisfactory and below the rating achieved by knee fusion, which scores a 60 on the HSS knee rating scale. This classification included knees in which the prosthesis had been removed or replaced and knees in which the improvement, if any, did not seem to justify the risk of arthroplasty.

Considering the entire group of 178 arthroplasties studied in the four different models (23 unicondylar, 60 Duocondylar, 50 Geometric, and 45 GUEPAR), the results were considered excellent in 47 (26%), good in 66 (37%), fair in 37 (21%), and poor in 28 (16%; Fig. 97-12). There was no statistically significant difference among the results obtained with each of the four prostheses studied. However, because it is easier to improve a bad knee than a relatively good one, the percentage of improvement was much greater with the GUEPAR than with the unicondylar (120% versus 45%).

Three specific problems were identified from this study: patellar pain, component loosening, and surgical technique. However, because the GUEPAR hinge was inserted into the worst knees originally, it gave the greatest percentage of improvement in the HSS knee rating scale. At the time of the study, the conclusion reached was that the GUEPAR prosthesis appeared superior in a number of ways. It had been selected for use in the most severely involved knees and yet equaled any of the other prostheses in the quality of results in rheumatoid arthritis and osteoarthritis. It also gave the lowest proportion of failures and was the only model to improve range of motion postoperatively. However, the potential problems of loosening and mechanical failure with the GUEPAR prosthesis were noted. More than 100 GUEPAR prostheses were used at the HSS almost 40 years ago, and these expected problems materialized to a large extent. Approximately 80% of the prostheses were loose clinically and radiographically at long-term follow-up, although they

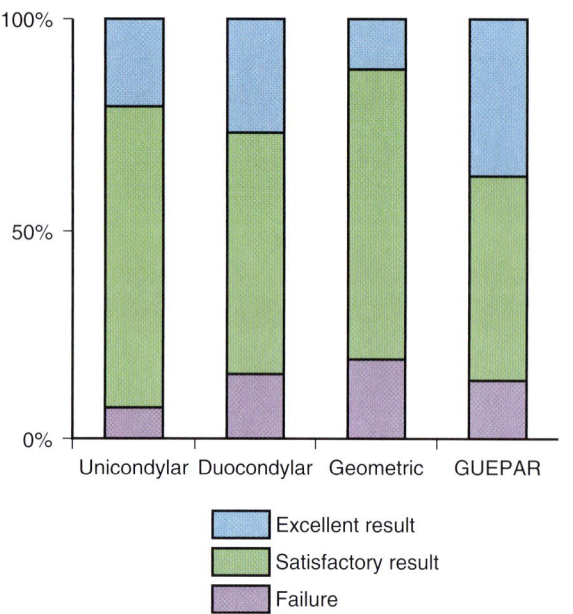

Figure 97-12. Graph showing the comparative results of four early prosthetic models.

are not necessarily symptomatic (Fig. 97-13A). There were also numerous cases of stem breakage (see Fig. 97-13B) and, as noted later, infection became a major problem. This study therefore reached some erroneous conclusions because of short follow-up—a point of great relevance today when many new prostheses are being used in patients with scant clinical follow-up to support their merits.

Patellar Pain

None of the four early prosthetic models studied made any provision for patellofemoral function. Patellectomy did not seem to offer a solution to the problem of patellofemoral arthritis (Fig. 97-14). In our early study, 38 patellectomies were performed in the group as a whole, 3 of which were done at a later date than the arthroplasty because of persistent patellar pain. Importantly, pain after patellectomy was as frequent as in patients in whom patellectomy had not been performed. In addition, patients who underwent patellectomy suffered from inadequacy of the extensor mechanism. In the GUEPAR group of 45 knees, pain on patellar compression was found in 22 on follow-up, and patellar erosion was observed in 5 patients. Patellar subluxation frequently occurred with the GUEPAR prosthesis, despite wide lateral release of the patellar retinaculum at the time of arthroplasty (Fig. 97-15). Nonetheless, the subluxation was often not apparent to the patient and was considered an incidental

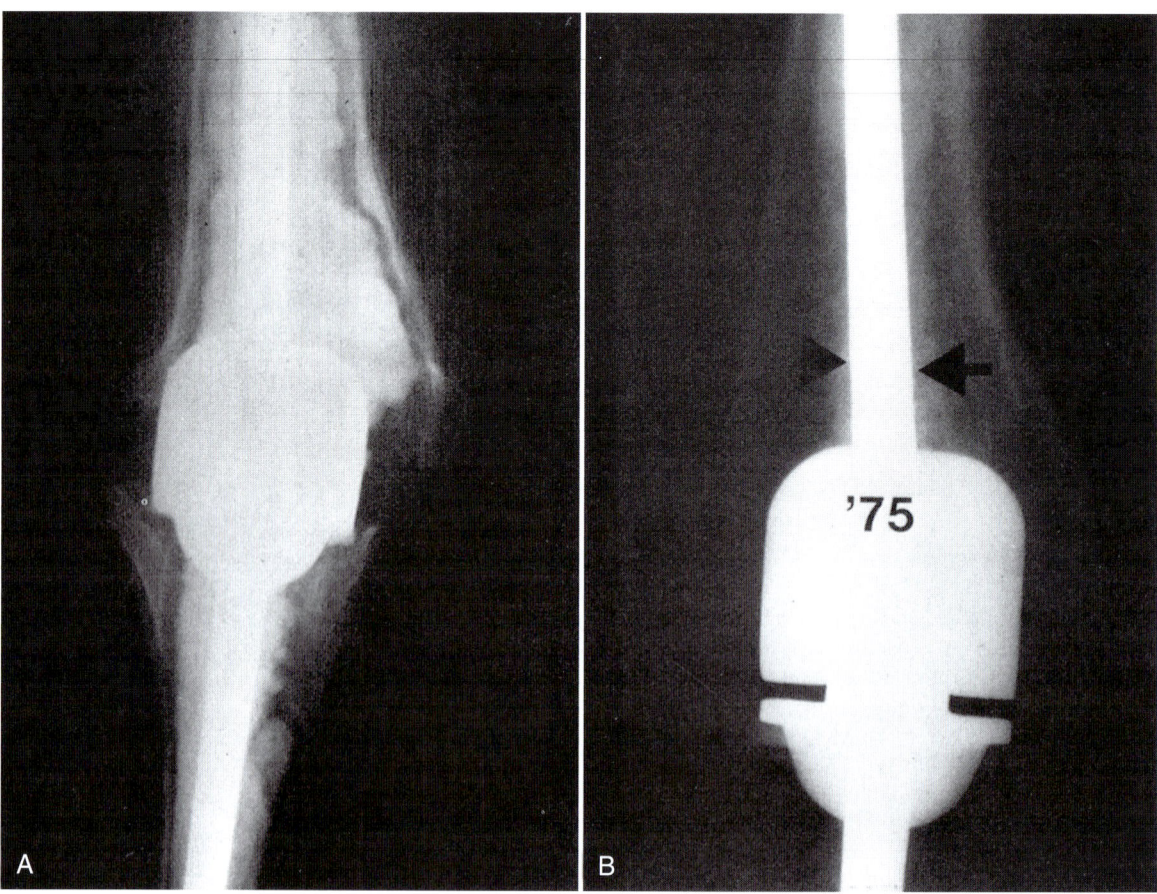

Figure 97-13. A, Radiograph of a grossly loose GUEPAR prosthesis 5 years after initial insertion. **B,** Stem breakage occurred with the GUEPAR prosthesis, usually at the site shown here in the radiograph, 5 cm proximal to the joint.

finding. Subluxation of the patella did not necessarily correlate with complaints of postoperative pain. However, with the Geometric prosthesis, 29 of 50 knees had pain on patellofemoral compression. Patellar subluxation was found in nine knees and all were painful.

Loosening

A radiolucent line surrounding the prosthetic components was seen with great frequency. With the condylar replacements, the radiolucency was usually observed around the tibial component. It was present in 70% of knees with the unicondylar, 50% with the Duocondylar, and 80% with the Geometric prosthesis. A radiolucent line was observed around the femoral component in 45% of the patients with a GUEPAR prosthesis. The radiolucent line was slightly more frequent in patients with osteoarthritis than in those with rheumatoid arthritis and it was observed in all knees with osteoarthritis in which the Geometric prosthesis was used. Radiolucent lines are by no means always symptomatic, but when complete, progressive, and associated with pain on weight bearing, they generally indicate failure of fixation. Our subsequent experience has shown that the incidence of partial radiolucencies for a particular prosthesis does not correlate with the eventual amount of component loosening. On the strength of a 10- to 12-year follow-up on one particular cemented prosthesis (the Total Condylar), we concluded that a detailed study of partial radiolucent lines about cemented knee replacements is worthless and a poor predictor of future failure (Fig. 97-16).

On the basis of early analysis of these data, it was clear that tibial loosening represented a failure in prosthetic design.

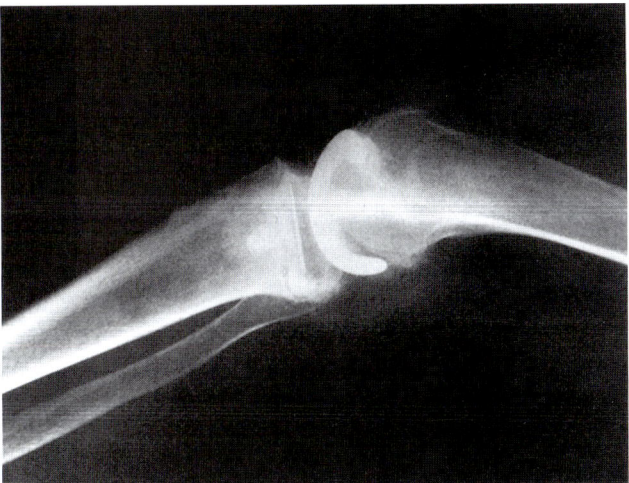

Figure 97-14. Patellectomy is not a satisfactory solution to patellofemoral pain. Patellectomy was performed in conjunction with the implantation of a unicondylar prosthesis.

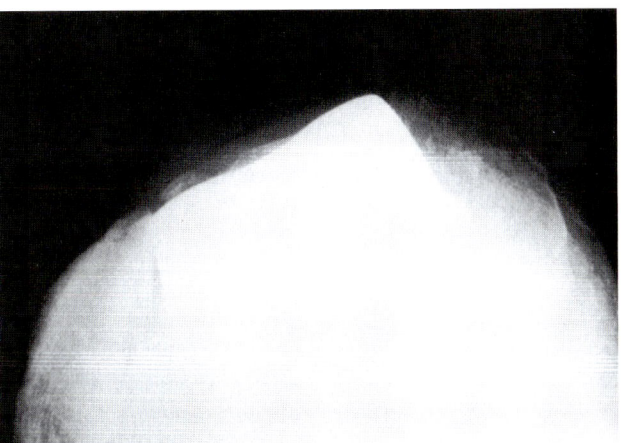

Figure 97-15. Patellar subluxation and dislocation often occurred with the GUEPAR prosthesis. It was not always symptomatic.

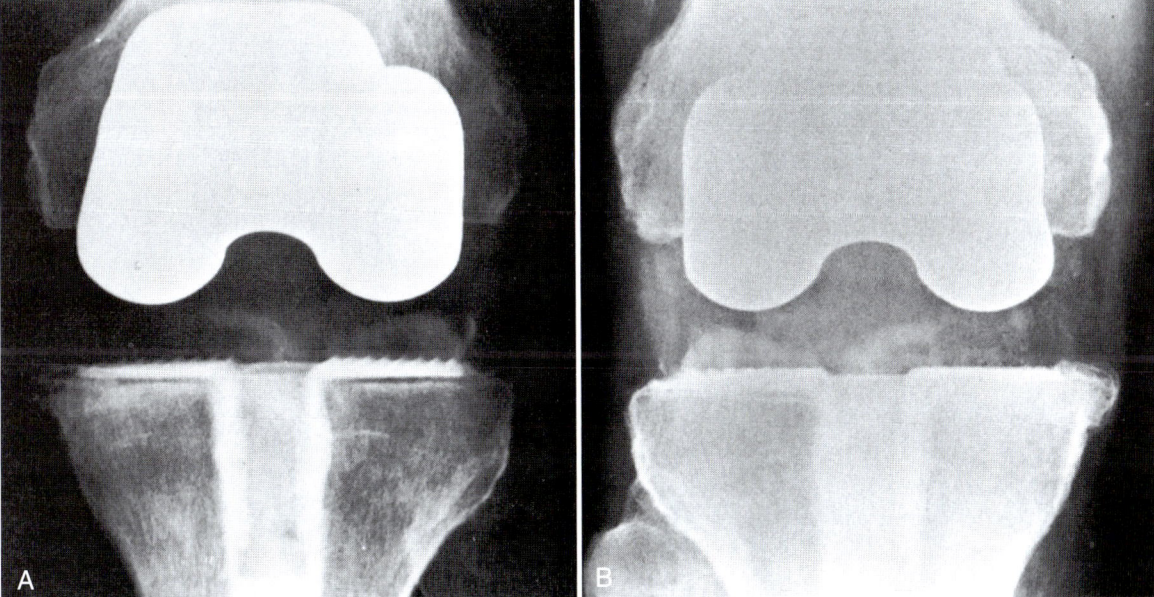

Figure 97-16. A, Radiograph taken 1 year after implantation shows a pronounced radiolucent line beneath the medial and lateral tibial plateaus. **B,** Radiograph of the same knee taken at 5 years shows a barely visible radiolucency.

The flat cancellous surface of the upper part of the tibia is not a suitable bed for a flat prosthetic component because of poor resistance to shear stress. Moreover, this bone is not of sufficient strength to resist subsidence of the tibial component, even if excavations are made to accommodate fixation fins or lugs on the bottom of the tibial prosthesis (Figs. 97-17 and 97-18). It was concluded that some form of cortical fixation would be essential for a successful TKR series.

Prosthesis Selection and Surgical Technique

Like many others, we initially believed in the concept of a graduated system, in which selection of a prosthesis depended on the severity of damage found in the arthritic knee (see Fig. 97-10). For example, knees with cartilage erosion restricted to one femorotibial compartment were replaced with a unicondylar prosthesis, whereas a hinged prosthesis was used in the most severely damaged and deformed knees. The bicondylar prosthesis occupied an intermediate position with respect to the severity of arthritis. Although the use of a hinged prosthesis is not technically demanding, the early condylar designs were difficult to insert and align, and there was very little margin for error. Obviously, the advantage of even the most sophisticated prosthetic design is lost if surgical

placement is incorrect. Furthermore, an inherent drawback in a graduated system of prostheses is that a model may be used for degrees of deformity exceeding the limits for which the prosthesis was intended. This error can itself be a cause of failure (e.g., dislocation; Fig. 97-19). Clearly, there is no purpose in selecting one prosthetic design over another unless some advantage can be shown. For example, in our comparative study, we did not find that the unicondylar prosthesis offers any advantage over bicondylar models. The merits of graduated knee systems still remain a source of debate.

Infection

Although deep periprosthetic infection was not a frequent cause of failure for the condylar designs, it has subsequently proved to be a major problem with the GUEPAR prosthesis. With further follow-up, 15 of 108 prostheses (14%) became infected (4 early and 8 late). There have been reports of similar occurrences in the literature.[12]

At the HSS, dissatisfaction with the early prostheses led to the design of the Total Condylar and Duopatellar prostheses, which were based on different concepts of how to manage the posterior collateral ligament (PCL).[232,245,252] During the 1980s, prosthetic characteristics diverged further and were generally linked to whether the prosthesis was designed to

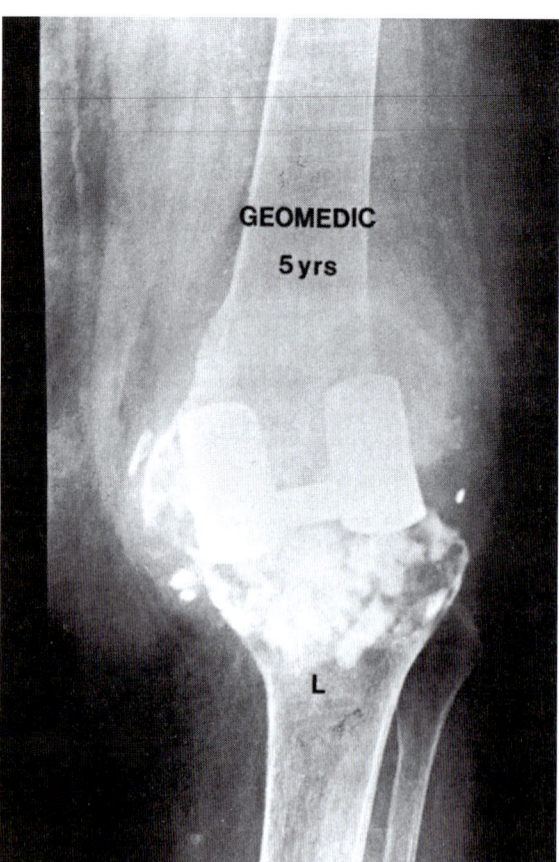

Figure 97-17. Failure of tibial fixation was a frequent problem with many early prosthetic designs. The problem was primarily attributable to collapse of the cancellous bone of the upper part of the tibia along with sinkage of the component.

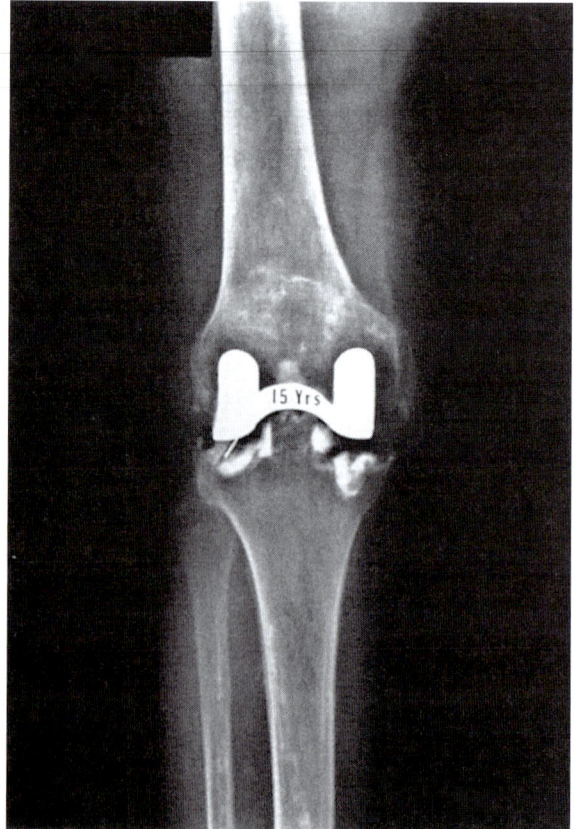

Figure 97-18. Radiograph of a 15-year follow-up of a Duocondylar prosthesis that had two separate tibial components. There is the appearance of osteopenia around the femoral component runners. The knee continued to function well.

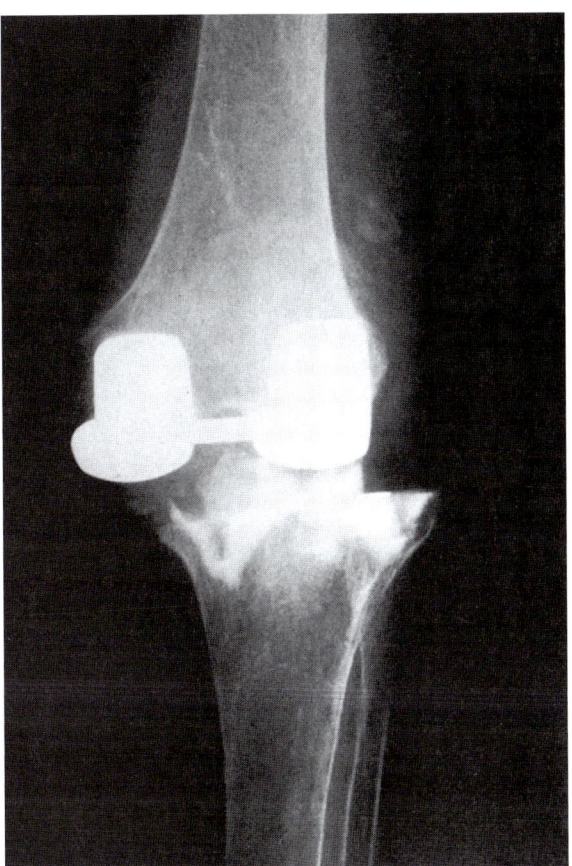

Figure 97-19. This Geometric prosthesis translocated and dislocated. This was the condition of the knee before the prosthesis was inserted and represents an error in prosthesis selection.

substitute for or preserve the PCL. However, during the 1990s, there was a convergence of prosthetic designs, particularly in the United States.

TYPES OF PROSTHESES

Most simply, a prosthesis can be a surface replacement or a constrained design. These two categories may be further subdivided. Surface replacements comprise unicondylar and bicondylar designs. Unicondylar prostheses are discussed elsewhere in this text.[*]

Bicondylar prostheses can be cruciate-retaining, cruciate-excising, or cruciate-substituting prostheses. Constrained prostheses can be hinged or unlinked. Most hinged devices are now designed to allow rotation in the axial plane while eliminating motion in the coronal plane. Although in original designs the load was transmitted solely through a metal axle that linked the femoral and tibial components, many contemporary designs allow for condylar load bearing between the femur and tibia, as found in surface replacement designs or, at a minimum, load sharing between the axle and femorotibial articulation. As discussed earlier, the primary characteristic of unlinked designs, such as the LCCK or PFC Sigma

TC3, is a cam and post mechanism, similar to that found in a PS prosthesis, but thicker and taller. This mechanism provides resistance not only to posterior translation but also to varus and valgus stress and rotation. Although these devices offer less constraint in the coronal plane than a hinged prosthesis, they are more constrained in the axial plane. Concerns with the high degree of rotational constraint in these fixed-bearing, unlinked constrained devices has led to the development of mobile-bearing, unlinked constrained prostheses. However, to date, there is still little information about which type of constrained device will prove superior in the long term.

Early Surface Replacement Designs

In the following sections, we discuss early surface replacement designs.[298] Supplemental information about the individual innovators and the tremendous advances in TKR during the early years of the modern era can be found in the three historical reviews by Robinson,[245] Ranawat,[232] and Scott[252] that should be compulsory reading for all students of knee arthroplasty. Much of the early debate about prosthesis design and the techniques used to implant the components, including how to address the cruciate ligaments, arose from conceptual differences among the pioneers about whether it was better to design a knee prosthesis from an anatomic or functional perspective. The current generation of prostheses has converged in many ways, with most designs incorporating characteristics from each category that seem to have optimized long-term outcomes—for example, side-specific femoral components with optimized trochlear geometries from the anatomic approach and the moderately conforming coronal and sagittal geometry that was more associated with the functional approach.

Total Condylar Prosthesis

Although originally coined as the name of a specific prosthesis, the term *total condylar prosthesis* has been used generically to describe a whole range of surface replacement prostheses that share general characteristics with the original (Fig. 97-20).[*]

The TCP, designed in 1973, was a true total replacement of the knee in that the patellofemoral joint was replaced as well as the femorotibial compartment. Designed from a functional perspective, the inherent geometry of the prosthesis was intended to substitute for the anatomic function of the cruciate ligaments, native articular geometry, and menisci. The salient features of the design are discussed in the following sections.[245]

Femoral Component. Made of cobalt chromium alloy, the femoral component contained a symmetrically grooved anterior flange that separated posteriorly into two symmetrical condyles, each of decreasing radius posteriorly, with a symmetrical convex curvature in the coronal plane.

Tibial Component. The tibial component was made of high-density polyethylene in one piece with two separate

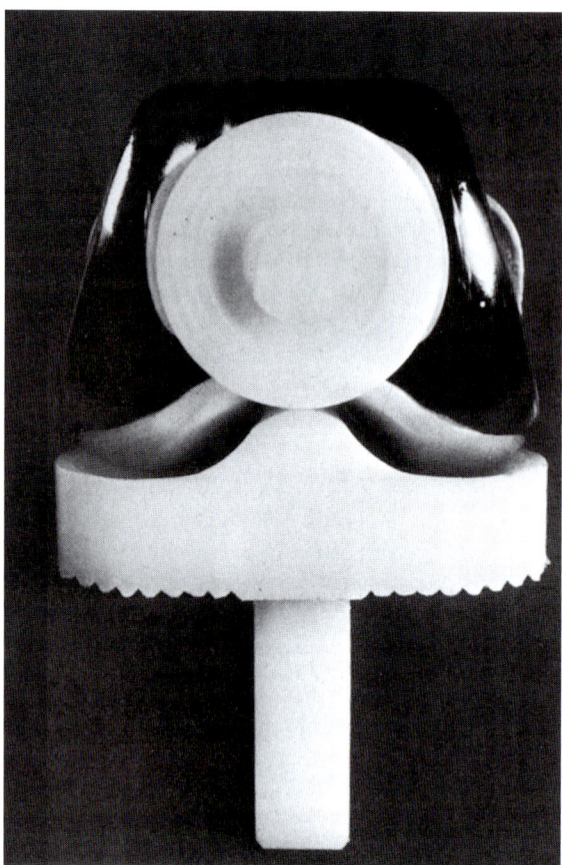

Figure 97-20. The Total Condylar Prosthesis.

biconcave tibial plateaus that mated (articulated) precisely with the femoral condyles in extension, thus permitting no rotation in this position. In flexion, the fit ceased to be exact and rotation and gliding motions were possible. The symmetrical tibial plateaus were separated by an intercondylar eminence designed to prevent translocation or sideways sliding movements. The peripheral margin of the articular concavities was of an even height anteriorly and posteriorly. The undersurface of the component had a central fixation peg 35 mm in length and 12.5 mm in width. The anterior margin of the peg was vertical but the posterior margin was oblique, thereby conforming with the posterior cortex of the tibia.

Patellar Component. Made of high-density polyethylene, the patellar component was dome-shaped on its articular surface, closely conforming to the curvature of the femoral flange. A dome was selected because this shape did not require rotary alignment as an anatomic prosthesis would. The bony surface of the prosthesis had a central, rectangular fixation peg.

Duopatellar Prosthesis

The Total Condylar Prosthesis was designed for cruciate excision. In contrast, the Duopatellar prosthesis,[81] a sibling prosthesis designed from an anatomic perspective at the HSS as a replacement for the Duocondylar model, was intended to preserve existing cruciate ligaments, particularly the PCL.[232,245,252] The general shape of the tibial runners was

anatomic in the sagittal plane. Coronally, the condyles were flat with a median curvature.

The anterior connecting bar of the Duocondylar prosthesis was extended into a femoral flange. The initial version of the Duopatellar model had two separate tibial plateaus identical to the Duocondylar design: flat in the sagittal plane, but with a median curvature coronally to prevent translocation. The deep surface was dovetailed for cement fixation. Later, the two components were joined, and a central fixation peg similar to that of the total condylar prosthesis was added. A PCL cutout was provided. The patellar component of the Duopatellar prosthesis was identical to that of the Total Condylar Prosthesis.

Cruciate Excision, Retention, and Substitution

The TCP and Duopatellar prosthesis were designed for cruciate excision and retention, respectively.[7,10,69,92,96] Subsequent modifications to the TCP incorporated a cam on the femoral component and a central post on the tibial polyethylene (Fig. 97-21). This cam and post mechanism was designed to act as a functional substitute for the PCL and produce femoral rollback during flexion. With the development of this so-called posterior-stabilized prosthesis, it was apparent that cruciate excision alone was not optimal. However, the relative merits of PCL retention versus PCL substitution have been debated vigorously within the orthopedic community for many years. The development of total knee prostheses has occurred along two distinct evolutionary paths based on these different principles.[245] The anatomic function of the cruciate ligaments, relative advantages and disadvantages of cruciate excision, and PCL retention versus PCL substitution will be reviewed here. It has also become clear that if the PCL is retained, the function of the ligament must be optimized through a balancing technique. Difficulties with balancing the PCL, as well as late PCL rupture leading to flexion instability, have led to the development of the so-called deep dish polyethylene inserts that are offered as part of many cruciate-retaining prosthesis systems. These inserts have moderately conforming articular surfaces in the coronal and sagittal planes, together with an anterior lip that limits paradoxical anterior translation of the femur on the tibia. This is one example of how prosthesis design has converged in the past 2 decades, thus making it more difficult to trace the origins of any particular design.

ANATOMIC FUNCTIONS OF THE CRUCIATE LIGAMENTS

One function of the cruciate ligaments, in addition to providing static anterior and posterior stability, is to impose certain movements on the joint surfaces relative to one another. The anterior cruciate ligament (ACL) is often absent in arthritic knees and has not been thought to be of much consequence in TKR. The importance of the ACL may have been underestimated inasmuch as unconstrained prostheses have increased sagittal plane laxity and fail more often when the ACL is absent.[313] Although the PCL is often attenuated in arthritic knees, it is usually present. It has been considered the collateral ligament for the medial compartment of the knee.[74] The PCL causes the femoral condyles to glide and roll

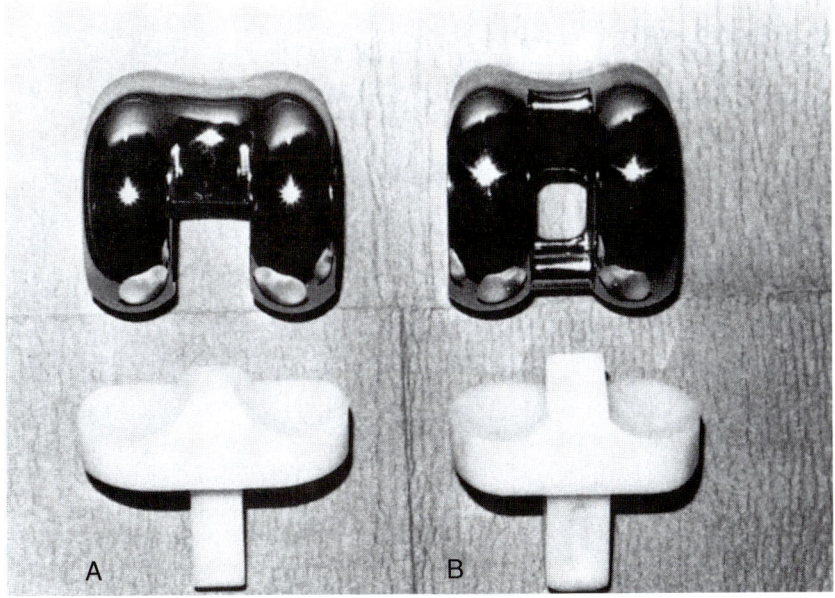

Figure 97-21. **A,** Total Condylar prosthesis. **B,** Posterior-Stabilized Condylar Knee, a newer derivative providing posterior cruciate substitution by means of a central cam mechanism. (From Insall JN, Lachiewicz PF, Burstein AH: The posterior stabilized condylar prosthesis: A modification of the total condylar design: two- to four-year clinical experience. J Bone Joint Surg Am 64:1317, 1982.)

back on the tibial plateau as the knee is flexed.[149] In a normal knee, the shape of the plateau does not restrain this motion and the laxity of the meniscal attachments allows the menisci to move posteriorly with the femur. This femoral rollback is crucial in prosthetic design. If the cruciates are excised, a more conforming tibial polyethylene component can be used to provide some degree of anterior and posterior stability. However, without the function of the PCL, femoral rollback will not occur, which theoretically limits the ultimate flexion that can be obtained. If the PCL is retained, the tibial surface must be flat or even sloped posteriorly (Fig. 97-22). If a more conforming component is used in these circumstances, posterior impingement will occur (Fig. 97-23). Substitution of the PCL with a cam and post mechanism not only re-creates femoral rollback but also allows a conforming articulation to be used without risk of posterior impingement. These considerations were reflected in the design of the Total Condylar, Duopatellar, Posterior-Stabilized, and various PCL-retaining (cruciate-retaining [CR]) prostheses.

ARGUMENTS FOR AND AGAINST CRUCIATE EXCISION

Arguments can be made in favor of and against cruciate excision, and will be presented here.

Arguments for Cruciate Excision

Correction of Deformity

Removal of the cruciate ligaments is an important element in the soft tissue release of fixed varus or valgus deformities. Correction of these deformities is therefore facilitated by cruciate excision. In addition, clearance of the intercondylar notch provides clear visualization of the posterior capsule, which facilitates release and osteophyte removal during correction of flexion deformities.

Simpler Technique

Release of the cruciate ligaments facilitates surgical exposure, especially in tight knees, which makes the procedure less demanding. It is also technically easier to cut straight across the tibia than around the cruciate insertions. These factors make it easier to make the correct bone cuts and achieve accurate placement of the prosthesis.

Wear

Cruciate excision allows the use of a more conforming articulation, which increases the contact area and reduces contact stress.

Arguments Against Cruciate Excision

Range of Motion

Without a functional PCL or PCL-substituting mechanism, rollback of the femoral component does not occur. This theoretically limits the ultimate flexion obtainable and was noted as a clinical limitation with the original cruciate-sacrificing prosthesis, the TCP.

Instability

Failure to achieve flexion and extension balance can result in anterior-posterior laxity that may exceed the stability imparted by the moderately conforming articular surfaces. Such laxity may lead to symptomatic instability.

Loosening

The increased conformity of the articular surfaces used in the TCP theoretically results in increased stress at the bone-cement-prosthesis interface, which provoked concern that it would ultimately cause loosening. However, as discussed later in the section on PCL substitution, these concerns have not become clinically significant.

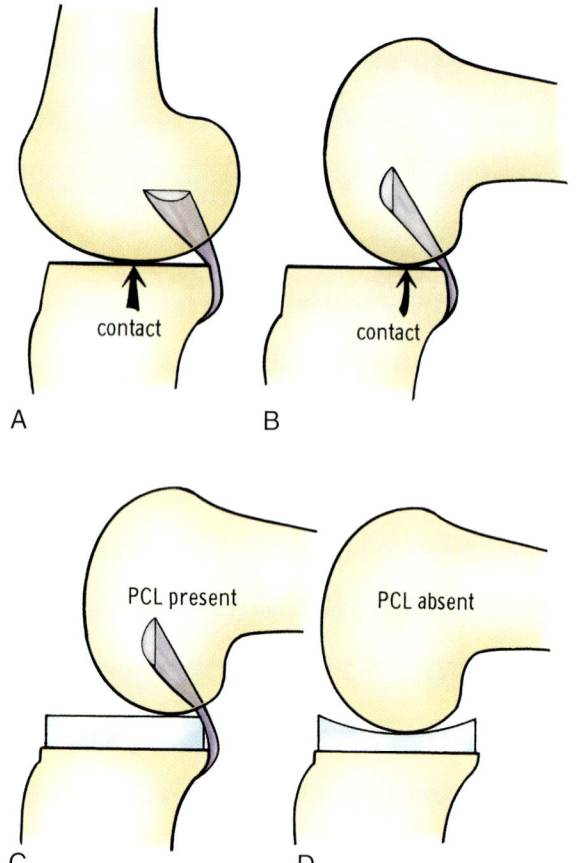

Figure 97-22. Effect of PCL retention on prosthetic design. **A, B,** Because of the rollback enforced by the PCL, the prosthetic tibial surface must be flat to allow this movement. **C, D,** When the PCL is absent, a dished tibial plateau is used.

POSTERIOR CRUCIATE LIGAMENT RETENTION VERSUS SUBSTITUTION

Kinematics

Retention of the PCL was initially believed to allow preservation of normal knee kinematics after TKR. In particular, preservation of the normal femoral rollback caused by tightening of the PCL, which acts to move the tibiofemoral contact point posteriorly during flexion, thereby increasing quadriceps efficiency and range of motion, was thought to be critical in activities such as stair climbing. The natural PCL was initially perceived to be better in performing this kinematic function than the cam and post mechanism used in PS knee prostheses. However, fluoroscopic studies by Stiehl and coauthors[285] and Dennis and colleagues[65] have demonstrated that CR prostheses do not replicate the kinematics of the normal knee. Instead, in many cases, a paradoxical roll forward of the femur occurs with anterior translation of the tibiofemoral contact area. This motion, which is the direct opposite of normal knee kinematics, may result from improper tension of the PCL (Fig. 97-24). Adverse consequences may include decreased flexion, reduced quadriceps efficiency, and posterior tibial polyethylene wear. In addition, Dennis and associates[65] have demonstrated that although PS prostheses do not completely reproduce normal knee kinematics, reliable rollback does occur. Surgeons who advocate the use of CR prostheses have emphasized the importance of balancing the PCL with techniques such as PCL release and recession.[244,255] However, the success of using these techniques to restore normal knee kinematics has still not been proven.

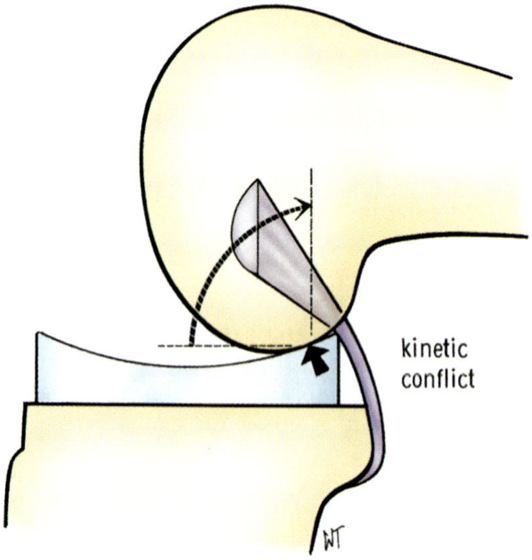

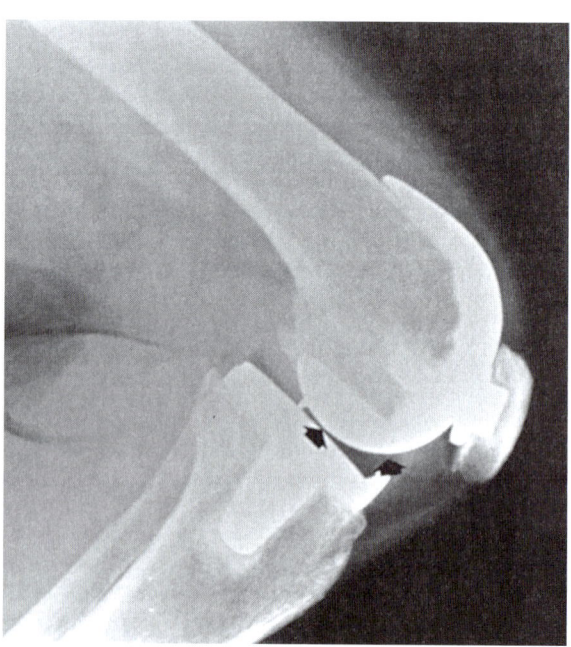

Figure 97-23. Kinematic conflict occurs if concepts are mismatched. In this case, the PCL is preserved with the use of a dished tibial component. Impingement occurs posteriorly with flexion.

Figure 97-24. Sagittal radiograph of a nonfunctional PCL. There has been roll-forward rather than rollback with knee flexion. The anterior margin of the femoral component abuts the anterior margin of the tibial component, as it does in a total condylar–type design.

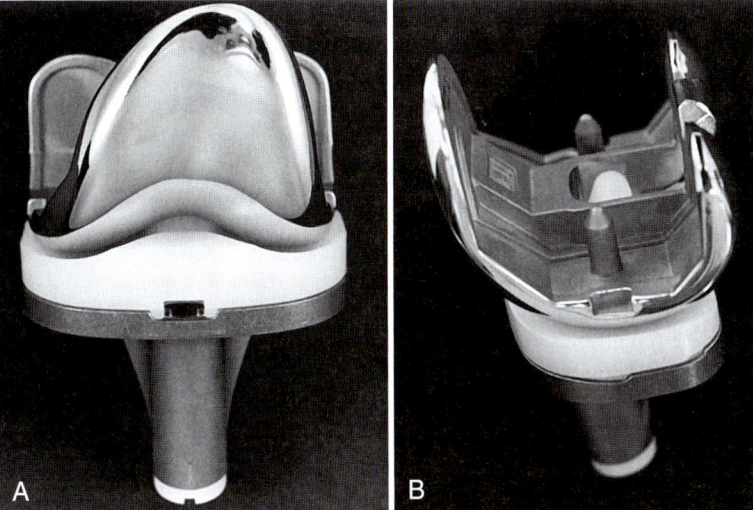

Figure 97-25. The Legacy PS prosthesis (Zimmer, Warsaw, Ind). **A,** Front view. **B,** Oblique view.

Range of Motion

Early experience with use of the cruciate-sacrificing TCP produced flexion of about 90 to 95 degrees, which is near the theoretical limit for this type of prosthesis. Improved flexion with PS and CR prostheses has been reported. Pooled data from numerous studies have demonstrated mean flexion of approximately 100 to 115 degrees with both types of prostheses.[24,220] Again, the importance of PCL recession and balancing in helping to produce optimal results with CR prostheses has been advocated.[244,255] With careful surgical technique, reliable flexion of 110 to 115 degrees should be obtainable with either type of prosthesis. However, because of the experience and attention that seem to be required to tension the PCL correctly, we believe that the PS prosthesis is less technically challenging and produces more consistent results. The consequences of inadequately tensioning the PCL have been reported. Arthroscopic release of a tight PCL seems to be successful in improving flexion for select patients with PCL-retaining prostheses.[318]

Modifications to the latest generation of PS prostheses, the Zimmer Nex Gen Legacy PS (LPS; Fig. 97-25), which is directly descended from the original Insall-Burstein Posterior-Stabilized (IB PS) knee, and before that the TCP, included redesign of the trochlea to accommodate the natural patella. This change necessitated posterior translation of the cam and post mechanism. As a result, the cam engages the post at approximately 70 degrees and then rides down the post, before eventually moving up the post with extreme flexion. This modification effectively increased the jump distance, thereby allowing greater flexion before dislocation. Further evolution of this device has included modifications to the posterior condyles to optimize the contact area in high flexion, as well as anterior scalloping of the polyethylene to reduce impingement on the extensor mechanism anteriorly. These changes have resulted in a new type of high flexion prosthesis, the Zimmer Nex Gen LPS Flex-Fixed, which is intended for use in patients with good preoperative motion in whom high postoperative flexion is anticipated (Fig. 97-26). Improvements in surgical technique, such as restoration of the posterior condylar offset and resection of posterior osteophytes, have also been emphasized in these cases to maximize

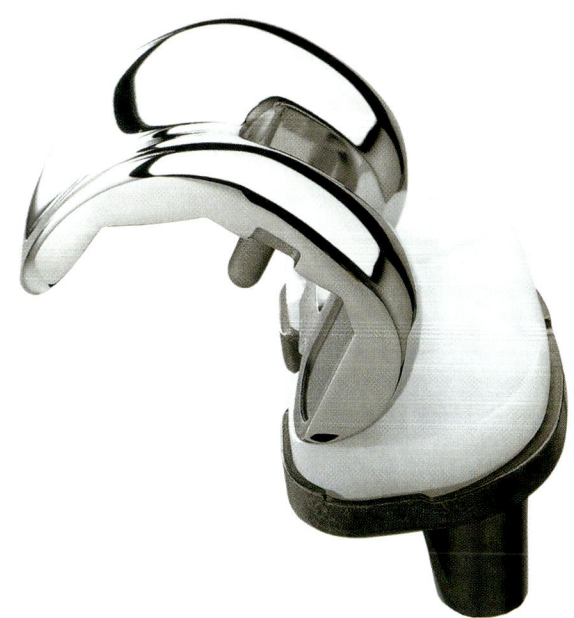

Figure 97-26. The LPS Flex prosthesis (Zimmer, Warsaw, Ind) has been optimized for use in patients with good preoperative motion to allow safer flexion.

postoperative motion. Similar design modifications have been made to other PS knee prostheses that are also intended for the high-flexion environment above 130 degrees, such as the Smith & Nephew Genesis II-HF, DePuy PFC Sigma PS and Biomet Vanguard PS prostheses, as well as to CR prostheses, such as the Zimmer Nex Gen CR Flex-Fixed.

Proprioception

Both cruciate ligaments contain mechanoreceptors, and therefore advocates of PCL retention have proposed that preserving the natural ligament would lead to superior proprioception after TKR. However, the current literature has not demonstrated a clear advantage. Simmons and associates[271] were unable to identify any advantage in proprioception in patients who had a CR prosthesis versus those with a PS prosthesis. Warren and coworkers[305] noted slightly different results. After TKR, all patients experienced improved proprioception regardless of whether a CR or PS prosthesis had been used. However, the improvement was greater in patients with a CR prosthesis. The improved proprioception in both groups was speculated to be caused by elimination of pain, restoration of articular congruity, and retensioning of the collateral ligaments and soft tissues. These inconclusive results may be to the result of the inherent qualities of the PCL in patients with arthritic knees. Kleinbart and colleagues[162] have observed significant degenerative changes in the PCLs of patients with arthritic knees that exceed those in age-matched controls. Therefore, a PCL that is preserved in a patient with a CR prosthesis is likely to be abnormal and should not be expected to function normally, either biomechanically or proprioceptively. The effects of PCL recession on the proprioceptive function of the ligament are not known.

Gait Analysis

Initial studies suggested that the mechanics of walking and stair climbing, in particular, is different in patients with CR and PCL-substituting prostheses.[7,155] Andriacchi and colleagues[7,9] have described a characteristic forward lean of the trunk with less knee flexion in patients with PCL-substituting prostheses during stair climbing when compared with patients

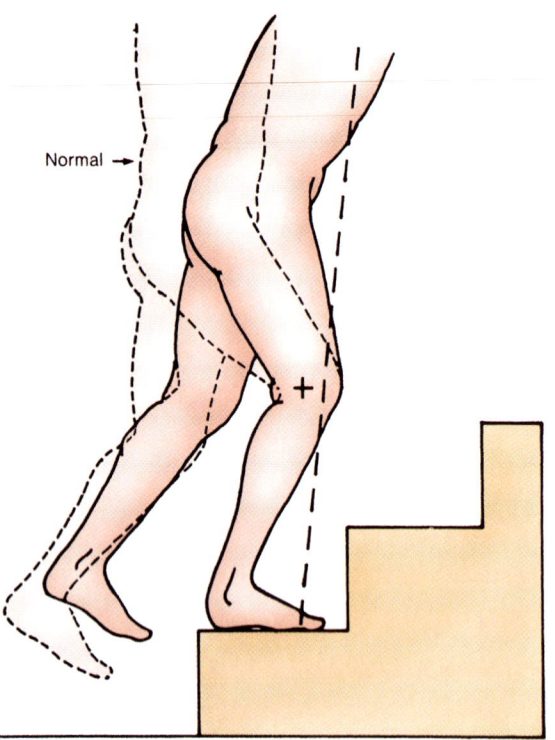

Figure 97-27. According to some gait analysis studies, there is a difference in stair climbing between cruciate-retaining and cruciate-sacrificing knee prostheses. It is reported that patients with the latter climb stairs with less knee flexion and a compensatory forward lean of the trunk. (From Andriacchi TP, Galante JO, Draganich LF: Relationship between knee extensor mechanics and function following total knee replacement. In Dorr LD [ed]: The knee: papers of the first scientific meeting of the knee society, Baltimore, 1985, University Park Press, p 83.)

with PCL-retaining prostheses (Fig. 97-27). This observation was suggested to represent a compensatory mechanism for the absence of the PCL. However, gait analyses in two studies have disputed these findings. Bolanos and coworkers[33] were unable to identify any significant differences in spatiotemporal gait parameters or knee range of motion during level walking or stair climbing in patients with CR or PS prostheses. Wilson and colleagues[320] also did not identify any differences in these parameters during stair climbing between patients with PS prostheses and normal age-matched controls. However, differences between patients after TKR and controls were identified during level walking and descending stairs. This evidence suggests that although gait patterns after TKR are different from those in normal controls, there is no clear effect of prosthesis type.

Correction of Deformity

Patients with significant preoperative fixed varus, valgus, or flexion deformities can be successfully managed with the use of CR prostheses. However, because the PCL is one deforming factor in these cases, careful balancing with PCL release or recession may be required to achieve flexion and extension space symmetry.[87,244,255] Balancing of the PCL may be difficult and is experience-dependent. The development of deep dish polyethylene inserts for use in cruciate-retaining prostheses when the PCL is impossible to tension accurately reflects the difficulties in accomplishing this task. Laskin[178] has reported inferior results in patients with fixed varus deformities exceeding 15 degrees in whom CR rather than PS designs were used. In most circumstances, we believe that the use of a PS prosthesis is technically less challenging and allows more reliable correction of the preoperative deformity. Failure to tension the PCL appropriately may lead to reduced flexion or flexion instability.[221,307,318]

Stability

The more conforming tibial insert and cam and post mechanisms of PS prostheses do not provide any constraint in the medial-lateral directions (Fig. 97-28). Neither the CR nor the PS prosthesis is designed to compensate for instability in this plane and therefore requires intact collateral ligaments. In the anterior and posterior directions, the inherent characteristics of the designs are different, and different problems are encountered if flexion-extension balance is not achieved. As noted, a less conforming tibial polyethylene insert should be used in CR prostheses because of the kinematic conflict that results during femoral rollback in flexion if a more conforming insert is used. If the PCL is functionally incompetent or stretches, posterior instability may occur because the minimally conforming or flat insert does little to prevent posterior translation of the femur. The phenomenon of symptomatic flexion instability in patients with CR prostheses as a result of an incompetent PCL has now gained more widespread recognition.[221,307] The consequences of overtensioning of the PCL have been discussed earlier. Biomechanical studies have suggested that it is difficult to obtain the appropriate tension in the PCL.[129,193] However, the results of techniques used to balance the PCL have not been directly evaluated.

Although PS prostheses eliminate the PCL as a factor in preventing adequate flexion-extension balancing, anterior

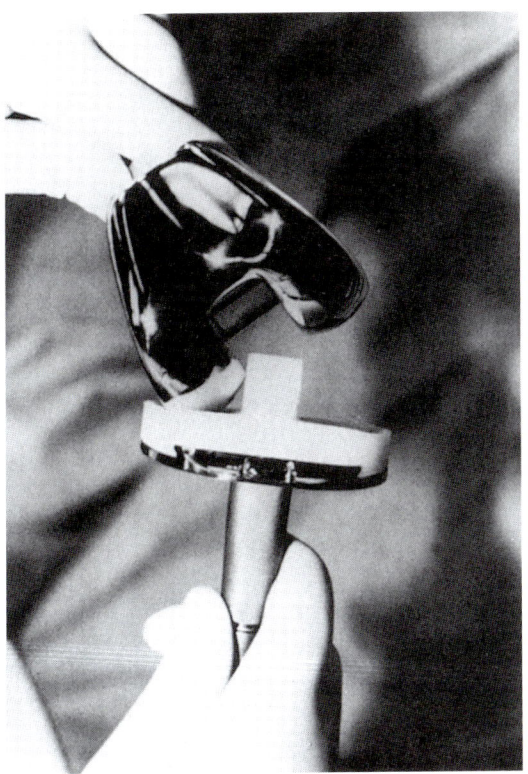

Figure 97-28. Posterior-stabilized prosthesis showing that the cam and post mechanism offers no restraint to varus or valgus stability.

and posterior instability can still occur. In some patients with significant flexion instability, the jump distance of the cam and post mechanism may be exceeded during extreme flexion and acute dislocation results (Fig. 97-29). In previous series, a dislocation rate of 2% to 3% was reported.[66,235] In one series, changes in design of the cam and post mechanism eliminated subsequent dislocations over a 2-year period.[235] Because of the uncertainties in achieving optimal tension in the PCL, we believe that PS prostheses produce more reliable long-term anterior-posterior stability.

Polyethylene Wear

Polyethylene wear in current PS designs that have moderately conforming articular surfaces has not been a major clinical problem in older, less active patients.[58,235] In contrast, the higher contact stress encountered in the unconstrained flat-on-flat articulations, in conjunction with the heat-pressed, thin polyethylene inserts used in CR prostheses during the 1980s, led to documented rapid wear.[31,76,157,291] Failure to balance the PCL may also result in severe posteromedial polyethylene wear. Based on these results, the more conforming surfaces of PS implants seem better suited to optimizing long-term wear (Fig. 97-30).

Loosening

The increased constraint imposed by the moderately conforming articular surfaces of PS prostheses was initially

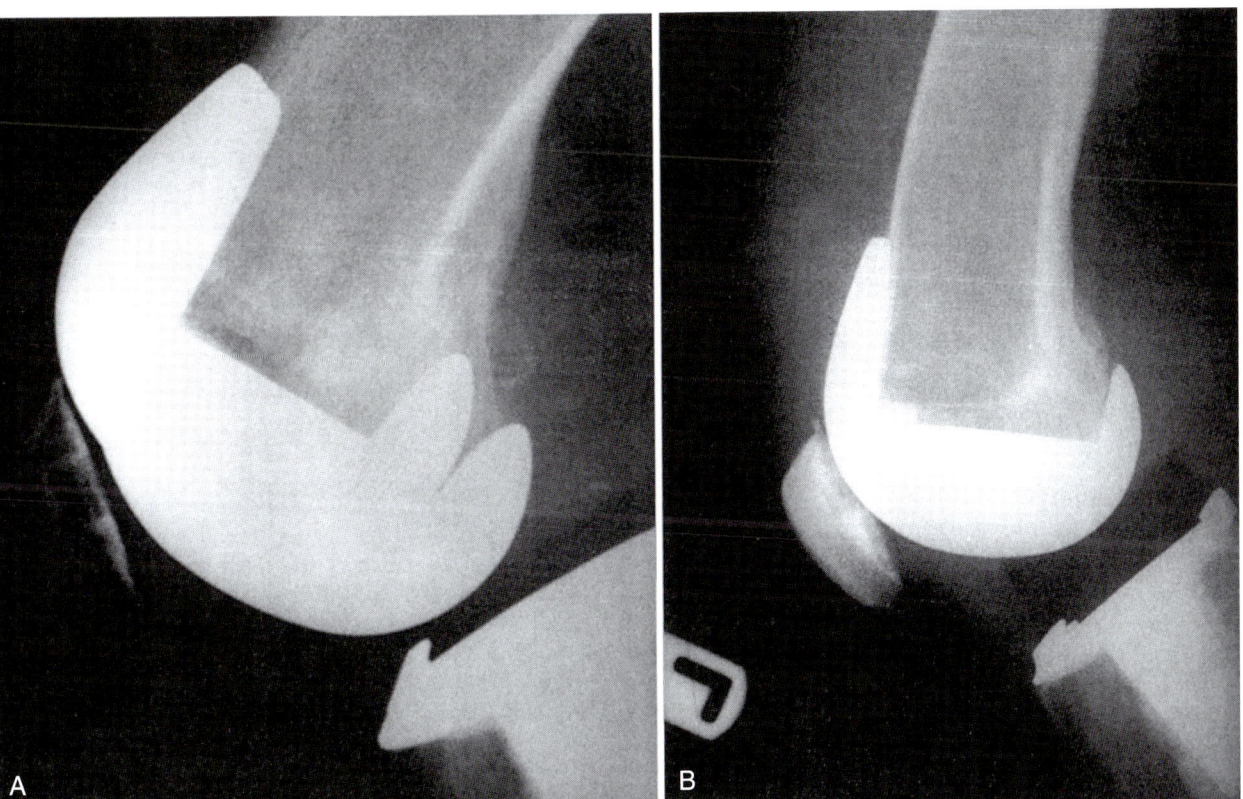

Figure 97-29. A, Radiograph of a dislocated posterior-stabilized prosthesis. The post of the tibial component has displaced posteriorly behind the cam of the femoral component. **B,** Radiograph after reduction.

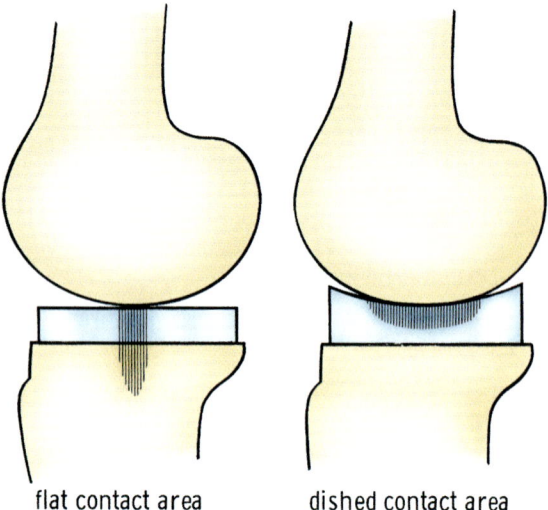

flat contact area   dished contact area

Figure 97-30. A dished component permits greater conformity, hence a larger contact area. The smaller contact area with a flat tibial component increases stress on the polyethylene.

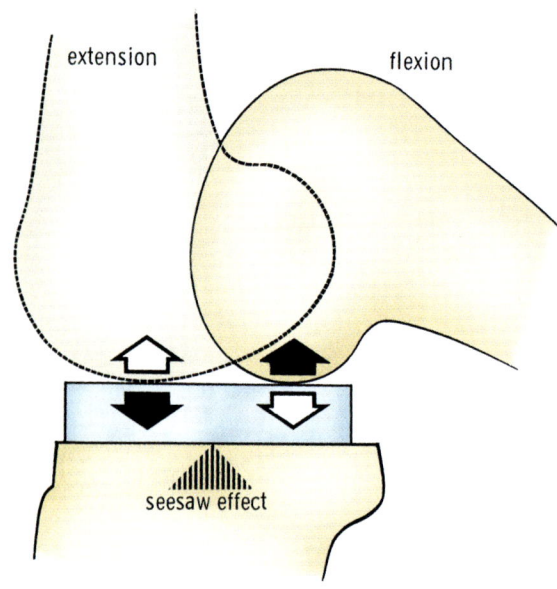

extension   flexion

seesaw effect

Figure 97-32. The seesaw effect. The back and forth movement on the tibial component caused by posterior cruciate ligament retention creates a rocking motion that may cause loosening.

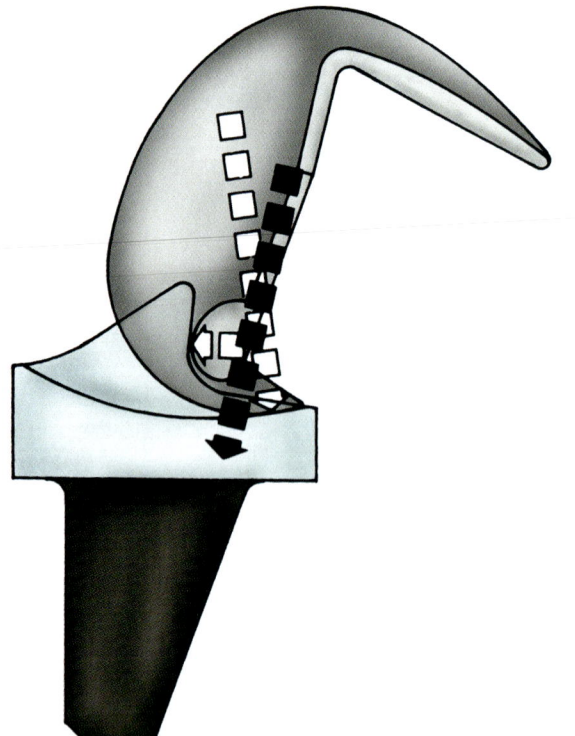

Figure 97-31. The cam mechanism of a posterior-stabilized knee simulates the function of the posterior cruciate ligament and causes rollback of the femur on the tibia with flexion. The resulting vector of forces passes distally through the fixation peg. (From Insall JN, Lachiewicz PF, Burstein AH: The posterior stabilized condylar prosthesis: a modification of the total condylar design: two- to four-year clinical experience. J Bone Joint Surg Am 64:1317, 1982.)

considered to be detrimental to long-term fixation at the cement-bone-prosthesis interface because of increased stress transmission versus the relatively less conforming CR prostheses. However, with proper design, this shear stress can be altered to forces that are compressive (Fig. 97-31).

A theoretical seesaw motion may occur in CR prostheses (Fig. 97-32). The rolling motion of the femur changes the metal-plastic contact point from anterior in extension to posterior in flexion. Thus, in extension, the anterior portion of the tibia is compressed and in flexion the situation is reversed. This alternating compression-distraction may theoretically affect long-term fixation.

Long-term follow-up studies have failed to identify a significant clinical problem caused by these theoretical concerns, with only rare cases of aseptic loosening with both types of prosthesis. In the senior author's (JI) experience with posterior-stabilized prostheses, no cases of aseptic loosening of the tibial component and only two cases of femoral component loosening have occurred in 165 primary TKRs at a mean of 10-year follow-up.[58] These results are similar to those obtained with CR designs. Malkani and associates[194] from the Mayo Clinic have reported a 96% survival rate at 10-year follow-up. In summary, at 10- to 15-year follow-up, there is little evidence to suggest that PS prostheses have an increased risk of aseptic loosening.

CURRENT PROSTHESIS DESIGN

During the past 15 years, early clear distinctions in prosthesis design between anatomic and functional concepts have, to a large degree, vanished and, at this point, many aspects of prosthesis design are common to a variety of prostheses. This not only includes articular surface geometry, but also fixation and bearing options. Insofar as possible, the types of currently available implants are discussed under broad headings in terms of similarities and differences. Specific implants and systems are presented within each category only as examples; certainly, the intent is not to present a comprehensive list of all current total knee prostheses marketed in the United States and elsewhere.

Fixed-Bearing, Surface Replacement Prostheses

Traditional Cruciate-Retaining and Posterior-Stabilized Prostheses

The prostheses described in the preceding sections have given rise to derivatives (Fig. 97-33). The TCP led to a series of PS prostheses initially developed by Insall and Burstein, including the IB PS prosthesis, and modular IB II (IB II PS) prosthesis.*

These devices then evolved into the Zimmer NexGen LPS prosthesis. Subsequently, although the basic elements of the LPS prosthesis have endured, line extensions have occurred to attempt to address specific issues noted with the initial device. A high-flexion variant, the Zimmer NexGen LPS

_____
*References 2, 3, 85, 111, 116, 135, 245, 259, 260, 282-284, and 314.

Flex-Fixed prosthesis, was introduced almost 10 years ago, with augmented posterior condyles to help decrease polyethylene contact pressures in higher flexion and a cam mechanism that was optimized for the high-flexion environment (Figs. 97-34 to 97-36; see Figs. 97-25, 97-26, and 97-28). More recently, a gender-optimized variant was added to the system (Zimmer Gender Solutions Nex Gen LPS High Flex knee), which has a narrower medial to lateral width, thinner anterior flange, and higher Q angle to the trochlear groove for a better match to the native female anatomy. In addition to the Nex Gen LPS prosthesis, the Press-Fit Condylar (PFC) PS and its successor, the PFC Sigma PS prosthesis (Fig. 97-37), were developed from the same TCP foundation, as were the Optetrak PS and Advance PS prostheses; the PCL-preserving Duopatellar prosthesis evolved into the Kinematic I and II and PFC CR prostheses (Fig. 97-38).[245,321]

During the consolidation of the PFC CR and PS variants under the PFC Sigma brand more than a decade ago, the coronal plane geometry of the CR and PS implants was made

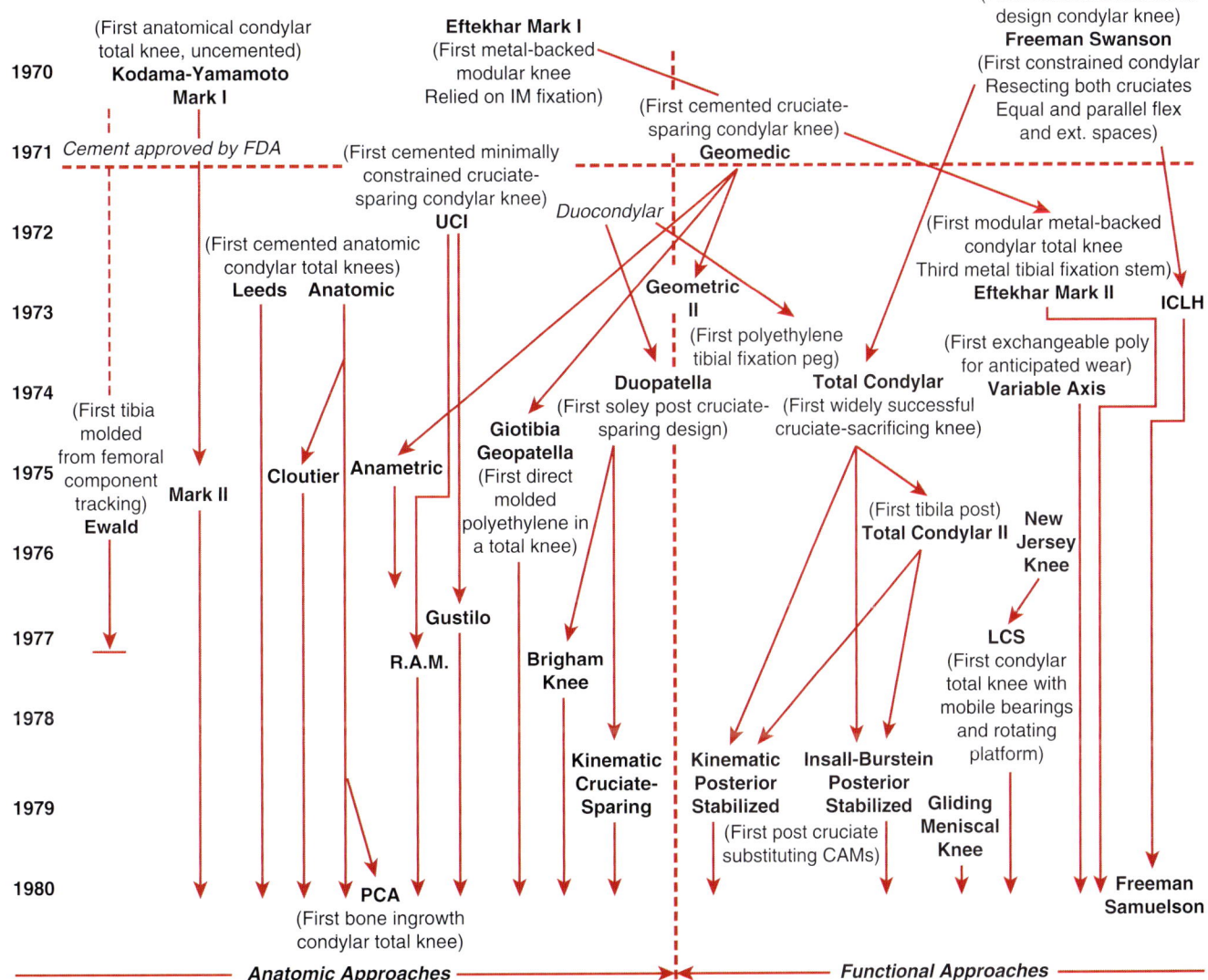

Figure 97-33. The evolution of the condylar total knee from 1970 to 1980. (Adapted from Robinson RP: The early innovators of today's resurfacing condylar knees. J Arthroplasty 20[Suppl 1]:2, 2005.)

identical.[252] This highlights the trend that has occurred over the past 15 years where, to some degree, prosthesis design has converged with several seemingly important elements becoming common, not only to CR and PS variants in the same implant system from one manufacturer, but also across manufacturers. These desirable features of fixed-bearing, surface replacement prostheses include the following: multiple sizing options to match a broader range of native anatomy better; side-specific femoral components with anatomically oriented trochlear grooves designed to accommodate native and resurfaced patellae; front-loading, modular, metal-backed tibial components for ease of potential revision and optimization of soft tissue balancing; moderately conforming round-on-round femorotibial geometry in the coronal plane to minimize edge loading and polyethylene wear; and a femoral component with the so-called J curve, multiradius sagittal plane geometry that is moderately to highly conforming during the early arc of flexion to optimize contact areas, but where the radius of curvature decreases toward the posterior condyles, which facilitates rollback and range of motion.[231] Examples of CR and PS knee prostheses that currently incorporate most or all of these concepts include the Zimmer Nex Gen, DePuy PFC Sigma, Smith & Nephew Genesis II, and Biomet Vanguard systems. Other systems, such as the Stryker Triathlon, Smith & Nephew Journey Bi-Cruciate Stabilized, and Wright Advance Medical Medial Pivot Knee,

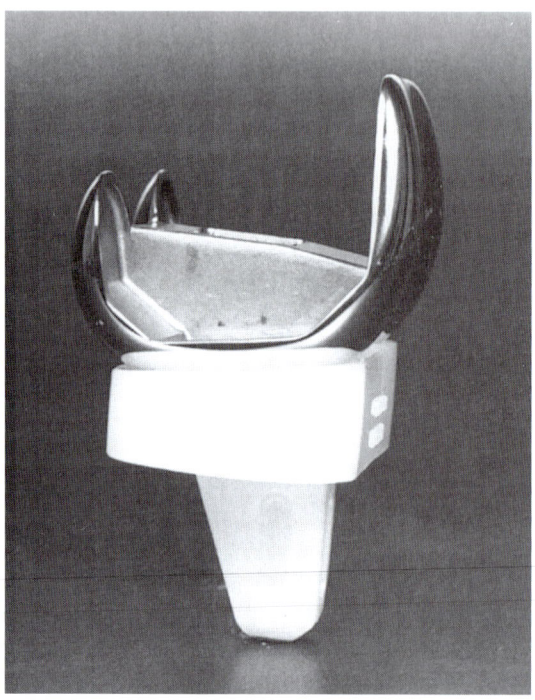

Figure 97-34. The original Insall-Burstein Posterior-Stabilized prosthesis.

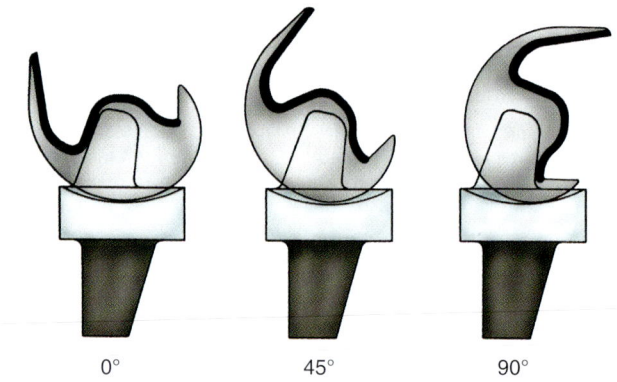

0°   45°   90°

Figure 97-36. The TCP II was a precursor of the posterior-stabilized knee that provided a passive stop against posterior displacement in flexion as well as a hyperextension stop in extension. (From Insall JN, Tria AJ, Scott WN: The total condylar knee prosthesis: the first five years. Clin Orthop Relat Res [145]:68, 1979.)

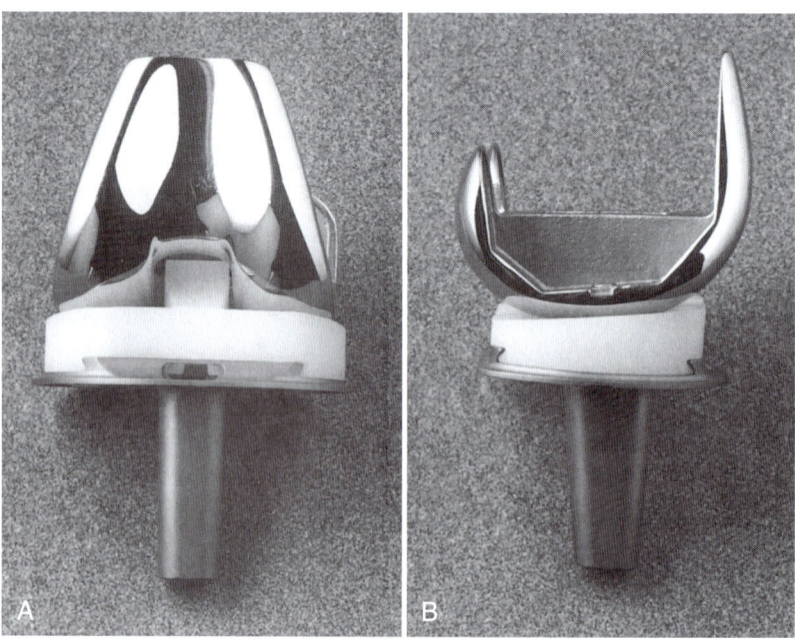

Figure 97-35. The modular Insall-Burstein II Posterior-Stabilized prosthesis. **A,** Front view. **B,** Side view.

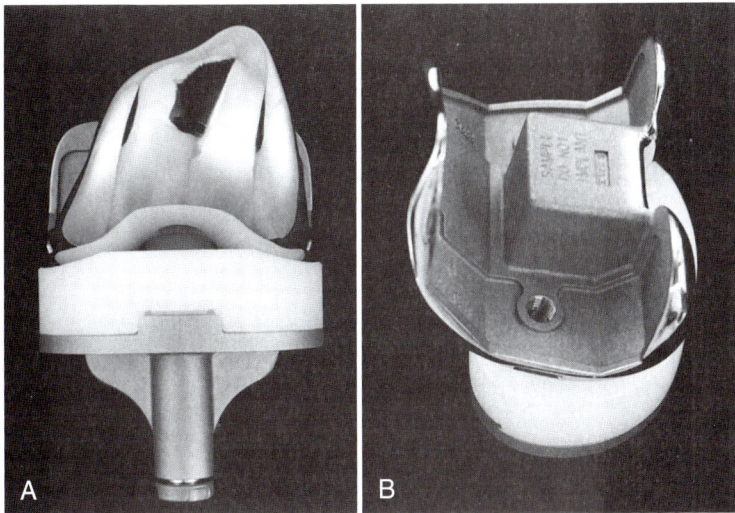

Figure 97-37. The PFC Sigma prosthesis (DePuy, Warsaw, Ind). **A,** Front view. **B,** Oblique view.

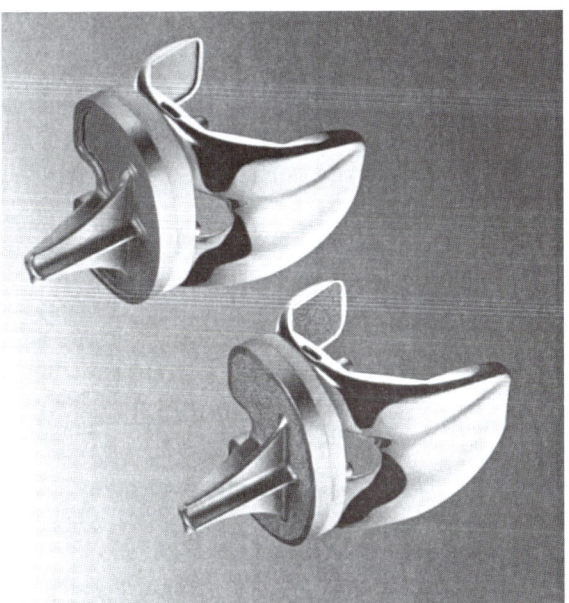

Figure 97-38. Press-Fit Condylar prosthesis.

incorporate alternative unique elements that theoretically change the function of the devices. The features of this later group of devices that are considered guided motion prostheses are described here.

Guided Motion Prostheses

Although traditional PS knees may be considered guided motion prostheses to some degree, the kinematics of traditional surface replacement prostheses is less rigidly dictated by the design than in the prostheses introduced during the past 10 years which are usually considered to be guided motion devices. Each of these devices has similar elements that attempt to compel the components to move in a specific way. Two common features include a femoral component with a single sagittal axis of rotation to at least 90 to 100 degrees of flexion, rather than the J curve noted earlier, and articular surfaces that are molded and shaped to encourage rotation and rollback of the lateral condyle on the tibia while

the medial femoral condyle remains relatively static. As noted in the previous section, most current traditional fixed-bearing surface replacement prostheses have a femoral component with posterior condylar geometry that incorporates a number of different axes of rotation. This effectively creates a decreasing sagittal radius of curvature of the posterior condyles, which facilitates rollback in flexion. However, although the J curve theoretically facilitates rollback and improves flexion, the decreasing radius of curvature reduces the contact area of the articulating surfaces as the knee flexes, which may lead to increased polyethylene stresses.[231] In most surface replacement designs, the effects of this J curve do not occur during the initial 30 to 40 degrees of flexion; therefore, the increased joint forces generated during the weight-bearing portion of the gait cycle are accommodated by articular surfaces with moderate to high combined coronal and sagittal plane conformity, which helps reduce potential wear. In addition to this problem with potential wear, the decreasing radius of curvature results in decreasing tension on the collateral ligaments as the knee flexes. This reduction in soft tissue tension has been implicated in the phenomenon described as midflexion instability, in which some patients experience pain and instability with activities performed with the knee in moderate flexion, such as stair climbing or rising from a chair.[304] This is a controversial subject; however, in a minority of modern fixed-bearing surface replacement prostheses, it has led to the incorporation of a fixed single sagittal radius of curvature through an extended arc of motion exceeding 90 to 100 degrees. The Stryker Triathlon prosthesis (Fig. 97-39), and the Scorpio knee that preceded it, along with the Wright Medical Technologies Advance Medial Pivot Knee, are designs that incorporate this concept of a single sagittal axis of rotation. However, at higher degrees of flexion, these devices actually incorporate a gradual reduction of the sagittal radius of curvature to allow better rollback. Other theoretical advantages of a prosthesis with a constant sagittal radius of curvature and a more posterior flexion-extension axis that lengthens the extensor moment arm are improved quadriceps function and reduced anterior knee pain.[192]

The second design element that is common to these guided motion devices, including the Wright Medical

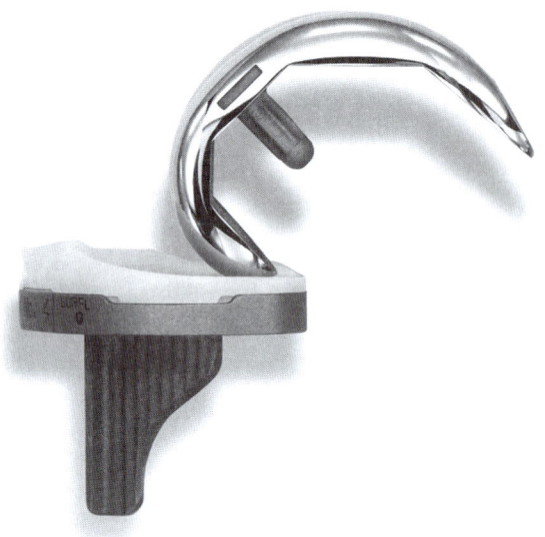

Figure 97-39. The Triathlon CR prosthesis. This device has a single sagittal radius of curvature from 10 to 110 degrees that is centered about the transepicondylar axis. This differs from the so-called J curve common to many surface replacement total condylar–type femoral components. (Courtesy Stryker, Mahwah, NJ.)

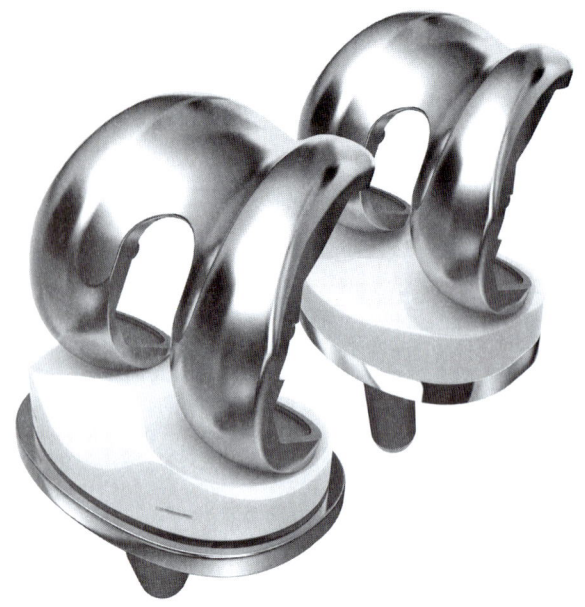

Figure 97-40. PFC Sigma CR150 High Flex Knee, mobile-bearing (front) and fixed-bearing (rear) variants. (Courtesy DePuy, Warsaw, Ind.)

Technologies Advance Medial Pivot Knee and Smith & Nephew Journey BCS Bi-Cruciate Stabilized Knee, is that the articular surfaces are manufactured in an attempt to replicate the kinematics of the normal knee. This is accomplished by encouraging the medial femoral condyle to rotate but remain relative static in the sagittal plan while the lateral condyle rotates, rolls back, and slides posteriorly on the tibial articular surface as the knee flexes. Although potential advantages have been attributed to the single sagittal axis of rotation and motion guided by the articular geometry, no long-term published data from prospective randomized studies are yet available to support or refute these assertions.

High-Flexion and Gender-Optimized Prostheses

Traditional surface replacement prostheses, both in CR and PS variants, have been associated with excellent clinical outcomes. However, despite successful pain relief and improvements in functional outcomes, the increased desire among patients to pursue activities associated with greater degrees of knee flexion, especially in certain Asian populations, have driven the development of knee prostheses designed to accommodate better and even facilitate higher degrees of flexion, exceeding 140 to 150 degrees. Design elements that have been used in many of these include the following: enhanced posterior condylar geometry of the femoral component to improve contact areas in high flexion, thereby reducing the risk of polyethylene wear; modifications to the anterior aspect of the tibial polyethylene insert to reduce the potential for extensor mechanism impingement in high flexion; and optimization of the cam-post design of PS variants to reduce the risk of dislocation in high flexion.[13,159,204,231] Examples of these optimized high-flexion variants of successful surface replacement prostheses include the Zimmer Nex Gen Flex-Fixed CR and PS implants (see Fig. 97-26), DePuy PFC Sigma CR150 High Flex Knee (Fig. 97-40), and Smith & Nephew Genesis II-HF.

To date, studies of high-flexion TKR prostheses have provided little data to support the theoretical advantages attributed to the optimized designs. In a recent meta-analysis, Ghandi and colleagues[100] noted that high-flexion designs are associated with improved range of motion (ROM) compared with traditional implants, but offer no clinical benefits. Similarly, Meneghini and associates[207] were unable to demonstrate any functional benefit from flexion more than 125 degrees after TKR. Studies of individual prostheses are also inconclusive. Kim and coworkers[160] have reported on a prospective randomized study of 50 patients who underwent simultaneous bilateral TKR with a standard fixed-bearing Zimmer NexGen LPS knee prosthesis on one side and a high-flexion, fixed-bearing NexGen LPS-Flex knee prosthesis on the opposite side. The Knee Society and HSS scores were not significantly different for either knee preoperatively or postoperatively. Moreover, there were no statistically significant differences in ROM at any time point preoperatively or postoperatively; at final follow-up, the standard prosthesis had a mean ROM of 135.8 degrees (range, 105 to 150 degrees) versus a mean of 135.8 degrees for the high-flexion prosthesis. The same authors have also reported their results from an identical prospective randomized study of 54 bilateral TKR patients comparing the Zimmer Nex Gen CR prosthesis on one side with the CR version of the NexGen Flex prosthesis on the other side.[159] Similar to their results demonstrated with the PS prostheses, no statistically significant differences in knee scores or ROM were identified between the two groups at any time, either preoperatively or postoperatively.

Similar results using the same implant system have also been reported from a second center in South Korea. In a trial of patients who had been randomized to receive the Zimmer fixed-bearing Nex Gen CR or the Nex Gen CR Flex-Fixed prosthesis, Seon and colleagues[262] did not identify any statistical differences in postoperative ROM between the two groups. In addition to these reports from Korea, similar results have been reported from Western patients with the same Zimmer NexGen prostheses. Nutton and associates[218] compared patients who had been randomized to receive a standard or high-flexion version of the Zimmer NexGen LPS fixed-bearing design. No significant differences in outcomes or knee flexion were noted between the two groups of patients. Published information on other high-flexion prostheses is even more limited. McCalden and coworkers[204] recently reported on a prospective randomized trial comparing the Smith & Nephew Genesis II PS fixed-bearing prosthesis with the high-flexion version of the same implant. At short-term follow-up, no differences in outcomes scores or ROM were demonstrated; at 2 years postoperatively the mean ROM for the standard prosthesis was 123 versus 124 degrees for the high-flexion variant. Therefore, there is no clear evidence currently that these fixed-bearing, high-flexion devices help obtain improved ROM or are associated with better clinical results at the 2- to 3-year range. However, it is possible that the theoretical improvements in contact area at high flexion may result in lower long-term wear and reduced rates of aseptic loosening and osteolysis.

In addition to surface replacement designs that have been optimized for the high-flexion environment, increased acknowledgment of the anthropomorphic variation that exists among different genders, races, and ethnic groups has also led to the introduction of optimized components that better accommodate these differences.*

These changes have chiefly involved modifications to the mediolateral to anteroposterior (AP) ratio of the femoral components that make the component narrower for any given AP dimension, as well as modifications to the orientation and thickness of the trochlear groove and anterior flange.[34,109,208] Examples of these modified prostheses include the Zimmer Gender Solutions Nex Gen High Flex CR and LPS prostheses, Zimmer Gender Solutions Natural Knee Flex System, and Wright Medical Technology Advance Stature Prostheses. In addition to modifications made to contemporary surface replacement prostheses, new knee implant systems have been introduced during the past decade that have attempted to embrace these concepts of expanded sizing options and high flexion from the initial product launch. Examples include the Biomet Vanguard knee system, Smith & Nephew Journey Bi-Cruciate Stabilized Knee, and Stryker Triathlon knee prostheses. Early results examining the use of these gender-optimized devices have been controversial. Whereas radiographic and anatomic studies have demonstrated the gender bias of standard implants toward white male anatomy, little data exist to date to support the contention that this bias has adversely affected clinical outcomes in white females or patients of other races.[56,119,189]

Cementless Fixation

Concerns about the long-term durability of cement fixation prompted the development of a variety of knee prostheses designed for cementless use during the 1980s. Because of theoretical concern about the increased stress transferred to the prosthesis-bone interface in PS designs that could potentially limit successful bone ingrowth, these uncemented devices were all designed to retain the PCL. The first design,

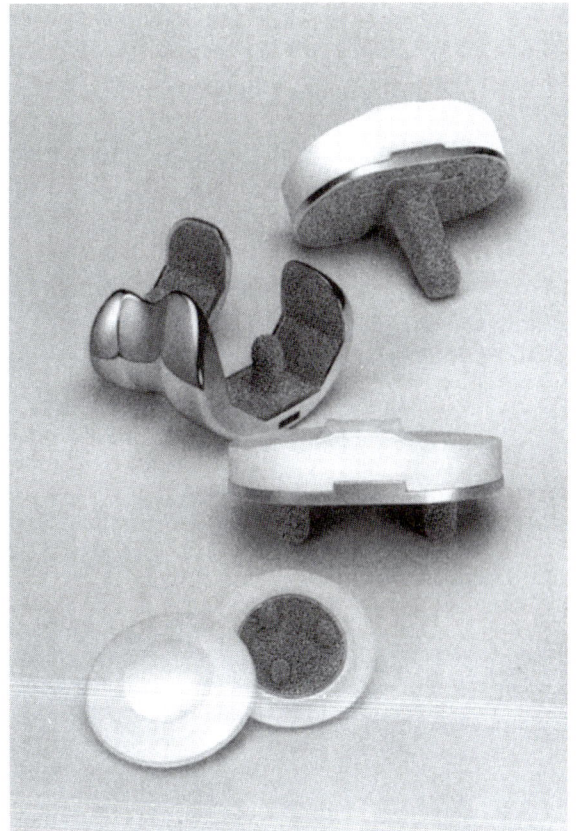

Figure 97-41. Porous Coated Anatomic prosthesis.

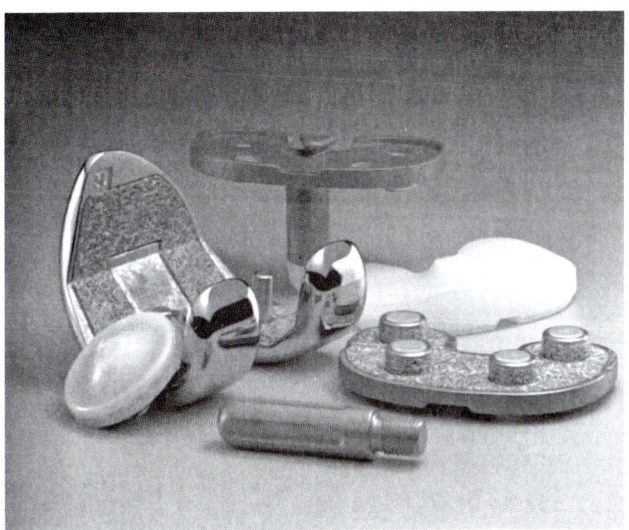

Figure 97-42. Miller-Galante prosthesis.

developed by David Hungerford, was the Porous Coated Anatomic (PCA) knee prosthesis (Fig. 97-41).*

Other examples included the Porous Coated Anatomic II, Miller-Galante (Fig. 97-42),[166,170,247] Miller-Galante II, Tricon M,[179,217] Genesis (Fig. 97-43), and Ortholoc prostheses.[315] The Freeman-Swanson prosthesis[96,98] was modified into the

---

*References 34, 109, 119, 167, 187, and 293.

*References 25, 54, 60, 67, 88, 124, 125, 163, 213, 246, 248, and 279.

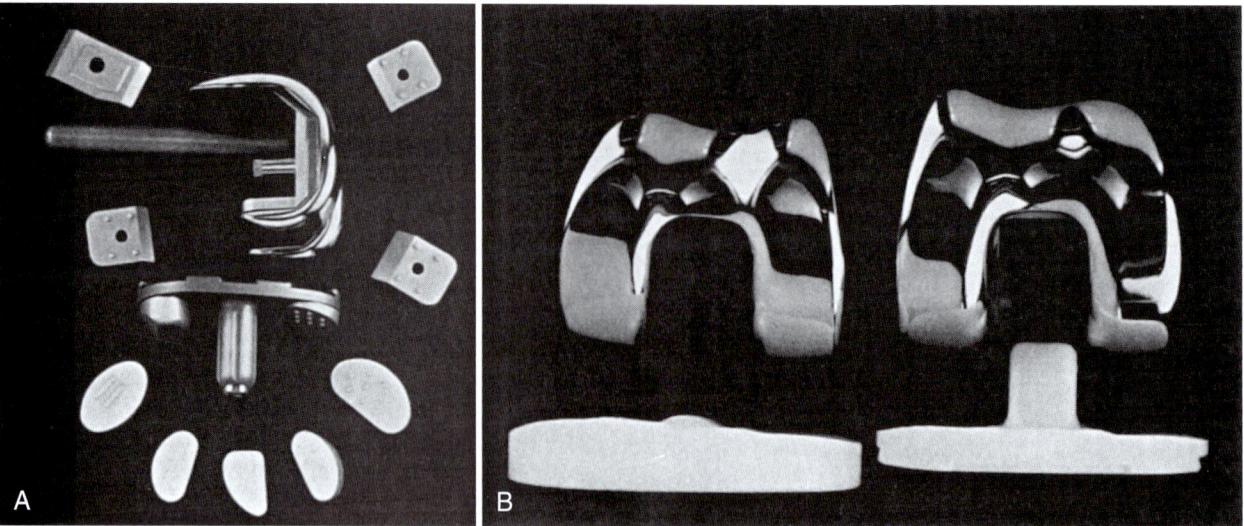

Figure 97-43. **A, B,** Genesis prosthesis.

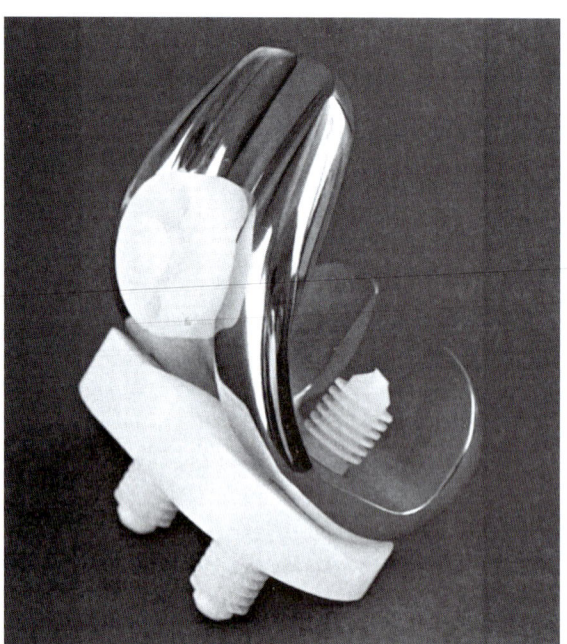

Figure 97-44. Freeman-Samuelson prosthesis. (Courtesy M.A.R. Freeman.)

Freeman-Samuelson prosthesis[93,94,249] (Fig. 97-44), which still used serrated polyethylene pegs for cementless fixation but offered a metal baseplate with intramedullary rods for the tibia and an intramedullary rod on the femoral component.

Unfortunately, the initial enthusiasm in some circles for these devices was not supported by the long-term results. Aseptic loosening and failure to achieve initial fixation, coupled with incidental problems related to the materials selected, as well as confounding problems caused by the flat-on-flat geometries used in most of these designs, led to higher failure rates than noted with comparable cemented prostheses during the first decade.[71,239] Consequently, these devices did not achieve widespread acceptance. More recently, the development of new bone ingrowth materials, especially those based on tantalum and other porous metal constructs,

has prompted renewed interest in this area. Many current CR and PS knee systems now offer uncemented fixation options for the femur, tibia, and patellar that can be used in conjunction with cemented components. Thus, the early division between cemented PS knees and uncemented CR knees is no longer pertinent and individual surgeons may choose fully cemented, fully uncemented, or hybrid components with CR or PS knees. However, at this time, long-term results of this next generation of uncemented and hybrid implants are not yet available.

Mobile-Bearing, Surface Replacement Prostheses

Conventional fixed-bearing knee prostheses have proved clinically successful, with favorable results at 10 to 15 years.[58,153,194] However, with only a few exceptions, these results were obtained in older, less active patient populations.[66,72] Concern exists regarding the long-term durability of current prostheses in younger, more demanding patients, especially regarding problems related to polyethylene wear and osteolysis. Polyethylene wear may be reduced by radical improvements in the inherent qualities of the material itself—for example, through cross linking or by decreasing the contact stress at the articular surfaces. Reduction in contact stress could be accomplished by increasing the conformity of the femoral component and polyethylene insert. However, because of the inherent trade-off between conformity and freedom of motion that exists in fixed-bearing prostheses, significant improvements in contact stress are not feasible. Mobile-bearing prosthesis represent a theoretically appealing solution to this problem.[130] A mobile bearing eliminates the relationship between articular conformity and freedom of rotation that exists in fixed-bearing prostheses because rotation occurs at the interface between the tibial baseplate and the undersurface of the polyethylene insert, and articular conformity is a property of the shape of the femoral component and superior surface of the polyethylene insert. Articular conformity can be maximized in a mobile-bearing prosthesis, thereby reducing contact stress and wear on the superior surface of the polyethylene while freedom of rotation is maintained.

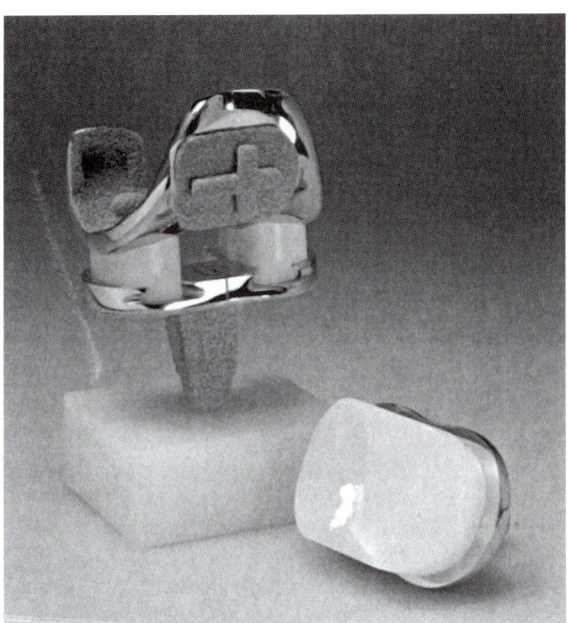

Figure 97-45. Low–Contact Stress prosthesis.

The many nuances of mobile-bearing prosthesis design and our interest in the development of these prostheses will be reviewed more thoroughly in a subsequent chapter. Briefly, the concepts behind these prostheses are not new, as borne out by the Oxford prostheses.*

In 1976, Goodfellow and O'Connor[107] introduced a bicondylar knee that attempted to solve the potential problem of polyethylene wear by providing a meniscal bearing—that is, a polyethylene tibial component that is fully congruent with the femoral component but free to move on a metallic tibial base tray. This concept hoped to provide the best possible wear characteristics with complete lack of constraint. The designers of the Oxford knee now recommend that this prosthesis be used only as a unicompartmental prosthesis when both the ACL and PCL are present and can be preserved. An absent ACL is now considered a contraindication to the Oxford knee. Buechel and associates[43-45] developed the meniscal-bearing concept into a series of prostheses known as the DePuy Low-Contact Stress (LCS) knee prostheses[26] (Fig. 97-45). These devices possess a femoral component similar to the TCP that was designed to be mated with a bicondylar meniscal-bearing tibial component that resembles that of the Oxford knee or, alternatively, a rotating platform for use when cruciate excision is indicated. There is also a metal-backed patellar component with a swiveling polyethylene surface of anatomic design.

Unlike the Oxford knee, the LCS model has a femoral component of decreasing radius posteriorly. Congruency is reduced when the knee is flexed so the contact area decreases in flexion, thereby losing a potential advantage of the original design.

A puzzle created by meniscal designs, particularly the Oxford model, was in deciding the position of the actual joint axis. Flexion takes place between the femur and superior surface of the polyethylene bearing, whereas anteroposterior sliding and rotation occur at the inferior surface (a position 8 to 10 mm distal to the true joint line). Whether this curious anomaly has clinical significance has not been studied extensively.

In Europe, a large number of other mobile-bearing knees have been in widespread clinical use for over a decade. In distinction, in the United States, the LCS prosthesis was the only available mobile-bearing knee until the merger of DePuy and Johnson & Johnson. This merger allowed the development of mobile-bearing variants of both the PFC Sigma CR and PS prostheses, along with high-flexion variants (see Fig. 97-40). Except for these notable exceptions, the complexity of gaining U.S. Food and Drug Administration (FDA) approval for new devices has restricted widespread introduction of other mobile-bearing prostheses. However, Zimmer recently introduced a mobile-bearing version of the Nex Gen LPS, along with a high-flexion variant, into the U.S. market. Important differences compared with the LCS and Sigma mobile-bearing prostheses are a more anterior pivot, a rotational stop that limits rotation to 20 degrees internally and externally, and a smaller contact area between the post of the metal base plate and the cutout of the polyethylene insert that allows rotation at the undersurface. Long-term follow-up will show whether these design features provide better long-term wear characteristics than contemporary fixed-bearing designs or the LCS-based mobile-bearing designs.

Although mobile-bearing prostheses have appealing theoretical advantages versus fixed-bearing knee designs, they are also associated with unique complications that result from their increased complexity. The movement that occurs on the proximal and distal surfaces of the polyethylene bearing introduces the potential for wear at both surfaces.[99] It remains unresolved whether the larger wear surfaces in mobile-bearing knees result in more total volumetric wear than in fixed-bearing knees. Also, there are concerns that the wear particles that are generated in mobile-bearing knees are smaller than those generated in fixed-bearing devices, and these smaller particles may be more likely to result in osteolysis than larger particles. However, in vivo analysis has failed to show a consistent result.[112] Another criticism of mobile-bearing designs is that some kinematic studies of in vivo prostheses have shown that little rotation is actually occurring at the undersurface of the polyethylene, effectively resulting in a fixed-bearing implant. In one recent study, almost 50% of the prostheses demonstrated axial rotation of 3 degrees or less with deep flexion.[306] Finally, dislocation of the bearings has also been reported.[26] Interestingly, in clinical practice, the potential advantages and disadvantages of mobile-bearing devices have not translated into convincingly better or worse outcomes versus those in fixed-bearing knees.[102,169,222,324] Prosthesis survivorship and clinical outcomes for the LCS prosthesis into the second decade and beyond are similar to the results noted with the best fixed-bearing CR and PS designs.*

Therefore, at this time, although the LCS prosthesis has proven successful in the clinical setting, after 3 decades of experience with mobile-bearing knees, they remain a niche product in North America.

Constrained Prostheses

Constrained Unlinked Prostheses

Constrained but unlinked prostheses are primarily intended for use in cases in which the medial and lateral soft tissue restraints about the knee have been compromised.[6,18,73,168] The original TCP III[55,68,120,152,158] evolved into the CCK prostheses, which in turn became the Zimmer LCCK prosthesis (Fig. 97-46). Improvements to the LCCK included the incorporation of the same features found on the third-generation PS prostheses, such as side-specific femoral components with anatomically oriented trochlear grooves, front-loading, modular, tibial polyethylene inserts, and an optimized cam and post mechanism. In addition, a full range of femoral and tibial augments and offset stem extensions added greater usefulness for the complex primary and revision cases. Constrained unlinked prostheses provide posterior stability and medial-lateral stability by means of an enlarged post that articulates closely with a femoral cam (Fig. 97-47). In

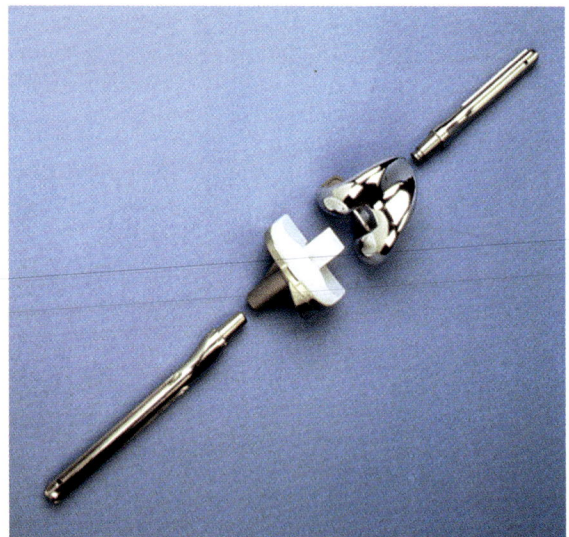

Figure 97-46. LCCK prosthesis. (Zimmer, Warsaw, Ind.)

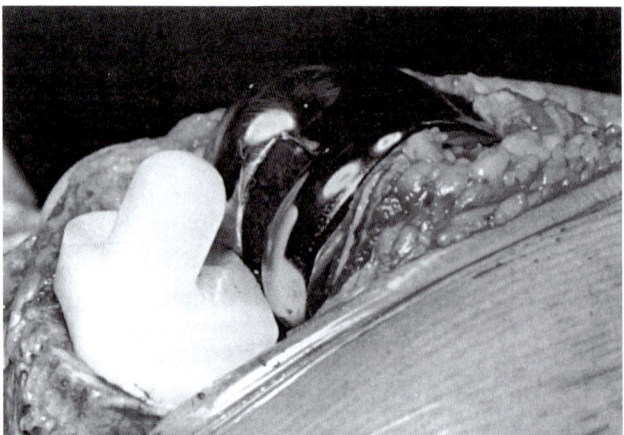

Figure 97-47. Articulation of the TCP III, a constrained condylar knee. A rectangular tibial post fits within a central femoral box or cavity, thereby providing varus and valgus stability as well as posterior restraint.

distinction to the post and cam of a PS prostheses, the augmented mechanisms in constrained prostheses also limit rotation. The theoretical advantages of constrained prostheses include improved stability but this comes with the risk of increased polyethylene wear and greater risk of loosening because of increased stress transmission to the prosthesis-cement-bone interface.

In its TCP III form, Donaldson and coworkers[68] found no loosening in 15 primary cases monitored for more than 2 years; all stems were cemented. The CCK was initially used primarily for revision cases, but based on this good experience with the TCP III in primary knees, these constrained devices have proved successful in managing difficult primary knees with predominantly valgus deformities in low-demand patients.[6,73,168] Avoidance of extensive release procedures and possible peroneal nerve complications has hastened recovery and lessened morbidity.

Although the clinical success of these devices has been demonstrated in difficult cases, potential risks remain. Therefore, in general, increased articular constraint is only used when the native soft tissues cannot be adequately balanced to provide medial and lateral stability. Importantly, the LCCK metal components can be used with a constrained polyethylene tibial insert or a standard PS polyethylene insert. Thus, during a difficult knee arthroplasty, if the LCCK metal components are inserted, an intraoperative decision can be made concerning the degree of constraint needed. When possible, we use a PS rather than a constrained tibial insert. It has been our practice to use stem extensions when using a constrained articulation in both the primary and revision settings, but good results with constrained implants without stem extensions used in the primary setting with good bone stock have also been reported at short-term to intermediate-term follow-up. In a study of 55 valgus knees that were managed without strict soft tissue balancing and a constrained unlinked prosthesis without stems, there were no cases of loosening or failures at a mean of 44.5 months.[6] Although stems potentially improve prosthesis fixation and help transfer stress from the prosthesis-cement-bone interfaces that may reduce long-term loosening rates, they increase the operative time, potentially increase fat embolization because of violation of the canal, are more difficult to remove at the time of revision, and add cost to the implant. At this time, long-term data are not available to answer the question of whether stems are necessary when a constrained prosthesis is used in a primary setting with good bone stock. However, in the revision setting, in which the bony surfaces of the femur and tibia have been compromised, stems of some variety should be used.

Numerous additional designs of constrained unlinked prostheses are now available. Many provide the full range of modular stems and augments along with both PS and constrained articulations that allow easy intraoperative management of bony and soft tissue problems in the complex primary and revision settings. These include the Zimmer LCCK, DePuy PFC Sigma TC3, Smith & Nephew Legion Revision, Biomet Vanguard SSK Revision, and Stryker Triathlon TS systems. One unique feature of the DePuy PFC Sigma TC3 system is the availability of a mobile-bearing tibial insert (M.B.T. revision tray; Fig. 97-48, which provides medial-lateral stability through the interaction of the cam and post but also allows rotational freedom through the undersurface

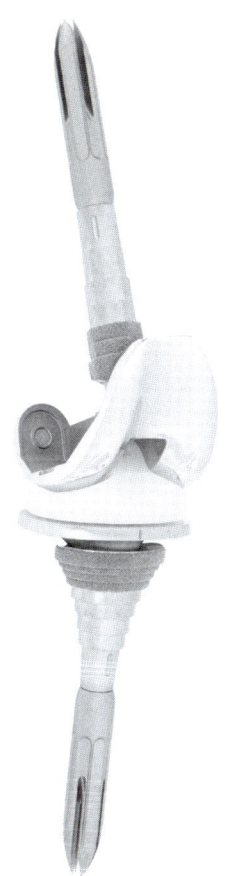

Figure 97-48. PFC Sigma TC3 prosthesis with the M.B.T mobile-bearing revision tray. (Courtesy DePuy, Warsaw, Ind.)

of the tibial bearing. Potential advantages include a reduction in polyethylene post wear and reduced transmission of stresses to the prosthesis-cement-bone interface. However, bearing dislocation is a potential disadvantage. At this time, no long-term data are available that clarify whether this mobile-bearing constrained articulation is associated with superior clinical results than the more traditional fixed-bearing constrained prostheses.

Constrained Rotating Hinge Prostheses

Early results with hinged devices, as previously noted, were not encouraging, with high rates of infection, loosening, and prosthesis failure. However, in parts of Europe, especially Germany, the use of hinged devices remained popular, even in primary TKR. Bohm and Holy[32] have reported excellent 20-year results with the Blauth prosthesis, a relatively simple early hinge prosthesis. With worst case survivorship exceeding 85% at 20 years, the results are comparable to the rates noted with surface replacement prostheses from the same era. Newer designs of hinged prostheses were developed to reduce the risk of loosening and improve the kinematics through the incorporation of rotating bearings that eliminated the rotational constraint of the earlier prostheses. Good results from Germany in primary knee replacement have also been reported with these more modern hinges.[224]

In North America, hinged devices were relegated to use in the worst cases of bone loss or ligamentous incompetence, often in the setting of oncologic reconstruction or multiply revised joints. Rand and colleagues[237] reported the results on

50 Kinematic Rotating-Hinge TKRs performed at the Mayo Clinic. The indications were ligamentous instability, loss of bone, or both. The follow-up was 50 months (range, 29 to 79 months). There were 14 excellent, 12 good, 5 fair, and 5 poor results. Progression of radiolucent lines was observed in 13 knees, and 5 knees probably had radiographic loosening. The rate of sepsis was 16%, patellar instability developed in 22%, and breakage of the implant occurred in 6%. In these patients, 74% of the operations were revisions—a first revision in 17, a second revision in 16, a third revision in 3, and a fourth revision in 1. The authors combined the incidence of complications reported for several series with a total of 1099 hinged implants. In these combined series, loosening was reported in 27% of knees, sepsis in 7%, and wound-healing problems in 5.5%. Based on this comparison, it was concluded that the Kinematic Rotating-Hinge prosthesis, although possessing theoretical advantages, gave no better results than the older nonrotating hinges. In a more recent report from the Mayo Clinic involving 69 Kinematic Rotating-Hinge knees at a mean of 75 months follow-up, the results were similar, with an overall complication rate of 32%, an infection rate of 14.5%, and component breakage in 10%.[281] Mechanical failures have also been reported by others.[136,156,237] Other centers in North America with experience using rotating hinge devices in the revision setting have also reported similar concerns with the same device, as well as other similar prostheses, such as the Finn Rotating hinged prosthesis.[226,311]

Regardless of these concerns, use of a hinged device remains the best option in some cases. Contemporary rotating hinged prostheses include the DePuy S-ROM Noiles (Fig. 97-49) and Limb Preservation System Rotating Hinges, Zimmer Nex Gen Rotating Hinge Knee (RHK), MOST Option System and Segmental System, Biomet Orthopedic Salvage System (OSS), and Stryker Global Modular Replacement System (GMRS). Many of these systems incorporate design features that have theoretical advantages over the older hinged devices. For example, the geometry of the femoral component in many systems is now more similar to contemporary surface replacement prostheses; in particular, the trochlear has been optimized to accommodate both native and resurfaced patellae. In addition, some newer designs allow for condylar load bearing between the femur and tibia, as found in surface replacement designs or, at a minimum, load sharing between the axle and femorotibial articulation. In distinction, many older hinge designs bore most of the load through the axle, which contributed to bushing wear and axle failure. It is likely that with improvements, these devices will be associated with better outcomes than previously noted but, unfortunately, the underlying limitations inherent to the multiply failed joint that these devices are used to address will dictate the overall complication rates. Nonetheless, early reports have suggested that superior outcomes will be achieved.[19,145]

GENERAL PROSTHETIC FEATURES

Interchangeability of Sizes

The natural variation that occurs between individual knee joints means that prosthetic components based on average dimensions do not always fit the femur and tibia of a particular joint equally well. Interchangeability of sizes, such that the femoral, tibial, and patellar components can be selected independently of each other according to the fit on their respective bones, becomes an attractive feature. Although it has long been possible to match patellar components with various femoral sizes, similar adaptability between the femoral and tibial components is a newer feature and one that is available to varying degrees in different systems. In some systems, a wide range of femoral and tibial sizes may be mated together, whereas in others each femur may only be combined with a limited number of tibial sizes, such as one size smaller or one size larger than the natural match. As with other aspects of knee arthroplasty, some compromises are involved, chiefly in regard to the degree of articular congruity or the inventory of parts that must be carried. Matching a smaller femur with a larger tibia (the usual combination) requires that the intercondylar distance or, more correctly, the bearing spacing between the femoral runners be constant for all sizes and that the tibial surface be almost flat. As we have seen, articulating a curved femur against a flat tibia produces a small contact patch, with the attendant disadvantage of high localized stress on the polyethylene. The contact patch can be enlarged by also flattening the femoral surfaces (Fig. 97-50). However, malalignment or any situation that leads to asymmetrical loading, even those occurring during the normal gait cycle, shifts the loading area to the periphery. This type of "edge" loading has been shown experimentally[22,298,300] to produce the greatest stress at the prosthesis-bone interface, perhaps offsetting any benefits obtained from more complete tibial coverage. To some degree, this compromise in congruity can be offset by increased inventory so that increased variety of polyethylene inserts can be manufactured to allow increased interchangeability.

Articular Geometry

Conforming joint surfaces should have the best wear resistance, particularly when the polyethylene is relatively thick.[22] However, conforming articulations, as noted, are not fully interchangeable, may conflict with PCL kinematics, and can theoretically cause greater fixation stress.

Thatcher and colleagues,[287] discussing inherent laxity in knee prostheses, have stated that laxity is a function of joint conformity. They believe that the implanted prosthesis should compensate for soft tissue structures that are deficient or removed. They think that the optimal laxity profile has

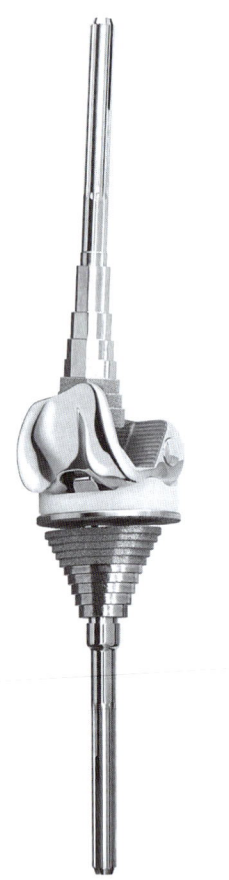

Figure 97-49. S-ROM Noiles Rotating Hinge prosthesis. (Courtesy DePuy, Warsaw, Ind.)

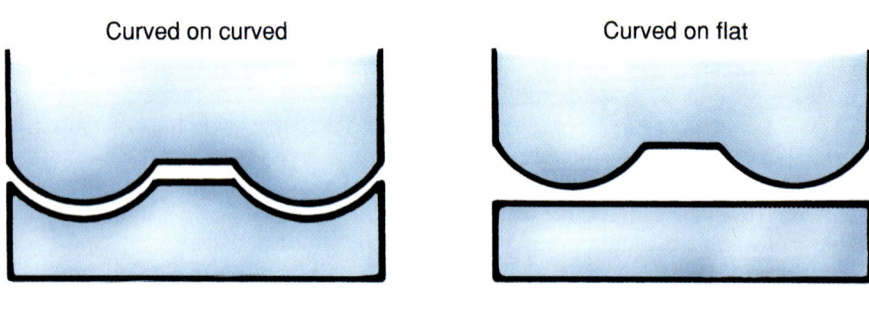

Curved on curved

Curved on flat

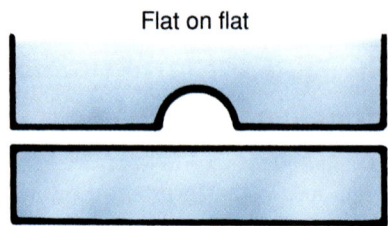

Flat on flat

Figure 97-50. The more conforming the articulation, the larger the contact area and the less stress on the polyethylene. In the frontal plane, curved-on-curved geometries are the best. Curved-on-flat geometry is the worst. Flat-on-flat surfaces can provide a good area of contact but are sensitive to edge loading whenever the prosthesis is loaded unevenly, such as in leaning or pivoting movements.

not yet been determined but suggest that the articular geometry should possess partial conformity, and comment on the classic inherent design compromise. The greater the conformity, the larger the contact area and the less the intrinsic stress and wear. However, conforming prostheses will create greater fixation stress, which may lead to loosening.

Wear is an increasing problem in TKR. Several factors have been implicated, including the quality of the polyethylene, manufacturing process, thickness of the tibial components, and articular geometry.[278] It is also true that in the best of circumstances, polyethylene is not an ideal bearing material,[323] but attempts to improve its performance have historically not been successful.[322] Many cases of severe wear and delamination of tibial components have been reported,[76,157] mainly involving thinner polyethylene components. Manufacturing processes (including heat-pressing[31] the polyethylene to give a smoother surface and gamma sterilization in air leading to free radical formation) have been indentified as detrimental factors in the development of polyethylene wear. In addition to these manufacturing issues, prosthesis design factors have certainly also contributed to this problem inasmuch as other prostheses manufactured using similar polyethylene treatments have not shown the same degree of damage. In particular, flat articular designs susceptible to edge loading and increased polyethylene stresses during condylar liftoff appear to be particularly susceptible. Finally, surgical technique is also important, with misalignment and instability potentially contributing to early failures. However, in general, more conforming round-on-round articular surfaces in the coronal plane that help reduce polyethylene stresses, particularly if condylar liftoff occurs, have become popular in a variety of CR and PS prostheses. As noted in the discussion on guided motion prostheses, considerable debate remains regarding whether a single axis or multiple axes of rotation in the sagittal plane is the optimal design. The J curve that results from the multiple axis of rotation theoretically optimizes flexion but results in decreasing contact areas as the knee flexes.

Design and Fixation of the Tibial Component

An important difference between prostheses is the method of tibial fixation.[186] The TCP and IB PS and Kinematic prostheses used a central peg. The PFC had a central trifin post. These prostheses are primarily designed for cement fixation. Long-term studies with a variety of cemented designs have shown tibial component loosening to be rare (Fig. 97-51).[58,153,194] Others that can be inserted with or without cement have two to four short studs, augmented in some cases by screws.

There is good evidence from early experience with knee arthroplasty that separate tibial components are susceptible to fixation failure. Neither an anterior bar nor the use of fixation studs is helpful. Extensive work has been performed to identify optimal design features.[23,299-301] Walker and colleagues[299] tested a variety of tibial components by applying compressive load with anteroposterior force, rotational torque, or varus-valgus moment (Fig. 97-52). The relative deflections, both compressive and distractive, were measured between the component and the bone. The fewest deflections occurred with one-piece metal components. Whether a

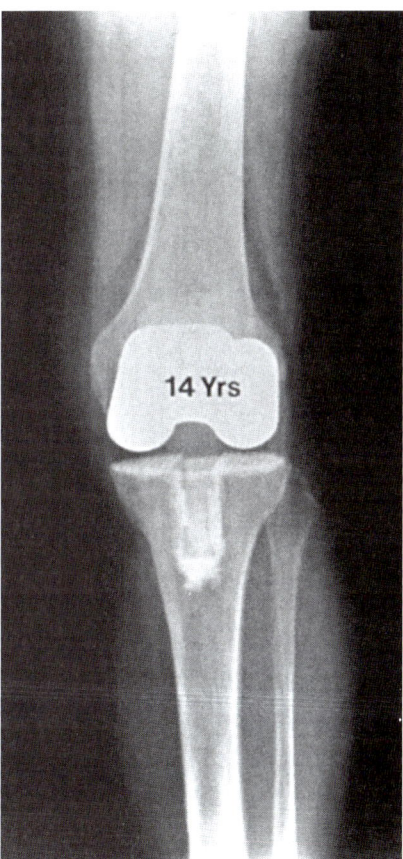

Figure 97-51. Radiograph of a Total Condylar Prosthesis 14 years postoperatively. Note the thin cement mantle clearly showing ridges in the cement caused by the design of the tibial polyethylene. There is no evidence of cracking or fragmentation of the cement. This type of appearance was seen frequently in the more than 10-year follow-up of this prosthesis and indicates that a thick cement mantle is unnecessary.

central peg or two lateral studs were used did not seem to make much difference. Thick plastic components behaved much like metal-backed ones, except when a cruciate cutout was made. Metal backing seems particularly desirable for cruciate-retaining implants.

Railton and associates[230] found metal backing of the polyethylene without a central stem to be of little value in enhancing fixation. They did not address the question of optimal stem length or the use of cement. Yamamoto and coworkers,[325] discussing the results of the Kodama-Yamamoto Mark II prosthesis, which has an all-polyethylene tibial component with four small studs and is inserted without cement, have expressed the opinion that a stem is unnecessary. They reported a 4.4% incidence of femoral loosening accompanied by tibial sinkage in some patients but cases with only tibial sinkage were not observed.

Lewis and colleagues[186] tested the fixation of six tibial component configurations by finite element analysis. They concluded that metal-backed, single-post designs provide the lowest system stress overall when cement is used.

Clinical data on implants using metal tray and small stud fixation are mostly applicable to cementless fixation. Computer simulations of bone remodeling around porous-coated implants[219] have demonstrated stress concentrations around

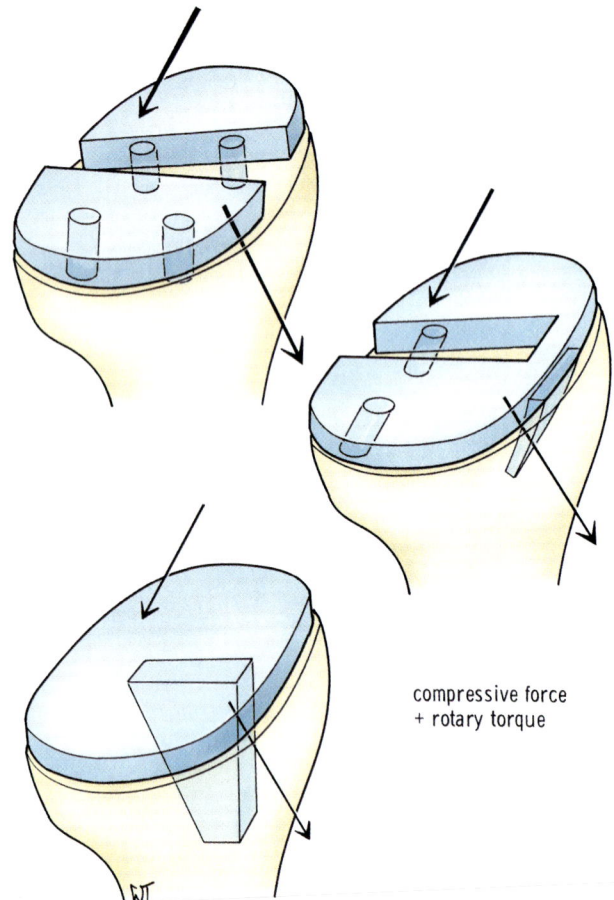

compressive force
+ rotary torque

Figure 97-52. Deflections at the bone-cement interface showing different configurations of the tibial component. (Courtesy Dr. Peter Walker.)

small tibial pegs. This resulted in denser bone, with a decrease in density in more peripheral locations. This finding agrees with the clinical observation that bone ingrowth occurs most predictably around fixation pegs. Walker and associates,[300] in a comparative study of uncemented tibial component designs, found that central stemmed and bladed designs perform better than short pegs placed near the periphery.

Support of the plastic by means of a metal tray or endoskeleton is certainly desirable when the bone of the upper part of the tibia is deficient (e.g., in severe erosive arthritis or revision operations), but when the bone is of good quality, metal backing may not offer an advantage. One-piece plastic components with a central peg have a low rate of loosening, but in 30% to 40% of cases, a partial radiolucency develops. For the most part, these radiolucencies appear within the first year, are nonprogressive, and are of dubious clinical significance. The addition of a metal tray reduces the incidence of radiolucency and also seems to reduce the incidence of late tibial loosening (Fig. 97-53).

Modular Augments and Stems

Modularity, in the sense under discussion, refers to the ability to add stems, augments, and wedges to standard components so that to a degree, the surgeon can make a custom prosthesis

intraoperatively (Fig. 97-54). Most manufacturers now offer a complete knee prosthesis system, such as the DePuy PFC Sigma TC 3, Biomet Vanguard SSK Revision System, Smith & Nephew Legion Revision System, Stryker Triathlon TS, and Zimmer LCCK, that offer all these modular components. Modularity is particularly useful for revision surgery when the bone deficiencies cannot be completely anticipated. It is also of value for primary knee replacement when dealing with bone defects.

Metal augments can be adapted to fit existing defects without the need to remove sclerotic areas to expose bleeding cancellous surfaces. In this sense, they can be considered as more conservative. If they fail, the bone deficiency is not made worse. The metal pieces are screwed or cemented to their components. Screw fixation, although mechanically satisfying, creates the possibility of metallic debris formation by micromotion (fretting). Cement may also not be the ideal bonding material between metal surfaces. At present, one or the other method must be used. Alternatives to metal augmentation include cement alone,[188] cement and screws,[242] and bone grafting.[41,177]

Prosthetic stems of varying lengths intended for use with and without cement are also an important part of modular knee systems. Early use of stems about the knee, especially cemented stems, had a stigma that was related to their use with hinges and other constrained models. However, Blauth and Hassenpflug[30] and Bohm and Holy[32] have reported continuing good results with the hinged knee prosthesis that bears Blauth's name. Reporting on the Stanmore hinge replacement, Lettin and coworkers[184,185] found 83% survivorship at 6 years (survivorship defined as prosthesis in situ), and Kaufer and Matthews[151] found an infection rate of 5% and revision rate of 15% for the spherocentric prosthesis monitored for an average of 8 years. Nonetheless, these reports appeared to be exceptions. In our experience, 15 of 108 GUEPAR prostheses became infected. All but four of them were late infections, and uncontrollable sepsis led to two above-the-knee amputations. Young[326] found that in a series of hinged prostheses, all had failed by the end of 10 years. Hui and Fitzgerald[123] reported an 11.7% infection rate in 77 GUEPAR arthroplasties monitored for 2 years or loger. They noted the difficulty of obtaining arthrodesis if the prosthesis has to be removed. Deburge and the Guepar group[64] had a failure rate of 34% with the GUEPAR prosthesis that was attributable to major complications. Grimer and colleagues[110] recommended against routine use of the Stanmore prosthesis as a primary arthroplasty. Of 103 Stanmore knee replacements, they had 7 cases of infection and 4 of fracture around the prosthesis that contributed to major complications. Eight knees were revised for aseptic loosening and a further 14 were found to have radiologic signs of loosening. There were two cases of amputation for fracture and sepsis. Only Wilson and associates[317] have reported favorable results over a long period with an uncemented Walldius prosthesis. The overall infection rate was 3.2% and clinical evidence of loosening occurred infrequently. The 20 knees monitored for an average of 10 years showed little evidence of progressive deterioration. They attribute this result to the absence of cement. Walldius[303] himself has written on 27 years' experience with his prosthesis and states that good results have been obtained in 80% of patients with a high degree of preoperative disability. No details were given.

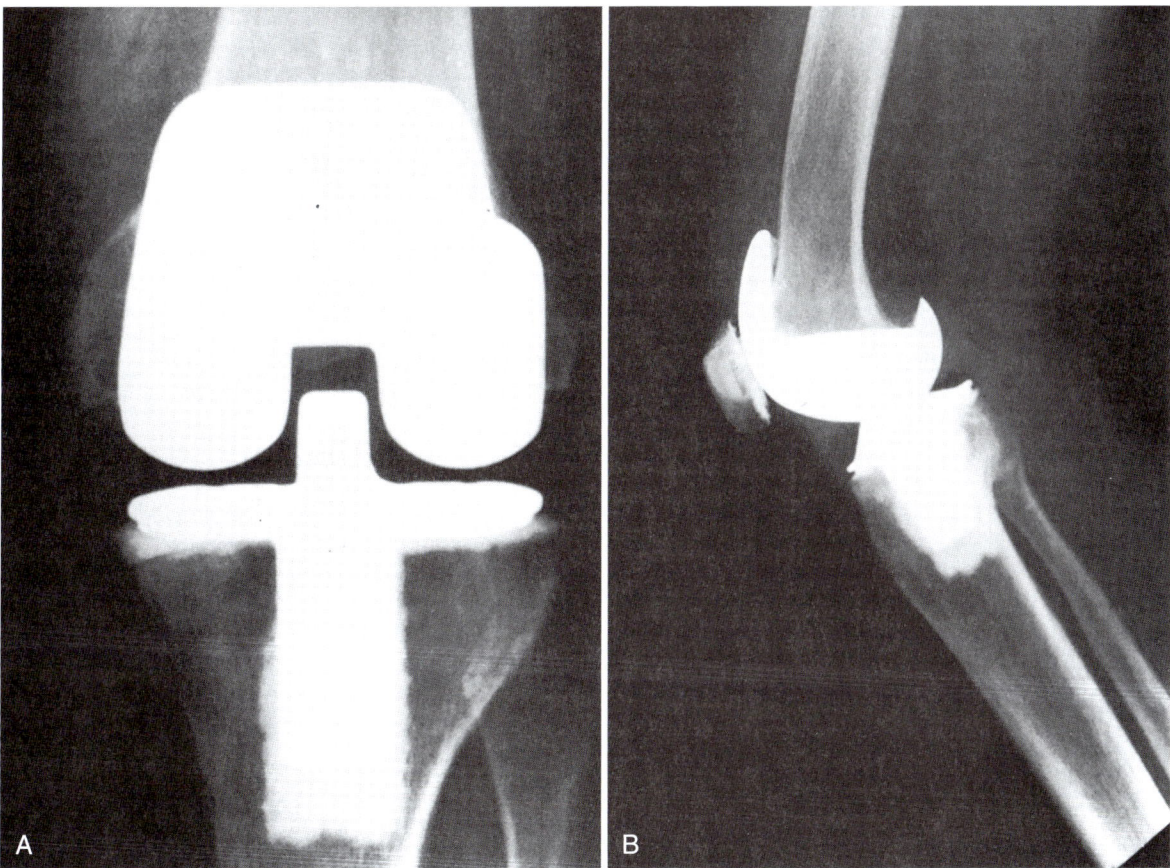

Figure 97-53. A, B, AP and lateral radiographs of a tibial component with an endoskeleton. Metal backing of this type reduces tibial loosening at long-term follow-up.

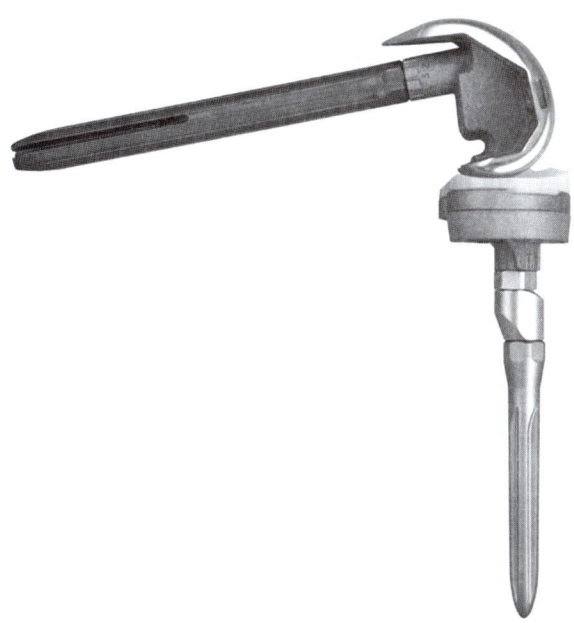

Figure 97-54. A, Contemporary modular revision knee system (Triathlon TS prosthesis). The components can be customized intraoperatively with a variety of straight or offset cemented or uncemented stems, augments, and PS or constrained tibial polyethylene inserts of varying thicknesses. (Courtesy Stryker, Mahwah, NJ.)

In assessing these results, it must be pointed out that all are related to constrained prostheses with cemented stems (except the Walldius) and the worst results were obtained with metal-on-metal–bearing surfaces, which generate large volumes of metallic debris.[228] Complete constraint of the degree provided by a hinge is rarely needed in knee arthroplasty, and lesser degrees of constraint, such as provided by the PFC Sigma TC3 or LCCK, do not seem to have particular disadvantages.[68] Murray and coworkers,[216] from the Mayo Clinic, have reported 5-year results with the use of cemented stems in conjunction with the Kinematic Stabilizer prosthesis in 40 revision TKRs. The incidence of radiolucent lines was 13% about the femoral stems and 32% about the tibial stems. However, most were incomplete, nonprogressive, and less than 1 mm. Only one femoral component and one tibial component were radiographically loose. Theoretical concerns regarding stress shielding were not noted in these cases. Longer term follow-up of the same cohort at 10 years, as reported by Whaley and colleagues,[312] has demonstrated continued good results with survival free of revision for any reason in 96% of these cases.

Similar results have also recently been reported from France, with no cases of stem loosening at a mean of 12.5 years postoperatively in a group of younger patients who had undergone knee reconstruction with a constrained prosthesis following oncologic resection.[171] Therefore, it appears that in this time frame, exceeding 10 years, cemented stems function adequately without significant complications. However, concerns regarding potential bone loss and increased surgical difficulty at revision remain. If the intention is merely to provide additional component support, in the case of deficient bone, stems need not be associated with constraint and do not need to be cemented.[210] The senior author (JI) has used uncemented stems since 1977 with both custom and modular components,[115] and Bertin and associates[27] have reported on Freeman's experience with uncemented stems in revision surgery. In neither report was there any increase in infection rate. Freeman used a stem of fixed diameter and did not attempt to obtain a press-fit (the so-called dangle stem; Fig. 97-55). Bertin and colleagues noted the development of radiopaque lines adjacent to the stem in 88% of cases. In our study, similar lines were observed about 67% of femoral rods and 69% of tibial rods, however, at a mean follow-up of 42 months, only 3% of the prostheses had failed because of loosening.[115] A sclerotic halo about the tip of the prosthesis has also been noted in some cases (Fig. 97-56).[27]

The importance of these findings is not fully understood but may be interpreted as evidence of the stem's function in resisting moments and load sharing. Although uncemented stems need not have rigid fixation in the shaft, the medial tilting and slight displacement noticed in one case suggest that press-fitting longer stems into the diaphysis is desirable, especially in patients with more extensive bone loss (Fig.

97-57). At a mean of 5 years, 9 months' follow-up, Shannon and coworkers[263] from the Mayo Clinic reported that 16% of the prostheses inserted with limited cement about the body of the implant and uncemented stems had been revised for aseptic loosening or were considered radiographically loose. In this series, it was noted that stems of varying lengths had been used but the failures were not subdivided by stem length. The higher failure rate noted in this series is different than the more favorable results previously noted from the same institution with cemented stems.[312] Fehring and colleagues[83] have also reported concerns regarding the use of short metaphyseal uncemented stems with cemented components in revision TKR. In their series of 95 uncemented metaphyseal stems at a minimum of 2-year follow-up, 10% were loose and 19% were considered possibly loose. In distinction, of the 107 cemented metaphyseal stems in the same report, 97% were considered stable, with only 7% possibly loose.[83] An additional benefit of diaphyseal engaging uncemented press fit stems compared with shorter metaphyseal stems is that unless there is an unusual anatomic variation, or prior deformity from trauma or osteotomy, diaphyseal engaging stems help restore anatomic alignment of the extremity. Based on current data, it is the surgeon's choice whether to use cemented or uncemented stems in revision TKR; however, it is clear that if uncemented stems are used, they should be longer diaphyseal engaging stems. Therefore, when we use

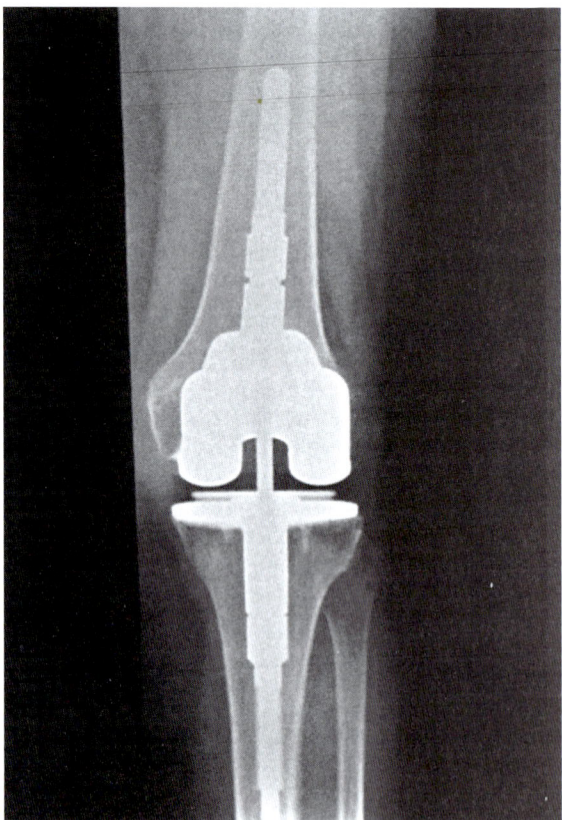

Figure 97-55. Radiograph of a knee prosthesis showing so-called dangle stems. These uncemented stems rest in the intramedullary canal and do not make contact with the cortices. Even so, roentgenographic stereophotogrammetric analysis data have shown that uncemented stems of this type on the tibial side have the lowest rates of migration and inducible displacement.

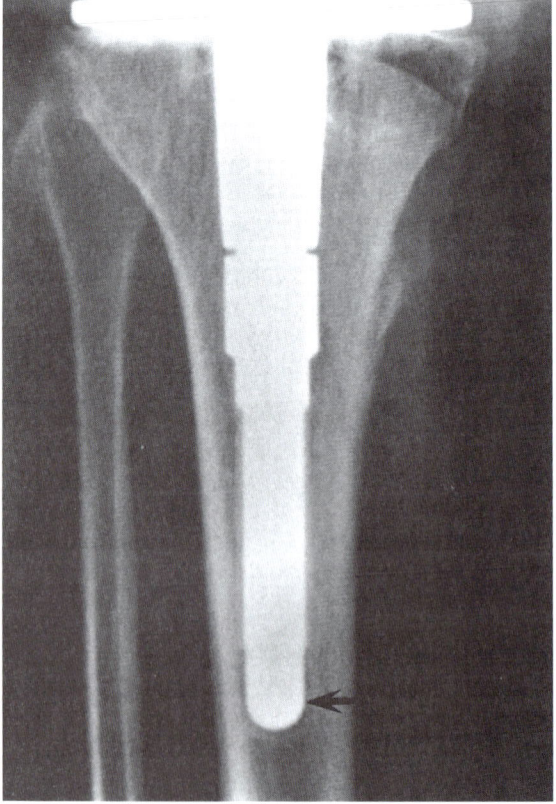

Figure 97-56. Radiograph showing sclerosis at the tip of an uncemented stem *(arrow)*. The interpretation of this finding, which is fairly constant, is arguable. In part, it is probably caused by bending of the more flexible bone, but it may also be indicative of the stem's role in resisting tilting movements.

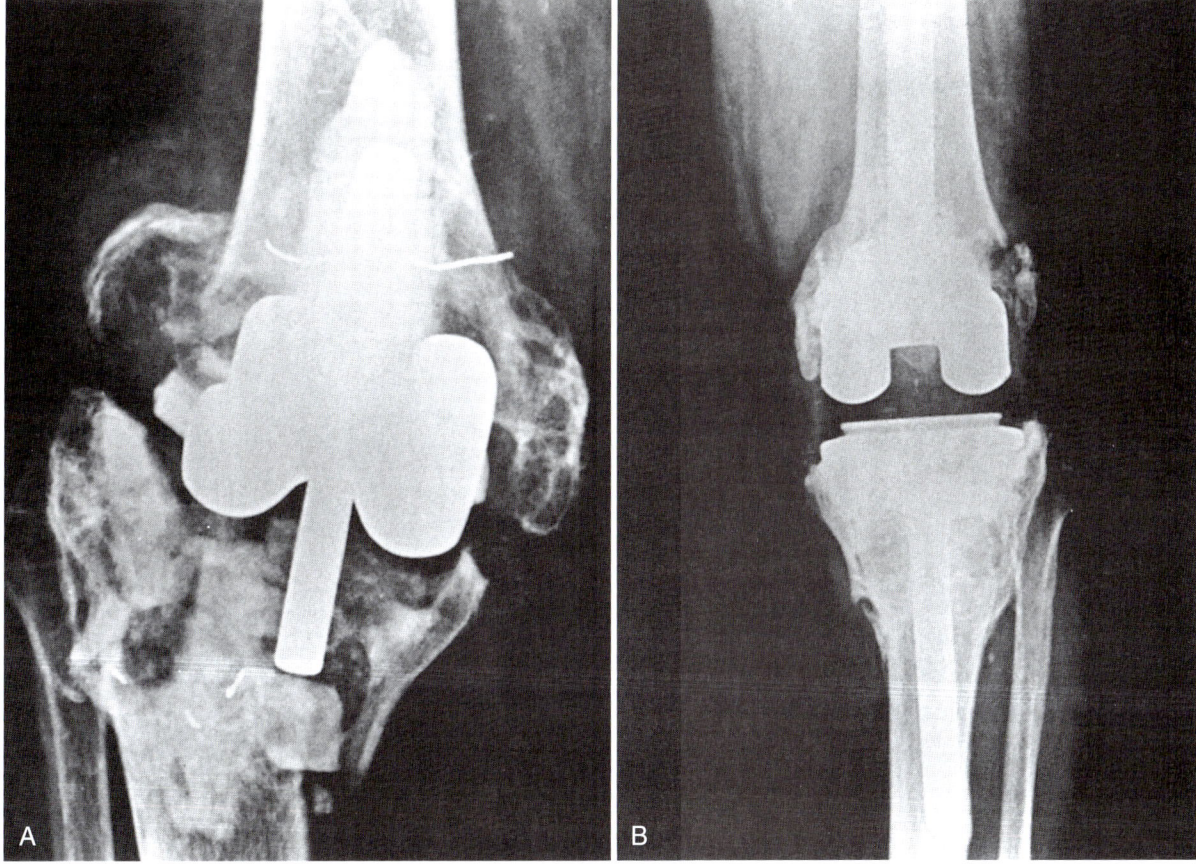

Figure 97-57. **A,** Failed Attenborough prosthesis with great loss of bone and fragmentation of the upper part of the tibia. **B,** Reconstruction with a custom prosthesis and a femoral head allograft in the tibia. The intramedullary rod was passed through a hole in the femoral head. Morcelized cancellous graft was used to fill in remaining defects. The custom rod was undersized and has migrated into slight varus and stabilized in this position. Some cortical reaction is seen. This indicates the need for precise sizing of the intramedullary rods for this type of revision case, an advantage of modular systems. However, this knee functioned well until the patient's death 8 years postoperatively.

uncemented stems in revision and reimplant surgery, we routinely use hand reamers to select a longer diaphyseal engaging stem that makes contact with the cortices, but we do not attempt to expand the canal. With the flexibility of current modular systems and the development of offset stems, this can routinely be accomplished without major difficulty.

Custom Prostheses

Modular components have greatly reduced the need for custom prostheses in primary and revision surgery. However, custom devices are occasionally needed, usually in our experience for cases in which a previous high tibial osteotomy has been performed. The problem in these knees occurs when the osteotomy has produced an offset in the diaphysis and a tibial stem is desired (Fig. 97-58). We have found that the development of offset stems as part of current modular prosthesis systems significantly reduces the number of custom components required.

Patellar Prostheses

Resurfacing

In rheumatoid arthritis the patella should always be replaced to remove all articular cartilage from the joint. Some surgeons

recommend selective resurfacing of the patella for patients with osteoarthritis.[256,269,275] Others think that the result is more predictable with routine patellar resurfacing (Fig. 97-59).[78,236,258,277] Undoubtedly, patellar resurfacing has its share of iatrogenic complications, such as fracture[288] and soft tissue overgrowth with impingement.[118] Fixation holes in the patella weaken its structure, central holes probably more so than peripheral ones (Fig. 97-60).

Configuration

Traditionally, most patellar components were dome-shaped. This configuration is not ideal because the convex contour might be expected to wear poorly on the basis of engineering experience—in an articulation, the softer material should be concave. A component that is anatomic (e.g., PCA and LCS) has a more desirable configuration in this respect but requires careful rotary alignment to prevent binding against the femur (Fig. 97-61). In addition, correct static alignment, even if achieved at surgery, may not predict the functional pull of the quadriceps in active use, and the more desirable wear characteristics can be offset by increased torque on the component caused by malalignment. The LCS patellar design attempts to solve this problem by having an anatomic polyethylene articulation swivel on a metal baseplate. This design has been in use for over almost 2 decades and is apparently very successful. The tendency of the universal patellar dome to

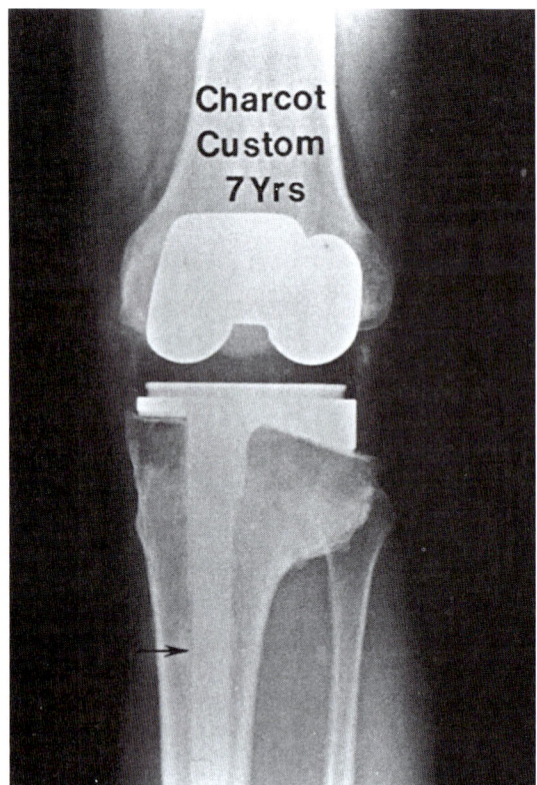

Figure 97-58. Radiograph of a custom prosthesis with a lateral wedge and offset stem. The prosthesis was designed for a patient with a neuropathic joint who had previously undergone high tibial osteotomy. The knee migrated into excessive valgus, leaving a lateral defect and an offset of the tibial diaphysis. A standard modular prosthesis would not have fit in this case.

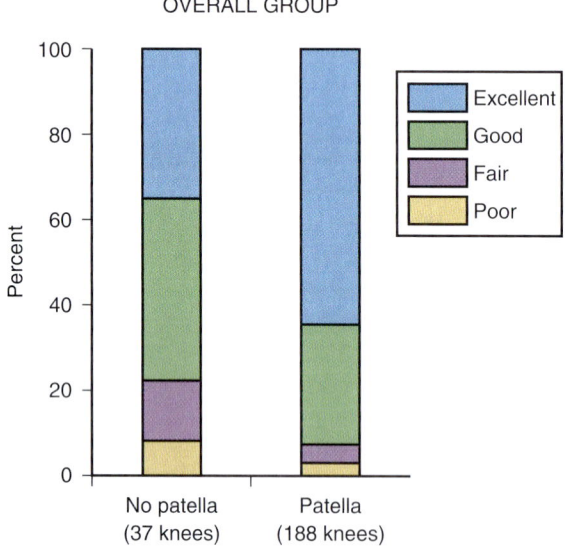

Figure 97-59. The clinical results are slightly better when a patellar component is used.

deform has led to the use of oval and sombrero shapes.[39] An oval patella provides greater coverage of the patellar bone and a sombrero shape theoretically has more attractive wear characteristics. Others have advocated inlaying the prosthesis into the central portion of the patellar bone[181] (Fig. 97-62),

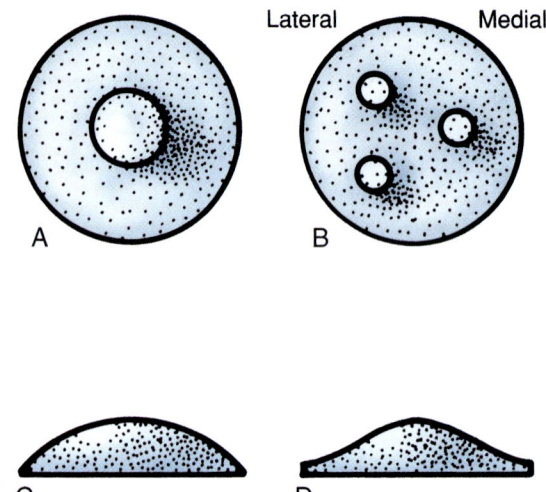

Figure 97-60. Patella shapes and methods of fixation. **A, C,** Dome patella with a central fixation lug. **B, D,** Sombrero patella with three fixation pegs.

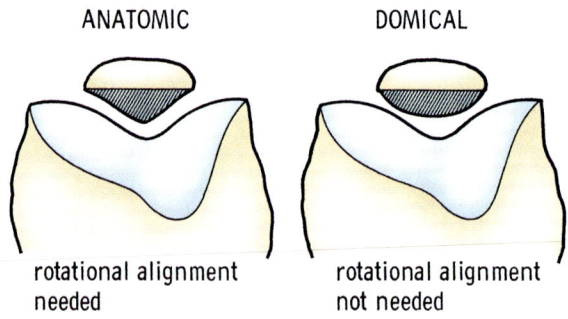

Figure 97-61. Rotational alignment is needed with a patellar replacement of anatomic shape.

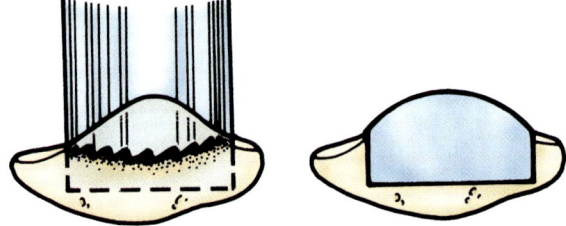

Figure 97-62. Insetting the patella allows greater thickness of polyethylene and the use of metal backing. There is a rim of peripheral exposed bone that can impinge against the femur.

stating that the peripheral bony rim in contact with the femoral condyles does not cause symptoms. If this is so, the inlay patella is attractive, but the concept does not appear to be entirely rational. In any event, wear with a dome-shaped patellar component has not been seen as a problem in long-term clinical studies, but retrieval analysis raises some cause for concern (Fig. 97-63).

Metal-Backed Patellar Component

Metal backing of the patellar component was inspired in part by the good experience with tibial component design and in part by the wish to obtain bone ingrowth.[88] It is now apparent that many early metal-backed patellae were designed with inadequate polyethylene thickness. This has resulted in catastrophic failures related to polyethylene dissociation from the baseplate and wear-through (Fig. 97-64).

It has proven difficult to design an onset patellar component with the necessary thickness of polyethylene to avoid wear-through without producing an unacceptably bulky component. This design difficulty caused a widespread return to all-polyethylene patellar components generally used with cement, although press-fit inlaid components have been used without cement.[29] The optimal patellar design remains uncertain.[59,181] A new generation of metal-backed patellae was introduced in the 2000s as a result of the development of new ingrowth materials. Porous trabecular metals offer excellent ingrowth potential and allow intrusion of the polyethylene into the metal backing, which not only creates an excellent bond but also allows the thickness of the polyethylene to be optimized. Currently, this new generation of metal-backed patellae represents only a small percentage of the patellar components used, with most comprised of cemented, all polyethylene domes, ovals, and sombrero-style onlay components.

Prosthetic Patellar Problems

However the patella is treated, patellofemoral symptoms on stair climbing and other flexed-knee activities remain a troublesome problem that is not yet fully resolved. Avoidance of a high shoulder profile of the femoral component in the junctional area between the flange and condylar runners in favor of a smooth, uniformly curved patellar sulcus reduces patellofemoral strain.[206] Technical factors, such as the orientation of the patellar osteotomy and thickness of the patellar prosthesis composite, are important, as is avoidance of patella infra as a result of proximal alteration of the prosthetic joint line.

Determining Whether the Patella Should Be Resurfaced

Some patellar problems can be avoided if the patellar prosthesis is omitted altogether (Fig. 97-65). Abraham and associates[1] studied 100 knees, 47 of which underwent patellar resurfacing, using Variable-Axis prosthesis. The two groups were similar in regard to diagnosis, age, and gender. They were unable to find significant differences between the two groups with regard to walking distance, ability to climb stairs, ability to rise from a chair, motion, extensor lag, and quadriceps strength. One patient in the resurfacing group required reoperation for subluxation, and two in the unresurfaced group required subsequent resurfacing. A number of other studies have noted similar findings. Keblish and coworkers[154]

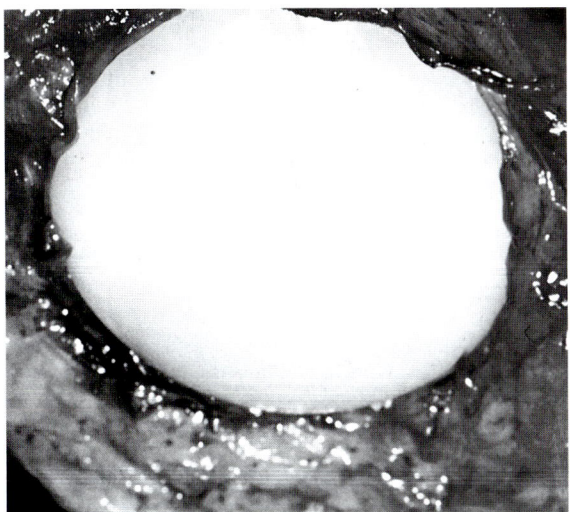

Figure 97-63. Patella showing considerable lateral polyethylene wear. This amount of polyethylene damage is unusual and was caused by lateral subluxation of the patella. Normally, only slighter flattening and deformation of dome-type patellae are noted.

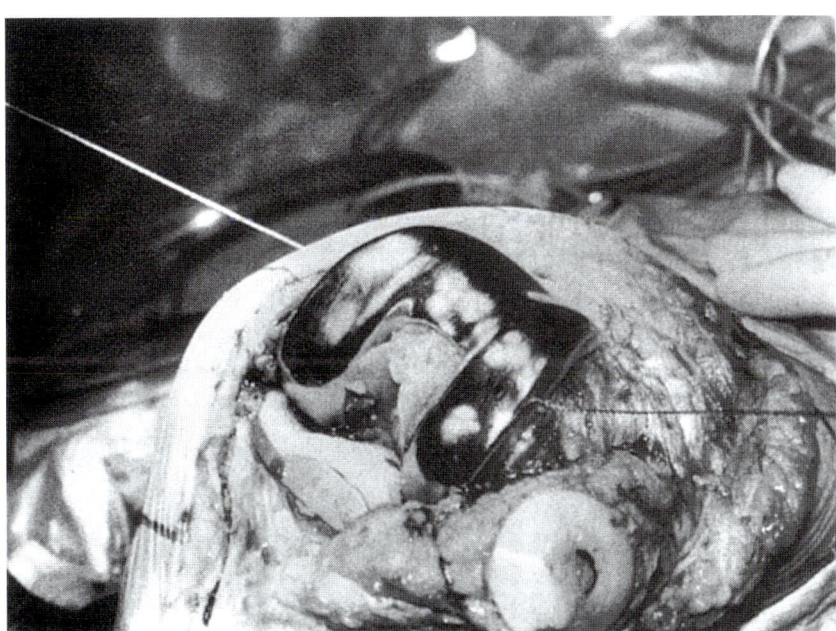

Figure 97-64. Kinematic prosthesis showing central wear-through of a metal-backed patellar component.

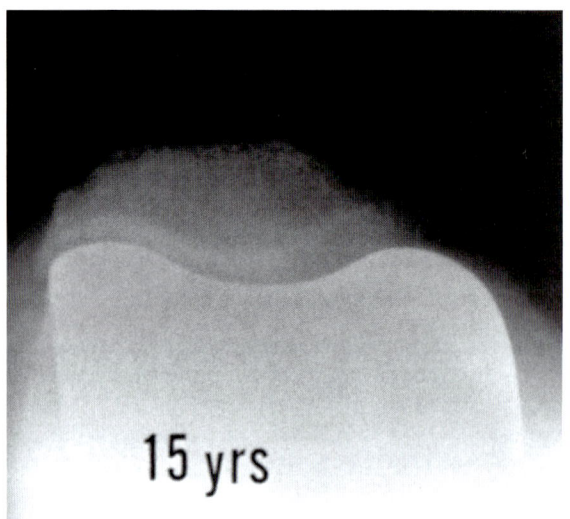

Figure 97-65. Skyline radiograph showing an unresurfaced patella 15 years postoperatively. In this case, the patella has remodeled to fit the femoral groove. The knee is functioning satisfactorily, has good function on stairs, and is pain-free. Unfortunately, this is not always the result with patellae that are left unresurfaced.

have reported on patients who underwent bilateral TKR with patellar resurfacing on one side and retention of the natural patella on the other. The patients expressed no preference between the two sides and there were no differences in stair climbing or the incidence of anterior knee pain. Barrack and colleagues[20] have also reported the results of a prospective randomized study on patellar resurfacing involving 86 patients. They were unable to detect differences in the overall Knee Society, pain, or function score, or in assessment of patellofemoral function. Although the results were not significantly different between the two groups, a clear difference in complications was noted. A significantly higher rate of reoperation was noted in the group in which the natural patella was retained, with a 12% prevalence of subsequent patellar resurfacing in this group. In distinction, there were no reoperations in the resurfaced group. Boyd and associates[37] also have reported that in early to midterm follow-up, increased complications occur in patients with a retained natural patella. At a mean of 3 years, the overall complication rate in the group with patellar resurfacing was 4% versus 12% in the unresurfaced group. Among patients with rheumatoid arthritis who had undergone patellar resurfacing, loosening of the patellar prosthesis occurred in 1%, whereas a 13% reoperation rate for subsequent resurfacing occurred in the group who initially had been left with the natural patella. Kajino and coworkers[148] noted superior pain relief in patients with rheumatoid arthritis after patellar resurfacing. Enis and associates[78] have also reported a slight preference in 25 patients with bilateral arthroplasties in whom the patella was resurfaced, with the Townley prosthesis implanted on one side but not the other. Most patients expressed a preference for the resurfaced side, which they found to be relatively pain-free and stronger during flexed-knee activities, such as stair climbing. However, the difference was not very great.

In a meta-analysis by Parvizi and coworkers,[223] similar findings were noted, with approximately a 10% risk of reoperation for subsequent patellar resurfacing and a greater risk

of anterior knee pain. Another meta-analysis also favored resurfacing but noted exceptions for which not resurfacing the patella could be considered, including in patients younger than 60 years, with minimal arthritic changes of the patella.[35] However, it is important to note that this issue of patellar resurfacing is still controversial and far from resolved, with conflicting results from prospective randomized studies. Two different studies by Burnett and colleagues[46,47] have reported no differences in outcomes, including reoperation rates, at 10-year follow-up.

Our experience suggests slightly better results after patellar resurfacing, particularly in patients with inflammatory arthritis. However, in certain cases, it may be preferable to leave the natural patella intact.[35] It may be advisable to omit patellar resurfacing in the following situations:

1. The patellar articular surface is almost normal.
2. The patient is obese. Stern and Insall[283] have shown that with resurfacing, pain and complications are more frequent in obese patients.
3. The patella is too small or eroded to accept a prosthesis.
4. The patient is young and active, which theoretically increases the risk of loosening and wear.

To allow the option to omit patellar resurfacing, it seems wise to design the femoral component to be compatible with the natural patella. Most current PS and CR resurfacing prostheses are available in side-specific configurations with an extended trochlea, which has a more gradual transition with the distal condyles to accommodate the natural patella as well as resurfaced patella.

Effect of Patellectomy on Total Knee Arthroplasty

Lennox and associates[182] have described 11 patients who underwent TKA after a previous patellectomy. Good to excellent results were obtained in 5 of the 11 knees as compared with 11 of 11 in a control group with intact patellae. They did not find that the presence or absence of the PCL was of importance. Two patients later underwent arthrodesis for continued complaints of pain. It was found that a patient who preoperatively had more than three previous operations with minimal or moderate tibiofemoral arthritic changes and with severely compromised quadriceps function was unlikely to achieve an acceptable result from TKA. Others have reported similar results in their studies of knee arthroplasty after patellectomy.[172,229]

The senior author's (JI) experience has been that when extensor mechanism function was good before knee arthroplasty, the result was also functionally satisfactory. However, postoperative pain from the patellar tendon area could not be predicted accurately.

KEY REFERENCES

Argenson JN, Scuderi GR, Komistek RD, et al: In vivo kinematic evaluation and design considerations related to high flexion in total knee arthroplasty. J Biomechanics 38:277, 2005.

Bohm P, Holy T: Is there a future for hinged prostheses in primary total knee arthroplasty? A 20-year survivorship analysis of the Blauth prosthesis. J Bone Joint Surg Br 80:302, 1998.

Colizza WA, Insall JN, Scuderi GR: The posterior stabilized total knee prosthesis: assessment of polyethylene damage and osteolysis after a ten-year-minimum follow-up. J Bone Joint Surg Am 77:1713, 1995.

Easley ME, Insall JN, Scuderi GR, Bullek DD: Primary constrained condylar knee arthroplasty for the arthritic valgus knee. Clin Orthop 380:58, 2000.

Fehring TK, Odum S, Olekson C, et al: Stem fixation in revision total knee arthroplasty. Clin Orthop Relat Res 416:217, 2003.

Greene KA: Gender-specific design in total knee arthroplasty. J Arthroplasty 22(Suppl 3):27, 2007.

Hitt K, Shurman JR II, Greene K, et al: Anthropometric measurements of the human knee: correlation to the sizing of current knee arthroplasty systems. J Bone Joint Surg Am 85:115, 2003.

Insall JN, Lachiewicz PF, Burstein AH: The posterior stabilized condylar prosthesis: a modification of the total condylar design: two to four-year clinical experience. J Bone Joint Surg Am 64:1317, 1982.

Insall JN, Ranawat CS, Aglietti P, et al: A comparison of four models of total knee replacement prostheses. J Bone Joint Surg Am 58:754, 1976.

Insall JN, Scott WN, Ranawat CS: The total condylar knee prosthesis: a report of two hundred and twenty cases. J Bone Joint Surg Am 61:173, 1979.

Pagnano MW, Cushner FD, Scott WN: Role of the posterior cruciate ligament in total knee arthroplasty. J Am Acad Orthop Surg 6:176, 1998.

Parvizi J, Rapuri VR, Saleh K, et al: Failure to resurface the patella during total knee arthroplasty may resulting more knee pain and secondary surgery. Clin Orthop Relat Res 438:191, 2005.

Robinson, RP: The early innovators of today's resurfacing condylar knees. J Arthroplasty 20(Suppl 1):2, 2005.

Springer BD, Hanssen AD, Sim FH, Lewallen DG: The kinematic rotating hinge prosthesis for complex knee arthroplasty. Clin Orthop 392:283, 2001.

Stiehl JB, Komistek RD, Dennis DA, et al: Fluoroscopic analysis of kinematics after posterior-cruciate–retaining knee arthroplasty. J Bone Joint Surg Br 77:884, 1995.

Full references for this chapter can be found on www.expertconsult.com.

Unicompartmental Knee Arthroplasty

Wolfgang Fitz and Richard D. Scott

John Repicci's introduction of minimally invasive techniques to unicompartmental knee arthroplasty (UKA) has led to renewed interest in UKA. Growth at triple the rate of total knee replacement (TKR) was observed over the past decade,[37] driven by the introduction of new technology. In 2004, mobile-bearing UKA was introduced to the United States; in 2006, a haptic guidance system and new adapted devices, as well as personalized UKA with prenavigated single-use instruments, further fueled this growth.

According to Frost and Sullivan (A. Shetty, personal communication, November 2009), the worldwide market for knee replacements in 2008 was $7.3 billion, with a total revenue of $3.21 billion in the United States alone. In 2008, 555,000 primary TKRs were performed in the United States, with projected annual growth rates between 5% and 6% over the next 5 years (Fig. 98-1). Although knee revisions will increase at annual rates of between 3% and 4% from 34,761 in 2008 to 44,500 in 2015, it is estimated that unicompartmental arthroplasty will stay at around 6% to 8% of primary knee replacements, already outnumbering the number of knee revisions. With better results and younger patients, a higher market share of UKA is possible.

Compared with TKR arthroplasty, unicompartmental replacement has the advantage of preserving both cruciate ligaments, yielding a knee with nearly normal kinematics.[22,38,49] A study of 42 patients with a bicompartmental or tricompartmental arthroplasty on one side and a unicompartmental replacement on the other showed that more patients preferred the unicompartmental side because it felt more like a normal knee and had better function.[8,31] More bone stock may be preserved with UKA. Theoretically, this should make conversion to TKR easier, should it become necessary. This advantage, however, was not initially supported by studies of revision of unicompartmental replacements.[3,23,32] Results of revision were not superior to those seen after revision of bicompartmental or tricompartmental replacement, and bone stock deficiency in the femoral condyle or the tibial plateau often had to be augmented with bone graft or special components. These deficiencies are frequently the result of poor surgical techniques or prostheses that unnecessarily invade the bone stock. More modern techniques using surface replacements on the femoral and tibial sides have made the procedure as conservative in practice as it is in theory, and conversions of failed UKA to total knee arthroplasty (TKA) demonstrate results similar to those seen with primary TKR.[24]

The concept of unicompartmental TKR is an attractive alternative to tibial osteotomy or tricompartmental replacement in the osteoarthritic patient with unicompartmental disease confirmed at arthrotomy.[14,22,49] As compared with osteotomy and TKR, unicompartmental arthroplasty has a higher initial success rate and fewer early complications.[18,43] Recovery is quicker and occurs with less blood loss, less pain, and better functional results. Survivorship analyses have been reported for tricompartmental replacement, indicating that survivorship with or without cruciate retention can be above 90% after 10 years of follow-up.[35,36,40,45] Early studies generated from unicompartmental series show that survivorship is not as good after 10 years, dropping into the 85% range.* However, these series were generated at a time when surgical techniques, implant design, and the quality of polyethylene were not yet perfected. Recent reports demonstrate that patients 60 years and younger have survivor rates above 90% at 10 years for fixed- and mobile-bearing UKA.[33,34] A randomized prospective study comparing TKR with unicompartmental knee replacement showed a 15-year survival rate of 89% for UKA and 79% for TKR. Patients undergoing UKA had better range of motion, were more satisfied, and were more active, with a comparable Bristol functioning score. The failure rate at 15 years of UKA was not higher than that seen with TKR.[30]

PATIENT SELECTION

The widespread use of arthroscopic treatment for osteoarthritis of the knee without large mechanical relevant meniscal tears has been questioned[21,28] and is not recommended. Osteotomy remains the procedure of choice in the young, very active patient with unicompartmental osteoarthritis. Internal derangement and its treatment in the younger subpopulation are not contraindications to osteotomy but may need to be relieved by an arthroscopic procedure before or after the osteotomy is performed. However, additional studies are needed to clarify the effectiveness of knee arthroscopy in this population. Subluxation and extreme angular deformity are contraindications to both osteotomy and unicompartmental replacement.

Currently, metallic interpositional arthroplasty is not recommended for the treatment of osteoarthritis,[1] although this treatment occasionally may be advisable for patients when osteotomy or knee arthroplasty is contraindicated.[10,42]

The ideal candidate for unicompartmental replacement is the unicompartmental osteoarthritic patient with an intact anterior cruciate ligament, preserved range of motion, a correctable deformity, no inflammatory arthritis, and an intact medial collateral ligament. Whether age, weight, and activity should be considered as part of the selection criteria for UKA has been a recurring topic in the literature for decades.

Although some authors reported no differences in outcomes regarding age,[29,33] others did describe such differences.[9,22] Certain fixed-bearing implants such as Miller-Galante and Marmor implants were reported not to have higher failure rates in heavier patients. This was confirmed by Cartier, Argenson, and Pennington.[2,7,33] Surovevic even

---

*References 5, 15, 26, 41, 46, and 48.

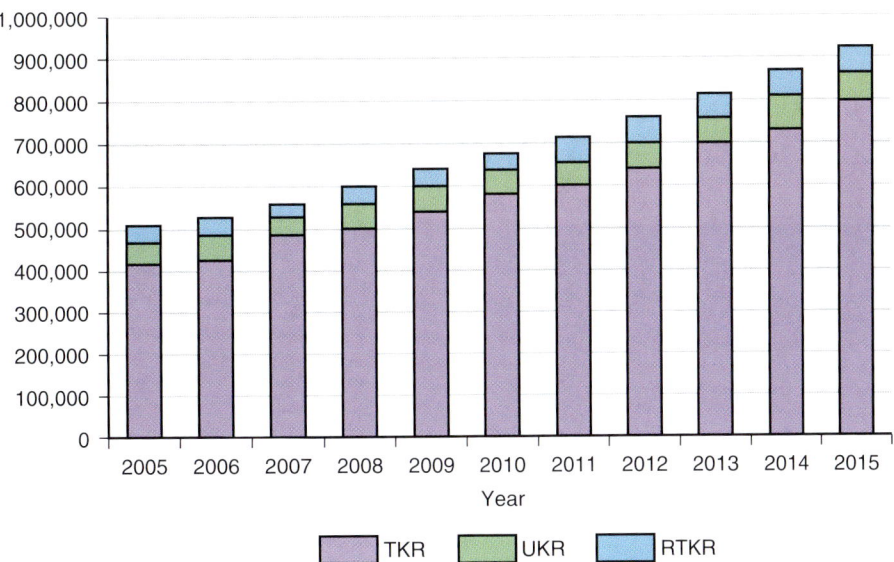

Figure 98-1. Predicted volume of primary unicompartmental knee arthroplasty (UKA), total knee arthroplasty (TKA), and revision total knee replacement (TKR) procedures over the coming years in the United States.

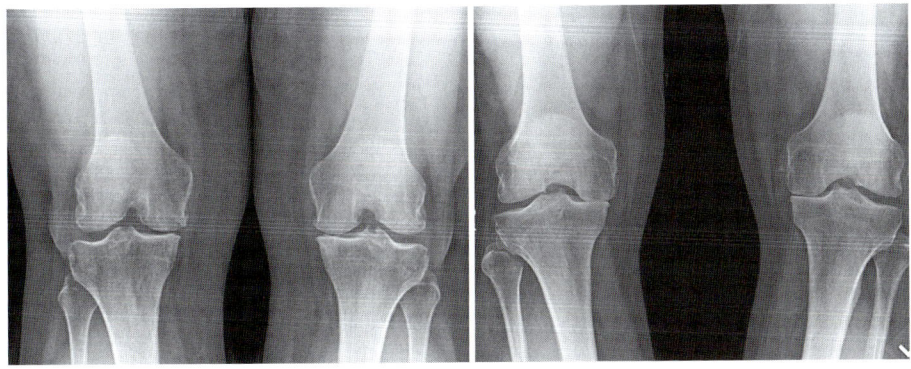

Figure 98-2. Anteroposterior (AP) standing and AP Rosenberg views of medial osteoarthritis.

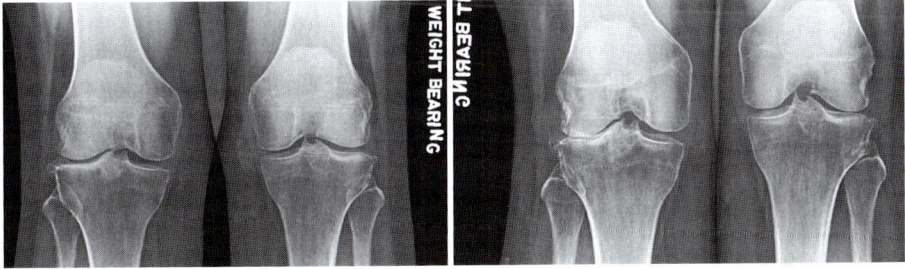

Figure 98-3. Anteroposterior (AP) standing and AP Rosenberg views are helpful in diagnosing lateral osteoarthritis.

extended the indication for UKA to a BMI of up to 42.[47] Berend reported higher failure rates in patients with a BMI above 32 in UKA using an all-polyethylene (PE) tibia.[4] Both implants (Repicci II, Biomet, Warsaw, Ind; Eius, Stryker Orthopedics, Mahwah, NJ) were all-PE whether they were an inlay or an onlay, but neither had a tibial keel.

Although most surgeons make their final decision on whether to use a UKA or a TKA at the time of surgery after arthrotomy,[22,43,49] special weight-bearing preoperative x-rays are helpful (Fig. 98-2). Standing posteroanterior standing views in extension and flexion (Rosenberg views) are nice screening tools for unicompartmental medial or lateral

osteoarthritis (Fig. 98-3). The standing lateral x-ray helps to identify an anteromedial wear pattern and is helpful in predicting whether the anterior cruciate ligament (ACL) is intact (Fig. 98-4).[20] Skyline views may demonstrate patellofemoral (PF) osteoarthritis (Fig. 98-5). PF eburnated bone is considered a contraindication to UKA.

Although a patient may be an ideal candidate for unicompartmental arthroplasty, as indicated by clinical examination and radiography, several contraindications may be discovered at the time of arthrotomy. We consider an absent ACL to be a significant (although not absolute) contraindication to unicompartmental replacement because this is usually

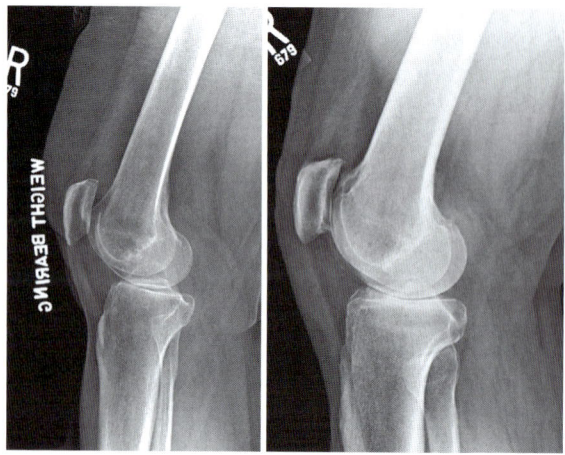

Figure 98-4. Lateral standing views are helpful in determining the medial wear pattern to predict anterior cruciate ligament (ACL) stability.

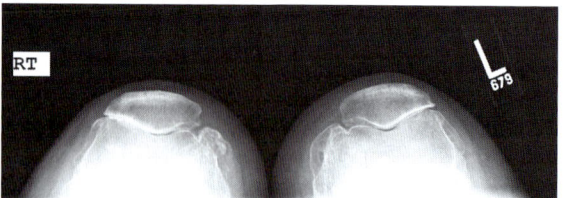

Figure 98-5. Bilateral skyline views screen for patellofemoral (PF) osteoarthritis.

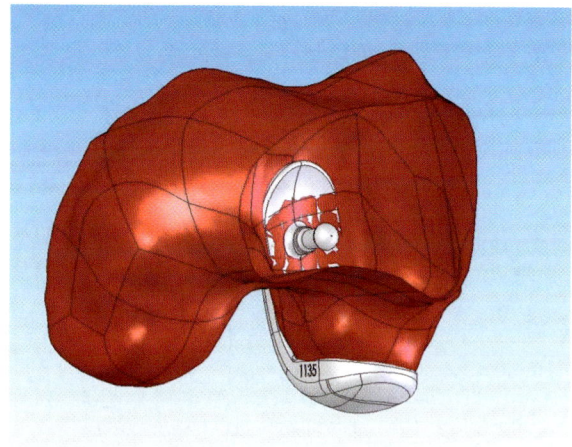

Figure 98-6. Tapering of the anterior edge of the femoral component underneath the subchondral bone decreases the risk of patellofemoral impingement.

IMPLANT DESIGN

Over the past two decades, many lessons have been learned concerning the ideal design of a unicompartmental arthroplasty. Many early femoral components were narrow in their mediolateral dimension and suffered a high incidence of subsidence of the component into the condylar bone.[41,43] The ideal component should be wide enough to maximally cap the resurfaced condyle, widely distributing weight-bearing forces and decreasing the chances of subsidence and loosening. For this reason, multiple sizes should be available to accommodate both small and large patients. Revision studies have shown the inadvisability of deeply invading the condyle with fixation methods.[3,23,32] Relatively small fixation lugs appear to be sufficient as long as two lugs or some sort of fin is present to gain rotational fixation. The posterior metallic condyle should fully cap the posterior condyle of the patient to allow physiologic range of motion without impingement and should be divergent to the femoral lugs to optimize cement pressurization against the posterior condyle during insertion. Also, the anterior femoral edge should taper below the subchondral bone, reducing the chance of patellar impingement. Figure 98-6 shows a personalized femoral component, where the anterior edge is tapered below the subchondral bone. It also demonstrates the anatomic restoration of the posterior condyle. Preferably, the femoral component can be supported on top of the distal subchondral bone without resection, but this requires sacrifice of more bone from the tibial side. The coronal articulating topography of the prosthetic components must also consist of a compromise. A flat surface on the femoral component articulating with a flat surface on the tibial component may potentially improve metal-to-plastic contact, but this is difficult to technically line up precisely enough to avoid edge contact throughout the range of motion. An articulating surface with a small radius of curvature articulating on the tibial side with a flat surface creates too much point contact. A femoral surface with a small radius of curvature matched to a similarly small radius on the tibial side can create too much constraint. The ideal surfaces of both components therefore are probably those with a relatively large radius of curvature that allows

accompanied by ligamentous laxity that eventually can promote lateral subluxation of the tibia on the femur and secondary opposite compartmental disease. If the tibial wear pattern remains in the anterior or central portion of the plateau, fixed-bearing UKA may be feasible, but little or no posterior tibial slope should be applied. Age and activity level need consideration, and mobile-bearing UKA should be avoided. Inspection of the opposite compartment and patellofemoral joint may show significant degenerative changes that make unicompartmental arthroplasty inadvisable.

As the disease progresses, varus knees reveal two typical findings. First, notch impingement of a tibial osteophyte anterior to the insertion of the ACL may result in a flexion contracture. After removal of this osteophyte, full extension may be restored. Second, the lateral spine may erode the medial aspect of the lateral femoral condyle secondary to central tibial subluxation. This chondral lesion is called a kissing lesion. If subluxation is great and the lesion large, bicompartmental or tricompartmental arthroplasty is advisable.

Mild chondromalacia with no eburnated bone in the opposite compartment can be accepted. A third contraindication discovered at the time of arthrotomy consists of a significant inflammatory component to the patient's disease. This may be seen in the form of a very strong synovial reaction or in the discovery of diffuse crystal deposits from gout or pseudogout. Deposits in the hyaline cartilage more than in the meniscus are of concern. Inflammatory disease in any form substantially increases the risk of secondary degeneration of the opposite compartment in subsequent years and remains a contraindication.

adequate metal-to-plastic contact without excessive constraint for fixed-bearing UKA.

In the sagittal plane, conformity at first might seem attractive to increase contact area and lower stresses that cause PE wear. Retrievals of worn unicompartmental tibial components have yielded important information regarding wear patterns and their implications for prosthetic design. It appears that the PE wear pattern tends to reproduce the preoperative wear pattern of the osteoarthritic knee.[27] As noted by White and associates,[50] this tends to be anterior and peripheral on the medial tibial plateau in a varus knee. Moving the femoral component more mesial may change this wear pattern and decrease the edge loading of the very medial aspect of the tibial component. This is even more important in mobile bearing, in that the meniscal bearing is driven through the position of the femoral component. Mesial placement (Fig. 98-7) of the femoral component keeps the meniscal bearing closer to the vertical rail and avoids soft tissue irritation of a subluxing meniscal bearing. If a fixed-bearing unicompartmental knee is too conforming, a higher incidence of component loosening is reported[17,44]; this applies for fixed-bearing UKA, but not for mobile-bearing UKA.

Thinner femoral components decrease femoral bone resection, and tibial resection is based on the composite thickness of metal-backed tibia and PE. Minimum tibial composite thicknesses are between 6 and 8 mm. Newer technologies may further decrease the minimal PE thickness, preserving more tibial bone stock.

Most tibial components have pegs or fins. Their placement should preserve tibial bone stock and should not compromise the posterior tibial cortex.

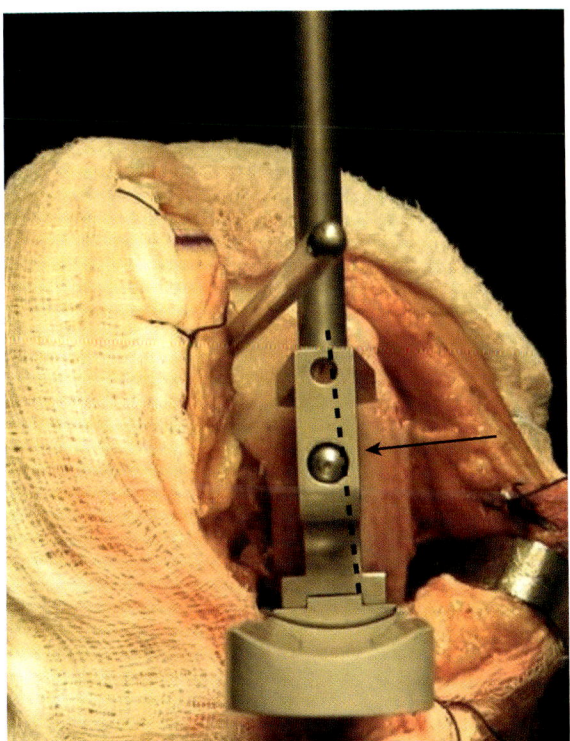

Figure 98-7. Mesial placement of the femoral component optimizes tracking of meniscal bearing in mobile-bearing unicompartmental knee arthroplasty (UKA).

The mobile- or meniscal-bearing articulation is an attractive way to maximize contact area and decrease contact stresses while avoiding excessive constraint.[12,13] This technique is technically demanding, and early failure rates are higher than 5%.[25] Ten-year results in patients 60 years of age and younger demonstrate no significant difference between mobile- and fixed-bearing UKA.[33,34]

The shape of the tibial component as it sits on the tibial plateau should probably be as anatomic as possible. This will maximize contact between the prosthesis and the bone and will widely distribute the weight-bearing forces to resist subsidence and loosening. An asymmetrical shape will be needed with right and left components. Optimal cortical coverage is difficult. Using computed tomography (CT) scans and computer-generated cuts 5 mm below the articular surface, standard implant edges lay up to 67% on cortical bone. Even with theoretically optimized implant designs, a maximum of 76% of the implant edge could lay on cortical bone.[11] As an alternative to overhanging implants or ill-fitting designs, personalized implants probably will play a large role in the future. Figure 98-8 shows bilateral personalized UKA demonstrating excellent anatomic fit.

Surgical Technique

Most surgeons use a short vertical skin incision from the top of the patella to the tibial tubercle and a short medial parapatellar arthrotomy. After the arthrotomy is performed and adequate exposure has been achieved, all three compartments of the knee are inspected carefully, and a final decision is made regarding whether the patient is ideally suited for UKA. The knee is positioned in 90 degrees of flexion, a bent Hohmann is placed lateral to the ACL, and the patella is pushed to the contralateral side. For a lateral UKA, the arthrotomy is performed from a medial or lateral arthrotomy. Most surgeons use a lateral parapatellar incision for a valgus deformity and lateral compartment arthroplasty[19]; others prefer a medial parapatellar approach.[39]

Exposure through a lateral arthrotomy is a little more difficult. Positioning the knee at 70 degrees reduces the tension of the patella and facilitates exposure. Usually, as lateral compartment osteoarthritis progresses, lateral subluxation of the tibia on the femur does not occur until the deformity is so severe that unicompartmental arthroplasty is not appropriate. The medial collateral ligament and the medial capsule gradually elongate as the valgus deformity progresses. With significant medial laxity, the knee can no longer be stabilized by unicompartmental arthroplasty. We found that a correctable deformity is actually a very good indicator as to whether a patient is suitable for lateral UKA.

In UKA, ligament releases are not necessary. In principle, overall knee alignment should be restored to the alignment that was present before cartilage loss occurred and should not be corrected to a fixed amount. Overcorrection should be avoided. Medially, adequate correction can be attained merely by removing the femoral and tibial osteophytes that tent up the medial collateral ligament and medial capsule. A formal medial ligament release is never recommended, because this need would imply that a varus deformity is present that is too great for unicompartmental arthroplasty (Fig. 98-9). A small Z-retractor around the tibial edge facilitates exposure and protects the medial collateral ligament.

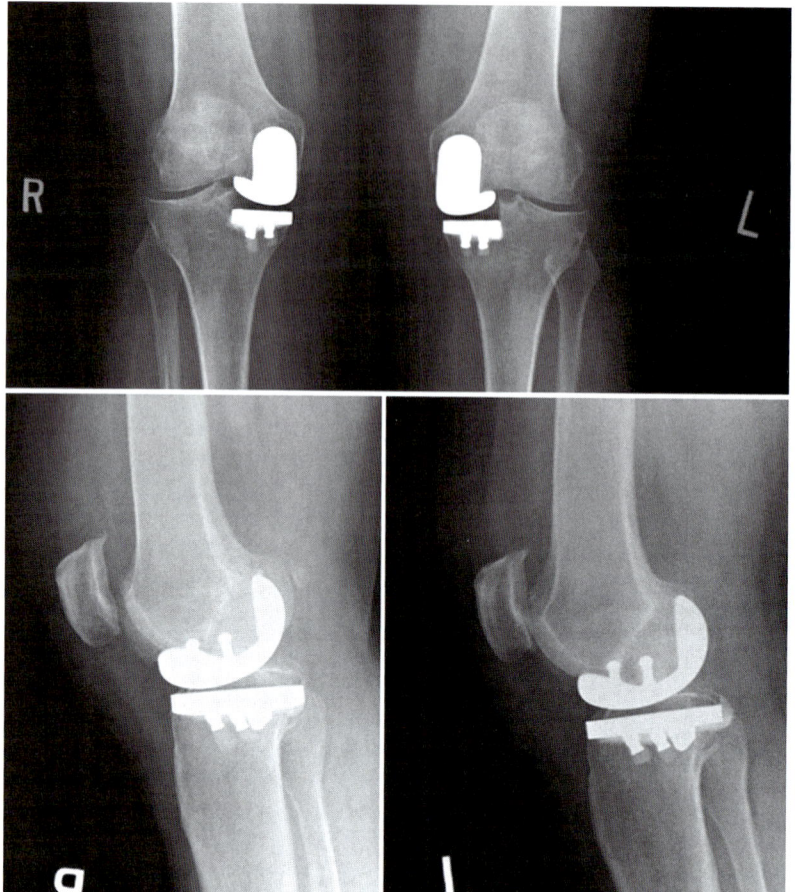

Figure 98-8. Anteroposterior (AP) and lateral views of bilateral medial personalized unicompartmental knee arthroplasty (UKA).

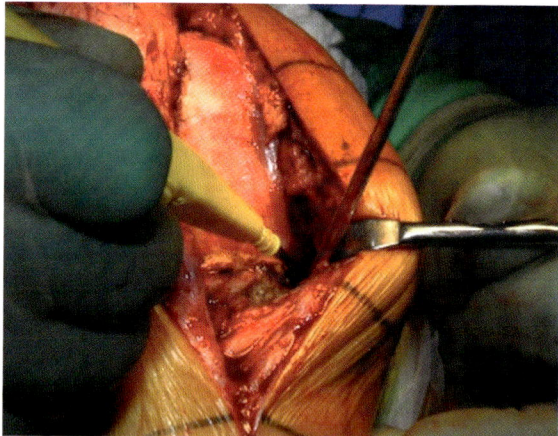

Figure 98-9. Removal of medial osteophytes without release of medial collateral ligament restores knee alignment.

Personalized implants provide images of the osteophytes that need to be removed (Fig. 98-10).

The extramedullary tibial alignment guide is best fixed to the tibia with one rather than two pins. This pin is placed lateral to the sagittal cut to avoid stress raisers and the potential for tibial stress fracture[6] (Fig. 98-11). Medial pins are not recommended.

Alternatively, a conservative tibial resection can be placed by preoperatively templating a conservative cut for a tibial

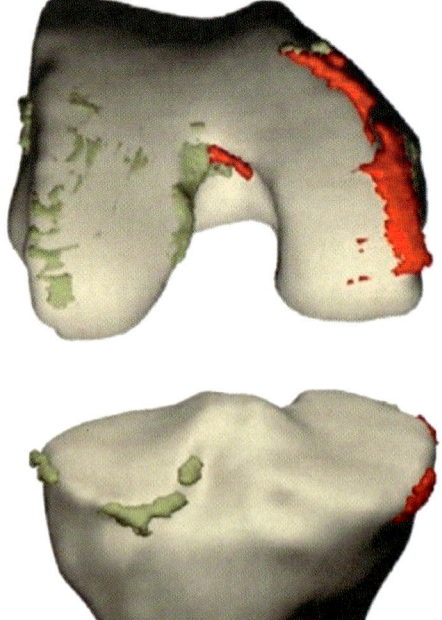

Figure 98-10. Personalized preoperative planning may facilitate surgical techniques for osteophyte removal.

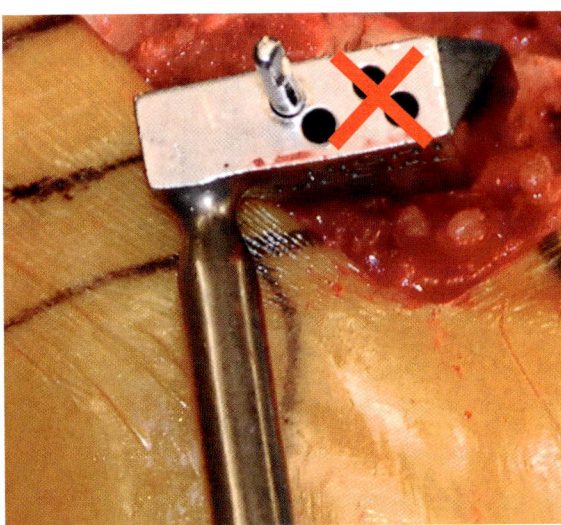

Figure 98-11. Fewer fixation pins decrease the risk of medial tibial plateau fracture.

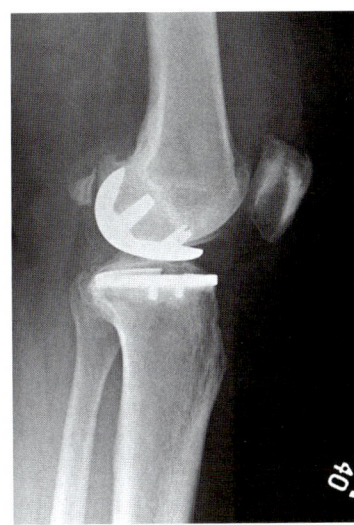

Figure 98-12. Flexion of the femoral component may cause patel-lofemoral impingement.

component based 8 to 10 mm from the normal lateral plateau. The surgeon then notes where this resection hits the medial tibial plateau. It remains to be clinically proven whether this conservative approach is superior to restoring the joint line.

In theory, the joint line should be restored. Assuming a tibial cartilage thickness of 3 mm and 2 mm of bone loss in the deepest portion, a total of 5 mm is lost. Given a tibial composite thickness of 8 mm, the difference of 3 mm has to be resected off the deepest tibial point. This does not apply if the medial collateral ligament is not intact. A stylus can help to determine the appropriate tibial resection. To avoid undermining of the ACL insertion, the sagittal tibial cut can be done first, leaving the saw blade just 1 mm below the cutting surface in situ. The blade should be about 2 mm lateral to the lateral edge of the medial condyle and in the ascending portion of the medial spine. Some implants are wider, and the sagittal cut has to be at the top of the medial spine. The direction of the sagittal cut is determined by the condyle itself, or by orienting the saw blade parallel to the wear pattern of the tibia or pointing it toward the center of the femoral head. A small Z-retractor is positioned along the joint line of the medial tibia to protect the medial collateral ligament. The natural slope is matched, but posterior slopes greater than 7 degrees are not recommended and should be reduced to decrease the strain of the ACL.[16] The cut is completed and the resected surface of the tibia removed and compared with tibial trial components for size determination. Now, the flexion gap is measured in millimeters using spacer blocks. The weight of the thigh has to be taken out of the equation by lifting the thigh with one arm up, if the knee is not operated in a hanging position. The block should slide between the medial femoral condyle and the resected tibia with little resistance. Rarely, the flexion gap is too loose. If an 8-mm-thick tibial component is used, a matching 8-mm spacer block should be used. The amount that needs to be resected off the posterior femoral condyle matches the thickness of the femoral component. By passing the 8-mm spacer block, we know that our flexion gap will be balanced.

The knee is brought into nearly full extension, and by applying some valgus stress for a medial UKA, the medial extension gap is measured with spacer blocks. Let's assume

that the extension gap measures 11 mm, and we implant a femoral component with a distal thickness of 6 mm. Tibial and femoral component thickness is 8 + 6 = 14 mm, plus desired joint play of 1 to 2 mm makes a total of 15 mm. Because we measured for the extension gap of 11 mm, we need to resect 4 mm off the distal femur when the femoral resection is linked to the tibial resection. It is important not to hyperextend or flex the knee to avoid flexion or extension of the femoral component. Figure 98-12 shows a femoral component with too much flexion, potentially causing patellofemoral impingement. Intramedullary femoral rods may help to avoid malpositioning. The same principle applies to the lateral side, with the difference that the lateral side is looser and should have more play. In extension, a laxity of around 2 to 3 mm should be achieved, whereas in 90 degrees flexion, a laxity of 4 to 6 mm is recommended.

The femoral cutting block should be moved toward the notch if possible, leaving about 1 to 2 mm of uncovered bone medially. This will move the contact point of the femur more mesial on the tibia in extension. In fixed-bearing UKAs, the wear pattern will be moved slightly more mesial, and in mobile-bearing UKAs, the meniscal bearing is closer to the vertical rail, decreasing the chance of overhang and soft tissue impingement medially. However, some designs without a tapered anterior end may be prone to patellar impingement, and one should be careful not to move the femoral component too far mesial.

On the lateral side, the tibial component should be moved medially to compensate for the more rounded geometry of the lateral tibial plateau. On the femoral side, the femoral component should be placed more laterally for optimal tracking. Sizing of the femoral component laterally is more difficult, because the lateral femoral condyle is shorter. Using the linea terminalis that separates the femoropatellar joint from the lateral tibiofemoral joint can be helpful. Single-radius designs or personalized components may address this issue best.

The tibial component should cover the tibial cortex without medial or posterior overhang. Using an arthroscopic probe, the anteroposterior length is measured and compared with tibial trials. If anteroposterior coverage is complete but medial overhang is noted, the sagittal cut should be moved

1 or 2 mm more laterally to achieve best coverage of the tibial surface. Authors prefer a laminar spreader to temporarily fix the tibial template to the tibia, rather than additional pin holes to further weaken the medial tibial plateau. We also recommend preserving the posterior tibial cortex and, if possible, leaving a 5-mm cancellous bone bridge anterior to it. On the femoral side, if the bone is sclerotic, a 2- to 3-mm drill bit can be used to improve cement bone interdigitation.

After trialing, the bony surfaces are washed and the components are cemented, starting with the tibia. One can initially pack the fixation holes with cement, while putting only a thin layer on the plateau. The remainder of the cement goes on the back of the tibial component, so that if it is inserted posteriorly first, any extruded cement will come forward. Using a trial insert, however, will allow access to any posterior extruded cement. Others prefer to insert the original PE before cementing the femoral component. Wound closure is performed in standard fashion. Some surgeons prefer periarticular injection of a mixture of Marcaine with Epi, Toradol, and Duramorph, if no contraindications apply.

New Technology in UKA

Although interest in traditional computer-assisted surgery in UKA has decreased since 2005, new technologies have emerged. Mako Surgical Corporation (Ft Lauderdale, Fla) introduced its "Makoplasty" to the United States in 2006. The system combines image-based (CT scan) computer navigation with a haptic-guided burring device that controls surgeons' movements through the use of tactile resistance technology. Virtual three-dimensional (3D) surface images are generated that are based on SolidWorks software technology (Dassault Systèmes SolidWorks Corp, Concord, Mass); these guide surgeons along their planned path (Fig. 98-13). Intraoperative adjustments can be made by balancing data to

facilitate optimal positioning of the implants. New unicompartmental components with rounded edges have been introduced to accommodate to the geometry of a round 6-mm burr. This is a passive robotic device that gives tactile, visual, and auditory feedback while allowing the cutting burr to function only in a predetermined 3D space as preoperatively defined. Early experiences include high accuracy of component placement and a short learning curve (M. Roche, Holy Cross Hospital, Fort Lauderdale, Fla, personal communication, November 2009).

A different approach was introduced by Conformis (Burlington, Mass) to simplify not only intraoperative registration, but the entire instrumentation and fit of the implants. Using preoperative high-resolution CT imaging of the affected knee and a few cuts through hip and ankle, the manufacture of prenavigated, single-use, personalized instrumentation with matching individualized implants can be accomplished. Although the instrumentation consists of autoclavable, 3D, printed nylon enhanced with metallic bushings and cutting surfaces, it is prenavigated and contains mechanical information related to the long axis of the leg. The femoral component is aligned along the mechanical axis, and the femoral pegs are pointing to the center of the femoral head. The tibial component is cut at a 90-degree angle to the coronal mechanical axis, and the medial slope is matched if it measures less than 7 degrees. If the slope is greater than 7 degrees, it is corrected to 7 degrees to reduce strain on the ACL. The slope of the lateral tibial component is matched individually. The instrumentation is delivered with the implants sterilized in a single box. It is a single-use formulation that eliminates processing, washing, sterilization, or storage. A new balancing system is incorporated into the instrumentation: after residual articular cartilage is removed from the affected compartment, personalized spacer blocks matching the tibial surface topography are inserted. Different thicknesses in 1-mm increments are provided until the

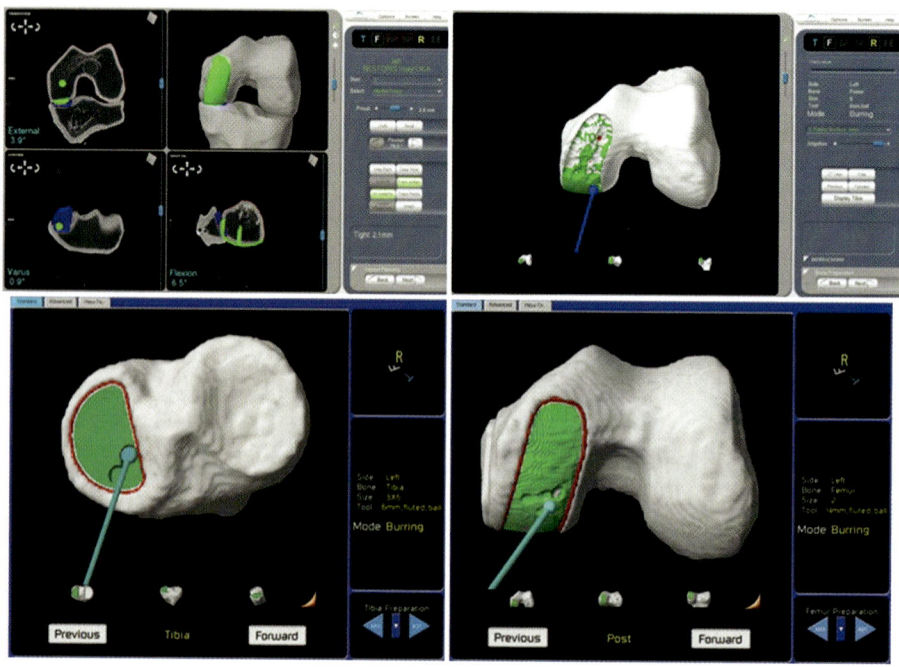

Figure 98-13. Intraoperative monitoring of component placement using a haptic robotic device.

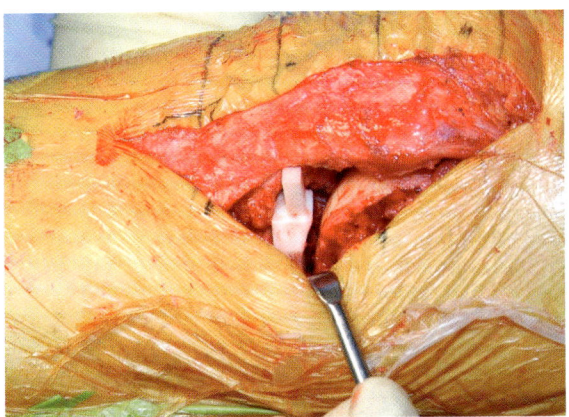

Figure 98-14. Various thicknesses of personalized balancing chips facilitate ligament balancing.

extension gap is balanced (Fig. 98-14). The thickness of the navigation chip determines the amount of bone removed from the tibia to accommodate for an 8-mm tibial component. The flexion gap is preserved by restoring the posterior femoral joint surface. The implants are individualized by matching the anatomy of femur and tibia. The anterior edge of the femoral component is tapered below the subchondral bone plate to avoid patellar impingement. Early experiences confirm a short learning curve and accurate implant placement.

POSTOPERATIVE REHABILITATION

Perioperative multimodal pain management in combination with periarticular infiltration of local anesthetics can facilitate a quick recovery with good pain control. In general, patients are allowed to bear weight as tolerated and to walk with an assistive device within a few days. Rehabilitation is less painful and is quicker than with TKR.

SUMMARY

Unicompartmental knee replacement continues to offer an attractive alternative to osteotomy or tricompartmental arthroplasty in selected unilateral osteoarthritic patients. Given the increased numbers of patients in need of joint replacement, UKA is an important treatment that outnumbers the revision knee replacements performed. With clinical results that are similar to those of TKA at 10 and 15 years, UKA offers a bone-sparing alternative along with preservation of both cruciate ligaments. It is feasible to consider UKA as the first prosthetic treatment for unilateral osteoarthritis in middle-aged patients, and likely as the last procedure in the elderly.

KEY REFERENCES

Cartier P, Sanouiller JL, Grelsamer RP: Unicompartmental knee arthroplasty surgery. J Arthroplasty 11:782, 1996.

Fitzpatrick C, Fitzpatrick D, Lee J, Auger D: Statistical design of unicompartmental tibial implants and comparison with current devices. The Knee 14:138–144, 2007.

Hernigou P, Deschamps G: Posterior slope of the tibial implant and the outcome of unicompartmental knee arthroplasty. J Bone Joint Surg Am 86:506–511, 2004.

Kirkley A, Birmingham TB, Litchfield RB, et al: A randomized trial of arthroscopic surgery for osteoarthritis of the knee. N Engl J Med 359:1097–1107, 2008.

Kozinn SC, Scott RD: Current concepts review: unicompartmental total arthroplasty. J Bone Joint Surg Am 71:145, 1989.

Marmor L: Unicompartmental knee arthroplasty: ten to thirteen year follow-up study. Clin Orthop Relat Res 226:24, 1987.

Moseley JB, O'Malley K, Petersen NJ, et al: A controlled trial of arthroscopic surgery for osteoarthritis of the knee. N Engl J Med 347:81, 2002.

Newman J, Pydisetty RV, Ackroyd C: Unicompartmental or total knee replacement: the 15-year results of a prospective randomised controlled trial. J Bone Joint Surg Br 91:52–57, 2009.

Pennington DW, Swienckowski JJ, Lutes WB, Drake GN: Unicompartmental knee arthroplasty in patients sixty years of age or younger. J Bone Joint Surg Am 85:1968–1973, 2003.

Price AJ, Dodd CA, Svard UG, Murray DW: Oxford medial unicompartmental knee arthroplasty in patients younger and older than 60 years of age. J Bone Joint Surg Br 87:1488–1492, 2005.

Riddle DL, Jiranek WA, McGlynn FJ: Yearly incidence of unicompartmental knee arthroplasty in the United States. J Arthroplasty 23:408–412, 2008.

Swienckowski JJ, Pennington DW: Unicompartmental arthroplasty in patients 60 years of age or younger: surgical technique. J Bone Joint Surg Am 86(Suppl 1):131–142, 2004.

Tabor OB Jr, Tabor OB: Unicompartmental arthroplasty: a long-term follow-up study. J Arthroplasty 13:373, 1998.

Full references for this chapter can be found on www.expertconsult.com.

Unicompartmental Knee Arthroplasty: A European Perspective

Jean-Noël Argenson and Sebastien Parratte

Isolated unicompartmental knee arthritis remains a challenging problem. Surgical management of unicompartmental knee arthritis includes conservative treatment such as arthroscopic débridement or high tibial osteotomy (HTO) and nonconservative treatment such as unicompartmental arthroplasty or total knee arthroplasty (TKA).[8,16] These procedures, however, have a finite lifespan in young and active patients and some concerns such as functional recovery and the possibility of returning to athletic activities should be considered.[26,29] During the last decade, enthusiasm for the use of HTO has declined.[2] It has been demonstrated that HTO remains an attractive conservative procedure to avoid knee prosthesis for patients younger than 50 years with a low-grade unicompartmental osteoarthritis and a varus knee. However, the HTO risk of failure increased dramatically for patients with osteoarthritis rated as Ahlback[1] grade 2 or higher. In these cases, nonconservative treatment should be considered, even in younger patients. Unicompartmental knee arthroplasty (UKA), which has been performed since the 1970s, may provide better physiologic function and quicker recovery compared with total knee arthroplasty and preserves the bone stock in a patient in whom only one compartment of the knee is affected.[11,12,21,32,40] Furthermore, patient satisfaction is greater because the knee feels more natural.

UKA has specific modes of failure, such as progression of the disease in the remaining compartments and polyethylene wear. In a recent survey of the American Association of Hip and Knee Surgeons,[10] UKA was the preferred procedure by 11.4% of surgeons for a 45-year-old active man and by 29.5% of surgeons for a 45-year-old active woman to manage a medial compartment arthritis, assuming a mechanical axis of 7 degrees of varus with an intact cruciate and mild patellofemoral symptoms. Improper patient selection combined with limited instrumentation and suboptimal designs may explain the less than satisfactory results originally published for UKA and the subsequent decreased interest, especially in the United States. Interest in UKA has been maintained in Europe since the first experience in the 1970s, and different new designs were developed in the 1980s.[15,18,35,37] Since the early 1990s, new implant designs have been introduced, with reliable instrumentation, which makes the procedure as reliable as TKA. With proper patient selection and a more reliable surgical technique, the 10-year results of modern UKA are now available and show survivorship greater than 90% after 10 years of follow-up. The other potential advantage over tricompartmental replacement is preservation of the bone stock in the remaining compartment and preservation of the ligaments.[4] Thus, modern UKA, as a conservative resurfacing arthroplasty of the knee, can preserve the cruciate mechanism, acting as a four-bar linkage guiding femorotibial movements.[4] In vivo kinematics studies performed in patients implanted with a UKA have shown a femorotibial pattern similar to that observed in the normal knee.

The most important evolution in UKA during the last decade is so-called mini-invasive surgery (MIS).[3,33] In regard to UKA, MIS is defined as the ability to implant components without an incision in the quadriceps tendon or the vastus medialis or lateralis, depending on the compartment to be replaced, and without everting the patella. Minimizing the trauma of the extensor mechanism should allow earlier walking and active muscle exercises. Repicci and Eberle[34] proposed this mini-incision for the implantation of unicompartmental components as a resurfacing procedure using limited instrumentation. With the advances in instrumentation over the last 5 years, it is possible to perform partial knee arthroplasty with cutting guides fixed only on the replaced compartment, thus preserving the integrity of the unaffected tibiofemoral compartment. New worldwide interest in UKA is the result of the possibilities of fast recovery and minimal surgical morbidity permitted by MIS and improvement in UKA design allowing greater and safer motion capabilities, especially for active patients who are candidates for a UKA.[8,9]

UNICOMPARTMENTAL KNEE ARTHROPLASTY: THE EUROPEAN EXPERIENCE

After the initial experience of Marmor in the United States in 1972, many variations of the Marmor Modular Knee were introduced in Europe at that time. Marmor published his own experience later, in the mid-1980s, but the concept of resurfacing the tibial and femoral sides of one femorotibial compartment gained great attention in several European countries.[25] The principles of these resurfacing systems were to minimize saw cuts by adapting the femoral component to the condyle and using an polyethylene tibial component inlay cemented in the subchondral tibial bone while preserving the cortical rim. The St. Georges Sled, mostly used in northern Europe, was based on the same concept. The second generation of Marmor-like designs introduced a metal backing of the tibia to bring modularity to the procedure and distribute the weight-bearing forces more uniformly on the cut surface of the plateau. Although the initial results seemed satisfactory in terms of a more friendly surgical technique, wear failure of the tibial plateau was attributed mainly to the use of 6-mm-thick polyethylene. It is now recognized that the minimum thickness should be 8 mm for flat-bearing designs.[6] Meanwhile, the Unicondylar Knee Prosthesis was used in the United States and Europe as an alternative to the Polycentric Knee or the Duocondylar design.[21] Resurfacing both tibiofemoral compartments of the knee while preserving the cruciate ligaments represented the first form of the Oxford mobile-bearing system developed by Goodfellow and O'Connor in 1978.[32] The concept was used for unicompartmental arthroplasty. It is based on a fully congruent mobile articulating surface, which aims to increase the area of contact and then reduce polyethylene wear. Measurement of retrieved bearings has shown a mean linear wear rate of 0.03 mm/yr or less (0.001 mm/yr) after normal function of the knee.[5]

In France, Cartier and Cheaib[12,13] introduced instrumentation specifically dedicated to UKA, promoting the concept that UKA was not a half-TKA and that the same type of persistent undercorrection of the deformity was suitable in opposition to the principle of TKA (Fig. 99-1A). These principles have been emphasized and accurately described by Kennedy and White[22] in their paper describing the postoperative targets in terms of angles restoration after UKA (see Fig. 99-1B).

The cutting jig systems brought the same type of instrumentation as that used for TKA, with posterior and chamfer cuts of the femoral condyle based on intramedullary instruments. The advantage of this type of instrumentation was to provide a reproducible surgical technique, allowing the component to be placed perpendicular to the mechanical axis as previously determined on preoperative radiographs. Most of these designs have been used widely in Europe and the United States since the late 1980s, and long-term follow-up of the Brigham, Duracon, PFC Uni, and Miller-Galante is now available through the Swedish Registry.[38] Independent publications also have reported survivorship comparable to that reported for TKA.[2,11,15,27,40] Most of this experience was realized using cemented components, which remain the current standard for UKA in Europe. The first reported use of porous-coated designs was not encouraging, but hydroxyapatite coating has gained limited acceptance in some European centers.

PATIENT SELECTION

The indications for UKA are painful osteoarthritis (OA) or osteonecrosis limited to one compartment of the knee associated with a significant loss of joint space on radiographs.[2,9,28,29] Results after UKA for osteonecrosis limited to one compartment of the knee (i.e., idiopathic or post-traumatic osteonecrosis) was comparable to those observed for OA at a mean of 12 years. Any type of inflammatory arthritis, such as rheumatoid arthritis, is recognized as a formal contraindication for UKA because this can be a cause of rapid degeneration of the unreplaced compartments. Mild chondrocalcinosis, which is mostly a radiographic finding, may be accepted as an indication to perform UKA, in contrast to the productive chondrocalcinosis often associated with cyclic effusion of the knee.

Age and Weight

Age and weight may still represent debatable issues as indications for UKA because the procedure is often presented as an alternative to osteotomy or TKA. As noted, and according to the results of previously published series, we do consider the HTO as an attractive and efficient conservative procedure for patient younger than 50 years with a low-grade unicompartmental osteoarthritis and a varus knee.[16] However, the HTO risk of failure increases dramatically for patients with osteoarthritis rated Ahlback grade 2 or higher, which is why in those cases we do consider UKA, even in younger patients.[31] Regarding age and based on the comparative results at 10 years of UKA and TKA, Scott and associates[40]

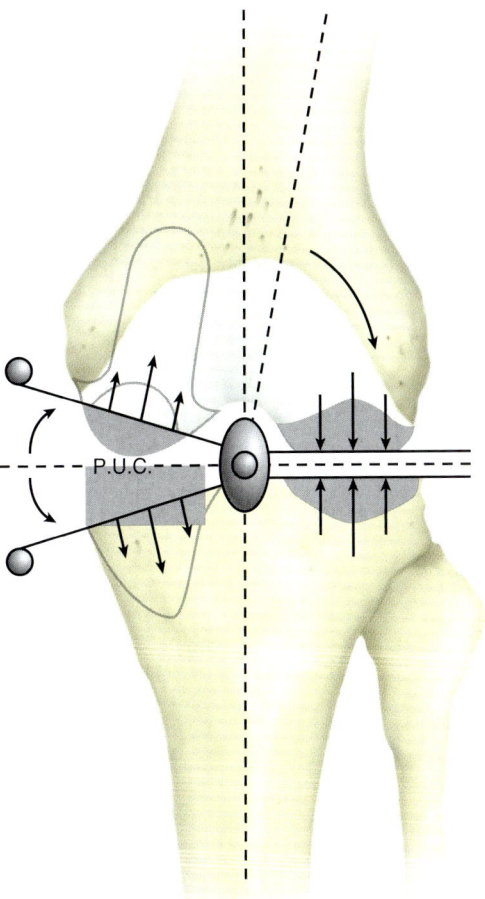

A

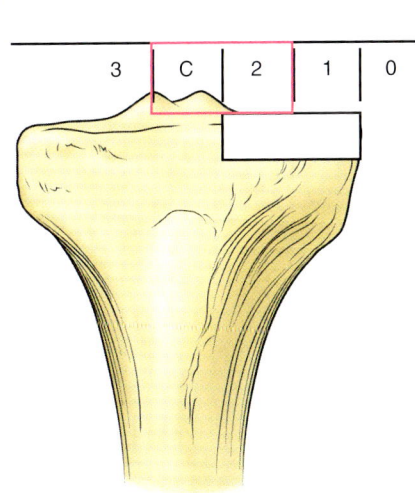

B   Kennedy classification

Figure 99-1. A, Diagram showing the mechanism of overcorrection leading to progression of osteoarthritis in the unreplaced compartment after UKA. **B,** These principles have been emphasized and accurately described by Kennedy and White[22] in their paper describing postoperative targets in terms of angles restoration after UKA.

considered that UKA now might assume a role in two groups of patients—middle-aged osteoarthritic patients (especially women undergoing a first arthroplasty) and osteoarthritic patients in their 80s octogenarians who are having their first and last arthroplasty. With survivorship studies of modern UKA comparable to those of TKA after the first decade, the selection process must be reconsidered; patients in their 60s and 70s would seem to have a greater chance of living out their lives with a TKA or UKA, which in any case would be easier to revise.[8,14] We recently reported very good survivorship in the younger than 50 years, despite greater polyethylene wear than for older patients as observed also after TKA.[29]

Early reports of UKA considered obesity as a relative contraindication for UKA, but more recent studies have found no correlation between weight and outcomes. We agree with the idea that wear related is more to activity than to weight.[6] Obesity itself is consequently not a contraindication.

Clinical Evaluation

The clinical examination of the knee before choosing UKA as a treatment option needs to focus on range of motion, with a minimum range of knee flexion of 100 degrees. A femoral contraction may be improved by only a few degrees after UKA and this should be recognized preoperatively. The clinical evaluation of the patellofemoral joint is also mandatory to seek out any type of anterior knee pain described by the patient during stair climbing and descending or during squatting. The stability of the joint must be evaluated carefully in the sagittal plane for the anterior cruciate ligament (ACL) and in the frontal plane using the results of specific tests. The unicompartmental implant fills the gap left by the worn cartilage, bringing the collateral ligament back to normal tension after the procedure. The clinical results of UKA using mobile-bearing meniscal or fixed-bearing prostheses and in vivo kinematics have highlighted the importance of a functional ACL for unicondylar knee replacement.[4] The clinical outcomes for sedentary patients with a probable secondary distention of the ACL have confirmed that proper clinical function of the knee may be achieved in these low-demand patients using fixed bearings, despite ACL deficiency. For these patients, we concur with the findings of Hernigou and Deschamps,[20] who studied the effects of posterior tibial slope on the outcome of UKA; they recommended avoiding a posterior slope more than 7 degrees when the ACL is absent at the time of implantation. For younger patients, a combined ACL-UKA surgery can be considered with good results in terms of pain and stability but with more limited range of motion as compared with isolated UKA (Fig. 99-2).

Radiologic Evaluation

Our radiologic analysis systematically includes anteroposterior (AP) and mediolateral (ML) views of the knee, full-length x-rays in bipedal and single-leg stance, varus and valgus stress radiographs, and skyline views at 30, 60, and 90 degrees of knee flexion.[17] On full-length x-rays, the angle between the mechanical and anatomic axes of the femur can be calculated and reproduced during the procedure at the time of the distal femoral cut. This also evaluates any extra-articular bony deformity that cannot be corrected by the

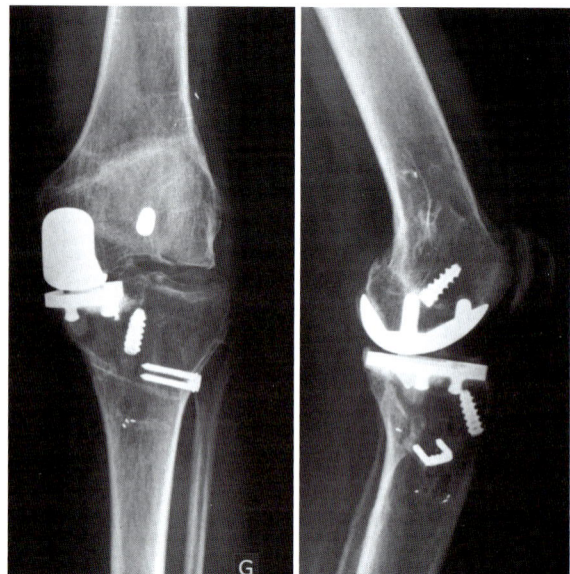

Figure 99-2. For younger patients, a combined ACL-UKA surgery can be considered with good results in terms of pain and stability but with more limited range of motion as compared with isolated UKA, as in this case at 12-year follow-up.

unicompartmental implant and searches for any femoral long hip stem that might require the use of a shorter intramedullary road or an extramedullary rod. Kozinn and Scott[23] first, and later others, suggested that UKA should be limited to preoperative varus or valgus deformity of the lower limb less than 15 degrees and that greater deformities might represent a contraindication for UKA, because the correction of such deformities may require collateral ligament release, which should not be performed when doing UKA because that could lead to frontal femorotibial subluxation. It is also important to consider any important metaphyseal varus deformity of the proximal tibia (>7 degrees) because, in these rare cases, combined or staged HTO-UKA surgery can be considered (Fig. 99-3).

Varus and valgus stress x-rays, performed with the patient supine using a dedicated knee stress system, are important—first to assess the presence of full-thickness articular cartilage in the uninvolved compartment and second to confirm the full correction of the deformity to neutral (Fig. 99-4).[17] In case of absence of insufficient or overcorrection of the deformity, this view indicates the need for soft tissue management and therefore the use of TKA. The lateral view of the joint confirms the absence of anterior tibial more than 10 mm, referencing the posterior edge of the tibial plateau, and shows that tibial erosion is limited to anterior and midportions of the tibial plateau. The height of the patella should also be analyzed because a patella baja will limit the exposure during MIS procedures.[9]

The radiographic analysis should ensure that there is no patellofemoral loss of joint space on skyline views at 30, 60, and 90 degrees of flexion. The presence of periarticular osteophytes may not be a contraindication for unicondylar replacement, and these osteophytes can be removed, even through a minimally invasive incision. Although the status of the patellofemoral joint is not a criterion of suitability for some, we now consider that the full loss of patellofemoral cartilage

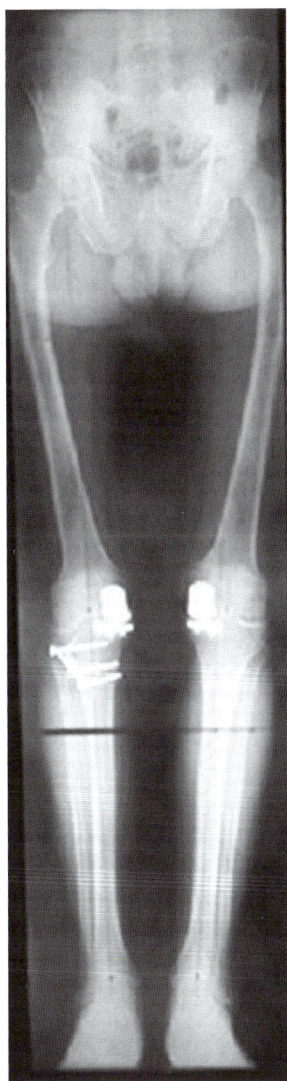

Figure 99-3. Staged opening wedge tibial osteotomy and UKA performed in a 46-year-old man who had a preoperative 8-degree metaphyseal varus deformity and a global varus deformity of 16 degrees. The patient returned to equestrian competition.

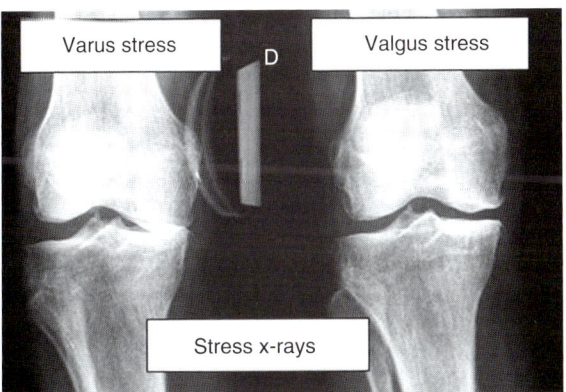

Figure 99-4. Varus and valgus stress x-rays, obtained with the patient supine using a dedicated knee stress system, are important to assess the presence of full-thickness articular cartilage in the uninvolved compartment and to confirm full correction of the deformity to neutral.

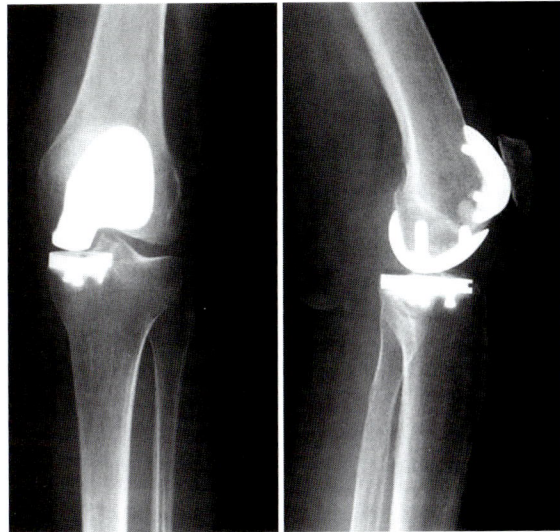

Figure 99-5. In cases of associated wear in the medial and patellofemoral compartments, bicompartmental arthroplasty combining medial UKA and patellofemoral arthroplasty can be considered during the same procedure. Shown here are the results at 2 years after bicompartmental arthroplasty in a 62-year-old woman. She returned to hiking.

is a contraindication for performing a unicondylar replacement. In these cases of associated wear in the medial and patellofemoral compartments, bicompartmental arthroplasty combining medial UKA and patellofemoral arthroplasty can be considered during the same procedure (Fig. 99-5).[30] When there is a question regarding the status of the ACL following the clinical examination, magnetic resonance imaging (MRI) may be useful to confirm that the ACL is intact.

Laskin,[24] in analyzing 300 knees undergoing TKA and evaluating the selection criteria presented by Kozinn and Scott,[23] found that 15% of their knees were eligible for UKA at intraoperative examination. This 15% rate of indication for UKA corresponds to figures reported in Europe, in contrast to the 6% rate of potential candidates for a UKA reported by Ritter and colleagues.[36]

SURGICAL TECHNIQUE

Approach

The procedure can be performed under general or epidural anesthesia on a routine operating table using a two-leg holder, one at the lateral aspect of the thigh and the other below the foot. The knee is flexed 90 degrees for the skin incision, the thigh tourniquet inflated, and the foot rests on the table. The length of the skin incision varies from 8 to 10 cm, depending on skin elasticity and patient morphotype. It is important to maintain proper visualization throughout the procedure and this in part depends on the variation in tissue elasticity. Sufficient visualization is required all throughout the entire procedure; this can be achieved by frequent extension-flexion manipulations to visualize the femoral or tibial side preferentially. When the anatomic structure or component is not properly visualized by shifting the position of the knee, it might be necessary to extend the size of the incision. One of the classic pitfalls of the procedure is related to the length of the incision, which should not be too small, particularly at the beginning of the learning curve. In fact, an insufficient exposure may lead to skin damage because of excessive tension, implant malposition, or inadequate knee balancing. The upper limit of the incision is the superior pole of the patella, extending distally toward the medial for a medial UKA or the lateral for a lateral UKA of the tibial tuberosity, but ending 2 cm under the joint line previously located (see video on the website). The proximal part of the incision is more essential for the procedure and two thirds of the incision should be located above the joint line. Once the synovial cavity is opened (see video on the website), the part of the fat pad in the way of the condyle is excised to visualize the condyle, ACL and corresponding tibial side of the tibial plateau properly. Then, it is important to note that the principles of ligament balancing as used in a TKA cannot be applied to UKA because the collateral ligaments should not be released in UKA. To protect the collateral ligament and perform the cuts safely, a dedicated curved, thin Homan retractor is placed on the medial or lateral side of the incision.

Before proceeding to the bone cuts or anything else, the first step is to bring the knee to 60 degrees of flexion to evaluate the joint by checking the resistance of the ACL with an appropriate hook and evaluating the state of the opposite tibiofemoral joint and patellofemoral joint (Fig. 99-6). The osteophytes are then removed on the medial or lateral side of the femoral condyle in the intercondylar notch to avoid late impingement with the ACL on the notch. This point is important to preserve the ACL and avoid the so-called Marie-Antoinette effect famous in Europe and related to the osteophytes developed in the intercondylar notch, which have a guillotine effect on the ACL (see video on the website). Finally, the osteophytes are also removed from around the patella and tibial plateau. After removing the peripherical osteophytes, there is a relative lengthening of the medial collateral ligament and capsule, allowing passive correction of the deformity.

Tibial Cut

Once the status of the patella, ACL, and opposite compartment have been checked, the next step is to progress to the bone cuts. It is important to remember that in UKA, the proper tension of the ligaments will be restored while filling the gap left by the worn cartilage with the unicompartmental components; therefore, UKA can be regarded as a surfacing procedure.

In our practice, the tibial cut is always performed first both for UKA and TKA; however, because the cuts are independent, surgery can start with the femoral side as well when considering the intramedullary technique for the femur. The entire procedure can be performed using extramedullary or intramedullary instrumentation. The extramedullary technique is based on the correction of the deformity of the leg in extension using an extramedullary rod that references the ankle and femoral head. This will determine the direction and level of the femoral distal cut performed first and link that parallel with the tibial cut made with the knee brought into flexion.

The tibial cut is made using an extramedullary rod (Fig. 99-7). The guide is placed distally around the ankle, with the

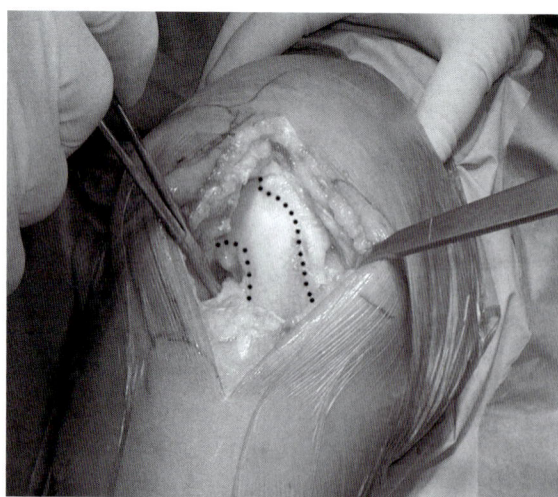

Figure 99-6. Operative view through a minimal incision shows the osteophytes to be removed and the ACL, with the knee at 45 degrees of flexion.

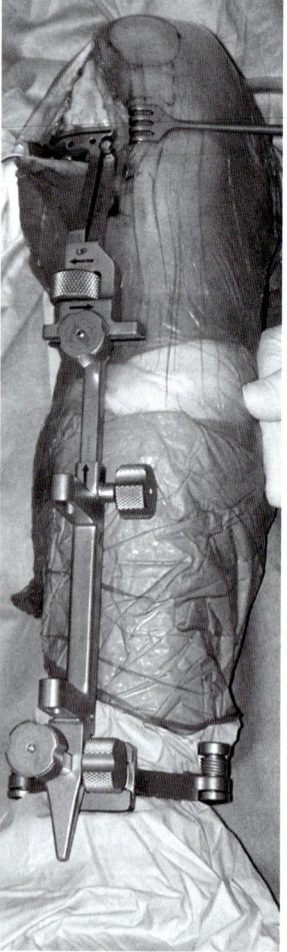

Figure 99-7. The tibial cut is made with an extramedullary cutting guide aligned on the tibial crest in the frontal plane and with a 5-degree posterior slope in the sagittal plane. The cutting jig is fixed on the superomedial part of the tibia (for a medial UKA).

axis of the guide lying slightly medial to the center of the ankle joint. The proximal part of the guide rests on the anterior tibia, pointing toward the axis of the tibial spines; with modern instrumentation, it is possible to have the cutting part of the guide resting only on the upper tibia (medial or lateral) to be resected. The diaphyseal part of the guide is parallel to the anterior tibial crest, and the anteroposterior position of the guide is adjusted distally to reproduce the natural upper tibial slope, usually between 5 and 7 degrees of posterior slope (see video on the website). The amount of resection is decided after using a 4-mm probe on the deepest part of the affected plateau, and particular care should be taken to define the level of the cut properly. To do so, it is important to control the level of resection using an angel wing probe to mimic the cut, not only on the anterior part of the plateau, but also on the posterior aspect (see video on the website). To complete the tibial cut, the sagittal tibial cut should be made. This could be done using one of the sagittal marks provided by the guide or made as a freehand cut. When the cut is made freehand, the cut should be aligned close to the tibial spine eminence. The anterior starting point is determined after checking the alignment of the edge of the femoral condyle on the tibial plateau when the knee is brought from flexion close to full extension. At this step, once again, particular care should be taken to protect the ACL (see video on the website).

Femoral Cut

The entrance hole of the distal femur for the intramedullary (IM) technique is centered above the roof of the intercondylar notch and prepared using an osteotome to conserve the cartilage. The drilling of the femoral medullary canal through a short incision often requires bringing the knee to 60 degrees of flexion. In fact, in flexion, the tension from the patella on the IM guide might induce incorrect alignment. Once the guide has been properly introduced, the distal femoral cut can be made by creating the angle between the anatomic and mechanical axis as previously calculated on the full weight-bearing view. This angle is usually 4 to 6 degrees. It is critical to protect the skin carefully at the proximal part of the incision while making this cut to avoid any skin damage (see video on the website). The amount of bone resected from the distal femur corresponds exactly, millimeter for millimeter, to the femoral prosthesis. The remainder of the femoral cuts (posterior cut and chamfers) will then be completed using the appropriate cutting block.

First, the size of the femoral implant should be determined using the cutting block. The size is determined once this femoral finishing guide is positioned on the distal femoral cut, looking for the best compromise between an anatomically centered position on the femoral condyle and a long axis perpendicular to the resected tibial plateau. The top of this finishing guide should be localized 1 to 2 mm above the deepest layer of the cartilage to avoid a potential notch between the femoral implant and patella. In other words, ideally, the femoral block should be slightly smaller anteriorly than the original femoral condyle (see video on the website). To control the mediolateral position of the femoral cutting guide, which determines the position of the final implant, the use of tibial referencing based on the previously made tibial cut is probably the best landmark. Because the divergence of

the medial condyle is different from one knee to another, checking the mediolateral position of the guide on the femoral condyle is also recommended. Once the posterior cut has been made and the cutting guide removed, removal of any posterior osteophytes is necessary using a curved osteotome to increase the range of flexion and avoid any posterior impingement with the polyethylene in high flexion (see video on the website).

Tibial Finishing and Trials

The size of the tibial tray should now be determined, obtaining the best compromise between maximal tibial coverage and overhang, which might induce pain. The AP size of the tibial plateau sometimes differs from the mediolateral one, especially for female knees, so different sizing trials are necessary to find the best compromise. It is important to keep the depth of the tibial cut as conservative as possible to take advantage of the strength of the tibial cortex and the increased area of contact proximally. The knee is then brought into maximal flexion and externally rotated. The final preparation of the tibia is completed with the appropriate guide, with the underlying keel impacted in the subchondral bone. Using a minimal incision, it is important to locate the posterior margin of the tibial plateau carefully to position the keel in the anteroposterior direction correctly. It is useful to precut the future location of the keel using a reciprocating saw blade or osteotom (see video on the website).

The flexion-extension gaps should be tested with the trial components in place, inserting a trial polyethylene liner. Common causes of impingement are residual bone eminence, incorrect position of the tibial or femoral component, or an oblique tibial cut. Once this has been verified, it is important at that step to look for a 2-mm protective laxity checked close to full extension to avoid any overcorrection of the deformity, which could lead to progression of osteoarthritis in the unreplaced compartment. On the other hand, important residual varus deformity should also be avoided, as recently reported, to minimize the risk of polyethylene wear when using flat polyethylene inserts.[6] The ideal correction, as measured on the postoperative full weight-bearing view, will probably consist of a tibiofemoral axis crossing the knee between the tibial spines and third of the tibial plateau for a medial UKA, as outlined by Kennedy and White[22] in their classification (Fig. 99-8). We cement all components for better fixation because long-term results suggest that loosening is not a common mode of failure with modern cemented, metal-backed components. The tibial component is cemented first, with the knee in full flexion and externally rotated for a medial UKA to improve the exposure of the medial compartment. When cementing the components, it is important to avoid leaving any cement at the posterior aspect of the knee; the use of a 90-degree curved probe is helpful to remove any posterior cement when using a minimal incision. Once the femoral implant has been cemented, bringing the knee close to extension helps remove any posterior cement, with the polyethylene inserted last (see video on the website). Patellar tracking should be checked before closing; the absence of patellar eversion during the procedure is helpful for that step. The tourniquet is released before closure to perform hemostasis adequately (see video on the website).

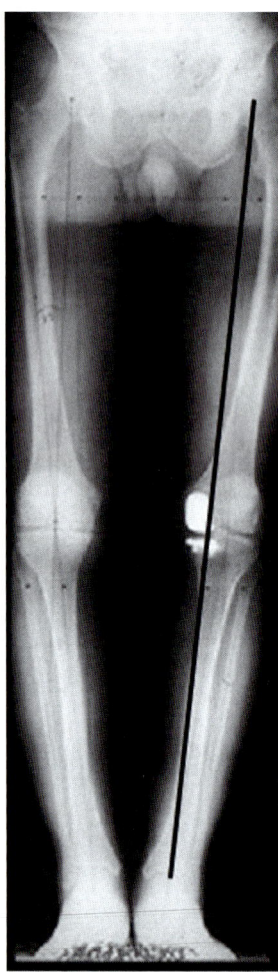

Figure 99-8. Full weight-bearing view of the limbs shows a hip-knee-ankle axis crossing the knee joint just medial to the tibial spines, leaving an undercorrected 3-degree varus deformity after a medial UKA.

Lateral Unicompartmental Replacement

The skin incision, using a minimal approach of the lateral compartment, needs to be lateral, especially at the distal portion, because of the frequent divergence of the lateral femoral condyle. When the lateral arthrotomy is performed, visualization of the joint is often easier than on the medial side because of the natural mobility of the lateral tibiofemoral joint. The tibial resection should stay minimal, because the disease is more often on the femoral side. In case of femoral dysplasia, it is often necessary to use a more proximodistal femoral cut.

The alignment of the femoral cutting guide on the tibial cut is crucial because of the natural shape of the lateral femoral condyle. It is frequently necessary to mark the correct alignment in extension rather than in flexion to avoid any medial edge loading and impingement between the femoral implant and tibial spines. The polyethylene insert is often thicker than for the medial side in case of femoral dysplasia, even if the principle of undercorrection of the deformity for all cases of lateral UKA remains the basis for successful long-term results.

In our practice, lateral UKA corresponds to 10% of the indications for UKA and our long-term results have confirmed those of previous studies, that lateral osteoarthritis can be treated successfully by unicondylar replacement.[7] The in vivo kinematic evaluation of patients implanted with lateral UKA has found a greater posterior displacement of the femorotibial contact point during flexion as compared with patients implanted with medial UKA.[4]

Postoperative Care

In our practice, one intra-articular drain is left for 36 hours. Postoperatively, immediate weight-bearing is recommended after the removal of the femoral nerve block catheter (left 12 hours postoperatively), protected by two crutches for 1 or 2 weeks. Manual range of motion physiotherapy is performed the day after surgery. Deep veinous thrombosis prevention is managed using mechanical devices and low-dose heparin for 3 weeks postoperatively.

OUTCOMES

Survivorship studies generated from early unicompartmental series have shown that survivorship rates at 10 years were decreasing into the 85% range. With better patient selection and reproducible instrumentation, more recent series have shown 10-year survivorship regularly at 90% or greater.[2] Many now also support the view that revision of a modern UKA is a relatively common and simple procedure.[14] Patients from the Swedish registry were more satisfied after revision of a failed UKA than after revision of TKA.[37]

Results With Mini-Invasive Surgery

This surgical technique combines the advantages of the limited incision in the extensor mechanism with the precision of modern and dedicated cutting guides.[9] Therefore, this MIS technique can be routinely performed with reliability (Fig. 99-9). Few reports are available at midterm follow-up for the evaluation of UKA performed through a mini-incision. After the initial description by Repicci and Eberle,[34] Romanowski and Repicci[39] evaluated a group of 136 knees implanted with UKA performed through a mini-incision at 8-year follow-up. The revision rate was 7%, including 3 of 10 for technical errors, and the revision time for osteoarthritis progression averaged 5 years. They suggested that the procedure was only temporary to relieve pain and improve function, with minimal morbidity. This suggestion contrasts with the long-term results reported for UKA performed through a conventional incision, with a survival rate greater than 94% at 10 or 13 years.[2,11] We believe that the results and technical errors reported by Romanowsky and Repicci highlight the difficulty of performing the procedure through a minimal incision if the visualization is not appropriate. Hamilton and colleagues[19] recently evaluated a group of 221 UKAs performed through a mini-incision and compared these cases with a previous group of 514 knees operated on with an open technique. They reported an overall revision rate for aseptic loosening of 3.7% in the mini-incision group compared with 1% in the group with the open technique. There is probably less tolerance in UKA compared with TKA in component malpositioning, and it is therefore critical to evaluate the radiographic position of components implanted with a limited incision carefully to provide the same reproducibility as the

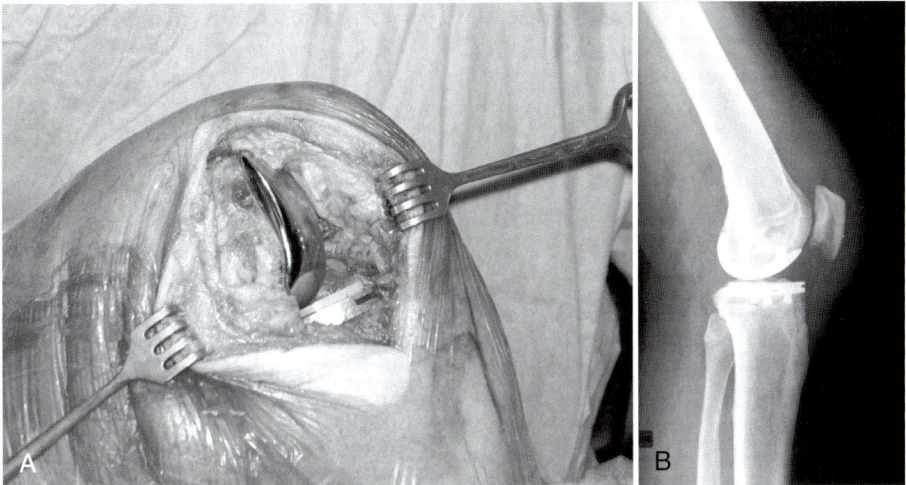

Figure 99-9. Intraoperative view **(A)** and postoperative sagittal radiograph **(B)** show a medial UKA implanted through an 8-cm skin incision and without disruption of the extensor mechanism.

open technique. There is no doubt that limiting or eliminating extensor mechanism disruption during the procedure provides more rapid recovery with less morbidity, as mentioned in the original report by Price and associates[31] using the Oxford knee. All the clinical and functional outcomes reports tend to show quicker recovery with limited pitfalls for patients implanted with UKA performed through a mini-incision. However, no study has yet evaluated implant survival at 10 years, commonly considered as the acceptable threshold for joint reconstruction procedures.

Results in Young Patients

In a study evaluating the results of UKA in those younger than 50 years, our results[29] suggested that the following: (1) UKA for unicompartmental arthritis is reliable for improving function in patients younger than 50 years and allowed a return to previous level of activities; (2) satisfying radiologic results can be achieved in terms of implant fixation and alignment and in restoring lower limb alignment; and (3) survivorship is acceptable but lower than the previously reported survivorship for older patients. In fact, revisions for polyethylene wear or progression of arthritis in the patellofemoral joint remain important concerns in altering the survivorship of the implant in this group of patients. Our experience has shown that knee function can be restored after UKA in patients younger than 50 years and UKA may be a reliable option for middle-aged patients; however, wear after 10 years remains a problem in this category of patients. In our series, four of the six revisions were related to polyethylene wear. We were unable to identify specific causes such as misalignment or body mass index in this group of patients to account for this wear. In the four cases, a direct exchange of the worn polyethylene insert for a new one was easily performed through a minimally invasive incision. Also, the functional results according to the Knee Society scores for these patients were comparable to those obtained for the unrevised patients at last follow-up. In our series, there was one case of osteoarthritis progression that required revision with a standard posterior stabilized TKA. Price and coworkers[31] reported a multicentric comparison between 512 patients older than 60 years and 53 patients younger than 60 years implanted with an Oxford UKA. The results of this comparison suggested that the Oxford medial UKA functions well and is durable in patients younger than 60 years, even if the calculated survivorship in this series was lower for the patients younger than 60 years (91% at 10 years in the <60-year group versus 96% in the >60-year group). UKA may be a reliable option for middle-aged patients, but wear after 10 years remains a problem in this category of patients.

Results of Lateral Unicompartmental Knee Arthroplasty

Unicompartmental femorotibial OA usually affects the medial compartment of the knee and, more rarely, the lateral compartment. In addition to osteotomy for correction of a valgus deformity, the surgical treatment of lateral femorotibial osteoarthritis includes TKA or UKA. The results of our study[8] have shown that lateral UKA can provide satisfying long-term clinical and radiologic results and the survivorship at 10, 16, and 22 years is comparable with the survivorship obtained for medial UKA in the literature. Our results at a maximum follow-up of 23 years ranged between the results of older and more recent studies of lateral UKA reported in the literature. Recent studies reported a very low failure rate, whereas the results of older series were more controversial. As noted, we observed a significant improvement of results over time, which is probably linked first to an improvement of patient selection, as illustrated by the two cases revised before 3 years for arthritis progression in the 1980s (group of patients operated on before 1989). A 21% failure rate was reported using the mobile-bearing Oxford unicompartmental prosthesis in the lateral compartment, with a 10% rate of bearing dislocation. This difference in the commonly reported excellent long-term results using the same implant for the medial compartment may be explained by the amount of femoral translation of the lateral condyle while the medial one remained fairly stationary. According to these results, and because of the biomechanical properties of the lateral compartment, fixed-bearing implants seem more appropriate.[7] Thus, two recent studies have shown more favorable results using fixed bearing UKA at midterm or long-and associates term follow-up. Although original reports comparing medial and lateral UKA were conflicting, the results of our series on patients treated surgically after 1989 were comparable with those reported recently and compare favorably with the results of medial UKA.

Results for Avascular Osteonecrosis of the Knee

In a retrospective study,[28] we analyzed the results of UKA for osteonecrosis using a modern implant and strict inclusion criteria, first regarding the limitation of the osteonecrosis to one compartment of the knee, even for cases of secondary osteonecrosis and, second, regarding the status of the uninvolved compartment, patellofemoral articulation, and ACL. The data suggest that UKA is reliable in osteonecrosis for alleviating pain and improving function, restoring proper lower limb mechanical axis, and achieving a durable survivorship at 12 years. Few studies have reported the results of a continuous series of UKA implanted for osteonecrosis.[28] A recent literature review has shown varying outcomes after UKA for spontaneous osteonecrosis of the knee and better outcomes with TKA. Nonetheless, the authors noted an improvement in outcome scores for the most recent series of UKA for osteonecrosis of the knee with strict selection criteria. These studies reported results of UKA only for spontaneous osteonecrosis.

The outcomes of UKA reported in our study for osteonecrosis are comparable with the average results of TKA for osteonecrosis, with a revision rate of 3% and a mean global knee score of 85 points. The 96.7% survival at 12 years is encouraging, and this favorable outcome may be related to different factors. Patient selection included osteonecrosis limited to a single femorotibial compartment, a fully correctable deformity on stress radiographs, a healthy patellofemoral joint, and an intact ACL. The second consideration may be related to the systematic use of cement in our series to fix the UKA components, as previously emphasized in TKA for osteonecrosis, with reported improvement in patient outcomes after TKA for osteonecrosis of the knee by using of cement with all components. Finally, the use of a bone-cutting device combined with a femoral component, including pegs, most often permitted a resection of the entire osteonecrotic lesion and secured the implant fixation in a healthy bone.

SUMMARY

Unicondylar knee replacement should not be considered as a temporary procedure; the 10-year survival can be as good as with TKA if patient selection and surgical principles are followed carefully. The advantages of UKA compared with TKA include retention of both cruciate ligaments, preservation of bone stock in the opposite compartment and patellofemoral joint, and better functional results. For young and active patients, a modern UKA represents a valid alternative to bridge the gap between high tibial osteotomy and TKA with isolated unicompartmental tibiofemoral noninflammatory disease (Ahlback grade 3 or higher). Although component loosening and progression of the arthritis in the remaining compartments has become rare with appropriate patient selection and adequate surgical technique, polyethylene wear, associated with a flat metal-backed component, remains a problem, particularly in the youngest, active, and heavy patients. The last decade's progress in terms of surgical technique, instrumentation, and implant designs have made unicompartmental arthroplasty the standard of treatment for patients with severe osteoarthritis limited to one tibiofemoral compartment.

KEY REFERENCES

Argenson JN, Chevrol-Benkeddache Y, Aubaniac JM: Modern unicompartmental knee arthroplasty with cement: a three to ten-year follow-up study. J Bone Joint Surg Am 84:2235–2239, 2002.

Argenson JN, Flecher X, Parratte S: [Mini-invasive implantation of an unicompartmental medial knee prosthesis.] Rev Chir Orthop Reparatrice Appar Mot 92:193–199, 2006.

Argenson JN, Komistek RD, Aubaniac JM, et al: In vivo determination of knee kinematics for subjects implanted with a unicompartmental arthroplasty. J Arthroplasty 17:1049–1054, 2002.

Argenson JN, Parratte S: The unicompartmental knee: design and technical considerations in minimizing wear. Clin Orthop Relat Res 452:137–142, 2006.

Argenson JN, Parratte S, Bertani A, et al: Long-term results with a lateral unicondylar replacement. Clin Orthop Relat Res 466: 2686–2693, 2008.

Argenson JN, Parratte S, Bertani A, et al: The new arthritic patient and arthroplasty treatment options. J Bone Joint Surg Am 91(Suppl 5):43–48, 2009.

Argenson JN, Parratte S, Flecher X, Aubaniac JM: Unicompartmental knee arthroplasty: technique through a mini-incision. Clin Orthop Relat Res (464):32–36, 2007.

Goodfellow J, O'Connor J, Murray DW: The Oxford meniscal unicompartmental knee. J Knee Surg 15:240–246, 2002.

Kennedy WR, White RP: Unicompartmental arthroplasty of the knee. Postoperative alignment and its influence on overall results. Clin Orthop Relat Res (221):278–285, 1987.

Kozinn SC, Scott R: Unicondylar knee arthroplasty. J Bone Joint Surg Am 71:145–150, 1989.

Parratte S, Argenson JN, Dumas J, Aubaniac JM: Unicompartmental knee arthroplasty for avascular osteonecrosis. Clin Orthop Relat Res 464:7–42, 2007.

Parratte S, Argenson JN, Pearce O, et al: Medial unicompartmental knee replacement in the under-50s. J Bone Joint Surg Br 91:351–356, 2009.

Parratte S, Pauly V, Aubaniac JM, Argenson JN: Survival of bicompartmental knee arthroplasty at 5 to 23 years. Clin Orthop Relat Res (468):64–72, 2010.

Price AJ, O'Connor JJ, Murray DW, et al: A history of Oxford unicompartmental knee arthroplasty. Orthopedics 30(5 Suppl):7–10, 2007.

Repicci JA: Mini-invasive knee unicompartmental arthroplasty: bone-sparing technique. Surg Technol Int 11:282–286, 2003.

Robertsson O, Knutson K, Lewold S, Lidgren L: The Swedish Knee Arthroplasty Register 1975-1997: an update with special emphasis on 41,223 knees operated on in 1988-1997. Acta Orthop Scand 72: 503–513, 2001.

Scott RD, Cobb AG, McQueary FG, Thornhill TS: Unicompartmental knee arthroplasty. Eight- to 12-year follow-up evaluation with survivorship analysis. Clin Orthop Relat Res (271):96–100, 1991.

Full references for this chapter can be found on www.expertconsult.com.

Unicompartmental Knee Arthroplasty: International Roundtable Discussion

Jean-Noël Argenson, David Murray, Thomas M. Coon, Gerard A. Engh, Richard A. Berger, Hong Zhang, and Richard D. Scott

Jean-Noël Argenson: Unicompartmental knee arthroplasty (UKA) has become a popular surgical technique. UKA represents the logical treatment option for an isolated femorotibial lesion of the knee. When the other compartments of the knee are preserved, there is no need to perform a total knee arthroplasty (TKA). When comparing the outcomes of UKA and TKA, several studies have shown that recovery is faster after UKA, and that patient satisfaction is greater, because the knee feels more natural. However, UKA has a specific mode of failure, which is progression of disease in unreplaced compartments. This might be related to surgical technique, but the most critical issue remains patient selection. Improper patient selection combined with limited instrumentation and suboptimal design may explain the less than satisfactory results originally published for UKA. However, in the United States, Europe, and Asia, indications have been more clearly defined, design and instrumentation have shown significant evolution, and the operation can be performed routinely using a minimally invasive technique. Therefore, it is interesting to share experiences within a group of international experts, which includes David Murray, Tom Coon, Jerry Engh, Richard Berger, Hong Zhang, and Richard Scott. Let us start this discussion with patient selection, which is critical for UKA. My own experience has shown that UKA is applicable mainly to osteoarthritis, and in some cases to avascular osteonecrosis. Dick, do you concur with that statement, and regarding osteoarthritis, what type of deformity in varus or in valgus do you think is suitable for UKA?

Richard Scott: I agree that UKA should be limited to patients with a noninflammatory, nonsystemic form of arthritis. I would add post-traumatic arthritis to your list, for example, lateral compartment degeneration that might follow a lateral plateau fracture.

UKA is contraindicated in RA (unless clearly "burned out") and in any patients with a history of inflammatory synovitis such as gout or pseudogout. The presence of radiographic chondrocalcinosis in the opposite compartment is a relative contraindication.

Severe deformity is a contraindication to UKA because it is difficult to correct. This is represented by more than 10 degrees of mechanical axis deviation in a varus knee, and by 5 to 7 degrees of deviation in a valgus knee. An attenuated medical collateral ligament (MCL) in a valgus knee is also a contraindication.

Jean-Noël Argenson: These indications clinically and radiographically speaking have been nicely outlined by Richard Scott for the femorotibial compartment; however, what about the third compartment represented by the patellofemoral joint (PFJ)? David, is it true to say that in Oxford it is very unlikely to have a UKA indication withdrawn because of the state of the patellofemoral joint?

David Murray: Indications for the mobile-bearing Oxford UKA are different from those for the fixed-bearing UKA. In early studies of the Oxford knee, it was found that the state of the PFJ did not influence the outcome. We therefore advised surgeons to ignore the PFJ and have implanted large numbers of Oxford knees, regardless of the state of the PFJ. As a result, we have been able to study in detail the effect of the PFJ on outcome. Our recent studies have confirmed that for medial UKA, the state of the PFJ can be ignored unless severe lateral PFJ arthritis with bone loss is present. In these rare cases, which involve combined medial tibiofemoral and lateral patellofemoral arthritis, a total knee replacement (TKR) should be implanted. Damage to the trochlear or medial part of the PFJ, however severe, should not be considered a contraindication to mobile-bearing UKA. In addition, anterior knee pain is not a contraindication.

Jean-Noël Argenson: Jerry, it is classical to assume that a functional anterior cruciate ligament (ACL) is mandatory for performing a UKA; however, both our kinematic evaluation of patients with flat fixed tibial bearings and the clinical outcomes of these sedentary patients with a probable secondary distention of the ACL have confirmed that correct clinical function of the knee may be achieved in these low-demand patients using fixed bearings, despite ACL deficiency. Based on your experience, what is your current attitude regarding the state of the ACL?

Jerry Engh: In most of my patients, an absent or attenuated ACL is not a contraindication to a fixed-bearing medial UKA. A patient who does not engage in running or twisting sporting activities and has no symptoms of knee instability prior to surgery will achieve a result similar to that of a patient with a functional ACL following medial unicompartmental arthroplasty.

Historically, patients with ACL deficiency have not done well with mobile-bearing implants. These implants failed by premature tibial component loosening, not by bearing dislocation. The load pattern on the tibial component is different in a knee with ACL deficiency. A mobile-bearing implant is more likely to experience eccentric loading that could cause loosening in a ligamentous deficient knee. In ACL-deficient knees, I prefer to reduce the anteroposterior (AP) slope of the tibial resection to tighten the flexion gap and reduce AP laxity.

Over the past 9 years, I have implanted UKAs in 87 patients (98 knees) with both attenuated (53 knees) and absent (45 knees) ACLs at the time of unicompartmental arthroplasty. Three of these patients died of causes unrelated to the arthroplasty without returning for 2-year follow-up. We revised five patients (six knees) for progression of disease (three knees), aseptic loosening (2 knees), and pain (1 knee). Fifty patients (56 knees) had clinical and radiographic follow-up at a mean of 40 months (range, 24 to 75 months). The mean American Knee Society Clinical Rating System (KS) Clinical Score of these patients was 92 points (range, 75 to 100 points), the mean KS Function Score was 84 points (range, 45 to 100 points), and the mean arc of motion was 127 degrees (range, 101 to 145 degrees). Patients reported less pain in the knee (89%), better function in the knee (88%), and overall satisfaction with the UKA (86%). No patient reported problems with knee instability.

Premature implant wear is another theoretical concern. In the laboratory, wear of polyethylene is increased with multidirectional sliding of metal on polyethylene. The same multidirectional sliding might occur in an ACL-deficient knee. However, I am unaware of any clinical studies that document accelerated wear in ACL-deficient knees.

Jean-Noël Argenson: Thanks Jerry, for reporting this experience, particularly in patients with no complaint of instability before the indication of UKA. Age and weight also represent debating issues for the indication of UKA, because the procedure is often presented as an alternative to osteotomy based on patient age. Our own experience shows that the best indication for osteotomy remains the young, heavy, active male patient with the presence of joint space and bony deformity. Regarding age and based on comparative results at 10 years after UKA and TKA, Richard Scott considered that UKA might assume its role in two groups of patients: middle-aged osteoarthritic patients and osteoarthritic octogenarians who are having their "first and last" arthroplasty. Dick, are there any changes in your current indications?

Richard Scott: I agree with you that osteotomy should always be considered in the young, heavy, active male patient. I still think that UKA is an excellent alternative to osteotomy in the middle-aged patient (especially female) compared with osteotomy. It leads to faster recovery, fewer complications, better longevity, and a better cosmetic result.

If revision should become necessary in the future, this is easy to accomplish following UKA as long as a conservative initial tibial resection has been performed.

I still advocate UKA in octogenarians as long as they are ideal (not borderline) candidates. Recovery is generally faster than after TKA, with better flexion, less medical morbidity, less need for transfusion, and better prosthetic survivorship than are seen with TKA.

Jean-Noël Argenson: I think we now have a more precise perception of the "ideal" patient candidate for a UKA regarding age, etiology, deformity, and state of the joint. Let us move to design considerations, because these might have a direct impact on knee function and on the types of activities performed by the patient following the procedure. The importance of full coverage of the condyle by the femoral component has been recently highlighted to allow full range of motion without impingement. Hong, how important are these activities in high flexion for the patients you have to treat, and more generally, in the Asian world?

Hong Zhang: In Asia, lifestyle and habits depend on religious beliefs, cultural background, and customs. Kneeling and cross-legged and squat positions are part of life for many Asian people when they pray, when they eat, when they get together and chat, and even when they go to the toilet. We understand that many patients expect to go back to their normal lifestyle after knee replacement, so achieving high flexion and full range of motion would be what surgeons strive for. However, although TKA has increased dramatically in Asian countries in recent years, the total number of UKAs performed is still very low. Riddle and colleagues reported that unicompartmental implants accounted for about 8% of all knee arthroplasty procedures in the United States in 2005 (Riddle D, Jiranek M, McGlynn F: Yearly incidence of unicompartmental knee arthroplasty in the United States. J Arthroplasty 23:408–412, 2008). But in Japan in 2007, UKA occurred in less than 1% of those with knee arthroplasty (data from 2007 yearly report of Yano Research Institute Ltd). In China, our UKA numbers are less than 1% as well (data from Beijing Jishuitan Hospital). Most of our patients present with end-stage arthritis when they come to us. It is very hard to find "ideal" patient candidates for UKA.

Jean-Noël Argenson: Yes, this is very true, and I do believe there are regional answers in terms of indications but also for designing philosophy. Rich, for this specific area related to designing considerations, metal backing of the tibial component is controversial because on one side, wear-through or enhanced polyethylene flow has been described with the use of metal backing, but on the other side, the modular tray allows polyethylene exchange without bone invasion through a limited incision. What is your experience?

Richard Berger: I believe that a modular metal-backed tibial component is superior to an all-polyethylene tibial component because of its ability to be easily replaced for wear and its superb long-term results. First, the modular polyethylene insert of a metal-backed component can be easily replaced if significant wear occurs. With an all-polyethylene component, if wear occurs, the entire component must be revised. Second, because a significant amount of polyethylene wear comes from third-body wear from retained cement, the modularity of a metal-backed component facilitates cement removal. Finally, great long-term results have been reported with the metal-backed component. We reported 11-year to 15-year results of UKA with a metal backing. Average follow-up was 13 years (range, 11 to 15 years). No component was radiographically loose, and no osteolysis was seen. Kaplan-Meier survival with loosening or revision for any reason was 98.0% ± 2.0% at 10 years, and 95.7% ± 4.3% at 15 years. Last, even though 64% of these cases had the thinnest polyethylene—only 5.7 mm of actual polyethylene—no revisions for polyethylene wear were performed.

Jean-Noël Argenson: I concur with this experience, including polyethylene liner exchange in UKA, and we have now a few cases at 5 years' follow-up after the exchange, extending then the overall survival of the UKA to more than 15 years, which is encouraging. However, polyethylene wear is one mode of failure of UKA, besides osteoarthritis progression, and it is multifactorial. Jerry, how important may material properties be in the issue of poly wear?

Jerry Engh: Polyethylene wear was the primary reason for failure of unicondylar arthroplasties when we were using polyethylene that was gamma-irradiated in air. Until the year 2000, 75% of the revisions at our institution were related directly to polyethylene wear. When we examined the revised implants in our lab, all of the gamma-irradiated components had some degree of delamination. During the same time interval, none of the nonirradiated implants were revised. The retrieval lab at Dartmouth reported a similar experience with nonirradiated polyethylene. A group of 16 retrieved unicondylar implants in situ after more than 15 years showed no evidence of fatigue-type wear.

Over the past 9 years at our institution, and since the industry shift to nongamma sterilization or sterilization in an inert environment, we have had no revisions of unicondylar implants for polyethylene wear. Therefore, in response to your question, the material properties appear to no longer be a major issue. However, I do have concern about implants irradiated in an inert environment without quenching of free radicals after the sterilization process. When retrieved components that have been irradiated in an inert environment were analyzed, it appears that oxidation in vivo is a real concern. If we have delayed oxidation only by sterilizing and vacuum packaging the components, polyethylene wear could re-emerge as a factor in the failure of UKAs with a longer time interval in situ.

Jean-Noël Argenson: Thanks for this update regarding properties issues. David, mobile bearings have been presented as the answer to polyethylene wear in UKA, and both retrieval studies and clinical outcomes with the Oxford knee have shown very limited wear. How different are the designing principles of a mobile-bearing meniscal knee in UKA?

David Murray: The Oxford knee was designed to minimize wear by reproducing the function of the normal meniscus. The meniscus, being compliant, achieves fully congruent contact in all positions with the femoral and tibial condyles, so contact stress and thus wear are low. In the artificial situation, because polyethylene cannot change shape, fully congruous contact can be achieved only by using a spherical femoral component. The Oxford knee therefore has a spherical femoral component, a flat tibial component, and an unconstrained bearing with a spherically concave upper surface and a flat lower surface. It has been shown to have very low wear (about 0.01 mm/yr), provided it has been implanted correctly without impingement. It is safe to use polyethylene as thin as 3 mm, so bone stock can be preserved. Unlike fixed-bearing designs, it can be used safely in young, heavy, active men. It also provides full flexion, which is important in Asian countries.

Jean-Noël Argenson: Thank you David, but what can be said to surgeons who are afraid of bearing dislocation and the difficulty of reproducing the surgical technique in every case?

David Murray: With phase 3 instrumentation, which is now generally used, the incidence of bearing dislocation following medial Oxford UKA is very low (less than 1%). So surgeons need not be unduly concerned. In contrast, the dislocation rate for lateral replacement has been high. We have therefore recommended that mobile bearings should not be used in the lateral compartment. However, short-term results of the new design of Oxford lateral UKA, which has a convex tibial component and a biconcave bearing, are encouraging with a low dislocation rate. In the future, this may be a good solution for lateral compartment arthritis.

The phase 3 instrumentation was designed for a minimally invasive approach and is relatively straightforward to use. It accurately balances the flexion and extension gaps. So, as well as preventing dislocation, it reliably restores knee kinematics and function to normal.

Jean-Noël Argenson: As mentioned by David, minimally invasive surgery (MIS) is now the routine approach for UKA without everting the patella, and I must say that the quality of patient recovery and implant positioning has been highly reproducible in our experience. Tom, what are your tricks

regarding the soft tissue environment to obtain adequate exposure of the knee?

Tom Coon: Good surgical exposure is critical to good results in UKA. It is desirable to avoid quadriceps muscle trauma to achieve the excellent rehabilitation results possible with the MIS technique. I have found that the best way to facilitate exposure is to use the medial retinacular "T," as recommended by Tria. This is done midway between the lower edge of the vastus medialis and the medial meniscus. It allows excellent visualization of the medial joint space for removal of osteophytes, placement of implants, or removal of cement, and it provides a good view of the medial tibia for assessment of the tibial slope, as well as for correct placement of the tibial cutting guide. In some cases, it may be useful to perform a medial patellar facetectomy as recommended by Repicci, although I have rarely found this to be necessary.

It is very useful also to utilize the "mobile window," that is, move the tissue opening from side to side or up and down, and to flex or extend the knee to tense or relax the extensor mechanism as necessary. Tibial exposure can be facilitated by the use of a leg holder, which allows the tibia to be fixed in internal or external rotation, thus allowing easy placement of instruments and implants.

Jean-Noël Argenson: Tom just showed us how to position correctly the tibial cutting guide in the frontal plane, but Hong, what about the tibial slope, which may be increased in some knees, and the direction of the sagittal cut at the upper surface of the tibia?

Hong Zhang: From my personal experience, I try to make a 5 to 7 degree tibial slope. This is the anatomic slope angle, and most manufacturers require the same slope angle as well. When I do my tibial plateau resection, I start with the vertical cut, made with the reciprocating saw. This step helps me confirm the lateral margin of the medial tibial plateau and the origin of the ACL to avoid damaging its fibers. Then I use a 12 mm wide oscillating saw blade to cut about a 2 mm thick plateau by naked eyes, without using the tibial saw guide. I find that without the tibial saw guide, it is more safe and accurate to finish the tibial cut, while not damaging the ACL.

Jean-Noël Argenson: I fully agree with this last point, and I usually bring the knee into extension at this step to decide where to start the vertical cut, according to where the lateral edge of the medial condyle will rest on the tibial plateau. Rich, do you think pin fixation may act as a stress raiser and increase the risk of tibial plateau fracture following UKA?

Richard Berger: Yes, pin fixation does act as a stress raiser, leading to fractures. Perioperatively, we had a high incidence (5%) of medial tibial plateau fractures in our series. This complication has been reported in other series but is rare. The high tibial fracture rate in our series was technique related. These fractures were related to the fixation pins for the tibial alignment guide, which were impacted without predrilling; furthermore, these pins were located in a row at the corner of the tibial resection—the area of greatest stress. Because we recognized the cause of these fractures, the tibial holes were predrilled and relocated; subsequently, tibial fractures have not occurred. Of note, fortunately these tibial fractures in our series did heal without adverse sequelae. Fractures of the medial tibial plateau fracture that were noted on the postoperative radiograph were treated nonoperatively and healed uneventfully. A fracture, when noted intraoperatively, was treated with screw fixation and also healed uneventfully.

Jean-Noël Argenson: Thank you Rich, for reporting this experience and, more important, for describing how such complications can be avoided. Moving now to the femoral component, I always found that mediolateral and rotational placement of the femoral implant was a critical issue in UKA, despite the type of design. Jerry, what is your own experience?

Jerry Engh: Component-to-component positioning is critical to avoid the two major causes of implant failure: aseptic loosening and implant wear. Abnormal medial-to-lateral positioning causes edge loading that can result in tibial bone collapse or aseptic loosening. Malrotation of the components increases contact stresses and accelerates implant wear.

The problem with component positioning relates to instrumentation and surgical technique, not to the design of the implant. Intramedullary instruments set the alignment of the components not to each other, but to the bone to which they are attached. This may or may not be correct for the rotation and translation of components.

The rotational alignment of the femoral component is dictated by the posterior condylar cut from the femur. If this cut is made in varus alignment to the patient's posterior femoral condyles, the femoral component will be internally rotated. When the knee is in full extension, this internal rotation can result in edge loading of the tibial component. Likewise, if the femoral component is centered on the femoral condyle, it may not articulate with the center of the tibial component. The femoral component should be positioned over the center of the tibial component.

I prefer setting the position of the femoral component relative to the center of the tibial component by using spacer blocks after the tibial resection to orient both the rotation and the translation of the femoral component. I use an extramedullary guide to resect the tibia; I then insert a spacer block to check the flexion/extension gap balance and tibial coverage. Next, I bring the knee to full extension and mark the front of the femur so that when the posterior condylar cut is made, the femur will be correctly oriented and centered on the tibial implant as referenced by this mark. With the knee flexed, I rotate the sizing/cutting guide and align the mark on the front of the femur before making the posterior condylar resection that will set the femoral implant properly.

Jean-Noël Argenson: David, is this true also for mobile bearings?

David Murray: One of the advantages of the mobile-bearing device is that component orientation is not critical. Because the femoral component is spherical, and because the contact area is large (6 cm^2), moderate amounts of component malalignment do not matter. We have found that 10 degrees of femoral component malalignment in all directions with 5 degrees of tibial component malalignment in all directions does not compromise the outcome. Therefore, the procedure is very forgiving, provided that the soft tissues are accurately balanced.

Jean-Noël Argenson: Dick, in my experience, lateral UKA is equally successful compared with medial UKA and represents 10% of my uni indications. How different can the surgical principles of lateral UKA be?

Richard Scott: My ratio of medial to lateral UKAs is also 10 to 1. This means that we all have less experience with lateral UKA, and it is technically more difficult than medial arthroplasty. Patellar impingement on the leading edge of the femoral component is more likely to occur. One must be careful to recess the leading edge of the femoral component to avoid this impingement. Little or no posterior slope should be applied to the tibial resection to avoid a postoperative posterior wear pattern. Medial-lateral incongruency is more likely, and one must err toward placing the femoral component laterally on the femoral condyle, and the tibial component medially on the tibial plateau.

Exposure for the arthroplasty can be attained through a short lateral arthroplasty or through a medial parapatellar approach, while sparing the anterior horn of the medial meniscus and subluxing or everting the patella. The medial approach allows easy intraoperative conversion to TKA if appropriate.

Jean-Noël Argenson: Yes, and following these considerations, our published results of lateral UKA compared equally with those reported for medial UKA. Tom, talking now about overall alignment of the limb, how different is the alignment goal following UKA compared with TKA?

Tom Coon: The generally accepted standard of alignment for the TKA is the neutral mechanical axis. This is done to promote equal loading of the tibial component and thus improve longevity of the implant. In the case of the UKA, longevity is promoted by slightly shifting the mechanical axis toward the implant to reduce the chance of progressive degeneration of the contralateral compartment. Toward this end, it is generally better practice to undercorrect the deformity by 1 or 2 degrees; this can be accomplished by filling the existing ligament envelope with an implant thickness sufficient to allow 1 to 2 mm laxity with the existing ligament, and by performing no ligament releases. This translates to undercorrection of 1 to 2 degrees, that is, a final varus of 3 to 5 degrees, or valgus of 7 to 8 degrees.

Jean-Noël Argenson: I also like observing the postoperative mechanical axis of the limb crossing the joint line somewhere between the tibial spines and the middle of my tibial plateau after UKA. Hong, because the possibilities of adjusting soft tissue tension are limited in UKA, what is your rationale for balancing flexion/extension gaps and choosing the appropriate insert thickness?

Hong Zhang: Because most UKA patients have mild varus or valgus deformity, with or without mild flexion contracture, we do not need to do too much soft tissue work during UKA surgery. For example, for 5 degrees of varus deformity, I will peel the medial tibial periosteum about 1 to 2 cm and completely remove the osteophytes and medial meniscus; this is sufficient for soft tissue release. Then I will follow the tibial and femoral cutting instructions to finish the bone cut and put the trail components in to test the tension of the flexion/extension gap. For fixed-bearing UKA, I will keep 1 mm open under the tension or flexion/extension position. I will also make sure that the mechanical alignment of the lower extremity is not overcorrected.

Jean-Noël Argenson: This 1 or 2 mm opening of the compartment is indeed probably a safe way to avoid overcorrection. Dick, what can be the role of computer-assisted surgery in the field of UKA?

Richard Scott: Computer-assisted surgery has promise for the future both in assessing alignment and in preparing the bony surfaces. I must confess that I presently have no personal experience with this technique. I find it to be too time consuming, too expensive, and un-necessary in most cases. I look forward to its eventual use, however, when these issues are resolved.

Jean-Noël Argenson: This is probably correct, and it will be interesting to follow the evolutions in the field of navigation and in using robotic assistance adapted to UKA. The 10-year results of UKA reveal that several centers regularly reported survival rates over 90% and very comparable with those of TKA. Results reported in national and community-based registries showed survivorship at 10 years around 88% for UKA compared with 94% for TKA. The same national registry in Sweden reported that patients are more satisfied after revision of a failed UKA than after revision of a TKA. Rich, it is now commonly supported that revision of a modern UKA is a simple procedure. Don't you think that this may play a role in differences reported by such registries?

Richard Berger: Yes. I think that we all see total knee patients who have some pain, or who are dissatisfied with their replacement; unless there is a definable and significant source of their pain, few of us recommend a revision. This is because a total knee revision is often a difficult procedure that has significant morbidity. Moreover, even with successful revision, the patient often has residual pain and some dysfunction. Therefore, we tell TKA patients who have pain or are dissatisfied that this is something they must learn to live with.

Conversely, the unicompartmental replacement patient who has some pain or who is dissatisfied, even without a definable or significant source of pain, often gets a conversion to a TKA. This is done because a conversion to a total knee is usually an easy procedure that does not have significant morbidity. Moreover, a successful conversion, as you have pointed out, often results in a perfectly functioning TKA. Therefore, we tell the UKA patient who has pain or is dissatisfied that a conversion to a TKA is warranted. It is a double standard that results in a higher revision rate for unicompartmental replacements than for total knee replacements.

Jean-Noël Argenson: Thanks Rich, for highlighting this point. Tom, what can be the role of the learning curve and providing courses on these results, since UKA is, by definition, a less frequently performed surgery than TKA?

Tom Coon: UKA is indeed less frequently performed than TKA, with UKA accounting for 10T to 25% of the knee replacement practice. For most surgeons who do them infrequently, learning centers are critical to allow improved confidence and better results with this technically demanding procedure. Specific implants have different technical requirements, and surgeons should avail themselves of widely available training courses, so that the nuances of each system to be used can be appreciated. Additionally, as was mentioned previously, newer techniques such as computer navigation and robotics can be learned and may help mitigate problems with earlier systems such as poor implant placement or alignment.

Jean-Noël Argenson: Since we have reached the end of this roundtable, I would like to thank all of you coming from different parts of the world for sharing your experiences with unicompartmental knee arthroplasty. We have been able to better define indications for the procedure, because many early failures are simply related to the wrong indications. Although surgical technique is now currently realized through MIS, this roundtable has explained ways of adhering to the well-established principle of undercorrection, because progression of osteoarthritis in the unreplaced compartment is a frequent mode of failure following UKA. Progress in instrumentation and in design has made the procedure an attractive solution for preserving both ligaments and cartilage for osteoarthritis limited to one femorotibial compartment of the knee.

Isolated patellofemoral arthritis can be the source of great pain and disability. Often, this clinical entity is treated effectively with nonsurgical interventions, such as weight reduction, physical therapy, and judicious use of injectable or oral medications. However, when the pain is refractory to these efforts, surgery may be considered. A number of surgical options have been used for patellofemoral arthritis, including arthroscopic débridement and lavage, patellar unloading procedures (e.g., tibial tubercle elevation or tibial tubercle anteromedialization), patellectomy, cartilage grafting techniques, patellar resurfacing, patellofemoral arthroplasty, and total knee arthroplasty. This chapter discusses the role of patellofemoral arthroplasty for isolated patellofemoral chondral degeneration. Results may be optimized by limiting the procedure to those patients with arthritis and pain localized to the anterior compartment of the knee and without significant patellar malalignment, by accurately aligning the prosthesis and balancing the soft tissues to optimize patellar tracking, and by using an implant that engages the patella within the trochlear groove but which has limited constraint and a sagittal radius of curvature that mates well with the native distal femur.

Whereas earlier design flaws predisposed to a relatively high rate of failures from patellar maltracking, catching, and anterior knee pain, newer and improved trochlear designs have reduced the incidence of patellofemoral dysfunction.[7,24,33,36] These improved outcomes, as well as an interest in single-compartment resurfacing, have led to growing enthusiasm for patellofemoral arthroplasty.

EPIDEMIOLOGY

Chondromalacia patella has been observed in 40% to 60% of patients at autopsy, and in 20% to 50% of patients at the time of arthrotomy for other diagnoses.[54] The prevalence of isolated patellofemoral arthritis is high, occurring in as many as 11% of men and 24% of women older than 55 years with symptomatic osteoarthritis of the knee in one study.[42] This gender predilection is undoubtedly related to the often subtle patellar malalignment and dysplasia that is common in women. The patellofemoral cartilage is also vulnerable to direct traumatic injury, considering its unprotected location in the body.

NONSURGICAL TREATMENT

Nonsurgical management is the mainstay of treatment for isolated patellofemoral arthritis; to be certain, it is the minority of patients who ultimately require an operation. A directed therapy program emphasizing short arc quadriceps strengthening, stretching of the lateral retinacular structures, and preservation of motion is frequently successful in mitigating symptoms. There is some evidence to suggest that vastus

medialis obliquus dysfunction may be associated with patellofemoral pain.[55] This serves to reinforce the importance of a directed strengthening program. When the anterior knee pain associated with patellofemoral arthrosis is refractory to months of nonoperative interventions, such as weight reduction, physical therapy, and judicious use of injectable or oral medications, surgery may be considered.

SURGICAL ALTERNATIVES

Arthroscopic Surgery

Arthroscopic options for patellofemoral chondromalacia and arthritis include lavage or débridement, with or without marrow stimulation. Arthroscopic débridement and lavage may be beneficial for those patients who have recurrent effusions by decreasing the debris load, which may be a source of inflammation. Furthermore, removal of an unstable chondral flap lesion on the patella or trochlear groove can improve the mechanical symptoms. However, these interventions have varied results, and patients should be counseled regarding the likelihood of only partial and temporary symptomatic relief and the persistence of functional limitations. The poor intrinsic healing capabilities of articular cartilage limit the value of arthroscopic treatments for patellofemoral arthritis, particularly in the absence of mechanical symptoms.

Federico and Reider[16] have analyzed a series of 36 patients who underwent arthroscopic chondroplasty for isolated chondromalacia patella without patellar malalignment. Those patients with traumatic chondromalacia had 60% good or excellent results compared with 41% good or excellent results in all others. Lateral retinacular release, after chondral degeneration has already occurred, is often ineffective in resolving anterior knee pain.[46] Schonholtz and Ling[50] performed chondroplasty for varying degrees of chondromalacia of the patella to remove loose fibrillation, but not to penetrate through subchondral bone or to débride intact cartilage. At a mean 40-month follow-up, the authors reported good to excellent results in 49% of patients and fair results in 44%. They noted that 78% of patients were satisfied and that the grade of chondromalacia did not correlate with the outcome. Marrow stimulation techniques, such as microfracture, have also fared relatively poorly in treating lesions of the patellofemoral articulation. The reparative fibrocartilage tissue, composed primarily of type I collagen, is incapable of withstanding the excessive shear stresses common to the patellofemoral articulation.

Tibial Tubercle Unloading Procedures

Anteromedialization of the tibial tubercle is a time-tested and well-established procedure for the treatment of patellar maltracking associated with patellofemoral malalignment.[18,20]

Although anteriorization of the tibial tubercle reduces the patellofemoral joint reaction forces by increasing the angle between the patellar tendon and quadriceps tendon and increases the lever arm for extensor mechanism function, medializing the tibial tubercle improves the Q angle and thereby decreases the strong lateral vectors acting on the patella. Combining these two components can therefore improve patellar tracking and relieve pain associated with subchondral overload of the lateral patellar facet. The obliquity of the tibial tubercle osteotomy allows for adjustment in the extent of anteriorization, and bone graft is not necessary. The angle can be adjusted to accommodate varying degrees of subluxation and articular cartilage damage. Although Fulkerson and colleagues[19] have reported excellent to good results in 89% of patients followed up for more than 5 years, no patients achieved excellent results and satisfaction was only 75% in the presence of substantial chondromalacia (Outerbridge grade III or IV).

Direct anteriorization of the tibial tubercle has also been advocated for patients with patellofemoral arthrosis when there is no patellar subluxation or malalignment. Symptom improvement with the classic Maquet osteotomy has ranged from 30% to 90%.[17,23,41] Biomechanical studies have demonstrated reductions in contact pressures; however, contact areas may shift proximally, paradoxically overloading the proximal portion of the patella in deep flexion.[11] The optimal patient to benefit from a Maquet osteotomy is one with posttraumatic arthrosis or chondromalacia involving the inferior half of the patella. Those patients with proximal arthrosis or diffuse patellofemoral arthrosis, and those with multiple prior patellofemoral surgeries, will have compromised outcomes. Its limited indications, unpredictable results, and risk of complications, such as wound necrosis or osteotomy nonunion, restrict the practical application of this procedure.

Cartilage Grafting

Autologous chondrocyte implantation for isolated patellar cartilage lesions has produced satisfactory results in approximately 75% of patients at 2- to 10-year follow-up.[10,44] Proponents advise that residual patellar malalignment is a common reason for failure of this technique and should therefore be addressed prior to or simultaneously with autologous chondrocyte implantation. Autologous osteochondral transplantation has been advocated by its innovator for patellofemoral lesions. Although the duration of follow-up is not clear, Hangody and Fules[21] have reported 79% satisfactory results in those with patellar and/or trochlear mosaicplasties.

Patellectomy

Patellectomy has been shown experimentally to reduce extension power by 25% to 60%, with a concomitant requisite increase in quadriceps force of 15% to 30% to achieve adequate extension torque.[8,26] Tibiofemoral joint reaction forces may increase by as much as 250%, explaining the propensity for tibiofemoral arthrosis after patellectomy.[15,25] Variable pain relief, residual quadriceps weakness, and secondary instability, with failures as high as 45%, relegate this to being a salvage procedure for the rare patient who does poorly with other more successful interventions. Additionally, results of total knee arthroplasty can be compromised

after patellectomy.[47] Therefore, patellectomy is less desirable than patellofemoral arthroplasty or total knee arthroplasty for the treatment of isolated patellofemoral arthrosis.

Total Knee Arthroplasty

Total knee arthroplasty is generally effective for older patients with isolated patellofemoral arthritis, yielding good and excellent results in 90% to 95% of patients at midterm follow up, although anterior knee pain has been reported in as many as 7% to 19% of patients.[29,45,48] In one study comparing total knee arthroplasty for isolated patellofemoral arthrosis to that for tricompartmental arthrosis, Knee Society scores, bipedal stair climbing capacity, and ability to rise from a seated position were all significantly better in the former group.[29] Given the predictably good results of total knee arthroplasty, it is preferable to patellofemoral arthroplasty in the older patient with isolated patellofemoral arthrosis. However, in younger patients with isolated patellofemoral arthrosis, patellofemoral arthroplasty may be favorable.

PATELLOFEMORAL ARTHROPLASTY

Patellofemoral arthroplasty (PFA) may be considered in the treatment algorithm for patients with localized patellofemoral arthrosis or severe recalcitrant chondromalacia (Fig. 101-1). Early designs resurfaced only the patella, using a metal implant and leaving the trochlea untouched. Although the patella is commonly more degenerated than the trochlea, results have been variable with this technique.[2,40] Recognition that residual anterior knee pain may have been related to trochlear chondromalacia, first-generation patellofemoral resurfacing arthroplasties were developed, using a polyethylene patellar component and metallic trochlear component.[9]

Patient Selection

The outcome of patellofemoral arthroplasty can be optimized by limiting its application to patients with isolated patellofemoral osteoarthrosis, post-traumatic arthrosis, or severe chondrosis (Outerbridge grade IV), and then only after an extended supervised program of nonoperative measures. Additionally, this option is best reserved for patients with isolated retropatellar and/or peripatellar pain and functional limitations, with considerable discomfort with provocative activities such as stair or hill ambulation, squatting, or prolonged sitting. The procedure should not be performed in patients with inflammatory arthritis or chondrocalcinosis involving the menisci or tibiofemoral chondral surfaces, nor should it be offered to patients with inappropriate expectations.[30,32,34,35] The presence of medial or lateral joint line pain suggests more diffuse chondral disease and should be considered as potential contraindications to isolated patellofemoral resurfacing. Alternative causes of anterior knee pain, such as patellar tendinitis, synovitis, patellar instability, sympathetic mediated pain, and pain referred from the back or ipsilateral hip, should be excluded, unless it appears that the pain is referred from the patellofermoral compartment.

Although it can be most effective for treating arthritis associated with patellofemoral dysplasia,[22] patellofemoral arthroplasty should be avoided in patients with considerable

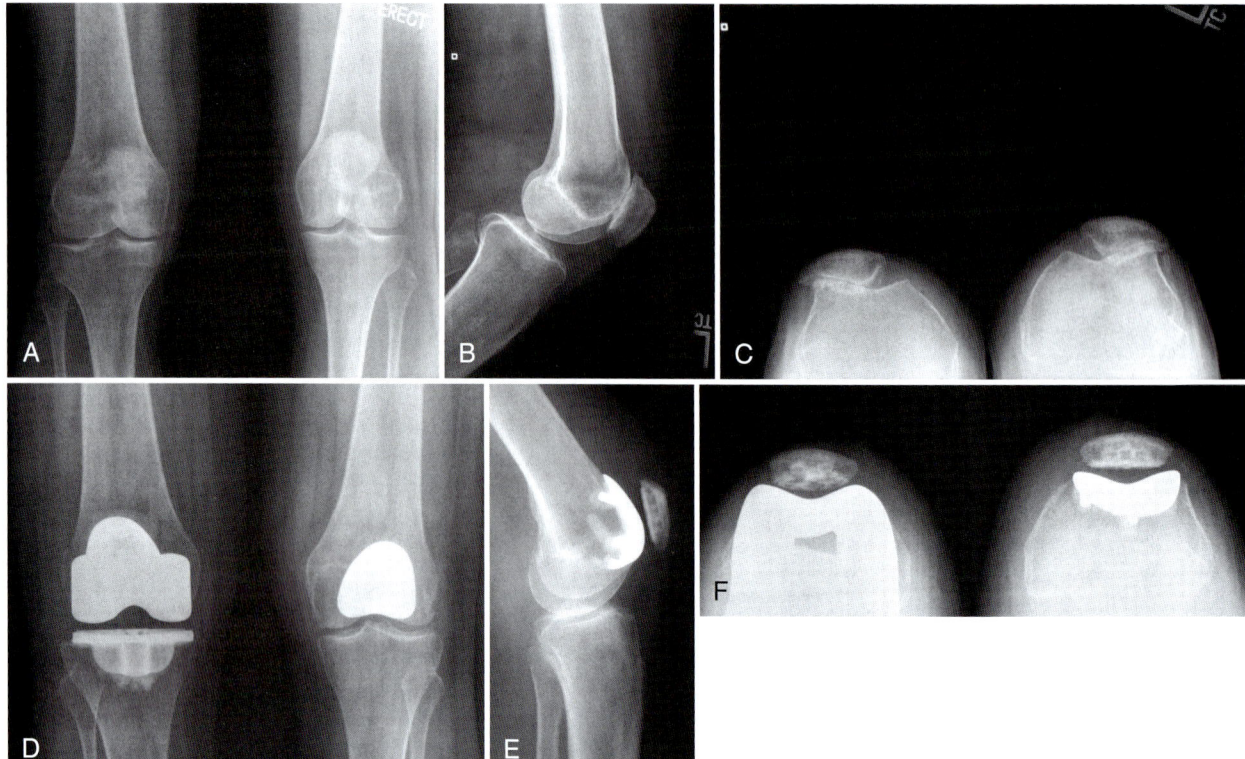

Figure 101-1. **A-C,** Weight-bearing anteroposterior, lateral, and axial radiographs demonstrating advanced patellofemoral arthrosis with sparing of the tibiofemoral compartments. **D-F,** Postoperative radiographs after a successful PFA.

patellar maltracking or malalignment, unless they are corrected. This is not to say, however, that moderate patellar tilt, observed on preoperative tangential radiographs or at the time of arthrotomy, should be considered contraindications for this procedure. In such cases, a lateral retinacular recession or release may be necessary at the time of arthroplasty.[32,34,38] Occasionally, for severe maltracking, a proximal realignment may be necessary. Persistent patellar subluxation may cause pain and snapping and potential polyethylene wear of the prosthesis. Patients with excessive Q angles should undergo tibial tubercle realignment before or during patellofemoral arthroplasty, although some trochlear prosthesis shapes may accommodate a slightly increased Q angle. Also, the presence of tibiofemoral arthrosis should discourage isolated patellofemoral arthroplasty. The presence of even focal grade III tibiofemoral chondromalacia can compromise the outcome after patellofemoral arthroplasty, although these patients will often acknowledge resolution of the most prominent component of pain. Combining patellofemoral arthroplasty with medial or lateral unicompartmental knee arthroplasty or autologous osteochondral grafting are sound considerations in these situations.[5,38]

Although there are intuitive concerns, there are no data available on whether obesity or cruciate ligament insufficiency put the PFA at risk for failure. There are no age criteria for PFA provided the other criteria are met.

Clinical Evaluation

Evaluation of the patient under consideration should be thorough to confirm that the pain is localized to the anterior compartment of the knee and that it emanates from the patellofemoral chondral surfaces and not soft tissues. This can usually be done by taking a detailed history of the problem and by performing a meticulous physical examination.

The key elements of the history that should be elaborated include whether there was previous trauma to the knee, a history of patellar dislocation, or prior patellofemoral problems. A history of recurrent atraumatic patellar dislocations may suggest considerable malalignment, which may need to be corrected. These patients may have severe trochlear flattening or even convexity, which can be improved with the trochlear component. A clear description of the location of the pain is important; discomfort anywhere but directly retropatellar, or just lateral or medial to the patella, will not be relieved with a PFA. Patellofemoral pain often is exacerbated by activities such as stair climbing and descent, ambulating on hills, standing from a seated position, sitting with the knee flexed, and squatting. Walking on level ground should not be as painful. A description of anterior crepitus is common. After establishing the location and quality of pain, it is important to ascertain whether there were previous interventions, such as physical therapy, weight reduction, medications, injections, or surgery.

With respect to the physical examination, pain on patellar inhibition testing, patellofemoral crepitus, and retropatellar knee pain with squatting are typical. Any associated medial or lateral tibiofemoral joint line tenderness should raise suspicion of more diffuse chondral disease, even in the presence of relatively normal radiographs, and may be a contraindication to isolated PFA. It is also essential to rule out other potential sources of anterior knee pain, such as pes anserinus bursitis, patellar tendinitis, prepatellar bursitis, instability, and pain referred from the ipsilateral hip or back. Careful assessment of patellar tracking and the Q angle also are important. As noted, even subtle tracking abnormalities and malalignment can predispose to inferior outcomes, particularly with certain designs. In patients with high Q angles, therefore, a tibial tubercle realignment procedure (anteromedialization) should be performed prior to or concurrent with PFA. Anterior or posterior cruciate ligament insufficiency is not a contraindication for this procedure; however, cruciate ligament reconstruction may be advisable to reduce the risk of anterior knee pain and instability and potentially to preserve the tibiofemoral articular cartilage.

Generally, weight-bearing radiographs are ample imaging studies. Standing anteroposterior and midflexion posteroanterior radiographs are critical to determine the presence of tibiofemoral arthritis. Mild squaring-off of the femoral condyles and even small marginal osteophytes may be accepted, provided that the patient is devoid of tibiofemoral pain with functional activities and on physical examination, and that there is minimal chondral degeneration during arthroscopy or arthrotomy. Lateral x-rays will occasionally demonstrate patellofemoral osteophytes, but usually are more useful in identifying whether there is patella alta or baja. Axial radiographs will demonstrate the position of the patella within the trochlear groove and the extent of arthritis, although on occasion there will be relative radiographic patellofemoral joint space preservation with minimal or no osteophytes, despite significant cartilage loss (see Fig. 101-1). Newer MRI sequences may be useful for evaluating patellofemoral arthrosis but, more importantly, can be used to evaluate the medial and lateral compartments for evidence of chondral wear. If committed to performing a PFA, patients should consent to autologous osteochondral grafting for associated focal condylar defects or unicompartmental knee arthroplasty as part of a bicompartmental resurfacing if there is more diffuse degeneration.[6,38] Photographs from prior arthroscopic treatment will provide valuable information regarding the extent of anterior compartment arthrosis and status of the tibiofemoral articular cartilage and menisci.

Surgical Technique

During arthrotomy, it is essential to avoid cutting normal articular cartilage or the menisci. Before proceeding with PFA, carefully inspect the entire joint to ensure that the tibiofemoral compartments are free of disease. As noted, if the weight-bearing condylar surfaces have a focal full-thickness cartilage defect, consider an autologous osteoarticular graft. If there is more diffuse medial or lateral compartment wear, consider a bicompartmental arthroplasty or a total knee arthroplasty.

In addition to the design features of some contemporary components, which have substantially improved patellar tracking, instrumentation has been developed that is low profile, accurate, and conducive to less invasive surgical techniques. Early-generation implants required freehand preparation of all bony surfaces, which contributed to inaccurate trochlear component alignment. Second-generation implants typically neither offered a means for preparing the distal femur for the intercondylar tail of the implant nor were they amenable to more contemporary, less invasive surgical

techniques, because they tended to be bulky. Newer systems have simplified the procedure and improved the anatomic mating of the implant to the articular surfaces of the transition zones.

The trochlear component should be externally rotated perpendicular to the anteroposterior axis of the femur (Whiteside axis) or parallel to the epicondylar axis to enhance patellar tracking.[33,34] Osteophytes bordering the intercondylar notch should be removed. The trochlear component should maximize coverage of the trochlea, without extending beyond the medial-lateral femoral margins anteriorly, encroaching on the weight-bearing surfaces of the tibiofemoral articulations, or overhanging into the intercondylar notch. The medial and lateral transitional edges of the prosthesis should be flush with or recessed approximately 1 mm from the adjacent condylar articular cartilage. The proximal edge should be flush with the anterior femoral cortex and the distal tip should be flush with the articular cartilage and not extend into the intercondylar notch. The patella is resurfaced by the same principles observed in total knee arthroplasty, restoring the original patellar thickness and medializing the component. The exposed cut surface of the lateral patella that is not covered by the patellar prosthesis is removed or beveled to avoid the potentially painful articulation on the trochlear prosthesis.[31] This may also enhance patellar tracking by releasing tension on the lateral retinaculum.

Assessment of patellar tracking is performed with the trial components in place. Attention is paid to identify patellar tilt, subluxation, or catching of the components. Patellar tilt and mild subluxation usually can be addressed successfully by performing a lateral retinacular recession or release. As noted, more severe extensor mechanism malalignment may require proximal or distal realignment.

Postoperative Management

Isometrics and range of motion exercises are started immediately. Use of a continuous passive motion machine during hospitalization (average, 1 or 3 days) may accelerate flexion recovery, but is probably not necessary for all patients. Full weight bearing is permitted immediately, with support of crutches and a cane until there is adequate recovery of quadriceps strength. In some circumstances, full recovery of quadriceps strength can take 6 months or longer, considering the severe preoperative quadriceps atrophy that is encountered in some patients with patellofemoral arthritis. Thromboembolism prophylaxis is used for 4 to 6 weeks and 24 hours of perioperative antibiotics is advisable. Appropriate precautions regarding antibiotic prophylaxis for dental procedures or other interventions should follow standard recommendations of the American Academy of Orthopaedic Surgeons.[22]

DESIGN FEATURES THAT AFFECT PATELLAR TRACKING

With few exceptions, the clinical results of PFA have improved as trochlear designs evolved over 30 years.[7,33,36,38] There are a variety of specific design features of the trochlear components that impact patellar tracking and the success of the patellofemoral arthroplasty, including the sagittal radius of curvature, proximal extension of the trochlear flange, thickness of the trochlear component, mediolateral width, and constraint of the trochlear groove. Additionally, whether they are onlay- or inlay-type designs and are asymmetrical or symmetrical also will affect patellofemoral performance.

The sagittal radius of curvature of some trochlear components, usually inlay-type designs such as the Lubinus, Richards types I and II, and Low-Contact Stress Patellofemoral Joint (LCS), are obtuse. It is difficult to implant these flush with both the anterior femoral cortex and medial, lateral, and distal margins of articular cartilage. The trochlear prostheses in those systems are therefore often implanted in a flexed position, leaving them prominent proximally, where they can cause patellar snapping, clunking, and maltracking when the patella transitions onto it (Fig. 101-2A). Other trochlear designs have a sagittal radius of curvature that is far more accommodating of most femora (see Fig. 101-2B). This allows flush implantation on the anterior femoral surface as well as on the intercondylar surface of the knee, without the need to flex the implant, thereby reducing the risk of patellar catching.

There is also variability in the mediolateral width of the anterior flange of available implants. Some are very narrow, a feature that is unforgiving of even subtle patellar subluxation and that can result in catching on the medial and lateral edges of the trochlear component (Fig. 101-3). Others are considerably broader (Fig. 101-4), covering almost the entire anterior surface of the distal femur. This latter feature allows a greater degree of freedom for patellar excursion and tracking; however, if the component is too wide, overhang into the soft tissues can cause painful soft tissue impingement and perhaps limit flexion.

The proximal extension of the trochlear flange on the anterior femur also differs among products (Figs. 101-5 and 101-6). Onlay implants are typically designed to extend considerably more proximally than the articular margin of the trochlear so that the patellar component articulates entirely with the trochlear component in extension. On the other hand, inlay designs, such as the Lubinus and LCS components, and custom designs, such as the Kinamed, do not

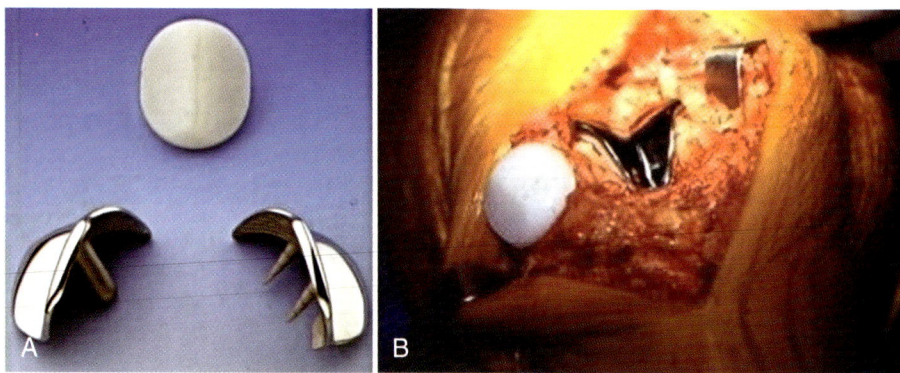

Figure 101-2. Richards types II and III PFAs. **A,** One central fixation lug. **B,** Three fixation spikes. (Courtesy Smith & Nephew, Memphis, Tenn.)

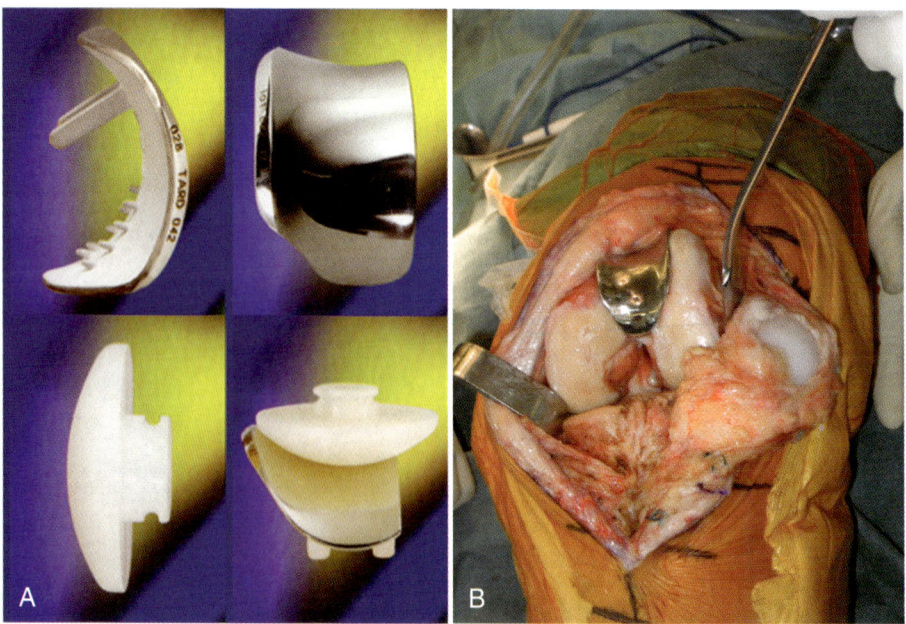

Figure 101-3. **A,** Autocentric PFA (DePuy, Warsaw, Ind.). **B,** Operative appearance of autocentric PFA 10 years after implantation. Revision to total knee arthroplasty was necessary because of progressive tibiofemoral arthrosis.

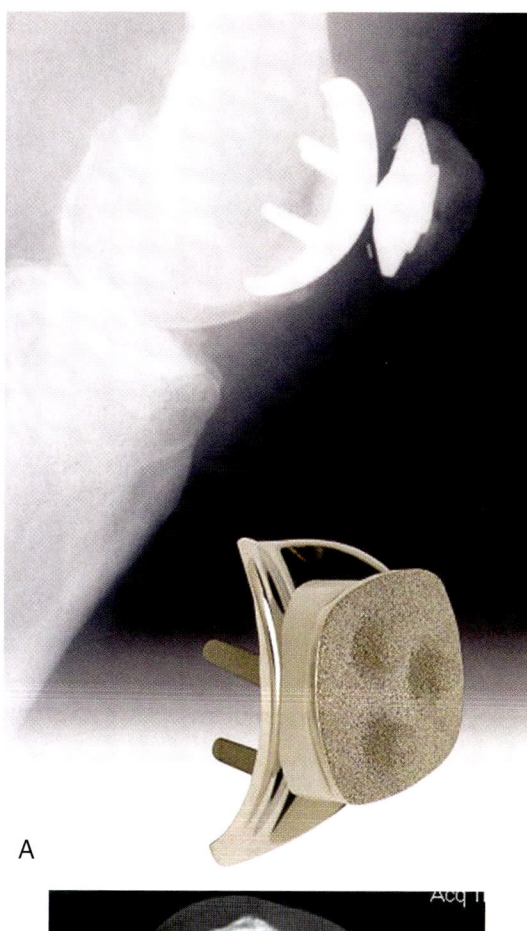

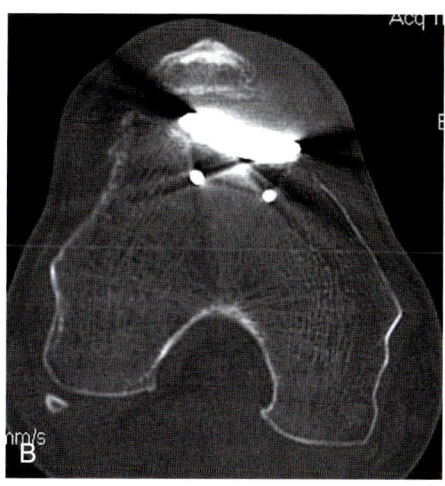

A

B

Figure 101-4. **A,** Low-Contact Stress Patellofemoral Joint. **B,** Axial CT scan of inlay-style implant demonstrating internal rotation relative to the anteroposterior axis of the distal femur, resulting in lateral patellar catching and subluxation. This was treated successfully with revision to an onlay-style implant, rotating the trochlear component perpendicular to the anteroposterior axis of the femur (DePuy, Warsaw, Ind).

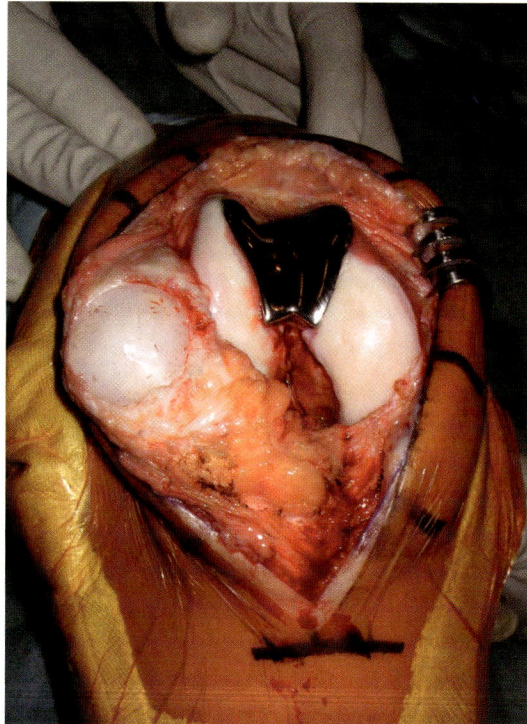

Figure 101-5. Lubinus PFA (Link, Hamburg, Germany).

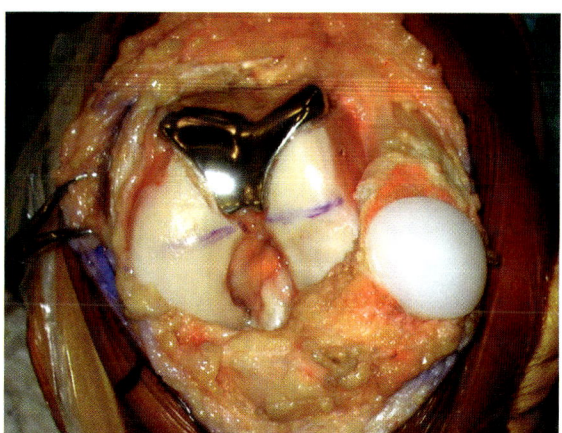

Figure 101-6. Avon patellofemoral arthroplasty (Stryker Orthopaedics, Mahwah, NJ).

extend proximally to the articular cartilage margin of the trochlea. The patellar prosthesis in these latter designs therefore articulates with the natural anterior femoral surface in full extension before it transitions onto the trochlear prosthesis. This predisposes them designs to catching and snapping in the initial 30 degrees of flexion, particularly if the trochlear prosthesis is flexed or offset anteriorly.

As noted, some trochlear designs are an inlay style, whereas others are an onlay-type component. The former design is inset into the trochlea and tends to be more bone-conserving; the latter is implanted flush with the anterior surface of the femoral cortex and removes the entire anterior trochlear surface. However, given the variability in distal anterior femoral morphology, inlayed trochlear components often do not mate accurately with the articular geometry of the trochlear region of the femur, resulting in offset on any of its edges. This typically results in patellar catching on the trochlear component, either proximally as the knee proceeds from extension to flexion or distally as the knee proceeds from deep flexion to extension. The onlay device is more suitable for a larger variation in trochlear geometries. Unlike the inlay designs, it can be used for patients with trochlear dysplasia without risk of having the component sit proud relative to the surrounding articular cartilage. It is my opinion that trying to inset a trochlear component into the bone is analogous to implanting a potato chip onto the anterior aspect of the knee. If the two surfaces are geometrically mated, the outcome will be absolutely perfect. However, if there is a mismatch, there is an increased risk for relative component malalignment and malposition relative to the articular surfaces, which is why patellar maltracking is more common with that style of implant. Additionally, the inlay trochlear design may also display greater variability in rotational alignment. By design, the component is rotated so that its medial and lateral edges are flush with the surrounding articular cartilage. Because most patients have a more prominent anterior lateral trochlear flange compared with the medial flange,

these inlay components are often implanted in internal rotation relative to the transepicondylar and anteroposterior axes of the distal femur. This predisposes to lateral patellar subluxation, which has been common with inlay style trochlear prostheses (see Fig. 101-1B).

CLINICAL RESULTS

Most series have reported good and excellent results in approximately 80% to 90% of cases at short-term and midterm follow-up (Table 101-1; Figs. 101-7 to 101-11). However, clinical results of patellofemoral arthroplasty are affected by trochlear component design features, as well as by patient selection and surgical technique.[7,33,36,38] Outcomes and patellofemoral performance have improved. The need for

Table 101-1 Results of Patellofemoral Arthroplasty

Study (Year)	Implant	No. of PFAs	Age (Yr)	Diagnosis (No. of Cases)	Duration of Follow-Up (Yr)	Good to Excellent Results (%)
Blazina et al (1979)[9]; see Fig. 101-7	Richards types I and II	57	39 (range, 19-81)	NA	2 (range, 8-42 mo)	NA
Arciero and Toomey (1988)[3]	Richards type II (14); CFS-Wright (11)	25	62 (range, 33-86)	OA (25); malalignment or instability (14)	5.3 (range, 3-9 yr)	85
Cartier et al (1990)[12]	Richards types II and III	72	65 (range, 23-89)	Dysplasia, grade IV chondromalacia (29); PTA (3); chondrocalcinosis (5)	4 (range, 2-12 yr)	85
Argenson et al (2009)[6]; see Fig. 101-8	Autocentric	66	57 (range, 19-82)	Dysplasia or dislocation (22); PTA (20); OA (24)	5.5 (range, 2-10 yr)	84
Krajca-Radcliffe and Coker (1996)[28]	Richards types I and II	16	64 (range, 42-84)	Primary OA (10) PTA (2) Recurrent dislocation (1)	5.8 (range, 2-18 yr)	88
Tauro et al (2001)[53]; see Fig. 101-9	Lubinus	62	66 (range, 50-87)	PTA (2); Primary OA (74)	7.5 (range 5-10 yr)	45
deWinter et al (2001)[14]	Richards type II	26	59 (range, 22-90)	Primary OA (17); Malalignment (8); PTA (1)	11 (range, 1-20 yr)	76
Ackroyd et al (2007)[1]; see Fig. 101-10	Avon	95	NA	NA	2-5 yr	83
Smith et al (2002)[52]	Lubinus	45	72 (range, 42-86)	Primary OA (44); PTA (1)	4 (range, 6 mo-7.5 yr)	69
Kooijman et al (2003)[27]	Richards type II	45	50 (range, 20-77)	OA (45)	17 (range, 15-21 yr)	86
Lonner (2004)[35]	Lubinus	30	38 (range, 34-51)	Primary OA (26); PTA (4); [s/p tibial tubercle realignment (10)]	4 (range, 2-6 yr)	84
Lonner (2004)[35]	Avon trochlea; Nexgen patella	25	44 (range, 28-59)	Primary OA (25); [s/p realignment (2)]	6 mo (range, 1 mo-1 yr)	96
Merchant (2004)[43]; see Fig. 101-11	LCS	15	49 (range, 30-81)	Chronic sublux or recurrent disloc'n with secondary DJD (13); chondrosis (2)	3.8 yr (range, 2.3-5.5 yr)	93
Sisto and Sarin (2006)[51]	Kinematch PFR	25	45 (range, 23-51)	OA (25) [s/p tibial tubercle elevation (6); s/p arthroscopic lateral release and débridement (13)]	73 mo (range, 32-119 mo)	100
Cartier et al (2005)[13]	Richards types II and III	79	60 (range, 36-81)	Dysplasia and patellar subluxation (70%); Primary OA (12%); Grade IV chondromalacia (7%); isolated chondrocalcinosis (6%); Post patella fracture (5%)	10 yr (range, 6-16 yr)	77
Argenson et al (1995)[4]	Autocentric	66	57 (range, 21-82)	Dysplasia or dislocation (21); PTA (18); OA (18)	16 yr (range, 12-20 yr)	NA
Ackroyd et al (2007)[1]	Avon	109	68 (range, 46-86)	OA (106); Dislocation (2); PTA (1)	5.2 yr (range, 5-8 yr)	80%

DJD, Degenerative joint disease; *NA,* not available; *OA,* osteoarthritis; *PTA,* post-traumatic arthritis; *s/p,* status post.

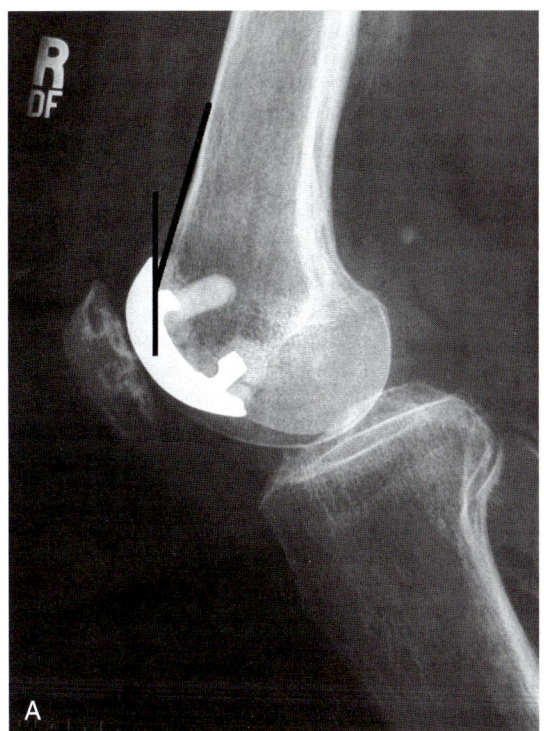

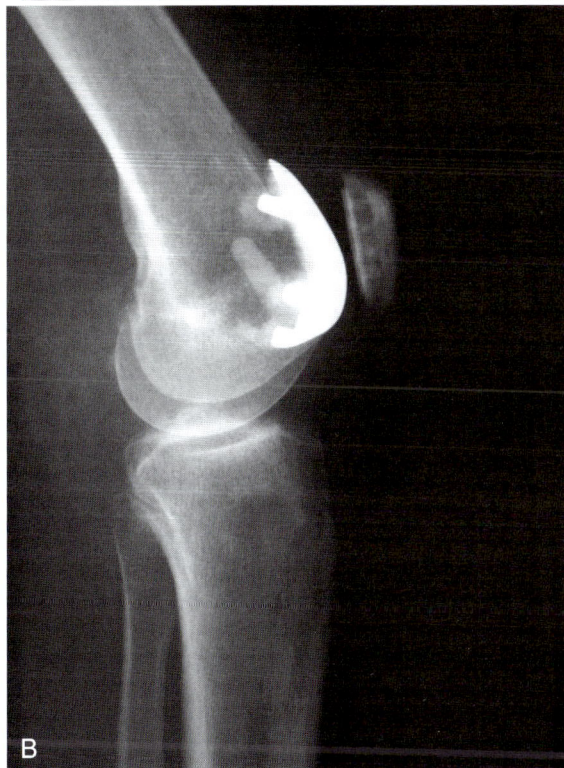

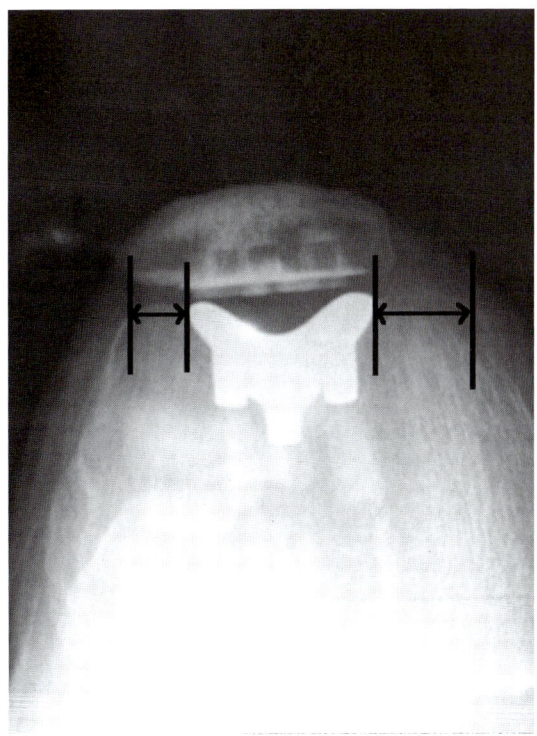

Figure 101-8. Axial radiograph of a large trochlear component inlay that is quite narrow. This increases the risk of subluxation with even small degrees of maltracking. There is little room for freedom of excursion. The *arrows* show the extent of uncapped cartilage anteriorly. (From Lonner JH: Patellofemoral arthroplasty: pros, cons, design considerations. Clin Orthop Relat Res (428):158–165, 2004.)

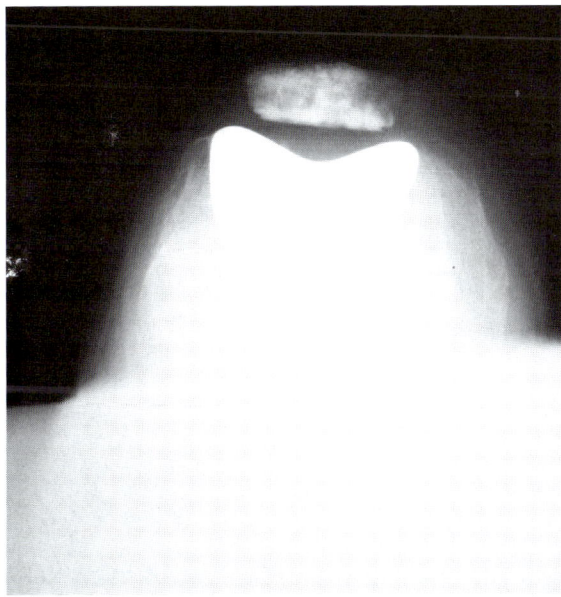

Figure 101-9. Broad anterior trochlear coverage provided by this onlay prosthesis accommodates patellar tracking. (From Lonner JH: Patellofemoral arthroplasty: the impact of design on outcomes. Orthop Clin N Am. 39:347–354, 2008.)

Figure 101-7. **A,** Lateral postoperative radiograph after PFA using an inlay prosthesis illustrates one of the potential problems with this design—namely, that the trochlear implant must be flexed, leaving it offset from the anterior femoral shaft, and making the patella prone to catching and subluxing. **B,** Postoperative radiographs after PFA using an onlay trochlear prosthesis. The postoperative lateral radiograph shows the implant to be flush with the anterior femoral cortex. The radius of curvature is approximately 90 degrees. (**A** from Lonner JH: Patellofemoral arthroplasty: pros, cons, design considerations. Clin Orthop Relat Res (428):158–165, 2004; **B** from Lonner JH: Patellofemoral arthroplasty: the impact of design on outcomes. Orthop Clin N Am. 39:347–354, 2008.)

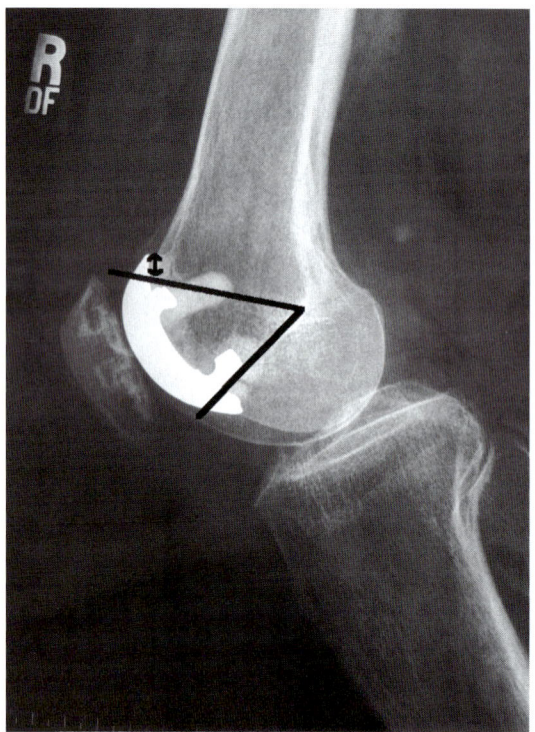

Figure 101-10. Limited proximal extension above the physeal scar predisposes this typical type of inlay style prosthesis to catching and subluxing as the patella transitions from the native femur onto the prosthesis in the initial 30 degrees of flexion. (From Lonner JH: Patellofemoral arthroplasty: pros, cons, design considerations. Clin Orthop Relat Res (428):158–165, 2004.)

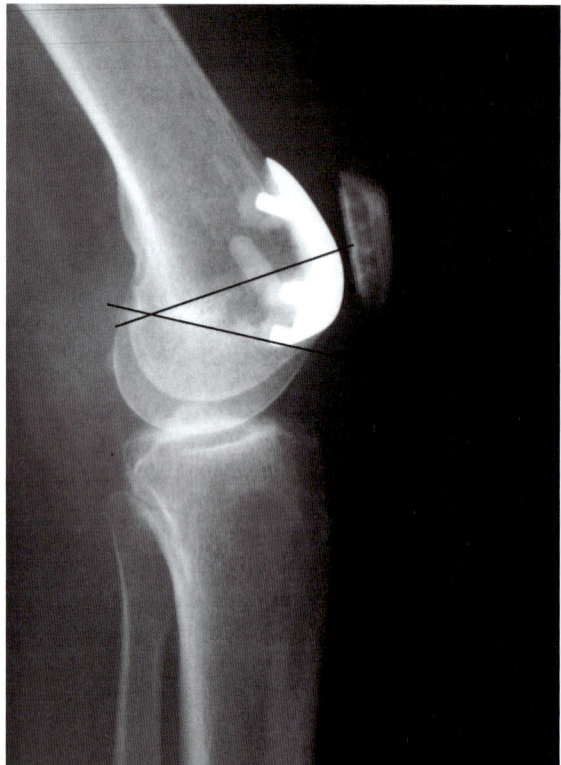

Figure 101-11. Greater proximal extension of this onlay trochlear implant above the physeal scar ensures that the patella articulates with the femoral prosthesis at all times in extension. (From Lonner JH: Patellofemoral arthroplasty: the impact of design on outcomes. Orthop Clin N Am. 39:347–354, 2008.)

secondary soft tissue surgery to enhance patellar tracking after patellofemoral arthroplasty has decreased because of trochlear design improvements that have occurred as first-, second-, and now third-generation implants have been developed. The radius of curvature, width, thickness, tracking angle, and extent of constraint of the trochlear component affect patellar tracking and outcomes. Contemporary designs have substantially reduced the incidence of patellofemoral complications, leaving tibiofemoral arthritis as the major source of failure of patellofemoral arthroplasties.

Blazina and colleagues[9] have reported 81% good results after a follow-up period of less than 2 years in 55 knees using a first-generation PFA with a trochlear implant constrained with a sharp trochlear groove. Thirty subsequent procedures were necessary in their series to realign the extensor mechanism or revise malpositioned components. Although the investigators credited technical errors as the reason for most secondary surgeries, component design—that is, trochlear constraint, an obtuse radius of curvature, and narrow implant width—most certainly contributed to the failures as well.

Cartier and associates[12] had 85% good or excellent results with 72 first-generation PFAs followed for an average of 4 years. There were numerous concomitant surgical procedures performed to enhance patellar tracking, including soft tissue realignment and tibial tubercle transfer. Longer term follow-up of those patients, at a mean of 10 years (range, 6 to 16 years) after surgery, found that results deteriorated over time, primarily because of the development of tibiofemoral arthritis. This is not surprising, given the average patient age of 60 years at the time of the initial PFA in that series. At most recent follow-up, 80% of those who retained their patellofemoral prostheses were pain-free and 20% had moderate or severe pain, primarily from tibiofemoral arthritis. Stair ambulation was considered normal in 91% of patients. No cases of patellar or trochlear loosening were identified. The authors noted that early failures peaked at 3 years and were related to inappropriate indications for the surgery, and presumably to patellar maltracking problems that could likely be traced to implant design quirks. They identified a later peak in failures in years 9 and 10 that corresponded to the development of symptomatic tibiofemoral osteoarthritis. The authors reported a survivorship of 75% at 11 years.[46] In another study, Kooijman and coworkers[27] reported an 86% long-term success rate with the same first-generation PFA, even though early secondary soft tissue surgery was necessary in 18% of patients and revision of the patellofemoral arthroplasty was necessary for catching, imbalance, or malposition in 16%.

In a consecutive series of 30 first-generation implants and 25 second-generation implants, I have found that results vary depending on which trochlear design is used.[38] The incidence of patellofemoral dysfunction, subluxation, catching, and substantial pain was reduced from 17% with earlier designs to less than 4% with more contemporary products. In another series,[24] 14 of the same first-generation patellofemoral implants were revised to a second-generation implant, which had a more favorable topography for patellar tracking. The causes of failure of the primary procedures were component malposition, subluxation, polyethylene wear, or overstuffing. After revision, there was statistically significant improvement in knee scores for patellar tracking at a mean 5-year follow-up. Mild femorotibial arthritis (Ahlback grade 1) was predictive of a poorer clinical outcome. At most recent follow-up, there was no evidence of wear, loosening, or subluxation. This study showed that significant improvement can be obtained when revising the failed patellofemoral arthroplasty with a more accommodating implant design, provided that there is no tibiofemoral arthritis.

Ackroyd and associates[1] have reported on 306 second-generation PFAs and found that patellar tracking was substantially improved compared with a first-generation implant. In that series, patellar subluxation occurred in 3% and residual anterior knee pain was noted in 4%; 4% required revision to total knee arthroplasty, mostly for tibiofemoral arthritis and none for mechanical loosening or wear.

Argenson and coworkers[4] have reported on 66 second-generation PFAs in patients with a mean age of 57 years and a mean follow-up of 16 years. Whereas most patients had substantial and sustained pain relief, 25% were revised to total knee arthroplasty (TKA) for tibiofemoral arthritis (mean, 7.3 years after PFA) and 14% for aseptic trochlear component loosening, many of which were uncemented (mean, 4.5 years after PFA). The authors reported the best results when the procedure was performed for post-traumatic patellofemoral arthritis or patellar subluxation and the least favorable in those with primary degenerative arthritis. The development of tibiofemoral arthritis was the most frequent cause of failure; however, at the time of initial PFA, 14% had concomitant tibiofemoral osteotomies for early arthritis, which confounds the results. In those who retained their PFAs at most recent follow-up, there were significant improvements in Knee Society scores. The authors continue to advocate for the procedure as an intermediate stage before TKA in the absence of tibiofemoral arthritis or coronal plane malalignment.

The Australian Orthopaedic Association National Joint Replacement Registry[7] has provided insight into the experience with and outcomes after PFA performed between 1999 and 2008. In that registry, 75.6% of the 977 PFAs performed in Australia were in women, usually patients younger than 55 years (37.5%) or between the ages of 55 and 64 years (29.1%). The tendency for revision after PFA varied among component types. For example, in that series, the cumulative 5-year revision rate was 18.1% with the Lubinus, 21.8% with the LCS, and 9.9% with the Avon. Data on some newer systems are not yet available in that registry. The registry does not clearly elucidate the mechanisms of failure and reasons for revision with each individual implant. However, the data do corroborate other studies that show a higher incidence of patellofemoral-related problems with some implants compared with others. The need for revision in that registry declined with increased patient age at the time of implantation.

My experience with more than 150 patellofemoral arthroplasties includes the use, most recently, of a third-generation prosthesis with enhanced design features to optimize patellar tracking and with fully instrumented bone preparation.[36] In an unpublished series of 67 PFAs that I performed using the Gender Solutions Patello-Femoral Joint (PFJ) system (Zimmer, Warsaw, Ind; Fig. 101-12), with a follow-up ranging from 6 months to 2.5 years, all patients had substantial improvement in anterior knee pain and ability to climb up and down stairs and stand from a chair, and there was statistically significant improvement in their Knee Society scores. There was one case of slight patellar subluxation noted on

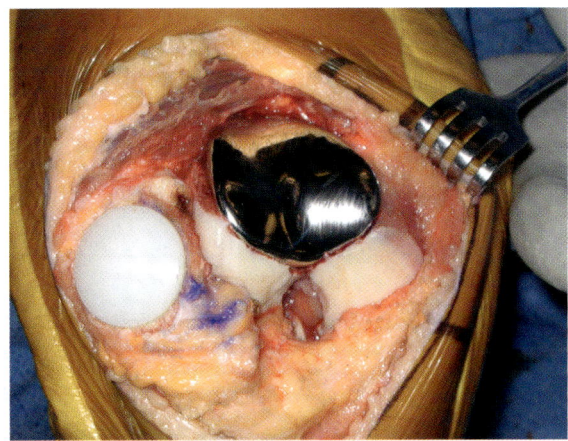

Figure 101-12. Gender Solutions Patello-Femoral Joint system (Zimmer, Warsaw, Ind).

routine postoperative radiographs caused by chronic weakness of the vastus medialis, which improved by 6 months postoperatively with an appropriate strengthening program, one iliotibial band snapping, and one recurrent hemarthrosis. One patient required manipulation under anesthesia 6 weeks after surgery and maintained 115 degrees of flexion at 6 months. There have been no failures from patellar catching, instability, or clinically apparent subluxation no mechanical failures at short-term follow-up.

COMPLICATIONS

As noted, early designs had a tendency to have a high incidence of patellar snapping and instability, requiring secondary surgery to realign the soft tissues or revise the trochlear prosthesis. These problems were often related to trochlear implant design features, as well as to soft tissue imbalance or extensor mechanism malalignment. Contemporary designs have substantially reduced the tendency for patellar maltracking or dysfunction because prosthetic trochlear geometries are more accommodating of patellar tracking, although even some contemporary inlay-style trochlear implants continue to have an inordinately high need for secondary surgeries or revision due to patellar catching and instability. According to the Australian National Joint Replacement Registry,[7] the revision rate for the LCS implant is higher than the Lubinus, with 4.8 revisions/100 observation years. These two designs are very similar. Contemporary onlay-style implants in that registry have a substantially lower likelihood of revision.

Although anterior knee pain and dysfunction from patellar instability resulting from soft tissue imbalance or component malalignment, were the major reported causes of failure with early PFA designs, these are much less common with some contemporary trochlear designs. A small percentage of patients will have mild anterior knee pain from soft tissue impingement but this occurs with a similar frequency as is seen with TKA. Late failures from component subsidence, polyethylene wear, or loosening may eventually develop in the long term, but these problems have been noted in less than 1% of published cases. Trochlear component loosening may be more common in cementless designs.[4,6]

The development of tibiofemoral arthritis is the most common failure mechanism with contemporary designs and, even in earlier designs that managed to avoid patellar instability, occurred in approximately 20% of knees at 15 years.[4,13,27] This is more common when the underlying diagnosis is primary osteoarthritis and less common in patellofemoral dysplasia or post-traumatic arthritis. If revision to TKA is necessary to treat progressive arthritis, the all-polyethylene patellar component can usually be retained if not worn or loose and standard total knee components can be used without the need for stems, augments, or bone graft, without compromising the results.[37,39] Arthrofibrosis is uncommon after patellofemoral arthroplasty. Although it has been reported with an incidence of 7.6% to 12% in two series, both included a number of patients who had undergone concomitant unicompartmental tibiofemoral arthroplasty, but did not mention whether the tendency for arthrofibrosis was increased in those with bicompartmental arthroplasty.[3,6]

Wear of the adjacent articular cartilage from articulation of the patellar prosthesis on the uncapped femoral cartilage is a concern after PFA. It has been established that the patellofemoral joint reaction forces increase in a normal knee from approximately 3.3 times body weight at 60 degrees of loaded flexion to 7.8 times body weight at 130 degrees of squatting.[49] Beyond 60 degrees, the edges of the patellar components or the cut, exposed lateral osseous patellar surface may begin to articulate, at least in part with the adjacent femoral condyles, as the trochlear components taper distally. This can predispose to wear of the exposed articular cartilage. Presently, there is no ideal bearing surface for the patella that can optimally articulate with both the femoral prosthesis and surrounding articular cartilage.

As with any arthroplasty procedure, infection and thromboembolic problems are potential complications, and standard prophylactic strategies should be followed.

SUMMARY

Patellofemoral arthroplasty can be an effective treatment alternative for patellofemoral arthritis resulting from primary osteoarthrosis, dysplasia, or post-traumatic arthrosis in patients with normal or correctable patella alignment and tracking.

PFA may provide patients with substantial pain relief of isolated patellofemoral arthrosis; however, the results can be affected by the geometric features of the trochlear component and technical issues. Residual instability may result in early failure, highlighting the importance of excluding those patients with uncorrectable patellar instability or

malalignment. Implant malposition, potentially hastened by particular designs, may also contribute to failures from maltracking and mechanical catching of the patella.[14,32,38] Sparing of the tibiofemoral compartments, menisci, and cruciate ligaments allows preservation of a more kinematically sound knee joint than total knee arthroplasty.

Although sparse, long-term data suggest that loosening of cemented trochlear and all-polyethylene patellar components is uncommon and the need for additional surgery for progressive tibiofemoral arthritis may be only approximately 25% at a mean of 15 years after PFA.[27] With emerging designs, the incidence of anterior knee pain after PFA should be comparable to that after total knee replacement surgery, approximately 4% to 7%.[29,45] Finally, even small amounts of tibiofemoral cartilage loss may compromise the results enough to warrant restricting this procedure to ideal candidate patients, although combining PFA with autologous osteochondral grafting for focal condylar defects or unicompartmental knee arthroplasty for associated medial or lateral arthritis may expand application of the procedure.

KEY REFERENCES

Ackroyd CE, Newman JH, Evans R, et al: The Avon patellofemoral arthroplasty. Five-year survivorship and functional results. J Bone Joint Surg Br 89:310–315, 2007.

Argenson JNA, Flecher X, Parratte S, Aubaniac JM: Patellofemoral arthroplasty: an update. Clin Orthop Relat Res 440:50–53, 2005.

Cartier P, Sanouiller JL, Khefacha A: Long-term results with the first patellofemoral prosthesis. Clin Orthop Relat Res 436:47–54, 2005.

Hendrix MRG, Ackroyd CE, Lonner JH: Revision patellofemoral arthroplasty: 3-7 year follow-up. J Arthrop 23:977–983, 2008.

Kooijman HJ, Driessen AP, van Horn JR: Long-term results of patellofemoral arthroplasty. J Bone Joint Surg Br 85:836–840, 2003.

Leadbetter WB, Seyler TM, Ragland PS, Mont MA: Indications, contraindications, and pitfalls of patellofemoral arthroplasty. J Bone Joint Surg Am 88(Suppl 4):122–137, 2006.

Lonner JH: Patellofemoral arthroplasty: pros, cons, design considerations. Clin Orthop Relat Res 428:158–165, 2004.

Lonner JH: Patellofemoral arthroplasty. J Am Acad Orthop Surg 15:495–506, 2007.

Lonner JH: Patellofemoral arthroplasty: the impact of design on outcomes. Orthop Clin N Am 39:347–354, 2008.

Lonner JH, Jasko JG, Booth RE: Revision of a failed patellofemoral arthroplasty to a total knee arthroplasty. J Bone Joint Surg Am 88:2337–2342, 2006.

Lonner JH, Mehta S, Booth RE: Ipsilateral patellofemoral arthroplasty and autogenous osteochondral femoral condylar transplantation. J Arthrop 22:1130–1136, 2007.

Sisto DJ Sarin VK: Custom patellofemoral arthroplasty of the knee. J Bone Joint Surg Am 88:1475–1480, 2006.

Tauro B, Ackroyd CE, Newman JH, Shah NA: The Lubinus patellofemoral arthroplasty. A five- to ten-year prospective study. J Bone Joint Surg Br 83:696–701, 2001.

Full references for this chapter can be found on www.expertconsult.com.

Bicompartmental Knee Arthroplasty

*Michael S. Shin, V. Karthik Jonna, and Alfred J. Tria, Jr.** *

Partial knee arthroplasty developed in the 1950s with devices such as the McKeever and MacIntosh implants.[8,16,17,19] Unicondylar arthroplasty (UKA)[†] and patellofemoral arthroplasty (PFA) prostheses[1,5,6] were used in the late 1970s and publications showed acceptable results at midterm follow-up. Some surgeons combined UKA and PFA when the pathology presented itself at the time of the surgical procedure. The results were once again acceptable at midterm follow-up and had the advantage of ligament preservation and improved proprioception. However, long-term follow-up showed a high revision rate.[2] As the total knee arthroplasty (TKA) designs improved, there was less interest in partial knee arthroplasty until Repicci and Eberle[21] Romanowski and Repicci[24] offered a smaller incision for UKA. Limited incisions for knee arthroplasty became more popular and partial knee arthroplasty became more common.[7,9]

The bicompartmental replacements from the early 1970s had some recognized advantages over TKA, including improved proprioception, easier range of motion, and faster recovery. However, the two separate implants removed a considerable amount of bone and the operative procedure was complex. Attempts were then made to combine the femoral resurfacing into one single component and there are presently two designs available. Rolston and colleagues[22,23] modified a previously existing TKA femoral component and combined this with a UKA-type tibial resurfacing (Journey-Deuce, Smith & Nephew, Memphis, Tenn). The prosthesis removes less bone and spares all the ligaments of the knee. A similar design is also available that makes cutting blocks based on preoperative computed tomography (CT) imaging of the involved knee. The blocks fit anatomically on the native femur and allow shaping of the surface for the implant (iDuo, Conformis, Burlington, Mass). The tibia is cut with more traditional instrumentation. These newer prosthetic designs borrow technology that has been developed for UKA and TKA. This chapter will review the status of the combined procedures and present the surgical technique for the single-piece femoral component.

HISTORICAL PERSPECTIVE

Partial arthroplasty of the knee started with the work of Marmor[18] in the early 1980s. The UKA that he designed replaced the medial aspect of the knee without interfering with the other two compartments. The early results were acceptable after some problems with the manufacturing were overcome; however, the approach did not become popular

among surgeons in the United States because of the increasing interest in TKA. Berger and associates[3,4] and Kozinn and Scott[12] maintained interest in UKA and developed newer designs in the late 1980s that began to show more promise for the technique. Long-term results are now available, which indicate that the prostheses mimic the results of current TKA for the first 10 years after surgery and may even be similar in the second decade.

Repicci's limited surgical approach in the 1990s increased interest in UKA and supported investigations into newer designs and minimally invasive surgical incisions. The instruments have continued to be modified, with some support from the field of navigation. There is even some interest in a robotic application to increase the degree of accuracy and, perhaps, improve on the long-term results.

PFA also dates back to the early 1980s, when attempts were made to resurface just the patellar side of the articulation in the belief that the patella was the more involved surface. A metallic implant was used, with only moderate success.[11] The implants were modified to include a metal trochlear surface and a polyethylene patella. The early designs did not include many sizes and the prostheses were not anatomically correct.[1] Krajca-Radcliffe and Coker[13] reported on 30 of 60 knees, with 2- to 18-year follow-up. The results were excellent or good in 84% of the cases. The anatomy was subsequently readdressed and, with modification of the implants, the more recent results are much improved but still do not come up to the level of the TKA.[15]

In the late 1980s, European surgeons who were performing partial knee arthroplasties looked at the other areas of the knee during surgery and sought to combine partial implants without moving to a total replacement. Argenson and coworkers[1] operated on 181 knees for primary patellofemoral disease and added a medial replacement in 57%. The early results were encouraging and similar to those of TKA in the first few years; however, there was a 30% revision rate into the second decade.[2] It was concluded that the results may have been compromised by limited early instrumentation and the combination of implants that were not entirely compatible. Cartier and colleagues[5] performed 87 PFAs and included a medial UKA in 36 knees (41%). They reported 86% excellent or good results with 2 to 12 years of follow-up.

Lonner[14] has continued to pursue bicompartmental replacement using two separate implants that are now more anatomically correct. Early results are encouraging but there is no long-term follow-up.

Rolston and coworkers[22] designed a single-piece femoral component that combined the femoral trochlear groove with the medial femoral condyle replacement. This articulated with a unicondylar type of tibial plateau insert and with an all-polyethylene patellar component. The instruments were designed to accommodate the complex nature of the femoral

---

*The senior author (AJT) is a consultant for Smith & Nephew Orthopaedics, Memphis, Tenn. Neither of the other authors received any benefits in relation to this article.
†References 3, 4, 10, 12, 18, and 20.

component; the tibial resection guide was a more traditional extramedullary instrument.

Based on a CT image of the knee, a second technology converts an individualized single-piece femoral component that resurfaces the diseased areas of the knee by using a custom-made shaping instrument that is also designed from the CT information. The tibial tray and patellar resurfacing are completed in a more traditional way with more standard instruments. This approach is very similar to the magnetic resonance imaging MRI patient-specific cutting blocks that are now available for TKA; however, the femoral component is manufactured as an individual custom design for each knee.

SURGICAL TECHNIQUE

The surgical techniques for the separate replacement of the patellofemoral joint and the medial tibiofemoral joint are presented elsewhere in this textbook and will not be reviewed again here. The two approaches can be combined at the same surgical sitting and are now more compatible with each other because of improvements in the anatomy. However, it does require planning by the operative surgeon and the patience to be sure that both implants are completed with equal precision.

The single-piece femoral components were developed in an attempt to simplify the surgical technique and make the operation similar to a TKA. The procedure can be performed through a limited, minimally invasive surgical approach if the surgeon is comfortable with the option (Fig. 102-1). Otherwise, a standard arthrotomy is acceptable. The tibial resection is performed using an extramedullary guide that is first set for the varus and valgus alignment with reference to the tibial shaft (Fig. 102-2). The depth is set at 2 mm below the deepest point on the medial articular surface. The sagittal alignment, or slope, should be between 5 and 7 degrees and is best if it is set to copy the preexisting tibial slope. Occasionally, a tibia will have a slope that is in excess of 10 degrees, especially in a patient of Eastern descent. It is best not to increase the slope above 10 degrees. If this angle is decreased, the flexion gap will be tightened and some adjustment will need to be made to match the extension gap.

The tibial resection is completed using a power saw for the vertical and horizontal cuts. A pin can be inserted through the cutting guide that protects the remaining tibial surface from any undercutting. After the cut is completed, a spacer

is placed into the knee in 90 degrees of flexion and in full extension (Fig. 102-3). The two gaps should be equal at this point. The most common presentation will be a flexion gap that is smaller than the extension gap because of a preexisting flexion contracture. This can be corrected by resecting more bone from the distal femur at the time of the distal resection. If the flexion gap is bigger than the extension gap, the slope of the tibial cut is usually too great and the slope should be decreased by removing bone from the anterior aspect of the tibial cut using the guide with a change in the slope.

After the gaps have been evaluated, the anteroposterior femoral axis (AP axis) is drawn on the surface of the femur for rotational reference and an intramedullary hole is made into the femoral canal just above the insertion of the posterior cruciate ligament at the base of the AP axis. The anterior femoral resection is performed with an instrument that is inserted over the intramedullary rod and set parallel to the AP axis (Fig. 102-4). The cut is made flush with the anterior femoral cortex, similar to the cut for a traditional TKA. The distal cut is made with another instrument that locks onto the intramedullary rod (Fig. 102-5). The depth is set on the medial side to equal the flexion gap and the angle of the distal cut is set with reference to the lateral femoral cortex. This is done so that the final cut will set the prosthesis flush with the lateral cortex and with the cartilaginous surface of the lateral femoral condyle. This cut is critical and is difficult to set to the exact depth.

After the distal femoral resection is completed, the space in flexion and full extension is again checked to ensure that

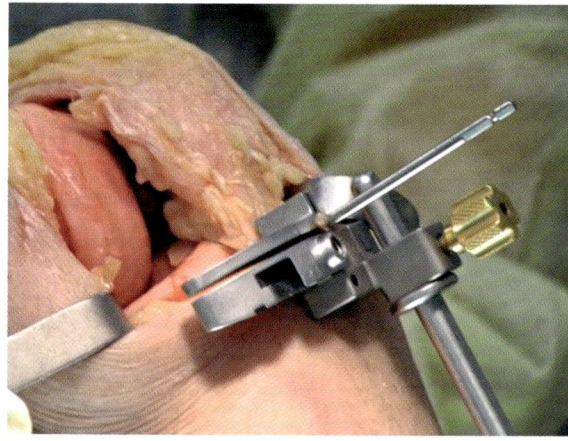

Figure 102-2. The extramedullary tibial guide references the medial tibial plateau surface.

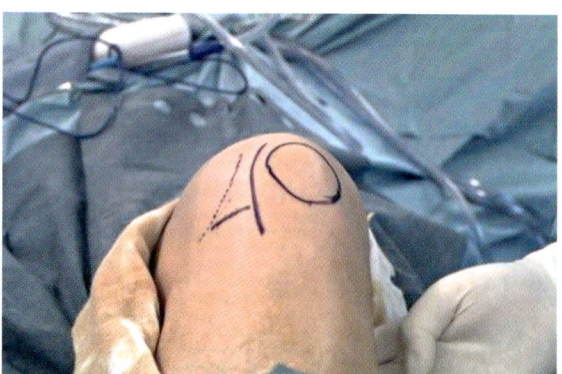

Figure 102-1. A minimally invasive medial incision can be used for this procedure.

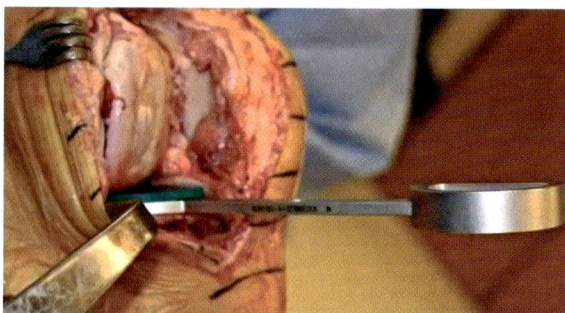

Figure 102-3. The spacer block is placed into the flexion gap and used as a reference for the extension gap.

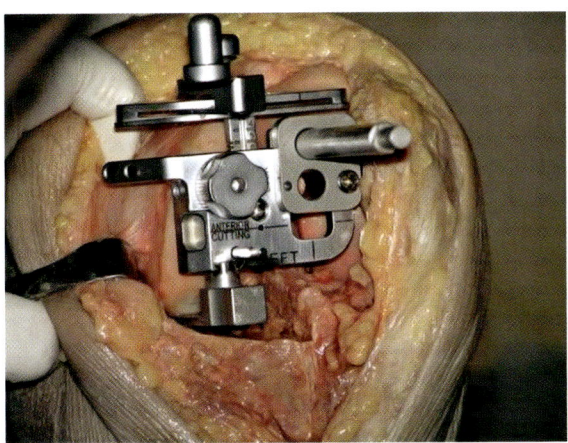

Figure 102-4. The first femoral guide references the posterior medial femoral condyle and sets the depth and rotation for the anterior cut.

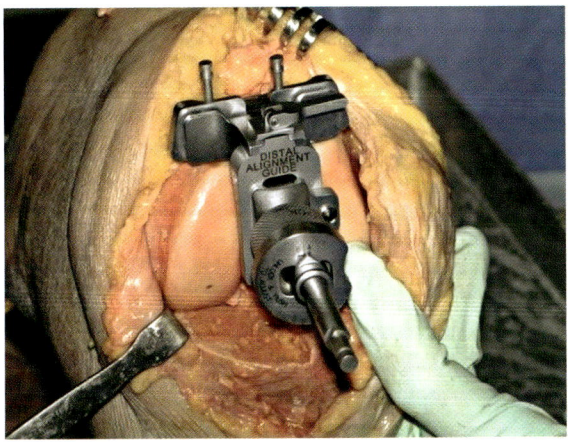

Figure 102-5. The distal femoral cut references the medial femoral condyle for the depth of resection and the lateral femoral cortex for the proper angulation.

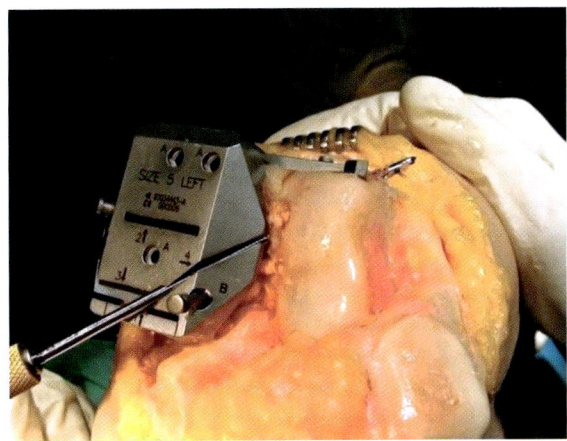

Figure 102-6. The femoral finishing block references the width of the medial femoral condyle and the lateral femoral cortex.

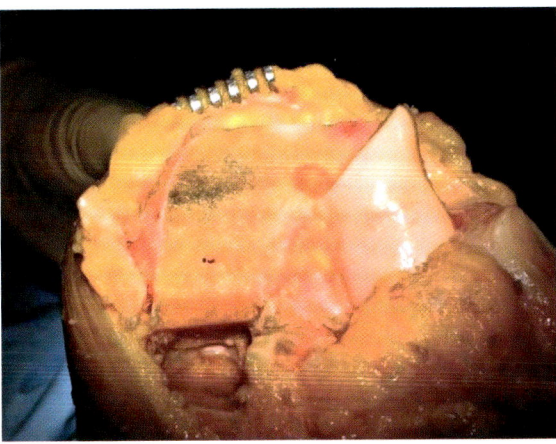

Figure 102-7. Finished cut surfaces of the femur.

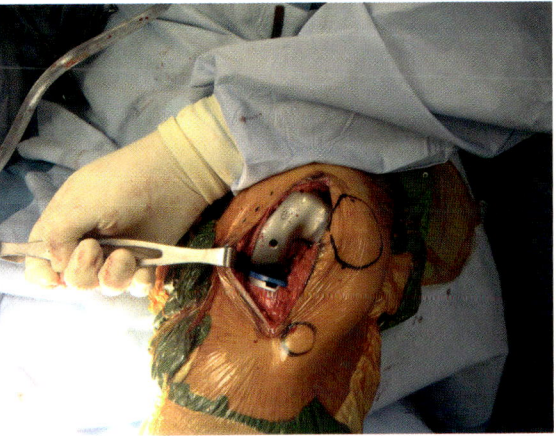

Figure 102-8. The trial components are positioned and the tracking, balance, and gap laxity are all evaluated.

the two are equal. If they are acceptable, the medial femoral condyle is sized by referring to the anteroposterior thickness. A finishing block is placed on the distal femoral cut surface and references the medial femoral condyle width and location of the lateral femoral cortex (Fig. 102-6). This is another step that is unique for the bicompartmental surgery and is not typical for TKA.

The final cuts are completed on the femoral side (Fig. 102-7). The tibial tray size is chosen and the trial components are inserted into the knee (Fig. 102-8). The patellar surface is resected with an oscillating saw or rotary blade and an onlay or inlay patellar component is positioned on the cut surface.

The knee is moved through a complete range of motion to evaluate the patellar tracking and the relationship of the medial femoral condyle to the tibial articular surface implant. The components are removed, the surfaces are lavaged, and all components are cemented in position at the same time.

The wound is closed over drains and a light dressing is applied so that motion can be instituted on the day of surgery. The patients are all anticoagulated and discharged within the first 2 to 3 days after surgery.

MATERIALS, METHODS, AND RESULTS

There has been only one report of results using the single piece femoral component with a minimum of 2-year follow-up. Tria and colleagues[25] studied 40 patients who underwent bicompartmental knee arthroplasty. The patients were chosen for the operation on the basis of the preoperative office interview, physical examination, and x-ray evaluation.

The patients were asked to indicate the location of their pain and its prevalence. If the pain was medial tibiofemoral with associated medial patellofemoral symptoms, the patient was considered a good candidate. The indications were very similar to those used for UKA but allowed more symptoms relating to the patellofemoral joint. Mild lateral tibiofemoral pain was acceptable if the patient was older than 75 years, but was not considered ideal. The older patient's symptom presentation was similar to the presentation of a patient who would usually undergo TKA rather than UKA. Global knee pain that was equally distributed in all areas of the knee was a definite contraindication, despite any physical examination and x-ray findings to the contrary.

The physical examination included medial tibiofemoral and patellofemoral tenderness. The clinical deformity did not exceed 10 degrees of varus or flexion contracture. When the varus deformity corrected to neutral with valgus stress, the knee was more ideal for the replacement. However, it was not absolutely necessary for the knee to be corrected. All ligaments were clinically intact. Some degree of anterior laxity related to anterior cruciate ligament deficiency was accepted but grade 4 instability was not included. Inflammatory arthritis and knees with previous ligament reconstructions or osteotomies were excluded.

The standing AP x-ray showed an anatomic varus deformity that was less than 10 degrees, with minimal translocation of the tibia beneath the femur. Patellofemoral arthritic changes of any extent were acceptable. Mild lateral osteoarthritic changes were considered acceptable. If there were changes in the lateral compartment, there should be no significant symptoms of pain or tenderness on physical examination.

The outpatient follow-up visits were at 2 weeks after surgery and then, 6 weeks, 3 months, 6 months, 1 year, and 2 years. X-rays were taken 2 weeks after surgery and then annually unless otherwise indicated by the clinical presentation.

There were 40 patients (17 men and 23 women). There were two bilateral operations, thus accounting for 42 knees. There were 16 right and 26 left knees. The average age of the patients was 70 years, with a range from 49 to 89 years. The average weight was 185 lb (84 kg), with a range from 114 lb (52 kg) to 262 lb (119 kg). The average body mass index (BMI) was 30 (range, 20 to 42). The average operative time (including surgery and anesthesia) was 114 minutes. The average tourniquet time was 68 minutes. The average cell saver blood return was 110 mL, with a hematocrit of 41%. There were no pulmonary emboli, proximal thigh deep vein thromboses, myocardial infarctions, infections, or mortalities. The average length of stay was 3 days (range, 1 to 6 days). The average preoperative flexion was 122 degrees (range, 115 to 130 degrees). The postoperative flexion at 2 to 4 weeks after surgery was 102 degrees and increased to 120 degrees at the last recorded office visit. The average preoperative anatomic axis was 3 degrees of varus and average postoperative axis was 2 degrees of valgus. The Knee Society score improved from 49 to 84 and the function score from 57 to 81.

One patient died after the first year of follow-up. One patient developed a subluxing patella in deep flexion at 6 weeks after the surgery. The components were not malaligned or internally rotated and there was no disruption of the medial retinacular closure. The patient was returned to the

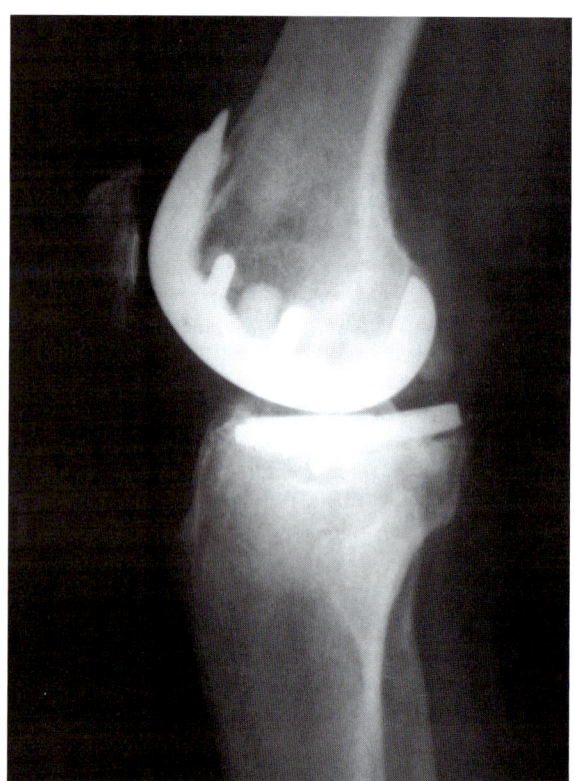

Figure 102-9. Lateral x-ray showing fracture of the tibial tray.

operating room for a lateral release and went on to have a good result.

Five knees have global pain (12%). One has been revised to a standard TKA, with a good result. At the time of the revision, the prosthesis did not appear to have any specific indicating factors for the failure. One patient was lost to follow-up and considered to be a revision. The remaining three patients continued to be followed but are expected to be revised. Persistent anterior knee pain was seen in 10 patients (24%). One tibial tray fractured in the coronal plane at 17 months after surgery, with initial pain that has resolved enough to avoid revision at this time (Fig. 102-9). One tray settled anteriorly at 20 months after surgery, with a reverse in the tibial slope (Fig. 102-10). The patient's pain is presently tolerable without revision.

SUMMARY

The results show a revision rate of 5% (one knee with global pain and one knee lost to follow-up for 2 of 42 knees) in the first 2 years, with another 12% (three knees with global pain, one knee with a tray fracture, and one knee with tray collapse [5 of 42 knees]) that might require revision in the near-future. None of the cases were technically overcorrected or malaligned. The incidence of anterior knee pain (24%; 10 of 42 knees) is high but has not led to any revisions to date.

The surgical results were studied for malalignment or overcorrection and there were no contributing factors. The one area of great difficulty in the surgical procedure was matching the remaining lateral femoral condyle surface to the surface of the femoral implant. One millimeter of separation or offset may lead to some patellofemoral symptoms but would not

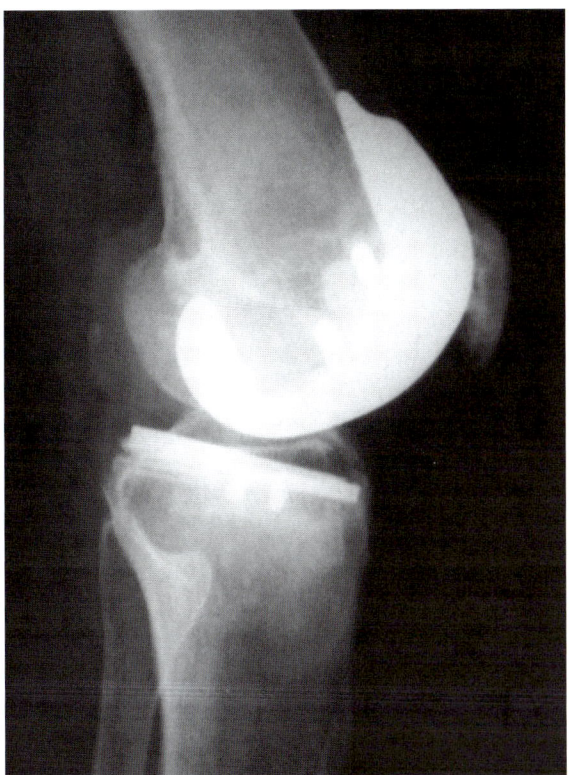

Figure 102-10. Lateral x-ray showing collapse of the tibial tray anteriorly, with reverse slope.

explain the cases with global knee pain. There are now newer instruments to position the femoral component and these may make a difference with respect to the lateral interface.

The prosthetic design may need to be revised. The tibial tray fracture occurred in the coronal plane, where the polyethylene slides into the posterior slot for the plastic. This is an area of a stress riser and the tray may need to be slightly thicker. The tibial tray that collapsed anteriorly might have been more solidly fixed if the pegs were slightly bigger.

The advantages of bicompartmental knee arthroplasty include preservation of the ligaments of the knee, less invasive surgery, and a quicker postoperative recovery. The knee should have more normal proprioception than TKA. Unfortunately, the clinical results have never been better than TKA with two separate implants or with a single-piece femoral component. It is surgically easier to perform a TKA or UKA than a bicompartmental replacement. With the present state of the art, however, we no longer perform bicompartmental arthroplasty.

KEY REFERENCES

Argenson JN, Guillaume JM, Aubaniac JM: Is there a place for patellofemoral arthroplasty? Clin Orthop Relat Res (321):162–167, 1995.

Argenson JN, Sebastian P, Aubaniac JM: The outcome of bicompartmental knee arthroplasty at 5- to 23-year follow-up. Presented at the Knee Society Annual Meeting, AAOS, Las Vegas, Nev, February 28, 2009.

Berger RA, Meneghini RM, Jacobs JJ, et al: Results of unicompartmental knee arthroplasty at a minimum of ten years of follow-up. J Bone Joint Surg Am 87:999–1006, 2005.

Cartier P, Sanouiller JL, Khefacha A: Long-term results with the first patellofemoral prosthesis, Clin Orthop Relat Res (436):47–54, 2005.

Chen AF, Alan RK, Redziniak DE, Tria AJ: Quadriceps sparing total knee arthroplasty: initial experience with two to four year results, J Bone Joint Surg Br 88:1448–1453, 2006.

Gesell MW, Tria AJ Jr: MIS unicondylar knee arthroplasty: surgical approach and early results. Clin Orthop Relat Res (428):53–60, 2004.

Goodfellow JW, Kershaw CJ, Benson MK, O'Connor JJ: The Oxford knee for unicompartmental osteoarthritis. The first 103 cases. J Bone Joint Surg Br 70:692–701, 1988.

Insall JN, Tria AJ, Aglietti P: Resurfacing of the patella. J Bone Joint Surg Am 62:933–936, 1980.

Kozinn SC, Scott R: Unicondylar knee arthroplasty. J Bone Joint Surg Am 71:145–150, 1989.

Lonner JH: Patellofemoral arthroplasty: the impact of design on outcomes. Orthop Clin North Am 39:347–354, 2008.

Marmor L: Marmor modular knee in unicompartmental disease. Minimum four-year follow-up. J Bone Joint Surg Am 61:347–353, 1979.

Price AJ, Webb J, Topf H, Dodd CAF, et al: Oxford Hip and Knee Group: rapid recovery after Oxford unicompartmental arthroplasty through a short incision. J Arthroplasty 16:970–976, 2001.

Repicci JA, Eberle RW: Minimally invasive surgical technique for unicondylar knee arthroplasty. J South Orthop Assoc 8:20–22, 1999.

Rolston L, Bresch J, Engh G, et al: Bicompartmental knee arthroplasty: a bone-sparing, ligament-sparing, and minimally invasive alternative for active patients. Orthopedics 30(Suppl):70–73, 2007.

Tria AJ, Shin MS, Jonna VK: Bicompartmental arthroplasty of the knee using a single piece femoral component. Presented at the Annual Closed Meeting of the Knee Society, October 9, 2009.

Full references for this chapter can be found on www.expertconsult.com.

Unicompartmental, Bicompartmental, or Tricompartmental Arthritis of the Knee: Algorithm for Surgical Management

Sridhar R. Rachala and Rafael J. Sierra

The knee joint is a modified hinge that can be arbitrarily divided into three compartments— medial, lateral, and patellofemoral. Arthritis from a surgical standpoint involves loss of articular cartilage, with narrowing of joint space. The loss of cartilage can be focal or more diffuse, with a more diffuse pattern seen commonly in degenerative arthritis. When this process is limited to only one compartment, it is defined as unicompartmental arthritis. Bicompartmental arthritis involves the medial or lateral compartment, with involvement of the patellofemoral compartment. Tricompartmental arthritis by definition involves all three compartments.

When faced with an articular pathology of the knee that has failed appropriate nonoperative management, the options for surgical management will include joint preservation and joint-sacrificing procedures. The former involves cartilage restoration procedures and/or osteotomies, done alone or in combination, and the latter involves a partial or a total knee replacement or arthrodesis of the knee. The goal of any of these procedures is primarily pain relief and secondarily improved function, with restoration of an active lifestyle.

The single most important factor in surgical decision making is the surgeon's philosophy and experience with nonarthroplasty or arthroplasty options. It is furthermore aided by numerous other factors, such as the age of the patient, extent and severity of articular pathology, clinical appearance and examination of the knee, and patient expectations with regards to activity, pain, and function. Although in some cases the decision may appear simple, in others all these factors must be taken into account to decide on the correct operation for the patient. The development of a fixed algorithm is therefore difficult.

Although the joint-preserving surgeries are less predictable,[12,14,25,26] when done with appropriate indications, they may afford long-term solutions with minimal need for activity restrictions. On the other hand, joint-sacrificing or replacement procedures are more predictable[5,6,19-21] in terms of pain relief but may need activity restrictions, especially in the young patient.

DEFINITIONS

- Total knee arthroplasty (TKA): Replacement of the tibiofemoral joint, with or without patellar resurfacing
- Partial knee arthroplasty (PKA): Replacement of one of the compartments of the tibiofemoral joint, with or without patellar resurfacing or replacement of the patellofemoral joint only
- Unicompartmental knee arthroplasty (UKA): One form of partial knee arthroplasty; involves replacement of the medial or lateral compartment
- Bicompartmental arthroplasty (BCA): Replacement of the medial or lateral compartment and the patellofemoral joint simultaneously

SURGICAL OPTIONS

Joint Preservation

The components of joint preservation include restoration of cartilage and restoration of alignment and joint stability. Restoring cartilage while leaving the limb malaligned or unstable is a setup for failure.

The ideal patient for a cartilage restoration is the young patient who has a focal cartilage defect with a well-aligned stable limb or one that can be aligned by an osteotomy procedure. It is also ideal for the patient with early arthritis who may require other concomitant procedures, such as meniscal allografts or anterior cruciate ligament (ACL) or posterior cruciate ligament (PCL) reconstruction.

Joint-Sacrificing Procedures

These include arthroplasty and arthrodesis. With the success of arthroplasty, the role of arthrodesis in the primary treatment of arthritis has become mostly obsolete, except for the patient with a native knee infection in whom this might still be an option.

PKA has gained popularity in the past decades as an alternative to TKA. As a group, historically it has been reserved for the relatively older patient with more advanced unicompartmental or bicompartmental arthritis but, with improvements in surgical design and technique, PKA is currently used for the younger patient as well. Also, for example, the middle-aged patient with limited disease who is active is also a good candidate for a PKA.[18]

TKA is the gold standard against which all procedures are compared. It traditionally has been described as the most predictable procedure for pain relief for any form of arthritis, either unicompartmental, bicompartmental, or tricompartmental. However, because of the sacrifice of the ACL and occasionally the PCL, it also the most kinematically different from a normal knee. Its best indication is for the patient with tricompartmental degenerative arthritis or in those knees with an inflammatory component to their arthritis.

FACTORS AFFECTING DECISION MAKING

These include severity and extent of the arthritis, clinical symptoms and examination of the knee, patient expectations, age, and previous surgery.

Severity and Extent of Arthritis

Inflammatory arthritis is a contraindication for osteotomy or PKA. The number of compartments involved and the severity of arthritic changes within them will determine the type of procedure that could be performed. Advanced cartilage loss is associated with poorer results after an osteotomy, and it would therefore be reasonable to recommend a realignment osteotomy for patients with isolated medial or lateral unicompartmental arthroplasty that is not end-stage,[24] or the extremely young patient (<40 years) with unicompartmental advanced arthritis. Severe unicompartmental arthritis of the tibiofemoral joint in middle-aged or older patients might benefit from PKA. The presence of tricompartmental arthritis would preclude a limited unicompartmental or bicompartmental replacement. The presence of either medial or lateral compartment arthritis with significant patellofemoral arthritis would be a reasonable indication for limited bicompartmental arthroplasty that replaces the medial or lateral and patellofemoral joint.

One of the most controversial subjects in TKA or PKA is the patellofemoral joint. Whether the patella should be replaced or not has been a matter of debate for years in patients undergoing TKA[4] and is currently controversial for patients undergoing PKA.

Radiographic evidence of arthritis without clinical symptoms emanating from the patellofemoral joint is currently not a contraindication for medial UKA. Furthermore, users of mobile-bearing designs do not believe that anterior knee pain in the presence of radiographic signs of patellofemoral arthritis—as long as there are no major grooves in the patellofemoral joint—is a contraindication to its use.[8,19] The designers have reported that patient symptoms improve after UKA as the patellofemoral joint is unloaded. In addition, long-term follow-up studies have shown low revision rates for progression of patellofemoral (PF) arthritis.[19] A similar scenario may apply to an osteotomy, especially a varus-producing distal femoral osteotomy, as PF joint kinematics are improved.[25]

However, the location of the patellar arthritis is important. Severe lateral patellar facet arthritis commonly requires replacement.[1a] Studies have shown that medial patellar facet arthritis may not be that critical and can be ignored when performing a medial UKA. This is not the case with lateral unicompartmental arthritis; if patellofemoral arthritis is present, then the patellofemoral joint should be replaced, most commonly in the form of TKA.

Clinical Symptoms and Examination

Some surgeons perform the single-digit test when assessing a patient for unicompartmental arthroplasty.[3] This is done by asking the patient to point with one finger at the area that generates the most pain. If the patient points to the medial, lateral, or patellofemoral joint and has all the other prerequisites on clinical examination for unicompartmental arthroplasty, the patient could be the best candidate for a PKA. The sensitivity and specificity of the single-digit test have not been determined, however, but for the surgeon with early experience using PKA, it may serve as a good way to screen for the best candidates for the procedure. In practice, referral patterns about the knee are highly variable and may have little clinical relevance to the location of the arthritis.

There are two critical examination findings that determine whether a patient is a good candidate for joint-preserving surgery, PKA, or TKA. In general terms, the presence of the anterior cruciate ligament and the ability to correct the deformity are important prerequisites[8,10] in patients for whom a PKA is considered.

Patients who have significant "touch me not" pain with tender points all over the knee may not be good candidates for any type of surgical intervention. The amount of deformity should be noted because patients with significant stiff deformities (varus >15 degrees or fixed flexion contracture >15 degrees) may be best treated with total knee arthroplasty, whereas patients with passively correctable deformities are better candidates for UKA or osteotomy. In our practice, patients who are believed to be candidates for unicompartmental arthroplasty undergo stress radiography with the knee flexed to 20 degrees to see whether the medial or lateral compartment can be corrected to a predisease state and whether the joint space in the contralateral compartment can be maintained.

Patient Expectations

The patient who wants to return to high-impact activities must be counseled about the possibility of early failure after arthroplasty. In this patient, especially if extremely young, an osteotomy should be entertained. Joint-preserving surgeries, however, are in general less predictable in regard to pain relief and in return of function when compared with arthroplasty options. There are data to suggest that some patients with UKA have achieved high levels of activity, but recommending that a patient undergo arthroplasty and go back to a high-impact sports activity would be acceptable for some surgeons.

Age

Although age was once thought to be a critical factor in decision making, it is currently not considered as such.[5,18] Younger patients, because of their higher activity level and life expectancy, are at higher risk for revision at some point in their lives but, if activity-limiting tricompartmental arthritis exists, this should not be ignored. There are long-term data to suggest that total knee arthroplasty is durable in the young patient[5]; however, these patients would likely benefit from less invasive arthroplasty techniques or osteotomy as long as tricompartmental arthroplasty does not exist. The extremely young patient, younger than 40 years, is likely the best candidate for osteotomy. The older patient (older than 40 years) is probably a good candidate for some form of arthroplasty, and PKA should be entertained as both temporizing and definitive management for this patient population.

Previous Surgery

Previous upper tibial osteotomy may be a relative contraindication to medial or lateral UKA if the knee has not failed back into its preoperative deformity. It has traditionally been described as an absolute contraindication for a mobile-bearing design used on the medial side.

LONG-TERM CLINICAL RESULTS OF SURGICAL OPTIONS

Osteotomy

An osteotomy helps by mechanically realigning the knee and unloading the affected compartment while relatively overloading the normal compartment. The review of the

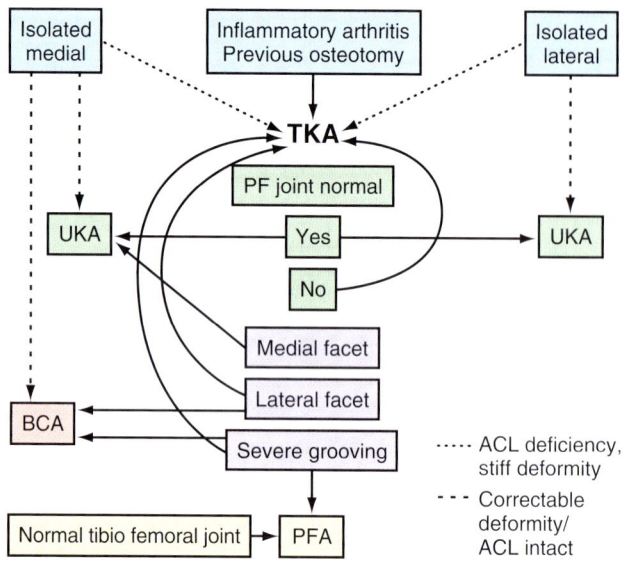

Figure 103-1 Depicted in this figure is our algorithmic approach to the patient with knee arthritis. The use of unicompartmental replacement has proven efficacy and durability in the literature, but the use of bicompartmental arthroplasty is in relatively early stages. We do not currently recommend it until further long-term studies are available, but it is included in this algorithm for completeness.

literature[23-26] shows that the results of this treatment deteriorate with time. Even in a best case scenario, the survivorship of the osteotomy is approximately 50% at 20 years.

Unicompartmental Knee Arthroplasty

Unicompartmental knee arthroplasty has the advantage of being a less invasive surgery, thereby aiding in a fast recovery period.[11,15] In addition, patients have a more natural feel to their knees because the kinematics of the knee are not altered.[17]

Unicompartmental arthroplasty is a surgical option in the middle-aged to older patient with advanced arthritis and symptoms largely confined to one or two compartments. Medial unicompartmental arthroplasty is an option in the patient with medial compartment arthritis with or without medial facet patellofemoral joint disease while lateral unicompartmental arthroplasty should only be entertained when isolated lateral compartment arthritis exists. Using fixed-bearing UKA, Berger and colleagues[2] have reported 96% survival and 92% good or excellent results at a minimum of 10 years. Using Oxford meniscal-bearing UKA, Price and associates[19] have reported a 15-year survival of 93% in 439 knees, with 91% good or excellent clinical results.

If a patient has isolated lateral compartment arthritis with no patellofemoral disease, a lateral unicompartmental arthroplasty may be a reasonable option, affording durable results.[1,9,13,16] However, the results in general are inferior when compared with those of medial UKA. If patellofemoral arthritis coexists with lateral unicompartmental disease, a total knee arthroplasty or bicompartmental arthroplasty would be indicated.

Bicompartmental Arthritis

A combined UKA and patellofemoral replacement can be done as a bicompartmental arthroplasty if there is medial or lateral uncompartmental arthritis with advanced patellofemoral arthritis. However, there are few studies to support this as a routine indication.[7,22]

Total Knee Arthroplasty

Total knee arthroplasty is the gold standard for the treatment of osteoarthritis and all other forms of surgical treatments are compared with it in terms of efficacy. Long-term follow-up studies of total knee replacement have shown 90%[20] good to excellent results and a 15-year survivorship of 92% to 93%,[5,6,20,21] with revision for any reason as an end point.

CONCLUSION

We have presented our algorithm for surgical management in Figure 103-1. For the extremely young patient with early-stage unicompartmental arthritis, osteotomy may be an option. Joint arthroplasty is the preferred treatment for patients with end-stage arthritis. Whether unicompartmental, bicompartmental, or tricompartmental replacement is performed is highly dependent on surgeon experience and philosophy. Our algorithm presents a decision tree approach for the surgeon who is interested in using PKA as an alternative to TKA.

KEY REFERENCES

Ashraf T, Newman JH, Evans RL, et al: Lateral unicompartmental knee replacement survivorship and clinical experience over 21 years. J Bone Joint Surg Br 84:1126-1130, 2002.

Berger RA, Meneghini RM, Jacobs JJ, et al: Results of unicompartmental knee arthroplasty at a minimum of 10 years follow-up. J Bone Joint Surg 87:999-1006, 2005.

Bert JM: Unicompartmental knee replacement. Orthop Clin North Am 36:513-522, 2005.

Burnett RS, Boone JL, Rosenzweig SD, et al: Patellar resurfacing compared with nonresurfacing in total knee arthroplasty. A concise follow-up of a randomized trial. J Bone Joint Surg Am 91:2562-2567, 2009.

Dixon MC, Brown RR, Parsch D, et al: Modular fixed-bearing total knee arthroplasty with retention of the posterior cruciate ligament. A study of patients followed for a minimum of fifteen years. J Bone Joint Surg Am 87:598-603, 2005.

Ohdera T, Tokunaga J, Kopayashi A: Unicompartmental knee arthroplasty for lateral gonarthrosis: midterm results. J Arthroplasty 16:196–200, 2001.

Patil S, Colwell CW Jr, Ezzet KA, et al: Can normal knee kinematics be restored with unicompartmental knee replacement? J Bone Joint Surg Am 87:332-338, 2005.

Pennington DW, Swienckowski JJ, Lutes WB, et al: Unicompartmental knee arthroplasty in patients sixty years of age or younger. J Bone Joint Surg Am 85:1968-1973, 2003.

Price AJ, Waite JC, Svard U: Long-term clinical results of the medial Oxford unicompartmental knee arthroplasty. Clin Orthop Relat Res (435):171-180, 2005.

Rasquinha VJ, Ranawat CS, Cervieri CL, et al: The press-fit condylar modular total knee system with a posterior cruciate-substituting design. A concise follow-up of a previous report. J Bone Joint Surg Am 88:1006-1010, 2006.

Rodricks DJ, Patil S, Pulido P, et al: Press-fit condylar design total knee arthroplasty. Fourteen- to seventeen-year follow-up. J Bone Joint Surg Am 89:89-95, 2007.

Rolston L, Siewert K: Assessment of knee alignment after bi-compartmental knee arthroplasty. J Arthroplasty 24:1111-1114, 2009.

Stukenborg-Colsman C, Wirth CJ, et al: High tibial osteotomy versus unicompartmental joint replacement in unicompartmental knee joint osteoarthritis: 7-10-year follow-up prospective randomized study. Knee 8:187-194, 2001.

Wang JW, Hsu CC: Distal femoral varus osteotomy for osteoarthritis of the knee. J Bone Joint Surg Am 87:127-133, 2005.

Full references for this chapter can be found on www.expertconsult.com.

Surgical Approaches in Total Knee Arthroplasty: Standard and MIS Techniques

Nilesh Patil, Michael P. Nett, Alfred Tria, Jr., and Giles R. Scuderi

Critical to exposing the knee during total knee arthroplasty is a complete understanding of the local anatomy, which is described in Chapter 1. With such knowledge, the pathologic condition, anatomy, and planned surgery can be correlated. Although well-defined soft tissue layers provide reproducible planes of dissection,[33,44,58] the blood supply to the skin should be respected, especially when previous incisions are present or multiple incisions are planned. Most of the blood supply to the skin arises from the saphenous artery and the descending geniculate artery on the medial side of the knee (Fig. 104-1).[18,60] The vessels perforate the deep fascia and form an anastomosis superficial to the deep fascia. Continuing through the subcutaneous fat to supply the epidermis, little communication occurs in the superficial layer. Therefore, dissection should be deep to the fascia to maintain the blood supply to the skin.[59] The blood supply to the skin should not be confused with the blood supply to the patella.

Many incisions and approaches to the knee joint were originally designed for open meniscectomy and reconstructive procedures before the advent of arthroscopy and are mainly of historical value.[1] The intent of this chapter is to detail the surgical approaches that are useful for total knee arthroplasty. Many planned approaches are extensile but have been modified for performing minimally invasive surgery.[20]

ANTERIOR APPROACHES

Skin Incisions

A straight anterior skin incision is extensile and can be extended proximally and distally to expose the distal end of the femur, the patella, and the proximal end of the tibia. This anterior incision allows exposure of the medial and lateral supporting structures and can be reopened if a reoperation is necessary. Through this skin incision, a medial parapatellar arthrotomy can be performed; this is the most versatile approach in that it allows the broadest exposure to the knee joint. Other arthrotomies, such as midvastus and subvastus approaches, are also performed through this skin incision and will be detailed in the following sections.

The anterior midline skin incision has provided a utilitarian extensile approach to the knee (Fig. 104-2). With proximal and distal extension of the skin incision, large flaps can be developed to expose the anterior, medial, and lateral supporting structures.[27] If the midline skin incision is moved medially, it will be parallel to Langer's cleavage lines and subject to less tension and disrupting force than would an anterior midline incision.[57] Incisions parallel to the cleavage lines heal faster, gain strength more quickly, and result in a finer scar.[31] No evidence indicates that this position creates any more hypoxia in the lateral skin margin than an anterior midline incision does.

The anterior Kocher U incision[31] and the Putti inverted U incision[42] have become obsolete, primarily because of complications associated with vascular compromise to the surrounding skin. The anterior transverse incision may be cosmetically pleasing, but it does not allow extensile exposure (see Fig. 104-2).[57]

ARTHROTOMY

The medial parapatellar arthrotomy, or anteromedial approach, has been the most used approach for exposure of the knee joint. It provides extensive exposure and is useful for open anterior cruciate ligament reconstruction, total knee replacement, and fixation of intra-articular fractures. Because this approach has been implicated in compromise of the patellar circulation (see Fig. 104-1C),[51,52] some authors have advocated the subvastus, midvastus, and trivector approaches for exposure of the knee joint. Whereas these approaches expose the knee from the medial side, the anterolateral approach exposes the knee joint from the lateral side. With careful planning and arthrotomy selection, the anterior aspect of the joint can be fully exposed with these arthrotomies.

MEDIAL PARAPATELLAR ARTHROTOMY

A medial parapatellar arthrotomy allows excellent exposure to most structures of the knee joint (Fig. 104-3). Von Langenbeck[57] originally described dissection of the vastus medialis from the quadriceps tendon with distal extension through the medial patellar retinaculum and along the patellar ligament. The synovium is divided in line with the capsular incision, and the fat pad is retracted or incised. Because dissection continues to the joint line, one must be aware of the anterior horn of the medial meniscus, as well as the transverse ligament between the medial and lateral menisci. Completion of this arthrotomy permits the patella to be everted or subluxated laterally. When the patella is dislocated and the knee is flexed, care should be taken to avoid avulsing the patellar tendon from the tibial tubercle. If difficulty is involved in dislocating the patella laterally, the proximal quadriceps tendon incision should be extended superiorly or the patellar tendon carefully reflected subperiosteally along the medial border of the tibial tubercle to its crest. The patellar tendon must not be detached from the tibial tubercle.

Insall[23] modified the split patella approach, as described by Sir Robert Jones, because of damage to the patellar articular surface (Fig. 104-4). The extensor mechanism is exposed through a midline skin incision, the quadriceps tendon is divided 8 to 10 cm above the patella, and the incision is continued distally in a straight line over the patella and along the medial border of the patellar tendon. The quadriceps expansion is peeled from the anterior surface of the patella

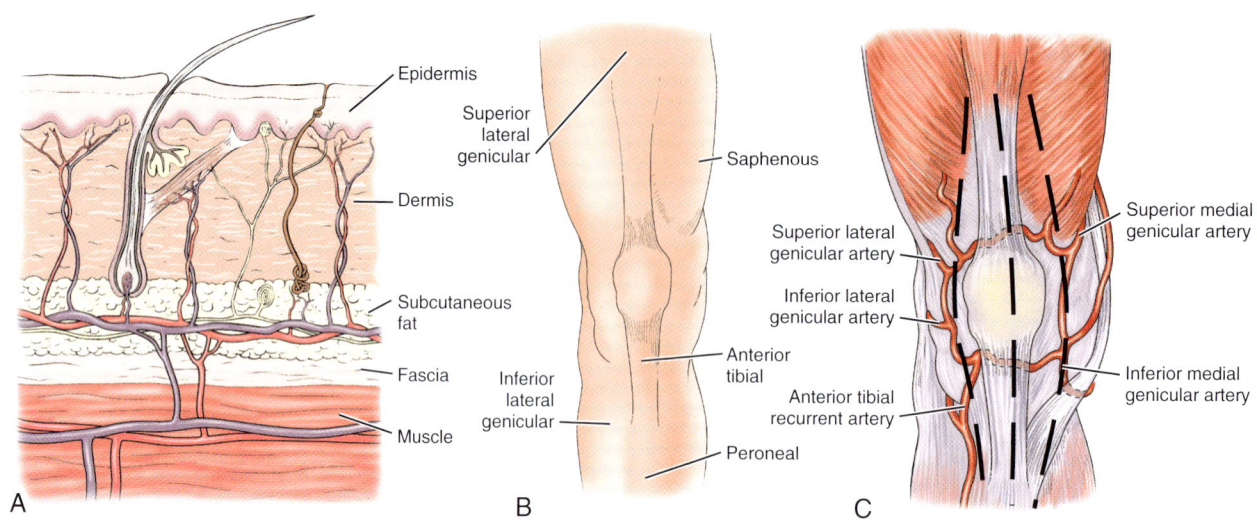

Figure 104-1. Blood supply to the knee. **A,** Microcirculation to the skin. **B,** Vessels contributing to the blood supply to the skin. **C,** Patellar blood supply. (**A** and **B,** Redrawn from Younger AS, Duncan CP, Masri BA: Surgical exposures in revision total knee arthroplasty. J Am Acad Orthop Surg 6:55, 1998; **C,** Redrawn from Scott WN: The knee, vol 1, St Louis, 1994, Mosby-Year Book, p 56.)

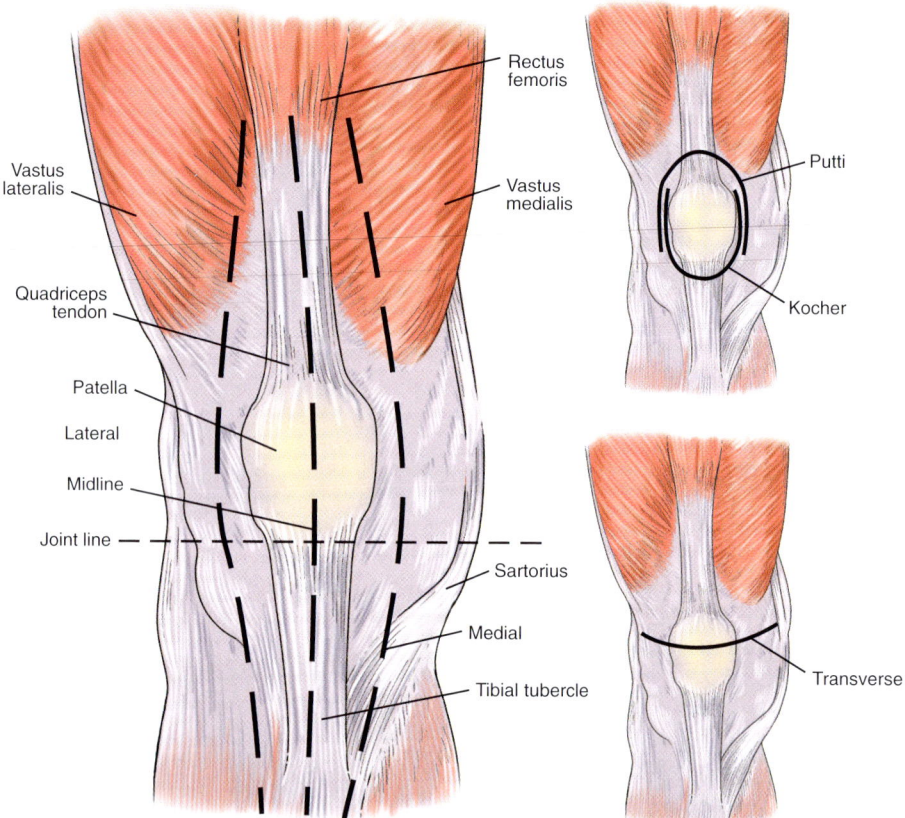

Figure 104-2. Anterior approaches to the knee. (Redrawn from Scott WN: The knee, vol 1, St Louis, 1994, Mosby-Year Book, p 56.)

by sharp dissection until the medial border of the patella is visualized. The synovium is divided, and the fat pad is split along the midline. The patella is then dislocated laterally. No internervous plane is used with this approach; however, both the rectus femoris and the vastus medialis are supplied by the femoral nerve proximal to this incision.

When the anteromedial approach is performed, the infrapatellar branch of the saphenous nerve comes into view

(see Fig. 104-4, *center*). The saphenous nerve travels posterior to the sartorius muscle and pierces the fascia between the tendons of the sartorius and gracilis muscles, where it becomes superficial to the medial aspect of the knee. At this level, the infrapatellar branch of the saphenous nerve arises to supply the skin over the anteromedial aspect of the knee. Kummel and Zazanis,[32] as well as Chambers,[7] noted variation of this infrapatellar branch and recommended protecting it at the

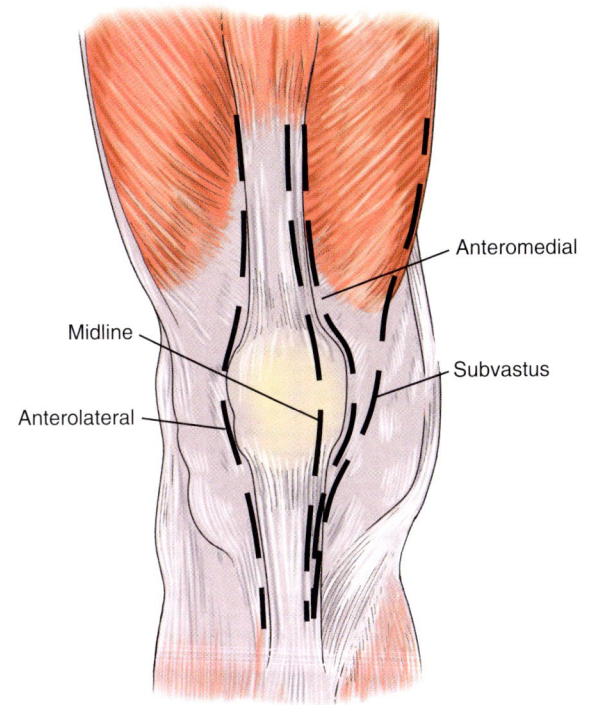

Figure 104-3. Preferred anterior approaches to the knee. (Redrawn from Scott WN: The knee, vol 1, St Louis, 1994, Mosby-Year Book, p 57.)

time of surgery to avoid painful neuromas. Insall et al[24] believed that neuroma formation is more related to the patient's temperament than to an actual pathologic condition.

SUBVASTUS APPROACH

The subvastus approach, which allows direct access to the anterior knee joint, has been heralded as being more anatomic than the medial parapatellar arthrotomy (Fig. 104-5).[21,39] The subvastus approach is applicable to most reconstructive procedures of the knee, with the exception of lateral unicompartmental replacement.

This approach uses a straight midline skin incision that is extended above and below the patella. After development of a medial subcutaneous flap, the lower border of the vastus medialis is visualized. Because the vastus medialis inserts into the superior medial aspect of the patella, the fascial sheath along the inferior border of the vastus medialis is incised from the patella down to the intermuscular septum. This incision separates the vastus medialis from the intermuscular septum. The arthrotomy then continues distally along the medial margin of the patella, with the medial retinaculum incised along the medial border of the patellar tendon and down onto the tibia. The vastus medialis then is peeled proximally, with blunt dissection, from the intermuscular septum. Care should be taken at this point to avoid injury to the neurovascular contents of Hunter's canal. To gain access to the joint, the capsule of the suprapatellar pouch should be divided to release the patella, which is everted or subluxated laterally as the knee is flexed.

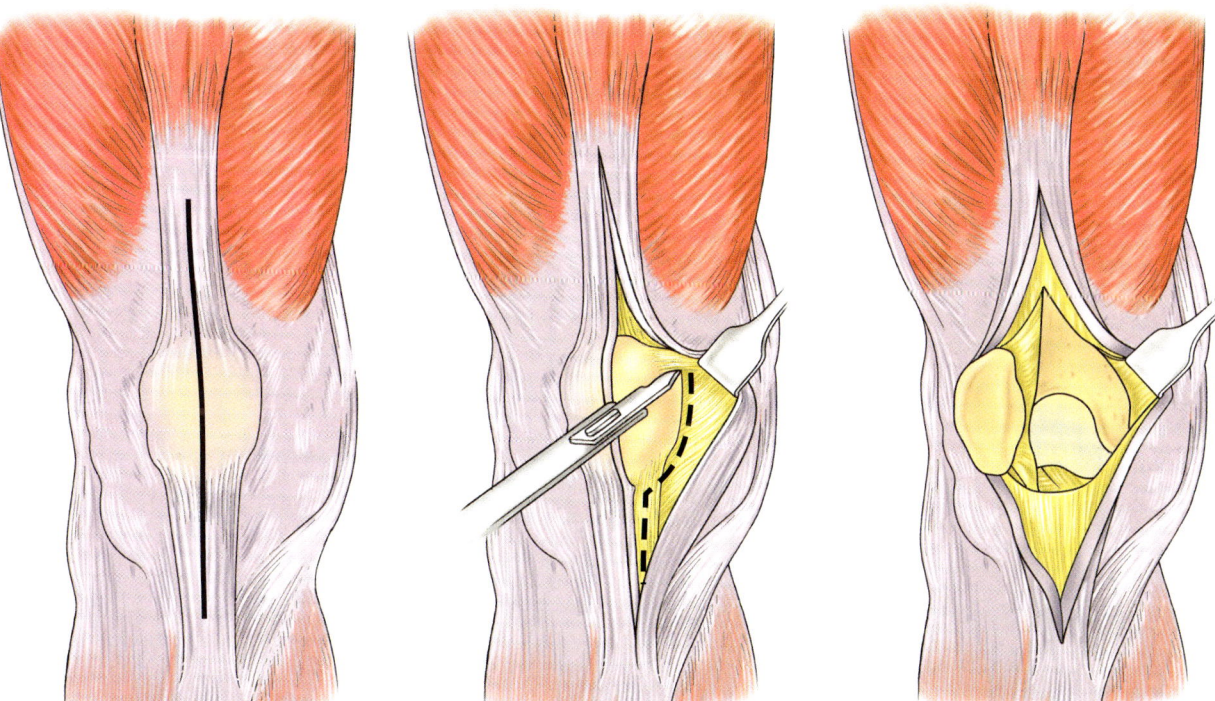

Figure 104-4. Insall's anterior approach. (Redrawn from Scott WN: The knee, vol 1, St Louis, 1994, Mosby-Year Book, p 57.)

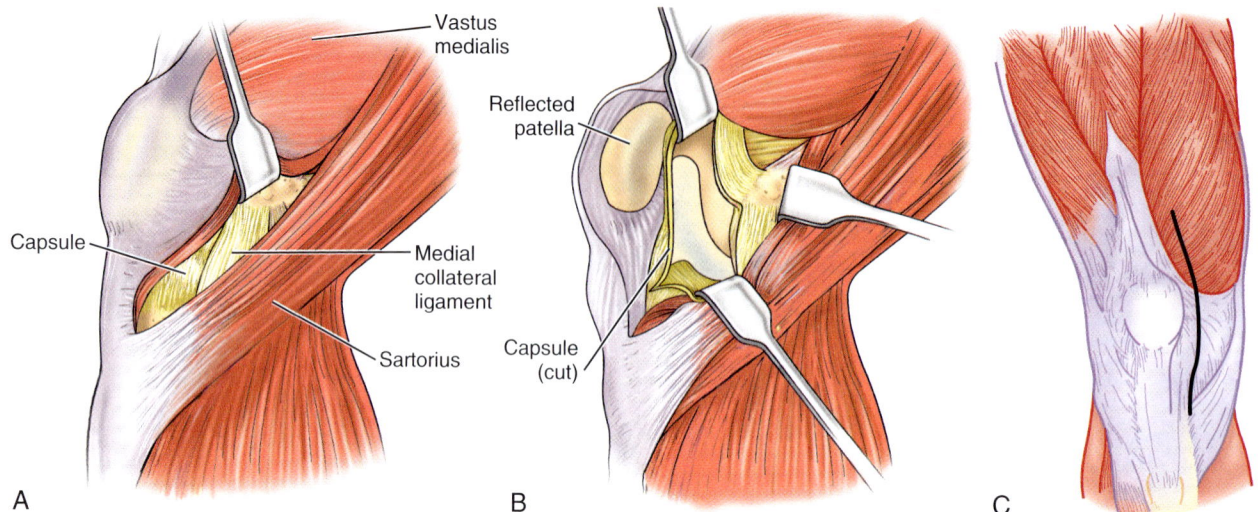

Figure 104-5. **A** and **B,** Subvastus approach. **C,** Trivector-retaining arthrotomy. (**A** and **B,** Redrawn from Scott WN: The knee, vol 1, St Louis, 1994, Mosby-Year Book, p 58; **C,** redrawn from Scuderi GR, Tria AJ: Surgical techniques in total knee arthroplasty, New York, 2002, Springer Verlag.)

MIDVASTUS APPROACH

The midvastus muscle-splitting approach is performed through a standard anterior midline skin incision. The incision is carried down through subcutaneous tissue and deep fascia to expose the quadriceps musculature. The vastus medialis is identified, along with split full thickness, parallel to its muscle fibers. The quadriceps tendon is not incised. The incision is extended to the superior medial corner of the patella and then is continued distally along the medial patella and the patellar tendon to the level of the tibial tubercle. As with the subvastus approach, the capsule of the suprapatellar pouch is divided, so that the patella can be everted or subluxated laterally. Advocates of this approach believe that it is easier to evert the patella with the midvastus approach than with the subvastus approach because of the reduced bulk of the vastus medialis. In addition, this approach splits the muscle well away from its neurovascular supply.[14]

TRIVECTOR-RETAINING ARTHROTOMY

The quadriceps musculature is exposed through an anterior midline skin incision. The trivector-retaining arthrotomy begins with transection of the vastus medialis obliquus muscle fibers 1.5 to 2 cm medial to the quadriceps tendon. Because the quadriceps tendon is not incised with this approach, the incision is extended distally 1 cm medial to the patella and the patellar tendon to the level of the tibial tubercle. It is recommended that this approach be performed with the knee flexed 90 to 110 degrees, so that the quadriceps musculature is under maximal tension during the incision. To evert the patella or subluxate it laterally, the capsule of the suprapatellar pouch must be divided.[5]

ANTEROLATERAL APPROACH

The anterolateral approach, as described by Kocher,[31] consists of a lateral capsular incision that begins approximately 8 cm proximal to the patella at the insertion of the vastus lateralis muscle into the quadriceps tendon and continues distally along the lateral retinaculum (see Fig. 104-3). The incision can be extended distally through the fat pad for visualization of the lateral compartment and ends just distal to the tibial tuberosity. This approach is less favorable than the anteromedial approach because it is more difficult to subluxate the patella medially than laterally.

LATERAL PARAPATELLAR APPROACH

The lateral parapatellar approach may be considered in total knee arthroplasty for fixed valgus deformities that are isolated or combined with flexion contracture or external tibial rotation. Fixed varus deformity represents the only relative contraindication.

In performing this approach, a curvilinear midline skin incision or a laterally placed anterior skin incision is made and extended distally over the lateral border of the tibial tubercle. The joint is entered through a lateral parapatellar incision that extends from the lateral border of the quadriceps tendon, over the lateral margin of the patella, and continues distally into the anterior compartment fascia, 1.5 cm from the tibial tubercle, and for a distance of 3 cm from the tibial tubercle. To dislocate the patella medially and expose the joint, a thin segment of the tubercle is osteotomized with the attached patellar tendon. A medial periosteal hinge is maintained along with the infrapatellar fat pad, which is used for later closure of the lateral retinacular defect.[6,29]

EXTENDED APPROACHES

Quadriceps Turndown

Coonse and Adams[12] originally described a quadriceps turndown. They used a paramedian skin incision that begins at the lower end of the quadriceps tendon along the patella and extends along the medial border of the patellar tendon. Skin flaps are developed, the quadriceps tendon is split down the middle, and about 1 cm above the patella the incision is swung both medially and laterally and continues along the patella and the patellar tendon. The patella and the patellar

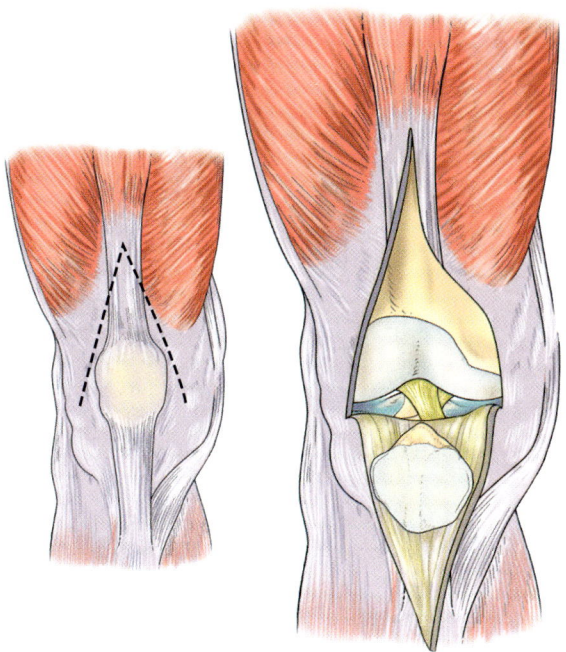

Figure 104-6. Coonse-Adams quadriceps turndown. (Redrawn from Scott WN: The knee, vol 1, St Louis, 1994, Mosby-Year Book, p 66.)

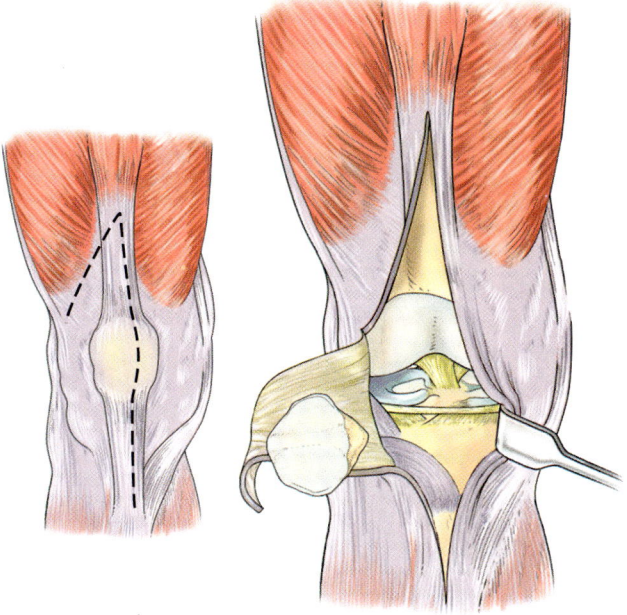

Figure 104-7. Modified Coonse-Adams quadriceps turndown. (Redrawn from Scott WN: The knee, vol 1, St Louis, 1994, Mosby-Year Book, p 66.)

tendon can be turned down to allow complete exposure of the joint (Fig. 104-6).

Further modification of the patellar turndown approach[26] involves the use of an anterior midline incision. A medial parapatellar arthrotomy is performed, and a second incision is made at an inclination of 45 degrees from the apex of the quadriceps tendon and extended laterally through the vastus lateralis and the upper portion of the iliotibial tract. This lateral incision stops short of the inferior lateral geniculate artery to preserve the blood supply (Fig. 104-7).

Quadriceps Snip

The full patellar turndown is now rarely necessary because cutting the quadriceps tendon proximally yields excellent soft tissue exposure, and functional reconstruction is possible (Fig. 104-8). This technique has been called the *quadriceps snip* by Insall.[26] Following a long medial parapatellar arthrotomy, an oblique incision is made at the proximal apex of the quadriceps tendon. This incision is approximately at a 45-degree angle across the quadriceps tendon and directly in line with the fibers of the vastus lateralis. This extended approach relieves tension on the extensor mechanism and the tibial tubercle. As the tibia is externally rotated and the patella subluxated laterally, the joint is exposed.

Tibial Tubercle Osteotomy

An anterior midline incision is made that extends 8 to 10 cm below the tibial tubercle. The medial parapatellar arthrotomy extends from 6 cm above the patella and distally along the tibial tubercle and anterior crest (Fig. 104-9). Whiteside and Ohl[58] used this exposure for difficult total knee arthroplasty, and they recommend using an oscillating saw to transect the tibial crest 8 to 10 cm below the tibial tubercle while

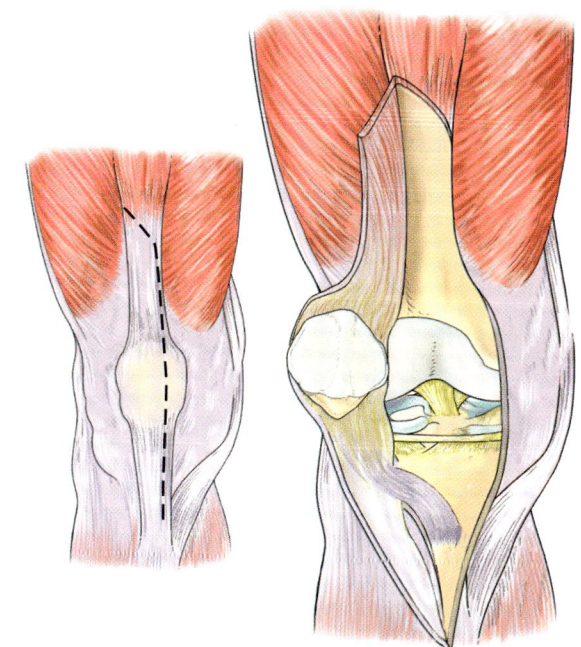

Figure 104-8. Insall's quadriceps snip. (Redrawn from Scott WN: The knee, vol 1, St Louis, 1994, Mosby-Year Book, p 67.)

elevating the tibial crest from the tibia. The lateral periosteum and musculature structures are left attached, as is the lateral aspect of the quadriceps mechanism. Fernandez[15] recommends tibial tubercle osteotomy for bicondylar tibial fractures. He uses a straight anterolateral parapatellar incision. Large medial and lateral subcutaneous flaps are developed. The osteotomy of the tibial tubercle is performed with an oscillating saw and osteotomes. The osteotomy is trapezoidal, 5 cm long, 2 cm wide, and 1.5 cm wide distally. Once the

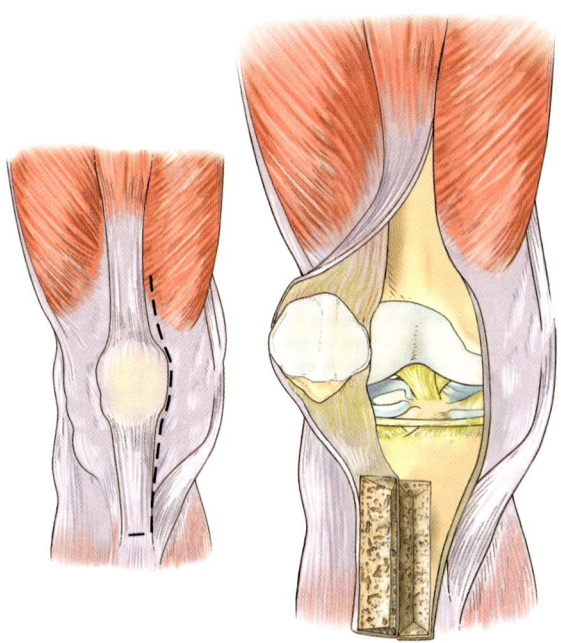

Figure 104-9. Anterior approach to the knee with osteotomy of the tibial tubercle. (Redrawn from Scott WN: The knee, vol 1, St Louis, 1994, Mosby–Year Book, p 67.)

tibial tubercle and the anterior tibial crest are freed, the entire extensor mechanism is elevated proximally, and the retropatellar fat pad is divided to expose the entire joint.

Minimally Invasive Total Knee Arthroplasty

Total knee arthroplasty (TKA) has been performed for decades by using a traditional extensile approach. Historically, surgical exposure was achieved through an 8- to 10-inch skin incision and a long medial parapatellar arthrotomy, although some authors used a midvastus[14] or a subvastus approach.[21] This was followed by extensive soft tissue dissection and eversion of the patella. With improvement in the techniques of ligament balancing, adjustments in the overall alignment, and flexion-extension gap equalization techniques, good to excellent clinical outcomes have been reported in long-term follow-up studies for TKA completed using an extensile approach.*

The introduction of minimally invasive surgery (MIS) for unicondylar knee replacement[45,47] encouraged interest in applying a similar approach to standard TKA. Various minimally invasive approaches, including limited medial parapatellar, limited midvastus, limited subvastus, and the quadriceps-sparing approach, are considered a continuum of traditional extensile approaches. The surgeon can shorten the skin incision as he or she becomes more familiar with the surgical technique, progressing along on the scale of complexity, and finally can become competent in performing quadriceps-sparing MIS TKA. The MIS approach can be easily converted to a traditional approach if required.

---

*References 10, 24, 25, 27, 37, 43, 46, 49, and 54.

Potential benefits of less invasive surgery include reduced blood loss, reduced pain, less morbidity, and faster recovery.[34,50,55] The primary objective in MIS TKA is to limit surgical dissection without compromising component position, ligament balancing, or overall limb alignment. Modification of TKA instrumentation has facilitated the procedure, but appropriate patient selection remains critical for a successful outcome. The ideal candidate for MIS TKA is a patient with minimal deformity and good preoperative motion, who is of small to average stature. Our patient selection preference has evolved to include patients with less than 15-degree varus, 20-degree valgus, or 10-degree flexion contracture, with a minimum of 90-degree range of motion. Short, thin females with low body mass index and narrow femurs are good candidates for this approach.[50] Muscular males with prominent vastus medialis and wider femurs often are better served by a more traditional approach. Patients with a compromised soft tissue envelope or a short patellar tendon, and those with severe deformities requiring extensive release, tend to need a standard approach. Moreover, patients with diabetes mellitus or rheumatoid or inflammatory arthritis and those who are obese tend to be less favorable candidates for MIS TKA.[55]

Limited Medial Parapatellar Arthrotomy

A limited parapatellar approach is useful in most cases because it involves little deviation from the traditional approach. It is popular because of its familiarity, simplicity, and excellent exposure of all three compartments of the knee. Additionally, it can be easily extended if a more extensile exposure is required, with little risk of skin or patellar tendon complications. This approach has four characteristic features: a small skin incision, a limited medial parapatellar arthrotomy, the use of a mobile window, and patellar subluxation instead of eversion.

A straight anterior midline skin incision of approximately 10 to 14 cm in length is made, extending from the superior pole of the patella to the tibial tubercle. Limited medial and lateral flaps are created by subcutaneous dissection to expose the extensor mechanism. Release of the deep fascia proximally beneath the skin aids mobilization of the skin throughout the procedure. Because of the elasticity of the skin, the skin incision usually stretches by 2 to 4 cm with knee flexion. This can be used to permit broader exposure. The planned arthrotomy path and the fat pad are injected with 30 mL 1% lidocaine with epinephrine. This has been shown to reduce perioperative blood loss when combined with a minimally invasive technique.[13]

The limited parapatellar arthrotomy is performed extending 2 to 4 cm into the quadriceps tendon proximal to the superior pole of patella, then curving around the medial border of the patella or straight over the medial aspect of the patella, and distally along the medial border of the patellar tendon (Fig. 104-10). The deep medial collateral ligament, the posteromedial capsule, and the semimembranosus tendon are elevated subperiosteally from the proximal tibia. The knee is flexed and the patella is subluxed laterally. The arthrotomy can be gradually extended proximally if difficulty is encountered in displacing the patella laterally. The supporting soft tissues are protected by careful placement of the retractors. The mobile window created by arthrotomy can be moved from medial to lateral and from superior to inferior as

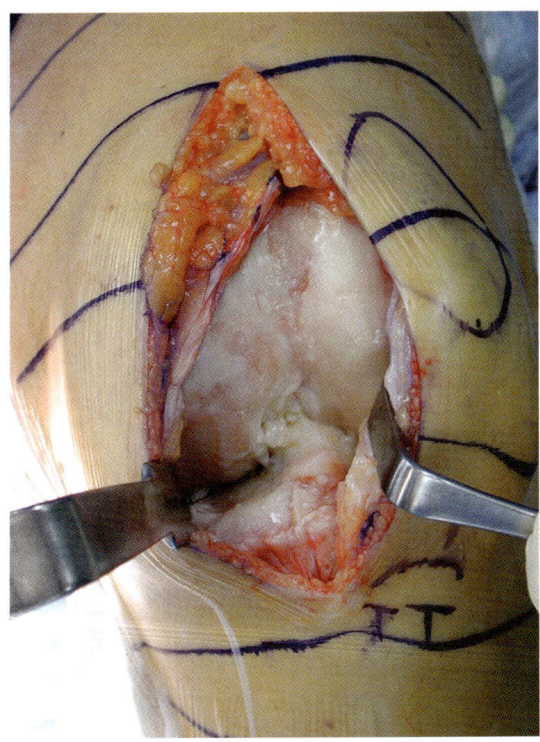

Figure 104-10. Limited medial parapatellar arthrotomy (minimally invasive surgery total knee arthroplasty [MIS TKA]).

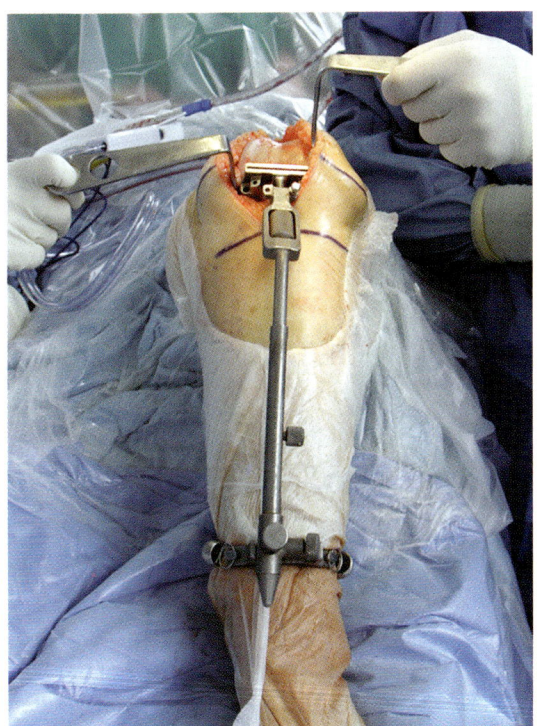

Figure 104-11. Tibial resection.

necessary to enable optimal exposure of the joint without application of undue pressure on the skin or the capsular tissues. It is recommended to extend the skin incision by 1 to 2 cm proximally or distally if excessive stretching of soft tissues is done to gain exposure without compromising wound healing.

Bone resection can be performed according to surgeon preference. We recommend cutting the tibia first because this enlarges the soft tissue envelope of the knee in flexion and extension, which provides better visualization of the knee. The tibial resection is performed in 90 degrees of flexion with an extramedullary cutting guide specially designed for MIS TKA (Fig. 104-11). Modified instrumentation, including alignment guides and cutting blocks, is utilized. Its altered geometry facilitates placement within a smaller soft tissue envelope. The retractors are placed appropriately to protect the collateral ligaments and the patellar tendon. The mobile window is moved medially and laterally during resection of the medial and lateral aspects of the tibia, respectively. Then the knee is brought into 60 to 70 degrees of flexion to remove the resected proximal tibial bone. The bone is removed after the roots of the medial and lateral menisci and the anterior and posterior cruciate ligaments have been cut. The resected tibial bone is externally rotated as the soft tissues are released.

Attention is then directed toward the femur. The knee is brought to 90 degrees of flexion, and a limited amount of synovial tissue and fat is resected from the anterior cortex. The distal femur is resected with an intramedullary cutting guide set at an appropriate valgus alignment (Fig. 104-12A). After the bone has been removed from the femur, the size and rotation of the femoral component are determined with the guide (Fig. 104-12B). The rotation is set with reference

to the posterior condyles (3 degrees external rotation) and is checked to ensure that it is parallel to the transepicondylar axis and perpendicular to Whiteside's line. The size closest to the measured femur is selected (Fig. 104-12C). Anterior and posterior cuts of the femur are made. At 90 degrees of flexion, the joint is distracted with laminar spreaders. This provides excellent exposure and facilitates removal of the menisci. The posterior cruciate ligament is resected if a posterior stabilized prosthesis is to be implanted. The flexion and extension gaps are measured and balanced with a spacer block. Appropriate medial or lateral soft tissue release is performed to balance the gaps. Subsequently, the femoral finishing cuts are made. The tibia is sized and prepared in appropriate rotation to accept the tibial component. Finally, the patella is prepared.

The additional laxity and space in the knee joint cavity following tibial and distal femoral resections allow patellar preparation with minimal extensor mechanism disruption. With the knee in extension or slight flexion, the patella is everted and resected to the appropriate depth. The provisional components are implanted in the following order: the knee is hyperflexed forward and externally rotated so that the trial tibial tray is introduced through the arthrotomy. The knee is brought back to 90 degrees of flexion, and the femoral component is impacted with distraction of the joint as the flexion space opens. The trial tibial insert is then inserted. A trial reduction is performed, and the knee is assessed for range of motion, alignment, ligament balance, and patellar tracking. If the trial tests are satisfactory, the provisional components are removed. The bone surfaces are prepared for cementation. The final tibial, femoral, and patellar components are cemented in sequential fashion. Anterior subluxation and external rotation of the tibia yield good exposure

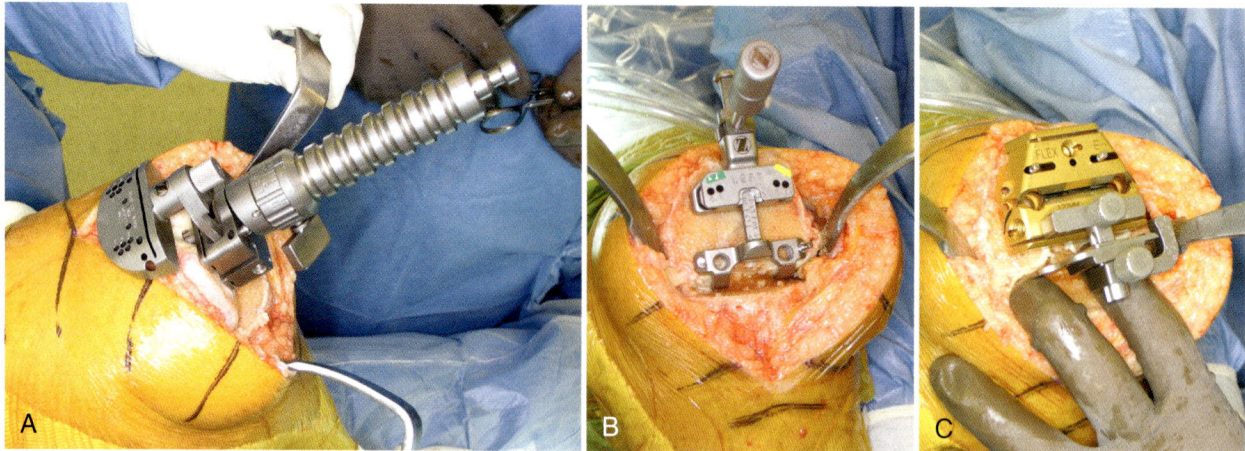

Figure 104-12. A, Distal femoral cutting guide. **B,** Femoral sizing guide. **C,** Femoral cutting block.

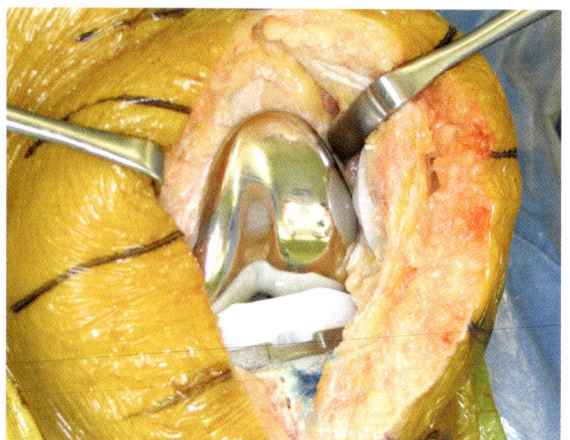

Figure 104-13. Final components implanted through a limited medial arthrotomy.

for cementing the tibial component in place. All excess cement is removed and the knee joint is reduced.

After the cement has hardened, the final tibial polyethylene component is inserted (Fig. 104-13). The wound is irrigated with antibiotic solution. The arthrotomy is closed over a suction drain with figure-of-eight absorbable Vicryl sutures. The sutures in the arthrotomy are placed in a slightly oblique fashion to use the vector pull of the vastus medialis muscle. The subcutaneous layer and the skin are closed in a routine manner.

Ample evidence indicates that MIS TKA is associated with decreased blood loss, leading to reduced transfusion requirements and improved postoperative motion.[34,50,55] In the author's experience, the minimally invasive approach has reduced the average length of incision by approximately 50% to an average length of 10 to 14 cm without adversely affecting the clinical outcome.[11] Tenholder and colleagues reported a consecutive series of 118 TKAs that included 69 patients reconstructed using an MIS approach and 49 patients reconstructed by a conventional approach. Better knee flexion and lower transfusion rates were observed in the MIS group. No differences in radiographic alignment and complication rates were noted between the two groups. A thin woman with low body mass index, a narrow femur and good preoperative knee

range of motion appeared to be the ideal patient for MIS TKA.[55]

In a recent study, Han and coworkers prospectively followed 30 patients undergoing simultaneous bilateral TKA. Patients were randomized into an MIS group (mini-medial parapatellar approach) or a conventional group. Functional recovery was faster in the MIS group for rehabilitation milestones such as walking without assistance and for improvement in range of motion.[19] Bonutti and associates reviewed clinical outcomes of 25 staged bilateral TKAs (50 knees) in which conventional TKA was performed on one knee, and a minimally invasive TKA was later performed on the contralateral side. Knee flexion and Knee Society objective scores were significantly greater in the minimally invasive group. Quadriceps muscle strength was statistically better in the MIS group at 12 weeks and at 1 year postoperatively, as demonstrated by isokinetic testing.[4] No difference in alignment was noted on radiographic analysis between the two approaches. Similar to any other surgical procedure, a learning curve is associated with MIS TKA. King and colleagues quantified the number of surgeries required to become proficient in minimally invasive TKA. They noted the learning curve for minimally invasive TKA was approximately 50 TKA procedures in the hands of high-volume arthroplasty surgeons, making this procedure a less desirable option for low-volume surgeons.[30]

LIMITED SUBVASTUS APPROACH

This approach takes advantage of the natural planes of dissection and minimizes patellofemoral instability by avoiding disruption of the extensor mechanism. The vastus medialis obliquus (VMO) inserts at a 50-degree angle relative to the long axis of the femur and extends to the midpole of the patella on the medial side.[41] It is imperative to clearly identify the inferior border of the VMO to preserve the entire quadriceps.

The arthrotomy is made along the inferior edge of the VMO down to the midpole of the patella. The arthrotomy is then extended straight distally along the medial border of the patella and the patellar tendon (Fig. 104-14). The VMO tendon and the patella are retracted laterally with a right-angled Hohmann retractor placed in the lateral gutter. The

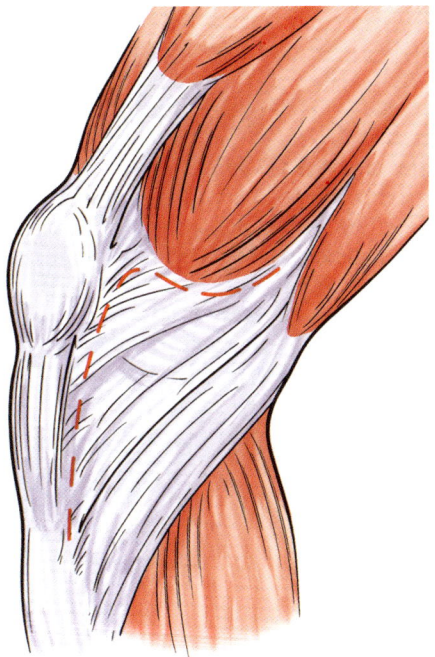

Figure 104-14. Subvastus approach.

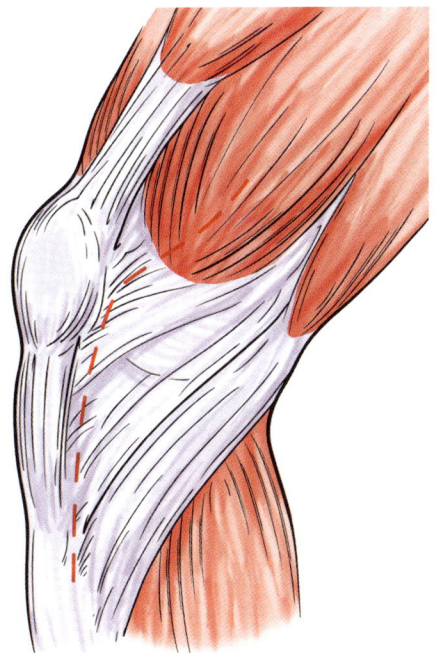

Figure 104-15. Midvastus approach.

knee is flexed to 90 degrees, providing good exposure of both distal femoral condyles. The TKA is performed in a similar fashion, as described earlier for limited medial parapatellar arthrotomy. Closure begins by reapproximating the corner of the capsular flap to the extensor mechanism at the midpole of the patella. Interrupted sutures are placed along the proximal limb of the arthrotomy. Care is taken to place the sutures through the fibrous tissue or the synovium attached to the distal surface or the undersurface of the VMO. Then the distal or vertical limb of the arthrotomy is closed with multiple interrupted sutures.

The MIS subvastus approach is not recommended in an obese patient or in a male patient with a large, prominent VMO. Patients with limited motion, a significant flexion contracture, and severe valgus alignment also are not amenable to this approach.[40] Moreover, patients with patella baja are poor candidates for the subvastus approach because of difficulty in translating the patella laterally. When this approach is performed, care must be taken while working in the subvastus region adjacent to the adductor tubercle because it contains the descending genicular artery and its branches, the intermuscular septal arteries, and the saphenous nerve.

In a prospective randomized study, Roysam and Oakley compared 46 MIS subvastus TKAs versus 43 TKAs performed through a traditional medial parapatellar approach. Clinical assessment revealed significantly earlier return of straight-leg raising (3.2 days vs. 5.8 days; $P < .001$), lower consumption of narcotics in the first week (78 mg vs. 102 mg; $P < .001$), less blood loss (527 mL vs. 748 mL; $P < .001$), and greater knee flexion at 1 week (78 degrees vs. 55 degrees; $P < .001$) in group II (subvastus approach).[48] In another study, Varela-Egocheaga and associates compared MIS subvastus TKA versus conventional TKA performed by the parapatellar approach. They noted superior Knee Society scores and range of motion at a minimum follow-up of 36 months in the MIS

group.[56] Functional recovery has been observed to be faster after a subvastus approach than after a medial parapatellar approach, as measured by isometric and isokinetic muscle strength.[8,53] Chang and colleagues noted greater peak torque in quadriceps strength at 6 months postoperatively and earlier normalization of hamstrings to quadriceps peak torque ratio after a subvastus approach compared with a medial parapatellar approach.[8] In a matched retrospective analysis of 120 patients, the mini-subvastus approach was associated with prolonged tourniquet time (average, 15 minutes) and two intraoperative complications. It was thought to be technically more challenging than a standard medial parapatellar approach. However, the mini-subvastus approach was associated with less blood loss, less postoperative pain, faster straight-leg raising, and better knee flexion. All patients, including those with complications, had good limb alignment and implant positioning.[3] In a recent randomized study, Aglietti and coworkers noted earlier straight-leg raising and better knee flexion at 10 and 30 days postoperatively with a mini-subvastus approach compared with a quadriceps-sparing technique. No difference in knee flexion was observed at 3 months' follow-up.[2]

MIDVASTUS APPROACH

Following an anterior midline skin incision, a medial arthrotomy is performed, beginning at the superior pole of the patella to the tibial tubercle distally. The VMO is identified, and an oblique 2 to 4 cm split is made sharply in line with the fibers at the level of the superior pole of the patella (Fig. 104-15). The patella is subluxated laterally as the knee is brought into flexion, and the procedure can be performed as described earlier. The fascia and the muscle fibers tend to split further as the knee is flexed upward. This has no adverse effect on outcome.

Exclusion criteria for the midvastus approach are similar to those for limited parapatellar arthrotomy. The midvastus approach preserves vascularity. Additionally, some reports have described improved patellar tracking.[35] Reported benefits of the midvastus approach include decreased postoperative pain, better quadriceps function, decreased blood loss, and shorter hospital stay.[16,17,35] Laskin and colleagues compared 32 MIS midvastus TKAs versus 26 TKAs done through a standard medial parapatellar approach. Improvements in knee scores were statistically higher in the MIS group at 6 weeks postoperatively. Additionally, the average visual analog pain score and the total amount of pain medication required were lower in the MIS group. Radiographic alignment and implant positioning were equally accurate in the two groups.[35] Similar encouraging clinical outcomes were noted in a recent retrospective analysis of 335 consecutive patients (391 TKAs). Range of motion was 111 degrees at 6 weeks, 121 degrees at 3 months, and 125 degrees at 1 and 2 years. Postoperative knee scores were greater than 95 in all patients. No increase in the rate of complication was noted with this approach.[17] Similarly, Karachalios and coworkers reported superior Oxford knee scores and knee function scores following MIS midvastus TKA compared with conventional TKA up to 9 months postoperatively. Patients in the MIS group had greater early knee flexion ($P = .04$) postoperatively compared with the conventional group.[27,28]

QUADRICEPS-SPARING SURGICAL APPROACH

Specialized instrumentation customized for side cutting is required for execution of this approach. These instruments can be used to cut in a medial-to-lateral direction, which allows incisions as small as 6 to 10 cm in length. Moreover, these instruments can be used with a limited parapatellar, mini-midvastus, or subvastus approach.

A curvilinear medial skin incision is made in a varus knee, extending from the superior pole of the patella to the tibial joint line (Fig. 104-16). The arthrotomy is made in line with the skin incision and may extend beneath the vastus medialis to improve exposure of the medial femoral condyle (Fig. 104-17). In the valgus knee, the incision can be made along the lateral aspect of the patella to the tibial joint line (Fig. 104-18). A vertical lateral parapatellar arthrotomy is performed,

and the iliotibial band is dissected from the tibial joint line in an anteroposterior direction (Fig. 104-19). After satisfactory exposure is achieved, the patella is resected using a freehand technique (Fig. 104-20). The patellar preparation can be completed at this stage.

The full composite thickness of the patella and the trial patellar button is compared with the native patellar thickness. The cut surface is then protected with a thin metal button. Early patellar resection gives the surgeon more room to work on the femoral and tibial cuts. An anteroposterior axis (Whiteside's line) is drawn along the distal femur. A drill hole is made in the femur just above the intercondylar notch along Whiteside's line. An intramedullary guide that

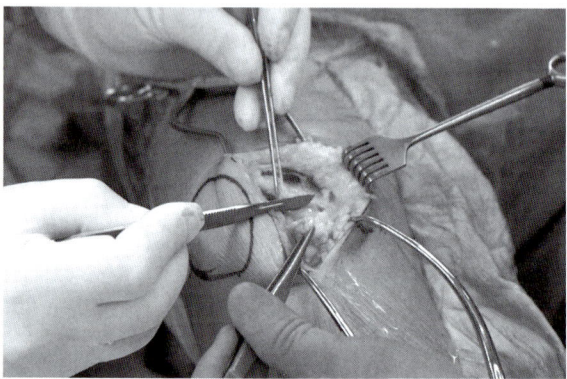

Figure 104-17. Surgical knife blade dissection beneath the vastus medialis.

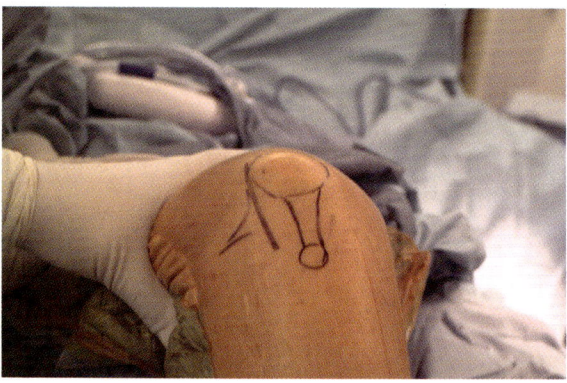

Figure 104-18. Lateral incision for valgus knee along the side of the patella to the tibial joint line.

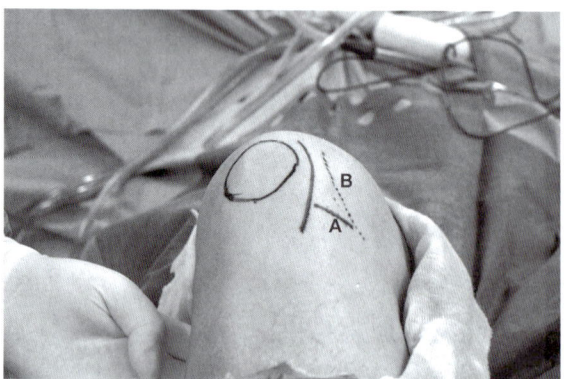

Figure 104-16. Medial incision in a varus knee. Line *A* represents the tibiofemoral joint line, and *B* outlines the margin of the medial femoral condyle.

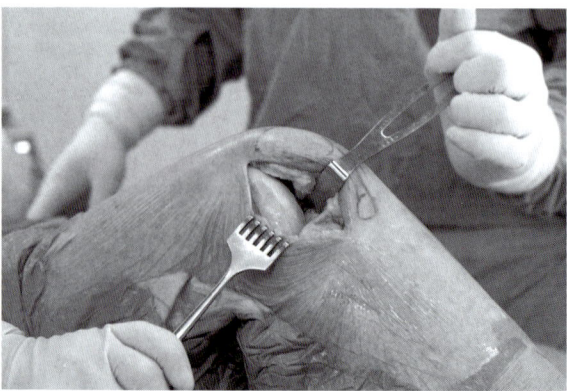

Figure 104-19. The iliotibial band is sharply elevated from the lateral aspect of the patella.

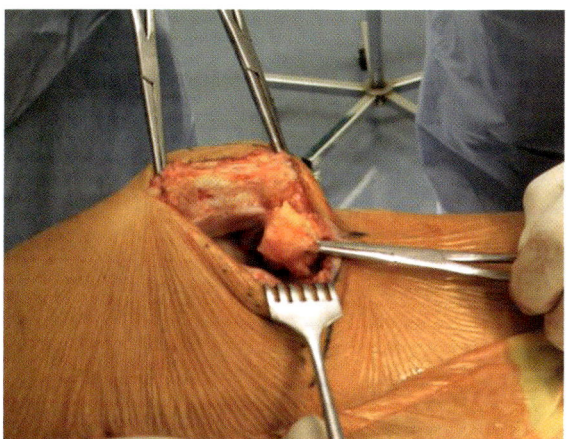

Figure 104-20. The fad pad is excised and the patellar surface is resected with a free-hand oscillating saw.

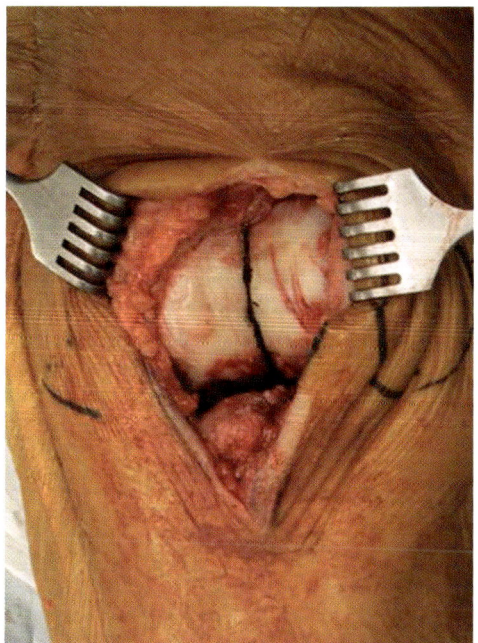

Figure 104-21. The anteroposterior axis (Whiteside's line) is drawn along the uncut femoral surface.

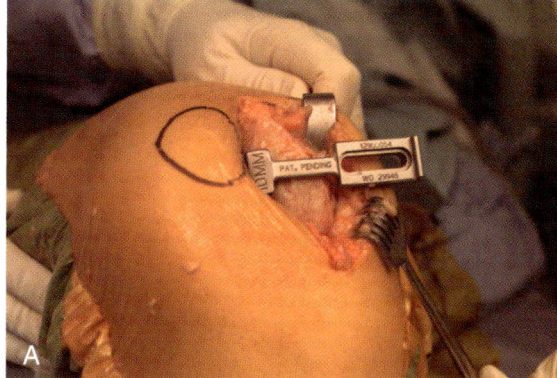

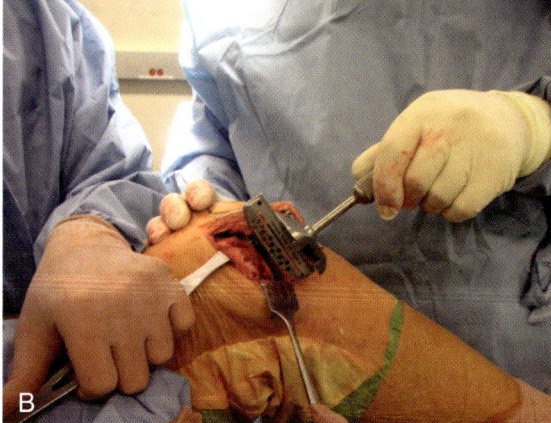

Figure 104-22. A, The intramedullary (IM) guide rests on the medial femoral condyle. **B,** The cutting block is attached to the IM guide, and distal femoral resection is performed from the medial side.

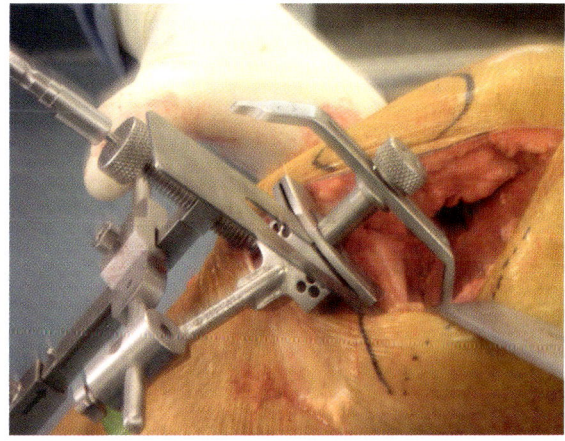

Figure 104-23. Extramedullary cutting guide with depth gauge sets the cutting block for proximal tibial resection.

references the medial femoral condyle is introduced into the femur (Fig. 104-21). A side cutting block is attached to the intramedullary guide, and a distal femoral resection is made across both condyles (Fig. 104-22). An extramedullary tibial cutting guide with a medially based cutting slot is centered on the tibial tubercle and secured with a threaded pin. The proximal tibial cut is performed after adjustment for varus/valgus, the posterior slope, and the depth of resection (Fig. 104-23). Care is taken to avoid injury to the posterior neurovascular structures, and the procedure is most often completed by dividing the resected bone into three pieces.

At this point, the extension space is evaluated with a spacer block and an extramedullary rod (Fig. 104-24). Appropriate medial or lateral release is performed to balance the space in extension. Then the knee is placed in 90 degrees of flexion, and the posterior referencing femoral guide is placed on the distal femur (Fig. 104-25). The guide is adjusted with

respect to the anteroposterior axis (Whiteside's line) to ensure accurate rotation of the femoral component. The guide is then pinned into place (Fig. 104-26). The knee is brought into full extension, and a gauge is attached to reference the anterior surface for determination of correct component size. An appropriate femoral finishing block is placed on the distal femur with the knee still in full extension. The femoral finishing block is attached to the reference plate in proper external rotation. After its proper positioning in the

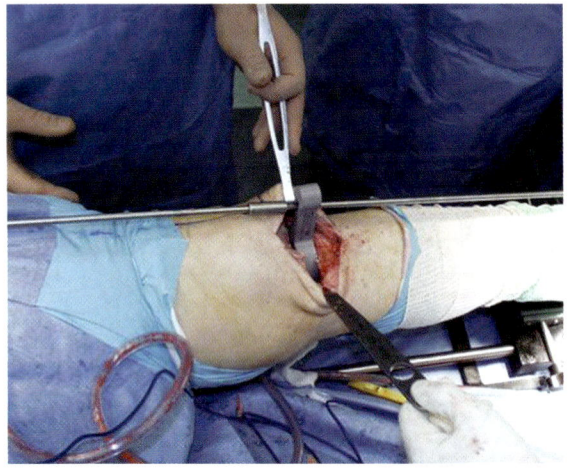

Figure 104-24. Extension space measured with a spacer block and an extramedullary rod.

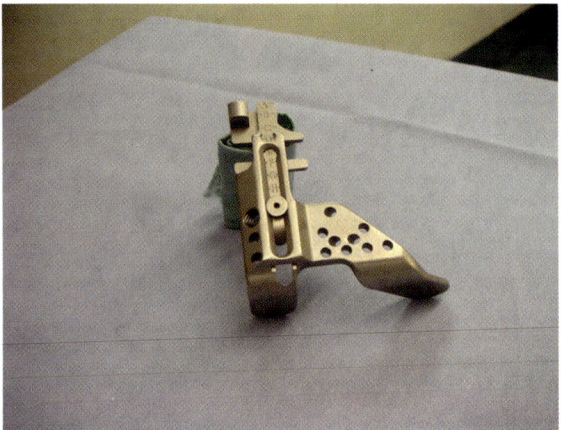

Figure 104-25. The femoral tower has two foot pads that reference the posterior aspect of the femoral condyles.

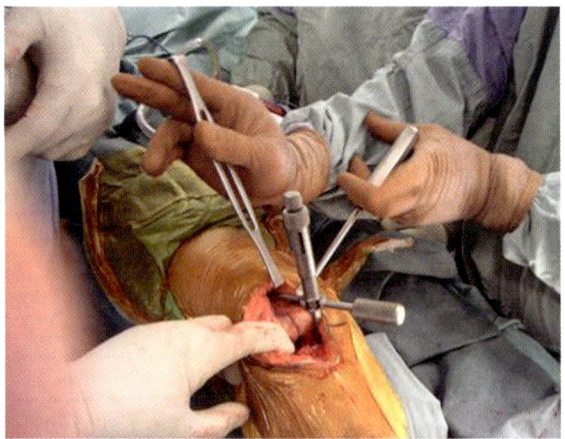

Figure 104-26. The probe identifies the size of the femur and the location of the anterior surface cut.

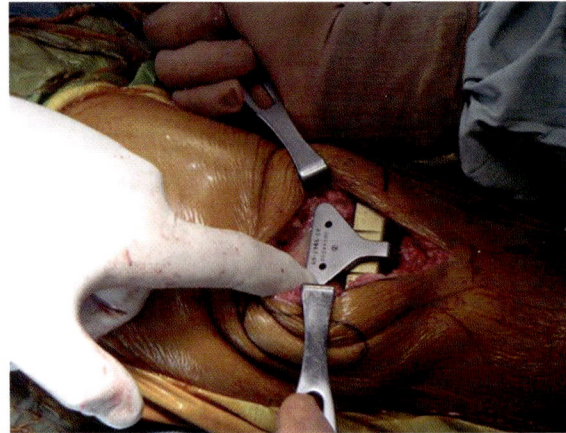

Figure 104-27. The femoral finishing block is attached to the plate that references the anterior femoral cut and is positioned in a medial-lateral direction in full extension.

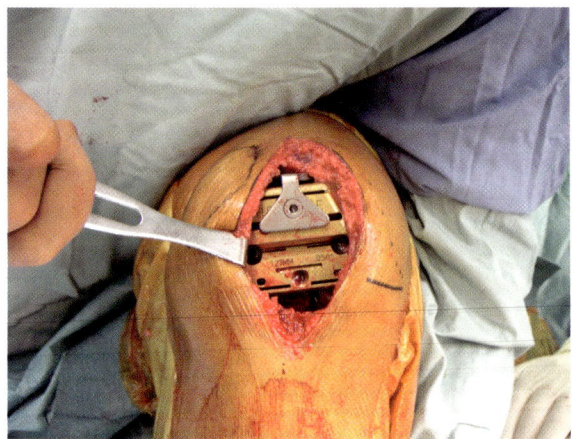

Figure 104-28. Femoral finishing cuts made with the knee in 90 degrees of flexion.

medial-lateral plane is ensured, the block is pinned into place (Fig. 104-27). Femoral cuts are performed with the knee in 90 degrees of flexion (Fig. 104-28). Flexion-extension gaps are compared and are balanced in traditional fashion if any discrepancy is noted. The remainder of the procedure is performed as described earlier. Knee position must be varied between 30 and 80 degrees of flexion during the procedure. The patella is subluxated laterally for implantation of the components.

Although the potential benefits of MIS TKA are realized with the quadriceps-sparing MIS approach using side-cutting instrumentation, this technique has been associated with relatively more complications compared with the other three MIS approaches.[9] Huang and associates reported on 2-year follow-up of quadriceps-sparing MIS TKA. The quadriceps-sparing MIS group had significantly faster recovery of quadriceps strength and knee flexion and had less pain during the first 2 postoperative weeks compared with the traditional group. However, nine radiographic outliers were identified in the MIS group and none in the standard group.[22] Similarly, in a recent randomized study, Martin and colleagues compared MIS TKA using side-cutting implant instrumentation and standard anteroposterior mini-incision instrumentation. In all, 50% of TKAs in each cohort were performed with computer-assisted navigation. Investigators found greater accuracy for limb and component alignment with standard mini-incision instrumentation compared with quadriceps-sparing side-cutting instrumentation. The navigation technique could not compensate for shortcomings of the side-cutting instrumentation.[38] In another recent study, Lin and coworkers noted a greater number of outliers for tibial and femoral component alignment in the quadriceps-sparing MIS TKA group compared with the MIS medial parapatellar TKA group.[36] However, no differences in short-term isokinetic peak muscle torque, postoperative pain, and functional outcomes were noted between the two approaches.

CONCLUSION

MIS TKA is not defined by the length of the incision or by the cosmetic result. True MIS TKA is defined by limited violation of anatomic structures about the knee. Exposure during MIS TKA should specifically avoid violation of the extensor mechanism and the suprapatellar pouch. The goal of MIS TKA is to reduce postoperative pain and promote faster recovery. To be successful, MIS TKA must not compromise surgical technique, accurate limb alignment, component positioning, soft tissue balancing, or longevity of the reconstruction. Appropriate patient selection as outlined previously is critical for the successful and safe execution of these approaches. An optimal MIS technique is expansible for situations in which the surgeon encounters difficulty and requires additional exposure. Extension of the arthrotomy into the quadriceps tendon and the vastus medialis produces variations of the quadriceps-sparing approach and can be considered part of the continuum of MIS TKA surgery.

The best way to become adept with MIS TKA may start by using MIS instrumentation during traditional TKA, gradually progressing to a mini-incision approach with increasing surgical experience.

KEY REFERENCES

Abbott LC, Carpenter WF: Surgical approaches to the knee joint. J Bone Joint Surg Am 27:277, 1945.

Bramlett KW: The trivector arthrotomy approach, AAOS Instructional Videotape, Rosemont, Ill, June 1994, American Academy of Orthopaedic Surgeons.

Chen AF, Alan RK, Redziniak DE, Tria AJ Jr: Quadriceps sparing total knee replacement: the initial experience with results at two to four years. J Bone Joint Surg Br 88:1448–1453, 2006.

Colizza WA, Insall JN, Scuderi GR: The posterior stabilized total knee prosthesis: assessment of polyethylene damage and osteolysis after a ten-year-minimum follow-up. J Bone Joint Surg Am 77:1713–1720, 1995.

Coonse KD, Adams JD: A new operative approach to the knee joint. Surg Gynecol Obstet 77:344, 1943.

Engh GA, Holt BT, Parks NL: A midvastus muscle-splitting approach for total knee arthroplasty. J Arthroplasty 12:322–331, 1997.

Haas SB, Manitta MA, Burdick P: Minimally invasive total knee arthroplasty: the mini midvastus approach. Clin Orthop Relat Res 452:112–116, 2006.

Henry AK: Extensile exposure, ed 2, Baltimore, 1970, Williams & Wilkins.

Hofmann AA, Plaster RL, Murdock LE: Subvastus (Southern) approach for primary total knee arthroplasty. Clin Orthop Relat Res 269:70–77, 1991.

Insall J: A midline approach to the knee. J Bone Joint Surg Am 53:1584, 1971.

Insall J, Ranawat CS, Scott WN, Walker P: Total condylar knee replacement: preliminary report. Clin Orthop Relat Res 120:149–154, 1976.

Insall J, Tria AJ, Scott WN: The total condylar knee prosthesis: the first 5 years. Clin Orthop Relat Res 145:68–77, 1979.

Insall JN, editor: Surgery of the knee, New York, 1984, Churchill Livingstone, pp 41–54.

Keblish PA: Valgus deformity in total knee arthroplasty: the lateral retinacular approach. Orthop Trans 9:28, 1985.

Kocher T: Textbook of operative surgery, ed 3, Stiles HJ, Paul CB (trans), London, 1911, Adam & Charles Black.

Mullen M: The subvastus approach for total knee arthroplasty. Tech Orthop 6:64, 1991.

Pagnano MW, Meneghini RM, Trousdale RT: Anatomy of the extensor mechanism in reference to quadriceps-sparing TKA. Clin Orthop Relat Res 452:102–105, 2006.

Scuderi GR: Minimally invasive total knee arthroplasty with limited medial parapatellar arthrotomy. Oper Tech Orthop 16:145–152, 2006.

Stern SH, Insall JN: Posterior stabilized prosthesis: results after follow-up of nine to twelve years. J Bone Joint Surg Am 74:980–986, 1992.

Tenholder M, Clarke HD, Scuderi GR: Minimal-incision total knee arthroplasty: the early clinical experience. Clin Orthop Relat Res 440:67–76, 2005.

Whiteside LA, Ohl MD: Tibial tubercle osteotomy for exposure of the difficult total knee arthroplasty. Clin Orthop Relat Res 206:6–9, 1990.

Full references for this chapter can be found on www.expertconsult.com.

Surgical Techniques and Instrumentation in Total Knee Arthroplasty

Thomas Parker Vail, Jason E. Lang, and C. Van Sikes, III

The surgical techniques and instrumentation in total knee arthroplasty discussed in this chapter are based on the remarkable vision and clarity of thought that was the trademark of John Insall. In the latest iteration of this foundational chapter, the authors have attempted to preserve Insall's important observations while expanding the discussion to include important intervening advances and new technology.

RELEVANT KNEE ANATOMY AND ALIGNMENT

Creating a plan for successful biomechanical reconstruction of the knee requires specific knowledge of an individual patient's anatomy that includes an understanding of alignment, ligamentous support, and skeletal anatomy at the knee, hip, and ankle. Thus, it is important to examine a patient in three positions: weightless, standing, and when walking. The weightless examination, with the patient seated or supine, allows careful assessment of ligament competence, range of motion, and passive patellar tracking. When the patient is standing, one can assess the overall axial alignment of the leg, the angle of the joint line in dual stance, and the static position of the patella. Walking the patient allows one to add a dynamic component to the examination, while observing the presence of antalgic movement, soft tissue impingement, and varus or valgus thrust during active single leg stance. Considerable variation is noted in body habitus, natural femoral anteversion, foot and ankle alignment, and patterns of gait, requiring caution in describing what is "normal." However, the following description represents consensus.[98,134]

Static Alignment

The mechanical axis of the leg (Fig. 105-1) is formed by a line that passes from the center of the hip through the center of the knee into the center of the ankle joint. The offset is the distance between the femoral shaft and the center of rotation of the hip, which is determined by the angle of the femoral neck and length of the neck and shaft of the femur. A valgus angle of 5 to 9 degrees between the femoral and tibial shafts allows the transverse axis of the knee joint to be perpendicular to the midline vertical axis of the body. Because the proximal-to-distal mechanical axis forms an angle of 3 degrees with the midline vertical axis of the body, there typically exists a 3-degree angle between the knee joint line and the axis of the tibial shaft, and a 10-degree angle between the joint line axis and the axis of the femoral shaft. Hungerford and Krackow[94] and Townley[204] have pointed out that the "normal" angle of proximal tibial varus is variable because of inherited and developmental anatomic factors such as pelvic

width, femoral neck varus, femoral and tibial bowing, physeal growth, and femoral length. Because of the fact that the mechanical axis passes through the medial compartment, and the transverse knee joint axis is in slight varus, the distribution of body weight when standing is more medial than lateral in most knees.[92,97,144,204]

Dynamic Alignment

During normal walking, the center of gravity of the body moves toward the supporting leg during each gait cycle. The leg typically will move toward the midline during single leg stance. However, the distribution of contact forces across the knee joint is not symmetrical; it is estimated that between 60% and 75% of these forces are carried by the medial compartment of the knee for reasons discussed in the previous section.[85,103,144]

Johnson and associates[103] noted that during normal walking, a greater medial load than predicted is observed because of the laterally directed ground reaction force. These forces do not rest on a perpendicular tibial plateau; the anatomic tibial plateau is sloped 2 to 10 degrees posterior and distally. However, when the menisci are taken into account, the cartilaginous articulation is not posteriorly sloped; only the bony surfaces give the appearance of posterior slope. Furthermore, the medial tibial subchondral bone is concave ("dished") relative to the more convex lateral tibial subchondral surface. Combined with the 3-degree angle of the tibial anatomic axis relative to the transverse knee axis, a varus moment is imparted during normal gait. This varus moment creates a lateral "thrust," which is resisted by the lateral stabilizing force arising from the capsule, the lateral collateral ligament (LCL), the cruciate ligaments, the ligamentum patellae, the popliteus, the posterior oblique ligament, and the iliotibial band (ITB).[134]

Abnormal patterns of gait can impact the loading of the knee joint. Muscle imbalance due to deconditioning or obesity can accentuate a varus thrust or cause the thighs to rub together during the swing phase of gait. Gait studies performed on obese patients have demonstrated locomotor adaptations, such as slower speed, shorter steps, increased double support time, and decreased knee range of motion. Additionally, Sharma and colleagues[189] reported on a correlation between body mass index (BMI) and osteoarthritis (OA) severity in knees with varus malalignment that was not seen in knees with valgus malalignment. Compensatory external rotation of the foot is a mechanism of unloading a painful medial compartment during stance. An extension moment moving the center of gravity anterior to the knee joint is a compensatory mechanism for quadriceps weakness that eventually can lead to laxity in the posterior capsule and the posterior cruciate ligament.

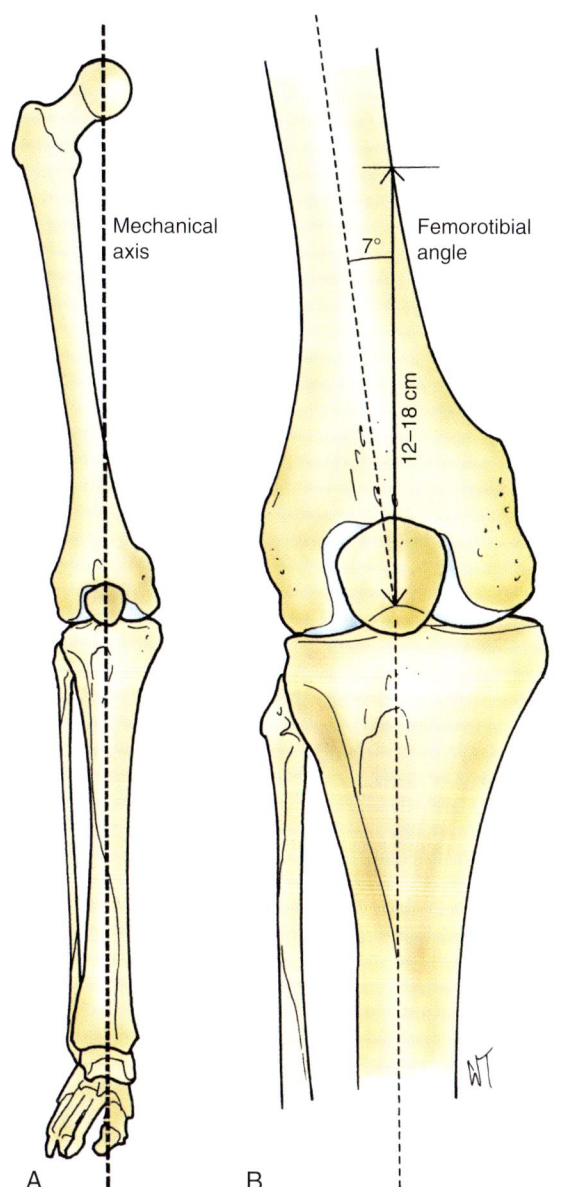

Figure 105-1. The mechanical axis usually corresponds to a femorotibial angle of about 7 degrees, and the mechanical axis intersects the medial femoral cortex 12 to 18 cm proximal to the knee.

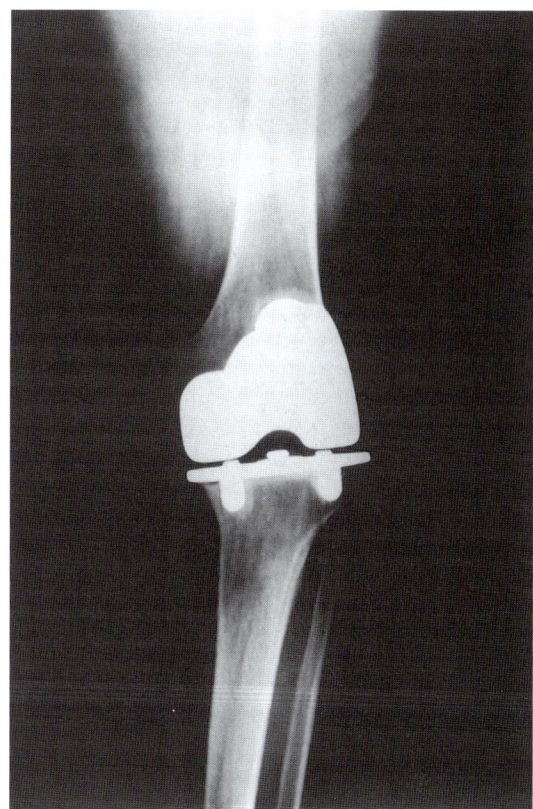

Figure 105-2. Radiograph of a prosthesis with a varus tibial cut. The instrument system designed for this prosthesis recommended a 3-degree tibial cut because this slope more closely duplicates normal anatomy. In practice, it often led to a greater and undesirable sloping cut to the tibia.

OBJECTIVES OF PROSTHETIC REPLACEMENT

The above description applies to the nonarthritic condition, but it must be appreciated that many patients developing OA of the knee have contributing anatomic variations such as habitual varus or valgus alignment. One must ask how closely prosthetic components should duplicate normal anatomy; for example, should the forces across a knee arthroplasty be borne predominantly by the medial compartment? How should the alignment of the prosthetic knee joint be changed to accommodate pathologic alterations in gait that are not restored to normal even after prosthetic replacement?

It was Insall's opinion that the objective of prosthetic replacement is to distribute contact stresses across the artificial joint as symmetrically as possible, avoiding overloading of one compartment. This philosophy can require altering an individual's prearthritic anatomy. For example, it is likely that many patients who develop medial compartment arthritis of the knee have been bowlegged, or have walked with a varus thrust, since childhood. Restoration of the prearthritic alignment, although "normal" for these people, would result in a component position of greater varus than is generally considered acceptable after knee arthroplasty.

Practical considerations have an impact on proper implant alignment. Given the human error factor, reproducibility during surgery is important. Instrumentation and careful operative technique can minimize the incidence of component malposition. Computer navigation of knee surgery has been shown to improve the accuracy of component positioning by reducing the incidence of alignment outliers,[32,41] but later studies demonstrated that this effect may be tied to the setting in which navigation is utilized. Carter and coworkers[26] demonstrated reduction in "outliers" with respect to number and severity when navigation was utilized in a low-volume, community-based practice, but recent studies from high-volume centers have found no statistical difference in component positioning or reduction in outliers through the use of navigation.[84,110] For most surgeons, it is easier to make a right-angle bone cut than an oblique one, and it is easier (and thus more reproducible) to make a cut across the upper tibia at right angles to the tibial shaft than to make a cut that is inclined 3 degrees medially and 10 degrees posteriorly (Fig. 105-2). Additionally, if angle cuts are not appropriately

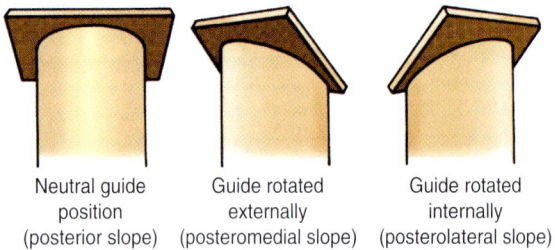

Neutral guide position (posterior slope)   Guide rotated externally (posteromedial slope)   Guide rotated internally (posterolateral slope)

Figure 105-3. Care must be taken when making a 10-degree posterior slope on the tibial cut. The guide must be placed in the neutral position. When it is externally rotated, a posteromedial slope (varus) will be produced. When the guide is internally rotated, a posterolateral slope (valgus) will result.

adjusted from a rotational perspective, further inaccuracy results; for example, an intended 10-degree posterior slope may result in a combination of posterior and valgus slope if the cutting guide is internally rotated (Fig. 105-3). Also, because referencing off of pathologic bone surfaces is likely to result in errors in both angular and rotational alignment due to loss of bone and absence of the soft tissue contribution to alignment, one might choose not to reproduce the original joint surfaces. In pathologic states, which in themselves create secondary changes in the ligaments, this difficulty is obviously compounded.

Insall believed that restoration of "normal" anatomy often was not achieved, and perhaps was not important to success. Evidence to support this assertion is that early models of knee prostheses were crude, often grossly mismatched in size because of a limited inventory of sizes, incompatible with ligamentous structures, and often inexpertly inserted. Many of these devices failed, but a surprising number not only worked well but continued to do so for many years, proving the human body's remarkable resilience (Fig. 105-4). As clinical experience increased, surgical expertise improved, and prosthetic design became more sophisticated, more durable, and more "natural" through designs that did not set up kinematic conflict with soft tissue structures. Today, in addition to painlessness, normality of feel, less invasive approaches, and a high level of function are often achieved. Nevertheless, total knee replacement is not universally successful, with some patients continuing to experience anterior knee pain, crepitation, or effusion despite dramatic functional improvement relative to the original pathologic state. Furthermore, some individuals, such as Middle Eastern and Asian patients who need significant knee flexion during prayer, require special design considerations.

Polyethylene wear continues to be a major clinical issue. Designers of knee implants have two possible routes to minimize wear potential: decreasing contact stresses or changing the mechanical properties of the bearing surface. Ideal "anatomic" highly conforming joint surfaces may conflict with the bioengineering requirements needed to reduce wear. In addition, modularity has introduced the potential for wear secondary to micromotion between the polyethylene insert and the tibial tray.[72,156,209,211] Recent studies have suggested that patterns of "backside wear" indicate differing mechanisms of wear at the two interfaces with a predominance of burnishing, dimpling, and deformation at the insert/tibial tray interface,[84,126] and other authors have investigated the wear patterns of the tibial post in posterior stabilized designs,

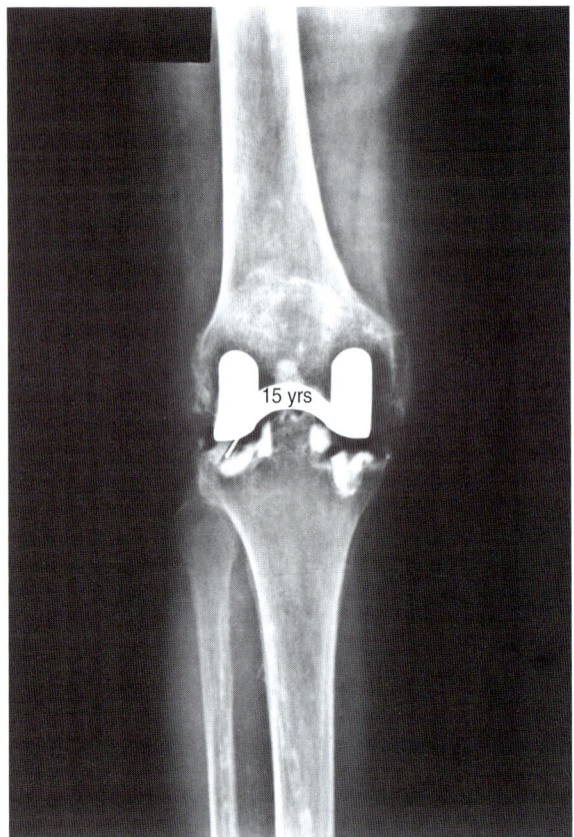

15 yrs

Figure 105-4. Radiograph of a 15-year follow-up of a duocondylar prosthesis with two separate tibial components. Osteopenia is apparent around the femoral component runners. The knee continued to function well.

noting that variations in wear are dependent on component design and degree of femoral flexion.[48] Despite the potential for increased wear debris generated by unintended backside movement, investigators have demonstrated that modular components can demonstrate comparable survivorship when compared with monoblock systems.[88] At least partial conformity between the articulating components in fixed-bearing designs is considered necessary to reduce high polyethylene stresses and to provide acceptable durability. Thus, all current fixed-bearing designs are compromises between conformity and mobility. Increasing conformity at the bearing surface can be combined with intended motion between the undersurface of the polyethylene and the tibial tray to reduce contact stress without adding constraint. This combination of conformity and motion is the theory that drives the mobile-bearing total knee concept. Polyethylene manufacturing techniques also play a role in determining the balance of conformity and durability. The cross-linking of polyethylene has proven safe and beneficial for decreasing wear rates.[89] When cross-linking is carried out in an oxygen-free environment (to reduce free radical formation), cross-linked polyethylene demonstrates lower rates of delamination or fracture.[40] Further advances in processing of polyethylene include combinations of cross-linking and annealing or heating the polyethylene past the melt point to retain even more of its original resistance to cracking and to address the issues of longevity associated with free radical formation.[208] The optimal balance between improvement in wear properties and reduction in mechanical properties such as elongation to fracture created by the cross-linking process still remains to be defined.

THEORIES OF SURGICAL TECHNIQUE

The development of implants and instruments led to two distinct surgical techniques during the early development of knee arthroplasty: the gap balancing technique and the measured resection technique.[51] Over time, instrument systems have adopted aspects of both philosophies, blurring the distinctions. The gap balancing technique was developed in conjunction with the design of cruciate substituting prostheses. The measured resection technique was developed by surgeons and designers who favor cruciate retention, emphasizing measured femoral and tibial resection as the primary consideration.

Gap Balancing Technique

The gap balancing technique[71,96,98] is used in conjunction with cruciate substituting prostheses and some cruciate retaining devices (often accompanied by posterior cruciate release from the posterior tibial insertion). Ligament releases (see later) are performed to correct fixed deformity, bringing the limb into approximate alignment before bone cuts are made (Fig. 105-5).

Although the technique is still favored by many surgeons today, the gap balancing technique was developed at a time when a limited number of anteroposterior femoral sizes were available, frequently dictating that a relatively small femoral component be fitted onto a larger distal femur. This scenario typically necessitated over-resection of the posterior femoral condyles to fit the implant on the end of the femur. To appropriately balance the flexion gap and avoid flexion instability due to the over-resected posterior condyles, less proximal

tibia was resected to fill the flexion gap at the risk of creating a tight extension gap. In fact, the largest available tibial polyethylene insert was approximately 15 mm during the era of the total condylar prosthesis. Leaving a substantial amount of proximal tibial bone was in accordance with the belief that the proximal tibial bone weakened significantly with resection greater than 5 mm. The gap technique is still used, but because most systems have a full complement of component sizes, posterior femoral over-resection is less likely, and the flexion gap may be balanced even with proximal tibial resection greater than 10 mm if required.

A particular sequence of steps in balancing the flexion gap was not deemed essential for the gap technique. The femur or tibia may be osteotomized first; the goal is to create a balanced flexion gap (Fig. 105-6). Insall traditionally would perform the tibial cut first, measure the flexion gap, and then make the distal femoral cut at a point such that the extension gap would match the flexion gap. The proximal tibial osteotomy is performed 10 mm below the least compromised articular cartilage (Fig. 105-7). A perpendicular tibial cut establishes proper limb alignment with reference to the distal femoral cut. Harada and coworkers[83] suggested that the proximal tibia weakens below a depth of 5 mm, prompting many surgeons to resect as little bone as possible and requiring the use of thinner polyethylene inserts at the risk of stress-related wear.[225] Clinical experience and later research on tibial bone strength[76] have supported a 10-mm cut below the joint line, obviating the need to use excessively thin polyethylene components. When the posterior cruciate ligament (PCL) was resected, the flexion gap would open up a few millimeters, often necessitating a distal femoral cut that would slightly elevate the joint line to match the flexion and extension gap. Insall would then proceed to balance the flexion gap by positioning the anteroposterior cut on the distal femur parallel to the tibial cut surface, often in line with the transepicondylar

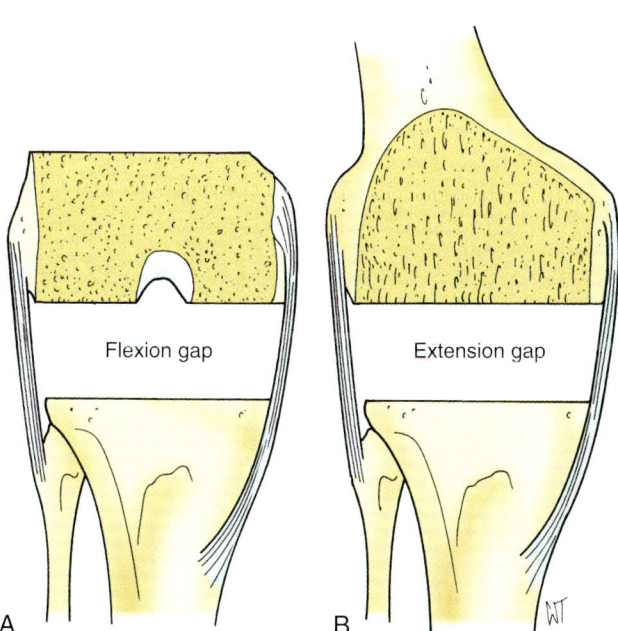

Figure 105-5. The extension gap must exactly equal the flexion gap.

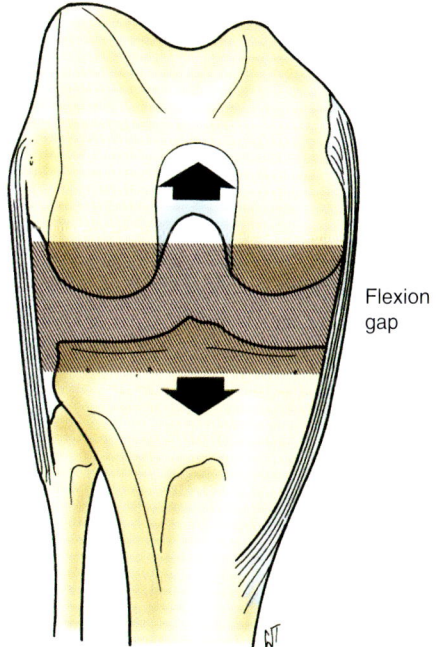

Figure 105-6. The flexion gap is created first by removing bone from the tibial plateaus and the posterior femoral condyles.

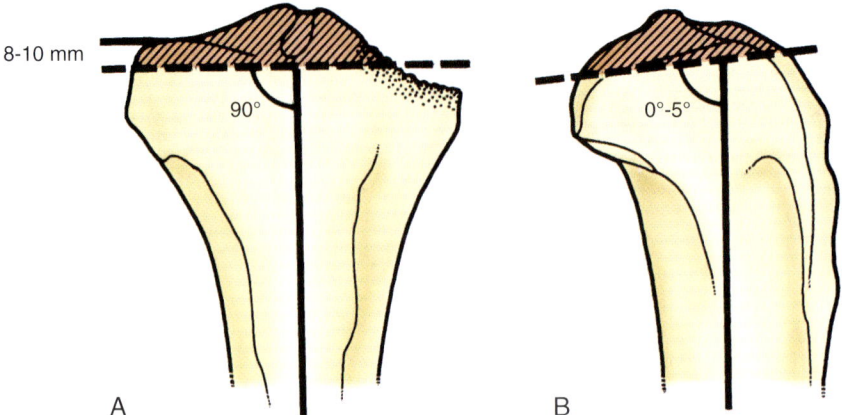

Figure 105-7. The correct cut on the tibia ignores defects and removes 10 mm from the normal side, cut at right angles to the long axis in the coronal plane **(A)** and sloped posteriorly no more than 5 degrees in the sagittal plane **(B)**.

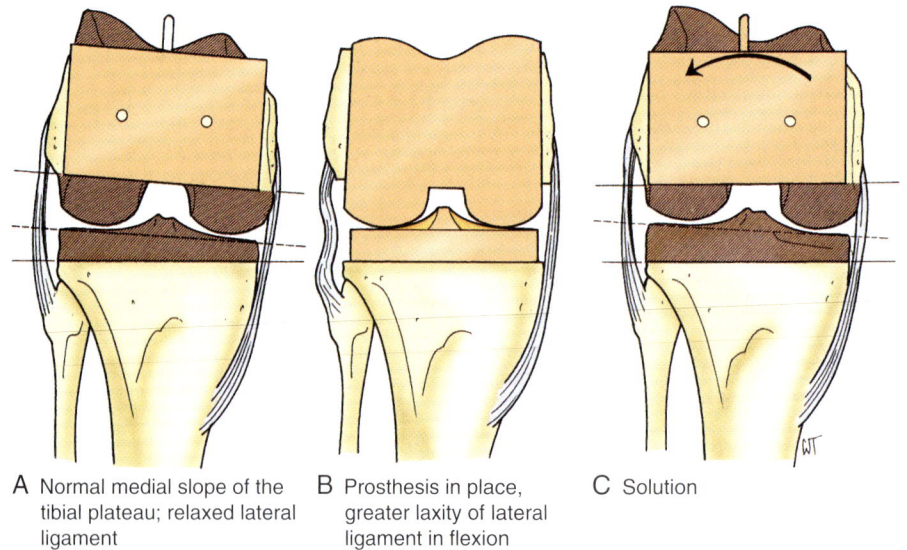

A Normal medial slope of the tibial plateau; relaxed lateral ligament

B Prosthesis in place, greater laxity of lateral ligament in flexion

C Solution

Figure 105-8. Imitating the normal anatomy results in lateral laxity in flexion.

axis. When the gap theory is applied to cruciate retaining designs, the PCL may be retained if it is appropriately balanced and the joint line position is restored with modular tibial inserts.

Rotational Alignment of the Femur

The rotational alignment of the femoral component is determined by the anatomy of the femur and is influenced to some degree by the condition of periarticular tissues. In a standard varus knee, when a medial release is not required for axial alignment, some external rotation of the femoral anteroposterior (AP) cutting block is needed to compensate for the normal medial inclination of the tibial plateau and the flexion laxity of the lateral ligamentous structures (Fig. 105-8). Only by this external rotation can a rectangular "flexion gap" be produced (Figs. 105-9 and 105-10). However, when a medial soft tissue release is done, a rectangular flexion gap is created by the ligament release itself, and the femoral template can be positioned anatomically relative to the epicondylar axis of the distal femur or the proximal tibial resection plane.

Proper femoral rotation is essential because inappropriate femoral component rotation may result in many downstream biomechanical issues such as flexion instability and patellofemoral maltracking problems.[8,15,164] Although an arbitrary external rotation of 3 degrees is often satisfactory,[68,163] several methods have been developed in an effort to accurately determine appropriate femoral rotation (Fig. 105-11):

1. Medial and lateral epicondyles[17,159]
2. Posterior femoral condyles[81]
3. AP femoral axis ("Whitesides' line")[9,218]
4. Tibial shaft axis[196]
5. Ligament tension

Femoral rotation is difficult to instrument precisely because of surface landmark inconsistencies and obscurities; the surgeon must form her or his own judgment upon taking many factors into account, making sure to err on the side of slight external rotation, *never* internal rotation.[8,15,164] The posterior condylar axis (PCA) is frequently used as the reference for femoral rotation; however, posterior condylar erosion as part of the arthritic process, particularly in the valgus knee,

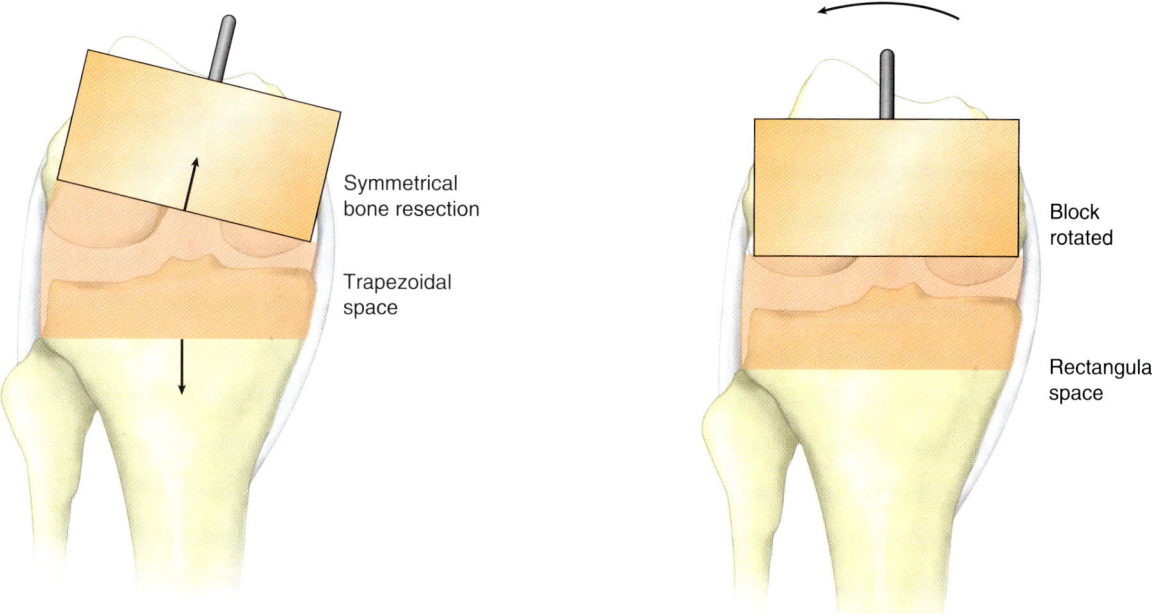

Symmetrical
bone resection

Trapezoidal
space

Block
rotated

Rectangular
space

Figure 105-9. In the osteoarthritic knee, lateral laxity is accentuated; when symmetrical bone is excised from the posterior femoral condyles, the resulting space on distraction is trapezoidal.

Figure 105-10. By externally rotating the femoral component and removing an asymmetrical amount of bone from the posterior femoral condyles, soft tissue length is equalized and the resulting space is rectangular.

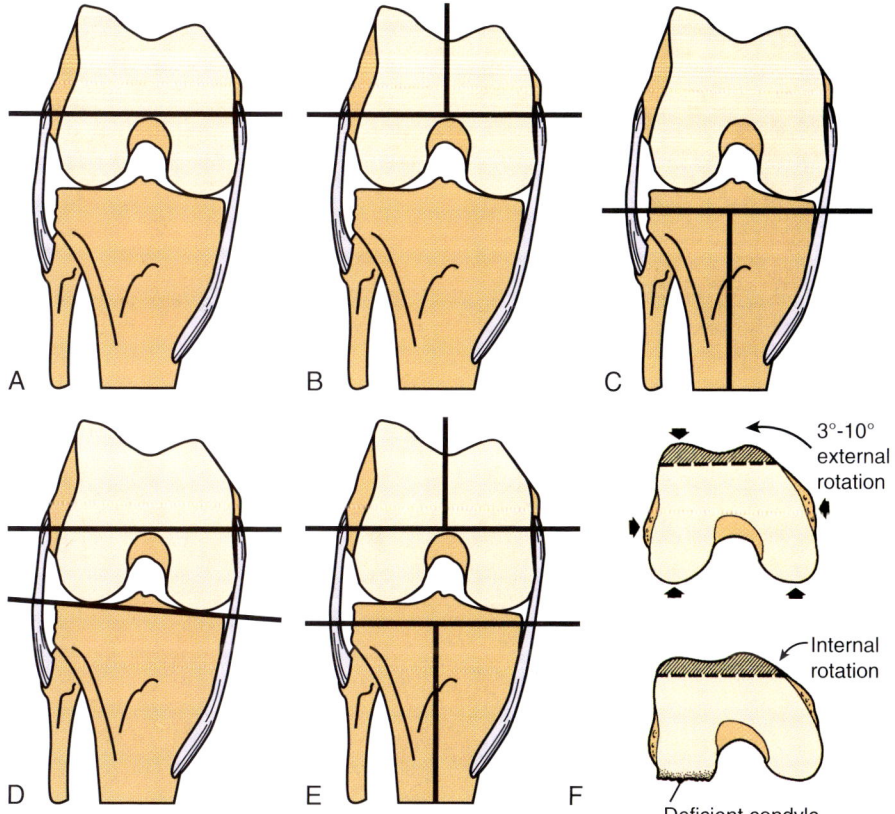

3°-10°
external
rotation

Internal
rotation

Deficient condyle

Figure 105-11. Reference points for rotational positioning of the femoral component include the epicondyles, the trochlear surface, the tibial shaft, and the posterior condyles. **A,** Transepicondylar axis. **B,** Anteroposterior trochlear sulcus ("Whiteside's line"). **C,** Tibial shaft axis. **D,** Posterior condylar angle. **E,** Transepicondylar axis is perpendicular to the anteroposterior sulcus line and the tibial shaft axis. **F,** When the posterior condyles are used for rotational reference, one must beware of erosion of the condyles. For example, in valgus knees, posterior erosion of the lateral femoral condyle is often present, which may result in internal rotation of the femoral component.

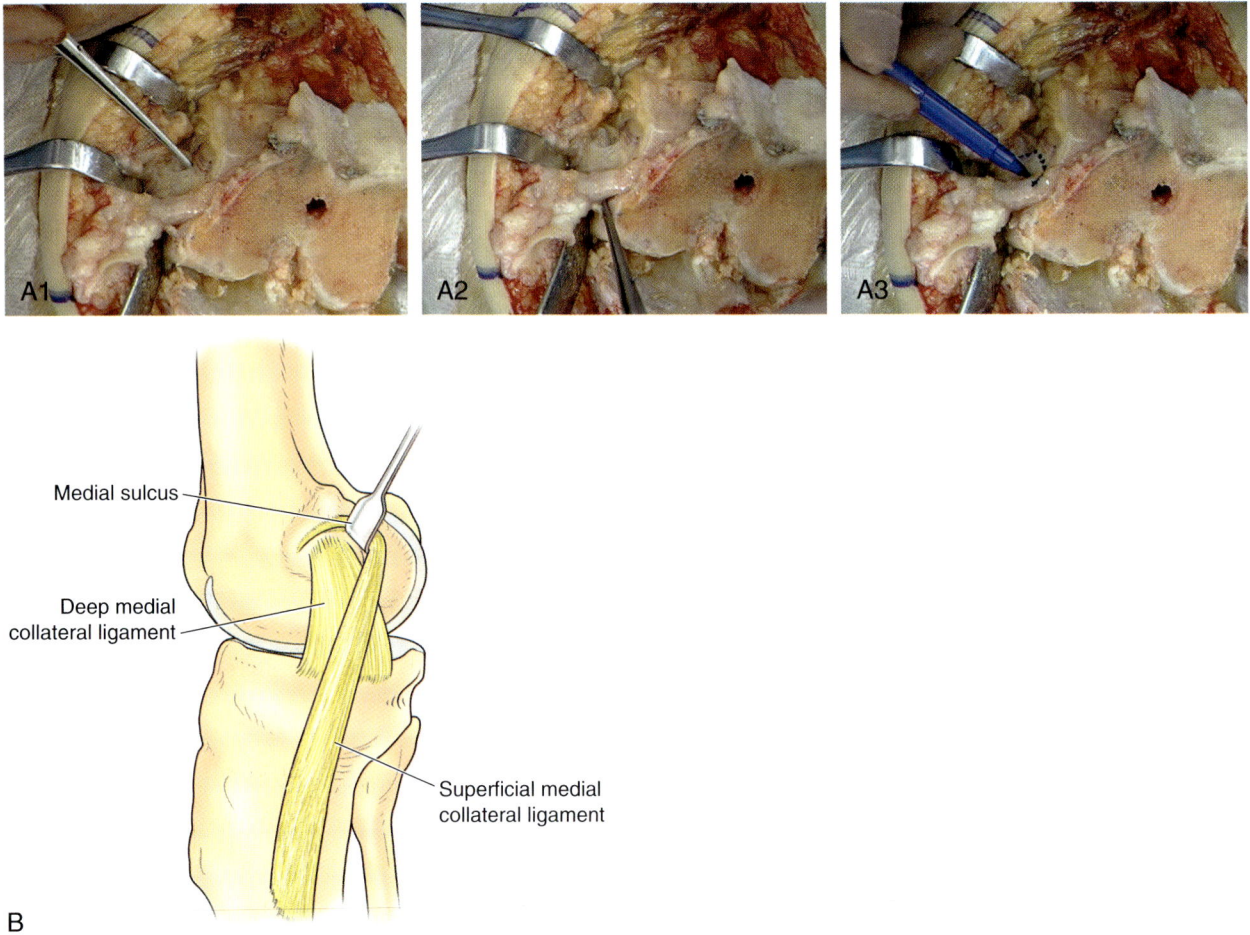

Figure 105-12. A, Intraoperative photos of the medial epicondyle. **A1,** Leash of vessels over the insertion of the superficial medial collateral ligament (MCL). **A2,** Instrument placed to define the insertion of the deep MCL. **A3,** Between the two MCL insertions, at the medial sulcus, the medial epicondyle is marked in a "bull's eye" fashion. **B,** Deep to the superficial MCL, the deep MCL overlies the medial sulcus, the palpable focus of the medial epicondyle.

often distorts this reference angle; and so, it probably should not be relied on as the sole method of determining femoral rotation.[81,196] The AP axis of the femoral sulcus, described by Whiteside and Arima,[9,218] has also been shown to be an accurate reference point for determining femoral rotation; however, it has been shown to be less reliable in cases of trochlear dysplasia and valgus deformity.[159] The tibial shaft axis has been described as an effective reference axis for defining femoral rotation.[196] Using the anatomic axis of the tibia is particularly useful because it should facilitate balancing the flexion space when perpendicular proximal tibial cuts are created and subsequently used as a reference for femoral component rotation.

Insall preferred the epicondylar axis as the reference that would most closely re-create the patient's natural femoral rotation.[17,159] The center of the medial epicondyle is located in a sulcus that lies between the proximal origin of the superficial deep medial collateral ligament (MCL) and the distal origin of the deep MCL. The medial epicondylar ridge at the origin of the superficial MCL can be identified by isolating the condylar vessels that lie proximal and anterior to the medial epicondylar ridge. From these vessels, the epicondylar ridge can be readily outlined; the center of this outline is the sulcus, which typically can be palpated without dissection

(Fig. 105-12). The lateral epicondyle is the most prominent point on the lateral aspect of the distal femur. Following the lateral condylar vessels (similar to the medial side) confirms the exact location of the lateral epicondyle, lying immediately distal to the vessels (Fig. 105-13). The line across the distal femur connecting the epicondyles with the knee flexed to 90 degrees is the epicondylar axis.

The benefit of having several different methods of assessing femoral rotation is that one or more can be used to confirm the surgeon's preferred method (Fig. 105-14). Several investigators have compared these various methods. Poilvache and associates[159] correlated the transepicondylar, anteroposterior, and posterior condylar axes. Berger and colleagues[17] and Griffin and coworkers[80] described the relationship of the epicondylar axis to the posterior condylar axis. Whiteside and Arima[9,218] defined the relationship of the anteroposterior and posterior condylar axes. Stiehl and associates[196] demonstrated that referencing from the tibial shaft axis is more accurate than referencing from the PCA. More recently, Katz and colleagues[107] found that using the transepicondylar axis was less predictable and resulted in excessive external rotation as compared with the AP axis and the balanced tension line. Fehring[65] reported rotational errors of at least 3 degrees occurring in 45% of patients when rotation was determined by fixed bony landmarks as compared with the balanced tension line. One study compared the use of the PCA and the transepicondylar axis (TEA) and demonstrated a decrease in the requirement for lateral retinacular release when the TEA was used: 56.9% with PCA reference versus 12.3% with TEA reference.[151]

As previously mentioned, the use of computer navigation has been proposed as a way to improve component position. In a study conducted to evaluate computer navigation as it relates to femoral rotation, it was reported that intraoperative decisions should be based on a combination of reference points, and that computer navigation alone suggested the incorrect femoral size in up to 50% of the cases reviewed. Furthermore, 34% of cases required intraoperative adjustments in rotation from the computer-modeled placement.[14] Ultimately, the determination of whether the rotation is "correct" will be made by considering all available anatomic references, ensuring proper tracking of the patella, and confirming unconstrained movement of the tibiofemoral articulation.

Anterior versus Posterior Referencing

Flexion Gap

In contrast to the early days, when gap balancing was developed, there exists now a larger range of femoral component sizes, with combinations of width and depth of the component allowing better matching of the patient's dimensions. Nevertheless, there will seldom be an exact match between the sagittal dimension of the femoral component and the actual size of the bone, necessitating some compromise to create a balanced knee. With anterior referencing, the size of the component is based on the amount of the posterior femoral condyle that is removed. Thus, the size of the flexion gap after the posterior condylar resection will differ from anatomic if the exact amount of resected condyle does not equal the amount replaced by the femoral implant. To create equal flexion and extension gaps, adjustments in the distal femoral resection (extension gap) may be necessary when the posterior condyles are over-resected. Over-resection of the posterior condyles can cause flexion instability, and under-resection can lead to excessive tightness in flexion, particularly when the PCL is preserved. Conversely, with posterior referencing (Fig. 105-15), the flexion gap is constant, but variability in sagittal size creates a risk of "notching" the anterior femoral cortex with an aggressive resection of bone, or of having the femoral flange sit anterior to the anterior femoral cortex when the component is larger than the bone. To compensate for in-between sizing when using anterior referencing, Insall recommended downsizing components and placing the femoral component in slight flexion (typically 3 degrees) to lessen the risk of anterior notching (Fig. 105-16). The same effect can be achieved if the instrument system creates a slightly divergent (as opposed to

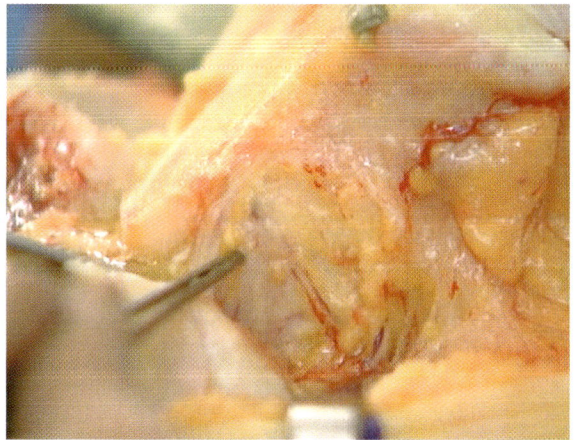

Figure 105-13. Intraoperative photo of the lateral epicondyle, the most prominent point on the distal lateral femur.

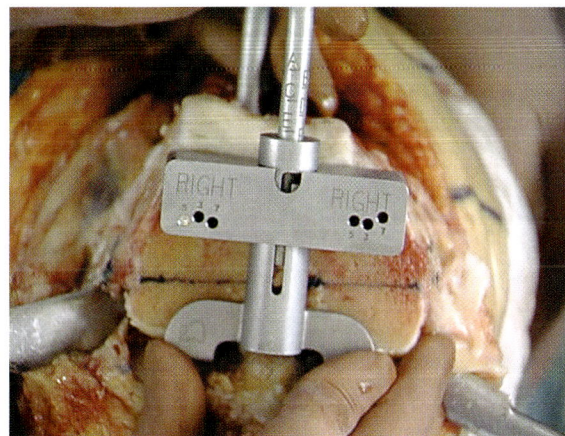

Figure 105-15. Instrument used for sagittal sizing of the femur.

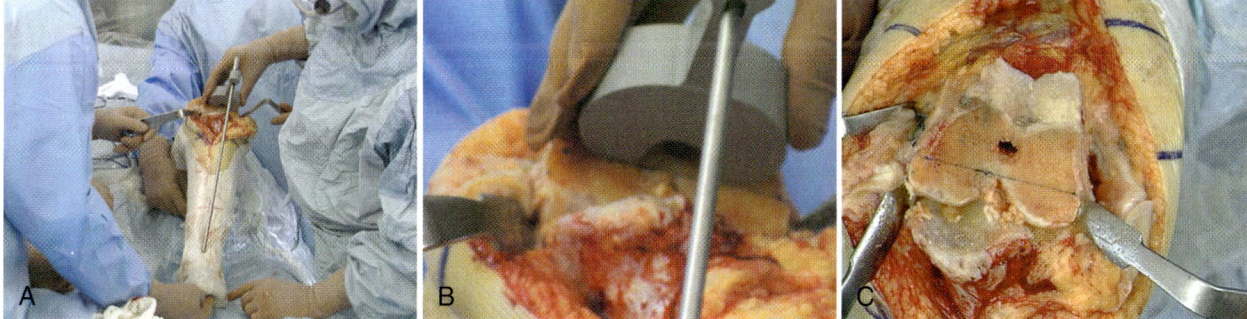

Figure 105-14. Confirming proper femoral rotation. **A,** Tibial shaft axis. **B,** Comparison of transepicondylar and tibial shaft axes. **C,** Transepicondylar axis.

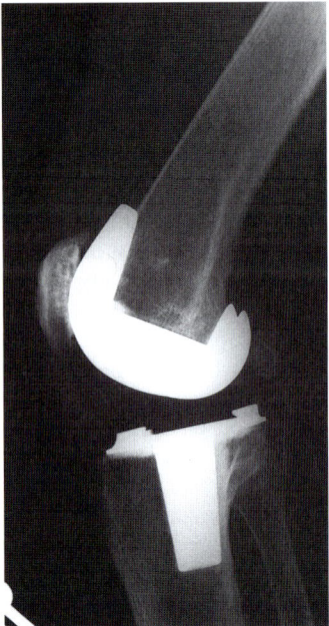

Figure 105-16. Lateral radiograph demonstrating the femoral component cemented in 3 degrees of flexion to avoid anterior notching of the femur.

parallel to the anterior cortex) anterior cut, also minimizing the risk of anterior femoral notching.

After the posterior condylar cut is made, the flexion gap between the surfaces of the posterior femoral condyles and proximal tibia is measured. Insall's original technique included spacer blocks to determine the gap size (Fig. 105-17). An alternative to static blocks is to use ligament tensor devices, ranging from something as simple as a lamina spreader to a more complicated sensor with a digitally calibrated read-out. The tensor technique measures soft tissue tension on the medial and lateral sides of the gap (Figs. 105-18 and 105-19). Using the tensor work flow, the proximal tibial cut is made first. The tensors then allow the surgeon to properly tension the flexion space and create a corresponding posterior condylar cut (Fig. 105-20). The size of the flexion space corresponds to the combined thickness of tibial and femoral components and determines the thickness of the tibial component required to stabilize the knee in flexion. If the flexion gap is not symmetrical, then additional ligament release procedures, as described later, may be necessary to establish flexion space symmetry. Alternatively, lack of flexion space symmetry may be the result of improper femoral rotation, requiring adjustment to correct rotation and balance the flexion gap.

Extension Gap

As with the flexion gap, sizing of the extension gap is performed using spacers or a tensioning device. For balancing gaps, the distal femoral osteotomy is performed after the

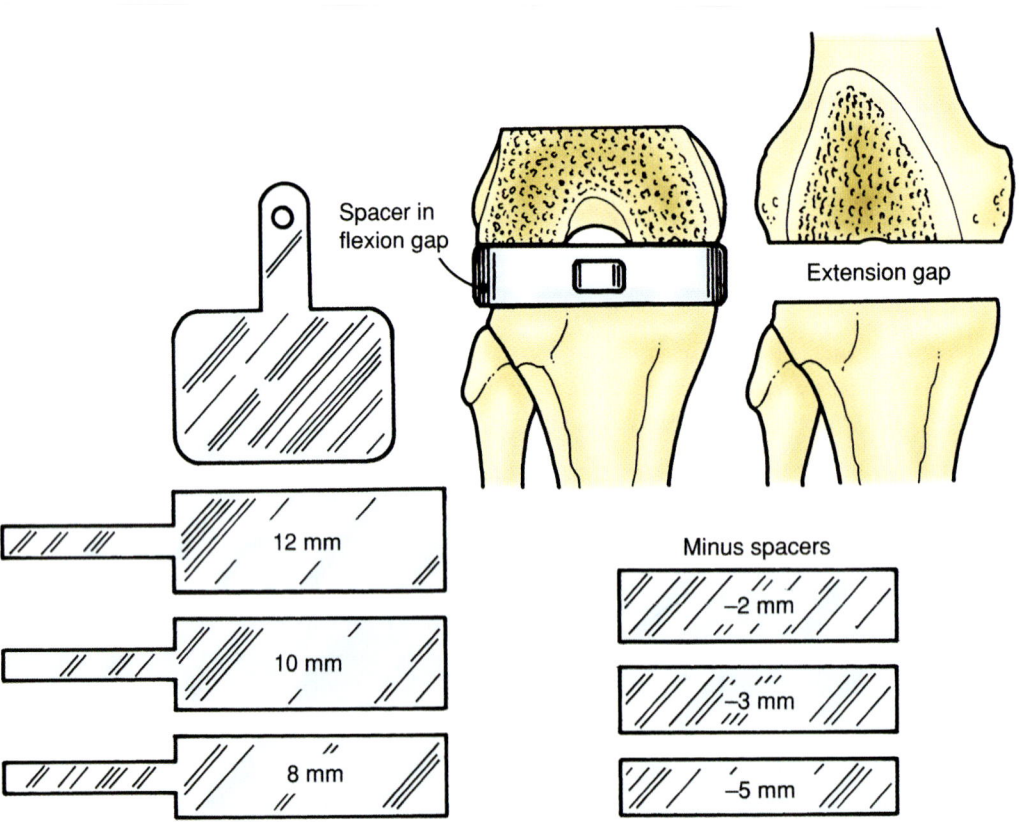

Figure 105-17. Flexion and extension gaps are assessed by a series of spacers. When the extension gap is smaller than the flexion gap, it must be equalized by resection of extra distal femoral bone. The amount needed is assessed using the spacer system. Minus spacers are available when the flexion gap requires the thinnest (8 mm) spacer.

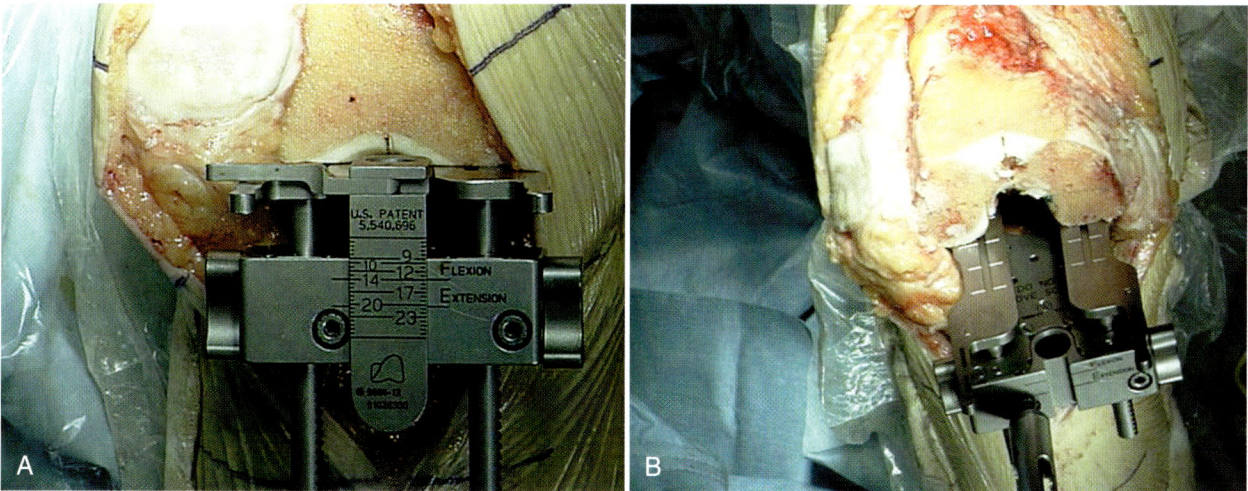

Figure 105-18. Close-up intraoperative view of a tensor. **A,** In extension. **B,** In flexion.

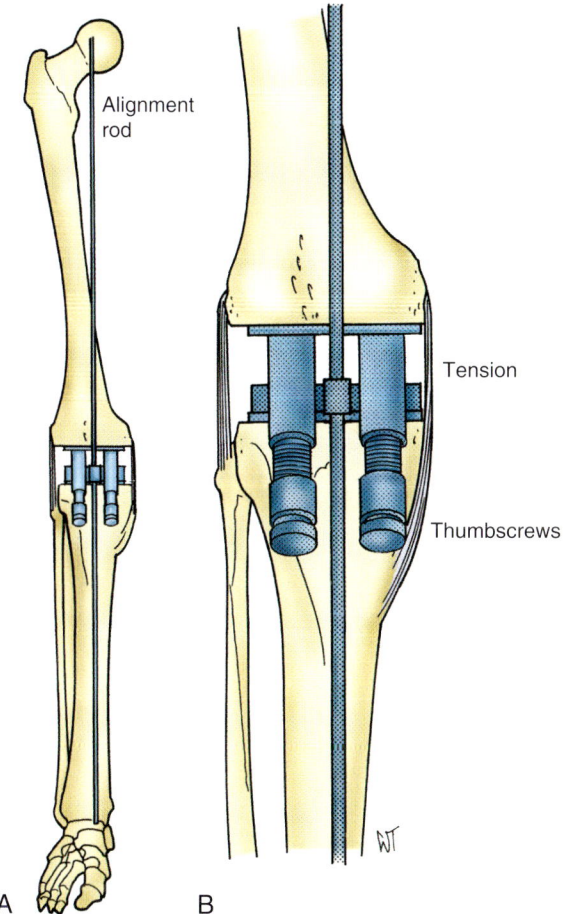

Figure 105-19. By adjusting the medial and lateral thumbscrews of the tensor, the alignment rod is brought into the mechanical axis.

proximal tibial cut is completed. The extension gap represents the combined thickness of the femoral component and the tibial component. With this concept in mind, the distal femoral resection is made to accommodate the thickness of both components, while matching the flexion gap

measurement. One approach to creating the proper distal femoral resection depth is to cut the distal femur at a predetermined level (usually 10 mm above the joint line) corresponding to the thickness of the femoral component alone (Fig. 105-21). The extension space so formed is then assessed with a spacer block or tensiometer, and the distal femur is recut when necessary to match the flexion gap (see Fig. 105-18). In this way, the amount of additional resection can be calculated from the difference between the thicknesses of the flexion block and the extension block. Cutting away more distal femur than the femoral component will ultimately replace should be minimized as it will elevate the joint line. When a preoperative flexion contracture contributes to gap imbalance, appropriate soft tissue balancing and posterior release should be performed before additional bone resection is considered.

An alternative to using a predetermined distal femoral resection is to cut the extension gap in one step based on the measured height of the flexion gap. When a one-step distal cut is performed, the knee is extended and axial traction is applied on the limb with a mechanical device such as a tensor (see Figs. 105-18 to 105-20). With the soft tissue under proper tension, the level of distal femoral osteotomy is determined by the thickness of spacer blocks that fit the flexion gap. A distal femoral osteotomy is performed at this level perpendicular to the mechanical axis and at a measured valgus angle relative to the anatomic axis of the femur (Figs. 105-22 through 105-24). The valgus cut on the distal femur relative to the anatomic axis is the difference between anatomic and mechanical axes, which can be measured using long cassette radiographs. Once again, the surgeon should recognize the fact that removing more distal bone than the femoral implant replaces will result in elevation of the joint line.

Pros and Cons of the Gap Balancing Technique

The essential philosophy of the gap technique is that it builds the joint line based on tension in the soft tissues after the initial soft tissue correction is performed. The soft tissue correction is performed first, and the measure gap resection is performed next. This technique can be applied universally to standard primary total knee arthroplasty (TKA), complex primary TKA with deformity, and revision TKA. In contrast

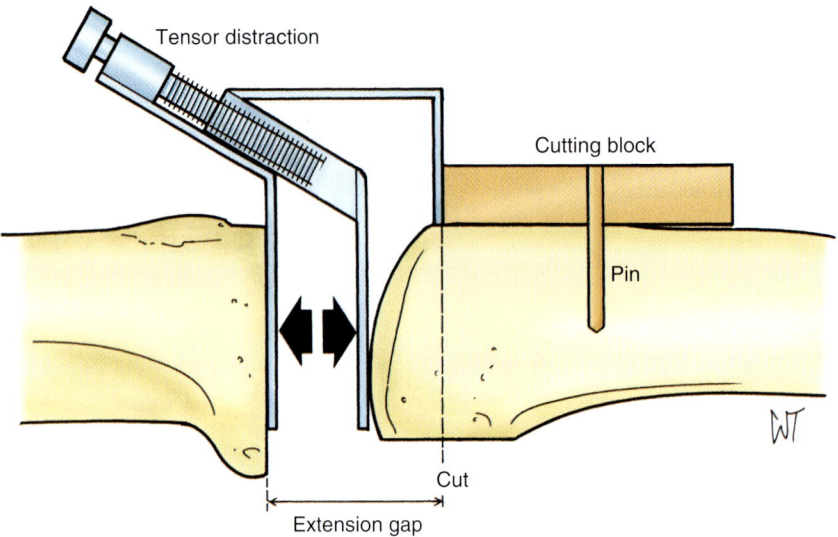

Figure 105-20. The distal femoral cutting guide is controlled by the tensor and is positioned to create an extension gap of the correct dimensions.

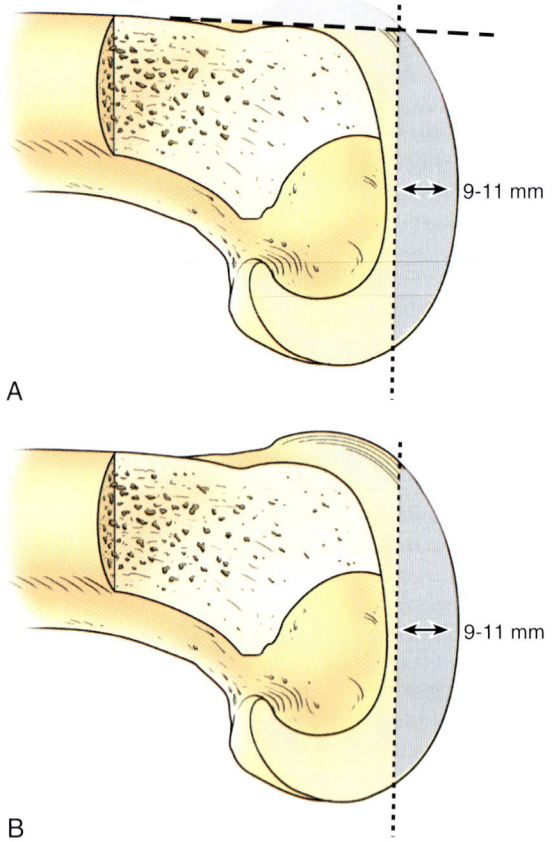

A

B

Figure 105-21. The thickness of the prosthesis, normally somewhere between 9 and 11 mm, is removed from the distal femur.

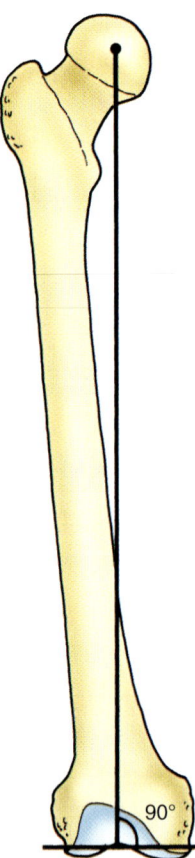

Figure 105-22. The distal femoral cut should be templated by measuring from the center of the femoral head to the center of the knee on a full-length radiograph of the femur. A second line passing into the intramedullary canal of the femur will indicate the angulation of the distal femoral cut.

to the measured resection method described next, the amount of bone removed from the femur may not equal the thickness of the femoral component. Rather, the amount of bone removed from the distal femur is determined by the flexion gap thickness.

Potential pitfalls of the gap technique include the following:

1. When the flexion gap size dictates a more aggressive distal femoral bone resection, the joint line may be moved proximally. This is most likely to happen when there is a preoperative flexion contracture, when a large flexion gap mandates resection of more distal femoral

bone than the femoral implant replaces, or when the chosen femoral component is smaller than the AP dimension of the femur, creating a large flexion gap. Joint line alteration can be minimized by correct femoral measurement, a full range of femoral component sizes, and posterior capsular release to correct a flexion contracture.

2. The method ensures soft tissue balance and correct tensioning in full extension and at 90 degrees of flexion, but midrange laxity may occur when a tight posterior capsule is not corrected. When the posterior contracture is not addressed, the extension gap balance is hinged upon the posterior capsule rather than the collateral ligaments. Thus, the collateral ligaments are not balanced throughout the range of motion, particularly in midflexion. Patients with midflexion laxity may report a loose knee or lack of confidence when descending stairs or walking on inclines.

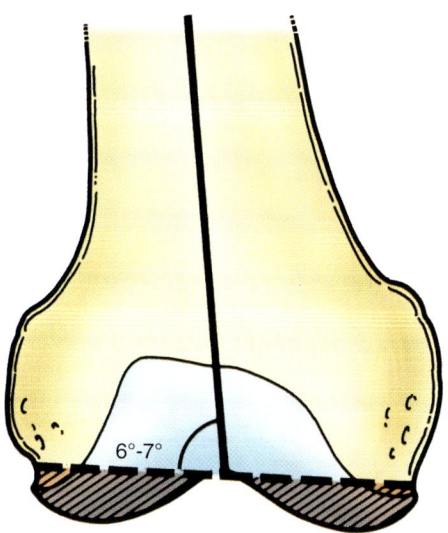

Figure 105-23. The distal femoral cut is normally aligned at 6 to 7 degrees of valgus from the intramedullary alignment rod.

Classic Measured Resection Technique

The second theory of surgical technique, the measured resection theory, begins with the philosophy of maintaining joint line position. This theory is predicated on the observation that a properly positioned joint line is essential to proper collateral ligament and cruciate ligament function, and consequently posterior cruciate retention.[136] Hungerford and Krackow developed the method of measured resection. This technique has been used in conjunction with principles of anatomic alignment, as well as the neutral tibial cut.[94,184]

Posterior Cruciate Ligament

Preservation of the PCL offers many potential advantages because this ligament is an important varus/valgus stabilizer of the knee; it is a strong structure that can absorb stresses that might otherwise be transmitted to the prosthesis-bone interface, can control the roll-back of the femur on the tibia that occurs with flexion, may be important for stair-climbing activities, and may have a proprioceptive function (although abnormal proprioception will not return to normal after knee replacement).

To function properly, the PCL must be accurately tensioned during knee replacement. If the PCL is too tight, this will promote excessive tibial roll-back, thereby impeding knee flexion, causing increased posterior stresses, and risking posterior polyethylene overload and anterior femoral component displacement. A tight PCL may also cause the knee to hinge "open like a book" (Fig. 105-25). Recognition of excess PCL tightness is possible by observing anterior tibial component "lift-off" with trial components (Fig. 105-26). Conversely, when the PCL is too loose, it does not control movement between the tibia and the femur (Fig. 105-27), allowing the femur to roll forward paradoxically (opposite of normal roll-back) in flexion, potentially limiting flexion by posterior impingement. The "slide-back" test has been described to assess for proper PCL tension following component positioning in rotating platform systems. The trial insert (without stabilizing post) is inserted and the knee flexed to 90 degrees. If the PCL is too tight, the insert moves posterior.

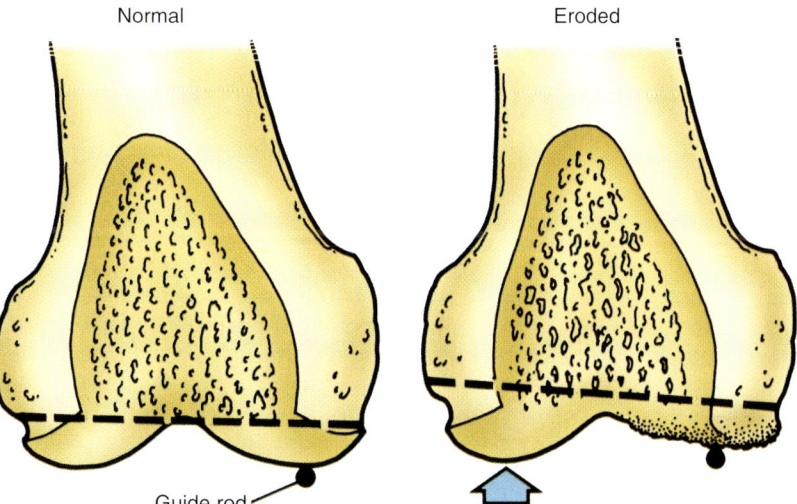

Normal   Eroded

Guide rod

Figure 105-24. Ideally, the amount of distal femoral resection should be judged from the normal side. When measurement is made from the medial femoral condyle, regardless of the pathology, extra distal femoral resection will occur.

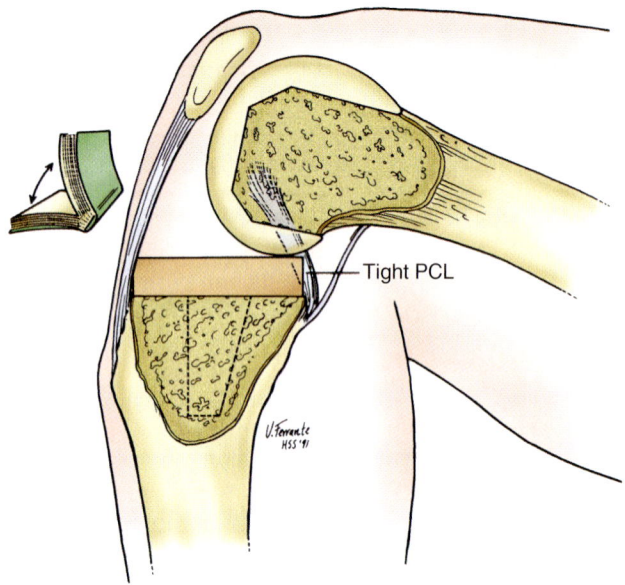

Figure 105-25. An overtight posterior cruciate ligament causes "booking." Excessive roll-back of the femur occurs, and the knee hinges open.

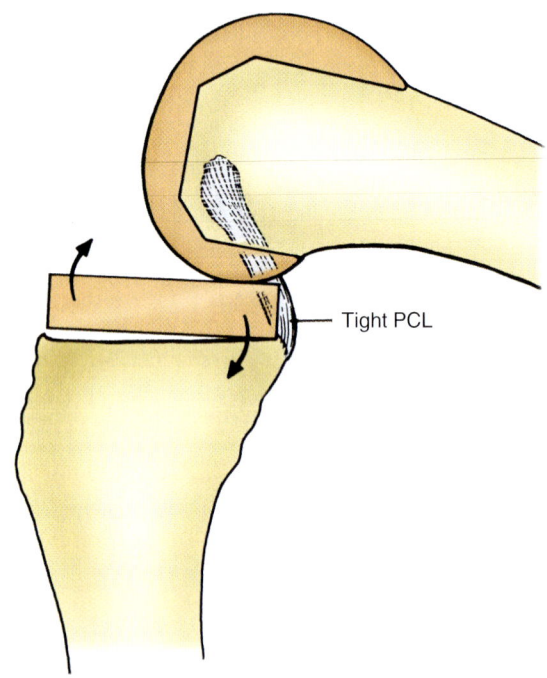

Figure 105-26. Method of demonstrating a tight posterior cruciate ligament intraoperatively. The tibial trial component does not have undersurface fixation, and the component lifts anteriorly.

Conversely, a PCL with excessive laxity will allow anterior migration of the insert. Best results have been reported with PCL tension adjusted to provide for 1 to 3 mm of posterior insert translation.[184]

Proper PCL tension is dependent upon maintaining the level of the joint line and the spatial relationship between the femur and the tibia. The ideal posterior cruciate retaining knee replacement would meet the following criteria:

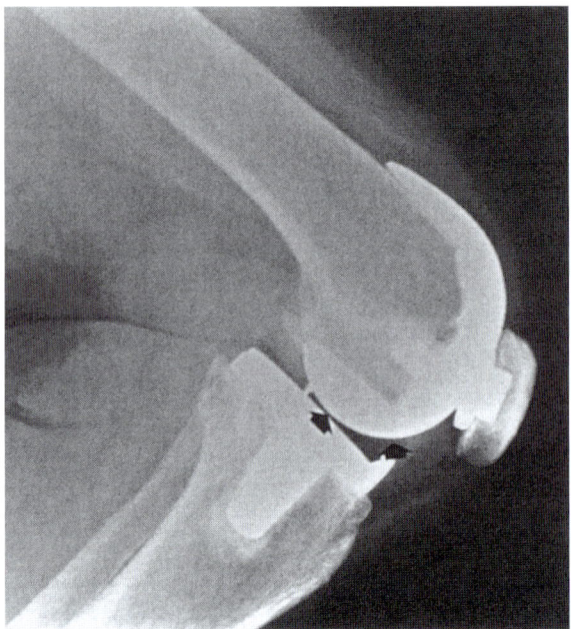

Figure 105-27. Sagittal radiograph of a "nonfunctional" posterior cruciate ligament. "Roll-forward" rather than "roll-back" is seen with knee flexion. The anterior margin of the femoral component abuts the anterior margin of the tibial component as it does in a total condylar-type design.

1. The joint line or axis is restored to its prearthritic condition.
2. The shape and size of the femoral condyles are restored to re-create the natural distal and posterior femoral cam effect.
3. The tibial plateau surface is sloped approximately 10 degrees posterior and approximately 3 degrees medial.
4. The tibial surface offers no impedance to rotation and gliding movements.

In practice, techniques that are aimed at preserving the PCL meet these requirements to varying degrees. The balance of the PCL remains a subjective assessment. Proper balancing even in the hands of experienced surgeons does not guarantee normal knee kinematics and tibial roll-back. A few systems mimic the medial slope of the normal tibia, and some cut the tibia at right angles to its shaft. However, all measured resection knee systems share the objective of closely preserving or restoring the anatomic joint line by referencing the distal femur. If this joint line preservation is achieved and the PCL is retained, the arc of motion should also be close to normal with correct ligament tensioning and optimal patellar tracking throughout the range of motion. Because patellofemoral dysfunction remains the cause of many unsatisfactory knee arthroplasties, maintenance of the anatomic joint line is potentially valuable. An optimal joint line avoids patella infera (Fig. 105-28). Further evidence comes from Figgie and colleagues,[68] who demonstrated that if the patella is not within a defined sagittal neutral zone (10 to 30 mm above the joint line), a greater number of patellar problems are observed (Fig. 105-29).

Successful PCL retention in TKA requires sustained function and proper initial balancing. Ligament balancing techniques have been developed that permit PCL retention when

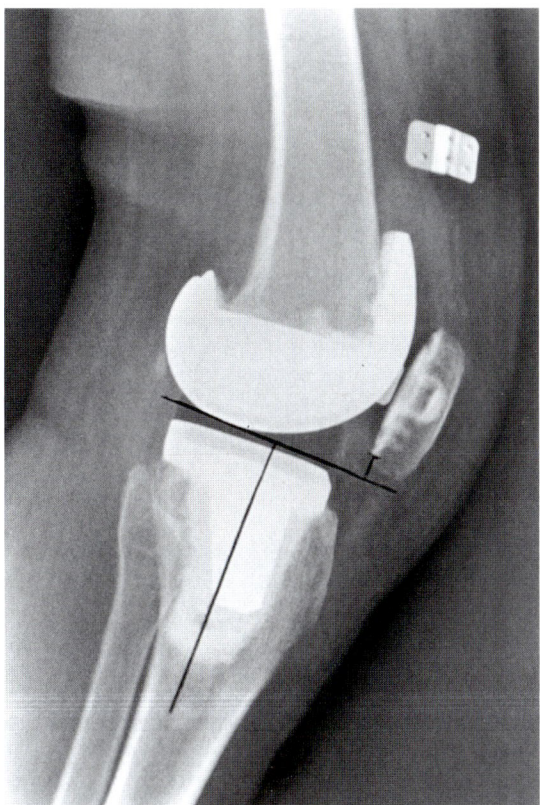

Figure 105-28. Lateral radiograph of a posterior stabilized prosthesis shows a patella infera. The distal pole of the patella lies just proximal to a projection of the joint line. Patella infera may be associated with increased frequency of patellar symptoms.

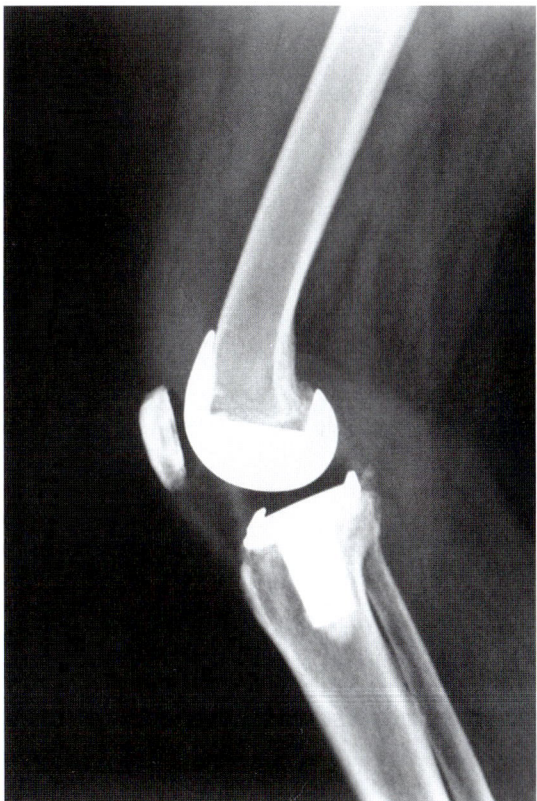

Figure 105-29. Lateral radiograph shows a satisfactory patellar position postoperatively. The patella lies in its normal position in relation to the joint line. The patellar prosthesis composite is of the correct thickness. Note the sclerosis that has developed in the remaining patellar bone. This is a common finding that develops several years postoperatively and is an example of Wolff's law.

the ligament is contracted but remains competent.[169,179,185] The technique is similar to the medial release performed for balancing varus deformity. A graduated PCL release (Fig. 105-30A) is performed from the posterior aspect of the tibia using a periosteal elevator until the PCL tension is deemed appropriate (see Fig. 105-30B). However, even for a skilled surgeon, it may be difficult to achieve the aims of successful PCL retention.[38] Although the PCL is typically intact in most arthritic knees,[183,186] the PCL can also degenerate and contract as part of the arthritic process,[5,112] rendering the ligament nonfunctional and making PCL retention not applicable in some arthritic knee deformities.[120,186] Likewise, the PCL occasionally becomes incompetent in the months or years after knee replacement, rendering the prosthesis unstable.[155,212] Using cine-radiography, Dennis et al demonstrated paradoxical roll-forward of the femur on the tibia as the knee flexes in apparently well-functioning knees with a retained PCL.[45] Follow-up studies by these investigators have reported improved and more consistent kinematics with an intact PCL when combined with an asymmetrical femoral component. More recent studies have even demonstrated reliable femoral roll-back with PCL retention in newer posterior stabilized designs.[27,113]

Anterior Cruciate Ligament

The anterior cruciate ligament (ACL) is an important functional element in the normal knee; its absence causes not only instability but an abnormal pattern of motion, including rotational and sliding movements (e.g., pivot shift). Together

with the PCL, the ACL forms a "four-bar linkage"[145] at the center of the knee, and the absence of either component destroys this mechanism. Abnormal sliding movements, in particular, can be expected when only the PCL is preserved.[43,44,109,197] *Cruciate retention* refers only to the PCL in the context of TKA. The ACL is sacrificed in most modern bicondylar total knee systems. Only a few knee prostheses are designed to preserve both cruciate ligaments. The bi-cruciate retaining meniscal-bearing Oxford knee is not recommended unless both ligaments are present.[78] In many arthritic knees, the ACL is damaged or absent, and most cruciate preserving systems advocate removal of the ACL.

Integrating the Measured Resection and Gap Techniques

From the previous discussion, it is apparent that philosophical differences exist between the gap balancing school of thought and the measured resection school of thought. The classic gap method emphasizes preservation of tibial bone and conforming joint surfaces, and accepts, when required, proximal migration of the joint surface to balance the gaps. The classic measured resection school of thought emphasizes preservation of the joint axis and accepts less congruence of the flexion and extension gaps. Flexion contractures, when present, are corrected by a combination of a posterior capsular release and stretching out of the remaining contracture with

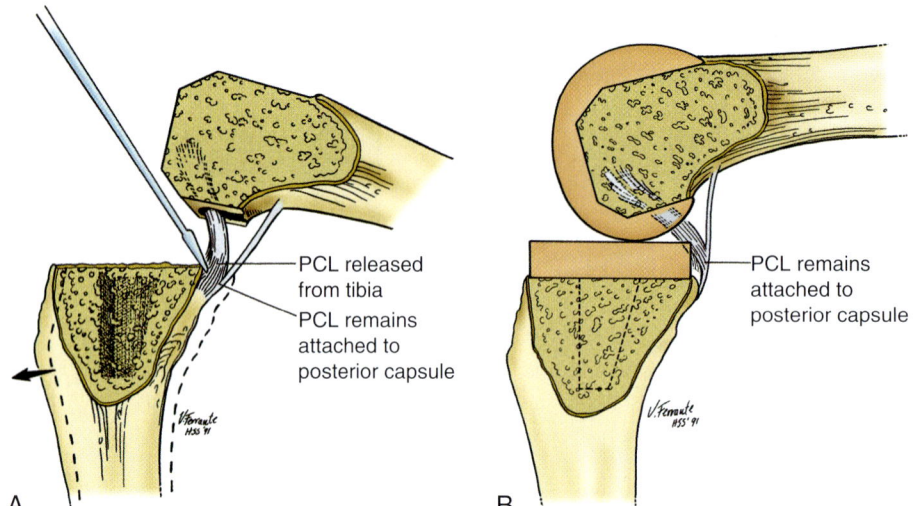

Figure 105-30. Posterior cruciate ligament (PCL) release from the posterior tibia lengthens a tight PCL. **A,** The release can be done progressively until correct tension is obtained. **B,** The PCL remains attached to the posterior capsule.

postoperative physiotherapy.[199] In contrast, the gap technique emphasizes the distal femoral bone resection in combination with posterior capsulotomy and PCL resection to accomplish intraoperative correction of flexion contractures, a principle emphasized by Insall.

The differing philosophies are also reflected in technique and instrument systems. Although the instruments used for making bone cuts are generally similar, gap systems depend on a tensor or a series of spacers, and *adjustment* cuts for extension balance are made on the distal femur. Ligament releases are generally performed before the bone cuts, or perhaps after the upper tibia resection and distal femoral preliminary valgus cut (technique using tensors or laminar spreaders). In contrast, measured resection systems osteotomize the tibia and femur independently, aiming to remove only enough bone to accommodate the components. The tensor or spacing function is performed by the components themselves, and ligament releases are done after the trial components have been inserted to achieve balance.

Despite obvious differences in philosophy, the distinctions between the gap and measured resection techniques have blurred with the evolution of surgical techniques. Methods of PCL recession or release have made the two techniques more similar. Because PCL release opens both flexion and extension gaps, measured resection used with PCL release creates larger gaps, especially in flexion.[106] In a clinical study of PCL resection, Kadoya measured an increase in the medial and lateral flexion gaps of 4.8 mm and 4.5 mm, respectively, as compared with increases in the medial and lateral extension gaps of 0.9 mm and 0.8 mm, respectively. Using fluoroscopic analysis, several investigators have demonstrated that femoral roll-back does not occur with flexion in cruciate retaining prostheses.[109,197] In fact, some authors report femoral roll-back similar to a natural knee using posterior stabilized prosthetic designs.[43,44] Furthermore, flat tibial surfaces are not a prerequisite for PCL retention.[185] In long-term follow-up evaluations of cruciate retaining knees with conforming articular surfaces, satisfactory results have been reported.[172,186,214] Therefore, completely flat tibial surfaces for PCL retaining designs are not necessary, and cupping of some

degree is acceptable (provided the PCL-driven roll-back is not overly constrained). If this degree of articular conformity is permissible and compatible with PCL retention, then a major objection (polyethylene wear) to retaining the PCL is negated.

The recent focus in knee replacement technique is on restoration of kinematics, not simply on the presence or absence of the PCL. More objective methods for deciding when the PCL is too tight or so loose as to be rendered nonfunctional are required. Some PCL retaining systems have *markers* on the trial components to indicate proper kinematics. When the PCL is not fulfilling its purpose within acceptable and defined limits, a PCL release may be performed or, alternatively, a posterior stabilized design may be adopted. Most newer knee systems afford flexibility by functioning as cruciate retaining or cruciate substituting systems, permitting an intraoperative switch to posterior stabilization when the PCL is deemed nonfunctional or detrimental.

Current Preference in Knee Balancing

The current preference in knee ligament balancing is a modified gap technique that has elements of both gap and measured resection methods. Insall advocated a blend of techniques whereby measured resections of both the distal femur and the proximal tibia are performed, avoiding the need for a variable distal femoral cut. Posterior referencing of the femoral condyles with some accommodation to a balanced flexion gap at the same time allows measured resection and balancing of the flexion gap as well. This measured resection combined with balancing of the flexion gap is facilitated by a larger inventory of femoral component sizes than existed when gap balancing was described, as well as a femoral component designed with a divergent anterior cut to minimize the risk of anterior femoral notching. Femoral component sizing and positioning remain critical to proper balancing. One should avoid allowing the femoral component to sit proud of the anterior femoral cortex, even to a minor degree (see Fig. 105-16). Because PCL release opens the flexion and extension gaps, modifications of the measured resection technique are possible. If the PCL is appropriately adjusted, strict adherence to anatomic alignment (varus tibial cut) is no longer required, and the classic alignment (perpendicular tibial cut) traditionally assigned to the gap technique can be applied. As noted previously, some degree of articular congruency that does not conflict with PCL kinematics is permissible, improving the prospects for longer-term polyethylene performance.

Summary of Modified Gap Technique

The modified gap technique can be performed by cutting either the femur or the tibia first. The femur first technique is done as follows:

1. Cut the distal femur in valgus relative to the anatomic axis (usually 4 to 6 degrees) using intramedullary guides at a predetermined level (usually 9 to 10 mm above the medial condyle, accommodating for bone deficiency).
2. Make a proximal tibial cut perpendicular to the anatomic axis using extramedullary guides.
3. Balance ligaments in extension.
4. Establish femoral rotation in flexion using the epicondylar axis, ligament tension, and the proximal tibial cut surface.
5. Cut the anterior and posterior femur.
   a. Posterior referencing: perform (1) 3-degree flexion cut (or divergent anterior cut) and (2) correct preoperative flexion contractures by posterior release
   b. Anterior referencing: avoid over-resection of the posterior condyles of the femur
6. Choose femoral component (downsize for in-between sizing).
7. Reassess ligament balance, midflexion balance, and posterior capsular tightness.
8. Adjust distal femoral cut to deal with extension gap tightness. (Note that under-resection of the distal femur is seldom needed.)

Tibia first technique is done as follows:

1. Perform initial ligament releases during the surgical approach.
2. Make a proximal tibial resection perpendicular to the mechanical axis using extramedullary guides. Resection depth is based on measurement of 10 mm below the normal surface or proportionately less below the deficient surface.
3. Cut the distal femur at a predetermined level, establishing the desired valgus angle.
4. Balance the knee in extension using a tensiometer or blocks.
5. Flex the knee to 90 degrees and create the AP cut after component sizing. Use all available information to create a balanced flexion gap, including epicondylar axis, posterior condylar axis, tibial cut plane, and Whiteside's line.
6. Reassess ligament balance, midflexion balance, and posterior capsular tightness.
7. Adjust distal femoral cut to deal with extension gap tightness.

PREOPERATIVE PLANNING

Full-length radiographs that show hip, knee, and ankle joints are desirable for preoperative planning but require special equipment. Standard radiographs showing the distal femoral

and proximal tibial anatomic axis serve as an acceptable alternative to long films when there is no history of prior bone instrumentation or trauma, or clinical suspicion of excessive bowing. Radiographs are position sensitive, requiring care to obtain the films in neutral rotation (Figs. 105-31 and 105-32).[102] Information concerning the angle of femoral and tibial cuts and the desired entry hole position (which may not be in the bone center) is obtained. Unusual shaft bowing is noted (Fig. 105-33). Unusual anatomic variations such as unusual canal size, angular malalignment, or previous surgery that could cause intraoperative difficulty are noted (Fig. 105-34).

EXPOSURE

Routine Exposure

Medial Parapatellar Approach

The medial parapatellar approach is the most common approach for TKA. A midline skin incision centered over the patella extends from the level of the tibial tuberosity to just above the patella. The incision is made sufficiently long to avoid traction on the skin edges during the procedure. Distally, the incision is placed approximately 1 cm medial to the tibial tubercle. The medial parapatellar arthrotomy through the capsule is made as straight as possible, usually crossing the medial border of the patella to avoid transecting longitudinal fibers of the extensor mechanism. Proximally, the capsular incision is positioned along the medial margin of the vastus medialis within 6 to 8 mm of its edge; distally, the arthrotomy parallels the patellar tendon approximately 5 to 10 mm medial to the tibial tubercle. A medial periosteal sleeve that includes the deep MCL is elevated from the tibia to allow the proximal tibia to be translated anteriorly and rotated externally. When the ACL is present, it is divided to improve the ease of this translation.

Techniques to Enhance Exposure in Standard Medial Parapatellar Approach

1. Elevation of the deep fibers of the MCL just below the tibial surface with posterior extension reflecting the medial capsule, the deep MCL, and the semimembranosus (Fig. 105-35). Extension of the posteromedial release allows hyperflexion and external rotation of the tibia, thereby enhancing exposure by rotating the tibia out from under the femur and moving the patella and extensor mechanism laterally.
2. Elevation of a small cuff of periosteum immediately adjacent to the patellar tendon insertion at the tibial tubercle. This diminishes the risk of patellar tendon avulsion during exposure.
3. Division of the lateral patellofemoral ligament, which permits slightly greater patellar eversion.
4. Excision of the fat pad. Although some surgeons perform a longitudinal split of the fat pad, excision of the fat pad can improve mobilization of the patella and minimize the potential for postoperative infrapatellar scar formation.
5. Separation of the capsule from the patella at the lateral osteochondral border of the patella.

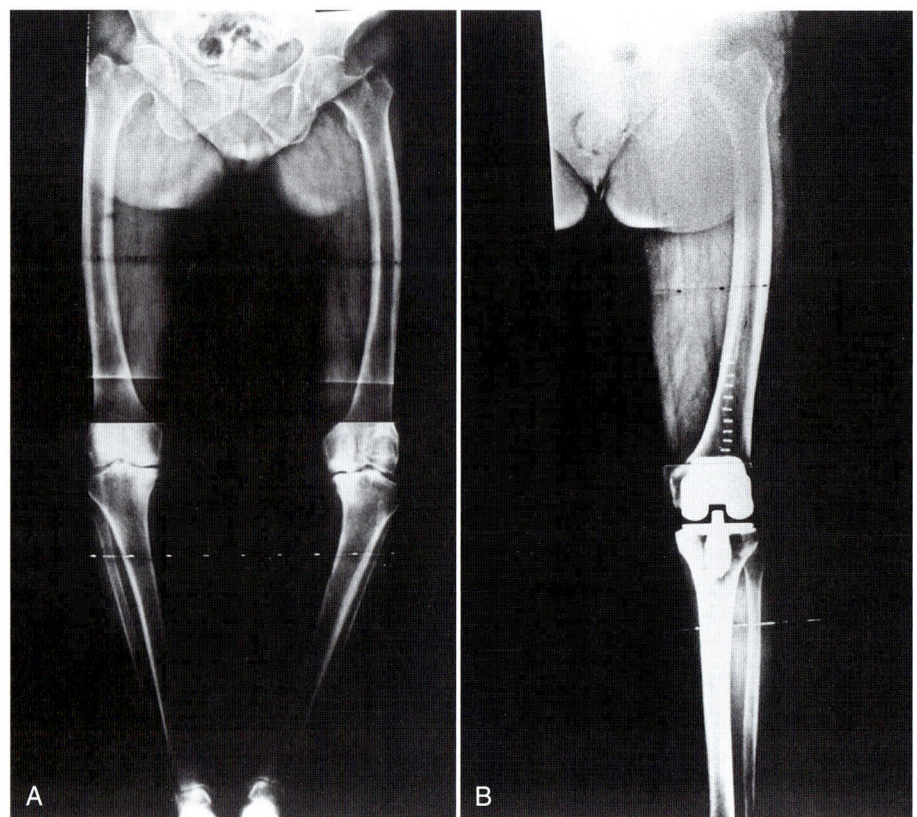

Figure 105-31. A, Long, 52-inch radiograph of a preoperative patient with varus osteoarthritis. From preoperative planning, a 14-degree valgus cut on the femur was predicted. **B,** Postoperative radiograph of the same patient. Extramedullary alignment check showed that the 14-degree prediction was grossly incorrect; in fact, the femur was resected at 7 degrees of valgus. Apparent lateral bowing was, in fact, excessive anterior bowing of the femur seen in a position of some external rotation.

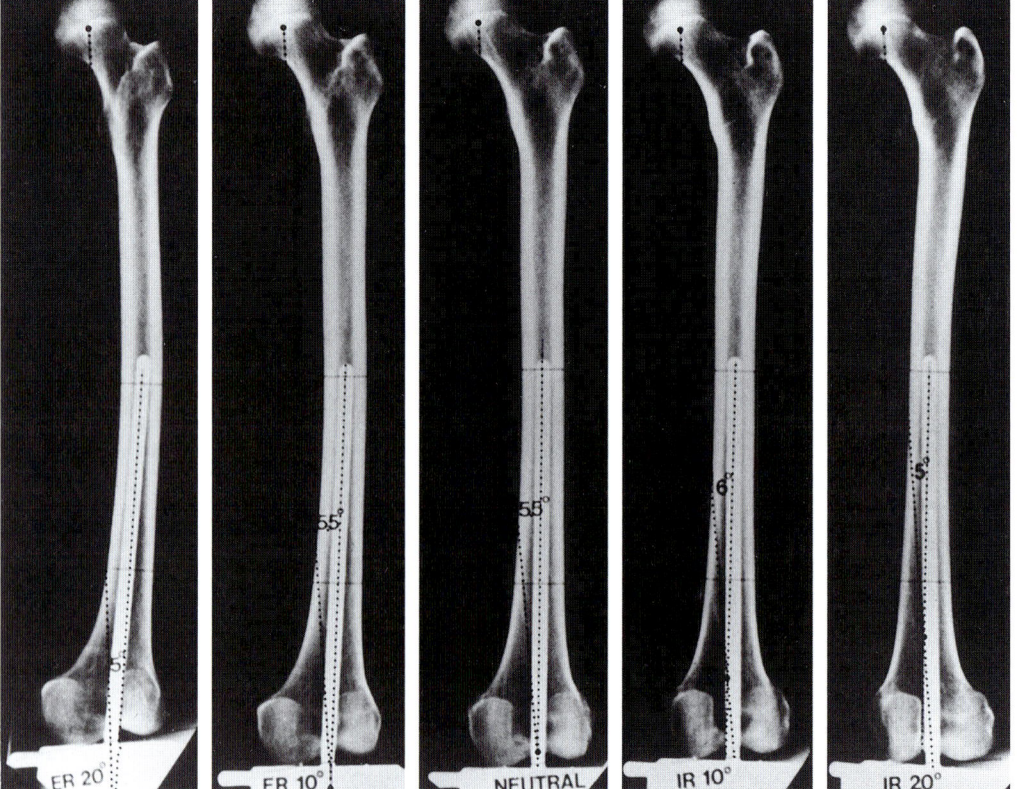

Figure 105-32. Radiographs of femur in internal and external rotation. It can be seen that internal rotation is perceived as medial bowing and external rotation as lateral bowing. This is a normal femur, and the effect would be accentuated if the femur had excessive anterior bowing.

6. Extension of the incision into the skin and the quadriceps proximally will also facilitate mobilization of the extensor mechanism and relieve skin tension in tight knees.

Other accepted methods of exposing the knee, such as the subvastus, vastus splitting, trivector, and lateral parapatellar methods, as well as the newer and unproven minimally invasive methods, are discussed elsewhere in this text.

Difficult Exposures

When a stiff or ankylosed knee is exposed, there is risk of avulsing the patellar ligament attachment to the tibial tubercle. If all aspects of the standard exposure are employed, with additional specific attention to areas of contracture, it is possible to minimize the risk of avulsion or damage to the extensor mechanism. When mobilizing the patella, it is important to perform releases to allow external rotation of the tibia, so that the patella can be subluxated laterally rather than

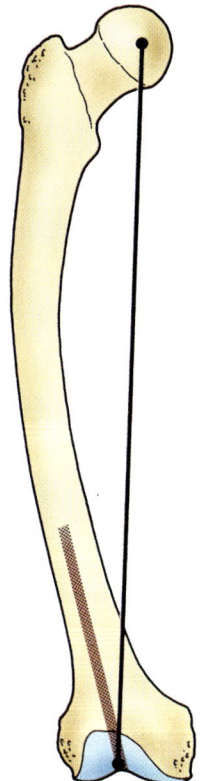

Figure 105-33. When the femur is bowed, the angle of the distal femoral cut will be increased. When templating the femur, beware of excessive valgus cuts, because bowing may represent external rotation of the femoral bone on the radiograph. An external alignment check is advisable.

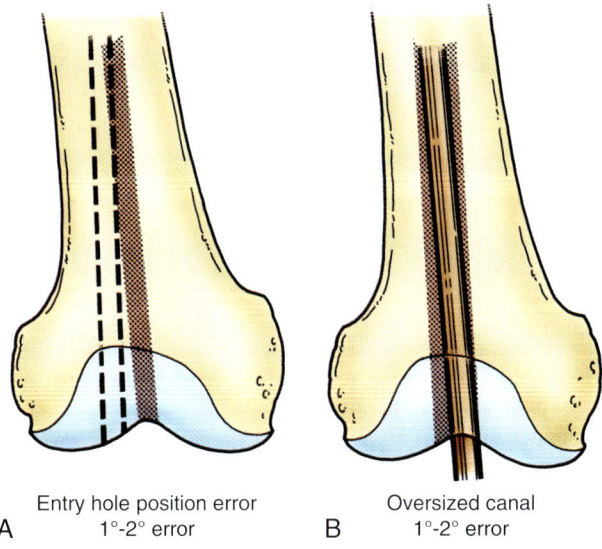

Entry hole position error
A   1°-2° error

Oversized canal
B   1°-2° error

Figure 105-34. Malposition of the entry hole into the femur introduces an error into the valgus cut. **A,** Lateral entry hole increases the valgus of the cut. **B,** Oversized canal allows the intramedullary rod to toggle, and a 1- to 2-degree error in both varus and valgus can be produced.

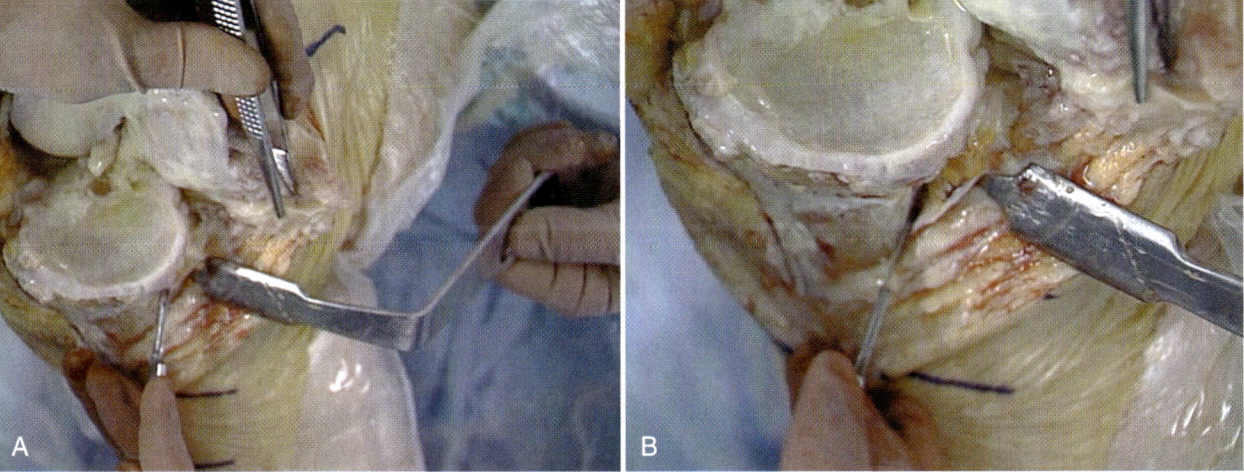

Figure 105-35. Routine exposure includes release of all soft tissues from the medial tibia at the joint line. A medial release involves distal stripping of the superficial medial collateral ligament, which was not performed in this case. **A,** Exposure to the posteromedial proximal tibia. **B,** Close-up view.

everted. This may entail creating a pocket in the lateral gutter for the patella if there is extensive scarring in the lateral gutter. Although it is common practice, the patella does not need to be everted except during patellar preparation with the knee extended. In addition to the standard releases, which include medial dissection around to the semimembranosus bursa, excision of the fat pad, and lateral release of the patella, one should expose the lateral tibial plateau, remove scar, and elevate the lateral capsule to the top of Gerdy's tubercle. The lateral dissection makes room for the patella, but should stay clear of the popliteal tendon insertion and the fibular collateral ligament. Elevation of the capsule around the osteoarticular border of the patella and longitudinal incision into a particularly fibrosed infrapatellar ligament can result in additional extensor mechanism flexibility. In more resistant cases of contracture or stiffness, more extensile exposures are required. Difficult surgical exposures are briefly reviewed here and are discussed in detail elsewhere in this text.

Rectus Snip

The rectus snip is the extensile proximal exposure described by Insall for the medial parapatellar approach.[73] The snip is performed (Fig. 105-36) as needed after other methods of patellar mobilization already described have been employed. The medial incision for the quad snip is the same as that described for the standard midline approach. At the apex of the quadriceps tendon, the arthrotomy is continued laterally across the thin proximal portion of the tendon into the vastus lateralis, dividing the rectus tendon superficially and the trilaminar tendon extensions of the vastus muscles deeply. More distally, a lateral retinacular patellar release may also be done at this stage if it is determined that the lateral retinaculum is sufficiently tight so as to pull the patella laterally or restrict knee bending. The superior lateral genicular vessels need to be identified and isolated as they run at the lower border of the vastus lateralis muscle. These vessels can sometimes be saved when identified and protected during the lateral release. An important feature of this approach is that none of the structures contributing to knee extension are transversely divided.

Tibial Tubercle Osteotomy

A tibial tubercle osteotomy can facilitate exposure of a stiff knee.[219] This technique requires that the fragment of bone osteotomized should be sufficiently large to enhance the potential for later healing back to the tibia (Fig. 105-37). The tibial fragment is opened on a lateral soft tissue hinge. A tibial fragment of sufficient size may be securely reattached by wires or screws at the conclusion of the operation, whereas small fragments in osteoporotic bone afford insufficient substance for successful reattachment. Whiteside[217] reported on use of this technique in 136 knees—both primary and revision TKAs. Complications were few, and no further release of the quadriceps mechanism was necessary in any procedure. However, Wolff and colleagues[222] reported a 23% complication rate when using a similar technique.

Subperiosteal Peel

In ankylosed knees, it may be necessary to perform a subperiosteal exposure of the femur or tibia. It is advisable to begin with a subperiosteal exposure of the medial tibia to

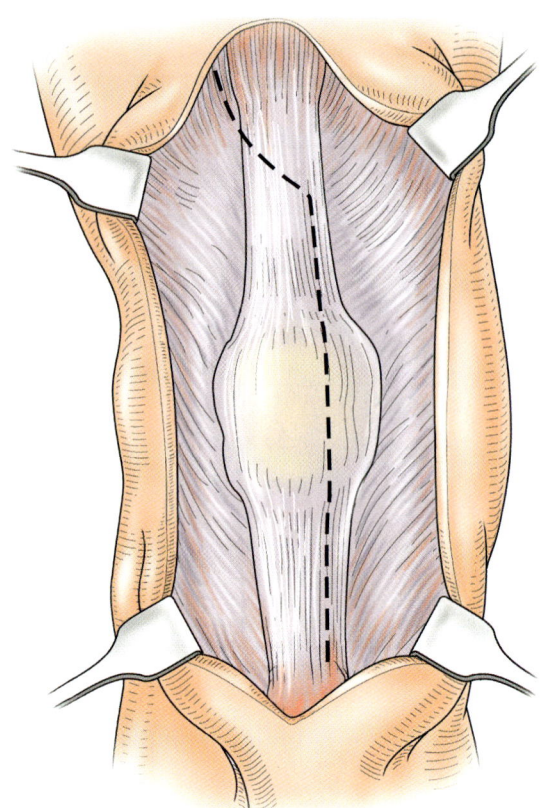

Figure 105-36. The rectus snip. The medial parapatellar incision is continued proximally across the apex of the rectus femoris tendon into the fibers of the vastus lateralis. Division of the rectus tendon in and of itself allows elasticity and takes stress off the patellar ligament insertion into the tibial tubercle. When combined with a lateral patellar release, but when a bridge of tissue consisting of the vastus lateralis insertion into the quadriceps tendon is retained, the result is equivalent to a quadriceps turndown.

mid-diaphysis while attempting to flex and externally rotate the knee, being careful not to avulse the femoral attachment of the MCL. If medial peel is not successful in creating adequate motion, the periosteum of the lower femur is incised, and the lower femur can be partially skeletonized by subperiosteal dissection (Fig. 105-38). The soft tissue envelope is peeled from the bone as a continuous sleeve and is retracted posterior, allowing the distal femur to be buttonholed forward. This exposure, combined with medial subperiosteal dissection of the upper tibia, allows the knee to be flexed without danger of damaging or tearing important soft tissue structures, which are often very fragile in an ankylosed knee because of prolonged lack of movement and physiologic stress. When the incision is closed, the soft tissue envelope falls back around the bones. This technique is useful for long-standing ankylosis of the knee and for reimplantation after infection.[141] Extensive exposures that result in medial-lateral instability patterns may occasionally require the use of increased articular constraint. The risk of extensive subperiosteal exposure is devascularization with subsequent osteonecrosis of the condyle. As such, extensive releases should be reserved for only the most extreme cases.

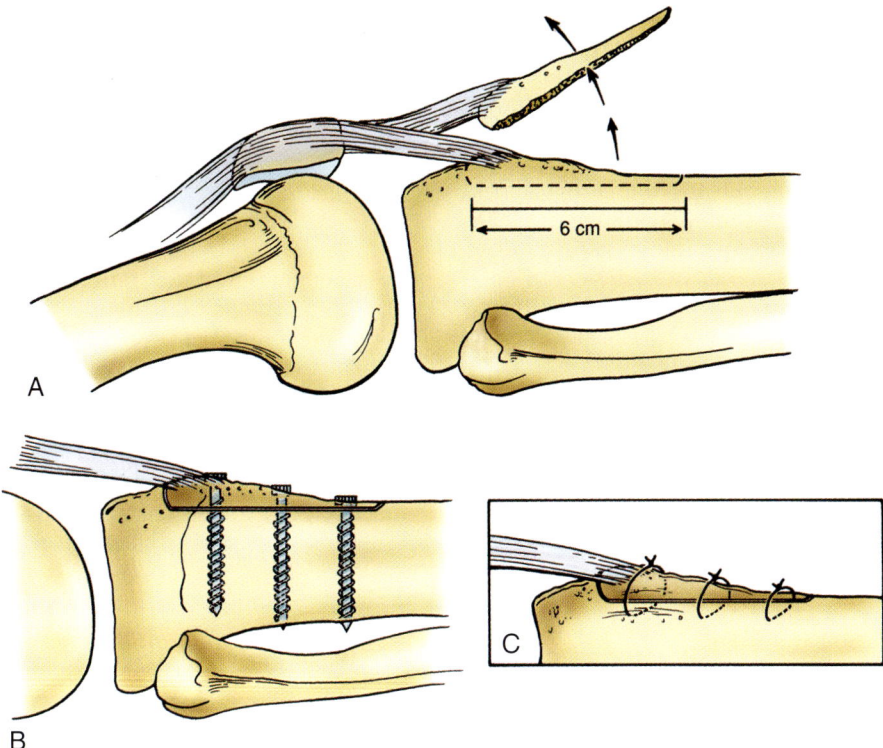

Figure 105-37. Method of exposure for difficult or ankylosed knees. **A,** Tibial tubercle is osteotomized by taking a large fragment of bone, at least 6 cm long. **B,** This allows firm reattachment with screws or wire sutures.

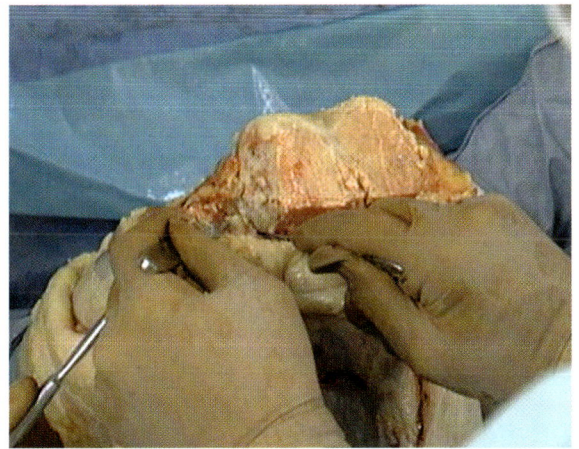

Figure 105-38. A skeletonized femur. The collateral ligaments, together with the adjacent periosteum of the distal femur, have been stripped posteriorly, allowing the distal femur to be buttonholed anteriorly. The soft tissues remain in continuity, and after the operation has been completed, the soft tissue sleeve remains intact, providing stability. This type of exposure, combined with subperiosteal stripping of the proximal tibia and quadriceps turndown or modification thereof, is very useful in dealing with ankylosed knees or reimplantation after infection.

Closure

Closure should be anatomic, with effort made to restore the longitudinal alignment of the medial and lateral soft tissues along the incision. Tissues should be approximated without being excessively tightened or imbricated. Closure of the knee in 45 degrees of flexion or greater will help to align the capsular incision using the shape of the incision or a transverse ink or cautery mark as a guide to alignment.[58,137] Insall routinely performed a modified vastus medialis obliquus (VMO) advancement, in which the medial soft tissue envelope is advanced several millimeters distal relative to the lateral soft tissues. Because the VMO is important in terminal extension, this advancement was meant to reduce the risk of a postoperative extension lag.

TECHNIQUES AND INSTRUMENTATION

Implant systems on the market today have similarities, differing only according to the two philosophies described previously. Thus, many of the instruments used in total knee replacement are similar. The advent of interest in minimally invasive and computer-navigated approaches has led to the downsizing of standard instrumentation and the development of alternative approaches such as making the distal femoral cut from a lateral approach. Such innovative ideas and concepts will require clinical testing and evaluation to determine accuracy, reproducibility, and performance before widespread adoption can be advocated.

Cutting Blocks

Bone cuts may be made from the free edge of the cutting block or through slotted capture guides. The slots may afford some degree of safety by limiting the excursion of saw blades; however, in practice they obscure the saw blade tip, potentially increasing the risk of compromising important structures such as the MCL, and sometimes leading to the creation of metal debris if the saw becomes confined. Although saw blades designed for the capture guides function well in the cutting slots, their cutting teeth are less efficient, because the teeth are designed with less offset to allow the blade to pass through the cutting slot (Fig. 105-39). When capture guides are used, it is important to lubricate surfaces and not to lever the saw blade against the guide to minimize the generation of metallic debris from the saw rubbing the cutting block. Milling frames are particularly useful in improving the accuracy of patellar preparation. Milling frames used in some systems to make the intercondylar cut create a smooth bone surface by their rotary blade action. Rotary blades have been shown to generate less heat than standard saw blades, thereby creating less damage to the cut bony surface.

Efficiency in femoral and tibial preparation has been advanced through improved instrumentation. Traditionally, multiple femoral cuts were made with individual cutting blocks. Newer universal cutting blocks allow multiple steps of bone surface preparation to be performed using a single block (Fig. 105-40). Most newer femoral cutting blocks provide slots for the anterior, posterior, and chamfer cuts, as well as guides for creation of the distal femoral lug holes. New technology has allowed introduction of cutting blocks prefabricated for an individual patient based on preoperative imaging and preplanned cuts. The accuracy, reliability, and economic feasibility of these designs are yet to be determined.

Alignment Guides

It is generally agreed that restoration of the mechanical axis of the limb should be achieved. Alignment is attained by making appropriate cuts on the femur and tibia, in addition to balancing the ligaments. Standard alignment guides may be placed according to external landmarks such as the anterosuperior iliac spine or the center of the hip joint[166] proximally and the ankle mortise distally (Fig. 105-41). Because these landmarks can sometimes be hard to identify, intramedullary guides have become popular for making the distal femoral osteotomy, and extramedullary guides for the proximal tibial resection.

Newer techniques of computer navigation utilize bone surface landmarks, which are registered in the computer utilizing a navigated stylus. An advantage of computer navigation is the potential to obviate the need to cannulate the medullary canal to achieve the desired mechanical alignment. Alignment is created by feeding data on surface topography into the computer using an instrumented stylus to map the bone surface. Once the bone contour is established by entering certain key points into the computer, the data are combined with data stored in the computer on standard tibial or femoral anatomy. This process of combining individual patient-derived data with stored data is called *morphing*. Computer morphing generates an image or likeness of the knee on the computer screen during surgery. From this hybrid of real data and stored data, the computer will proceed to direct the surgeon regarding accuracy of alignment.

Method of Alignment

Classic Method

Either the tibial or the femoral osteotomy may be performed first (Fig. 105-42). The valgus cut at the distal femur in theory

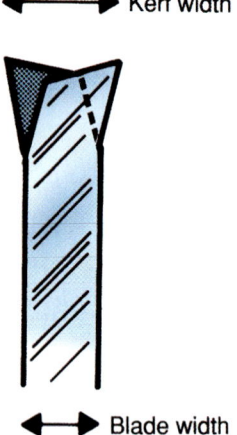

Kerf width

Blade width

Figure 105-39. Saws with cutting slots must use appropriately designed blades with reduced offset to the cutting tips so that kerf width and slot width are nearly the same, thus reducing "slot."

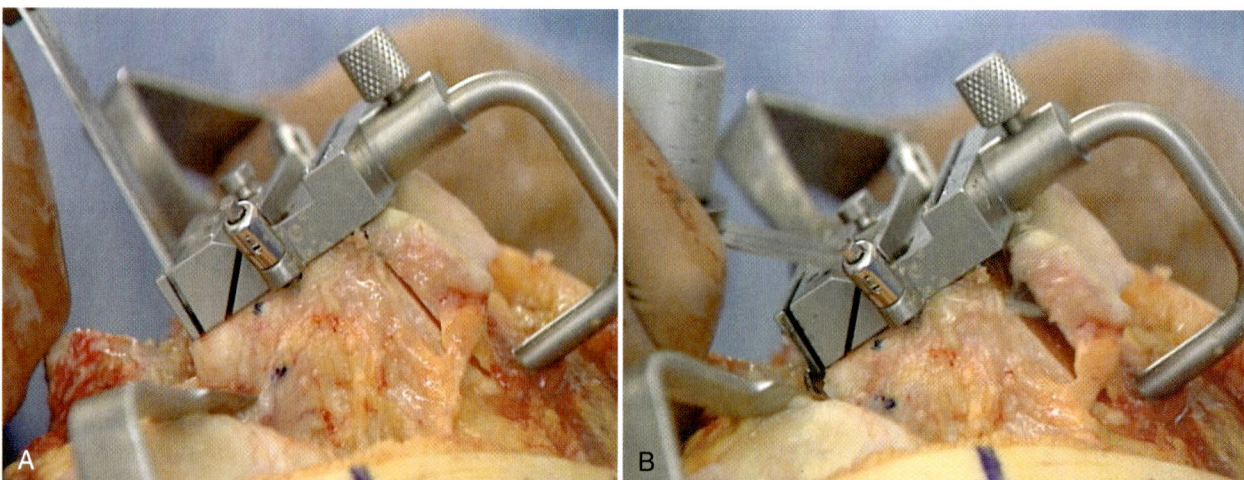

Figure 105-40. Universal femoral cutting block. **A,** Anteroposterior cuts. **B,** Chamfer cuts.

is the difference between the anatomic and mechanical axes, created using the femoral shaft as the anatomic reference. The distal femoral valgus can be varied depending on the patient's body habitus, generally falling around 5 to 6 degrees of valgus. Valgus knees are generally cut in 4 to 5 degrees of valgus, whereas varus and normally aligned knees are cut at 5 to 6 degrees of valgus. In obese patients, it is important to limit the amount of valgus to 5 degrees to avoid contact between the medial knee soft tissues. The tibial cut is always made neutral to the tibial anatomic axis.[129] Hsu and associates[91] confirmed that 7 degrees of femoral valgus matched with 0 degrees of proximal tibial alignment resulted in the most even load distribution across a total condylar knee prosthesis. Ample evidence suggests that a varus tibial cut not only results in uneven stress distribution in the proximal tibia[79] but also leads to premature clinical failure.[170]

Anatomic Method

In an attempt to re-create natural knee kinematics with a PCL retaining prosthesis, Hungerford and Kenna used an anatomic method (Fig. 105-43) of lower limb alignment for TKA.[93] Femoral valgus is set at an anatomic 9 to 10 degrees, and the tibial cut is made in 2 to 3 degrees of varus, thereby creating an anatomic 6 to 7 degrees of lower extremity valgus. Hsu and colleagues[91] demonstrated that these angles produce even load distribution across the knee joint in a cruciate retaining design. As noted previously, if the surgeon is not experienced in this technique, intentional varus tibial cuts can easily result in excessive tibial varus, creating uneven load distribution and ligament imbalance.

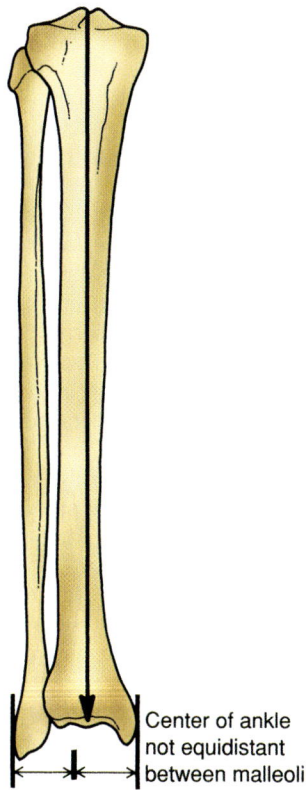

Figure 105-41. Center of the knee. Center of the talus axis lies a few millimeters medial to the center point between the malleoli.

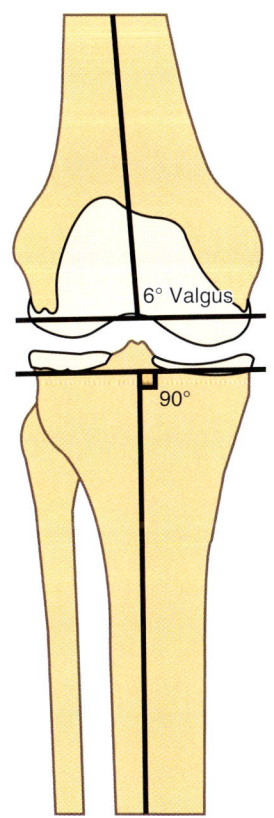

Figure 105-42. Classic alignment.

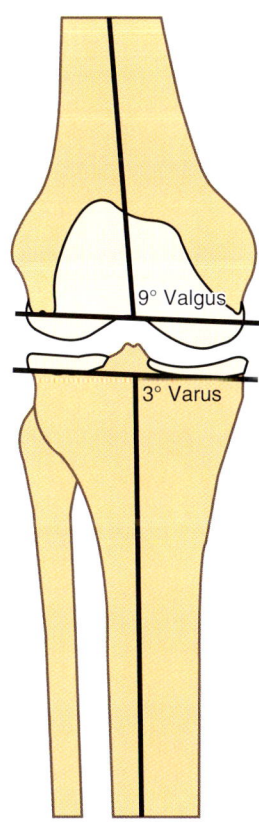

Figure 105-43. Anatomic alignment.

Tibial Guides

Background

Most systems continue to use an extramedullary guide for the upper tibial osteotomy. Advocates of intramedullary tibial guides maintain that a rod of sufficient length reaching well into the tibial diaphysis will reliably align the tibial-cutting guide when there is no bow or offset to the tibial shaft. One potential pitfall of the intramedullary technique is that the shape of the tibia is inconsistent. Additionally, as for any intramedullary guide, the entry point is critical to alignment. Templating to determine the proper entry point for the tibial guide on the tibial surface will minimize the risk of creating a varus tibial cut based on a medial entry point and a bowed tibia. A central entry hole often will cause the intramedullary rod to impact against the tibial cortex (usually lateral), and placing the entry hole so that this does not happen alters the angle of the proximal guide (Fig. 105-44).

The extramedullary tibial guide is placed on the leg using surface landmarks. The distal end of the guide attaches above the ankle, while the proximal end is pinned to the center of the proximal tibia, generally at the medial one third of the tibial tubercle. Most guides allow adjustment at the ankle in both mediolateral and anteroposterior directions. The center of the ankle does not exactly correspond to the midpoint between the malleoli but instead is slightly medial to this point (5 to 10 mm) (see Fig. 105-41). The anteroposterior

distal guide adjustment controls the posterior slope of the proximal tibial cut. The posterior slope of the proximal tibia may also be incorporated into the tibial osteotomy. As noted previously, we favor an essentially perpendicular cut relative to the tibial shaft. However, some systems, especially cruciate retaining designs and some mobile bearing knee designs, function more effectively with posterior slope. The 7 degrees of posterior slope is anatomic when the subchondral bone is considered, but when the posterior menisci are taken into consideration, the proximal tibial surface is actually perpendicular to the shaft (Fig. 105-45).

In obese patients, anteroposterior guide adjustment at the ankle may be necessary to make the guide parallel to the tibial shaft. Locating the proper proximal position of the extramedullary guide may be difficult; the natural tendency is to place the guide medially, producing a varus cut. Mobilization of the infrapatellar ligament combined with a lower profile lateral plateau cutting surface will facilitate placement of the tibial guide. By referencing off the tibial plateau center, the tibial shaft axis, and the center of the ankle, proper alignment for the proximal tibial osteotomy is usually possible. Several investigators have demonstrated that extramedullary and intramedullary systems are equally accurate in establishing tibial alignment.[42,122] However, intramedullary instrumentation forfeits some of its accuracy in the face of tibial bowing or offset of the tibial shaft, especially when used for valgus knees. Simmons and coworkers[192] noted that accuracy for intramedullary tibial alignment systems was 83% for varus knees versus 37% for valgus knees; they attributed the poor accuracy to tibial bowing observed in two thirds of valgus knees.

Authors' Preferred Technique of Tibial Preparation

The upper tibial osteotomy is made at right angles to the tibial shaft both in the coronal plane and sloped posterior

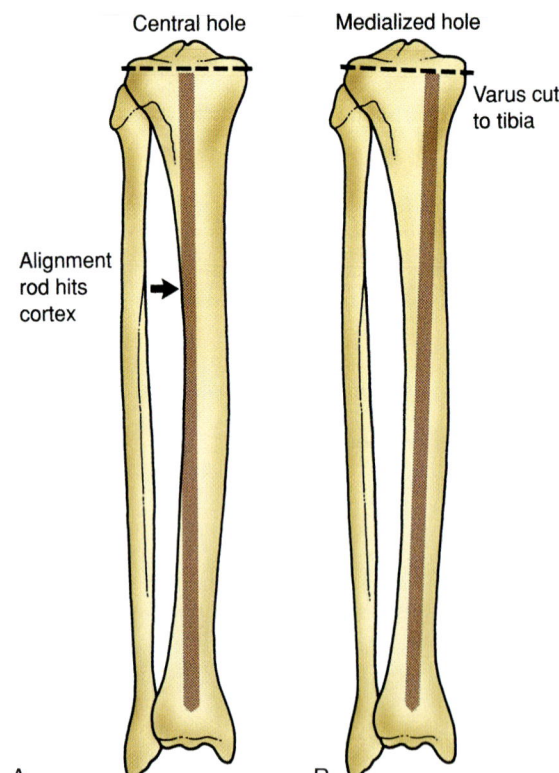

Figure 105-44. Intramedullary guides are not satisfactory when the tibia is bowed. **A,** The guide passed through a central hole abuts the lateral cortex. **B,** To pass the guide down the shaft to the ankle, the entry hole has to be medialized. This produces a varus cut to the tibia.

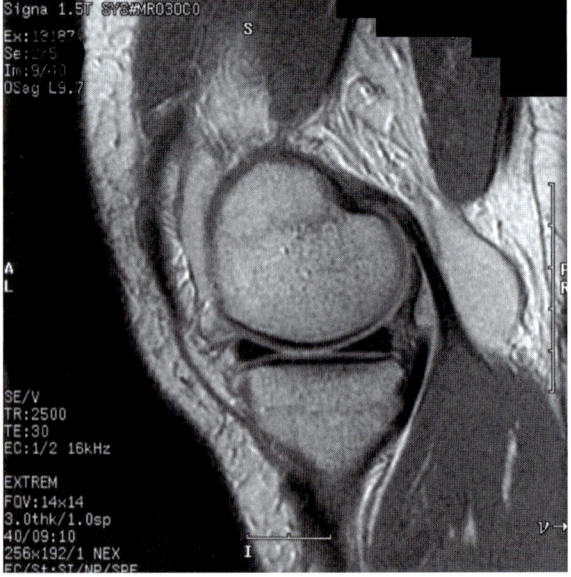

Figure 105-45. Lateral magnetic resonance image of the knee demonstrating that the posterior slope is present when the subchondral surface is considered; however, with the menisci intact, the 5 to 7 degrees of "physiologic posterior slope" is reduced to essentially neutral.

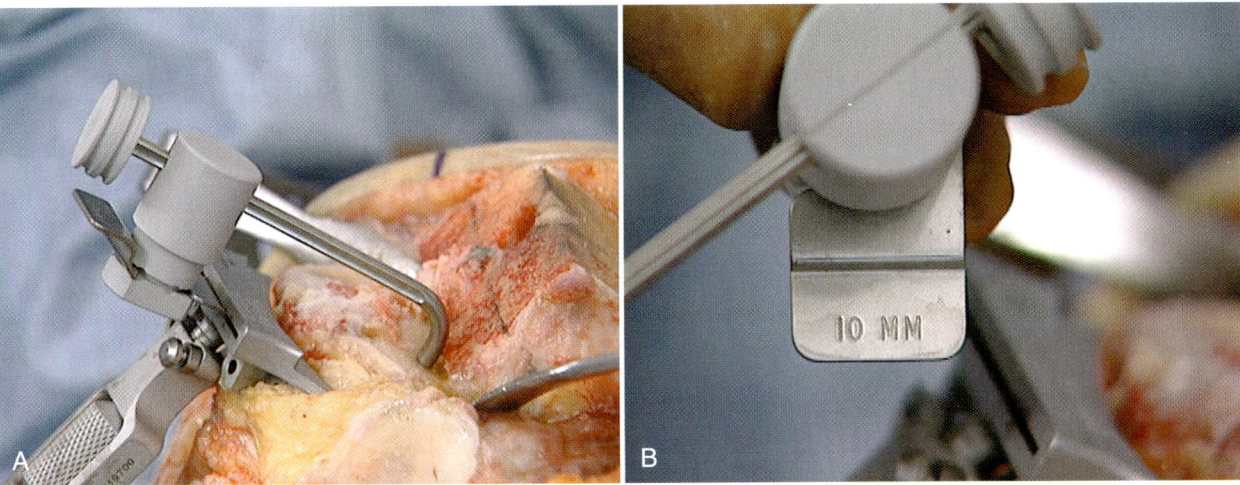

Figure 105-46. **A,** Intraoperative photo of the stylus used to determine the amount of proximal tibial bone resection. **B,** In this case, a 10-mm resection is measured off the least affected articular surface.

about 3 to 5 degrees in the sagittal plane. The extramedullary guide is provisionally secured to the tibia in alignment with the medial third of the tibial tuberosity, the tibial shaft, the center of the tibial plateau, and the middle of the ankle. Adjustments to the tibial cutting block are then performed at the ankle. The depth of proximal tibial resection is determined such that enough bone is removed to accommodate the tibial component (with a 10-mm polyethylene insert being the desired lower limit in modular tibial components, and 8 mm being the lower limit with all polyethylene components). Given the few additional millimeters of laxity produced following PCL excision, 1 cm of proximal tibia is excised to accommodate at least a 10-mm tibial component when a cruciate substituting knee is performed. The 10 mm of resection is typically measured using a stylus placed on the articular surface with the most residual cartilage; alternatively, the stylus can measure 2 mm of resection from the most eroded articular surface (Fig. 105-46). The cutting block is then fixed, and the proximal tibial osteotomy is performed. Although studies have shown that resection of up to 20 mm from the least involved side of the joint is acceptable,[76] care must be taken to avoid detaching the ITB at the level of Gerdy's tubercle.

Femoral Guides

Background

Intramedullary femoral alignment to determine the angle of the distal femoral cut is generally favored because reliable external landmarks are not readily palpable. The thigh musculature, obesity, and surgical drapes make defining femoral shaft orientation difficult. Multiple investigations have demonstrated that both intramedullary and extramedullary alignment systems are accurate; however, most studies suggest that intramedullary femoral alignment systems are more commonly used because of limitations of extramedullary alignment as noted previously.[133] Femoral alignment can be determined using intramedullary methods and confirmed with extramedullary methods if any uncertainty exists (e.g.,

unusual femoral bowing, wide or obstructed intramedullary canal).

Preoperative radiographic evaluation with a three-joint view allows identification of extra-articular deformity, such as abnormal femoral bowing. A strong correlation has been noted between the mechanical axis and the anatomic axis obtained with standard radiographs in the absence of extra-articular deformity.[117] Rotation of the femur in the preoperative full-length radiograph can create a false impression of varus or valgus bowing (Fig. 105-47). With extra-articular deformity, the starting hole position for femoral canal access can be altered slightly to properly position the intramedullary guide. However, when an extra-articular deformity prevents passage of a standard femoral guide, then a modified (shorter) intramedullary alignment rod may be used, provided that the distal segment of the femoral canal that serves as a reference is oriented to achieve proper component alignment. A disadvantage of intramedullary guides is that if the angle of entry or the starting point into the canal is incorrect, the intramedullary rod may contact the femoral cortices rather than pass directly into the center of the diaphysis (see Fig. 105-34). If the rod contacts the lateral cortex, the valgus angle may be reduced, and if the medial cortex is contacted, the valgus angle may be increased.

Depending on the particular instrument system and arthritic pattern, an intramedullary rod may cause the distal femoral cutting block to contact the medial (valgus knee) or the lateral (varus knee) condyle first. If attempts are made to fully seat the instrumentation on both condyles, errors in the distal femoral cut may occur. For example, in valgus knees (associated with lateral femoral condylar erosion), the distal femoral cutting block attachment typically contacts the medial femoral condyle first. If the surgeon allows the instrumentation to contact both condyles in this situation, the valgus angle of the distal femoral cut will be exaggerated. To avoid such errors, the surgeon must be aware of the arthritic pattern and use the intramedullary guide to establish proper positioning of the distal femoral cutting block, even if the instrumentation contacts only a single condyle (see Fig. 105-24). Asymmetrical distal femoral resections are very common,

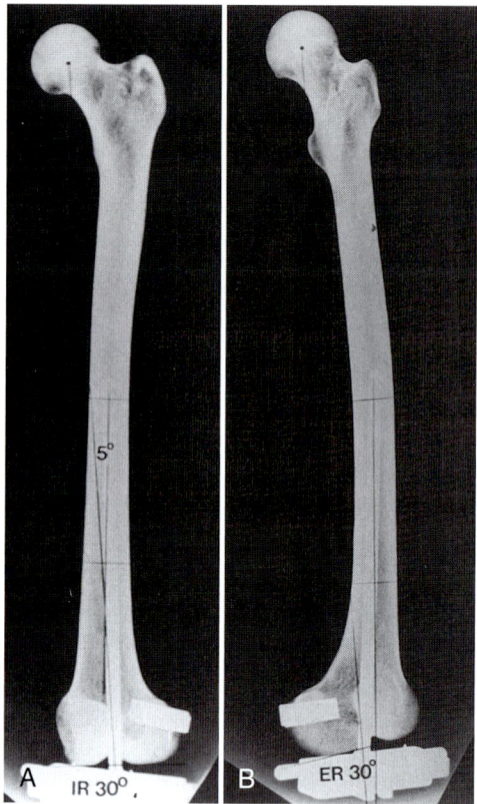

Figure 105-47. Radiographs of femur in **(A)** internal and **(B)** external rotation. It can be seen that internal rotation is perceived as medial bowing, and external rotation as lateral bowing. This is a normal femur, and the effect would be accentuated if the femur had excessive anterior bowing.

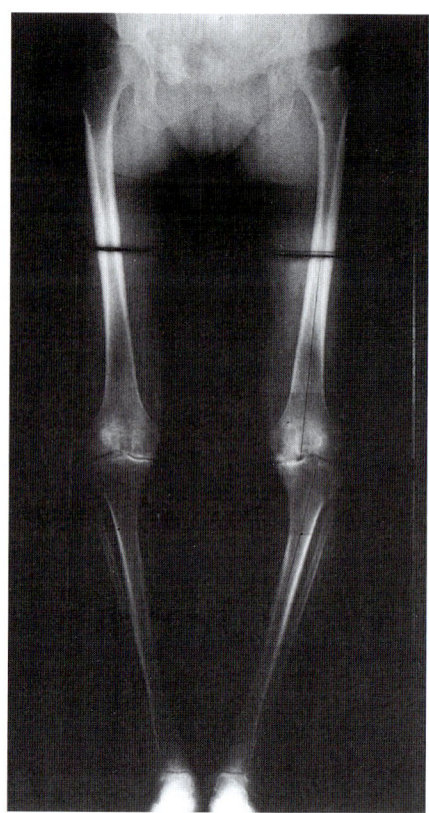

Figure 105-48. A 52-inch radiograph shows the positions of entry holes from preoperative templating. Note that the femoral entry hole is slightly medial, and that the tibial entry hole is slightly lateral.

serving to correct the angular deformity rather than re-create the deformity with a symmetrical bone resection.

Authors' Preferred Technique of Femoral Preparation

The entering hole for a femoral intramedullary guide is made about 1 cm anterior to the origin of the PCL, although this position can be adjusted to accommodate any abnormalities noted on preoperative radiographs; usually the entry hole is directed slightly medially toward the top of the intercondylar notch (Fig. 105-48). Overdrilling the entry to 12 mm is recommended because of increased intramedullary pressure during intramedullary rod insertion; use of a fluted rather than a round intramedullary rod has also been shown to diminish intramedullary pressure during rod insertion.[165] The distal femoral osteotomy guide is attached to the intramedullary guide at an angle derived from the preoperative radiograph; normally, this is 5 to 7 degrees, representing the difference between the mechanical and anatomic axes of the femur. When intramedullary assessment appears unreliable, an extramedullary rod should be used to confirm that the proposed osteotomy is appropriate. When this step provides conflicting information, the preoperative radiographs should be re-evaluated; rarely, intraoperative radiographic determination of the proper femoral valgus angle is necessary.

The distal femoral osteotomy is made by removing precisely the amount of bone that will be replaced by the femoral prosthesis. Some systems measure this amount from the

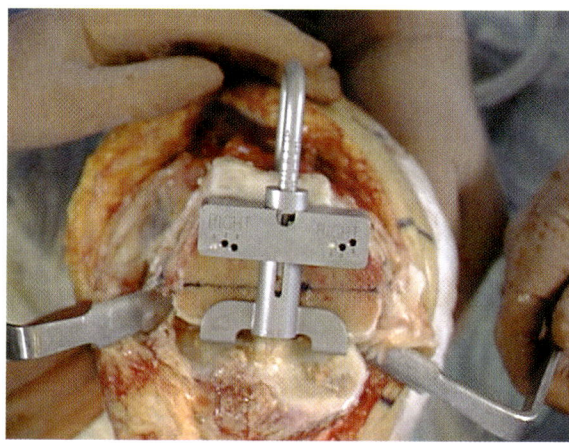

Figure 105-49. Sizing the femoral condyle.

uninvolved condyle, whereas others key off the medial femoral condyle, regardless of the knee pathology (see Fig. 105-24). Generally, the surgeon can make a choice regarding the depth of the distal femoral resection. It is important to keep in mind that any resection above that which is replaced by the prosthesis will result in a corresponding elevation of the joint line. Once the distal osteotomy is completed, appropriate templates are used to size the distal femur and perform anterior and posterior femoral resections (Fig. 105-49). Rotational alignment is adjusted when the femoral template is positioned by marking the epicondylar axis on the distal femoral surface (Figs. 105-50 and 105-51).

For cruciate substituting prostheses, flexion and extension gaps can be measured with spacers or tensiometers, with additional distal femoral bone removal performed when the extension gap is tighter than the flexion gap (Fig. 105-52A and B). Measured resection of the distal femur will rarely warrant readjustment (typically only with severe flexion contractures). Adjustment cuts should be made before the chamfer cuts (Fig. 105-52B and C). Chamfer, notch, and fixation holes are made on the distal femur (Fig. 105-53) and the proximal tibia (Fig. 105-54). A flexion contracture due to posterior capsular contracture or a narrow extension gap should be corrected in favor of accepting an overly thin polyethylene liner (Fig. 105-55). Flexion of the femoral component will more readily lead to anterior impingement, and a thinner tibial insert can lead to accelerated polyethylene wear.

Rotational Positioning of Prosthetic Components

Rotational alignment of the femoral component is based on the epicondylar axis. Rotational positioning of the tibial component can be based on the posterior surface of the cut tibia, the anterior surface of the tibia, the tibial tubercle, and the ankle mortise. Assessment can be done with the knee in flexion, in extension, or in both as the knee is passed through a range of movement with trial components in place.

When the tibial component rotation is determined with the knee flexed, the rotation can be related to the anterior surface of the tibia and to the position of the tibial tubercle, which should lie slightly lateral to the midposition of the component (Fig. 105-56). Reference is then made to the ankle and to the position of the malleoli, which should lie approximately 30 degrees externally rotated to the tibial component position. An alignment rod can be suspended from the tibial guide to view the relationship between the tibial component and the ankle joint. When a symmetrical tibial

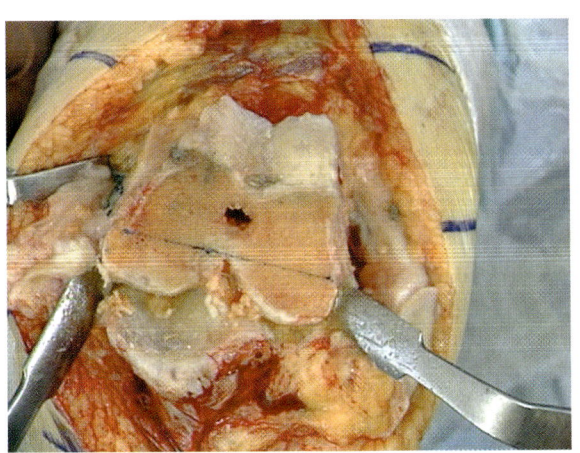

Figure 105-50. Intraoperative photograph demonstrating the epicondylar axis drawn across the cut distal femoral surface.

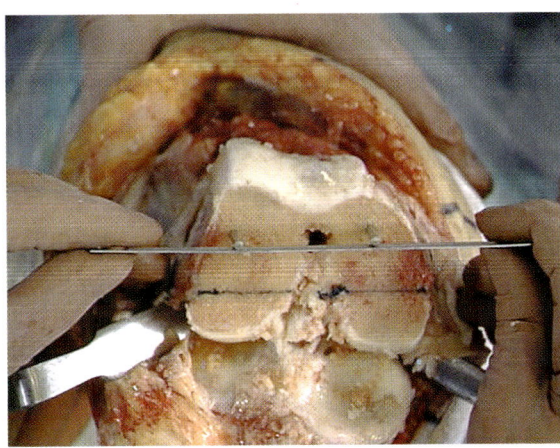

Figure 105-51. The instrumentation is aligned with the epicondylar axis (pins are parallel to the epicondylar axis, as indicated by a ruler placed across them).

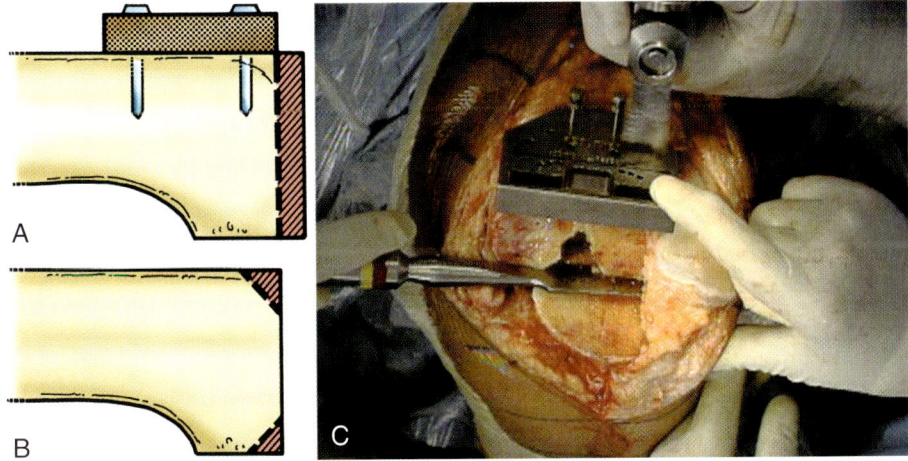

Figure 105-52. **A,** Femoral recutting should be done before the chamfer cuts are made—an important reason for incorporating spacers into the system. It is simple to remove 2 to 3 mm from the end of the distal femur. **B,** When the femur has been sculpted to receive the prosthesis, recutting is much more complex. **C,** The distal femoral recutter, allowing 2, 3, and 5 mm of additional resection. (The cut tibial surface should be protected.)

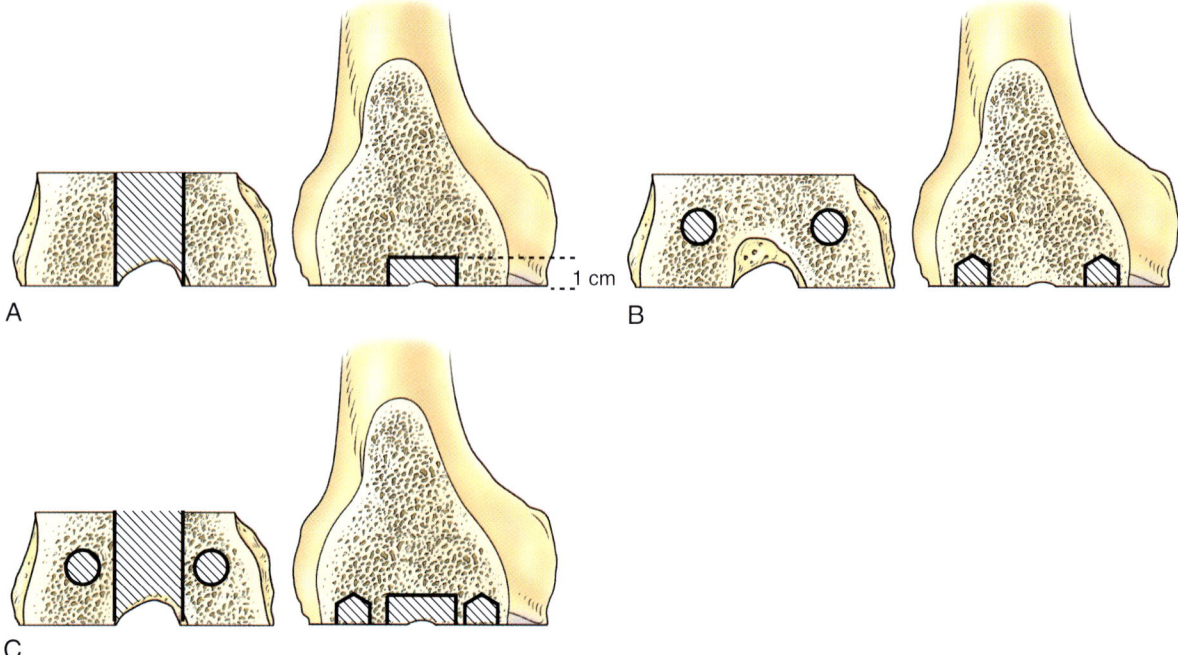

Figure 105-53. Femoral fixation can be enhanced by a central box usually found with **(A)** posterior stabilized designs, **(B)** medial and lateral fixation lugs, or **(C)** both.

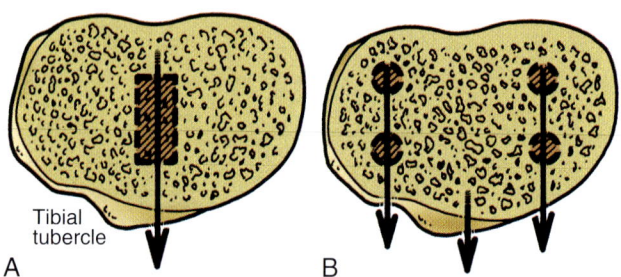

Figure 105-54. A, Alignment of the tibial component is projected at a point slightly medial to the tibial tubercle. **B,** Alignment of a symmetrical component with the posterior margin of the tibial plateau usually will result in some internal rotation of the tibial component. One should err on the side of external rotation.

component is used, some overhang is often noted posterolaterally (Fig. 105-57), because the medial tibial plateau is larger than the lateral; for this reason, we do not favor using the posterior margins of the tibial plateau as alignment landmarks.

Rotational alignment can also be assessed in extension, allowing the tibial component position to be related to the patellar groove of the femoral component, the tibial tubercle, and the ankle mortise. With the femoral trial prosthesis in position, a range of motion is performed and patellar tracking is observed before the final fixation holes for the tibial component are made. A tibial trial component without fixation pegs allows the component to find its correct position. This type of component positioning is subject to error introduced by the person holding the leg, the tourniquet on the thigh, and flexion gap tightness. Using the anatomy of the proximal tibia and ankle eliminates these potential errors in rotational positioning. Tibial tray malrotation is detrimental to patellar tracking, especially with excessive internal rotation of the

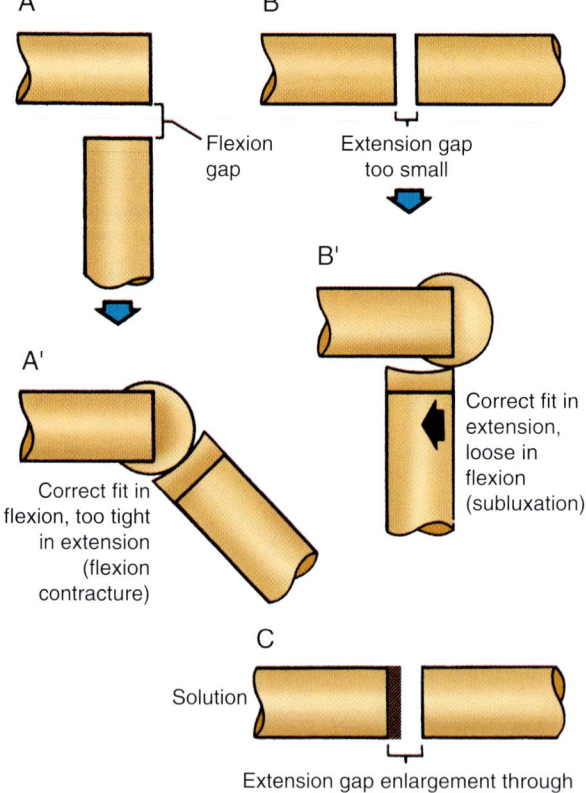

Figure 105-55. Unequal gap size is a frequent technical error. When the extension gap is too small, the knee will not fully extend; if a thinner tibial component is used, the prosthesis will be too loose in flexion. The solution is to excise more bone from the distal femur.

tibial component. Excessive internal rotation of the tibial component increases the risk of patellar subluxation.[15] Conversely, excessive external tibial component rotation may also result in abnormal tracking of the patella,[149] as well as a kinematic conflict in the femorotibial articulation such as notch-cam impingement in a cruciate substituting design.

Mediolateral Positioning of Prosthetic Components

The medial-lateral positioning of both femoral and tibial components is important. Generally, components should be positioned anatomically on their respective bones without overhang. Overhang can create pain and predispose to stiffness due to capsular stretching. For prosthesis systems that allow separate sizing of the femur and tibia (interchangeable components), the tibial component selected will normally and precisely coincide with the resected tibial plateau. However, for some cruciate substituting designs, the option exists for some medial or lateral translation of the tibial component. This option is useful when marginal bony defects exist, to reduce the size of the bony defect (Fig. 105-58). On

the femoral side, the component ideally should coincide with the resected margin of the lateral femoral condyle. The femoral components should not be placed medially because of consequent stress on the lateral patellar retinaculum. Newer component systems allow for standard and narrow options to match the coronal and sagittal dimensions more exactly.

Patellar Cuts and Cutting Guides

The goal of the patellar osteotomy is a patellar cut that facilitates central tracking of the patella and minimal tilt while accurately restoring patellar height (Fig. 105-59). The patellar osteotomy is perhaps the most difficult to instrument and still is often done by freehand technique with an oscillating saw used to resect the articular surface (Fig. 105-60 and 105-61).[128] Reaming or patellar milling devices[77] (Fig. 105-62) used for inset patellar components are also effective in establishing the proper resection level for onset patellar components. Caliper measurements of the patellar size after resection should be equal to or slightly less than the original thickness of the patellar bone (Fig. 105-63).

Patellar resurfacing is generally recommended in patients with osteoarthrosis involving the patellofemoral joint, crystalline disease, or inflammatory arthropathy[162]; however, the patella does not have to be resurfaced. Investigators have

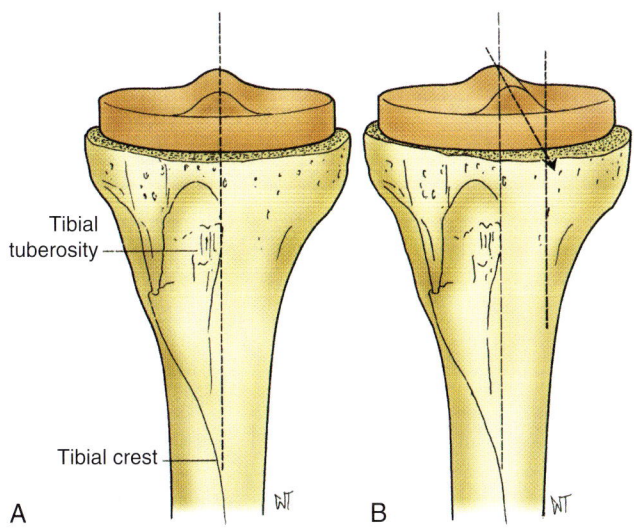

Figure 105-56. The tibial component should be aligned with the tibial tubercle. **A,** Correct position. **B,** Tibial component internally rotated on the tibia.

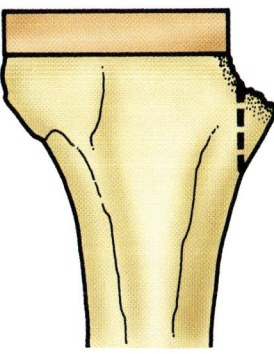

Figure 105-58. Lateralization of the tibial component can be done with cruciate substituting designs. The tibia is deliberately undersized and is placed at the lateral margin of the tibia. The medial defect is reduced, and overhanging bone can be excised vertically.

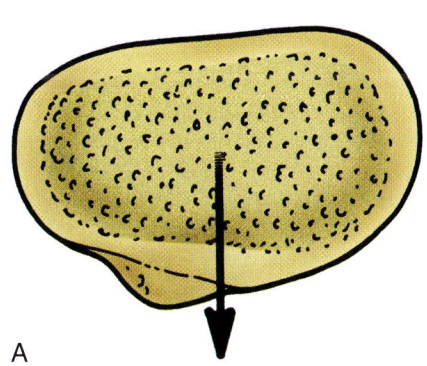

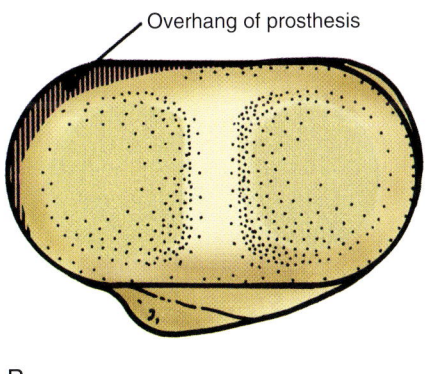

Figure 105-57. A and **B,** With a symmetrical component, some degree of posterolateral overhang of the prosthesis is expected.

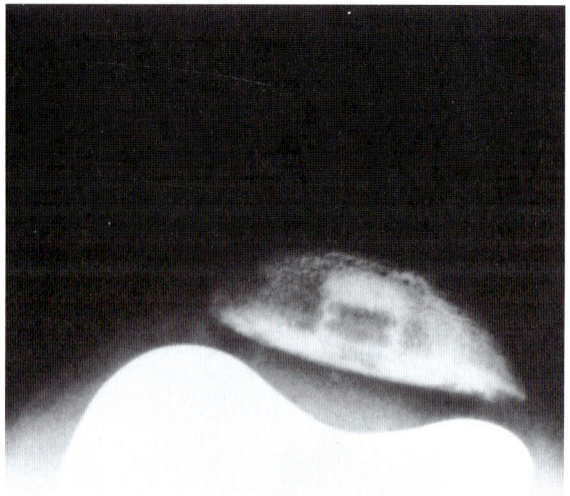

Figure 105-59. Radiograph shows a patellar component with "ideal" patellar tracking, orientation, and thickness.

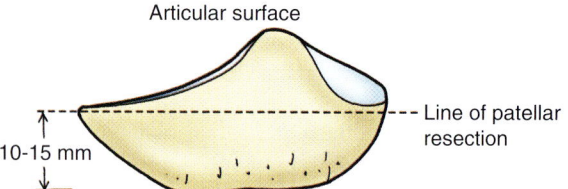

Figure 105-60. The line of patellar resection.

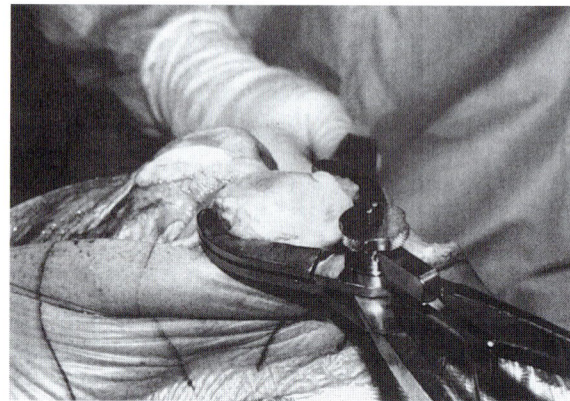

Figure 105-61. A slotted patellar cutting guide. The depth of the resection is selected by the knurl knob. The jaws grasp the patella, and the slots direct the cutting blade.

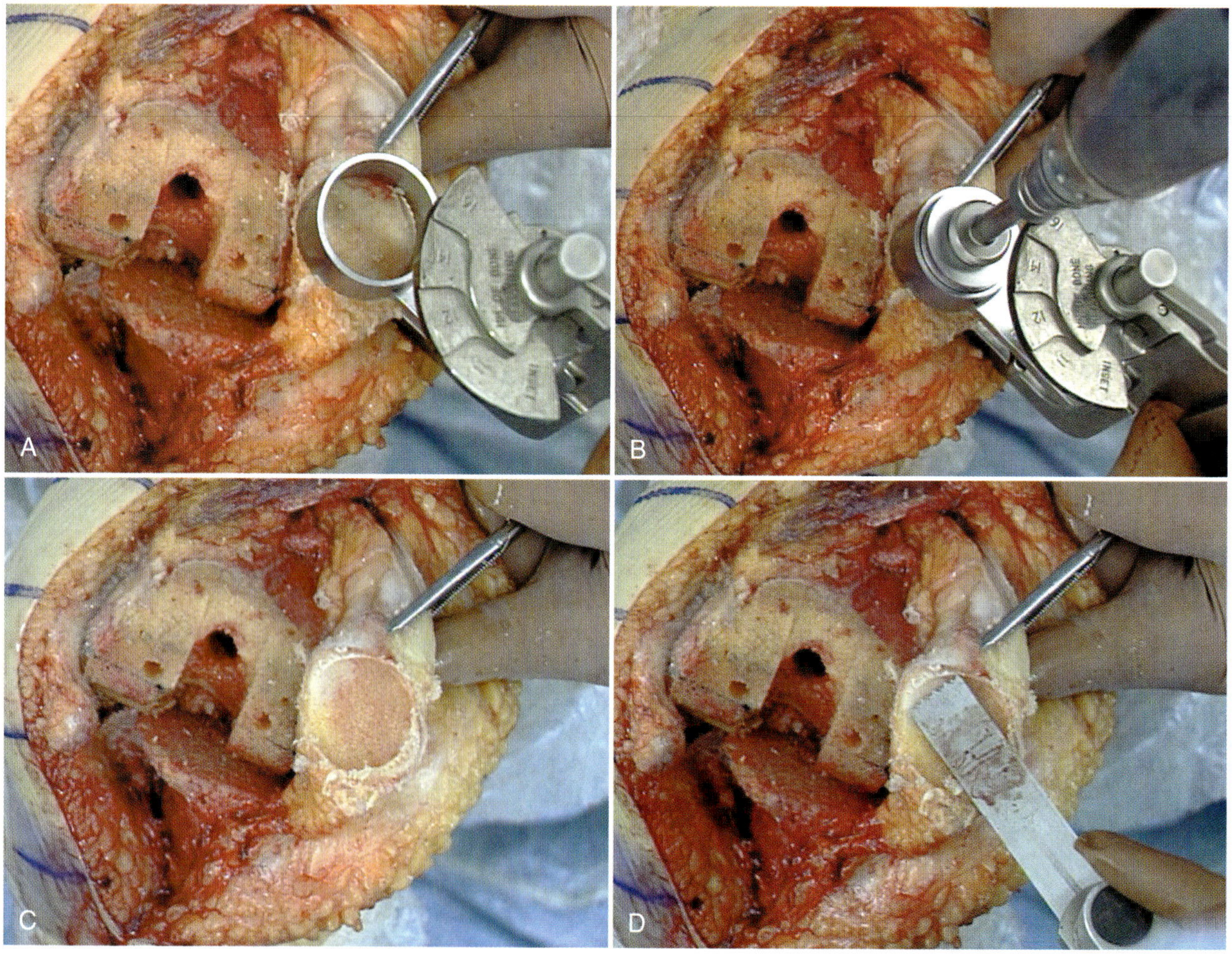

Figure 105-62. Although the reamer is traditionally used for insetting patellar components, it may also be used in creating an accurate flat cut for an onset component. **A,** Patellar clamp balanced on the patella. **B,** Reamer positioned within the clamp. **C,** Patella reamed to desired resection level. **D,** Resection completed with the saw blade.

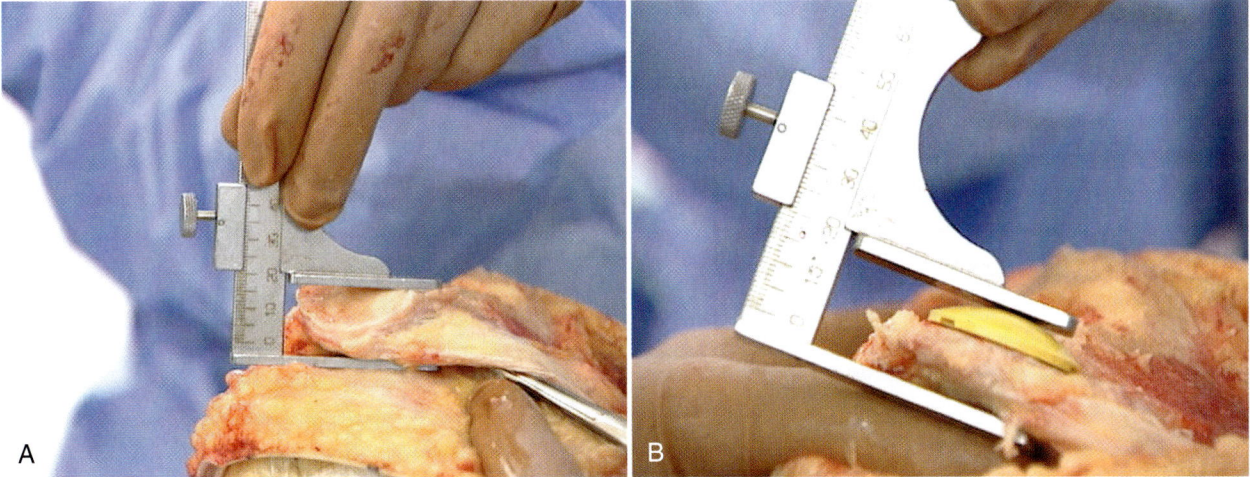

Figure 105-63. **A** and **B,** Caliber measurements of patellar thickness should be made before and after patellar osteotomy. The thickness of the patellar composite should not be increased; rather, a thickness of 2 to 3 mm less is preferred. Between 10 and 15 mm of patellar bone should remain.

reported acceptable results without patellar resurfacing,* especially when the patellar articular cartilage has limited articular wear. On the other hand, extreme patellar articular erosion makes use of a patellar component difficult or impossible in some cases. In these cases, contouring of the residual patellar bone (*patelloplasty*) is performed. TKA without patellar resurfacing in these patients has been reported with satisfactory results on short-term follow-up.[135,162] However, a study with follow-up at 8.5 years on nonresurfaced patellae showed progressive patellofemoral arthritis and maltracking in 40% of patients studied.[190]

Recent prospective, randomized trials have supported patellar resurfacing. Waters and Bentley (JBJS-A 2003)[213] randomized 514 primary TKAs to have the patella resurfaced or retained. The incidence of anterior knee pain was significantly higher in the nonresurfacing group (25.1%) as compared with the resurfaced group (5.3%), and 10 of 11 patients undergoing secondary resurfacing for anterior knee pain experienced complete relief. A prospective randomized study by Wood and colleagues[223] also showed a significant difference in anterior knee pain between resurfaced and nonresurfaced groups, although 10% of patients in the resurfacing group underwent a revision or reoperation involving the patellofemoral joint, as compared with 12% in the nonresurfacing group.

Lug or fixation holes are made into the patella. Most designers currently favor 3- to 4-mm holes placed in a triangular fashion rather than at a larger, centrally placed fixation point (Fig. 105-64). A small, centralized single-peg inset design has also functioned well.[118] A round, dome patellar prosthesis should be positioned to the medial side of the oblong patellar osteotomy and sized by the superoinferior dimension of the bone (Fig. 105-65). The median ridge of the patella is a useful reference point for centering the component, given that the medial facet is shorter and more acutely sloped than the lateral patellar facet. Insetting designs of 28 or 32 mm in diameter have been tried with some success (Fig. 105-66). These designs require central reaming of the

patella, leaving the periphery intact. Studies focused on appropriate sizing of patellar inserts have identified a relationship between patellar thickness and knee flexion in cases where increasing thickness by 2-mm increments led to a 3-degree decrease in intraoperative flexion but did not affect patellar subluxation or tilt.[13] Inadvertent patellar fracture can be avoided by adequately lubricating the reamer, firmly grasping the patella during reaming, and not resecting an excessive amount of patellar bone.

FITTING OF TRIAL COMPONENTS

Fitting of trial components is done when all of the initial bone cuts are completed. Stability and alignment are checked in both flexion and extension. For cruciate substituting designs with balanced gaps, little further adjustment should be required. For cruciate retaining prostheses, ligament balancing is done at this stage, using with different thicknesses of tibial trial components until satisfactory stability is obtained. When the PCL is spared, particular attention must be paid to the PCL balance. Excessive tightness of the PCL can be detected by noting a tight flexion gap with excessive femoral roll-back. On the contrary, a loose PCL will allow roll-forward of the femur on the tibia as the knee is flexed, resulting in posterior impingement. PCL recession can be performed by completing intrasubstance ligament lengthening, or by elevating the ligament off the tibial insertion. At this stage, if optimal balance cannot be obtained, it is wise to make an intraoperative change to a PCL substituting design.

Patellar Tracking and Position

When the correct tibial component thickness has been selected, patellar tracking is observed with the patellar component in place. The "no thumb" test is applied: the patella should track with its medial border in contact with the femoral component throughout the range of motion without the surgeon maintaining it in this position manually (Fig. 105-67). It is permissible to take the slack out of the quadriceps tendon by applying longitudinal tension (Fig. 105-68)

*References 10, 11, 18, 19, and 135.

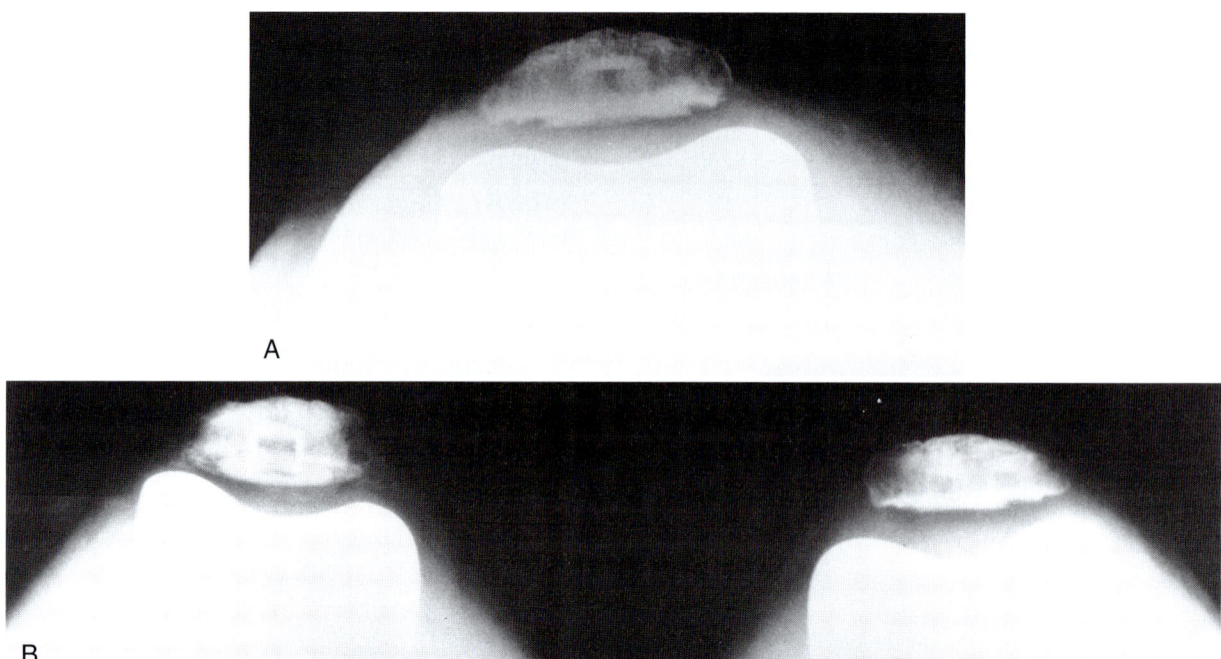

Figure 105-64. A, Merchant's view radiograph of a well-aligned and well-positioned polyethylene patellar implant. The thickness of the bone polyethylene composite restores the original thickness of the patellar bone. **B,** Patellar implants done some years apart. On the left, the patellar cut was made by eye and a single-peg patellar implant was used. The patella is too thick, and the patellar osteotomy is not quite symmetrical. On the right, the arthroplasty was done more recently, a slotted patellar cutting guide was used, and a three-peg patellar implant was inserted. Although there is a slight tilt, the patellar cut is symmetrical, and the patellar thickness is correct.

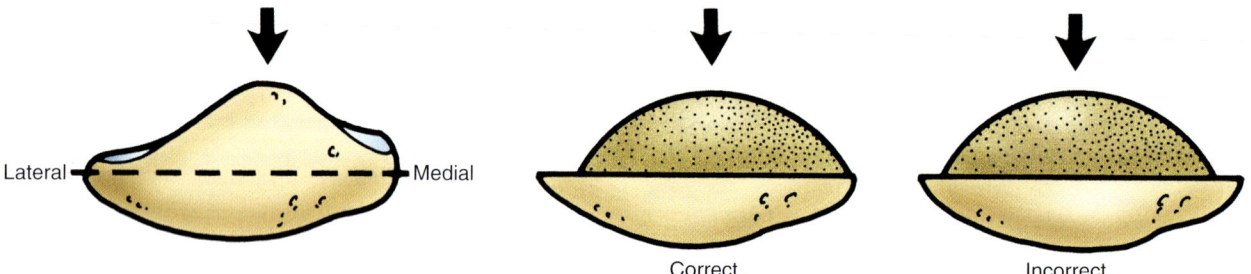

Figure 105-65. With a conventional patellar dome onset on the patella, the component should be medialized. This has the advantage of placing the apex of the dome in the correct position for patellar tracking but has the disadvantage of leaving peripheral lateral bone exposed.

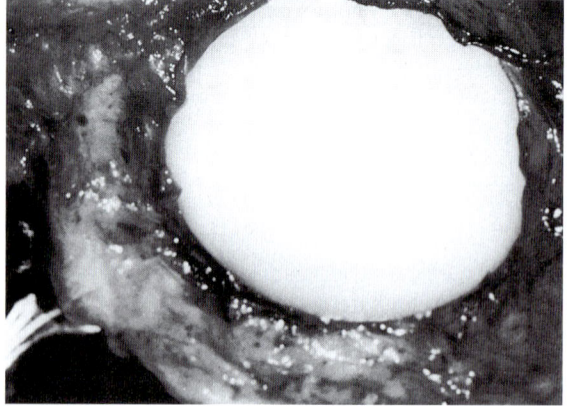

Figure 105-66. Insetting the patella allows greater thickness of polyethylene and use of metal backing. A rim of peripheral exposed bone can impinge against the femur.

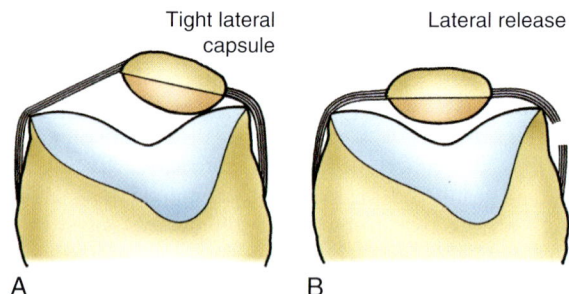

Figure 105-67. If the patella does not track smoothly without a tendency to displace, a lateral release is done.

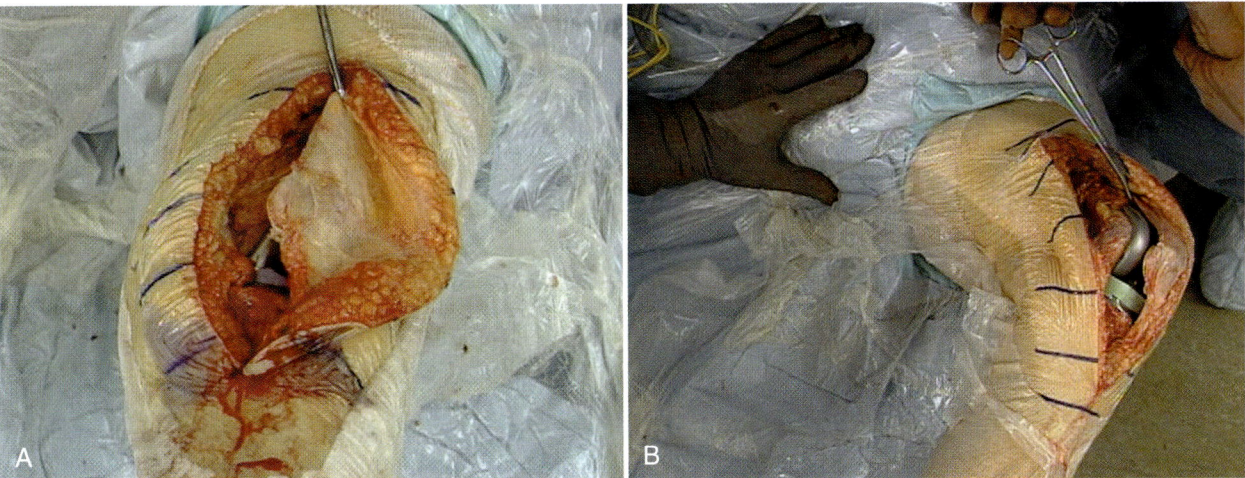

Figure 105-68. **A** and **B,** When patellar traction is assessed, the "rule of no thumb" must be observed, but it is advisable to take longitudinal slack out of the extensor mechanism because, on bringing the knee from flexion into extension, the patellar ligament tends to buckle and can cause a misleading lateral tilt to the patella.

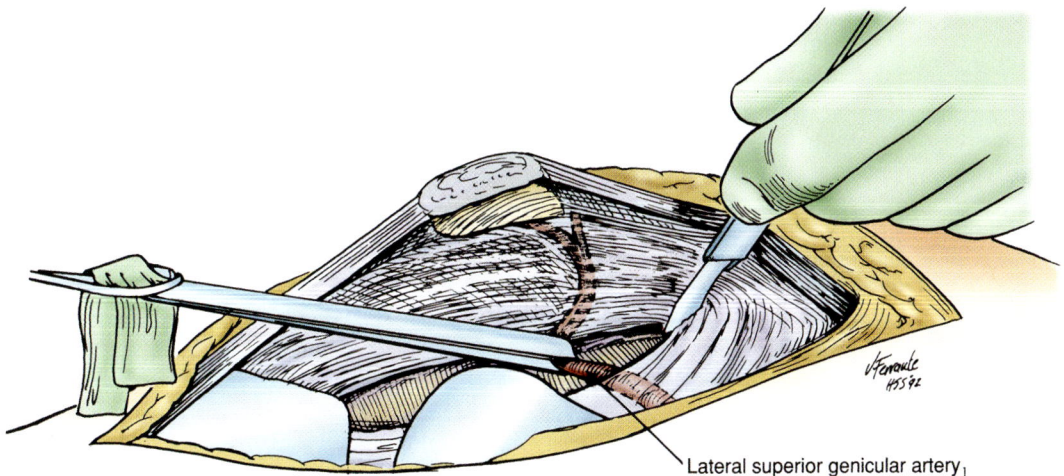

Lateral superior genicular artery₁

Figure 105-69. The patellar release is performed vertically about 1 inch from the lateral border of the patella from inside out while the lateral genicular vessels are retracted and preserved. The release may include the lower fibers of the vastus lateralis.

or by using a single stitch or towel clip to reapproximate the vastus medialis to the proximal patellar margin. If this suture ruptures, or if there is any doubt about patellar tracking, a lateral retinacular release is considered. Because the "no thumb" technique may be a particularly stringent test of patellar tracking, one should consider the status of the tourniquet and other factors that might impact patellar movement during trial testing.

Testing of patellar tracking with the tourniquet deflated will give a better assessment of patellar tracking and may decrease the number of lateral releases performed.[127] Another method of checking lateral retinacular tightness is to subluxate the patellar component over the medial femoral condyle with the knee in extension. If the patella can be subluxated one half of its diameter over the medial femoral condyle, then the retinaculum likely is not too tight. If it is determined that the patella will not track properly when the assessments already mentioned are used, a lateral retinacular release is performed. After the lateral superior genicular vessels (Fig. 105-69), which can be found distal to the lower border of the vastus lateralis, have been isolated and protected, a lateral

retinacular release is done from inside out approximately 1 to 2 cm from the lateral patellar margin (Fig. 105-70).

The patellar position in the sagittal plane is also important, but it is for the most part determined by the bone cuts of the femur and tibia. There is a tendency toward producing patella infera when the joint line is elevated or a thick tibial component is required. Observation of a postoperative patella infera may also be related to fibrosis around the infrapatellar ligament.[114] In the end, tracking of the patella is impacted by every step in the knee replacement procedure. If the patella does not track properly, the size, rotation, translation, and balance of every component must be considered and reassessed.

CEMENTED VERSUS UNCEMENTED FIXATION

Long-term follow-up studies of cemented TKA have consistently demonstrated successful clinical results and survivorship, particularly when used in combination with a posterior stabilized design (Fig. 105-71A).[35,46,187,194] Cemented designs

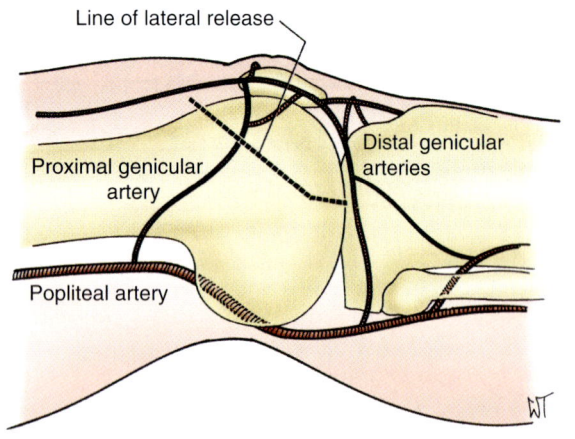

Figure 105-70. The lateral release is done obliquely to preserve the distal genicular arteries.

afford the benefit that slight incongruities of the bone-prosthesis interface can be eliminated with the cement, whereas cementless prostheses require almost perfect bone cut congruency to optimize bony ingrowth with available materials for cementless fixation. Failure of early cemented TKA designs was most likely a result of excessive prosthetic tibiofemoral constraint, concerns over polymethylmethacrylate degradation, bone-cement interface deterioration, and resultant third-body wear. This experience led to the development of minimally constrained, PCL retaining TKA designs that featured cementless fixation.[93] The limitation of cementless total knee design has been related to unreliable bone ingrowth secondary to incongruity, movement at the bone-prosthesis interface, or heightened requirements for both exact bone cuts and prosthetic stability for bone ingrowth to occur on the tibial side.

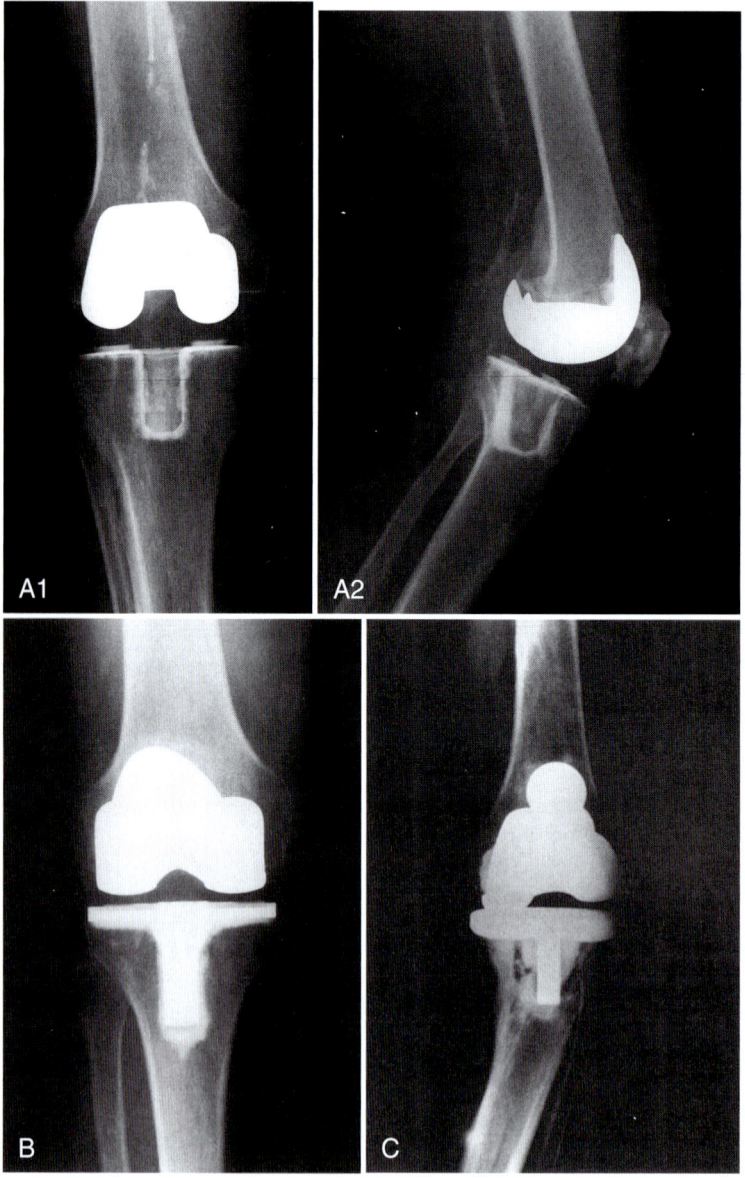

Figure 105-71. **A,** Anteroposterior and lateral radiographs of an Insall-Burstein I prosthesis at 19-year follow-up. **B,** Radiograph of a knee prosthesis that has been correctly cemented. The amount of cement is minimal. This type of cement fixation is obtained by using cement in the doughy stage. **C,** Radiograph of a knee prosthesis showing undesirable cement technique. In addition to varus positioning, excessive cement is noted in the proximal tibia and around the stem.

Although initial results of cementless and cemented TKA were comparable, a decline in satisfactory results was observed with cementless fixation.[4,142,148] Berger and colleagues[16] published in 2001 that his group was abandoning cementless fixation in TKA because of an unacceptable aseptic loosening rate (8%) and a 12% incidence of osteolytic lesions around screw holes. PCL retention with thin, flat polyethylene inserts frequently used in the past in combination with cementless designs created high-contact stresses, resulting in polyethylene wear and osteolysis.* However, all failures of cementless TKA cannot be attributed to PCL retention and nonconforming polyethylene inserts alone. Cement fixation appears to provide an advantage in durability over currently available press-fit techniques. In a prospective comparison of cemented and cementless fixation using the same implant, Duffy and coworkers[54] demonstrated better durability of femoral and tibial fixation with cemented techniques. At an average follow-up of 10 years, survival rates of cemented prostheses were 94% versus 72% for the uncemented group. Although these results suggest that cementless fixation alone is responsible for a higher failure rate, failure of cementless TKA is probably multifactorial. Knee implants designed for cementless use will require not only rethinking of design and instrumentation, but also new materials to improve the chances for bone ingrowth. Highly porous metals may offer this possibility, with recent new data suggesting better durability and reliability of bone ingrowth into cementless tibial components.

Retrieval studies of cementless components revealed minimal bone ingrowth, resulting in component loosening and migration. To enhance fixation, pegs were added to the distal femoral component and screws to the tibial component. Although femoral component fixation improved, screw osteolysis was observed under the tibial component, resulting in proximal tibial bone resorption without enhancing bone ingrowth.[61,125] Smooth tracks on the undersurface of the tibial baseplate, screw holes in the tibial baseplate itself, and drill holes in bone serve as conduits that permit polyethylene debris to reach the cancellous tibial surface.[216] Despite dramatic cases of osteolysis with some cementless knee designs, the use of cement in TKA does not eliminate the risk of osteolysis. Cases of severe osteolysis have been observed in cemented TKA.† Osteolysis has been related to polyethylene quality and backside wear issues accelerated by poor polyethylene locking mechanisms in cemented TKA.

Renewed efforts in cementless total knee design have resulted in the development of methods to improve bony ingrowth, including uniform porous coating of the tibial baseplate that is not recessed,[216] use of highly porous tantalum tibial baseplate, and fixation enhanced by hydroxyapatite (HA).[154,155] O'Keefe and associates reported excellent 5-year follow-up results in 125 knees implanted with a partially cemented porus tantalum monoblock implant with uncemented pegs. In this series, no patients were lost to follow-up, and the implant demonstrated 100% survivorship with regard to loosening and no observed osteolysis.[153] Akizuki and colleagues[3] reported on a series of 32 HA-coated TKAs at 7-year follow-up. By 6 months after implantation, no radiographic

clear zones surrounded the prostheses. Clinically, patients were doing well with no reported revisions. One patient died 2 years after implantation of her prosthesis, and autopsy showed bone tissue at 77.7% of the interface. Results reported by Murty and coworkers[147] on HA-coated femoral components showed 94% survivorship at 7- and 10-year follow-up. Ritter et al's [172] cemented cruciate retaining total condylar knees and the series of cemented cruciate retaining TKAs described by Scott and associates[183] approached results with cemented posterior stabilized designs.

More recently, Nilsson and associates[152] reported 2-year follow-up data for a randomized trial comparing cement fixation versus uncemented HA-coated tibial components and recommended the use of uncemented HA-coated implants without screw fixation based on equal survivorship and implant migration at 2 years for each implant. Improvements in design have enhanced results in cementless TKA as well; Whiteside's[214] series of cementless, cruciate retaining prostheses with conforming articular surfaces and intramedullary alignment techniques common to posterior stabilized cemented designs demonstrated outcomes matching those of cemented cruciate substituting prostheses. Buechel et al[23] also reported excellent results at 18 years using a cementless mobile-bearing knee design. Although these and more recent articles report promising results with new uncemented implants,[6,35,87] the literature continues to support improved survival of cemented components,[75] and this will be the gold standard by which other techniques are measured.

Cement Technique

Cement fixation is achieved as polymethylmethacrylate penetrates the porous cancellous bony surfaces, creating a mechanical interlock. Pulsatile lavage is used to remove blood, fat, and debris, and proper cleaning of the cancellous bone permits uninhibited penetration of cement.[173] Cement should be applied to bone digitally in the doughy tactile state, which allows for easy handling and manual pressurization (see Fig. 105-71B and C). Insall believed that centrifugation is unnecessary in TKA because the cement layer is thin and air bubbles escape readily. Walker et al[207] determined that the ideal cement penetration into bone is 3 to 4 mm; however, caution should be exercised in softer rheumatoid bone, where deeper penetration may occur. In contrast, sclerotic surfaces frequently encountered in OA may be drilled. Drilling of bone surfaces is performed with a 2-mm drill and should be limited to no more than 3 to 4 mm in drill depth, because deeper cement penetration transfers the bone-cement interface away from the tibial surface into the cancellous bone, where tibial bone strength tends to be less.

MANAGEMENT OF INSTABILITY OR DEFORMITY

Principles

In most arthritic knees, some degree of instability, deformity, contracture, or a combination of these elements will be found.[33,100] Deformity and instability can be created by asymmetrical loss of articular cartilage, resulting in collateral, capsular, and cruciate imbalance. Contracture of soft tissues is a secondary change that generally arises as a consequence of

---

*References 21, 67, 104, 180, and 198.
†References 31, 80, 158, 164, and 175.

trauma or long-standing angular malalignment. Variations in anatomy such as tibia vara or a diminutive lateral femoral condyle can also contribute to angular abnormalities that should be corrected at the time of total knee replacement. Although some minor degree of postoperative ligament asymmetry may be tolerated, it is better to obtain near-perfect stability, avoiding persistent contracture while accepting small amounts of laxity through surgical technique.

Although several investigators have suggested that residual malalignment is not detrimental to the outcome of TKA,[39,63,174,193] other authors have demonstrated that malalignment has a negative influence on long-term results of TKA.* These investigations suggest that the most important factor for maintaining satisfactory long-term outcome in TKA is anatomic alignment, which depends significantly on ligamentous balance and accurate bone resection. Although bone cuts can be made to establish anatomic alignment, proper ligamentous balance is required to maintain alignment throughout the range of motion. In a polyethylene retrieval study, Wasielewski and associates[210] noted that increased wear occurred when preoperative varus or valgus was present. Polyethylene wear and cold flow tended to be greater in the tightest prearthroplasty compartment, most frequently when ligament releases were inadequate.

Instability of the arthritic knee may be viewed as symmetrical or asymmetrical. Symmetrical instability is a result of erosion of cartilage or bone without associated adaptive ligamentous changes. This type of deformity is common in early arthritis of the knee and can be corrected under active reciprocal stress during physical examination. Standard surgical techniques that create symmetrical flexion and extension gaps are typically adequate to restore ligamentous balance (Fig. 105-72). Asymmetrical instability, common to advanced knee arthritis and presenting with a fixed deformity on physical examination, occurs when bone and cartilage compromise

*References 24, 79, 90, 91, 101, 124, 143, 170, 204, and 221.

is associated with adaptive ligamentous change (Figs. 105-73 and 105-74). These adaptive changes present as a continuum of deformity and may include contracture on the concave side of the joint with or without associated ligament laxity on the convex side of the deformed joint. Standard surgical technique and prosthesis spacing prove inadequate in balancing asymmetrical instability because of fixed ligament changes. Ligament release and ligament balancing are required to address this type of advanced deformity.

Operative management of asymmetrical instability and contracture cannot be accomplished by bone cuts alone. Although postoperative bracing has been described for the management of instability following TKA, it is seldom

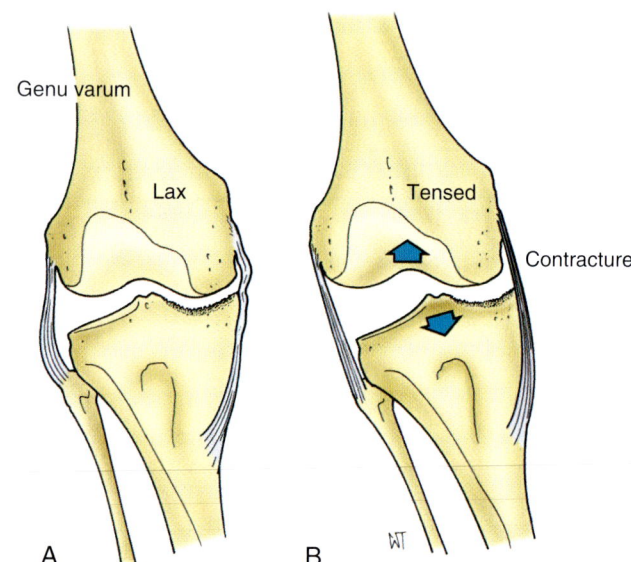

Figure 105-73. Asymmetrical instability in varus. The medial ligament is shorter than the lateral ligament.

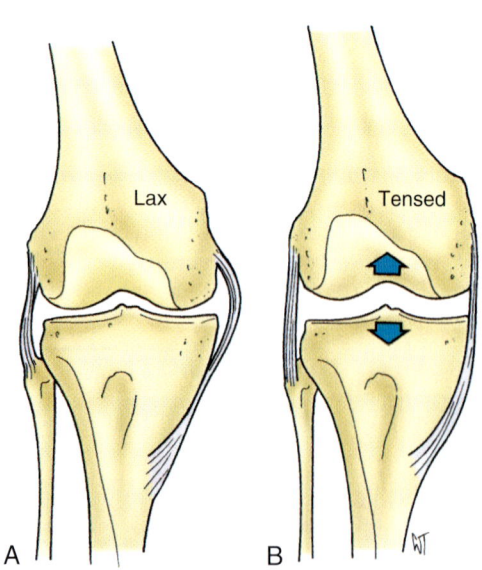

Figure 105-72. Symmetrical instability. The ligaments, although lax, are of equal length. Both alignment and stability are restored by tensioning the ligaments.

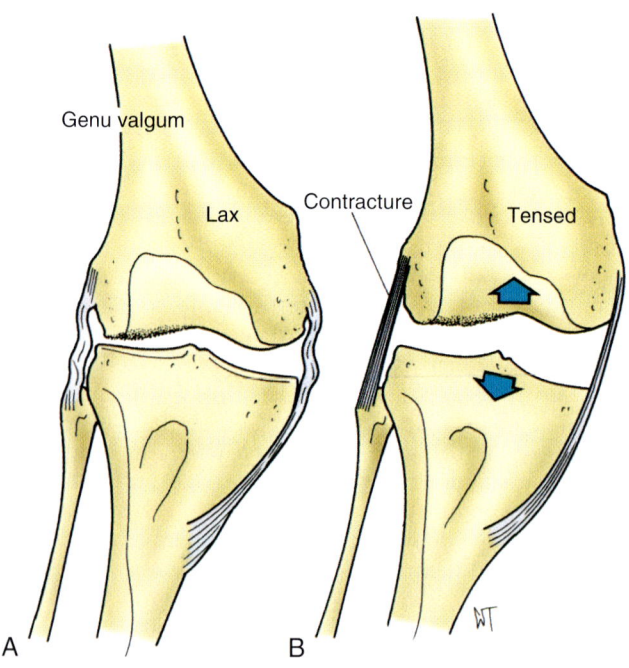

Figure 105-74. Asymmetrical instability in valgus.

optimal. Bracing is a treatment for ligament instability, not a treatment for ligament contracture. Two surgical methods have been described for correction of asymmetrical instability. The two surgical methods are used together or in combination, depending on the type of ligament deformity present. The first technique is a controlled ligament release from the contracted concave side of the deformity; the second technique consists of ligament advancement on the attenuated convex side. Ligament release of the contracted structures is adequate for correction of most deformities, although there are limits to the amount of correction that can be gained with ligament release. This statement is particularly true for valgus deformities, in which the amount of correction and release of structures on the lateral side of the knee is restricted by fear of stretching the peroneal nerve. Conversely, one cannot balance a knee simply by releasing the contracted side of the knee when the opposing ligaments are stretched to the point of being incompetent. Nevertheless, every attempt should be made to balance the knee before increasing the degree of constraint in TKA, especially in younger, active patients. When a ligament is incompetent, repair of the incompetent ligament or use of a more constrained knee design will be required. When extreme deformity cannot be balanced with controlled ligament release, options for treatment include bracing of instability, reconstruction of the incompetent ligament, and adding increased articular constraint (such as a constrained condylar knee [CCK or TC3]) that provides for collateral ligament substitution (Figs. 105-75 through 105-77).

Asymmetrical Varus Instability

Pathophysiology

Varus deformity is defined as any preoperative femorotibial angle less than naturally occurring anatomic valgus. This definition is not absolute because of the variability of human limb alignment; in patients with habitual genu varum, this malalignment is typically exaggerated. Generally, TKA in patients with arthritis and habitual genu varum involves realignment to physiologic valgus. Moderate to severe varus has been arbitrarily defined as greater than 15 to 20 degrees of varus deviation from the mechanical axis.[120,200]

Development of asymmetrical varus instability typically follows a sequence with loss of medial compartment bone and cartilage imparting a varus moment to the joint. The varus moment combined with the attendant periarticular inflammation associated with the arthritic process ultimately results in pathologic fibrosis and contracture of the MCL. Bony deficits in a varus knee typically occur on the medial tibial plateau, although both the medial tibia and the femur may develop deficits in advanced disease. The MCL contracture is worsened by medial osteoarthritic overgrowth pressing outward from the joint on the ligament, thereby causing relative shortening. Eventually, the effect of contracture of the MCL is a fixed varus deformity (Fig. 105-78; see also Fig. 105-73). Simultaneously, adaptive elongating changes occur in the LCL and capsule, resulting in attenuation of these lateral soft tissue structures. This combination of elements

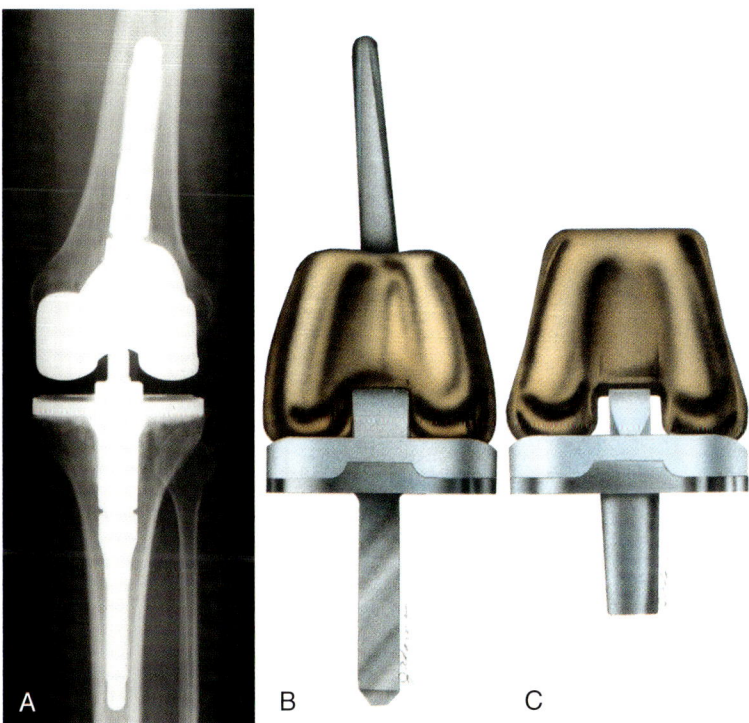

Figure 105-75. Constrained condylar knee prosthesis. **A,** Radiograph. **B,** The constrained condylar device uses an unlinked constrained design that places limitations on varus/valgus deflection, anteroposterior displacement, and rotation within the flexion-extension axis of the knee. Restriction of varus/valgus deflection and rotation is provided by a large tibial spine within an intracondylar femoral box, while posterior subluxation is prevented by engagement of the spine on the femoral cam. **C,** Posterior stabilized device. Nonlinked, semiconstrained posterior stabilized devices prevent posterior subluxation via a tibial spine that engages a femoral cam. Slight rotational constraint is afforded by the degree of conformity of the femorotibial articulation. (**B** and **C,** From Scott WN: The knee, vol 2, St Louis, 1994, Mosby–Year Book, p 1308.)

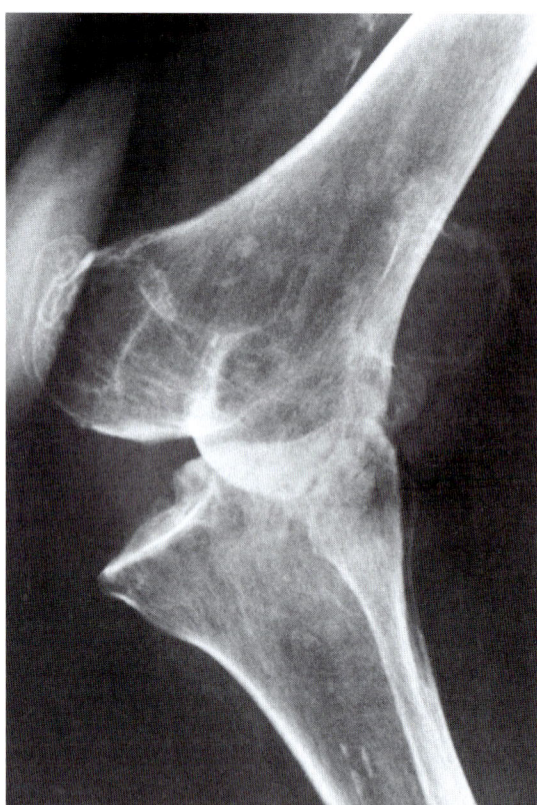

Figure 105-76. Radiograph of a very unstable valgus knee. This degree of ligamentous instability cannot be managed by any type of ligament release. Reconstruction will involve a medial ligament tightening procedure or a constrained prosthesis.

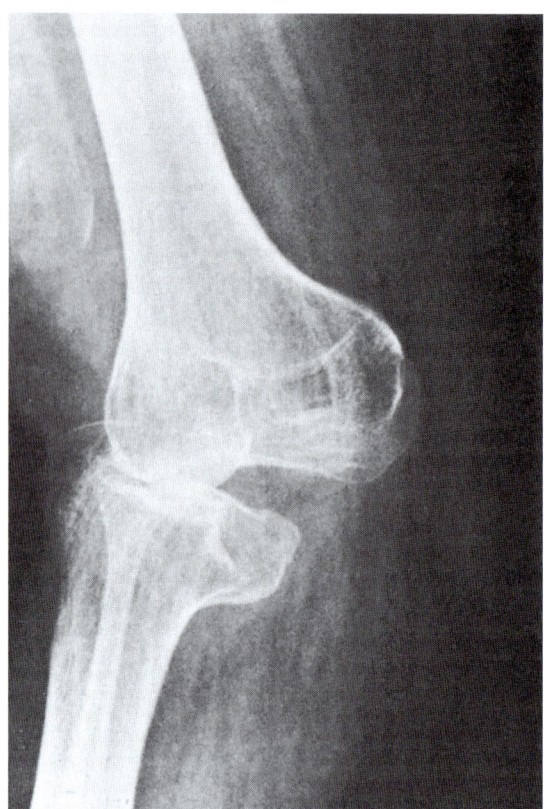

Figure 105-77. In this valgus knee, although the medial ligament is not absent, it is so elongated that soft tissue balancing by lateral release is impractical. This is an indication for a constrained prosthesis.

results in a *lateral thrust* or *varus thrust* of the knee that is observed during the stance phase of walking. Varus contracture may also be associated with a flexion contracture (described later).

MANAGEMENT OF VARUS DEFORMITY

Principles

MCL release is essential to achieve soft balance in TKA with fixed varus deformity. Several authors have shown that residual varus deformity in TKA increases the failure rate.* Sambatakakis and colleagues[178] described a radiographic *wedge sign* characteristic of incompletely corrected varus deformity hinging on a tight medial ligament; this finding has been confirmed by Laskin[120] and correlates with Insall's observation that most TKA failures occur because of medial tibial collapse related to recurrence of the preoperative deformity.

Some studies have suggested that moderate to severe varus deformity warrants PCL resection because of its contribution to varus malalignment. Alexiades and coworkers[5] showed that without the counterbalance of the ACL, the PCL tends to contract. Dennis and associates[45] demonstrated that retaining the PCL may not result in the desired femoral roll-back, nor does it prevent condylar lift-off during knee flexion. Laskin et al[120,121] (Fig. 105-79) reported that for fixed varus

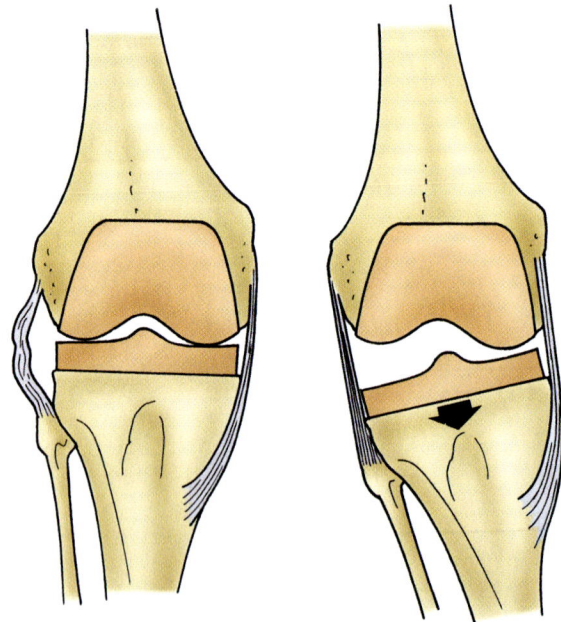

Figure 105-78. The medial ligament was not released; hence, asymmetrical instability remains.

deformities exceeding 15 degrees, the best results in terms of pain relief, correction, and range of motion are obtained by excision of the PCL and use of a cruciate substituting prosthesis. Teeny and colleagues[200] noted that 40% of knees with preoperative varus tended to remain in varus; their series

*References 24, 90, 91, 101, 124, 143, 204, 210, and 221.

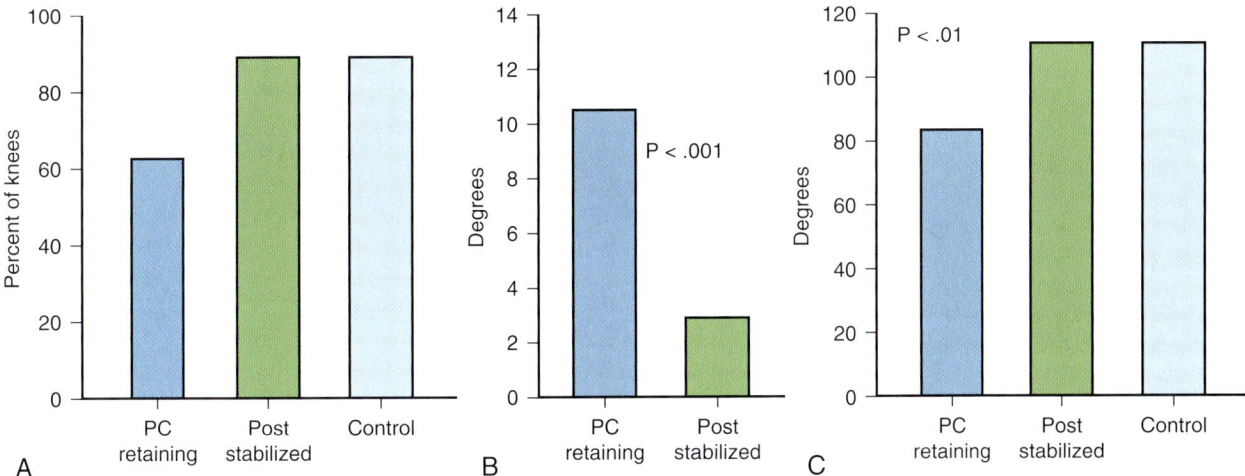

Figure 105-79. Bar graphs showing **(A)** percentage of knees accurately aligned, **(B)** residual flexion contracture (average), and **(C)** average range of motion in knees with greater than 15 degrees of fixed varus deformity. The parameters studied were equivalent to those for a group of control knees (without significant deformity) in which a cruciate retaining prosthesis was used. Cruciate retention in deformed knees led to a less satisfactory correction of alignment and flexion contracture and an inferior range of motion.

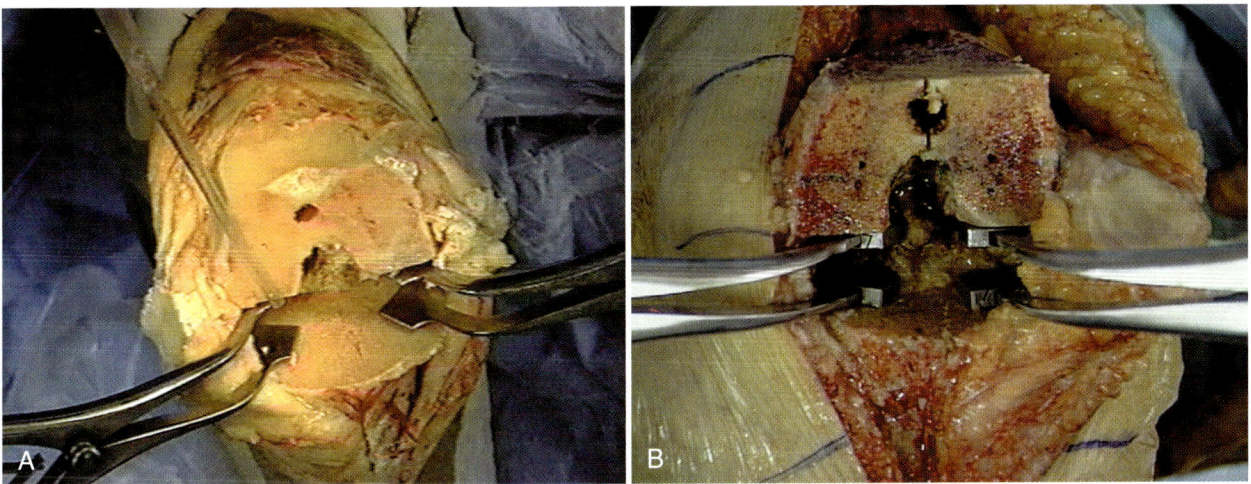

Figure 105-80. **A** and **B**, Laminar spreaders are useful in monitoring soft tissue balance and the performance of ligament releases.

included more than 50% of knees with cruciate retaining prostheses. Both Laskin[120] and Teeny and coworkers[200] observed that functional outcomes of varus knees approached but did not equal the results of nondeformed knees.

Conversely, Ritter and associates[168a] reported on his group's series of 82 patients undergoing PCL retaining TKA with greater than or equal to 20 degrees of preoperative deformity, both varus and valgus. Their results showed no difference in knee score, postoperative alignment, or revision rate as compared with a group of patients with smaller preoperative deformity. Similarly, Kubiak and colleagues[117a] reported on a series of cruciate retaining TKAs with at least 15 degrees of preoperative coronal plane deformity that showed 93% revision-free survival at 10 years. Both of these studies conclude that with proper balancing of the soft tissues, a PCL retaining TKA provides very good long-term outcomes.

Technique

Ligament balance is achieved by progressively releasing the medial soft tissues until they reach the length of the lateral ligamentous structures. The extent of the release can be monitored by periodically inserting lamina spreaders (Fig. 105-80) or using a ligament tensiometer to judge alignment with the aligning rod or plumb line. The endpoint of the release is a stable position in which a plumb line will extend from the hip through the center of the knee to the ankle joint. Computer navigation of TKA also allows the possibility of a real-time assessment of knee alignment and balance during the course of a ligament release. Component placement can also affect angular deformity. Scott has described the use of a downsized tibial component with lateral translation of the component, along with removal of a portion of the medial tibial plateau to correct rigid varus deformity. If the PCL is tethering the release, it should be excised or lengthened by posterior release from the tibia or recession from the femur. In a measured resection technique, ligament release will be done partially during the approach and after the initial proximal tibial and distal femoral bone cuts have been made; for cruciate substituting designs done with gap balancing, ligament releases will also be done during the approach and after the tibial cut has been made. The cruciate

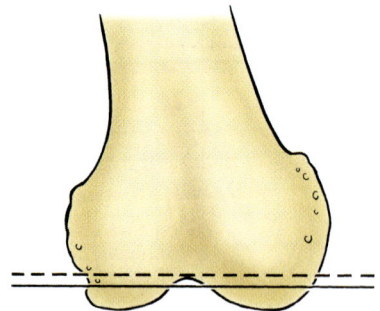
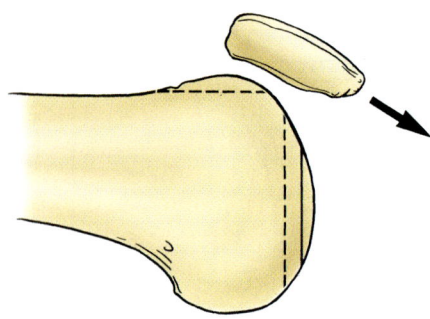

Figure 105-81. In cases with considerable ligamentous laxity, an under-resection of the distal femur may be preferable. The standard femoral resection will necessitate a thicker tibial component to take up the slack in the soft tissues and may cause distal migration of the patella. By under-resecting the femur, desirable patellar position is maintained.

substituting gap balancing technique was favored by Insall for very large deformities, because laxity in the knee joint after release may occasionally dictate an under-resection of the distal femur to accurately balance the knee (Fig. 105-81). A full MCL release not only will correct fixed varus but also will open the medial space in flexion (whereas the normal knee in flexion has more lateral than medial laxity). Flexion gap symmetry is influenced by medial release. Attention to the importance of gap balancing and joint line preservation dictates that femoral component rotational alignment should be determined relative to both femoral anatomy and ligament balance.

The medial release (Fig. 105-82) is done in steps by first removing medial osteophytes from the femur and tibia, including the protruding flare of the tibial plateau, and raising a sleeve of soft tissue from the upper medial tibia that is allowed to slide proximally. The sleeve consists of periosteum, deep medial ligament, superficial medial ligament, and insertion of the pes anserinus tendons. More posterior, at the joint surface, the sleeve is continuous with the semimembranosus insertion and the posterior capsule. Distally, the release may include the deep fascia investing soleus and popliteus muscles. The sleeve is made by stripping the periosteum medially from the tibia 10 to 15 cm distal to the standard arthrotomy. The knee is flexed, and the tibia is progressively externally rotated to gain posterior access. The distal attachment of the superficial medial ligament can be left intact in moderate deformities. When this is not enough, the release is continued posteriorly and distally by further subperiosteal stripping of the superficial fibers of the MCL. Thereby, correction of deformity occurs in a graduated manner and is aided by the intermittent stretching action of a medial laminar spreader. With progressive release, no discontinuity between the medial soft tissue structures is noted, but rather a progressive separation of the periosteal layer from the tibia at a point distal to the MCL attachment to the tibia (Fig. 105-83). The result is balancing, with some overall lengthening of the limb (the amount of lengthening depends on the degree of preoperative stretching of the lateral structures). The released medial soft tissues ideally should give way gradually rather than with an obvious "pop," which would indicate that the distal insertion of the ligament has been forcibly separated from its tibial attachment, or that a transverse disruption of a medial structure has occurred.

To gain access with the lamina spreader, the proximal tibial osteotomy may be done first. When varus is combined with flexion contracture, it is helpful to divide transversely the medial portion of the posterior capsule, or alternatively to elevate the capsule from both the posterior tibia and the posteromedial femur. Laterally, the posterior capsule is often sufficiently stretched to the point that it does not contribute to a flexion contracture. Posterior osteophytes should be removed. The occasional need for under-resection of the femur should be carefully judged before too much bone is removed, as the distal femur can always be recut. Such a situation may arise in a varus knee when the lateral structures are stretched and the medial structures are released to balance those structures, thereby increasing the height of the extension gap. When proper release and balancing is performed, mobilization can be started immediately, and walking with full weight bearing is permitted as tolerated.

Ligament advancement procedures have also been described to correct varus deformity.[200] In the rare case when varus knees cannot be fully corrected with medial release and are associated with lateral laxity, consideration may be given to lateral ligament reconstruction.

ASYMMETRICAL VALGUS INSTABILITY

Pathophysiology

Valgus deformity is defined as malalignment exceeding natural femorotibial valgus orientation, typically greater than 7 to 10 degrees.[140,195,215] Krackow et al classified valgus deformity into three distinct types.[116] Type I involves lateral femoral bone loss, lateral soft tissue contracture, and intact medial soft tissues. Type II is type I with lengthened medial soft tissues. Type III is severe valgus deformity with malpositioning of the proximal tibial joint line (e.g., secondary to high tibial osteotomy).

In the valgus knee, the lateral soft tissue structures, including the LCL, ITB, and lateral capsule, contract, while the medial soft tissues become stretched. The lateral femoral condyle has been shown to be frequently dysplastic in the valgus deformity; therefore most of the bony deficit occurs on the femoral side.[195] However, in advanced disease, cartilage and bone erosion may be observed on the tibial side as well. In long-standing deformity, lateral contracture and medial lengthening become permanent (see Fig. 105-74). This combination of pathologies may result in a *medial thrust* during gait. Similar to varus deformities, valgus contractures may be associated with a flexion contracture. However, presumably

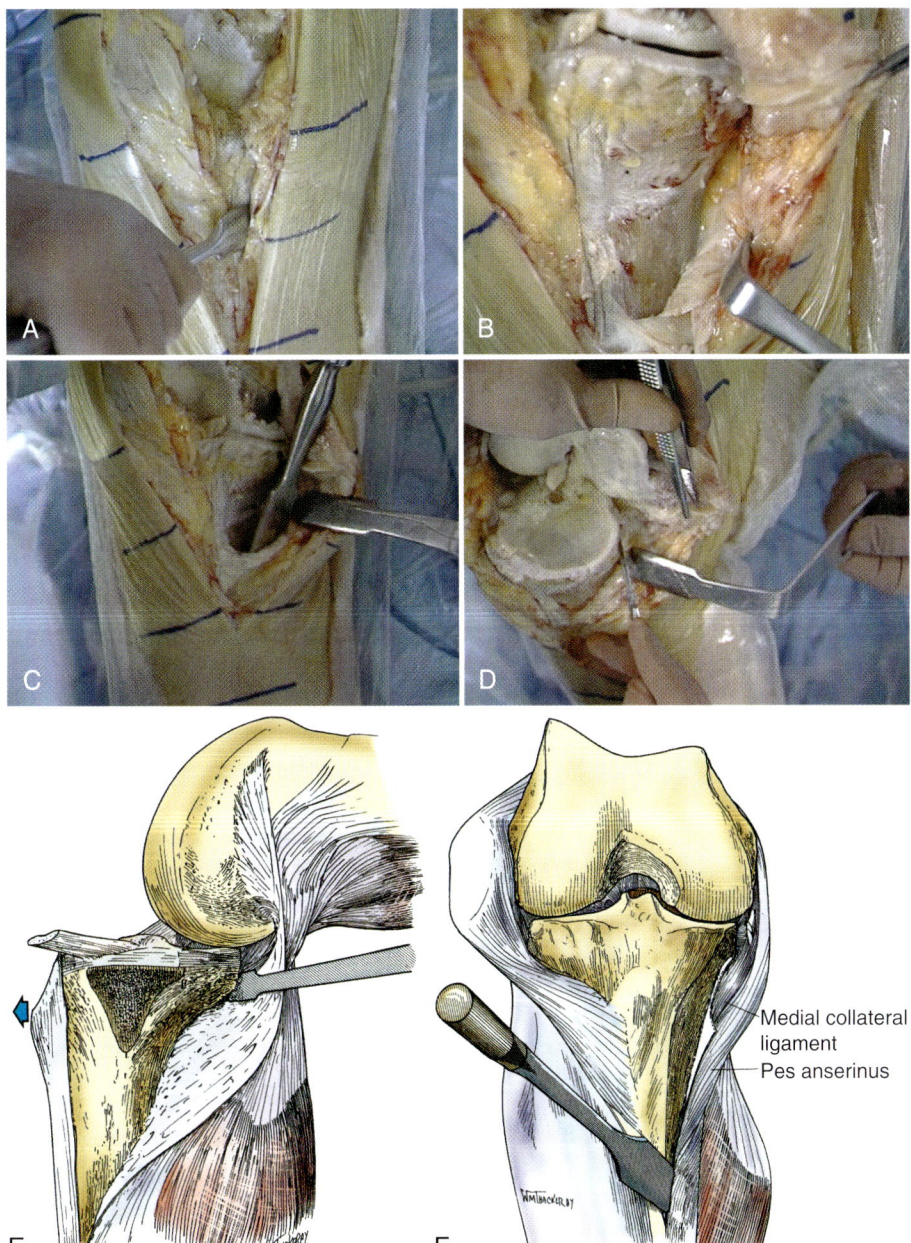

Figure 105-82. Varus release. **A** and **B,** The exposure is begun with subperiosteal stripping beneath the superficial medial collateral ligament. **C,** Completed release. Only the superficial medial collateral ligament remains intact, but this too can become detached if necessary. **D,** The tibia is externally rotated with a complete posteromedial release. **E,** Graphic illustration demonstrating complete release of the deep and superficial medial collateral ligament, and the semimembranous. **F,** Subperiosteal elevation of the medial collateral ligament and pes anserinius tendom completes the full medial release.

because of contracture of the ITB, a fixed external rotation deformity often accompanies asymmetrical valgus instability, particularly in patients with inflammatory arthritis.

Management

Principles

Valgus release traditionally has been performed by elevating the lateral capsule, LCL, arcuate ligament, popliteus tendon, lateral femoral periosteum, distal ITB, and adjacent lateral intermuscular septum from their bony attachments. Except for the ITB, release is performed from the lateral femoral condyle; the ITB is released from Gerdy's tubercle. Because

desired postoperative alignment is physiologic valgus, some degree of lateral laxity after an extensive lateral release is typically well tolerated. The sequence of lateral release has been the focus of some controversy.* Insall described the management of lesser deformities with simple release of the ITB from its insertion on Gerdy's tubercle (Fig. 105-84). For moderate to severe fixed deformities, the lateral femoral condyle would be stripped of its soft tissue attachments proximally for about 9 cm, and at this level the periosteum, the iliotibial tract, and the lateral intramuscular septum would be

---

*References 1, 21, 108, 123, 140, 195, and 215.

transversely divided from inside out (Figs. 105-85 and 105-86). Any part of the lateral intramuscular septum that remained attached to the distal femur was divided longitudinally until the entire flap was free to slide. Although such an extensive release generally corrects any severity of deformity, posterolateral flexion instability may occur postoperatively.[97,140] Furthermore, case reports have described extensive soft tissue stripping that has devascularized the lateral femoral condyle, resulting in osteonecrosis.

Because of the risk of posterolateral instability (and osteonecrosis) following extensive soft tissue stripping from the lateral femoral condyle, stab-incision[140] and pie-crusting techniques were developed and have become the methods of choice. These techniques permit a graduated intra-articular

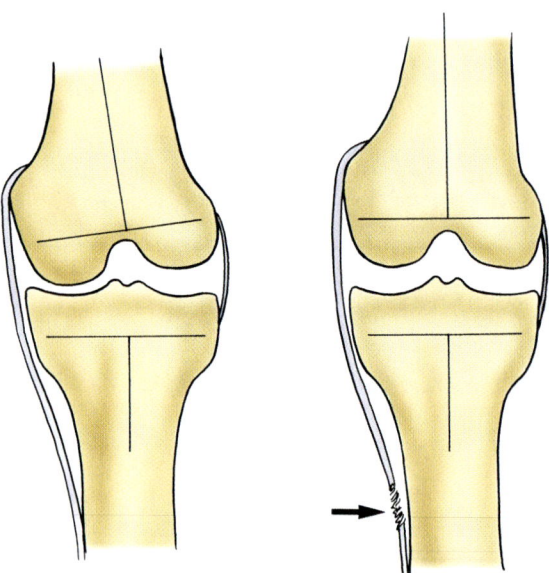

Figure 105-83. The ideal medial collateral ligament (MCL) release occurs distal to the insertion of the ligament into the tibia through the periosteum and in continuity with the MCL. At this level, a controlled release is obtained.

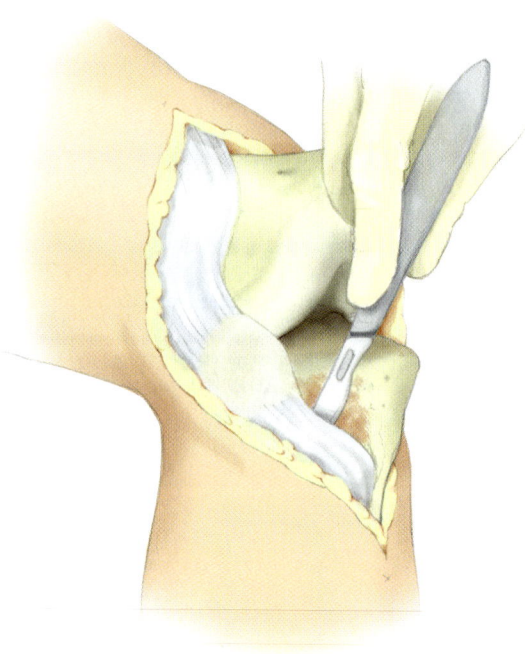

Figure 105-84. First stage of a lateral release. The iliotibial band is separated from its attachment to Gerdy's tubercle and capsular attachments from the lateral margin of the tibia.

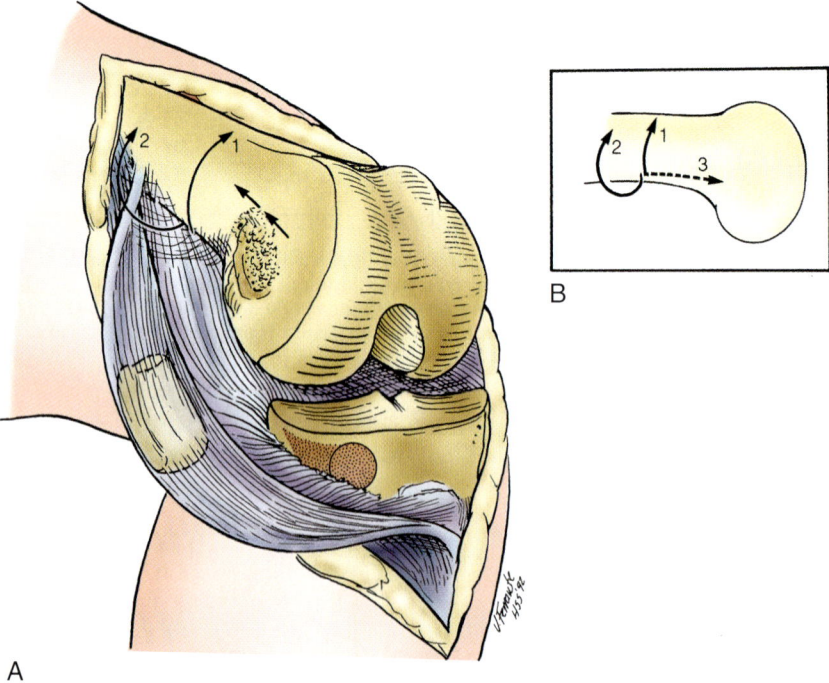

A

B

Figure 105-85. A, Additional stages of lateral release include raising a flap from the lateral femoral condyle to a point 3 inches proximal to the joint. **B,** The periosteum is incised transversely *(1)*; the lateral intramuscular septum and the proximal iliotibial tract are divided transversely at the same level *(2)*; and the remaining distal attachment of the lateral intramuscular septum is divided vertically and separated from the femur *(3)*.

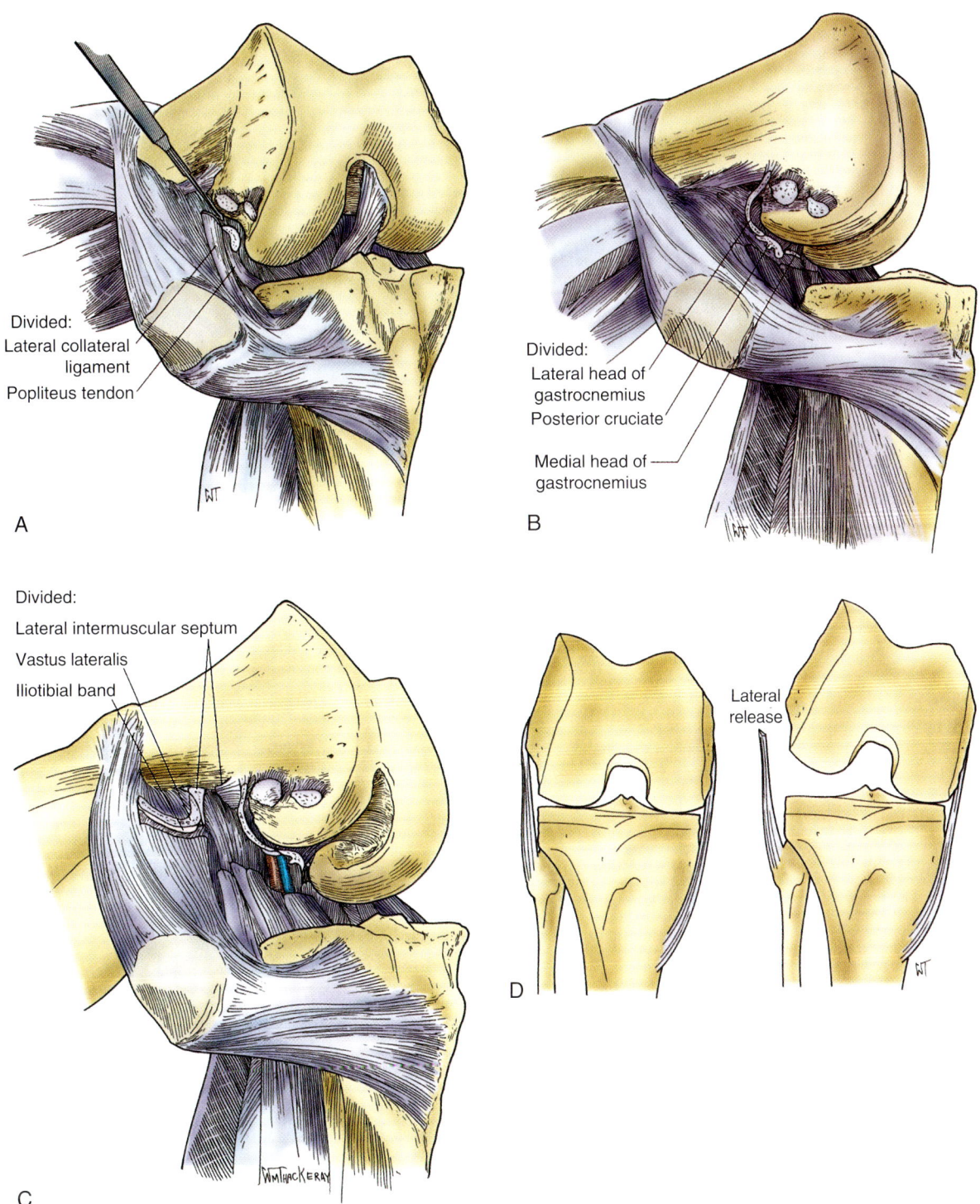

Figure 105-86. **A** through **C,** Valgus release is done on the femur, completely releasing the soft tissues from the lateral femoral condyle and, if necessary, transversely dividing the iliotibial band. **D,** After lateral release for the correction of valgus, the knee is always inherently unstable in flexion. A lateral rotary instability may develop that will be exacerbated if any malrotation of the tibial component occurs.

release of the posterolateral capsule and ITB. Although both techniques involve transverse punctures (pie-crusting) of the ITB well above the joint line and some degree of transverse release of the posterolateral capsule, the stab-incision technique includes a more extensive transverse release of the arcuate complex immediately above the joint line and posterior to the ITB (Fig. 105-87). Releasing at the joint line

leaves only the LCL for lateral restraint; perforations of the lateral capsule and ITB above the joint line in combination with a limited transverse posterolateral capsular release maintain greater soft tissue continuity. Both techniques typically allow for preservation of the popliteus tendon, affording greater stability to the posterolateral corner. Whereas Miyasaka and coworkers[140] observed a 24%

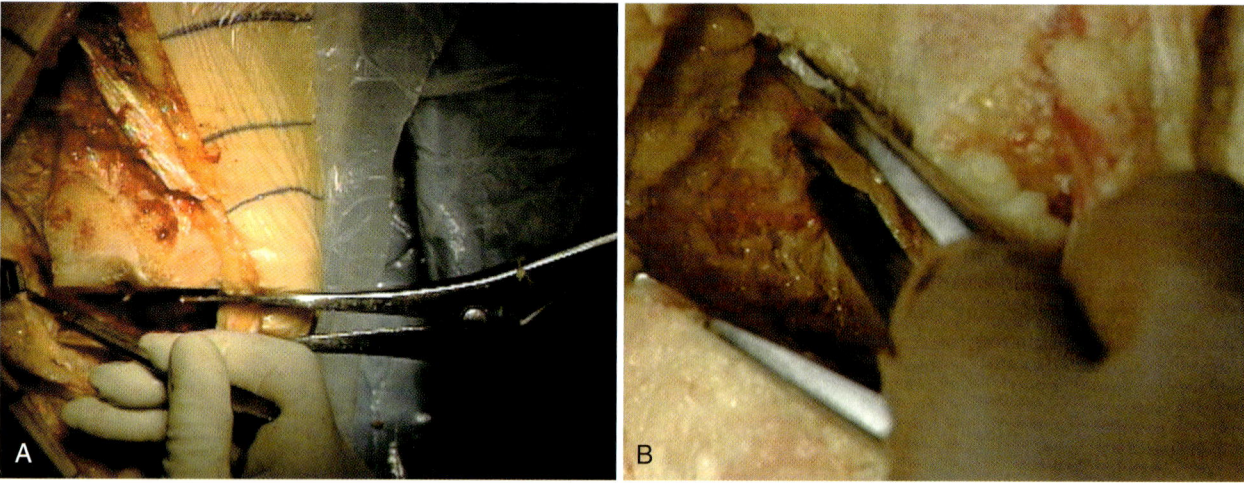

Figure 105-87. Intraoperative photo of lateral release using the "pie-crusting" technique. **A,** Joint distracted using a laminar spreader placed medially. **B,** Close-up view of multiple intra-articular punctures in the contracted lateral soft tissues proximal to the joint line.

incidence of posterolateral instability with extensive lateral femoral condylar release for valgus deformity, by using the stab-incision technique they limited the incidence to 6%, similar to what Insall described. Correction of valgus deformity in TKA has been associated with patellofemoral instability due to lateral tethering of the patella and peroneal palsy due to stretching of the nerve. The incidence of patellofemoral instability has been reported to be as high as 4%[123]; however, the incidence using the stab-incision technique and preserving the popliteus has been reported as low as 0%.[140] Although the overall incidence of peroneal nerve palsy after TKA has been estimated as less than 1%, the incidence in valgus knees has been reported at 3% to 4%.[116,195] In a recent investigation using the stab-incision technique, no cases of peroneal nerve compromise were observed.[140] Clinical outcomes in patient series where the pie-crusting technique has been used to correct valgus deformity in TKA have shown positive results. Clarke and associates[32a] reported excellent Knee Society scores and range of motion and no cases of postoperative instability in a series of 24 patients who underwent TKA with a valgus preoperative deformity corrected with the pie-crusting technique. Aglietti and colleagues[1a] reported the 5-year follow-up on 53 patients who underwent correction of valgus deformity at the time of TKA using the pie-crusting technique. Coronal alignment was within 5 degrees of neutral in 96% of knees; one patient had transient peroneal nerve palsy, one patient had varus instability, and no revisions were reported.

In elderly patients and in those with low physical demands, the use of articular constraint may avoid postoperative morbidity. In Insall's series of primary constrained implants (with up to 10 years of follow-up), uniform success has been reported without prosthetic loosening, indicating that this approach may be a reasonable option in selected cases.

Technique

Pie-Crusting Method (Insall)

The knee is approached through a standard midline incision and a standard medial parapatellar capsular approach. Femoral and tibial bone cuts are made to gain access and to create

congruent surfaces to assess gap symmetry. Because erosion occurs on the lateral femoral condyle in long-standing valgus malalignment, bone resection from the lateral condyle is often minimal. Appropriate femoral rotation is imperative to ensure proper balancing in flexion. Referencing off of the posterior condyles often is not reliable because of posterior condylar erosion. Insall believed that the PCL often contributed to the deformity, which led him to recommend a posterior stabilized design for valgus knees.[97,140] Other studies have reported good outcome in valgus TKA with preservation of the PCL and appropriate soft tissue balancing. The posterolateral capsule and arcuate complex lateral to the popliteus are cut transversely at the level of the tibial cut, and titrated intra-articular and extra-articular releases of the lateral capsule at the tibial insertion and the ITB at Gerdy's tubercle are performed using a knife blade. This technique is performed with a moderate amount of stress in the lateral compartment using a laminar spreader or ligament tensiometer. Multiple stab incisions are made in the contracted lateral soft tissues (particularly the ITB and the portion of the arcuate complex below the popliteus that tends to tether the popliteus tendon) within and above the joint until the deformity is corrected (see Fig. 105-87A and B). Spacer blocks are frequently used to check the balance to avoid overcorrection. As noted previously, the popliteus and the LCL are preserved if possible to limit posterolateral instability in flexion. A cadaver study by Mihalko and Krackow (JOA 2000) highlights the risk of injury to the peroneal nerve during this technique. In their study, the peroneal nerve was found to be between 6 and 12 mm (less than the depth of a no. 11 blade [16 mm]) from the surface of the posterolateral corner in full extension.

Correction Through a Lateral Parapatellar Approach

Keblish[108] and Buechel[22] have described a three-step lateral release through a lateral parapatellar approach for severe valgus deformity. The tibial tubercle is osteotomized and reflected medially, retaining a medial periosteal hinge. The infrapatellar fat pad is maintained on the patellar tendon to

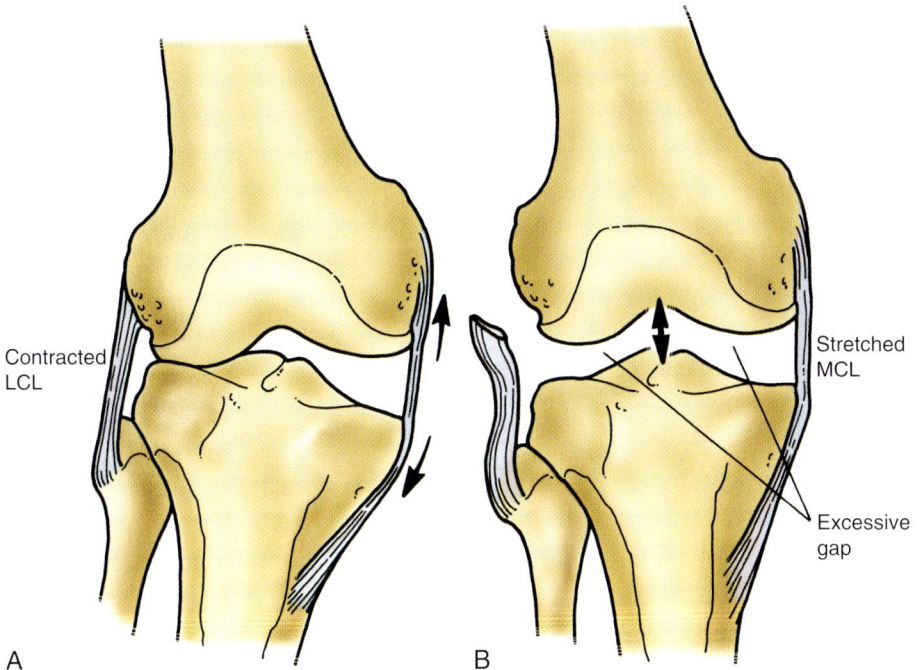

Figure 105-88. **A** and **B,** There are limits to ligament balancing. In this case, the medial collateral ligament is stretched beyond its normal length, and after lateral release, the knee will be distracted abnormally. Stabilizing this knee with thicker components involves actual lengthening of the limb, and there are clearly limits to how much lengthening can be tolerated without damage to the neurovascular structures.

facilitate closing of the lateral retinacular defect. The three steps of lateral release are as follows:

1. The anterior compartment musculature and the iliotibial tract are elevated from Gerdy's tubercle to the level of the fibular head. The amount of correction is tested at this point.
2. With the knee flexed to 90 degrees, the LCL and the popliteus are elevated as a subperiosteal flap based proximally on the lateral femoral shaft. If needed, the entire periosteum is elevated. If the peroneal nerve is observed to subluxate, then the fibular head is resected.
3. With the knee maintained at 90 degrees of flexion, the entire periosteum of the fibular head is elevated while the peroneal nerve at the fibular neck is protected, and the fibular head is resected. The extension position of the peroneal nerve is checked to ensure that the nerve is situated in the space created by femoral head resection.

As emphasized by Buechel,[22] the lateral instability that occurs in flexion with extensive lateral release can be corrected with compensatory femoral component external rotation. Patellar tracking must be carefully assessed after adjustment is made for femoral component rotation.

Ligament Advancement or Tightening

Ligament advancement or tightening is rare in TKA. Krackow[115] has described techniques for ligament tightening for both medial and lateral soft tissues and estimates that he has performed them in 1% to 2% of knee replacements. In the correction of a valgus knee, a lateral ligament release may allow overlengthening of perhaps 5 mm to compensate for

5 mm of stretching of the MCL (Fig. 105-88). However, when MCL elongation is 10 mm or greater, it simply is not possible to achieve this much stretching by lateral release alone. The same argument can be applied to varus deformities, although there are differences (notably that there is no counterpart to the peroneal nerve). It is possible to overlengthen the medial side a greater extent and, provided axial alignment is correct, some degree of lateral laxity is tolerable. As a rule of thumb, lateral laxity is acceptable provided the knee alignment cannot be passively brought into varus with the knee extended. The MCL can be tightened by proximal or distal advancement. This type of soft tissue reconstruction may have merit for overconstrained prostheses in younger patients. In support of Krackow's methods, Healy and colleagues[86] reported success with lateral soft tissue release and proximal MCL advancement with bone plug recession into the medial femoral condyle to correct valgus deformity in a small group of patients.

Medial and Lateral Proximal Advancement. Krackow[115] has described a method whereby the proximal attachment of the MCL to the medial femoral epicondyle is detached from the bone over a fairly wide area (Fig. 105-89). The flap of tissue is advanced to a more proximal and slightly anterior position. It is secured by passing an interlocking stitch through the flap and tying this tightly over a proximally placed screw and washer, with further augmentation using a staple placed into the area of the original femoral condyle (Fig. 105-90). Engh and Ammeen[59] have described the use of an epicondylar osteotomy with advancement of a ligament and bone block for correction of varus deformities; Healy's method[86] involves recession of the MCL attachment in its anatomic position at

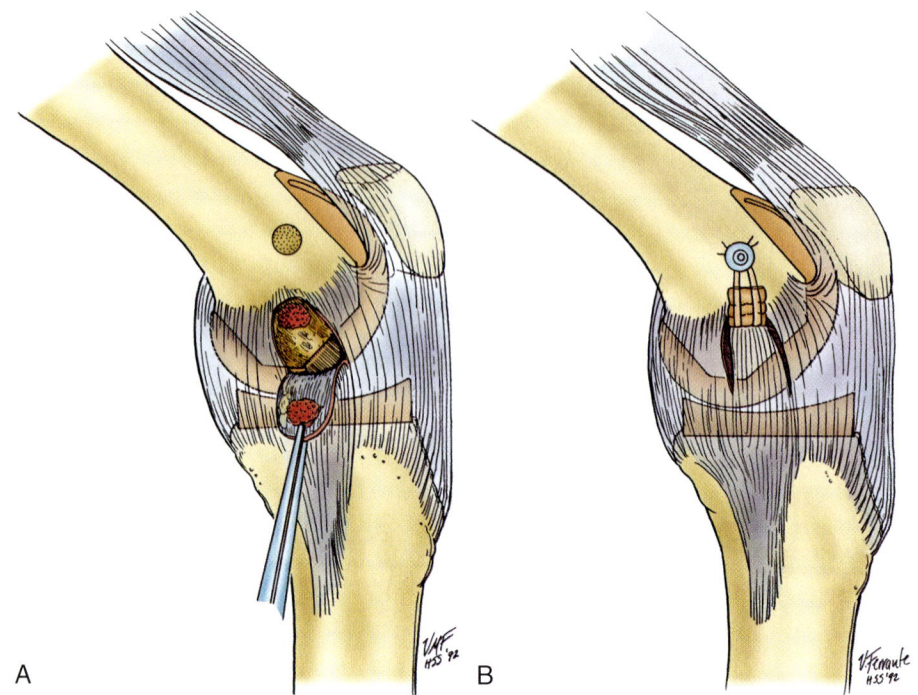

Figure 105-89. Krackow's technique of proximal medial collateral ligament (MCL) advancement. **A,** The proximal attachment of the MCL is removed en bloc without bone. A screw and washer are placed proximal and slightly anterior. **B,** Using the locking loop ligament fixation suture, the MCL is tightened proximally by tying the sutures around the screw and washer, which is then tightened. A second screw may be placed through the new attachment of the MCL.

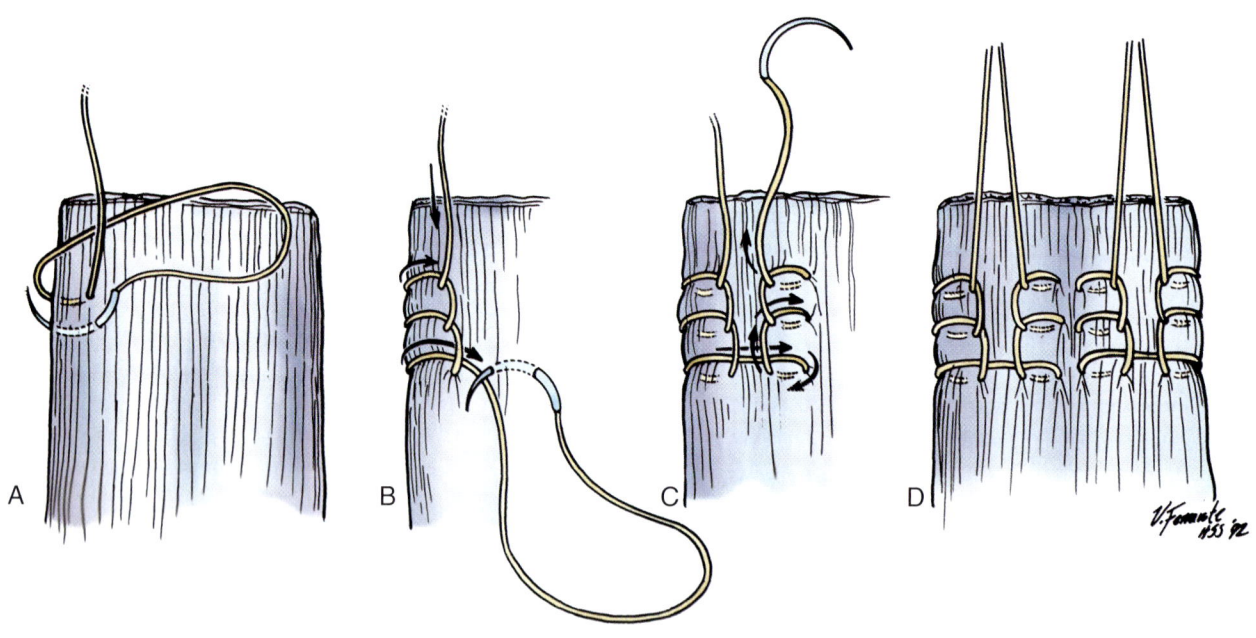

Figure 105-90. A through **D,** Krackow's locking loop ligament fixation suture.

the medial femoral condyle, rather than translocation of the proximal ligament (Figs. 105-91 through 105-96). The recessed proximal bone plug is secured over a bony bridge or button on the lateral side. For lax lateral structures, Krackow's method has been described for the varus knee; reports describing Healy's method of proximal recession of the LCL are not available.

FLEXION CONTRACTURE

Pathophysiology

Flexion contractures involve the posterior capsule, the PCL, and the musculotendinous units crossing the posterior aspect of the knee joint. In OA, the deformity is typically limited

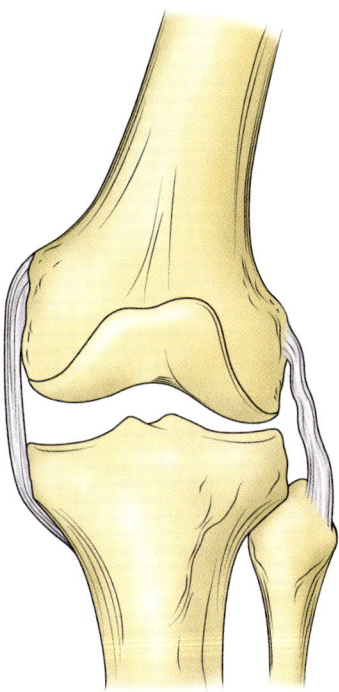

Figure 105-91. Valgus deformity with lateral contracture and medial laxity. (Illustration redrawn from Lahey Clinic, Burlington, Mass.)

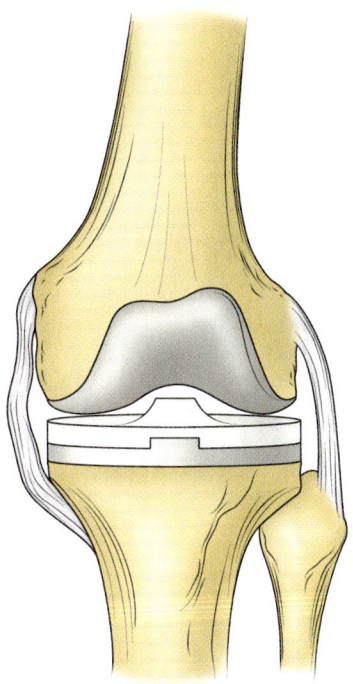

Figure 105-92. After lateral release, with total knee arthroplasty trials in place, the medial collateral ligament is lax. (Illustration redrawn from Lahey Clinic, Burlington, Mass.)

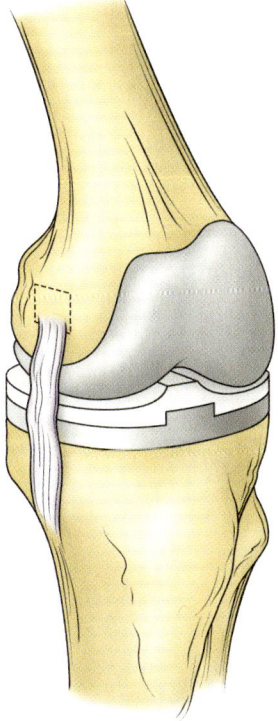

Figure 105-93. The proximal insertion of the medial collateral ligament is elevated with a bone plug. (Illustration redrawn from Lahey Clinic, Burlington, Mass.)

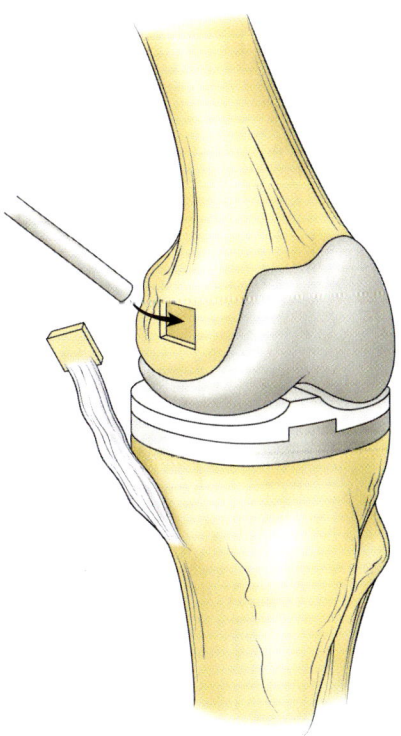

Figure 105-94. The metaphyseal bone at the epicondyle is recessed with a bone tamp. (Illustration redrawn from Lahey Clinic, Burlington, Mass.)

to soft tissue contracture associated with posterior compartment osteophytes (Fig. 105-97), whereas in inflammatory arthritis, flexion contracture may result in significant posterior femoral condylar erosion (Fig. 105-98). Extreme posterior femoral condylar erosion generally occurs in patients who have been unable to walk and have developed fixed flexion deformities that may exceed 90 degrees. Because of posterior condylar erosion, in addition to posterior capsular contracture, flexion contracture may be paradoxically associated with flexion instability. This situation represents a considerable technical challenge and typically warrants application of revision TKA principles.

Several authors have suggested that full intraoperative correction of flexion contractures in TKA is not essential because postoperative correction is possible[70,138,199] and clinical outcome is not affected by residual flexion contractures of up to 30 degrees.[138,201] In contrast, Firestone and colleagues[70] reported that if a flexion contracture remains at the completion of TKA, then the residual deformity will persist and worsen with time, especially if the PCL is preserved. Ritter and coworkers similarly found that a postoperative flexion contracture was associated with poorer postoperative outcomes. The current consensus among knee surgeons is that flexion contractures should be corrected to the maximum extent possible at the time of TKA.

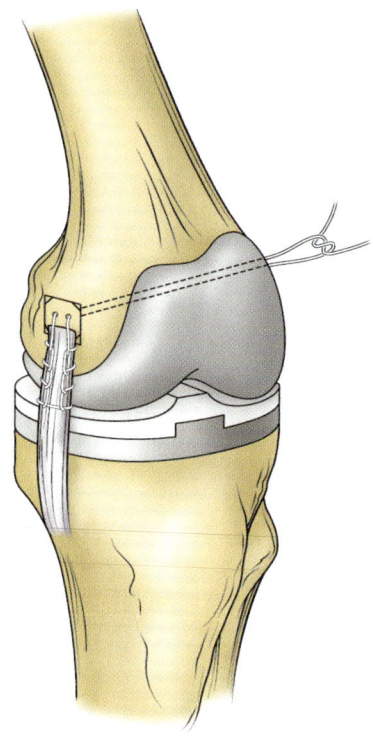

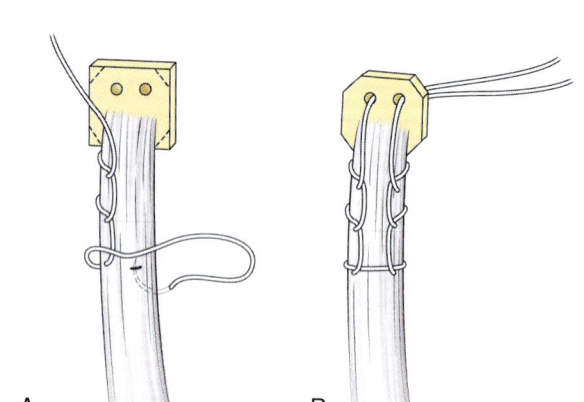

Figure 105-95. **A,** The medial collateral ligament bone plug is prepared for recession into the medial femoral condyle. **B,** A Krackow ligament suture is placed in the medial collateral ligament. (Illustration redrawn from Lahey Clinic, Burlington, Mass.)

Figure 105-96. The medial collateral ligament bone plug is recessed and advanced in an isometric position. The ligament suture is tied over a bony bridge or a button on the lateral cortex. (Illustration redrawn from Lahey Clinic, Burlington, Mass.)

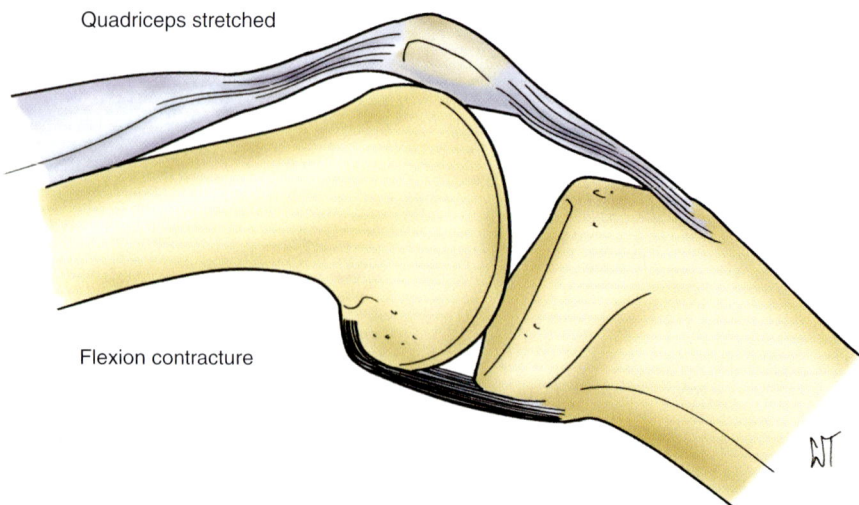

Quadriceps stretched

Flexion contracture

Figure 105-97. In a flexion contracture, the posterior capsule is shortened and adherent.

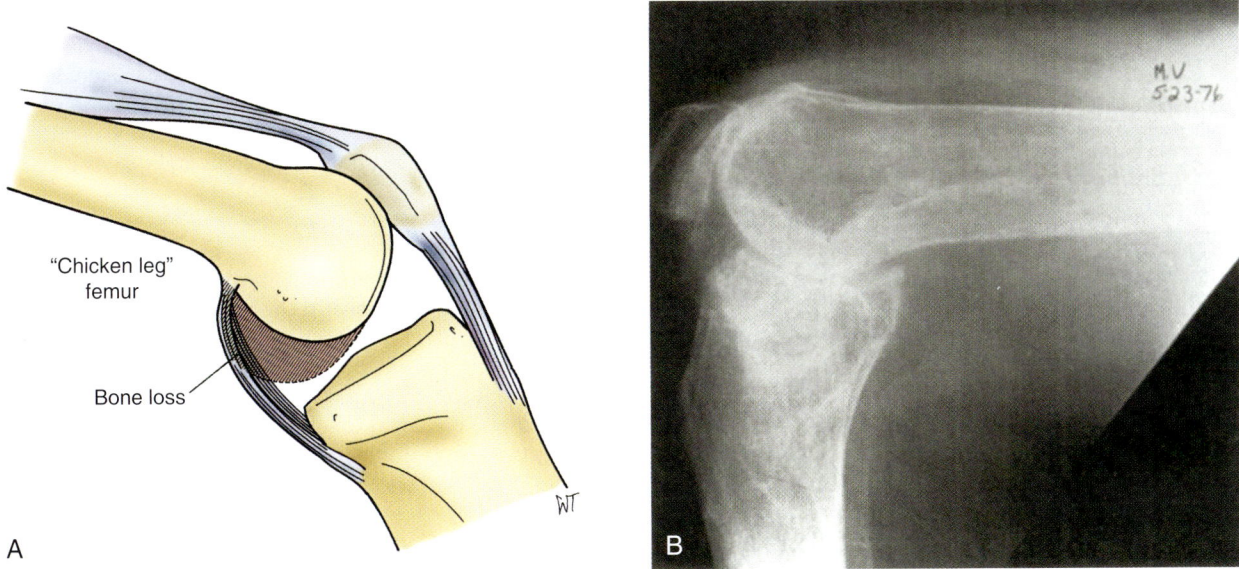

Figure 105-98. **A,** In rheumatoid arthritis, excessive loss of bone is evident on the posterior aspect of the femoral condyles. **B,** Lateral radiograph showing this condition. Unless the condition is recognized and the technique adjusted for it, flexion instability will result.

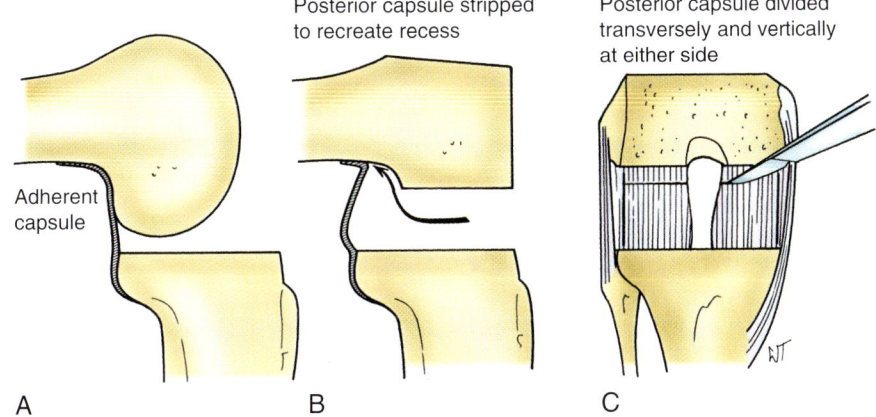

Figure 105-99. Posterior capsulotomy for flexion contracture. **A,** The posterior capsule is adherent. **B,** The original recess is re-established. **C,** The cruciate ligaments have already been excised; only the medial and lateral parts of the posterior capsule need division. Often the underlying gastrocnemii are adherent and must be divided as well. At the margin of the collateral ligaments, vertical incisions must be made in the capsule.

Technique for Release of Flexion Contracture

Posterior capsular release should be done after the bone cuts. Until the bone cuts are made, posterior visualization is impeded by the posterior femoral condyles. Initially, distal femoral and proximal tibial bone cuts should be conservative. Small flexion contractures can be reduced by removal of posterior osteophytes and elevation of the posterior capsule (Fig. 105-99).[199,201] Correction by bone resection from the distal femur alone unbalances the collateral ligaments so that stability in extension is provided by the tight posterior capsule, resulting in kinematic abnormalities. Posterior capsulotomy is the preferred method for moderate to severe contractures and should be performed with the knee flexed. First, the shortened posterior capsule is elevated from the central posterior aspect of the femur at the top of the intercondylar notch. Next, the medial and lateral capsule is elevated in a subperiosteal plane off the back of the femur. In more resistant cases, the capsule may be cut transversely and may be separated from collateral structures by vertical incisions made at the medial and lateral corners. Resection of the PCL may be necessary in severe flexion contracture cases and aids in division of the midline fibers. After the capsulotomy and posterior release, the trial knee components are inserted, and the knee is brought into as much extension as possible. If extension is still not complete, further bone can be removed from the distal femur. This procedure may require use of a constrained prosthesis when the collateral ligaments are removed from their origins, because extreme cases may require resection of so much bone that the knee becomes completely unbalanced. Surgery is followed by aggressive range of motion with an emphasis on extension in the immediate postoperative period.

EXTENSION CONTRACTURE ("STIFF KNEE")

Overview

Primary TKA in stiff and ankylosed knees, although technically demanding, has been shown to provide excellent pain relief and to significantly improve range of motion.[2,141,146] Stiff knees are typically defined as having less than 50 degrees of motion; ankylosed knees have essentially no motion (Fig. 105-100). Montgomery and associates[141] studied 82 stiff or ankylosed knees in 71 patients at an average follow-up of 5.3 years. Investigators noted an average Hospital for Special Surgery (HSS) knee score improvement of from 38 to 80 points and an average arc of motion improvement of from 36 degrees to 93 degrees. All prostheses were posterior stabilized, with most being nonconstrained. Only one quadricepsplasty was necessary. Two patients with flexion-valgus deformities developed peroneal nerve palsies that resolved spontaneously, and one patient had an inferior pole of the patellar fracture managed conservatively. This investigation is reflective of previous, smaller series,[2,146] although one series reported that quadricepsplasty was required in 42% of cases. More recently, Kim and colleagues[110] presented a series of 86 stiff knees undergoing TKA. This group also showed improvement in range of motion and in knee ratings, along with a 12% complication rate, most commonly related to skin necrosis.

Technique

The approach, as described by Montgomery and coworkers, is made using a midline longitudinal incision and a medial parapatellar arthrotomy. Typically, the techniques described in "Difficult Exposures" are necessary. Eversion of the patella is generally challenging and may not be possible or necessary. Early release of the lateral retinaculum and lateral patellofemoral ligaments is commonly performed. Soft tissue releases are performed in the same fashion as they are for the varus, valgus, and flexion deformities described earlier; however, extensive soft tissue releases are routinely required. In varus knees, an extensile proximal medial tibial release is performed, whereas valgus knees are managed with lateral release, occasionally including elevation of the LCL off the femoral side. Flexion contractures require posterior capsule release; because of its contribution to contractures, Insall

favored excision of the PCL. Occasionally, complete subperiosteal reflection of the soft tissues from the distal femur (femoral peel) is necessary (see Fig. 105-38). Adequate bone cuts are then made to create balanced flexion and extension gaps. Despite extensive releases, constrained prostheses typically are not required unless ligament stability is forfeited.

CORRECTION OF GENU RECURVATUM

Genu recurvatum is an uncommon deformity that is seldom severe except in poliomyelitis or certain soft tissue abnormalities such as Ehlers-Danlos. Operative correction is obtained by under-resection of the bone ends and use of thicker components. However, paralytic types tend to recur. Krackow[115] has described a technique whereby the proximal ligament insertions are transferred proximally and posteriorly; this repositioning causes the collateral ligaments to tighten in extension. Postoperative bracing or the use of a heel wedge to promote a flexion moment may enhance chances for success. Recurrent cases of recurvatum may constitute one of the few indications for the use of a hinged implant or a similarly constrained prosthesis. Occasionally after a previous tibial osteotomy, recurvatum will be noted because of deformity of the tibia itself (tibial recurvatum) (Fig. 105-101). The anterior cortices have impacted, and the result is an anterior slope to the tibia. This should be evident from a study of the radiographs, and the level of the tibial cut should be adjusted accordingly.

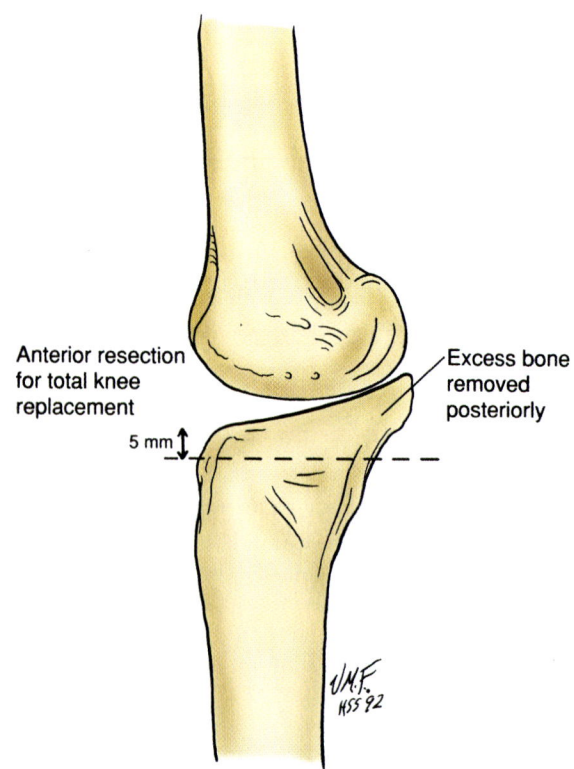

Figure 105-101. Tibial recurvatum after high tibial osteotomy. The osteotomy has healed with the distal fragment extended on the proximal, resulting in an anterior tilt to the anterior surface. Unless care is taken in performing the tibial resection for total knee replacement, excessive bone may be removed.

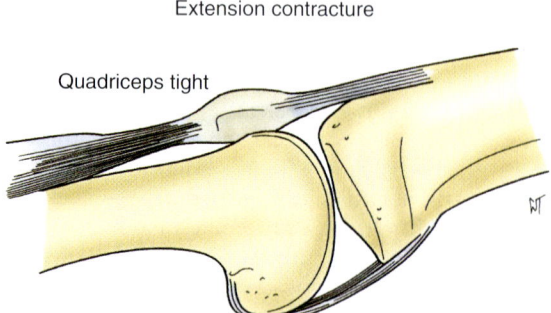

Figure 105-100. In an extension contracture, not only are intra-articular adhesions present, but the quadriceps muscle itself is shortened and tight.

MANAGEMENT OF BONE DEFECTS

Principles

Although bone defects are more common in revision TKA, they do occur in primary TKA. Causes of bone defects in primary TKA include erosion secondary to angular arthritic change, inflammatory arthritis, osteonecrosis, and fracture. Bone defects in primary TKA are typically asymmetrical and peripheral, although contained deficiencies caused by cyst formation may occur. The base of contained and peripheral defects in primary TKA typically comprises condensed sclerotic bone, in contrast to revision surgery, in which removal of components often leaves osteopenic surfaces. A major concern with tibial defects is that subchondral bone strength diminishes substantially distal to the subchondral plate.[12,83,95] Several authors have advised that the level of lateral tibial resection should not exceed 1 cm to avoid compromising implant durability,[52,160] yet others have demonstrated that proximal tibial bone strength is adequate to 20 mm.[76]

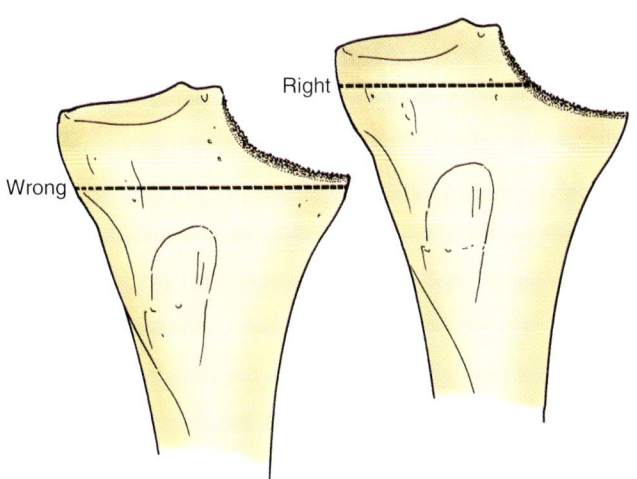

Figure 105-102. When asymmetrical bone loss occurs from the upper tibia, the tibial resection must not be too distal, but rather must be at the usual level.

Management

Various techniques are available to compensate for bone defects in primary TKA, including (1) translation of the component away from a defect, (2) lower tibial resection, (3) cement filling, (4) autologous bone graft, (5) allograft, (6) wedges or augments, and (7) custom implants. Use of stems in primary TKA is necessary when bone grafting is required or when the bone defect compromises fixation and renders the resurfacing component unstable without the added support of intramedullary fixation.

Lower Tibial Resection

A lower tibial resection is often effective in elimination of bony defects (Fig. 105-102). The limit of a lower tibial resection is the insertion of the ITB and infrapatellar ligament. When more than 10 mm of bone is removed, the resection must be proximal to Gerdy's tubercle, or else ITB function may be compromised. Additionally, a lower tibial resection will complicate component fit because of the natural taper of the tibia, necessitating the use of a smaller tibial component or tapered tibial augments.

Lateral Translation

Lateralizing a smaller tibial component may effectively eliminate a bony defect (see Fig. 105-58) by removing any contact of the implant with the defect.[99,129] However, the largest tibial tray size and polyethylene insert should always be favored to create the largest reasonable contact surface to distribute load.

Cement Filling

Lotke and associates[131] and Ritter[167] demonstrated satisfactory long-term results with cement fill (Fig. 105-103), provided tibial bone defects are no deeper than 20 mm and involve less than 50% of either plateau. Despite these results, other authors recommend that use of cement should be limited to smaller peripheral defects that do not compromise tibial component support, because biomechanical testing suggests that cement fill with or without screw reinforcement is an inferior method of defect management.[21] Clinical results have demonstrated that radiolucent lines are commonly observed under defects filled with cement.[50,100] Furthermore,

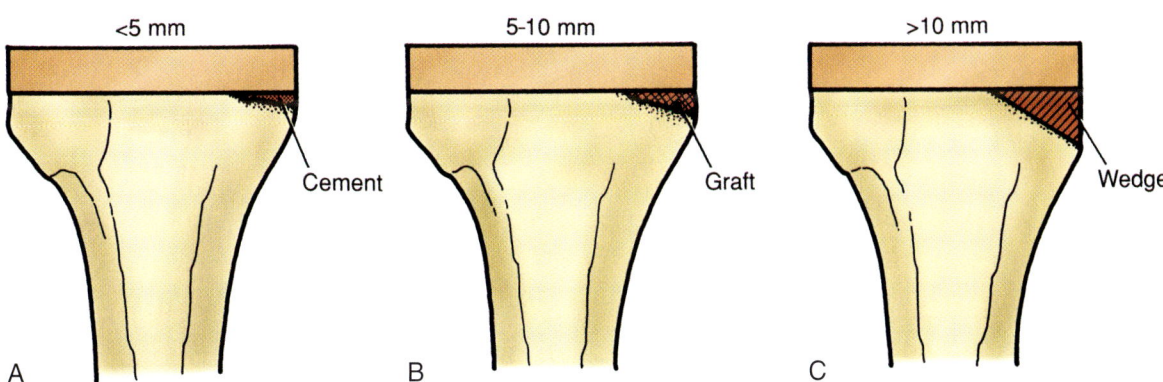

Figure 105-103. Bone defects are frequently seen in the medial tibia. It is incorrect to make the tibial cut at the base of the defect. It is correct to resect a normal amount from the upper tibia and fill the remaining defect. **A,** Defects smaller than 5 mm can be filled with cement. **B,** Defects between 5 and 10 mm are suitable for bone grafting. **C,** Defects larger than 10 mm are best treated with a metal wedge or augment.

larger volumes of cement introduce the risk of thermal necrosis of the cement-bone interface, and net cement shrinkage during polymerization may diminish the cement-prosthesis and cement-bone interface contact areas[21] (Fig. 105-104).

Bone Grafting

Autologous bone and allograft (Figs. 105-105 through 105-107) are readily available in primary TKA. Both have demonstrated high rates of incorporation that are particularly important in reestablishing proximal tibial bone strength and restoring bone stock, should revision surgery be required. Autografting generally is favored because of its osteoinductive properties and lack of potential disease transmission. Bone graft is typically used when the size criteria for cement fill are exceeded. Dorr and coworkers[53] identified criteria that promote improved outcome, as follows: (1) creation of a viable/bleeding bed of host bone, (2) proper fit and finish of

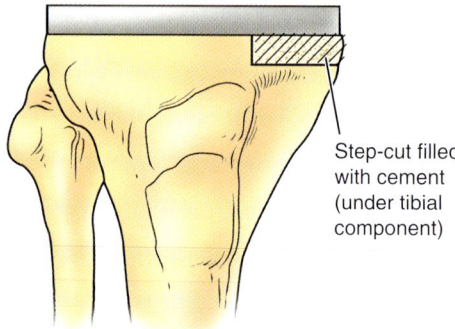

Step-cut filled with cement (under tibial component)

Figure 105-104. Step-cut technique for cement filling of a peripheral proximal tibial defect.

graft in host bed, (3) complete coverage of graft by the component to avoid graft resorption secondary to stress shielding, (4) optimal alignment of components for even load distribution, (5) limited weight bearing when larger grafts are used to allow for graft union, and (6) grafts protected with stems when required. Advantages of bone graft include its availability, its adaptability to size or shape of defect, and its biologic compatibility.[188]

Although contained defects are easily filled with bone graft, peripheral defects are more challenging. Several techniques have been developed using bone available during surgery from other areas of the knee to address peripheral defects. Dorr and associates[53] described success with a technique in which the peripheral defect is converted into a single oblique cut at the base of the deficiency and is filled using bone from the larger distal femoral condylar resection. The graft is secured to the oblique surface using screw fixation (see Fig. 105-106). Altcheck and colleagues[7] reported good to excellent results at an average follow-up of 4 years in 14 patients with severe angular deformity managed with this technique. All grafts had consolidated without evidence of collapse, resorption, or prosthetic subsidence. In contrast, Laskin[119] used the resected posterior femoral condyles as bone graft to fill tibial defects and concluded after a 5-year follow-up review that the long-term prognosis for this method of bone grafting was not satisfactory.

Insall originally described the inlay autogeneic bone-grafting technique. An interference fit for a contoured bone graft is created by converting the dish-shaped peripheral defect into a trapezoidal shape (see Fig. 105-107). Because of the interlocking fit, this method of bone grafting does not require fixation. Windsor et al[220] and later Scuderi et al[188] reviewed 26 primary TKAs treated using this technique, reporting 96% good to excellent results at an average

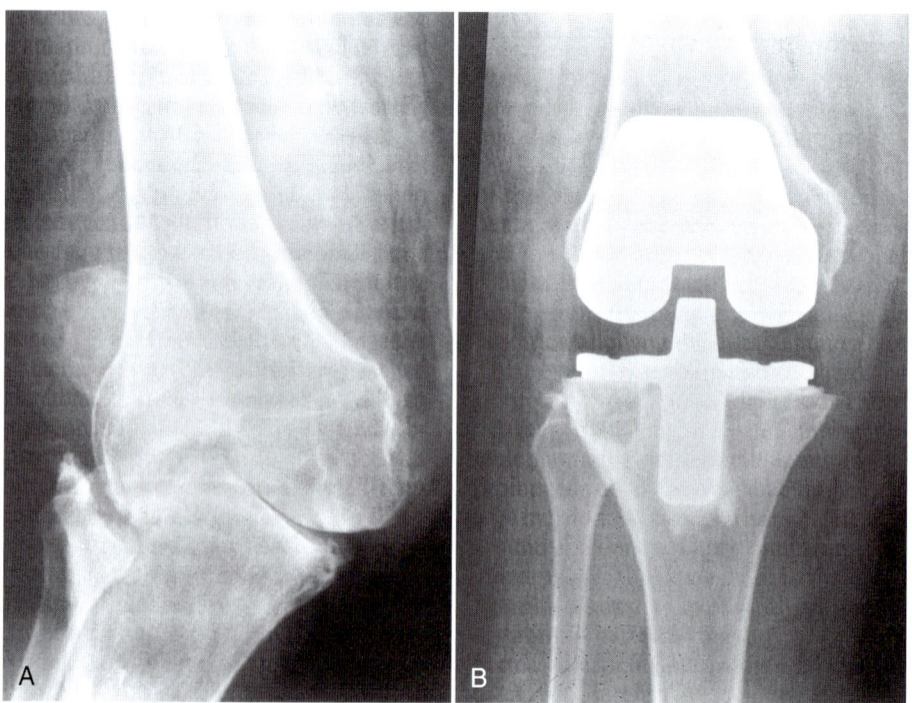

Figure 105-105. **A,** Radiograph showing large defect in lateral tibial plateau. **B,** Radiograph showing appearance after packing defect with cancellous bone graft. The graft can be autologous or homologous.

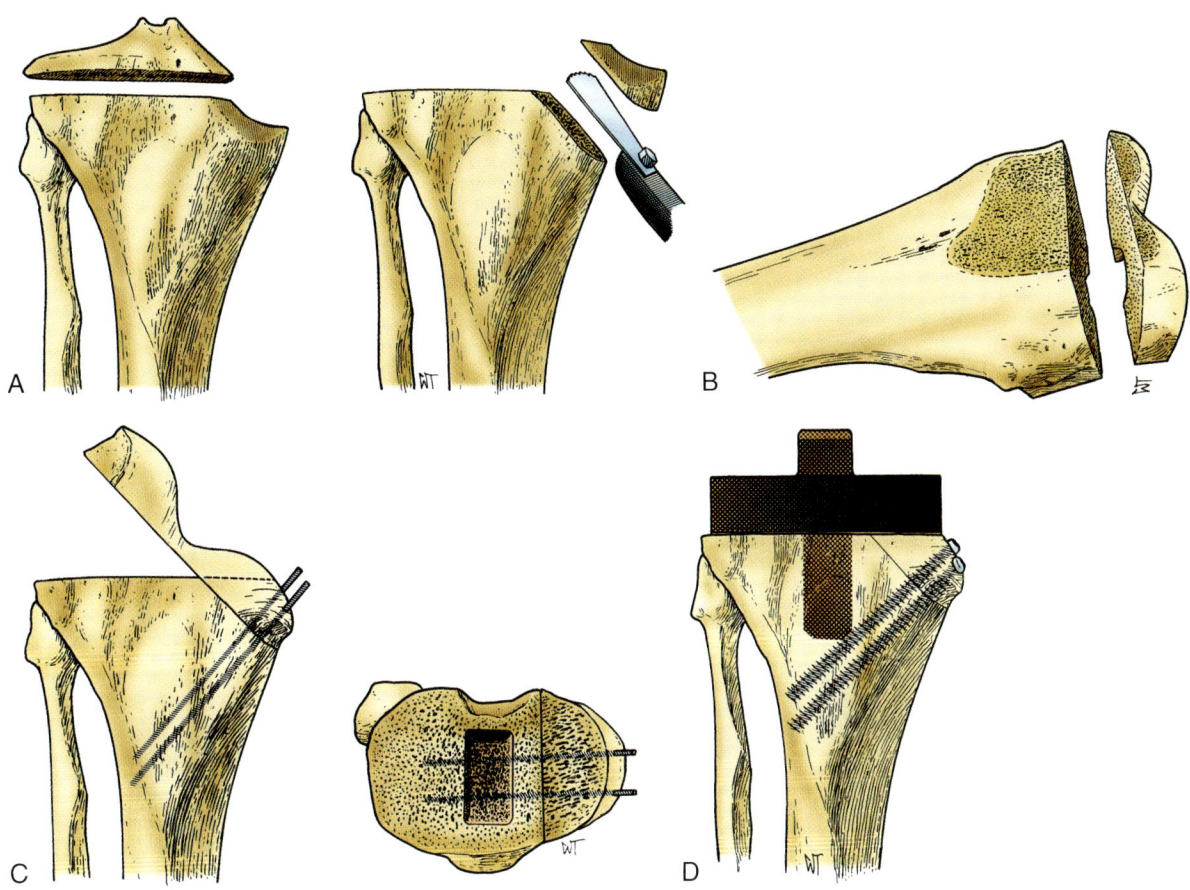

Figure 105-106. Bone graft technique. **A,** The tibia is resected at the usual level, leaving a medial defect. The sclerotic bone at the base of the defect is removed with a saw, exposing cancellous bone. **B,** The bone graft is obtained from the distal femoral resection. **C,** The femoral condyle is applied to the defect temporarily with Kirschner wires. The graft is resected at the level of the tibial cut. **D,** Kirschner wires are replaced by screws, and the tibial component is in place. (From Behrens JC, Walker PS, Shoji H: Variation in strength and structure of cancellous bone at the knee. J Biomech 7:201, 1974.)

follow-up of 3 years. Graft position medially or laterally did not influence the results. With restoration of anatomic knee alignment, no tibial component loosened and one medial bone graft collapsed.

Custom Prostheses and Metal Wedge Augmentation

Metal wedge augmentation permits intraoperative construction of a custom implant to address a bone defect, affording load transfer from the implant to the bone.[156] Custom prostheses (Figs. 105-108 through 105-111) are an option for dealing with larger defects[21]; however, custom prostheses have limitations of practicality and cost. Defects of less than 25 mm can be managed effectively with metal wedge augmentation.[20] Custom prostheses may be required for larger defects. Brooks and coworkers[21] demonstrated that metal wedge augmentation of tibial trays provided support similar to that provided by custom prostheses. Augments are available in triangular and rectangular shapes, in both cemented and cementless options. Although the mechanical support afforded by triangular[28] and rectangular wedges has been shown to be similar,[203] load transfer across a larger defect probably is best managed with a rectangular block[66] and stem augmentation[22,203] (see Fig. 105-109). Modular augments do introduce the potential for interface fretting; however, reports

have described good results using wedges attached with screw fixation.[181] In the series of Pagnano and associates of 24 primary cemented TKAs performed using metal wedge augmentation for tibial bone deficiency, clinical results were 96% good to excellent at an average follow-up of approximately 5 years.[156] Radiolucent lines at the cement-bone interface beneath the metal wedge were noted in 13 of 24 knees. Longer-term consequences of the radiolucencies are not known.

Authors' Preferred Method in the Management of Bone Defects

Tibial Defects

Contained Defects. When the bony defect, cavity, or cyst is enclosed within the bone, it is known as a contained defect. The treatment of choice is bone grafting, using local bone graft from the osteotomies. In the rare event that local autograft is insufficient, supplementary allograft may be added.

Peripheral Defects. Peripheral defects typically are located in the posteromedial aspect of the tibial plateau. Although small and intermediate-size defects are relatively shallow and elliptical and are bound anteriorly, medially, and posteriorly

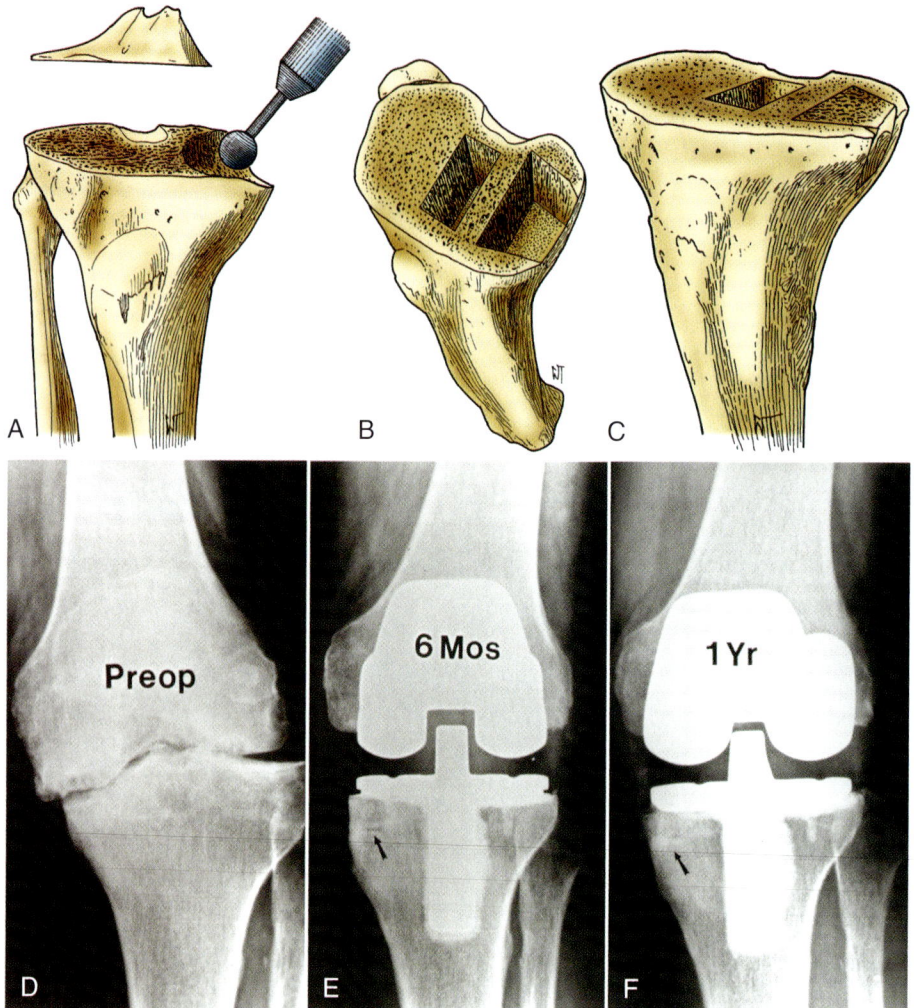

Figure 105-107. Autogenous tibial bone graft technique. **A,** The tibial defect is resected at the standard level. The remaining medial defect is reshaped with a burr. **B,** A trapezoidal defect is formed medially; usually, intact bone is present anteriorly and posteriorly to make this possible. **C,** A self-locking bone graft is fashioned to fit into the trapezoidal defect. The bone graft can be obtained through local resection in the knee; in the case of the posterior stabilized prosthesis, bone removed from the intercondylar notch serves as an ideal source. **D,** Preoperative radiograph of a medial defect. **E,** Radiograph taken 6 months after medial bone grafting using the interlocking technique. **F,** Bone graft after 1 year; arthroplasty appears to be fully incorporated.

by a solid rim of cortical bone, severe defects have a steeper pitch and may involve the entire medial plateau. Several management options are available:

1. If possible, translate the tibial tray away from the location of the peripheral defect. Although simple and attractive, this method results in use of a smaller polyethylene tray that may not distribute load as effectively as a larger tibial tray (see Fig. 105-58).[94,99]

2. If not deeper than 10 mm, the defect can be eliminated by resecting the tibia at a lower level. However, when a larger defect is present, the tibial resection can be increased up to 12 to 14 mm (see Fig. 105-102).

3. Defects smaller than 5 mm can be managed with cement. Cement performance can be enhanced by converting the dished defect into a rectangular shape with a horizontal base and three vertical borders. The defect base should be cleaned to permit cement interdigitation (see Fig. 105-103).

4. For defects measuring between 6 and 10 mm after the proximal tibial osteotomy is performed, bone graft is

utilized through the technique described by Dorr et al.[53] The inlay bone-grafting method[188] is preferred because it allows for an interference fit of the graft and does not require fixation that may interfere with tibial stem placement (see Fig. 105-107).

In situations with massive defects, alternative sources of bone graft (allograft) or metal augmentation are utilized. When bone can be used, the bone block is tapped into place and should fit snugly into the defect to prevent cement from entering the graft-tibia interface. In the technique of Dorr and colleagues, the anterior and posterior margins of the defect are excised to create a single oblique cut to the base of the tibial deficiency.[53] The base of the cut should comprise a bleeding cancellous surface. To fill this defect, local autograft is obtained from the larger condyle of the distal femoral resection that is rotated so that its cancellous surface is matched to the cancellous surface of the tibial defect. The junction of intact tibia and graft is occluded with supplemental bone graft to prevent cement from entering the space between the graft and the tibia.

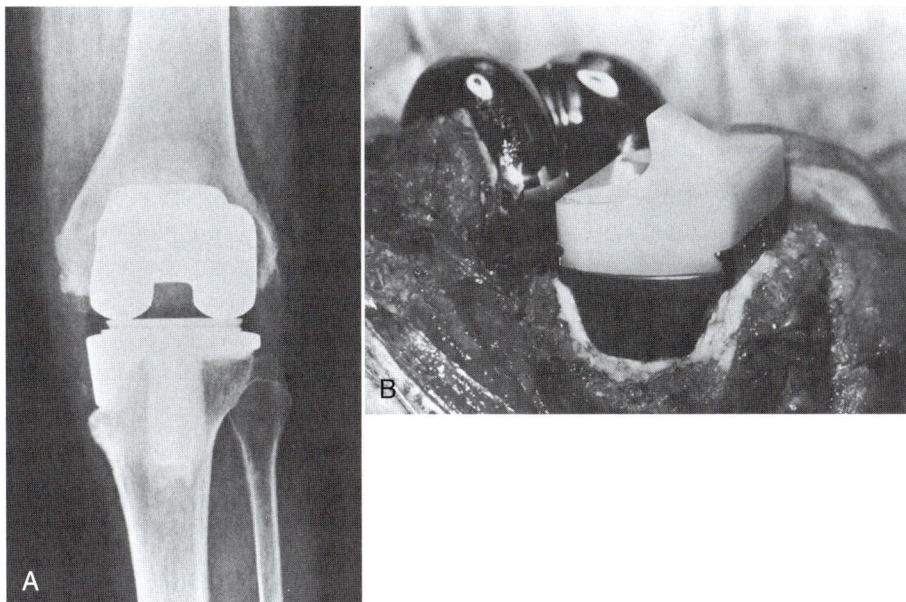

Figure 105-108. **A** and **B,** Asymmetrical bone loss should be compensated for by an asymmetrical tibial component.

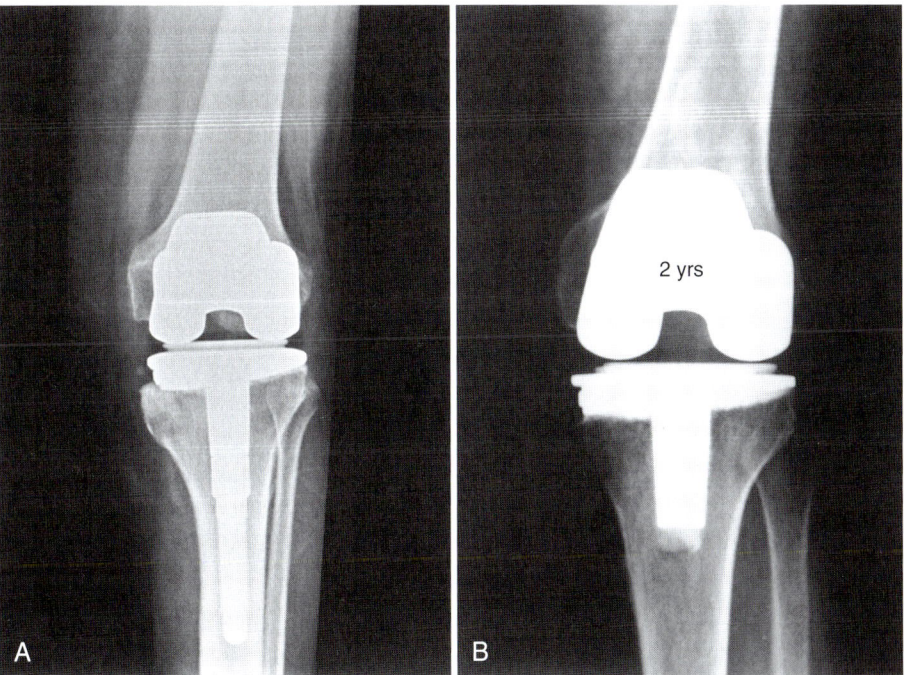

2 yrs

Figure 105-109. **A,** Full wedge applied to a tibial component for a medial tibial defect. In this case, an uncemented stem has been added. **B,** Full wedge applied to a tibial component. No stem extension has been added. It is not known at present whether a stem extension is necessary to resist possible shearing effects.

5. When inlay bone grafting with autogenous graft is not feasible, modular wedges or blocks attached to resurfacing prostheses may be used. To diminish shear forces, an intramedullary stem is added to the tibial component when a full or half oblique wedge is used.

Distal Femoral Defects

Contained Defects. Contained femoral defects are managed in the same manner as contained tibial defects.

Peripheral Defects. Surface or peripheral defects of the femur are categorized as (1) affecting the chamfer cuts, (2) affecting the distal surface, or (3) causing major bone loss. Loss of femoral condylar bone is most frequently observed in valgus deformities when the lateral femoral condyle is dysplastic. As with the tibia, defects can be managed with cement, bone graft, and metal augments.

Femoral deficiencies can be viewed in increasing stages of bone loss.

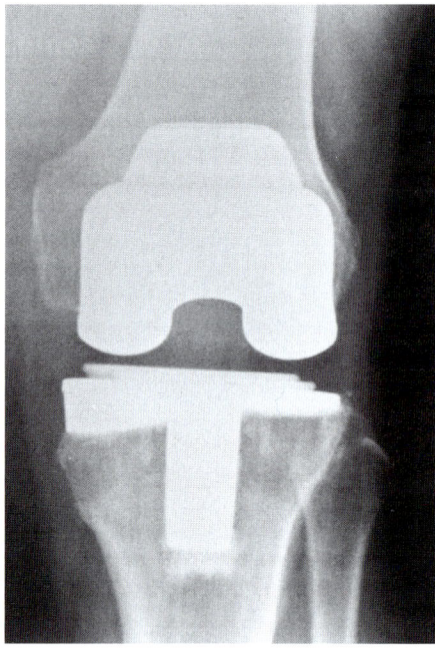

Figure 105-110. A modular medial wedge is attached to the prosthesis to fill a medial defect in the tibia.

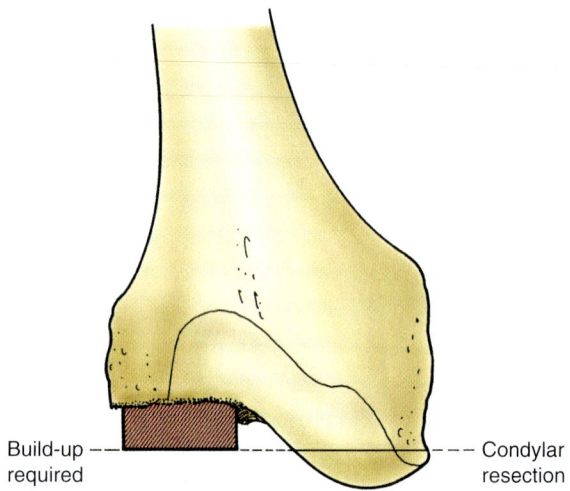

Figure 105-111. In some valgus knees, the level of femoral resection may pass distal to the lateral femoral condyle. Lateral augmentation of the femoral component is required.

- *Stage 1*
  Stage 1 is observed when the femoral osteotomy includes a portion of the lateral distal femur, but contouring to accommodate the femoral component results in chamfer "air cuts" anteriorly and posteriorly. In our experience, cement fill is acceptable for filling anterior and posterior spaces between bone and prosthesis. The sclerotic bone surface should be prepared to accept cement interdigitation.
- *Stage 2*
  Stage 2 occurs when the level of the femoral osteotomy passes distal to the lateral femoral condyle even without chamfer cuts. In this situation, cement fill typically is unsatisfactory unless combined with a femoral stem

extension. Even in this instance, a metal augment to the distal femur is preferred.
- *Stage 3*
  Stage 3 refers to massive bone loss of one femoral condyle. Substantial bone loss can be managed with allograft or metal block augmentation, which has been shown to incorporate well but requires a period of non–weight bearing postoperatively and a femoral stem extension. The advantage of allograft is that if a revision is required, bone stock may be partially restored. Metal augments allow quicker rehabilitation without restricted weight bearing. Posterior augmentation without distal augmentation is required in cases of posterolateral deficiency. This unusual situation is encountered in the rheumatoid patient with long-standing flexion contracture that results in posterior condylar erosion, and in cases of combined valgus and flexion deformity. Most cases requiring posterior augmentation are also deficient distally. In general, optimized collateral ligament stability and restoration of normal anatomy is preferable to the use of constrained prostheses.

INTRAOPERATIVE PROBLEMS AND THEIR SOLUTIONS (INSALL)

Many of the basic elements of technique, bone cutting, soft tissue balancing, and overall alignment have already been addressed. A few intraoperative situations remain to be discussed (Fig. 105-112):

1. The flexion gap is too small to admit the thinnest tibial component. If spacers are used, this error will be identified early on. It may be caused by under-resection of the proximal tibia or oversizing of the femoral component. Therefore, the size of the tibial fragment should be measured, and if 7 to 8 mm has already been removed from the normal side, then the problem lies in oversizing of the femur, and it will be necessary to recut the posterior femoral condyles so that one size smaller can be used.

2. The flexion gap is unequal—that is, tighter medially or laterally. The cause is an error in the tibial cut into varus or valgus, malrotation of the femoral component, or excessive ligament release. If the cause is either of the first two or insufficient release of a contracted structure, it should be corrected. However, sometimes the necessary medial or lateral release will cause an asymmetrical flexion gap that must be accepted. A larger than normal medial gap is not of clinical consequence, but an excessive lateral gap can lead to posterolateral subluxation. The soft tissues must be given time to adhere, which means pursuing postoperative flexion rehabilitation less vigorously than normal.

3. The extension gap is larger than the flexion gap (Fig. 105-113). This unusual situation is created by standard bone resection in a knee with excessive ligamentous laxity. A tensor obviates this occurrence because the need for femoral under-resection will be indicated; if one has committed to a standard femoral cut, the solution is to augment the distal femur (a thicker tibial component cannot be used because the flexion gap will not admit it). Augments on the distal femur usually require the use of a stemmed femoral component to get

Flexion   Extension

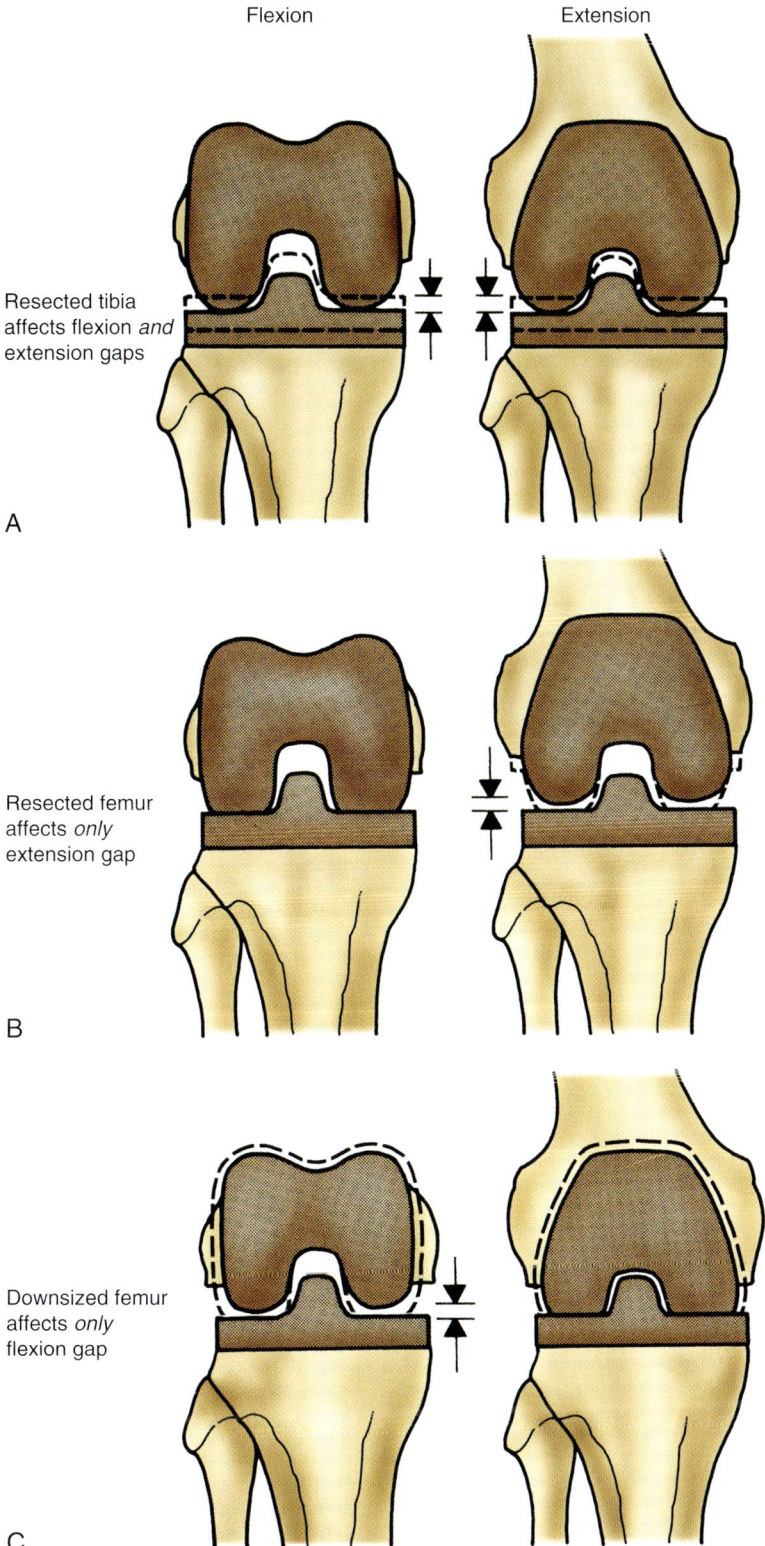

Resected tibia
affects flexion *and*
extension gaps

A

Resected femur
affects *only*
extension gap

B

Downsized femur
affects *only*
flexion gap

C

Figure 105-112. The effect of bone cuts on prosthetic fit. **A,** The level of tibial resection affects flexion and extension gaps equally. Under-resection of the tibia will make the joint tight in both positions. Over-resection of the tibia can be compensated for by using a thicker tibial component. **B,** Distal resection of the femur affects only the extension gap, which may cause instability in extension. If the knee is too tight in flexion to admit a thicker tibial component, distal femoral buildup is the solution. **C,** Over-resection of the femur in the sagittal plane affects only the flexion gap, causing laxity in flexion. This cannot be overcome by a thicker tibial component because the knee will be too tight in extension. A solution is *(1)* to restore the proper sagittal dimension of the femur by using a larger femoral component with a posterior buildup, or *(2)* to resect additional distal femur. The former is preferred.

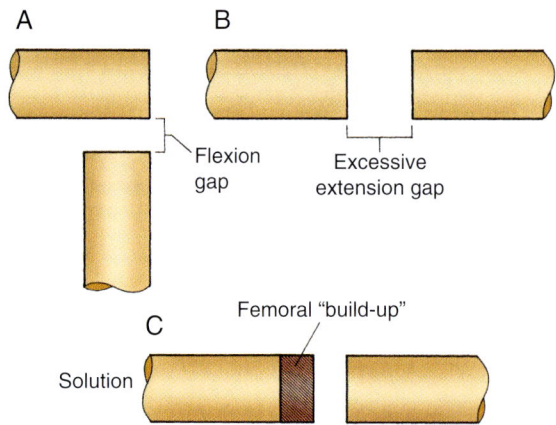

Figure 105-113. When the extension gap is too large, equalization cannot be attained by further bone resection. The prosthesis must be built up on the femoral side.

proper fixation. The laxity must be symmetrical and limited to a few millimeters of passive motion. No "thrust" on weight bearing is permissible. Conversely, the components should not be so tight as to produce a flexion contracture.

4. The patella cannot be made to track in spite of an extensive lateral retinacular release. Causes include (1) femoral malrotation, (2) tibial malrotation, and (3) an overly thick patella. The latter two causes are readily correctable, but the first is more difficult and will result in a poor fit of the femoral component. Recutting the femur in additional external rotation and adding a posterolateral augment can remedy the first situation. A stemmed component and cement are needed to attain adequate fixation.

5. Alignment, fit, and motion with the trial components are satisfactory, but this is not so when the final components are inserted. There are several reasons for this:

   a. The knee does not reach full extension. The probable explanation is that the femoral component has been put on flexed, so it is sitting proud of the bone. This problem has been virtually eliminated with the use of pegs that engage the femur, ensuring proper sagittal position of the femoral component. Careful placement of the final component is required when pegs are not available.

   b. The knee is too loose in extension after satisfactory trial reduction. This can happen even with a proper fit because the finished components are polished and become slightly less bulky than the trials; adjustment to the thickness of the tibial component will remedy the situation. A more serious occurrence is when the femoral component has been driven into soft rheumatoid or osteoporotic bone. A thicker tibial component may upset the flexion-extension balance, and a stemmed femoral component, possibly with augments, may be needed to restore the proper femoral position.

   c. Varus/valgus alignment and balance are incorrect. This is also due to compacting of one or the other of the components (usually the femoral component) asymmetrically into soft bone. The correction is the same as previously described. When the final

cementation is performed, it is important to hold the leg so it does not fall into the preoperative deformity or create component lift-off while the cement hardens.

   d. Patellar tracking is unsatisfactory. The cause is insertion of the final components in a different position to the trials. This usually happens when the bone is soft, and it is most likely to happen when a central stem tibial design is used and the tibial component is allowed to spin into internal rotation. It is, of course, correctable but can be prevented if the position of the tibial trial on the tibia is marked with methylene blue, so that the surgeon can be certain that both the trial and the final components are correctly inserted.

   e. Excessive bleeding occurs. Opinions differ about the timing of tourniquet release or even on whether to release it at all. Studies have showed blood loss to be similar with and without tourniquet release. Tourniquet release serves two purposes: (1) occasional profuse bleeding, usually from the lateral genicular artery, can be secured (see Figure 105-48), and (2) blood flow may not return through an arteriosclerotic femoral artery when the tourniquet is let down. This is usually due to clotting in the femoral artery, and if treated early has an uneventful outcome. Release of the tourniquet alerts the surgeon to this possibility, whereas identification of this potentially catastrophic event may be delayed in the recovery room.

AFTERCARE OF TOTAL KNEE ARTHROPLASTY

At the conclusion of the operation, a bulky cotton dressing or compression stocking is applied to limit extremity swelling. A postoperative drain is left in place for approximately 24 to 36 hours. The bulky dressing is removed on the first postoperative day. Some surgeons prefer to apply a lighter dressing and to initiate continuous passive motion in the recovery room, with use of simultaneous continuous passive motion machines in bilateral cases. The patient is encouraged to flex the knee as much as is tolerated; recent investigations suggest that high flexion in the immediate postoperative period accelerates postoperative rehabilitation and is not associated with wound complications.[105]

With a cemented knee, full weight bearing under the supervision of a therapist is allowed on the first or second postoperative day. Some surgeons recommend protected weight bearing even when cement is used from the perspective of patient comfort. Progression of walking is variable and age dependent, and walking is initially done with a walker until the patient is steady enough to use canes. General muscle exercises are for the feet and ankles, and isometric exercises are for the thigh and buttock muscles. Bicycle exercises are most useful as soon as the patient has sufficient flexion. Particularly motivated patients are placed on a "fast track" and will initiate ambulation on the afternoon of surgery. Regional anesthesia has improved pain management. The ideal block is titrated to allow motor function while moderating pain, allowing for rapid conversion to oral pain medication and avoidance of intravenous or intramuscular narcotics. Care must be taken to protect patients from falls when femoral nerve blocks and other peripheral nerve blocks are employed.

EMERGING TECHNOLOGIES IN SURGICAL TECHNIQUE

Minimally Invasive Total Knee Arthroplasty

Recent experience with minimally invasive surgery for unicondylar knee arthroplasty has stimulated interest in applying those basic principles to total knee replacement. The goals of minimally invasive surgery include patient satisfaction, less patient discomfort, less intraoperative blood loss, fewer inpatient days, and faster recovery, without compromising outcome. These goals are currently being investigated through such techniques as a less extensive arthrotomy, smaller cutting jigs, and instrumentation that allows cuts to be made without everting the patella. Tria and Coon[206] published early results from their series of 70 minimally invasive TKAs showing trends toward decreased blood loss and hospital stay, with no statistical difference in radiographic alignment of the components when compared with a group of patients with a standard arthrotomy.

Sustained interest in this approach will require demonstration of the positive treatment benefits, because limitations and potential drawbacks such as component malposition, retained cement, poor wound healing, and infection have been reported in association with minimally invasive procedures. Future directions for investigation into this technique include guidelines for patient selection (e.g., degree of deformity, leg circumference, patients who can tolerate longer surgical times), quantification of blood loss between different techniques, and development of a clinical tool to measure the hypothetical faster recovery.

Computer-Assisted Surgery

Computer-assisted navigation in TKA is an emerging technology that seeks to improve clinical outcome and implant survival by improving the reliability of bone cuts and component positioning. Computer-assisted navigation systems attempt to eliminate outliers in component positioning. Three main types of systems are available: image-free navigation, image-based navigation, and robotic systems. Image-free systems use information regarding range of motion and position of the lower extremity, gathered intraoperatively, to assist with component placement. Image-based navigation uses information obtained from preoperative computer tomography on intraoperative fluoroscopy. Robotic systems use machines to guide the surgeon during portions of the procedure.

Over the past several years, as the technology has gone through a number of upgrades and improvements, studies in the literature have compared results from computer-assisted surgery versus those of conventional techniques. Chauhan and associates[29] performed a prospective randomized trial on 70 patients to compare these two methods, using an image-free navigation system and postoperatively evaluating alignment using a computed tomography (CT) protocol. That study showed statistically significant improvements in the computer-assisted group with varus/valgus and rotational alignment of the femoral component, as well as varus/valgus rotation and a posterior slope of the tibial component. Computer-assisted surgery took an average of 13 minutes longer but resulted in statistically significantly less blood loss. Although studies such as this one have shown improved accuracy, the impact of computer-assisted navigation on long-term clinical outcomes and implant survival remains unproven.

KEY REFERENCES

Berger RA, Crossett LS, Jacobs JJ, et al: Malrotation causing patellofemoral complications after total knee arthroplasty. Clin Orthop Relat Res 356:144, 1998.

Berger RA, Rubash HE, Seel MJ, et al: Determining the rotational alignment of the femoral component in total knee arthroplasty using the epicondylar axis. Clin Orthop Relat Res 286:40, 1993.

Chen F, Krackow KA: Management of tibial defects in total knee arthroplasty: a biomechanical study. Clin Orthop Relat Res 305:249, 1994.

Dennis DA, Komistek RD, Mahfouz MR: In vivo fluoroscopic analysis of fixed-bearing total knee replacements. Clin Orthop Relat Res 410:114, 2003.

Fehring TK, Peindl RD, Humble RS, et al: Modular tibial augmentations in total knee arthroplasty. Clin Orthop Relat Res 327:207, 1996.

Kim YH, Kim JS, Choi Y, Kwon OR. Computer-assisted surgical navigation does not improve the alignment and orientation of the components in total knee arthroplasty. J Bone Joint Surg Am 91:14, 2009.

Nagamine R, Whiteside LA, White SE, et al: Patellar tracking after total knee arthroplasty: the effect of tibial tray malrotation and articular surface configuration. Clin Orthop Relat Res 304:262, 1994.

Pagnano MW, Hanssen AD, Lewallen DG, et al: Flexion instability after primary posterior cruciate retaining total knee arthroplasty. Clin Orthop Relat Res 356:39, 1998.

Poilvache PL, Insall HN, Scuderi GR, et al: Rotational landmarks and sizing of the distal femur in total arthroplasty. Clin Orthop Relat Res 331:35, 1996.

Ritter MA, Faris PM, Keating EM, Meding JB: Postoperative alignment of total knee replacement: its effect on survival. Clin Orthop Relat Res 299:153, 1994.

Ritter MA, Stringer EA: Predictive range of motion after total knee replacement. Clin Orthop Relat Res 143:115, 1979.

Scott RD, Chmell MJ: Balancing the posterior cruciate ligament during cruciate-retaining fixed and mobile-bearing total knee arthroplasty: description of the pull-out lift-off and slide-back tests. J Arthroplasty 23:605, 2008.

Wasielewski RC, Galante JO, Leighty RM, et al: Wear patterns on retrieved polyethylene tibial inserts and their relationship to technical considerations during total knee arthroplasty. Clin Orthop Relat Res 299:31, 1994.

Whiteside LA: Correction of ligament and bone defects in total arthroplasty of the severely valgus knee. Clin Orthop Relat Res 288:234, 1993.

Whiteside LA, Ohl MD: Tibial tubercle osteotomy for exposure of the difficult total knee arthroplasty. Clin Orthop Relat Res 260:6, 1990.

Full references for this chapter can be found on www.expertconsult.com.

Correction of Fixed Deformities With Total Knee Arthroplasty

Andrea Baldini and Paolo Aglietti

Correction of deformity is a main goal after total knee arthroplasty (TKA). Full correction means reestablishment of a neutral mechanical axis with a balanced ligamentous envelope of the joint. When deformity is fixed and nonreducible, correction is more difficult to achieve. In arthritic knees, deformity becomes fixed when the disease is at a late stage of its natural history. Some degree of bone erosion is often present at the concave side of the deformity, where ligaments and knee capsule are contracted. Bone erosion or condylar dysplasia usually involves one knee compartment, leading to an asymmetrical configuration of the joint relative to the flexion-extension axis of the knee. The opposite, convex side of the joint is affected by tension forces and may be stretched to varying degrees. Fixed deformities are rarely limited to a single plane. Significant varus or valgus malalignment on the coronal plane is very often associated with sagittal plane (e.g., flexion contracture) and torsional deformities. Correction of the deformity with the TKA procedure should be done as completely as possible, because no residual degree of a fixed deformity will be successfully addressed by postoperative means.

PREOPERATIVE PLANNING

Clinical Assessment

It is helpful to recognize preoperatively the abnormal gait patterns of patients with fixed deformities of the knee. Patients with varus knees and high adduction moments without flexion contracture, experiencing an evident lateral thrust at heel strike, will show elongated lateral soft tissues intraoperatively. The medial release that these deformities need to match the elongated lateral side will generate automatic opening of the flexion and extension gaps. Standard tibial bone resection in this scenario will result in larger gaps, which need to be filled by thicker polyethylene inserts.

Patients with valgus knees and a planovalgus foot walking with a high abduction moment at the knee are prone to stretch the medial collateral ligament after TKA if not overcorrected, and if the foot deformity is not addressed by surgery or insoles.[22] In bilateral fixed valgus deformity after one side is corrected with TKA, the other valgus nonoperated knee may push the operated leg in a high adduction moment. If a nonconstrained implant was used and an extensive lateral release was performed, the adduction moment created by the contralateral limb may predispose to a varus angulation, as in a windswept deformity. In bilateral significant fixed flexion contracture deformity, when one side is addressed by TKA, the other flexed and shortened limb will drive the operated leg in flexion again. Careful planning with bilateral simultaneous or short-term staged procedures, when possible, and precautions against flexion contracture recurrence are mandatory. Neuromuscular disorders with low or absent

quadriceps activity remain a relative contraindication to TKA; if a patient with this disorder undergoes a TKA procedure, the surgeon will have to address the patient's need to walk with some residual recurvatum while working with the biomechanical properties of the implant.

Radiographic Assessment

The surgeon should identify the presence and magnitude of osteophytes. If prominent, they may tent capsule and ligaments enough to avoid correctability of the deformity. Osteophyte removal may sometimes be sufficient to achieve balance. Beware of significant fixed flexion deformities without associated hypertrophic osteophytes. In this scenario, the surgeon may need more extensile soft tissue work on the posterior capsule and gastrocnemius insertions.

Extra-articular diaphyseal or metadiaphyseal deformities are often associated with the development of fixed deformities at the knee joint. Preoperative planning should analyze the possibility of correcting the deformity at the joint level with generous bone resections and ligament releases, or whether a combined osteotomy is needed.

Intra-articular bone deformities can be recognized preoperatively. Ipoplasia of the lateral femoral condyle in valgus knees and the possible need for augmentation should be identified. With ipertrophic medial femoral condyles in knees with a metaphyseal varus deformity, a preoperative kneeling view or computed tomography (CT) scan may prove beneficial to establish the amount of rotational correction needed to achieve a stable and rectangular flexion gap.[23,27]

The femoral entry point for intramedullary instruments should be planned on both coronal and sagittal x-ray views to avoid mistakes in the amount of angular correction achieved. A common mistake in large canals is to use a low entry point and the wrong reaming direction in the sagittal plane, resulting in a flexed position of the femoral component.

FIXED VARUS DEFORMITY

Techniques described to correct fixed varus deformity include the so-called gap technique and the measured resection technique.[10,13] Differences between these two techniques are presented in Table 106-1. As described by Whiteside and associates, correction of a varus knee with the gap technique may result in residual varus alignment in flexion.[11,29] A 90-degree resection of the tibia without, or with minimal, medial collateral release is followed by soft tissue tension in flexion using tensiometers, which internally rotate the femur (Fig. 106-1A and B). A rectangular flexion gap is then obtained with an externally rotated femoral bone resection parallel to the tibia (see Fig. 106-1B). When the femur derotates in its original position, the knee joint in flexion will be malaligned again in varus (see Fig. 106-1C). Our technique of choice is a combination of the gap technique and the measured resection technique as described by Insall.[14] Standard bone resections are performed with different bone landmarks in extension and flexion, while contracted ligaments are released incrementally. Gap equalization is then checked with laminar spreaders, blocks, and trial components.[14]

Table 106-1 Main Technical Differences Between Soft Tissue Tension and Measured Resection Techniques

	TECHNIQUES	
	Soft Tissue Tension (Gap Technique)	Measured Resections
Tibia first	Yes	Independent
Ligament release	No to minimal	As needed
Femoral bone resection	Variable	Fixed

Bone resections are performed according to the preoperative template on the long wb films. Tibial cutting jig positioning should be done according to the talus center distally and the plateau-to-anatomic axis intersection proximally. In constitutional metaphyseal varus deformities, the proximal center of the tibial cutting jig is usually facing the lateral tibial plateau spine (Fig. 106-2). On the femoral side, angulation of the intramedullary cutting guide for valgus correction is established by measuring the divergence between the anatomic and mechanical femoral axes. Failure in achieving varus correction to neutral ±3 degrees is related to a greater incidence of loosening at medium- to long-term follow-up.[4]

As part of the approach, some initial medial release is performed. With the knee joint in slight flexion, incision of the anterior horn of the medial meniscus allows subperiosteal elevation of a medial flap of tissue, which includes the meniscotibial fibers of the deep medial collateral ligament (MCL). Proximal tibial insertion of the superficial MCL is often involved in the subperiosteal elevation of the medial soft

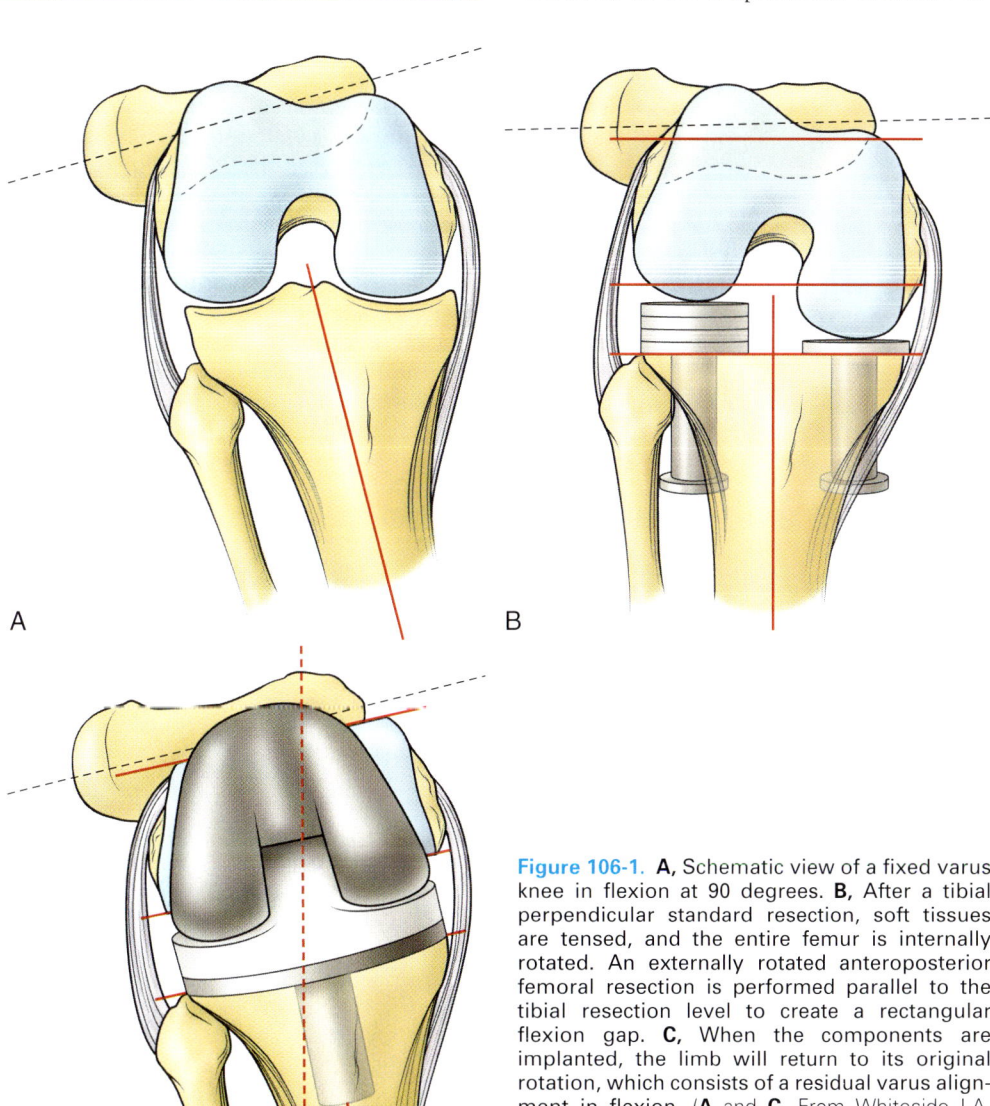

A

B

C

Figure 106-1. A, Schematic view of a fixed varus knee in flexion at 90 degrees. **B,** After a tibial perpendicular standard resection, soft tissues are tensed, and the entire femur is internally rotated. An externally rotated anteroposterior femoral resection is performed parallel to the tibial resection level to create a rectangular flexion gap. **C,** When the components are implanted, the limb will return to its original rotation, which consists of a residual varus alignment in flexion. (**A** and **C,** From Whiteside LA, Saeki K, Mihalko WM: Functional medial ligament balancing in total knee arthroplasty. Clin Orthop Relat Res 380:45–57, 2000; Whiteside LA: Varus knee. In Ligament balancing in total knee arthroplasty: an instructional manual, Berlin, 2004, Springer-Verlag, pp 32–62.)

tissue flap as part of the exposure.[19] The second step is to sublux the tibia forward in flexion and external rotation (the so-called RanSall maneuver, from its originators Ranawat and Insall). In advanced deformities, the worn tibial medial plateau develops a concave "pagoda" shape in which the femoral condyle is embedded, leading to a difficult tibial

dislocation maneuver that may arm the MCL. In these cases, we suggest violating the posterior tibial osteophyte with the tibia still in situ by using a straight osteotome between femur and tibia at 90 degrees of flexion (Fig. 106-3). After joint exposure, both tibial and femoral osteophytes are removed. Proximal tibial and distal femoral cuts are performed. Anteroposterior femoral resections are performed with a rotational position of the cutting jig, according to multiple bone landmarks such as the Whiteside line, the transepicondylar axis, and the posterior condylar line. In cases where more than 3 degrees of external rotation with respect to the posterior condylar line is required, we suggest switching the pivot point of the cutting guide from the center of the knee, as usual, to the medial condyle.[26] Pivoting the femoral guide at the center of the femur would create an over-resection of the posterior medial femoral condyle, which may lead to excessive "paradoxical" opening of the medial gap in flexion in a varus knee (Fig. 106-4A and B). The stretched lateral compartment will be better filled in flexion and anterolateral notching will be avoided if few degrees of flexion in the distal femoral cut are applied.

We prefer to remove the posterior cruciate ligament (PCL) and to use a posterior substituting implant for these advanced deformities. We believe that the PCL is part of these deformities. By removing the PCL, it is easier to address complex ligament balancing and to guarantee a reproducible, nonerratic postoperative pattern of kinematics.[20] Only in advanced flexion contracture will PCL removal selectively open the flexion gap farther. This 2 to 3 mm gap opening can be filled by adding a few degrees of flexion to the femoral component, and by switching the femoral component rotational pivot point from central to medial.[3]

Calibrated laminar spreaders and spacer blocks can now be used to check gap symmetry both in flexion and in

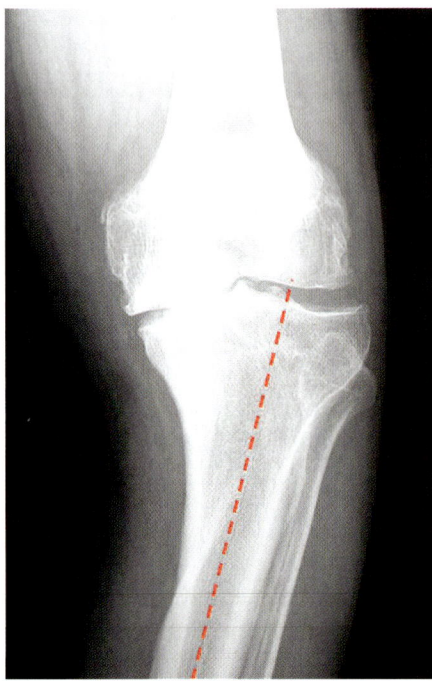

Figure 106-2. In metaphyseal varus deformed knees, anatomic and mechanical axes of the tibia have their proximal centers at the lateral tibial spine level.

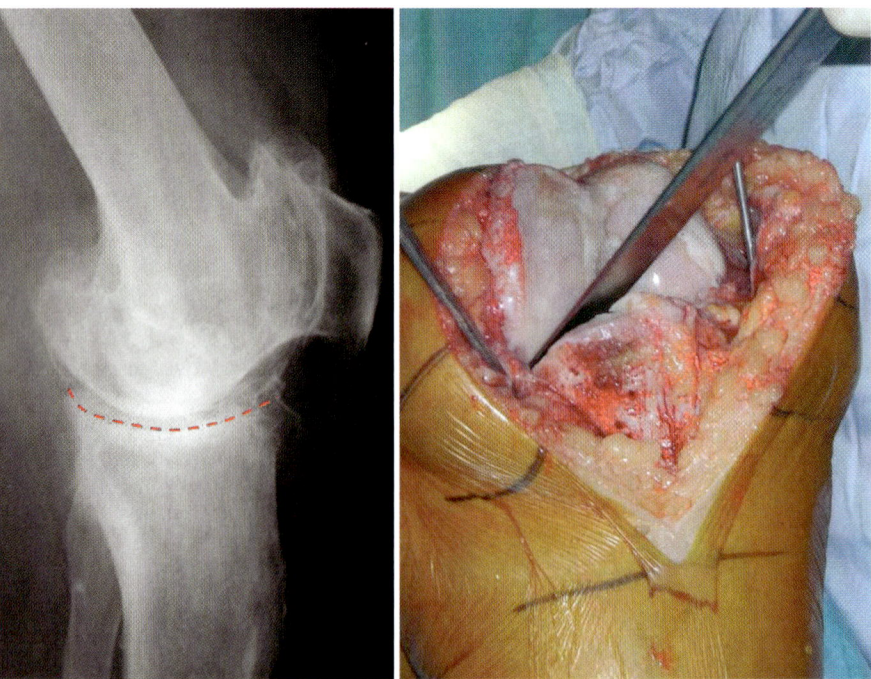

Figure 106-3. Advanced medial wear in varus knees may produce a sagittal "pagoda-shaped" deformity, with the medial femoral condyle embedded in the worn medial tibial plateau. Posterior tibial osteophytes, which constrain anterior tibial dislocation, can be violated using a straight osteotome with the tibia still in situ.

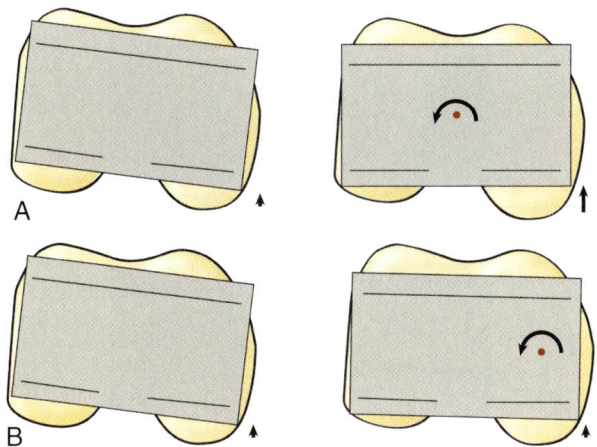

Figure 106-4. **A,** Femoral external rotation with a central pivot decreases the amount of posterior lateral condyle resection and increases the amount of posterior medial condyle resection. **B,** If the femoral resection guide pivot point is medially based, the posterior medial resection will not change with external rotation.

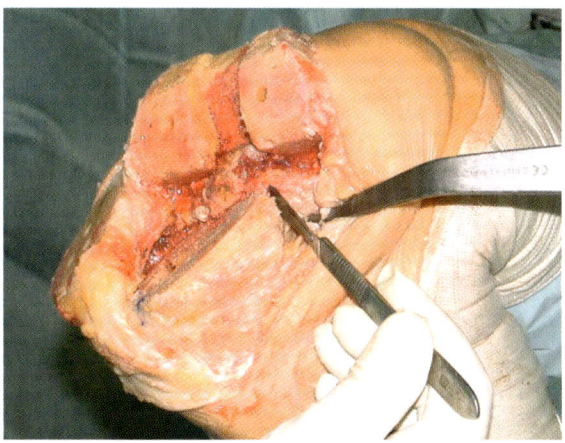

Figure 106-5. Semimembranosus tendon subperiosteal release with the knee joint in "figure four," with combined flexion, adduction, and external rotation.

extension. In fixed deformities, it is common, in this phase of the procedure, to face the need for additional medial release for residual varus in extension. This is particularly evident if a combined fixed flexion deformity is present. The following soft tissue structures will be involved in the incremental medial release to balance the extension gap: the posterior capsule, the posteromedial corner with the posterior oblique ligament (POL), the semimembranosus (SM) direct tibial insertion, and the posterior fibers of the superficial MCL (Table 106-2).[30] All these structures can be released with the knee in flexion. Using laminar spreaders, the posterior capsule can be addressed by a periosteal elevator from the femoral side. By holding the knee in deep flexion and applying a posterior drawer to the proximal tibia, it is possible to access the femoral insertion of the posterior capsule with a periosteal elevator. The posteromedial corner of the knee is safely exposed while the joint is held in the "figure four" position, with the foot externally rotated (Fig. 106-5). All of the tibial medial metaphysis is easily exposed, progressively involving the POL and SM insertions up to the posterior midline. If some residual medial tension remains, the distal insertion of the superficial MCL can be released from its posterior aspect in flexion or in extension. To reach this distal broad insertion, the elevator should be deepened distally on the tibial diaphysis at least 8 to 10 cm from the joint line. Alternatively, the MCL could be pie-crusted with a 16-gauge needle with multiple punctures, but progression of this type of release is not always achievable.[9] In advanced fixed varus deformities, it is helpful to select a relatively small tibial size to lateralize the tibial component and remove the exposed medial sclerotic bone, which is tenting the medial structures both in extension and in flexion (Fig. 106-6).[7] The resultant effect is similar to osteophyte removal, with a reduced need for ligamentous release. Paradoxical medial gap opening in flexion after ligament balancing may now indicate a technical mistake. The surgeon should recheck for a possible excessive external femoral rotation, a varus tibial resection, or full-thickness damage to the superficial MCL.

With trial components inserted, a final flexion-extension balance check is performed. Cases with preoperative advanced

Table 106-2 Medial and Lateral Soft Tissue Structures of the Knee and Their Involvement in Flexion and Extension Gap Tension

	Extension Gap	Flexion Gap
Medial Structures		
Superficial MCL (anterior fibers)	−	+
Superficial MCL (posterior fibers)	+	−
Deep MCL	+	+
Posterior oblique ligament	+	−
Semimembranosus tendon	+	−
Pes anserinus tendons	+	−
Posteromedial capsule	+	−
Medial gastrocnemius head	+	−
Lateral Structures		
Iliotibial band	+	−
Anterior iliotibial band fibers + Lateral retinaculum	−	+
Popliteal tendon	−	+
Lateral collateral ligament	+	+
Biceps tendon	+	−
Posterolateral capsule	+	−
Lateral gastrocnemius head	+	−

MCL, Medial collateral ligament.

disease showing lateral tibiofemoral subluxation and rotational deformity may experience popliteal tendon retraction, which snaps over the lateral femoral component condyle during flexion-extension. The popliteal tendon insertion can be partially released from its femoral attachment to avoid postoperative painful lateral snapping symptoms.

FIXED VALGUS DEFORMITY

Classification of deformity for valgus knees considers a fixed noncorrectable deformity with some medial soft tissue stretching as type II.[17] Type III valgus deformity is severe osseous deformity seen after a prior osteotomy with an incompetent medial soft tissue sleeve. We believe it is possible to safely

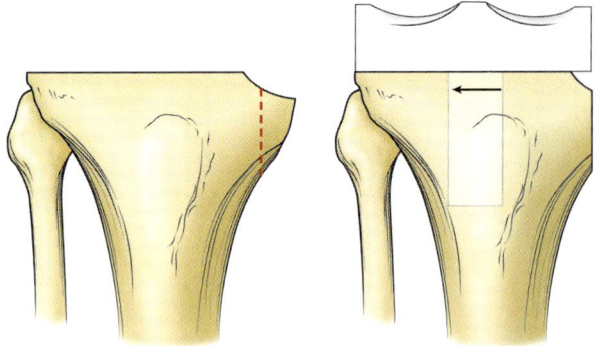

Figure 106-6. Tibial component undersizing and lateralization. The resultant effect is to reduce the amount of medial bone defect while decreasing tension on the medial soft tissue sleeve. (From Dixon MC, Parsch D, Brown RR, Scott RD: The correction of severe varus deformity in total knee arthroplasty by tibial component downsizing and resection of uncapped proximal medial bone. J Arthroplasty 19:19–22, 2004.)

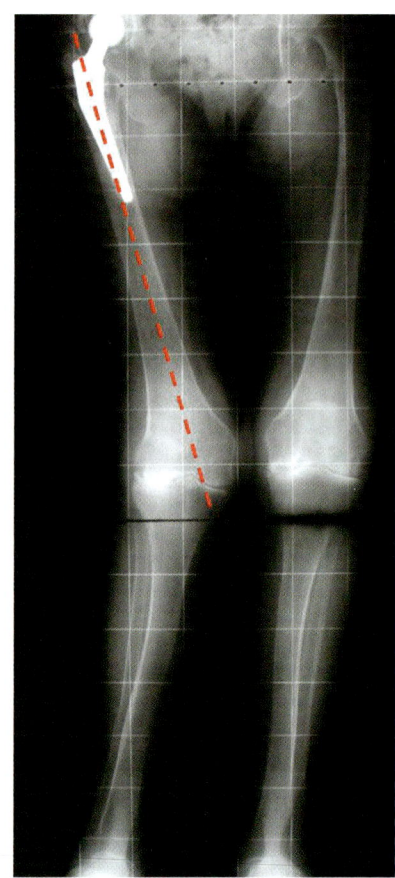

Figure 106-7. Femoral entry point in valgus deformity may be more medial than usual if lateral diaphyseal bowing occurs.

address all valgus deformity from a medial parapatellar approach. Some surgeons advocate the need for a lateral approach to these deformities to directly access contracted structures and to preserve the blood supply to the patella.[15] We do not support the use of a lateral approach because the surgeon is facing the joint with an unusual view, which can be misleading. Extensile approaches such as tibial tubercle osteotomy are needed to expose difficult cases without damaging the patellar tendon. Distal capsular closure difficulties are frequent and may predispose to postoperative skin problems, even when the fat pad tissue is used as a capsular patch. From the lateral side, it is not possible to perform a medial soft tissue retensioning procedure if needed. Moreover, in cases of failure requiring revision, the knee should receive a parallel medial capsulotomy. A review of all the literature on valgus deformities approached through a medial parapatellar capsulotomy reveals only one paper reporting a significant occurrence (2 of 25 cases) of patellar necrosis.[21] In this study, a lateral retinacular release was performed in all 25 cases without preserving the superior lateral geniculate artery.[21]

Bone resection levels and directions should be planned preoperatively. A distal femoral bone cut is performed with a slight overcorrection to avoid recurrence of medial soft tissue stretching. We suggest planning the degree of correction, but most often, we select the option of 4 degrees for the distal femoral cut. Attention is paid to entering the femoral canal from the appropriate entry point, which is often more medial than usual in cases with femoral diaphyseal valgus bowing (Fig. 106-7). Because of hypoplasia of the lateral femoral condyle, distal and posterior lateral resections usually remove a minimal amount of bone or no bone at all. We suggest starting bone resections from the femoral side in valgus deformities. Through a medial capsulotomy, the knee joint should be exposed without the need to perform the usual subperiosteal peel of the deep MCL around the medial tibial metaphysis. Once the distal and posterior femoral condyles are resected, the tibia can be easily exposed with less risk for MCL disruption caused by the RanSall maneuver.

Tibial resection is performed perpendicular to the mechanical axis, as usual. Conservative femoral and tibial resections are performed in cases of recurvatum or medial soft tissue

stretching to allow soft tissue balancing without elevating the joint line or creating an extension gap that is too large.

Anteroposterior (AP) femoral bone resections are performed using all available rotational landmarks, with a special focus on the epicondyles, which are not affected by the disease. The posterior condylar angle is increased as the result of lateral condyle hypoplasia and wear, thus requiring additional degrees of external rotation related to the posterior condylar line. This correction, if performed using a central pivot of the AP resection guide, will generate a greater resection of the posterior medial femoral condyle, which may lead to medial laxity in flexion. Medializing the pivot point of the cutting guide, as described earlier, will limit the amount of medial resection (see Fig. 106-4A and B).

Valgus knees usually are more deformed in extension than in flexion. This makes the posterior capsule and the iliotibial band (ITB) the most frequently contracted structures.[28] The lateral collateral ligament (LCL) is also contracted in more than 50% of cases, and the popliteal tendon is less commonly involved.[21]

Our preferred lateral release technique is the so-called pie-crusting technique, performed with multiple punctures.[24] With the knee in extension and the laminar spreader distracting the femorotibial joint space, the contracted structures are palpated. A no. 15 small blade is used to perform a capsular incision at the level of the tibial bone cut of the posterior capsule, following the lateral corner anterior to the popliteal tendon (Fig. 106-8). Care is taken at this time to avoid cutting the popliteal tendon, which is always preserved.

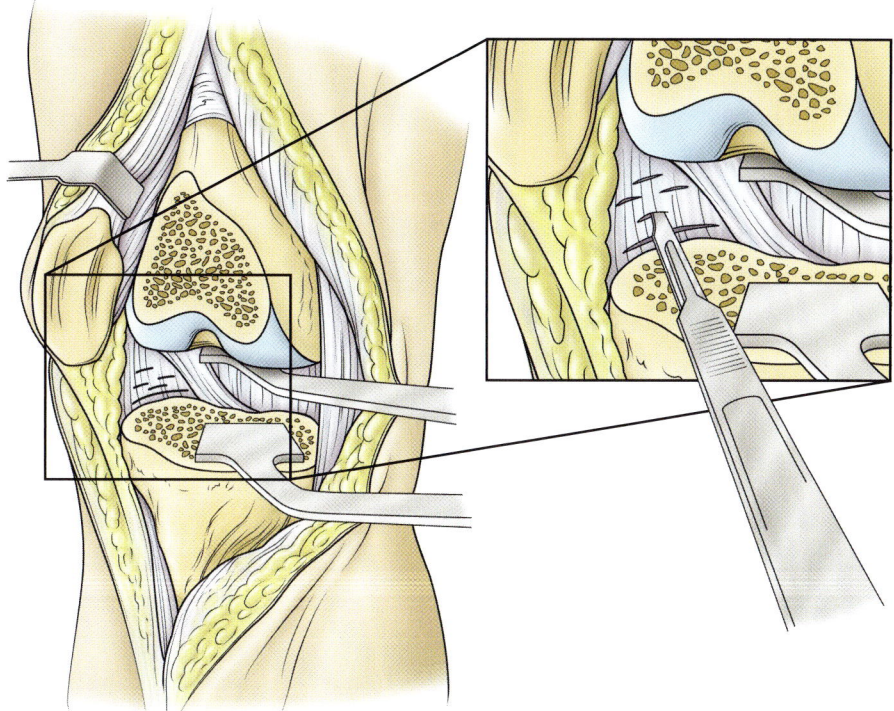

Figure 106-8. Illustration of the "pie-crusting" technique for valgus deformity. While the laminar spreader is distracting the knee joint in extension, a longitudinal incision is made in the posterolateral capsule, along with multiple punctures, with a small blade in the iliotibial band. (From Clarke HD, Schwartz JB, Math KR, Scuderi GR: Anatomic risk of peroneal nerve injury with the "pie crust" technique for valgus release in total knee arthroplasty. J Arthroplasty 19:40–44, 2004.)

Resection of the popliteal tendon in valgus deformity leads to uncontrolled knee instability in flexion. A cadaveric study with incremental lateral soft tissue sectioning clearly showed the sudden flexion gap increase after the popliteal tendon was involved.[18]

The pie-crusting release is then performed in a progressive manner with multiple horizontal stab incisions involving the ITB at the tibial resection level, and continuing proximally as needed, with the aim of reaching a rectangular gap (Fig. 106-9). The LCL is sometimes involved in the pie-crusting, if needed. The transverse incision and the multiple stab incisions through the lateral structures should be made with only the tip of the knife blade, and soft tissue penetration should be limited to 5 mm or less, particularly in patients with small legs, to avoid direct peroneal nerve damage, as has been revealed by magnetic resonance and cadaveric studies.[5,6]

Results with this technique were analyzed by Aglietti and colleagues in 48 patients with 53 valgus knees who underwent TKA and were followed a minimum of 5 years (mean, 8 years; range, 5 to 12 years).[1] A fixed-bearing posterior-stabilized implant or an ultracongruent mobile-bearing implant was used. A lateral patellofemoral retinacular release was performed in 67% of cases. One transient postoperative peroneal nerve palsy, which spontaneously recovered, was observed. In 51 of 53 knees (96%), alignment within 5 degrees from neutral was achieved. One patient had varus instability in extension. None of the components was revised. In this series, the pie-crusting technique reliably corrected moderate to severe fixed valgus deformity, with a low

complication rate and reasonable midterm results. Multiple punctures allowed gradual stretching of the lateral soft tissues and preservation of the popliteal tendon, reducing the risk of posterolateral instability.[1]

The medial convex side of the deformity needs to be addressed when medial soft tissue stretching is significant, with a medial compartment opening in extension of 15 mm or more. In this scenario, even minimal bone resection creates a medial gap larger than 25 mm, which would require an extensive lateral release and raising the joint line with the use of a thick polyethylene insert. Possible solutions include medial soft tissue retensioning and the use of a varus-valgus constrained implant. Krackow and coworkers described MCL advancement off the tibial side, and the same authors described MCL midsubstance division and imbrication to equalize the joint gaps.[16,17] Healy and associates described recessing the origin of the MCL with a bone block from the femoral epicondyles.[12] Although these procedures are technically demanding and may affect ligament strength and isometricity, they may be necessary to equalize joint gaps to achieve stability without the use of a varus-valgus constrained implant, particularly in a young, active patient.

Use of a stemmed varus-valgus constrained (VVC) condylar implant for fixed valgus deformities has produced excellent results at mid- to long-term follow-up.[8] Biomechanical analysis of VVC implants showed no difference in stresses at the bone-implant interface between stemmed and nonstemmed VVCs given adequate metaphyseal bone stock.[25] We recently reviewed our midterm clinical results with 70

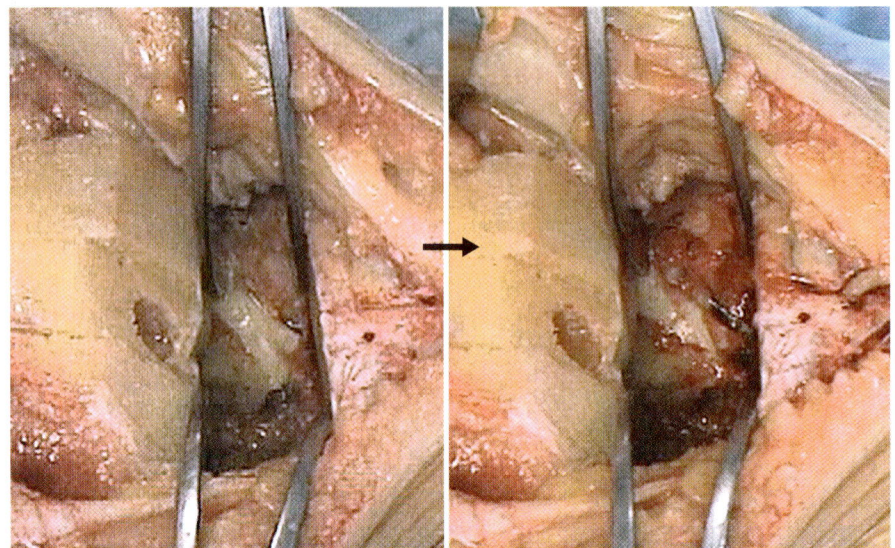

Figure 106-9. Intraoperative picture shows the extension gap of a valgus knee before *(left)* and after *(right)* lateral release is performed with multiple punctures. Gap symmetry is attained, and the popliteal tendon is preserved.

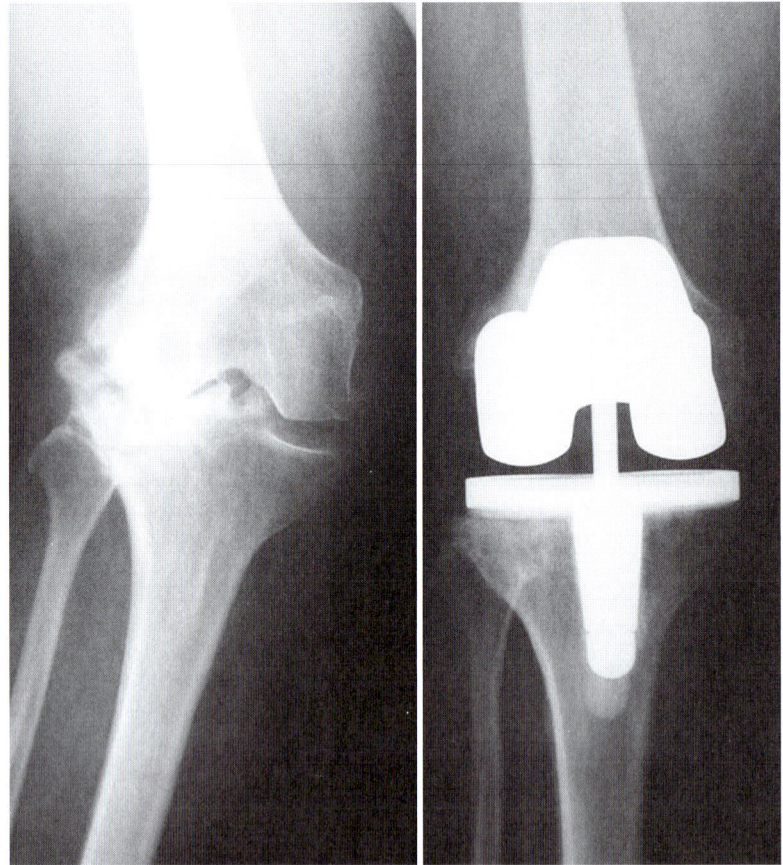

Figure 106-10. Preoperative *(left)* and postoperative *(right)* anteroposterior x-ray views of a severe valgus deformity treated by total knee arthroplasty (TKA) with a nonstemmed varus-valgus constrained implant at 6 years' follow-up. (From Anderson JA, Baldini A, MacDonald JH, et al: Primary constrained condylar knee arthroplasty without stem extensions for the valgus knee. Clin Orthop Relat Res 442:199–203, 2006.)

consecutive primary nonstemmed VVC implants for severe valgus deformity (Fig. 106-10).[2] From 1998 to 2001, 70 non-stemmed constrained TKAs were performed in 61 patients with knees in 15 degrees valgus or greater. Forty-nine patients (55 knees) were followed for 44.5 months (range, 2 to 6

years). Outcome was assessed using the Knee Society scoring system. Knee Society scores and functional scores improved from 34 points and 40 points to 93 points and 74 points, respectively. No radiographic loosening or wear was found. No peroneal nerve palsies were noted, and no patients had flexion or medial instability. One patient with a preoperative chronically dislocated patella had a postoperative recurrence of the dislocation. Constrained condylar knee implants in patients with severe valgus deformity resulted in excellent pain relief and improved function, without substantial complications at midterm follow-up and without diaphyseal–engaging stem extensions.[2]

CONCLUSIONS

The need to balance the soft tissue sleeve of the knee to create rectangular gaps is well recognized as a critical step in TKA. Multiple techniques are available for use in addressing the soft tissue imbalance that arises in fixed deformities during primary TKA. Correction of angular deformity with ligament release is done variably by different techniques, with little scientific evidence to support any of them. The few scientific studies that have been done have examined the influence on knees from cadavers without fixed deformity, or they have reported clinical outcomes of TKA cases following correction of fixed deformity. Correction of fixed deformity by separate bone resection and ligamentous release requires a thorough understanding of the underlying pathology. Extensive ligamentous releases are often required, but they should be performed in a progressive manner with recognition of which of the contracted structures is responsible for extension or flexion gap tensions. When extensive ligamentous releases are performed, resection of the PCL and implantation of a PCL-substituting prosthesis may be advisable to obtain more reproducible kinematics. The deformity should be completely corrected intraoperatively, and the knee should be balanced with an unconstrained implant most of the time. If residual ligamentous laxity is present by the end of the procedure, a VVC implant type with a relatively low threshold for elderly patients should be selected. Advanced fixed deformities with a combined flexion contracture may develop postoperative complications at a higher rate than minor deformities usually do. Careful surgical technique and postoperative monitoring are mandatory in these demanding cases.

KEY REFERENCES

Aglietti P, Lup D, Cuomo P, et al: Total knee arthroplasty using a pie-crusting technique for valgus deformity. Clin Orthop Relat Res 464:73–77, 2007.

Anderson JA, Baldini A, MacDonald JH, et al: Primary constrained condylar knee arthroplasty without stem extensions for the valgus knee. Clin Orthop Relat Res 442:199–203, 2006.

Baldini A, Scuderi GR, Aglietti P, et al: Flexion-extension gap changes during total knee arthroplasty: effect of posterior cruciate ligament and posterior osteophytes removal. J Knee Surg 17:69–72, 2004.

Berend ME, Ritter MA, Meding JB, et al: Tibial component failure mechanisms in total knee arthroplasty. Clin Orthop Relat Res 428:26–34, 2004.

Bruzzone M, Ranawat A, Castoldi F, et al: The risk of direct peroneal nerve injury using the Ranawat "inside-out" lateral release technique in valgus total knee arthroplasty. J Arthroplasty 25:161–165, 2010.

Clarke HD, Schwartz JB, Math KR, Scuderi GR: Anatomic risk of peroneal nerve injury with the "pie crust" technique for valgus release in total knee arthroplasty. J Arthroplasty 19:40–44, 2004.

Dixon MC, Parsch D, Brown RR, Scott RD: The correction of severe varus deformity in total knee arthroplasty by tibial component downsizing and resection of uncapped proximal medial bone. J Arthroplasty 19:19–22, 2004.

Hanada H, Whiteside LA, Steiger J, et al: Bone landmarks are more reliable than tensioned gaps in TKA component alignment. Clin Orthop Relat Res 462:137–142, 2007.

Keblish PA: The lateral approach to the valgus knee: surgical technique and analysis of 53 cases with over two-year follow-up evaluation. Clin Orthop Relat Res 271:52–62, 1991.

Krackow KA, Jones MM, Teeny SM, Hungerford DS: Primary total knee arthroplasty in patients with fixed valgus deformity. Clin Orthop Relat Res 273:9–18, 1991.

LaPrade RF, Engebretsen AH, Ly TV, et al: The anatomy of the medial part of the knee. J Bone Joint Surg Am 89:2000–2010, 2007.

Laurencin CT, Scott RD, Volatile TB, Gebhardt EM: Total knee replacement in severe valgus deformity. Am J Knee Surg 5:135–139, 1992.

Ranawat AS, Ranawat CS, Elkus M, et al: Total knee arthroplasty for severe valgus deformity: surgical technique. J Bone Joint Surg Am 87(Suppl 1 Pt 2):271–284, 2005.

Scott RD: Primary total knee arthroplasty surgical technique. In Scott RD, editor: Total knee arthroplasty, Philadelphia, 2006, Saunders Elsevier, pp 20–38.

Whiteside LA: Varus knee. In Ligament balancing in total knee arthroplasty: an instructional manual, Berlin, 2004, Springer-Verlag, pp 32–62.

Full references for this chapter can be found on www.expertconsult.com.

Chapter 107

Cemented Total Knee Arthroplasty: The Gold Standard

Bryan D. Springer and J. Bohannon Mason

Total knee arthroplasty (TKA) is one of the most successful surgical procedures in medical history. A condylar design with good cementing technique is considered the gold standard in TKA. Many implants today should reasonably be expected to function well for the remaining life of the patient.

Despite the success of cemented condylar knee replacements, many surgeons have advocated a change to cementless fixation for their total knee patients. The impetus for this change is to try to improve on current results, particularly as they relate to longevity in young patients. The purpose of this chapter is to look critically at the available evidence to determine what type of fixation is best for our total knee patients. An evidence-based analysis of the current literature regarding knee fixation should help define the role for cemented and cementless knee fixation.

EVOLUTION OF CEMENTLESS FIXATION

Cementless fixation was developed as a response to early failures of total hip arthroplasty (THA) in young patients. Cemented total hips did poorly in this subset of patients. Dorr et al reported a 67% revision rate in patients undergoing cemented total hips who were younger than 45 years of age.[9] Ranawat et al reported a 30% radiographic loosening rate in patients who had cemented total hips between ages 40 and 60.[28] Sullivan et al looked at 90 patients with an 18-year follow-up, all of whom were younger than 50 years old, and found that 50% of the acetabular components loosened, while 8% of the stems loosened.[36] In an effort to improve the long-term results of hip replacement, cementless fixation was offered as a potential solution. The transition from cemented total hip arthroplasty to cementless total hip arthroplasty in young patients has been truly successful. Tapered or extensively coated cementless femoral hip implants have demonstrated outstanding clinical results at long-term follow-up. In addition, the success and durability of modern cementless femoral components in young patients are well documented.[35] At this point in time, many authors would suggest that total hip fixation is a solved problem.

The success of cementless hip fixation in young patients led to increased interest in cementless fixation in knee replacement. Proponents of cementless fixation in TKA believe that biologic fixation has the potential to achieve a more durable bond of the implant to the bone, and hence improved success over cemented fixation. In addition, the introduction of newer, more porous metals for fixation in TKA has the potential to provide more reliable ingrowth than was previously achieved with cementless TKA.

RATIONALE FOR THE USE OF CEMENTLESS TOTAL KNEE ARTHROPLASTY

With the success of cemented condylar TKA, one must critically look at the potential advantages of cementless TKA design prior to widespread introduction of this technology. What advantages does it offer, and what potential problems with cemented TKA are we trying to improve upon? The purported advantages of cementless total knee fixation include shorter operative time, elimination of cement as a cause of third body polyethylene wear, ease of revision should failure occur, and improved longevity for our younger patients.

Reduced operative time is probably the most seductive reason for a surgeon to use this technology. By eliminating the 15 to 20 minutes per case needed for polymerization of the cement, the surgeon can complete the procedure in a timely manner. In the age of diminishing reimbursement, this certainly is enticing. In addition, elimination of cement from the surgical procedure removes a possible source of third body wear. Retained cement has been shown to be a leading factor in the damage of retrieved polyethylene inserts and has the potential to be a source of increased polyethylene wear and osteolysis.[7,22,27,37]

Another potential advantage of cementless knee fixation is ease of revision. In the absence of cement interdigitation, component removal is simplified. The interface between the host bone and the prosthesis is divided, and there is no need to remove embedded cement fragments. Additionally, when porous implants have failed to show ingrowth, removal is easily accomplished with disruption of the fibrous membrane. The resultant bone is usually a sclerotic bed that can be prepared for revision implants with only a few millimeters of bone resection. However, data have shown that the results of revision of a failed cementless implant to a cemented construct are similar to those of a failed cemented knee revised with cement.[13]

The main advantage of cementless fixation in young patients is the potential for improved longevity. With improved success of TKA, indications are being expanded to younger patients. Concern remains regarding the durability and longevity of a cemented TKA in the young, more physically demanding patient population. In addition, recent demographic data suggest that by 2011, nearly 50% of all TKAs will be performed in patients younger than age 65.[26] These factors are the driving force behind the evolution to cementless total knee fixation.

Once a cementless implant becomes osseously integrated, it is extremely rare for it to subsequently loosen. This outcome certainly is attractive for our younger patients. In contrast, concern has arisen that the bone-cement interface has the potential for late deterioration, especially in young, active patients. Although this failure mechanism is possible, it occurs infrequently. It must be recognized that a cemented knee replacement is loaded primarily in compression—a force well tolerated at the bone-cement interface. This is distinctly different from hip replacement in which the forces on the cement-bone interface are a combination of tension, compression, and shear. Although such forces can lead to early failure in young, active hip patients, little evidence in the literature substantiates that deterioration of this interface is a significant problem in young, cemented knee replacement patients.[6,8,12,30,32]

Results of Cemented Total Knee Arthroplasty

To justify this change to a cementless design, we first must analyze the currently available data on cemented TKA to determine whether in fact change is necessary. Second, we must determine whether cementless designs eliminate concerns associated with cemented TKA. An evidence-based approach to the current literature offers the best opportunity to do so. To date, true long-term prospective studies comparing the results of cemented versus cementless TKA are scarce and fail to show the advantages of a cementless design.[1]

The long-term results of cemented TKA in all age groups are outstanding (Fig. 107-1). Without stratifying for age, multiple published articles cite a greater than 90% success rate. Scuderi et al, looking at 1200 posterior stabilized knees, had

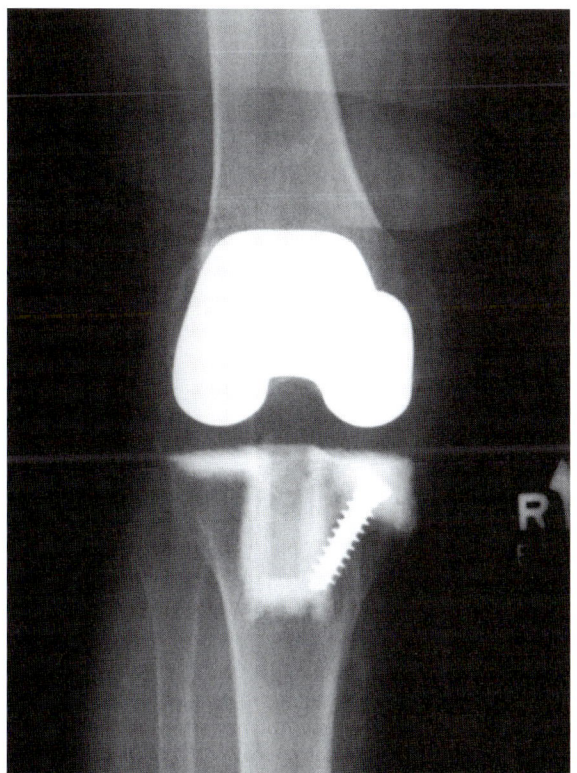

Figure 107-1. A 22-year follow-up of a cemented total knee arthroplasty with pristine interfaces and no evidence of polyethylene wear or osteolysis.

98% good or excellent results.[33] Ranawat et al, reporting on a 14-year survivorship of cemented total knee replacement, described a 95% success rate.[29] Font-Rodriguez et al, upon evaluating more than 2000 posterior stabilized metal-backed knees at 14 years' follow-up, noted a success rate of 98%.[16]

Thus a cemented TKA performed in an elderly patient should have a service life longer than the life of the patient, barring technical failure or infection. However, the true test of longevity consists of examining the results of cemented total knee replacement in studies stratified for age.

Cemented Total Knee Arthroplasty in Young Patients

Initial reports of mid- to long-term results of cemented condylar knee design in young patients have been encouraging. Ranawat reported a 94% ten-year survivorship in patients younger than 55 years of age using cemented fixation.[30] Gill reported 98% good or excellent results at 10 years in his cemented total knee patients younger than 55 years,[19] Diduch et al, in evaluating 118 patients younger than 55 had 94% good or excellent results at 8 years using cemented fixation.[8]

More recent reports have echoed these results, indicating the continued durability of a cemented condylar knee design in a young, high-demand patient population. Ritter and colleagues reported on 207 cemented cruciate-retaining TKA patients younger than age 55.[32] The survival rate at 12 years was 94.8%. Duffy and coworkers reported a 96% survivorship at 10 years using a Press-Fit condylar prosthesis (Depuy, Warsaw, Ind) on patients younger than 55 years.[12] No revisions for aseptic loosening were required.

The results of cemented fixation in this demanding patient subset are encouraging and fail to substantiate the theory of cement interface deterioration over time. Therefore, the rationale that there is a mandate for change caused by poor results of cemented fixation in young total knee patients is not substantiated by long-term data.

COMPARATIVE LITERATURE: CEMENT VERSUS CEMENTLESS

Numerous studies reported in the literature directly compared cemented fixation versus cementless fixation in TKA.[11,17] Rand and associates looked at more than 11,000 TKAs and performed a survivorship analysis at 10 years. When cemented fixation was used, 92% of total knees were successful, compared with only 61% successful without cement (P < .001).[31] Barrack and colleagues examined 82 cementless rotating platform knees and compared them with 76 cemented rotating platform mobile-bearing knees.[2] Eight percent of cementless knees were revised, and no cemented knees were revised. The cementless knees had significantly lower Knee Society scores. Gioe et al evaluated 5760 knees treated with various implants and methods of fixation and found that cementless total knees had the lowest survival rate of all implants reviewed.[20] Berger and coworkers, in evaluating 131 cementless total knees at a mean follow-up of 11 years, found that 8% of the tibial components never achieved ingrowth.[3] The authors of this article and designers of this implant commented that they have abandoned cementless fixation in TKA. Duffy and colleagues and Gioe and coworkers reported the results in a community-based registry on TKA in patients younger than 55 years.[21] Patients were implanted with 1047 joints of three predominant designs by 48 surgeons in four hospitals associated with a community joint registry. The mean age for this cohort was 49.8 years, and 62.8% (657/1047) of the patients were female. A total of 73 revisions were performed—5.6% (37/653) in women and 9.2% (36/394) in men. Cemented TKAs performed best, with a cumulative revision rate of 15.5%, compared with 34.1% in cementless designs. Eighty-five percent of cemented TKA implants survived at 14 years in the population younger than 55 years, and cementless designs were an independent risk factor for revision.

HYBRID FIXATON TECHNIQUES

Two so-called hybrid techniques are currently used clinically:
1. Cementing the tibial component while leaving the femoral component cementless
2. Partial cementation of the tibial component, that is, cementing the baseplate and leaving the tibial stem cementless

Neither of these hybrid fixation methods has evidence-based literature support.

Campbell and associates looked at 74 hybrid total knees in which the tibia was cemented and the femur was left cementless.[5] They found femoral component survivorship to be only 87%. These authors concluded that cementless femoral fixation is unreliable, and that this type of hybrid fixation should be abandoned. Gioe et al evaluated 5760 knees and found that cemented metal-backed components had 96% survival, while hybrid total knee replacements had only an 89% success rate.[20] Gao and colleagues performed a small, prospective, randomized study of cementless femoral components.[18] At short-term follow-up, the cementless design offers no advantage over a cemented femoral component. The magnitude and pattern of migration as measured by RSA did not differ significantly between cemented and uncemented fixation during the 2-year follow-up, nor were any differences noted between groups in terms of clinical outcome.

In addition, biomechanical studies do not support the use of partial cementation of the tibial stem. Bert and McShane found that tibial trays treated with partial cementation had significantly more micromotion compared with fully cemented constructs.[4] Jazrawi and associates confirmed this in their laboratory finding that cemented metaphyseal engaging stems had significantly less tray motion than cementless constructs of the same length.[24]

FAILURE MODES IN TOTAL KNEE ARTHROPLASTY

The rationale for cementless TKA fixation hinges on more reliable fixation and decreased risk of aseptic loosening. Patients who have undergone total knee replacement expect at least 10 to 15 years of in-service life before subsequent revision surgery becomes necessary. If one looks critically at the modes of failure seen in cemented TKA, aseptic loosening is an uncommon mode of failure and thus may not justify the use of a cementless design.

Fehring and colleagues analyzed the mechanisms of failure in patients requiring revision surgery within 5 years of their index arthroplasty.[15] From a revision TKA dataset of 440 knees, the authors found that 63% of patients were revised within 5 years of their index arthroplasty. The key reasons for these revisions included infection, poor surgical technique, and poor surgeon judgment. Thirty-seven percent of early failures among those patients revised within 5 years occurred because of infection. Twenty-six percent of cases failed because of instability. Thirteen percent of patients were revised within 5 years because of failure of cementless fixation. In contrast, only 3% of early failures were the result of aseptic loosening of a cemented implant. Dominant modes of failure within the first 5 years included infection, instability, and fibrous ingrowth of cementless implants. If all patients in this early failure group would have been routinely cemented and would have had proper ligamentous balancing, the overall failure rate would have decreased by 40%, and the overall number of revisions would have decreased by 25%.

DIAGNOSIS OF FAILED CEMENTLESS KNEES

Results of TKA are generally good. However, a certain subset of patients, despite excellent radiographic results, do not do well. Multiple reasons are known for failure of a TKA.[15,34] The diagnosis of aseptic loosening as a source of pain and failure can be elusive.[10,23,25] Plain radiographs are helpful and can be diagnostic of aseptic loosening, but even slight obliquity of the film can obscure radiolucent lines adjacent to the prosthesis.[10] Plain radiographs with a divergence of the beam of only 3 degrees from a plane parallel to the bone-implant interface will not detect a 2 mm lucent line beneath the tibial component.

Fluoroscopic radiographs of the knee may be used to facilitate evaluation of aseptic loosening in patients with cementless total knees. Fluoroscopic guidance allows one to position the x-ray beam parallel to the bone-prosthesis interface, so that the presence and extent of radiolucent lines beneath a cementless component can be measured[14] (Fig. 107-2).

In contrast to failed cemented TKA in which cement fragmentation may be evident and the cement-bone interface is not close to the obscuring metal of the implant, the interface beneath a cementless implant may be more difficult to

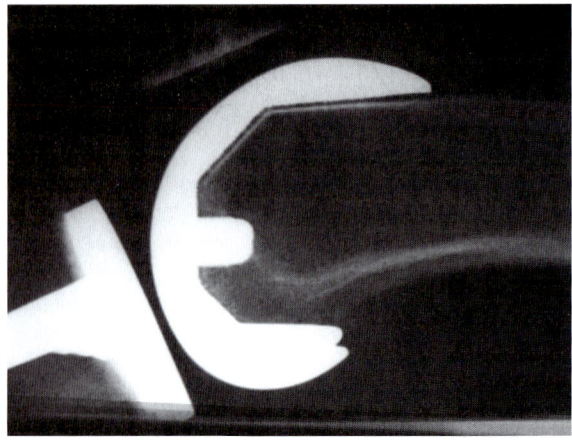

Figure 107-2. Fluoroscopic view of a cementless total knee depicting failure of ingrowth.

assess. The porous surface may obscure a demarcation line, and sclerosis beneath a fixed porous implant can be confused with consolidation and spot welds.

In cementless knee arthroplasty, the presence of any line between implant and bone shows lack of bony incorporation in that area. If such lines are extensive or progressive, this implant is loose and may be the source of symptoms.[14] Undoubtedly, there are patients who lack bony ingrowth yet function well with a fibrously ingrown implant. However, if a patient presents with a painful TKA and normal-appearing x-rays and has start-up pain, fluoroscopic views are indicated. If fluoroscopic radiographs corroborate a problem with the interfaces, chances for successful revision are good.[13]

CONCLUSION

Much interest is being generated in the arena of cementless TKA fixation. With the purported advantages of less operative time, easier revision, and the potential for improved survivorship, especially in younger patients, this approach has some theoretical appeal. In addition, the advent of new porous surfaces that allow more rapid and reliable bony ingrowth has the potential to improve current results and address some of the concerns associated with previous cementless designs.

We have presented in this chapter a systematic review of currently available literature on cemented and cementless TKA. It is clear that the results of cemented TKA are excellent, and that durable long-term results can be achieved in all patient populations. In addition, the issue of aseptic loosening in cemented TKA design is minimal, thereby undermining the rationale for the use of a cementless design. Although continued research efforts are important in the evaluation of cementless designs and their application in arthroplasty, a cemented TKA must still be considered the gold standard.

KEY REFERENCES

Baker PN, Khaw FM, Kirk LM: A randomised controlled trial of cemented versus cementless press-fit condylar total knee replacement: 15-year survival analysis. J Bone Joint Surg Br 89:1608–1614, 2007.

Barrack RL, Nakamura SJ, Hopkins SG, Rosenzweig S: Winner of the 2003 James A. Rand Young Investigator's Award: early failure of cementless mobile-bearing total knee arthroplasty. J Arthroplasty 19(7 Suppl 2):101–106, 2004.

Berger RA, Lyon JH, Jacobs JJ, et al: Problems with cementless total knee arthroplasty at 11 years followup. Clin Orthop Relat Res 392:196–207, 2001.

Campbell MD, Duffy GP, Trousdale RT: Femoral component failure in hybrid total knee arthroplasty. Clin Orthop Relat Res 356:58–65, 1998.

Fehring TK, Griffin WL: Revision of failed cementless total knee implants with cement. Clin Orthop Relat Res 356:34–38, 1998.

Fehring TK, McAvoy G: Fluoroscopic evaluation of the painful total knee arthroplasty. Clin Orthop Relat Res 331:226–233, 1996.

Fehring TK, Odum S, Griffin WL, et al: Early failures in total knee arthroplasty. Clin Orthop Relat Res 392:315–318, 2001.

Font-Rodriguez DE, Scuderi GR, Insall JN: Survivorship of cemented total knee arthroplasty. Clin Orthop Relat Res 345:79–86, 1997.

Furnes O, Espehaug B, Lie SA, et al: Early failures among 7,174 primary total knee replacements: a follow-up study from the Norwegian Arthroplasty Register 1994-2000. Acta Orthop Scand 73:117–129, 2002.

Gao F, Henricson A, Nilsson KG: Cemented versus uncemented fixation of the femoral component of the NexGen CR total knee replacement in patients younger than 60 years: a prospective randomised controlled RSA study. Knee 16:200–206, 2009.

Gill GS, Chan KC, Mills DM: 5- to 18-year follow-up study of cemented total knee arthroplasty for patients 55 years old or younger. J Arthroplasty 12:49–55, 1997.

Gioe TJ, Killeen KK, Grimm K, et al: Why are total knee replacements revised? Analysis of early revision in a community knee implant registry. Clin Orthop Relat Res 428:100–106, 2004.

Gioe TJ, Novak C, Sinner P, et al: Knee arthroplasty in the young patient: survival in a community registry. Clin Orthop Relat Res 464:83–87, 2007.

Rand JA, Trousdale RT, Ilstrup DM, Harmsen WS: Factors affecting the durability of primary total knee prostheses. J Bone Joint Surg Am 85:259–265, 2003.

Sharkey PF, Hozack WJ, Rothman RH, et al: Insall Award paper: why are total knee arthroplasties failing today? Clin Orthop Relat Res 404:7–13, 2002.

Full references for this chapter can be found on www.expertconsult.com.

Cementless Total Knee Designs

Leo A. Whiteside

HISTORY

Cement use in arthroplasty remains a controversial issue and has decreased sharply in total hip, total shoulder, and total ankle arthroplasty. Although cement fixation still is widely used in the knee, new studies report remarkable success with the osteointegration technique, and some new porous metal materials appear promising.[7,17,68] Many cemented total knee replacement designs introduced through the years have failed and have been removed from the market. Those that remain are the few select designs that have performed reasonably well because of specific design characteristics, including a well-fixed tibial component with an effective stem, multiple sizes of femoral components, a generous curvature on each femoral condyle, and a conforming polyethylene surface with a large articular contact surface area.[22] With the advent of new instruments, these cemented implants, even when placed by inexperienced arthroplasty surgeons, have had a high rate of success. Cement fixation, however, remains a source of consternation for implant designers. Attempts to produce a cemented all-polyethylene tibial component resulted in a loosening rate in excess of 20% at 5 years,[14] and the use of cemented total knee replacement in younger, active patients resulted in high failure because of loosening.[29,42] One of the engineering considerations that has not been addressed satisfactorily is fixation of the cement mantle to the metal substrate; this is especially important for the metal-backed tibial component.

The primary goal of noncemented fixation of total joint arthroplasty is to improve the longevity of the implant. Many cementless designs were unsuccessful even at early follow-up periods, but others have been highly successful. In fact, the femoral component in almost all cementless designs reliably achieves fixation to bone and commonly is used in hybrid total knee arthroplasty.[25] The tibial component in cementless total knee arthroplasty, as in cemented arthroplasty, has been the greatest source of problems related to fixation because most designs have begun with inadequate fixation.

Quality of fixation and load transfer characteristics of the implant-bone interface are two of the most important factors in determining implant longevity. Implants must be designed to apply load in compression to ensure bone hypertrophy and avoid shear or tensile failure of the interface between the porous surface and the base metal. The fixation system must achieve the best immediate fixation possible to allow early weight bearing.

Fixation of the femoral component generally has not been as difficult as that of the tibial component, but femoral component design is far from simple. Weight bearing with the knee in extension can generate high shear stress at the anterior and posterior flange surfaces if the surfaces are adherent to bone.[53] Weight bearing in flexion can generate high shear stress at the distal surfaces if the bone is not seated

posteriorly and the component is not fixed rigidly against shear loading.[53]

Load transfer characteristics of the femoral component observed in a clinical radiographic study[66] are predictable from the study of Walker and associates[53] on fixation of the femoral component. If the anterior and posterior flange surfaces of the femoral component are bonded to bone, the femoral shaft transfers weight-bearing load in the form of shear stress through the flange surfaces during weight bearing in extension, but the load can be transferred to the distal surfaces in the form of compressive stress if the anterior and posterior flange surfaces are not bonded to bone. Compressive loading is desirable because it encourages ossification at the porous metal-bone interface and promotes hypertrophy of adjacent cancellous bone. Whiteside and Pafford found that gaps at the distal surface failed to close and developed a surrounding halo of cancellous bone atrophy, but this is not surprising because the hypertrophy produced by compressive loading on either side of the gap leads to stiffening of the bone and thus increases its ability to transfer load.[66] As the load is transferred in increasing proportion through hypertrophic bone, atrophic bone overlying the gap becomes less capable of bearing load, thus transferring more load to areas that contact the metal surface. It is difficult to see how load sharing and equalization of stress could be expected to occur, and it is not surprising that gaps, when carefully scrutinized, were seldom seen to close. Current designs incorporate anterior porous coating to ensure early complete bonding of bone to metal and accept higher shear stress on the anterior flange surfaces. This is acceptable because of improvement in the bonding strength of the porous metal surface to the bare metal. The distal stress relief that occurs because of this design feature is deemed preferable to the anterior femoral osteolysis that can occur if this surface is left unbonded to bone.[68]

Walker and colleagues[53] further predicted that unbonding of the posterior flange surfaces would cause stress relief of these surfaces during weight bearing in flexion. In the study by Whiteside and Pafford,[66] all specimens showed evidence of greater hypertrophy at the posterior bevel and posterior flange surfaces than at any other surface. The observed pattern of cancellous hypertrophy suggested that weight-bearing loads were transmitted primarily in compression through the cancellous bone and through the interfaces of both components. The smooth posterior femoral flange surface did not appear to affect posterior femoral condylar hypertrophy. Smooth flange surfaces and smooth stem and pegs on the femoral component did not appear to bear significant axial load.

The tibial component traditionally has been considered to present the major load transfer and fixation problems. Adherence of the stem and pegs to supporting cancellous bone may cause proximal stress shielding, as well as high shear stress at the bone-prosthesis interface and high bending stress in the stem.[36] According to Murase and coworkers[36] in a study of cemented designs, the best configuration to achieve stability and yet avoid proximal stress shielding included a short central stem for toggle control. Tibial component fixation systems without a central stem do not achieve adequate toggle control to prevent lift-off and sinking of the tibial component in response to an eccentrically applied load.[1,27,28,44,54] Although some current designs do not incorporate stems or peripheral stems, these principles have not changed, and they must be considered in modern implant design. Eccentric and tangential loading also causes shear stress at the interface between bone and the undersurface of the tray, and these stresses must be considered in implant design.*

Load transfer in the tibia is important when bone quality and stress relief osteopenia are considered. Low-strain readings around the peripheral rim correspond to peripheral atrophy seen in a radiographic study, and the area of high-strain readings on the metaphyseal flare corresponds to the area where the hypertrophic cancellous bone joined the metaphyseal cortex.[66] These findings suggest that tibial load bearing causes primarily compressive stress, and that the load is transferred through the cancellous bone to the cortical bone of the tibial metaphysis, to a certain extent bypassing the proximal peripheral rim of the tibia. High strain in the anterolateral area of the tibia suggests that the bone surface in this area deforms to a greater extent than do other areas after total knee arthroplasty.

In the medial condylar area, the bone is denser than in the central condylar area and therefore is more capable of transferring axial load.[66] The relatively soft cancellous bone in the upper surface of the tibia[23] makes this area especially vulnerable to compressive failure, and the need for a stem on the tibial tray to protect this area is abundantly documented in the biomechanical literature. Bartel and coworkers[1] demonstrated in a finite element analysis that prostheses without a stem are likely to sink into soft areas of the tibial surface when the component is loaded eccentrically. Walker and associates[53] and Lewis and colleagues[28] found in separate studies that fixation of the tibial component was best achieved by a rigid tray and a central metal stem. Results of the study by Bartel and coworkers[1] also suggest that peripheral contact between the tray and the cortex of the upper part of the tibia would alleviate this problem of sinking. However, the peripheral rim of the proximal end of the tibia does not have a true cortex,[56] and the hardest bone is not arranged around the periphery but instead is usually found on the medial and lateral posterior surfaces and medially just beneath the articular cartilage. Therefore, a finite element model that includes a substantial cortex probably would predict inappropriate benefits from rim contact with the upper tibial surface. All tibiae in the study in which sinking of the tibial component occurred had good rim contact.

The loading pattern of the tibia during normal gait is complex. Although eccentric anterior and posterior loading occurred during weight bearing in flexion and extension in Whiteside and Pafford's study,[66] no attempt was made to quantify this effect. In general, it appeared possible to achieve reliable fixation of the femoral and tibial components without

clinically significant stress shielding in the distal femur or the proximal tibia.

Applying a rigid metal tray to a flat surface of cancellous bone does not provide adequate resistance to compressive failure of cancellous bone, lift-off of the opposite side, or toggling micromotion of the component. When early results showed problems with fixation, stems and peripheral screws began to appear on these implant designs. Biomechanical studies clearly indicated that peripheral screws and stems on the tibial component were highly effective, and that micromotion of the tray was unacceptably large without these fixation-enhancing features.[34,51] An aspect of tibial component fixation that is commonly overlooked but is probably the most important is preparation of the upper tibial surface. Small surface irregularities and incongruities can have a devastating effect on fixation, but this aspect of fixation has received little attention in most cementless tibial component designs.

Biomechanical studies have shown that when tibial components are fixed to the bone surface with only short pegs, they sink on the loaded side and lift off on the opposite side.[51] Both stems and screws were effective in controlling sinking and lift-off in the study by Volz and associates.[51] Radiographic and histologic studies have shown that bone ingrowth into a tibial tray is infrequent,[9] which suggests that micromotion may be unacceptably large. Achieving rigid initial fixation is the most important factor in promoting bone ingrowth. Miura and colleagues[34] evaluated the effects of screws through the tibial tray and a sleeve on the stem to improve fixation of the tibial component. Bone strength was a major factor in preventing subsidence and micromotion. Without mechanical fixation, poor bone quality was associated with unacceptably large micromovement. The anterolateral portion showed the least bone strength in the proximal tibial surface. Hvid and Hansen reported that bone strength at the anterolateral and intercondylar regions was very low.[21]

In a study by Miura and coworkers,[34] screws were effective in controlling micromovement under axial and shear loading. When components with screws were compared with those without screws, lift-off was found to be reduced by more than 90%. Screws shifted the tilting center lines posteriorly. This finding suggested that the main effect of the screws was to prevent lift-off. Screws also ensured initial bone-implant contact. Miura and associates reported that they frequently observed the component to settle on the tibial surface when the screws were tightened. Screws did not eliminate micromotion under axial loads, but they did change the pattern of micromotion. Without screws, micromotion was associated with lift-off and sinking, whereas with screws, sinking and lift-off were minimized, but downward bending of the tray was significantly greater. Although it is uncertain how much micromotion is acceptable while bone ingrowth occurs, it should be minimized as much as possible. A material with an elastic modulus similar to that of cancellous bone may be optimal for stress distribution beneath the tibial tray, but it may also increase the micromotion caused by bending. Results of the study by Miura and colleagues[34] suggest that techniques to lessen bending of the tibial tray minimize micromotion. Mechanisms to prevent bending of the tibial tray might include a material with a higher elastic modulus and the addition of an arch to support the tibial tray.

---

*References 16, 24, 26, 33, 35, and 55.

The mechanical effect of a tight stem appeared in the study of Miura and coworkers[34] to improve the keel effect by packing surrounding soft cancellous bone and thus improving the press-fit effect, increasing the surface area, and placing the stem closer to the inner surface of the posterior cortex. Use of a tight stem alone was effective in preventing lift-off and sinking under axial loads, but the use of screws had overriding effects on sinking and subsidence. Addition of the stem to a screwed-down tibial component had a small (but statistically significant) effect in controlling lift-off. The location of the tilting axis varied with each specimen and with each group. The effect of screws was to shift the tilting axis posteriorly in comparison with groups without screws. This is an important mechanical effect and is probably a result of the resistance to lift-off afforded by the screws. If lift-off was unchecked, the tilting axis shifted toward the point of load application, thus decreasing the area through which the load was transferred. This increased pressure and aggravated sinking.

DESIGN-RELATED FAILURE

Implant materials and design features that have occurred coincidentally with cementless total knee replacement designs and are responsible for implant failure are flat polyethylene,[5] heat-pressed polyethylene,[4] and patch porous-coated surfaces.[62] The combination of these features, along with poor quality assurance of polyethylene and gamma irradiation of this material, has caused remarkable wear problems that have led to clinically significant osteolysis.[12,49,58,62] This type of wear and osteolysis is not a function of the fixation method; instead, it is caused by design features that have incidentally been associated with cementless fixation.

Femoral Component Design

Fracture of the metal femoral component has rarely been a problem in the development of total knee designs, but those that fractured were usually cementless designs that generated excessive stress through an attempt to conserve bone. Stress in noncemented knees is different from that generated in knees fixed with cement,[53,66] and these differences in point and direction of load application may focus high stress on critical cross-sectional dimensions. Porous coating decreases the strength of metal implants because it thins the cross-sectional dimension, especially at corners and junction areas, where the metal may already be at critical dimensions.

When the Ortholoc II knee femoral component was designed in the mid-1980s, a double porous bead layer was applied to the inner surface for cementless fixation.[65] This design was changed soon thereafter to a single layer of beads to improve strength characteristics because within a year of implantation, the manufacturer received reports that fracture of the femoral component had occurred in the design with a double layer of beads, especially those of smaller size (Figs. 108-1 to 108-3). In the author's series of 613 Ortholoc II prostheses with a double bead layer on the femoral component, four fractures occurred. All four implants fractured at

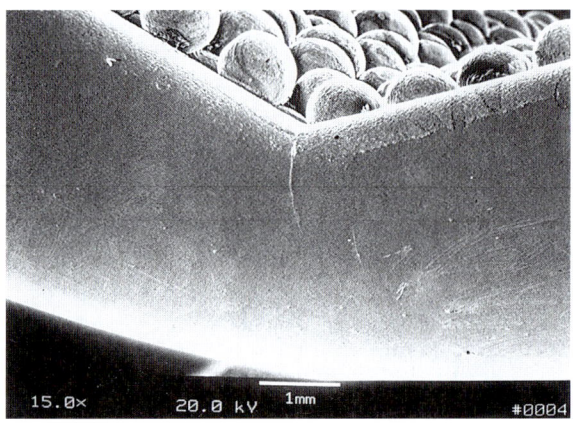

Figure 108-2. A crack originated from the inner beaded surface at the junction between the posterior bevel and the distal surface of the nonfractured lateral side in a femoral condyle. (From Whiteside LA, Fosco DR, Brooks JG Jr: Fracture of the femoral component in cementless total knee arthroplasty. Clin Orthop Relat Res 286:75, 1993.)

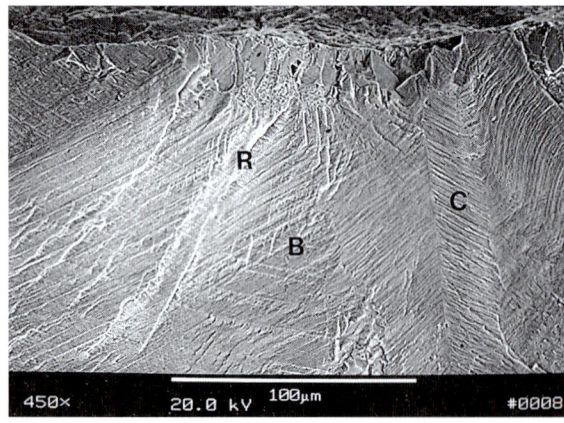

Figure 108-1. Beach marks *(B)* on the fractured surface of an Ortholoc II femoral component. The concentric beach mark lines converge at a point on the inner surface of the implant where the crack initiated. Radial lines *(R)* were found on all fractured surfaces. They are oriented in a radial pattern from the point of crack initiation on the inner beaded surface of the component. Chevron zones *(C)* were found consistently on the fractured surface. These markings are typical of bending fatigue failure. (From Whiteside LA, Fosco DR, Brooks JG Jr: Fracture of the femoral component in cementless total knee arthroplasty. Clin Orthop Relat Res 286:74, 1993.)

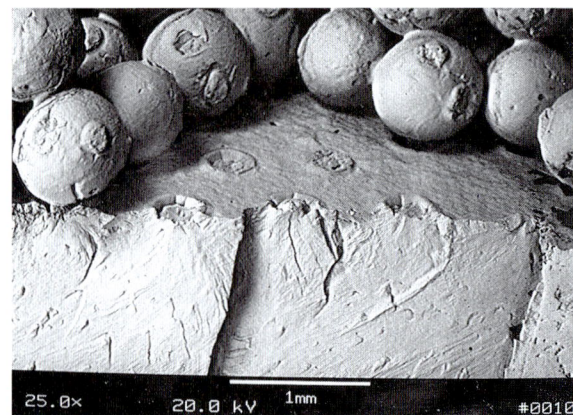

Figure 108-3. Scanning electron micrograph of the inner beaded surface. The fracture joint remnants of several bead craters can be seen. (From Whiteside LA, Fosco DR, Brooks JG Jr: Fracture of the femoral component in cementless total knee arthroplasty. Clin Orthop Relat Res 286:76, 1993.)

the junction between the posterior bevel and the distal surface of the medial femoral condyle.[65]

When a geometric design is shaped with a saw to fit into a curved surface that follows the normal contours of the knee surface, thin sections are formed at the corners. Thin metal at this critical area predisposes the piece to fracture, and porous coating of the inner surface requires that these critical sections be thinned even further. The sintering process can degrade the quality of the base metal itself, thus weakening the implant, and the notch effect caused by the porous coating can be important in weakening the implant if the porous surface is loaded in tension.

Loads applied to the outer surface of the implant by body weight and muscle force cause bending moments that tend to close the implant and apply tensile stress to the outer surface. However, loads applied to the inner surface are likely to have the opposite effect. If the anterior and posterior surfaces are not allowed to adhere to bone, load is borne on the distal surfaces preferentially.[53,66] Because the Ortholoc II femoral component was designed to avoid axial load bearing by its anterior and posterior flange surfaces, surgical technique that over-resected the distal surface in relation to the bevel surfaces could have resulted in load bearing exclusively through the inner bevel surfaces. If the implant contacted only the anterior and posterior bevel surfaces and was not also adherent to the surfaces, a wedge would be created, and the femoral component would straighten slightly with weight-bearing loads. Application of these cyclic bending loads on the distal portion of the implant probably produced a bending moment that generated tensile load on the inner surfaces.

Surgical bone preparation of the femoral surface for the Ortholoc II implant apparently created a mechanical environment that exposed the porous inner surface to tensile load. Although the inner surface of the femoral component generally is not considered to be the site of significant tensile stress, the combination of cementless technique and smaller implant size predisposed implants with a double layer of beads to fracture.

Tibial Component Design

An inflammatory response to particulate debris has been identified as the primary cause of osteolysis in total knee arthroplasty.[40] Debris contained within the joint minimally affects the surrounding bone, but once it gains access, the osteolytic attack is aggressive. Design features of implants that allow particulate debris access to the bone include the configuration of the porous coating, the stability of the locking mechanism that secures the polyethylene articulating surface to the tibial tray, and the amount of intra-articular pressure within the joint.

Smooth metal surfaces that separate pads of porous coating have been shown in experimental and clinical studies to produce metaphyseal and diaphyseal osteolytic lesions by conducting debris into areas of bone that are not protected by the synovial membrane particle transfer system that captures wear debris and transfers it to the local lymphatic system.[6,12,30,57,69] Although these osteolytic lesions have been ascribed to cementless fixation and to the use of screws,[12] they are rare unless the tibial component design includes patch porous coating on the undersurface of the tray, inadequate

fixation of the tibial component, and mechanisms that produce large amounts of particulate debris in the knee. As has been seen in cementless total hip arthroplasty, osteolysis occurs when patches of porous coating on the implant are separated by smooth metal surfaces. These smooth metal surfaces form fibrous tissue bridges that conduct polyethylene debris and joint fluid to the diaphyseal endosteal area, where no mechanism exists to diminish the inflammatory response. Porous coated patches on the Harris-Galante cementless total hip femoral prosthesis appeared to be the cause of a high rate of femoral diaphyseal osteolysis, regardless of the method of fixation to bone.[30,69]

This phenomenon can be explained by a study conducted by Ward and associates,[57] in which the porous coating around the extraosseous portion of proximal tibial prostheses was observed to seal the bone-cement interface from invasion by polyethylene debris, whereas prostheses with smooth surfaces connecting the joint to the bone-cement interface had high rates of osteolysis and loosening.

This observation also was supported in a laboratory study by Bobyn and colleagues,[6] who reported the effects of porous coating and smooth metal surfaces on migration of particulate debris from the joint cavity in rabbits. Partially porous coated rods readily conducted polyethylene debris from the knee joint into the medullary canal of the femur, but circumferentially porous coated rods had bone and tissue penetration into the porous coating that acted as a barrier to migration of the polyethylene debris.

The Ortholoc Modular tibial component (Wright Medical Technology, Arlington, Tenn), which has patches of porous coating separated by smooth metal bridges on its undersurface, was clinically compared with the Ortholoc II tibial component (Wright Medical Technology), which has continuous porous coating on the undersurface. The rate of osteolysis was found to be statistically significantly greater in knees with the patch porous coating design (Fig. 108-4).[62] Osteolysis did not occur around the tibial stem or pegs in 675

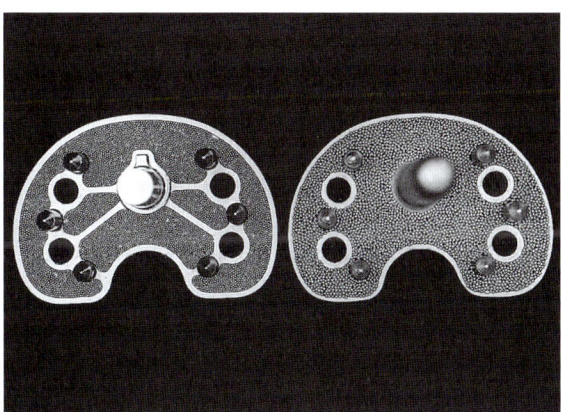

Figure 108-4. Undersurfaces of the Ortholoc Modular *(left)* and Ortholoc II *(right)* tibial components. The Ortholoc Modular has smooth metal bridges around the pegs and screw holes that converge on the central stem. Porous coating covers the entire undersurface of the Ortholoc II component. No bridges of smooth metal connect the joint cavity or screw holes to the smooth stem. (From Whiteside LA: Effect of porous-coating configuration on tibial osteolysis after total knee arthroplasty. Clin Orthop Relat Res 321:93, 1995.)

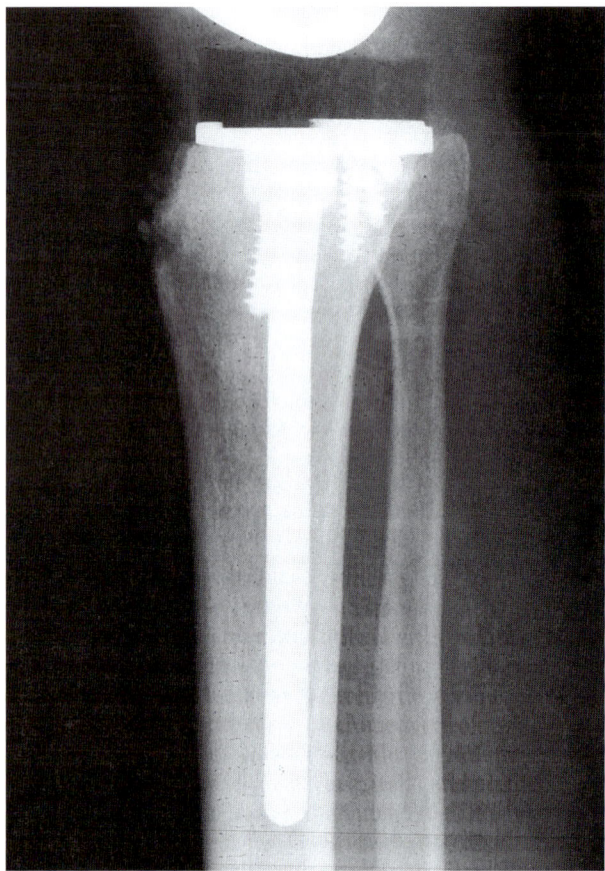

Figure 108-5. Lateral radiograph of an Ortholoc Modular tibial component 1 month after surgery. No sign of osteolysis is evident around the stem, screws, or pegs. (From Whiteside LA: Effect of porous-coating configuration on tibial osteolysis after total knee arthroplasty. Clin Orthop Relat Res 321:95, 1995.)

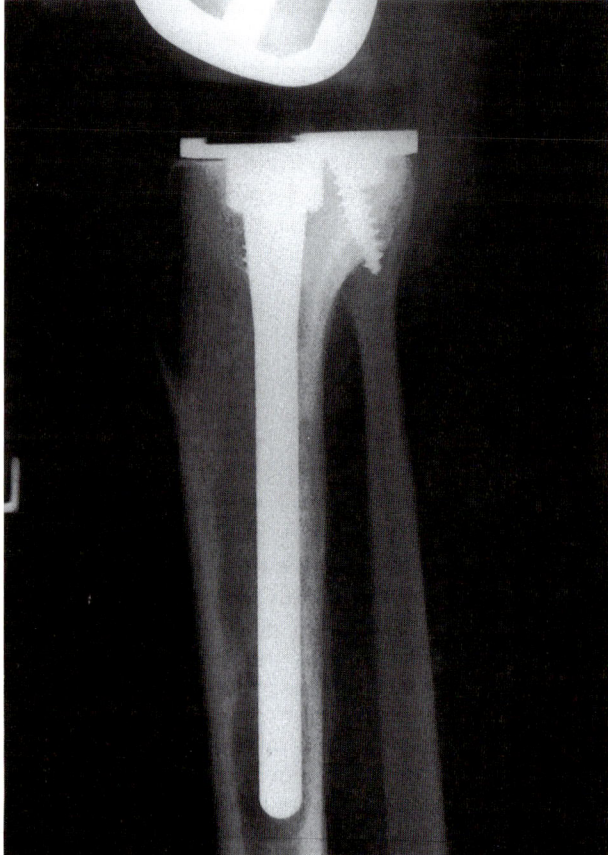

Figure 108-6. Lateral radiograph of an Ortholoc Modular tibial component with osteolysis surrounding the 150 cm stem 2 years after surgery. No evidence of osteolysis is present around the screws or pegs. (From Whiteside LA: Effect of porous-coating configuration on tibial osteolysis after total knee arthroplasty. Clin Orthop Relat Res 321:95, 1995.)

patients whose knees were replaced with the Ortholoc II design, but three nonprogressive osteolytic lesions were found around screws on postoperative radiographs. Partial radiolucency was seen beneath the tibial surface in 27 knees. None have been revised for osteolysis. In contrast, radiographically detectable osteolysis was seen around the tibial stem in 28 (23%) of 124 Ortholoc Modular total knee prostheses with long (150 mm) stems (Figs. 108-5 and 108-6). Of those 28, none had radiographically identifiable osteolysis around the screws or pegs, but 15 (54%) had partial radiolucent lines that extended beneath at least half the tray on the anteroposterior or lateral view, and 4 (14%) had radiolucency beneath the entire tibial surface on either radiographic view. An additional 15 (12%) of 124 knees had radiographically identifiable radiolucency around the stem. Radiographically detectable osteolysis was seen around the tibial stem in 19 (17%) of 112 Ortholoc Modular total knee prostheses with short (75 mm) stems. Thirty (27%) knees had radiolucent lines that extended halfway across the undersurface of the tray, and 9 (8%) knees had complete radiolucent lines under the tray on the anteroposterior or lateral radiographic view.

Two Ortholoc Modular knees (one with a short-stem prosthesis, one with a long-stem prosthesis) underwent revision for progressive osteolytic defects around the stem. The knee

with a short stem had severe, persistent pain, whereas the knee with a long stem had no pain. Both knees had hypertrophic synovial tissue that filled the cyst around the stem and connected freely with the undersurface of the tibial tray and the joint cavity, following along the smooth metal surfaces between porous coated patches. Histologic analysis of biopsy tissue revealed abundant polyethylene-laden macrophages and free polyethylene particles throughout the tissue, but no metallic debris (Fig. 108-7).

It was postulated that the gasket effect of the continuous porous coating on the Ortholoc II tibial tray prevented access of uncontained polyethylene debris and joint fluid to surrounding bone. However, in knees with an Ortholoc Modular component, the smooth metal bridges connecting the screw holes and joint cavity with the stem provided access for migration of fluid and debris to the diaphyseal medullary canal. In biopsy specimens taken from the two knees that underwent revision, polyethylene debris was present around the stems and in all osteolytic cysts.

Polyethylene Locking Mechanism

The design of the locking mechanism that secures the polyethylene articulating surface to the tibial component appears

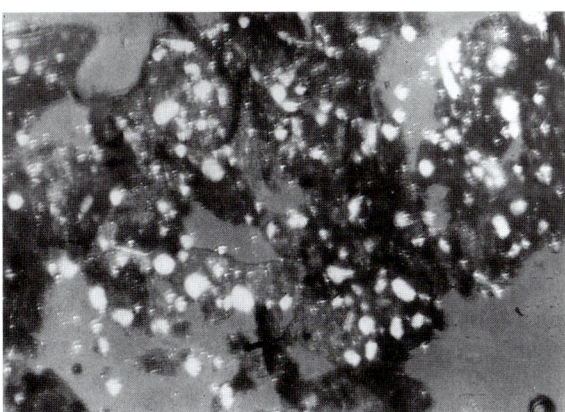

Figure 108-7. Photomicrograph of a histologic section under polarized light. Abundant polyethylene-laden macrophages and free polyethylene particles are present throughout the tissue. No metal debris could be found (original magnification ×100). (From Whiteside LA: Effect of porous-coating configuration on tibial osteolysis after total knee arthroplasty. Clin Orthop Relat Res 321:96, 1995.)

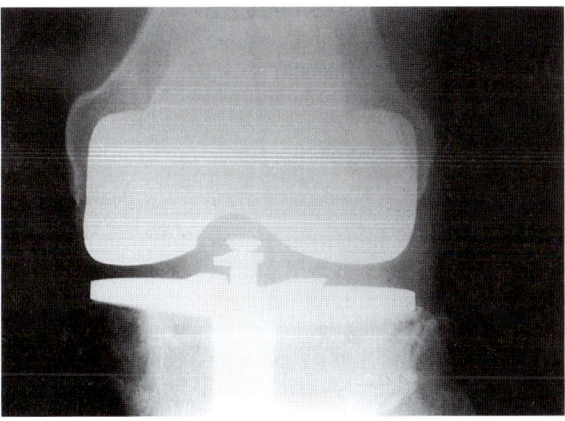

Figure 108-8. Radiograph of a knee with evidence of osteolysis in the femur and tibia. At the time of revision surgery, the locking mechanism of the polyethylene to the tibial component was found to allow at least 1 mm of micromotion between components, thus creating a pumping action that forced joint fluid into surrounding tissue.

to be another factor in migration of debris from the joint to surrounding bone stock. In a study of four failed knee implants (one Synatomic, three AMK; DePuy, Warsaw, Ind) retrieved at the time of revision surgery for osteolysis, gross motion of more than 1 mm between the polyethylene piece and the metal component was observed. Osteolysis had appeared on radiographs between 18 and 36 months after the original implantation and progressed rapidly (Fig. 108-8). At the time of revision surgery, a connection between the joint cavity and the intraosseous cyst was always found at the synovial attachment to the bone in implants fixed with or without screws. The bone-cement interface was eroded severely in the two cemented tibial components. In the two cases in which prostheses were fixed with a cementless technique, the bone-metal interface remained intact, but the synovial fluid and inflamed synovial tissue attacked the bone at the synovial attachment. Severe wear was found in three tibial

components, and the cysts were filled with a thick, friable, synovial pannus. The other knee had no visible sign of wear. Pumping of the loose polyethylene appeared to create a pressure wave in the synovial fluid that was conducted directly to the capsular attachment to bone.[31]

A laboratory study was undertaken in retrieved knees whose implants were intact to simulate the piston-like motion of a loose locking mechanism and to determine the amount of hydrostatic pressure generated at the interface. Polyethylene articulating components with locking tabs removed were tested first to simulate a loose locking mechanism; they then were exchanged for components with locking tabs intact to simulate a secure locking mechanism. The pressure measured beneath the anteromedial screw hole was nearly the same as or higher than intra-articular pressure in the knees with a mobile polyethylene component, whereas pressure beneath the screw hole was a fraction of the intra-articular pressure in knees with a fixed polyethylene component. Clearly secure fixation of the polyethylene component is an important part of implant design. Loose polyethylene components cause high wear and high hydraulic pressure at the bone-implant interface. Both of these effects markedly increase the incidence of osteolysis.[10]

Intra-articular Pressure

Regarding the effect of hydraulic pressure created by a poorly fixed locking mechanism, bone cysts and tissue necrosis are thought to occur as a result of joint fluid forced under high pressure through cartilage defects into subchondral bone. Intra-articular pressure was measured in the laboratory in 10 normal knees and 10 knees retrieved at autopsy with total knee implants intact. Testing conditions were set to determine whether the pressure was high enough during range of motion and with effusion to force reactive joint fluid and particulate debris into surrounding tissue and bone and cause osteolysis. Although normal and retrieved knees had similar trends in intra-articular pressure throughout range of motion, retrieved knees had statistically significantly higher intra-articular pressure at every flexion angle except 30 degrees without effusion. Joint pressure was especially high in the suprapatellar and posterior regions of retrieved knees, and significantly more time was required for it to diminish compared with pressure in normal knees. Pressure in the retrieved knees was occasionally high enough to cause tissue necrosis and bone cysts, which may suggest a mechanism for osteolytic cyst formation around components, even when wear is minimal.

The amount or size of particulate debris therefore does not appear to matter as much in the progression of osteolysis as does free access to the joint. Ortholoc Modular knees revised for osteolysis did not show severe polyethylene wear, and knees with radiographically detectable osteolysis did not appear to have radiographic evidence of severe wear.[62] In knees retrieved for gross motion between the polyethylene articulating surface and the tibial tray, destruction of bone was present even without severe component wear.[31] Clearly, the environment in the knee after total knee arthroplasty is highly conducive to osteolysis, and every effort should be made to design implants so that the interfaces between bone and metal and between polyethylene and metal are fixed securely and sealed.

Patellar Design

Attempts to produce a metal-backed cementless patellar component led to further problems that were unrelated to a specific method of fixation but nonetheless were attributed to cementless technology. Wear through the polyethylene to the metal backing and subsequent contamination of the articular surface with metal and polyethylene debris led to further damage of already compromised tibial polyethylene components and also to massive osteolysis and loss of bone stock. This cascade of events is often attributed to cementless fixation of the femoral and tibial components, whereas it really indicates that the design concepts and performance of the patellar component were poor. It is clear that the patellar surface is difficult to replace with a cemented or a cementless component, and use of metal backing on a thin polyethylene patellar component is a treacherous undertaking.

INSTRUMENTATION

The instrumentation that has made cemented arthroplasty successful for most surgeons was developed primarily to ensure correct alignment for cementless knee replacement.[20,67] Aside from instrumentation, many of the principles that resulted in successful cemented knee arthroplasty were not applied to the newer cementless components. Early in the process, developers often stated that implants designed for cemented installation could not simply be porous coated and then used for cementless fixation to bone. In fact, that was exactly what should have been done. Ignoring established criteria of successful total knee arthroplasty design led to experimentation in design that culminated in poor short-term and catastrophic long-term results of many of the early cementless knee components. Early failure of cemented tibial components led to extensive research on fixation of the tibial component, and finally the published literature arrived at a consensus that the cancellous bone of the upper part of the tibia was incapable of supporting the tibial component unless an effective stem was incorporated into the design. Nevertheless, most of the early cementless designs did not have a stem and failed to achieve adequate peripheral fixation of the tibial component to the cancellous-cortical structure of the upper tibia. It is not surprising that large numbers of these tibial components loosened, requiring revision arthroplasty.

RESULTS

Results of cementless total knee replacement since the mid-1980s have proved to be highly dependent on design. Prostheses with excellent fixation of the tibial component, minimal constraint at the articular surface, or both have had very low rates of loosening and have been reliable in all age groups and in cases of inflammatory and degenerative arthritic conditions. Fifteen-year survival rates of the Ortholoc total knee replacement[63] and the LCS[8] (DePuy) are similar in terms of loosening and wear. The Natural Knee (Intermedics Orthopaedics, Austin, Tex) has also continued to deliver excellent clinical results with cementless fixation techniques.[19] The Performance total knee design (Biomet, Warsaw, Ind) and the PFC total knee design (Johnson & Johnson Orthopaedics, Raynham, Mass) have been reported to perform similarly when fixed with cemented or

osteointegrated techniques. These five knee systems have varying combinations of excellent initial fixation, low articular surface constraint, and precise preparation of the upper tibial surface.

A study of 10-year results with cemented and cementless techniques for the AGC (Biomet) knee implant revealed no differences in loosening, pain, or knee scores with the two fixation methods. It is important to note that in this study, the most difficult patients—young, active, male patients—all underwent the cementless technique.[2] The PFC knee design was evaluated in a randomized, prospective study comparing cemented and cementless fixation.[32] Clinical performance was virtually identical, but radiolucent lines were found to be significantly more likely to occur in cemented components. The status of cementless total knee arthroplasty is now at the same point that it was 10 to 15 years after its introduction. The design characteristics that consistently lead to success are now well known, and the surgical procedure is effective when performed by surgeons who are expert in its use.

Cemented total knee replacement is fairly consistently successful but has not yet become standardized. Some authors recommend superficial penetration of cement into the surface of the bone,[22] whereas others recommend deep penetration. Some authors recommend cementing only the tibial component,[26] whereas others recommend that all components be cemented.[22] Although many reports of excellent long-term results with cemented all-polyethylene tibial components are available in the literature, efforts to design an all-polyethylene tibial component that is reliable with full cement technique have been fraught with fixation problems. One clinical review reported that 18% of patients had to undergo revision or experienced gross loosening 1 year after surgery.[14] Although this finding may be related to the articular surface design and to the flatness of the femoral component surface, the reasons have not been fully established, and other subtle features of cemented total knee replacement design may make it less than completely reliable.

Close evaluation of published long-term results reveals a rapid fall in prosthetic survival rate after 10 years in service,[37,42] especially in heavy, active patients, who begin to show radiographic evidence of failure as early as 4 years after surgery.[42] One group reported a good 10-year survival rate (approximately 94%) when revision for loosening was considered the endpoint, but when the endpoint represented moderate pain, loosening, or revision, the survival rate dropped to 84% at 10 years.[37] Worsening results in their series over the 10-year period were caused by progressively increasing pain, instability, and deformity. This suggests that implants gradually loosen, move, and migrate. This explanation was supported in a report on motion of the tibial component of radiographically intact cemented total condylar knee arthroplasties.[46] In this study, 27 cemented knee arthroplasties were evaluated for motion between the tibial component and bone during varus-valgus stress testing. The least amount of motion was 0.2 mm, and the greatest amount was 2.1 mm. All knees had detectable motion between cement and bone.

Because the bone-cement interface is subject to progressive osteolytic attack, and this attack is especially rapid in cement interfaces with cancellous bone, as is the case with the acetabular component in total hip arthroplasty,[48] it is not unlikely that the bone-cement interface in total knee arthroplasty is undermined during the first few years and develops a fibrous tissue interface without a surrounding sclerotic margin. Early studies comparing migration of cemented implants with that of cementless ones implanted by means of the radiostereophotogrammetry technique revealed less migration in cemented components. However, as these studies progress and as the more effective cementless tibial component techniques are evaluated, it appears that progressive migration is minimized as reliably with the cementless technique when a stem and screws are used.[45] Reports comparing the current cementless technique with cemented fixation of the tibial component showed progressive migration of cemented components over the 5-year observation period, whereas cementless implants ceased to migrate during the first year.[39] All these results suggest that the interface between porous metal and bone is stable and reliable. As in the hip, once ingrowth occurs, loosening is rare on long-term follow-up.

CEMENTLESS REVISION AND BONE RECONSTRUCTION IN TOTAL KNEE REPLACEMENT

Of the few modern-design cementless implants that require revision, most have good bone stock and seldom need major bone grafting or cementing to restore bone stock and achieve stability.[64] The bone-implant interface has been remarkably benign, even in cases with severe patellar wear and massive contamination of the joint by metal and particulate polyethylene debris.

In patients who have massive bone loss, the cementless technique has been used successfully in revision arthroplasty of previously cemented or noncemented knees.[47,60,61,64] Bone deficit has been managed with block and morselized grafting techniques in combination with various implant systems. Even though larger defects are commonly thought to require a block allograft and a specially designed prosthesis,[50] a high rate of success has been reported with morselized grafting and a regular prosthesis.[47,60,61,64]

Although it may seem that bone loss around the knee joint would cause irreversible laxity and chronic instability, the capsular structures remain highly functional. A simple surgical procedure can restore the joint surface and achieve ligament stability. However, injury and chronic deformity usually do cause adaptive changes in fibrous tissue structures about the knee, so reconstruction of the femur and tibia to their original lengths may not be possible. As in knees with prolonged flexion contracture, permanent shortening of posterior capsular structures occurs to accommodate the sinking implants; therefore, restoration of stability requires bringing the ligaments to correct tension in flexion and extension, with the joint surface in a new position to accommodate these changes in length of the ligaments.

When total knee arthroplasty fails, cancellous bone in the distal femur and the proximal tibia has usually been damaged severely or destroyed completely, such that a sclerotic shell with large peripheral deficits is left. In most cases, however, enough diaphyseal cortical structure remains intact above and below the knee to allow implants with long stems to be used to engage this bone. The articular surfaces can then be augmented to rest on the rim of the deficient femoral and tibial metaphyses. The capsular ligaments can be tensioned so that constrained implants are seldom necessary.

Operative Procedure

The operative procedure includes complete removal of the implant and cement, débridement of the reactive membrane, and curettage to expose viable bone at all accessible surfaces. The medullary canals of the femur and tibia are reamed to accept an implant with a stem length of at least 150 mm, sized to fit tightly into the diaphyseal isthmus over a 2 to 4 cm length. The metaphyseal bone surface is prepared to accept seating of the femoral and tibial components over at least 25% of the rim circumference, and an effort is made to seat the femoral component posteriorly against substantial bone structure. Three thicknesses of femoral component are generally available for each size of implant in modern revision total knee arthroplasty systems, as are tibial thicknesses from 10 to 35 mm (Fig. 108-9). Posteriorly thickened femoral components make it possible to seat the implant posteriorly on bone. The porous surface of the metaphyseal component should seat on stable cortical or dense cancellous bone, but in many cases, this is inadequate. Bone surface contact against porous metal and long-term fixation must be augmented with porous coated stems to bypass metaphyseal defects, as is commonly done in revision total hip replacement. Implants must be designed with fatigue strength adequate to sustain long-term out-of-plane loading and bending moments, and a

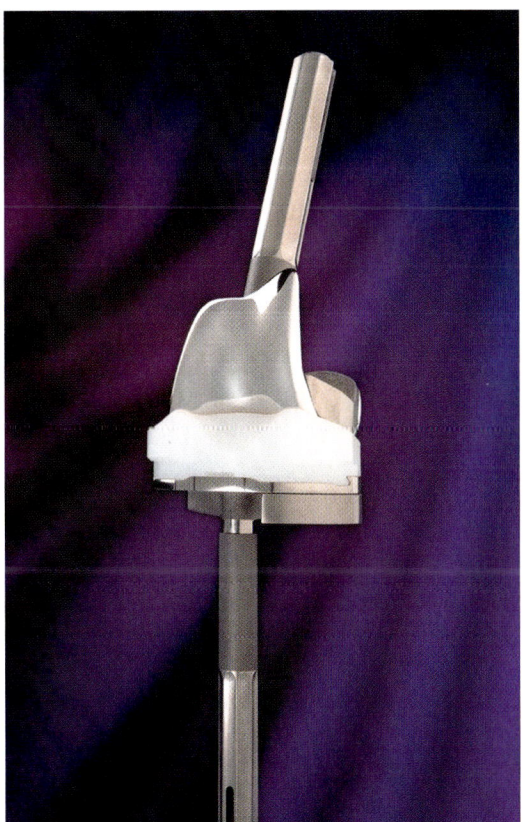

Figure 108-9. The Profix revision total knee replacement system (Smith and Nephew, Memphis, Tenn) features femoral and tibial components with a long stem for stability, posterodistal, and distal-only wedges on the femoral component for severe structural bone loss, and conforming polyethylene with anterior buildup for anteroposterior stability.

variety of space-occupying augments are necessary to link the metaphyseal bone to the articular implant.

Rationale

Cancellous and cortical bone loss after failure of total knee arthroplasty may require replacement with allograft; although block allografts have been advocated for such large deficits, the described morselized grafting technique obviates the more expensive, prolonged, and complicated preparation of a solid allograft. Use of morselized allograft was developed in conjunction with stem-stabilized augmented implants that allow rigid fixation and adjustment of joint surface position, and it was found that revision for loosening seldom was needed.[60,61] The ready availability of morselized allograft and its history of clinical success led to its use for reconstruction of bone defects. Granulated allograft bone that is smaller than the 0.5 to 1 cm pieces advocated is often resorbed and removed by the inflammatory process.[15] Pieces larger than those advocated are much more difficult to construct, are slower to ossify, and are slower to incorporate.[13] Rapid healing and ossification occurred in the reported series, probably because the implants were stable and the allograft was surrounded by viable bone (Figs. 108-10 to 108-13).[64]

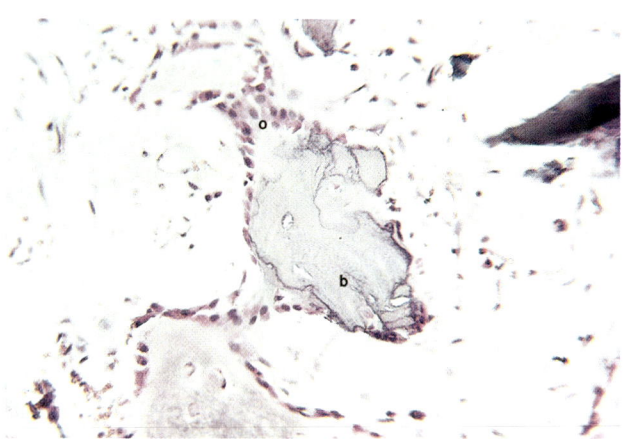

Figure 108-10. Photograph of a histologic section from a 3 week postoperative biopsy specimen. Granules of demineralized bone *(b)* are visible and are surrounded by plump osteoblasts *(o)* and new osteoid. Vascular stroma is present throughout the allografted area. No histologic evidence of bone resorption is seen (hematoxylin-eosin stain; original magnification ×160). (From Whiteside LA: Results: cementless. In Rorabeck CH, Engh GA [eds]: Revision total knee arthroplasty, Baltimore, 1997, Williams & Wilkins, p 456.)

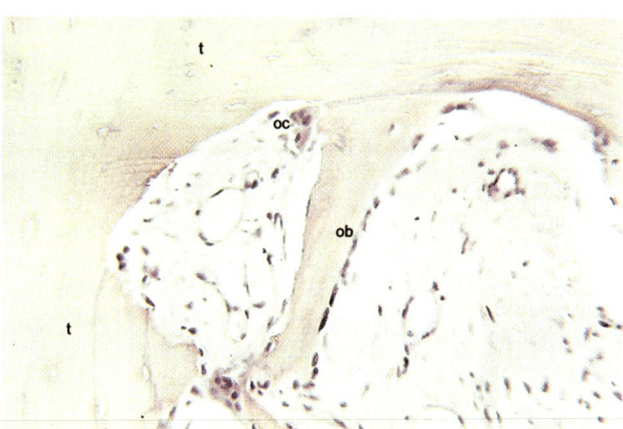

Figure 108-11. Photograph of a histologic section from a 3 month biopsy specimen. Dead trabeculae *(t)* are still abundant. Osteoclasts *(oc)* and new osteoid with osteoblasts *(ob)* are evident adjacent to the allograft. The allografted area contains multiple sites of bone resorption. New osteoid is often found on one surface of a trabecula with osteoclastic resorption on the opposite surface. Osteoblasts at this interval are flatter and less numerous than in the 3 week biopsy specimen (hematoxylin-eosin stain; original magnification ×160). (From Whiteside LA: Results: cementless. In Rorabeck CH, Engh GA [eds]: Revision total knee arthroplasty, Baltimore, 1997, Williams & Wilkins, p 456.)

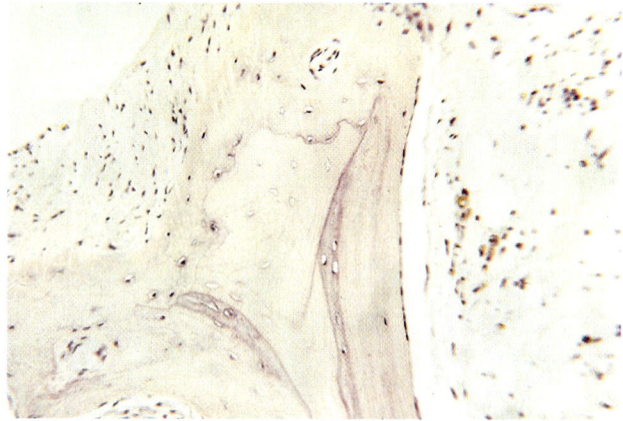

Figure 108-12. Photograph of a histologic section from a 21 month biopsy specimen. Mature lamellar bone and disorganized woven bone surround the allograft. The bone remodeling rate in the allografted area has decreased significantly. Trabeculae are now completely entombed by mature or woven bone. Bone remodeling has decreased, and osteoblastic or osteoclastic activity is directed toward new bone, not toward the allograft (hematoxylin-eosin stain; original magnification ×100). (From Whiteside LA: Results: cementless. In Rorabeck CH, Engh GA [eds]: Revision total knee arthroplasty, Baltimore, 1997, Williams & Wilkins, p 457.)

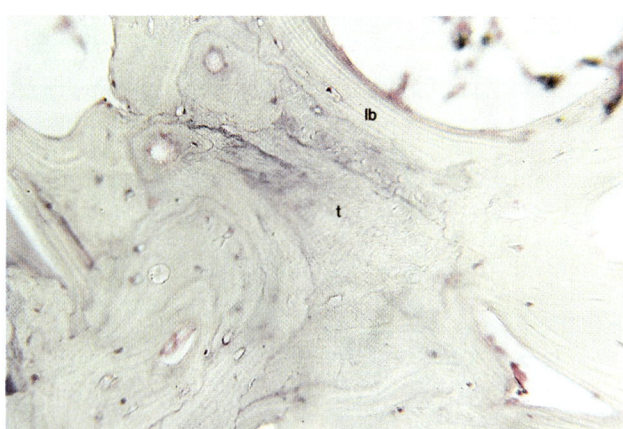

Figure 108-13. Photograph of a histologic section from a 37 month biopsy specimen. Entombed trabeculae *(t)* are present throughout the allograft. The visible allograft is completely encased by mature lamellar bone *(lb)*. Bone remodeling continues at normal levels. Few osteoclasts are found, and minimal evidence of osteoblastic activity is seen (hematoxylin-eosin stain; original magnification ×100). (From Whiteside LA: Results: cementless. In Rorabeck CH, Engh GA [eds]: Revision total knee arthroplasty, Baltimore, 1997, Williams & Wilkins, p 457.)

Although morselized cancellous allograft is osteoconductive rather than osteoinductive, it can serve as scaffolding for new bone formation. Demineralized bone added to the morselized allograft provides the osteoinductive stimulus and probably augments healing of failed hinge cases in which massive defects are encountered. Bone formation appears to begin early and progresses slowly through the first 18 months to 2 years. Findings from biopsy specimens taken from patients undergoing this treatment program suggest that the graft is fully mature by 3 years after surgery.[64] Most of the bone visible in the grafted areas is a combination of entombed allograft trabeculae and new lamellar bone, thus indicating that bone graft healing plus maturation of morselized cancellous allograft fortified with demineralized bone powder is similar to the mechanism of fracture callous formation. Structurally reliable bone is produced to support the implant and can be used in the event that a revision operation is required.

Bone-Grafting Procedure

Fresh-frozen allograft with morsels measuring 0.5 to 1 cm in diameter is soaked for 5 to 10 minutes in normal saline with the addition of polymyxin 500,000 U, bacitracin 50,000 U, and cefazolin 1 g/L. Ten milliliters of powdered demineralized cancellous bone is added to each 30 mL of fresh-frozen cancellous allograft. The bone defects are packed with this mixture, and the implants are impacted to seat on the remnant of viable bone, while the morselized bone graft is gently compacted. The morselized bone is not a weight-bearing structure and is meant to encourage bone regeneration in deficient metaphyseal bone stock. Actual weight bearing in the early postoperative period is accomplished through direct contact with metaphyseal cortical and cancellous bone, and in the long term through load sharing between the porous stem and metaphyseal bone contact.

Clinical Results

In a clinical review of 62 patients managed with this operative and bone-grafting treatment program, all patients except one had significant improvement in postoperative pain scores in comparison with preoperative scores, and 82.6% of patients were pain free at the 1 year postoperative follow-up visit (Figs. 108-14 to 108-16). Although the complication rate was high (22.5% of patients required repeated surgical treatment), only two patients required repeated revision for implant loosening. Pain was eliminated in one patient and was reduced to mild in the other.[64] Longer-term follow-up recently has added more information about the need for superior fatigue strength and more extensively porous coated metaphyseal augments and stems. Follow-up past 10 years is revealing fracture of the Morse taper stem in porous coated cast femoral components and loosening of components that have small amounts of porous coating in contact with bone[59] (Figs. 108-17 to 108-23). These mechanical problems of fixation and long-term durability of the implant are solved best with porous systems that allow for bone-ingrowth fixation in the diaphysis, as well as in the remaining metaphyseal bone. This strategy has provided the most reliable fixation of the femoral component in revision total hip arthroplasty.[3,11] Engh's et al early work with a fully porous coated cobalt-chromium stem demonstrated the high success

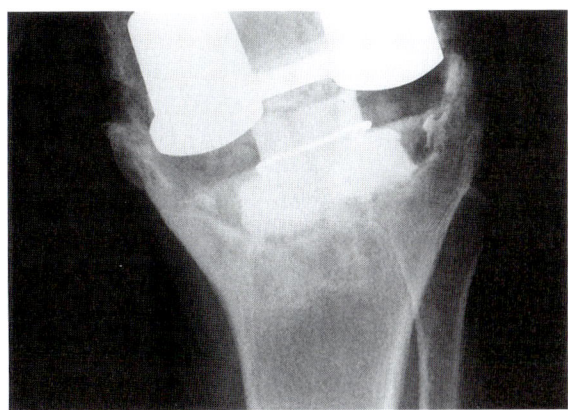

Figure 108-14. Preoperative radiograph of a left knee with a failed cemented component. Massive central and peripheral bone loss has occurred. (From Whiteside LA, Bicalho PS: Radiologic and histologic analysis of morselized allograft in revision total knee replacement. Clin Orthop Relat Res 357:152, 1998.)

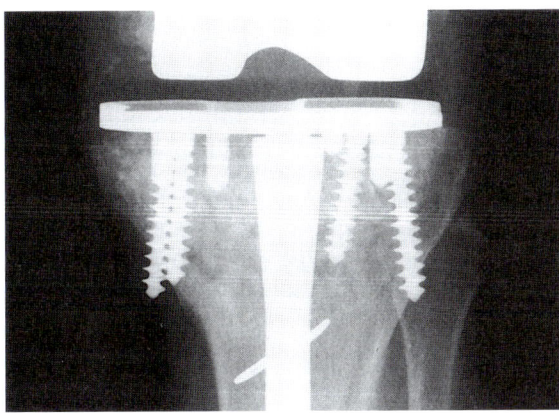

Figure 108-15. Radiograph, 1 month after surgery, of the knee shown in Figure 90-10. Tibial grafting with morselized allograft fills the defect. The lateral edge of the tibial tray is resting on bone. The stem prevents the medial edge from sinking into the allograft. (From Whiteside LA, Bicalho PS: Radiologic and histologic analysis of morselized allograft in revision total knee replacement. Clin Orthop Relat Res 357:152, 1998.)

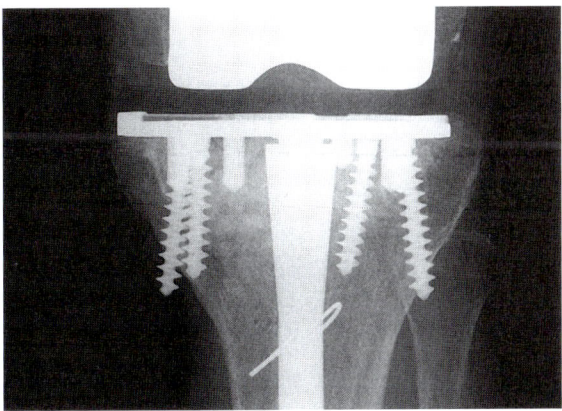

Figure 108-16. Radiograph, 7 years after surgery, of the knee shown in Figure 90-10. The graft has ossified, and trabecular bone is evident along the medial side of the tibia. (From Whiteside LA, Bicalho PS: Radiologic and histologic analysis of morselized allograft in revision total knee replacement. Clin Orthop Relat Res 357:152, 1998.)

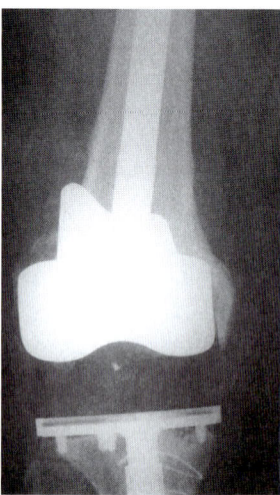

Figure 108-17. Anteroposterior radiograph of total knee revision case 12 years postoperatively. The lateral condyle was seated on the distal femoral surface, and the medial was grafted with allograft. The allograft failed, leaving the medial femoral condyle unsupported. Stem fracture occurred approximately 1 month prior to the time this radiograph was taken. (From Rapp SM: Surgeons find porous-coated TKA revision stems provide good fixation and build bone. Orthopedics Today 29:7, 2009.)

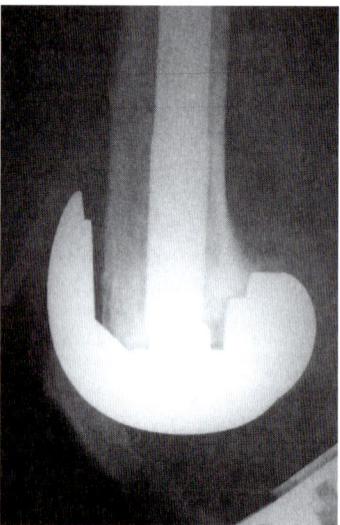

Figure 108-18. Lateral radiograph of the same knee. Destruction of bone is apparent. Both posterior femoral condylar bone structures have been destroyed, and the distal surface of the femur is severely damaged. (From Rapp SM: Surgeons find porous-coated TKA revision stems provide good fixation and build bone. Orthopedics Today 29:7, 2009.)

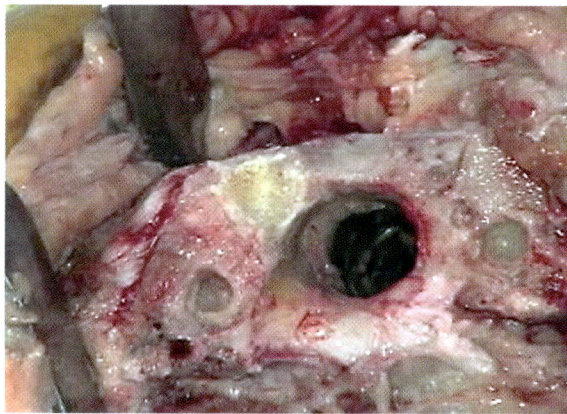

Figure 108-19. Intraoperative photograph of the distal femur of the same knee. The medial femoral condyle is much more severely damaged by loosening of the implants. (From Rapp SM: Surgeons find porous-coated TKA revision stems provide good fixation and build bone. Orthopedics Today 29:7, 2009.)

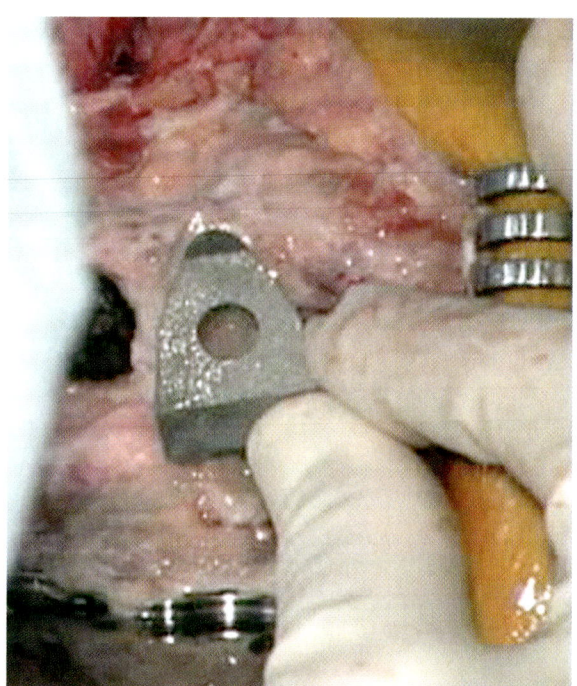

Figure 108-20. An L-shaped porous buildup module is being positioned against the deficient bone surface. (From Rapp SM: Surgeons find porous-coated TKA revision stems provide good fixation and build bone. Orthopedics Today 29:7, 2009.)

rate and effective long-term fixation that can be achieved with intramedullary diaphyseal osteointegration, which allows the deficient metaphyseal bone to be bypassed.[11] Flexible titanium stems such as those used by Wagner and Wagner[52] allow the load to be shared between the diaphysis and the metaphysis and even encourage recovery of metaphyseal bone stock. Regardless of the quality of fixation of and the degree of recovery of bone stock, implants must be designed for long-term fatigue resistance. This is especially challenging with porous coated implants because the sintering process weakens the base implant material. Plasma spray and arc deposition processes do not require heating to near-melting temperature and therefore do not weaken the base metal. New porous metal manufacturing techniques produce a porous surface that is an integral part of the base metal and are likely to further improve the strength of the revision constructs and the osteointegration potential of the surface.

SUMMARY

A cementless total knee replacement operation can be performed quickly and effectively, the results are reliable and durable, and complications are relatively easy to handle.

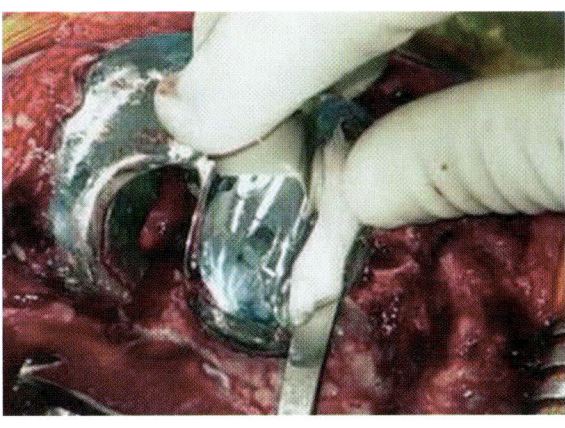

Figure 108-21. The femoral component with porous stem has been seated on the lateral bone stock, using a standard porous augment for the lateral femoral condyle. The porous augment is held against the deficient medial femoral condylar bone surface, and the gap between the augment and the femoral component is filled with acrylic cement to make a custom augment. (From Rapp SM: Surgeons find porous-coated TKA revision stems provide good fixation and build bone. Orthopedics Today 29:7, 2009.)

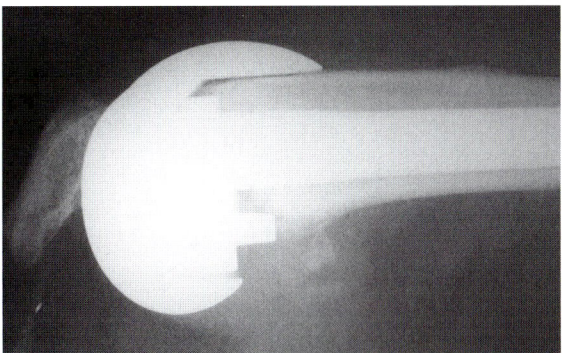

Figure 108-23. Lateral radiograph of the same knee showing the medial augment that contacts the deficient bone stock with its porous surface and is cemented to the main femoral component with acrylic cement. (From Rapp SM: Surgeons find porous-coated TKA revision stems provide good fixation and build bone. Orthopedics Today 29:7, 2009.)

Advanced biomaterials that improve osteointegration of porous interfaces will certainly broaden the scope of cementless fixation techniques in total knee arthroplasty. Hydroxyapatite added to the porous surface has already proved successful, even in implants that are not otherwise very effective.[18,38,41,43] Highly porous metal surfaces have stimulated interest in primary and revision arthroplasty and will make osteointegration more attractive.

In revision total knee arthroplasty, the cementless technique is especially effective if certain issues are addressed. Adequate rigidity of fixation must be achieved with long-stemmed implants seated on structurally reliable bone, and bone graft material should have osteoinductive properties.

Durability of the implants remains a significant clinical concern, and structural design, as well as strength of materials, will continue to present challenges to implant designers and surgeons. The strength of the porous material used to produce the porous surface is very important, especially if the material is to be made into structural support devices to replace missing bone. Late fatigue fracture of primary and revision components continues to be a clinical issue. As total knee replacement evolves, continued care will be necessary to ensure adequate fatigue resistance, as well as reliable osteointegration.

KEY REFERENCES

Bobyn JD, Poggie RA, Krygier JJ, et al: Clinical validation of a structural porous tantalum biomaterial for adult reconstruction. J Bone Joint Surg Am 86(Suppl 2):123, 2004.

Engh GA, Dwyer KA, Hanes CK: Polyethylene wear of metal-backed tibial components in total and unicompartmental knee prostheses. J Bone Joint Surg Br 74:9, 1992.

Harrington IJ: A bioengineering analysis of force actions at the knee in normal and pathological gait. Biomed Eng 11:167, 1976.

Helm AT, Kerin C, Ghalayini SR, McLauchlan GJ: Preliminary results of an uncemented trabecular metal tibial component in total knee arthroplasty. J Arthroplasty 24:941, 2009.

Kostuik JP, Schmidt O, Harris WR, et al: A study of weight transmission through the knee joint with applied varus and valgus loads. Clin Orthop Relat Res 108:95, 1975.

Nilsson KG, Karrholm J: Increased varus-valgus tilting of screw-fixated knee prostheses: stereoradiographic study of uncemented versus cemented tibial components. J Arthroplasty 8:529, 1993.

Ryd L: The role of roentgen stereophotogrammetric analysis (RSA) in knee surgery. Am J Knee Surg 5:44, 1992.

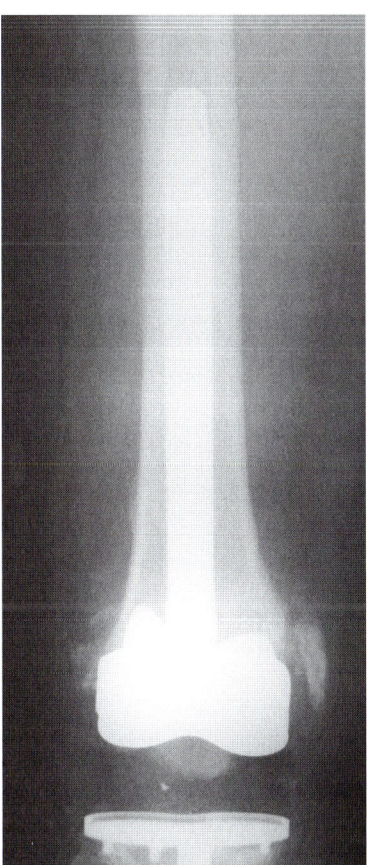

Figure 108-22. Anteroposterior radiograph of the same knee with a view of the porous titanium stem engaging the medullary canal. Correct alignment and position of the joint surface have been re-established. (From Rapp SM: Surgeons find porous-coated TKA revision stems provide good fixation and build bone. Orthopedics Today 29:7, 2009.)

Samuelson K: Bone grafting and noncemented revision arthroplasty of the knee. Clin Orthop Relat Res 226:93, 1988.

Walker PS, Granholm J, Lowrey R: The fixation of femoral components of condylar knee prostheses. Eng Med 11:135, 1982.

White SE, Tanner MG, Whiteside LA: Effects of sterilization on wear in total knee arthroplasty. Clin Orthop Relat Res 331:164, 1996.

Whiteside LA: Effect of porous-coating configuration on tibial osteolysis after total knee arthroplasty. Clin Orthop Relat Res 321:92, 1995.

Whiteside LA: Long-term followup of the bone-ingrowth Ortholoc knee system without a metal-backed patella. Clin Orthop Relat Res 388:77, 2001.

Whiteside LA: Cementless fixation in revision total knee arthroplasty. Clin Orthop Relat Res 446:140, 2006.

Whiteside LA: Anatomical landmarks for an intramedullary alignment system for total knee replacement. Orthop Trans 7:546, 1983.

Whiteside LA, Vigano RA: Young and heavy patients with a cementless TKA do as well as older and lightweight patients. Clin Orthop Relat Res 464:93, 2007.

Full references for this chapter can be found on www.expertconsult.com.

Posterior Cruciate Ligament Retention in Total Knee Arthroplasty

Aaron G. Rosenberg

The debate over whether to preserve the posterior cruciate ligament (PCL) in total knee arthroplasty (TKA), so-called cruciate-retaining (CR), or to substitute for it, so-called posterior stabilized (PS), continues to engage orthopedists. Although multiple differing design philosophies have come and gone over the past several decades, no consensus has been reached as to which knee is preferable. Several factors account for this. First, no clear benefits or drawbacks are apparent for either type of implant to the extent that either is clearly superior. In addition, multiple confounding factors are present in the comparative evaluation of implants (e.g., function, patient satisfaction, implant longevity, complication rates), as well as the influence of tradition in the implant choices of most surgeons, which makes comparison difficult. However, it should be noted that of primary importance in understanding the debate over implant choice in knee replacement is the difficulty of "hitting" a moving target.

Analysis of the available data is limited by two issues. First, the implants we now use are frequently different in both big and small (but perhaps no less important) ways from those reported on in most of the long-term follow-up studies. Second, these longer-term studies may reflect a significantly different patient population than that currently presenting for knee replacement. In the early decades of knee arthroplasty surgery, some series reflected as many as half of patients having inflammatory (most commonly rheumatoid) arthritis.[35] Young age, large size, primary or secondary degenerative osteoarthritis, and what were considered high physical activity demands generally were not thought to be ideal indications for TKA. Concerns about implant longevity, as well as a relatively higher complication rate and fear of early failure, led many surgeons to delay arthroplasty of the knee until more advanced disease was present, along with a lower likelihood that the patient would stress the implant construct.

Advances in implant design, surgical technique, and rehabilitative procedures, following careful critical assessment of results, have led to systematic improvement in the quality and consistency of TKA results, such that better pain relief, improved function, and better longevity can be expected for most patients undergoing TKA. These advances have given surgeons the confidence to offer knee replacement to afflicted individuals not previously deemed sufficiently debilitated or aged to warrant the risk. Current indications have subsequently expanded to younger and less severely affected individuals. Thus the surgeon must be aware of the fact that data in the literature may reflect implant and patient types that are not identical to those seen in today's practice.

PS designs (discussed in Chapter 11) have been suggested to offer easier correction of deformity without concern for obtaining appropriate tension on the PCL, a more conforming polyethylene surface that results in decreased polyethylene wear, and more reliable rollback of the femur on the tibia in flexion.[58] Proponents of the PS design note the more widespread clinical usefulness in that it can be used in knees without a PCL,[36] as well as the potential benefit of avoiding late posterior instability from PCL rupture, which has been reported in osteoarthritic patients[49] and in those with inflammatory arthritis.[41,45]

Proponents of CR[3,4,7,14,28] have suggested that advantages include preservation of an important central stabilizing ligamentous structure, transfer of stress to a functional ligament rather than a mechanical structure with subsequent reduction in wear and fixation stress, more consistent preservation of the joint line,[29] improvement in stair climbing ability,[4] and greater conservation of bone. In addition, problems that appear to be unique to PS designs—patellar clunk and post breakage and wear—are absent from CR designs.[42,44] Finally, the concept of simply resurfacing the joint and maintaining as much of the normal structures structure as possible is a philosophically appealing one, and indeed clinical data support both the quality and the longevity of the CR TKA.

RESULTS OF PCL-RETAINING TKA

Long-term series of many different CR TKA systems demonstrate excellent longevity and clinical results.* These results reflect 3 decades of evolving implant designs, which have corrected some of the problems noted in previous implant designs and materials and have reflected improvements in surgical technique and understanding of the technical requirements of implanting a knee that retains the PCL. These include improved patellofemoral design characteristics; better understanding of modularity, locking mechanisms, and the adverse effects of back-side wear; improved understanding of the relationship between implant surface kinematics and normal knee function and motion requirements; and improved manufacturing and sterilization of polyethylene. Although earlier studies of older-generation CR systems frequently showed 10-year survivorship of 90%, newer-generation systems have demonstrated improved 10-year survivorship to 96% to 100%.†

Aseptic loosening as a mode of failure is relatively rare in both CR and PS TKA, with no clear advantage seen for either type.[21,37,60] However, a relative weakness in much of the literature is that it reflects single surgeon series (frequently performed by the implant designer or in an academic setting by individuals who perform high volumes of TKA) and so is less likely to give a balanced view of a particular knee's performance, hence the importance of registry studies and large database reviews. The few of these that are available do show differences in outcome by implant type.

---

*References 7, 11, 16, 24, 32, 34, 43, 50, 55, 56, 59, and 65.
†References 1, 7, 10, 11, 30, 57, and 59.

A study of all primary TKAs performed at the Mayo Clinic over a 22-year period noted several trends.[54] Overall survivorship of 84% at 15 years was a significant improvement from the 69% noted in an earlier study from the same institution. Significant risk factors for failure included young age, male gender, noninflammatory arthritis, and the use of metal-backed patellae. Of note with regard to survival of CR versus PS implants, the 10-year survival rate of the CR TKA group was 91% as compared with 76% with posteriorly stabilized designs.

Additional multicenter investigational cohort studies support this finding. Heck and associates[69] reported a survey of 563 TKAs performed by 43 community surgeons and found that one of the factors related to maximal performance was PCL retention; in addition, the annual reoperation rate was 0.43 per year with CR knees as opposed to 0.51 in the PS design. Both studies indicated that CR implants have better long-term survivorship than PS implants.

FUNCTIONAL COMPARISONS

Several studies claim that sensitive function measures show better performance in deep flexion for the CR knee[23]; however, no substantial body of evidence indicates that sacrifice, substitution, or retention leads to consistently "better" knee function.[37,38] Multiple studies have noted no difference between the two in ultimate range of motion or in traditional knee outcome ratings. Studies comparing patients with a CR TKA on one side and a PS on the other have failed to reveal a persistent patient preference for one TKA type over the other.[9,13,60,61]

KINEMATICS

In the normal knee, the PCL serves several functions. It guides rollback of the femoral condyles on the tibial plateau during flexion, thereby allowing the posterior condyles to "clear" the posterior aspect of the tibia in high degrees of flexion and improving the mechanical efficiency of the extensor mechanism.[3] From the standpoint of stability, it prevents posterior subluxation of the tibia on the femur in flexion, while playing a strong secondary role in varus/valgus stability with the knee in flexion.

The history of knee arthroplasty is replete with studies evaluating the kinematic performance of total knee replacement in vivo. Multiple techniques have been used, and multiple claims promoted.* Indeed, controversy continues regarding the ability of the surgeon to successfully preserve the PCL in a way that is clinically meaningful. Several authors have claimed that maintaining PCL function following TKA is impossible, and that the kinematic demands of PCL retention require design considerations contrary to maximizing implant longevity.[36]

In the late 1990s, Komistek, Dennis, Steihl and coworkers studied in vivo knee performance in flexion by measuring rollback of the femur on the tibia in PS and CR knees via digital analysis of video fluoroscopy. Their initial studies showed a consistent pattern of anterior translation of the femur on the tibia in flexion in all CR knees studied.[25–27,46,62]

This finding was the reverse of the expected rollback of the femur and was termed paradoxical motion (Fig. 109-1A and B). These reports implied that no evidence suggested that the retained PCL was functioning in its expected role. It should be noted that these studies did not describe the surgical technique employed or the type of CR knee used. Yet the same group subsequently demonstrated that preservation of the PCL, combined with appropriate implant design, preserves femoral rollback in a study of an unselected group of CR TKAs performed by a single surgeon using a standardized technique with the use of a specific implant design, specific instrumentation, and a specific technique to adjust PCL tension.[12] In this group of 20 patients, all but one demonstrated essentially normal patterns of femoral rollback. More

FEMUR POSITION ON THE TIBIA DURING A DEEP KNEE BEND

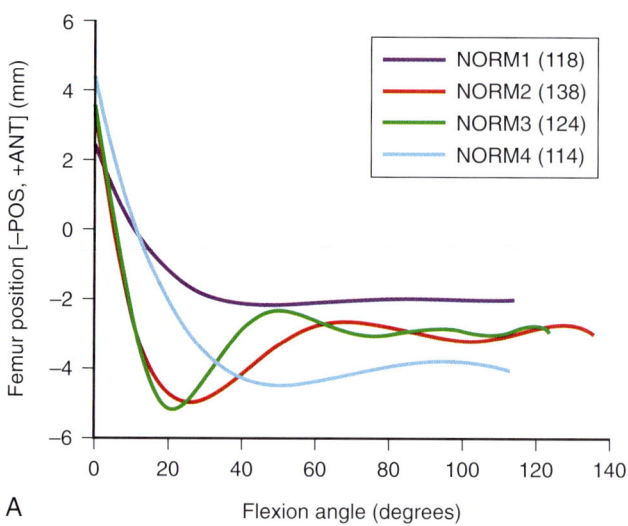

FEMUR POSITION ON THE TIBIA DURING A DEEP KNEE BEND

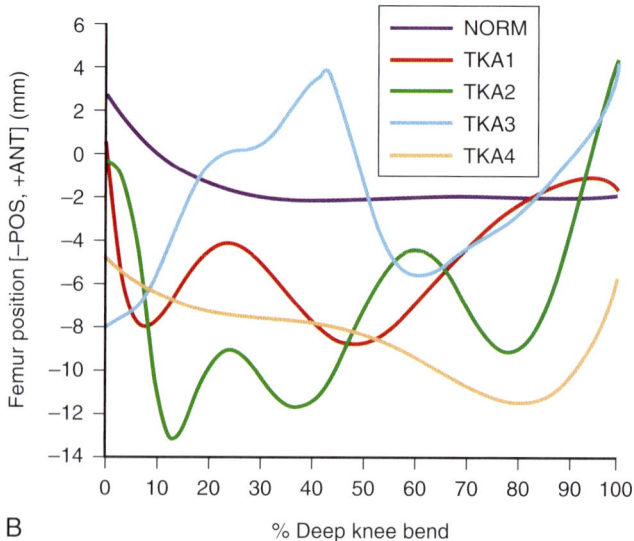

Figure 109-1. Paradoxical anterior motion of many cases of posterior cruciate–retaining total knee arthroplasty (CR TKA). **A,** Groups of normal knees demonstrating normal femoral rollback. **B,** Groups of CR TKA demonstrating paradoxical anterior motion of femur on tibia in deep knee bend.

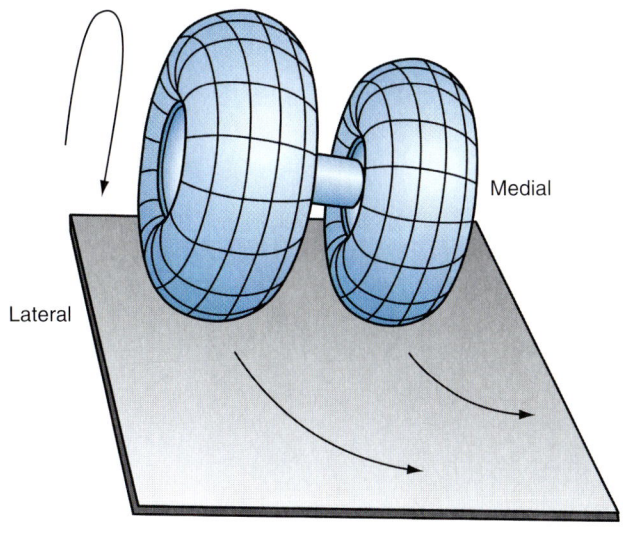

Figure 109-2. NexGen kinematics with a larger radius of curvature of the lateral condyle.

recent studies of the same implant design, implanted by three different surgeons using differing techniques,[40] revealed consistent rollback in all patients, thus indicating that these findings are not surgeon dependent, but rather are influenced by component design and technique. Results strongly implied that routine PCL preservation could be accomplished with functionally appropriate tensioning.

Additionally, Banks and associates[6] used three-dimensional kinematic assessment with fluoroscopy in a group of total knee replacements with intact PCLs that had essentially normal axial rotation and condylar translation; those with a post-and-cam substitution and no PCL had the smallest in vivo range of rotation and translation.

Of course, the articular surfaces must be designed to be compatible with normal femoral rollback. The "normal" rollback in the CR knees studied by Komistek and colleagues featured differing femoral condylar radii (Fig. 109-2). The differential radii allow the femoral component to roll posteriorly to a greater degree on the lateral side, as in the normal knee.[12,40] On the tibial side, a slightly flattened design in the sagittal plane takes advantage of the retained ligament, allowing the femur to both roll back and rotate in a relatively normal fashion. At the same time, significant congruence in the frontal plane allows stress in the polyethylene to be minimized, thus reducing long-term wear. It is clear that the geometry of articular surfaces affects motion-bearing surface strain and wear.[47,51]

PCL-RETAINING VERSUS PCL-SUBSTITUTING DESIGNS

Clinical Comparisons

Range of Motion

Numerous studies comparing CR and PS TKA have found no differences between the two in ultimate range of motion.[9,19,28]

Functional Studies

The theoretical advantage of improved proprioception attained by retaining the PCL was claimed by Warren and colleagues,[66] but most investigators have reported no difference in proprioception between the two types of TKA.[18,61] This may be due in part to the fact that the PCL in osteoarthritic knees has been shown to be more commonly histologically abnormal in comparison with control groups,[39] which may render the PCL less able to provide proprioception.

Although early studies demonstrated more normal stair climbing patterns and improvement in CR TKA,[4] several studies have shown no difference.[28,60] Conditt and coworkers[23] found poorer functional scores on squatting, kneeling, and gardening in patients with PS knees. They suggested that the PCL offers better functional capacity in higher-demand activities, especially those involving deep knee flexion. Unfortunately, like so many studies, this represents the results of one surgeon using one specific technique and one specific CR and PS implant system; thus, it cannot be thought to validate the claim that these findings can be generalized to other implants, surgeons, or patient groups.

Bilateral Studies

Numerous studies have compared patients with a CR TKA on one side and a PS TKA on the other.[9,13,21,60] These studies have not demonstrated a persistent patient preference for one TKA type over another.

Polyethylene Wear

The earliest CR designs featured polyethylene of relatively poor quality, resulting in higher rates of wear. Problems included the use of excessively thin and heat-pressed plastic, as well as the addition of calcium stearate. Over time, other manufacturing and sterilization techniques were shown to affect wear. These problems have since been addressed, and increased wear rates have not been seen with newer designs. However, poor soft tissue balancing in a CR TKA can result in tightness of the PCL in flexion, which can lead to posterior polyethylene wear.[64,69] Problems of instability and post dislocation can be seen in PS TKA as well if the soft tissues are not balanced.[58] This delineates the importance of soft tissue balancing, no matter what type of TKA is performed.

Correction of Deformity

Proponents of PS TKA have argued that larger deformities present difficulty with soft tissue balancing and are more easily balanced with a PS TKA. Although this can certainly be the case, some authors have used CR TKA in the setting of significant preoperative deformity and have had good results.[11,31] If the deformity is severe enough, flexion/extension mismatches or collateral ligamentous insufficiency often necessitates that even PS TKA is insufficient, and that more constrained knee replacements or even hinged TKA is necessary (Figs. 109-3A and B and 109-4A–C).

Aseptic Loosening

Rates of aseptic loosening of both CR and PS TKA remain low in modern designs, implanted with good cement technique, soft tissue balance, and alignment. No advantage for either type of TKA is apparent with regard to aseptic loosening rates.

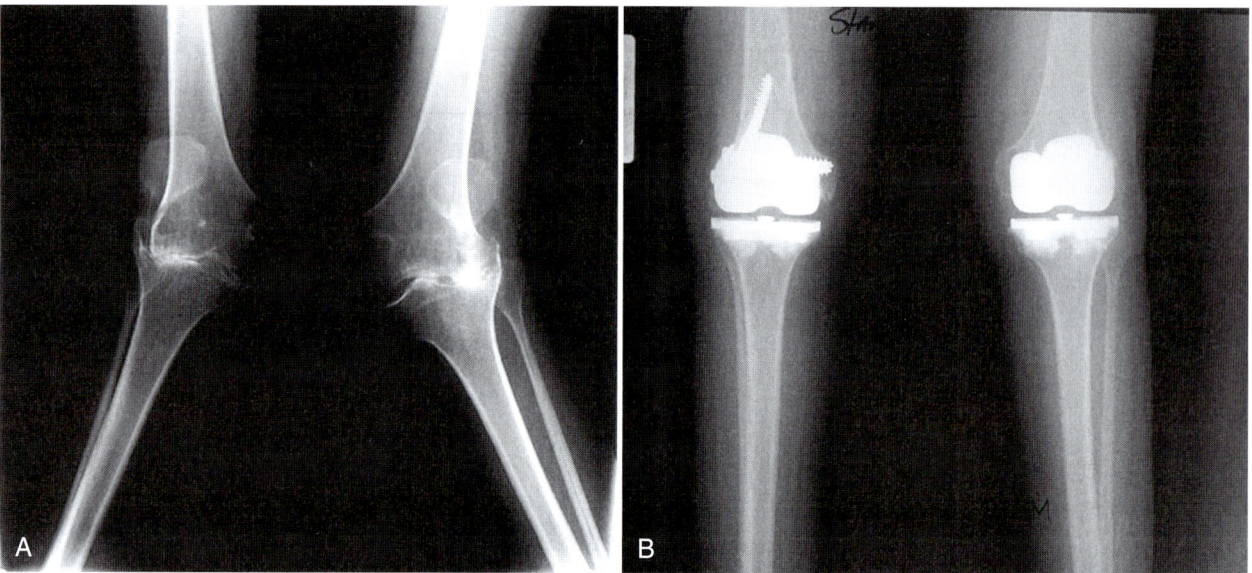

Figure 109-3. **A** and **B**, Correction of a large valgus deformity with a posterior cruciate–retaining total knee arthroplasty. In **A**, note severe bilateral valgus deformities. In **B**, note correction of valgus deformity with cruciate-retaining total knee arthroplasty.

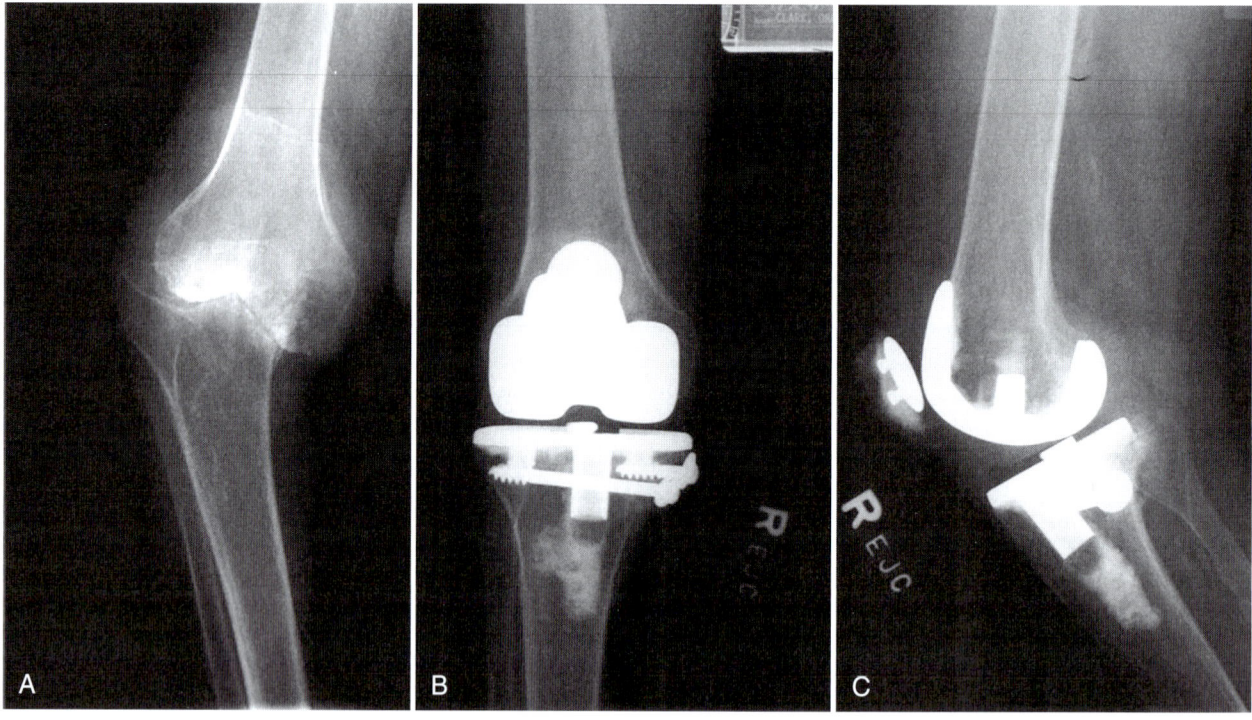

Figure 109-4. Correction of large varus deformity with a posterior cruciate–retaining total knee arthroplasty. **A**, Large varus deformity. **B**, Anteroposterior (AP) and **(C)** lateral films of correction of deformity with cruciate-retaining total knee arthroplasty.

Inflammatory Arthritis

It has been suggested that PS TKA is the proper choice in patients with inflammatory arthritides such as rheumatoid arthritis because of perceived attenuation of the ligament often noted in these patients. Many authors also feared that late rupture of the PCL could lead to late posterior instability.[41] However, Archibeck et al[5] demonstrated 95% good or excellent results in 46 knees of rheumatoid patients treated with CR TKA at an average of 10.5 years. Of note, in only one patient did posterior instability develop as a late complication. Similar findings were noted by Dennis et al.[24] These studies suggest that treating rheumatoid patients with knee arthritis by CR TKA yields excellent results.

POTENTIAL ADVANTAGES OF POSTERIOR CRUCIATE RETENTION

Maintenance of a Central Stabilizer

It is often said that TKA is a soft tissue operation. It is the contention of the CR surgeon that it is inappropriate to remove an essential soft tissue structure when retaining it makes the soft tissue portion of the operation easier. How so? The intact PCL functions as an important secondary stabilizer. When the PCL is preserved, it not only resists posterior subluxation forces, it also serves as a secondary stabilizer that resists varus/valgus instability. As opposed to the standard PS technique, which requires maintaining a relatively tight flexion gap (to prevent cam-post subluxation), CR TKA provides a natural means of balancing the flexion space after collateral ligament release. When large collateral ligament releases are required, there is less flexion instability than in cases in which the cruciate is removed. Consequently, flexion/extension gap balancing is simplified.

Maintenance of Joint Line Position

Perhaps of equal importance, functioning of the preserved PCL requires strict maintenance of the joint line to allow for appropriate tensioning of the PCL through range of motion. One potential problem that has been noted with PS knees is elevation of the joint line. Elevation greater than 8 mm has been found to significantly affect knee kinematics and has been correlated with patellofemoral symptoms and the need for revision.[33] Retention of the PCL requires strict maintenance of the joint line[29]; thus rarely is joint line elevation a problem in CR TKA.

Patellar Clunk Syndrome

Traditional PS designs have included a rather abrupt transition from the patellofemoral groove to the intercondylar box. Although recent designs minimize such transitions, PS TKA can still result in this complication. It generally is not seen in CR TKA.[1,42,51]

Avoidance of the Stress Inherent in Posterior Cruciate–Substituting Knees

In CR TKA, the PCL acts as a central stabilizer to absorb force and prevent posterior subluxation. Absorption of deforming force by the ligament may protect the fixation interface from such stress and prolong long-term fixation, in addition to eliminating the need for a mechanical structure (the cam-and-post mechanism) to absorb this force. In PS TKA, the spine/cam mechanism must resist posterior force, which can result in post wear.[17,53] O'Rourke and associates[49] noted relatively high rates of osteolysis in PS knees at intermediate follow-up and raised the question of increased polyethylene wear from the post. Wasielewski[67] raised the possibility that shear force can be higher in PS knees and in knee replacements with more conforming polyethylene inserts, also more commonly found in PS knees. Such shear force is noted at the modular articulation with the tibial baseplate; increases therefore could contribute to increased back-side wear. Scott and Volatile likewise noted the

possibility of increased loosening rates in PS TKA secondary to increased interface stress.[58] Post wear and post fracture can also occur with PS TKA and can lead to osteolysis and/or failure of the TKA.[22,48] A poorly balanced PS TKA can result in post dislocation. These problems are not encountered in CR TKA.

SURGICAL TECHNIQUE AND IMPLANT DESIGN

The primary focus of PCL retention in TKA is preservation of the PCL with re-creation of an environment that maintains appropriate ligament tension during function through the range of motion. To preserve the PCL, it must be recognized that the ligament inserts distal to the articular surface of the tibia by 5 to 10 mm, and during the tibial preparation, one should pay special attention to preserving the insertion. Some surgeons do this by placing an osteotome in front of the PCL insertion during the tibial cut. Another option includes leaving a small block of bone anterior to the PCL insertion (Fig. 109-5).

Three important features of surgical technique lead to appropriate tensioning of the PCL. All of these involve accurate restoration of the flexion space in which the PCL functions. First, the femoral component size should be chosen to reproduce the anteroposterior (AP) dimension of the native posterior femoral condyles. Provision of a large number of femoral AP sizes makes PCL balancing through measured resection techniques easier. Having a choice of widths for every AP size makes selection of the appropriate implant easier.

Second, the joint line can be reproduced by attending to two details. The first involves resecting at least as much tibial bone from the healthy side of the tibia (lateral in the varus knee and medial in the valgus knee) as will be replaced by the smallest thickness of tibial component. This prevents inadvertent elevation of the joint line in two ways. If a maximum of 5 mm is taken from the healthy side of the tibia and is replaced with a 10 mm component, the joint line will have been moved proximally by 5 mm. The second technique is to be sure that full extension is achieved by appropriate soft tissue releases and not by taking excessive distal femur to enlarge the extension gap. The greater the amount of distal

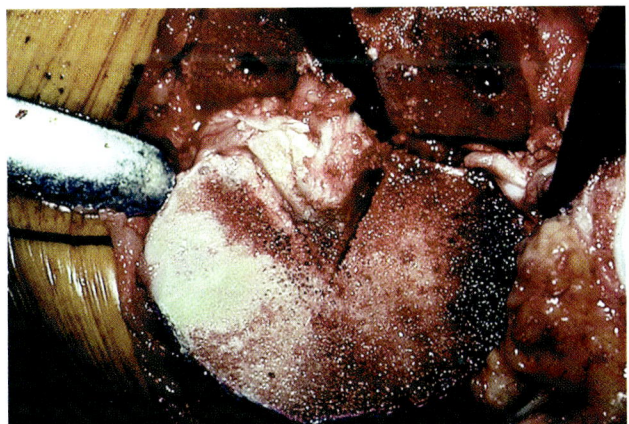

Figure 109-5. Bone block preserved for the posterior cruciate ligament.

femoral resection, the more the joint line is relatively elevated, and the greater the likelihood that tension on the PCL will be inappropriate.

Third, it is equally important to re-create the natural degree of the patient's posterior tibial slope so as to avoid excessive tightness in flexion. If this slope is not re-established, the posterior aspect of the tibial component will be placed too far proximal relative to the patient's original joint line, which will result in excessive tightness in the PCL during flexion. This can cause excessive rollback with a "nutcracker" effect and high contact pressure in the posterior part of the tibial articulation. Polyethylene wear may be increased in this setting; perhaps equally important, the range of motion can be limited. Both of these situations are undesirable and can be eliminated by reproducing the normal tibial slope. If the prosthesis is designed to be inserted with a posterior inclination to the plane of resection, this must be surgically performed. Most tibial components are designed in this fashion.

After preparing the femur and the tibia, the surgeon must look for signs that the ligament may be too loose or too tight during the trial reduction.[20] This assessment is made with the knee in flexion—the position in which the ligament is placed under tension. Excessive tightness in flexion is evidenced by several signs: the trial base plate (if unrestricted by a post embedded in the tibia) may lift off from the tibial cut anteriorly; the femoral component may be pushed anteriorly off the distal femoral cut as the knee is brought into flexion; rollback of the femur on the tibia may be observed to be occurring too far posteriorly, with flexion indicating excessive tension in the PCL; and finally, the ligament tension can be palpated directly and assessed during the trial reduction (Fig. 109-6). An insufficiently tensioned ligament can also be

assessed by palpation or by performing a posterior drawer test or observing a typical posterior sag.

Of course, tightness in flexion may simply indicate an unbalanced flexion/extension gap, and so correction of this tightness should be appraised with attention to appropriate filling of the extension gap as well. Assuming that the extension gap is well filled (there is no recurvatum or flexion contracture), one must actually assess the tension in the PCL to determine whether or not it is the sole contributor to flexion tightness. If the PCL is found to be too tight with the previously mentioned methods, this may reflect insufficient tibial slope; tightness should be checked before further attempts are made to alter PCL tension.

If the slope is appropriate and the implant system has a femoral downsizing capability (so-called minus sizing), this is where the smaller AP dimension of the femoral component will decrease tension on a tight PCL. Alternatively, when the PCL is found to be too tight with these methods of evaluation, the tibia can be moderately subluxed anteriorly, while the PCL is gradually released from the tibial insertion subperiosteally.

Occasionally, severe deformity may require release of the PCL, because contracture of the ligament is actually part of the pathology (generally moderate or severe sagittal plane alignment abnormalities combined with flexion contracture); in these cases and in the revision setting, substitution seems a most reasonable alternative. However, Worland and associates[68] demonstrated that patients' subjective and objective results were not compromised if flexion gap filling was appropriate as measured by acceptable KT-1000 measurements at follow-up in TKAs with PCL recession. The claimed advantages of this approach are that the patient's joint line is not changed, and the rest of the knee kinematics is preserved. If "excessive recession" is observed, the surgeon must accurately assess the knee's AP stability and select an ultra-congruent (AP motion restricting) polyethylene or must convert to a PS knee.

Several considerations must be kept in mind when the surgeon converts to a PS-substituting implant after initially preparing for a CR implant. Paradoxically, the most serious potential complication in converting to a PS knee is instability of the cam-and-post mechanism. This may occur through a combination of factors that produce a well-functioning CR knee but may sabotage the PS knee: a relatively excessive posterior tibial slope and the general principle of downsizing the femoral component when between sizes. Combined with relative flexion and collateral ligament instability, this may result in an underfilled flexion gap, and with flexion and varus or valgus stress (depending on the side of collateral instability), the post may slip under the cam. Increasing the filling of the flexion gap is likely to solve the problem, and the surgeon must keep this in mind when converting from the CR to the PS.

In cases in which the ligament is a part of the ligament contracture pathology (generally moderate or severe sagittal plane alignment abnormalities combined with flexion contracture) and in the revision setting, PCL substitution seems to be the most reasonable alternative. Additional settings in which PS designs are appropriate include a patellectomized knee,[8] a knee with complex deformity after proximal tibial osteotomy,[2] and a knee with severe inflammatory changes that have affected the integrity of the ligament itself.[5]

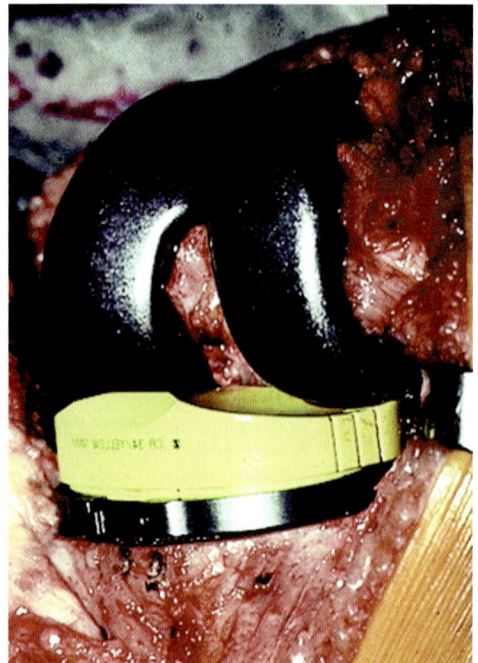

Figure 109-6. Tightness in flexion on this prosthesis can be checked at 90 degrees of flexion. Note the anterior lift-off of the polyethylene insert and the anterior position of the tibia, indicating excess posterior cruciate ligament tightness in flexion.

CONCLUSION

The concept of simply resurfacing the joint and maintaining as much of the native (healthy?) structure as possible is a philosophically appealing one. However, retention of the PCL necessitates understanding the differences required in surgical technique and component design (and occasionally patient selection) for successful performance of this procedure. Multiple femoral sizes are needed to allow PCL balancing through measured resection techniques. The posterior slope must be reconstituted to allow a balanced PCL in flexion. Improvements in component design now allow improved kinematics with improved femoral rollback. These advances in design and surgical technique have led to great success in previous outcome studies and lend promise for ever-improving functional outcomes among patients in the future. In the near future, these improvements will help meet the increased demand for TKA in the younger, more active, more demanding patient with increased life expectancy.

KEY REFERENCES

Barrington JW, Sah A, Malchau H, Burke DW: Contemporary cruciate-retaining total knee arthroplasty with a pegged tibial baseplate: results at a minimum of ten years. J Bone Joint Surg Am 91:874–878, 2009.

Bellemans J, Robijns F, Duerkinckx J, et al: The influence of tibial slope on maximal flexion after total knee arthroplasty. Knee Surg Sports Traumatol Arthrosc 13:193–196, 2005.

Berger RA, Rosenberg AG, Barden RM, et al: Long-term followup of the Miller-Galante total knee replacement. Clin Orthop Relat Res 388:58–67, 2001.

Bozic KJ, Kinder J, Menegini M, et al: Implant survivorship and complication rates after total knee arthroplasty with a third-generation cemented system: 5 to 8 years followup. Clin Orthop Relat Res 430:117–124, 2005.

Chaudhary R, Beaupré LA, Johnston DW: Knee range of motion during the first two years after use of posterior cruciate-stabilizing or posterior cruciate-retaining total knee prostheses: a randomized clinical trial. J Bone Joint Surg Am 12:2579–2586, 2008.

Clarke HD, Math KR, Scuderi GR: Polyethylene post failure in posterior stabilized total knee arthroplasty. J Arthroplasty 19:652–657, 2004.

Conditt MA, Noble PC, Bertolusso R, et al: The PCL significantly affects the functional outcome of total knee arthroplasty. J Arthroplasty 19(7 Suppl 2):107–112, 2004.

Ginsel BL, Banks S, Verdonschot N, Hodge WA: Improving maximum flexion with a posterior cruciate retaining total knee arthroplasty: a fluoroscopic study. Acta Orthop Belg 75:801–807, 2009.

Jacobs WC, Clement DJ, Wymenga AB: Retention versus sacrifice of the posterior cruciate ligament in total knee replacement for treatment of osteoarthritis and rheumatoid arthritis. Cochrane Database Syst Rev 19(4), 2005.

Kim YH, Choi Y, Kwon OR, Kim JS: Functional outcome and range of motion of high-flexion posterior cruciate-retaining and high-flexion posterior cruciate-substituting total knee prostheses: a prospective, randomized study. J Bone Joint Surg Am 91:753–760, 2009.

Komistek RD, Mahfouz MK, Bertin KC, et al: In vivo determination of TKA kinematics: the NexGen prosthesis with and without a PCL—a multicenter analysis. J Arthroplasty 23:41–50, 2008.

Niki Y, Mochizuki T, Momohara S, et al: Factors affecting anteroposterior instability following cruciate-retaining total knee arthroplasty in patients with rheumatoid arthritis. Knee 15:26–30, 2008.

Omori G, Onda N, Shimura M, et al: The effect of geometry of the tibial polyethylene insert on the tibiofemoral contact kinematics in advance medial pivot total knee arthroplasty. J Orthop Sci 14:754–760, 2009.

Pagnano M, Scuderi G: Rationale for posterior cruciate substituting knee arthroplasty. J Orthop Surg. Available at: FindArticles.com./p/articles/miqa3794/is200112/ain90007247/. Accessed April 25, 2010.

Ploegmakers MJ, Ginsel B, Meijerink HJ, et al: Physical examination and in vivo kinematics in two posterior cruciate ligament retaining total knee arthroplasty designs. Knee 17:204–209, 2010.

Wright RJ, Sledge CB, Poss R, et al: Patient-reported outcome and survivorship after Kinemax total knee arthroplasty. J Bone Joint Surg Am 86:2464–2470, 2004.

Full references for this chapter can be found on www.expertconsult.com.

Chapter 110

Posterior Cruciate Sacrificing Total Knee Arthroplasty

Aaron A. Hofmann and Jeremy McCandless

Debate continues regarding the posterior cruciate ligament (PCL) in total knee arthroplasty (TKA). Good long-term data exist both radiographically and clinically for PCL sparing and PCL substituting types of implants.[7,20] Some surgeons routinely sacrifice the PCL, and others routinely spare the PCL. Some surgeons make an intraoperative decision based on intraoperative findings. National trends from the previous decade in which most knee arthroplasties were performed with PCL retaining–type implants have changed to a more recent trend of PCL substituting implants with a post and cam mechanism, or sacrificing and substituting with a highly conforming deep dish polyethylene.[17]

This author represents the group of surgeons who make an intraoperative decision to spare or sacrifice the PCL. The algorithm followed closely matches that suggested by Lombardi and associates.[13] Initial attempts in straightforward TKA are to spare the PCL, with the exception of a few notable clinical situations. Significant initial malalignment greater than 15 degrees in varus or valgus or significant flexion contracture precludes the ability to sufficiently balance soft tissues and expose the joint with PCL retention.[9,21] Inflammatory arthropathies are also known for late failure of PCL after initial retention.[1,10] Prior patellectomy disrupts the normal kinematics of the knee and yields inferior results if PCL retention is chosen.[15] Similarly, inferior results have been detected in prior high tibial osteotomy patients who do not have a PCL substituting implant.[26]

SPARING THE PCL

Salvage of the PCL provides possible kinematic and proprioceptive benefits. However, concerns with regard to salvage of the PCL have been raised. The kinematic benefit of cruciate retaining arthroplasty appears to be absent on fluoroscopic analysis.[25] One magnetic resonance imaging (MRI)-based study demonstrated that tibial bone cuts interrupted the PCL to a significant degree most of the time.[24] Late failure of a retained PCL leading to revision is described as occurring in up to 2% of cases in one series.[1,18] Histologically, the PCL is abnormal in a significant number of arthritic knees.[19] These findings and others show why this author recommends protecting the PCL (Fig. 110-1) with an osteotome if it is to be saved, and proving its stability before selecting PCL retaining or substituting final components.

SACRIFICING THE PCL

If a unique clinical indication for PCL sacrifice exists (as mentioned earlier), or if the PCL is proven not to be sufficiently stable, some form of sagittal plane motion stability is required. Currently, two techniques are available for stabilizing the sagittal motion of the tibia during flexion after PCL sacrificing primary TKA: (1) posterior stabilized polyethylene

utilizing a posterior middle intercondylar tibial post that articulates with a cam on the femoral component during flexion to reproduce femoral roll-back; and (2) posterior stabilization utilizing deeply dished, highly congruent anterior lipped polyethylene that has an anterior polyethylene buildup in a highly conforming fashion, which prevents posterior translation of the tibia on the femur. This author utilizes the deeply dished highly congruent anterior lipped method if the PCL is to be sacrificed.

Posterior Stabilized Polyethylene Prosthesis

The posterior stabilized condylar prosthesis was introduced in 1978 with specific goals of preventing tibial subluxation, improving range of motion, and improving stair-climbing ability.[6] Design theory included lengthening the effective moment arm of the quadriceps by forcing the contact point of the femur more posterior, giving a mechanical advantage over previous designs.[6] Long-term results are good with the posterior stabilized design, but specific clinical problems are associated with this design.

Patellar clunk syndrome was a significant problem with early designs of posterior stabilized TKA. The long intercondylar notch of the femoral cam and post mechanism allows fibrous tissue overgrowth proximal to the patella. Impingement and occasional painful snapping occur upon extension of the knee.[5] Subsequent design changes to the femoral component have minimized this problem. This painful and frequent cause of reoperation is still associated with cam and post posterior stabilized components.

Post breakage and wear is another complication that occurs uniquely to posterior stabilized implants. The tibial post, which functions to keep femoral contact points posterior on the tibia, is impacted repetitively by the femoral cam through normal use. Loads of 8 to 10 times body weight have been recorded with chair rise. The small surface area of contact between cam and post yields a significant concentration of stress. The post can break; this has been documented in case reports for both conventional polyethylene and highly cross-linked polyethylene.[2,22] The tibial post serves as an additional source of wear contributing to osteolysis.[21]

Complications

Complications of posterior stabilized implants occur on the femoral side as well. The cam of the femur that articulates with the post requires more bone to be removed from the intercondylar notch than other designs. This results in bone loss that may complicate revision surgery. Case reports of fracture between the condyles as a result of intercondylar bone loss are a matter of concern.[14]

The femoral cam of posterior stabilized implants can be dislocated and can become lodged anteriorly (Fig. 110-2).

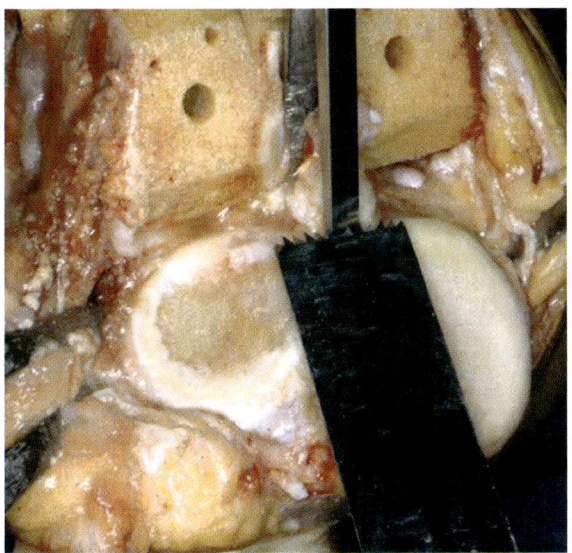

Figure 110-1. An osteotome is used to protect the posterior cruciate ligament if it is to be spared.

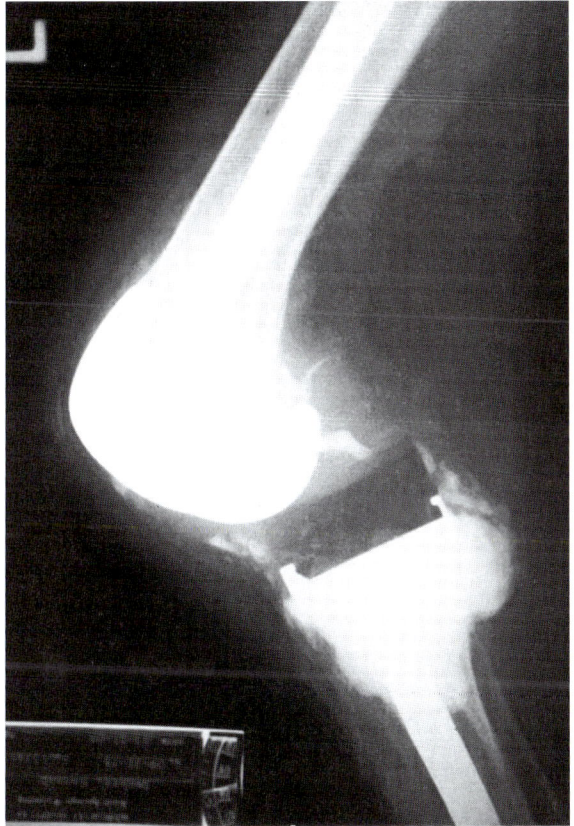

Figure 110-2. Total knee arthroplasty with dislocated cam and post form of posterior stabilization.

The tibial post engages the femoral cam at approximately 60 to 75 degrees of flexion. No contact or posterior stabilization occurs during this early range of motion (ROM). Soft tissue imbalance may yield laxity that allows dislocation to occur.[15] If this occurs, closed reduction and/or revision may be required.

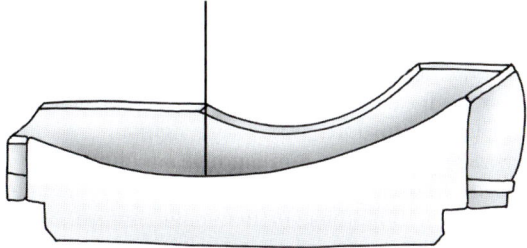

Figure 110-3. The null point, or femoral resting point, is 4 to 6 mm posterior to the midline.

Anterior Polyethylene Buildup Alternative

The current anterior buildup deeply dished alternative to the cam and post form of stabilization was developed out of necessity. A particularly difficult case involving a long-stemmed revision was reported in 1991 in a patient with Parkinson's disease who had persistent dislocation of the standard congruent insert. Because his medical health would not allow a prolonged revision operation, an alternative solution was sought. A custom polyethylene insert of highly conforming nature with an anterior buildup of 12.5 mm was designed. This insert was subsequently placed in production for use with the Natural Knee system (Zimmer, Warsaw, Ind) as the ultracongruent posterior stabilized polyethylene. Since that time, this concept has been incorporated into at least six other TKA systems.

The ultracongruent deep dished anterior buildup alternative for PCL sacrificing TKA has several advantages. First, no additional femoral inventory is needed if the PCL is sacrificed or saved. Stabilization of the femur is maintained in flexion and stair climbing. The anterior buildup maintains the tibial and femoral anteroposterior relationship throughout the arc of motion. There is no need for a long intercondylar femoral notch for a cam mechanism that reduces bone loss at primary operation and reduces risk of iatrogenic femoral fracture. Additionally, lack of a long trochlear notch prevents abnormal fibrous tissue formation with the theoretical advantage of preventing patellar clunk. Less stress concentration occurs on the tibial polyethylene than on the posts of posterior stabilized implants because of the highly conforming nature of the ultracongruent anterior lip stabilized polyethylene. No "forced" roll-back occurs via a cam and post mechanism; however, the null point or resting position of the femur on the tibia is posterior to midline by 4 to 6 mm and then operates as a ball-in-socket rotation point (Fig. 110-3). Dislocation of this design has not been reported.

Disadvantages

Theoretical disadvantages of ultracongruent anterior buildup polyethylene have been described.[14] In early flexion, less rotational laxity is noted than with cam and post posterior stabilization. This has been theorized to transmit greater shear stress to the tibia-bone interface and to create early loosening; however, this has not been our experience. Rotational freedom of the femur on the tibia is maintained with ±7.5 degrees of rotational freedom. The study of kinematics has demonstrated in cadaveric specimens an increase in quadriceps force (approximately 25 lb) to extend the knee with anterior buildup versus cam and post–type posterior stabilization.[14] This is most likely due to lack of full posterior translation that a post would provide through deep flexion to give the quadriceps lever arm maximal advantage. Quadriceps rehabilitation preoperatively and postoperatively has negated this potential negative effect.

A misconception about ultracongruent anterior buildup polyethylene bears discussion. When the total condylar knee prosthesis was designed and implanted, lack of optimal flexion was noted with a deeply dished polyethylene. Several studies since then have published on the dramatic improvement in knee flexion that occurs with posterior stabilized knees. It is clear that the deeply dished tibial component on the total condylar knee was suffering from a high posterior lip of the polyethylene and was impacting the posterior femur at lower levels of flexion than the posterior stabilized component. Ultracongruent and other anterior buildup posterior stabilization–type polyethylenes have a low posterior lip, and our experience suggests that flexion is comparable between cruciate retaining and cruciate sacrificing implants.

Study Results

Results of the first 100 ultracongruent inserts[4] compared with a control group of PCL sparing prostheses have been published. Goals of the study were to see whether patellar complications were avoided if the radiographic tibial interface was maintained, and to assess for differences in range of motion between the two groups. No patellar complications were reported in this study group. Two revisions of the ultracongruent insert occurred during the average 60-month follow-up; these were likely due to cementless fixation of the modular tibial baseplate. No difference in range of motion was noted between the two groups relative to preoperative motion.

Others have reported similar midterm results with anterior buildup posterior stabilizing PCL sacrificing arthroplasty.[23] Laskin and associates performed a randomized prospective study comparing anterior buildup posterior stabilization versus posterior stabilization with PCL sacrifice in all. No difference between the two groups in terms of range of motion, stair climbing, pain, knee scores, anterior knee pain, and stability was detected in that study.[11]

CONCLUSION

Total knee arthroplasty enjoys excellent survivorship and functional outcomes, regardless of posterior cruciate ligament status. There are clear indications to sacrifice the PCL to achieve the desired goal. Two ways of achieving stability of the tibiofemoral relationship after PCL sacrifice are known: posterior stabilized post and cam designs, and anterior buildup deeply dished highly congruent designs. Dished highly congruent stabilization may avoid some of the problems that post and cam–type posterior stabilized designs have encountered, with similar radiographic, functional, and clinical outcomes.

KEY REFERENCES

Archibeck MJ, Berger RA, Barden RM, et al: Posterior cruciate ligament-retaining total knee arthroplasty in patients with rheumatoid arthritis. J Bone Joint Surg Am 83:1231–1236, 2001.

Hofmann AA, Tkach TK, Evanich CJ, Camargo MP: Posterior stabilization in total knee arthroplasty with use of an ultracongruent polyethylene insert. J Arthroplasty 15:576–583, 2000.

Jacobs W, Clement DJ, Wymenga AB: Retention versus sacrifice of the posterior cruciate ligament in total knee replacement for treatment of osteoarthritis and rheumatoid arthritis. Cochrane Database Syst Rev (4):CD004803, 2005.

Laskin R: The Insall Award. Total knee replacement with posterior cruciate ligament retention in patients with a fixed varus deformity. Clin Orthop Relat Res 331:29–34, 1996.

Laskin RS, Maruyama Y, Villanueva M, Bourne R: Deep-dish congruent tibial component use in total knee arthroplasty: a randomized prospective study. Clin Orthop Relat Res 380:36–44, 2000.

Lombardi AV, Mallory T, Fada R, et al: An algorithm for the posterior cruciate ligament in total knee arthroplasty. Clin Orthop Relat Res 392:75–87, 2001.

Mont M, Booth R, Laskin R, et al: The spectrum of prosthesis design for primary total knee arthroplasty. Instr Course Lect 52:397–407, 2003.

Mullaji A, Marawar S, Simha M, Jindal G: Cruciate ligaments in arthritic knees: a histologic study with radiologic correlation. J Arthroplasty 23:567–572, 2008.

NIH Consensus Panel: NIH consensus statement on total knee replacement, December 8–10, 2003. J Bone Joint Surg Am 86:1328–1335, 2004.

Peters C, Mohr RA, Bachus K: Primary total knee arthroplasty in the valgus knee: creating a balanced soft tissue envelope. J Arthroplasty 16:721–729, 2001.

Sathappan S, Wasserman B, Jaffe W, et al: Midterm results of primary total knee arthroplasty using a dished polyethylene insert with a recessed or resected posterior cruciate ligament. J Arthroplasty 21:1012–1016, 2006.

Shannon F, Cronin J, Cleary M, et al: The posterior cruciate ligament-preserving total knee replacement: do we "preserve" it? A radiological study. J Bone Joint Surg Br 89:766–771, 2007.

Full references for this chapter can be found on www.expertconsult.com.

Chapter 111

Posterior Cruciate Ligament–Substituting Total Knee Arthroplasty

Michael P. Nett, Gregory J. Roehrig, Giles R. Scuderi, and W. Norman Scott

Posterior cruciate substitution in total knee arthroplasty gathered momentum and popularity as the pioneering surgeons and design teams improved on their prototypes. Today, surgeons that prefer this principle and technique over cruciate retention believe that the anterior and posterior cruciate ligaments (ACL, PCL) are histologically abnormal and therefore compromised in arthritic knees.[4,16,37] Furthermore, these surgeons believe that it is difficult to balance the PCL appropriately while maintaining its functional integrity and ability to accomplish near-normal femoral rollback.[7]

An understanding of the history behind the current posterior-substituting prostheses on the market, key design concepts, important surgical principles and techniques will aid surgeons in providing well-functioning, durable, total knee replacements. This chapter will first address the time line and progression of posterior-substituting components, from the earliest years to the currently available designs. The surgical technique and clinical results will then be reviewed.

The terms *posterior-substituting* and *posterior-stabilized* have been used interchangeably for many years. For clarity in this chapter, posterior-stabilized will be reserved to describe the Hospital for Special Surgery implant that originally bore this name in 1978. Posterior-substituting will be used to reference this entire style of total knee design.

EVOLUTION OF POSTERIOR CRUCIATE LIGAMENT–SUBSTITUTING KNEE ARTHROPLASTY

The Insall Group

The early years of knee arthroplasty saw multiple designs and design modifications. The unicondylar design was applied, in fact doubled, to yield the duocondylar prosthesis. Other designs that were studied at that time at the Hospital for Special Surgery (1971-1973) included the Geometric and the Gueper. These prostheses yielded good to excellent results in about 50% of patients. Problems included patellar pain, which led to the development of the duopatellar knee, and loosening of the components.

The next significant advancement was achieved with the original total condylar prosthesis which was cruciate-sacrificing, not PCL-substituting. It was a semiconstrained, nonlinked, cemented design that involved excising both cruciate ligaments. First implanted in 1974, this cobalt-chrome femoral component had a symmetrical anterior flange and groove, two symmetrical condyles in the coronal plane, and a smaller radius of curvature posteriorly in the sagittal plane. The tibial component was a single piece of high-density polyethylene with biconcave articular surfaces, offering some stability.[50] It was fully conforming in extension and less conforming in flexion to allow for more rotation and gliding of the femur. The small intercondylar eminence helped prevent

translation movement, and the 35- × 12.5-mm tibial peg helped achieve fixation. The patella was a dome-shaped, central peg, high-density polyethylene design.

Complete cruciate ligament excision accomplished greater exposure and allowed for easier correction of fixed deformities. Without an intact ACL and PCL, the knee design relied on the congruity of the articular surfaces and integrity and balance of the collateral ligaments for stability. With well-balanced flexion and extension gaps, the collateral ligaments will tighten as the femoral component translates anteriorly, up the conforming tibial well, preventing dislocation. This concept, designed with the input of engineer Peter Walker and surgeons John Insall and Chitranjan Ranawat, was termed the *uphill principle*. The femoral component was intended to articulate centrally on the tibial component surface, with no rollback built into the design. This original total condylar knee proved to be a durable, sound design,[31] but not without problems. Patients rarely achieved more than 90 degrees of flexion and, on occasion, the tibia would subluxate if the flexion gap was not adequately balanced, especially descending stairs. Such issues could potentially be resolved with a new prosthetic design that spared or substituted for the PCL.

Insall-Burstein I Posterior-Stabilized Prosthesis

To address the posterior subluxation and instability that would sometimes occur with the total condylar prosthesis, a central tibial post was added. This modification, however, proved to be an imperfect solution, as the specifics of the design and the hyperextension stop led to tibial edge loading and loosening.[64] In 1976, Al Burstein joined John Insall at the Hospital for Special Surgery where they combined their experience, insight, and innovation to develop a posterior-stabilized knee that would substitute for the PCL, allow for complete correction of deformity, reproduce femoral rollback, improve flexion stability, and increase knee flexion.

The first-generation Insall-Burstein prosthesis (IB I) was first implanted in 1978. The tibiofemoral contact point was shifted from a more central location to a more posterior point,[32] resulting in a greater distance or hill to climb before the femur subluxates anteriorly. An intercondylar femoral cam was added to the design to replicate femoral rollback. It engaged the tibial post at approximately 70 degrees of flexion and, as the cam climbed the post, the tibiofemoral contact point shifted more posteriorly until approximately 115 degrees of flexion. These features, along with the increased conformity and 3-degree posterior slope of the all-polyethylene tibial component, helped the IB I achieve great success and durability.

Importantly, the Insall-Burstein prosthesis substituted for the PCL, not the collateral ligaments. Gap balancing was critical to prevent anterior tibial subluxation. The spine-cam mechanism did not articulate in extension and therefore provided no additional medial-lateral stability. Stability was dependent on the integrity and balance of the collateral ligaments and somewhat influenced by the conformity of the tibiofemoral surfaces. An insufficient collateral ligament would necessitate a design with more inherent constraint.

During the 1980s, the IB I went through some design modifications. Research on load transmission to the tibia concluded that metal backing of the tibial component would improve this factor and the all-polyethylene design was replaced at the Hospital for Special Surgery by 1981. Carbon reinforcement of the polyethylene was introduced with the hope of increasing its strength and durability, but it did not achieve the anticipated success, early failures were reported, and this alteration was abandoned. In the mid-1980s, the femoral component underwent a few improvements. The anterior flange was deepened and rounded to allow for better patellar tracking and a smoother transition as the patellar-femoral contact point moved toward the distal runners with increasing flexion. Also, additional femoral component sizes became available, reducing the amount of mismatch between the prosthesis and distal femur.

Insall-Burstein II Posterior-Stabilized Prosthesis

The Insall-Burstein I posterior stabilized knee underwent more significant modifications in the late 1980s to yield the Insall-Burstein II. Intramedullary instruments assisted the surgeon in obtaining appropriate alignment in a reproducible and accurate manner. The original tension device for determining equal and rectangular flexion and extension gaps was replaced with a technique using spacer blocks. The concept of modularity was expanded to include multiple sizes for the femoral and tibial components, different polyethylene thicknesses, intramedullary stems, and wedges to address defects.

Additional changes were made to enhance femoral rollback, thereby improving flexion. Reports of component dislocation arose, especially in knees with preoperative valgus alignment or those that achieved a high degree of postoperative flexion. Consequently, additional modifications of the tibial insert included positioning the tibial post more anteriorly and increasing its height. This posterior-substituting design proved to be a functionally sound concept that performed well for more than a decade before it evolved further (Fig. 111-1).

NexGen Legacy

The Zimmer NexGen Legacy (Zimmer, Warsaw, Ind) prosthesis was, in fact, the next generation in the line of posterior-stabilized knee components. This prosthesis and its new instrumentation became available in the mid-1990s. One of the key improvements in design was anatomic right and left femoral components. The tibial components were symmetrical and therefore universal. In addition, the lateral flange of the femur was enhanced and the trochlea deepened to facilitate proper patellofemoral tracking and kinematics further.

Previous posterior-stabilized designs, including the Insall-Burstein prostheses, would occasionally experience inadvertent flexion of the femoral component during implantation. This would lead to gapping between the anterior cortex of the femur and anterior flange of the component. Attempts to correct this intraoperatively, if noticed, could result in a gap between the posterior condyles of the native femur and posterior condyles of the component. The addition of femoral lugs to the NexGen design assisted the surgeon during cementation and helped prevent unwanted flexion of the femoral component.

An expanded array of instruments became available with the NexGen Legacy prosthesis. These include epicondylar instruments to assist with femoral component rotation, anterior and posterior referencing size guides, and instruments to prepare the femur and tibia using a milling technique instead of the traditional cutting blocks and oscillating saw (Fig. 111-2).

NexGen Legacy High-Flexion and Gender-Optimized Implants

The increased desire by patients to pursue activities associated with greater degrees of knee flexion, as well as acknowledgment of the important cultural requirements in certain Asian populations, have driven the development high-flexion knee prostheses. These implants are designed to exceed 140 to 150 degrees of flexion compared with the 120 degrees permitted by traditional designs. To accommodate higher flexion, these design modifications include enhanced posterior condylar geometry of the femoral component, which improves contact areas in high flexion, thereby reducing the risk of polyethylene wear.[6] In addition, modifications to the anterior aspect of the tibial polyethylene insert were made to

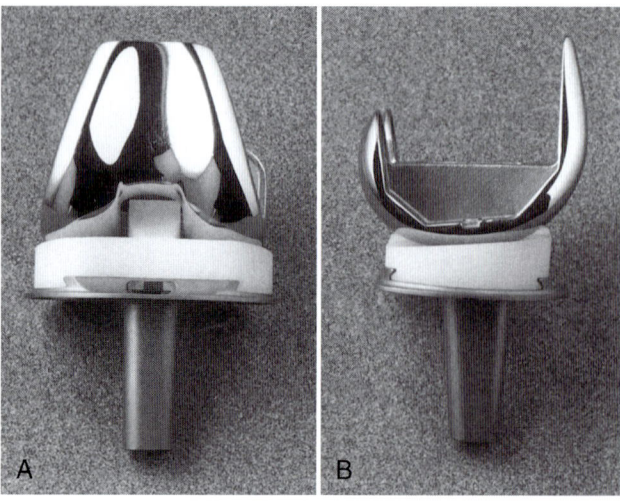

Figure 111-1. Insall-Burstein II prosthesis.

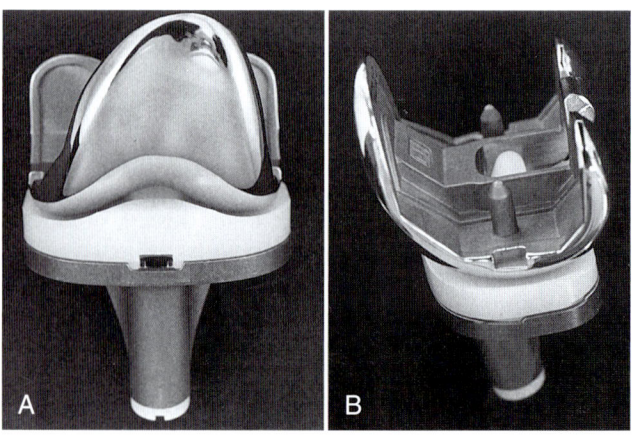

Figure 111-2. Zimmer NexGen prosthesis.

reduce the potential for extensor mechanism impingement in high flexion. Finally the cam-post design of posterior-stabilizing (PS) variants was optimized to reduce the risk of dislocation in high flexion. To date, studies of high-flexion total knee replacement (TKR) prostheses have provided little data to support the theoretical advantages attributed to the optimized designs. In a recent meta-analysis, Ghandi and associates[25] have noted that high flexion designs were associated with improved ROM compared with traditional implants, but offered no clinical benefits. Meneghini and coworkers[52] have confirmed the lack of any functional benefit with flexion more than 125 degrees after TKR.

An example of a high-flexion design is the Zimmer NexGen Flex-Fixed PS implant, a modification of the NexGen legacy prosthesis. Studies of the NexGen Flex-Fixed PS implant are inconclusive. Kim and colleagues[36] have reported on a prospective randomized study of 50 patients who underwent simultaneous bilateral TKR with a standard fixed-bearing Zimmer NexGen LPS knee prosthesis on one side and a high-flexion, fixed-bearing NexGen LPS-Flex knee prosthesis on the opposite side. The Knee Society and Hospital for Special Surgery (HSS) scores were not significantly different for either knee, either pre- or postoperatively. Moreover, there were no statistically significant differences in range of motion (ROM) at any time point pre- or postoperatively; at final follow-up, the standard prosthesis had a mean ROM of 135.8 degrees (range, 105 to 150 degrees) versus a mean of 135.8 degrees for the high-flexion prosthesis. A similar study was published by Nutton and associates.[56] They compared patients who had been randomized to receive a standard or high-flexion version of the Zimmer NexGen LPS fixed-bearing design. Again, no significant differences in outcomes or knee flexion were noted between the two groups of patients.

Shortly after the development of high-flexion designs, increased acknowledgment of the anthropomorphic variation that exists among humans of different genders, races, and ethnic origins led to the introduction of gender-optimized components.[26] These gender-specific components included modifications of the mediolateral to anteroposterior ratio of the femoral components, as well as to the orientation and thickness of the trochlear groove and anterior flange. An example of a gender-specific implant is the Zimmer Gender Solutions NexGen High Flex LPS prosthesis. This implant is a further modification of the NexGen Legacy. Results examining the use of gender-optimized devices remain controversial. Although radiographic and anatomic studies have demonstrated the gender bias of standard implants toward white male anatomy, little data exist to date to support that this bias has adversely affected clinical outcomes in white females or patients of other races.[49]

Other Current Posterior Cruciate Ligament–Substituting Implants

The outstanding performance of the Insall-Burstein device prompted the other total knee prosthesis manufacturers and their engineers to incorporate a PCL-substituting design into their product lines.

PFC Sigma

DePuy (Raynham, Mass) developed this comprehensive knee arthroplasty system with modularity in mind. The femoral

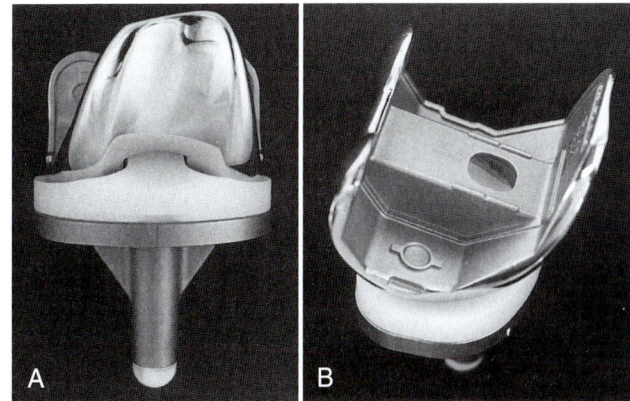

Figure 111-3. Depuy Johnson & Johnson PFC prosthesis.

component can be mated with a tibial tray of the same size, or one size larger or smaller, providing three choices for every femur size. This is meant to help optimize contact at the implant-implant interfaces and implant-bone interfaces.

The versatile tibial tray was designed to accept a PCL-retaining, PCL-supplementing, or PCL-substituting polyethylene insert of varying thicknesses. In addition, the tray can be augmented with wedges, blocks, and stems if bone loss or poor bone quality dictates. More recently, a tibial rotating platform design was released. The goals of this concept are improvement in rotational biomechanics (20 degrees of supported internal and external rotation in deep flexion), reduction of backside wear, and lower peak stresses on the condyles because of tibiofemoral self-alignment (Fig. 111-3).

Genesis II

The Genesis II total knee (Smith & Nephew, Andover, Mass) was designed as a comprehensive knee system with a modern PCL-substituting option. The components are designed to be versatile and allow the femoral prosthesis to mate with four different-sized tibial components. An additional feature is the elongation and lateralization of the femoral component's trochlear groove to maximize contact with the patella throughout the arc of motion (full contact through 85 degrees of flexion).

An innovative design concept used in the Genesis II is the design of the femoral component's posterior condyles. Most conventional knee system designs require external rotation of the femoral component to achieve a trapezoidal flexion gap. External rotation of the femoral cut results in more bone resected from the posterior medial femur than from the posterior lateral femur. The asymmetrical femoral bone resections help compensate for the traditional asymmetrical tibial resection that occurs with a perpendicular tibial cut. This traditional cut results in more bone resected from the lateral than from the medial tibial plateau. Thus, in the traditional method of component implantation, the bone cuts counterbalance each other and result in a rectangular flexion space. Traditional components are designed for this and have symmetrical posterior femoral condyles.

The Genesis II does not us external rotation of the femoral component and, consequently, the posteromedial femoral condyle is thinner than the posterolateral condyle. The designers hoped to minimize some of the theoretical limitations associated with traditional external femoral rotation

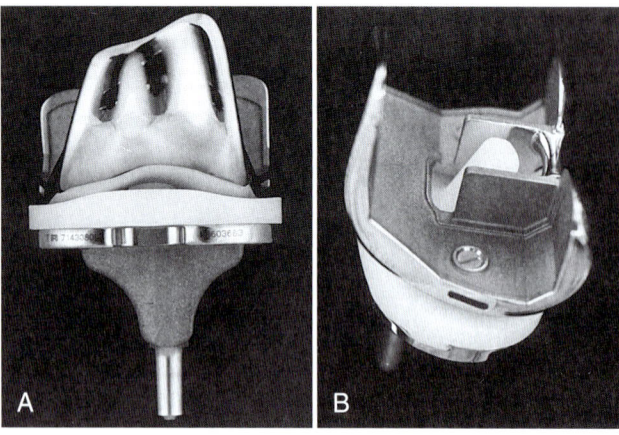

Figure 111-4. Smith & Nephew Genesis II prosthesis.

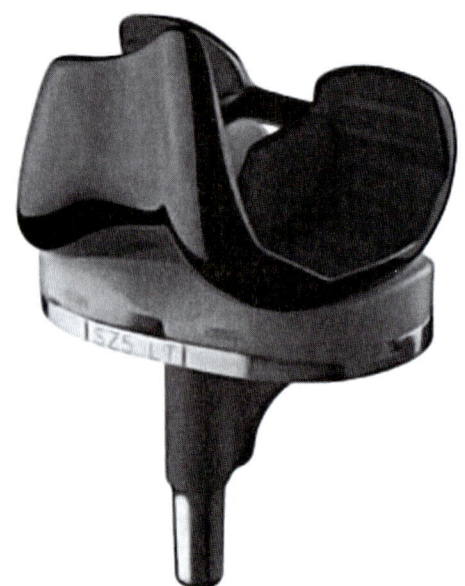

Figure 111-5. Smith & Nephew Journey prosthesis.

including unnecessary anterolateral femoral bone removal, rotational malalignment of the femoral and tibial components, and excessive medial patellar tracking at high flexion angles. Conceptually, the flexion space remains balanced because the smaller medial posterior condyle compensates for the smaller posterior medial flexion space.

Stability of the Genesis II PCL-substituting knee depends on both the component's articular geometry and the spine-cam interaction. The implants are designed to articulate freely through the first 60 degrees of flexion, with stability dependent on the surface geometry and soft tissue balance. Spine-cam engagement occurs at 60 to 70 degrees of knee flexion (Fig. 111-4).

Journey

In an effort to reproduce more normal knee function, Smith & Nephew used analyses and comparisons of the geometry and kinematics of the normal knee and conventional total knee arthroplasty (TKA) systems. The Journey Bi-Cruciate Stabilized Knee System is designed to replicate PCL and ACL function, accommodate deep flexion, induce normal tibiofemoral axial rotation, and provide proper patellar tracking throughout the entire range of flexion. The femoral component is made of oxidized zirconium for enhanced durability.

The medial condyle has been placed more distally than the lateral condyle, thereby creating a 3-degree physiologic joint line. The lateral distal condyle is thinner than the medial, but posterior offset is maintained on both sides. Other new design features include a tibial articular surface with a medial sulcus near the anteroposterior (AP) midline and a thicker lateral compartment with a convex surface in the sagittal plane. The femoral component has both anterior and posterior cams to enhance anterior-posterior stability and replicate the ACL and PCL.

In this effort to reproduce more anatomic knee motion, there are 5 degrees of screw-home designed in the Journey articulation as the knee comes to full extension. With progressive flexion, the forces of the extensor mechanism on the femur and the convex shape of the lateral tibial plateau yield external axial rotation of the femur, posterior femoral translation and rollback, and a slight medial pivot (Fig. 111-5).

Vanguard

Vanguard, the newest complete knee system from Biomet (Warsaw, Ind) offers 10 femoral component sizes and 9 tibial tray sizes. The femur comes in an open or closed box design and has a conservative bone resection for the intercondylar box. The posterior cam has been extended to minimize dislocation in deep flexion. The trochlear groove was deepened and lengthened in an effort to maximize patellar tracking and contact during deep flexion.

The tibial component is available in a monoblock design with a compression-molded polyethylene articular surface. If conversion to modularity is necessary, a removable bearing wedge allows for the polyethylene to be removed and the monoblock component to be rendered modular. The standard tibial tray has a locking clip that allows for compressive loading of the locking mechanism to minimize micromotion between the tray and the polyethylene.

The Vanguard system provides a spectrum of constraint from the standard PS insert, to the PS+, to the Super Stabilized Knee (SSK), to the SSK Constrained. These different polyethylene inserts allow for varying degrees of rotation, post height, and varus-valgus constraint (Fig. 111-6).

Triathlon

The Stryker Triathlon total knee arthroplasty system (Stryker Orthopaedics, Mahwah, NJ) was designed with the common goals of improved motion, increased flexion, greater sizing options, and minimization of wear. The femoral component radius of curvature was centered at the transepicondylar axis and designed to be more anatomic between 10 and 110 degrees. The central edges of the posterior condyles were tapered and the articular surface of the polyethylene was precisely machined to allow for approximately 20 degrees of tibiofemoral rotation. An anthropometric study was used to optimize the tibial and femoral sizing options. A 7-degree flexion cut was built into the anterior flange so that the femoral component could be downsized when necessary, with

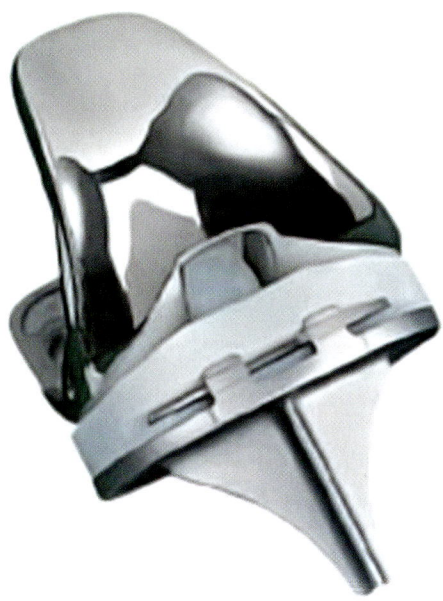

Figure 111-6. Biomet Vanguard prosthesis.

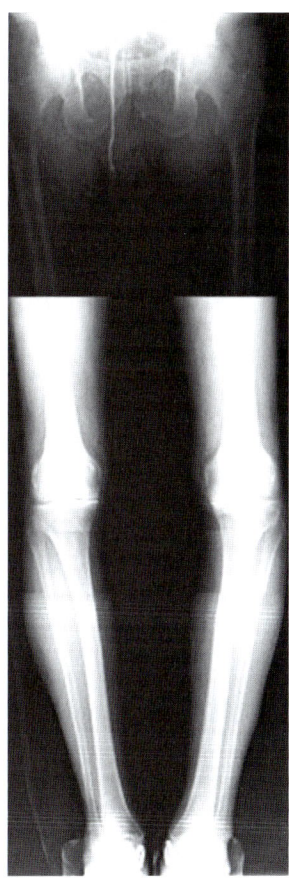

Figure 111-8. Full-length standing hip to ankle view is helpful in preoperative templating and in determining overall limb alignment.

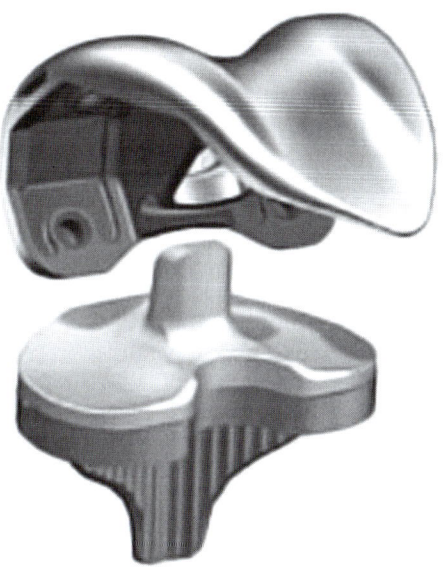

Figure 111-7. Stryker Triathlon prosthesis.

a reduced chance of femoral notching. The tibial component was designed with a central inset island to improve the ease of insertion and stability of the polyethylene component. This feature, along with the surface geometry mentioned earlier, aim to minimize micromotion and backside wear (Fig. 111-7).

SURGICAL TECHNIQUE

The primary objectives of total knee arthroplasty are to relieve pain, improve function, correct deformity, and minimize the need for reoperation. The basic surgical technique for implanting PCL-substituting prostheses has been well documented.[30,32] The intraoperative goal is a well-aligned, well-fixed prosthesis with coronal balance, an equal flexion and extension gap, and constant collateral ligament stability

throughout the full range of motion. The postoperative mechanical axis is to be in the central portion of the knee. This will result in load sharing equally by the medial and the lateral compartments to minimize polyethylene wear and improve longevity.

As implant sizes expanded and instrumentation improved, Insall advocated a modified gap technique combining aspects of both measured resection and the gap technique of TKA.[70] Tensors used to balance the collateral ligaments and align the knee were replaced with more sophisticated intramedullary instrumentation and spacer blocks. However, despite evolution of the technique and instrumentation, the basic concepts of the posterior-stabilized knee remain virtually unchanged.

The modern surgical technique begins with thorough preoperative planning. AP, lateral, and Merchant view radiographs are obtained. Templating for size is performed with traditional templates or with a digital templating system. A hip to ankle full-length radiograph provides additional critical information (Fig. 111-8). This includes the preoperative anatomic and mechanical axis, preoperative deformity, presence of hardware from prior surgery, and status of the ipsilateral hip. Ensuring that there is nothing to preclude the use of intramedullary instrumentation will help avoid intraoperative surprises. The surgeon may choose the angle of distal femoral resection from the measured difference between the anatomic and mechanical axis of the femur (Fig. 111-9). Other surgeons prefer using 6 degrees for varus knees and

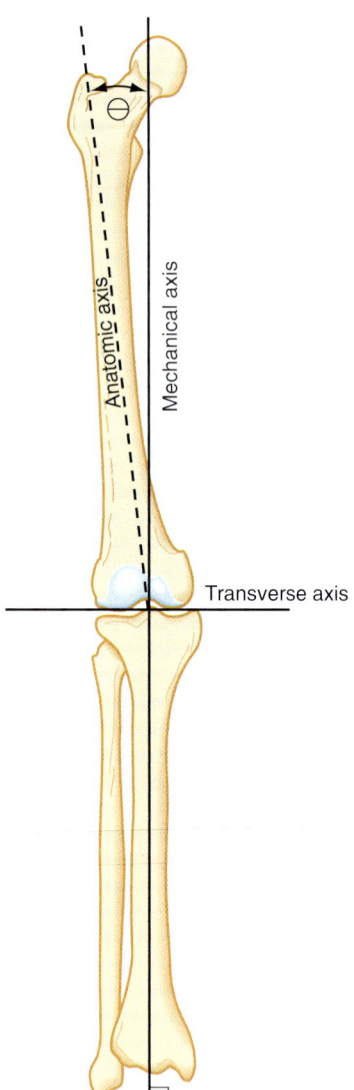

Figure 111-9. Calculating the angle between the anatomic and mechanical axes.

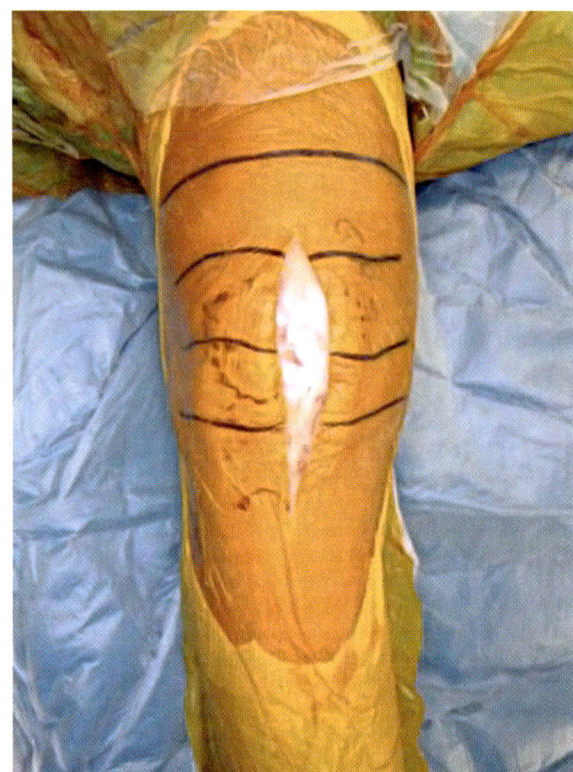

Figure 111-10. A straight anterior midline incision is made from just proximal to the superior pole of the patella, extending 10 to 14 cm distally to the medial aspect of the tibial tubercle.

5 degrees for valgus knees or patients with larger thighs. Finally, a line is drawn perpendicular to the mechanical axis of the tibia, noting the estimated amount of bone to be resected from the medial and lateral aspects of the tibia.

A bump is placed under the operative leg and secured to the operative table to help support the knee at 90 degrees of flexion. The contralateral leg is secured loosely to the operative table. A Foley catheter is placed. A tourniquet is placed high on the thigh and elevated after the limb is exsanguinated.

The knee is exposed with a straight anterior skin incision extending from the medial aspect of the tibial tubercle to two fingerbreadths proximal to the superior patellar pole (Fig. 111-10). Full-thickness subcutaneous flaps are developed, and 30 mL of 1% lidocaine with epinephrine is injected along the planned arthrotomy site to reduce intraoperative blood loss. A straight medial parapatellar capsular incision is used for the arthrotomy. A portion of the fat pad and genu articularis is excised to improve exposure. The periosteum of the proximal medial tibia is raised in a continuous layer off the tibia. Caution is used to avoid excessive medial dissection in the valgus knee. Laterally, a small cuff of periosteum is raised in continuity with the patellar ligament to provide some protection against tibial tubercle avulsion. The knee is assessed for a coronal fixed deformity. In the varus knee with a fixed deformity, a medial release may be performed at this point using the ¼-inch straight osteotome to elevate the superficial and deep fibers of the medial collateral ligament in continuity[35] (Fig. 111-11). The knee is flexed and the patella is allowed to subluxate laterally (Fig. 111-12). Routine patellar eversion is not necessary.[65]

With the knee in the flexed position, the ACL is transected off the tibia surface. The tibia is now subluxed anteriorly. It is sometimes necessary, especially on varus knees, to continue the release of the structures off the posteromedial aspect of the tibia, including a portion of the semimembranosus, to allow adequate tibial subluxation.[35]

After adequate exposure has been achieved, attention is turned to the bone cuts. Proceeding with the tibial cut opens the flexion and extension gaps and further facilitates exposure. The tibia may be cut with an extramedullary or intramedullary guide system, depending on the surgeon's preference and the knee anatomy. More frequently, an extramedullary guide is used during primary total knee arthroplasty (Fig. 111-13). The ideal cut is 90 degrees to the mechanical axis of the tibia, with a slight posterior slope in the anteroposterior plane. A skim cut is performed on the side with more severe wear and only 5 to 9 mm of bone is removed from the normal side. This is extremely important in patients with preoperative valgus deformity or obese females. In these patients, not only will excessive bone resection place the tibial component in a weaker cancellous bone bed, but it can lead to run way

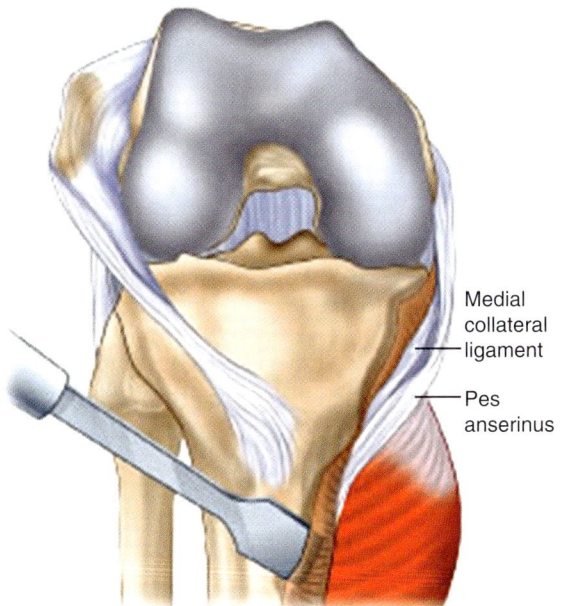

Medial collateral ligament

Pes anserinus

Figure 111-11. The correction of a fixed varus deformity may require subperiosteal release of the superficial medial collateral ligament. The preferred technique is elevation with a ¾-inch straight osteotome.

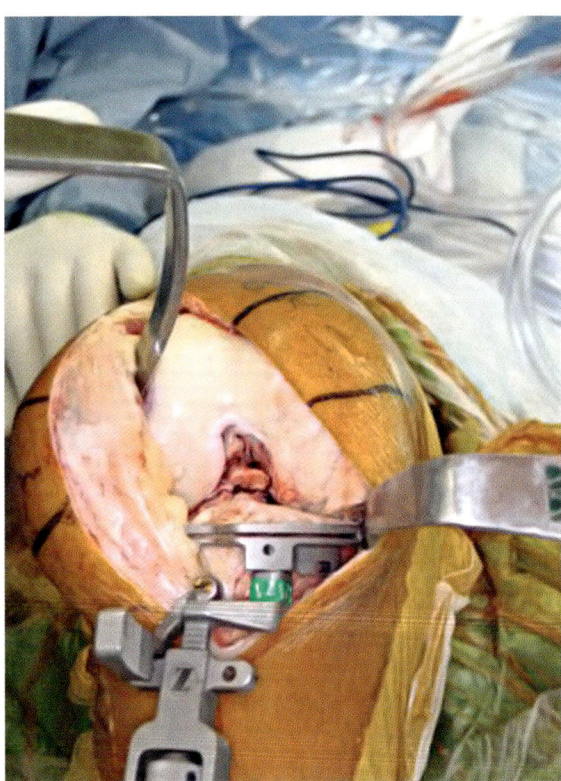

Figure 111-13. The extramedullary tibial cutting guide is placed perpendicular to the mechanical axis of the tibia. Medial offset tibial guides accommodate smaller incisions.

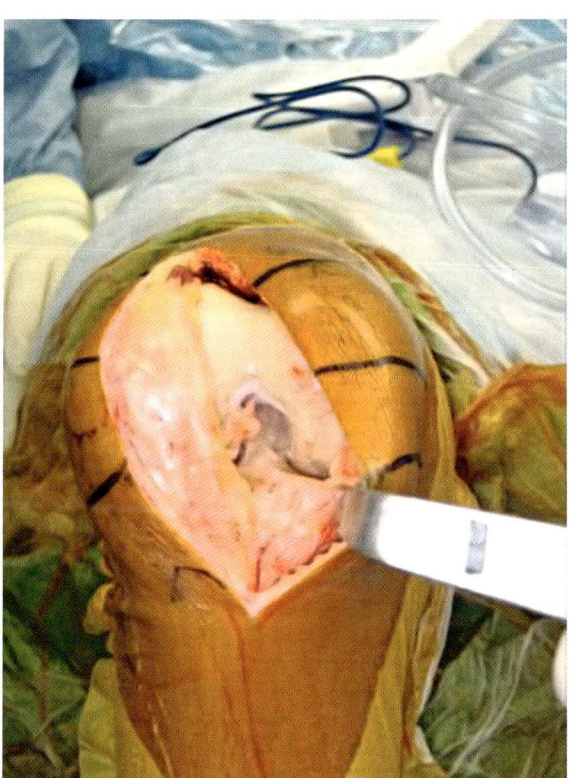

Figure 111-12. Excellent exposure can be obtained without routine patella eversion. The patella is allowed to sublux laterally as the knee is flexed to 90 degrees.

instability, requiring large polyethylene inserts or increased constraint. Additional tibial bone can easily be removed at a later stage of the procedure if the extension and flexion gaps are found to be too tight following the necessary ligament releases.

Attention is then turned to the femur. A small intramedullary hole is made to gain access to the femoral canal. This hole should be slightly (3 to 5 mm) medial to the center of the femoral groove to allow easy drilling of the intramedullary portion of the femur. The entry point can be more accurately determined using full-length radiographs and noting the point of intersection between the mechanical and anatomic axes of the femur. Because of concern regarding physiologic changes associated with intramedullary instrumentation, the hole is routinely vented by overdrilling the hole with a step drill and using a fluted intramedullary rod.[21] This helps reduce intramedullary pressure during the placement of subsequent intramedullary guides. The femoral alignment guide is then inserted into this intramedullary channel. It should be set for the proper side and valgus angle (frequently 5 or 6 degrees) as determined by preoperative radiographs (Fig. 111-14).

For most knees, the standard cutting block is attached to the intramedullary femoral alignment guide before its insertion in the femoral canal. Most flexion contractures can be managed with standard bone cuts and soft tissue releases. However, for knees with a significant preoperative flexion deformity (>30 degrees), it may be beneficial to resect an additional 3 mm of distal femoral bone initially.[66] This can be accomplished by removal of the standard cutting block, which will allow for this additional distal bone resection. At this point, the femoral alignment guide is inserted into the

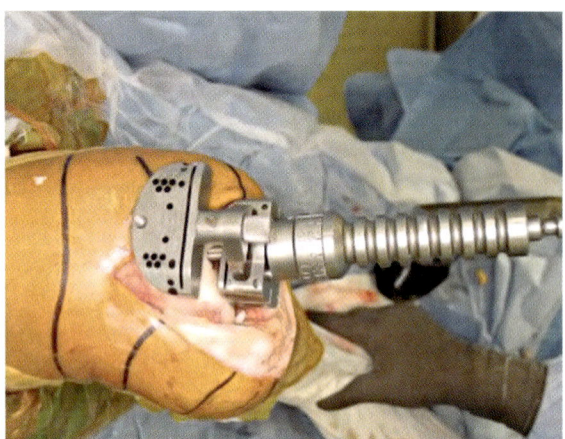

Figure 111-14. The femoral intramedullary guide is in place. A standard distal femoral cutting guide with 3 degrees of built-in flexion is used for the routine total knee arthroplasty. Additional femoral resection may be required in patients with a preoperative flexion contracture >20 degrees.

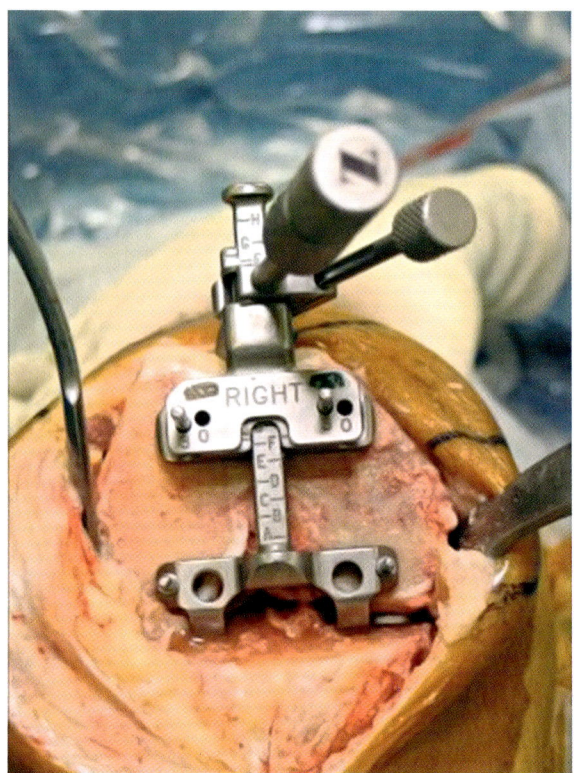

Figure 111-15. The anteroposterior sizing guide is pinned into place. For a varus knee, the femoral rotation is set at 3 degrees of external rotation. For the valgus knee with a deficient lateral femoral condyle, it may be necessary to increase the external rotation of the femoral component when referenced from the posterior femoral condyles.

intramedullary canal. Although this step does not set the final rotation of the femoral component, it is useful to place the guide carefully to achieve reasonable rotation of the distal femoral cut. The epicondylar axis can be used to aid in optimizing this rotation. Desired rotation is neutral to slight external rotation to ensure that the posterior femoral condylar cut will parallel the cut surface of the proximal tibia. In addition, slight external rotation will also enhance tracking of the patella.

After the intramedullary alignment guide is placed within the femoral canal, the femoral cutting block is attached to the 3-degree distal placement guide. They are then both inserted into the intramedullary alignment guide until the cutting block rests on the anterior femoral cortex. Making the distal femoral cut in 3 degrees of flexion helps avoid anterior cortical notching and allows the surgeon to downsize the femoral component, if necessary.[70] Two pins are placed in the femoral cutting block for the 0-mm resection. Finally, the distal placement guide is loosened and a slap hammer is used to remove the distal placement guide and intramedullary femoral alignment guide. The distal femur is then cut through the cutting slot in the femoral cutting block (see Fig. 111-14).

The next step is sizing and establishing rotation of the femoral component. The AP sizing guide is used to determine which of the component sizes will yield the best reconstructive result. Ideally, the body of the guide will contact the resected distal femur. Both of the guide's feet should rest on the posterior femoral condyles. The guide is then pinned to the distal femur with two short threaded pins (Fig. 111-15). The guide's anterior boom should contact the anterior cortex of the femur. The boom should be positioned so that it does not contact abnormal bony anatomy, such as an osteophyte or a depression. Occasionally, large anterior osteophytes must be removed to ensure accurate sizing. The ideal position to determine the size is with the boom at the beginning of the upslope of the lateral trochlear ridge. The femoral size should then be read directly from the guide. If the guide falls between sizes, the closest size is chosen. The boom can be adjusted (normally by moving it medially or more proximally) until the guide directly aligns with a size. This

maneuver essentially allows the AP sizing guide to be used in a posterior referencing manner. By adjusting the boom, the surgeon can optimize the AP position of the implant using strict anterior or posterior referencing, or a combination of both techniques. Two headless holding pins are placed in the AP sizing guide's holes. These pins are used to establish the AP position of the femoral component as well as to place it in 3 degrees of external rotation (referenced from the posterior condyles; see Fig. 111-15). The pins should be checked to ensure that they are parallel to the epicondylar axis. If the headless pins do not align with the epicondylar axis, the pins should be fine-tuned (commonly, the lateral one is adjusted) so that the pins and axis correspond. With severe valgus deformity and a deficient posterolateral femoral condyle, the surgeon may choose to increase the external rotation to 5 degrees when referenced from the posterior condyles.

At this point, the correct size of four-in-one femoral finishing guide (as determined by the previous AP sizing guide) is placed onto the distal femur over the already positioned headless pins (Fig. 111-16). The four-in-one femoral finishing guide is then pinned to the distal femur. The distal femur is cut in a sequential order. The collateral ligaments must be protected during this step to avoid iatrogenic injury.

Laminar spreaders are then inserted into the lateral joint space with the knee flexed to 90 degrees. The intercondylar notch is examined. Osteophytes are removed with a 1/4-inch straight osteotome to expose the notch fully. The ACL is excised directly off its femoral attachment. The PCL is then

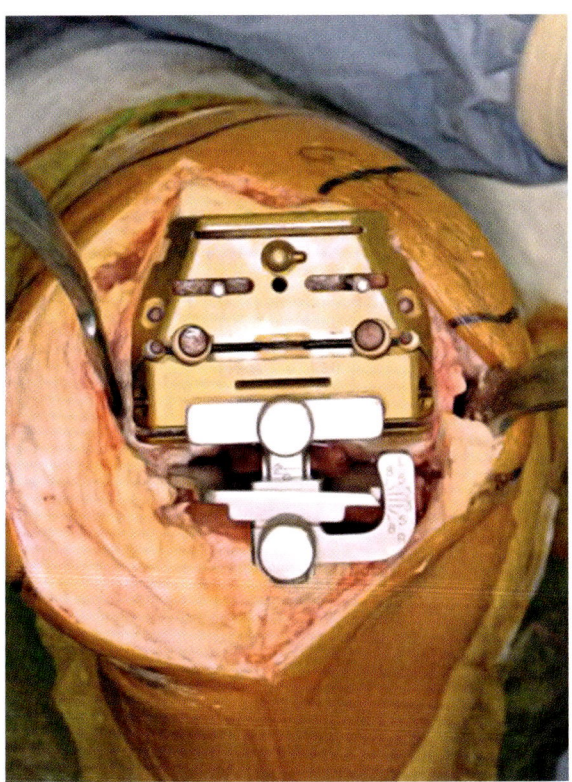

Figure 111-16. The four-in-one femoral guide corresponding to the appropriate size is pinned to the distal femur. The anterior, posterior, and chamfer femoral cuts are made.

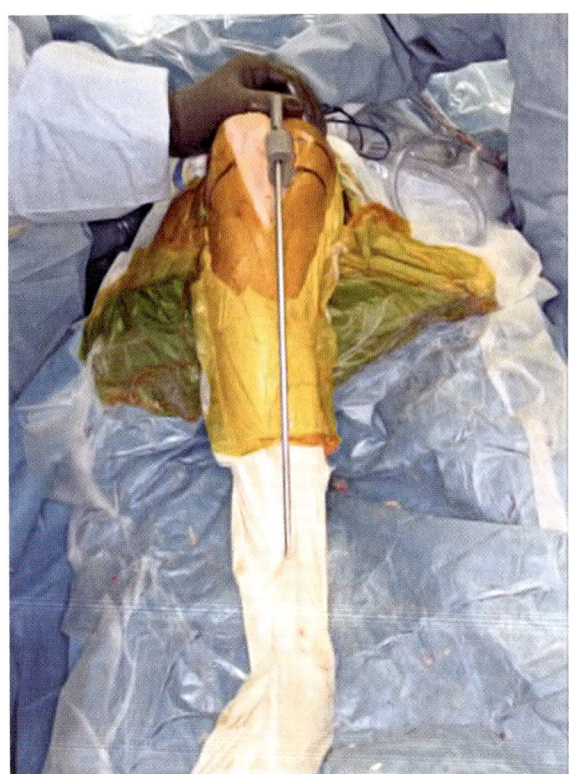

Figure 111-17. A spacer block and drop rod are inserted into the flexion space. Alignment of the tibia cut is confirmed. If the drop rod is not centered over the talus, the tibial cut is revisited to ensure appropriate alignment of the tibial component.

excised off its femoral attachment and followed to the posterior horn of the lateral meniscus. The medial meniscus is removed with care to avoid injury to the deep medial collateral ligament. Any remaining posterior osteophytes are removed from the posteromedial femoral condyle with a curved ¼-inch osteotome. A second set of laminar spreaders are placed in the medial joint space and the lateral laminar spreaders are removed. Remnants of lateral meniscus are removed with the PCL attached. Any remaining posterior osteophytes are removed from the posterolateral femoral condyle with a curved ¼-inch osteotome.

Next, the flexion and extension gaps are carefully measured and balanced. Various spacer blocks are used in the flexed knee until proper soft tissue balance is achieved. An alignment rod is placed through the end of a block and checked to ensure that its distal end aligns with the center of the ankle (Fig. 111-17). Malalignment of the rod is corrected by adjusting the proximal tibial bone cut. With the correct size block inserted to balance soft tissue tension in flexion adequately, the knee is brought into extension (Fig. 111-18).

At this point in the operative procedure, the collateral ligaments should be assessed to ensure correct knee balance. With the spacer block in place, a varus and valgus stress is applied. Spacing and collateral ligament tension must be symmetrical. In general, there are three situations that the surgeon will face:

1. *Neutral knee:* Knees with a preoperative alignment between 0 and 10 degrees are usually relatively easy to balance. In most cases, no further releases are required

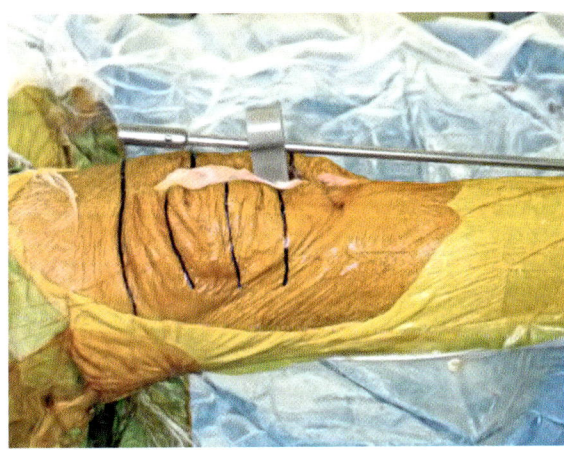

Figure 111-18. With the correct size of block inserted to balance soft tissue tension in flexion adequately, the knee is brought into extension. Collateral ligaments should be assessed to ensure correct knee balance. With the spacer block in place, a varus and valgus stress is applied. The appropriate soft tissue releases are performed to ensure symmetric collateral ligament tension.

other than those done initially to achieve adequate exposure.

2. *Varus knee:* In general, knees with a severe varus deformity require a more extensive medial release. An osteotome is used to strip the distal insertion of the superficial medial collateral ligament subperiosteally. If necessary, the deep portion of the medial collateral ligament and a portion of the semimembranosus insertion on the

tibia are often released while the foot is externally rotated.

3. *Valgus knee:* Knees with more than 10 degrees of anatomic valgus often require release of the lateral structures. There are multiple methods for performing the ligamentous releases necessary for balancing valgus knees. Currently, a laminar spreader is used to tension the tight lateral structures. These are then sequentially released using multiple stab wounds with a no. 15 blade in a "pie crust" manner. In addition, it may be necessary to perform a lateral retinacular release in knees with a severe valgus deformity. This can also enhance ligamentous balance and improve patellar tracking.

After appropriate coronal soft tissue balancing is performed, flexion and extension gap balance is assessed with the spacer block in place. If the knee does not fully extend with the spacer block necessary to fill the flexion gap, the posterior capsule can be carefully released off the posterior aspect of the femur in a subperiosteal manner. Following posterior capsule release, if the knee still does not reach full extension, the optional distal femoral resector is used to remove additional bone until full extension is achieved. Bone from the distal femur can be resected back to the insertion of the collateral ligaments. but this is rarely indicated; it raises the joint line and is undesirable. However, it is imperative that additional femoral resection be undertaken if required to achieve full knee extension. The alternative choice of using a thinner tibial tray is unacceptable because it will result in laxity in flexion and increase the chance of flexion instability and knee dislocation.

After the soft tissues are adequately balanced, the remaining bone cuts are completed. An intercondylar notch cutting guide that corresponds to the chosen size is used (Fig. 111-19). This determines the correct position of the femoral component mediolaterally. In general, the guide should be placed slightly lateral to the midpoint in the mediolateral plane, without any overhang. The intercondylar guide should not be placed medially. Lateral placement of the notch guide decreases the chances of intraoperative fracture of the medial femoral condyle and enhances patellar tracking by reducing the Q angle. Gender-specific components with reduced mediolateral dimensions may be more appropriate if the standard intercondylar guide demonstrates medial and lateral overhang. The appropriate decision to use a gender component frequently becomes apparent during this step. Bone from the intercondylar notch can be removed with a mill, oscillating saw, reciprocating saw, or osteotome. If the chamfer cuts have not already been made, the anterior and posterior chamfer cuts can also be made through slots in the intercondylar notch guide. In addition, the femoral lugholes are now drilled.

Attention is returned to the tibia. The largest tibial template that fits on the resected proximal tibia without overhang is chosen (Fig. 111-20). Alignment of the tibial resection can be assessed again with a drop rod placed through the handle of the tibial template. Final adjustments to the tibial cut are made at this point. The template is then carefully placed to ensure correct tibial component rotation. The template should align with the anterior aspect of the tibia, with the handle pointing to the medial third of the tibial tubercle. Care is taken to place the template as posteriorly as possible. Correct rotation of the template, coupled with a posterior

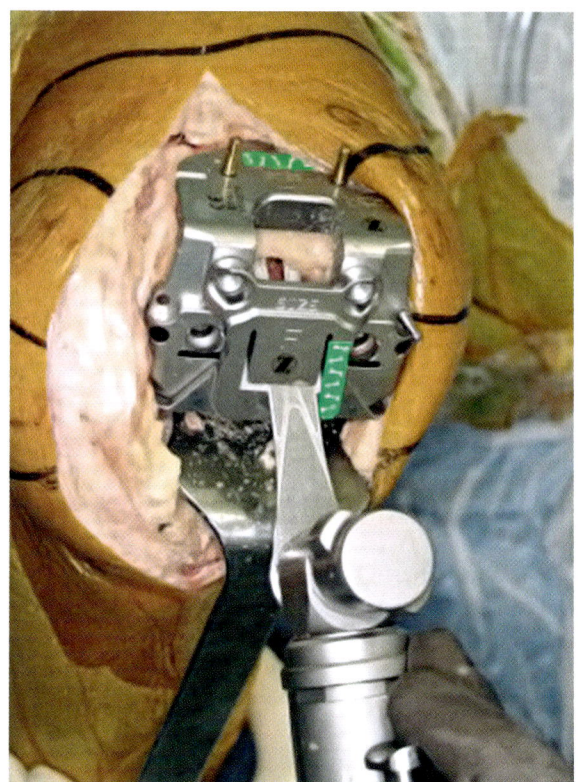

Figure 111-19. After balancing the knee, the final finishing cuts are made on the distal femur.

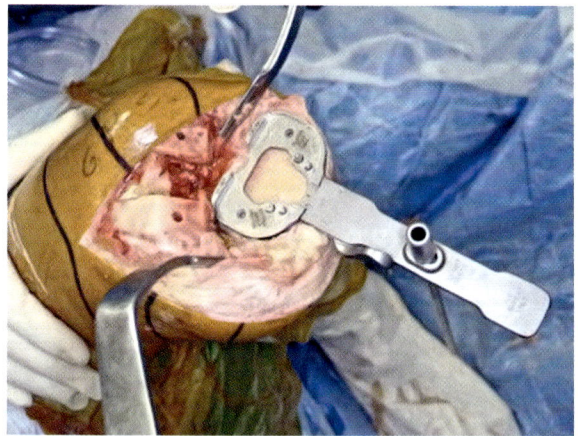

Figure 111-20. The tibia is sized and prepared to accept the final component.

placement, often causes slight overhang in the posterior lateral corner, which is acceptable. After the template is positioned and pinned in place, the tibial stem hole is prepared. This is done by first drilling through the tibial drill guide and then completing tibial preparation with impaction of the appropriately sized tibial broach. The trial tibial component is gently impacted into place.

Attention is turned to the patella. Synovium around the patella is carefully débrided to minimize the patellar clunk syndrome.[28,30] This is especially important in the region of the quadriceps tendon. The width of the patella is assessed with calipers; the aim is to restore the prosthesis-bone composite to the same width as the preresection patellar bone. Usually, the bone is prepared with an oscillating saw aligned with a patellar clamp or a patellar reaming system. The remaining patellar bone should be more than 12 mm to minimize the risk of fracture.[69]

After preparation of the host patellar bone, the appropriate-size and position of the patellar implant is chosen. The patellar component should be medialized to reduce the Q angle, but overhang must be avoided. Fixation holes are fashioned compatible with the prosthetic patellar design used. A trial component is put in place and thickness is once again assessed. This new thickness should be within 1 to 2 mm of the original width. If it is too thick, additional bone is resected.

At this point, the trial femoral component is put in place, as well as the trial insert. The knee is checked to ensure adequate balance of the collateral ligaments. The knee is inspected with regard to limb alignment. Finally, full ROM, without flexion contracture, excessive tightness, or laxity, is ensured.

Patellar tracking is assessed. The patella should track smoothly without lateral tilt or subluxation. The use of towel clips or thumb pressure should not be necessary in most cases. If the patella is noted to subluxate laterally, ensure that component rotation is appropriate. If subluxation persists despite appropriate component positioning and rotation, a retinacular release is performed. If a tourniquet is used, the tracking should be rechecked with the tourniquet down before considering lateral retinacular release. After the release is performed, the tracking of the patella is rechecked.

The trial components are removed. The bone surfaces are copiously irrigated and subsequently thoroughly dried. The components are cemented in place in one or two stages. The tibial component is cemented first. The femoral and patellar components are cemented with a second batch of cement (Fig. 111-21). Pressure is maintained on the components as the cement polymerizes, and excess cement is trimmed away. The final tibial insert is snapped into place. Stability, alignment, and ROM are again confirmed. The knee is copiously irrigated and the arthrotomy carefully closed over a reinfusion drain. After the skin is closed, a sterile dressing is applied and the patient is transferred to the recovery room.

CLINICAL RESULTS OF POSTERIOR CRUCIATE LIGAMENT–SUBSTITUTING DESIGNS

Insall-Burstein Posterior-Stabilized Prosthesis and Its Descendants

Insall Group Experience

The early cruciate-sacrificing design of the total condylar knee prosthesis provided excellent results. Insall and colleagues[34] reported on the 3- to 5-year results on the first consecutive 200 arthroplasties performed in 183 patients. Although 93% of knees were rated excellent or good, the complications, including four cases of posterior subluxation, highlighted the role for cruciate substitution. With evolution of design, the Insall-Burstein prosthesis incorporated posterior cruciate substitution.

Stern and Insall[67] have reported on the 9- to 12-year results of the original Insall-Burstein prosthesis with an

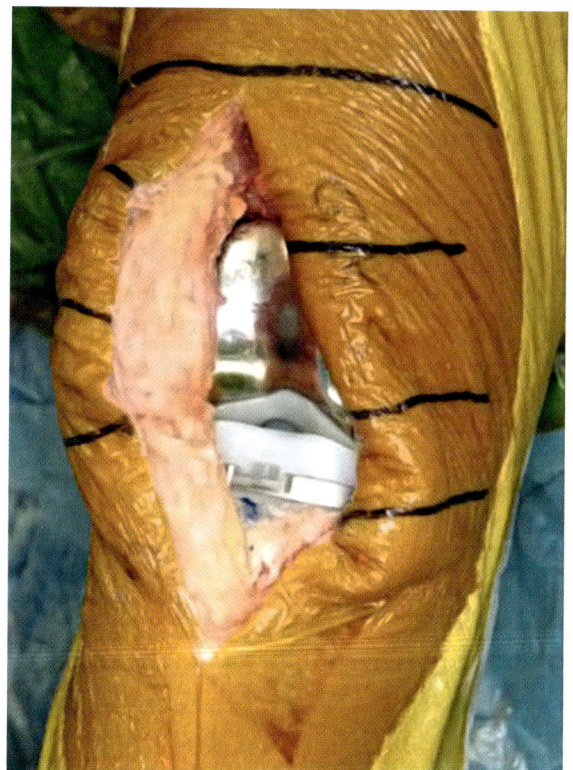

Figure 111-21. The final components are cemented in place with the final polyethylene insert.

all-polyethylene tibial component. Of 289 arthroplasties inserted at the Hospital for Special Surgery, 180 knees in 139 patients were available for review, with excellent or good results in 87%. Of the poor results, 14 knees required revision surgery; 9 knees were revised successfully for aseptic loosening of the femoral component (3 knees) or tibial component (6 knees), and 5 knees developed deep prosthetic infections and were treated with a two-stage procedure. The average annual rate of failure was 0.4%, with a 12-year cumulative success of 94% with an all-polyethylene tibial component.

Colizza and associates[15] then reported on the long-term results of Insall-Burstein PS prosthesis with a metal-backed tibial component; 101 knees in 74 patients were examined at a mean follow-up time of 10.8 years. The Hospital for Special Surgery results were good to excellent in 96%. In this cohort, with a monoblock metal-backed tibial component, no cases of tibial component loosening were seen.

Modularity of the tibial component was introduced with the Insall-Burstein II prosthesis in 1987. The addition of modularity was attractive to surgeons because it simplified the procedure and allowed intraoperative fine tuning. However, concerns began to arise that polyethylene wear on the backside of the tibial component (backside wear) would lead to osteolysis. Brassard and coworkers[10] have addressed the question of whether modularity affects clinical success with a long-term evaluation comparing the modular Insall-Burstein II prosthesis with the monoblock Insall-Burstein I. They compared the results over 10-year follow-up for 101 Insall-Burstein I knees with 117 Insall-Burstein II knees. Excellent or good results were seen in 96% and 95% of patients, respectively. The radiographic review demonstrated no cases of massive osteolysis, but the authors mentioned that three knees had local minimally progressive lesions, which were not clinically significant. This series of monoblock metal-backed tibial components had an overall incidence of tibial component radiolucent lines of 11%, compared with 26% seen with the modular tibial component. All radiolucent lines were nonprogressive and asymptomatic. Therefore, the introduction of modularity to this particular implant did not appear to raise concerns about osteolysis.

In other long-term studies of the Insall-Burstein posterior prosthesis with a metal-backed tibial component, best and worst case scenarios were noted.[10,15] The best case scenario revealed a cumulative success of 96.4% at 11 years. In distinction, the worst case scenario considered knees that were lost to follow-up time as failures; this yielded a cumulative success of 92.6% at 11 years. A further testimony to implant durability is a 94% survivorship at 18 years in an active patient population younger than 55 years with a PS prosthesis.[20]

The Insall-Burstein II prosthesis then evolved into the NexGen Legacy PS (LPS) prosthesis in 1987. Modifications to patellofemoral geometry and the cam and post mechanism were made. In addition, left and right femoral components were introduced. The initial cohort of patients with the NexGen prosthesis has been reviewed.[22] In this study, 233 patients underwent 279 primary total knee arthroplasties between August 1997 and December 1999. Eleven patients (11 knees) subsequently died, and 22 patients (23 knees) were excluded because of severe medical disability. Patients with severe medical conditions included those known to be alive with the prosthesis still in place but for whom no meaningful assessment of knee scores could be made after communication with a family member. Inclusion of this group of 22 patients may have lowered the overall knee scores, but the incomplete data precluded adequate analysis. Telephone contact was able to determine that none of these patients required revision and the prosthesis seemed to be functioning well. An additional seven patients (seven knees) were lost to follow-up despite use of a professional search firm. Thus, 193 patients with 238 knees (85%) were available for analysis. The mean age at the time of surgery was 66 years. The mean duration of follow-up time was 48 months (range, 24 to 72 months).

Preoperatively, the mean arc of motion was 107 degrees, compared with 117 degrees at the latest follow-up examination. The mean preoperative Knee Society score was 48 points compared with 96 points at the latest follow-up examination. The mean Knee Society functional score was 83 points at the latest follow-up examination. Radiographic evaluation revealed an incidence of minor radiolucent lines of 4%, which was of no clinical significance. No evidence of loosening, osteolysis, or polyethylene wear was seen. Three patients (1%) developed late deep infections. Six patients (3%) required early manipulation under anesthesia for arthrofibrosis. There were no cases of patellar dislocation, patellar clunk, or posterior dislocation.[22]

More recent modifications to the NexGen LPS prosthesis include a gender-specific prosthesis, high-flexion implants, and the addition of mobile bearings. The gender-specific prosthesis includes modification of the mediolateral-anteroposterior aspect ratio and the patellofemoral geometry. Long and associates[48] have demonstrated a significant decrease in lateral release rate with use of the gender-specific LPS femoral component. In 159 consecutive TKAs, the lateral

release rate decreased from 16.5% to 4.3% when using the gender component compared with the standard femoral component in women. The high-flexion design includes modification to the cam-spine mechanism, deepening of the anterior patellar cutout on the tibial articulating surface, and extension of the posterior condyles on the femoral component. These changes make high flexion safe, if achieved.[47] In addition, high postoperative range of motion has been shown to correlate with improved patient-rated outcomes. Interest, therefore, remains devoted to improving knee flexion.[5] Finally, mobile bearings have been shown to improve knee kinematics and polyethylene wear, but clinical performance and longevity appear equivocal.[11,19] Although these design changes likely improve clinical outcomes, further studies are needed.

Other Experiences

Aglietti and coworkers[2] have reviewed their results at a minimum of 10 years with 99 IB posterior-stabilized prostheses; 39 knees were in patients who had died before the 10-year follow-up and 4 were removed or revised, leaving 56 knees for evaluation at an average of 12 years. There were 58% excellent, 25% good, 7% fair, and 10% poor results. Knee flexion average 106 degrees. Of the six (10%) failures, four were attributable to aseptic component loosening; none was attributable to polyethylene wear. With revision as the end point, 10-year survivorship was 92%.

The same group then reviewed their results at a minimum of 5 years with 92 IB II posterior-stabilized prostheses.[29] At an average follow-up of 7.5 years (range 5 to 9 years), 97% of patients demonstrated good to excellent Knee Society scores. Survivorship analysis showed a success rate of 98.9% and 90.9% best and worst case scenarios, respectively, at 8 years.

Thadani and colleagues[68] have reviewed their results of the IB I metal-backed PS prosthesis at a minimum of 10 years; 100 TKAs were performed in 86 consecutive patients. Of these, 36 were in patients who had died and 2 were in patients who were weak. Of the remaining 62 knees, 54 were evaluated directly and 8 by telephone at an average of 10.8 years. No patients were lost to follow-up. At latest follow-up, 64% were rated as excellent, 18% as good, 7% as fair, and 11% as poor, which included six failures. Flexion averaged 111 degrees. Excluding the failures, the average Knee Society clinical score was 91.6. Of the six failures, two were secondary to sepsis, two secondary to nonspecific pain, one secondary to patellar wear and fracture, and one because of aseptic tibial component loosening. Polyethylene wear was specifically examined in this study and no implant demonstrated significant polyethylene wear or failure. There were seven patellar fractures; four required additional surgery and the remaining three were asymptomatic and discovered incidentally at routine follow-up. Using revision as the end point, 12-year survivorship averaged 92%.

Abdeen and associates[1] have published a 15- to 19-year follow-up of the same group of patients. Of this group, 55 patients (66 knees) had died and 29 patients were available for clinical or telephone follow-up. No additional knees required revision. With revision as the end point, the survival was 92.4% at 19 years. It was concluded that "the prosthesis is likely to outlive the patients when classic indications for age and activity are respected."

Vince and coworkers[72] also followed 100 IB II prostheses prospectively; 51 knees were evaluated at 10 or more years with Knee Society scores and radiographs and 14 were evaluated by telephone. An additional 6 knees required revision, and 29 were in patients who died. None were lost. Complete revision surgery was performed for instability (two knees), sepsis (two), loosening from osteolysis (one), and stiffness (one). Twelve patients required reoperation without revision of the tibia or femoral components—patellar revision for loosening (one), patellectomy for fracture (one), polyethylene exchange for dislocation of the spine-cam mechanism (three) and for dissociation (one), and arthroscopic resection of scar from the quadriceps tendon in six (patellar clunk). One case of tibial osteolysis occurred in the IB II. The problem of patellar fractures was decreased significantly in the IB II group, probably as a result of smoothing the anterior trochlear groove. Tibiofemoral dislocation occurred in three IB II prostheses.

Li and colleagues[43] reported their experience with an IB II prosthesis in 1999. Of 146 knees, 94 were reviewed at a mean of 10 years. HSS scores were excellent or good in 79%, fair in 14%, and poor in 7%. The average Knee Society score was 87. Knee flexion improved from an average of 88 degrees preoperatively to 100 degrees after arthroplasty, considerably less than has been expected from this device. The 10-year survivorship was 92.35, using revision as the end point, and there were 9 failures.

Lachiewicz and Soileau[41] performed a prospective consecutive study of 193 knees in 131 patients who were managed with the modular IB II PS total knee prosthesis by 1 surgeon. The mean age of the patients at the time of surgery was 68 years, and the mean duration of follow-up was 7 years (range, 5 to 14 years). Clinical evaluation was performed with the use of standard knee scoring systems. Radiographs were evaluated for the presence of radiolucent lines, osteolysis, and loosening. The overall result (as determined by HSS knee scores) was rated as excellent for 112 knees, good for 60, fair for 15, and poor for 6. The mean postoperative flexion was 112 degrees. No clinical or radiographic loosening of the tibial component was noted. Eight knees had osteolytic lesions of the tibia. Thin, incomplete, nonprogressive radiolucent lines were noted around 30 tibial components (16%). There were three reoperations.

Lachiewicz and Soileau then reported results on the same cohort 5 years later.[40] With a mean follow-up of 12 years (range, 10 to 18 years), two additional knees were revised for mechanical failure. With mechanical failure as an end point, the 15-year survival was 96.8%. Overall survival rate was 90.6% at 15 years.

Oliver and associates[59] have reported the clinical and radiographic outcomes of a consecutive series of 138 hydroxyapatite-coated IB II total knee replacements, with a mean follow-up of 11 years (range, 10 to 13 years). The patients were entered into a prospective study and all living patients (76 knees) were evaluated. The HSS knee score was obtained for comparison with the preoperative situation. No patient was lost to follow-up. Radiographic assessment revealed no loosening. Seven prostheses have been revised, giving a cumulative survival rate of 93% at 13 years.

Bozic and coworkers[9] have reviewed their experience with NexGen TKA system. Of 334 consecutive primary TKAs,

148 knees were NexGen Legacy posterior-stabilized prostheses. A minimum 5-year follow-up was available for 130 of these knees. The 5- and 8-year survivorships for the posterior-stabilized prosthesis were 100% and 94.6%, respectively. The revision rate was 1.5%, with only one knee being revised for aseptic failure. There were no cases of patellar dislocation, patellar clunk, or posterior dislocation.

Other Posterior Cruciate Ligament–Substituting Knee Results

There have been some reports on the results of PCL-substituting designs other than the Insall-Burstein posterior-stabilized prosthesis.

Press-Fit Condylar Posterior-Stabilized Design

Ranawat and colleagues[63] have reviewed the results of 150 consecutive primary total knee replacements (118 patients) performed between 1988 and 1990. There were 16 bilateral procedures. All the knees in this study were PCL-substituting Press-Fit Condylar modular knees implanted with the use of cement. The predominant diagnosis was osteoarthritis in 98 patients (83%). Mean age at the time of the index procedure was 70 years (range, 29 to 85 years); 125 knees were observed for a mean of 4.8 years (range, 3.8 to 6.2 years). The clinical results were excellent for 103 knees (82%), good for 13 (10%), fair for 3 (2%), and poor for 6 (5%). At the most recent follow-up, the Knee Society's average functional score was 78 points (range, 0 to 100 points), and the average knee score was 93 points (range, 57 to 100 points). The mean preoperative range of motion increased from 107 to 111 degrees after arthroplasty. The rate of survival was 97% at 6 years. Three revision operations were necessary: two of these were for infection, and one was for femorotibial instability. Patellofemoral symptoms were noted in 8% (10 knees). It was concluded that the PCL-substituting PFC modular knee system results in excellent relief of pain, excellent range of motion, and restoration of function, with a low prevalence of patellofemoral problems.

Kinematic Stabilizer Prosthesis

Hanssen and Rand[27] have reported on the Mayo Clinic experience with the Kinematic Stabilizer prosthesis. The Kinematic Stabilizer has a central tibial post in the femoral housing, restraining anterior as well as posterior motion of the tibia between 0 and 30 degrees of flexion. Past 30 degrees of flexion, as in the Insall-Burstein prosthesis, the substituting mechanism replaces only the function of the PCL in enhancing femoral rollback. Neither design substitutes for the collateral ligament. In this study, 79 arthroplasties (66 patients) with an average follow-up of 37 months were reported. There were 53 revisions and 26 primary arthroplasties in the series. Postoperatively, of the entire group, 34 knees (43%) were rated excellent, 33 (42%), good, 7 (9%), fair, and 5 (6%), poor. However, in this group of arthroplasties, most underwent revision procedures. Separate analysis of the results of the 26 knees undergoing index procedures revealed 54% with excellent results, 38% good, 4% fair, and 4% poor. Postoperative motion averaged 101 degrees. Small (1- to 2-mm) tibial radiolucent lines were seen in 29% of the knees. Overall, five knees required removal, two for deep sepsis, two for instability, and one for tibial component malposition. Only one revision was required for instability in the group undergoing primary total knee arthroplasty.

Scorpio Prosthesis

Kolisek and Barnes[39] have reported on a series of 103 consecutive primary TKAs performed on 101 patients using the Scorpio PS knee system (Stryker Orthopaedics). The Scorpio knee was designed with a single sagittal radius and a more posterior center of rotation to reduce compressive forces across the patellofemoral joint. At a mean follow-up of 5.25 years, good to excellent HSS scores were exhibited in 96.1%. Mean ROM improved from a preoperative level of 96.5 to 124.5 degrees postoperatively. Four patients reported anterior knee pain. The complication rate was 4.9%. This included one postoperative patellar fracture, one deep infection, one wound complication, one case of excessive knee pain, and one transient peroneal nerve palsy.

Mahoney and Kinsey[50] have published results by a single surgeon on a series of 1030 consecutive cemented TKAs performed with the Scorpio PS prosthesis. At a mean follow-up of 7 years (range, 5 to 9.5 years), 32 knees required revision. The mean time to revision was 2.4 years (range, 0.1 to 8.2 years). The leading cause of failure was deep infection (11 of 32 knees). The Kaplan-Meier survivorship with revision as an end point was 95.8%. With aseptic loosening as the end point, the survivorship was 98.6%.

COMPLICATIONS OF POSTERIOR CRUCIATE LIGAMENT SUBSTITUTION

Certain complications have arisen with PCL-substituting total knee designs that can at least in part be attributed to this type of knee replacement. These include component dislocation, intercondylar fractures, patellar fractures, patellar clunk syndrome, and tibial spine wear and breakage.

Dislocations

As increasingly deep flexion was experienced with PCL-substituting designs, there were cases of the tibial spine riding underneath the femoral cam with subluxation of the flexed knee and painful locking of the joint.[33] A knee with a dislocated implant normally presents acutely with inability to extend. In many cases, the patients are unable to explain the exact mechanism, or the position of the knee, when the actual dislocation occurred. In fact, this problem can occur during sleep, causing the patient to awaken with an acute inability to extend the knee. On physical examination, an obvious knee deformity is commonly found. Radiographs reveal the femoral cam translated anterior to the polyethylene tibial spine. Often, the spine can be reduced by hyperflexion of the knee and application of an anterior drawer.

Reports of dislocations have included knees implanted with the Insall-Burstein Posterior-PS prosthesis,[23,33,46] IB II prosthesis,[14,44,55,73] Kinemax posterior substituting prosthesis[58] or Kinematic II Stabilizer prosthesis (Stryker Orthopaedics),[24] and other designs.[73] It is not surprising that this problem has been seen most commonly with the Insall-Burstein and Kinematic II Stabilizer designs because they have the longest track record with the PCL-substituting concept.

Dislocations have been described in knees with a preoperative valgus alignment and in those after patellectomy.[14,23,24,44,58] Although preoperative valgus appears to increase the incidence of this problem, it can also occur in varus knees. There is some controversy over whether the actual component dislocation occurs with the knee in mild flexion with a straight posterior mechanism or occurs at high flexion angles with a combination of posterior and rotatory stress.[46]

Lombardi and associates[44] have analyzed the incidence of dislocations in 3032 primary knees implanted with the Insall-Burstein prosthesis series. The incidence of this problem was rare with the original Insall-Burstein PS prosthesis (0.2%, or 1 in 494). However, with the advent of the IB II prosthesis, the problem became more apparent (2.5%, or 1 in 40). Knees that dislocated were found to have achieved statistically significant higher average flexion (118 degrees) compared with control knees (105 degrees; $P < .001$). In addition, they tended to reach high flexion angles rapidly in the postoperative period. In response to this problem, the tibial plastic was modified by raising the tibial spine and moving it anteriorly. This increased the inherent stability of the component and decreased the incidence of dislocation (0.2%, or 1 in 656).

Combining the two most recent articles on a third-generation prosthesis, the NexGen Legacy posterior-stabilized implant, rates of dislocation continue to decrease.[9,22] In 323 knees with up to 8-year follow-up, no dislocations were reported. This likely represents an improvement in implant design and a better understanding of flexion instability and the role of soft tissue balance.

A computer analysis of this phenomenon analyzed the propensity of PCL-substituting knee components to dislocate in the sagittal plane.[18] Kocmond and coworkers[38] have defined a dislocation safety factor (DSF) as the jump distance between the bottom of the femoral cam and the top of the tibial spine. The DSF was found to vary with the knee flexion angle. For knees with the Insall-Burstein PCL-substitution mechanism, the DSF increases as knee flexion increases and peaks at about 70 degrees. Knee flexion beyond this angle causes the DSF to decrease and theoretically increases the risk of dislocation. Many contemporary designs have attempted to minimize the risk of dislocation by ensuring a DSF equal to or greater than that of the original Insall-Burstein Posterior-Stabilized prosthesis at high flexion angles.

The lesson with respect to arthroplasty design is simple. Sometimes, very small changes, on the order of millimeters, can result in catastrophic complications. Not all spine mechanisms are the same. In general, to prevent knee dislocations, it is imperative that the surgeon balance the knee in both flexion and extension, with a special emphasis on knees with a preoperative valgus alignment. In addition, it may be undesirable to achieve large flexion angles (more than 115 degrees) in the first postoperative week.

Intercondylar Fractures

Femoral fractures, although a relatively rare occurrence, can occur at the time of knee arthroplasty. Because PCL-substituting components require the removal of extra bone from the intercondylar region, the possibility of distal femoral fracture with this technique is increased. Risk factors for fractures include inadequate, as well as excessive, intercondylar bone notch resection. Although it is self-evident that excessive bone removal results directly in stress risers and deficient bone, the risks associated with incomplete bone resection are not as clear-cut. Nonetheless, if insufficient notch bone is removed, the intercondylar region of the femoral component (or trial) can act like a wedge during insertion and induce a distal femoral fracture. It is imperative to remove enough bone to allow full seating of the cam. When placing the trial femoral component, forceful impaction should never be used. To ensure adequate bony resection, never undercut the femoral condyles. Although this complication has been reported, the exact incidence of this phenomenon has not been well defined. Lombardi and colleagues[45] have described the risk factors, which include osteopenic bone, improper bone cuts, an eccentric box cut for the posterior stabilized prosthesis, overimpaction of the femoral component, and misplacement of the trial component.

Lombardi and associates[45] reported on this complication in comparing two large series of PCL-substituting knees. In this report, 898 nonconsecutive primary knee arthroplasties performed with a PCL-substituting prosthesis were compared with a second nonconsecutive series of 532 PCL-substituting knee arthroplasties. In the second series, an intercondylar sizing guide was used to confirm the intercondylar resection size. In the initial series, 40 distal femoral fractures were noted (approximate rate, 1:22; nondisplaced, 35; displaced, 5). This was in contrast to the second series, in which only one displaced fracture was noted (rate, 1:532). The rate difference between the two series was statistically significant. The authors advocated careful resection technique and intercondylar notch size verification to minimize this complication. Of note, no change in postoperative rehabilitation was required for patients identified with a nondisplaced intercondylar fracture or those with an intercondylar fracture treated with intraoperative stabilization.

Patellar Fractures

The initial follow-up of the original Insall-Burstein Posterior-Stabilized knee demonstrated a high patellar fracture prevalence. The AP dimensions and shape of the femoral component tended to be full to accommodate the spine-cam mechanism in the Insall-Burstein Posterior-Stabilized prosthesis. This pushed the patella anteriorly and presumably increased forces, which may have been responsible for a relatively higher rate of patellar fractures. In 10 cadaver knee specimens, Matsuda and coworkers[51] demonstrated significantly higher contact stresses in the unresurfaced patella when compared with the normal knee throughout the flexion arc for several implants, including the Insall-Burstein Posterior-Stabilized prosthesis. They noted that in flexion exceeding 105 degrees, patellofemoral contact occurred in two small patches. They concluded that the forces could be normalized by extending the trochlear groove farther posteriorly and were less concerned with the anterior prominence of the component. The groove of the IB II was deepened potentially to decrease patella fractures and other patella problems. Other posterior-stabilized knees have been designed with a single sagittal radius and a more posterior center of rotation to reduce compressive forces across the patellofemoral joint.[39]

Larson and Lachiewicz[42] have concluded that many patellar complications with the IB Posterior-Stabilized prosthesis could be avoided by a careful surgical technique. This includes appropriate rotation of the femur and tibia, adequate patellar resection, débridement of peripatellar synovium, and proper evaluation of patellar tracking before wound closure. They studied 118 arthroplasties at 2 to 8 years and found that no knee required reoperation for the patellofemoral joint. Mean flexion of 112 degrees was comparable to other studies with this device, and they had no cases of patellar clunk syndrome and no subluxations. There were three patellar fractures (2.5%) treated without surgery. Even this small number of fractures might be expected to improve with changes to the femoral prosthesis. It was concluded that the total patellofemoral complication rate in the series was 4.2%. This was superior to the 11% that has generally been described, of which 7% were actually fractures.

With improved design, surgical technique, and more favorable patellofemoral geometry, it is likely that the incidence of patellar fracture will continue to decrease. Ortiguera and Berry[60] found an incidence of periprosthetic fracture of the patella to be only 0.68% following modern TKA. Additionally, when combining the two most recent articles on 323 knees treated with the NexGen Legacy posterior-stabilized implant, no patellar fractures were reported with up to 8-year follow-up.[9,22] This again likely represents an improvement in implant design and better surgical technique.

Patellar Clunk Syndrome and Synovial Entrapment

The deeper flexion provided by the initial Insall-Burstein stabilized design enabled the quadriceps tendon to extend beyond the trochlear groove of the femoral component. If the anterior edge of the femoral component terminates abruptly, synovium or scar residing on the tendon falls into the intercondylar groove. If this has occurred, the same tissue must ride up out of the intercondylar area and "jump" back up onto the femoral trochlea as the patient extends her or his knee. Within a few months after the arthroplasty, the offending (or offended) tissue hypertrophies and becomes rubbery. This creates the painful and noisy complication that has been described as patellar clunk. Historically, a case of patellar catching was mentioned by Insall in his original report on the posterior-stabilized knee. However, Hozack and colleagues[28] appear to be the first authors to define the term *patellar clunk syndrome*. They described a prominent fibrous nodule at the junction of the proximal patellar pole and quadriceps tendon. They believed that during flexion, this fibrous nodule would enter the femoral component's intercondylar notch but not restrict flexion. However, as the knee extended, the nodule would remain within the notch while the rest of the extensor mechanism slid proximally. At 30 to 45 degrees of flexion, the tension on the fibrous nodule would be sufficient to cause the nodule to jerk out of the notch as it returned to its normal position. This sudden displacement would cause the audible and palpable clunk found with this entity.

Synovial entrapment or hyperplasia is a similar entity but less well-described syndrome.[61] It is caused by similar hypertrophy of soft tissue in the same location, but without a discrete nodule. Rather than a clunk or catch, the patient experiences pain and crepitus, typically with active knee extension from a 90-degree flexed position. This typically occurs during stair climbing or rising from a chair.

The original IB design had a high incidence of patellar clunk, up to 21%. This is likely related to the femorotrochlear geometry—a short trochlea with a sharp transition into the intercondylar notch.[3,13] Changes to the sagittal geometry of the femoral component in the IB II reduced the incidence to approximately 3% to 8%, but did not eliminate the problem. Finally, with the introduction of the NexGen Legacy prosthesis in 1997, one of the main areas of focus was the patellofemoral articulation and the reduction of patellofemoral complications. The side-specific components, with anatomic oriented trochlear grooves, lengthening and deepening of the femoral trochlea, and an increase in the number of femoral sizes, all helped reduce the incidence of patellar entrapment syndromes. In 238 knees reconstructed with the NexGen legacy prosthesis, no cases of patellar clunk or synovial entrapment were seen with 24- to 72-month follow-up.

Treatment recommendations for patellar clunk syndrome and synovial entrapment have included physical therapy, surgical removal of the nodule, patellar prosthesis revision, open resection through a limited lateral incision, and arthroscopic débridement.[8,28,53,71] Pollock and associates[61] have reviewed the prevalence of synovial entrapment with three different cam-post designs. Those with proximally positioned or wide femoral boxes were more likely to have a higher prevalence of this problem.

Beight and coworkers[8] have reported on 14 operative procedures (11 arthroscopic débridements and 3 patellar component revisions) performed in 12 patients. As in other reports, they found a suprapatellar fibrous nodule that wedged into the intercondylar notch during flexion and dislodged as the knee extended, causing the clunk. They noted that the symptoms resolved after nodule excision. However, four of the knees treated with arthroscopic débridement had recurrence of symptoms. None of the knees that underwent arthrotomy and patellar button revisions had recurrence. The authors recommended a treatment protocol that commenced with a short course of nonoperative physical therapy, although they acknowledged that the results were disappointing. Arthroscopic débridement was suggested for knees without radiographic component abnormalities. Arthrotomy was suggested for recurrent clunks or malpositioned or loose components.

The Mayo Clinic[17] has recently reported on a series of 25 patients who underwent arthroscopic treatment of patellar clunk syndrome (15 knees) or patellofemoral synovial hyperplasia (10 knees). After surgery, patient reported knee pain and crepitus but Knee Society knee and function scores improved in both groups. It was concluded that arthroscopic débridement of symptomatic patellofemoral synovium after TKA is a safe and effective procedure.

Tibial Spine Wear and Breakage

There has been a recent focus on the spine-cam mechanism in some posterior-stabilized prostheses as a source of wear debris. Mikulak and colleagues[54] have reported unanticipated aseptic loosening and osteolysis with the posterior-stabilized model of the Press-Fit Condylar implant. They found that 16 of 557 (2.9%) had been revised for osteolysis from 37 to 89

months after surgery. Retrieval analysis demonstrated damage to the lateral and medial walls of the tibial spine. There was also damage to the inferior surface of the articular polyethylene inserts.

Similar findings were reported by Puloski and associates.[62] Their study, by contrast, was a retrieval analysis of a variety of failed posterior-stabilized implants. Wear was quantified on the tibial posts of all retrievals, including those revised for reinfection. They were unable to conclude that this wear mode was responsible for the failures but cautioned that the interaction between the spine and the cam is not an "innocuous articulation."

Callaghan and coworkers[12,57] have studied this phenomenon extensively. When they recognized osteolysis around IB II modular components, as well as Press-Fit Condylar PS modular components, they began performing retrieval analyses. In their cases, the patients were able to hyperextend slightly and most had bilateral implants. They hypothesized that impingement on the anterior post by the femoral cam causes wear damage to the post and transmits rotational stresses to the modular inserts, generating backside wear. Avoiding flexion of the femoral component and posterior slope in the proximal tibial resection should help eliminate the problem. In addition, cam-post designs should allow for hyperextension before impingement occurs.

CONCLUSION

The potential of the PCL-substituting type of knee design continues to evolve. In general, it has allowed the surgeon to perform a reproducible operation in almost all arthritic knees, no matter what the cause of the disease and how involved and complex the deformity of the knee. The recent modifications in prosthetic design and surgical technique have addressed most of the early concerns involving patellofemoral complication and tibiofemoral dislocation. Although many advancements has been made, there is still potential for functional and clinical improvements with the newer designs that are now and will become available in the future.

KEY REFERENCES

Abdeen AR, Collen SB, Vince KG: Fifteen-year to 19-year follow-up of the Insall-Burstein-1 total knee arthroplasty. J Arthroplasty 25:173, 2010.

Aglietti P, Buzzi R, De Felice R, Giron F: The Insall-Burstein total knee replacement in osteoarthritis: a 10-year minimal follow-up. J Arthroplasty 14:560, 1999.

Callaghan JJ, O'Rourke MR, Goetz DD, et al: Tibial post impingement in posterior-stabilized total knee arthroplasty. Clin Orthop Relat Res 404:83, 2002.

Clarke HD, Fuchs R, Scuderi GR, et al: The influence of femoral component design in the elimination of patellar clunk in posterior-stabilized total knee arthroplasty. J Arthroplasty 21:167, 2006.

Fuchs R, Mills EL, Clarke HD, et al: A third-generation, posterior stabilized knee prosthesis: early results after follow-up of 2 to 6 years. J Arthroplasty 21:821, 2006.

Indelli PF, Aglietti P, Buzzi R, Baldini A: The Insall-Burstein II prosthesis: a 5- to 9-year follow-up study in osteoarthritic knees. J Arthroplasty 17:544, 2002.

Insall JN: Technique of total knee replacement. Instr Course Lect 30:324, 1981.

Insall JN, Lachiewicz PF, Burstein AH: The posterior stabilized condylar prosthesis: a modification of the total condylar design. Two to four-year clinical experience. J Bone Joint Surg Am 64:1317, 1982.

Insall J, Scott WN, Ranawat CS: The total condylar knee prosthesis. A report of two hundred and twenty cases. J Bone Joint Surg Am 61:173–180, 1979.

Lachiewicz PF, Soileau ES: The rates of osteolysis and loosening associated with a modular posterior stabilized knee replacement: results at five to fourteen years. J Bone Joint Surg Am 86:525, 2004.

Lachiewicz PF, Soileau ES: Fifteen-year survival and osteolysis associated with a modular posterior stabilized knee replacement. A concise follow-up of a previous report. J Bone Joint Surg Am 91:1419, 2009.

Larson CM, Lachiewicz PF: Patellofemoral complications with the Insall-Burstein II posterior-stabilized total knee arthroplasty. J Arthroplasty 14:288, 1999.

Ritter MA, Campbell E, Faris PM, Keating EM: Long-term survival analysis of the posterior cruciate condylar total knee arthroplasty. A 10-year evaluation. J Arthroplasty 4:293, 1989.

Stern SH, Insall JN: Posterior stabilized prosthesis: results after follow-up of nine to twelve years. J Bone Joint Surg Am 74:980, 1992.

Full references for this chapter can be found on www.expertconsult.com.

Mobile-Bearing Total Knee Arthroplasty

Raymond H. Kim and Douglas A. Dennis

Indications for total knee arthroplasty (TKA) have expanded as prosthetic designs, implant materials, and surgical techniques have improved. Although early total knee designs were generally reserved for older and sedentary patients with debilitating pain and loss of function, excellent clinical results with 10- to 15-year outcomes have encouraged many surgeons to consider performing TKA on younger patients, who have higher activity demands.[10-12,15,20,55,58] Patient expectations for increased function and longer survivorship following TKA continue to drive advances in both surgical technique and component design. Integrating established and successful TKA design concepts with the current kinematic and biomechanical discoveries will continue to answer the public's demand for improvements in TKA stability, function, component longevity, and patient satisfaction. One successful design concept that has evolved over the last 3 decades to meet the increased demands is the development of the mobile-bearing TKA. The careful integration of clinical and laboratory studies has led to advances in development of mobile-bearing TKA systems.

DESIGN RATIONALE OF MOBILE-BEARING TOTAL KNEE ARTHROPLASTY

Early TKAs were performed prior to comprehensive understanding of the importance of alignment and soft tissue balancing. First-generation instruments were used that lacked alignment guides or size-specific cutting blocks. Early clinical TKA failures often resulted from malalignment, instability, and the use of implants with excessive prosthetic constraint. Although increased constraint provided by hinged or extremely conforming unlinked TKA systems improved the stability of TKA, the torsional, coronal, and sagittal stresses normally shared by the surrounding soft tissue–stabilizing structures were transferred through the implant to the fixation interface,[5] resulting in premature TKA failure secondary to aseptic component loosening.* Biomechanical studies have also shown that highly conforming fixed-bearing TKA designs are intolerant of higher rotational and anteroposterior translational kinematic motion patterns that are commonly encountered after TKA, with increased polyethylene wear frequently observed.[17,27,41,43,65] Subsurface polyethylene stresses experienced in situations of malalignment have also been shown to be significantly higher in highly conforming fixed-bearing TKA systems than in less conforming fixed-bearing or highly conforming mobile-bearing TKA designs.[17,43,65]

Understanding that the highly constrained implant designs of the 1970s increased the risk of early aseptic loosening, the next generation of implant designs was subsequently developed that relied more on the load-sharing and stabilizing roles of the native soft tissue structures. This was accomplished by reducing articular conformity constraint, which typically incorporated the use of round-on-flat or flat-on-flat articular geometries. These designs allowed for rotation and multiplane translation to occur at the articulating interface and relied more on the surrounding soft tissue structures than conformity of the articular surfaces for stability and dispersion of the applied loads.

Although these low-conformity TKA designs significantly reduced stresses transmitted to the fixation interface, this also decreased the contact area between the femoral component and polyethylene-bearing surface. The lower the conformity at the articulating countersurfaces, the less the contact area between these surfaces. Decreased articular congruity increases detrimental subsurface contact stresses experienced by the polyethylene and also increases the amount of cross-shear stresses, which risks accelerated polyethylene wear. The use of round-on-flat and flat-on-flat bearings produces point and line loading conditions at the articular interface, respectively, with an overall reduction in contact area through which polyethylene loads are distributed. Because the contact stress experienced at the polyethylene surface is inversely proportional to the degree of conformity between the femoral condyles and tibial polyethylene insert, reduction of contact area with low-conformity designs led to accelerated polyethylene wear and subsequent premature TKA failure.[42,60]

Fluoroscopic kinematic evaluations of round-on-flat and flat-on-flat articulations have also demonstrated an increased incidence of paradoxical anterior femoral translation during deep flexion, instead of controlled posterior femoral rollback, and reverse axial rotation patterns. These abnormal kinematic patterns are likely secondary to a reduction in articular conformity with resulting instability.* This paradoxical motion produces detrimental cyclical tensile shear stresses at the articulating surface, further increasing the risk of accelerated polyethylene wear.[5,14]

Strategies to reduce polyethylene wear include the use of thicker polyethylene bearings,[5,6] improvements in polyethylene locking mechanisms of modular tibial components to reduce potential backside wear,[29,56,66] the use of improved sterilization techniques,† returning to the use of TKA designs with increased articular surface conformity, and the use of mobile-bearing TKA systems.[10-12,15,48,53]

As noted, an important component design concept for reducing contact stresses at the articulating surface and effectively reducing polyethylene wear is increasing the articular conformity. The higher the conformity of the articular surfaces, the lower the amount of cross-shear stresses, the greater the articular surface contact area, the less the subsurface polyethylene contact stress per unit area, and subsequently

---

*References 9, 19, 23, 28, 36, and 37.

*References 3, 21, 23, 24, 26, and 28.
†References 4, 8, 13, 18, 46, and 67.

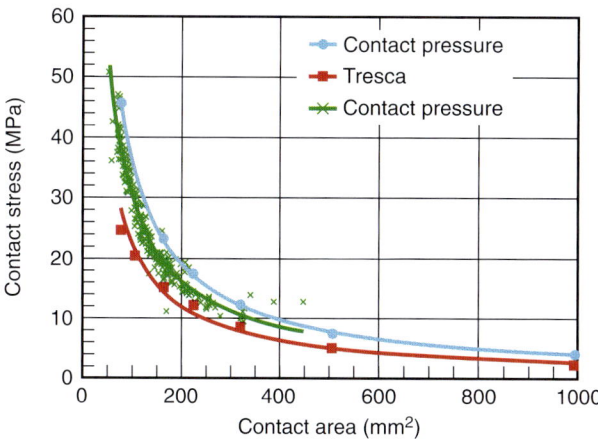

Figure 112-1. Graph demonstrating experimental and finite element analyses of polyethylene contact area (mm²) and resultant contact stresses (MPa). (From Rullkoetter PJ, Gabriel SM, Colleran DP, et al: The relationship between contact stress and contact area with implications for TKR evaluation and design, Transactions of the 45th Annual Meeting, Orthopaedic Research Society, Feb 1-4, 1999, Anaheion, CA, p. 974.)

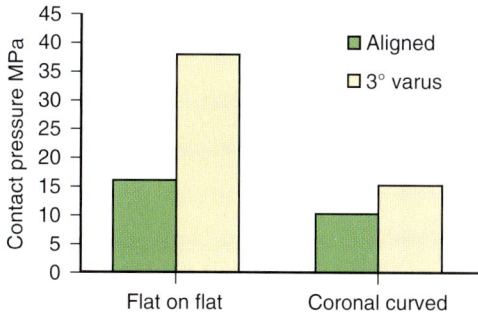

Figure 112-2. TekScan analysis demonstrating peak polyethylene contact stresses (MPa) of low (flat-on-flat) versus high (coronal curved) conformity TKA designs in neutral and 3-degree varus alignment. (From Medscape: [http://www.medscape.com/viewprogram/3133].)

the less polyethylene wear seen. Analyses of contact area versus contact stress have demonstrated a dramatic reduction of contact stress as the contact area is increased. Because of the logarithmic relationship between contact area and stress, increasing the contact area beyond 350 to 400 mm² reduces contact stresses further but to a substantially lesser degree[57] (Fig. 112-1). Conformity can be achieved in multiple planes. In contrast to total hip arthroplasty, in which conformity may be achieved in all planes, the focus in TKA is primarily on achieving sagittal and coronal plane conformity. It has been demonstrated that increasing coronal plane conformity is the most critical plane to reduce peak polyethylene stresses, particularly in the presence of femoral condylar liftoff.[5,27,41,59]

BIOMECHANICAL ADVANTAGES OF A MOBILE-BEARING TOTAL KNEE ARTHROPLASTY

The increased sagittal plane conformity typically present in most mobile-bearing TKA designs provides the opportunity of improved control of anteroposterior translation, with reduced paradoxical anterior femoral translation, particularly when tested during gait.[26,64] The increased coronal plane conformity typically present in mobile-bearing TKA also increases the contact area and lessens the increased contact stresses that are present if femoral condylar liftoff occurs.[5,27,41,59] This has been observed using TekScan analysis.[61] During testing of a flat-on-flat design in good alignment with equal loading of each condyle, peak polyethylene stresses reach approximately 16 MPa. When the same design is loaded in 3 degrees of varus malalignment, shifting the load to one condyle, as occurs with femoral condylar liftoff, the peak stresses dramatically increase to 38 MPa, far exceeding the yield strength of polyethylene (20 to 22 MPa). Similar testing performed with a TKA design with increased coronal conformity has demonstrated peak polyethylene stresses increasing only to 16 MPa with varus loading conditions (Fig. 112-2). Numerous studies have shown that the increased conformity in mobile-bearing designs substantially increases contact area and reduces

contact stresses, which should reduce the rate of polyethylene wear.[14,33,49,61,65]

Greenwald and Heim[33] have demonstrated contact areas of mobile-bearing TKA during gait range from approximately 400 to 800 mm² which minimizes contact stresses to 14 MPa or less (Fig. 112-3). This magnitude of contact area is substantially greater than what is typically seen in most fixed-bearing TKA designs (200 to 250 mm²; Fig. 112-4) Other finite element evaluations have similarly demonstrated reduced polyethylene contact stresses as a direct result of increased contact area, further supporting the observations of Greenwald and Heim.[7,47,50] The advantage of this increase in contact area is reflected in knee simulator wear studies of fixed- versus mobile-bearing TKA. McNulty and colleagues[45] and McEwen and associates,[44] in separate laboratory evaluations, both demonstrated significantly diminished polyethylene wear rates with highly conforming rotating platform designs when compared with similarly designed fixed-bearing systems. In the McNulty study, a 94% wear reduction was observed when analyzing a highly conforming rotating platform design versus a similar fixed-bearing TKA design, whereas the McEwen study noted over a fourfold reduction in wear with testing of a rotating platform TKA (Fig. 112-5).

Most rotating platform systems use a flat tibial tray–polyethylene countersurface that allows freedom of the polyethylene insert to rotate around a central post on a highly polished, cobalt-chrome surface with a very low surface roughness. In vivo fluoroscopic kinematic studies conducted with two commonly implanted rotating platform designs (LCS RP and PFC Sigma RP, DePuy, Warsaw, Ind) have confirmed that polyethylene bearing rotation predictably occurred in all subjects tested.[25,40] To evaluate the polyethylene-bearing position, four metallic beads were inserted at known positions into each bearing by the implant manufacturer, because the polyethylene would otherwise be transparent during fluoroscopy. Computer-assisted design (CAD) models were then created for the polyethylene inserts with the four strategically placed beads. Using a CAD model-fitting algorithm, the orientation of the femoral component and tibial tray were initially determined. The polyethylene insert was then made transparent and only the four beads were visible in the CAD model. The best fit with the CAD model of the four metallic beads onto the four beads visible

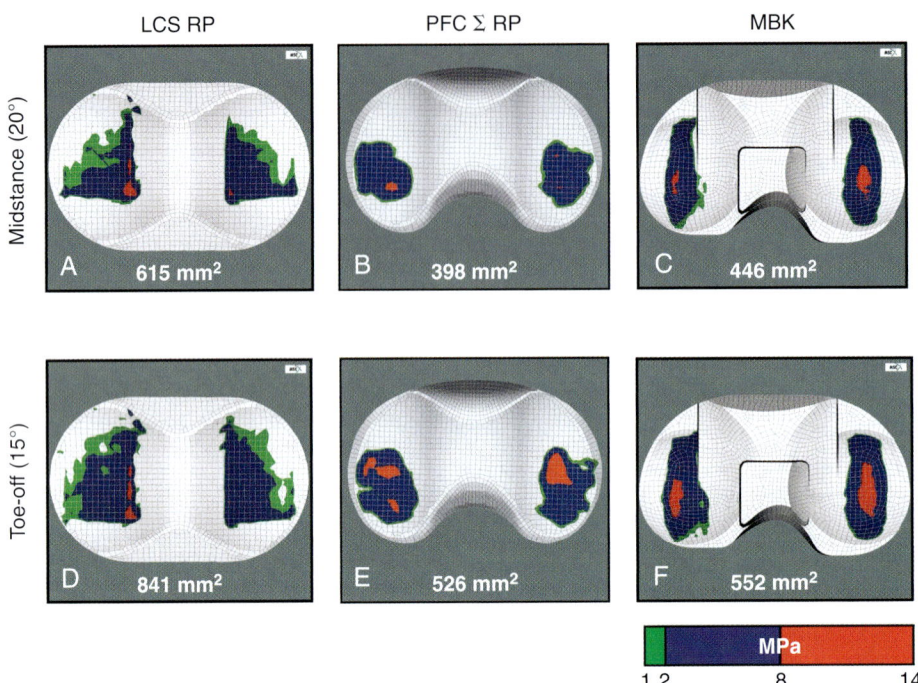

Figure 112-3. Contact area and stress analysis demonstrating high polyethylene contact areas (mm²) and low peak stresses (MPa) of three mobile-bearing TKA designs.[33] (From Greenwald AS, Heim CS: Mobile-bearing knee systems: ultra-high molecular weight polyethylene wear and design issues. Instr Course Lect 54:195–205, 2005.)

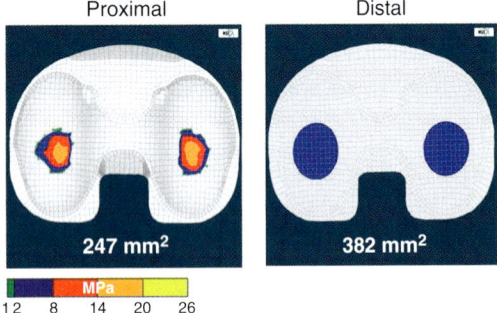

Figure 112-4. Contact area and stress analysis demonstrating a lower polyethylene contact area (mm²) and higher peak stress (MPa) in a fixed-bearing TKA design.[33] (From Greenwald AS, Heim CS: Mobile-bearing knee systems: ultra-high molecular weight polyethylene wear and design issues. Instr Course Lect 54:195–205, 2005.)

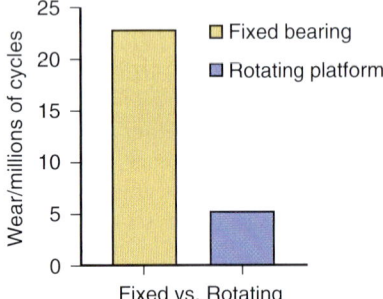

Figure 112-5. Histogram of a high kinematic knee simulator analysis comparing polyethylene wear (mg)/million cycles in a rotating platform versus a fixed-bearing TKA. (From Mobile Bearing Total Knee Arthroplasty, Medscape: [http://www.medscape.com/viewprogram/3133, 2004].)

in the fluoroscopic image was then determined using the same automated computer model-fitting process (Fig. 112-6). Once the process determined the best-fit match, the polyethylene insert could be visualized and axial rotation measurements of the rotating platform bearing relative to the femoral component and tibial tray were determined. These analyses have demonstrated that most axial rotation in these rotating platform designs occurs at the polyethylene bearing–tibial tray interface as the polyethylene bearing "follows" the rotation of the femoral component.[28]

All rotating platform knee designs, however, are not the same kinematically. Garling and coworkers[32] performed a similar fluoroscopic kinematic evaluation of 10 rheumatoid patients implanted with a different rotating platform TKA (NexGen LPS mobile, Zimmer, Warsaw, Ind) and found that the femoral component underwent greater axial rotation than the mobile polyethylene-bearing insert, suggesting that the femoral component was sliding on the top of the insert. They concluded that this finding was possibly attributed to the limited articular conformity in this design, an anterior pivot point for the rotating platform, insert impingement, or fibrous tissue caught between the insert and tibial tray. Therefore, the kinematic finding of polyethylene-bearing rotation in conjunction with the femoral component is a design-specific condition.

Rotation of the rotating platform polyethylene insert with the femoral component, independent of the rotation of the firmly fixed tibial tray, creates the potential for self-alignment of the polyethylene bearing with the femoral component. Self-alignment is advantageous for optimizing the kinematics of the prosthesis, reducing cross-shear stresses experienced by the polyethylene bearing surface, and maintaining acceptable stresses on posterior cruciate–substituting tibial posts. This self-aligning behavior with a highly conforming design has

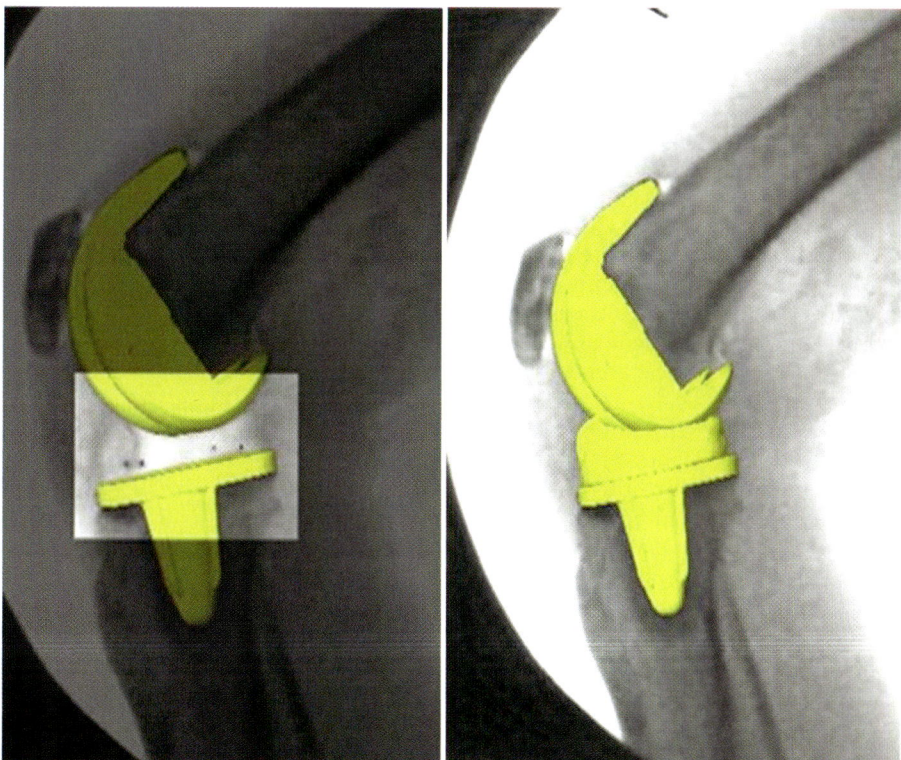

Figure 112-6. Fluoroscopic images demonstrating strategically placed metallic beads within a rotating platform polyethylene insert *(left)* and the computer-automated model-fitting process *(right)* used to determine polyethylene bearing mobility. (From Mobile Bearing Total Knee Arthroplasty, Medscape: [http://www.medscape.com/viewprogram/3133, 2004].)

been shown to maintain large, centrally located surface contact areas at the femorotibial articulation during flexion-extension and axial rotation of the knee,[65] which is much more difficult to achieve in fixed-bearing TKA designs.

An additional advantage of the self-aligning feature of rotating platform TKA systems is facilitation of central patellar tracking. In a fixed-bearing TKA, if substantial malrotation of the tibial component relative to the femoral component is present (especially tibial component internal rotation), the tibial tubercle can become lateralized, enhancing the risk of patellar subluxation. A rotating platform design, through bearing rotation, typically provides for greater self-correction of the component malalignment, allowing better centralization of the extensor mechanism. We have reviewed 1318 consecutive primary TKA performed by the senior author (DAD) over a 6-year period.[68] All subjects were implanted using a single posterior-stabilized knee design (Sigma Press-Fit Condylar, DePuy). The femoral and patellar components were identical and the tibial component type was a mobile-bearing rotating platform tibial design or a fixed-bearing tibial design (all-polyethylene or modular metal-backed tibial component). The selection of a fixed-versus mobile-bearing TKA was primarily based on patient age, with subjects younger than 70 years receiving a mobile-bearing TKA. Mobile-bearing TKA devices were implanted in 940 cases (71.3%; 940 of 1318) and fixed-bearing knees were implanted in 378 cases (28.7%; 378 of 1318). The overall prevalence of lateral release was 7.9% (104 of 1318 knees). The incidence of lateral release in the fixed-bearing group (14.3%; 54 of 378) was found to be significantly higher

($P < .0001$) than in the mobile-bearing group (5.3%; 50 of 940).

The magnitude of axial rotation occurring during deep flexion activities is an important factor in knee implant design. An in vivo fluoroscopic evaluation of over 1000 TKAs incorporating 33 different fixed- and mobile-bearing TKA designs has demonstrated that most TKAs will experience less than 10 degrees of axial rotation with normal postoperative activities.[24] However, in this large multicenter analysis, a number of subjects experienced normal or reverse axial rotational magnitudes greater than 20 degrees during these same activities, which are beyond the rotational boundaries of most fixed-bearing TKA designs. Therefore, mobile-bearing TKA designs that provide more freedom of rotation should reduce rotational polyethylene impingement, with the potential for reduction of polyethylene wear. In addition, studies examining the contribution of posterior cruciate–substituting (PS) polyethylene post wear to TKA failure have shown that excessive axial rotation in PS fixed-bearing designs can predispose to premature polyethylene wear and compromise the integrity of the central post.[54] This occurs because of lateral and medial post impingement with attempted excessive rotation of a fixed square tibial polyethylene post in a fixed femoral intercondylar housing. The freedom of rotation present in rotating platform designs allow them to adapt to a greater range of axial rotation without creation of rotational impingement and wear on posterior cruciate–stabilizing posts.

The additional polyethylene-metal interface at the undersurface of the polyethylene bearing has raised concerns about the generation of additional polyethylene particles and accelerated polyethylene wear. With fixed-bearing TKA systems, backside polyethylene motion against a rough tibial tray that is not designed to accommodate motion has shown significant polyethylene wear and subsequent periprosthetic osteolysis.[29,56,66] In rotating platform systems, a rotating yet flat polyethylene bearing is matched against a highly polished, cobalt-chromium surface with extremely low surface roughness. To date, backside polyethylene wear has not emerged as a clinically significant issue in rotating platform designs. Retrieval studies that have physically examined the backside bearing surface of rotating platform polyethylene inserts have reported only limited evidence of significant undersurface wear.[35,36]

One explanation for the lack of clinically significant backside polyethylene wear is the decoupling of multidirectional motions occurring at the articular interfaces with rotating platform TKA designs.[44,46] In fixed-bearing systems, all rotational, translational, and flexion-extension motion patterns are experienced at a single (superior) articular surface. Therefore, the superior aspect of a fixed-bearing polyethylene insert experiences multidirectional motion pathways. In a rotating platform design that allows no anteroposterior translation, the inferior, or tibial tray–polyethylene countersurface, is designed to experience purely rotational (reciprocal-unidirectional) motion patterns. In mobile-bearing designs in which the polyethylene bearing tracks with the femoral component,[25,40] the superior articular surface (femoral component–polyethylene interface) primarily experiences flexion-extension (reciprocal-unidirectional) motion because rotation is occurring on the inferior aspect of the bearing. Pooley and Tabor[52] have reported that when high-density polyethylene is subjected to unidirectional sliding, the molecules tend to align along the direction of sliding, resulting in lowering of the coefficient of friction, potentially reducing wear of the material. Conversely, when the material is exposed to multidirectional wear pathways, increased cross-shear stresses are created that accelerate polyethylene wear. Additional laboratory studies have shown that the multidirectional shear stresses typically experienced at the single polyethylene interface in fixed-bearing systems may contribute to the generation of 4 to 10 times the polyethylene wear experienced at the unidirectional interfaces in rotating platform designs.[39,48] Therefore, the use of rotating platform TKA designs can reduce polyethylene wear by decoupling multidirectional motions to more monodirectional motion patterns at two differing interfaces, thus reducing cross-shear stresses and wear occurring at both interfaces (Fig. 112-7).

Concern that polyethylene wear microparticulate debris created in mobile bearing designs will result in increased osteolysis has yet to be observed. Fisher and colleagues[31] have analyzed wear debris created in fixed-bearing and rotating platform TKA designs in a knee simulator analysis under high kinematic conditions, attempting to simulate the activity patterns of the younger patient. They observed no differences in microparticulate size but thought that the osteolytic potential was much higher in fixed-bearing designs because of substantially more debris particle generation observed in the fixed-bearing TKA subgroup.

In contrast to a purely rotating platform TKA design, there are other mobile-bearing TKA systems that permit

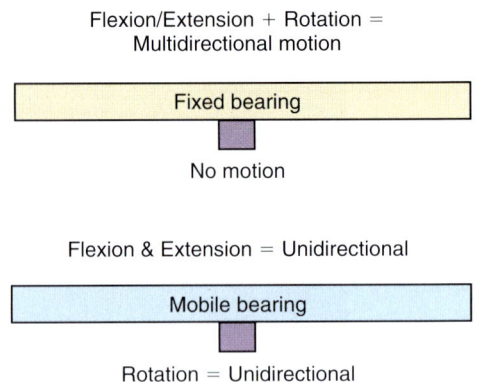

Flexion/Extension + Rotation = Multidirectional motion

Fixed bearing

No motion

Flexion & Extension = Unidirectional

Mobile bearing

Rotation = Unidirectional

Figure 112-7. Diagram illustrating the decoupling of multidirectional motions found on the superior aspect of a fixed polyethylene bearing to monodirectional motion patterns occurring at two articulating interfaces (superior and inferior) of a rotating platform polyethylene bearing. (From McEwen HM, Barnett PI, Bell CJ, et al: The influence of design, materials and kinematics on the in vitro wear of total knee replacements. J Biomech 38:357–365, 2005.)

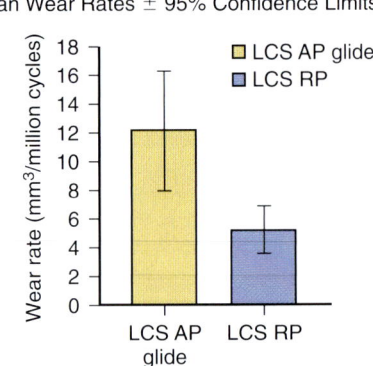

Mean Wear Rates ± 95% Confidence Limits

Figure 112-8. Histogram of a knee simulator analysis comparing polyethylene wear (mg)/million cycles of a rotating platform (LCS RP) versus a mobile-bearing TKA, which allows both rotation and anteroposterior translation (LCS AP Glide). (From Jennings LM, Galvin AL, McEwen HM, Fisher J: The influence of design on the wear of mobile bearing total knee replacements. ORS poster no. 2002. Presented at the 54th Annual Meeting of the Orthopaedic Research Society, San Francisco, March 2-5, 2008.)

rotation and anteroposterior translation to occur on the inferior aspect of the polyethylene bearing. In these designs, the inferior aspect of the polyethylene bearing is exposed to multidirectional motion patterns. Jennings and associates[38] have compared wear of a rotating platform TKA (LCS RP; DePuy) in a knee simulator wear analysis and at 5 million cycles, observed over twice the amount of polyethylene wear in the LCS AP Glide TKA (Fig. 112-8). Therefore, close follow-up evaluation of this type of mobile-bearing TKA is merited to see whether premature failure caused by backside wear occurs secondary to the multidirectional motion on the inferior aspect of the mobile polyethylene bearing.

SURGICAL TECHNIQUE

The surgical goals and techniques used (e.g., alignment, bone resection, ligamentous balancing) for the implantation of a mobile-bearing TKA are typically no different from those used with fixed-bearing TKA systems. Soft tissue balancing, creation of equal flexion and extension gaps, and precise component positioning are extremely important in both fixed- and mobile-bearing TKA systems.

Extension and flexion gap balance is of particular importance with the use of a mobile-bearing TKA because imbalance risks bearing dislocation or spin-out, in which the polyethylene bearing is no longer congruous with the femoral component. Gap balance can be achieved by several methods. We use a spacer block to evaluate and balance the extension gap initially prior to addressing the flexion gap and the directly related femoral component rotation. Proper rotation of the femoral component is essential to obtain a balanced flexion gap. Numerous methods are available to assist in gaining correct rotation of the femoral component.[1,2,30,51,69]

These include use of the following: (1) cutting jigs that automatically rotate the femoral component three or more degrees externally relative to the posterior condylar axis; (2) femoral component placement either parallel to the transepicondylar axis or perpendicular to the anteroposterior axis; and (3) a gap balancing method in which the femoral component is placed parallel to the tibial resection, with each collateral ligament equally tensioned (Fig. 112-9). All methods have been shown to have potential shortcomings and it is prudent to use a combination of femoral component rotational methods. With the use of mobile-bearing TKA systems, we have found that the use of a gap balancing method with some type of tensioning device (e.g., laminar spreaders, spacer blocks, specific gap-tensioning device) to tension the flexion gap while femoral component rotation is determined provides the most reliable and reproducible balance and tension of the flexion gap.[22] Specific gap-tensioning devices provide an additional advantage of facilitating equalization of the flexion gap width to the previously established extension gap (Fig. 112-10). These tensioning devices have been specifically designed to allow measurements (width and tension) obtained from a balanced extension gap to determine and direct flexion gap resections and femoral component rotation. Obtaining 1 to 2 mm of medial and lateral laxity in flexion is desired with the use of mobile-bearing TKA systems. Inability to obtain flexion-extension gap balance or substantial incompetence of the collateral ligamentous structures should prompt consideration of using

a fixed-bearing TKA to lessen the risk of polyethylene bearing instability.

CLINICAL RESULTS

As noted, mobile bearings in TKA offer the advantage of allowing increased implant conformity and contact area while reducing stresses to the fixation interface. The rotating platform TKA design allows rotation through the tibial tray–polyethylene-bearing articulation and effectively minimizes the torsional stresses to the fixation interface that have been associated with fixed-bearing TKA implants.[3] This claim is supported by excellent long-term clinical results, with low loosening rates reported in numerous studies of mobile-bearing TKA. Callaghan and coworkers[15] have reported 15-year clinical outcome of the LCS rotating platform design and observed no failures secondary to loosening, osteolysis, or wear. In the early combined experience with both the LCS meniscal bearing and rotating platform systems (DePuy), Buechel and Pappas[10] have reported 95.1% and 98.2% (cemented and cementless) good to excellent results, with a follow-up duration of 10 years. When evaluating only the rotating platform LCS system, Buechel and associates[11,12] have reported survivorship rates of 97.7% and 98.3% (cemented and cementless) at both 10 and 20 years, with end points defined as revision for any mechanical reason or poor clinical knee scores. Survivorship of the cementless LCS rotating platform system with loosening as the end point was observed to be 99.4% at 20 years. Sorrels and Stiehl[62] have reported similar excellent outcomes with a 90.3% survivorship at a 13-year follow-up duration. Various studies evaluating primary TKA using the rotating platform design reported no evidence of radiographic loosening, even at 20-year radiographic follow-up, and reported that revision TKA was required in only 0% to 0.2% because of aseptic loosening.[5]

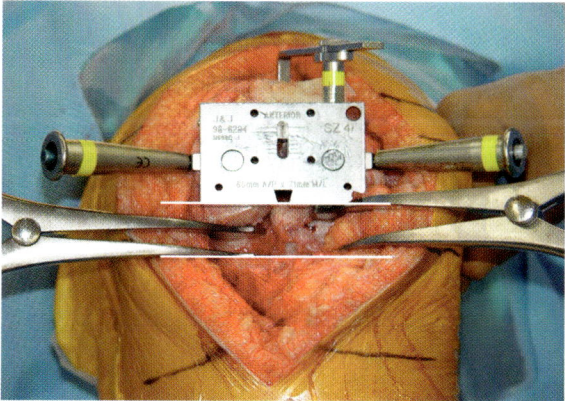

Figure 112-9. Intraoperative photograph of an equalized flexion gap achieved by placement of the anteroposterior femoral cutting jig parallel to the tibial resection, with each collateral ligament equally tensioned using laminar spreaders.

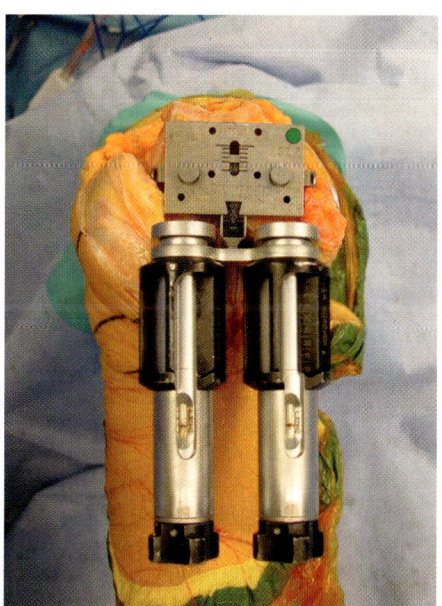

Figure 112-10. Intraoperative photograph of a flexion-extension gap balancer (Knee Balancer, DePuy) placed into the flexion gap to determine gap symmetry, width, and tension.

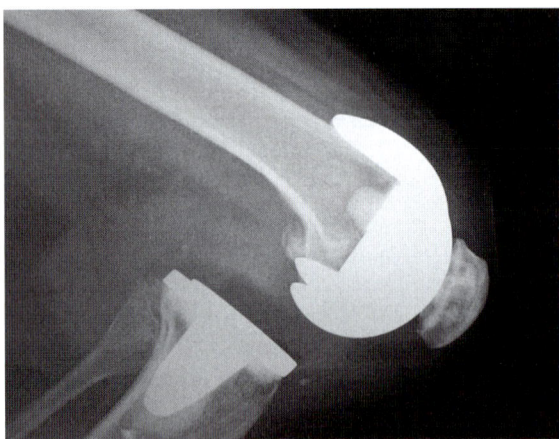

Figure 112-11. Lateral radiograph demonstrating a polyethylene bearing spin-out of a rotating platform TKA.

Reports of polyethylene bearing spin-out in rotating platform TKA have traditionally described this phenomenon as occurring during deep knee flexion (Fig. 112-11). Usually, the polyethylene bearing rotates 90 degrees around its central axis in the tibial tray as the posterolateral polyethylene lip slips posteriorly underneath the lateral femoral condyle and the anteromedial polyethylene lip slips anteriorly underneath the medial femoral condyle. This complication is usually reducible via a closed reduction but may require operative reduction in rare cases. Although this is a legitimate concern with the use of rotating platform designs, the highest incidence of bearing spin-out (3.3% [5 of 149] to 12% [2 of 17])[9,12] has been associated with early outcome evaluations of rotating platform TKA, when attention to flexion gap tension and balance was less emphasized. Advances in component design, surgical implantation instrumentation, increased understanding of the importance of flexion and extension gap tension and balance, accurate ligamentous balancing, and proper femoral component rotation have decreased the incidence of bearing instability following mobile-bearing TKA. Several outcome evaluations have reported a 0% to 2.2% incidence of bearing spin-out in primary TKA at up to 20 years following the operative procedure.[11,15,35]

We performed a recent meta-analysis to determine the clinical outcomes of mobile-bearing TKA.[16] After an extensive literature search, 19 reports met the criteria for analysis, which included 3482 knees implanted with a mobile-bearing TKA. Types of mobile-bearing knees included rotating platform knees (RP group), meniscus-bearing knees (MeBe group), and mobile-bearing designs that allowed bearing rotation as well as anteroposterior translation (APGR group). The purpose of the meta-analysis was to determine the bearing complications rate, survivorship, range of motion, clinical knee scores, and component loosening rate for subjects implanted with a mobile-bearing TKA. With regard to bearing complication rates, implants placed prior to 1995 displayed higher bearing instability rates (1.6%) in contrast to those placed after 1995 (0.1%), likely secondary to improved surgical technique; 15-year survivorship of the RP group was 96.4%. The average arc of motion improved 12.5 degrees in the RP group, 10.1 degrees in the MeBe group, and 6.7 degrees in the APGR group. Knee Society scores improved 62.6 points in the RP group, 62.0 points in the MeBe group,

and 65.6 points in the APGR group. Radiographic component loosening rates for the entire study group was observed to be low, 0.33%.

MOBILE-BEARING USE IN REVISION TOTAL KNEE ARTHROPLASTY

Revision TKA presents numerous additional challenges beyond those in the primary arthroplasty setting. Significant bone loss secondary to osteolysis or iatrogenic removal is commonly encountered. As a result, fixation naturally becomes increasingly difficult in the context of diminished bone stock. Disrupted or unbalanced soft tissue supporting structures may also be encountered, which often requires the use of revision components with increased prosthetic constraint. Although increased constraint can substitute for ligamentous instability, it often increases stresses at the fixation interface, which may lead to premature component loosening and increased polyethylene post wear secondary to increased torque on the constraining mechanism. Potential advantages of use of mobile-bearings in the revision TKA setting include reduction in polyethylene wear, decreasing fixation stresses, and protection of the constraining mechanisms.

Between January 2000 and November 2006, a total of 341 revision TKA procedures were performed by three surgeons at our institution. Of the 341 revisions, 143 revisions (137 patients) were performed using a mobile-bearing TKA system (PFC Sigma and LCS posterior-stabilized rotating platform implants; DePuy). The factors used to determine the use of a mobile-bearing implant design were patient age, activity requirements, longevity expectations, and ability to achieve both a symmetrical extension and flexion gap balance, as we deemed appropriate. Mobile-bearing revisions represented 42% (143 of 341 knees) of all the revision TKA procedures that we performed at our institution. Indications for revision for the 143 knees included instability (50 knees) (Fig. 112-12), loosening (45 knees), failed unicompartmental knee replacement (16 knees), infection reimplantation (13 knees), arthrofibrosis (10 knees), polyethylene wear with osteolysis (3 knees), chronic hemarthrosis (3 knees), failed patellofemoral replacements (2 knees), and nonunion of a supracondylar femur fracture (1 knee). A posterior-stabilized rotating platform insert was used in 88 knees, whereas a constrained condylar rotating platform prosthesis was implanted in 55 knees.

Patients were followed with a clinical and radiographic protocol. With a minimum follow-up of 2 years, 126 knees in 122 patients were available for evaluation and the mean follow-up was 3.6 years (range, 2 to 8 years). The average flexion improved from 100.4 to 117.1 degrees. The Knee Society clinical scores improved from 48.4 preoperatively to 89 points postoperatively; the Knee Society functional scores improved from 49.3 points preoperatively to a mean of 79.2 points at the latest follow-up evaluation. There were no cases of bearing instability and no revision procedures were required for prosthetic loosening. Longer follow-up is necessary to see whether the theoretical benefits of mobile-bearing use in revision TKA is clinically observed.

CONCLUSION

The use of mobile-bearing TKA allows the incorporation of increased coronal and sagittal implant conformity without an

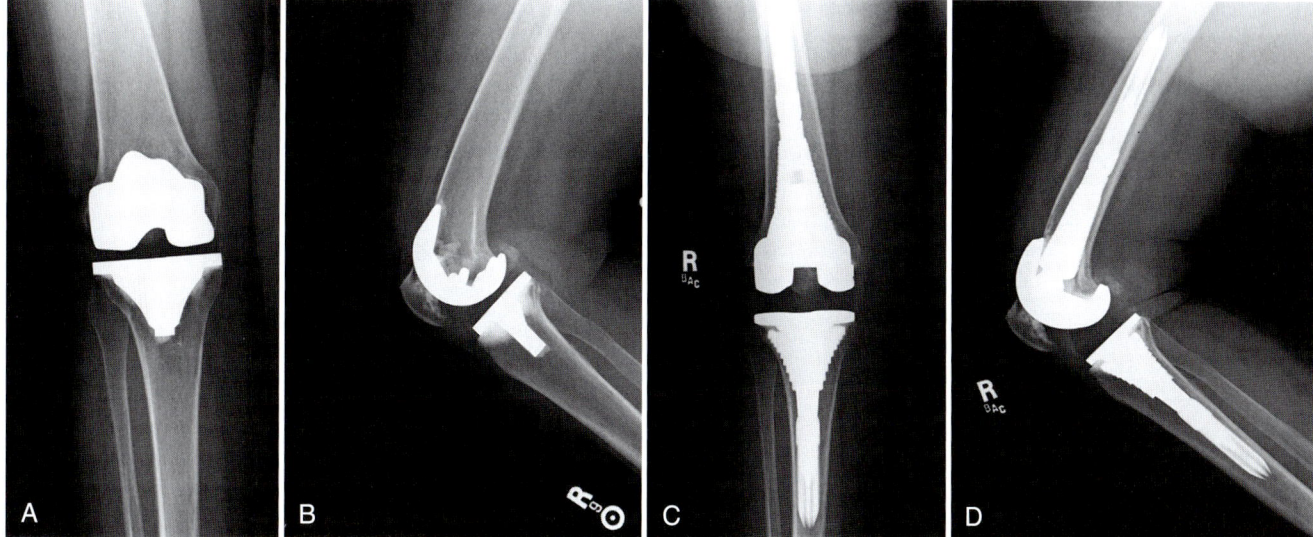

Figure 112-12. **A** and **B,** Preoperative anteroposterior (**A**) and lateral (**B**) radiographs of a failed total knee caused by disabling instability. **C** and **D,** Postoperative anteroposterior (**C**) and lateral (**D**) radiographs following revision TKA with posterior-stabilized mobile-bearing components.

associated increase in fixation interface stresses and resultant aseptic loosening. The increase in sagittal conformity has resulted in more predictable and controlled anteroposterior motion, and increased coronal conformity prevents excessively high polyethylene stresses if femoral condylar liftoff occurs. The overall increase in conformity also increases surface contact area, decreases subsurface polyethylene stresses, and should ultimately decrease polyethylene wear.

The rotating articulation is more forgiving of tibial component rotational malalignment and patient outliers who demonstrate excessive axial rotation following TKA. It facilitates some correction of patellar alignment through optimization of the Q angle. Rotation of the polyethylene insert with the femoral component also minimizes medial and lateral tibial post wear in situations in which a posterior-stabilizing system has been used.

The kinematics of mobile-bearing TKA, however, are not perfect. There are still situations in which femoral condylar liftoff and reverse rotational patterns occur,[28,63] and paradoxical anterior sliding during deep flexion can occur in nonstabilized designs.[34] Future goals include the development of mobile-bearing TKA designs that create better control of bearing mobility patterns.

The exact indications for the use of the mobile-bearing TKA are still unclear. Clinically, fixed-bearing and mobile-bearing TKA systems have performed similarly in outcome studies.*

However, because of the potential for reduced polyethylene wear and enhanced fixation longevity, mobile-bearing TKA designs are to be considered, particularly for younger and higher demand patients with longer life expectancies. Rotational polyethylene post wear seen in fixed-bearing posterior-stabilized systems should be minimized in rotating platform designs and may be another indication for mobile-bearing TKA use. Finally, rotating platform TKA systems

should be considered in revision or extremely complicated primary TKA situations in which constrained or hinged components are needed. Rotating platform designs would help reduce the high torque stresses typically seen at the fixation and hinge interfaces when using a fixed-bearing TKA system.

Although mobile-bearing TKA designs demonstrate a number of favorable features when compared with fixed-bearing systems, it is important to remember that not all mobile-bearing systems are the same. Differences exist in the condylar geometry and bearing mobility patterns. To date, the purely rotating platform design has emerged as the most clinically successful, reliable, and predictable among mobile-bearing designs. Future studies are indicated to determine and compare the kinematic and clinical effects associated with multidirectional (anteroposterior translation and bearing rotation) versus unidirectional (rotation-only) mobile-bearing TKA systems.

KEY REFERENCES

Beuchel FF, Sr: Long-term follow-up after mobile-bearing total knee replacement. Clin Orthop Relat Res (404):40–50, 2002.

Buechel FF, Sr, Buechel FF, Jr, Pappas MJ, et al: Twenty-year evaluation of the New Jersey LCS rotating platform knee replacement. J Knee Surg 15:84–89, 2002.

Callaghan JJ, O'Rourke MR, Iossi MF, et al: Cemented rotating-platform total knee replacement. A concise follow-up, at a minimum of fifteen years, of a previous report. J Bone Joint Surg Am 87:1995–1998, 2005.

Cheng CK, Huang CH, Liau JJ, et al: The influence of surgical malalignment on the contact pressures of fixed and mobile bearing knee prostheses—a biomechanical study. Clin Biomech 18:231–236, 2003.

Dennis DA, Komistek RD, Mahfouz MR, et al: Multicenter determination of in vivo kinematics after total knee arthroplasty. Clin Orthop Relat Res (416):37–57, 2003.

Dennis DA, Komistek RD, Mahfouz MR, et al: Mobile-bearing total knee arthroplasty: do the polyethylene bearings rotate? Clin Orthop Relat Res (440):88–95, 2005.

Fisher J, McEwen H, Tipper J, et al: Wear-simulation analysis of rotating-platform mobile-bearing knees. Orthopedics 29(Suppl):S36–S41, 2006.

Garling EH, Kaptein BL, Nelissen RG, Valstar ER: Limited rotation of the mobile-bearing in a rotating platform total knee prosthesis. J Biomech 40(Suppl 1):S25–S30, 2007.

---

*References 10-12, 15, 20, 55, 58, and 62.

Greenwald AS, Heim CS: Mobile-bearing knee systems: ultra-high molecular weight polyethylene wear and design issues. Instr Course Lect 54:195–205, 2005.

Komistek RD, Dennis DA, Mahfouz MR, et al: In vivo polyethylene-bearing mobility is maintained in posterior stabilized total knee arthroplasty. Clin Orthop Relat Res (428):207–213, 2004.

McEwen HM, Barnett PI, Bell CJ, et al: The influence of design, materials and kinematics on the in vitro wear of total knee replacements. J Biomech 38:357–365, 2005.

Pooley C, Tabor D: Friction and molecular structure: the behaviour of some thermoplastics. Proc R Soc Lond A 329:251, 1972.

Sorrels RB, Stiehl JB: Long-term outcomes of a rotating platform mobile bearing prosthesis after TKA. J Arthroplasty 19:255, 2004.

Stukenborg-Coleman C, Ostermeier S, Hurschler C, et al: Tibiofemoral contact stress after total knee arthroplasty: comparison of fixed and mobile-bearing inlay designs. Acta Orthop Scand 73:638–646, 2002.

Yang CC, McFadden LA, Dennis DA, et al: Lateral retinacular release rates in mobile-versus fixed-bearing TKA. Clin Orthop Relat Res (466):2656–2661, 2008.

Full references for this chapter can be found on www.expertconsult.com.

Patellar Resurfacing in Total Knee Arthroplasty

Oliver S. Schindler

For a long time, the patella was wrongfully marginalized and merely considered as an afterthought during total knee arthroplasty (TKA). Even today, patella resurfacing is often thrown in for good measure without proper understanding of the functional interplay among arthroplasty components. The patella should be recognized as an integral part of any TKA. The clinician must be aware that judicious surgical management of the patella will not only affect patient satisfaction but occupies a pivotal role in the success or failure of TKA.

When contemplating treatment for conditions affecting the patellofemoral joint (PFJ), clinicians must understand the anatomy, biomechanics, and kinematics of the knee and locomotor system. Without such understanding, it is difficult to appreciate the implications associated with the surgical and conservative treatment modalities. This is of particular importance in the consideration of patellar resurfacing in TKA, because surgically imposed changes may have significant effects on the performance and behavior of the PFJ. The appreciation of the consequences of the mechanical environment on the behavior of the PFJ are of particular importance in the attempt to develop knee replacement systems that provide a high level of patient satisfaction combined with clinical long-term success.

NATIVE PATELLOFEMORAL JOINT

Kinematics

Kinematics of the knee joint characterizes the relative motion that exists between femur, tibia, and patella. The patella is considered a sesamoid bone implanted within the tendon of the extensor mechanism. Arguably, the most important function of the patella is its role in facilitating extension of the knee by enhancing quadriceps efficiency through increasing the distance of the extensor apparatus from the axis of flexion and extension.[128] The patella exerts a mechanical advantage by acting as a fulcrum, thus anteriorly displacing the line of pull and increasing the moment arm of the quadriceps muscle force in relation to the center of rotation of the knee. In doing so, the patella may enhance the force of extension by as much as 50% throughout the entire range of motion.[285] In addition, the patella allows for the distribution of the reaction force on the femur by increasing the contact area during knee flexion. It also acts as a guide for the extensor mechanism by centralizing the divergent pull from the four muscles of the quadriceps and transmitting these forces to the patellar tendon. Together with the anatomic shape of the patellofemoral articulation, this protects the extensor apparatus from dislocating.

When the knee is extended, the tightening quadriceps pulls the patella upward until the upper border reaches beyond the femoral trochlea groove. So long as the line of gravity falls behind the center axis of the knee joint when standing upright, the quadriceps must contract to neutralize the rotatory effect of gravity on the knee, which would otherwise force it into flexion. As soon as the line of gravity falls within or in front of the knee, which usually occurs in full extension or hyperextension, the quadriceps becomes relaxed. The quadriceps apparatus, being oblique in its angulation toward the patella and patellar tendon, creates a line of pull with an outwardly directed horizontal component when contracted. The angle between the line of pull and patellar tendon is often referred to as the Q angle, which measures on average between 10 and 20 degrees (Fig. 113-1).[91] In coronal and axial planes, this gives rise to a tendency of the patella to slip outward over the lateral femoral condyle, giving a resultant force in the lateral direction.[92,316] To offset this propensity, the lateral condyle projects farther forward, whereas the fibers of vastus medialis that secure the patella medially extend farther distally compared with those of the vastus lateralis.[285] In addition, the tibia derotates during the first 30 degrees of flexion, essentially reversing the screw-home mechanism and significantly reducing the Q angle, which in turn also decreases the lateral vector.[35,92,111,203] Because of a lack of mechanical engagement and the presence of lateral force vectors, the patella is most vulnerable in the early flexion range. Even at 30 degrees of knee flexion, the patella will not have fully engaged into the trochlea groove and the effect of the Q angle may not have neutralized. Walker[316] has conceded that in the midrange of flexion, the condition for lateral stability of the patella is that the angle of inclination of the lateral trochlear groove is larger than the Q angle.

Contact Areas

With the knee in full extension, the patella is usually out of contact with the trochlear groove. Depending on the length of the patellar tendon, the patella is drawn into the trochlea from a slight lateral position and gains contact with the femur between 10 and 20 degrees. The contact begins with the inferior margin of the patella and moves proximally as flexion proceeds. Beyond 30 degrees, the patella settles into the deepening trochlear groove, where it is further stabilized by the quadriceps and patellar tendon force. During flexion and extension, the patella presents an excursion of 5 to 7.4 cm in the sagittal plane, whereas the distance between the lower pole of the patella and tibial tuberosity remains constant.[35,93,276]

The patellofemoral contact area extends from the medial margin of the medial facet to the lateral margin of the lateral facet as a broad band of contact moving from distal to proximal.[3,110,112,301] At 60 degrees of flexion, the contact is across the center, at 90 degrees of flexion the contact is toward the superior pole and, beyond 90 degrees, the patella, lying across the medial and lateral condyles, is forming two separate contact areas[131,140] (Figs. 113-2 and 113-3). Ficat and Hungerford[92] have described this movement of the patella in the coronal plane during flexion as a "gentle curve with its concavity facing laterally." Studies of the tracking pattern of the natural patella have confirmed that the patella rotates as much as 15 degrees in relation to the femur at flexion angles beyond 50 degrees, tilts in a mediolateral direction in the axial plane, and undergoes medial displacement of up to 4° during early knee flexion, and lateral displacement of up to 8° during high flexion beyond 60°.[156,247,309,310]

In the transverse or axial plane, as seen on skyline radiographs, the patella is perfectly congruent with the trochlea, ensuring its medial and lateral stability. Longitudinal sectioning of the patella has confirmed that the patella adopts almost a flat surface in the sagittal plane, making it perfectly unconstrained as far as its anatomic form is concerned.[142,166] The form of the patella provides stability against lateral subluxation but does not impede it from rocking around its transverse axis to the point at which the resultant of the PFJ reaction force is perpendicular to the contact surface.

As with the location of patellofemoral contact areas, the size of the contact areas is highly dependent on knee position. From 20 to 60 degrees of flexion, the average contact area increases linearly from approximately 150 to 480 mm².[2,3,302] It then remains almost constant up to approximately 90 degrees of flexion, after which a linear reduction occurs.[112,139] Because of the drastically changed contact pattern beyond 100 degrees, when the patella leaves the trochlea, straddling the intercondylar notch, contact areas may fall well below 100 mm² at full flexion (see Fig. 113-3). Subsequently, only a certain proportion of the retropatellar surface will be in contact with the femur at any one time. Matthews and associates[196] have shown that on average only 19% of the patella-bearing surface is engaged at 30 degrees of flexion, 29% at 60 degrees, 28% at 90 degrees, and 13% at 120 degrees.

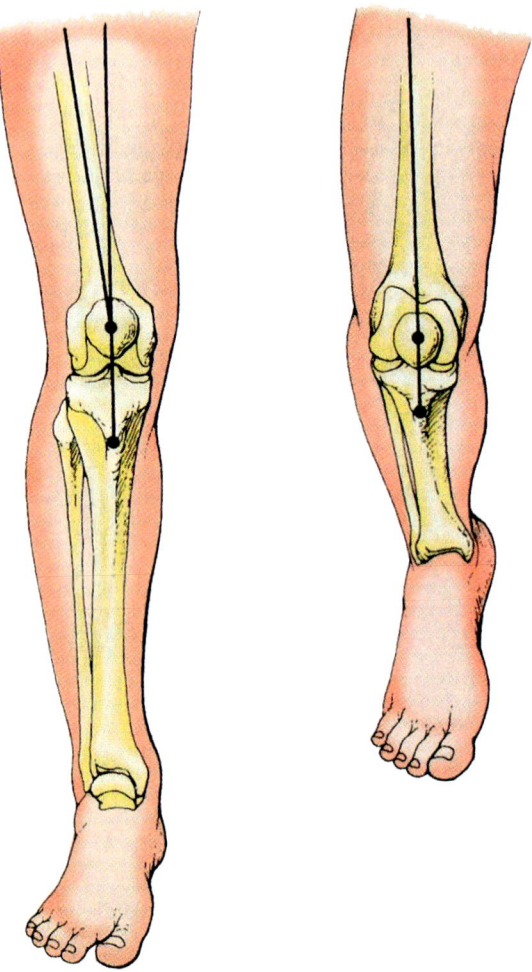

Figure 113-1. The quadriceps angle (Q angle), a measure of the overall rotational alignment of the lower leg, is affected by the knee flexion angle. As the knee progresses from full extension into flexion the tibia rotates internally, reversing the screw-home mechanism, reducing the Q angle, and assisting in centralizing patellar tracking. (Adapted from Tria AJ Jr, Klein KS: An illustrated guide to the knee, New York, 1992, Churchill Livingstone.)

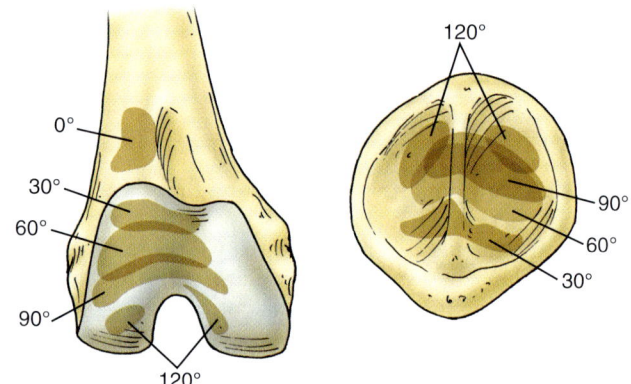

Figure 113-3. Patellofemoral contact areas at various degrees of knee flexion based on an applied quadriceps force of 1110 N (250 pounds). (From Walker PS: Human joints and their artificial replacement, Springfield, Ill, 1977, Charles C Thomas.)

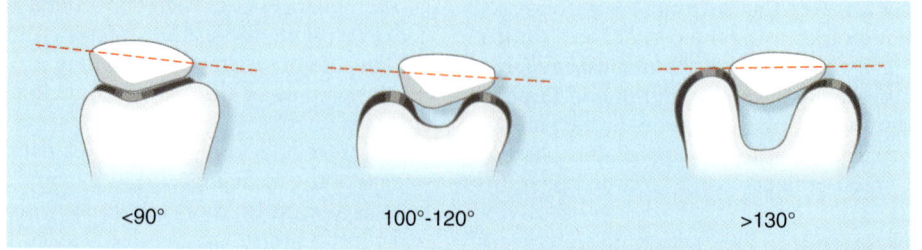

Figure 113-2. Bifurcation of patellofemoral contact area beyond 100 degrees of knee flexion leads to a significant decrease in patellofemoral contact area. (Adapted from Hehne HJ: Das patellofemoralgelenk [The patellofemoral joint], Stuttgart, Germany, 1983, Enke.)

Biomechanics

Much attention has been given to define the force transmission in the PFJ. For ease of calculation, it is sufficiently accurate to consider that these forces lie in a sagittal plane. The patellofemoral reaction (or compressive) force (PRF) is acting perpendicular to the articulating surface of the patella and is equal and opposite to the resultant of the patellar tendon and quadriceps forces (Fig. 113-4). With increasing flexion, the line of reaction moves upward, leading to an increase in PRF for the following reasons. As the angle between the patellar tendon and quadriceps becomes more acute, the resultant force vector increases. With knee flexion, effective lever arms of the femur and tibia increase, requiring greater quadriceps power to resist the flexion moment of the body weight (BW). Close to extension, the PRF is only about one third of the quadriceps force, whereas beyond 60 degrees of flexion, the patellar force is about 1.25 times the quadriceps force.[316]

The most important variable in the calculation of static forces is the distance between the line of body weight (center of gravity) and PFJ. Changes of posture in the sagittal plane (leaning forward or backward) will alter this distance and lead to substantial differences in static force transmission, whereas changes in the coronal plane will exert little influence.[16,66] In full extension, the center of gravity usually falls anterior to the knee and moment arms become 0; hence, no forces will be acting on the PFJ. In this situation the body is instinctively balanced by compensatory deviations of its different parts creating a condition of unstable equilibrium. Whenever the line of body weight is moved away from the PFJ in a posterior direction, muscle activity and tension in the patellar and quadriceps tendon increase to maintain position, resulting in higher PRFs.

During normal activities requiring flexion under load, hip flexion is also present, thus bringing the center of gravity forward and shortening the femoral lever arm. This relationship is exemplified by the patient with quadriceps weakness who can rise from a chair by leaning forward, bringing the center of gravity closer to the knee. Similarly, there are significant differences in patellofemoral compressive forces when ascending and descending stairs (Fig. 113-5). Predicted force values for stair ascent range from 1.8 to 2.3 × BW, compared with those for stair descent of 2.9 to 6 × BW[8,223] (Table 113-1). The increased values on descending are a result of the center of gravity being moved further backward behind the PFJ, as the body adopts a more upright position to maintain balance.[17,18,261] Force transmission in the PFJ is therefore dependent on the relationship between the center of gravity of the body and knee flexion angle, and calculations should not be based on the length of the femur and position of the hip joint per se.[16]

The quadriceps tendon abuts onto the proximal aspect of the femoral trochlea in midrange of knee flexion, allowing compressive forces to become divided between the tendofemoral and patellofemoral contact areas.[18,93,102,214] This phenomenon, described as the "turn-round" of forces, represents an elegant way of maintaining relatively constant unit load under a mechanical situation in which total load is increasing[112] (see Fig. 113-4). The efficacy of the turn-round of the divided forces is dependent on the length and altitude of the patella, and it takes effect between 50 and 90 degrees of flexion.[16] According to measurements obtained by Hehne,[131] the contact area of the quadriceps tendon is significantly larger compared with the contact area of the PFJ. At 90 degrees, the quadriceps contact area was one to two

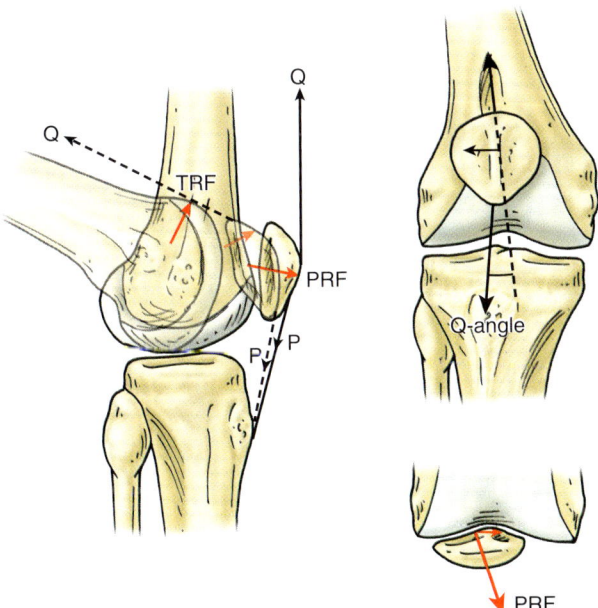

Figure 113-4. The PRF bisects the angle made by the quadriceps and patellar tendon forces and moves upward on the patella with flexion. The TRF occurs through engagement of the quadriceps tendon with the femoral trochlea at 50 to 90 degrees of flexion (turn-round of forces), providing a load-sharing function to the patella. In the coronal and axial views, the sideways component is balanced by the reaction occurring on the slope of the femoral trochlea. (Adapted and redrawn from Walker PS: Contact areas and load transmission in the knee. In American Academy of Orthopaedic Surgeons: Symposium on reconstructive surgery of the knee, St. Louis, 1978, Mosby, pp 26–36 and Walker PS: Human joints and their artificial replacement, Springfield, Ill, 1977, Charles C Thomas.)

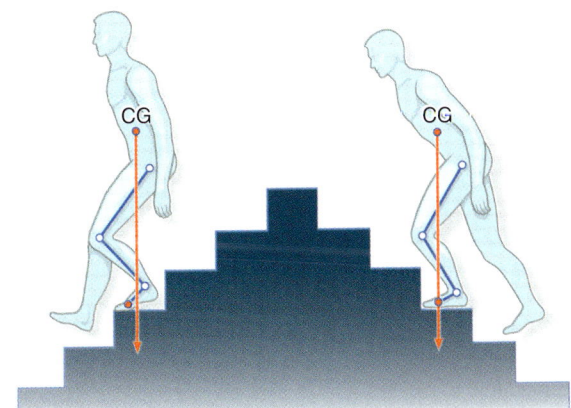

Figure 113-5. The center of gravity (CG) is positioned almost in line with the patellofemoral joint during stair ascent; thus moment arms of the femur and tibia are relatively short and the PRF is low. During stair descent, the CG is positioned further behind the PFJ, creating longer moment arms and leading to an increase in the PRF. (From Schindler OS, Scott WN: Basic kinematics and biomechanics of the patello-femoral joint. Part 1: The native patella. Acta Orthop Belg [in press].)

Table 113-1 Patellofemoral Joint Reaction Forces For Various Activities*

Study (Year)	Activity	Body Weight (kg)	Knee Flexion Angle (Degrees)	Peak PRF (*N*)	Peak PRF (× BW)
Bresler and Frankel (1950)[38]	Level walking	71	20	840	1.2
Ericson and Nisell (1987)[85]	Cycling	71	83	905	1.3
Nisell (1985)[214]	Lifting (12.8-kg box)	77	90	1600	2.2
Andriacchi et al (1980)[8]	Stair ascent	71	65	1500	2.1
Smidt (1973)[276]	Isometric quad contraction	82	75	2127	2.6
Kelley et al (1976)[162]	Rising from a chair	—	90	3800	5.5
Kaufman et al (1991)[158]	Isokinetic exercise	81	70	—	5.1
Andriacchi et al (1980)[8]	Stair descent	71	60	4000	5.7
Huberti and Hayes (1984)[139]	Isometric extension	—	90	4600	6.5
Dahlqvist et al (1982)[63]	Ascending from squat	—	140	—	6.0
Dahlqvist et al (1982)[63]	Descending from squat	—	140	—	7.6
Winter (1983)[329]	Jogging	72	50	—	7.7
Wahrenberg et al (1978)[314]	Kicking	76	100	5800	7.8
Smith (1972)[277]	Jumping	—	—	—	20
Nisell (1985)[214]	Quadriceps tendon rupture	—	—	10,900-18,300	14.4-24.2
Zernicke et al (1977)[336]	Patellar tendon rupture	—	90	—	25

*Results should be viewed with due regard to the complexity of the problem and with knowledge of the assumptions that must necessarily be made in obtaining them.

times larger, at 120 degrees two to three times larger, and at 140 degrees three to four times larger than the patellofemoral contact area. Huberti and Hayes[139] have calculated average tendofemoral reaction forces (TRFs) at 120 degrees of flexion as approximately 550 N, whereas PRFs at the same degree of knee flexion measured on average 1600 N, indicating a TRF-to-PRF ratio of 1 : 3. This may partly explain the higher frequency of chondromalacia in patella alta, because tendofemoral contact may be eliminated or substantially decreased, creating an increase in PRF.[148,168]

Static measurements of PRFs show an almost linear increase, with values ranging from 0.2 × BW at 10 degrees to 12.9 × BW at 135 degrees.* In vivo PRFs vary and are dependent on the type of activity performed. Predicted force values range from 0.6 × BW for level walking to 7.7 × BW for jogging and 20 × BW for jumping.[158,214,223,277,329]

Reaction forces during cycling are generally lower than those generated through daily activities and most other athletic activities. Ericson and Nisell[85] were able to show that the magnitude of joint forces is almost independent of body weight, but increases with workload and reduced seat height. TRF rose to 295 N at 108 degrees of knee flexion, whereas PRF peaked at 83 degrees with 905 N. Anterior knee pain (AKP) during cycling is therefore more likely to occur if the seat position is kept low, because this will increase knee flexion angles throughout all stages of the revolution.[73] Cycling should be considered a recommended activity for most patients following knee arthroplasty, especially those who are obese, but proper attention should be given to the level of workload and seat height (see Table 113-1).

When considering the magnitude of PRF, it has to be remembered that this force acts through an area that varies with knee flexion.[190,301,316] Thus, an increase in PRF does not necessarily assume an increase in patellofemoral pressure. The patellofemoral contact area is small near full extension

of the knee, indicating that patellofemoral pressure is higher for the same magnitude of PRF. Subsequently, patellofemoral pressure near extension may be relatively high, although the compressive force appears to be comparatively low.[214]

To obtain a rough estimate of the resulting contact pressures in the PFJ, the mean pressure is calculated by dividing patellofemoral force values by the patellofemoral contact area. Calculated patellofemoral contact pressure values, dependent on activity and knee flexion angle, range from 1.28 to 12.6 N/mm^2.[139,196] A man of 71 kg (696 N) climbing stairs would generate a patellofemoral compressive force of 1754 N equivalent to 2.5 × BW and experience patellofemoral pressures between 3.73 and 6.87 N/mm^2. Women have smaller knees and hence shorter patellar tendon moment arms than men. Subsequently, the PRF increases by up to 20% for the same knee-extending moment, which would explain the somewhat higher frequency of patellofemoral disorders in women.[214]

Denham and Bishop[66] have shown that the PRF exceeds the tibiofemoral reaction force in angles above 25 degrees. At almost full knee flexion, these values rise to almost 150% of the forces passing through the tibiofemoral joint. It is therefore not surprising that the cartilaginous cover of the patellofemoral articulation is the thickest in the body and allows the transmission of forces to the subchondral bone in such a way that the pain threshold of the richly innervated bone is not surpassed.[92] The articulating surfaces are able to adapt to the changing surface contours because of the viscoelastic properties of cartilage, which allow for its deformation under load and subsequent increase in pressure-transmitting area. This process is time-dependent and pressure values will thus be different for short-term and long-term loading. The measured values of patellofemoral pressure should therefore be regarded as reference values only, because pressure-transmitting areas of the PFJ increase with increasing load and duration of loading.[16,110,131,196,302] This may explain why peak stresses of up to 20 times body weight can be tolerated

*References 16, 102, 139, 190, 226, and 276.

without causing lasting damage, because they are applied for only very short periods of time, whereas long-term application of such loads would invariably lead to cartilage breakdown.

HISTORY OF PATELLAR RESURFACING

The earliest types of total knee arthroplasties were pure tibiofemoral replacements, primarily designed to treat severe axial deformities and intractable knee pain in patients affected by tuberculosis or rheumatoid arthritis.[106,273,319] The procedure was seen as an alternative to arthrodesis and performed in patients of extremely low demand, for whom any improvement in pain relief or mobility level was considered a success.[321]

The PFJ remained largely ignored until the end of the 1960s, with most hinged knee arthroplasties failing to provide an anterior femoral flange as an articulating surface to accommodate for physiologic patellar tracking.[132,273,319] In these earlier designs, the patella usually impinged with the anterior ridge of the proximal margin of the femoral component, which was not countersunk to the level of the retained part of the proximal trochlea.[86,191,234,321] This incongruity between prosthetic femoral and native patellar surface created an articulation of poor geometry, which often led to patellar erosion and deformity, prompting some surgeons to promote patellectomy actively as part of the surgical procedure.[335] Through the increase in patellofemoral complications and extensor mechanism failures, clinicians became aware of the shortcomings of available knee implants in providing for normal patellofemoral function. Design changes were introduced based on proximal extension of the femoral component and creation of a trochlear groove in an attempt to emulate the anatomic shape of the femur, whereas the patella itself maintained its "Cinderella" status.[62,206,263,270] A case in point was the Duocondylar prosthesis, which did not provide for the PFJ and yielding mixed results, with many patients suffering anterior knee discomfort. Changes in the design through the addition of a trochlear flange improved clinical outcome results dramatically by allowing the natural patella to articulate with the femoral component throughout the entire range of flexion.

Continuing disenchantment with the unpredictability of clinical results, however, encouraged some clinicians to experiment with replacement of the retropatellar surface.[3,120,123] Hanslik,[123,124] in 1969, reported the use of a modified version of the McKeever patellar prosthesis made of high-density polyethylene, which was combined with the hinged arthroplasty by Young.[335] Hanslik was critical of the replacement designs available at that time and stressed the importance of patellar preservation for enhancing the functional outcome. Between 1969 and 1973, 46 TKAs with a patellar prosthesis were implanted, mostly for end-stage osteoarthritis. Short-term results indicated that the great majority of patients were walking unaided, with only slight or no pain.

The first recorded patellar resurfacing combined with a nonconstrained condylar-type replacement arthroplasty was performed by Groeneveld and colleagues in 1970[118-120] (Fig. 113-6). They adopted the low-friction principle popularized by Charnley when combining a femoral mould arthroplasty with tibial polyethylene disks and a three-pegged anatomic

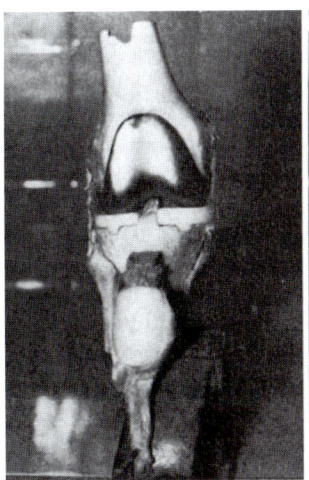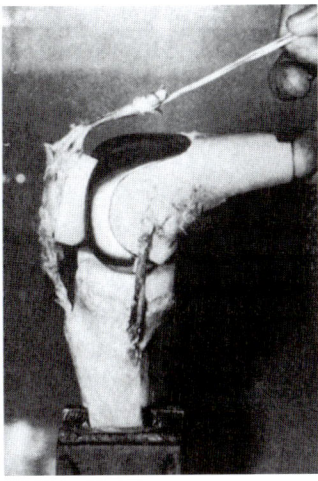

Figure 113-6. First-generation patellar component. This three-peg, all-polyethylene anatomic design was used in combination with the Münster-TKA between 1970 and 1973. (From Groeneveld HB, Schöllner D, Bantjes A, Feijen J: Eine Kniegelenkstotalendoprothese unter Erhalt der Kreuz und Seitenbänder. [Total knee arthroplasty with preservation of cruciate and collateral ligaments.] Z. Orthop 109:599–607, 1971.)

polyethylene patellar component. At 2-year follow-up, 64% of patients with a replaced patella had excellent or good results compared with 46% in whom the patella was left unresurfaced. The authors expressed uncertainty about the long-term survival of the patellar implant and thought that patellar resurfacing should be reserved for cases of persistent pain and only used in combination with a patella-friendly femoral component.

Gunston and MacKenzie[121] developed a patellofemoral arthroplasty designed to work in conjunction with the polycentric knee system in response to the inability to alleviate AKP, despite patellectomy. A stainless steel patellar button articulating with a grooved polyethylene track placed into the trochlea was used between 1973 and 1976 in several knees, with satisfactory initial results. Gunston was, however, aware that the additional prosthetic components would increase the possibility of complications and therefore urged it not to be used indiscriminately.

At the Hospital of Special Surgery, Insall, Ranawat, Scott, and Walker started to develop the duopatellar and total condylar prosthesis, the first complete prosthetic system allowing for optional resurfacing of the patella.[152,235,318] A dome-shaped polyethylene patellar design was chosen because of its simplicity and to prevent binding in the femoral groove. Their first tricompartmental total condylar replacement was implanted in October 1974 by Ranawat et al.[3,150,235] Other designs followed and, by the beginning of the 1980s, almost all available knee replacement systems had provisions for patellar resurfacing.[117,141,173,318]

Many different patellar surface designs became established, but despite the relative clinical success of cemented, all-polyethylene patellar components, metal-backed patellar implants were introduced in the early 1980s. Metal backing was initially applied to polyethylene acetabular and tibial components to improve load transfer and bending resistance, in addition to allowing for the application of porous metal surfaces for biologic anchoring.[20,243,317] Concerns about the failure of cemented prosthesis through loosening and bone resorption, erroneously thought to be caused by an adverse biologic response to methylmethacrylate, added to the enthusiasm for cementless fixation and the use of porous-coated patellar implants.[141,327] The principal advantages of metal backing, however, were applied to the patella without clinical justification.[236] Problems of polyethylene deformation and wear, fatigue fracture, and component dissociation through locking mechanism failure led to the rapid demise of the metal-backed patella, which by the end of the decade was almost universally abandoned[22,236,258,292] (Fig. 113-7).

All-polyethylene dome-shaped patellar components have since experienced a renaissance and have been used in conjunction with the vast majority of currently available knee arthroplasties. Their obvious disadvantages appear to be outweighed by their simplicity in design, ease of application, and relative forgiveness. Improvements in patellofemoral implant design and geometry have led to a reduction in PFJ-related complications but have so far been unable to eradicate them completely.[59]

PATELLAR IMPLANT DESIGN

Matthews and colleagues have assessed the load-bearing characteristics of the patellofemoral joint and remarked that "high patellofemoral load values, small patellofemoral contact areas, and resultant high stress magnitudes indicate the need for caution in the design and development of a patellofemoral component for total joint replacement prosthesis."[196] These comments remain applicable even today, with retrieval analysis of patellar components and the significant failure rate of metal-backed patellar designs underscoring the extreme mechanical environment in which these implants are expected to perform (Fig. 113-8).

It should be remembered that patellar tracking, contact area, and pressure distribution are significantly different between native and prosthetic knees.[146,288] The configuration and mechanical features to be considered in the design of the prosthetic PFJ should include functional range of motion in multiaxial planes, stability, fixation, dimensions, load transfer areas, and materials.[117] A successful patellofemoral articulation must be designed to function under high-stress

conditions, over a long period of time, because ground reaction, gravitational, ligamentous, and muscular forces all act to produce significant compressive, shear, and torsional loads. Thus, both design and materials used must at least be compatible with mechanical forces generally encountered during daily activities.

Patellar and femoral components in TKA are inextricably linked and function as a unit. The configuration of this unit has been a matter of ongoing debate, indicating that the ideal combination is yet to be determined. For example, increasing the congruency of the patellofemoral articulation reduces peak stresses on the surface level of the components but, in turn, increases shear stresses at the patellar fixation site. From a wear point of view, an increase in component conformity would appear advantageous.[21] Overconstraining the joint, however, is incompatible with secure fixation and freedom of motion. It is therefore reasonable to suggest a compromise solution that provides partially conforming surfaces that may satisfy reasonable motion, laxity, and stability between patella and femur. This concept of partial patellofemoral conformity has been incorporated successfully into most knee implant systems, but some mobile-bearing devices have defied science and have performed well, despite highly congruent surface geometries.[43,153,161]

The myriad of patellar components currently available reflects the lack of consensus with respect to the ideal design (see Fig. 113-8). Persistent attempts to implement design changes are often influenced by reported complications, such as the high failure rate of metal backing. Such changes are often based more on the absence of a satisfactory alternative than an indication that continued refinements are leading to improved results. Currently, central fixation lugs are less common because of the increased risk of patellar fracture associated with this particular design.[58,267] Fixation lugs placed peripherally are subject to less stress than lugs placed centrally, especially if oriented in a transverse direction.[55,170]

Articular surface geometries of patellar components vary greatly but can be classified into four basic shapes—convex or dome-shaped, modified dome-shaped with peripheral concavity (also known as Mexican hat, sombrero type), cylindrical or saddle-shaped, and anatomic[164] (see Fig. 113-8). Every implant design bears particular advantages regarding conformity, stability, forgiveness, and wear pattern, with none ultimately being superior. However, advantages attributed to a particular design, such as the dome-shaped patella, should not be generalized to all domes because the behavior of a specific patellar component is directly dependent on a number of variables, with the surface geometry of the mating femoral component being the most important.* Apart from component positioning and alignment, other factors, such as patient demographics and clinical function, will influence the performance and longevity of the PFJ.[129]

Dome-Shaped Patella

The great majority of currently available patellar components are of the all-polyethylene dome-shaped type (Fig. 113-9; see also Fig. 113-14). Dome-shaped components usually articulate congruently with the trochlear groove in extension

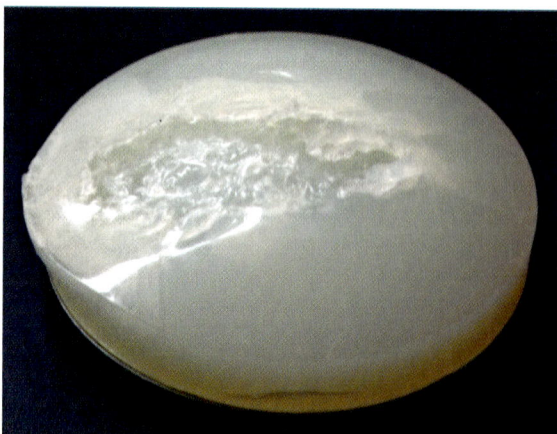

Figure 113-7. Retrieved patellar component showing severe polyethylene wear and delamination. (Courtesy Professor Wolfgang Plitz, Laboratory of Biomechanics, Ludwig-Maximilian University, Munich, Germany.)

---

*References 56, 75, 200, 296, 297, and 334.

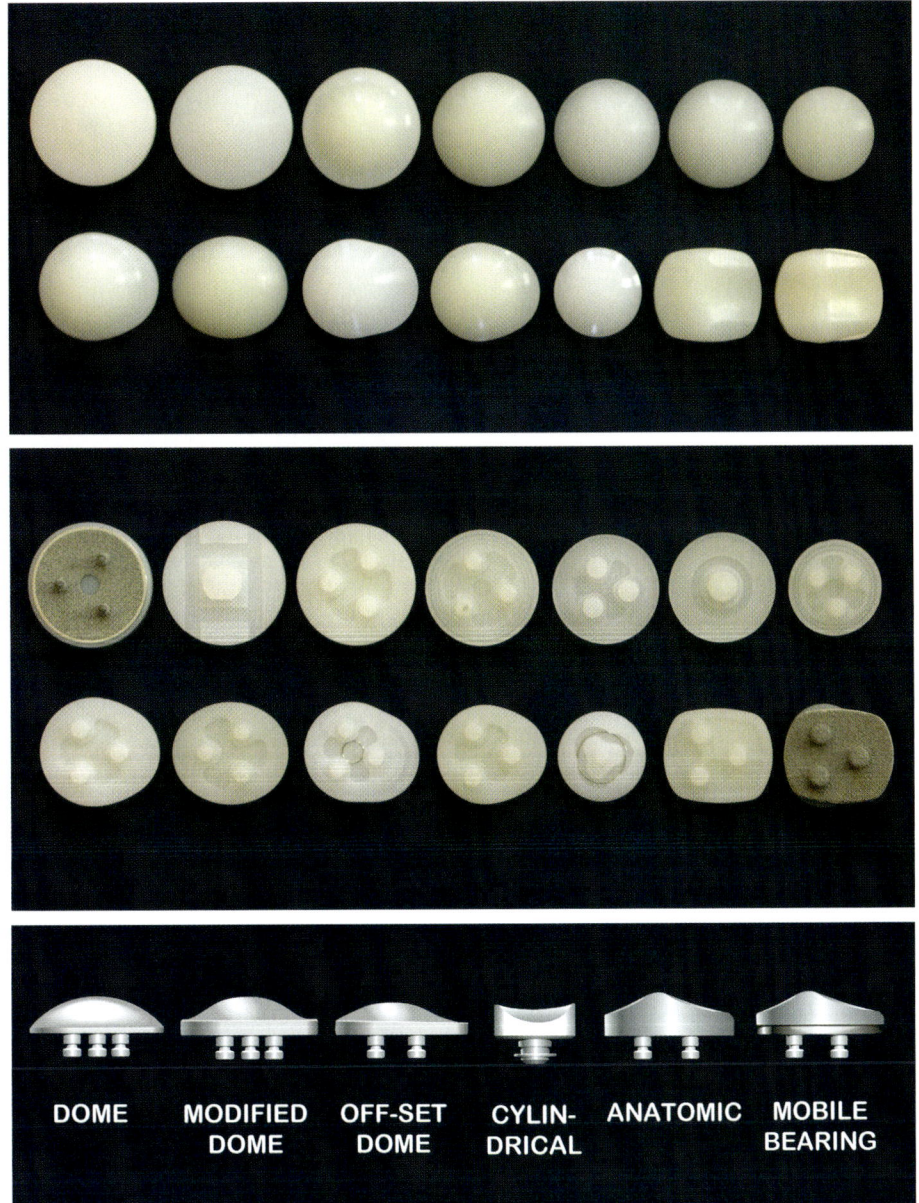

Figure 113-8. A, Lateral positioning of the patellar implant will tighten the lateral retinacular structures and may provoke lateral subluxation. **B,** Moderate medialization will re-create the asymmetrical contours of the native retro-patellar high point, centralize quadriceps tendon and patellar reaction force and improve patellar tracking. **C,** Overzealous medial positioning of the patellar implant may create lateral patellar tilt through off centre positioning of the quadriceps tendon force.

but may be exposed to high stresses and point contact in flexion, when the patella comes into contact with the convexities of the femoral condyles. Some of these problems have been addressed successfully through design adaptations of femoral condylar and trochlear geometries. Extension of the trochlear groove concavity onto the inner portion of the femoral condyles has allowed for an increase of patellofemoral congruency in flexion. In addition, the round-on-round shape of the articulation permits patellar tilt to occur without excessive edge loading, a problem associated with modified dome-shaped and anatomic patellar devices. However, failure of cemented, all-polyethylene dome-shaped

patellar components is not uncommon; this has been attributed to the exposure of increase shear stresses in vivo, especially in malpositioned components.[22,98,137,331]

Modified Dome-Shaped Patella

In an attempt to increase the contact area in flexion, the standard dome patella was modified by adding a concave circumferential extension, allowing it to match the curve of the femoral condyles in the frontal plane more closely (Fig. 113-10). The modified dome-shaped patella, also known as Mexican or sombrero hat, improves the articulation with

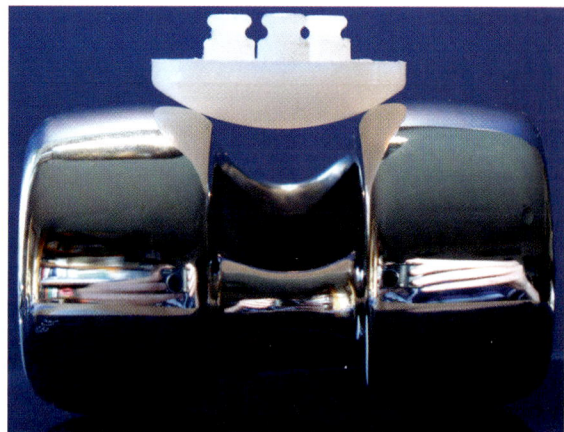

Figure 113-9. Point contact between dome-shaped patellar implant and relatively nonconforming femoral component at higher flexion.

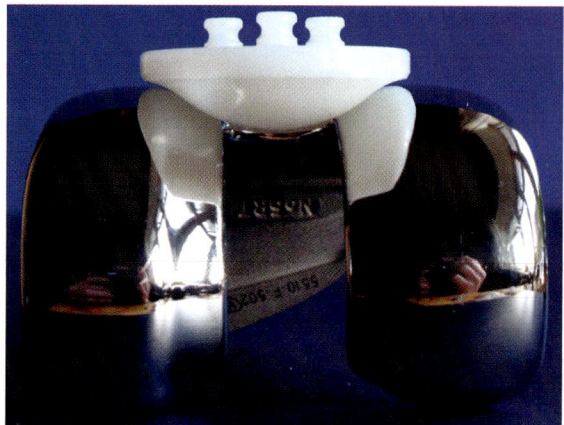

Figure 113-10. Modified dome-shaped (Mexican hat, sombrero type) patella. The trochlear groove shape is extended onto the femoral condyles to increase metal to plastic contact at higher flexion angles (Triathlon, Stryker).

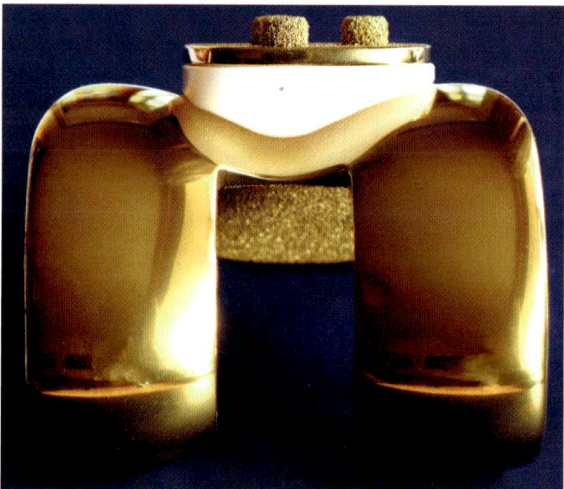

Figure 113-11. Anatomically shaped, rotating platform patellar component emulating the asymmetrical shape of the native patella. Both the patella and femoral condyle provide conforming surface configuration (Buechel-Pappas, Endotec, Orlando, Fla).

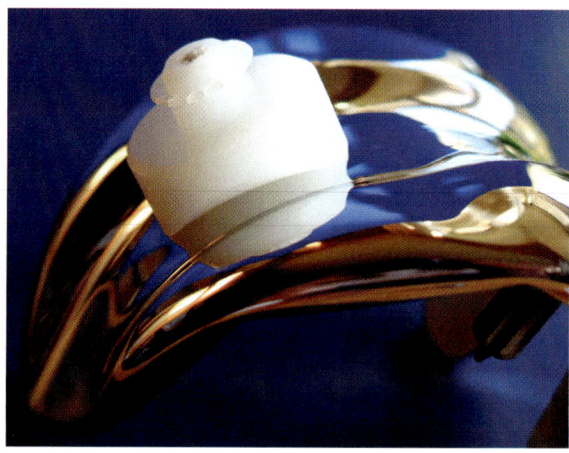

Figure 113-12. Cylindrical patellar component is a highly congruent design with close-matching patellofemoral geometry in both sagittal and coronal planes (Medial Rotation Knee, Finsbury, Leatherhead, England).

the convexities of the femoral condyles in the intercondylar notch beyond 90 degrees of flexion by increasing metal to plastic contact. Hsu and Walker[136] have compared the wear pattern of the all-polyethylene dome and modified dome-shaped patellar components in an experimental study. They found that increasing the conformity in the frontal plane increases the life of the component on a wear simulator by more than 20 times. The authors, however, raise concern that the amount of conformity that is acceptable must be considered in relation to patellar motion path, which is affected by rotation, tilt, and sideways shift.[247,309]

Anatomically Shaped Patella

Prostheses with an anatomic surface profile have lateral and medial facets and bear certain theoretical advantages. They maximize the contact area, thereby minimizing contact pressures, and create a more conforming articulation, thus decreasing the risk of subluxation.[43,44,141] A variety of anatomically shaped patella implants have been available over the years, including a mobile-bearing variant (Fig. 113-11;

see Fig. 113-8). Unfortunately, however, anatomically shaped patellar prostheses are more sensitive to malpositioning and hence more difficult to implant.[185] Thus, only a few anatomic patella implants remain commercially available, with most being discontinued in favor of more forgiving designs.

Cylindrical Patella

The cylindrical or saddle-shaped patellar component occupies a fringe position in TKA and is offered by only a few manufacturers (Fig. 113-12). The initial idea was developed by Freeman et al in the late 1970s[99,100]; they attempted to combine a high level of congruency and large contact area throughout the flexion range, with freedom of motion in the coronal plane but without compromising component stability. Because of the design specifics, the patella becomes highly dependent on a close-matching geometry of the femoral component in the sagittal plane, hence requiring a femoral trochlea of single radius.[167] The diameter of the patellar component is reduced to 25 to 30 mm, allowing the implant to be recessed into the patella, similar to the inlay technique (see later). Subsequently, the remaining patellar rim participates in articulating with the femoral component and further contributes to stress dissipation. The patellar implant possesses a central peg with a collar and can be used with or without cement. If left uncemented, the implant retains the ability to self-center and to rotate, as has been observed in revision situations for reasons unrelated to the patella.[14] Although fibrous ingrowth may eventually halt this process, the implant is likely to have adopted favorable alignment by this time.[308] Despite its relative rotational constraints, the design concept has provided patellofemoral survival rates of 96% to 98.4% at 10 years.[188] Concerns that preservation of cartilage at the patellar rim may negatively affect pain perception has so far not been confirmed.[188]

Mobile-Bearing Patella

A different biomechanical concept was conceived with the anatomically shaped, mobile-bearing, metal-backed patella[43,44] (see Fig. 113-11). The design rationale is based on the same principle as that of rotating platform tibial components. The clinical performance record of mobile-bearing patellae has been surprisingly good. Although not generally affected by complications otherwise associated with metal-backed prostheses, failures caused by fracture, wear, and dissociation of the polyethylene element have been described.[138] Reported survival rates of up to 99.5% at 12 years are attributed to the high conformity and low stresses permitted by the mobile-bearing articulation.[153] The absence of significant backside wear in mobile patellar bearings has led some clinicians to believe that these devices may not actually rotate in service. It has been speculated that the advantages of mobile-bearing patellae may be their ability to compensate for variations in surgical alignment by rotating into a preferential position after engagement with the femoral component, and simply to remain there.[200]

Metal-Backed Patellar Components

Metal backing became fashionable in the early 1980s. It has since largely been abandoned, with the exception of some uncemented fixed-bearing designs (e.g., Townley TKO System, Biopro, Port Huron, Minn; Foundation Knee, DJO Surgical, Austin, Tex; Natural Knee II, Zimmer, Warsaw, Ind) and rotating platform anatomic designs (e.g., LCS, DePuy Orthopaedics, Warsaw, Ind; AMC, Corin USA, Tampa, Fla; ROCC, Biomet, Warsaw, Ind; Buechel-Pappas, Endotec, Orlando, Fla). Adding a stiff metal layer to the back surface of the polyethylene patella was thought to improve load transfer and protect the fixation interface.[20,317] To accomplish the addition of metal backing to the patellar component without increasing its overall thickness, substantial reduction in polyethylene thickness is required.[21] These changes in implant design create an increase in contact stresses because of the rigidity of the metal substrate. Subsequently, polyethylene deformation through cold flow, fracture, and dissociation of the polyethylene layer from the metal backing have been observed in retrieved components[96,180,292] (see Fig. 113-7).

KINEMATICS AND BIOMECHANICS OF THE PATELLOFEMORAL JOINT IN TOTAL KNEE ARTHROPLASTY

The mechanical environment of the replaced PFJ differs from the natural knee. The contact area of the prosthetic PFJ measures, at best, no more than 40% of the contact area established for the native knee.[164,295,332] Measurements obtained experimentally vary widely and depend on the technical setup and level of compressive force applied during testing. For dome-shaped designs, contact areas range from 13 to 162 mm^2, with the highest values usually observed between 90 and 120 degrees of knee flexion.[207] Values for anatomic, cylindrical, and modified dome-shaped patellar components also vary but, because of the increased level of conformity, are generally higher when compared with their dome counterpart.[127,193,287]

One of the major challenges for the resurfaced patella is its resistance to wear, despite being biomechanically disadvantaged by having a small contact area through which high contact pressures are transferred. Patellar components are exposed to compressive and shear forces during knee flexion, increasing their risk of damage and failure, especially in patients of high demand and with increased postoperative flexion.[79,217] Up to 75 degrees of knee flexion, the contact area between the prosthetic patella and femur is relatively large and contact pressures generally low. Beyond this point, bifurcation of patellofemoral contact creates two distinctly separated contact areas on the medial and lateral extremities of the articulating surface of the patella, straddling the intercondylar notch[131] (Fig. 113-13). The transition from

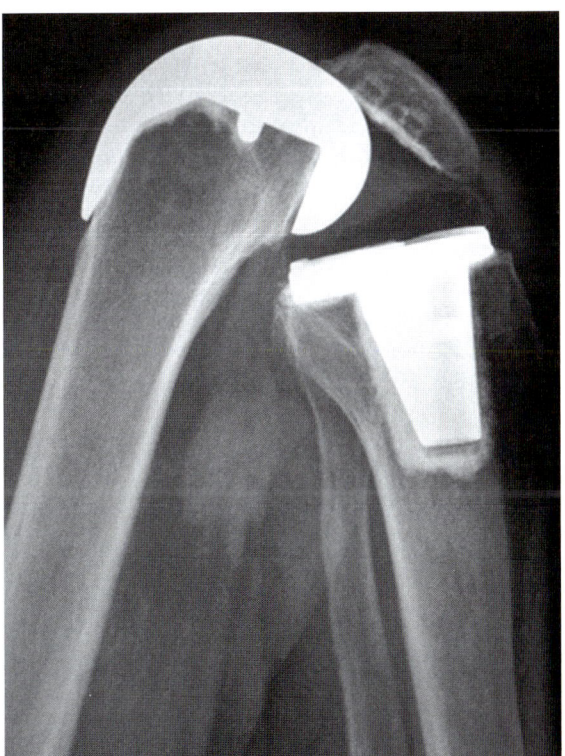

Figure 113-13. Lateral roentgenogram showing TKA in vivo in full flexion. The patella has left the trochlear groove and is resting against the inner portion of the femoral condyles, leading to bifurcation of the patellofemoral contact area.

a one-point to a two-point contact is associated with an overall decrease in contact area, whereas patellofemoral compressive forces and contact pressure increase almost exponentially. The direct influence of this transition in contact area on the wear pattern can be observed in retrieved patellar components, which often demonstrate deformation and development of characteristic facets at the margin of the polyethylene patellar surface.[136,198,200] Such changes may be described as a wearing-in phenomenon, as it demonstrates the ability of the patellar component to accommodate non-conformity by creeping in ways to reduce contact stresses (see Fig. 113-15).

We know that in level walking, the PFJ is exposed to compressive forces of up to $1.2 \times BW$, whereas activities such as descending stairs and rising from a chair may create forces up to $5.7 \times BW$.[38,162] The intensity of these stresses is directly influenced by the contact stress at the surface of the bearing, which is in part largely a function of implant design and surface conformity. During level walking, an activity most frequent for most patients, lower patellofemoral forces and more central contact areas indicate that failure of the patellar component is unlikely to occur. In contrast, the higher ranges of flexion seen when ascending and descending stairs and rising from a chair accompanied by high patellofemoral forces, and therefore are more likely to lead to patellar component wear and subsequent failure[8] (see Figs. 113-5 and 113-13).

Matsuda and coworkers[193] have assessed patellofemoral contact stress and contact area in TKA by comparing the native knee with a dome-shaped nonconforming patella, anatomically conforming patella, and unresurfaced patella. Values for patellofemoral peak contact stress and contact area remained almost at the level of the native knee if the patella was left unresurfaced. Following patellar resurfacing, patellofemoral contact stress rose beyond yield strength for ultra–high-molecular-weight polyethylene (UHMWPE), with an average increase of 200%, whereas the patellofemoral contact area decreased on average by 60%. There was no statistically significant difference between conforming and nonconforming patellar components; thus, neither design assumed superiority. It was concluded that although the effect of metal action on cartilage was uncertain, the option of leaving the patella without a prosthetic component remains an attractive one, especially if the patella is well preserved. In a similar study, McLain and Bargar[198] reported a threefold rise in anterior patellar strain at knee flexion angles beyond 30 degrees in TKAs with dome-shaped patellar components when compared with the native knee.

Stiehl and associates[290] have assessed patellar kinematic pattern and demonstrated that patellar axis rotation, which compares the angle between the patellar tendon and sagittal axis of the patella, increases with flexion in TKAs beyond the levels observed in normal knees. The contact position between the dome-shaped and anatomically shaped patellar components showed greater variability compared with the normal knee, with the average contact position for the resurfaced patella lying more superior and tilt angles being significantly increased. The kinematic behavior of an anatomically shaped or unresurfaced patella more closely resembled the native knee, compared to that observed with dome shaped patellar designs.

The effects of the three-dimensional movement path on domed, modified domed, anatomic, and rotating patellar designs were investigated by Kim and associates[163] in a cadaver model. They exposed specimens to mediolateral tilt, shift, and rotation and measured changes in contact area. Under optimal tracking conditions, contact areas of the dome-shaped patella were significantly smaller compared with the modified dome and anatomic designs. When exposed to three-dimensional movements, however, the contact areas of the dome-shaped patella were significantly greater, indicating enhanced forgiveness regarding patellar malpositioning, whereas modified dome-shaped and anatomic components appeared more sensitive to patellar malalignment (Fig. 113-14).

The level of conformity between femoral and patellar components influences the joint's ability to tolerate natural variations in motion, potentially limiting the patella's ability to follow its natural movement path.[247,289,290,309] If such motion is insufficient, shear forces will arise. Toleration of these variations in motion hence requires a level of nonconformity in order to establish "equilibrium of forces." High conformity within the patellofemoral articulation clearly limits flexibility in terms of component positioning. Malalignment is known to impart additional shear forces on the patella and its fixation site increasing the risk of subsequent

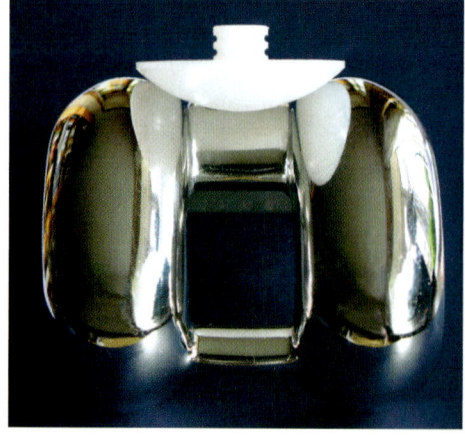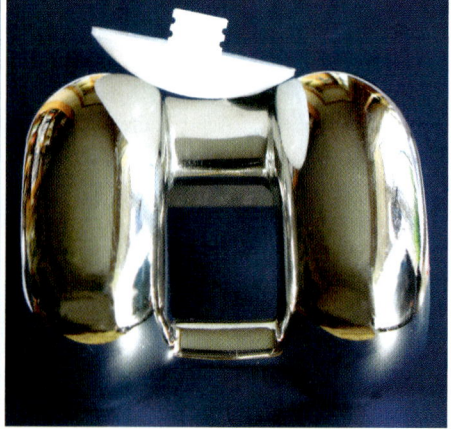

Figure 113-14. Dome-shaped patellar designs can compensate for a limited degree of patellar tilt and rotation by maintaining acceptable contact congruency (Insall-Burstein II, Zimmer, Warsaw, Ind).

component failure. This has been shown by MacCollum and Karpman,[185] who reported complications in 18 of 75 fixed-bearing anatomic patellar components, which included subluxation in 10, fracture in 5, tendon rupture in 2, and implant loosening in 1.[300,306]

Potential advantages of low contact stresses in conforming designs may be offset by an increase in constraint, resulting in deleterious effects on patellar wear and fixation. This typically leads to a compromise in which the conformity and therefore contact area are reduced to avoid overconstraining the joint. However, the question of how much contact area to sacrifice and how to best achieve that compromise remains unanswered. As a general trend, most clinicians shy away from anatomic patella implants and, for ease of application, prefer the more forgiving dome-shaped designs.[235,252]

Material Science of Ultra–High-Molecular-Weight Polyethylene in Patellar Implants

Because of the great disparity between moduli and strength of cobalt-chrome alloys on one hand and UHMWPE on the other, wear is primarily observed on the polymeric side of the prosthetic patellofemoral articulation (Fig. 113-15; see Fig. 113-7). Notwithstanding its limitations, UHMWPE has evolved as the material of choice for the patellar component, based on the low-friction principle of Charnley. Mechanical properties of UHMWPE are far from being ideal, with yield strength being affected by the level of molecular weight, degree of cross linking, and sterilization method. Uniaxial yield strength of UHMWPE, which equals the lowest stress at which the material undergoes plastic deformation, is estimated at 21 to 23 MPa (1 MPa = 1 N/mm²), according to manufacturer's guidelines.[21,59,248,284] Some manufacturers have expressed concern if such stresses are applied on a regular basis. For machinery applications, repeated maximum contact stresses of no more than 10 MPa have now been recommended, a value identical to the yield strength estimated for

articular cartilage.[245] These values are based on room temperature, whereas the strength of UHMWP may be reduced by up to 25% at body temperature; therefore, values of 5 MPa may be more appropriate for use in vivo.[43]

In vitro contact stress analysis has confirmed that all-polyethylene dome-shaped patellar components produce contact pressures from 20 to 30 MPa in extension, increasing to 36 to 100 MPa at 90 to 120 degrees of knee flexion, therefore exceeding the yield strength of UHMWPE by up to 400%.[145,164,200,332] Anatomically shaped rotating platform patellar components produced significantly lower values, mostly remaining below the yield strength of UHMWP.[59] Wear simulator studies have further confirmed that congruent patellar components (modified dome-shaped and anatomic) exhibit significantly lower rates of creep and wear than dome-shaped designs, again indicating that conformity is critical to wear resistance and protection against post–yield deformation[134,136] (see Fig. 113-15).

Viscoelastic properties of surface cartilage allow for its deformation under load and subsequent increase in pressure-transmitting area. Because of differences in elastic modulus between cartilage and UHMWPE, the prosthetic patella, however, has limited ability to change its surface contact area through variations in patellofemoral load.[26,131,136,200] Xu and associates[332] were able to demonstrate the effect of patella resurfacing on contact area and pressure in cadaveric knees. The mean contact area between 30 and 120 degrees of flexion in the nonresurfaced PFJ ranged from 70 to 150 mm², whereas peak patellar contact pressures did not exceed 12 MPa. Once resurfaced, the mean contact area decreased almost 10-fold to 10 to 15 mm², creating a dramatic increase in patellar contact pressure values of 50 to 100 MPa. Steubben and associates[287] have carried out biomechanical studies assessing patellar surface contact area, compressive forces, and contact pressure using different prosthetic models.[54,207] They found that patellofemoral contact pressure values at knee flexion angles beyond 45 degrees exceeded polyethylene yield strength in all tested components, with peak measurements of up to 75 N/mm² (75 MPa). Results were not a true function of contact area and contact pressure, signaling the importance of design features in the dissipation of contact forces across the PFJ.

Greenwald and colleagues have measured the distribution of patellofemoral surface stresses by mapping areas above and below the tensile yield strength of polyethylene.[116,287] All implants—whether dome-shaped, modified dome-shaped, or anatomic—demonstrated material yielding over their range of flexion. The results indicated the importance of appreciating the location of the yield areas within a given patellar component, because rim-loaded contact areas above yield are more likely to deform and wear. It may thus be conceivable that polymer integrity is not determined primarily on the size of the contact area, but rather on the extent of the surface within this region, which exceeds yield conditions.

Subsequently, contact stresses above the yield strength do not necessarily lead to catastrophic failure, as demonstrated by the large number of relatively undamaged retrievals. As highest values of contact stress are experienced during flexion, variations in a patient's activity may not expose the patellar component to large cyclic loads frequently enough to accumulate damage. McNamara and coworkers[200] have considered the constraining effect of the surrounding polyethylene as

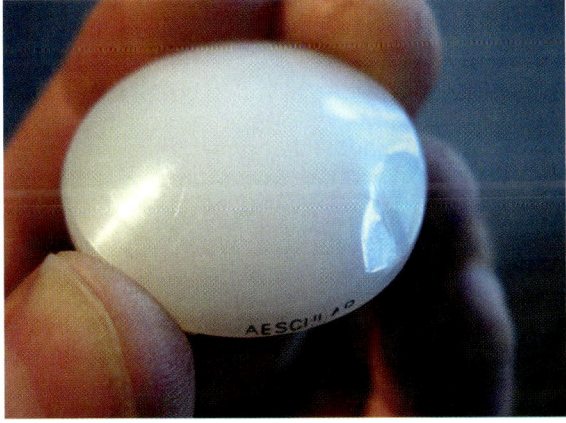

Figure 113-15. Focal area of polyethylene deformation in retrieved patellar component. This is created through point contact of the patellar component with femoral condyles at higher knee flexion angles. It is often seen as part of a wearing-in process in partially congruent patellofemoral articulations. (Courtesy Professor Wolfgang Plitz, Laboratory of Biomechanics, Ludwig-Maximilian University, Munich, Germany.)

responsible for this phenomenon. Yield in polyethylene is characterized by plastic deformation rather than brittle failure, which explains why nonconforming patellar components are capable of wearing in.[26] Such surface adaptation has been demonstrated to produce characteristic facets at the margin of the patellar component, increasing the contact area particularly in flexion when there is least congruency between the patella and condyles[136] (see Figs. 113-9 and 113-15). Although reduction in contact stresses of 23% to 58% through increased conformity have been reported, contact stress values remain above the UHMWP yield strength.[59,127] Elbert and associates[79] were surprised that despite reduction in overall component thickness, stress values did not increase. In their opinion, changes in geometry and contact area dominate the response of the deformed component, overriding the effect on the stresses of the decreased thickness. Analysis of Von Mises stress, a yielding criterion based on a combination of principle stresses occurring within the material, has revealed that most stresses above yield strength occur 1 to 2 mm below the articulating surface area in the newly manufactured component; however, in retrieved components, Von Mises stress remains near yielding through the depth of the implant.[207,328] Because of subsurface stresses, permanent deformation may be expected to continue, even when the component has worn in. Collier and associates[59] have noted that all-polyethylene patellar components do not solve this problem because of distinct biomedical and biomechanical disadvantages of UHMWPE as a bearing surface. In the absence of a suitable alternative however, UHMWPE is here to stay, at least for the foreseeable future.

Femoral Component Design

The patella, whether native or prosthetic, cannot be considered separately because it works in direct partnership with the femoral component. Contact areas are highly dependent on the congruency of the PFJ articulation at all angles of knee flexion, whereas motion constraints of the patella are terminated by the surface geometry of the femoral component and by the balance of soft tissue forces. Bartel and associates[20] have demonstrated the importance of conformity in prosthetic design to increase contact area and decrease contact stress. Current femoral prostheses display a wide variation in design features in regard to length, depth and orientation of the trochlear groove, sagittal radius, and axial geometry.[75,297,334] Anatomically shaped femoral components appear to be particularly suitable if articulating against the nonresurfaced patella, which will be referred to as patella-friendly from this point on[161,296] (Fig. 113-16). They provide for increased conformity between the native patella and femur and demand minimal biologic patellar remodeling.[43,161,325] Nonanatomic designs are those in which the trochlear groove is concave spherical and designed to accommodate a nonanatomic patella, usually of dome-shaped design. Proximal extension of the femoral flange will help capture the patella during early flexion, whereas extension of the concave shape of the trochlear groove onto the inner aspects of the femoral condyles will allow for increased metal to plastic contact at higher flexion angles (see Figs. 113-10 and 113-14).[54,56,227,264,297]

The effect of valgus alignment of the trochlear groove compared with symmetrical designs on shear stresses has been

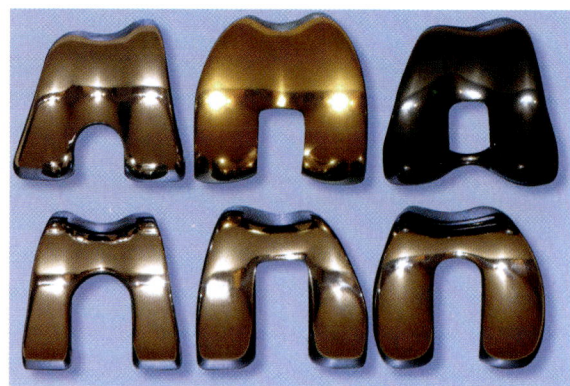

Figure 113-16. Various levels of 'patella-friendly' design features in six different femoral components. Relatively patella-friendly designs *(top row)* with asymmetrical, anatomic femoral groove, elevated lateral trochlear flange, and distal extension of trochlear groove (modified Ortholoc, Wright Medical, Arlington, Tenn; Buechel-Pappas, Endotec; Journey PS, Smith & Nephew, Memphis, Tenn). Relatively patella-unfriendly designs *(bottom row)* with symmetrical, shallow, and short trochlear groove *(left to right:* Ortholoc, Dow Corning Wright; AGC, Biomet, Warsaw, Ind; Townley TKO, Biopro, Port Huron, Mich). (Ortholoc femoral components courtesy Leo Whiteside, Missouri Bone & Joint Research Foundation, St Louis.)

investigated with mixed results. Asymmetrical trochlear groove designs are thought to provide earlier patellar capture through prominence of the lateral flange and to decrease the predominant valgus force vector, thus reducing patella shear.[75] In some reports, reduction in lateral shear forces of up to 10% were observed, whereas others saw no effect or even a shift toward the generation of medial shear forces.[56,227,297] The exact clinical advantages of asymmetrical designs have remained largely theoretical, with no compelling clinical proof of their effectiveness.[318]

The importance of femoral component design and its influence on patellofemoral performance have been highlighted by Theiss and associates[297] based on the clinical results of two arthroplasty designs with distinct differences in trochlear geometry. A 14-fold decrease in patella-related complications was observed when using a patella-friendly design with an extended anterior flange and a deeper and wider trochlear groove. It was concluded that the more proximal capture of the patella in a deeper groove, with more gradual proximal to distal transition, appears advantageous in reducing patella morbidity. Yoshii and associates[334] used an experimental model and demonstrated that specific femoral design changes, including deepening and distal extension of the trochlear groove, improve patella tracking compared with an unmodified femoral component.

Lateral forces acting at the patellofemoral articulation increase with knee flexion[14] (see Fig. 113-4). The magnitude of the lateral forces, which are dependent on valgus alignment, Q angle, and soft tissue balance may, if excessive, cause patellar subluxation and contribute to component failure. Steubben and associates[287] have investigated the resistance offered to lateral subluxation of the resurfaced patella by defining the intrinsic lateral stability of various patellofemoral designs. They found that the forces required to cause lateral displacement were at or above those measured for the native knee, and highly dependent on the interaction

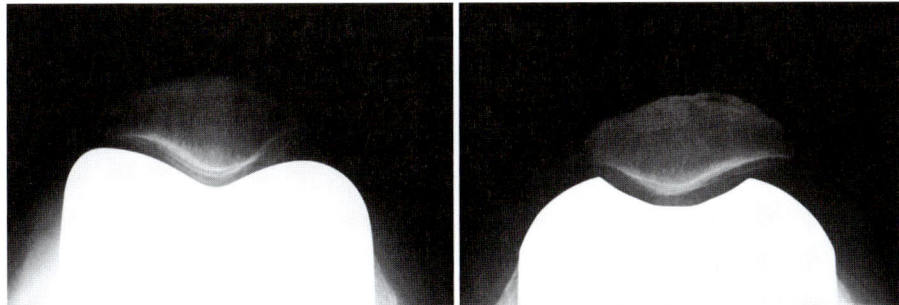

Figure 113-17. Skyline radiographs showing an anatomically shaped "patella-friendly" femoral component design (*left,* LCS [DePuy Orthopaedics, Warsaw, Ind]) compared with a nonanatomic design (*right,* Optetrak [Exactech, Gainsville, Fla]).

of condylar and patellar surface geometry. Their results highlighted that appropriate design changes can significantly increase resistance to patellar subluxation.

Unresurfaced Patella

Following bicompartmental knee arthroplasty, the nonresurfaced patella becomes exposed to the metallic surface of the femoral component. Because of differences in the modulus of elasticity, the articular surface of the patella must adapt to the geometry of the opposing surface by bedding in.[161] This process of remodeling, which has been termed *stress contouring,* produces a gradual adaptation of the retropatellar surface and subchondral bone plate to the trochlear shape.[280] Keblish and associates[161] have noted that minimal remodeling is required if the patella is exposed to an anatomic design with a constant radius of curvature and uniform femoral geometry, whereas excessive remodeling is observed in nonanatomic designs (Fig. 113-17). The remodeling process is time-dependent and not seen on axial radiographs much before 2 years after implantation.

Tanzer and associates[296] have studied the effect of femoral component designs on the contact and tracking characteristics of the unresurfaced patella in TKA. They noted substantial alterations in patellofemoral contact areas, contact pressures, and tracking at higher flexion angles when the native patella was articulating with a prosthetic femoral component. Although the percentage of patellofemoral contact area compared with the native knee is markedly reduced with increasing knee flexion, with measured values of 79% at 60 degrees, 69% at 90 degrees, and 65% at 105 degrees, it remains well above those measured for the prosthetic patella.

The surface geometries of some prosthetic femoral components, particularly those of posterior-stabilized design, appear incompatible with the native patella, because the apex of the retropatellar ridge may impinge on the prosthetic intercondylar notch beyond 90 degrees of knee flexion. Patellar deformation and wear are likely consequences and, in the case of significant patellar tilt, displacement of the patella into the notch becomes possible.[198] Distal extension of the trochlea and shortening of the intercondylar notch have been shown to safeguard patellar support beyond 90 degrees of knee flexion.[334] Such design modifications are therefore important if one considers leaving the patella unresurfaced. Most current femoral components present a surface geometry designed to articulate with a designated patellar component but are ill equipped to accommodate the native patella. Specific efforts

are required to improve patellar kinematics by creating a femoral component that conforms to the normal trochlear and intercondylar notch topography, and that takes the geometry of the native patella into account.[325] Only then would we be in a position to offer prostheses dedicated to be used with the native patella, compared with the mostly inadequate femoral designs currently available.

Effect of Cruciate Retention or Substitution

Moment arms affecting the patellar are dependent on the distance between the PFJ and the axis of flexion and extension of the femoral component. They are increased if the axis is deviated posteriorly from its physiologic position. Femoral rollback facilitates this process and represents a characteristic feature of normal knee kinematics. Increased rollback effectively lengthens the patellar moment arm thus increasing the efficacy of the extensor mechanism. D'Lima and associates[75] have investigated the influence of various degrees of posterior femoral rollback on patellofemoral compressive forces. Femoral rollback resulting from PCL preservation produced reductions in patellofemoral compressive forces of up to 7% throughout knee flexion, whereas the effect in PCL-substituting devices only became noticeable after cam-post engagement, with a maximum effect recorded at 85 degrees of knee flexion. Miller and colleagues,[205] in an earlier study comparing PCL-retaining with PCL-substituting arthroplasties, failed to note femoral rollback when the PCL was retained. They stipulated that the absence of the anterior cruciate ligament may render the PCL ineffective, which may explain the appearance of paradoxical movements (reverse rollback)[75] observed on fluoroscopic investigation.[68-70] Although PCL substitution kept patellofemoral forces close to the level of the native knee, a lateral release became necessary in 50% of knees, raising potential concerns about an increase in patellofemoral stress through ligamentous tension. This concept has also been expressed by Ranawat and Sculco[233,235] who raised concern that femoral rollback, through a cam and post mechanism, as in posterior-stabilizing designs, or through a functional posterior cruciate ligament (PCL), may increase tensile forces across the patella in flexion. Overstuffing will tighten the extensor mechanism, and increase anterior patellar strain and PRF, with the likely consequences of loss of flexion, patellar implant failure, and fracture.[78,204,235,303] Overall patellar thickness following resurfacing should therefore not exceed preoperative values. With regard to clinical outcomes, Waters and Bentley[320] have assessed the occurrence of postoperative anterior knee pain in 327 cruciate-substituting and 147 cruciate-retaining TKAs, but found no significant difference.

PATELLECTOMY AND ALTERNATIVES

In the first half of the 20th century excision of the patella was heralded by most surgeons as the treatment of choice for debilitating and intractable anterior knee pain, patellar dislocation, and fracture.[41,322] Most cases were usually affected by rheumatoid or osteoarthritis but removal of this "somewhat mysterious bone," as described by Bruce and Walsmley in 1942,[42] was also used for various other disabilities because of the apparent innocuous nature of the procedure. Some surgeons even went as far as removing the patella as part of a suitable alternative to displacement of the patella in arthrotomy of the knee; it is fair to say that especially those cases not affected by fracture or degenerative disease of the patella often ended up being worse.[186] The general consensus on the appropriateness of patellectomy was so deeply entrenched in the surgical ranks that it prevented Bruce and Walmsley from completing their study on the subject. Both authors recognized the unjust globalized approach to patellectomy and its widespread abuse when they concluded their investigations by saying that "The whole question requires further study, however, and the outbreak of hostilities prevented this part of the investigation being pursued to a definite conclusion."[42] This conclusion, however was soon to come, in part through new scientific evidence but more so through discouraging clinical results disclosed in long-term follow-up studies.[71,151]

Anterior knee pain was a design-related complication common with early hinge arthroplasties. However, rather than addressing the problem by improving the design, the initial response was to promote patellectomy as part of the arthroplasty procedure.[273,335] Insall and associates[150] reported on four different prosthetic models used in the early 1970s, none of which made any provision to accommodate the patella. Out of 178 patients, 35 received a patellectomy at the time of arthroplasty and complaints of pain after patellectomy were as frequent from those patients as from patients in whom patellectomy was not performed.

Apart from failing to alleviate anterior knee pain reliably, removal of the patella creates added biomechanical disadvantages by decreasing the lever arm and extensor torque of the quadriceps mechanism, leaving most patients with measurable weakness.[2,71,157,175,293] Haxton[128] demonstrated that this decrease in lever arm is particularly noticeable in the more extended knee positions, when the patella would normally move out of the intercondylar fossa onto the femoral trochlea. Although patellectomy improves the efficiency of the extensor mechanism at higher flexion angles, in the daily flexion range, between 0 and 90 degrees, extensor power is greatly reduced.[101,122] Increases in TRF and subsequent joint degeneration have also been reported following patellectomy.[102] The surgeon contemplating patellectomy must thus be aware that the biomechanical effect of the loss of the fulcrum is the increased strength requirements of the quadriceps to provide extensor stability. Seriously disabled patients may not be able to develop sufficient quadriceps strength to provide this necessary extensor force.[6]

Today, patellectomy in knee arthroplasty patients has largely been abandoned as a routine measure and remains reserved for the treatment of severe comminuted fractures, advanced osteonecrosis, and tumors.[2,238,240] In the treatment of comminuted fractures, total patellectomy is reserved for patients with loose patellar implants who present significant extensor lag and for whom reconstruction is unattainable.[115] The general consensus has been to preserve the patella, even in revision situations in which severe bone loss may compromise its integrity. In situations in which less than 10 mm of bone remains, preservation of the patellar remnant avoids the need for reconstitution of the extensor mechanism and retains some of its residual lever arm.[83]

If patellectomy is performed, the technique of Compere has proven popular, with longitudinal shelling out of bone fragments and formation of a tube by suturing the medial and lateral edges of the rectus tendon together.[61] Alternative measures are the use of biconvex, all-polyethylene patellar components, trabecular metal inlays, or bone grafting of the patellar defect.[125,213,240] The biconvex patella requires at least 10 mm of bone stock and a 70% circumferential rim of bone equal to the thickness of the peripheral edge to provide for adequate cement fixation. Trabecular metal components allow for cementless fixation because of their osteoconductive properties. Medium-term results, despite a reported incidence of fracture through the patella remnant in up to 15% of cases, are promising. Trabecular metal facilitates excellent bonding to the patellar shell, even with less than 10 mm of bone remaining but, as with cancellous bone grafting, sufficient peripatellar blood supply is required to promote bone ingrowth.[211] However, inferior results are to be expected if most of the fixation surface is composed of soft tissue and if the blood supply to the patella is substantially compromised.[250]

SURGICAL TECHNIQUE

The patella functions in a complex arrangement between the extensor mechanism and tibiofemoral articulation. Its performance as a fulcrum of the quadriceps apparatus is not only influenced by implant design, but also depends on the positional relationship between patellar, femoral, and tibial components and on overall leg alignment. Surgical decisions may compensate for implant design limitations but conversely may also exacerbate them. Unless all these factors work in unison, satisfactory patellar tracking cannot be achieved. Proper patellofemoral function is ultimately dependent on good and reproducible surgical technique and an understanding of the principles of biomechanics of the PFJ in TKA. Re-creation of physiologic leg alignment, Q angle, and joint line, appropriate component rotation, and balancing of the extensor mechanism are the key ingredients of successful surgery.

The Q angle, however, remains the most significant factor influencing patellar tracking. Any increase of the Q angle beyond normal limits will lateralize patellar tracking and could lead to patellar subluxation. Maltracking of the patella is often the manifestation of a technical error or a combination of minor errors and, according to Pagnano and Kelly,[219] should be considered a red flag. Proceeding directly with a lateral retinacular release may improve patellar tracking but should only be considered once the surgeon is satisfied that there are no errors in rotational, translational, or angular alignment of the arthroplasty components.

Femoral Positioning

The patella is particularly sensitive to malrotation of the prosthetic implants of the femur and tibia.[10,107] It is generally accepted that placing the femoral component in approximately 3 to 5 degrees of external rotation, relative to the posterior condylar axis, improves patellar tracking and proximal engagement.[212] External rotation moves the trochlear groove toward the natural position of the patella, thereby relaxing the lateral retinacular structures and reducing the lateral force vector acting on the patella. Second, it also corrects any mismatch in the flexion-extension gap created through cutting the proximal tibia perpendicularly to its long axis, rather than emulating its natural varus alignment. This can be achieved through the relative thickness of bone removed from the posterior femoral condyles, but care must be taken to establish a rectangular flexion gap; otherwise, knee stability in flexion may be compromised. Any instrumentation for distal femoral preparation that references femoral component rotation on the posterior condyles would, if left unadjusted, place the femur in internal rotation relative to the transepicondylar axis. Posterior condylar referencing therefore requires the surgeon to dial in a degree of external rotation to achieve parallel cuts to the transepicondylar axis (TEA), which has created what is referred to as external femoral rotation. Whiteside and coworkers[211] have found the patellar tracking pattern and contact areas to be most normal when the femoral implant is externally rotated by approximately 5 degrees in relation to the PCA.[10] External rotation angles beyond 5 degrees, however, appear to have a detrimental effect on the spatial position of the patella in the trochlea.[13] Because of the variability in the relationship between the posterior condylar axis (PCA) and TEA, this technique carries certain dangers. Although the main difference between the two axes is 3 degrees of internal rotation, the range is 0 to 10 degrees, with higher values for valgus knees.[219] The risk of femoral malrotation is thus higher in the valgus knee, especially if a somewhat hypoplastic posterior lateral femoral condyle has been used as a reference for rotational alignment when making anteroposterior cuts. The situation is usually compounded because the internally rotated femur necessitates subsequent internal rotation of the tibial component to establish rotational tibiofemoral congruency, thus creating excessive external rotation of the tibial tuberosity and patellar maltracking.

Because the TEA represents the functional flexion-extension axis of the knee, it has been established as the ideal reference point for femoral component orientation.[24,144,230] Studies have confirmed improved patellar kinematics and a significant reduction of patellofemoral shear forces when the femoral component is placed parallel to the TEA as compared with internal or external rotation.[75,205]

As an alternative reference to the TEA, the anteroposterior axis, or Whiteside's line (WL), drawn from the base of the trochlear groove to the center of the intercondylar notch, may be used to establish femoral rotational alignment.[12] Current technique encourages clinicians to use TEA and WL to place the femoral component in neutral rotation with respect to those landmarks (Fig. 113-18).

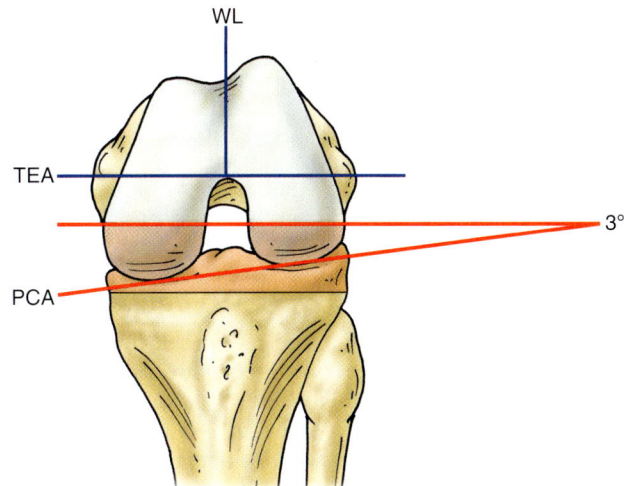

Figure 113-18. The TEA and the anteroposterior axis (WL), are used as reference guides for femoral component rotation and have shown to be more reliable than the PCA. (Adapted from Krackow KA: The technique of total knee arthroplasty. St Louis, 1990, Mosby.)

Alignment of the femoral component in the sagittal plane also requires attention. Placing the femoral component in flexion creates liftoff of the anterior flange and patellar impingement with the proximal lip of the trochlear groove at lower knee flexion angles. Patellar component wear, loosening, subluxation, and catastrophic failure may be the consequence. Excessive extension of the femoral implant will displace the extensor mechanism anteriorly, increasing retinacular tension and patellofemoral compressive force. The result is a potential decrease in range of motion and an increased risk of patellar fracture.

In the frontal plane, mediolateral positioning of the femoral component will influence patellar kinematics. Rhoads and associates[247] have found that laterally translated femoral implants demonstrate improved patellar tracking compared with those placed centrally or medially onto the distal femur. The ideal position can be achieved by placing the center of the femoral component immediately lateral to the midline of the intercondylar notch. Excessive lateral translation must be avoided, because it enhances the risk of implant overhang and impingement with the lateral retinaculum, PCL, and popliteus tendon.

Tibial Positioning

Rotational alignment of the tibial component is equally critical in preventing patellar maltracking and instability.[209] The center of the anterior portion of the tibial baseplate should be aligned with the tibial crest, which is equivalent to the medial third of the tibial tubercle. This will create relative external rotation and lateral translation of the tibial component, improving extensor mechanism stability by internally rotating the tibial tubercle and decreasing the Q angle. Appropriate rotation can be determined by using a stemless tibial trial component, which will adopt optimal rotational positioning once the knee has been put through a full range of motion. Tibiofemoral compression is to be avoided during this maneuver because it inhibits free rotation of the tibial baseplate. The clinician must be aware that if dynamic positioning suggests excessive internal or external rotation, reassessment of femoral component orientation is required (Fig. 113-19).

Internal rotation of the tibial component has been implicated as the leading cause of patellar instability and may occur as a result of inadequate exposure of the lateral tibial plateau, particularly if the knee is approached through a minimally invasive medial incision.[25] Barrack and associates[19] found that in patients suffering anterior knee pain after TKA, the tibial component was on average in 6.2 degrees of internal rotation, compared with 0.4 degrees in the control group. Berger and associates[25] assessed 30 knee arthroplasties affected by patellar tracking abnormalities by relating the level of lateralized patellar tracking to the degree of combined internal rotation of the femoral and tibial components. Combined internal rotation of 1 to 4 degrees resulted in lateralized patellar tracking and tilt, 3 to 8 degrees in patellar subluxation, and 7 to 17 degrees in frank patellar dislocation.

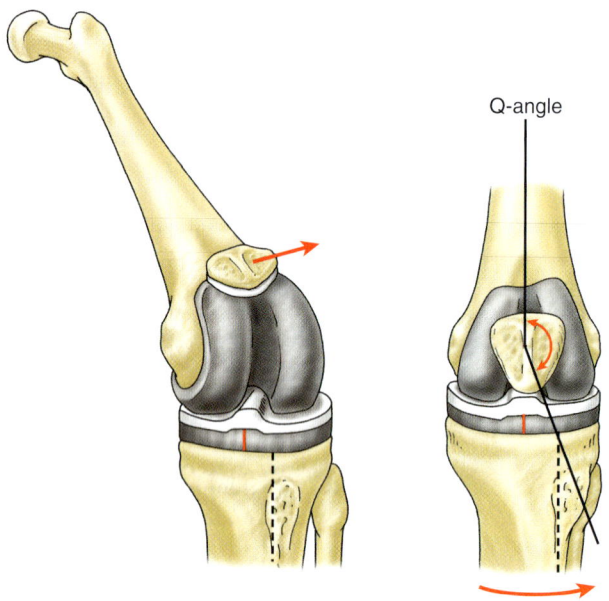

Figure 113-19. Internal rotation of the tibial component will increase the Q angle and may lead to patellar maltracking and instability. (Adapted from Rand JA [ed]: Total knee arthroplasty, New York, 1993, Raven Press.)

The degree of conformity of the articulating surfaces between the tibial and femoral components may determine the rotational position of the tibia. This is particularly evident in fully conforming prostheses in which condylar geometry drives kinematic function, forcing the tibia to rotate in unison with the femoral component during the terminal degrees of extension. However, if the articular surfaces are nonconforming, the tibial rotational position is far less dependent on component position and instead is guided by ligament tension.[324] It is therefore not surprising that Nagamine and associates[209] were able to show that up to 15 degrees of malrotation of an unconstrained tibial tray did not affect patella tracking compared with a semiconstrained implant. The potential benefits on the PFJ, however, may be outweighed by detrimental tibiofemoral kinematics displayed in fluoroscopic investigations of flat-on-flat condylar arthroplasty designs.[288] Some controversy surrounds the potential benefits of mobile-bearing total knee designs on the patellofemoral mechanism. Some clinical studies were able to show a decrease in the rate of lateral retinacular release, improvements in patellar tracking, and reduction in patellofemoral contact stresses thought to be caused by the implant's self-aligning properties.[49,259] Others, however, have failed to confirm such clinical advantages over their fixed-bearing counterparts.[221]

If positional abnormalities of any of the prosthetic components are suspected, radiographs will most likely suffice to assess abnormalities in the frontal or sagittal plane. However, rotational malalignment is best determined by computed tomography (CT)[25,307] (Fig. 113-20).

Axial Leg Alignment

The key is to reestablish physiologic leg alignment, which varies between 5 and 7 degrees of anatomic valgus.[303] Any increase in valgus angle beyond 7 degrees will increase the Q angle and therefore contribute to patellar maltracking. Long-term follow-up studies have shown that prosthetic survival is not compromised if leg alignment is restored within 2.4 to 7.2 degrees of anatomic valgus.[88] There is a higher probability to place the femoral component in excessive valgus if the knee is affected by preoperative valgus malalignment, especially if the lateral femoral condyle is deficient.[219] Even if compensated for by a tibial component placed into varus, this is still likely to create abnormal patellofemoral kinematics.

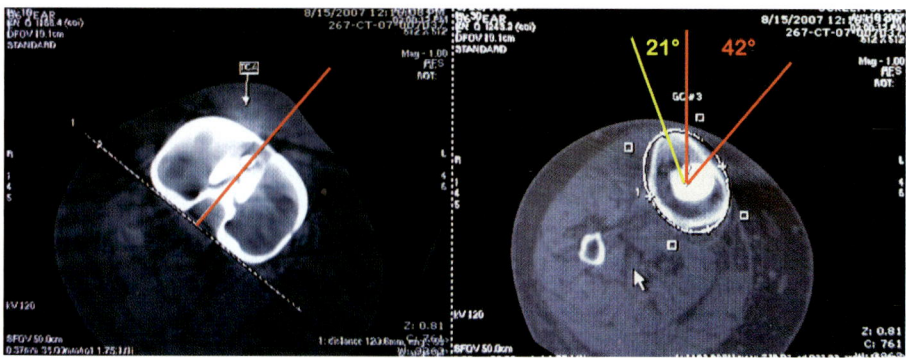

Figure 113-20. Axial CT sequence showing the tibial component placed in 63 degrees of internal rotation from the center of the tibial tuberosity and in 42 degrees from its ideal position at the medial third of the tubercle.

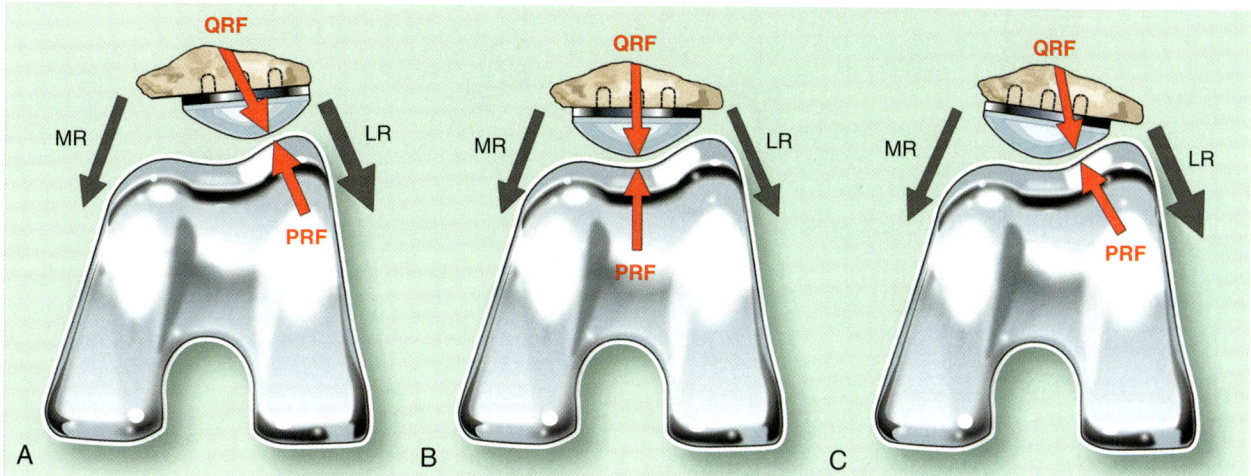

Figure 113-21. A, Lateral positioning of the patellar implant will tighten the lateral retinacular structures and may provoke lateral sub-luxation. **B,** Moderate medialization will re-create the asymmetrical contours of the native retro-patellar high point, centralize quadriceps tendon and patellar reaction force and improve patellar tracking. **C,** Overzealous medial positioning of the patellar implant may create lateral patellar tilt through off centre positioning of the quadriceps tendon force.

Patellar Preparation and Component Alignment

The normal patella has an asymmetrical shape with the prominent articular ridge, which separates medial and lateral facets, located toward its medial aspect. The patellar bone should be resected parallel to its anterior surface to create a uniformly thick remnant, which usually requires removal of considerably more bone from the medial aspect of the patella. Proper patellar exposure and appropriate removal of surrounding soft tissues will allow for better visualization and judgment of the cutting level. Failure to appreciate the asymmetry of the patella may lead to the removal of equal amounts of bone from the medial and lateral facets, creating an oblique cutting surface. Such errors in preparation have been shown to increase the risk of patellar tilt and maltrack-ing.[67,184,239] In a series of 300 knee arthroplasties, Pagnano and Trousdale[220] found that 21 had the patella asymmetrically resurfaced. At a mean follow-up of 7.5 years, 11 (51%) of these cases were affected by patellofemoral complications requiring revision.

Placement of the patellar component in a more medial position relative to the center of the retropatellar surface is considered beneficial because it emulates the medialized posi-tion of the native retropatellar eminence (Fig. 113-21). Medialization of the patellar component by 2 mm reduces peak lateral shear force by 10 to 15 N, but a corresponding medial shear force was noted at knee flexion angles below 25 degrees.[75] Radiographic results of medialized insertion of patellar prosthesis have confirmed the effect on lateralization of the bony structure of the patella, which is thought to decrease lateral shear forces and decrease the likelihood of patellar subluxation.[334] In clinical series, the rate of lateral retinacular release was 13% to 17% when the patellar com-ponent was placed medially compared with 46% to 48% when placed centrally onto the retropatellar surface.[133,179] Anglin and associates[9] have measured the impact of various levels of patellar component medialization on patellar kine-matics and force distribution in a cadaver model. A signifi-cant reduction of patellofemoral contact force above

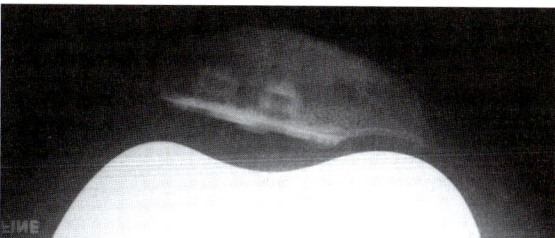

Figure 113-22. Lateral patellar facet impingement through failure to perform appropriate soft tissue balancing and lateral facetectomy.

60 degrees of knee flexion occurred with increasing medializa-tion of the patellar component. At the same time, however, the researchers noted that the more the patellar was medial-ized, the more it tended to tilt laterally relative to the femur. Biomechanically, the tendency to lateral tilt is thought to result from the mediolateral moment created when the exten-sor mechanism, positioned centrally on the patella and acting posteriorly, becomes off-center from the patellar implant after medialization. To take advantage of reduced contact force while containing the level of lateral patellar tilt, the authors recommended to medialize the patella by no more than 2.5 mm. Overzealous medialization has been shown to leave excessive bone on the exposed lateral patellar facet, poten-tially creating painful contact with the femoral condyle[76] (Fig. 113-22). It is therefore recommended to chamfer the patellar rim to reduce risk of bony impingement.[181]

An equivalent effect to medialization of the patella implant may, in many respects, be achievable by lateralizing the femoral component in terms of both reducing tension in the lateral retinaculum and reducing the Q angle. The prin-ciple advantage of changing the femoral rather than patellar component position lies in reducing the risk of patellar tilt, because the extensor mechanism would remain centered on the patella. The final decision should rest with the intra-operative assessment prior to the definitive placement of the implants.

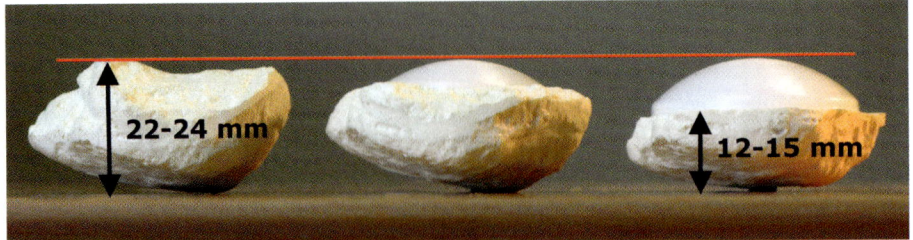

Figure 113-23. Maintaining patellar height after patella resurfacing using inlay *(middle)* and onlay *(right)* technique. Preparation of the patella should aim to preserve between 12 to 15 mm of bone.

Patellar Thickness

It is important to re-create physiologic patella thickness after resurfacing. This may be difficult if the patella is affected by advanced degenerative change, severe deformation, or erosion, all of which will invariably distort the surface anatomy. Under those circumstances, one should aim at reestablishing average patellar height, which in men and women is surprisingly constant, with values ranging from 22 to 24 mm[57] (Fig. 113-23). Greenfield and associates[114] reduced the incidence of lateral retinacular release from 55% to 12% by ensuring that the overall patellar thickness was less than or equal to that of the native patella.

It would therefore appear satisfactory to keep the composite height (total height of patellar shell plus patellar implant) of the patella slightly below the level of the native patella. Reducing the overall thickness by 1 to 2 mm in an attempt to improve patellar tracking has been recommended by some.[219] Furthermore, there are some biomechanical data supporting this concept. Reithmeier and Plitz[244] have shown that lowering the effective patellar component height allows for the load-sharing effect of the quadriceps tendon (turn-round phenomenon; see earlier) to commence at lower knee flexion angles, resulting in a linear reduction in force ratio between patellofemoral and quadriceps forces. Care should be taken not to compromise the structural integrity of the remaining patellar bone shell, because removal of excessive bone during the resurfacing procedure will weaken the patella, making it prone to fracture.[246] This will also predispose the patellar component to loosening, especially if the underlying bone structure is poor. Ideally, one should aim to preserve approximately 15 mm of patellar bone, but it appears that many surgeons consider 12 mm to be the cutoff point, below which the patella may be left unresurfaced[27] (Fig. 113-24).

Particular problems have been observed when patellar composite thickness exceeds preoperative values. This will create overstuffing of the PFJ, with subsequent increases in retinacular tension, anterior patellar strain, and PRF, leading to patellar tilt and subluxation.[283] Overall flexion may be reduced and the risk of patellar component failure and fracture increased.[78,204,246]

Joint Line

Maintenance of the joint line and patellar height has been shown to be an important factor in re-creating normal patellofemoral kinematics.[4] Raising or lowering the joint line will create secondary patella baja or alta, respectively. In cases of patella baja, the patellofemoral compressive forces will be

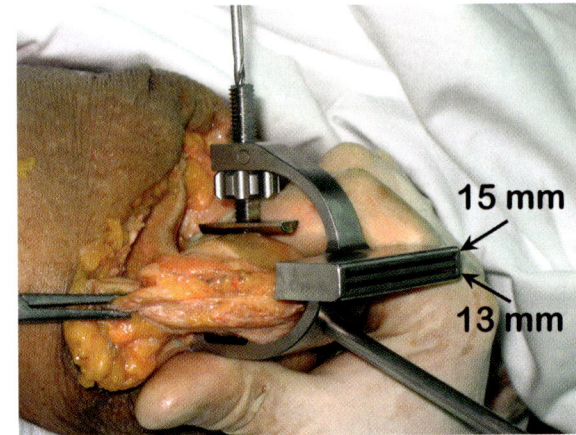

Figure 113-24. Patellar resection guide that allows for a set amount of patellar bone to remain. (Courtesy Dr. Andrea Baldini, Florence, Italy.)

increased during early knee flexion and overall range of motion is often compromised. Patella alta is generally less common and often developmental rather than secondary to surgery. It is primarily associated with patellar instability and subluxation.

Applying the correct surgical technique using these measures will assist in the reduction of lateral forces acting on the patella, leading to improved patellar tracking, and are thought to assist in reducing the need for lateral retinacular release.

Inlay versus Onlay

The patellar component may be placed onto the retropatellar surface (onlay) or inserted into a reamed cavity (inlay), with many manufacturers offering both alternatives (Figs. 113-25 and 113-26). It has been suggested that inlay patellar components provide greater composite strength between the implant and patella and may decrease the amount of patellar tilt and shift.[100,171,174] However, insetting the patellar component is not without risks because overzealous removal of subchondral cancellous bone may weaken the patella, increasing its susceptibility to fracture. Therefore, the preservation of a minimum of 15 mm of bone has been recommended to minimize surface strain on the patella.[154,246] In a comparison of 20 onlay patellar resurfacing prostheses with 20 inlay prostheses, Gomes and associates[109] saw less patellar tilt and better overall patellar alignment in patients with inlay implants. In a cadaver study, Ezzet and associates[87] observed similarities in patellar kinematics among implant types. However, inlay components showed a higher tendency to

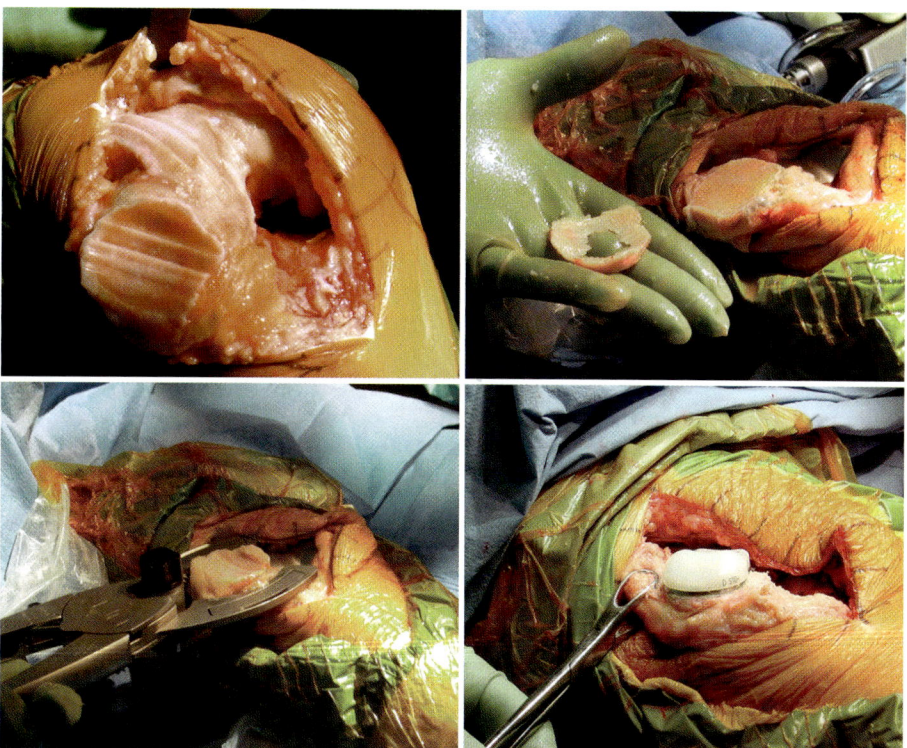

Figure 113-25. Patellar preparation using an onlay, cemented, anatomic patellar component. A conservative patellar cut compensates for severe retropatellar bone loss caused by advanced degenerative disease.

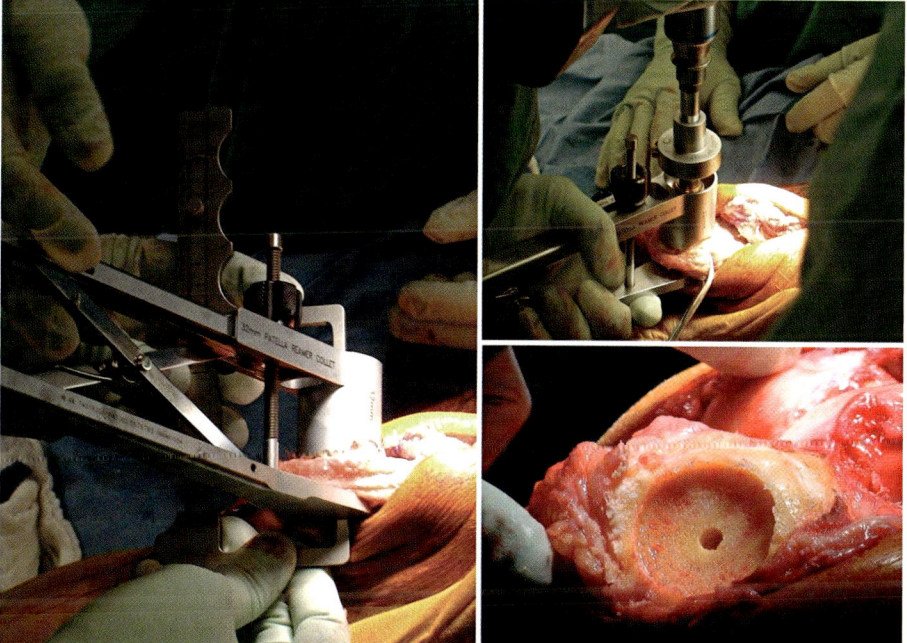

Figure 113-26. Patellar preparation using inlay technique requires a round single-peg component. The thickness is calibrated with a caliper prior to reaming.

lateral shift and tilt, although the differences did not reach statistical significance. Rand and Gustilo[241] have retrospectively compared 116 inlay and 135 onlay patellar components using an identical total knee system. At the time of surgery, 79% of onlay implants required lateral release, compared with only 28% of the knees with an inlay patella. At a mean follow-up of 2.3 years, they noticed that patellar tilt and subluxation were less common with the inlay design, which

led them to conclude that insertion of the patellar implant (inlay) results in better ability to centralize the extensor mechanism.

Lateral Release

A lateral release may become necessary if, after placement of all implants, the patella shows a tendency to lateral tracking or subluxation. Although the reason for such tracking abnormalities often remains obscure, it is paramount to assess the arthroplasty components for potential malalignment before contemplating lateral retinacular release. It is recommended that patellar tracking should be assessed at a point during surgery when trial components are assembled, because minor adjustments are still relatively easy to perform at this stage. Once tibial and femoral components have been cemented into place or press-fitted onto the bony surfaces, failure to correct patellar tracking may result in formal revision.

Most surgeons release the lateral patellofemoral ligament routinely when performing a medial parapatellar approach because it assists in exposure and eversion of the patella and allows for correction of minor tracking abnormalities.[219,263] It is worthwhile to check the integrity of the lateral patellofemoral ligament, because division of this structure alone may render a more formal lateral release unnecessary.

Scott's "rule of no thumb test" is widely used in the assessment of patellar tracking and in the decision making process, whether or not lateral release may be required.[263] The test is performed before closure of the medial capsule. If the patella tracks well throughout the full flexion arc without the surgeon holding the patella located in the trochlear groove with his or her thumb, no lateral release is necessary. If the patella tends to sublux or even dislocate without counteracting pressure from the thumb, the lateral retinaculum should be release in a staged fashion until the patella is stabilized. This technique has been criticized by some who believe that it may overestimate the need for lateral release if a medial parapatellar approach is used.[30,216,219] Other techniques, such as the towel clip test and one-stitch or single-suture test, have been described, claiming certain advantages, but merely represent variations on a theme.[11,232] Briard[39] has described the kissing rule, implying that if in deep flexion the medial surface of the patella does not touch the medial condyle of the femoral component, a lateral retinacular release is indicated. Tourniquet release is thought to provide a more realistic appreciation of patellar tracking and has been shown to reduce the number of lateral releases otherwise performed by up to 31%.[143,172] Dynamic forces may also favor lateral patellar tracking, but unfortunately these are outside the realm of clinical assessment during surgery.[29]

Although the technique of performing a lateral release is simple, much debate exists about the potential morbidity associated with it. The all-inside technique is favored by the great majority of surgeons because it avoids the creation of a cutaneous flap and, with it, potential wound-healing problems. The knee should be extended during the maneuver and the patella retracted anteriorly or everted halfway. Keeping the retinaculum under tension helps define the various soft tissue planes and may assist in identifying the lateral superior and inferior genicular arteries (Fig. 113-27). The incision is made approximately 1 to 2 cm lateral to the patellar margin, dividing the synovium, capsule, and retinacular fibers up to the subcutaneous fat. The release is performed in stages, with the clinician assessing patellar tracking regularly and therefore tailoring the amount of tissue released to the requirements. An extensive release may start distally to the joint line close to the fascia lata attachment onto Gerdy's tubercle, reaching up proximally to the junction of the vastus lateralis. Care should be taken not to buttonhole the incision through

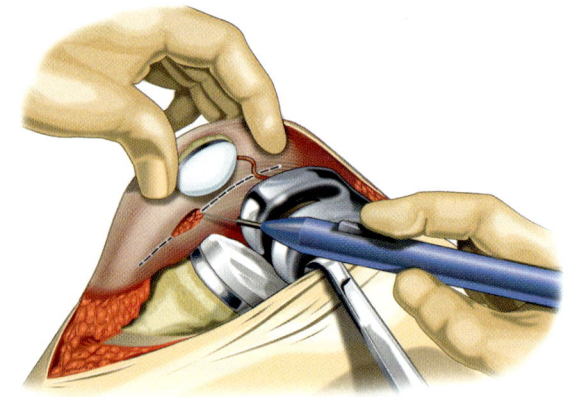

Figure 113-27. Identification and protection of the lateral superior genicular artery prior to performing a lateral retinacular release will help preserve blood supply to the patella.

the skin, a problem associated with the use of electrocautery in thin patients. The procedure itself carries some morbidity, including postoperative swelling, bruising, and hemarthrosis, most of which is related to inadequate hemostasis.

Much has been written about the importance of preserving the patellar blood supply, in particular the superior genicular artery, when performing a lateral release. The medial genicular vessels are obviously sacrificed as part of the medial parapatellar approach to the knee, whereas the lateral inferior genicular artery is often compromised during excision of the lateral meniscus, leaving the lateral superior genicular artery as the main source of circulation to the patella.[305] The vessel can be found close to the superior pole of the patella and, if identified, should be isolated through blunt dissection and protected during the release procedure[269] (see Fig. 113-27). However, it is not always possible to preserve the lateral superior genicular artery and provide adequate release at the same time. Under those circumstances, it may be advantageous to leave the lateral skin flap intact without separating skin from subcutaneous tissue; this is thought to preserve superficial vessels and ensure nourishment to the patellar bone from the overlying skin.[251]

The importance of the preservation of the lateral superior genicular artery remains open to debate. Accessory blood supply through the anterior vascular plexus, Hoffa's fat pad, and patellar and quadriceps tendon may be sufficient to maintain patellar viability, but there is evidence of temporary devascularization of the patellar bone after surgery.[199,277,323] Although most of the consequences arising from the sacrifice of the lateral genicular vessels are theoretical in nature, direct clinical complications, including avascular necrosis, patellar fracture, and wound-healing problems, have been reported.[201,304] In a series of 1146 TKAs, Ritter and associates[253] observed patella fractures in 5.4% of patients who had undergone lateral release compared with 2.4% in those who had not.

The surgical approach may also influence patellar tracking. A reduced incidence of lateral release has been shown with the midvastus and subvastus approach compared with a standard medial parapatellar incision.[30,82,195] This should be viewed against an increase in medial patellar tilt associated with a muscle-splitting approach.[30] However, no difference in the rate of lateral release or patellar function was observed if

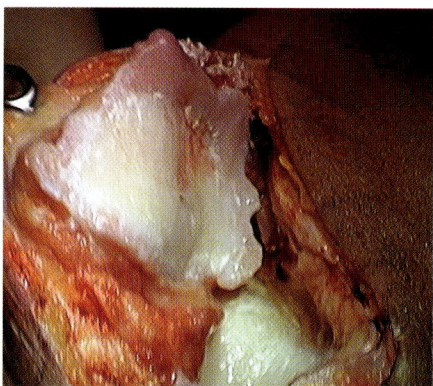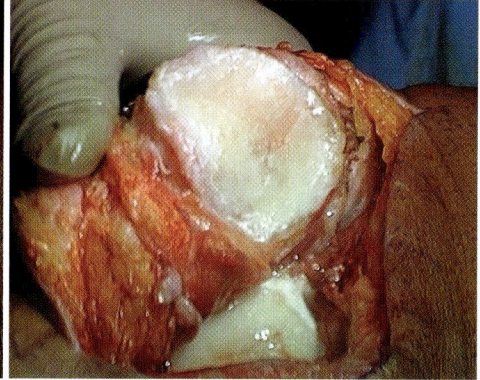

Figure 113-28. Patelloplasty is advisable if the patella is left unresurfaced. Marginal osteophytes are excised, circumferential synovium is cauterized and, if necessary, facets are reshaped to improve patellar seating on the femoral component.

a modified medial parapatellar approach was used instead.[159] This approach is directed into the musculotendinous junction of the vastus medialis, leaving the quadriceps tendon intact.

Wachtl and Jakob[313] have described a lateral patellar osteotomy as an alternative surgical procedure to the traditional retinacular release. The lateral patellar facet is exposed through eversion of the patella, 7 to 9 mm of the lateral border is resected using an oscillating saw, and the bony fragment are removed by subperiosteal dissection. The authors claim that the lateral patellar ligamentous structures are thus decompressed, relaxing the lateral retinaculum and making a formal release unnecessary. In their series of 76 patients, none required a lateral retinacular release, but 15% presented a degree of lateral patellar tilt.

Overall, the potential complications of a lateral retinacular release should be viewed in light of the detrimental long-term effects of patellar maltracking and subluxation on patellar component survival and AKP. Most clinicians would agree that the advantages by far outweigh the consequences of those complications.

Patelloplasty

Patelloplasty is recommended if the clinician decides not to resurface the patella. The procedure is essentially designed to re create a patellar shape and surface configuration similar to the native patella. It involves the removal of any marginal osteophytes from the periphery and, in case of significant patellar deformation, a lateral facetectomy. Areas of eburnization are shaved or exposed to transcortical Pridie drilling to encourage fibrocartilage ingrowth[147,160,161,231] (Fig. 113-28). The surrounding patellar meniscus and excessive synovial tissue are generally excised to avoid soft tissue impingement. Some surgeons promote circumferential thermocoagulation, thought to create a level of sensory denervation, in an attempt to combat postoperative AKP.[160]

PATELLA-RELATED COMPLICATIONS IN TOTAL KNEE ARTHROPLASTY

The advent of patellar resurfacing inadvertently introduced a new and different set of complications to the clinician performing TKA. Failures associated with the PFJ are multifactorial and may be related to patient selection, surgical technique, and implant design. The most common reason for patellar complications and premature patellar failure, however, are patellar maltracking and instability arising from surgical misjudgement and mismanagement. Patellar complications include patellar fracture, implant loosening and dissociation, soft tissue impingement (e.g. patellar clunk syndrome), and extensor mechanism disruption (Fig. 113-29).

Nevertheless, the component design, material choice, and manufacturing process may have a significant effect on performance, longevity, and potential complications, as has been observed through high failure rates of metal-backed and carbon fiber–reinforced UHMWPE patellar components. Problems arising through gamma sterilization in air and poststerilization oxidation and degradation have been recognized and addressed through changes in the sterilization process and awareness of the detrimental effect of prolonged shelf life.[60,197,249]

Patellar Fracture

Periprosthetic fractures of the patella are generally rare, with reported figures ranging from 0.5% to 5.2% following patellar resurfacing and 0.05% in the unresurfaced patella.* Although such fractures may result from trauma or from a complication during primary or revision surgery, most appear to occur spontaneously.[149,201,267] The Danish knee arthroplasty registry[64] has recorded an intraoperative patellar fracture rate of 0.2% in 38,759 primary total knee arthroplasties, likely caused by improper surgical technique, overresection of patellar bone, or weakened patellar bone structure from osteopenia or inflammatory arthropathy.

Compromise in patellar vascularity through medial arthrotomy combined with lateral retinacular release is thought to be a major factor in the cause of patellar fractures, but its clinical significance remains unclear. Some series have demonstrated a relationship between avascularity and fracture,[51,152,253] but others have failed to do so.[94,218,251] Nevertheless, the fear of causing vascular impairment to the patella prompted Cameron and Fedorkow[51] to promote access to the knee through a lateral parapatellar approach after they had observed a fracture rate of 21.4%. Scintigraphic assessment

*References 40, 108, 113, 217, 253, and 299.

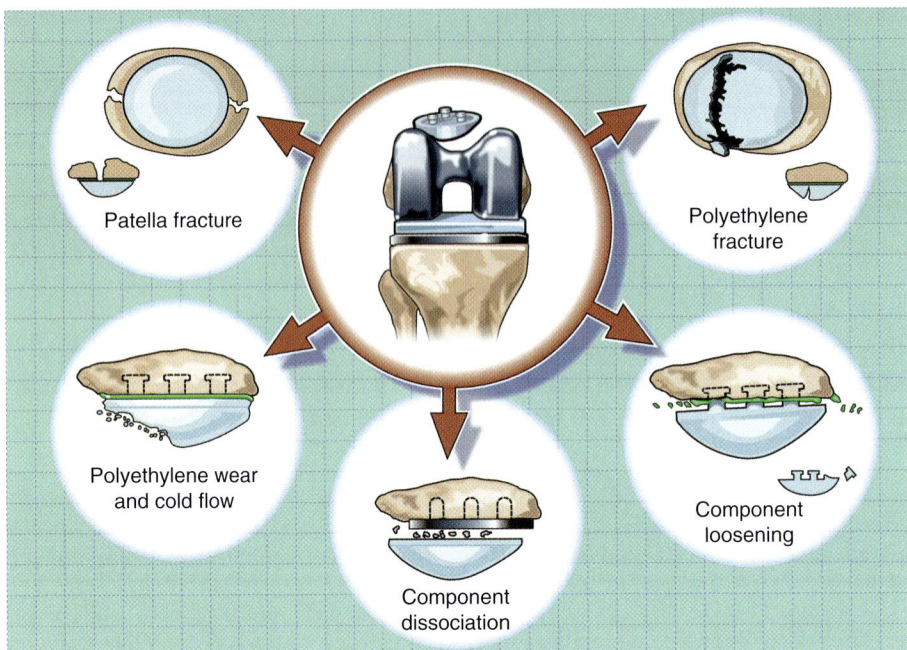

Figure 113-29. Various modes of failure mechanisms to which a prosthetic patella may be exposed when maltracking. (Adapted and redrawn from Keblish PA, Greenwald SA: Patella retention vs patella resurfacing in total knee arthroplasty. The patella: the unresolved problem in TKA. Presented at the 41st Annual Meeting of the American Academy of Orthopaedic Surgeons, Anaheim, Cal, 1991.)

of the patella following lateral release has confirmed a noticeable reduction in tracer uptake as early as 7 to 10 days following surgery, with a return to a normal appearance after 8 to 12 weeks. These changes are thought to represent transient patellar hypovascularity, which has been observed in up to 40% of cases.[224,269] Such temporary ischemia infrequently results in clinical problems, especially if viewed against the overall number of lateral releases performed. Its clinical relevance remains debatable.

The literature conveys an array of other potentially causative factors, including technical errors (e.g., patellar maltracking secondary to implant malalignment, excessive or asymmetrical patellar bone resection, thermal necrosis through cement polymerization), patient demographics (male gender, obesity [with BMI >30 kg/m^2], knee flexion >95 degrees, high activity level), and implant design (large patellar component ≥37 mm diameter, inlay patellar design, large central fixation peg, posterior-stabilizing implant).* Large single central fixation pegs, common in earlier implant designs, have been a major design factor associated with patellar fracture and implant loosening.[40,51] Most modern knee implant systems feature three-peg patellar components, which although not entirely free of problems, have generally performed better and are currently considered the gold standard.[67,170,192,272] With regard to the influence of posterior-stabilizing implant designs on patellar fracture incidence, it has been suggested, that anterior displacement of the tibia may increase the distance from the origin to the insertion of the extensor mechanism, leading to an increase in anterior patellor strain with increasing knee flexion.[233,235] The effect

is perpetuated if the composite height of the patella is excessive because tension may exceed the yield strength of patellar bone.[312]

In the Mayo Clinic classification, fractures are divided into three types according to implant stability and integrity of extensor mechanism.[217] In type I, the patellar implant is stable and the extensor mechanism is intact; in type II, the extensor mechanism is disrupted; and in type III, the patellar implant is loose but the extensor mechanism remains intact. Type III fractures are further subdivided into type IIIa, indicating reasonable remaining bone stock, and type IIIb, in which the bone stock is either poor, with an overall thickness of less than 10 mm, or where there is significant patellar comminution.

A large proportion of patellar fractures are asymptomatic. Ortiguera and Berry[217] have diagnosed 78 fractures in 12,464 total knee arthroplasties, 44 of which were asymptomatic and discovered incidentally during postoperative follow-up. Treatment in those cases was therefore mostly conservative. Surgical intervention may be necessary when the patellar component is loose or dislodged, provided that the patient is sufficiently symptomatic, but becomes essential in cases of extensor mechanism disruption. For type I fractures, the authors recommended immobilization in cylinder cast for 6 weeks; type II fractures are often suitable for tension band wiring and retinacular repair. In type III, the patellar implant should be retrieved and not replaced initially because it could interfere with fracture healing. Reconstitution of the extensor mechanism has precedence over patellar reconstruction. If patellar fixation is not feasible because of the severity of comminution, patellectomy may represent an acceptable option. In this study, Ortiguera and Berry reported complication rates of 56% in patients treated operatively, 90% of whom required a further surgical procedure compared with a

*References 58, 77, 108, 149, 184, 201, 217, 272, 303, and 326.

complication rate of less than 10% in patients treated conservatively.

In the management of patellar fractures, the clinician must evaluate the underlying cause and eradicate any associated pathology. Malalignment of the femoral or tibial component should be rectified at the time of patellar fixation or component revision to avoid recurrence. Conservative management, however, should be considered whenever possible, because the risk of complications is high. Most authors support prolonged immobilization in extension, followed by gradual mobilization in a hinged brace. Even if overall range of movement is likely to be compromised in the long term, healing should take precedence over motion in these difficult cases.[68,217,237]

Patellar Implant Wear and Loosening

Loosening of the patellar component with or without displacement is reported to occur in 0.6% to 4.8% of cases.[40,67] As with patellar fracture, patients may be asymptomatic and rarely require surgical intervention unless the component has become dislodged or mechanical symptoms occur. The frequency of patellar component loosening has decreased significantly since the discontinuance of metal-backed patellar components in the early 1990s, which were notorious for developing wear and loosening[22,180,292] (see Fig. 113-7). Meding and associates[201] have reviewed 8531 cruciate-retaining TKAs using a cemented, dome-shaped patellar component with a central peg. At an average follow-up of 7 years (range, 2 to 22 years), they found radiographic evidence of patellar loosening in 409 cases (4.8%). In this series, obesity placed the patella at 6.3 times the risk of loosening, followed by lateral release at 3.8 times, elevated joint line at 2.2 times, and flexion beyond 100 degrees at 2.1 times. Other factors identified included poor remaining bone stock, asymmetrical patellar resection, small fixation pegs, inadequate implant fixation, patellar maltracking secondary to component malalignment, osteonecrosis, and osteolysis.[23,182] Signs of patellar component loosening can usually be depicted on plain axial and sagittal radiographs. Occasionally, however, these may be inconclusive and arthroscopic assessment may become indicated. In low-demand patients, simple patellar component retrieval and patelloplasty using an arthroscopic burr may suffice, whereas in all others patellar component revision may be indicated.

Wear is a common feature in patellar implants because of the unfavorable mechanical environment of the patellofemoral articulation. The in vivo wear pattern of patellar implants is highly dependent on the inherent mechanical properties of the materials (e.g., UHMWPE, polymethylmethacrylate [PMMA]), the interaction between patellar and femoral components, and the external forces acting on them. The mechanical performance of the various designs is best assessed from observations made on retrieval components, which have shown considerable degree of wear and deformation.[72,96,134,200] The level of wear damage appears to increase with patient's weight, postoperative range of motion, and how long the component has been implanted. It is therefore of interest to note that despite patellofemoral compressive forces exceeding the yield strength of UHMWPE, catastrophic wear or component fractures are seen infrequently and have not become endemic.

Soft Tissue Impingement and Patellar Clunk Syndrome

Any redundant or proliferative synovial tissue, intra-articular fibrotic scar tissue, and/or Hoffa's fat pad may become impinged between the patellar and femoral components and act as a mechanical impediment. Such impingement often leads to just minor clicking but, if severe, mechanical symptoms of locking, catching, popping, and giving way, associated with various degrees of discomfort or pain, can occur. Late-onset patellar maltracking may be caused by the proliferation of granulation tissue or the development of fibrous adhesions tethering the patella during joint movement. Such tissue growth is thought to originate from exposed cancellous bone at the margins of the components or through chronic irritation of the synovium against prosthetic prominences. Insall and associates[149] first described peripatellar synovial hypertrophy as a cause of symptomatic patellar clicking and catching in posterior-stabilized TKAs. In 1989, Hozack and associates[135] coined the term *patellar clunk syndrome*, referring to a painful catching sensation on knee extension. The cause of this syndrome was found to be a prominent fibrous nodule at the junction between the proximal patellar pole and distal quadriceps tendon, which became entrapped in the intercondylar housing of a posterior-stabilized femoral component between 30 and 45 degrees of knee flexion (Fig. 113-30). The syndrome is primarily seen with cruciate-substituting designs but may also occur when femoral components with sharp transition zones between the trochlear groove and intercondylar notch are used. Lucas and coworkers[183] have reported an incidence of patellar clunk syndrome of 3.5% in a series of 900 TKAs using the Insall-Burstein II prosthetic design. An impingement problem of a similar type was highlighted by Pettine and Bryan.[228] They described painful loss of flexion caused by infrapatellar fibrous tissue that had filled the intercondylar notch.

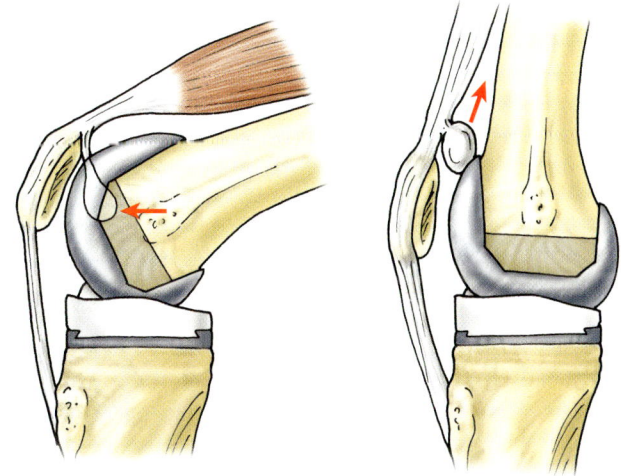

Figure 113-30. Patellar clunk syndrome. A nodule of fibrous tissue becomes entrapped in the housing of a posterior-stabilized TKA during flexion. Patients experience a painful clunk sensation when the nodule exits the housing during extension. (Adapted from Scuderi GR, DeMuth BC: Management of patellar tendon disruption in total knee arthroplasty. In Scuderi GR, Tria AJ Jr [eds]: Surgical techniques in total knee arthroplasty, New York, 2002, Springer.)

For the treatment of painful soft tissue impingement, conservative measures, including ultrasound application and deep friction massage, should be used initially. Quadriceps strengthening using the stationary bike may prove beneficial because it mechanically softens and autodébrides the lesion through repetitive motion. If nonoperative management fails, open or arthroscopic excision of the tissue growth is usually curative.[74,299,311]

Patellar Instability and Dislocation

Patellar instability represents a serious problem in TKA and is responsible for a number of associated complications, making it the most common reason for secondary surgery, including revision.[40,53,206] The patella may be affected by maltracking, intermittent subluxation or even dislocation and the effect of these problems on the patient's mobility level can be considerable (Fig. 113-31). Patients may present with a plethora of symptoms, ranging from mild discomfort to pain, weakness, giving way, and locking.

The cause of patellar instability can generally be traced to improper patient selection, implant design, or surgical technique.[237,238] Patient factors include preoperative valgus malalignment, patellar subluxation, and severe patellofemoral degeneration, which have all been associated with an increased prevalence of lateral retinacular release and postoperative patellar maltracking.[236,286]

The effect of implant design on patellofemoral stability is well recognized.[287,324] Femoral components featuring a symmetrical and shallow trochlear groove with an abrupt sagittal radius have been shown to create abnormal patellar kinematics and increase the risk of patellar maltracking.[227,297,334] Campbell and associates[53] have reviewed 289 knee arthroplasties with a shallow and narrow trochlea and found that out of 20 revisions, 14 were required for patellar maltracking.

Technical errors relating to surgical misjudgment are common reasons for patellar instability.[219] Residual valgus limb malalignment, patella alta, excessive internal rotation of the femoral or tibial component, medial translation of the femoral component, valgus alignment of the femoral component (even if the overall limb alignment appears neutral), asymmetrical patellar resection, lateral placement of the patellar button, excessive patellar composite thickness, improper soft tissue balancing, and failure to perform a lateral release have all been shown to exert a detrimental effect on patellar tracking.[39,40,51,107,204] Failure to appreciate and correct such problems at the time of surgery will invariably lead to patellofemoral complications.

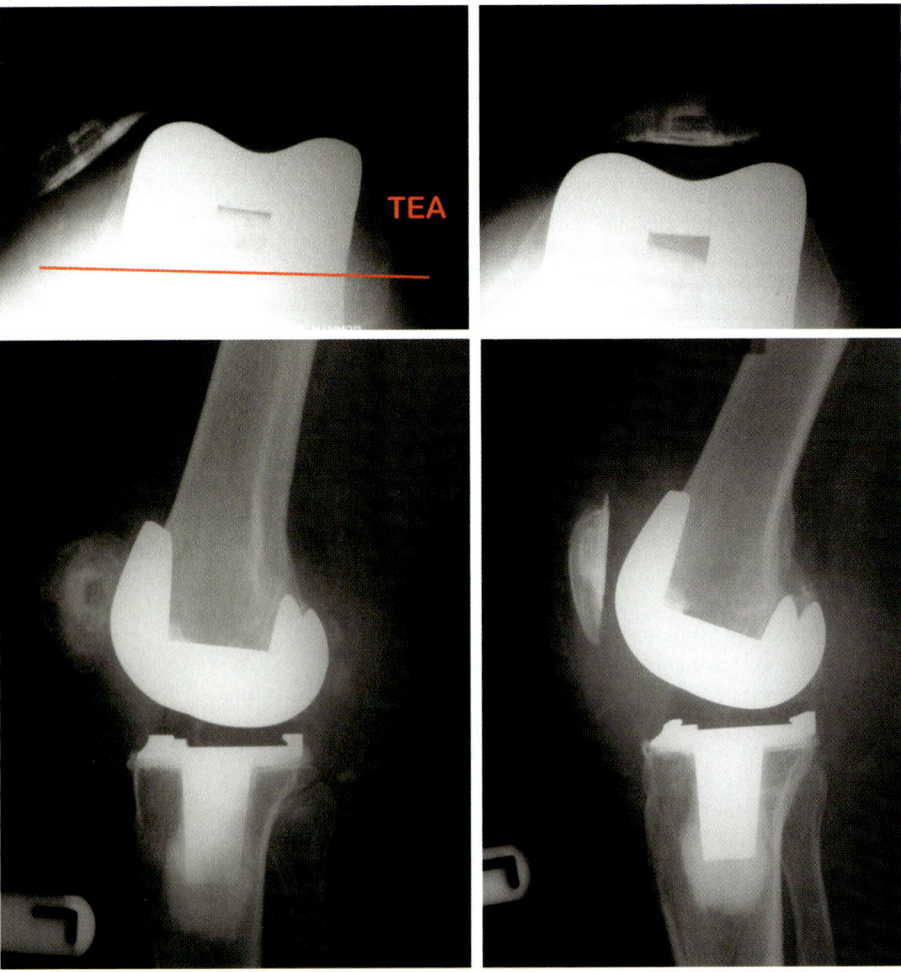

Figure 113-31. Lateral dislocation of the patella following TKA. Isolated patellar component revision and extensor mechanism realignment have proved sufficient in establishing satisfactory patellar tracking, despite slight femoral component internal rotation.

The treatment of patellar instability must address the underlying cause. A high degree of suspicion is often necessary during the investigation process to detect subtle abnormalities. Simple clinical examination can often provide vital clues. Excessive internal rotation of the femoral component can easily be spotted through noticeable valgus of the lower limb in knee flexion. Similarly, internal rotation of the tibial component will affect the foot progression angle and the patient may present with an out-toeing gait on the affected side.

Axial radiographs (Merchant or skyline view), especially if taken at less than 45 degrees, are often able to confirm the level of patellar malpositioning and subluxation and degree of patellar tilt (Fig. 113-31). Excessive knee flexion should be avoided because patellofemoral maltracking is best demonstrated at earlier degrees of knee flexion. CT is required if component malpositioning is suspected[25,307] (see Fig. 113-20).

If the symptoms associated with these abnormalities are subtle, a nonoperative treatment approach should be considered, focusing on physiotherapeutic measures. Those measures usually include strengthening of the vastus medialis, stretching of the iliotibial band, McConnell taping, and use of a patellar stabilization brace. If this treatment approach remains unsuccessful, surgical intervention becomes necessary.

A maltracking, laterally subluxing patella can be assessed arthroscopically using a 70-degree arthroscope, which is introduced through a superolateral portal, placed approximately 3 to 4 cm proximal to the upper border of the patella.[291] This will allow for precise judgment on the passive patellar movement path during flexion and extension. A lateral release can, if deemed necessary, be performed under direct vision until patellar positioning appears acceptable. In more severe cases, in which patella positioning is unresponsive to the aforementioned measures and component malpositioning has been excluded, medial soft tissue imbrication, vastus medialis advancement, or tibial tuberosity transfer should be taken into consideration (in that order)[236,237] (see Fig. 113-31). In cases of significant implant malpositioning, component revision may become necessary.

Extensor Mechanism Disruption

Rupture of the patellar or quadriceps tendon is an unlikely complication following TKA, with a reported incidence for patellar tendon rupture of 0.22% to 2.5% and for quadriceps tendon rupture of 0.1%.[40,67,185,236] Factors associated with tendon ruptures are significant preoperative flexion contracture and angular deformities, difficult surgical exposure, obese patients, revision surgery, arthrofibrosis, quadriceps release (quadriceps snip), and extensive lateral retinacular release.[218,242] Systemic disease such as diabetes mellitus, chronic renal insufficiency, Parkinson's disease, gout, morbid obesity, and multiple intra-articular steroid injections will predispose patients to tendon ruptures and should always be considered, particularly if the rupture occurs spontaneously. Quadriceps tendon ruptures may be amenable to conservative management, especially in low-demand patients using prolonged brace immobilization; otherwise, direct suture repair using the Scuderi turndown technique has been recommended.[31,32] Repair of patellar tendon ruptures is extremely challenging and treatment results are often discouraging and fraught with

complications. Direct suture repair is often unsuccessful, as highlighted by Rand and associates,[242] who reported a 75% failure rate and a 25% infection rate after primary suture repair. Consideration should be given to the use of some form of augmentation.[268] Autogenous semitendinosus tendon graft, patellar tendon or Achilles tendon allograft, or rerouting of a fascia lata strip have all been recommended.[218] If necessary, the repair can be secured further with a figure-of-eight tension band wire loop. If the viability of the repair tissue is compromised a medial gastrocnemius flap may be advantageous but carries the disadvantage of poor cosmetic appearance and weakness of plantar flexion. The literature supports a prolonged period of bracing and protection from extremes of motion and impact activities for 3 to 6 months following surgery. Functional outcomes are often disappointing, with a residual extensor lag to be expected in most cases. Allograft reconstruction of the extensor mechanism, as popularized by Emerson and colleagues,[81] remains controversial. In a series of 36 patients receiving an extensor mechanism allograft, Nazarian and Booth[212] reported eight graft reruptures requiring revision. Two patients were considered failures, an extensor lag was present in 15 patients, and the average Knee Society Function Score measured 68.

ADVANTAGES AND DRAWBACKS OF PATELLAR RESURFACING

In 1836, Malgaigne wrote, "When one searches among the past or present authors for the origins of doctrines generally accepted today concerning dislocation of the patella, one is surprised to find among them such disagreement and such a dearth of facts with such an abundance of opinions."[187] Although focusing on a slightly different subject matter, Malgaigne's views strongly characterize the diversity of opinions expressed in the debate about patella resurfacing in TKA to date. In Krackow's opinion,[165] the issue for or against patellar resurfacing has become analogous to topics of religion and politics.

Three basic strategies have evolved—always to resurface, never to resurface, or to resurface the patella selectively. Clinicians who prefer patellar resurfacing claim reduced incidence of postoperative AKP, avoidance of secondary resurfacing, higher patient satisfaction, better overall function, and low complication rate.[177,235,267,320] They also argue that the procedure is relatively inexpensive and not time-consuming when performed during a standard TKA. The articulation between cartilage and metal is considered nonphysiologic, and prolonged exposure to high compressive forces is believed to cause cartilage erosion.[97] So far, however, no conclusive evidence exists that the patella that is affected by such degradation becomes symptomatic.[178,281] The proportion of the overall revision rates attributable to the resurfaced patella have decreased over the past 25 years, from almost 50% in the 1980s to approximately 12% today.[40,271] The prevalence of patellofemoral complications has also decreased significantly and currently is approximately 4%.[19,36,169,330]

Those in support of nonresurfacing claim conservation of patellar bone, reduced likelihood of patellar osteonecrosis, more physiologic patellofemoral kinematics, ability to withstand high patellofemoral forces, especially in younger and more active patients without the concern of prosthetic wear or failure, and ease of resurfacing in case of recalcitrant

AKP.[1,51,89,161] Particular emphasis is placed on the avoidance of intraoperative and postoperative complications associated with patellar resurfacing, which include patellar fracture, implant wear, loosening, and dissociation.[22,67,68,160]

Selective resurfacing attempts to identify those who are thought to have an improved clinical outcome with patellar resurfacing while avoiding potential complications associated with unnecessary resurfacing.[40,178,228,264,281] Favorable patient selection criteria for patella retention include younger patients (<65 years) with reasonably well-preserved retropatellar cartilage, absence of crystalline disease, central patellar tracking, and use of a patella-friendly femoral component. Kim and associates[163] have reported a 97.5% survival rate in unresurfaced TKAs at 10 years when these selection criteria were applied.

Some argument exists about the indication for patellar resurfacing in patients affected by inflammatory arthropathies. Sledge and Ewald[275] have suggested that failure to resurface the patellar in rheumatoid arthritis (RA) may allow continued release of sequestered antigen from the retained cartilage, resulting in recurrent inflammation. Concerns about an ongoing inflammatory process, however, have remained largely theoretical and, although some studies have recommended routine resurfacing for all RA patients,[19,178,229,263] others have not reported any ill effects, despite patellar retention.*

When resurfacing the patella, the surgeon is required to adhere to strict surgical principles to reproduce patellar thickness, preserve patellar blood supply, and achieve appropriate positioning of all implant components, with balanced soft tissue to allow for central patellar tracking.[165,219,258] When not resurfacing the patella, the choice of prosthetic design with a patella-friendly femoral component becomes critical to success.[33,194,295,297]

Anterior Knee Pain and Patellar Resurfacing

The high incidence of AKP in early arthroplasty designs without a patellar component led initially to recommendations for universal patellar resurfacing.[51,152,235,281] The move toward universally replacing the patella, however, attracted a different spectrum of complications. Problems such as patellar maltracking and subluxation, component wear and loosening, patellar fracture, extensor mechanism failure, and AKP have been reported in 4% to 35% of cases, even when using contemporary total knee designs. Therefore, selective resurfacing of the patella has been popularized by some clinicians, mainly based on patient's weight, presence of preoperative AKP, and degree of patellar degeneration.†

The incidence of AKP following TKA shows wide variations, with reported figures of 0 degrees to 47% in patients with patellar resurfacing and 0 degrees to 43% in those patients in whom the patella is retained.‡ These variations are likely to be caused by differences in pain assessment, patient selection, surgical technique, and implant design. Scott and Kim[265] have indicated that regardless of the management of the patella, clinicians can expect approximately

10% of patients to be affected by significant AKP after TKA, a finding that has been confirmed through prospective observational studies.[7,37,80,130]

A significant number of clinical studies have shown that patients undergoing patellar resurfacing are less likely to be affected by AKP and overall are more satisfied.* However, it is still controversial whether patients with a nonresurfaced patella really suffer more pain than those who have been resurfaced. Robertsson and associates[255] have reviewed data of 27,372 patients from the Swedish Knee Registry and found that 15% of patients with a resurfaced patella were generally dissatisfied, compared with 19% of those in whom the patella was retained. However, patients with patellar resurfacing became less satisfied with their knee over time, whereas satisfaction ratings in those without resurfacing remained unchanged. It was concluded that the benefit of the patellar component diminishes with time and that the need for secondary resurfacing may be balanced by the need for revision of failed patellar components.[256]

Studies on the subject of patellar resurfacing have been diverse, using a variety of assessment tools, and have not consisted of identical study designs. Their methodologic limitations prevent a direct comparison of like with like, and therefore have done little to reduce the insurmountable divide between clinicians who promote resurfacing and those who do not.

The great debate about the pros and cons of patellar resurfacing revolve around a lack of understanding about why some patients may suffer AKP after knee arthroplasty and others may not, irrespective of preoperative symptoms and patellar resurfacing.[19,225] Even though many clinicians believe that in the presence of preoperative symptoms resurfacing should be considered, the scientific basis for such action is missing, because no conclusive evidence currently exists. In a randomized controlled trial, Barrack and associates[19] have found that 28% of patients without AKP before resurfacing suffered AKP after surgery. Similarly, 9% of patients with preoperative AKP continued having pain postoperatively, despite resurfacing. In the group in whom the patella was retained, 23% continued suffering pain and new pain developed in 14%. Hasegawa and Ohashi[126] have followed 78 unresurfaced TKAs for 12 years; of these, 17 knees (22%) developed patellar subluxation and lateral facet erosion, but only 4 of these (5%) experienced pain.

It is simplistic to attribute all AKP to the patella, because various conditions may be responsible for the development of discomfort projected in and around the patellofemoral articulation. Soft tissue affliction (e.g., peripatellar tendinopathy, bursitis, impinging Hoffa's fat pad, synovial folds and plicae, scar tissue bands, neuromas, Sudek dystrophy, complex regional pain syndrome), bony abnormalities (e.g., Sinding-Larsen-Johansson syndrome, stress fracture, retained osteophytes, impinging loose bodies), and patellar maltracking have all been implicated as potential causes of AKP, and should be excluded before treatment is initiated.[45,46,260]

Predictors of Anterior Knee Pain

Predictors for postoperative AKP have been suggested but few, such as obesity and flexion contracture, have been

*References 1, 36, 65, 84, 126, and 274.
†References 1, 126, 161, 178, 229, 263, and 274.
‡References 36, 46, 52, 90, 95, 126, 155, 177, 229, 320, and 333.

*References 36, 51, 84, 155, 222, 262, and 320.

reliably identified.[129,229] Most clinical studies have failed to depict differences between knees affected by AKP and those that are not. Soudry and coworkers[281] were unable to define a correlation between the degree of cartilage damage and the level of pain or quality of result in patients whose knees had been left unresurfaced. Elson and Brenkel[80] prospectively assessed 602 primary TKAs and found mild pain in 8% and moderate to severe pain in 5% of knees. Age was delineated as the only reliable predictor of pain, with patients younger than 60 years being more than twice as likely to be affected. Results from randomized controlled trials have shown no association among obesity, preoperative AKP, degree of chondromalacia or chondrolysis, lateral release, and occurrence of postoperative AKP.[19,52,279] Height and weight, but not BMI, have been indicated as being predictive of anterior pain and revision in resurfaced patellae, which is thought to be caused by increased lever arms and patellofemoral forces.[46,330] Waters and Bentley[320] assessed 514 knees randomized for patellar resurfacing and found no difference between knees with AKP and those without in regard to age, weight, gender, lateral release, cruciate retention or sacrifice, and whether the knees were affected by osteoarthritis or RA.

Despite resurfacing or nonresurfacing of the patella, the prevalence of AKP remains high. Combined with the fact that such pain often fails to respond to secondary resurfacing, it has been suggested that underlying patient, implant, or surgical factors, other than patellar resurfacing, may have a significant impact on the presence of AKP following TKA.[19,144] Figgie and associates[95] have shown that AKP was present in 23 of 75 TKAs in which the implants were positioned outside the ideal alignment compared with no AKP in 41 knees in which the components were positioned correctly.

Implant design has been shown to have a major effect on patellar kinematics and it is therefore conceivable that such an effect may influence the development of postoperative AKP.[126,295,334] Most femoral components are designed to articulate with a designated patellar prosthesis. Articulation between the native patella and prosthetic femur may induce potential problems in terms of abnormal contact and tracking characteristics.[167,297,325] It has been speculated that AKP in patients in whom the patella has been left unresurfaced may be secondary to altered patellar biomechanics and femoral component configuration.[36,194,280]

The importance of design issues has been highlighted by a group from the University of Western Australia, who conducted two randomized controlled studies with almost identical study design in which the only major variable was the type of prosthesis used. In the first study, by Wood and coworkers,[330] a relatively patella-unfriendly design was used, featuring flat condyles with a shallow and angular trochlear groove. In the second study, by Smith and associates,[278] a relatively patella-friendly design was used, characterized by a deepened trochlear groove with curved transition toward the femoral condyles. Comparing the outcome for nonresurfaced patients, it would appear that the rate of postoperative AKP decreased from 31% to 21%, the reoperation rate for patellofemoral complications decreased from 12% to 1.2%, and the Knee Society score increased by 11 points. With this in mind, the reported results from clinical studies should be viewed as being design-specific and reliable only for the implant studied. Some older and often retrospective studies have featured implant designs that have now been

altered or discontinued, which substantially impairs their validity.

However, despite proper patient and implant selection and good surgical technique, the inability to determine with any degree of certainty whether a patient may be affected by AKP, regardless of the treatment of the patella, remains a surgical conundrum and demands further investigation.

Secondary Resurfacing

The number of revisions for pain is higher if the patella is left unresurfaced and involves the insertion of patellar components in up to 10% of cases.[36,84,229,281] This is thought to reflect the higher incidence of AKP in patients with patellar retention. In a significant proportion of these patients, symptoms will remain unchanged despite secondary resurfacing or revision arthroplasty, and satisfactory outcomes are expected in no more than 50% to 60% of cases.* Even after successful secondary resurfacing, recurrence of symptoms may be as high as 55%.

Spencer and associates[282] have reviewed 28 patients who had undergone secondary patellar resurfacing for persistent AKP. Patient satisfaction was assessed at a mean of 28 months postoperatively, resulting in 59% feeling improved, 34% feeling the same, and 7% feeling worse. In a similar study, Garcia and colleagues[104] reviewed 17 cases of isolated patellar resurfacing, of which 53% of patients were asymptomatic and satisfied and 47% continued to be affected by AKP and were unsatisfied. It would appear reasonable to suggest that failure to improve in patients following secondary resurfacing may indicate a multifactorial cause or a different cause of pain other than the PFJ altogether.

Ahmad and associates[5] have recently suggested three-phase bone scintigraphy as an assessment tool in an attempt to distinguish patients who are likely to benefit from secondary resurfacing. Increased tracer uptake of the patella in patients with localized AKP appeared predictive of symptomatic pain relief following secondary patellar resurfacing. Overall numbers, however, were small, hence further research is needed to confirm the value of scintigraphy in assessing and treating AKP in this specific group of patients. If a patient with a nonresurfaced patella presents with AKP, secondary resurfacing, despite its limited success, remains an available option and potential remedy. Conversely, there are fewer options available for the treatment of patients with AKP whose patella has already been resurfaced. Isolated patellar component revision for pain is not generally recommended because the clinical outcome is uncertain. Furthermore, patellar revision is not an innocuous procedure and should be approached with utmost caution because of frequent complications.[28,176] It could therefore be argued that if this clinical situation occurs, in which a patient is affected by AKP following primary patellar resurfacing, the surgeon is less likely to proceed with a revision procedure. This would partly explain the higher proportion of revisions in nonresurfaced knee arthroplasties.

Revisions for patellofemoral symptoms are mostly performed relatively soon after the index procedure, whereas revisions for wear or loosening of the patellar implant usually

---

*References 19, 53, 104, 167, 188, 254, and 282.

Table 113-2 Randomized, Controlled Clinical Trials Comparing Patellar Resurfacing With Nonresurfacing in Total Knee Arthroplasty

Study (Year)	TKA Implant Type	Patellar Implant	No. of Cases NR/RS	Follow-Up (Yr)	PAIN (%)		ROP (%)		KSS		Investigator's Comments
					NR	RS	NR	RS	NR	RS	
Partio and Wirz (1995)[222]	PFC CR	Modified dome	50/50	2.5	22	2	0	0	169	170	RS better
Feller et al (1996)[89]	PCA	Offset dome	20/20	3	n.s.	n.s.	0	5	(89)*	(86)*	NR better
Schroeder-Boersch et al (1998)[262]	Duracon	Onlay	20/20	4.8	20	10	10	5	150	163	RS better
Barrack et al (2001)[19]	MG-II CR	Modified dome	60/58	5	17	19	12	0	169	162	No difference
Fengler (2001)[90]	PFC	Dome (inlay)	68/68	1	0	0	0	0	147	138	NR better
Wood et al (2002)[330]	MG-II CR	n.s.	128/92	4	31	16	12	10	152	157	RS better
Waters and Bentley (2003)[320]	PFC CR/PS	Dome	231/243	5.3	25.1	5.3	4.8	1.2	162	167	RS better
Burnett et al (2004)[46]	AMK CR	Dome	48/42	10.8	25	37	6	2	146	145	No difference
Gildone et al (2005)[105]	NexGen PS	Dome	28/28	2	21	0	0	0	178	178	RS better
Myles et al (2006)[208]	LCS RP	Anatomic	25/25	1.75	n.s.	n.s.	0	0	162	147	No difference
Campbell et al (2006)[52]	MG-II CR	Modified dome	54/46	10	43	47	3.7	2.2	136†	138†	No difference
Burnett et al (2007)[47]	MG-II CR	Modified dome	32/32	10	17.3	16.5	6.2	3.1	148	146	No difference
Smith et al (2008)[279]	Profix	Dome (inlay)	86/73	4.4	21	30	1.2	1.4	163	152	No difference
Burnett et al (2009)[48]	MG-II CR	Modified dome	60/58	10	16	21	12	3	155	146	No difference
Totals			910/855	5	21.5	17.0	4.8	2.3	157	155	

CR, Cruciate-retaining; *CS*, cruciate-sacrificing; *KSS*, Knee Society score; *LCS*, low-contact stress; *MG*, Miller-Galante; *NR*, nonresurfaced; *n.s.*, not specified; *PCA*, porous-coated anatomic; *PFC*, press-fit condylar; *PS*, posterior-stabilized; *RP*, rotating platform; *RS*, resurfaced.
*Hospital for Special Surgery (HSS) score.
†4-year results.

occur much later. Putting this in perspective with the finding that patients who have had their patella resurfaced are, at least initially, more satisfied with their knee, one might suggest a more liberal use of patellar resurfacing, at least for older patients.

National Arthroplasty Registries

National joint registries are a valuable source of information because they include a large number of patients. Unfortunately, data collection is of variable quality and does not cover all aspects of treatment and complications surrounding the treatment of the PFJ in TKA.[254] The frequency of implanting a patellar component varies greatly among countries. According to the Swedish Knee Arthroplasty Register, patellar resurfacing as part of a TKA is performed in less than 10% of cases by Swedish surgeons.[294] In Norway, the local arthroplasty registry has indicated that surgeons resurface the patella in 35% of cases, whereas secondary resurfacing for AKP is performed in 1.8% of cases.[215,103] Reported figures from the Australian Arthroplasty Registry have suggested that in Australia, patellar resurfacing has increased from as low as 41.5% in 2005 to 47.0% in 2009, whilst pain represents the reason for revision in 6.5% of all nonresurfaced TKAs.[15] According to data from the Danish Knee Arthroplasty Registry, Danish

surgeons use a patellar component in almost 65% of knee arthroplasties.[64]

Randomized Controlled Trials

The controversy surrounding the need for patellar resurfacing at the time of TKA has been fueled by differing results derived from clinical studies and historic data. Unfortunately, most studies are retrospective and use redundant implant designs. Randomized, controlled, prospective trials have tried to address these shortcomings, but variations in patient assessment and study design remain and continue to impair their comparability.

A meta-analysis of 14 randomized controlled trials (RCTs) revealed a total of 855 knees that were treated with patellar resurfacing at the time of TKA, compared with 910 knees in which the patella was left unresurfaced (Table 113-2).* The average follow-up period was 5 years (range, 1 to 10.8 years). Postoperative AKP was present in 21.5% of unresurfaced and 17.0% of resurfaced patellae. Knee Society scores of 157 in unresurfaced and 155 in resurfaced patellae were recorded. Patellar complications led to a reoperation rate of 4.8% in

---

*References 19, 46-48, 52, 89, 90, 105, 208, 222, 262, 279, 310, and 330.

Table 113-3 Comparisons of Patellar Resurfacing versus Nonresurfacing in Patients With Bilateral Total Knee Arthroplasties

Study (Year)	TKA Type	Patellar Implant	Type of Trial	No. of Cases	Follow-Up (Yr)	PREFERENCE (%)			Investigator's Comments
						RS	NR	None	
Shoji et al (1989)[274]	Yoshino-Shoji total condylar CS	n.s.	Prospective	35	2	23	29	48	Routine resurfacing not advisable
Enis et al (1990)[84]	Townley	Dome, metal-backed	Prospective	20	3.3	45	15	40	Better pain relief with resurfacing
Levitsky et al (1993)[178]	n.s	n.s.	Retrospective	13	7.5	46	8	46	Patellar retention acceptable if selection criteria applied
Keblish et al (1994)[161]	LCS RP	Anatomic RP	Prospective	30	5.2	30	23	47	Patellar retention acceptable with patella-friendly implant
Barrack et al (2001)[19]	MG-II CR	Modified dome	Randomized	23	5	21	29	50	Anterior knee pain unrelated to patellar resurfacing
Waters and Bentley (2003)[320]	PFC CR/CS	Dome	Randomized	35	5.3	51	11	37	Patellar resurfacing preferred
Peng et al (2003)[225]	NexGen/MG-II	Dome	Prospective	35	3.2	28	26	46	No difference
Burnett et al (2007)[47]	MG-II CR	Modified dome	Randomized	32	10	37	22	41	Equivalent clinical results
Smith et al (2008)[279]	Profix	Dome (inlay)	Randomized	16	4.4	—	—	100	No benefit of patellar resurfacing over nonresurfacing
Total				239	5.1	31	18	51	

CR, Cruciate-retaining; *CS,* cruciate-sacrificing; *LCS,* low-contact stress; *MG,* Miller-Galante; *NR,* nonresurfaced; *n.s.,* not specified; *PCA,* porous-coated anatomic; *PFC,* press-fit condylar; *PS,* posterior-stabilized; *RP,* rotating platform; *RS,* resurfaced.

unresurfaced and 2.3% in resurfaced patellae. Overall, seven studies were unable to define a clinically significant difference between resurfacing and nonresurfacing in patients' function and their perception of pain,* two studies showed slight preference toward nonresurfacing[89,90] and, in five studies, resurfacing appeared superior over nonresurfacing.[106,222,262,320,330]

Some of these studies have examined knee function in more detail by assessing the patient's ability to climb stairs. Bourne and associates,[34] who devised a 30-second stair-climbing test, found no statistically significant difference at 2-year follow-up between patients with and without patellar resurfacing. The same group of patients was again reviewed at 10 years, by which time those with patella resurfacing climbed on average 20 stairs compared with 31 stairs in the nonresurfaced group, a difference that reached statistical significance.[46] Similar findings were reported by Feller and associates,[89] who found that stair-climbing ability in the nonresurfaced patient group was significantly better compared with those with patellar resurfacing. Two RCTs found no significant difference regarding the performance of functional tasks between resurfaced and nonresurfaced patients,[105,279] whereas two other RCTs showed a trend toward increased pain with stair ascent and descent if the patella was left unresurfaced, although values did not reach statistical significance.[52,330]

Two randomized, controlled biomechanical studies looked at functional range of movement and walking gait pattern.[208,278] Both studies were unable to find any clinically relevant differences between resurfaced and nonresurfaced knees, but highlighted discrepancies in kinematics compared with normal individuals.

Bilateral Studies

Nine studies represent a comparative assessment of patients who received bilateral total knee arthroplasties with patellar resurfacing performed on one side only (Table 113-3).* A meta-analysis of these studies revealed a total of 239 patients followed up for 2 to 10 years (average, 5.1 years). In all studies, satisfaction was assessed by asking patients which knee they prefer. The resurfaced side was favored by 31% of patients, the nonresurfaced side was favored by 18%, and 51% expressed no preference for either knee.

Outlook

The orthopedic community is deeply divided regarding the issue of patellar resurfacing, and the argument for or against patellar resurfacing remains unresolved. Opponents of resurfacing contend that the native patella provides better patellar tracking, improved clinical function, and avoids implant-related complications, whereas proponents of resurfacing argue that patients have less pain, are overall more satisfied, and the need for secondary resurfacing is avoided.

*References 19, 46-48, 52, 208, and 279.

*References 19, 47, 84, 161, 178, 225, 274, 279, and 320.

Clinicians have to weigh the possible risk of secondary patellar resurfacing for anterior pain against an increased probability of complications arising from patellar resurfacing, such as patellar component wear, loosening, infection, and fracture.

The literature can be confusing because it provides evidence to support both sides of the argument. Recent evidence-based research and meta-analyses have failed to draw clear conclusions and therefore have been unable to provide clinicians with specific guidance.[50,202] Symptoms originating from the patellofemoral joint following knee arthroplasty are rarely severe enough to justify revision but may be sufficient to spoil an otherwise satisfactory result. Our knowledge of indicators that would reliably identify those patients who may develop AKP and how best to treat them to avoid dissatisfaction remains deficient. Selective resurfacing has been suggested as a possible compromise but evidence regarding the validity of selection criteria remains elusive, and the decision when to resurface is often based on intuitive reasoning alone.

Awareness of the importance of proper component alignment and the effects of malpositioning on the PFJ are paramount in achieving long-term success, regardless as to whether the patella is resurfaced or not. Surgical technique and implant design have been unequivocally identified as major factors in influencing clinical outcome. Their improvements have further reduced the incidence of AKP and patella-related complications. However, too many questions remain unanswered, and it appears that we are still a long way from an unambiguous agreement on best practice with regard to patellar resurfacing. Until then, it may be tempting to follow the advice of the Roman poet Ovid who, in 20 BC, said, *"In medio tutissimus ibis,"* meaning "he who will be safest may take the middle ground."

KEY REFERENCES

Barrack RL, Bertot AJ, Wolfe MW, et al: Patellar resurfacing in total knee arthroplasty: a prospective randomised double blinded study with five to seven years of follow-up. J Bone Joint Surg Am 83:1376–1381, 2001.

Berger RA, Crossett LS, Jacobs JJ, Rubash HE: Malrotation causing patellofemoral complications after total knee arthroplasty. Clin Orthop Relat Res 356:144–153, 1998.

Berry DJ, Rand JA: Isolated patellar component revision of total knee arthroplasty. Clin Orthop Relat Res 286:110–115, 1993.

Bourne RB, Burnett RSJ: The consequences of not resurfacing the patella. Clin Orthop Relat Res 428:166–169, 2004.

Burnett RS, Bourne RB: Indications for patellar resurfacing in total knee arthroplasty. Instr Course Lect 53:167–186, 2004.

Burnett RSJ, Boone JL, Rosenzweig SD, et al: Patellar resurfacing compared with nonresurfacing in total knee arthroplasty. A concise follow-up of a randomized trial. J Bone Joint Surg Am 91:2562–2567, 2009.

Calvisi V, Camillieri G, Luparelli S: Resurfacing versus nonresurfacing the patella in total knee arthroplasty: a critical appraisal of the available evidence. Arch Orthop Trauma Surg 129:1261–1270, 2009.

Campbell DG, Duncan WW, Ashworth M, et al: Patellar resurfacing in total knee arthroplasty: a ten year randomised prospective trial. J Bone Joint Surg Br 88:734–739, 2006.

Collier JP, McNamara JL, Suprenant VA, et al: All-polyethylene components are not the answer. Clin Orthop Relat Res 273:198–203, 1991.

D'Lima D, Chen PC, Kester MA, Colwell Jr, CW: Impact on patellofemoral design on patellofemoral forces and polyethylene stresses. J Bone Joint Surg Am 85:85–93, 2003.

Elbert K, Bartel D, Wright T: The effect of conformity on stresses in dome-shaped polyethylene patellar components. Clin Orthop Relat Res 317:71–75, 1995.

Hsu H-P, Walker PS: Wear and deformation of patellar components in total knee arthroplasty. Clin Orthop Relat Res 246:260–265, 1989.

Kim BS, Reitman RD, Schai PA, Scott RD: Selective patellar nonresurfacing in total knee arthroplasty. 10-year results. Clin Orthop Relat Res 367:81–88, 1999.

McNamara JL, Collier JP, Mayor MB, Jensen RE: A comparison of contact pressures in tibial and patellar total knee components before and after service in vivo. Clin Orthop Relat Res 299:104–113, 1994.

Meding JB, Fish MD, Berend ME, et al: Predicting patellar failure after total knee arthroplasty. Clin Orthop Relat Res 466:2769–2774, 2008.

Meneghini RM: Should the patella be resurfaced in primary total knee arthroplasty? An evidence-based analysis. J Arthroplasty 23(Suppl 1):11–14:2008.

Morra EA, Greenwald AS: Patello-femoral replacement polymer stress during daily activities: a finite element study. J Bone Joint Surg Am 88:213–216, 2006.

Ortiguera CJ, Berry DJ: Patellar fracture after total knee arthroplasty. J Bone Joint Surg Am 84:532–540, 2002.

Pagnano MW: Patellar tendon and quadriceps tendon tears after total knee arthroplasty. J Knee Surg 16:242–247, 2003.

Rand JA: Current concept review: the patellofemoral joint in total knee arthroplasty. J Bone Joint Surg Am 76:612–620, 1994.

Rand JA: Extensor mechanism complications following total knee arthroplasty. J Bone Joint Surg Am 86:2062–2072, 2004.

Rhoads DD, Nobel PC, Reuben JD, et al: The effect of femoral component position on patella tracking after total knee arthroplasty. Clin Orthop Relat Res 260:43–51, 1990.

Sheth NP, Pedowitz DI, Lonner JH: Current concepts review. Periprosthetic patellar fracture. J Bone Joint Surg Am 89:2285–2296, 2007.

Smith AJ, Wood DJ, Li M-G: Total knee replacement with and without patellar resurfacing: a prospective randomised trial using the Profix total knee system. J Bone Joint Surg Br 90:43–49, 2008.

Steubben CM, Postak PD, Greenwald AS: Mechanical characteristics of patellofemoral replacements. Presented at the 43rd Annual Meeting of the American Academy of Orthopaedic Surgeons, San Francisco, 1993.

Theiss SM, Kitziger KJ, Lotke PS, Lotke PA: Component design affecting patellofemoral complications after total knee replacement. Clin Orthop Relat Res 326:183–187, 1996.

Yoshii T, Whiteside LA, Anouchi YS: The effect of patella button placement and femoral design on patellar tracking in total knee arthroplasty. Clin Orthop Relat Res 275:211–219, 1992.

Full references for this chapter can be found on www.expertconsult.com.

Chapter 114

Total Knee Arthroplasty—Which Implant Do I Prefer for my Patients? International Roundtable Discussion

Steve Haas, John Callaghan, Bruno Violante, Christopher Hulet,
James B. Stiehl, Aaron G. Rosenberg, Hong Zhang, and Thomas Thornhill

Dr. Rosenberg: Although multiple differing design philosophies have come and gone over the past several decades, in many cases no consensus has been reached as to which features are preferable. There are multiple confounding factors in the comparative evaluation of implants (e.g., function, patient satisfaction, implant longevity, complication rates), as well as the influence of tradition in the implant choices of most surgeons that make comparisons difficult. Why do debates continue on such matters as whether to preserve the posterior cruciate ligament (PCL) in total knee arthroplasty (TKA), so-called cruciate-retaining (CR), or to substitute for it with a posterior-stabilized (PS) knee, to use mobile versus fixed bearings, and to use cemented or cementless fixation?

I think it's important to keep in mind the changes in implant design as well as surgical technique made as a result of evaluating early outcomes, and that for the most part these have led to systematic improvements in the quality and consistency of TKA. The implants we use now are different in important ways from those reported on in most long term follow-up studies. These longer term studies also reflect a significantly different patient population than that currently presenting for knee replacement.[11] Historically, concerns about implant longevity, as well as relatively higher complication rates, along with the fear of early failure, led many surgeons to delay arthroplasty until more advanced disease was present. These advances have given surgeons the confidence to offer knee replacements to younger and less severely affected individuals who were not previously considered sufficiently debilitated or aged to warrant the risk. In the modern era, younger age, larger size, and what were considered high physical activity demands are much more common in all of our practices. Thus, the surgeon must be aware of the fact that data in the literature may reflect both implants and patient types that are not identical to those seen in today's practice. In addition, we are getting better at mobilizing our patients by reducing postoperative pain.[7]

It is my pleasure to have these experienced TKA surgeons gathered from around the world to share their thoughts on contemporary total knee issues with us: Steve Haas, Bruno Violante, Hong Zhang, Christopher Hulet, James Stiehl, and John Callaghan.

Let's start by discussing the evolution of our implant choices. Dr. Callaghan, what is the current TKA of choice in your practice, how did you come to use this particular knee, and how has your thinking evolved?

Dr. Callaghan: I have been in practice for 26 years and, in the first 5, I used posterior CR designs in patients with smaller deformities and PS designs in larger deformities. As time went along, I decided that I could not really make definite cut-offs on when to go from CR to PS, so for standardization and predictability, I went to using posterior-stabilized designs in all patients. It was also during this time that there was

some question about rollback kinematics in CR designs. In addition, with the difficult patient population that I operate on at a state university, I believe it is essential to perform one operation and see how that works in the long term.

We now have 15-year survivorship of the PFC knee (DePuy, Warsaw, Ind) that I have been using and, other than a few infections, most of which were hematogenous, the only failures were related to polyethylene wear. This particular implant had an issue with the polyethylene used in the early to mid-1900s and we and others have reported this. Hence, in summary, I use a posterior-stabilized design because it allows me to feel comfortable that I have provided the best operation for patients with little as well as maximum deformity. I think the survivorship is similar to cruciate-retaining designs of the same brand. I do, however, think that the literature is clouded because of the variance in polyethylenes used in the late 1980s and 1990s. The implant I use allows for fixed- or mobile-bearing options and I have gone to using the mobile-bearing design for 60% of knees.

Dr. Rosenberg: Dr. Stiehl, I know your experience is quite similar.

Dr. Stiehl: My initial experience for over 15 years was with posterior cruciate–retaining implants. Back in the 1980s, I saw numerous implant failures caused by excessive wear, patellar failure, and loss of fixation. I was then heavily influenced by fluoroscopic kinematic studies that I performed beginning in 1992 and subsequently published extensively. My early experience was with a flat-on-flat condylar design that used radiation-sterilized polyethylene.

As I learned more about the deleterious effects of sliding and ploughing wear on polyethylene surfaces, kinematic issues such as poor femoral condylar rollback in many patients, and femoral condylar liftoff with activity, I began to use a posterior cruciate–sacrificing mobile-bearing implant. These implants seemed immune to these problems from long-term studies, and typically offered higher ranges of motion with activity.

Following my early kinematic studies, I sought methods, such as flexion ligament balancing, that appeared to limit the problems of instability and wear that were often seen with posterior cruciate–retaining, fixed-bearing knees implanted with measured resection methods. I remember a brief conversation with one of the prominent originators of posterior cruciate–retaining implants when I asked if he had seen significant laxity in the lateral compartment in deep flexion. He explained that he witnessed that phenomenon commonly but never recognized a clinical problem with it. He may be correct in his answer to this day, but the kinematics that I could demonstrate on weight-bearing fluoroscopy were truly scary (Fig. 114-1).

Dr. Rosenberg: Dr. Zhang, isn't your experience affected by implant availability?

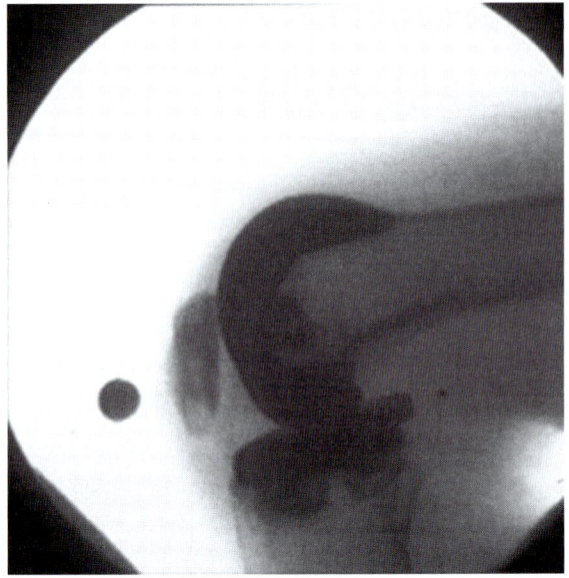

Figure 114-1. Lateral fluoroscopic image of a total knee in maximum flexion. Note the degree to which one of the femoral condyles has lifted off from the tibia.

Dr. Zhang: Because there are almost no CR implants available in China, almost all implants I have used are PS fixed or mobile bearing. However, I have had the chance to use different knee implants from different companies. I have used Innex (Zimmer, Winterthur, Switzerland), Insall-Burstein II (IB II, Zimmer, Warsaw, Ind), NexGen LPS and LPS-flex II (Zimmer), Scorpio and NRG (Stryker, Mahwah, NJ), LCS, PFC, PFC-RP, and PFC-RPF (DePuy, Warsaw Ind), and Genesis-II (Smith & Nephew, Memphis, Tenn). In China knee arthroplasty, surgery has only become popular in the past 5 years; in 2001, our department did 55 total knees, but last year we did almost 1000. Although I can't report on longevity and survivorship, in my experience different implants have shown different function and outcomes.

Dr. Rosenberg: Dr. Violante, I remember going to Italy 20 years ago and was struck by the state of the art in TKA, clearly somewhat behind the United States. But, what a difference 2 decades have made!

Dr. Violante: The story of the TKA in Europe is quite different than that in North America. Despite the popularity of total hip arthroplasty in the 1980s and 1990s, there was a lack of acceptance of total knee arthroplasty. During that period, proximal tibial osteotomy was the standard treatment for knee osteoarthritis. The most common indications for a total knee were failed osteotomies or real disasters in terms of deformity and function.

In the early 1990s, I started with a CR design (Genesis, Smith & Nephew), which required managing the PCL, which might be loose, tight, or appropriately balanced. Loose was more desirable in the presence of an optimal flexion space, but a tight PCL led to bad outcomes with lack of flexion, pain, and early tibial loosening.

Because of this early experience and looking more to the anatomy of the knee, I shifted toward a PS design (IB II, Zimmer) to eliminate the PCL management problem and to work on a more easily reproduced surgical technique and more reliable outcomes. So, from the early 1990s I used the

IB II and in 1997, switched to the LPS NexGen Legacy (Zimmer), also designed by John Insall.

Dr. Rosenberg: Dr. Violante, like Dr. Callaghan and Dr. Stiehl, made the move from CR to PS. Dr. Hulet, what has been your experience?

Dr. Hulet: In the early 1980s and 1990s, we used the IB II knee system and the Kinemax knee. But, in 1994, we developed a new prosthesis in France, which was called the Jade TR prosthesis (Howmedica [Stryker Orthopaedics], Mahwah, NJ). It was a complete system with the PCL either sacrificed or retained. There was also a revision system with stems and wedges. We do not resurface the patella in our practice. The trochlear design accommodates the shape of the patella and the needed posterior translation during knee flexion.

Dr. Rosenberg: Dr. Hulet, I think this is an important point that most knee systems have both CR and PS implants but, Dr. Haas, you have some experience with bicruciate-substituting knee design.

Dr. Haas: For many years, I used the Genesis II knee system (Smith & Nephew). This system provided excellent results. I have used primarily the high-flexion version of the Genesis II posterior-stabilized knee. This provided excellent clinical results. However, as more of my patients were doing higher levels of activity, such as tennis, skiing, and competitive golf, I wanted to have a knee arthroplasty that would provide normal rotational motions of the knee in addition to high flexion. I currently choose to use the Journey Knee (Smith & Nephew) as my main implant of choice. I use this system because my practice involves a large number of younger active patients. Many of the features of the Genesis II system were incorporated into the Journey Knee and this system restores near-normal kinematics and allows for a high level of function.

Dr. Rosenberg: My own experience has been primarily with cruciate-retaining arthroplasty. Early on I used the Miller-Galante I (Zimmer) with both cemented and cementless fixation but found that although my cemented implants almost never loosened, my cementless tibias failed to obtain ingrowth at about a 3% rate.[17] I subsequently began cementing everyone by the late 1980s and, at longer term follow-up, the cementless cohort had loosenings of the tibial component that the cemented components just did not have.[4] The implant had a unique tibial component that featured four small pegs and had no conventional keel. Although our initial experience demonstrated a high rate of metal-backed patellar failures,[16] wear, lysis, and component loosening have ever been an issue, even in our long-term follow-up of that implant.[5] The lessons learned from that experience led to the MG II (Zimmer), which featured a deepened trochlear sulcus, all-polyethylene patella of improved design, and minor modifications of the articular surface configuration of the polyethylene in the sagittal plane.

We have not yet talked much about fixed versus mobile bearings. Dr. Stiehl, I know that you have done a lot of research and given a lot of thought to this.

Dr. Stiehl: I would state categorically that I now use mobile bearings in all primary patients and in virtually all settings. This choice is then divided into two groups. For patients who I consider at high risk for long-term wear problems and loss of fixation, I will perform the classic LCS (DePuy), posterior cruciate–sacrificing or rotating platform mobile-bearing, usually without resurfacing of the patella. Specifically, those patients are under 65, desiring a normal functional outcome, with the ability to perform many sports including tennis, golf, snow skiing, horseback riding, power walking, and moderate lifting in occupational settings. The second group consists of patients who are at lower risk for long-term failure including most patients over 65 or those with severe bone loss or pre-operative deformities with loss of motion. These patients generally desire to decrease pain, improve motion, and kneel without restriction. This group receives the Nexgen LPS High Flex (Zimmer), a mobile-bearing posterior cruciate–stabilized design, often without resurfacing of the patella. These patients are told that they may accomplish very high range of motion and have a higher likelihood of feeling normal on stairs than with other choices.

Dr. Rosenberg: I think the whole issue of mobile bearings is an interesting one, but my impression is that there are no published data, at least at intermediate follow-up, that show lower revision rates, better function, or longevity. So, where are the advantages?

Dr. Stiehl: I believe that mobile bearings offer two very notable features that enhance the potential outcome. First, I am convinced that the bearing surfaces have better wear performance with higher surface contact. The high contact forces seen with limited surface contact were indigenous to flat-on-flat designs. This idea is supported by numerous wear studies and observations made from large numbers of implant retrievals.

Second, the problem of tibial tray malrotation on implantation is eliminated with mobile bearings.[22] The knee has the normal function of tibial internal rotation that occurs with flexion. This can be distorted or eliminated in the diseased state. Combined with anatomic variation, there are few reliable landmarks that predict the position of the tibial base plate position in all comers. Add the challenge of placing a tibial tray correctly through smaller surgical incisions that have become the fashion of the day, and you have a problem that cannot be eliminated, even with the experiences of several thousand total joint procedures.

Mobile-bearing polyethylene adds an important safety factor, in my view. I recently published my retrospective experience evaluating preoperative and postoperative tibial rotation measured with computer navigation, and found that fixed trays tended to be more internally placed and had less internal rotation with flexion compared with the mobile-bearing knees.[22]

Dr. Rosenberg: Dr. Zhang, is the mobile bearing harder to implant?

Dr. Zhang: Whether or not an implant is easy to put in depends on the surgeon's surgical experience and the implantation equipment. Most PS prostheses are easy to put in if the manufacturer's instructions and surgical steps are followed. However, it is a little more complicated to achieve a good balance of the soft tissue and prosthesis stability for mobile-bearing implantation, such as LCS or Innex. The learning curve is longer for mobile-bearing TKA.

Dr. Stiehl: Mobile-bearing implants do have the notorious clinical experience of bearing spin-out or dislocation if the prosthetic ligament balancing is not adequate (Fig. 114-2). Both implants that I use are particularly stable if a reasonable surgical technique is performed and I can confess not one single bearing dislocation with 15 years of clinical

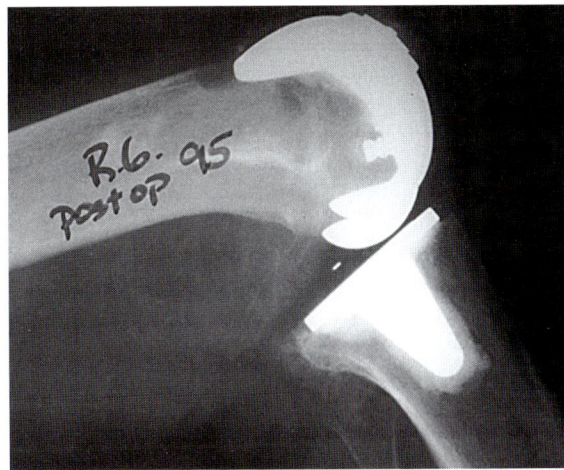

Figure 114-2. Lateral radiograph of a mobile-bearing total knee with a dislocated bearing. Note the lateral view of the femoral component abutting the dislocated polyethylene just posterior to it.

experience. Early on, I avoided mobile bearings in valgus deformities over 20 degrees and, in some severe varus deformities, deferred to a fixed-bearing, posterior-stabilized device, as would be done in total knee revision arthroplasties. Today, I would use the LCS (DePuy) mobile rotating platform or the LPS High Flex mobile (Zimmer) with impunity in any primary total knee setting. The LPS actually has a spin-out stop to limit rotation over 20 degrees in one plane and might be safer for the community surgeon.

I would stongly discourage surgeons from using a measured resection method with a mobile-bearing device. Although measured resection may work in straight forward cases with little deformity, it will fail if there is poor ligament balancing after correction of marked deformity or bone defect and the gaps are not appropriately matched. Mobile-bearing implants are not for the occasional knee surgeon, but more appropriate for the engaged surgeon who is willing to learn from experienced technicians, as I did with my first few.

Dr. Rosenberg: Dr. Callaghan, are you wedded to fixed or mobile bearings in the majority of your primary knees?

Dr. Callaghan: One of the specific advantages of the current implant I use is the fact that I can use a fixed-bearing or mobile-bearing option. In addition, the fixed-bearing option has a polished tray, which I believe has the potential benefit of decreasing backside wear. However, this has never been proven in the literature. It also allows for using a more constrained component. The mobile-bearing design allows for more conformity of the polyethylene to the femoral component, with potential for decreasing wear. This is why I use it in the younger patients instead of the fixed-bearing design, which is not as conforming.

Being as it allows for both fixed bearing as well as mobile bearing the implant I use allows for much versatility. In patients with large valgus deformities, I am a little more apt to use the fixed-bearing design as well as in cases that have tremendous range of motion—that is, more than 140 degrees as I would imagine the patient's femoral runners run past the tibial inserts which are only designed to obtain 120 degrees of flexion.

Dr. Rosenberg: What about bearing spin-out? Dr. Callaghan, have you had any experience with this phenomenon?

Dr. Callaghan: Although I have not had a bearing spin-out with a PS component, it still is a concern with mobile-bearing knees. The capability of the system that I use allows the surgeon to use constraint, whether it be a fixed or mobile bearing. This helps me in the consideration of which of these two implants I use. In a younger patient, if I am going to use constraint, I will tend to use a mobile-bearing design, which I hope will lead to less issues with loosening of the implants.

I have personally reviewed minimum 20-year follow-ups of mobile-bearing designs, performed with polyethylene gamma-irradiated in air, and have seen no loosening over that period. Although the average age of the patients at the time of surgery was 70 years old, I have gained more confidence in believing that these devices have potential for greater long-term durability in the most kinematically challenging patients.

Dr. Rosenberg: Dr. Violante, please tell us what you believe to be the specific advantages of the current implant you use and how its design features compare with previous implants you used.

Dr. Violante: With the exception of the post-cam mechanism, the difference between the IB II (Zimmer) and the LPS NexGen Legacy (Zimmer) is substantial. With the IB II, patellar clunk, caused by the soft tissue impingement between the infrapatellar scar and the femoral trochlea–box junction during flexion, was seen occasionally.[15] With the LPS NexGen, asymmetrical femoral components were introduced and, along with this, changes in the patellofemoral geometry with a deeper and prolonged trochlear groove, obliquely oriented by 7 degrees, and smoother transition of the distal femoral condylar geometry to achieve better patellar tracking, patellofemoral kinematics, and reduced patellar clunk.[10] More femoral component sizes and more accurate shaping of the native femur also helped reduce patellofemoral overstuffing.

The polyethylene tibial fixation was subject to micromovements, with subsequent backside polyethylene wear as a cause of tibia lysis in the IB II. In the NexGen Legacy, the polyethylene was compression-molded and gamma-sterilized in inert gas and the polyethylene locking mechanism was reinforced with a posterior dovetail mechanism and peripheral anterior compression.

The cam and post mechanism was also optimized to reduce the risk of posterior dislocation and was moved posteriorly so that the cam engages the post at 75 degrees. High-flexion, specific design geometry variations were made so the patient could safely bend up to 155 degrees.[19,20]

Dr. Rosenberg: I was involved with the development of the same system (NexGen) but focused on the cruciate-retaining side. We were building on the improved results we had experienced going from the Miller-Galante I to the Miller-Galante II (Zimmer) and after having developed a lot of confidence in PCL retention at that point in time. The results with PCL retention in the MG II appeared to be much better than those reported for multiple other devices. Thus, the NexGen CR retained the kinematic advantages we thought were inherent in the shape of the femoral and tibial articulating surfaces but added a lot of attractive design features related to component sizing, matching, and deepening of the trochlea to improve patellofemoral kinematics, and to other features.

Over time, we made modifications to the implant by creating the Flex design, which allowed for more precise tensioning of the PCL by introducing a larger number of anteroposterior sized implants, and then the Gender design, which allowed for better overall femoral component size matching, medially and laterally, to the individual patient. However, it was particularly gratifying when the kinematic studies that Dr. Stiehl had helped develop demonstrated that our implant design actually produced normal-appearing femoral rollback and minimized liftoff, in comparison to all the other CR designs that Dennis and colleagues[12] had tested.

Dr. Stiehl, what are the distinguishing features of your current implant choice?

Dr. Stiehl: My choice of the DePuy LCS Mobile and the NexGen LPS High Flex Mobile relies on two specific advantages that I perceive to have guided my overall technical approach. I believe that the mobile feature allows for dramatically increased articulation surface areas over older flat-on-flat designs that arose in my early years and were developed with posterior cruciate–retaining methods. The original predicted advantage of mobile-bearing devices was decreased wear, which was based on diminished contact surface forces that may be exaggerated by sliding and ploughing point contact. What I find ironic is that my current choices were conceived and perfected well before these interim devices, and are now emerging as contemporary replacements of those improved options.

The second important advantage is the ability to correct errors with tibial tray placement in terms of rotational position because the device self-corrects with final ligament tension. I have studied this problem extensively with computer navigation and believe that the tibial tray position for a given patient is highly variable and can be affected by anatomic variation, degree of arthritic deformity, and surgical technique.

Dr. Rosenberg: Dr. Zhang, you have used a lot of different implants. What are your particular findings?

Dr. Zhang: I am very interested in bone conservation. The Scorpio, NRG, LCS, and Innex remove very little bone when shaping the femoral intracondylar box whereas the PFC and PFC-RP require removal of a bigger piece of bone. The difference is significant.

Dr. Hulet: The Jade system TKA can be used with PS constraint or PCL retention. It features a molded polyethylene (PE) insert with curved geometry for the femoral component. The tibial component theoretically allows for normal femoral rollback. The geometry and dimensions of the femoral component reproduce the normal femur based on a medial pivot design with a single radius curve for the femoral condyle. The geometry of the femoral component should restore normal kinematics and also reproduce normal ligament tension in both extension and flexion. The tibial tray is flat and the PE insert needs to be compatible with femoral rollback (curved-on-curved). The PE insert in both designs is symmetrical, such as the design of the femoral condyles for both the PCL-substituting or PCL-retaining version. We used cement fixation for both components.

Dr. Haas: The Journey system concept is fundamentally a resurfacing-type arthroplasty with a completely left- and right-sided anatomically shaped femur, with medial distal and posterior condyles 2 mm thicker than the lateral distal and posterior condyles. The anterior flange is also thinner medially and thicker laterally because the implant is placed in external rotation. The tibia is similarly asymmetrical to mimic the thickness and shape of the cut bone and reproduce the natural shape of the tibia. These features allow more consistent joint line restoration and result in less tension in the patellofemoral articulation.

The tibial base plate is also asymmetrical. It allows increased tibial coverage and leads to more accurate rotational alignment. The anatomic shape of the base plate also helps avoid posterolateral overhang, which makes minimally invasive insertion easier. Although there is high coronal conformity medially and laterally, the sagittal conformity is greater on the medial tibial plateau compared to the lateral tibial plateau. This differential geometry helps promote more natural rotational motions with a screw-home mechanism in extension and lateral rollback in flexion.

Dr. Rosenberg: Dr. Violante, what sort of clinical results are available on the Nex Gen LPS?

Dr. Violante: There are as yet no long-term published follow-up data on function, outcomes, longevity, and radiographs but at up to 6-year follow the LPS NexGen showed better results than the IB II. In an early series of 279 knees from August 1997 to December 1998, all made by senior surgeons (Drs. Insall, Scott, and Scuderi), with a mean follow-up of 48 months, the mean Knee Society score for 238 knees was 96 points at the latest follow-up, with no case of patellar clunk, maltracking, or posterior dislocation. There was no radiographic evidence of loosening or osteolysis and no revisions performed or recommended for loosening, osteolysis, instability, or PE wear. Some radiographic evidence of radiolucent lines no larger than 1 mm located at the tibial component in zone 1 was observed in about 4% of cases not associated with any clinical symptoms.[10]

Dr. Rosenberg: That certainly seems acceptable! Our own results with the NexGen CR at 10-year minimum follow-up[18] have been published on a cohort of 161 patients with 179 cemented TKAs in whom the patella was resurfaced; we had originally reported on them at 5 years.[6] Of these, 40 patients had died and 8 were lost, leaving 113 patients with 126 knees. Survivorship at a minimum of 10 years, using revision for any reason, was 98% and, with revision for aseptic loosening, it was 100%. Three knees were revised—one each for infection, periprosthetic fracture, and arthrofibrosis. There were no r-operations for patellar component problems or wear and neither lysis nor aseptic loosening were seen. Interestingly, both the Australian and Swedish arthroplasty registry seem to confirm these findings, noting the lowest cumulative revision rates for this implant in both countries.

Dr. Hulet, what about the Jade system?

Dr. Hulet: We began to use this design in 1996 and recently at the last Effort (European Federation) Meeting in Nice, in 2008; we have published the results of our first 122 cases with 10-year follow-up.[1] These were cemented PCL-sparing, with the patella resurfaced in only eight cases. No reoperation was performed for patellar pain. There were no early complications. The mean Knee Society score was 90 points, with mean motion of 109 degrees. The mean Knee Society function score was 85 points, with survival of 95% at 9.5 years (Kaplan-Meier method), considering all reasons for removal, and 99.4% for removal for aseptic loosening.

Dr. Rosenberg: Dr. Haas, what sort of results have been reported with the Journey knee?

Dr. Haas: Victor and Ries have recently reported excellent clinical results in the Journey knee, with a 30-degree improvement in average range of motion. In addition, in vivo kinematic evaluations have shown consistent and reproducible flexion and rotational motions. Komistek has performed several in vivo two- and three-dimensional fluoroscopic studies and has shown that patients with Journey BCS TKA "consistently experience kinematic patterns similar to that of the normal knee." Studies by Komestek and Catani have shown a normal pattern of knee rotation without significant paradoxical anterior sliding commonly seen in TKA. Greenwald has performed a kinematic analysis of several contemporary TKA designs and found that " the Journey most closely replicated the healthy un-operated knee kinematics."

Dr. Rosenberg: I am consistently intrigued by reports of TKA without patellar resurfacing; to me this seems more like a hemiarthroplasty at the patellofemoral joint. We have a great deal of experience with hemiarthroplasty at other joints and the results are consistently inferior to what Charnley has demonstrated at the hip and has also been found in most other joints. That is, replacing both sides of the articulation generally results in better pain relief and function than replacing only one side of the joint and letting it articulate with native cartilage or what remains of it.

Dr. Stiehl: I believe that mobile-bearing devices optimize the patellofemoral articulation. This is a controversial problem and there are numerous conflicting ideas about how to manage the patella in total knees. In favor of the mobile-bearing method is that flexion gap balance must be very precise and anatomic, close to the normal 2 to 3 mm. I believe that this will optimize the patellar tracking as the knee goes into deep flexion.[21] A number of authors, including myself, have minimized the problem of abnormal femoral rotation that could occur by using flexion-based tensor instruments (Figs. 114-3 and 114-4).

However, I must add that late pain and arthrofibrosis remain concerns. I published a study on the occurrence of arthrofibrosis in mobile LCS knees in which there was exaggerated femoral component internal rotation in the coronal

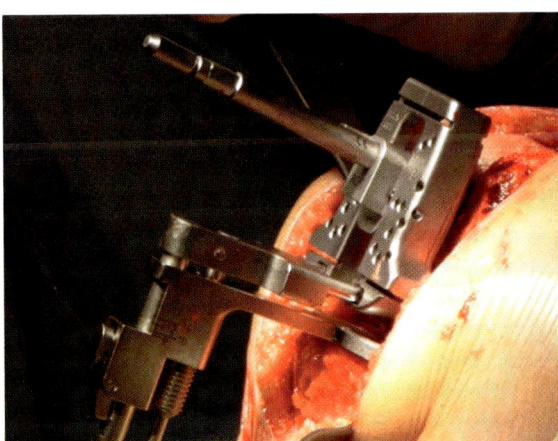

Figure 114-3. Lateral view of the tensioning device used to create a rectangular flexion gap. The device rests on the cut surface of the proximal tibia.

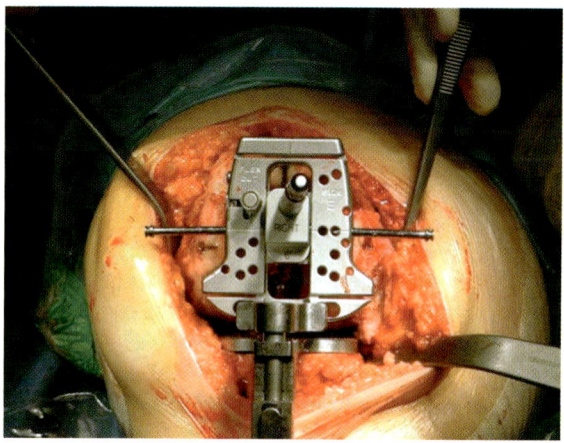

Figure 114-4. AP view of the tensioning device seen in Figure 114-3. Outrigger pins are used to check anterior and posterior femoral cut alignment, which controls femoral rotation, with reference to the epicondyles of the femur.

plane.[8] On the other hand, the international experience with the LCS has been that patellar implant failures are very rare and most LCS surgeons, including myself, have moved away from patellar resurfacing in most cases, except if there is inflammatory arthritis, severe patellar bone loss, or the workmen's compensation knee problem. Although abnormal femoral component rotation may exacerbate patellar problems, I believe functional laxity problems in the lateral compartment in flexion that result from posterior cruciate–retaining techniques are much more problematic.

Finally, for cases with exposed cartilage and advanced chondromalacia determined at the time of surgery, my choice of patellar resurfacing is the dome patella, but most other patients are unresurfaced. All patients who are likely to have no patellar resurfacing are asked preoperatively if they want to be able to kneel and have no restrictions on deep knee bends. I explain my implant choices with reference to the extensive documented experience without patellar resurfacing in the orthopedic surgery literature, and that I keep the option for patellar resurfacing if problems develop after surgery.

Dr. Rosenberg: Dr. Zhang, what is your experience in China?

Dr. Zhang: Because I do not replace the patella in most patients, I find that patellar clunk is rare. I have had only one patient receiving arthroscopic treatment to solve this problem. However, patellar crepitus is a common phenomenon in some prostheses and is very prosthesis-dependent. Scorpio and PFC are the prostheses that seem to cause more crepitus, in my experience. In extreme cases, you can hear the crepitus even from a distance. LCS and LPS are the least problematic from this point. However, even with crepitus, patients usually do not complain of anterior knee pain. The patellofemoral articulation of NexGen, LCS, and Genesis II prostheses are more smooth and congruent, and they have distinguished advantage in my experience compared with other prostheses. Up to now I have seen no severe anterior knee pain cases that need further patellar replacement surgery. Now, if I choose the Scorpio or PFC, I will replace the patella.

Dr. Rosenberg: Dr. Callaghan, where do you stand on patellar resurfacing?

Dr. Callaghan: I do resurface all my patellas with a domed patella. I think that the dome patella with a larger superior-inferior distance may help in diminishing the patella grind that is seen with posterior cruciate–substituting designs. I also use the largest size patella component that the patellar bone can accommodate. I think this may have also decreased my incidence of crepitance.

Dr. Rosenberg: Dr. Violante, I know that leaving the patella unresurfaced is much more common in Europe.

Dr. Violante: A big advantage of the LPS NexGen compared with the IB II consists of the freedom of patellar management. In Europe, the unresurfaced patella technique is a very strong philosophy and the LPS NexGen has an excellent femoral trochlea to accommodate the native patella. I've therefore been changing my patellar management, shifting from 100% patellar resurfacing with the IB II to 40% with the LPS NexGen. I resurface the patella only in the presence of patellar maltracking or predominant patellofemoral joint (PFJ) disease. The LPS NexGen also gives me the opportunity to use a high-flexion design with an extended radius of the posterior femur condyles, which increases the passive and weight-bearing flexion.

Dr. Rosenberg: I know that in my practice the specifics of surgical technique have evolved significantly, and I think we all would agree that rather than implant design, surgical technique is more important in influencing short-term success. Dr. Hulet, how do you visualize implantation of the knee?

Dr. Hulet: There are three gaps to consider in TKA—the anterior gap (the patellofemoral joint), the femorotibial gap in extension, and the femorotibial gap in flexion. They should be all rectangular with good ligament tension to allow good range of motion with stability in extension and also in flexion to avoid liftoff. This is a more functional than anatomic approach and is gap-based, rather than the measured resection technique developed by Hungerford.

The Jade system TKA is a prosthesis with the bone cut made in an adequate soft tissue envelope. This is achieved with a ligament tensor and depends on cuts in flexion but not in extension, while allowing for a compromise between mobility and stability.

Dr. Stiehl: I also have become a strong proponent of flexion-based tensor methods as the best option for recreating optimized knee kinematics after total knee replacement. Again, this method was Insall's early approach, but required that all ligament balancing be done in extension before any bone cuts were made. The method was used originally for posterior cruciate–sacrificing and posterior-stabilized implants, but actually has been done successfully with posterior cruciate– and bicruciate-retaining methods.

Of historical note, this approach went out of favor with the introduction of femoral measured resection methods that were favored by posterior cruciate–retaining surgeons. Those surgeons focused on the bone cuts to achieve optimum alignment and kinematics, using ligament balancing as finishing step to get the desired result. For the mobile-bearing surgeon, perfect gap balance in flexion is the end game. This is because so many bad things happen if flexion balancing is not perfect.[23]

Dr. Callaghan: I am actually not big on using any specific instruments. As long as I have a tibial cutting jig to give me a flat surface perpendicular to the tibial shaft, as well as distal femoral cutting jigs that allow me to modify the femoral

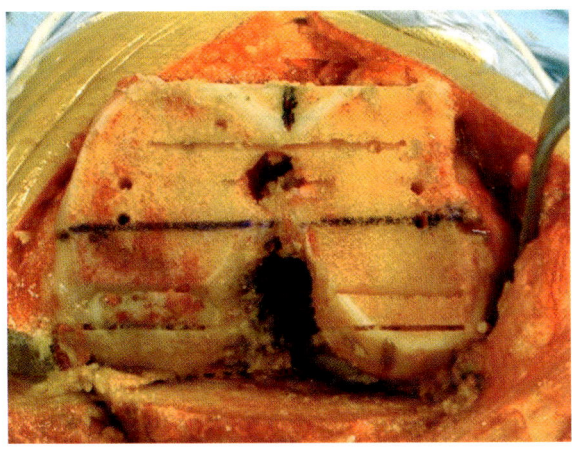

Figure 114-5. Intraoperative view of the previously cut surface of the distal femur. The marker lines in the trochlea remain from the creation of Whiteside's line and the perpendicular drawn in reference to it. Both anterior and posterior chamfer cut lines are visible, as are the relative thicknesses of the bone removed from the medial and lateral aspects of the posterior femoral condyles. See Figures 114-6 and 114-7.

component position, this is all I really need other than anterior-posterior and chamfer cutting blocks, which I can reference off the anterior aspect of the femur. As far as my surgical procedure, I use a combination of gap balancing and measured resections. I anterior-reference my femoral sizing and I use the epicondyles for rotation.

I start with getting an extension gap and then match the flexion gap to that extension gap. I use the epicondyles (Fig. 114-5) mainly, as well as Whiteside's line, for my femoral rotation and I check my tibial rotation both in extension and flexion using the tibial tubercle as a landmark. I fix all the components with cement.

Dr. Hulet: Understanding technique requires understanding the degree of pathology.[13,14] Thus, preoperative planning with long-extremity x-rays, anteroposterior (AP) and profile views in weight-bearing position, along with stress x-rays to analyze both bony deformity and the soft tissue envelope to determine the degree of laxity of the medial or the lateral side or the extent of ligament contracture, are important. The Société Orthopédique de l'Ouest (SOO) classification described in 2003 by Burdin and myself has four grades, which allow for better understanding of the degree of pathology.

In grade 1, the clinical deformity is reducible and there is no laxity on the convexity of the deformation. This deformity is only caused by bony wear. The prosthesis can be placed in the soft tissue envelope without any difficulties.

In grade 2, the deformity is no longer reducible on the concavity side and shows no laxity on the convex side. A release will be required during surgery to achieve good ligament balancing.

In grade 3, the deformity is reducible on the concave side but laxity on the convex side increases the deformity. There is a symmetrical instability that should be taken care of during the procedure. In a varus knee, this creates difficulties in maintaining the height of the joint line and questions arise regarding the PCL preservation or substitution.

In grade 4, the deformed joint is not reducible. There is contracture on the convex side of the joint associated with ligament laxity on the convex side of the deformed joint.

This is the most complicated situation. TKA is a permanent compromise between alignment, mobility, and stability.

Our instruments create a distal femoral resection perpendicular to the mechanical axis with an intramedullary guide. The bony resection removes the thickness of the femoral component while the tibial resection is perpendicular to the mechanical axis. A rectangular extension gap is thus created with reference to the healthy component. The extension gap should be rectangular. There are then no difficulties and there is no need to release the concave side of the deformity. The PCL can be preserved.

If the gap is trapezoidal (with a longer side on the lateral side in a varus knee or medial side in a valgus knee) appropriate release will be required as necessary. If he is trapezoidal, gap is longer on the lateral side in a varus knee, this situation is more complex and may be tolerated or the medial side could be further released but in this situation a greater space is created. It is also possible to tighten the lateral side. Posterior femoral resection is performed according to femoral component rotation using a combination of ligament tension balancing, Whiteside's line and the epicondylar axis (Figs. 114-6 and 114-7; see Fig. 114-5). Finally, the extension gap should equal the flexion gap.

Dr. Violante: I have progressively reduced my capsular incision and have been reducing joint subluxation, working in more extension to reduce the early postoperative soft tissue inflammatory response. I use a tenser and spacer blocks in the standard way, avoiding any ligament discrepancy or excessive soft tissue lengthening to avoid influencing the joint line.

In 2002, I switched from the femur-first to tibia-first approach. The tibial cut is the classic 90-degree coronal cut, with a sagittal cut of around 5 degrees. The reason I adopted the tibia-first approach is that as a single cut, it is easiest to make and to correct and, once correct, represents the base and the reference point for all future cuts, including creating equal flexion and extension gaps. It also gives information on implant thickness, facilitates estimating the need for soft tissue releases, and facilitates orientation of the transepicondylar axis parallel to the neutrally cut tibia in both flexion and extension, the most important point in balancing a PS knee.

For femoral rotation, I use both bone and soft tissue references (see Fig. 114-5). I like my femoral cuts to show that the transepicondylar line is parallel to the tibial cut and the posterior condylar cut, with more posterior medial condyle resected than posterior lateral condyle (see Fig. 114-6).

Dr. Rosenberg: Dr. Hulet, is there anything different in your technique?

Dr. Hulet: Rotational alignment of the femur requires assessing the distal femoral anatomy and the flexion gap, specifically the condition of the medial soft tissues in varus knees and the lateral soft tissues in valgus knees, to obtain a rectangular flexion gap similar to the extension gap obtained after proximal tibial and distal femoral resection. We do not use the posterior femoral condylar reference frame to perform a symmetrical bone resection. This technique tends to create a trapezoidal flexion gap and also excessive femoral internal rotation. Also, there is large variation in the medial and lateral epicondyles.[24]

So, we use a combination of two methods—the AP femoral axis, also known as Whiteside's line, and a ligament-tensioning technique with an active spacer or tensor. First,

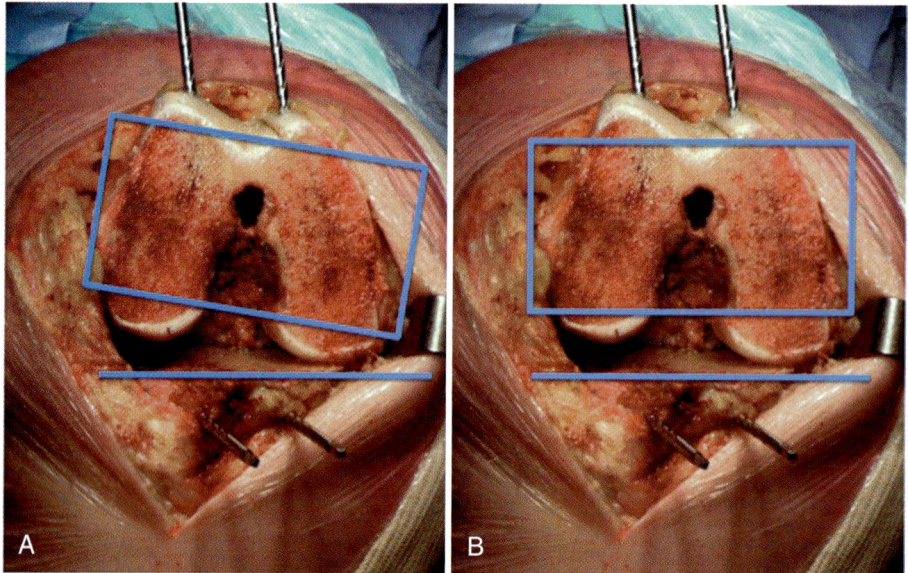

Figure 114-6. Anterior views of the cut surface of the distal femur. **A,** If the collateral ligaments are appropriately balanced, removal of equal bone thickness from the medial and lateral aspects of the posterior femoral condyles will result in the trapezoidal flexion space. This is seen by the blue lines, which represent the cut proximal tibial surface and position of the femoral component adjusted to remove equal bone from the medial and lateral posterior femoral condyles. **B,** Appropriate rotation of the femoral component (in line with the epicondylar axis) results in significantly different amounts of posterior condylar bone removed from the medial and lateral sides.

we check the rectangularity of the extension gap with the tensor. Then, we flex the knee at 90 degrees and increase the lateral gap in flexion below the lateral femoral condyle to produce some external rotation. Ligament symmetry and stability are then tested at 90 degres of flexion to avoid liftoff. In each case, we adapt external femoral rotation from 1 to 5 degrees, depending on the bony anatomy and soft tissue deformity (see Fig. 114-7).

Dr. Rosenberg: Dr. Haas, is there anything different in the way you approach technique as opposed to our international colleagues?

Dr. Haas: My implantation philosophy has changed over the last few decades in that I currently perform minimally invasive surgery on almost all patients. Modern minimally invasive instruments are not only smaller but more anatomically shaped and have facilitated this. Our data show improved range of motion and function during the postoperative period. I am also currently using patient-matched instruments, which allow for preoperative computer planning along with more rapid and efficient surgery. They may also increase accuracy, although this has not been proven at this time.

Dr. Rosenberg: Over the last decade, we have significantly increasesd our understanding of bearing surfaces and how they relate to wear. Essentially, all manufacturers have changed their polyethylene, if not in formulation at least in sterilization techniques. Dr. Stiehl, what is your impression of current bearing surfaces?

Dr. Stiehl: I believe that the two methods that have optimized wear couples currently have been precise machine polishing of chrome cobalt surfaces in mobile bearings and the use of improved polyethylene. These avoid the old sources of failure, such as radiation sterilization and calcium stearate inclusion needed for ram extruding, in favor of ethylene oxide sterilization and compression molding methods. I remain unconvinced regarding the highly cross-linked

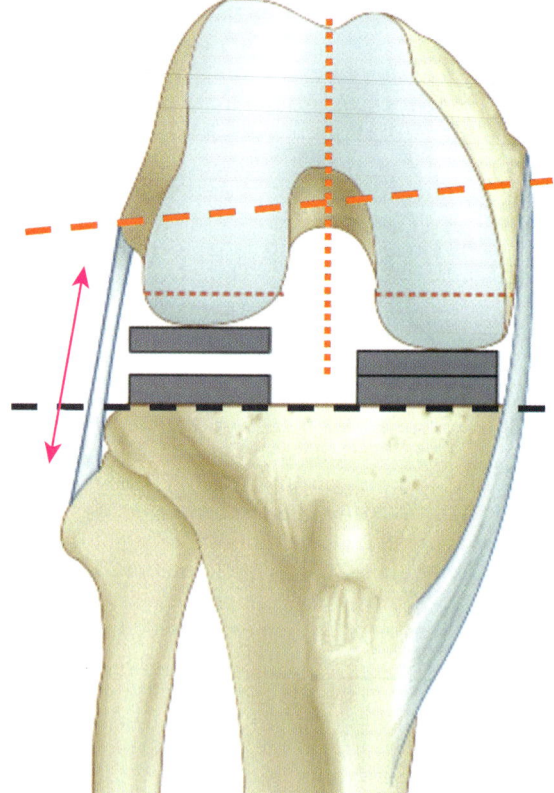

Figure 114-7. Schematic representation of Figure 114-6B, with the tensioning device represented in grey. As seen here, release of the tight lateral structure will allow the femur to rotate (clockwise in this right knee) as the lateral paddles of the tensioner are spread apart. If the cutting block for the femoral component is allowed to rotate freely about the cephalocaudad axis, the posterior condylar bone cuts will produce a rectangular flexion space but will remove unequal amounts of bone from the medial and lateral aspects of the posterior femoral condyles.

polyethylene that may increase implant stiffness as a negative wear factor, although the strength may be better.

Dr. Rosenberg: Dr. Callaghan, you have had experience with good polyethylene and bad.

Dr. Callaghan: I used polyethylene gamma-irradiated in air through the mid-1990s and into the present decade, until gamma irradiated in an inert environment became available, at which time I switched. I have personally reviewed minimum 20-year follow-ups of mobile-bearing designs that were performed with polyethylene gamma-irradiated in air and have demonstrated no loosening over the 20-year period—although the average age of the patients at the time of surgery was 70 years. So, I have gained more confidence in believing that the mobile-bearing devices in the most kinematically challenging patients have potential for greater long-term durability.

I now use a moderately cross-linked polyethylene for fixed bearings, and I would also use it if it were available in the mobile bearing. Frankly, now that cross-linked polyethylene is available for the fixed-bearing design, I tend to use it in a slightly younger population, although when the patient is younger than 55 years, all patients get mobile bearings.

Dr. Rosenberg: Dr. Haas, you prefer to attack this issue on the metal side as well.

Dr. Haas: The choice of bearing surfaces is crucial, especially given active patients. For patients 65 and younger or those active and older than 65, I choose to use an oxidized zirconium femoral component, Oxinium (Smith & Nephew, Andover, Mass). Numerous studies have shown that this hybrid ceramic-metal component has significantly lower wear. Because the ceramic surface is much harder than that of chrome cobalt, it is more scratch-resistant. Several studies have shown that scratches develop with normal use of a chrome cobalt component, and retrieved femoral components have significantly greater polyethylene wear compared with new chrome cobalt components. We performed a retrieval analysis with a matched pair analysis comparing identical chrome cobalt with Oxinium articulations and found significantly less scratching of the femoral component and less polyethylene wear with the Oxinium femur.

Dr. Rosenberg: Dr. Violante, do you have any other comments on modern design innovations that you have been using?

Dr. Violante: One of the latest innovations in the geometry of the knee implant itself is the gender femur design. This represents an evolutionary change made to improve the fit of the component to the female femur. Three-dimensional morphometric analysis has shown that female arthritic knees are narrower on the mediolateral (ML) dimension than their male counterparts, with a significantly greater AP/ML ratio than in males. Other differences include the thickness of the AP trochlear dimension and the Q angle. The gender solution femur offers a higher Q angle at 10 degrees, lateralized patellar tracking, a thinner anterior trochlear femoral dimension, and a reduced ML midbox size. For a PS surgeon, this means avoiding component overhang when upsizing is required.

Dr. Rosenberg: Dr. Zhang, what else stands out for you in choosing an implant for your practice?

Dr. Zhang: I take into consideration which implants allow for easy postoperative rehabilitation, and in my experience the LPS Flex and Genesis II are the prostheses that allow for

easiest postoperative rehabilitation. With the same instruction and assistance, it is much easier for patients to return to normal gait and range of motion (ROM) with less patellas crepitus and anterior knee pain. From my personal experience, most patients are very satisfied with the TKA outcome. If considering prosthesis and patient outcome, I prefer to choose the LPS, Genesis II, or LCS for my patients.

Dr. Rosenberg: Dr. Callaghan, could you review your implant design philosophy?

Dr. Callaghan: Over the 26 years I've been in practice, I have gone from using cruciate-retaining designs for patients with less deformity and cruciate-substituting designs for patients with larger deformities to using posterior cruciate–substituting designs in all patients. In my experience, this has allowed for a more predictable operation.

The implant I use allows for both fixed- as well as mobile-bearing designs and thus can result in much versatility. In patients with large valgus deformities, I am a little more apt to use the fixed-bearing design, as well as in patients who have tremendous range of motion—that is, more than 140 degrees—because I can imagine the patient's femoral runners sliding past the tibial inserts, which are only designed to obtain 120 degrees of flexion.

Although I have not had a bearing spinout with a PS component, it still is a concern of mine with mobile-bearing knees. This feature of the system allows the surgeon to use constraint, whether it be a fixed- or mobile-bearing constraint, which helps in deciding which of these two implants to use. In a younger patient, if I am going to use more constraint, I tend to use a mobile-bearing design, which I hope will lead to less loosening of the implant.

Dr. Rosenberg: Dr. Violante, are there settings where you prefer a mobile bearing?

Dr. Violante: Personally, I think that this LPS design allows for the surgeon to get the most reproducible results possible with a standard and well done surgical technique, and represents the best compromise possible when converting damaged knee anatomy to an artificial anatomy. The balance existing between longevity and a high functional result is hard to attain if we forget the compromises we are required to make.

In the osteoporotic patient with a small mediolateral femoral size and poor patellar bone quality, which represents two thirds of my female patients, I use a mobile platform design with rotational freedom for the ultracongruent PS polyethylene and a bone-sparing femoral resection (Innex, Zimmer, Winterthur). I can follow the PS philosophy but avoid cutting out the intercondylar bone. I also believe that the mobile platform is more patella-forgiving. I think that the ultracongruent polyethylene design helps restore the stability of the knee in rheumatoid and osteoporotic patients, which can represent a challenge for ligament balancing. Another potential advantage is a lower incidence of femur fracture and lower torque forces.

Dr. Rosenberg: Dr. Haas, please summarize your thoughts for us.

Dr. Haas: The Journey Knee can be used in most patients, but is ideally suited for the active patient, especially those younger than 60 years. These patients are most likely to benefit from the natural kinematics, rotation, and flexion. Patients with severe deformity, especially valgus more than 20 degrees, often require extensive ligament releases and so are less likely to regain normal kinematics and may require additional constraint.

Dr. Rosenberg: Gentlemen, thank you for your time and sharing your experience with us.

KEY REFERENCES

Arabori M, Matsui N, Kuroda R, et al: Posterior condylar offset and flexion in posterior cruciate–retaining and posterior-stabilized TKA. J Orthop Sci 13:46, 2008.

Bellemans J, Banks S, Victor J, et al: Fluoroscopic analysis of the kinematics of deep flexion in total knee arthroplasty. Influence of posterior condylar offset. J Bone Joint Surg Br 84:50, 2002.

Bozic KJ, Kinder J, Menegini M, et al: Implant survivorship and complication rates after total knee arthroplasty with a third-generation cemented system: 5 to 8 years follow-up. Clin Orthop Relat Res 435:277, 2005.

Clarke HD, Fuchs R, Scuderi GR, et al: The influence of femoral component design in the elimination of patellar clunck in posterior-stabilized total knee arthroplasty. J Arthroplasty 21:167, 2006.

Crowninshield RD, Rosenberg AG, Sporer SM: Changing demographics of patients with total joint replacement. Clin Orthop Relat Res 443:266, 2006.

Victor J: Rotational alignment of the distal femur: a literature review. Orthop Traumatol Surg Res 95:365, 2009.

Full references for this chapter can be found on www.expertconsult.com.

Chapter 115

Computer Navigation in Primary Total Knee Arthroplasty

James B. Stiehl

Numerous authors have investigated outcomes following total knee arthroplasty (TKA), finding that malalignment greater than 3 degrees resulted in a significantly higher potential for mechanical loosening and implant failure. Petersen and Engh investigated the radiographic results of 50 patients who underwent primary TKA with conventional methods, noting a 26% failure to achieve alignment within the optimum of 3 degrees of varus or valgus from the mechanical axis.[34] Jeffery and associates noted satisfactory postoperative coronal alignment (mechanical axis deviation less than 3 degrees) in 68% of their TKAs. In operated knees with mechanical axis deviation greater than 3 degrees in the coronal plane, a mechanical loosening rate of 24% occurred at 8 years, as opposed to 3% mechanical loosening for normally aligned knees.[16] Berend and colleagues investigated tibial component failure mechanisms, noting that malalignment of the tibial component at more than 3 degrees of varus increased the odds of failure.[4]

Computer-assisted navigation of TKA has been shown to produce improved mechanical axis alignment in the clinical setting and offers significant advantages, particularly in cases with severe deformity resulting from long-standing arthritis or traumatic causes.* Access to bony landmarks with open procedures has made TKA navigation a very feasible system when imageless referencing protocols are used. After the original navigation system was developed in 1991 by Dr. Stephane Lavallee at the University of Grenoble for anterior cruciate ligament reconstruction, Saragaglia and coworkers introduced the first kinematic navigation protocol for determining the centers of the hip and ankle; this paved the way for a reproducible and simple imageless approach.[38] Optical tracking has been the primary data accrual method for most current systems.[1,8,11,13,26] This review discusses the basis of that technology, clinical methods, and outcomes offered by current methods of computer navigation in TKA. Additionally, problem areas that have shown limited acceptance of this technology are addressed by the introduction of a system that makes navigation a simple and limited surgical tool customized to the individual needs of each surgeon.

COMPONENTS OF A COMPUTER NAVIGATION SYSTEM

Three elements are required for computer navigation: (1) the computer platform; (2) the tracking system; and (3) the group of dynamic reference bases (DRBs) that constitute the target objects of the navigation procedure. These target objects include the patient's bones, the surgical instruments, and the implants used in the surgical procedure. Important choices regarding each of these components face the practicing surgeon, who must decide from a variety of options. The surgeon should be knowledgeable about possible sources of measurement error that may be demonstrated by a computer navigation system.

Computer Platform

The most basic component of a computer navigation system is the computer on which the system relies for coordination of inputs from the surgical field, mathematical interpretation of the datasets, and display of the resultant information on a monitor. Currently utilized systems require hardware capable of a robust, real-time calculation. Commonly, this results in pairing of powerful microprocessors and software platforms based on Windows or Linux systems. These base operating systems are considered more responsive and stable for the use of mission critical applications. The measurement system is designed in such a fashion that the three-dimensional position of objects or targets in the operative field can be determined with low rates of error—much as a global positioning satellite system would function. Computer platforms may be considered closed, or proprietary, if the navigation provides support limited to a specific implant system or surgical technique. The other possibility is an open system that is more general and allows, for example, a software protocol to support the implantation of total knee implants from different manufacturers. The advantage of a proprietary system is that more elaborate representations are usually supported such that virtual implant sizing to a virtual reconstruction of the patient's anatomy can be performed.

A typical capital system will have a rolling cart with computer, keyboard, mouse, LCD monitor, foot pedal activator, and optical tracking camera. The optical camera may be placed on a boom or a separate tower to allow placement in its appropriate position during the operative procedure. The optical camera system typically will have two charged-coupled device (CCD) receivers that will pick up laser impulses from an active tracker or reflected beam from passive balls attached to a passive tracker. Portable options have been developed that allow similar hardware and applications but with smaller desktop computers and microcameras or tracking devices that may be quickly assembled from a suitcase. This allows manufacturers' representatives to conveniently bring in a full navigation system for limited one-time use as a service that may be purchased by the hospital. This option is a great opportunity for the surgeon who is new to computer navigation and who may not be committed to asking his hospital to make the several hundred thousand dollar (U.S.) purchase of a capital system. It is an excellent option for low-volume surgeons and hospitals that may not have resources to afford the large investment for more permanent systems, in that

---

*References 2, 3, 5-7, 9, 14, 15, 18, 20, 24, 32, 33, 35, 38, 39, 42, 48, 49, and 51.

it provides similar technology to perform computer-aided surgery.

Tracking Technologies

An important element of any computer navigation system is the mechanism or technology chosen to track the target or object. The basic elements are trackers that may be attached to the patient's bones or surgical instruments. These trackers are then used in an environment that consists of a camera, electromagnetic coil, or ultrasonic probe that will pick up laser or electromagnetic pulses that originate from the trackers. Recently, video monitoring has been added as a "real-time" tracking option, but this method has not reached significant clinical application.

Optical tracking systems require two or three CCD cameras to pick up laser impulses from the trackers that are recognized by a minimum of three and possibly four or five active emitters or passive reflective balls. The computer calculates the three-dimensional position of the trackers based on recognition of the spatial footprint of the tracker emitters. The footprint of each tracker is unique and allows differentiation of bones, instruments, and implants. Conventional optical cameras function by being placed 6 to 8 feet from the object trackers, and must have an unobstructed "line of sight" to the trackers. This requires that operating personnel must be aware of this relationship, but if positioning is optimal, staff readily adapt to the requirement. Clinical validation studies of optical tracking systems have demonstrated very high reliability and accuracy with a typical translational error of 0.25 mm.[23,35,52] This absolute measurement error increases trigonometrically with increasing distance from the camera.[43]

Electromagnetic (EM) tracking relies on small trackers that create an electromagnetic impulse that is recognized by an electromagnetic coil placed 20 to 30 inches away.[29] These trackers may be placed inside the wound but require small wires that go directly to the computer system for activation. The magnetic coil then measures interference created by the tracker as it moves within the electromagnetic field. The disadvantage of current electromagnetic tracking systems is distortion of the field created by ferrous metals that are inherently magnetic, but any metal such as brass and copper and even nonmetals such as Kevlar may interfere. Current computer algorithms have been calibrated to shut down the system if distortion is recognized. However, the EM approach still remains vulnerable to many other potentially distorting fields that are found in the typical operating room. Clinical validation studies have identified this problem, and although the electromagnetic system seems to perform with the precision of current optical systems at the 0.5 mm level, the occasional outlier may be off by several degrees, which makes this method less reliable.[1,11,13,24]

Referencing Methods

For the surgeon, referencing of target objects is the most significant problem and requires a thorough knowledge of both the technology and the desired anatomic points to be matched on the virtual computer model. The process basically is to define points in space with a tracker that can be triangulated by the tracking system. For surgical instruments, a referencing tool allows the surgeon to capture the "marked" instrument such as a pointer probe. The precision of the instrument will be within 250 to 500 μ of error.[23] Imageless referencing is possible if the targeted objects are directly visible, and is most applicable in TKA. Numerous studies have demonstrated the efficacy of imageless referencing as compared with conventional instrumentation for TKA, but these results depend on the expertise of the surgeon to choose the correct reference points.[19] Computer algorithms are written with the assumption that the ideal point will be selected. For example, referencing of one universal total knee protocol prescribes that the femoral center is chosen as a point that is under the roof of the intercondylar notch and lies on both the transepicondylar line and the anteroposterior axis of Whiteside. Deviation from this "ideal" point adds error.

Kinematic referencing in TKA as pioneered by Lavallee has been a novel innovation for determining the center of the hip and ankle joints, markedly simplifying this procedure.[38] Because the hip joint is not directly visible, a method was needed by which to accurately reference the hip center. This was accomplished by tracking the femur with the optical camera as the femur was rotated in a circular motion. The movement of the tracker described the base of a cone, which when projected to its zenith closely approximates the center of the hip joint. The computer algorithm calculates the root mean square error or the standard deviation, which must fall within a limited range for the computer to accept the hip center reference point.

A secondary method of referencing is bone *morphing*, which involves selecting hundreds of surface match points by "painting" the bone with the pointer probe.[46,47] This method does not require the segmented three-dimensional model typical of computed tomography (CT) but uses a virtual model that is then constructed by the computer algorithm. The virtual image created allows enhanced capabilities such as prosthetic sizing, "live" bone resection, and kinematic assessment. However, this additional technology usually adds time and complexity to the operative procedure and may limit the surgeon's choice of prosthetic implants. One current morph technology is to limit the referenced areas to small patches. For example, surgeons find difficulty referencing the femoral posterior condyle in finding the most posterior or dorsal position. This process can be simplified and made much more precise by morphing a small patch, allowing the computer to find the optimum position.

Ultrasound image capture is a newer method of referencing that is evolving as a potential technique whereby multimodal referencing is performed.[8,26] Depending on frequency and the acoustical properties of the object, point localization is accurate to submillimeter levels on the order of 0.25 to 0.75 mm with ultrasound, whether it is 2-dimensional, 2.5-dimensional, or 3-dimensional in the modality of image capture. Segmentation is possible when this image may be matched with a preoperative CT image or even an intraoperative "bone morphed" image. However, the clinical applications remain limited for a variety of reasons. Definition of baseline anatomic points is difficult with ultrasound, which creates an error on the order of 2 to 5 mm, which is unacceptable for clinical practice. However, the promise of ultrasound is that it can be done through the tissues intraoperatively without the need for skin incision or radiation exposure.

CLINICAL METHODS

The specifics of navigation referencing constitute an important element of the technique and bear detailed description. Tracker placement requires rigid fixation of the dynamic reference base to the femur and tibia, because any movement creates error. Current systems have validation check points that may be established and then remeasured throughout the procedure to monitor tracker error. Recent studies have favored two pins of 3 mm diameter.[28] It is important to note that single pins of 5 mm and bicortical placement should be avoided, as incidental fractures have been described. Placement of the femoral pins in the medial femoral condyle or in a percutaneous transepicondylar position avoids the potential for neurovascular injury[43] (Fig. 115-1). Hip center determination is done using the kinematic method originally described by Saragaglia et al.[38]

Anatomic referencing of the patient's landmark, the most critical step for the surgeon, requires a thorough understanding of what the system's software engineers had in mind when they designed the system. This becomes the most likely source of error. For typical referencing, the computer definition of the femoral center is a point under the roof of the intercondylar notch that is in the middle of the intercondylar notch and lies in the anteroposterior axis of Whiteside (Fig. 115-2). From dissections, this point also lies directly on the transepicondylar axis of the distal femur. The surgical epicondyle depression is the reference for the medial epicondyle, and the lateral epicondyle is the most prominent point of that landmark.

For the tibial reference, the tibial center is defined as the bisection of the transverse tibial axis. The transverse tibial axis is a line that connects the anteroposterior midpoints of the medial and lateral condylar surfaces. The tibial center approximates the lateral insertion of the anterior cruciate ligament (Fig. 115-3). The anteroposterior tibial axis is a perpendicular extension of the tibial center of the transverse tibial axis. This point typically matches the extension of the femoral anteroposterior axis that may be extended onto the anterior surface of the tibia. Great care must be taken to determine the tibial center, as this will affect both coronal and sagittal plane measurements. The posterior condylar axis of the tibia is 3 to 4 degrees external to the transverse tibial axis. The center of the tibial tubercle is typically about 18 degrees external to the anteroposterior axis of the tibia. Finally, the transverse tibial axis should nearly approximate the transepicondylar axis with regard to coupled rotation. The center of the distal tibia is determined by picking points that center over the medial and lateral malleoli—the transmalleolar axis. The computer algorithm then kinematically picks a point on the transmalleolar axis that is 40% from the most medial point.

Once referenced, the computer system may be used to assess each step in the surgical technique. For the beginning surgeon, the logical method is to perform the standard surgical technique using the computer as an adjunct to conventional instrumentation. This allows the surgeon to become comfortable with the navigated measurements and eliminates the early risk of error from inexperience. With practice, the surgeon will learn to depend on the increased precision of the navigated steps, and may be able to make cuts even without conventional instruments. The computer, which becomes an excellent source of information regarding the surgical procedure, will teach the surgeon about the potential measurement errors that may occur with his conventional techniques.

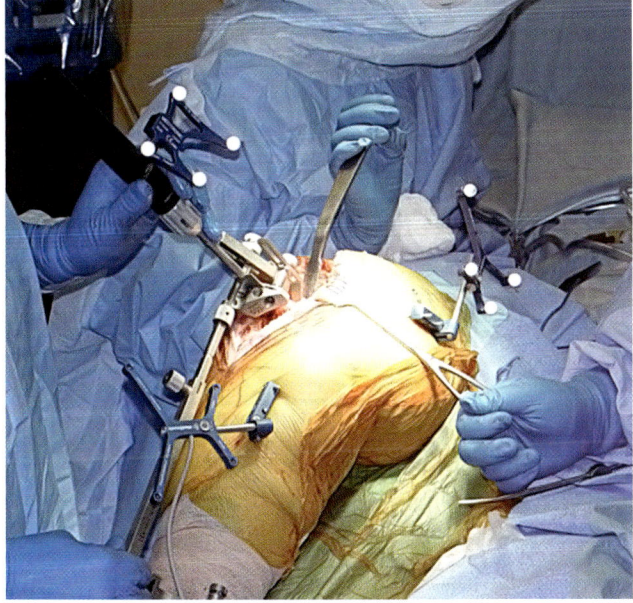

Figure 115-1. Typical navigation of the proximal tibial cut using a cut guide dynamic reference base (DRB) placed in a conventional instrument guide slot. Note the medial percutaneous placement of femoral and tibial tracker pins.

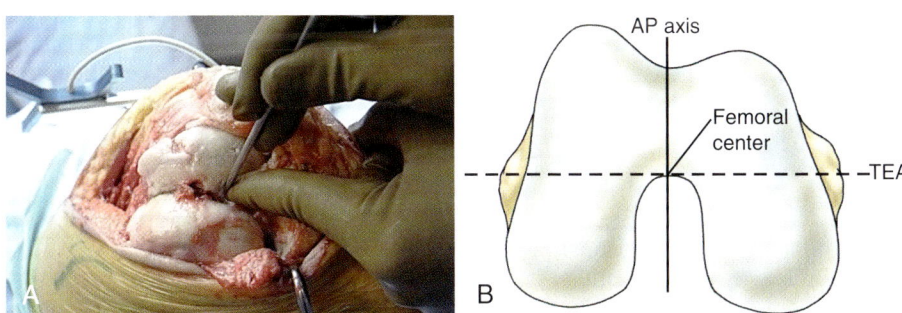

Figure 115-2. A, Referencing of the femoral center places the touch point at the center of the roof of the intercondylar notch in line with the anteroposterior line of Whiteside. **B,** Diagrammatic representation demonstrates the relationship of the femoral center, transepicondylar axis, and anteroposterior line of Whiteside.

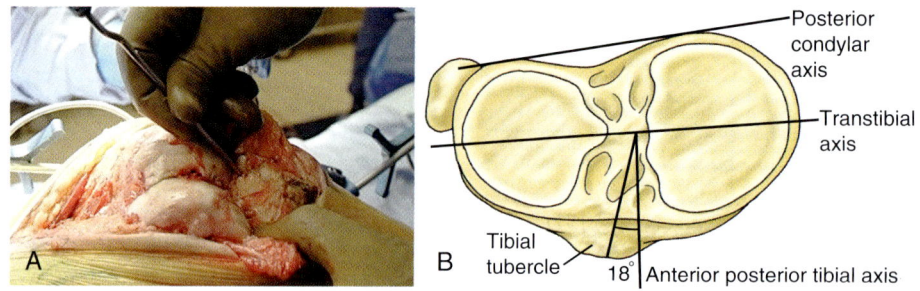

Figure 115-3. A, Referencing of the tibial center places the touch point at the tibial center, which is the intersection of the transtibial and anteroposterior axes. **B,** Diagrammatic representation demonstrates landmarks of the proximal tibia, including posterior condylar axis, transtibial axis (line bisecting the midpoints of the medial and lateral tibial plateaus), tibial center (bisects the transtibial axis), anteroposterior tibial axis (perpendicular anterior projection of the tibial center from the transtibial axis), and tibial tubercle (which is 18 degrees lateral to the anteroposterior axis).

Table 115-1 Clinical Studies That Compare Conventional Manual Surgical Techniques With Computer Navigation in Placing Limb Alignment Within ±3 Degrees of the Mechanical Axis of the Lower Extremity

Author	N	Navigated, %	Conventional, %	% Difference
Haaker et al, 2005[14]	100	96	75	21
Sparmann et al, 2003[42]	120	98	78	20
Victor and Hoste, 2004[51]	50	100	74	27
Jenny et al, 2005[20]	235	97	74	23
Jenny and Boeri, 2001[18]	30, 30	83	70	17
Kim et al, 2005[24]	69, 78	78	58	20
Perlick et al, 2004[32,33]	40	93	75	28
Seon and Song, 2005[39]	47, 50	96	76	20
Bathis et al, 2004[3]	160	96	78	18
Perlick et al, 2004[32,33]	50	92	72	20
Hart et al, 2003[15]	60	88	70	18
Anderson et al, 2005[2]	116, 51	95	84	11
		93 (average)	74 ($P < .001$)	20

CLINICAL OUTCOMES

Literature Review

Computer-assisted alignment devices were developed to improve the positioning of implants during TKA. Early data on the use of these image-free optical tracking systems appeared positive with improved mechanical alignment, frontal and sagittal femoral axis alignment, and frontal tibial axis alignment. Furthermore, no studies have demonstrated increased complications compared with hand-guided techniques. Yau and associates compared the combined intraobserver error for image-free acquisition of reference landmarks during TKA, finding that the maximum combined error for the coronal plane mechanical axis alignment was 1.32 degrees.[53] Perlick and colleagues compared an image-free navigation system versus a conventional method using an intramedullary femoral guide and an extramedullary tibial guide. They reported postoperative mechanical alignment to be within 3 degrees varus or valgus in 96% of navigation cases versus 78% in the conventional group.[32] Sparmann and coworkers determined that an image-free navigation system produces significant improvement in mechanical alignment, frontal and sagittal femoral alignment, and frontal tibial alignment ($P < .0001$) compared with a hand-guided technique. Postoperative mechanical alignment was within 3

degrees varus or valgus in 87% of the conventional group versus 100% of the navigation group.[42] A significant number of studies have compared the use of imageless computer-assisted navigation versus conventional methods for TKA. All studies demonstrated a statistically significant improvement in terms of placing the final mechanical alignment of the knee within 3 degrees of the ideal mechanical axis. Furthermore, we noted that 93% of overall cases from these studies reached this level of precision with computer navigation compared with 73% when conventional methods were used (Table 115-1).

Results of assessment of the transepicondylar axis or the anteroposterior axis of Whiteside are inconsistent as compared with mechanical axis alignment. This most likely reflects the difficulty involved in reproducibly picking the epicondylar or anteroposterior axis landmarks. Prior studies have confirmed this problem, finding a large amount of variability in the basic anatomic landmark and in the ability of the surgeon to clinically define the structure.* The problem with using the anteroposterior axis for computer navigation referencing can easily be understood by the fact that distances for landmarking are very short. Slight errors in judgment can

---

*References 12, 17, 30, 37, 41, and 50.

be off by several degrees. This contrasts with mechanical axis landmarking, in which an error of just 1 degree will require a point matching mistake of at least 5 mm. Yau and associates found that errors in the transepicondylar axis could be as high as 9 degrees.[54] Restrepo and colleagues reported that the fixed posterior condylar axis reference could result in malalignment of more than 5 degrees in 17% of cases as compared with other rotational axes.[36] Siston and coworkers suggested that improvement is needed in determining femoral alignment accuracy.[40]

Other image acquisition and tracking methods are available, beyond the current standard imageless total knee systems; these include CT, fluoroscopy, and electromagnetic tracking. Perlick and associates compared CT with imageless referencing methods in TKA and found that 92% with CT versus 97% with imageless systems produced TKA mechanical axis alignment less than 3 degrees.[33] Victor and Hoste used fluoroscopic image acquisition in a randomized study with TKA to find that 100% of navigated knees had mechanical alignment within ±3 degrees, while 73% of conventional TKAs were within ±3 degrees.[51]

Blood loss has been significantly reduced with the use of computer navigation and avoidance of intramedullary rods. Kalairag and coworkers were able to reduce mean blood loss from 1747 mL to 1351 mL by using pin-placed trackers instead of intramedullary guided femur and tibia jigs; this represented a significant difference in 60 patients.[22] Kalairag and associates performed a transcranial Doppler study on 14 patients, finding that all patients who had undergone intramedullary instrumentation of the femur and tibia with conventional TKA had documented intracranial microemboli compared with only 50% of those who had undergone procedures in which only intracortical tracking pins had been placed.[21] However, Kim and colleagues could not find a significant difference with fat or bone marrow embolization when comparing navigation with conventional instrumentation.[25]

Navigation with minimally invasive total knee approaches has been shown to offer some advantages. Dutton and associates demonstrated that with a minimally invasive technique, 92% of patients were within the ±3 degrees target with navigation as opposed to 68% with conventional instruments. Although navigation increased operating room time by 24 minutes, both length of hospital stay and functional recovery at 1 month were improved by the method.[10] Stiehl et al were able to show that increased navigation time could be diminished by using a custom computer protocol for the specific surgeon, and noted that navigation actually had a 10-minute average shorter duration compared with conventional instrument techniques.[45] Nowac and colleagues studied cost-effectiveness with computer navigation and suggested that the typical added cost of $1500 for navigation would need to be reduced to less than $629 for the method to become effective in decreasing the morbidity shown with poorer total knee alignment.[31]

EVOLUTIONARY TECHNOLOGIES

We have alluded to our recent efforts to develop a futuristic system that provides the surgeon with a highly accurate tool that may be abbreviated or customized to his particular needs. Most contemporary systems are "one size fits all," and the

surgeon not only must learn the navigation system but often will need to change his own approach, which he may have painstakingly developed over several years. He may not have great skills with the computer, nor the inclination to struggle through the learning curve needed for this technology. We are developing a very limited system with a laptop computer and a compact camera that may be placed directly into the surgical field (Figs. 115-4 and 115-5). More important, we want the system to be customized for each surgeon, such that he may develop his own custom protocol. The number of navigated steps, their order in the software protocol, and actual surgical field screen views are developed by each individual surgeon with help from a manufacturer's representative. By navigating only the critical steps in the procedure, we believe the surgeon improves the accuracy of the surgical procedure with the strength of the technology; this technique may be more efficient than the use of conventional manual instruments.

Our new PICO station has limited, legible numbers with appropriate screen prompts or diagrams to enhance the flow. This focus came from our middle-aged surgeons, who were having trouble reading screens that were 6 to 8 feet away. We were told that each surgeon was looking for a certain number

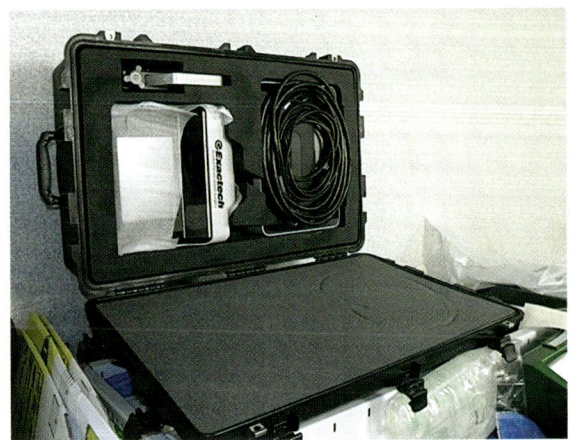

Figure 115-4. Example of the new PICO system (Blue Orthopaedics SAS, Grenoble France), which has a compact camera and computer designed to be placed within the operative field.

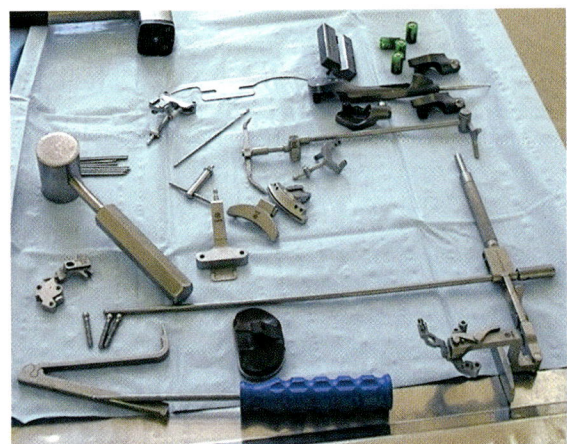

Figure 115-5. Note the typical position of the computer screen and camera at the head of the table in the operative field.

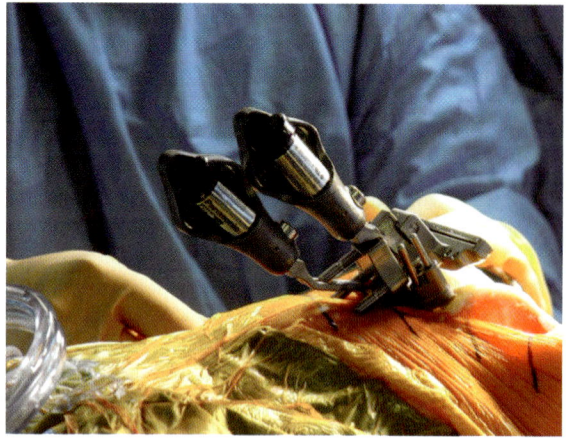

Figure 115-6. PICO haptic robot will position the proximal tibial cut guide and uses active battery-powered tracker dynamic reference bases (DRBs) attached to the base block and the tibial cut guide. Note that no additional tracker or pin sites are needed.

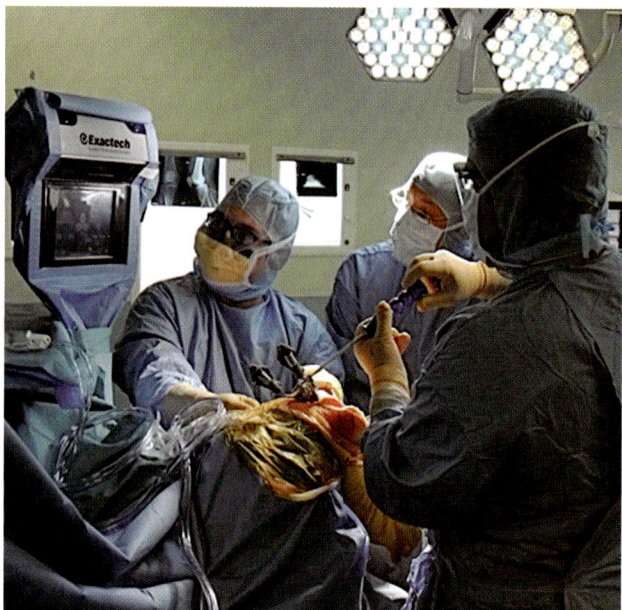

Figure 115-7. PICO robotic screwdriver turns threads of the cut guide the specified number of turns to precisely place the cut guide in the appropriate position.

for a step, thus our effort to limit the screen to only that number could be found on the screen in 1 to 2 seconds. Ergonomics is important for the surgeon, and we developed a small battery-powered active tracker that could be attached directly to a cutting block or prosthetic trial. This enhances the surgeon's ability to avoid separate tracking DRBs because the trackers are placed directly onto his instruments. Furthermore, it enables the possibility of pinless registration, or registration that does not require placement of separate pin pods.

We have developed a haptic robot that will interface with our current system (Figs. 115-6 and 115-7). This robot comes in the form of a battery-powered screwdriver that is enabled by the computer software to turn a certain number of screw thread turns to place a series of cutting block screws into the exact position created by the computer software protocol.

This system favors minimally invasive cutting blocks, has all of the technology improvements noted earlier, and avoids intramedullary device placement, but it significantly shortens surgical time by removing the guesswork of the procedure.

DISCUSSION

In conclusion, computer-assisted navigation offers significant advantages for improving the precision of surgical technique with TKA. This review has attempted to clarify the general nature of the technology and to point out the strengths and weaknesses of various approaches. Improved mechanical axis alignment is the signal refinement offered to TKA; this may also be applied to unicondylar and revision arthroplasty. Navigation provides the ability to assess ligamentous balance and overall kinematics after prosthetic reconstruction. However, certain elements such as determining the femoral and tibial rotational axes are less precise with current applications. One must consider that constant technology evolution is occurring, but the overall advantages of computer navigation in TKA have been recognized and will not change substantially in the near future.

KEY REFERENCES

Dutton JA, Yeo SJ, Yang KY, et al: Computer-assisted minimally invasive total knee arthroplasty compared with standard total knee arthroplasty: a prospective, randomized study. J Bone Joint Surg Am 90:2–9, 2008.

Jeffery R, Morris R, Denham R: Coronal alignment after total knee replacement. J Bone Joint Surg Br 73:709–714, 1991.

Jenny JY, Boeri C: Low reproducibility of the intra-operative measurement of the transepicondylar axis during total knee replacement. Acta Orthop Scand 75:74–77, 2004.

Jenny JY, Clemens U, Kohler S, et al: Consistency of implantation of a total knee arthroplasty with a non-image-based navigation system: a case-control study of 235 cases compared with 235 conventionally implanted prostheses. J Arthroplasty 20:832–839, 2005.

Kalairaj Y, Cossey AJ, Verall GM, Ludbrook G, Spriggins AJ: Are systemic emboli reduced in computer assisted surgery? J Bone Joint Surg Br 88:198–202, 2005.

Kalairaj Y, Simpson P, Cossey AJ, Verrall GM, Spriggins AJ: Blood loss after total knee arthroplasty: effects of computer assisted surgery. J Bone Joint Surg Br 87:1480–1482, 2005.

Kim YH, Kim JS, Hong KS, Kim YJ, Kim JH: Prevalence of fat embolism after total knee arthroplasty performed with or without computer navigation. J Bone Joint Surg Am 90:123–128, 2008.

Moon YW, Seo JG, Lim SJ, Yang JH: Variability in femoral component rotation reference axes measured during navigation-assisted total knee arthroplasty using gap technique. J Arthroplasty 25:238–243, 2010.

Nowac EJ, Silverstein MD, Bozic KJ: The cost-effectiveness of computer-assisted navigation in total knee arthroplasty. J Bone Joint Surg Am 89:2389–2397, 2007.

Petersen T, Engh G: Radiographic assessment of knee alignment after total knee arthroplasty. J Arthroplasty 3:67–72, 1988.

Pitto RP, Graydon AJ, Bradley L, et al: Accuracy of computer-assisted navigation system for total knee replacement. J Bone Joint Surg Br 88:601–605, 2006.

Siston RA, Cromie MJ, Gold GE, et al: Averaging different alignment axes improves femoral rotational alignment in computer-navigated total knee arthroplasty. J Bone Joint Surg Am 90:2098–2104, 2008.

Siston RA, Patel JJ, Goodman SB, Delp SL, Giori NJ: The variability of femoral rotational alignment in total knee arthroplasty. J Bone Joint Surg Am 87:2276–2280, 2005.

Sparmann M, Wolke B, Czupalla H, Banzer D, Zink A: Positioning of total knee arthroplasty with and without navigation support: a prospective, randomised study. J Bone Joint Surg Br 85:830–835, 2003.

Victor J, Hoste D: Image-based computer-assisted total knee arthroplasty leads to lower variability in coronal alignment. Clin Orthop Relat Res 428:131–139, 2004.

Full references for this chapter can be found on www.expertconsult.com.

Chapter 116

Computer-Navigated Total Knee Arthroplasty

S. David Stulberg

Computer-assisted surgery (CAS) has emerged as one of the most important technologies in orthopedic surgery, and many of the initial applications have focused on adult reconstructive surgery of the knee. The goals of this chapter are as follows: (1) provide a brief history of CAS of the knee and the evolution of basic concepts; (2) present the rationale for the use of CAS in knee surgery; (3) describe the hardware and software components of CAS systems; (4) illustrate the measured resection technique for total knee replacement surgery; and (5) present CAS applications in knee surgery that will be available in the near future.

HISTORY OF COMPUTER-ASSISTED KNEE SURGERY AND EVOLUTION OF BASIC CONCEPTS

Although a large volume of important work that became the foundation for computer-assisted knee surgery was being carried out throughout the 20th century, the initial clinical applications for knee surgery began in the 1980s.[109] In 1986, Kaiura, from the University of Washington presented a thesis on robotic-assisted total knee arthroplasty (TKA).[39,62] This work led to the design of one of the first computer robotic assistive systems for TKA, described by Matsen and colleagues[86] in 1993.[137] In the early 1990s, Kienzle and associates[65] and Stulberg[134] also described a computer-assisted robotic total knee replacement system. The desired position of the femoral and tibial cutting blocks was determined on a three-dimensional model derived from a computed tomography (CT) scan obtained preoperatively. The robot was secured to the operating table and to the bones and then positioned a drill to make holes for the pins over which the femoral and tibial cutting blocks were placed. The surgeon then performed the cuts with a standard oscillating saw. The accuracy of block placement with this system was within 1 mm and 1 degree. This work also introduced a method for determining the center of the femoral head by means of a kinematic registration technique. This technique was subsequently incorporated into all current navigation systems. Dynamic reference frames that were tracked by a camera were placed on the femur and the hip was put through a range of motion. The center of the sphere described during the circumduction maneuver represented the center of the femoral head.

By the early 1990s, the principles on which current computer-assisted total knee replacement systems are based had been established and validated, and important steps had been taken to identify how critical anatomic landmarks for knee surgery could be accurately acquired. It was, however, apparent to those working on these projects at that time, especially orthopedic surgeons, that robotic-based computer-assisted systems were too cumbersome, complex, and potentially too unsafe to be of substantial use to an active knee replacement surgeon in the foreseeable future.

Surgical navigation systems, however, appeared then to offer an attractive alternative to a field such as knee surgery, which could benefit from the accuracy provided by computer-assisted techniques without having to deal with the drawbacks and complexity of robots. These systems allowed intraoperative tracking of the position of the surgical tools and the bones to which they were attached. The surgeon, not a robot, could control all phases of the procedure.

The rapid evolution of surgical navigation systems to support the performance of knee surgery was made possible by the availability, in the early 1990s, of optical and electromagnetic tracking systems (Fig. 116-1). Optical tracking systems have played a special role in the development of surgical navigation systems for knee surgery because of their accuracy and reliability. These tracking systems, also referred to as optical localizers, have charge-coupled devices (CCDs, or cameras) mounted on a rigid frame. These cameras measure the position and orientation of multiple tracking markers, also called trackers, or rigid bodies. Each tracker incorporates a set of light-emitting diodes (LEDs), or reflective spheres, mounted in precise relative positions. These trackers can be affixed to bones, tools, and implants. The optical tracker is therefore able to monitor the precise position of these objects at any point during the surgical procedure.

During the first half of the 1990s, a great deal of basic research was performed to develop surgical navigation systems using these optical tracking systems.[109] The first clinical applications incorporating these efforts began in 1995 in the field of spine surgery. Although these applications were based on the acquisition of anatomic information by means of preoperative imaging techniques, they were the basis for the development in the late 1990s of the image-free systems currently most widely used in knee surgery.

Four types of surgical navigation models are used in computer-assisted orthopedic surgery: (1) preoperative image–based (e.g., CT scans)[68,75]; (2) intraoperative image–based (e.g., fluoroscopy)[84,85]; (3) image-free; and (4) individual templating.[37,75,93,112,130] The anatomic information on which the surgical plan is made is acquired differently in each model. Although each model has its advantages and drawbacks, the image-free method for acquiring critical anatomic information has proved to be most amenable to the methods used currently to perform knee surgery. This method was first used clinically in 1993 to place grafts during anterior cruciate ligament (ACL) surgery.[109] Image-free navigation was subsequently applied to TKA surgery by Leitner and colleagues.[80] The first image-free computer-assisted TKA was performed in Grenoble, France, by Picard and associates in 1997.[107] The system used became the first commercially available image-free navigation system for knee reconstructive surgery (the OrthoPilot).[106] It identified critical anatomic landmarks using both kinematic (e.g., femoral circumduction, as described by Kienzle and coworkers in 1989[65]) and surface registration

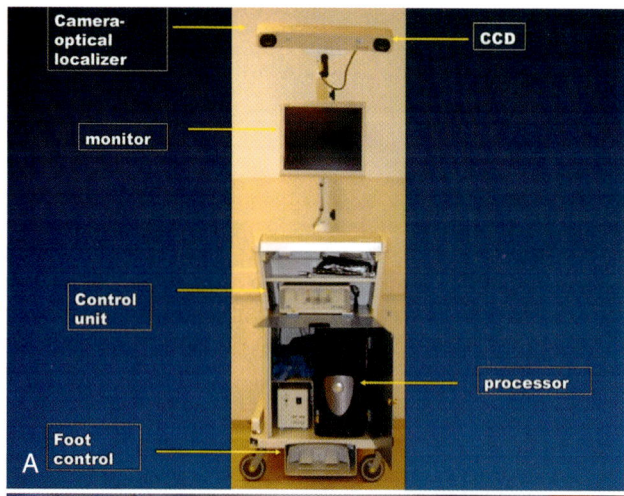

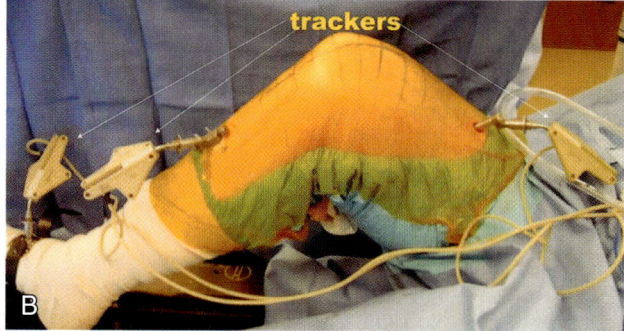

Figure 116-1. **A,** Typical image-free computer-assisted hardware system consisting of an optical tracker with charged-coupled devices (CCDs—the cameras), computer monitor, control unit and processor, and foot control system for communication between the surgeon and the system. **B,** Active trackers (also called rigid bodies or fiducials) attached to bicortical screws rigidly fixed to the femur and tibia.

techniques. Krackow and colleagues[74] subsequently developed surgical navigation systems based on these concepts. There are now a large number of image-free navigation systems available for use with almost every total knee system.

Although the foundations for the CAS systems currently being used in knee surgery began to be developed a century ago, actual systems available for clinical use have been available for less than 10 years. The rapid emergence of these systems suggests that current models will undergo substantial evolution and modification in the next few years.

RATIONALE FOR USE

Successful surgical reconstruction of the knee requires proper patient selection, appropriate perioperative management, correct implant selection, and accurate surgical technique. The consequences of performing a knee reconstruction inaccurately have been well documented for TKA, unicondylar arthroplasty, ACL reconstruction, and high tibial osteotomy.*

Although mechanical instrumentation has significantly increased the accuracy and reliability with which knee reconstructions are performed, errors in implant and limb alignment continue to occur, even when the procedures are performed by experienced surgeons. Moreover, the accuracy with which these procedures are performed is dependent on the knowledge and experience of the surgeon and the frequency with which the surgeon performs the procedure. CAS techniques have been developed to address the inherent limitations of mechanical instrumentation. The goals of integrating CAS with knee reconstruction techniques are to increase the accuracy of these procedures and reduce the proportion of alignment outliers that occur when these procedures are performed.

A surgeon can only use computer-assisted navigation safely and effectively if he or she is familiar with and comfortable with the procedure's goals and the surgical techniques necessary to achieve those goals. Numerous reports have confirmed that when surgeons experienced in the manual performance of the knee reconstruction procedure use CAS techniques, average implant and limb alignment is improved and the incidence of outliers is reduced.* Moreover, a recent study has indicated that when experienced surgeons and coworkers use techniques to perform knee reconstructive procedures, their ability to perform these procedures manually improves.[145]

Errors can occur at numerous points during the performance of a knee reconstruction. Placement of the cutting blocks or ligament alignment jigs may be inaccurate. Attachment of these tools to bone may produce an error in their placement. The actual performance of the cut or drilling of the hole may be inaccurate (e.g., the saw blade may deflect). The final insertion of the implant may be inaccurate. Mechanical instrumentation does not provide a method for checking the accuracy of each of these steps of a knee reconstructive procedure. Another goal of integrating CAS with knee reconstruction is to provide the surgeon with a means to measure the accuracy with which each step of the procedure is performed.

Knee reconstructive procedures attempt to align limbs and implants correctly. They also seek to restore appropriate kinematic relationships and ligamentous stability to the knee.

Mechanical instrumentation cannot measure the precision with which knee kinematics and ligament stability are restored. CAS techniques make it possible to determine the presurgical kinematic relationships and ligamentous stability of the knee and help guide the surgeon to restore desired kinematic relationships and ligamentous balance.

Finally, CAS provides a unique and unprecedented opportunity to train residents and orthopedic surgeons to perform knee reconstruction procedures accurately.[95,140,148] CAS as a training tool has now been used more frequently. Applications have been developed and are now being used to allow surgeons to carry out self-assessment evaluation of their surgical skills for performing TKA and ACL surgery. Applications are also being developed to test the skills of surgeons and residents to learn various knee reconstruction procedures.

---

*References 2, 4, 5, 11, 17, 29, 30, 35, 36, 41, 45, 46, 48-51, 54, 59, 77-79, 81, 90, 95, 96, 98, 104, 105, 113-116, 123, 129, 146, 147, 149, 151, and 152.

*References 1, 3, 7, 9, 10, 13, 14, 16, 18, 19, 21, 22, 24, 25, 31, 33, 42-44, 56, 58, 64, 66, 68, 69, 87, 89, 90, 97, 100, 111, 118, 121, 122, 125, 128, 133, and 154.

Possibly, the most compelling rationale for applying CAS to knee reconstruction will prove to be the potential to revolutionize how surgeons develop and evaluate their surgical skills.

HARDWARE AND SOFTWARE REQUIREMENTS

A detailed description of the hardware and software needed to perform computer-assisted reconstructive knee surgery is beyond the scope of this chapter. However, it is important that knee surgeons understand the basic components of a computer-assisted orthopedic system so that they can use the system correctly, safely, and efficiently and make intelligent choices regarding the appropriateness of various systems for their surgical needs.

Hardware

Hardware devices common to CAS systems are (1) imaging devices; (2) computers, peripherals, and interfaces to allow them to function in the operating room; and (3) localizers and trackers (see Fig. 116-1).

Imaging Devices

The imaging devices that are currently available for use with computer-assisted orthopedic surgery systems include CT, magnetic resonance imaging (MRI), and fluoroscopy machines. These devices are used to acquire the anatomic information on which a presurgical or intraoperative surgical plan is formulated. This plan becomes the basis for the placement of cutting tools intraoperatively and for establishing the alignment and stability of the knee. Although potentially extremely useful for knee reconstruction surgery, especially for robotic or customized surgery, imaging devices as currently used with CAS knee systems have been perceived by surgeons as adding additional and cumbersome steps to well-established knee procedures without providing significant benefits. Consequently, image-free, computer-assisted systems have emerged as the most desired form of CAS for knee reconstruction. As a result, the role of imaging when image-free CAS systems are used remains largely identical to its role when CAS is not used. Imaging is used preoperatively to develop a plan (e.g., applying a goniometer on a long, standing anteroposterior [AP] radiograph to determine the desired frontal alignment) and postoperatively to assess the results of the procedure.

Computers, Peripherals, and Interfaces

The computers used in CAS are obviously the core of these systems. They integrate information from medical images, implant data, intraoperative tracking, and surgical plans to guide the surgeon in the performance of a knee procedure. The speed of computing, memory, storage capacity, and communication ability with peripherals have reached a level where even midrange, less expensive personal computers can satisfy the needs of image-free CAS knee applications. All current CAS knee applications use a range of platforms based usually on the UNIX or Windows operating systems. It is likely that applications will soon be written on the open Linux operating system. The computers are currently mounted on transportable carts (or operating room booms)

that include the computer, monitor, keyboard, mouse, power transformer and isolation unit, and tracker controller unit with ports to plug in the tracker and tracking markers. Communication between the surgeon and computer is necessary for continuous monitoring of the procedure. This can be accomplished with single or double foot pedals, keypads, touch screens, pointer-integrated controls, or voice-activated controls (see Fig. 116-1A).

Localizers and Trackers

A CAS knee navigation system can be thought of as an aiming device that enables real-time visualization of surgical action with an image of the operated structures. For this navigation to occur, it is necessary that the position and orientation of an instrument be visualized with respect to the anatomic structures to which it is attached. Although this objective could be met by attaching tools to a rigid multilinked arm attached to a pedestal, such a device would be unsuitable for knee surgery, in which the limb must be freely moved. Therefore, contactless systems are used to communicate between the extremity and computer system. Information can be transmitted by infrared light, electromagnetic field, or ultrasound. Each method has its advantages and drawbacks. All these methods allow several objects (e.g., two bones) to be viewed simultaneously.

Optical Localization

Optical localization via infrared light is currently the most widely used method of communication between the operated extremity and computer. Two types of optical tracking are used, active and passive. Systems with active tracking use markers (also called trackers, or rigid bodies) with LEDs that send out light pulses to a camera (optical localizer). Three or (for redundancy) more of these LEDs are attached to screws or wires that are rigidly attached to the femur and tibia. The camera system to which the light is sent consists of two planar or three linear CCDs that are rigidly mounted onto a solid housing (Polaris, Northern Digital, Ontario, Canada, is a commonly used camera system). Passive systems use reflecting spheres placed on tracking markers that are attached to screws or pins rigidly implanted in the femur and tibia. Infrared flashes sent by LED arrays on the camera housing illuminate the spheres. The two planar or three linear CCDs observe the reflections and interpolate the spatial location of each light source. It is important for the surgeon and staff to realize that the arrays on the tracking markers, whether active or passive, are specific to each CAS system. One company's trackers cannot be used on another company's CAS system, even though the trackers may appear to be similar (see Fig. 116-1).

The advantages of optical localizing systems are that they are reliable, flexible, and highly accurate and have good operating room compatibility. A disadvantage of these systems is that it is necessary to provide free line of sight between the LED spheres and the CCD arrays on the camera (optical localizer). Active trackers may require cables to power and synchronize the LEDs. These cables may be cumbersome. Active trackers can be driven by batteries, which eliminates the need for cables, but these batteries require recharging, thus making their use for sequential procedures more difficult. Passive trackers do not require cords. However, automatic tool identification is more difficult for passive systems because all spheres in view reflect the light flashes equally. Unique identification of each tracker is possible with the sequentially pulsed LEDs of active trackers. The reflecting spheres must constantly be kept clean to obtain accurate signal transmission. Moreover, the spheres are disposable and therefore a source of additional expense for each procedure.

Magnetic Fields

Magnetic fields can be used to measure the position and orientation of objects in space. A generator coil is used to erect a homogeneous magnetic field. Specially designed coils can be implanted into the femur and tibia or attached to tools. These coils measure the changes in magnetic field characteristics during performance of the procedure. The computer can integrate these changes with the implant data and surgical plans to guide the surgeon in the performance of a knee procedure. These systems have a number of potential advantages. The equipment (coils) attached to the bones and tools can be small, and the accuracy of many systems is very good. The need for a camera and its associated line of sight requirement is eliminated. However, the presence of ferromagnetic items such as implants, instruments, and operating room equipment made of steel can disturb precise measurements dramatically and unpredictably. Moreover, the coils are disposable and therefore a source of additional expense for each procedure.

Ultrasound Systems

Ultrasonic-based navigation systems measure how long a sound impulse needs to travel between the emitter and microphone. Calculation of the position of each tracked object is based on the speed of sound. Although technically feasible, these systems require delicate calibration. Precision depends on the speed of sound, which may vary with differences in temperature. Sterilization of ultrasonic equipment can also be difficult.[83]

Software

The function of software in CAS systems is to integrate medical images and mathematic algorithms with surgical tools and surgical techniques. A relatively small number of software components underlie most CAS image-free systems. These components include registration, navigation, procedure guidance, and safety.

Image-free CAS knee systems use as their preoperative plan the concepts of limb and implant alignment that are currently used with manual instrumentation (e.g., restoration of the mechanical axis). To accomplish this, anatomic and kinematic information about a patient must be transmitted to the software on the computer and geometrically transformed by registration algorithms. Because bones are rigid and assumed to be unlikely to deform during the procedure, the algorithms used are termed *rigid*. These algorithms also require that the trackers attached to bones do not move during the procedure. Fiducial-based registration is a type of rigid registration. Therefore, the objects to which the LEDs are attached may be referred to as fiducials, trackers, or rigid bodies. Fiducial registration requires that at least three sets of markers be implanted into each bone or attached to each tool to determine the object's position and orientation. Therefore, each tracker must have at least three LEDs or reflecting spheres. Some CAS knee systems currently use shaped-based registration as an alternative to fiducial-based registration. These systems measure the shape of the bone surface intraoperatively and match the acquired shape to a surface model created from medical images stored in the computer. The registration process for image-free knee navigation systems requires that information be acquired via kinematic techniques (e.g., circumducting the leg to determine the center of the femoral head) or surface registration techniques (e.g., touching bone landmarks with a probe).

Once the software takes anatomic and kinematic input from the extremity and geometrically transforms it, the surgeon is presented with a user interface that depicts the steps of the knee procedure in sequence. One of the most important objectives of software development in CAS knee applications is to depict procedure sequences that are familiar to surgeons and with which they have previously become comfortable using manual instrumentation.

MEASURED GAP RESECTION TECHNIQUE

A surgeon can only use computer-assisted navigation safely and effectively if he or she is familiar with and comfortable with the procedure's goals and surgical techniques necessary to achieve those goals. The goals of TKA surgery are to align the extremity and implant(s) accurately and to produce a stable, balanced knee joint. These goals can be achieved using one of two surgical strategies: (1) a gap balancing approach, in which equal collateral ligament tension in flexion and extension is sought prior to and as a guide to final bone cuts; or (2) a measured gap resection approach, in which bone landmarks are used to guide resections equal to the distal and posterior thicknesses of the femoral component. Collateral ligaments are then balanced with the trial implants in place. If done properly, the two techniques should produce identical results with regard to stability and alignment. A navigation system for assisting the performance of a total knee replacement should provide separate software programs to support each surgical approach. Surgeons should use the approach with which they are most familiar and comfortable.

Ligaments function properly with the desired isometry in the measured resection technique if the origin of the collateral ligaments is at or closely related to the axis of tibiofemoral flexion-extension. For circular condylar femoral geometry and dished tibial plateau geometry, the centers of femoral rotation coincide with the centers of the femoral surface geometry. It is essential to the optimum performance of the measured resection technique that the size of the femoral implant closely approximates the size of the femur. It is important to realize that the measured resection technique can be carried out by starting with a femoral or tibial resection. The femoral implant size and rotation can be determined using a posterior referencing or anterior referencing technique. Navigation software should allow the surgeon to choose among these options.

Preferred Approach

I prefer the navigated measured resection approach for the following reasons:

1. It is easier and faster for me to perform than the gap balancing technique.

2. It is consistent with the way I perform a TKA using manual techniques.
3. The instrumentation is most compatible with less invasive surgical approaches.
4. It places the implants in consistent positions with regard to the bones.
5. It allows accurate reproducible alignment of the extremity and implants.
6. Its use has been associated with very little need for soft tissue releases.
7. It allows for an accurate assessment of ligament tension with actual trials firmly in position.

Although the measured resection technique can be performed accurately beginning on either the femur or tibia, I prefer to start the procedure on the femur for the following reasons:

1. Exposure of the distal femur for initial resections is relatively easy and can be accomplished with the leg in relative extension.
2. Removal of the resected distal femoral fragment is relatively easy in comparison to removal of the proximal tibia fragment. As a result, there may be less tendency to overresect the tibia once access is made possible by the femoral resection.
3. Knowledge of the thickness of resection of the distal and posterior femur helps in planning the tibial resection.

Although the measured resection technique can be performed accurately using an anterior or posterior referencing approach to establish the size and rotation of the femur, I prefer the anterior referencing approach because the posterior condylar anatomy is highly variable and unpredictable and locating consistent posterior condylar points is not reliable. As a result, the posterior condylar line is not a reliable guide for establishing the rotation or size of the femoral component. Moreover, precise placement of the femoral implant on the anterior cortex is difficult with the posterior referencing technique. The accuracy of this technique is further compromised if less invasive approaches are used that may make access to the posterior condyles even more difficult. The anterior referencing approach allows the anterior cortex of the femur to be identified accurately and makes precise rotational alignment of the femoral component using the plane of patellar tracking possible. However, if the anterior referencing technique is used, it is critical that an accurate determination of femoral component size be made before positioning the alignment guide. Both navigation and manual tools should be used to make this determination.

Surgical Technique

The computer-assisted measured gap resection technique follows the steps that a surgeon normally takes during the manual performance of a TKA using this approach. Pins are placed in the femur and tibia to hold the passive or active trackers (Fig. 116-2A). The skin incision is then made in routine fashion for the approach favored by the surgeon (see Fig. 116-2B). Kinematic (Fig. 116-3) and surface (Fig. 116-4) registration are then performed to establish the location of critical anatomic landmarks. The eventual femoral rotation is established by marking the path of the patella (Fig. 116-5). The distal femoral alignment guide is positioned using navigation to establish desired varus-valgus and flexion-extension

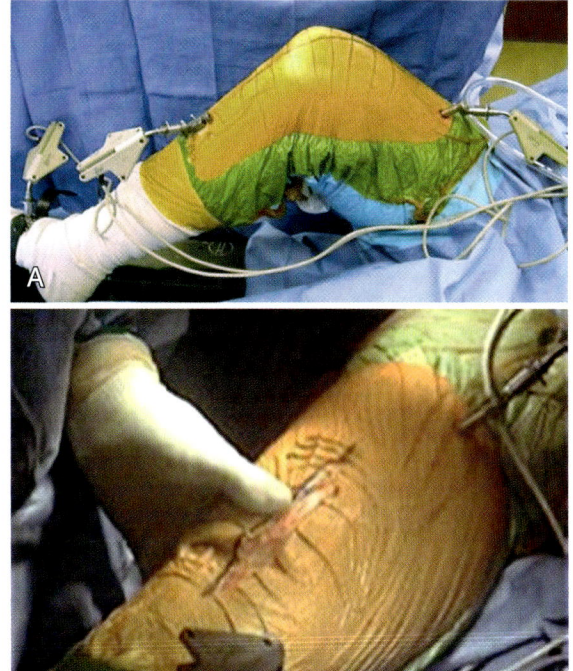

Figure 116-2. A, Cortical pins in distal femur and proximal tibia with trackers attached. **B,** Skin incision from top of patella to tibial tubercle.

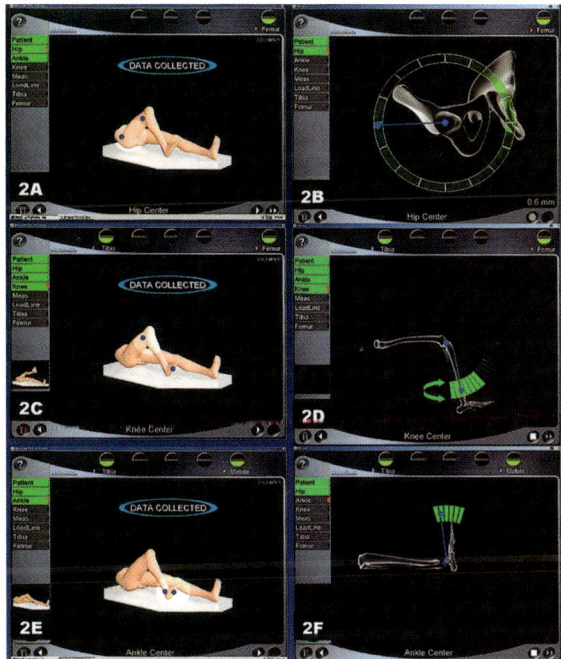

Figure 116-3. A-F, Registration of the kinematic centers of the hip, knee, and ankle joints.

and depth of the femoral resection, which is then performed (Figs. 116-6 and 116-7). The anterior femoral and posterior condylar points acquired during the navigation registration process are used to determine the desired femoral component size. The AP position and rotation of the 4-in-1 cutting

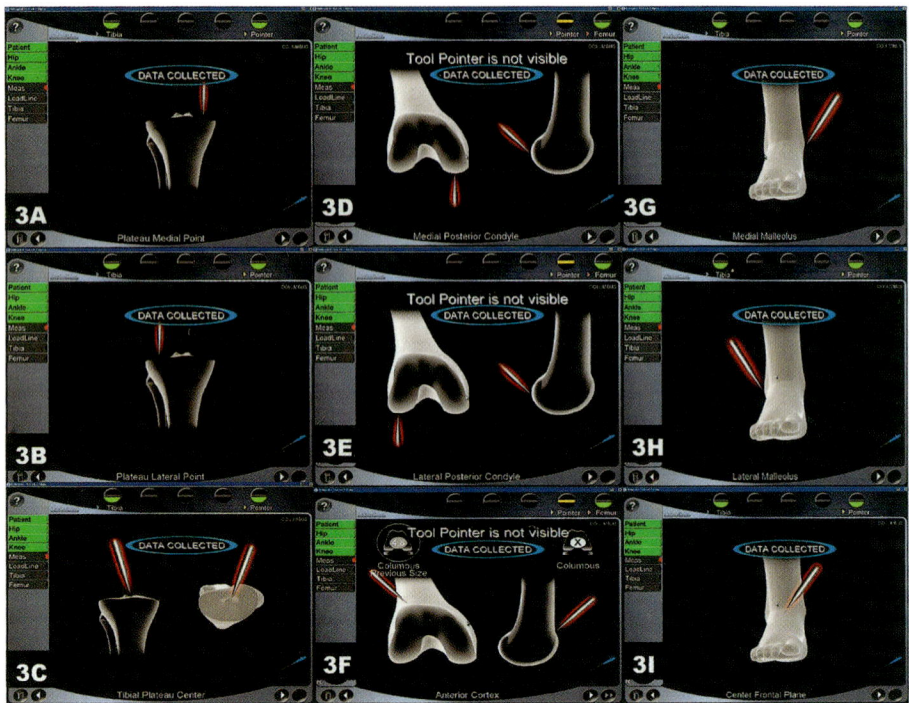

Figure 116-4. A-I, Surface registration the distal femur, proximal tibia, and ankle joint.

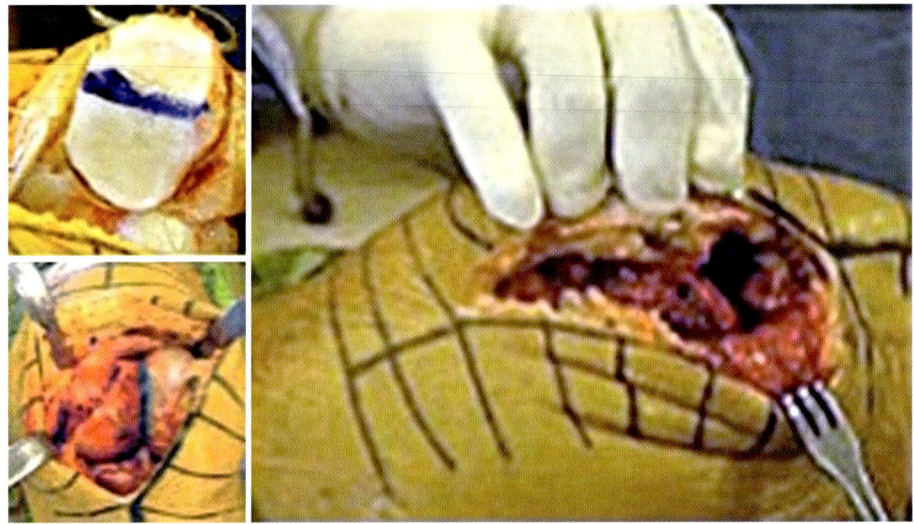

Figure 116-5. Establishing the path of patellar tracking.

block are established using the anterior referencing navigation guide (Fig. 116-8). The desired position of the tibial cutting block is established using the navigation system (Fig. 116-9). The size and symmetry of the flexion and extension gap are measured (Fig. 116-10). A trial reduction is performed and final implants are selected and inserted. Final balance, alignment, and range of motion are measured and recorded using the navigation system. Final patellar tracking is assessed (Fig. 116-11).

Summary

There is still some debate as to whether computer-assisted surgical techniques achieve a more accurately performed

TKA than manual procedures,[67,82,92,153] but a fair assessment of the current status of CAS TKA is that it is clearly helpful but not necessarily essential for producing an accurate, optimally functional, durable, and successful TKA. Moreover, there are certain clinical situations (e.g., the presence of intramedullary hardware in the femur or of a significant femoral or tibial diaphyseal deformity) for which CAS techniques are uniquely helpful. It is still uncertain whether a CAS TKA is associated with improved or more optimal clinical or kinematic knee function in the short or long term.[32,63] The impact of CAS TKA on the ultimate durability of total knee implants is also unknown.

However, the experience with CAS in the last 10 years has established that its value is much greater than simply

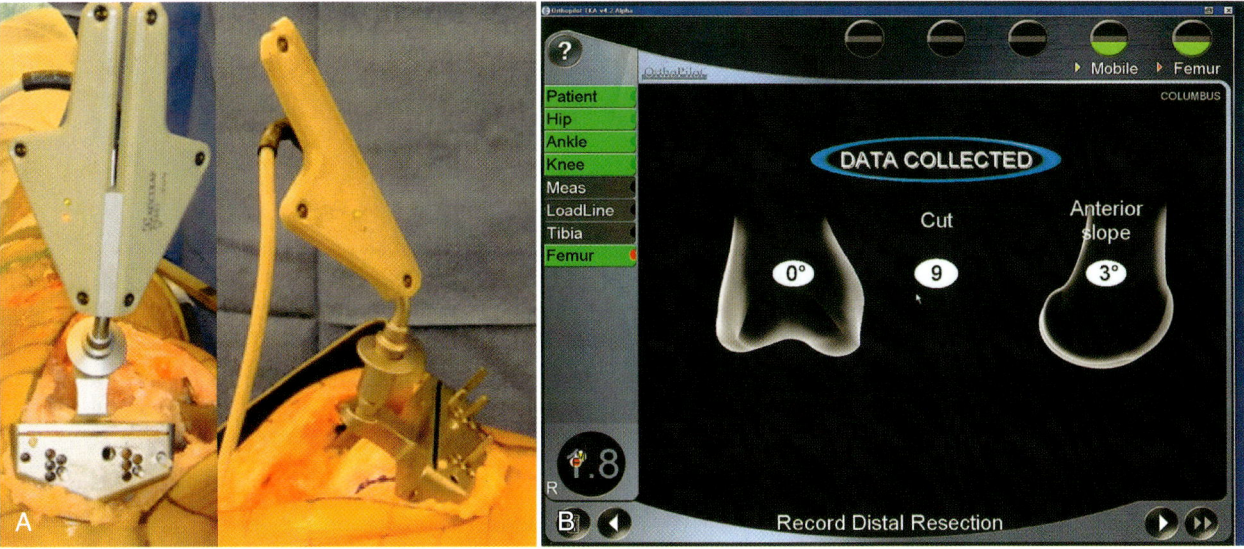

Figure 116-6. **A** and **B,** Distal femoral resection using navigation to guide frontal and sagittal alignment and depth of cut.

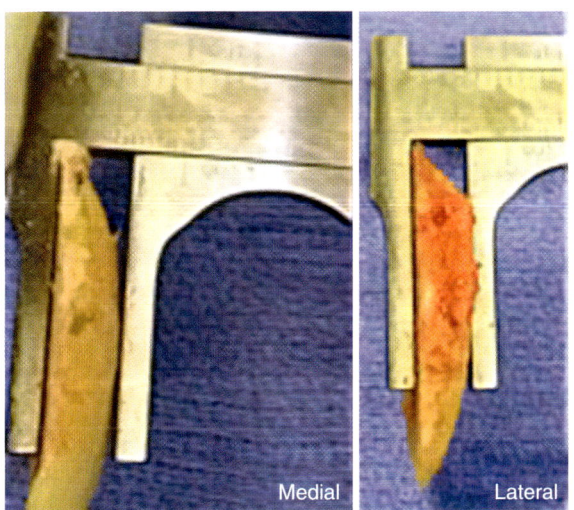

Figure 116-7. Thickness of distal cuts medially and laterally. The distal condyle with the greatest thickness should equal the thickness of the distal condyle of the implant.

making possible the performance of an accurate knee procedure. CAS can be used in the following ways: (1) as an adjunctive technology for minimally invasive TKA surgery; (2) as an important and potentially revolutionary teaching tool for knee reconstructive procedures; and (3) essential platform for the evolution of emerging CAS-based knee surgical technologies, including robotic-assisted surgery and patient-specific implants and instruments. These technologies are based on and, in many ways, are extensions of the navigation technologies that have been developed and used in the past decade. It is essential that these new technologies be evaluated carefully and critically and applied safely and accurately. Surgeons who are familiar and comfortable with current navigation technologies are in the best position to examine and initiate the use of these new CAS-based technologies. Because these technologies make direct control of the procedure less transparent than CAS navigation techniques, the potential for inadvertently introducing error into

a knee procedure is greater. For example, custom-made implants or instruments require that the devices be made accurately and used precisely. As currently conceived, the devices do not allow the surgeon to confirm intraoperatively the accuracy of the devices. However, surgeons who combine the use of navigation with the application of these devices can check the accuracy with which they were designed and applied. The emergence of new CAS-based surgical technologies is an exciting and natural development of CAS-based navigation technologies. Their emergence requires that surgeons obtain a clear understanding of the principles underlying their development and use.

UNICOMPARTMENTAL ARTHROPLASTY, ANTERIOR CRUCIATE LIGAMENT RECONSTRUCTION, AND HIGH TIBIAL OSTEOTOMY

The application of CAS to unicompartmental knee arthroplasty (UKA), ACL reconstruction, and high tibial osteotomy (HTO) is still in a relatively early stage of development. However, initial reports by the developers of these applications are extremely encouraging.* As with CAS TKA studies, these initial reports have indicated that the overall accuracy of implant and limb alignment is improved, the accuracy of individual implant alignment is increased, and the incidence of outliers is reduced when CAS techniques are used. Acceptance of these CAS applications for knee surgery is likely to be more widespread in the next few years.

FUTURE CONSIDERATIONS

There is surprisingly wide acceptance of the concept that navigation systems will become an accepted part of the knee surgeon's armamentarium. However, until the systems become more surgeon-friendly, less cumbersome, more efficient, and

---

*References 27, 28, 31, 33, 53, 56, 57, 60, 61, 70, 103, 108, and 120.

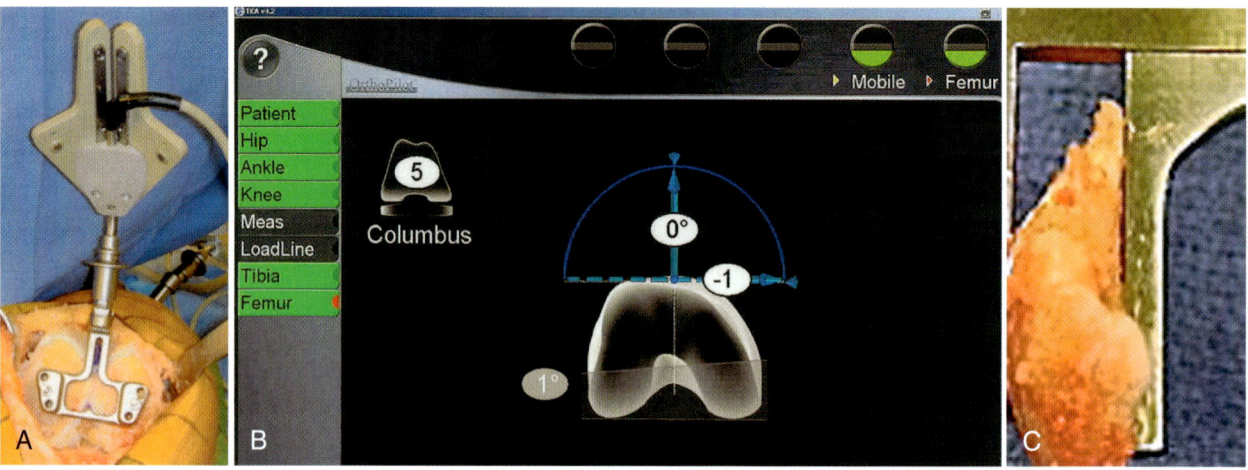

Figure 116-8. A-C, The size, rotation, and anteroposterior position of the 4-in-1 cutting block are established. The posterior resection thickness should equal the thickness of the posterior condyle of the implant.

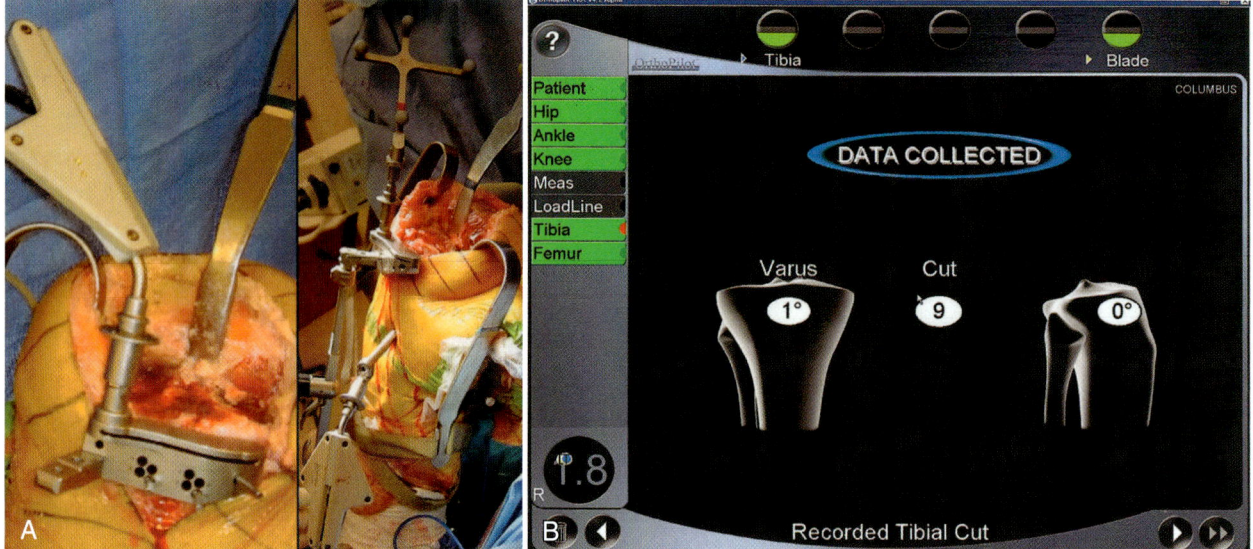

Figure 116-9. Align proximal tibial cutting block, carry out resection, and check accuracy of the cut.

less expensive, the widespread acceptance of CAS by knee surgeons may be limited. Many developments currently in progress may accelerate this acceptance.

CAS systems will continue to be refined to allow multiple knee procedures (e.g., TKA, UKA, ACL reconstruction, HTO) to be performed by a single CAS unit with a common set of computer hardware and software and common user interface. These knee suites will facilitate the use of a single CAS system by surgeons performing a wide range of knee procedures.[136] The effort expended to learn how to use one system for one application will not need to be repeated when the same system is used for other knee applications. The use of a single CAS system to perform multiple knee procedures will also make the substantial financial outlay required for these units more justifiable.

The price of the hardware components of CAS systems is also likely to decrease significantly. As the number of users of CAS technologies increases, the source of hardware components (e.g., optical trackers) will increase and thus put downward pressure on prices. The consolidation of orthopedic companies has resulted in each one offering the full array of knee procedures, from arthroscopy to complex arthroplasty reconstructions. As these companies integrate and support the CAS systems for these procedures, the cost of these units to hospitals should also decrease.

Developments that are most likely to increase the use of CAS systems by knee surgeons are those that further integrate surgeons' current techniques with navigation techniques. Wireless systems using a technology such as electromagnetism would eliminate the current aggravation of having to maintain a line of sight between the computer and operated extremity, decrease the bulkiness of current navigation equipment, and reduce concerns regarding intraoperative tracker movement, bone fracture, or neurovascular injuries. However, as these systems become available, their safety and accuracy must be confirmed. They must be equal in safety and accuracy to the optical systems currently available.

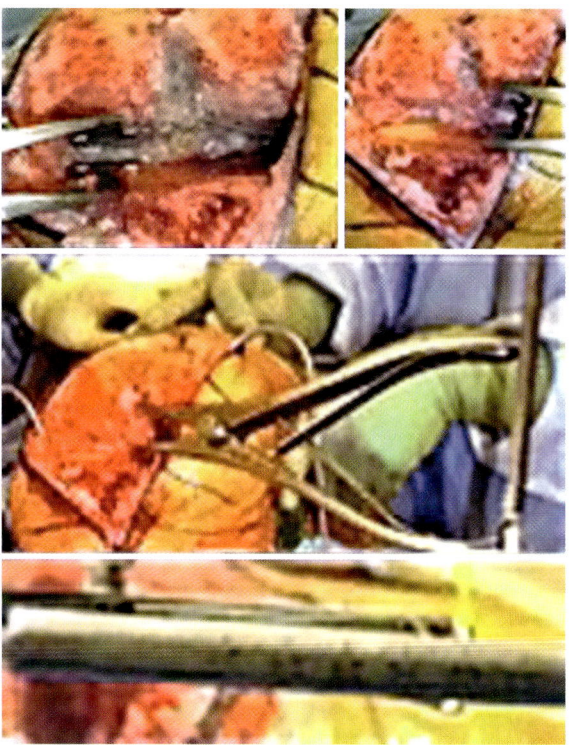

Figure 116-10. Check the size and symmetry of the flexion and extension gaps.

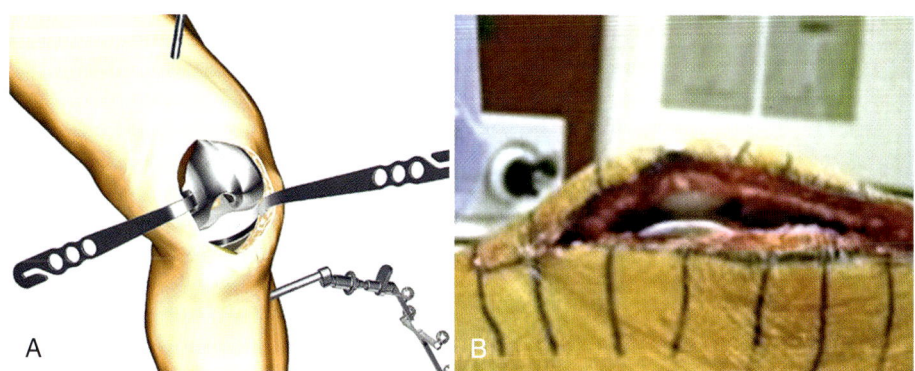

Figure 116-11. A, Implants inserted. **B,** Patellar tracking assessed.

Perhaps the most immediate benefit of CAS knee systems will be the development of more accurate mechanical tools. The influence of CAS on mechanical instrumentation is already being felt. Most knee surgery systems now require that cutting blocks be affixed to bone with power-driven pins. Anterior referencing for the establishment of femoral rotation is increasing in popularity. Jigs have been developed to improve the positioning of cutting blocks in the sagittal plane, the source of the most consistent error in TKA implant and limb alignment.

The widespread interest in minimally invasive arthroplasty surgery is focusing surgeons' attention on the importance of retaining accurate implant and limb alignment as the exposure of surgical anatomy is reduced.[150] Techniques using nonfrontal resection planes (e.g., quadrant-sparing medial approach) are making clear how the position of an implant in one plane critically affects its position in all other planes.[138] CAS systems can greatly facilitate the evolution of

minimally invasive knee surgery procedures. However, CAS hardware and software must be configured to support the minimally invasive systems that are being developed safely, accurately, and efficiently.

KEY REFERENCES

Anderson KC, Buehler KC, Markel DC: Computer assisted navigation in total knee arthroplasty: comparison with conventional methods. J Arthroplasty 20(Suppl 3):132–138, 2005.

Bauwens K, Matthes GT, Wich M, et al: Navigated total knee replacement. A meta-analysis. J Bone Joint Surg Am 89:261–269, 2007.

Chauhan SK, Scott RG, Breidahl W, Beaver RJ: Computer-assisted knee arthroplasty versus a conventional jig-based technique. A randomized, prospective trial. J Bone Joint Surg Br 86:372–377, 2004.

Delp SL, Stulberg SD, Davies B, et al: Computer-assisted knee replacement. Clin Orthop Relat Res 354:49–56, 1998.

Jenny JY, Boeri C: Navigated implantation of total knee prostheses: a comparison with conventional techniques. Orthop Ihre Grenzgeb 139:117–119, 2001.

Kim YH, Kim JS, Choi Y, Kwon OR: Computer-assisted surgical navigation does not improve the alignment and orientation of the components in total knee arthroplasty. J Bone Joint Surg Am 91:14–19, 2009.

Klos TVS, Habets RJE, Banks AZ, et al: Computer assistance in arthroscopic anterior cruciate ligament reconstruction. In DiGioia AM, Jaramaz B, Picard R, Nolte PL, editors: Computer and robotic assisted knee and hip surgery, Oxford, 2004, Oxford University Press, pp 229–234.

Koyonos L, Granieri M, Stulberg SD: At what steps in performance of a TKA do errors occur when manual instrumentation is used? Presented at the Annual Meeting of the American Academy of Orthopaedic Surgeons, Washington, DC, February 23–27, 2005.

Stulberg SD, Yaffe MA, Koo SS: Computer-assisted surgery versus manual total knee arthroplasty: a case-controlled study. J Bone Joint Surg Am 88:47–54, 2006.

Weng YJ, Hsu RWW, Hsu WH: Comparison of computer-assisted navigation and conventional instrumentation for bilateral total knee arthoplasty. J Arthroplasty 24:668–673, 2009.

Full references for this chapter can be found on www.expertconsult.com.

Chapter 117

Imageless Computer Navigation in Total Knee Arthroplasty: The Simpler Wave of the Future

Aaron A. Hofmann and Jeremy McCandless

The use of computer-based systems during total knee arthroplasty (TKA) has become more readily accepted during recent years. Computer-assisted surgery for total knee replacement was first approved for use in the United States in 2001. Since its introduction, this technology has expanded rapidly, and several different types of navigation systems have been developed by several different manufacturers. Each new version of the software has incorporated increasingly sophisticated analysis modules to allow not only accurate alignment of the limb and component position but also assessment of ligament balance and knee kinematics.[45] An increasing number of references in the orthopedic literature are reporting on computer-assisted techniques and early outcomes with these techniques.* Each system affords surgeons the opportunity to maximize clinical outcomes by perfecting the surgical technique. Specifically, component alignment during the procedure must be optimized.[20,21,31]

The significance of component and limb alignment has been extensively studied since the earliest days of TKA. Several early references in the knee arthroplasty literature focusing on outcome and experience with TKA underscore the importance of alignment.[2,29,37] Alignment errors in TKA greater than 3 degrees can be associated with poorer outcomes and accelerated failure. Rotation of the femoral and tibial components has a strong influence on patellar tracking, and malrotation of components can lead to patellofemoral complications.[8] Hungerford and Krackow proposed that technical perfection of alignment and component position should be the goals for TKA.[20] Insall found that most failures in TKA could be attributed to incorrect ligament balance or incorrect alignment.[21] Moreland's experience in TKA yielded similar findings and led him to state that component alignment was the most important factor influencing postoperative loosening and instability.[31] The real promise with computer navigation may be its potential to help surgeons avoid outliers when using standard instruments (Fig. 117-1). Outliers represent patients who fall outside the accepted values for alignment. Conventional techniques that use extramedullary alignment guides or intramedullary rods for component orientation can result in component malalignment.[15,34] The computer-assisted technique allows errors to be verified and corrected intraoperatively. Even an experienced surgeon can attain improved results (Tables 117-1 and 117-2).

Numerous studies already support the use of computer-assisted systems in knee arthroplasty. In 1999, Krackow and associates published a technique that used computer assistance to determine proper mechanical axis alignment during TKA.[26] Jenny and Boeri compared a navigation system with a surgeon-controlled operative technique in 60 TKAs.[23] Radiographic evaluation demonstrated improved accuracy of

implantation in the computer-assisted group. Bathis and colleagues showed that computer-assisted TKA gave better correction of alignment of the leg and orientation of the components than the conventional technique did.[3] If implant longevity, pain relief, and function are related to the accuracy with which a TKA is performed, mechanical instrumentation does not result in a high incidence of accuracy when each step of the procedure is measured.[42] Computer-assisted TKA allows more reproducible component positioning, avoids outliers in alignment errors, and assists with soft tissue balancing.

The incidence of fat embolism syndrome from instrumenting the medullary canal during cemented or cementless TKA is not negligible.[25,30] Kim found that fat embolism was seen in 65 patients (65%) with a bilateral TKA and in 46 patients (46%) with a unilateral TKA.[25] Comparative studies between conventional and computer-assisted surgery have been performed to look at embolism occurrence via Doppler or echocardiography studies. It has been shown using this method that computer-assisted surgery significantly decreases the occurrence of embolic events.[12,24] With computer-assisted surgery, violation of the medullary canal is avoided, thereby reducing the occurrence of embolic events.

Computer-assisted systems generally can be grouped into three different types: image-based navigation systems, robotic systems, and image-free navigation systems. Image-based systems require preoperative computed tomography (CT) scans, whereas image-free navigation systems gain all necessary information intraoperatively during a registration process. Computer-integrated instrumentation incorporates highly accurate measurement devices to locate joint centers, track surgical tools, and confirm alignment of prosthetic components. Image-based knee replacement provides a three-dimensional preoperative plan that guides placement of the cutting blocks and prosthetic components. Robot-assisted knee replacement allows one to machine bones accurately without the use of standard cutting blocks. Image-free navigation allows real-time evaluation of deformity and bone cuts and is becoming the standard for computer-assisted knee surgery.

IMAGE-BASED SYSTEMS

In image-based total knee replacement, the procedure begins with preoperative planning. To create the preoperative plan, three-dimensional computer models of the patient's femur and tibia are constructed from CT or fluoroscopic data. Once computer models of the bones have been created, planning software orients the tibial and femoral components and calculates bone resections that align the mechanical axis of the limb and produce the intended implant contact. An intraoperative system determines the position and orientation of the patient's femur and tibia and guides placement of the cutting

---

*References 2, 3, 6, 9, 11, 15, 24, 29, 34, 35, 39, 42, and 48.

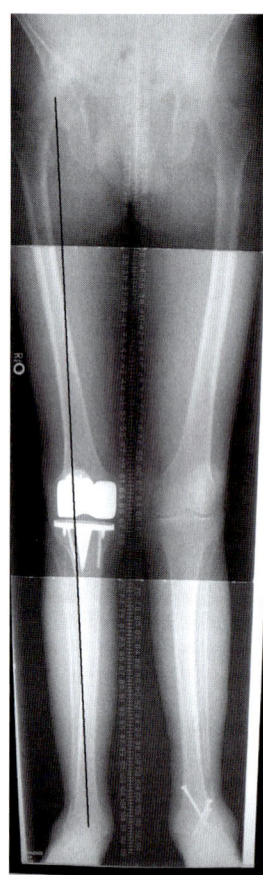

Figure 117-1. Long, standing radiograph of malpositioned total knee arthroplasty components performed with standard instruments.

jigs so that resections determined in the preoperative plan can be made.[14] Image-based navigation systems include the fluoroscope unit and the CT scanner. Frequent use of the fluoroscope in an operation presents a potential radiation hazard to the surgical staff and patient. A technique known as virtual fluoroscopy enhances the fluoroscope's capability for image-guided surgery by optically tracking the position of the C-arm, the surgical instruments, and the patient. Virtuality is achieved by the overlay of surgical instruments onto one or more previously captured fluoroscopic images. A key benefit of virtual fluoroscopy is that it considerably reduces the radiation hazard.[36]

CT scan navigation has shown good results in surgeons' hands. Chauhan and coworkers demonstrated that computer-assisted total knee replacement via CT navigation techniques resulted in better alignment of the femoral component and the posterior slope of the tibial component in rotation and flexion and better matching of the femoral and tibial components in rotation in a cadaver model.[10] Perlick and associates implanted 100 TKAs with the computer-assisted technique (50 knees) or the conventional approach (50 knees). Accuracy of implantation was determined on postoperative long-leg coronal and lateral radiographs. A postoperative leg axis between 3 degrees varus and 3 degrees valgus was achieved in 46 patients in the group with computer-assisted implantation and in 36 patients in the control group ($P = .01$). A significant difference was noted in femoral component alignment in the frontal plane. Investigators concluded that the

CT-based navigation system improves the accuracy of TKA, but that higher cost and time-consuming planning mean that its use will be limited to special cases.[35]

In image-based knee replacement, analysis of the three-dimensional image data allows the surgeon to determine the size of the implant preoperatively, thereby potentially reducing inventory. Image-based systems also allow comparison of actual placement of the implants relative to planned placement. Radiation exposure from CT or fluoroscope sources in image-based navigation remains a significant concern for both patient and surgeon.

ROBOT-ASSISTED SURGERY

Robot-assisted knee replacement was designed to improve the accuracy and precision of bone resection. Robot-assisted surgery can aid in drilling alignment holes for conventional cutting blocks to make femoral and tibial bone cuts. Robot assistance also provides the capability to machine bone surfaces for alignment or for contact areas for bone ingrowth. The earlier version of these robotic systems used industrial robots, which are not suitable or designed for use in the operating room.[39] Similar to image-guided knee replacement, robot-assisted surgery has the advantage of providing preoperative imaging, modeling, and planning. The machining capability of a robot may provide a more accurate fit between prosthesis and bone, thus making the use of cement unnecessary in certain cases because of the ability to control milling heads and minimize temperature increases noted with the conventional saw technique. One mechanism being used to minimize the discomfort that surgeons feel regarding robotic surgery is robotically assisted surgery. A surgeon may template an implant using computer navigation, and the surgeon's hand controls a burr that machines a location in the bone for it. Errant strokes with the burr at the terminal end of the robotic arm are controlled by a mechanical block (haptic feedback). Bellemans and associates described their initial results with 25 robot-assisted primary knee arthroplasties. They achieved excellent results with alignment, yet they point out that cost, the learning curve, and excessive tourniquet time (>100 minutes) are significant obstacles that remain to be overcome.[6]

IMAGE-FREE NAVIGATION SYSTEMS

Image-free navigation systems use mechanical instruments that are enhanced by their integration with accurate measuring equipment. Current image-free navigation systems are predominantly using infrared or electromagnetic tracking technology (Fig. 117-2).[47] Reference frames or trackers are used to locate the limb in space (Fig. 117-3). These trackers or frames can be attached to bones and to surgical instruments to track the position and orientation of each surgical tool relative to the bone. The computer workstation displays the position of the cutting blocks relative to the desired position. Once the jig is oriented properly, it is secured in position, and bone cuts are made with a standard saw.[13]

The author compared alignment between 50 TKAs performed with an imageless computer navigation system— Navitrack System-Optical Total Knee Replacement CT-Less device (Orthosoft, Montreal, Quebec, Canada) or Medtronic Trio system (Louisville, Colo) (see Fig. 117-3)—and 50

Table 117-1 Standard Instrumentation—Accuracy of Alignment*

Author	Technique	Study Size	Results
Engh and Petersen[16]	Intramedullary	72 TKAs	Femoral component position
	Extramedullary		IM: 35/40 (87.5%) within ±3 degrees of goal
			EM: 22/32 (68.8%) within ±3 degrees of goal
			Tibiofemoral alignment
			IM: 88% correct
			EM: 73% correct
Dennis et al[15]	Intramedullary	120 TKAs	Tibial component position
	Extramedullary		IM: 72% within ±2 degrees of goal
			EM: 88% within ±2 degrees of goal
Teter et al[46]	Intramedullary	352 TKAs	Tibial component position
	Extramedullary		IM: 94% within ±4 degrees of goal
			EM: 92% within ±4 degrees of goal
Teter et al[46]	Intramedullary	201 TKAs	Femoral component position
			IM: 91.5% within ±4 degrees of goal
Lam & Shakespeare[28]	Intramedullary	362 TKAs	Femoral component position
			IM: 92% within ±3 degrees of goal
Jeffcote & Shakespeare[22]	Extramedullary	350 TKAs	Tibial component position
			IM: 96.3% within ±2 degrees of goal
Bolognesi & Hofmann[9]	CAS	100 TKAs	Femoral component position
	Intramedullary		CAS: 98% within ±3 degrees of goal
	Extramedullary		IM: 90% within ±3 degrees of goal
			Tibial component position
			CAS: 100% within ±3 degrees of goal
			EM: 92% within ±3 degrees of goal

CAS, Computer-assisted system; *EM*, extramedullary; *IM*, intramedullary; *TKA*, total knee arthroplasty.
　*Composite table of published results for standard instrumentation. Results of the current study are included for the purpose of comparison.

Table 117-2 Comparative Studies—Computer-Assisted Technique versus Standard Instrumentation*

Author	System	Technique	Study Size	Results
Jenny & Boeri[23]	Orthopilot	CAS	30 TKAs	Tibiofemoral alignment
		Standard	30 TKAs	CAS: 25/30 within ±3 degrees of goal
				Standard: 21/30 within ±3 degrees of goal
Sparmann et al[40]	Stryker	CAS	240 TKAs	Tibiofemoral alignment
		Standard		CAS > Standard
Hart et al[18]	Orthopilot	CAS	60 TKAs	Tibiofemoral alignment
		Standard	60 TKAs	CAS: 53/60 within ±2 degrees of goal
				Standard: 42/60 within ±2 degrees of goal
Bathis et al[4]	BrainLab	CAS	50 TKAs	Tibiofemoral alignment
		Standard	50 TKAs	CAS: 48/50 within ±3 degrees of goal
				Standard: 38/50 within ±3 degrees of goal
Bolognesi & Hofmann[9]	Orthosoft	CAS	50 TKAs	Tibiofemoral alignment
		Standard	50 TKAs	CAS: 45/50 within ±3 degrees of goal
				Standard: 43/50 within ±3 degrees of goal

CAS, Computer-assisted system; *TKA*, total knee arthroplasty.
　*Composite table of published results for studies comparing a computer-assisted technique with a standard instrumentation technique. Results of the current study are included for the purpose of comparison.

TKAs performed with standard instrumentation. The purpose of the study was to compare postoperative component alignment between two groups of 50 TKAs, all performed by a single surgeon. The same surgeon used a posterior-referencing TKA system (Natural Knee, Zimmer, Warsaw, Ind) in all cases. Long, standing radiographs were collected at 6 weeks'

follow-up and were measured for component orientation. When the navigation system was used, 98% (49/50) of all femoral components and 100% (50/50) of all tibial components were placed within ±3 degrees of the radiographic goal position. In the standard instrumentation group, accuracy was decreased to 90% (45/50) and 92% (46/50) within ±3

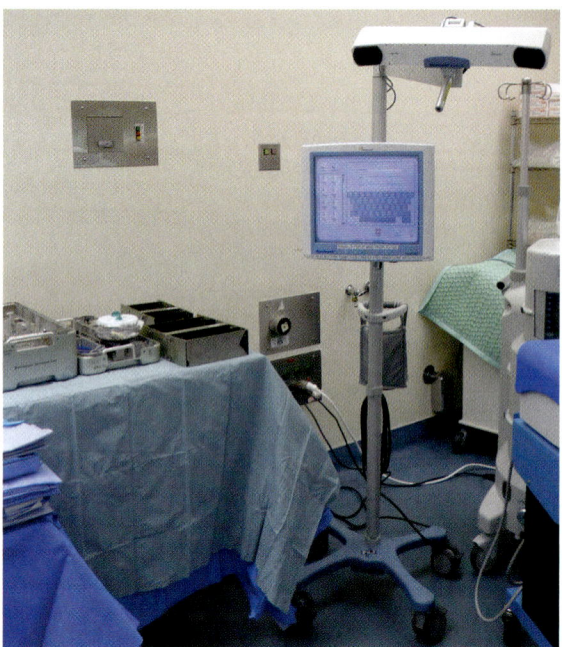

Figure 117-2. An imageless computer navigation system showing the computer screen and infrared camera.

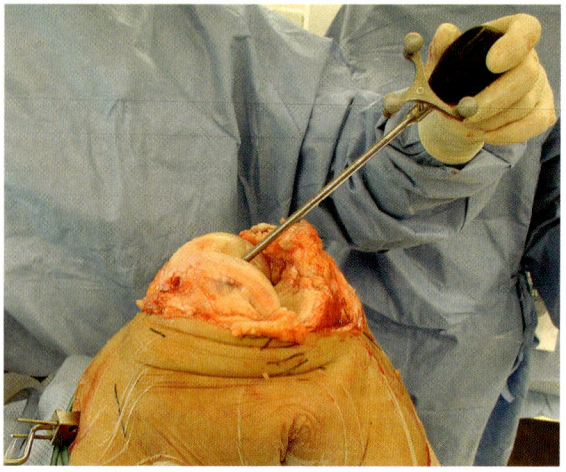

Figure 117-3. Trackers are placed on the femur and tibia to allow the computer to assess the limb in space. A pointer is used to identify a few additional registration points.

degrees, respectively. A significant difference in standard deviations was observed for the navigated cases and the conventional cases when femoral ($P = .016$) and tibial ($P = .013$) component position was considered. Average tourniquet time was 68 minutes in the navigated group and 57 minutes in the conventional group.[9] Chauhan and coworkers showed that computer-assisted surgery took slightly longer, with a mean increase of 13 minutes ($P = .0001$).[11]

This imageless navigation system is straightforward and simple with only a few additional steps needed for tracker placement and validation of bone cuts. The authors use a technique that allows intraoperative flexibility to abandon computer navigation at any point by utilizing conventional instrumentation confirmed by computer navigation. This technique has been simplified over time to minimize redundancy and maximize operating room efficiency. The

Navitrack System-Optical Total Knee Replacement CT-Less device consists of a computer workstation, an optical tracking system, surgical instruments, and tracking devices. Tracking devices are affixed to a free tracker and a pointing instrument, which allows these instruments to be tracked and displayed in real-time on a monitor. The surgical technique is very straightforward. The knee is exposed via a standard medial parapatellar, midvastus, or subvastus approach, depending on the surgeon's preference. Intraoperatively, tracking devices are attached to the femur and to the tibia; this allows them to also be displayed in real-time on the monitor. The lower extremity is held in extension during placement of the femoral trackers. Two partially threaded $\frac{1}{8}$-inch Steinmann pins are placed in unicortical fashion so that they slightly engage the second cortex of the femur. The inset screws in the tracker are tightened to secure the tracker to the pins. A similar technique is used to place two pins distally on the anteromedial aspect of the tibia for placement of the tibial tracker.

The hip is taken through a range of motion to establish the center of rotation of the femoral head. Fourteen points are documented during this motion analysis to compute the location of the center of the femoral head. The pointer instrument is then used to digitize the entry point of the femur in the intercondylar notch 2 mm above the fibers of the posterior cruciate ligament (PCL). The posterior referencing guide with the claws attached is placed on the distal femur to reference the two posterior condyles because the Natural Knee II (Zimmer) system is a posterior-referencing system. The tracking device with claws is positioned in the desired 5 degrees of flexion on the distal femur while contact with the posterior condyles is maintained as a posterior reference. The registration of the femur is now complete. Tibial registration begins with registration of the mechanical axis of the tibia, which is roughly in the footprint of the anterior cruciate ligament (ACL). Registration of the medial third of the tibial tubercle and the posterior tibia registers an anteroposterior axis. Finally, registration of the most prominent point of the medial and lateral malleoli completes registration of the tibia for the computer. Once these points are entered, the intraoperative deformity can be determined and evaluated. The varus/valgus deformity, as well as the flexion/extension deformity, can be saved on the system. At this point, the surgeon can make an evaluation of how correctable the deformity is in real-time with numeric values appearing on the computer module. This capability gives the surgeon valuable information for planning soft tissue balancing strategies.

Femoral preparation is begun by minimally impacting a cruciate spike into the distal femoral entry point without penetration or violation of the actual canal (Fig. 117-4). Conventional instrumentation in the form of a distal femoral cutting jig is then placed over the spike, which alternatively could be placed over an intramedullary rod for non–computer navigated arthroplasty. A tracker attached to the cutting block assesses flexion and varus/valgus based on registration data from the initial computer calibration. The distal femoral cutting guide is pinned into place after it is confirmed that the computer alignment is correct. After the distal femoral cut, the free tracker can assess and validate the varus/valgus and flexion angle of the cut (Fig. 117-5). The goal of flexion is 5.0 degrees to account for the anterior bow of the femur. Further modification of the cut can be

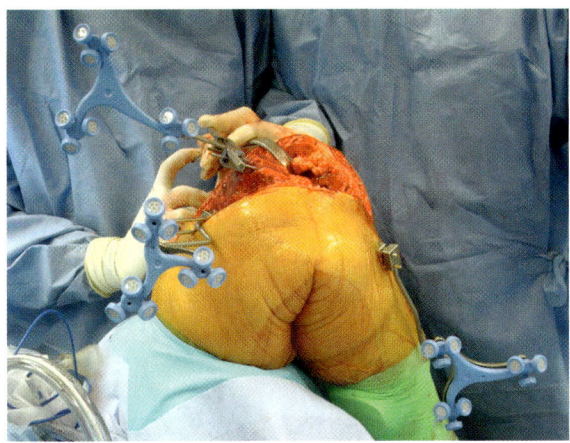

Figure 117-4. When conventional cutting blocks are used, navigation of the saw capture verifies alignment of distal femoral and proximal tibial cuts to allow fine-tuning of the position.

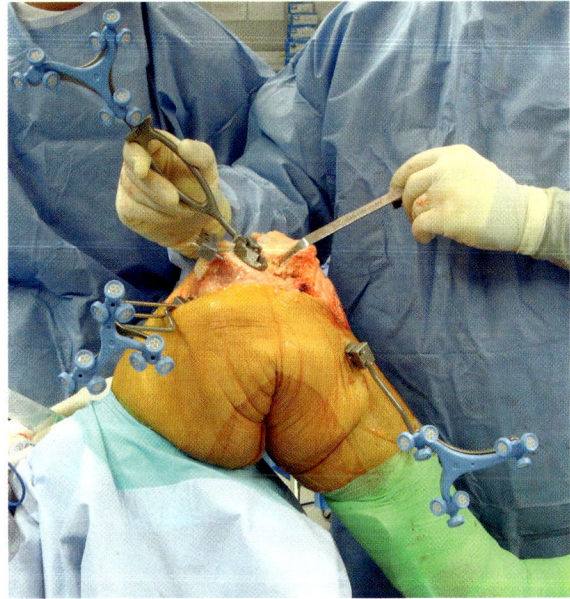

Figure 117-5. Validation of cut is performed with a tracker designed to fit against the flat surface of cut bone.

made if it is unsatisfactory at this point. The remainder of femoral preparation proceeds in conventional fashion with anteroposterior and chamfer cuts.

Attention is then directed to the tibia. Rotation, slope, and varus/valgus orientation are established by positioning the conventional extramedullary tibial cutting guide. A tracker device is then placed in the saw capture slot, and the computer guides the actual varus/valgus and slope of the standard tibial cutting system. After the cut is completed, the free tracker with claws attached is placed on the flat tibial surface to compare the planned cut with the final result. Additional modifications, if necessary, can be done at this point.

Trial components can then be placed, and the navigation system can evaluate flexion and extension of the knee, as well as the overall alignment axis. The surgeon can evaluate the soft tissue balancing that has been achieved by manual varus/valgus stress testing. The range of motion of the knee and

overall hip-knee-ankle alignment can be documented by the system at the time of trial reduction, and again at final component placement. When a cemented technique is used, fine-tuning can be performed during cement setup. This allows for further adjustment of varus/valgus alignment, as well as flexion/extension relationships. All this information can be saved on the system as data points to determine how effectively the deformity was corrected. Threaded pins used for the trackers are removed from the femur and the tibia at the time of wound closure.

The authors believe that some features of this imageless computer navigation system may be advantageous over other computer-assisted systems. The system is truly imageless; therefore there is no need for preoperative CT imaging or intraoperative fluoroscopy to allow navigation. Another advantage of the system is the fact that it incorporates standard cutting blocks and cutting guides from a preexisting total knee design (Natural Knee II) with a proven clinical track record.[19] The current set has only a few additional instruments (see Fig. 117-5). In addition, violation of the intramedullary canal is avoided with this instrumentation. Navigation may lead to improved component survivorship in the long term and a reduction in the complications associated with embolic phenomena that occur with intramedullary instruments.

Radiographic comparison between image-based and image-free navigation systems was conducted by Bathis and associates. A total of 130 patients underwent TKA with a CT-based or a CT-free module of the BrainLAB Vector-Vision Navigation System (Westchester, Ill). Postoperative leg alignment and component orientation were determined on long-leg coronal and lateral radiographs. Sixty of 65 patients in the CT-based group and 63 of 65 patients in the CT-free group had a postoperative leg axis between 3 degrees varus/valgus. No significant differences were found for varus/valgus orientation of the femoral and tibial components.[3] A similar study by Zumstein and colleagues was performed in 2006 to evaluate alignment by comparing image-based, image-free, and conventional techniques. Investigators demonstrated significant improvement in femoral component positioning with both image-based and image-free navigation, at 92% and 97%, respectively, within ±3 degrees of goal, compared with 80% with conventional techniques. In this study, image-free navigation performed better than image-based navigation in terms of femoral component alignment.[48]

It is important to realize that computer navigation systems are not all the same, and that they cannot be relied on independently. As with all techniques, they can certainly have imperfections. Stulberg and coworkers reported significant concerns about the registration accuracy of software for the OrthoPilot system.[43] It was thought that the biggest variable leading to inaccuracy was the surgical technique. Their experience indicated that approximately 10 procedures were required to develop a reliable registration technique. However, the software is constantly being upgraded to allow easier operation of the system, thus facilitating the procedures necessary for data input and understanding. In addition, standard instrumentation can be used to validate computer information before the actual bone cuts are made. Some concern about bone fractures has arisen as a result of tracker placement in the femur or tibia. The authors have not seen this complication in their patient population with unicortical placement of threaded pins.

CONCLUSION

The cost associated with use of any of the systems just described is not minimal at this time. New equipment, including robots, modules, trackers, and computers, along with expenditures for CT scans and fluoroscopy, increases the cost of the operative procedure. Over time, however, prices will become more competitive between the manufacturing companies, and more compact computer systems will become available.

The success of total knee replacement depends on several factors, including patient selection, prosthesis design and choice, soft tissue balancing, and alignment of the limb. Proper rotational and translational alignment of the femoral and tibial components, as well as the limb, is an important factor that can influence the outcome of knee replacement. A reduction in wear and component loosening and an increase in functional performance will be the result.

We predict that computer-assisted surgical techniques will be considered part of the standard of care for primary TKA in the future. Computer-integrated instruments that combine standard cutting guides with highly accurate measurement equipment are a natural extension of current techniques and offer several potential advantages. Improved accuracy has the potential to provide a very real advantage over more traditional techniques. Use of a navigation system provides improved alignment accuracy and can help avoid femoral malrotation and errors in axial alignment.[41] Long-term studies are required to confirm that this improvement in technique will lead to decreased rates of component revision and improved outcomes. The authors believe that computer navigation improves component position while minimizing outliers and makes a good surgeon even better.

Acknowledgment. The authors would like to acknowledge the contributions of Dr. Amit Lahav to the previous version of this chapter.

KEY REFERENCES

Bargren JH, Blaha JD, Freeman MA: Alignment in total knee arthroplasty: correlated biomechanical and clinical observations. Clin Orthop Relat Res 173:178–183, 1983.

Bathis H, Perlick L, Tingart M, et al: Alignment in total knee arthroplasty: a comparison of computer-assisted surgery with the conventional technique. J Bone Joint Surg Br 86:682–687, 2004.

Bellemans J, Vandenneucker H, Vanlauwe J, et al: Robot-assisted total knee arthroplasty. Clin Orthop Relat Res 464:111–116, 2007.

Bolognesi M, Hofmann A: Computer navigation versus standard instrumentation for TKA: a single-surgeon experience. Clin Orthop Relat Res 440:162–169, 2005.

Chauhan SK, Scott RG, Breidahl W, et al: Computer-assisted knee arthroplasty versus a conventional jig-based technique: a randomised, prospective trial. J Bone Joint Surg Br 86:372–377, 2004.

Dennis DA, Channer M, Susman MH, et al: Intramedullary versus extramedullary tibial alignment systems in total knee arthroplasty. J Arthroplasty 8:43–47, 1993.

Kalairajah Y, Cossey AJ, Verrrall GM, et al: Are systemic emboli reduced in computer-assisted knee surgery? A prospective, randomised, clinical trial. J Bone Joint Surg Br 88:198–202, 2006.

Lotke PA, Ecker ML: Influence of positioning of prosthesis in total knee replacement. J Bone Joint Surg Am 59:77–79, 1977.

Novotny J, Gonzalez MH, Amirouche FM, et al: Geometric analysis of potential error in using femoral intramedullary guides in total knee arthroplasty. J Arthroplasty 16:641–647, 2001.

Perlick L, Bathis H, Tingart M, et al: Navigation in total-knee arthroplasty: CT-based implantation compared with the conventional technique. Acta Orthop Scand 75:464–470, 2004.

Siston R, Giori N, Goodman S, et al: Surgical navigation for total knee arthroplasty: a perspective. J Biomech 40:728–735, 2007.

Stulberg SD: How accurate is current TKR instrumentation? Clin Orthop Relat Res 416:177–184, 2003.

Zumstein A, Frauchiger L, Wyss D, et al: Is restricted femoral navigation sufficient for accuracy of total knee arthroplasty? Clin Orthop Relat Res 451:80–86, 2006.

Full references for this chapter can be found on www.expertconsult.com.

Since the first uses of navigation appeared in orthopedics in the late 1990s, much has changed in terms of application, expectations, and options.* More information that has become available on failure allows the surgeon to refine accuracy in avoiding mechanical misalignment and in using individual components to reduce shear and eccentric loading.[5-7,11] Computer-assisted navigation (CAS) is one tool that now is more available, user-friendly, and versatile, and increasingly less expensive.

The most common system by far is infrared (IR). Trackers are designed to reflect IR signals from the camera receiver assembly. The limit of intercept or transmission of signals received is bound to a 135- to 100-degree arc or azimuth depending on the system. This mandates the array to be placed in the sweet spot of the best transmission power. Because of the physics of signal resolution and accuracy, the wider the separation of reflector balls of the tracker array, the more accurate the system. This mandates a minimum acceptable downsizing of the array, which many times is obtrusive to surgical exposure and is easily caught on instruments in the field of exposure. This necessitates placing the array in a remote area by using one or more pins to ensure secure fixation. However, this may result in soft issue tethering or injury when the extremity is moved.

Because of problems involving fixation, signal acquisition, and signal disruption by operating room (OR) personnel, thought was given to a non–line-of-sight signal that would be powerful enough to penetrate soft tissue, yet would not be prone to radiation such as that found in x-rays or fluoroscopy.[8] Electromagnetic (EM) CAS provided this full-radius reception without radiation exposure. EM CAS was first used for neurosurgical and ear, nose, and throat (ENT) applications in pediatric cranial surgery, where 360-degree coordinate measurements and minute three-axis navigation are necessary.[20]

Many of the drawbacks of early EM technology arose from stability of the signal, outside interference, and speed of computer computation of positional changes. However, with the advent of improved transmitters, magnetic flux generators referred to as localizers and receivers, and dynamic reference frames (DRFs) with multiple magnetic coils, signal accuracy has improved to the same level of accuracy as the industry standard of IR. Achieving this level of accuracy allows EM tracking to have status equivalent to that of traditional line-of-sight IR navigation systems while maintaining signal strength through soft tissues.

PHYSICS BEHIND ELECTROMAGNETIC NAVIGATION

By creating a low-intensity magnetic field, copper coil sensor receivers (DRFs) are able to read the strength received from

*References 1, 4, 10, 16-18, 21, 22, 25, and 33.

the electromagnetic field and produce a microcurrent. This field is produced by a transmitter or localizer that runs off of AC or DC current. Usually, these localizers are made by combining three or more coils that produce magnetic strength in an intermittent fashion, so as to constantly produce an oscillating or varied field, which imparts stronger sensitivity for receiver reception. The magnetic field is generally one gauss (0.0001 Tesla). A DRF placed in a particular position away from a magnetic field will transmit varied electric current depending on its position in relationship to field strength. However, the electric current produced is based on changes in the magnetic field, as well as in its intensity, hence the rationale behind a pulsed or oscillating field. The coil positioned in a parallel direction in relation to the field produces the maximum strength, whereas 90-degree polarization negates the electric current produced. With knowledge of field strength, computer calculations can determine its direction (Fig. 118-1). The system then can locate and orient the position of the receiver by the electric current it receives from one or more coils. A coil may measure not only field strength, but also the direction of the magnetic field, such that the XYZ position can be determined. It can also compute pitch and yaw, which is better known as 5 degrees of freedom. However, the sixth degree or role cannot be determined without two or more receiver coils to obtain this final dimension of orientation. Therefore, DRFs in an orthopedic setting will always have two coils. If an additional coil is used, it can fine-tune or can be a reference for the two primary coils to improve accuracy.

Transmitter coils, or field strength generators, are merely solenoids that are powered through the use of AC or DC current. Both types of technology have inherent advantages and disadvantages. Although DC is simple, it is not as accurate as AC because the sample size of the signal is reduced. Also, the magnet necessary to power the system is somewhat obtrusive in an operative field. AC technology uses audiofrequency wave energy to transmit to the receiver coil. The receiver coil works in much the same way as a transformer, in that it consists of loops of wire that create a small electric current. Through this oscillation system, a time sequence for frequency-multiplexed transmission of multiple magnets can create a more consistent and sustaining magnetic field that is less susceptible to outside interferences, such as metal, or environmental factors of other electromagnetic sources. It also is more prone to be misread by DRFs; therefore outside interferences are capable of disrupting accuracy. In the AC system using three-coil technology, computation is significantly more complex in terms of mathematical determination of the positions of instruments because of the oscillation, creating a more robust network of signals from the higher number of measured signal transmissions per second.[15] Yet as a result of increased signal sampling, the CAS system has enhanced sensitivity. Additionally, the magnet necessary to power the system is somewhat obtrusive in an operative field.

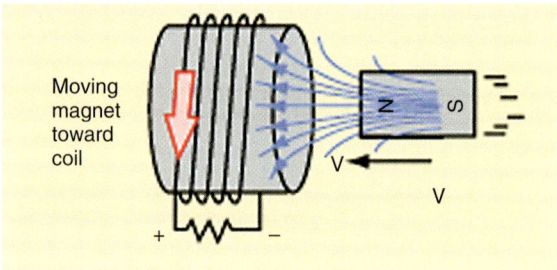

Figure 118-1. The soft iron inside the coil creates a magnetic field when the current is flowing. On the right is the receiver or dynamic reference frame (DRF), which creates the maximum current when the coil orientation is parallel in the field. These resultant formulas describe the energy of both.

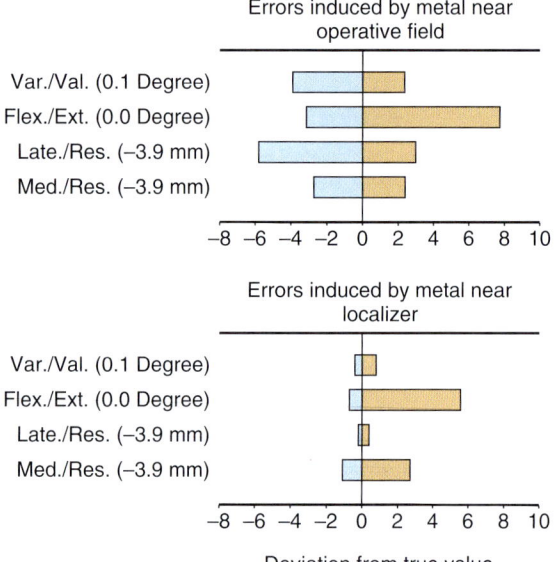

Figure 118-2. This graph shows the electromagnetic (EM) interference created when a mallet is placed near the operative field *(upper panel)* and the localizer *(lower panel)*. *Flex./Ext.,* Flexion/extension angle; *Late./Res.,* lateral resection depth; *Med./Res.,* medial resection depth; *Var./Val.,* varus/valgus angle. *Dark bars,* Minimal deviation; *light bars,* maximal deviation.

Multiple coils can reduce the size of the transmitter but can increase the computation time and the speed of localization. As such, AC technology is currently the gold standard.

DC technology uses coils powered by a direct current source. These coils are cycled sequentially and are subsequently read by the receiver coil. However, magnetic fields do not couple energy into loops of wire; therefore, they require a "hall effect" sensor, or flex gait technology. This flex gait technology refers to a much larger and more expensive sensor or receiver, which sometimes interferes with navigation issues in a surgical setting.

Originally, it was believed that DC current systems would offer the advantage of less interference from metal and other conductive distortions. However, in practice, the effect is a creation of fields from remote metal sources, which actually distort the navigation more than in a pulsed AC system. Because of these issues, AC technology has been adopted as the standard (Fig. 118-2).

Once a signal is activated, a pulse field is oscillated at 30 Hz and is sampled by the computer 10 times per second.

This measurement is averaged for the update on a second-by-second basis, providing the surgeon with the measured value currently displayed on the monitor screen.

Industry standards currently mandate ±1 mm in localization accuracy and ±1 degree of error in angle accuracy. Another term that is commonly used is *root mean square (RMS) error.* This is the normalization (always a positive value) of absolute deviation in values obtained by a measure, and it defines errors in system accuracy. Currently, the industry standard RMS error is ±4 mm of the center of the femoral head. This equals 1 degree of error at the level of the knee, which is well within the realm of human hand-held jigs. In actuality, many systems are much more accurate than the industry standard; however, to aid in simplicity at the time of surgery, decimal point accuracy is rounded up or down to make navigation more simplified. In actuality, the systems currently available in some cases are dummied down to 1 degree or 1 mm to provide more simplified navigation for surgeons.

Part of the exceptional accuracy of the systems stems from the aforementioned transmitter field generation system. However, additional precision has been achieved by smart instruments, which have defined read only memory (ROM) values. When the computer recognizes a particular distinctive discrete sensor that has its own ROM chip, the device, when powered up, can be individually calibrated to the highest level of accuracy without the need for user interaction. Although single-coil navigation is possible, incorporation of a second or third coil makes accuracy and precision of the system even better defined. Despite these measures to enhance accuracy, it is important to realize that the bench-tested accuracy of any system is only as good as the environment in which it is used. Soft tissue shifts, environmental factors of metal or magnetic distortion, and surgical tactile accuracy all play a large role in the intraoperative accuracy of any system.[16]

Sources of Distortion

Inherent in any magnetic system is interference from other objects in the environment. These can be classified into two general areas: conductive and ferric.

Conductive distortion is produced by a transmission source that creates a current in a conductive metal that results in a "parasitic" field. Examples of this are most steels and aluminum and any other highly conductive metals. Because titanium is only partially conductive, it remains relatively unable to affect the field of a nearby coil generation. Even carbon-containing Kevlar and other synthetic fibers can create some small conductivity and therefore are subject to small distortion if placed directly into the transmission field.

Ferrous interference is the more frequently referenced and better understood concept, especially given our understanding of magnetic resonance imaging (MRI) interferences. Any object to which a simple magnet is attracted can be considered ferrous. Generally, the stronger the attraction, the more ferrous is the metal. Therefore, steels such as the 400 Series and 17-4 stainless are highly ferrous. Because aluminum and titanium cobalt chrome are not as ferrous, they tend not to "bend" the magnetic field and therefore create less distortion. The effects of ferrous metals are seen in both AC and DC systems. However, AC CAS is least affected by remote ferrous interference (Fig. 118-3).

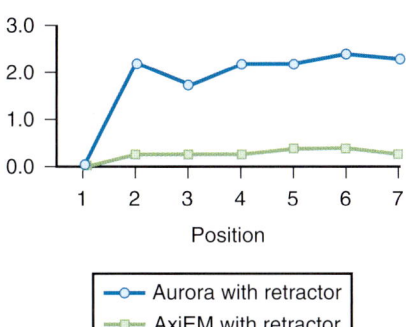

METALLIC DISTORTION ERROR

	AxiEM	Aurora
Mean	0.71	1.30
Standard deviation	0.34	0.96
99% Confidence Int.	1.74	4.17
Max	1.59	4.31

Figure 118-3. Distortion from metallic interference is different depending on DC versus AC transmitter field production.

Cons of EM

Just as the line of sight interferes with traditional IR navigation, EM navigation can be influenced by outside sources. One of the most important disruptions comes from ferromagnetic interference. When these objects pass between the localizer and the DRFs, a signal change is created that prevents the receiving coils from acquiring adequate flux or field strength, and this could create erroneous values. To prevent this, sophisticated signal strength quality monitors in software are incorporated to turn off the CAS on screen measures while these reception voids are experienced. This is absolutely imperative if one is engaged in the program, to prevent a surgeon from relying on an aging reading that does not represent a real-time, accurate reception value.

Other signal disrupters include some metals that may interfere with reception strength. Examples are aluminum, copper, and stainless steel (see Fig. 118-3). Yet some metals, such as the 300-series stainless (303, 316 L), cobalt chrome, and all of the titanium alloys, have a surprisingly low interference constant.

As long as these more disruptive metals are kept removed from the immediate field of the generator/receiver environment, maintaining adequate and accurate signal strength does not seem to be a problem. For example, despite the massive content of aluminum and steel in the operating table, adequate reception of the signal can be maintained, especially with the knee in its typical surgical position in flexion, which places it away from these interfering metals. This metallurgical interference has been eliminated with the use of EM-friendly instruments, as can be seen in previous trials of EM tracking, with which unstable signals were often encountered.

Edge-of-distortion interference is another form of potential error unique to EM navigation. As disruptive fields encroach on the navigation field, cancellation or signal instability can result from ferromagnetic electric or other magnetic

influences. This has been dealt with by computers that detect aberrant signal-to-noise ratios. The computer can detect this "clipping" of detected strength versus what it should be at the distance to the field when disruption occurs. At this point, the computer shuts down or creates an off-signal status, and the system defaults to "no readings." IR systems do not experience the same disruption because the signal usually is completely blocked by blockage of the IR beam; however, they too go to a blank mode of service if transmission ceases or becomes weakened.

Magnetic signals created by the localizer, along with their receivers, are sensitive to movement. Therefore, ridged or steady dampening movement during acquisition or measurement improves the speed of data registry. If any movement is noted in the localizer, response time on the DRF is lengthened. It is important to stabilize motion by placing the localizer on a firm platform or support.

With knowledge of metal and magnetic interference, our understanding of the environment for successful electromagnetic navigation has improved. A number of axioms have evolved, including the following:

- Maximizing proximity of the localizer to the operative field by 15 to 25 cm
- Instrumentation selection of titanium or cobalt chrome to minimize ferrous disruption
- Minimization of metal between the transmitter and the receiver coils, no matter what the metal type, to a distance greater than 10 cm.

With recent advancements in sensitivity and distortion, many of these nuisances of signal disruption have been eliminated. Nonetheless, as the environment of extraneous metal influence becomes more pristine, reception and speed of the computer response are improved.

Safety of magnetism exposure is the subject of an age-old debate and has not been completely elucidated even now.[24] Because its uses have transcended application to bone and tissue ingrowth, cartilage generation, or pain relief, no published studies have reported detrimental effects. Disruption of the field may thwart proper activation or engagement of cardiac monitoring and pacemaker capabilities. Difficulties within the confines of cardiac defibrillation and pulsing are being addressed by pacemaker-tolerant circuitry currently built into many pacemakers. This has not been an issue in any reported cases.

Error and Accuracy

CAS can be evaluated on the basis of numerous measurements of accuracy. Although federal guidelines mandate limits of ±1 degree and ±1 mm of translation accuracy before 510K approval is issued, most systems are able to measure with reasonable accuracy sub-degree and sub-millimeter values.

These measures are subject to other errors as well, such as edge of distortion, whereby interference increases as an object gets closer to the transmitter-receiver field. Drift can also occur as voltage, temperature, or circuitry relationships fluctuate.

Acquisition speed, or the time required to capture, read, and calculate a receiver, varies with different systems. Additionally, processing speeds of computers linked to software modifications influence acquisition speed. Sampling may be instantaneous; however, most systems use a mean or average to acquire position values before the program allows the screen to display numeric readings. To minimize delay during position readings, EM CAS samples the most accurate values when localizers and DRFs are not moving. Also, the software responds more rapidly if sampling of positions is consistent and is not drifting. In this way, averaging software is not forced to exclude data or to average high RMS values.

Finally, there is the human time factor. In a series of monitored patients, EM CAS revealed that average care time increased by 10 minutes. This was divided into three components: application, acquisition computation, and data collection. Of the 10 minutes required, the human portion (computation) was by far the most time consuming of the CAS time burden.[19]

If a numeric representation of varus/valgus is placed on the screen, it takes longer for the human mind to respond accurately to correct or to comprehend than if it is graphically displayed as a target or bull's eye. Although it is imperative to have confirming numeric values to accurately document final position, the speed of acquisition and of comprehension is greatly reduced for surgeons who are not colinked to target graphics.

USE AND TECHNIQUE

If one is familiar with the typical IR tracking system, graduating to an EM system will prove to be not only easy, but also gratifying. Because of the small size of the DRFs, continuous unobstructed 360 degrees of visibility, and downsizing of instruments, EM systems provide an easier platform that is virtually invisible in the operative field (Fig. 118-4).

Although a technique such as IR involves affixing two DRFs to the area about the knee, unlike IR, EM DRFs are completely inboard to the incision. The femoral tracker is placed beneath the VMO inferior margin of the vastus medialis off the articular surface to avoid disruption from the femoral component or cutting guides (Fig. 118-5). The tibial DRF is placed on the medial tibial flair (again, inboard to the incision) low enough to avoid disruption by cutting guide impingement, yet out from the canal so as not to catch the stem of the tibial tray or its corresponding preparatory instruments (Fig. 118-6).

Once these are affixed, waypoints are inputted and the hip center is acquired through repeated circumduction of the hip. The magnetic field emitter must remain very steady during this phase. Digitized waypoints are required by a DRF-incorporated stylus (Fig. 118-7); these are single-point, not multiple-point, acquisition waypoints and include the following:

Medial posterior condyle	Medial tibial plateau
Lateral posterior condyle	Lateral tibial plateau
Medial distal condyle	Tibial eminence
Lateral distal condyle	Tibial tendon insertion
Anterior notch	Medial malleolus
Whiteside's line	Lateral malleolus

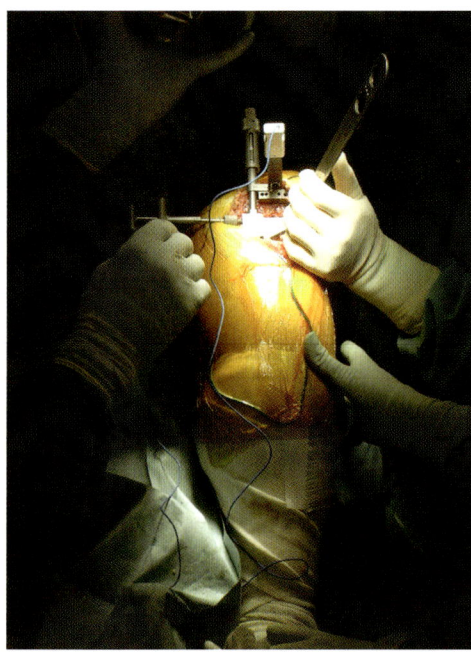

Figure 118-5. Typical subvastus and tibial plateau placement of dynamic reference frames (DRFs) on a minimally invasive surgery (MIS) incision.

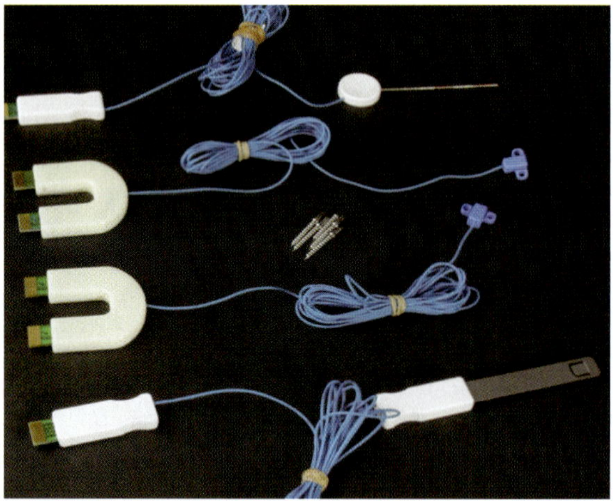

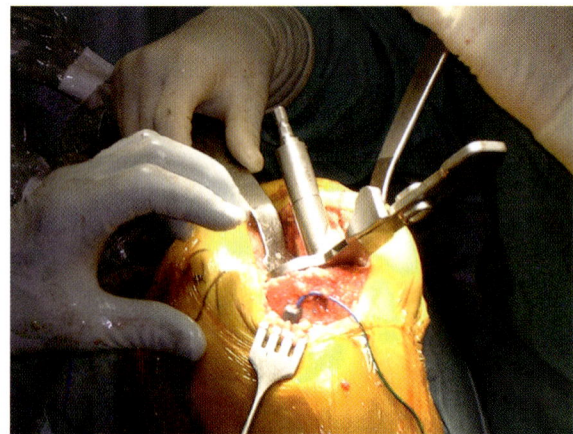

Figure 118-6. An electromagnetic (EM) pointer probe, two dynamic reference frames (DRFs)—one for femur, one for tibia— and a paddle probe with 8 degrees of freedom capability.

Figure 118-4. Transmitter coils or dynamic reference frame (DRF) in order from top to bottom consists of stylus, femoral and tibial trackers, and paddle probe.

The localizer is generally about the size of three tennis balls. This can be cumbersome at first, but eventually the surgical team works around it as if it is not there. If it interferes with surgical techniques, it can be moved away or completely out of the field when not in use.

Most navigation systems have capabilities of verification of kinematics coordinating before any cuts are made. This not only instills confidence in establishing the playing field of presurgical knee deformity and ranges, it also assists in future soft tissue releases and corrected resection requirements necessary to regain the best postoperative function of the knee. As the sequence of resections proceeds, the program can be customized to follow an intuitive path of steps to prepare the surgeon for navigating each step. Then, smart cutting jigs or paddle probes, which fit into saw capture guides, allow for nonintramedullary preparation of the distal femur or proximal tibia (see Figs. 118-7 and 118-8). Prediction of size for optimal femoral sizing without violation of the anterior cortex or notching is graphically displayed before bone is resected (Fig. 118-9). This ensures proper restoration of the joint line and equal, adequate extension and flexion gap distances for proper joint ligament isometry. Referencing posteriorly or anteriorly when exposure allows during sequences of articular resections makes acquisition more accurate (Fig. 118-10). Freshening up unsatisfactory cuts to perfect alignment is easily done because the surgeon can maintain an interactive, constant feedback of instruments without losing reception of navigational signals when the surgeon or assistants are in the way of the receiver. Gap distance measurements available in this system provide true center point tibia-to-femur values, which allow the surgeon actual real-time numeric millimeter values of condyle-to-tibial plateau distance in four simultaneously displayed flexion angles. This then enhances confidence in making prudent judgments of joint laxity in all positions, while intraoperative corrections can be made to balance ligaments (Fig. 118-11). EM CAS gives excellent insight into potential midflexion laxity because it provides distance separation under load at any orientation or position that is automatically recorded as a maximum excursion under load. Once cementing is complete, final verification can be recorded, even in a revision long-stem implant, because DRFs are superficial to the canal. Data entered and on-screen shots are then downloaded to a disk from the computer and are made available for PowerPoint, patient, and/or research use.

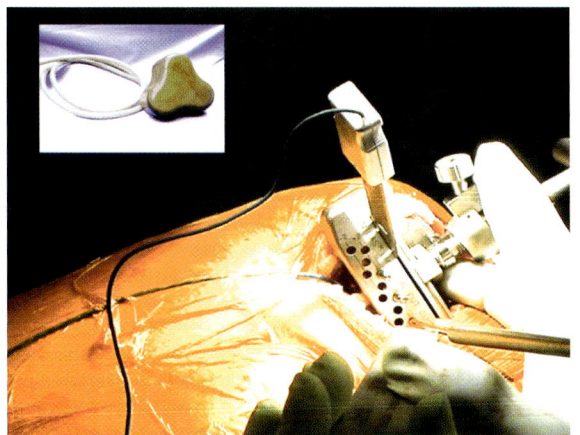

Figure 118-7. Typical operative setup with field triangular transmitter in the background and paddle probe inserted to measure proximal tibial resection angles.

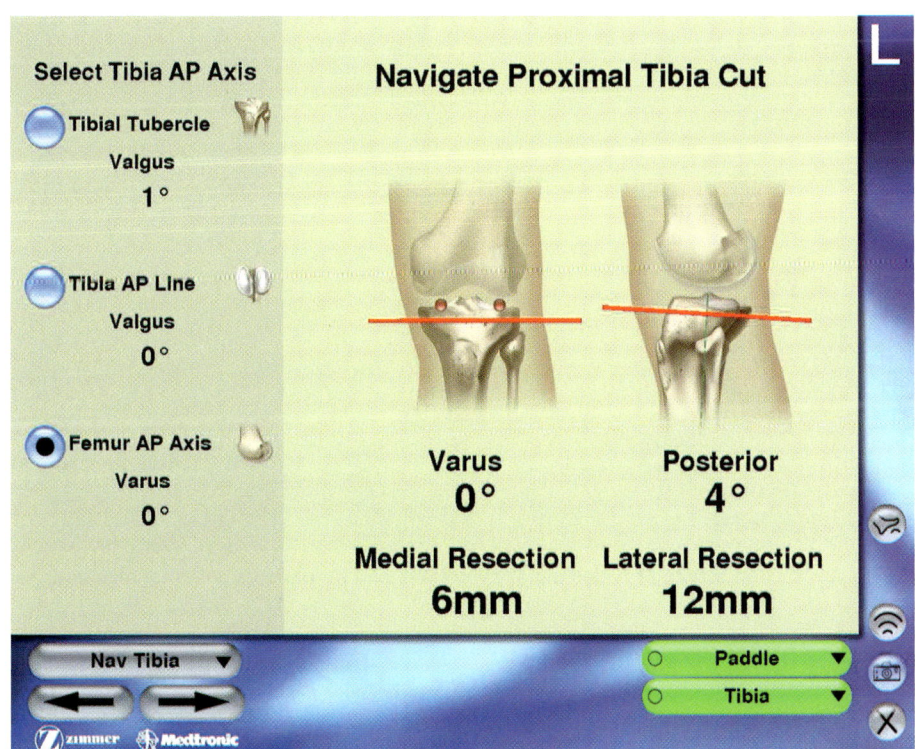

Figure 118-8. Distal femoral resection screen with angles and level in millimeters represented.

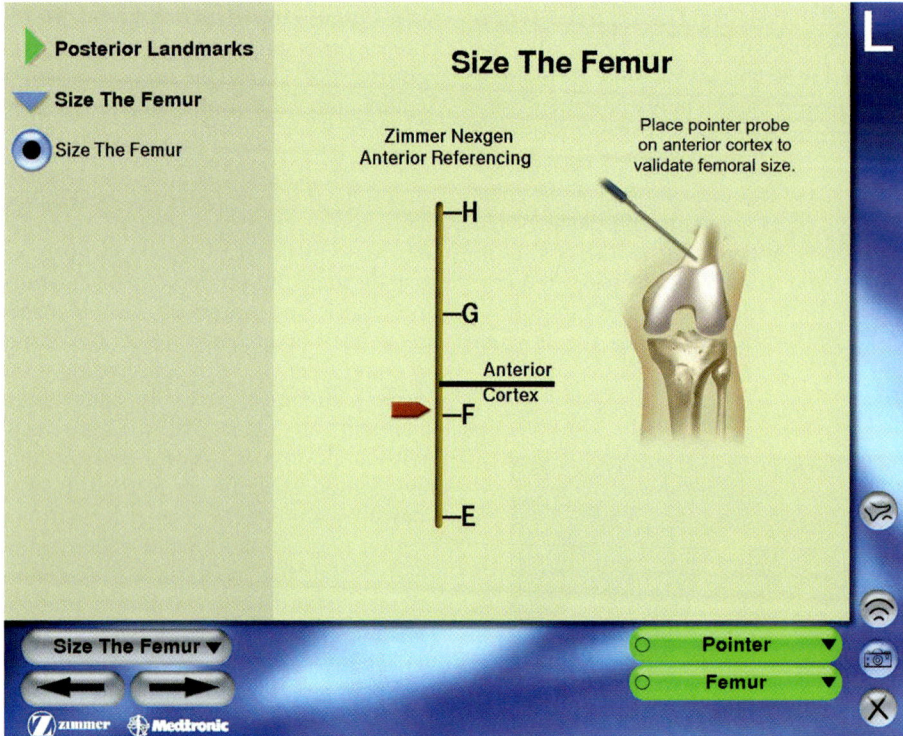

Figure 118-9. Femoral prediction "best size" based on computer-assisted navigation (CAS) measurements.

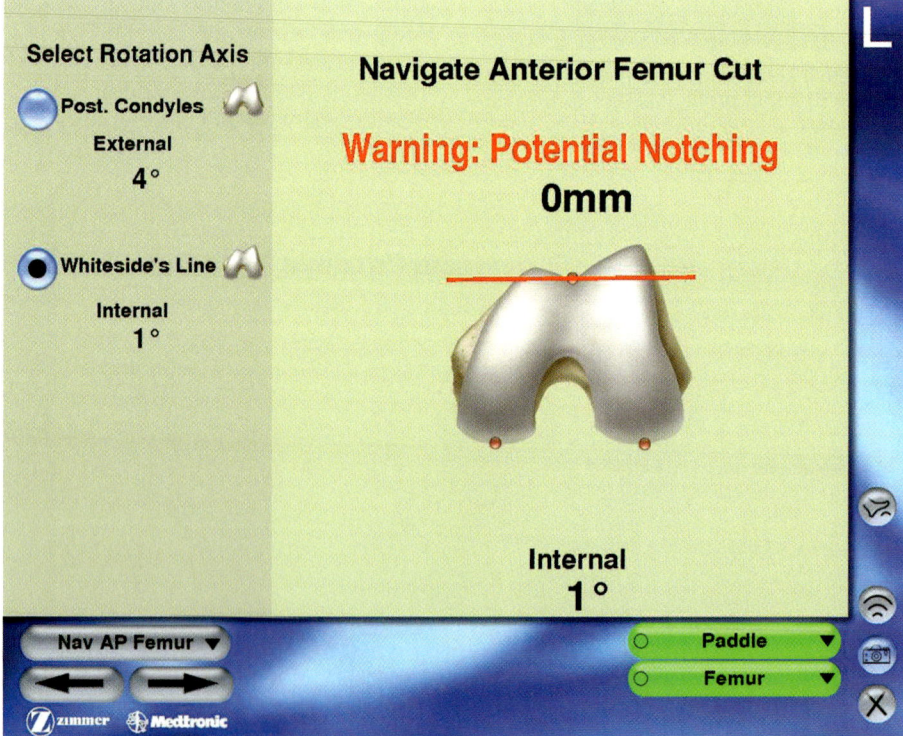

Figure 118-10. Tibial resection screen provides pictorial updates and numeric values of angles and resection levels.

ADVANTAGES OF EM NAVIGATION

One of the most frustrating problems with traditional IR trackers is the bone and soft tissue trauma they create. Because of the intense lever arm on the big reflective arrays, ridged bicortical nonrotary stability is mandatory to achieve and requires large ridged pins. These have been reported to induce scar tissue or lesions if hit during the procedure around pen sites (which defeats the intent of CAS); this sometimes is referred to as *navigation disease*.

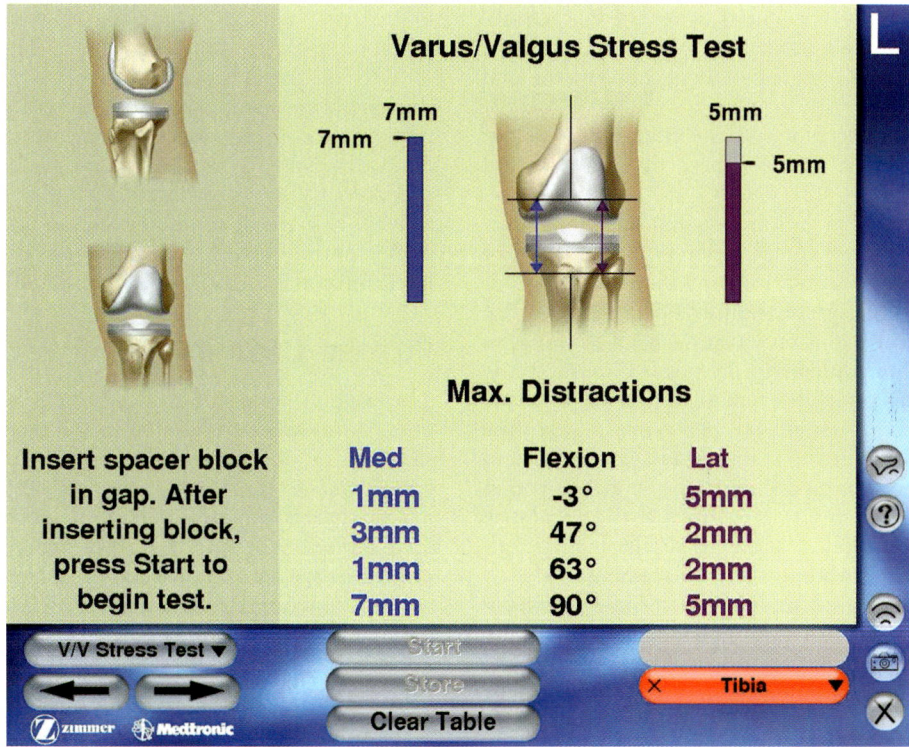

Figure 118-11. Gap distance measurement.

Additionally, large, bicortical, multiple-hole violation of bone has been implicated in fractures postoperatively, leading many to look for single, smaller fixation options away from rigid tracker framers. EM CAS is still not without risk. We reported four fractures of the medial tibia on our first 400 knees when using concentrated DRF and saw capture pins in the medial cortex. This has been eliminated by downsizing of DRFs to single cortical mounts and by reducing medial pin penetration of the cortex on the medial tibia such as lateralizing cutting blocks to the central tibia. Additionally, use of stemmed tibias in osteoporotic patients has reduced fracture incidence over the past 200 total knee replacements (TKRs).

The single most enjoyable aspect of EM tracking over traditional IR is the disappearance of the assistant's or surgeon's signal interference from the signal or camera boom. Those familiar with IR CAS can attest to the frustration of difficulties in reception of signals, which only are made worse by an untimely signal fade at the precise moment the surgeon can least afford it.[14] EM tracking simplifies this with the ability to see through the assistant, surgeon, and patient. With EM-friendly instruments and retractors, less disruption to the signal occurs, and this lessens the constraint on the working environment.

Because of lack of interference from outside the operative field and seeing through personnel, mobile DRFs such as paddles provide instantaneous real-time verification of the accuracy of a cut without having to reposition trackers such as in the case of ER CAS. Subsequent revision cuts are made intelligently rather than by cumbersome jigs where complex angles or anatomic variations could result in errors.*

The single most important provision EM brings to the table is the ability to navigate minimally invasive surgery (MIS). Whether or not one is an advocate of smaller incisions, the invasive destructive nature of four or more bicortical pins takes away much of what an MIS total joint can provide. When even a small incision allows placement of DRFs without extending the incision, exceptional guidance can be achieved without interference or alternation of exposure.[11] If one believes that precision is to implant sarvival as important as minimization of tissue trauma is to patient satisfaction, then EM is the tool that allows this marriage.[26] Critical evaluation of a series of TKRs reveals that the mean target value that the surgeon believes is ideal may not be the same.[29,31] For example, in our series of the first 458 knees, the mean mechanical value using EM CAS was 1.03 degrees more valgus than targeted, even though 92% of our patients were ±3 degrees from 6 degrees valgus. This was also the case in the other series, where although precision of CAS created an acceptable alignment, a subtle shift to valgus was noted.[6,28] What this says is simply that one might consider getting more out of CAS by "trimming" or re-aiming the target through a shift of target values of CAS. When we retargeted to 1.0 degree more of varus on the femur, alignment accuracy rose to 98%.[19]

The following features are available on the EM CAS system. This represents a wish list that any CAS surgeon should desire in any system, whether IR or EM:

1. Lessened frequency of outliers for acceptable angulation and alignment is achieved.
2. Documentation of presurgical and postsurgical kinematics is given as a spontaneously available permanent record or as a retrievable digital file.
3. Analytic cataloguing and recall are provided for research purposes.

---

*References 2, 3, 8, 13, 15, and 30.

4. Refinement of the first cut is a perfect cut. Unobstructed CAS measurements make it possible to monitor the actual progress of a cut, not just the end result.

5. Revision of cut inaccuracy is done more easily without cumbersome recut jigs or their invasive fixation anchors.

6. The femoral canal violation inducing a possible intraoperative pulmonary complication of fat embolism or bleeding is avoided.

7. A predictive measure of the intraoperative template of a best fit scenario is provided.

8. Gap distance measurements are possible in obtaining a variety of flexion angles, making it possible to check and refine flexion extension gaps so as to optimize range without giving up stability. This is available in the first part of the procedure for osteophyl resection and/or at the conclusion to verify soft tissue balance with documentation of achieved results in true millimeter measures, not angular displacement.

9. Rotational mating of the femoral-to-tibial prosthesis in the anatomic axis of motion is achieved. Flexibility in assigning proper axis rotation can be by Whiteside, kinematic flexion, anterior trochlea, posterior condyle, or a combination of these.

10. Given inherent disagreement on correct positions of the epicondylar axis from limited exposure to the epicondyles in MIS knee exposures, reliance on other guidance systems is mandatory.[32] The CAS system must give the surgeon a choice of femoral axis positions. This provides an avenue to achieve this.

As with any CAS, EM has other hidden advantages. Prosthesis-specific inventory reduction by instrumentation simplification or elimination has been the added benefit of CAS. Eventually, this not only may improve provisional inventory, it may also ease the burden on staff and personnel. Reduction in tray count, complexity of the instrument turnover, and time is a means of reducing cost. It is realistic to expect cost reduction; shifting of cost from the hospital, surgeon, or patient may eventually be realized.

With all the glitz and glamor of bringing a computer into the operating room, we as surgeons have a duty to avoid implying to our patients that our using the computer automatically makes us better surgeons than those not using the technology. Only decades of review will truly tell the result of what this era of computer technology did to improve our understanding of knee mechanics and whether that translated into more durable and functional knees.[8]

FUTURE USES OF EM

The brightest aspect of EM technology is its seemingly innocuous, nonobtrusive presence in the operative field. As incisions shrink, so will the patience of surgeons to be saddled with cumbersome technology that lengthens their day or makes their job more difficult. By short-circuiting steps in knee replacement with the use of smart jigs, smart drills, and prosthesis-specific knowledge-based programs, researchers will make knee replacement much easier in the coming decade. The procedure should become less time-consuming as refinements are made in the software to intuitively lead the surgeon. In refining precision to a more consistent product, accuracy, which has never been an issue in computer-assisted surgery, is complemented and assured.[23]

To provide the same service while reducing hospital, physician, and implant costs, technology must continue to be refined and expedited to better assist the surgeons of tomorrow. If computerization can accomplish in the private health care sector the same efficiency it has in the field of business, all of us will benefit (Fig. 118-12).

Virtual reality and augmented reality may continue to be developed in the years to come. With the use of data-gathering gloves and head or eyeglass displays, more flexible tracking and navigating can be achieved. Wireless military applications may prove to be the next technology from which CAS may borrow. Through microchip and nanotechnology

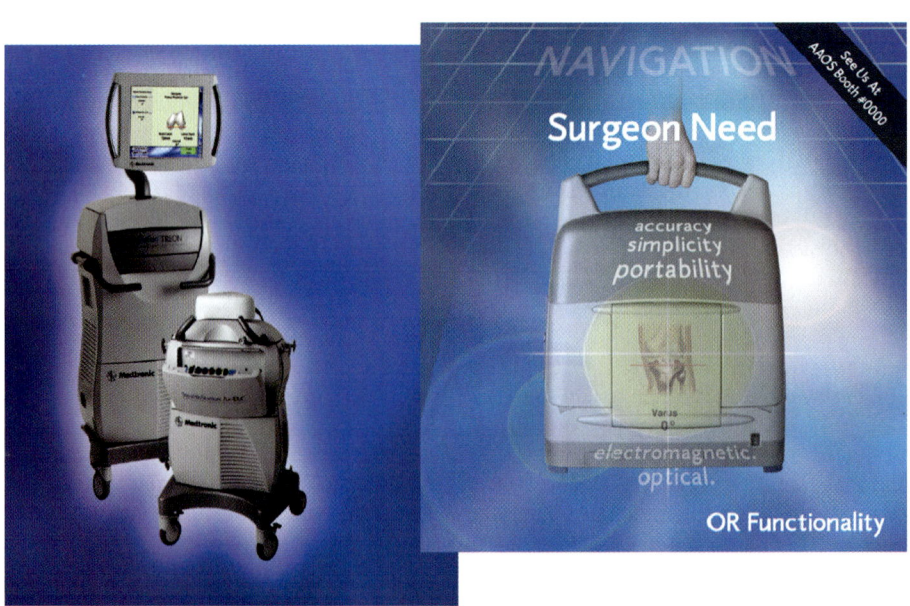

Figure 118-12. Then and now technology reflecting some trends seen in today's downsizing of computers.

research, this field continues to flourish toward reaching more imaginative and hard-to-fathom goals, such as procedures to correct skeletal deformity and revision trauma surgery. Linking heads-up displays (now found in many production vehicle windshields) to heads-down displays (on eyeglasses) and using GPS-like guidance (EM CAS) are examples of the plethora of technology that remains to be explored. These aids are likely to enhance operative efficiency and accuracy for the surgeon. They will also reduce the length of procedures and make recovery far easier for patients.

KEY REFERENCES

Anderson KC: Computer assisted navigation in total knee arthroplasty: comparison with conventional methods. J Arthroscopy 20:132–138, 2005.

Asano T, Akugi M, Nakamura T: Functional flexion extension axis of the knee corresponds to the surgical epicondylar axis. J Arthroscopy 20:1060–1066, 2005.

Berend KR, et al: Avoiding the potential pitfalls of minimally invasive total knee surgery. Orthopedics 28:11, 2005.

Chauahon SK, et al: Computer-assisted knee arthroplasty is better than a conventional jig-based technique in terms of component alignment. J Bone Joint Surg Am 86:11, 2004.

Fang DM, Ritter MA, Davis KE: Coronal alignment in TKR, just how important is it? J Arthroplasty 24:39–43, 2009.

Fehring TK, et al: Early failures in total knee arthroplasty. Clin Orthop Relat Res 392:315–318, 2001.

Gioe TJ, et al: Why are total knee replacements revised? Clin Orthop Relat Res 428:100–106, 2004.

International Commission on Non-Ionizing Radiation Protection (ICNIRP): Guidelines for limiting exposure to time varying electric, magnetic and electromagnetic fields (up to 300 GHz). Health Physics 74:494–522, 1998.

Jenny JY, et al: Consistency of implantation of a total knee arthroplasty with a non-image-based navigation system, a case-control study of 235 cases compared with 235 conventionally implanted prostheses. J Arthroplasty 20:832–839, 2005.

Kim SJ, et al: Computer assisted navigation in total knee arthroplasty: improved coronal alignment. J Arthroplasty 20:123–131, 2005.

Sharkey PR, et al: "Why are total knee arthroplasties failing today?" Clin Orthop Relat Res 404:7–13, 2002.

Sparmann M, et al: Positioning of total knee arthroplasty with and without navigation support, a prospective randomised study. J Bone Joint Surg Br 85:830–835, 2003.

Van Damme G, et al: What should the surgeon aim for when performing computer assisted total knee arthroplasty? J Bone Joint Surg Am 87:52–58, 2005.

Victor J, Hoste D: Image-based computer-assisted total knee arthroplasty leads to lower variability in coronal alignment. Clin Orthop Relat Res 428:131–139, 2004.

Wagner A, et al: Quantitative analysis of factors affecting intraoperative precision and stability of optoelectronic and electromagnetic tracking systems. Med Phys 29:905–912, 2002.

Yau WP, et al: Intraobserver errors in obtaining visually selected anatomic landmarks during registration process in nonimage-based navigation-assisted total knee arthroplasty, a cadaveric experiment. J Arthroplasty 20:5, 2005.

Full references for this chapter can be found on www.expertconsult.com.

Management of Extra-articular Deformity in Total Knee Arthroplasty With Navigation

J. Bohannon Mason and Thomas K. Fehring

Total knee arthroplasty is challenging in the presence of extra-articular deformity as the anatomic landmarks may be altered, traditional instrumentation may not be applicable, and ligament balance may be compromised. Additionally, with prior surgery, complicating hardware may be present. The ability to obtain a neutral mechanical axis is reported to be central to the long-term survival of total knee replacements.[18,33,46,48] Extra-articular deformities, particularly of the femur, require placement of implants often at odds with the usual referenced bone landmarks to achieve a summed mechanical axis that is neutral and perpendicular to the ground at the joint line.[11,32] The intramedullary canal used to assist with femoral component alignment instrumentation may be blocked by callus from a malunited fracture or filled with hardware. The diaphyseal canal additionally may be offset from the metaphysis, resulting in sagittal or coronal plane deformities.

These deformities are not new, and surgeons for the past 30 years have attempted to compensate for them with "best guess" measure and cut techniques, or with more sophisticated alignment systems.[3,27,40] In recent years, imageless computer-assisted navigation systems have been developed that allow surgeons to accurately plan and execute bone resections in total knee arthroplasty based on a virtual mechanical axis.[20,29,31] Numerous studies have shown the accuracy of this navigation technology, often reporting fewer outliers in sagittal and coronal plane alignment compared with manual conventional total knee instrumentation.[2,9,10,16,30,43] Although debate over the utility of computer-assisted total knee for routine total knee surgery continues, focusing on the cost of the technology, surgical time investment, and the impact of error reduction on revision rates,[34,42,49] one distinct area of benefit of computer-assisted navigation is help with the management of extra-articular deformity.

EXTRA-ARTICULAR DEFORMITIES: INTRA-ARTICULAR VERSUS EXTRA-ARTICULAR CORRECTION

Painful arthritis resulting in the need for total knee replacement may occur in association with extra-articular deformity of the femur or tibia. These deformities are typically the result of prior trauma with malunited fractures, but they can result from other conditions such as prior corrective osteotomies and metabolic conditions such as Blount's, Paget's, tertiary syphilis, or rickets.[47] Often, the surgeon is forced to consider the possible presence of confounding hardware or a tortuous relationship of the diaphysis to the metaphysis, which may prevent the passage of intramedullary guide instrumentation or may complicate the placement of stems required for secondary stabilization of the implant (Fig. 119-1).

Strategies for management of extra-articular deformity include performing simultaneous corrective osteotomies at the time of total knee, with restoration of the diaphyseal-to-metaphyseal relationship,[12,26,36,37] or correction of the deformity within the joint via corrective bone resections and subsequent soft tissue balancing to allow implant stability throughout the motion arc of the knee.[47] The latter strategy, intra-articular correction with soft tissue balancing, is appealing because it is more efficient for the surgeon. It does not require creating an osteotomy that needs to be stabilized and heal. If, however, the degree of deformity would require a bone resection that extends to the epicondylar attachment of the collateral ligaments, then ligament integrity would be lost and constraining implants required.[15,36] A more optimal strategy in this case is corrective osteotomy (Fig. 119-2A-C).

Some authors have argued that when deformities of the distal femur or proximal tibia exceed 15 degrees, because of the difficulty associated with simultaneous osteotomy and total knee replacement, corrective osteotomies should be performed and allowed to heal before total knee replacement surgery is performed.[8,39] Wang and Wang[47] reported on 15 patients with extra-articular deformities and arthritis treated with total knee replacement using intra-articular bone resections and soft tissue releases to achieve correction of mechanical alignment. These authors stressed the need for long-standing films to outline the deformity. Using line drawings, they determined whether the intra-articular bone resection necessary to correct the mechanical axis of the extremity would pass through the insertion of the collateral ligaments. Successful intra-articular correction was attained when coronal plane resections were less than 20 degrees and/or sagittal plane resections less than 25 degrees in the femur, or less than 30 degrees in coronal plane alignment of the tibia.

Wolff and colleagues[50] stressed the relationship between degree of deformity and distance from the joint line. The closer the deformity apex is to the joint line, the greater is the impact on soft tissue releases necessary for balancing. Additionally, the authors noted that deformities of the tibia are easier to correct at the time of total joint replacement than those of the femur before the ligaments are balanced. Compensatory wedge resections necessary for axial correction of femoral deformities result in an asymmetrical extension space, with reduced impact on flexion balance. In contrast, correction of tibial deformity by compensatory wedge resection equally impacts flexion and extension spaces. Finally, varus deformities that cannot be completely balanced via intra-articular correction and soft tissue releases produce subtle lateral laxity that can be tolerated if the alignment is proper. In contrast, valgus deformity that cannot be completely balanced leads to medial laxity, which is much less well tolerated.[50] These authors also concluded that in cases of extreme deformity wherein intra-articular resection is

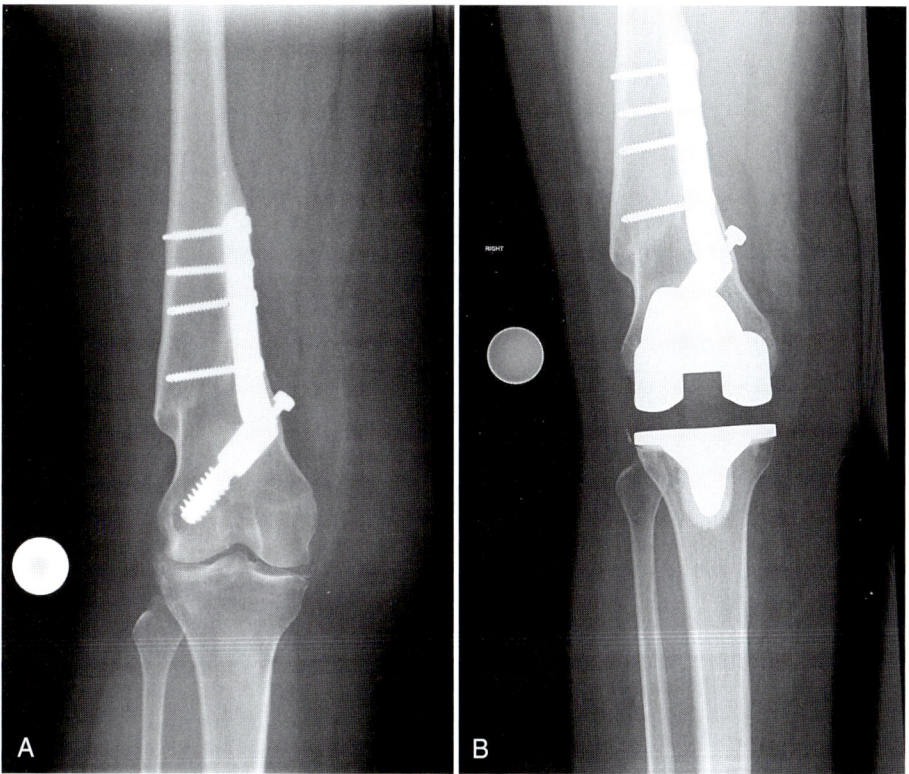

Figure 119-1. A, Anteroposterior radiograph of a patient with translational deformity status post osteotomy of the distal femur. **B,** Utilizing intraoperative navigation, the axial alignment was corrected to neutral. Traditional instrumentation would be difficult to use because of the femoral deformity and the retained hardware.

unlikely to yield satisfactory ligament balance, extra-articular osteotomy is indicated.

With coronal plane deformity of less than 20 degrees in the femur or less than 30 degrees in the tibia, intra-articular correction with total knee replacement is advantageous.[26,28,50] One-stage correction of these deformities eliminates the risks associated with a possible second incision for the osteotomy, nonunion of the osteotomy, the need for osteotomy-stabilizing hardware, and potential delay in rehabilitation related to the osteotomy. For these reasons, when possible, one-stage intra-articular correction is preferable to performing a correction osteotomy.

RATIONALE FOR TOTAL KNEE ARTHROPLASTY WITH NAVIGATION IN THE MANAGEMENT OF EXTRA-ARTICULAR DEFORMITIES ABOUT THE KNEE

Optimal component alignment and positioning are critical to the long-term clinical success of total knee replacement.[4,18,38] Failure to achieve optimal positioning of prosthetic knee implants can result in instability, increased pain, decreased range of motion, increased polyethylene wear, and implant loosening.[5,14,17,22,41] The challenges of alignment and positioning in routine total knee replacement surgery and its association with compromised results when these goals are not achieved have led to the development of numerous systems and alignment guides designed to achieve neutral mechanical alignment and correct component rotation.

These mechanical alignment systems include intramedullary and extramedullary guide rod systems that have inherent limitations in accuracy.[24,45] Despite surgical experience and improved mechanical alignment devices, errors in postoperative alignment in total knee surgery still occur.[44] Optical navigation systems—so-called imageless navigation—have become readily available in operating theaters around the world. Endorsement in multiple centers has allowed evaluation of the accuracy of the navigation systems, as well as comparative assessment versus manual instrumentation. Meta-analysis of available data suggests that these systems can deliver coronal and sagittal plane alignment that is superior to that attained with manual instrumentation.[29]

Although adoption of computer-assisted navigation for routine total knee replacement is hampered by the cost of the instrumentation, operative time requirements, and the paucity of literature linking its use to improved clinical outcomes,[42] the value of this technology is uniquely leveraged when patients present with extra-articular deformity, retained hardware, or both (Fig. 119-3A and B). With computer-assisted navigation systems, the mechanical axis for the femur is determined irrespective of the bone between the femoral head and the central portion of the distal femur, and similarly between the central aspect of the tibia and the ankle. By virtually linking these points through imageless navigation, a mechanical axis is automatically calculated. In contrast, conventional instrumentation in the presence of obstructing hardware, a tortuous medullary canal, or complete occlusion of the medullary canal would require extramedullary alignment devices, osteotomy, or removal of the obstructing hardware. Digital mapping of the hip center of rotation, articular

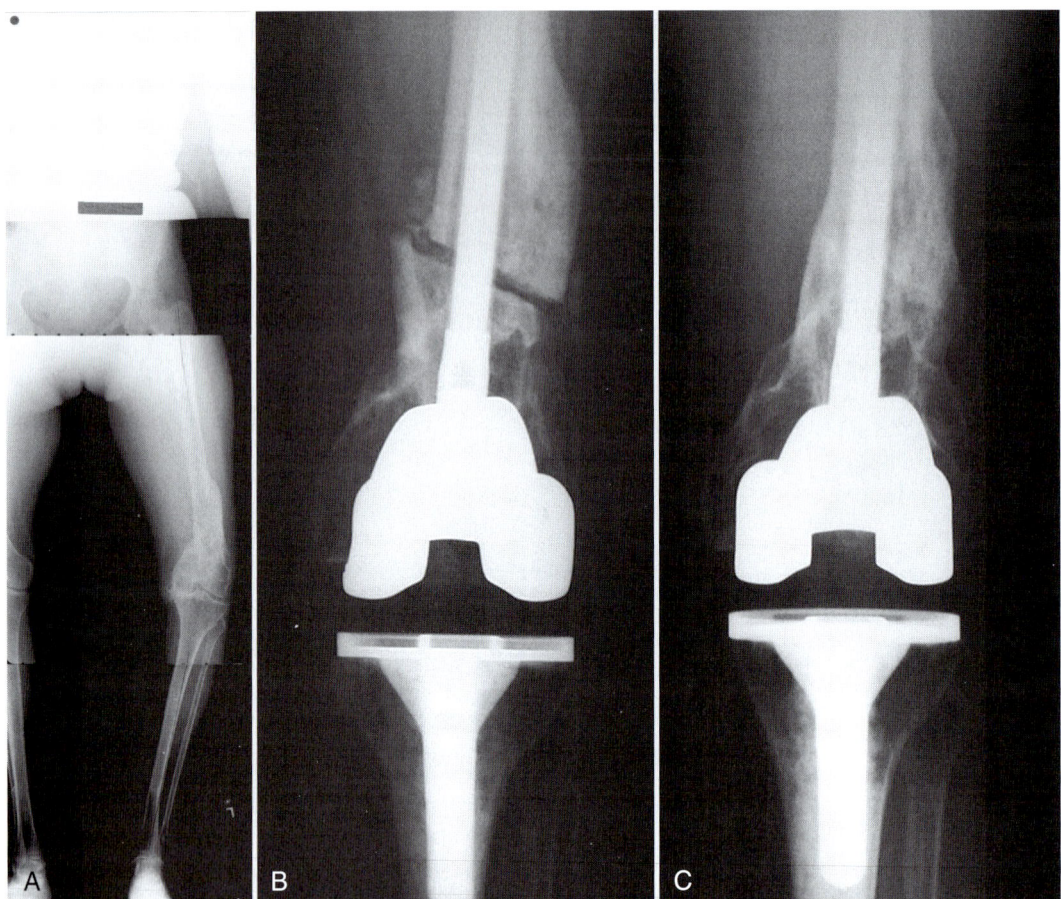

Figure 119-2. **A,** Anteroposterior (AP) radiograph showing coronal plane deformity due to a malunited distal femoral fracture. Intra-articular correction would sacrifice the integrity of the lateral collateral ligament. **B,** Navigation-assisted distal femoral osteotomy is stabilized with a fluted press-fit stem. **C,** Three-year postoperative AP radiograph showing union of the osteotomy.

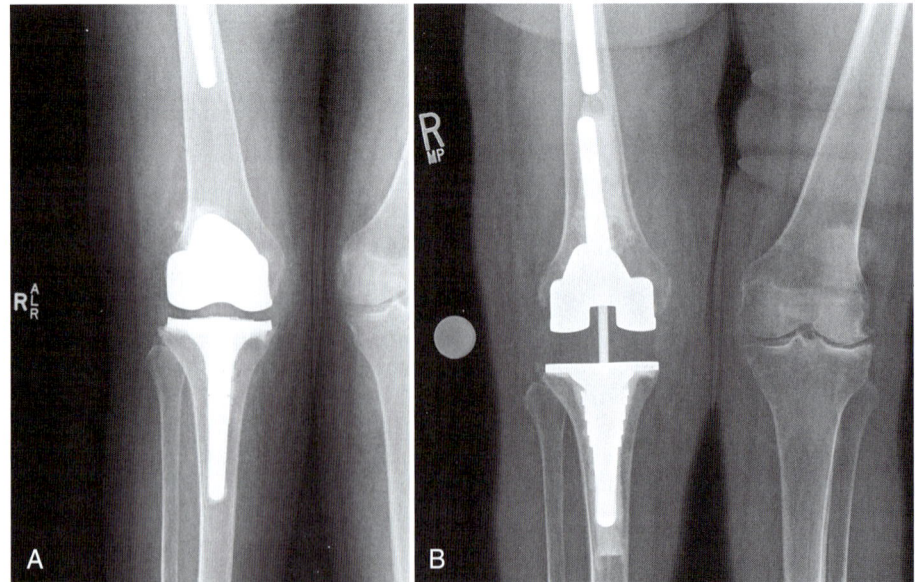

Figure 119-3. **A,** Anteroposterior radiograph of a patient with a failed total knee arthroplasty due to valgus instability. **B,** Navigation was helpful in this revision situation because the femoral canal was blocked from a femoral hip stem.

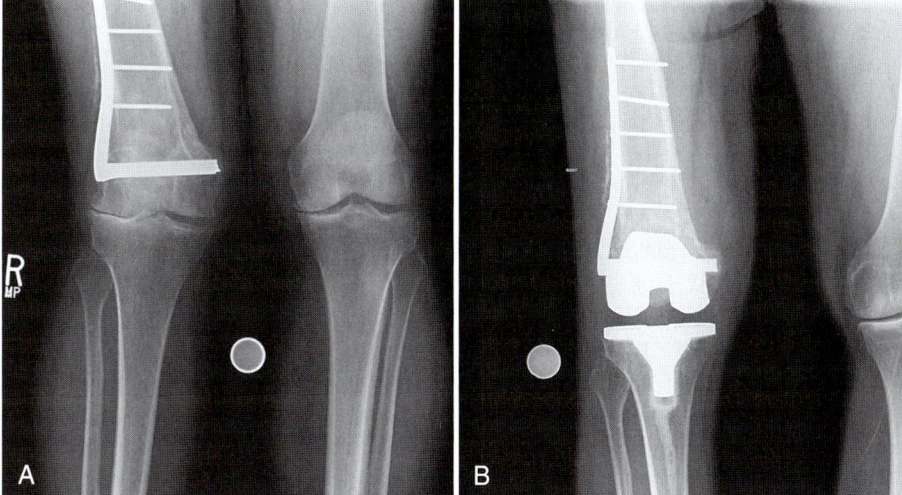

Figure 119-4. **A,** Hardware from prior surgery can present a challenge to traditional alignment instrumentation. **B,** Computer-assisted navigation was used, obviating the need for increased surgical exposure and hardware removal.

portions of the knee, and the ankle center offers the surgeon a clinical solution to the obstacles associated with extra-articular deformity.

In the relatively common presentation of patients with arthritis of the knee and retained hardware, the advantage of navigation is unique (Fig. 119-4A and B). Two scenarios may present. The first is hardware that for structural reasons may not be removed and that obstructs the use of conventional intramedullary instrumentation. In the second presentation, removal of the hardware is structurally feasible but requires greater surgical exposure, operative time, and risk to the patient. In these cases, navigation may represent a better option for the surgeon.

SURGICAL TECHNIQUE: NAVIGATION FOR EXTRA-ARTICULAR DEFORMITIES NOT REQUIRING OSTEOTOMY

Standard midline incision and medial parapatellar arthrotomy are recommended to facilitate any extensile approaches required. Imageless navigation requires placement of reference arrays, either active emitting or passive reflective (manufacturer dependent), which present a stereographic series of at least three points that the computer can record. Biopic cameras record the location of the position of the array, and using trigometric algorithms can fix and follow the points, and hence the bone, in space. The bone model is created by registering the center of the femoral head as the central rotation point when the femur is taken through a range of motion and a series of distal points are collected with a stylus, which is also visible to the computer. The center of the distal femur, the condylar morphology, and the epicondylar axis are typically collected. The tibia is modeled in a similar fashion; after collecting the central axis point within the footprint of the anterior cruciate ligament and surface points defining the medial and lateral tibial plateaus, the surgeon estimates the anterior-to-posterior axis of the proximal tibia and uses the malleoli to establish the ankle center.

The mechanical axis of the extremity prior to bone resection can then be recorded. Standard navigation cutting guides are used to perform a distal femoral resection perpendicular to the mechanical axis of the femur; the proximal tibial resection is performed at 90 degrees to the long axis of the tibia. Soft tissue releases are governed by the residual soft tissue tension, which can be assessed with a tensioning device, with lamina spreaders, or manually. Releases proceed until a rectangular extension gap is obtained.

In cases with deformity primarily in the coronal plane, rotational alignment of the femoral component may be based on routine landmarks such as the transverse epicondylar axis. Unfortunately, in patients with extra-articular deformities, simple coronal deformity is uncommon, often corrupted by rotational deformities. The correct rotational position of the femoral implant is perpendicular to the resected surface of the proximal tibia when the knee is flexed and the ligaments are tensed. Consequently, after sufficient releases are obtained in extension to create a rectangular extension space, classic gap balancing techniques are utilized to obtain femoral rotation in flexion, while tensioning the collateral ligaments at 90 degrees of flexion and making anterior and posterior femoral cuts parallel to the tibial cut. Most navigation balancing algorithms assist the surgeon in referencing the femoral rotation to the resected tibial plane. Once femoral rotation is determined, femoral bone resections are completed (Fig. 119-5).

SURGICAL TECHNIQUE: NAVIGATION FOR EXTRA-ARTICULAR DEFORMITIES REQUIRING OSTEOTOMY

As discussed previously, the amount of bone resection necessary to correct extremity alignment to a neutral mechanical axis is positively related to the degree of deformity and is inversely related to the distance of the deformity from the joint line.[50] In instances where preoperative planning indicates that the scale of bone resection required to correct femoral coronal plane alignment would result in resection of the origin of either collateral ligament, or exceeds 30 degrees of correction within the tibia, an associated osteotomy should be considered.[47] The surgical technique used for navigation

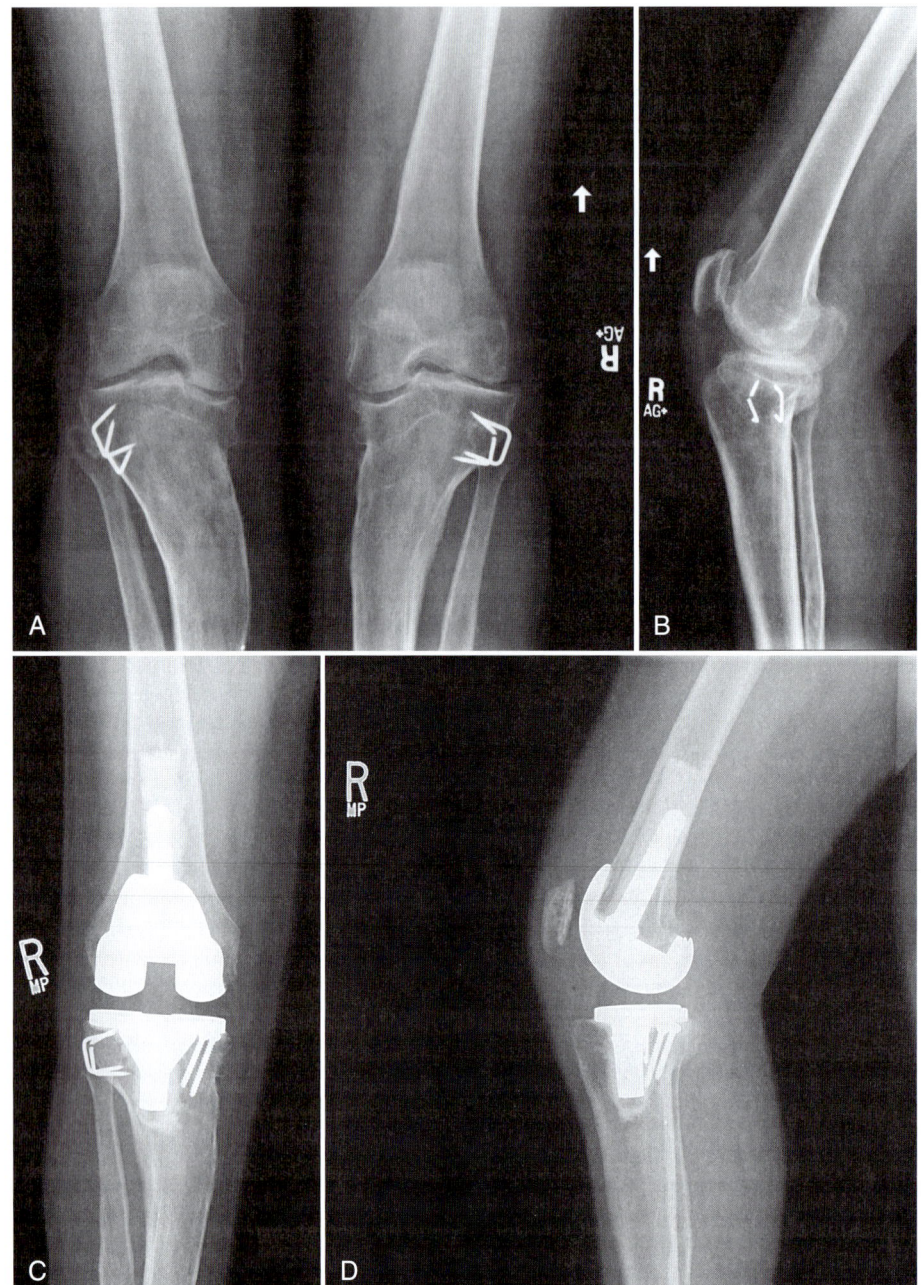

Figure 119-5. A, Anteroposterior (AP) radiograph of a 68-year-old male with profound deformity of the proximal tibia post osteotomy and prior fracture. **B,** Lateral radiograph showing sagittal plane deformity of the proximal tibia. **C,** AP postoperative film of the same patient. Navigation was helpful to establish neutral axial alignment despite the significant tibial deformity. **D,** Lateral postoperative radiograph.

in these cases varies from that used in intra-articular correction, because the optical tracking reference to the osteotomized bone segment can be lost after the osteotomy is performed.

When an osteotomy of the femur is anticipated, the femoral array should be placed proximal to the planned osteotomy. Pins generally should be unicortical to avoid interference with stabilizing intramedullary stems if used. Surgical approach and registration of the bone are identical to those of navigation techniques used for deformity when no osteotomy is required. Soft tissue releases are minimized because alignment correction is achieved via the osteotomy proximal

to capsular and collateral ligament origins. First, the navigated tibial resection is performed perpendicular to the long axis of the tibia (Fig. 119-6A-D). Next, with the extremity in extension, the collateral ligaments are tensed with lamina spreaders or a commercial tensioning device. With equal tension medially and laterally, the mechanical axis of the extremity is recorded by the navigation system. The degree of mechanical axis error from neutral is noted, and a corresponding resection of the distal femur is performed parallel to the proximal tibial resection (coplanar if the tibia is resected at 0 degrees of slope). In appropriate circumstances, biplanar correction through the osteotomy is facilitated by

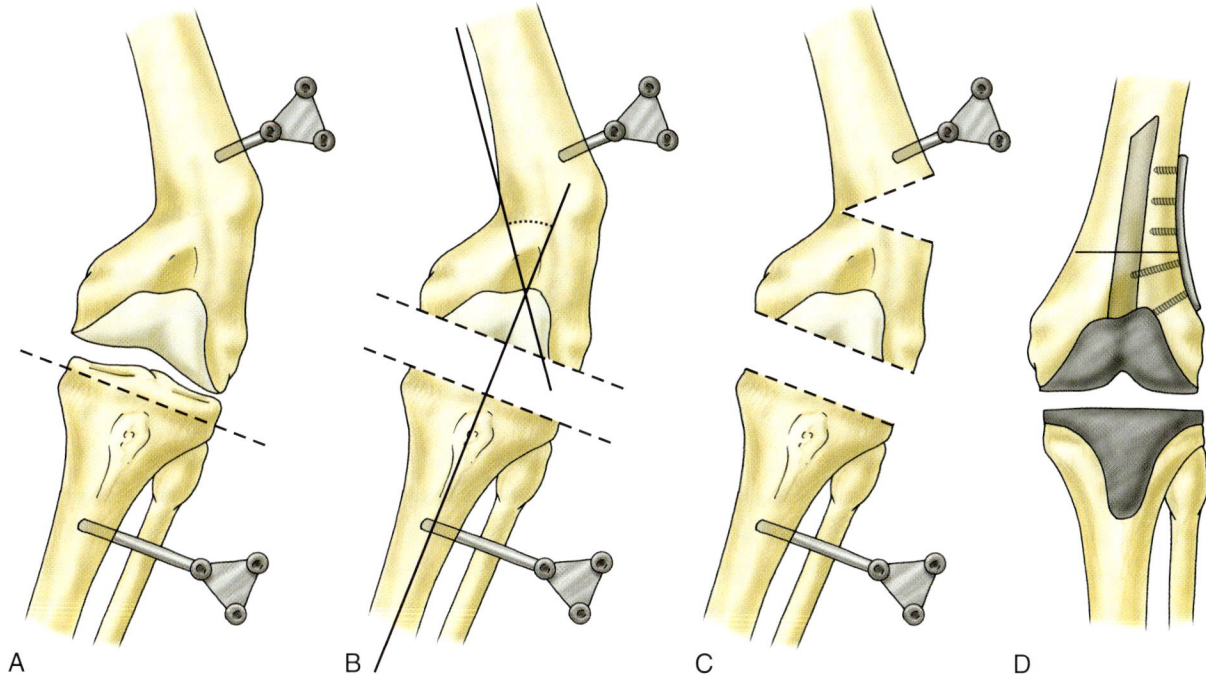

A   B   C   D

Figure 119-6. **A,** Sequence of surgical steps for navigation-assisted distal femoral osteotomy for severe extra-articular deformity. The array of the femur is positioned proximal to the planned osteotomy. The proximal tibial resection is performed at 90 degrees to the long axis of the tibia. **B,** The collateral ligaments are tensioned in extension, and the overall limb alignment is recorded. A distal femoral resection of appropriate depth was navigated and made parallel to the proximal tibial resection. **C,** The difference between the overall limb alignment and a neutral mechanical axis is the angle of the corrective osteotomy. The plane orientation tool in most navigation systems is used to navigate the angle for the osteotomy. **D,** The osteotomy is collapsed and stabilized. The surgeon should note the rotational alignment of the femur before performing the osteotomy.

the bone model created from registration of the bone anatomy. In such cases, the anterior cortex of the distal femur is referenced to the sagittal axis of the femur, and this angular difference is considered in the osteotomy. Once performed, the osteotomy is collapsed and stabilized with medullary reamers and/or bone clamps, while the remaining femoral resections are completed. Rotational alignment should be clearly marked on the femoral bone traversing the osteotomy before the osteotomy is performed. The correct mechanical axis can be confirmed with trial components in place.

Navigated alignment correction when a tibial osteotomy is anticipated for extra-articular deformity is similar to the technique for the femur but differs in the sequence of resections. In these cases, again, minimal soft tissue releases are required. The tibial array is secured to the tibia in the diaphyseal region, below the osteotomy site, which is at the metaphyseal-diaphyseal junction, distal to the medial collateral ligament insertion and the tubercle. After completion of the femoral bone cuts, the extremity again is brought to full extension, and the collateral ligaments are tensioned. Axial alignment of the distorted extremity is recorded with the navigation system. The proximal tibial resection is performed with the navigated cutting guides at the "angle of error" of the extremity (Fig. 119-7A-D). This resection plane is parallel to the distal resected femur, creating a rectangular extension space. A wedge osteotomy of equal angle is removed from the tibia at the metaphyseal-diaphyseal junction. The osteotomy is collapsed and stabilized with a tightly reamed, fluted tibial stem. In cases of extreme tibial correction, a fibular osteotomy additionally may be required.

Results of Navigation for Extra-articular Deformity

Klein and associates[21] first reported on the use of navigation-assisted TKA in patients with extra-articular deformity, retained hardware preventing standard intramedullary alignment instrumentation, or intramedullary implants. In this case series of 5 patients, collected from the senior author's experience with more than 500 primary and revision total knees over 2 years, total knee arthroplasty was successfully completed with navigation. The mechanical axis was restored to within 1 degree of neutral in four of five patients, and to within 2 degrees in the fifth. Klein and colleagues recognized that the risks associated with hardware removal, including multiple surgeries, multiple incisions or elevation of larger flaps to gain access to remove hardware, and creation of stress risers in the bone after removal of screws (which potentially requires additional support such as addition of stems, struts, or IM rods), were obviated with the use of navigation.

We reported on 16 patients requiring total knee arthroplasty for advanced osteoarthritis, in whom navigation was used to achieve alignment.[15] Standard intramedullary alignment guides could not be used because of angular deformity, obliteration of the canal, or use of intramedullary hardware, or when standard intramedullary guides were believed to be clinically contraindicated (prior osteomyelitis or severe cardiopulmonary compromise). Nine of 16 patients had severe extra-articular deformities. The mechanical axis was accurately restored in eight of these nine. We concluded that in

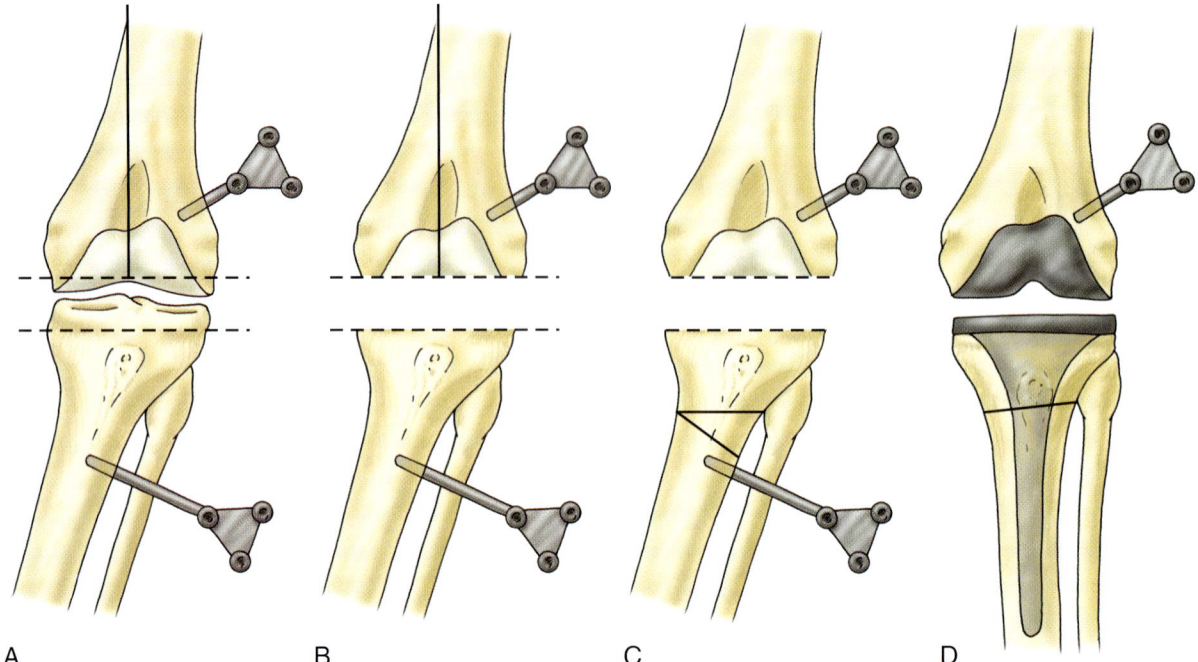

A   B   C   D

Figure 119-7. A, Navigation arrays are placed distal to the anticipated osteotomy. **B,** Distal femoral resection is performed as usual. The proximal tibial resection is performed parallel to the distal femoral resection after tensioning of the collateral ligament structures in extension. **C,** The resultant angle of "error" between extremity positions in extension, with collateral ligament tension equilibrated, is the angle of the wedge osteotomy. (Technical note: Spacer blocks are useful in stabilizing the extremity while the osteotomy is navigated.) **D,** The osteotomy is performed distal to the tibial tubercle and collateral insertions, and is transfixed with a tight diaphyseal fitting stem. (Technical note: The distal navigation array may need to be removed before the stem is placed.)

such patients, navigation was of direct benefit for both the surgeon and the patient.

Chou and associates[11] reported a single case of femoral deformity due to malunited distal femur with a coronal plane angulation of 15 degrees of varus and a sagittal plane angulation of 8.7 degrees. Navigation was "feasible and satisfactory" in this patient; however, the postoperative component position was not reported. The mechanical axis resulted in 1 degree of varus. Kim and colleagues[19] reported a series of four patients with severe extra-articular femoral deformities managed with navigation-assisted minimally invasive knee arthroplasty. The authors argued that the advantages of minimally invasive knee surgery (MIS), namely, decreased pain, faster recovery, and improved function,[1,6,23,25] justified the potential reported disadvantages, including improper component alignment and orientation due to inadequate exposure.[1,13] Investigators postulated that the increased accuracy of computer-assisted surgery may compensate for the possible alignment complications associated with MIS. Mean mechanical axis alignment improved from 15.1 degrees to 0.3 degrees (range, −1.2 to 0.5 degrees), and no complications were related to the MIS technique or the use of navigation. Additionally, significant improvement in function, Knee Society score, and SF-36 score was reported.

Bottros and coworkers[7] reported a series of nine knees (seven patients) with femoral extra-articular deformities severe enough to prevent the use of standard intramedullary alignment rods and advanced osteoarthritis necessitating total knee replacement. With the use of imageless navigation, the mean mechanical axis deviation postoperatively was 1.3 degrees (range, −0.2 to 2.5 degrees). The authors reported

clinical outcomes, noting improvement in Knee Society score from a mean of 62 preoperatively to 92 postoperatively and in function scores (from 52 to 83; $P < .05$) and range of motion (from a mean of 4 to 74 degrees to 0.6 to 98 degrees; $P < .05$) at 12 months' follow-up. Despite distorted anatomic landmarks and extra-articular femoral deformity, navigation was a useful and accurate tool for patients.

The largest reported series to date of extra-articular deformities about the knee corrected with the assistance of computer navigation was reported by Mullaji and Shetty,[32] who managed 40 severe extra-articular deformities in 34 patients. Twenty-two were femoral deformities, and 18 were tibial. The mean deformity was 9.3 degrees. Three of the 40 patients required simultaneous corrective osteotomy. In addition to reporting sagittal plane correction to a mean mechanical axis deviation of 1 degree (standard deviation, 1.4 degrees), the authors described similarly accurate results for coronal plane alignment postoperatively, noting that this is the only report on excessive coronal plane alignment complicating total knee arthroplasty managed with computer-assisted navigation. In contrast to the series of patients reported by Papadopoulos and colleagues,[35] who were treated with simultaneous corrective osteotomy (investigators saw increased risk of restricted motion and 50% of patients without optimal component position or axial alignment in the absence of computer navigation assistance), Mullaji noted no complications in patients treated with an osteotomy. Other authors have highlighted the challenges of simultaneous corrective osteotomy at the time of total knee replacement, including risks of nonunion, arthrofibrosis, infection, and pulmonary embolism.[26] Consequently, Mullaji notes that surgeons undertaking simultaneous corrective osteotomies with navigation assistance should be well versed in navigation before they apply combined techniques.

CONCLUSIONS

Total knee arthroplasty in the presence of extra-articular deformity has always been a challenge, because the typical alignment references are frequently absent or distorted, and traditional alignment guides cannot be used accurately because of hardware, malunion, or metabolic conditions. Computer-assisted surgical navigation offers a new tool for surgeons who undertake these difficult cases, allowing intraoperative spatial feedback to the operating surgeon that can be used to orient bone resections and occasionally osteotomies. Emerging data suggest that computer navigation in the clinical setting of total knee replacement surgery can be used to accurately align implants with the mechanical axis in the coronal and sagittal planes. Extension of these navigation techniques to difficult cases with extra-articular deformity is only logical, as traditional tools for alignment are often precluded by the deformity itself. As clinical data are accumulated via case series and more rigorous studies, intraoperative computer-assisted navigation will remain a useful adjunctive in these difficult cases.

KEY REFERENCES

Bottros J, Klika AK, Lee HH, et al: The use of navigation in total knee arthroplasty for patients with extra-articular deformity. J Arthroplasty 23:74, 2008.

Chou WY, Ko JY, Wang CJ, et al: Navigation-assisted total knee arthroplasty for a knee with malunion of the distal femur. J Arthroplasty 23:8, 2008.

Fehring TK, Mason JB, Moskal J, et al: When computer-assisted knee replacement is the best alternative. Clin Orthop Relat Res 452:132, 2006.

Kim K, Ramteke AA, Bae DK: Navigation-assisted minimal invasive total knee arthroplasty in patients with extra-articular femoral deformity. J Arthroplasty 25:658, 2010.

Lonner JH, Siliski JM, Lotke PA: Simultaneous femoral osteotomy and total knee arthroplasty for treatment of osteoarthritis associated with severe extra-articular deformity. J Bone Joint Surg Am 82:342, 2000.

Mann JW III: Total knee replacement with associated extra-articular angular deformity of the femur. In Scuderi GR, Tria AJ Jr, editors: Surgical techniques in total knee arthroplasty, New York, 2002, Springer-Verlag, p 636.

Mason JB, Fehring TK, Estok R, et al: Meta-analysis of alignment outcomes in computer-assisted total knee arthroplasty surgery. J Arthroplasty 22:1097, 2007.

Matziolis G, Krocker D, Weiss U, et al: A prospective, randomized study of computer-assisted and conventional total knee arthroplasty: three-dimensional evaluation of implant alignment and rotation. J Bone Joint Surg Am 89:236, 2007.

Mullaji A, Shetty GM: Computer-assisted total knee arthroplasty for arthritis with extra-articular deformity. J Arthroplasty 24:8, 2009.

Papadopoulos EC, Parvizi J, Lai CH, et al: Total knee arthroplasty following prior distal femoral fracture. Knee 9:267, 2002.

Papagelopoulos PJ, Karachalios T, Themistocleous GS, et al: Total knee arthroplasty in patients with pre-existing fracture deformity. Orthopedics 30:373, 2007.

Radke S, Radke J: Total knee arthroplasty in combination with a one-stage tibial osteotomy: a technique for correction of a gonarthrosis with a severe (>15 degrees) tibial extra-articular deformity. J Arthroplasty 17:533, 2002.

Slover JD, Tosteson A, Bozic KJ, et al: Impact of hospital volume on the economic value of computer navigation for total knee replacement. J Bone Joint Surg Am 90:1492, 2008.

Sparmann M, Wolke B, Czupalla H, et al: Positioning of total knee arthroplasty with and without navigation support: a prospective, randomized study. J Bone Joint Surg Br 85:830, 2003.

Wang JW, Wang CJ: Total knee arthroplasty for arthritis of the knee with extra-articular deformity. J Bone Joint Surg Am 84:1769, 2002.

Full references for this chapter can be found on www.expertconsult.com.

Chapter 120

Custom-Made Cutting Guides for Total Knee Arthroplasty

Mahmoud Hafez

Custom-made cutting guides is a new concept of using computer-assisted preoperative planning to provide patient-specific instruments that could replace conventional instrumentation systems. Preoperative computed tomography (CT) or magnetic resonance imaging (MRI) scans are acquired and imported to a special software system that has three-dimensional data of the total knee arthroplasty (TKA) implant to be used. Planning and possibly virtual surgery is performed on the computer before it is done on real patients. This includes sizing, alignment, bone cutting, and verification of optimal implantation and positioning. As described later ("Summary of the Technique"), two virtual templates are designed and transformed into physical guides using rapid prototyping technology. Information built into the guides can be transferred to the patient's knee, and surgeons can use these guides or conventional cutting blocks. TKA can then be done without using intra- or extramedullary guides (Fig. 120-1). This revolutionary technique is considered to be an important step in the development of TKA since the introduction of instrumentation systems in the 1970s.

COMPUTER-ASSISTED ORTHOPEDIC SURGERY

The application of computer technology in medicine has been progressing rapidly since the introduction of CT scanning. Computer-assisted surgery (CAS) started with navigation and robotics; computer-assisted orthopedic surgery (CAOS) involves several other devices that can improve the accuracy and reproducibility of surgical techniques, provide objective means for preoperative planning and measurement of surgical performance, and supply powerful training tools. TKA, like many other orthopedic procedures, is well suited for the diversity of CAOS applications.

CAOS is defined as the use of computer-enabled technology at any stage (pre-, intra-, and postoperative) in the surgical management of orthopedic conditions using various systems (active, semiactive, passive or hybrid) and delivering several applications, including planning, simulation, guidance, robotic, telesurgery, and/or training.[13] Also, previous classification of CAOS focused on robotics and navigation.[34] There are several CAOS techniques that extend far beyond the narrow categories of robotics and navigation. Hafez and colleagues have described a more comprehensive classification for CAOS systems based on their functionality and clinical use.[9] This includes six main categories, which are then subgrouped on a technical basis (Table 120-1). This classification could be extended because future devices can later be added under new categories or subcategories. It has made it easier for orthopedic surgeons to comprehend the complexity of surgical robots and the differences in their mechanisms of action and functionality. Currently, there has been an increasing number of developed robots, up to 159 surgical robots in

the literature.[36] The orthopedic robots are subcategorized here only as industrial, hand-held, or bone-mounted based on mechanism of action and ergonomics. Robots actively perform surgical actions, whereas navigation acts as a position tracking device and information system, subclassified based on the mechanism of action related to imaging requirements. Hybrids combine features of robotic and navigation, subclassified in a similar way as navigation.

Templating (category 4) provides guidance and/or tooling, subclassified based on the mechanism of action of the templates. Simulation (category 5) provides a rehearsal of surgical procedure that improves visualization for surgeons and trainees through intuitive user interfaces (with or without interactive animation). These are subclassified based on the mechanism of action and how the data are manipulated. The preoperative digital templating software used by surgeons to size and plan hip and knee arthroplasty is an example of a planning simulator; it is the most clinically used modality representing simulation.[17] Telesurgery (category 6) allows the surgeon to operate or mentor other surgeons remotely but it is not yet developed to where it can be exploited and used in clinical practice.

Robotics, Navigation, and Early Templating Techniques

Navigation techniques for TKA are now the most popular CAOS system in surgical use. This modality is passive and does not perform any steps of the surgical procedure. Instead, it provides the surgeon with intraoperative measurements and feedback. The three different types of navigation systems have been used in TKA but image-free systems are the most commonly used. Several authors have reported the better accuracy of navigation systems in TKA.[1,2,4,22] Robotic techniques have been less popular and the earlier, large industrial robots that were used for hip and knee arthroplasty have been withdrawn from clinical practice.[14] Recently, a newer version of has been orthopedic robots are gaining popularity and been used in unicompartmental arthroplasty[7] and then TKA.

Templating and custom-made guides is a type of CAOS in category 4 in Table 120-1. It involves image-based preoperative planning, followed by the production of templates that match the surface geometry of the patient's bony structures. The templates are designed to transfer the preoperative planning to the intraoperative performance. The production machines range from computer numeric-controlled (CNC) to a more sophisticated technology of rapid prototyping (RP), which acts as a three-dimensional printer to produce physical objects from the three-dimensional computer-aided designs (virtual templates). RP acts by joining together liquid, powder, and sheet materials, producing complex templates in the form of plastic or metals. The medical applications of this technology started in the late 1970s, with modeling and

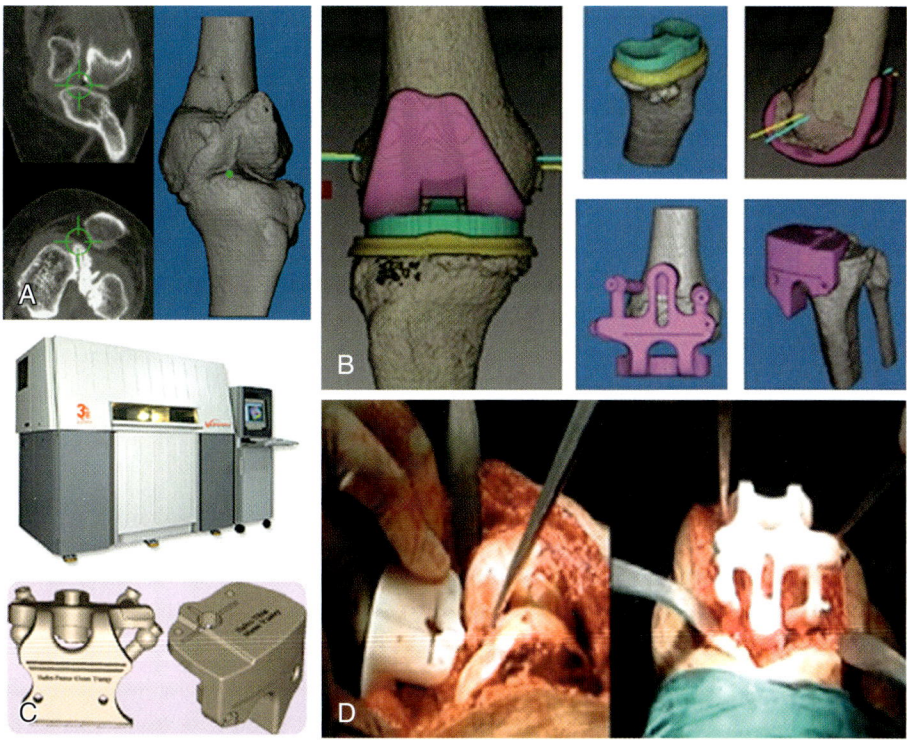

Figure 120-1. Custom-made cutting guides. **A,** Step 1, CT scan following a special protocol. **B,** Step 2, Preoperative planning—sizing, alignment, and implant positioning; design of cutting guides and simulation. **C,** Step 3, rapid prototyping machine that produces the femoral and tibial cutting guides. **D,** Step 4, TKA is done using two cutting blocks without conventional instruments.

Table 120-1 Classification of Computer-Assisted Orthopedic Surgery (CAOS) Systems

CATEGORY		Subcategory (Based on Mechanism of Action)
No.	Name	
1	Robotics	Industrial Hand-held Bone-mounted
2	Navigation	Image-free Image-based (preoperative) Fluoroscopy-based (intraoperative)
3	Hybrid techniques	Image-free and image-based
4	Templating	Guide (pin positioning) Instrument (cutting block) or tool (implant)
5	Simulation	Planning simulators (templating software) Virtual reality and augmented reality
6	Telesurgery	Telepresence Telementoring

computer-aided design and computer-aided manufacturing (CAD-CAM) producing custom prostheses.[3] The earliest surgical reports of using RP technology came from the dentistry and maxillofacial fields.[18] In orthopedics, this technology was used in pelvic, spinal, trauma, osteotomy, and knee surgery.[32,35] These applications ranged from a simple printing of anatomic models using CT images to more sophisticated preoperative planning to produce surgical guides, such as those reported

by Radermacher and associates.[37] This developed further to the currently used custom-made cutting guides, with more specific software allowing a complete planning of TKA based on preoperative imaging and the CAD files of the TKA prosthesis.[11-13] Thus, templates or cutting guides are produced that can completely replace TKA conventional instruments.

History of Custom-Made Guides

In 2004, Hafez and coworkers[12] reported a new technique of using two-piece custom-made cutting guides instead of conventional instrumentation to perform TKA. Preoperative computer-assisted CT-based planning was used to design the templates (femoral and tibial cutting blocks) that were successfully used for 17 experimental cases (14 cadaveric and 3 plastic knee specimens) without resorting to conventional jigs. This work started in 2001 and the concept of this new technique was presented by these authors as a poster at a 2002 meeting of the International Society of Technology in Arthroplasty. A complete description of the technique, including the principles and experimental use for 45 TKAs, was presented by Hafez and associates in 2006,[11] naming the technique patient-specific templating.[10,13] Although the term *custom-made cutting guides* is very popular now, the term *templating* is more scientific and descriptive from technical and engineering aspects. This is because the technique involves preoperative planning with sizing, alignment, cutting, and verification of implant positioning and surgical simulation, and then the production of patient-specific templates. These templates can be used as guides, cutting blocks, instruments, or tools and the concept is applicable to other procedures in orthopedics (e.g., total hip arthroplasty [THA], osteotomy, spine surgery) or other specialties such as dental and maxillofacial surgery, in which template would be more relevant than cutting guides.

Although our work on custom-made cutting guides started in early 2001, the clinical application started toward the end of the decade. When the first successful cadaveric procedure was done in 2001, it was perceived that a new era of TKA was about to begin. The technique evolved over time and modified gradually until it reached its optimal accuracy and applicability in 2004. Although the success and the revolutionary nature of this technique were obvious, it was difficult at that time to apply the technique clinically because of several reasons. New techniques are not easily accepted by senior surgeons, reviewers, and health care systems, particularly when it competes with a time-honored technique such as conventional jig systems. I used to present the custom-made cutting guide as an alternative technique to conventional instrumentation (CI); the latter was the gold standard and the only technique available for most surgeons, and was the state of the art instrumentation for many implant companies. Conversely, there was no interest from implant companies to exploit the idea because of the unlucky coincidence with the emerging navigation systems at that time. Custom-made guides were considered by some implant companies as a competitor to navigational TKA, which was their marketing tool. The delay in clinical application allowed the laboratory work to continue until 2006, with the technique validated by testing its reliability and intraobserver and interobserver variation.[10,15]

In 2008, Howell and colleagues[20] reported the first clinical application of custom-made cutting guides, named the Otis knee. They used MRI rather than CT scanning and based the position of the implants on kinematic rather than mechanical alignment. Then, the concept of custom-made cutting guides was exploited by all major manufacturers but with some modifications, such as using MRI instead of CT and using the templates as a guide to locate conventional cutting blocks (i.e., pin locator). MRI has the theoretical advantages of detecting cartilage and being a radiation-free imaging modality. However, CT scanning was found to be more practical because of the limitations of MRI, such as difficult segmentation, certain contraindications (e.g., the presence of pacemaker, implants), and obesity. The other limitations, of different degrees according to different health care systems, are cost, long waiting list, reimbursement, and other logistical considerations. In addition, most commercially available MRI-based systems have approximately a 6-week interval from the time of acquiring the MRI scans until the templates are delivered to the hospital. This may carry the risk of anatomic changes to the knee as a result of daily activities or any abnormal loading during this long delay, thus resulting in intraoperative malpositioning of the templates and subsequently implant malalignment. The same errors of malpositioning of the templates can occur because of errors in bone segmentation with MRI, which is less likely to occur with CT. These types of errors have already been reported.[26] Our CT-based software system was easy to use. This allowed surgeons themselves to do the preoperative planning and designing of the templates, unlike MRI-based systems, which have to be done planned and designed by experienced technicians

because of the need to do manual segmentation of the images. For CT-based systems, the segmentation is done automatically by the software.

The other modification of using the template as a pin locator was defeating the objective of the custom-made cutting guide technique, which is meant to replace conventional instrumentation and eliminate all the drawbacks mentioned in next section. Using templates as a pin locator means adding extra pieces of instruments to conventional instrumentation and mixing principles, which could lead to unexpected errors.

RATIONALE FOR USE

There are several reasons why TKA techniques and their outcomes need to be improved. Several authors[1,2,4,23] have outlined the rationale for using CAOS techniques in general, which is mainly to improve the accuracy of TKA. This may apply to computer-assisted, custom-made cutting guides without the drawbacks of navigation and robotics. Moreover, the cutting guide technique is an alternative to conventional instruments and can overcome the deficiencies in conventional techniques; these disadvantages are explained by the following.

Plain radiography is the routine preoperative imaging modality for conventional TKA and is usually done in the form of short leg x-ray. Plain radiographs have limited accuracy.[25,29] Ten degrees of knee flexion and 20 degrees of external to 25 degrees of internal rotation can cause significant differences in knee alignment measurements. The knee has a complex three-dimensional anatomy, so planning, alignment measurement, and bone cutting have to be done in a three-dimensional fashion. The ability to understand the three-dimensional complexity of the knee is variable and depends on the surgeon's experiences. Surgeons make intraoperative decisions based on what they visualize (eyeballing), which is usually focused on one plane. The accuracy of visual inspection by surgeons is limited, especially when using ill-defined or inconsistent operative landmarks, such as the center of the femoral head, center of the ankle, or epicondylar axis. These errors are even greater when dealing with obese patients or in the presence of bony abnormalities. Minor errors in bone cutting, such as posterior sloping of the tibial cut and posterior femoral cut, can affect the flexion gap and errors in tibial and distal femoral cuts can affect the joint line level. Intraoperatively, it is usually difficult to determine the normal level of the joint line accurately. The recent introduction of minimally invasive surgery (MIS) has made it more difficult to visualize the knee joint or even to visualize the bone completely during cutting.

CI systems are relatively complex tools with numerous jigs and fixtures and their use is time-consuming. They need setting up before surgery, assembling and dismantling during surgery, and washing and sterilization afterward for reuse in subsequent procedures. For example, a demonstration kit for a standard size 3 primary TKA (PFC Sigma, DePuy, Warsaw, Ind) has 84 different pieces. Most primary prostheses have various options—fixed-bearing, mobile-bearing, cruciate-substituting, cruciate-retaining. There are different sizes (average, six sizes) of implants for each of these options, with additional pieces of instruments to fit the different sizes and different options. It is more common to add extra pieces of instruments or more complex sets (e.g., modified sets, MIS or revision instruments). Every implant has its own instrumentation system and, in the same hospital, there could be several different systems. A report from England has revealed more than 30 TKA prostheses in use.[28] This may overload hospital inventory, sterilization services and nurses' learning curves, and increase operating room time. The conventional instrumentation set is packed in several trays (at least four) requiring one or two additional carrying tables, which need to be positioned as close to the surgeon and nurse as possible, but the environment is often not ergonomically efficient. In addition, the tables usually are in the way of the surgical assistant(s). There is generally a lack of space and these trays may cross the zone of the laminar flow. The complexity of CI systems may adversely affect the performance of nurses, trainees, and low-volume surgeons. In one report, 50% of TKA procedures were done in the United States by surgeons who perform about six procedures/year.[27] Also, these drawbacks may affect high-volume surgeons, who may want to perform 10 joint replacement procedures or more in a single day, leading to exhaustion, with higher risk of errors because of unforeseen circumstances or the complexity of cases. Furthermore, in developing countries, in which TKA procedures are not common, most surgeons and hospitals have a low volume of arthroplasty procedures. Implant manufacturers cannot permanently store their instrumentation systems in such hospitals; rather, they provide the instruments on a loan basis and the cost is offset toward the cost of the implants.

CI systems can be invasive and hazardous. The use of alignment guides involves the violation of intramedullary (IM) canals. This can lead to a higher risk of bleeding,[4,23] infection,[30] and fat embolism.[24] The numerous pieces of CI systems are metallic and some have sharp edges, spokes, or pins. They may require drilling to attach them to bone at different steps of the procedure. These metallic edges and pins require careful handling and can potentially cause sharp injuries to the surgeon or patient. There are risks related to the long operative time, such as longer tourniquet time, contamination, longer rehabilitation, and anesthetic complications. In a retrospective analysis of postoperative complications of 17,644 TKA procedures, it was found that extended surgery time increased the rate of hematoma and infection.[6] The repeated use of conventional instruments carries a theoretical risk of contamination.

CI systems, including medullary guides, are used to guide several steps of a TKA, such as sizing, alignment measurement, and bone cutting. These steps are dependent on each other and this could lead to the accumulation of errors that might occasionally pass unnoticed. Most of these steps or actions (bone cuts) are irreversible. For example, the surgeon may correct the inaccurate bone cutting by making unplanned soft tissue release. Overzealous soft tissue release on one side will lead to imbalance and the surgeon may then have to release the other side, which might lead to laxity and instability. Femoral intramedullary guides are used by most surgeons, but this technique may not be suitable for patients with significant extra-articular deformities, marked bowing, and those with prior surgery or fractures. Several other authors have reported different sources of errors from using IM guides.[42] It was noted that the anatomic axis exits the distal femur at an average of 6.6 mm medial to the center of the

femoral notch, whereas most implant manufacturers recommend making the entry point at the center of the femoral notch. Other sources of errors include using short rods that do not reach the isthmus of the femur or tibia, using thin rods in large IM canals, or placing a straight rod in a deformed bone.

The average bone geometry of white patients has been used for designing most CI systems, which may vary even among patients of the same ethnic origin. Nagamine and associates[31] have reported several anatomic variations in 133 Japanese patients with knee osteoarthritis (OA). They found proximal tibia vara, lateral offset of the tibial shaft with respect to the center of the tibial plateau, and external rotation of the femoral component of more than 3 degrees in 20% of patients. In 2000, Tang and coworkers[43] reported that Chinese patients require 5 degrees of external rotation of their femoral component to obtain a rectangular flexion gap as compared with the commonly reported 3 degrees of external rotation. The accuracy of using conventional instrumentation for sizing is also questionable.[21] It is not uncommon to have a mismatch between sizing of the femoral anteroposterior (AP) and mediolateral (ML) dimensions, leading to overhang or not enough coverage. Deformities and bone loss can make sizing somewhat difficult. Selecting a smaller size implant means cutting more bone and, once the bone is cut, it cannot be reattached. Bone cutting for a smaller size implant results in more bone cut posteriorly than distally, creating a wider flexion gap. The correction of this imbalance may lead to a series of compromises; more bone is removed distally with elevation of the joint line, there is excessive soft tissue release, or both can occur, requiring a thicker tibial insert. Undersizing may also result in femoral notching.

Alternative techniques, such as navigation and robotics, have been developed. Although conventional surgical instrumentation have been repeatedly modified, it appears that further refinements are unlikely to overcome their inherent drawbacks, such as the multiplicity of instruments and medullary canal perforation. Thus, a practical alternative to CI systems is required. The recent introduction of CAOS, particularly navigation, into surgical practice has allowed surgeons to evaluate its accuracy objectively; it has been proved to be superior to conventional instrumentation systems.[1,2,4,22] However, navigation techniques still require the use of conventional instruments for making the various bone cuts and they even require additional instruments and the insertion of pins, onto which tracking instruments are attached. This doubling of instrumentation systems (navigational and conventional) is costly and could overload hospital inventory, sterilization services, and operating room time. They may also increase the number of decisions that have to be made by the surgeon. There is a growing need to introduce ergonomics in the surgical workplace,[41] which is more difficult to achieve with bulky navigational or robotic devices. Furthermore, navigation and robotics require registration and tracking with a continuous line of sight. The overwhelming intraoperative information from navigation systems may confuse the surgeon and complicate the decision making process. These techniques can ultimately take senior surgeons away from their comfort zone and interrupt their learning curve. The rate of complications may increase during the early stages of learning the technique. All these drawbacks have limited the broad clinical application of robotics and navigation techniques. There is a need for alternative techniques that are simple, less invasive, less expensive, and accurate, with minimal drawbacks.

SURGICAL PROCEDURES

Hardware and Software Requirements

The technique requires preoperative imaging (CT or MRI), a personal computer with the specific software needed, and a production machine, such as rapid prototyping. For commercially available techniques, surgeons usually request the required imaging technique according to the protocol provided by the implant manufacturers, who usually perform the planning and production of the cutting guides by themselves. The guides are then delivered to the surgeon. With some techniques, the surgeon may have access to carry out or approve the preoperative planning, either on line over the Internet or directly on a computer that has the specific software installed.

Summary of the Technique

The technique involves the use of computer-assisted preoperative planning to provide patient-specific instruments that could replace CI systems. Preoperative CT or MRI scans are imported into a special software system that has three-dimensional data of the TKA implant to be used. Planning and possibly virtual surgery is performed on the computer before it is done on real patients. This includes sizing, alignment, bone cutting, and verification of optimal implantation and positioning. Two virtual templates (femoral and tibial cutting guides) are designed and then transformed into physical guides using rapid prototyping technology. The guides have built-in information about the preoperative planning, which can be transferred to the patient's knee when the guides are positioned on the matching surfaces of the distal femur and proximal tibia. Then, surgeons can use these guides to make all necessary cuts or guide the position of conventional cutting blocks using locating pins. These patient-specific guides should be used once because they are designed based on the surfacing matching of the patient CT scan. TKA can then be done without using sizing or alignment jigs (intra- or extramedullary). The patient's initials, hospital number, and sides of the knee should be engraved on the cutting guides (see Fig. 120-1).

Imaging

Three-dimensional image of the knee is required via CT or MRI, along with data on the mechanical axis of the leg (hip to ankle). The latter can be obtained using the same three-dimensional imaging (CT or MRI of the hip and ankle region) or AP and lateral views of the whole leg using a CT scanogram (topogram). This technique does not require mechanical data because it relies on kinematic alignment based on the information obtained from the knee joint with the goal of restoring the natural prearthritic alignment of the limb. This approach is controversial; all other techniques using custom-made cutting guides rely on the mechanical axis, which is a standard parameter. Because every manufacturers has different software, a special protocol is thus required

for image acquisition. Surgeons have to follow the protocol specified for the implant they are going to use; otherwise, images might not be accepted by the software and become useless. Surgeons may have to use certain radiologic centers that are registered for this service. Regardless of the imaging protocol used, the image of the knee joint should be with 1-mm thick slices and 1-mm spacing, which is the minimum requirement for accurate reconstruction of the joint.

Preoperative Planning

Special CAD software is required, with information about the implant to be used in the form of three-dimensional(CAD) files of different sizes of tibial and femoral components. Preoperative images (CT or MRI) will be imported by the software and reconstructed. Thus, the anatomy of the knee is created and displayed in three dimensions, with the ability to rotate and tilt the image to view all its aspects (front, back, and sides) at any angle.

Default planning is based on the standard parameters, such as 3 degrees of external rotation for the posterior femoral cut and 0 degrees for coronal tibial cut. The surgeon's preference can also be added to the default, such as 5 degrees of posterior slope in the tibial cut. The default parameters can be changed according to the specific nature of the case or the surgeon's preference.

Sizing of the femoral and tibial components is done automatically by the system and can be verified to avoid anteroposterior and mediolateral mismatching or any implant overhang in any plane. The planning can reveal information that would not be available to the surgeon during actual surgery, such as posterior tibial overhang or femoral notching. Alignment (angles and rotation) and bone resection are planned according to the set default for eight standard parameters—femoral coronal alignment, femoral saggital alignment, femoral rotation, level of distal femoral cutting, tibial coronal alignment, tibial saggital alignment, tibial rotation, and level of tibial cutting. Surgeons may have a role in preoperative planning, either by performing the planning or by approving it through an interactive website.

Production of Cutting Guides

This step requires a special production machine; the most sophisticated machine is rapid prototyping, which can print the cutting guides based on the virtual design created by the planning software. The guides are made of specific plastic materials that should be biocompatible and durable enough to withstand the heat of sterilization (e.g., autoclave) and the contact with surgical instruments, such as power drills and saws. The most popular material used by many implant manufacturers is polyamide. The cutting guides produced are delivered to the hospital, autoclaved, and then used for the specific patient. It is technically possible to produce a plastic knee model specific to the patient based on the patient's CT or MRI scans. The surgeon can use this model to simulate the positioning of the guides before doing the actual surgery.

Using Cutting Guides in the Operating Room

The surgical steps are significantly reduced to three steps—fit, pin, and cut. It is extremely important that surgeons check the individual details engraved on the cutting guides (e.g., patient's initial, number, and side of surgery) to make sure that they are matching the patient to be operated on. This should be done as a habit similar to the routine practice for checking blood bags before blood transfusion.

The design of the cutting guides is based on the approach to be used, such as MIS or the standard medial parapatellar approach. For other approaches, osteophytes should not be removed because they may be used as a reference for positioning cutting guides. The femoral and tibial guides (one at a time) are positioned over the respective bone following their unique surface matching. The guide should fit into one single position without rocking and with no other possibility for a different position. This step is critical and surgeons should double-check to make sure that the single unique position is found so that they can proceed with no hesitation.

Because these guides are based on the morphology of the patient's knee, they should fit into the optimal position without using any alignment jigs to guide them. Femoral guides are usually used first, giving more space for the tibial cutting guide to be placed over the tibial plateau. Fixation pins are inserted through the guides into the bone, similar to what is done with conventional cutting guides to provide stability during bone cutting. Avoid using damaged or bent pins. Because the sizing of the implant is predetermined, no sizing jigs are needed. Also, there is no need for alignment guides such as extramedullary or intramedullary guides because the cutting guides are uniquely positioned, following the mechanical axis; this has been predetermined during preoperative planning. There are two different schools of thought, one for pin placement and the other for cutting guides.

Pin Placement Technique

In this case, the surgeon uses the guides just to insert locating pins for reference cuts, which are distal and anteroposterior femoral cuts and then a proximal tibial cut. Once the pins are inserted, the guide will be removed and the corresponding conventional cutting block inserted over the locating pins to allow the surgeon to make the necessary cuts. In this technique, no cuts are done through the custom-made guides. For example, Signature (Biomet, Warsaw, Ind) is a pin placement technique (Fig. 120-2 and Table 120-2).

Cutting Guide Technique

In this case, the surgeon uses the custom-made guides to carry out all actions that require a machine, such as cutting and drilling, without resorting to conventional cutting blocks. For example, the femoral cutting guide are used to make all five cuts (distal, anterior, posterior, anterior chamfer, and posterior chamfer) in addition to lug holes. Also, surgeons can make the proximal tibial cut, the stem and the keel, through the tibial cutting guide. Traditional saw blades and drill bits of the appropriate diameter are used to make the various bone cuts and holes for the lugs, stem, and keel. Unless otherwise indicated by the manufacturer, the order for bone cutting is usually distal femoral and then the four femoral cuts, followed by the tibial cut. For example, my preferred technique is the best example for cutting guides (see Table 120-2 and Fig. 120-2).

Some implant manufacturers provide guides that can be used for pin placement or for cutting according to surgeons'

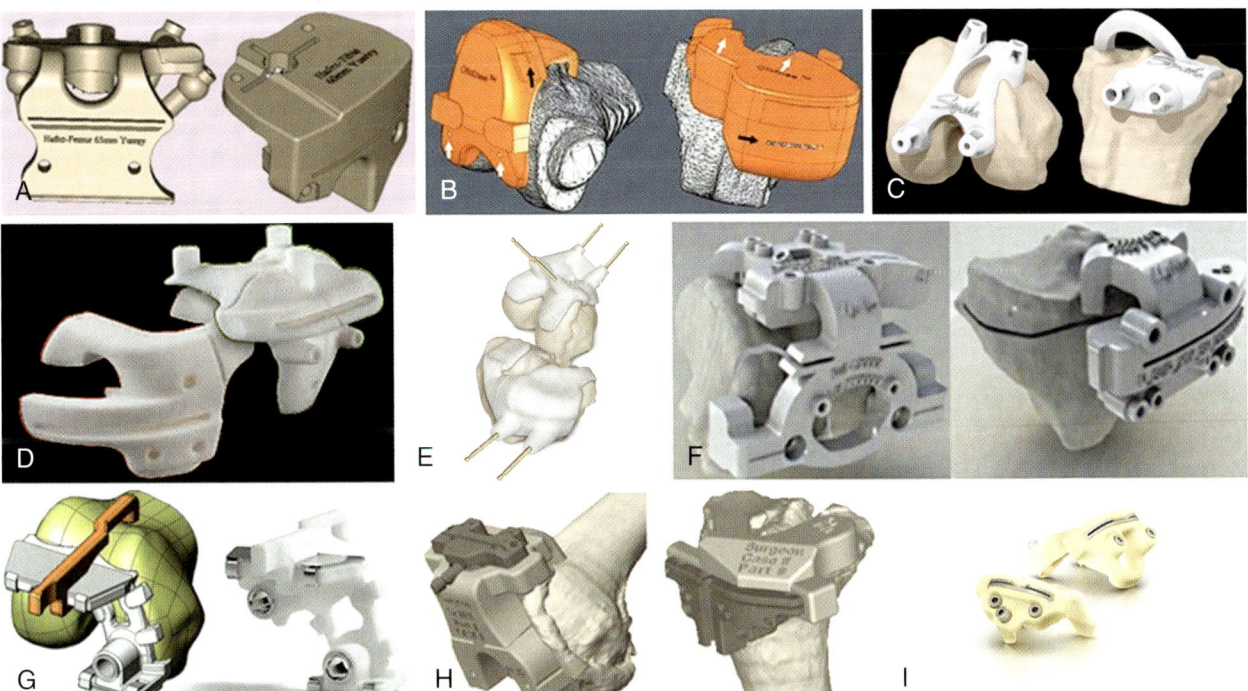

Figure 120-2. Models of the currently available custom made cutting guides for TKR. **A,** Author's Technique "Patient Specific Templating." **B,** Stryker OtisKnee (Kalamazoo, MI, USA). **C,** Biomet Signature (Warsaw, IN, USA). **D,** Smith & Nephew Visionaire (London, United Kingdom). **E,** Zimmer Patient Specific Instruments (Warsaw, IN, USA). **F,** Medacta MyKnee (San Pietro, Switzerland). **G,** ConforMIS iJig (Burlington, MA, USA). **H,** Wright Prophecy (Arlington, TN, USA). **I,** DePuy TruMatch (Warsaw, IN, USA).

Table 120-2 Currently Available Custom-Made Cutting Guides for Total Knee Replacement

Supplier	Author's Technique (classic)	MANUFACTURER							
		Stryker	Biomet	Smith & Nephew	Zimmer	Medacta	ConforMIS	Wright Medical	DePuy
Cutting Guides	Patient Specific Templating	OtisKnee	Signature	Visionaire	Patient Specific Instruments	MyKnee	iJig	Prophecy	TruMatch
Implant name	Open plat form (any implant)	Triathlon	Vangaurd	1. JOURNEY BCS 2. LEGION 3. GENESIS II	1. Gender Solutions 2. NexGen	1. GMK System 2. Cinétique 3. Evolis	iUni G2 iDuo G2	1. ADVANCE 2. EVOLUTION	Sigma
Functionality	Cutting guide	Cutting guide	Pin locator	Cutting guide	Pin locator	Dual	Dual	Both types	Cutting guide
Need for CI	No	No info	Yes	Yes	Yes	Yes	No info	Yes	Yes
Guide Material	Polyamide	Dupont Delrin	Polyamide	No info	Polyamide	Polyamide	No info	Polyamide	RenShape (polyurethane)
Scan Type	CT	MRI	MRI	MRI or x-ray	MRI	CT or MRI	MRI or CT	CT or MRI	CT
Scan protocol	CT scan of knee + Scanogram from Hip to ankle	Knee scan only	MRI of hip, knee, and ankle	No info	hip, ankle, and knee	No info	Spiral scans of hip, ankle, and knee	CT: Hip, femoral shaft, ankle, and knee MRI: hip, ankle, and knee	Entire leg scan or separate hip, ankle, and knee scans
Software	Materialise SurgiTaix	OtisMed	Vanguard (Materialise Mimics)	No info	Materialise	No Info	ConforMIS iFit	No info	Trumatch
Starting Year (published laboratory or clinical work)	2002	2008	2008	2009	2010	2009	2008	2009	2009

preference. For example, MyKnee (Medacta, Castel San Pietro, Switzerland) provides the two options of pin placement and cutting guides (see Table 120-2 and Fig. 120-2).

CURRENT TECHNIQUES

Author's Preferred Technique

My classic technique is not restricted to a single implant manufacturer; rather, it is an open platform that can be applied to any TKA prosthesis, provided that implant manufacturers are willing to provide the CAD files of their prostheses for preoperative planning. A special consent form for this procedure is obtained from all patients after explaining the technique verbally and providing an information sheet with a visual demonstration describing the technique in detail. This description is written in simple language and included risks and hazards in addition to benefits. Every patient has had a CT scan of the knee and a long-leg scanogram (topogram) extending into the hip and the ankle in AP and lateral projections following a specific protocol. An appointment for surgery is scheduled to be in 2 to 3 weeks' time.

Figure 120-1 illustrates the steps for this technique, including CT scanning, reconstruction of three-dimensional images, sizing and alignment of prosthetic components, template design, and surgical simulation. The virtually designed cutting guides are transferred to the production machine via electronic mail. The femoral and tibial cutting guides are produced using an SLS rapid prototyping machine (3D Systems, Valencia, Calif) and polyamide (nylon). The production service is done outside the hospital (outsourcing by private firms) without the need to buy the expensive machine. The patient's initials, side of the knee, and surgeon's name (with or without a code number) were engraved on the body of the templates. The cutting guides were autoclaved in the hospital and the operating room staff was informed about the size of the tibial and femoral implant to be used, and that conventional instruments are not required.

The knee is exposed through a medial parapatellar approach, with the use of a tourniquet but without a drain at the end. The femoral cutting guide is positioned first, making sure that all locating probes in the undersurface of the guide are touching the distal femur centrally, medially, and laterally at the same time. Once this unique single position is achieved, the guide is fixed by fixation pins passing through drill guides in the femoral cutting guide. An angel wing could be used to verify the amount of bone to be removed distally and anteriorly. Saw blades of an appropriate thickness are inserted first into the slit for the distal cut and the cut bone is removed through the gap between the cutting block and distal femur. The same approach is used for the anterior, posterior, and chamfer cuts. Lug holes can also be made through the cutting guide. The tibial cutting guide is positioned over the tibial plateau and the anteromedial surface of the proximal tibia, close to patellar tendon insertion after clearance of soft tissues in this area. The position is verified based on surface matching and ensuring that there is no other chance of having more than one matching position. The cutting guide is fixed by fixation pins from the front and optionally from the top. An angel wing is used to verify the amount of bone cutting, the cut is made through the slit, and the cut bone is removed from the

medial or lateral side. The stem and keel are prepared through the corresponding hole and slit at the top of the tibial cutting guide, thus determining the rotation of the tibial implant. The cutting guides are removed and trial implants are used in a similar way to trial implantation in conventional TKA. The surgeon can then perform soft-tissue release as needed. Trial implants are made of durabl plastic material similar to those of cutting guides (mostly polyamide).

Other Techniques

In the last few years, the principle of this novel technique has been used and commercialized by major implant manufacturers. Several versions were released under different names for custom-made cutting guide techniques, such as custom-made cutting guides, custom-fit total knee, patient-specific cutting guides, shape-fit, and true match. The technique has been gradually spreading over the last 2 years; by the end of 2010, there were approximately 5000 procedures being done every month. Few orthopedic surgeons have reported their early clinical results.[20,26,40] However, the validation of this technique and the reliability of intraoperative positioning of these templates still has not been reported by their developers or users. Table 120-2 and Figure 120-2 show the information available about each technique at the time of this writing.

CLINICAL APPLICATIONS

Although custom-made cutting guides were clinically applied without U.S. Food and Drug Administration (FDA) approval based on the assumption that these instruments are class I. Now, FDA is considering these instruments to be class 2 and requiring all companies to reclassify them from the class 1 to class 2 designation.

Indications

All patients selected for TKA who can undergo CT or MRI are indicated for this technique. Some patients are not suitable for MRI, such as obese, medically unfit, and claustrophobic patients and those with a pacemaker. Those patients could undergo for CT-based procedures. There are no known contraindications, apart from the theoretical risk of allergy to the material of the cutting guides. However, the technique is limited by some logistic considerations, which may lead to a delay of several weeks until the cutting guides are produced and delivered to the surgeon, unlike conventional TKA instrumentation, which can be used any time. This current limitation will restrict the use of the technique to certain cases rather than being extended for routine use.

Absolute indications for using custom-made cutting guides include the following:
- Extra-articular deformities
- Retained hardware such as nails or plates and screws
- When IM instrumentation is problematic
- Bleeding tendency, such as hemophilia
- Medically unfit patients and anesthetic risk
- Severe OA with bone loss and articular deformities
- Abnormal anatomy
- Obese patients
- Risk of infection

In some of these cases (e.g., extra-articular deformities), conventional TKA techniques are difficult and risky to use or cannot be used at all. The clinical trial should adopt a graduated approach. During the early learning curve, the surgeon(s) can perform this technique on patient-specific plastic knee models that can be produced by a rapid prototyping machine based on the patient's own CT scans. Thus, the surgeon can see the results of surgery before using the custom-made cutting guide technique on real patients. The surgeon can position the templates over the bone to test the ease and accuracy of positioning and mark the level and inclination of bone cutting on the bone. After this is done, conventional instruments can be used for comparison and evaluation of the proposed cuts. Navigation techniques (if available) can be used in a similar manner to that used for the reliability testing to measure the accuracy of this technique (see later). Once the surgeon develops confidence with this technique, it can be used for bone cutting, without resorting to conventional instrumentation. Simple instruments, such as angel wings, can be used to mark the level of bone cutting for visual inspection and confirmation by the surgeon before real cuts. With an improved learning curve, possibly after five cases, the surgeon(s) may proceed to a comparative trial.

Published Clinical Studies

The concept of custom-made cutting guides has been exploited by different companies. The reported clinical results of commercial systems have confirmed the clinical applicability of this technique. Although one report has revealed suboptimal clinical results and criticized the technique, the other reports have shown good clinical results with the same technique. Klatt and associates[26] have used an image-free navigation system to evaluate the recommended custom-made cuts and alignment of the components and found that they were more than 3 degrees of the mechanical axis. Spencer and coworkers[40] have reported the results of 21 patients with custom-fit TKAs who were compared with a matching cohort of 30 patients with previous conventional TKAs. In the custom-fit series, there was a mean decrease in operative time of 14% and an average deviation from the mechanical axis of 1.2 degrees of varus. The authors concluded that the "technique appeared to be a safe procedure for uncomplicated cases of osteoarthritis." Howell and colleagues[20] have reported the results of 48 consecutive patients treated with the custom-fit technique; they showed rapidly returned function, restored motion, stability, and postoperative good mechanical axis alignment, high patient satisfaction, and an acceptable clinical outcome. None of their cases required soft tissue (collateral ligament or retinacular) release. In their series, there were three tibial guides and three femoral guides that were not positioned properly. Their retrospective analysis attributed the cause of poor positioning to a random error by the technician who was aligning the MRI. They also conducted a similar retrospective analysis for the cases reported by Klatt and associates[26] and found a similar type of errors caused by the technician, who malaligned the MRI in two of four knees in that pilot study. They concluded that the poor results reported by Klatt and coworkers were caused by poor positioning of the guides (templates) that affected the position of the components because of an MRI alignment error, which was not a known problem when the surgeries were performed.

I have reported on the clinical application of the custom-made cutting guides based on CT scanning.[8,15] The details of this technique have been explained earlier. The difference from previous studies involves the complexity and difficulty of these cases. They were divided into five different unusual categories of patients: (1) extra-articular deformities; (2) bleeding tendencies; (3) bilateral deep venous thrombosis (DVT) and/or pulmonary embolism; (4) bilateral TKA in patients seeking short recovery; and (5) medically unfit patients (usually cardiorespiratory compromise). Patients with these problems were refused conventional TKA or denied the procedure by anesthetists or other arthroplasty surgeons. In all cases, the custom-made cutting guides were successfully applied, with preplanning and without using CI. Neither intramedullary guides nor alignment rods were used. Preoperative sizing was accurate in all cases. A tourniquet was used routinely but no drains were used. No reported intraoperative or postoperative complications occurred with any patient, and there were no reports of postoperative confusion or respiratory symptoms to indicate fat embolism. Postoperative recovery was uneventful, and all patients had full extension and more than 100 degrees of flexion.

There were specific and unusual scenarios for some cases. In category 1 patients, a preoperative radiograph (Fig. 120-3) showed no room or trajectory for the insertion of femoral intramedullary guides or conventional jigs following the anatomic axis. Figure 120-4 shows the reconstructed CT scan of this case, ready for preoperative planning and positioning of the guides, and based on mechanical rather than anatomic axes. Figure 120-5 shows the final planning, ready to be approved by the surgeon, verifying sizing, alignment, implant positioning, and bone cutting. It also reveals an important piece of information about the shape of the femoral and tibial cutting guides and how they should be positioned during surgery. This should guide the surgeon while positing the cutting guides on real patients. A printed copy of the final plan should accompany the surgeon in the operating room.

The relatively most difficult and time-consuming step of this technique was the positioning of the cutting guides over the bone (Fig. 120-6). However, this step was guided by the printed copy of the final planning (see Fig. 120-5). The longest time of positioning was 5 minutes for each guide. The matching of the template to the respective bone was satisfactory. In patients who had severe flexion deformity of more than 30 degrees, two femoral cutting guides had to be designed to provide a second option for excessive distal cutting. The optional guide was used intraoperatively and proved to be optimal for these cases. CT scanning had to be repeated for patients who did not follow the protocol (e.g., moving during scanning) and also for some patients who had TKA on the other side because of the interference caused by the knee prosthesis in the contralateral knee, which was supposed to be bent and not kept straight during scanning.

ACCURACY AND VALIDATION

Laboratory Testing

A literature search at the time of this writing revealed no published data on laboratory validation for custom-made cutting guides, apart from the experimental trial

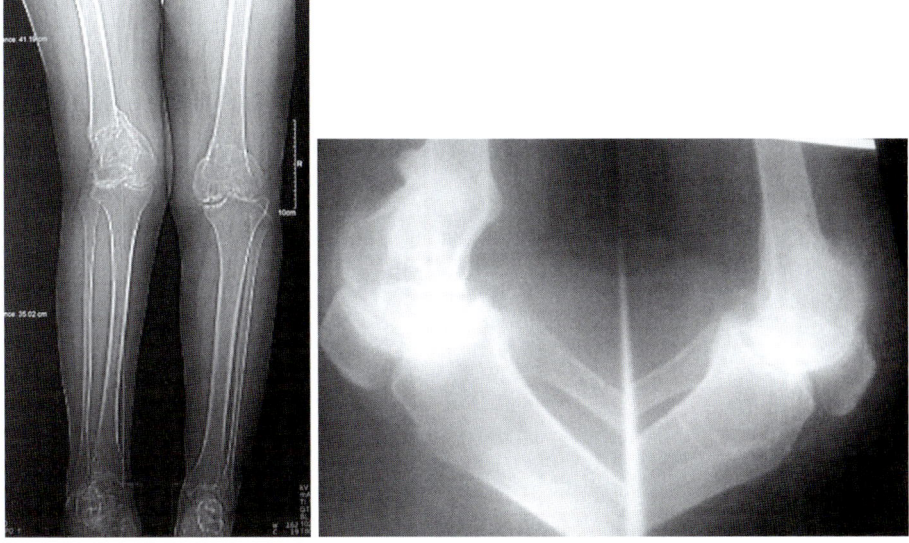

Figure 120-3. Preoperative long leg x-ray of patient with knee OA with extra-articular deformities.

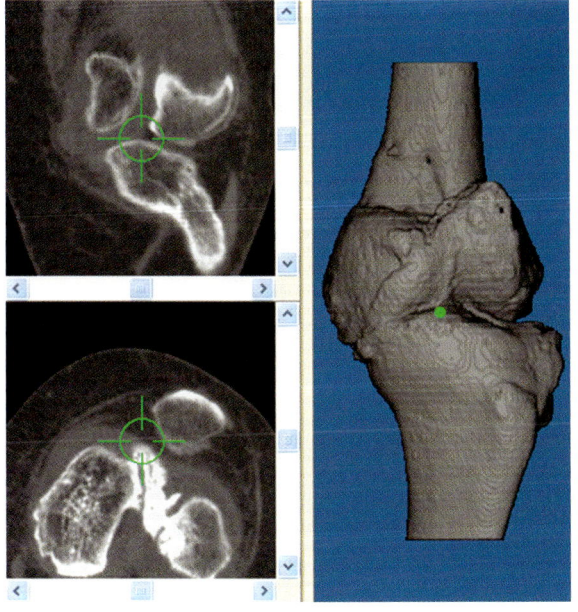

Figure 120-4. CT scan reconstructed and ready for preoperative planning.

and reliability testing that I and my colleagues have reported.[11,13,15] In the experimental trial, the patient-specific templates (custom-made cutting guides) were used to perform 45 total knee arthroplasties on 16 cadaveric and 29 plastic knees, including a comparative trial against conventional instrumentations (PFC, DePuy, Warsaw, Ind). All operations were performed using patient-specific templates, with no conventional instrumentations or intramedullary perforation. The mean time for bone cutting was 9 minutes with a surgical assistant and 11 minutes without an assistant. Computer-assisted analyses of six random CT scans showed mean errors for alignment and bone resection within 1.7 degrees and 0.8 mm (maximum, 2.3 degrees and 1.2 mm, respectively). Patient-specific templates were found to be a practical alternative to conventional instrumentations. The level of

accuracy and reliability of this technique were better than that reported for conventional techniques,[38,42] which had errors of more than 3 degrees. This level of accuracy also compares favorably with the results of navigation (within 3 degrees).[1,2,22] Laboratory validation experiments were performed by five observers, myself and four independent observers who were not familiar with the custom-made cutting guide technique (new users). The experiment was conducted using a plastic knee specimen (foam cortical shell, model 1151, Sawbones, Mamlö, Sweden). The planning for TKA was based on the PFC prosthesis (DePuy) and electronic implant data was imported to the planning system.

As illustrated in Figure 120-1, the typical steps for the custom-made cutting guide technique include CT scanning, reconstruction of three-dimensional images, sizing and alignment of prosthetic components, template design, surgical simulation, and finally production of patient-specific templates using SLS RP machines (3D Systems). The primary outcome measure was alignment and level of bone cutting, as determined by the position of the templates. A navigation system (VectorVision, BrainLab, Heimstetten, Germany) was used only as a measurement tool for the template positioning by the observers without playing any role in guiding them. An independent assessor recorded the measurements that were displayed on the navigation monitor. Kappa statistics was used to analyze qualitative data and quantitative analysis was performed using Friedman's repeat measure, nonparametric analysis of variance (ANOVA), and the Kruskal-Wallis ANOVA. Interobserver and intraobserver concordance were tested using the Kendall coefficient of concordance. Correlation between the results of the study observers was done using the Pearson moment correlation test (r). A probability value (P value) less than .05 was considered significant.

The results of this study showed a satisfactory level of accuracy for new users, with a mean alignment error of 0.67 degrees (maximum, 2.5 degrees). The mean error for bone cutting was 0.32 mm (maximum, 1 mm). For qualitative analysis, it was apparent (without even using kappa statistics) that all measured values were within 3 degrees, indicating complete interobserver and intraobserver agreement. For

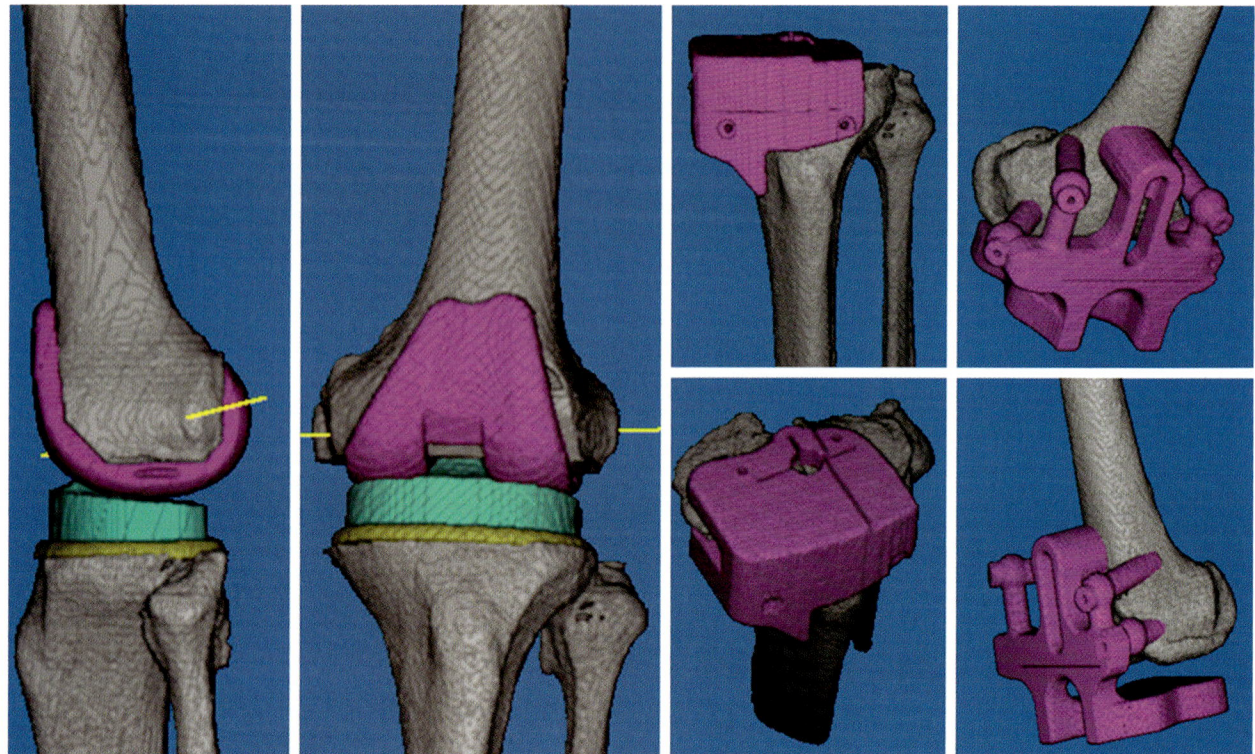

Figure 120-5. Final plan showing sizing, alignment, and implant positioning and cutting guides designed and positioned to match the patient's anatomy.

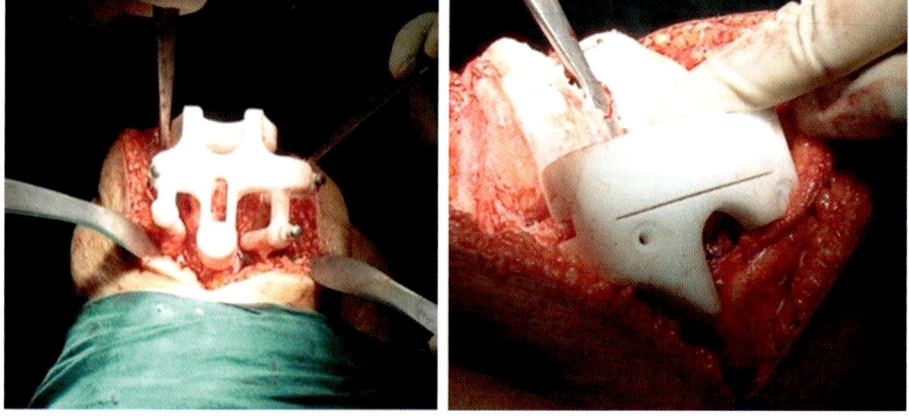

Figure 120-6. Cutting guides positioned over the bone based on surface matching.

quantitative analysis using the Friedman test and Kendall concordance coefficient, there was an overall significant agreement between observers ($P < .05$). The concordance coefficient was high, indicating a considerable interobserver agreement for all measured parameters except the femoral cutting level, which had a relatively low concordance coefficient. Comparison between different recorded measurements for the same observer (intraobserver variation test) showed significant agreement ($P < .003$) and the concordance coefficient was very high. This means that there was no difference after repeating the same test by the same observer and that there was a considerable intraobserver agreement.

This laboratory study showed that the positioning of the templates was reliable, because there was no significant

intraobserver and interobserver variation for alignment or levels of bone cutting in the femur and tibia. The observers found the custom-made cutting guide to be user-friendly and could be uniquely positioned and held with one hand. They were able to do the experiments without assistants.

Clinical Validations and Outcomes

To date, there is no level 1 evidence study published on the clinical outcome of custom-made cutting guides. Therefore, clinical validation is required before recommending this technique for routine use. There have been only a few clinical studies published with favorable clinical outcome,[15,20,40] and all were reported by developers of the technique. There is one report with unfavorable results.[26] The previous section on clinical application noted the results of these studies in more detail. I have conducted a prospective comparative trial[17] among custom-made cutting guides, navigation, and conventional techniques in 60 patients on whom I had performed TKA. The full statistical analysis of the results is not ready at this time. However, the alignment in all cases was within 3 degrees of error, compared with the optimal planned alignment. There were no complications on short-term follow-up. The conventional technique had the advantage of being the default technique, and all those involved in the surgical procedure were familiar with it. The navigational technique had accurate and comprehensive documentation of intraoperative performance and measurements. This clinical study showed the superiority of custom-made cutting guides over conventional instrumentation. It eliminated medullary guides, reduced operative time, and provided better accuracy. It was a simple, less expensive technique, with no need for registration or tracking, so it was better than navigation for TKA. The technique was used in straightforward TKA and in complex cases of extra-articular deformities (see Fig. 120-3) and unsuitable patients, such as those with bleeding tendency or a previous history of DVT and pulmonary embolism.

ADVANTAGES AND DISADVANTAGES

Benefits

Considering all the drawbacks noted for of CI, navigation, and robotic techniques, it appears that the proposed custom-made cutting guide technique is relatively easier to use, less invasive, time-saving, and inexpensive. It confines the computer-assisted work to the preoperative stage and provides the surgeon with a two-piece instrumentation system (femoral and tibial templates) but no bulky equipment. The technique requires no registration or tracking and can be used by surgeons who have no prior experience with CAS. It shares some of the capabilities of CAS, particularly the high accuracy of CT-based planning.[25] The results of this technique have demonstrated a level of accuracy (error <3 degrees) that compares favorably with that of navigation techniques.[4,5]

There are several benefits of this technique. Some are already proven and others are still theoretical, as follows:

- Three-dimensional planning and better visualization of abnormal anatomy
- Preoperative sizing and identification of expected problems
- Performing and viewing the results of surgery before performing it on real patients
- No conventional instruments and no problems with inventory, storage, setup, installation, washing, sterilization, and packing; easier handling and less risk of losing and damaging pieces
- Significant reduction of operative steps (sizing, alignment, and cutting) by shifting intraoperative steps to preoperative stage, thus, improving operating room performance and efficiency, with a positive effect on health care systems
- Short learning curve for surgeons and nurses and reduced need for training on CI
- Significant reduction of operative time, useful for patients and surgeons

- No violation of intramedullary canals, with less risk of fat embolism and bleeding
- Possibly less risk of infection because of shorter operative time, including anesthesia and tourniquet time, no repeated use of instruments, no IM perforation
- Cost reduction—reducing costs of instruments ($30,000 to $100,000), sterilization and packing, long operative time, training, and complications caused by CI
- Accurate implant positioning
- Can allow procedures that could not be done before using conventional surgery

Examples include patients with extra-articular deformities, in whom conventional intramedullary rods cannot be used.[16] Such patients are traditionally treated by osteotomy and then TKA when the osteotomy has healed. Custom-made cutting guide allow the correction of the deformity at the knee level during TKA, saving the trouble of another procedure (osteotomy). CAOS techniques in general can provide more accurate preoperative planning in cases of multiplane deformities.[33] The first case in our series showed the capability of CT-based three-dimensional planning for the severely deformed knee and the simplicity of doing TKA without using intramedullary guides, as compared with the difficulties of using conventional techniques in such cases.

- Extends the indications for bilateral TKA
- Less complications (bleeding and infection) for hemophiliacs and those with other bleeding tendencies
- Less operative risk for medically unfit patients with high anesthetic risk because of associated cardiorespiratory disease and comorbidities
- Reduces the need for tourniquet, drains, and blood transfusions
- Potential to be used as a training tool, allowing complete planning of surgery with three-dimensional simulation that facilitates identification and correction of errors in real time

Also, it allows the measurement of surgical performance by comparing postoperative images with the recorded preoperative planning. Rapid prototyping machines can produce a patient-specific model of the knee joint based on the CT scan data of the patient. Thus, the surgeon can perform TKA on the patient's model and evaluate the results before operating on the real patient.

- Optimal solution for use in developing countries and in places in which knee OA and extra-articular deformities are prevalent (e.g., Middle East, Far East)

In these areas, there is a huge unmet need for TKAs; the ratio of TKA procedures done annually in Egypt as compared with England, which have almost the same population, is as low as 1:20. The reason is multifactorial and related to the economy, complexity of cases, cultural fear of surgery and complications, and lack of structured training. Hospitals in these countries usually do not stock implants and do not own conventional instrumentation systems, so they have to be lent for each case. Also, CT scans are relatively inexpensive and useful for complex cases.

Drawbacks

The technique has known drawbacks, such as the following:

- It requires imaging that is not a routine requirement for conventional TKAs.

Some patients are not suitable for MRI scans (e.g., obese, medically unfit, and claustrophobic patients and those with pacemakers); the segmentation of bone from MRI images is more difficult as compared with CT scans. However, MRI is safe and its images have the advantage of visualizing the articular cartilage, a feature that CT scans lack. Also, the radiation risk of CT scans cannot be ignored. The radiation dose for a knee CT scan is approximately 1.2 mSv, which is relatively low as compared with the dose for a lumbar spine plain radiograph (1.3 mSv).[32] Attempts have been made to develop low-cost, low-radiation CT scan devices.[39] Even with conventional CT scanners, certain protocols for knee CT scans may result in reducing the dose to 0.1 mSv.[19]

- Unlike navigation, templating techniques do not normally provide intraoperative measurements, because sizing, alignment, and bone cutting are determined preoperatively.
- There is an extra cost for this technique as a result of imaging and the process of making the custom-made guides.

Over the short term, this extra cost will be paid by the patient or care provider but over the long term, the technique could be cost-effective.

- Lack of support for soft tissue balancing

However, in conventional techniques, surgeons use their own judgment to perform soft tissue balancing. Moreover, the accurate preoperative sizing and alignment in this technique should lead to precise bone cutting, which will diminish the need for soft tissue release.

- Change of the routine practice of TKA by shifting certain surgical steps from the intraoperative to the preoperative stage

Some surgeons might not tolerate such a change because they like to make the necessary measurements and adjustments intraoperatively on a stepwise basis.

- Unknown allergy to the material of the cutting guides

Polyamide is the most popular material used for producing cutting guides. This material has been licensed for short-term tissue exposure (i.e., to be used as an instrument but not as an implant). Shedding as a result of machine work and contact between metals and plastics may occur. The short- and long-term risks are unknown. So far, there have been no reported problems with the short-term experience in using these materials in orthopedics and the long-term experience of their use in maxillofacial and dental surgery.

Pitfalls and Complications

The following issues need to be considered. When using CT scanning as an imaging modality, dimensions and measurements will be based on bone, with no information on cartilage thickness. MRI segmentation is difficult, time-consuming, and may cause errors. As noted in an earlier section in more detail ("Published Clinical Studies"), positioning of the templates is the most critical step in this technique and is a significant source of errors. Retrospective analyses[20] have shown malalignment errors; these produced unacceptable results because of poor positioning of the guides (templates),[26] which affected the position of the components. This problem was not recognized at the time the surgeries were performed.

The reported errors of positioning templates (custom guides) in MRI-based techniques[20,40] confirm the rationale and clinical relevance of our study,[15] which aimed to validate this technique and test the reliability of template positioning. We believe that laboratory validation with reliability testing should be done before introducing new techniques for clinical use. This study tested intraobserver and interobserver variability; this has not been reported previously for other similar cutting guide techniques. The published results for other custom-made cutting guide techniques have been reported with no data on the results for new users.

FUTURE DIRECTIONS

From the technical point of view, computer technologies are fast progressing and computer-aided designing and manufacturing software systems are becoming increasingly more sophisticated and powerful. Rapid prototyping machines are frequently modified to add more features, such as the ability to produce complex tools. There are now new generations of compact RP machines that are as small as an office PC printer. These compact machines can be purchased by hospitals and stored inside the operating room, radiology department, or outpatient clinic. This will allow imaging, planning, and template production to be done at one site, saving time and resources. Other imaging modalities may be used in the future, such as three-dimensional radiography.[39]

Applications for Challenging Cases

In addition to the promising results of this study and the demonstrated benefits of the custom-made cutting guide technique, there are potential benefits that can be investigated and exploited in the future, such as the following:

Minimally Invasive Surgery

The custom-made cutting guide is more amenable to minimally invasive techniques, because it uses two-piece instruments and obviates the need for using IM guides. The current size and shape of the templates can be further reduced to fit into the minimally invasive approaches. The recent trend of combining MIS and CAS may prove to be more practical with the use of the custom-made cutting guide technique. However, the problems of inserting the templates and observing the process of positioning and surface matching through small incisions have to be overcome.

Complex Total Knee Arthroplasty

The custom-made cutting guide technique would be useful for patients with complex deformed knees and revision surgery and for young active patients, with the additional benefits of preserving bone stock by quantifying the volume of removed bone during planning and before actual surgery. In revision surgery, the cost of implants is much higher and the complexity of the surgery much greater, so the advantages of the custom-made cutting guide technique, with its preoperative planning, become more important and the costs become less significant.

Patients Susceptible to Infection

Theoretically, the custom-made cutting guide can reduce the risk of contamination and infection by avoiding intramedullary perforation, shortening tourniquet time, and eliminating the reusable numerous instruments that have multiple holes and canals. The custom-made cutting guide can further reduce the risk of infection by reducing bleeding and hematoma formation. Unlike navigation techniques, the custom-made cutting guide does not require tracking or the insertion of pins to the femur and tibial, which has a risk of pin track infection. The custom-made cutting guide technique may prove useful for TKA in certain patients who are susceptible to infections such as HIV or those susceptible to infection and bleeding, such as hemophilia. Reusable instruments also carry the theoretical risk of spreading serious diseases, such as variant Creutzfeldt-Jakob Disease; these instruments require extraordinarily high levels of sterilization. The custom-made cutting guide has the advantage of being a single-use instrument.

Applications for Other Surgical Procedures

The custom-made cutting guide technique has the potential to be used for other procedures, such as unicompartmental, bicondylar—a new procedure to replace the medial and lateral compartments only while preserving the anterior and posterior cruciate ligaments, and patellofemoral arthroplasty, which require a higher level of accuracy and less invasive approaches. The same can be applied to hip resurfacing. The custom-made cutting guide technique for these procedures might be easier to learn and perform and can provide a better environment for training in TKA.

Use of Custom-Made Cutting Guides For Training

The technique can serve as a powerful and inexpensive training tool. The preoperative planning software can be installed in desktop and laptop computers with modest cost. The software may provide the opportunity for surgeons in training to practice on the preoperative planning of TKA, including sizing, measuring alignment and rotation, and performing virtual bone cutting. The surgical simulation allows the identification and analysis of errors in three-dimensional planes and in real time. It also provides training for cognitive and motor skills, allowing repetitive practice, committing errors and correcting them. For workshops on plastic bones, RP machines can produce reusable metallic templates that are specific to the plastic knee model, thus avoiding the need to keep producing new templates for each practice. The custom-made cutting guide technique itself requires less training as compared with conventional instrumentation, because it is easier to use and involves only a few intraoperative steps. With further modification and refining of the custom-made cutting guide technique and its combination with MIS approaches, it may prove possible to achieve the ideal TKA procedure.

CONCLUSIONS

Conventional instrumentation systems consist of numerous pieces of jigs and fixtures that are cumbersome because they require set-up, assembly, dismantling, and cleaning, which are time-consuming. Alignment guides perforate medullary canals, leading to a higher risk of bleeding, infection, and fat embolism. Reusable instruments carry a theoretical risk of contamination and may overload hospital inventory and sterilization services. The accuracy of conventional instrumentation has been questioned by many authors. Since the introduction of these systems in the 1970s, they have been modified repeatedly but without radical changes or substitutes. Robotics and navigation had the potential to replace such systems but their application was limited by cost and complexity.

The custom-made cutting guide is a revolutionary step in the development of TKA. This new concept exploits the capability of using computer-assisted preoperative planning software to provide patient-specific instruments that could replace conventional instrumentation systems. Preoperative CT or MRI images are acquired and imported to a special software system that has three-dimensional data of the TKA implant to be used. Planning and possibly virtual surgery is performed on the computer before it is done on real patients. This includes sizing, alignment, bone cutting, and verification of optimal implantation and positioning. Two virtual templates, femoral and tibial cutting guides, are designed and then transformed into physical guides using rapid prototyping technology. The guides have built-in information of the preoperative planning that can be transferred to the patient's knee when the guides are positioned on the matching surfaces of the distal femur and proximal tibia. Then, surgeons can use these guides to make all necessary cuts or to guide the position of the conventional cutting blocks. These patient-specific guides should be used once because they are designed based on the surfacing matching of the patient's anatomy. TKA can then be done without using IM or extra medullary guides.

The technique has several advantages over conventional instrumentation and can be used for complex cases of extraarticular deformities and unsuitable patients. It eliminates medullary guides, reduces operative time, and provides better accuracy. It is a simple, less expensive technique that can be an alternative to navigation for TKA. However, further clinical studies with level 1 evidence are needed to confirm the results of limited clinical studies. Until this is done, the custom-made cutting guide technique should be used with caution and ideally should be confined to clinical trials.

Acknowledgments. The assistance of the staff in the following institutions is greatly appreciated: October 6 University Hospital, Cairo; Helmholtz-Institute of Biomedical Engineering, Aachen, Germany; Institute for Computer-Assisted Orthopedic Surgery (ICAOS), Western Pennsylvania Hospital, Pittsburgh; and the Bioengineering Division, Academic Unit of Musculoskeletal and Rehabilitation Medicine, University of Leeds, Leeds, England.

KEY REFERENCES

Bauwens K, Matthes G, Wich M, et al: Navigated total knee replacement. A meta-analysis. J Bone Joint Surg Am 89:261–269, 2007.

Claus AM, Bosing-Schwenklengs M, Scharf H-P: Risk-profiling in knee arthroplasty based on postoperative complications of 17,644 arthroplasties. Paper presented at the 7th European Federation of National Associations of Orthopaedics and Traumatology Congress, Lisbon, June 4–7, 2005.

Hafez MA: Custom-made cutting guides, navigation and conventional techniques for TKR: a comparative study. Paper presented at the Proceedings of the 4th International Arthroplasty Conference, Sharm El Sheikh, Egypt, January 2011.

Hafez MA, Chelule KL, Seedhom BB, Sherman KP: Computer-assisted total knee replacement: could a two-piece custom template replace the complex conventional instrumentations? Comput Aided Surg 9:93–94, 2004.

Hafez MA, Chelule KL, Seedhom BB, Sherman KP: Computer-assisted total knee arthroplasty using patient-specific templating. Clin Orthop Relat Res 444:184–192, 2006.

Hafez MA, Chelule KL, Seedhom BB, Sherman KP: Computer-assisted total knee arthroplasty using patient-specific templates: The custom-made cutting guides. In Stiehl JB, Konermann WH, Haaker RG, DiGioia AM, editors: Navigation and MIS in orthopedics, Heidelberg, Germany, 2007, Springer, pp 182–188.

Hafez MA, Jaramaz B, DiGioia AM, III: Computer-assisted surgery of the knee: an overview. In Insall JN, Scott N, editors: Surgery of the knee, ed 4, New York, 2006, Churchill Livingstone, pp 1655–1674.

Hafez MA, Jaramaz B, DiGioia AM: Alternatives to navigation. In Navigation and MIS in orthopaedics, Springer, 2006, pp 580–587.

Howell SM, Kuznik K, Hull ML, Siston RA: Results of an initial experience with custom-fit positioning total knee arthroplasty in a series of 48 patients. Orthopedics 31:857–863, 2008.

Kalairajah Y, Simpson D, Cossey AJ, et al: Blood loss after total knee replacement: effects of computer-assisted surgery. J Bone Joint Surg Br 87:1480–1482, 2005.

Kim YH: Incidence of fat embolism syndrome after cemented or cementless bilateral simultaneous and unilateral total knee arthroplasty. J Arthroplasty 16:730–739, 2001.

Kinzel V, Scaddan M, Bradley B, Shakespeare D: Varus/valgus alignment of the femur in total knee arthroplasty: can accuracy be improved by preoperative CT scanning? Knee 11:197–201, 2004.

Klatt BA, Goyal N, Austin MS, Hozack WJ: Custom-fit total knee arthroplasty (Otis knee) results in malalignment. J Arthroplasty 23:637–638, 2008.

Liow RY, Murray DW: Which primary total knee replacement? A review of currently available TKR in the United Kingdom. Ann R Coll Surg Engl 79:335–340, 1997.

Spencer BA, Mont MA, McGrath MS, et al: Initial experience with custom-fit total knee replacement: intra-operative events and long-leg coronal alignment. Int Orthop 33:1571–1575, 2009.

Full references for this chapter can be found on www.expertconsult.com.

Kinematic Alignment in Total Knee Arthroplasty

Stephen M. Howell and Maury L. Hull

The most important predictor of clinical outcome in total knee arthroplasty (TKA) is placement of the femoral and tibial components. Prior to the advent of kinematic alignment, the placement of components was based on the widely accepted principles of classic mechanical alignment, as follows: (1) aligning the femoral component perpendicular to the mechanical axis of the femur; (2) aligning the tibial component perpendicular to the mechanical axis of the tibia; (3) adjusting the anterior-posterior and internal-external rotation positions of the femoral component so that the extension and flexion gaps are equal; and (4) releasing ligaments when necessary to restore motion and balance the knee. In kinematic alignment, the principles for placing the components are different from those of classic mechanical alignment, as follows: (1) coaligning the transverse axis of the best-fitting femoral component with the primary transverse axis in the femur about which the tibia flexes and extends; (2) removing osteophytes to restore ligament length motion and stability; and (3) placing the tibial component so that the longitudinal axis of the tibia is perpendicular to the transverse axis in the femur, about which the tibia flexes and extends.

Kinematic alignment can prevent the loss of flexion and extension, stiffness, instability, pain, and prolonged recovery associated with mechanical alignment.[16,17] Kinematic alignment of the femoral component is confirmed intraoperatively by comparing the symmetry of the thickness of the distal medial, distal lateral, posterior medial, and posterior lateral femoral bone resections after measuring the thickness of the resections with calipers and after correcting for cartilage wear, bone wear, and kerf (i.e., the bone removed by the saw blade). Once kinematic alignment of the femoral component is confirmed, restoring motion and balancing the total knee arthroplasty is simplified by following a stepwise algorithm. The algorithm consists of four steps—removing osteophytes, adjusting the plane of the tibial cut, releasing the posterior capsule from the femur, and medializing or lateralizing the tibial component.

This chapter reviews the history and definition of kinematic alignment with patient-specific guides, highlights the inherent disadvantages of mechanical alignment that kinematic alignment strives to avoid, describes the planning, outlines the algorithm for restoring motion and balancing the kinematically aligned TKA, provides an overview of the surgical technique of kinematic alignment with patient-specific cutting guides and unconventional use of conventional instruments, addresses theoretical concerns of kinematic alignment, and reviews clinical studies showing the early benefits of kinematically aligning the TKA.

HISTORY AND DEFINITION OF KINEMATIC ALIGNMENT

The biomechanical rationale for kinematic alignment is traced to Hollister and colleagues' classic research on the kinematics of the knee.[12] Kinematics refers to the relative relationship of the femur, patella, and tibia at any angle of flexion, without force applied to the knee. The joint surface, menisci, and ligament structures determine the normal kinematic relationship among the femur, patella, and tibia. The center of the femoral head and center of the ankle, which are used by conventional and computer-assisted instruments to align a TKA mechanically, have no bearing on the kinematics of the knee.[10,11,14,15]

Three axes govern the movement of the patella and tibia with respect to the femur, and understanding how the placement of the femoral and tibial components affects the interrelationship of these axes is the key to kinematically aligning a TKA (Fig. 121-1). The primary axis is a transverse axis in the femur about which the tibia flexes and extends. It passes through the center of a circle fit to the articular surface of the femoral condyles from 10 to 160 degrees of flexion.[7,10-12] There is a second transverse axis in the femur about which the patella flexes and extends that is parallel, proximal, and anterior to the transverse axis in the femur about which the tibia flexes and extends. The third axis is a longitudinal axis in the tibia about which the tibia internally and externally rotates on the femur that is perpendicular to each of the two transverse axes in the femur. Although each of the three axes is aligned parallel or perpendicular to one another, none are aligned orthogonally to the three anatomic planes, which means that the axis cannot be found with imaging studies performed in the sagittal, coronal, and axial planes.[15]

The goal for kinematically aligning the femoral component is to coalign the transverse axis of a symmetrical femoral component with the primary transverse axis in the femur about which the tibia flexes and extends (Fig. 121-2).[7,10-12,14] Because there is no clinically important asymmetry between the medial and lateral femoral condyles in the varus and valgus knee with end-stage osteoarthritis, a symmetrical, single-radius femoral component is an optimal design for replicating knee kinematics.

The principle for kinematically aligning the femoral component to the femur is the simple step of shape-matching the femoral component to the articular surface of the femur on a three-dimensional model of the knee that has been restored to normal by filling in the worn articular surface. Shape matching the femoral component to the femur coaligns the transverse axis of the femoral component with the primary transverse axis in the femur about which the tibia flexes and extends, which is requisite to restoring the normal interrelationships among the three axes.[13,16]

In contrast to the simplicity of kinematically aligning the femoral component, kinematically aligning the tibial component involves several steps. The first step is to align the anterior-posterior axis of the tibial component perpendicular to the transverse axis in the femoral component, which has previously been coaligned to the primary transverse axis in

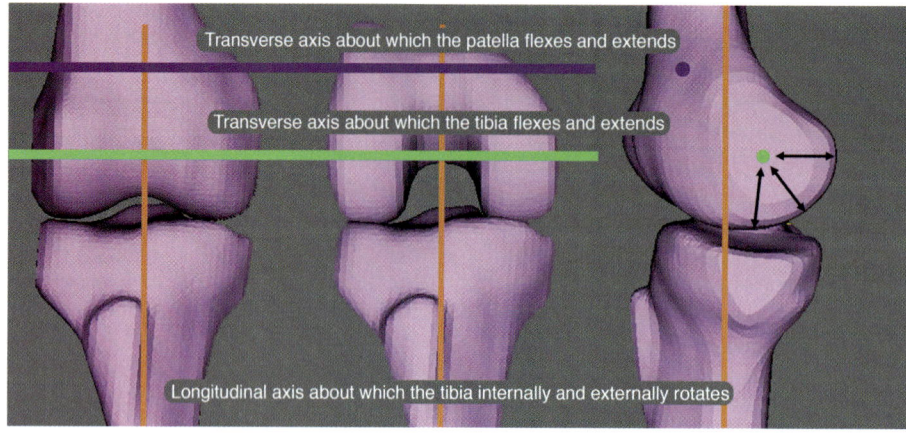

Figure 121-1. Interrelationship of the three kinematic axes in a right knee. **A,** Coronal projection with the knee in extension. **B,** Axial projection of the femur with the knee in 90 degrees of flexion. **C,** Lateral projection with the knee in extension. The primary transverse axis in the femur about which the tibia flexes and extends passes through the center point of the best-fit circles of the medial and lateral femoral condyles *(green line and circle),* which is equidistant from the articular surface of the *condyles (double-headed black arrows).* A second transverse axis in the femur about which the patella flexes and extends axis *(magenta line and circle)* is oriented parallel, proximally, and anteriorly to the transverse axis in the femur about which the tibia flexes and extends. A third longitudinal axis in the tibia *(vertical orange line)* about which the tibia rotates on the femur internally and externally is oriented perpendicular to both transverse axes in the femur.

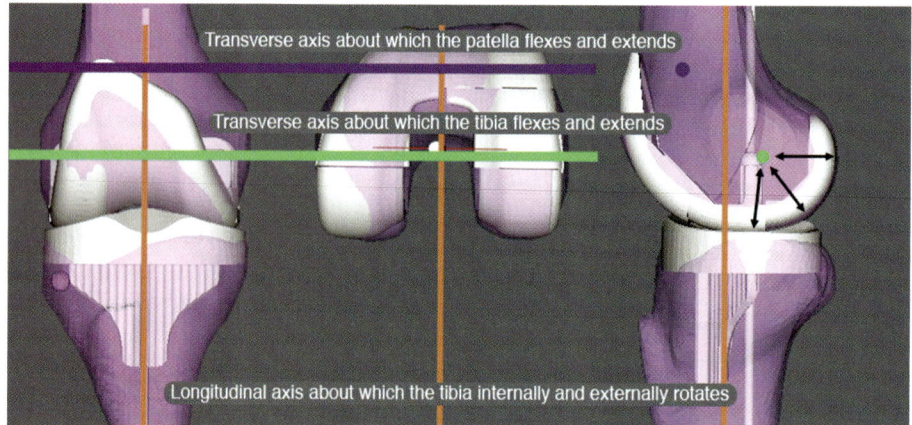

Figure 121-2. Single-radius femoral component of a right knee *(silver)* shape-matched to the femur of a normal knee model *(pink).* Shape matching the femoral component to the femur is the critical step in kinematically aligning the knee and in reestablishing the orthogonal interrelationships among the three kinematic axes. A kinematically aligned femoral component greatly simplifies the step-wise algorithm for identifying the correct options for restoring motion and balance to the knee before cementation of the components. The principle for kinematically aligning the tibial component to the femoral component is to align the anterior-posterior axis of the tibial component perpendicular to the transverse axis in the femur and femoral component. The principle for kinematically aligning the tibia to the tibial component is to accept the assumption that the internal-external rotational relationship between the femur and tibia is normal in a non–weight-bearing MRI scan and then center the tibia under the center of the tibial component.

the femur about which the tibia flexes and extends by the shape-matching step.[1,7] The second step is to align the tibia to the tibial component kinematically, which is based on the assumption that the internal-external rotational relationship between the femur and tibia is normal in a magnetic resonance imaging (MRI) scan of the non–weight-bearing knee with end-stage osteoarthritis. The assumption that the internal-external rotational relationship is normal in the non–weight-bearing knee with end-stage osteoarthritis is inferred from the layer of joint fluid that is consistently seen separating the worn articular surface between the femur and tibia on the MRI scan of the knee. Both the layer of joint fluid and the image of a non–weight-bearing knee indicate that there is no contact between the worn femur and tibia and no transmission of force across the knee to malrotate the

tibia on the femur. The final step is aligning the center of the tibia under the center of the tibial component.

With a goal of improving on the 20% prevalence of patient dissatisfaction from mechanically aligned TKA with conventional and computer-assisted instruments,[3,5] we began developing the method for performing kinematic alignment with patient-specific femoral and tibial cutting guides in 2005. We developed software that creates a three-dimensional model of the arthritic knee from a non–weight-bearing MRI or computed tomography (CT) arthrogram of the knee (OtisKnee, OtisMed, Alameda, Calif; http://www.otismed.com). Additional software transforms the arthritic knee model to a normal knee model and then kinematically aligns the components by shape-matching the best-fitting femoral and tibial components to the normal

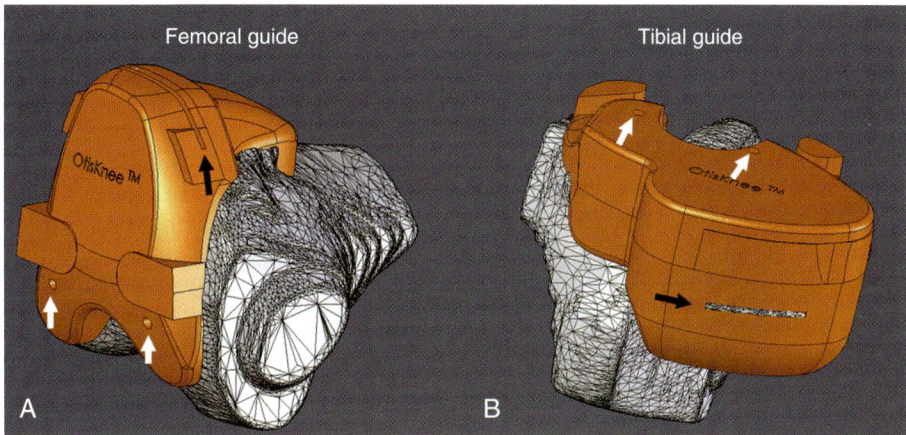

Figure 121-3. Femoral **(A)** and tibial **(B)** patient-specific cutting guides *(orange)* on the arthritic knee model (right knee). The saw slot *(black arrow)* in each guide sets the proximal-distal, flexion-extension, and varus-valgus degrees of freedom of each component. The two holes *(white arrows)* in each guide set the internal-external rotation, anterior-posterior, and medial-lateral degrees of freedom of each component.

knee model. The three-dimensional position of each component is then transferred from the normal knee to the arthritic knee model. Patient-specific cutting guides that incorporate the cut planes of each component and that reference the arthritic knee model are made to fit the patient's femur and tibia (Fig. 121-3). The cutting guides are used intraoperatively to transfer the six degrees of freedom (6DOF) positions of the femoral and tibial components from the computer to the patient—varus-valgus, internal-external rotation, flexion-extension, anterior-posterior, proximal-distal, and medial-lateral.[13,14,16,25]

The first use of patient-specific cutting guides to align a TKA kinematically was in January 2006. As of August 2009, 23,000 kinematically aligned TKAs had been implanted with patient-specific cutting guides nationwide with the lead author (SMH) implanting over 700. From September through December 2009, he implanted 116 kinematically aligned TKAs with unconventional use of conventional instruments instead of patient-specific cutting guides. This 4-year developmental and clinical experience, which is admittedly limited in terms of long-term follow-up, forms the basis for the concepts shared in this chapter with the primary goals of stimulating debate and advancing the understanding of kinematic alignment of total knee arthroplasty.

ADVANTAGES OF KINEMATIC ALIGNMENT OVER MECHANICAL ALIGNMENT

Studies from the United Kingdom and Canada that reviewed more than 10,000 patients at 1 year following mechanically aligned TKA with conventional instruments and contemporary components have shown that one of five patients are not satisfied because of continued pain and poor function in activities of daily living (ADLs).[3,5] The use of computer-assisted surgery has improved the mechanical alignment compared with conventional surgery, but has not improved the clinical outcome (much to the dismay of proponents of computer-assisted surgery).[2,9,21,26] Therefore, a mechanically aligned TKA, whether performed with conventional instruments or computer assistance, has an unacceptably high prevalence of continued pain, poor function in ADLs, and

patient dissatisfaction, which means that there is ample room for improvement.

For the kinematics of a TKA to be the same as a normal knee, the three-dimensional placements of the femoral and tibial components have to be chosen so that the orientation of the three kinematic axes is unchanged from that of the normal knee. None of these axes can be found by referencing the transepicondylar axis, center of the femoral head, and center of the ankle with the use of conventional or computer-assisted instruments.[1,10,15] There is a 5-degree average difference (range, 2 to 11 degrees) between the transepicondylar and primary transverse axes in the femur about which the tibia flexes and extends, which means that referencing the transepicondylar axis substantially changes the joint line from normal in the axial plane.[11] Of normal subjects, 98% do not have a neutral hip-knee-ankle axis because the longitudinal shape of the femur and tibia are unrelated and variable among subjects, which means that referencing the center of the femoral head and of the ankle changes the joint line in the coronal plane.[12] Changing the joint line of the femur from normal in the axial and/or coronal planes using instruments that align components to the transepicondylar axis, center of the femoral head, and center of the ankle kinematically malalign the knee and may explain the midrange instability reported in TKA (Fig. 121-4).[7] Because mechanical alignment kinematically malaligns the knee, we hypothesized that kinematic alignment would reduce the high prevalence of persistent pain, poor function in ADLs, and patient dissatisfaction after mechanically aligned TKA with conventional and computer-assisted instruments.[16,25]

PLANNING KINEMATIC ALIGNMENT WITH PATIENT-SPECIFIC CUTTING GUIDES

Protocol for Aligning and Performing Magnetic Resonance Imaging of the Knee

For kinematic alignment, the projection of the knee in the MRI scan has to be customized to the patient's knee position in the MRI scanner so that the oblique sagittal image plane is perpendicular to the primary axis in the femur about which the tibia flexes and extends. A patient that has a painful osteoarthritic knee should be allowed to choose a position for the leg that is comfortable so that he or she does not inadvertently move the knee during image acquisition and cause

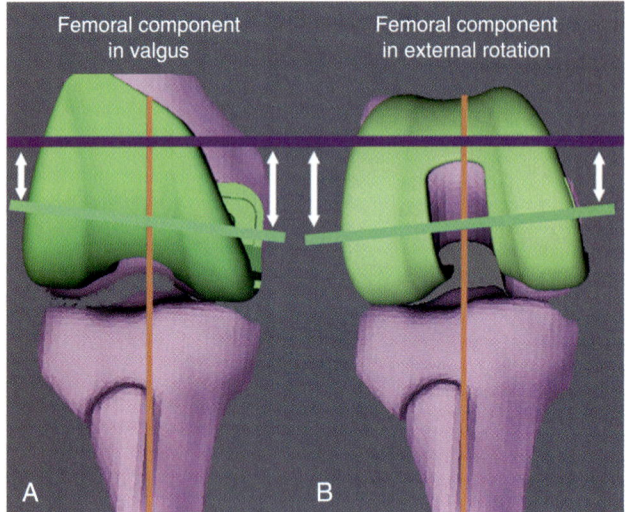

Figure 121-4. Illustration of how a femoral component not shape-matched to the articular surface of the normal knee in the coronal plane **(A)** or the axial plane **(B)** kinematically malaligns the knee. Placing the femoral component in more valgus (or varus) than normal **(A)** tilts the transverse axis in the femoral component *(green line)* so that it is no longer parallel to the primary transverse axis in the femur about which the patella flexes and extends *(magenta line)*, nor is it perpendicular to the longitudinal axis in the tibia *(orange)*, which kinematically malaligns the movement of the patella on the femur and the tibia on the femur. Placing the femoral component in more external rotation (or internal rotation) than normal **(B)** tilts the transverse axis in the femoral component *(green line)* so that it is no longer parallel to the transverse axis in the femur nor is it perpendicular to the longitudinal axis in the tibia *(orange)*, which kinematically malaligns the movement of the patella on the femur and the tibia on the femur. Tilting the femoral component in just one plane or in opposite directions in the coronal and axial planes creates an uncorrectable ligament imbalance *(white arrows)*. In this right knee, valgus positioning of the femoral component loosens the lateral side in extension **(A)** and external rotation of the femoral component worsens the ligament balance by tightening the lateral side in flexion **(B)**. The only way to maintain ligament balance throughout the motion arc is to shape-match the femoral component to the femur.

a motion artifact. The knee with a severe varus or valgus deformity or flexion contracture can be successfully imaged without forcing the knee into extension or an uncomfortable rotation by customizing the projection of the knee in the coronal and axial planes.

The following are contraindications for MRI of the knee for patient-specific cutting guides: (1) presence of a pacemaker; (2) movement of the knee during image acquisition because of inability to follow instructions, tremor, and claustrophobia; (3) obese knee that prevents the use of a dedicated knee coil; (4) hardware about the knee that distorts the image and subsequent three-dimensional model; and (5) metal in the body that might move in the magnetic field (e.g., brain aneurysm clips, metal in the eye, shrapnel near vital structures).

The following is a description of the suggested MRI technique, which relies on the use of coronal and axial locator images to obtain nonorthogonal, oblique, sagittal images perpendicular to the primary transverse axis in the femur about which the tibia flexes and extends (Fig. 121-5).[14] A nonorthogonal, oblique, sagittal MRI scan of the treated knee is obtained using a 1.5- or 3.0-T scanner and dedicated knee coil. The plane for the nonorthogonal, oblique, sagittal scan is based on the use of coronal and axial locator images. These images are used to align the image plane perpendicular to the primary transverse axis in the femur about which the tibia flexes and extends, which projects the femoral condyles approximately in the same plane that the tibia flexes and extends about the femur. Coronal, axial, and sagittal high-resolution locator images are obtained using a 4-mm slice thickness, 1-mm spacing/gap, 256 × 128 matrix, one number of excitations (NEX), and 24-cm field of view (FOV), which yield nine slices in all three planes.

The locator image in the coronal plane that shows the largest projection of the distal femoral condyles is used to adjust the varus-valgus orientation of the plane of the nonorthogonal, oblique, sagittal scan. The nonorthogonal, oblique, sagittal scan plane is aligned perpendicular to a line connecting the cortical-cancellous bone interface of the distal femoral condyles on the locator image in the coronal plane. The locator image in the axial plane that shows the largest projection of the posterior femoral condyles is used to adjust the axial rotation of the plane of the nonorthogonal, oblique, sagittal scan. The nonorthogonal, oblique, sagittal

Figure 121-5. Illustration of the coronal **(A)** and axial **(B)** localizers, femoral joint line *(thick white line)*, transverse axis in the femur about which the tibia flexes and extends *(green line)*, and plane for the nonorthogonal, oblique, sagittal scan *(thin parallel lines)*. Aligning the nonorthogonal, oblique, sagittal scan perpendicular to the distal femoral joint line *(thick white line)* in the coronal localizer and the posterior femoral joint line *(thick white line)* in the axial localizer aligns the nonorthogonal, oblique, sagittal scan perpendicular to the transverse axis in the femur about which the tibia flexes and extends *(green line)*, which projects the femoral condyles as a circle in the same plane that the tibia flexes and extends about the femur.

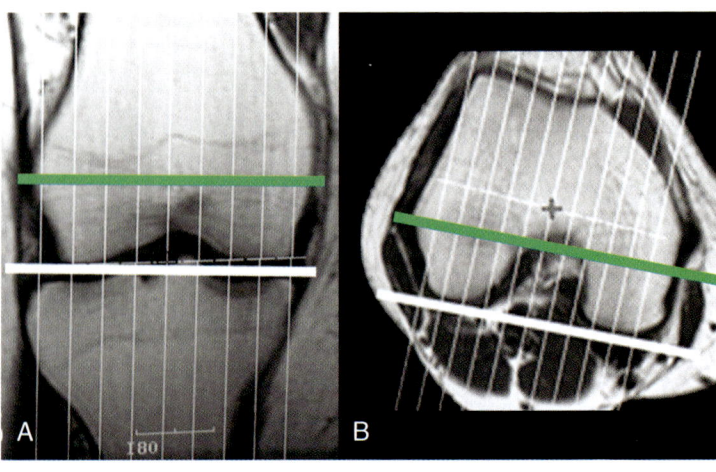

scan plane is aligned perpendicular to a line connecting the cortical-cancellous bone interface of the posterior femoral condyles in the locator image in the axial plane. Because the contour of the posterior femoral condyles from 10 to 160 degrees forms a single radius of curvature, and because the primary transverse axis in the femur about which the tibia flexes and extends is equidistant from the distal and posterior articular surfaces of the femoral condyles, the femoral condyles are projected as circular in the nonorthogonal, oblique, sagittal imaging plane and perpendicular to the primary transverse axis in the femur about which the tibia flexes and extends.[10,11,14]

A nonorthogonal, oblique, sagittal scan is then acquired of the knee, which is subsequently processed with software to generate a three-dimensional model of the knee. The scanning parameters are selected to provide contrast among fat, joint fluid, cartilage, degenerative and normal menisci, and subchondral, cancellous, and cortical bone. For a 1.5-T scanner and a dedicated knee coil (General Electric Medical Systems, Milwaukee, Wisc), we use these parameters: FRFSE PD, 30 to 35 TE, 2800 to 3400 TR, 31.25-Hz bandwidth, and minimum of two excitations using a 16-cm field of view centered at the joint line of the knee, 512 × 512 matrix, 2-mm slice thickness, with no spacing or gap. The length of each side of a pixel in the oblique sagittal image is 0.31 mm.[14]

Generation of Three-Dimensional Arthritic and Normal Knee Models

Kinematic alignment of the femoral and tibial components begins with a three-dimensional arthritic knee model generated from the MRI scans, from 44 to 60 slices, depending on the width of the knee (Fig. 121-6). Proprietary software segments the femur, tibia, articular cartilage, and osteophytes from each image and meshes the images together to form a

three-dimensional model of the arthritic knee (OtisMed). A series of steps is applied to the arthritic knee model to create a normal knee model. The articular surface of the arthritic knee model is transformed into a knee with a normal articular surface by filling articular defects. Osteophytes are removed to restore ligament length and restore a normal shape to the knee. The normal knee model is then aligned in the coronal plane by adjusting the varus-valgus rotation and proximal-distal position of the tibia until the distance between the femoral and tibial articular surfaces is equal medially and laterally.[13,16] This process of creating a normal knee from an arthritic knee by filling defects, removing osteophytes to restore ligament length, and reestablishing a symmetrical medial-lateral joint space borrows from the well-established principles used to align the mobile-bearing unicompartmental knee replacement (i.e., Oxford Knee).

Shape-Matching Femoral and Tibial Components

The three-dimensional model of the femoral and tibial component that best fits the normal knee model is selected by proprietary software (see Fig. 121-2). Algorithms shape-match the femoral component to the restored articular surface of the femur in the normal knee model from 10 to 160 degrees, which kinematically aligns the femoral component by coaligning the transverse axis of the femoral component with the primary transverse axis in the femur about which the tibia flexes and extends. The internal-external rotation of the anterior-posterior axis of the tibial component is set perpendicular to the transverse axis of the femur and femoral component, which kinematically aligns the tibial component to the femoral component. The tibia is centered under the tibial component, which kinematically aligns the tibia to the tibial component.[1,7,10,12] In theory, kinematic alignment restores the normal parallel and perpendicular interrelationship among the three kinematic axes of the prearthritic knee.[14]

Function, Design, and Machining of Patient-Specific Cutting Guides

A common function of all patient-specific cutting femoral and tibial cutting guides, whether they are made to align the TKA kinematically or mechanically, is to transfer the position of each component in three-dimensional space accurately from the computer to the operating room (see Fig. 121-3). Each cutting guide sets 6DOF positions of the component in three-dimensional space, which is comprised of three rotations—flexion-extension, varus-valgus, and internal-external—and three translations—(proximal-distal, anterior-posterior, and medial-lateral). When osteophyte removal changes the dimensions of the femur and tibia, the surgeon has the option to adjust the medial-lateral position of the femoral and tibial components visually.

The patient-specific cutting guides are designed to be small enough to fit in the knee using minimally invasive incisions, yet large enough to register enough knee topography so that the surgeon accurately seats the guide in the intended position. In the event that a cutting guide is inadvertently dropped on the floor, the guide must be sturdy enough to avoid breakage and retain its cavitary shape during resterilization with heat. Rapid manufacturing is required to make the

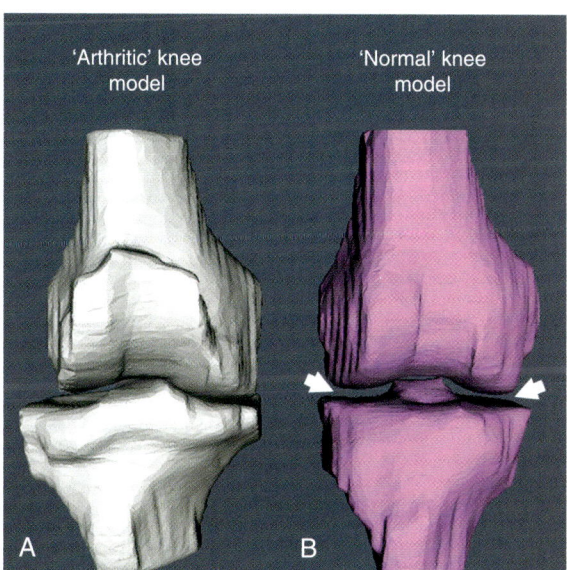

Figure 121-6. Illustration of the arthritic knee model **(A)** and normal knee model **(B)** created with software from an MRI scan of the knee. The software creates the normal knee model from the arthritic knee model by removing osteophytes, filling in worn joint surfaces, centering the tibia under the femur, and reestablishing an equal medial and lateral joint space *(white arrows).*

production of patient-specific cutting guides cost-effective and to limit the turnaround time between receiving the MRI scan and shipping the finished guides. Currently, the turnaround time varies from 10 to 20 business days, depending on the manufacturer, but with future technologic improvements, might only be 1 day.

Patient-specific femoral and tibial cutting guides are machined to fit the arthritic knee model using a biocompatible plastic (polyoxymethylene [POM], Delrin). The cut planes corresponding to the positions of the femoral and tibial components in the normal knee model are transferred to the arthritic knee model. There is one saw slot and four holes for fixation pins in each guide (see Fig. 121-3). The saw slot sets the proximal-distal, flexion-extension, and varus-valgus degrees of freedom of each of the femoral and tibial components. The two pinholes on the articular surface of each guide set the anterior-posterior and internal-external rotation degrees of freedom of each of the femoral and tibial components. The two pinholes on the articular surface of each guide are used to pin the guide to the knee and also reference the conventional chamfer block and tibial component alignment instrument. The two pinholes on the anterior surface of each guide are used to pin the guide to the knee; they also accept the conventional distal femoral and proximal tibial cutting guides for the surgeon who prefers to use the conventional cutting block instead of the saw slot in the patient-specific guide. Hence, each guide provides the surgeon with the size and position of the femoral and tibial components and efficiently and accurately transfers the 6DOF position of each component from the computer to the patient.*

---

*References 1, 2, 6, 7, 9, and 13.

ALGORITHM FOR RESTORING MOTION AND BALANCING THE KINEMATICALLY ALIGNED TOTAL KNEE ARTHROPLASTY

The algorithm for determining the stepwise corrections to restore motion and balance to the knee before cementation of the components is greatly simplified by first aligning the femoral component kinematically (Fig. 121-7). Kinematic alignment of the femoral component is confirmed intraoperatively by comparing the symmetry of the thickness of the distal medial, distal lateral, posterior medial, and posterior lateral femoral bone resections after measuring the thickness of the resections with calipers and after correcting for cartilage wear, bone wear, and saw blade kerf. After correction, the thickness of each bone resection should equal the thickness of the condyle of the femoral component. For example, if a femoral component 8 mm thick and a saw blade 1.25 to 1.37 mm thick are used, then each bone resection should be 6.5 mm thick when there is no cartilage wear or bone wear.

Predicting the thickness of each bone resection is more complicated in the arthritic femur in which there is preexisting focal cartilage wear (typically, 1 to 2 mm) and occasionally bone wear (usually no more than 1 mm). The resection thickness can be predicted preoperatively from a biplanar, rotationally controlled MRI scan, which is carefully viewed to reveal the location and amount of wear (Fig. 121-8).[14] After selecting the image that projects the largest radius of each femoral condyle using image analysis software (OsiriX DICOM Viewer, Dicom Solutions, Irvine, Calif; www.osirixviewer.com), the thickness of the cartilage on the distal and posterior surface of the unworn and worn condyles is measured in millimeters. The difference in thickness between the worn and unworn condyle is computed in millimeters and

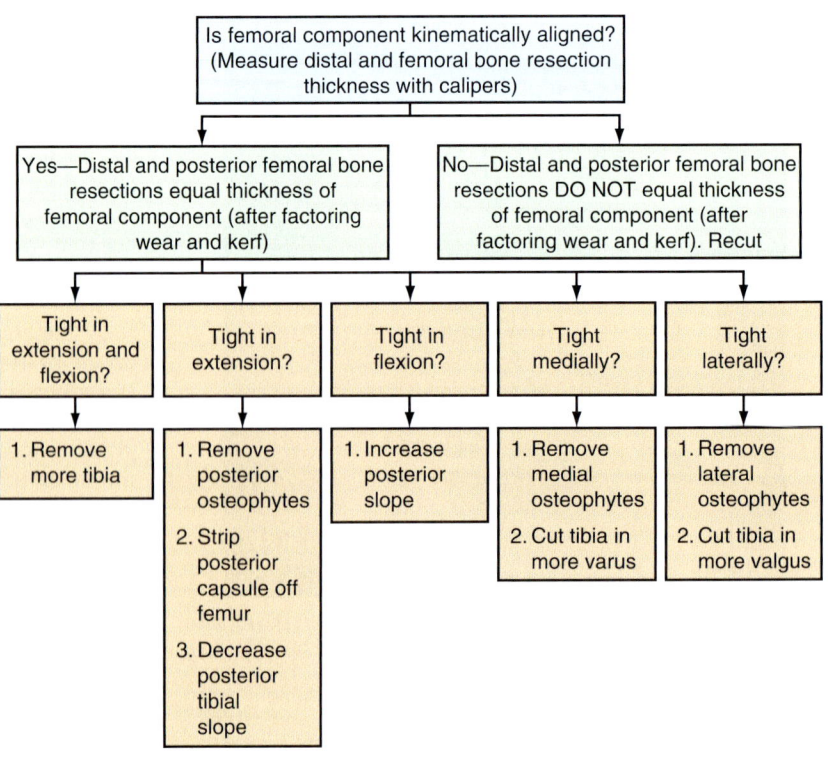

Figure 121-7. Algorithm for restoring motion and balancing the kinematically aligned TKA.

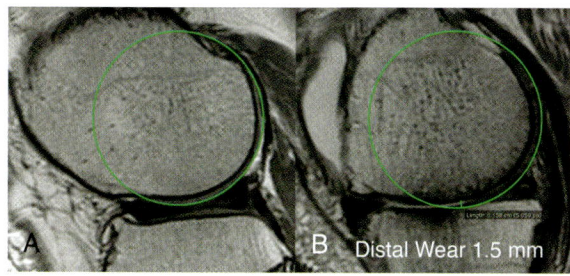

Figure 121-8. Illustration of a circle fit to the unworn lateral femoral condyle **(A)** and worn medial femoral condyle **(B)**. On the medial side, the wear on the distal medial femoral condyle measures 1.5 mm and there is no wear on the posterior medial femoral condyle. For an 8-mm-thick femoral condyle, the thickness of the distal medial resection should be 5 mm and the thickness of the posterior medial, distal lateral, and posterior lateral resection should be 6.5 mm. The femoral component is kinematically aligned when the thicknesses of each femoral resection are equal and equal to the thickness of the femoral component, after correcting for cartilage wear, bone wear, and saw blade kerf.

used to determine the location and amount of correction needed for the worn condyle.

In a varus osteoarthritic knee, which typically has 2 mm of distal and 1 mm of posterior cartilage wear, the distal medial resection should be 4.5 mm thick and the distal lateral resection should be 6.5 mm, which give a 2-degree correction in the coronal plane (Fig. 121-9). The posterior medial resection should be 5.5 mm thick and the posterior lateral resection should be 6.5 mm thick, which gives a 1-degree correction in the axial plane. If the planned and executed cuts do not match, fine adjustments in the varus-valgus, internal-external rotation, proximal-distal, and anterior-posterior positions of the femoral component should be made. Accounting for cartilage wear, bone wear, and saw blade kerf when selecting the distal and posterior cut planes is needed to correct coronal and axial malrotation. This is also needed to set the varus-valgus and internal-external rotation and flexion-extension, proximal-distal, anterior-posterior, and medial-lateral positions of the femoral component so that the femoral component is shape-matched to a restored articular surface. When a single-radius femoral component is used, shape-matching the femoral component to a restored articular surface on the femur coaligns the transverse axis of the femoral component with the primary transverse axis of the femur about which the tibia flexes and extends and kinematically aligns the knee.[16,17]

Once the femoral component is kinematically aligned, all subsequent steps to restore motion and balance the knee are limited to just four options—removing osteophytes, adjusting the plane of the tibial cut, releasing the posterior capsule from the femur, and medializing or lateralizing the tibial component. To determine which options are needed to restore motion and balance the knee, the knee is examined with trial components with the aim of deciding whether the knee fully flexes and extends and whether anterior-posterior and varus-valgus stability are acceptable at 30-degree intervals, from full extension to flexion. If the knee lacks extension and lacks flexion but has anterior-posterior and varus-valgus stability throughout the motion arc, then remove more tibia. If the knee lacks extension but fully flexes and has anterior-posterior and varus-valgus stability throughout the motion arc, then

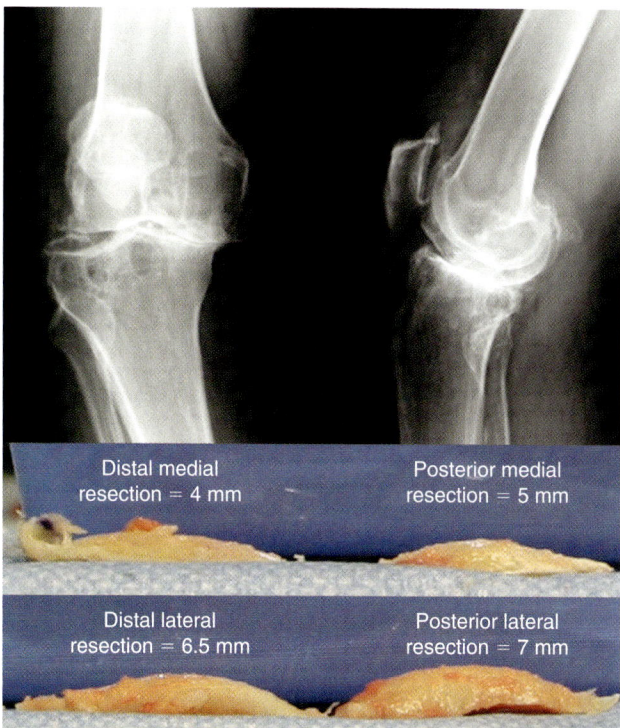

Figure 121-9. Illustration of a weight-bearing anteroposterior and lateral radiograph of a right knee with varus osteoarthritis *(top)* and the distal medial, posterior medial, distal lateral, and posterior lateral bone resections with their measured thickness in millimeters (mm; *bottom*). The distal medial resection is 4.5 mm thick and the distal lateral resection is 6.5 mm, which gives a 2-degree correction in the coronal plane. The posterior medial resection is 5 mm thick and the posterior lateral resection is 7 mm thick, which gives a 2-degree correction in the axial plane. To align an 8-mm-thick femoral component kinematically, each resection should be 6.5 mm thick after accounting for cartilage and bone wear and saw blade kerf, which is 1.25 to 1.5 mm thick, depending on the thickness of the saw blade.

remove posterior osteophytes and release the posterior capsule. If removal of the posterior osteophytes and releasing the posterior capsule are ineffective, decrease the posterior slope on the tibia.

We do not recommend additional resection of bone from the distal femur to restore extension unless the distal bone resection is 2 mm or more thinner than the posterior bone resection. The penalty from additional resection of bone from the distal femur is proximal movement of the femoral component, primary transverse axis of the femur, and joint line, which kinematically malaligns the knee and limits flexion.[24] If the knee lacks flexion but fully extends and has anterior-posterior and varus-valgus stability throughout the motion arc, then increase the posterior slope on the tibia. We have not found the need to recess or release the posterior cruciate ligament (PCL) to increase flexion. If the knee is tight medially throughout the motion arc, then remove all medial osteophytes. If the medial tightness persists after removing medial osteophytes from the tibia and femur, recut the tibia in 1 to 2 degrees more varus as long as the overall alignment of the limb will be acceptable. If the medial tightness persists after recutting, medialize the tibia on the tibial component and remove any bone from the tibia that extends beyond the tibial component[19] (Fig. 121-10). If the knee is tight laterally

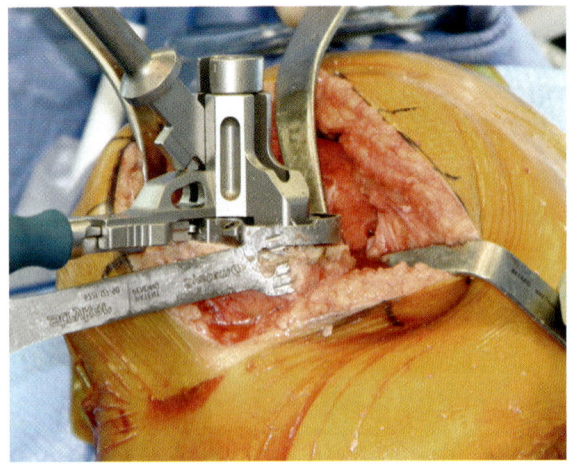

Figure 121-10. Intraoperative photograph of a right knee showing the tibia medialized on the trial base plate and a saw-trimming bone extending beyond the component to reduce medial tightness. The decision to medialize the tibia on the tibial component was made because of medial tightness that persisted after removing osteophytes from the medial femur and tibia, and after verifying that the plane of the varus-varus cut of the tibia was correct. This sequence of steps restores motion, stability, and alignment without releasing the medial collateral ligament in the knee with varus deformity caused by osteoarthritis.

throughout the motion arc, remove all lateral osteophytes. If the lateral tightness persists after removing lateral osteophytes from the tibia and femur, recut the tibia in 1 to 2 degrees more valgus as long as the overall alignment of the limb will be acceptable. If the PCL ligament is insufficient because of inadvertent release or incompetency and there is anterior-posterior and varus-valgus instability in 90 degrees of flexion but not in full extension, resect 2 mm of bone from the distal femur and use a 2-mm thicker liner. If the knee still has anterior-posterior and varus-valgus instability in 90 degrees of flexion, use a liner with an increased anterior slope or a posterior-stabilized component.

SURGICAL TECHNIQUES

Patient-Specific Cutting Guides

The range of motion and magnitude of varus-valgus deformity are assessed under anesthesia. A knee with a varus or valgus deformity is typically corrected by a thorough removal of medial or lateral femoral and tibial osteophytes, respectively.[16,25] A knee with a flexion contracture of 10 degrees or more is typically corrected by removal of posterior osteophytes and posterior capsule release from the femur; this rarely requires additional resection of bone from the femur.[24]

The operating room technician, circulating nurse, and surgeon should each cross-check the information etched on the patient-specific femoral and tibial cutting guides before anesthetizing the patient. Each guide has the name of the surgeon, patient initials and date of birth, component size, and an inscription of R or L, which indicates the side of the knee being operated on. The operating room technician and circulating nurse should also verify that they have sterilized the patient-specific cutting guides, correct subset of conventional instruments, and trial components that match the size determined by computer planning (Fig. 121-11). The use of

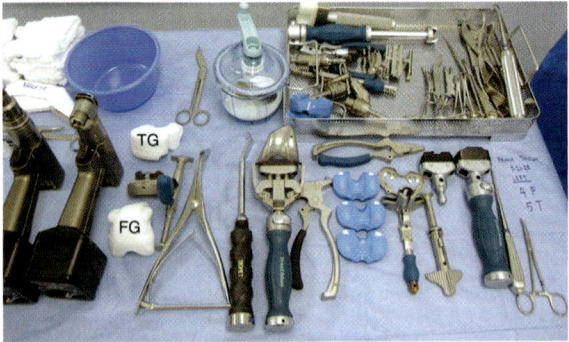

Figure 121-11. Photograph of the scrub table shows that one tray of instruments is needed to perform a kinematic TKA with patient-specific cutting guides. The patient-specific femoral guide (FG) and tibial guide (TG) are sterilized with the instruments and trial components that match the size of the components to be used, as determined by computer planning.

patient-specific cutting guides reduces the number of instrument trays from eight to one, which decreases operating time, room turnover time, and cost of processing instruments.[16]

A midvastus approach without patellar eversion gives an adequate exposure for using the patient-specific cutting guides. Fat is removed from the anterior surface of the femur proximal to the trochlear groove, as are any prominent osteophytes extending from the proximal trochlea. The patient-specific femoral guide is seated on the anterior cortex and trochlear groove, and centered mediolaterally on the distal femur (Fig. 121-12). The guide is secured with two articular and two anterior pins. The saw slot sets the varus-valgus, flexion-extension, and proximal-distal positions of the femoral component. The medial and the lateral distal pins are sequentially removed as the distal cut is made. Alternatively, the patient-specific femoral guide can be removed and the conventional distal femoral cutting guide can be placed over the two anterior pins, which allows visual assessment of the thickness of the distal resections before the cuts are made.

The thickness of each distal femoral resection is measured with a caliper. The symmetry between the distal resections is assessed using the stepwise algorithm and minor corrections are made when the symmetry is not correct. The chamfer guide from the conventional set of instruments that corresponds to the size of the femoral component determined by preoperative planning is inserted into the two articular pinholes. The chamfer guide sets the internal-external rotation, anterior-posterior, and medial-lateral positions of the femoral component. The two posterior femoral resections are made before the anterior and chamfer cuts, and the thickness of each resection is measured with calipers. The symmetry between the two posterior resections and between the two posterior and two distal resections is assessed using the algorithm, and minor corrections are made when the symmetry is not correct. An intramedullary alignment rod is not used because the wide variability in the longitudinal shape of the femur makes use of the center of the femoral head an unreliable landmark, and because referencing the center of the femoral head kinematically malaligns the knee.[10,11,15]

The tibia is exposed by preserving the insertion of the PCL and by removing both menisci. With the tibia dislocated anteromedially, the patient-specific tibial guide is seated on the articular surface and anteromedial cortex of the tibia. The

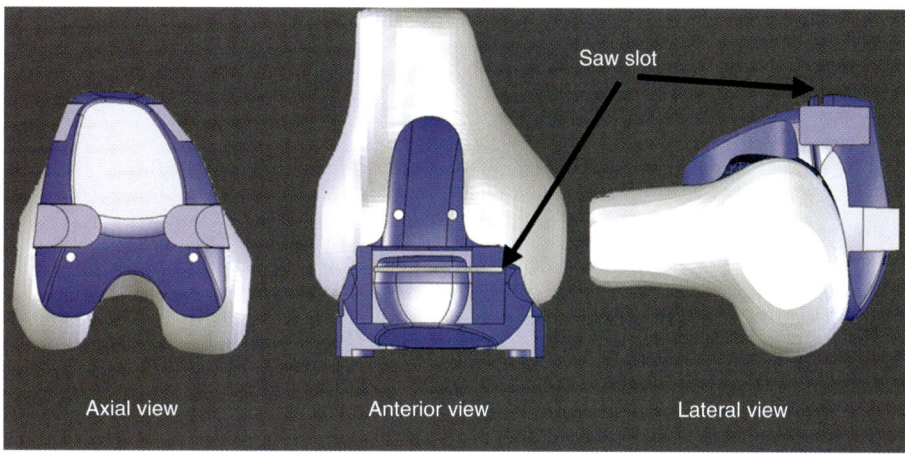

Figure 121-12. Illustration of the right knee showing axial, anterior, and lateral views of the patient-specific femoral guide on the normal knee model. The saw slot sets the varus-valgus, flexion-extension, and proximal-distal degrees of freedom of the femoral component. The axial view shows two articular pinholes through which pins are drilled to fix the femoral guide. After making the distal femoral resections, these two holes are used to position the conventional chamfer block, which sets the internal-external rotation, anterior-posterior, and medial-lateral positions of the femoral component. The anterior view shows two pinholes through which pins are drilled to fix the femoral guide. A conventional distal femoral cutting guide can be placed over these two pins to make the distal cut for the surgeon who wants to assess the thickness of each distal resection before making the cut.

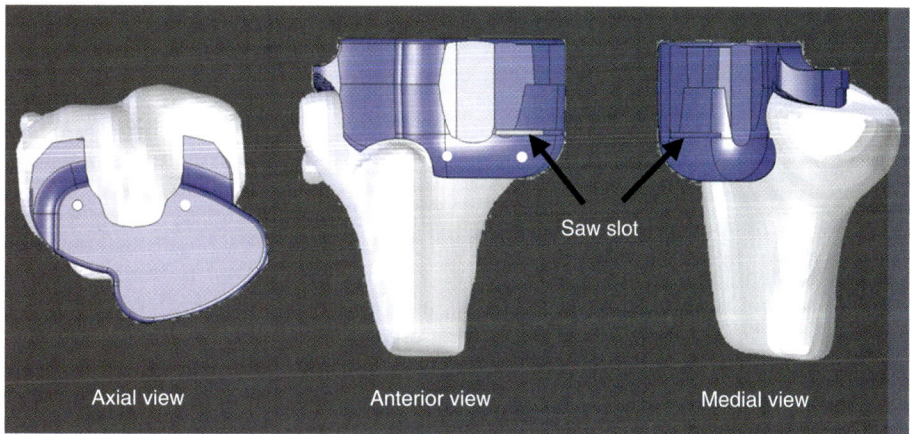

Figure 121-13. Illustration of a right knee showing axial, anterior, and medial views of the patient-specific tibial guide on the normal knee model. The saw slot sets the varus-valgus, flexion-extension, and proximal-distal position of the tibial component. The axial view shows two articular pinholes through which pins are drilled to fix the tibial guide. After making the tibial resection, these two holes are used to align the tibial positioning guide, which sets the internal-external rotation, anterior-posterior, and medial lateral positions of the tibial component. The anterior view shows two pinholes through which pins are drilled to fix the tibial guide. A conventional tibial cutting guide can be placed over these two pins for the surgeon who wants to assess the thickness and slope of the tibial resection before making the cut.

guide is secured with two articular and two anterior pins (Fig. 121-13). The medial and lateral articular pins are sequentially removed as the tibial cut is made. Alternatively, the patient-specific tibial guide can be removed and the conventional tibial guide can be placed over the two anterior pins to assess the thickness and slope of the tibial resection before making the cut. The medial-lateral thickness and anterior-posterior slope of the resected portion of the tibia are examined. The thickness of the worn side should be thinner than the unworn side by the amount of wear. After removing the resected portion of the tibia, the anterior-posterior slope of the proximal tibia should be neutral and conservative, which helps preserve the insertion of the PCL and tibial bone. A long-alignment rod is not used to check the varus-valgus

orientation of the tibial cut because the wide variability in the longitudinal shape of the tibia makes the use of the center of the ankle an unreliable landmark, and because referencing the center of the ankle kinematically malaligns the knee.[15]

The trial reduction is used to assess the range of motion and anterior-posterior and varus-valgus stability at 30-degree intervals, from full extension to flexion. Any loss of motion, instability, or tightness is noted and corrected using the algorithm. Correction of a flexion contracture rarely requires additional resection of distal femur as long as the sequence of removing posterior osteophytes, stripping the posterior capsule from the femur, and ensuring that the tibial cut is neutral and not sloped posteriorly is followed.[24] The sequence of complete removal of medial osteophytes, moving the tibia medially on the tibial component and removing more medial tibia,[22] and cutting the tibia in 1 to 2 degrees of varus corrects almost all knees with varus deformity and medial tightness without releasing the medial ligaments. The sequence of complete removal of lateral osteophytes (and, if necessary, then recutting the tibia in 1 to 2 degrees of valgus) corrects almost all knees with valgus deformity and lateral tightness without releasing the medial ligaments.[16] The step of ensuring that the tibial cut is neutral and not anteriorly sloped corrects most knees with loss of flexion.

The articular pinholes made by drilling through the tibial guide are used to set the internal-external rotation of the tibial component on the tibia. We prefer to use the articular pinholes to set internal-external rotation because of the following factors: (1) medial-lateral location of the tibial tubercle is an inconsistent landmark (ranges 32 to 47 mm from the medial tibia); (2) the range of movement or floating trial technique, which allows the tibial component to orient itself in the best position relative to the femoral component gives widely variable results; and (3) registration of anatomic landmarks with conventional and computer-assisted techniques is not repeatable.[18,23] The tibial template, corresponding to the size of the tibial component, is aligned with the articular pinholes. Small, 1- to 2-mm medial-lateral and anterior-posterior translation adjustments may be required to center the tibia on the tibial component. In the varus knee, moving the tibia medially on the tibial component and removing more medial tibia is effective for restoring coronal alignment and eliminating medial tightness.[22]

Unconventional Use of Conventional Instruments

In September 2009, the OtisMed patient-specific cutting guides became unavailable in the United States because of a U.S. Food and Drug Administration (FDA) classification issue. Accordingly, the senior author (SMH) developed a method to align the knee kinematically using a preoperative rotationally controlled MRI scan and using conventional total knee arthroplasty instruments unconventionally. We term this procedure *manual kinematic alignment* because the cut planes are selected and assessed manually without using patient-specific cutting guides.

Manual kinematic alignment requires preoperative planning to determine the location and amount of cartilage and bone wear on the femur. The thickness of each femoral bone resection is predicted by measuring the amount of cartilage and bone wear in millimeters from a nonorthogonal, oblique, sagittal MRI scan (see Fig. 121-8). A knee with end-stage varus osteoarthritis typically has 2 mm of distal wear and 1 mm of posterior wear confined to the medial femoral condyle; a knee with end-stage valgus osteoarthritis typically has 2 mm of distal wear and 2 mm of posterior wear confined to the lateral femoral condyle.

The surgical technique for manual kinematic alignment is the same as the surgical technique for kinematic alignment with patient-specific guides, regarding exposure, assessing and correcting motion, and addressing tightness and instability. The principle for kinematically aligning the femoral component is to remove the correct amount of bone and cartilage from the distal and posterior femur after accounting for wear and saw blade kerf, so that the total thickness of the missing and removed tissue matches the thickness of the femoral component. The location for the distal femoral cut is selected by manually positioning the conventional femoral guide on the distal surface of the femur, just posterior to the apex of the notch, without using an intramedullary rod (Fig. 121-14). The intramedullary rod is not used because it can kinematically malalign the femoral component because of the longitudinal shape of the femur being variable among subjects.[7]

The conventional femoral guide is placed flush on the unworn side and pinned, and then the guide is manually raised away from the worn side according to the thickness of the wear (typically, 2 mm) and pinned. The proximal-distal

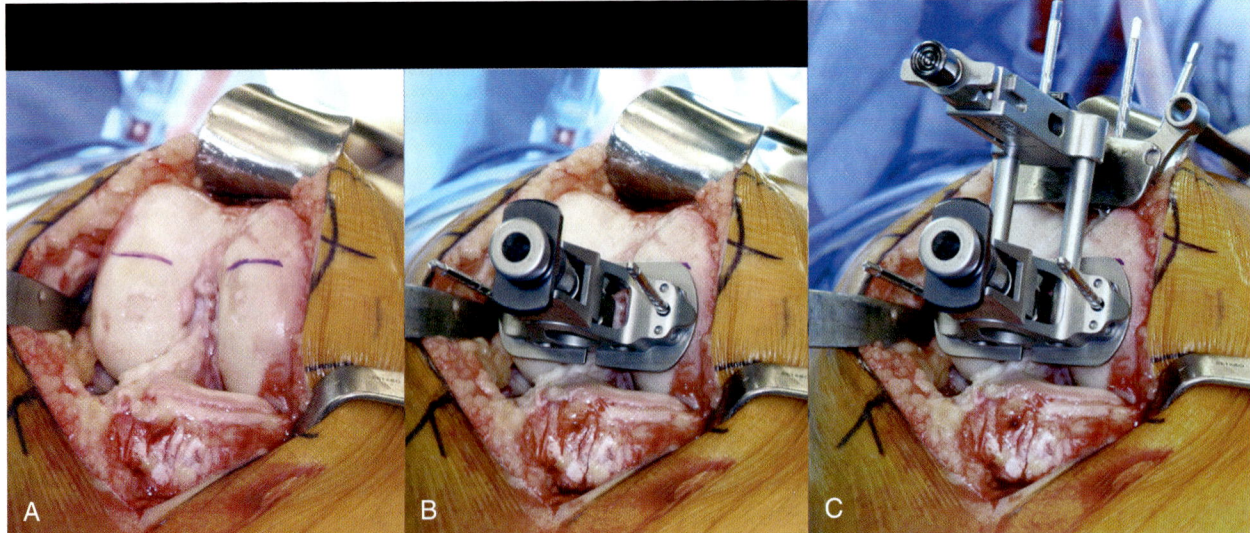

Figure 121-14. Photographs of a right knee showing the distal femur with the anterior boundary of the notch marked by blue lines **(A)**, the conventional distal femoral guide pinned to the femur posterior to the anterior boundary of the notch **(B)**, and the cutting guide attached to the conventional distal femoral guide **(C)**. The conventional femoral guide is placed flush on the unworn side and manually raised away from the worn side according to the thickness of the wear (typically, 2 mm) and pinned.

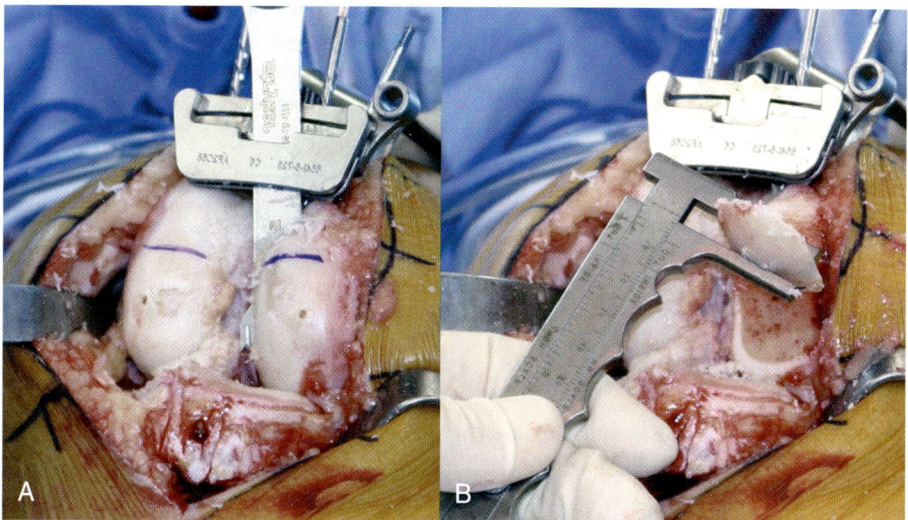

Figure 121-15. Photographs of a right knee showing the distal medial resection **(A)** and the caliper measurement of the thickness of the resection **(B)**. The thickness of each distal femoral resection should be 6.5 ± 1 mm thick after correcting for cartilage wear, bone wear, and saw blade kerf.

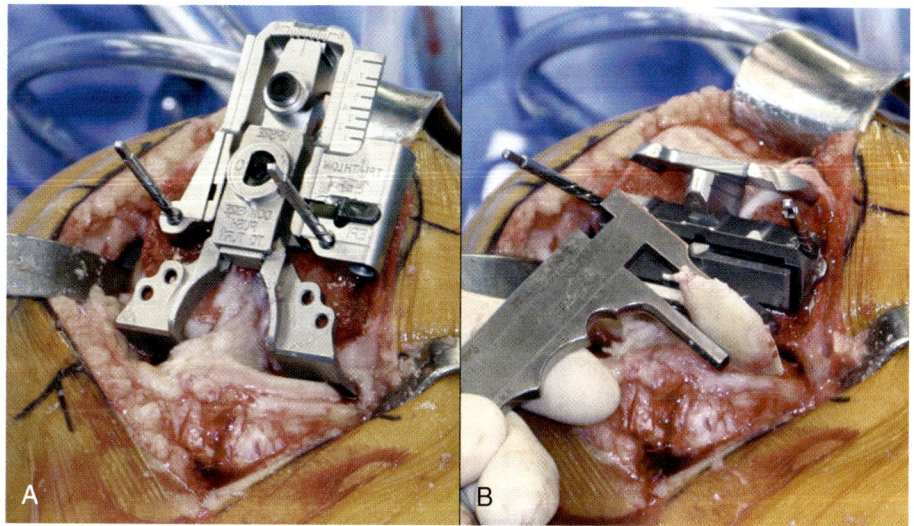

Figure 121-16. Photographs of a right knee showing the positioning of the conventional posterior referencing guide set at 0 degrees of rotation **(A)** and the caliper measurement of the posteromedial resection **(B)**. Each posterior femoral resection should be 6.5 ± 1 mm thick after correcting for cartilage wear, bone wear, and saw blade kerf. Small internal-external rotational adjustments can be made without compromising the fit of the femoral component if the posterior resections are made and measured before making the anterior and chamfer resections.

setting on the proximal extension of the conventional femoral guide is set to match the thickness of the femoral component and the cutting block portion is pinned to the anterior surface of the femur. The distal femoral resection is made, and each distal bone resection is measured with calipers (Fig. 121-15). The worn side should be 4 to 5 mm thick and the unworn side should be 6 to 7 mm thick when an 8-mm thick femoral component is used. A parallel cutting guide is used to adjust the thickness of the distal femoral cut when the difference between the predicted and actual thickness of each distal resection is 2 mm or more. The location for the posterior femoral cut is selected with the conventional posterior referencing guide set at neutral rotation. The conventional posterior referencing guide is placed flush on the

unworn side and pinned. The guide is then manually raised away from the worn condyle equal to the amount of wear (typically, 1 to 2 mm) and pinned (Fig. 121-16). The chamfer block matching the size of the best-fitting femoral component is placed in the pinholes. The posterior cuts are made before making the anterior and chamfer cuts, and each posterior resection is measured with calipers. The worn side should be 4 to 5 mm thick and the unworn side 6 to 7 mm thick. If the difference between the predicted and actual thickness of each distal resection is 2 mm or more, the internal-external rotation and anterior-posterior positions of the chamfer guide are adjusted to correct the posterior femoral cut.

The principle for kinematically aligning the tibial component is to set the tibial cut plane so that the worn side of the

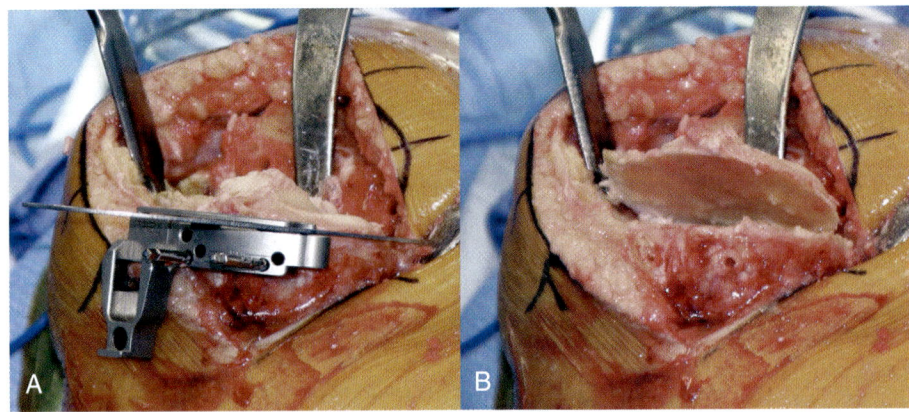

Figure 121-17. Photographs of a right knee showing the positioning of the conventional tibial cutting guide with an angel wing placed in the slot to assess the proximal-distal and anterior-posterior slopes of the tibial cut (**A**). The plane of the conventional tibial cutting guide is manually positioned so that the proximal-distal location of the tibial cut plane is conservative and the anterior-posterior slope of the tibial cut plane is neutral. The varus-valgus orientation of the tibial cut plane is adjusted until the worn side of the resected portion of the tibia is thinner than the unworn side by the amount of wear. **B**, The conservative tibial resection shows that more anterior bone is removed than posterior bone, which places the tibial component in neutral slope and preserves the insertion of the posterior cruciate ligament.

resected portion of the tibia is thinner than the unworn side by the amount of wear, and the anterior-posterior slope is neutral and conservative, which helps preserve the insertion of the posterior cruciate ligament. An angel wing is placed in the slot of the conventional tibial cutting guide (Fig. 121-17). The plane of the conventional tibial cutting guide is manually positioned so that the proximal-distal location of the tibial cut plane is conservative and the anterior-posterior slope of the tibial cut plane is neutral. One pin is placed in the conventional tibial cutting guide, which sets the proximal-distal and anterior-posterior slopes. The varus-valgus orientation of the tibial cut plane is adjusted by rotating the conventional tibial cutting guide until the worn side of the resected portion of the tibia is thinner than the unworn side by the amount of wear. The conventional tibial cutting guide is pinned to the tibia and the tibial cut is made. A long-alignment rod is not used to check the varus-valgus orientation of the tibial cut because the wide variability in the longitudinal shape of the tibia makes the use of the center of the ankle an unreliable landmark, and because referencing the center of the ankle kinematically malaligns the knee.[7] The alignment of the limb is visually inspected during the trial reduction and varus-valgus adjustments of the tibial resection are made if the limb appears malaligned.

THEORETICAL CONCERNS

One theoretical concern is whether the hip-knee-ankle axis of the kinematically aligned TKA is different from a TKA mechanically aligned with conventional and computer-assisted instrumentation. A source of this concern was a pilot study, in September 2006, of four knees treated with patient-specific cutting guides at the request of an implant company to evaluate the first-time use of their knee component before commercial release. The authors of this pilot study suggested that kinematically aligned knees were malaligned in the coronal plane.[20]

Although the primary goal of kinematic alignment is to restore knee kinematics and not to restore a neutral or 0-degree hip-knee-ankle axis, two other studies have shown

that kinematic alignment does not malalign the limb in the coronal plane, as suggested by Klatt and associates[20] in their study of four subjects.[16] One level III study, consisting of 21 subjects, found an average hip-knee-ankle axis of 1.2 degree varus,[25] which was closer to the 0-degree mechanical axis and had less fewer outliers outside the range of 0 ± 3 degrees than many previously reported results using conventional and computer-assisted techniques.[25] A second level III study, consisting of 48 subjects, found an average hip-knee-ankle axis of 1.4 degrees valgus, which is within the range of 0 ± 3 degrees. A level I prospective, double-blinded, randomized clinical trial is underway to further clarify the differences in limb alignment between the kinematically aligned knee with patient-specific cutting guides and mechanical alignment with conventional instruments.[8] However, on the basis of these level III studies, the hip-knee-ankle axis of the kinematically aligned TKA is similar to that of conventional and computer-assisted techniques.

Although there is a widely held opinion that a neutral hip-knee-ankle axis will result in better TKA survivorship, the mid- or long-term scientific support for this contention is surprisingly weak. Every study that has been considered evidence to support this contention is limited for various reasons. Six of seven published studies used short-leg radiographs, which cannot accurately assess the hip-knee-ankle axis.[15,27] In the one study that used long-leg radiographs, a rudimentary implant design consisted of a noncondylar roller and trough design that was implanted with primitive instrumentation (Denham Knee).[2,23a] A recent study of the survivorship of a modern implant design with better instrumentation in 395 knees has shown that factors other than the mechanical axis are more important for determining survivorship at 15 years, which suggests that the surgical goal of restoring a 0-degree hip-knee-ankle axis should be revisited. The study indicated that the group with a hip-knee-ankle axis outside the range of 0 ± 3 degrees, which consisted of 25% of the knees, had a threefold better survivorship at 15 years than the group with a hip-knee-ankle axis inside the range of 0 ± 3 degrees, which consisted of 75% of the knees, a finding that starkly contrasts with the study of the Denham

Knee.[2] The better survivorship of so-called outliers, with modern implant design and modern instrumentation, might be the result of better balancing of the knee and restoration of normal kinematics. Studies have shown that release of the collateral ligaments is not needed with kinematic alignment,[17,25] which may explain why kinematic alignment restores more normal contact kinematics than mechanical alignment, with the potential for better mid- and long-term survivorship.[13]

A second theoretical concern is whether the process of kinematic alignment that begins with performing MRI of the knee and ends with surgical implantation of the components consistently aligns the knee kinematically. There are many sources of error in the process, including the quality of the MRI image (i.e., proper biplanar alignment, high signal-to-noise ratio, no motion artifact), generation of the arthritic and normal knee models, shape fitting of the components, manufacturing the patient-specific cutting guides, and the surgeon using the guides in the operating room. Although some studies have shown that the process is reliable,[16,17,25] we believe that there is still a need to follow the algorithm intraoperatively to verify that the actual and predicted thickness of each bone resection is correct and, when necessary, to make adjustments in component position before cementing.

EARLY CLINICAL BENEFITS

As of December 2009, the clinical experience with kinematic alignment spanned 4 years and comprised 23,000 knees, which is sufficient to determine whether there are any early clinical benefits or failures associated with kinematic alignment. We have prospectively used a handheld computer (OrthoSight, Conshohocken, Pa; www.orthosight.com) to eliminate interviewer bias that patients self-administer to respond to a survey of queries consisting of custom questions, Oxford score, Short Form Health Survey (12 items; SF-12), and Knee Society score. Patients spend an average of 8 to 10 minutes preoperatively and postoperatively filling out the survey in the waiting room, which has improved our office efficiency. The handheld computer is used intraoperatively to record operative time, ligament releases, bone recuts, guide fit, and whether the implanted component matches the size of the planned component.[16,17]

The perioperative data suggest that kinematic alignment may lessen the surgical stress experienced by the patient, shorten the recovery time, and increase the rate of return to ADLs. The average operative duration of 53 minutes is less than the average reported operative times for conventional (73 minutes) and computer-assisted (90 minutes) approaches.[16,25,26] Currently, our average operative duration is 30 minutes with patient-specific cutting guides and 36 minutes with the unconventional use of conventional instruments. Transfusions are infrequent, which is attributed to not releasing collateral and retinacular soft tissue releases. Fat emboli have not occurred because intramedullary rods are not used with either kinematic alignment technique. The hospital stay of 2 nights is short, with 98% of patients discharged to home rather than to a rehabilitation facility. At 4 to 5 weeks postoperatively, 80% of patients walk without a cane, 54% drive a car, 88% notice that their knee functions better than before surgery, 94% judge the treated knee as normal or almost normal, and 98% judge the alignment of their limb as "just right." In terms of patient response to standardized questionnaires, by 4 to 5 weeks patients experience less pain than before surgery and show significant improvements in 11 of 12 activities evaluated by the Oxford score, SF-12 physical score, knee function score, and Knee Society score.[17] A level I prospective, double-blinded, randomized clinical trial is underway to clarify further the differences in early recovery between the kinematically aligned knee with patient-specific cutting guides and mechanical alignment with conventional instruments.[8]

SUMMARY

The primary goals of this chapter were to stimulate debate and advance the understanding of kinematic alignment of TKA. Kinematic alignment offers a much-needed alternative to mechanical alignment because mechanical alignment with conventional and computer-assisted techniques has a prevalence of patient dissatisfaction (20%) because of continued pain and poor function in ADLs. Kinematic alignment does not malalign the hip-knee-ankle axis. The early success of the kinematically aligned TKA (OtisKnee) has been recognized by the implant manufacturing industry. Most major implant manufacturers have since developed patient-specific cutting guides, but these guides align the limb mechanically and do not align the knee kinematically. As of the end of 2009, the available patient-specific cutting guides that mechanically align the limb are Signature (Biomet, Warsaw Ind), Visionaire (Smith & Nephew, Memphis, Tenn), Prophecy (Wright Medical Technology, Arlington, Tenn), and Tru-Match (DePuy Orthopaedics, Warsaw, Ind). We have recognized that there is a need for level I studies to clarify differences in limb alignment and early recovery between the kinematically aligned knee with patient-specific cutting guides and mechanical alignment with conventional and computer-assisted instruments, and we await the publication of the registered level I study that is currently underway.[8] We also want to emphasize that level I studies are also needed to determine whether patient-specific cutting guides that mechanically align the limb improve on the high prevalence of patient dissatisfaction with mechanically aligned TKAs implanted with conventional and computer-assisted instruments.

KEY REFERENCES

Alden KJ, Pagnano MW: Computer-assisted surgery: a wine before its time. Orthopedics 31:936–939, 2008.

Baker PN, van der Meulen JH, Lewsey J, Gregg PJ: The role of pain and function in determining patient satisfaction after total knee replacement. Data from the National Joint Registry for England and Wales. J Bone Joint Surg Br 89:893–900, 2007.

Coughlin KM, Incavo SJ, Churchill DL, Beynnon BD: Tibial axis and patellar position relative to the femoral epicondylar axis during squatting. J Arthroplasty 18:1048–1055, 2003.

Dossett GH: Total knee replacement study using standard cutting guide vs. Otismed MRI generated cutting guide, Phoenix, Ariz, 2010, Department of Veterans Affairs.

Eckhoff D, Hogan C, DiMatteo L, et al: Difference between the epicondylar and cylindrical axis of the knee. Clin Orthop Relat Res 461:238–244, 2007.

Eckhoff DG, Bach JM, Spitzer VM, et al: Three-dimensional mechanics, kinematics, and morphology of the knee viewed in virtual reality. J Bone Joint Surg Am 87(Suppl 2):71–80, 2005.

Hollister AM, Jatana S, Singh AK, et al: The axes of rotation of the knee. Clin Orthop Relat Res 290:259–268, 1993.

Howell SM, Hodapp EE, Kuznik K, Hull ML: In vivo adduction and reverse axial rotation (external) of the tibial component can be minimized. Orthopedics 32:319, 2009.

Howell SM, Howell SJ, Hull ML: Assessment of the radii of the medial and lateral femoral condyles in varus and valgus knees with osteoarthritis. J Bone Joint Surg Am 92:98–104, 2010.

Howell SM, Kuznik K, Hull ML, Siston RA: Results of an initial experience with custom-fit positioning total knee arthroplasty in a series of 48 patients. Orthopedics 31:857–863, 2008.

Howell SM, Kuznik K, Hull ML, Siston RA: Longitudinal shapes of the tibia and femur are unrelated and variable. Clin Orthop Relat Res 468:1142–1148, 2010.

Howell SM, Rogers SL: Method for quantifying patient expectations and early recovery after total knee arthroplasty. Orthopedics 32:884–890, 2009.

Matziolis G, Krocker D, Weiss U, et al: A prospective, randomized study of computer-assisted and conventional total knee arthroplasty. Three-dimensional evaluation of implant alignment and rotation. J Bone Joint Surg Am 89:236–243, 2007.

Smith C, Chen J, Howell SM, Hull ML: An in vivo study of the effect of distal femoral resection on passive knee extension. J Arthroplasty 25:1137–1142, 2010.

Spencer BA, Mont MA, McGrath MS, et al: Initial experience with custom-fit total knee replacement: intra-operative events and long-leg coronal alignment. Int Orthop 33:1571–1575, 2009.

Full references for this chapter can be found on www.expertconsult.com.

Chapter 122

Robotics in Total Knee Arthroplasty

Sabine Mai, Werner E. Siebert, and Peter F. Heeckt

Degenerative joint disease of the knee is treated with total knee arthroplasty (TKA) after conservative therapy options have been exhausted. However, despite conscientious planning and carefully performed procedures, surgeons are often unsatisfied with implant alignment. Various studies have described significant axial or rotational malalignment, and mediolateral and ventrodorsal tilt.[2,3,15,26] Seemingly small displacements of 2.5 mm potentially alter the range of motion by as much as 20 degrees.[8] None of the contemporary improvements in implant design and instrumentation have alleviated these problems.

To improve precision in surgery, robotic systems were developed. Robots are able to position and move tools accurately, thereby reducing human error. These systems rely on preoperative imaging, registration, and planning. The first clinical use was reported in 1985 in the field of neurosurgery.[16] In 1992, orthopedic surgeons started using robot systems for total hip arthroplasty.[4] The active surgical robot CASPAR (*c*omputer-*a*ssisted *s*urgical *p*lanning *a*nd *r*obotics) was initially adapted for total hip arthroplasty and for anterior cruciate ligament repair.[20] Later it was developed for total knee arthroplasty. The first robot-assisted knee replacement with this system was performed in March 2000 at the Kassel Orthopedic Hospital (Kassel, Germany). A total of 108 consecutive procedures were performed at this institution and followed up for at least 5 years in a prospective study.[25]

SURGICAL TECHNIQUE

Robot-assisted TKA consists of the placement of fiducial markers, computed tomography (CT) scanning, preoperative planning, and surgery.

Placement of Fiducial Markers

To facilitate orientation, the robot requires placement of femoral and tibial pins that serve as fiducial markers for each bone (Fig. 122-1). The robot uses these pins for spatial orientation and performs geometric calculations based on their location.

Computed Tomography Scanning and Preoperative Planning

After the pins have been placed, a helical CT scan is obtained. Particular attention is paid to the areas of the femoral head, pins, knee, and ankle. The CT data are then transferred into the computer-based planning station. The technical quality of the scan is automatically checked and the pin position is verified. The surgeon identifies specific anatomic landmarks. The anatomic and mechanical axes of the femur and tibia are then calculated in the frontal and sagittal planes. The joint line, epicondylar twist, torsion of the tibia, and relationship

of the dorsal part of the tibia and condylar line serve as additional important parameters.

The system allows the user to select and position a specific implant in different sizes. With computer-assisted planning, the strong interdependence of all parameters, including the mechanical axes, becomes evident. Implant fit can be accurately assessed by scrolling through the scan. Unintentional notching can easily be avoided. All angles and possible geometric translations are displayed on the video screen during the planning procedure (Fig. 122-2). The system informs the user about the expected change in extension and flexion gaps and the resulting ligament tension. After positioning the implants, the milling areas are specified in order to protect the surrounding soft tissue. As a last step, the system prints out an overview of the final plan. All data are stored on a PC card and transferred to the robot control unit before surgery.

Robot-Assisted Surgery

A conventional median incision with parapatellar approach to the knee joint is used. The knee joint is secured by a transfemoral and transtibial self-cutting screw to a specially designed frame. This rigid frame is also used for fixation of self-holding soft tissue retractors. To control for unwanted micromovements of the leg during robotic surgery, rigid bodies with light-emitting diodes (LEDs) are firmly attached to the frame. The LED signal is constantly monitored by an infrared camera system, which will automatically shut off the robot in the event of excessive motion (Fig. 122-3). After registration of the fiducial markers, robotic milling is started by the surgeon. The cutting tool is equipped with internal water cooling and irrigation. A splash guard helps keep the operative field and LEDs dry and clean (Fig. 122-4). Milling heads are changed during the procedure, depending on the type of cut to be made. Varying with the size of the implant and bone density, the entire milling procedure takes approximately 18 minutes. If required, it is possible to revert to conventional manual technique at any point during surgery.

The resulting bone surfaces are accurately shaped and smooth (Fig. 122-5). After the fixation frame and pins are removed, soft tissues are balanced and the components of the implant are inserted. In this study, we started with the cemented LC Search Evolution knee system (Aesculap, Tuttlingen, Germany) in the robotic group because this was the first knee implant system geometry that was loaded into the planning software.

Patients and Methods

A total of 108 knees were operated using the CASPAR robot system. The following cruciate-retaining implant designs were used: 70 Search Evolution (Aesculap), 31 PFC Sigma (DePuy Orthopaedics, Warsaw, Ind), and 7 Genesis (Smith

& Nephew, Andover, Mass). Of these, 55 were implanted with both components being cemented (Figs. 122-6 and 122-7), 46 implants were hybrids (tibia cemented, femur cementless), and 7 were completely cementless (Fig. 122-8). The average age of the patients (74 women, 34 men) was 66 years (range, 37 to 87 years). Patients were clinically evaluated before and after surgery according to their Knee Society score.[12] All patients were followed up at intervals of 3, 6, 12, 24, and 60 months after surgery. No patients were lost to follow-up.

Before and 2 weeks after surgery, standing long-leg anteroposterior roentgenograms were taken of all patients to control for correct alignment. The mechanical leg axis was measured on these films and directly compared with the preoperative plan.

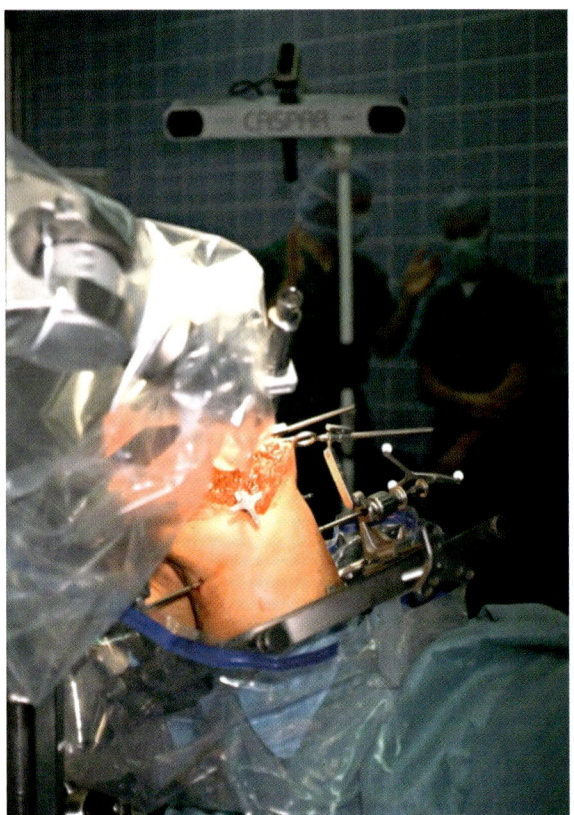

Figure 122-3. View of the working robot. Unwanted motion is detected by an infrared camera system, as seen in the background, and corresponding rigid bodies fixed to the frame, as seen in the foreground.

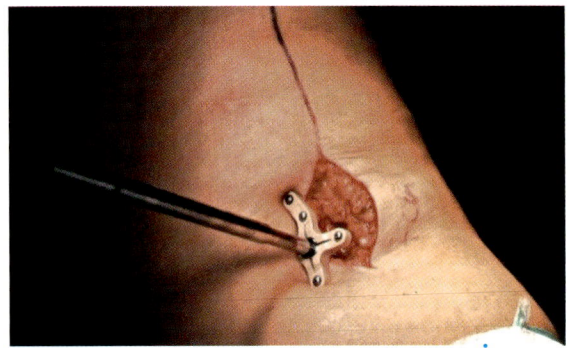

Figure 122-1. Fastening of the special CT cross on the tibial pin.

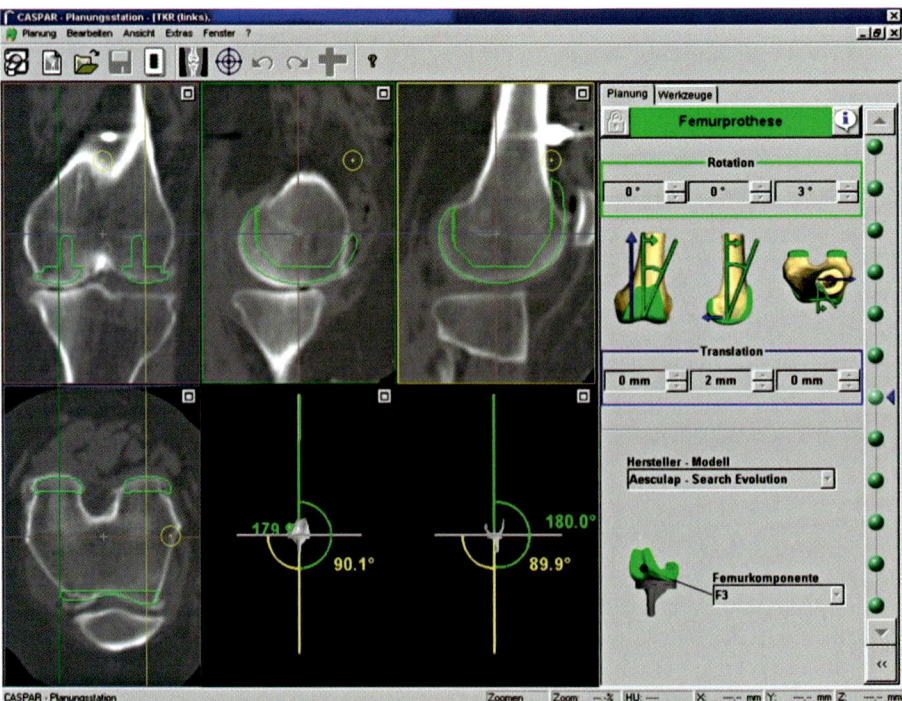

Figure 122-2. Original screen shot from the planning station showing the PC-based planning of the femoral component and the resulting mechanical leg axis.

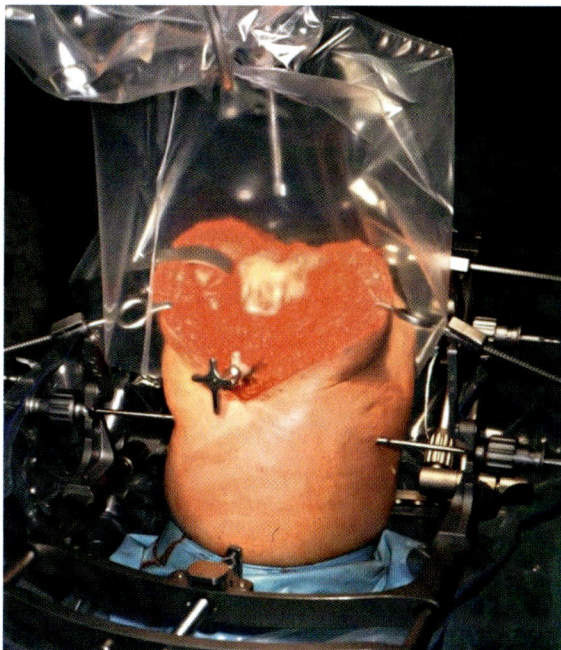

Figure 122-4. Knee securely fixed with cutting tool and splash guard in place just before femoral milling action commences. The tibial registration cross is still in place at the distal end of the incision.

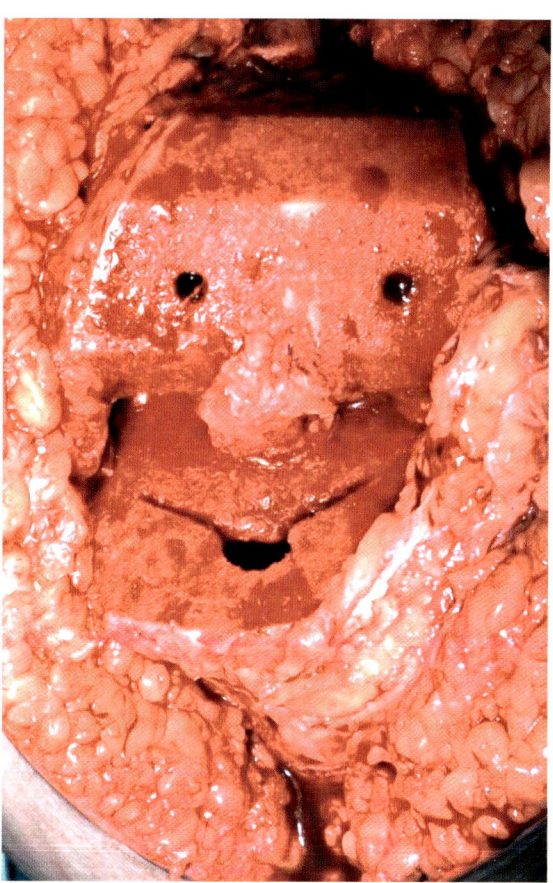

Figure 122-5. Final tibial and femoral bone surfaces with preserved posterior cruciate ligament.

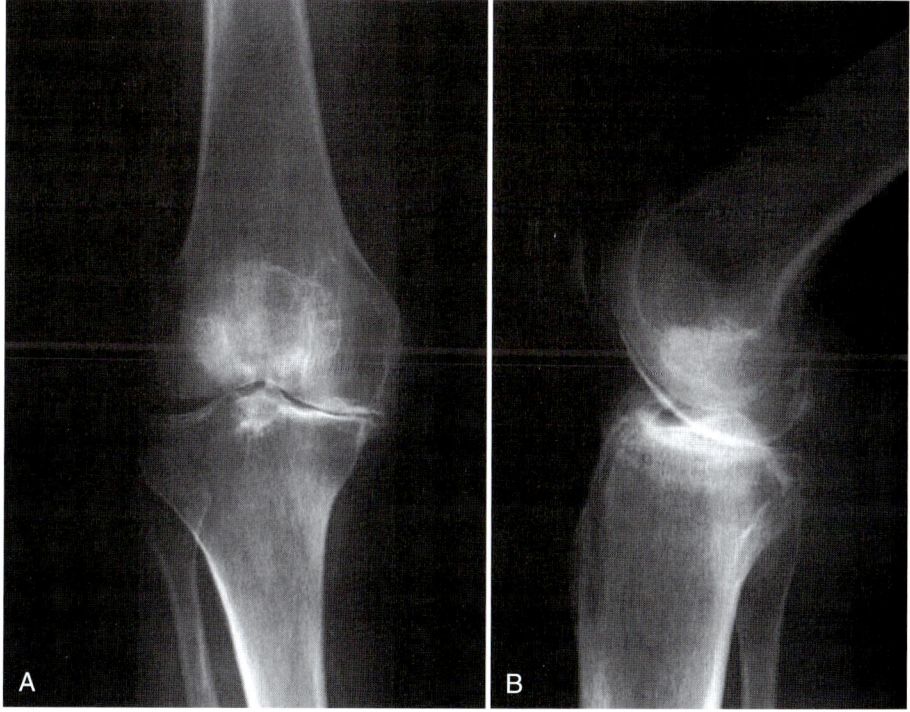

Figure 122-6. Anteroposterior **(A)** and lateral **(B)** x-rays of a patient with medial gonarthrosis before robotic TKA.

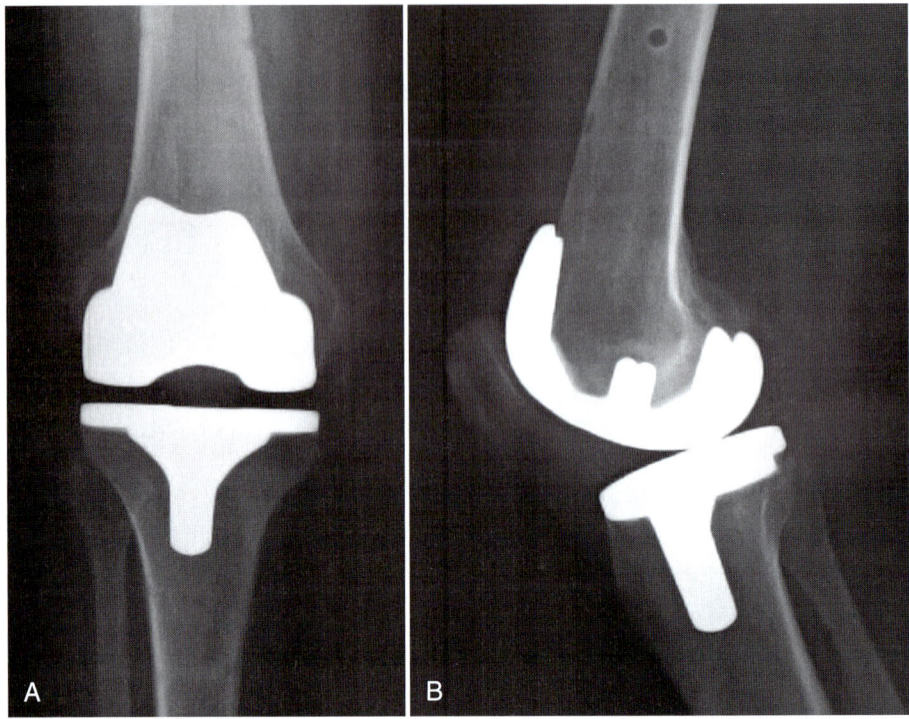

Figure 122-7. Anteroposterior **(A)** and lateral **(B)** x-rays of the same patient after robotic TKA. (Courtesy Search Evolutioner, Aesculap, Tuttlingen, Germany.)

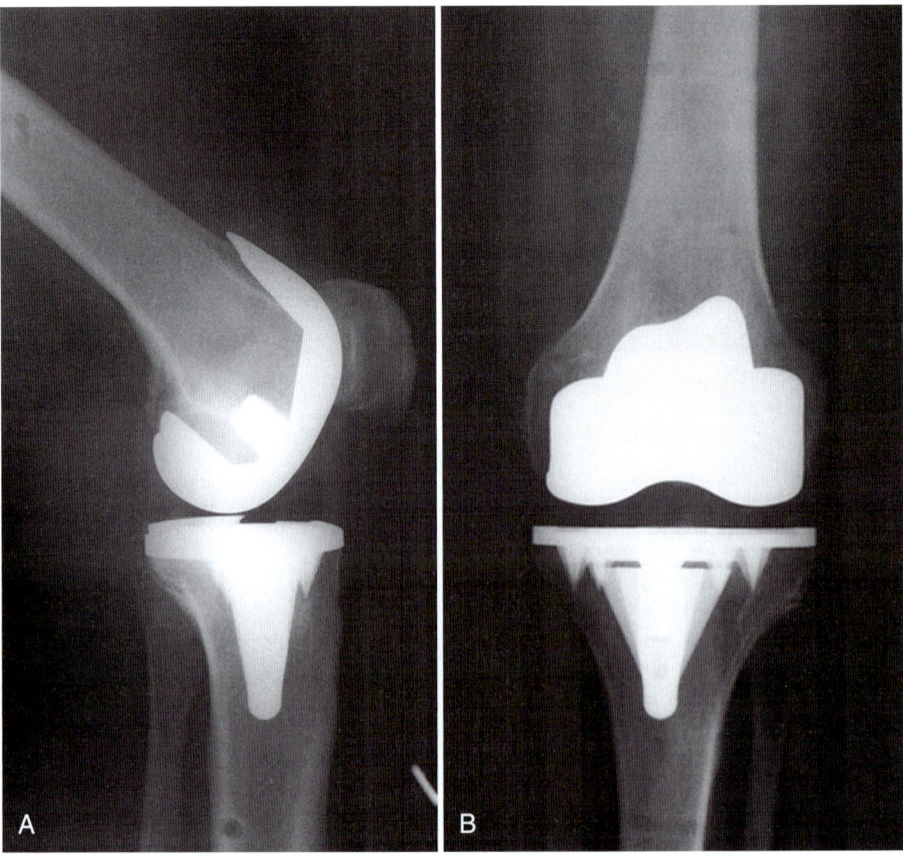

Figure 122-8. Anteroposterior **(A)** and lateral **(B)** x-rays of the same patient after robotic TKA (Genesis).

Data were statistically analyzed by using a two-tailed Student's t-test. Statistical significance was assumed at a P value less than 0.01.

RESULTS

General Observations and Complications

Operating time for the 108 robotic cases averaged 137 minutes (range, 80 to 200 minutes). At discharge, all patients had 90 degrees or more of flexion. No major adverse events directly related to the CASPAR System have been noted.

A minor complication occurred in one patient. Because of a defective registration marker, the femoral milling process could not be completed as planned. Full correction was achieved by converting to manual technique. Three patients had superficial infections at one of the sites at which the fiducial marker pins had been fixed to the bone. All infections resolved under conservative management.

Postoperative Tibiofemoral Alignment

In the computerized preoperative planning procedure, the mechanical axis was routinely corrected to a tibiofemoral angle of 0 degrees. The overall mean difference between preoperative plan and postoperative result for tibiofemoral alignment was 0.8 degrees, with a standard deviation of 1.0 degrees and a range of 0 to 3 degrees. Also, the joint lines in relation to the position of the femoral and tibial components were in good alignment. In 2004, Decking and colleagues[5] proved with postoperative CT scans the accuracy of this system in all planes—frontal, sagittal, and transverse. The mean tibiofemoral angle in a comparable manual group (NexGen CR Prosthesis, Zimmer, Warsaw, Ind) was 2.6 degrees, with a standard deviation of 2.2 degrees and a range of 0 to 7 degrees. In this study, 18 patients (35%) had a deviation of more than 3 degrees, with a maximum of 7 degrees. The exact distribution of varus and valgus deviations of the

mechanical axis is shown in Figure 122-9. The difference in tibiofemoral alignment was highly significant (P < .0001).

Knee Society Score

The Knee Society score is divided into the knee score and function score. The patient can achieve a maximum of 100 points in each category. We have found that the difference between the preoperative and postoperative scores is significant (Fig. 122-10). Unfortunately, comorbidities and increasing age influence the outcome so that for these patients, the full score declines and they continue to lose functional capabilities, as noted in the scores at 24 and 60 months postoperatively (Fig. 122-11).

CONCLUSIONS

Various experimental active and semiactive robotic systems have been developed to improve the accuracy of implant alignment.[10] To our knowledge, this is the only clinical report

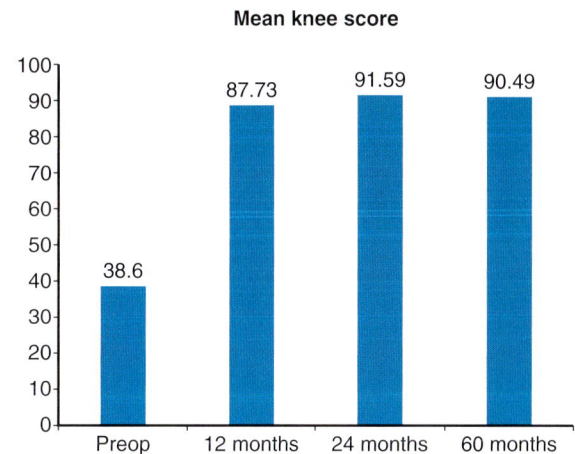

Figure 122-10. Comparison of knee scores preoperatively and 60 months postoperatively is highly significant in robot-assisted TKA.

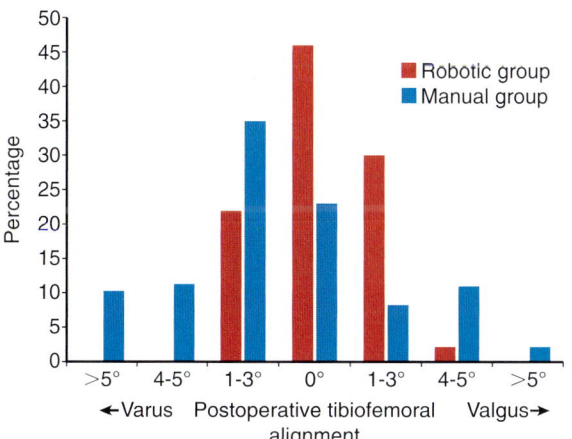

Figure 122-9. Postoperative tibiofemoral angles of patients after manual and robotic TKAs. Measured values show a much broader variation of varus or valgus angles after manual TKA compared with robotic technique (P < .0001).

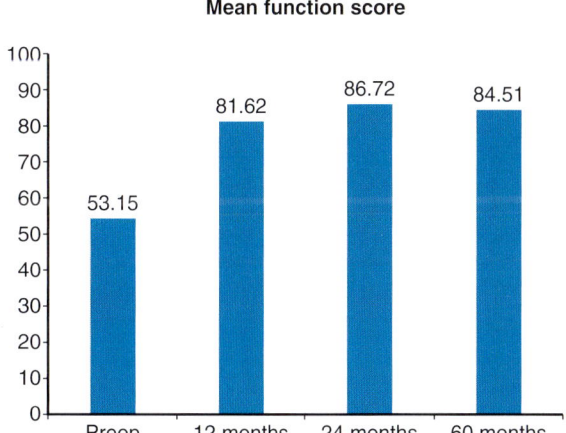

Figure 122-11. Comparison of Knee Society function scores preoperatively and 60 months postoperatively is highly significant in robot-assisted TKA. Declination between 24 and 60 months because of old age.

Box 122-1 Advantages of Robot-Assisted Surgery

- Exact preoperative planning and transfer to the robot
- High precision and safey
- Better mechanical axis
- Reduced bone loss
- Exact milling process
- Precision of implantation less dependent on experience and skill of surgeon

Box 122-2 Disadvantages of Robot-Assisted Surgery

- Additional cost
- Increased planning time
- Longer operation time
- Soft tissue balancing dependent on experience of surgeon
- Additional pins required
- Rigid leg fixation
- Additional CT scans needed

of robotic TKA in a large series of consecutive patients with a 5-year follow-up.

Our results clearly demonstrate that after a short learning period, the active system allows the surgeon to execute the preoperative plan precisely, with a mean error less than 1 degree, and achieve satisfactory to very good results regarding tibiofemoral alignment in over 95% of cases compared with approximately 65% with manual technique. Aglietti and coworkers[3] have reported that most conventionally operated patients end up with a mean valgus angle of 9.6 degrees (range, 2 to 16 degrees). Correct tibiofemoral alignment seems to be particularly important, because it is generally agreed that axial deviation and imprecise implantation may lead to early loosening of implant components.[6,7,17,23] An axial deviation of more than 3 degrees, or Maquet's line not passing through the middle third of the implant, is considered the most frequent cause of early TKA failure.[9,11,13,22] The results of alignment after robotic TKA are not only superior to the results with conventional technique, but also to the results of computer-assisted navigated TKA. Miehlke and colleagues[18] have found that 63% of patients have an acceptable tibiofemoral alignment within the 2-degree varus-valgus range after navigated TKA. More than 4 degrees of deviation, with a maximum error of 7 degrees, was observed in almost 7% of the navigated patients. This indicates that although computer-assisted navigation yields superior results to manual technique, it is still inferior to robotic technique regarding orientation of the prosthetic components.

In contrast to the CASPAR system, navigation systems for TKA still depend on intramedullary and extramedullary guides, which might be an important cause of potential errors in axial alignment.[19] Another benefit of the robotic technique might be the accurate planning of the milling track and type of cutting used. This should result in a reduced risk for injury of ligaments, vessels, and nerves, which are undoubtedly endangered by manually directed oscillating saws. For example, the osseous insertion of the posterior cruciate ligament can always be preserved. Implants fit more exactly because the milled surfaces are always precisely flat, a matter of particular importance when cementless systems are used. Finally, the amount of removed bony substance can be minimized, which could facilitate later revision surgery.

There are certain advantages and disadvantages in robot assisted surgery (Boxes 122-1 and 122-2). Robotic systems hold great promise in assisting surgeons to perform difficult procedures with a high degree of accuracy and repeatability. Preoperative plans can reliably be translated into clinical reality with the help of a robotic device. The CASPAR system fulfilled these requirements, but also had major drawbacks, such as added costs, need for additional surgery and

CT imaging, and increased time for preoperative planning and surgery. Being a modified industrial robot—that is, used for computer chip production in a clean room environment—the CASPAR system represents a cumbersome piece of capital equipment, which for many hospitals is difficult to purchase and maintain. Despite excellent clinical results, in particular in the area of knee arthroplasty, the CASPAR robot did not become a commercial success and the manufacturer stopped production and sales in 2001. Other robotic systems are currently being clinically investigated. Passive robotic systems that leave more control to the surgeon but limit the surgeon's path and range of milling and cutting seem to be ideal candidates for future clinical use, especially when combined with real-time computer navigation.[1,14,24]

KEY REFERENCES

Aglietti P, Buzzi R, Gaudenzi A: Patellofemoral functional results and complications with the posterior stabilized total condylar knee prosthesis. J Arthroplasty 3:17, 1988.

Decking J, Theis C, Achenbach T, et al: Robotic total knee arthroplasty: the accuracy of CT-based component placement. Acta Orthop Sand 75:573, 2004.

Ecker ML, Lotke PA, Sindsor RE, Cella JP: Long-term results after total condylar knee arthroplasty. Significance of radiolucent lines. Clin Orthop Relat Res 216:151, 1987.

Feng EL, Stuhlberg SD, Wixon RL: Progressive subluxation and polyethylene wear in total knee replacements with flat articular surfaces. Clin Orthop Relat Res 299:60, 1994.

Garg A, Walker PS: Prediction of total knee motion using a three-dimensional computer graphics model. J Biochem 23:45, 1990.

Howe RD, Matsuoka Y: Robotics for surgery. Annu Rev Biomed Eng 1:211, 1999.

Insall JN, Binzzir R, Soudry M, Mestriner LA: Total knee arthroplasty. Clin Orthop Relat Res 192:13, 1985.

Insall JN, Dorr LD, Scott R, Scott WN: Rationale of the knee society clinical rating system. Clin Orthop Relat Res 248:13, 1989.

Jakopec M, Harris SJ, Rodriguez Y, Baena F, et al: The first clinical application of a "hands-on" robotic knee surgery system. Comput Aided Surg 6:329, 2001.

Jeffery RS, Morris RW, Denham RA: Coronal alignment after total knee replacement J Bone Joint Surg Br 73:709, 1991.

Miehlke RK, Clemens U, Kershally S: Computer-integrated instrumentation in knee arthroplasty—a comparative study of conventional and computerized technique. Presented at the Fourth Annual North American Program on Computer Assisted Orthopaedic Surgery, Pittsburgh, Pa, June 15-17, 2000.

Nuño-Siebrecht N, Tanzer M, Bobyn JD: Potential errors in axial alignment using intramedullary instrumentation for total knee arthroplasty. J Arthroplasty 15:228, 2000.

Ranawat CS, Adjei OB: Survivorship analysis and results of total condylar knee arthroplasty. Clin Orthop Relat Res 323:168, 1988.

Siebert W, Mai S, Kober R, Heeckt PF: Technique and first clinical results of robot-assisted total knee replacement Knee 9:173, 2002.

Tew M, Waugh W: Tibiofemoral alignment and the results of knee replacement. J Bone Joint Surg Br 67:551, 1985.

Full references for this chapter can be found on www.expertconsult.com.

Computer-Assisted Navigation: Minimally Invasive Surgery for Total Knee Replacement

David R. Lionberger

Much of the hesitation in using minimally invasive surgery (MIS) in total knee replacement (TKR) evolves from coping with the complexities of a smaller incision without visual cues. When using a constrained exposure, reliance on instruments rather than direct visual reference is paramount. Second, sequencing to augment exposure becomes important to afford better access. If one adds deformity or increased body mass to the equation the traditional visual references, angular and translational position is compromised. Such dependence on traditional instruments, which rely on some degree of visually estimating cuts, may result in less dependable accuracy.[3-5,10,12,16]

Computer-assisted surgery (CAS), also known as surgical navigation, becomes necessary to reclaim lost visual reference and confirm accuracy lost in MIS exposure.[17] If the surgeon avoids the use of small incisions because of lost accuracy, the addition of CAS can allay concerns about this deficiency. Although doubt still exists in regard to the efficacy of CAS to improve performances, this accuracy ensures the surgeon that the extra step of precision has been taken.* The confidence gained in achieving accuracy with documentation easily overcomes any reticence of a short learning curve in adoption of this technology.

However, there are other factors in addition to the time required to learn the systems. Lack of confidence in believing what the instruments are reading can hinder surgical progress.[15] Although some readings are often not realistic or believable, the computer is usually smarter than the surgeon. Once reliance and confidence in CAS have been achieved, less time is spent using traditional instruments to confirm readings and more rapid surgery can be performed.

I have used every system on the market in an effort to provide a global review of the advantages and disadvantages of all systems discussed in this chapter. This will be based on the latest available software and not what is under development. The system that might be most efficacious in an institution is dependent on factors such as TKR systems, incision size, preference in operating room configuration, and data desired be used on the CAS monitor. Just by reading this chapter identifies you as a surgeon willing to consider using technology to afford a better result, and for that there is no wrong answer.

CHOICES IN SYSTEMS

Infrared Computer-Assisted Surgery

Infrared (IR) CAS not only holds the competitive edge for acceptance, it also represents the bulk of available products available worldwide. In terms of signal strength and stability,

---

*References 1, 2, 6, 8, 11, 13, and 14.

IR CAS is clearly the most advantageous. These advantages include an abundance of proprietary choices, software versatility for multiple TKR systems, and ease of use.

Tracker Mounting Options

With the exception of one system (Aesculap, Center Valley, Pa), all now have gone to a dual- or multiple-pin fixation format positioned out of the incision opposite the surgeon's side. Pins are placed at dedicated distances so that they will accommodate the tracker mounting block. Only one system (Stryker Orthopaedics, Mahwah, NJ) has the provision for a third pin to be inserted divergently or nonparallel. For most systems, parallel is the norm, using $\frac{1}{8}$-inch self-drilling or self-tapping threaded pins in varied lengths.

The surgeon's preferences of the operative side is the usual mandate for where to place the reflective tracker array. Whether using active or passive reflections, transmissions require constant visual reference to CAS data or the transmitter tower while working. Therefore, if the surgeon operates from the opposite side, as is my preference (stands on the left of the patient for a right TKR), trackers should face to the right of the patient. The other option is to face the trackers over the shoulder of the surgeon, which creates the dilemma of constantly dodging the receiver tower. Although trackers are traditionally inserted on the lateral tibia and femur, my preference is to insert the tracker array on the medial tibia and distal femur to view the CAS screen from the opposite side. This limits the choice of systems or may mandate modification in the system's software for side prioritization and CAS programming.

Lateral Monitor and Medial Pin Insertion Option

The tibia insertion point is best started at or approximately 4 cm below the tibial tubercle to avoid cutting jig interference and remain free of the incision access. The pins are inserted with the first pin bicortically applied at a 45- to 60-degree angle off the anterior crest of the anteroposterior (AP) plane of the tibia and the second pin rotated sufficiently to allow just enough room for the tracker array to clear the drapes and the crest of the tibia (Fig. 123-1). Some tracker pin blocks allow multiaxial rotation, so the exact rotation may not be necessary. However, fixed tracker blocks require some attention to rotation and elevation.

The femoral tracker may be applied intraincisionally by first installing the distal pin 2 cm above the medial epicondyle at a 10- to 20-degree angle off the midsaggital plane. This first pin is the best bicortical pin fixation and therefore is the first inserted—plus, it uses two single cortical screws, not pins. Pins are inserted at 45-degree knee flexion so as to minimize tethering forces from the vastus medialis and skin edges. This first pin should also capture a supracondylar ridge of bone above the lateral epicondyle on the lateral femur. The second pin can be applied by single cortical or bicortical

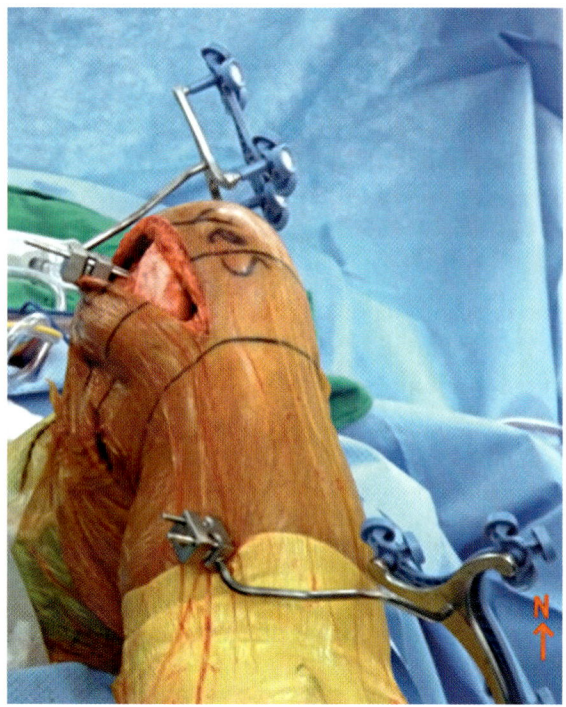

Figure 123-1. IR trackers in place for a left medial approach, with surgeon positioned to right of patient. Note the dorsal fin configuration for best reception in any leg position.

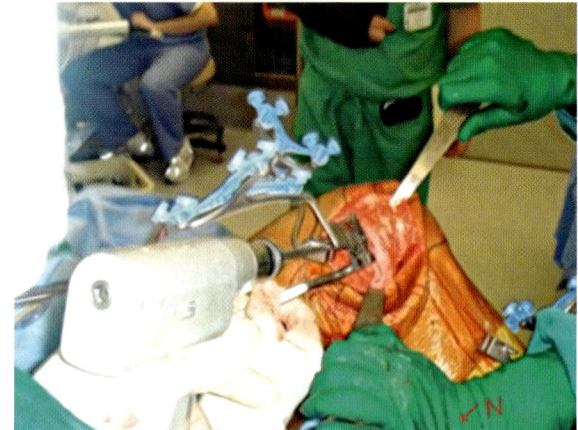

Figure 123-2. Freehand navigation of distal femoral cut. The drill acts as a stabilizer for less drastic fine tuning of varus-valgus flexion-extension.

penetration. If the first pin is firm, the need for bicortical fixation is not so important. However, if the patient is osteoporotic or there is a suspicion of less firm fixation on the distal pin, the stabilization is achieved through the second pin and bicortical fixation is imperative. Care must be taken to allow for optional exposure to prevent the vastus medialis oblique (VMO) and skin flaps from deforming the pins, which would cause aberrant values from the CAS system. If tethering occurs, such as in muscular males, one must extend the incision or readings will be in error because of pin deflection in flexion.

Medial Monitor and Lateral Pin Option

Some systems (e.g., ORTHOsoft, Zimmer, Warsaw, Ind), have no provisions for medial mounting of the tracker arrays and therefore the surgeon is compelled to affix them to the lateral side. Although tibial pins are not generally a problem, the femoral side can be a potential source of vascular injury. The femoral vessels coursing into the adductor canal have not reached the posterior position on the lower femur until the lower third of the femur; therefore, mounting trackers in an interiorly rotated position may place the upper pins in an intersection with the femoral artery. To avoid, this remember to proceed in a more anterior saggital direction on the upper pin and midsaggital on the lower pins while taking care not to penetrate the cortices by any pins. As noted, you may only need one bicortical pin because the second often serves as a derotation pin. There is little to disturb fixation on the lateral thigh, so these pins rarely lose fixation.

In all systems, tracker arrays should be adjusted to face the emitter, similar to the dorsal fin of a fish. Hence, the reflection surface will be planar to the AP axis with a 10-degree convergence and a 20-degree elevation for the best view.

Intraincisional Considerations

The temptation for almost every MIS-trained surgeon is to see how small one can make the incision and still get the job done. With reliance and confidence in CAS as the primary source of navigation, the surgeon can be more accurate in achieving that goal. The next question is whether one can keep the tracker pins inboard to the incision, or at least include one tracker assembly inside the wound margins.

Although it is possible to keep all pins inbound, there are two prerequisites. The system must have a medial pin application and a pin footprint of no more than a 2-cm separation between pins (Galileo Plus and Medtronics; see later). Anything with a wide tracker base will likely require a second small percutaneous incision to maintain the tissue-sparing look of a MIS incision. A small pinhole can be used, which may be just the right mix for many surgeons.

The greatest obstacle comes with the reduced room for accessing cutting jigs. This commits one to a freehand cut on the femur and tibia or modifying current cutting jigs to lie over and behind the view of the trackers to make the cuts. My preference is to use a freehand cut with a small two-pin block on the femur (Fig. 123-2). This is done by holding the cutting block in one hand, with a paddle array in the cutting slot. The other hand holds a pin or screw on a drill, which provides a means of fine correction of varus-valgus once resection depth is established.

On the tibial side, some cutting jigs set up in an elevated position (BrainLAB, Munich, Germany; ORTHOsoft). This affords just enough maneuvering room that a three-axis adjustment is possible over the top of the tracker array. However, the space is tight, thereby making the importance of proper tracker placement paramount to prevent the frustration of inadequate room for cutting jigs. Most importantly, the cutting jig needs firm fixation on the tibia to reduce saw blade drift and the need for corrective cuts.

Sequencing Changes

When MIS TKR was first introduced, femoral preparation followed by the tibia was taught. There are three reasons why this is no longer applicable. First, bone removal of the tibia-first cut is sometimes difficult without the hard cortical surface of the femur to pry against to remove it in osteoporotic patients. Second, many surgeons prefer basing all future cuts on the rectangular flexion-extension gap of their tibial cut. This facilitates the ability of the surgeon to achieve some visual confirmation if one doesn't want to take the time for cumbersome tensometer or gap distance measures. Finally, and most importantly, without the tibial cut removed, there is no easy way to see the lateral posterior femoral condyle to assess femoral waypoints or wear asymmetry to acquire valid computer baseline data adequately. Many systems lack the software to proceed without this waypoint identified or the posterior-based cutting blocks must be forcibly placed, which is subject to error. My suggestion is that unless the surgeon is firmly committed to a femur-first resection, he or she should become comfortable with the tibia-first approach, because this will be the direction toward which most systems will be moving.

Surgical Technique

With the incision completed and trackers in place, the femoral head center is acquired. This is done by concentric circle overlap software or multiple cone intersection points added, depending on the system. Next, waypoints for the tibia are acquired and the tibia is resected.

This is undoubtedly the most difficult part of the procedure, but all the following steps hinge on access gained from the proximal tibial approach. When performing this, the knee is flexed to 90 degrees and tactile sensation provides the primary end point of saw blade excursion. A wide patellar retractor (fat fork) is placed laterally, a forked retractor posteriorly, and a cruciate or Hohmann retractor on the medial side to protect the medial collateral ligaments. In large patients, 80 mm is the furthest excursion of the saw blade to the poster lateral corner, although 60 mm is adequate for women. The posterior retractor protects the popliteal structures. Use caution not to abrade the patellar tendon anteriorly with the blade oscillations because it can cut as easily by the edge as it does on the cutting end. When sawing is complete, a twist of the saw is usually enough to pop the remaining capsule free of any bound bony tissue. For large patients with marginal osteophytes or for osteoporotic individuals, blade twisting to elevate the respected bone may not be sufficient, or worse yet can mash the tibial metaphases. I use a 1.5-inch osteotome gently inserted across the osteotomy and then a second ¾-inch inserted on top. This provides protection to the tibia to prevent penetration into the soft cancelous bed from the distraction maneuver. The ¾-inch osteotome is twisted with a pliers or the back of a locked Cocker, to dislodge the bone enough which aids in the initially freeing of the fragment (Fig. 123-3).

Next, the fragment is elevated with a sweetheart (Lewin) clamp) on the anterior medial edge while a Hohmann retractor resting on the posterior condyle is levered forward, thereby freeing the medial portion enough to see the posterior capsule, cruciate, and soft tissue. Cutting free these structures leaves the last remaining hold, which is the posterior lateral meniscus. Once the popliteal meniscal complex is cut, the entire tibial fragment can be rotated free in a progressive role-out manner rather than an anterior drawer removal.

If the patient is large or the fragment stubborn, just bisect it at the notch, using an osteotome to remove the medial and then the lateral fragment; this is the easiest method (see earlier). If even this leaves an incomplete resection, I often

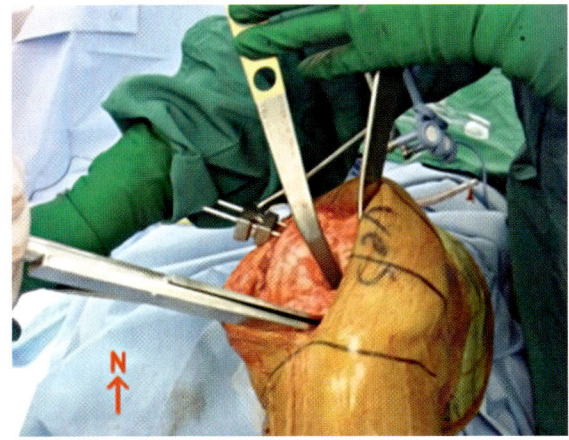

Figure 123-3. Retractors are in place in the posterior proximal fragment to pry it forward. Once free, the sweetheart clamp is used to apply added pressure to role out the fragment laterally while freeing posterior meniscal attachments.

will extend the knee to get slack in the collaterals to remove any remaining large fragments. However, this is not the final clean-out, so don't waste time looking for a little debris. All you want is a metaphyseal platform big enough to support a paddle tracker to confirm proper resection angles and heights. If you are within approximately 1 degree, you can proceed. If not, I usually make a corrective sanding or blade pass with the saw and do not verify the accuracy after the correction. Remember, you are already three times better with navigation than with traditional instruments, when there was no valid way to check cuts except cumbersome alignment rods, which are subject to rotation.

This now makes the femoral waypoint acquisition ready by viewing the posterior condyles or using the posterior referencing rotation jigs. Note first any abrasive wear or skid marks in relation to Whiteside's line. This can be an important clue to an aberrant trajectory of true knee flexion rather than anatomic points. Once the computer has inputted waypoints on the femoral rotation, anterior cortex, and distal condylar surface, the distal femur can be resected. A freehand jig is my preference, but it takes some practice to keep the three axes in perspective on CAS monitors (see Fig. 123-3). As noted, be sure that your jig tracker is in the dorsal or saggital plane and not oblique to prevent composite angle changes. I start with the on-screen crosshairs to get varus-valgus roughed in. Then, while holding the cutting guide on the medial side of the femur in one hand, move it to the approximate calculated femoral resection (10 mm in most systems). I use the formula of 10 mm + = 1 mm resection for every 4-degree lag of extension noted preoperatively to achieve adequate flexion contracture correction. I have found this to be an accurate guide for providing adequate extension in patients with flexion contractures not corrected by osteophyte removal, similar to other authors.[2]

Orient the cutting block first by using the graphic lines on AP and lateral monitor pictures to line up the block crudely. Then, slide the block to the proper resection level and push (not drill) a pin to hold the rough position of the same capture. While monitoring numbers to fine-tune all angles try not to fall into the trap of "perfect numbers." Choose your own ideal target but try not to chase numbers and hence waste time. Remember, CAS is capable of improving accuracy by 3 fold (+/– 3 degrees human site VS. +/– 1 degree CAS). However even CAS has accuracy limits which are not improved by spending excessive time on small degree variations of 1 degree off target values. My personal limits are 0-1 degree accept, 2 degrees think about, and >3 degrees fix or change. If, when anchoring the block, the drill deviates the saw capture, put a second pin in while overcorrecting in the plane opposite to the pin deflection. The spring effect usually results in a stabilization to the target value originally sought. Remember, large femurs invariably result in excessive varus over the CAS value because the saw blade drift undercuts the lateral and more distant condyle. This should achieve a first-time correct cut, but I still verify my cuts. If the monitor CAS value is still off by 1 or 2 degrees, don't unpin the guide. Instead, force-feed the saw blade to achieve the ideal angles; one can generally correct for small errors.

Next, the femoral finishing block is applied and rotated to the proper 3- to 4-degree external rotation of posterior condyles (or 0 degrees if using Whiteside's line). I use the computer to reference the anterior notch status. This is faster than using posterior reference guides, and most systems have on-screen notch and rotation values available. If size was predicted, I prefer to undersize if between sizes. Edge to edge coverage without overhang is the goal, which is best based on visual reference.

Once the block is positioned with convergent or multiple pins, a check for proper midline positioning is done. If the block somehow is too far medial or lateral, I skip drilling peg holes and cut the notch to the side minus the correction desired to side-slip the block to correct any miscentered placement. In this way, you still obtain precise rotational and AP cuts while providing a final centering of the implant in the medial lateral plane.

The knee is now ready for final clean-up in extension (Fig. 123-4). I prefer a large laminar spreader to separate the bone ends if a more elaborate foot holder is not available. I pay particular attention to three problem bleed areas. The first is the inferior genicular vessel to the lateral meniscus, just adjacent to the popliteus tendon. Second is the posterior cruciate found in the top of the box cut or in the notch. The final active vessel is the medial inferior genicular vessel to the medial meniscus and capsule. Even if I see no active bleeding, I generally use a Bovie or Bipolar (high-frequency bipolar unit) in these regions while the tourniquet is down. Then the

capsule is injected. Avoid the popliteal corner because of the proximity of the peroneal nerve. I use an injection cocktail of 15 mL of 0.5% ropivacaine (Naropin), 100 mL of 0.2% ropivicaine, 0.5 mL of epinephrine 1/1000, a 30-mg solution of ketorolac (Toradol), and 10 mg of morphine sulfate. As a natural depot, the pes anserinus is injected with 10 to 15 mL while the remaining 25-mL allotment is placed in the muscle tissue and medial capsule, near the pes anserinus insertion.

Implants are now installed, with the femur first. A fat fork or wide Hohmann retractor goes over the lateral condyle to protect the patella so the femur can be viewed. The round retractor goes medially. Once the femur is checked for adequate seating, the tibial inserts are inserted. I start with the plastic provisional without the metal tray. I do this for one reason—speed. For example, using a 14-mm plastic insert for a 3-mm tray height could result in a tight 12 mm or loose 10 mm when using the real 10-mm insert on a metal tray. You do not have to go through the mental calculations, but the upshot is that you don't need to worry about the insert riding on the edge of the tray, which would cause an erroneous read. The manufacturer can supply a chart for reference that can be hung next to the x-rays until you get used to carrying out the procedure in this way.

Now, check computer readings and document unassisted full extension and flexion. If not correct, do traditional up and down sizing where appropriate. Remember, a varus or valgus knee with uncorrected soft tissue balance may be cut perfectly but tensioned unequally. It is at this point that I make appropriate osteophyte and soft tissue corrections. Some systems would mandate releases at the beginning of the case but I find this unreliable until all cuts and exposures have been made. Only when a surgeon starts monitoring equalization of varus-valgus tension test results can he or she appreciate of how unbalanced knees can be, even with all osteophytes removed. CAS makes all surgeons very honest in this regard.

Before removing the tray, mark the middle of the anterior center on the tibia with a Bovie or marker to ensure tray congruence with the femur in extension. I have yet to see a trustworthy, meaningful, femoral-tibial tray rotation value given by the CAS systems currently available. This is more a directional validation number used by all software to calculate flexion and alignment values. Direct visualization still appears to be the best way to verify component congruence in extension, even if using a mobile tray. Repeat the same retractor placements for the tibial base plate as with the original resection. CAS tracker pins are now removed, using the pin driver, unless you desire to navigate through cementing, which is not my recommendation. At this point the tourniquet goes up for the first time after 2 minutes of elevation by the assistant to drain pooled blood. Cleaning of the surface is done in a routine fashion and component insertion can be done in the usual manner.

Low-viscosity cement is my preference, with a bevel cut on the cement gun outlet. This can put cement under pressure in a wide surface of the tibia and is easier to direct a thin, 2-mm film of cement to the tray. When these are combined with a similar 2-mm cement layer on the implant, there is often no cement to have to clean while ensuring that water and debris don't become sandwiched between the cement fixation (Fig. 123-5). If stems are used, they are inserted via the manufacturer's protocol. My preference is a two-part drop-down modular stem, which gives a little more anchor to the tray and may provide protection from tibial stress

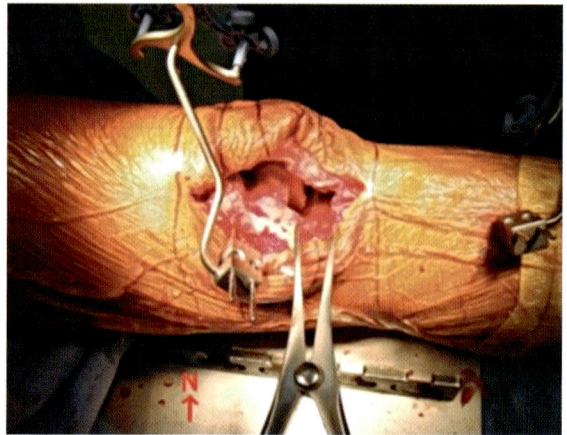

Figure 123-4. Laminar spreader in place allows for less obstructed view of the posterior joint and does not interfere with trackers.

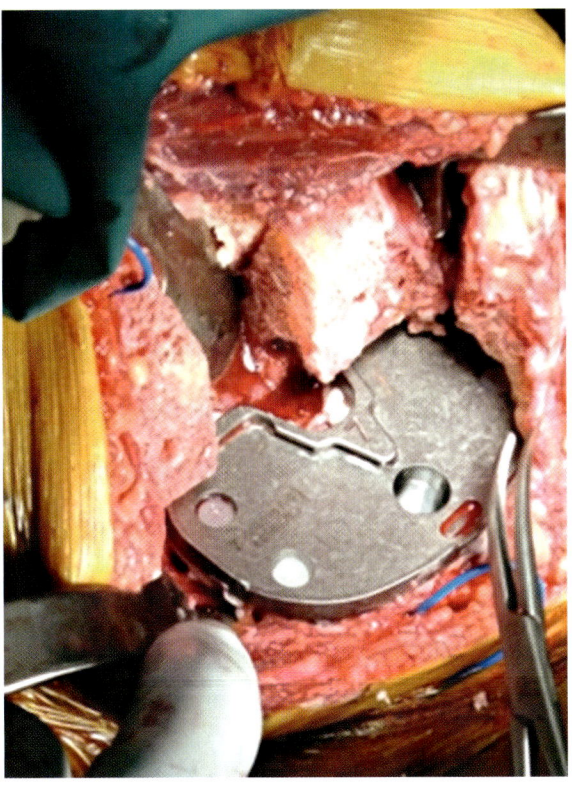

Figure 123-5. Retractor position of the tibia tray starts with the medial collateral ligament (MCL), posterior cruciate ligament (PCL), and lateral fat fork, with optional hemostat to prevent soft tissue drift under the tray. The fat fork is being moved to the lateral femur to make ready for the next step.

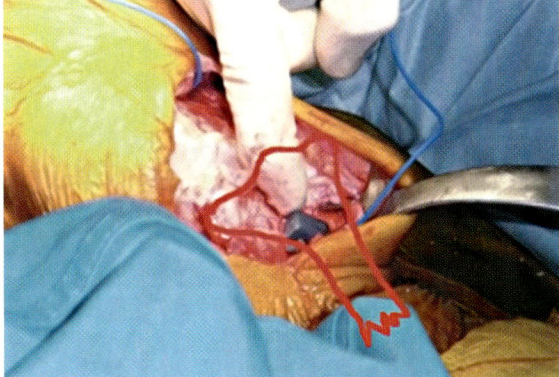

Figure 123-6. Tibia DRF is inserted anterior to the insertion of the pes anserinus, with adequate distance below the future tibial resection line to fit cutting jigs into position.

fractures from jig anchor points. This is much easier to use than a fixed keel. If using other, less friendly, MIS nonmodular trays, I have found it easier to insert these with tibial resection in the 12- to 14-mm range because this provides a little more room to insert longer keels.

The femur is then inserted using the same 2-mm cement thickness on the implant, but with no cement on the femur. The tray is inserted, followed by the patella, and remaining clean-up is completed.

I suture the knee in flexion with the tourniquet still up until 12 minutes, or until the closure is complete. A new easy option is a barbed locking monofilament, a no. 2 Quill (Ethicon, Somerville, NJ), from the center of the incision to the outside of either end of the capsule. If the patella was originally subluxed, a more nonabsorbable suture reconstruction with a release may be necessary. Subcutaneous closure is done by running a 2-0 Quill barbed suture or 2-0 monocryl suture approximately 1 cm apart to ensure tight closure. The final skin closure is completed by using a 4-0 monocryl subcuticular stitch and Dermabond (Ethicon) to seal the surface. I don't use a drain but always use elevation, and actively stress this throughout the first 2 weeks of postoperative rehabilitation.

Electromagnetic Computer-Assisted Surgery

The major difference in electromagnetic (EM) over IR CAS is the ability to place trackers or dynamic reference frames (DRFs) inbound to the incision (Fig. 123-6). This allows

more room to navigate the saw captures and perform surgery in the absence of external IR tracking arrays. Although this appears satisfactory, the disadvantage is that reception is often disrupted because of metal interference. The following discussion will describe how to perform a MIS TKR without the frustration of signal disruption.

Dynamic Reference Frame Installation

The best leg holder is a sandbag anchored at the upper malleolus area on the operating table to minimize metal interference. However, a Kevlar or fiberglass Alverado leg holder is an acceptable but expensive alternative. Incisions for MIS are done in the usual manner when it comes to installing the DRF. For the femoral side, the first screw is positioned in the medial posterior ridge of bone on the hard cortical ridge of the adduction magnus insertion. I use the supplied driver with the first screw in the proximal hole of the DRF and palpate the posterior femur. Then I move it anteriorly enough to capture the cortical bone. The second screw, as in the IR CAS, can be placed anywhere in the softer anterior bone to act as an antirotation fix.

Similarly, the tibial DRF is first affixed in the pes anserinus insertion along the harder posterior bone (Fig. 123-7). The second more proximal derotation screw is placed at 1.5 cm below the estimated future resection level of the tibia in the softer cancellous tibial flair. Angle screws are used parallel to the tibial resection and posteriorly to provide more room for future stem preparation if you plan on navigating through the cementing phase. With practice, the power drill can complete the tightening, but the hand tightener is safer to use until a feel for torque resistance is acquired to prevent stripping the screw threads.

Techniques to enhance reception of signal from the localizer or magnetic field generator is the next step to learn. There are basically two cardinal or primary positions that receive signals over the disruptive influence of a ferric environment of metal cutting blocks and cutting jigs. On the femur, the best localizer placement is the 11 and 1 o'clock positions on the right and left knees, respectively, with a distance of 15 to 20 cm. On the tibia, the 7 and 5 o'clock positions on the right and left knees, respectively, will maximize stubborn metal influence disruption (Fig. 123-8).

Femoral and tibial preparation can then be done with MIS user-friendly cutting jigs. Tibial resection is performed using an extramedullary swivel tibial saw capture; the femur uses a

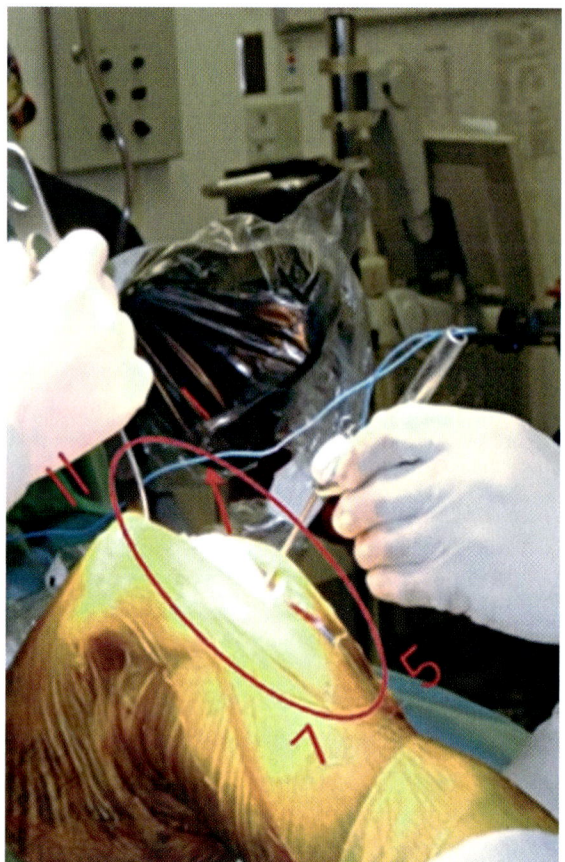

Figure 123-7. Localizer in the 1 o'clock position, which is the most sensitive position to transmit tracking power to the femoral and tibial DRFs with implant provisionals installed.

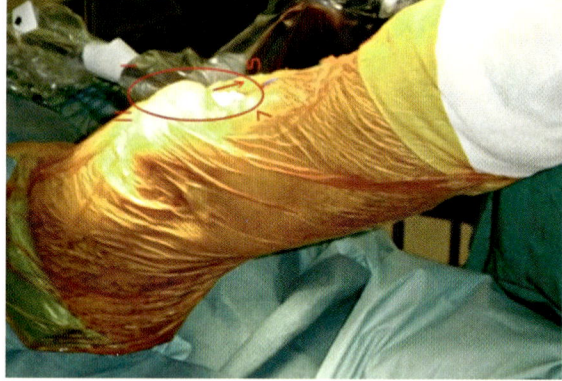

Figure 123-8. Localizer shown in one of four more cardinal areas best suited to transmit tracking power for the DRFs to transmit. Note the leg being elevated away from potential metal interference of the operating room table. A left knee is shown with the localizer in the 5 o'clock position depicted on the superimposed clock face, which provides the best tibial reception, and the 1 o'clock position for femoral reception.

versatile ball navigation jig, which allows 3 degrees of adjustment (Fig. 123-9). I use this secondary position of the localizer on the front of the thigh (10 to 20 cm above the patella) in 80% of cuts.

Because of the metal interference of the large cutting blocks, it may not always be easy to view all positions with a completely assembled provisional arthroplasty. One trick to

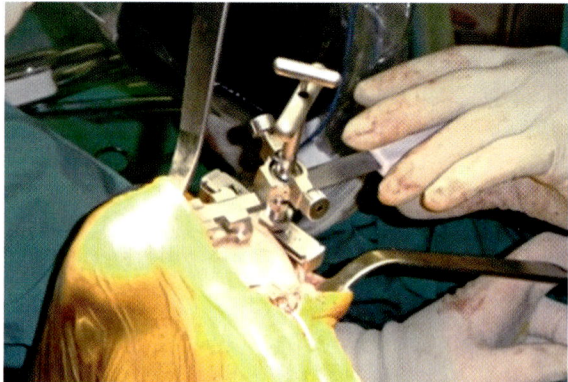

Figure 123-9. Ball navigation jig mounted in the distal femur with the EM paddle probe used as guidance. The jig allows one to navigate in varus-valgus and flexion-extension while depth resection is controlled by the screw T at the top of the jig.

reduce metal interference is to use the plastic tibial provisional (see earlier) without the metal tray in the ligament gap and alignment testing. This works well by using the localizer above the femur in the 1 and 11 o'clock positions at a distance of 15 to 20 cm from the DRF unless the patient requires a large or oversized component. Sometimes, because of the metal, spacer blacks are the only alternative. Once the kinematics are recorded and alignment is satisfactory, I remove the DRF and follow through with the same closure as described in the IR section (see earlier).

The EM CAS is the most difficult system to use. However, once one masters the subtle position requirements, the unencumbered noninvasive surgical environment it affords is unequaled by any IR system that I have used.

Summary

As noted, I prefer not to check alignment after cementing the components. However, as one uses CAS, a careful evaluation of patients may reveal subtle consistencies. In a review of my first 458 patients, EM CAS consistently showed a 1- to 1.5-degree valgus shift. As a result, when I use this unit, I always correct or trim for a 1-degree extra varus femoral cut or a 1.5-degree varus femoral and 0.5-degree valgus tibial cut to make up for this, given recent evidence of failure in varus tibial tray placements.[7] Different IR systems may yield similar results. One tendency is to overimpact the lateral side because of an obscured view, which may result from surgical error rather than CAS error. In any case, fine-tuning through CAS is an easy option for the surgeon. I also prefer to put the knee in 3 to 5 degrees of hyperextension when testing the knee ranges with provisionals. I have found that this cuts down on extension lags and does not result in a hyperextension laxity problem. Accuracy in TKR can be obtained by trimming or fine-tuning CAS and will produce better results more often than when using traditional procedures.

SPECIFIC PROPRIETARY FEATURES

Aesculap

Aesculap has the only single-pin (screw) tracker application available, which appears firm and secure while providing a fast insertion. The downside to one screw is that it may bend or rotate under load on the femoral side if the soft tissue is tensioned too high. The trackers are only mountable on one side (lateral), making viewing for some surgeons difficult. Although not as MIS-friendly as some systems, the active- or passive-mounted trackers connect easily with the best quick connections to dedicated cutting jigs. Active trackers' azimuth of reception is in the 100-degree range, with a tendency for fluid or blood debris sensitivity. Version 4.2 provides one of the most state of the art gap testing for preresection balance systems of any CAS tested. It provides exceptional information on true millimeter displacement of medial and lateral gap distance, as well as predictive component planning and resultant distance relative to a posterior reference starting point for those interested in balancing ligaments before implantation. It is retrievable to recheck after provisionals are in but requires some on-screen maneuvering. Universal application is available; however, this provides only rudimentary navigation, without a ligament balance option. Waypoint acquisition is made more cumbersome by multiple redundant functional and point digitization for dual-reference averaging. The hip center acquisition is also one of the slowest available because of the fixed radial clock face design for waypoint input. Previous screen review is not available. Although pictures are not taken automatically, there is an optional floor mouse, which unlike any other system makes hands-free picture taking possible. Data retrieval is cumbersome and no disc drive is available on the machine tested, only a USB port. The CAS station is physically the biggest on the market if storage is an issue.

BrainLAB

This system is operationally a DePuy-product and therefore is specific to sizing and positioning of their implant only. Trackers may only be mounted extraincisionally. Mounts allow for 4-mm pin fixation versatility, rather than the more standard 3-mm pin fixation; also, flexible base mounts allow for lateral or medial tracker positions. Passive trackers are very debris-sensitive; however, the reception range, if clean, is 8 feet, making it one of the longest range machines. Mechanical alignment with individual component AP and saggital readings are available universally; however, recall on screen requires direct monitor input. There is no universal guidance for other TKR systems but it is well mated to the DuPuy implant (DePuy Orthopaedics, Warsaw, Ind). Screen layout is the most robust and realistic. However, usable information is difficult to focus on because of the overabundance of numbers. One has to navigate between flexion angles, making gap distance comparisons difficult between flexion ranges. Gap distance measures are expressed in user-friendly millimeter measurements. The longer version of the software mandates balancing ligaments before cuts are complete, which may be cumbersome to some surgeons who want the postimplantation option. On the other hand, the ease of recall of archived data is among the best in regard to ease of access and the large amount of data obtained. Reception of signals by ball reflectors is 125 degrees but is debris-sensitive. Software is procedure-mandated and is not flexible in sequence changes that were not previously planned. One has to reboot to change sequence order, which will require all new landmarks. There are three different CAS units

available, ranging from a single-stand portable unit to larger separable units, which make the system easier to use in the operating room, no matter the size constraints.

Medtronic

Universal application of the version 2.4 system (Medtronic, Minneapolis) is available with IR for all TKR systems whereas the EM CAS provides sizing only for the Zimmer TKR. Only medial pin insertion for IR CAS is currently available. The EM CAS system has no localizer to track directional priorities or limits but signal disruption from metal interference is a common limitation of the system. All angles and rotations are universally available in one screen for each specific angle of flexion. The surgeon can carry out direct gap distance comparisons through the entire flexion range, which gives it the easiest use of gap distance balance data available in any of the CAS systems tested. The gap values registered are true distinct medial and lateral measured values, rather than mathematically based on rotation. Distance measures appear at the provisional insertion stage of the procedure, not at the preresection stage. The screen display is easy to use and flexible to cross-reference to the preoperative deformity values, making tibial and femoral resection calculations faster than with other systems. Acquisition of waypoints is the fastest of the systems tested with the notable exception of the femoral hip center, which can at times be slow or impossible to achieve if pelvic movement is not dampened in those with a high body mass index (BMI). This makes the overall speed of the system one of the slowest when ferric disruption from provisional implants are figured into the equation. Pictures of screen shots are not available remotely, except through touch screen button entry. Each case is automatically archived and is retrieved in an easy to use PowerPoint file format.

ORTHOsoft

Lateral pin insertion is the only insertion side available, with no provision for medial tracker placement. A universal knee application is used to provide for all angles and rotations. Gap distance ligament balance measures are expressed in degrees, not the more familiar and usable millimeter values. The screen display is flexible and easy to read. Sequence changes are easy to make in order of procedure or waypoints. Acquisition of waypoints is slow and temperamental because of limited instrumentation for an actual MIS application system. This is especially true of the distal femur and posterior femoral waypoints, which do not allow measurement of valgus-varus deformity of 6 degrees or more, which is common in a large adult reconstructive practice. Although the system has a remote picture-taking capability via the stylus, it is cumbersome and slow; it probably is more practical to use the on-screen option. It has good archived storage capacity, but retrieval of data is difficult for research or patient use. The reception of the signal azimuth is 135 degrees, with undoubtedly the best debris-resistant reflectors of those tested on the market today, including all active systems.

Galileo Plus

The Galileo Plus IR MIS version 2.0 (Smith & Nephew, Andover, Mass) offers the only IR intraincisional dual-screw tibial and femoral mounts for tracker anchors. Mounting via a MIS incision is more feasible, while avoiding diaphyseal pins, making tracker insertion the most MIS-friendly of the IR systems. This CAS system expresses gap measures in angles, not millimeter separation. Acquisition is the fastest of tested units; they are specific to Smith & Nephew TKR and therefore have no universal application to other knee systems. Older reflector balls are used, so resection is difficult if they get soiled with blood, but the reception azimuth is a respectable 125 degrees. The screen display is among the most basic, yet direct. Reviews and cross references to preoperative deformity are not currently available, and previous screen shots were extremely difficult to retrieve. Data are recorded in and retrieved in an easy to use PowerPoint file format.

Stryker

Pin application is possible in the medial or lateral side, with versatile angular (nonparallel) pin mounts available. All angles and rotation readings are available for any implant, but sizing is specific for Stryker implants. The system provides a variety of cutting jigs from the fixed-pin multiaxial adjustable to the more demanding freehand variety (my preference). The reception azimuth, even for active trackers, is narrower than most (100 degrees), but graphics and monitor display are easy to use and exceptionally simple. Trackers cannot be used inside the incision because of 3-cm spacing on the tracker pins, forcing extraincisional MIS use. Customization for surgical sequence changes is easy but must be done before starting. Waypoint acquisition is slower than most, mainly because of the multiple-point acquisition rather than single-point entry, which in some cases cannot be overridden. MIS application is slightly difficult to accomplish without excessive stress on soft tissues. Gap distances are not measured in segregated medial and lateral separation but rather as middle absolute separation from the joint surface, making their use of limited value. Balance of ligaments is displayed in a complex histogram graphic rather than set distances at any angle. There is universal application for other TKR systems. The screen display is robust and easy to use. However, preoperative data stress test results cannot be easily obtained unless preoperative stress testing is done for soft tissue release before any resection, making this feature difficult to use for interpretive value. Remote picture shots are possible but not easy for the surgeon; therefore, on-screen activation is easier. Copying and data archiving are done automatically but the file is an Adobe tif format, which is difficult to use for research, patient's viewing, or documentation.

KEY REFERENCES

Asano T, Akagi M, Nakamura T: The functional flexion-extension axis of the knee corresponds to the surgical epicondyar axis. J Arthroplasty 20:1060–1067, 2005.

Bengs BC, Scott RD: The effect of distal femoral resection on passive knee extension in posterior cruciate ligament retaining total knee arthroplasty. J Arthroplasty 21:161–166, 2006.

Berend KR, Lombardi A, Jr: Avoiding the potential pitfalls of minimally invasive total knee surgery. Orthopedics 28:1326–1330, 2005.

Berry DJ: Computer-assisted knee arthroplasty is better than a conventional jig-based technique in terms of component alignment. J Bone Joint Surg Am 86:2573. 2004.

Chin PL, Yang KY, Yeo SJ, Lo NN: Randomized control trial comparing radiographic total knee arthroplasty implant placement using computer navigation versus conventional technique. J Arthroplasty 20:618–626, 2005.

Damme GV, Defoort K, Ducoulombier Y, et al: What should the surgeon aim for when performing computer-assisted total knee arthroplasty? J Bone Joint Surg Am 87(Suppl 2):52–58, 2005.

Fang DM, Ritter MA, Davis KE: Coronal alignment in total knee arthroplasty. J Arthroplasty 24:39–42, 2009.

Gioe TJ, Killeen KK, Grimm K, et al: Why are total knee replacements revised? Clin Orthop Relat Res 428:100–106, 2004.

Incavo SJ, Coughlin KM, Beynnon BD: Femoral component sizing in total knee arthroplasty: size matched resection versus flexion space balancing. J Arthroplasty 19:493–497, 2004.

Jeffrey RS, Morris RW, Denham RA: Coronal alignment after total knee replacement. J Bone Joint Surg Br 73:709–714, 1991.

Jenny JV, Clemens U, Kohler S, et al: Consistency of implantation of a total knee arthroplasty with a non-image-based navigation system: a case-control study of 235 cases compared with 235 conventionally implanted prostheses. J Arthroplasty 20:832–839, 2005.

Kim S, MacDonald M, Hernandez J, Wixson R: Computer-assisted navigation in total knee arthroplasty: improved coronal alignment. J Arthroplasty 20(Suppl 3):123–131, 2005.

Rottman SJ, Dvorkin M, Gold D: Extramedullary versus intramedullary tibial alignment guides for total knee arthroplasty. Orthopedics 28:1445–1448, 2005.

Sparmann M, Wolke B, Czupalla H, et al: Positioning of total knee arthroplasty with and without navigation support. A prospective, randomised study. J Bone Joint Surg Br 85:830–835, 2003.

Yau WP, Leung A, Chiu KY, et al: Intraobserver errors in obtaining visually selected anatomic landmarks during registration process in nonimage-based navigation-assisted total knee arthroplasty: a cadaveric experiment. J Arthroplasty 20:591–601, 2005.

Full references for this chapter can be found on www.expertconsult.com.

Advanced Technologies in Performing Total Knee Arthroplasty: Roundtable Discussion

Moderator: Thomas K. Fehring, Participants: Keith R. Berend, Siegfried Hofmann, Adolph V. Lombardi, Jess H. Lonner, Shuichi Matsuda, and Michael D. Ries

The purpose of this chapter is to investigate some of the new technologic advances and surgical techniques in the field of knee arthroplasty. We have assembled an internationally renowned faculty with vast clinical and research experience to help answer some of the important questions in knee surgery today.

Our participating arthroplasty surgeons for this roundtable discussion are Keith R. Berend from New Albany, Ohio; Thomas K. Fehring from Charlotte, North Carolina; Siegfried Hofmann from Stolzalpe, Austria; Adolph Lombardi from New Albany, Ohio; Jess Lonner from Philadelphia; Shuichi Matsuda from Fukuoka City, Japan; and Michael Ries from San Francisco.

MINIMALLY INVASIVE SURGERY: DR. RIES AND DR. BEREND

Dr. Fehring: Minimally invasive total knee surgery was introduced about 5 years ago as a means to diminish pain and hasten rehabilitation. As problems with alignment, proper ligamentous balance, and wound healing have arisen since its inception, enthusiasm for this technique has waned.

Dr. Ries, is there still a place for minimally invasive techniques at this time?

Dr. Ries: The real risks and benefits of minimally invasive total knee arthroplasty (TKA) have been obscured by the effects of marketing minimally invasive surgery (MIS) TKA in clinical practice with broad claims about the benefits and little acknowledgment of risks. However, most studies of MIS compared with conventional TKA generally indicate that there can be some early benefit of faster recovery, a higher risk of complications, and no long-term benefit.[10,14,24,26]

Prior to the introduction of minimally invasive surgery, I believe most surgeons, myself included, were trained to use a standard incision size and approach for all patients. I had used an incision from approximately 4 fingerbreadths above the patella to 2 cm distal to the tibial tubercle. Although this incision size may be necessary in obese patients, TKA can be safely performed in thin patients with good range of motion (ROM) and minimal deformity through a smaller incision.

The experience of MIS for me has been to emphasize the concept that the same incision length is not needed for all patients. I now begin my surgery with an incision from the superior pole of the patella to the tibial tubercle. If I am having any difficulty with the surgery, I then extend the incision. I consider minimally invasive surgery as the smallest incision that can be used to safely perform the TKA. When patients ask if I use MIS, I reply, "Yes, I use it routinely," and I repeat my definition of it. In my experience, this approach has provided a very satisfactory end to the discussion for both the surgeon and patient.

Dr. Fehring: Is there an ideal candidate for minimally invasive total knee surgery?

Dr. Berend: I firmly believe that no total knee arthroplasty is as minimally invasive as the minimal operation would be to perform a compartmental arthroplasty with preservation of any normal structures. Therefore, in most knees, total knee arthroplasty is by definition not minimal. Assuming that we agree that minimally invasive total knee arthroplasty is likely a misnomer, the ideal candidate for less invasive arthroplasty would be a patient with minimal deformity, a supple flexible knee, and good range of motion. Patients with mild valgus deformity and mild lateral patellar subluxation appears to be the easiest patients to begin learning and gaining experience with the techniques for less invasive total knee surgery. Patients in whom concerns over less invasive techniques exist would be those with patella baja, previous surgery to the knee, significant intra-articular and extra-articular deformity, morbidly obese patients, and patients with previous issues of wound healing.

Dr. Fehring: What is your preferred approach to a normal-sized patient with minimal deformity?

Dr. Ries: I begin the surgery with the knee flexed 30 to 40 degrees, making an incision from the superior pole of the patella to the tibial tubercle, and raise a relatively wide medial skin and subcutaneous tissue flap and a smaller lateral flap. I believe it's very important to dissect the subfascial plane carefully and maintain the full thickness of the subcutaneous layer to preserve the vascularity of the soft tissue flaps. I then make a medial parapatellar arthrotomy and dissect the medial tibial soft tissue sleeve subperiosteally to the midcoronal plane. Mid- or subvastus approaches have not been particularly useful for me in that these require more tension on the extensor mechanism to sublux the patella and can result in trauma to the vastus medialis. I then flex the knee fully, which retracts the proximal skin and subcutaneous soft tissues and exposes the rectus tendon. I extend the proximal arthrotomy into the rectus tendon, remove some portions of the fat pad that impinge into the knee, release the tibial insertion of the fat pad and lateral meniscus, and sublux the patella laterally without eversion.

I prefer to make the distal femoral cut first, followed by the tibial cut, and check the size of my extension space and alignment with a spacer block. Then I proceed with the remaining femoral cuts and TKA. The most helpful MIS technique for me has been the concept of a mobile window. I flex the knee fully while working on the tibia, place the knee at 90 degrees while working on the distal femur, and extend the knee to 60 to 80 degrees while working on the anterior femur.

Dr. Fehring: What is your preferred approach, Dr. Berend?

Dr. Berend: My preferred approach to a normal size patient with a minimal deformity would be to perform a less invasive, small incision, a modified mini-Tri-Vector. Through this approach, the vastus medialis is taken down from the extensor mechanism and the rectus tendon of the quadriceps is not involved in the dissection.

Dr. Berend, is there any evidence-based literature that documents improved function or quicker rehabilitation with MIS techniques?

Dr. Berend: There is clear evidence-based literature that supports the fact that partial knee arthroplasty does allow for quicker rehabilitation compared with total knee arthroplasty. Lombardi and colleagues,[30] in a retrospective study, has shown that patients undergoing partial knee arthroplasty recovered significantly faster than those undergoing a total knee arthroplasty. In terms of less invasive approaches to total knee arthroplasty as compared with standard approaches, the perioperative care of the patient is likely the most important factor. If we truly isolate the surgical technique away from the perioperative care protocols, recent literature from Tsuji and associates[52] has shown that MIS TKA patients have an earlier, faster recovery than traditional total knee arthroplasty patients. In another recent, well-designed study, Dalury and coworkers[15] have demonstrated that the invasiveness of the procedure as measured by the amount of tibial translation and patellar eversion does not affect the early postoperative recovery period after total knee arthroplasty. Therefore, it should be concluded that there are multiple factors at play when looking at the improved function and quicker rehabilitation with MIS techniques.

Dr. Ries, do you agree?

Dr. Ries: Most publications on this topic consist of observational case series, single-cohort studies, and expert opinions.[10] However, several randomized prospective studies have been done that indicate either no benefit of MIS or faster recovery of early knee function in the MIS group.[24,26] Long-term benefits of MIS have not been demonstrated and there can be a greater risk of complications with MIS surgery.[14]

CUSTOM IMPLANTS AND INSTRUMENTATION: DR. BEREND AND DR. LOMBARDI

Dr. Fehring: A recent advance in knee arthroplasty has been the use of computed tomography (CT) or magnetic resonance imaging (MRI) data to make patient-specific implants and instruments. This technology is now offered by a number of orthopedic manufacturers.

Dr. Lombardi, what are the clinical advantages of this technique versus traditional total knee arthroplasty?

Dr. Lombardi: The use of CT or MRI data to make patient-specific implants and instruments has a number of clinical advantages. First and foremost, it takes preoperative planning to a totally different level. It requires the orthopedic surgeon to evaluate a three-dimensional model of each patient and develop a sophisticated preoperative plan. Restoration of the mechanical axis has been shown to be the key to success in total knee arthroplasty, especially with reference to enhanced durability.[7,13,32] The use of patient-specific guides has been shown to decrease the number of outliers and therefore enhance the quality of the reconstruction.[28] Obtaining the appropriate rotation of the femoral component at the time of surgical intervention has been shown to be keenly important to the success of the arthroplasty, especially with respect to

the patellofemoral articulation.[25] With the three-dimensional reconstruction of the patient's anatomy, the transepicondylar axis can be adequately identified in the preoperative plan. Computer navigation doesn't offer the same degree of accuracy with respect to femoral component rotation. The use of patient-specific guides requires less instrumentation and, therefore, there is less potential for contamination of the surgical field. The use of patient-specific guides does not require violation of the femoral canal or the placement of pins in the femur and tibia. Finally, the operative intervention can be performed more efficiently with patient-specific guides because many decisions have been performed prior to the commencement of the surgical procedure.

Dr. Fehring: Do you share this enthusiasm?

Dr. Berend: Clinical advantages to any patient-specific technology are somewhat abstract at this time. It is, however, logical to assume that any instrumentation that allows more accurate implantation of the total knee arthroplasty device may reduce the incidence of either outliers or early failure. When comparing the MRI custom implant and instrumentation technology to that of traditional total knee arthroplasty, the bar has been set extremely high through previous implant and instrument designs and surgical techniques. However, the clinical advantages may be in more accurate implantation, possibly allowing for a lower incidence of early and midterm failure.

It has been our experience that custom MRI-based cutting guides for total knee arthroplasty have been advantageous in efficiency in the operating room and accuracy of femoral and tibial preparation.

Dr. Fehring: What are the economic implications of this technique versus traditional knee arthroplasty?

Dr. Berend: The economic implications are significant—the cost of the MRI, the establishment and creation of the custom instruments, and potentially the creation of custom implants. All add increased cost to an already expensive procedure. Extrapolating this to surgical navigation for total knee arthroplasty, we have shown that when compared with navigation, the use of this technology is much more cost-effective because of decreased operative time. However, compared with traditional knee arthroplasty, there are significant increases in cost. If this technology is able to reduce outliers and reduce the failure rate of total knee arthroplasty, the economic impact may be positive.

Dr. Fehring: Can we afford this in an era of declining health care resources?

Dr. Lombardi: Economic implications of the use of CT or MRI data to make patient-specific implants and guides involve the actual cost of this technology. Patients will need to obtain a preoperative CT or MRI scan. There is a cost associated with this. Furthermore, this information will be used to create a three-dimensional model and a patient-specific guide. The current economic burden for this technology is between $1000 and $1500 per case. The economic justification for this technique involves the following:

1. Hopefully, patient-specific guides will decrease the number of outliers with respect to restoration of the mechanical axis and attainment of appropriate femoral component rotation. If this is true, this should correlate with improved clinical results, a decrease in the number of failures, and savings to the ultimate cost of health care.

2. The appropriate component sizes are determined preoperatively. Knowledge of the sizes will significantly decrease the inventory burden of the hospitals, which should translate into an economic benefit, not only for the hospital but also for the manufacturer.

3. The use of the patient-specific guide significantly streamlines the number of instruments required to perform the operative intervention. The savings in operative intervention time combined with turnover time could allow the surgeon to be more efficient and possibly perform additional surgical procedures per day in the same operating room.

Dr. Fehring: Concerns about this technique have been voiced by surgeons who consider knee arthroplasty a soft tissue operation. This technique seems to focus solely on bony anatomy. What are your thoughts about this concern?

Dr. Lombardi: It is a well-known fact that the satisfactory performance of a total knee arthroplasty is a combination of bony resection and appropriate soft tissue reconstruction. The keys to success appear to be restoration of the mechanical axis and effective balance of the flexion-extension gap. Traditionally, surgeons have been offered a combination of intramedullary and extramedullary alignment guides to perform the appropriate bony resections. Computer navigation has also assisted the surgeon in performing the appropriate bony resections and has served to eliminate outliers.[37] Neither technique has specifically addressed soft tissue balance. The use of patient-specific guides brings the bony resections to a different level. It allows the surgeon to perform very precise resections and obtain appropriate alignment to reconstruct the mechanical axis and to position the femoral component appropriately with respect to rotation. These guides do not eliminate the need for the surgeon to be a surgeon and balance the soft tissues. However, it provides them with a set of instruments that are more accurate and less invasive than either the conventional instruments or computer navigation. With these guides, the surgeon can competently perform the bony resections and spend more time in balancing the soft tissues.

Dr. Fehring: Is this technique appropriate for severe deformities?

Dr. Berend: We have yet to determine whether this technique is appropriate for severe deformities. It would appear that it may be beneficial because our technique uses the mechanical axis. It may therefore be extremely helpful in these difficult cases. Time and experience will have to tell us whether this is true.

BEARING SURFACE ISSUES: DR. MATSUDA AND DR. RIES

Dr. Fehring: A number of different strategies have been used to diminish wear and osteolysis in total knee arthroplasty. Rotating platforms have been used for many years with the theoretical advantage of diminishing wear. Clinical studies documenting this improvement in wear are lacking; however, the theoretical advantage of linear wear at the articular surface and undersurface of the polyethylene remain encouraging. Countersurface wear through the use of ceramic-coated implants also has enticing theoretical advantages.

Dr. Ries: In your practice, do you use mobile bearings or alternative bearings to improve wear characteristics in your total knee patients?

The benefit of mobile bearings was most apparent when ultra–high-molecular-weight polyethylene (UHMWPE) was sterilized by gamma irradiation in air. Fixed-bearing, relatively nonconforming tibial components typically failed as a result of fatigue wear mechanisms (delamination and pitting). Nonconforming designs with low contact areas are associated with high contact stresses and, when coupled with the diminished ductility, wear resistance, and fatigue strength of UHMWPE, fatigue mechanisms occurred. Mobile bearings have highly conforming articular surfaces, which results in lower contact stresses. Fatigue failure of UHMWPE that was gamma-irradiated in air with mobile bearings has been extremely uncommon. Although wear can occur at both the upper and lower articulating surfaces of the tibial insert, the contact areas are high, resulting in contact stresses that are sufficiently low to reduce fatigue wear substantially. However, gamma-irradiated in air sterilization of UHMWPE was abandoned by manufacturers in the mid-1990s. Failure caused by fatigue wear (delamination and pitting) does not appear to be a clinical problem with currently available conventional UHMWPE tibial inserts (gamma-irradiated in an inert atmosphere, ethylene oxide, or gas plasma–sterilized). Therefore, it is not clear if there is much of a benefit to the use of mobile bearings with currently available conventional UHMWPE.

Wear is increased by counterface roughening, which can occur in vivo. This is why titanium, which is a relatively soft material, is not used as a bearing surface. Cobalt-chrome used in total knee femoral components is generally cast, which is not as hard as the forged cobalt-chrome used in total hip femoral heads. Cobalt-chrome femoral components in TKA can roughen during in vivo use. Surface hardening treatments such as diffusion hardening or ion bombardment can increase the hardness of the counterface. Ceramics are extremely scratch-resistant, but monolithic ceramics are brittle and can fracture in vivo. I use an oxidized zirconium femoral component, which has a ceramic surface and the strength of a metal, to reduce in vivo counterface roughening and wear. The only disadvantage I see with this material is that it costs more than cobalt-chrome.

Dr. Fehring: Is there any evidence-based literature that would support the use of these newer technologies?

Dr. Mastsuda: I have not seen any randomized control studies demonstrating better wear performance in the clinical use of mobile bearings or alternative bearings. I am currently doing a randomized control trial (RCT) using an identical design for both mobile and fixed bearings. This study has not shown any improvement with mobile bearings in wear or loosening at 5 years of follow-up.[38]

Dr. Fehring: Why don't we have an evidence-based answer for this question?

Dr. Ries: Evidence-based literature to support use of alternative bearings in TKA is lacking for several reasons. Evidence-based medicine generally requires that a statistically significant clinical outcome be demonstrated in randomized prospective studies between new and conventional technologies. However, differences in outcomes related to wear are not apparent for many years. By the time a clinical outcome such as failure caused by wear and osteolysis is demonstrated, the technology may be outdated and potentially newer and better technologies have been developed. In an effort to provide the best care for our patients, many of our clinical decisions are not based on evidence-based literature. There is a large body of literature demonstrating high survivorship with mobile bearings used with gamma-irradiated in air sterilized UHMWPE. I would expect that mobile bearings with currently available conventional UHMWPE will also have excellent long-term survivorship because conventional UHMWPE (gamma-irradiated in an inert environment, ethylene oxide, or gas plasma–sterilized) has more favorable wear behavior than UHMWPE that has been sterilized by gamma irradiation in air. However, it is not clear if currently available mobile bearings will provide an advantage over fixed bearings used with currently available conventional UHMWPE, because fatigue failure is unlikely to occur with either design.

There is a large body of in vitro wear testing data to support the use of a ceramic counterface in TKA, and the literature indicates that no adverse effects have occurred from the use of oxidized zirconium in TKA.[48-50] However, long-term clinical studies that demonstrate an advantage of a hardened counterface compared with a cast cobalt-chrome counterface are not available. Although wear can be measured radiographically in total hip arthroplasty (THA), there are no reliable radiographic methods to measure wear in TKA. Evidence-based studies that demonstrate an effect of new technology on wear in TKA will require an assessment of clinical failure caused by wear as an outcome measure. Because failure caused by wear occurs after many years of in vivo use, well-controlled, large, long-term clinical studies will be needed to determine the effects accurately of new technologies intended to reduce wear in TKA.

Dr. Fehring: Who is the most appropriate candidate for an alternative bearing surface or a mobile bearing?

Dr. Matsuda: I think that the most appropriate candidates for mobile bearings would be young, active patients requiring high flexion. Theoretically, we can expect low wear from these implants and young patients would benefit from this during their extended postoperative period.

Dr. Fehring: Do you concur?

Dr. Ries: The results of TKA with conventional materials can generally be expected to provide excellent survivorship of greater than 90% at 10 years. For older or inactive patients who would not be expected to outlive the longevity of their TKA, an alternative bearing is not necessary to reduce wear further.

However, because these technologies are also associated with increased costs, the technology is best suited for young active patients who may develop wear-related failure in their lifetime with the use of conventional materials.

CROSS-LINKED POLYETHYLENE: DR. BEREND AND DR. RIES

Dr. Fehring: Cross-linked polyethylene has become the gold standard in hip arthroplasty. Clinical studies have verified the improved wear characteristics of cross-linked polyethylene in the hip. To date, such studies with regard to knee arthroplasty are lacking. Concern about the use of cross-linked polyethylene in the knee revolves around the mechanical toughness of cross-linked polyethylene in a different kinematic environment from hip arthroplasty.

What is different about the stress on the polyethylene in the knee versus the hip and why are mechanical properties of the plastic important in the knee?

Dr. Ries: The hip is a fully conforming joint with a large contact area. This results in low contact stresses, whereas the contact area in the knee is smaller and associated with higher contact stresses. The higher contact stresses in the knee have contributed to delamination and pitting observed with the use of UHMWPE that was gamma-irradiated in air and produce larger wear particles than in THA.

In THA, high stresses can also develop at the liner-locking mechanism from impingement of the neck on the acetabular rim. In high-flexion TKAs, cam post contact and femoral rollback in deep flexion results in increased stress on the post and insert baseplate locking mechanism. High strength and ductility of the UHMWPE are needed in TKA to minimize the risk of fatigue failure (delamination and pitting) and catastrophic failure of the posterior-stabilized (PS) post or insert baseplate locking mechanism.

Dr. Fehring: What concerns you most about using cross-linked polyethylene in the knee?

Dr. Berend: I have some concerns about post integrity. We know from some of the early experiences with cross-linked polyethylene in the hip that brittleness and crack propagation are significant issues, depending on the manufacturing process. In addition, in vivo oxidation may occur in some of the materials available. Therefore, the mechanical properties of the plastic may become extremely important in a PS or constrained-type knee design.

Dr. Fehring: Do you use cross-linked polyethylene in your practice today, and why or why not?

Dr. Berend: I'm just beginning to use cross-linked polyethylene in the knee as the newest generation of cross-linked polyethylene has become available. The new generation involves cross linking the polyethylene and then doping the material with tocopherol (vitamin E) to reduce the oxidation potential. Early biomechanical testing shows that the yield and tensile strength are unaffected by this manufacturing process, but the resistance to wear is significantly improved. Although this is an early experience, we have to be very vigilant with following these patients for any type of mechanical complication, early failure, or significant midterm issues with polyethylene degradation.

Dr. Fehring: How about you, Dr. Ries?

Dr. Ries: The clinical experience with the use of highly cross-linked UHMWPE in THA has been very good. Radiographic studies consistently demonstrate reduced femoral head penetration into the acetabular liner. However, occasional rim fractures have also been reported.[20,22,51] These appear to result from neck impingement and cantilever stresses on an unsupported elevated section of the rim above the metal shell. The post of a PS TKA also represents an area of unsupported UHMWPE when contacted by the cam, which could result in fracture. PS post fractures have occurred in vivo with both sterilized UHMWPE gamma-irradiated in air and gamma-irradiated in an inert atmosphere.[3,12] Because I routinely use a TKA having a cam-post mechanism, I have not used highly cross-linked UHMWPE in my TKA patients. However, there is a potential benefit of improved abrasion resistance and little risk of fracture using highly cross-linked UHMWPE in a posterior cruciate–retaining TKA because there is no cam-post mechanism.[23]

Dr. Fehring: Are there patients for whom we should routinely use cross-linked polyethylene and, conversely, are there patients for whom we should avoid this type of polyethylene?

Dr. Ries: The experience from the use of highly cross-linked UHMWPE in THA and in vitro wear simulator studies in TKA indicate that wear in TKA can be reduced with the use of highly cross-linked UHMWPE. However, highly cross-linked UHMWPE has diminished mechanical properties compared with conventional UHMWPE. This risk needs to be assessed to determine if the risk-benefit ratio with the use of highly cross-linked UHMWPE in TKA is favorable.

In TKA, the stresses on the insert–baseplate locking mechanism would be expected to be higher with the use of a cam-post mechanism. For cruciate-retaining (CR) designs in which the anteroposterior (AP) tibiofemoral position is controlled more by ligaments and dynamic muscular forces, the insert locking mechanism stresses and risk of mechanical failure with the use of highly cross-linked UHMWPE would be expected to be low. For CR designs, the use of highly cross-linked UHMWPE appears to be safe.[23] For younger, more active patients who may experience failure because of wear and require future revision surgery, the use of highly cross-linked UHMWPE in CR TKA has a favorable risk-benefit ratio. For cam-post designs, it is difficult to assess the level of risk of post or insert locking mechanism failure. Modular implants with more articular constraint and cam-post mechanisms should be evaluated to determine if the insert-baseplate locking mechanisms and post designs are sufficient to be used with highly cross-linked UHMWPE. Highly cross-linked UHMWPE in these implants should probably be reserved more for young patients at high risk of failure because of wear and avoided in patients at high risk of failure because of mechanical overload, such as overweight active patients, until more information is available about the safety of these designs when used with highly cross-linked UHMWPE.

COMPUTER-ASSISTED SURGERY AND ROBOTICS: DR. LONNER AND DR. MATSUDA

Dr. Fehring: Computer-assisted surgery (CAS) and robotics have recently been advocated as ways to improve surgical accuracy and improve alignment and, in some types of CAS, work flows aid in soft tissue balance. Controversy exists over the cost-effectiveness of this technology and whether improvement in surgical accuracy and alignment will lead to improved functional results.

In your practice, do you use CAS or robotic surgery for your patients, and why?

Dr. Matsuda: I do use CT-based computer navigation for my patients. In my practice, and in the literature, it has been shown that navigation achieved better alignment than conventional methods.[39,42] With the use of CT scanning, higher accuracy of rotational alignment can be achieved.[40] Previous studies have shown that 4 to 5 degrees of malalignment has been correlated with poor clinical results. Therefore, I believe that the use of CT-based navigation would improve wear performance and decrease mechanical loosening.

Dr. Fehring: Do you use CAS or robotics?

Dr. Lonner: I use robotic assistance for unicompartmental knee arthroplasty (UKA; unicondylar arthroplasty). The use

of robotic instrumentation improves the accuracy of bone preparation. The current robotic technology available in the United States is semiautonomous, meaning that the surgeon controls the robotic arm, but the tip of the burr is constrained by the system within the predetermined area on the bones. The improved accuracy of bone preparation is expected to improve durability of the implants. I do not use CAS with conventional cutting techniques for UKA or TKA.

Dr. Fehring: Have you noticed a functional improvement in your patients since using CAS or robotics, respectively?

Dr. Matsuda: Honestly, I have not noticed any functional improvement in range of motion, recovery, muscle strength, or gait by using computer navigation. Only a few studies[13,33] have shown the efficacy of computer navigation for improving knee function in the short term.

Dr. Fehring: What about robotics, Dr. Lonner—any functional improvement?

Dr. Lonner: I have noticed improved functional outcomes with robotic-assisted techniques, with more rapid recovery. This may be to the result of the diminished soft tissue trauma compared with the use of conventional cutting guides. However, no study has been done that demonstrates whether there is any functional difference in early outcomes after UKA using robotic arm technology or conventional techniques.

Dr. Fehring: As reimbursement continues to diminish, there is economic pressure to improve efficiency as well as to increase procedure throughput.

Dr. Lonner, how long do robotics add to the length of the procedure, and how do you rationalize this in an era of diminishing reimbursement?

Dr. Lonner: The learning curve with the robotic arm technology that I am currently using is very short. The time can be reduced considerably by creating a system of efficiency that includes working with a staff that is familiar with the setup of the system. If a surgeon operates in one room, however, the setup time can be an extra 20 to 40 minutes. This may not be much longer than the setup time when conventional instrumentation sets are used. If a surgeon has the luxury of staggering cases between two rooms, ideally the setup is done while the surgeon is in the second room. The surgical time is not significantly different than when using conventional instrumentation. There is a small additional billable fee for use of navigation that many insurers honor.

Dr. Fehring: What about CAS?

Dr. Matsuda: Computer navigation adds approximately 15 minutes in my practice. I do two or three total knee surgeries per day and, in this situation, lengthening 15 minutes of surgery time does not affect my surgery schedule. For high-volume surgeons, however, the use of navigation would decrease the number of surgeries.

PARTIAL COMPARTMENT REPLACEMENT: DR. HOFMANN AND DR. LONNER

Dr. Fehring: Partial joint replacement has undergone a resurgence in interest in the last few years. Proponents of unicondylar arthroplasty have debated whether patellofemoral arthritis was a contraindication to this procedure.

Dr. Hofmann, Do you think that patellofemoral arthritis is a contraindication to unicondylar arthroplasty?

Dr. Hofmann: The role of patellofemoral arthritis in unicondylar arthroplasty in the published literature is still controversial, ranging from "it is not a problem"[6] to "clear contraindication."[9] To the best of my knowledge, there is no prospective randomized study available that would help solve this problem. In my own practice, I base my decision on clinical symptoms, a functional weight-bearing patella axial view,[4] and intraoperative findings (not more than diffuse grade I or focal grade II chondromalacia at the trochlea and patella). If one of these three findings is present, I would go directly to a TKA.

Dr. Fehring: What is your philosophy?

Dr. Lonner: In years past, I would not have considered a unicompartmental arthroplasty in a patient who had anterior knee pain and/or radiographic patellofemoral (PF) arthritis. In recent years, however, my approach has changed slightly. If a patient has anterior knee pain with any activities (but particularly stairs, sitting, hills), I would perform a UKA unless I could establish that the anterior pain is not emanating from the medial (or lateral) compartments. If a patient has advanced PF arthritis, I would not offer an isolated UKA because of the risk of early and accelerated PF pain. I'd be more likely in the situation of advanced medial and patellofemoral arthritis to combine a UKA with a PF arthroplasty (PFA). If a patient has no anterior knee pain with activities, climbs stairs and hills comfortably, and has no patellofemoral pain with compression testing, then I would perform an isolated UKA even if there is a small area of focal grade IV chondromalacia.

Dr. Fehring: Do you prefer a traditional total knee or a bicompartmental prosthesis if the medial compartment and patellofemoral joint are arthritic?

Dr. Lonner: My preference has become a modular bicompartmental arthroplasty for bicompartmental disease, provided the other tibiofemoral compartment has no symptoms, the deformity is minimal, there is no flexion contracture (less than 5 degrees), good ROM and stability, and no bony deficiency. Once you start to see varus more than 10 degrees and valgus greater than 15 degrees or flexion contractures, the deformity is often uncorrectable and is better managed with a TKA. A patient who has had a bicompartmental arthroplasty often believes that a bicompartmental arthroplasty is more normal-feeling than a TKA. I also prefer it as a bone- and ligament-conserving alternative to TKA so if it fails, revision can be done with greater ease.

Dr. Fehring: Do you agree?

Dr. Hofmann: In this situation, I perform a conventional TKA. The reason why we have not started with the bicompartmental solution are the poor to medium outcomes of these combined procedures in the literature.[44] Furthermore, they are technically very demanding. If we cannot correct the pathologic biomechanics that have caused the failure of the natural patellofemoral joint, the replacement will fail again.

Dr. Fehring: Is there a role for isolated patellofemoral arthroplasty and who would you consider the ideal candidate?

Dr. Hofmann: About 5% to 10% of our patients (mainly female) have isolated patellofemoral arthritis. It is well known that TKA with and without patellar replacement works well in these patients.[16] Nevertheless, it does not seem to be the best solution to replace a well-functioning tibiofemoral joint without arthritis to solve isolated patellofemoral problems. So far, the outcome of the patellofemoral replacement procedures show wide variation and are not as consistent as TKA.[18] This might be the reason why most surgeons still perform a TKA in this situation.

We strongly believe that the overall unsatisfactory results of this procedure is caused by the lack of biomechanical understanding of the failure mechanism of the natural joint. Furthermore, the surgical technique and implant designs are not addressing the different causes sufficiently.

Dr. Fehring: Dr. Lonner, I believe you are a strong proponent of patellofemoral arthroplasty. Please explain its role in your practice.

Dr. Lonner: There is a role for isolated PF arthroplasty. The ideal candidate is a patient with isolated anterior knee pain or medial or lateral peripatellar pain caused by patellofemoral osteoarthritis or post-traumatic arthritis. It is not appropriate for inflammatory arthritis or chondrocalcinosis because of the potential for tibiofemoral or soft tissue pain that can compromise the outcome. It can be most effective for arthritis that has occurred as a sequela of patellofemoral dysplasia, but should be avoided in patients with considerable maltracking or malalignment, unless they can be corrected. Mild patellar subluxation or tilt can be corrected during patellofemoral arthroplasty with appropriate component rotational and axial alignment as well as a lateral retinacular release, but large Q angles (>20 degrees in women and >15 degrees in men), measured preoperatively, should be corrected first with tibial tubercle anteromedialization. Newer trochlear component designs may accommodate slightly more patellar malalignment but, in general, a PF prosthesis should not be called on to stabilize the patella. As little as grade III tibiofemoral chondromalacia can result in discomfort after patellofemoral arthroplasty. This procedure must be used with caution in this situation. This procedure is contraindicated in cases with advanced tibiofemoral chondromalacia or arthrosis observed at the time of arthrotomy or on review of photographs from prior arthroscopic surgery. Although arthroscopic assessment can be helpful, there is no data that identify whether it is necessary prior to patellofemoral arthroplasty. Newer MRI technologies improve the ability to assess preoperatively the integrity of the articular cartilage of the weight-bearing surfaces of the tibiofemoral joints. There are no data currently available regarding whether a cruciate ligament deficiency or obesity will predispose to premature failure of patellofemoral arthroplasty. It should generally be avoided in patients with medial and lateral joint line pain and morbid obesity. There is no age restriction, provided the patient fits the criteria noted.

UNICONDYLAR ARTHROPLASTY: DR. LONNER AND DR. LOMBARDI

Dr. Fehring: Arthroplasty surgeons use registry data to help with clinical decision making. Recently, some large registries have reported early failure rates as well as diminished survival of unicondylar arthroplasty.

Dr. Lombardi, please review these and give your thoughts.

Dr. Lombardi: After a spike in unicondylar arthroplasty about 5 years ago, there seems to be a decrease in the numbers of unicondylar replacements being performed, now approaching traditional levels. Indeed, several years ago, there was an initial spike in enthusiasm with unicompartmental knee arthroplasty. This spike was fueled by a number of factors. Perhaps the most important factor was the desire to perform minimally invasive surgical procedures. John Repicci identified that unicompartmental knee arthroplasty could be performed with small incisions and without subluxing the patella. He noted that this diminution in iatrogenic trauma to the suprapatellar pouch enhanced postoperative physiotherapy and decreased the number of postoperative physical therapy sessions required for the patient to obtain a satisfactory range of motion. Repicci's limited surgical approach was coupled with enhancements in prosthetic design and in surgical technique.[47] Furthermore, the Nuffield Orthopaedic Centre expanded the indications[21] for unicompartmental knee arthroplasty beyond the limited scope dictated by the Kozinn and Scott indications.[27] These improvements led to the approval by the U.S. Food and Drug Administration (FDA) of a mobile-bearing unicompartmental knee arthroplasty system. In their wisdom, the FDA required that all surgeons wishing to perform the mobile-bearing unicompartmental knee arthroplasty be trained with a specific training program. Orthopedists responded by attending these training programs and increasing the number of unicompartmental knee arthroplasties performed.

However, although over the past year there has been a decrease in the number of unicompartmental knee arthroplasties performed, it has not returned to its traditional level. Three factors are thought to contribute to this decline: First, not all patients are extremely satisfied with a unicompartmental knee arthroplasty. Frequently, patients develop a pes anserinus bursitis and require conservative care with ultrasound and phonophoresis or corticosteroid injections. These symptoms resolve in a 12- to 18-month period. However, if these patients are not satisfied with waiting, they may seek second opinions and undergo revision or conversion to a total knee arthroplasty. Some surgeons are reluctant to deal with these patients and, therefore, have decreased the number of unicompartmental knee arthroplasties that they perform. The second reason for the decrease in the number of unicompartmental knee arthroplasties may be related to the current economic crisis. Because these patients tend to be younger patients with private insurance, they often fear that loss of time from work may equate to a loss of their job. Therefore, they have become more tolerant and willing to postpone their surgical intervention. The third factor may also be financial. Orthopedists are compensated less for a unicompartmental knee arthroplasty than for a total knee arthroplasty, despite the fact that the technique is more surgically demanding. Therefore, some orthopedists have discontinued their use of unicompartmental knee arthroplasty.

Dr. Fehring: What percentage of arthritic knee patients in your practice do you think are candidates for this procedure?

Dr. Lonner: Overuse of the technology can be problematic. Appropriate patient selection is important to avoid early failures from preventable issues, such as the presence of patellofemoral arthritis. In the future, younger patients may come in for UKA rather than waiting until they are old enough for TKA. Surgeons are using osteotomies less in practice now, and instead are considering UKA more frequently. In my practice, 10% to 12% is unicondylar arthroplasty. Combining UKA with PF arthroplasty will likely expand the indications for use to 20% to 30% of our knee arthroplasty patients.

Dr. Fehring: What about your practice, Dr. Lombardi?

Dr. Lombardi: Historically, the percentage of patients presenting with arthritic knees who are candidates for unicompartmental knee arthroplasty has been approximately 5%. With the expanded indications based on the Nuffield Orthopaedic Centre experience, the Nuffield surgeons noted that as many as 30% of their patients may be candidates for unicompartmental knee arthroplasty.[5,41,46,50] In my current practice, the percentage of patients presenting with arthritic knees who are candidates for unicompartmental knee arthroplasty is approximately 10%.

Dr. Fehring: Who is the ideal unicondylar candidate?

Dr. Lonner: The classic recommendations are attributed to Kozinn and Scott,[27] who advocated restricting unicompartmental arthroplasty to low-demand patients older than 60 years with unicompartmental osteoarthritis or focal osteonecrosis. Additionally, they recommended that patients weigh less than 82 kg (181 lb), have a minimum 90-degree flexion arc and flexion contracture of less than 5 degrees, an angular deformity not exceeding 10 degrees of varus or 15 degrees of valgus (both of which should be correctable to neutral passively after removal of osteophytes), an intact anterior cruciate ligament, and no pain or exposed bone in the patellofemoral or opposite tibiofemoral compartment.

More recently, the indications for unicompartmental arthroplasty have expanded to include younger and more active patients. Obese patients have been shown to have compromised outcomes, although unicompartmental arthroplasty is a reasonable option for patients who are only mildly obese. I would not advocate the procedure for morbidly obese patients. Incompetence of the anterior cruciate ligament (ACL) may cause abnormal knee kinematics and anterior tibial subluxation, which will typically result in posterior tibial wear. However, although ACL insufficiency had historically been considered an absolute contraindication to UKA, it is now considered a reasonable option if there is limited functional instability and the area of femoral contact on the tibia in extension and the location of the tibiofemoral arthritis are anterior. Minimizing the tibial slope in the ACL-deficient knee during UKA is critical, however, to ensure durability.

Significant subchondral bone loss caused by a large cyst or extensive focal osteonecrosis with structural compromise may predispose the knee to component subsidence and should thus be considered a contraindication to unicompartmental arthroplasty. Additionally, UKA should be restricted to those without inflammatory arthritis and crystalline arthropathy (e.g., gout, chondrocalcinosis), because these can increase the risk of pain and accelerated degeneration of the remaining compartments of the knee. Patient with areas of grade IV chondromalacia in other compartments of the knee should also not be considered candidates for unicompartmental arthroplasty. However, lesser stages of chondromalacia should not be considered contraindications unless the patient reports pain in those compartments.

It is a point of debate whether the presence of patellofemoral arthritis is a contraindication to the performance of unicompartmental arthroplasty. The classic indications suggest that no more than grade III patellofemoral chondromalacia should be present. However, recent studies with a mobile-bearing medial unicompartmental arthroplasty design have suggested that the presence of preoperative patellofemoral arthritis and patellofemoral symptoms are not a contraindication to unicompartmental arthroplasty and, in fact, do not adversely affect the outcomes. This has not been corroborated with fixed-bearing designs or in other studies, and further investigation will be necessary to determine the role of patellofemoral symptoms or arthritis on UKA outcomes.

Dr. Fehring: In your opinion, is this an operation for the very young and very old or is it applicable to all age groups?

Dr. Lombardi: In my opinion, this operation is applicable to all age groups. It is certainly indicated for the very young and the very old. Having said this, there is no reason that the middle-aged patient is not also an ideal candidate. Unicondylar knee arthroplasty treats the patient's symptoms and gives the patient a knee that feels more normal.[43]

KINEMATICS: DR. MATSUDA, DR. HOFMANN, AND DR. RIES

Dr. Fehring: There has been a trend in knee arthroplasty design recently to mimic normal knee kinematics in an attempt to improve function and lessen anterior knee pain.

Dr. Ries, what design modifications can help make a knee replacement more closely resemble the kinematics of a normal knee?

Dr. Ries: ACL-retaining TKAs have been used in the past and were abandoned because of problems of implant breakage, loosening, and stiffness. However, the kinematics after ACL-retaining TKA were relatively normal.[2] There are a number of anatomic differences between the normal and replaced knee that contribute to the abnormal kinematics that is typically observed after TKA. Posterior stability and posterior cruciate ligament (PCL) function can be achieved with a posterior cam-post mechanism. However, anterior stability to replicate ACL function requires a different mechanism, such as an anterior cam-post mechanism or highly conforming tibiofemoral joint articular surfaces.

During flexion, the femur rolls back on the tibia and rotates externally. The lateral tibial plateau of the normal knee is relatively convex while the medial plateau is more concave to permit this motion. Femoral external rotation during knee flexion after TKA can be achieved with an asymmetrical cam-post mechanism to drive more lateral than medial rollback. A more anatomic polyethylene insert, where the medial plateau is more conforming, coupled with a posteriorly sloped lateral plateau may improve kinematic function.

Dr. Fehring: Is there a design that is superior?

Dr. Hofmann: The knee is the most complex joint and its biomechanics are still not understood completely. Dynamic MRI, three-dimensional computer models and in vivo fluoroscopy have significantly improved our knowledge in the last few years. A number of sophisticated designs, including medial and lateral pivoting, single-radius, different mobile bearings, and ACL- and PCL-substituting knees have been brought on the market in the last decade. To the best of my knowledge, it has never been proven that one of these new designs has shown clinically better function or patient satisfaction.

Dr. Fehring: In your opinion, can a knee replacement without an anterior cruciate mimic normal knee kinematics?

Dr. Hofmann: Normal knee kinematics is possible only when a sufficient medial-lateral cruciate ligament and ACL-PCL are present. During the last 20 years, there has been controversy among surgeons who wish to have natural biomechanics and those who prefer simple and reproducible biomechanics after TKA. Because the ACL is resected in almost all our TKAs, the kinematics will never not be normal again. In ACL-insufficient knees, the center of axial rotation is moving from medial to lateral. Nevertheless, medial and lateral pivoting knees have not been shown to produce better biomechanics. The new design of anterior and posterior substitution with guided motion is an interesting biomechanical concept. However, I doubt that this will show clinically relevant better biomechanics.

Dr. Fehring: What is your opinion?

Dr. Ries: Kinematic studies of conventional PCL-retaining TKAs have demonstrated paradoxical motion, in which the femur is positioned relatively posteriorly on the tibia in extension and, during knee flexion, the femur translates anteriorly.[17] The posterior cam-post mechanism of a PS TKA prevents anterior femoral translation in flexion. However, lack of an ACL contributes to the posterior position of the femur on the tibia in extension. Anterior stability can be achieved during knee extension with an anterior cam-post mechanism in which the anterior part of the PS box engages with the anterior side of a PS post to prevent anterior tibial translation in extension.[11,53]

Dr. Fehring: How can the cam-post mechanism in a posterior-stabilized knee drive normal knee kinematics?

Dr. Matsuda: The cam-post mechanism can drive near-normal posterior rollback of the femur and an anterior cam can give anterior stability. I do not think, however, that the post can control rotational movement. Axial rotation differs among patients because of different rotational alignment, muscle force, or soft tissue balancing. Therefore, the cam-post mechanism should accommodate rotational movement rather than control rotational movement. A round-on-round shape at the post-cam mechanism in the axial plane or mobile-bearing prosthesis should be used to avoid edge loading.[1]

Dr. Fehring: Can the shape of the cam-post mechanism help?

Dr. Ries: The posterior cam drives posterior rollback of the femoral condyles on the tibia during flexion, but typically does not control rotation. For normal kinematics to be achieved, the lateral condylar rollback needs to be greater than the medial condylar rollback, which produces femoral external rotation or a screw-home mechanism. Asymmetry in the geometry of the cam or post in which the lateral side of the cam is wider than the medial side can drive more lateral than medial femoral rollback during knee flexion.

Dr. Fehring: Assuming a knee can be manufactured that can mimic normal knee kinematics, can implantation be forgiving enough to the variety of surgical techniques and skill sets in the marketplace?

Dr. Hofmann: From my own experience during surgery and teaching, there is a clear correlation between design and surgical technique. The more sophisticated the design, the less forgiving is the surgical technique. The two classic designs with fixed-bearing PS and mobile rotating platforms have shown during the last 2 decades that they offer simple biomechanics but forgiving technique. Furthermore we do not operate on biomechanical normal knees in most cases. It begs the question of whether severe arthritic knees ever go back to normal biomechanics.

In TKA, 90% of the success is the surgeon and her or his instruments, and only 10% the design. On the other hand, about 20% of our patients with TKA are not satisfied. Furthermore, the early revision rates within the first years is still unacceptably high and the curve has not changed significantly during the last 2 decades. Training and education are much more important than striving for more sophisticated designs. If every knee surgeon would follow the 10 basic principles for TKA, the satisfaction rate would immediately increase.

REHABILITATION PROTOCOLS AND PAIN MANAGEMENT: DR. HOFMANN AND DR. LOMBARDI

Dr. Fehring: One of the true clinical improvements in knee arthroplasty is the area of perioperative pain management and accelerated rehabilitation. A variety of spinal and regional anesthetic techniques have allowed us to avoid the side effects of general anesthesia as well as improve postoperative pain control. Adequate oral analgesics have allowed patients to avoid the sedative effects of parenteral narcotics and participate in their rehabilitation more quickly.

Dr. Lombardi, in your center, what do you use for anesthesia for your routine knee arthroplasty patients?

Dr. Lombard: Perhaps the single most important outcome from the whole minimally invasive movement has been an enhanced understanding of the multimodal approach to pain management of patients undergoing arthroplasty. Enhancement of our perioperative pain management protocols has resulted in accelerated rehabilitation.[8,29,31,35,36]

At our facility, most patients undergoing total and partial knee arthroplasty are treated with a single-shot spinal anesthetic. This consists of a combination of bupivacaine and morphine injection (Duramorph). The bupivacaine affords the immediate perioperative anesthetic and the morphine results in sustained analgesia for a period of 12 to 24 hours. Prophylactic antiemetics are administered in the form of dexamethasone, ondansetron, and a scopolamine patch. The use of this perioperative anesthesia allows for effective pain relief without motor blockade. Patients are therefore able to participate in physiotherapy within several hours of the operative procedure. On the day of surgery, patients perform active range of motion and ambulate with assistive devices. This has resulted in a decrease in length of stay, with our current average length of stay being less than 2 days.

Dr. Fehring: At our center, we use femoral nerve catheters along with single-shot sciatic nerve blocks routinely. Patients are pain-free the first 18 hours or so and require no narcotics during this period. After the blocks wear off, the patient is maintained on oral narcotics. In my opinion, these blocks have been the greatest advance in pain management in my career.

Dr. Hofmann, what analgesics do you use perioperatively?

Dr. Hofmann: We have developed a perioperative multimodality pain management program (PMP). This includes local infiltration anaesthesia (LIA) and sophisticated oral pain management.[45] The principles of this regime are oral administration at the right time and high doses of non-narcotic pain

killers to optimize the use of oral narcotics. This includes celecoxib and ondansetron for the prevention of perioperative nausea and vomiting. Both are started before surgery, as well as metamizol and low-dose hydromorphone. The pain medication is standardized for all patients and administered at 7 AM and 7 PM.

Immediately after surgery, and until discharge, the patients are actively asked three times a day (9 AM, 2 PM, and 9 PM) about their pain level using the visual analogue scale (VAS) by the nursing staff. Whenever the VAS score is more than 3, standardized rescue medication is administered within 10 minutes. In a prospective study on 100 consecutive TKAs, the effectiveness and practicability of this PMP was studied; 8% of patients had to be excluded because of contraindications or organization problems. In the remaining 92 patients, the average VAS at any time was 2.8 and no patient had a VAS score higher than 5. The subjective results for the patients were excellent and negative side effects were seen in only 6% of patients.

Dr. Fehring: Do you use intra-articular injections?

Dr. Lombardi: We have used and continue to use intra-articular injections. Our data, along with that of others, has demonstrated the benefit of the use of intra-articular injections with respect to the multimodal approach to pain management of the patient undergoing total knee arthroplasty.[47,52,53] Although these authors have demonstrated the benefit of intra-articular injections, there has been no consensus on the ideal medications or dosage that should be used. What is clear is that the injections must be delivered directly into the soft tissue rather than simply an intra-articular injection, which bathes the soft tissues. Our current intra-articular injection is 60 mL of 0.5% ropivacaine with 0.5 mg of epinephrine. In patients with normal renal function, 30 mg of ketorolac is added. The injection is administered throughout all the soft tissues in and around the knee. Therefore, our multimodal approach to perioperative pain management involves the use of a long-acting oral narcotic, oxycodone, combined with an anti-inflammatory, celecoxib. A single-shot spinal is administered with an acute anesthetic, bupivacaine, and a long-acting analgesic, Duramorph. Perioperative breakthrough pain is treated with intravenous narcotics, such as hydromorphone (Dilaudid). Patients are then transitioned to oxycodone and hydrocodone.

Dr. Fehring: Comment on your thoughts concerning the feasibility of outpatient knee arthroplasty.

Dr. Lombardi: Total knee arthroplasty represents a significant operative intervention. Patients undergoing this procedure should be evaluated preoperatively by an appropriate medical team and their preoperative medical status should be optimized. Effective multimodal pain management protocols should be established. The key to success of these protocols is management of the patient's pain without motor blockade so that the patient can participate in physiotherapy and rehabilitation. Using this protocol, we find that over 50% of our patients are able to be discharged on postoperative day 1. Therefore, it is feasible that this group of patients could be treated in an outpatient setting. Patients enrolled in outpatient total knee arthroplasty would have to undergo intensive preoperative screening. These patients should have optimization of their medical status with a thorough preoperative medical clearance. They should represent a group of patients with minimal medical comorbidities. They should have a high tolerance to pain and should not have been managed preoperatively with narcotics. They require preoperative education and should attend preoperative physiotherapy. They also require a very involved and engaged caretaker who will be there to assist them on discharge. If these criteria are met, then it is possible to consider outpatient total knee arthroplasty.

Dr. Fehring: Do you agree?

Dr. Hofmann: Outpatient TKA has been tried at several places. I do not think that this makes sense. More than 80% of all complications after TKA occur within the first 4 days. This would have a significant impact on patients' safety and outcome. Furthermore, the logistics for outpatient TKA are difficult and expensive. In my country, the patients would not accept this outpatient service. MIS unicondylar knees show significant less trauma and bleeding and might benefit from an outpatient service in selected cases with sophisticated pain management.

KEY REFERENCES

Andriacchi TP, Galante JO, Fermier RW: The influence of total knee replacement design on walking and stair climbing. J Bone Joint Surg Am 64:1328, 1982.

Berger RA, Nedeff DD, Barden RM, et al: Unicompartmental knee arthroplasty. Clinical experience at 6- to 10-year followup. Clin Orthop Relat Res 367:50, 1999.

Bozic K, Beringer D: Economic considerations in minimally invasive total knee arthroplasty. Clin Orthop Relat Res 463:20, 2007.

Catani F, Innocenti B, Belvedere C, et al: The Mark Coventry Award: Articular contact estimation in TKA using in vivo kinematics and finite element analysis. Clin Orthop Relat Res 468:19, 2010.

Choong PF, Dowsey PF, Stoney JD: Does accurate anatomical alignment result in better function and quality of life? Comparing conventional and computer-assisted total knee arthroplasty. J Arthroplasty 24:560, 2009.

Dalury D, Dennis D: Minimal incision total knee arthroplasty can increase risk of component malalignment. Clin Orthop Relat Res 440:71, 2005.

Dennis DA, Komistek RD, Mahfouz MR, et al: Multicenter determination of in vivo kinematics after total knee arthroplasty. Clin Orthop Relat Res 416:37−57, 2003.

Mason JB, Fehring TK, Estok R, et al: Meta-analysis of alignment outcomes in computer-assisted total knee arthroplasty. J Arthroplasty 22:1097, 2007.

Mizu-uchi H, Matsuda S, Miura H, et al: The evaluation of post-operative alignment in total knee replacement using a CT-based navigation system. J Bone Joint Surg Br 90:1025, 2008.

Murray DW, Goodfellow JW, O'Connor JJ: The Oxford medial unicompartmental arthroplasty: a ten-year survival study. J Bone Joint Surg Br 80:983, 1998.

Noble PC, Gordon MJ, Weiss JM, et al: Does total knee replacement restore normal knee function? Clin Orthop Relat Res 431:157, 2005.

Ries MD, Salehi A, Widding K, Hunter G: Polyethylene wear performance of oxidized zirconium and cobalt-chromium knee components under abrasive conditions. J Bone Joint Surg Am 84:S129, 2002.

Full references for this chapter can be found on www.expertconsult.com.

Complications of Total Knee Arthroplasty

Saurabh Khakharia, Michael P. Nett, Christopher A. Hajnik, and Giles R. Scuderi

GENERAL COMPLICATIONS

The results following total knee arthroplasty (TKA) are excellent. The literature demonstrates over 90% survivorship at 20 years with a well-performed arthroplasty. Despite routine excellent outcomes, as with any substantial surgery, complications occur. With the newly initiated Surgical Care Improvement Project (SCIP) initiative, emphasis has been placed on avoiding preventable complications during the perioperative period. This chapter will focus on management of complications but avoidance and prevention will also be discussed.

Prevention of medical complications begins with the preoperative evaluation. Prior to total knee arthroplasty, the patient should be evaluated by the primary care physician for preoperative medical clearance. The orthopedic surgeon is also responsible for reviewing the medical history and should note the comorbidities that must be addressed to minimize the chance of complication. Memtsoudis et al[151] has recently reported on in-hospital complications, including mortality, following unilateral, bilateral, and revision total knee arthroplasty. Over 4 million discharges were evaluated with regard to patient demographics, comorbidities, and in-hospital stay. Complications and mortality of each procedure were compared. In this series, in-hospital mortality was highest for patients who had bilateral total knee arthroplasty (0.5%) whereas the lowest mortality rate was associated with unicompartmental TKA (0.3%). It was interesting to note that revision total knee arthroplasties had a similarly low mortality rate of 0.3%. The overall complication rate during hospitalization was highest for bilateral total knee arthroplasties, 12.2%, but the rate for in-hospital complications following unicompartmental TKA was still 8.2%.

A patient's medical history should be reviewed carefully if bilateral TKA is contemplated. Although several studies have demonstrated success in bilateral procedures, numerous studies have demonstrated the higher risk of complication.[28,50] Younger patients in good health seem to tolerate a bilateral procedure with little increased risk. However, older or obese patients, and those with an extensive medical or cardiac history, should be discouraged from considering a bilateral procedure. If a bilateral procedure is performed, postoperative monitoring should be considered.

SYSTEMIC COMPLICATIONS

Thromboembolism

DVT occurs in approximately 50% of unilateral cases and in 75% of bilateral cases when no prophylaxis is used. Although DVT occurs mainly in the calf veins (Fig. 125-1), life-threatening emboli do not arise from this region. In contrast to the situation after total hip arthroplasty (THA), isolated proximal vein thrombosis does not seem to occur after knee surgery, despite the possible trauma of a pneumatic tourniquet.

Some have argued that distal thrombosis can be ignored, provided that the patient convalesces normally and is not confined to bed for a lengthy period. We believe that this view is too optimistic, although we concede that the risk of a fatal thromboembolus is small and is lower than that after THA. In a prospective review of 527 TKAs in 499 patients, Khaw and colleagues,[118] using no prophylaxis other than antithrombotic stockings and relatively early (48 hours) mobilization, found only one death in 3 months from pulmonary embolism (0.19%). This patient had bilateral TKA and had a myocardial infarction 1 day postoperatively, with the subsequent pulmonary embolus occurring 22 days postoperatively. Seven other patients (1.3%) developed symptomatic pulmonary embolism and were treated with anticoagulation, without sequelae. This low incidence of fatal pulmonary embolism has been supported in other studies by Stulberg and associates (0%),[214] Stringer and coworkers (0%),[213] Khaw and colleagues (0.2%),[118] and Ansari and associates (0.4%).[4] Fatal emboli do occur, however, and three patients died as a result of emboli in the first 400 arthroplasties performed at the Hospital for Special Surgery. No specific prophylaxis was used at that time; the cause of death was confirmed by autopsy in all cases. In addition, we believe that the incidence of fatal pulmonary emboli is underestimated. A certain proportion of calf clots propagate proximally to form the more dangerous clots in the popliteal and femoral veins. This process takes time, however, and the major risk period for a fatal pulmonary embolism after TKA may be in weeks 3 and 4 postsurgery; this is in contrast to what occurs after THA, in which a clot in the proximal veins may be found in 20% of cases after the first week. Because most TKA patients now are discharged after hospitalization of 2 to 3 days, sudden death at home in a patient having no clinical evidence of vein thrombosis may be attributed to myocardial infarction.

Calf clots may not in themselves be important, but should be regarded as a harbinger of more proximal clotting. Haas and coworkers[85] have studied 1329 patients with 1697 TKAs. Thrombosis was found in 808 patients (61%); 53% had thrombosis of the calf vein and 8% had thrombosis of the proximal veins. The lung scans of 60 patients (4.5%) were positive, and symptomatic pulmonary emboli occurred in 14 patients (1.1%). All these patients received aspirin as prophylaxis. Venography was performed between postoperative days 4 and 6. A perfusion lung scan obtained on postoperative day 5 to 7 was compared with a preoperative baseline perfusion lung scan. Thrombosis of the calf vein was treated with warfarin (Coumadin); the dosage was adjusted to maintain a prothrombin time at approximately 1.5 times control. Only patients with symptomatic proximal thrombi or symptomatic pulmonary emboli were fully anticoagulated with intravenous

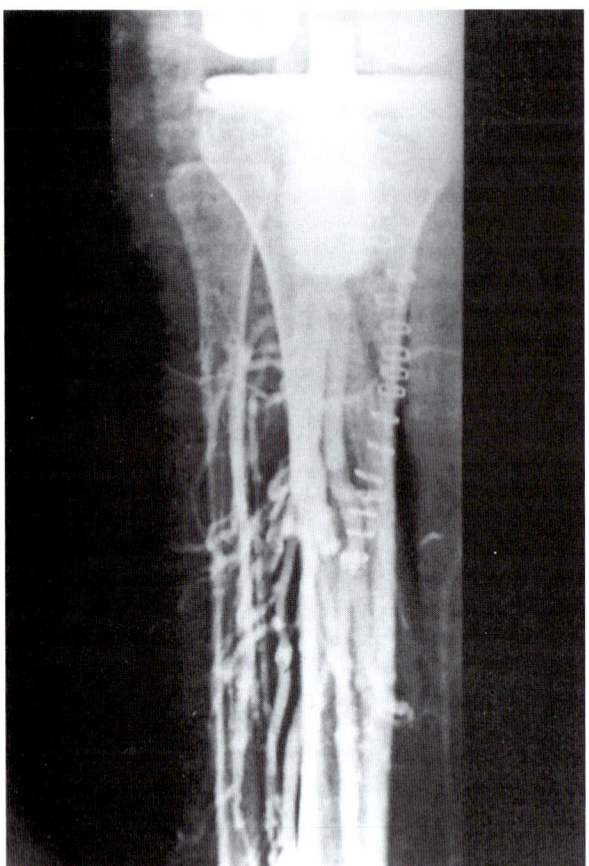

Figure 125-1. Venogram showing clots in the calf veins.

heparin. Although the natural history of thromboembolic disease was altered by prophylaxis and treatment, 6.5% of patients with calf thrombi had a positive lung scan and 1.6% had symptomatic pulmonary emboli. This finding was compared with patients who had no venographic evidence of deep vein thrombosis (DVT), of whom 1.9% had a positive lung scan and 0.2% had symptomatic pulmonary emboli. Statistical significances for the difference in lung scan and pulmonary embolus results were $P = .001$ and $P = .034$, respectively. Patients with calf or proximal thrombi were found to have similar rates of positive lung scans and symptomatic pulmonary emboli.

The risk of symptomatic and fatal pulmonary embolism is of greatest concern. Without prophylaxis, the rates of pulmonary embolism and fatal pulmonary embolism range from 1% to 28% and 0.1% to 2.0%, respectively.[74] From six randomized studies comparing low-molecular-weight heparin (LMWH) with warfarin, the total rate of DVT was 33% for patients who received LMWH compared with 48% for patients who received warfarin. Similarly, the rate of proximal DVT was 7.1% and 10.4% for patients who received LMWH and warfarin, respectively. Barrett and colleagues[11] have reviewed 122,385 U.S. Medicare enrollees who had a TKA in 2000. Pulmonary embolism developed in the first 3 months in 0.81% of patients who had a unilateral TKA compared with 1.44% of patients who had undergone a simultaneous bilateral TKA.

The discussion of appropriate DVT prophylaxis is covered elsewhere in this text and is beyond the scope of this chapter.

Many questions concerning how best to effect thromboprophylaxis in the orthopedic setting remain unanswered, and our (likely unobtainable) need for an ideal strategy combining complete efficacy with absolute safety remains unmet. However, we should not permit such questions and needs from obscuring fundamental truths made clear by intense research over the past several decades: (1) venous thromboembolism (VTE) is a known and serious complication of total joint arthroplasty; (2) evidence-based thromboprophylaxis works; (3) the orthopedic community needs to improve compliance with available guidelines and work on reaching a consensus.

Protocol for Patients With Documented Thromboembolic Disease

Positive Venography or Ultrasound

Patients with calf, popliteal, or femoral thrombi are treated with warfarin for 6 weeks. Asymptomatic pulmonary emboli are treated in the same manner. Symptomatic proximal thrombi and symptomatic pulmonary emboli are treated with heparin until the effect of the warfarin is established.[225] Based on the discretion of the individual medical consultant, heparin treatment intravenously may be continued for 1 week. Intravenous heparin carries an extreme risk of local bleeding complications and, in our opinion, should be used only in potentially life-threatening situations. This policy sometimes may cause conflict among medical advisors, who often may wish to use heparin in less threatening circumstances. Orthopedic surgeons should preemptively discuss and establish a policy and guidelines within their own institution on which surgeons and medical consultants can agree.

Greenfield Filter

A Greenfield filter should be considered when pulmonary embolism occurs despite therapeutic warfarin prophylaxis, when warfarin is contraindicated in a high-risk patient, or when complications develop as a result of anticoagulation. Vaughn and associates[222] have reported on its use in 66 patients and found the technique to be safe, easy, and effective. They inserted the filter preoperatively in 42 patients who were considered at high risk for pulmonary embolus (group I) and postoperatively in 24 patients (group II). The preferred site of insertion was by way of the right internal jugular vein, and a vascular surgeon carried out the implantations. One patient in group II died of a massive pulmonary embolism 3 days after implantation. At follow-up, none of the remaining patients experienced migration of the filter, and there was no evidence of postphlebitic syndrome or chronic symptomatic edema of the lower extremity.

Fat Embolism Syndrome

The diagnosis of fat embolism can be elusive,[20,32,56,64,160] and we suspect that the condition often may pass unrecognized as the cause of transient confusional states after surgery. The syndrome results from the embolization of fat and other debris from the femur or tibia that travels mostly to the lungs. The initial effects in the lungs are mechanical, with an increase in perfusion pressure, engorgement of the vessels in the lungs, and secondary right-sided heart strain. In the presence of hypovolemic shock, the patient may die from acute right-sided heart failure. The delayed effects of fat embolism occur after 48 to 72 hours because of the chemical effects of fat. The pulmonary tissue secretes lipase, which hydrolyzes fat into free fatty acids and glycerol. These free fatty acids increase capillary permeability, cause destruction of alveolar architecture, and damage lung surfactant. The end result of all these changes is hypoxia.[183]

Clinical findings of fat embolism syndrome include tachypnea, dyspnea, profuse tracheobronchial secretions, apprehension, anxiety, delirium, confusion, unconsciousness, and petechial hemorrhage. Laboratory findings are hypoxemia on arterial blood gas testing and thrombocytopenia lower than 150,000 mm^3. Treatment is supportive. Mechanical ventilation may be required in advanced cases. Corticosteroids may be beneficial in diminishing the inflammatory response from the chemical effects of fat emboli.[174]

Monto and coworkers,[160] in a review of the literature, reported 19 cases with 9 deaths. Of the 19 cases, 15 were associated with long-stem cemented prostheses, such as the Guepar hinge. Four cases were associated with total condylar arthroplasty. One case was associated with intramedullary instrumentation. Fahmy and colleagues[64] have shown human intramedullary (IM) femoral canal pressures of 500 to 1000 mm Hg generated by using standard alignment rod techniques. Venting the canal did not lower the canal pressure significantly. IM pressures were maintained within normal limits only by overdrilling the femoral canal and gently placing the guide rod. Copious irrigation of the IM canal with pulsatile lavage, suction of marrow contents after irrigation, and use of fluted rods to assist the egress of bone marrow elements may reduce the intramedullary pressure. The use of a pneumatic tourniquet does not protect against fat embolism and, with the popularity of IM guidance systems for femoral and tibial components, an increase in the incidence of fat embolism syndrome may be expected. The surgeon should consider avoiding routine instrumentation of the IM canals of the femur and tibia in bilateral cases.

Young-Hood and Kim and colleagues[121] have compared the prevalence of fat embolism after TKA in 160 patients (210 knees) with navigation and 160 patients (210 knees) without navigation. They found no significant difference in the intraoperative and postoperative hemodynamic values between the groups. A higher prevalence of fat embolism was seen (60% vs. 41%) in patients with higher triglyceride levels. However, in contrast, Kalairajah and colleagues[113] have demonstrated a significant reduction in the number of cranial fat emboli in a group treated with computer-assisted TKA compared with a group treated with TKA using standard IM instrumentation.

LOCAL COMPLICATIONS

Wound Drainage and Delayed Wound Healing

Soft tissue considerations must always be at the forefront when planning surgical intervention. This is especially true for high-risk patients, including those with prior incisions. Although several plastic surgery techniques are available to treat wound complications, much of the damage is already done once the complication occurs. Even the best outcomes of salvage techniques following wound failure result in functional loss and cosmetic deficit. Therefore, the surgeon's primary goal should be to avoid postoperative wound complications. Despite appropriate planning and meticulous technique, however, wound complications will occur. The orthopedic surgeon must work in conjunction with the plastic surgeon and be aware of the nonsurgical and surgical techniques available to minimize functional loss. Inappropriate management of postoperative skin problems can result in failure of the reconstruction, deep infection, a nonfunctioning extremity, amputation, and/or a potentially life-threatening situation.

Preoperative Considerations

General Overview

The knee has a thin, overlying soft tissue envelope that must be protective, well vascularized, and supple enough to allow for the large degrees of stretch and shear required for a functional range of motion (ROM). Although most TKAs can be performed with standard protocols, an understanding of when to apply specific soft tissue management principles is required. Preoperative evaluation for TKA should include not only a complete history and physical examination, including radiographic and clinical assessment of the degree of deformity and joint space narrowing, but also a thorough history and evaluation of the skin. Systemic concerns include vascular compromise, obesity, malnutrition, prolonged corticosteroid or nonsteroidal anti-inflammatory drug use, diabetes mellitus, an immunocompromised state, and a history of smoking.* Local factors that affect wound healing include the inability to incorporate a previous incision into the planned incision, a small skin bridge between the previous incision and the planned incision, local radiation or burns, and dense or adherent scar tissue. Other local factors may play a role as well. The correction of severe deformity may make subsequent closure difficult. Special caution should be used in patients with severe varus and rotational deformity because, as the deformity is corrected, there may not be enough skin to close the inferior aspect of the wound over the subcutaneous surface of tibia. Prior trauma may also play a role because of previously placed skin incisions, significant scarring, and loss of skin mobility.

Preoperative consultation regarding medical optimization and early plastic surgery consultation for soft tissue management should be considered in any complex case. Not only will this help minimize complication, but it will help ensure comprehensive involvement should complications be encountered.

Planning the Skin Incision

Previous anterior incisions present a concern regarding both the planned approach and healing potential of the skin and underlying tissue. A balance must be achieved between the ability to expose the knee through a prior incision and avoiding extensive undermining of the subcutaneous flaps. A clear history of the previous incision should be obtained, including the age of the wound, subcutaneous dissection and procedure performed, and any wound complications encountered. The previous surgical reports often provide critical information.

---

*References 48, 54, 84, 110, 191, 234, and 237.

Understanding of the local anatomy and blood supply is also necessary. Terminal branches of the peripatellar anastomotic ring of arteries are responsible for most of the blood supply to the anterior skin and subcutaneous tissues. This occurs through a subdermal plexus supplied by arterioles in the subcutaneous fascia. Thus, flap formation over the anterior aspect of the knee must be limited and performed deep to the subcutaneous fascia. A midline skin incision is optimal and should be used whenever possible. This approach reduces the dimensions of the lateral skin flap at which lower skin oxygen tension is noted. Previous longitudinal incisions can be used safely. Some degree of modification is often required to incorporate previous paramedian incisions. If multiple parallel longitudinal incisions exist, the most lateral incision is chosen, because the predominant blood supply enters medially. Johnson[108] has shown a reduction in oxygenation of the skin in the lateral region after skin incisions about the knee by the measurement of transcutaneous oxygen. Clarke and associates[37] also have described decreased oxygen tension in the incisional skin margins when using tourniquets. This hypoxia increased with tourniquet tightness. The recommended pressure is 125 mm Hg above the mean blood pressure.

Transverse skin incisions, such as those from previous patellar surgery or osteotomy, can be safely approached at a 90-degree angle. Short oblique incisions, such as from previous meniscectomies, can often be ignored. Caution should be exercised when crossing longer oblique incisions or oblique incisions that cross the midline, because crossing these incisions may result in a narrow point at which the incisions intersect. When the planned surgical incision and prior incision create an angle of less than 60 degrees, alternative techniques should be considered.

Alternative Techniques

If the previous skin incision cannot be incorporated and there are other concerns, several techniques can be considered. One option is the sham incision. This technique has limited applications today; we mention it here mainly for historic reasons. A sham incision involves making the planned skin incision, performing the necessary subcutaneous dissection, developing flaps, closing the wound, and then waiting a period of time to observe how the wound heals. This provides information regarding the ability of the tissues to heal and creates a so-called delay phenomenon, with increased local perfusion. If the sham incision heals, then the TKA can proceed as planned 1 to 3 weeks later. Disadvantages to this approach include the need for two procedures and, in patients in whom the sham incision does not heal, the need for further prearthroplasty management but with more limited options.

Another option is prophylactic flap coverage. The best candidates for prophylactic flap coverage are patients with prior skin graft, local irradiation, or densely adherent scar tissue. The choice of flap depends on the location of the lesion, extent of coverage required, and status of the limb. Most lesions can be covered adequately with a medial or lateral gastrocnemius muscle flap or myocutaneous flap. Lesions proximal to the superior pole of the patella may require a free flap. The principles involve excision of the area of concern followed by soft tissue coverage. A minimum of 12 weeks should be allowed between coverage and subsequent arthroplasty. Available data demonstrate successful outcomes

in most patients. However, because the indications for this procedure are few, results are extremely limited.

Indications for Soft Tissue Expansion

Our preferred technique is soft tissue expansion. Soft tissue expanders are indicated when insufficient or inadequate soft tissue is present for wound healing. This may occur with multiple crossing and combined incisions, previous skin grafts or flaps, or severe preoperative deformity, or when expanded soft tissue coverage is required. For example, when an extensor mechanism allograft as well as a TKA is to be performed, the added bulk of the extensor mechanism reconstruction may necessitate soft tissue expansion, and 8 to 10 weeks must be allocated for this procedure. Good long-term results have been reported from our institution. Soft tissue expansion is discussed elsewhere in this text.

Postoperative Considerations

Appropriate postoperative wound management depends on the severity and timing of the complication. The failure of the soft tissues to heal following TKA has serious effects. Careful examination at the time of the first dressing change can often alert the clinician to a potentially problematic wound. Early indications may include ecchymosis, blistering, and persistent or large amounts of wound drainage. The goal is early intervention, when possible, to prevent further wound breakdown and complication.

Serosanguineous drainage from the incision is common and is a cause for concern only when the drainage is profuse and persistent. If there is no purulence or erythema, initial management should be a compression dressing, immobilization, and observation. Wound healing takes precedence over motion. When there is drainage, antibiotic therapy is controversial because it may mask a deep infection, making it difficult to identify the causative organism. We recommend consulting with an infectious disease specialist and administering intravenous antibiotics only in select cases. This is a matter of clinical judgment, but we do not consider antibiotics in these circumstances wrong if clinical suspicion for a deep infection is low. Prolonged and persistent serosanguineous drainage raises the issue of a capsular defect, which should be surgically repaired. Some authors recommend that if drainage does not stop after 5 days of appropriate treatment, an open débridement should be performed.

Local Care

Local care measures begin with frequent dressing changes, elevation of the extremity, and limiting mobilization, including ROM activities. When a wound is identified to be at risk in the early postoperative period, we routinely discontinue continuous passive motion, apply a compressive dressing, place the knee in an immobilizer, and institute physical therapy. When superficial epidermal loss occurs in an area smaller than 2 to 3 cm^2, several modified dressing protocols can be instituted to protect the underlying tissues and allow for secondary healing (Fig. 125-2). These include antibacterial ointments or gels and enzymatic débriding agents. During this phase, we may consider temporary discontinuation of the anticoagulant agent, because a hematoma related to overaggressive anticoagulation can be devastating at this stage of healing. The use of mechanical devices for DVT prophylaxis should be considered until the wound stabilizes.

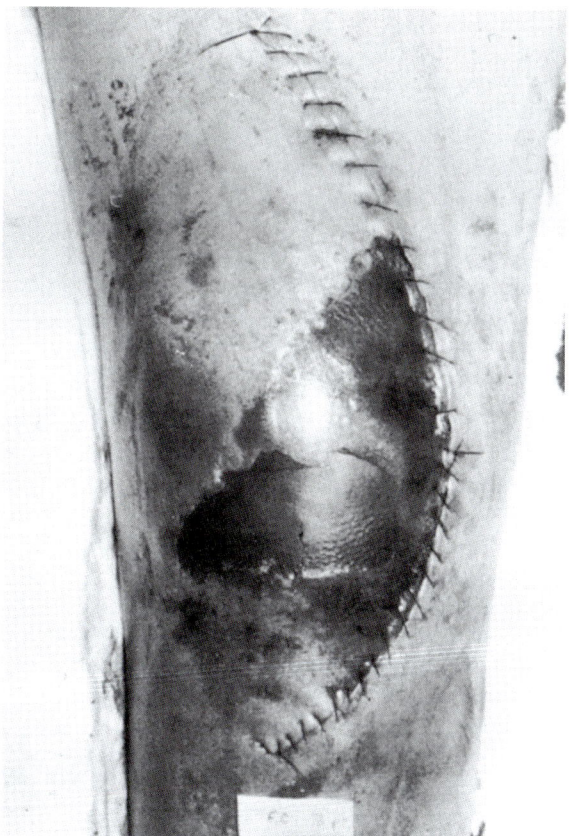

Figure 125-2. Because of its subcutaneous position, skin necrosis is a particular hazard in knee joint replacement. Overaggressive débridement can lead to deep infection. When necrosis occurs, the knee should be immobilized until the eschar separates.

Irrigation and Débridement

Early surgical intervention may be helpful and is indicated in certain situations. In cases of imminent wound compromise caused by a large or expanding hematoma or prolonged wound drainage beyond 1 week postoperatively, early surgical interventions should be considered. The goal of irrigation and débridement (I&D) is to prevent further wound breakdown and deep infection. Studies have shown that each day of persistent drainage greatly increases the risk of wound infection. In addition, other studies have shown a lower incidence of deep infection when postoperative hematoma or persistent drainage is treated with I&D versus nonsurgical management.

Burnett and coworkers[30] have reported that the rates of surgical site complications necessitating readmission, irrigation and débridement of hematoma and the wound, or prolonged hospitalization for wound drainage are 4.7%, 3.4%, and 5.1%, respectively. Wound drainage occurred for 4 to 7 days after 9.3% of the procedures and for more than 7 days after 9.3% of the procedures, with more than 7 days of drainage being highly predictive of readmission and wound reoperation.

Once the decision is made to proceed with surgery, the patient is taken to the operating room expediently. The setup is the same as with the index arthroplasty. Thorough I&D is performed. Deep cultures should be obtained to direct antibiotic therapy, if indicated. If an opening in the arthrotomy exists, or if the hematoma is deep to the arthrotomy, then the entire prosthesis should be exposed and irrigated and a polyethylene liner exchange is performed. It is best to assume that deep infection is present and perform a thorough I&D with antibiotic irrigation. After hemostasis is obtained, the wound is closed in a layered fashion over a drain. A compressive dressing is applied. Occasionally, when a tension-free closure cannot be obtained, a gastrocnemius muscle flap may be necessary. This should be anticipated before surgery. Appropriate accommodations should be made preoperatively, including the involvement of a plastic surgeon.

Postoperatively, the limb is elevated while ROM and chemical DVT prophylaxis are initially held. Broad-spectrum antibiotics are given until pending cultures are final. An infectious disease consultation is obtained for patients in whom infection is suspected or cultures return positive. Decisions regarding range of motion, DVT prophylaxis, and continued antibiotic therapy are made on an individual basis.

Galat and colleagues,[72] in their study of 17,784 primary TKAs, have reported that the rate of early return to surgery for wound complication is 0.33%. They found that the 2-year cumulative probabilities of major subsequent surgery (component resection, muscle flap coverage, or amputation) and deep infection were 5.3% and 6.0%, respectively, in the knees with early surgical treatment of wound complications as compared with 0.6% and 0.8%, respectively, for knees without early surgical intervention. The overall prosthesis salvage rate was 98%, but obviously results are inferior compared with those of patients without early wound complication.

Hematoma

A current debate exists between appropriate VTE guidelines following TKA. Although discussed elsewhere in this text, the debate centers around the incidents of postoperative hematoma. Given the nature of a TKA with numerous bone cuts, intramedullary canal violation, and soft tissue releases, it is no surprise that postoperative hematomas can occur. Symptoms include not only intense palpable hemarthrosis around the knee but can also be accompanied by skin discoloration, bruising, increased pain, decreased ROM, and wound drainage.

Wound drainage is of particular concern. Weiss and Krackow[278] have described an increased rate of knee infection with prolonged wound drainage. Patel and associates[173] have evaluated factors that lead to prolonged drainage in the postoperative period. The authors have demonstrated that an increase in the initial postoperative drainage in the recovery room was most indicative for further drainage on days 2, 3, 4, and 5. In other words, better control in the immediate postoperative period, with less postoperative recovery room drainage, led to less wound drainage on subsequent hospitalization days. Limiting blood loss in the recovery room begins in the operating room (OR). Plugging of the intramedullary canal can help decrease initial blood loss as can cauterization of known sources of bleeding, such as genicular vessels and the posterior capsule[49] (Fig. 125-3). Intraoperative tourniquet deflation has not been shown to decrease blood loss; in fact, some studies have shown an increase in blood loss when this is performed.[182] The appropriate timing of tourniquet release remains debated, even among surgeons at our institution. The improved designs of TKA and improved surgical techniques have led to improved

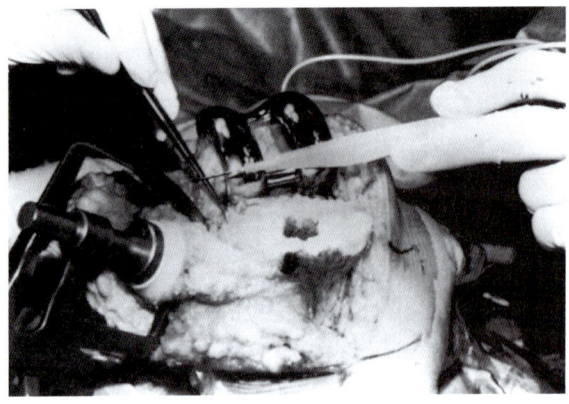

Figure 125-3. Cauterization of the lateral genicular artery. Unless this artery is visible, it is advisable to release the tourniquet before closure so that the vessel can be clearly identified. It is the major source of dangerous postoperative bleeding.

patellar tracking, resulting in less wound drainage when the lateral release is avoided. At our institution, we use a multimodal approach to minimizing intraoperative bleeding, including a smaller quadriceps-sparing incision, meticulous surgical technique, lidocaine and epinephrine injection, bipolar sealer device, and a topical fibrin spray.

When postoperative hematoma occurs, a period of immobilization and observation is permissible, and many hematomas subside spontaneously. If bleeding continues, as evidenced by tense and painful swelling, the knee must be reopened and the source of the bleeding identified (an argument for intraoperative tourniquet release). Probing and squeezing the wound to evacuate a hematoma are not recommended because this could lead to retrograde contamination. Indications for surgical evacuation of a hematoma include skin compromise, wound dehiscence, impending skin necrosis, leakage through the incision, persistent sanguineous drainage, and pain. Galat and associates[71] have studied 42 TKA patients matched with 42 control subjects. They found that the rate of return to surgery within 30 days for evacuation of a postoperative hematoma was 0.24%. The 2-year rates of a subsequent major operation or deep periprosthetic infection in the study group were 12.3% and 13.6%, respectively and 0.9% and 1.4%, respectively, in the control group.

Skin Necrosis

Postoperative soft tissue and skin necrosis should be handled early and aggressively. Treatment options for Small areas (<4 cm), especially over the patella or more proximal, include healing by secondary intention, split-thickness skin grafts, or local fasciocutaneous flaps. Small areas (<4 cm), especially over the patella or proximal, may be treated by secondary intention healing, split-thickness skin grafts, or local fasciocutaneous flaps. Skin loss over the patellar tendon or tibial tubercle is best treated with muscle flap coverage; usually, the medial head of the gastrocnemius rotator flap is adequate.

VASCULAR COMPLICATIONS

Arterial complications are rare,[130,185] and the preoperative absence of peripheral pulses has not been regarded as a contraindication to surgery, provided that the capillary circulation was adequate. Vascular complication has been reported in 0.03% to 0.2% of cases.[47] Injury to the popliteal artery can occur during resection of the proximal tibia or posterior femoral condyles and while releasing the posterior capsule or posterior collateral ligament (PCL). Failure to remove protruding cement from the back of the tibia can also cause direct damage or thermal injury.

Da Silva and Sobel[51] have reported on 19 patients with TKA-related popliteal artery injury. Of these, 84% (16/19) of patients had full recoveries. Limb loss occurred in 2 of 19 patients (10.5%). Parvizi and coworkers[172] collected data on 13,517 patients undergoing total joint arthroplasty and reported 16 vascular injuries (0.1%). Eleven injuries occurred after TKA and five after THA. Of the 16 patients, 8 (50%) had launched a legal suit against the operating surgeon. Abularrage and colleagues,[1] in their prospective study of 41,633 patients, evaluated the predictors of lower extremity arterial injury after TKA or THA. They found that the revision procedures and African American race were statistically significant predictors of arterial injury.

Numerous studies have reported arteriovenous fistula formation, arterial aneurysm, and pseudoaneurysm following TKA. A possible reason may be an unrecognized injury to the perigenicular vessels, leading to hemarthrosis. Most present within 6 months of surgery but some may be delayed. In a case reported by Sharma and associates,[210] three large hemorrhagic effusions occurred 4 weeks after total knee replacement (TKR). An arteriogram revealed a pseudoaneurysm filling from the inferior medial genicular artery. Ibrahim and coworkers[102] have reported two cases of pseudoaneurysm after TKR, presenting after 5 days and 1 month, respectively. The first patient was successfully embolized and the second patient was treated by injecting a solution of thrombin into the pseudoaneurysm to produce immediate thrombosis without impairing flow across the vessel. Sandoval and colleagues[202] have reported a case of popliteal pseudoaneurysm following TKA. Open vascular surgery with resection of the pseudoaneurysm and end to end bypass of contralateral saphenous vein graft was successfully performed. Their possible explanation was perforation of the anterior wall of the popliteal artery during the TKA. Haddad and associates[86] have reported a case of recurrent hemarthrosis following TKR after a previous dome tibial osteotomy for medial compartment osteoarthritis. Recurrent hemarthrosis in this case was secondary to arteriovenous (AV) fistula of the peroneal artery at the site of the previous fibular osteotomy. Thomas and coworkers[218] have reported an iatrogenic popliteal AV fistula 3 years after TKA. This was successfully treated by resection of the fistula and direct repair of the artery and vein.

Acute arterial occlusion can be seen after TKA. Rates in the literature have been reported from 0.03% to 0.17%.[125] Possible causes include manual manipulation to reduce a flexion contracture[58,147] and the use of tourniquet. Pressure on a preexisting atheromatous plaque may cause release of the plaque, which is then lodged into a more distal artery. Gregory and colleagues[81] have reported a case of an 81-year-old patient with acute arterial occlusion 9 days after TKA. This was successfully treated by urgent surgical embolectomy.

It is important to determine and document the presence of peripheral vascular disease, arterial calcifications, and popliteal aneurysm preoperatively (Fig. 125-4). Absolute vascular contraindications for performing a TKA include the

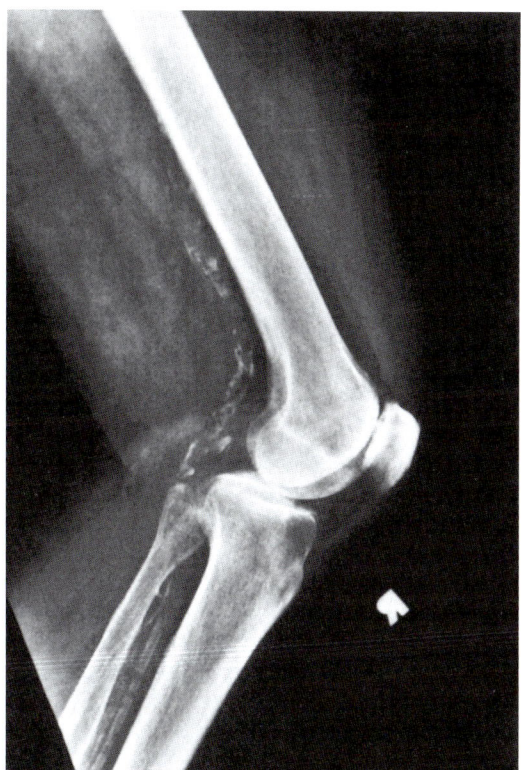

Figure 125-4. Lateral radiograph showing extensive calcification in the femoral, popliteal, posterotibial, posterior tibial, and peroneal arteries. Although this patient had palpable peripheral pulses, knee surgery may result in arterial occlusion by a dislodged clot. Some investigators recommend avoiding a tourniquet. The patient should be watched closely after surgery for evidence of arterial insufficiency.

presence of verified vascular claudication with minimal or no activity, active skin ulcerations secondary to arterial insufficiency or venous stasis, and ischemia or frank necrosis in the toes. Others have cautioned against the use of a tourniquet after previous bypass surgery.

When there is concern about the circulation, we recommend preoperative evaluation by a vascular surgeon. The operation should be scheduled at a time of day when consultant advice is available postoperatively so that prompt investigation with arteriography can be done if the state of the circulation is in doubt. Prompt embolectomy usually restores the circulation. Prolonged observation of postoperative vascular insufficiency is justified only in a setting of extreme vigilance and under the guidance of a vascular surgeon.

NERVE PALSY AND NEUROLOGIC COMPLICATIONS

Anatomy of the Peroneal Nerve

The peroneal nerve is composed of fibers from the dorsal portion of the L4 and L5 and S1 and S2 nerves. As the nerve courses down from the thigh, it curves laterally behind the head of the fibula to reach the two heads of the peroneus longus. The nerve flattens as it passes between these two heads, separating the bundles and exposing unprotected nutrient vessels. The nerve then curves around the neck of

the fibula and divides into deep and superficial branches. The deep peroneal nerve continues under the extensor digitorum longus, along the anterior aspect of the intraosseous membrane. It sends motor branches to the tibialis anterior, extensor digitorum longus, extensor hallucis longus, and peroneus tertius. The nerve continues distally, ending in the medial and lateral terminal branches, which, among other functions, supply sensation to the first web space of the foot.

The superficial peroneal nerve passes distally between the peronei and extensor digitorum longus. Motor branches are given off to the peroneus longus and peroneus brevis. In the lower third of the leg, the nerve branches into the medial and intermediate dorsal cutaneous nerves. These terminal branches complete the sensory innervation of the feet. Bruzzone and associates[26] identified anatomic landmarks after 20 cadaveric knee dissections and defined a danger zone and a safe zone to avoid common peroneal nerve injury when performing the inside-out release technique of the posterior-lateral corner during TKA. During the release of the posterior-lateral capsule, the nerve was identified to be at risk in the triangle defined by the popliteus tendon, tibial cut surface, and most posterior fibers of the iliotibial band (danger zone), but not during "pie-crusting" of the iliotibial band (safe zone). They also defined the average distance from the nerve to the posterior-lateral corner of the tibia and to the posterior border of the iliotibial band as 13.5 and 35.8 mm, respectively.

Postoperative Clinical Findings

Peroneal nerve palsy is an infrequent but worrisome complication after TKA. The incidence is higher in revision cases than primary TKA. The prevalence of peroneal nerve palsy has been reported many times in the literature. Mont and coworkers[157] have reviewed the literature and found the cumulative prevalence to be 0.58% (74 of 12,784). Asp and Rand[6] reported an incidence of 0.3% in 8754 TKAs performed at the Mayo Clinic. Yacub and colleagues,[240] in their retrospective study of 14,979 patients, reported a 0.01% incidence of nerve injury after TKA. They noted a 10-fold difference in nerve injury rates between diabetic and nondiabetic patients, 0.11% versus 0.01%, respectively.

Numerous causes for nerve palsy have been described, but they are most commonly associated with the correction of severe flexion and valgus deformity or a combination of the two. The following factors contribute to the development of peroneal nerve palsy: (1) stretching of the nerve in valgus and flexion contractures; (2) fascial compression of the nerve and its vascular supply; (3) direct pressure from the postoperative dressing; and (4) epidural anesthesia. In rare idiopathic cases, none of the mechanisms listed seem to apply. Factors that have not been found to be associated with peroneal nerve palsy include age, gender, type of arthritis, and duration of tourniquet. Idusuyi and Morrey[103] performed 10,321 TKAs from 1979 through 1992 at the Mayo Clinic and reported 32 postoperative peroneal nerve palsies. The factors associated with peroneal nerve palsies in this series were epidural anesthesia for postoperative pain control, previous laminectomy, and preoperative valgus deformity. The relative risk for patients who had previous proximal tibial osteotomy was doubled but was not statistically significant.

In patients with severe combined deformities, the large soft tissue dissections required to balance the deformities may be responsible for increased traction or vascular compromise to the nerve. The alternative method of bone sacrifice to correct large deformities, although appealing because of elimination of the need for obtaining soft tissue balance, does not entirely avoid peroneal nerve palsy. The bone-sacrificing method also leaves a residual, permanent, leg-length discrepancy that may be associated with an extensor lag because of relative lengthening of the quadriceps mechanism. When ligament balance is not attempted, a constrained prosthesis is needed. In younger patients, this may lead to eventual loosening, although, with the constrained condylar prosthesis, this has not yet been seen in our practice. In older patients at high risk for peroneal nerve palsy, the use of the constrained condylar knee is a suitable alternative. These patients recover much more rapidly than after major release procedures and, because of their age, the risk of ultimate loosening is less concerning.

Although it is sometimes necessary to splint the knee in extension after correction of a severe flexion contracture, evidence of nerve palsy demands immediate removal of the splints and flexion of the knee. If this is done promptly, complete recovery can be expected. In the case of varus deformities, splinting is not necessary. For severe valgus deformity (>20 degrees), one may consider splinting the patient with the knee in 30 degrees of flexion. Nerve function is then monitored closely when the surgical dressing is removed on postoperative day 2. Tight dressings that might press directly on the peroneal nerve should also be avoided.

Postoperative dressings that are too tight or improperly padded can cause direct pressure on the peroneal nerve, causing nerve palsy. Beller and associates,[15] in their study, described a double crush syndrome, which includes unrecognized pressure on the peroneal nerve caused by continuous epidural anesthesia and an axonal lesion from the pressure of the pneumatic tourniquet. To prevent a peroneal lesion after TKA while using continuous epidural anaesthesia, they recommended limiting the pneumatic tourniquet pressure to 320 mm Hg and ensuring pressure-free positioning of the operated leg.

Asp and Rand[6] performed 8998 arthroplasties and reported 26 nerve palsies. They noted that complete recovery was more likely when the palsy was initially incomplete. Dressing removal and flexion of the knee on diagnosis did not always help. The time of presentation of the problem varied from discovery in the recovery room to postoperative day 6. The motor fibers of the tibialis anterior and extensor hallucis longus muscles were affected in all cases; a sensory deficit was noticed in 20 patients (87%). The peroneus longus muscle was affected in nine patients (39%). Electromyographic evaluation showed a diffuse motor neuropathy in the mild cases and denervation potentials in muscles supplied by the deep branch of the common peroneal nerve in the more severely involved cases. The treatment rendered on discovery of these findings varied according to the discretion of the surgeon involved. The most frequent therapeutic measure was to loosen the Robert Jones dressing and place the knee in a more flexed position. In two cases, this maneuver brought immediate improvement of motor and sensory deficits. The time interval between discovery and the beginning of the return of function ranged from immediately in the two cases

mentioned to 6 months. Motor improvement occurred first, with sensory return lagging behind.

Omeroglu and coworkers[166] have reported the case of 46-year-old rheumatoid patient with bilateral peroneal nerve palsy on the second postoperative day after simultaneous bilateral TKA. Electromyographic studies revealed bilateral axonotmesis. Complete motor recovery was seen on both sides within 6 months, although sensory deficit was present on one side at 2 years postoperatively. They reported preoperative severe flexion contracture and epidural anesthesia as the risk factors for the development of the nerve palsy in this patient.

Treatment and Results

The treatment of chronic peroneal nerve palsy usually consists of an ankle-foot orthosis for a footdrop and passive ankle ROM to prevent an equinus deformity. Complete recovery of a peroneal palsy is rare. The recovery seen is usually partial, with sensory deficits that may be permanent; residual motor deficits are not usually of clinical significance. Occasional marked weakness, especially of the great toe extensor, may be seen. In Asp and Rand's study[6] of 26 postoperative peroneal palsies, palsies were complete in 18 and incomplete in 8. Of these patients, 23 had motor and sensory deficits and 3 had only motor deficits. At 5-year follow-up, recovery was complete for 13 palsies and partial for 12. Complete recovery was more likely in palsies that were initially incomplete.

Although most investigators support nonoperative treatment of this complication, others disagree. Krackow and colleagues[129] treated five patients with operative exploration and decompression of the peroneal nerve for a postoperative palsy. The procedure was performed 5 to 45 months after the index TKA. All patients have shown improved nerve function, and 4 of 5 patients had full peroneal nerve recovery. All patients were able to discontinue their ankle-foot orthosis.

MECHANICAL COMPLICATIONS

Instability

Instability is a common cause of mechanical failure of TKA. Instability accounts for 10% to 22% of TKA failures requiring revision.* The direction of instability at the tibiofemoral articulation can occur in the coronal (varus-valgus) plane, sagittal (anteroposterior) plane, or as a combination of planes. Early instability may be a result of malalignment of the components, failure to restore the mechanical axis of the limb, imbalance of the flexion-extension space, intraoperative or postoperative rupture of the medial collateral ligament (MCL), or posterior PCL rupture with cruciate-retaining designs. Commonly, late instability is secondary to polyethylene wear. Asymmetrical polyethylene wear related to malalignment can result in relative lengthening of the collateral ligament on the involved side and subsequent coronal instability. In patients with cruciate-retaining knees, it is not uncommon for the PCL to elongate or attenuate. This can lead to progressive polyethylene wear and late sagittal plane instability. However, late sagittal plane instability is seen not

---

*References 24, 167, 170, 224, 241, and 242.

only with cruciate-retaining designs, because significant wear or fracture of the tibial polyethylene post in posterior-stabilized knees may result in late sagittal plane instability.[207] Instability after knee arthroplasty can be subdivided into three types—extension instability, flexion instability, and genu recurvatum.

Extension Instability

Symmetrical Instability

Symmetrical extension instability occurs when the extension space is not filled by the thickness of the components. This can be caused by overresection of the tibia or the distal femur.[24] Although overresection of the tibia results in equally large flexion and extensions gaps, excessive resection from the distal femur results in asymmetrical flexion and extension gaps. If overresection of the tibia is recognized intraoperatively, it can be easily managed by increasing the size of the polyethylene insert. Similarly, if a postoperative TKA is noted to be equally loose in flexion and extension, one option is revision surgery with a polyethylene exchange to a larger insert. Overresection of the distal femur creates a much different scenario. With overresection of the distal femur, the joint line is elevated. This creates a larger extension gap compared with the flexion gap. By simply increasing the size of the tibial insert, the result will be a knee that is too tight in flexion. The elevated joint line will also affect patellar tracking and limit flexion, and may result in midflexion instability[170] (Fig. 125-5). It is best in these cases to restore the joint line by adding distal femoral augmentation.

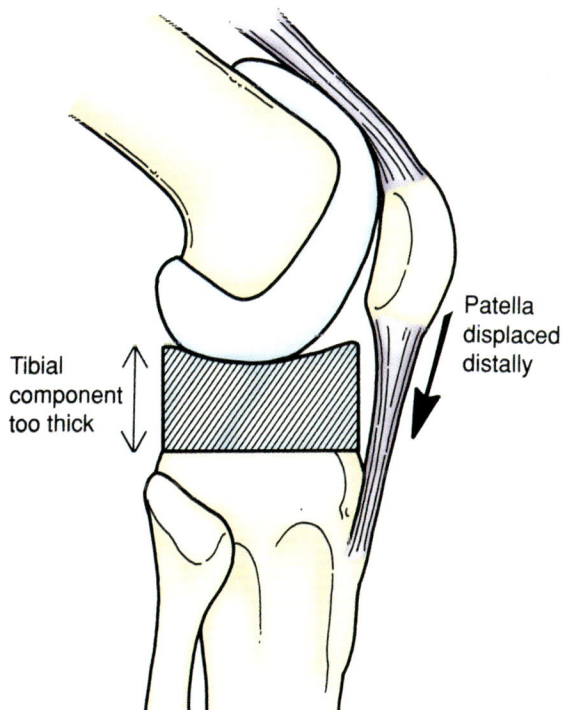

Figure 125-5. If an extra thick tibial component is needed to stabilize the knee, the patella is displaced distally, causing a patella infra. Undersizing of the femoral component in the sagittal plane and anterior malpositioning are possible causes. Excessive distal resection of the femur moving the joint line proximally is another cause.

Asymmetrical Instability

Asymmetrical extension instability is frequently encountered. Following the femoral and tibial preparation, the extension and flexion gaps must be assessed. An asymmetrical extension gap in the face of appropriate bony resection is most often caused by inadequate correction of the preoperative deformity.[24,170] Preoperative varus deformity is the most common soft tissue deformity. The shortening or tightening of the medial structures, including the superficial MCL, must be recognized. Often, these tightened structures are not sufficiently released and the deformity is not completely corrected (Fig. 125-6). This will lead to progressing varus deformity with increased medial joint line stresses, accelerated polyethylene wear, and stretching out of the soft tissue structures on the lateral side. The asymmetrical extension gap must be recognized intraoperatively and an appropriate subperiosteal elevated of the superficial MCL performed, as described by Insall and associates.[105] They thought that valgus instability from overrelease of the medial structures during correction of a fixed varus deformity was rare.

Knees with asymmetrical extension instability may also result from undercorrection of a preoperative valgus deformity.[170] Excessively tight lateral structures, including the lateral collateral ligament (LCL) and iliotibial band (ITB), if left uncorrected, will lead to recurrence of the valgus deformity and increased lateral joint line forces. Currently, the most commonly used technique to correct preoperative valgus deformity without causing lateral instability has been described by Insall and associates[105] as the "pie-crust" technique. This is recommended for patients with a preoperative valgus deformity of less than 20 degrees.[3] Clarke and coworkers[36] have published results of 24 TKAs with preoperative valgus deformity ranging from 9 to 30 degrees. The deformity was corrected using the "pie-crust" technique and the knee was reconstructed with a posterior-stabilized prosthesis. This series reported complete correction of the deformity and no instability in all cases. In patients with more than 20 degrees of valgus deformity, the risks of iatrogenic peroneal nerve injury must be considered.[59] The surgeon may consider the use of a constrained condylar design in much older patients, whereas increased constraint in younger patients should be avoided unless absolutely necessary.

Extension instability can result secondary to iatrogenic injury of the collateral ligaments (Fig. 125-7). The excursion of large oscillating saw blades was studied and found to be greater than the width of the medial and lateral femoral condyles in the female knee.[59] Meticulous attention must be paid to the position of retractors during femoral and tibial resection. Also, iatrogenic collateral ligament injury can be produced during aggressive testing of varus-valgus stability or with attempts to reduce the polyethylene insert in an excessively tight knee. With iatrogenic injury to the MCL, most authors advocate a direct repair with Krackow-pattern suturing. If primary repair is insufficient, augmentation can be performed using the hamstring tendons. Finally, a constrained condylar design can be used to provide additional stability while the repair heals. Several studies have demonstrated good outcomes without the use of increased constraint or tissue augmentation. Leopold and coworkers[137] have demonstrated good to excellent results in 100% of 16 TKAs treated with direct repair of an iatrogenically injured MCL,

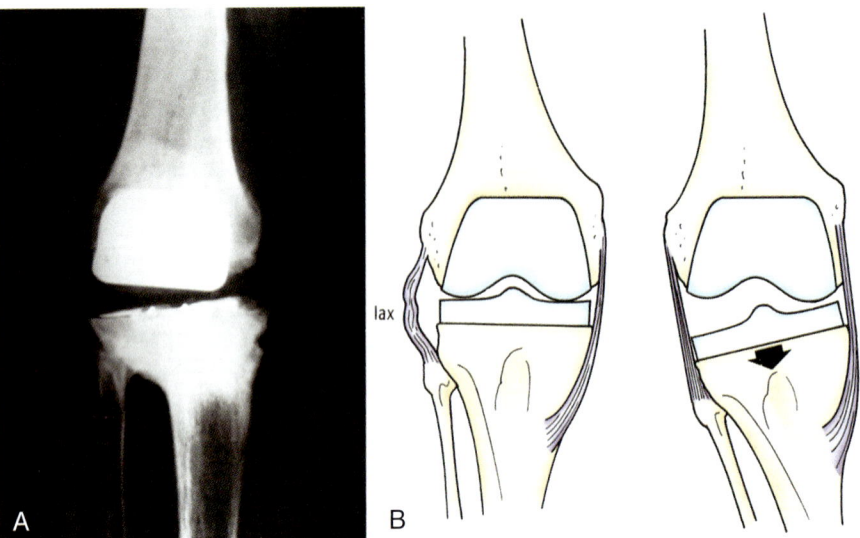

Figure 125-6. A, This arthroplasty is unstable, but not because of a ligament deficiency. **B,** The medial ligament was not released; an asymmetrical instability remains.

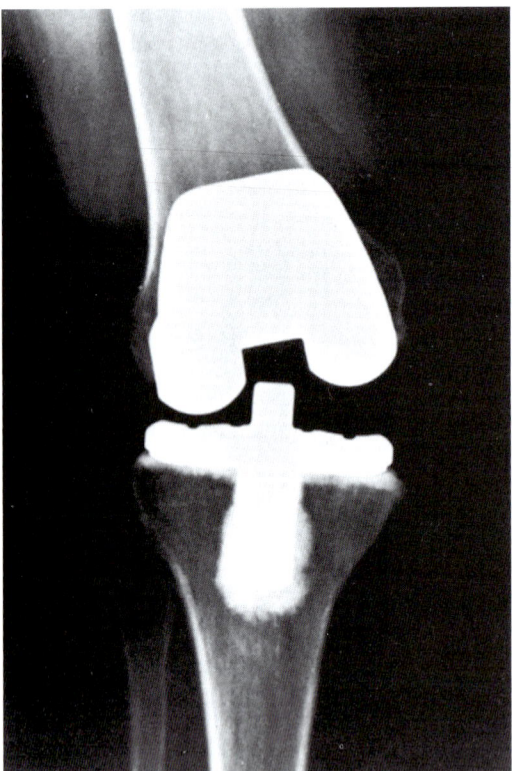

Figure 125-7. Radiograph showing the instability that results from a transected medial collateral ligament. This is not the result of an overzealous medial release.

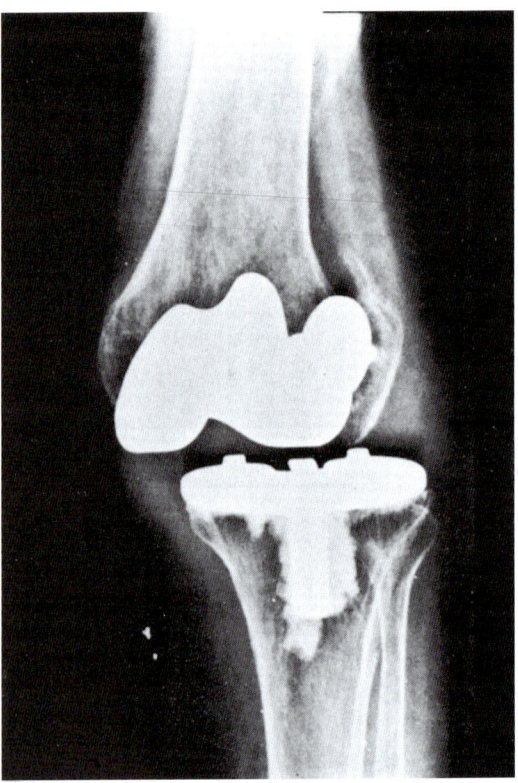

Figure 125-8. AP radiograph of a knee with flexion instability. With the knee in flexion, a posterolateral dislocation is observed. This dislocation is caused by inequality between the flexion and extension gaps, and the PCL is not sufficient to provide stability, particularly when the prosthesis is unconstrained.

reconstruction using a cruciate-retaining implant, and postoperative bracing for 6 weeks. More recently, Koo and Choi[126] performed a retrospective review of 15 TKAs treated conservatively for intraoperative iatrogenic detachment of the MCL from the tibia. Specifically, no increased constraint, bracing, or ligament reconstruction was performed. No significant difference was seen between MCL-intact TKAs and the knees with iatrogenic MCL injury with a minimum of 2-year follow-up.

Flexion Instability

Flexion instability results from inadequate filling of the flexion gap or attenuation of the PCL following cruciate-retaining TKA. Flexion instability is now a well-recognized cause of TKA failure (Fig. 125-8). Early flexion instability is likely secondary to gap imbalance, with or without laxity of a collateral ligament[170] (Fig. 125-9). Late flexion instability can occur in cruciate-retaining and posterior-stabilized TKAs, but the cause is different. In patients with cruciate-retaining knees, it is not uncommon for the PCL to elongate or attenuate. This can lead to progressive polyethylene wear and late flexion instability.[167] Late flexion instability in posterior-stabilized knees may result from significant wear or fracture of the tibial polyethylene post.[207] Symptoms can range from a vague sense of instability and recurrent effusions to frank dislocation. Flexion instability is best assessed with the knee in 90 degrees of flexion while the patient sits on the end of the examination table.

Frank dislocation following posterior-stabilized TKA is a rare complication[204] (Fig. 125-10). Improved prosthetic design with increased jump distances have reduced this complication to well below 0.5%.[170] Although the posterior-stabilized prosthesis can resist direct posterior translation, deep flexion combined with a varus or valgus stress can lead to posterior dislocation of the tibia. Patients who are at highest risk are those who have had the correction of a large valgus deformity and quickly regained their ROM during the postoperative period. The dislocated TKA can continue to function well following closed reduction under anesthesia; however, subsequent dislocation may occur. Recurrent dislocation requires revision to a larger polyethylene insert, if the extension gap permits, or component revision to a constrained condylar design.

More commonly, posterior stabilized knees may be symptomatic because of flexion instability but not demonstrate dislocation.[204] Patients report a sense of instability, recurrent effusion, periarticular tenderness, and difficulty ambulating on stairs. The diagnosis is made on clinical examination with the knee flexed at 90 degrees. Schwab and colleagues[204] have reviewed 1370 revision TKAs performed at the Mayo Clinic (Rochester, Minn). Ten revisions were performed for flexion instability. Eight (80%) had successful outcomes following revision of both components and appropriate balancing of the flexion and extension gaps. The excessively large flexion gap was frequently managed by upsizing the femoral component following posterior femoral augmentation.

Similarly, cruciate-retaining (CR) knees can be symptomatic because of flexion instability without dislocation. Patients again report a sense of instability, recurrent effusion, periarticular tenderness, pes anserine tenderness, and difficulty ambulating on stairs. Additionally, on physical examination, a posterior sag and positive posterior drawer may be readily apparent. Pagnano and associates[167] have reported two types of causes for flexion instability following CR TKA. The first type creates an excessive flexion gap by surgical error. This can occur by undersizing the femoral component, which results in overresection of the posterior femoral condyles and a reduction in the femoral offset. Alternatively, the creation of excessive tibial slope can result in a knee that is well balanced in extension but remains loose in flexion. The second

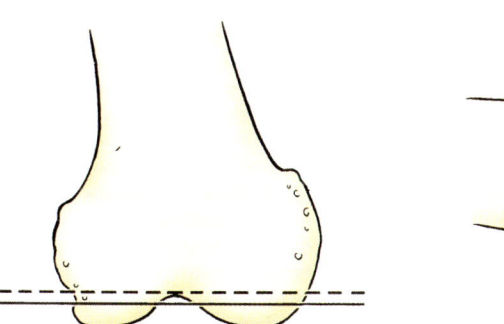
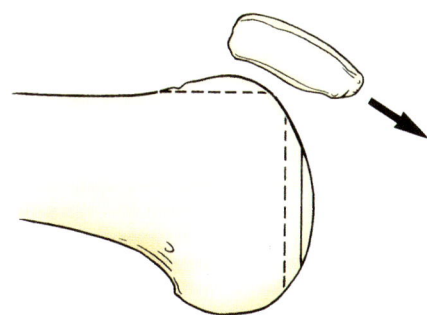

Figure 125-9. In cases with considerable ligamentous laxity, an underresection of the distal femur may be preferable. The standard femoral resection necessitates a thicker tibial component to take up the slack in the soft tissues and may cause distal migration of the patella. By underresecting the femur, a desirable patellar position is maintained.

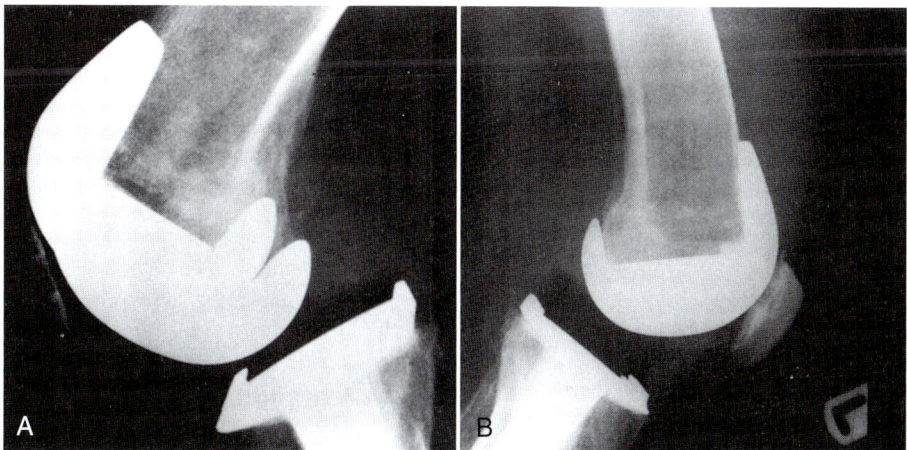

Figure 125-10. A, Posterior dislocation of a PS prosthesis. **B,** After reduction.

type involves late failure of the PCL and late instability. Other causes may include polyethylene wear, synovitis, iatrogenic PCL injury, traumatic PCL rupture, and an excessively tight flexion gap and PCL rupture following aggressive ROM exercises.

Treatment of CR knees with flexion instability most often involves revision arthroplasty to a posterior-stabilized (PS) design.[170] At the time of revision, a larger femoral component is frequently used following posterior femoral augmentation. This improves posterior femoral offset and reduces the size of the flexion gap. Attention must also be paid to the tibial slope. If excessive posterior slope is present preoperatively, this must be addressed with revision of the tibial resection. Careful balancing of the flexion and extension gaps is then performed. Pagnano and associates[167] have demonstrated successful outcomes following revision of a CR knee with flexion instability to a well-balanced PS design in 19 of 22 knees (86%).

Genu Recurvatum

Genu recurvatum, or hyperextension, is difficult to manage and therefore is best prevented during primary TKA. Because genu recurvatum is known to recur in patients with certain neuromuscular disorders, the cause of the hyperextension deformity must be elucidated thoroughly before surgery. In the absence of neuromuscular disease, however, hyperextension deformities tend not to recur after TKA. In the remainder of cases, recurvatum was likely present at the end of the index procedure as a result of excessively loose collateral ligaments and failure to fill the extension gap.[148]

Recurvatum before TKA is rare and is most often associated with neuromuscular diseases, including poliomyelitis.[148] Patients with neuromuscular disease and significant quadriceps weakness rely on hyperextension of the knee to prevent limb collapse during the stance phase of gait. In the absence of neuromuscular disease, recurvatum may develop in patients with a fixed valgus deformity associated with a contracted ITB or in patients with rheumatoid arthritis. Patients at risk and those with preoperative hyperextension must be recognized so that appropriate considerations can be made.

Several options have been described to prevent the recurrence of recurvatum when performing a TKA in a patient with preoperative recurvatum. One option is to use a rotating hinged component with an extension stop. Giori and Lewallen[76] reviewed the Mayo Clinic experience performing TKA in patients with poliomyelitis. They recommended the use of a rotating hinged prosthesis in patients with less than antigravity quadriceps strength. Jordan and coworkers[111] more recently demonstrated 95% good to excellent results in 15 TKAs performed in patients with poliomyelitis using a PS or constrained condylar design. Unlike the results published by Giori and Lewallen,[76] their results did not deteriorate with worsening quadriceps strength. Anterior-posterior stability was restored in all 15 patients. Only one patient required a hinged implant for reconstruction. The discrepancy in results remains unclear. Caution should remain when treating patients with less than antigravity quadriceps function.

A second alternative for patients with preoperative recurvatum is to underresect the distal femur. This will result in a relatively smaller extension gap. Then, by filling the flexion gap with the largest polyethylene insert possible, the knee will have a slight flexion contracture,[170] which will prevent hyperextension. Finally, others have recommended repositioning the collateral ligaments more posteriorly to re-create the normal tightening action as full extension of the knee is achieved. The largest series available of patients with preoperative recurvatum without neuromuscular disorder has suggested that increased constraint, thicker components, and collateral ligament transfer are not necessary. Meding and colleagues[149] published results of 57 TKAs performed on patients with at least 5 degrees of flexion contracture in the absence of neuromuscular disease. Using a CR design, they corrected the hyperextension deformity in 98% of knees. All but two knees (5%) reached full extension at the end of the procedure. With an average 4.5-year follow-up, only two knees had a hyperextension deformity. Both these knees demonstrated residual medial instability immediately following insertion of the prosthesis.

Inadequate Motion

Arthrofibrosis is the most common cause of stiffness following TKA. The incidence ranges from 1.2% to 17%. Inadequate motion has several causes, including patient-related factors, surgical factors, and postoperative complications. Patient factors include preoperative ROM (most important risk factor), preoperative diagnosis (e.g., juvenile rheumatoid arthritis, ankylosing spondylitis, post-traumatic arthrosis, previous septic arthritis), body habits, and patient personality, such as depressed patients, or patients with a low threshold for pain.[164,208,209] Fisher and associates,[70] in their study of 1024 TKAs, identified patient-related factors contributing to poor results. The authors identified female gender, higher body mass index (BMI), previous knee surgery, disability status, diabetes mellitus, pulmonary disease, and depression as being significantly associated with the risk of having stiffness or pain at 1 year after surgery, despite the presence of well-aligned, well-fixed components.

Stiffness not only limits the patient's function but also predisposes the patient to pain. The cause is often unclear. Correct component position is critical, and the internal rotation of the femoral component and patellar maltracking must be avoided because they can contribute to a painful knee with limited ROM. It is also thought that certain factors may predispose an individual to the formation of abundant scar tissue, resulting in arthrofibrosis and limited motion. Pereira and coworkers[175] compared those patients with those with an acceptable ROM following arthroplasty procedures. No kinematic factors could be identified as the cause of stiffness in these patients. Lang and colleagues[134] recently looked at preoperative and postoperative ROMs for a contralateral TKA in patients with a history of a stiff TKA. They found that the range of motion was not significantly different than a control group at 2-year follow up, but the rate of manipulation was 26.7% in the study group compared with 8% in the control group. They demonstrated that good results could be obtained in the contralateral knee of patients with a history of arthrofibrosis but that there is a predisposition for the need of manipulation. Some patients may be more prone to keloid formation and may also be prone to arthrofibrosis. Abundant keloid or scar tissue results in decreased ROM. Another risk factor is an abnormal response to pain or poorly controlled pain, which limits postoperative rehabilitation. New emphasis on intraoperative injections and multimodal anesthesia may help make progress toward avoidance of a stiff knee because of poorly controlled pain.

Scott[205] has recently reviewed stiffness associated with TKA and discussed factors such as patient diagnosis, preoperative range of motion, prosthetic geometry, surgical technique, intraoperative range of motion, capsular closure, postoperative rehabilitation, and wound healing factors, which they considered as all playing a role in the development of a stiff knee. Ipsilateral hip degenerative joint disease (DJD) can also lead to the stiffness through persistent pain and limitations with regard to participation in therapy.

If the stiff knee fails to resolve after adjustments in pain medication and physical therapy, manipulations can be considered. This is done usually at the 6-week period, when adequate wound healing has occurred. The hip is gently flexed to 90 degrees and gentle flexion is applied. Manipulations tend to be more successful for poor flexion, although mild improvement can be made in extension. Yercan and coworkers[243] have evaluated 1188 knee arthroplasties with a prevalence of stiffness of 5.3%. The average premanipulation range of motion was 67 degrees and improved to 117 degrees after manipulation. It should be noted that motion at follow-up was better for those who had manipulation early compared with those who had it done later. Kim and colleagues[119] have evaluated stiffness after TKA. In their series, stiffness was associated with knees having a preoperative flexion contracture of 15 degrees or less than 75 degrees of flexion. The prevalence of stiffness was 1.3%. Recently, Rubinstein and DeHaan[197] reported the results and incidence of manipulation for primary knee arthroplasty. In this study, 37 of 800 TKAs were manipulated, with a 4.6% incidence of stiffness; the ROM improved from 68 to 109 degrees postmanipulation. Keating and associates[117] found no difference between patients who had undergone manipulation before and after 12 weeks in 113 knees, with an average flexion of 70 degrees. Namba and Inacio[162] studied 102 patients who had undergone manipulation under anesthesia within 90 days after TKA and 93 patients who had undergone manipulation more than 90 days after TKA. Manipulation was found to improve the ROM and function in both groups, although greater gains were observed in the early-manipulation group. The authors recommended manipulation for the treatment of stiffness after TKA, even if it was delayed beyond 90 days.

In cases of a stiff knee that does not respond to manipulation, the results of arthroscopic lysis of adhesions have been reported. These findings are rather controversial in the literature. Numerous authors have reported significant improvement, but some have reported poor results.[206] Court and colleagues[46] have described the results of arthroscopic arthrolysis after a TKR procedure. In this procedure, retinacular releases were performed medially and laterally and patella mobility was restored. Regional anesthesia was continued postarthroscopy to allow for intensive mobilization and early ROM. They recommended that this arthroscopic arthrolysis be done from 3 to 6 months after the knee replacement for better results. Best results are obtained in the case of isolated patellofemoral fibrosis. Bocell and coworkers[22] reported an increase in postoperative ROM in 43% of patients, Williams and associates[233] reported an average increase in ROM of 30.6 degrees whereas Mont and coworkers[159] reported an average improvement of 31 degrees in 94% of patients. In the case of severe ROM limitation, arthroscopic treatment alone is less

effective. Cates and Schmidt have evaluated the stiff TKA.[32a] They found that manipulation is most successful in patients within 8 weeks with full extension and at least 90 degrees of flexion prior to manipulation. Patients with large flexion contractures were less successfully treated with manipulation.

For those with significant flexion contracture who did not respond to more conservative management, open lysis is a final option before revision arthroplasty. However, open arthrolysis and isolated tibial insert exchange have not been successful in the Mayo Clinic series. Babis et al reported on a series of severely stiff knees treated between 1992 and 1998 and seven knees were identified that underwent isolated tibial insert exchange and open arthrolysis.[8] Unfortunately, isolated tibial insert exchange with arthrolysis and débridement did not yield significant improvement in this group of patients. Hutchinson and colleagues[99] reported an increase in ROM from 55 to 91 degrees 6 months after open arthrolysis, and Pretzsch and Dippold[179] showed an increase in knee flexion from 46 to 90 degrees and a decrease in flexion contracture from 11 to 7 degrees. In contrast, Babis and colleagues[8] have reported poor results with open arthrolysis and polyethylene exchange for stiff knees with fixed and well-aligned prosthetic components. More recently, Della Valle and colleagues[53] described their results with open arthrolysis with lysis of adhesions. Their emphasis was on access to the posterior capsule to regain full extension. With this technique, significant increases in range of motion were noted.

Prosthetic Loosening

Aseptic loosening of knee implants is multifactorial in regard to cause. The causes include but are not limited to malalignment of the prosthesis, higher BMI, small tibial components, higher potential stresses, polyethylene wear, and osteolysis.[16] Recently, a rapid increase in loosening of total knee components has been seen. Hossain and associates[92] reviewed 349 revision TKAs (343 patients) and reported aseptic loosening in 14.9% patients undergoing revision TKA and 1.4% in patients undergoing rerevision TKA. Piedade and coworkers[177] have compared 944 primary TKAs without surgical revision (890 patients) and 22 primary TKAs (22 patients) that had revision TKA secondary to aseptic failure. They reported that component loosening was one of the most common causes—50%—for revision in their study.

Tibial Component

There is reason to believe that the high failure rate caused by tibial component loosening (Fig. 125-11) represents a design problem that is now on the way to being solved (Fig. 125-12). High rates of loosening have been reported with polycentric, geometric, and early Freeman-Swanson designs. In addition to loosening, plastic deformation and cold flow were reported with the original University of California at Irvine (UCI) prosthesis, indicating that the rigidity of polyethylene can be compromised by excessively thin components and generous cruciate cutouts. Modifications to the tibial components were made in subsequent designs. The total condylar prosthesis had a one-piece tibial component and a central fixation peg, and no component loosening was seen in 220 knees monitored for 3 to 5 years. Reports from the Brigham and Women's Hospital in Boston[238] on the

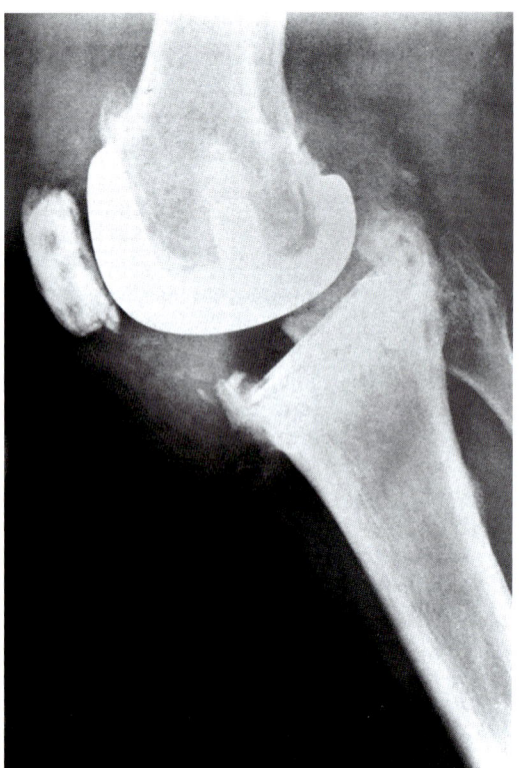

Figure 125-11. Flat tibial components, although of one piece, are inadequately supported by the cancellous bone of the upper tibia and are susceptible to sinkage, usually in an anterior or medial direction.

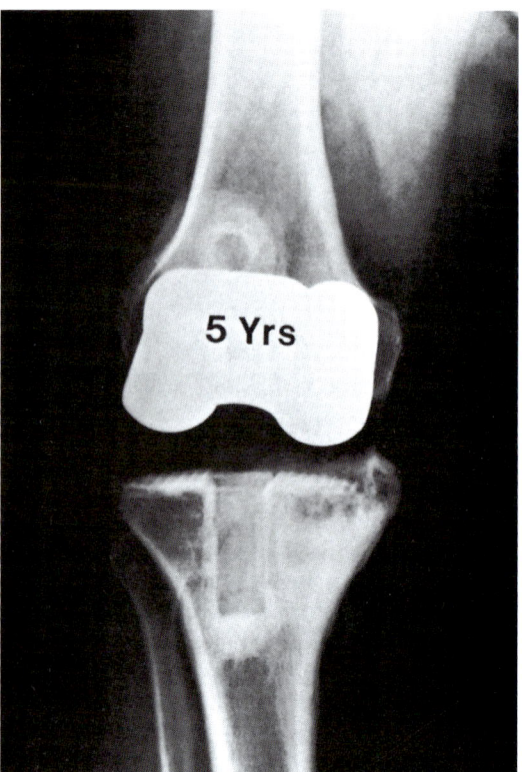

Figure 125-13. The importance of axial alignment. This total condylar knee prosthesis was positioned at surgery in slight varus, which gradually increased over a 5-year period. Collapse of the medial bone support with distortion of the polyethylene can be seen.

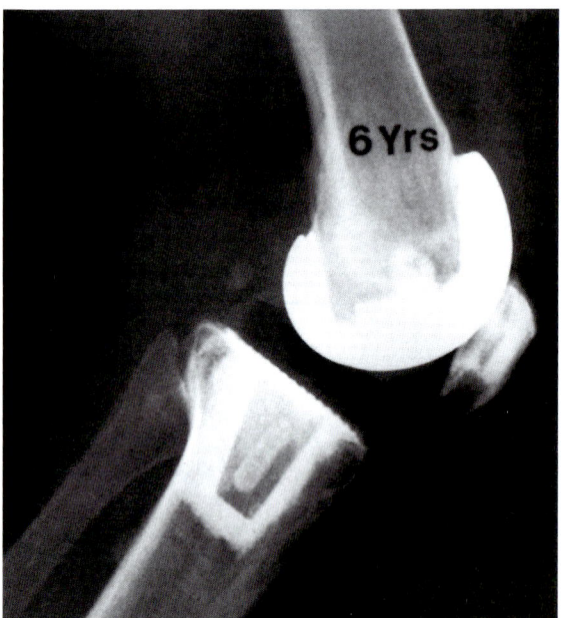

Figure 125-12. The addition of a central fixation peg to the tibial component almost eliminates tibial component loosening.

PCL-retaining, but otherwise similar, Kinematic prosthesis also have shown aseptic loosening to be negligible.

Malalignment and malposition should be related to mechanical loosening and are perhaps the leading cause (Figs. 125-13 and 125-14). There is some evidence for this. Lotke

and Ecker[143] have shown a correlation between malalignment and radiolucent lines and Hvid and Nielsen[101] confirmed these findings. Dorr and Boiardo[55] stated that "prosthetic alignment is the most important factor influencing postoperative loosening and instability." Hsu and coworkers[94] and Hsu and colleagues[96] were unable to show an association between varus positioning and component loosening, however, and Smith and colleagues,[211] using a cemented total condylar prosthesis, could find no relationship between radiolucent lines or loosening and component position. Cornell and associates,[45] also using the total condylar prosthesis, did find a correlation between radiolucency (although not loosening) and varus positioning. Tew and Waugh[217] found the association between positioning and loosening to be inconclusive. There are possible explanations for these discrepancies. Loosening rates for modern prostheses are low, and not all prostheses that are positioned in varus loosen. The identification and interpretation of radiolucent lines are confusing to the point that their analysis is probably meaningless (Fig. 125-15), unless the radiolucency is complete and progressive, a circumstance usually accompanied by clinical symptoms (Fig. 125-16). Analyzing the modes of failure in revision TKA, Mulhall and coworkers[161] identified polyethylene wear as a late mode of failure that may occur after an 11-year mean TKA revision interval. In addition, implant malalignment was reported in 9% of TKA loosening cases.

The use of metal-backed tibial components has further reduced the incidence of tibial loosening, presumably by more evenly distributing stress. The earliest version of

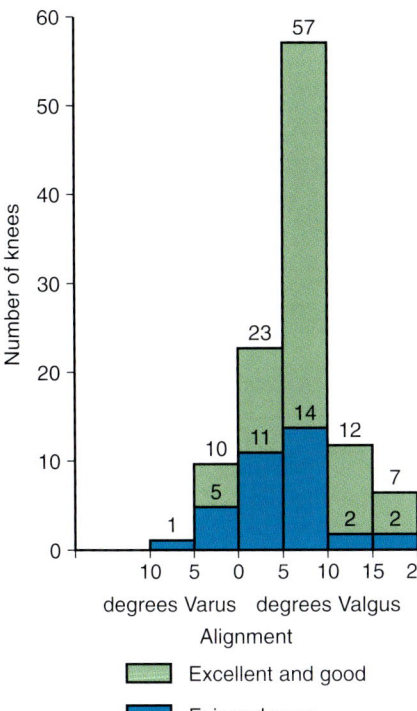

Figure 125-14. Bar graph showing the relationship between post-operative alignment and the clinical rating. The best results were obtained in knees aligned between 5 and 15 degrees of valgus. However, the relationship between alignment and the clinical result is by no means absolute. (From Insall J, Hood RW, Vanni M: The correction of knee alignment in 225 consecutive total condylar knee replacements. Clin Orthop Relat Res [160]:94, 1981.)

the posterior stabilized knee had an all-polyethylene tibial component and, at 9- to 12-year follow-up, a 3% tibial loosening rate was recorded.[212] More recently, a minimum 10-year study[38] of the same prosthesis with a metal-backed tibial component indicated no tibial loosening and no complete radiolucent lines. Partial radiolucent lines were seen in 50% of the all-polyethylene components compared with 10% of the metal-backed components. Faris and colleagues[65] have described an unacceptably high failure rate of 30% at 10 years in all-polyethylene tibial components with a coronal flat on flat design. All components failed beneath the medial tibial plateau, with bony collapse and medial tibial subsidence. It was thought that all-polyethylene tibial component success rates are highly design-specific and should be used with more conforming designs. Gioe and associates[75] reported the 8- to 12-year follow-up of congruent all-polyethylene tibial components with a modular metal-backed tibial component of the same design. Ten-year survivorship of the all-polyethylene tibial component was 91.6% with revision for any reason and 100% for aseptic loosening. The metal-backed tibial component survivorship was 88.9% with revision for any reason and 94.3% for aseptic loosening. Lachiewicz and coworkers,[132] in their study of 193 knees (131 patients) with the modular Insall-Burstein II PS total knee prosthesis, noted thin, incomplete, nonprogressive radiolucent lines around 30 tibial components (16%). No clinical or radiographic loosening of the tibial component was noted. Parsch and colleagues[171] reported on long-term survivorship and clinical outcomes for the Sigma PFC total knee arthroplasty (PFC-TKA; DePuy Orthopaedics, Warsaw, Ind) in a series of 141 TKAs with a mean follow-up of 13 years. With aseptic loosening of the implant as the end point, the 10- and 14-year survival rates were 97%.

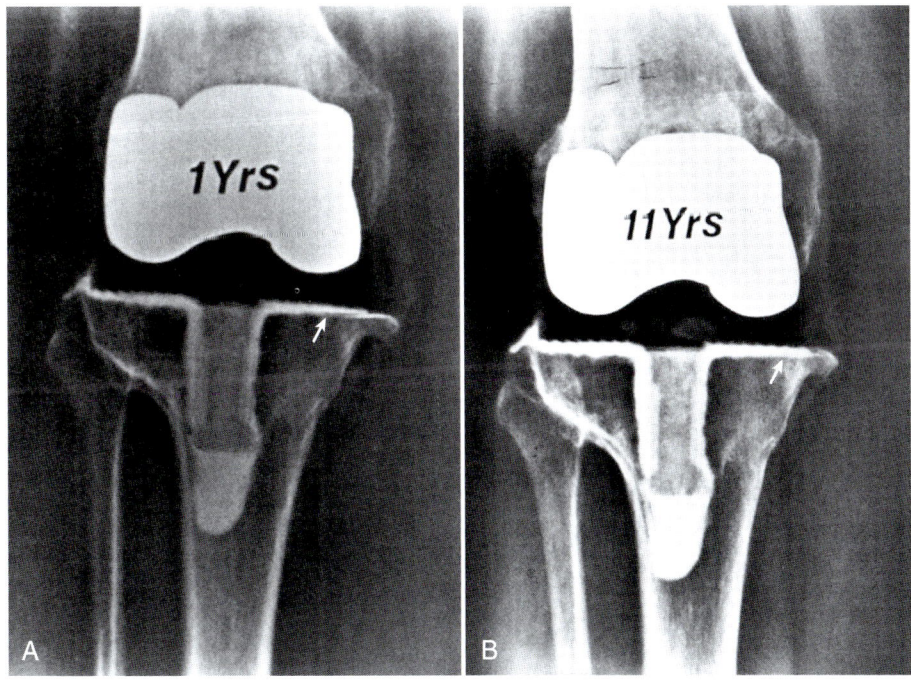

Figure 125-15. **A,** Small partial radiolucency beneath the medial tibial plateau. **B,** The radiolucency is barely perceptible 10 years later, probably because of a slight difference in projection.

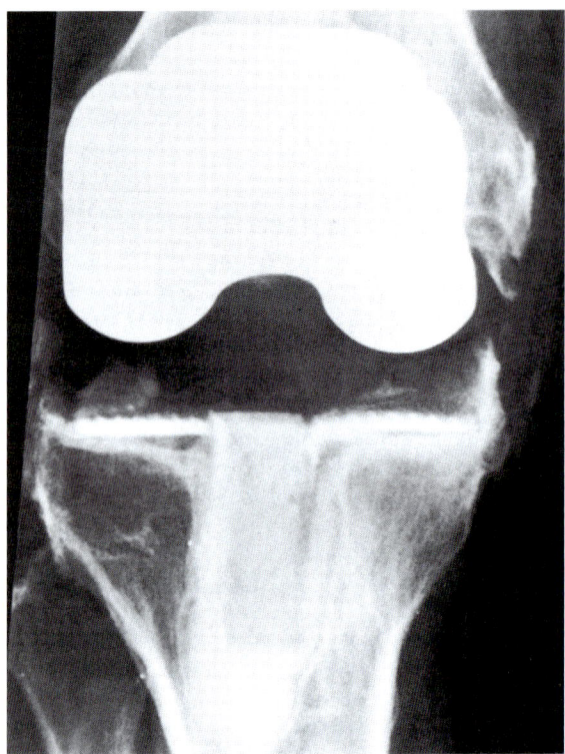

Figure 125-16. With the total condylar prosthesis, a complete radiolucency is attributed to low-grade infection until proven otherwise.

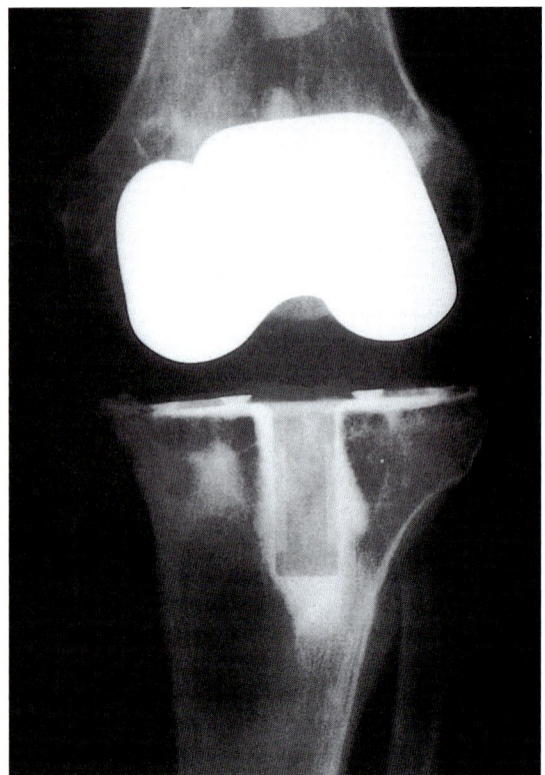

Figure 125-17. Radiograph showing an example of osteolysis involving a prosthesis.

The underlying mechanism of loosening is also of interest. Miller[154] has indicated that the process is initiated by micromotion between the component and bone, postulating that micromotion could be reduced or eliminated by improving the interlock between cement and cancellous bone. This argument, similar to others in joint arthroplasty, may apply more to hip prostheses than to knee prostheses. Another possible mechanism of loosening is that the components sink or subside into the bone. Seitz and associates,[209] using computed tomography (CT), noted a loss of bone density for several months after knee arthroplasty, coupled with a tendency for the implant to migrate in a mediolateral direction. Periprosthetic osteolysis is another cause of component loosening (Fig. 125-17). The tibia is the more common site, but there have been documented cases in the literature involving femoral and tibial components. Osteolysis is discussed in more detail in the next section.

Ryd and coworkers[198-201,220] have extensively studied fixation of knee prostheses in vivo using roentgenographic stereogrammetric analysis. This technique was developed in Lund, Sweden in 1974 and applied to various orthopedic problems, such as spinal fusion stability, healing of tibial osteotomy, and skeletal growth patterns. It also has been used for assessing hip joint prosthetic loosening. In the knee, three or more tantalum balls of 0.8-mm diameter are implanted into the tibial metaphysis, using a special instrument with a needle and piston. Markers also are introduced approximately 3 mm into the polyethylene tibial component from underneath, using holes made with a dentist's drill. The postoperative reference examination, using a biplanar radiographic technique (Fig. 125-18), is carried out on the supine patient

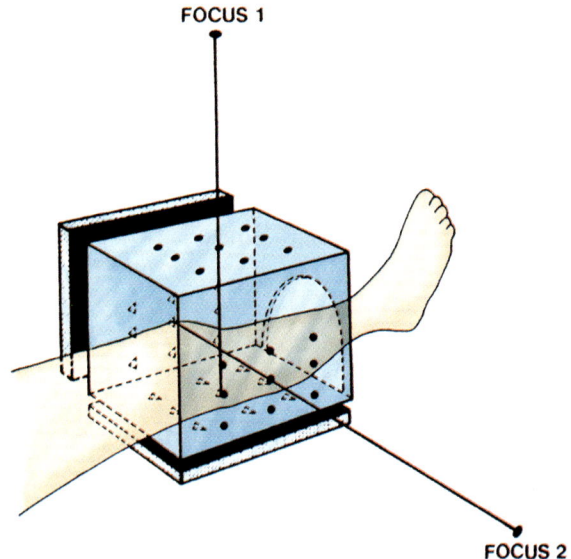

Figure 125-18. Biplanar radiographic setup for roentgenographic stereogrammetric analysis of the knee joint. (From Ryd L, Boegard T, Egund N, et al: Migration of the tibial component in successful unicompartmental knee arthroplasty: a clinical, radiographic, and roentgen stereophotogrammetric study. Acta Orthop Scand 54:408, 1983.)

before the operated leg has become weight bearing. The follow-up examination is carried out with the patient standing on the operated leg only. Rotations about the transverse and sagittal axes were the only movements determined. The initial study was performed on Marmor unicondylar replacements, all of which were clinically successful. The study indicated that none of the prostheses were rigidly fixed to the skeleton, and a degree of micromotion and migration occurred. There was some pattern to migration. Of the six patients studied, five showed posterior and downward migration and four showed medial tilting away from the central axis of the knee.

Subsequent studies have been performed with cemented and uncemented prostheses, with similar results. Migration was greatest in the first year, after which it tended to stabilize; the direction tended to be medial, posterior, and downward. The mode of fixation was important and migration was greater for uncemented prostheses. The magnitude was approximately 1 mm for a cemented total condylar prosthesis and 2.6 mm for an uncemented porous-coated anatomic (PCA) prosthesis. In another study, the same authors examined 26 patients randomized to cemented or cementless TKA.[220] Using a similar study design, they found the migration between the two groups to be similar. At 1 year, the cemented tibial migration was 1 ± 0.2 mm compared with 1.4 ± 0.22 mm for the cementless TKA. Ryd and Linder[200] have published a description of the bone-cement interface in three well-functioning unicondylar replacements that initially had been shown to migrate by roentgenographic stereogrammetric analysis. The three prostheses were removed for reasons other than fixation. The tibial components were solidly fixed to the bone. The three interfaces had a similar distribution of fibrous tissue and fibrocartilage. The peripheral 5 to 10 mm consisted of fibrous tissue, whereas the remainder of the supporting tissue was fibrocartilage. This layer of cartilage always rested on bone, sometimes with a seam of osteoid sandwiched between the bone and cartilage. The bone underneath the cartilage was vital. There was a total absence of any cellular reaction in the fibrocartilage.

Ryd and associates'[198-201,220] studies have shown that there is no such thing as rigid fixation between prosthesis and bone, and that the normal situation allows some degree of micromotion. Prostheses move or migrate a certain amount early on and then, in most cases, stabilize into a state of equilibrium, which is compatible with satisfactory long-term function. The normal interface between cement and bone consists of fibrocartilage and fibrous tissue, with little cellular reaction. This interface probably corresponds with thin stable radiolucencies that can be identified in long-term studies of well-functioning knee arthroplasties. Hvid and Nielsen[100,101] have concluded that bone strength may be crucial from the point of view of fatigue. Consequently, it can be argued that excessive penetration of cement into the cancellous bone of the knee may be undesirable. It is unlikely that bone trabeculae enclosed within a massive amount of cement remain viable; although the initial mechanical interlock may be improved, the long-term effect may be to transfer the interface to a more distal area of the tibia and into an area in which the strength of the bone is weaker. If one believes this argument, cement penetration should be minimal; 2 to 3 mm is ideal.[226] The theoretical argument coincides with clinical observations. Long-term studies of prostheses using old-fashioned cement techniques that gave little bone penetration have shown extremely good survival. For about 2 years, roughly encompassing 1984 and 1985, we sought greater cement penetration using low-viscosity cement[154]; however, after realizing that our earlier patients continued to function

well, we returned to the earlier cement techniques. Most of our metal-backed tibial components have been fixed, using a thin layer of cement with little attempt to penetrate the cancellous bone.

Alignment is more crucial in cementless knees because cement fixation is not present to help protect against excessive point loading, which may occur with malalignment. With cement fixation, load is distributed more evenly across the tibia, even when malalignment is present. Without cement fixation, this even distribution of load is not present, and a point-load situation is created, which causes necrosis of bone under the overloaded tibial component. Also, without the protective effect of cement fixation, failure of fixation at the opposite condyle occurs from excessive tension at the interface.[57] Ritter and Meneghini[194] have reviewed 73 cementless TKAs (AGC, Biomet, Warsaw, Ind). They found that survivorship for aseptic loosening of any component was 76.4% at 20 years, and two tibial components failed because of of aseptic loosening at 1.1 and 2.2 years.

Femoral Component

Loosening of femoral components is uncommon, whether cemented or uncemented. When it does occur, however, it follows a particular pattern in which the bone resorbs posteriorly, allowing the femur to migrate anteriorly and rotate into flexion (Fig. 125-19). King and Scott[123] described a series of 15 loose, cemented, duopatellar femoral prostheses. The incidence of femoral loosening was not stated but, in one series at the Hospital for Special Surgery, there were 6 femoral loosenings in 430 cemented arthroplasties (1.4%) over a 15-year follow-up period. The mechanism of loosening was similar to that described by King and Scott, who thought that the lack of posterior femoral support as a result of osteoporotic bone or poor technique was the cause. In this region, cancellous bone hypertrophy was reported by Whiteside and Pafford[232]; this region of the femur is most likely to be highly stressed.

Patellar Component

Loosening of the patellar component is associated most often with patellar fractures or with dissociation of polyethylene and metal-backed components. Loosening of cemented all-polyethylene patellae in other circumstances is infrequent. The incidence of patellar component loosening is approximately 1% but has been reported to be as high as 3%.[238] Loosening of the patella was more common with the small central lug but, more recently, the tripod configuration of three small peripheral lugs has become popular. Mason and coworkers[146] have reported no loose patellar components among 577 tripod configuration patellae at an average of 3 years.

Firestone and colleagues[69] found loosening rates of 0.6% to 11.1% in several cementless patellar component designs. Factors associated with loosening include insertion of the prosthesis with cement into worn or sclerotic bone, malpositioning of the patellar component, subluxation, fracture or avascular necrosis of the patella, osteoporosis, asymmetrical resection, loosening of other prosthetic components, and lack of osseous growth into the porous coating.[188,228] Reduction in the rate of loosening of the patellar component requires improved bone preparation and cementing techniques, proper patellar resection, avoidance of asymmetrical or excessive bone removal, and central patellar tracking.[7]

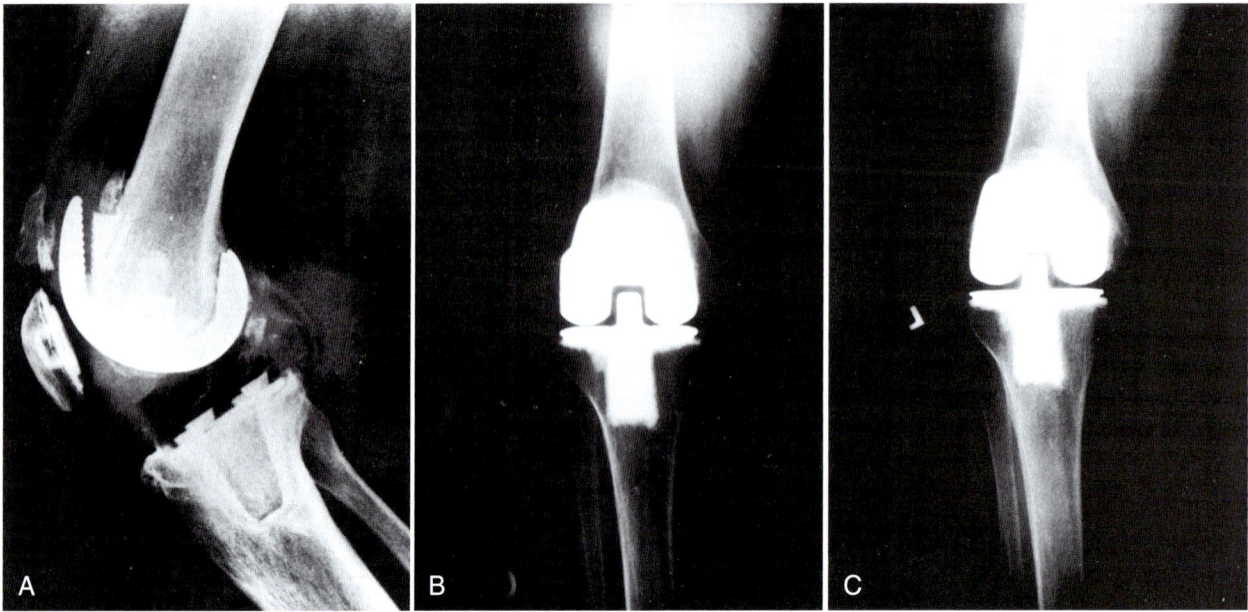

Figure 125-19. A, Radiograph showing a typical example of femoral loosening. In the lateral view, the femur has migrated anteriorly and moved into a flexed position as a result of resorption of posterior bone. **B, C,** The diagnosis of femoral loosening in the AP view is not always easy to make. The femur tends to migrate proximally so that there is the appearance of bone overgrowth medially or laterally. In this case, the diagnosis of loosening was made because a change in position into varus was noted and was confirmed by overlapping the radiographs.

Osteolysis

Osteolysis is well documented in the THA literature in response to particulate debris, and it has shown a rapid increase more recently in the TKA literature. The cause of osteolysis in the knee is the same as in the hip—inflammatory response to particulate debris.

Osteolysis has been reported to be associated with the polyethylene stock and sterilization method, tibial modularity and backside wear, design of the PS tibial post, patient factors (e.g., age, activity level), and surgical factors.[18,60,163,227] Lachiewicz and associates,[132] at a mean of 12 years (range, 10 to 18 years), reported 7% osteolysis. This study indicated an association between younger patient age and radiographic evidence of osteolysis.

Collier and coworkers[43] reviewed 365 PCR-TKAs and found that the prevalence of osteolysis at 5 to 10 years was 34% when polyethylene sterilized with gamma radiation in air was used on a grit-blasted titanium base; the prevalence was 9% when polyethylene sterilized with gamma radiation in air or polyethylene that had been sterilized with gas plasma was used on a polished cobalt-chromium (Co-Cr) base. Their analysis has shown that the osteolysis is associated with male gender, the use of a grit-blasted titanium tibial base, three polyethylene-related factors (variety from which it had been machined, sterilization method, and shelf age), and femoral component hyperextension.

The incidence of osteolysis around a knee replacement is difficult to assess for many reasons. First, obtaining an accurate radiographic assessment at the interface is difficult. For example, if there is tibial osteolysis below the tray, and the x-ray angle is from slightly above the joint, this lysis may be missed. Engh and colleagues[61] indicated that femoral lesions are more difficult to recognize. Femoral lesions are often hidden by the femoral component on the radiograph.

Posterior femoral condyle overlap and the central box of PS components limit complete evaluation of femoral condyles on lateral radiographs. Whereas the anterior flange of the component may hide lesions on the anteroposterior (AP) image, Miura and associates[156] have reported that the oblique posterior femoral condylar radiographic view is significantly better than a true lateral view for the detection of radiolucencies.

Reish and coworkers[189] have determined the accuracy of plain radiography in detecting osteolytic lesions around total knee prostheses compared with multidetector CT. They studied 31 patients diagnosed with periprosthetic osteolysis by plain radiography and multidetector CT after TKA. They reported that plain radiographs are inadequate for evaluating periprosthetic osteolysis in TKA, with only 8 of 48 lesions (17%) detected by multidetector CT visible on the standard radiographs.

Another reason for the difficulty in assessing the incidence of osteolysis is the length of follow-up. Ezzet and colleagues[63] reported a strong correlation between length of follow-up and the prevalence of osteolysis. Before 24 months, no cases of osteolysis were identified, between 24 and 60 months, the incidence was 15%, and at follow-up longer than 60 months, the incidence was 39%.[181]

The cause of the particulate debris, which contributes to osteolysis, remains controversial. Small particles are generated from the articular surface, tibial post impingement in PS knees, backside wear in all modular designs, and backside wear in mobile-bearing knees. It is apparent, however, that osteolysis is extremely rare in monoblock tibial designs, especially with net shape–molded components. Particulate debris displaced from the articular and backside surfaces of tibial polyethylene inserts is considered to be a predominant cause. Polishing the tibial baseplate counterface, polyethylene sterilization by gamma radiation in an inert gas environment, and nonradiation sterilization methods have reduced loss of polyethylene debris and may yield a more fatigue-resistant bearing surface. Collier and associates[42] also investigated the factors of the backside interface and polyethylene sterilization method in a study of 365 CR TKAs (Anatomic Modular Knee; DePuy) with minimum 5-year follow-up. They reported a significant reduction in the prevalence of osteolysis, from 24% to 2%, when transition was made to a polished baseplate and away from gamma irradiation in air.

Histologic analysis of synovial tissue and osteolytic tissue has been performed. The synovial tissue of knees associated with osteolysis shows subsynovial infiltrates consisting of histiocytes and giant cells.[176] Polyethylene and metal particulate debris have been found in specimens. The size of the debris and type of material are both important. Polyethylene particles smaller than 3 μm are usually engulfed by giant cells. Polyethylene particles larger than 3 μm are found in the cytoplasm of histiocytes and occasionally within giant cells. Larger particles of metal (≈5 μm) usually elicit little cellular response. Histologic examinations of osteolytic tissue have revealed a hypercellular membrane consisting of sheets of histiocytes and occasional giant cells. There is no necrosis and little associated vascularity.

The presentation of a patient with osteolysis varies. Most patients with well-fixed components are asymptomatic. Others present with symptoms of boggy synovitis. Mild or moderate diffuse pain may occur with activity, especially in patients in whom the tibial component is unstable. The radiographic criteria for diagnosis of osteolysis, as proposed by Peters and coworkers,[176] included a lytic osseous defect that extends beyond the limits of that potentially caused by loosening of the implant alone, absence of cancellous bone trabeculae, and geographic demarcation by a shell of bone. Accelerated polyethylene wear and the subsequent osteolysis can give rise to aseptic loosening, periprosthetic fracture, recurrent painful effusions, and polyethylene fractures, which can necessitate or complicate revision surgery.

TKA produces greater wear of the polyethylene surface than THA, yet less osteolysis is seen compared with THA. Engh and colleagues[61] have described four factors that could explain this phenomenon. First is the size of the particles produced, which is related to the type of wear (i.e., delamination and abrasion in TKA); this releases large fragments of polyethylene, rarely seen in THA. Large particles produced in the TKA are relatively bioinert. Second, the synovial cavity of the knee is the most extensive of any synovial joint in the body and has greater capacity to engulf and digest wear debris (i.e., greater resistance to osteolysis). Third, the fixation interface with polymethylmethacrylate (PMMA) is a better seal to potential debris than PMMA in a THA. Fourth, the shear and tensile stresses on PMMA may be less at the knee than at the hip. The modulus of elasticity of PMMA is relatively close to that of the cancellous bone of the upper tibia and tibial component. The decreased amount of stress and fatigue means decreased fracture of the cement mantle, which leads to decreased access for debris to the bone-cement interface.

When osteolysis appears around a TKA, it usually appears on the tibial side; this is probably a multifactorial event. Peters and associates[176] have suggested three possible causative factors for this:

1. Gravity and weight bearing through the medial side of the knee tend to localize the particulate polyethylene on the tibial side.
2. On the femoral side, if the osteolytic process is initiated along the implant-bone interface, the flanges of the femoral implant tend to obscure a radiographic diagnosis.
3. The addition of screws to the tibial implant provides avenues for the migration of debris into metaphyseal bone.

The treatment of osteolysis around a TKA is controversial. If the implant is stable, and the patient is asymptomatic, one can observe the patient with serial x-ray films on a yearly basis. If the patient is symptomatic or the prosthesis is grossly loose, there are several different options. For patients who are symptomatic with a well-fixed modular prosthesis and excessive polyethylene, one can débride the lesion with a curette, pack the defect with a morcellized bone graft, and exchange the polyethylene. Exchange of the bearing surface in TKA offers several potential benefits compared with complete component revision, including the preservation of bone stock, reduced complexity, reduced cost, and potentially easier patient recovery. Because polyethylene wear and osteolysis are increasingly indicated as reasons for revision, the prospect of less complicated isolated insert exchange is an attractive option. Griffin and coworkers[82] have evaluated the results of isolated polyethylene exchange for wear and/or osteolysis in 68 press-fit condylar TKAs at the mean 44 months and had 11 failures (16.2%). Failures included aseptic loosening in 10 knees and infection in 1. They reported an 84% success rate with modular polyethylene exchange and the lack of progression of osteolytic lesions in the 97% of knees. O'Brien and associates[165] reported that osteolytic lesions resolved in the 17 of 18 hips studied at a mean of 3 years after the postexchange procedure. Similarly, Maloney and coworkers[145] reported that osteolytic lesions resolved in one third of 40 hips treated with isolated liner exchange; in the remaining two thirds of hips, the lesions reduced in size at a mean of 3.5 years following isolated liner exchange. Engh and colleagues[61] either changed out the polyethylene or performed removal of screws, curettage, and polyethylene exchange. They reported good results, with no tibial defects progressing and no development of new lesions.

If the components are grossly loose, revision of the components is in order. Because the defects are always larger in situ than they appear on film, a full armamentarium of revision instruments should be ready. In most cases, allografts and the full complement of modular augments should be available. In Engh and associates' series,[61] in which the components were revised and structural allografts were used, four of five patients had excellent fixation interfaces at 2 years. There were no lucencies and no graft resorption. One patient with rheumatoid arthritis had a 1- to 2-mm radiolucency beneath the tibial plateau without change in component alignment. The patient was pain-free at 6 years. Robinson and associates[195] reported on 17 revisions performed for osteolysis. The original method of component fixation was a mixture of hybrid fixation, including both cemented and cementless implants. The average time interval from the index surgery to radiographic evidence of osteolysis was 56 months. The prostheses used in the treatment of these 17 revisions were PS implants in 65% of cases and a constrained implant in 30%. Osteolytic defects were reconstructed with cement only in 47%, allograft in 30%, and metallic wedges in 35%. No follow-up or outcome data were available from this series. Kim and coworkers[122] reported the prevalence of osteolysis after simultaneous bilateral fixed-bearing and mobile-bearing TKAs in young patients. Osteolysis was identified in radiographs and CT scans in 6 knees (10%) in the anatomic molecular knee fixed bearing prosthesis (Depuy, Warsaw, Ind) group and 4 knees (7%) in the low contact stress mobile meniseal bearing prosthesis (Depuy, Warsaw, Ind) group. Kim and colleagues[120] also studied 62 patients who underwent simultaneous bilateral TKAs, with a unidirectional prosthesis implanted in one knee and a multidirectional prosthesis in the other. No differences in preoperative and postoperative knee and functional scores were seen. No patients had detectable tibial polyethylene liner wear or osteolysis.

Component Breakage

Breakage of components is rare[23,56,109] and usually restricted to hinges and linked designs.[111] Breakage is manifest by instability, pain, and deformity, but does not always call for immediate revision. Historically, one of our patients had a fracture of the femoral stem associated with an episode of transient pain 3 years after the arthroplasty. Although some instability was present, this patient functioned at a high level with little or no pain for another 5 years before revision became necessary for an increasing varus deformity.

Mechanical failure in surface replacement is rare. We encountered three fractured femoral components in the early version of the unicondylar and duocondylar prostheses. In these, the femoral runner was made of considerably thinner metal than that used on subsequent designs, and it is not expected that similar fatigue failure will be seen in current models. Fracture of unicondylar metal components also has been reported.[23] Whiteside and associates[229] examined fracture of femoral components in cementless TKAs. They compared 6172 Ortholoc II femoral components (Wright Medical Technology, Arlington, Tenn) with double-bead layers with 16,230 Ortholoc II femoral components with single-bead layers for fracture of components. They found a total of 32 fractured femoral components, of which 31 were in the double-bead layers. The overall minimum rate of failure for the double-bead layers was 0.42, whereas for the single-bead layer it was 0.006. They found that all the failures occurred at the junction between one of the level surfaces and the distal surface of the implant.

Fracture of the metallic tibial tray has been reported on isolated occasions.[56,138] Subsequently, in these designs, the metal tray was strengthened, particularly in the region of the posterior cruciate cutout. We have not seen a metal tray fracture in a cruciate-substituting design.

Polyethylene fractures are generally wear-related, as with late catastrophic failure of the tibial inserts of modular components. However, catastrophic fractures of the tibial post in posterior PS and constrained designs have been reported. Although these failures seem to occur predominantly in designs that do not provide adequate anterior clearances, which results in anterior post impingement in hyperextension, they have been reported in newer designs as well.[112,135,139] They also may occur as a result of overflexion of the femoral component or inadequate posterior slope of the tibial component. Thus, the importance of surgical technique relative to component positioning cannot be overemphasized. Even neutral intraoperative saggital positioning of components is biased toward clinical hyperextension. This is because the combination of the anterior bow of the femur and the anterior-posterior slope of the tibial resection results in approximately 10 degrees of relative component hyperextension when the knee is placed in full extension.[10] As the femoral component moves from flexion to hyperextension, the intercondylar notch may contact the anterior region of the tibial eminence or tibial post, depending on the design of the implant (i.e., PCL-retaining vs. PCL-substituting). If impingement occurs, fracture, significant polyethylene wear, or both may follow.[22,104,142]

Factors inherent to the polyethylene may also predispose it to fracture. Ionizing radiation improves the adhesive and abrasive wear resistance of polyethylene by producing cross linkages[192] and a recent retrospective study has demonstrated that highly cross-linked polyethylene is safe for use in TKA.[88] However, in an oxygen environment, ionizing radiation can create free radicals that embrittle polyethylene through oxidation. Modern techniques such as vacuum processing, heat annealing, and remelting have been devised to avoid or eliminate these free radicals. However, it is interesting to note that if oxidation has occurred prior to implantation, it is likely to continue in vivo as the polyethylene implant is exposed to oxygen-containing body fluids.[131] In total hip arthroplasty, the clinical effects of in vivo oxidation have been negligible, presumably because the ball and socket interface affords a degree of protection to most of the polyethylene component. In these cases, in vivo oxidation is most severe at the rim of the liner. For TKA, the implications are more severe because the tibial eminence or post is constantly bathed in synovial fluid. This may account for the high rate of early postoperative tibial post breakage reported by Bal and coworkers[9] for polyethylene implants sterilized with gamma radiation in an oxygen environment.

Component Wear

Retrieval analysis of removed total joint implants consistently has revealed polyethylene particles in the synovium.[29,78,79,155,181] In addition, acrylic debris and occasionally metallic particles have been seen. Inspection of the removed components often reveals embedded cement particles in the polyethylene component with scratching, pitting, and burnishing of the articular surface. Distortion of the polyethylene and gross deformation of the component as a result of cold flow (Fig. 125-20) also may occur; this is particularly likely when the tibial polyethylene component is thin. Some earlier designs had a component that was deliberately made thin to minimize bone removal and often had a cruciate cutout. This combination sometimes led to gross distortion and deformation, which contributed to loosening of the component (the early UCI design was prone to this type of failure). It is now considered that unless the component is reinforced with a metal tray, a minimum thickness of 8 mm is desirable.

Metal femoral components may be observed to have scratches in the highly polished articular surface in more than 50% of retrieved specimens. It is believed that some of the debris is generated from free cement particles that have become trapped between the articular surfaces. Careful

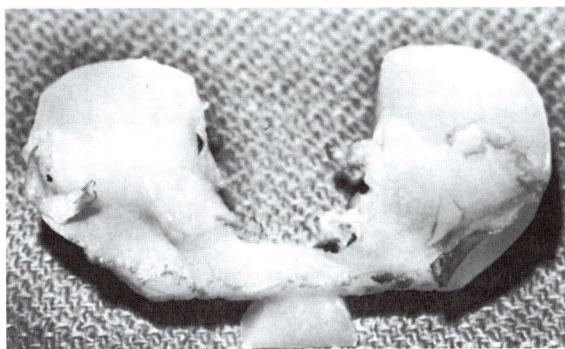

Figure 125-20. Retrieved geometric tibial component showing severe wear.

surgical technique can lessen cement entrapment; however, even in the absence of evidence of cement or body wear, polyethylene failure at the articular surface may be observed. This failure is manifested by pitting, scratching, burnishing, and abrasion of the surface. The amount of surface failure is highly correlated with the level of patient activity, body weight, and length of implantation and seems to be more than that noted in retrieval analysis of total hip implants.[90]

The type of motion occurring in the articulation is also important. Sliding as opposed to rolling movements causes much greater wear, especially of the delamination type. The kinematic conditions in the joint seem to be of paramount importance.[21] Uncomforming flat surfaces, together with lax ligaments, predispose to various sliding motions.

The durability of a spherically convex polyethylene patellar implant may be questioned in that this shape theoretically causes more wear. Retrieval analysis at the Hospital for Special Surgery of 20 patellar buttons[91] did not indicate that the rate of wear is greater than that of the tibial plateau. However, there was some deformation of the polyethylene, usually with elongation in the long axis and some flattening of the convex shape where it articulates with the femoral component. Figgie[68] has examined all-polyethylene dome patellar components and found a positive correlation between the amount of polyethylene damage and the ROM achieved postoperatively.

Metal backing of patellar components did not improve the wear performance characteristics, but rather led to an increase in wear-related complications.[17,13,147,196,215] Up to ten times serum levels of titanium, aluminum, and vanadium were measured in patients with metal on metal contact after metal-backed patellar failure.[216] These extreme levels of debris have been associated with extensive osteolysis and periarticular soft tissue cysts and masses.[33]

Hsu and Walker[95] more recently studied wear patterns in patellar components. They found that wear occurred regardless of the design shape, although wear was most rapid in dome-shaped patellae with metal inlays. A dome-shaped patella is only in line contact with the femur until approximately 70 degrees of flexion, after which the patella contacts peripherally with the condylar runners. Contouring the shape of the patella (central convexity and peripheral concavity) greatly improved the wear characteristics, which was better still when the component was metal-backed. Even with optimal shape and metal backing, however, wear-through was ultimately predicted because of design constraints on the

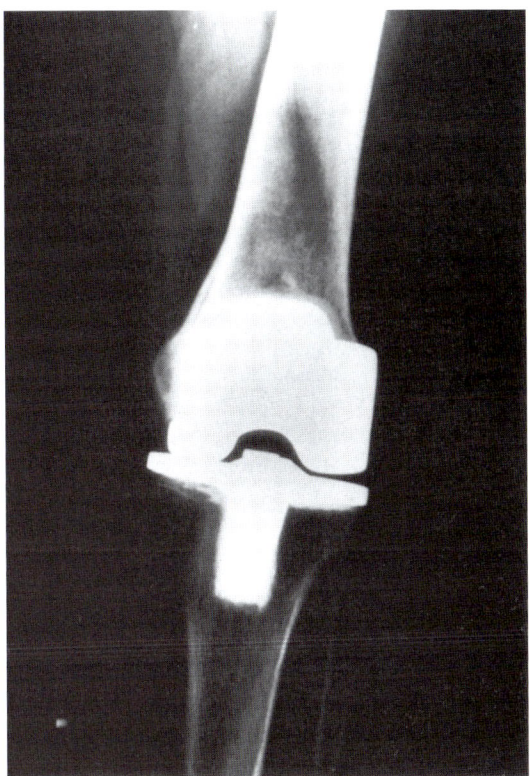

Figure 125-21. Radiograph of a Kinematic prosthesis 5 years postoperatively showing wear-through of the medial tibia.

thickness of the polyethylene (approximately 3 mm). It was concluded that onset patellar replacements with metal backing should not be used at this time. Inlaying the patellar component allows a thicker layer of plastic, which may be an improvement from the wear point of view, but does not allow polyethylene resurfacing at the margins of the patella, the regions that are subject to the greatest contact pressures when the knee is flexed. There has been a general return to cemented all-polyethylene patellar components, although agreement on this point is not uniform.[44]

Tibial polyethylene wear has emerged as a major clinical problem,[39,61,77,141] particularly with designs having flat tibial surfaces and thin polyethylene.[34] Isolated cases of wear-through initially were reported for the porous-coated anatomic prosthesis[60] and the variable axis prosthesis. In the cases described, the medial polyethylene wore through to the metal baseplate (Fig. 125-21). The original thickness of the components was about 5 mm. These were treated by replacing the polyethylene insert with a thicker one. Posterior wear-through to metal has been seen on the Robert Brigham unicondylar design on 6-mm components[127,128] and on the posterior polyethylene of Kinematic components, in which it was judged that excessive femoral rollback had occurred.

Wear damage to polyethylene is influenced by clinical and design factors.[193] Studies performed on tibial components of a single design have shown significant correlation between the amount of polyethylene damage to the articulating surface and patient weight and the length of implantation of the component.[239] Greater wear damage also has been found in patients who achieved better ambulatory status postoperatively.

Other factors also influence the wear characteristics of polyethylene. Polyethylene inserts are currently manufactured by compression molding of resin or machining of ram-extruded bars. Of these two processes, compression molding seems to provide greater resistance to articular[236] and backside wear,[140] although data are limited. Polyethylene has traditionally been sterilized with gamma radiation or gas plasma. Postproduction irradiation of polyethylene was serendipitously found to induce cross linking, which imparts statistically lower wear rates than conventional non–cross-linked polyethylene. In laboratory trials, this benefit is maintained across different rotating and fixed-bearing total knee designs.[221] However, the free radicals formed by irradiation in air can adversely affect the polyethylene through oxidation. In an in vivo wear analysis performed at the Anderson Orthopaedic Research Institute, wear rates were significantly greater for polyethylene components radiation-sterilized in air versus those sterilized in inert gas.[41] These findings have been confirmed by a recent survivorship analysis as well. Griffin and colleagues[83] compared the incidence of wear-related failure between two cohorts of patients who had received identical modular tibial trays and polyethylene sterilized by different methods. The polyethylene implants sterilized in air demonstrated an 87% 10-year survivorship whereas those sterilized in an oxygen-free environment demonstrated a 97% 10-year survivorship. The locking mechanism for modular designs is also a factor in reducing wear. A recent retrieval analysis of three different total knee designs at the Hospital for Special Surgery found a lower incidence of backside wear for polyethylene components that were locked to the tibial baseplate with a peripheral capture mechanism as opposed to partial dovetailing or pinning.[106] Finally, shelf life longer than 1.5 years is another independent variable that negatively influences wear.[40]

With the increased modularity afforded by metal tibial trays, undersurface or backside wear has become a recognized entity.[169] This problem is caused by micromotion between the polyethylene insert and the tray (usually made of titanium), causing particulate polyethylene debris to accumulate. In uncemented trays, the debris can filter down the screw holes, initiating osteolysis. Studies have documented that under physiologic loading, modular designs have motion between the tray and polyethylene insert, regardless of the locking mechanism.[168] Wasielewski and colleagues[227] examined 67 polyethylene tibial inserts from cementless TKAs retrieved at autopsy or revision surgery. The mean implantation time was 62.8 months. Polyethylene cold flow and abrasive wear on the monoarticulating insert surface (undersurface) were assigned a wear severity score (grades 0 to 4). The investigators found that severe grade 4 wear of the tibial insert undersurface was associated with tibial metaphyseal osteolysis or osteolysis around fixation screws. Time in situ was statistically related to grade 4 undersurface wear and tibial metaphyseal osteolysis.

Lessons learned from the polished undersurface of the mobile-bearing designs are being applied to fixed platform designs. Polishing the tibial baseplate may help lessen the extent of backside wear for fixed-bearing designs as well. In a laboratory trial, material and surface factors were found to influence backside wear. In fixed-bearing designs, polished titanium has slightly better wear characteristics than polished Co-Cr in decreasing the polyethylene wear, but both polished surfaces provide substantial benefits over their traditional nonpolished counterparts.[19]

Much attention has been placed on the development of mobile bearing designs. Despite theoretical benefits, an in vitro wear study comparing mobile- and fixed-bearing options of the same implant at over 6 million cycles failed to demonstrate statistically significant improvement.[87] Although previous retrieval analysis of mobile-bearing designs has not shown excessive wear of the back insert surface or tibial metaphyseal osteolysis,[27] more recent analysis has demonstrated that the articular surface of mobile-bearing designs remains vulnerable to wear, in addition to the independent inferior surface.[73] When compared with fixed-bearing designs, mobile-bearing knees seem to trade improved articular-sided wear characteristics for more serious backside wear.[144] On close inspection of retrieved implants, mobile-bearing designs are more susceptible to burnishing and scratching of the undersurface than fixed-bearing designs, and a higher incidence of burnishing is also noted on the articular surface.[62]

Meniscal-bearing designs, such as the Oxford and LCS (low contact stress), are theoretically the least liable to wear, but the possibility of dislocation of the bearings offsets the advantage to some extent.[14] Although backside wear seems decreased in these designs, it does occur and has been reported as a cause of bearing dislocation and catastrophic polyethylene failure.[97,98]

Landy and Walker[133] have examined 90 retrieved knee prostheses with implant times of up to 10 years. Polyethylene wear was much greater than that seen in wear studies of acetabular components in total hip prostheses (Fig. 125-22).

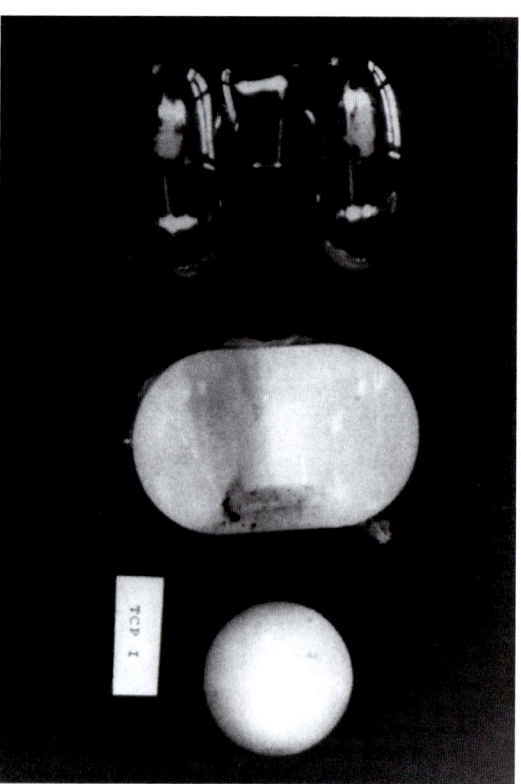

Figure 125-22. Retrieved total condylar prosthesis removed because of infection after having been implanted for 7 years in an active patient. The appearance of the tibial component shows some burnishing and a few small pits. The patellar component shows slight flattening in one area. There is no other evidence of cold flow, delamination, or cracking of the polyethylene.

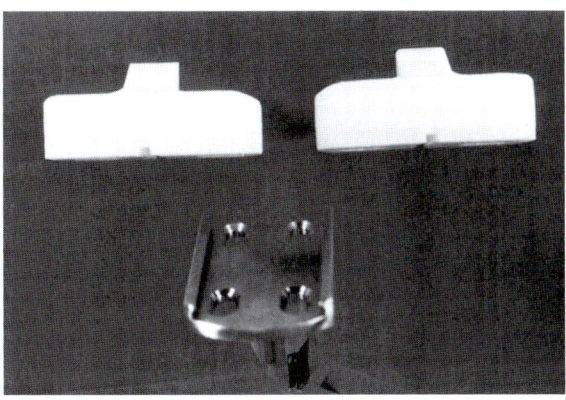

Figure 125-23. Metal tray support of the polyethylene prevents deformation.

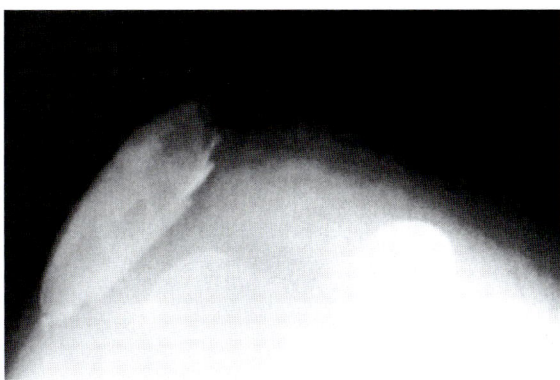

Figure 125-24. Gross rotary malposition of the tibial component leads to patellar dislocation.

Abrasion, burnishing, and deformation were seen in approximately 90 of the components. Cement particles embedded in the surface were found in about half. Delamination, the most severe form of polyethylene degradation, was found in 37 prostheses. Eight flat unicondylar components, which had the longest mean implant times (7.8 years), showed the most severe delamination. Twelve dished unicondylar components (6.3-year implant time) showed less delamination. Six one-piece tibial components, with a mean wear time of 4.3 years, showed much less delamination, almost entirely restricted to the central margin. There was considerable variation in the range of molecular weights between manufacturers and even between different components from the same manufacturer; the wear score for compression-molded components was higher than for other components.

The widespread adoption of metal-backed tibial components reduces deformation (Fig. 125-23), but the extra thickness of the metal is obtained at the expense of greater tibial resection or thinner polyethylene. Apel and associates[5] have found that thicker (>10 mm) all-polyethylene components behaved similarly to metal-backed components. For this and economic reasons, we believe there may be some interest in returning to all-polyethylene components or monoblock metal-back tibial augments; however, based on high failure rates of flat on flat, all-polyethylene components, all-polyethylene components are extremely design-sensitive. They should be used only after long-term clinical data accumulation.[136]

PATELLAR COMPLICATIONS

Subluxation and Dislocation

Various technical and design factors may contribute to subluxation and dislocation of the patella (Fig. 125-24).*

Depth of the Femoral Trochlea

The design of the femoral sulcus is a compromise. A shallow sulcus predisposes the patella to instability, but an overly deep sulcus offers excessive constraint to the patella, which may lead to patellar component loosening and patellar fracture.

---

*References 17, 25, 80, 124, 141, 152, and 184.

Position of the Femoral Component

Placement of the femoral component in internal rotation increases the lateral soft tissue tension as the knee is flexed.[190] As noted, some degree of external rotation is preferred (Fig. 125-25). We use the epicondylar axis to set the femoral rotation.

Malrotation of the Tibial Component

Internal rotation of the tibial component gives an external placement of the tibial tubercle, increasing the quadriceps angle and contributing to patellar instability. Malrotation of the tibial component is often the result of inadequate exposure. Sufficient dissection around the tibia to displace the tibial surface anteriorly provides the best visualization of the various landmarks for tibial component placement (Fig. 125-26).

Overall Valgus Alignment

Excessive valgus position increases the quadriceps angle. Reports have suggested that patellar instability often occurs in knees that were originally valgus.

Tight Lateral Retinaculum

A tight lateral retinaculum can contribute to patellar dislocation. Patellar tracking problems after TKA have been reported to occur with an incidence of 29%.[107] Subluxation is more common than dislocation.[17] Patients usually complain of anterior knee pain or gross subluxation or dislocation. The treatment of this complication depends on its cause. A patient with mild subluxation and a weak vastus medialis would benefit from intense physical therapy. The components could be malpositioned or malaligned, which could be determined preoperatively with a CT scan (Fig. 125-27). If this is the cause, a revision would be appropriate. In most cases, the treatment is a lateral retinaculum release, sometimes in conjunction with a proximal realignment. We do not recommend a tibial tubercle transposition because of its high complication rate.

Results of surgical treatment for patellar instability are good for combined lateral release and proximal realignment procedures. Grace and Rand[80] studied 25 knees with symptomatic lateral patellar instability after TKA. The knees were treated by one of three methods—proximal realignment, combined proximal and distal realignment, or component

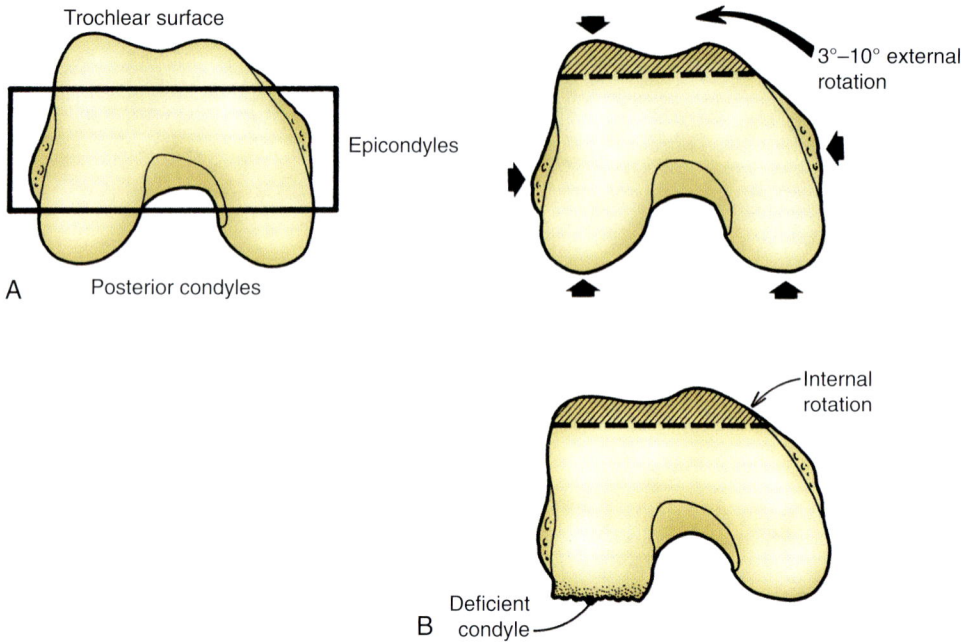

Figure 125-25. A, B, Internal rotation of the femoral component is a cause of patellar dislocation. The component always should be in slight external rotation.

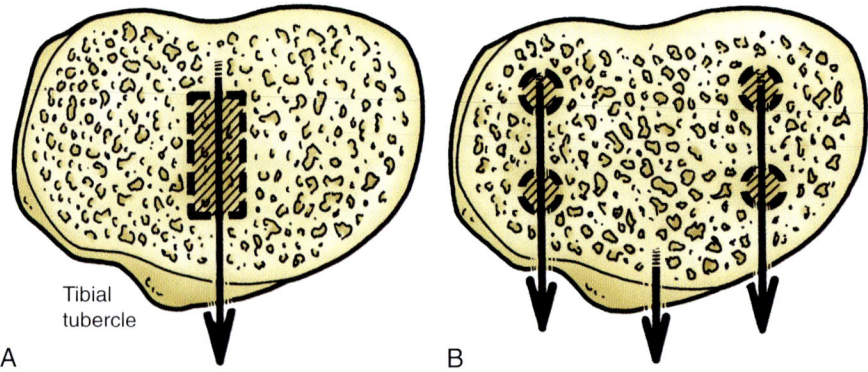

Figure 125-26. A, B, Alignment of the tibial component is projected at a point slightly medial to the tibial tubercle. Alignment of a symmetrical component with the posterior margin of the tibial plateau usually results in some internal rotation of the tibial component. One should err on the side of external rotation.

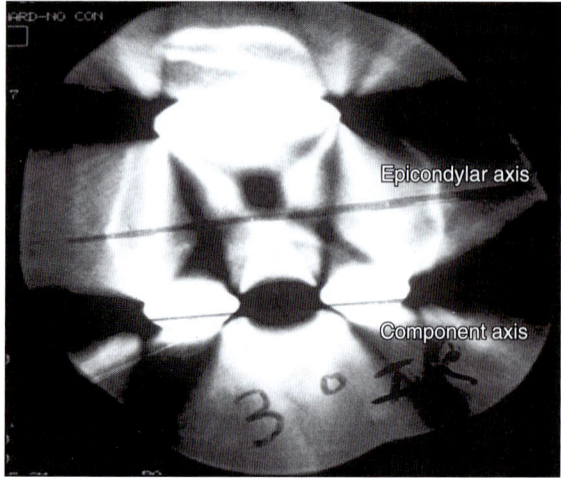

Figure 125-27. CT scan demonstrating 3 degrees of internal rotation of the femoral component compared with reference line through the epicondylar axis.

revision. At 50-month follow-up, 20 knees had normal patellar tracking and 5 had recurrent instability. Two of nine patients who had a combined realignment had patellar tendon rupture. The authors recommended proximal realignment alone in the absence of component malposition. If the component is malpositioned, component revision should be performed.

Merkow and coworkers[152] have reported their experience at the Hospital for Special Surgery. Between 1974 and 1982, 12 dislocations occurred in 11 patients. Trauma was the cause of dislocation in three knees, incorrect tracking of the patella in six, and malrotation of the tibial component in three. Many of the knees were in valgus preoperatively. Dislocations occurred in four different prosthetic designs, suggesting that in this series, design was not a factor. Unrestrained tibial rotation has been described as predisposing to patellar dislocation by others. Whiteside and colleagues[230] have maintained that the degree of tibial rotation is determined by the ligaments, provided that the ligaments are correctly tensioned during surgery. They noted that rotational constraint in the prosthesis is unnecessary and may predispose to loosening. We believe, however, that knees with initial external rotation deformities of the tibia are managed more easily by a design with rotational constraint, and this feature is useful in managing a patellar dislocation that has already occurred. Altering the rotational position of the tibial component in a design with some constraint is the equivalent to transferring the tibial tubercle.

In Merkow and associates' series,[152] the patellar dislocation was managed by proximal realignment in 10 cases, lateral release in 1 case, and proximal realignment and revision of the tibial component into a more desirable externally rotated position in 1 case. None of the dislocations recurred, and transposition of the tibial tubercle was required in none. We agree with Rand and Bryan[187] that tibial tubercle transposition is inadvisable after TKA because the bone quality is often poor, and the proportion of complications is high. Wolff and coworkers[235] and Whiteside and Ohl[231] have claimed that tibial tubercle transposition is effective with good technique. They recommended taking a relatively large fragment of the tibial tubercle so that secure fixation with screws is attainable.

Soft Tissue Impingement

In 1982, we described a case in which a fibrous nodule was excised from the suprapatellar region of the quadriceps tendon. This nodule gave rise to what has become known as the patellar clunk syndrome (Fig. 125-28),[14,93,219,223] most commonly associated with the use of a PS prosthesis.

The deeper flexion provided by the initial Insall-Burstein (IB) stabilized design enabled the quadriceps tendon to extend beyond the trochlear groove of the femoral component. If the anterior edge of the femoral component terminates abruptly, synovium or scar residing on the tendon falls into the intercondylar groove. If this has occurred, the same tissue must ride up out of the intercondylar area and jump back up onto the femoral trochlea as the patient extends her or his knee. Within a few months after the arthroplasty, the offending (or offended) tissue hypertrophies and becomes rubbery. This creates the painful and noisy complication that has been described as patellar clunk. Historically, a case of patellar catching was mentioned by Insall in his original report on the PS knee. However, Hozack and colleagues appeared to be the first to define the term *patellar clunk syndrome*.[93] They described a prominent fibrous nodule at the junction of the proximal patellar pole and quadriceps tendon. They believed that during flexion, this fibrous nodule would enter the femoral component's intercondylar notch but not restrict flexion. However, as the knee extended, the nodule would remain within the notch while the rest of the extensor mechanism slid proximally. At 30 to 45 degrees of flexion, the tension on the fibrous nodule would be sufficient to cause the nodule to jerk out of the notch as it returned to its normal position. This sudden displacement would cause the audible and palpable clunk found with this entity.

Synovial entrapment or hyperplasia is a similar entity but a less well-described syndrome.[178] It is caused by similar hypertrophy of soft tissue in the same location, but without a discrete nodule. Rather than a clunk or catch, the patient

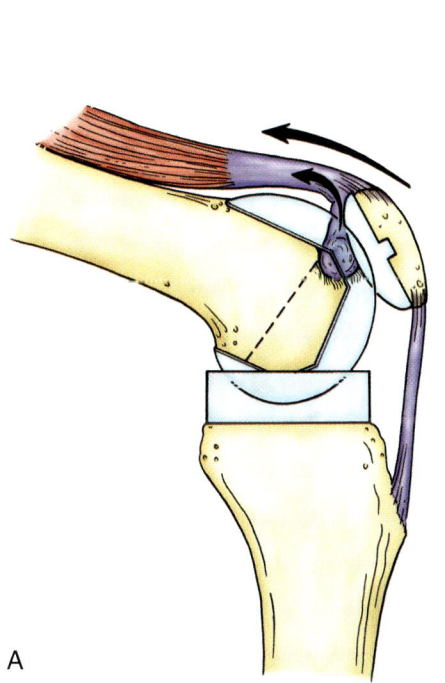
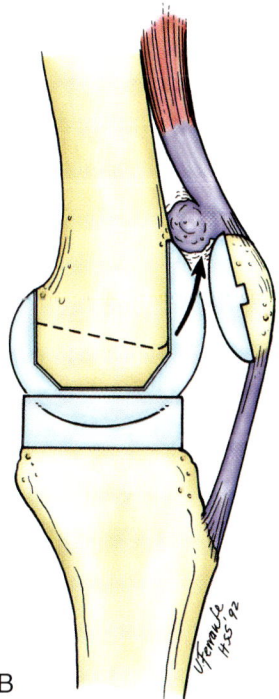

A B

Figure 125-28. A and **B,** Patellar clunk syndrome. The cause of this peculiar symptom is a suprapatellar mass of synovium and fibrous tissue that forms a nodule, which is caught between the patella and femoral component. This nodule typically forms at between 60 and 45 degrees of flexion and can result in locking of the knee in this position. As the knee is brought into terminal extension, the patella can be seen to pop and the nodule is released from its entrapped position. The symptom can be cured by arthroscopic removal of the fibrous nodule.

experiences pain and crepitus, typically with active knee extension from a 90-degree flexed position. This typically occurs during stair climbing or rising from a chair.

The original IB design had a high incidence of patellar clunk, up to 21%. This is likely related to the femorotrochlear geometry, a short trochlea with a sharp transition into the intercondylar notch.[2,35] Changes to the sagittal geometry of the femoral component in the IB II reduced the incidence to approximately 3% to 8%, but did not eliminate the problem. Finally, with the introduction of the NexGen Legacy prosthesis (Zimmer, Warsaw, Ind) in 1997, one of the main areas of focus was the patellofemoral articulation and the reduction of patellofemoral complications. The side-specific components with anatomically oriented trochlear grooves, lengthening and deepening of the femoral trochlea, and an increase in the number of femoral sizes all helped reduce the incidence of patellar entrapment syndromes. In 238 knees reconstructed with the NexGen Legacy prosthesis, no cases of patellar clunk or synovial entrapment were seen with 24- to 72-month follow-up.

Treatment recommendations for patellar clunk syndrome and synovial entrapment have included physical therapy, surgical removal of the nodule, patellar prosthesis revision, open resection through a limited lateral incision, and arthroscopic débridement.[14,93,153,223] Pollock and associates[178] have reviewed the prevalence of synovial entrapment with three different cam-post designs. Those with proximally positioned or wide femoral boxes were more likely to have a higher prevalence of this problem.

Beight and coworkers[14] have reported on 14 operative procedures (11 arthroscopic débridements and three patellar component revisions) performed in 12 patients. As in other reports, they found a suprapatellar fibrous nodule that wedged into the intercondylar notch during flexion and dislodged as the knee extended, causing the clunk. It was found that the symptoms resolved after nodule excision. However, four of the knees treated with arthroscopic débridement had recurrence of symptoms. None of the knees that underwent arthrotomy and patellar button revisions had recurrence. The recommended treatment protocol commenced with a short course of nonoperative physical therapy, although it was acknowledged that these results were disappointing. Arthroscopic débridement was suggested for knees without radiographic component abnormalities. Arthrotomy was suggested for recurrent clunks or malpositioned or loose components.

Researchers at the Mayo Clinic have recently reported on a series of 25 patients who underwent arthroscopic treatment of patellar clunk syndrome (15 knees) or patellofemoral synovial hyperplasia (10 knees).[52] After surgery, patients reported knee pain and crepitus, and as well as Knee Society knee and function scores improved in both groups. It was concluded that arthroscopic débridement of symptomatic patellofemoral synovium after TKA is a safe and effective procedure.

UNEXPLAINED PAIN

A certain proportion of patients continue to complain of pain for which there is no apparent explanation. Sometimes, the arthroplasty is objectively functioning well and has a good ROM. The pain may be present continuously or mainly at rest. For example, one of our patients was able to walk considerable distances and climb stairs normally without difficulty. He complained of severe pain when sitting and, because his occupation involved frequent flying, this was a considerable problem for him. Complaints of pain may be associated with lack of motion or flexion contracture, although the components appeared to be well seated and well positioned. We estimate the incidence of these cases to be approximately 1 in 300 arthroplasties. The cause is usually difficult to show. There is an overlap with reflex sympathetic dystrophy,[116] particularly in patients who have restricted motion. It may seem, in retrospect, that the preoperative symptoms were worse than the pathologic condition of the knee. Some type of material allergy has been suspected but never proved, although in one of our patients with a loose metal on metal hinge prosthesis, we were able to show a skin allergy to cobalt chloride. Low-grade infection is always a possibility.

In the management of these patients, infection must be excluded as much as possible. Aspiration should be attempted, and if sufficient fluid is obtained, cultures can be quite reliable; 90% of our infected knees have been diagnosed by culture of the aspirate. Bone scintigraphy[89,114,180] also may be useful, although technetium-99m scanning after TKA yields highly variable results[203] in that asymptomatic knees may continue to have abnormal scans indefinitely. Indium scanning[186] was found to be 85% reliable in 18 infected knees. In a group of 20 knees with aseptic loosening, however, the scan results were not given.

When reflex sympathetic dystrophy is suspected, sympathetic block should be tried. If the response is good, a lumbar sympathectomy should be considered.

A 1996 study[158] examined the role of exploratory surgery in unexplained pain in TKA. In this study, 27 patients underwent exploration of their TKA secondary to severe debilitating pain of an unknown origin. They were divided into two groups—patients with ROM less than 80 degrees and patients with ROM greater than 80 degrees. At final follow-up, there were 11 excellent and good results (41%) and 16 fair or poor results (59%). Of the 15 patients with decreased ROM, 9 (60%) had good or excellent results. The ROM arc improved from a preoperative 43-degree average to an 81-degree average. For the pain-only group, there were only two excellent or good results (17%). If a problem was identified at surgery, only 3 of 12 knees (25%) had successful outcomes. This study highlights the frustration of performing surgery on patients for unexplained pain. Even when the authors identified a problem at the time of surgery and corrected it, they only had a 25% success rate.

If the workup of a painful TKA is negative, one must consider obtaining fluoroscopically assisted radiographs. In this way, near-perfect perpendicular radiographs can be obtained to evaluate any radiolucencies, especially under the tibial tray. In one study that examined painful TKA without explanation,[67] fluoroscopic evaluation was used to study the knees. The authors had 20 patients referred to them for pain and disability after TKA, with normal-appearing radiographs. All 20 patients had fluoroscopic radiographs obtained. In 14 of 20 patients, the diagnosis of aseptic loosening was made with the new radiographs. Each of the patients considered to have a loose component at fluoroscopy did have a loose component at revision. Each patient improved after revision, with an increase in Hospital for Special Surgery score of 26 points.

Great caution is recommended when deciding to revise a knee without good explanation of the pain and, in most cases, the condition of the patient is unimproved or is worse after revision, unless a convincing intraoperative cause is found. Sometimes, overgrown soft tissues or an interposed meniscal fragment is found. Because these conditions can be managed without arthrotomy, an arthroscopic examination is recommended before revision is attempted.

Nonarticular causes of knee pain, including referred pain, should also be kept in mind when performing the clinical examination. Hip and lumbar spine pathology must be ruled out as the underlying cause of pain. Less recognized causes are patellar clunk, lateral patellar facet irritation, irritation from retained osteophytes, extruded bone cement, popliteus tendon dysfunction, and collateral ligament irritation caused by medial tibial displacement. Hypertrophic pulmonary osteoarthropathy as an unusual cause of late pain and effusion has been reported.[150]

Primary malignant neoplasms and metastatic disease have been described in association with total joint arthroplasty.[3] Cases of patients with periprosthetic non-Hodgkin's lymphoma, bronchogenic carcinoma, gastric carcinoma, and squamous cell carcinoma of the lung have been described in relation to THA.[31,150] Fehring and Hamilton[66] have reported a case of a 73-year-old patient with continued severe pain following TKA. Synovial biopsy revealed metastatic adenocarcinoma from colon. Therefore, a thorough history and physical examination should be done to identify the nature and cause of the pain. It is important that this phenomenon be considered in older patients when other causes have been ruled out.

KEY REFERENCES

Ayers DC, Dennis DA, Johanson NA, et al: Common complications of total knee arthroplasty. J Bone Joint Surg Am 79:278, 1997.

Berry DJ: Recognizing and identifying osteolysis around total knee arthroplasty. Instr Course Lect 53:261, 2004.

Brassard MF, Insall JN, Scuderi GR, Faris PM: Complications of total knee arthroplasty. In Scott WN, editor: Insall & Scott surgery of the knee, vol 2, ed 4, Philadelphia, 2006, Churchill Livingstone-Elsevier, pp 1716–1760.

Clarke HD, Fuchs R, Scuderi GR, et al: Clinical results in valgus total knee arthroplasty with the "pie crust" technique of lateral soft tissue releases. J Arthroplasty 20:1010, 2005.

Cushner FD: Transfusion avoidance in orthopedic surgery. J Cardiothorac Vasc Anesth 18(Suppl):29S, 2004.

Maloney WJ, Paprosky W, Engh CA, Rubash H: Surgical treatment of pelvic osteolysis. Clin Orthop Relat Res 393:78, 2001.

Meding JB, Keating EM, Ritter MA, et al: Genu recurvatum in total knee replacement. Clin Orthop Relat Res 416:64, 2003.

Mont MA, Serna FK, Krackow KA, et al: Exploration of radiographically normal total knee replacements for unexplained pain. Clin Orthop 331:216, 1996.

Pagnano MW, Hanssen AD, Lewallen DG, Stuart MJ: Flexion instability after primary posterior cruciate retaining total knee arthroplasty. Clin Orthop Relat Res 356:39, 1998.

Rand JA, Brown ML: The value of indium 111 leukocyte scanning in the evaluation of painful or infected total knee arthroplasties. Clin Orthop 259:179, 1990.

Scuderi GR: Revision total knee arthroplasty: how much constraint is enough? Clin Orthop Relat Res 392:300, 2001.

Whiteside LA, Ohl MD: Tibial tubercle osteotomy for exposure of the difficult total knee arthroplasty. Clin Orthop Relat Res 260:6, 1990.

Full references for this chapter can be found on www.expertconsult.com.

Extensile Surgical Exposures for Revision Total Knee Replacement

Christopher R. Gooding, Donald S. Garbuz, and Bassam A. Masri

Adequate exposure is one of the most common difficulties encountered in revision knee arthroplasty. Choosing the correct surgical approach while having a comprehensive understanding of the anatomic pitfalls allows the surgeon to proceed safely and achieve a successful outcome for the patient.[36] Wound edge necrosis and extensor mechanism rupture are significant complications that can adversely affect the outcome of revision knee surgery.[29] Such complications can be avoided with judicious preoperative planning and knowledge of safe approaches to exposing a failed knee arthroplasty. Great care must also be taken in protecting the collateral ligaments, which are at particular risk at the level of the joint line and posterolaterally, where neurovascular structures are in close proximity to the joint. Careful attention must be paid to those patients with previous incisions, because they are at risk of wound breakdown; it can also be particularly difficult to gain adequate exposure in those with restricted range of movement. Other comorbidities may have implications as well, such as vasculitis, which can occur with polyarthropathies such as rheumatoid arthritis. These patients are at risk of poor wound healing and skin edge necrosis. The risk of deep infection is further increased in patients with renal failure, acquired immunodeficiency syndrome with a CD4 count of 200 or lower, diabetes, psoriasis, and rheumatologic conditions such as rheumatoid arthritis and systemic lupus erythematosus.[42]

Extensile surgical exposure by excision of unwanted scar tissue, rectus snip, tibial tubercle osteotomy, medial epicondylar osteotomy, or a quadriceps myocutaneous approach can provide sufficient exposure of the implants and at the same time can avoid significant patellar tendon disruption.

ANATOMY

Sufficient exposure is essential to allow removal of implants, along with soft tissue balancing and management of bone loss in the revision setting. Only with a comprehensive understanding of the anatomy can adequate exposure be achieved without damaging the skin, extensor mechanism, collateral ligaments, remaining bone stock, and neurovascular structures. Specifically, knowledge of the blood supply to the skin can help reduce the risk of skin necrosis, and any deep dissection requires identification of the extensor mechanism, followed by dissection around it. Particular attention should be paid to the blood supply of the patella to avoid the possibility of avascular necrosis. At the level of the joint line, the collateral ligaments are at risk. If these are damaged, resulting in compromise of varus/valgus stability, a hinged knee prosthesis may be the only option for achieving adequate stability. This outcome can be avoided with sufficient knowledge of their location in the knee.

The blood supply to the skin overlying the knee is well understood because of the results of a cadaveric study conducted by Haertsch and associates.[16] Anastomosis of blood vessels immediately superficial to the deep fascia that are fed by perforating vessels from below the fascia is noted. From this anastomosis, blood vessels course their way through the subcutaneous fat and supply the dermis and epidermis. No such anastomoses are seen within the dermal layers; hence, extensive dissection superficial to the deep fascia will disrupt the blood supply to the skin, increasing the risk for areas of ischemia and necrosis. Therefore, if most of the dissection in exposing the knee is kept below the fascial layer, the skin's blood supply is less likely to be compromised.

Large skin flaps should be avoided to reduce the chances of compromising the arterial blood supply to the skin.

The origin of the blood supply to the skin overlying the knee is asymmetrical. Perforators arise mostly from the medial aspect of the knee from the saphenous artery and the descending geniculate artery. If a midline incision is already present, this should be used for the revision. Although this is the situation in most cases, other incisions may occasionally be present. A previous transverse skin incision obviously cannot be avoided and should be crossed at 90 degrees.[40] However, creating a skin flap with an acute angle of less than 60 degrees at the intersection of the incisions risks compromising the blood supply and should be avoided. If a previous oblique incision is present, it should be crossed at as close to 90 degrees as possible, and the incision can be curved away from the intersection if necessary.

If multiple longitudinal incisions are in close proximity, then the most lateral incision should be used, while preserving the blood supply medially.[7] If this is not possible, then the surgeon should aim to leave an intact skin bridge of approximately 6 cm between the previous incisions and the new one.

The area of skin that is particularly vulnerable during revision surgery is the anteromedial aspect of the proximal tibia, because of limited soft tissue cover deep to the skin. Careful attention should be paid to this area postoperatively and rapid intervention instigated should problems arise because of the risk of deep infection (Fig. 126-1). Should skin necrosis occur, skin grafting alone is rarely successful because of the limited muscle coverage. In this scenario, a medial gastrocnemius rotation flap is a good option when additional soft tissue coverage is required.* This should be done as early as possible, because delay may lead to infection.

The skin over the patella also has a somewhat tenuous blood supply, because it is separated from the patella by the prepatellar bursa, through which very few blood vessels pass.

---

*References 1, 6, 21, 22, 24, 25, 27, 30, and 31.

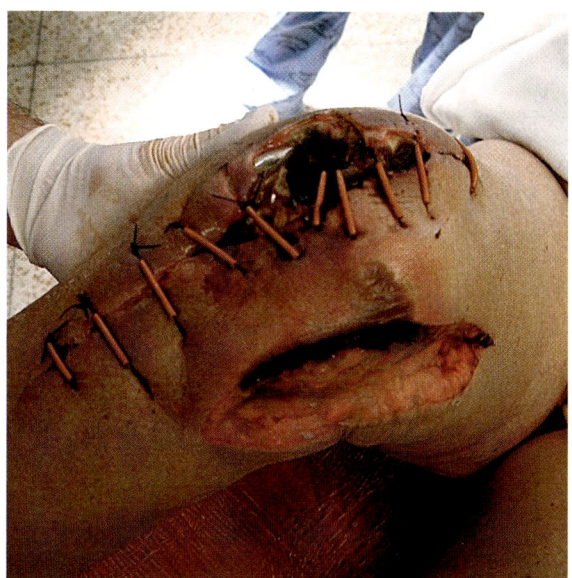

Figure 126-1. Photograph showing a necrotic wound post total knee arthroplasty.

The blood supply to the patella forms a plexus of arteries surrounding it supplied by the descending geniculate, superior medial, inferior medial, superior lateral, and inferior lateral geniculate arteries and the anterior tibial recurrent artery.[18,19,34] From this plexus, branches arise in front of the patella; these include the infrapatellar artery and the oblique prepatellar artery, which is found within the infrapatellar fat pad. The distal pole of the patella receives its blood supply inferiorly,[34] and the remaining patella receives its blood supply from vessels that penetrate it over the middle third of its anterior surface. The standard medial parapatellar approach will interrupt the contribution from the medial vessels to the plexus, and excision of the lateral meniscus at the index operation will compromise the inferior lateral geniculate artery. Similarly, when the infrapatellar fat pad is excised, the superior lateral geniculate artery[18] and the branches of the recurrent anterior tibial artery may be interrupted. If a lateral release has also been performed, then the blood supply to the patella can potentially become somewhat tenuous. An increased incidence of patellar avascular necrosis with its subsequent fragmentation has been observed with lateral release and sacrifice of the superior lateral geniculate artery.[32] The superior lateral geniculate artery is found running horizontally and immediately distal to the inferior border of the vastus lateralis muscle. When a lateral release is performed from within the knee joint, great care must be taken to try to preserve this vessel and thus avoid compromising the blood supply to the patella. It is advisable to avoid a release from "outside-in" because this involves considerable undermining of the lateral skin edge with the inherent risk of causing skin edge necrosis.

Identifying the collateral ligaments, as well as the capsular structures found laterally, medially, and posteriorly, is an important step in the surgical exposure of revision knee surgery.[18] The medial collateral ligament is a flat, triangular band that courses its way from the medial femoral epicondyle, just distal to the adductor tubercle, and inserts into the tibia 2 cm distal to the joint line. Its anterior margin forms the vertical base of the triangle; the posterior apex of the triangle blends with the capsule and is attached to the medial meniscus. Above its distal attachment, the ligament is crossed by the tendons of sartorius, gracilis, and semitendinosus with a bursa interposed. The superficial medial collateral ligament, along with the pes anserinus, inserts more distally. The semimembranosus tendon inserts into the posterior aspect of the medial tibial condyle. From this attachment, it gives off three expansions. One passes anteriorly along the medial surface of the condyle deep to the deep medial collateral ligament. The second expansion passes obliquely and superiorly to the lateral femoral epicondyle and is called the oblique popliteal ligament. The third expansion forms a thick, strong fascial layer overlying the popliteus and inserts into posterior aspect of the tibia along the soleal line.

The lateral collateral ligament is a cordlike structure that arises from the lateral epicondyle, below the lateral head of the gastrocnemius and above the tendon of popliteus. It inserts into the head of the fibula overlapped by the biceps femoris tendon, along with its interposing bursa. The lateral collateral ligament at the level of the joint line is superficial to the popliteus tendon. The posterior capsule of the knee joint is firmly attached to the femur immediately above the condyles and deep to the medial and lateral heads of the gastrocnemius. One option in knees with a fixed flexion deformity is to carefully strip off the capsule from the back of the femur at this level.

During revision knee surgery, the posterior cruciate ligament is commonly divided. For those patients who had a posterior cruciate sacrificing knee arthroplasty as their primary operation, the ligament will have already been resected. If the posterior cruciate ligament is intact, it is found immediately anterior to the joint capsule; it arises from the intercondylar notch of the femur and descends posteriorly and laterally to insert on the posterior aspect of the tibia. When the posterior cruciate ligament is divided, great care must be taken during its dissection not to penetrate the posterior capsule and cause a neurovascular injury. The safest place to resect the ligament is at the level of its femoral origin.

The popliteal artery is the deepest of the large neurovascular structures throughout its course through the popliteal fossa. It extends from the hiatus in the adductor magnus (a hand's breadth above the knee) to the fibrous arch in the soleus (a hand's breadth below the knee). It enters the fossa on the medial side of the femur and lies deep and medial to the sciatic nerve and its vertical continuation, the tibial nerve. As it descends through the popliteal fossa, it follows a somewhat convex course laterally, so it then lies lateral to the tibial nerve. The popliteal vein, meanwhile, lies between the artery and the nerve throughout its course through the popliteal fossa. The anterior relations of the popliteal artery starting superiorly include the posterior aspect of the femur, followed by the oblique popliteal ligament; at the level of the knee joint, it is separated from the posterior capsule behind the posterior horn of the lateral meniscus by a thin layer of fat, and then farther inferiorly in the fascia overlying the popliteus muscle, it disappears under the fibrous arch of the soleus. The popliteal artery is tethered by its geniculate branches to the posterior aspect of the capsule. Any division of the capsule in this vicinity can damage these branches; as a result, subperiosteal elevation of the capsule off the back of the femur or tibia medially and laterally is considered safer.

Knee flexion offers no protection for the popliteal artery, as it remains tethered to the posterior capsule at the level of the knee joint.[43] From the neurologic point of view, the peroneal nerve is at greater risk during revision surgery than the tibial nerve. Damage to the peroneal nerve can occur from traction (especially if the normal mechanical axis is restored in a valgus knee), compression, and laceration. The common peroneal nerve descends on the lateral aspect of the joint and initially is medial to the biceps tendon; it then courses just behind its insertion on the fibular head.[36] It is at particular risk from lateral release or during release of the biceps tendon; for this reason, such a procedure is best avoided.

PREOPERATIVE ASSESSMENT

Careful preoperative evaluation of a patient before a revision total knee replacement is contemplated involves obtaining a thorough history and performing a comprehensive examination. Additional investigations, including laboratory tests and radiographs, should be requested. A surgical plan should be created, so that any additional components, instruments, and bone grafting materials that are needed can be preordered.

History

The history should include a review of any possible wound healing problems, previous nerve injury, or weakness of knee extension, which may suggest disruption of the extensor mechanism. A history of knee stiffness should precipitate further questioning as to the duration of stiffness or loss of motion, as this can affect the choice of surgical approach used. Specific questions regarding infection should be asked, specifically if the knee wound from the primary operation took a long time to heal, or if it was complicated by prolonged drainage or a "superficial" infection. Within the systemic inquiry, information regarding peripheral vascular disease is helpful, as it may point to other possible causes of the patient's pain, but it is also relevant as to the risk of developing wound necrosis and a postoperative ischemic limb.[28]

During the examination, the location and shape of surgical scars should be carefully assessed (Fig. 126-2). The general

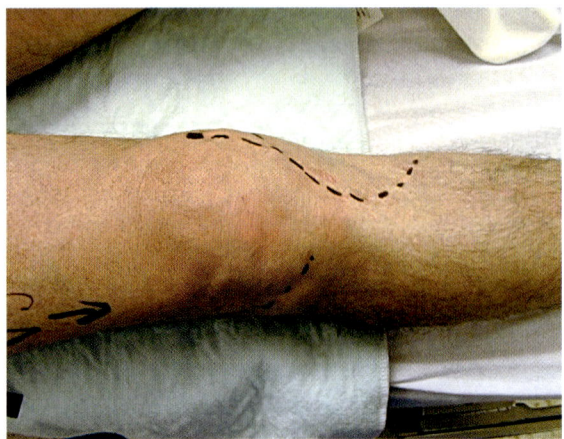

Figure 126-2. Preoperatively, all surgical incisions should be clearly marked with an indelible marker.

health of the skin and its capillary return in the vicinity of the planned incision should be reviewed. Discoloration of the wound edge at the previous incision with hemosiderin may suggest previous wound healing problems. The range of motion should be carefully checked before any revision knee replacement is performed. A stiff knee will likely require extensile maneuvers to achieve safe exposure. Any patient with less than 70 degrees of flexion is a likely candidate for extensile exposure.

A knee that has been infected is associated with increased scar formation resulting in stiffness, which can also increase the risk of patellar tendon avulsion.[15] Neurovascular status should be inspected, and if there is any doubt as to the blood supply distally, additional imaging studies should be requested, along with the opinion of a vascular surgeon. Poor venous return can also be a problem and may cause tissue ischemia and wound breakdown secondary to venous engorgement. If any wound issues are envisaged, preoperative review by a plastic surgeon can be timely. Some plastic surgeons may advise creating a flap before the revision is undertaken, although this is uncommon. Occasionally, tissue expanders can be used to increase the amount of skin available for closure.[14,20,26,33]

Radiographs, including a weight-bearing anteroposterior view of the lower limbs and lateral, skyline, and notch views of the affected knee, should be requested. This will facilitate surgical planning in terms of components needed and choice of surgical exposure. Radiographs should be evaluated for the presence of retained hardware within the tibia, such as large amounts of cement, a broken stem, or screws that may make insertion of a revision stem difficult. These scenarios may necessitate a tibial tubercle osteotomy. Evidence of patella alta is suggestive of patellar tendon rupture; alternatively, patella baja may suggest a quadriceps tendon disruption, particularly if a small avulsion fragment of the superior pole of the patella is seen proximal to the patella on the lateral radiograph. However, this is a rare event. More commonly, patella baja is related to scarring, previous surgery such as proximal tibial osteotomy, or an elevated joint line caused by the previous knee replacement.

PRINCIPLES OF EXPOSURE

Exposure to the knee can be considered as "unleashing" the extensor mechanism.[8] The four leashes acting on the extensor mechanism through the patella are lateral, medial, distal, and proximal. The two minor leashes are the medial and lateral retinacular structures and capsule, together with the insertion of the vasti. The two major leashes are the quadriceps tendon proximally and the patellar tendon distally. It is the major leashes that are often involved in extensile approaches in revision total knee arthroplasty. Most revisions can be orchestrated through the standard medial parapatellar approach with slight modifications such as the quadriceps snip,[13] as well as complete intra-articular excision of scar tissue. In a knee that has had a number of revisions and is stiff, and in which exposure is predicted to be difficult, a more extensile exposure can be performed proximally—a patellar turndown[2,35]—or distally—a tibial tubercle osteotomy.[38,39] In all cases, the choice of exposure is made in a stepwise manner, starting with the medial parapatellar approach and progressing as required.

INITIAL EXPOSURE

Following the medial parapatellar approach, wide resection of the intra-articular scar is performed by clearing any fibrous adhesions in the suprapatellar pouch and lateral and medial gutters, as well as by exposing the proximal tibia. The surgeon should then proceed to dissect subperiosteally the medial structures off the proximal tibia. The medial retinaculum and the deep medial collateral ligament should be elevated subperiosteally from the medial aspect of the tibia around to the semimembranous insertion. By externally rotating, the flexed tibia will further aid the exposure. If more of a medial release is needed, then the subperiosteal dissection should be extended distally on the medial side of the tibia, with care taken to avoid complete release of the superficial medial collateral ligament; otherwise a more constrained prosthesis will be needed. The insertion of the patellar tendon into the tibial tubercle should not be disturbed. Next, the interval between the patellar tendon anteriorly and the fibrous tissue directly posteriorly should be identified. Once a plane is established, the fibrous tissue should be removed from the inferior patella distal to the insertion of the patellar tendon to the tubercle. This procedure should enable the patella to be subluxed. It is our practice to never evert the patella because of risk of damage to the patellar tendon. A similar procedure is then performed on the quadriceps tendon, where the suprapatellar pouch is denuded of scar tissue, as are the medial and lateral gutters. This frees up the distal femur and is an essential technique in the stiff knee. It is sensible, however, to leave a thin periosteal layer on the femur to prevent excessive bleeding from the venous plexus that exists between the bone and its periosteum, and to prevent the formation of heterotopic ossification. At this stage, the modular polyethylene tibial liner can be removed, and the surgeon can proceed with the revision.

EXTENSILE EXPOSURES

If the exposure is still difficult, a number of extensile exposures can be utilized with varying morbidities and degrees of difficulty. They are divided into proximal and distal. Proximal exposures include rectus snip, quadriceps turndown, medial epicondylar osteotomy, and femoral peel; the distal exposure is the tibial tubercle osteotomy.

RECTUS SNIP

The rectus snip is a relatively straightforward method of improving the exposure.[4,13] This procedure should relieve tension on the patella. It is performed by extending the incision within the quadriceps tendon obliquely at 45 degrees. The incision starts distal-medial, follows a 45-degree oblique line, and ends proximally-laterally across the quadriceps tendon (Fig. 126-3). Care is taken to maintain some of the vastus lateralis with the lateral retinaculum and patella; otherwise the vastus lateralis will be defunctioned. The vastus medialis and the portion of rectus femoris attached to the medial retinaculum are unaffected. Performing an oblique snip as opposed to a transverse snip means that at closure, the tendon is closed from side to side, rather than from end to end, which could weaken the tendon and increase the risk of extensor tendon disruption. Postoperative rehabilitation

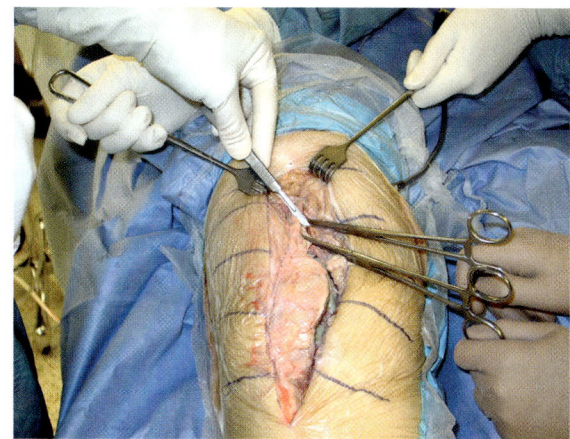

Figure 126-3. Intraoperative photograph demonstrating the rectus snip. Note that the tendon is cut at a 45-degree angle, thus avoiding an end-to-end repair at the time of closure.

can follow similar guidelines as those used for the standard medial parapatellar approach.

Results of the rectus snip have shown that this procedure does not adversely affect the overall outcome following a revision knee arthroplasty.[5,13] Garvin's[13] results showed no compromise of the extensor mechanism, and among 16 patients who were reviewed, no complications were reported. All 16 patients had a good or excellent result based on the Hospital for Special Surgery Knee Score. The authors mentioned that four patients returned to their preoperative work and had no limitations to their activity level. However, postoperatively, five patients developed a fixed flexion contracture that averaged 7 degrees. No cases of an extensor lag were reported. Of the 16 patients, 14 reported an improvement in knee motion by an average of 38 degrees. The authors also performed objective testing to assess patients' peak torque and work. They reported that peak torque was statistically significantly less in the operated knee than in the unoperated knee, as one would expect. However, the difference in work between the two knees did not reach statistical significance. In comparing a knee that had had a rectus snip as part of its exposure versus a knee that had undergone a standard medial parapatellar arthrotomy, no difference in peak torque or work was noted.[13] The authors of this study concluded that it was the preoperative condition that influenced the isokinetic testing results, and not the exposure.

In a more recent study, Meek and associates[23] reviewed 107 patients who underwent a revision knee arthroplasty with a mean follow-up of 40.5 months. A standard medial parapatellar approach was performed in 57 patients and a rectus snip in 50. The two groups were matched for age, sex, and comorbidity scores. No statistically significant difference was noted between the two groups based on Western Ontario and McMaster Universities Arthritis Index (WOMAC) function, pain, stiffness, and satisfaction scores. The authors concluded that the rectus snip has no effect on outcome.

Barrack and colleagues[5] reviewed 123 revision total knee arthroplasties with a 2- to 4-year follow-up. Among 31 patients who had undergone a rectus snip as part of their exposure, no difference in terms of clinical outcome was noted compared with those who had a medial parapatellar approach. Range of motion, extensor lag, patellofemoral pain, and patient satisfaction all were comparable, although the authors of this study did note that patients who underwent a quadriceps snip had better Knee Society scores than patients who had a tibial tubercle osteotomy or a quadriceps turndown during the same period.

Very few complications have been reported with the rectus snip as an extensile exposure. In a study comparing a quadriceps snip with the standard medial parapatellar approach, no statistically significant difference was observed in terms of outcome, and no associated complications were reported.[23] However, care must be taken when performing this procedure to ensure that the snip is made at the oblique angle of 45 degrees, thus avoiding an end-to-end repair, which is less likely to heal and as a result could lead to extensor lag or disruption.

V-Y QUADRICEPSPLASTY OR QUADRICEPS TURNDOWN

The main indication for this approach is severe stiffness that requires lengthening of the extensor mechanism at the time of revision knee replacement. If this is considered, however, the patient has to be warned that a substantial extensor lag may result. A medial parapatellar approach is performed in the standard fashion, then the incision is extended laterally from the superior extent of the medial parapatellar incision, at a 45-degree angle inferolaterally in the lateral retinaculum, to the level of the tibia (Fig. 126-4).[17] Although this puts the blood supply to the patella at risk, Insall and coworkers maintained that the blood supply to the patella is preserved via the superior lateral geniculate artery and the vessels within the remaining fat pad supplying the patella inferiorly.[17] With this approach, there is the option of lengthening the quadriceps tendon, if indicated, by converting the inverted V-shaped incision into an inverted Y. This is a modification of the more traditional Coonse-Adams technique because the disadvantage with the earlier approach is that it cannot be extended from a standard medial parapatellar incision. Scott and associates[35] modified Insall's approach further by taking the lateral extension of the incision inferior to the edge of the vastus lateralis through its tendinous insertion, rather than through the lateral retinaculum. This approach puts the superior lateral geniculate artery at less risk of compromise. However,

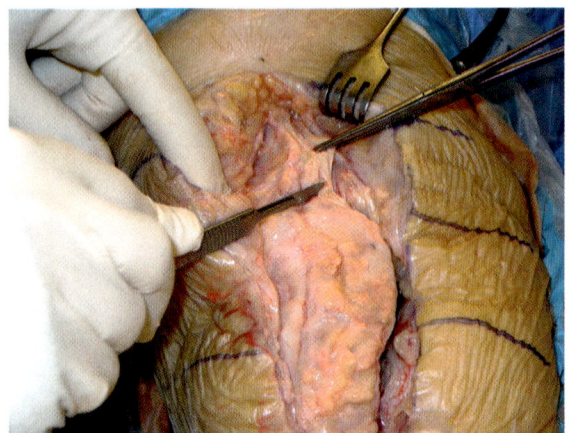

Figure 126-4. Intraoperative photograph demonstrating the quadriceps turndown. Note the angle of the incision of the quadriceps tendon.

Ritter and colleagues[32] have questioned whether preservation of the superior geniculate artery has any bearing on whether the patella undergoes avascular necrosis.

When it comes to closure, the lateral retinaculum can be left unrepaired as a lateral release. Patients are advised to avoid active extension postoperatively for 6 weeks.[9] Some have advocated that the knee should be protected for 2 weeks before flexion is permitted, to allow the repair to partially heal before the patient is mobilized.[17] Others have recommended that patients should be put on a continuous passive motion machine immediately postoperatively with flexion up to 30 degrees.[35] In our opinion, this exposure is performed to allow greater motion, and restricting motion postoperatively will potentially mitigate the positive effect of the operation. Although this is a rare operation in our hands, we recommend immediate motion.

Scott and coworkers[35] reported on seven patients with limited preoperative motion who had a modified V-Y quadricepsplasty technique as part of their exposure. The average increase in flexion was 49 degrees, and the average extension lag postoperatively was 8 degrees.

Trousdale and associates[37] reviewed 16 knees in 14 patients who had a total knee arthroplasty with a V-Y quadricepsplasty as part of their exposure. However, 10 knees had a revision arthroplasty and 6 knees had a primary arthroplasty. Using the Hospital for Special Surgery Knee Score, 2 patients were judged as excellent, 10 good, 2 fair, and 2 poor. The mean range of motion was 4 to 85 degrees. Biomechanical testing did show statistically significant weakness in extension compared with the contralateral side at test speeds of 120, 180, and 240 degrees per second in those patients who had an unoperated contralateral knee. Other test speeds also showed some weakness in extension, but this did not reach statistical significance. The authors also compared the V-Y quadricepsplasty versus a standard medial parapatellar approach and showed that the extensor mechanism was weaker in the former but not to a significant degree, but this may be related to the small sample size. The authors concluded that a V-Y quadricepsplasty can give a good result with near normal active extension but with some moderate weakness, and added that knee scores reflect the difficult challenges in this particular patient group.

Potential complications following this technique include the theoretical risk to the blood supply of the patella. Aglietti attempted to reduce this risk by modifying the technique[3] by preserving the inferior lateral geniculate artery and maintaining the integrity of the vastus medialis. Della Valle[8] reflected that in a multiply operated knee, the inferior lateral geniculate artery may already be compromised, and as a result this approach may lead to avascular necrosis of the patella with subsequent fragmentation and extensor mechanism dysfunction.

TIBIAL TUBERCLE OSTEOTOMY

Dolin[10] first described the use of a tibial tubercle osteotomy in total knee arthroplasty. The approach was subsequently modified by Whiteside, who helped to popularize the technique.[38,39] It is performed by making an incision in the periosteum between 8 and 10 cm in length, 1 cm medial to the tibial tubercle. A cortical cut is made medial to the tuberosity with an oscillating saw; a distal cut is also made, which can be a transverse or a tapered cut. A curved or tapered distal cut may be more attractive to help reduce the risk of tibial fracture. A similar cut is made proximally using a curved osteotome or a reciprocating saw. An osteotomy through the area of the cortex lateral to the tubercle is gently performed, without disrupting the lateral periosteum. The aim is to have a tibial tubercle fragment that is greater than 2 cm wide and more than 1 cm thick and 8 to 10 cm long. By gently cracking the lateral cortex and leaving the overlying soft tissues intact, the osteotomy fragment remains attached laterally via a soft tissue hinge that can be everted laterally (Fig. 126-5). The osteotomized tibial tubercle can be reattached with two or three cerclage wires, which are passed around the lateral edge of the tubercle and back onto the tibial crest. By angling the wires at 45 degrees inferiorly from proximal-lateral to distal-medial, the osteotomy fragment is pulled distally. The wires are passed within the tibial canal behind the stem and are inserted before the stem is inserted. They can be tightened once the tibial component is in place (Figs. 126-6 and 126-7). Dolin[10] originally described the technique using a screw to reattach the tubercle, but concerns were raised that there was a potential for the osteotomy fragment to pull off, hence Whiteside's modification as described previously.[39] This approach is helpful if there are difficulties in exposing the tibial canal, or if a proximal extensile approach is insufficient. Postoperatively, patients can be fully weight-bearing and can flex their knee as tolerated.[39] To avoid a tibial fracture, it is important to use a stem that is long enough to bypass the osteotomy.

Whiteside[39] reported on 71 knees that had a tibial tubercle osteotomy as part of their exposure for a difficult total knee arthroplasty with a follow-up period of 1 to 5 years. All patients were reported to heal without a problem, and no significant complications occurred. The mean postoperative flexion was reported as 97 degrees. Of these 71 patients, none had an extensor lag, and the mean fixed flexion contracture was 2.5 degrees. In a report 5 years later, the same author reviewed 136 total knee arthroplasties in which an exposure utilizing an extended tibial tubercle and a tibial crest osteotomy was performed. Of those 136 arthroplasties, 26 were primaries, 76 revisions, 10 repeated revisions, 19 infected, and 5 repeated revisions for infection. The mean range of

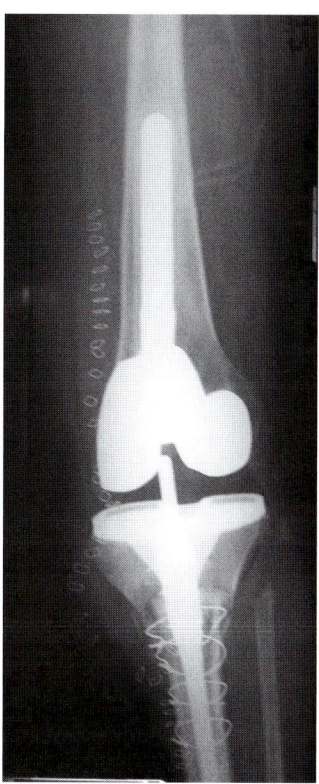

Figure 126-6. Postoperative anteroposterior radiograph following complex revision of a total knee arthroplasty, using a proximal tibial allograft and a tibial tubercle osteotomy to gain exposure.

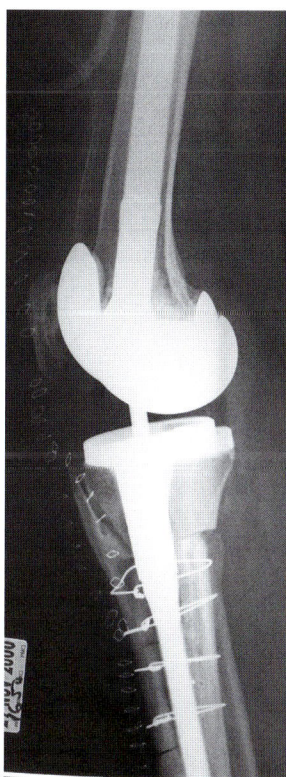

Figure 126-7. Postoperative lateral radiograph following a tibial tubercle osteotomy to gain adequate exposure in a long-stem revision total knee arthroplasty.

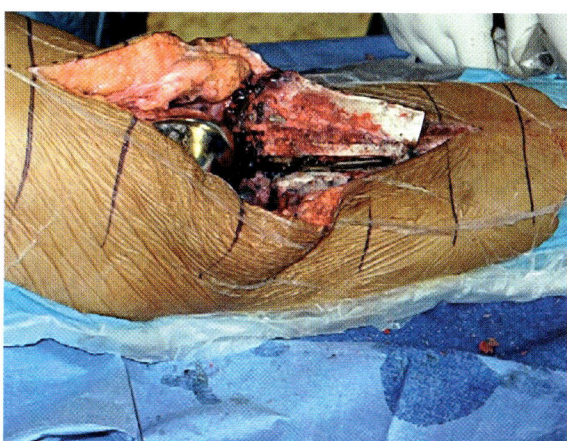

Figure 126-5. Intraoperative photograph demonstrating a tibial tubercle osteotomy. Note that the bone fragment remains attached to the tibia via a lateral soft tissue hinge.

motion at 2 years postoperatively was 93.7 degrees (range, 15 to 140 degrees). Two knees were reported to have an extensor lag, although this was noted preoperatively. No compromise of quadriceps function was observed in any of the patients.

After the quadriceps snip, the two most popular extensile approaches are the tibial tubercle osteotomy and the quadriceps turndown. Barrack[5] reviewed both of these procedures and concluded that the quadriceps turndown cohort had a significantly increased range of motion compared with those patients who underwent the tibial tubercle osteotomy. Although the tibial tubercle osteotomy cohort did have less of a problem with an extensor lag, a greater number of patients had difficulty kneeling and stooping, and a larger number of patients believed that their surgery was unsuccessful in relieving their pain and returning them to normal activities.

Complications associated with the tibial tubercle osteotomy include proximal displacement of the osteotomized tuberosity and tibial shaft fractures. As a prophylactic measure, it would seem prudent to bypass the distal extent of the osteotomy with a stemmed tibial component by at least two diaphyseal diameters.

Whiteside[38] reported that of a total of 136 knee arthroplasties that had a tibial tubercle osteotomy as part of the exposure, 2 cases involved proximal avulsion of the tuberosity. Three patients had to have their wires removed because of pain. Two tibial fractures occurred in one patient who had a diabetic Charcot arthropathy, and one tibial fracture was reported in a patient who had a subsequent manipulation after open adhesiolysis. Wolff and associates[41] reported on 26 tibial tubercle osteotomies with a complication rate related to the osteotomy of 23%, including an extensor lag with extensor tendon disruption in 5 knees and wound healing problems in 4 knees.

FEMORAL PEEL

This technique starts with a standard medial parapatellar approach. Dissection is continued around the medial and lateral sides of the femur subperiosteally to include the origins of the medial and lateral collateral ligaments. Posteriorly, the capsule is stripped off the femur, so that the distal femur is completely exposed.[40] The obvious risk of this technique is causing avascular necrosis of the distal end of the femur; for this reason, it is rarely used in the revision knee arthroplasty setting and is more likely to be used for excising neoplastic lesions from the distal femur.

MEDIAL EPICONDYLAR OSTEOTOMY

This technique was first described by Engh and colleagues[11,12] in 1997. The knee is initially exposed via a medial parapatellar approach. Then, the superficial medial collateral ligament and the structures superior to the medial epicondyle are raised as one continuous flap with the medial epicondyle as a fragment of bone within it. This fragment of bone should measure approximately 1 cm in thickness and should also include the adductor tubercle. Dissection is continued around the femur and the tibia posteriorly and laterally. The knee is fully exposed by externally rotating and applying a valgus force on the tibia relative to the femur. The medial epicondyle osteotomy fragment then is reattached to the femur with screws, staples, or sutures. The knee is closed in standard fashion.

SUMMARY

Revision of a total knee arthroplasty can be a challenge to the knee surgeon. A comprehensive understanding of the anatomic nuances of extensile approaches to the knee is essential in achieving a good outcome for the patient. This starts with the choice of skin incision and awareness of its blood supply, thereby avoiding any potential complications of wound necrosis and subsequent breakdown. Often sufficient exposure can be achieved by simply excising the scar tissue that forms within the joint following a knee arthroplasty. If this fails to gain adequate exposure, then a quadriceps snip can be performed with no additional morbidity, if it is performed carefully. A V-Y quadricepsplasty can be useful if a rectus snip does not allow sufficient exposure. Reasonable results have been reported[2,5,35,37] and probably justify conservative use of this extensile approach, particularly if lengthening of the quadriceps tendon is required. In Barrack's study comparing extensile exposures,[5] the V-Y quadricepsplasty group had greater range of movement but a higher incidence of an extensor lag compared with the tibial tuberosity osteotomy group. However, patients who underwent a tibial tubercle osteotomy were less satisfied postoperatively than those who had had a V-Y quadricepsplasty.

To date, no prospectively randomized studies have compared the different extensile exposures, which would help to further delineate the differences between these techniques, particularly given the importance of the surgical approach in revision total knee arthroplasty.

KEY REFERENCES

Aglietti P, Buzzi R, D'Andria S, Scrobe F: Quadricepsplasty with the V-Y incision in total knee arthroplasty. Ital J Orthop Traumatol 17:23–29, 1991.

Aglietti P, Windsor RE, Buzzi R, Insall JN: Arthroplasty for the stiff or ankylosed knee. J Arthroplasty 4:1–5, 1989.

Arsht SJ, Scuderi GR: The quadriceps snip for exposing the stiff knee. J Knee Surg 16:55–57, 2003.

Barrack RL, Smith P, Munn B, Engh G, Rorabeck C: The Ranawat Award. Comparison of surgical approaches in total knee arthroplasty. Clin Orthop Relat Res 356:16–21, 1998.

Della Valle CJ, Berger RA, Rosenberg AG: Surgical exposures in revision total knee arthroplasty. Clin Orthop Relat Res 446:59–68, 2006.

Engh GA: Medial epicondylar osteotomy: a technique used with primary and revision total knee arthroplasty to improve surgical exposure and correct varus deformity. Instr Course Lect 48:153–156, 1999.

Garvin KL, Scuderi G, Insall JN: Evolution of the quadriceps snip. Clin Orthop Relat Res 321:131–137, 1995.

Meek RMD, Greidanus NV, McGraw RW, Masri BA: The extensile rectus snip exposure in revision of total knee arthroplasty. J Bone Joint Surg Br 85:1120–1122, 2003.

Scott RD, Siliski JM: The use of a modified V-Y quadricepsplasty during total knee replacement to gain exposure and improve flexion in the ankylosed knee. Orthopedics 8:45–48, 1985.

Trousdale RT, Hanssen AD, Rand JA, Cahalan TD: V-Y quadricepsplasty in total knee arthroplasty. Clin Orthop Relat Res 286:48–55, 1993.

Whiteside LA: Exposure in difficult total knee arthroplasty using tibial tubercle osteotomy. Clin Orthop Relat Res 321:32–35, 1995.

Whiteside LA, Ohl MD: Tibial tubercle osteotomy for exposure of the difficult total knee arthroplasty. Clin Orthop Relat Res 260:6–9, 1990.

Wolff AM, Hungerford DS, Krackow KA, Jacobs MA: Osteotomy of the tibial tubercle during total knee replacement: a report of twenty-six cases. J Bone Joint Surg Am 71:848–852, 1989.

Younger AS, Duncan CP, Masri BA: Surgical exposures in revision total knee arthroplasty. J Am Acad Orthop Surg 6:55–64, 1998.

Full references for this chapter can be found on www.expertconsult.com.

Revision of Aseptic Failed Total Knee Arthroplasty

Michael P. Nett and Giles R. Scuderi

Although the durability of total knee arthroplasty (TKA) with current techniques and implants is well established, failure still occurs as a result of instability, stiffness, component loosening or malposition, periprosthetic fracture, component breakage, polyethylene wear, and osteolysis. The number of primary total knee arthroplasties performed annually continues to rise rapidly.[38] With a much larger population of patients having undergone primary total knee arthroplasty, the number of patients requiring revision arthroplasty will also rise, despite improvements in technique, implant design, and biomaterials.[38] When failure occurs and revision is contemplated, the surgeon must recognize that revision TKA is a complex procedure that requires skill and meticulous technique to restore a predictable outcome. Preoperative evaluation should identify the cause of failure to improve the likelihood of a successful outcome.[34,47] Once the cause of failure has been identified, revision surgery is performed expediently. Consideration must be given to the incision and approach, management of soft tissues, techniques of implant removal, balancing of ligaments and flexion/extension gaps, management of bone loss, tensioning and alignment of the extensor mechanism, and choice of the appropriate revision implant. The objective of revision arthroplasty is similar to that of primary surgery: to have a well-aligned limb with a stable and securely fixed implant that allows restoration of function and reduction in pain.

INDICATIONS FOR REVISION

Mechanical Failure

Indications for revision arthroplasty include mechanical failure, malalignment, stiffness, fracture, and infection. Mechanical failure is often due to technical error at the time of primary arthroplasty.[34] Mechanical failure includes aseptic loosening, polyethylene wear, osteolysis, instability, and extensor mechanism dysfunction.[73] If the components are loose or have shifted position, failure is inevitable and revision surgery should be performed expediently.[34] Similarly, revision is imperative with polyethylene wear-through of the tibia insert or a metal-backed patellar component. Delay will only result in additional metallic debris and massive metallic synovitis.

Osteolysis is one of the leading causes of late reoperation in patients who undergo total knee arthroplasty. The extent of osteolysis is often underappreciated with routine radiographs. Computed tomography (CT) or magnetic resonance imaging (MRI) can be obtained to more accurately image the osteolytic lesion and to determine the extent of bone loss.[58] Small, asymptomatic osteolytic lesions warrant close observation and possibly medical management with bisphosphonates and calcium supplementation.[27] Large, progressive, or symptomatic lesions are addressed with revision arthroplasty

ranging from simple polyethylene insert exchange to full component revision with structural bone graft or porous metal augments, depending on polyethylene availability, specific implant reliability, and extent of bone loss.[44]

Instability is another common cause of mechanical failure of TKA. The direction of instability at the tibiofemoral articulation can occur in the coronal (varus/valgus) plane, in the sagittal (anteroposterior) plane, or as a combination of planes. Early instability may result from malalignment of the components, failure to restore the mechanical axis of the limb, or imbalance of the flexion/extension space, as is often the case with midflexion instability.[49] Other common causes of early instability include intraoperative or postoperative rupture of the medial collateral ligament (MCL) or posterior cruciate ligament (PCL) with cruciate-retaining designs. Commonly, late instability occurs secondary to polyethylene wear. Asymmetrical polyethylene wear related to malalignment can result in relative lengthening of the collateral ligament on the involved side and subsequent coronal instability. In patients with cruciate-retaining knees, it is not uncommon for the PCL to elongate or attenuate. This can lead to progressive polyethylene wear and late sagittal plane instability.[40] However, late sagittal plane instability is seen not only with cruciate-retaining designs. Significant wear or fracture of the tibial polyethylene post in posterior stabilized knees may result in late sagittal plane instability.[55] Nonoperative management plays a small role in managing instability in TKA. Stability can often be achieved with a revision arthroplasty utilizing a posterior stabilized design. A constrained condylar design may be necessary to address collateral insufficiency or flexion and extension gap imbalance. Occasionally, a hinged design may be indicated and should be readily available.[62]

Extensor mechanism dysfunction remains a cause of failure in TKA. Extensor mechanism dysfunction consists of maltracking, instability, polyethylene wear, and prosthetic loosening. Unfavorable prosthetic design and error in surgical technique lead to patellar maltracking, which may result in tilt, wear, loosening, subluxation, frank instability, or patellar fracture.[32] With improved prosthetic design and a better understanding of appropriate component position, the percentage of TKA failures related to extensor mechanism dysfunction is likely less than historical figures. Extensor mechanism failure responds poorly to nonoperative management and requires isolated component revision, extensor mechanism realignment, or complete component revision depending on the cause of failure.

Stiffness

Stiffness is a disabling problem following TKA. Stiffness is often associated with a decrease in functional capacity and increased pain. Before revision arthroplasty is performed for stiffness, the cause should be determined and the extrinsic sources addressed. Extrinsic sources include but are not limited to osteoarthritis of the ipsilateral hip, muscle rigidity secondary to neurologic injury, and heterotopic ossification. After exclusion of an extrinsic source, the intrinsic origin should be determined. Intrinsic causes include infection, overstuffing of the patellofemoral joint, an oversized femoral component, an excessively tight flexion or extension gap, component malposition or malrotation, a tight posterior cruciate ligament, and arthrofibrosis. If an intrinsic cause is identified and infection is ruled out, revision arthroplasty can be performed. The role of isolated arthrolysis and polyethylene component downsizing in patients with a stiff arthroplasty and well-fixed, well-aligned components remains unclear. Poor results with a high complication rate and no significant improvement in range of motion or pain were demonstrated with this approach in 7 carefully selected patients with 4-year average follow-up.[2] Single-component revision may be successful in the stiff total knee with an oversized femoral prosthesis or a single malpositioned component.[29,41] However, revision of both components is usually necessary.[29] Full component revision is likely to provide improved results, but improvement in range of motion and level of pain has been shown to be modest in the hands of experienced surgeons despite meticulous patient selection.[29,51]

Periprosthetic Fracture

Periprosthetic fracture remains a problematic complication following arthroplasty. It is estimated that 0.3% to 2.5% of patients will sustain a periprosthetic fracture as a complication of TKA.[17] Patient-specific factors, including rheumatoid arthritis, osteopenic bone, and osteolysis, and technique-specific factors, such as anterior femoral cortical notching, have been implicated as potential causes of periprosthetic fracture. Frequently, fractures occur in the supracondylar area above a well-fixed implant.[33] Fractures of the tibia are much less common and frequently are associated with implant loosening.[20] In general, patients with fractures around loose implants are best treated with revision TKA, whereas those with fractures around well-fixed implants should be considered for open reduction and internal fixation.[17]

Infection

Deep infection remains one of the most devastating and challenging complications of TKA. It is estimated that by 2030, 65.5% of all revisions will be performed secondary to infection.[38] Currently, the risk of postoperative infection after TKR is 0.4% to 2.0%.[31] Appropriate treatment for acute infection remains debatable and depends on organism virulence, host factors, and time from onset to surgical intervention.[61,66] Chronic infection is treated most appropriately with two-stage reimplantation, including removal of components, débridement, and placement of a cement spacer, followed by 6 to 8 weeks of intravenous antibiotics and reimplantation once the infection has been eradicated[31] (Fig. 127-1). Complete discussion of the management of periprosthetic infection is beyond the scope of this chapter.

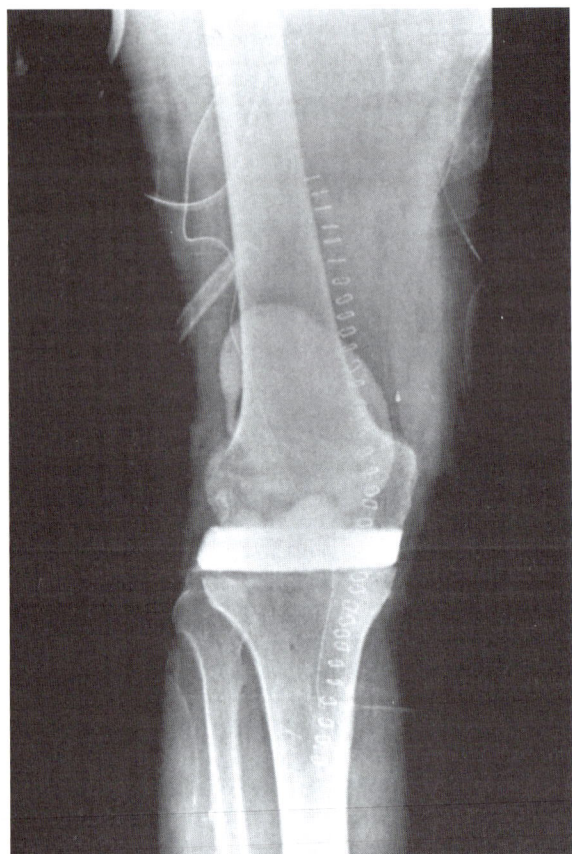

Figure 127-1. Radiograph showing antibiotic-impregnated cement spacers used after removal of an infected implant. The use of spacers contributes to eradicating infection and enhancing patient comfort and makes reimplantation technically easier. Routinely, 3 to 4 g each of vancomycin and tobramycin is utilized per batch of cement for creation of the spacer. Placement of intramedullary "dowels" should be considered.

PREOPERATIVE ASSESSMENT

History and Physical Examination

It is important to use a systematic diagnostic approach when evaluating the patient with a painful TKA. A thorough history and physical examination is an essential part of the preoperative evaluation and often can alert the surgeon to the possible cause of failure. An appropriately directed history may reveal critical issues that suggest infection, including delayed wound healing, prolonged drainage, fever, chills, night sweats, remote sources for hematogenous infection, such as urinary tract infection, or a recent invasive procedure, including dental work. It is also valuable to assess the pain pattern. An arthroplasty that was never pain free may lead the clinician to suspect nonarticular sources of pain, infection, or instability. A history of initial functional improvement followed by late onset of pain or dysfunction may suggest component loosening, late instability, or a hematogenously based infection. A history of start-up pain can suggest mechanical failure and implant loosening; persistent pain despite inactivity may suggest infection, regional pain syndrome, or tumor.

The wound and skin should be carefully evaluated for evidence of local infection or peripheral vascular disease.

Meticulous palpation for point tenderness can lead to a diagnosis of tendinitis, bursitis, or cutaneous neuroma.[12] Physical examination of the hip and spine can reveal sources of referred pain, including ipsilateral hip arthritis or radiculopathy. Evaluation of the knee with regard to range of motion, stability, alignment, patellar tracking, and the presence of an effusion may provide additional evidence of local infection, malalignment, instability, stiffness, or extensor mechanism dysfunction.

Laboratory Evaluation

All patients presenting with a painful TKA should have a complete blood count with differential (CBC), erythrocyte sedimentation rate (ESR), and C-reactive protein (CRP). The CBC is often normal even in the presence of infection. Any elevation in laboratory values should raise the clinician's suspicion for infection. Routine use of additional laboratory tests, including serum interleukin-6, procalcitonin, and tumor necrosis factor-alpha, in making the diagnosis of infection has yet to be implemented, but may play a role in the near future.[6]

Aspiration is advisable whenever joint fluid is present.[12] The aspirate should be examined for signs of purulence, bleeding, metallic or polyethylene debris, or change in viscosity. The fluid is then sent for cell count, gram stain, and aerobic, anaerobic, and fungal culture. A synovial fluid leukocyte differential of greater than 65% neutrophils has a sensitivity of 97% and a specificity of 98% for diagnosing prosthetic joint infection; a leukocyte count greater than 1.7 $\times 10^3/\mu L$ has a sensitivity of 94% and a specificity of 88%.[67] Ghanem and associates[23] reported similar results and recommend a cut-off of greater than 64% neutrophils and a leukocyte count greater than $1.1 \times 10^3/\mu L$, which demonstrated a combined positive predictive value of 98.6%.[23]

Radiographic Evaluation

Routine standing anteroposterior (AP) and lateral radiographs should be obtained and evaluated for component position, fixation, and sizing. Any evidence of osteolysis, polyethylene wear, component failure, loosening, or migration is noted. The most recent radiographs are compared with initial postoperative films to address concerns of subtle component migration, progressive radiolucent lines, or progressive osteolysis. A Merchant view is also essential in evaluating the patellofemoral articulation and extensor mechanism tracking. Obtaining a full-length hip-to-ankle film has several advantages. This film can be evaluated for sources of referred pain from the ipsilateral hip, including degenerative joint disease and stress fracture. It allows more accurate assessment of alignment of the involved limb and can detect distant osseous problems such as malunion, tumor, stress fracture, orthopedic hardware, or an adjacent joint arthroplasty that may be the source of pain or may interfere with a planned revision.[12] Additional radiographic views may be warranted in specific scenarios. Fluoroscopically positioned radiographs can be used to image the implant fixation interface tangentially and allow the diagnosis of subtle component loosening.[18] Oblique radiographs have been shown to enhance visualization of the periprosthetic bone and to facilitate diagnosis of early osteolysis, especially with posterior stabilized implants.[48] Stress radiographs are not routinely needed, but

may assist in diagnosing subtle ligamentous instability or PCL deficiency.[14]

Advanced Imaging

Computed tomography (CT) is used to more accurately diagnose and size periprosthetic osteolysis related to polyethylene wear. This can facilitate preoperative planning with regard to the management of bone loss during revision arthroplasty. Reish and colleagues[58] demonstrated that standard radiographs detected 17% of osteolytic lesions diagnosed by multidetector CT in 31 patients. CT is an effective and accurate way to measure tibial and femoral component rotation.[58] This may be most appropriate in the preoperative evaluation of patients with extensor mechanism complications, including patellofemoral pain, excessive tilt, maltracking, subluxation, or dislocation.

Recent modifications of MRI pulse sequence parameters have permitted imaging of arthroplasty with significantly less artifact. MRI allows imaging of the surrounding soft tissue envelope, including nerves, tendons, and ligaments. As well, MRI can be a useful tool to detect and quantify particle disease, osteolysis, synovitis, and prosthetic infection.[54] The exact role of MRI in evaluating the painful TKA has not yet been determined; however, it is likely that MRI will play a larger role in the future as imaging abilities continue to improve.

Nuclear medicine scans play an undefined role in evaluating the painful or failed TKA. Commonly used scans include the Tc-99m–labeled bone scan, the [111]gallium Ga-67 scan, the indium-labeled white blood cell scan, and the sulfur colloid bone marrow scan. Positive scans indicate loosening, stress fracture, infection, or complex regional pain syndrome. Nuclear scans typically provide high sensitivity but variable specificity. A Tc-99m–labeled bone scan may be positive up to 2 years following a successful arthroplasty that may limit its role in evaluation of the recently postoperative patient. Smith and associates[64] reviewed the use of [99]Tc[m]-MDP in evaluating 80 painful TKAs. They demonstrated low specificity (75.9%) and a positive predictive value (64.9%). Specifically, 33% of patients with an abnormal scan had a normal TKA with further follow-up. However, a negative bone scintigram has proved reassuring. In Smith's study, the sensitivity and negative predictive value were 92.3% and 95.0%, respectively. [111]Indium-labeled white blood cell scans are used most often in evaluation for infection. Rand and colleagues[57] evaluated 18 infected and 20 noninfected TKAs with [111]indium scan. They demonstrated a sensitivity and specificity of 83% and 85%, respectively, along with a diagnostic accuracy of 84%. Similarly, Scher and coworkers[60] observed 84% accuracy and a 95% negative predictive value for the prediction of infection in 143 arthroplasty patients evaluated with [111]indium leukocyte scan. As demonstrated, a positive [111]indium scan is by itself nonspecific and can be positive because of marrow redistribution around a prosthesis. Therefore, the [111]indium scan has been combined with a Tc-99m sulfur colloid scan to scan bone marrow. Incongruent uptake of the two is highly suggestive of infection.[64] Palestro and associates[52] demonstrated greater diagnostic accuracy (95%) with combined labeled leukocyte and sulfur colloid marrow imaging compared with that of labeled leukocyte scintigraphy alone (78%).

Preoperative Planning

Preoperative planning is essential for successful revision surgery. The exact mode for failure of the prior arthroplasty must be identified.[34,73] The diagnosis of infection in the vast majority of cases is established prior to the procedure, so intraoperative "surprises" are rare.[73] The original operative report is obtained and reviewed whenever possible. This provides information regarding the previous approach, prior soft tissue management, including releases, and implant-specific information, including manufacturer, design, and size. This is particularly important if single-component revision is being entertained. Thought is given to the type of prosthesis and the amount of constraint that will be required for revision.[62] Any special components must be ordered in advance. The surgeon attempts to quantify the extent of bone loss and osteolysis present with the knowledge that it is often underestimated. The need for structural bone graft, augments, wedges, porous metal metaphyseal cones, and stems is anticipated, and they are made readily available during the revision. Preoperative templating for selected revision components can be helpful. This is essential in cases where extra-articular deformity or osseous pathology is present that may require osteotomy or may interfere with stem fixation. Revision components should be modular to allow intraoperative attachment of augments, wedges, and stems. The revision proceeds more predictably when the cruciate ligaments are excised and both posterior stabilized and constrained condylar designs are available. Ligament stability and integrity of the extensor mechanism are assessed. If ligament stability is compromised, at the time of revision a hinged prosthesis is kept readily available. A compromised soft tissue envelope due to impaired skin viability or previous incision may warrant a plastic surgery consultation; occasionally, soft tissue expansion or a soft tissue flap will be required.[25,45]

SURGICAL TECHNIQUE

Exposure

The surgical approach most often utilizes the previous surgical incision. In cases with multiple longitudinal prior incisions, the most lateral and anterior incision is used to preserve the blood supply to the medial aspect of the lateral skin flap.[36] Attempts to maintain a minimum skin bridge of 6 cm between parallel incisions are recommended. Previous transverse incisions that cannot be avoided are crossed at 90 degrees if possible, but certainly at no less than 60 degrees. Soft tissue expanders can be considered in cases with multiple crossing incisions or densely adherent soft tissue.[45] Subcutaneous dissection is carried out in a limited manner, and flaps are kept as thick as possible to avoid ischemia. A medial parapatellar arthrotomy is performed. Synovial fluid is obtained as the first intraoperative culture. In revision arthroplasty with good preoperative motion, a medial subperiosteal exposure that allows the tibia to be externally rotated and anteriorly subluxed is usually sufficient for exposure. This is incorporated into a medial release if needed for soft tissue release and balancing. In revision for infection or arthrofibrosis, or during two stage reimplantation, a quadriceps snip may be anticipated and is performed early to prevent injury to the tibial tubercle and extensor mechanism[63] (Fig. 127-2). The quadriceps snip is a

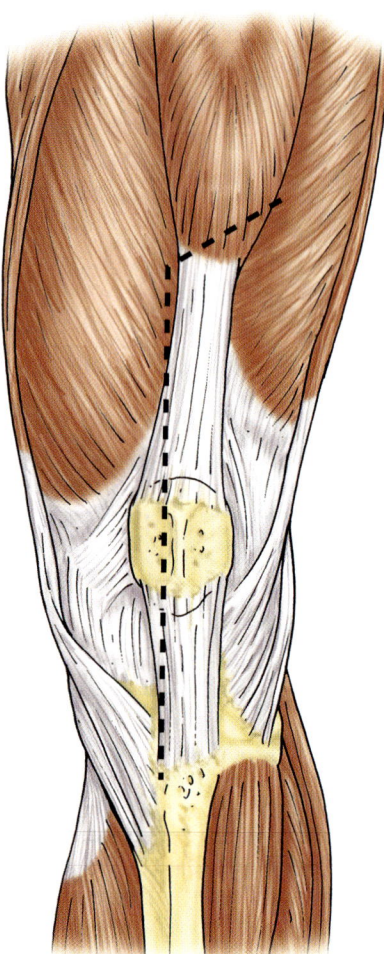

Figure 127-2. A quadriceps snip is a versatile technique used to provide expansile exposure without requiring a change in the postoperative protocol.

versatile exposure that is used in a majority of revisions requiring extensile exposure; it does not require alteration of the postoperative weight-bearing protocol. When quadriceps snip does not allow adequate exposure, tibial tubercle osteotomy or a "banana peel" release of the patellar tendon can be considered[39,71] (Fig. 127-3). A long osteotomy as described by Whiteside and Ohl[71] is particularly useful in patients with marked patella baja, or to assist with removal of long cemented stems and well-fixed ingrowth components. A "step-cut" is performed at the most proximal aspect of the osteotomy. This allows more secure fixation and helps prevent proximal escape of the fragment. Care is taken to maintain the lateral soft tissue attachments to the osteotomized bone and to hinge the osteotomy open. This facilitates closure and maintains fragment vascularity. The fragment is repaired utilizing cerclage wires or two screws.[71] With secure fixation, the postoperative weight-bearing protocol does not have to be altered. An alternative technique for additional exposure is V-Y quadricepsplasty.[1,63] V-Y quadricepsplasty provides excellent exposure and allows lengthening of the extensor mechanism if needed. Quadicepsplasty necessitates postoperative immobilization in extension and may result in extensor lag. For patients with rigid deformity and arthrofibrosis, a femoral peel may be necessary. Because this procedure involves complete

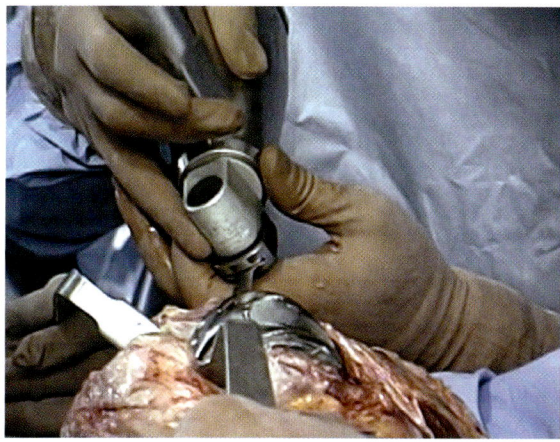

Figure 127-4. A flexible saw blade is placed along the cement/prosthesis interface and is moved parallel to the component to avoid cutting into the bone.

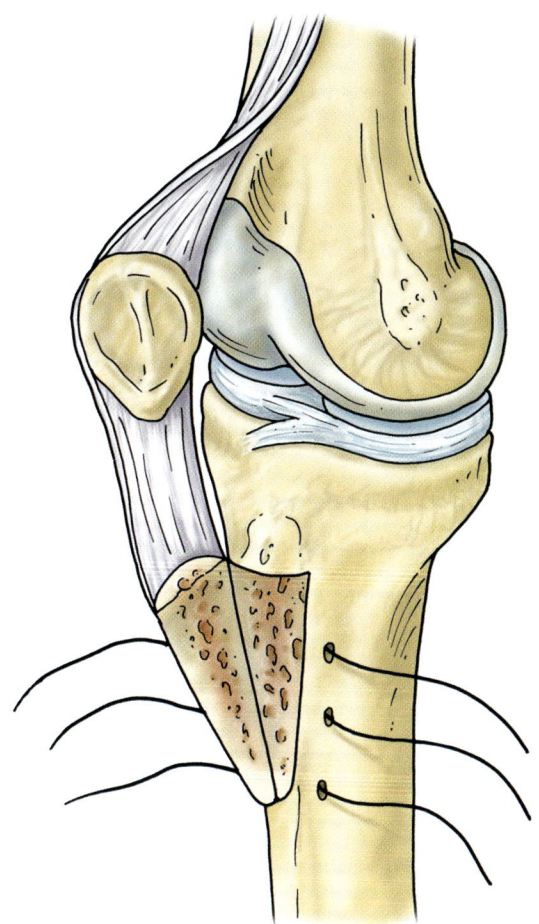

Figure 127-3. When additional exposure is needed, or in cases with severe patella baja or a stemmed cemented tibial component, a tibial tubercle osteotomy may be beneficial.

release of the medial and lateral supporting structures, use of a constrained design will be necessary.

Fixed angular deformities are often encountered during revision arthroplasty and are addressed during the exposure. A fixed varus deformity is corrected with subperiosteal release of deep and superficial portions of the MCL and the pes anserine insertion.[37] The distal insertion of the superficial MCL is elevated subperiosteally in an incremental fashion with a straight ¼-inch osteotome. Finally, while the tibia is externally rotated, the semimembranosus and posterior capsule are released off the posteromedial aspect of the tibia.[37] This results in skeletonization of the proximal medial tibia. A fixed valgus deformity is less common in the revision setting, but if encountered, it must be addressed. Mild valgus deformity of less than 20 degrees may be addressed with the lateral "pie-crust" technique.[10] Severe valgus deformities of greater than 20 degrees necessitate complete release of the lateral supporting structures from the femoral condyle with a subperiosteal peel or a lateral epicondylar osteotomy.

Débridement

Débridement of the suprapatellar and parapatellar regions is performed routinely. The medial and lateral gutters are

re-created and cleared of all fibrous tissue. This facilitates exposure and removes debris of polyethylene, polymethyl-methacrylate, and bone fragments. If the synovium is hypertrophic from reaction to intra-articular polyethylene and metal debris, a complete synovectomy is performed. The synovectomy also facilitates exposure of the joint.

Removal of Components

When operative inspection reveals granulation tissue, necrotic tissue, or other evidence of infection, the components should be removed, thorough débridement performed, and frozen section tissue examined. Evidence of acute inflammation is a reason for aborting the procedure until microbacterial cultures are available. Closing the wound over an antibiotic-impregnated polymethylmethacrylate spacer makes subsequent reentry of the knee easier in the event that cultures prove negative.

Revision operations are being performed increasingly for reasons other than loosening. Removal of well-fixed components can be difficult, especially if they are porous coated or have long cemented stems. Initially, all soft tissue is cleared from the bone/cement/prosthesis interface. Special instruments can facilitate component removal. If a modular tibial component is present, the polyethylene insert is removed first to open both flexion and extension spaces. This aids in obtaining additional exposure. The polyethylene insert is removed using manufacturer-specific tools for extraction, or by passing a straight osteotome between the insert and the tibial component. The femoral component is subsequently removed. A microsagittal saw blade is placed along the cement/prosthesis interface and is moved parallel to the component to avoid cutting into the bone (Fig. 127-4). Thin flexible osteotomes are then passed around the periphery of the component to separate the component at the cement/prosthesis interface and leave the underlying bone intact (Fig. 127-5A and B). Once the adhesion between component and cement is broken, a femoral component extraction tool is used to gently remove the femoral prosthesis (Fig. 127-6). If the procedure is performed properly, the cement is left behind still attached to the bone with minimal bone loss from

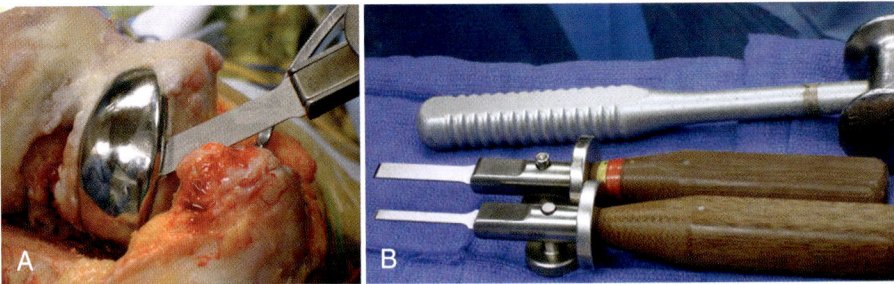

Figure 127-5. A and **B,** Flexible osteotomes are passed parallel to the femoral component at the cement/prosthesis interface. These flexible osteotomes are much less likely to crush the underlying host bone, minimizing iatrogenic bone loss.

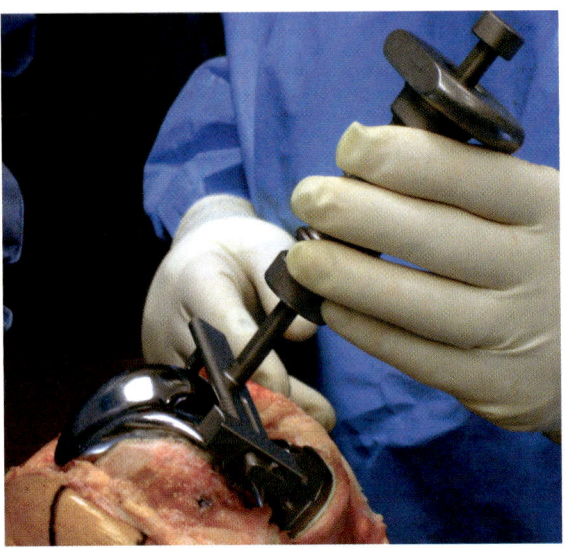

Figure 127-6. A sliding hammer is used to extract the femoral component once the bond at the cement/prosthesis interface is loosened.

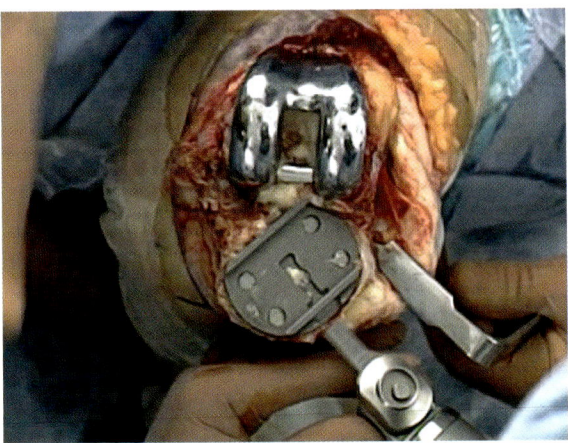

Figure 127-7. The microsagittal saw is passed beneath and parallel to the tibial component. Caution should be used to avoid digging into the tibial bone and causing unnecessary iatrogenic bone loss.

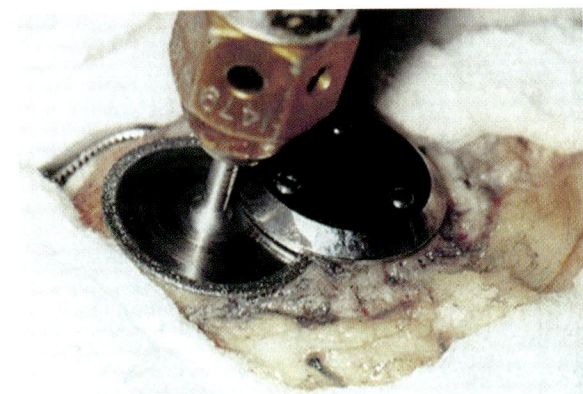

Figure 127-8. Removal of a well-fixed metal-backed patellar component with a diamond-edged saw blade.

implant removal. The cement is then removed by cracking it with a small osteotome in a mosaic pattern.

The tibial component is addressed next. All polyethylene components are separated from the tibial surface with a microsagittal saw that cuts across any polyethylene pegs or stems that are subsequently removed. Metal-backed tibial components are approached in a similar manner as the femoral component. The microsagittal saw is passed beneath and parallel to the tibial component (Fig. 127-7). Caution should be used to avoid digging into the tibial bone and causing unnecessary iatrogenic bone loss. Due to exposure, separating the tibial component from the cement mantle is most difficult on the posterolateral aspect of the tibia. Tibial exposure is improved by external rotation of the tibia and release of the semimembranosus and posterior capsule. The posterolateral aspect of the component is then reached by passing the microsagittal saw and thin flexible osteotomes under the posteromedial aspect of the tray to the posterolateral side. Once the bond is broken between the cement and the component, a manufacturer specific extractor or the femoral component extractor is used to gently lift the component from the tibia. An osteotome is used to crack the remaining cement in a mosaic pattern.

A well-fixed, compatible patellar component that tracks well is left in place.[3,28] All polyethylene patellar components

are removed by cutting between the cement/component interface with an oscillating saw. The saw cuts across the pegs, which are subsequently removed with a small burr or drill bit. Metal-backed patellar components are more difficult to remove. A high-speed diamond-edged saw may be necessary to remove a well-fixed uncemented metal-backed patellar component[13] (Fig. 127-8).

After the components are removed, the bone surfaces are cleaned of cement, debris, and granulation tissue (Fig. 127-9). The bone ends are "freshened-up" in preparation for cement fixation of the revision component. In the revision setting in which infection has been ruled out, well-fixed cement in the canals that does not impact component stem placement can be left in place to avoid unnecessary iatrogenic bone loss or perforation of the canal. Removal of a cemented porous-coated prosthesis can be a difficult task, especially with stems designed for bone ingrowth. It may be necessary in this scenario to disassemble the components to gain access to the stems (Fig. 127-10).

Reconstruction

After removal of the components and thorough débridement comes time to rebuild the knee. The basic principle of revision arthroplasty involves creating a kinematically stable arthroplasty that is well fixed and well aligned. The key is to create equal flexion and extension gaps. Often this is not readily achieved, and adjustments need to be made. The surgeon must understand that adjustments made on the femoral side can affect the knee in flexion or extension, whereas adjustments on the tibial side will affect both. Reconstruction is approached using a three-step method: (1) re-create the flat tibial surface, (2) re-create the femur and rebuild the flexion space, and (3) rebuild the extension space.[8]

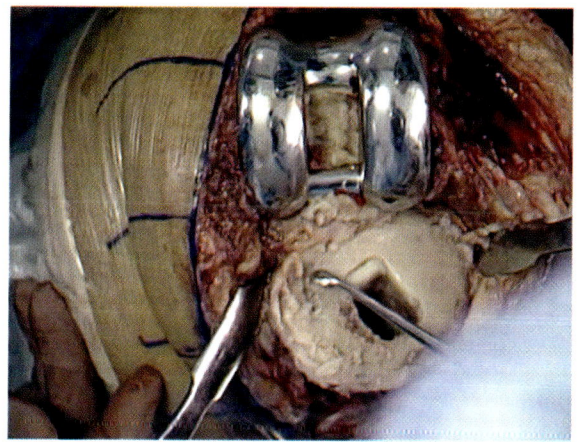

Figure 127-9. After removal of the components, retained cement and debris are removed with curettes, osteotomes, and a rongeur.

Re-create the Tibia

The tibia is the foundation of the revision arthroplasty and is addressed first to establish the platform on which the subsequent arthroplasty is built.[8] Because the tibia affects the knee in both extension and flexion, a flat surface that is perpendicular to the mechanical axis must be created. If stems on the tibial component are to be used, the intramedullary canal often provides an excellent guide to re-creating a flat, perpendicular surface. Augmentation is utilized to re-create the proximal tibia to support the perpendicular, flat tibial surface as close to the original height of the tibia as possible. This will provide the surgeon with more options for choosing the appropriate polyethylene insert to balance flexion and extension gaps. Modular augments, wedges, blocks, or structural allograft may be needed (Fig. 127-11). In knees with severe tibial bone loss, modular tibial cones are utilized to reconstruct the proximal end of the tibia[1] (Fig. 127-12). Care is taken to position the tibial component in the proper rotation using the tibial tubercle and the anteromedial aspect of the tibia as reference points.

Re-create the Femur

Size the Femur

Choosing the correct size of components is an essential step. Femoral component sizing specifically influences the flexion space by restoring the anteroposterior dimensions and the posterior condylar offset of the femur. It is helpful to preoperatively procure the operative notes from the previous procedure. Another useful preoperative step is to template the opposite side to obtain a relative idea of the size. Look at the size of the femoral component that is being removed, and determine whether it is appropriate. The remaining bone should be templated in the anteroposterior plane. Posterior bone loss usually occurs, so templating intraoperatively runs the risk of undersizing the femoral component (Fig. 127-13). The epicondylar width of the femur can also be helpful in selecting the appropriate femoral size.

The danger in selecting an excessively small femoral component is that this will fail to restore posterior femoral offset and will compromise flexion stability. It is better to select a larger femoral component and augment the posterior condyles to restore the anteroposterior dimension. Bone loss usually is most significant in the posterior femoral condyle

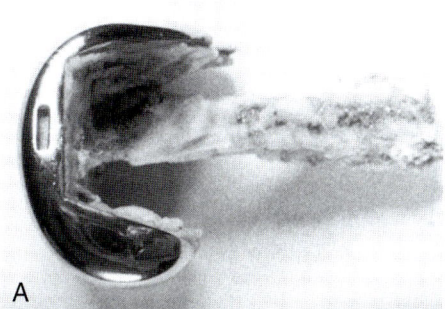

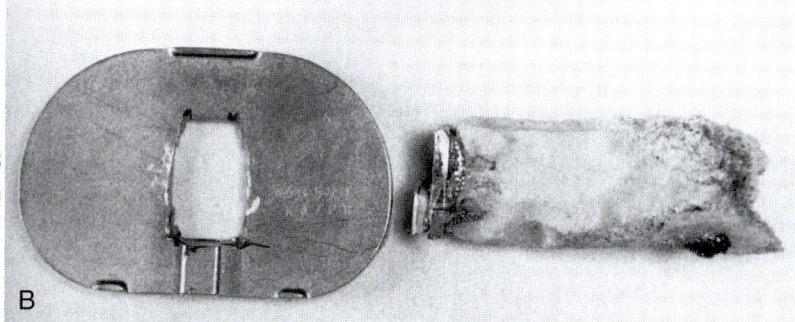

Figure 127-10. Photograph shows porous cemented components that were removed because of infection. This task was very difficult and resulted in some bone loss on the posterior surface of both the femur and the tibia. The tibial component could not be extracted until the central peg had been cut from the baseplate with a diamond-tipped saw.

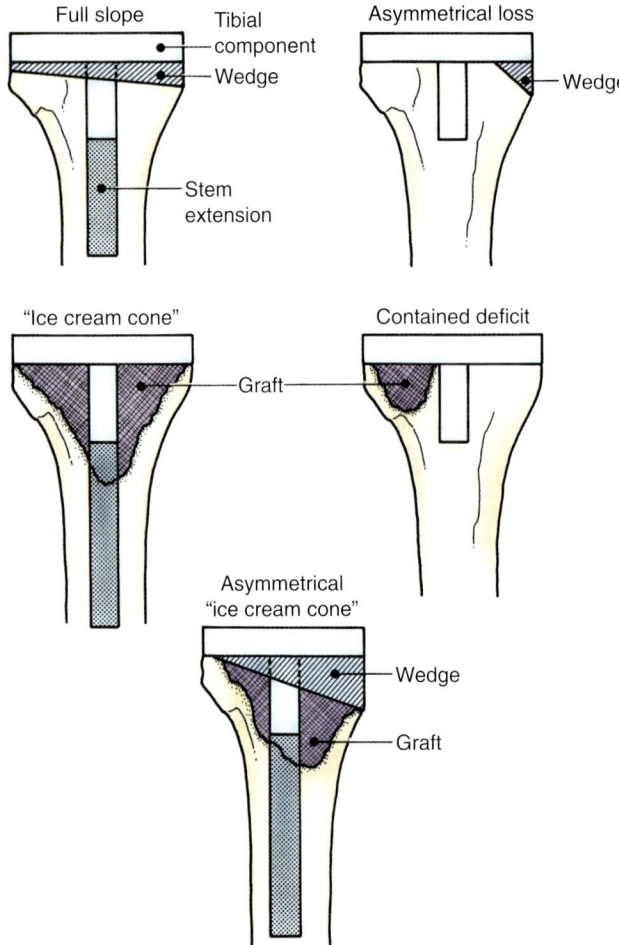

Figure 127-11. Reconstruction of tibial defects. Symmetrical tibial deficiency can be compensated for by thicker tibial polyethylene. Stem extension is usually advisable.

area, but anterior femoral bone loss can occur and can influence sizing, especially sizing of the femoral component in the sagittal position (Fig. 127-14).

Femoral Component Rotation

Correct rotation of the femoral component is vital to knee kinematics and patellar tracking. The best way to determine rotation is to identify the medial and lateral epicondyles and establish the epicondylar axis. Rotational adjustments should be made to the residual distal femur, with shaving of bone from the anterolateral and posteromedial aspects of the femur usually required if the previous component was rotated internally. To ensure correct femoral component rotation, the posterolateral condyle generally has to be augmented. If a posterior stabilized or similar prosthesis is used, the intercondylar notch is prepared 90 degrees to the epicondylar axis. In cases of severe bone loss, the epicondyles may not be available. The tibial platform is then used as a reference for femoral component rotation with the knee at 90 degrees of flexion.

Distal Femur Position

The key to this step is restoring the distance from the joint line, distally and posteriorly. The epicondyles are a useful landmark from which to determine the joint line, which on

average is 25 mm from the lateral epicondyle and 30 mm from the medial epicondyle. Because the tibial cut is established at 90 degrees to the tibial mechanical axis, the joint line of a prosthetic knee of average size is 30 mm from both epicondyles.

After the appropriate joint line has been determined, the femoral component can be set provisionally to reestablish the distal joint line. Symmetrical distal femoral augments are used on both medial and lateral sides if there is symmetrical bone loss, or if the joint line has been previously elevated (Fig. 127-15). Unilateral distal augmentation or asymmetrical augmentation is utilized to accommodate asymmetrical femoral bone loss. Treatment of femoral bone loss depends on the severity of the deficiency and consists of cement, metal augmentation, modular cones, structural allograft, and distal femoral replacement[16,56] (Fig. 127-16). The distance from the epicondyles to the posterior joint line is similar to that to the distal joint line and is helpful in confirming the correct femoral component size.

Because this step is provisional, no bone should be resected to fit the augments until the final position and size of the femoral component have been determined. Additional adjustments to the position and size of the femoral component may be needed as the flexion and extension gaps are balanced.

Rebuild the Flexion Space

Balance the Flexion Space

This step requires choosing the correct tibial polyethylene articulation. With the provisional femoral component in place, the thickest tibial polyethylene surface that fills the flexion space is inserted on the provisional tibial tray (Fig. 127-17).

Rebuild the Extension Space

The knee is brought into extension with the tibial insert in place. If the knee can be fully extended and the gaps are equal and stable, the polyethylene insert is correctly sized and the femoral augments are finalized. Minor adjustments can be made to the polyethylene insert to achieve this goal. When an imbalance in the flexion and extension gaps is present, additional adjustments are required. Several possible basic scenarios[8] are detailed below and in Table 127-1:

1. If the knee is too tight in both flexion and extension, reducing the thickness of the tibial component may be sufficient to balance the knee.
2. If the knee is tight in flexion but acceptable in extension, there are two options:
   a. Check the sagittal position of the femoral component. If it is positioned too posteriorly, consider using an offset femoral stem extension. This will move the femoral component more anteriorly. Be careful to avoid overstuffing the patellofemoral joint, because this will adversely affect motion and patellofemoral tracking.
   b. Downsize the femoral component.
3. If the knee is tight in flexion and loose in extension, consider the following three options:
   a. Check the sagittal position of the femoral component as in point 2, and consider using a thicker tibial component.

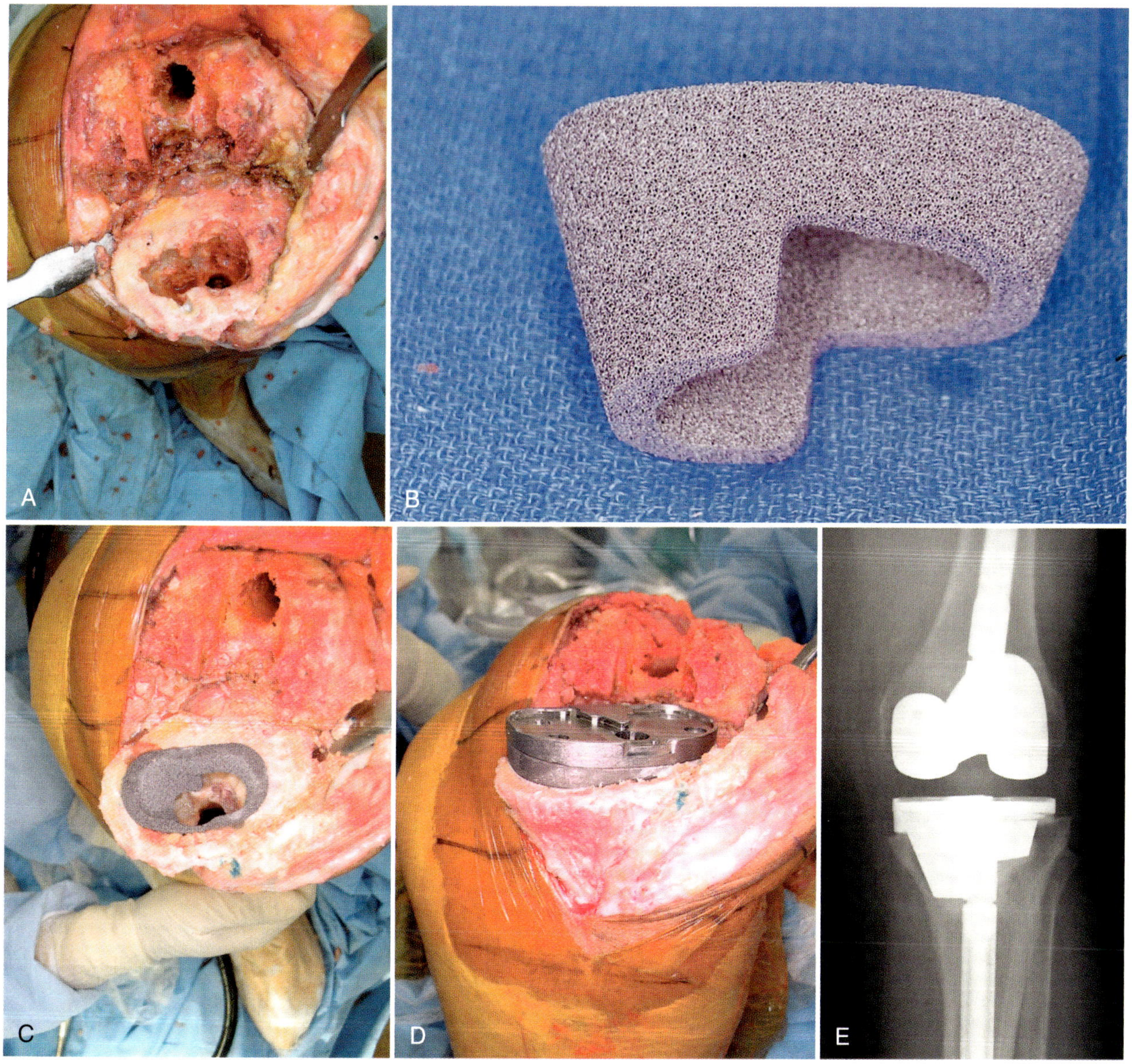

Figure 127-12. A trabecular metal cone is used to manage severe bone loss of the proximal tibia in revision total knee arthroplasty.

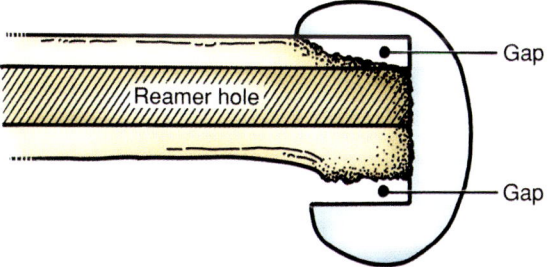

Figure 127-13. The revision femoral component must be sized from measurements of the opposite knee or estimated from the removed components. Typically, gaps will be noted anteriorly and posteriorly.

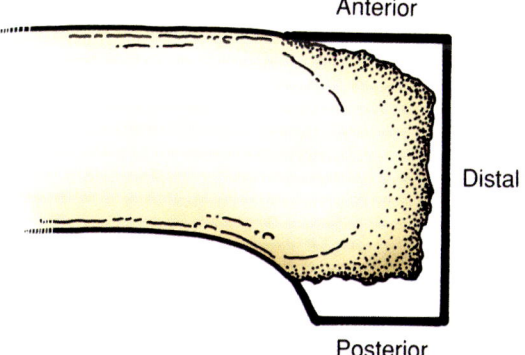

Figure 127-14. Typical bone loss after removal of a femoral component. Distal, anterior, and posterior bone deficiencies are illustrated.

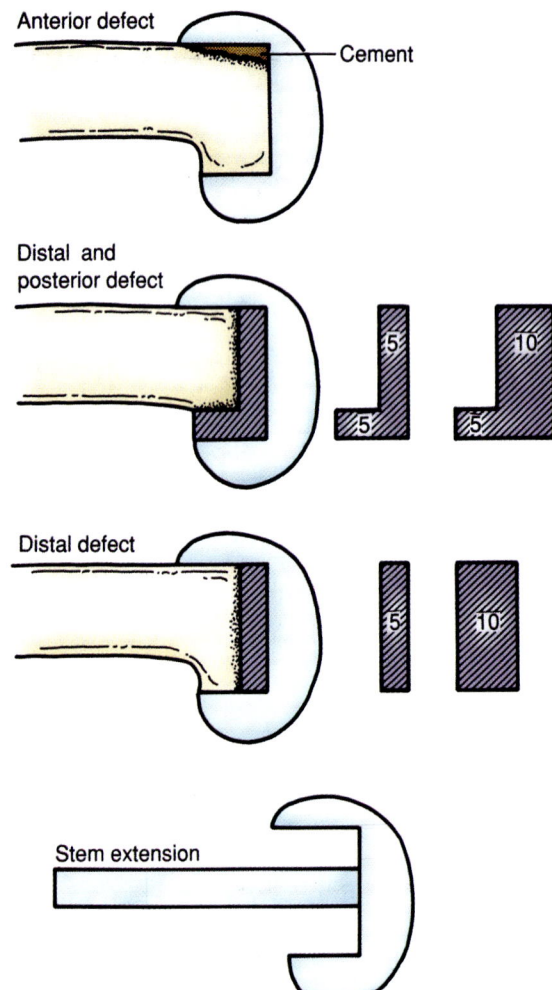

Figure 127-15. Augmentation of the distal end of the femur. The revision femoral component should have a stem extension; usually, both distal and posterior augments are required, although the amount of augmentation at each site may differ. Thus, 5 mm may be sufficient posteriorly, although distal augmentation of 10 mm could be required. This can be judged by considering the spacers needed in flexion and extension and the amount of distal augmentation necessary to restore the joint line.

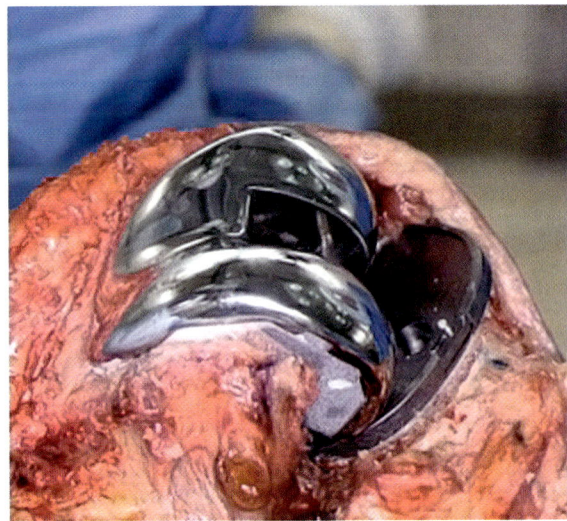

Figure 127-16. Final revision components demonstrating distal and femoral augmentation to restore the joint line and fill the flexion gap.

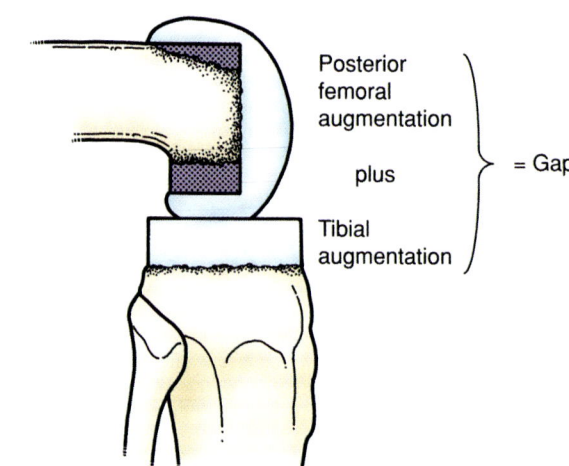

Figure 127-17. During reconstruction, the flexion gap is restored by a combination of posterior femoral and tibial augmentation.

b. Downsize the femoral component, and use a thicker tibial component.

c. If the femoral component is the correct size, increase the distal femoral augmentation until the extension gap is equal to the flexion gap. A thinner tibial component may be required to balance the knee. Be careful to not move the joint line too far distally, because this will adversely affect patellar tracking.

4. If the knee is acceptable in flexion but tight in extension, there are two options:

a. Reduce the distal femoral augmentation or resect more distal femoral bone. This will move the femoral component more proximally and increase the extension space.

b. If a preoperative flexion contracture is present, release the posterior capsule, preferably from the femur.

5. If flexion and extension gaps are equal, no further adjustments are necessary.

6. If the knee is acceptable in flexion and loose in extension, the solution is to augment the distal end of the femur so that the extension gap requires the same amount of tibial polyethylene as the flexion gap.

7. The most common problem is that the flexion space is larger than the extension space. If the knee is loose in flexion and tight in extension, the solution is to go through a series of checks and adjustments.

a. Check the sagittal position of the femoral component. If it is positioned too anteriorly, consider using an offset femoral stem extension. This will move the femoral component more posteriorly and reduce the flexion space.

b. Check the distal position of the femoral component. Consider reducing the distal augmentation or resecting more distal femoral bone.

c. Check the femoral component size. If it appears to be too small, consider choosing the next larger size, but be careful to not oversize the femur.

Table 127-1 Nine-Point Grid for Balancing Flexion and Extension Gaps in Revision Total Knee Arthroplasty

		EXTENSION SPACE		
		Tight	**OK**	**Loose**
FLEXION SPACE	**Tight**	• Reduce the thickness of the tibial insert. • Remove symmetrical tibial augments if present.	• Downsize the femoral component. • Use an offset stem to adjust the sagittal position of the femoral component more anteriorly.	• Add distal femoral augmentation. • Downsize the femoral component and use a thicker insert. • If possible, use an offset stem to adjust the sagittal position of the femoral component more anteriorly, and use a thicker tibial insert.

	OK	• Mild flexion contracture:
		  • Subperiosteal posterior capsule release
		• Severe contracture:
		  • Reduce the distal femoral augmentation.
		   or
		  • Resect additional distal femur.
			• Balanced gaps	• Add additional distal femoral augmentation.

	Loose	• First, address the distal position of the femoral component:
		  • Remove distal augmentation.
		  • Resect additional distal femur.
		• Next, adjust the sagittal position of the femoral component. If possible, use an offset stem to move the component posteriorly.
		• If the femoral component is undersized, increase the size of the femoral component.
			• Adjust the sagittal position of the femoral component. If possible, use an offset stem to move the component posteriorly.
			• If the femoral component is undersized, increase the size of the femoral component.
				• Increase the thickness of the tibial insert.
				• Add symmetrical tibial augmentation.

d. If the previous maneuvers fail to balance the gaps, a constrained condylar knee (CCK) articulation may be needed.

e. Depending on the experience of the surgeon, collateral ligament advancement and reconstruction may be considered.

8. If the knee is loose in flexion and acceptable in extension, moving the femoral component proximally and using a thicker tibial component may solve the problem. If this does not balance the knee, the options in point 7 should be considered.

9. If the knee is symmetrically loose in flexion and extension, a thicker tibial component will solve the problem.

Management of Bone Loss

Bone loss is frequently encountered during revision arthroplasty. Even unicompartmental replacements can leave substantial asymmetrical bone deficiencies (Fig. 127-18). Osteolysis is often more expansive than anticipated. The keys to management of intraoperative bone loss are anticipation and preoperative preparation. At the time of revision, all materials for reconstruction, including wedges, blocks, allografts, metaphyseal cones, and special components, are available.

Bone defects have been classified in numerous ways.[16,27,59] They can be classified as contained, uncontained, or a combination (Figs. 127-19 and 127-20). Contained defects have an intact cortical rim, while uncontained defects involve segmental bone loss with no remaining cortex. Treatment for bone loss depends largely on two factors: (1) whether the defect is contained or uncontained, and (2) the size of the defect. Small (<5 mm) contained defects are easily managed with cement or morselized bone graft. Small uncontained defects often are not large enough to adversely affect

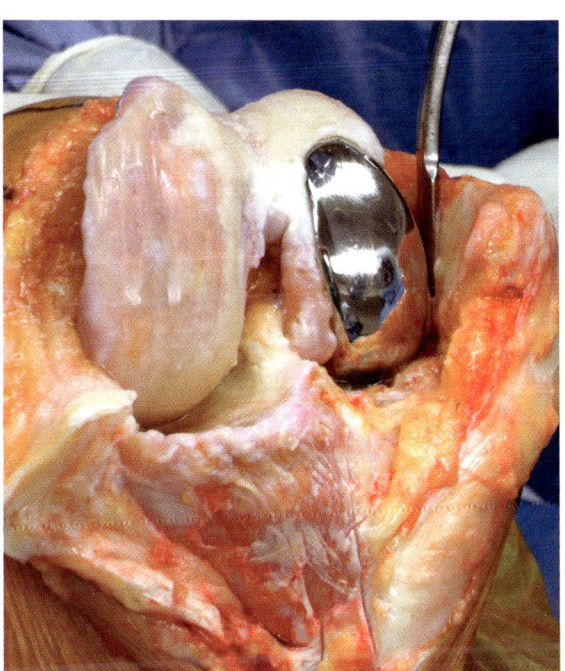

Figure 127-18. The most common reason for failure of unicondylar replacement is progressive arthritis of unreplaced compartments of the knee. Free or embedded particles of acrylic cement are frequently found.

component stability. They have been managed historically with cement and screws, but can be managed well with cement alone.[9] Large (>10 mm) contained cavitary defects can be managed with autogenous or allogenic bone graft. If the contained defect is large enough to compromise support of the implant, then impaction grafting, structural allograft,

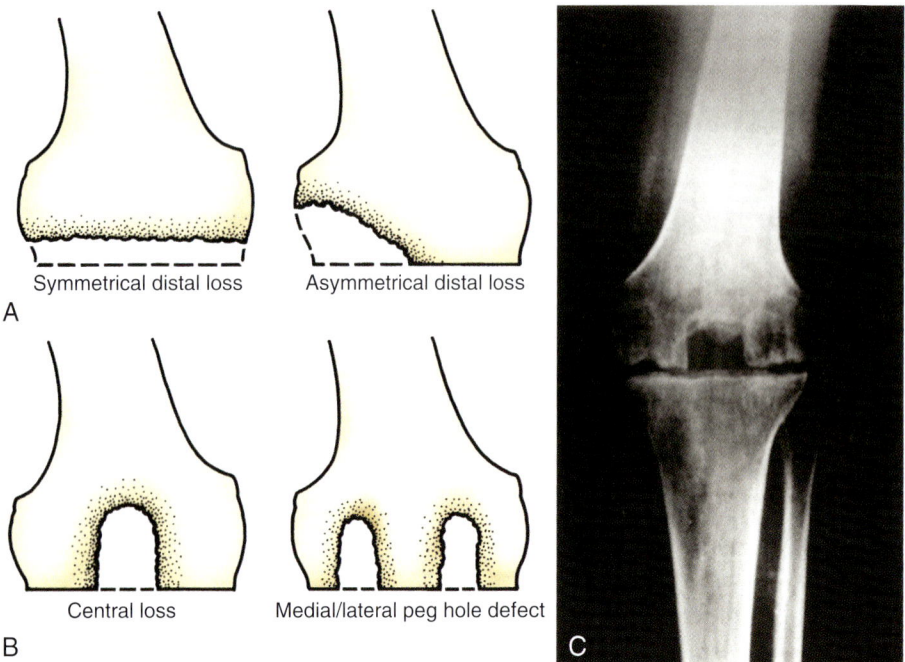

Figure 127-19. A, In the coronal plane, distal femoral bone loss may be symmetrical or asymmetrical. **B,** Contained defects may be created by central or peripheral fixation lugs. **C,** Radiograph shows defects left after removal of the prosthesis, with a central box on the femur and a central stem on the tibia. Note the good preservation of medial and lateral bone.

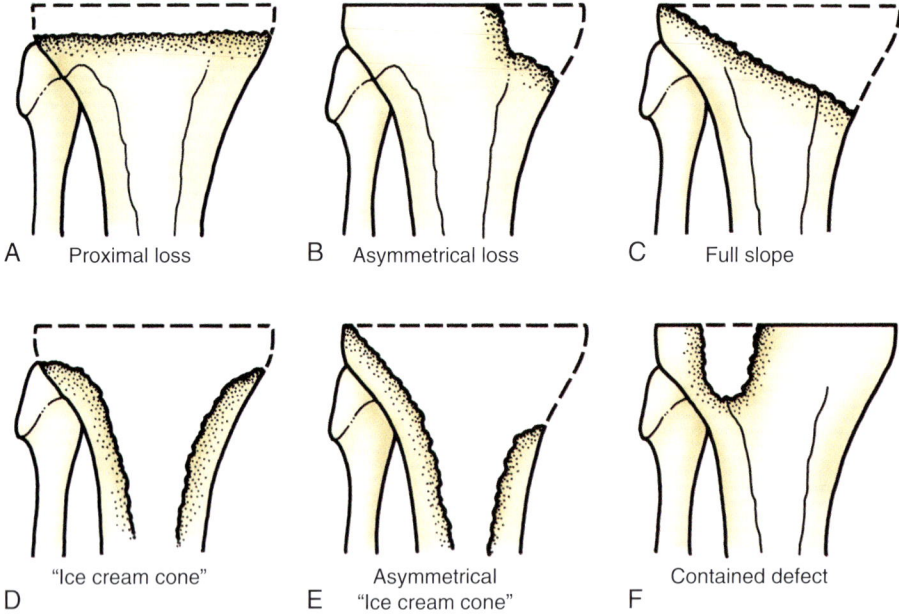

Figure 127-20. Patterns of tibial bone loss. **A,** Proximal loss. **B,** Asymmetrical loss. **C,** Full slope. **D,** "Ice cream cone." **E,** Asymmetrical "ice cream cone." **F,** Contained defect.

or metaphyseal cones should be considered.[56] Intermediate (5 to 10 mm) uncontained defects are managed well with modular wedges. Large uncontained defects often affect component stability and are best managed with modular augments, structural allograft, or metaphyseal filling cones.[56] The Anderson Orthopaedic Research Institute (AORI) classification scheme is useful and descriptive, and allows independent classification of the femoral and tibial sides.[59] Management

of the bone defect based on the AORI scheme is detailed in Figure 127-21.

Type 1 defects have healthy cancellous bone with an undamaged metaphyseal segment and no evidence of component subsidence or osteolysis. Type 1 defects most often are managed using cement or occasionally metal augments. Type 2 defects may or may not have a healthy cancellous bed of bone, the metaphyseal flare is shortened, and mild to

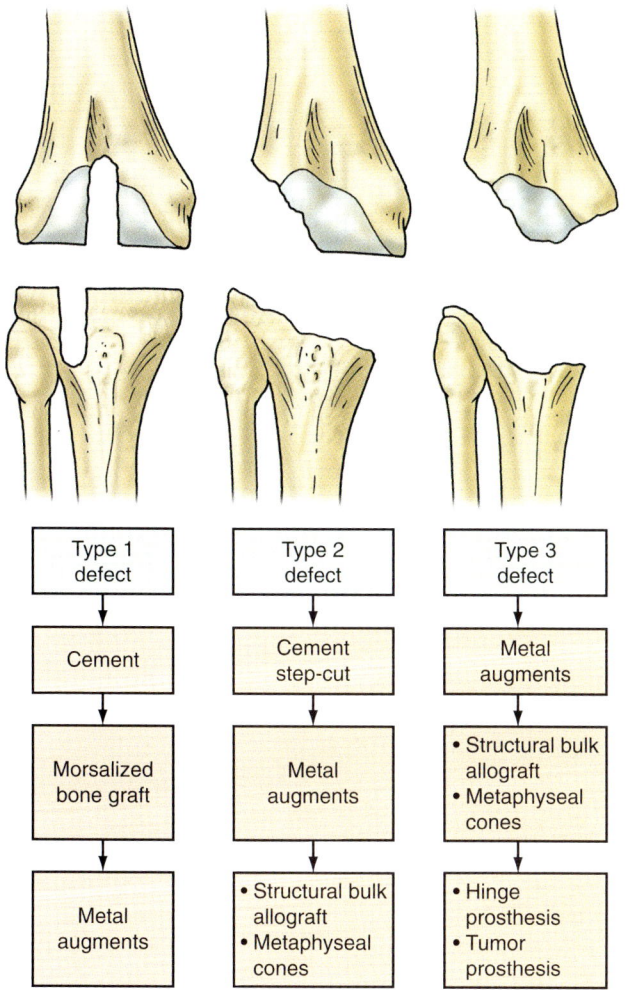

Type 1 defect	Type 2 defect	Type 3 defect
Cement	Cement step-cut	Metal augments
Morsalized bone graft	Metal augments	• Structural bulk allograft • Metaphyseal cones
Metal augments	• Structural bulk allograft • Metaphyseal cones	• Hinge prosthesis • Tumor prosthesis

Figure 127-21. Managing bone loss in revision in total knee arthroplasty.

moderate evidence of component subsidence and osteolysis is found. Type 2 defects are managed with cement, metal augments, or morselized and structural allograft, depending on intraoperative assessment. Typically, type 2 defects are ideal for modular metal augmentation.[28] Type 3 defects have a deficient metaphyseal segment at or above the levels of the epicondyles on the femur and at or below the level of the tubercle on the tibia. Considerable component subsidence and osteolysis are noted with type 3 defects. Type 3 defects typically are managed with metal augmentation, impaction grafting, structural allograft, and constrained condylar prostheses. Rarely, alternative components including allograft/prosthetic composite or a hinged prosthesis may be required, depending on the involvement of the epicondyles and the status of the collateral ligaments. In the AORI scheme, each type is subdivided into "A" for one condyle or one side of the tibial plateau involved, and "B" for bicondylar or total plateau involvement. The classification of bone loss should be performed intraoperatively after component removal.

Metal augmentation as part of modern modular revision systems is an effective and convenient modality to manage bone loss; however, it is not used without concern. Brooks and associates compared five different techniques in the treatment of wedge-shaped proximal tibial defects. They

concluded that a metal wedge was an acceptable alternative to a custom-made component for reconstruction of tibial bone stock defects.[9] Brand and colleagues[7] reported good results with use of a metal wedge for proximal tibial defects. In their series, 22 knees (20 patients) were monitored for an average of 37 months. No failures and no loosening of tibial components were reported. However, a 27% incidence of nonprogressive radiolucent lines was described. None of these patients required revision surgery, and all but one patient was pain free. Although the literature currently does not support these concerns, with reported 84% to 98% good or excellent results, theoretical disadvantages include undersurface wear between the augment and the component and dissociation of the augments.[28]

The use of morselized allograft to manage bone loss remains a viable option and has several advantages. Advantages include biocompatibility, versatility, cost-effectiveness, and restoration of bone stock. However, some disadvantages are known, including graft availability, late resorption, infection, and risk of disease transmission.[7] An absolute contraindication to allograft is infection; relative contraindications include immunosuppression, metabolic bone disorders, neuropathic arthropathy, and a deficient extensor mechanism. The use of allograft to manage bony defects has had some encouraging results for small and large defects. Whiteside[70] used morselized allograft for localized areas of bone defects in 56 cementless revisions. All 56 knees demonstrated increased density in the grafted zone. For larger defects, Wilde and coworkers[72] reported their results on 12 knees. Five of the knees had contained defects and seven had an uncontained defect; all were treated with structural allograft. Radiographs demonstrated complete incorporation of the graft in 11 of 12 knees at an average of 23 months after surgery. Single-photon emission computed tomography scans showed uniform activity in the area of the graft in four of the five knees that were studied.

For more extensive bone loss, including AORI type 2B and three bone defects, structural allografts, impaction grafting, and metallic prosthetic augments are frequently utilized. Structural allografts, which have been used for decades in revision TKA, allow the surgeon to create intraoperatively constructs of any size or shape to fill the defect. These provide excellent initial support for the revision implant and, with biologic integration with host bone, will provide long-term support and will restore bone stock for future revision arthroplasty. Specific disadvantages of structural allografts include prolonged operative time required to shape the graft, limited availability of large allografts, nonunion, delayed union, graft resorption or collapse, and graft infection or disease transmission.[11] Dennis and associates[15] reported encouraging early clinical results and a high allograft/host union rate with use of structural allograft composite in revision knee arthroplasty. Unfortunately, midterm follow-up is not as promising. A recent study of 70 allografts demonstrated revision-free survival of 80% and 75% at 5 and 10 years, respectively.[4] Allograft failures (8 of 16) and infection (5 of 16) were responsible for 13 of 16 revisions during the follow-up period.

Impaction grafting is well established in revision total hip arthroplasty. Theoretically, impaction of morselized graft allows more rapid and complete revascularization compared with large structural allograft. Based on success in revision hip arthroplasty, surgeons have used impaction grafting to manage contained and uncontained defects in revision knee arthroplasty.[43] Although impaction grafting alone can be utilized in contained defects, uncontained defects usually require wire mesh to contain the graft. Advantages of impaction grafting include cost-effectiveness, restoration of bone stock, and the ability to accommodate defects of varying shapes and sizes. Disadvantages include technical difficulty, graft resorption, intraoperative fracture, disease transmission, and prolonged operative time spent fashioning mesh and impacting graft. Lotke and colleagues[43] reported no mechanical failures with impaction grafting in 42 patients with 2- to 7-year (average, 3.8-year) follow-up. Two infections and two late periprosthetic fractures were reported. All radiographs demonstrated incorporation and remodeling of the bone graft. Because of these encouraging results, the authors continue to use impaction grafting as their procedure of choice for managing large bone defects in revision knee arthroplasty.

More severe type 2 and most type 3 defects typically require more support than is offered by traditional wedge or block augments. Porous metaphyseal filling cone augments not only have the potential for long-term biologic fixation but can be utilized to fill large defects and to provide additional structural support without some of the concerns associated with structural allograft[1] (see Fig. 127-20). Modularity of cone augments allows accommodation for defects of various shapes and sizes without the added time and complexity associated with impaction grafting or shaping of structural allografts. In addition, issues of graft resorption, disease transmission, and graft fracture or failure are avoided. Early reports demonstrate excellent short-term follow-up with evidence of osseointegration and no mechanical failure in a combined 25 patients with 12- to 47-month follow-up.[46,56] Long and Scuderi[42] reported the results of 16 revision TKAs with tibial cones used to manage severe type 2 and 3 tibial bone defects. With minimum and average follow-up of 24 and 31 months, respectively, no mechanical failures occurred, and all radiographs demonstrated stable osseointegration into the cones. Larger studies with longer follow-up are needed, but these augments appear to provide a viable alternative to structural allograft and impaction grafting.

MANAGEMENT OF THE PATELLA

After insertion of the trial components for a final check, patellar tracking is assessed. Lateral patellar release and balancing may be necessary, but proper femoral and tibial component rotation should be confirmed before it is assumed that a release is necessary. If augments have been chosen appropriately and the joint line restored, the patellar position will be in the "neutral zone." If the patella is out of the "neutral zone," then alteration or redistribution of the augments may be necessary (Fig. 127-22). Awareness of preoperative patellar position is essential. If patella baja was present preoperatively secondary to patellar tendon shortening, the patellar position will be difficult to alter. Here, patella baja may have to be accepted. Occasionally, patella baja is so severe that the patellar component articulates with the tibial insert. Attempts to lengthen the patellar tendon or to advance the tubercle should be avoided. One alternative is to remove the patellar prosthesis and reduce the size of the remaining patellar bone.[8]

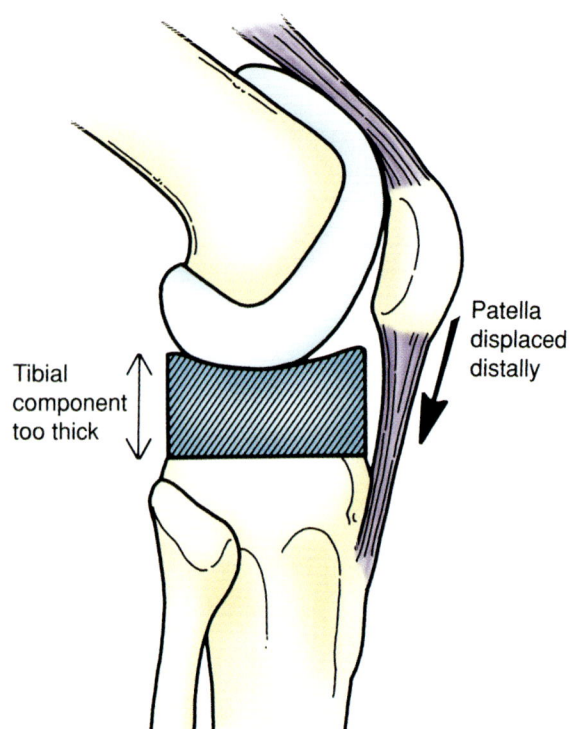

Figure 127-22. If an extra-thick tibial component is needed to stabilize the knee, the patella is displaced distally, thereby causing patella infra. Undersizing of the femoral component in the sagittal plane and anterior malpositioning are possible causes. Excessive distal resection of the femur in which the joint line is moved proximally is another cause.

Frequently, the patellar component is retained during revision arthroplasty.[28] If the patellar component is well fixed, compatible with the design of the prosthesis to be reimplanted, and tracks well, it may remain in place.[3,28] If the patellar component necessitates removal, the decision to implant a new prosthetic patella component depends on the patellar position and the remaining bone stock. In most cases, a new three-peg cemented component can be implanted. Consider omitting the patellar prosthesis when the patellar bone is insufficient (<12 mm thick), or when the remaining bone quality is extremely poor. Trim the remaining patellar bone with an oscillating saw while performing a *patelloplasty*; this will allow the patella to fit well in the femoral sulcus.[8]

If the remaining patellar bone stock is insufficient for placement of a patellar component, aside from patelloplasty, alternative reconstruction options exist. Hanssen[30] described packing bone graft in the remaining patellar shell, which then is covered with a local soft tissue sleeve. This technique appears to result in bone graft remodeling, appropriate patellar tracking, and restoration of patellar bone stock. Trabecular metal augments are also available (Fig. 127-23). If a remaining shell of bone is present, these augments may be sutured in place and can support a cemented patellar component.[50]

Use of Stem Extensions

Stem extensions are almost universally utilized in revision arthroplasty. Femoral and tibial bone quality is compromised to a variable degree, and stems act to offload and reduce

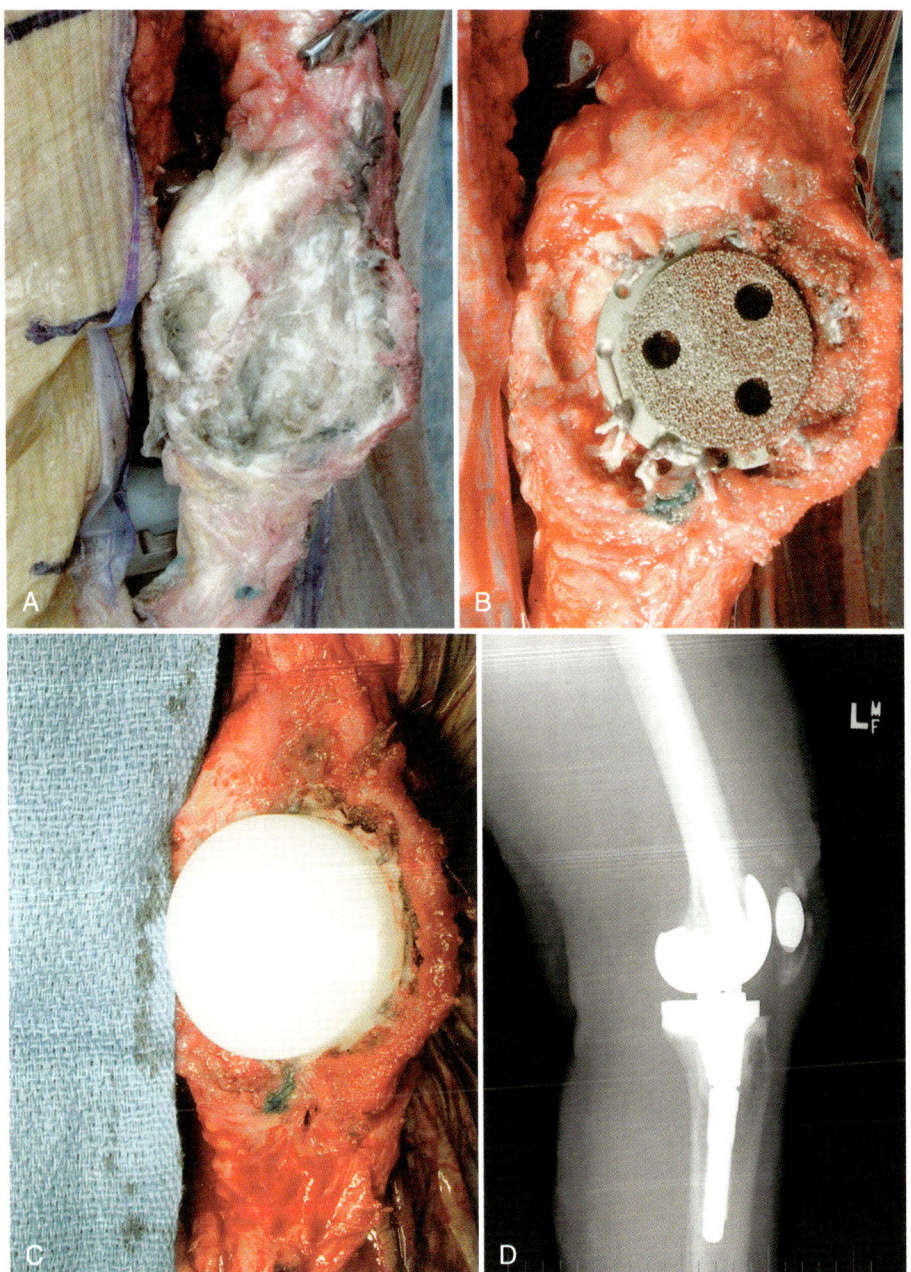

Figure 127-23. A trabecular metal patella is used to reconstruct the patellar component when only a shell of patellar bone remains.

interface stresses. Offset stems are also helpful because they can better align the implant on the metaphysis (Fig. 127-24). Debate continues regarding the use of uncemented compared with cemented stems. Short-stem extensions (25 to 30 mm), which do not engage the diaphysis, should be cemented. Similarly, long and narrow-diameter stems, which are not canal filling, should be cemented. Fehring and colleagues[19] reviewed 202 metaphyseal-engaging stems in 113 revision TKAs and demonstrated an advantage of cementing metaphyseal-engaging stems. However, longer modular stem extensions, which are canal filling and diaphyseal engaging, can be used in a tight press-fit manner. Wood and coworkers[74] published their results of 135 revision TKAs performed using a press-fit technique (press-fit diaphyseal fixation and cemented metaphyseal fixation). Kaplan-Meier survivorship analysis at 12 years revealed a 98% probability of survival free of revision for aseptic loosening. This involves cementing the core prosthesis and inserting diaphyseal-engaging stem extensions in a tight press-fit manner, allowing establishment of limb alignment, offloading interface stresses, and easier removal, while long-term fixation is attained by cementing the core prosthesis.

Constraint in Revision Arthroplasty

It is most desirable to utilize the least amount of constraint necessary (Fig. 127-25).[62] This will minimize forces on bone/cement/prosthesis interfaces and theoretically will minimize the rate of aseptic loosening. Therefore, in most revisions, a posterior stabilized articulation is used.

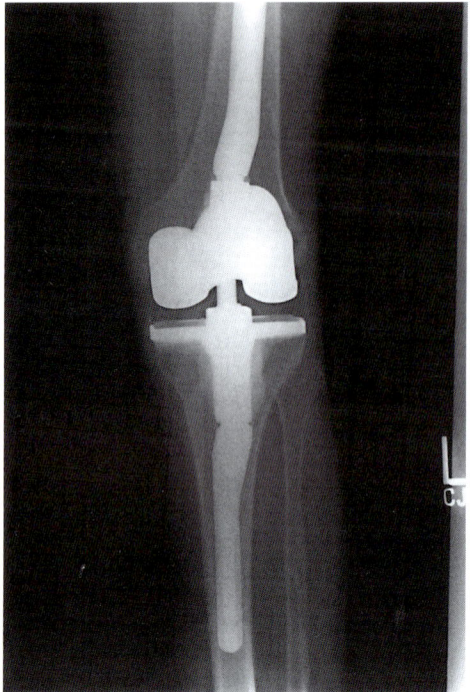

Figure 127-24. Offset stem extensions in revision arthroplasty.

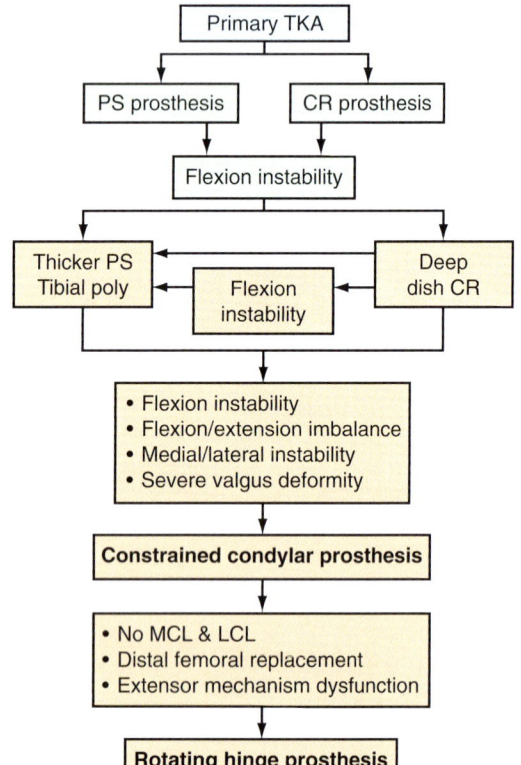

Figure 127-25. Constraint in revision total knee arthroplasty.

When additional constraint is needed over a posterior stabilized prosthesis, a nonlinked CCK design is used. Concern over accelerated component loosening and wear related to increased constraint has not been supported by the available literature. Font-Rodriguez and associates[21] reported

a 7-year survivorship of 98% in a cohort of 64 knees. Similarly, Trousdale and colleagues[68] reported 80% survivorship at 15.3 years following revision TKA in 20 patients using an earlier design of the CCK. Although every effort is made to minimize constraint during revision TKA, when necessary, a nonlinked CCK design can be used with apparently little detriment to long-term survival.

At times, even a constrained implant will not provide adequate stability. In these cases, a hinged implant should be kept available during revision surgery. Hinged implants are indicated in patients with global instability, a deficient extensor mechanism, or severe bone loss after fracture or during tumor reconstruction.[62]

Final Preparation

The bone surfaces are cleaned with pulsatile lavage. Note that in most revision cases, even with considerable bone loss, the margins of the defect will consist of sclerotic bone or irregular contours. This bone is the strongest available and should not be removed or drilled, and no attempt should be made to obtain a cancellous surface. Even when this is possible, the quality of the bone may be poor and inadequate for providing proper prosthetic support.

The final components are assembled, selected modular augments and wedges are fixed with screws or cement according to the designer's intention, and intramedullary stems are attached. It is recommended that these stems be 1 mm larger than stems used for the trial reduction to get the firmest possible fit.

Cementing

Cementing the interface and the core prosthesis ensures that the prosthesis will fit perfectly on the inherently irregular surface. Cement serves to level the bone ends and causes even loading beneath the prosthesis. Implant fixation is provided by the shape of the component and the press-fit intramedullary stems. If metaphyseal cones are utilized, they are impacted prior to cementation. The interface of the cone is grafted and protected from cement extrusion.

Two batches of cement are utilized for each component during standard revision TKA. Commercially prepared antibiotic-impregnated cement is utilized. Alternatively, 1 g of tobramycin powder may be added per bag of cement. With high-viscosity cement in the "doughy" phase, the surface of the tibia and the undersurface of the core tibial prosthesis are coated. Handling the cement in the "doughy" phase allows easy cement manipulation and avoids leakage of the cement into the intramedullary canal. Coating the surface of the bone and the implant produces a cement/cement interface during the curing process. Cement is prevented from entering the tibial canal. The component is gradually impacted into place. Excess cement is removed periodically to allow excellent visualization to ensure proper component rotation and depth. The rotational position of the trial tibial component is marked with methylene blue to serve as a reference during impaction of the final component.

Cement for the femoral side is then mixed. If the final femoral component is going to "float" on cement, it may be useful to mark the desired position of the anterior flange with the trial components in place. This will serve as a reference during impaction of the final femoral component. Cement is applied again to the surface of the distal femur and the underside of the core prosthesis in a "doughy" condition. The prosthesis is inserted and is gently impacted into the bone. Cement is prevented from entering the femoral canal. Excess cement is removed.

A clean laparotomy sponge is placed in the joint space between the final implants. The knee is extended, and attention is turned to the patella. The patellar component, when used, is cemented and held in place with a clamp until the cement is cured.

Once the cement is cured, the tourniquet is let down. Meticulous hemostasis is obtained. The previously selected tibial insert is trialed. The knee should be able to reach full extension. Varus/valgus stability is checked at full extension and throughout the arc of motion. Patellar tracking is reassessed. Flexion stability is checked at 90 degrees of flexion with the patella reduced by applying an anterior and posterior draw. If the surgeon is satisfied with the thickness of the trial insert, the knee is copiously irrigated and the final insert is impacted into place. Minor adjustments to the thickness of the tibial insert can be made at this time if necessary.

Aftercare

Aftercare for revision surgery does not differ from that indicated for primary cases, except with extensive bone grafting, which would require some protection in weight bearing. Even with the use of a quadriceps snip or a tibial tubercle osteotomy, we still progress with range-of-motion and strengthening exercises. If any question arises regarding fixation of the tibial tubercle osteotomy, motion and quadriceps exercises are limited for 6 to 8 weeks, or until the osteotomy is healed.

RESULTS OF REVISION SURGERY

Historical Results

Techniques for revision arthroplasty continue to evolve. A majority of available long-term results involve cases in which techniques were used that are not applicable today. As customized implants, metal augments, wedges, stems, and allograft techniques are refined, long-term results should continue to improve.

Bertin and associates[5] were the first to report results of revision TKA with the use of uncemented stems. A total of 24 revision arthroplasties performed using the Imperial College of London Hospital (ICLH) prosthesis with a mean follow-up of 18 months showed no radiographic evidence of subsidence or failure and 91% satisfactory relief of preoperative pain. These results, if anything, were better than those reported with primary arthroplasty. This experience led Freeman (personal communication) to use similar stems for all of his replacements.

The Hospital for Special Surgery published results using custom implants, augments, wedges, and stems.[69] This group reported an infection rate of 5% and an overall mechanical loosening rate of 3%. It is interesting to note that all mechanical failures occurred in knees reconstructed with short, cemented stems, and no knees reconstructed with long uncemented stems loosened. Of the noncemented stems, 96% showed a sclerotic halo around the stem and, in most cases,

cortical reaction at the distal tip of the stem. This study highlighted the difficulty of accurate preoperative templating based on radiographs. Problems of sizing and fit occurred intraoperatively with the custom prosthesis. This, in part, led to the newer concept of modular design.

In 1982, Insall and Dethmers[34] reported 89% good to excellent results in 72 cemented revision TKAs with a minimum of 2 years of follow-up. This was the earliest report in which results of revision arthroplasty approached those of primary arthroplasty. Fewer excellent and more good results were described than in a primary arthroplasty series. Compared with primary knee arthroplasty, the authors noted a much higher incidence of radiolucent lines and a greater number of postoperative extensor mechanism problems. The short follow-up and high incidence of radiolucent lines were matters of concern regarding the longevity of the revision arthroplasties.

Goldberg and colleagues[26] reported the results of 65 consecutive revision TKAs performed for mechanical failure. The types of implants used included total condylar, posterior stabilized, total condylar III, and a kinematic rotating-hinge prosthesis. In this series, 46% of the knees were considered excellent or good, and 42% were poor or failures. The infection rate was 4.5%, and multiple revisions did poorly.

Jacobs and coworkers reviewed 24 patients with 28 failed TKAs replaced with porous-coated anatomic components.[35] Good and excellent results were achieved in 68%, along with three failures. Patients who underwent revision operations for severe pain or who had no clearly definable problem were not improved. Friedman and coworkers[22] presented the results of 137 revision total knees at the Brigham and Women's Hospital in Boston. Function instability, motion, and pain all improved after revision, but improvements were significantly less than those seen after primary total knee replacement. A third of the patients still walked with crutches, with a walker, or not at all. Loosening was the most common reason for failure. The clinical success rate was 63% for a single revision, and the failure rate at 5 years was 5.8%.

Contemporary Results With Uncemented Stems

The results of our own experience with CCK components and uncemented stems have been examined.[28] A total of 68 revision operations were reported, and follow-up ranged from 2 to 10 years. Excellent and good results were obtained in 56 knees, with 11 poor results. Further revision was performed on six knees, all because of infection. A posterior stabilized tibial insert was used in 49 knees, 43 (88%) of which achieved excellent and good results, with 4 additional revisions. The CCK tibial insert was needed to give greater stability in 18 knees, and 13 (72%) knees were rated excellent and good, with 2 additional revisions. The overall infection rate was high (9%), which confirms the wisdom of avoiding intramedullary cement. Survivorship analysis of this group of patients was calculated to be 80% at 10 years—a figure less satisfactory than in a similar analysis performed on total condylar and posterior stabilized prostheses (90% and 94%, respectively). Thus, even with so-called modern techniques, the results of revision surgery are understandably less satisfactory than those of primary arthroplasty.

In 2002, Gofton and associates[24] reported results utilizing uncemented stem fixation for 89 revisions. With an average of 5.9 years (range, 4.1 to 8.6 years) of follow-up, they demonstrated a Kaplan-Meier survivorship of 93.5% at 8.6 years. Four poor outcomes were reported, and five patients required subsequent revision for aseptic loosening (two), infection (one), arthrofibrosis (one), and instability (one).

In 2005, Peters and colleagues[53] reported on 50 consecutive revisions in 47 patients with uncemented stems. At an average of 36 months (range, 24 to 96 months) of follow-up, 88% good to excellent results were described. No patients demonstrated aseptic loosening. One patient had a poor outcome requiring an above-knee amputation for diabetic ulcers. Four patients (9%) developed deep infection, again highlighting the advantage of easier component removal with uncemented rather than cemented stem extensions.

As previously mentioned, Wood and coworkers[74] published results on 135 revisions with uncemented stems. Minimum follow-up was 2 years (mean, 5 years; range, 2 to 12 years). A total of 36 knees in 31 patients were lost to follow-up because of patient death. Of the remaining patients, six required subsequent revision for infection (two), instability secondary to MCL rupture (two), and aseptic loosening (two). Kaplan-Meier survivorship free of re-revision was 87% at 12 years. Kaplan-Meier survivorship free of re-revision or radiographic loosening was 82% at 12 years. It is impressive that Kaplan-Meier survivorship with aseptic loosening as an indication for re-revision was 98% at 12 years.

The point made by Jacobs and associates[35] about poor results of revision surgery performed for pain, without clear definition of the reason, is well taken and cannot be overemphasized. Our own experience confirms this, although we understand how difficult it is to manage a patient with a painful arthroplasty. The temptation to "give it a go" is sometimes irresistible, but the result most likely will be failure.

CUSTOM COMPONENTS

Since the introduction of modularity, custom components have a limited role in revision knee arthroplasty. A custom prosthesis can be considered if one of the following conditions prevails:

1. The bone is so oversized or undersized that standard components will not fit.
2. Stems are needed to enhance fixation, but bone shapes preclude the use of standard devices (e.g., when a fracture malunion occurs adjacent to the prosthesis [Fig. 127-26] or an offset stem is needed because of peculiarities in intramedullary alignment [Fig. 127-27]; shorter modular stem extensions and offset stems also provide a solution to this problem [Fig. 127-28]).
3. The size or location of bone loss cannot be accommodated by standard augments.

Otherwise, custom components should be avoided for the following reasons:

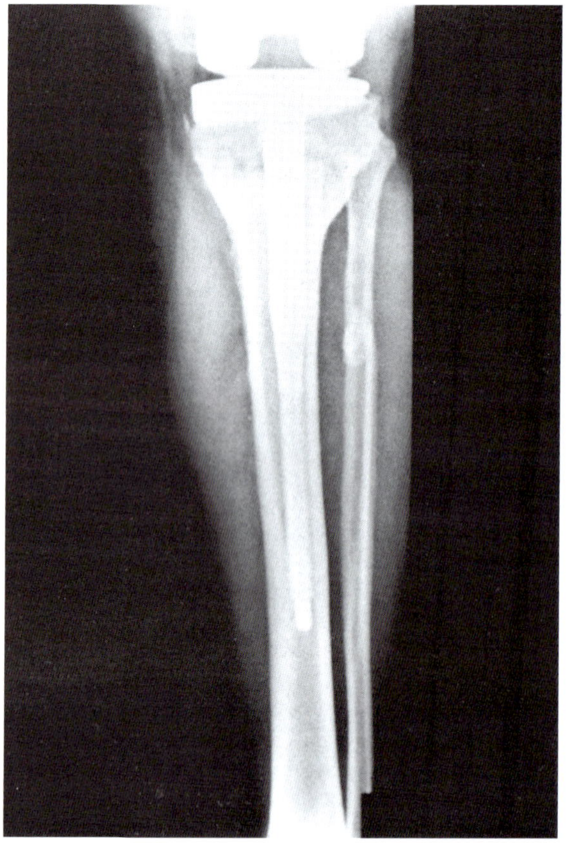

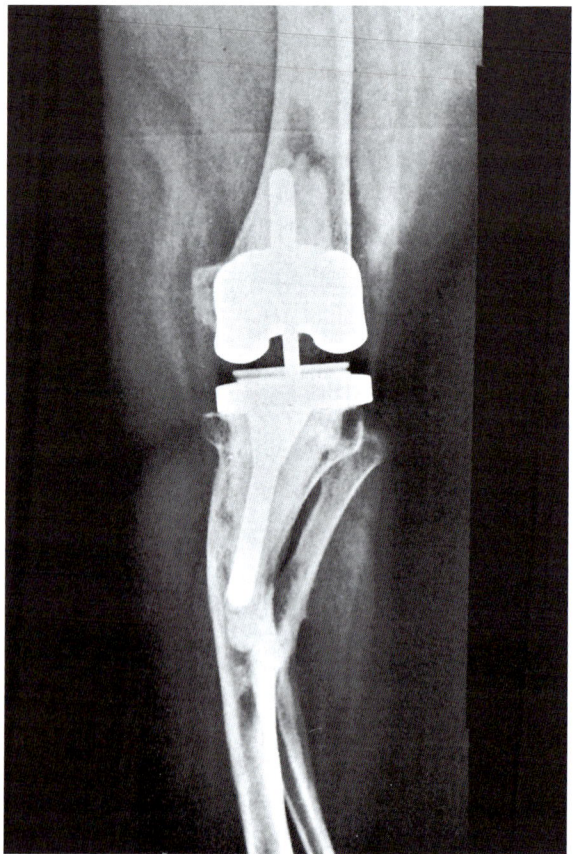

Figure 127-26. A long-stemmed tibial component is used during reconstruction following nonunion of an upper tibial osteotomy.

Figure 127-27. Severe proximal tibia deformity precludes the use of standard stems for tibial reconstruction. A custom, angulated tibial stem is used to eliminate the need for a corrective tibial osteotomy.

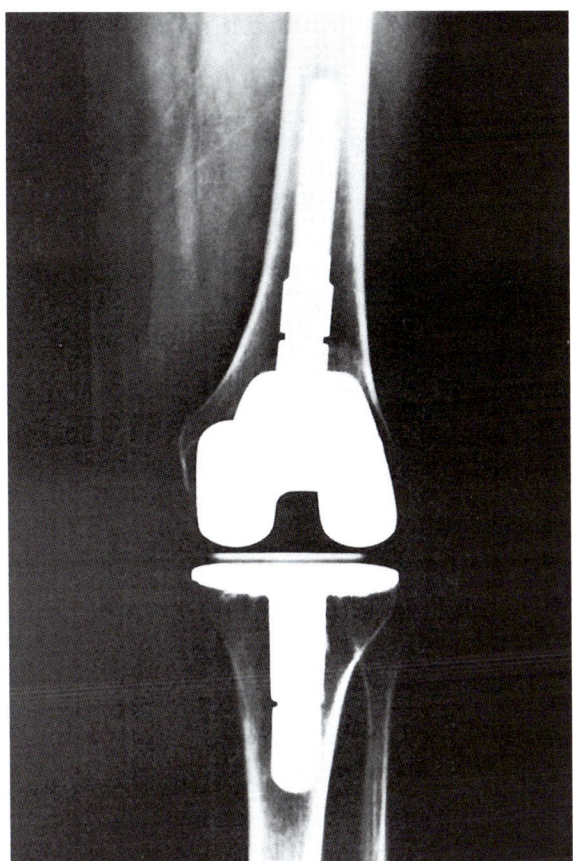

Figure 127-28. Radiograph of a "stubby" stem extension on the tibial component. The "stubby" stem impinges against the lateral cortex of the tibia. If a longer stem extension had been used, the tibial component would have tilted into valgus. Alternatively, the whole component could be medialized, but this would result in medial overhang of the prosthesis. In this case, an offset stem is required.

1. No instruments have been designed for implanting custom components.
2. Use of a custom component does not provide sizing options intraoperatively.

Generally, the high degree of modularity available with today's knee systems has obviated what little need there is for custom components.

SUMMARY

Revision TKA is not straightforward and is not technically easy. Instruments and guides are not as useful as they are for primary surgery. The surgeon needs to develop a good understanding of the principles of revision arthroplasty, and thorough preoperative planning is necessary. Even in the hands of experienced, well-prepared surgeons, complications and failures may occur.

Suarez and colleagues[65] asked the question, "Why do revision knee arthroplasties fail?" In their retrospective review of 566 revision knee arthroplasties, 12% failed at an average of 40.1 months. Predominant reasons for failure included infection (46%), aseptic loosening (19%), and instability (13%). Knees revised for infection had a fourfold higher re-revision rate (21%) compared with those revised for aseptic loosening (4.3%).

Use of a systematic approach to revision TKA can minimize failure. The surgeon must identify the reason for implant failure, rule out infection, and develop a preoperative plan. Optimal exposure, meticulous management of soft tissues, and knowledge of the techniques are essential. Minimizing bone loss, managing bone defects, and reconstructing the gaps while balancing soft tissues are the critical steps. Finally, adequate fixation is attained and the appropriate amount of constraint is utilized. Adhering to these steps will help the clinician to achieve a well-aligned limb with a stable and securely fixed implant that allows restoration of function.

KEY REFERENCES

Brassard MF, Insall JN, Scuderi GR: Revision of aseptic failed total knee arthroplasty. In Scott WN editor: Surgery of the knee, ed 4, Philadelphia, 2006, Churchill Livingstone Elsevier, 1761–1781.

Dennis DA: Evaluation of the painful total knee arthroplasty. J Arthroplasty 19(4 Suppl 1):35–40, 2004.

Engh GA, Ammeen DJ: Periprosthetic fractures adjacent to total knee implants: treatment and clinical results. Instr Course Lect 47:437–448, 1998.

Fehring TK, McAvoy G: Fluoroscopic evaluation of the painful total knee arthroplasty. Clin Orthop Relat Res 331:226–233, 1996.

Fehring TK, Odum S, Olekson C, et al: Stem fixation in revision total knee arthroplasty: a comparative analysis. Clin Orthop Relat Res 416:217–224, 2003.

Haas SB, Insall JN, Montgomery W III, Windsor RE: Revision total knee arthroplasty with use of modular components with stems inserted without cement. J Bone Joint Surg Am 77:1700–1707, 1995.

Haidukewych GJ, Jacofsky DJ, Pagnano MW, Trousdale RT: Functional results after revision of well-fixed components for stiffness after primary total knee arthroplasty. J Arthroplasty 20:133–138, 2005.

Hanssen AD, Rand JD: Evaluation and treatment of infection at the site of a total hip or knee arthroplasty. Instr Course Lect 48:111–122, 1999.

Hanssen AH, Pagnano MW: Revision of failed patellar components. Instr Course Lect 53:201–206, 2004.

Long WJ, Scuderi GR: Porous tantalum cones for large metaphyseal tibial defects in revision total knee arthroplasty: a minimum 2 year follow-up. J Arthroplasty 24:1086–1092, 2009.

Lucey SD, Scuderi GR, Kelly MA, Insall JN: A practical approach to dealing with bone loss in revision total knee arthroplasty. Orthopedics 23:1036–1041, 2000.

Meneghini RM, Lewallen DG, Hanssen AD: Use of porous tantalum metaphyseal cones for severe tibial bone loss during revision total knee replacement. J Bone Joint Surg Am 90:78–84, 2008.

Mont MA, Serna FK, Krackow KA, et al: Exploration of radiographically normal total knee replacements for unexplained pain. Clin Orthop Relat Res 331:216–219, 1996.

Scuderi GR: Revision total knee arthroplasty: how much constraint is enough? Clin Orthop Relat Res 392:300–305, 2001.

Scuderi GR, Insall JN: Revision total knee arthroplasty with cemented fixation. Tech Orthop 7:96–105, 1993.

Whiteside LA, Ohl MD: Tibial tubercle osteotomy for exposure of the difficult total knee arthroplasty. Clin Orthop Relat Res 206:6–9, 1990.

Full references for this chapter can be found on www.expertconsult.com.

The Infected Total Knee Replacement

Erik P. Severson and Arlen D. Hanssen

Deep infection remains one of the most challenging complications following total knee replacement (TKR). The complexity and duration of treatment often impart dramatic physical, emotional, and financial costs for the patient and the treating physician(s).[98] As the incidence rate of primary TKR continues to accelerate, it has been suggested that the demand for primary TKR is expected to grow by 673% in the year 2030.[57] Although the incidence of deep infection after TKA remains relatively low, these workload projections suggest an associated increase in the number of infected knee arthroplasties requiring treatment.

In the face of an increasing prevalence of TKR, intensified efforts at infection prevention seem logical to reduce the overall burden of prosthetic joint infection (PJI). As an overview, prevention of PJI relies upon augmentation of the host response, optimization of the wound environment, and reduction of bacterial contamination in the preoperative, intraoperative, and postoperative time periods.[41] In addition to these prevention efforts, a thorough understanding of the principles of proper diagnosis and treatment of the infected TKR is essential. Diagnostic and treatment principles for an infected TKR are often complex and require an individualized approach because of the multitude of variables affecting the final treatment outcome. These variables include the type of offending microorganism, the attendant host comorbidities, and the severity of damage to the local soft tissues and bone, as well as the level of expertise of available medical care.

In general, treatment of periprosthetic knee infection has become more standardized over the past several decades, primarily in terms of the approach toward routine use of high-dose local antibiotics and appropriate delay prior to reimplantation. However, indications for reinsertion of a new prosthesis after treatment for infection have liberalized significantly, so that the likelihood of successful treatment outcome or cure remains remarkably similar to that reported by early investigators, who used much more rigid patient selection criteria.[50]

INCIDENCE, RISK FACTORS, AND PREVENTION

Although the incidence rates of infection following TKR appear to have fallen over the past several decades, the reported incidence varies in many studies. Much of this variability is inherent in the relatively small numbers of patients studied and in the differences in patient populations described in these reports. As a result, the expected incidence varies widely according to risk factors present in the patient population and the expertise of providers being studied. For example, in 69,663 Medicare patients undergoing elective TKA, the incidence of PJI within 2 years was 1.55%, whereas the incidence occurring between 2 and 10 years was an additional 0.46%.[59] In another report, with a different patient population, the rate of infected knee arthroplasties was 0.92%; in this study, urban nonteaching hospitals experienced the highest burden of infection (1.26%) compared with those in a rural setting (0.69%) and urban teaching hospitals (0.77%).[58] Thus, any study reporting on the incidence of deep infection following TKR requires extensive stratification of patient risk factors and comorbidities, and an adequate description of the setting in which the procedures were performed.

Many inherent patient risk factors are known to predispose toward postoperative deep infection. Host factors include a diagnosis of rheumatoid arthritis,[12,52,120] skin ulcers,[120] diabetes mellitus,[31,88] a history of malignancy,[7] obesity,[88] a history of smoking,[88] renal or liver transplantation,[103] HIV-positive status,[87,109] prior open knee surgery or periarticular fracture,[52] and prior septic arthritis or adjacent osteomyelitis.[53] It is incumbent on the physician to be cognizant of these risk factors and to incorporate adequate screening measures and efforts to identify these risk factors into a disciplined preoperative evaluation process that facilitates optimization of host variables when possible.

Every effort should be made to incorporate differences in surgical technique and treatment algorithms that minimize the effects of these risk factors. For example, patients on immunosuppressive therapy should be optimized by altering or stopping their medications in the perioperative time period. A recent review summarized current recommendations for perioperative management of the more common antirheumatoid medications (Table 128-1).[49] Other risk factors, potentially under the influence of the surgeon in the perioperative time period, that seem to predispose toward an increased incidence of deep infection include an increased international normalized ratio (INR) in the postoperative period,[74] hematoma requiring reoperation,[35] early wound healing complications,[7,36] recent intra-articular injection of corticosteroid,[85] and prolonged operative time.[7,89]

Proper use of antibiotic prophylaxis represents the single most effective method of reducing infection in total joint arthroplasty.[46] Optimization of the surgical environment with proper surgical protocols is beyond the scope of this chapter but is clearly under the influence of the surgeon and operating room personnel (Table 128-2).[41,78] Use of low-dose antibiotic-loaded bone cement (ABLC) represents an additional surgeon-directed prevention measure for reduction of infection in high-risk patients and in revision surgery.[52] Frequent irrigation, careful surgical technique, and excellent wound closure are important variables under the surgeon's control.

Hematogenous infection of TKR in the early postoperative period, or many years after prosthetic replacement, is often influenced by the surgeon through education efforts made with arthroplasty patients. The rate of bacteremia after invasive procedures appears highest with oral procedures, followed by genitourinary manipulation, and lowest in

Table 128-1 Perioperative Antirheumatoid Medication Recommendations

Medication	Important Drug Interactions	Comments
Corticosteroids	Corticosteroid use with fluoroquinolones increases the risk of tendon rupture. Antifungal agents and clarithromycin may increase levels of corticosteroids.	Perioperative use depends on the level of potential surgical stress.
Methotrexate	Methotrexate along with intravenous penicillins may lead to neutropenia.	Continue perioperatively for all procedures. Consider withholding 1 to 2 doses of methotrexate for patients with poorly controlled diabetes; the elderly; and those with liver, kidney, or lung disease who are undergoing moderate or intensive procedures.
Leflunomide	Leflunomide may elevate levels of warfarin and rifampin.	Continue for minor procedures. Withhold 1 to 2 days before moderate and intensive procedures, and restart 1 to 2 weeks later.
Sulfasalazine	May increase INR in patients on warfarin	Continue for all procedures.
Hydroxychloroquine	None	Continue for all procedures.
TNF antagonists	Avoid live vaccines in patients taking these agents; otherwise, no significant perioperative drug–drug interactions are known.	Continue for minor procedures. For moderate to intensive procedures, withhold etanercept for 1 week, and plan surgery for the end of the dosing interval for adalumimab and infliximab. Restart 10 to 14 days postoperatively.
IL-1 antagonist	None	Continue for minor procedures. Withhold 1 to 2 days before surgery and restart 10 days postoperatively for moderate to intensive procedures.

From Howe CR, Gardner GC, Kadel NJ: Perioperative medication management for the patient with rheumatoid arthritis. J Am Acad Orthop Surg 14:544–551, 2006.
IL, Interleukin; *INR*, international normalized ratio; *TNF*, tumor necrosis factor.

Table 128-2 Prevention of Deep Prosthetic Infection

	Preoperative Period	Operative Period	Postoperative Period
Host	Altered immune system Immunosuppressive medications Diabetes mellitus Rheumatoid arthritis Advanced age Malnutrition Anesthetic risk	Anesthetic agents Transfusions	Rheumatoid arthritis Altered immune system
Bacteria	Urinary tract infection Skin ulcers Poor dental hygiene Preoperative shaving Preoperative showers Prolonged hospitalization	Instrument sterilization Operating room traffic Personnel ("dispersers") Face masks/hoods Exhaust suits Laminar airflow Ultraviolet light Prophylactic antibiotics Antibiotic-impregnated PMMA Skin preparation Gloves Drapes/gowns Wound irrigants Sucker tips Splash basins	Antibiotic prophylaxis Urinary tract management Invasive procedures Remote sites of infection Clean dental procedures
Wound	Extensive scarring Prior surgery Prior infection Obesity Vascular disease Anatomic site Condition of skin	Duration of procedure Surgical technique Sutures Implant selection Antibiotic impregnated PMMA Bone graft Surgical drains Wound closure	Postoperative hematoma Wound drainage Skin necrosis Reoperation Loose prosthesis Particulate debris

From Morrey BF, An K-N: Joint replacement arthroplasty, Philadelphia, 2003, Churchill Livingstone, p 1192, with permission from Mayo Foundation for Medical Education and Research; Hanssen AD, Osmon DR, Nelson CL: Prevention of deep periprosthetic joint infection. Instr Course Lect 46:555–567, 1997.
PMMA, Polymethylmethacrylate cement.

association with gastrointestinal procedures.[29] In general, invasive procedures that potentially cause bacteremia should simply be avoided in the first 3 to 6 months after TKR. In a retrospective review of late infections, seven cases were strongly linked to a dental procedure.[115] Predisposing factors in these patients included risk factors such as rheumatoid arthritis or diabetes mellitus with dental procedure duration greater than 75 minutes.

The American Academy of Orthopaedic Surgeons (AAOS) no longer has published guidelines for the use of prophylactic antibiotics for high-risk patients undergoing a procedure considered at high risk for bacteremia. Rather, the AAOS has provided this information in the format of an information statement because of the position that evidence-based literature on this topic is insufficient to meet the criteria of an established guideline. Information included within this information statement, entitled "Antibiotic Prophylaxis for Bacteremia in Patients With Joint Replacements," can be obtained by request from the AAOS.

MICROBIOLOGY AND DIAGNOSIS

An appreciation of microbial pathophysiology is essential to the accurate diagnosis and subsequent treatment of infected TKR. As strange as it may seem, no criteria for the definitive diagnosis of PJI have attained universal agreement.[82] Although many authors have suggested that positive cultures are required to make the diagnosis, it is well recognized that some true prosthetic infections are culture negative. In one report of 897 episodes of PJI, 60 (7%) occurred in patients for whom this was the initial episode of culture-negative results.[9] The 5-year estimate of survival free of treatment failure was 94% for patients treated with two-stage exchange and 71% for patients treated with débridement and prosthetic retention. Culture-negative PJI has been reported to be as high as 19%.[88]

Our current definition of prosthetic infection includes a combination of clinical signs and symptoms, histologic analysis of tissue, and results of cultures. The diagnosis of definite infection is made if evaluation of the knee establishes at least one of the following criteria: (1) two or more cultures obtained by aspiration or deep tissue specimens obtained at surgery yield the same organism, (2) histopathologic evaluation of intra-articular tissue reveals changes in acute inflammation, (3) gross purulence is observed at the time of surgery, or (4) an actively discharging sinus tract is evident.[43]

It seems reasonable to assume that optimal treatment outcomes are achieved by accurately identifying the offending microorganism(s) whenever possible and enacting directed treatment strategies. Multiple reports have documented the distribution of microorganisms involved.* In most series, gram-positive organisms predominate; however, it is important to remember that polymicrobial infections represent approximately 9% of cases of infected TKR.[88] It is also important to note that in the current era, many investigators are observing an increasing incidence of resistant organisms.[86]

Methicillin-resistant *Staphylococcus aureus* (MRSA) and methicillin-resistant *Staphylococcus epidermidis* (MRSE) have emerged as common nosocomial pathogens often requiring

complex antibiotics and potentially inferior treatment outcomes. In a study of 35 infected TKRs, those infected with methicillin-sensitive organisms demonstrated a treatment success rate of 89% compared with only 18% treatment success in those with methicillin-resistant infection.[55] In contrast, a multicenter study of 37 patients with a resistant organism found only 24% with reinfection, with most of these reinfections caused by a different organism.[75] These authors believe that two-stage reimplantation remains a viable treatment option for patients who have an infection with a resistant organism at the site of a TKR.

Periprosthetic fungal infections fortunately are rare, with *Candida* being the predominant species identified.[91] A review of 10 cases documented successful treatment in 8 of 10 patients with appropriate antifungal therapy and two-stage reimplantation. Prosthetic joint infection due to *Mycobacterium tuberculosis* is also rare.[8] To decrease the risk of reactivation of quiescent tuberculous infection, consideration should be given to preoperative or perioperative antituberculous prophylaxis.

Identification and diagnosis of biofilm organisms via traditional culture methods have lacked optimal sensitivity and specificity.[107] Basically, several strategies can be used to address these organisms. Culture-independent molecular methods have been developed to improve the diagnosis of prosthetic joint infection in the research setting. Detection of 16S ribosomal deoxyribonucleic acid by polymerase chain reaction is just one example.[69] One of the primary problems with this approach is the relative difficulty associated with excellent sensitivity of these techniques leading to false-positive test results.

An alternative strategy employs culturing of samples obtained from the prosthesis by sonication of explanted prostheses to dislodge adherent bacteria from the prosthesis.[108] In this study, culture of samples obtained by sonication of prostheses was more sensitive than that of conventional periprosthetic tissue culture for the microbiologic diagnosis of prosthetic hip and knee infection, especially in patients who had received antimicrobial therapy within 14 days before surgery. This technique is now used in our institution as a matter of common clinical practice to improve the detection of organisms causing PJI.

Definitive diagnosis requires a heightened sense of suspicion on the part of the clinician in both early and delayed presentations following surgery. A thorough history, physical examination, plain radiographs, arthrocentesis, and hematologic studies should be considered routine parts of the infection workup. Radionuclide studies are rarely required to make the diagnosis of infection.

Timing of the clinical presentation is a critical factor in the identification and implementation of the correct treatment strategy. These various clinical presentations have been characterized and classified as a useful guide to selecting the most appropriate treatment option for infected TKR (Table 128-3).[99]

In this classification, postoperative infections diagnosed by positive intraoperative cultures after revision arthroplasty are generally low-virulence organisms such as coagulase-negative staphylococci and *Propionibacterium* spp.[68] Five-year survival free of treatment failure for the 16 episodes was 89%. These results suggest a favorable outcome of prosthetic joint infections caused by low-virulence pathogens initially

---

*References 15, 38, 40, 43, 50, 88, and 111.

Table 128-3 Classification System of Prosthetic Joint Infection: Time to Onset of Infection Dictates Treatment

	Type 1	Type 2	Type 3	Type 4
Timing of diagnosis	Positive intraoperative cultures	Early postoperative infection	Acute hematogenous infection	Late (chronic) infection
Definition	Two or more positive cultures at surgery	Infection occurs within first month after surgery	Hematogenous seeding of previously well-functioning arthroplasty	Chronic indolent clinical course; infection present for longer than 1 month
Treatment	Appropriate antibiotics	Attempt at débridement with prosthesis salvage	Attempt at débridement with prosthesis salvage or prosthesis removal	Prosthesis removal

From Segawa H, Tsukayama DT, Kyle RF, Becker DA, Gustilo RB: Infection after total knee arthroplasty: a retrospective study of the treatment of eighty-one infections. J Bone Joint Surg Am 81:1434–1445, 1999.

diagnosed as positive intraoperative cultures after revision arthroplasty.

For the remaining clinical presentations, rapid and expedient diagnosis is essential to prevent the delay of diagnosis, which could result in diagnosis of a late or chronic infection that could have been identified and treated as an early infection. Pain is the most common presenting symptom. Persistent wound drainage is strongly suggestive of infection and probably should be treated with arthrotomy, débridement, and irrigation within the first several weeks after surgery.[117] Cultures of serous wound drainage are difficult to interpret and potentially misleading and therefore are discouraged. Empirical antibiotic use for persistent wound drainage should be avoided, as this only suppresses the clinical symptoms of infection and potentially delays diagnosis, eliminating the possibility of treatment of the infection without removal of the prosthesis.[17,73,97,105]

Diagnosis of early postoperative infection is typically confirmed by joint arthrocentesis, as the erythrocyte sedimentation rate (ESR) and C-reactive protein (CRP) levels are nonspecific in the early postoperative period. CRP levels after TKR peak on postoperative day number two and decrease to preoperative baseline levels as early as 1 week but typically at 14 to 21 days postoperatively.[11,60,118] In the early postoperative period, assertive management of delayed wound healing or marginal skin necrosis by débridement of necrotic skin and primary wound closure is preferable to empirical antibiotic treatment, prolonged observation, and eventual development of deep infection.[62]

An acute hematogenous infection typically presents with sudden onset of pain or stiffness in a previously well-functioning arthroplasty.[5] Specific risk factors for a hematogenous infection, such as a remote source of infection or a recent invasive procedure causing significant bacteremia, should be identified.[66] The severity of symptoms with pain, effusion, and restricted range of knee motion in this setting facilitates rapid diagnosis. Although ESR and CRP are typically elevated in these patients, the cornerstone of diagnosis is arthrocentesis with evaluation of the aspirate by gram stain, quantitative leukocyte count, and culture for aerobic and anaerobic bacteria. Empirical antibiotics for the unexplained painful prosthesis, without attempts at definitive diagnosis, unfortunately are commonly given; this approach only complicates subsequent efforts to diagnose deep infection.

A vast majority of patients with an infected total knee arthroplasty (TKA) are diagnosed in the subacute or chronic setting. Historical factors such as persistent pain since the

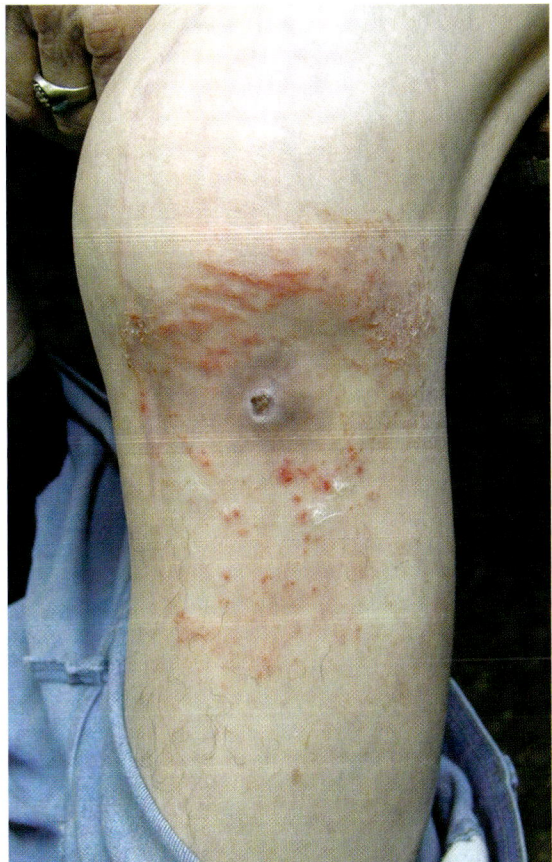

Figure 128-1. Photograph of a chronic sinus tract over the anterolateral aspect of the knee joint in a patient with a chronically infected total knee replacement.

arthroplasty, prolonged postoperative wound drainage (Fig. 128-1), antibiotic treatment for difficulties with primary wound healing, and knee stiffness despite extensive rehabilitation efforts may be indicative of deep infection. Sequential comparison of plain radiographs may reveal progressive radiolucencies, focal osteopenia or osteolysis of subchondral bone, and periosteal new bone formation (Fig. 128-2).[79] Additional studies should include CRP, ESR, and aspiration of the affected TKR. When elevated, CRP and ESR are obtained not only for diagnosis but to serve as baseline values for comparison with testing obtained during and after treatment.

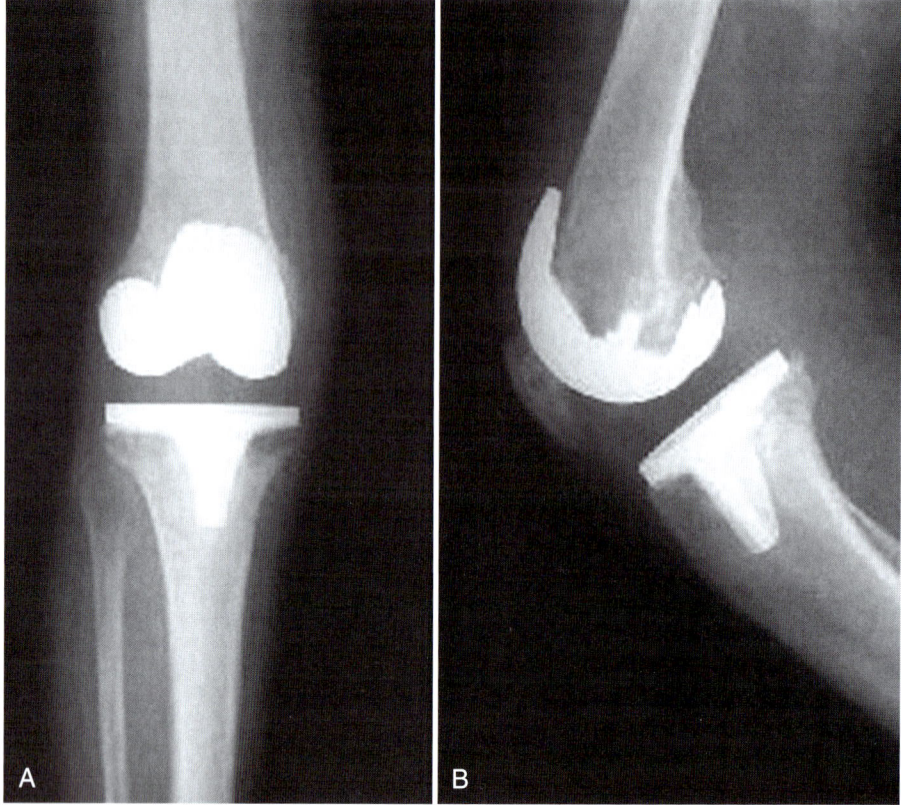

Figure 128-2. **A,** Anteroposterior and **(B)** lateral radiographs of a patient with a chronically infected total knee arthroplasty. Radiolucencies at the bone/cement interface, which typically are late findings in periprosthetic infection, can be seen inferior to the tibial component on both views.

In our opinion, arthrocentesis is considered an essential element of the workup and evaluation of a suspected deep periprosthetic infection. Synovial fluid analysis and culture enable identification of microorganisms, and knowledge of the synovial fluid cell count and differential provides an additional data point for diagnosis. Although these values may resemble a native joint infection in the acute hematogenous infection (neutrophil differential >90% and total nucleated cell counts >50,000/μL), it is important to note that most chronic TKR infections are associated with much lower values.[37,70,106]

Based on our experience, a synovial fluid leukocyte differential of >65% neutrophils (or a leukocyte count of >1.7 × 10³/μL) is a sensitive and specific test for the diagnosis of prosthetic knee infection in patients without underlying inflammatory joint disease.[106] Patients should have all antibiotics discontinued several weeks prior to aspiration, as this oversight frequently accounts for the inability to isolate organisms.[4] Use of molecular genetic diagnostic methods with joint aspirates, such as the polymerase chain reaction technique, is potentially promising, but these remain experimental modalities for diagnosis of infected joint arthroplasty.[24,69] The use of radioisotope scans to facilitate diagnosis of the chronically infected knee prosthesis is only occasionally useful.[67,94,96]

Despite all reasonable efforts to diagnose infection preoperatively, intraoperative evaluation of surgical tissue specimens may be necessary to confirm the diagnosis in difficult cases. The gram stain is notoriously unreliable, with a high percentage of false-negative results and an extremely low sensitivity.[2,26] Frozen section testing to detect infection has been widely used with variable accuracy and results.[25,33,64,80,83] Variability is likely accounted for by differences in technique, sampling errors during retrieval of tissue samples, pathologist experience, and the definition used to declare the presence of infection. Analysis of intraoperative frozen section is a reasonable and reliable method when an accomplished and experienced pathologist evaluates appropriate tissue samples.

Although quantitative assessment is difficult, the surgeon's intraoperative assessment is very helpful, and if there is any reason to suspect deep infection, one should obtain multiple tissue specimens for culture and sensitivity testing. In this setting, a careful review of the history, ESR, and CRP, when combined with the results of preoperative synovial fluid analysis and interpretation of tissue by the pathologist, will often allow determination of whether or not infection is likely.

TREATMENT

Variables that must be considered before treatment is initiated include (1) determination of whether the infection is superficial or deep; (2) the duration of time elapsed between arthroplasty and diagnosis; (3) identification of host factors that may adversely affect treatment of the infection; (4) appraisal of the soft tissue envelope surrounding the knee, specifically, the integrity of the extensor mechanism; (5) determination of whether the implant is loose or well fixed; (6) consideration of the pathogen(s) responsible for the infection; (7) the physician's ability to provide the proper level of required care; and (8) careful assessment of the patient's expectations and functional requirements.

Treatment goals for the infected TKA include eradication of infection, alleviation of pain, and maintenance of a functional extremity. Basic treatment options include (1) antibiotic suppression, (2) open débridement, (3) reimplantation of another prosthesis, (4) arthrodesis, (5) resection arthroplasty, and (6) amputation. With the exception of chronic antibiotic suppression, which does not eliminate infection, the cornerstone treatment principles of these treatment options include thorough surgical débridement combined with appropriate use of antibiotics and optimization of the host response. When confronted with an infected TKR, the treating physician should start by considering the question of whether or not the prosthesis can be retained, or if prosthesis removal is required to treat the infection.

TREATMENT METHODS WHEREBY THE PROSTHESIS IS RETAINED

Antibiotic Suppression

Antibiotic treatment alone will not eliminate deep periprosthetic infection but can be used as suppressive treatment when the following criteria are met: (1) prosthesis removal is not feasible (usually because of a medical condition that precludes an operative procedure), (2) the microorganism has low virulence, (3) the microorganism is susceptible to an oral antibiotic, (4) the antibiotic can be tolerated without serious toxicity, and (5) the prosthesis is not loose.[112] The presence of other joint arthroplasties or a cardiac valvular prosthesis is a relatively strong contraindication to this treatment approach.

In a multicenter study, antibiotic suppression was successful in only 40 of 225 knees (18%).[6] Combining several series reveals that antibiotic suppression was successful in 62 (24 %) of 261 knees.[42] Use of a combined regimen of rifampin with a quinolone has been reported to be more successful than treatment with a single antibiotic.[28] Despite the fact that most patients fail to meet all of these selection criteria, antibiotic suppression is commonly practiced, and this practice unfortunately prolongs the presence of infection and often complicates subsequent treatment attempts. Long-term antibiotic suppression should be initiated rarely and should be considered only when all treatment criteria are met.

Débridement With Prosthesis Retention

Open débridement may be indicated for the occasional acute infection in the early postoperative period (type II) or for acute hematogenous infection (type III) of a securely fixed and functional prosthesis. Suggested criteria for this treatment technique include (1) short duration of symptoms of infection (less than 2 weeks), (2) susceptible gram-positive organisms, (3) absence of prolonged postoperative drainage or a draining sinus tract, and (4) no prosthetic loosening or

radiographic evidence of infection.[18] Again, a relative contraindication for débridement and attempted salvage of the prosthesis is the presence of other joint replacements or of a cardiac valvular prosthesis.

Results of débridement are difficult to determine because of differences in microbiology and subsequent antibiotic management, variability in time to treatment, quality of the soft tissue envelope, extent and completeness of débridement, status of implant fixation, and the criteria for success in each report. A multicenter study reported a success rate of only 19.5% with open débridement of 154 knees.[6] In another literature review, a success rate of 32.6% was reported in 530 infected TKRs treated with open débridement and component retention.[101] Factors identified with failure of open débridement included postoperative drainage longer than 2 weeks in duration, existence of a sinus tract at débridement, hinged prostheses, and immunocompromised hosts.[101]

The importance of the timing of débridement in relationship to the onset of symptoms or the period of time elapsed since insertion of the prosthesis cannot be overemphasized.[17,76,97,99,104] In a study of 24 infected TKRs treated with open débridement and component retention, a success rate of 100% was reported in the early postoperative infection group (type 2) and 71% in the acute hematogenous group with duration of symptoms less than 30 days.[76] These authors emphasized the strict selection criteria, with patients demonstrating evidence of infection for less than 30 days.[76] It is clear that débridement with prosthesis retention should not be attempted in patients with chronic infection.[14,54,99]

As just detailed, expeditious treatment provided as soon as possible after the diagnosis of infection has been established is a matter of paramount concern. This is particularly true for S. aureus, as delay beyond 48 hours after onset of symptoms resulted in a significant decrease in the success rate.[18] The specific organism and its virulence are significant predictors of success following open débridement. It is well documented that S. aureus prosthetic joint infection is associated with the lowest success rate following débridement.[23,97,120] Débridement attempts for resistant organisms are particularly unsuccessful, with a cure rate of only 18%.[16]

In contrast, in a report of 19 cases of infection with penicillin-susceptible streptococcal species, in which all surgical débridement procedures occurred within 10 days of symptom onset, treatment was successful in 89.5% of cases.[73] In a recent report, only 1 (8%) of 13 patients infected with S. aureus was successfully treated, compared with 10 (56%) of 18 patients with S. epidermidis or a streptococcal species.[23]

Arthroscopy is not recommended as a method of débridement for the infected TKR, because the inability to perform satisfactory débridement of modular implants between the tibial tray and the polyethylene insert impairs success. In a series of 16 infected TKRs treated by arthroscopic débridement within the first 7 days after onset of symptoms, only 6 (38%) of the knees were successfully treated.[114] These results were significantly worse than the 71% success rate obtained with open débridement of 24 TKRs, also performed by these authors.[76] One of the primary reasons for recommending against arthroscopic débridement is that once arthroscopy is performed and subsequent antibiotics are started, failure of treatment with this approach extends the timeline, so that failure occurs long enough after the onset of symptoms that prosthesis removal is required.

TREATMENT METHODS WHEREBY THE PROSTHESIS IS REMOVED

Resection Arthroplasty

Definitive resection arthroplasty implies implant removal with no intention of subsequent knee reconstruction. The ideal candidate for definitive resection arthroplasty is a patient with polyarticular rheumatoid arthritis with limited ambulatory demands, which allow the patient to sit more readily than is feasible with a knee arthrodesis. Patients with less disability are likely to be less satisfied with a resection arthroplasty.[52] The primary disadvantage of resection arthroplasty is the frequent occurrence of knee instability associated with pain during transfer or ambulation.

Three basic fundamentals of the operative technique include (1) initial débridement and removal of all infected tissue and foreign material; (2) temporary fixation with pins or sutures to maintain alignment and apposition of the tibia and femur; and (3) cast immobilization, permitting weight bearing, for at least 6 months. Although resection arthroplasty usually achieves satisfactory resolution of infection, most patients experience some pain, have knee instability, and have limited ambulatory capacity. Definitive resection arthroplasty is rarely utilized in the current era.

Arthrodesis

Traditionally, arthrodesis was considered the standard treatment option for an infected TKR because of the excellent potential for resolving infection, alleviating pain, and providing stable knee function. These advantages are offset by elimination of knee motion, which often makes sitting and other activities cumbersome. Currently, the functional limitations of an arthrodesis seem to be poorly tolerated and unacceptable to most patients. In a report of 30 patients who underwent conversion of a spontaneous ankylosis or a formal arthrodesis to a TKA, 17 patients had attempted suicide preoperatively because of unhappiness regarding the affected extremity.[56] Before arthrodesis is recommended, a detailed discussion should be carried out with the patient regarding the physical limitations and functional restrictions imparted to the patient who undergoes a knee arthrodesis.

Indications for knee arthrodesis with failed TKA include (1) individuals with high functional demands, (2) single-joint disease, (3) young patient age, (4) extensor mechanism disruption, (5) a poor soft tissue envelope requiring extensive soft tissue reconstruction, (6) systemic immunocompromise, and (7) microorganisms requiring highly toxic antibiotic therapy or resistant to conventional antibiotics.[42] Relative contraindications include (1) bilateral knee disease, (2) ipsilateral ankle or hip disease, (3) severe segmental bone loss, and (4) contralateral extremity amputation.

Fixation techniques most commonly used for knee arthrodesis include external fixation, internal fixation with an intramedullary nail, and dual-plate fixation. The type of prior knee implant, the extent of bone deficiency, and the arthrodesis technique used affect the success of knee arthrodesis following TKA.[21,27,42]

Inherent complications of arthrodesis following TKA include nonunion, recurrent infection, and ipsilateral limb fracture, with the most frequent being nonunion. Causes of nonunion include bone deficiency, persistent infection, poor bone apposition, malalignment, and inadequate immobilization.[42] Specific complications associated with the external fixation technique include neurovascular injury during pin insertion, pin site infection, and fracture through pin sites; complications have been reported in 20% to 65% of patients.[93] Complications inherent to intramedullary nailing include nail breakage and nail migration; complications associated with intramedullary nailing for arthrodesis have been reported in 40% to 56% of cases.[93]

In a recent report of 85 consecutive patients who underwent knee arthrodesis for an infected TKR, external fixation achieved successful fusion in 41 of 61 patients and was associated with a 4.9% rate of deep infection.[65] Fusion was successful in 23 of 24 patients with intramedullary (IM) nailing and was associated with an 8.3% rate of deep infection. Differences between fusion and infection rates with these two techniques were not statistically significant. Thirty-four patients (40%) had complications. The primary message from this report is that knee arthrodesis remains a reasonable salvage alternative for some difficult cases of infected TKR, and one must consider the risks of both nonunion and infection when choosing the fixation method in this setting. IM nailing appears to show a higher trend toward successful union but has a higher risk of recurrent infection when compared with external fixation knee arthrodesis.

Amputation

Patients with an infected TKR commonly express fear of eventual amputation. Amputation is rarely indicated except in cases of life-threatening systemic sepsis or persistent local infection associated with massive bone loss. Amputation is estimated to occur in less than 5% of patients treated for an infected TKA.[42] Factors most commonly leading to amputation include multiple revision attempts for chronic infection, severe bone loss, and intractable pain.[51] Consideration of arthrodesis earlier in the treatment process, when bone stock is adequate, rather than repeated attempts at revision surgery in the presence of chronic infection helps reduce the incidence of amputation following failed TKR.

Amputation should be performed at a level that maximizes function yet facilitates eradication of infection. Many patients have a cavernous bone defect of the distal femur, and local muscle transposition of the gastrocnemius muscles during the amputation procedure can be extremely helpful for dead space management, as well as for optimizing the soft tissue envelope of the amputation stump. Following amputation, many elderly patients remain limited ambulators or are non-ambulatory because of the increased energy expenditure required for walking.

Of 23 patients treated with above-the-knee amputation for a failed TKA, only 7 (30%) could ambulate regularly, 20 of the 23 (87%) used a wheelchair for part of the day, and 12 (52%) were confined to the wheelchair.[92] In another report, the prevalence of 25 above-the-knee amputations done for causes related to TKR was 0.36%.[100] Functional outcomes after amputation performed above a TKR were poor. Nine of the 25 limbs were fitted with an above-the-knee prosthesis, but only 5 patients were walking even to a limited degree with the prosthesis at the time of the last follow-up.

Reimplantation

Reimplantation, or reinsertion of another prosthesis, is currently the primary accepted method of treatment for patients with an infected TKR.[19] Generally accepted contraindications for insertion of another prosthesis include (1) persistent or recalcitrant infection, (2) medical conditions that prevent multiple reconstructive procedures, (3) extensor mechanism disruption, and (4) a poor soft tissue envelope about the knee joint.[42]

The optimal duration and route of antibiotic delivery for treatment of the infected knee arthroplasty have not been clearly determined. A 4- to 6-week course of intravenous antibiotics prior to reimplantation has yielded excellent success rates and represents the most commonly accepted clinical standard.[38,50,121] Ultimately, the duration of antibiotic therapy most likely should be individualized for each patient based on the virulence of the microorganism, the patient's comorbidities, and whether antibiotic-impregnated spacers or beads are also being used to deliver adjunctive antibiotics.

Reimplantation can be performed as a direct-exchange technique, or by delayed reinsertion of the new prosthesis (two-stage approach) after antibiotic therapy. In a review of direct-exchange arthroplasty using ABLC, successful control of infection was documented in 33 of 37 (89.2%) infected TKRs.[101] These authors suggest that factors associated with successful direct exchange include (1) infection by gram-positive organisms, (2) absence of sinus formation, (3) use of antibiotic-impregnated bone cement for the new prosthesis, and (4) a prolonged 12-week course of antibiotic therapy.[101] It is important to note that reports analyzed by these authors focus primarily on patients treated in the 1980s, and in the current era of drug-resistant organisms and severe bone loss, direct-exchange techniques are indicated only in groups of patients highly selected by arthroplasty surgeons familiar with the treatment of periprosthetic infection.

Two-Stage Reimplantation

The rate of successful eradication of infection at the site of an infected TKA with a modern, two-stage protocol ranges from 85% to 95%, depending on the duration of follow-up.* The exact time delay before reimplantation has not been established. Initially, a poor success rate (57%) was reported when 14 patients were treated with insertion of a new prosthesis within several weeks after removal of the infected knee prosthesis.[95] In contrast, the two-stage reimplantation protocol proposed by Insall has been a highly effective method of treatment.[50] This protocol consists of soft tissue débridement and removal of the infected prosthesis and cement, followed by 6 weeks of intravenous antibiotics and subsequent reimplantation. The success of this protocol was confirmed in a follow-up report of 64 infected TKRs.[38] These early reports established the commonly accepted time delay of 6 weeks before reimplantation; however, it is important to note that

ABLC was not used in the form of spacers or for prosthetic fixation.

Many subsequent reports have used ABLC spacers in the interval between removal of the infected prosthesis and eventual reimplantation, and many have used antibiotic-loaded cement for prosthesis fixation at reimplantation.[42] Use of antibiotic-impregnated cement for prosthesis fixation has been reported to exert a beneficial effect at the time of reimplantation.[43] Among 89 infected TKRs treated by reimplantation, ABLC for prosthesis fixation was a significant treatment variable, as 7 (28%) of 25 knees without the use of ABLC developed reinfection compared with only 3 (4.7%) of 64 knees with ABLC for prosthesis fixation. This difference was statistically significant irrespective of the duration of intravenous antibiotics ($P = .0025$).[43]

Use of adjunctive antibiotic delivery provided by the ABLC gradually led to decreased antibiotic duration and shorter time delays prior to reimplantation.[42] Although some investigators have shortened this time frame to several weeks, large prospective trials are necessary to settle the issue.

ANTIBIOTIC CEMENT SPACERS

During the time after resection of the infected TKA, prior to eventual reimplantation of another prosthesis, local antibiotics are delivered via static or articulating spacer blocks. Many reports have used antibiotic ratios of only 1 g of antibiotic per 40-g batch of bone cement in the ABLC.[42,43,120] Currently, most investigators use higher dosage ratios, such as 4 to 6 g of antibiotics per 40-g batch of bone cement.[39,44,90] Low-dose ABLC (<2 g antibiotic/40 g cement) should be used for prophylaxis in reimplantation or in primary TKAs in high-risk patients, or for prosthesis fixation at reimplantation.[44] The higher dosage ratios of antibiotic cement should be reserved for the treatment of active infection with spacers, as greater than 4.5 g of antibiotic powder substantially diminishes the mechanical strength of bone cement and should not be used for prosthesis fixation.[44,102]

Antibiotic elution is highly dependent on bone cement porosity, and mixing high doses of powdered antibiotics creates considerable cement porosity, facilitating increased antibiotic elution for at least 4 weeks.[44] Combining two antibiotics in bone cement will improve elution of both antibiotics, and the two most commonly used antibiotics in clinical practice are vancomycin and tobramycin.[42] The use of at least 3.6 g of tobramycin and 1 g of vancomycin per package of bone cement is recommended to obtain effective elution levels.[71,90] Local levels of antibiotic elution typically far exceed the levels observed in serum during parenteral antibiotic administration.[44] Up to 12 g of antibiotics per 40-g batch of bone cement may be added without prohibiting cement polymerization.[1] The systemic safety of high-dose ABLC for the infected TKR has been established.[102]

The primary functions of block spacers include delivery of local antimicrobial agents and maintenance of collateral ligament length.[13] Potential disadvantages of block spacers include the presence of a foreign body and bone loss incurred while awaiting reimplantation.[20] Essentially, the different types of block spacers include a simple tibiofemoral block, the molded arthrodesis block, articulating mobile spacers, and medullary dowels. The simple tibiofemoral block was the original spacer block that was pre-formed and then inserted

---

*References 9, 39, 40, 61, 99, and 110.

into the tibiofemoral space after the cement had polymerized. These blocks were shaped as simple "hockey pucks" or "L-shaped" spacers inserted into the tibiofemoral space. Additional antibiotic beads or thin disks were often placed into the suprapatellar pouch or lateral gutters. Difficulties with this type of block spacer included inability to match the surfaces of the block with the irregular surfaces of the distal femur and proximal tibia, subluxation of the bony surfaces off of the spacer surface, instances of extensor mechanism necrosis, wound breakdown, and progressive bone loss.[20]

The molded arthrodesis block method avoids some of the difficulties encountered with pre-formed spacer blocks.[44] These spacers are fabricated so that the cement is placed within the knee in a doughy state and are polymerized within the knee so that the cement can conform to the irregular contour of the femur and tibia (Fig. 128-3). This macrointerdigitation of the cement into bone defects and the intercondylar notch with extension into the medullary canals and suprapatellar pouch creates stability of the knee joint. This stability is helpful for patient comfort and prevents the difficulties of spacer migration and progressive bone erosion. Removal of these spacers requires fragmentation of the spacer into several large pieces with an osteotome at the time of reimplantation.

The mobile articulating spacer technique allows the patient to place the knee through a range of motion during

the time period following prosthesis removal and insertion of the new prosthesis.[39,48] These spacers, originally facsimiles of antibiotic-impregnated cement shaped into femoral and tibial components, allowed knee motion through articulation of the acrylic cement surfaces.[39] Eventually, a system of molds was developed to incorporate small metal runners and polyethylene tibial trays, so that cement surfaces were not articulating against each other.[39] One alternative has been to sterilize the prosthesis just removed and then incorporate the femoral component and tibial tray into the antibiotic-loaded spacer.[48]

The theoretical advantages of mobile articulating spacers include the potential for improved functional outcomes and better range of motion; yet conclusive results in this regard have not been realized.[30,34] In a series of 55 patients—25 with solid spacers and 30 with mobile articulating spacers—no difference between the two groups was observed with respect to knee scores or final range of motion.[34] In a recent report of two-stage reimplantation comparing 26 septic TKAs treated with a static antibiotic spacer versus a group of 22 septic TKAs treated with mobile articulating spacers, no difference in reinfection rates was found between groups at 36 months.[30] Although the mobile articulating spacer group demonstrated significantly better average range of motion (107.8 degrees) than the static spacer group (93.7 degrees) at final follow-up, it should be noted that the patient groups were not similar, and that the block spacer group represents an historical control group.[30]

Articulating spacers appear to simplify surgical exposure at reimplantation for many surgeons. A recent trend toward the use of mobile spacers that incorporate cement against cement of the articulating surfaces is worrisome, as this abrasion causes cement debris, and anecdotally, some of these cases are associated with extensive scar formation at the time of reimplantation. Regardless of whether a static or mobile articulating antibiotic-loaded spacer is utilized, strong consideration should be given to insertion of antibiotic cement into the canals (see Fig. 128-6).[44] Extension of the infectious process into the medullary canals of the femur or tibia is seen in roughly one third of infected knee replacements without stems.[72] Insertion of antibiotic-impregnated medullary dowels is preferable to insertion of ABLC beads, as these beads often are extremely difficult to remove at reimplantation. A tapered cement dowel fashioned from the nozzle of a cement gun provides an excellent size and shape for insertion into, and subsequently for removal from, the medullary canal.[44]

To date, no significant differences have been noted between knee scores, functional scores, and range of motion arcs when knees are analyzed according to the length of delay, the type of knee prosthesis used at reimplantation, or the use of a block cement spacer as compared with a mobile articulating spacer.[43] The final functional result appears to be more dependent on the patient's overall medical and musculoskeletal functional status.[116] Despite lack of evidence for improved functional outcomes with the use of spacers, the advantages of mechanical stability for the patient and the reduction of difficulty with surgical exposure at reimplantation have led to common acceptance and use of these ABLC spacers. Block spacers should be supplemented by external immobilization, such as a brace or cast, as the patient awaits the reimplantation. Patients with mobile articulating spacers are encouraged to participate in range-of-motion exercises and are allowed

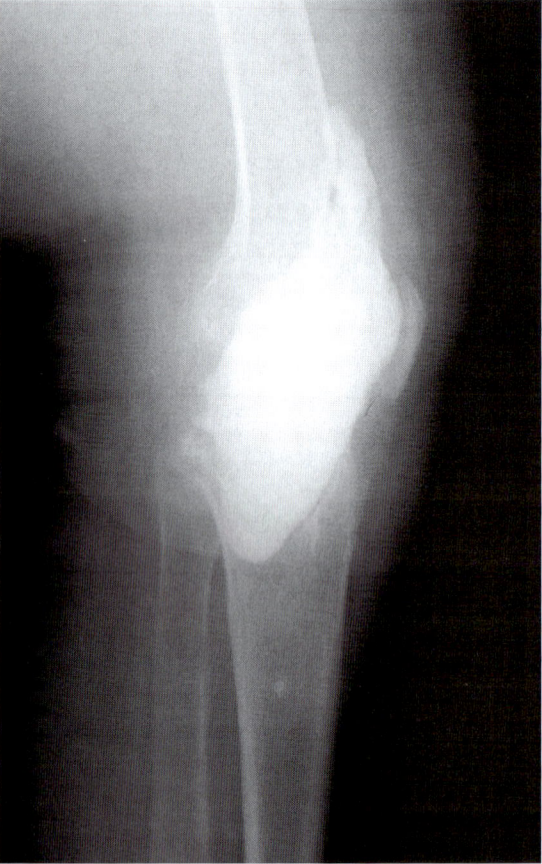

Figure 128-3. Lateral radiograph of a static antibiotic cement spacer, molded to conform to the femoral and tibial osseous surfaces with extension into the suprapatellar pouch to prevent scarring and adhesion of the extensor mechanism to the anterior femur.

up to 50% partial weight bearing.[39] Patients with bilateral infected TKRs are excellent candidates for the use of articulating mobile ABLC spacers.[122]

TIME PERIOD BETWEEN RESECTION AND REIMPLANTATION

Patients undergoing two-stage reimplantation are typically anemic, and 88% require allogeneic blood transfusions, particularly because the two surgeries are temporally close.[84] The presence of infection precludes traditional alternatives such as reinfusion or autologous blood donation, thus novel blood management practices are required in this patient population. A total of 39 patients with 39 consecutive two-stage reimplantations were enrolled in a prospective study to determine whether the use of recombinant human erythropoietin could lower allogeneic transfusion requirements.[22] When compared with a group of 81 patients not receiving recombinant human erythropoietin, the requirement for transfusion was significantly lowered ($P < .001$). Among patients receiving recombinant human erythropoietin, 52% avoided transfusion for the entire time period encompassing both stages of reimplantation.[22]

One of the most important issues for both patient and surgeon is the determination of when it is safe and appropriate to proceed with reimplantation. In just 4 or 6 weeks, ESRs are not expected to normalize; however, the trend should suggest that values obtained just before reimplantation have improved.[42] CRP levels typically normalize by the twenty-first day after surgery, and if the levels remain elevated, this may suggest the presence of persistent infection.[11,42,118] Open biopsy or aspiration for culture and sensitivity has been suggested before proceeding with reimplantation.[77] However, a recent study reported 8 false-negative aspirations out of 32 resection TKAs with antibiotic spacers after 6 weeks of IV antibiotics prior to reimplantation.[63] The authors report that preoperative aspiration prior to reimplantation has a sensitivity of 0%, a positive predictive value of 0%, and an accuracy of 71% and cannot be recommended for routine use.

It is preferable to utilize intraoperative decision making based on the appearance of the knee joint supplemented by analysis of frozen sections. However, it is important to recognize that this method requires considerable experience on the part of the surgeon and the pathologist, and the presence of spacers or beads may alter the appearance of the tissues at reimplantation.[25] In this study, analysis of frozen sections at reimplantation to determine the presence of infection had a sensitivity of 25%, a specificity of 98%, a positive predictive value of 50%, a negative predictive value of 95%, and an accuracy of 94%.[25] If concern arises about the presence of persistent infection, it is prudent to perform another débridement, insert new ABLC spacers, close the wound, and await the results of culture and sensitivity testing.

RESULTS OF REIMPLANTATION

Mid-term to long-term results of reimplantation are beginning to emerge in the literature.[38,40] Both of these delayed reimplantation protocols, with a mean 7-year follow-up, reported that 9% of knees required component removal for infection, and 6% were revised secondary to aseptic loosening. A recent report, at average 5-year follow-up of 46 infected

TKRs, documented a 93.5% success rate with no difference in failure rates between methicillin-sensitive and methicillin-resistant organisms.[113] These results suggest that the high likelihood of success after two-stage reimplantation for infected TKA is well maintained through long-term follow-up, and that two-stage reimplantation is an acceptable treatment of choice for infections involving resistant and virulent organisms, with a modest rate of reinfection.

STAGED REIMPLANTATION SURGICAL TECHNIQUE

Thorough and complete débridement is paramount to ensure treatment success in staged reimplantation of an infected TKR. Careful placement of the skin incision is critical, and when multiple prior incisions are present, the most lateral, longitudinal midline incision is recommended. Excision of heavily scarred tissue back to healthy tissue is advised, as is excision of all sinus tracts. Subcutaneous tissue flap elevation during the approach should be minimized. A formal arthrotomy is preferred through a medial parapatellar arthrotomy, and subperiosteal release of the deep medial collateral ligament allows external rotation of the tibia necessary for adequate exposure (Fig. 128-4). Removal of tibial polyethylene is recommended at this point, as this decreases tension in the joint and releases tension of the extensor mechanism.

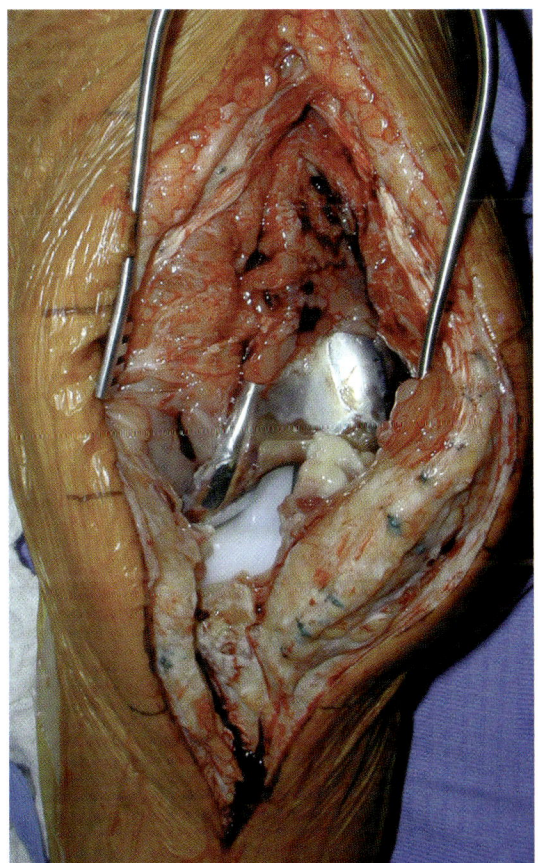

Figure 128-4. Medial parapatellar arthrotomy in a patient undergoing resection of an infected total knee arthroplasty. Gross purulent material and prominent synovial proliferation are visualized throughout the knee.

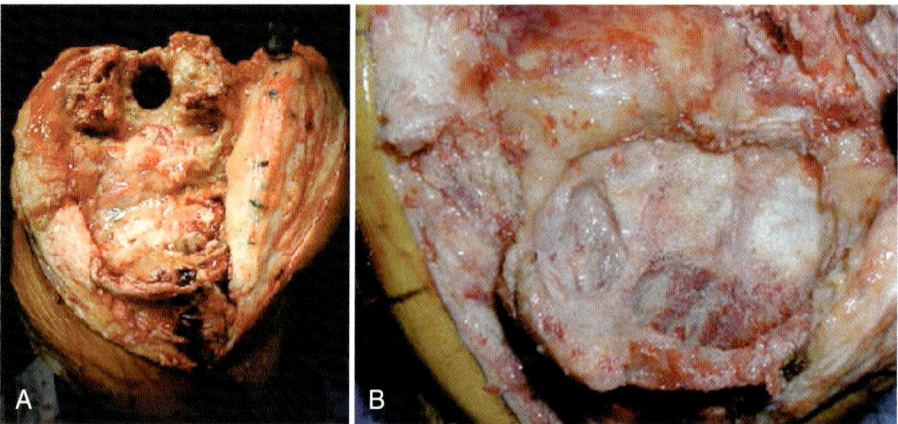

Figure 128-5. A, Intraoperative picture of infected total knee arthroplasty after initial resection of the prosthetic components, demonstrating grossly purulent material lining the synovium and bone surfaces. **B,** Proximal tibia after thorough débridement of purulent debris and necrotic bone, revealing a clean viable bony surface for future implantation of a tibial component.

Eversion of the patella can be extremely difficult and dangerous during exposure of the infected TKR and is generally considered unnecessary. Adequate external rotation of the tibia allows lateral translation and subluxation of the extensor mechanism, minimizes the need for lateral retinacular release, and avoids undue tension on the patellar tendon insertion. If additional exposure is necessary, a quadriceps snip may be utilized, as a formal V-Y turndown and a tibial tubercle osteotomy are avoided if at all possible because of the potential for extensor mechanism necrosis in this setting.

The femoral, tibial, and patellar components are carefully removed to preserve as much viable bone stock as possible. Particular attention is paid to meticulous removal of all cement particles and debris, as well as to débridement of any osteolytic defects and nonviable bone. The tibial and femoral intramedullary canals are thoroughly débrided when implants with stems are removed; however, it is not uncommon for the infectious process to extend into the medullary canals even in the absence of medullary stems. The final step in the débridement process consists of synovectomy and scar excision of the suprapatellar pouch, medial and lateral gutters, and posterior capsular region. It is helpful to perform this step at the end of the resection and débridement, as cement and particulate debris may fall into these areas during removal of the prosthetic components. These fragments are easily identified and removed along with the synovium and scar tissue during the synovectomy. It is critical to perform a meticulous and thorough débridement and synovial excision (Fig. 128-5) of viable bone and soft tissue. It is also imperative to attain access and thoroughly débride the posterior aspect of the knee, as this represents a frequent location for missed cement particles and foreign material. Three to five tissue samples are routinely sent for culture and sensitivity testing.

The knee joint is copiously irrigated and preparation made for placement of the ABLC spacer. The antibiotic cement is mixed and placed into the tibiofemoral space in the final stages of polymerization to prevent solid interdigitation into the bone; it is gently molded to the contour of the distal femur and proximal tibia. Intramedullary antibiotic cement dowels, when used, are inserted prior to insertion of the tibiofemoral spacer (Fig. 128-6). The cement from the tibiofemoral spacer is extended into the suprapatellar space, as this

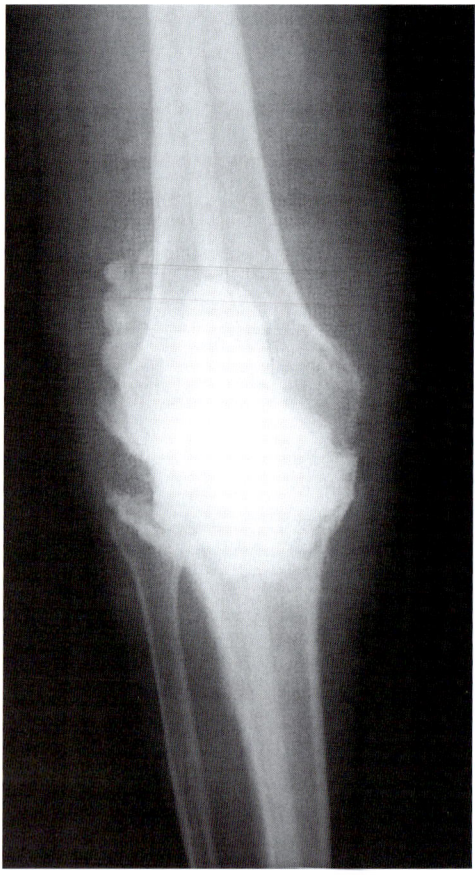

Figure 128-6. Anteroposterior radiograph of a static spacer with antibiotic-loaded bone cement (ABLC) medullary cement dowels extending into the femoral and tibial canals.

effectively maintains the length of the extensor mechanism by minimizing scarring and contracture against the anterior femur (Fig. 128-7). The wound is closed meticulously over drains. Capsular closure is accomplished with a large absorbable monofilament suture, and the skin is closed with large monofilament retention sutures and smaller interrupted skin sutures. The importance of perfect epidermal apposition to facilitate primary wound healing cannot be overemphasized.

The surgical approach at reimplantation is typically more difficult than at the time of implant removal. As previously mentioned, extensive subperiosteal release of the deep medial collateral ligament from the tibia facilitates anterolateral subluxation of the tibia and lateral translation of the patella and extensor mechanism. If removal of the spacer is difficult, the

cement spacer is removed in pieces with an osteotome. Forcible removal of block spacers can result in a periprosthetic fracture of the femur or tibia. Thorough débridement of any residual nonviable synovium and scar tissue is performed, as is débridement of necrotic bone. Attention then is turned to insertion of the implants.

Great care should be taken to place the femoral and tibial components in the correct rotation. Use of the transepicondylar axis is helpful for preventing inadvertent placement of the femoral component into relative internal rotation. Reimplantation knee arthroplasty often is associated with ligamentous and osseous defects that require implant systems with a more constrained design to achieve stability.[10] Stemmed prosthetic components are typically used in this setting to augment prosthesis fixation against stresses transferred to the associated interfaces from increased constraint. Although the use of uncemented implants has been recommended for reimplantation, the benefit of antibiotic cement for prosthesis fixation should be strongly considered in the setting of previous periprosthetic infection (Fig. 128-8).[43,119] Unless one chooses to use an uncemented implant, bone graft is rarely required for reimplantation arthroplasty. Bone graft is avoided by the use of other alternatives such as modular wedges or filling of bone defects with ABLC.

Occasionally after insertion of the new prosthesis, it is difficult to close the soft tissue envelope. Leaving the patellar shell unresurfaced facilitates capsular closure in this setting. Simultaneous use of a gastrocnemius rotational flap to achieve wound closure during the reimplantation procedure has also been reported.[43,72,119] Another alternative for patients with

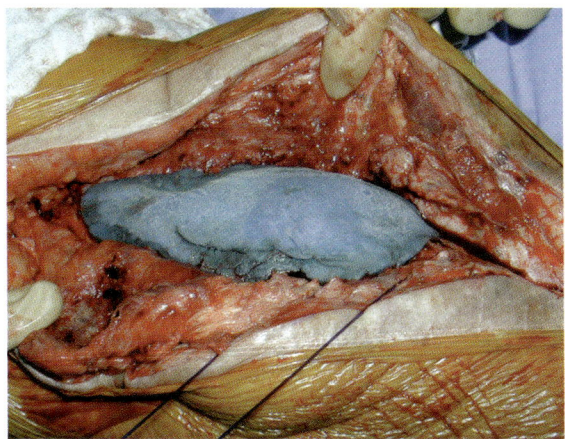

Figure 128-7. Intraoperative photograph of a static molded antibiotic cement spacer inserted after resection of an infected total knee arthroplasty. Notice the extension into the suprapatellar region to prevent adhesion of the extensor mechanism to the anterior femur.

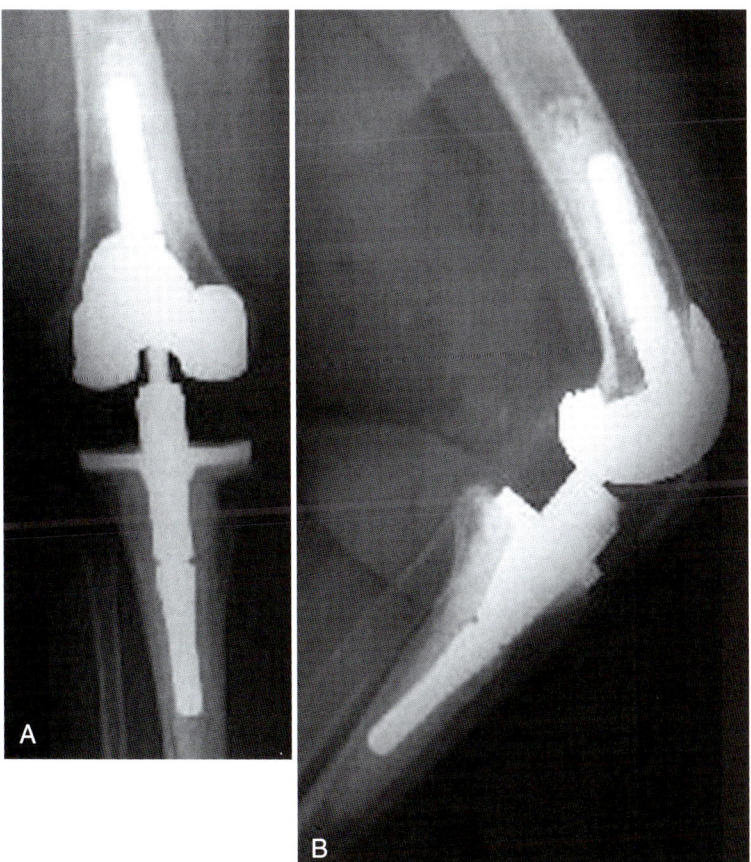

Figure 128-8. A, Anteroposterior and **(B)** lateral radiographs of a reimplantation total knee arthroplasty utilizing a semiconstrained prosthetic design. The femoral and tibial stems were cemented with low-dose antibiotic-loaded bone cement (ABLC) using gentamicin and vancomycin.

multiple skin incisions or a tightly scarred soft tissue envelope is gradual soft tissue expansion prior to reimplantation.[38,81] This procedure has allowed successful wound closure and avoids the use of soft tissue muscle transposition.

REINFECTION AFTER REIMPLANTATION

Reinfection is more likely when an infected revision TKA rather than an infected primary TKA is treated.[47] These patients have greater bone loss and compromise of the soft tissue envelope. Although reimplantation has become a commonly accepted treatment modality for the infected knee prosthesis, the poor outcome of patients who develop reinfection following reimplantation can be devastating. Among 24 knees treated for reinfection after reimplantation, the final outcome included 10 knees with a successful knee arthrodesis, 5 patients with infected prostheses maintained on suppressive oral antibiotics, 4 above-the-knee amputations, 3 persistent pseudarthroses, 1 resection arthroplasty, and 1 uninfected total knee prosthesis.[45]

A report of 12 patients who acquired another infection in the reimplantation knee differs from these findings.[3] Three knees were treated by arthrodesis, whereas nine knees underwent another salvage attempt with implant removal, débridement, 6 weeks of parenteral antibiotics, and reimplantation. At an average of 31 months' follow-up, the average Knee Society knee score was 79, the average functional score was 73, and no instance of recurrent infection had occurred.[3] Despite these differing viewpoints, the difficulties encountered in obtaining a healed wound, completing a successful knee arthrodesis, and successfully eradicating infection with nonprosthetic salvage procedures after failed reimplantation are considerable. The morbidity and increased likelihood of amputation associated with reinfection must be carefully considered and presented to the patient before additional attempts at reimplantation are undertaken.

KEY REFERENCES

Berbari EF, Marculescu C, Sia I, et al: Culture-negative prosthetic joint infection. Clin Infect Dis 45:1113–1119, 2007.
Bongartz T, Halligan CS, Osmon DR, et al: Incidence and risk factors of prosthetic joint infection after total hip or knee replacement in patients with rheumatoid arthritis. Arthritis Rheum 59:1713–1720, 2008.
Bradbury T, Fehring TK, Taunton M, et al: The fate of acute methicillin-resistant *Staphylococcus aureus* periprosthetic knee infections treated by open debridement and retention of components. J Arthroplasty 24(6 Suppl):101–104, 2009.
Burnett RS, Kelly MA, Hanssen AD, Barrack RL: Technique and timing of two-stage exchange for infection in TKA. Clin Orthop Relat Res 464:164–178, 2007.
Deirmengian C, Lonner JH, Booth RE, Jr: The Mark Coventry Award. White blood cell gene expression: a new approach toward the study and diagnosis of infection. Clin Orthop Relat Res 440:38–44, 2005.
Galat DD, McGovern SC, Hanssen AD, et al: Early return to surgery for evacuation of a postoperative hematoma after primary total knee arthroplasty. J Bone Joint Surg Am 90:2331–2336, 2008.
Galat DD, McGovern SC, Larson DR, et al: Surgical treatment of early wound complications following primary total knee arthroplasty. J Bone Joint Surg Am 91:48–54, 2009.
Ghanem E, Parvizi J, Burnett RS, et al: Cell count and differential of aspirated fluid in the diagnosis of infection at the site of total knee arthroplasty. J Bone Joint Surg Am 90:1637–1643, 2008.
Haleem AA, Berry DJ, Hanssen AD: Mid-term to long-term followup of two-stage reimplantation for infected total knee arthroplasty. Clin Orthop Relat Res 428:35–39, 2004.
Jamsen E, Huhtala H, Puolakka T, Moilanen T: Risk factors for infection after knee arthroplasty: a register-based analysis of 43,149 cases. J Bone Joint Surg Am 91:38–47, 2009.
Kilgus DJ, Howe DJ, Strang A: Results of periprosthetic hip and knee infections caused by resistant bacteria. Clin Orthop Relat Res 404:116–124, 2002.
Kurtz SM, Lau E, Schmier J, et al: Infection burden for hip and knee arthroplasty in the United States. J Arthroplasty 23:984–991, 2008.
Kurtz SM, Ong KL, Lau E, et al: Prosthetic joint infection risk after TKA in the Medicare population. Clin Orthop Relat Res 468:52–56, 2010.
Leone JM, Hanssen AD: Management of infection at the site of a total knee arthroplasty. J Bone Joint Surg Am 87:2335–2348, 2005.
Marculescu CE, Berbari EF, Hanssen AD, Steckelberg JM, Osmon DR: Prosthetic joint infection diagnosed postoperatively by intraoperative culture. Clin Orthop Relat Res 439:38–42, 2005.
Meehan AM, Osmon DR, Duffy MC, Hanssen AD, Keating MR: Outcome of penicillin-susceptible streptococcal prosthetic joint infection treated with debridement and retention of the prosthesis. Clin Infect Dis 36:845–849, 2003.
Mittal Y, Fehring TK, Hanssen A, et al: Two-stage reimplantation for periprosthetic knee infection involving resistant organisms. J Bone Joint Surg Am 89:1227–1231, 2007.
Parvizi J, Bender B, Saleh KJ, et al: Resistant organisms in infected total knee arthroplasty: occurrence, prevention, and treatment regimens. Instr Course Lect 58:271–278, 2009.
Sierra RJ, Trousdale RT, Pagnano MW: Above-the-knee amputation after a total knee replacement: prevalence, etiology, and functional outcome. J Bone Joint Surg Am 85:1000–1004, 2003.
Trampuz A, Piper KE, Jacobson MJ, et al: Sonication of removed hip and knee prostheses for diagnosis of infection. N Engl J Med 357:654–663, 2007.

Full references for this chapter can be found on www.expertconsult.com.

Instability in Total Knee Arthroplasty

James A. Browne, Sebastien Parratte, and Mark W. Pagnano

It has been said that total knee arthroplasty is a soft tissue procedure. Creating rectangular gaps and balancing the soft tissue envelope around the knee are recognized as prerequisites for successful and durable outcomes following total knee arthroplasty. Ligamentous instability is increasingly recognized as a common mode of prosthetic knee failure. Reports in the literature suggest that instability is a reason for 10% to 22% of total knee revisions.* Early failure in the first 5 years following the index arthroplasty is common when stability is not achieved,[6] and instability is second only to infection as the cause of revision surgery less than 2 years after the index operation.[35]

The clinical presentation of instability is variable and the symptoms must be clarified. Symptoms may be apparent immediately after the index arthroplasty or may manifest late and largely depend on the underlying cause of instability. It has been noted that the patient's report of "instability" does not make the diagnosis.[37] Buckling and giving way can have many causes, including pain, fixed flexion contracture of the knee, quadriceps weakness, and patellar dislocation.[37] Whereas gross instability may present with frank dislocation, subtle mechanical instability often presents with vague complaints of anterior knee pain, recurrent effusions, soft tissue tenderness to palpation, and above average range of motion.[29] Patients with subtle instability may also note difficulty in starting ambulation after being seated.

An accurate history is important in determining the factors that led to failure. Considerations include obtaining information on the original diagnosis that precipitated the knee replacement, any preoperative deformity or contracture, previous knee procedures, type of prosthesis, the specifics of the operative technique for knee replacement, the postoperative rehabilitation program, and any trauma to the knee after surgery.[37,43,44] Extra-articular deformity, neuromuscular pathology, and large surgical corrections with ligament releases all have been cited as risk factors that predispose to postoperative instability.[37] Obesity has also been reported as a risk factor for intraoperative collateral ligament injury and complicates both intraoperative and postoperative assessment of soft tissue balance.[42]

The patient's complaints must be carefully reconciled with objective physical examination findings. The physical examination requires assessment of generalized ligamentous laxity and muscle strength. Observation of gait may reveal a varus or valgus thrust and may suggest coronal plane instability. The knee should be examined for anteroposterior and varus/valgus stability and symmetry in extension, 30 degrees of flexion, and 90 degrees of flexion. Subtle instability may be challenging to appreciate if the patient is guarding. Flexion laxity is often most evident when an anterior or posterior

drawer test is performed with the patient sitting and the knee flexed to 90 degrees.[29] The precise amount of laxity and translation that is considered pathologic has not been defined. However, reproduction of a patient's symptoms during laxity testing is at least suggestive of a pathologic link. An above average range of motion may be observed commonly in an unstable knee replacement.[29] The integrity of the extensor mechanism should be assessed as a potential cause of global instability. Aspiration of synovial fluid from the knee may reveal hemarthrosis with elevated red blood cell counts.[32]

A complete set of radiographs, including full-length weight-bearing views, should be obtained. The size and position of the components should be assessed and the mechanical and anatomic axes determined. Weight-bearing views may stress and accentuate the instability (Fig. 129-1). Apparent instability may be readily explained by component wear or loosening, implant breakage, fracture, and bone loss (Fig. 129-2).[37] A large modular tibial insert often suggests problems with intraoperative balancing. Ligament attenuation may have occurred as the result of component overhang. Stress radiographs may provide an objective way to diagnose prosthetic knee instability, although they are rarely used in our clinical practice.

True mechanical instability may be a result of improper surgical technique, poor prosthesis design, incorrect positioning of the implants, and overall limb alignment problems. Instability may be categorized into three types: extension instability, flexion instability, and genu recurvatum or hyperextension deformity. Extension and flexion instability are further subdivided into asymmetrical or symmetrical. The exact nature of the instability should be determined before revision surgery is performed.

EXTENSION INSTABILITY: SYMMETRICAL

Symmetrical extension instability occurs when medial and lateral collateral ligament tensions are lax in extension. In this relatively rare situation, the combined thickness of the components is not sufficient to restore physiologic tension to the ligaments in extension only; this has been termed *instability due to bone resection*.[43,44] Excessive bone removal from the femur will selectively increase the extension gap without altering the flexion gap; this is termed *gap inequality*.[17]

Management of isolated symmetrical extension instability caused by excessive femoral bone loss can be challenging. A thicker tibial insert will not solve the problem. Increasing the tibial insert thickness will elevate the joint line and excessively tighten the flexion space (Fig. 129-3).[37,44] Elevation of the joint line can adversely affect knee kinematics (particularly the patellofemoral joint) and lead to worse clinical outcomes.[31] Distal femoral augments should be used to move the joint line distally. Such augments are available in most contemporary revision total knee systems.

---

*References 3, 7, 15, 16, 36, 43, and 44.

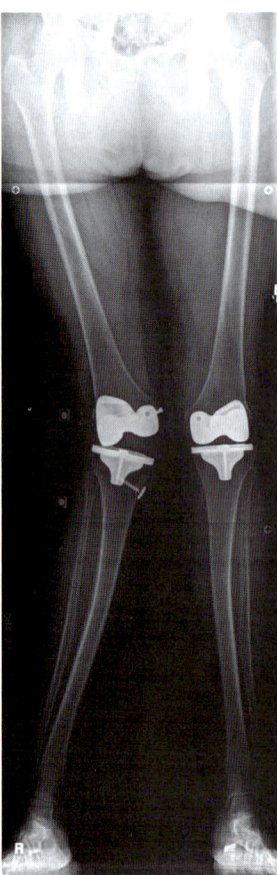

Figure 129-1. Full-length weight-bearing view of a patient with instability of the right knee secondary to medial collateral ligament insufficiency. The patient failed an attempt at allograft reconstruction and required revision to a constrained implant.

EXTENSION INSTABILITY: ASYMMETRICAL

Asymmetrical extension instability is much more common than symmetrical extension instability.[30] This situation is typically related to preoperative angular deformity of the knee and is caused by persistent or iatrogenic ligamentous asymmetry after the knee is replaced (Fig. 129-4).[29,30,37,44] Fear of creating iatrogenic ligamentous instability in the opposite direction is a frequent reason for incomplete ligament balancing and undercorrection of deformity.

In the case of a varus knee, concerns about over-releasing the medial collateral ligament can leave the knee tight on the medial side—a situation exacerbated by leaving the limb alignment in varus.[29,37,44] Excessive medial collateral ligament tension and varus malalignment can result in medial overload with polyethylene wear and further stretching out of the lateral ligaments.[29,37,44] Recurrence of deformity may occur postoperatively. An appropriate medial release as originally described by Insall and associates should be performed when necessary.[15] A thicker tibial insert may be required following medial release to restore tension in the collateral ligaments. Lateral collateral ligament advancement can be considered if complete medial release fails to balance the knee.[18]

Asymmetrical extension instability may result from undercorrection of a valgus knee deformity. Failure to appropriately release contracted lateral tissues will leave laxity or redundancy in the medial collateral ligament. The medial collateral ligament has no ability to tighten over time, and the valgus deformity will recur.[37,43] Minimal laxity of the medial collateral ligament should therefore be accepted. Sequential lateral ligament release approaches[12,15] have been associated with frequent over-release of the lateral soft tissues.[27] As a result, the "pie-crust" multiple puncture technique has gained

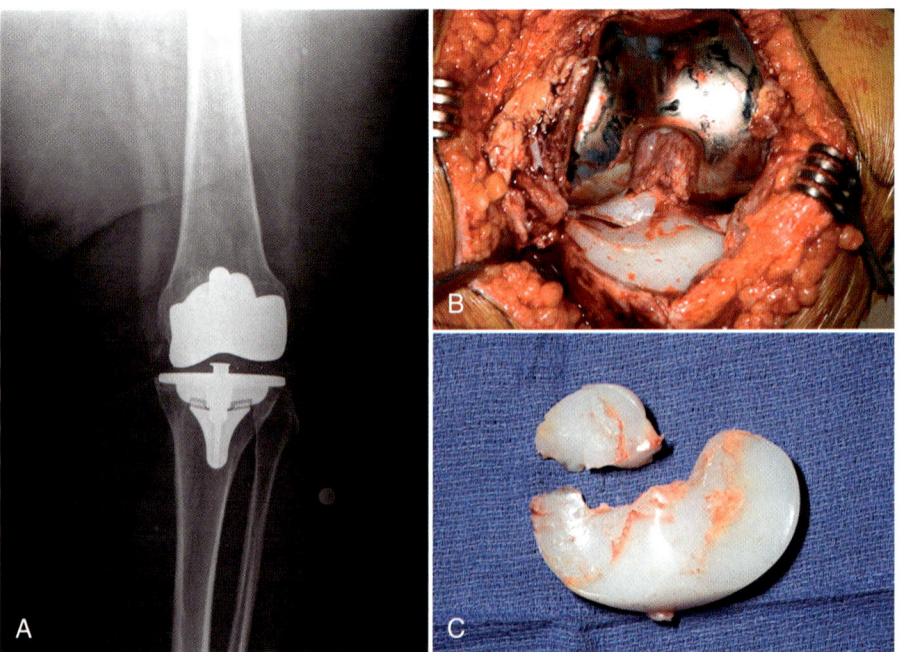

Figure 129-2. A, Anteroposterior radiograph of an obese patient with an unstable left total knee arthroplasty. Note varus positioning of the components and lack of parallelism between the distal femoral component and tibial tray. **B** and **C,** Intraoperative photographs at the time of revision demonstrating medial overload with wear and catastrophic failure of the polyethylene.

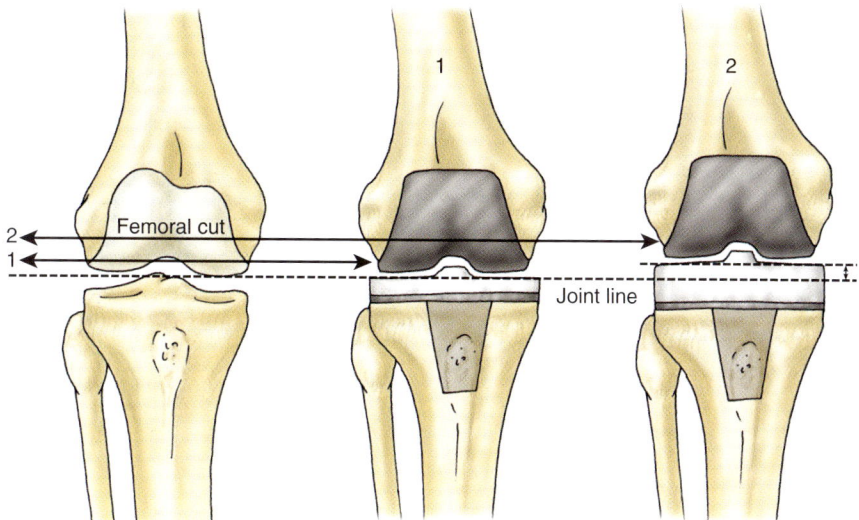

Figure 129-3. Excessive bone removal from the distal part of the femur cannot be managed with the use of a thicker tibial insert, which will elevate the joint line and excessively tighten the flexion space. (Reprinted with permission from Vail TP, Lang JE: Surgical techniques and instrumentation in total knee arthroplasty. In Insall JN, Scott WN [eds]: Surgery of the knee, ed 4, vol 2, Baltimore, Md, 2006, Churchill Livingstone, pp 1455–1521.)

widespread use.[4,27] To check for an over-released lateral side, the trials can be inserted and the knee placed in a "figure-of-four" position (90 degrees of knee flexion while the surgeon holds the foot and allows the hip and knee to maximally externally rotate). If the post of a posterior stabilized insert subluxates from the femoral housing, a thicker or more constrained tibial insert should be used.[4]

Complete correction of severe valgus deformity incurs the risk of peroneal nerve stretch.[5] Satisfactory results have been reported with intentional deformity undercorrection and the use of a varus/valgus constrained implant to compensate for residual medial collateral ligament laxity.[5] This approach carries the theoretical concern that a constrained implant will impart additional stresses to the implant and fixation interfaces and should be reserved for elderly, lower demand patients.

Intraoperative iatrogenic collateral ligament injury can occur, most commonly when the proximal tibia is cut. Vigorous attempts to assess stability intraoperatively can lead to ligament stretch or rupture, typically of the medial collateral ligament. Surgical reapproximation of the ligament is the recommended approach.[21] The hamstring tendons may be used to augment the repair, and a condylar constrained implant may be used to enhance stability.[5,21] Postoperative bracing may help reduce stresses on the healing ligament.[21]

FLEXION INSTABILITY: SYMMETRICAL

Symmetrical flexion instability is likely under-reported as the diagnosis can be elusive. This distinct clinical entity can occur with both posterior stabilized and cruciate retaining designs and is characterized by painful subluxation of the tibia on the femur. This situation is often seen in patients in whom the total knee prosthesis is well aligned axially and well fixed.[29] Manifestations of flexion instability differ depending on the cause of the problem and the implant design.

A large flexion gap may result from inadequate filling with the implant, often due to under-resection of the distal femur in an attempt to avoid elevating the joint line. In this scenario, the surgeon will typically preferentially balance the resulting tight extension gap at the expense of a loose flexion gap. With trials in place, the tibia should have less than 5 mm of anteroposterior translation when the knee is tested intraoperatively at 90 degrees of flexion with the patella reduced.[30] The "figure-of-four" position, as described earlier, can be used to establish that the knee will not dislocate.

Dislocation of a posterior stabilized total knee arthroplasty is rare but dramatic, with a reported incidence between 0% and 0.5%.[9,14,22] If the flexion gap is large enough, the cam mechanism may jump over the post, resulting in posterior dislocation of the tibia on the femur. Dislocation typically occurs with marked knee flexion plus a valgus or varus stress (such as occurs when crossing the legs to put on socks or shoes).[8] At-risk patients include those who had correction of a large valgus deformity, particularly if they quickly regained knee flexion postoperatively.[34] First-time dislocations should be treated with closed reduction, a trial of bracing, and avoidance of the activity that induced the dislocation, although severe laxity will often lead to repeated dislocations. Mobile-bearing designs may require open reduction.[13] Recurrent dislocation may require revision with thicker polyethylene (if the extension space permits). A constrained condylar implant may be helpful but will not prevent repeat dislocation in the setting of continued gap imbalance (Fig. 129-5). The "Figure 4" maneuver can be used to assess correction of the instability.

Posterior stabilized total knee replacements can be symptomatically unstable in flexion without dislocating. Schwab and colleagues described a typical constellation of symptoms and physical findings, including a sense of instability without giving way, recurrent knee effusions, multiple areas of soft tissue tenderness about the knee, and substantial anterior

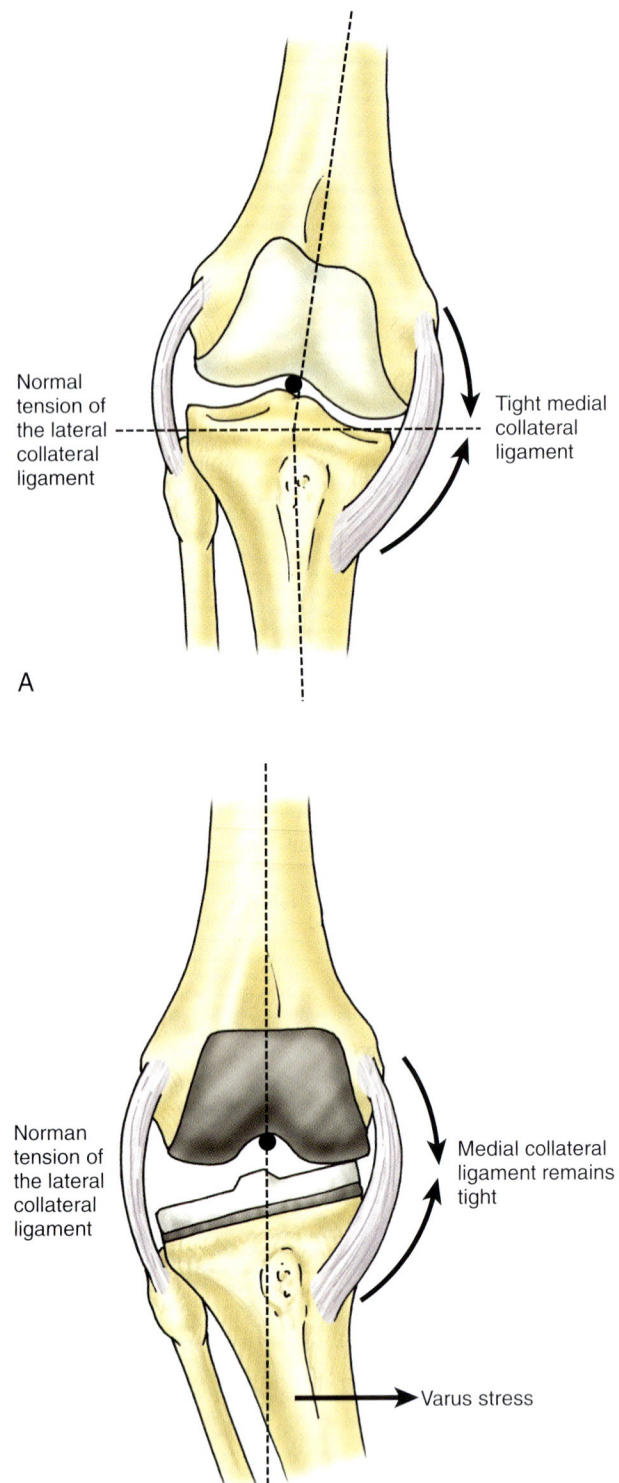

A

B

Figure 129-4. **A,** Example of a varus knee with a contracted medial collateral ligament that has been incompletely released. **B,** The medial collateral ligament remains tight, and the lateral collateral ligament is subsequently lax. (Reprinted with permission from Vail TP, Lang JE: Surgical techniques and instrumentation in total knee arthroplasty. In Insall JN, Scott WN [eds]: Surgery of the knee, ed 4, vol 2, Baltimore, Md, 2006, Churchill Livingstone, pp 1455–1521.)

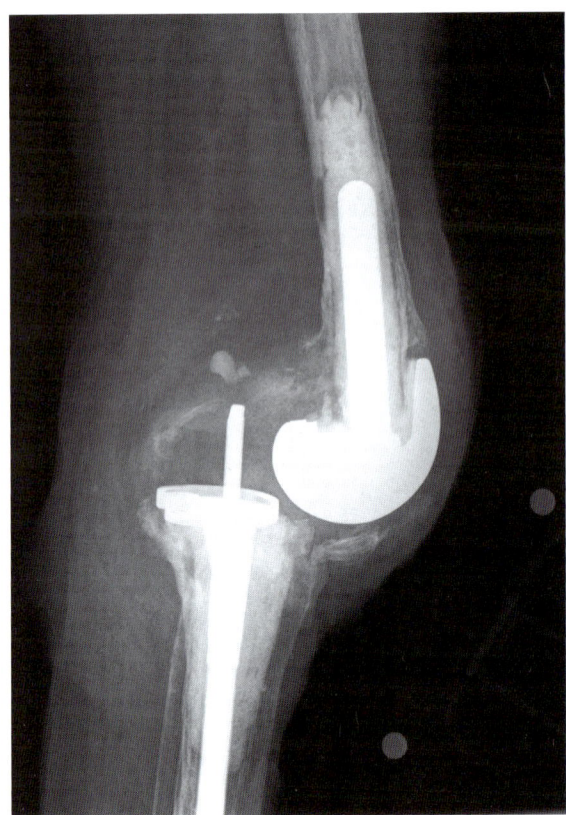

Figure 129-5. Revision to a constrained posterior stabilized implant can result in dislocation if the flexion gap is not balanced.

tibial translation at 90 degrees of flexion.[34] They reported reliable results in alleviating pain, improving stability, and improving patient satisfaction in 10 patients following revision, usually with a larger femoral component and posterior femoral augmentation.

Flexion instability after cruciate retaining total knee arthroplasty has been well described but likely remains underdiagnosed.[29] The clinical presentation is similar to that described previously for posterior stabilized knee designs. Typically, this occurs in knees with well-fixed, well-positioned implants.[29] A posterior sag or drawer sign is often observed (Fig. 129-6). Visible anterior translation of the tibia on the femur while the leg is extended from a seated, 90-degree flexed position may be present.[40] The knee is usually stable to varus and valgus stress in extension. Multiple causes of flexion instability after cruciate retaining total knee arthroplasty are possible (Table 129-1). A tibial liner with a flat sagittal plane contour offers little resistance to anteroposterior translation and may contribute to flexion instability.

Early flexion instability is often the result of technical error. Undersizing the femoral component in the anteroposterior dimension will decrease the posterior offset and selectively increase the flexion gap. Postoperative lateral radiographs may suggest over-resection of the posterior condyles compared with preoperative views. Excessive tibial slope will lead to a total knee that is well balanced in extension but loose in flexion (Fig. 129-7). This scenario puts the posterior cruciate ligament at risk for iatrogenic injury. In these cases, revision surgery should focus on rebalancing the

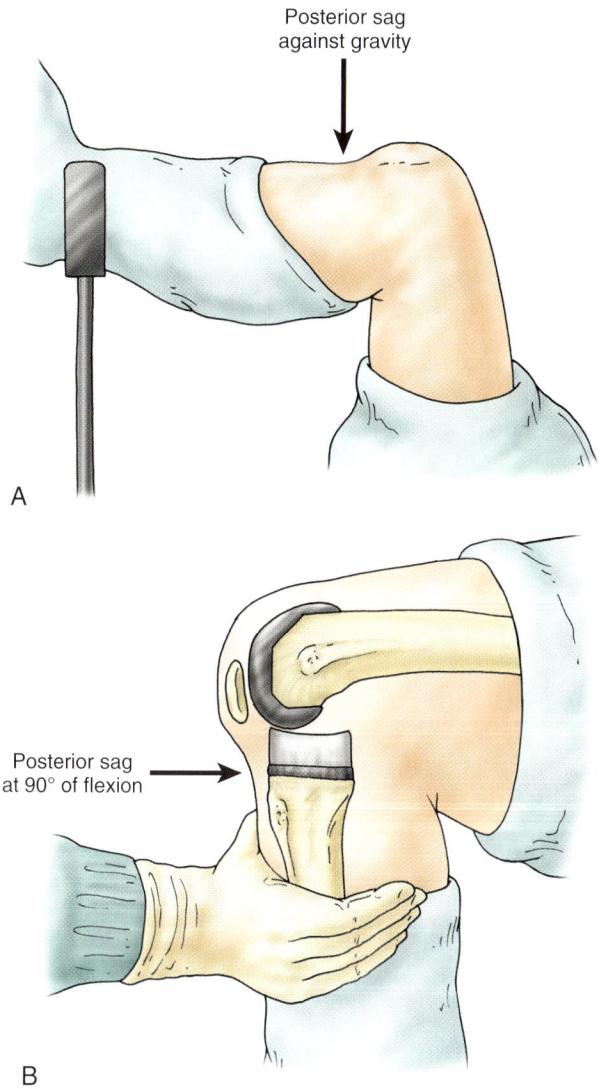

A

B

Figure 129-6. **A,** A posterior sag at 90 degrees of flexion is typically observed with flexion instability. **B,** A posterior drawer sign is also commonly observed. On a lateral radiograph, the tibia can be subluxated posteriorly beyond the anterior lip of the tibial insert. (Reproduced with permission from Pagnano MW, Hanssen AD, Lewallen DA, Stuart MJ: Flexion instability after primary posterior cruciate retaining total knee arthroplasty. Clin Orthop Relat Res [356]:39–46, 1998.)

Posterior sag against gravity

Posterior sag at 90° of flexion

knee; converting to a posterior-stabilized implant design is typically the most reliable approach.

Injury to the posterior cruciate ligament can manifest as early or late flexion instability. Direct iatrogenic injury at the time of knee replacement may lead to early failure. Leaving the flexion space excessively tight can lead to early indirect iatrogenic failure of the posterior cruciate ligament. Patients with a tight knee in flexion may work aggressively to regain motion in the postoperative period and rupture the posterior cruciate ligament. These patients often recall a specific event when a pop or snap occurs in concert with a sudden increase in motion. Late instability may be observed when

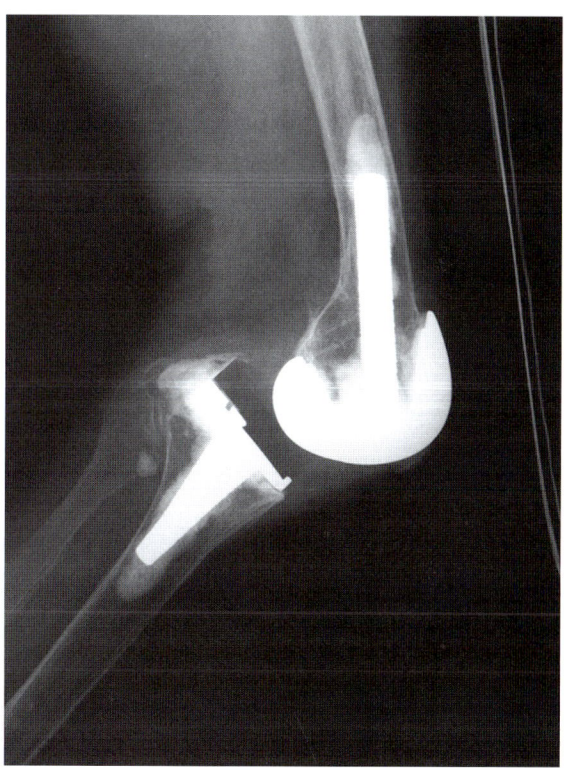

Figure 129-7. Flexion instability with posterior translation of the tibia occurring several years after revision knee replacement in a patient with a previous patellectomy. A flat polyethylene liner has exacerbated the instability.

Table 129-1 Causes of Flexion Instability After Cruciate Retaining Total Knee Arthroplasty

Cause of Flexion Instability	Presentation of Clinical Symptoms	Considerations	Revision Solution
Undersized femoral component	Early	Encouraged by anterior referencing	Use larger femoral components, posterior augments
Excessive tibial slope	Early	Puts PCL at risk for iatrogenic damage	Recut tibia and rebalance, convert to PS implant
Acute rupture of PCL	Variable	Flexion space too tight after TKA	Rebalance and convert to PS implant
Attritional rupture of PCL	Late	Attrition of PCL or reactivation of inflammatory arthritis	Revise to PS implant
Posteromedial polyethylene wear	Late	Functionally increases the flexion space, synovitis	Perform isolated polyethylene exchange or complete revision

PCL, Posterior cruciate ligament; *PS,* posterior stabilized; *TKA,* total knee arthroplasty.

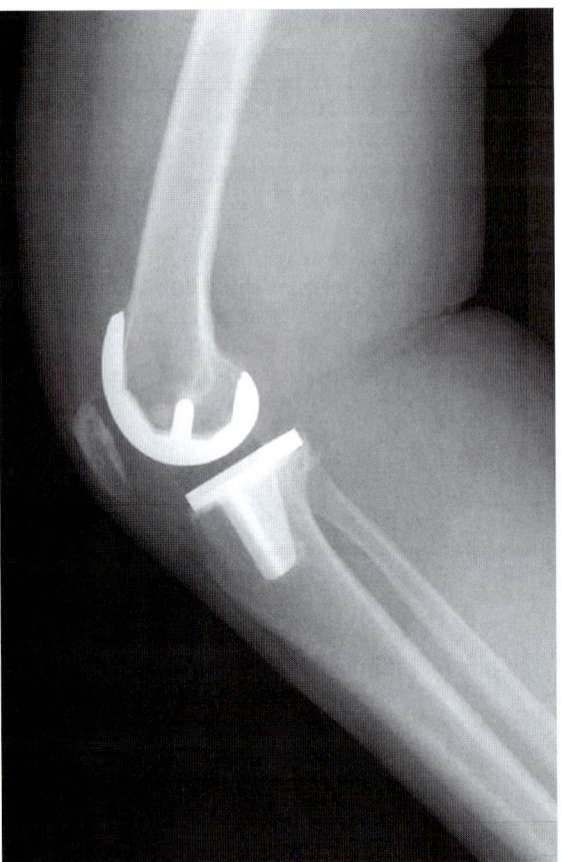

Figure 129-8. Excessive posterior slope (16 degrees in this example) can lead to symptomatic flexion instability.

the posterior cruciate ligament deteriorates from age-related changes or following reactivation of inflammatory disease (Fig. 129-8).[28] Posterior instability with incapacitating anterior knee pain and swelling has been reported in 8% of patients following cruciate retaining knees.[40] In patients with rheumatoid arthritis, late instability has been reported in 2% to 15% of knees at long-term follow-up using cruciate retaining implants.[1,10,26,28]

Initial treatment options include quadriceps strengthening and local modalities for tenderness and swelling. Bracing may afford some symptomatic relief. However, nonoperative treatment generally has not been successful in our experience. Operative management is often required for patients with incapacitating symptoms and marked disability.[1,26,29]

Operative management with isolated tibial polyethylene exchange is inherently appealing as it minimizes blood loss, bone loss, and operative time. However, this approach should be used with caution. Upsizing the liner does not address the underlying imbalance between flexion and extension gaps and therefore is not recommended. A high rate of failure has been reported with revision operations that included only insertion of a thicker tibial polyethylene.[1,29] One exception may occur when posteromedial polyethylene liner wear has functionally increased the flexion space, resulting in instability.

Conversion to a posterior stabilized design is the preferred approach when a cruciate retaining implant is revised for flexion instability; it facilitates balancing of flexion and extension spaces. Careful attention must be directed toward gap balancing, as converting to a posterior stabilized prosthesis alone is likely to fail. In a series from our institution, 19 of 22 knees revised in this manner were satisfactorily improved.[29]

FLEXION INSTABILITY: ASYMMETRICAL

The extent to which mild isolated collateral ligament asymmetry in flexion without dislocation is symptomatic is unclear.[17] A rectangular flexion gap is created by a combination of posterior condylar resection, femoral component rotation, and/or ligament release. Femoral component malrotation may result in patellofemoral malalignment, an asymmetrical trapezoidal flexion gap, and asymmetrical collateral laxity in flexion.[20,33] Appropriate femoral component rotation remains a source of some debate, with so-called gap balancing surgeons advocating rotation of the femur to create a rectangular gap via bone cuts, and other surgeons favoring femoral rotation set to anatomic landmarks (often the transepicondylar axis) with rectangular gap symmetry subsequently created by selective ligament release.

The clinical implications of asymmetrical flexion instability are unclear. Whiteside, Krakow, and others have advocated setting femoral component rotation with bony landmarks and accepting slight soft tissue asymmetry.[17,41] However, Laskin found increased range of flexion and less medial tibial pain with a rectangular flexion space compared with an asymmetrical trapezoidal gap.[20] Large medial release with a resultant grossly asymmetrical flexion gap may lead to dislocation of the tibial component but may otherwise be asymptomatic.

MIDFLEXION INSTABILITY

The concept of midflexion instability is contentious, and the condition remains to be fully defined as a distinct clinical entity. Coronal plane instability due to collateral ligament imbalance may be masked by tightness of the posterior capsule in full extension and may be experienced by the patient in early flexion. Patients may also experience true flexion instability earlier in the flexion arc.

In a cadaveric study, Martin and Whiteside found a significant increase in varus/valgus laxity during midflexion when the femoral component was positioned 5 mm proximally and 5 mm anteriorly.[23] Although collateral ligament tension appeared appropriate in full extension and 90 degrees of flexion, alteration in position of the joint line appeared to alter ligament tension at intermediate angles. The authors suggested that this midrange laxity leads to progressive stretching of secondary restraints and increased instability over time. Accelerated polyethylene wear can also occur as a result.[2]

Femoral component sagittal plane design may play a role in collateral ligament isometry in midflexion. In response to the traditional view that multiple instantaneous centers of flexion and extension rotation exist in the knee, femoral components have been traditionally designed with multiple radii of rotation. However, as our understanding of knee kinematics has changed, some systems have been designed with a single radius of rotation. The shift from a longer to a shorter radius within a multiple-radius design has been reported to cause temporary varus/valgus instability during knee flexion between 30 degrees and 45 degrees.[38] Corresponding functional performance differences have been reported,[39] although additional studies are required to determine the clinical significance of this finding.

Despite various descriptions of midflexion instability following primary total knee arthroplasty, no studies have been performed to evaluate approaches to treatment. Although this has not been proven, extrapolation from flexion instability would suggest that nonoperative management is likely to be unsuccessful in the patient with significant symptoms. No data are available on the outcomes of revision total knee arthroplasty for midflexion instability.

Midflexion instability has been described in revision total knee arthroplasty as rotational instability with combined external rotation and valgus stress in a knee flexed between 45 degrees and 90 degrees.[24] Anterior medial collateral ligament attenuation, femoral-tibial articular geometry, and tibial postfemoral box geometry were reported to contribute to this instability.

RECURVATUM OR HYPEREXTENSION DEFORMITY

Preoperative recurvatum in the primary total knee arthroplasty setting is rare and most commonly occurs in patients with neuromuscular disease.[19,25] Patients with true quadriceps weakness, such as those with polio, will compensate by ambulating with the knee locked in hyperextension, the so-call back knee gait. Patients with a fixed valgus deformity and an isolated iliotibial band contracture may demonstrate recurvatum. This is a classic contraindication to total knee arthroplasty,[37] and surgery should be approached with caution. Postoperatively, the patient with marked quadriceps weakness will continue to force the knee into hyperextension to stabilize the joint during stance, resulting in progressive recurvatum. Consideration should be given to under-resection or augmentation of the distal femur to move the joint line distally, with the knee left with a slight flexion contracture at the conclusion of the procedure (Fig. 129-9). Alternatively, the femoral origins of the collateral ligaments

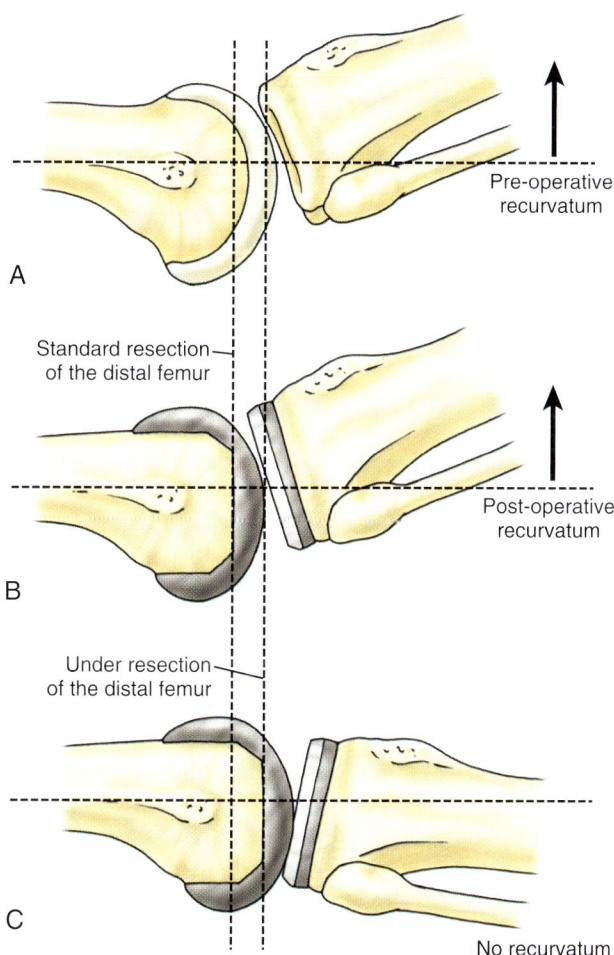

Figure 129-9. Consideration should be given to under-resection of the distal femur at the time of total knee arthroplasty in the patient with **(A)** hyperextension, because **(B)** standard resection will leave the patient with a postoperative recurvatum deformity. It is reasonable to leave the knee with **(C)** a slight flexion contracture at the conclusion of the procedure. (Reprinted with permission from Vail TP, Lang JE: Surgical techniques and instrumentation in total knee arthroplasty. In Insall JN, Scott WN [eds]: Surgery of the knee, ed 4, vol 2, Baltimore, Md, 2006, Churchill Livingstone, pp 1455–1521.)

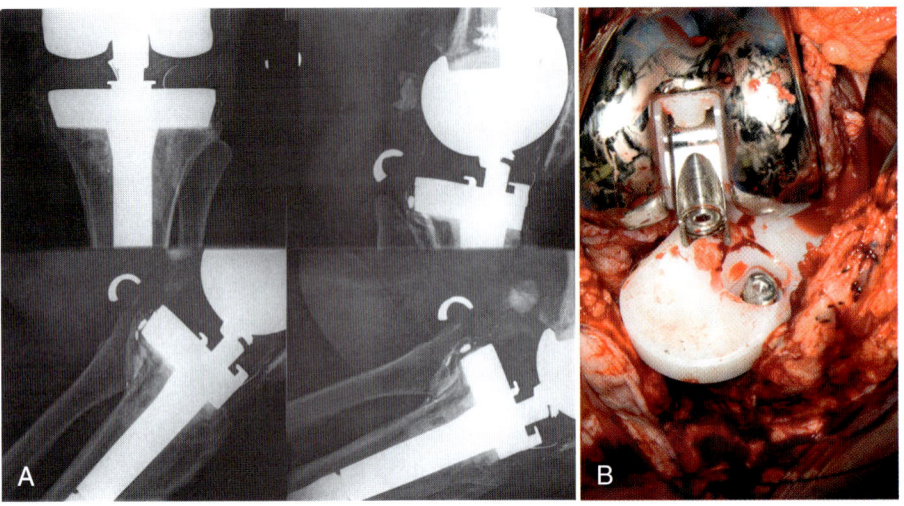

Figure 129-10. A, Radiographs of a broken hinged revision total knee arthroplasty secondary to hyperextension. Note the metallic density in the posterior aspect of the knee. The patient was morbidly obese. **B,** Intraoperative photograph shows the fractured hinge, necessitating complete femoral revision with distalization of the joint line.

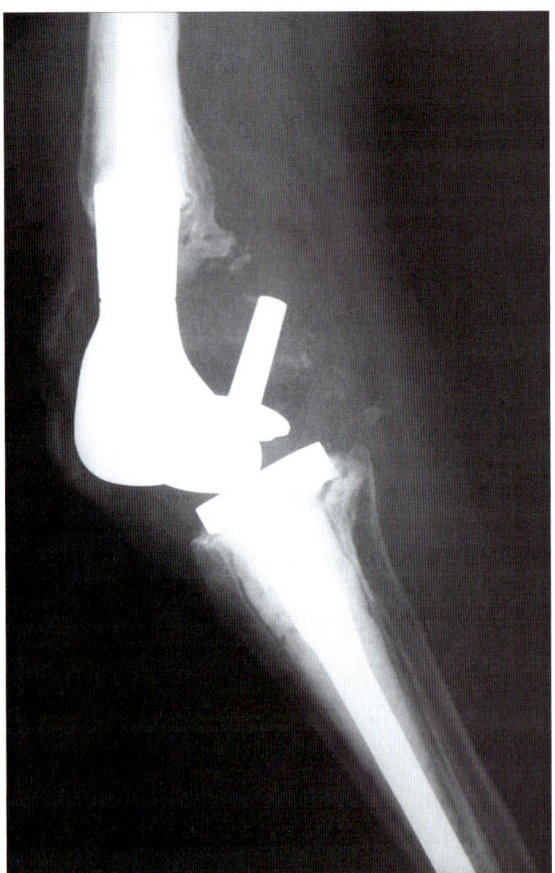

Figure 129-11. A dislocated hinged revision total knee arthroplasty. The hinge mechanism became disassociated from the tibial component in deep knee flexion.

may be moved proximally and posteriorly to re-create normal tightening action during full extension of the knee.[19] The cam action of the prosthesis with a curved insert combined with collateral ligament transfer can prevent recurvatum.

Once established, a recurvatum deformity following primary total knee arthroplasty is difficult to treat. A rotating-hinge total knee prosthesis with an extension stop has been advocated in patients with failed implants or quadriceps lacking antigravity strength.[11] Although this can provide a satisfactory solution, continued hyperextension may lead to mechanical failure of the hinge, particularly in obese patients (Fig. 129-10). With some designs, persistently lax soft tissues in flexion may allow the hinge mechanism to dislocate from the tibial component (Fig. 129-11).

KEY REFERENCES

Callaghan JJ, O'Rourke MR, Saleh KJ: Why knees fail: lessons learned. J Arthroplasty 19(4 Suppl 1):31–34, 2004.

Clarke HD, Fuchs R, Scuderi GR, et al: Clinical results in valgus total knee arthroplasty with the "pie crust" technique of lateral soft tissue releases. J Arthroplasty 20:1010–1014, 2005.

Easley ME, Insall JN, Scuderi GR, Bullek DD: Primary constrained condylar knee arthroplasty for the arthritic valgus knee. Clin Orthop Relat Res 380:58–64, 2000.

Giori NJ, Lewallen DG: Total knee arthroplasty in limbs affected by poliomyelitis. J Bone Joint Surg Am 84:1157–1161, 2002.

Insall JN, Binazzi R, Soudry M, Mestriner LA: Total knee arthroplasty. Clin Orthop Relat Res 192:13–22, 1985.

Krackow KA, Weiss AP: Recurvatum deformity complicating performance of total knee arthroplasty: a brief note. J Bone Joint Surg Am 72:268–271, 1990.

Laskin RS: Flexion space configuration in total knee arthroplasty. J Arthroplasty 10:657–660, 1995.

Leopold SS, McStay C, Klafeta K, et al: Primary repair of intraoperative disruption of the medial collateral ligament during total knee arthroplasty. J Bone Joint Surg Am 83:86–91, 2001.

Pagnano MW, Hanssen AD, Lewallen DG, Stuart MJ: Flexion instability after primary posterior cruciate retaining total knee arthroplasty. Clin Orthop Relat Res 356:39–46, 1998.

Parratte S, Pagnano MW: Instability after total knee arthroplasty. J Bone Joint Surg Am 90:184–194, 2008.

Raab GE, Fehring TK, Odum SM, et al: Aspiration as an aid to the diagnosis of prosthetic knee instability. Orthopedics 32:318, 2009.

Schwab JH, Haidukewych GJ, Hanssen AD, et al: Flexion instability without dislocation after posterior stabilized total knees. Clin Orthop Relat Res 440:96–100, 2005.

Sharkey PF, Hozack WJ, Rothman RH, et al: Insall Award paper. Why are total knee arthroplasties failing today? Clin Orthop Relat Res 404:7–13, 2002.

Vince KG, Abdeen A, Sugimori T: The unstable total knee arthroplasty: causes and cures. J Arthroplasty 21(4 Suppl 1):44–49, 2006.

Winiarsky R, Barth P, Lotke P: Total knee arthroplasty in morbidly obese patients. J Bone Joint Surg Am 80:1770–1774, 1998.

Full references for this chapter can be found on www.expertconsult.com.

Management of Bone Defects in Revision Total Knee Arthroscopy: Augments, Structural and Impaction Grafts, and Cones

R. Michael Meneghini and Arlen D. Hanssen

Bone loss may be encountered in a multitude of scenarios during revision total knee arthroplasty (TKA), such as osteolysis, infection, and component subsidence, and is a challenge to the joint replacement surgeon. Appropriate reconstructive techniques are dictated by the quantity and location of tibial and/or femoral bone loss. Reconstructive strategies include fill with cement and screws, block augments, impaction or bulk allografts, and newly developed highly porous metaphyseal cones. This chapter details the indications, basic surgical techniques, and available clinical results for these reconstructive strategies.

BACKGROUND

Reconstruction of large bony defects in the femur and tibia during revision knee replacement remains a challenging clinical problem. Smaller bone defects have been traditionally and effectively treated with limited quantities of morselized cancellous bone graft,[3,27] cement augmented with screw fixation,[1,11,28,29] or modular augments attached to revision prosthetic implants.[4,14] Large or massive bone defects require more extensive reconstructive efforts and have been managed traditionally with the use of large structural allografts,* impaction bone grafting techniques with or without mesh augmentation,[17,32,33,36] fabrication of custom prosthetic components,[8] or specialized hinged knee components.[15] Despite the multitude of utilized treatment methods, the best reconstructive technique for bone defects during revision knee replacement has not been clearly determined.[8]

Preoperative Planning

In revision knee arthroplasties with bone deficiency, it is helpful to determine several important variables to establish the requirements of reconstruction. Good quality anteroposterior, lateral, and patellar views are usually sufficient for assessment of bone loss in the large majority of cases; however, tomograms are occasionally helpful. It is often stated that the magnitude of bone loss observed on preoperative radiographs vastly underestimates the true magnitude of bone loss discovered intraoperatively. This tenet is particularly true of bone loss associated with osteolysis secondary to wear debris. If a lateral radiograph of the knee obtained before the original arthroplasty was performed is unavailable, a lateral radiograph of the opposite knee is valuable to determine the appropriate anteroposterior dimension of the knee. A true lateral radiograph, obtained with fluoroscopically positioning, may occasionally be useful for accurate assessment of the anteroposterior dimensions of the femur.

Bone loss in the four primary areas of typical occurrence assessed. The severity and location of bone loss and the quality of remaining bone should be assessed. The location of the joint line is marked and noted. The optimal joint line position is roughly 2 cm below the origin of the medial collateral ligament and 2.5 cm below the prominence of the lateral epicondyle. In some knees, particularly those with *flexion instability*, the prosthetic joint line may actually be lower than the anatomic joint line, which usually suggests that additional distal femoral resection will be required during the revision procedure to balance flexion and extension spaces.

BONE LOSS ASSESSMENT AND CLASSIFICATION

The critical step in determining the appropriate reconstruction method in revision total knee replacement (TKR) is to accurately determine the quantity, location, and extent of bone loss. This is done after meticulous removal of failed tibial and femoral implants, with careful attention to existing bone preservation. Once the components have been removed, it is important to determine whether the defects are contained or uncontained (segmental). In addition, the location of supportive bone that surrounds the bone loss is essential and will dictate the type and size of augmentation that is required. Smaller contained defects can be treated with cement fill with screw augmentation or with morselized allograft fill, particularly in older patients. However, larger uncontained defects typically require larger reconstructive measures such as modular block augments, bulk allograft, or highly porous metal metaphyseal cones.

A common system of categorizing bone defects in revision knee arthroplasty is the Anderson Orthopaedic Research Institute Bone Defect Classification.[8] This system permits communication and comparison of knees between different institutions and also allows preoperative and postoperative classification and management recommendations for specific bone defect severities. In this bone defect classification, type 1 defects describe only minor and contained cancellous bony defects within either tibial plateau, type 2A defects include moderate to severe cancellous and/or cortical bone defects of only one tibial plateau, type 2B defects consist of moderate to severe cancellous bone defects of both tibial plateaus and/or segmental cortical defects of one tibial plateau, and type 3 defects describe combined cavitary and segmental bone loss in both tibial plateaus.

RECONSTRUCTION WITH CEMENT AND SCREWS

Cement used as a reconstructive augment has the attraction of being simple, inexpensive, and efficient, as the revision

---

*References 7, 9, 10, 13, 14, 21-23, 31, and 34.

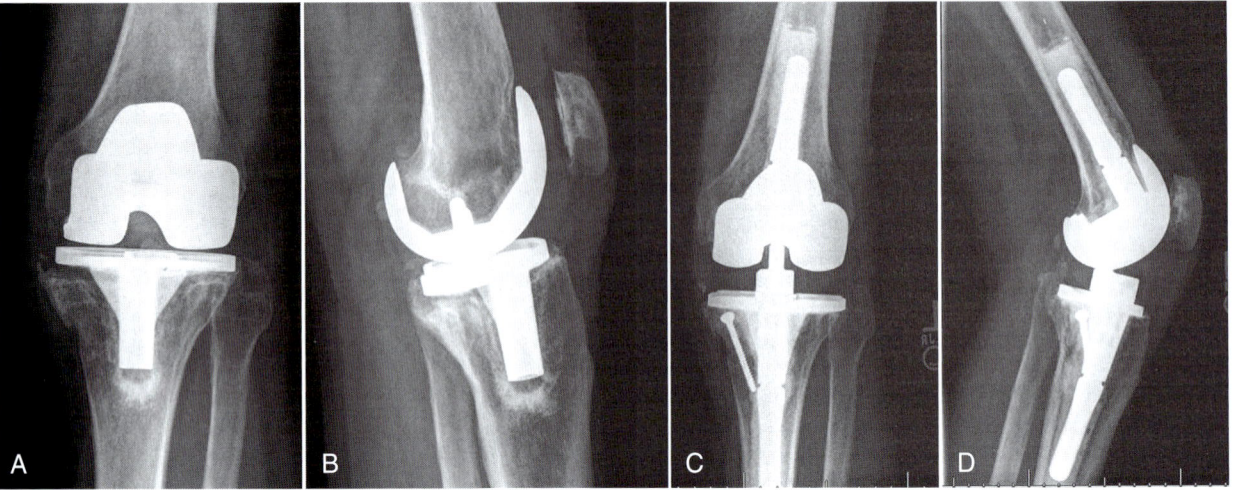

Figure 130-1. A, Anteroposterior (AP) and **(B)** lateral radiographs of contained medial tibial bone defect secondary to osteolysis. **C,** AP and **(D)** lateral radiographs of the reconstruction utilizing cement fill with screw augmentation at 12 months' follow-up. Note the screw head well below and without contact with the tibial tray.

knee arthroplasty is already utilizing the material for fixation in most instances. This reconstruction method is typically indicated for smaller contained defects measuring less than 5 mm in depth,[1,11] although some authors have advocated its use in larger defects with excellent clinical results.[28,29] When cement is used for defects in revision knee arthroplasty, augmentation with bone screws is typically recommended to enhance the biomechanical properties of the construct (Fig. 130-1). In addition, if the patient is young and active, it may be more advantageous to utilize morselized allograft to restore bone stock in these types of defects.

Surgical Technique

The surgical technique begins with tibial or femoral provisional or freshening cuts. Once these are performed, a more accurate assessment of the defect is possible. Meticulous débridement of the defect is performed with removal of all fibrous tissue that would impede adequate interdigitation of the cement and create suboptimal fixation. Sclerotic bone surfaces are frequently encountered in revision surgeries; these must be roughened with a small drill or a burr. Once the defect is clearly delineated and prepared, the location of remaining bone is identified for adequate screw fixation. Sloping surfaces are converted to step-shaped to minimize the quantity of shear forces acting on the cement, as cement is known to be much more biomechanically stable and supportive in compression. If the defect is of minimal depth, it may be filled with cement alone during cementation of the standard revision tibial or femoral components. If defects are larger, or if the surgeon is uncertain, reinforcement with screw augmentation is recommended. Once the bone defect has been adequately prepared for cement, titanium, self-tapping cancellous bone screws are placed into the host metaphyseal bone and are advanced so that the heads are positioned below the level of the eventual tibial tray or femoral component. Titanium screws are typically used to prevent galvanic corrosion that occurs with dissimilar metals, because a majority of tibial baseplates are composed of titanium. Once the screw is in position, the trial components are inserted to ensure that there is no contact of the screw head with the prosthesis. Once the cement has been mixed and is in a doughy state, it is placed into the defect and around the screw heads and is pressurized by hand. The final prosthesis is then placed and cement is allowed to cure with removal of the excess.

Clinical Results

Satisfactory midterm results have been reported with the use of screws and cement for bone defects in TKA. Ritter and associates[28] reported on 57 TKRs with large (9 ± 5 mm) medial tibial defects reconstructed with screws and cement at an average of 6.1 years' follow-up.[28] Although nonprogressive radiolucent lines were common and were seen in 27%, no cases of tibial component loosening, component failure, or cement failure were reported. In a subsequent report by the same authors, 125 TKAs that utilized screws and cement to fill large medial tibial defects secondary to severe varus deformities were reported at a mean of 7.9 years' follow-up.[29] The authors reported two failures that occurred as the result of medial tibial collapse at 5 and 10 years, respectively, but no other failure or loosening was observed in the remainder of the cohort. However, this was a series of primary knee arthroplasties without the typical stem extensions used in revision knee arthroplasty to augment fixation and prevent medial collapse in the setting of bone deficiency and suboptimal bone quality. Therefore, in smaller and contained defects such as those encountered in revision knee arthroplasty, particularly in older or less active patients, the use of screws and cement is a viable and successful method of reconstruction that is inexpensive, relatively simple, and efficient.

RECONSTRUCTION WITH MORSELIZED ALLOGRAFT

Bone loss in revision knee arthroplasty can be treated reliably and successfully with morselized cancellous allograft and has

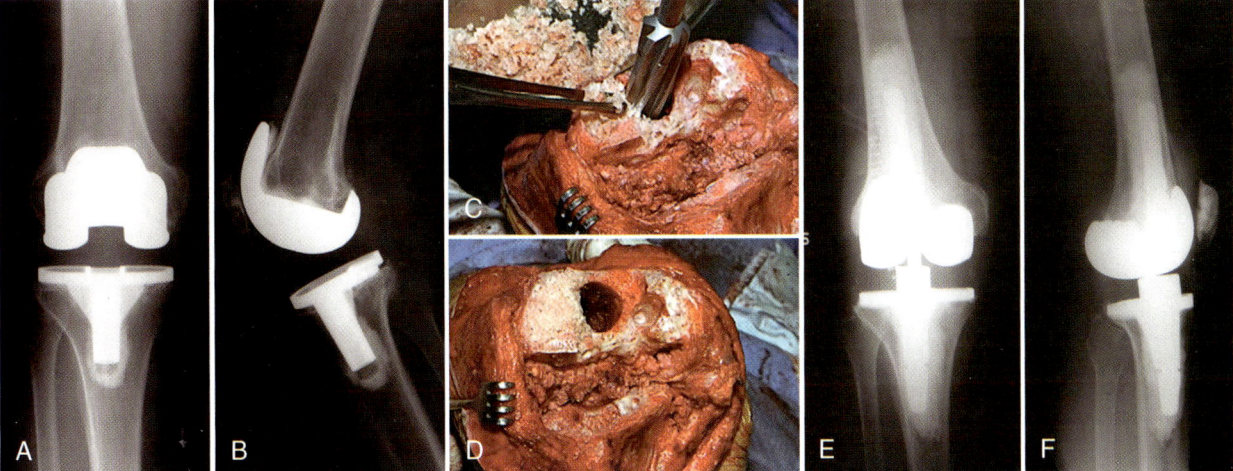

Figure 130-2. A, Anteroposterior (AP) and **(B)** lateral radiographs of failed total knee replacement (TKR) with severe femoral bone loss in the lateral condyle secondary to osteolysis. **C,** Intraoperative picture of impaction grafting using the intramedullary reamer to facilitate compaction of morselized allograft into the defect. **D,** Removal of the reamer after morselized allograft compaction demonstrating complete fill and reconstitution of the contained defect. **E,** AP and **(F)** lateral radiographs of the revision TKR in parts **A** and **B** demonstrating the reconstituted lateral femoral defect bypassed with an intramedullary stem.

an established clinical track record.* This method typically is reserved for contained defects (Fig. 130-2) and is particularly attractive for younger patients, in whom restoration of deficient bone stock is a priority given the potential for future reconstructive surgeries. Biologically, morselized cancellous allograft appears to incorporate similarly to cancellous autograft, albeit at a much slower rate. It is also beneficial to have a well-vascularized recipient bed to facilitate incorporation of the allograft bone; if a highly sclerotic defect is encountered, it may be beneficial to burr away the sclerotic bone to underlying cancellous and vascular bone, or conversely to use another reconstruction method such as a block augment. Furthermore, if the defect is large and segmental, although some authors have reported adequate results with impaction allografting,[17,18] reconstruction with more robust structural augments such as metal blocks, bulk allograft, or metaphyseal porous metal cones typically will produce more biomechanically stable constructs.

Surgical Technique

As with all reconstructive techniques, the surgical technique of utilizing morselized allograft to fill contained defects requires meticulous débridement of the defect with careful attention to removal of all fibrous tissue. Careful attention is paid to preparation of a vascular bed for allograft incorporation to host bone and long-term bone reconstruction. Once the defect is adequately débrided, prepared, and confirmed to be contained with supporting peripheral structures, the morselized allograft can be inserted into the defect. It is also preferential to grind up any larger pieces into a fine morselized consistency to facilitate the development of biologic and structural properties. It is helpful to place an adequately sized reamer or trial stem into the medullary canal to impact

the morselized allograft material around the reamer; this facilitates compaction of the graft to optimize its ability to provide structural support (see Fig. 130-2C and D). Once this is complete, the reamer is removed, and the final implant is inserted with an intramedullary stem for supplemental support.

Clinical Results

Midterm results are available for the technique of impaction allograft reconstruction in revision total knee arthroplasty. Lotke and associates[18] prospectively studied the midterm results of 48 consecutive revision TKAs with substantial bone loss treated with impaction allograft. At an average follow-up of 3.8 years, no mechanical failures of the revisions were reported, and all radiographs demonstrated incorporation and remodeling of the bone graft. Six complications were reported among the 42 revisions available for follow-up (14%): 2 periprosthetic fractures, 1 early infection salvaged with irrigation and antibiotics, 1 late infection resulting in fusion, and 2 patellar clunk syndromes. Although the authors concede that the technique is time consuming and technically demanding, they advocate impaction grafting for bone loss in revision TKA.[18] Whiteside and colleagues[37] reported on 63 patients who underwent revision knee arthroplasty using morselized cancellous allograft to fill large femoral and/or tibial defects. Firm seating of the components on a rim of viable bone and rigid fixation with a medullary stem were achieved in all cases. Fourteen reoperations occurred, and a biopsy specimen taken from the central portion of the allograft revealed evidence of active new bone formation. Evidence of healing, bone maturation, and formation of trabeculae was observed on all radiographs at 1-year follow-up. Two patients in this series required revision surgery for aseptic loosening, and the authors believed that both had greatly improved bone stock, so new implants could be applied with minor additional grafting.[37]

*References 5, 17, 18, 30, 35, and 37.

RECONSTRUCTION WITH BULK ALLOGRAFT

Bulk allograft has been used frequently to reconstruct large bone defects with the intention of providing mechanical support and reconstituting bone, which certainly are considered advantages of this technique. Bulk allograft is typically indicated for defects that are larger than 1.5 cm in depth and that exceed the dimensions of typical metal block augments accompanying most revision total knee systems (Fig. 130-3). The advantage of bulk allograft is the potential for bone reconstitution, particularly in young patients, for whom this goal is of great importance with the likelihood of multiple future surgeries and reconstructions. Potential drawbacks include the potential for graft resorption, collapse, and graft–host nonunion. Patient factors such as health status, physiologic age, bone quality, and activity must be weighed heavily when use of this reconstructive technique over other reconstruction strategies such as porous metal cones is considered.

Surgical Technique

The technique involves shaping the defect to accept a bulk allograft, most commonly a femoral head. Shaping can be done with a high-speed burr or acetabular reamers. As with morselized allograft, it is beneficial to ensure that the allograft bone is in contact with the vascularized host bone, as opposed to the dense and frequently avascular sclerotic bone encountered in many revision knee defects. Once in place, the graft is secured to the host bone with threaded Steinmann pins or screws (see Fig. 130-3C). It is advantageous to countersink the screw heads to avoid metal–metal contact with the prosthesis and the subsequent galvanic corrosion that can occur. The tibial (or femoral) surface is then shaped accordingly either free hand or with use of the knee revision system alignment cutting guides, and supplemental stem fixation with or without cement is used to bypass the reconstructed defect (see Fig. 130-3D and E).

Clinical Results

Recently, Engh and Ammeen reported on a series of 46 revision TKRs with reconstruction of massive tibial defects using bulk allograft.[9] The authors reported only 4 failures—2 for infection—at a mean of 95 months' follow-up with no evidence of graft collapse and recommend using bulk allograft for large tibial defects.[9] However, resorption and collapse of the allograft has been a matter of concern for other authors.[7,22] In a series of 52 revision TKRs with bulk allograft followed prospectively, Clatworthy and coworkers reported that 13 knee replacements failed, yielding a 75% success rate at 97

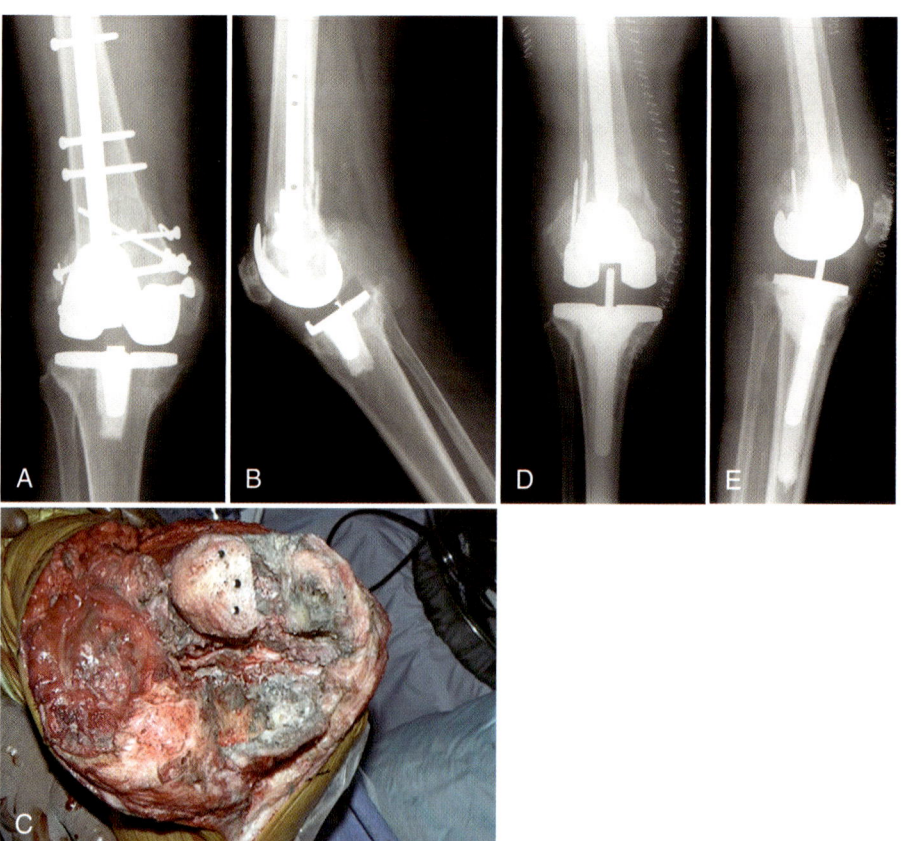

Figure 130-3. **A,** Anteroposterior (AP) and **(B)** lateral radiographs of failed total knee replacement (TKR) with severe femoral bone loss in the lateral condyle secondary to failed fixation of a periprosthetic femur fracture. **C,** Intraoperative picture of bulk femoral head allograft secured with three threaded Steinmann pins. **D,** AP and **(E)** lateral radiographs of the revision TKR in parts **A** and **B** demonstrating lateral femoral condyle bulk allograft bypasses supplemented with an intramedullary stem.

months' follow-up. Five knees had graft resorption resulting in implant loosening, and two knees showed nonunion between the host bone and the allograft. The survival rate of the allografts was 72% at 10 years.[7] In a 2009 retrospective study from the Mayo Clinic, authors reviewed 65 knees that underwent revision knee arthroplasty with bulk allograft for large bone defects and reported a 10-year revision-free survivorship of 76%. Sixteen patients (22.8%) had failed reconstructions and underwent additional surgery; 8 of 16 cases were due to allograft failure, and 3 to failure of a component unsupported by allograft.[2] These reports support the use of bulk allograft for severe tibial or femoral bone defects in revision knee arthroplasty, yet also highlight the need for a more durable reconstruction method to facilitate long-term success and avoid the complications inherent to the allograft, namely, graft nonunion and resorption.

RECONSTRUCTION WITH MODULAR BLOCKS OR WEDGES

Modular blocks and wedges are indicated in small to moderate segmental tibial and femoral defects (Figs. 130-4 and 130-5). Modular metal blocks have the advantages of being versatile and relatively technically straightforward without requiring osseointegration. Therefore they are particularly useful in older and less active patients, yet they have the disadvantage of not restoring bone stock. A majority of revision total knee systems have numerous shapes and sizes of augments for both the tibia and the femur; this facilitates restoration of the joint line and proper balancing of the knee in a relatively efficient manner.

Surgical Technique

The surgical technique of using modular metal blocks or wedges is relatively straightforward. Once the location and the extent of the defects have been determined, the size and shape of the augment that best fits that defect is selected. In the tibia, wedges or blocks may be used, and most knee

revision systems have alignment and cutting guides that prepare the bone for a nearly exact fit with the prosthesis. Although modular tibial wedges were designed to accommodate the frequently encountered defect seen in varus collapse of the medial tibia, legitimate concern has arisen that wedges subject the interface cement to shear forces that are not favorable over to the cement over the long term. Therefore, many surgeons will remove a bit more bone and convert a wedge-shaped defect into one that will accept a block augment, so that the cement interface is subjected to predominantly compressive loads, which are much more favorable to cement over the long term. Furthermore, it has been shown that block augments are superior to wedges biomechanically in creating an overall more stable and rigid tibial construct.[6] It is helpful to use intramedullary instrumentation to align the tibial cut perpendicular to the mechanical axis of the tibia; the associated cutting guide will guide the 1- to 2-mm "skim" or "freshening" cut on each plateau to enact the least amount of bone removal, while removing bone to accept the exact size and shape of the augment. It is also important to determine the proper tibial component rotation, which is typically aligned with the medial one third of the tibial tubercle, so that the sagittal cut of the block augment will seat in the corresponding correct rotational position (see Fig. 130-5D). Once the cuts have been made, sclerotic bone is roughened to facilitate cement interdigitation, and the final tibial component with stem extension is placed.

Several factors are unique to the femoral component preparation for modular block augments. First, a majority of augments are block shaped, and they come in a variety of sizes distally and posteriorly to accommodate the most commonly encountered areas of bone loss encountered in revision knee arthroplasty. Once the tibial platform has been reconstructed, as is typically the initial step in performing a revision TKA, the thickness of these augments can be altered to correctly position the femoral component with regard to balancing the flexion and extension gaps. For example, if the extension space is larger than the flexion space, distal augmentation may be used to balance the knee; this emphasizes the importance of determining the correct balance of the knee before making any femoral augment cuts that may compromise the surgeon's ability to properly balance the knee. Conversely, if the flexion gap is larger than the extension gap, which is the more commonly encountered scenario, upsizing the femoral component and using thicker posterior augments to maintain bone contact and fixation will facilitate proper knee balancing. As with the tibia, correct alignment of the distal femoral cuts typically should be determined with the use of intramedullary alignment guides that also have associated cutting guides for correct placement and sizing of augments. The final and critical step in femoral component position is determining the correct femoral component rotation; this should align the implant with the transepicondylar axis as determined by the medial and lateral epicondyles. Frequently, a larger posterior augment will be required laterally compared with the medial side to avoid placement of the femoral component in relative internal rotation, which is deleterious for patellar tracking and overall knee balance. Again, once the bone preparation is complete, the final modular augments are applied to the femoral component and are implanted with cement to bony surfaces that have been adequately prepared to facilitate cement interlock.

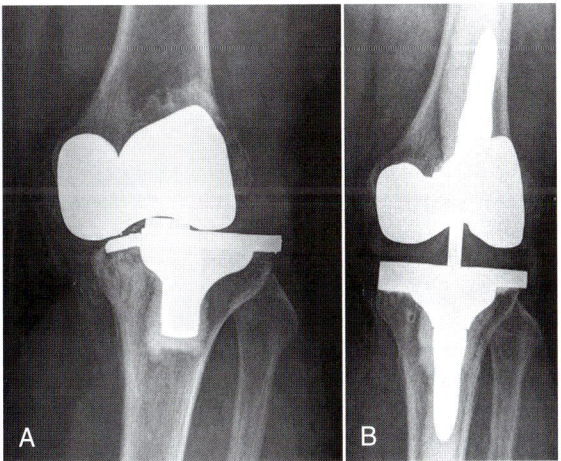

Figure 130-4. A, Anteroposterior (AP) radiograph of a failed total knee replacement (TKR) secondary to medial tibial collapse, with a broken tibial baseplate creating a moderate medial tibial defect. **B,** AP radiograph of the revision TKR reconstruction with a block augment and a cemented stem extension.

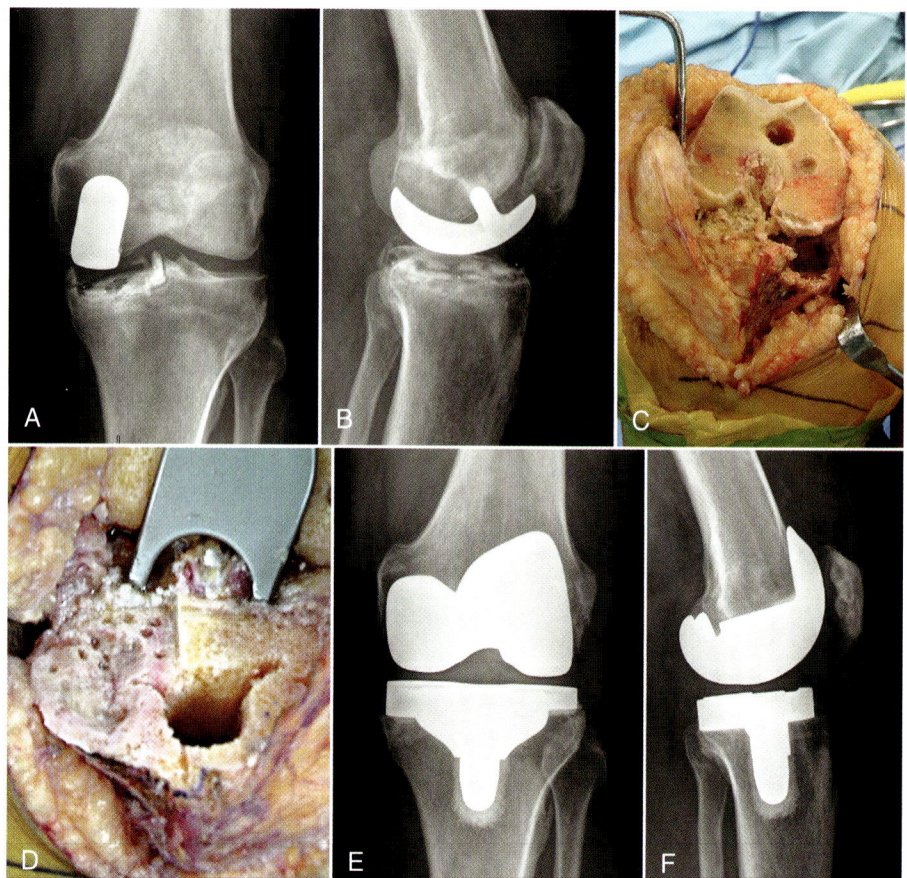

Figure 130-5. A, Anteroposterior (AP) and **(B)** lateral radiographs of failed unicompartmental arthroplasty with moderate tibial bone loss. **C,** Intraoperative picture of moderate tibial defect. **D,** Intraoperative picture demonstrating correct alignment of the sagittal step cut for the block augment to correctly align the tibial component rotation with the tibial tubercle. **E,** AP and **(F)** lateral radiographs of the revision total knee replacement in parts **A** and **B** demonstrating reconstruction with a cemented block augment and a small cemented stem extension.

Clinical Results

Several studies have reported successful midterm results with modular metal augments in revision knee arthroplasty.[12,24,26] Patel and associates[24] reported 5- to 10-year results of 102 revision knee arthroplasties in patients with type 2 defects treated with augments and stems, who were studied prospectively. Average follow-up was 7 years (range, 5 to 11 years); nonprogressive radiolucent lines were observed around the augment in 14% of knees, but they were not associated with decreased survivorship or increased failure of the implants. Overall survivorship of the components was 92% at 11 years.[24] Rand prospectively studied 41 consecutive revision TKAs with modular augmentation.[26] Modular augments were used for the distal femur alone in 2 knees, for posterior condyles of the femur alone in 16, and both distally and posteriorly in 12 knees. Tibial augmentation was used in 13 knees. At a mean of 3 years' follow-up, 96% of the knees demonstrated good to excellent results, and no cases of aseptic loosening were reported.[26]

RECONSTRUCTION WITH POROUS METAL METAPHYSEAL CONES

Recently, highly porous metal metaphyseal cones have been developed and used for large tibial and femoral defects and were designed to avoid the incidence of nonunion and resorption associated with bulk allograft reconstructions. Highly porous metals, particularly porous tantalum, are biomaterials that offer several potential advantages over traditional materials, including low stiffness, high porosity, and high coefficient of friction. The design intent for these porous tantalum metaphyseal cones was to address the variable patterns of severe tibial bone loss encountered during revision knee arthroplasty, in addition to providing mechanical support with biologic integration and avoiding allograft nonunion and resorption. Short-term evidence now supports the use of these implants in the reconstruction of large tibial defects in revision TKA.[16,19,20,25]

Indications for use of highly porous metaphyseal cones are similar to traditional indications for bulk allograft and include large contained or uncontained tibial or femoral bony defects in a failed TKR due to instability, osteolysis, infection, or aseptic loosening. The defect is typically larger than one that can be appropriately reconstructed with traditional modular blocks or wedges. Defects can be classified with the Anderson Orthopaedic Research Institute Bone Defect Classification, and porous metaphyseal cones are typically indicated for type 2 and type 3 defects, which are characterized by moderate to severe cancellous and/or cortical defects. The surgeon should keep in mind, however, that contained defects with a substantial supportive cortical rim may be more appropriate for impaction grafting, particularly in younger patients, and small uncontained defects measuring less than 5 to 10 mm in depth and isolated to one tibial plateau likely will be more amenable to standard metal blocks.

Alternatively, reconstruction of large tibial or femoral defects in young patients may be more appropriately performed with bulk allograft in an attempt to reconstitute bone stock for future revision surgery. Furthermore, large defects in patients with insufficient bone support or the potential for osseointegration may be amenable to reconstruction with custom prostheses or tumor megaprostheses.

Surgical Technique

The quantity and location of remaining cortical and cancellous bone must be noted and considered in the final assessment of whether porous metal metaphyseal cones are indicated to augment the reconstruction. The most common tibial scenario appropriate for porous metaphyseal cones is

typically a severe contained or uncontained medial tibial plateau bony defect with varying amounts of lateral tibial plateau remaining for structural support (Fig. 130-6). The most common femoral defect appropriate for porous metal cones is a severe medial and lateral condyle cancellous bone deficiency with intact, yet minimally supportive, cortical rim. Assessment should include the anticipated appropriate size and shape of the porous metaphyseal cone with respect to its fit within the tibial or femoral metaphysis, as well as its tentative location and placement as required to reconstitute the proximal tibial or distal femoral supporting surface. Visual inspection of the metaphyseal region and associated defects is performed with respect to the fit of the trabecular metal (TM) cone trial, and a high-speed burr is used to contour the metaphyseal bone to accommodate the TM cone trial, with maximal bone contact and stability possible. The surgeon should not be overly concerned with stability of the smooth plastic trials, as the actual implant will have better interference fit and stability because of the frictional resistance of the porous tantalum surface.

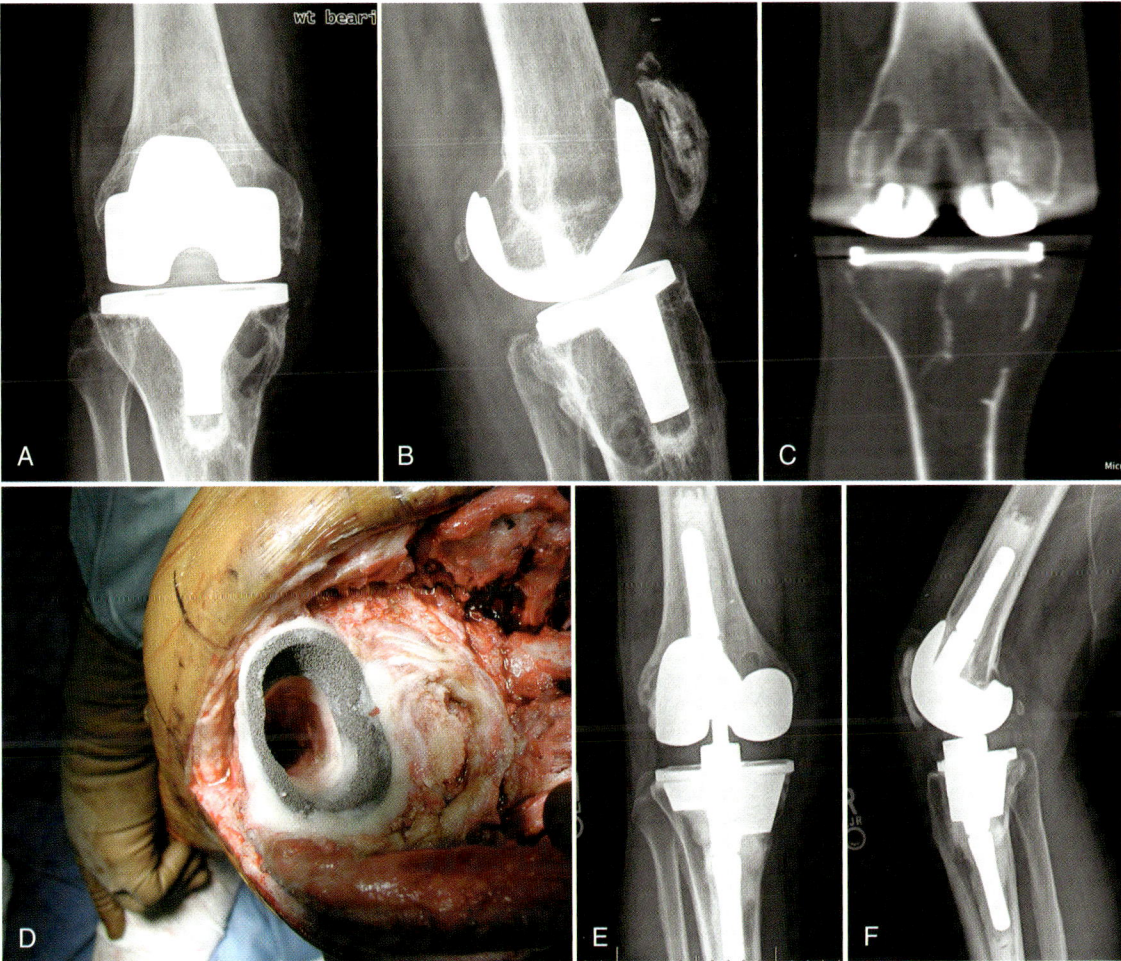

Figure 130-6. **A,** Anteroposterior (AP) and **(B)** lateral radiographs of failed total knee replacement (TKR) with severe tibial bone loss due to medial tibial osteolysis. **C,** Computed tomography (CT) scan demonstrating significant osteolytic defect in the medial tibia with cortical disruption. **D,** Intraoperative picture of severe tibial defect containing the highly porous tantalum metaphyseal cone implanted into the tibial defect with allograft bone putty impacted around the periphery between the surrounding tibial metaphyses. **E,** AP and **(F)** lateral radiographs of the revision TKR in parts **A** and **B** demonstrating the porous metal metaphyseal cone and its intimate contact with the surrounding tibial bone while supporting the tibial component at 14 months' follow-up.

The appropriate size and shape of the porous tantalum cone are chosen, and the final implant is impacted carefully in the tibial or femoral metaphysis with size-specific impactors. To minimize the chance of intraoperative periprosthetic fracture, the surgeon should be careful of overly aggressive impaction of the final implant. Tibial and femoral metaphyseal bone in the revision setting typically is sclerotic, damaged, mechanically weak, and prone to inadvertent fracture. The frictional coefficient of the actual porous tantalum implant will create greater resistance to insertion and subsequent stability. Once the porous metal cone is in its final and stable position, any areas or voids between the periphery of the porous tantalum cone and the adjacent bone of the proximal tibia are filled with morselized cancellous bone or putty to prevent egress of bone cement between cone and host bone during cementation of the stemmed component (see Fig. 130-6C). Also, the surgeon should be aware that the rotation of the final implant is not dependent on the final rotation of the femoral or tibial components, as porous metal cones are designed to fit within the defect to reconstitute the metaphyseal platform. Typically, room within the porous metal cone is sufficient to allow rotation of the tibial and femoral components into correct position to optimize stability and patellofemoral mechanics, but this rotational freedom varies among implant systems.

The tibial and/or femoral revision prosthetic component is inserted through the cone using cementless or cemented stem extensions. With either type of stem fixation, polymethylmethacrylate is placed between the porous cone and the tray and the proximal keel of the tibial component, and/or between the box and augments of the femoral component. It is advantageous to contour and smooth the curing cement around the exterior of any exposed porous tantalum material, such as occurs in the area of uncontained defects, particularly in the vicinity of the medical collateral ligament (MCL). This helps to minimize postoperative medial knee pain that can occur as the result of local irritation of soft tissues intended to be mobile, such as the MCL, against the high frictional surface of the porous tantalum. Once the cement has hardened, the remainder of the surgical procedure is carried out in standard fashion with insertion of the appropriate polyethylene insert and meticulous wound closure.

Postoperative care of revision knee arthroplasty patients who have reconstructions utilizing porous tantalum metaphyseal cones is not different from that provided for those undergoing a standard revision TKA. Patients are allowed to bear weight as tolerated based on implant stability and the quality of the reconstruction. If the surgeon achieves an inherently stable porous metaphyseal cone and a final implant construct, the patient is allowed to bear weight as tolerated. If it is suspected that the mechanical stability of the construct is tenuous, the patient is kept at partial weight bearing for 6 weeks, and radiographs are obtained at that follow-up interval. If no evidence of implant or construct migration is found, the patient is allowed to progress to weight bearing as tolerated.

Clinical Results

Early outcomes with highly porous metaphyseal cones utilized in large tibial defects for revision TKA have been reported by multiple authors.[16,19] Meneghini and associates[19] reported a series of 15 revision knee arthroplasties that were performed with a porous metal metaphyseal tibial cone and were followed for a minimum of 2 years. All tibial cones were found to be osseointegrated radiographically and clinically at final follow-up, with no reported failures in this initial series. In a series of 16 revision TKAs with severe tibial defects, Long and Scuderi[16] reported good results with osseointegration of the porous tantalum cone in 14 of 16 cases at a minimum 2-year follow-up. Two metaphyseal cones required removal for recurrent sepsis and were found to be well fixed at surgery. These early results are equivalent to those obtained with bulk allograft, custom implants, or large modular metal augments at the same time interval. Further clinical and radiographic follow-up will provide insight into the long-term durability of these highly porous augments.

KEY REFERENCES

Bauman RD, Lewallen DG, Hanssen AD: Limitations of structural allograft in revision total knee arthroplasty. Clin Orthop Relat Res 467:818–824, 2009.

Benjamin J, Engh G, Parsley B, et al: Morselized bone grafting of defects in revision total knee arthroplasty. Clin Orthop Relat Res 392:62–67, 2001.

Clatworthy MG, Ballance J, Brick GW, et al: The use of structural allograft for uncontained defects in revision total knee arthroplasty: a minimum five-year review. J Bone Joint Surg Am 83:404–411, 2001.

Engh GA, Ammeen DJ: Bone loss with revision total knee arthroplasty: defect classification and alternatives for reconstruction. Instr Course Lect 48:167–175, 1999.

Engh GA, Ammeen DJ: Use of structural allograft in revision total knee arthroplasty in knees with severe tibial bone loss. J Bone Joint Surg Am 89:2640–2647, 2007.

Hockman DE, Ammeen D, Engh GA: Augments and allografts in revision total knee arthroplasty: usage and outcome using one modular revision prosthesis. J Arthroplasty 20:35–41, 2005.

Long WJ, Scuderi GR: Porous tantalum cones for large metaphyseal tibial defects in revision total knee arthroplasty: a minimum 2-year follow-up. J Arthroplasty 24:1086–1092, 2009.

Lotke PA, Carolan GF, Puri N: Impaction grafting for bone defects in revision total knee arthroplasty. Clin Orthop Relat Res 446:99–103, 2006.

Meneghini RM, Lewallen DG, Hanssen AD: Use of porous tantalum metaphyseal cones for severe tibial bone loss during revision total knee replacement. J Bone Joint Surg Am 90:78–84, 2008.

Meneghini RM, Lewallen DG, Hanssen AD: Use of porous tantalum metaphyseal cones for severe tibial bone loss during revision total knee replacement: surgical technique. J Bone Joint Surg Am 91(Suppl 2 Pt 1):131–138, 2009.

Patel JV, Masonis JL, Guerin J, et al: The fate of augments to treat type-2 bone defects in revision knee arthroplasty. J Bone Joint Surg Br 86:195–199, 2004.

Radnay CS, Scuderi GR: Management of bone loss: augments, cones, offset stems. Clin Orthop Relat Res 446:83–92, 2006.

Ries MD: Impacted cancellous autograft for contained bone defects in total knee arthroplasty. Am J Knee Surg 9:51–54, 1996.

Ritter MA: Screw and cement fixation of large defects in total knee arthroplasty. J Arthroplasty 1:125–130, 1986.

Toms AD, Barker RL, Jones RS, et al: Impaction bone-grafting in revision joint replacement surgery. J Bone Joint Surg Am 86:2050–2060, 2004.

Full references for this chapter can be found on www.expertconsult.com.

Chapter 131

Patellar Revision

James A. Browne and Mark W. Pagnano

Management of the patella at the time of revision knee arthroplasty can be challenging. The optimal approach depends on a host of factors, including the design, wear, and fixation status of the existing component, along with the quantity and quality of the remaining patellar bone stock. Treatment can be particularly difficult if the patellar component is loose, malpositioned, or damaged. Whereas bone defects of the tibia and femur are well addressed with typical stems, augments, cones, and wedges available in contemporary revision knee implant systems, treatment options for the patella are limited. This is problematic given that mild to moderate compromise of patellar bone stock is often encountered at the time of revision total knee arthroplasty.

Reasons for compromised patellar bone at the time of revision are numerous, with iatrogenic causes being common. Over-resection or asymmetrical resection of the patella can compromise the residual bone stock and limit reconstructive options. Excessive medial malpositioning of the patellar component with osseous impingement and lateral subluxation of the remaining patella on the femoral component can lead to bony erosion or can cause implant loosening and migration.[4,29] Bone fragmentation and compromise of fixation can be caused by disruption of the vascular supply to the patella from extensive lateral dissection or retinacular release.[4] Loose patellar components can lead to bony erosion. Berend and associates reported a 4.2% loosening rate in 4287 all-polyethylene patellar components, with a mean time to loosening of 2.6 years, although only a minority went on to revision.[4]

Osteolysis is another cause of patellar bone loss. Wear debris is most commonly generated from the tibiofemoral articulation but can also come from the patellofemoral articulation. Increased wear of the patellar polyethylene implant is seen in cases of high contact loading with low conformity of patellar and trochlear geometries.[17] Maltracking of the patella may create high-contact loading forces and may lead to wear.[10] Polyethylene patellar components sterilized with gamma irradiation in air have been associated with failure due to wear,[26] as have metal-backed patellar implants.[3]

Whether the patellar revision is done for an isolated problem or as part of a revision in which other components are being revised, a number of treatment options are available. An algorithm for direct management is presented in Figure 131-1 and will be discussed later in this chapter.

THE WELL-FIXED PATELLA

The patellar component is often well fixed at the time of revision knee arthroplasty, and retention of this component is an attractive option when certain criteria are met. This approach is simple and avoids the potential morbidity of removal of a well-fixed implant and catastrophic compromise of the extensor mechanism.[22] Patellar component retention

is feasible in many cases of aseptic revision total knee arthroplasty. In contrast, the patellar component should always be removed at the time of one-stage or two-stage revision done for deep prosthetic infection.

A well-fixed patellar component must be compatible with the prosthetic design of the rest of the knee to consider retention. The surgeon is often faced with the dilemma of leaving a patellar component that is mismatched with the implants used for revision of the femur and tibia. Patellar tracking can be used to gauge the appropriateness of leaving the patellar implant. Proper tracking ensures that the patellar component geometry is reasonably compatible with the femoral trochlear design, that it has been implanted in an appropriate position, and that the overall patellar height is acceptable. Care must be taken to ensure that lateral subluxation of the patellar component has not resulted from an internally rotated femoral component, likely the greatest iatrogenic cause of maltracking in the revision setting.[22] A patellar component that is technically poor, from the asymmetrical resection of bone or from overstuffing of the patellofemoral articulation, is an indication for removal.

Concerns about subtle mismatches in geometry and conformity between patellar and femoral components from different manufacturers have not been shown to lead to deleterious clinical results.[26] Looking at 73 total knee revisions, Barrack and associates[2] reported that retaining a well-fixed patellar component gives equivalent short-term clinical results and patient satisfaction compared with those obtained by successfully reimplanting a new patellar component. Lonner and colleagues[26] reported similar good results with retention of a well-positioned, stable, all-polyethylene patellar component in 202 revisions, provided that the polyethylene was not oxidized.

Catastrophic wear or substantial surface damage to the patellar implant is a clear indication for revision. However, minimal wear may be acceptable. Quantifying the exact amount of acceptable wear or deformation for component retention is impossible; the surgeon may consider patient age and activity level in that decision. Given that forces generated at the prosthetic patellofemoral joint are often greater than the yield strength of polyethylene,[30] there is likely to be some wear or deformation of most patellar implants, and mild damage should not be an indication to revise all components.[22] Late failure due to wear from retained patellar components has been reported when the polyethylene was sterilized with gamma irradiation in air; revision should be considered in the presence of obvious oxidation.[26]

Many authors have stated that the presence of a metal-backed patellar implant is an indication for revision because of the poor track record and high rate of failure of many of these designs.[3,13,25,37] A review of metal-backed patellar components suggested that most large series reported a failure rate of approximately 6% to 8%, with late failures seen commonly at 6 or 8 years secondary to polyethylene wear and exposure of the metal backing.[37] However, others have argued that a well-fixed, undamaged, metal-backed component can be left in place with a reasonable expectation of success.[2] Some mobile-bearing metal-backed patellae have a good track record and may allow for isolated patella–polyethylene exchange in selected cases. Certain metal-backed patellae are extremely difficult to remove, and doing so risks removal of significant bone and fracture. The surgeon must assess the potential risk of future failure due to a retained metal-backed component against the morbidity associated with patellar revision. It seems reasonable to retain a metal-backed patellar component when other criteria for component retention are met, particularly when the remaining bone stock is poor.[16]

PATELLAR COMPONENT REMOVAL

A malpositioned, damaged, or significantly worn patellar component will require revision. The markedly loose component presents little challenge. However, removal of a well-fixed implant must be performed with caution to minimize bone loss and avoid catastrophic extensor mechanism compromise.

An all-polyethylene component can be removed by separating the implant from the cement base with an osteotome or saw. Alternatively, a burr may be used to section the polyethylene, with subsequent piecemeal removal of the implant. Any residual cement can be removed in standard fashion by recutting the patella or by using osteotomes, a burr, or a reamer.

A well-fixed metal-backed implant can be difficult to remove, and removal performed haphazardly risks bone loss or fracture. A diamond wheel cutting tool is often useful in separating the baseplate from the underlying host bone (Fig. 131-2).[11] If the metal-backed design includes lugs, they are typically well ingrown and can be removed with a fine-tipped high-speed burr after removal of the baseplate. Alternatively, it is reasonable to consider leaving well-fixed lugs and covering them with the new patellar implant during aseptic revision. This can be accomplished by varying lug design (e.g., by using a central peg design when revising a three-pegged component) or by slightly repositioning the lugs when the host patellar bone allows.

PATELLAR COMPONENT REVISION

Usually, it is technically feasible and reasonable to implant a revision patellar component when only mild or moderate bone loss is encountered. Although the exact thickness of bone required for an onlay all-polyethylene patellar component has not been precisely defined, a uniform thickness of 10 to 12 mm has been described as adequate.[35] A traditional onlay component may be used by preparing a flat surface and drilling new lug holes in the remnant bone. Meticulous removal of fibrous tissue and good cementation technique are important. Prior defects from lug holes and areas of cavitary bone loss can be filled with cement. An implant that matches the design of the femoral component should be used.

When a patellar implant fails, isolated patellar revision has been associated with disappointing results and a relatively high rate of recurrent failure.[5,24] This is likely due to an incomplete understanding of the mechanism of patellar failure, which is often multifactorial and includes component rotation, relative "overstuffing" of the anterior compartment, lateral placement of the patellar component, and residual tightness of the lateral retinacular structures.[24]

Berry and Rand reported on 42 knees that underwent isolated revision of the patellar implant.[5] A relatively high complication rate was seen, including five late patellar fractures and a 19% reoperation rate directly related to the extensor mechanism. Adequate vascularity and thickness of the

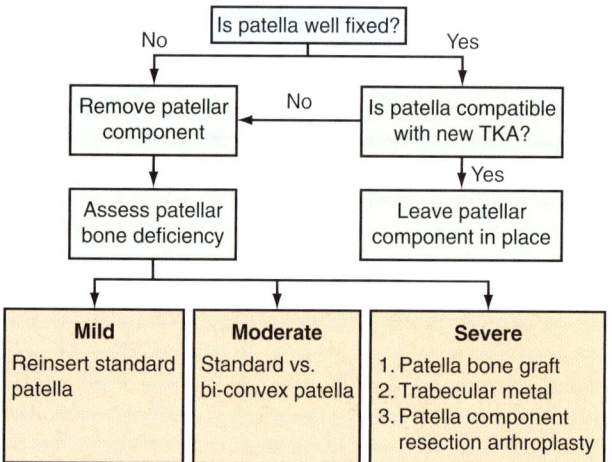

Figure 131-1. Algorithm to guide management of the patella at the time of revision knee arthroplasty. See text for details.

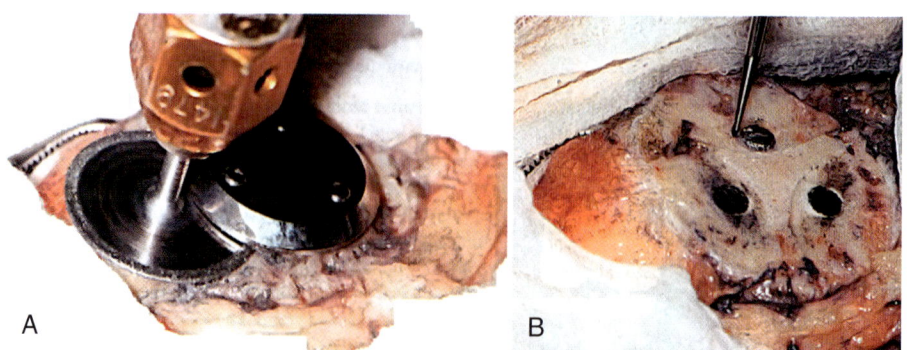

Figure 131-2. A, A diamond wheel cutting tool can be used to separate a metal-backed patellar component from the underlying host bone. **B,** If the metal-backed design includes lugs, they are typically well ingrown and can be removed with a fine-tipped high-speed burr after removal of the baseplate.

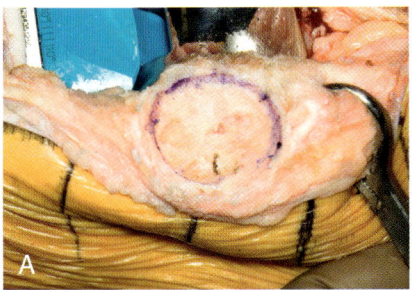
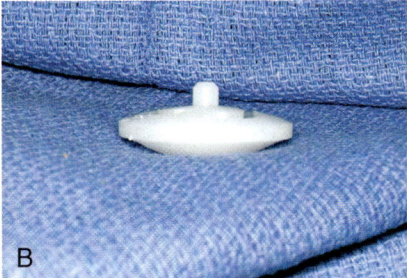
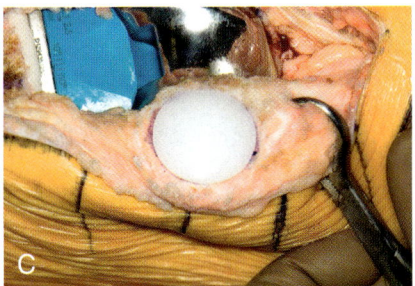

Figure 131-3. A, Intraoperative photograph following removal of a loose patellar component. The peripheral rim of bone *(outlined)* is intact with a central cavitary defect. **B,** A biconvex patella with a single central peg was used in this case to fill the defect and restore patellar height. **C,** The final construct is shown.

residual bone stock were felt to be important factors in a durable outcome. Other studies have reported worse outcomes following isolated patellar procedures compared with those who had undergone concomitant femoral revision.[34]

An inset biconvex patella may be used when an intact rim of bone remains but central cavitary bone loss is too great to provide support for a traditional onlay button (Fig. 131-3). Restoration of the composite thickness of the patella may be achieved with a thick but small-diameter button.[16] The biconvex design allows for successful implantation in the patella with as little as 5 mm of central bone, although residual thickness less than 6 mm has been associated with fracture and implant failure.[12,18] Published clinical results of this technique have generally been good with few complications reported at midterm follow-up.[18,27] In a recent report of 89 revision biconvex patellar implants, 2 cases of aseptic loosening and fracture were seen in association with avascular necrosis, to give a 98% survival rate at 10 years and 86% at 14 years.[12] Absence of a supportive rim of bone was thought to be a risk factor for radiographic loosening. The authors concluded that the presence of vascular bone was an important determinant in the satisfactory outcome of revision with a biconvex component.

SEVERE BONE LOSS

Severe bone loss, defined as residual bone stock insufficient for reimplantation of a prosthesis, has been reported to occur in 10% of revision total knees.[15] Most authors consider an absolute thickness less than 8 to 10 mm to be a contraindication to patellar revision,[37] although satisfactory results have been reported with a biconvex patella with central bone stock as little as 2 mm.[18] The typical patellar remnant consists of a thin bony shell with an intact anterior cortex and variable amounts of patellar rim.[15] Little cancellous bone usually remains.

A number of options are available for the management of severe bone loss. Traditional approaches in this setting have included patellectomy or resection arthroplasty (patelloplasty).[15] Alternative techniques such as bone grafting and porous metal augmentation have been described in an attempt to improve clinical results. The respective advantages, disadvantages, and outcomes of these techniques will be reviewed.

Patellectomy

Patellectomy has been generally condemned for poor clinical results in revision total knee arthroplasty.[16] Inferior outcomes

following primary total knee arthroplasty in patients with prior patellectomy have been well reported,[19] and although data are lacking for patellectomy at the time of revision, extrapolation of these poor results has led to the recommendation to restore or augment the deficient or absent patella in an attempt to optimize function.

Chang and coworkers[9] retrospectively reviewed 8 patients who underwent patellectomy for comminuted patellar fracture following total knee arthroplasty. Four patients had mild extensor lags at final examination, but all were less than 10 degrees. Instability and quadriceps tendon rupture each were seen in 1 patient, and functional results were poor. The authors urge that caution should be taken in considering patellectomy following total knee arthroplasty.

Resection Arthroplasty

Resection arthroplasty, or patelloplasty, is a simple approach whereby the patellar bone remnant is left unresurfaced. Unlike patellectomy, this approach maintains a fulcrum for knee extension. The remnant bone should be reshaped to remove sharp edges and rebalanced to optimize tracking. The benefits of this approach, namely, ease of technique and low cost, must be weighed against the potential morbidity of fracture, maltracking, osteonecrosis, stiffness, extensor lag, and knee pain.[33]

Pagnano and associates[33] reviewed 34 knees that were treated with patelloplasty when the patellar thickness was less than 10 mm and the bone stock precluded adequate implant fixation. Clinical results were modest. Twenty-six patients were satisfied with the results of their revision operation, and 5 were dissatisfied. However, mild or moderate anterior knee pain persisted in one third of these patients. Complications included fracture, recurvatum, extensor lag, flexion contracture, and stiffness. Fragmentation and lateral subluxation of the patellar remnant are common findings (Fig. 131-4). Although the clinical results are somewhat unpredictable, Lavernia and colleagues[23] reported that this technique does appear to avoid untoward associations with patellectomy such as quadriceps lag and extension weakness and should be considered an acceptable strategy.

A number of studies have attempted to retrospectively compare the results of resection arthroplasty versus patellar component revision. Barrack and coworkers[1] reported that 21 cases treated with patelloplasty had a higher percentage of worse clinical outcomes and dissatisfaction compared with 92 cases treated with reimplantation of a patellar component. However, a selection bias was clearly present, with the resection group having a significantly lower preoperative knee score. The authors acknowledge that patelloplasty may be an indicator of a more complicated and complex revision, and thus a lower-quality result may be expected compared with patellar reimplantation. Masri and associates,[28] in a retrospective matched cohort study, found that presence or absence of a patellar implant did not appear to affect pain, function, or satisfaction outcome after revision total knee arthroplasty, again suggesting that other variables are more important in determining outcome.

One variation of patelloplasty involves a midline sagittal osteotomy of the patella to improve contour and tracking.[40] The so-called gull-wing greenstick osteotomy is performed by creating medial and lateral wings to form a convex patellar surface for articulation with the concavity of the femoral trochlear groove. This gives a V-shaped appearance on the

patellar radiographic view. Successful early results of this technique have been reported in 12 patients with good bony healing, acceptable tracking, and no significant complications.[20]

Bone Grafting

Techniques used to bone graft the severely deficient patella have been developed in an attempt to address some of the disadvantages of resection arthroplasty. Potential restoration of bone stock is a distinct advantage of these approaches. Two major categories of bone grafting have been identified: structural bone grafting and cancellous bone augmentation.

Structural autogenous bone grafting was first described by Buechel to address patients with prior patellectomy.[6] The technique involves harvesting iliac crest autograft, fashioning it in the shape of a patella, and sewing it into a subsynovial pouch for stabilization at the previous anatomic position of the patella. In cases where a patellar shell remains, autologous monocortical iliac crest graft can be shaped, opposed to the patellar remnant, and secured with screws.[38] Donor site morbidity is a clear disadvantage of autogenous bone grafting, and limited clinical reports make the outcome of these procedures uncertain.

The use of structural allograft has also been reported. Clinical results have been poor with the use of patellar autografts in the setting of total knee arthroplasty and prior patellectomy.[7] A high rate of complications, including graft resorption, does not justify routine use of this procedure.

Hanssen has reported the use of cancellous bone grafting of the deficient patella.[15] Building upon earlier work by Cave and Rowe,[8] this straightforward procedure involves the use of a soft tissue flap to contain morcelized autograft within the residual patellar bone shell (Fig. 131-5). The tissue flap functions as an interposition arthroplasty against the femoral

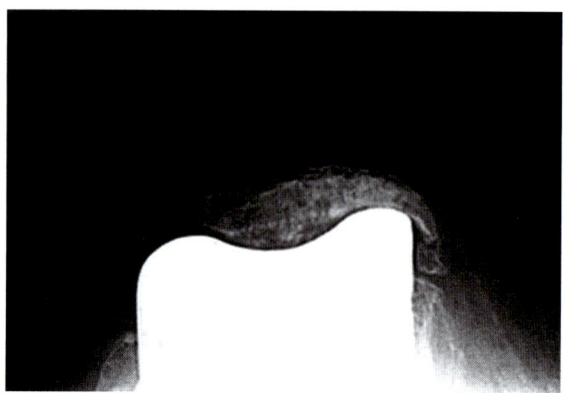

Figure 131-4. The remnant bone often remodels to the lateral condyle of the femoral component following resection arthroplasty.

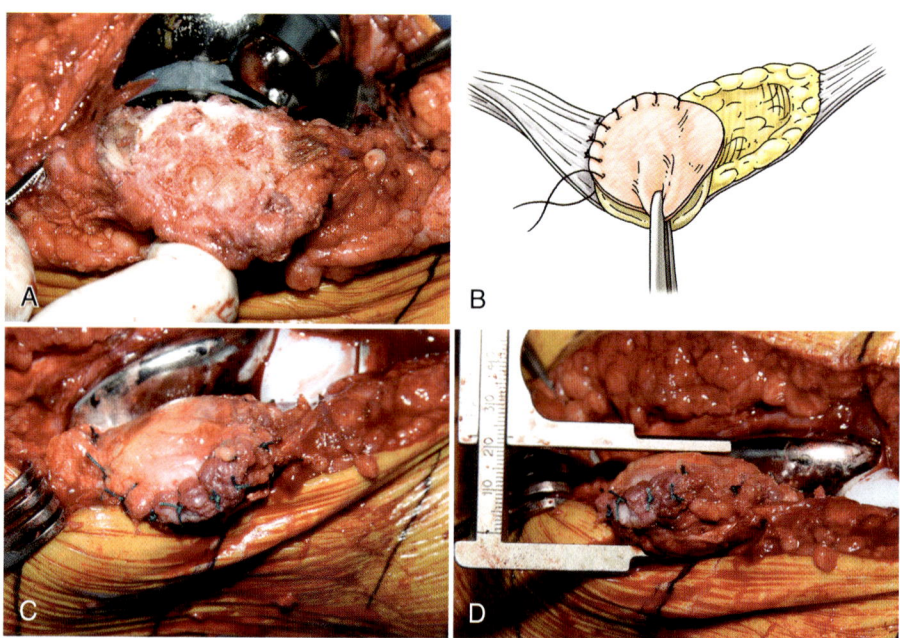

Figure 131-5. A, Intraoperative photograph of a severely deficient patella without adequate bone to support an implant. **B,** This patella was treated with Hanssen's bone grafting technique, in which a soft tissue graft is sutured to the remnant bony rim and peripatellar tissue to act as a pouch for bone grafting. **C,** Photograph following graft impaction and closure of the pouch with sutures. **D,** This technique allows for restoration of patellar height.

trochlea and allows the contained bone graft to undergo molding and compression during range of motion.[16] Following preparation of the patellar shell, the peripatellar fibrotic tissue on the undersurface of the quadriceps tendon is elevated, turned down, and secured to the periphery of the patella using multiple nonabsorbable sutures. Fascia lata may also be used for the flap, if needed. This creates a pouch into which the bone graft is inserted through a small purse-string opening. Tight impaction of the graft is performed to restore patellar height (typically between 20 and 25 mm), and the small opening in the flap is closed.

Early clinical results of this technique are promising. Hanssen reported significant improvement in pain and function knee scores in 9 patients at a mean follow-up of 3 years.[15] Patellar height ranged from 7 to 9 mm at the time of bone grafting. Minimal loss in patellar height was observed following the procedure (mean 22 mm on the immediate postoperative radiograph, compared with 19.7 mm at the time of most recent follow-up). Both cancellous autograft and allograft were seen to work successfully. Although one patient in this series had no evidence of revascularization at a subsequent operation, we have observed incorporation and gross bleeding of the graft when using this technique (Fig. 131-6). With successful reconstitution of bone stock, the potential for future resurfacing exists.

Trabecular Metal Baseplate

Trabecular metal, a biomaterial fabricated from porous tantalum, has been used to fabricate an implant to address severe bone deficiency of the patella (Fig. 131-7). The design concept is analogous to the structural bone graft previously described.[16] The implant allows augmentation of patellar height by filling the central defect with metal. The flat

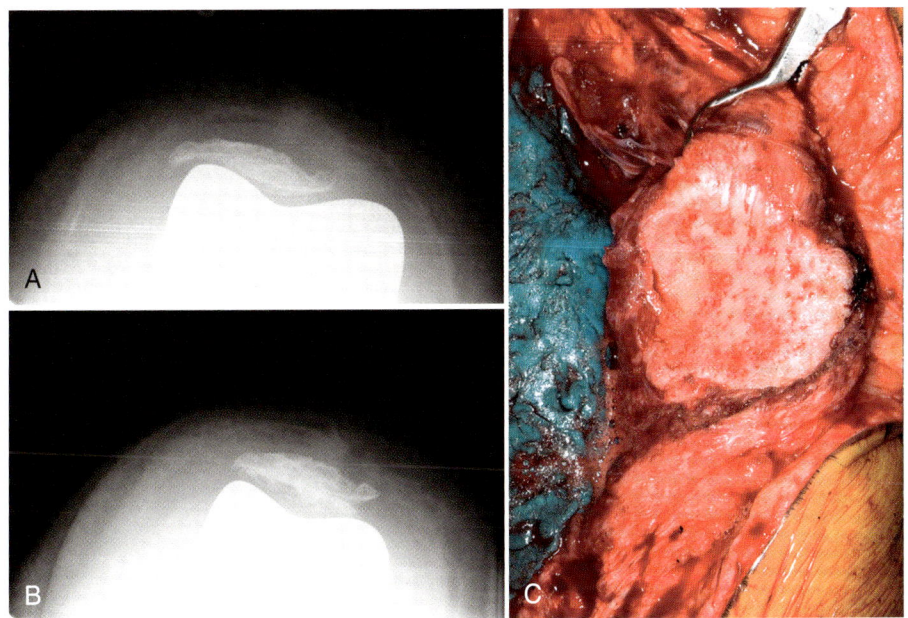

Figure 131-6. A, Preoperative and **(B)** postoperative radiographs 18 months after cancellous bone grafting of the patella show restoration and maintenance of patellar height. This patient subsequently developed a deep infection that required a two-stage revision. **C,** An intraoperative radiograph at the time of resection arthroplasty revealed viable bleeding bone with reconstitution of patellar bone stock measuring 14 mm in thickness.

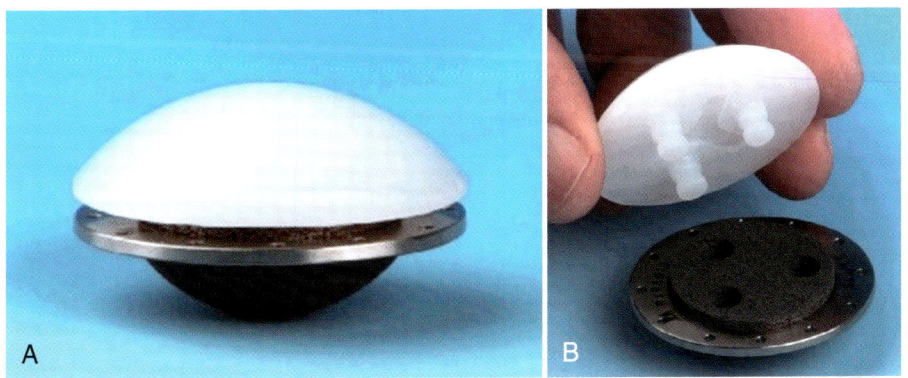

Figure 131-7. A, The trabecular porous metal baseplate is dome shaped for apposition to the patellar shell. **B,** The opposite surface has lug holes for cementation of the all-polyethylene component. (Reproduced with permission from Hanssen AD, Pagnano MW: Revision of failed patellar components. In Greene WB [ed]: Instructional course lectures, vol 53, Rosemont, Ill, 2004, American Academy of Orthopaedic Surgeons.)

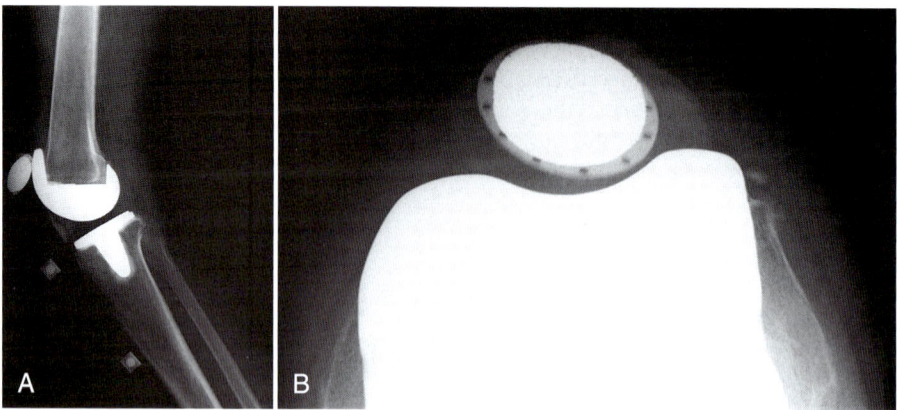

Figure 131-8. Some amount of residual bone stock appears to be required for fixation of the trabecular metal implant. **A,** Lateral and **(B)** patellar radiographs demonstrating migration of a trabecular metal patella that was sutured into the quadriceps tendon in a patient with prior patellectomy.

articular-sided surface of the patella has three holes by which to accept cementation of an all-polyethylene component. The patellar shell is prepared for the augment with domed reamers, and the augment is subsequently secured with sutures through a peripheral titanium ring.

Several series using this trabecular metal patellar implant have been published.[21,31,32,36,39] The importance of adequate residual bone stock for fixation has been recognized by multiple authors. When 50% or more of the patellar implant is covered, results have been good, with stable fixation and good patient satisfaction.[31,36] Reports suggest that, when fixation is possible, this option may compare favorably with patellar resection arthroplasty in the short term.

However, when soft tissue (quadriceps tendon) is used for fixation of the implant, results have been consistently poor (Fig. 131-8). Ries and colleagues[36] reported loosening and early migration of the patellar implant in 100% of cases with no host–bone contact, two of which went on to necrosis and discontinuity of the extensor mechanism. Similarly high rates of loosening and universally poor results were reported by Kwong and Desai in patients with previous patellectomies.[21] Despite experimental studies suggesting rapid and robust soft tissue ingrowth into porous tantalum,[14] this implant does not appear to provide predictable stability or clinical results when applied directly to tendon alone.

CONCLUSION

Most revision total knee arthroplasties will be best served with retention of a well-fixed, compatible patellar component. When the patellar component requires removal, assessment of bone deficiency is crucial in guiding subsequent treatment options. Multiple different approaches used to address severe bone loss attest to the complexity and difficulty of this situation. In an attempt to address the modest clinical results of patellar resection arthroplasty, several techniques have been described, including the gull-wing osteotomy, cancellous bone grafting, and the trabecular metal implant. Early results of these procedures are encouraging in this challenging situation. The underlying goal for any patellar revision is to ensure proper patellar tracking while avoiding iatrogenic morbidity.

KEY REFERENCES

Barrack RL, Rorabeck C, Partington P, et al: The results of retaining a well-fixed patellar component in revision total knee arthroplasty. J Arthroplasty 15:413–417, 2000.

Berend ME, Ritter MA, Keating EM, et al: The failure of all-polyethylene patellar components in total knee replacement. Clin Orthop Relat Res 388:105–111, 2001.

Berry DJ, Rand JA: Isolated patellar component revision of total knee arthroplasty. Clin Orthop Relat Res 286:110–115, 1993.

Hanssen AD: Bone-grafting for severe patellar bone loss during revision knee arthroplasty. J Bone Joint Surg Am 83:171–176, 2001.

Leopold SS, Silverton CD, Barden RM, Rosenberg AG: Isolated revision of the patellar component in total knee arthroplasty. J Bone Joint Surg Am 85:41–47, 2003.

Ries MD, Cabalo A, Bozic KJ, Anderson M: Porous tantalum patellar augmentation: the importance of residual bone stock. Clin Orthop Relat Res 452:166–170, 2006.

Full references for this chapter can be found on www.expertconsult.com.

Chapter 132

Patellar Fractures in Total Knee Arthroplasty

Daniel J. Berry

Extensor mechanism problems frequently are cited as among the most common reasons for failure after total knee arthroplasty (TKA).[21,22,26] This may have changed as surgeons have learned more about the importance of tibial and femoral rotational alignment,[1] patellar component and trochlear groove design, and optimal patellar resurfacing techniques. Nevertheless, patellar fractures still occur after TKA.[2,3] About half of patellar fractures heal without major consequence; unfortunately those that do not often are associated with serious problems.[17] Patellar fracture after TKA occurs far more commonly in resurfaced than in non-resurfaced patellae. A large proportion of fractures occur in the absence of a clear traumatic event. This chapter reviews risk factors for fracture, fracture classification, fracture results, and techniques of fracture management.

Prevalence and Risk Factors for Patellar Fracture

The prevalence of patellar fracture varies in different series, with most reports describing between 0.5% and 6% for resurfaced patellae.* The prevalence is higher after revision TKA.[2] Prevalence probably varies according to many factors, including patient demographics, implant design, and surgical technique. The reported prevalence also undoubtedly varies in part in terms of completeness of follow-up for this complication. As surgeons and implant designers have become more aware of what causes extensor mechanism problems and how to prevent them, there is reason to believe that the incidence of patellar fracture has declined or shall decline.

The strongest risk fracture for patellar fracture is resurfacing of the patella.[16,36] Grace and Sim[16] reported that the risk of fracture of non-resurfaced patellae was only 0.05%. Gender is a risk factor for fracture, and unlike most periprosthetic fractures, men are at higher risk for fracture than women. In the series of Ortiguera,[28] the overall prevalence of fracture in 12,246 consecutive TKAs was 0.68%. The prevalence was 0.40% in women, but 1.01% in men. One possible reason for the higher incidence in men could be the capability to generate greater quadriceps forces. Analysis of large patient groups by Meding and associates[27] from Indiana and Tamachote and colleagues[39] from the Mayo Clinic has demonstrated that increased body mass index (BMI) is a risk factor for fracture. Diagnosis leading to TKA and age at TKA have not yet been demonstrated to be major risk factors for patellar fracture.

Most patellar fractures are not associated with a substantial traumatic event. In the series of Ortiguera,[28] 11 of 78 fractures were associated with a blow to the knee, 6 occurred as the patient stood from sitting, 5 spontaneously while walking, 3 with knee hyperflexion, and 2 in patients with previous patellar subluxation; notably, in 48 patients, no clear event leading to fracture was recognized.

Technical and design factors also probably affect risk of fracture. Revision arthroplasty patients are at higher risk than primary TKA patients. The thickness of the patella probably affects risk, and both very thin and very thick resurfaced patellae are at increased risk. Thin patellae are likely at risk because of bone weakness. Erak and coworkers[13] reported that fractures were more common in revision TKA with an inset "biconvex" patellar component when the patellar remnant measured less than 6 mm in thickness.

Some patellar fractures clearly appear to occur in the presence of patellar osteonecrosis, but a clear link between lateral retinacular release and patellar fracture has not been established, and papers have been published both for and against an association.[25,31-33,37] Lateral retinacular release has been shown by scintigraphy methods[30] to produce transient patellar hypovascularity. However, Kusuma and associates[23] evaluated 1108 consecutive TKAs, of which 314 had a lateral retinacular release, and reported no cases of patellar fracture.

Malalignment of the limb and of tibial and femoral implants has clearly been shown to increase patellar fracture risk.[14] In Ortiguera's series,[28] 76% of patients had a major limb or implant axial malalignment and 6% a minor malalignment by Figge's criteria.[14] Seventeen of 18 patients in Tria's series[41] had a minor malalignment. In recent years, the strong relationship between malrotation of tibial and femoral implants and extensor mechanism complications, including patellar fractures, has increasingly been demonstrated.[1] Certain femoral component designs with a boxy configuration on lateral projection may have been associated with higher patellar fracture risk. Patellae of certain designs,[43] including some components with a large central peg (as opposed to a three-anchoring-peg design), also may be associated with increased fracture risk.[24]

Little has been written about the chronology of patellar fractures after TKA, but they seem to occur most often in the first several years after TKA.[9] Ortiguera and Berry[28] reported that 82% of fractures occurred in the first 3 years after TKA, with 46% recognized in the first year. In the series of 18 fractures reported by Tria and colleagues,[41] fractures occurred from 3 to 22 months postoperatively, with a mean at 11 months postoperatively.

Classification

Several different classification schemes for patellar fractures around TKA have been proposed[35] (Figs. 132-1 and 132-2). The classification of Goldberg and coworkers[15] considers fracture pattern, extensor mechanism disruption, and patellar subluxation. Type I fractures do not have disruptions of the extensor mechanism or implant fixation; type II fractures do have disruption of the extensor mechanism or implant

---

*References 2, 6, 7, 10, 18, 26, 27, and 42.

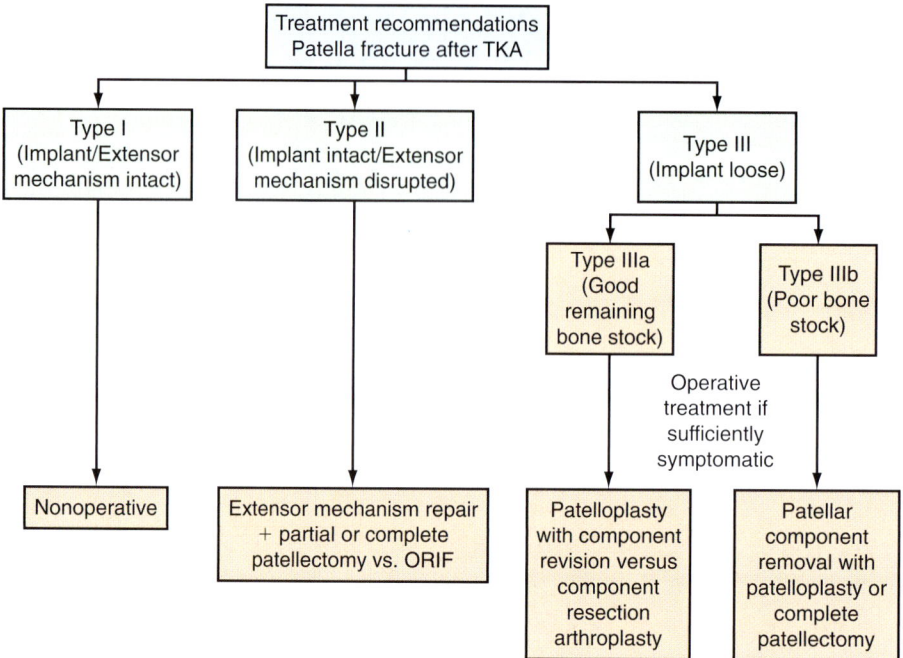

Figure 132-1. Classification and treatment algorithm proposed by Ortiguera and Berry.[28]

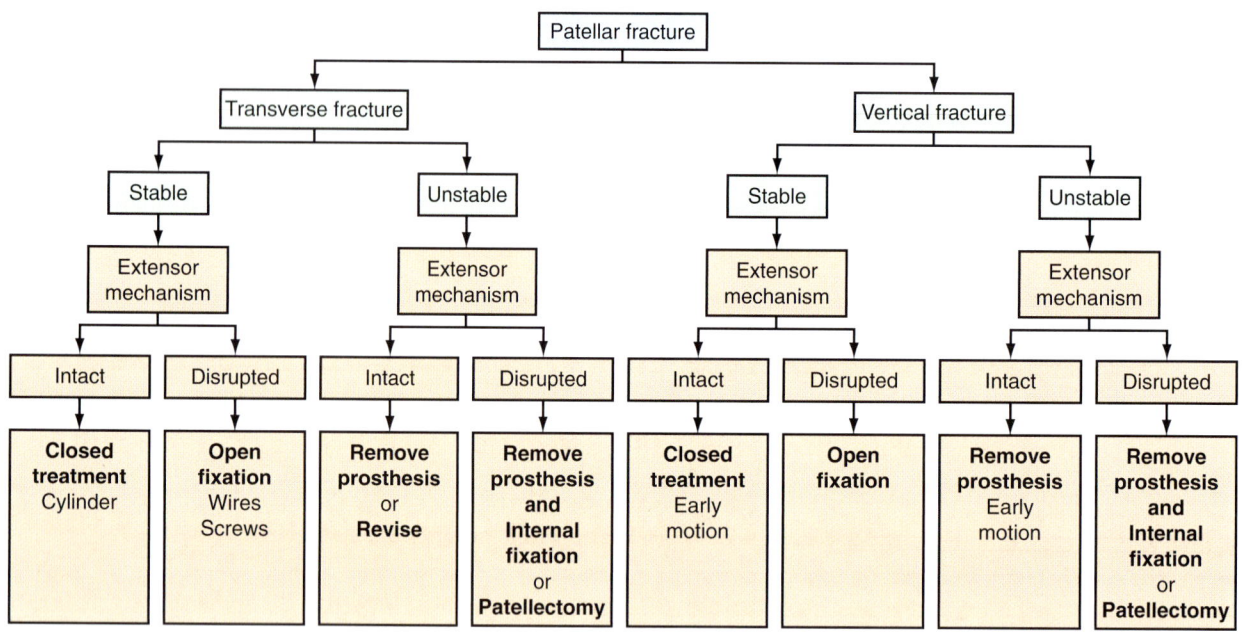

Figure 132-2. Classification and treatment algorithm proposed by Rorabeck and colleagues.[34]

fixation; type IIIa fractures have a disrupted extensor mechanism with an inferior patellar pole fracture; type IIIb fractures have the same characteristics as IIIa but with an intact extensor mechanism; and type 4 fractures are patellar fracture-dislocations. Hozack and associates[19] used a classification that included fracture displacement, presence or absence of extensor lag, fracture location, and failure of previous treatment.

The classification of Ortiguera and Berry[28] (Table 132-1) focuses on three main factors: integrity of the extensor mechanism, fixation status of the patellar implant, and remaining patellar bone stock. Type I fractures have an intact extensor mechanism and a fixed patellar component, type II fractures

Table 132-1 Classification of Periprosthetic Patellar Tracking According to Ortiguera

Type	
Type I	Extensor mechanism intact; patellar implant well fixed
Type II	Extensor mechanism disrupted
Type IIIa	Patellar implant loose; patellar bone stock allows revision
Type IIIb	Patellar implant loose; patellar bone stock does not allow revision

From Ortiguera CJ, Berry DJ: Patellar fracture after total knee arthroplasty. J Bone Joint Surg Am 84:532–540, 2002.

have a functionally disrupted extensor mechanism, and type III fractures have a loose implant but an intact extensor mechanism. Type III fractures are further subdivided as IIIa (satisfactory remaining bone stock for patellar component revision) and IIIb (unsatisfactory remaining bone stock for patellar component revision).

RESULTS

Minimally displaced or nondisplaced fractures with an intact extensor mechanism commonly are successfully treated nonoperatively with satisfactory results. Ortiguera and Berry[28] reported that all but 1 of 38 such fractures were treated successfully without operation. In the series of Parvizi and associates,[29] six of seven patients with such fractures had good results with nonoperative (cast or brace) treatment. In Goldberg's series,[15] good results of treatment also were seen in 16 patients with an intact extensor mechanism.

Fractures associated with a disrupted extensor mechanism have had the poorest results. In the series of Ortiguera and Berry[28] 11 of 12 patients with this type of fracture were treated operatively, and complications occurred in 6 of these patients. Only one of six patients treated with open reduction and internal fixation went on to bone-to-bone healing of the patella, and three of four patients treated with fragment excision and tendon advancement to bone had complications necessitating reoperation. Seven of the 12 patients had residual pain, weakness, or extensor mechanism instability. In the series of Goldberg and colleagues,[15] five of eight patients with an inferior pole fracture and a disrupted extensor mechanism had poor results. Keating and coworkers[20] reported on 17 patients with a disrupted extensor mechanism: 2 were treated with open reduction and internal fixation, and neither healed.

For fractures associated with a loose patellar component, results vary considerably. In the series of Ortiguera and Berry[28] a few patients with sufficient bone stock for patellar component revision (2 of 28 fractures with a loose implant) did well, as did many patients with sufficiently fewer symptoms to allow nonoperative treatment of this fracture type. When patients required resection arthroplasty and partial or complete patellectomy, the results were less satisfying: six of eight knees treated with resection arthroplasty and partial patellectomy remained symptomatic, and two of three knees treated with patellectomy remained symptomatic. Goldberg and colleagues[15] reported poor results in four of six patients with a loose patellar component. Keating and coworkers[20] reported that infection developed in four of nine patients treated with patellar component excision for an extruded patellar component in association with patellar fracture. Chang and associates[8] reported on 9 knees treated with patellectomy for comminuted patellar fracture after TKA: 2 of 12 patients had a complication of extensor mechanism disruption, 2 were unable to use stairs, and 4 patients had some mild extensor lag (less than 10 degrees). They concluded that patellectomy often provided satisfactory pain relief, but that functional results were often poor.

Treatment

A number of different fracture treatment algorithms have been proposed based on different fracture classification

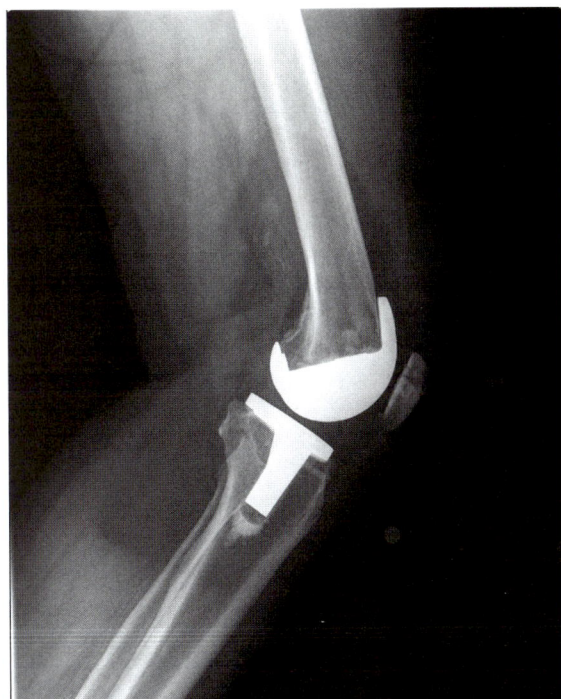

Figure 132-3. Nondisplaced patellar fracture (Ortiguera type I) that occurred 2 years following total knee arthroplasty. The patient was treated nonoperatively with a good result.

methods.[4,5,34] The Ortiguera classification method may be used as a framework for treatment of periprosthetic patellar fractures.

Type I Fractures

A great majority of type I fractures may be treated nonoperatively with a good likelihood of a favorable result (Fig. 132-3). At the time of presentation, the orthopedist should attempt to understand the time frame during which the fracture occurred. In many patients, these fractures occur spontaneously and are asymptomatic, and the first time they are found is on a routine follow-up radiograph. If it appears that the fracture is not acute and that it occurred at an indeterminate time in the past, discussion of the finding with the patient followed by observation alone is appropriate for most asymptomatic or minimally symptomatic patients. For acute fractures, the goal is to prevent notable displacement that could lead to functional extensor mechanism disruption. In most cases, this means protection or immobilization with a knee immobilizer or a cast for about 6 weeks. Depending on the clinical course and serial radiographic findings, the patient may progress to gentle passive motion of the knee at some point during the first 6 weeks of treatment in selected cases. The more at risk for displacement the fracture, the more cautious the orthopedist should be in progression of range-of-motion and active quadriceps activities. Many fractures will go on to bony healing, others to fibrous healing with an intact extensor mechanism; most eventually will be asymptomatic.

Type II Fractures

As discussed in the "Results" section of this chapter (earlier), type II fractures with a disrupted extensor mechanism are associated with a high rate of treatment-related complications. This finding likely relates in part to the difficulty of gaining good internal fixation and union of the thin, sometimes dysvascular, resurfaced patella, and to the risk of infection or other complications when operation is pursued. In some cases, despite a widely displaced patellar fracture, patients may have reasonable extensor mechanism power and little extensor lag because of intact medial and lateral retinacular soft tissues through which the quadriceps can transmit force (Fig. 132-4). In some such patients, after careful discussion of the pros and cons with the patient, nonoperative management may be elected.[12] Nonoperative management also may be chosen in some very low-demand elderly patients and patients with other very serious medical problems, even when the extensor mechanism is notably functionally deficient; however, this decision should not be taken lightly because of the substantial long-term functional deficit that is likely to occur.

Most surgeons prefer to treat many patients with a type II fracture operatively in an attempt to restore extensor mechanism continuity.[3,38] When large fracture fragments with satisfactory vascularity are present, internal fixation using tension band wiring methods (often with addition of stabilizing adjunctive K-wires or cannulated screws) may be considered. When only a small fragment of the proximal or distal pole of the patella is present, the surgeon may choose tendon advancement methods and fixation of the tendon to patellar bone with nonabsorbable sutures passed through small-diameter longitudinal drill holes in the patella, using Krackow-style stitches in the advanced tendon. A temporary protective wire or suture passed over the superior patella and

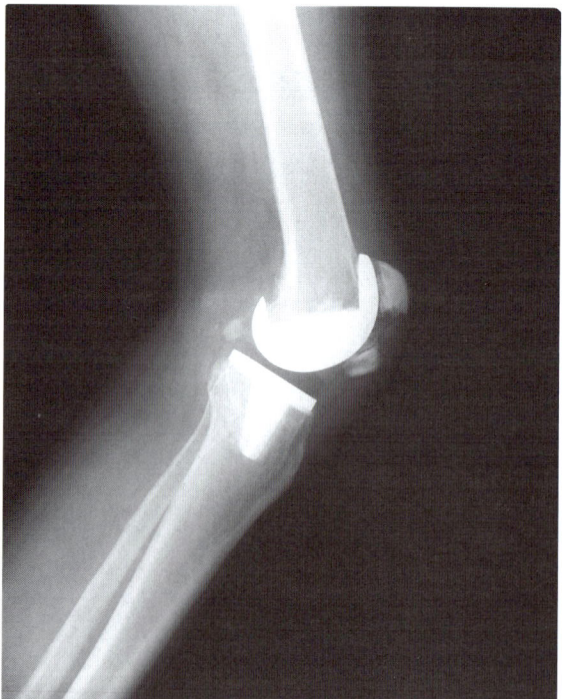

Figure 132-4. Displaced patellar fracture (Ortiguera type II) 1 year following total knee arthroplasty. The patient had a surprisingly modest extension lag (15 degrees) and because of multiple comorbidities was treated nonoperatively.

through a drill hole in the tibial tubercle may be considered for patients with patellar tendon advancements. Whether the displaced patellar fracture is treated with internal fixation or tendon advancement, the surgeon should be aware that fixation and healing failure represent a serious threat to successful surgical outcome, and generous postoperative protection is justified, even at the risk of loss of some knee motion. Infection remains an ever-present risk when operative management of patellar fractures is employed, and all efforts to minimize infection risk, with appropriate antibiotic use, careful soft tissue handling, and maintenance of tissue vascularity are recommended.

Some type II fractures present as chronic problems with long-standing extensor mechanism disruption.[40] In cases for which operative management is chosen, whole extensor mechanism allograft replacement or augmentation techniques (with quadriceps-patella-patellar tendon-tibial tubercle bone block or Achilles tendon with bone block) may be considered. Although technically challenging, such reconstructions can successfully restore extensor mechanism function to very disabled patients. Details of this method of reconstruction are discussed elsewhere in this textbook.

Type III Fractures

Many fractures of this type are minimally displaced and can be treated initially with nonoperative measures, as described earlier for type I fractures. If nonoperative measures fail because of ongoing pain and/or dysfunction related to the fracture or the loose implant, then operative treatment may be considered. For most Ortiguera type IIIa fractures, this involves patellar component revision to solve the problem of the loose implant. So long as the extensor mechanism remains intact (i.e., the fracture has not become a type II fracture), nonessential fragments of the patella may be ignored, debrided, or excised, depending on their location and their value to extensor mechanism continuity.

Ortiguera type IIIb fractures often occur in the setting of a previously revised patella or osteonecrosis of the patella. Fortunately, some are insufficiently symptomatic to require reoperation, and, in consultation with the patient, nonoperative measures and observation may be elected. The main options for more symptomatic patients include patellar component resection arthroplasty, patellar component resection arthroplasty with reshaping or excision of some patellar fracture fragments, or patellectomy. In most cases, one of the first two methods will be chosen as initial treatment, with patellectomy (discussed later) reserved for failure of one of these two methods. At operation, the surgeon should remove not only the loose patellar component, but also the loose bone fragments and any cement retained on the posterior patellar surface. Patellectomy after TKA is usually considered a treatment method of last resort, but it can be successful in highly selected circumstances, such as persistent pain with a dysvascular, highly fragmented, chronic patellar fracture. The extensor mechanism tube method of Compere et al[11] is favored because it provides a strong residual extensor mechanism, helps with extensor mechanism tracking, and provides extensor mechanism bulk, which helps restore the quadriceps lever arm and creates a cosmetically more normal appearing knee contour.

At the time of operation for any type III fracture, the surgeon should be prepared to perform a polyethylene insert exchange (for modular implants), because loosening of the patella often leads to third body debris damage to the polyethylene. The surgeon must strive to optimize extensor mechanism tracking. It is important to note that the surgeon should evaluate whether notable tibial or femoral implant malposition or malrotation is present as an underlying and predisposing condition for the fracture and should consider whether tibial/femoral component revision is warranted.

KEY REFERENCES

Berger RA, Crossett LS, Jacobs JJ, Rubash HE: Malrotation causing patellofemoral complications after total knee arthroplasty. Clin Orthop Relat Res 356:144–153, 1998.

Berry DJ: Epidemiology: hip and knee. Orthop Clin N Am 30:183–190, 1999.

Burnett RS, Bourne RB: Periprosthetic fractures of the tibia and patella in total knee arthroplasty. Instr Course Lect 53:217–235, 2004.

Compere CL, Hill JA, Lewinnek GE, et al: A new method of patellectomy for patellofemoral arthritis. J Bone Joint Surg Am 61:714–718, 1979.

Dennis DA: Periprosthetic fractures following total knee arthroplasty. Instr Course Lect 50:379–389, 2001.

Figgie HE, III, Goldberg VM, Figgie MP, et al: The effect of alignment of the implant on fractures of the patella after condylar total knee arthroplasty. J Bone Joint Surg Am 71:1031–1039, 1989.

Goldberg VM, Figgie HE, III, Inglis AE, et al: Patellar fracture type and prognosis in condylar total knee arthroplasty. Clin Orthop Relat Res 236:115–122, 1988.

Keating EM, Haas G, Meding JB: Patella fracture after post total knee replacements. Clin Orthop Relat Res 416:93–97, 2003.

Kelly M: Extensor mechanism complications in total knee arthroplasty. Instr Course Lect 53:193–199, 2004.

Meding JB, Fish MD, Berend ME, Ritter MA, Keating EM: Predicting patellar failure after total knee arthroplasty. Clin Orthop Relat Res 466:2769–2774, 2008.

Ortiguera CJ, Berry DJ: Patellar fracture after total knee arthroplasty. J Bone Joint Surg Am 84:532–540, 2002.

Parvizi J, Kim KI, Oliashirazi A, Ong A, Sharkey PF: Periprosthetic patellar fractures. Clin Orthop Relat Res 446:161–166, 2006.

Ritter MA, Pierce MJ, Zhou HL, et al: Patellar complications (total knee arthroplasty): effect of lateral release and thickness. Clin Orthop Relat Res 367:149–157, 1999.

Rorabeck CH, Taylor JW: Classification of periprosthetic fractures complicating total knee arthroplasty. Orthop Clin N Am 30:209–214, 1999.

Sheth NP, Pedowitz DI, Lonner JH: Periprosthetic patellar fractures. J Bone Joint Surg Am 89:2285–2296, 2007.

Full references for this chapter can be found on www.expertconsult.com.

Chapter 133

Extensor Mechanism Disruption After Total Knee Arthroplasty

Kelly G. Vince and Martin Bédard

Disruption of the extensor mechanism after total knee arthroplasty (TKA), although still feared, should not be considered untreatable. Demanding but proven surgical techniques can restore durable function. Nonetheless, extensor loss still rivals deep infection as the worst outcome of a knee replacement and the challenge is clear—this structure sustains huge tensile loads.[120]

The true scale of ruptured extensor mechanism complicating TKA is difficult to quantify. In 1999, Aracil et al[2] reported 5 cases out of 312 primary TKAs (1.6%). The relative contribution of extensor failure in failed TKAs varies. Data from the 2006 North American Knee Arthroplasty Revision Study identified 6 revisions of 290 that were done for a ruptured extensor (2.1%).[92] One study reported in 1999 that significant extensor lag—from rupture, patella baja, or patellectomy—accounted for 6.6% of revisions.[99] The results of first-revision arthroplasty for a ruptured extensor mechanism are inferior to revision knee arthroplasty in general, and this complication is particularly problematic in failed revision knee arthroplasty surgery.[104]

Although extensor mechanism rupture is a recognized cause of knee arthroplasty failure,[76,111] it does not appear in most national joint registries. Data from Australia list up to 27 categories of failure requiring revision arthroplasty, but not extensor mechanism deficiency.[4,5] The New Zealand Registry[79] lists 19 modes of failure and a British community registry[41] lists 11, but neither specifies extensor mechanism rupture. Our understanding would improve if this mode of failure were included in diagnostic schemes of how knees fail.[77]

Extensor mechanism complications, including maltracking, patellar component wear and loosening, patellar fracture, and extensor rupture, have all been reviewed.* This chapter, like other reviews, focuses exclusively on problems that separate the quadriceps muscle from the tibial tubercle.[†]

ANATOMIC LOCATION OF EXTENSOR RUPTURE

Although we generally think of the patellar tendon when extensor rupture complicates TKA, failure may occur anywhere from the quadriceps muscle to the tibial tubercle. The anatomic location (quadriceps tendon, patellar bone, or patellar tendon) has implications for prevention, prognosis, and treatment (Fig. 133-1). Transverse patellar fractures that disrupt the extensor mechanism are usefully included with

soft tissue ruptures because the usual fracture care is not applicable in the presence of an arthroplasty. If extensor rupture is associated with sepsis[18,33,34,68,78] or instability,[75,98] more complex procedures, including concurrent revision, will be required (Fig. 133-2).

QUADRICEPS TENDON RUPTURE

Incidence and Prevention

The quadriceps tendon is the least common site of extensor disruption. Lynch and colleagues[69] have cited a 1.1% incidence (3 of 281) of quadriceps tendon rupture after TKA. This figure, from 1987, is probably high by current standards. Dobbs and associates[31] have identified 24 of 23,800 primary TKA patients (0.1%) from the Mayo Clinic with a partial or complete quadriceps tendon rupture. The actual risk nationwide probably lies somewhere between 0.1% and 1.0%.

Systemic factors beyond the control of the surgeon may increase the risk for quadriceps tendon rupture. Rheumatoid arthritis,[36] diabetes mellitus, chronic renal failure, obesity, and hyperthyroidism are risk factors for quadriceps tendon rupture, with or without knee arthroplasty.[31,46,102,105] Aggressive resection of patellar bone at the time of resurfacing may compromise the attachment of the quadriceps tendon to the patellae; a lateral patellar retinacular release that extends proximally and then medially across the tendon may increase the risk.[69] Patellectomy to treat complications of TKA has resulted in quadriceps tendon rupture in two of nine cases.[23]

An insidious cause of quadriceps tendon rupture may be the location and orientation of the arthrotomy. If the popular medial parapatellar approach strays transversely across the quadriceps tendon, especially if it is close to the proximal part of the patella, many if not all the longitudinal fibers of the tendon will be transected, with little soft tissue for repair. Such an arthrotomy will be held together only by sutures until the surgery heals (Fig. 133-3).

An arthrotomy that transects the quadriceps tendon medially to laterally has been recommended (called the wandering resident approach because of its inadvertent origins) for difficult exposures.[48] It seems best, with this approach, to cross the tendon proximally to the patella to maintain a long section for side to side closure. In this respect, the wandering resident approach resembles the quadriceps snip,[3,7,39,47,74] which does not seem to risk quadriceps tendon rupture. Ideally, none of the longitudinal fibers in the structures (e.g., quadriceps tendon, patella, patellar tendon and its attachments to the patella and the tibia) that resist the huge tensile force in normal knee function would be transected by the surgical approach.[51]

---

*References 29, 58, 72, 83, 85, 86, 103, and 112.
[†]References 8, 30, 32, 69, 82, 85, 100, and 101.

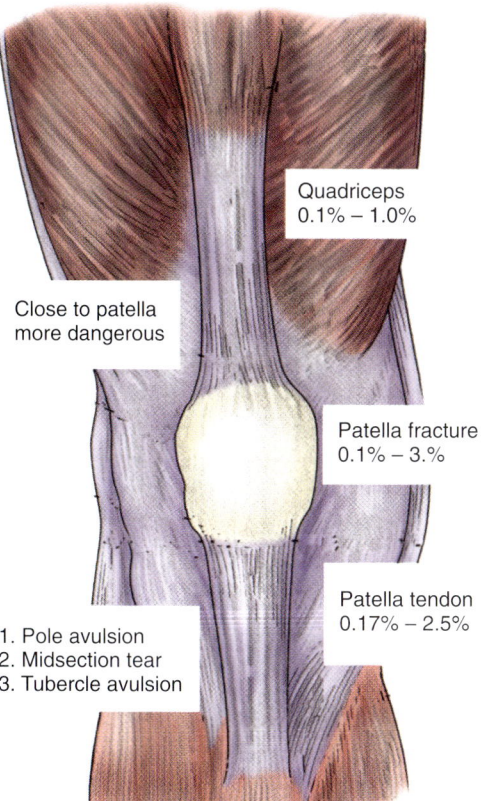

Quadriceps
0.1% – 1.0%

Close to patella
more dangerous

Patella fracture
0.1% – 3.%

Patella tendon
0.17% – 2.5%

1. Pole avulsion
2. Midsection tear
3. Tubercle avulsion

Figure 133-1. The incidence of extensor mechanism rupture after TKA is difficult to quantify. Quadriceps tendon rupture may be easier to treat unless the rupture is transverse and close to the superior pole of the patella. Not all patellar fractures result in rupture of the extensor mechanism, but it may be the most common cause of extensor lag. Inferior rupture may result from avulsion of the patellar tendon from the patella, a midsubstance tear, or avulsion from the tibial tubercle. These are always problematic.

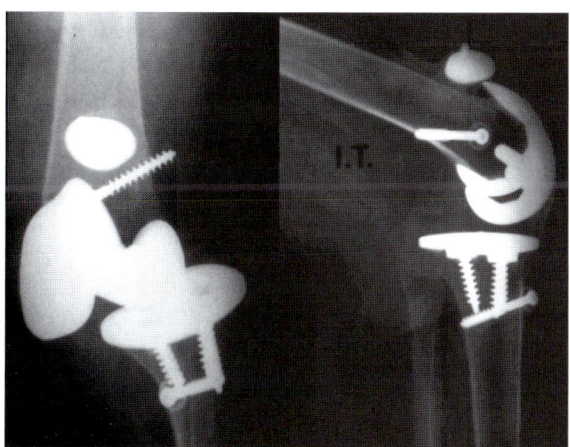

Figure 133-2. Radiographs of an older patient with a ruptured patellar tendon and dislocated knee. Sometimes, the extensor mechanism is the last structure holding an unstable knee together. This case, like many, clearly requires revision arthroplasty in addition to extensor mechanism allograft reconstruction.

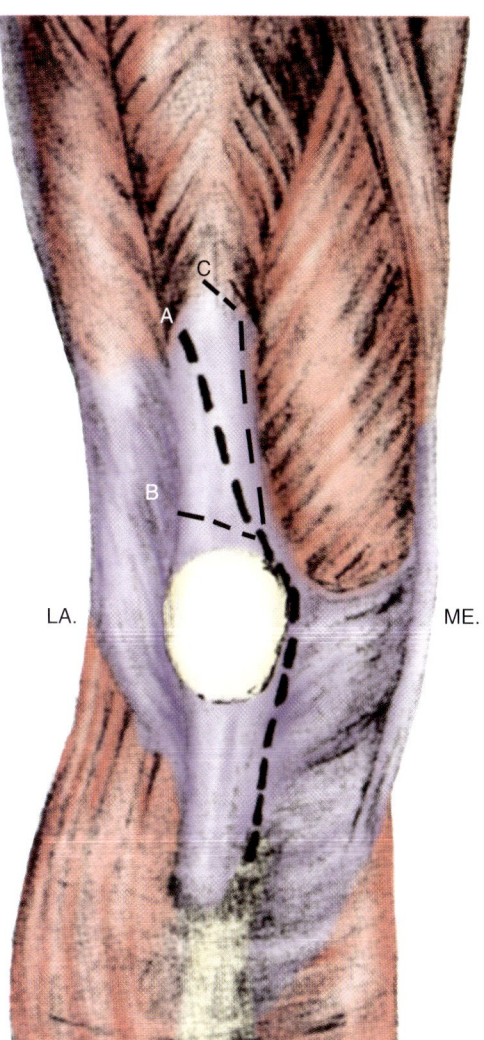

LA.   ME.

Figure 133-3. Line *A* depicts the wandering resident arthrotomy, recommended for difficult exposure. Line *C* is the standard snip exposure, which is easily and safely created from a standard medial approach. Line *B* is to be avoided. The more horizontal the arthrotomy, and the closer to the patella, the more likely is a chronic extensor mechanism rupture that cannot easily be repaired. (From Hendel D, Weisbort M, Garti A: Wandering resident surgical exposure for 1- or 2-stage revision arthroplasty in stiff aseptic and septic knee arthroplasty. J Arthroplasty 19:757–759, 2004.)

Treatment

Few quadriceps tendon ruptures after TKA have been reported. A technique described by Scuderi[95] in 1958 for the treatment of quadriceps tendon rupture in the absence of knee arthroplasty (turning the superficial portion of the tendon back down onto the patella) was applied successfully by Fernandez-Baillo and colleagues[36] to a TKA patient. This repair was reinforced with Dacron tape and the knee immobilized in a cast for 6 weeks. Sinha and coworkers[100] have described attempted primary repair and Achilles tendon reconstruction for ruptured quadriceps tendons, with mixed results. The Leeds-Keio prosthetic ligament has been used[2] and extensor mechanism allografts, originally described for insufficiency resulting from patellectomy and rupture or avulsion of the patellar tendon, work well to repair the quadriceps tendon (Fig. 133-4).[18,32,78]

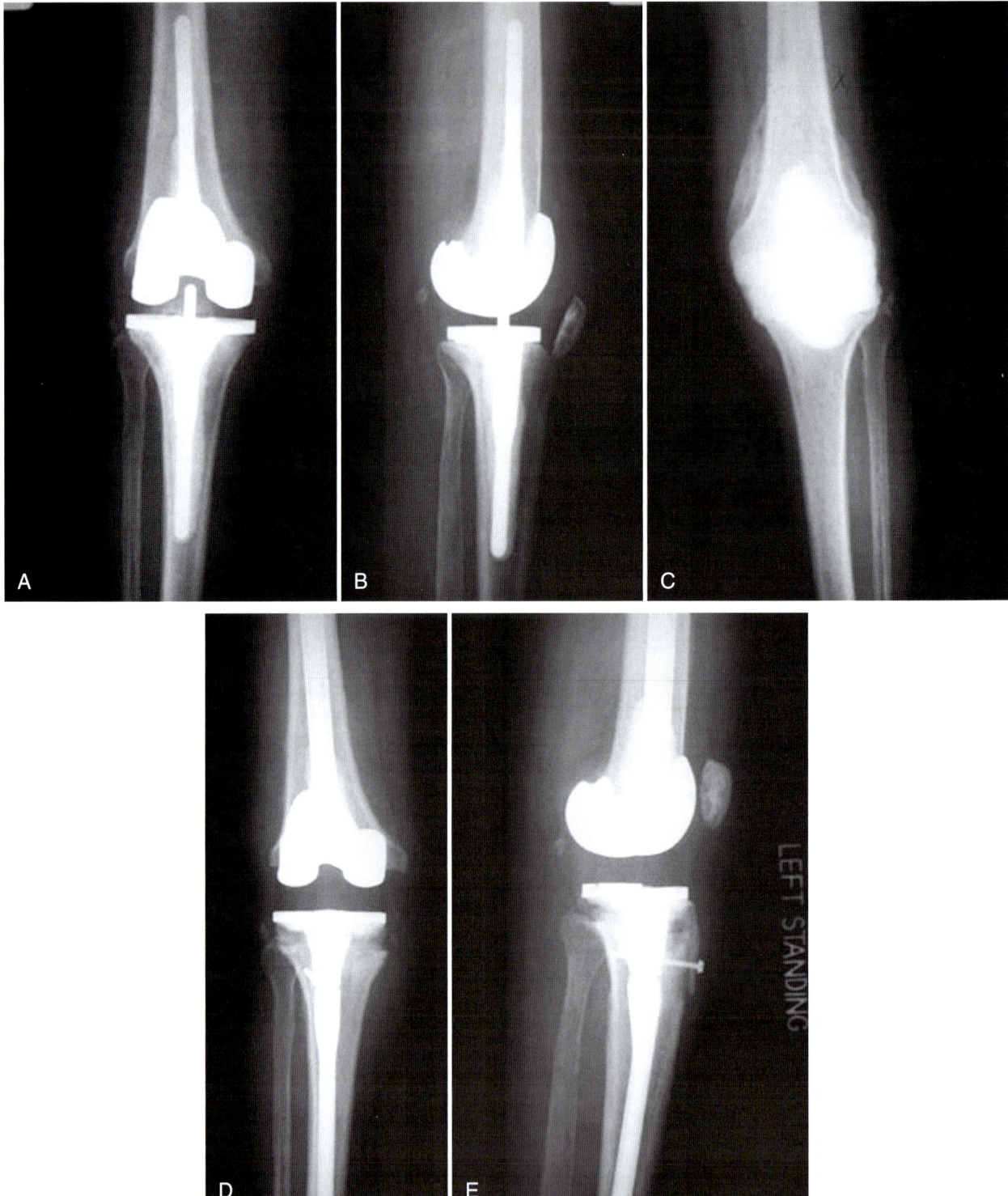

Figure 133-4. Combined proximal tibial and extensor mechanism allograft for ruptured quadriceps tendon and infection. **A, B,** Anteroposterior (AP) and lateral radiographs of a failed revision TKA with extreme patella baja–patella infra as a result of a chronic quadriceps mechanism tear. **C,** Resection arthroplasty and nonarticulating, antibiotic-impregnated polymethylmethacrylate spacer block. **D,** AP radiograph of a second revision reimplantation TKA with a proximal tibial allograft and attached extensor mechanism allograft. **E,** Lateral radiograph with a single screw to resist avulsion of the tubercle.

Dobbs and colleagues[31] reported good results with conservative treatment of partial quadriceps tendon tears. By contrast, 7 of 11 complete tears treated surgically, without supplementary biologic tissue, suffered poor outcomes and a high complication rate. The technique in 10 was adapted from Scuderi's 1958 surgery,[95] with or without drill holes in the patella; 2 were reinforced with Marlex mesh (CR Bard, Murray Hill, NJ), which is recommended and illustrated in that report. Complications in the surgical cases were legion: four with rerupture, one with recurvatum (suggesting extensor insufficiency) and instability, and two with deep periprosthetic infection necessitating resection arthroplasty that ended in amputation for one patient. Motion was maintained in the four successful cases, with 0 to 10 degrees of extensor lag and flexion ranging from 60 to 125 degrees. In one patient, a revision knee arthroplasty was performed concurrently. The results with extensor mechanism allograft reconstruction are superior.[78]

INCIDENCE AND PREVENTION OF TRANSVERSE PATELLAR FRACTURES

Patellar fractures complicating TKA usually do not interrupt the extensor mechanism. The common vertical fracture can often be treated without surgery unless a patellar component has loosened. Some of these fractures may result from rotational positioning problems of the tibial and femoral components.[13,72,73,103] Improved implant design and surgical techniques make old information regarding causes and incidence irrelevant. Sinha and colleagues[100,101] have indicated that the incidence of all patellar fractures after TKA ranges from 0.27%[116] to 5.4%. The incidence with the original Insall-Burstein posterior-stabilized prosthesis was as high as 8.4%, attributable to larger (thicker) patellar components, prominent anterior trochlear groove, increased flexion, and higher level of activity.[52,94] Most of those fractures, however, were longitudinal, without disruption of the extensor.

All studies of patellar fracture after TKA have concluded that transverse fractures with extensor mechanism disruption (and extensor mechanism lag) are uniquely problematic. Goldberg and colleagues,[43] in a 1988 report, segregated patellar fractures after arthroplasty by anatomic site. Goldberg types II (fractures involving the implant-cement interface or quadriceps mechanism) and IIIA (inferior pole fracture with patellar ligament rupture) resulted in extensor discontinuity and accounted for 6 of 36 (16.7%) and 8 of 36 (22.2%) patellar fractures in their series, respectively, establishing that over one third of all patellar fractures disrupted the extensor in that era.

More recently, Keating and colleagues[58] identified 177 patellar fractures in 4583 TKAs (3.9%). They segregated them into four groups: (1) 22 vertical fractures with a well-fixed implant and an intact extensor mechanism; (2) 21 with disruption of the extensor mechanism of less than 1 cm; (3) 17 with disruption of the extensor by more than 1 cm; and (4) 114 with a loose component but an intact extensor mechanism. Accordingly, only in group 3, 17 of 4583 cases had a ruptured extensor (0.37%) with the patellar fracture. Ortiguera and Berry[81] have identified 85 fractures after 12,464 TKAs (0.68%) at the Mayo Clinic. Only 12 fractures (0.09%) were associated with extensor mechanism rupture.

The incidence of patellar fractures has decreased with time, as has concomitant extensor mechanism rupture, confirming that few surgeons will encounter this difficult problem. Both recent studies have clearly indicated that the best results, no matter which type of fracture, occur when conservative management is feasible. The results of surgical fixation were poor.

RISK FACTORS FOR EXTENSOR MECHANISM DISRUPTION THROUGH THE PATELLA

Much of the discussion on risk factors for patellar fracture after TKA is conjectural and falls into the following categories: (1) patellar maltracking and avascular necrosis (including the effect of lateral patellar retinacular release, fat pad excision, and thermal necrosis from cement); (2) weak or damaged bone and tendon (osteoporosis, revision surgery, excessive bone resection, clamping of tendon, bone cysts); (3) component design (prominent femoral trochlea, thick patellar prosthesis, size and alignment of patellar fixation holes); and (4) large tensile force in the extensor mechanism (male gender, patient size and activity, manipulation under general anesthesia, degree of flexion).

Sinha and associates,[100] in their careful review of patellar fractures, found three factors, that statistically increased the risk for patella fracture: resurfacing, lateral patellar retinacular release, and revision surgery. Several trends have emerged, including a decreased incidence of all nonseptic complications (including patellar fractures and patellar tendon ruptures) and growing evidence that resurfacing delivers, on average, slightly better pain relief.[89] Data from three representative studies have illustrated this trend,[61,114,117] arguing against leaving the patella unresurfaced for fear of complications and in favor of better implant designs and superior surgical technique. Extensor mechanism maltracking probably heightens the risk for all patellar complications, including fracture.[72] If internal rotation of the femoral and/or tibial components is at the root of a patellar fracture, most treatments short of revision arthroplasty are likely to produce poor results. Hozack and coworkers[49] reviewed their patellar fractures in 1988, predating studies that link internally rotated components and patellar complications.[13,16] Revision surgeries were not usually done and the results, consistent with subsequent studies on the surgical treatment of extensor mechanism rupture through the patella, were poor.[57,81]

Whether avascular necrosis or patellar maltracking has a greater impact on the development of patellar fractures is unknown. Avascular necrosis of the patella is more frequent after lateral patellar retinacular release.[96] However, lateral releases are performed for maltracking, which usually results from internal rotation positioning of tibial and/or femoral components. Does the release itself cause avascular necrosis and fracture, or does maltracking cause the lateral portion of the patella to dislocate, separating itself from that portion of the patellar component that wants to stay in the trochlear groove?[46,91,93]

The statistical significance of lateral patellar retinacular release was indicated by Healy and colleagues in 1995,[46] Scott and associates in 1982,[93] and Tria and coworkers in 1994.[106] Again, it is difficult to argue against performing lateral release and even more difficult to discern whether this effect originates from avascularity, maltracking, or a combination of the two. In general, with improved designs, greater understanding of the importance of rotational positioning of femoral and tibial components, and improved surgical approaches,[15] the incidence of lateral patellar retinacular release has decreased dramatically in clinical practice.

Component positioning is certainly the factor most directly under the control of the surgeon. Other factors postulated but unproven to increase the risk for fracture via avascular necrosis include compromise of the patellar blood supply by excision of the infrapatellar fat pad and thermal necrosis of bone from the heat of polymethylmethacrylate cement as it polymerizes.[26,44]

Progressive compromise of patellar circulation after medial arthrotomy, fat pad resection, and then lateral patellar retinacular release was quantified by laser Doppler to be 30.6% of normal.[50] In a hydrogen washout study, the same surgical sequence demonstrated reduction to 17% of control.[80] The threshold at which a patella necroses has not been established. Although the fat pad contributes to the blood supply of the patella, the link has not been established between patellar fracture and its removal. Many surgeons routinely excise it, without an apparent increase in patellar fractures, much less disruption of the extensor mechanism. Cadaver studies have demonstrated that the prepatellar or anterior blood supply is very important.[56]

Thermal necrosis may result from polymerization of polymethylmethacrylate bone cement, but to a depth that is unlikely to result in structural impairment. In fact, when this effect is avoided with uncemented patellar implants, the incidence of patellar fracture is higher.[46,91] Bone saws create high temperature in bone.[66]

Bone may be weakened not only by avascular necrosis but also as a result of overresection for patellar resurfacing by osteoporosis, osteoarthritic cysts, and previous fracture. The implications for fracture of weakened bone cannot be refuted. In general, surgeons have been encouraged to resect an amount of bone equal in thickness to the known thickness of the polyethylene patellar component.

A frequent concern is that a thicker resurfaced patella will result in a stiff knee. A biomechanical test measured a 22% increase in anterior patellar strain with a conventional resurfacing prosthesis and a 28% increase with an inset-style patellar prosthesis. Increased strain is likely to increase the risk for fracture. Progressive overresection of bone was significantly more detrimental with inset designs.[118]

The final statistically significant feature associated with patellar fractures is revision surgery. Grace and Sim[44] found patellar fractures in 3 of 495 revision knee arthroplasties (0.61%) and 9 of 7754 primary replacements (0.12%; $P < .05$). Multiple surgeries have a deleterious effect by virtue of thinner, weaker, often osteolytic patellar bone, compromised vascularity, and poor flexion. This can be improved with attention to detail in the surgical approach.[97]

PATELLAR FRACTURES: TREATMENT

Patellar fractures must be treated differently when they complicate a TKA. Without an arthroplasty, the patella is a normal size and shape and blood supply is intact, and it is important to reestablish articular congruence. Consequently,

tension band wiring based on the principles of Pauwel is appropriate.[27] The fracture fragments are held by two parallel wires, around which 18-gauge stainless steel wire is wrapped in a figure-of-eight and then tightened. This induces a force vector across the anterior aspect of the patella that may be strong enough to create a gap on the articular side. With knee flexion, the femoral condyle theoretically compresses the gap and forces the fracture fragments together.[107] Conceptually, tension should be converted to compression, but this mechanism has been difficult to validate in experimental models.[115]

A resurfaced patella, by contrast, cannot be expected, even theoretically, to benefit from tension band wiring. There is barely enough room to admit the parallel wires. The deep surface of the bone, usually forced together by tension banding, no longer exists, and thus the principles are not applicable. Furthermore, if the patella was not avascular at the time of fracture, there is a strong possibility that the surgical approach has compromised the blood supply, so important for fracture healing. Simply stated, tension band wiring is not recommended for patellar fractures complicating knee arthroplasty (Figs. 133-5 and 133-6).

Despite fracture displacement, loose patellar prostheses, and even an acute extensor lag, it is useful to temporize before fixing a fractured resurfaced patella. The knee joint can usually be immobilized in extension and reevaluated within 2 to 4 weeks. Many of these patellae, although relatively avascular and fragmented, may consolidate without surgery (Fig. 133-7). Immediate intervention can only remove the loose component and perhaps cerclage the residual bone fragments, and has been associated with poor results.

A persistent lag or a loose component after 4 to 6 weeks clarifies the need for surgery. If the lag improves, surgery can be limited to removal or revision of a loose button. Prerevision computed tomography (CT) scanning may help determine whether the rotational positioning of the tibial and femoral components would indicate revision to improve tracking.[13]

Keating and colleagues[57] have observed that four of nine patients with patellar fractures and loose components suffered infection after simple removal of the components. Both patients in whom open reduction plus internal fixation was performed ended with nonunion. They recommended nonoperative treatment and acknowledged the advantage of patellectomy with repair of the residual tendon. Ortiguera and Berry[81] have described 12 patellar fractures with extensor disruption out of 85 that complicated knee arthroplasty. One patient treated with prolonged immobilization (and no surgery) was pain-free, with a 5-degree lag. Of six who underwent open reduction and internal fixation, one patella united. Five had partial patellectomies and tendon advancement to bone, with three requiring additional surgery. Six of the 12 suffered complications; 5 underwent reoperations, and 7 had pain, patellar instability (suggesting tibial or femoral internal rotation), or extensor weakness. Both of these studies illustrate examples of catastrophically failed tension band wiring.

A fixation device for inferior pole avulsion fractures of the patella (in the absence of knee replacement), the basket plate, has been described.[58] As yet unreported in the presence of a knee replacement, it risks failure for many of the same reasons as tension band wiring—limited bone stock and avascularity. Although cerclage fixation has been recommended

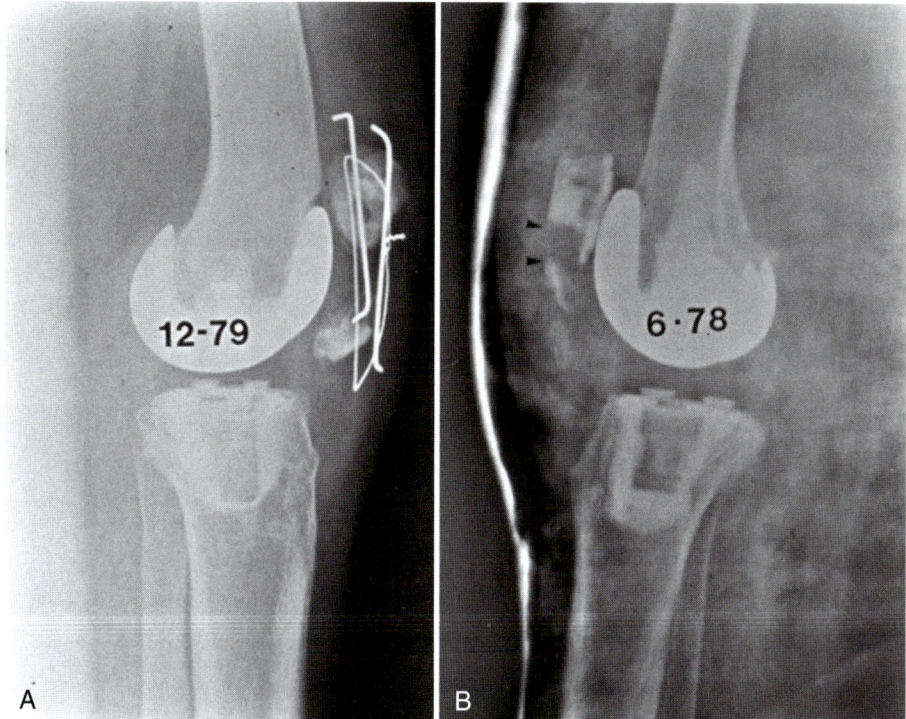

Figure 133-5. The problem of tension band wiring in fractured TKA patellae has been appreciated for many years. **A,** Lateral radiograph (dated December 1979) showing failed tension band wiring of a transverse patellar fracture that in many ways is equivalent to a ruptured patellar tendon. **B,** Lateral radiograph (dated June 1978) of a TKA immobilized in plaster after an inferior pole fracture of the patella resulting in an extensor lag. This is good initial treatment and will succeed in many cases.

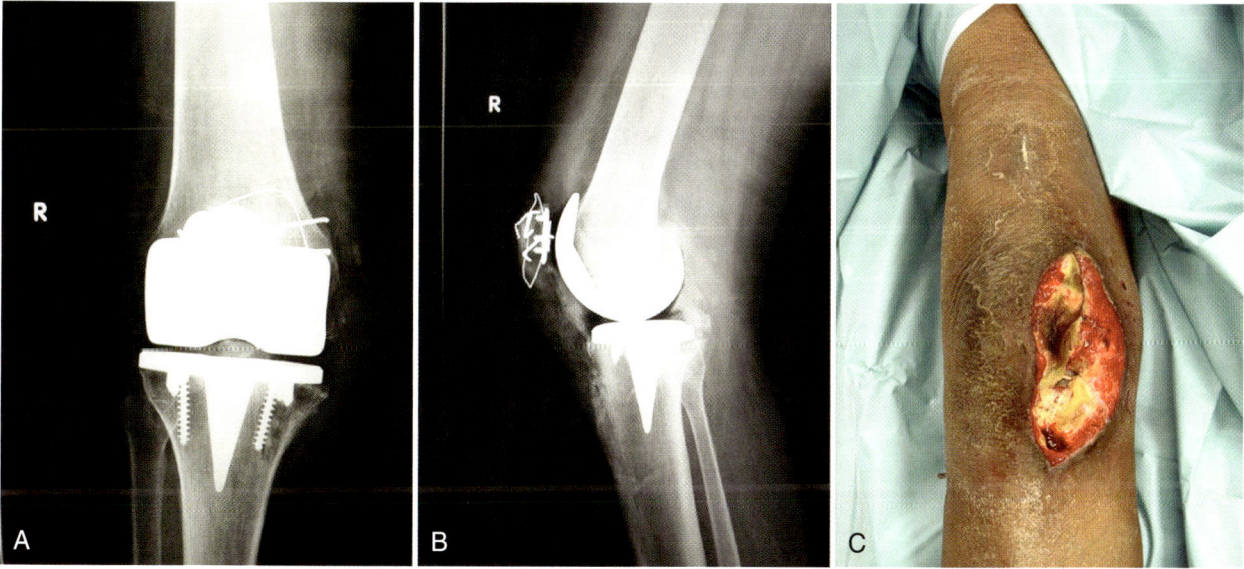

Figure 133-6. A, AP radiograph of a primary TKA showing wiring of an acute intraoperative fracture or an old fibrous union during primary TKA. **B,** Lateral radiograph showing cerclage fixation and an inferior third transverse fracture. **C,** The fixation wires eroded through the skin and led to infection with profound soft tissue loss.

for patellar fractures with an extensor lag, no data substantiate this recommendation, other than the abysmal results with tension band wiring. The ultimate recourse will be reconstruction with an extensor mechanism allograft, something that if considered earlier in the treatment of these patients, may avoid the complications of multiple procedures (Fig. 133-8). The technique can be modified, as will be described later in the case of the patellectomy patient, to safeguard the patient's own patellar tendon attachment to bone should the graft fail.

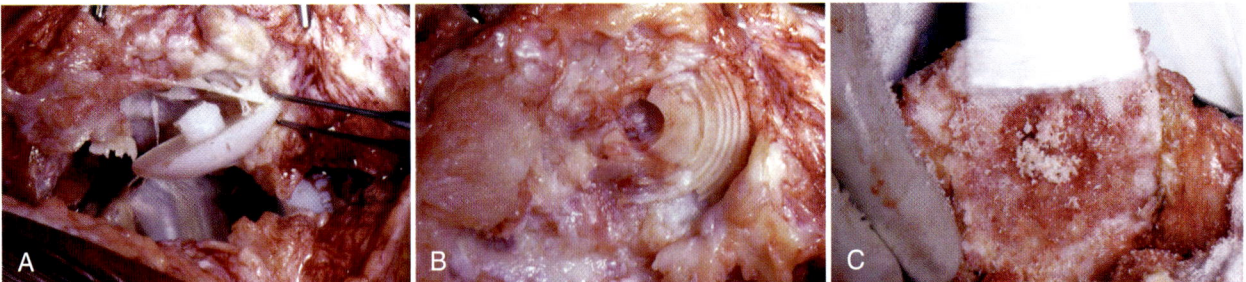

Figure 133-7. **A,** Comminuted patellar fracture, a loose patellar button, and an extensor lag. **B,** Cast immobilization allowed the fracture fragments to coalesce. The residual cement mantle is apparent. **C,** The healed fragments were thick enough to allow resurfacing. Acute surgical intervention is unlikely to have succeeded.

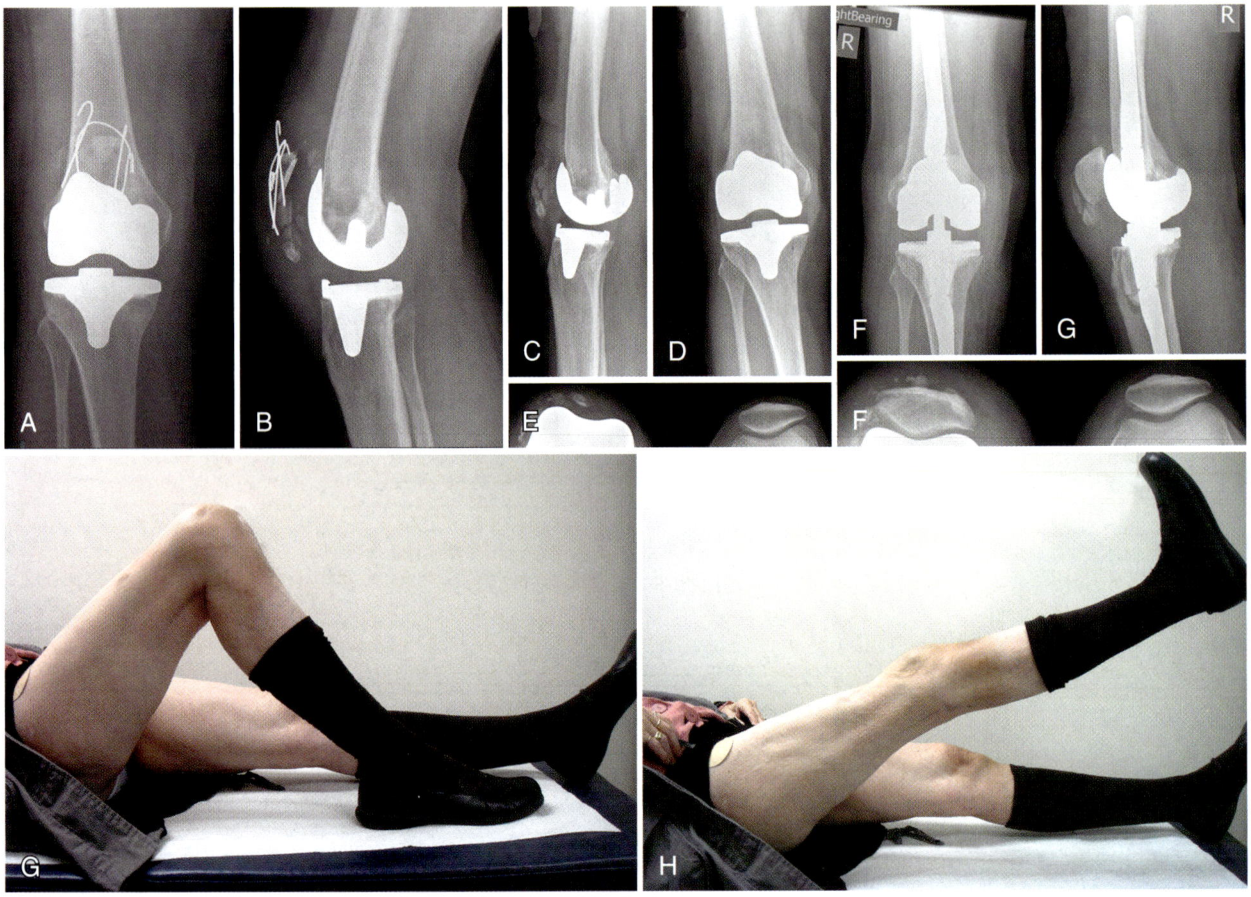

Figure 133-8. AP **(A)** and lateral **(B)** radiographs of failed tension band wiring of a transverse patellar fracture that occurred within 1 year after primary TKA and resulted in debilitating extensor lag. Lateral **(C)** and AP **(D)** radiographs after patellectomy. Significant lag persists. **E,** Patellofemoral radiograph shows tendency of patellar fragments to sublux laterally implying some degree of internal rotation position of the tibial and/or femoral components. AP **(F)** and lateral **(G)** radiographs after revision with nonlinked constrained implants and concurrent extensor mechanism allograft. Note that the allograft tibial tubercle has been implanted into the medullary canal with the technique to preserve the patient's original extensor integrity. **F,** Centrally tracking, large graft from donor, more easily fixed with the implanted technique. **G,** Flexion past 90 degrees. **H,** Improvement of extensor power.

PATELLAR TENDON RUPTURE AND AVULSION

Risk Factors

Patellar tendon rupture or avulsion has been reported in 0.17% to 2.5%[22,69,87,92] of patients with TKA. Careful attention to detail during difficult exposures with the extensor mechanism tenolysis approach should spare the patellar tendon and its attachment to the tibia.[97] Aracil and associates[2] reported patellar tendon disruptions with TKA for ankylosed knees, revisions, after distal realignment procedures, and after a Maquet osteotomy. Some surgeons recommend the insertion of a pin or Kirschner wire (K wire) through the patellar tendon and into the tubercle to protect it during difficult exposures. Although a useful reminder to exercise caution, inordinate force will tear the tendon through the pin. Medial rather than midline arthrotomies will stay to the side of the patellar tendon, whereas arthrotomies that divide any portion of the tendon necessarily elevate some of its insertion to bone, a partial rupture from the outset.

Treatment

Because of its relative rarity, large studies have not been conducted and the ideal treatment is uncertain. Conventional wisdom once recommended arthrodesis in these cases, but the resulting disability is severe. More functional reconstructions have been described, including one chronic, neglected patellar tendon rupture in the presence of severe osteoarthritis that was treated by patellectomy and TKA with advancement of the tendon.[24] Only proximal patellar tendon ruptures would be structurally amenable to this treatment; flexion may be restricted and the considerable benefit of the patellar fulcrum would be lost.

The typical appearance of midsubstance patellar tendon ruptures in TKA-attenuated fibrous tissue stretched over the usual area of the patellar tendon will surprise surgeons[35] accustomed to the mop ends of acute ruptures in the absence of a TKA. Simply put, the very strong tensile bands of collagen have suffered plastic deformation and are gone, and attempts to shorten and repair the residual structure without supplementary tissue are tempting but futile.

Surgeons have sutured the end of the avulsed tendon into a trough in the tubercle and supplemented the repair with cerclage wiring.[1] Fujikawa and coworkers[37] treated 25 ruptures with a Leeds-Keio synthetic ligament with good results in the 18 that they assessed. Aracil and colleagues[2] also reported success with this device.

Other techniques, studied in limited numbers, include reconstructions with semitendinosus,[22] fascia lata (Fig. 133-9), Dacron 4-mm vascular grafts (U.S. Catheter and Instrument, Glen Falls, NY), and bovine xenografts.[91] Zanotti and associates[119] have described success with the bone–patellar tendon–bone complex used for anterior cruciate ligament reconstructions. The patella was fused to the proximal end of the tibia in an unusual case of ruptured patellar tendon complicating a TKA in the presence of metabolic bone disease.[59] Recently, a quadriceps tendon was successfully turned down to repair what must have been a proximal patellar tendon rupture.

EXTENSOR MECHANISM ALLOGRAFTS

Indications

Reconstruction with an intact allograft consisting of the tibial tubercle, patellar tendon, patella, and quadriceps tendon (Fig. 133-10) was first reported by Emerson and coworkers in 1990.[36] Several studies of this and related techniques have established important surgical principles (Table 133-1). Five series have been studied—Dallas,[33,34] Philadelphia,[78] Chicago,[17,18,68] St. Louis,[11,19] and Los Angeles.[12] Three cases with good results have been reported from Omaha.[84]

These patients were slightly older than the mean for most series of TKAs, but similar to those for revision TKAs. Extensor allografts have been used for disruptions anywhere from the tibial tubercle to the quadriceps tendon, but most have been used for ruptures between the tubercle and patella. Up to 25% of allografts have been used in patellectomy patients, beginning with the first report.[18,33,34,78] There is another case of an extensor graft for a patellectomy patient, with a similar but modified technique.[65] Extensor allografts are used from 10% to 20% of the time for unhealed patellar fractures with a debilitating lag (and some of the patellectomy patients originated as patellar fractures). Quadriceps tendon ruptures have been treated successfully with extensor mechanism allografts in some series but not attempted in others.

Some series have reported allografting at the time of the primary TKA for concomitant osteoarthritis and chronic extensor rupture,[33,34] but most procedures are for failed extensors in primary or revision TKA. Unusual indications include extensor reconstruction when a knee fusion has been converted to a TKA[19] and TKA with severe patella infra.[17]

Infection makes any difficult situation worse, and there is good reason to recommend arthrodesis for an infected arthroplasty without an extensor mechanism. In the most comprehensive report of treating infected TKAs, which included patients revised up until 1994 (the Mayo Clinic experience), did not include the combination of extensor mechanism rupture with sepsis,[45] presumably because these patients were not admitted to the treatment protocol. In a state of the art review of treatment for infected TKAs, the same group included the state of the extensor mechanism as one of eight major considerations as to whether reimplantation is reasonable and recommended fusion when the extensor is ruptured and the TKA infected.[67]

Nonetheless, allograft reconstruction is feasible after prior sepsis. With successful healing of a two-stage reimplantation protocol, Emerson and colleagues[33] performed one graft as a third stage. Grafting at the time of reimplantation comprised 17% to 32% of cases in other series.[12,18,68] In the largest experience, 2 of 13 patients with an allograft after a two-stage reimplantation became reinfected and proceeded to an above-knee amputation.[78]

Technical Considerations

Resurfacing of Allograft Patella

Resurfacing an allograft patella is considered unnecessary. In their original patients, Emerson and associates[33,34] resurfaced all allograft patellae. By 1990, 31% were resurfaced with an all-polyethylene component and 69% with metal-backed buttons. In their 1994 report, 60% of their patellae were resurfaced with an all-polyethylene component and only 40% with metal-backed implants. Complications related to the patellar components developed in 2 of their original 15 patients (13.3%). One patient had catastrophic wear of a metal-backed component. It was revised to an all-polyethylene component that sustained a nondisplaced patellar fracture. In the second patient, loosening of a cemented all-polyethylene component resulted in mechanical problems. They were the first to question the need to resurface the insensate allograft patella and to warn of complications. Resurfacing is not currently considered part of the extensor mechanism allograft technique, with the possible exception of reconstruction with

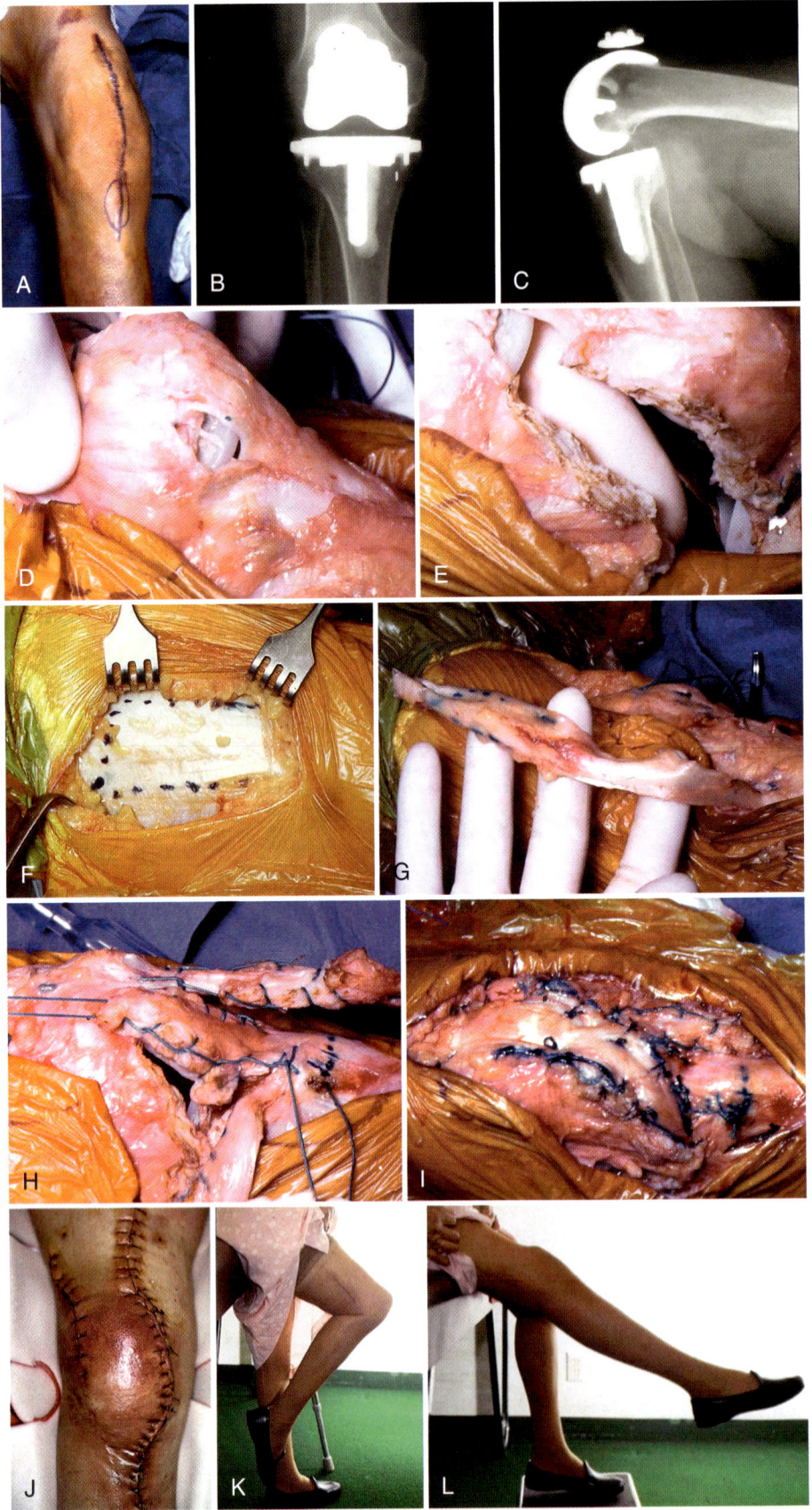

Figure 133-9. Reconstruction with patient's fascia latae left attached to Gerdy's tubercle. This is an alternate treatment, from 1992, predating the extensor mechanism allograft. **A,** Clinical photograph demonstrating that in this patient who suffered a patellar tendon rupture, the incision lies close to the tubercle and may have compromised the medial portion of the tendon in the surgical approach. AP **(B)** and **(C)** lateral radiographs showing severe patella alta. **D,** Surgical exposure shows the typical attenuated condition of the patellar tendon. The structure has suffered plastic deformation such that shortening and repair alone would not be expected to sustain the loads from the extensor mechanism. **E,** Nonetheless, in addition to augmentation with tensor fascia latae, a step cut was performed in the residual tendon so that it could be shortened. **F,** A separate incision over the more proximal tensor fascia latae (TFL), with the area of graft marked. **G,** Once harvested, it is pulled distally under the skin, but left attached to Gerdy's tubercle. **H,** The step cut of residual, stretched patellar tendon is overlapped—the medial portion *(red arrow)* is pulled distally and the lateral half *(yellow arrow)* pulled proximally. This repair is reinforced with a Krackow ligament stitch. The TFL *(green arrow)* will be applied on top of the repair. **I,** The reconstruction is complete with the TFL *(blue arrow)* sutured over top of the patellar tendon. **J,** Early postoperative radiograph shows a long incision for the revision and, to retrieve the quadriceps from the thigh, a shorter lateral incision is used to harvest the TFL. The proximity of these two incisions, jeopardizing wound healing was a major factor in abandoning this approach in favor of the extensor mechanism allograft. **K, L,** Once healed (note scar), functional results were highly satisfactory.

a graft from the contralateral side, where an implant surface improves congruence (Fig. 133-11).

Freeze-Dried versus Fresh-Frozen Allograft

In 1994, Emerson and coworkers[34] reported complications with freeze-dried irradiated allografts. Their series consisted of nine freeze-dried allografts and six fresh-frozen allografts. Although they did not condemn freeze-dried allografts, they questioned their strength.

Subsequent series implanted only fresh-frozen allografts, which have also been subject to complications. Leopold and

colleagues[68] reported a 14.0% rupture in their fresh-frozen allografts, Nazarian and Booth[78] reported 6%, and Burnett and associates[18] reported 29%; Nazarian and Booth[78] reported that 17% failed at the quadriceps tendon anastomosis, whereas Burnett and coworkers[18] experienced an 8% incidence of the same failure. In analyzing their failed reconstructions, Leopold and colleagues[68] reported that 29% of allografts exhibited attenuation of the quadriceps tendon and 14% demonstrated attenuation of the patellar tendon; they attributed the failures to inadequate tension at the time of implantation.

Graft Tension

When Emerson and associates[33] first reported this technique in 1990, they recommended tensioning the graft so that 60 degrees of knee flexion could be obtained with gravity while the patient was anesthetized on the operating table. They reported an overall failure rate of 44% with this technique. Of these patients, 33% had a residual extensor lag averaging 28.3 degrees. In 1999, Leopold and coworkers[68] reported that 100% of their patients exhibited a residual extensor lag averaging 59.0 degrees.

Nazarian and Booth,[78] in their report of 40 reconstructions earlier that same year, had sutured the allograft under maximal tension with the knee in full extension. Furthermore, the patients were cast-immobilized in extension for 6 weeks. They reported an overall failure rate of 22%, with 42.0% exhibiting a residual extensor lag averaging 13.0 degrees.

In 2004 (from the same unit as Leopold), Burnett and colleagues[18] retrospectively compared their 7 original patients

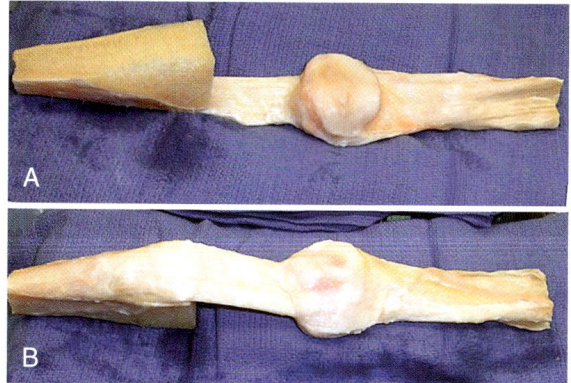

Figure 133-10. **A,** Articular surface of the allograft specimen. To the left is the tibial tubercle, not yet completely shaped for implantation. **B,** Superficial surface of the graft, with quadriceps tendon attached.

Table 133-1 Reconstruction With an Intact Allograft

Study (Year)	No. of Patients in Study	Technique	Age (Yr)	Follow-Up (Mo)	Patellectomy	Patellar Tendon Rupture, Avulsion	Patellar Fracture	Quadriceps Tendon Rupture	Convert Fusion, Patella Inframe
			MEAN (RANGE)		INDICATIONS (%)				
Emerson et al (1990)[33]	13	Extensor allograft	74 (36-81)	10 (6-57)	30.8	69.2	0	0	0
Emerson et al (1994)[34]	9	Extensor allograft	69 (36-81)	49 (28-96)	26.7	73.3	0	0	0
Nazarian and Booth (1999)[78]	40	Extensor allograft	71(NA)	43 (21-120)	15	55	10	20	0
Leopold et al (1999)[68]	7	Extensor allograft	73 (62-82)	39 (6-115)	0	85.7	14.3	0	0
Burnett et al (2004)[18]	13	Extensor allograft	64 (51-77)	37 (27-46)	23.1	53.8	0	15.4	7.7
Barrack et al (2003)[11]	14	Extensor allograft	61 (NA)	42 (24-60)	0	71.4	28.6	0	0
Burnett et al (2006)[19]	19	Extensor allograft and Achilles tendon allograft	66 (51-81)	56 (24-96)	0	68.4	26.3	0	7.7
Bedard and Vince (2009)[12]	24	Extensor allograft	67.2 (48-79)	28.5	33	29	33	4	0
Crossett et al (2002)[28]	9	Achilles tendon allograft	70 (57-81)	28 (16-36)	0	100	0	0	0

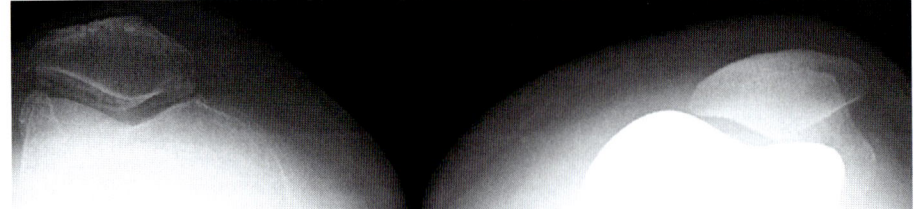

Figure 133-11. Patellofemoral radiograph of a successful extensor mechanism allograft procedure with restoration of function, using a right patella on a left TKA. These grafts are difficult to acquire and may not be labeled as to side. It is difficult to ascertain the side until the specimen is thawed but feasible to use the graft on the contralateral side. Poor congruence may be helped with resurfacing.

with 13 patients later treated by extensor mechanism reconstruction as described by Nazarian and Booth.[78] All patients in the first group had failed, with average extensor lags of 59.0 degrees and average knee scores of 52. In contrast, all those in the second group were successes, with an average extensor lag of 4.3 degrees and an average knee score of 88. It was concluded that placing the graft under tight tension with the knee in full extension dramatically improves the results. Although the grafts themselves might stretch, there is probably more elongation from a quadriceps muscle that has been chronically retracted, scarred, and shortened in the thigh.

Standard Surgical Technique

The extensor mechanism allograft technique is applicable to the widest range of clinical scenarios and has been studied more extensively than any other technique. Excellent descriptions of this technique are available in print[17] and video.[88] Advanced planning is essential because fresh-frozen grafts may be difficult to obtain.[108] In many cases, other problems will have contributed to the extensor complications (instability or maltracking) or resulted from the chronic extensor lag (recurvatum). Accordingly, concurrent revision arthroplasty may be necessary. Preoperative CT scanning to quantify the rotational position of components is instructive.[10,13]

The skin incision should follow an existing scar. When the patellar tendon or its bony attachments have been completely disrupted, the arthrotomy is made directly over the center of the tubercle. This allows the residual soft tissue and periosteum to be split, elevated medially and laterally, and perhaps closed over the top of the tubercle graft.

When revision arthroplasty is necessary, it is completed with standard technique, before the allograft is installed.[17] The method of allograft tubercle fixation should be selected before completing the revision to maintain the option of passing wires around the tibial stem extension.[78] The location of the trough, cerclage, and end of any intramedullary stem extension should be planned prior to revision to ensure that stress risers are not concentrated in one location (Fig. 133-12). The allograft tubercle bone will usually have to be reduced in width so that it fits into a trough on the host bone. If too wide, the medial and lateral cortices of the host tibia will be destroyed.

The dimensions of the allograft tubercle can be marked on the host. A transverse piece of host tibial bone should be preserved proximally to the graft and distally to the tibial prosthesis to enhance fixation. The location of the graft tubercle determines the height of the patella relative to the

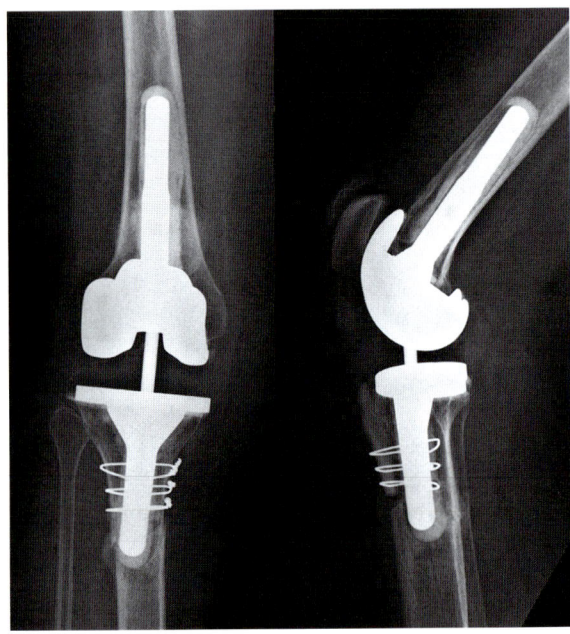

Figure 133-12. AP and lateral radiograph showing a revision TKA with extensor mechanism allograft compromised by the confluence of cerclage wires, trough for the allograft tubercle, and tip of a metaphyseal length stem. A relatively nondisplaced fracture has occurred and the graft tubercle, fixed with wires has migrated proximally. These risks may be mitigated with an intramedullary tubercle fixation, a longer stem, and perhaps screws.

femoral component and should be located carefully, because the donor may have been a different size and gender than the recipient.

Shaping graft bone is facilitated by having the saw held firmly and immobile by an assistant, with the blade in a vertical position. The surgeon can move the bone block into the blade for shaping (Fig. 133-13). Saws with finer teeth will work most efficiently; large teeth break the graft or make it difficult to hold. An oblique cut on the proximal surface of the graft (making the anterior cortex shorter than the deeper surface) will enable it to wedge into the trough under a cortical bridge. This is comparable to the step cut that has been studied in the laboratory by Davis and coworkers, providing a physical obstacle to proximal migration of the tubercle. The standard procedure has been well described (Fig. 133-14).

The trough should be very slightly, more narrow than the graft, and a mallet will be required for impaction. Wires can be placed around the tibial stem extension[78] (if revision arthroplasty is being done) or through drill holes.[11]

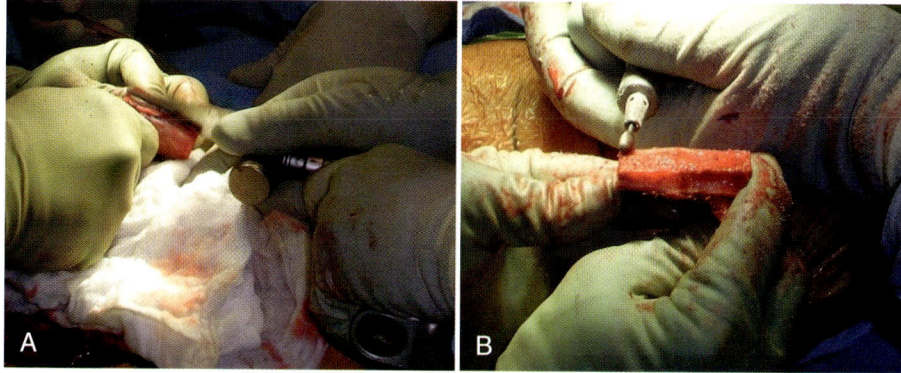

Figure 133-13. **A,** Although a microsagittal saw is ideal for shaping the trough in the host tibia, the graft may be shaped with an oscillating saw, provided the blade is relatively short and the teeth fine. This is most easily done by having the assistant *(right)* hold the saw rigidly and in a vertical position, braced on the operating table. The surgeon then advances the specimen into the saw *(left)*. **B,** Fine shaping with the burr is performed more conventionally, with the specimen held rigidly. The low-speed burr often gives the surgeon a superior sense of touch.

Alternately, one could use small-fragment lag screws or a combination of a locking fit of the graft into the host proximally, one screw distally, a fine-gauge stainless steel wire around the screw, crossed anteriorly, and passed through a transverse hole in the host tibia. Because screws can erode through the skin, it may be advantageous to countersink them when possible. At other times, depending on graft strength and configuration, washers may be required (Fig. 133-15).

There is no general agreement on the technique for the proximal anastomosis, except that the extensor mechanism should be very tight in extension. Having been installed tightly, the reconnected extensor graft will bend very little (0 to 30 degrees) when the leg is lifted (from under the thigh) during surgery. Remember that the detached quadriceps muscle has been retracted up into the thigh, often for many months, and stretching may be explained by the muscle slowly returning to its previous length and position.

In our experience, the two layers of the quadriceps may be separated in the midline, on the medial and lateral sides, to sandwich the allograft tendon (superficial to the rectus medius and deep to the rectus femoris) between them. This maximizes surface contact area for healing. The entire graft (patellar tendon, patella, and quadriceps tendon) is placed inside the knee joint, deep to the capsule and extensor mechanism. The only exception to this may be a portion of the anterior surface of the graft tubercle, for which it is simply not possible to cover it completely with periosteum (Fig. 133-16). It should be clear that autograft, fundamentally dead bone, cannot be expected to substitute for the joint capsule anywhere.

Two sets of heavy suture may be used for the proximal junction, one for position and the other to resist tensile load. The first, so-called pants over vest sutures, bring the quadriceps muscle distally and tightly over the graft quadriceps tendon. The second set is comprised of two ligament stitches with strong anchorage on both graft and host to resist the longitudinal forces in the reconstruction.[63,64]

Very heavy (e.g., no. 5) nonresorbable suture is passed down from the outside of the knee, through the top of the host quadriceps tendon at a relatively proximal location, and down to the superficial surface of graft tendon. It passes through the graft and exits on its deep surface, where the needle now faces the anterior femur or femoral component. If the host quadriceps tendon has been split into rectus femoris and rectus intermedius, the suture is carried through the anterior surface of the rectus intermedius and then back up through each level to lie adjacent to the entry point on the superficial surface of the host quadriceps tendon. If the host quadriceps tendon has not been split, the suture goes down through the rectus femoris and then the allograft quadriceps, at which point it reverses 180 degrees and comes back to the surface.

This suture is clamped but not tied because would make it difficult to place other similar sutures. At least four, and preferably six, will be positioned to establish preliminary fixation and extensor mechanism tension. Although many surgeons would perform a patellectomy, the residual host patella, if present, can be useful. The prosthesis is removed and the bone prepared with a small acetabular reamer to make the deep surface concave. The residual patella can be sutured to the allograft patella, with heavy suture, through drill holes in both. Drill holes in the graft patella, if used, should be on the periphery and oriented obliquely, medially, and laterally to avoid compromise to the graft. This technique helps identify how distally the host extensor should be pulled and provides a bone to bone junction that could strengthen the proximal junction.

Krackow-style sutures can be placed along the edges of the graft quadriceps tendon, one medially and one laterally, and continued proximally into the host for longitudinal strength.[63,64] The ends are tied to each other proximally and distally. The arthrotomy is closed over the top of the graft, usually with absorbable no. 1 sutures.

The knee is placed in a bulky, padded cotton dressing (Jones dressing), often with plaster reinforcement for several days, at which point some surgeons would apply a long-leg cast. Our preference is a hinged knee brace with drop locks for ambulation and dial locks for gentle passive motion up to a predetermined limit, usually about 30 degrees after the first 2 weeks. This brace is useful for 3 months as the limits of the

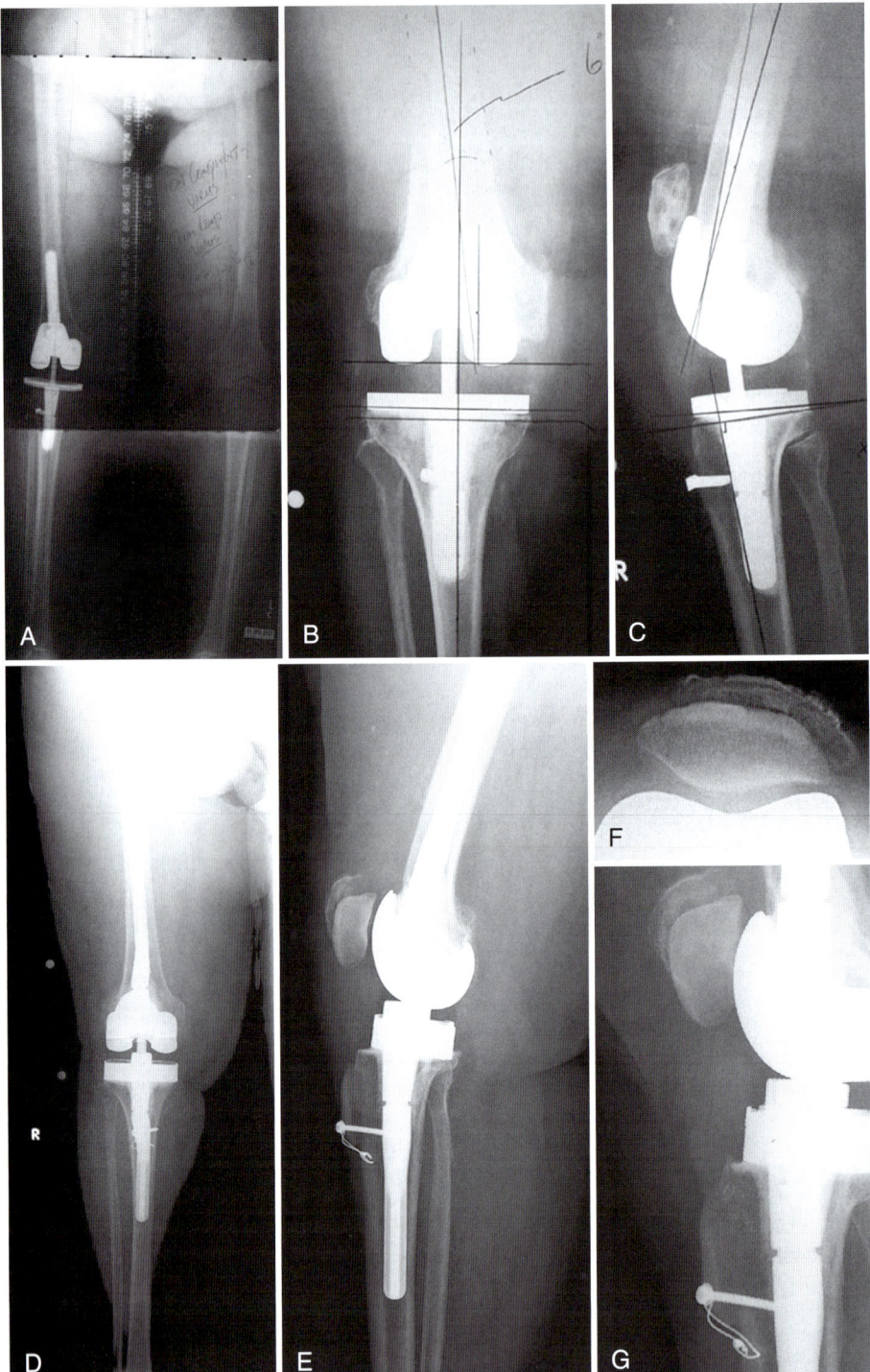

Figure 133-14. Radiographs depicting a patellar tendon avulsed during revision arthroplasty and referred for allograft reconstruction. **A,** Full-length radiographs of the failed revision demonstrate greater than desired valgus alignment, consistent with the valgus instability reported by the patient. **B,** AP and lateral (**C**) radiographs. The conventional cassette does not fully reveal the problem of valgus alignment. The tell-tale staple, rarely effective in maintaining the patellar tendon, suggests that the problem occurred during surgery. **D,** Post–second revision long-leg radiograph shows subtle but important reduction of valgus alignment with restoration of stability. An offset metaphyseal length stem has been used to assist with fixation and alignment. **E,** Lateral radiograph a few months after the second revision show the graft tubercle locked into the trough on the host tibia. The proximal end of the graft has been angled to wedge under the host proximal tibia and secure fixation has been achieved with one screw and a wire looped around it. **F,** The anterior shell of the host patella has been retained. This assists positioning and tensioning of the host extensor and may enhance union of the proximal junction. **G,** Lateral radiograph showing integration of the grafted tubercle more than 2 years after the reconstruction.

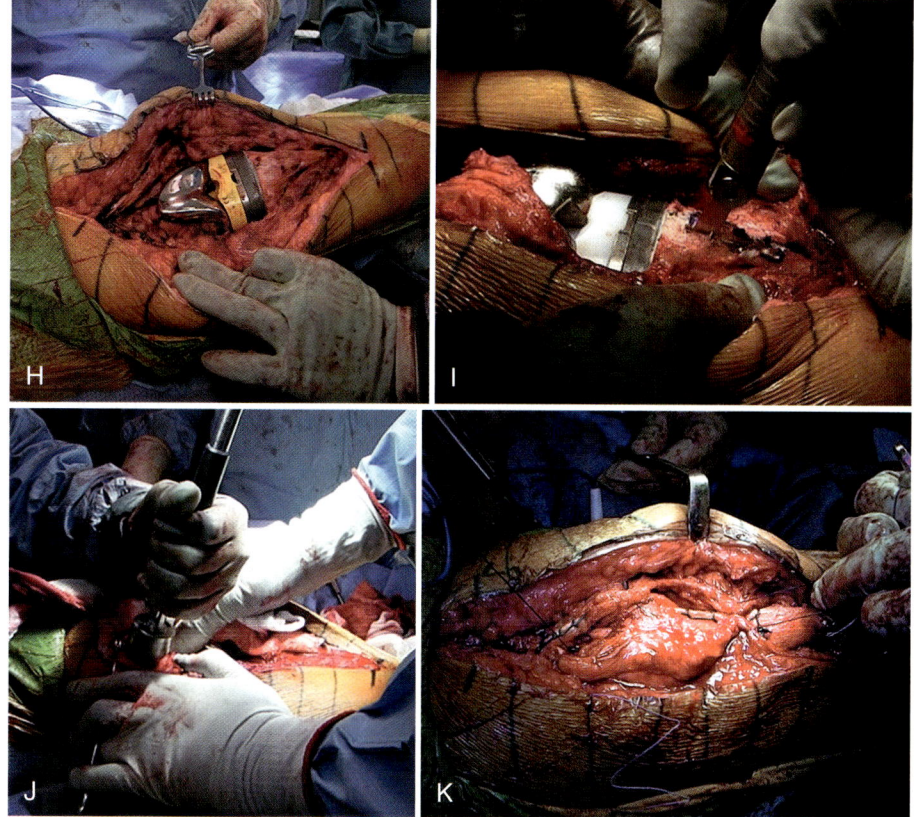

Figure 133-14, cont'd. H, Intraoperative photographs with the tubercle *(right)* and quadriceps *(left),* showing trial components for the revision TKA in place, ready to implant the actual prosthesis and then the allograft. Note how the exposure for this standard technique necessarily removes all residual soft tissue for the anterior aspect of the tubercle. **I,** A microsagittal saw is ideal for creating the trough on the host tubercle. **J,** Acetabular reamers are useful to create a concavity on the deep surface of the host patella so that it may fit more congruently on top of the graft, which must be implanted inside the joint deep to the host extensor. **K,** Approximately three pairs of pants over vest sutures to achieve full tension in the extensor with the knee extended, plus a pair of Krackow ligament stitches to dissipate tensile load. All soft tissues should be closed over the graft as much as possible.

dial lock are increased. Active extension is prohibited for about 12 weeks, and crutches or a walker is necessary.

Recent Modifications to Standard Technique

With the goal of strengthening the proximal connection of the graft to host, Malhotra and colleagues have described a technique for interlocking the host and graft patellae to reduce dependence on the tendinous junction (Fig. 133-17). This would only be feasible for ruptures distal to the patella and it necessitates bringing the graft anterior to host tissues as the transition is made from the patellar tendon to patella. The graft would then be covered by subcutaneous tissue alone. Others have used flat but longer allograft tubercle. The technique would be easier, and presumably the length of the graft would help resist the tendency for proximal migration.[65] Their description of the technique does not explicitly state that the host tissue was closed over the top of the quadriceps tendon graft, but rather that the whole stretched extensor was excised and that the proximal tendon of the allograft was sutured into the quadriceps tendon defect. Expecting the graft to function as part of the capsule is cause for concern.

Alternative Techniques

Distal Fixation by Graft Tubercle Implantation

We have developed the allograft tubercle implantation technique to expedite surgery, preserve the patient's residual patellar tendon attachment, and maximize soft tissue coverage of avascular graft. These are specifically advantageous after patellectomy. When the extensor is intact but lax because of patellectomy or patellar fracture, but contributes to a modest (but disabling) lag of 15 or more degrees, the standard surgical technique requires that the patient's patellar tendon insertion be removed to implant the graft tubercle. Unfortunately, if the allograft fails, the situation will be worse. An earlier modification to the standard technique removed the host tubercle, flush with the tibial cortex, to expose the area needed for the trough. At closure, this cortical portion of the host tubercle, in continuity with the patellar tendon, was closed over the graft and secured with screws (Fig. 133-18). Another modification was spurred by a desire to retain the patient's residual extensor, facilitate soft tissue coverage, and contend with large grafts to be used in smaller patients. The larger graft may not fit between the cortices of the proximal tibia without compromising or breaking the essential trough for fixation. The following technique, implanting the graft tubercle with a tibial component, is only

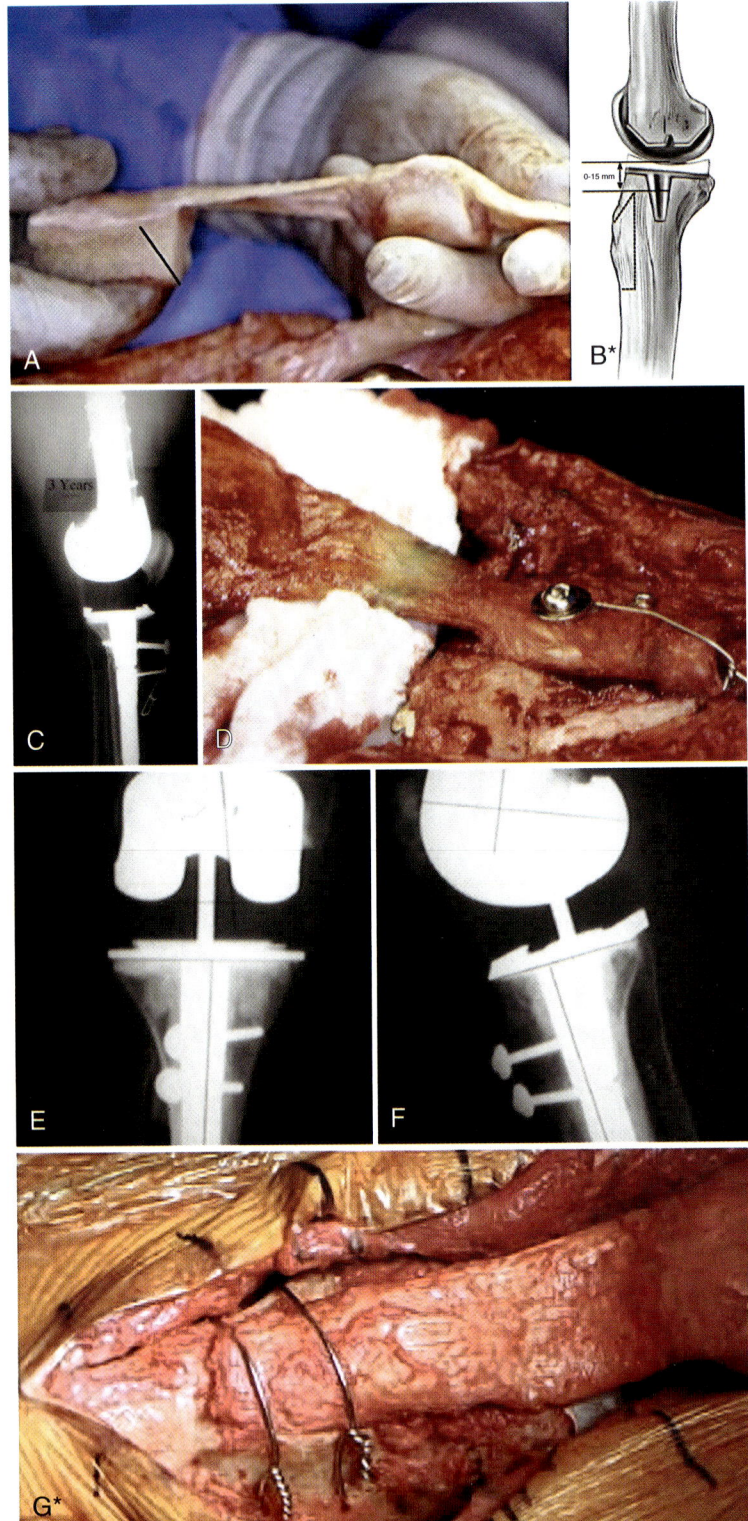

Figure 133-15. Allograft technique: options for distal fixation. **A,** Irrespective of the method of distal fixation with the standard technique, the proximal part of the tubercle graft must lock under the trough in the host bone. The *black line* indicates the oblique cut that should be made on the graft to lock into the trough in the patient tubercle **(B)**. **C, D,** Modification of the standard technique using one or two screws with wire. **E,** AP and lateral **(F)** radiographs showing double screws. This gives excellent resistance to proximal migration, but screw heads can be troublesome and the graft may not be wide enough to accommodate screws without splitting. **G,** Widely favored technique of wires. These may be placed around the stem at the time of revision. (**B, G** From Burnett RS, Berger RA, Paprosky WG, et al: Extensor mechanism allograft reconstruction after total knee arthroplasty. A comparison of two techniques. J Bone Joint Surg Am. 2004;86:2694–2699.)

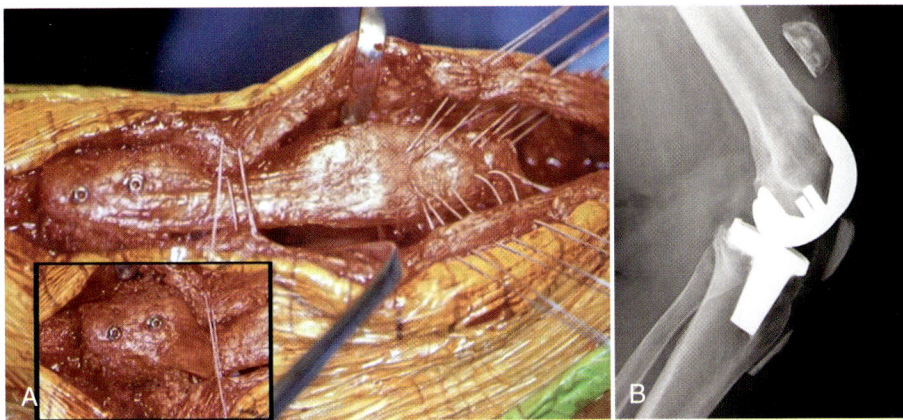

Figure 133-16. Ideally, the graft should be completely covered by the joint capsule and periosteum, not just skin and subcutaneous tissue. **A,** This may be difficult at times because of the bulk of the graft tubercle and the paucity of tissue over the tibial tubercle. *Inset,* As sutures are tightened, we see how difficult it may be to cover completely. **B,** Misguided and failed technique. The host patella (resurfaced) is in an extremely proximal position, indicating the reconstruction has failed. A sliver of graft tibial tubercle has been applied to the anterior surface of the host tubercle without any attempt to lock it in place—and presumably after placing it on top of the host extensor. It seems not to have migrated because the proximal junction failed rapidly. The grafted patella lies ineffectually at the level of the joint line. This contravenes the principles of extensor mechanism allograft reconstruction.

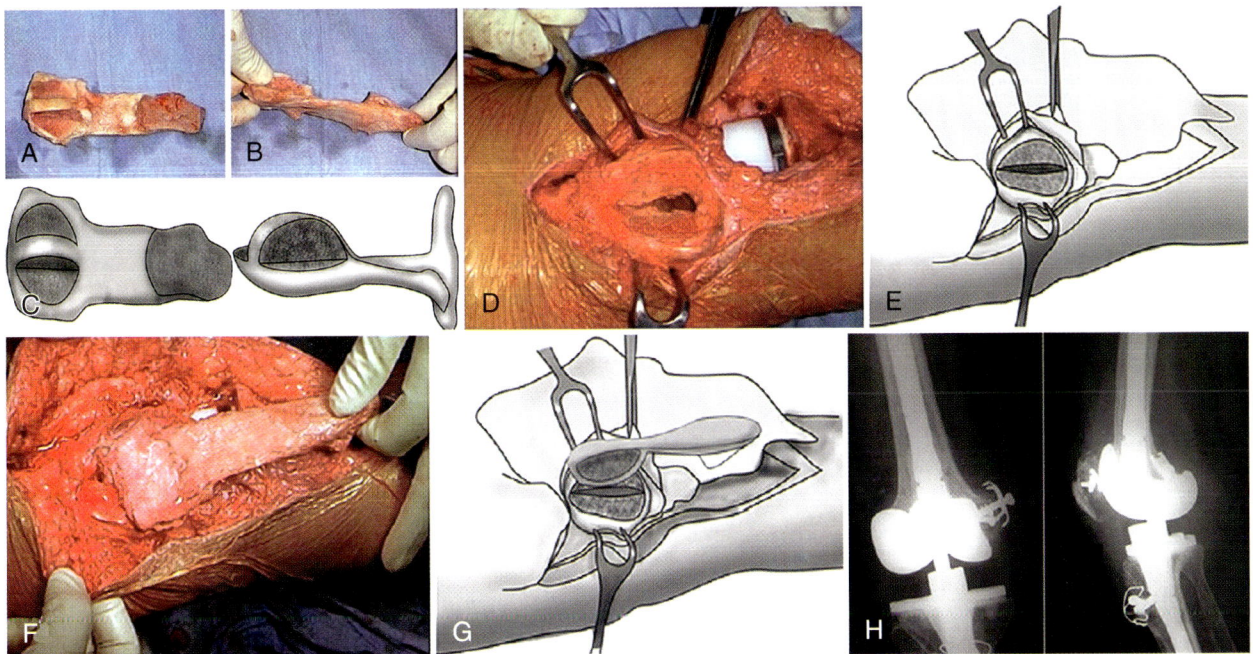

Figure 133-17. Technique for bony union between host and grafted patella. **A-C,** Graft prepared by removing quadriceps tendon and excavating lateral and medial facets to create a central bony ridge that will fit into **D** and **E,** a corresponding groove in the anterior aspect of the host patella. **F, G,** This leaves the patellar graft in a subcutaneous position, where the risk of infection may be increased. It would be unwise to expect the graft to function as part of the capsule. **H,** Postoperative AP and lateral radiographs. Hardware in the patella itself risks the complications of fixation of patellar fractures in TKA.

feasible when concurrent revision (or primary) arthroplasty is indicated (Fig. 133-19A, B). This is a frequent occurrence because chronic extensor insufficiency is often accompanied by instability—in particular, recurvatum.

After removal of failed implants before implantation, the allograft bone block is prepared with a saw and high-speed burr to match the deepest surface of the graft to the anterior aspect of the tibial keel (see Fig. 133-19C, D). The patellar height is adjusted by the amount of bone left on the graft between the

tibial tray and insertion of the patellar tendon (see Fig. 133-19E). The revision follows standard technique.[109]

A high-speed burr is then used to shape the anterior portion of the proximal tibial canal, just deep to the tubercle, to receive the allograft bone block (see Fig. 133-19F). Trial reduction is performed with the allograft in its final position to confirm that the tibial component will seat. Fixation is supplemented with intramedullary stem extensions, preferably offset to manage the asymmetry of the tibia.

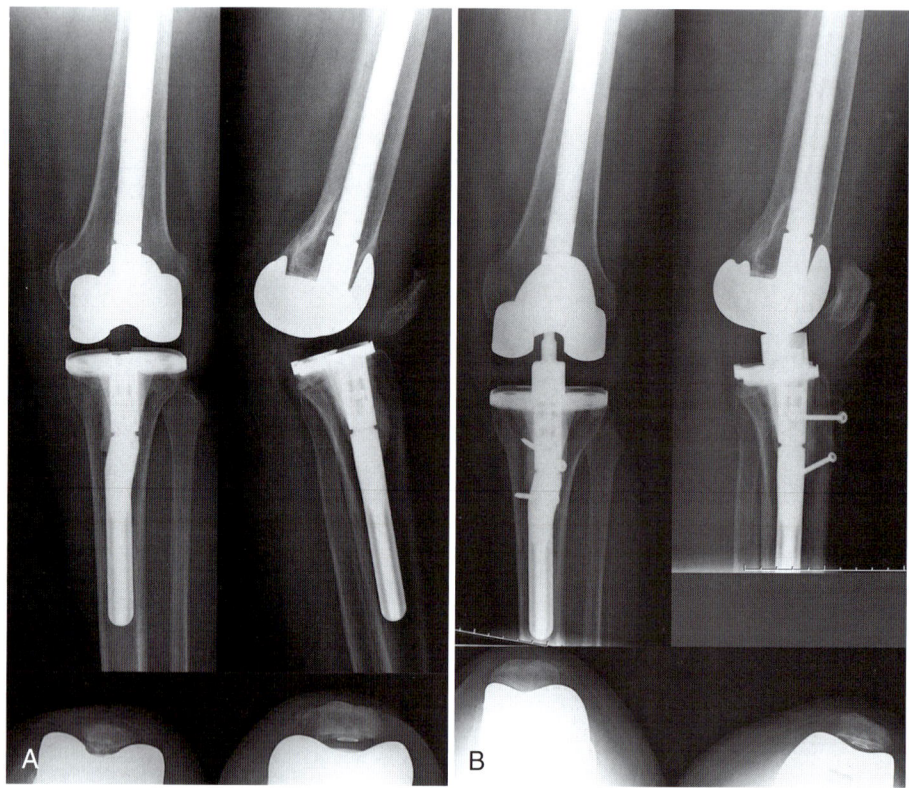

Figure 133-18. A, B, Our modified technique to preserve a patient's residual extensor mechanism without concurrent revision arthroplasty. **A,** AP, lateral, and Merchant radiographs of patient with revision TKA complicated by severe extensor mechanism insufficiency subsequent to remote partial patellectomy, spinal stenosis, and obesity. Like the polio patient with quadriceps compromise, the patient has suffered progressive recurvatum deformity. Patellar remnant *(left)* tracks centrally. **B,** AP, lateral, and Merchant radiographs after exchange of tibial polyethylene insert to a thicker and constrained implant plus an extensor mechanism allograft. The patellar allograft *(left)* tracks centrally. Intraoperative photographs demonstrate technique in **A** and **B. C,** Standard medial arthrotomy to preserve residual extensor mechanism (compare Fig. 133-14*H*), followed by a saw cut in the lateral to medial plane to remove the anterior cortical portion of the host tubercle. This saw cut does not extend proximally to the prosthesis. **D,** Instead, a portion of proximal bone is left to resist proximal migration of the graft (see **G**). Buttress created by a small transverse osteotomy. **E,** A wide osteotome elevates the anterior tibial cortex. **F,** Standard trough is created to receive allograft. **G,** Patient's extensor, which is functionally deficient but not ruptured, has been reflected laterally. When placed back on top of the allograft, the original extensor is still functional, important if the graft resorbs. **H,** Graft is impacted with mallet, emphasizing the importance of a very tight fit of the graft in the tibial trough. **I-L,** The allograft patella will be covered completely by host tissue.

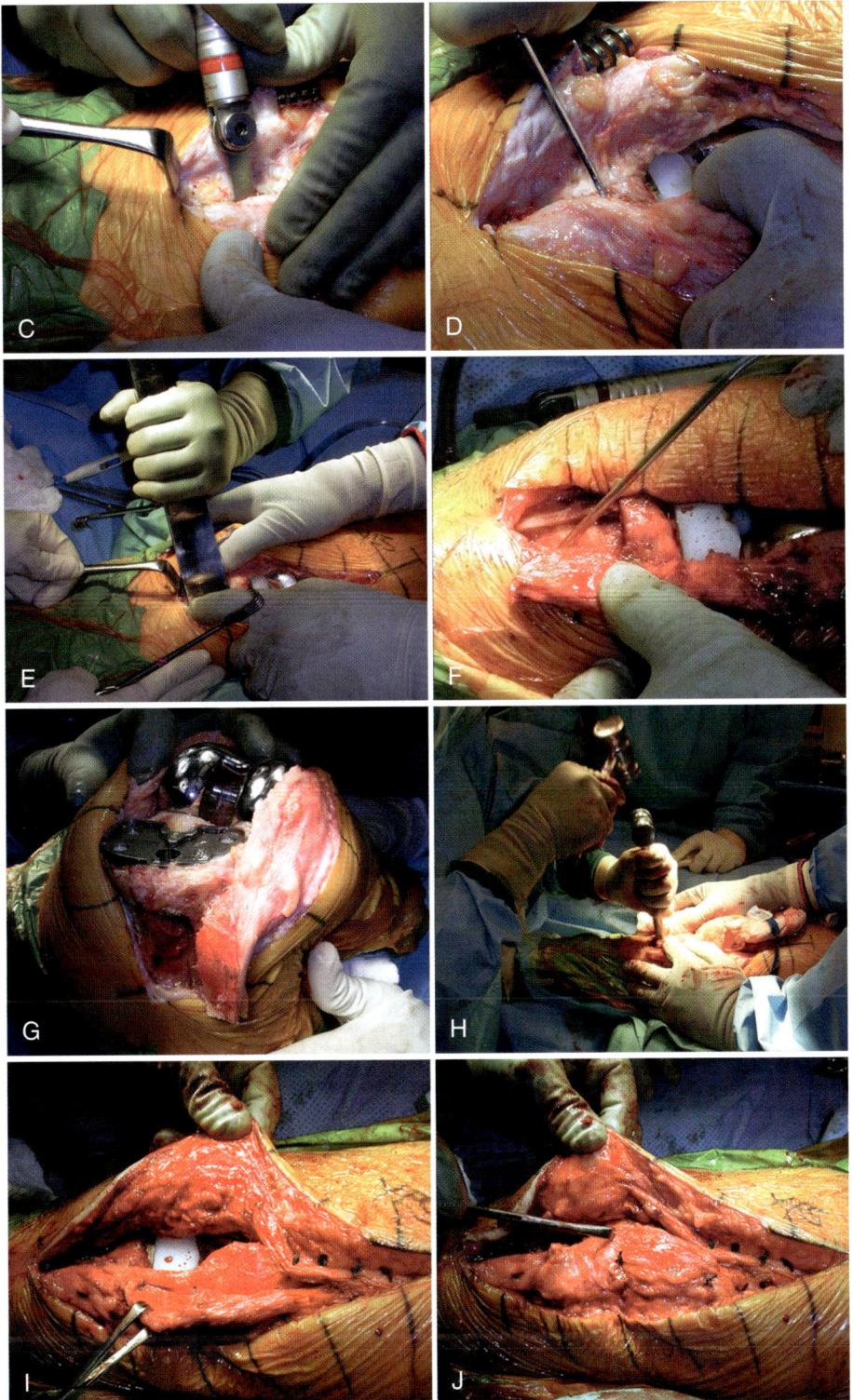

Figure 133-18, cont'd.

Continued

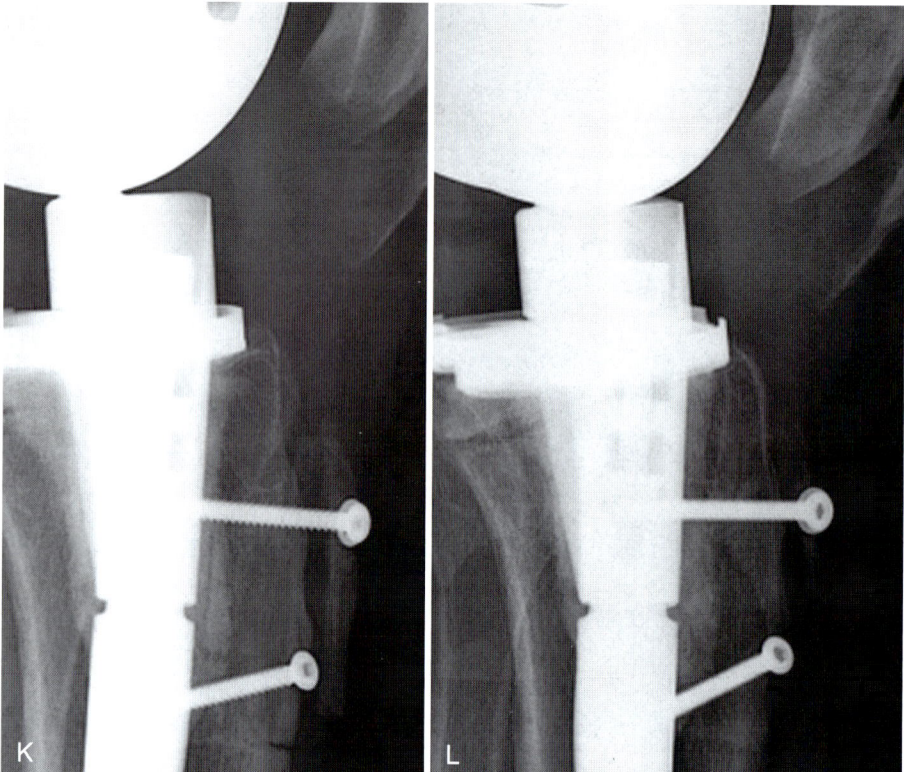

Figure 133-18, cont'd.

The graft sits in the medullary canal, its anterior surface against the endosteal side of the host tubercle. Cementing and implanting are performed as for any revision. Bone cement is first applied to the proximal cut bone surface. The prosthetic stem extension is positioned in the canal and held proud by 3 to 4 cm. A cement gun introduces cement into the proximal portion of the canal and the anterior surface of the tibial keel. The presence of the stem extension will prohibit cement from going down the canal (see Fig. 133-19G). The component is driven into final position with a mallet and impactor.

The allograft tubercle has been implanted with the tibial component and the proximal tendinous junction is secured with the standard technique. The patient's own extensor mechanism has not been disrupted, and there is usually good tissue to close over the top of the graft.

Augmented Technique: Combined Proximal Tibial Allograft and Extensor Mechanism Allograft

Large proximal tibial defects and extensor mechanism rupture may be treated with an allograft that includes the proximal tibial bone, as well as the tendons and patella.[9] A recent small series has been reported by surgeons apparently unaware of its prior description. This technique addresses several important problems, including the challenge of creating a trough for a grafted tubercle when the proximal tibia is deficient. The alternative, less appealing solution to extreme proximal tibial bone loss is the Achilles allograft, anchored distally to the anatomic tubercle.[19]

Achilles Tendon Allograft

The first report of extensor mechanism reconstruction with an Achilles tendon allograft appeared in 1998 by Wascher and Summa.[113] In 2002, Crossett and coworkers[28] published a series of extensor mechanism reconstructions with an allograft Achilles tendon and an attached calcaneal bone block. The study included nine patients, average age 70 years, with an average follow-up of 28 months. We may reasonably compare these results with those described by Nazarian and Booth,[78] who studied 40 patients, average age 71 years, and average follow-up of 43 months. Patellar tendon rupture accounted for 100% and 55% of the extensor mechanism disruptions in these studies,[28,78] respectively. Both surgical techniques tighten the graft in full extension. The extensor mechanism allograft is placed at the deepest level, inside the knee. The Achilles technique, however, repairs the damaged tendon first and then lays the graft on top of it, where it rests in the subcutaneous layer.

The extensor allograft series includes more chronic ruptures and patients with multiple previous surgeries, including failed extensor repairs. The Achilles graft was used in two of nine patients as treatment for an intraoperative rupture. Postoperative mean knee scores were 81[28] and 75[78] points; 70% and 60% of patients achieved full active extension in the Achilles tendon group and the extensor mechanism group, respectively. Crossett and associates[28] reported that 30% had a residual extensor lag with an average magnitude of 3.0 degrees, whereas Nazarian and Booth[78] reported that 40% of their patients had a residual lag averaging 13.0 degrees. Both

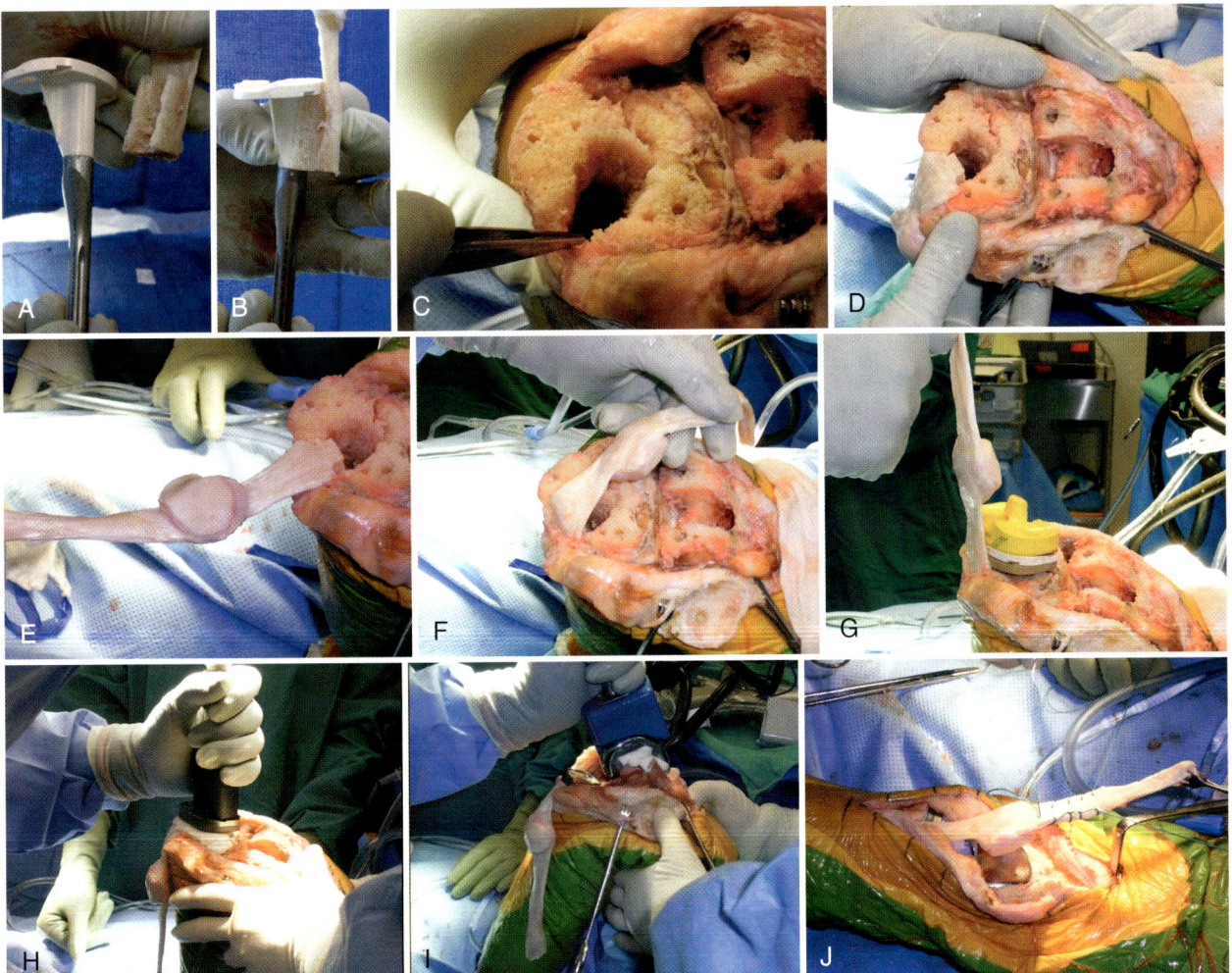

Figure 133-19. Our second modification, the implanted tubercle technique, for extensor mechanism allograft reconstruction of the patellectomy patient, with concurrent revision. **A, B,** The allograft tubercle is shaped with a hand-held burr to match the contour of the anterior aspect of the revision tibial component. The location at which the graft contacts the undersurface of the tibial component must be adjusted to control the eventual height of the patella relative to the femoral component and joint line. This step should be performed after the trial components are in place to assess the joint line height, but before the actual components are implanted. **C,** The anterior aspect of the medullary canal is shaped with the burr, leaving the cortical bone intact but making space to accommodate the graft. **D-F,** Graft is positioned in canal. **G,** Trial tibial component is placed to ensure adequate space and correct height of graft. **H,** Tibial component is implanted with graft in place. No cement is allowed between the graft and the host bone. **I,** Femoral component implanted. **J,** Standard proximal anastomosis performed.

groups reported that 22% of patients required revision of the extensor mechanism reconstruction. The Achilles tendon graft was not used in patellectomy or patella fracture patients.

Barrack and coworkers[11] have described very good results after eight Achilles tendon allograft and six extensor mechanism allograft reconstructions (Fig. 133-20). They recommended the Achilles graft for quadriceps ruptures and the extensor mechanism allograft for disruptions of the patella or patellar tendon.

Autogenous Semitendinosus Reconstruction

In 1992, Cadambi and Engh[22] reported their experience with reconstructing patellar ligament disruption after TKA with an autogenous semitendinosus graft. No case included rupture proximal to the inferior pole of the patella. They reported seven cases at an average of 30 months after surgery. The average age of their patients at the time of reconstruction was

78 years. Their average postoperative knee score was 73 points (Nazarian and Booth,[78] 75 points), and the average postoperative knee flexion was 80 degrees (Nazarian and Booth,[78] 98 degrees). Of their patients, 70% continued to have a residual extension lag averaging 4.4 degrees (Nazarian and Booth,[78] 40% and 13.0 degrees). Fifty percent had a flexion contracture averaging 5.4 degrees. None required repeat surgery or were considered failures. No patient had an extensor lag more than 10 degrees. Further reports with this or similar[35,53] techniques are scant and there has been no sequential follow-up from the original group. Extensor allografting has been reported for failed semitendinosus procedures,[78] but not the converse. This technique may be best suited to the reconstruction of intraoperative tears.

Gastrocnemius Flap

Malawer and Price,[70,71] in resecting tumors about the knee in the early 1980s, reported a variety of techniques for

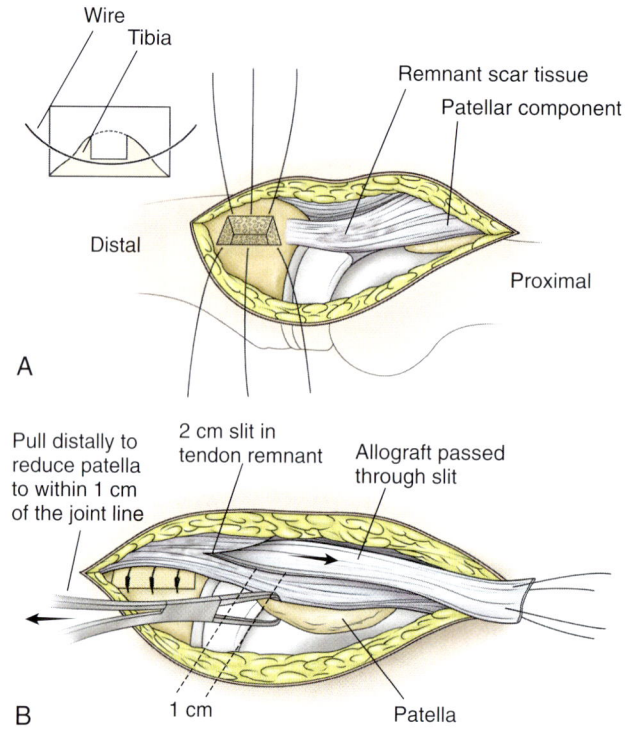

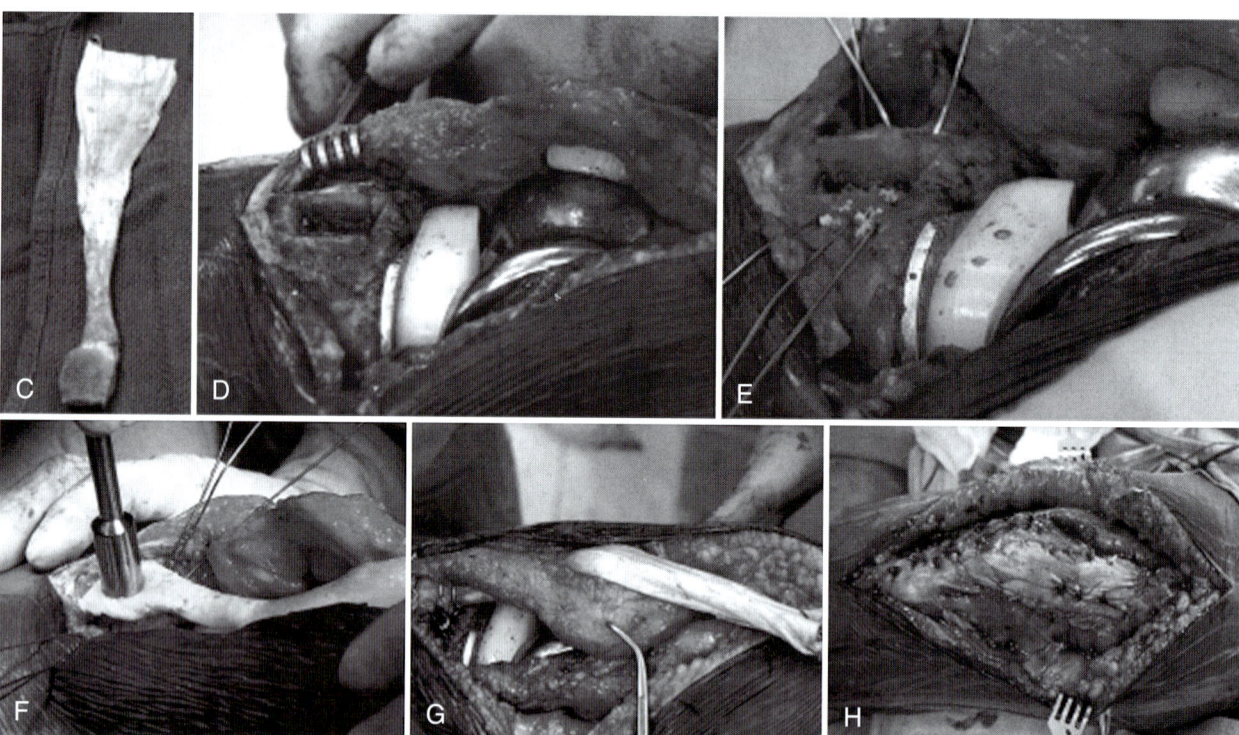

Figure 133-20. **A,** Schematic illustrations of Achilles tendon allograft reconstruction show bone trough preparation with cable passage. **B,** The scar tissue lateral to the disrupted patellar tendon is retained. A slit incision is created in the remnant of scar tissue or remaining host patellar tendon, and the allograft Achilles tendon is brought through this slit, over the host patella, and sewn into the proximal quadriceps extensor mechanism. **C-H,** Technique of Achilles tendon allograft reconstruction. **C,** Achilles tendon fresh-frozen allograft is harvested, with an attached calcaneal bone block. **D,** A generous bone block is later cut to size for the tibial insertion. The host tibial trough is prepared to accept the allograft bone block. The trough is typically 1.5 cm wide × 2.5 cm long × 1.5 cm deep, and is just medial to the host tibial tubercle. **E,** The trough is created smaller than the allograft to allow for a press fit of the slightly oversized allograft bone block. Three wires or cables are passed beneath the floor of the host tibial trough for allograft fixation **F,** The allograft is tamped into place and the wires are tightened (**G**). **H,** The allograft tendon is passed through a slit in the lateral retinaculum (posterior and lateral) to the host patellar tendon remnant and then pulled proximally anterior to the host patella. The allograft is tensioned and sewn into the host quadriceps mechanism with Ethibond suture. (From Burnett, 2005.)

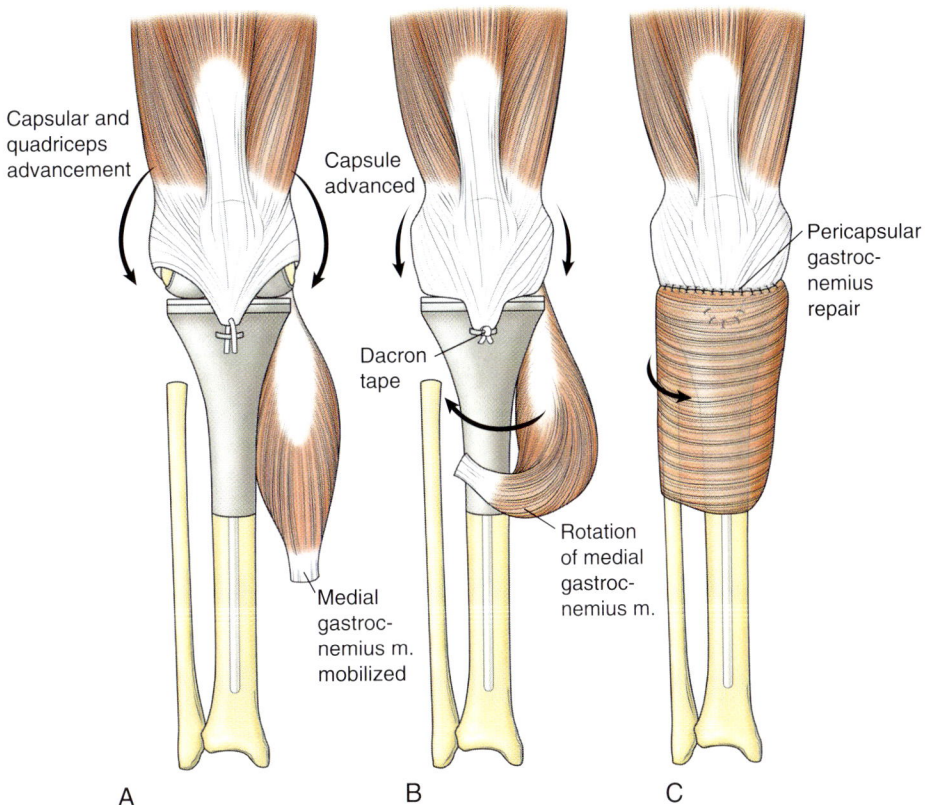

Figure 133-21. Gastrocnemius flap technique for surgical reconstruction of the patella and extensor mechanism, as originally applied to tumor resection. The patellar tendon and extensor mechanism are attached to the prosthesis with Dacron tape under the appropriate tension and then sutured to the transferred gastrocnemius. (From Malawer, 1989.)

reconnecting the patellar tendon to the tibia, if tumor margins required that it be removed when a limb salvage arthroplasty was implanted (Fig. 133-21). They believed that reattachment of the patellar tendon to the prosthesis plus reinforcement with an autologous bone graft and a gastrocnemius flap was reliable.[14] A similar technique has been described in detail, largely for tumor surgery by Kollender and colleagues,[62] using a third of the quadriceps tendon and supplemented with Gore-Tex for enhancement before being covered with the gastrocnemius (Fig. 133-22).

Gastrocnemius flaps that include a portion of the Achilles tendon have been rotated into place and used to reconstruct the patellar and quadriceps tendons.[21] Jaureguito and colleagues,[54] in 1997, described seven patients whose ruptured extensor mechanisms were reconstructed in this way. The residual patellar tendon was sutured to the transposed gastrocnemius muscle and, when the quadriceps had ruptured, a portion of the Achilles tendon was extended up over the knee to the distal remnant of tendon. Six were available for assessment 26 to 41 months after reconstruction. All patients who had required a walker preoperatively ambulated with or without a cane, and wheelchair patients progressed to the use of a walker. Two of them had previously undergone patellectomy. One of the coauthors of the original report has collaborated on a more recent review of the technique.[42] This procedure is useful for patients, often infected, in need of a gastrocnemius flap for soft tissue coverage. The lateral gastrocnemius has also been used.[25] Restoration of the patellar fulcrum, an appealing part of the extensor mechanism

allograft, is not part of this procedure unless the flap is combined with an allograft.

Later, Busfield and colleagues[21] reported a similar experience for a ruptured extensor mechanism in seven patients with a TKA, plus an additional two with no arthroplasty but a ruptured extensor and previous septic arthritis. In four patients, an Achilles tendon allograft had already failed and in two the arthroplasty had become infected. Some patients were infected with human immunodeficiency virus or had hemophilia or diabetes. One died after surgery and another, with reflex sympathetic dystrophy, elected to have an above-knee amputation. A third, originally with an arthroplasty as conversion of an arthrodesis, suffered late wound problems requiring a free flap. The technique is promising and was reserved in this series for the most severely disabled and medically compromised individuals.

Concurrent semitendinosus tendon reconstruction and gastrocnemius flap has recently been reported by Roidis and associates.[90] Given the large forces on the extensor and the challenge of wound healing, this procedure has the advantage of a relatively less plastic ligamentous junction and new, vascularized muscle tissue.

DECIDING ON WHICH TREATMENT TO CHOOSE

When extensor rupture arises emergently, during primary or revision surgery, allograft material may not be available and this option may not have been discussed with the

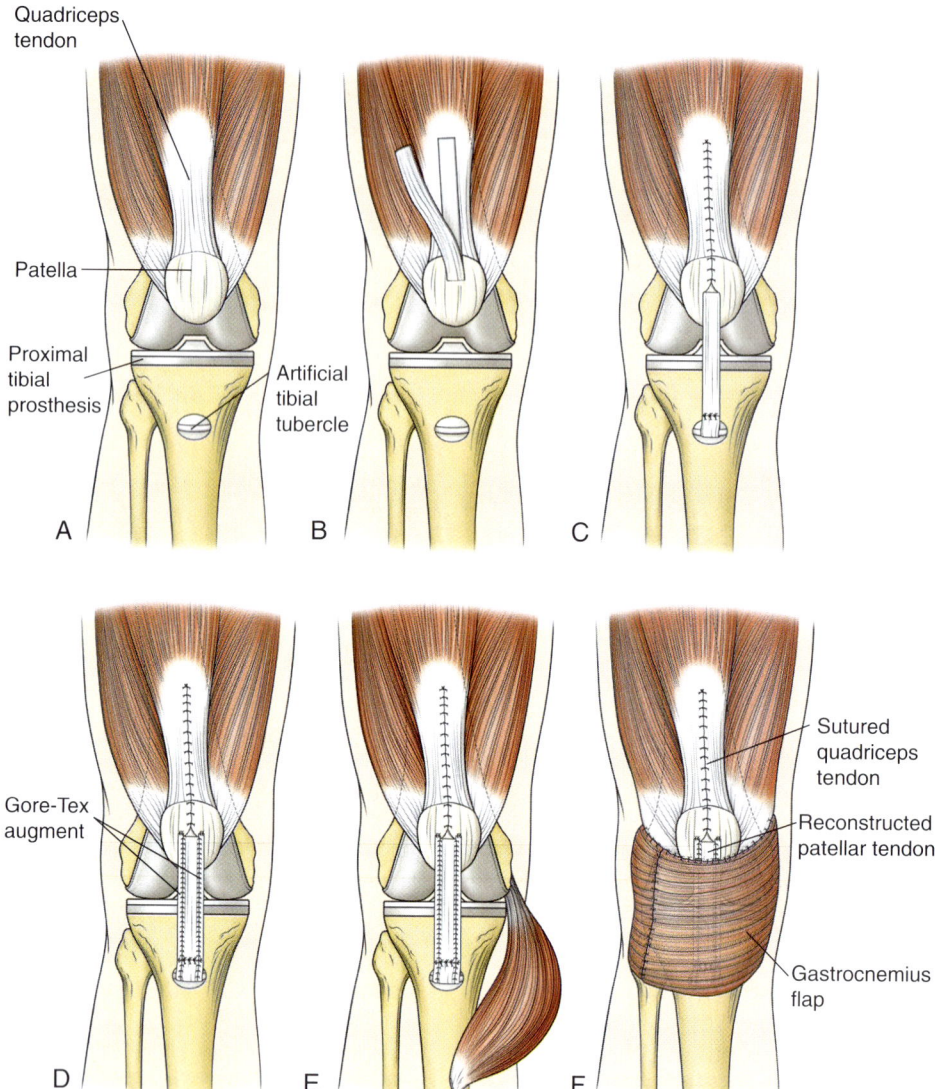

Figure 133-22. Secondary reconstruction of the extensor mechanism. **A,** Disrupted extensor. **B,** Reconstruction of the patellar tendon with the medial third of the quadriceps tendon and patellar retinaculum. **C,** Quadriceps tendon and patellar retinaculum looped over the artificial tibial tubercle and sutured. **D,** Augmentation of the newly formed extensor mechanism with two Gore-Tex strips. **E,** Mechanical and biologic reinforcement of the extensor mechanism is provided by a gastrocnemius flap. **F,** Reconstructed extensor mechanism. (From Kollender Y, Bender B, Weinbroum AA, et al: Secondary reconstruction of the extensor mechanism using part of the quadriceps tendon, patellar retinaculum, and Gore-Tex strips after proximal tibial resection. J Arthroplasty 19:354–360, 2004.)

patient. The incipient quadriceps rupture at this stage may go unrecognized. True avulsion of the quadriceps tendon from the patella would be unlikely and suture repair will help with secure healing, taking care to anchor the lateral side of the arthrotomy proximally and distally to the medial side. Krackow-type ligament stitches are useful and can continue through drill holes in the patella. The superficial quadriceps might be turned down over the patella and supplemented with Marlex mesh.

Bipartite patellae and fibrous unions of old fractures can be problematic. In both situations, the patellae can be left unresurfaced and internal fixation is inadvisable, unless the fracture fragments have separated in surgery. Gelinas and Ries[40] encountered a vertical patellar fracture in a revision patella weakened by osteolysis and opted for cerclage and implantation of a cemented prosthetic button. Alternatively,

this configuration can be bone-grafted and left as the so-called gull wing osteotomy.[38,60,110]

Transverse fractures would be more likely during revision arthroplasties because of osteolysis. No studies are available, but cerclage wiring or a patellectomy with repair of the tendon might be advisable. New patellar implants made of porous elemental tantalum in conjunction with cerclage wiring may provide a useful option. Immediate extensor mechanism allografting would also be reasonable, but these grafts are rarely available immediately outside of large centers and this option should be included in the preoperative consent.

Intraoperative rupture or avulsion of the patellar tendon is more common and represented two of nine cases treated with Achilles tendon allograft.[28] Alternately, very heavy sutures with a Krackow-type stitch may be applied to either side of the patellar tendon, up and over the patella (sometimes through oblique drill holes) and anchored proximally in the quadriceps tendon by tying to each other. The same sutures can be woven, much like a shoelace, through transverse drill holes under the tibial tubercle and tied to each other. Distal reattachment with staples jeopardizes wound healing. Autogenous grafting with the semitendinosus is possible but might not have been discussed with the patient prior to surgery.

Prior to any reconstruction of chronic extensor deficiency, the same systematic and comprehensive preoperative evaluation is essential.[109] Concurrent revision is often helpful; just because the extensor has ruptured does not mean that the arthroplasty may not also be infected or unstable. Extensor reconstructions of unsound arthroplasties are doomed.

It may seem difficult to choose a procedure for the chronic rupture, given the many possibilities. Simple repairs and reattachments with staples or screws have high failure rates. Reconstruction with autogenous structures or allograft substitutes are now preferred and, whatever the location, because tensile loads are considerable, the linkage of the quadriceps muscle to the tibial tubercle cannot be very elastic. Comprehensive algorithms have been derived from the literature after a review of six cases.[92]

When the quadriceps tendon has been disrupted, the Achilles graft can be long enough to extend from the tubercle

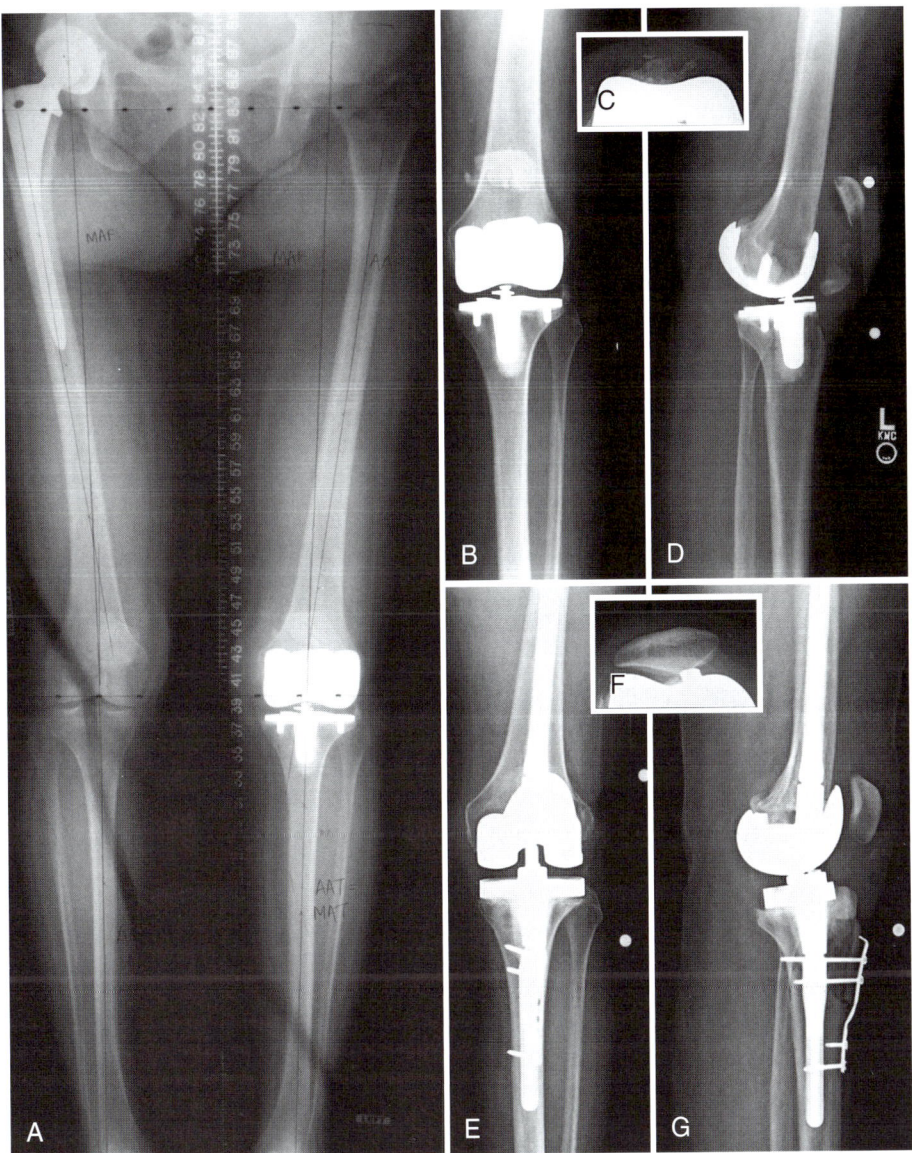

Figure 133-23. Technique for repeat extensor mechanism allograft reconstruction after failure of distal fixation. **A,** Full-length radiograph showing slight valgus mechanical axis of primary TKA that was complicated by transverse patellar fracture. **B-D,** After multiple unsuccessful attempts on the part of the surgeon to fix the fracture, the proximal fragment is high-riding and the patella tracks centrally **(E, F).** The original revision was performed with a concurrent extensor mechanism allograft reconstruction that failed at the tibial junction (not shown). The proximal buttress and tibial trough were compromised, so the extensor graft procedure shown here was performed with a technique similar to that in Figure 133-18. **G,** Graft was implanted deep to all capsular tissue and fixation enhanced with a one-third tubular plate that has been cut proximally, through the proximal border of the screw holes, so that the metal on both sides of the screw holes could be bent at 90 degrees and form a hook to grasp the graft better.

up and over the patella to the quadriceps. Because the host patella is retained, the graft will necessarily have to be placed on the superficial surface of the patella and, in most cases, will be anchored to the tibia in a way that disrupts the host patellar tendon. For patellar fractures and disruptions distal to the patella, we have found that nothing works as well as allograft tissue and replication of the patellar fulcrum—that is, the extensor mechanism allograft.

REPAIRING FAILED RECONSTRUCTIONS

Aseptic failures have most commonly been treated with extensor mechanism allografts, irrespective of the original surgery. Although successful grafts demonstrate extraordinary infiltration of host tissue into the graft tendon,[20] the most common site of failure is the proximal junction, followed by the graft itself and then the distal junction. Most of these failures will require new graft material and not simple resuturing. Distal failure may require supplementary fixation because the trough in the patient tubercle will have been compromised. A modified small-fragment plate may be beneficial (Fig. 133-23).

Septic failure of an allograft reconstruction, in particular if the patient has already been through a two-stage reimplantation protocol, is dire. A second two-stage reimplantation protocol is only recommended for selected patients,[6] which usually would not include the failed extensor mechanism patient.

Although arthrodesis is the logical alternative to arthroplasty, there may be too little bone by the time a patient agrees to fusion. The infection will have to be eradicated, which usually means removal of all foreign material, including the grafted tubercle. No matter how well it has incorporated, it is a sequestrum.

Most of these patients, older and ill, have experienced multiple disappointing operations and extended therapy with sometimes toxic antibiotics. Septic failure of an extensor mechanism allograft, especially in the presence of extensive bone loss, may best be treated with an above-knee amputation. The prosthesis has the advantage of flexion, which facilitates riding in a car or plane. This highlights the serious implications of a ruptured extensor mechanism, still one of the most feared complications in knee arthroplasty surgery.

KEY REFERENCES

Barrack RL, Lyons T: Proximal tibia—extensor mechanism composite allograft for revision TKA with chronic patellar tendon rupture. Acta Orthop Scand 71:419–421, 2000.

Barrack RL, Stanley T, Allen Butler R: Treating extensor mechanism disruption after total knee arthroplasty. Clin Orthop Relat Res 416:98–104, 2003.

Berger RA, Crossett LS, Jacobs JJ, Rubash HE: Malrotation causing patellofemoral complications after total knee arthroplasty. Clin Orthop Relat Res 356:144–153, 1998.

Burnett RS, Berger RA, Della Valle CJ, et al: Extensor mechanism allograft reconstruction after total knee arthroplasty. J Bone Joint Surg Am 87(Suppl 1 Pt 2):175–194, 2005.

Burnett RS, Berger RA, Paprosky WG, et al: Extensor mechanism allograft reconstruction after total knee arthroplasty. A comparison of two techniques. J Bone Joint Surg Am 86:2694–2699, 2004.

Burnett RS, Butler RA, Barrack RL: Extensor mechanism allograft reconstruction in TKA at a mean of 56 months. Clin Orthop Relat Res 452:159–165, 2006.

Cadambi A, Engh GA: Use of a semitendinosus tendon autogenous graft for rupture of the patellar ligament after total knee arthroplasty. A report of seven cases. J Bone Joint Surg Am 74:974–979, 1992.

Crossett LS, Sinha RK, Sechriest VF, Rubash HE: Reconstruction of a ruptured patellar tendon with achilles tendon allograft following total knee arthroplasty. J Bone Joint Surg Am 84:1354–1361, 2002.

Dobbs RE, Hanssen AD, Lewallen DG, Pagnano MW: Quadriceps tendon rupture after total knee arthroplasty. Prevalence, complications, and outcomes. J Bone Joint Surg Am 87:37–45, 2005.

Emerson RH, Jr, Head WC, Malinin TI: Extensor mechanism reconstruction with an allograft after total knee arthroplasty. Clin Orthop 303:79–85, 1994.

Jaureguito JW, Dubois CM, Smith SR, et al: Medial gastrocnemius transposition flap for the treatment of disruption of the extensor mechanism after total knee arthroplasty. J Bone Joint Surg Am 79:866–873, 1997.

Keating EM, Haas G, Meding JB: Patella fracture after post total knee replacements. Clin Orthop 416:93–97, 2003.

Leopold SS, Greidanus N, Paprosky WG, et al: High rate of failure of allograft reconstruction of the extensor mechanism after total knee arthroplasty. J Bone Joint Surg Am 81:1574–1579, 1999.

Nazarian DG, Booth RE, Jr: Extensor mechanism allografts in total knee arthroplasty. Clin Orthop 367:123–129, 1999.

Full references for this chapter can be found on www.expertconsult.com.

Economics of Total Knee Arthroplasty

Adam J. Rana and William L. Healy

SECTION 13

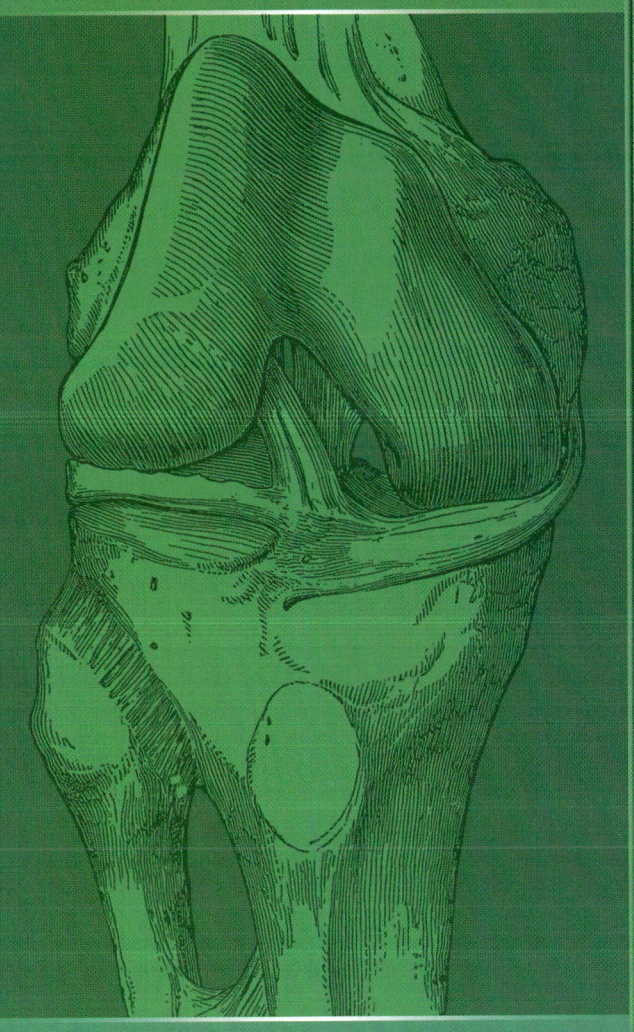

Medical/Surgical Considerations in Managing the Total Knee Replacement Patient

Chapter 135

Perioperative Management of the Patient With Coronary Stents

Ezra Deutsch

Chapter 136

American Academy of Orthopaedic Surgeons Guidelines

Paul F. Lachiewicz

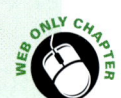

Chapter 137

Prevention of Venous Thromboembolism in Knee Surgery: Limitations of Aspirin and Mechanical Devices

John P. Fletcher

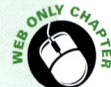

Chapter 138

Venous Thromboembolism Prophylaxis After Knee Surgery: The European Approach

David Warwick

Chapter 139

Thromboembolic Disease and Unicompartmental Knee Arthroplasty

Keith R. Berend, Adolph V. Lombardi, Jr., and Michael J. Morris

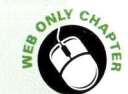

Chapter 140

Treatment of Hematoma and Hemarthrosis Following Total Knee Arthroplasty

Fred D. Cushner and Michael P. Nett

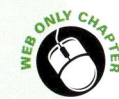

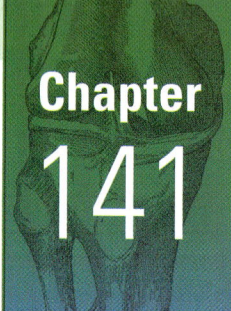

Chapter 141

Multimodal Approach to Transfusion Avoidance and Blood Loss Management in Total Knee Arthroplasty

Michael P. Nett, William J. Long, and Fred D. Cushner

WEB ONLY CHAPTER

RISK OF INFECTION

RISK FACTORS FOR TRANSFUSION

PREOPERATIVE BLOOD MANAGEMENT
Preoperative Autologous Donations
Use of Erythropoietins
Insall-Scott Institute Protocol

INTRAOPERATIVE BLOOD MANAGEMENT
Acute Normovolemic Hemodilution
Intraoperative Blood Salvage
Hypotensive Anesthesia
Tissue Hemostasis
Pharmacologic Strategies

POSTOPERATIVE MANAGEMENT
Drain Usage
Special Situations

CONCLUSION

Chapter 142

Advances in Anticoagulation for Total Joint Arthroplasty— The Newer Agents

Richard J. Friedman

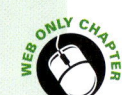

WEB ONLY CHAPTER

DIRECT FACTOR Xa INHIBITORS
Mode of Action
Apixaban
Rivaroxaban

DIRECT THROMBIN INHIBITORS
Mode of Action
Dabigatran Etexilate

OTHER ANTICOAGULANTS IN DEVELOPMENT

CONCLUSIONS

Chapter 143

Advances in Mechanical Compression Devices

Andrew I. Spitzer

WEB ONLY CHAPTER

MECHANICAL DEVICES

THE ROLE OF MECHANICAL COMPRESSION AFTER TKA

EMERGING TECHNOLOGY

SUMMARY AND RECOMMENDATIONS

Chapter 144

Prevention of Thrombophlebitis and Pulmonary Embolism in Total Knee Arthroplasty

Richard J. Friedman

KNEE SURGERY AND THROMBOTIC RISK

OPTIONS FOR THROMBOPROPHYLAXIS IN KNEE SURGERY
Pharmacologic Thromboprophylaxis
Mechanical Thromboprophylaxis

THROMBOPROPHYLAXIS IN KNEE ARTHROSCOPY

THROMBOPROPHYLAXIS IN TRAUMA SURGERY

RISK STRATIFICATION

DURATION OF THROMBOPROPHYLAXIS

EIGHTH ACCP GUIDELINES FOR KNEE SURGERY PATIENTS

AAOS GUIDELINES FOR KNEE SURGERY PATIENTS

CONCLUSIONS

Chapter 145

A Multimodal Approach to Pain Management in Total Joint Arthroplasty

Asokumar Buvanendran, Bryan S. Williams, and Craig J. Della Valle

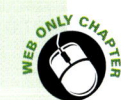

ACUTE PAIN MEDICINE SERVICE

NSAIDs, COX-2 INHIBITORS, AND ACETAMINOPHEN
Nonselective NSAIDs
Ketorolac

Acetaminophen
COX-2 Inhibitors
Gabapentinoids
Ketamine

OPIOIDS

INTERVENTIONAL TECHNIQUES
Regional Blockade
Periarticular Infiltration

PROTOCOL

CONCLUSION

Chapter 146

Pain Management: The Surgeon's Approach

Kelly Stets and Jose Rodriguez

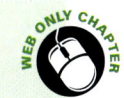

ANXIETY REDUCTION

PREEMPTIVE ANALGESIA

REGIONAL ANESTHESIA AND BLOCKS

INTRAOPERATIVE INTERVENTIONS
Local Injection/Tissue
 Infiltration

PACU AND IMMEDIATE POSTOPERATIVE PERIOD

SUMMARY

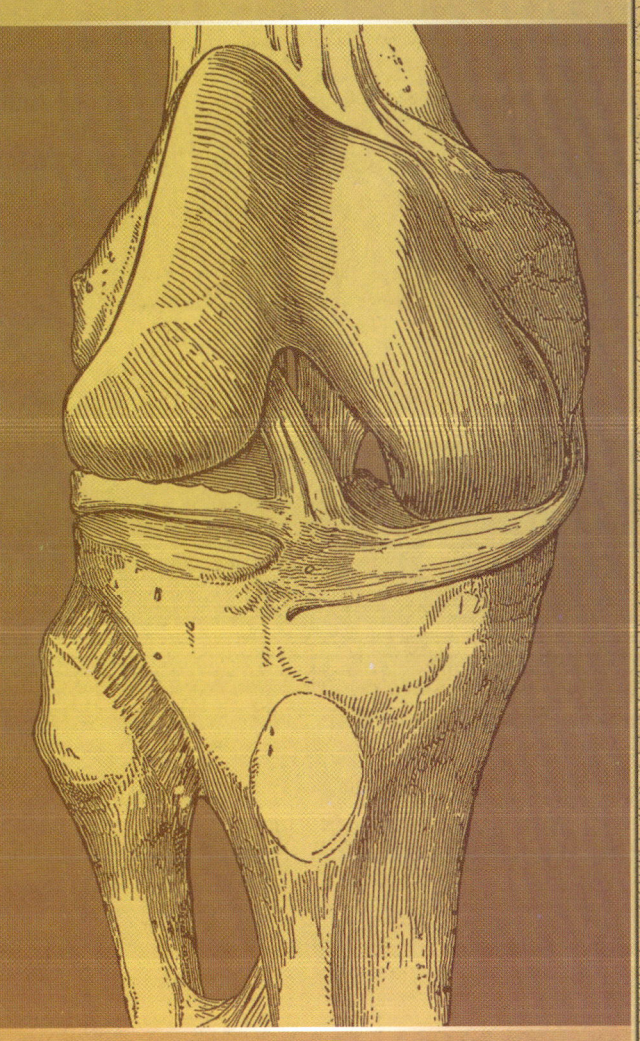

**Tumors About
the Knee**

Chapter 147

Evaluation of the Patient With a Bone Lesion About the Knee

Ginger E. Holt

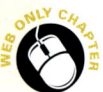

Chapter 148

Surgical Treatment of Benign Bone Lesions

R. Lor Randall and Nicholas P. Webber

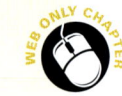

Chapter 149

Surgical Management of Malignant Bone Tumors Around the Knee

Michael D. Neel

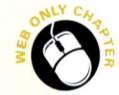

Chapter 150

Allograft Prosthetic Composite Reconstruction of the Knee

Christopher P. Beauchamp and Ian D. Dickey

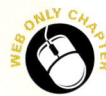

Chapter 151

Megaprostheses for Reconstruction Following Tumor Resection About the Knee

Mary I. O'Connor

Chapter 152

Metastatic Disease About the Knee: Evaluation and Surgical Treatment

Timothy A. Damron

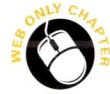

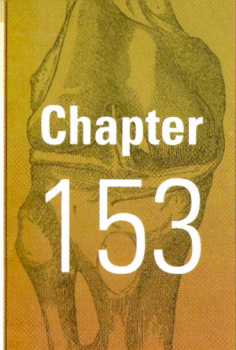

Chapter 153

Soft Tissue Tumors of the Knee

Kimberly Templeton

Note: Page numbers followed by "f" refer to illustrations; followed by "t" refer to tables; followed by "b" refer to boxes; and preceded "e" refer to web-only content.

1423